BRAUNWALD'S

HEART DISEASE

A TEXTBOOK OF CARDIOVASCULAR MEDICINE

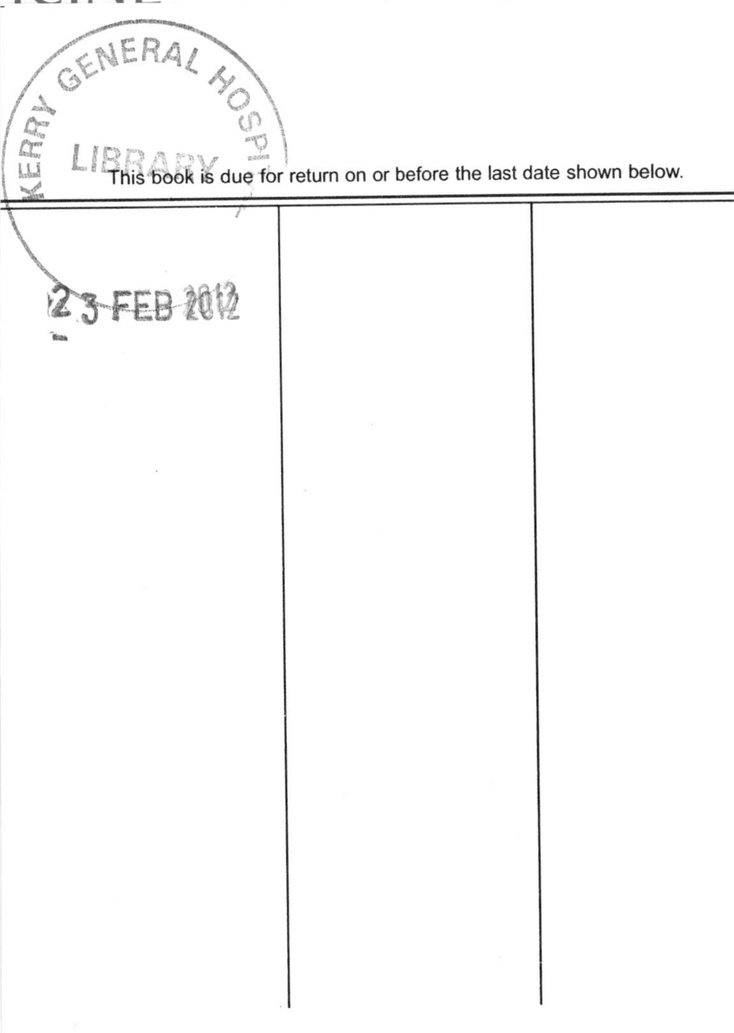

Edited by

Douglas P. Zipes, MD, MACC

Distinguished Professor of Medicine, Pharmacology, and Toxicology
Director, Division of Cardiology and the Krannert Institute of Cardiology
Indiana University School of Medicine
Indianapolis, Indiana

Peter Libby, MD

Mallinckrodt Professor of Medicine
Harvard Medical School
Chief, Cardiovascular Division
Brigham and Women's Hospital
Boston, Massachusetts

Robert O. Bonow, MD

Goldberg Distinguished Professor of Cardiology
Northwestern University Feinberg School of Medicine
Chief, Division of Cardiology
Northwestern Memorial Hospital
Chicago, Illinois

Eugene Braunwald, MD, MD (Hon), ScD (Hon), FRCP

Distinguished Hersey Professor of Medicine
Harvard Medical School
Chairman, TIMI Study Group
Brigham and Women's Hospital
Boston, Massachusetts

VOLUME 2

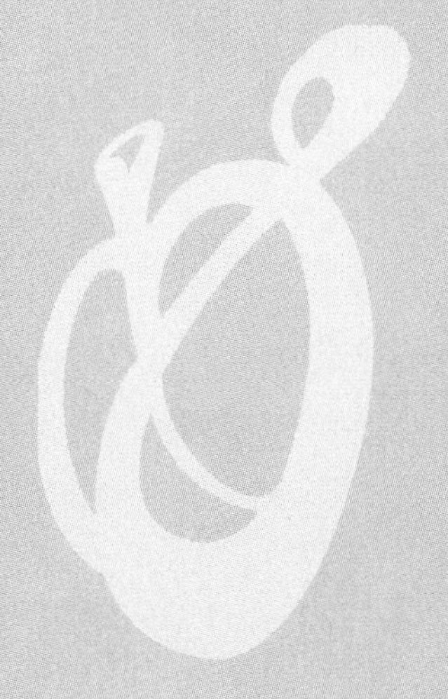

BRAUNWALD'S HEART DISEASE

A TEXTBOOK OF CARDIOVASCULAR MEDICINE

7th Edition

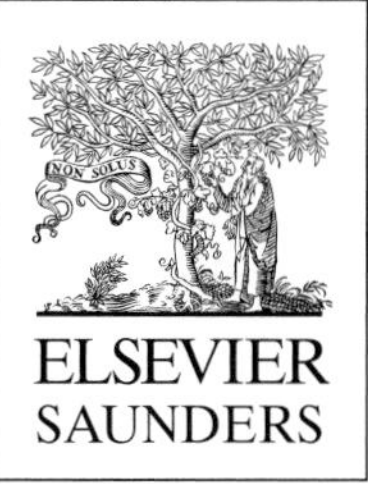

ELSEVIER
SAUNDERS

The Curtis Center
170 S Independence Mall W 300E
Philadelphia, Pennsylvania 19106

BRAUNWALD'S HEART DISEASE: A Textbook of Cardiovascular Medicine, Seventh Edition

Two-volume set	0-7216-0509-5
Single volume	0-7216-0479-X
Two-volume e-dition	1-4160-00038-0
Single volume e-dition	1-4160-00014-3
International edition	0-8089-2305-6
Indian edition	0-8089-2334-X

NOTICE

Medicine is an ever-changing field. Standard safety precautions must be followed, but as new research and clinical experience broaden our knowledge, changes in treatment and drug therapy may become necessary or appropriate. Readers are advised to check the most current product information provided by the manufacturer of each drug to be administered to verify the recommended dose, the method and duration of administration, and contraindications. It is the responsibility of the licensed prescriber, relying on experience and knowledge of the patient, to determine dosages and the best treatment for each individual patient. Neither the publisher nor the authors assume any liability for any injury and/or damage to persons or property arising from this publication.

Library of Congress Cataloging-in-Publication Data

Braunwald's heart disease : a textbook of cardiovascular medicine / [edited by] Douglas P. Zipes . . . [et al.].—7th ed.
p. ; cm.
Rev. ed. of: Heart disease / edited by Eugene Braunwald, Douglas P. Zipes, Peter Libby. 6th ed. 2001.
Includes bibliographical references and index.
ISBN 0-7216-0509-5 (2 vol. set)—ISBN 0-7216-0479-X (Single vol.)—ISBN 0-8089-2305-6 (International ed.)
1. Heart—Diseases. 2. Cardiology. I. Title: Heart disease. II. Zipes, Douglas P. III. Braunwald, Eugene—Heart disease.
[DNLM: 1. Heart Diseases. 2. Cardiovascular Diseases. WG 210 B825 2005]
RC681.H36 2005
616.1′2—dc22 2004050808

Publishing Director: Anne Lenehan
Managing Editor, Developmental Editorial: Deborah Thorp
Publishing Services Manager: Frank Polizzano
Senior Project Manager: Robin E. Davis
Design Manager: Steven Stave

Printed in the United States of America.

Last digit is the print number: 9 8 7 6 5 4 3 2 1

To:

Joan, Debra, Jeffrey, and David

Beryl, Oliver, and Brigitte

Pat, Rob, and Sam

Elaine, Karen, Allison, and Jill

CONTRIBUTORS

Stephan Achenbach, MD
Assistant Professor of Medicine and Cardiology, Friedrich-Alexander University School of Medicine; Staff Cardiologist, Division of Cardiology, Department of Medicine, University Hospital Erlangen, Erlangen, Germany
Computed Tomography of the Heart

David H. Adams, MD
Marie-Josée and Henry R. Kravis Professor and Chair, Department of Cardiothoracic Surgery, Mount Sinai Medical Center, New York, New York
Medical Management of the Patient Undergoing Cardiac Surgery

Elliott M. Antman, MD
Professor of Medicine, Harvard Medical School; Director, Samuel A. Levine Cardiac Unit, Brigham and Women's Hospital, Boston, Massachusetts
ST-Elevation Myocardial Infarction: Pathology, Pathophysiology, and Clinical Features; ST-Elevation Myocardial Infarction: Management; Medical Management of the Patient Undergoing Cardiac Surgery

Karen Antman, MD
Deputy Director for Translational and Clinical Sciences, National Cancer Institute, National Institutes of Health, Bethesda, Maryland
The Patient with Cardiovascular Disease and Cancer

Piero Anversa, MD
Professor, Department of Medicine, Cardiovascular Research Institute, New York Medical College, Valhalla, New York
Myocardial Regeneration

William F. Armstrong, MD
Professor of Medicine, University of Michigan; Associate Clinical Chief, Division of Cardiology, Associate Chair, Department of Internal Medicine, University of Michigan Health System, Ann Arbor, Michigan
Echocardiography

Donald S. Baim, MD
Professor of Medicine, Harvard Medical School; Director, Center for Integration of Medicine and Innovative Technology, Partners Healthcare System and Brigham and Women's Hospital, Boston, Massachusetts
Percutaneous Coronary and Valvular Intervention

Leora B. Balsam, MD
Resident in Surgery, Department of Surgery, Stanford University School of Medicine, Stanford, California
Heart Transplantation

Arthur J. Barsky, MD
Professor of Psychiatry, Harvard Medical School; Director, Psychiatric Research, Brigham and Women's Hospital, Boston, Massachusetts
Psychiatric and Behavioral Aspects of Cardiovascular Disease

Kenneth Lee Baughman, MD
Professor of Medicine, Harvard Medical School; Director, Advanced Heart Disease Section, Brigham and Women's Hospital, Boston, Massachusetts
Myocarditis

Joshua A. Beckman, MS, MD
Assistant Professor of Medicine, Harvard Medical School; Associate Physician, Cardiovascular Division, Brigham and Women's Hospital, Boston, Massachusetts
Diabetes Mellitus, the Metabolic Syndrome, and Atherosclerotic Vascular Disease

George A. Beller, MD
Ruth C. Heede Professor of Cardiology and Professor of Medicine, University of Virginia School of Medicine; Department of Internal Medicine, Cardiovascular Division, University of Virginia Health System, Charlottesville, Virginia
Relative Merits of Cardiac Diagnostic Techniques

Michael A. Bettman, MD
Professor of Radiology, Dartmouth Medical School, Hanover, New Hampshire
The Chest Radiograph in Cardiovascular Disease

Robert O. Bonow, MD
Goldberg Distinguished Professor of Cardiology, Northwestern University Feinberg School of Medicine; Chief, Division of Cardiology, Northwestern Memorial Hospital, Chicago, Illinois
Care of Patients with End-Stage Heart Disease; Nuclear Cardiology; Cardiac Catheterization; Valvular Heart Disease

Eugene Braunwald, MD, MD (Hon), ScD (Hon), FRCP
Distinguished Hersey Professor of Medicine, Harvard Medical School; Chairman, TIMI Study Group, Brigham and Women's Hospital, Boston, Massachusetts
The History; Physical Examination of the Heart and Circulation; Pathophysiology of Heart Failure; Clinical Aspects of Heart Failure; Pulmonary Edema, High-Output Failure; ST-Elevation Myocardial Infarction: Pathology, Pathophysiology, and Clinical Features; Unstable Angina and Non–ST Elevation Myocardial Infarction; Chronic Coronary Artery Disease; Valvular Heart Disease; The Cardiomyopathies

Michael R. Bristow, MD, PhD
Professor of Medicine and Head, Division of Cardiology, University of Colorado Health Sciences Center, Denver, Colorado
Drugs in the Treatment of Heart Failure; Management of Heart Failure

Hugh Calkins, MD, FACC, FAHA
Professor of Medicine, Johns Hopkins University School of Medicine; Director, Arrhythmia Service and Clinical Electrophysiology Laboratory, Johns Hopkins Hospital, Baltimore, Maryland
Hypotension and Syncope

Christopher P. Cannon, MD
Associate Professor of Medicine, Harvard Medical School; Senior Investigator, TIMI Study Group, Cardiovascular Division, Brigham and Women's Hospital, Boston, Massachusetts
Approach to the Patient with Chest Pain; Unstable Angina and Non–ST Elevation Myocardial Infarction

John D. Carroll, MD
Professor of Medicine, Division of Cardiology, University of Colorado Health Sciences Center; Director, Cardiac and Vascular Center and Director, Interventional Cardiology, University of Colorado Hospital, Denver, Colorado
Assessment of Normal and Abnormal Cardiac Function

Agustin Castellanos, MD
Professor of Medicine, University of Miami School of Medicine; Director, Clinical Electrophysiology, University of Miami/Jackson Memorial Medical Center, Miami, Florida
Cardiac Arrest and Sudden Cardiac Death

Bernard R. Chaitman, MD
Professor of Medicine and Director, Cardiovascular Research, St. Louis University School of Medicine, St. Louis, Missouri
Exercise Stress Testing

Jonathan M. Chen, MD
Assistant Professor of Surgery, Columbia University College of Physicians and Surgeons; Attending Surgeon, New York Presbyterian Hospital, New York, New York
Assisted Circulation in the Treatment of Heart Failure

Wilson S. Colucci, MD, FACC
Thomas J. Ryan Professor of Medicine; Professor of Physiology; Director, Myocardial Biology Unit, Boston University School of Medicine; Chief, Cardiovascular Medicine, Boston Medical Center, Boston, Massachusetts
Pathophysiology of Heart Failure; Clinical Aspects of Heart Failure; Pulmonary Edema, High-Output Failure; Primary Tumors of the Heart

Mark A. Creager, MD
Professor of Medicine, Harvard Medical School; Director, Vascular Center; Simon C. Fireman Scholar in Cardiovascular Medicine, Brigham and Women's Hospital, Boston, Massachusetts
Diabetes Mellitus, the Metabolic Syndrome, and Atherosclerotic Vascular Disease; Peripheral Arterial Diseases

Adnan S. Dajani, MD
Professor Emeritus of Pediatrics, Wayne State University School of Medicine; Director Emeritus, Division of Infectious Diseases, Children's Hospital of Michigan, Detroit, Michigan
Rheumatic Fever

Werner G. Daniel, MD
Professor of Medicine and Cardiology, Friedrich-Alexander School of Medicine; Division of Cardiology, Department of Medicine, University Hospital Erlangen, Erlangen, Germany
Computed Tomography of the Heart

Charles J. Davidson, MD
Professor of Medicine, Northwestern University Feinberg School of Medicine; Chief, Cardiac Catheterization Laboratories, Northwestern Memorial Hospital, Chicago, Illinois
Cardiac Catheterization

Vasken Dilsizian, MD
Professor of Medicine and Radiology, University of Maryland School of Medicine; Director of Cardiovascular Nuclear Medicine and Cardiac Positron Emission Tomography, University of Maryland Medical Center, Baltimore, Maryland
Nuclear Cardiology

Pamela S. Douglas, MD
Ursula Geller Professor of Medicine, Chief, Cardiovascular Medicine, Duke University Medical Center, Durham, North Carolina
Cardiovascular Disease in Women

Kim A. Eagle, MD
Albion Walter Hewlett Professor of Internal Medicine; Chief, Clinical Cardiology; Clinical Director, Cardiovascular Center, University of Michigan Health System, Ann Arbor, Michigan
Anesthesia and Noncardiac Surgery in Patients with Heart Disease

Andrew C. Eisenhauer, MD
Assistant Professor of Medicine and Radiology, Harvard Medical School; Director, Interventional Cardiovascular Medicine Service, Brigham and Women's Hospital, Boston, Massachusetts
Endovascular Treatment of Noncoronary Obstructive Vascular Disease

Uri Elkayam, MD
Professor of Medicine, University of Southern California Keck School of Medicine, Los Angeles, California
Pregnancy and Cardiovascular Disease

Linda L. Emanuel, MD, PhD
Buehler Professor of Geriatric Medicine and Director, Buehler Center of Aging, Northwestern University Feinberg School of Medicine, Chicago, Illinois
Care of Patients with End-Stage Heart Disease

Anthony L. Estrera, MD
Assistant Professor of Cardiothoracic and Vascular Surgery, University of Texas Health Science Center, Houston, Texas
Traumatic Heart Disease

Farzan Filsoufi, MD
Assistant Professor of Cardiothoracic Surgery, Mount Sinai School of Medicine, New York, New York
Medical Management of the Patient Undergoing Cardiac Surgery

Stacy D. Fisher, MD
Department of Cardiology, Sinai Hospital of Baltimore, Johns Hopkins University; Mid-Atlantic Cardiovascular Associates, Baltimore, Maryland
Cardiovascular Abnormalities in HIV-Infected Individuals

Lee A. Fleisher, MD, FACC
Professor of Anesthesia and Medicine, University of Pennsylvania School of Medicine; Chair, Department of Anesthesia, University of Pennsylvania Health System, Philadelphia, Pennsylvania
Anesthesia and Noncardiac Surgery in Patients with Heart Disease

J. Michael Gaziano, MD, MPH
Associate Professor of Medicine, Harvard Medical School; Chief, Division of Aging, Brigham and Women's Hospital; Director, Massachusetts Veterans Epidemiology and Research Information Center (MAVERIC), Boston VA Healthcare Systems, Boston, Massachusetts
Global Burden of Cardiovascular Disease; Primary and Secondary Prevention of Coronary Heart Disease

Jacques Genest, MD
Professor of Medicine, McGill University; Chief, Cardiology, McGill University Medical Center, Montréal, Québec, Canada
Lipoprotein Disorders and Cardiovascular Disease

Bernard J. Gersh, MD, DPhil, FRCP
Professor of Medicine, Mayo College of Medicine; Consultant, Division of Cardiovascular Diseases, Mayo Clinic, Rochester, Minnesota
Chronic Coronary Artery Disease

Michael M. Givertz, MD
Assistant Professor of Medicine, Harvard Medical School; Co-Director, Cardiomyopathy and Heart Failure Program, Brigham and Women's Hospital, Boston, Massachusetts
Clinical Aspects of Heart Failure; Pulmonary Edema, High-Output Failure

Ary L. Goldberger, MD
Associate Professor of Medicine, Harvard Medical School; Director, Margret and H. A. Rey Laboratory for Nonlinear Dynamics in Physiology and Medicine, Beth Israel Deaconess Medical Center, Boston, Massachusetts
Electrocardiography

Samuel Z. Goldhaber, MD
Associate Professor of Medicine, Harvard Medical School; Staff Cardiologist and Director, Venous Thromboembolism Research Group; Director, Anticoagulation Service, Brigham and Women's Hospital, Boston, Massachusetts
Pulmonary Embolism

Antonio M. Gotto, Jr., MD, DPhil
Stephen and Suzanne Weiss Dean, Provost for Medical Affairs, Professor of Medicine, Weill Medical College of Cornell University, New York, New York
Lipoprotein Disorders and Cardiovascular Disease

William J. Groh, MD, MPH
Associate Professor of Medicine, Indiana University School of Medicine, Indianapolis, Indiana
Neurological Disorders and Cardiovascular Disease

David L. Hayes, MD
Professor of Medicine, Mayo Medical School, Mayo Clinic College of Medicine; Chair, Division of Cardiovascular Diseases and Internal Medicine, Mayo Clinic, Rochester, Minnesota
Cardiac Pacemakers and Cardioverter-Defibrillators

Otto M. Hess, MD
Professor of Cardiology, Swiss Cardiovascular Center, University Hospital, Bern, Switzerland
Assessment of Normal and Abnormal Cardiac Function

L. David Hillis, MD
Professor and Vice Chair, Department of Medicine; James M. Wooten Chair in Cardiology, University of Texas Southwestern Medical Center, Dallas, Texas
Toxins and the Heart

Mark A. Hlatky, MD
Professor of Health Research and Policy and Professor of Cardiovascular Medicine, Stanford University School of Medicine; Attending Physician, Stanford University Medical Center, Stanford, California
Economics and Cardiovascular Disease

Gary S. Hoffman, MS, MD
Professor of Medicine, Cleveland Clinic Lerner College of Medicine of Case Western Reserve University; Professor of Medicine and Harold C. Schott Chair of Rheumatic and Immunologic Diseases; Director, Center for Vasculitis Care and Research, Cleveland Clinic, Cleveland, Ohio
Rheumatic Diseases and the Cardiovascular System

David R. Holmes, Jr., MD
Professor of Medicine, Mayo Clinic College of Medicine; Consultant, Mayo Clinic Saint Marys Hospital, Rochester, Minnesota
Primary Percutaneous Coronary Intervention in the Management of Acute Myocardial Infarction

Sharon A. Hunt, MD
Professor of Cardiovascular Medicine, Stanford University Medical Center, Stanford, California
Heart Transplantation

Eric M. Isselbacher, MD
Assistant Professor of Medicine, Harvard Medical School; Co-Director, Thoracic Aortic Center, Director, Cardiac Unit Associates, Massachusetts General Hospital, Boston, Massachusetts
Diseases of the Aorta

Samer Kabbani, MD
Assistant Professor of Medicine, University of Vermont College of Medicine; Attending Cardiologist, Fletcher Allen Health Care, Burlington, Vermont
Pericardial Diseases

Norman M. Kaplan, MD
Clinical Professor of Internal Medicine, University of Texas Southwestern Medical Center, Dallas, Texas
Systemic Hypertension: Mechanisms and Diagnosis; Systemic Hypertension: Therapy

Adolf W. Karchmer, MD
Professor of Medicine, Harvard Medical School; Chief, Division of Infectious Diseases, Beth Israel Deaconess Medical Center, Boston, Massachusetts
Infective Endocarditis

Morton J. Kern, MD
Professor of Medicine, Saint Louis University School of Medicine; Director, Cardiac Catheterization Laboratory, Saint Louis University Hospital, St. Louis, Missouri
Coronary Blood Flow and Myocardial Ischemia

Irwin Klein, MD
Professor of Medicine, New York University School of Medicine, New York, New York; Chief, Division of Endocrinology, North Shore University Hospital, Mannasset, New York
Endocrine Disorders and Cardiovascular Disease

Barbara A. Konkle, MD
Associate Professor of Medicine and of Pathology and Laboratory Medicine; Director, Penn Comprehensive Hemophilia and Thrombosis Program, University of Pennsylvania School of Medicine and Health System, Philadelphia, Pennsylvania
Hemostasis, Thrombosis, Fibrinolysis, and Cardiovascular Disease

Peter C. Kouretas, MD, PhD
Cardiothoracic Transplantation Fellow, Department of Cardiothoracic Surgery, Stanford University School of Medicine; Staff Physician and Clinical Instructor, Stanford University Hospital, Stanford, California
Heart Transplantation

Ronald M. Krauss, MD
Adjunct Professor, Department of Nutritional Sciences, University of California, Berkeley, Berkeley, California; Senior Scientist and Director, Atherosclerosis Research, Children's Hospital Oakland Research Institute, Oakland, California
Nutrition and Cardiovascular Disease

Meir H. Kryger, MD, FRCPC
Professor of Medicine, University of Manitoba Department of Medicine; Director, Sleep Disorders Centre, St. Boniface Hospital Research Centre, Winnipeg, Manitoba, Canada
Sleep Disorders and Cardiovascular Disease

Richard E. Kuntz, MD
Associate Professor of Medicine and Chief, Division of Clinical Biometrics, Harvard Medical School, Boston, Massachusetts
Percutaneous Coronary and Valvular Intervention

Gary E. Lane, MD
Assistant Professor, Mayo Medical School; Director, Cardiac Catheterization Laboratory, Mayo Clinic St. Luke's Hospital, Jacksonville, Florida
Primary Percutaneous Coronary Intervention in the Management of Acute Myocardial Infarction

Richard A. Lange, MD
Professor of Medicine and E. Cowles Andrus Professor of Cardiology, Johns Hopkins University School of Medicine, Baltimore, Maryland
Toxins and the Heart

Thomas H. Lee, MSc, MD
Professor of Medicine, Harvard Medical School; Network President, Partners Healthcare System, Boston, Massachusetts
Measurement and Improvement of Quality of Cardiovascular Care; Guidelines: Electrocardiography; Guidelines: Exercise Stress Testing; Guidelines: Use of Echocardiography; Guidelines: Nuclear Cardiology; Guidelines: Management of Heart Failure; Guidelines: Ambulatory Electrocardiography and Electrophysiological Testing; Guidelines: Cardiac Pacemakers and Cardioverter-Defibrillators; Guidelines: Treatment of Hypertension; Approach to the Patient with Chest Pain; Guidelines: Primary Percutaneous Coronary Intervention in Acute Myocardial Infarction; Guidelines: Unstable Angina; Guidelines: Chronic Stable Angina; Guidelines: Percutaneous Coronary and Valvular Intervention; Guidelines: Management of Valvular Heart Disease; Guidelines: Infective Endocarditis; Guidelines: Pregnancy; Guidelines: Reducing Cardiac Risk with Noncardiac Surgery

Annarosa Leri, MD
Associate Professor, Department of Medicine, Cardiovascular Research Institute, New York Medical College, Valhalla, New York
Myocardial Regeneration

Martin M. LeWinter, MD
Professor of Medicine and of Molecular Physiology and Biophysics, University of Vermont College of Medicine; Director, Heart Failure Program, Fletcher Allen Health Care, Burlington, Vermont
Pericardial Diseases

Peter Libby, MD
Mallinckrodt Professor of Medicine, Harvard Medical School; Chief, Cardiovascular Division, Brigham and Women's Hospital, Boston, Massachusetts
The Vascular Biology of Atherosclerosis; Risk Factors for Atherothrombotic Disease; Lipoprotein Disorders and Cardiovascular Disease; Diabetes Mellitus, the Metabolic Syndrome, and Atherosclerotic Vascular Disease; Peripheral Arterial Diseases

Stuart Linas, MD
Professor of Medicine, University of Colorado Health Sciences Center; Chief, Nephrology, Denver Health, Denver, Colorado
Drugs in the Treatment of Heart Failure

Steven E. Lipshultz, MD
Professor and Chair, Department of Pediatrics; Professor of Medicine and of Epidemiology and Public Health, University of Miami School of Medicine; Chief of Staff, Holtz Children's Hospital of the University of Miami–Jackson Memorial Medical Center, Miami, Florida
Cardiovascular Abnormalities in HIV-Infected Individuals

Brian D. Lowes, MD
Associate Professor of Medicine, University of Colorado Health Sciences Center; Director, Heart Failure Program, University Hospital, Denver, Colorado
Management of Heart Failure

Brian F. Mandell, MD, PhD
Professor of Medicine, Cleveland Clinic Lerner College of Medicine of Case Western Reserve University; Vice Chair of Medicine for Education, Cleveland Clinic, Cleveland, Ohio
Rheumatic Diseases and the Cardiovascular System

JoAnn E. Manson, MD, DrPH
Professor of Medicine and Elizabeth F. Brigham Professor of Women's Health, Harvard Medical School; Chief, Division of Preventive Medicine, Co-Director, Connors Center for Women's Health and Gender Biology, Brigham and Women's Hospital, Boston, Massachusetts
Primary and Secondary Prevention of Coronary Heart Disease

Daniel B. Mark, MD, MPH
Professor of Medicine, Duke University Medical Center; Director, Outcomes Research, Duke Clinical Research Institute, Durham, North Carolina
Economics and Cardiovascular Disease

Andrew R. Marks, MD
Professor and Chair, Department of Physiology and Cellular Biophysics; Professor of Medicine; Clyde and Helen Wu Professor of Molecular Cardiology, Columbia University College of Physicians and Surgeons
The Patient with Cardiovascular Disease and Cancer

Barry J. Maron, MD
Director, Hypertrophic Cardiomyopathy Center, Minneapolis Heart Institute Foundation, Minneapolis, Minnesota; Adjunct Professor of Medicine, Tufts University School of Medicine, Boston, Massachusetts
Cardiovascular Disease in Athletes

Kenneth L. Mattox, MD
Professor and Vice Chair, Michael E. DeBakey Department of Surgery, Baylor College of Medicine; Chief of Surgery Service and Chief of Staff, Ben Taub General Hospital, Houston, Texas
Traumatic Heart Disease

Peter A. McCullough, MD, MPH
Consultant Cardiologist and Chief, Division of Nutrition and Preventive Medicine, William Beaumont Hospital, Royal Oak, Michigan
Interface Between Renal Disease and Cardiovascular Illness

Vallerie V. McLaughlin, MD
Associate Professor of Medicine and Director, Pulmonary Hypertension Program, University of Michigan Health System, Ann Arbor, Michigan
Pulmonary Hypertension

John M. Miller, MD
Professor of Medicine, Indiana University School of Medicine; Director, Clinical Cardiac Electrophysiology, Clarian Health System, Indianapolis, Indiana
Diagnosis of Cardiac Arrhythmias; Therapy for Cardiac Arrhythmias

David M. Mirvis, MD
Professor and Director, Center for Health Services Research, University of Tennessee, Memphis, Tennessee
Electrocardiography

David A. Morrow, MD, MPH
Assistant Professor of Medicine, Harvard Medical School; Associate Physician, Brigham and Women's Hospital, Boston, Massachusetts
Chronic Coronary Artery Disease

Robert J. Myerburg, MD
Professor of Medicine and Physiology, University of Miami School of Medicine; Director, Division of Cardiology, University of Miami–Jackson Memorial Hospital, Miami, Florida
Cardiac Arrest and Sudden Cardiac Death

Elizabeth G. Nabel, MD
Scientific Director, National Heart, Lung, and Blood Institute, National Institutes of Health, Bethesda, Maryland
Principles of Cardiovascular Molecular Biology and Genetics

Yoshifumi Naka, MD, PhD
Herbert Irving Assistant Professor of Surgery, Division of Cardiothoracic Surgery, Columbia University College of Physicians and Surgeons; Adjunct Assistant Professor of Cardiothoracic Surgery, Cornell University Weill Medical College; Director, Cardiac Transplantation and Mechanical Circulatory Support Program, Division of Cardiothoracic Surgery, New York Presbyterian Hospital, New York, New York
Assisted Circulation in the Treatment of Heart Failure

Carlo Napolitano, MD, PhD
Senior Scientist, Molecular Cardiology Laboratories, IRCCS Fondazione S. Maugeri, Pavia, Italy
Genetics of Cardiac Arrhythmias

Richard W. Nesto, MD
Associate Professor of Medicine, Harvard Medical School, Boston; Chair, Department of Cardiovascular Medicine, Lahey Clinic Medical Center, Burlington, Massachusetts
Diabetes and Heart Disease

Jeffrey E. Olgin, MD
Associate Professor in Residence and Chief, Cardiac Electrophysiology, University of California, San Francisco, School of Medicine, San Francisco, California
Specific Arrhythmias: Diagnosis and Treatment

Lionel H. Opie, MD, DPhil, DSc, MD (Hon)
Director, Hatter Institute and Cape Heart Center, Faculty of Health Sciences, University of Cape Town; Senior Physician, Department of Medicine, Groote Schuur Hospital, Cape Town, South Africa
Mechanisms of Cardiac Contraction and Relaxation

Richard C. Pasternak, MD
Associate Professor of Medicine, Harvard Medical School; Director, Preventive Cardiology and Cardiac Rehabilitation, Massachusetts General Hospital, Boston, Massachusetts
Comprehensive Rehabilitation of Patients with Cardiovascular Disease

Dudley Pennell, MD, FRCP, FACC, FESC
Professor of Cardiology, Imperial College; Director, Cardiovascular Magnetic Resonance Unit, Royal Brompton Hospital, London, United Kingdom
Cardiovascular Magnetic Resonance

Joseph K. Perloff, MD
Streisand/American Heart Association Professor of Medicine and Pediatrics, Emeritus, Founding Director, Ahmanson/UCLA Adult Congenital Heart Disease Center, David Geffen School of Medicine at UCLA; Los Angeles, California
Physical Examination of the Heart and Circulation

Jeffrey J. Popma, MD
Associate Professor of Medicine, Harvard Medical School; Director, Interventional Cardiology, Brigham and Women's Hospital, Boston, Massachusetts
Coronary Angiography and Intravascular Ultrasound Imaging; Percutaneous Coronary and Valvular Intervention

J. David Port, PhD
Associate Professor of Medicine and Pharmacology, University of Colorado Health Sciences Center, Denver, Colorado
Drugs in the Treatment of Heart Failure

Silvia G. Priori, MD, PhD
Associate Professor, University of Pavia School of Cardiology; Director of Molecular Cardiology, IRCCS Fondazione S. Maugeri, Pavia, Italy
Genetics of Cardiac Arrhythmias

Reed E. Pyeritz, MD, PhD
Professor of Medicine and Genetics, Chief, Division of Medical Genetics, University of Pennsylvania School of Medicine, Philadelphia, Pennsylvania
Genetics and Cardiovascular Disease

Andrew N. Redington, MD, MBBS, MRCP(UK), FRCP(UK), FRCPC
University of Toronto; Head, Division of Cardiology, Hospital for Sick Children, Toronto, Ontario, Canada
Congenital Heart Disease

Stuart Rich, MD
Professor of Medicine and Director, Center for Pulmonary Heart Disease, Rush Medical College, Chicago, Illinois
Pulmonary Hypertension

Paul M. Ridker, MD, MPH
Eugene Braunwald Professor of Medicine, Harvard Medical School; Director, Center for Cardiovascular Disease Prevention, Brigham and Women's Hospital, Boston, Massachusetts
Risk Factors for Atherothrombotic Disease; Primary and Secondary Prevention of Coronary Heart Disease

Robert C. Robbins, MD
Associate Professor, Department of Cardiothoracic Surgery, Stanford University School of Medicine and Stanford Hospital, Stanford, California
Heart Transplantation

David Robertson, MD
Elton Yates Professor of Medicine, Pharmacology, and Neurology; Director, General Clinical Research Center, Vanderbilt University School of Medicine, Nashville, Tennessee
Cardiovascular Manifestations of Autonomic Disorders

Rose Marie Robertson, MD
Professor of Medicine, Vanderbilt University School of Medicine; Chief Science Officer, American Heart Association, Nashville, Tennessee
Cardiovascular Manifestations of Autonomic Disorders

Dan M. Roden, MD
Professor of Medicine and Pharmacology and Director, Division of Clinical Pharmacology, Vanderbilt University School of Medicine, Nashville, Tennessee
The Principles of Drug Therapy

Eric A. Rose, MD
Morris and Rose Milstein/Johnson & Johnson Professor and Chair, Department of Surgery; Surgeon-in-Chief, Columbia University College of Physicians and Surgeons; Director, Surgical Service, New York Presbyterian Hospital, New York, New York
Assisted Circulation in the Treatment of Heart Failure

Kenneth Rosenfield, MD
Lecturer on Medicine, Harvard Medical School; Director, Cardiac and Vascular Invasive Services, Massachusetts General Hospital, Boston, Massachusetts
Endovascular Treatment of Noncoronary Obstructive Vascular Disease

Michael Rubart, MD
Assistant Scientist, Indiana University School of Medicine, Indianapolis, Indiana
Genesis of Cardiac Arrhythmias: Electrophysiological Considerations

Marc S. Sabatine, MD, MPH
Instructor in Medicine, Harvard Medical School; Associate Physician, Cardiovascular Division, Brigham and Women's Hospital, Boston, Massachusetts
Primary Tumors of the Heart

Andrew I. Schafer, MD
Frank Wister Thomas Professor and Chair, Department of Medicine, University of Pennsylvania School of Medicine and Health System, Philadelphia, Pennsylvania
Hemostasis, Thrombosis, Fibrinolysis, and Cardiovascular Disease

Frederick J. Schoen, MD, PhD
Professor of Pathology and Health Sciences and Technology, Harvard Medical School; Executive Vice Chair, Department of Pathology, Brigham and Women's Hospital, Boston Massachusetts
Primary Tumors of the Heart

J. Sanford Schwartz, MD
Professor of Medicine and Health Management and Economics, University of Pennsylvania School of Medicine and The Wharton School, Philadelphia, Pennsylvania
Clinical Decision-Making in Cardiology

Janice B. Schwartz, MD
Clinical Professor of Medicine, Divisions of Cardiology and Clinical Pharmacology, University of California, San Francisco, School of Medicine; Director, Research, Jewish Home of San Francisco, San Francisco, California
Cardiovascular Disease in the Elderly

Peter J. Schwartz, MD
Professor of Cardiology, University of Pavia, Pavia, Italy
Genetics of Cardiac Arrhythmias

Jeffrey F. Smallhorn, MBBS, FRACP, FRCPC
University of Toronto; Hospital for Sick Children, Toronto, Ontario, Canada
Congenital Heart Disease

Nancy K. Sweitzer, MD, PhD
Assistant Professor of Medicine, University of Wisconsin Medical School; Director, Heart Failure Program, University of Wisconsin Hospital and Clinics, Madison, Wisconsin
Cardiovascular Disease in Women

Judith Therrien, MD, FRCPC
McGill University, Department of Medicine; Sir Mortimer B. Davis Jewish General Hospital, Montréal, Québec, Canada
Congenital Heart Disease

James E. Udelson, MD
Associate Professor of Medicine and Radiology, Tufts University School of Medicine; Associate Chief, Division of Cardiology; Director, Nuclear Cardiology; Co-Director, Heart Failure Center, Tufts–New England Medical Center, Boston, Massachusetts
Nuclear Cardiology

Matthew J. Wall, Jr., MD
Professor, Michael E. DeBakey Department of Surgery, Baylor College of Medicine; Deputy Chief of Surgery, Chief of Cardiothoracic Surgery, Ben Taub General Hospital, Houston, Texas
Traumatic Heart Disease

Gary D. Webb, MD, FRCPC
Bitove Family Professor of Adult Congenital Heart Disease and Professor of Medicine, University of Toronto; Director, Toronto Congenital Cardiac Centre for Adults, Toronto General Hospital, Toronto, Ontario, Canada
Congenital Heart Disease

Joshua Wynne, MD, MBA, MPH
Professor of Medicine, Wayne State University; Attending Physician, Detroit Medical Center, Detroit, Michigan
The Cardiomyopathies; Myocarditis

Clyde W. Yancy, MD
Professor of Medicine (Cardiology) and Medical Director, Heart Failure and Heart Transplantation, University of Texas Southwestern Medical Center; Associate Dean of Clinical Affairs, St. Paul University Hospital, Dallas, Texas
Heart Disease in Varied Populations

Douglas P. Zipes, MD, MACC
Distinguished Professor of Medicine, Pharmacology, and Toxicology, Director, Division of Cardiology and the Krannert Institute of Cardiology, Indiana University School of Medicine, Indianapolis, Indiana
Genesis of Cardiac Arrhythmias: Electrophysiological Considerations; Diagnosis of Cardiac Arrhythmias; Therapy for Cardiac Arrhythmias; Cardiac Pacemakers and Cardioverter-Defibrillators; Specific Arrhythmias: Diagnosis and Treatment; Hypotension and Syncope; Cardiovascular Disease in the Elderly; Neurological Disorders and Cardiovascular Disease

PREFACE

The preface to the previous (sixth) edition of *Heart Disease* began, "The accelerating advances in cardiology since the publication of the fifth edition of *Heart Disease* have required the most extensive changes yet made in any revision." That statement applies with even greater emphasis to this edition. The exponential growth curve of new knowledge has never been steeper, and the seventh edition of *Braunwald's Heart Disease* has been created to meet that challenge.

The appearance of the book has been changed radically: the cover shows a holographic MRI of a heart, alternating between systole and diastole, and the pages within are in full color, both to enhance reader appeal and to make figures and images more realistic and understandable. We now have an e-dition that provides electronic access to the entire book and enables the reader to download any figures or tables to his or her own computer and to use them in a PowerPoint format for lectures. The book contains 569 tables and 1503 figures, and the accompanying CD contains additional images and video clips. Finding a particular fact can be done with a flip of a finger in the e-dition, as a reader can electronically scan pages, facts, figures, and references. We recognize that books published on a four-year cycle cannot hope to keep current with the incredible pace of new observations. Therefore, by scanning and summarizing the important articles in the literature, and posting those commentaries on the e-dition site, we will update the e-dition *weekly*. Updates will be keyed to related book content. Finally, having recognized the important issues of professionalism and ethics, for the first time we have included an index listing of potential conflict of interest associations for all contributors.

The contents of this edition have also been comprehensively upgraded. As expected, all of the 51 chapters in the sixth edition that have been retained for the current edition have been thoroughly revised and updated. In addition, 36 new chapters have been included, whose topics range from clinical decision-making to cardiovascular manifestations of autonomic disorders. Fifty-seven new authors have made contributions. Thus, the state-of-the-art information serving as the foundation of the text's intellectual vitality has been retained and strengthened in this edition. Bibliographic citations have been generally limited to sources published in 1998 or later, to avoid the accretion of references that can consume valuable pages without offering the utility of fresh content. Earlier references can be obtained from the reviews cited and from previous editions. We continue to present an understanding of basic mechanisms underlying disease states, but we also emphasize the practical evaluation and treatment of patients with these problems, as well as provide a compendium of current guidelines for the reader's convenience.

Part I includes the general considerations of cardiovascular disease, with chapters on the global burden, economics, *clinical decision making,** *assessment of quality of cardiac care, principles of drug therapy*, and *care of patients with end-stage heart disease.*

Part II continues the tradition of the previous edition, emphasizing history and physical examination, electrocardiography, exercise stress testing, and echocardiography. However, recognizing the increasing importance of new imaging techniques, we include new chapters on *radiology of the heart and great vessels, nuclear cardiology, magnetic resonance imaging, computed tomography*, cardiac catheterization, and coronary angiography and intravascular ultrasonography, as well as a chapter that places the various imaging modalities into perspective.

Heart failure has emerged as one of the most important problems in cardiology, as is reflected in **Part III**. It comprises a chapter on understanding mechanisms of cardiac contraction, *assessment of cardiac function*, pathophysiology of heart failure and its clinical aspects, two chapters on pharmacological treatment, and chapters on *assisted circulation* and *transplantation.*

Almost a quarter of all deaths in the U.S. are due to sudden death, most commonly from a rhythm disturbance, and **Part IV** deals with that issue, beginning with the genesis of arrhythmias. We have a new chapter addressing the growing importance of *genetics and arrhythmias*, and then continue with diagnosis, treatment, pacemakers and defibrillators, specific arrhythmias, cardiac arrest, and syncope.

Preventive cardiology is a mainstay of the cardiologist's role, and we devote multiple chapters to this important initiative in **Part V**, including the biology of atherogenesis, risk factors, hypertension (two chapters), lipoprotein disorders, *diabetes, nutrition*, prevention of coronary heart disease, and *rehabilitation.* In view of the growing importance of diabetes in the practice of cardiology, the current edition now includes a new chapter devoted to the vascular complications of this common condition.

Part VI includes the section on coronary disease, which accounts for the vast majority of heart disease in developed countries. The chapters include *understanding coronary blood flow and ischemia, approach to the patient with chest pain*, pathophysiology, clinical features, and management of ST-segment elevation myocardial infarction (MI), *percutaneous coronary intervention in MI*, unstable angina and non–ST-elevation MI, *chronic coronary artery disease, diabetes and heart disease*, percutaneous coronary and valvular intervention, aortic diseases, peripheral vascular diseases, and *endovascular treatment of noncoronary obstructive vascular disease.*

The rest of the book addresses somewhat less common, but still very important, problems. **Part VII** includes chapters on *congenital heart disease*, valvular heart disease, infective endocarditis, cardiomyopathies, *myocarditis*, HIV and the heart, *toxins*, primary cardiac tumors, *pericardial diseases*, traumatic heart disease, pulmonary embolism and pulmonary hypertension, and *sleep disorders.* **Part VIII** focuses on aspects of molecular biology and genetics. The chapters include *general principles of molecular biology needed by physicians*, genetics, and *myocardial regeneration.*

Part IX focuses on special populations of patients with cardiovascular disease, including *elderly patients, women*, pregnant patients, athletes, patients undergoing cardiac and *noncardiac surgery*, and patients belonging to *varied populations.* **Part X** fills remaining gaps by including cardiovascular disease and disorders of other organs, such as *endocrine disorders*, hematologic issues, rheumatic fever and rheumatic diseases, *oncologic disorders*, behavioral issues, neurological disorders, *renal disorders*, and *autonomic dysfunction.*

Companion volumes continue to supplement the information in *Braunwald's Heart Disease*, and they now include

*New chapters indicated in italics.

Heart Disease Review and Assessment, sixth edition (Lilly), Cardiovascular Therapeutics, second edition (Antman), Molecular Basis of Cardiovascular Disease, second edition (Chien), Clinical Trials in Heart Disease, second edition (Manson), Heart Failure (Mann), Marcus' Cardiac Imaging, second edition (Skorton), Acute Coronary Syndromes (Theroux), and Clinical Cardiovascular Imaging (St. John Sutton and Rutherford). Companion volumes in other areas of cardiology are planned for the near future. The seventh edition of *Braunwald's Heart Disease* continues to serve as the anchor for this collection of books, all of which help the busy scientist and clinician keep up with contemporary issues in cardiovascular diseases.

As always, the goal of this textbook is to educate, stimulate, and serve as a resource for all professionals caring for patients with cardiovascular disease. We are certain that the e-dition will add significant value to accomplishing that end. We could not have accomplished this goal without the help of our editorial associates, Janet Hutcheson, Karen Williams, Cynthia Escobedo, and Kathryn Saxon. The staff at Elsevier has been extremely supportive, and has tolerated our frequent requests for changes to make the book even better. To our editor, Anne Lenehan, developmental editor, Deborah Thorp, and project manager, Robin Davis, we give our thanks.

On the cover is a holographic magnetic resonance image of a cross section of the heart of Dr. Saptarsi Haldar in end-systole and end-diastole courtesy of Dr. Raymond Kwong, both of Brigham and Women's Hospital, reproduced with both of their permissions.

Finally, we thank you, the reader, from medical student to skilled clinician, for showing support for this textbook over the years. You, and our patients, are the driving forces to make this the kind of effort that contributes meaningfully to the education of cardiovascular specialists.

Douglas P. Zipes

Peter Libby

Robert O. Bonow

Eugene Braunwald

2004

PREFACE *Adapted from the First Edition*

Cardiovascular disease is the greatest scourge affecting the industrialized nations. As with previous scourges—bubonic plague, yellow fever, and smallpox—cardiovascular disease not only strikes down a significant fraction of the population without warning but also causes prolonged suffering and disability in an even larger number. In the United States alone, despite recent encouraging declines, cardiovascular disease is still responsible for almost 1 million fatalities each year and more than half of all deaths; almost 5 million persons afflicted with cardiovascular disease are hospitalized each year. The cost of these diseases in terms of human suffering and of material resources is almost incalculable. Fortunately, research focusing on the causes, diagnosis, treatment, and prevention of heart disease is moving ahead rapidly.

In order to provide a comprehensive, authoritative text in a field that has become as broad and deep as cardiovascular medicine, I chose to enlist the aid of a number of able colleagues. However, I hoped that my personal involvement in the writing of about half of the book would make it possible to minimize the fragmentation, gaps, inconsistencies, organizational difficulties, and impersonal tone that sometimes plague multiauthored texts.

Since the early part of the 20th century, clinical cardiology has had a particularly strong foundation in the basic sciences of physiology and pharmacology. More recently, the disciplines of molecular biology, genetics, developmental biology, biophysics, biochemistry, experimental pathology, and bioengineering have also begun to provide critically important information about cardiac function and malfunction. Although *Heart Disease: A Textbook of Cardiovascular Medicine* is primarily a clinical treatise and not a textbook of fundamental cardiovascular science, an effort has been made to explain, in some detail, the scientific bases of cardiovascular diseases.

Eugene Braunwald, 1980

CONTENTS

PART VII ■ Diseases of the Heart, Pericardium, and Pulmonary Vasculature Bed 1489

PART VIII ■ Molecular Biology and Genetics 1849

PART IX ■ Cardiovascular Disease in Special Populations 1925

PART VI

Atherosclerotic Cardiovascular Disease

CHAPTER 44

Coronary Blood Flow and Myocardial Ischemia

Morton J. Kern*

The coronary circulation supplies the heart with oxygen and nutrients to maintain cardiac function and thus supply the remainder of the body with blood. The systemic metabolic needs may change rapidly and widely, thus requiring rapid adaptation of cardiac function and coronary blood flow. Imbalance in myocardial oxygen demand and supply can produce myocardial ischemia with contractile cardiac dysfunction, arrhythmias, infarction, and possibly death. Knowledge of the coronary anatomy and flow mechanics of different regions helps us understand the clinical presentations of myocardial ischemia.

The flow through the coronary arteries is pulsatile, with characteristic phasic systolic and diastolic flow components. Systolic compression of the intramural coronary vessels causes mean systolic arterial flow to be reduced relative to diastolic flow, despite having a higher systolic driving pressure. The systolic flow wave has rapid, brief retrograde responses corresponding to phasic myocardial compliance over the cardiac cycle. Diastolic flow occurs during the relaxation phase after myocardial contraction with an abrupt increase above systolic levels and a gradual decline parallel with that of aortic diastolic pressure.

Intramural coronary blood volume changes during each heartbeat, with the myocardium acting as a capacitance circuit to accommodate the volume change brought about by muscular contraction. Coronary venous flow is out of phase with coronary arterial flow, occurring predominantly in systole and nearly absent during diastole. The arterial and venous pulsatile flow characteristics describing the heart as a pump are dependent on intramyocardial compliance. The capacity of the pump as reservoir is controlled by resistance arterioles to coronary vascular inflow, whereas outlet resistance is related to intramural cardiac veins. The intramyocardial capillary resistance influences both arterial and venous responses but predominantly acts in concert with outlet resistance. The coronary blood flow not only is phasic but also varies with the type of vessel and location in the myocardium. The nonlinear and time-dependent behavior of coronary flow may not be negligible under specific experimental or clinical conditions.

Myocardial Oxygen Supply and Demand Relationship

The basic concept of the myocardial supply and demand relationship is that for any given oxygen need, the heart will be supplied with a sufficient quantity to prevent underperfusion leading to ischemia or infarction. Myocardial oxygen demand (MVO_2) has been indexed by the product of systolic aortic pressure and systolic duration. Myocardial oxygen supply (flow) can be indexed by the product of diastolic time and mean diastolic pressure. Figure 44–1 displays major factors of the supply-and-demand relationship.

The heart, an aerobic organ, relies almost exclusively on the oxidation of substrates for energy generation. It can develop only a small oxygen debt. In a steady state, MVO_2 provides an accurate measure of its total metabolism. MVO_2 correlates directly with the fraction of energy derived from the metabolism of fatty acids, which varies directly with the arterial concentration of fatty acids and inversely with that of glucose and insulin. The total metabolism of the arrested, quiescent heart is only a small fraction of that of the working organ. The MVO_2 of the beating canine heart ranges from 8 to 15 ml/min/100 gm, whereas the MVO_2 of the noncontracting heart is approximately 1.5 ml/min/100 gm, an amount required for those physiological processes

*Portions of this chapter have been taken and incorporated from Drs. Peter Ganz and William Ganz, coauthors of this chapter in the sixth edition of this book.

FiO2
Hgb
Fe++
Oxygen carrying capacity
SUPPLY
DEMAND
Heart rate
Contractility
Ventricular wall tension
Coronary blood flow
Diastolic flow
Resistances
R1 epicardial
R2 precapillary
R3 microvascular
Regulation
Metabolic control
Endothelial function
Autoregulation
Neurohumeral factors
Myogenic and
Extravascular compressive forces

FIGURE 44–1 Factors influencing myocardial oxygen supply and demand. FiO_2 = fraction of inspired oxygen; Hgb = hemoglobin.

not directly associated with contraction. Increases in the frequency of depolarization of the noncontracting heart are accompanied by only small increases in MVO_2 (Table 44–1).

Determinants of Myocardial Oxygen Demand

The three major determinants of MVO_2 are heart rate, myocardial contractility, and myocardial wall tension or stress.[1] Additional factors are shown in Table 44–2.

TABLE 44–1 Myocardial O_2 Consumption Components*
Total 6-8 ml/min/100 gm
Distribution Basal, 20% Electrical, 1% Volume work, 15% Pressure work, 64%
Effects on MVo2 of 50% Increase In Wall stress, 25% Contractility, 45% Pressure work, 50% Heart rate, 50% Volume work, 4%

From Gould KL: Coronary Artery Stenosis. New York, Elsevier, 1991, p 8.
*The table demonstrates the dominant contribution to myocardial O_2 consumption (MVO_2) made by pressure work and prominent effects of increasing pressure work and heart rate on MVO_2.

TABLE 44–2 Determinants of Myocardial O_2 Consumption
Heart rate
Contractile state
Tension development
Activation
Depolarization
Direct metabolic effect of catecholamines
Family history of coronary artery disease
Fatty acid uptake
Maintenance of active state
Maintenance of cell viability in basal state
Shortening against a load (Fenn effect)

Heart Rate

Heart rate is the most important determinant of MVO_2. When heart rate doubles, myocardial oxygen uptake approximately doubles. Heart rate is a dominant factor in the supply-demand ratio for two reasons: (1) increases in heart rate also increase oxygen consumption and (2) increases in heart rate reduce subendocardial coronary flow due to diminution of the diastolic filling period. As demonstrated by Spaan,[2] subendocardial ischemia occurs during tachycardia because of a declining MVO_2–heart rate slope, whereas the relationship between increasing demand (tachycardia) and maximal flow for the subepicardium is relatively stable (Fig. 44–2).

Myocardial Contractility

MVO_2 is determined by the summed responses relating contractility and generated pressure on a per-beat basis. The net effect of positive inotropic stimuli (e.g., Ca^{2+} and catecholamines) on MVO_2 is the result of two major determinants that change in opposite directions in the intact heart. These are *wall tension*, which declines as a consequence of reduction in heart size, and *myocardial contractility*, which, by definition, is augmented by inotropic stimuli. In the failing, dilated ventricle, the increased contractility reduces the left ventricular pressure and volume. On the basis of the Laplace relation, the reduction in ventricular volume leads to a reduction in myocardial tension, which reduces MVO_2. However, the decrease in MVO_2 that might be expected to result from falling ventricular wall tension is opposed by the increase in

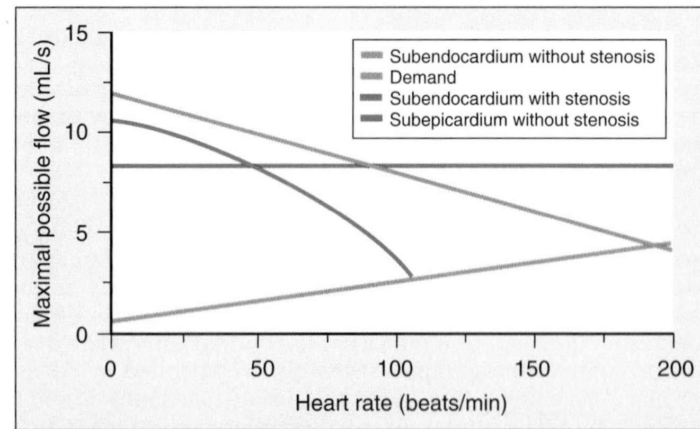

FIGURE 44–2 Schematic representation of the effect of heart rate on myocardial blood flow: The myocardial oxygen demand for unit weight of tissue is similar for the two layers in the heart, but the maximum flow at the subendocardium decreases with heart rate faster than the demand increases, especially in the presence of the stenosis. The maximum flow curve for the subepicardium in the presence of a stenosis has not been drawn. (Modified from Spaan JAE, Piek JJ, Siebes M: Coronary circulation and hemodynamics. *In* Kurachi Y, Terzic A, Cohen M, et al [eds]: Heart Physiology and Pathophysiology. 4th ed. Boston, Academic Press, 2001.)

contractility, which tends to augment MVO_2. Thus, the change in MVO_2 consequent to an inotropic stimulus depends on the extent to which intramyocardial tension is reduced in relation to the extent to which contractility is augmented. In the absence of heart failure, drugs that stimulate myocardial contractility elevate MVO_2 because heart size and therefore wall tension are not reduced substantially and do not offset the effect of the stimulation of contractility. The increase in MVO_2 produced by positive inotropic agents, such as Ca^{2+} and epinephrine, results from the energy costs of enhanced excitation-contraction coupling.

Myocardial Wall Tension

Myocardial tension developed during systole is proportionate to the aortic pressure, myocardial fibril length, and ventricular volume. MVO_2 doubles as mean aortic pressure increases from 75 to 175 mm Hg, at constant heart rate and stroke volume. The myocardial inotropic state determines ventricular performance independent of preload and afterload and increases 30% when the rate of pressure development in the left ventricle (dP/dt) is doubled, such as occurs following extrasystolic potentiation or by norepinephrine when heart rate, aortic pressure, and cardiac output are maintained constant. Comparing the relative effects of ventricular pressure, stroke volume, and heart rate on MVO_2, it was found that ventricular pressure development is a key determinant of MVO_2. MVO_2 per beat correlated well with the area under the left ventricular pressure curve (time × pressure), termed the *tension-time index.*[2,3] Subsequently, the myocardial wall tension–time integral was found to be a more accurate determinant of MVO_2 than is the developed pressure. An augmentation of *heart rate* elevates MVO_2 by increasing the frequency of tension development per unit time, as well as by increasing contractility.

MVO_2 is also influenced by the degree of myocardial shortening during stroke volume ejection, although less than by tension development. The systolic pressure-rate product (also known as the *double product*) can be used as an estimate of MVO_2 in a clinical setting, such as exercise or pacing tachycardia, recognizing the limited accuracy. MVO_2 closely correlates with the left ventricular systolic pressure–volume loop area (the external mechanical work) and the end-systolic elastic potential energy in the ventricular wall (the area enclosed by the systolic pressure–volume trajectory, and the E_{max} line) (Fig. 44–3).

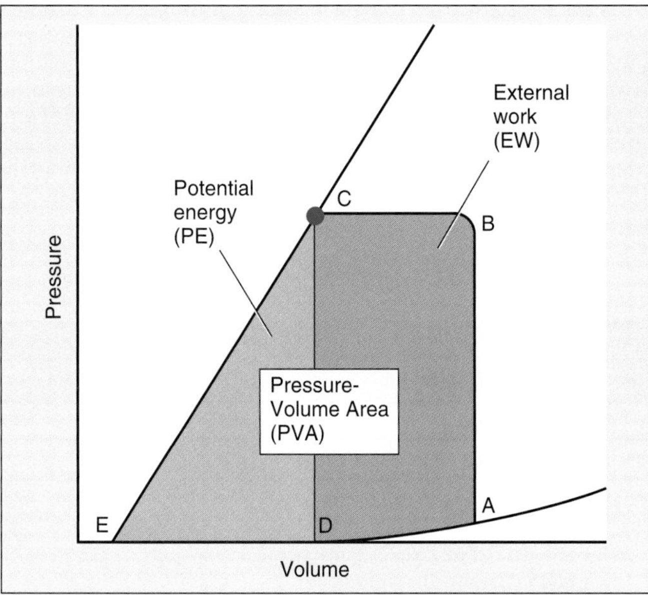

FIGURE 44–3 Myocardial oxygen consumption correlates with the left ventricular pressure-volume area (PVA). PVA is the area in the pressure-volume (PV) diagram that is circumscribed by the end-systolic PV line (E-C), the end-diastolic PV relation curve (D-A), and the systolic segment of the PV trajectory (E-A-B-C-E). PVA consists of the external work (EW) performed during systole and the end-systolic elastic potential energy (PE) stored in the ventricular wall at end-systole. EW is the area within the PV loop trajectory (A-B-C-D-A), and PE is the area between the end-systolic PV line and the end-diastolic PV relation curve to the left of EW (E-C-D-E). (From Kameyama T, Asanoi H, Ishizaka S, et al: Energy conversion efficiency in human left ventricle. Circulation 85:988, 1992.)

Determinants of Myocardial Oxygen Supply

Myocardial oxygen supply is provided by the coronary arterial and capillary inflow and a satisfactory capability of hemoglobin to transport and deliver oxygen to the myocardial cells. A breakdown in any link of this chain can result in an inadequate myocardial oxygen supply.

OXYGEN TRANSPORT AND DELIVERY. Satisfactory oxygen transport and delivery require an adequate inspired quantity of oxygen and red blood cells with normally functioning hemoglobins. Hypoxia from pneumonia or carbon monoxide overdose, anemia, or hemoglobinopathies can produce myocardial ischemia despite adequate coronary blood flow.

REGULATION OF CORONARY BLOOD FLOW AND RESISTANCE. Approximately 75 percent of total coronary resistance occurs in the arterial system, which comprises conductance (R1), prearteriolar (R2), and arteriolar and intramyocardial capillary vessels (R3).[4] Normal epicardial coronary arteries in humans are typically 0.3 to 5 mm in caliber and do not offer appreciable resistance to blood flow. Even at the highest level of blood flow, there is no detectable resistance that would manifest as a pressure drop along the length of human epicardial arteries.[5] Normally, large epicardial vessel resistance (R1) is trivial until atherosclerotic obstructions compromise the lumen. During systole, the blood volume increases approximately 25 percent as antegrade flow from the aorta enters and retrograde flow is squeezed from the myocardial vessels. Elastic energy of the vessel wall during systole is transformed into blood kinetic energy at the beginning of diastole. Since most of the vessel wall comprises a muscular media that responds to changes in aortic pressure and modulates coronary tone in response to flow-mediated endothelium-dependent vasodilators, circulating vasoactive substance, and neurostimuli, conductive activity is impaired when vascular wall disease is present. Large conduit arteries are unaffected by myocardial metabolites because of their extramural location.

Precapillary arterioles (R2) are resistive vessels connecting epicardial to myocardial capillaries and are the principal controllers of coronary blood flow.[4] Precapillary arterioles (100 to 500 μm in size) contribute approximately 25 to 35 percent of total coronary resistance (Fig. 44–4). The prearteriolar resistance function maintains driving pressure at the origin of the precapillary arterioles within a preset autoregulatory pressure range. This regulatory function is also mediated by myogenic autoregulation and flow-dependent vasodilation related to shear stress.

Distal precapillary arteriolar vessels are the main site of *metabolic* regulation of coronary blood flow. These vessels (<100 μm in diameter) are responsible for 40 to 50 percent of coronary flow resistance. The distal arteriolar tone is modulated by neurogenic stimuli and local vasoactive products. In some settings, the effects of vasoconstrictor stimuli are strong enough to induce myocardial ischemia unopposed by locally released myocardial vasodilatory metabolites.

The dense network of about 4000 capillaries per square millimeter ensures that each myocyte is adjacent to a capillary. Capillaries are not uniformly patent because precapillary sphincters regulate flow according to the needs of the myocardium. This capillary density is reduced in the presence of ventricular hypertrophy. Several conditions, such as left ventricular hypertrophy, myocardial ischemia, or diabetes can impair the microcirculatory resistance (R3), blunting the maximal absolute increase in coronary flow in times of increased oxygen demand. Increased R3 resistance may also be associated with elevated resting blood flow above that expected for the existing MVO_2, resulting in reduced coronary flow reserve.

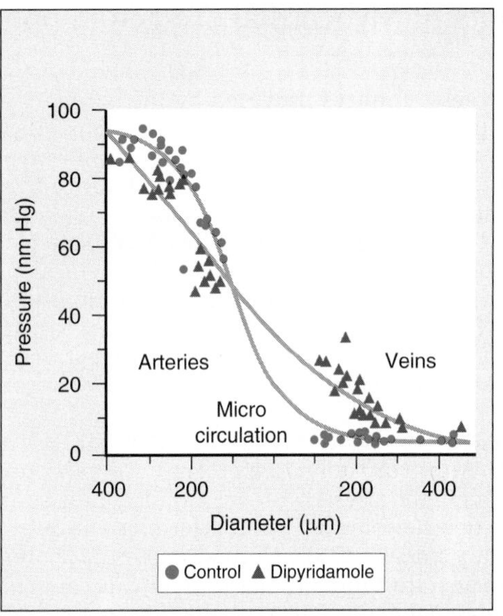

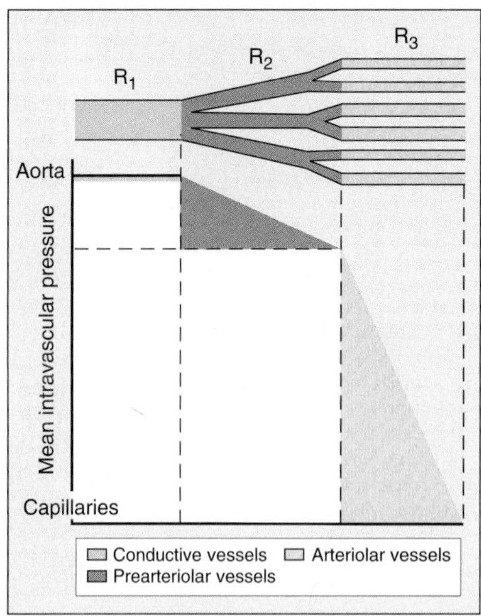

FIGURE 44–4 **A,** Pressure distribution as a function of vessel diameter in the cat. **B,** Schematic representation of the coronary arterial system and its subdivisions. Resistance to blood flow is highest in the arteriolar bed, in which vasodilator activity is under myocardial metabolic regulation. Prearteriolar vessels also contribute to coronary resistance but are not influenced by direct metabolic control. The prearteriolar vessels function to maintain pressure at the origin of the arterioles within a narrow range under varying aortic pressure and coronary flow. The conductive vessels provide negligible resistance to flow. (**A,** From Chilian WM, Layne SM, Klausner ED, et al: Redistribution of coronary microvascular resistance produced by dipyridamole. Am J Physiol 256:H383-390, 1989. **B,** From Maseri A: Ischemic Heart Disease. New York, Churchill Livingstone, 1995.)

Control heterogeneity of the coronary resistance vessels has been demonstrated with specialized resistance vessel functions according to their size.[4] For example, in the smallest arterioles (<30 μm), metabolic vasodilation occurs predominantly, whereas intermediate arterioles (30 to 60 μm) are the principal site of myogenic regulation. The large arterioles (100 to 150 μm) appear to be the sites of flow-mediated dilation.[6] A system of multiple functional "valves" permits fine control of the coronary circulation. The smallest arterioles dilate during metabolic stress, resulting in reduced microvascular resistance and increased myocardial perfusion. As the upstream arteriolar pressure decreases owing to a fall in distending pressure across a stenosis, myogenic dilation of slightly larger arterioles upstream occurs and causes an additional decrease in resistance. Increased flow in the largest arterioles augments shear stress and triggers flow-mediated dilation, further reducing the resistance of this network. Thus, coronary arterioles appear to have specialized regulatory elements along their length that operate "in series" in an integrated manner.

As in any vascular bed, blood flow to the myocardium depends on the coronary artery driving pressure and the resistance offered by the resistance components. Coronary vascular resistance, in turn, is regulated by several interrelated control mechanisms that include myocardial metabolism (metabolic control), endothelial (and other humoral) control, autoregulation, myogenic control, extravascular compressive forces, and neural control. These control mechanisms may be impaired in disease states, thereby contributing to the development of myocardial ischemia (Tables 44–3 and 44–4).

TABLE 44–3 Regulation of Coronary Circulation

Mechanism	Effector
Autoregulation	Intrinsic vasoconstrictor tone
Perfusion pressure	Aortic or poststenotic pressure
Metabolic activity	Exercise, ischemia
Myocardial compression and myogenic mechanisms	Systolic-diastolic interaction
Neural control	Sympathetic, parasympathetic, pain
Endothelium	EDRF, EDCF
Pharmacologic	Dipyridaimole, adenosine, acetylcholine, α, β, agonists and antagonists, and so forth

EDRF = endothelial-derived relaxing factor; EDCF = endothelial-derived constricting factor.
Modified from Gould L: Coronary Artery Stenosis and Reversing Atherosclerosis. 2nd ed. New York, Arnold and Oxford University Press, 1998.

TABLE 44–4 Mediators of Coronary Vasodilation*

Stimulus	Epicardial Arteries	Arterioles, Increased Flow
Acetylcholine	*Nitric oxide*	*Endothelial*
Flow shear	*Endothelial*	*Nitric oxide*
Exercise	*Nitric oxide*, neural	*Metabolic*, nitric oxide, neural
Pacing	*Nitric oxide*	*Nitric oxide*, metabolic
Ischemia or hypoxia	*Metabolic*, nitric oxide	*Metabolic*, nitric oxide
Perfusion pressure	*Myogenic*	*Myogenic*
Reactive hyperemia	*Myogenic*, flow shear	*Myogenic*, flow shear, metabolic, nitric oxide, prostacycline
Dipyridamole, adenosine	No direct effect	*Direct dilator*, nitric oxide
Nitroglycerine	*Direct dilator*	No direct effect
Collaterals	—	*Nitric oxide*, prostaglandin

From Gould L: Coronary Artery Stenosis and Reversing Atherosclerosis. 2nd ed. New York, Arnold and Oxford University Press, 1998.
*Italics, primary mechanism followed by secondary or contributing mechanisms; endothelial, unknown mediator, not oxide; metabolic, unknown mediators or mechanisms but in part mediated by adenosine.

Endothelial Function

The vascular endothelium performs an array of homeostatic functions within normal blood vessels. Located between the blood lumen and the vascular smooth muscle cells, the endothelium is a monolayer of cells capable of transducing blood-borne signals, sensing mechanical forces within the lumen, and regulating vascular tone through the production of a variety of vasoactive humoral factors (Table 44–5; see also Fig. 37–14).[7] Endothelium produces both potent vasodilators, such as endothelium-derived relaxing factor (EDRF), nitric oxide (NO), prostacyclin, and endothelium-derived hyperpolarizing factor (EDHF), and vasoconstrictors, such as endothelin 1 (ET-1). Normally, the endothelium promotes vasodilatory functions in response to a variety of systemic, neurohumoral, and mechanical stimuli. Inappropriate vasoconstriction characterizes the vascular response in patients with endothelial dysfunction.[8]

An imbalance among the endothelium-derived counteracting vasoactive factors occurs in vascular segments damaged early in the atherosclerotic process. Dysfunctional endothelium, common in patients with cardiovascular risk factors, leads to disturbances in coronary blood flow, promoting myocardial ischemia, and accelerating the evolution of atherosclerosis and thrombosis.[9]

Endothelium-dependent vasodilation not only operates in large (conductance) arteries, but is also an important mechanism that controls dilation in small (resistance) vessels. Although atherosclerosis does not directly involve resistance vessels, coronary risk factors markedly impair resistance vessel responses to endothelium-dependent vasodilator stimuli.[8] Endothelial dysfunction in resistance vessels may be an important factor in preventing increases in coronary blood flow during times of augmented metabolic stress. Impaired endothelium-dependent dilation of coronary resistance vessels also accounts for some of the cases of syndrome X (patients with normal coronary angiography, chest pain, and evidence of stress-induced myocardial ischemia).[10] For example, in normal subjects, exercise induces coronary vasodilation, whereas in patients with atherosclerotic coronary artery disease and stable angina, exercise produces paradoxical vasoconstriction typically at the site of coronary stenoses or mildly irregular arterial segments. Vasomotor changes during exercise parallel the responses observed to the endothelium-dependent agent, acetylcholine. Paradoxical constriction of atherosclerotic coronary arteries has also been observed with mental stress, the cold pressor test, and tachycardia,[11] conditions normally activating the sympathetic nervous system, increasing circulating catecholamines and coronary blood flow secondary to a rise in MV_{O_2}. The loss of endothelium-dependent dilation occurs early in atherosclerosis, even prior to its detection by angiography, and is related to risk factors for atherosclerosis (Table 44–6).[12] Oxidized low-density lipoprotein (LDL) and small, dense LDL particles reduce NO synthase.[2] Degradation of chylomicrons and very low-density lipoprotein produce highly atherogenic remnant particles associated with endothelial dysfunction and reduced NO.[13]

ENDOTHELIUM-DERIVED RELAXING FACTORS. In healthy arteries, endothelium-dependent vasodilation predominates over direct smooth muscle vasoconstriction. EDRF is produced from an intact endothelium and mediates acetylcholine-induced vasodilation.[14] EDRF has been identified as the NO radical formed in endothelial cells from L-arginine by the action of NO synthase (Fig. 44–5).[15] The activity of the reaction is also controlled by calcium and calmodulin. NO diffuses into smooth muscle cells activating intracellular guanylate cyclase, increasing cyclic guanosine monophosphate (GMP), and consequently decreasing intracellular calcium. Once released from endothelial cells, NO has a very short half-life due to interaction with other free radicals in tissues, principally superoxide, and is destroyed after entering red blood cells to react with oxyhemoglobin. Endothelium-dependent vasodilation by NO secretion in healthy human epicardial arteries can be inhibited by specifically blocking NO synthesis with N^G-monomethyl-L-arginine (L-NMMA).[16]

TABLE 44–5 Autocrine and Paracrine Substances Released from the Endothelium

Type of Substance	Specific Substances
Vasodilators	NO, prostacyclin, endothelium-derived hyperpolarizing factor, bradykinin, adrenomedullin, C-natriuretic peptide
Vasoconstrictors	ET-1, angiotensin II, thromboxane A_2, oxidant radicals, prostaglandin H_2
Antiproliferative	NO, prostacyclin, transforming growth factor-β, heparin sulfate
Proproliferative	ET-1, angiotensin II, oxidant radicals, platelet-derived growth factor, basic fibroblast growth factor, insulin-like growth factor, interleukins
Antithrombotic	NO, prostacyclin, plasminogen activator, protein C, tissue factor inhibitor, von Willebrand factor
Prothrombotic	ET-1, oxidant radicals, plasminogen-activator inhibitor-1, thromboxane A_2, fibrinogen, tissue factor
Inflammatory markers	CAMs (P- and E-selectin, ICAM, VCAM) chemokines, nuclear factor κB
Permeability	Receptor for advanced glycosylation end-products
Angiogenesis	Vascular endothelial growth factor

CAM = cellular adhesion molecule; ET = endothelin 1; ICAM = intercellular adhesion molecule; NO = nitric oxide; VCAM = vascular cellular adhesion molecule.

Modified from Verma S, Anderson T: Fundamentals of endothelial function for the clinical cardiologist. Circulation 105:546-549, 2002.

TABLE 44–6 Risk Factors Associated with Impaired Endothelium-Dependent Vasodilation

Dyslipidemia
Hypertension
Diabetes mellitus
Cigarette smoking
Menopause
Hyperhomocysteinemia
Aging
Family history of coronary artery disease
Mutations in eNOS

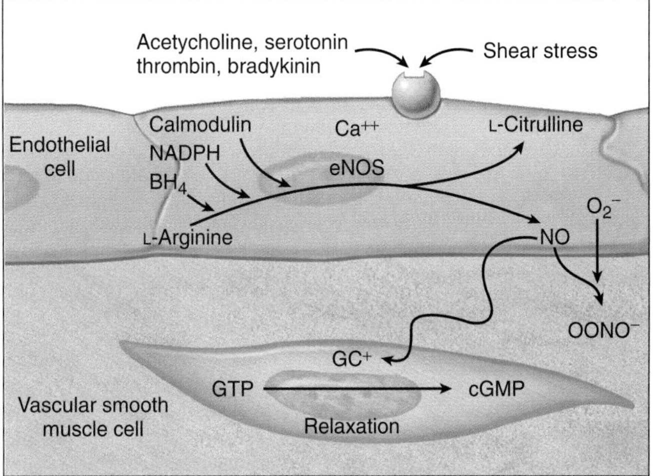

FIGURE 44–5 Endothelial cell production of nitric oxide (NO) by the action of nitric oxide synthase (eNOS) on L-arginine. This reaction requires a number of cofactors such as tetrahydrobiopterin (BH_4), calmodulin, and NADPH. eNOS stimulation by vasodilator agonists or shear stress is mediated by rise in intracellular calcium (Ca^{2+}). NO may be broken down by free radicals (O_2^-), producing peroxinitrite ($OONO^-$), which is vasoinactive. NO acts on vascular smooth muscle cells to cause relaxation by activating guanylate cyclase (GC^+), thereby increasing intracellular cyclic guanosine monophosphate (cGMP).

The release of NO is stimulated by products of thrombosis (thrombin), aggregating platelets (serotonin, adenosine diphosphate [ADP]), other chemical stimuli (histamine, bradykinin), and increased shear stress with flow-mediated vasodilation. In contrast to NO, the nitrovasodilators (e.g., nitroglycerin, nitroprusside) and prostacyclin act independently of the endothelium and directly on vascular smooth muscle.[7] Adenosine elicits both endothelium-independent and endothelium-dependent vasodilation; at high concentration of adenosine, endothelium-independent dilation dominates.

NO also inhibits the recruitment and differentiation of inflammatory cells by inhibiting the production of chemoattractant cytokines, leukocyte adhesion molecules, and factors encouraging the differentiation of monocytes into macrophages. Reductions in NO are associated with activation of potentially vulnerable atherosclerotic plaques and acute coronary syndromes.[17]

Endothelium-dependent vasodilation also occurs by hyperpolarizing the underlying smooth muscle through activation of Ca^{2+}-activated K^+ channels, a response attributed to a diffusible factor termed *EDHF* (also known as *11,12-epoxyeicosatrienoic acid*).[18] EDHF appears to be far more important in small arterioles than in larger conduit arteries.[19] It is released by many of the same stimuli that stimulate NO, including acetylcholine, bradykinin, substance P, and shear stress. Although there may be more than one EDHF molecule, cytochrome P450–dependent metabolites of arachidonic acid, especially the epoxide EDHF, also act as mediators of endothelium-dependent hyperpolarization and have antiinflammatory properties. NO inhibits the production of EDHF. A decrease in NO bioavailability maintains endothelial vasodilator function by upregulation of EDHF.[19]

ENDOTHELIUM-DERIVED CONSTRICTING FACTORS. The endothelium not only mediates vasodilation but also is a source of vasoconstrictor factors, the best characterized being the endothelins. ET-1 is a 21-amino-acid peptide that has a potent vasoconstrictor activity. Two other isoforms of ET have been discovered (ET-2 and ET-3), but endothelium produces only ET-1. Beginning with a large precursor molecule, preproendothelin is converted by the action of endothelin-converting enzyme to the fully active ET-1.[20]

Unlike NO, which can be released rapidly in response to vasodilator stimuli and then inactivated within seconds, ET-1–mediated constriction is slow in onset and lasts over minutes to hours. Agents that stimulate ET-1, such as thrombin, angiotensin II, epinephrine, or vasopressin, do so by de novo transcription of messenger RNA. ET-1 contributes to the regulation of vascular tone primarily by exerting a tonic vasoconstrictor influence and stimulates smooth muscle proliferation, vascular remodeling, and leukocyte adhesion and recruitment.[21] Plasma concentrations of ET-1 are elevated in a number of cardiovascular disorders including hypercholesterolemia, hypertension, atherosclerosis, acute myocardial infarction, and congestive heart failure.[21] Oxidized LDL associated with vulnerable plaque activators is a potent stimulus to ET-1 synthesis. ET-1 exerts its vascular effects by binding to two specific receptors named ET-A and ET-B. ET-A receptors are present on vascular smooth muscle cells and promote vasoconstriction and smooth muscle proliferation. ET-B receptors are located on endothelial cells, where they mediate endothelium-dependent dilation by releasing NO, and also on smooth muscle cells, where they mediate constriction.[22]

ENDOTHELIAL FUNCTION TESTING. Endothelial function can be tested by examining the angiographic vasodilatory responses to intracoronary infusions of endothelial-dependent and -independent vasodilators. The infusion of acetylcholine evokes an endothelium-dependent NO-mediated vasodilatory response. In patients with endothelial dysfunction the normal vasodilatory response is blunted or paradoxic vasoconstriction occurs. Endothelial function of microvascular reserve is assessed by intracoronary Doppler flow velocity measurements during intracoronary infusions of acetylcholine and adenosine for endothelial-dependent and -independent responses, respectively.

Noninvasive assessments of coronary endothelial function, evaluating coronary epicardial blood flow and microcirculatory responses, have been obtained by Doppler echocardiography, positron-emission tomography, and phase-contrast magnetic resonance imaging. The most widely used noninvasive method to assess endothelial function of the peripheral circulation is brachial artery reactive hyperemia obtained during upper arm arterial occlusion and release. Normal endothelial function produces flow-mediated vasodilation of the arterial diameter assessed by continuous ultrasound scanning. Peripheral vascular resistance using strain-gauge venous impedance plethysmography examines forearm blood flow in response to intraarterial administration of vascular agonist into the brachial artery. Brachial artery responses have been generally related to coronary endothelial function. (Fig. 44-6 illustrates changes in coronary diameter and flow during endothelial function testing.) Abnormal endothelial responses can be restored by treatment with angiotensin-converting enzyme inhibitors, antioxidants, and the oral administration of L-arginine.[23] Table 44-7 lists strategies to counter endothelial dysfunction.

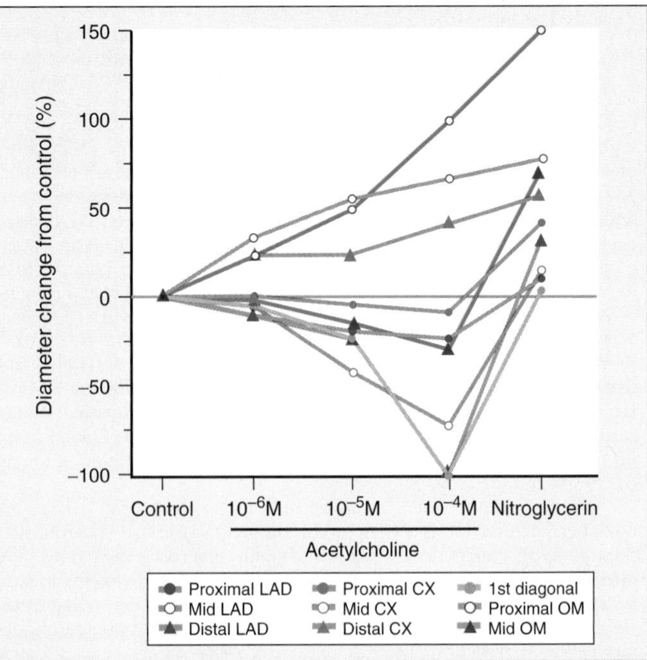

FIGURE 44–6 Heterogeneous responses of coronary artery diameter to the intracoronary acetylcholine in a patient with coronary artery disease. CX = circumflex artery; LAD = left anterior descending [coronary artery]; OM = obtuse marginal artery. (From El-Tamini H, Mansour M, Wargovich TJ, et al: Constrictor and dilator responses to intracoronary acetylcholine in adjacent segments of the same coronary artery in patients with coronary artery disease. Circulation 89:45-51, 1994.)

Autoregulation

Foremost in the control of coronary blood flow is the fundamental relationship that myocardial oxygen supply rises and falls in response to the oxygen (energy) demands of the myocardium. Sudden alterations in systemic hemodynamics are matched with abrupt and transitory changes in blood flow, promptly returning to the resting steady state after activity has ceased. The ability to maintain myocardial perfusion at constant levels in the face of changing driving pressure is termed *autoregulation* (Fig. 44–7). Autoregulation maintains coronary perfusion at relatively constant levels over a wide range of mean aortic pressure from130 to 40 mm Hg in experimental animals and humans.[24] When aortic pressure exceeds its upper or lower limits, coronary blood flow precipitously declines or increases proportionately. Normally functioning autoregulation prevents myocardial ischemia at rest. When reduced perfusion pressure distal to stenoses is not compensated by autoregulatory dilation of the resistance vessels, ischemia occurs. Chronic hypertension and left ventricular hypertrophy narrow the range of autoregulation, especially in the subendocardium. In some patients, exhaustion of subendocardial autoregulation may lead to ischemia in the absence of a significant coronary stenosis.

Systemic hypotension can lower perfusion pressure below the critical lower limit of effective autoregulation, producing myocardial ischemia that increases left ventricular filling pressure, further reducing the coronary perfusion gradient. Hypotension begets a deteriorating, self-perpetuating ischemic spiral, especially deadly in patients with critical coronary stenoses, such as those with left main or with three-vessel coronary disease. Augmenting coronary (diastolic)

TABLE 44–7 Conditions Associated with Impaired Endothelial Function, Strategies to Counter Endothelial Dysfunction, and Surrogate Soluble Markers of Endothelial Dysfunction

Conditions associated with impaired endothelial function	Atherosclerosis, hypercholesterolemia, high LDL-C, low HDL-C, high lipoprotein (a), small dense LDL-C, oxidized LDL-C, hypertension, high homocysteine, aging, vasculitis, preeclampsia, metabolic syndrome, variant angina, diabetes, active smoking, passive smoking, ischemia-reperfusion, transplant atherosclerosis, cardiopulmonary bypass, postmenopause, Kawasaki disease, Chagas disease, family history CAD, infections, depression, inactivity, obesity, renal failure, increased CRP, congestive heart failure, left ventricular hypertrophy, postprandial state
Interventions to improve endothelial function	ACE inhibitors, angiotensin receptor blockers, endothelin blockers, statins, tetrahydrobiopterin, folates, exercise, improving insulin sensitivity, LDL reduction, HDL augmentation, antioxidants, estrogen, L-arginine, desferoxamine, glutathione, homocysteine reduction, lowering CRP, reducing free fatty acid flux
Soluble surrogate markers of endothelial dysfunction	CAMs, von Willbebrand factor, ET-1, nitrites, asymmetric dimethylarginine, CRP, tissue plasminogen activator, fibrinogen, amyloid A

Modified from Verma S, Anderson T: Fundamentals of endothelial function for the clinical cardiologist. Circulation 105:546-549, 2002.
ACE = angiotensin-converting enzyme; CAM = cellular adhesion molecule; CAD = coronary artery disease; CRP = C-reactive protein; ET = endothelin; HDL = high-density lipoprotein; LDL = low-density lipoprotein.

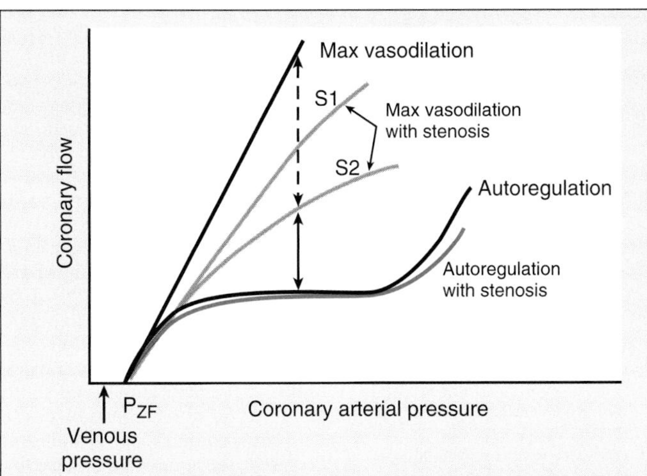

FIGURE 44–7 Coronary pressure-flow relations with and without stenosis. Autoregulation of flow at rest without stenosis and maximal vasodilation without stenosis are indicated in black lines. S1 has mild stenosis compared to S2. The solid arrow illustrates the reduced coronary flow reserve related to the presence of a severe stenosis. The dashed arrow indicates the dilatory reserve loss because of the stenosis. P_{ZF} is pressure at zero flow. (From Spaan JAE, Piek JJ, Siebes M: Coronary circulation and hemodynamics. *In* Kurachi Y, Terzic A, Cohen M, et al [eds]: Heart Physiology and Pathophysiology. 4th ed. Boston, Academic Press, 2001.)

perfusion pressure with intraaortic balloon pumping in this setting restores coronary pressure so that autoregulation is reestablished and the cycle of myocardial ischemia may be attenuated or terminated.

Metabolic Regulation

Coronary blood flow is closely coupled to MVO_2 in normal hearts because (1) the myocardium depends almost entirely on aerobic metabolism; (2) the myocardial oxygen extraction saturation is very high as evidenced by low coronary venous oxygen saturation (25 to 30 percent at rest); and (3) oxygen stores in the heart are meager. Potent vasodilator agents such as NO, adenosine, and dipyridamole can relax vascular smooth muscle in coronary arterioles and can attenuate autoregulation. Release of intrinsic vasodilators links myocardial oxygen supply to demand.

ADENOSINE. Adenosine, the principal mediator of coronary blood flow and local metabolic regulation, is formed by degradation of adenine nucleotides. Degradation occurs when adenosine triphosphate (ATP) utilization exceeds the capacity of myocardial cells to resynthesize high-energy phosphate compounds (a process dependent on mitochondrial oxidative phosphorylation). This results in the production of adenosine monophosphate (AMP). The enzyme 5′-nucleotidase is responsible for the formation of adenosine from AMP (Fig. 44–8). Accordingly, adenosine diffuses from myocytes into the interstitial fluid and the coronary venous effluent. Adenosine is a powerful coronary dilator, and its production increases during an imbalance in the oxygen supply-to-demand ratio. The rise in the interstitial concentration of adenosine parallels the increase in coronary blood flow. The inhibition of adenosine, either by its destruction by adenosine deaminase or by administration of adenosine receptor antagonists, does not always reduce the magnitude of the hyperemia in response to metabolic stimuli in animals or humans.[25] Adenosine is certainly not the *only* vasoactive factor involved in the metabolic regulation of coronary blood flow. NO, vasodilator prostaglandins, ATP-sensitive K^+ channels (K^+-ATP channels), and myocardial oxygen and carbon dioxide tensions also contribute to metabolic regulation.

NITRIC OXIDE AND OTHER METABOLIC MEDIATORS. NO increases blood flow in response to metabolic stimuli. Inhibition of NO reduces the magnitude of metabolic dilation in animals and in the peripheral and coronary circulation in humans.[25] Metabolic stimuli augment NO production by at least two mechanisms: (1) hypoxia-stimulated release of NO from the endothelium and (2) coronary flow–mediated vasodilation. Although hypoxia may initiate hyperemia, flow-mediated dilation sustains and amplifies it.

Prostaglandins and K^+-ATP channels also act in concert to regulate coronary flow in response to metabolic needs.[26] A loss or inhibition of one mediator is compensated for by upregulation of others. Although the inhibition of K^+-ATP channels, adenosine, and NO individually have, at most, a modest effect on the increase in coronary blood flow during exercise in dogs, inhibition of all three simultaneously nearly abolishes the flow increase.[27]

Neural and Neurohumeral Control

Neural control of the coronary circulation complements local metabolic, autoregulatory, and endothelial mechanisms.[28] Epicardial arteries and coronary arterioles are innervated by sympathetic and parasympathetic fibers, with extensive adrenergic and muscarinic receptor supply (Table 44-8). In addition to acetylcholine and norepinephrine, nonadrenergic and noncholinergic neurotransmitters have been identified modulating adrenergic and cholinergic output.[28,29] These substances include purines (ATP), amines (serotonin and dopamine), and peptides (neuropeptide Y, calcitonin-gene related peptide [CGRP], substance P, and vasoactive intestinal peptide). Neuropeptide Y released during sympathetic nerve stimulation causes ischemia by microvascular constriction. Intracoronary infusion of CGRP and substance P cause release of EDRF and dose-dependent vasodilation of epicardial vessels equivalent to that produced by nitrates.[30]

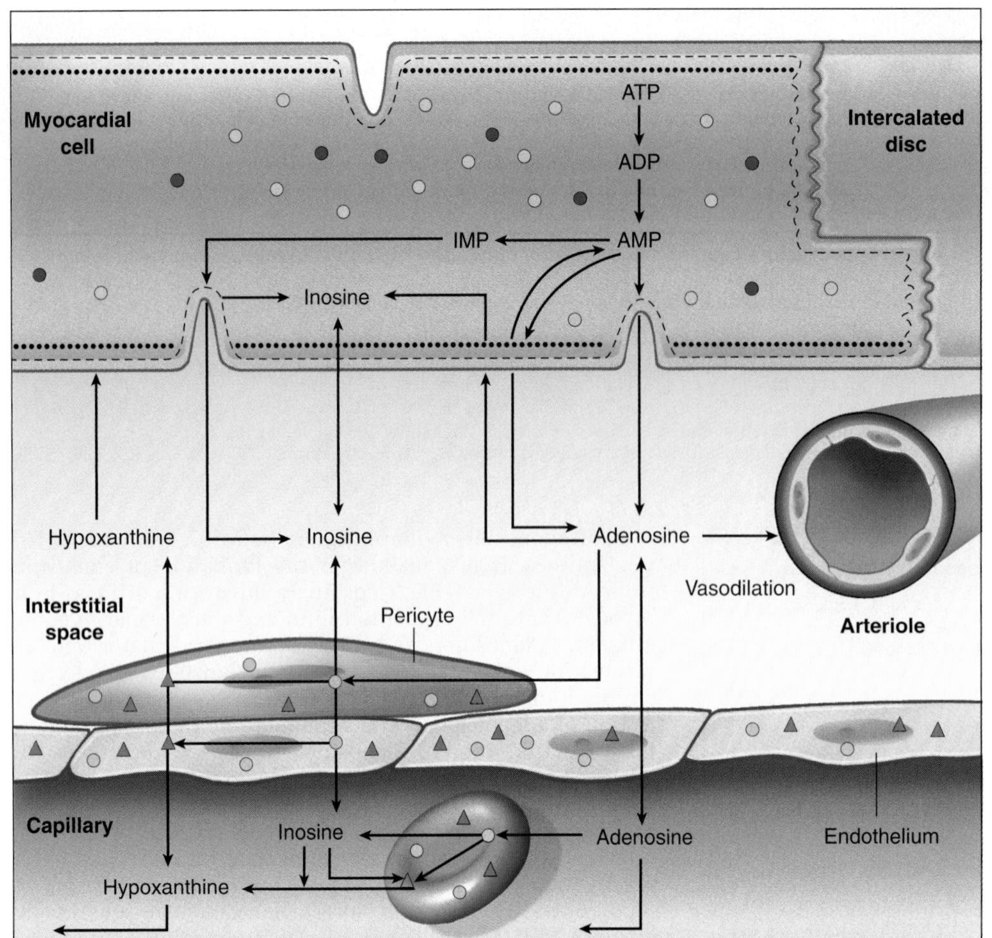

FIGURE 44–8 Schematic depiction of a myocardial interstitial space, an arteriole, and a capillary with the localization of enzymes involved in the formation and fate of adenosine. Adenosine formed by 5′-nucleotidase from adenosine monophosphate (AMP) (which in turn arises from adenosine triphosphate) can enter the interstitial space. There it can induce arteriolar dilation and reenter the myocardial cell, where it is either phosphorylated to AMP by adenosine kinase or deaminated to inosine monophosphate (IMP) by adenosine deaminase, or it can enter the capillaries and leave the tissue. A large fraction of adenosine that crosses the capillary wall is deaminated to inosine, which in turn is split to hypoxanthine and ribose-1-PO_4 by nucleoside phosphorylase located in the endothelial cells, pericytes, and erythrocytes. Most of the adenosine is taken up by the myocardial cells. Adenosine escaping into the circulation is largely in the form of inosine and hypoxanthine. Because adenylic acid deaminase (which deaminates AMP to IMP) is in low concentration in heart muscle, the major degradative pathway from AMP is by means of dephosphorylation to adenosine. Open circles = adenosine deaminase; closed circles = adenylic acid deaminase; triangles = nucleoside phosphorylase; dashed lines = 5′-nucleotidase; dotted lines = adenosine kinase. (From Berne RM, Rubio R: Coronary circulation. *In* Berne RM, Sperelakis N, Geiger SR [eds]: Handbook of Physiology, Section 2. The Cardiovascular System. Bethesda, MD, American Physiological Society, 1979, p 924.)

SYMPATHETIC CONTROL. The effect of stimulation of the adrenergic system depends on the net result of alpha- and beta-receptor activation, with alpha-mediated vasoconstriction normally balanced by $beta_1$-mediated vasodilation (Table 44–9). In the presence of beta-adrenoreceptor antagonists, electrical activation of sympathetic fibers results in coronary vasoconstriction mediated by alpha receptors and attenuated by alpha-adrenergic antagonists. Alpha-adrenergic vasoconstriction competes with metabolic regulation.[31]

Reflex alpha-adrenergic vasoconstriction occurs in response to hypotension mediated through the carotid baroreceptor reflex, which produces activation of sympathetic fibers and inhibition of vagal discharge. The resultant increase in MVo_2 and blood flow is countered by alpha-adrenergic–mediated vasoconstriction. This restraint imposed by the alpha-adrenergic system results in increased myocardial oxygen extraction. In humans, alpha-adrenergic coronary constriction can be demonstrated by activation of another reflex sympathetic pathway by the cold pressor test and its potentiation by pretreatment with beta-adrenergic blockade and attenuation by selective $alpha_1$-adrenergic antagonism. Selective $alpha_1$-adrenergic and $alpha_2$-adrenergic blockade improves coronary vasodilation and reserve after epicardial stenting by increasing both the epicardial vasodilation and flow velocity, suggesting that the adrenergic system may limit the vasodilatory capacity in patients with coronary artery disease.[32]

Alpha-adrenergic coronary vasoconstriction has also been observed during exercise in conscious dogs wherein myocardial oxygen delivery increased markedly but not maximally, because the increase in blood flow was blunted by alpha-adrenergic activation. The apparent

TABLE 44–8 Neural Control of Coronary Blood Flow

	Neural	Metabolic
Parasympathetic Vagal stimulation CSP vagotonic Bezold-Jarish reflex	Vasodilation flow ↑	HR, BP ↓, vasoconstrict, flow ↓
Sympathetic Alpha stimulation Beta stimulation Stellectomy relieves chronic alpha constrictor tone	 Vasoconstriction flow ↓ Vasodilation flow ↑ (β_2)	 BP ↑, vasodilation, flow ↑ HR, contractility ↑ dilation, flow (β_1)
Metabolic	Overrides neural control, but alpha constriction limits vasolation	

BP = blood pressure; CSP = carotid sinus pressure; HR = heart rate.
Modified from Gould L: coronary Artery Stenosis and Reversing Atherosclerosis, 2nd ed. Arnold and Oxford University Press, New York, 1998.

TABLE 44–9 Actions of the Sympathetic Neural Systems

Receptor	Site	Action
β_1	Myocardium SA, AV nodes	Increased contractility Increased heart rate and conduction
β_2	Coronary arterioles Peripheral arterioles Large coronary arteries Peripheral arterioles Lungs	Vasodilation Vasodilation Bronchodilation
α	Large coronary arteries Coronary arterioles Peripheral arterioles	Vasoconstriction Vasoconstriction Vasoconstriction

AV = atrioventricular; SA = sinoatrial.

paradox of sympathetic coronary constriction during exercise results in the favorable transmural distribution of blood in the left ventricular wall away from the endocardium. Recently, a genetic link to alpha-adrenergic coronary vasoconstriction has been demonstrated,[33] and a genetic predisposition to alpha$_2$-adrenergic coronary vasoconstriction has been identified as a risk factor for fatal myocardial infarction and sudden death.[34]

Beta-receptor activation leads to coronary vasodilation under experimental conditions during which adrenergic activation does not alter MVO_2. This vasodilation is mediated predominantly by a beta$_1$ receptor in conduit arteries and by beta$_2$ receptors in resistance arterioles.[28]

PARASYMPATHETIC CONTROL. When MVO_2 is held constant, stimulation of the parasympathetic nervous system releases acetylcholine, leading to vasodilation of the epicardial arteries. Although the small release of acetylcholine from nerve terminals occurs at the medial-adventitial junction, sufficient amount diffuses to stimulate the endothelium.

Myogenic Control and Extravascular Compressive Forces

Arteriolar smooth muscle reacts to increased intraluminal pressure by contracting. The consequent augmentation of resistance tends to return blood flow toward normal despite the higher perfusion pressure. This regulatory mechanism, referred to as *myogenic control*, is important in some vascular beds. Although myogenic responses are present in coronary resistance arteries, their contribution to autoregulation is relatively small.[35]

Because systolic ventricular wall contraction compresses intramyocardial vessels, most of the coronary blood flow to the left ventricle occurs during diastole. At peak systole, there is detectable retrograde flow in the coronary arteries, particularly in the intramural and small epicardial arteries.[36] The extravascular systolic compressive force has two components. The first is left ventricular systolic intracavitary pressure, which is transmitted fully to the subendocardium but declines to almost zero near the epicardial surface. The second, and perhaps even more important, component is the vascular narrowing caused by compression and bending of vascular arterioles coursing through the ventricular wall as the heart contracts. The effect of systole on reducing myocardial perfusion is particularly important when systolic intraventricular pressure exceeds coronary perfusion pressure, as may occur with valvular or subvalvular aortic stenosis, or with severe aortic regurgitation.[37] Extravascular compressive forces are magnified when coronary vascular tone is diminished after arteriolar vasodilation or during metabolic vasodilation associated with exercise.

Because compressive forces exerted by the right ventricle are far smaller than those of the left ventricle, right ventricular perfusion is reduced but not interrupted during systole. When the right ventricular systolic pressure is elevated by disease (e.g., pulmonic stenosis), the phasic blood flow pattern of the arteries perfusing the right ventricle resembles that of the left ventricle.

Transmural Distribution of Myocardial Blood Flow

Extravascular compressive forces are greater in the subendocardium than in the subepicardial layer (Fig. 44–9). Subendocardial arterioles are particularly susceptible to compression as they arborize from long, transmural vessels. Therefore, *systolic* flow is reduced more in the subendocardium than the subepicardium. Nevertheless, in conscious dogs under resting physiological conditions, the ratio of endocardial to epicardial flow averaged throughout the cardiac cycle is approximately 1.25:1 due to preferential dilation of the

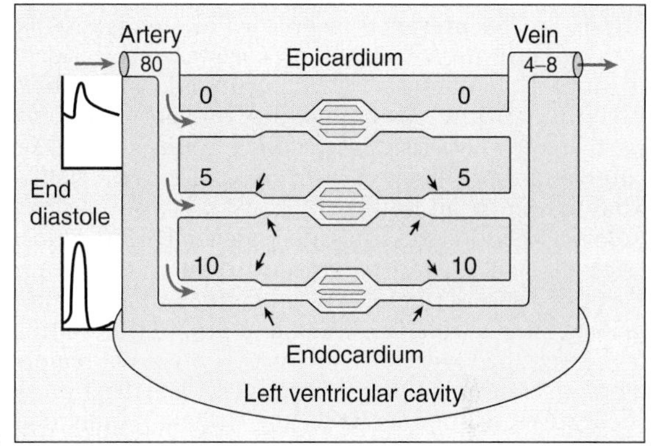

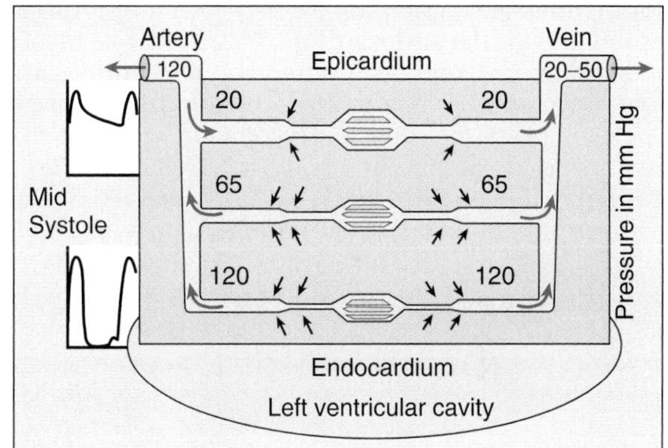

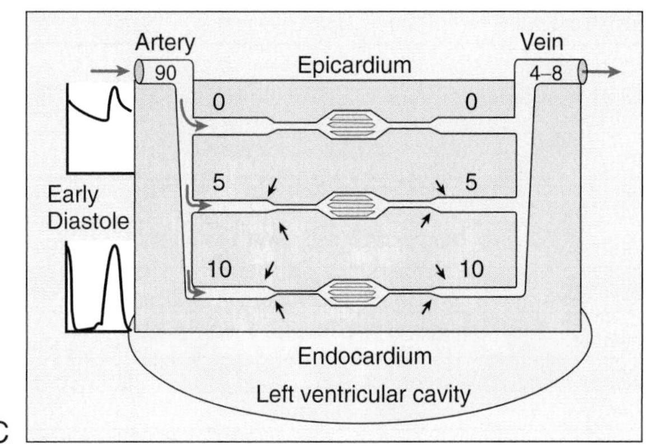

FIGURE 44–9 **A** to **C,** Changes in interstitial and intravascular pressure in vessel flow across left ventricular free wall during the cardiac cycle. During systole, interstitial tissue pressures are greater in subendocardium than in subepicardium. The subendocardial vessels are squeezed more than subepicardial vessels at the end of systole and take longer to resume full diastolic dimension. In the presence of low perfusion pressure, subendocardial flow is impaired by reduced diastolic time, especially with tachycardia and by elevated left ventricular diastolic pressure. (**A** to **C,** Modified from Hoffman JIE, Baer RW, Hanley FL, et al: Regulation of transmural myocardial blood flow. J Biochem Eng 107:2, 1985.)

subendocardial arterioles, causing a large increase in diastolic flow in the subendocardium. The greater subendocardial blood flow appears to be secondary to the wall stress (and therefore oxygen consumption per unit weight).[38]

The subendocardium is more vulnerable to ischemic damage than the mid-myocardium or subepicardium. Epicardial coronary stenoses are associated with reductions in the subendocardial-to-subepicardial flow ratio.[38] When coronary arteries were constricted sufficiently to reduce total coronary flow to approximately 40 percent of control, endocardial-to-epicardial flow ratio fell from 1.16 at baseline to 0.37. This pattern of redistribution of flow away from the endocardium is further exaggerated during exercise, mental stress, and pacing-induced tachycardia. Potent arteriolar vasodilators, such as dipyridamole or adenosine, also cause redistribution of blood flow from the endocardium to the epicardium. In the presence of epicardial stenoses, this transmural redistribution leads to a "coronary steal," or vertical diversion of blood away from the subendocardial layer with flow falling below resting values. Severe left ventricular hypertrophy, as well as heart failure with elevated left ventricular end-diastolic pressure, may also reduce the endocardial-to-epicardial flow ratio.

A low subendocardial-to-subepicardial flow ratio can be increased by elevation of aortic pressure, which preferentially increases perfusion of subendocardial region whose arterioles are maximally dilated and are, in this setting, pressure dependent. Overperfusion of the epicardial region is prevented by autoregulatory arteriolar constriction. Potent vasoconstrictors such as ET-1 and alpha-adrenergic agonists or inhibitors of adenosine-induced arteriolar dilation such as theophylline cause arteriolar constriction and redistribution of blood flow to the endocardium.[38,39] As long as the absolute blood flow is not reduced appreciably, these measures may lessen myocardial ischemia. Reduction of MVO_2, for example by beta blockers, also decreases epicardial blood flow and increases perfusion pressure and flow to the ischemic subendocardial region. Table 44–10 compares characteristics of the subepicardial and subendocardial circulatory responses.

TABLE 44–10 Characteristics of Subendocardium and Subepicardium

Variable	Subendocardium	Subepicardium
Wall stress	++	+
VO_2	++	+
Tissue PO_2	+	++
Perfusion pressure	+	++
SVO_2, ATP	+	++
Lactate	++	+
Flow reserve	+	++
Resistance	+	++
Capillaries open, systolic flow decrease	+++	+
Due to compression, diastolic flow increase	+	++
Due to resistance	++	+
Mean flow (equal)	++	++

Strength of effects: + = mild; ++ = moderate; +++ = prominent or large.
ATP = adenosine triphosphate.
Modified from Gould L: Coronary Artery Stenosis and Reversing Atherosclerosis. 2nd ed. New York, Arnold and Oxford University Press, 1998.

Influence of a Stenosis on Coronary Blood Flow

A stenosis produces resistance to blood flow related directly to the morphologic features of the stenosis. Resistance to flow changes exponentially with lumen cross-sectional area (the most commonly used measure of severity) and linearly with lesion length. Additional factors contributing to resistance include the shape of the entrance and exit orifices, vessel stiffness, and distensibility of the diseased segment (permitting active or passive vasomotion) and the variable lumen obstruction that may be superimposed by platelet aggregation and thrombosis compromising lumen area, a process active in acute coronary syndromes.

As blood traverses a stenosis, pressure (energy) is lost, resulting in a pressure gradient (ΔP) across the stenosis. Using a simplified Bernoulli formula of fluid dynamics (Fig. 44–10), pressure loss across a stenosis can be estimated as follows:

$$\Delta P = fQ + sQ^2 \quad (1)$$

$$\Delta P = \frac{1.8 \bullet Q}{d^4_{sten}} + \frac{6.1 \bullet Q^2}{d^4_{sten}} \quad (2)$$

where ΔP is the pressure drop across a stenosis in millimeters of mercury, Q is the flow across the stenosis in milliliters per second, and d_{sten} is the minimal diameter of the stenosis lumen in millimeters. In equation 1, the first term (f) accounts energy losses due to viscous friction between laminar layers of fluid.

$$f = \frac{8\pi\mu L}{A_s^2}$$

where A_s is the stenotic segment cross-sectional area, μ is the blood viscosity, and L is the stenosis length.

In equation 1, the second term (s) reflects energy loss when normal arterial flow is transformed first to high-velocity flow in the stenosis and then to the turbulent nonlaminar distal flow eddies at the exit from the stenosis (inertia and expansion).

$$s = \frac{\rho}{2}\left[\frac{1}{A_s} - \frac{1}{A_n}\right]^2$$

where ρ is the blood density, and A_n represents the normal artery cross-sectional area. This results in energy loss due to flow separation and disturbed laminar flow.

As described by the Bernoulli formula (equation 1), the separation energy loss term (s) increases with the *square* of the

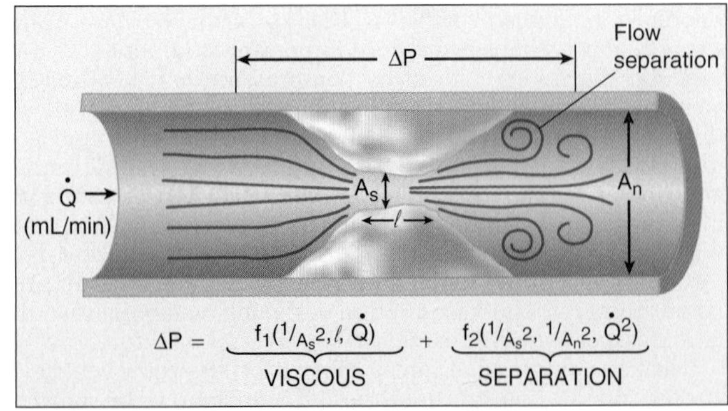

FIGURE 44–10 Diagrammatic illustration of the Bernoulli equation. ΔP = pressure gradient; A_s = area of the stenosis; A_n = area of the normal segment; L = stenosis length; $\dot{Q}$ = flow; f_1 = viscous factor; f_2 = separation factor. See text for details.

flow while viscous energy loss (f) becomes negligible. Thus, increases in coronary blood flow augment the associated pressure gradient in an exponential manner (Fig. 44–11). Despite augmentation of coronary blood flow, the increasing pressure loss across the stenosis reduces myocardial perfusion pressure and lowers the threshold for myocardial ischemia relative to demand.[40]

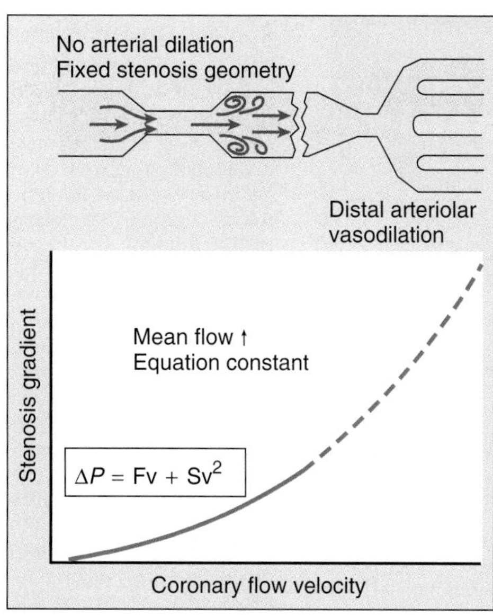

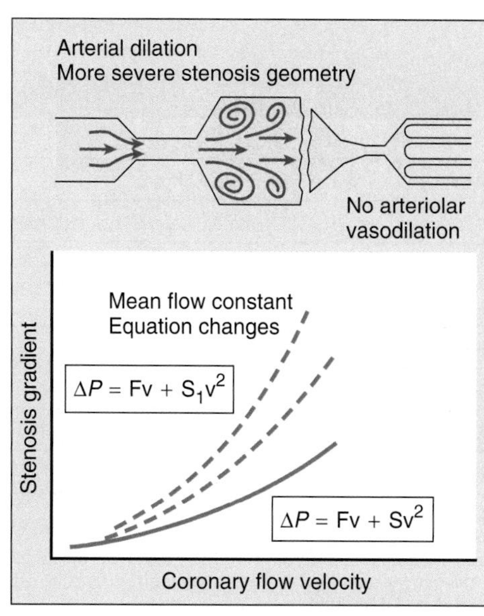

FIGURE 44–11 Conceptional diagrams of the effects of distal arteriolar vasodilation and proximal epicardial vasodilation on the geometry of the stenosis and pressure gradient (ΔP)–velocity relationship. With arteriolar vasodilation alone, stenosis geometry is constant and ΔP increases proportionally with velocity, V, according to the Bernoulli equation. With large epicardial artery vasodilation, the relative percent stenosis would become worse since the stenotic segment would remain fixed while the adjacent normal segment of the artery would become larger. The angle of divergence of flow exiting the lesion would become greater; consequently, greater pressure loss due to flow separation would occur, increasing the gradient-velocity curve. The separation coefficient would likewise increase from S to S_1. (From Gould L: Pressure-flow characteristics of coronary stenoses in unsedated dogs at rest and during coronary vasodilation. Circ Res 43:242-253, 1978.)

Factors Influencing Resistance Across a Stenosis

At any level of blood flow, the single most important determinant of stenosis resistance is the minimum diameter of the stenosis. The transstenotic pressure drop is inversely proportional to the *fourth* power of the lumen radius. As a consequence, in a severe stenosis, relatively small changes in luminal diameter (such as caused by active or passive vasomotion or transient obstruction by thrombus) can produce marked hemodynamic effects. For example, when the diameter stenosis is increased from 80 to 90 percent, the resistance of a stenosis rises nearly threefold. For most stenoses, the length of the narrowing has only a modest effect on its physiological significance. However, in very long, narrowed segments, significant turbulence occurs along the walls of the stenotic segment, and energy is dissipated as heat when eddies form and impact on the vessel wall. A preserved arc of vascular smooth muscle in some diseased arteries may be compliant and subject to dynamic changes that can alter luminal caliber and stenosis resistance. Dynamic changes in stenosis severity and resistance can also occur passively in response to changes in intraluminal distending pressure, or selective dilation of distal resistance vessels with agents such as dipyridamole. A single pressure-flow curve thus cannot be applied to a compliant or dynamic stenosis, because the pressure-flow relationship moves over a family of curves reflecting altered stenosis diameter and variable distending pressure. Despite the theoretical concerns, coronary artery pressures always remain positive, and collapse of distal segments is unlikely when intracoronary pressure is high due to microvascular compression.

The physiological effect of a coronary stenosis also depends on the degree to which the resistance to flow can be compensated by dilation of the microcirculation distal to the stenosis. *Resting* coronary flow is not impeded by mild or moderate stenoses and is maintained by normal vasodilatory regulation of the microcirculation. Resting coronary blood flow remains constant up to the point where an epicardial coronary constriction exceeds 85 to 90 percent of the normal segment diameter. However, unlike resting flow, *maximal* hyperemic coronary blood flow begins to decline when diameter stenosis exceeds 45 to 60 percent (Fig. 44–12). The capacity to increase coronary blood flow in response to a hyperemic stimulus, called *coronary flow reserve* (CFR), is abolished when diameter stenosis exceeds 90 percent. Factors responsible for reduced CFR in the absence of epicardial stenosis are shown in Table 44–11.

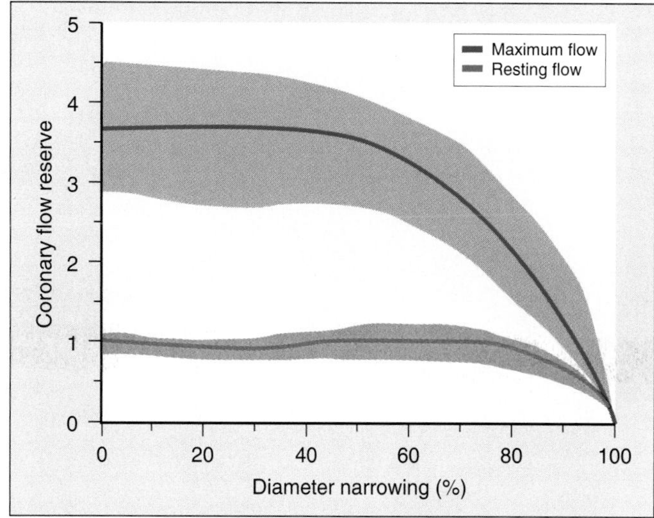

FIGURE 44–12 Coronary flow reserve expressed as the ratio of maximum to resting flow plotted as a function of percent diameter narrowing. With progressive narrowing, resting flow does not change (magenta line) whereas maximum potential increase in flow (blue line) and coronary flow reserve begin to be impaired at approximately 50 percent diameter narrowing. The shaded area represents the limits of variability of data about the mean. (From Gould KL, Lipscomb K, Hamilton GW: Physiologic basis for assessing critical coronary stenosis: Instantaneous flow response and regional distribution during coronary hyperemia as measures of coronary flow reserve. Am J Cardiol 33:87-94, 1974.)

CORONARY PRESSURE AND FLOW FOR THE PHYSIOLOGICAL ASSESSMENT OF A CORONARY STENOSIS

The limitations of angiography to determine the functional significance of an intermediate coronary stenosis can be overcome by measurements of coronary blood flow and pressure as estimates of coronary reserve. These measurements provide important information that complements the anatomical (most often angiographic) evaluation and facilitates clinical decision making. The hemodynamic significance of a given stenosis in humans can be measured by the pressure-flow relationship using sensor angioplasty guidewires.[41]

TABLE 44–11 Factors Responsible for Microvascular Disease and the Reduction of Coronary Flow Reserve

Abnormal vascular reactivity
Abnormal myocardial metabolism
Abnormal sensitivity toward vasoactive substances
Coronary vasospasm
Myocardial infarction
Hypertrophy
Vasculitis syndromes
Hypertension
Diabetes
Recurrent ischemia

From Baumgart D, Haude M, Liu F, et al: Current concepts of coronary flow reserve for clinical decision making during cardiac catheterization. Am Heart J 136:136-149, 1998.

Coronary Hyperemia

The myocardium can increase coronary flow from its basal level to a maximal flow in response to physiology or pharmacological stimuli. The most basic form of CFR is *reactive hyperemia* produced by transient severe myocardial ischemia, which produces maximal coronary dilation and a marked increase in coronary flow. Reactive hyperemia follows an occlusion as short as 200 milliseconds. *Maximal reactive hyperemia* follows coronary occlusion of 20 seconds. Longer occlusion increases the duration but not the amplitude of the hyperemic response. Reactive hyperemia is a response partly driven by metabolic regulation, fulfilling a requirement to repay oxygen debt. However, the hyperemic response is less pronounced when coronary arteries are perfused with deoxygenated blood for the same duration, suggesting that factors other than hypoxia, such as the local accumulation of adenosine, prostacyclin, and NO, stimulate the hyperemic response. At maximal hyperemia, autoregulation is also abolished and coronary blood flow is directly related to the driving pressure. Therefore, maximal hyperemic coronary blood flow is closely dependent on the coronary arterial pressure at the time of the measurement, a fact that is used in the derivation of pressure-derived fractional flow reserve of the myocardium (see later).

Three types of stimuli have been used to elicit maximal coronary blood flow in humans: (1) transient coronary occlusion during angioplasty (reactive hyperemia); (2) pharmacological vasodilators; and (3) metabolic stress. Adenosine, dipyridamole, and papaverine are the principal pharmacological vasodilators used to elicit coronary hyperemia. Adenosine, the most commonly used agent in the catheterization laboratory, can be administered by the intravenous or intracoronary route. Adenosine is benign in the appropriate dosages (20 to 30 μg in the right coronary artery or 30 to 50 μg in the left coronary artery or infused intravenously at 140 μg/kg/min) (Fig. 44–13). In a small (8 percent) percentage of patients, maximal coronary hyperemia may require higher (>50 μg) intracoronary adenosine doses.[42] Intravenous dobutamine (10 to 40 μg/kg/min) can also produce maximal hyperemia without modifying the angiographic area of the epicardial stenosis.[43]

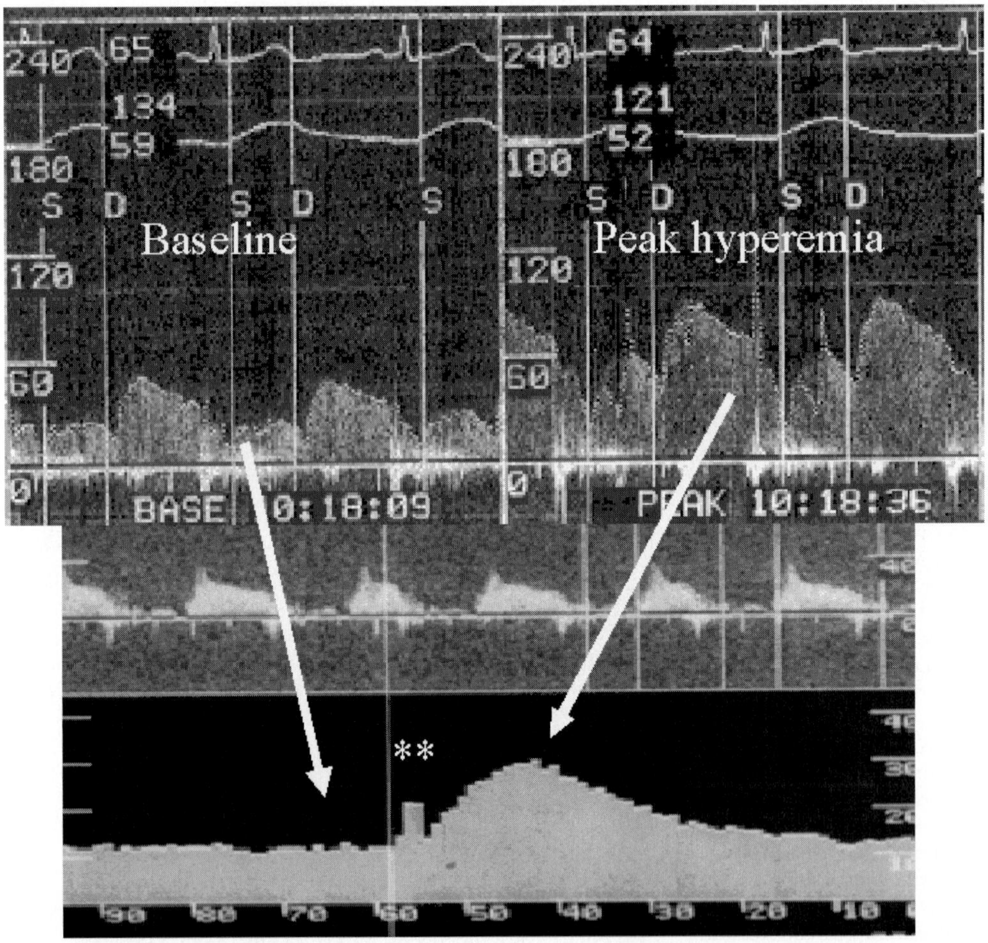

FIGURE 44–13 Coronary Doppler flow velocity signals used for the measurement of coronary flow velocity reserve in the cardiac catheterization laboratory. **Top panel,** Divided into the baseline (left) and the peak hyperemic velocity (right) signals, phasic flow-velocity tracing is demarcated by systolic (S) and diastolic (D) markers, corresponding to the electrocardiogram and aortic pressure at top of panels. Diastolic flow normally predominates over systolic flow. (Flow velocity scale is 0 to 240 cm/sec). **Bottom panel,** Continuous trend plot of average peak velocity (APV) showing the baseline and time course of peak hyperemia. The effect of an intracoronary bolus of adenosine (**) can be seen by the rapid increase in APV. The phasic peak hyperemic velocity signal was captured and displayed in the upper right panel. (The APV trend plot scale is from 0 to 60 cm/sec, with a time base of 0 to 90 seconds). In this example, baseline flow is 13 cm/sec and peak hyperemic flow is 30 cm/sec, for a coronary flow reserve of 2.3.

Measurement of Coronary Flow Reserve

CFR is defined as the ratio of maximal to basal coronary flow. CFR measures the ability of the two components of myocardial perfusion, namely the epicardial stenosis resistance and the microvascular resistance, to achieve maximal blood flow. There are two methods available to measure coronary blood flow in the catheterization laboratory: intracoronary Doppler flow velocity[41] and coronary thermodilution.[44]

Coronary Doppler measures the velocity of red blood cells moving past the ultrasound emitter/receiver on the end of a Doppler-tipped angioplasty guidewire. Velocity is determined from the frequency shift, defined by the Doppler equation (see Chap. 11). Volumetric flow is the product of vessel area (square centimeters) and flow velocity (centimeters per second) yielding a value in cubic centimeter per second. Absolute Doppler flow velocities represent changes in volumetric coronary flow when the vessel cross-sectional area remains constant over the measurement period. Compared to volumetric measurements, velocity may underestimate the volumetric CFR in some vessels that demonstrate intact endothelial-mediated vasodilation. The coronary thermodilution technique uses thermistors on a pressure-sensor angioplasty guidewire and measures the arrival time of room temperature saline bolus indicator injections through the guiding catheter into the coronary artery.[44] When combined with poststenotic pressure measurements, CFR measurements can provide a complete description of the pressure-flow relationship and the response of the microcirculation.

Normal CFR in young patients with normal arteries by intravascular ultrasound commonly exceeds 3.0.[45] In patients with chest pain undergoing cardiac catheterization with angiographically normal vessels, the CFR averages 2.7 ± 0.6[46] and is related, in part, to comorbid conditions such as hyperlipidemia, hypertension, or diabetes mellitus. Changes in heart rate, blood pressure, and contractility alter CFR by changing resting basal flow or maximal hyperemic flow or both. Tachycardia increases basal flow, reducing CFR. Increasing mean arterial pressure reduces maximal vasodilation, reducing hyperemic flow more than basal flow. CFR may be reduced in patients with normal coronary arteries who have essential hypertension or aortic stenosis. Diabetes mellitus also reduces CFR, especially in patients with diabetic retinopathy, due to reduced volumetric coronary blood flow (velocity × vessel cross-sectional area) during hyperemia and higher baseline flow compared to nondiabetic control subjects.[47]

RELATIVE CORONARY FLOW VELOCITY. Because CFR is the summed response of the major two coronary flow resistances, an abnormal value cannot distinguish between increased epicardial resistance or microvascular flow impairment (Fig. 44–14). To identify the resistance level, a relative CFR (rCFR) can be calculated as the ratio of maximal flow in the coronary with stenosis (Q^S) to flow in a normal coronary without stenosis (Q^N), assuming basal flows are the same. It was shown that rCFR is independent of the aortic pressure and heart rate pressure product and was well suited to assess the physiological significance of coronary stenoses. Using coronary flow velocity in the catheterization laboratory, rCFR is defined as the ratio of CFR_{target} to CFR in an angiographically normal reference vessel,

$$rCFR = (Q^S/Q_{base})/(Q^N/Q_{base}) = CFR_{target}/CFR_{reference}$$

and assumes both that basal flow in the two vessels is similar and that the microcirculatory response is uniform in the regions measured. A normal range for rCFR is 0.8 to 1.0. rCFR but cannot be used in patients with three-vessel coronary disease who have no suitable reference vessel. Because it relies on the assumption that the microvascular circulation is uniformly distributed, rCFR is of no value in patients with myocardial infarction, in patients with left ventricular regional dysfunction, or patients in whom the microcirculatory responses are heterogeneous. Because of the inherent difficulties and variability of both absolute and relative coronary flow velocity measurements, pressure-derived measurements are the preferred invasive method of physiological stenosis assessment.[48]

PRESSURE-DERIVED FRACTIONAL FLOW RESERVE OF THE MYOCARDIUM. Using coronary pressure distal to a stenosis measured at constant and minimal myocardial resistances (i.e., maximal hyperemia), Pijls and associates[49] derived an estimate of the percentage of normal coronary blood flow expected to go through a stenotic artery. This pressure-derived ratio is called the fractional flow reserve (FFR) and can be subdivided into three components describing the flow contributions by the coronary artery, the myocardium, and the collateral supply. FFR of the coronary artery (FFR_{cor}) is defined as the maximum coronary artery flow in the presence of a stenosis divided by the normal theoretical maximum flow of the artery (i.e., the maximum flow in that artery if no stenosis were present). Similarly, FFR of the myocardium (FFR_{myo}) is defined as maximum myocardial (artery and bed) blood flow distal to an epicardial stenosis divided by its value if no epicardial stenosis were present. Stated another way, FFR represents that fraction of normal maximum flow that remains despite the presence of an epicardial lesion (Fig. 44–15). The difference between FFR_{myo} and FFR_{cor} is FFR of the collateral flow (see later).

The FFR of a coronary artery and its dependent myocardium can be calculated by the following equations:

(1) $$FFR_{cor} = (P_d - P_w)/(P_a - P_w)$$
(2) $$FFR_{myo} = (P_d - P_v)/(P_a - P_v)$$
(3) $$FFR_{collateral} = FFR_{myo} - FFR_{cor}$$

where P_a, P_d, and P_w are pressures of the aorta, distal artery, and coronary wedge (during balloon occlusion), respectively, taken at maximum vasodilation, and P_v is venous or right atrial pressure. Because FFR_{cor} uses P_w, it can be calculated only during balloon coronary angioplasty. However, FFR_{myo} can be calculated during diagnostic procedures (Fig. 44–16). FFR reflects both antegrade and collateral myocardial perfusion rather than merely transstenotic pressure loss (i.e., a stenosis pressure gradient). Because it is calculated only at peak hyperemia, FFR is differentiated from CFR by being largely independent of basal flow, driving pressure, heart rate, systemic blood pressure, or status of the microcirculation.[50]

The FFR, but not the resting pressure or hyperemic pressure gradient, is strongly related to provocable myocardial ischemia demonstrated by comparisons to different clinical stress testing modalities in patients with stable angina. The nonischemic threshold value of FFR is greater than 0.75 (Fig. 44–17). In patients with an abnormal microcirculation, it can be argued that a normal FFR indicates the conduit resistance is not a major contributing factor to perfusion impairment and that focal conduit enlargement (e.g., stenting) would not restore normal perfusion.

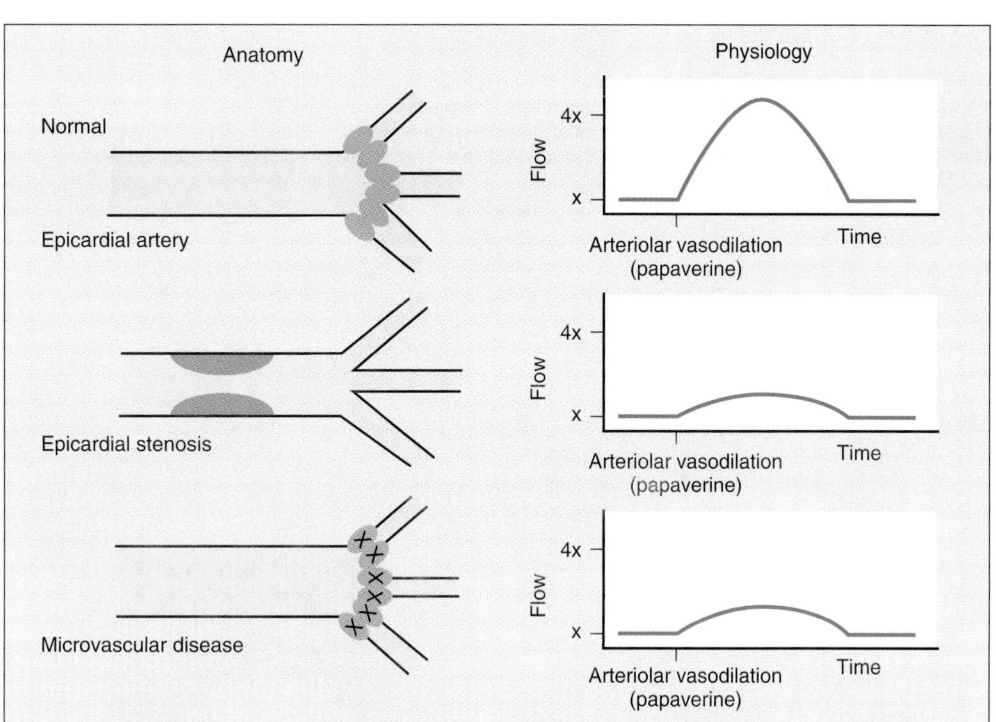

FIGURE 44–14 Interaction of the two major components of coronary flow reserve. **Top,** The two components—the epicardial artery and microcirculation—when both are normal, produce a normal coronary flow velocity reserve that is more than three times basal flow. **Middle,** With an epicardial stenosis and normal microcirculation, coronary flow reserve is impaired. **Bottom,** With microvascular disease and a normal epicardial, coronary artery flow reserve is also impaired. Coronary flow reserve alone thus cannot differentiate between an epicardial stenosis and an impaired microvascular disease. X = impaired microcirculation. (Modified from Wilson RF, Laxson DD: Caveat emptor: A clinician's guide to assessing the physiologic significance of arterial stenoses. Cathet Cardiovasc Diagn 29:93-98, 1993.)

n

s

n′

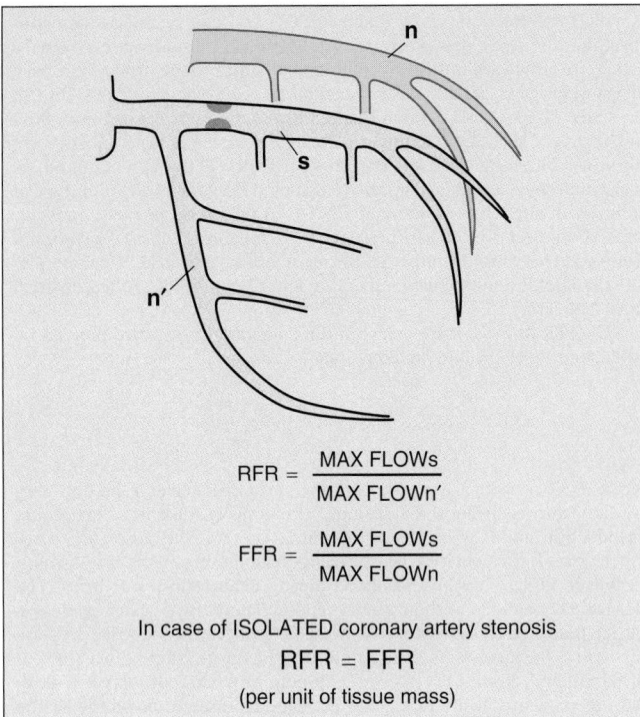

$$RFR = \frac{\text{MAX FLOWs}}{\text{MAX FLOWn}'}$$

$$FFR = \frac{\text{MAX FLOWs}}{\text{MAX FLOWn}}$$

In case of ISOLATED coronary artery stenosis

RFR = FFR

(per unit of tissue mass)

FIGURE 44–15 Diagram of an artery illustrating the rationale of comparing relative and fractional myocardial flow reserve. The relative flow reserve RFR) is the ratio of hyperemic flow in the anterior region (depending on the stenotic left anterior descending (LAD) coronary artery) to the hyperemic flow in the normal region (depending on the left circumflex coronary artery). The myocardial fractional flow reserve (FFR) is the ratio of hyperemic flow in the anterior region (depending on the stenotic LAD coronary artery) to hyperemic flow in that same region in the hypothetical case of a normal LAD coronary artery (faint lines). These measurements are derived from the mean pressure distal to the stenosis divided by the mean pressure proximal to the stenosis at maximal hyperemia. In the case of a similar decrease of myocardial resistance during hyperemia in the LAD area and the left circumflex area, the value of both the relative and the fractional myocardial flow reserves should be identical. n = the hypothetical normal left anterior descending coronary artery; n′ = normal left circumflex coronary artery; s = stenotic left anterior descending coronary artery. (From De Bruyne B, Banohuin T, Melin J, et al: Coronary flow reserve calculated from pressure measurements in humans: Validation with positron emission tomography. Circulation 89:1013-1022, 1994.)

FFR is thus specific for stenosis resistance and by design excludes the assessment and influence of the microcirculation.

SIMULTANEOUS PRESSURE-FLOW VELOCITY (P-V) RELATIONSHIPS. In a manner similar to that proposed by Gould and colleagues (see Fig. 44-16), Marques and coworkers[51] demonstrated the pressure-velocity flow (P-V) relationships characterizing mild, moderate, and severe human coronary stenoses.The P-V data also demonstrated that the variability of microvascular resistance possibly contributed to discrepancies between FFR and coronary blood flow velocity reserve in intermediate coronary lesions (Fig. 44-18)[52] with concordance between FFR and CFR occurring in 73 percent of patients. Minimum microvascular resistance (the ratio of mean distal pressure to average peak blood flow velocity during hyperemia) was significantly higher in patients with FFR greater than 0.75 and CFR less than 2.0.A hyperemic stenosis resistance index (defined as the ratio of hyperemic stenosis pressure gradient [mean aortic—mean distal pressure] divided by hyperemic average peak

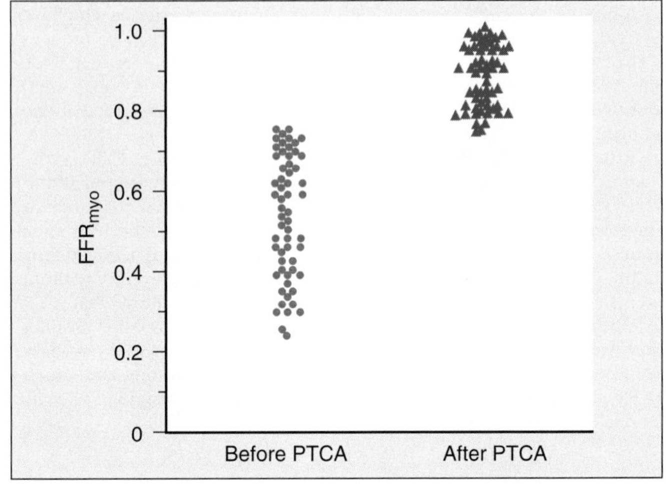

FIGURE 44–17 Values of fractional flow reserve of the myocardium (FFR_{myo}) before and after percutaneous transluminal coronary angioplasty (PTCA). Values associated with proven myocardial ischemia are indicated by magenta circles, and values definitely not associated with ischemia are indicated by blue triangles. The threshold of FFR below which exertional ischemia is observed and above which no ischemia occurs is 0.74. (From Pijls NH, De Bruyne B, Peels K, et al: Measurement of fractional flow reserve to assess the functional severity of coronary artery stenoses. N Engl J Med 334:1703-1708, 1996.)

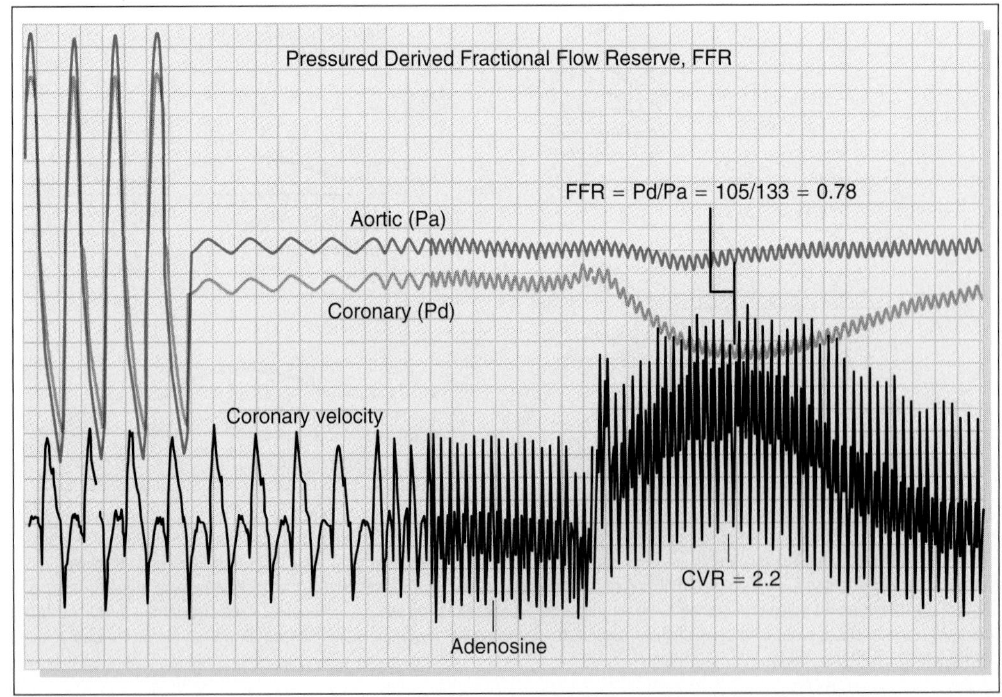

FIGURE 44–16 Pressure and flow velocity signals obtained in a patient with intermediate severity of coronary artery disease. A coronary flow velocity tracing is used to demonstrate timing of coronary hyperemia and coronary vasodilatory reserve (CVR). Mean aortic (P_a) and distal coronary pressures (P_d) during adenosine hyperemia are used to compute fractional flow reserve (FFR). FFR = 0.78 when CVR = 2.2. (Courtesy of B. DeBruyne.)

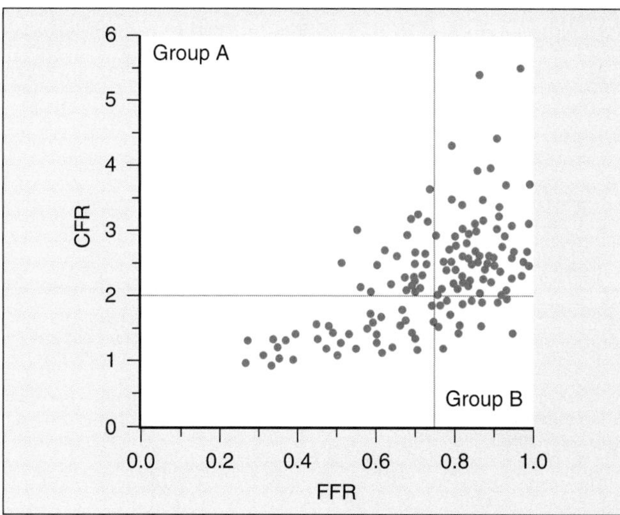

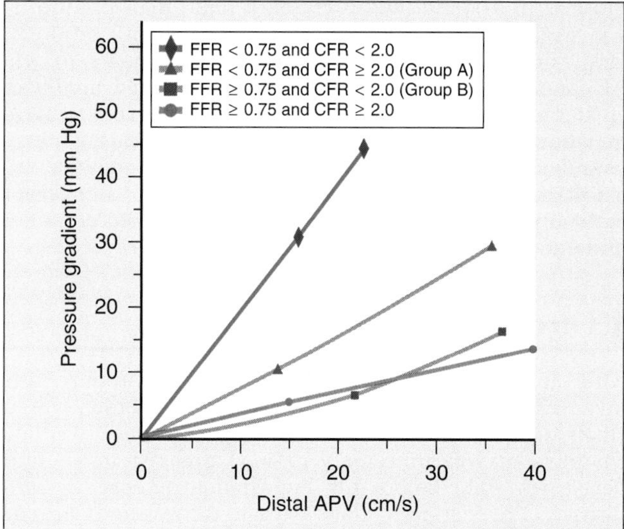

FIGURE 44–18 Comparison of fractional flow reserve (FFR) and coronary flow reserve (CFR) in 150 patients. Data are categorized on the basis of threshold values. **A,** Group A, FFR < 0.75 and CFR > 2.0, and Group B, FFR > 0.75 and CFR ≤ 2. **B,** Pressure gradient-flow velocity relation showing average data at baseline and hyperemia for all groups. APV = average peak velocity. (**A** and **B,** From Meuwissen M, Chamuleau S, Siebes M, et al: Role of variability in microvascular resistance on fractional flow reserve and coronary blood flow velocity reserve in intermediate coronary lesions. Circulation 103:184-187, 2001.)

velocity [APV]) was determined to be more specific for agreement with perfusion imaging by single-photon emission tomography in lesions with discordant FFR and CFR.[53] Thus, combined P-V measurements are needed to describe the contribution of both the epicardial and microvascular resistance to myocardial perfusion.

Clinical Outcomes of Coronary Blood Flow Measurements

Strong correlations exist between inducible myocardial ischemia by stress testing and FFR or CFR. An FFR less than 0.75 or abnormal CFR (<2.0) identified physiologically significant stenoses associated with inducible myocardial ischemia, with high (>90 percent) sensitivity, specificity, positive predictive value, and overall accuracy.[41,50,53-55] FFR or CFR values above the ischemic thresholds have been used safely to defer coronary interventions for intermediate stenoses, with clinical event rates of less than 10 percent over a 2-year follow-up period.[56-59]

Percutaneous intervention of lesions with normal FFR has a worse outcome than when such patients are treated medically. Bech and associates[59] studied 325 patients with intermediate coronary stenosis without documented myocardial ischemia. When FFR was greater than 0.75, patients were randomly assigned to a deferral group ($n = 91$) or a performance group ($n = 90$). If FFR was less than 0.75, percutaneous transluminal coronary angioplasty (PTCA) was performed as planned (reference group, $n = 144$). At clinical follow-up to 24 months, the event-free survival was higher in the deferral than in the performance group (89 percent vs. 83 percent) and significantly lower in the reference group (78 percent). FFR identified those patients in whom percutaneous coronary intervention (PCI) provides no additional clinical benefit (Fig. 44–19).

The AHA/ACC recommendations[60] for use of physiological measurements during invasive procedures are provided in Table 44–12.

DIFFUSE ATHEROSCLEROSIS. Coronary arteries without focal stenosis are generally considered non–flow limiting. A diffusely diseased atherosclerotic coronary artery can be viewed as a series of branching units diverting and gradually distributing flow and reducing pressure longitudinally along the conduit. In such a vessel, a reduced CFR is not associated with any single location of stenotic pressure loss. Diffuse atherosclerosis, rather than a focal narrowing, is characterized by a continuous and gradual pressure recovery from distal to proximal without a localized abrupt increase in pressure related to an isolated stenosis. De Bruyne and colleagues[5] examined FFR in normal arteries and in atherosclerotic nonstenotic arteries. FFR in the normal group was 0.97 ± 0.02 but was significantly lower, 0.89 ± 0.08, in the diffuse disease group indicating significant arterial resistance without focal obstruction. In 8 percent of arteries in the diffusely diseased group FFR was less than 0.75, well below the ischemic

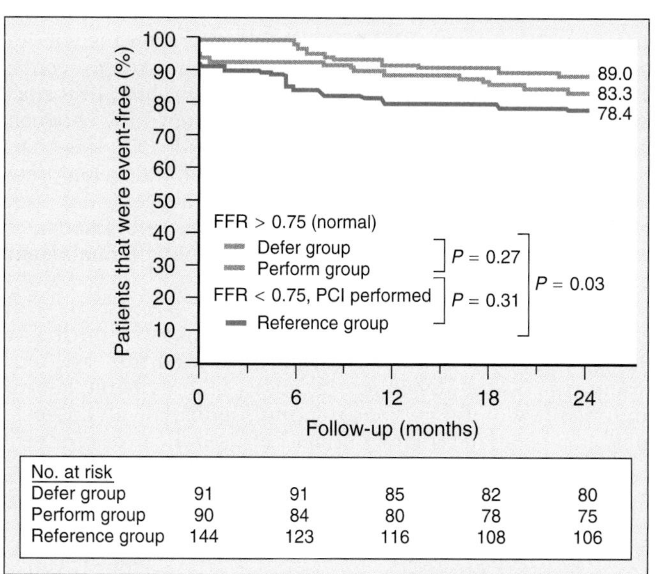

No. at risk					
Defer group	91	91	85	82	80
Perform group	90	84	80	78	75
Reference group	144	123	116	108	106

FIGURE 44–19 Clinical outcome of deferring or treating patients with intermediate stenosis and fractional flow reserve (FFR) > 0.75. Event-free Kaplan-Meier curves for three strategies are shown. The top curve are patients with intermediate coronary stenosis with FFR > 0.75 and in whom intervention was deferred (blue). The bottom curve is the reference group (magenta) in whom FFR was < 0.75 and percutaneous coronary intervention (PCI) was performed. The middle curve is the group of patients with FFR > 0.75 who had PCI performed (brown). In a follow-up over 2 years, events were higher in the FFR > 0.75 PCI-perform group than in the PCI-deferred group. PCI offered no advantage in terms of events or symptom relief to these patients. (From Bech GJW, De Bruyne B, Pijls NHJ, et al: Fractional flow reserve to determine the appropriateness of angioplasty in moderate coronary stenosis: A randomized trial. Circulation 103:2928-2934, 2001.)

TABLE 44–12 Recommendations for Intracoronary Physiologic Measurements (Doppler Ultrasound, FFR)

Class	Indication	Level of Evidence
IIa	1. Assessment of the physiological effects of intermediate coronary stenosis (33-70% luminal narrowing) in patients with anginal symptoms. Coronary pressure (FFR) of Doppler velocimetry may also be useful as an alternative to performing noninvasive functional testing (e.g., when the functional study is absent or ambiguous) to determine whether an intervention is warranted	B
IIb	1. Evaluation of the success of percutaneous coronary revascularization in restoring flow reserve and to predict the risk of restenosis	C
	2. Evaluation of patients with anginal symptoms without an apparent angiographic culprit lesion	C
III	1. Routine assessment of the severity of angiographic disease in patients with a positive, unequivocal noninvasive function study	C

FFR = fractional flow reserve.

From Smith SC Jr, Dove JT, Jacobs AK, et al: ACC/AHA guidelines for percutaneous coronary intervention (revision of the 1993 PTCA Guidelines)—executive summary. A report of the American College of Cardiology/American Heart Association Task Force on Practice Guidelines (committee to revise the 1993 guidelines for percutaneous transluminal coronary angioplasty. J Am Coll Cardiol 37:2215-2238, 2001).

threshold (Fig. 44–20). In this setting, mechanical therapy to treat a presumed focal flow limiting plaque would be futile. Diffuse atherosclerosis also explains persistently abnormal perfusion imaging studies in some patients despite unobstructed proximal coronary artery segments.

PERCUTANEOUS CORONARY INTERVENTIONS (see Chap. 52). Sequential flow velocity data have confirmed that the normalization of CFR occurring in only 50 percent of patients after PTCA alone was due to angiographically unapparent residual lumen obstruction. CFR may normalize in 80 percent of patients after stenting, corresponding to improved lumen area as the mechanism responsible for improved coronary blood flow. The remaining 20 percent of patients with widely patent stents had impaired CFR (<2.0) attributed to microvascular disease and/or transient emboli from PCI. A low postprocedural CFR has been associated with a worse periprocedural outcome.

FFR after *stenting* also predicts adverse cardiac events at follow-up. In a multicenter study, Pijls and coworkers[61] examined FFR and clinical outcomes in 750 patients 6 months after stent placement. FFR immediately after stenting was an independent variable related to all adverse cardiac events. The event rate was 5 percent in patients in whom FFR normalized, 6 percent in patients with poststent FFR between 0.90 and 0.95, and 20 percent in those with FFR less than 0.90. In patients with FFR less than 0.80, the event rate was 30 percent (Fig. 44–21). These data suggest that lack of normalization of FFR and diffuse disease are associated with worse long-term outcome independent of final stent diameter.

ACUTE MYOCARDIAL INFARCTION (see Chap. 46). Measurements of coronary blood flow or pressure during or immediately after acute myocardial infarction may not represent true lesion physiology because of the dynamic nature and recovery of the microcirculation. De Bruyne and associates[62] demonstrated that a normal FFR is indicative of reversal of myocardial perfusion defects in patients with acute myocardial infarction after 6 days. Excluding false-positive and -negative studies, the corresponding sensitivity, specificity, and predictive accuracy of FFR values were 87 percent, 100 percent, and 94 percent, respectively. An FFR greater than 0.75 distinguished patients after myocardial infarction with negative perfusion scintigraphic imaging (Fig. 44–22).

Postinfarction viability is associated with preservation of the microcirculation as reflected by phasic flow velocity characteristics (Fig. 44–23). Phasic coronary blood flow characteristics correlate with myocardial recovery after rescue PCI for acute myocardial infarction[63-65] and differentiated patients with Thrombolysis in Myocardial Infarction (TIMI)-2 versus TIMI-3 angiographic flow. Patients with reduced APV and prolonged diastolic deceleration time and small diastolic-to-systolic velocity ratio had better left ventricular recovery than those with systolic flow reversal, a rapid deceleration time, and negative diastolic-to-systolic flow velocity ratio. Similarly, after acute myocardial infarction, patients in whom APV increased after only a transient decline had significantly greater left ventricular systolic functional recovery than those in whom the APV progressively decreased throughout the next day.[66] These findings suggest that maneuvers that might maintain or augment coronary blood flow (e.g., an intraaortic balloon pumping or adenosine) could be monitored to determine the impact on myocardial salvage.

Coronary Collateral Circulation

After total or near-total occlusion of a coronary artery, myocardial perfusion occurs by way of collaterals—vascular channels that interconnect epicardial arteries.[67] Collateral channels may form acutely or may preexist in an underdeveloped state before the appearance of coronary artery disease. Preexisting collaterals are thin-walled structures ranging in diameter from 20 to 200 µm, with a variable density among different species. Preexisting collaterals are normally closed and nonfunctional because no pressure gradient exists to drive flow between the arteries they connect. After coronary occlusion, the distal pressure drops precipitously and preexisting collaterals open virtually instantly.

Collateral Growth and Function

The transformation of preexisting collaterals into mature collaterals, called *arteriogenesis,* occurs in three stages. The initial stage (first 24 hours) involves *passive widening* of the preexisting channels, facilitating increased flow. Endothelial cells become *activated* by increased blood flow velocity and shear stress and secrete proteolytic enzymes that fragment the basement membrane and dissolve extracellular matrix (an essential process in the upcoming migration of endothelial cells).[68] Shear stress induces widespread functional changes in the endothelium, many of which reflect new gene expression, including upregulation of leukocyte adhesion molecules and production of proinflammatory cytokines (monocyte chemoattractant protein-1, tumor necrosis factor-alpha, granulocyte-macrophage colony-stimulating factor).[68,69]

The second stage (1 day to 3 weeks) is characterized by *inflammation and cellular proliferation.* Monocytes migrate into the vascular wall and secrete cytokines and growth factors. Over several weeks, proliferating endothelial and smooth muscle cells arrange themselves into circular and longitudinal layers. During these first two phases, the luminal diameter of collateral channels increases nearly 10-fold. The third stage of collateral maturation (3 weeks to 6 months) involves thickening of the vessel wall due to *deposition of extracellular matrix* and further cellular proliferation in part stimulated by a variety of growth factors.[70] This is balanced by inhibitory factors such as angiostatin (a fragment of plasminogen), endostatin (a proteolytic fragment of collagen) and thrombospondin-1.[71] The mature collateral vessel may reach 1 mm in luminal

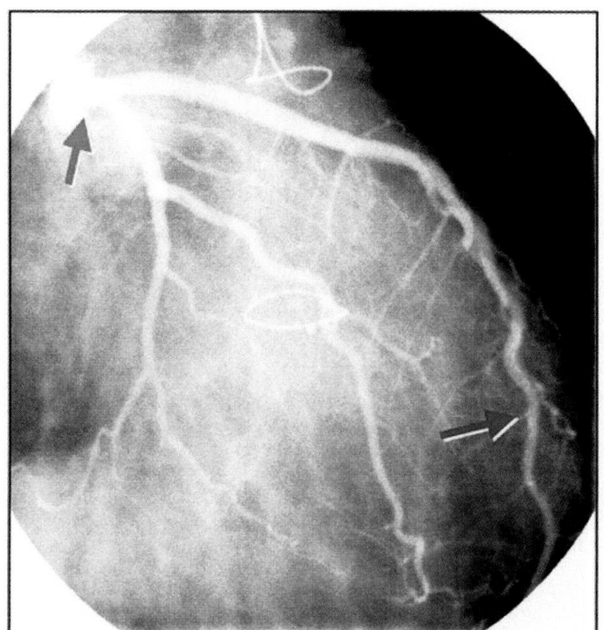

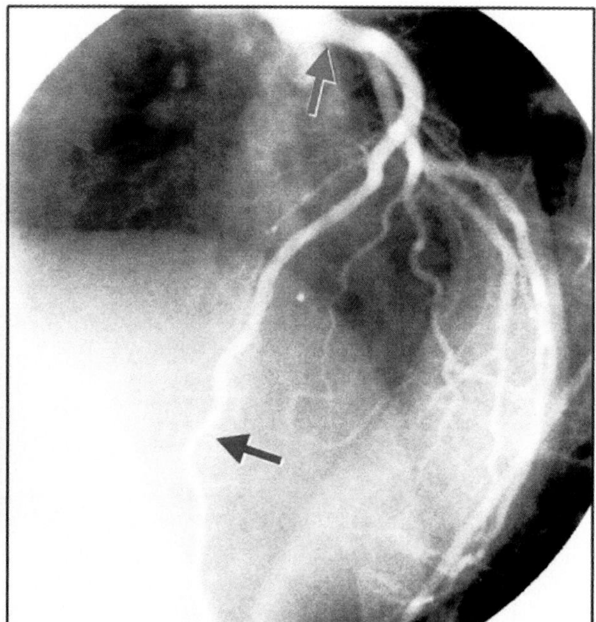

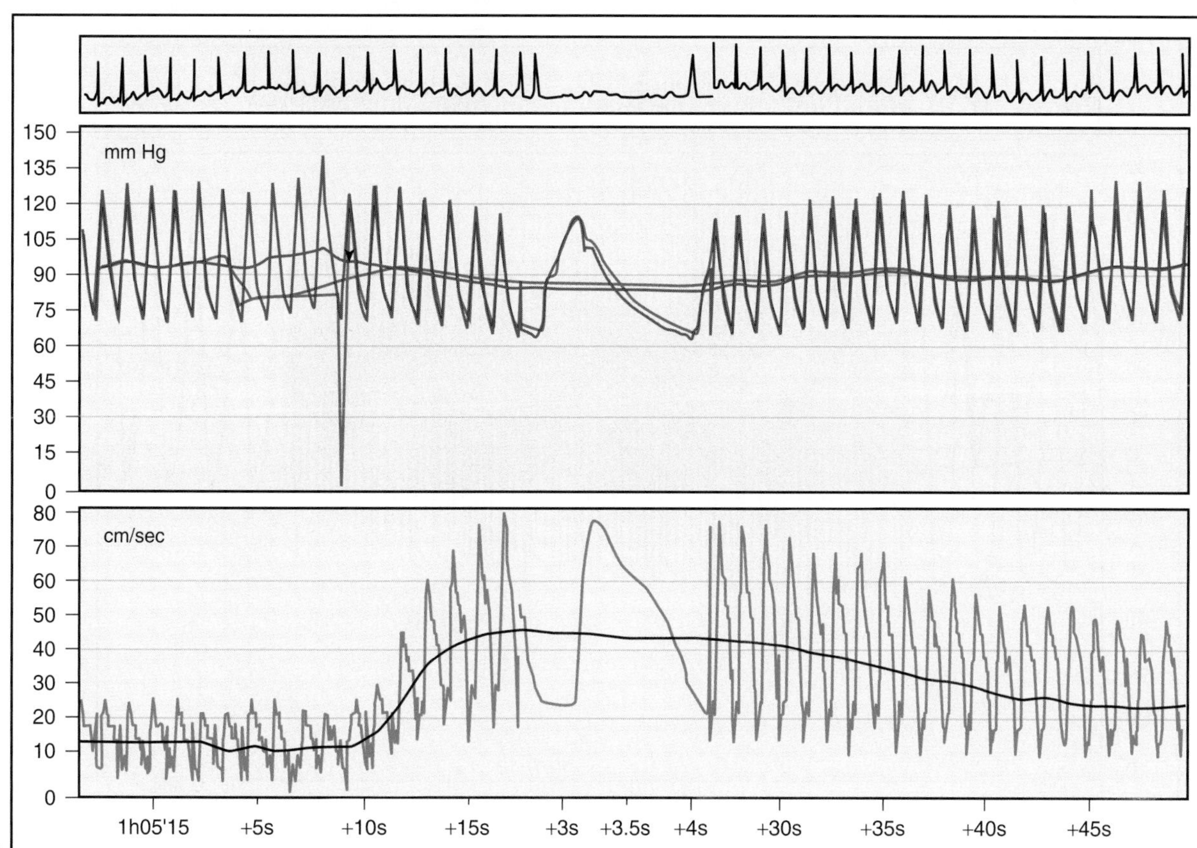

FIGURE 44–20 **A,** Angiograms **(upper panels),** aortic and distal coronary pressures **(middle panel),** and coronary flow velocity data **(bottom panel)** in a normal coronary artery. Coronary pressure (blue curve) and aortic pressure (magenta curve) remain identically matched during maximal hyperemia in arteries without evidence of atherosclerosis, indicating normal fractional flow reserve (FFR). The black curve in the **bottom panel** is average peak velocity. Red and blue arrows in the angiograms indicate locations of the red and blue pressure measurements, respectively.

Continued

diameter. Its three-layer structure is nearly indistinguishable from a normal coronary artery of the same size.[67,69]

The severity of coronary obstruction is a critical determinant of the development of coronary collateral channels. In patients, coronary collaterals do not develop until a coronary stenosis of at least 70 percent diameter narrowing is present. The same risk factors that predispose to atherosclerosis may limit the formation of collateral pathways. For example, patients with diabetes mellitus have an impaired ability to develop collateral blood vessels in the setting of obstructive coronary artery disease.[72]

The mature coronary collaterals can appreciably dilate or constrict in response to vasoactive stimuli. Conditions that reduce endothelium-derived NO, including coronary risk factors, may reduce the dilator reserve of coronary collaterals, a condition correctable by the administration of exogenous nitrates.[73] Coronary collaterals can mitigate the severity of myocardial ischemia and, in acute myocardial infarction,

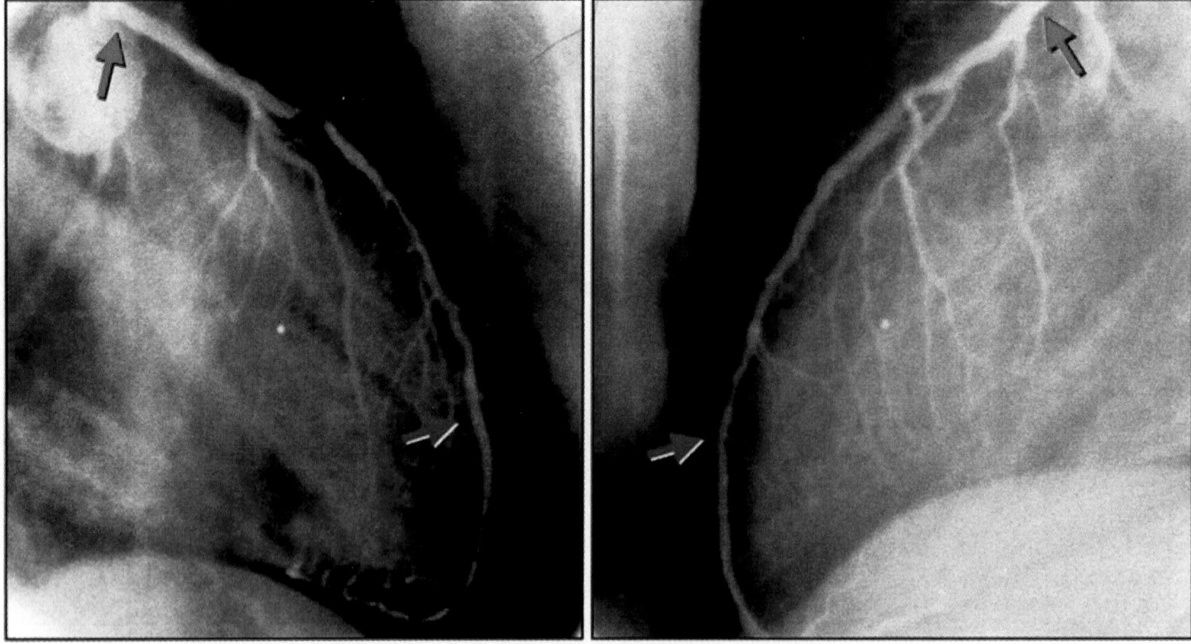

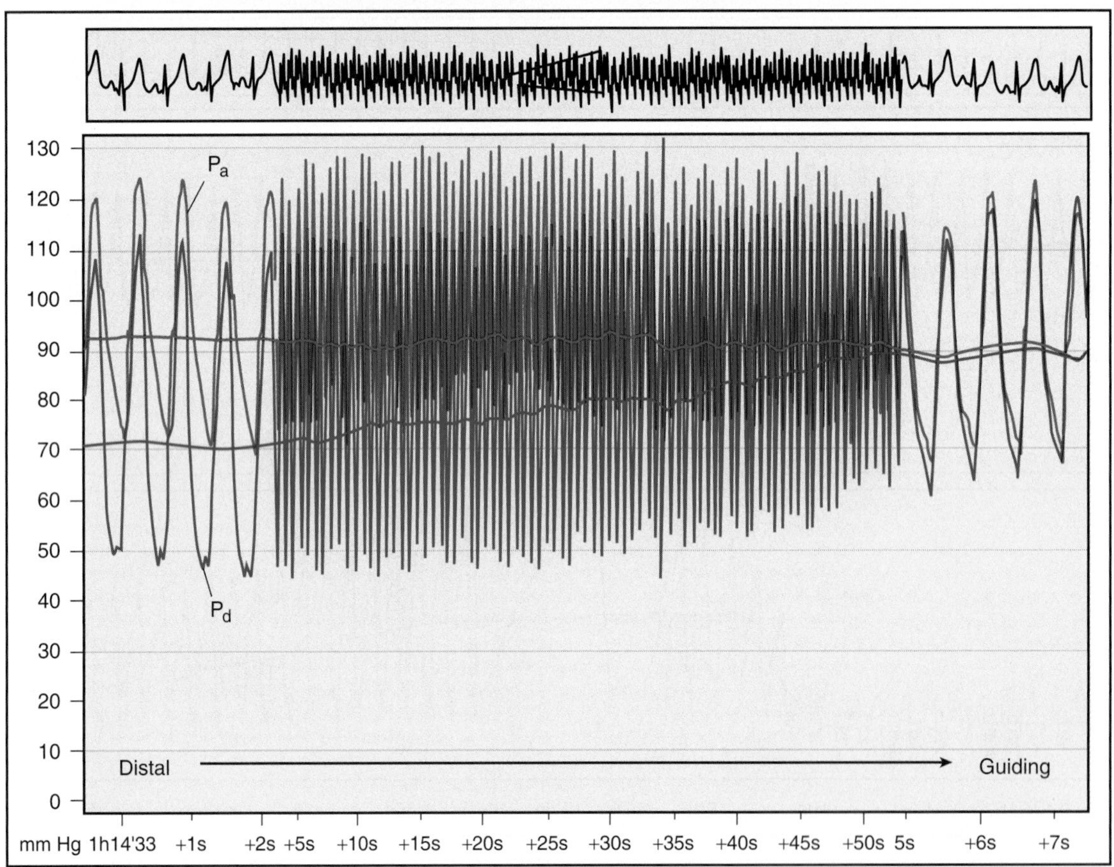

FIGURE 44–20, cont'd **B,** Example of a 44-year-old man with stable angina pectoris. A tight stenosis in the mid-right coronary artery was treated by angioplasty. The coronary angiogram of the left anterior descending coronary artery **(upper panels)** did not show any focal stenosis, but luminal irregularities suggested diffuse atherosclerosis. Aortic (Pa) and distal coronary (Pd) pressures recordings **(lower panel)** during adenosine-induced maximal hyperemia show a pressure gradient of 23 mm Hg (corresponding to an FFR of 0.76) when the pressure sensor is located in the distal left anterior descending coronary artery. This pressure gradient indicates that the diffusely atherosclerotic artery is responsible for approximately one-fourth of the total resistance to blood flow. When the sensor is slowly pulled back, a graded, continuous increase in distal coronary pressure is observed, which indicates diffuse atherosclerosis, not focal stenosis. The exact locations of aortic and distal coronary pressure measurements are indicated by the red and blue arrows, respectively.

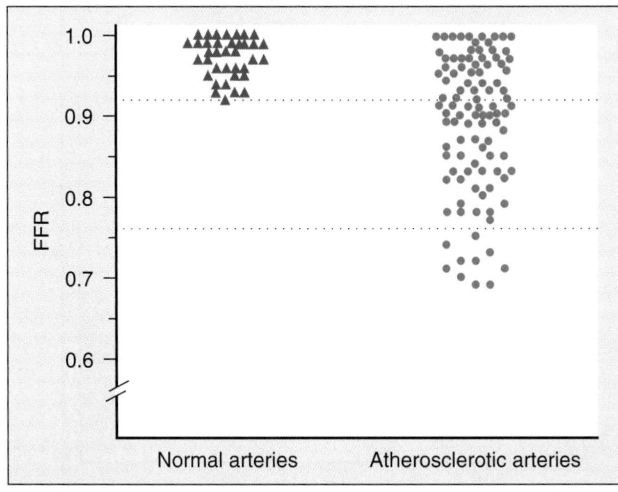

FIGURE 44–20, cont'd C, Graphs of individual values of FFR in normal arteries and in atherosclerotic coronary arteries without focal stenosis on arteriogram. The upper dotted line indicates the lowest value of FFR in normal coronary arteries. The lower dotted line indicates the threshold level of greater than 0.75. (From De Bruyne B, Hersbach F, Pijls NHJ, et al: Abnormal epicardial coronary resistance in patients with diffuse atherosclerosis but "normal" coronary angiography. Circulation 104:2401-2406, 2001.)

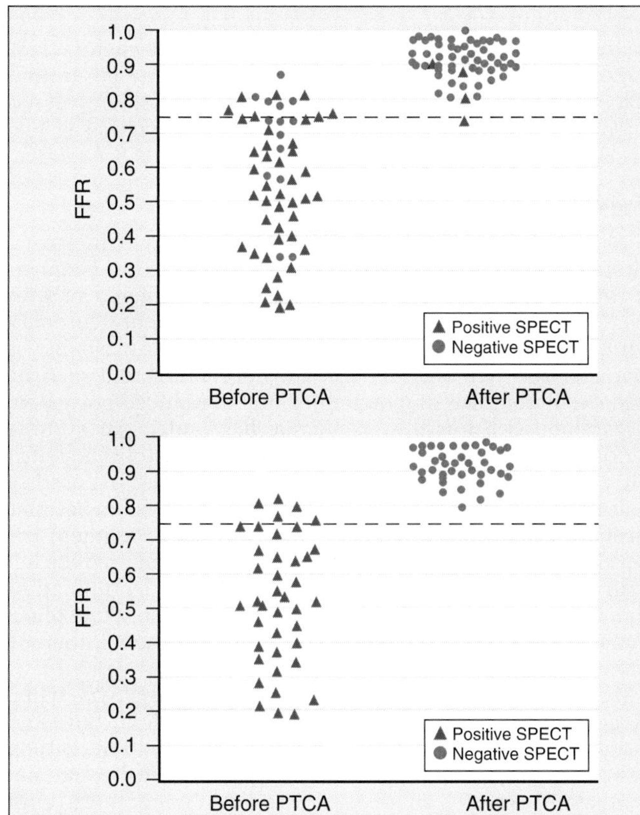

FIGURE 44–22 Fractional flow reserve (FFR) in patients after myocardial infarction. Values of FFR before and after percutaneous transluminal coronary angioplasty (PTCA) according to results of sestamibi single-photon emission computed tomography (SPECT) myocardial perfusion imaging in the patient population as a whole **(top)** and in patients with truly positive and negative SPECT imaging **(bottom)**. (From De Bruyne B, Pijls NHJ, Bartunek J, et al: Fractional flow reserve in patients with prior myocardial infarction. Circulation 104:157-162, 2001.)

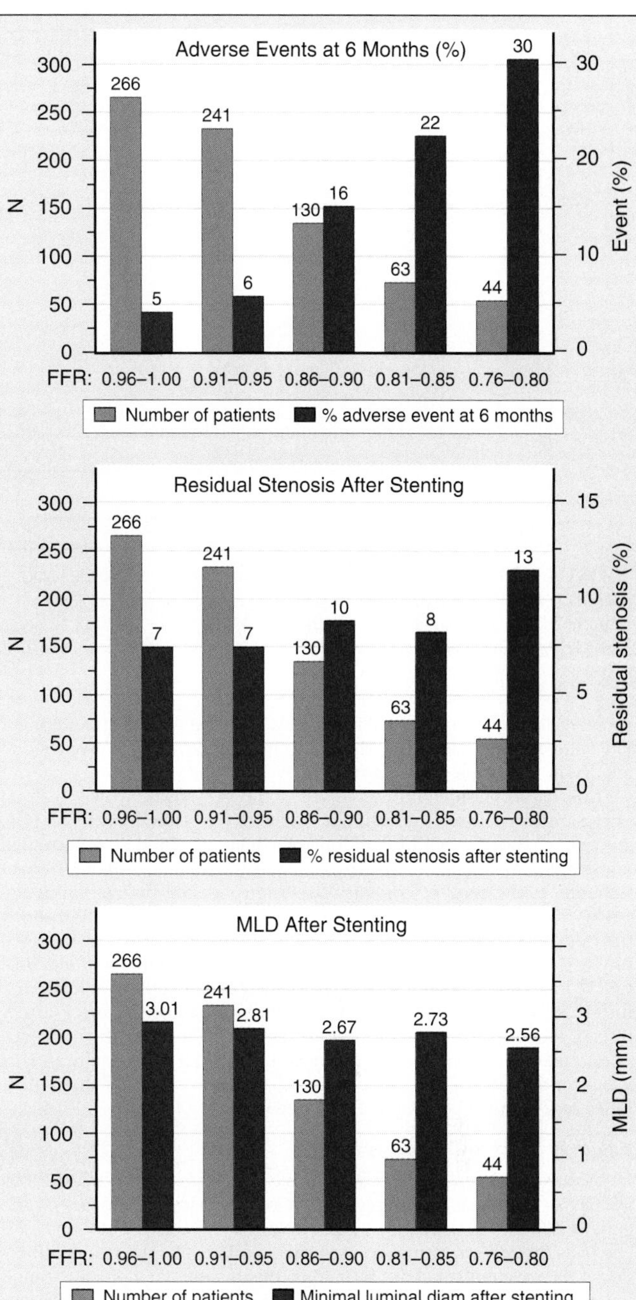

FIGURE 44–21 Clinical outcome of stenting and relationship to fractional flow reserve (FFR) in the FFR-post Stent Registry, involving 750 patients. **Top,** Distribution of the study population over the five FFR categories. A strong inverse correlation was present between FFR after stenting and event rate at 6-month follow-up. **Middle,** Distribution of percent residual stenosis in the five FFR categories. **Bottom,** Minimal luminal diameter (MLD) in the five FFR categories. (From Pijls NHJ, Klauss V, Siebert U, et al: Coronary pressure measurement after stenting predicts adverse events at follow-up: A multicenter registry. Circulation 105:2950-2954, 2002.)

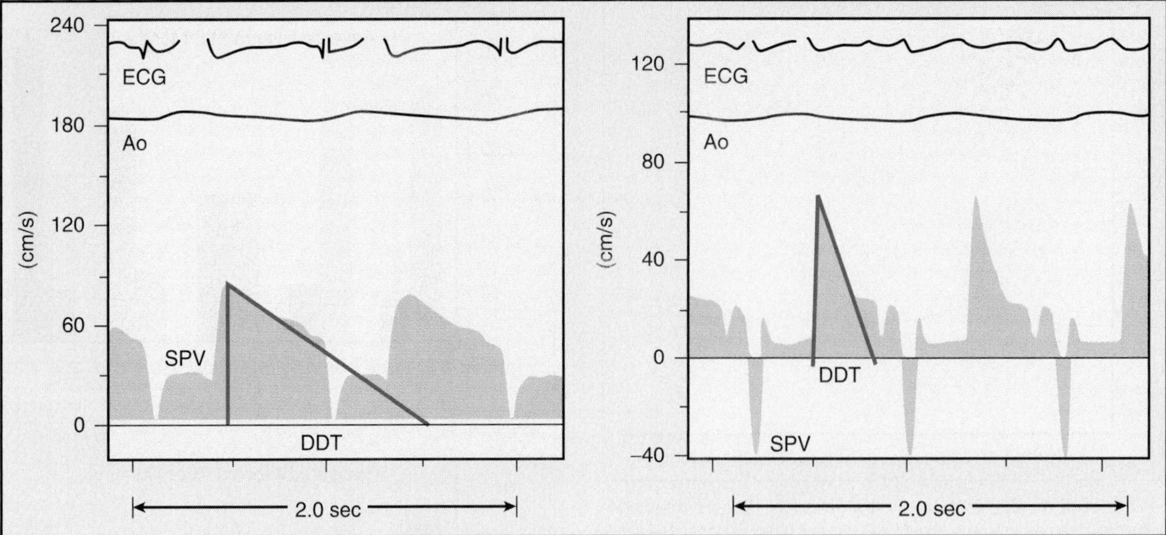

FIGURE 44–23 Phasic flow velocity signals in two patients with acute myocardial infarction demonstrating diastolic deceleration time (DDT) and systolic peak velocity (SPV). A rapid DDT and the presence of systolic flow reversal (negative SPV), as shown in the **right panel,** is associated with poor myocardial functional recovery after infarction. ECG = electrocardiogram; Ao = aorta. (From Yamamuro A, Akasaka T, Tamita K, et al: Coronary flow velocity pattern immediately after percutaneous coronary intervention as a predictor of complications and in-hospital survival after acute myocardial infarction. Circulation 106:3051-3056, 2002.)

provide significant myocardial blood flow, decrease infarct size, improve left ventricular function, reduce the likelihood of left ventricular aneurysm formation, and improve survival.

Coronary pressure and flow distal to the site of angioplasty balloon occlusion can be used to quantitate recruitable collateral perfusion (Fig. 44-24).[74,75] Patients in whom recruitable collateral blood flow exceeded 28 percent of normal maximal myocardial blood flow were free of ischemia at the time of coronary occlusion induced by balloon angioplasty.[76] This approach has also shown that collateral circulation rarely provides blood flow increases adequate to meet the MVO_2 of maximal physical exercise; it is typically limited to less than 50 percent of maximal CFR.[74] In addition, quantitatively determined collateral flow is related to future ischemic events.[75] In 403 patients with stable coronary artery disease followed over a 2-year period (Fig. 44-25), those with well-developed collateral supply, (collateral flow index > 0.25) had substantially significantly reduced events compared to those with collateral flow index less than 0.25 (2 percent vs 9 percent).

Arteriogenesis and Angiogenesis

In contrast to *arteriogenesis*, which refers to formation of mature collaterals by enlargement of preexisting rudimentary collaterals, *angiogenesis* refers to *sprouting of new vessels* from preexisting blood vessels and usually results in formation of smaller, capillary-like structures. Subendocardial collaterals may be formed in this manner. Angiogenic stimuli initiate activation of endothelial cells of capillaries or postcapillary venules. This results in local vasodilation, increased vascular permeability, and degradation of the basement membrane. Migration and proliferation of endothelial cells occur with formation of capillary sprouts. Further endothelial proliferation elongates the sprouts, and adjacent sprouts connect to form capillary loops that can carry blood flow. Maturation of the sprouts is associated with deposition of basement membrane.[68]

Angiogenic growth factors can promote formation of new collateral channels in animal models of peripheral and myocardial ischemia. The angiogenic growth factors used in these studies, administered as recombinant protein or by gene transfer, included vascular endothelial growth factor, fibroblast growth factors 1 and 2, hepatocyte growth factor, and hypoxia inducible factor 1. Each of these growth factors can stimulate the critical steps in angiogenesis, including endothelial activation and mitogenesis and upregulation of matrix proteins and matrix proteinases.[77]

In *therapeutic angiogenesis*, exogenous angiogenic growth factors (or genes encoding these growth factors) are administered to stimulate neovascularization of ischemic issues.[77] Therapeutic angiogenesis has since been carried out successfully in several animal species for the treatment of peripheral ischemia. Whether vessels formed in this manner arise from preexisting rudimentary collaterals by arteriogenesis or whether they are vessels newly formed by angiogenesis remains to be determined.

Myocardial Ischemia

Historically, ischemia has been defined as tissue anemia (lack of red blood cells) due to obstruction of arterial inflow. Myocardial ischemia is characterized by an imbalance between myocardial oxygen supply and demand (see Fig. 44–1).

Supply Ischemia

A reduction of arterial blood flow secondary to increased coronary vascular tone (vasospasm) or obstruction (stenosis or thrombus formation) results in *supply ischemia* or *low-flow ischemia* and is often associated with acute coronary syndromes or myocardial infarction. Low-flow ischemia is characterized not only by oxygen deprivation but also by inadequate removal of metabolites due to reduced perfusion. In patients with low-flow ischemia, left ventricular systolic performance is lower and left ventricular diastolic distensibility greater than when the same patients were exposed to high-flow ischemia or hypoxia. This response occurs because coronary flow and perfusion pressure normally augment left ventricular systolic performance (Gregg effect) and reduce left ventricular diastolic distensibility (Salisbury effect). In addition, buildup of tissue metabolites, especially inorganic phosphate, reduces calcium sensitivity of myofilaments, thereby diminishing contractility.

Myocardial ischemia may also be caused by *hypoxia*, when oxygen supply is reduced despite adequate blood flow and tissue perfusion. It may be present in asphyxiation, carbon monoxide poisoning, cyanotic congenital heart disease, cor pulmonale, severe anemia, or hemoglobinopathies with reduced oxygen-carrying capacity.

Demand Ischemia

In the presence of severe chronic coronary obstruction with relatively fixed coronary blood flow, an increase in MVO_2 due to exercise, tachycardia, or emotion with insufficient increases in coronary blood flow produces *demand ischemia* or *high-flow ischemia*. Demand ischemia is generally associated with episodes of chronic stable angina. In most clinical presentations, myocardial ischemia usually results from both an increase in oxygen demand and a reduction in myocardial oxygen supply. These mechanisms may act singly or in combination in the same patient at the same or during different episodes of ischemia.

Effects of Ischemia and the Ischemic Cascade

The heart has virtually no stores of oxygen and relies almost entirely on aerobic metabolism to provide for its high rate of energy expenditure. Within seconds of coronary occlusion, myocardial oxygen tension rapidly falls and left ventricular dysfunction occurs. Impairment of systolic and diastolic function are likely related to alterations in intracellular calcium handling. Ischemic regional asynergy may be so extensive that the uninvolved myocardium cannot sustain the normal hemodynamic function, resulting in systolic heart failure. Ischemia changes myocardial stiffness, shifting the diastolic pressure-volume relationship, adding to left ventricular diastolic failure, increasing the resistance to ventricular filling, elevating ventricular filling pressures, and ultimately causing symptoms of pulmonary congestion.

When an epicardial stenosis limits coronary blood flow, compensatory mechanisms are activated to preserve myocardial perfusion. Distal vessels dilate in response to reduced transmural perfusion pressure and release of metabolic vasodilators, and these newly released vasodilatory stimuli enhance flow from preexisting collateral connections. Subendocardial blood flow diminishes because of the higher intramyocardial forces acting on vessels in this region. The subendocardium has less vasodilatory reserve and is thus unable to compensate completely for the fall in coronary perfusion pressure. Subsequently, subendocardial ischemia reduces ventricular contractile force, ultimately stretching and paradoxically elongating the myocardium during ventricular systole. The depression of contractile force during moderate ischemia appears to be mediated by cardiac myocyte K^+-ATP channels. Adenosine stimulates opening of these channels. Although the energy balance may return to normal with recovery of phosphocreatine, contractile function usually remains depressed.

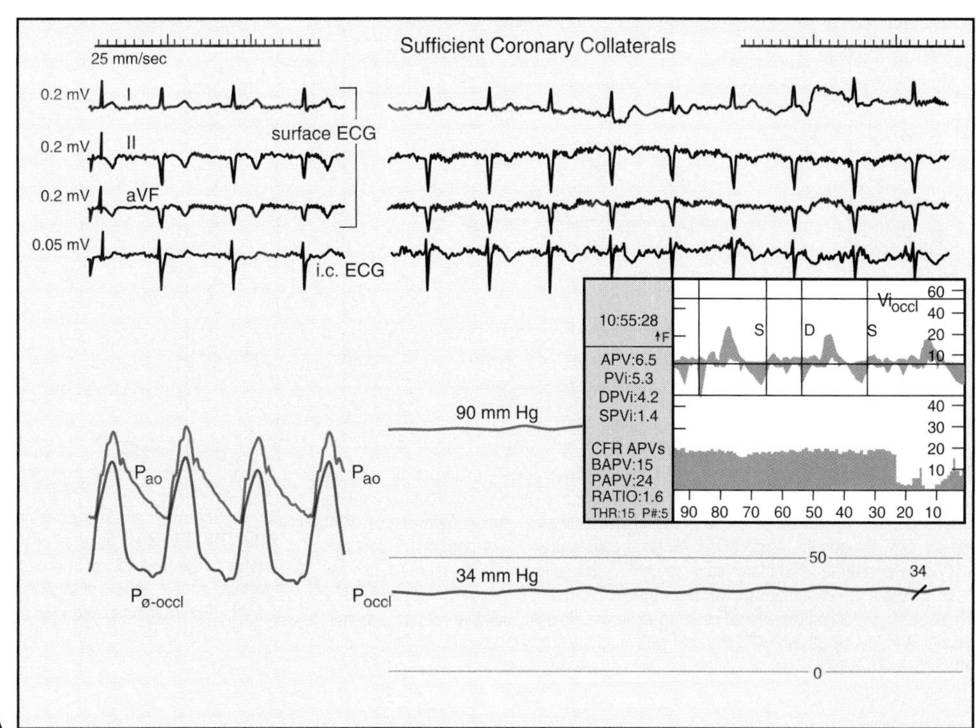

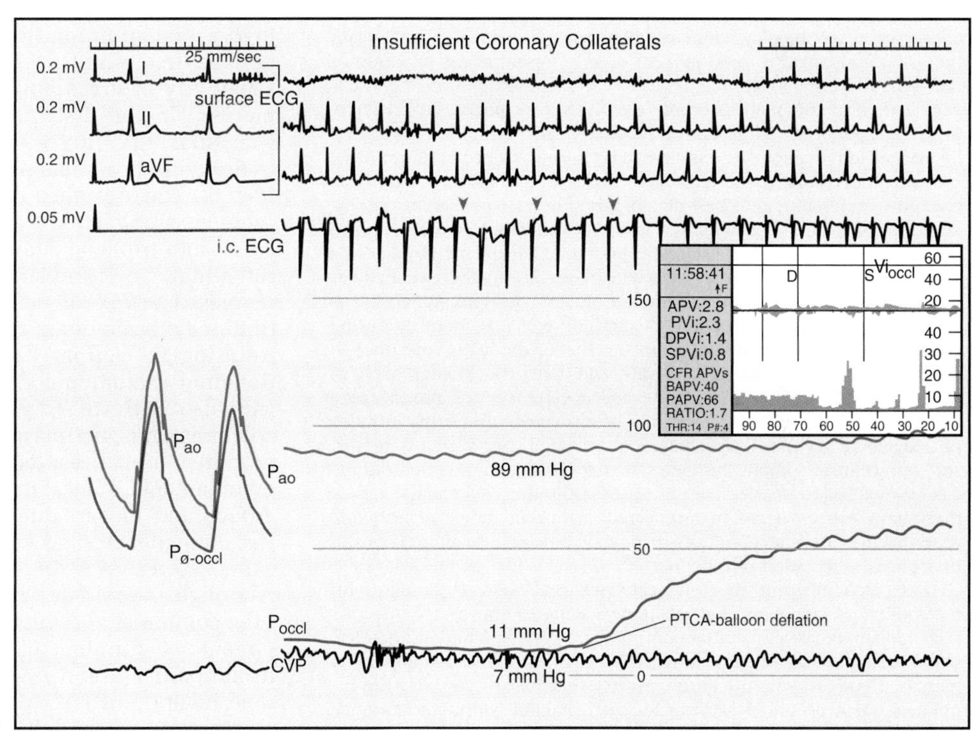

FIGURE 44–24 Pressure and flow tracings during balloon occlusion in two patients, one with sufficient collaterals **(A)** and one with insufficient collaterals **(B)**. Note that the coronary balloon occlusion pressure in the patient with sufficient collaterals is 34 mm Hg with maintained distal flow velocity. The patient with insufficient collaterals has an occlusion pressure of 11 mm Hg and reduced distal coronary occlusion pressure. P_{ao} = aortic guide catheter pressure; P_{occl} = distal coronary pressure during balloon occlusion; Vi_{occl} = distal flow velocity integral during balloon occlusion; CVP = central venous pressure; i.c. = intracoronary; ECG = electrocardiogram; PTCA = percutaneous transluminal coronary angioplasty; AVP = average peak velocity. (From Seiler C, Fleisch M, Billinger M, Meier B: Simultaneous intracoronary velocity- and pressure-derived assessment of adenosine-induced collateral hemodynamics in patients with one- to two-vessel coronary artery disease. J Am Coll Cardiol 34:1985-1994, 1999.)

The sudden cessation of myocardial blood flow due to occlusion of an epicardial artery is followed by predictable physiologic and metabolic changes within seconds following the occlusion. Myocardial energy metabolism immediately shifts from aerobic or mitochondrial metabolism to anaerobic glycolysis in a few seconds as underperfused tissue consumes oxygen from oxyhemoglobin and oxymyoglobin. Simultaneous with energy depletion, myocardial contraction diminishes and then stops. The myocardium elongates rather than shortens with each subsequent systole. The cellular membrane potential decreases and ischemic electrocardiographic abnormalities appear.[78,79]

Anaerobic glycolysis provides 80 percent of new high-energy phosphates in the ischemic zone. As this is insufficient to meet energy demands, high-energy phosphate stores decrease. Tissue ATP is metabo-

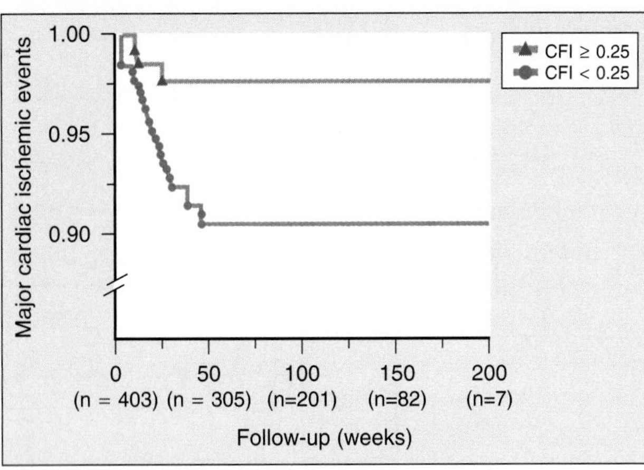

FIGURE 44–25 Clinical outcome in patients with sufficient collateral flow index (CFI): Cumulative event rate analysis and time to occurrence of major adverse cardiac events (death, myocardial infarction, and unstable angina) during follow-up of 200 weeks. Only 3 patients (2 percent) with good collaterals, but 24 patients (9 percent) with poor collaterals, had major adverse cardiac ischemic events during the first year after successful percutaneous coronary intervention. (From Billinger M, Kloos P, Eberli FR, et al: Physiologically assessed coronary collateral flow and adverse cardiac ischemic events: A follow-up study in 403 patients with coronary artery disease. J Am Coll Cardiol 40:1545-1550, 2002.)

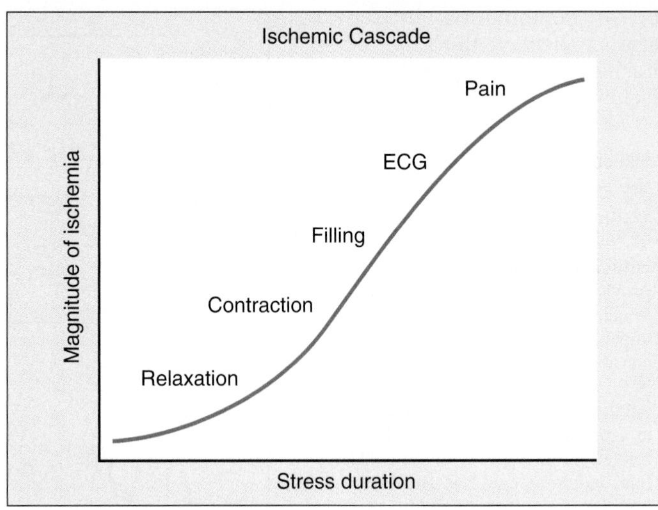

FIGURE 44–26 Schema of the ischemic cascade. The events (on the vertical) are related to the time course of occurrence on the horizontal. The first changes of ischemia are biochemical, followed by diastolic dysfunction, systolic dysfunction, electrocardiographic (ECG) changes, and ultimately angina.

lized and ADP accumulates. Creatinine phosphate, a source of high energy, decreases quickly, whereas ATP is more gradually metabolized. In reversible ischemia, 75 to 80 percent of ATP present at the initiation of the ischemic event is depleted. Because glucose trapped in the extracellular fluid is minimal, anaerobic glycolysis uses glucose-1-phosphate from glycogenolysis as its active substrate. Lactate and its associated hydrogen ion accumulate immediately during ischemia. Continued ischemia decreases tissue glycogen stores and increases anaerobic glycolysis, releasing glucose-1-phosphate, glucose-6-phosphate, alpha-glycerophosphate, and lactate. ADP is rapidly generated, whereas rephosphorylation of the adenine nucleotide pool to ATP is retarded by acidosis and lactate. During ischemia, adenosine diffuses into the extracellular fluid and is removed from the adenine nucleotide pool. Adenosine is further degraded to inosine and hypoxanthine, which accumulate during ischemia, resulting in a reduction of the size of the adenosine pool to 30 to 40 percent of its initial levels. Additional metabolites such as bradykinin, opioids, norepinephrine, and angiotensin are also released and participate in receptor activation of myocytes, stimulating intracellular signaling systems. Intracellular ionic calcium rises during ischemia, and intracellular sodium competes to expel calcium via the sodium-calcium exchange system. During reperfusion after ischemia, many of these basic processes can be attenuated or reduced; however, ischemic reperfusion is associated with its own set of biochemical alterations and only partial restoration of function.[78,79]

Thus, ischemia produces a typical cascade of events beginning with metabolic and biochemical alternations leading to impaired ventricular relaxation and diastolic dysfunction, impaired systolic function, and electrocardiographic abnormalities with ST segment alterations, followed by increased end-diastolic pressure with left ventricular dyssynchrony, hypokinesis, akinesis, and dyskinesis and, lastly, painful symptoms of angina (Fig. 44–26). The sequence of hemodynamic and electrocardiographic events can be reproduced by transient epicardial coronary artery occlusion during angioplasty or during spontaneous coronary vasospasm.

Myocardial Stunning and Hibernation

A brief episode of severe ischemia may produce prolonged myocardial dysfunction with a gradual return of contractile activity, a condition termed *myocardial stunning*. Myocardial stunning is represented by persistent regional dysfunction at a time when chest pain, ST segment deviation, and regional perfusion have recovered.[75,79] In patients with a myocardial infarction (with and without thrombolytic therapy), stunned myocardium lies adjacent to infarcted myocardium. Improvement in ventricular function occurs gradually over the course of days to weeks. Myocardial stunning is also an important feature of unstable angina.[80]

There are three major mechanisms in the pathogenesis of myocardial stunning (Fig. 44–27): (1) generation of oxygen-derived free radicals, (2) calcium overload, and (3) reduced sensitivity of myofilaments to calcium and loss of myofilaments.[78] In the first minutes of reperfusion after transient ischemia, the increased production of superoxide and hydroxyl radicals inactivate enzymes and cause lipid peroxidation. The presumed targets of oxygen-derived free radicals include sarcolemmal Na^+,K^+-ATPase and calcium-stimulated adenosine triphosphatase (ATPase) and, in the sarcoplasmic reticulum, calcium-stimulated ATPase. The result is increased influx of calcium through the sarcolemma and diminished calcium reuptake by the sarcoplasmic reticulum, resulting in cellular calcium overload and, ultimately, in impaired excitation-contraction coupling. Calcium overload can also activate enzymes that further damage the sarcolemma and sarcoplasmic reticulum. Ischemia followed by reperfusion also results in decreased calcium sensitivity of myofilaments, at least in part due to oxidation of critical thiol groups and in part due to partial proteolysis of troponin.[81] Recent evidence suggests that calcium overload may activate calpains, resulting in selective proteolysis of myofibrils.[79] Although antioxidants are effective, they do not prevent stunning completely because of two postulated interrelated components of stunning: an ischemic component not responsive to antioxidants and a second, larger component related to reperfusion.[78]

Impaired resting left ventricular function due to chronically reduced coronary blood flow that can be restored by revascularization has been attributed to *myocardial hibernation*. Even some akinetic segments can occasionally regain systolic contraction after revascularization. Conceptually, hibernation represents a condition in which the myocardium reduces its contractility (and hence its MV_{O_2}) to match reduced perfusion, thereby preserving cellular viability. Hibernating myocardium is present in approximately one-third of patients with coronary artery disease and impaired left ventricular function. The time course of recovery of hibernating myocardium after revascularization is quite variable, ranging from days to months. Slower recovery is typically associated with longer duration of hibernation. Revascularization can be effective whether achieved by coronary bypass grafting or by coronary angioplasty.[82]

Dysfunctional, hibernating myocardium can be identified by noninvasive methods such as echocardiography, nuclear perfusion imaging, and magnetic resonance imaging (see Chaps. 11, 13, and 14). This has significant practical importance because revascularization can improve left ventricular function, alleviate symptoms of heart failure, and, in the long term, forestall myocardial necrosis. Features of ischemia, stunning, and hibernation are summarized in Table 44–13.

Myocardial Necrosis

Unrelieved ischemia produces cell death. Because energy requirements, rates of metabolic activity, and oxygen extraction are greatest in the subendocardium, the subendocardium is the most susceptible region to ischemic injury and necrosis.[83] Severely ischemic myocardium undergoes necrosis first in the subendocardium, beginning as early as 15 to 20 minutes after coronary artery occlusion. Necrosis progresses toward the epicardium in a wavefront, gradually involving the less severely ischemic outer epicardial layers. The progression of the wavefront is slowed by the presence of residual blood flow when the coronary occlusion is incomplete or when mature collaterals are present at the time of occlusion. The wavefront conversely is accelerated when myocardial ischemia is unusually severe or when collateral blood flow is low, MVO_2 is high, or marked arterial hypotension is present (e.g., in patients in cardiogenic shock). In dogs with acute coronary occlusion, the subendocardial lateral boundaries of myocardial infarcts are established early in the first hour, whereas the myocardial infarct enlarges in the transmural direction over 4 to 6 hours, a finding similarly noted in humans. The recognition of the time-dependent progression of necrosis is the basis of timely interventions to salvage myocardium.[83,84]

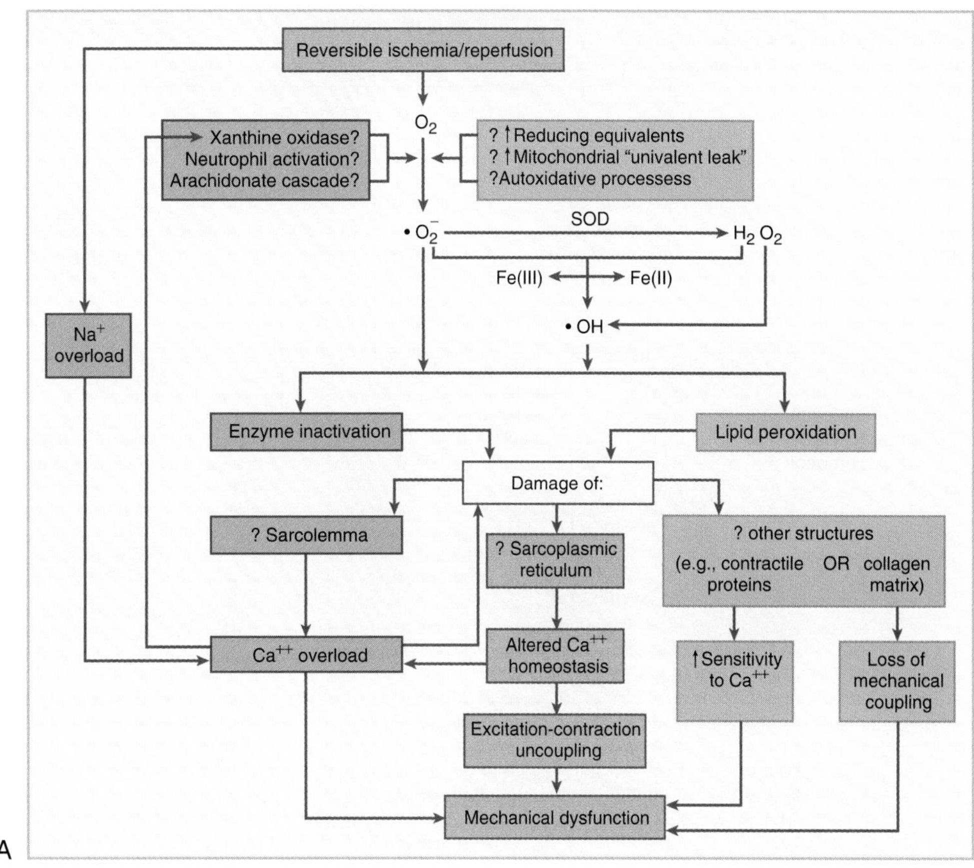

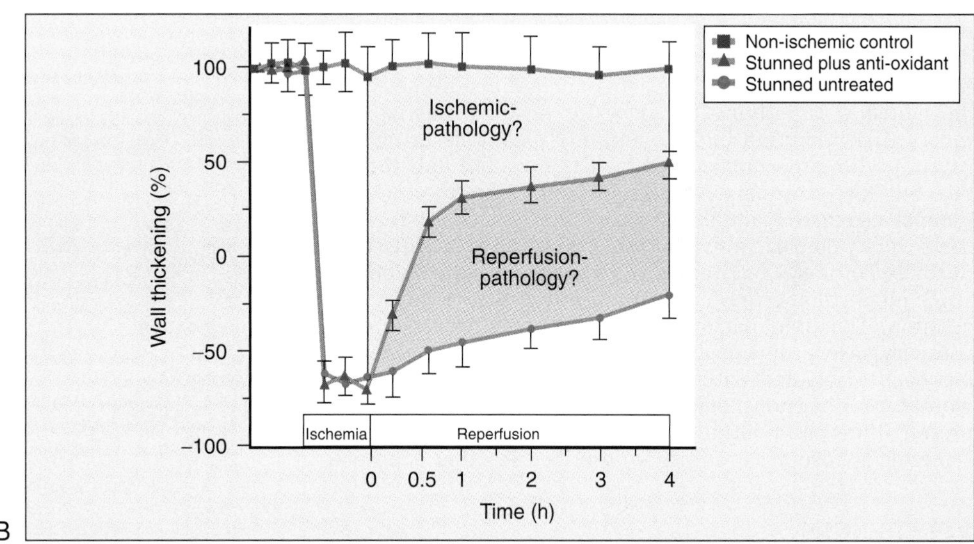

FIGURE 44–27 **A,** Illustration of proposed mechanisms of postischemic myocardial dysfunction integrating the mechanisms into three major hypotheses involving calcium overload, increased sensitivity to calcium, and loss of mechanical coupling. SOD = sodium oxide dismutase. **B,** Components of postischemic dysfunction: myocardial stunning probably arises from the additive effects of a reperfusion-induced pathology (magenta shading) of the contractile deficit, which can be restored through the use of antioxidant intervention transiently at the time of reperfusion. The second component (blue shading) incorporates pathology from which the heart is slowly recovering together with additional reperfusion-induced components not amenable to intervention. (Adapted from Hearse DJ: Stunning: A radical re-view. Cardiovasc Drugs Ther 5:853, 1991; Opie LH [ed]: Stunning, Hibernation, and Calcium in Myocardial Ischemia and Reperfusion Loss in Massachusetts. Dordrecht, Kluwer, 1992, pp 10-55; and Kloner RA, Bolli R, Marban E, et al: Medical and cellular implications of stunning, hibernation, and preconditioning: An NHLBI workshop. Circulation 97:1848-1867, 1998.)

The clinical presentations of myocardial ischemia are reflective of distinct pathogenic mechanisms. Clinical syndromes are often but not always associated with anginal pain and include chronic stable angina, unstable angina, variant (vasospastic) angina, and myocardial infarction (Fig. 44–28) (see Chaps. 46, 49, and 50). Atherosclerotic coronary stenosis is the most common cause of myocardial ischemia because of the high disease prevalence. Acute thrombosis superimposed on atherosclerotic plaque is associated with acute

TABLE 44–13 Features of Ischemia, Stunning, and Hibernation

Variable	Coronary Blood Flow	Lactate Production	Contractile Function
Ischemia/infarction	Markedly reduced/absent	Yes	Impaired transiently or permanently Recovers after relief of ischemia
Stunning	Preserved	No	Impaired, improved by inotropic with patent artery stimulation Recovers spontaneously
Hibernation	Reduced with abnormal myocardium	No	Impaired; recovery after revascularization

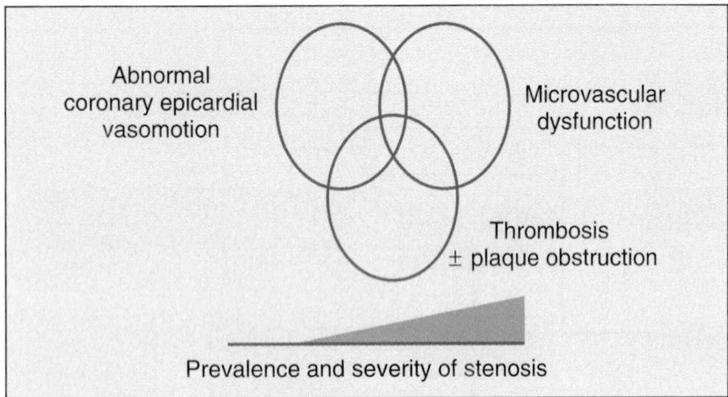

FIGURE 44–28 Pathophysiological components of myocardial ischemia. Different clinical ischemic syndromes result from fixed obstruction to coronary blood flow by atherosclerotic plaques, thrombosis, and/or coronary vasoconstriction of epicardial or microvascular vessels. These events may occur together or separately. (Modified from Maseri A, Crea F, Lanza GA, et al: Coronary vasoconstriction: Where do we stand in 1999? An important, multifaceted but elusive role. Cardiologia 44:115, 1999.)

myocardial infarction and unstable anginal syndromes. The mechanisms underlying the onset of unstable angina and myocardial infarction include not only plaque fissuring and rupture with superimposed platelet aggregation and thrombus but also coronary vasoconstriction. The products of platelet aggregation and thrombosis dilate normal arteries but can severely constrict the atherosclerotic artery. Patients with unstable coronary syndromes and complex plaques demonstrate augmented release of serotonin into the coronary circulation. Dynamic narrowing of coronary arteries due to coronary vasospasms or dynamic reduction in stenosis areas has been associated with cocaine use, cigarette smoking in women, or other nonspecific neurogenic stimuli. The clinical presentations and findings of the different myocardial ischemic syndromes are further described in other chapters.

REFERENCES

Myocardial Oxygen Supply and Demand Relationship

1. Braunwald E: Myocardial oxygen consumption: The quest for its determinants and some clinical fallout. J Am Coll Cardiol 35:45B, 2000.
2. Spaan JAE: Coronary Blood Flow: Mechanics, Distribution, and Control. Dordrecht, Netherlands, Kluwer, 1991.
3. Kal JE, Van Wezel HB, Vergroesen I: A critical appraisal of the rate pressure product as index of myocardial oxygen consumption for the study of metabolic coronary flow regulation. Int J Cardiol 71:141-148, 1999.
4. Chilian WM: Coronary microcirculation in health and disease: Summary of an NHLBI workshop. Circulation 95:522-528, 1997.
5. De Bruyne B, Hersbach F, Pijls NHJ, et al: Abnormal epicardial coronary resistance in patients with diffuse atherosclerosis but "normal" coronary angiography. Circulation 104:2401-2406, 2001.
6. Stepp DW, Nishikawa Y, Chilian WM: Regulation of shear stress in the canine coronary microcirculation. Circulation 100:1555-1561, 1999.

Endothelial Function

7. Mombouli JV, Vanhoutte PM: Endothelial dysfunction: From physiology to therapy. J Mol Cell Cardiol 31:61-74, 1999.
8. Verman S, Anderson TJ: Fundamentals of endothelial function for the clinical cardiologist. Circulation 105:546-549, 2002.
9. Selwyn AP, Kinlay S, Libby P, Ganz P: Atherogenic lipids, vascular dysfunction, and clinical signs of ischemic heart disease. Circulation 95:5-7, 1997.
10. Hasdai D, Gibbons RJ, Holmes DR Jr, et al: Coronary endothelial dysfunction in humans is associated with myocardial perfusion defects. Circulation 96:3390-3395, 1997.
11. Drexler H: Endothelial dysfunction: Clinical implications. Prog Cardiovasc Dis 39:287-324, 1997.
12. Thorne S, Mullen MJ, Clarkson P, et al: Early endothelial dysfunction in adults at risk from atherosclerosis: Different responses to L-arginine. J Am Coll Cardiol 32:110-116, 1998.
13. Inoue T, Saniabadi AR, Matsunaga R, et al: Impaired endothelium-dependent acetylcholine-induced coronary artery relaxation in patients with high serum remnant lipoprotein particles. Atherosclerosis 139:363-367, 1998.
14. Xu WM, Liu LZ: Nitric oxide: From a mysterious labile factor to the molecule of the Nobel Prize. Recent progress in nitric oxide research. Cell Res 8:251-258, 1998.
15. Moncada S: Nitric oxide: Discovery and impact on clinical medicine. J R Soc Med 92:164-169, 1999.
16. Ignarro LJ, Cirino G, Casini A, Napoli C: Nitric oxide as a signaling molecule in the vascular system: An overview. J Cardiovasc Pharmacol 34:879-886, 1999.
17. Lee RT, Libby P: The unstable atheroma. Arterioscler Thromb Vasc Biol 17:1859-1867, 1997.
18. Quilley J, Fulton D, McGiff JC: Hyperpolarizing factors. Biochem Pharmacol 54:1059-1070, 1997.
19. Bauersachs J, Popp R, Fleming I, Busse R: Nitric oxide and endothelium-derived hyperpolarizing factor: Formation and interactions. Prostaglandins Leukot Essent Fatty Acids 57:439-446, 1997.
20. Ortega Mateo A, de Artinano AA: Highlights on endothelins: A review. Pharmacol Res 36:339-351, 1997.
21. Kelly JJ, Whitworth JA: Endothelin-1 as a mediator in cardiovascular disease. Clin Exp Pharmacol Physiol 26:158-161, 1999.
22. Verhaar MC, Strachan FE, Newby DE, et al: Endothelin A receptor antagonist–mediated vasodilatation is attenuated by inhibition of nitric oxide synthesis and by endothelin-B receptor blockade. Circulation 97:752-756, 1998.
23. Heitzer T, Schlinzig T, Krohn K, et al: Endothelial dysfunction, oxidative stress, and risk of cardiovascular events in patients with coronary artery disease. Circulation 104:2673-2678, 2001.

Autoregulation

24. Pijls NHJ, De Bruyne B: Coronary Pressure. Dordrecht, Netherlands, Kluwer, 1997, pp 12-13.
25. Yada T, Richmond KN, Van Bibber R, et al: Role of adenosine in local metabolic coronary vasodilation. Am J Physiol 276:H1425-H1433, 1999.
26. Duffy SJ, Castle SF, Harper RW, Meredith IT: Contribution of vasodilator prostanoids and nitric oxide to resting flow, metabolic vasodilation, and flow-mediated dilation in human coronary circulation. Circulation 100:1951-1957, 1999.
27. Ishibashi Y, Duncker DJ, Zhang J, Bache RJ: ATP-sensitive K^+ channels, adenosine, and nitric oxide–mediated mechanisms account for coronary vasodilation during exercise. Circ Res 82:346-359, 1998.
28. Feigl EO: Neural control of coronary blood flow. J Vasc Res 35:85-92, 1998.
29. Saetrum OO, Gulbenkian S, Edvinsson L: Innervation and effects of vasoactive substances in the coronary circulation. Eur Heart J 18:1556, 1997.
30. Tanaka E, Mori H, Chujo M, et al: Coronary vasoconstrictive effects of neuropeptide Y and their modulation by the ATP-sensitive potassium channel in anesthetized dogs. J Am Coll Cardiol 29:1380, 1997.
31. Heusch G; Baumgart D, Camici P, et al: Alpha-adrenergic coronary vasoconstriction and myocardial ischemia in humans. Circulation 101:689, 2000.
32. Gregorini L, Marco J, Farah B, et al: Effects of selective α_1- and α_2-adrenergic blockade on coronary flow reserve after coronary stenting. Circulation 106:2901-2907, 2002.
33. Heusch G, Erbel R, Siffert W: Genetic determinants of coronary vasomotor in humans. Am J Physiol Heart Circ Physiol 281:H1465, 2001.
34. Snapir A, Mikkelsson J, Perola M, et al: Variation in the $alpha_2$-B adrenoceptor gene as a risk factor for pre-hospital fatal myocardial infarction and sudden death. J Am Coll Cardiol 41:190-194, 2003.
35. Rajagopalan S, Dube S, Canty JM Jr: Regulation of coronary diameter by myogenic mechanisms in arterial microvessels greater than 100 microns in diameter. Am J Physiol 268:H788-H793, 1995.
36. Morita K, Mori H, Tsujioka K, et al: Alpha-adrenergic vasoconstriction reduces systolic retrograde coronary blood flow. Am J Physiol 273:H2746-H2755, 1997.

37. Zhang J, Duncker DJ, Ya X, et al: Effect of left ventricular hypertrophy secondary to chronic pressure overload on transmural myocardial 2-deoxyglucose uptake: A ^{31}P NMR spectroscopic study. Circulation 92:1274-1283, 1995.
38. Duncker DJ, Traverse JH, Ishibashi Y, Bache RJ: Effect of NO on transmural distribution of blood flow in hypertrophied left ventricle during exercise. Am J Physiol 276:H1305-H1312, 1999.
39. Duncker DJ, Ishibashi Y, Bache RJ: Effect of treadmill exercise on transmural distribution of blood flow in hypertrophied left ventricle. Am J Physiol 275:H1274-H1282, 1998.

Influence of a Stenosis on Coronary Blood Flow

40. Siebes M, Campbell CS, D'Argenio DZ: Fluid dynamics of a partially collapsible stenosis in a flow model of the coronary circulation. ASME J Biomech Eng 118:489-497, 1996.
41. Kern M: Curriculum in interventional cardiology: Coronary pressure and flow measurements in the cardiac catheterization laboratory. Cathet Cardiovasc Intervent 54:378-400, 2002.
42. Jeremias A, Whitbourn RJ, Filardo SD, et al: Adequacy of intracoronary versus intravenous adenosine-induced maximal coronary hyperemia for fractional flow reserve measurements. Am Heart J 140:651-657, 2000.
43. Bartunek J, Winjs W, Heyndrickx GR, de Bruyne B: Effects of dobutamine on coronary stenosis: Physiology and morphology comparison with intracoronary adenosine. Circulation 100:243-249, 1999.
44. Pijls NH, De Bruyne B, Smith L, et al: Coronary thermodilution to assess flow reserve: Validation in humans. Circulation 105:2482-2486, 2002.
45. Baumgart D, Haude M, Liu F, et al: Current concepts of coronary flow reserve for clinical decision making during cardiac catheterization. Am Heart J 136:136-149, 1998.
46. Kern MJ, Bach RG, Mechem C, et al: Variations in normal coronary vasodilatory reserve stratified by artery, gender, heart transplantation and coronary artery disease. J Am Coll Cardiol 28:1154-1160, 1996.
47. Akasaka T, Yoshida K, Hozumi T, et al: Retinopathy identifies marked restriction of coronary flow reserve in patients with diabetes mellitus. J Am Coll Cardiol 30:935-941, 1997.

Measurement of Coronary Flow Reserve

48. Kern MJ: Coronary physiology revisited: Practical insights from the cardiac catheterization laboratory. Circulation 101:1344-1351, 2000.
49. Pijls NH, Van Gelder B, Van der Voort P, et al: Fractional flow reserve: A useful index to evaluate the influence of an epicardial coronary stenosis on myocardial blood flow. Circulation 92:3183-3193, 1995.
50. De Bruyne B, Bartunek J, Sys SU, et al: Simultaneous coronary pressure and flow velocity measurements in humans: Feasibility, reproducibility, and hemodynamic dependence of coronary flow velocity reserve, hyperemic flow versus pressure slope index, and fractional flow reserve. Circulation 94:1842-1849, 1996.
51. Marques KMJ, Spruijt HJ, Boer C, et al: The diastolic flow-pressure gradient relation in coronary stenoses in humans. J Am Coll Cardiol 39:1630-1636, 2002.
52. Meuwissen M, Chamuleau S, Siebes M, et al: Role of variability in microvascular resistance on fractional flow reserve and coronary blood flow velocity reserve in intermediate coronary lesions. Circulation 103:184-187, 2001.
53. Meuwissen M, Siebes M, Chamuleau SAJ, et al: Hyperemic stenosis resistance index for evaluation of functional coronary lesion severity. Circulation 106:441-446, 2002.
54. Pijls NH, De Bruyne B, Peels K, et al: Measurement of fractional flow reserve to assess the functional severity of coronary artery stenoses. N Engl J Med 334:1703-1708, 1996.
55. Chamuleau SAJ, Meuwissen M, van Eck-Smit BLF, et al: Fractional flow reserve, absolute and relative coronary blood flow velocity reserve in relation to the results of technetium-99m sestamibi single-photon emission computed tomography in patients with two-vessel coronary artery disease. J Am Coll Cardiol 37:1316-1322, 2001.
56. Kern MJ, Donohue TJ, Aguirre FV, et al: Clinical outcome of deferring angioplasty in patients with normal translesional pressure-flow velocity measurements. J Am Coll Cardiol 25:178-187, 1995.
57. Bech GJ, De Bruyne B, Bonnier HJRM, et al: Long-term follow-up after deferral of percutaneous transluminal coronary angioplasty of intermediate stenosis on the basis of coronary pressure measurement. J Am Coll Cardiol 31:841-847, 1998.
58. Bech GJW, Pijls NHJ, De Bruyne B, et al: Usefulness of fractional flow reserve to predict clinical outcome after balloon angioplasty. Circulation 99:883-888, 1999.
59. Bech GJW, De Bruyne B, Pijls NHJ, et al: Fractional flow reserve to determine the appropriateness of angioplasty in moderate coronary stenosis: A randomized trial. Circulation 103:2928-2934, 2001.
60. Smith SC Jr, Dove JT, Jacobs AK, et al: ACC/AHA guidelines for percutaneous coronary intervention (revision of the 1993 PTCA guidelines)—executive summary. A report of the American College of Cardiology/American Heart Association Task Force on Practice Guidelines (committee to revise the 1993 guidelines for percutaneous transluminal coronary angioplasty. J Am Coll Cardiol 37:2215-2238, 2001.
61. Pijls NHJ, Klauss V, Siebert U, et al: Coronary pressure measurement after stenting predicts adverse events at follow-up: A multicenter registry. Circulation 105:2950-2954, 2002.
62. De Bruyne B, Pijls NHJ, Bartunek J, et al: Fractional flow reserve in patients with prior myocardial infarction. Circulation 104:157-162, 2001.
63. Akasaka T, Yoshida K, Kawamoto T, et al: Relation of phasic coronary flow velocity characteristics with TIMI perfusion grade and myocardial recovery after primary percutaneous transluminal coronary angioplasty and rescue stenting. Circulation 101:2361-2367, 2000.
64. Yamamuro A, Akasaka T, Tamita K, et al: Coronary flow velocity pattern immediately after percutaneous coronary intervention as a predictor of complications and in-hospital survival after acute myocardial infarction. Circulation 106:3051-3056, 2002.
65. Kawamoto T, Yoshida K, Akasaka T, et al: Can coronary blood flow velocity pattern after primary percutaneous transluminal coronary angiography predict recovery of regional left ventricular function in patients with acute myocardial infarction? Circulation 100:339-345, 1999.
66. Tsunoda T, Nakamura M, Wakatsuki T, et al: The pattern of alteration in flow velocity in the recanalized artery is related to left ventricular recovery in patients with acute infarction and successful direct balloon angioplasty. J Am Coll Cardiol 32:338-344, 1998.

Coronary Collateral Circulation

67. Schaper W, Ito WD: Molecular mechanisms of coronary collateral vessel growth. Circ Res 79:911-919, 1996.
68. Pepper MS: Manipulating angiogenesis: From basic science to the bedside. Arterioscler Thromb Vasc Biol 17:605-619, 1997.
69. Wolf C, Cai WJ, Vosschulte R, et al: Vascular remodeling and altered protein expression during growth of coronary collateral arteries. J Mol Cell Cardiol 30:2291-2305, 1998.
70. Stetler-Stevenson WG: Matrix metalloproteinases in angiogenesis: A moving target for therapeutic intervention. J Clin Invest 103:1237-1241, 1999.
71. Majno G: Chronic inflammation: Links with angiogenesis and wound healing. Am J Pathol 153:1035-1039, 1998.
72. Schaper W, Buschmann I: Collateral circulation and diabetes. Circulation 99:2224-2226, 1999.
73. Klassen CL, Traverse JH, Bache RJ: Nitroglycerin dilates coronary collateral vessels during exercise after blockade of endogenous NO production. Am J Physiol 277:H918-H923, 1999.
74. Pijls NH, Bech GJ, el Gamal MI, et al: Quantification of recruitable coronary collateral blood flow in conscious humans and its potential to predict future ischemic events. J Am Coll Cardiol 25:1522-1528, 1995.
75. Billinger M, Kloos P, Eberli FR, et al: Physiologically assessed coronary collateral flow and adverse cardiac ischemic events: A follow-up study in 403 patients with coronary artery disease. J Am Coll Cardiol 40:1545-1550, 2002.
76. Seiler C, Fleisch M, Billinger M, Meier B: Simultaneous intracoronary velocity- and pressure-derived assessment of adenosine-induced collateral hemodynamics in patients with one- to two-vessel coronary artery disease. J Am Coll Cardiol 34:1985-1994, 1999.
77. Isner JM, Asahara T: Angiogenesis and vasculogenesis as therapeutic strategies for postnatal neovascularization. J Clin Invest 103:1231-1236, 1999.

Myocardial Ischemia

78. Kloner RA, Bolli R, Marban E, et al: Medical and cellular implications of stunning, hibernation, and preconditioning: An NHLBI workshop. Circulation 97:1848-1867, 1998.
79. Bolli R, Marban E: Molecular and cellular mechanisms of myocardial stunning. Physiol Rev 79:609-634, 1999.
80. Gerber BL, Wijns W, Vanoverschelde JL, et al: Myocardial perfusion and oxygen consumption in reperfused noninfarcted dysfunctional myocardium after unstable angina: Direct evidence for myocardial stunning in humans. J Am Coll Cardiol 34:1939-1946, 1999.
81. Perez NG, Marban E, Cingolani HE: Preservation of myofilament calcium responsiveness underlies protection against myocardial stunning by ischemic preconditioning. Cardiovasc Res 42:636-643, 1999.
82. Elsasser A, Schlepper M, Klovekorn WP, et al: Hibernating myocardium: An incomplete adaptation to ischemia. Circulation 96:2920-2931, 1997.
83. Bogaert J, Maes A, Van de Werf F, et al: Functional recovery of subepicardial myocardial tissue in transmural myocardial infarction after successful reperfusion: An important contribution to the improvement of regional and global left ventricular function. Circulation 99:36-43, 1999.
84. Jennings RB, Steenbergen C Jr, Reimer KA: Myocardial ischemia and reperfusion. Monogr Pathol 37:47-80, 1995.

CHAPTER 45

Approach to the Patient with Chest Pain

Thomas H. Lee • Christopher P. Cannon

Acute chest pain remains a difficult challenge for clinicians, and the percentage of patients who present to the emergency department with acute chest pain and are then admitted to the hospital may be increasing.[1-4] The reasons for caution include short-term mortality rates that are about twice as high for patients with acute myocardial infarction (MI) who are mistakenly discharged from the emergency department compared to what would be expected if they were admitted.[5,6] The legal costs that result from missed diagnoses of MI represent the largest category of losses from emergency medicine malpractice litigation.[7] For patients with low risks of complications, however, these concerns must be balanced against the costs and inconvenience that accompany admission to the hospital, and the risks of complications from tests and procedures with a low probability of improving patient outcomes.

Several advances in recent years have enhanced the accuracy and efficiency of the evaluation of patients with acute chest pain.[8] These advances include better serum markers for myocardial injury; decision aids to stratify patients according to their risks of complications; early and even immediate exercise testing and radionuclide scanning for lower risk patient subsets; and use of chest pain units and critical pathways for efficient and rapid evaluations of lower risk patients.

Causes of Acute Chest Pain

In a typical population of patients presenting for evaluation of acute chest pain in emergency departments, about 20 percent have acute MI or unstable angina.[5] A small percentage have other life-threatening problems, such as pulmonary embolism or acute aortic dissection, but most are discharged without a diagnosis or with a diagnosis of a noncardiac condition. These noncardiac conditions include musculoskeletal syndromes, disorders of abdominal viscera, and psychological conditions (Table 45–1).

MYOCARDIAL ISCHEMIA OR INFARCTION (see Chaps. 46 and 49). The most common serious cause of acute chest discomfort is myocardial ischemia or infarction, which occurs when the myocardial oxygen supply is inadequate compared to myocardial oxygen needs. Myocardial ischemia usually occurs in the setting of coronary atherosclerosis but also may reflect dynamic components of coronary vascular resistance. Coronary spasm can occur in normal coronary arteries, or, in patients with coronary disease, near atherosclerotic plaques and in smaller coronary arterioles (see Chap. 49). Other, less common causes of impaired coronary blood flow include syndromes that compromise the orifices of the coronary arteries or the arteries themselves, such as syphilitic aortitis, collagen-vascular diseases, aortic dissection, myocardial bridges, or congenital abnormalities of the coronary arteries.

Ischemic chest pain also can result from any disease process that causes occlusion of a coronary artery, such as thrombosis arising at the site of a ruptured atherosclerotic plaque. Other potential causes include coronary artery emboli such as may occur in patients with infectious or noninfectious endocarditis, or a clot in the left atrium or left ventricle.

Myocardial ischemia can be precipitated by conditions that cause a mismatch between the perfusion pressure within the coronary arteries and myocardial oxygen demand, such as aortic stenosis, aortic regurgitation, or hypertrophic cardiomyopathy. Increases in heart rate can markedly exacerbate ischemia in such patients because, even while oxygen demand is rising, myocardial perfusion falls due to a reduction in the proportion of time that the heart is in diastole, thereby decreasing the available time for coronary perfusion. Other clinical conditions can worsen oxygen delivery and/or raise oxygen need, although they generally cause myocardial ischemia and chest pain only when accompanied by coronary atherosclerosis. Such conditions include anemia, sepsis, and thyrotoxicosis.

The classic manifestation of ischemia is angina, which is usually described as a heavy chest pressure or squeezing, a "burning" feeling, or difficulty breathing. It is often associated with radiation to the left shoulder, neck, or arm. It typically builds in intensity over a period of a few minutes. The pain may begin with exercise or psychological stress, but acute coronary syndromes most commonly occur without obvious precipitating factors.

"Atypical" descriptions of chest pain reduce the likelihood that the symptoms represent myocardial ischemia or injury. The American College of Cardiology and the American Heart Association (ACC/AHA) guidelines list the following as pain descriptions that are *not* characteristic of myocardial ischemia[9]:

- Pleuritic pain (i.e., sharp or knife-like pain brought on by respiratory movements or cough)
- Primary or sole location of discomfort in the middle or lower abdominal region
- Pain that may be localized at the tip of one finger, particularly over the left ventricular (LV) apex
- Pain reproduced with movement or palpation of the chest wall or arms
- Constant pain that persists for many hours
- Very brief episodes of pain that last a few seconds or less
- Pain that radiates into the lower extremities

TABLE 45–1 Common Causes of Acute Chest Pain

System	Syndrome	Clinical description	Key Distinguishing Features
Cardiac	Angina	Retrosternal chest pressure, burning, or heaviness; radiating occasionally to neck, jaw, epigastrium, shoulders, or left arm	Precipitated by exercise, cold weather, or emotional stress; duration <2-10 minutes.
	Rest or unstable angina	Same as angina, but may be more severe	Usually <20 minutes; lower tolerance for exertion
	Acute myocardial infarction	Same as angina, but may be more severe	Sudden onset, usually lasting 30 minutes or longer. Often associated with shortness of breath, weakness, nausea, vomiting
	Pericarditis	Sharp, pleuritic pain aggravated by changes in position; highly variable duration	Pericardial friction rub
Vascular	Aortic dissection	Excruciating, ripping pain of sudden onset in anterior of chest, often radiating to back	Marked severity of unrelenting pain; usually occurs in setting of hypertension or underlying connective tissue disorder such as Marfan syndrome
	Pulmonary embolism	Sudden onset of dyspnea and pain, usually pleuritic with pulmonary infarction	Dyspnea, tachypnea, tachycardia, and signs of right heart failure
	Pulmonary hypertension	Substernal chest pressure, exacerbated by exertion	Pain associated with dyspnea and signs of pulmonary hypertension
Pulmonary	Pleuritis and/or pneumonia	Pleuritic pain, usually brief, over involved area	Pain pleuritic and lateral to midline, associated with dyspnea
	Tracheobronchitis	Burning discomfort in midline	Midline location, associated with coughing
	Spontaneous pneumothorax	Sudden onset of unilateral pleuritic pain, with dyspnea	Abrupt onset of dyspnea and pain
Gastrointestinal	Esophageal reflux	Burning substernal and epigastric discomfort, 10-60 minutes in duration	Aggravated by large meal and postprandial recumbency; relieved by antacid
	Peptic ulcer	Prolonged epigastric or substernal burning	Relieved by antacid or food
	Gallbladder disease	Prolonged epigastric, right upper quadrant pain	Unprovoked or following meal
	Pancreatitis	Prolonged, intense epigastric and substernal pain	Risk factors including alcohol, hypertriglyceridemia, and medications
Musculoskeletal	Costochondritis	Sudden onset of intense fleeting pain	May be reproduced by pressure over affected joint; occasional patients have swelling and inflammation over costochondral joint
	Cervical disc disease	Sudden onset of fleeting pain	May be reproduced with movement of neck
Infectious	Herpes zoster	Prolonged burning pain in dermatomal distribution	Vesicular rash, dermatomal distribution
Psychological	Panic disorder	Chest tightness or aching, often accompanied by dyspnea and lasting 30 minutes or more, unrelated to exertion or movement	Patient may have other evidence of emotional disorder

However, data from large populations of patients with acute chest pain indicate that acute coronary syndromes occur in patients with atypical symptoms with sufficient frequency that no single factor should be used to exclude the diagnosis of acute ischemia heart disease.[10]

PERICARDIAL DISEASE (see Chap. 64). The visceral surface of the pericardium is insensitive to pain, as is most of the parietal surface. Therefore, noninfectious causes of pericarditis (such as uremia) usually cause little or no pain. In contrast, infectious pericarditis nearly always involves surrounding pulmonary pleura, so that patients typically experience pleuritic pain with breathing, coughing, and changes in position. Swallowing may induce the pain because of the proximity of the esophagus to the posterior heart. Because the central diaphragm receives its sensory supply from the phrenic nerve, and the phrenic nerve arises from the third to fifth cervical segments of the spinal cord, pain from infectious pericarditis is frequently felt in the shoulders and neck. Involvement of the more lateral diaphragm can lead to symptoms in the upper abdomen and back, creating confusion with pancreatitis or cholecystitis. Pericarditis occasionally causes a steady, crushing substernal pain that is similar to that of acute myocardial infarction.[11]

VASCULAR DISEASE. Acute aortic dissection (see Chap. 53) usually is accompanied by sudden onset of excruciating, ripping pain, the location of which reflects the site and progression of the dissection.[12] Ascending aortic dissections tend to manifest with pain in the midline of the anterior chest, and posterior descending aortic dissections manifest with pain in the back of the chest. Aortic dissections usually occur in the presence of risk factors that include hypertension, pregnancy, atherosclerosis, and other conditions that lead to degeneration of the aortic media, such as Marfan and Ehlers-Danlos syndromes.

Pulmonary emboli (see Chap. 66) may be asymptomatic but often cause sudden onset of dyspnea and pleuritic chest pain.[13] Massive pulmonary emboli tend to cause severe and persistent substernal pain, which is believed to be due to distention of the pulmonary artery. Smaller emboli that lead to pulmonary infarction can cause lateral pleuritic chest pain. Hemodynamically significant pulmonary emboli may cause hypotension, syncope, and signs of right heart failure.

Pulmonary hypertension (see Chap. 67) can cause chest pain similar to angina pectoris, presumably because of right heart hypertrophy and ischemia.[14]

PULMONARY. Pulmonary conditions that cause chest pain usually produce dyspnea and pleuritic symptoms, the location of which reflect the site of pulmonary disease.[15] Tracheobronchitis tends to be associated with a burning midline pain,[16] whereas pneumonia can produce pain over the involved lung. The pain of a pneumothorax is sudden in onset and is usually accompanied by dyspnea.

GASTROINTESTINAL. Irritation of the esophagus by acid reflux can produce a burning discomfort that is exacerbated by alcohol, aspirin, and some foods. Symptoms often are worsened by a recumbent position and relieved by sitting upright and by acid-reducing therapies.[17] Esophageal spasm can produce a squeezing chest discomfort similar to that of angina.[18] Mallory-Weiss tears of the esophagus can occur in patients who have had prolonged vomiting episodes.

Chest pain due to ulcer disease usually occurs 60 to 90 minutes after meals and is typically relieved rapidly by acid-reducing therapies. This pain is usually epigastric in location but can radiate into the chest and shoulders.

Cholecystitis produces a wide range of pain syndromes and usually causes right upper quadrant abdominal pain. Chest and back pain due to cholecystitis is not unusual, however. The pain is often described as aching or colicky. Pancreatitis typically causes an intense aching epigastric pain that may radiate to the back. Relief through acid-reducing therapies is limited.

MUSCULOSKELETAL AND OTHER CAUSES. Chest pain can be caused by musculoskeletal disorders involving the chest wall, such as costochondritis, or by conditions affecting the nerves of the chest wall, such as cervical disc disease or herpes zoster. Musculoskeletal syndromes causing chest pain are often induced by direct pressure over the affected area or by movement of the patient's neck. The pain itself can be fleeting, or a dull ache that lasts for hours.

Panic syndrome is a major cause of chest discomfort among emergency department patients.[19] The symptoms typically include chest tightness, often accompanied by shortness of breath and a sense of anxiety, and generally lasting for 30 minutes or more.

CLINICAL EVALUATION. When evaluating patients with acute chest pain, the clinician must address a series of issues related to prognosis and immediate management. Even before trying to arrive at a definite diagnosis, high-priority questions include the following:

- *Clinical stability:* Is the patient in need of immediate treatment of circulatory collapse or respiratory insufficiency?
- *Immediate prognosis:* If the patient is currently clinically stable, what is the risk that the patient has a life-threatening condition, such as an acute coronary syndrome, pulmonary embolism, or aortic dissection?
- *Safety of triage options:* If the risks of life-threatening conditions are low, would it be safe to discharge the patient for outpatient management, or should the patient have further testing and/or observation to guide management?

Initial Assessment

The evaluation of the patient with acute chest pain actually begins before the physician sees the patient, and its effectiveness depends on the actions of office staff and other nonphysician personnel. Guidelines from the ACC/AHA[9] (see Guidelines section of Chap. 49) emphasize that patients with symptoms consistent with acute coronary syndromes should *not* be evaluated solely over the telephone but should be referred to facilities that allow evaluation by a physician and the recording of a 12-lead electrocardiogram.[19] These guidelines also recommend strong consideration of immediate referral to an emergency department or a specialized chest pain unit for patients with suspected acute coronary syndrome with chest discomfort at rest for more than 20 minutes, hemodynamic instability, or recent syncope or presyncope. Transport as a passenger in a private vehicle is considered an acceptable alternative to an emergency vehicle only if the wait would lead to a delay of greater than 20 to 30 minutes.

The National Heart Attack Alert Program guidelines recommend that patients with the following chief complaints should have immediate assessment by triage nurses and should be referred for further evaluation[20]:

- Chest pain, pressure, tightness, or heaviness; pain that radiates to neck, jaw, shoulders, back, or one or both arms
- Indigestion or "heartburn"; nausea and/or vomiting associated with chest discomfort
- Persistent shortness of breath
- Weakness, dizziness, lightheadedness, loss of consciousness

EXAMINATION. If the patient is not in immediate need of interventions because of circulatory collapse or respiratory insufficiency, the physician's assessment should begin with a clinical history that captures the characteristics of pain, the time of onset, and the duration of symptoms and an examination that emphasizes vital signs and cardiovascular status. This evaluation should be focused on screening for the most common life-threatening conditions: acute myocardial infarction, pulmonary embolism, and acute aortic dissection (see Table 45–1). Although information on coronary risk factors can help clinicians in the assessment of whether a patient has coronary artery disease, available data indicate that such information has limited ability to improve risk stratification of patients with acute chest pain, presumably because the probability of acute complications is dominated by other factors, such as the presence or absence of evidence of ischemia on the electrocardiogram.[3] Younger patients have a lower risk of acute coronary syndrome[21] but should be screened with greater care for histories of recent cocaine use (see Chap. 62).[22]

ELECTROCARDIOGRAM. The most important single source of data, the electrocardiogram, should be obtained within 10 minutes after presentation in patients with ongoing chest discomfort and as rapidly as possible in patients who have a history of chest discomfort consistent with acute coronary syndrome but whose discomfort has resolved by the time of evaluation,[19] to permit identification of patients who might benefit from primary angioplasty or thrombolytic therapy. When the electrocardiogram shows ST-segment changes or T-wave abnormalities that are consistent with the presence of ischemia and are not known to be old, discharging the patient home without further evaluation is hazardous both clinically and legally. The prevalence of acute MI is 80 percent among patients with 1 mm or more of new ST-segment elevation and 20 percent among patients with ST-segment depression or T-wave inversion not known to be old. However, if the electrocardiogram does not show changes consistent with ischemia, the risk of acute MI is about 4 percent among patients with a history of coronary artery disease and 2 percent among patients with no such history.[8] Failure to perform an electrocardiogram is one of the most important factors in malpractice losses related to patients with acute chest pain, followed by failure to interpret the electrocardiogram correctly.

For patients with a moderate or high probability of acute coronary syndromes, physicians usually perform assays of markers of myocardial injury such as the cardiac troponins T or I (cTnT or cTnI) or creatine kinase MB isoenzyme (CK-MB). Many hospital laboratories perform these tests on a "stat" basis, and point of care ("bedside") assays for these markers are now widely available; thus, results are often available to inform initial management decisions (see Chap. 46).

Studies of the diagnostic performance of cTnI or cTnT or CK-MB indicate that when any of these test findings are abnormal, the patient has a high likelihood of having an acute coronary syndrome (Fig. 45–1; Tables 45–2 and 45–3). The more challenging issues in the interpretation of these test findings during the initial evaluation of acute chest pain are (1) the frequency and causes of false-positive results; (2) the prognostic implications of abnormal test results; and (3) the interpretation of single values of these tests, such as are available during the initial evaluation of acute chest pain.

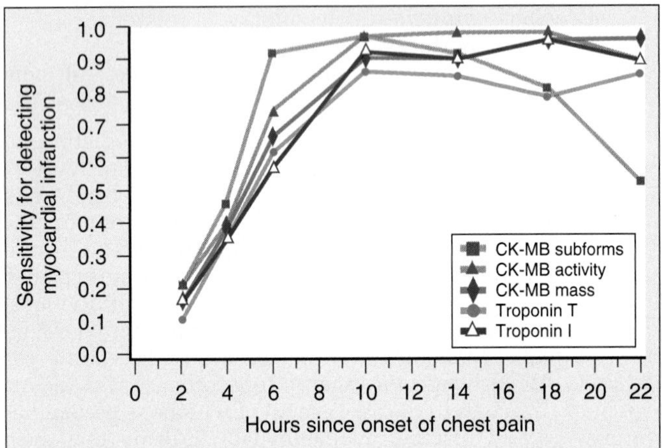

FIGURE 45–1 Diagnostic sensitivity of macromolecular markers of myocardial infarction according to the length of time from the onset of chest pain. CK-MB = creatine kinase MB isoenzyme. (Data from Zimmerman J, Fromm R, Meyer D, et al: Diagnostic marker cooperative study for the diagnosis of myocardial infarction. Circulation 99:1671, 1999.)

DIAGNOSTIC PERFORMANCE. Studies of the major assays used to evaluate patients with acute chest pain (CK-MB, cTnI, and cTnT) indicate that with serial sampling, these agents all have excellent sensitivity for detection of acute MI.[23-29] Cardiac troponin abnormalities persist for several days after myocardial injury; hence, after 24 hours from symptom onset, these assays are significantly more sensitive than CK-MB. The oldest of these three assays, CK-MB, provides the benchmark against which the other two are evaluated. Meta-analysis of published data indicate that CK-MB mass has a clinical sensitivity for acute myocardial infarction of 97 percent and specificity of 90 percent.[30]

Creatine Kinase MB Isoenzyme. The dissemination of the radioimmunoassay for CK-MB (versus the older activity assay and electrophoretic assays) have greatly reduced false-positive rates; measured CK-MB with the mass assay can be reliably assumed to represent true CK-MB. However, noncardiac muscle frequently has trace amounts of true CK-MB, and these amounts are increased in patients with conditions that cause chronic muscle destruction and regeneration, such as muscular dystrophy or high performance athletics (e.g., marathon running).[31] CK-MB elevations are particularly common in emergency department patients, who have higher rates of histories of alcohol abuse or trauma.

In addition to the problem of "false-positive" CK-MB results due to CK-MB from noncardiac sources, clinicians also struggle with uncertainty as to whether the amount of CK-MB measured represents a pathological elevation. Although there is no physiological basis for such an index, many clinicians calculate a "CK-MB mass index" dividing the CK-MB mass level by the total CK activity level. Ratios greater than 2.5 percent are considered suggestive of myocardial damage.[32] This ratio may be inaccurate when (1) high levels of total CK are present because of skeletal muscle injury, (2) chronic skeletal muscle injuries release greater amounts of CK-MB, and (3) total CK measurements are within normal reference range for the laboratory and while the CK-MB level is elevated.[33]

For several years, there has been investigative interest in CK-MB isoforms as a possible refinement to measurement of CK-MB. CK-MB exists in only one form in myocardial tissue (CK-MB2) but is modified in plasma so that another isoform (CK-MB1) also exists. An absolute level of CK-MB2 greater

TABLE 45–2 Likelihood that Signs and Symptoms Represent an Acute Coronary Syndrome

Feature	High Likelihood (any of the following)	Intermediate Likelihood (absence of high-likelihood features and presence of any of the following)	Low Likelihood (absence of high- or intermediate-likelihood features but may have any of the following)
History	• Chest or left arm pain or discomfort as chief symptom reproducing prior documented angina • Known history of coronary artery disease, including myocardial infarction	• Chest or left arm pain or discomfort as chief symptom • Age >70 years • Male sex • Diabetes mellitus	• Probable ischemic symptoms in absence of any of the intermediate likelihood characteristics • Recent cocaine use
Examination	• Transient mitral regurgitation, hypotension, diaphoresis, pulmonary edema, or rales	• Extracardiac vascular disease	• Chest discomfort reproduced by palpation
Electrocardiogram	• New, or presumably new, transient ST-segment deviation (≥0.05 mV) or T-wave inversion (≥0.2 mV) with symptoms	• Fixed Q waves • Abnormal ST segments or T waves not documented to be new	• T-wave flattening or inversion in leads with dominant R waves • Normal ECG
Cardiac markers	Elevated cardiac TnI, TnT, or CK-MB	Normal	Normal

From Fleet RP, Dupuis G, Marchand A, et al: ACC/AHA 2002 guideline update for the management of patients with unstable angina and non–ST-segment elevation myocardial infarction: Summary article. A report of the American College of Cardiology/American Heart Association Task Force on Practice Guidelines (Committee on the Management of Patients With Unstable Angina). Circulation 106:1893, 2002.

TABLE 45–3 Short-Term Risk of Death or Nonfatal Myocardial Ischemia in Patients with Unstable Angina

Feature	High Likelihood (any of the following)	Intermediate Likelihood (absence of high-likelihood features and presence of any of the following)	Low Likelihood (absence of high- or intermediate-likelihood features but may have any of the following)
History	Accelerating tempo of ischemic symptoms in preceding 48 hours	Prior MI, peripheral or cerebrovascular disease, or CABG; prior aspirin use	
Character of pain	Prolonged ongoing (>20 minutes) rest pain	• Prolonged (>20 min) rest angina, now resolved, with moderate or high likelihood of coronary artery disease • Rest angina (<20 min) or relieved with rest or sublingual NTG	New-onset or progressive Canadian Cardiovacular System Class III or IV angina the past 2 weeks without prolonged (>20 min) rest pain but with moderate or high likelihood of coronary artery disease
Clinical findings	• Pulmonary edema, most likely due to ischemia • New or worsening mitral regurgitation murmur • S_3 or new/worsening rales • Hypotension, bradycardia, tachycardia • Age >75 years	Age >70 years	
Electrocardiogram	• Angina at rest with transient ST-segment changes >0.05 mV • Bundle-branch block, new or presumed new • Sustained ventricular tachycardia	• T-wave inversions >0.2 mV • Pathological Q waves	• Normal or unchanged ECG during an episode of chest discomfort
Cardiac markers	Elevated (e.g., TnT or TnI >0.1 ng/ml)	Slightly elevated (e.g., TnT >0.01 but <0.1 ng/ml)	Normal

CABG = coronary artery bypass grafting; ECG = electrocardiogram; MI = myocardial infarction; NTG = nitroglycerin.
From Fleet RP, Dupuis G, Marchand A, et al: ACC/AHA 2002 guideline update for the management of patients with unstable angina and non–ST-segment elevation myocardial infarction: Summary article. A report of the American College of Cardiology/American Heart Association Task Force on Practice Guidelines (Committee on the Management of Patients With Unstable Angina). Circulation 106:1893, 2002.

than 1 U/liter and a ratio of CK-MB2 to CK-MB1 greater than 1.5 indicates fresh release of CK-MB and, when measured within the first 6 hours of symptoms, has better sensitivity for MI than conventional CK-MB assays.[34] The CK-MB isoform assay is not widely available, however, and, as is true of the conventional CK-MB assay, suffers from lack of specificity of CK-MB to myocardial tissues.

Troponins. The troponins T and I are encoded by different genes in cardiac muscle, slow skeletal muscle, and fast skeletal muscle; hence, the assays that were developed for the cardiac troponins are more specific than CK-MB for myocardial injury. Assessment of the diagnostic performance of the cardiac troponin assays is complicated by the known limitations of the CK-MB assay, which, by necessity, is used to determine whether newer assays have provided a misleading result. Using combinations of clinical criteria including CK-MB data, cardiac troponins have had good but not perfect sensitivity (84 to 89 percent) for detecting acute MIs.[25,27] cTnI and cTnT have been described as having a lower specificity for MI than the traditional CK-MB assays, but these findings may be due to greater sensitivity for smaller degrees of myocardial damage than can be detected with CK-MB assays.

Because the cardiac troponins are highly specific to myocardial tissues, "false-positive" elevations usually represent myocardial damage from causes other than coronary artery disease. Such damage may occur with myopericarditis, trauma, congestive heart failure, pulmonary embolus, and sepsis. Elevated levels of cardiac troponins have been reported in patients with renal disease and connective tissue diseases.[35,36] In patients with acute coronary syndromes, even minor elevations of cTnI and cTnT have been shown to identify patients with an increased risk of complications who benefit from aggressive management strategies.[37]

Rapid bedside assays for cTnT and cTnI using whole blood samples yield results that are in close agreement with serum cTnT concentrations measured by the standard enzyme immunoassay.[28,38,39] For example, in one multicenter study, 95 percent of all samples with cTnT concentration below 0.3 ng/ml were negative on the bedside assay, and 99 percent of samples above 0.3 ng/ml were positive.[38] In this study, the "gray zone" in which the bedside assay was not perfect extended from 0.1 to 0.5 ng/ml. A bedside assay for cTnI has also been reported to have diagnostic efficacy comparable to the standard enzyme-linked immunosorbent assay (ELISA).[39] One of the few studies that assessed both rapid cardiac troponin assays found that 94 percent of patients with MI had a positive cTnT result at least within 6 hours from the onset of chest pain and all had a positive cTnI result; the specificities were 89 percent and 83 percent, respectively.[25] Hence, diagnostic performance with the two cardiac troponins appears essentially the same.

Myoglobin. Serum myoglobin has long interested clinicians as a potential aid to early detection of MI, because this smaller molecule diffuses through interstitial fluids more rapidly after cell death than the larger CK and troponin molecules. It therefore becomes abnormal as early as 30 minutes after myocardial injury. However, myoglobin is not specific to myocardial tissue, so false-positive rates in emergency department populations are high.

Prognostic Implications of Test Results. Abnormal levels of CK-MB, cTnI, and cTnT are predictors of increased risk of complications (see Tables 45–2 and 45–3).[25,40-44] Even if patients do not have CK-MB elevations, cTnI and cTnT are useful for early risk stratification in patients with acute chest pain, particularly those without ST-segment elevation.[40] For example, in the GUSTO-IIa troponin T substudy, which enrolled patients with acute ischemic syndromes, patients with elevated cTnT at baseline had a 30-day mortality rate of 10 percent, compared with 5 percent in patients with late positive cTnT levels (8-16 hours) and 0 percent in those with persistently normal cTnT results.[44] The prognostic value of cTnI seems to be comparable to that of cTnT in patients with unstable angina.[45]

Test Performance of Single Assays. Although high sensitivities and specificities for diagnosis of myocardial injury can be achieved for several assays through serial sampling, the diagnostic performance of a single value of any of these tests is not nearly as good. A single CK-MB value in emergency department patients with acute chest pain has a sensitivity for detecting acute MI of 34 percent and a specificity of 88 percent[46]; a single value of cTnI has a sensitivity of about 40 percent.[27]

The diagnostic performance of single values of these tests is influenced considerably by the time elapsed since the onset of symptoms. For example, a single CK-MB mass or troponin drawn within 4 hours of the onset of symptoms has a sensitivity of less than 25 percent.[27,46,47] However, single values of CK-MB mass and troponins that are drawn more than 12 hours after the onset of symptoms have sensitivities for myocardial infarction in the range of 70 to 90 percent.

INTERPRETATION OF TESTS: RELATIONSHIP BETWEEN PRETEST PROBABILITY AND POSTTEST PROBABILITY. As is true of most tests in medicine, results should be interpreted in the context of the patient's overall probability of having the diagnosis of interest. Thus, a normal result on a test or series of tests in a patient with a high clinical probability of acute coronary syndrome does not exclude this diagnosis, although it raises the question of whether any myocardial injury may have occurred several days previously. Similarly, an abnormal test result in a patient with a low probability of coronary disease does not necessarily mean that the patient has had myocardial injury, although it may suggest that a reassessment of the patient's clinical data is in order.

To formalize such analyses, cardiac markers can be interpreted in a bayesian framework in which pretest probabilities are modified by test results (Fig. 45–2). These calculations of posttest probabilities assume that the sensitivity and specificity of serial sampling of CK-MB mass values, for example, in patients presenting within 24 hours of the onset of symptoms are about 95 percent (see Fig. 45–2A). In contrast, the impact of single CK-MB mass results on patients' probabilities of coronary disease is quite modest (see Fig. 45–2B). These analyses assume a sensitivity of 56 percent and a specificity of 98 percent for single CK-MB mass values greater than 5 ng/ml at admission.[27]

TESTING STRATEGY. Guidelines from the ACC/AHA recommend measurement of biomarkers of cardiac injury in patients with symptoms that are consistent with acute coronary syndromes (Table 45–4).[19] Implicit is this recommendation is recognition that patients with very low probability of acute coronary syndrome should not undergo measurement of biomarkers, because of the possibility that false-positive results will lead to unnecessary hospitalizations, tests, procedures, and their complications. Because single values of these assays have limited sensitivity for detecting myocardial injury, a single negative biomarker does not really "rule out" myocardial injury for these low-risk patients.

The ACC/AHA guidelines recommend that cTnI or cTnT are the preferred first-line markers but note that CK-MB (by mass assay) is an acceptable alternative. The preference for cardiac troponins reflects the greater specificity of these markers compared with CK-MB and the prognostic value of troponin elevations in the presence of normal CK-MB levels. If the initial set of markers is negative in patients who have presented within the first 6 hours of the onset of pain, the

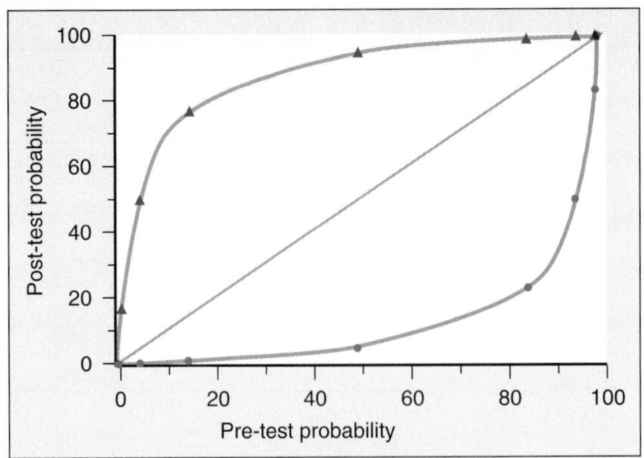

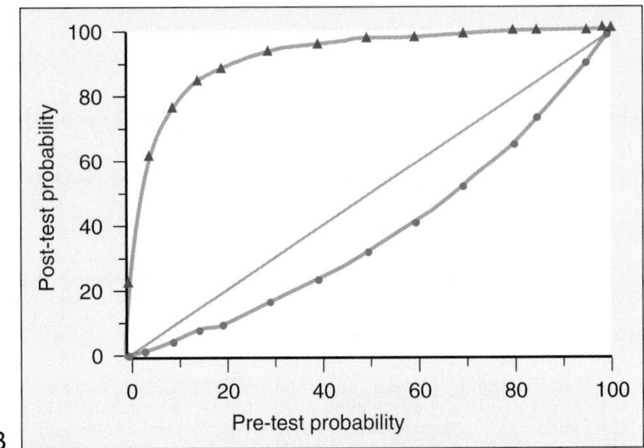

FIGURE 45–2 Effect of serial CK-MB results **(A)** and single CK-MB values **(B)** on the probability of acute myocardial infarction. The pretest probabilities, as marked along the *x* axis, can be derived through use of computerized algorithms, personal experience, or analysis of published data. Posttest probabilities are plotted on the *y* axis. The curves correspond to posttest probabilities of infarction with normal (magenta) or elevated (blue) creatine kinase MB isoenzyme (CK-MB) results, assuming a 95 percent sensitivity and 95 percent specificity for serial sampling of CK-MB levels.

guidelines recommend that another sample should be drawn in the 6- to 12-hour time frame.

Initial Risk Stratification

For patients with chest pain, the initial risk stratification focuses on the safety of various triage and testing options. These options include the following:

- Immediate treatment of acute coronary syndrome with invasive therapy or thrombolytic agents
- Admission to a coronary care or other intensive care unit
- Admission to an intermediate care facility with central electrocardiographic monitoring, such as chest pain units
- Further data collection, such as via immediate exercise testing or radionuclide imaging
- Discharge to home

The decision among these options is made on the basis of information from the history, physical examination, electrocardiogram, and, for patients with suspected acute coronary syndrome, one or more sets of biomarkers for myocardial injury. Key factors suggesting a high risk of acute coronary syndrome and its complications include prolonged or accelerating ischemic symptoms; evidence of congestive heart

TABLE 45–4 ACC/AHA Recommendations for Early Risk Stratification

	Indication	Level of Evidence
Class I (indicated)	1. A determination should be made in all patients with chest discomfort of the likelihood of acute ischemia caused by CAD as high, intermediate, or low.	C
	2. Patients who present with chest discomfort should undergo early risk stratification that focuses on anginal symptoms, physical findings, ECG findings, and biomarkers of cardiac injury.	B
	3. A 12-lead ECG should be obtained immediately (within 10 min) in patients with ongoing chest discomfort and as rapidly as possible in patients who have a history of chest discomfort consistent with ACS but whose discomfort has resolved by the time of evaluation.	C
	4. Biomarkers of cardiac injury should be measured in all patients who present with chest discomfort consistent with ACS. A cardiac-specific troponin is the preferred marker, and if available, it should be measured in all patients. CK-MB by mass assay is also acceptable. In patients with negative cardiac markers within 6 hr of the onset of pain, another sample should be drawn in the 6- to 12-hr time frame (e.g., at 9 hr after the onset of symptoms).	C
Class IIa (good supportive evidence)	For patients who present within 6 hr of the onset of symptoms, an early marker of cardiac injury (e.g., myoglobin or CK-MB subforms) should be considered in addition to a cardiac troponin.	C
Class IIb (weak supportive evidence)	C-reactive protein and other markers of inflammation should be measured.	B
Class III (not indicated)	Total CK (without MB), aspartate aminotransferase (AST, SGOT), beta-hydroxybutyric dehydrogenase, and/or lactate dehydrogenase should be the markers for the detection of myocardial injury in patients with chest discomfort suggestive of ACS.	C

ACS = acute coronary syndrome; CAD = coronary artery disease; CK-MB = creatine kinase MB isoenzyme; ECG = electrocardiogram.
From Braunwald E, Antman EM, Beasley JW, et al: ACC/AHA 2002 guideline update for the management of patients with unstable angina and non–ST-segment elevation myocardial infarction: Summary article. A report of the American College of Cardiology/American Heart Association Task Force on Practice Guidelines (Committee on the Management of Patients With Unstable Angina). Circulation 106:1893, 2002.

failure on physical examination; electrocardiographic abnormalities consistent with ischemia that are not known to be old, and elevated markers for myocardial injury (see Tables 45–2 and 45–3). The association of these findings with risks of complications is discussed in Chapters 46 and 49. This discussion focuses on the ability of various data to improve initial patient management.

Clinical History

Other factors from the history contribute to risk stratification in addition to the assessment of whether the patient's symptoms are consistent with myocardial ischemia, and whether the duration and pattern of symptoms suggest an elevated risk for complications (see Tables 45–2 and 45–3). A prior history of myocardial infarction is associated not only with a high risk of obstructive coronary disease but also with an increased risk of multivessel disease.[48] Women with suspected acute coronary syndrome are less likely to have coronary disease than are men with similar clinical presentations, and, when coronary disease is present, it tends to be less severe.[49,50] Older patients, particularly beyond 70 years of age, have a higher risk for coronary disease and higher risk for adverse outcomes.[51]

Information on traditional risk factors, especially diabetes, can help identify high-risk patients among those with acute coronary syndrome. However, risk factor data are of relatively little value in the diagnosis of patients with acute ischemia after consideration of other data from the history, electrocardiogram, and cardiac markers.[51] Thus, ACC/AHA guidelines recommend that these data should *not* be used to determine whether a patient should be admitted.[19] Similarly, the guidelines note that a family history of premature coronary disease is *not* a useful indicator of diagnosis or prognosis for patients with acute chest pain.

The Physical Examination

The initial examination of patients with acute chest pain is directed toward identifying potential precipitating causes of myocardial ischemia[52] (e.g., uncontrolled hypertension); important comorbid conditions (e.g., chronic obstructive pulmonary disease); and evidence of hemodynamic complications (e.g., congestive heart failure, new mitral regurgitation, or hypotension). The ACC/AHA guidelines recommend that every patient with suspected acute coronary syndrome have blood pressure measured in both arms, as well as documentation of heart rate and temperature and a thorough cardiovascular and chest examination. The examination of the peripheral vessels should include assessment of the presence of bruits or pulse deficits that might suggest extracardiac vascular disease.

For patients whose clinical presentations are not suggestive of myocardial ischemia, the search for noncoronary causes of chest pain should focus first on potentially life-threatening issues (aortic dissection, pulmonary embolism), and then turn to the possibility of other cardiac (e.g., pericarditis) and noncardiac (e.g., esophageal discomfort) diagnoses. Aortic dissection is suggested by pulse deficits or a new murmur of aortic regurgitation in the presence of back or midline anterior chest pain. Differences in breath sounds in the presence of acute dyspnea and pleuritic chest pain raises the possibility of pneumothorax. Tachycardia and tachypnea may be the major manifestations of pulmonary embolism on physical examination.

The Electrocardiogram

The electrocardiogram provides critical information for both diagnosis and prognosis (see Tables 45–2 and 45–3), particularly when a tracing is obtained during episodes of pain. New persistent or transient ST-segment changes (≥0.05 mV) that develop during a symptomatic episode at rest and resolve when the symptoms resolve strongly suggest acute ischemia and severe coronary disease. Nonspecific ST-segment and T-wave changes are usually defined as lesser amounts of ST-segment deviation or T-wave inversion of less than or equal to 0.2 mV and are less helpful in risk stratification. A completely normal electrocardiogram (ECG) does not exclude the possibility of acute coronary syndrome; about 1 to 6 percent of such patients with acute chest pain are subsequently found to have acute MI, although the prognosis of patients with a normal or near-normal ECG is better than that of patients with clearly abnormal ECGs at presentation.[53,54]

The availability of a prior ECG improves diagnostic accuracy and is associated with a reduced rate of admission for patients with abnormal baseline tracings.[55] Serial ECG tracings improve the clinician's ability to diagnose acute MI,[56] particularly if combined with serial measurement of cardiac markers.[57] Continuous ECG monitoring to detect ST-segment shifts is technically feasible, but the contribution to patient management is uncertain.[19,58]

Decision Aids

Multivariate algorithms have been developed and prospectively validated with the goal of improving the stratification of risk in patients with acute chest pain. These algorithms can be used to estimate the probability for individual patients of acute myocardial infarction,[2] acute ischemic heart disease,[1,4] or the risk of major cardiac complications.[3] These algorithms have been used mainly to identify patients who are at low risk for complications and who therefore do not require admission to the hospital or coronary care unit.

A prospectively validated algorithm for prediction of risk of complications requiring intensive care unit care[3] is presented as a flow chart in Figure 45–3. In this algorithm, patients with suspected myocardial infarction on ECG are immediately classified as having a high risk (>16 percent) of major complications within the next 72 hours. Patients whose ECGs are consistent with ischemia but not infarction are then classified as intermediate (approximately 8 percent) or high risk for complications depending on the presence or absence of clinical risk factors, including systolic blood pressure below 100 mm Hg; bilateral rales heard above the bases; and known unstable ischemic heart disease (defined as worsening of previously stable angina, a new onset of angina after infarction or after a coronary revascularization procedure, or pain that was the same as that associated with a prior MI). These same risk factors are used to stratify patients without ischemic changes on their ECGs.

Validated algorithms for prediction of acute ischemic heart disease and the risks and benefits of thrombolytic therapy have been incorporated into computerized reports of electrocardiograms to help clinicians make decisions about admission[4] and to help them assess the risks and benefits of using thrombolytic therapy in individual cases.[59] In a multicenter randomized trial, an intervention in which information about the expected impact of the use of thrombolytic therapy on the electrocardiogram led to an increase in the use of thrombolytic therapy for women (from 18 to 22 percent) and was associated with an improvement in timeliness of treatment.

Prospective trials indicate that these algorithms have little effect in the routine clinical practice of clinicians who have not received training in their use.[4,60,61] Among the reasons that practicing physicians do not use algorithms are that they are too busy, are unsure of their value, or are concerned about the legal and clinical consequences of inappropriately discharging patients who are subsequently found to have had MI.[61,62]

Immediate Management

The ACC/AHA guidelines suggest an approach to the immediate management of patients with possible acute coronary syndrome (ACS) that integrates information from the history, physical examination, 12-lead ECG, and initial cardiac marker tests to assign patients to four categories: noncardiac diagnosis, chronic stable angina, possible ACS, and definite ACS (Fig. 45–4). In this algorithm, patients with ST elevation are triaged immediately for reperfusion therapy, according to ACC/AHA guidelines for acute MI. For patients with acute coronary syndrome who have ST or T wave changes, ongoing pain, positive cardiac markers, or hemodynamic abnormalities, admission to hospital for management of acute ischemia is recommended. Cost-effectiveness analyses support triage of such patients to the coronary care unit for their initial care.[63] For patients with possible or definite acute coronary syndrome who do not have diagnostic electrocardiograms and whose initial serum cardiac markers are within normal limits, observation in a chest pain unit or other nonintensive care facility is appropriate.[19]

Chest Pain Protocols and Units

Until the 1980s, most patients with suspected acute coronary syndrome were triaged to coronary care units, where they underwent 2 to 3 days of "rule out MI" evaluations.[64] In the last two decades, however, economic pressures and advances in risk stratification have led many institutions to develop "critical pathways" to standardize management of lower risk patients with acute chest pain.[65] These critical pathways make explicit the timing and sequence of key tests and triage decisions.

The main elements of a typical chest pain critical pathway are included in the bottom part of Figure 45–4. According to the ACC/AHA recommendations,[19] patients with a low risk of acute coronary syndrome or associated complications can be observed for 4 to 8 hours while undergoing electrocardiographic monitoring and serial measurement of cardiac markers. Patients who develop evidence of ischemia or other indicators of increased risk should be admitted to the coronary care unit for further manage-

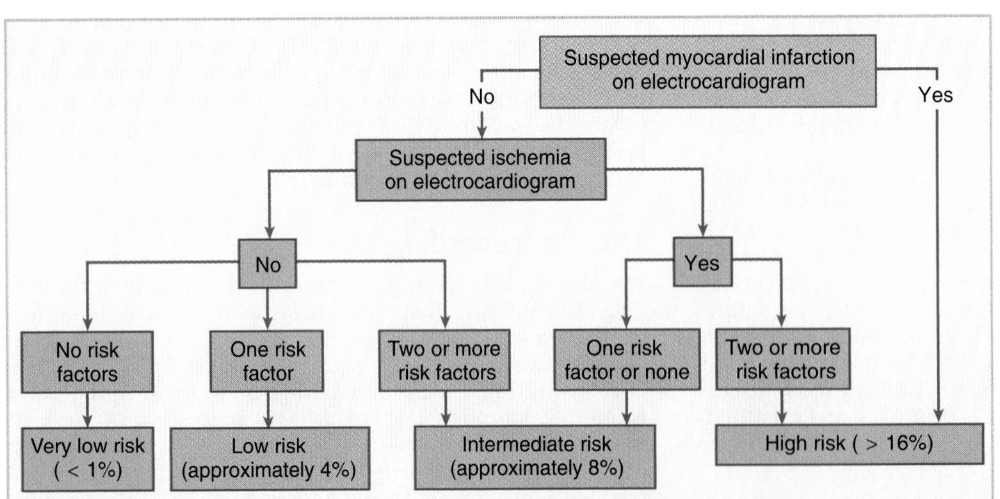

FIGURE 45–3 Derivation and validation of four groups into which patients can be categorized according to risk of major cardiac events within 72 hours after admission. (From Goldman L, Cook EF, Johnson PA, et al: Prediction of the need for intensive care in patients who come to emergency departments with acute chest pain. N Engl J Med 334:1498, 1966.)

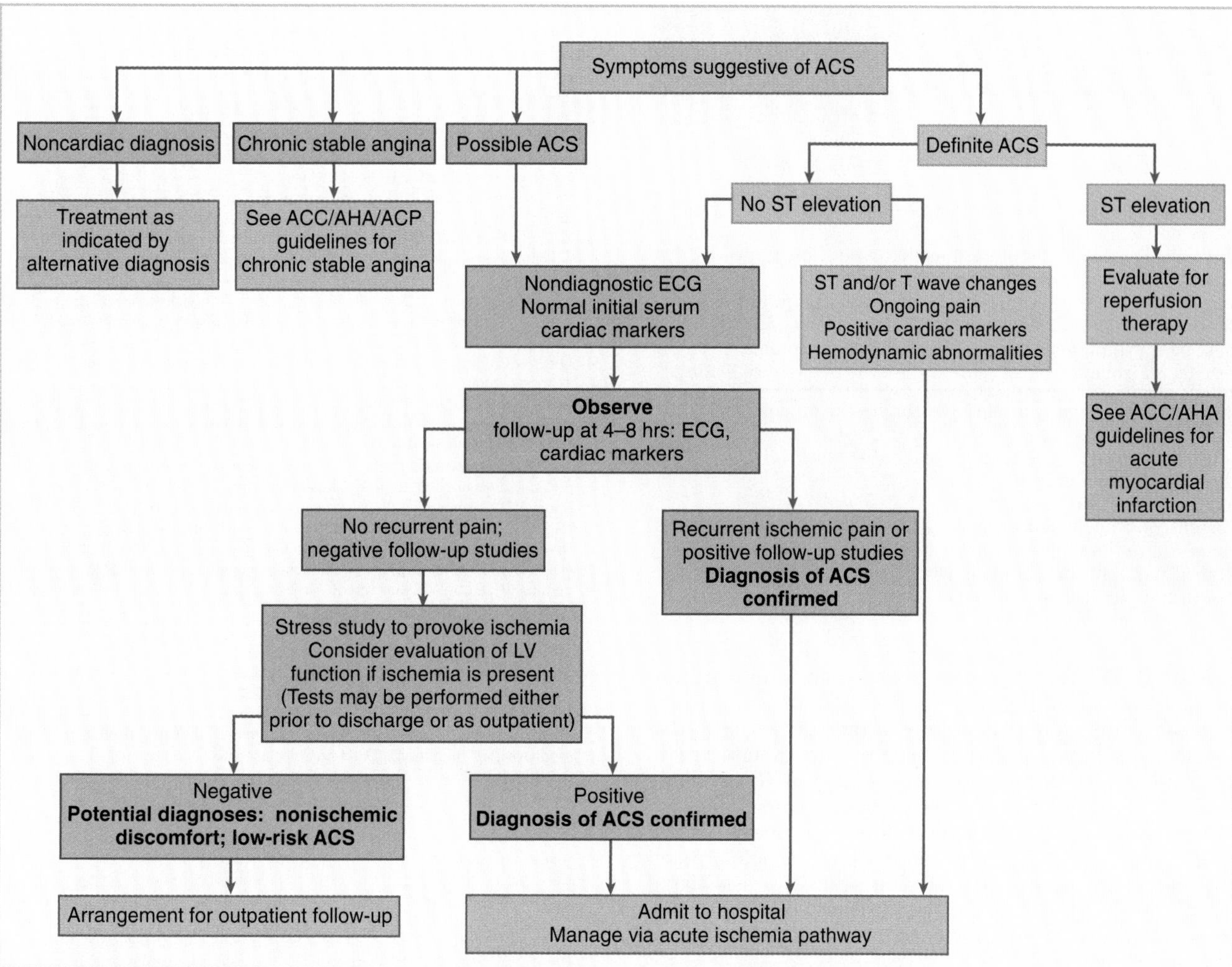

FIGURE 45–4 Algorithm for evaluation and management of patients suspected of having acute coronary syndrome (ACS). (From Braunwald E, Antman EM, Beasley JW, et al: ACC/AHA guideline update for the management of patients with unstable angina and non-ST-segment elevation myocardial infarction—Summary article 2002: A report of the American College of Cardiology/American Heart Association Task Force on Practice Guidelines [Committee on the Management of Patients With Unstable Angina]. Circulation 106:1893, 2002.)

ment. Patients who do not develop recurrent pain or other predictors of increased risk can be triaged for early noninvasive testing (see below) either before or after discharge.

To enhance the efficiency and reliability of implementation of such chest pain protocols, many hospitals triage low-risk patients with chest pain to special chest pain units.[66-69] These units are often adjacent to or in emergency departments but are sometimes located elsewhere in the hospital. In most such units, the rate of MI has been about 1 to 2 percent. These units have proved safe and cost-saving sites of care for low-risk patients[68,69] because fewer personnel are involved than in coronary-care units and there is an explicit emphasis on a protocol-driven approach.

Chest pain units are also sometimes used for intermediate-risk patients, such as patients with a prior history of coronary disease but no other high-risk predictors. In one community-based randomized trial, patients with unstable angina and an overall intermediate risk of complications had similar outcomes and lower costs if they were triaged to a chest pain unit versus conventional hospital management.

Early Noninvasive Testing

TREADMILL ELECTROCARDIOGRAPHY. A major goal of the initial short period of observation of low-risk patients in chest pain units is to determine whether performance of exercise testing or other noninvasive tests is safe. Treadmill exercise electrocardiography is an inexpensive test that is available at many hospitals 7 days per week and beyond traditional laboratory hours, and prospective data indicate that early exercise test results provide reliable prognostic information for low-risk patient populations. Most studies have used the Bruce or modified Bruce treadmill protocol. One study found that, among low-risk patients who had exercise testing within 48 hours of presentation for acute chest pain, the 6-month event rate among 195 patients with a negative test was 2 percent, in contrast to a rate of 15 percent among patients with a positive or equivocal test result.[70]

Studies have shown that patients who have a low clinical risk of complications can safely undergo exercise testing within 6 to 12 hours after presentation at the hospital[66-68] or even immediately.[71] In general, protocols for early or immediate exercise testing exclude patients with electrocardiographic changes consistent with ischemia not known to be old, ongoing chest pain, or evidence of congestive heart failure. Analyses of pooled data suggest that the prevalence of coronary disease in populations undergoing early exercise testing averages about 5 percent, and that the rate of adverse events is negligible.[66] Indications and contraindications for exercise ECG testing in the emergency department from an Advisory Statement from the American Heart Association are summarized in Table 45–5.[66]

TABLE 45–5 Indications and Contraindications for Exercise Electrocardiographic Testing in the Emergency Department

Requirements before exercise ECG testing that should be considered in the emergency department setting

- Two sets of cardiac enzymes at 4-hr intervals should be normal.
- ECG at the time of presentation, and preexercise 12-lead ECG shows no significant change.
- Absence of rest ECG abnormalities that would preclude accurate assessment of the exercise ECG.
- From admission to the time results are available from the second set of cardiac enzymes: patient asymptomatic, lessening chest pain symptoms, or persistent atypical symptoms.
- Absence of ischemic chest pain at the time of exercise testing.

Contraindications to exercise ECG testing in the emergency department setting

- New or evolving ECG abnormalities on the rest tracing.
- Abnormal cardiac enzymes.
- Inability to perform exercise.
- Worsening or persistent ischemic chest pain symptoms from admission to the time of exercise testing.
- Clinical risk profiling indicating imminent coronary angiography is likely.

IMAGING TESTS. Stress echocardiography or radionuclide scans are the preferred noninvasive testing modalities for patients who cannot undergo treadmill ECG testing due to physical disability or ECGs that do lend themselves to interpretation. Imaging technologies are less readily available and more expensive than exercise electrocardiography but have increased sensitivity for detection of coronary disease and the ability to quantify the extent of jeopardized myocardium. High-risk rest perfusion scans are associated with an increased risk of major cardiac complications, whereas patients with low-risk scans have low 30 day cardiac event rates (<2 percent).[72,73]

In addition to stress imaging studies to detect provokable ischemia, rest radionuclide scans also can help determine whether a patient's symptoms represent myocardial ischemia.[74] In a multicenter prospective randomized trial of 2475 adult emergency department patients with chest pain or other symptoms suggestive of acute cardiac ischemia and with normal or nondiagnostic initial ECG results, patients were randomly assigned to receive either the usual evaluation strategy or the usual strategy supplemented with results from acute resting myocardial perfusion imaging.[74] The availability of scan results did not influence management of patients with acute MI or unstable angina, but rates of hospitalization for patients without acute cardiac ischemia were reduced among patients who underwent scanning (52 to 42 percent).

Echocardiography can also be used with and without physical stress to detect wall-motion abnormalities consistent with myocardial ischemia.[75,76] The presence of induced or baseline regional wall motion abnormalities is associated with worse prognosis. Cost-effectiveness analyses indicated that radionuclide imaging, stress echocardiography, and prompt coronary angiography may all be appropriate for diagnosing coronary artery disease in some subgroups of patients,[77,78] but guidelines recommend exercise electrocardiography as the preferred first-line test.[15,66]

REFERENCES

Causes of Chest Pain

1. Pozen MW, D'Agostino RB, Selker HP, et al: A predictive instrument to improve coronary-care unit admission practices in acute ischemic heart disease: A prospective multicenter clinical trial. N Engl J Med 310:1273, 1984.
2. Goldman L, Cook EF, Brand DA, et al: A computer protocol to predict myocardial infarction in emergency department patients with chest pain. N Engl J Med 318:797, 1988.
3. Goldman L, Cook EF, Johnson PA, et al: Prediction of the need for intensive care in patients who come to emergency departments with acute chest pain. N Engl J Med 334:1498, 1996.
4. Selker HP, Beshansky JR, Griffith JL, et al: Use of the acute cardiac ischemic time-insensitive predictive instrument (ACI-TIPI) to assist with triage of patients with chest pain or other symptoms suggestive of acute cardiac ischemia: A multicenter, controlled clinical trial. Ann Intern Med 129:845, 1998.
5. Pope JH, Aufderheide TP, Ruthazer R, et al: Missed diagnoses of acute cardiac ischemia in the emergency department. N Engl J Med 342:1163, 2000.
6. Lee TH, Rouan GW, Weisberg MC, et al: Clinical characteristics and natural history of patients with acute myocardial infarction sent home from the emergency room. Am J Cardiol 60:219, 1987.
7. Rusnak RA, Stair TO, Hansen K, Fastow JS: Litigation against the emergency physician: Common features in cases of missed myocardial infarction. Ann Emerg Med 18:1029, 1989.
8. Lee TH, Goldman L: Evaluation of the patient with acute chest pain. N Engl J Med 342:1187, 2000.
9. Braunwald E, Antman EM, Beasley JW, et al: ACC/AHA guidelines for the management of patients with unstable angina and non-ST-segment elevation myocardial infarction. J Am Coll Cardiol 36:970, 2000.
10. Lee TH, Cook EF, Weisberg M, et al: Acute chest pain in the emergency room: Identification and examination of low risk patients. Arch Intern Med 145:65, 1985.
11. Spodick D: Acute pericarditis: Current concepts and practice. JAMA 289:1150, 2003.
12. Hagan PG, Nienaber CA, Isselbacher EM, et al: The International Registry of Acute Aortic Dissection (IRAD): New insights into an old disease. JAMA 283:897, 2000.
13. Goldhaber SZ: Medical progress: Pulmonary embolism. N Engl J Med 339:93, 1998.
14. Fedulla PF, Auger WR, Kerr KM, Rubin LJ: Chronic thromboembolic pulmonary hypertension. N Engl J Med 345:1465, 2001.
15. Halm EA, Tierstein AS: Management of community-acquired pneumonia. N Engl J Med 347:2039, 2002.
16. Long W, Tate RB, Neuman M, et al: Respiratory symptoms in a susceptible population due to burning of agricultural residue. Chest 113:351, 1998.
17. Pandak WM, Arezo S, Everett S, et al: Short course of omeprazole: A better first diagnostic approach to noncardiac chest pain than endoscopy, manometry, or 24-hour esophageal pH monitoring. J Clin Gastroenterol 35:307, 2002.
18. Spechler SJ, Castell DO: Classification of oesophageal motility abnormalities. Gut 49:145, 2001.
19. Fleet RP, Dupuis G, Marchand A, et al: ACC/AHA 2002 guideline update for the management of patients with unstable angina and non-ST-segment elevation myocardial infarction: Summary article: A report of the American College of Cardiology/American Heart Association Task Force on Practice Guidelines (Committee on the Management of Patients With Unstable Angina). Circulation 106:1893, 2002.
20. National Heart Attack Alert Program: Emergency department: Rapid identification and treatment of patients with acute myocardial infarction. US Department of Health and Human Services, US Public Health Service, National Institutes of Health, National Heart, Lung, and Blood Institute; September 1993; NIH Publication No. 93-3278.
21. Walker NJ, Sites FD, Shofer FS, Hollander JE: Characteristics and outcomes of young adults who present to the emergency department with chest pain. Acad Emerg Med 8:703, 2001.
22. Lange RA, Hillis LD: Cardiovascular complications of cocaine use. N Engl J Med 345:351, 2001.
23. Antman EM, Tanasijevic MJ, Thompson B, et al: Cardiac-specific troponin I levels to predict the risk of mortality in patients with acute coronary syndromes. N Engl J Med 335:1342, 1996.
24. Newby LK, Christenson RH, Ohman EM, et al: Value of serial troponin T measures for early and late risk stratification in patients with acute coronary syndromes. Circulation 98:1853, 1998.
25. Hamm CW, Goldmann BU, Heeschen C, et al: Emergency room triage of patients with acute chest pain by means of rapid testing for cardiac troponin T or troponin I. N Engl J Med 337:1648, 1997.
26. Zimmerman J, Fromm R, Meyer D, et al: Diagnostic marker cooperative study for the diagnosis of myocardial infarction. Circulation 99:1671, 1999.
27. Polanczyk CA, Lee TH, Cook EF, et al: Cardiac troponin I as a predictor of major cardiac events in emergency department patients with acute chest pain. J Am Coll Cardiol 32:8, 1998.
28. Antman EM, Grudzien C, Sacks DB: Evaluation of a rapid bedside assay for detection of serum cardiac troponin T. JAMA 273:1279, 1995.
29. Polanczyk CA, Johnson PA, Cook EF, Lee TH: A proposed strategy for utilization of creatine kinase-MB and troponin I in the evaluation of acute chest pain. Am J Cardiol 83:1175, 1999.
30. Christenson RH, Duh SH: Evidence based approach to practice guides and decision thresholds for cardiac markers. Scand J Clin Lab Invest Suppl 230:90, 1999.
31. Lee TH, Goldman L: Serum enzyme assays in the diagnosis of myocardial infarction. Recommendations based on a quantitative analysis. Ann Intern Med 105:221, 1986.
32. Pearson JR, Carrea F: Evaluation of the clinical usefulness of a chemiluminometric method for measuring creatine kinase MB. Clin Chem 36:1809, 1990.
33. Adams JE, Abendschein DR, Jaffe AS: Biochemical markers of myocardial injury: Is MB creatine kinase the choice for the 1990s? Circulation 88:750, 1993.
34. Puleo PR, Meyer D, Warthen C, et al: Use of a rapid assay of subforms of creatine kinase-MB to diagnose or rule out acute myocardial infarction. N Engl J Med 331:561, 1994.
35. Mockel M, Schindler R, Knorr L, et al: Prognostic value of cardiac troponin T and I elevations in renal disease patients without acute coronary syndromes: A 9-month outcome analysis. Nephrol Dial Transplant 14:1489, 1999.
36. Krahn J, Parry DM, Leroux M, Dalton J: High percentage of false positive cardiac troponin I results in patients with rheumatoid factor. Clin Biochem 32:477, 1999.

37. Morrow DA, Cannon CP, Rifai N, et al: Ability of minor elevations of troponins I and T to predict benefit from an early invasive strategy in patients with unstable angina and non-ST elevation myocardial infarction. JAMA 286:2405, 2001.
38. Collinson PO, Gerhardt W, Katus HA, et al: Multicentre evaluation of an immunological rapid test for the detection of troponin T in whole blood samples. Eur J Clin Chem Clin Biochem 34:591, 1996.
39. Heeschen C, Goldman BU, Moeller RH, Hamm CW: Analytical performance and clinical application of a new rapid bedside assay for the detection of serum cardiac troponin I. Clin Chem 44:1925, 1998.
40. Hoekstra JW, Hedges JR, Gibler WB, et al: Emergency department CK-MB: A predictor of ischemic complications. Acad Emerg Med 1:17, 1994.
41. Galvani M, Ottani F, Ferrini D, et al: Prognostic influence of elevated values of cardiac troponin I in patients with unstable angina. Circulation 95:2053, 1997.
42. Hillis GS, Taggart P, Dalsey WC, Mangione A: Utility of cardiac troponin I, creatine kinase-MB (mass), myosin light chain 1, and myoglobin in the early in-hospital triage of "high risk" patients with chest pain. Heart 82:614, 1999.
43. Ohman EM, Armstrong PW, Christenson RH, et al: Cardiac troponin T levels for risk stratification in acute myocardial ischemia. GUSTO IIA Investigators. N Engl J Med 335:1333, 1996.
44. Newby LK, Christenson RH, Ohman EM, et al: Value of serial troponin T measures for early and late risk stratification in patients with acute coronary syndromes. Circulation 1998:1853, 1998.
45. Luscher MS, Thygesen K, Ravkilde J, Heickendorff L: Applicability of cardiac troponin T and I for early risk stratification in unstable coronary artery disease. TRIM Study Group. Thrombin Inhibition in Myocardial ischemia. Circulation 96:2578, 1997.
46. Lee TH, Weisberg MC, Cook EF, et al: Evaluation of creatine kinase and creatine kinase-MB for diagnosing myocardial infarction: Clinical impact in the emergency room. Arch Intern Med 147:115, 1987.
47. Brogan GX Jr, Hollander JE, McCuskey CF, et al: Evaluation of a new assay for cardiac troponin I vs creatine kinase-MB for the diagnosis of acute myocardial infarction. Biochemical Markers for Acute Myocardial Ischemia (BAMI) Study Group. Acad Emerg Med 4:6, 1997.

Initial Risk Stratification

48. Brieger DB, Mak KH, White HD, et al: Benefit of early sustained reperfusion in patients with prior myocardial infarction (the GUSTO-I trial). Global Utilization of Streptokinase and TPA for Occluded Arteries. Am J Cardiol 81:282, 1998.
49. Hochman JS, Tamis JE, Thompson TD, et al, for the Global Use of Strategies to Open Occluded Coronary Arteries in Acute Coronary Syndromes IIb Investigators: Sex, clinical presentation, and outcome in patients with acute coronary syndromes. N Engl J Med 341:226, 1999.
50. Hochman JS, McCabe CH, Stone PH, et al, for the TIMI Investigators: Thrombolysis In Myocardial Infarction: Outcome and profile of women and men presenting with acute coronary syndromes: a report from TIMI IIIB. J Am Coll Cardiol 30:141, 1997.
51. White HD, Barbash GI, Califf RM, et al: Age and outcome with contemporary thrombolytic therapy: Results from the GUSTO-I trial. Global Utilization of Streptokinase and TPA for Occluded coronary arteries trial. Circulation 94:1826, 1996.
52. Jayes RLJ, Beshansky JR, D'Agostino RB, Selker HP: Do patients' coronary risk factor reports predict acute cardiac ischemia in the emergency department? A multicenter study. J Clin Epidemiol 45:621, 1992.
53. Rouan GW, Lee TH, Cook EF, et al: Clinical characteristics and outcome of acute myocardial infarction in patients with initially normal or nonspecific electrocardiograms (a report from the Multicenter Chest Pain Study). Am J Cardiol 64:1087, 1989.
54. Slater DK, Hlatky MA, Mark DB, et al: Outcome in suspected acute myocardial infarction with normal or minimally abnormal admission electrocardiographic findings. Am J Cardiol 60:766, 1987.
55. Lee TH, Cook EF, Weisberg MC, et al: Impact of the availability of a prior electrocardiogram on the triage of the patient with acute chest pain. J Gen Intern Med 5:381, 1990.
56. Kudenchuk PJ, Maynard C, Cobb LA, et al: Utility of the prehospital electrocardiogram in diagnosing acute coronary syndromes: The Myocardial Infarction Triage and Intervention (MITI) Project. J Am Coll Cardiol 32:17, 1998.
57. Hedges JR, Young GP, Henkel GF, et al: Serial ECGs are less accurate than serial CK-MB results for emergency department diagnosis of myocardial infarction. Ann Emerg Med 21:1445, 1992.
58. Patel DJ, Knight CJ, Holdright DR, et al: Long-term prognosis in unstable angina: The importance of early risk stratification using continuous ST segment monitoring. Eur Heart J 19:240, 1998.
59. Selker HP, Beshansky JR, Griffith JL, for the TPI Trial Investigators: Use of the electrocardiograph-based thrombolytic predictive instrument to assist thrombolytic and reperfusion therapy for acute myocardial infarction: A multicenter, randomized, controlled, clinical effectiveness trial. Ann Intern Med 137:87, 2002.
60. Corey GA, Merenstein JH: Applying the acute ischemic heart disease predictive instrument. J Fam Pract 25:127, 1987.
61. Pearson SD, Goldman L, Garcia TB, et al: Physician response to a prediction rule for the triage of emergency department patients with chest pain. J Gen Intern Med 9:241, 1994.
62. Lee TH, Pearson SD, Johnson PA, et al: Failure of information as an intervention to modify clinical management: A time-series trial in patients with acute chest pain. Ann Intern Med 122:434, 1995.

Immediate Management

63. Tosteson ANA, Goldman L, Udvarhelyi IS, Lee TH: Cost-effectiveness of a coronary care unit versus an intermediate care unit for emergency department patients with chest pain. Circulation 94:143, 1996.
64. Lee TH, Goldman L: The coronary care unit turns 25: Historical trends and future directions. Ann Intern Med 108:887, 1988.
65. Nichol G, Walls R, Goldman L, et al: A critical pathway for management of patients with acute chest pain who are at low risk for myocardial ischemia: Recommendations and potential impact. Ann Intern Med 127:996, 1997.
66. Stein RA, Chaitman BR, Balady GJ, et al: Safety and utility of exercise testing in emergency room chest pain centers: An advisory from the Committee on Exercise, Rehabilitation, and Prevention, Council on Clinical Cardiology, American Heart Association. Circulation 102:1463, 2000.
67. Farkouh ME, Smars PA, Reeder GS, et al: A clinical trial of a chest-pain observation unit for patients with unstable angina. N Engl J Med 339:1882, 1998.
68. Gibler WB, Runyon JP, Levy RC, et al: A rapid diagnostic and treatment center for patients with chest pain in the emergency department. Ann Emerg Med 25:1, 1995.
69. Gomez MA, Anderson JL, Karagounis LA, et al: An emergency department-based protocol for rapidly ruling out myocardial ischemia reduces hospital time and expense: Results of a randomized study (ROMIO). J Am Coll Cardiol 28:25, 1996.
70. Polanczyk CA, Johnson PA, Hartley LH, et al: Clinical correlates and prognostic significance of early negative exercise tolerance test in patients with acute chest pain seen in the hospital emergency department. Am J Cardiol 81:288, 1998.
71. Lewis WR, Amsterdam EA, Turnipseed S, Kirk JD: Immediate exercise testing of low risk patients with known coronary artery disease presenting to the emergency department with chest pain. J Am Coll Cardiol 33:1843, 1999.
72. Hilton TC, Fulmer H, Abuan T, et al: Ninety-day follow-up of patients in the emergency department with chest pain who undergo initial single-photon emission computed tomographic perfusion scintigraphy with technetium 99m-labeled sestamibi. J Nucl Cardiol 3:308, 1996.
73. Kontos MC, Jesse RL, Schmidt KL, et al: Value of acute rest sestamibi perfusion imaging for evaluation of patients admitted to the emergency department with chest pain. J Am Coll Cardiol 30:976, 1997.
74. Udelson JE, Beshansky JR, Ballin DS, et al: Myocardial perfusion imaging for evaluation and triage of patients with suspected acute cardiac ischemia: A randomized controlled trial. JAMA 288:2693, 2002.
75. Colon PJ III, Mobarek SK, Milani RV, et al: Prognostic value of stress echocardiography in the evaluation of atypical chest pain patients without known coronary artery disease. Am J Cardiol 81:545, 1998.
76. Fleischmann KE, Lee TH, Come PC, et al: Echocardiographic predictors of complications in patients with chest pain. Am J Cardiol 79:292, 1997.
77. Kuntz KM, Fleischmann KE, Hunink MG, Douglas PS: Cost-effectiveness of diagnostic strategies for patients with chest pain. Ann Intern Med 130:709, 1999.
78. Garber AM, Solomon NA: Cost-effectiveness of alternative test strategies for the diagnosis of coronary artery disease. Ann Intern Med 130:719, 1999.

CHAPTER 46

ST-Elevation Myocardial Infarction: Pathology, Pathophysiology, and Clinical Features

Elliott M. Antman • Eugene Braunwald

Definition

The *pathological* diagnosis of myocardial infarction (MI) requires evidence of myocyte cell death as a consequence of prolonged ischemia. Characteristic findings include coagulation necrosis and contraction band necrosis, often with patchy areas of myocytolysis at the periphery of the infarct. The *clinical* diagnosis of MI requires an integrated assessment of the history with some combination of indirect evidence of myocardial necrosis using biochemical, electrocardiographic, and imaging modalities (Table 46–1). The sensitivity and specificity of the various clinical tools for diagnosing MI vary considerably, and at varying times after the onset of the infarction.

Epidemiological reports from the World Heath Organization and American Heart Association beginning in the late 1950s required the presence of at least two of the following: characteristic symptoms, electrocardiographic changes, and a typical rise and fall in biochemical markers for the diagnosis of myocardial infarction.[1] This epidemiological approach was then generally adopted in routine clinical practice, although the rigor with which clinicians apply the electrocardiographic and biochemical criteria for infarction varies considerably.

Since the original epidemiological efforts, considerable advances have occurred in the electrocardiographic and biochemical aspects of the definition of infarction. The electrocardiographic criteria for MI were codified and scoring systems were developed for estimation of infarct size.[2] Biochemical assays became available for markers more specific for cardiac damage. Thus, assays for lactic dehydrogenase and creatine kinase activity (CK) have been superseded by mass assays for the MB fraction of CK and immunoassays for cardiac-specific troponins. The cardiac-specific troponin assays have nearly absolute myocardial tissue specificity and have become the preferred biomarker for diagnosing MI. Advances in the techniques for diagnosing MI, especially the introduction of assays for cardiac-specific troponins, were the impetus for a consensus document published jointly by the European Society of Cardiology and the American College of Cardiology.[2] The main features of the revised definition of MI are summarized in Table 46–2. The revised definition of MI has important implications not only for clinical care of patients but also for tracking epidemiological trends, public policy, and clinical trials.[3,4] The paradigm shift to cardiac-specific troponins as the markers of choice for the diagnosis of MI requires new cutoff values for cardiac injury. The term *normal range* has been replaced by *upper reference limit*, defined as the 99th percentile of a normal reference control group.[5]

As discussed later, the contemporary approach to patients presenting with ischemic discomfort is to consider that they are experiencing an acute coronary syndrome. The 12-lead electrocardiogram (ECG) is pivotal for segregating patients into those presenting with ST-segment elevation, the subject of Chapters 46 through 48, and those presenting without ST-segment elevation, the subject of Chapter 49.[6] Although the revised definition of MI has greater impact on the non-ST-segment elevation end of the acute coronary syndrome spectrum (i.e., distinction between unstable angina and non-ST-segment elevation MI), the issues are also pertinent to discussion of ST-segment elevation myocardial infarction (STEMI).

Changing Patterns in Clinical Care

Despite impressive advances in diagnosis and management over the last four decades, STEMI continues to be a major public health problem in the industrialized world and is becoming an increasingly important problem in developing countries (see Chap. 1).[7,8] In the United States, nearly 1.0 million patients annually suffer from an acute MI.[9] More than 1 million patients with suspected acute MI are admitted yearly to coronary care units in the United States.[9]

TABLE 46–1 Aspects of Diagnosis of Myocardial Infarction by Different Techniques

Pathology	Myocardial cell death
Biochemistry	Markers of myocardial cell death recovered from blood samples
Electrocardiography	Evidence of myocardial ischemia (ST and T wave abnormalities) Evidence of loss of electrically functioning cardiac tissue (Q waves)
Imaging	Reduction or loss of tissue perfusion Cardiac wall motion abnormalities

Adapted from Alpert JS, Thygesen K, Antman E, et al: Myocardial infarction redefined—A consensus document of The Joint European Society of Cardiology/American College of Cardiology Committee for the redefinition of myocardial infarction. J Am Coll Cardiol 36:959, 2000.

TABLE 46–2 Revised Definition of Myocardial Infarction (MI)

Criteria for acute, evolving, or recent MI
Either one of the following criteria satisfies the diagnosis for an acute, evolving, or recent MI:
1. Typical rise and gradual fall (troponin) or more rapid rise and fall (CK-MB) of biochemical markers of myocardial necrosis with at least one of the following: a. Ischemic symptoms b. Development of pathologic Q waves on the ECG reading c. ECG changes indicative of ischemia (ST-segment elevation or depression) d. Coronary artery intervention (e.g., coronary angioplasty)
2. Pathological findings of an acute MI
Criteria for established MI
Either of the following criteria satisfies the diagnosis for established MI:
1. Development of new pathological Q waves on serial ECG readings. The patient may or may not remember previous symptoms. Biochemical markers of myocardial necrosis may have normalized, depending on the length of time that has passed since the infarct developed.
2. Pathological findings of a healed or healing MI

CK = creatine kinase; ECG = electrocardiographic.

From Alpert JS, Thygesen K, Antman E, et al: Myocardial infarction redefined—A consensus document of The Joint European Society of Cardiology/American College of Cardiology Committee for the redefinition of myocardial infarction. J Am Coll Cardiol 36:959, 2000.

The development of STEMI is a fatal event in approximately one-third of patients, with about half of the deaths occurring within 1 hour of the event from ventricular tachyarrhythmias. Because STEMI can strike an individual during the most productive years, it can have profound deleterious psychosocial and economic ramifications.

Of particular concern from a global perspective are projections from the World Heart Federation that the burden of disease in developing countries will become similar to those now afflicting developed countries.[9] Given the wide disparity of available resources to treat STEMI in developing countries, major efforts are needed on an international level to strengthen primary prevention programs at the community level.[10]

IMPROVEMENTS IN OUTCOME

A steady decline in the mortality rate from STEMI has been observed across several population groups since 1960.[11] This drop in mortality appears to be caused by a fall in the incidence of STEMI (replaced in part by an increase in the rate of unstable angina/non-ST-segment elevation MI[12]) and a fall in the case fatality rate once STEMI has occurred.[13]

Several phases in the management of patients have contributed to the decline in mortality from STEMI.[14] The "clinical observation phase" of coronary care consumed the first half of the 20th century and focused on a detailed recording of physical and laboratory findings, whereas treatment consisted of strict bed rest and sedation. Subsequently, the "coronary care unit phase" began in the mid-1960s and was notable for detailed analysis and vigorous management of cardiac arrhythmias. The "high-technology phase" was ushered in by the introduction of the pulmonary artery balloon flotation catheter, setting the stage for bedside hemodynamic monitoring and more precise management of heart failure and cardiogenic shock associated with STEMI. A battery of tests, sometimes providing overlapping information, was developed during the high-technology phase. The modern "reperfusion era" of coronary care was introduced by intracoronary and then intravenous fibrinolysis, increased use of aspirin, and development of primary percutaneous coronary intervention (PCI).

Driven in large part by the need for cost-saving measures, contemporary care of patients with STEMI has entered the "evidence-based coronary care phase" and is becoming increasingly influenced by managed care systems and guidelines for clinical practice (see Chap. 47, Guidelines).[15] Coronary care practice is better equipped than other fields of cardiovascular medicine to face this transition from pathophysiologically based decision-making to evidence-based decision-making, given the rich data base of patients with suspected STEMI studied in clinical trials and registries and efforts at summarizing a vast amount of data using meta-analysis.[16] New therapies for STEMI are being evaluated not only for evidence of safety and efficacy but also for their cost-effectiveness in caring for patients and their impact on quality of life. However, despite an abundance of cost-effectiveness information using data from clinical trials, clinicians weighing the risk-benefit ratio of any given intervention at the bedside of an individual patient may have difficulty applying the findings for several reasons: uncertainty about whether the benefits observed in a strictly defined trial population are applicable to a wider selection of patients, limited data on specific subgroups, variations in the absolute level of baseline risk, and variations in patient preferences.[17]

LIMITATIONS OF CURRENT THERAPY. Despite the gratifying success of medical therapy for STEMI, several observations indicate that considerable room for improvement exists. The short-term mortality rate of patients with STEMI who receive aggressive pharmacological reperfusion therapy as part of a randomized trial is in the range of 6.5 to 7.0 percent,[18] whereas observational data bases suggest that the mortality rate in STEMI patients in the community is 15 to 20 percent.[19] In part, this difference relates to the selection of patients without serious comorbidities for clinical trials.

Although the survival of elderly patients (>65 years of age) after STEMI has improved significantly, advanced age consistently emerges as one of the principal determinants of mortality in patients with STEMI.[20] Despite reluctance to use potentially life-saving drug therapies in elderly patients, cardiac catheterization and other invasive procedures are being performed more commonly at some point during hospitalization in elderly patients with STEMI. Nevertheless, evidence suggests that the greatest reductions in mortality for elderly patients are derived from those strategies employed during the first 24 hours, a time frame in which prompt and appropriate use of life-saving pharmacotherapy is of paramount importance, emphasizing the need to extend advances in drug therapy for STEMI to the elderly.[16]

Despite trends toward greater use of mortality-reducing therapies such as fibrinolytics, aspirin, and beta-adrenoceptor blockers in patients with STEMI, these drugs still appear to be underutilized.[17] Considerable variation exists in practice patterns for management of patients with STEMI.[21] Mortality rates for STEMI are lower in hospitals with a high clinical volume, a high rate of invasive procedures, and a top ranking in quality reports (see Chap. 4).[22,23] Variation has also been observed in the treatment patterns of certain population subgroups with STEMI, notably women and blacks. Although the unadjusted rates of fibrinolytic use and referral for cardiac catheterization and angioplasty are lower and unadjusted mortality rates are higher in women with STEMI, gender differences are less apparent (but may not disappear entirely) once adjustment is made for baseline variables such as comorbidities and age (see Chap. 73).[19] Of interest, after STEMI, younger women but not older women have higher rates of in-hospital mortality than men of the same age.[24]

Pathology

Almost all MIs result from coronary atherosclerosis, generally with superimposed coronary thrombosis. Nonatherogenic forms of coronary artery disease are discussed later in this chapter and causes of STEMI without coronary atherosclerosis are shown in Table 46–3.

Prior to the fibrinolytic era, clinicians typically divided patients with MI into those suffering a Q-wave and those suffering a non-Q-wave infarct, based on the evolution of the pattern on the ECG over several days. The term *Q-wave infarction* was frequently considered to be virtually synonymous with *transmural infarction*, whereas *non-Q-wave infarctions* were often referred to as *subendocardial infarctions*. Phibbs summarized the arguments that previous distinctions between Q-wave infarction and non-Q-wave infarctions were based on erroneous interpretation of pathological data and should not serve as the basis for designing therapy.[25] A more suitable framework based on pathophysiology is referred to as the *acute coronary syndromes* (Fig. 46–1).

Plaque

Slowly accruing high-grade stenoses of epicardial coronary arteries can progress to complete occlusion but do not usually precipitate STEMI, probably because of the development of a

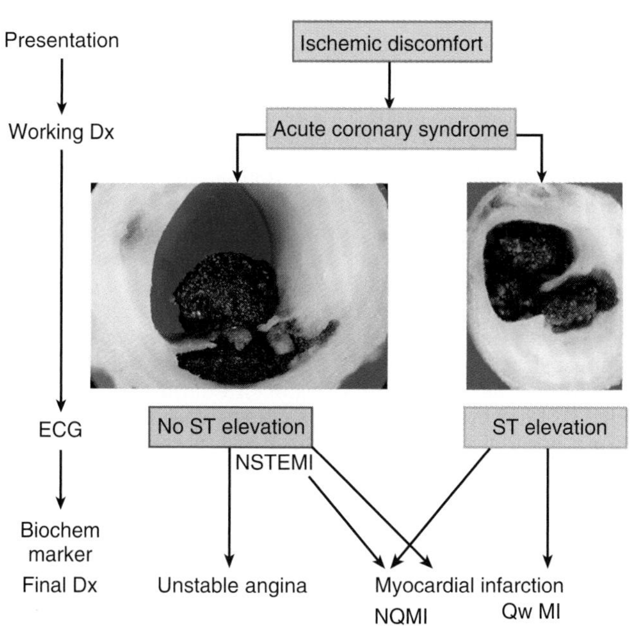

FIGURE 46–1 Nomenclature of acute coronary syndromes. Patients with ischemic discomfort present with or without ST-segment elevation on the electrocardiogram (ECG). The majority of patients with ST-segment elevation ultimately develop a Q wave acute myocardial infarction (QwMI), whereas a minority develop a non-Q-wave myocardial infarction (NQMI). Patients who present without ST-segment elevation are either experiencing unstable angina or a non-ST-segment elevation myocardial infarction (NSTEMI). The distinction between these two diagnoses is ultimately made based on the presence or absence of a cardiac biomarker detected in the blood. Most patients with NSTEMI do not evolve a Q wave on the 12-lead ECG and are subsequently referred to as having sustained an NQMI; only a minority of NSTEMI patients develop a Q wave MI and are later diagnosed as Q wave MI. The spectrum of clinical conditions ranging from unstable angina to non-Q wave MI constitutes the acute coronary syndromes. (From Braunwald E, Antman EM, Beasley JW, et al: ACC/AHA guidelines for the management of patients with unstable angina: A report of the American College of Cardiology/American Heart Association Task Force on Practice Guidelines [Committee on the Management of Patients With Unstable Angina]. J Am Coll Cardiol 36:970, 2000.)

TABLE 46–3 Causes of Myocardial Infarction without Coronary Atherosclerosis
Coronary Artery Disease Other than Atherosclerosis
Arteritis
Luetic
Granulomatous (Takayasu disease)
Polyarteritis nodosa
Mucocutaneous lymph node (Kawasaki) syndrome
Disseminated lupus erythematosus
Rheumatoid spondylitis
Ankylosing spondylitis
Trauma to coronary arteries
Laceration
Thrombosis
Iatrogenic
Radiation (radiation therapy for neoplasia)
Coronary mural thickening with metabolic disease or intimal proliferative disease
Mucopolysaccharidoses (Hurler disease)
Homocysteinuria
Fabry disease
Amyloidosis
Juvenile intimal sclerosis (idiopathic arterial calcification of infancy
Intimal hyperplasia associated with contraceptive steroids or with the postpartum period
Pseudoxanthoma elasticum
Coronary fibrosis caused by radiation therapy
Luminal narrowing by other mechanisms
Spasm of coronary arteries (Prinzmetal angina with normal coronary arteries)
Spasm after nitroglycerin withdrawal
Dissection of the aorta
Dissection of the coronary artery
Emboli to Coronary Arteries
Infective endocarditis
Nonbacterial thrombotic endocarditis
Prolapse of mitral valve
Mural thrombus from left atrium, left ventricle, or pulmonary veins
Prosthetic valve emboli
Cardiac myxoma
Associated with cardiopulmonary bypass surgery and coronary arteriography
Paradoxical emboli
Parpillary fibroelastoma of the aortic valve ("fixed embolus")
Thrombi from intracardiac catheters or guidewires
Congenital Coronary Artery Anomalies
Anomalous origin of left coronary from pulmonary artery
Left coronary artery from anterior sinus of Valsalva
Coronary arteriovenous and arteriocameral fistulas
Coronary artery aneurysms
Myocardial Oxygen Demand-Supply Disproportion
Aortic stenosis, all forms
Incomplete differentiation of the aortic valve
Aortic insufficiency
Carbon monoxide poisoning
Thyrotoxicosis
Prolonged hypotension
Hematological (in situ Thrombosis)
Polycythemia vera
Thrombocytosis
Disseminated intravascular coagulation
Hypercoagulability, thrombosis, thrombocytopenic purpura
Miscellaneous
Cocaine abuse
Myocardial contusion
Myocardial infarction with normal coronary arteries
Complication of cardiac catheterization

Modified from Cheitlin MD, McAllister HA, de Castro CM: Myocardial infarction without atherosclerosis. JAMA 231:951, 1975. Copyright 1975, American Medical Association.

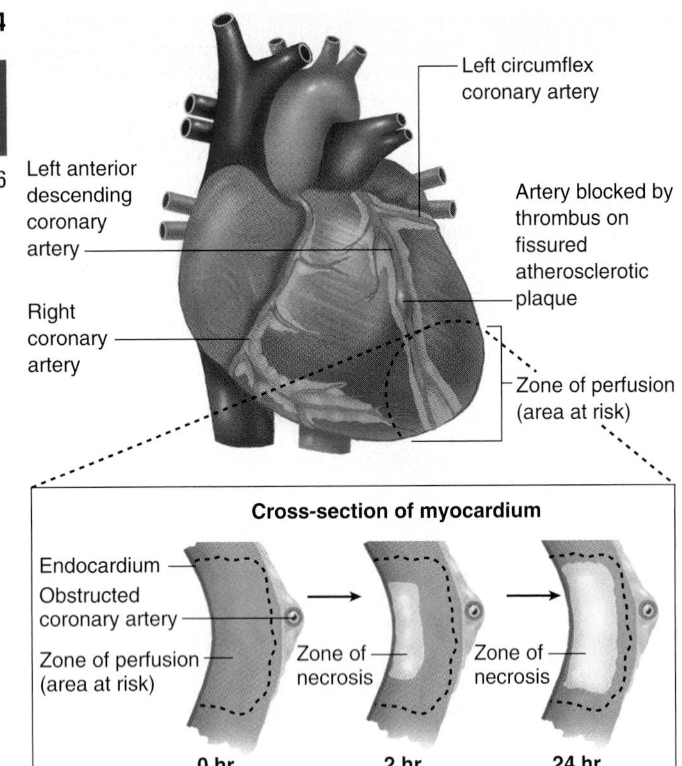

FIGURE 46–2 Schematic representation of the progression of myocardial necrosis after coronary artery occlusion. Necrosis begins in a small zone of the myocardium beneath the endocardial surface in the center of the ischemic zone. This entire region of myocardium (dashed outline) depends on the occluded vessel for perfusion and is the area at risk. Note that a very narrow zone of myocardium immediately beneath the endocardium is spared from necrosis because it can be oxygenated by diffusion from the ventricle. (From Schoen FJ: The heart. *In* Cotran RS, Kumar V, Collins T [eds]: Pathologic Basis of Disease. 6th ed. Philadelphia, WB Saunders, 1999, p 557.)

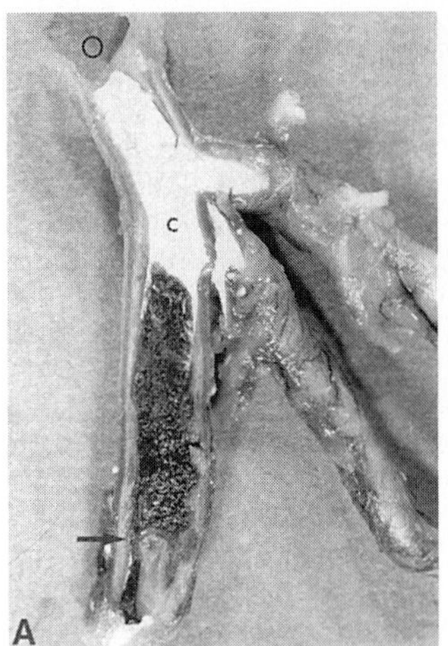

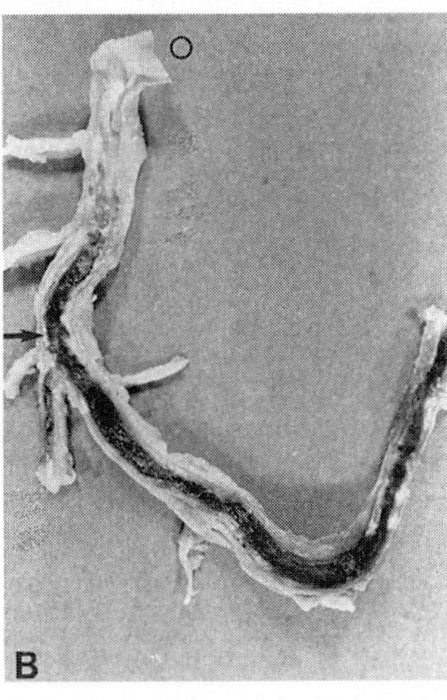

FIGURE 46–3 Thrombus propagation. **A,** Left anterior descending coronary artery cut open longitudinally, showing a dark (red) stagnation thrombosis propagating upstream from the initiating rupture/platelet-rich thrombus at the arrow. In this case, the thrombus has propagated proximally up to the nearest major side branch (the first diagonal branch). **B,** The right coronary artery cut open longitudinally, showing a huge stagnation thrombosis propagating downstream from the initiating rupture/platelet-rich thrombus at the arrow. Unlike upstream thrombus propagation, downstream propagation may, as in this case, occlude major side branches. c = contrast medium injected postmortem; O = coronary ostium. (From Falk E: Coronary thrombosis: Pathogenesis and clinical manifestations. Am J Cardiol 68:28B, 1991.)

rich collateral network over time. However, during the natural evolution of atherosclerotic plaques, especially those that are lipid-laden, an abrupt and catastrophic transition can occur, characterized by plaque disruption. Some patients have a systemic predisposition to plaque disruption that is independent of traditional risk factors.[16,26,27] After plaque disruption, there is exposure of substances that promote platelet activation and aggregation, thrombin generation, and ultimately thrombus formation.[28,29] The resultant thrombus that is formed interrupts blood flow and leads to an imbalance between oxygen supply and demand and, if this imbalance is severe and persistent, to myocardial necrosis (Fig. 46–2).

COMPOSITION OF PLAQUES. At autopsy, the atherosclerotic plaque of patients who died of STEMI is composed primarily of fibrous tissue of varying density and cellularity with superimposed thrombus. Calcium, lipid-laden foam cells, and extracellular lipid each constitutes 5 to 10 percent of the remaining area. The atherosclerotic plaques that are associated with thrombosis and a total occlusion, located in infarct-related vessels, are generally more complex and irregular than those in vessels not associated with STEMI. Histological studies of these lesions often reveal plaque rupture or erosion. Coronary arterial thrombi responsible for STEMI are approximately 1 cm in length in most cases, adhere to the luminal surface of an artery, and are composed of platelets, fibrin, erythrocytes, and leukocytes (Fig. 46–3). The composition of the thrombus may vary at different levels: a white thrombus is composed of platelets, fibrin, or both, and a red thrombus is composed of erythrocytes, fibrin, platelets, and leukocytes.[27] Early thrombi are usually small and nonocclusive and are composed predominantly of platelets.

PLAQUE FISSURING AND DISRUPTION. In atherosclerotic plaques prone to disruption, there is an increased rate of formation of metalloproteinase enzymes such as collagenase, gelatinase, and stromelysin that degrade components of the protective interstitial matrix.[26] These proteinases can be elaborated by activated macrophages and mast cells that have been shown to accumulate in high concentration at the site of atheromatous erosions and plaque disruption in patients who died of STEMI.[26] Examination of specimens from atherectomy reveals a much higher content of macrophages and tissue factor in patients with unstable angina or STEMI compared with patients with chronic stable angina.[30] In addition to these structural aspects of vulnerable or high-risk plaques, stresses induced by intraluminal pressure, coronary vasomotor tone, tachycardia (cyclic stretching and compression), and disruption of nutrient vessels combine to produce plaque disruption at the margin of the fibrous cap near an adjacent plaque-free segment of the coronary artery wall (shoulder region of plaque).[28] A number of key physiological parameters such as systolic blood pressure, heart rate, blood viscosity, endogenous tissue plasminogen activator (t-PA) activity, plasminogen activator inhibitor-1 (PAI-1) levels, plasma cortisol levels, and plasma epinephrine levels that exhibit circadian and seasonal variations are increased at times of stress. They act in concert to produce a heightened propensity to plaque disruption and coronary thrombosis, yielding the clustering of STEMI in the early morning hours, and especially in the winter and after natural disasters.[31]

Acute Coronary Syndromes

When plaque disruption occurs, a sufficient quantity of thrombogenic substances is exposed, and the coronary artery lumen may become obstructed by a combination of platelet aggregates, fibrin, and red blood cells (see Fig. 46–3). An adequate collateral network that prevents necrosis from occurring can result in clinically silent episodes of coronary occlusion. Disruption of plaques is now considered to be the common pathophysiological substrate of the acute coronary syndromes (ACS) (see Fig. 46–1).[16] Characteristically, such completely occlusive thrombi lead to a large zone of necrosis involving the full or nearly full thickness of the ventricular wall in the myocardial bed subtended by the affected coronary artery and typically produce ST elevation on the ECG (see Fig. 46–2). The infarction process alters the sequence of depolarization ultimately reflected as changes in the surface of QRS.[25] The most characteristic change in the QRS that develops in about 75 percent of patients initially presenting with ST elevation is the evolution of Q waves in the leads overlying the infarct zone—leading to the term *Q-wave infarction* (see Fig. 46–1). In about 25 percent of patients presenting with ST elevation, no Q waves develop,[32] but other abnormalities of the QRS complex are frequently seen such as diminution in R wave height and notching or splintering of the QRS. Patients presenting without ST elevation are initially diagnosed as suffering either from a non-ST-elevation MI (NSTEMI) or unstable angina (see Fig. 46–1 and Chap. 49).

The ACS spectrum concept, organized around a common pathophysiological substrate, is a useful framework for developing therapeutic strategies.[15] Patients presenting with persistent ST-segment elevation are candidates for reperfusion therapy (either pharmacological or catheter-based) to restore flow in the occluded epicardial infarct-related artery. ACS patients presenting without ST segment elevation are not candidates for pharmacological reperfusion but should receive antiischemic therapy, often followed by PCI. Antithrombin therapy and antiplatelet therapy should be administered to all patients with ACS regardless of the presence or absence of ST-segment elevation. Thus, the 12-lead ECG remains at the center of the decision pathway for management of patients with ACS to distinguish between presentations with ST elevation and without ST elevation (see Fig. 46–1).[12] The ECG lacks sufficient sensitivity and specificity to permit reliable distinction of transmural from subendocardial infarcts. Categorization of patients into those with Q-wave and those with non-Q-wave infarction pattern is best conceived of as only a crude guide to the extent of ventricular damage—prognostic considerations must take into account other important factors, such as whether the ECG abnormality is due to a first infarct versus subsequent infarct, the location of infarction (anterior versus inferior), infarct size, and demographic factors such as patient age.[25]

The Heart Muscle

Gross Pathology

On gross inspection, MI can be divided into two major types: transmural infarcts, in which myocardial necrosis involves the full thickness (or nearly full thickness) of the ventricular wall, and subendocardial (nontransmural) infarcts, in which the necrosis involves the subendocardium, the intramural myocardium, or both without extending all the way through the ventricular wall to the epicardium (Fig. 46–4).

An occlusive coronary thrombosis appears to be far more common when the infarction is transmural and localized to the distribution of a single coronary artery (see Fig. 46–3). Nontransmural infarctions, however, frequently occur in the presence of severely narrowed but still patent coronary arteries. Patchy nontransmural infarction may arise from thrombolysis or PCI of an originally occlusive thrombus with restoration of blood flow *before* the wavefront of necrosis has extended from the subendocardium across the full thickness of the ventricular wall (see Fig. 46–2). Paradoxically, before their infarction, patients with nontransmural infarcts have,

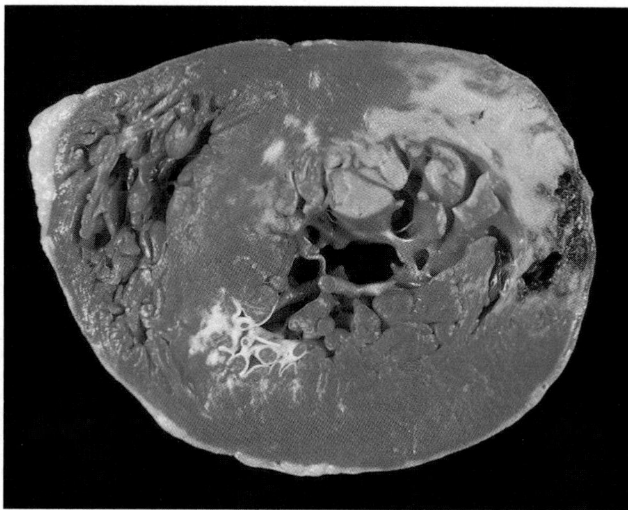

FIGURE 46–4 Acute myocardial infarction, predominantly of the posterolateral left ventricle, demonstrated histochemically by a lack of staining by the triphenyltetrazolium chloride (TTC) stain in areas of necrosis. The staining defect is due to the enzyme leakage that follows cell death. Note the myocardial hemorrhage at one edge of the infarct that was associated with cardiac rupture, and the anterior scar (lower left), indicative of old infarct. (Specimen oriented with posterior wall at top.) (From Schoen FJ: The heart. *In* Cotran RS, Kumar V, Collins T [eds]: Pathologic Basis of Disease. 6th ed. Philadelphia, WB Saunders, 1999, p 559.)

on average, a more severe stenosis in the infarct-related coronary artery than do patients suffering from transmural infarcts. This finding suggests that a more severe obstruction occurring before coronary occlusion protects against the development of transmural infarction, perhaps by fostering the development of collateral circulation. It also accords with the concept that less severely stenotic but lipid-laden plaques with a fragile cap are responsible for the abrupt presentation of ST-segment elevation that may evolve to transmural infarctions.

THE FIRST HOURS. Gross alterations of the myocardium are difficult to identify until at least 6 to 12 hours have elapsed following the onset of necrosis (Fig. 46–5). However, a variety of histochemical stains can be used to identify zones of necrosis that can be discerned after only 2 to 3 hours. Tissue slices of suspected infarct sites are immersed in a solution of triphenyltetrazolium chloride (TTC), which stains viable myocardium brick red (because of preserved dehydrogenase enzymes that form a red formazan precipitate) and leaves the infarcted region pale as a result of failure of uptake of the vital dye (see Fig. 46-4). The nitroblue tetrazolium (NBT) staining technique can similarly distinguish viable zones of myocardium, which stain dark blue, from necrotic areas of myocardium that therefore remain uncolored and identifiable. Other approaches include autofluorescence staining, immunohistochemical analysis, and, more recently, special DNA staining techniques to identify apoptotic bodies in myocardial sections.[33]

THE FIRST DAYS. Initially, the myocardium in the affected region may appear pale and slightly swollen. Eighteen to 36 hours after the onset of the infarct, the myocardium is tan or reddish purple (due to trapped erythrocytes), with a serofibrinous exudate evident on the epicardium in transmural infarcts. These changes persist for approximately 48 hours; the infarct then turns gray, and fine yellow lines, secondary to neutrophilic infiltration, appear at its periphery. This zone gradually widens and during the next few days extends throughout the infarct.

THE FIRST WEEKS. Eight to 10 days after infarction, the thickness of the cardiac wall in the area of the infarct is reduced as necrotic muscle is removed by mononuclear cells.

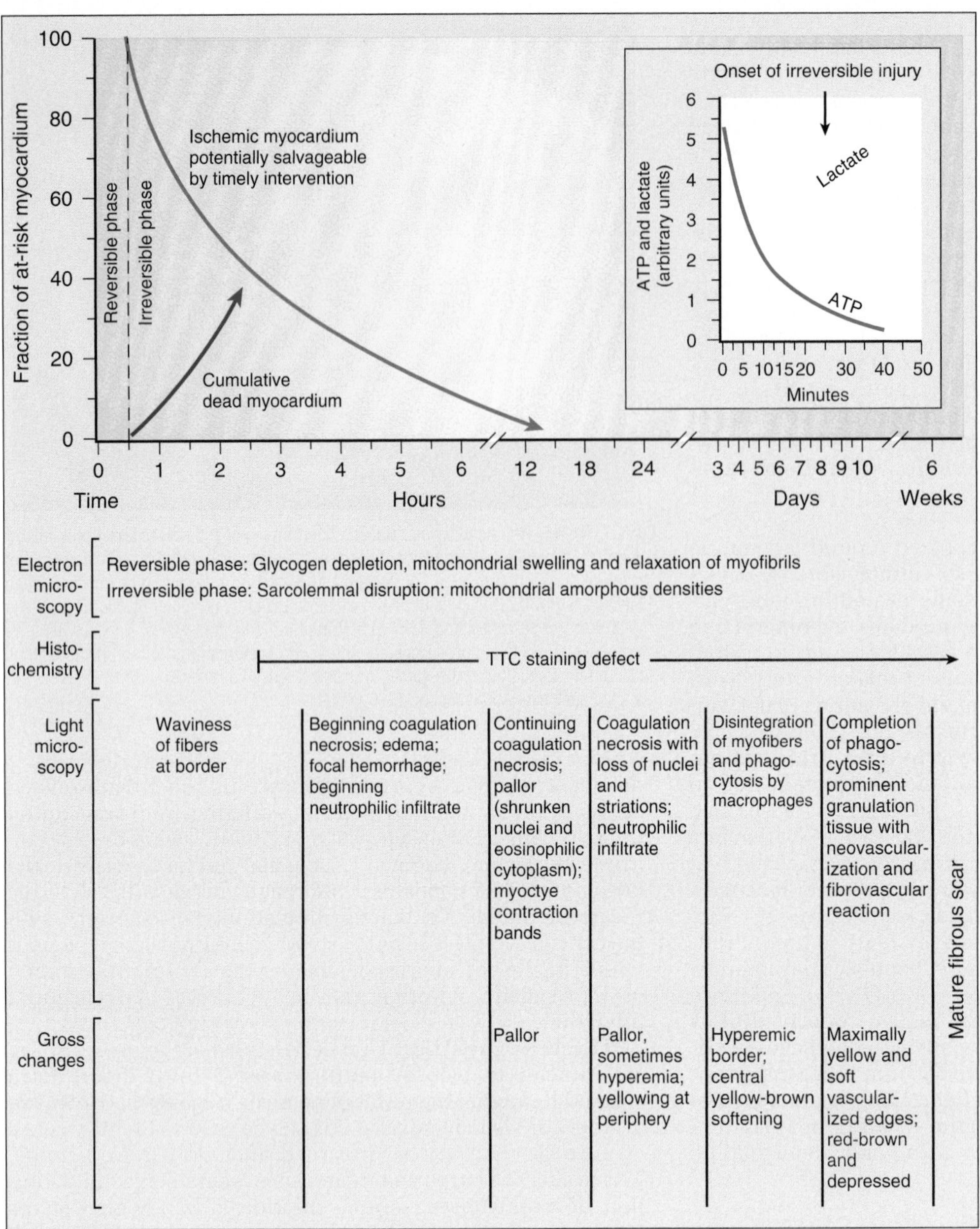

FIGURE 46–5 Temporal sequence of early biochemical, ultrastructural, histochemical, and histological findings after onset of myocardial infarction. At the top of the figure are schematically shown the time frames for early and late reperfusion of the myocardium supplied by an occluded coronary artery. For approximately $^1/_2$ hour after the onset of even the most severe ischemia, myocardial injury is potentially reversible; after that there is progressive loss of viability that is complete by 6 to 12 hours. The benefits of reperfusion (both early and late) are greatest when it is achieved early, with progressively smaller benefits occurring as reperfusion is delayed. ATP = adenosine triphosphate; TTC = triphenyltetrazolium chloride. (From Schoen FJ: Pathologic considerations of the surgery of adult heart disease. *In* Edmunds LH [ed]: Cardiac Surgery in the Adult. New York, McGraw Hill, 1997, p 85.)

The cut surface of an infarct of this age is yellow, surrounded by a reddish purple band of granulation tissue that extends through the necrotic tissue by 3 to 4 weeks. Commencing at this time and extending over the next 2 to 3 months, the infarcted area gradually acquires a gelatinous, ground-glass, gray appearance, eventually converting into a shrunken, thin, firm scar, which whitens and firms progressively with time (see Fig. 46–4).[34] This process begins at the periphery of the infarct and gradually moves centrally. The endocardium below the infarct increases in thickness and becomes gray and opaque.

Histological and Ultrastructural Changes

LIGHT MICROSCOPY

In some infarcts, a pattern of wavy myocardial fibers may be seen as early as 1 to 3 hours after onset, especially at the periphery of the infarct (Figs. 46–5 and 46–6). It is hypothesized that wavy fibers result from the stretching and buckling of noncontractile fibers as forces are transmitted to them from adjacent viable contractile fibers.[34] After 8 hours, edema of the interstitium becomes evident, as do increased fatty deposits in the muscle fibers, along with infiltration of neutrophilic polymorphonuclear leukocytes and red blood cells. Muscle cell nuclei become pyknotic and then undergo karyolysis, and small blood vessels undergo necrosis.

By 24 hours, there is clumping of the cytoplasm and loss of cross-striations, with appearance of focal hyalinization and irregular cross-bands in the involved myocardial fibers. The nuclei become pyknotic and sometimes even disappear. The myocardial capillaries in the involved region dilate, and polymorphonuclear leukocytes accumulate, first at the periphery and then in the center of the infarct. During the first 3 days, the interstitial tissue becomes edematous and red blood cells may extravasate (see Fig. 46–5). Generally, on about the fourth day after infarction, removal of necrotic fibers by macrophages begins, again commencing at the periphery (see Figs. 46–5 and 46–6). Later, lymphocytes, macrophages, and fibroblasts infiltrate between myocytes, which become fragmented. At 8 days, the necrotic muscle fibers have become dissolved; by about 10 days, the number of polymorphonuclear leukocytes is reduced, and granulation tissue first appears at the periphery (see Figs. 46–5 and 46–6). Ingrowth of blood vessels and fibroblasts continues, along with removal of necrotic muscle cells, until the fourth to sixth week after infarction, by which time much of the necrotic myocardium has been removed. This process continues along with increasing collagenization of the infarcted area. By the sixth week, the infarcted area has usually been converted into a firm connective tissue scar with interspersed intact muscle fibers (see Figs. 46–5 and 46–6).

PATTERNS OF MYOCARDIAL NECROSIS

COAGULATION NECROSIS. This results from severe, persistent ischemia and is usually present in the central region of infarcts, which results in the arrest of muscle cells in the relaxed state and the passive stretching of ischemic muscle cells. On light microscopy, the myofibrils are stretched, many with nuclear pyknosis, vascular congestion, and healing by phagocytosis of necrotic muscle cells (see Fig. 46–5). There is evidence of mitochondrial damage with prominent amorphous (flocculent) densities but no calcification.

NECROSIS WITH CONTRACTION BANDS. This form of myocardial necrosis, also termed *contraction band necrosis* or *coagulative myocytolysis*, results primarily from severe ischemia followed by reflow.[34] It is characterized by hypercontracted myofibrils with contraction bands and mitochondrial damage, frequently with calcification, marked vascular congestion, and healing by lysis of muscle cells. It is caused by increased Ca^{2+} influx into dying cells, resulting in the arrest of cells in the contracted state. It is seen in the periphery of large infarcts and is present to a greater extent in nontransmural than in transmural infarcts. The entire infarct may show this form of necrosis after reperfusion (Figs. 46-6 and 46-7).[35] The presence of contraction band necrosis in a large segment of the infarcts of patients who did not receive reperfusion therapy suggests that reperfusion through spontaneous fibrinolysis and/or the release of spasm have occurred.

MYOCYTOLYSIS. Ischemia without necrosis generally causes no acute changes that are visible by light microscopy. However, severe prolonged ischemia can cause myocyte vacuolization, often termed *myocytolysis*. Prolonged severe ischemia, which is potentially reversible, causes cloudy swelling, as well as hydropic, vascular, and fatty degeneration. Frequently seen at the borders of an infarct as well as in patchy areas of infarction in patients with chronic ischemic heart disease, myocytolysis is characterized by edema and cell swelling, lysis of myofibrils and nuclei, no neutrophilic response, and healing by lysis and phagocytosis of necrotic myocytes and ultimately scar formation.

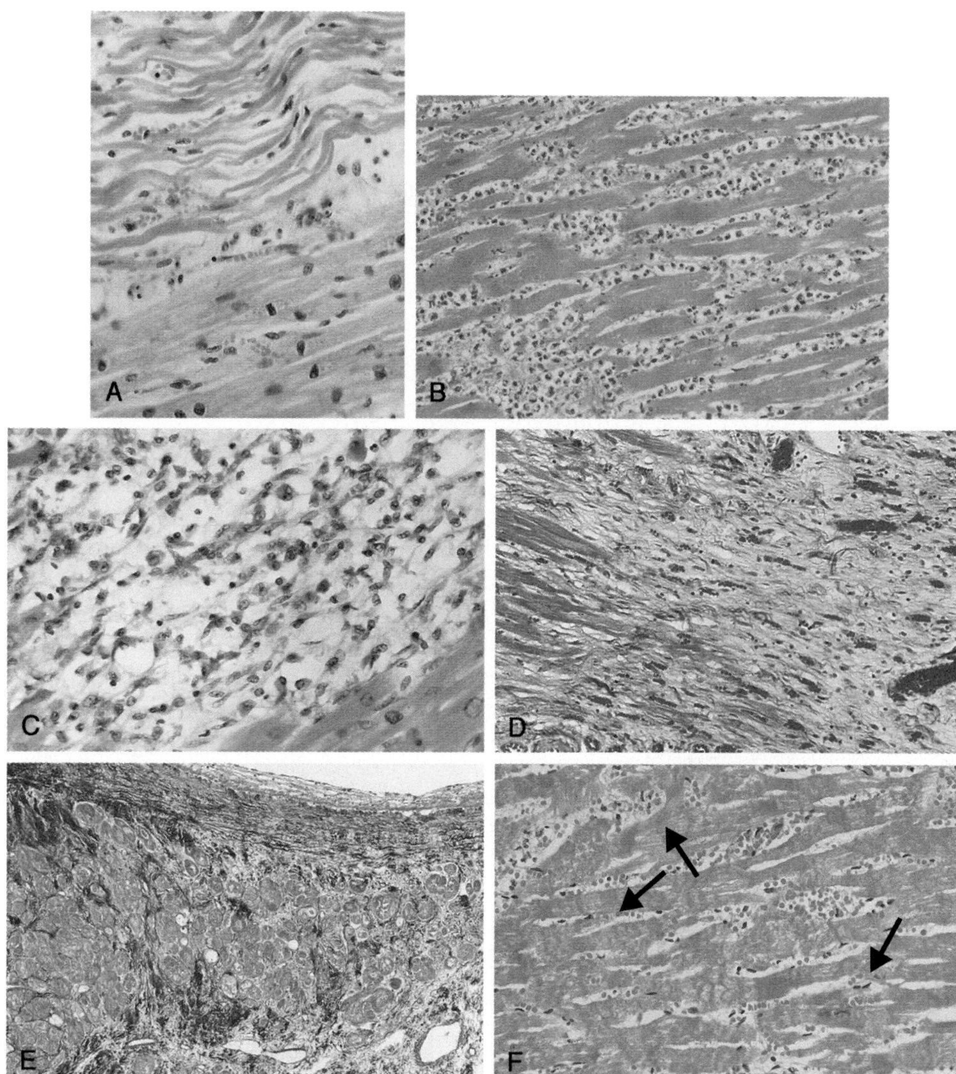

FIGURE 46–6 Microscopic features of myocardial infarction. **A,** One-day-old infarct showing coagulative necrosis, wavy fibers with elongation, and narrowing, compared with adjacent normal fibers (lower right). Widened spaces between the dead fibers contain edema fluid and scattered neutrophils. **B,** Dense polymorphonuclear leukocytic infiltrate in an area of acute myocardial infarction of 3 to 4 days' duration. **C,** Nearly complete removal of necrotic myocytes by phagocytosis (approximately 7 to 10 days). **D,** Granulation tissue with a rich vascular network and early collagen deposition, approximately 3 weeks after infarction. **E,** Well-healed myocardial infarct with replacement of the necrotic fibers by dense collagenous scar. A few residual cardiac muscle cells are present. (In **D** and **E,** collagen is highlighted as blue in this Masson trichrome stain). **F,** Myocardial necrosis with hemorrhage and contraction bands, visible as dark bands spanning some myofibers (arrows). This is the characteristic appearance of markedly ischemic myocardium that has been reperfused. (From Schoen FJ: The heart. *In* Cotran RS, Kumar V, Collins T [eds]: Pathologic Basis of Disease. 6th ed. Philadelphia, WB Saunders, 1999, pp 560-561.)

ELECTRON MICROSCOPY

In experimental infarction, the earliest ultrastructural changes in cardiac muscle following ligation of a coronary artery, noted within 20 minutes, consist of reduction in the size and number of glycogen granules, intracellular edema, and swelling and distortion of the transverse tubular system, the sarcoplasmic reticulum, and the mitochondria (see Fig. 46-5).[33] These early changes are reversible. Changes after 60 minutes of occlusion include myocardial cell swelling, swelling and internal disruption of mitochondria, and development of amorphous, flocculent aggregation and margination of nuclear chromatin, and relaxation of myofibrils. After 20 minutes to 2 hours of ischemia, changes in some cells become irreversible, and there is progression of these alterations; additional changes include indistinct tight junctions at the intercalated discs, swollen sacs of the sarcoplasmic reticulum at the level of the A band, greatly enlarged mitochondria with few cristae, thinning and fractionation of myofilaments, disappearance of the heterochromatin, rarefaction of the euchromatin and peripheral aggregation of chromatin in the nucleus, disorientation of myofibrils, and clumping of mitochondria. Cells irreversibly damaged by ischemia are usually swollen, with an enlarged sarcoplasmic space; the sarcolemma may peel off the cells, defects in the plasma membrane may appear, and the mitochondria are fragmented. The swollen mitochondria obtained from ischemic myocardium contain deposits of calcium phosphate and amorphous matrix densities. Many of these changes become more intense when blood flow is restored.[34]

MODIFICATION OF PATHOLOGICAL CHANGES BY REPERFUSION

When reperfusion of myocardium undergoing the evolutionary changes from ischemia to infarction occurs sufficiently early (i.e., within 15 to 20 minutes), it can successfully prevent necrosis from developing. Beyond this early stage, the number of salvaged myocytes and therefore the amount of salvaged myocardial tissue (area of necrosis/area at risk) is directly related to the length of time the coronary artery has been totally occluded, the level of myocardial oxygen consumption, and the collateral blood flow (see Fig. 46-7). Typical pathological findings of reperfused infarcts include a histological mixture of necrosis, hemorrhage within zones of irreversibly injured myocytes, coagulative necrosis with contraction bands, and distorted architecture of the cells in the reperfused zone (see Fig. 46-7).[33] After reperfusion, mitochondria in nonviable myocytes may develop deposits of calcium phosphate. Reperfusion of infarcted myocardium also accelerates the washout of intracellular proteins ("serum cardiac markers"), producing an exaggerated and early peak value of substances such as CK-MB and cardiac-specific troponin T and I (see Fig. 46-5).[36]

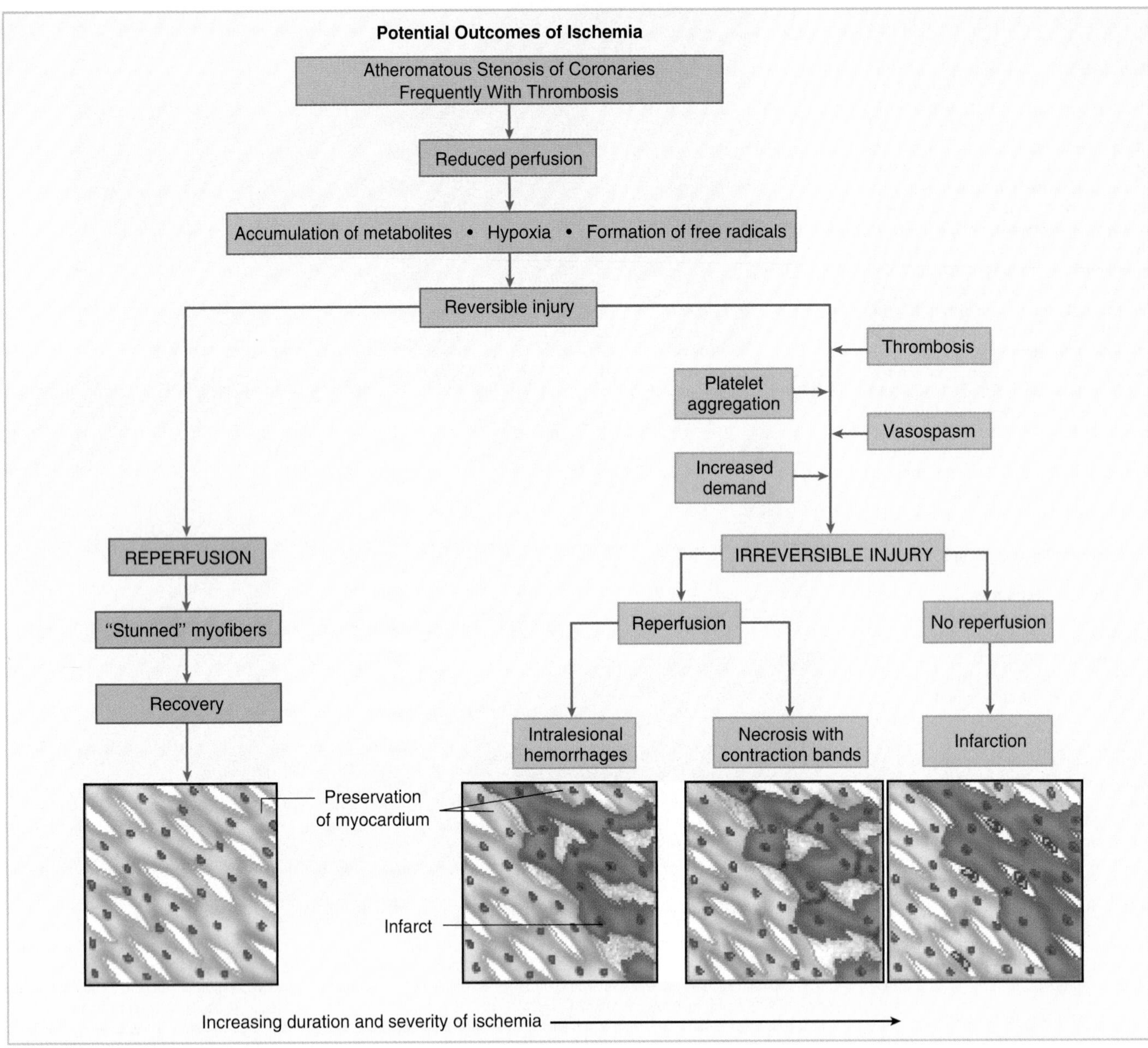

FIGURE 46–7 Several potential outcomes of reversible and irreversible ischemic injury to the myocardium. (From Schoen FJ: The heart. *In* Cotran RS, Kumar V, Robbins SL [eds]: Pathologic Basis of Disease. 5th ed. Philadelphia, WB Saunders, 1994, p 538.)

CORONARY ANATOMY AND LOCATION OF INFARCTION

In more than 75 percent of patients with STEMI who come to autopsy, more than one coronary artery is severely narrowed. Approximately one-half of patients with STEMI have critical obstruction (to less than 25 percent of luminal area) of all three coronary arteries, whereas the remainder are equally divided between those having one-vessel disease and those having two-vessel disease. Coronary arteriographic studies in surviving patients show that a higher percentage have one-vessel disease. Angiographic studies performed in the earliest hours of STEMI have revealed approximately a 90 percent incidence of total occlusion of the infarct-related vessel.[37] Recanalization from spontaneous thrombolysis as well as attrition due to some mortality among those patients with total occlusion results in a diminishing incidence of angiographically totally occluded vessels in the period following the onset of MI (Fig. 46–8). Pharmacological thrombolysis markedly increases the proportion of patients with a patent infarct-related artery early after STEMI (see Fig. 46–8).

A STEMI with transmural necrosis occurs distal to an acutely totally occluded coronary artery with thrombus superimposed on a ruptured plaque. The converse is not the case, however, in that chronic total occlusion of a coronary artery is not always associated with MI. Collateral blood flow and other factors—such as the level of myocardial metabolism, the presence and location of stenoses in other coronary arteries, the rate of development of the obstruction, and the quantity of myocardium supplied by the obstructed vessel—all influence the viability of myocardial cells distal to the occlusion. In many series of patients studied at necropsy or by coronary arteriography, a small number (5 percent) of patients with STEMI are found to have normal coronary vessels. In these patients, an embolus that has lysed, a transiently occlusive platelet aggregate, or a prolonged episode of severe coronary spasm may have been responsible for the reduction in coronary flow.

Studies of patients who ultimately develop STEMI after having undergone coronary angiography at some time before its occurrence have been helpful in clarifying coronary anatomy before infarction. Although high-grade stenoses, when present, more frequently lead to STEMI than do less severe lesions, the majority of occlusions actually occur in vessels with a previously identified stenosis of less than 50 percent on angiograms performed months to years earlier. This finding supports the

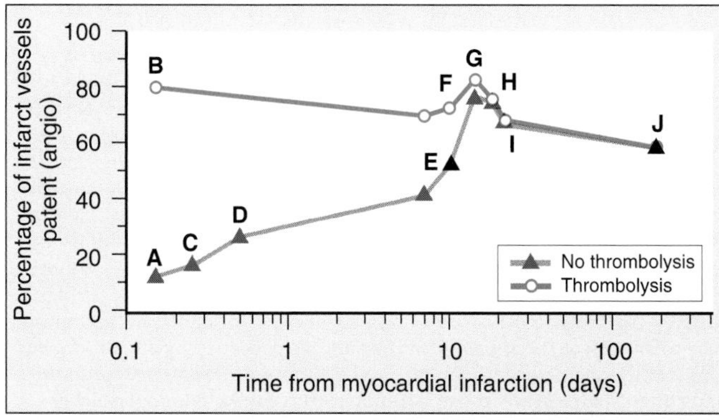

FIGURE 46–8 Comparison of angiographically documented infarct-related coronary artery patency rates in 10 separate clinical studies and time from myocardial infarction as modulated by early administration of a thrombolytic agent versus nonthrombolytic (conventional) therapy. The *x*-axis is a semilogarithmic scale of time in days from myocardial infarction. Note that the difference in patency rates becomes diminishingly small within the first 2 to 3 weeks after infarction. (From Rumberg JA, Gersh BJ: Coronary artery patency and left ventricular remodeling after myocardial infarction: Mechanisms and mechanics. *In* Califf RM, Mark DB, Wagner GS [eds]: Acute Coronary Care. St. Louis, Mosby-Year Book, 1995, p 122.)

concept that STEMI occurs as a result of sudden thrombotic occlusion at the site of rupture of previously nonobstructive but lipid-rich plaques.

When an area of the ventricle is perfused by collateral vessels, an infarct may occur at a distance from a coronary occlusion. For example, following the gradual obliteration of the lumen of the right coronary artery, the inferior wall of the left ventricle can be kept viable by collateral vessels arising from the left anterior descending coronary artery. Later, an occlusion of the left anterior descending artery may cause an infarct of the diaphragmatic wall.

RIGHT VENTRICULAR INFARCTION. Approximately 50 percent of patients with inferior infarction have some involvement of the right ventricle.[38] Among these patients, right ventricular infarction occurs exclusively in those with transmural infarction of the inferoposterior wall and the posterior portion of the septum. Right ventricular infarction almost invariably develops in association with infarction of the adjacent septum and left ventricular myocardium, but isolated infarction of the right ventricle is seen in 3 to 5 percent of autopsy-proven cases of MI (Fig. 46–9).

Regardless of whether it is combined with involvement of the left ventricle, right ventricular infarction is generally associated with obstructive lesions of the right coronary artery. However, right ventricular infarction occurs less commonly than would be anticipated from the frequency of atherosclerotic lesions involving the right coronary artery. This discrepancy probably can be explained by the lower oxygen demands of the right ventricle, because right ventricular infarcts occur more commonly in conditions associated with increased right ventricular oxygen needs such as pulmonary hypertension and right ventricular hypertrophy. Moreover, the intercoronary collateral system of the right ventricle is richer than that of the left, and the thinness of the right ventricular wall allows the chamber to derive some nutrition from the blood within the right ventricular cavity. Therefore, the right ventricle can sustain long periods of ischemia but still demonstrate excellent recovery of contractile function after reperfusion.[39]

ATRIAL INFARCTION. This can be seen in up to 10 percent of patients with STEMI if PR-segment displacement is used as the criterion for atrial infarction. Although isolated atrial infarction is observed in 3.5 percent of autopsies of patients with STEMI, it often occurs in conjunction with ventricular infarction and can cause rupture of the atrial wall.[40] This type of infarct is more common on the right side

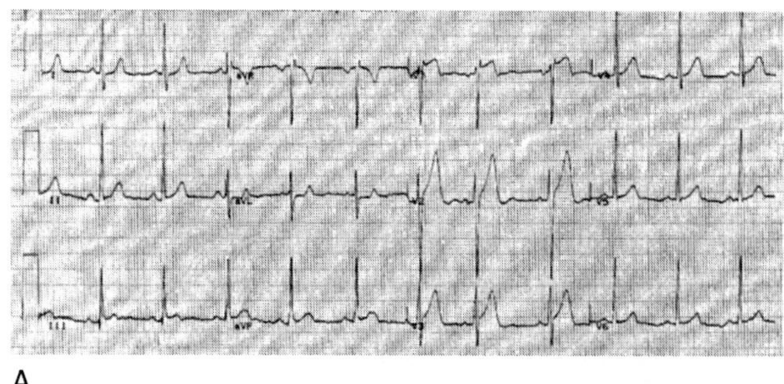

A

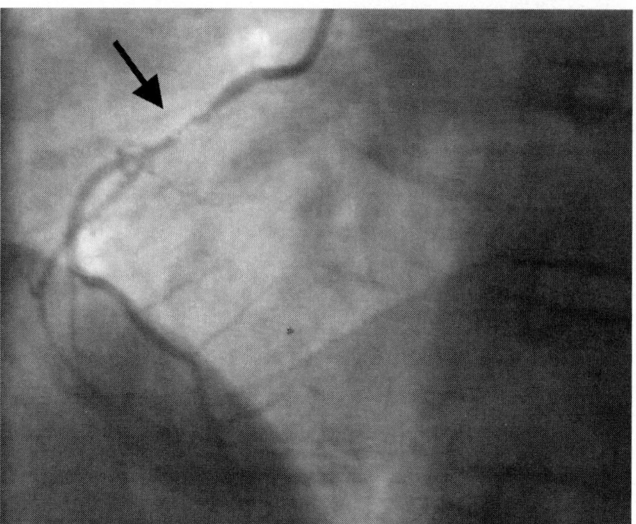

B

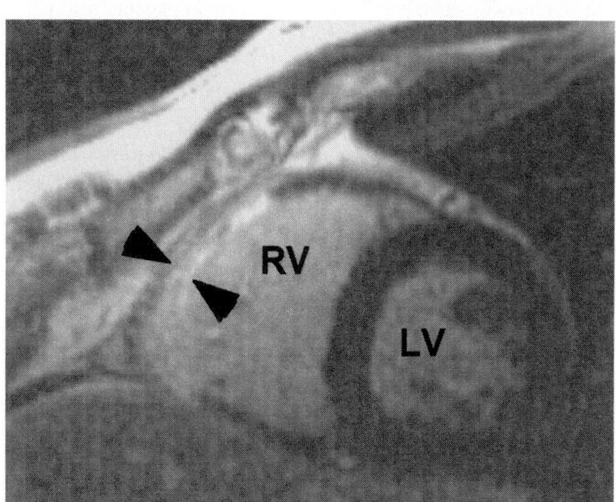

C

FIGURE 46–9 A 47-year-old man with no prior history of cardiac disease presented to an outside hospital describing "an awesome feeling that just sat in my chest" associated with bilateral arm weakness. The initial electrocardiogram **(A)** revealed ST-segment elevation in the right precordial leads and to a lesser extent in the inferior leads. The patient was treated with fibrinolytic therapy and transferred for catheterization. Angiography revealed a tight stenosis of a proximal nondominant right coronary artery (**B,** arrow) without significant disease in the left coronary artery. Contrast-enhanced cardiac magnetic resonance imaging **(C)** demonstrated delayed hyperenhancement consistent with injury of the right ventricle (RV) with distinct involvement of the right ventricular free wall (arrowhead), sparing the left ventricle (LV) as well as the right ventricular apex. The patient remained hemodynamically stable throughout his hospital course and was discharged home. (From Finn AV, Antman EM: Images in clinical medicine. Isolated right ventricular infarction. N Engl J Med, 349:1636, 2003.)

than on the left side, occurs more frequently in the atrial appendages than in the lateral or posterior walls of the atrium, and can result in thrombus formation. The difference in incidence between right and left atrial infarction might be explained by the considerably higher oxygen content of left atrial blood. Atrial infarction is frequently accompanied by atrial arrhythmias.[41] It has also been reported to be associated with reduced secretion of atrial natriuretic peptide and a low cardiac output syndrome when right ventricular infarction coexists.

COLLATERAL CIRCULATION IN ACUTE MYOCARDIAL INFARCTION (see Chap. 50)

The coronary collateral circulation is particularly well developed in patients with (1) coronary occlusive disease, especially when it is severe, with the reduction of the luminal cross-sectional area by more than 75 percent in one or more major vessels; (2) chronic hypoxia, as occurs in cases of severe anemia, chronic obstructive pulmonary disease, and cyanotic congenital heart disease; and (3) left ventricular hypertrophy, which intensifies coronary collaterals.

The magnitude of coronary collateral flow is one of the principal determinants of infarct size. Indeed, it is rather common for patients with abundant collaterals to have totally occluded coronary arteries without evidence of infarction in the distribution of that artery; thus, the survival of the myocardium distal to such occlusions must depend on collateral blood flow. Even if collateral perfusion existing at the time of coronary occlusion is not successful in preventing infarction, it may still exert a beneficial effect by preventing the formation of a left ventricular aneurysm. Some collaterals are seen in nearly 40 percent of patients with an acute total occlusion, and more begin to appear soon after the total occlusion occurs.[37] It is likely that the presence of a high-grade stenosis (90 percent), possibly with periods of intermittent total occlusion, permits the development of collaterals that remain only as potential conduits until a total occlusion occurs or recurs. Total occlusion then brings these channels into full operation.[42]

The incidence of collaterals 1 to 2 weeks after STEMI varies considerably and may be as high as 75 to 100 percent in patients with persistent occlusion of the infarct vessel, or as low as 17 to 42 percent in patients with subtotal occlusion.

NONATHEROSCLEROTIC CAUSES OF ACUTE MYOCARDIAL INFARCTION

Numerous pathological processes other than atherosclerosis can involve the coronary arteries and result in STEMI (see Table 46–3). For example, coronary arterial occlusions can result from embolization of a coronary artery. Emboli most frequently lodge in the distribution of the left anterior descending coronary artery, commonly in the distal epicardial and intramural branches. The causes of coronary embolism are numerous: infective endocarditis and nonbacterial thrombotic endocarditis (see Chap. 58), mural thrombi, prosthetic valves, neoplasms, air that is introduced at the time of cardiac surgery, and calcium deposits from manipulation of calcified valves at operation. In situ thrombosis of coronary arteries can occur secondary to chest wall trauma (see Chap. 65).

A variety of inflammatory processes can be responsible for coronary artery abnormalities, some of which mimic atherosclerotic disease and may predispose to true atherosclerosis. Epidemiological evidence suggests that viral infections, particularly with coxsackie B, may be an uncommon cause of MI. Viral illnesses precede MI occasionally in young persons who are later shown to have normal coronary arteries.

Syphilitic aortitis can produce marked narrowing or occlusion of one or both coronary ostia, whereas Takayasu arteritis can result in obstruction of the coronary arteries (see Chap. 53). Necrotizing arteritis, polyarteritis nodosa, mucocutaneous lymph node syndrome (Kawasaki disease), systemic lupus erythematosus (see Chap. 82), and giant cell arteritis can cause coronary occlusion. Therapeutic levels of mediastinal radiation can cause thickening and hyalinization of the walls of coronary arteries, with subsequent infarction. MI can also be the result of coronary arterial involvement in patients with amyloidosis (see Chap. 59), Hurler syndrome, pseudoxanthoma elasticum, and homocystinuria.

As cocaine abuse has become more common, reports of MI after the use of cocaine have appeared with increasing frequency (see Chap. 62). Cocaine can cause MI in patients with normal coronary arteries, preexisting MI, documented coronary artery disease, or coronary artery spasm.

MYOCARDIAL INFARCTION WITH ANGIOGRAPHICALLY NORMAL CORONARY VESSELS

Approximately 6 percent of all patients with STEMI and perhaps four times that percentage of patients with this diagnosis younger than 35 years of age do not have coronary atherosclerosis demonstrated by coronary arteriography or at autopsy.[37] Perhaps half of the patients of this group, in turn, have a variety of other lesions involving the coronary vessels or myocardium (see Table 46–3), whereas the others have no detectable coronary obstructive lesions. Patients with STEMI and normal coronary arteries tend to be young and to have relatively few coronary risk factors, except that they often have a history of cigarette smoking. Usually they have no history of angina pectoris prior to the infarction. The infarction in these patients is usually not preceded by any prodrome, but the clinical, laboratory, and ECG features of STEMI are otherwise indistinguishable from those present in the overwhelming majority of patients with STEMI who have classic obstructive atherosclerotic coronary artery disease. In patients who recover, areas of localized dyskinesis and hypokinesis can often be demonstrated by left ventricular angiography. Many of these cases are caused by coronary artery spasm and/or thrombosis, perhaps with underlying endothelial dysfunction or small plaques that are not apparent on coronary angiography.

Additional suggested causes include (1) coronary emboli (perhaps from a small mural thrombus, a prolapsed mitral valve, or a myxoma); (2) coronary artery disease in vessels too small to be visualized by coronary arteriography or coronary arterial thrombosis with subsequent recanalization; (3) a variety of hematological disorders causing in situ thrombosis in the presence of normal coronary arteries (polycythemia vera, cyanotic heart disease with polycythemia, sickle cell anemia, disseminated intravascular coagulation, thrombocytosis, and thrombotic thrombocytopenic purpura); augmented oxygen demand (thyrotoxicosis, amphetamine use); (5) hypotension secondary to sepsis, blood loss, or pharmacological agents; and (6) anatomical variations such as anomalous origin of a coronary artery (see Chap. 56), coronary arteriovenous fistula (see Chap. 56), or a myocardial bridge (see Chap. 18).

PROGNOSIS. The long-term outlook for patients who have survived a STEMI with angiographically normal coronary vessels on arteriography appears to be substantially better than for patients with STEMI and obstructive coronary artery disease. After recovery from the initial infarct, recurrent infarction, heart failure, and death are unusual in patients with normal coronary arteries. Indeed, most of these patients have normal exercise ECGs and only a minority develop angina pectoris.

Pathophysiology

Left Ventricular Function

Systolic Function

Upon interruption of antegrade flow in an epicardial coronary artery, the zone of myocardium supplied by that vessel immediately loses its ability to shorten and perform contractile work. Four abnormal contraction patterns develop in sequence: (1) dyssynchrony, that is, dissociation in the time course of contraction of adjacent segments; (2) hypokinesis, reduction in the extent of shortening; (3) akinesis, cessation of shortening; and (4) dyskinesis, paradoxical expansion, and systolic bulging.[43,44] Accompanying dysfunction of the infarcting segment initially is hyperkinesis of the remaining normal myocardium. The early hyperkinesis of the noninfarcted zones is thought to be the result of acute compensatory mechanisms, including increased activity of the sympathetic nervous system and the Frank-Starling mechanism. A portion of this compensatory hyperkinesis is ineffective work because contraction of the noninfarcted segments of myocardium causes dyskinesis of the infarct zone. Increased motion of the noninfarcted region subsides within 2 weeks of infarction, during which time some degree of recovery can be seen in the infarct region as well, particularly if reperfusion of the infarcted area occurs and myocardial stunning diminishes.

Patients with STEMI often also show reduced myocardial contractile function in noninfarcted zones. This may result from previous obstruction of the coronary artery supplying the noninfarcted region of the ventricle and loss of collaterals from the freshly occluded infarct-related vessel, a condition that has been termed *ischemia at a distance*.[45] Conversely, the presence of collaterals developing before STEMI may allow for greater preservation of regional systolic function in an area of distribution of the occluded artery and improvement in left ventricular ejection fraction early after infarction.

If a sufficient quantity of myocardium undergoes ischemic injury, left ventricular pump function becomes depressed; cardiac output, stroke volume, blood pressure, and peak dP/dt are reduced[44]; and end-systolic volume is increased. The degree to which end-systolic volume increases is perhaps the most powerful predictor of mortality following STEMI.[46] Paradoxical systolic expansion of an area of ventricular myocardium further decreases left ventricular stroke volume. As necrotic myocytes slip past each other, the infarct zone thins and elongates, especially in patients with large anterior infarcts, leading to infarct expansion. As the ventricle dilates during the first few hours to days after infarction, regional and global wall stress increase according to Laplace's law. In some patients, a vicious circle of dilation begetting further dilation is initiated.[47] The degree of ventricular dilation, which depends closely on infarct size, patency of the infarct-related artery,[48,49] and activation of the local renin-angiotensin system in the noninfarcted portion of the ventricle, can be favorably modified by angiotensin-converting enzyme (ACE) inhibition therapy, even in the absence of symptomatic left ventricular dysfunction.[50]

With the passage of time, edema and cellular infiltration and ultimately fibrosis increase the stiffness of the infarcted myocardium back to and beyond control values. Increasing stiffness in the infarcted zone of myocardium improves left ventricular function because it prevents paradoxical systolic wall motion (dyskinesia).

The likelihood of developing clinical symptoms such as dyspnea and ultimately a shock-like state correlate with specific parameters of left ventricular function. The earliest abnormality is a reduction in diastolic compliance (see later), which can be observed with infarcts that involve only 8 percent of the total left ventricle on angiographic examination. When the abnormally contracting segment exceeds 15 percent, the ejection fraction may be reduced and elevations of left ventricular end-diastolic pressure and volume occur. The risk of developing physical signs and symptoms of left ventricular failure also increase proportionally to increasing areas of abnormal left ventricular wall motion.[44] Clinical heart failure accompanies areas of abnormal contraction exceeding 25 percent, and cardiogenic shock, often fatal, accompanies loss of more than 40 percent of the left ventricular myocardium.

Unless infarct extension occurs, some improvement in wall motion takes place during the healing phase, as recovery of function occurs in initially reversibly injured (stunned) myocardium (Fig. 46–7). Regardless of the age of the infarct, patients who continue to demonstrate abnormal wall motion of 20 to 25 percent of the left ventricle are likely to manifest hemodynamic signs of left ventricular failure.

Diastolic Function

The diastolic properties of the left ventricle (see Chap. 21) are altered in infarcted and ischemic myocardium. These changes are associated with a decrease in the peak rate of decline in left ventricular pressure [peak (−)dP/dt], an increase in the time constant of the fall in left ventricular pressure, and an initial rise in left ventricular end-diastolic pressure. Over a period of several weeks, end-diastolic volume increases and diastolic pressure begins to fall toward normal. As with impairment of systolic function, the magnitude of the diastolic abnormality appears to be related to the size of the infarct.

Circulatory Regulation

The abnormality in circulatory regulation that is present in patients with STEMI is diagrammed in Figure 46–10. The process begins with an anatomical or functional obstruction in the coronary vascular bed, which results in regional myocardial ischemia and, if the ischemia persists, in infarction. If the infarct is of sufficient size, it depresses overall left

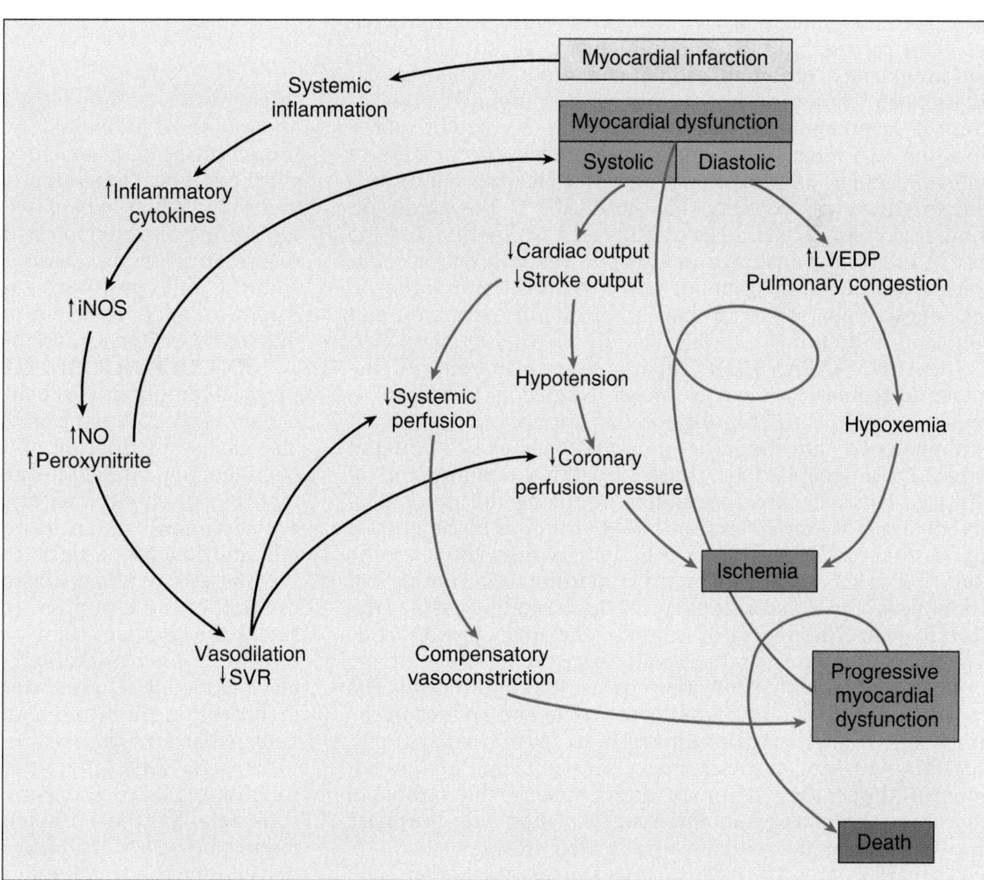

FIGURE 46–10 Classic shock paradigm is shown in black. The influence of the inflammatory response syndrome initiated by a large myocardial infarction is illustrated in red. LVEDP = left ventricular end-diastolic pressure. (From Hochman J: Cardiogenic shock complicating acute myocardial infarction: Expanding the paradigm. Circulation 107:2998, 2003.)

ventricular function so that left ventricular stroke volume falls and filling pressures rise. A marked depression of left ventricular stroke volume ultimately lowers aortic pressure and reduces coronary perfusion pressure; this condition may intensify myocardial ischemia and thereby initiate a vicious circle (see Fig. 46–10). Systemic inflammation leads to the release of cytokines that contribute to vasodilation and a fall in systemic vascular resistance.[51]

The inability of the left ventricle to empty normally also leads to an increased preload; that is, it dilates the well-perfused, normally functioning portion of the left ventricle. This compensatory mechanism tends to restore stroke volume to normal levels, but at the expense of a reduced ejection fraction. The dilation of the left ventricle also elevates ventricular afterload, however, because Laplace's law dictates that at any given arterial pressure, the dilated ventricle must develop a higher wall tension. This increased afterload not only depresses left ventricular stroke volume but also elevates myocardial oxygen consumption, which in turn intensifies myocardial ischemia. When regional myocardial dysfunction is limited and the function of the remainder of the left ventricle is normal, compensatory mechanisms sustain overall left ventricular function. If a large portion of the left ventricle becomes necrotic, pump failure occurs; that is, overall left ventricular function becomes so depressed that the circulation cannot be sustained despite the dilation of the remaining viable portion of the ventricle.

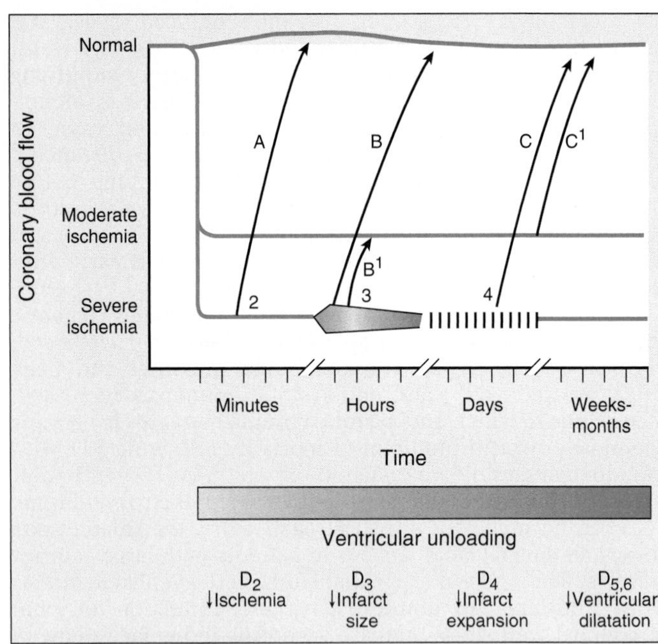

FIGURE 46–11 Therapeutic maneuvers in various stages of ischemia and infarction. Severely ischemic tissue (2) may be reperfused, thereby averting myocardial infarction (A). Infarcting tissue (3) may be reperfused, leading to sparing of myocardial tissue (B). If blood flow is restored only in part B, the myocardium may remain noncontractile although viable, that is, hibernating. After completion of the infarct (4), late reperfusion (C) may still be useful. Mechanical reperfusion of moderately ischemic myocardium (C) may restore contractility of hibernating myocardium to normal. Ventricular unloading may be useful throughout the preinfarct and postinfarct periods. Unloading may reduce ischemia (D_2), infarct size (D_3), infarct expansion (D_4), and ventricular dilatation ($D_{5,6}$). (From Braunwald E, Pfeffer MA: Ventricular enlargement and remodeling following acute myocardial infarction: Mechanisms and management. Am J Cardiol 68:4D, 1991.)

Ventricular Remodeling

As a consequence of STEMI, the changes in left ventricular size, shape, and thickness involving both the infarcted and the noninfarcted segments of the ventricle described earlier occur and are collectively referred to as *ventricular remodeling*. This process, in turn, can influence ventricular function and prognosis.[47] A combination of changes in left ventricular dilation and hypertrophy of residual noninfarcted myocardium is responsible for remodeling. After the size of infarction, the two most important factors driving the process of left ventricular dilation are ventricular loading conditions and infarct artery patency (Fig. 46–11).[47,49,52] Elevated ventricular pressure contributes to increased wall stress and the risk of infarct expansion, and a patent infarct artery accelerates myocardial scar formation and increases tissue turgor in the infarct zone, reducing the risk of infarct expansion and ventricular dilation.

INFARCT EXPANSION. An increase in the size of the infarcted segment, known as *infarct expansion*, is defined as "acute dilation and thinning of the area of infarction not explained by additional myocardial necrosis."[53] Infarct expansion appears to be caused by (1) a combination of slippage between muscle bundles, reducing the number of myocytes across the infarct wall; (2) disruption of the normal myocardial cells; and (3) tissue loss within the necrotic zone.[53] It is characterized by disproportionate thinning and dilation of the infarct zone prior to formation of a firm, fibrotic scar. The degree of infarct expansion appears to be related to the preinfarction wall thickness, with existing hypertrophy possibly protecting against infarct thinning. The apex is the thinnest region of the ventricle and an area of the heart that is particularly vulnerable to infarct expansion.[54] Infarction of the apex secondary to occlusion of the left anterior descending coronary artery causes the radius of curvature at the apex to increase, exposing this normally thin region to a marked elevation in wall stress.

When it is present, infarct expansion is associated with both a higher mortality and a higher incidence of nonfatal complications, such as heart failure and ventricular aneurysm. Infarct expansion has been noted in more than three-fourths of the hearts of patients succumbing to STEMI and one-third to one-half of all patients with anterior Q-wave infarctions. Infarct expansion is best recognized echocardiographically as elongation of the noncontractile region of the ventricle. When expansion is severe enough to cause symptoms, the most characteristic clinical finding is deterioration of systolic function associated with new or louder gallop sounds and new or worsening pulmonary congestion. Rupture of the ventricle may be considered to be a consequence of extreme infarct expansion.

VENTRICULAR DILATION. Although infarct expansion plays an important role in the ventricular remodeling that occurs early following myocardial infarction, remodeling is also caused by dilation of the viable portion of the ventricle, commencing immediately after STEMI and progressing for months or years thereafter (see Fig. 46–11). Dilation may be accompanied by a shift of the pressure-volume curve of the left ventricle to the right, resulting in a larger left ventricular volume at any given diastolic pressure (see Chap. 21). This dilation of the noninfarct zone can be viewed as a compensatory mechanism that maintains stroke volume in the face of a large infarction. However, ventricular dilation is also associated with nonuniform repolarization of the myocardium that predisposes the patient to life-threatening ventricular arrhythmias.

After STEMI, an extra load is placed on the residual functioning myocardium, a load that presumably is responsible for the compensatory hypertrophy of the uninfarcted myocardium. This hypertrophy could help to compensate for the functional impairment caused by the infarct and may be responsible for some of the hemodynamic improvement seen in the months after infarction in some patients.

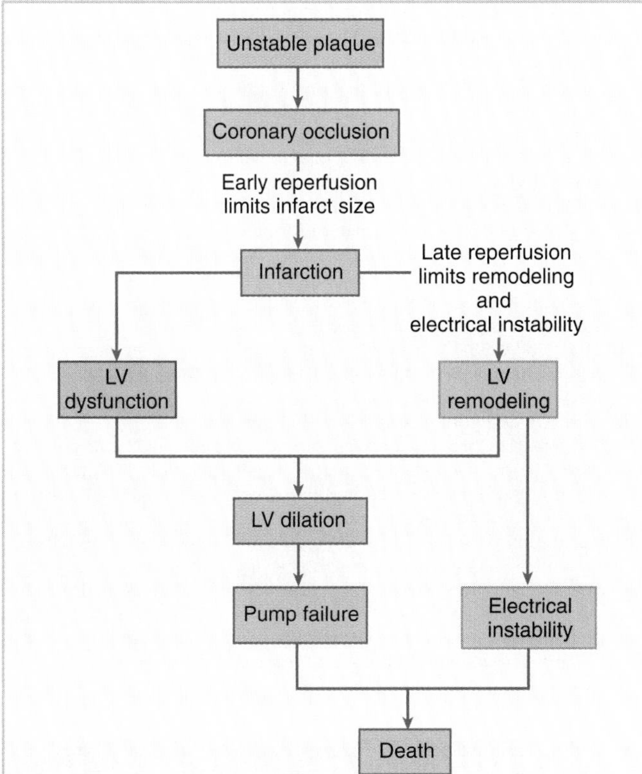

FIGURE 46–12 Flow chart showing postulated sequence of events from an unstable atherosclerotic plaque to death. The original paradigm emphasizing early reperfusion is shown at the left; the expanded paradigm illustrating the benefits of late reperfusion is shown at the right. LV = left ventricular. (Modified from Kim CB, Braunwald E: Potential benefits of late reperfusion of infarcted myocardium: The open artery hypothesis. Circulation 88:2426, 1993. Copyright 1993 American Heart Association.)

EFFECTS OF TREATMENT. Ventricular remodeling after STEMI can be affected by several factors, the first of which is infarct size (see Fig. 46–11). Acute reperfusion and other measures to restrict the extent of myocardial necrosis limit the increase in ventricular volume after STEMI, and evidence suggests that an open infarct artery per se, achieved even late after coronary occlusion, also attenuates ventricular enlargement (Fig. 46–12).[49] The second factor is scar formation in the infarct. Glucocorticosteroids and nonsteroidal antiinflammatory agents given early after MI can cause scar thinning and greater infarct expansion, whereas ACE inhibitors[47] attenuate ventricular enlargement (see Figs. 46–11 and 46–12). Additional beneficial consequences of inhibition of angiotensin II that may contribute to myocardial protection include attenuation of endothelial dysfunction and direct antiatherogenic effects.[55]

Pathophysiology of Other Organ Systems

PULMONARY FUNCTION

Changes in pulmonary gas exchange, ventilation, and distribution of perfusion occur with STEMI. There is an inverse relationship between arterial oxygen tension and pulmonary artery diastolic pressure. This suggests that increased pulmonary capillary hydrostatic pressure leads to interstitial edema, which results in arteriolar and bronchiolar compression that ultimately causes perfusion of poorly ventilated alveoli with resultant hypoxemia (see Chap. 22). In addition to hypoxemia, there is a fall in diffusing capacity. Hyperventilation often occurs in patients with STEMI and may cause hypocapnia and respiratory alkalosis, particularly in restless, anxious patients with pain. With reversal of heart failure, hypoxemia and intrapulmonary shunting diminish.

INCREASE IN INTERSTITIAL WATER. A positive correlation has been demonstrated between pulmonary extravascular (interstitial) water content, left ventricular filling pressure, and the clinical signs and symptoms of left ventricular failure. The increase in pulmonary extravascular water may be responsible for the alterations in pulmonary mechanics observed in patients with STEMI; that is, reduction of airway conductance, pulmonary compliance, forced expiratory volume and midexpiratory flow rate, and an increase in closing volume, the last presumably related to the widespread closure of small, dependent airways during the first 3 days after STEMI. Ultimately, severe increases in extravascular water may lead to pulmonary edema. Recovery of left ventricular function or diuresis reduces back to normal the abnormally elevated values for closing volumes, such as the lung volume at which airway closure commences.

The "closing volume" can encroach on and sometimes exceed functional residual volume. This can lead to arterial hypoxemia by the shunting of blood through alveoli that are not well ventilated.

REDUCTION OF VITAL CAPACITY. Virtually all lung volume indices—total lung capacity, functional residual capacity, and residual volume, as well as vital capacity—fall in the presence of STEMI.[56] These reductions correlate with the elevations of left-sided filling pressures and are most probably due to increases in pulmonary extravascular water. Lung volumes, oxygenation, and airway resistance all return toward normal by the time of hospital discharge for most patients. Increased pulmonary venous pressure also results in redistribution of pulmonary blood flow from the bases to the apices of the lung in patients with STEMI, altering the relationship between ventilation and perfusion. At follow-up examination 3 to 25 weeks after STEMI, however, the ventilation-perfusion relationship has usually returned to normal or almost so.

REDUCTION OF AFFINITY OF HEMOGLOBIN FOR OXYGEN. In patients with MI, particularly when complicated by left ventricular failure or cardiogenic shock, the affinity of hemoglobin for oxygen is reduced; that is, the P_{50} is increased. The increase in P_{50} results from increased levels of erythrocyte 2,3-diphosphoglycerate (2,3-DPG), which constitutes an important compensatory mechanism, responsible for an estimated 18 percent increase in oxygen release from oxyhemoglobin in patients with cardiogenic shock.

ENDOCRINE FUNCTION

PANCREAS. Hyperglycemia and impaired glucose tolerance are common in patients with STEMI. Although the absolute levels of blood insulin are often in the normal range, they are usually inappropriately low for the level of blood sugar, and there may be relative insulin resistance as well. Patients with cardiogenic shock often demonstrate marked hyperglycemia and depressed levels of circulating insulin, often with complete suppression of insulin secretion in response to tolbutamide. These abnormalities in insulin secretion and the resultant impaired glucose tolerance appear to be secondary to a reduction in pancreatic blood flow as a consequence of splanchnic vasoconstriction accompanying severe left ventricular failure. In addition, increased activity of the sympathetic nervous system with augmented circulating catecholamines inhibits insulin secretion and augments glycogenolysis, also contributing to the elevation of blood sugar.[57]

Glucose appears to be a more favorable energy source than free fatty acids for the ischemic myocardium by more efficiently replenishing the Krebs cycle and stimulating contractile performance.[58] Because hypoxic heart muscle derives a considerable portion of its energy from the metabolism of glucose (see Chap. 19) and because insulin is essential for the uptake of glucose by the myocardium as well as for myocardial protein synthesis and inhibition of lysosomal activity, the deleterious effects of insulin deficiency are clear. These metabolic considerations, combined with epidemiological observations that diabetic patients have a markedly worse prognosis, have served as the foundation for efforts to more aggressively administer insulin-glucose infusions to diabetic patients with STEMI.

ADRENAL MEDULLA. Excessive secretion of catecholamines produces many of the characteristic signs and symptoms of STEMI. The plasma and urinary catecholamine levels are highest during the first 24 hours after the onset of chest pain,[57] with the greatest rise in plasma catecholamine secretion occurring during the first hour after the onset of STEMI. These high levels of circulating catecholamines in patients with STEMI correlate with the occurrence of serious arrhythmias and result in an increase in myocardial oxygen consumption, both directly and indirectly, as a consequence of catecholamine-induced elevation of circulating free fatty acids. As might be anticipated, the concentration of circulating catecholamines correlates with the extent of myocardial damage and incidence of cardiogenic shock, as well as both early and late mortality rates.

Circulating catecholamines enhance platelet aggregation; when this occurs in the coronary microcirculation, the release of the potent local vasoconstrictor thromboxane A_2 may further impair cardiac perfusion. The marked increase in sympathetic activity associated with STEMI serves as the foundation for beta-adrenoceptor blocker regimens in the acute phase.

LOCAL MYOCARDIAL AND SYSTEMIC RENIN-ANGIOTENSIN SYSTEM. Noninfarcted regions of the myocardium appear to exhibit activation of the tissue renin-angiotensin system with increased angiotensin II production. Both locally and systemically generated angiotensin II can stimulate the production of various growth factors, such as platelet-derived growth factor and transforming growth factor, that promote compensatory hypertrophy in the noninfarcted myocardium as well as control the structure and tone of the infarct-related coronary and other myocardial vessels. Additional potential actions of angiotensin II that have a more negative impact on the infarction process include release of endothelin, PAI-1, and aldosterone, which may cause vasoconstriction, impaired fibrinolysis, and increased sodium retention, respectively. Inhibition of generation of circulating and tissue angiotensin II is one of the proposed mechanisms of benefit from ACE inhibitors in STEMI.

NATRIURETIC PEPTIDES. The peptides atrial natriuretic factor (ANF) and N-terminal pro-ANF are released from cardiac atria in response to elevation of atrial pressure. Brain natriuretic peptide (BNP), originally isolated from porcine brain, has been shown to be secreted by human ventricular myocardium (see Chap. 21). It appears to be released early after STEMI, peaking at about 16 hours. Patients with anterior infarction, lower cardiac index, and more significant congestive heart failure after STEMI have higher levels of BNP and also show a second peak of BNP release about 5 days after infarction. These intriguing observations suggest that BNP levels may be a marker of the degree of left ventricular dysfunction in patients with STEMI and that markedly elevated levels of BNP correlate with a worse prognosis.[59-61]

ADRENAL CORTEX. Plasma and urinary 17-hydroxycorticosteroids and ketosteroids, as well as aldosterone, are also markedly elevated in patients with STEMI.[57] Their concentrations correlate directly with the peak level of serum CK, implying that the stress imposed by larger infarcts is associated with greater secretion of adrenal steroids. The magnitude of the elevation of cortisol correlates with infarct size and mortality. Glucocorticosteroids also contribute to the impairment of glucose tolerance.

THYROID GLAND. Although patients with STEMI are generally euthyroid clinically, there is evidence of a transient decrease in serum triiodothyronine (T_3) levels, a fall that is most marked on about the third day after the infarct. This fall in T_3 is usually accompanied by a rise in reverse T_3, with variable changes or no change in thyroxine (T_4) and thyroid-stimulating hormone (TSH) levels. The alteration in peripheral T_4 metabolism appears to correlate with infarct size and may be mediated by the rise in endogenous levels of cortisol that accompanies STEMI.

RENAL FUNCTION

Both prerenal azotemia and acute renal failure can complicate the marked reduction of cardiac output that occurs in cardiogenic shock. On the other hand, an increase in circulating atrial natriuretic peptide occurs following STEMI, which is correlated with the severity of left ventricular failure. An increase in natriuretic peptide is also found when right ventricular infarction accompanies inferior wall infarction, suggesting that this hormone may play a role in the hypotension that accompanies right ventricular infarction.

HEMATOLOGICAL FUNCTION

PLATELETS. STEMI generally occurs in the presence of extensive coronary and systemic atherosclerotic plaques, which may serve as the site for the formation of platelet aggregates, a sequence that has been suggested as the initial step in the process of coronary thrombosis, coronary occlusion, and subsequent MI. Circulating platelets are hyperaggregable in patients with STEMI. Platelets from STEMI patients have an increased propensity for aggregation locally in the area of a disrupted plaque and also release vasoactive substances such as thromboxane A_2.[27]

HEMOSTATIC MARKERS. Elevated levels of serum fibrinogen degradation products, an end-product of thrombosis, as well as release of distinctive proteins when platelets are activated, such as platelet factor 4 and beta-thromboglobulin, have been reported in some patients with STEMI. Fibrinopeptide A, a protein released from fibrin by thrombin, is a marker of ongoing thrombosis and is increased during the early hours of STEMI. Marked elevation of hemostatic markers such as FPA, TAT, and F1&2 is associated with an increased risk of mortality in STEMI patients[62] (see Chap. 80). The interpretation of the coagulation tests in patients with STEMI may be complicated by elevated blood levels of catecholamines, concomitant shock, and/or pulmonary embolism, conditions that are all capable of altering various tests of platelet and coagulation function.

LEUKOCYTES. STEMI is usually accompanied by leukocytosis, which is related to the magnitude of the necrotic process, elevated glucocorticoid levels, and possibly inflammation in the coronary arteries. The magnitude of elevation of the leukocyte count is associated with in-hospital mortality after STEMI.[63] Activation of neutrophils may produce important intermediates, such as leukotriene B_4 and oxygen free radicals, which have important microcirculatory effects.

BLOOD VISCOSITY. Clinical and epidemiological studies suggest that several hemostatic and hemorheological factors (e.g., fibrinogen, factor VII, plasma viscosity, hematocrit, red blood cell aggregation, total white blood cell count) are involved in the pathophysiology of atherosclerosis and also play an integral role in acute thrombotic events. An increase in blood viscosity also occurs in patients with STEMI. During the first few days after infarction, this is mainly attributable to hemoconcentration, but later the increases in plasma viscosity and red blood cell aggregation correlate with elevated serum concentrations of alpha$_2$-globulin and fibrinogen, which are nonspecific reactions to tissue necrosis and are also responsible for the elevated sedimentation rate characteristic of STEMI. The high values of blood viscosity indices are observed most frequently in patients with complications such as left ventricular failure, cardiogenic shock, and thromboembolism.

Clinical Features

Predisposing Factors

The risk factors for atherosclerotic coronary artery disease are discussed in Chapter 36.

In as many as one-half of patients with STEMI, a precipitating factor or prodromal symptoms can be identified. Evidence suggests that unusually heavy exercise (particularly in fatigued or emotionally stressed, habitually inactive patients) may play a role in precipitating STEMI.[64] Such infarctions could be the result of marked increases in myocardial oxygen consumption in the presence of severe coronary arterial narrowing. Patients with known coronary disease who have been hospitalized for treatment of an acute coronary syndrome–related event and who subsequently report a high level of stress in their life have an increased risk of rehospitalization for cardiovascular reasons and also for "hard" events such as death and myocardial infarction.

Accelerating angina and rest angina, two patterns of unstable angina, may culminate in STEMI (see Fig. 46–1). Noncardiac surgical procedures have also been noted as precursors of STEMI. Perioperative risk stratification and the use of beta blockers may reduce the likelihood of STEMI and cardiac-related mortality (see Chap. 77).[65] Reduced myocardial perfusion secondary to hypotension (e.g., hemorrhagic or septic shock) and increased myocardial oxygen demands secondary to aortic stenosis, fever, tachycardia, and agitation can also be responsible for myocardial necrosis. Other factors reported as predisposing to STEMI include respiratory infections, hypoxemia of any cause, pulmonary embolism, hypoglycemia, administration of ergot preparations, use of cocaine, sympathomimetics, serum sickness, allergy, and, on rare occasion, wasp stings. In patients with Prinzmetal angina (see Chap. 49), STEMI may develop in the territory of the coronary artery that repeatedly undergoes spasm.[66] Rarely, munition workers exposed to high concentrations of nitroglycerin develop MI when they are withdrawn from this exposure, suggesting that it is caused by vasospasm.

CIRCADIAN PERIODICITY. An analysis of a large number of patients hospitalized with MI, studied as a part of the Multicenter Investigation of Limitation of Infarct Size (MILIS), revealed a pronounced circadian periodicity for the time of onset of STEMI, with peak incidence of events between 6 AM and 12 noon. This observation has been confirmed repeatedly.[64] Circadian rhythms affect many physiological and biochemical parameters; the early morning hours are associated with rises in plasma catecholamines and cortisol and increases in platelet aggregability.[67] Interestingly, the characteristic circadian peak was *absent* in patients receiving beta blocker or aspirin before their presentation with STEMI. The concept of "triggering" a STEMI is a complex one and likely involves the superimposition of multiple factors such as time of day, season, and the stress of natural disasters.[64]

History

PRODROMAL SYMPTOMS. Despite advances in the laboratory detection of STEMI, the patient's history remains of substantial value in establishing a diagnosis. The prodrome is usually characterized by chest discomfort, resembling classic angina pectoris, but it occurs at rest or with less activity than usual and can therefore be classified as unstable angina. However, it is often not disturbing enough to induce patients to seek medical attention, and if they do, they may not be hospitalized. A feeling of general malaise or frank exhaustion often accompanies other symptoms preceding STEMI.

NATURE OF THE PAIN (see Chap. 7). The pain of STEMI is variable in intensity; in most patients, it is severe and in some instances intolerable. The pain is prolonged, usually lasting for more than 30 minutes and frequently for a number of hours. The discomfort is described as constricting, crushing, oppressing, or compressing; often the patient complains of a sensation of a heavy weight or a squeezing in the chest. Although the discomfort is typically described as a choking, vise-like, or heavy pain, it can also be characterized as a stabbing, knife-like, boring, or burning discomfort. The pain is usually retrosternal in location, spreading frequently to both sides of the anterior chest, with predilection for the left side. Often the pain radiates down the ulnar aspect of the left arm, producing a tingling sensation in the left wrist, hand, and fingers. Some patients note only a dull ache or numbness of the wrists in association with severe substernal or precordial discomfort. In some instances, the pain of STEMI may begin in the epigastrium and simulate a variety of abdominal disorders, a fact that often causes STEMI to be misdiagnosed as "indigestion." In other patients, the discomfort of STEMI radiates to the shoulders, upper extremities, neck, jaw, and interscapular region, again usually favoring the left side. In patients with preexisting angina pectoris, the pain of infarction usually resembles that of angina with respect to location. However, it is generally much more severe, lasts longer, and is not relieved by rest and nitroglycerin.

The pain of STEMI may have disappeared by the time the physician first encounters the patient (or the patient reaches the hospital), or it may persist for many hours. Opiates, in particular morphine, usually relieve the pain. Both angina pectoris and the pain of STEMI are thought to arise from nerve endings in ischemic or injured, but not necrotic, myocardium. Thus, in cases of STEMI, stimulation of nerve fibers in an ischemic zone of myocardium surrounding the necrotic central area of infarction probably gives rise to the pain.

The pain often disappears suddenly and completely when blood flow to the infarct territory is restored. In patients in whom reocclusion occurs after thrombolysis, pain recurs if the initial reperfusion has left viable myocardium. Thus, what has previously been thought of as the "pain of infarction," sometimes lasting for many hours, probably represents pain caused by ongoing ischemia. The recognition that pain implies ischemia and not infarction heightens the importance of seeking ways to relieve the ischemia, for which the pain is a marker. This finding suggests that the clinician should not be complacent about ongoing cardiac pain under any circumstances. In some patients, particularly the elderly, STEMI is manifested clinically not by chest pain but rather by symptoms of acute left ventricular failure and chest tightness or by marked weakness or frank syncope. These symptoms may be accompanied by diaphoresis, nausea, and vomiting.

OTHER SYMPTOMS. Nausea and vomiting may occur, presumably owing to activation of the vagal reflex or to stimulation of left ventricular receptors as part of the Bezold-Jarisch reflex. These symptoms occur more commonly in patients with inferior STEMI than in those with anterior STEMI. Moreover, nausea and vomiting are common side effects of opiates. When the pain of STEMI is epigastric in location and is associated with nausea and vomiting, the clinical picture can easily be confused with that of acute cholecystitis, gastritis, or peptic ulcer. Occasionally, a patient complains of diarrhea or a violent urge to evacuate the bowels during the acute phase of STEMI. Other symptoms include feelings of profound weakness, dizziness, palpitations, cold perspiration, and a sense of impending doom. On occasion, symptoms arising from an episode of cerebral embolism or other systemic arterial embolism are the first signs of STEMI. The aforementioned symptoms may or may not be accompanied by chest pain.

Differential Diagnosis

The pain of STEMI may simulate the pain of acute pericarditis (see Chap. 64), which is usually associated with some pleuritic features: it is aggravated by respiratory movements and coughing and often involves the shoulder, ridge of the trapezius, and neck. An important feature that distinguishes pericardial pain from ischemic discomfort is that ischemic discomfort never radiates to the trapezius ridge, a characteristic site of radiation of pericardial pain.[68] Pleural pain is usually sharp, knife-like, and aggravated in a cyclical fashion by each breath, which distinguishes it from the deep, dull, steady pain of STEMI. Pulmonary embolism (see Chap. 66) generally produces pain laterally in the chest, is often pleuritic in nature, and may be associated with hemoptysis. The pain due to acute aortic dissection (see Chap. 53) is usually localized to the center of the chest, is extremely severe and described by the patient as a "ripping" or "tearing" sensation, is at its maximal intensity shortly after onset, persists for many hours, and often radiates to the back or the lower extremities. Often one or more major arterial pulses are absent. Pain arising from the costochondral and chondrosternal articulations may be associated with localized swelling and redness; it is usually sharp and "darting" and is characterized by marked localized tenderness. Episodes of retrosternal discomfort induced by peristalsis in patients with increased esophageal stiffness and also episodes of sustained esophageal contraction can mimic the pain of STEMI.[69]

SILENT STEMI AND ATYPICAL PRESENTATION. Nonfatal STEMI can be unrecognized by the patient and discovered only on subsequent routine electrocardiographic or postmortem examinations. Of these unrecognized infarctions, approximately half are truly silent, with the patients unable to recall any symptoms whatsoever. The other half of patients with so-called silent infarction can recall an event characterized by symptoms compatible with acute infarction when leading questions are posed after the electrocardiographic abnormalities are discovered. Unrecognized or silent infarction occurs more commonly in patients without antecedent angina pectoris and in patients with diabetes and hypertension.[70] Silent STEMI is often followed by silent ischemia (see Chap. 50). The prognoses of patients with silent and symptomatic presentations of STEMI appear to be similar.

Atypical presentations of STEMI include the following: (1) heart failure, that is, dyspnea without pain beginning de novo or worsening of established failure; (2) classic angina pectoris without a particularly severe or prolonged episode; (3) atypical location of the pain; (4) central nervous system manifestations, resembling those of stroke, secondary to a sharp reduction in cardiac output in a patient with cerebral arteriosclerosis; (5) apprehension and nervousness; (6) sudden mania or psychosis; (7) syncope; (8) overwhelming weakness; (9) acute indigestion; and (10) peripheral embolization.

Physical Examination

GENERAL APPEARANCE. Patients suffering STEMI often appear anxious and in considerable distress. An anguished facial expression is common, and—in contrast to patients with severe angina pectoris, who often lie, sit, or stand still, recognizing that all forms of activity increase the discomfort—some patients suffering STEMI may be restless and move about in an effort to find a comfortable position. They often massage or clutch their chests and frequently describe their pain with a clenched fist held against the sternum (the Levine sign, named after Dr. Samuel A. Levine). In patients with left ventricular failure and sympathetic stimulation, cold perspiration and skin pallor may be evident; they typically sit or are propped up in bed, gasping for breath. Between breaths, they may complain of chest discomfort or a feeling of suffocation. Cough productive of frothy, pink, or blood-streaked sputum is common.

Patients in cardiogenic shock often lie listlessly, making few if any spontaneous movements. The skin is cool and clammy, with a bluish or mottled color over the extremities, and there is marked facial pallor with severe cyanosis of the lips and nailbeds. Depending on the degree of cerebral perfusion, the patient in shock may converse normally or may evidence confusion and disorientation.

HEART RATE. The heart rate can vary from a marked bradycardia to a rapid regular or irregular tachycardia, depending on the underlying rhythm and the degree of left ventricular failure. Most commonly, the pulse is rapid and regular initially (sinus tachycardia at 100 to 110 beats/min), slowing as the patient's pain and anxiety are relieved; premature ventricular beats are common, occurring in more than 95 percent of patients evaluated within the first 4 hours after the onset of symptoms.

BLOOD PRESSURE. The majority of patients with uncomplicated STEMI are normotensive, although the reduced stroke volume accompanying the tachycardia can cause declines in systolic and pulse pressures and elevation of diastolic pressure. Among previously normotensive patients, a hypertensive response occasionally is seen during the first few hours, with the arterial pressure exceeding 160/90 mm Hg, presumably as a consequence of adrenergic discharge secondary to pain anxiety and agitation. It is common for previously hypertensive patients to become normotensive without treatment after STEMI, although many of these previously hypertensive patients eventually regain their elevated levels of blood pressure, generally 3 to 6 months after infarction. In patients with massive infarction, arterial pressure falls acutely, owing to left ventricular dysfunction and venous pooling secondary to administration of morphine or nitrates or both; as recovery occurs, the arterial pressure tends to return to preinfarction levels.

Patients in cardiogenic shock by definition have systolic pressures below 90 mm Hg and evidence of end-organ hypoperfusion. However, hypotension alone does not necessarily signify cardiogenic shock, because some patients with inferior infarction in whom the Bezold-Jarisch reflex is activated may also transiently have systolic blood pressure below 90 mm Hg. Their hypotension eventually resolves spontaneously, although the process can be accelerated by intravenous atropine (0.5-1.0 mg) and assumption of the Trendelenburg position. Other patients who are initially only slightly hypotensive may demonstrate gradually falling blood pressures with progressive reduction in cardiac output over several hours or days as they develop cardiogenic shock as a consequence of increasing ischemia and extension of infarction (see Fig. 46–10). Evidence of autonomic hyperactivity is common, varying in type with the location of the infarction. At some time in their initial presentation, more than half of patients with inferior STEMI have evidence of excess parasympathetic stimulation, with hypotension, bradycardia, or both, whereas about half of patients with anterior STEMI show signs of sympathetic excess, having hypertension, tachycardia, or both.[71]

TEMPERATURE AND RESPIRATION. Most patients with extensive STEMI develop fever, a nonspecific response to tissue necrosis, within 24 to 48 hours of the onset of infarction. Body temperature often begins to rise within 4 to 8 hours after the onset of infarction, and rectal temperature may reach 38.3° to 38.9° C (101°-102° F). Fever usually resolves by the fourth or fifth day after infarction.

The respiratory rate may be slightly elevated soon after the development of STEMI; in patients without heart failure, it results from anxiety and pain because it returns to normal with treatment of physical and psychological discomfort. In patients with left ventricular failure, the respiratory rate correlates with the severity of failure; patients with pulmonary edema may have respiratory rates exceeding 40 per minute. However, the respiratory rate is not necessarily elevated in patients with cardiogenic shock. Cheyne-Stokes (periodic) respiration (see Chap. 8) may occur in elderly individuals with cardiogenic shock and heart failure, particularly after opiate therapy and in the presence of cerebrovascular disease.

JUGULAR VENOUS PULSE. The height and contour of the jugular venous pulse reflect right atrial and right ventricular diastolic pressures (see Chap. 8). Because these pressures are usually normal or only slightly elevated in patients with STEMI (even in the presence of mild to moderate left ventricular failure), it is not surprising that usually the jugular venous pulse fails to show any abnormalities. The *a* wave may be prominent in patients with pulmonary hypertension secondary to left ventricular failure or reduced compliance. In contrast, right ventricular infarction (whether or not it accompanies left ventricular infarction) often results in marked jugular venous distention and, when it is complicated by necrosis or ischemia of right ventricular papillary muscles, tall *c-v* waves of tricuspid regurgitation are evident. In patients with STEMI and cardiogenic shock, the jugular venous pressure is usually elevated. In patients with STEMI, hypotension, and hypoperfusion (findings that may resemble those of patients with cardiogenic shock) but who have flat neck veins, it is likely that the depression of left ventricular performance may be related, at least in part, to hypovolemia. The differentiation can be made only by assessing left ventricular performance using echocardiography or by measuring left ventricular filling pressure with a pulmonary artery flotation catheter.

CAROTID PULSE. Palpation of the carotid arterial pulse provides a clue to the left ventricular stroke volume; a small pulse suggests a reduced stroke volume, whereas a sharp, brief upstroke is often observed in patients with mitral regurgitation or ruptured ventricular septum with a left-to-right shunt. Pulsus alternans reflects severe left ventricular dysfunction.

THE CHEST. Moist rales are audible in patients who develop left ventricular failure and/or a reduction of left ventricular compliance with STEMI. Diffuse wheezing can present in patients with severe left ventricular failure. Cough with hemoptysis, suggesting pulmonary embolism with infarction, can also occur. In 1967, Killip proposed a prognostic classification scheme based on the presence and severity of rales detected in patients presenting with STEMI.[72] Class I patients are free of rales and a third heart sound. Class II patients have rales but only to a mild to moderate degree (<50 percent of lung fields) and may or may not have an S_3. Patients in class III have rales in more than half of each lung field and frequently have pulmonary edema. Finally, class IV patients are in cardiogenic shock. Despite overall improvement in mortality rate in each class, compared with data observed during the original development of the classification scheme, the classification scheme remains useful today as evidenced by data from large MI trials of STEMI patients.[18,73]

Cardiac Examination

PALPATION. Despite severe symptoms and extensive myocardial damage, the findings on examination of the heart may be quite unremarkable in patients with STEMI. Palpation of the precordium may yield normal findings, but in patients with transmural STEMI, it more commonly reveals a presystolic pulsation, synchronous with an audible fourth heart sound, reflecting a vigorous left atrial contraction filling a ventricle with reduced compliance. In the presence of left ventricular systolic dysfunction, an outward movement of the left ventricle can be palpated in early diastole, coincident with a third heart sound.

AUSCULTATION (see Chap. 8). The heart sounds, particularly the first sound, are frequently muffled and occasionally inaudible immediately after the infarct, and their intensity increases during convalescence. A soft first heart sound may also reflect prolongation of the P-R interval. Patients with marked ventricular dysfunction and/or left bundle branch block may have paradoxical splitting of the second heart sound.

A fourth heart sound is almost universally present in patients in sinus rhythm with STEMI and is usually best heard between the left sternal border and the apex. This sound reflects the atrial contribution to ventricular filling and is particularly prominent in STEMI patients due to a reduction in left ventricular compliance and elevation of left ventricular end-diastolic pressure, even in the absence of left ventricular systolic dysfunction. This finding is of limited diagnostic value because it is commonly audible in most patients with chronic ischemic heart disease and is recordable, although not often audible, in many normal subjects older than 45 years.

A third heart sound in patients with STEMI usually reflects severe left ventricular dysfunction with elevated ventricular filling pressure. It is caused by rapid deceleration of transmitral blood flow during protodiastolic filling of the left ventricle with resultant oscillations of the cardiohemic system (i.e., myocardium and stream of blood flowing from left atrium to left ventricle) and is usually heard in patients with large infarctions. This sound is detected best at the apex, with the patient in the left lateral recumbent position, and is more common in patients with transmural anterior infarctions than in those with inferior or nontransmural infarctions. A third heart sound may be caused not only by left ventricular failure but also by increased inflow into the left ventricle, as occurs when mitral regurgitation or ventricular septal defect complicates STEMI (see Chap. 8). Third and fourth heart sounds emanating from the left ventricle are heard best at the apex; in patients with right ventricular infarcts, these sounds can be heard along the left sternal border and are intensified by inspiration.

Systolic murmurs, transient or persistent, are commonly audible in patients with STEMI and generally result from mitral regurgitation secondary to dysfunction of the mitral valve apparatus (papillary muscle dysfunction, left ventricular dilation). A new, prominent, apical holosystolic murmur, accompanied by a thrill, may represent rupture of a head of a papillary muscle. The findings in cases of rupture of the interventricular septum are similar, although the murmur and thrill are usually most prominent along the left sternal border and may be audible at the right sternal border as well. The systolic murmur of tricuspid regurgitation (caused by right ventricular failure due to pulmonary hypertension and/or right ventricular infarction or by infarction of a right ventricular papillary muscle) is also heard along the left sternal border. It is characteristically intensified by inspiration and is accompanied by a prominent *c-v* wave in the jugular venous pulse and a right ventricular fourth sound.

Pericardial friction rubs may be heard in patients with STEMI, especially those sustaining large transmural infarctions.[68] Rubs are notorious for their evanescence and hence are probably even more common than reported; frequent auscultation in patients with transmural infarction often results in the discovery of a rub that might otherwise have gone unnoticed. Although friction rubs can be heard within 24 hours or as late as 2 weeks after the onset of infarction, most commonly they are noted on the second or third day.[68] Occasionally, in patients with extensive infarction, a loud rub can be heard for many days. Patients with STEMI and a pericardial friction rub may have a pericardial effusion on echocardiographic study, but only rarely are the classic electrocardiographic changes of pericarditis seen.[68] Delayed onset of the rub and the associated discomfort of pericarditis (as late as 3 months post infarction) are characteristic of the now rare post-myocardial infarction (Dressler) syndrome.

Pericardial rubs are most readily audible along the left sternal border or just inside the point of maximal impulse. Loud rubs may be audible over the entire precordium and even over the back. Occasionally, only the systolic portion of a rub is heard; it can be confused with a systolic murmur, and the diagnosis of rupture of the ventricular septum or mitral regurgitation may be incorrectly considered.

OTHER FINDINGS

FUNDI. Hypertension, diabetes, and generalized atherosclerosis commonly accompany STEMI, and because these conditions can produce characteristic changes in the fundus, a funduscopic examination may provide information concerning the underlying vascular status; this is particularly useful in patients unable to provide a detailed history.

ABDOMEN. As already noted, in patients with STEMI, particularly in an inferior location with diaphragmatic irritation, the pain may be localized to the epigastrium or the right upper quadrant. Pain in the abdomen associated with nausea, vomiting, restlessness, and even abdominal distention is often interpreted by patients as a sign of "indigestion," resulting in self-medication with antacids, and it can suggest an acute abdominal process to the physician. Right heart failure, characterized by hepatomegaly and a positive abdominojugular reflux, is unusual in patients with acute left ventricular infarction but does occur in patients with severe and prolonged left ventricular failure or right ventricular infarction.

EXTREMITIES. Coronary atherosclerosis is often associated with systemic atherosclerosis, and therefore patients with STEMI commonly have a history of intermittent claudication and demonstrate physical findings of peripheral vascular disease. Thus, diminished peripheral arterial pulses, loss of hair, and atrophic skin in the lower extremities are noted frequently in patients with coronary artery disease. Peripheral edema is a manifestation of right ventricular failure and, like congestive hepatomegaly, is unusual in patients with acute left ventricular infarction. Cyanosis of the nailbeds is common in patients with severe left ventricular failure and is particularly striking in patients with cardiogenic shock.

NEUROPSYCHIATRIC FINDINGS. Except for the altered mental status that occurs in patients with STEMI who have a markedly reduced cardiac output and cerebral hypoperfusion, the neurological examination findings are normal unless the patient has suffered cerebral embolism secondary to a mural thrombus. The coincidence between these two conditions can be explained by systemic hypotension due to STEMI precipitating a cerebral infarction and the converse, as well as by mural emboli from the left ventricle causing cerebral emboli.

Patients with STEMI often exhibit alterations of the emotional state, including intense anxiety, denial, and depression. Medical staff caring for STEMI patients must be sensitive to changes in the patient's emotional state; a calm, professional atmosphere, with thorough explanations of equipment and prognosis, can help alleviate the distress associated with STEMI.

Laboratory Findings

Serum Markers of Cardiac Damage

The classic World Health Organization (WHO) criteria for the diagnosis of MI require that at least two of the following three elements be present: a history of ischemic-type chest discomfort, evolutionary changes on serially obtained ECG tracings, and a rise and fall in serum cardiac markers.[74] There is considerable variability in the pattern of presentation of MI with respect to these three elements, as exemplified by the following statistics. ST-segment elevation and Q waves on the ECG, two features that are highly indicative of MI, are seen in only about half of MI cases on presentation. Approximately one-fourth of patients with MI do not present with classic chest pain, and the event would go unrecognized unless an ECG were recorded fortuitously in temporal proximity to the infarction or permanent pathological Q waves are seen on later tracings. Nondiagnostic ECGs are recorded in approximately half of patients presenting to emergency departments with chest pain suspicious for MI who ultimately are shown to have an MI. Among patients admitted to the hospital with a chest pain syndrome, fewer than 20 percent are subsequently diagnosed as having had an MI. In the majority of patients, therefore, clinicians must obtain serum cardiac marker measurements at periodic intervals to either establish or exclude the diagnosis of MI; such measurements can also be useful for a rough quantitation of the size of infarction.

The availability of serum cardiac markers with markedly enhanced sensitivity for myocardial damage enables clinicians to diagnose MI in about an additional one-third of patients who would not have fulfilled criteria for MI in the past.[75] The increased use of more sensitive biomarkers of MI combined with more precise imaging techniques has necessitated establishment of new criteria for MI (see Table 46–2).

As myocytes become necrotic, the integrity of the sarcolemmal membrane is compromised and intracellular macromolecules (serum cardiac markers) begin to diffuse into the cardiac interstitium and ultimately into the microvasculature and lymphatics in the region of the infarct (Fig. 46–13 and Table 46–4).[76] The rate of appearance of these macromolecules in the peripheral circulation depends on several factors, including intracellular location, molecular weight, local blood and lymphatic flow, and the rate of elimination from the blood.[76]

Given the accelerated pace of decision-making in patients with acute coronary syndromes and emphasis on reduction of length of hospital stay, there is considerable interest in evaluating new serum cardiac markers, shortening assay time in the central chemistry laboratory, and designing rapid whole blood bedside assays.[77] For optimal specificity, a serum marker of MI should be present in high concentration in the myocardium and be absent from nonmyocardial tissue and serum. For optimal sensitivity, it should be rapidly released

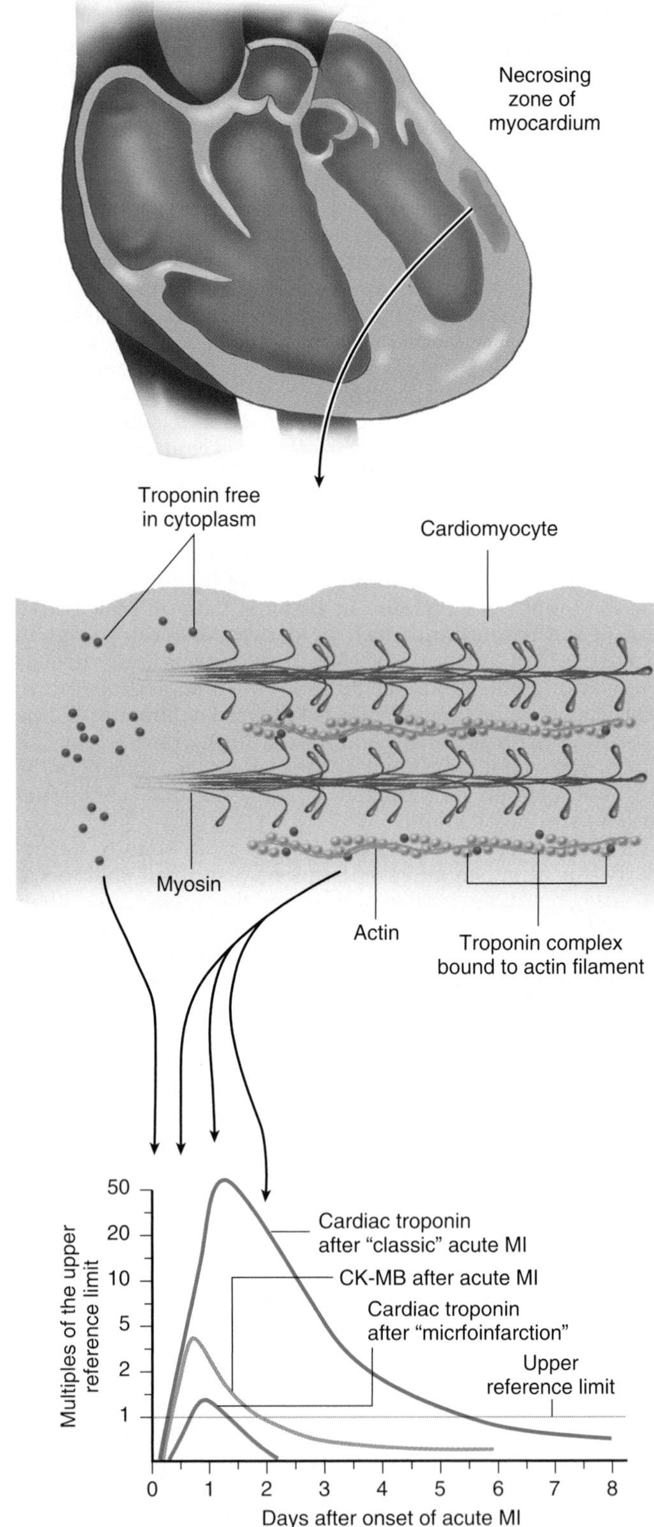

FIGURE 46–13 The zone of necrosing myocardium is shown at the top of the figure, followed in the middle portion of the figure by a diagram of a cardiomyocyte that is in the process of releasing biomarkers. Most troponin exists as a tripartite complex of C, I, and T components that are bound to actin filaments, although a small amount of troponin is free in the cytoplasm. After disruption of the sarcolemmal membrane of the cardiomyocyte, the cytoplasmic pool of troponin is released first (left-most arrow in bottom portion of figure), followed by a more protracted release from the disintegrating myofilaments that may continue for several days (three-headed arrow). Cardiac troponin levels rise to about 20 to 50 times the upper reference limit (the 99th percentile of values in a reference control group) in patients who have a "classic" acute myocardial infarction (MI) and sustain sufficient myocardial necrosis to result in abnormally elevated levels of the MB fraction of creatine kinase (CK-MB). Clinicians can now diagnose episodes of microinfarction by sensitive assays that detect cardiac troponin elevations above the upper reference limit, even though CK-MB levels may still be in the normal reference range (not shown). (From Antman EM: Decision making with cardiac troponin tests. N Engl J Med 346:2079, 2002.)

TABLE 46–4 Molecular Biomarkers for the Evaluation of Patients with ST-Elevation Myocardial Infarction

Biomarker	Molecular Weight (D)	Range of Times to Initial Elevation (h)	Mean Time to Peak Elevations (Nonreperfused)	Time to Return to Normal Range
Frequently used in clinical practice				
MB-CK	86,000	3-12	24 h	48-72 h
cTnI	23,500	3-12	24 h	5-10 d
cTnT	33,000	3-12	12 h-2 d	5-14 d
Infrequently used in clinical practice				
Myoglobin	17,800	1-4	6-7 h	24 h
MB-CK tissue isoform	86,000	2-6	18 h	Unknown
MM-CK tissue isoform	86,000	1-6	12 h	38 h

*Increased sensitivity can be achieved with sampling every 6 or 8 h.

CP = chest pain; cTnI = cardiac troponin I; cTnT = cardiac troponin T; MB-CK = MB isoenzyme of creatine kinase (CK); MM-CK = MM isoenzyme of CK.

Modified from Adams J III, Abendschein D, Jaffe A: Biochemical markers of myocardial injury. Is MB creatine kinase the choice for the 1990s? Circulation 1993;88: 750. Copyright 1993 American Heart Association.

into the blood after myocardial injury, and there should be a stoichiometric relationship between the plasma level of the marker and the extent of myocardial injury. For ease of clinical use, the marker should persist in blood for an appropriate length of time to provide a convenient diagnostic time window (see Table 46–4). Finally, the assay methodology should be inexpensive and easy to use.[78]

CREATINE KINASE. Serum CK activity exceeds the normal range within 4 to 8 hours after the onset of STEMI and declines to normal within 2 to 3 days (see Fig. 46–13). Although the peak CK occurs on average at about 24 hours, peak levels occur earlier in patients who have had reperfusion as a result of the administration of fibrinolytic therapy or mechanical recanalization (as well as in patients with early spontaneous fibrinolysis). Because the time-activity curve of serum CK is influenced by reperfusion, and because reperfusion itself influences infarct size, reperfusion interferes with estimation of infarct size by enzyme analysis (Fig. 46–14).[79]

Although elevation of the serum CK concentration is a sensitive enzymatic detector of STEMI that is routinely available in most hospitals,[80] important drawbacks include false-positive results in patients with muscle disease, alcohol intoxication, diabetes mellitus, skeletal muscle trauma, vigorous exercise, convulsions, intramuscular injections, thoracic outlet syndrome, and pulmonary embolism.[80]

CREATINE KINASE ISOENZYMES. Three isoenzymes of CK (MM, BB, and MB) have been identified by electrophoresis. Extracts of brain and kidney contain predominantly the BB isoenzyme; skeletal muscle contains principally MM but does contain some MB (1 to 3 percent); and both MM and MB isoenzymes are present in cardiac muscle. The MB isoenzymes of CK can also be present in minor quantities in the small intestine, tongue, diaphragm, uterus, and prostate. Strenuous exercise, particularly in trained long-distance runners or professional athletes, can cause elevation of both total CK and CK-MB.[81] Since CK-MB can be detected in the blood of healthy subjects, the cutoff value for abnormal elevation of CK-MB is usually set a few units above the upper reference limit for a given laboratory (see Fig. 46–13).[80] Despite the fact that small quantities of CK-MB isoenzyme are found in tissues other than the heart, elevated levels of CK-MB may be considered, for practical purposes, to be the result of MI (except in the case of trauma or surgery on the aforementioned organs).

Creatine kinase MB is analyzed in most laboratories by highly sensitive and specific enzyme immunoassays that utilize monoclonal antibodies directed against CK-MB.[80] Mass assays report results in nanograms per milliliter rather than units per milliliter and have been confirmed to be more

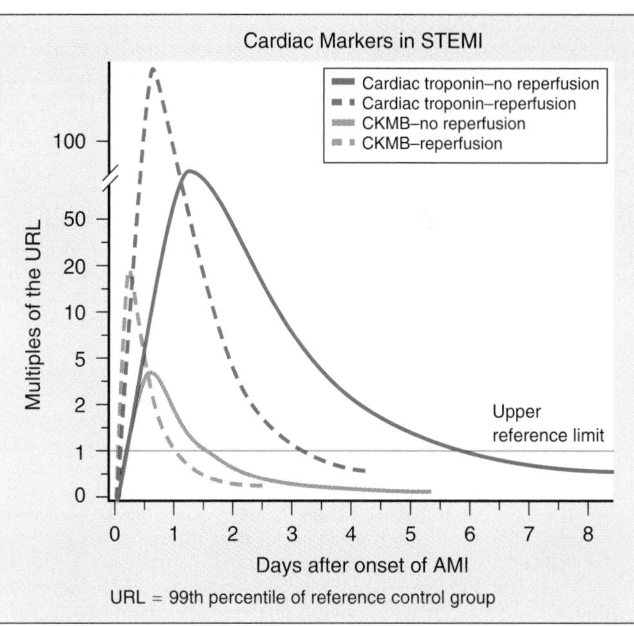

FIGURE 46–14 The kinetics of release of creatine kinase MB (CKMB) and cardiac troponin in patients who do not undergo reperfusion are shown in the solid green and red curves as multiples of the upper reference limit (URL). Note that when patients with ST-segment elevation myocardial infarction (STEMI) undergo reperfusion, as depicted in the dashed green and red curves, the cardiac biomarkers are detected sooner, rise to a higher peak value, but decline more rapidly, resulting in a smaller area under the curve and limitation of infarct size. AMI = acute myocardial infarction. (Adapted from Alpert JS, Thygesen K, Antman E, Bassand JP: Myocardial infarction redefined—A consensus document of The Joint European Society of Cardiology/American College of Cardiology Committee for the redefinition of myocardial infarction. J Am Coll Cardiol 36:959, 2000; and from Wu AH, Apple FS, Gibler WB, et al: National Academy of Clinical Biochemistry Standards of Laboratory Practice: Recommendations for the use of cardiac markers in coronary artery diseases. Clin Chem 45:1104, 1999.)

accurate than CK-MB activity assays, especially in patients presenting within 4 hours of the onset of STEMI. It has been proposed that a ratio (relative index) of CK-MB mass to CK activity of about 2.5 is indicative of a myocardial rather than a skeletal source of the CK-MB elevation. Although this ratio may be satisfied by many patients with STEMI, it is inaccurate in several circumstances: (1) when high levels of total CK are present because of skeletal muscle injury (a large quantity of CK-MB must be released from the myocardium to satisfy criteria); (2) when chronic skeletal muscle injury releases large amounts of CK-MB; and (3) when total CK measurements are within the normal reference range for the laboratory and CK-MB is elevated (possibly indicating that a microinfarction has occurred). Patients with minimally elevated CK-MB and normal CK have a prognosis that is generally worse than that for patients with suspected MI but no CK-MB elevation. Elevation of CK-MB following PCI is associated with increased late (1-3 years) cardiac mortality.[82]

Clinicians should not rely on measurements of CK and CK-MB at a single point in time but instead should evaluate the temporal rise and fall of serially obtained values; skeletal muscle release of CK-MB generally remains elevated for a longer time than myocardial release of CK-MB and produces a "plateau" pattern of CK-MB values over several days, in contrast to the shorter time course of skeletal muscle CK-MB elevation, as depicted in Figure 46–13. Of note, since cardiac-specific troponins I and T (cTnI and cTnT) (see Fig. 46–13 and Tables 46–2 and 46–3) accurately distinguish skeletal from cardiac muscle damage, the troponins are now considered the preferred biomarker for diagnosing MI.[76]

In addition to STEMI secondary to coronary obstruction, other forms of injury to cardiac muscle, such as those resulting from myocarditis, trauma, cardiac catheterization, shock, and cardiac surgery, may also produce elevated serum CK-MB levels.[80] These latter causes of elevation of serum CK-MB values can usually be readily distinguished from STEMI by the clinical setting.

CREATINE KINASE ISOFORMS. Isoforms of the MM and MB isoenzymes have been identified.[83] These are subtypes of the individual isoenzymes and are formed in the circulation when the enzyme carboxypeptidase cleaves lysine residues from the carboxy terminus of the myocardial forms of the enzyme (CK-MM3 and CK-MB2), producing isoforms with a different electrophoretic mobility (CK-MM2, CK-MM1, and CK-MB1). Certain isoforms appear to be released into the blood quite rapidly, perhaps as soon as 1 hour, after the onset of infarction. An absolute level of CK-MB2 isoform greater than 1.0 U/liter or a ratio of CK-MB2 to CK-MB1 greater than 2.5 has a sensitivity for diagnosing MI of 46.4 percent at 4 hours and of 91.5 percent at 6 hours.[84] A rapid high-voltage electrophoretic assay for these isoforms is available, and results from experienced research laboratories suggest that it could permit early identification of patients with MI and early detection of successful reperfusion (peak CK-MB2/CK-MB1 > 3.8 at 2 hours), but controversy exists about the utility of CK isoforms in general clinical practice.[78]

MYOGLOBIN. This low-molecular-weight heme protein is released into the circulation from injured myocardial cells and can be detected within a few hours after the onset of infarction (see Table 46-3). Peak levels of serum myoglobin are reached considerably earlier (1 to 4 hours) than peak values of serum CK.[85] Because of its lack of cardiac specificity, an isolated measurement of myoglobin within the first 4 to 8 hours after the onset of chest discomfort in patients with a nondiagnostic ECG should not be relied upon to make the diagnosis of MI but should be supplemented by a more cardiac-specific marker such as cTnI or cTnT (see Table 46-3).[86]

In contrast to CK, myoglobin is readily excreted into the urine. A more rapid rise in serum myoglobin has been observed after reperfusion, and its measurement has been suggested as a useful index of successful reperfusion[79,87,88] and even infarct size. In patients presenting less than 6 hours from symptom onset and with ST elevation in whom the diagnosis of STEMI is not in doubt, an elevated myoglobin level is associated with an increased risk of mortality.[89] The adverse prognostic significance of an elevated myoglobin level at presentation is probably due to a combination of a large amount of myocardial damage and a delay of at least several hours from onset of symptoms to blood sampling.

CARDIAC-SPECIFIC TROPONINS. The troponin complex consists of three subunits that regulate the calcium-mediated contractile process of striated muscle. These include troponin C, which binds Ca^{2+}; troponin I (TnI), which binds to actin and inhibits actin-myosin interactions; and troponin T (TnT), which binds to tropomyosin, thereby attaching the troponin complex to the thin filament. Although the majority of TnT is incorporated in the troponin complex, approximately 6 percent is dissolved in the cytosol; about 2 to 3 percent of TnI is found in a cytosolic pool.

Although both TnT and TnI are present in cardiac and skeletal muscle, they are encoded by different genes and the amino acid sequence differs. This permits the production of antibodies that are specific for the cardiac form (cTnT and cTnI) and has led to the development of quantitative assays for cTnT and cTnI that have been approved by the Food and Drug Administration for clinical use[76] (see Fig. 46–13 and Table 46–4). Several studies have confirmed the reliability of these new quantitative assays for detecting myocardial injury, and measurement of cTnT or cTnI is now at the center of a new diagnostic criteria for STEMI.[90,91] Qualitative, rapid, bedside assays for cTnT and cTnI have also been approved for diagnosing MI.[92]

When interpreting the results of assays for cTnT or cTnI, clinicians must be cognizant of several analytical issues. The first-generation assay for cTnT exhibited some nonspecific binding to skeletal muscle troponin, but this was corrected in subsequent generations of assays.[93] The cTnT assays are produced by a single manufacturer, leading to relative uniformity of cutoffs, whereas several manufacturers produce cTnI assays. The majority of cTnI released into the bloodstream in patients with STEMI is complexed with cardiac troponin C.[94] Variations in the cutoff concentration for abnormal levels of cTnI in the clinically available immunoassays may be due in part to different specificities of the antibodies used for detecting free and complexed cTnI.[94] Thus, when using the measurement of cTnI for diagnosing STEMI, clinicians should apply the cutoff values for the particular assay used in their laboratory.[95] For both cTnT and cTnI, the definition of an abnormally increased level is a value exceeding that of 99 percent of a reference control group.[90]

Cutoff Values. Because cTnT or cTnI is not detected in the peripheral circulation under normal circumstances, the cutoff value for these analytes may be set only slightly above the "noise" level of the assay. Furthermore, whereas CK-MB usually increases 10- to 20-fold above the upper limit of the reference range, cTnT and cTnI typically increase more than 20 times above the reference range. These features of the cardiac-specific troponin assays provide an improved signal-to-noise ratio, enabling the detection of even minor degrees of myocardial necrosis.[96] In patients with MI, cTnT and cTnI first begin to rise above the upper reference limit by 3 hours from the onset of chest pain. Due to a continuous release from a degenerating contractile apparatus in necrotic myocytes, elevations of cTnI may persist for 7 to 10 days after MI; elevations of cTnT may persist for up to 10 to 14 days. The prolonged time course of elevation of cTnT and cTnI is advantageous for the late diagnosis of MI (see Fig. 46–13).

Patients with STEMI who undergo successful recanalization of the infarct-related artery have a rapid release of cardiac troponins that may be useful as an indicator of reperfusion, although myoglobin appears slightly more efficient in this regard (see Fig. 46–14).[79,97]

Troponin versus CK-MB. When comparing the diagnostic efficiency of the cardiac troponins versus CK-MB for MI, it is important to bear in mind that the troponin assays are probably capable of detecting episodes of myocardial necrosis that are below the detection limit of the current CK-MB assays, leading to a number of "false-positive" cases of troponin elevations if CK-MB is used as the gold standard. The somewhat vague terms *minor myocardial damage* and *microinfarction* have been used to describe the pathological process in patients who have a chest pain syndrome and elevated cardiac troponin but in whom CK-MB is in the normal range.[98] From a clinical perspective, it is desirable to have diagnostic tests for MI with increased sensitivity to increase the number of MI cases identified and increased specificity to reduce the number of cases incorrectly diagnosed and treated for MI. In addition, cardiac troponin measurements have been shown to have prognostic value for identifying patients with an acute coronary syndrome at risk for adverse clinical outcomes and who also exhibit enhanced responsiveness to new therapies such as glycoprotein IIb/IIIa inhibitors and low-molecular-weight heparins. The prognostic value of the troponins is independent of other risk factors such as age and ECG abnormalities, as well as the measurement of classic biomarkers such as CK-MB.[76]

Interpretation of Troponin Elevations. Balanced against the advantages of the troponins for improved detection of MI and prognostication of risk are the epidemiological, social, and health care delivery implications of assigning a diagnosis of MI to a larger cohort of patients than was the case in an earlier era (see Table 46–2).[99] Revised criteria for MI have an impact on our ability to monitor trends in the incidence of MI and draw comparisons with previous observations, on the psychological status of the patient, on patients' ability to obtain driving and pilot licenses, on disability applications, and on hospital reimbursement.[90] There is no clear solution to these issues.

Recommendations for Measurement of Serum Markers

It seems reasonable for clinicians to measure either cTnT or cTnI in patients with suspected MI. From a cost-effectiveness perspective, it is unnecessary to measure both a cardiac-specific troponin and CK-MB at all time points.[100] Routine diagnosis of MI can be accomplished within 12 hours using CK-MB, cTnT, or cTnI by obtaining measurements approximately every 8 to 12 hours (see Table 46–2). Retrospective diagnosis or diagnosis of MI in the presence of skeletal muscle injury is more readily accomplished with cTnT or cTnI.

Although serum cardiac markers have been used successfully to stratify patients for risk of cardiac events when the presenting ECG does not show ST elevation, bedside assays for troponin or myoglobin either alone or in combination with the ECG also are useful for stratifying risk in patients with STEMI.[89,101]

OTHER LABORATORY MEASUREMENTS

Numerous nonspecific manifestations can be recognized in patients with STEMI. Although they are not generally employed in establishing the diagnosis, awareness of their coexistence with infarction is important to avoid misinterpretation or erroneous diagnosis of other disorders.

SERUM LIPIDS. These are often determined in patients with STEMI. However, the results may be misleading because numerous factors that can alter the values are operating at the time of the patient's admission to the hospital. Serum triglycerides are affected by caloric intake, intravenous glucose, and recumbency.

During the first 24 to 48 hours after admission, total cholesterol and high-density lipoprotein (HDL) cholesterol remain at or near baseline values but generally fall precipitously after that. The fall in HDL cholesterol after STEMI is greater than the fall in total cholesterol; thus, the ratio of total cholesterol to HDL cholesterol is no longer useful for risk assessment early after MI. A lipid profile should be obtained on all STEMI patients who are admitted within 24 to 48 hours of symptoms. Based on the success of lipid-lowering therapy in primary and secondary prevention studies and evidence that hypolipidemic therapy improves endothelial function and inhibits thrombus formation,[102] it has been argued that early management of serum lipids in patients hospitalized for STEMI is advisable.[103,104] For patients admitted beyond 24 to 48 hours, more accurate determinations of serum lipid levels are obtained about 8 weeks after the infarction has occurred.

HEMATOLOGICAL FINDINGS. The elevation of the white blood cell count usually develops within 2 hours after the onset of chest pain, reaches a peak 2 to 4 days after infarction, and returns to normal in 1 week; the peak white blood cell count usually ranges between 12 and 15×10^3/ml but occasionally rises to as high as 20×10^3/ml in patients with large STEMI. Often there is an increase in the percentage of polymorphonuclear leukocytes and a shift of the differential count to band forms. An epidemiological association has been reported indicating a worse angiographic appearance of culprit lesions and increased risk of adverse clinical outcomes the higher the white blood cell count at presentation with an acute coronary syndrome.[63,105]

The erythrocyte sedimentation rate (ESR) is usually normal during the first day or two after infarction, even though fever and leukocytosis may be present. It then rises to a peak on the fourth or fifth day and may remain elevated for several weeks. The increase in the ESR is secondary to elevated plasma alpha$_2$-globulin fibrinogen, but the peak does not correlate well with the size of the infarction or with the prognosis. The hematocrit often increases during the first few days after infarction as a consequence of hemoconcentration. Although an elevated C-reactive protein (CRP) level appears to identify patients at increased risk of coronary heart disease, evidence also exists that in patients presenting with STEMI, an elevated CRP is associated with worse angiographic appearance of the infarct artery and a greater likelihood of developing heart failure.[106,107]

Electrocardiography (see Chap. 9)

In the majority of patients with STEMI, some change can be documented when serial ECGs are compared. However, many factors limit the ability of the ECG to diagnose and localize MI: the extent of myocardial injury, the age of the infarct, its location, the presence of conduction defects, the presence of previous infarcts or acute pericarditis, changes in electrolyte concentrations, and the administration of cardioactive drugs. Changes in the ST segment and T wave are quite nonspecific and may occur in a variety of conditions, including stable and unstable angina pectoris, ventricular hypertrophy, acute and chronic pericarditis, myocarditis, early repolarization, electrolyte imbalance, shock, and metabolic disorders and following the administration of digitalis. Serial ECGs may be of considerable aid in differentiating these conditions from STEMI. Transient changes favor angina or electrolyte disturbances, whereas persistent changes argue for infarction if other causes such as shock, administration of digitalis, and persistent metabolic disorders can be eliminated. Nevertheless, serial standard 12-lead ECGs remain a potent and extremely clinically useful method for the detection and localization of MI.[108] Analysis of the constellation of ECG leads showing ST elevation may also be useful for identifying the site of occlusion in the infarct artery.[108] The extent of ST deviation on the ECG, location of infarction, and QRS duration correlate with risk of adverse outcomes.[109] Even when left bundle branch block is present on the ECG, MI can be diagnosed when striking ST segment deviation is present beyond that which can be explained by the conduction defect.[108] In addition to the diagnostic and prognostic information contained within the 12-lead ECG, it also provides valuable noninvasive information about the success of reperfusion for STEMI (see Chap. 47).[108,110]

Although general agreement exists on electrocardiographic and vectorcardiographic criteria for the recognition of infarction of the anterior and inferior myocardial walls, less agreement is found on criteria for lateral and posterior infarcts[111]; in this area, even the terminology can be confusing. It has been reported that patients with an abnormal R wave in V_1 (0.04 sec in duration and/or R/S ratio ≥ 1 in the absence of preexcitation or right ventricular hypertrophy) with inferior or lateral Q waves have an increased incidence of isolated occlusion of a dominant left circumflex coronary artery without collateral circulation; such patients have a lower ejection fraction, increased end-systolic volume, and higher complication rate than patients with inferior infarction due to isolated occlusion of the right coronary artery.

More sophisticated forms of ECG recordings, including high-resolution electrocardiography, body surface potential mapping of ST segments, and continuous vectorcardiography, have all been reported in small series of patients to augment the 12-lead ECG in diagnosing MI, but the lack of ready availability of equipment and the special expertise required limits the use of these techniques.

Although most patients continue to demonstrate the ECG changes from an infarction for the rest of their lives, particularly if they evolve Q waves, in a substantial minority the typical changes disappear, Q waves can regress, and the ECG can even return to normal after a number of years. Under many circumstances, Q-wave patterns simulate MI. Conditions that may mimic the electrocardiographic features of MI by producing a pattern of "pseudoinfarction" include ventricular hypertrophy, conduction disturbances, preexcitation, primary myocardial disease, pneumothorax, pulmonary embolus, amyloid heart disease, primary and metastatic tumors of the heart, traumatic heart disease, intracranial hemorrhage, hyperkalemia, pericarditis, early repolarization, and cardiac involvement with sarcoidosis.

Q-WAVE AND NON-Q-WAVE INFARCTION. As noted earlier, the presence or absence of Q waves on the surface ECG does not reliably predict the distinction between transmural and nontransmural (subendocardial) MI.[25] Q waves on the ECG signify abnormal electrical activity but are not synonymous with irreversible myocardial damage. Also, the absence of Q waves may simply reflect the insensitivity of the standard 12-lead ECG, especially in the posterior zones of the left ventricle. True pathological subendocardial MI, as recognized at autopsy, is seen with ST-segment depression and/or T-wave changes only about 50 percent of the time.[112] Angiographic studies in MI patients without ST-segment elevation show a higher incidence of subtotal occlusion of the culprit coronary vessel and greater collateral flow to the infarct zone. Observational data suggest that MI without ST-segment elevation is seen more commonly in elderly patients and patients with a prior MI.

ISCHEMIA AT A DISTANCE. Patients with new Q waves and ST-segment elevation diagnostic for STEMI in one territory often have ST-segment depression in other territories. These additional ST-segment changes are caused either by ischemia in a territory other than the area of infarction, termed *ischemia at a distance*, or by reciprocal electrical phenomena. A good deal of attention has been directed to associated ST-segment depression in the anterior leads, when it occurs in patients with acute inferior STEMI. However, despite the clinical importance of differentiation among causes of anterior ST-segment depression in such patients, including anterior ischemia, posterior wall infarction, and true reciprocal changes, such a differentiation cannot be made reliably by electrocardiographic or even vectorcardiographic techniques. Although precordial ST-segment depression is more commonly associated with extensive infarction of the posterior, lateral, or inferior septal segments, rather than anterior wall subendocardial ischemia, imaging techniques such as two-dimensional echocardiography are necessary to ascertain whether an anterior wall motion abnormality is present.[113] Regardless of whether the anterior ST-segment changes reflect anterior wall ischemia or are reciprocal to changes elsewhere, this finding, as with ischemia at a distance, implies a poorer prognosis than if such changes were not present.[114]

RIGHT VENTRICULAR INFARCTION. ST-segment elevation in right precordial leads (V_1, V_3R-V_6R) is a relatively sensitive and specific sign of right ventricular infarction.[108,115] Occasionally, ST-segment elevation in leads V_2 and V_3 is due to acute right ventricular infarction; this appears to occur only when the injury to the left inferior wall is minimal.[116–118] Usually, the concurrent inferior wall injury suppresses this anterior ST-segment elevation resulting from right ventricular injury. Likewise, right ventricular infarction appears to reduce the anterior ST-segment depression often observed with inferior wall myocardial infarction. A QS or QR pattern in leads V_3R and/or V_4R also suggests right ventricular myocardial necrosis but has less predictive accuracy than ST-segment elevation in these leads.

ATRIAL INFARCTION. The most common electrocardiographic patterns are depression or elevation of the PR segment, alterations in the contour of the P wave, and abnormal atrial rhythms, including atrial flutter, atrial fibrillation, wandering atrial pacemaker, and atrioventricular nodal rhythm.[40]

Imaging

Roentgenography (see Chap. 12)

The initial chest roentgenogram in patients with STEMI is almost invariably a portable film obtained in the emergency room or the coronary care unit. When present, prominent pulmonary vascular markings on the roentgenogram reflect elevated left ventricular end-diastolic pressure, but significant temporal discrepancies can occur because of what have been termed *diagnostic lags* and *post-therapeutic lags*. Up to 12 hours can elapse before pulmonary edema accumulates after ventricular filling pressure has become elevated. The post-therapeutic phase lag represents a longer time interval; up to 2 days are required for pulmonary edema to resorb and the radiographic signs of pulmonary congestion to clear after ventricular filling pressure has returned toward normal. The degree of congestion and the size of the left side of the heart on the chest film are useful for defining groups of patients with STEMI who are at increased risk of dying after the acute event.[119]

Echocardiography (see Chap. 11)

TWO-DIMENSIONAL ECHOCARDIOGRAPHY. The relative portability of echocardiographic equipment makes this technique ideal for the assessment of patients with MI hospitalized in the coronary care unit or even in the emergency department before admission.[113] In patients with chest pain compatible with MI but with a nondiagnostic ECG, the finding on echocardiography of a distinct region of disordered contraction can be helpful diagnostically because it supports the diagnosis of myocardial ischemia. Echocardiography is also useful in evaluating patients with chest pain and a nondiagnostic ECG who are suspected of having an aortic dissection. The identification of an intimal flap consistent with an aortic dissection is a critical observation because it represents a major contraindication to fibrinolytic therapy (see Chap. 47).

Areas of abnormal regional wall motion are observed almost universally in patients with MI, and the degree of wall motion abnormality can be categorized with a semiquantitative wall motion score index. Of note, abnormal wall motion is less often noted echocardiographically when the infarction is small and the age of regional wall motion abnormality cannot always be determined. Left ventricular function estimated from two-dimensional echocardiograms correlates well with measurements from angiography and is useful in establishing prognosis after MI.[113] Furthermore, the early use of echocardiography can aid in the early detection of potentially viable but stunned myocardium (contractile reserve), residual provocable ischemia, patients at risk for the development of congestive heart failure after MI, and mechanical complications of MI.[113]

Although transthoracic imaging is adequate in most patients, occasional patients have poor echo windows, especially if they are undergoing mechanical ventilation. In such patients, transesophageal echocardiography can be safely performed and can be useful in evaluating ventricular septal defects and papillary muscle dysfunction.[120]

DOPPLER ECHOCARDIOGRAPHY. This technique (see Chap. 11) allows assessment of blood flow in the cardiac chambers and across cardiac valves. Used in conjunction with two-dimensional echocardiography, it is helpful in detecting and assessing the severity of mitral or tricuspid regurgitation after STEMI. Identification of the site of acute ventricular septal rupture, quantification of shunt flow across the resulting defect, and assessment of acute cardiac tamponade are also possible.[120,121]

Other Imaging Modalities

COMPUTED TOMOGRAPHY (see Chap. 15). This technique can provide useful cross-sectional information in patients with MI. In addition to the assessment of cavity dimensions and wall thickness, left ventricular aneurysms can be detected, and, of particular importance in patients with STEMI, intracardiac thrombi can be identified. Although cardiac computed tomography is a less convenient technique, it probably is more sensitive for thrombus detection than is echocardiography.

MAGNETIC RESONANCE IMAGING (see Chap. 14). In addition to localizing and sizing the area of infarction, magnetic resonance imaging techniques are capable of early recognition of MI and of providing an assessment of the severity of the ischemic insult. This modality is attractive because of its ability to assess perfusion of infarcted and noninfarcted tissue as well as of reperfused myocardium; to identify areas of jeopardized but not infarcted myocardium; to identify myocardial edema, fibrosis, wall thinning, and hypertrophy; to assess ventricular chamber size and segmental wall motion; and to identify the temporal transition between ischemia and infarction.[122] It has limited practical application, however, because of the need to transport patients with MI to the magnetic resonance imaging facility.

NUCLEAR IMAGING (see Chap. 13). Radionuclide angiography, perfusion imaging, infarct-avid scintigraphy, and positron emission tomography have been used to evaluate patients with STEMI.[123] Nuclear cardiac imaging techniques can be useful for detecting MI; assessing infarct size, collateral flow, and jeopardized myocardium; determining the effects of the infarct on ventricular function; and establishing prognosis of patients with STEMI.[123] However, the necessity of moving a critically ill patient from the coronary care unit (CCU) to the nuclear medicine department limits their practical application unless a portable gamma camera is available. Cardiac radionuclide imaging for the diagnosis of MI should be restricted to special limited situations in which the triad of clinical history, ECG findings, and serum marker measurements is unavailable or unreliable.

Estimation of Infarct Size

ELECTROCARDIOGRAPHY. Interest in limiting infarct size, in large part because of the recognition that the quantity of myocardium infarcted has important prognostic implications, has focused attention on the accurate determination of MI size. The sum of ST-segment elevations measured from multiple precordial leads correlates with the extent of myocardial injury in patients with anterior MI.[108] QRS scoring systems and planar or vectorcardiographic techniques to estimate infarct size have also been developed. Although they demonstrate good correlations with infarct size at autopsy and with enzymatic estimates, formal sizing of infarcts by ECG technique is not necessary in most patients. Of note, however, there is a relationship between the number of ECG leads showing ST-segment elevation and mortality rate: patients with 8 or 9 of 12 leads with ST-segment elevation have three to four times the mortality of those with only 2 or 3 leads with ST-segment elevation. The duration of ischemia time as estimated from continuous ST-segment monitoring is correlated with infarct size, the ratio of infarct size to area at risk, and the extent of regional wall motion abnormality observed subsequently.[124]

SERUM CARDIAC MARKERS. To estimate infarct size by analysis of serum cardiac markers, it is necessary to account for the quantity of the marker lost from the myocardium, its volume of distribution, and its release ratio.[125] Serial measurements of proteins released by necrotic myocardium are helpful in determining MI size. Clinically, the peak CK or CK-MB provides an approximate estimate of infarct size and is widely used prognostically. In the prethrombotic era, quantification of the cumulative release of CK or CK-MB correlated with other techniques for estimating infarct size in vivo as well as with the area of necrosis at autopsy. However, coronary artery reperfusion dramatically changes the wash-out kinetics of CK and other markers from myocardium, resulting in early and exaggerated peak levels and limiting the usefulness of such curves as a measure of infarct size.

NONINVASIVE IMAGING TECHNIQUES. Echocardiography (see Chap. 11), radionuclide scintigraphy (see Chap. 13),[123] computed tomography (see Chap. 15), and magnetic resonance imaging (see Chap. 14) have all been utilized for the clinical and experimental assessment of infarct size. Infarct-avid scintigraphy and myocardial perfusion imaging have been used to quantify infarct size. Estimation of infarct size by quantitative tomographic ^{99m}Tc-sestamibi imaging appears to be less limited by ventricular geometry and can distinguish small infarcts and ischemia from infarcted myocardium more readily than other noninvasive methods.[126] Tomography has improved on planar techniques employing technetium-99m pyrophosphate to image MI.[127] Contrast-enhanced magnetic resonance imaging has been helpful in demonstrating the regional heterogeneity of infarction patterns in patients with persistently occluded infarct arteries versus those with successfully reperfused vessels.[128]

REFERENCES

1. Luepker RV, Apple FS, Christenson RH, et al: Case definitions for acute coronary disease in epidemiology and clinical research studies. Circulation 108:2543, 2003.
2. Alpert JS, Thygesen K, Antman E, et al: Myocardial infarction redefined: A consensus document of The Joint European Society of Cardiology/American College of Cardiology Committee for the redefinition of myocardial infarction. J Am Coll Cardiol 36:959, 2000.
3. Newby LK, Alpert JS, Ohman EM, et al: Changing the diagnosis of acute myocardial infarction: Implications for practice and clinical investigators. Am Heart J 144:957, 2002.
4. White HD: Things ain't what they used to be: Impact of a new definition of myocardial infarction. Am Heart J 144:933, 2002.
5. Apple FS, Wu AHB, Jaffe AS: European Society of Cardiology and American College of Cardiology guidelines for the redefinition of myocardial infarction: How to use existing assays clinically and for clinical trials. Am Heart J 144:981, 2002.
6. Hamm CW, Bertrand M, Braunwald E: Acute coronary syndrome without ST elevation: Implementation of new guidelines. Lancet 358:1533, 2001.
7. Rogers WJ, Canto JG, Lambrew CT, et al: Temporal trends in the treatment of over 1.5 million patients with myocardial infarction in the US from 1990 through 1999: The National Registry of Myocardial Infarction 1, 2 and 3. J Am Coll Cardiol 36:2056, 2000.
8. Kesteloot H, Sans S, Kromhout D: Evolution of all-causes and cardiovascular mortality in the age-group 75-84 years in Europe during the period 1970-1996: A comparison with worldwide changes. Eur Heart J 23:384, 2002.
9. American Heart Association: Heart Disease and Stroke Statistics—2004 Update. Dallas, American Heart Association, 2003.
10. Ezzati M, Vander Hoorn S, Rodgers A, et al: Estimates of global and regional potential health gains from reducing multiple major risk factors. Lancet 362:271, 2003.
11. Tunstall-Pedoe H, Mahonen M, Tolonen H, et al: Contribution of trends in survival and coronary-event rates to changes in coronary heart disease mortality: 10-year results from 37 WHO MONICA Project populations. Lancet 353:1547, 1999.
12. Braunwald E, Antman EM, Beasley JW, et al: ACC/AHA 2002 guideline update for the management of patients with unstable angina and non-ST-segment elevation myocardial infarction—summary article: A report of the American College of Cardiology/American Heart Association task force on practice guidelines (Committee on the Management of Patients With Unstable Angina). J Am Coll Cardiol 40:1366, 2002.
13. Tunstall-Pedoe H, Vanuzzo D, Hobbs M, et al: Estimation of contribution of changes in coronary care to improving survival, event rates, and coronary heart disease mortality across the WHO MONICA Project populations. Lancet 355:688, 2000.
14. Braunwald E, Antman EM: Evidence-based coronary care. Ann Intern Med 126:551, 1997.
15. Antman EM, et al: ACC/AHA Guidelines for the Management of Patients with ST-Elevation Myocardial Infarction. 2004 (http://www.acc.org/clinical/guidelines/stemi/index.htm).

16. Boersma E, Mercado N, Poldermans D, et al: Acute myocardial infarction. Lancet 361:847, 2003.
17. Burwen DR, Galusha DH, Lewis JM, et al: National and state trends in quality of care for acute myocardial infarction between 1994-1995 and 1998-1999: The medicare health care quality improvement program. Arch Intern Med 163:1430, 2003.
18. Assessment of the Safety and Efficacy of a New Thrombolytic Regimen (ASSENT)-3 Investigators: Efficacy and safety of tenecteplase in combination with enoxaparin, abciximab, or unfractionated heparin: The ASSENT-3 randomised trial in acute myocardial infarction. Lancet 358:605, 2001.
19. Canto JG, Rogers WJ, Chandra NC, et al: The association of sex and payer status on management and subsequent survival in acute myocardial infarction. Arch Intern Med 162:587, 2002.
20. White HD: Thrombolytic therapy in the elderly. Lancet 356:2028, 2000.
21. Krumholz HM, Chen J, Rathore SS, et al: Regional variation in the treatment and outcomes of myocardial infarction: Investigating New England's advantage. Am Heart J 146:242, 2003.
22. Thiemann DR, Coresh J, Oetgen WJ, et al: The association between hospital volume and survival after acute myocardial infarction in elderly patients. N Engl J Med 340:1640, 1999.
23. Chen J, Radford MJ, Wang Y, et al: Do "America's Best Hospitals" perform better for acute myocardial infarction? N Engl J Med 340:286, 1999.
24. Vaccarino V, Parsons L, Every NR, et al: Sex-based differences in early mortality after myocardial infarction. National Registry of Myocardial Infarction 2 Participants. N Engl J Med 341:217, 1999.
25. Phibbs B, Marcus F, Marriott HJC, et al: Q-wave versus non-Q wave myocardial infarction: A meaningless distinction. J Am Coll Cardiol 33:576, 1999.

Pathology

26. Libby P: Current concepts of the pathogenesis of the acute coronary syndromes. Circulation 104:365, 2001.
27. Fuster V, Corti R, Fayad ZA, et al: Integration of vascular biology and magnetic resonance imaging in the understanding of atherothrombosis and acute coronary syndromes. J Thromb Haemost 1:1410, 2003.
28. Malek AM, Alper SL, Izumo S: Hemodynamic shear stress and its role in atherosclerosis. JAMA 282:2035, 1999.
29. Rosenberg RD, Aird WC: Vascular-bed-specific hemostasis and hypercoagulable states. N Engl J Med 340:1555, 1999.
30. Ardissino D, Merlini PA, Ariens R, et al: Tissue-factor antigen and activity in human coronary atherosclerotic plaques. Lancet 349:769, 1997.
31. Kloner RA, Leor J: Natural disaster plus wake-up time: A deadly combination of triggers. Am Heart J 137:779, 1999.
32. Goodman SG, Langer A, Ross AM, et al: Non-Q-wave versus Q-wave myocardial infarction after thrombolytic therapy: Angiographic and prognostic insights from the global utilization of streptokinase and tissue plasminogen activator for occluded coronary arteries-I angiographic substudy. GUSTO-I Angiographic Investigators. Circulation 97:444, 1998.
33. Vargas SO, Sampson BA, Schoen FJ: Pathologic detection of early myocardial infarction: A critical review of the evolution and usefulness of modern techniques. Mod Pathol 12:635, 1999.
34. Schoen FJ: The heart. *In* Cotran FS, Kumar V, Collins T (eds): Pathologic Basis of Disease. 7th ed. Philadelphia, WB Saunders, 2004.
35. Kloner RA, Ellis SG, Lange R, et al: Studies of experimental coronary artery reperfusion: Effects on infarct size, myocardial function, biochemistry, ultrastructure and microvascular damage. Circulation 68:15, 1983.
36. Lehrke S, Giannitsis E, Steen H, et al: Cardiac troponin T in ST-segment elevation acute myocardial infarction revisited. Cardiovasc Toxicol 1:99, 2001.
37. DeWood MA, Spores J, Notske RN, et al: Prevalence of total coronary artery occlusion during the early hours of transmural myocardial infarction. N Engl J Med 303:897, 1980.
38. Ozdemir K, Altunkeser BB, Icli A, et al: New parameters in identification of right ventricular myocardial infarction and proximal right coronary artery lesion. Chest 124:219, 2003.
39. Bowers TR, O'Neill WW, Grines C, et al: Effect of reperfusion on biventricular function and survival after right ventricular infarction. N Engl J Med 338:933, 1998.
40. Neven K, Crijns H, Gorgels A: Atrial infarction: A neglected electrocardiographic sign with important clinical implications. J Cardiovasc Electrophysiol 14:306, 2003.
41. Kyriakidis M, Barbetseas J, Antonopoulos A, et al: Early atrial arrhythmias in acute myocardial infarction. Role of the sinus node artery. Chest 101:944, 1992.
42. Fujita M, Nakae I, Kihara Y, et al: Determinants of collateral development in patients with acute myocardial infarction. Clin Cardiol 22:595, 1999.

Pathophysiology

43. Swan HJC, Forrester JS, Diamond G, et al: Hemodynamic spectrum of myocardial infarction and cardiogenic shock. Circulation 45:1097, 1972.
44. Forrester JS, Wyatt HL, Daluz PL, et al: Functional significance of regional ischemic contraction abnormalities. Circulation 54:64, 1976.
45. Schuster EH, Bulkley BH: Ischemia at a distance after acute myocardial infarction: A cause of early postinfarction angina. Circulation 62:509, 1980.
46. White HD, Norris RM, Brown MA, et al: Left ventricular end-systolic volume as the major determinant of survival after recovery from myocardial infarction. Circulation 76:44, 1987.
47. Pfeffer MA, Braunwald E: Ventricular remodeling after myocardial infarction. Experimental observations and clinical implications. Circulation 81:1161, 1990.
48. Sadanandan S, Buller CE, Menon V, et al: The late open artery hypothesis—A decade later. Am Heart J 142:411, 2001.
49. Braunwald E, Kim CB: Late establishment of patency of the infarct-related artery. *In* Julian D, Braunwald E (eds): Acute Myocardial Infarction. London, WB Saunders, 1994, pp 147-162.
50. Pfeffer MA, Lamas GA, Vaughan DE, et al: Effect of captopril on progressive ventricular dilatation after anterior myocardial infarction. N Engl J Med 319:80, 1988.
51. Hochman JS: Cardiogenic shock complicating acute myocardial infarction: Expanding the paradigm. Circulation 107:2998, 2003.
52. Pfeffer JM, Pfeffer MA, Fletcher PJ, et al: Progressive ventricular remodeling in rat with myocardial infarction. Am J Physiol 260:H1406, 1991.
53. Weisman HF, Bush DE, Mannisi JA, et al: Cellular mechanisms of myocardial infarct expansion. Circulation 78:186, 1988.
54. Pfeffer MA: Left ventricular remodeling after acute myocardial infarction. Ann Rev Med 46:455, 1995.
55. Schmermund A, Lerman LO, Ritman EL, et al: Cardiac production of angiotensin II and its pharmacologic inhibition: Effects on the coronary circulation. Mayo Clin Proc 74:503, 1999.
56. Gray BA, Hyde RW, Hodges M, et al: Alterations in lung volume and pulmonary function in relation to hemodynamic changes in acute myocardial infarction. Circulation 59:551, 1979.
57. Ceremuzynski L: Hormonal and metabolic reactions evoked by acute myocardial infarction. Circulation Res 48:767, 1981.
58. Sack MN, Yellon DM: Insulin therapy as an adjunct to reperfusion after acute coronary ischemia: A proposed direct myocardial cell survival effect independent of metabolic modulation. J Am Coll Cardiol 41:1404, 2003.
59. Stein BC, Levin RI: Natriuretic peptides: Physiology, therapeutic potential, and risk stratification in ischemic heart disease. Am Heart J 135:914, 1998.
60. de Lemos JA, Morrow DA, Bentley JH, et al: The prognostic value of B-type natriuretic peptide in patients with acute coronary syndromes. N Engl J Med 345:1014, 2001.
61. Morrow DA, Braunwald E: Future of biomarkers in acute coronary syndromes: Moving toward a multimarker strategy. Circulation 108:250, 2003.
62. Li YH, Teng JK, Tsai WC, et al: Prognostic significance of elevated hemostatic markers in patients with acute myocardial infarction. J Am Coll Cardiol 33:1543, 1999.
63. Sabatine MS, Morrow DA, Cannon CP, et al: Relationship between baseline white blood cell count and degree of coronary artery disease and mortality in patients with acute coronary syndromes: A TACTICS-TIMI 18 (Treat Angina with Aggrastat and determine Cost of Therapy with an Invasive or Conservative Strategy-Thrombolysis in Myocardial Infarction 18 trial) substudy. J Am Coll Cardiol 40:1761, 2002.

Clinical Features

64. Singh JP, Muller JE: Triggers to acute coronary syndromes. *In* Theroux P (ed): Acute Coronary Syndromes: A Companion to Braunwald's Heart Disease. Philadelphia, WB Saunders, 2003, pp 108-118.
65. Eagle KA, Berger PB, Calkins H, et al: ACC/AHA guideline update for perioperative cardiovascular evaluation for noncardiac surgery—Executive summary: A report of the American College of Cardiology/American Heart Association Task Force on Practice Guidelines (Committee to Update the 1996 Guidelines on Perioperative Cardiovascular Evaluation for Noncardiac Surgery). J Am Coll Cardiol 39:542, 2002.
66. Maseri A, L'Abbate A, Baroldi G, et al: Coronary vasospasm as a possible cause of myocardial infarction. N Engl J Med 299:1271, 1978.
67. Muller JE, Abela GS, Nesto RW, et al: Triggers, acute risk factors and vulnerable plaques: The lexicon of a new frontier. J Am Coll Cardiol 23:809, 1994.
68. Spodick DH: Pericardial complications of myocardial infarction. *In* Francis GS, Alpert JS (eds): Coronary Care. 2nd ed. Boston, Little, Brown & Company, 1995, pp 333-341.
69. Balaban DH, Yamamoto Y, Liu J, et al: Sustained esophageal contraction: A marker of esophageal chest pain identified by intraluminal ultrasonography. Gastroenterology 116:29, 1999.
70. McGuire DK, Granger CB: Diabetes and ischemic heart disease. Am Heart J 138:366, 1999.
71. Webb SW, Adgey AA, Pantridge JF: Autonomic disturbance at onset of acute myocardial infarction. BMJ 818:89, 1982.
72. Killip T, Kimball JT: Treatment of myocardial infarction in a coronary care unit: A two year experience with 250 patients. Am J Cardiol 20:457, 1967.
73. Magnesium in Coronaries (MAGIC) Trial Investigators: Early administration of intravenous magnesium to high-risk patients with acute myocardial infarction in the Magnesium in Coronaries (MAGIC) Trial: A randomised controlled trial. Lancet 360:1189, 2002.
74. Pedoe-Tunstall H, Kuulasmaa K, Amouyel P, et al: Myocardial infarction and coronary deaths in the World Health Organization MONICA Project. Circulation 90:583, 1994.
75. Ravkilde J, Horder M, Gerhardt W, et al: Diagnostic performance and prognostic value of serum troponin T in suspected acute myocardial infarction. Scand J Clin Lab Invest 53:677, 1993.
76. Antman EM: Decision making with cardiac troponin tests. N Engl J Med 346:2079, 2002.
77. Hamm CW: Cardiac biomarkers for rapid evaluation of chest pain. Circulation 104:1454, 2001.
78. Penttila K, Koukkunen H, Halinen M, et al: Myoglobin, creatine kinase MB isoforms and creatine kinase MB mass in early diagnosis of myocardial infarction in patients with acute chest pain. Clin Biochem 35:647, 2002.
79. French JK, Ramanathan K, Stewart JT, et al: A score predicts failure of reperfusion after fibrinolytic therapy for acute myocardial infarction. Am Heart J 145:508, 2003.
80. Apple FS, Quist HE, Doyle PJ, et al: Plasma 99th percentile reference limits for cardiac troponin and creatine kinase MB mass for use with European Society of Cardiology/American College of Cardiology consensus recommendations. Clin Chem 49:1331, 2003.
81. Apple FS: Tissue specificity of cardiac troponin I, cardiac troponin T and creatine kinase-MB. Clin Chim Acta 284:151, 1999.

82. Gibson CM, Murphy SA, Marble SJ, et al: Relationship of creatine kinase-myocardial band release to thrombolysis in myocardial infarction perfusion grade after intracoronary stent placement: An ESPRIT substudy. Am Heart J 143:106, 2002.
83. Roberts R, Kleiman N: Earlier diagnosis and treatment of acute myocardial infarction necessitates the need for a "new diagnostic mind-set." Circulation 89:872, 1994.
84. Zimmerman J, Fromm R, Meyer D, et al: Diagnostic marker cooperative study for the diagnosis of myocardial infarction. Circulation 99:1671, 1999.
85. Apple FS: Creatine kinase isoforms and myoglobin: Early detection of myocardial infarction and reperfusion. Coron Artery Dis 10:75, 1999.
86. Wu AH, Apple FS, Gibler WB, et al: National Academy of Clinical Biochemistry Standards of Laboratory Practice: Recommendations for the use of cardiac markers in coronary artery diseases. Clin Chem 45:1104, 1999.
87. de Lemos JA, Morrow DA, Gibson CM, et al: Early noninvasive detection of failed epicardial reperfusion after fibrinolytic therapy. Am J Cardiol 88:353, 2001.
88. Srinivas VS, Cannon CP, Gibson CM, et al: Myoglobin levels at 12 hours identify patients at low risk for 30-day mortality after thrombolysis in acute myocardial infarction: A Thrombolysis in Myocardial Infarction 10B substudy. Am Heart J 142:29, 2001.
89. de Lemos JA, Antman EM, Giugliano RP, et al: Very early risk stratification after thrombolytic therapy with a bedside myoglobin assay and the 12-lead electrocardiogram. Am Heart J 140:373, 2000.
90. Alpert JS, Thygesen K, Antman E, Bassand JP: Myocardial infarction redefined—A consensus document of the Joint European Society of Cardiology/American College of Cardiology Committee for the redefinition of myocardial infarction. J Am Coll Cardiol 36:959, 2000.
91. Jaffe AS, Ravkilde J, Roberts R, et al: It's time for a change to a troponin standard. Circulation 102:1216, 2000.
92. Apple FS, Murakami MM, Jesse RL, et al: Near-bedside whole-blood cardiac troponin I assay for risk assessment of patients with acute coronary syndromes. Clin Chem 48:1784, 2002.
93. Aviles RJ, Askari AT, Lindahl B, et al: Troponin T levels in patients with acute coronary syndromes, with or without renal dysfunction. N Engl J Med 346:2047, 2002.
94. Katrukha AG, Bereznikova AV, Esakova TV, et al: Troponin I is released in bloodstream of patients with acute myocardial infarction not in free form but as complex. Clin Chem 43:1379, 1997.
95. Cheitlin MD, Khayam-Bashi H: Biomarkers of myocardial infarction: Finding the right cut-off point. Cardiol Rev 9:323, 2001.
96. Antman EM, Grudzien C, Sacks DB: Evaluation of a rapid bedside assay for detection of serum cardiac troponin T. JAMA 273:1279, 1995.
97. Tanasijevic MJ, Cannon CP, Antman EM, et al: Myoglobin, creatine-kinase-MB and cardiac troponin-I 60-minute ratios predict infarct-related artery patency after thrombolysis for acute myocardial infarction: Results from the Thrombolysis in Myocardial Infarction study (TIMI) 10B. J Am Coll Cardiol 34:739, 1999.
98. Panteghini M, Apple FS, Christenson RH, et al: Use of biochemical markers in acute coronary syndromes. IFCC Scientific Division, Committee on Standardization of Markers of Cardiac Damage. International Federation of Clinical Chemistry. Clin Chem Lab Med 37:687, 1999.
99. Apple FS, Wu AH: Myocardial infarction redefined: Role of cardiac troponin testing. Clin Chem 47:377, 2001.
100. Collinson PO, Stubbs PJ, Kessler AC: Multicentre evaluation of the diagnostic value of cardiac troponin T, CK-MB mass, and myoglobin for assessing patients with suspected acute coronary syndromes in routine clinical practice. Heart 89:280, 2003.
101. Ohman EM, Armstrong PW, White HD, et al: Risk stratification with a point-of-care cardiac troponin T test in acute myocardial infarction. Am J Cardiol 84:1281, 1999.
102. Wolfrum S, Jensen KS, Liao JK: Endothelium-dependent effects of statins. Arterioscler Thromb Vasc Biol 23:729, 2003.
103. Teo KK, Burton JR: Who should receive HMG CoA reductase inhibitors? Drugs 62:1707, 2002.
104. MRC/BHF Heart Protection Study of cholesterol lowering with simvastatin in 20,536 high-risk individuals: A randomised placebo-controlled trial. Lancet 360:7, 2002.
105. Barron HV, Cannon CP, Murphy SA, et al: Association between white blood cell count, epicardial blood flow, myocardial perfusion, and clinical outcomes in the setting of acute myocardial infarction: A thrombolysis in myocardial infarction 10 substudy. Circulation 102:2329, 2000.
106. Berton G, Cordiano R, Palmieri R, et al: C-reactive protein in acute myocardial infarction: Association with heart failure. Am Heart J 145:1094, 2003.
107. Sano T, Tanaka A, Namba M, et al: C-reactive protein and lesion morphology in patients with acute myocardial infarction. Circulation 108:282, 2003.

Electrocardiography

108. Zimetbaum PJ, Josephson ME: Use of the electrocardiogram in acute myocardial infarction. N Engl J Med 348:933, 2003.
109. Manes C, Pfeffer MA, Rutherford JD, et al: Value of the electrocardiogram in predicting left ventricular enlargement and dysfunction after myocardial infarction. Am J Med 114:99, 2003.
110. Feldman LJ, Coste P, Furber A, et al: Incomplete resolution of ST-segment elevation is a marker of transient microcirculatory dysfunction after stenting for acute myocardial infarction. Circulation 107:2684, 2003.
111. Cooksey JD, Dunn M, Massie E: Clinical Vectorcardiography and Electrocardiography. 2nd ed. Chicago, Year Book Medical Publishers, 1977.
112. Levine HD: Subendocardial infarction in retrospect: Pathologic, cardiographic, and ancillary features. Circulation 72:790, 1985.
113. Cheitlin MD, Armstrong WF, Aurigemma GP, et al: ACC/AHA/ASE 2003 guideline update for the clinical application of echocardiography: A report of the American College of Cardiology/American Heart Association Task Force on Practice Guidelines (ACC/AHA/ASE Committee to Update the 1997 Guidelines on the Clinical Application of Echocardiography). American College of Cardiology, 2003. (http://www.acc.org/clinical/guidelines/echocardiography/dirIndex.htm)
114. Mirvis DM: Physiologic bases for anterior ST segment depression in patients with acute inferior wall myocardial infarction. Am Heart J 116:1308, 1988.
115. Lopez-Sendon J, Coma-Canella I, Alcasena S, et al: Electrocardiographic findings in acute right ventricular infarction: Sensitivity and specificity of electrocardiographic alterations in right precordial leads V4R, V3R, V1, V2, and V3. J Am Coll Cardiol 6:1273, 1985.
116. Geft IL, Shah PK, Rodriguez L, et al: ST elevations in leads V1 to V5 may be caused by right coronary artery occlusion and acute right ventricular infarction. Am J Cardiol 53:991, 1984.
117. Acikel M, Yilmaz M, Bozkurt E, et al: ST segment elevation in leads V1 to V3 due to isolated right ventricular branch occlusion during primary right coronary angioplasty. Catheter Cardiovasc Interv 60:32, 2003.
118. Finn AV, Antman EM: Images in clinical medicine. Isolated right ventricular infarction. N Engl J Med 349:1636, 2003.

Imaging

119. Brattler A, Karliner JS, Higgins CB, et al: The initial chest x-ray in acute myocardial infarction: Prediction of early and late mortality and survival. Circulation 61:1004, 1980.
120. Reimold SC, Antman EM: Noninvasive cardiac imaging in chest pain syndromes. J Thrombosis Thrombolysis 6:239, 1998.
121. Spodick DH: Acute cardiac tamponade. N Engl J Med 349:684, 2003.
122. Pohost GM, Hung L, Doyle M: Clinical use of cardiovascular magnetic resonance. Circulation 108:647, 2003.
123. Klocke FJ, Baird MG, Bateman TM, et al: ACC/AHA/ASNC guidelines for the clinical use of cardiac radionuclide imaging: A report of the American College of Cardiology/American Heart Association Task Force on Practice Guidelines (ACC/AHA/ASNC Committee to Revise the 1995 Guidelines for the Clinical Use of Radionuclide Imaging). American College of Cardiology, 2003 (http://www.acc.org/clinical/guidelines/radio/dirIndex.htm).
124. Krucoff MW, Johanson P, Crater SW, et al: The clinical utility of serial and continuous ST-segment recovery in patients with acute ST elevation myocardial infarction: Assessing the dynamics of epicardial and myocardial reperfusion. Circulation 2004, in press.
125. Adams J III, Abendschein D, Jaffe A: Biochemical markers of myocardial injury. Is MB creatine kinase the choice for the 1990s? Circulation 88:750, 1993.
126. Gibbons RJ, Miller TD, Christian TF: Infarct size measured by single photon emission computed tomographic imaging with (99m)Tc-sestamibi : A measure of the efficacy of therapy in acute myocardial infarction. Circulation 101:101, 2000.
127. Kopecky SL, Aviles RJ, Bell MR, et al: A randomized, double-blinded, placebo -controlled, dose-ranging study measuring the effect of an adenosine agonist on infarct size reduction in patients undergoing primary percutaneous transluminal coronary angioplasty: The ADMIRE (AmP579 Delivery for Myocardial Infarction REduction) study. Am Heart J 146:146, 2003.
128. Kwong RY, Yucel EK: Computed tomography and magnetic resonance imaging. Circulation 108:e104, 2003.

CHAPTER 47

ST-Elevation Myocardial Infarction: Management

Elliott M. Antman

Although considerable advances have been made in the process of care for patients with ST-elevation myocardial infarction (STEMI), room for improvement exists, especially in special populations such as the very elderly and members of ethnic minority groups.[1-4] It is useful to organize a discussion of the phases of management of STEMI along the chronology of the interface of clinicians with the patient. Primary and secondary prevention of STEMI are discussed in Chapter 42. Treatment at the time of onset of STEMI (prehospital issues, initial recognition and management in the emergency department, reperfusion), hospital management (medications, arrhythmics, complications, preparation for discharge), and secondary prevention of STEMI are discussed in this chapter. The reader is referred to Chapter 48 for a discussion of percutaneous coronary intervention (PCI) in patients with STEMI.

PREHOSPITAL CARE. The prehospital care of patients with suspected STEMI is a crucial element bearing directly on the likelihood of survival. Most deaths associated with STEMI occur within the first hour of its onset and are usually due to ventricular fibrillation (see Chap. 32). Accordingly, the importance of the immediate implementation of definitive resuscitative efforts and of rapidly transporting the patient to a hospital cannot be overemphasized. Major components of the delay from the onset of symptoms consistent with acute myocardial infarction to reperfusion include the following[5]: (1) the time for the patient to recognize the seriousness of the problem and seek medical attention; (2) prehospital evaluation, treatment, and transportation; (3) the time for diagnostic measures and initiation of treatment in the hospital (e.g., "door-to-needle" time for patients receiving a thrombolytic agent and "door-to-balloon" time for patients undergoing a catheter-based reperfusion strategy); and (4) the time from initiation of treatment to restoration of flow (Fig. 47–1).

Patient-related factors that correlate with a longer time to the decision to seek medical attention include older age, female gender, African-American race, low socioeconomic status, low emotional or somatic awareness, history of angina, diabetes, or both, consulting a spouse or other relative, and consulting a physician.[5,6] Health care professionals should heighten the level of awareness of patients at risk for STEMI (e.g., those with hypertension, diabetes, history of angina pectoris).[5,7] They should review and reinforce with patients and their families the need to seek urgent medical attention for a pattern of symptoms including chest discomfort, extreme fatigue, and dyspnea, especially if accompanied by diaphoresis, lightheadedness, palpitations, or a sense of impending doom.[8,9] Although many patients shun such discussions and tend to minimize the likelihood of ever needing emergency cardiac treatment, emphasis should be placed on the prevention and treatment of potentially fatal arrhythmias as well as salvage of the jeopardized myocardium by reperfusion, for which time is crucial.[8] Patients should also be instructed in the proper use of sublingual nitroglycerin and to call 911 emergency services if the ischemic-type discomfort persists for more than 5 minutes.[10,11]

EMERGENCY MEDICAL SERVICES (EMS) SYSTEMS. These have three major components: emergency medical dispatch, first response, and EMS ambulance response. Ongoing efforts to shorten the time to treatment of patients with STEMI include improvement in the medical dispatch component by expanding 911 coverage, providing automated external defibrillators to first responders, placing automated external defibrillators in critical public locations, and greater coordination of EMS ambulance response.[12,13] Well-equipped ambulances and helicopters staffed by personnel trained in the acute care of the STEMI patient allow definitive therapy to commence while the patient is being transported to the hospital (Table 47–1). To be used effectively, they must be placed strategically within a community, and excellent radio communication systems must be available. These units should be equipped with battery-operated monitoring equipment, a DC defibrillator, oxygen, endotracheal tubes and suction apparatus, and commonly used cardiovascular drugs. Radiotelemetry systems that allow transmission of the electrocardiographic (ECG) signal to a medical control officer are highly desirable to facilitate triage of STEMI patients and are becoming increasingly available in many communities (Fig. 47–2). Observations of simple variables such as age, heart rate, and blood pressure permit initial classification of patients into high- or low-risk subgroups.[14]

In addition to prompt defibrillation, the efficacy of prehospital care appears to depend on several factors, including early relief of pain with its deleterious physiological sequelae, reduction of excessive activity of the autonomic nervous system, and abolition of prelethal arrhythmias, such as ventricular tachycardia. However, these efforts must not inhibit rapid transfer to the hospital (see Fig. 47–2).

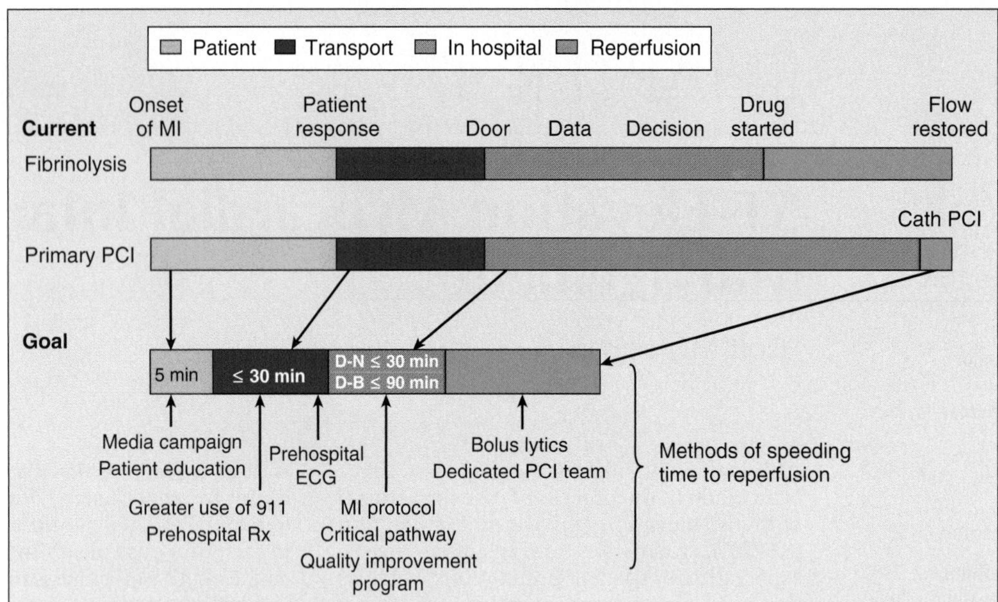

FIGURE 47–1 Major components of time delay between onset of infarction and restoration of flow in the infarct-related artery. Plotted sequentially from left to right are the time for patients to recognize symptoms and seek medical attention, transportation to the hospital, in-hospital decision-making and implementation of reperfusion strategy, and time for restoration of flow once the reperfusion strategy has been initiated. The time to initiate fibrinolytic therapy is the "door-to-needle" (D-N) time; this is followed by the period of time required for pharmacological restoration of flow. More time is required to move the patient to the catheterization laboratory for a percutaneous coronary interventional (PCI) procedure, referred to as the "door-to-balloon" (D-B) time, but restoration of flow in the epicardial infarct-related artery occurs promptly after PCI. At the bottom are shown a variety of methods for speeding the time to reperfusion along with the goals for the time intervals for the various components of the time delay. (Adapted from Cannon CP, Antman EM, Walls R, Braunwald E: Time as adjunctive agent to thrombolytic therapy. J Thromb Thrombolysis 1:27, 1994.)

TABLE 47–1 Reperfusion Checklist for Evaluation of the STEMI Patient

Step One: Has patient experienced chest discomfort for **greater than** 15 min and **less than** 12 hr?

YES → Step Two

NO → STOP

Step Two: Are there contraindications to fibrinolysis?
If ANY of the following are CHECKED, fibrinolysis ***MAY*** be contraindicated.

Systolic blood pressure greater than 180 mm Hg	■ **YES**	NO
Diastolic blood pressure greater than 110 mm Hg	■ **YES**	NO
Right vs. left arm systolic blood pressure difference greater than 15 mm Hg	■ **YES**	NO
History of structural central nervous system disease	■ **YES**	NO
Significant closed head/facial trauma within the previous 3 mo	■ **YES**	NO
Recent (within 6 wk) major trauma, surgery (including laser eye surgery), gastrointestinal or genitourinary bleed	■ **YES**	NO
Bleeding or clotting problem on blood thinners	■ **YES**	NO
CPR more than 10 min	■ **YES**	NO
Pregnant female	■ **YES**	NO
Serious systemic disease (e.g., advanced/terminal cancer, severe liver or kidney disease)	■ **YES**	NO

Step Three: Does the patient have severe heart failure or cardiogenic shock such that percutaneous coronary intervention is preferable?

Pulmonary edema (rales greater than halfway up)	■ YES	**NO**
Systemic hypoperfusion (cold, clammy)	■ YES	**NO**

From Antman EM, et al: ACC/AHA Guidelines for the Management of Patients with ST-Elevation Myocardial Infarction, 2004 (http://www.acc.org/clinical/guidelines/stemi/index.htm).

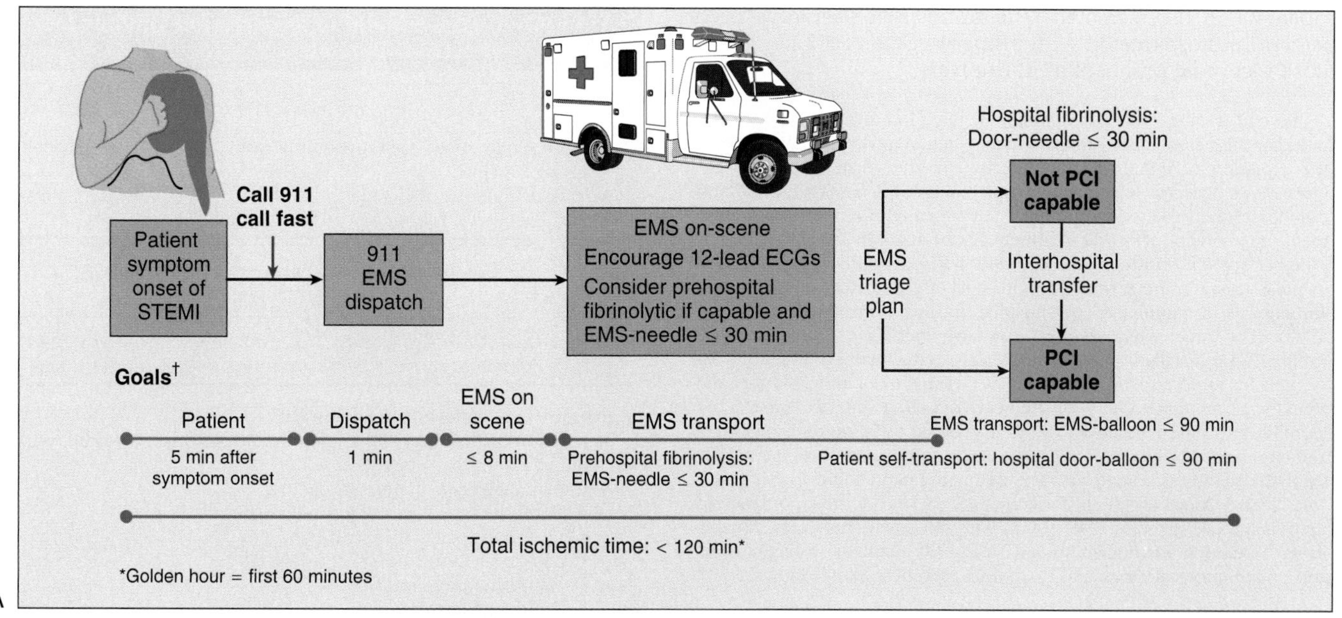

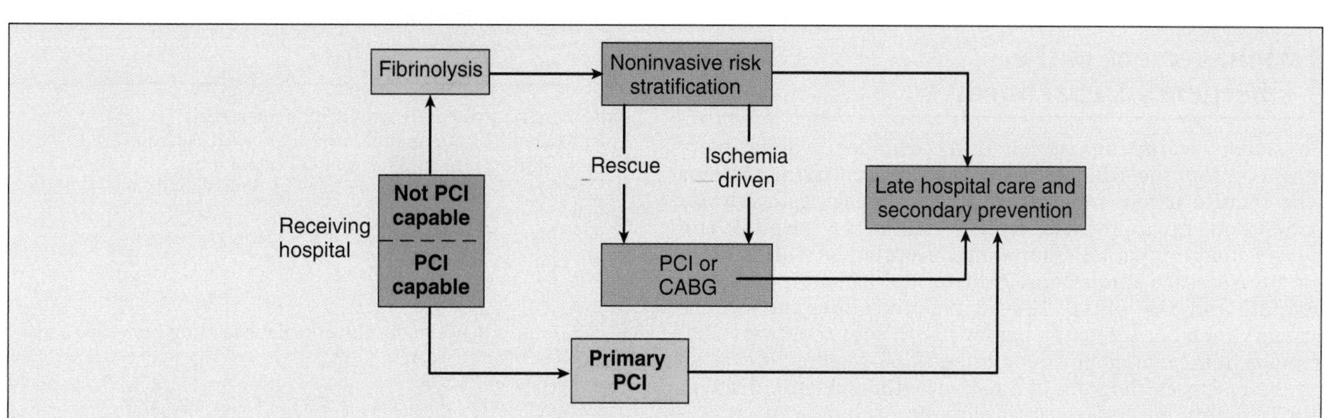

FIGURE 47–2 Options for transportation of STEMI patients and initial reperfusion treatment. Reperfusion in patients with STEMI can be accomplished by the pharmacological (fibrinolysis) or catheter-based (primary PCI) approaches. Implementation of these strategies varies based on the mode of transportation of the patient and capabilities at the receiving hospital. **A,** Patient transported by emergency medical services (EMS) after calling 911. Transport time to the hospital is variable from case to case, but the goal is to keep total ischemic time less than 120 minutes. There are three possibilities. (1) If EMS has fibrinolytic capability and the patient qualifies for therapy, prehospital fibrinolysis should be started within 30 minutes of EMS arrival on scene. (2) If EMS is not capable of administering prehospital fibrinolysis and the patient is transported to a non-PCI capable hospital, the hospital door-to-needle time should be less than or equal to 30 minutes for patients in whom fibrinolysis is indicated. (3) If EMS is not capable of administering prehospital fibrinolysis and the patient is transported to a PCI-capable hospital, the hospital door-to-balloon time should be less than or equal to 90 minutes.

Interhospital transfer. It is also appropriate to consider emergency interhospital transfer of the patient to a PCI-capable hospital for mechanical revascularization if (1) there is a contraindication to fibrinolysis; (2) PCI can be initiated promptly (≤90 min after the patient presented to the initial receiving hospital or ≤60 min compared to when fibrinolysis could be initiated at the initial receiving hospital; (3) fibrinolysis is administered and is unsuccessful (i.e., "rescue PCI"). Secondary nonemergency interhospital transfer can be considered for recurrent ischemia **(B)**.

Patient self-transport. Patient self-transportation is discouraged. If the patient arrives at a non-PCI-capable hospital, the door-to-needle time should be 30 minutes or less. If the patient arrives at a PCI-capable hospital, the door-to-balloon time should be 90 minutes or less. The treatment options and time recommendations after first hospital arrival are the same.

B, For patients who receive fibrinolysis, noninvasive risk stratification is recommended to identify the need for rescue PCI (failed fibrinolysis) or ischemia drive PCI. Regardless of the initial method of reperfusion treatment, all patients should receive late hospital care and secondary prevention of STEMI.

†The medical system goal is to facilitate rapid recognition and treatment of patients with STEMI such that door-to-needle (or EMS-to-needle) for initiation of fibrinolytic therapy can be achieved within 30 minutes or that door-to-balloon (or EMS-to-balloon) or PCI can be achieved within 90 minutes. These goals should not be understood as "ideal" times, but rather the longest times that should be considered acceptable for a given system. Systems that are able to achieve even more rapid times for treatment of patients with STEMI should be encouraged. (Adapted from Armstrong PW, Collen D, Antman E: Fibrinolysis for acute myocardial infarction: The future is here and now. Circulation 107:2533, 2003; and Antman EM, et al: ACC/AHA Guidelines for the Management of Patients with ST-Elevation Myocardial Infarction, 2004 [http://www.acc.org/clinical/guidelines/stemi/index.html]).

PREHOSPITAL FIBRINOLYSIS. The potential benefits of prehospital versus in-hospital fibrinolysis have been evaluated in several randomized trials. Although none of the individual trials showed a significant reduction in mortality with prehospital-initiated thrombolytic therapy, there was a generally consistent observation of benefit from earlier treatment, and a meta-analysis of all the available trials demonstrated a 17 percent reduction in mortality.[15] The CAPTIM trial reported a trend toward a lower rate of mortality among STEMI patients receiving prehospital fibrinolysis as compared with primary PCI, especially if patients were treated within 2 hours of the onset of symptoms.[16,17] Additional support for the benefit of prehospital lysis is found in a report from a French registry of STEMI patients treated less than 12 hours from the onset of symptoms; the 1-month mortality rate was 14.7 percent in patients who did not receive reperfusion,

9 percent in those treated with in-hospital fibrinolysis, 7.9 percent in those treated with primary PCI, and 3.2 percent in those receiving prehospital fibrinolysis.[18]

Several factors must be weighed when communities consider whether their ambulances and emergency transport vehicles should have the capability to initiate fibrinolytic therapy. The greatest reduction in mortality is observed when reperfusion can be initiated within 60 to 90 minutes of the onset of symptoms.[19] Streamlining of emergency department triage practices so that treatment can be started within 30 minutes, when coupled with the 15- to 30-minute transport time that is common in most urban centers, may be more cost-effective than equipping all ambulances to administer prehospital fibrinolytic therapy (see Fig. 47-2).[7] The latter would require extensive training of personnel (see Table 47-1), installation of computer-assisted electrocardiography or systems for radio transmission of the ECG signal to a central station, and stocking of medicine kits with the necessary drug supplies. In selected communities where transport delays may be 60 to 90 minutes or longer and experienced personnel are available on ambulances, prehospital fibrinolytic therapy is beneficial.[20] Therefore, prehospital fibrinolysis is reasonable in settings in which physicians are present in the ambulance or there is a well-organized EMS system with full-time paramedics, capability for obtaining and transmitting 12-lead ECG readings from the field, and on-line medical command to authorize prehospital fibrinolysis.

Management in the Emergency Department

Physicians evaluating patients in the emergency department must confront the difficult task of rapidly identifying patients who require urgent reperfusion therapy, triaging lower risk patients to the appropriate facility within the hospital, and not discharging patients home inappropriately while avoiding unnecessary admissions. A history of ischemic-type discomfort and the initial 12-lead electrocardiogram are the primary tools for screening patients with acute coronary syndromes in the emergency department.[21] ST segment elevation on the electrocardiogram of a patient with ischemic discomfort is highly suggestive of thrombotic occlusion of an epicardial coronary artery, and its presence should serve as the trigger for a well-rehearsed sequence of rapid assessment of the patient for contraindications to fibrinolysis and initiation of a reperfusion strategy (Tables 47–2 and 47–3).[7] Since the 12-lead electrocardiogram is at the center of the decision pathway for initiation of reperfusion therapy, it should be obtained promptly (≤10 minutes) in patients presenting with ischemic discomfort.

Because lethal arrhythmias can occur suddenly in patients with STEMI, all patients should be attached to a bedside ECG monitor and intravenous access obtained for infusion of 5 percent dextrose in water. If the initial ECG reading shows ST segment elevation of 1 mm or more in at least two contiguous leads or a new or presumably new left bundle branch block, the patient should be evaluated immediately for a reperfusion strategy. Critical factors to be considered when selecting a reperfusion strategy include (1) the time elapsed since the onset of symptoms, (2) the risk associated with STEMI, (3) the risk of administering fibrinolysis, and (4) the time required to initiate an invasive strategy (see Table 47–2). There is controversy about which form of reperfusion therapy is superior. A detailed discussion of the issues is found later in this chapter.

Given the importance of time to reperfusion,[13] the concept of medical system goals has arisen. Benchmarks for medical systems to use when assessing the quality of their performance are a door-to-needle time of ≤30 minutes for initiation of fibrinolytic therapy and a door-to-balloon time of ≤90 minutes for PCI (see Fig. 47–2).[7] With increasing sophistication of EMS systems, it is possible to initiate the process of evaluation/implementation of a reperfusion strategy even before the patient arrives in the emergency department. For those patients transported by ambulance, the medical system goals can be restated as an EMS-to-needle time of ≤30 minutes for initiation of fibrinolysis and an EMS-to-balloon time of ≤90 minutes for initiation of PCI (see Fig. 47–2).[7,22] An intriguing proposal that may also facilitate care of patients with STEMI is the development of regionalized centers for care of patients with acute ischemic heart disease.[23] Implementation of such "centers of excellence" requires a coordinated commitment of multiple components of the health care system—a formidable challenge, but one that many authorities believe is a vital step toward improvement of care of patients with STEMI.[24]

Patients with an initial ECG reading that reveals new or presumably new ST segment depression and/or T wave inversion, while not considered candidates for thrombolytic therapy, should be treated as though they are suffering from myocardial infarction without ST elevation or unstable

TABLE 47–2 Assessment of Reperfusion Options for STEMI Patients

Step 1: Assess time and risk.

- Time since onset of symptoms
- Risk of STEMI
- Risk of fibrinolysis
- Time required for transport to a skilled PCI lab

Step 2: Determine if fibrinolysis or invasive strategy is preferred.

- *If presentation is less than 3 hr and there is no delay to an invasive strategy, there is no preference for either strategy.*

Fibrinolysis is generally preferred if:

- Early presentation (≤ 3hr from symptom onset and delay to invasive strategy) (see below)
- Invasive strategy is not an option
  - Catheterization lab occupied or not available
  - Vascular access difficulties
  - Lack of access to a skilled PCI lab†‡
- Delay to invasive strategy
  - Prolonged transport
  - (Door-to-Balloon)–(Door-to-Needle) more than 1 hr*§
  - Medical contact-to-balloon or door-to-balloon more than 90 min

An invasive strategy is generally preferred if:

- Skilled PCI lab available with surgical backup
  - Skilled PCI lab is available, defined by:†‡
  - Medical contact-to-balloon or door-to-balloon less than 90 min
  - (Door-to-Balloon)–(Door-to-Needle) less than 1 hr*
- High risk from STEMI
  - Cardiogenic shock
  - Killip class ≥ 3
- Contraindications to fibrinolysis including increased risk of bleeding and ICH
- Late presentation
  - Symptom onset was more than 3 hr ago
- Diagnosis of STEMI is in doubt

*Applies to fibrin-specific agents.
†Operator experience greater than a total of 75 primary PCI cases/yr.
‡Team experience greater than a total of 36 primary PCI cases/yr.
§This calculation implies that the estimated delay to the implementation of the invasive strategy is greater than 1 hr versus initiation of fibrinolytic therapy immediately.
ICH = intracranial hemorrhage; PCI = percutaneous coronary intervention; STEMI = ST-elevation myocardial infarction.
From Antman EM, et al: ACC/AHA Guidelines for the Management of Patients with ST-Elevation Myocardial Infarction. 2004 (http://www.acc.org/clinical/guidelines/stemi/index.htm).

TABLE 47–3 Contraindications and Cautions for Fibrinolytic Use in STEMI*

Absolute contraindications

- Any prior intracranial hemorrhage
- Known structural cerebral vascular lesion (e.g., arteriovenous malformation)
- Known malignant intracranial neoplasm (primary or metastatic)
- Ischemic stroke within 3 months EXCEPT acute ischemic stroke within 3 hours
- Suspected aortic dissection
- Active bleeding or bleeding diathesis (excluding menses)
- Significant closed head or facial trauma within 3 months

Relative contraindications

- History of chronic severe poorly controlled hypertension
- Severe uncontrolled hypertension on presentation (SBP greater than 180 or DBP greater than 110 Hg)†
- History of prior ischemic stroke greater than 3 months, dementia, or known intracranial pathology not covered in contraindications
- Traumatic or prolonged (more than 10 min) CPR or major surgery (less than 3 wk)
- Recent (within 2-4 weeks) internal bleeding
- Noncompressible vascular punctures
- For streptokinase/anistreplase: prior exposure (more than 5 days ago) or prior allergic reaction to these agents
- Pregnancy
- Active peptic ulcer
- Current use of anticoagulants: the higher the INR, the higher the risk of bleeding

CPR = cardiopulmonary resuscitation; DBP = diastolic blood pressure; INR = international normalized ratio; SBP = systolic blood pressure; STEMI = ST-elevation myocardial infarction.

From Antman EM, et al: ACC/AHA Guidelines for the Management of Patients with ST-Elevation Myocardial Infarction. 2004 (http://www.acc.org/clinical/guidelines/stemi/index.htm).

*Viewed as advisory for clinical decision-making and may not be all-inclusive or definitive.

†Could be an absolute contraindication in low-risk patients with myocardial infarction.

angina (a distinction to be made subsequently after scrutiny of serial electrocardiograms and serum cardiac marker measurements) (see Chaps. 46 and 49).

In patients with a clinical history suggestive of STEMI (see Chap. 46) and an initial nondiagnostic ECG reading (i.e., no ST segment deviation or T wave inversion), serial tracings should be obtained while the patients are being evaluated in the emergency department. Emergency department staff can be alerted to the sudden development of ST segment elevation by periodic visual inspection of the bedside ECG monitor, by continuous ST segment recording, or by auditory alarms when the ST segment deviation exceeds programmed limits. Decision aids such as computer-based diagnostic algorithms, identification of high-risk clinical indicators, rapid determination of cardiac serum markers, two-dimensional echocardiographic screening for regional wall motion abnormalities, and myocardial perfusion imaging are of greatest clinical utility when the ECG reading is nondiagnostic. In an effort to improve the cost-effectiveness of care of patients with a chest pain syndrome, nondiagnostic ECG reading, and low suspicion of myocardial infarction but in whom the diagnosis has not been entirely excluded, many medical centers have developed critical pathways that involve a coronary observation unit with a goal of ruling out myocardial infarction in less than 12 hours.[25]

General Treatment Measures

ASPIRIN. This agent not only is useful for the primary prevention of vascular events (see Chap. 42) but is also effective across the entire spectrum of acute coronary syndromes and forms part of the initial management strategy for patients with suspected STEMI. The pharmacology of aspirin is presented in Chapter 80. The goal of aspirin treatment is to quickly block formation of thromboxane A_2 in platelets by cyclooxygenase inhibition. Because low doses (40 to 80 mg) take several days to achieve full antiplatelet effect, at least 162 to 325 mg should be administered acutely in the emergency department.[7] To achieve therapeutic blood levels rapidly, the patient should chew the tablet, thus promoting buccal absorption rather than absorption through the gastric mucosa.

CONTROL OF CARDIAC PAIN. Analgesia is an important element of management of STEMI patients in the emergency department. Often there is a tendency to underdose the patient for fear of obscuring response to antiischemic or reperfusion therapy. This should be avoided, because pain contributes to the heightened sympathetic activity that is particularly prominent during the early phase of STEMI. Control of cardiac pain is typically accomplished with a combination of nitrates, analgesics (e.g., morphine), oxygen, and beta-adrenoceptor blockers. Similar pharmacological principles apply in the coronary care unit, where many of the therapies discussed herein are continued after initial dosing in the emergency department. Because the pain associated with STEMI is related to ongoing ischemia, many interventions that act to improve the oxygen supply-demand relationship (by either increasing supply or decreasing demand) have a functional analgesic effect.

Analgesics. Although a wide variety of analgesic agents has been used to treat the pain associated with STEMI, including meperidine, pentazocine, and morphine, morphine remains the drug of choice, except in patients with well-documented morphine hypersensitivity. Four to 8 mg should be administered intravenously and doses of 2 to 8 mg repeated at intervals of 5 to 15 minutes until the pain is relieved or evident toxicity—hypotension, depression of respiration, or severe vomiting—precludes further administration of the drug. In some patients, remarkably large cumulative doses of morphine (2-3 mg/kg) may be required and are usually tolerated.

The reduction of anxiety resulting from morphine diminishes the patient's restlessness and the activity of the autonomic nervous system, with a consequent reduction of the heart's metabolic demands. The beneficial effect of morphine in patients with pulmonary edema is unequivocal and may be related to several factors, including peripheral arterial and venous dilation (particularly among patients with excessive sympathoadrenal activity), reduction of the work of breathing, and slowing of heart rate secondary to combined withdrawal of sympathetic tone and augmentation of vagal tone.

Hypotension following the administration of nitroglycerin and morphine can be minimized by maintaining the patient in a supine position and elevating the lower extremities if systolic arterial pressure declines below 100 mm Hg. Such positioning is undesirable in the presence of pulmonary edema, but morphine rarely produces hypotension under these circumstances. The concomitant administration of atropine in doses of 0.5 to 1.5 mg intravenously may be helpful in reducing the excessive vagomimetic effects of morphine, particularly when hypotension and bradycardia are present before it is administered.[7] Respiratory depression is an unusual complication of morphine in the presence of severe pain or pulmonary edema, but as the patient's cardiovascular status improves, impairment of ventilation may supervene. It can be treated with naloxone, in doses of 0.1 to 0.2 mg intravenously initially, repeated after 15 minutes if necessary. Nausea and vomiting may be troublesome side effects of large doses of morphine and can be treated with a phenothiazine.

Nitrates. By virtue of their ability to enhance coronary blood flow by coronary vasodilation and to decrease ventricular preload by increasing venous capacitance, sublingual nitrates are indicated for most patients with an acute coronary syndrome. At present, the only groups of patients with STEMI in whom sublingual nitroglycerin should *not* be given are those with inferior myocardial infarction and suspected right ventricular infarction[26] or marked hypotension (systolic pressure < 90 mm Hg), especially if accompanied by bradycardia.

Once it is ascertained that hypotension is not present, a sublingual nitroglycerin tablet should be administered and the patient observed carefully for improvement in symptoms or change in hemodynamics. If an initial dose is well tolerated and appears to be of benefit, further nitrates should be administered, with monitoring of the vital signs. Even small doses can produce sudden hypotension and bradycardia, a reaction that can be life-threatening but can usually be easily reversed with intravenous atropine if it is recognized quickly. Long-acting oral nitrate preparations should be avoided in the very early course of STEMI because of the frequently changing hemodynamic status of the patient. In patients with a prolonged period of waxing and waning chest pain, intravenous nitroglycerin may be of benefit in controlling symptoms and correcting ischemia, but frequent monitoring of blood pressure is required.

Beta-Adrenoceptor Blockers. These drugs relieve pain, reduce the need for analgesics in many patients, and reduce infarct size. A popular and relatively safe protocol for the use of a beta blocker in this situation is as follows. (1) Patients with heart failure (rales > 10 cm up from diaphragm), hypotension (blood pressure < 90 mm Hg), bradycardia (heart rate < 60 beats/min), or heart block (PR interval > 0.24 sec) are first excluded. (2) Metoprolol is given in three 5-mg boluses. (3) Patients are observed for 2 to 5 minutes after each bolus, and if the heart rate falls below 60 beats/min or systolic blood pressure falls below 100 mm Hg, no further drug is given; a total of three intravenous doses (15 mg) is administered. (4) If hemodynamic stability continues, 15 minutes after the last intravenous dose, the patient is begun on oral metoprolol, 50 mg every 6 hours for 2 days, then switched to 100 mg twice daily. An infusion of an extremely short-acting beta blocker, esmolol (50 to 250 mg/kg/min), may be useful in patients with relative contraindications to beta blockade in whom heart rate slowing is considered highly desirable.

Oxygen. Hypoxemia can occur in patients with STEMI and is usually secondary to ventilation-perfusion abnormalities that are sequelae of left ventricular failure; pneumonia and intrinsic pulmonary disease are additional causes of hypoxemia. It is common practice to treat all patients hospitalized with STEMI with oxygen for at least 24 to 48 hours, based on the empirical assumption of hypoxia and evidence that increased oxygen in the inspired air may protect ischemic myocardium. However, this practice may not be cost-effective. Augmentation of the fraction of oxygen in the inspired air does not elevate oxygen delivery significantly in patients who are not hypoxemic. Furthermore, it may increase systemic vascular resistance and arterial pressure and thereby lower cardiac output slightly.

In view of these considerations, arterial oxygen saturation can be estimated by pulse oximetry (an increasingly available technology), and oxygen therapy can be omitted if it is normal. On the other hand, oxygen should be administered to patients with STEMI when arterial hypoxemia is clinically evident or can be documented by measurement (e.g., SaO_2 < 90 percent).[7] In these patients, serial arterial blood gas measurements can be employed to follow the efficacy of oxygen therapy. The delivery of 2 to 4 liters/min of 100 percent oxygen by mask or nasal prongs for 6 to 12 hours is satisfactory for most patients with mild hypoxemia. If arterial oxygenation is still depressed on this regimen, the flow rate may have to be increased, and other causes for hypoxemia should be sought. In patients with pulmonary edema, endotracheal intubation and positive-pressure controlled ventilation may be necessary.

Limitation of Infarct Size

Infarct size is an important determinant of prognosis in patients with STEMI. Patients who succumb from cardiogenic shock generally exhibit either a single massive infarct or a small to moderate-sized infarct superimposed on multiple prior infarctions.[27] Survivors with large infarcts frequently exhibit late impairment of ventricular function, and the long-term mortality rate is higher than for survivors with small infarcts, who tend not to develop cardiac decompensation.[27]

In view of the prognostic importance of infarct size, the concept that modification of infarct size is possible has attracted a great deal of experimental and clinical attention (see Fig. 46–12).[13,28] Efforts to limit the size of the infarct have been divided among several different (sometimes overlapping) approaches: (1) early reperfusion, (2) reduction of myocardial energy demands, (3) manipulation of sources of energy production in the myocardium, and (4) prevention of reperfusion injury. Although early reperfusion ("time-dependent effect of reperfusion") has been the major focus of modern management strategies for STEMI, it is important to note that in addition to the limitation of infarct size, late reperfusion of ischemic myocardium may convey several benefits that contribute to mortality reduction ("time-independent effect of reperfusion") (see Fig. 46–12).[29]

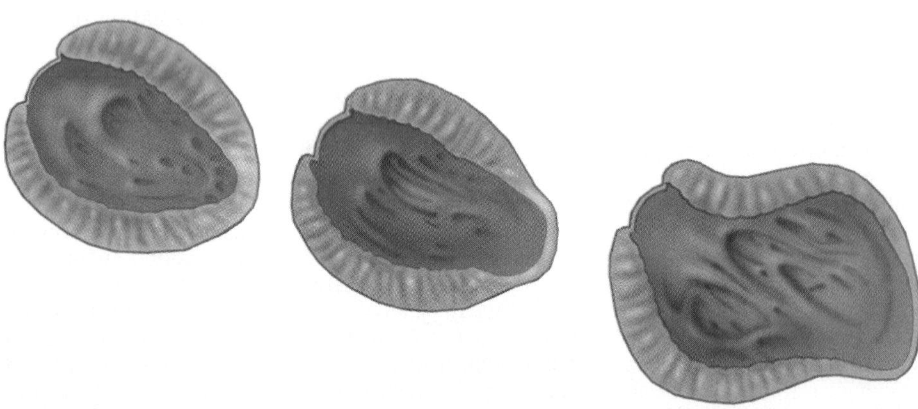

FIGURE 47–3 Remodeling of left ventricle after ST segment elevation myocardial infarction (STEMI). On the left is shown an apical STEMI (white zone of left ventricle). Over time, the infarct zone elongates and thins. Progressive remodeling of the left ventricle occurs (center and right images) ultimately converting the left ventricle from an oval shape to a spherical shape. Pharmacological and catheter-based reperfusion strategies for STEMI have a favorable impact on this process by minimizing the extent of myocardial necrosis (left) through prompt restoration of flow in the epicardial infarct vessel. (Adapted from McMurray JJV, Pfeffer MA (eds): Heart Failure Updates. London, Martin Dunitz, 2003.)

THE DYNAMIC NATURE OF INFARCTION. STEMI is a dynamic process that does not occur instantaneously but evolves over hours. The fate of jeopardized, ischemic tissue can be affected favorably by interventions that restore myocardial perfusion, reduce microvascular damage in the infarct zone, reduce myocardial oxygen requirements, inhibit accumulation of or facilitate wash-out of noxious metabolites, augment the availability of substrate for anaerobic metabolism, or blunt the effects of mediators of injury that compromise the structure and function of intracellular organelles and constituents of cell membranes.[30-32] Strong evidence in experimental animals and suggestive evidence in patients indicate that ischemic preconditioning, a form of endogenous protection against STEMI (see Chap. 19), prior to sustained coronary occlusion decreases infarct size and is associated with a more favorable outcome, with decreased risk of extension of infarction and recurrent ischemic events. Brief episodes of ischemia in one coronary vascular bed may precondition myocardium in a remote zone, attenuating the size of infarction in the latter when sustained coronary occlusion occurs.[33]

The perfusion of the myocardium in the infarct zone appears to be reduced maximally immediately following coronary occlusion. Up to one-third of patients develop spontaneous recanalization of an occluded infarct-related artery beginning at 12 to 24 hours. This delayed spontaneous reperfusion has been associated with improvement of left ventricular function because it improves healing of infarcted tissue, prevents ventricular remodeling, and reperfuses hibernating myocardium. However, to *maximize* the amount of salvaged myocardium by *accelerating* the process of reperfusion and also implementing it in those patients who would otherwise have an occluded infarct-related artery, the strategies of pharmacologically induced and catheter-based reperfusion of the infarct vessel have been developed (Fig. 47-3) (see Chap. 48).

Additional factors that may contribute to limitation of infarct size in association with reperfusion include relief of coronary spasm, prevention of damage to the microvasculature, improved systemic hemodynamics (augmentation of coronary perfusion pressure and reduced left ventricular end-diastolic pressure), and development of collateral circulation. The prompt implementation of measures designed to protect ischemic myocardium and support myocardial perfusion may provide sufficient time for the development of anatomical and physiological compensatory mechanisms that limit the ultimate extent of infarction (see Fig. 46-3). It is possible that interventions designed to protect ischemic myocardium during the initial event may also reduce the incidence of extension of infarction or early reinfarction.

ROUTINE MEASURES FOR INFARCT SIZE LIMITATION. Although reperfusion of ischemic myocardium is the most important technique for limiting infarct size, several routine measures to accomplish this goal are applicable to all patients with STEMI, whether or not reperfusion therapy is prescribed. The treatment strategies discussed in this section can be initiated in the emergency department and then continued in the coronary care unit.

It is important to maintain an optimal balance between myocardial oxygen supply and demand so that as much as possible of the jeopardized zone of the myocardium surrounding the most profoundly ischemic zones of the infarct can be salvaged. During the period before irreversible injury has occurred, myocardial oxygen consumption should be minimized by maintaining the patient at rest, physically and emotionally, and by utilizing mild sedation and a quiet atmosphere that may lower heart rate, a major determinant of myocardial oxygen consumption. If the patient was receiving a beta-adrenoceptor blocking agent at the time the clinical manifestations of the infarction commenced, the drug should be continued unless a specific contraindication develops, such as left ventricular systolic failure or bradyarrhythmia. Marked sinus bradycardia (heart rate less than approximately 50 beats/min) and the frequently coexisting hypotension should be treated with postural maneuvers (the Trendelenburg position) to increase central blood volume and atropine and electrical pacing, but not with isoproterenol. On the other hand, the routine administration of atropine, with the resultant increase in heart rate, to patients without serious bradycardia is contraindicated. All forms of tachyarrhythmias require prompt treatment because they increase myocardial oxygen needs.[7]

Congestive heart failure should be treated promptly. Given their multiple beneficial actions in STEMI patients, inhibitors of the renin-angiotensin-aldosterone system are indicated in the treatment of congestive heart failure associated with STEMI unless the patient is hypotensive. Inotropic agents such as isoproterenol that increase myocardial oxygen consumption should be avoided.

As discussed earlier, arterial oxygenation should be restored to normal in patients with hypoxemia, such as occurs in patients with chronic pulmonary disease, pneumonia, or left ventricular failure. Oxygen-enriched air should be administered to patients with hypoxemia, and bronchodilators and expectorants should be used when indicated. Severe anemia, which can also extend the area of ischemic injury, should be corrected by the cautious administration of packed red blood cells, accompanied by a diuretic if there is any evidence of left ventricular failure. Associated conditions, particularly infections and the accompanying tachycardia, fever, and elevated myocardial oxygen needs, require immediate attention.

Systolic arterial pressure should not be allowed to deviate by more than approximately 25 to 30 mm Hg from the patient's usual level unless marked hypertension had been present before the onset of STEMI. It is likely that each patient has an optimal range of arterial pressure; as coronary perfusion pressure deviates from this level, the unfavorable balance between oxygen supply (which is related to coronary perfusion pressure) and myocardial oxygen demand (which is related to ventricular wall tension) that ensues increases the extent of ischemic injury.

Reperfusion Therapy

GENERAL CONCEPTS. Although late spontaneous reperfusion occurs in some patients, persistent thrombotic occlusion is present in the majority of patients with STEMI while the myocardium is undergoing necrosis.[34] Timely reperfusion of jeopardized myocardium represents the most effective way of restoring the balance between myocardial oxygen supply and demand. When fibrinolysis is administered, the extent of protection appears to be related directly to the rapidity with which reperfusion is implemented after the onset of coronary occlusion.[34] Evidence exists to suggest that the extent of myocardial salvage when reperfusion is achieved with PCI (including stent deployment) is less time dependent than that for fibrinolysis.[28] The mechanisms underlying the therapy-dependent influence of time-to-treatment on myocardial salvage are not clear but probably include restoration of full antegrade flow in the infarct artery with PCI and decreasing efficacy of fibrinolytic agents as coronary thrombi mature with the passage of time.[28] It should be noted, however, that analyses adjusting for baseline risk demonstrate a statistically significant increase in mortality with progressive delays between the onset of symptoms and PCI.[35] For every 30-minute delay from symptom onset to PCI, there is an 8 percent increase in the relative risk of 1-year mortality (Fig. 47-4).[36]

In some patients, particularly those with cardiogenic shock, tissue damage occurs in a "stuttering" manner rather than abruptly, a condition that might more properly be termed *subacute infarction*. This concept of the nature of the infarction process, as well as the observation that the incidence of complications of STEMI in both the early and late postinfarction periods is a function of infarct size, underscores the need for careful history-taking to ascertain whether the patient appears to have had repetitive cycles of sponta-

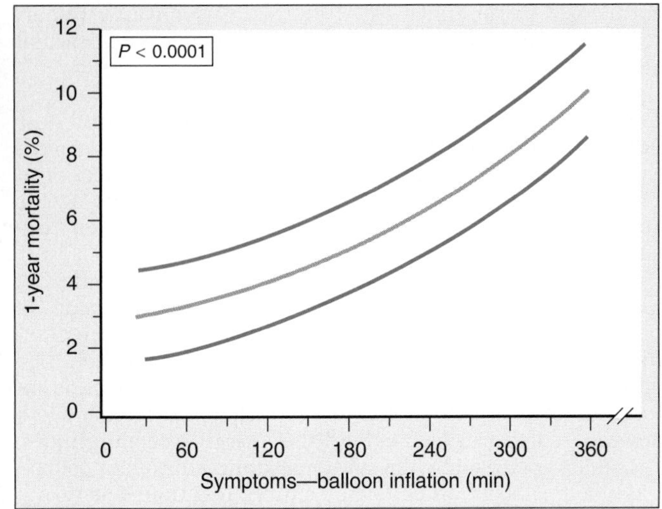

FIGURE 47–4 Importance of time to reperfusion in patients undergoing primary percutaneous coronary intervention (PCI) for ST segment elevation myocardial infarction (STEMI). This plot is based on the pooled data from 1791 patients undergoing primary PCI for STEMI. After adjusting for baseline risk, there is a curvilinear relationship between the time elapsed from the onset of symptoms to balloon inflation and the rate of mortality at 1 year. For every 30-minute delay from onset of symptoms to primary PCI, there is an 8 percent increase in the relative risk of 1-year mortality. (From De Luca G, Suryapranata H, Ottervanger JP, et al: Time-delay to treatment and mortality in primary angioplasty for acute myocardial infarction: Every minute counts. Circulation 109:1223, 2004.)

neous reperfusion and reocclusion. "Fixing" the time of onset of the infarction process in such patients can be difficult. In such patients with waxing and waning ischemic discomfort, a rigid time interval from the first episode of pain should not be used when determining whether a patient is "outside the window" for benefit from acute reperfusion therapy.

PATHOPHYSIOLOGY OF MYOCARDIAL REPERFUSION. Prevention of cell death by the restoration of blood flow depends on the severity and duration of preexisting ischemia. Substantial experimental and clinical evidence exists indicating that the earlier blood flow is restored, the more favorably influenced are recovery of left ventricular systolic function, improvement in diastolic function, and reduction in overall mortality.[19] Collateral coronary vessels also appear to play a role in the resultant left ventricular function following reperfusion.[37] They provide sufficient perfusion of myocardium to retard cell death and are probably of greater importance in patients having reperfusion later rather than 1 to 2 hours after coronary occlusion.

Even after successful reperfusion and despite the absence of irreversible myocardial damage, a period of postischemic contractile dysfunction can occur—a phenomenon referred to as *myocardial stunning.*[38] Periods of myocardial stunning are well described in experimental animals but have also been confirmed in STEMI patients using positron emission tomography (PET) scanning after percutaneous transluminal coronary angiography (PTCA) to measure myocardial blood flow and oxygen consumption.[39]

REPERFUSION INJURY

The process of reperfusion, although beneficial in terms of myocardial salvage, may come at a cost due to a process known as *reperfusion injury.* Kloner has summarized the data on the four types of reperfusion injury that have been observed in experimental animals. These consist of (1) lethal reperfusion injury—a term referring to reperfusion-induced death of cells that were still viable at the time of restoration of coronary blood flow; (2) vascular reperfusion injury—progressive damage to the microvasculature such that there is an expanding area of no reflow and loss of coronary vasodilatory reserve[40]; (3) stunned myocardium—salvaged myocytes display a prolonged period of contractile dysfunction following restoration of blood flow owing to abnormalities of intracellular biochemistry leading to reduced energy production; and (4) reperfusion arrhythmias—bursts of ventricular tachycardia and on occasion ventricular fibrillation that occur within seconds of reperfusion. The available evidence suggests that vascular reperfusion injury, stunning, and reperfusion arrhythmias can all occur in patients with acute myocardial infarction. The concept of lethal reperfusion injury of potentially salvageable myocardium remains controversial, both in experimental animals and in patients.[41]

Reperfusion increases the cell swelling that occurs with ischemia. Reperfusion of the myocardium in which the microvasculature is damaged leads to the creation of a hemorrhagic infarct (see Fig. 46-6). Fibrinolytic therapy appears more likely to produce hemorrhagic infarction than reperfusion by mechanical means. Although concern has been raised that this hemorrhage may lead to extension of the infarct, this does not appear to be the case. Histological study of patients not surviving in spite of successful reperfusion has revealed hemorrhagic infarcts, but this hemorrhage usually does not extend beyond the area of necrosis.[41]

PROTECTION AGAINST REPERFUSION INJURY. A variety of adjunctive approaches have been taken to protect the myocardium against injury that occurs after reperfusion: (1) preservation of microvascular integrity by using antiplatelet agents and antithrombins to minimize embolization of atheroembolic debris[42,43]; (2) prevention of inflammatory damage[31,44-47]; and (3) metabolic support of the ischemic myocardium.[48-50] The effectiveness of agents directed against reperfusion injury rapidly declines the later they are administered after reperfusion; eventually, no beneficial effect is detectable in animal models after 45 to 60 minutes of reperfusion has elapsed.[48]

REPERFUSION ARRHYTHMIAS

Transient sinus bradycardia occurs in many patients with inferior infarcts at the time of acute reperfusion; it is most often accompanied by some degree of hypotension. This combination of hypotension and bradycardia with a sudden increase in coronary flow has been ascribed to the activation of the Bezold-Jarisch reflex.[51] Premature ventricular contractions, accelerated idioventricular rhythm, and nonsustained ventricular tachycardia are also seen commonly following successful reperfusion. In experimental animals with STEMI, ventricular fibrillation occurs shortly after reperfusion, but this arrhythmia is not as frequent in patients as in the experimental setting. Although some investigators have postulated that early afterdepolarizations participate in the genesis of reperfusion ventricular arrhythmias, early afterdepolarizations are present both during ischemia and during reperfusion and are therefore unlikely to be involved in the development of reperfusion ventricular tachycardia or fibrillation.

When present, rhythm disturbances may actually be a marker of successful restoration of coronary flow. However, although reperfusion arrhythmias have a high sensitivity for detecting successful reperfusion, the high incidence of identical rhythm disturbances in patients without successful coronary artery reperfusion limits their specificity for detection of restoration of coronary blood flow. In general, clinical features are poor markers of reperfusion, with no single clinical finding or constellation of findings being reliably predictive of angiographically demonstrated coronary artery patency.[52]

Although reperfusion arrhythmias may show a temporal clustering at the time of restoration of coronary blood flow in patients with successful fibrinolysis, the overall incidence of such arrhythmias appears to be similar in patients not receiving a thrombolytic agent who may develop these arrhythmias as a consequence of spontaneous coronary artery reperfusion or the evolution of the infarct process itself. These considerations, as well as the fact that the brief "electrical storm" occurring at the time of reperfusion is generally innocuous, indicate that no prophylactic antiarrhythmic therapy is necessary when thrombolytics are prescribed.

LATE ESTABLISHMENT OF PATENCY OF THE INFARCT VESSEL

It has been suggested that improved survival and ventricular function after successful reperfusion are not due entirely to limitation of infarct size (see Fig. 46-12).[53] Both experimental and clinical evidence indicate that the benefits of a patent artery include a favorable effect on ventricular remodeling (improved healing of infarcted tissue and prevention of infarct expansion), enhancement of collateral flow, improvement in diastolic and systolic function, increased electrical stability, and reduced long-term mortality. Late reperfusion of the artery perfusing an infarction provides a vascular scaffolding in the infarct zone and increases the influx of inflammatory cells that participate in the formation of a mature fibrous scar. The vascular scaffold and firmer myocardial scar prevent infarct segment lengthening and decrease the tendency to infarct expansion and aneurysm formation.[29] Poorly contracting or noncontracting myocardium in a zone that is supplied by a stenosed infarct-related artery with slow antegrade perfusion may still contain viable myocytes. This situation is referred to as *hibernating myocardium*,[54] and its function can be improved by PCI to augment flow in the infarct-related artery. Late reperfusion of the infarct-related artery by thrombolysis or late restoration of flow via PCI enhances the electrical stability of the infarcted zone and is probably related to the reduced incidence of ventricular fibrillation and of automatic firing of implantable cardioverter-defibrillator devices.[53] The beneficial effect of late reperfusion of the infarct-related artery is independent of left ventricular function and other mortality-reducing therapies such as angiotensin-converting enzyme (ACE) inhibitors. Several clinical trials are testing the benefits of late reperfusion of an occluded infarct artery in asymptomatic patients (see Fig. 46-12).[29,55]

SUMMARY OF EFFECTS OF MYOCARDIAL REPERFUSION. Rupture of an unstable plaque in the culprit vessel produces complete occlusion of the infarct-related coronary artery. STEMI occurs with the ensuing development of left ventricular dilation and ultimate death through a combination of pump failure and electrical instability (Fig. 47–3; see also Fig. 46–12). Early reperfusion shortens the duration of coronary occlusion, minimizes the degree of ultimate left ventricular dysfunction and dilation, and reduces the probability that the STEMI patient will develop pump failure or malignant ventricular tachyarrhythmias.[34,56] Late reperfusion may favorably affect the process of infarct healing and minimize left ventricular remodeling and the ultimate development of pump dysfunction and electrical instability.[57]

Coronary Fibrinolysis

Many years elapsed between the first report of intracoronary clot lysis in an experimental animal and the widespread use of fibrinolytic agents in patients with STEMI. With publication of the first GISSI trial of more than 11,000 patients in 1986, in which intravenous streptokinase was shown to result in a significant reduction in the rate of mortality in patients treated within 6 hours of the onset of symptoms, the use of fibrinolytic therapy in cases of STEMI was established.[34] It is now clear that fibrinolysis recanalizes thrombotic occlusion associated with STEMI, and restoration of coronary flow reduces infarct size and improves myocardial function and survival over both the short and the long terms.[58] The majority of the mortality benefit seen at 10-year follow-up in the GISSI trial was obtained prior to hospital discharge, since no survival difference was seen in fibrinolysed and control patients discharged alive except for those treated within the first hour after onset of symptoms.[59]

INTRACORONARY THROMBOLYSIS. Clinical investigation of pharmacological reperfusion of ischemic myocardium initially focused on intracoronary thrombolysis in the early hours of STEMI. Because of the delay involved in catheterizing patients with STEMI, current consensus is that intracoronary administration of fibrinolytic therapy should be reserved for the rare situation in which a patient develops coronary thrombosis during the course of an angiographic procedure and in whom either a coronary catheter is already in place or such placement is easily and rapidly achieved. In contemporary practice, however, such patients are more likely to be treated by PCI (see Chap. 48).

INTRAVENOUS FIBRINOLYSIS

TIMI Flow Grade. To provide a level of standardization for comparison of the various regimens, most investigators describe the flow in the infarct vessel according to the Thrombolysis in Myocardial Infarction trial (TIMI) grading system: grade 0 is complete occlusion of the infarct related artery; grade 1, some penetration of the contrast material beyond the point of obstruction but without perfusion of the distal coronary bed; grade 2, perfusion of the entire infarct vessel into the distal bed but with delayed flow compared with a normal artery; and grade 3, full perfusion of the infarct vessel with normal flow.[60,61] When evaluating reports of angiographic studies of fibrinolytic agents, it must be kept in mind that only in studies in which a pretreatment coronary arteriogram documents occlusion of the culprit vessel can the term *recanalization* be applied if flow is restored. If the status of the culprit vessel is not known prior to treatment, the only fact that can be stated with certainty is the *patency rate* of the vessel at the moment the contrast material is injected. This snapshot in time does not reflect the fluctuating status of flow in the infarct vessel that characteristically undergoes repeated cycles of patency and reocclusion, as has been documented angiographically and by continuous ST segment monitoring.

Issues of the fluctuating nature of patency of the infarct-related artery notwithstanding, the majority of angiographic studies of reperfusion regimens for STEMI used an assessment of the TIMI flow grade at 90 or preferably 60 minutes after the start of fibrinolytic therapy.[62]

Initially, TIMI grade 2 and grade 3 flows were lumped into the favorable category of coronary patency that was compared with a combined TIMI grade 0 and grade 1 flow in an unfavorable category of persistent occlusion. It has been learned, however, that TIMI grade 2 flow should not be combined with grade 3 flow because it has been recognized that TIMI grade 3 flow is far superior to grade 2 in terms of infarct size reduction and both short-term and long-term mortality benefit.[30] Therefore, TIMI grade 3 flow should be considered to be the goal when assessing flow in the epicardial infarct artery (Fig. 47–5).[30]

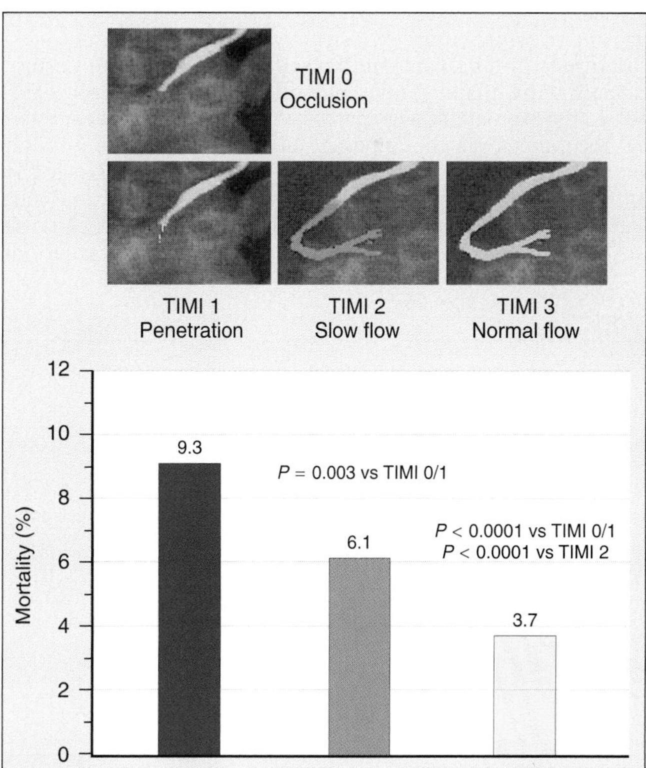

FIGURE 47–5 Correlation of TIMI flow grade and mortality. A pooled analysis of data from 5498 patients in several angiographic trials of reperfusion for ST elevation myocardial infarction showed a gradient of mortality when the angiographic findings were stratified by TIMI flow grade. Patients with TIMI 0 or TIMI 1 flow had the highest rate of mortality; TIMI 2 flow was associated with an intermediate rate of mortality; the lowest rate of mortality was observed in patients with TIMI 3 flow. (Dr. Michael Gibson, personal communication.)

THE TIMI FRAME COUNT. In an effort to provide a more quantitative statement of the briskness of coronary blood flow in the infarct artery and also to account for differences in the size and length of vessels (e.g., left anterior descending versus right coronary artery) and interobserver variability, Gibson and coworkers developed the *TIMI frame count*—a simple count of the number of angiographic frames elapsed until the contrast material arrives in the distal bed of the vessel of interest. This is an objective and quantitative index of coronary blood flow, is an independent predictor of in-hospital mortality from STEMI, and also discriminates patients with TIMI grade 3 flow into low- and high-risk groups.[63] Using the TIMI frame count, Gibson and coworkers determined that the following were univariate predictors of delayed coronary blood flow following fibrinolytic administration: a greater percentage diameter stenosis, a decreased minimum lumen diameter, a greater percentage of the culprit artery distal to stenosis, and the presence of delayed achievement of patency, a culprit artery location in the left coronary circulation, pulsatile flow (i.e., reversible flow in systole), or intraluminal thrombus.[64] The TIMI frame count can also be used to quantitate coronary blood flow (cc's per second) calculated at

$$21 \div (\text{observed TIMI frame count}) \times 1.7$$

(based on Doppler velocity wire data showing that normal flow equals 1.7 cm^3 per second, which is proportional to 21 frames). The relationship between calculated coronary perfusion and mortality for patients treated with fibrinolytics and primary PCI is illustrated in Figure 47–6.

MYOCARDIAL PERFUSION. Despite intense interest in the development of reperfusion regimens that normalize flow in the epicardial infarct-related artery, the real goal of reperfusion in patients with STEMI is to improve myocardial perfusion in the infarct zone. Of course, myocardial perfusion cannot be improved adequately without restoration of flow in the occluded infarct-related artery. However, even patients with TIMI grade 3 flow may not achieve adequate myocardial perfusion. The two major impediments to normalization of myocardial perfusion are microvascular damage (Fig. 47–7) and reperfusion injury.[30] Obstruction of the distal microvasculature in the downstream bed of the infarct-related artery is caused by platelet microemboli and thrombi. Microembolization of platelet aggregates may actually be exacerbated by fibrinolysis via the exposure of clot-bound thrombin, an extremely potent platelet agonist. Spasm can also occur in the microvasculature due to the release of substances from activated platelets such as serotonin and thromboxane A_2. Reperfusion injury results in cellular edema, free radical formation, and calcium overload. In addition, cytokine activation leads to neutrophil accumulation and inflammatory mediators that contribute to tissue injury.

Several techniques have been used to evaluate the adequacy of myocardial perfusion. Electrocardiographic ST segment resolution is a strong predictor of outcome in STEMI patients but is a better predictor of an occluded than of a patent infarct-related artery.[65,66] Absence of early ST segment resolution after angiographically successful primary PCI identifies patients with a higher risk of left ventricular dysfunction and mortality, presumably because of microvascular damage in the infarct zone. Thus, the 12-lead electrocardiogram is a marker of the biological integrity of myocytes in the infarct zone and can reflect inadequate myocardial perfusion even in the presence of TIMI 3 flow.[40,67] Given the dynamic nature of coronary occlusion, it has been proposed that continuous ST segment monitoring is more informative than static 12-lead ECG recordings, but practical limitations have prevented continuous ST monitoring from widespread clinical application.[66] Defects in perfusion patterns seen with myocardial contrast echocardiography correlate with regional wall motion abnormalities and lack of myocardial viability on dobutamine stress echocardiography. A practical limitation to myocardial contrast echocardiography is the need for intracoronary injection of echo contrast, although this can be circumvented by the availability of new echo contrast agents that can be injected intravenously. Doppler flow wire studies, magnetic resonance imaging, and nuclear imaging with positron emission tomography have also been used to define abnormalities of myocardial perfusion (Fig. 47–8).[30]

A new angiographic method for assessing myocardial perfusion has also been introduced by Gibson and colleagues: the TIMI myocardial perfusion grade (see Fig. 47–9). Abnormalities of increasing myocardial perfusion as assessed by the TIMI myocardial perfusion grade correlate with mortality risk even after adjusting for the presence of TIMI grade 3 flow or a normal TIMI frame count.[68]

Effect of Fibrinolytic Therapy on Mortality

There is no doubt that early intravenous fibrinolysis improve survival in patients with STEMI.[58] Mortality varies considerably depending on the patients included for study and the adjunctive therapies employed. The benefit of fibrinolytic therapy appears to be greatest when agents are administered as early as possible, with the most dramatic results when the drug is given less than 2 hours after symptoms begin.[69]

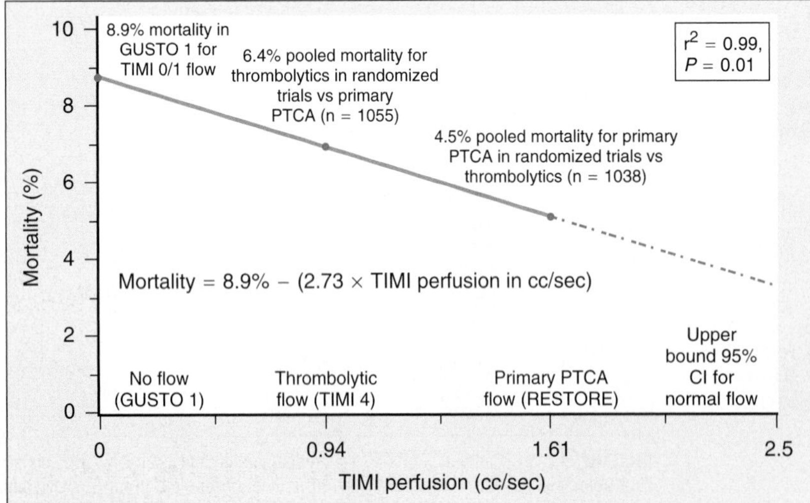

FIGURE 47–6 Relationship between coronary blood flow and mortality rate in patients with acute myocardial infarction. (From Gibson CM: Primary angioplasty, rescue angioplasty, and new devices. *In* Hennekens CH [ed]: Clinical Trials in Cardiovascular Disease: A Companion to Braunwald's Heart Disease. Philadelphia, WB Saunders, 1999, p 194.)

The Fibrinolytic Therapy Trialists' Collaborative Group (FTT) has performed a comprehensive overview of nine trials of thrombolytic therapy, each of which enrolled more than 1000 patients (Fig. 47-10).[19] The database for the FTT overview consisted of 58,600 patients, including 6177 (10.5 percent) who died, 564 (1.0 percent) who sustained a stroke, and 436 (0.7 percent) who sustained major noncerebral bleeds. The absolute mortality rates for the control and fibrinolytic groups stratified by presenting features are shown in Figure 47-10. The overall results indicated an 18 percent reduction in short-term mortality, but as much as a 25 percent reduction in mortality for the subset of 45,000 patients with ST segment elevation or bundle branch block. Two trials, LATE and EMERAS, viewed together provide evidence that a mortality reduction may still be observed in patients treated with thrombolytic agents between 6 and 12 hours from the onset of ischemic symptoms. The data from LATE and EMERAS and the FTT overview form the basis for extending the window of treatment with fibrinolytics up to 12 hours from the onset of symptoms. Boersma and

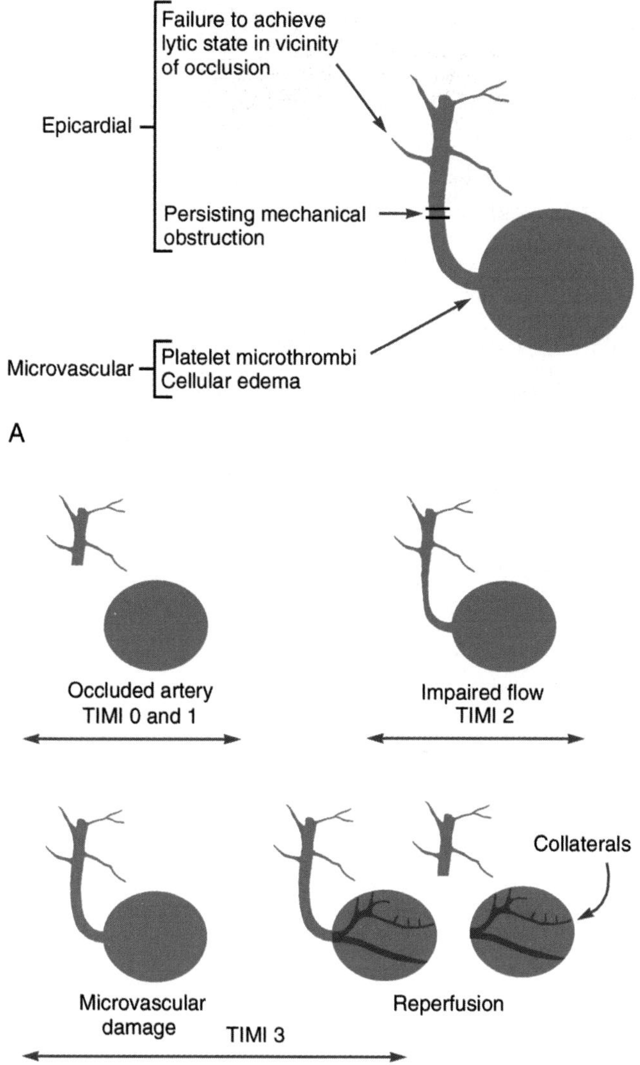

FIGURE 47–7 Patterns of response to fibrinolysis. **A,** Failure of epicardial reperfusion can occur due to failure to induce a lytic state or due to mechanical factors at the site of occlusion. Failure of microvascular reperfusion is due to a combination of platelet microthrombi followed by endothelial swelling and myocardial edema ("no reflow"). **B,** Fibrinolysis may fail due to persistent occlusion of the epicardial infarct-related artery (TIMI grades 0 and 1), patency of an epicardial artery in the presence of impaired (TIMI grade 2) flow, or microvascular occlusion in the presence of angiographically normal (TIMI grade 3) flow. Successful reperfusion requires a patent artery with an intact microvascular network. Conversely, reperfusion may occur despite an occluded epicardial artery due to the presence of collateral arteries. (From Davies CH, Ormerod OJ: Failed coronary thrombolysis. Lancet 351:1191, 1998.)

colleagues pooled the trials in the FTT overview, two smaller studies with data on time to randomization, and 11 additional trials of more than 100 patients. Patients were divided into six time categories from symptom onset to randomization. A nonlinear relationship of treatment benefit to time was observed, with the greatest benefit occurring in the first 1 to 2 hours from the onset of symptoms (Fig. 47–11).[69]

The mortality effect of fibrinolytic therapy in elderly patients is of considerable interest and controversy. Although patients older than 75 years of age were initially excluded from randomized trials of fibrinolytic therapy, they now constitute about 15 percent of the patients studied in contemporary megatrials of fibrinolysis and about 35 percent of patients analyzed in registries of STEMI patients.[70-72] Barriers to initiation of therapy in older patients with STEMI include a protracted period of delay in seeking medical care, a lower incidence of ischemic discomfort and greater incidence of atypical symptoms and concomitant illnesses, and an increased incidence of nondiagnostic ECG readings.[7] Younger patients with STEMI achieve a slightly greater relative reduction in mortality compared with elderly patients, but the higher absolute mortality in the elderly results in similar absolute mortality reductions. Thus, as seen in Figure 47–10, there was a 26 percent decrease in mortality in patients who were younger than 55 years of age (11 lives saved per 1000 with thrombolytic therapy) and a 4 percent reduction in mortality in patients older than 75 years of age (10 lives saved per 1000 treated).[73] Data from a Swedish national registry in patients 75 years of age or older with a first STEMI support the use of fibrinolysis in the elderly in that there was a 13 percent relative risk reduction (p = 0.001) in the composite of mortality and cerebral bleeding at 1 year compared to no fibrinolysis (Fig. 47–12).[72]

Other important baseline characteristics that have an impact on the mortality effect of fibrinolytic therapy include the vital signs at presentation and the presence of diabetes mellitus (see Fig. 47–10). For example, there was an 18 percent decrease in mortality for patients presenting with a systolic pressure less than 100 mm Hg (62 lives saved per 1000 treated), compared with a 12 percent reduction in mortality for patients with a systolic pressure of 175 mm Hg or more (10 lives saved per 1000 treated). Patients with a history of diabetes mellitus experienced a mortality reduction of 21 percent (37 lives saved per 1000 treated), compared with a mortality reduction of 15 percent (15 lives saved per 1000 treated) in patients without a history of diabetes.

A number of models have been developed to integrate the many clinical variables that affect a patient's mortality risk before administration of fibrinolytic therapy. A convenient, simple, bedside risk-scoring system for predicting 30-day mortality at presentation for fibrinolytic-eligible patients with STEMI was developed by Morrow and associates using the InTIME-II trial database (Fig. 47–13).[74,75] However, modeling of mortality risk cannot cover all clinical scenarios and should not substitute for clinical judgment in individual cases. For example, patients with inferior STEMI who might

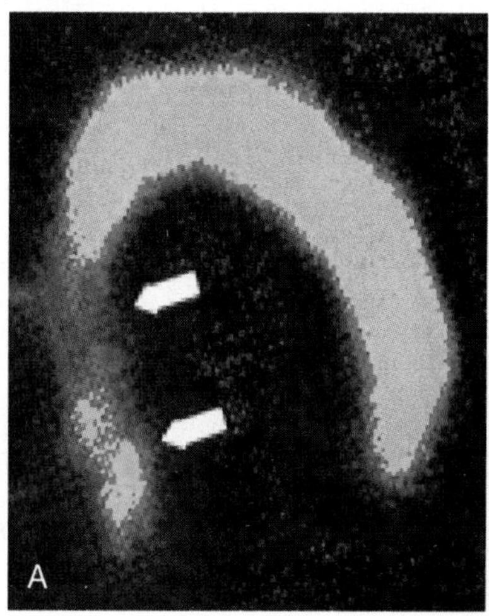

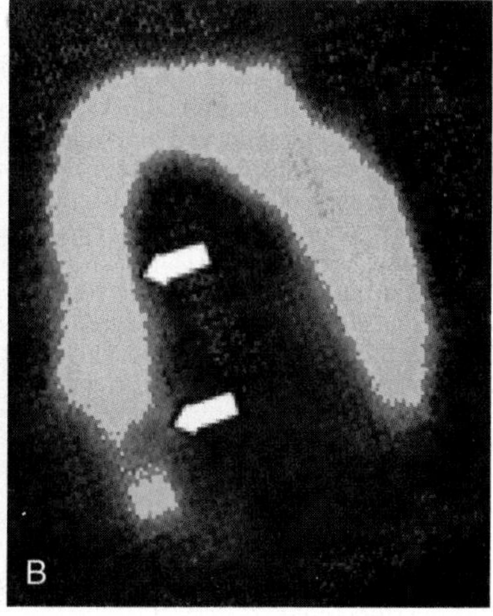

FIGURE 47–8 Myocardial perfusion in a case of acute myocardial infarction. **A,** ^{99m}Tc-sestamibi single-photon emission computed tomography (SPECT) before reperfusion; vertical long axis slice; reduced tracer uptake of basal inferior left ventricular myocardium (arrows). **B,** ^{99m}Tc-sestamibi SPECT 7 days after stenting of left circumflex coronary artery; nearly normal tracer uptake of basal inferior left ventricular myocardium. (From Horcher J, Blasini R, Martinoff S, et al: Myocardial perfusion in acute coronary syndrome. Circulation 99:e15, 1999.)

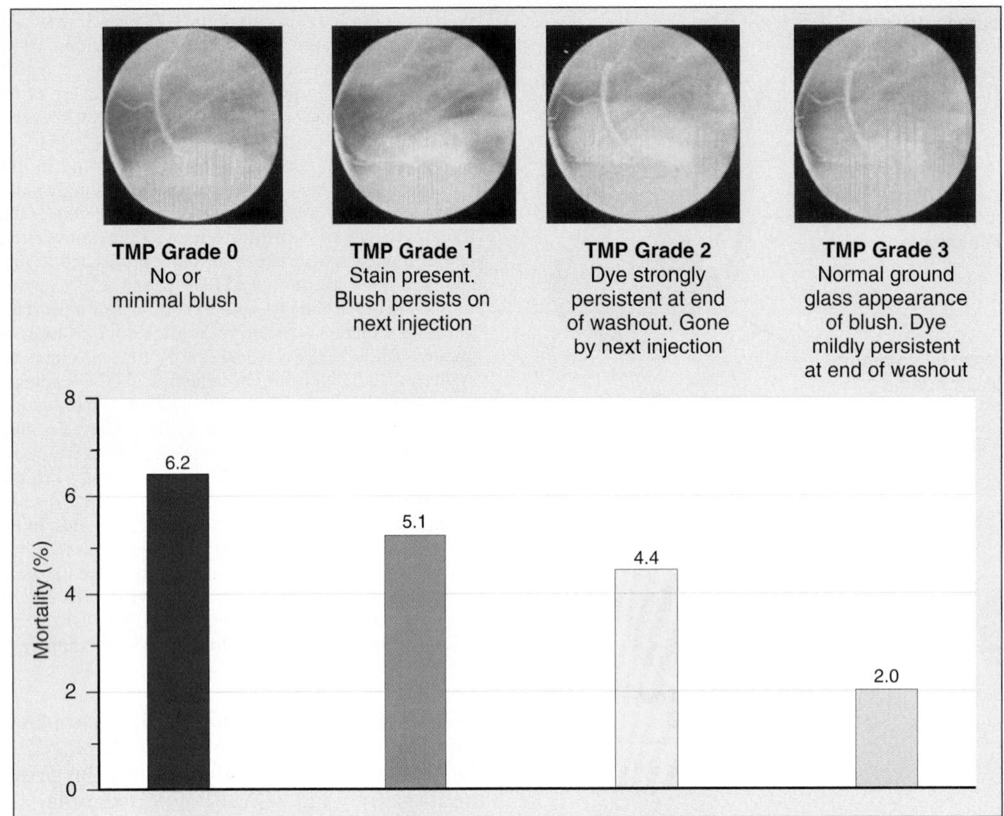

FIGURE 47–9 Relationship between TIMI myocardial perfusion grade and mortality. TIMI myocardial perfusion grade 0 or no perfusion of the myocardium is associated with the highest rate of mortality. If the stain of the myocardium is present (grade 1), mortality is also high. A reduction in mortality is seen if the dye enters the microvasculature but is still persistent at the end of the washout phase (grade 2). The lowest mortality rate is observed in those patients with normal perfusion (grade 3) where the dye is minimally persistent at the end of the washout phase. (From Gibson CM, Murphy SA, Rizzo MJ, et al: Relationship between TIMI frame count and clinical outcomes after thrombolytic administration. Thrombolysis In Myocardial Infarction [TIMI] Study Group. Circulation 99:1945, 1999.)

otherwise be considered to have a low risk of mortality and for whom many physicians have questioned the benefits of fibrinolytic therapy might be in a much higher mortality risk subgroup if their inferior infarction is associated with right ventricular infarction, precordial ST segment depression, or ST segment elevation in the lateral precordial leads.

The short-term survival benefit enjoyed by patients who receive fibrinolytic therapy is maintained over the 1- to 10-year follow-up.[59] Room for improvement remains, however, given reports of reocclusion rates of the infarct-related artery as high as 10 percent in hospital and up to 30 percent by 3 months,[76] and reinfarction rates as high as 9.5 percent within 6 weeks in fibrinolytic-treated patients.[77]

COMPARISON OF FIBRINOLYTIC AGENTS (see Chap. 80)

Some comparative features of the approved fibrinolytic agents for intravenous therapy are presented in Table 47–4.

The tissue plasminogen activator (t-PA) molecule contains the following five domains: finger, epidermal growth factor, kringle 1 and kringle 2, and serum protease (Fig. 47–14).[78] In the absence of fibrin, t-PA is a weak plasminogen activator; fibrin provides a scaffold on which t-PA and plasminogen are held in such a way that the catalytic efficiency for plasminogen activation of t-PA is increased many-fold. Plasma clearance of t-PA is mediated to a varying degree by residues in each of the domains except the serine protease domain, which is responsible for the enzymatic activity of t-PA. The accelerated dose regimen of t-PA over 90 minutes produces more rapid thrombolysis than the standard 3-hour infusion of t-PA. The recommended dosage regimen for t-PA is a 15 mg intravenous bolus followed by an infusion of 0.75 mg/kg (maximum 50 mg) over 30 minutes, and then an infusion of 0.5 mg/kg (maximum 35 mg) over 60 minutes.

Modifications of the basic t-PA structure have been made to yield a group of third-generation fibrinolytics (see Fig. 47–14 and Table 47–4). A common feature among the third-generation fibrinolytics is prolonged plasma clearance, allowing them to be administered as a bolus rather than the bolus and double-infusion technique by which accelerated-dose t-PA is administered.[78]

RETEPLASE. This is a recombinant deletion mutant form of t-PA lacking the finger, epidermal growth factor, and kringle 1 domains as well as the carbohydrate side chains (see Fig. 47–14 and Table 47–4).

The GUSTO III trial compared the 10 + 10 unit regimen of reteplase with accelerated t-PA in 15,059 patients.[79] The 30-day mortality rate was 7.47 percent in the reteplase group and 7.24 percent in the t-PA group corresponding to an absolute difference of 0.23 percent with a 95 percent confidence interval of −0.66 to +1.1 percent. The results of GUSTO III did not demonstrate superiority of reteplase over t-PA, and, using a 1 percent absolute difference as a boundary for equivalence, the mortality results also do not formally demonstrate equivalence.[80,81] The intracranial hemorrhage rate was 0.91 percent with reteplase and 0.87 percent with t-PA. The secondary composite endpoint of net clinical benefit (death or disabling stroke) was 7.89 percent with reteplase and 7.91 percent with accelerated t-PA. Although GUSTO III did not fulfill formal criteria for equivalence of reteplase and t-PA, many clinicians consider the two agents to be therapeutically similar and consider the double bolus method of administration of reteplase to be an advantage over t-PA.

TENECTEPLASE. Tenecteplase is a mutant of t-PA with specific amino acid substitutions in the kringle 1 domain and

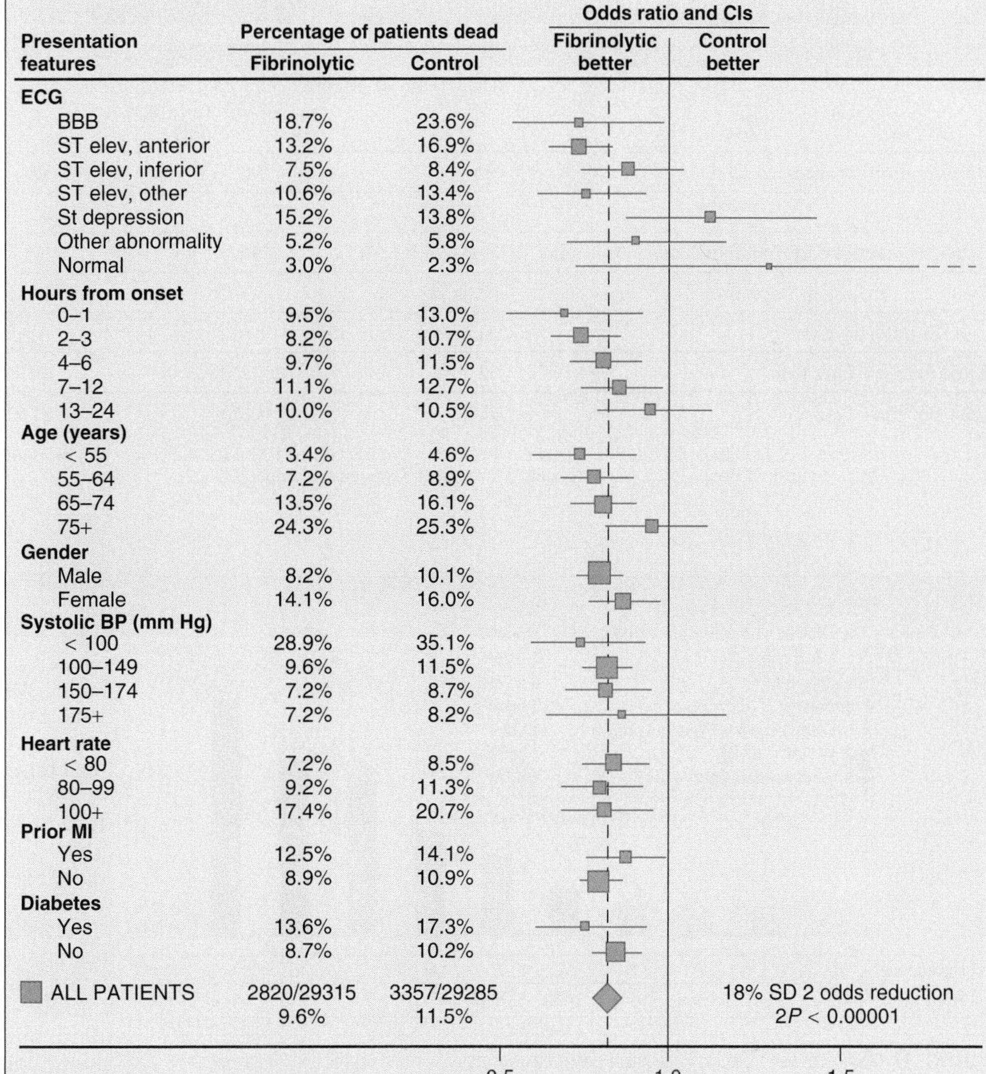

Presentation features
Percentage of patients dead
Fibrinolytic
Control
Odds ratio and CIs
Fibrinolytic better
Control better
ECG
BBB 18.7% 23.6%
ST elev, anterior 13.2% 16.9%
ST elev, inferior 7.5% 8.4%
ST elev, other 10.6% 13.4%
St depression 15.2% 13.8%
Other abnormality 5.2% 5.8%
Normal 3.0% 2.3%
Hours from onset
0–1 9.5% 13.0%
2–3 8.2% 10.7%
4–6 9.7% 11.5%
7–12 11.1% 12.7%
13–24 10.0% 10.5%
Age (years)
< 55 3.4% 4.6%
55–64 7.2% 8.9%
65–74 13.5% 16.1%
75+ 24.3% 25.3%
Gender
Male 8.2% 10.1%
Female 14.1% 16.0%
Systolic BP (mm Hg)
< 100 28.9% 35.1%
100–149 9.6% 11.5%
150–174 7.2% 8.7%
175+ 7.2% 8.2%
Heart rate
< 80 7.2% 8.5%
80–99 9.2% 11.3%
100+ 17.4% 20.7%
Prior MI
Yes 12.5% 14.1%
No 8.9% 10.9%
Diabetes
Yes 13.6% 17.3%
No 8.7% 10.2%
ALL PATIENTS 2820/29315 9.6% 3357/29285 11.5%
18% SD 2 odds reduction
2P < 0.00001
0.5
1.0
1.5

FIGURE 47–10 Mortality differences during days 0 to 35 subdivided by presentation features in a collaborative overview of results from nine trials of thrombolytic therapy. The absolute mortality rates are shown for fibrinolytic and control groups in the center portion of the figure for each of the clinical features at presentation listed on the left side of the figure. The ratio of the odds of death in the fibrinolytic group to that in the control group is shown for each subdivision (colored square), along with its 99 percent confidence interval (horizontal line). The summary odds ratio at the bottom of the figure corresponds to an 18 percent proportional reduction in 35-day mortality and is highly statistically significant. This translates to a reduction of 18 deaths per 1000 patients treated with thrombolytic agents. (From Fibrinolytic Therapy Trialists' [FTT] Collaborative Group: Indications for fibrinolytic therapy in suspected acute myocardial infarction: Collaborative overview of mortality and major morbidity results from all randomized trials of more than 1000 patients. Lancet 343:311, 1994. Copyright by The Lancet Ltd.)

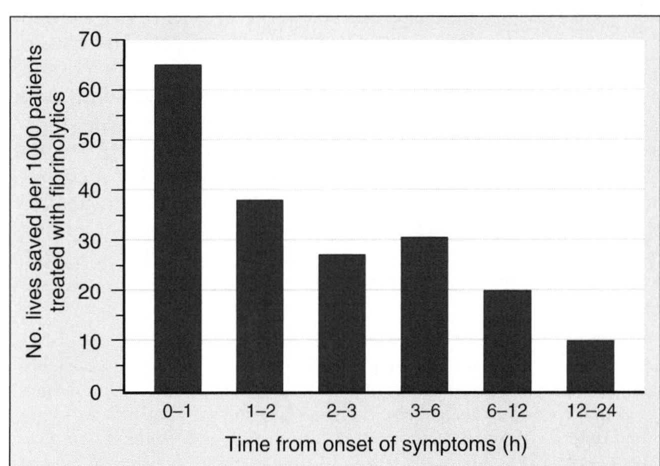

FIGURE 47–11 Importance of time to reperfusion in patients receiving fibrinolytic therapy for ST segment elevation myocardial infarction. The data from 22 trials of fibrinolytic therapy were pooled and the findings stratified by the six time categories shown in the figure. The number of lives saved per 1000 patients treated with fibrinolytics compared with placebo is greatest the earlier treatment is initiated after the onset of symptoms and this decreases in a nonlinear fashion with incremental time delays. Since the life-saving effect of fibrinolysis is maximal in the first hour from onset of symptoms, this has been referred to as the "golden hour" for pharmacological reperfusion. (From Boersma E, Maas AC, Deckers JW, et al: Early thrombolytic treatment in acute myocardial infarction: Reappraisal of the golden hour. Lancet 348:771, 1996.)

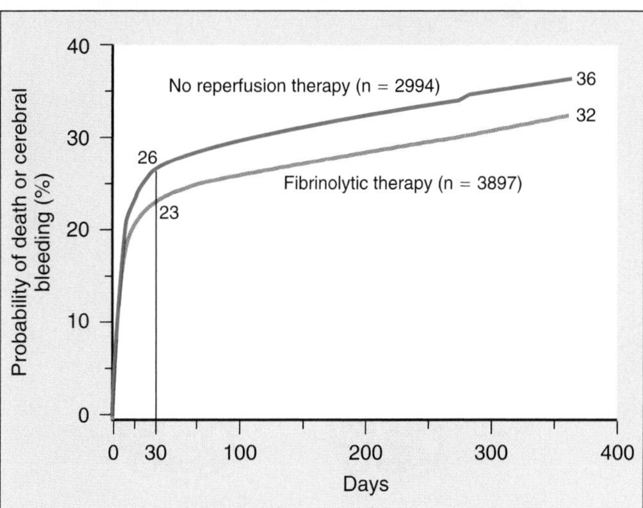

FIGURE 47–12 Probability of death or cerebral bleeding in elderly patients with ST segment elevation myocardial infarction. Patients older than 75 years of age entered in a Swedish national registry had significantly lower rates of death or cerebral bleeding if they received fibrinolytic therapy compared to no reperfusion therapy. The adjusted relative risk of death or cerebral bleeding through 1 year was 0.87 (0.80-0.94; $p = 0.001$). (From Stenestrand U, Wallentin L: Fibrinolytic therapy in patients 75 years and older with ST-segment-elevation myocardial infarction: One-year follow-up of a large prospective cohort. Arch Intern Med 163:965, 2003.)

TABLE 47–4 Comparison of Approved Fibrinolytic Agents

	Streptokinase	Alteplase	Reteplase	TNK-t-PA
Dose	1.5 MU in 30-60 min	Up to 100 mg in 90 min (based on weight)	10 U × 2 each over 2 min	30-50 mg based on weight*
Bolus administration	No	No	Yes	Yes
Antigenic	Yes	No	No	No
Allergic reactions (hypotension most common)	Yes	No	No	No
Systemic fibrinogen depletion	Marked	Mild	Moderate	Minimal
90-min patency rates (%)	Approximately 50	Approximately 75	Approximately 75	Approximately 75†
TIMI grade 3 flow (%)	32	54	60	63
Cost per dose (U.S. $)‡	568	2750	2750	2750 for 50 mg

Data from *Armstrong PW, Collen D: Circulation 103:2862, 2001; †Cannon CP, Gibson CM, McCabe CH, et al: Circulation 98:2805, 1998; and ‡Medical Economics Staff: 2001 Drug Topics Red Book. 105th ed. Montvale, NJ, Medical Economics Company, 2001.

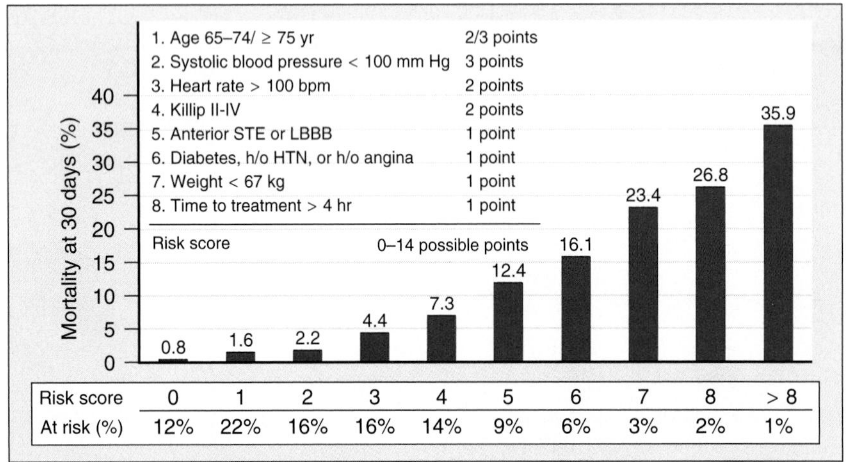

FIGURE 47–13 TIMI risk score for ST segment elevation myocardial infarction predicting 30-day mortality. h/o = history of; HTN = hypertension; LBBB = left bundle branch block; STE = ST segment elevation. (From Morrow DA, Antman EM, Charlesworth A, et al: The TIMI risk score for ST elevation myocardial infarction: A convenient, bedside, clinical score for risk assessment at presentation: An InTIME II substudy. Circulation 102:2031, 2000.)

protease domain introduced to decrease plasma clearance, increase fibrin specificity, and reduce sensitivity to plasminogen activator inhibitor-1 (see Fig. 47–14 and Table 47–4). The phase II angiographic dose-ranging studies TIMI 10A and TIMI 10B helped to define the optimum dose of tenecteplase with respect to efficacy.[82,83] An analysis comparing the weight-adjusted dose of tenecteplase compared with TIMI grade 3 flow indicated that a dose of 0.53 mg/kg was optimal for achieving high rates of TIMI grade 3 flow.[83] The safety of tenecteplase was evaluated in both TIMI 10B and another large phase II clinical trial called ASSENT 1.[84]

ASSENT 2 was a randomized, double-blind, phase III equivalence trial comparing single bolus tenecteplase with accelerated dose t-PA in 16,949 patients.[85] The 30-day mortality rate with tenecteplase was 6.179 percent and with t-PA it was 6.151 percent ($p = 0.0059$ for equivalence). The rate of intracranial hemorrhage was 0.93 percent with tenecteplase and 0.94 percent with t-PA. Major bleeding occurred in 4.66 percent of tenecteplase-treated patients compared with 5.94 percent of t-PA-treated patients (peak was 0.0002). There was no specific subgroup of patients in whom tenecteplase or t-PA was significantly better, with the exception of patients treated after 4 hours from the onset of symptoms, among whom the mortality rate was 7.0 percent with tenecteplase and 9.2 percent with t-PA ($p = 0.018$).

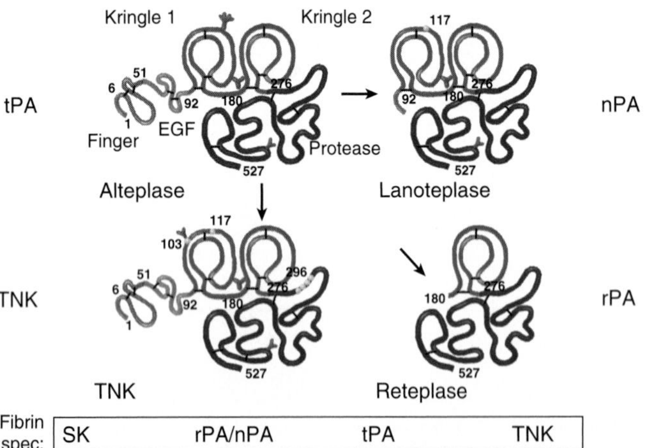

FIGURE 47–14 Molecular structure of alteplase (tPA), lanoteplase (nPA), reteplase (rPA), and tenecteplase (TNK). Streptokinase is the least fibrin-specific thrombolytic agent in clinical use; the progressive increase in relative fibrin specificity for the various thrombolytics is shown at the bottom. (Modified from Brener SJ, Topol EJ: Third-generation thrombolytic agents for acute myocardial infarction. *In* Topol EJ [ed.]: Acute Coronary Syndromes. New York, Marcel Dekker, 1998, p 169.)

OTHER FIBRINOLYTIC AGENTS. *Lanoteplase* is a novel plasminogen activator that is a mutant of t-PA lacking the finger and epidermal growth factor domains and also containing an amino acid substitution in the kringle 1 domain, leading to deletion of a glycosylation site (see Fig. 47–14). InTIME-II was a phase III double-blind equivalence trial in 15,078 patients comparing 120 kU/kg of lanoteplase with 100 mg of accelerated-dose t-PA. The 30-day mortality rate was 6.61 percent in the t-PA group and 6.75 percent in the lanoteplase group (RR, 1.02; $p = 0.075$ for equivalence).[86] The intracranial hemorrhage rate was 0.64 percent for t-PA and 1.12 percent for lanoteplase ($p = 0.004$). Because of the increased rate of intracranial hemorrhage with lanoteplase compared to t-PA in the dose studied, it is no longer being pursued for clinical development.

Urokinase is used on rare occasion as an intracoronary infusion (6000 IU/min) to an average cumulative dose of 5,000,000 IU to lyse intracoronary thrombi that are believed to be responsible for an evolving STEMI.

Anistreplase, usually administered in a dose of 30 mg over 2 to 5 minutes intravenously, has a side-effect profile similar to that of streptokinase, a patency profile similar to that of conventional-dose t-PA, and a mortality benefit similar to that of streptokinase or t-PA (double-chain form, duteplase). The lack of any compelling advantages (other than bolus administration) and costs higher than streptokinase have relegated anistreplase to an extremely infrequently prescribed drug for acute myocardial infarction in the United States.

Staphylokinase is a highly fibrin-specific plasminogen activator that requires priming on the surface of a clot. A pegylated, recombinant form of staphylokinase has been shown to yield TIMI grade 3 flow rates similar to those obtained with t-PA.[87]

Effect on Left Ventricular Function

Although precise measurements of infarct size would be an ideal endpoint for clinical reperfusion studies, such measures have been found to be impractical. Attempts to use left ventricular ejection fraction as a surrogate for infarct size have not been productive because little difference is seen in ejection fraction between treatment groups that show a significant difference in mortality. Methods of assessing left ventricular function, such as end-systolic volume or quantitative echocardiography, are more revealing because patients with smaller volumes and better preserved ventricular shape have an improved survival. The myocardial salvage index, defined as the difference between an initial perfusion defect (e.g., by sestamibi scintigraphy) and final perfusion defect, is a useful means for comparing the effectiveness of reperfusion therapies.[28]

As with survival, improvement in global left ventricular function is related to the time of fibrinolytic treatment, with greatest improvement occurring with earliest therapy.[28] Greater improvement in left ventricular function has been reported with anterior than with inferior infarcts. The angiographic substudy in GUSTO I reported detailed regional wall motion analyses stratified by thrombolytic regimen.[88] Patients who received the accelerated t-PA regimen had significantly less depression of regional wall motion in the ischemic zone, as evidenced by fewer abnormal chords when their ventricular silhouettes were subjected to segmental wall motion analysis. In addition, this patient group tended to have a slightly higher global ejection fraction and slightly reduced end-systolic volume index at 90 minutes following initiation of thrombolytic therapy. The totality of the data presented in the GUSTO I angiographic substudy[88] is consistent with the hypothesis that more rapid and complete restoration of normal coronary blood flow in the infarct-related artery with t-PA was associated with an improvement in regional and global left ventricular function (presumably through greater myocardial salvage in the ischemic zone) and that this difference in function compared with that obtained with streptokinase may have contributed to the mortality differences observed at 30 days and beyond.

Complications of Fibrinolytic Therapy

Recent (<1 year) exposure to streptococci or streptokinase produces some degree of antibody-mediated resistance to streptokinase (and anistreplase) in most patients. Although this is of clinical consequence only rarely, it is recommended that patients not receive streptokinase for STEMI if they have been treated with a streptokinase product within the last year. Bleeding complications are, of course, most common and potentially the most serious. Most bleeding is relatively minor with all agents, with more serious episodes occurring in patients requiring invasive procedures.[89] Intracranial hemorrhage is the most serious complication of fibrinolytic therapy; its frequency varies with the clinical characteristics of the patient and the fibrinolytic agent prescribed (Fig. 47–15).[7]

There have been reports of an "early hazard" with fibrinolytic therapy, that is, an excess of deaths in the first 24 hours in fibrinolytic-treated patients compared with control subjects (especially in elderly patients treated more than 12 hours).[19] However, this excess early mortality is more than offset by the deaths prevented beyond the first day, culminating in an 18 percent (range, 13 to 23 percent) reduction in mortality by 35 days.[19] The mechanisms responsible for this

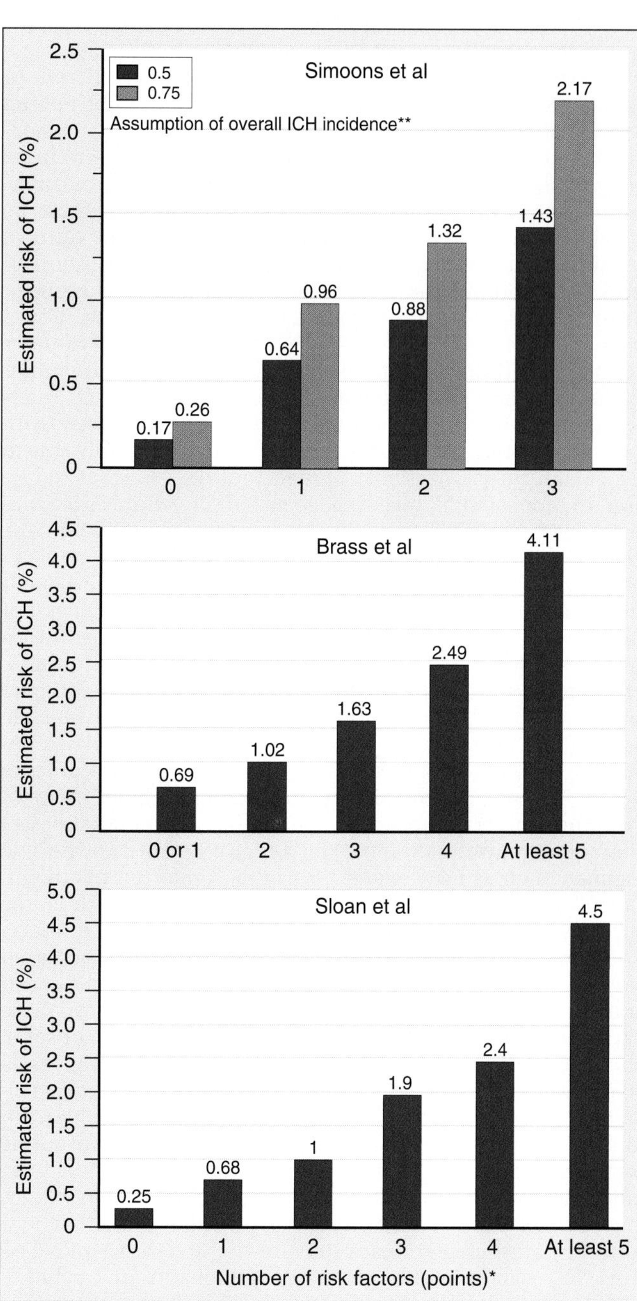

FIGURE 47–15 Estimation of risk of intracranial hemorrhage (ICH) with fibrinolysis. *The number of risk factors is the sum of the points based on criteria established in the studies shown. Although the exact risk factors varied among the studies, common risk factors across all the studies include increased age, low body weight, and hypertension on admission. **If the overall incidence of ICH is assumed to be 0.75 percent, patients without risk factors who receive streptokinase have a 0.26 percent probability of ICH. The risk is 0.96, 1.32, and 21.7 percent in patients with one, two, or three risk factors, respectively. See references for further discussion. (Data from Simoons et al: Lancet 342:1523, 1993; Brass et al: Stroke 31:1802, 2000; Sloan et al: J Am Coll Cardiol:37(Suppl A):372A, 2001.)

early hazard are not clear but probably are multiple, including an increased risk of myocardial rupture (particularly in the elderly), fatal intracranial hemorrhage,[90] inadequate myocardial reperfusion resulting in pump failure and cardiogenic shock,[91] and possible reperfusion injury of reperfused myocardium. Reports of more unusual complications such as splenic rupture, aortic dissection, and cholesterol embolization have also appeared.

Recommendations for Fibrinolytic Therapy

NET CLINICAL BENEFIT OF FIBRINOLYSIS. Perhaps one of the most important messages from all of the available evidence is that fibrinolytic therapy is underutilized in patients with STEMI.[92] Hesitancy in prescribing a fibrinolytic agent is often the result of uncertainty about the risk of bleeding. Patients with a higher baseline risk of mortality are more likely to benefit from fibrinolytic therapy. Against the mortality benefit associated with fibrinolytic therapy must be weighed the excess risk of stroke. Using the net clinical benefit composite endpoint of 30-day mortality or nonfatal stroke, a small but statistically significant benefit is seen for accelerated-dose t-PA compared with streptokinase. Given the data from the GUSTO 3 and ASSENT-2 trials, it appears that the net clinical benefit of accelerated-dose t-PA is similar to that obtained with reteplase or tenecteplase.[79,85] Of interest, the rate of noncerebral major bleeding was lower with tenecteplase than t-PA in the ASSENT-2 trial, possibly due to the greater fibrin specificity of tenecteplase.[85] Further reduction in noncerebral bleeding occurred in ASSENT-3 compared with ASSENT-2, probably due to a reduction in the dose of unfractionated heparin used in ASSENT-3.[93]

CHOICE OF AGENT. Analysis of the net clinical benefit and cost-effectiveness of t-PA versus streptokinase does not easily yield recommendations for treatment because clinicians must weigh the risk of mortality and the risk of intracranial hemorrhage when confronting a fibrinolytic-eligible patient with STEMI; additional considerations may be the constraints placed on physicians' therapeutic decision-making by the health care system in which they are practicing. In the subgroup of patients presenting within 4 hours of symptom onset, the speed of reperfusion of the infarct vessel is of paramount importance, and a high-intensity fibrinolytic regimen such as accelerated t-PA is the preferred treatment, except in those individuals in whom the risk of death is low (e.g., a young patient with a small inferior myocardial infarction) and the risk of intracranial hemorrhage is increased (e.g., acute hypertension), in whom streptokinase and accelerated t-PA are approximately equivalent choices. For those patients presenting between 4 and 12 hours after the onset of chest discomfort, the speed of reperfusion of the infarct vessel is of lesser importance, and therefore streptokinase and accelerated t-PA are generally equivalent options, given the difference in costs. Of note, for those patients presenting between 4 and 12 hours from symptom onset with a low mortality risk but an increased risk of intracranial hemorrhage (e.g., elderly patients with inferior myocardial infarction, systolic pressure greater than 100 mm Hg, and heart rate less than 100 beats/min), streptokinase is probably preferable to t-PA because of cost considerations if fibrinolytic therapy is prescribed at all in such patients.

In those patients considered appropriate candidates for fibrinolysis and in whom t-PA would have been selected as the agent of choice in the past, we believe clinicians should now consider using a bolus thrombolytic such as reteplase or tenecteplase. The rationale for this recommendation is that bolus fibrinolysis has the advantage of ease of administration, a lower chance of medication errors (and the associated increase in mortality when such medication errors occur), and less noncerebral bleeding and also offers the potential for prehospital treatment.[94,95]

LATE THERAPY. No mortality benefit was demonstrated in the LATE and EMERAS trials when fibrinolytics were routinely administered to patients between 12 and 24 hours, although we believe it is still reasonable to consider fibrinolytic therapy in appropriately selected patients with persistent symptoms and ST elevation on the electrocardiogram beyond 12 hours. Persistent chest pain late after the onset of symptoms correlates with a higher incidence of collateral or antegrade flow in the infarct zone and is therefore a marker for patients with viable myocardium that might be salvaged. Because elderly patients treated with fibrinolytic agents more than 12 hours after the onset of symptoms are at increased risk of cardiac rupture, it is our practice to restrict late fibrinolytic administration to younger patients (<65 years) with ongoing ischemia, especially those with large anterior infarctions. The elderly patient with ongoing ischemic symptoms but presenting late (>12 hours) is probably better managed with PCI (see Chap. 48) than with fibrinolytic therapy.

Before the institution of fibrinolytic therapy, consideration should be given to the patient's need for intravascular catheterization, as would be required for the placement of an arterial pressure monitoring line, a pulmonary artery catheter for hemodynamic monitoring, or a temporary transvenous pacemaker. If any of these are required, ideally they should be placed as expeditiously as possible *before* infusion of the fibrinolytic agent. If such procedures require an additional delay of more than 30 minutes, they should be deferred as long as possible after fibrinolytic therapy is begun. In the early hours after institution of fibrinolytic therapy, such catheterization should be performed only if crucial to the patient's survival, and then sites where excessive bleeding can be controlled should be chosen (e.g., subclavian vein catheterization should be avoided).

As noted earlier, all patients with suspected STEMI should receive aspirin (160-325 mg) regardless of the fibrinolytic agent prescribed. Aspirin should be continued indefinitely. The issues surrounding antithrombin therapy as an adjunct to thrombolysis are complex and are discussed in detail in a subsequent section.

Catheter-Based Reperfusion Strategies

Reperfusion of the infarct artery can also be achieved by a catheter-based strategy. This approach has evolved from passage of a balloon catheter over a guidewire to now include potent antiplatelet therapy (intravenous glycoprotein IIb/IIIa inhibitors, thienopyridines) and coronary stents.[56] When PCI is used in lieu of fibrinolytic therapy, it is referred to as direct or primary PCI. When fibrinolysis has failed to reperfuse the infarct vessel, or a severe stenosis is present in the infarct vessel, a rescue PCI can be performed. A more conservative approach of elective PCI can be used to manage STEMI patients only when spontaneous or exercise-provoked ischemia occurs, whether or not they have received a previous course of fibrinolytic therapy. Discussion of the use of PCI in STEMI patients and recommendations for catheter-based reperfusion strategies are found in Chapter 48.

SURGICAL REPERFUSION. Despite the extensive improvement in intraoperative preservation with cardioplegia and hypothermia and numerous surgical techniques (see Chap. 76), it is not logistically possible to provide surgical reperfusion in a timely fashion. Therefore, patients with STEMI who are candidates for reperfusion routinely receive either fibrinolysis or PCI. However, about 10 to 20 percent of STEMI patients are currently referred for coronary bypass grafting for one of the following indications: persistent or recurrent chest pain despite fibrinolysis or PCI, high-risk coronary anatomy (e.g., left main stenosis) discovered at catheterization, or a complication of STEMI such as ventricular septal rupture or severe mitral regurgitation due to papillary muscle dysfunction. Patients with STEMI with continued severe ischemic and hemodynamic instability are likely to benefit from emergency revascularization. PCI with stenting as needed is the preferable technique when revascularization is needed in the first 48 to 72 hours following STEMI; surgery should be reserved for patients in whom PCI has been unsuccessful or whose anatomy dictates the need for coronary artery bypass grafting, such as patients with left main or extensive multivessel coronary artery disease.

Patients undergoing successful fibrinolysis but with important residual stenoses, who on anatomical grounds are more suitable for surgical revascularization than for PCI, have undergone coronary artery bypass grafting with quite low rates of mortality (about 4 percent) and morbidity, *provided* that they are operated on more than 24 hours from STEMI; those patients requiring urgent or emergency coronary artery bypass grafting within 24 to 48 hours of acute myocardial infarction have mortality rates between 12 and 15 percent.[96] When surgery is performed under urgent conditions with active and ongoing ischemia or cardiogenic shock, the operative mortality rate rises steeply.

Selection of Reperfusion Strategy

Despite strong evidence in the literature that prompt use of reperfusion therapy improves survival of STEMI patients, room for improvement exists, since reperfusion therapy is underutilized and often not administered soon after presentation.[92,97] Considerable controversy exists about the optimum form of reperfusion therapy.[98] An important factor that continues to fuel this controversy is the dynamic and rapidly changing evidence base regarding the best approach to reperfusion for patients with STEMI. With respect to pharmacological reperfusion, new fibrinolytic agents, modified dosing regimens, and combinations of adjunctive treatments have produced a continuous process of refinement and improvement in medical measures to restore flow in the infarct artery (Fig. 47–16). From the perspective of PCI, improvements in catheterization laboratory facilities, new forms of stents, and distal embolization protection devices have dramatically improved the efficacy and safety of PCI for patients with STEMI (see Chap. 48). Improvements in pharmacological and PCI-based reperfusion strategies rapidly make prior studies less relevant to contemporary practice. In addition, progressive reductions in mortality from STEMI have made it increasingly difficult to conduct clinical trials of a practical size. Investigators frequently use composite endpoints that combine mortality with nonfatal events such as recurrent myocardial infarction, recurrent ischemia, or target vessel revascularization.

In a pooled analysis of 23 randomized trials comparing PCI versus fibrinolysis for STEMI over both the short and the long terms, PCI was superior to fibrinolysis for almost all of the endpoints analyzed (see Fig. 48–2).[99] However, the absolute risk difference between the two reperfusion strategies varied depending on the endpoint; this translates into a wide range of patients who need to be treated (or who are harmed) to prevent one event using PCI as compared with fibrinolysis as the reperfusion strategy for patients with STEMI.

Several issues should be considered in selecting the type of reperfusion therapy:

1. *Time from the onset of symptoms to initiation of fibrinolytic therapy*: This is an important predictor of infarct size and patient outcome.[66] Schomig and colleagues reported that the influence of time-to-treatment interval on myocardial salvage in patients with STEMI depends on the type of reper-

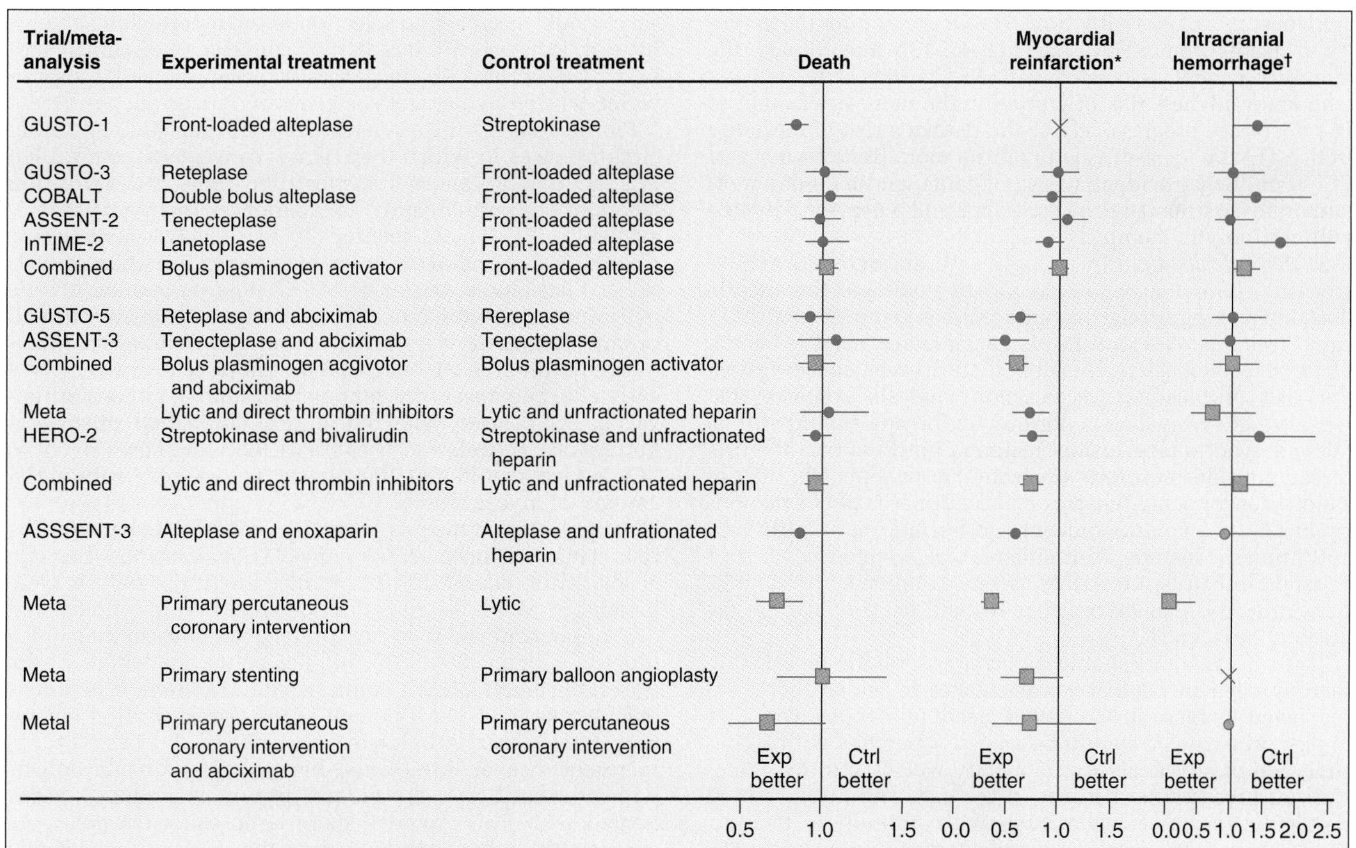

FIGURE 47–16 Relative treatment effect associated with several acute reperfusion modalities in patients presenting with ST segment elevation myocardial infarction (STEMI). Data are odds ratios and 95 percent confidence intervals. (Modified from Boersma E, Mercado N, Poldermans, et al: Acute myocardial infarction. Lancet 361:851, 2003.)

fusion therapy.[28] Patients who were treated with fibrinolysis less than 165 minutes, 165 to 280 minutes, and more than 280 minutes from the onset of symptoms had final infarct sizes of 13.6 percent, 20.2 percent, and 24.0 percent of the left ventricle; in patients treated with stenting, the final infarct sizes were 10.1 percent, 9.4 percent, and 11.1 percent, respectively, in the same time intervals. Despite the time-dependent increase in infarct size in patients treated with fibrinolysis and the more stable pattern of smaller infarcts in patients treated with PCI, no consistent time-dependent pattern was seen in clinical outcomes with either reperfusion strategy.[28] The lack of a consistent relationship between infarct size and clinical outcomes regardless of reperfusion strategy suggests that a complex interplay of multiple factors determines the likelihood of clinical events. While infarct size is one such factor, others include the coexistence of obstructions in noninfarct-related coronary arteries, the level of electrical stability of the myocardium, the extent of left ventricular remodeling, and the number of medications prescribed following STEMI as well as the patient's response to them. Thus, for patients treated by fibrinolysis or PCI, time from the onset of symptoms is an important predictor of mortality, underscoring the need for prompt reperfusion, whichever strategy is selected (see Figs. 47–1 and 47–2).[35–36,69]

2. *Risk of the STEMI*: Patients presenting with cardiogenic shock have an improved 1-year survival chance if they are treated with an early revascularization strategy (PCI and/or coronary artery bypass grafting as indicated).[100] Observational data from the Second National Registry of Myocardial Infarction also suggests the superiority of PCI compared with fibrinolysis for patients presenting with a condition of a Killip class ≥ II.[101] Kent and associates performed an analysis to test whether subgroups of patients with STEMI with a high risk of mortality might be especially likely to benefit from PCI and those at lower risk might be less likely to benefit.[102] Patients at highest risk of mortality from STEMI account for the majority of deaths from STEMI (see Fig. 47–13). Accordingly, the mortality benefit associated with PCI is largest in patients who are at highest risk of mortality; the mortality benefit of PCI decreases progressively as the patient's risk of mortality from STEMI decreases, such that the mortality advantage of PCI is no longer evident among patients whose 30-day mortality rate is estimated to be between 2 and 3 percent if treated with fibrinolytic therapy.[102]

3. *Risk of bleeding*: In patients with an increased risk of bleeding, particularly intracranial hemorrhage, therapeutic decision making strongly favors a PCI-based reperfusion strategy[103] (see Fig. 47–15). If PCI is unavailable, then the benefit of pharmacological reperfusion should be balanced against the risk of bleeding. A decision analysis suggests that when no PCI is available, fibrinolytic therapy should still be favored over no reperfusion treatment until the risk of a life-threatening bleed exceeds 4 percent. For patients who are not candidates for acute reperfusion because of lack of availability of PCI and contraindications to fibrinolysis, aspirin and antithrombin therapy with either unfractionated heparin or enoxaparin can be prescribed. There is no benefit to amplifying the antiplatelet regimen by adding tirofiban to the medical regimen.[104]

Thus, every effort should be made to provide reperfusion therapy even in clinical circumstances in which there is a perceived increase in the risk of bleeding. Arrangements for urgent primary PCI should be made for patients with a constellation of advanced age, low body weight, and hypertension on presentation because of the substantially increased risk of intracranial hemorrhage with fibrinolytic therapy. When the estimated delay to implementation of primary PCI is substantial (much greater than 90 minutes), fibrinolysis (with a fibrin-specific agent) may be preferable to no reperfusion therapy in such patients when the risk from the STEMI is high (e.g., anterior infarction with hemodynamic compromise). In the setting of absolute contraindications to fibrinolysis (see Table 47–3) and lack of access to PCI facilities, antithrombin therapy with unfractionated heparin or enoxaparin and antiplatelet therapy with aspirin should be prescribed because of the small but finite chance (10 percent) of restoration of TIMI grade 3 flow in the infarct vessel and decreasing the chance of thrombotic complications of STEMI.[88]

4. *Time required for transportation to a skilled PCI center*: The greatest operational impediment to routine implementation of a PCI reperfusion strategy is the delay required for transportation to a skilled PCI center (see Figs. 47–1 and 47–2).[98] Although several trials reported that referral to a PCI center was superior to fibrinolysis administered in a local hospital, such studies were conducted in dedicated health care systems with extremely short transportation and door-to-balloon times at the PCI centers.[105-107] Evidence exists to suggest that for every 10 minutes of delay to perform primary PCI versus administration of fibrinolytic therapy, there is a 1 percent absolute reduction in the mortality difference originally favoring primary PCI.[108] Thus, a 1-hour delay for initiation of primary PCI may equalize the mortality benefit of primary PCI versus administration of fibrin-specific fibrinolytic therapy.

Circumstances in which fibrinolysis or PCI is the preferred reperfusion strategy are summarized in Table 47–2. The assessment of reperfusion options for STEMI is a two-step process. Step one involves the integrated assessment of the time since onset of symptoms (see Figs. 47–4 and 47–11), risk of STEMI (see Fig. 47–13), risk of bleeding if fibrinolysis were to be administered (see Fig. 47–15), and time required for transportation to a skilled PCI center (see Fig. 47–4 and Chap. 48). The complexities of clinical medicine do not permit the decision-making to be reduced to a simple equation or "one size fits all" approach to selection of the reperfusion strategy. Instead, for step two, it is best to conceive of circumstances in which fibrinolysis is generally preferred and those in which an invasive strategy is generally preferred.

Fibrinolysis is the preferred reperfusion strategy under circumstances in which there is no ready access to a skilled PCI facility (prolonged transportation time, catheterization laboratory occupied, only inexperienced operator/team is available), PCI is not technically feasible (vascular access difficulties), or the decision-making favors initiation of lysis rather than risking the delay to PCI (door-to-balloon time is >90 minutes, the difference between door-to-balloon time and prompt initiation of lysis with a fibrin-specific agent [door-to-needle time] is >1 hour). When the patient presents very early after the onset of symptoms (<3 hours), either fibrinolysis or PCI is acceptable, but in most clinical circumstances fibrinolysis is preferred because of the anticipated delay to PCI, which would put the patient at risk of a substantial amount of myocardium.

An invasive strategy is generally preferred, the greater the risk. This risk may be from the STEMI itself (cardiogenic shock, Killip class ≥ II) or from bleeding if fibrinolysis were prescribed. When a skilled PCI operator/team is available and can implement an invasive strategy without undue delay (door-to-balloon time < 90 minutes or within 1 hour of the time a fibrinolytic agent could be administered), it is preferable to take the STEMI patient to the catheterization laboratory rather than administer fibrinolysis. Because of the increased risk of intracranial hemorrhage with fibrinolysis with advanced age, the elderly patient is probably better treated with PCI, provided there is no excessive delay. As coronary thrombi mature over time, they become increasingly resistant to fibrinolysis. Thus, PCI is the preferred reperfusion strategy if more than 3 hours have elapsed from the onset of symptoms, again assuming there is no significant delay in the anticipated time to balloon inflation (see Fig. 47–4). Finally, when the diagnosis is in doubt, an invasive strategy is clearly the preferred strategy, since it not only provides key diagnostic information regarding the patient's symptoms but does so without the risk of intracranial hemorrhage associated with fibrinolysis.

Antithrombin and Antiplatelet Therapy

Antithrombin Therapy

The rationale for administering antithrombin therapy acutely in STEMI patients includes prevention of deep venous thrombosis, pulmonary embolism, ventricular thrombus formation, and cerebral embolization. In addition, establishing and maintaining patency of the infarct-related artery, whether or not a patient receives fibrinolytic therapy, is another common rationale for antithrombin therapy in cases of STEMI (Fig. 47–17).

EFFECT ON MORTALITY. Randomized trials in STEMI patients conducted in the prefibrinolytic era showed that the risks of pulmonary embolism, stroke, and reinfarction were reduced in patients who received intravenous heparin, providing the support for prescription of heparin to STEMI patients not treated with fibrinolytic therapy. With the introduction of the fibrinolytic era and, importantly, after the publication of the ISIS-2 trial,[109] the situation became more complicated because of strong evidence of a substantial mortality reduction with aspirin alone and confusing and conflicting data regarding the risk-benefit ratio of heparin used as an adjunct to aspirin or in combination with aspirin and a fibrinolytic agent. For every 1000 patients treated with heparin compared with aspirin alone, there are 5 fewer deaths ($p = 0.03$) and 3 fewer recurrent infarctions ($p = 0.04$), at the expense of 3 more major bleeds ($p < 0.001$).[110] Nonrandomized subgroup analyses from the LATE trial of 2821 patients who received t-PA showed a 35-day mortality rate of 7.6 percent when intravenous heparin was administered, compared with 10.4 percent when no heparin was given. Heparin was administered as adjunctive therapy in randomized trials of reteplase and tenecteplase under the supposition that those agents were more fibrin-specific than streptokinase and required concomitant use of heparin.[84,111]

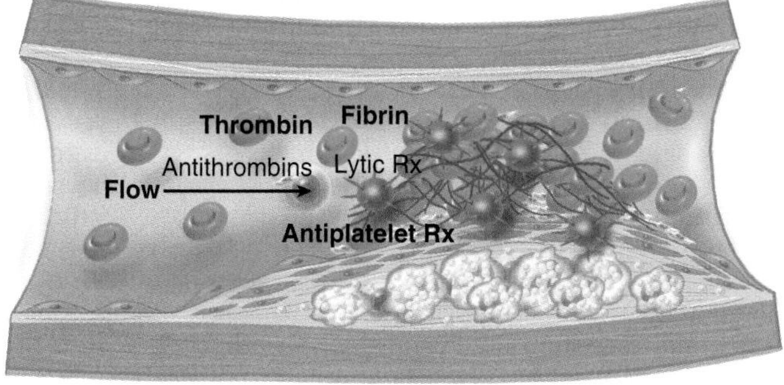

FIGURE 47–17 Pharmacological dissolution of thrombus in infarct-related artery. This figure shows a schematic view of a longitudinal section of an infarct-related artery at the level of the obstructive thrombus. Following rupture of a vulnerable plaque (bottom center), the coagulation cascade is activated, ultimately leading to the deposition of fibrin strands (blue curvilinear arcs); platelets are activated and begin to aggregate (transition from flat discs representing inactive platelets to green spiked ball elements representing activated and aggregating platelets). The mesh of fibrin strands and platelet aggregates obstructs flow (normally moving from left to right) in the infarct-related artery; this would correspond to TIMI grade 0 on angiography. Pharmacological reperfusion is a multipronged approach consisting of fibrinolytic agents that digest fibrin, antithrombins that prevent the formation of thrombin and inhibit the activity of thrombin that is formed, and antiplatelet therapy. (Courtesy of Luke Wells, The Exeter Group.)

OTHER EFFECTS. A number of angiographic studies have examined the role of heparin therapy in establishing and maintaining patency of the infarct-related artery in patients with STEMI. Comparison of these trials is difficult because of potentially important differences in study design, including whether aspirin was administered along with heparin, the fibrinolytic agent that was administered, and variations in the time of diagnostic coronary arteriography. Although the evidence favoring the use of heparin for enhancing patency of the infarct artery when a fibrin-specific fibrinolytic agent is prescribed is not conclusive, the suggestion of a mortality benefit and amelioration of the pattern of left ventricular thrombus (less protuberant) that develops after STEMI indicates it is prudent to use heparin for at least 48 hours after fibrinolysis and to maintain an activated partial thromboplastin time (aPTT) target of one-and-a-half to two times that of control.[7,112]

Although heparin may induce thrombocytopenia through an immunological mechanism, this is seen only rarely, probably occurring in only 2 to 3 percent of patients.[113] The most serious complication of antithrombotic therapy is bleeding, especially intracranial hemorrhage, when fibrinolytic agents are prescribed. Major hemorrhagic events occur more frequently in patients of low body weight, advanced age, female gender, marked prolongation of the aPTT (greater than 90 to 100 seconds), and the performance of invasive procedures.[112] Frequent monitoring of the aPTT (facilitated by use of a bedside testing device) reduces the risk of major hemorrhagic complications in patients treated with heparin. It should be noted, however, that during the first 12 hours following fibrinolytic therapy, the aPTT may be elevated from the fibrinolytic agent alone (particularly if streptokinase is administered), making it difficult to accurately interpret the effects of a heparin infusion on the patient's coagulation status.

NEW ANTITHROMBOTIC AGENTS

Potential disadvantages of unfractionated heparin include dependency on antithrombin III for inhibition of thrombin activity, sensitivity to platelet factor 4, inability to inhibit clot-bound thrombin, marked interpatient variability in therapeutic response, and the need for frequent aPTT monitoring. In an effort to circumvent these disadvantages of unfractionated heparin, there has been interest in the development of novel antithrombotic compounds.[114]

HIRUDIN AND BIVALIRUDIN. Direct thrombin inhibitors such as hirudin or bivalirudin have not been shown to reduce mortality compared with heparin when used as adjuncts to fibrinolysis.[115,116] While recurrent myocardial infarction is reduced by 25 to 30 percent compared with heparin, this benefit is primarily observed during the period of administration of the direct thrombin inhibitor and decreases in magnitude over time. In addition, both hirudin and bivalirudin have been associated with higher rates of major bleeding versus heparin when used with fibrinolytic agents.[115,116]

LOW-MOLECULAR-WEIGHT HEPARINS. These are formed by controlled enzymatic or chemical depolymerization, producing chains of glycosaminoglycans of varying length but with a mean molecular weight of approximately 5000.[114] Advantages of low-molecular-weight heparins include a stable, reliable anticoagulant effect, high bioavailability, permitting administration via the subcutaneous route, and a high antiXa:antiIIa ratio, producing blockade of the coagulation cascade in an upstream location, resulting in a marked decrement in thrombin generation. Compared with unfractionated heparin, the rate of early (60-90 minutes) reperfusion of the infarct artery, either assessed angiographically or by noninvasive means, is not enhanced by administration of a low-molecular-weight heparin.[117-119] However, the rates of reocclusion of the infarct artery, reinfarction, or recurrent ischemic events appear to be reduced by low-molecular-weight heparins.

The ASSENT-3 trial compared unfractionated heparin with enoxaparin (30 mg intravenous bolus followed by subcutaneous injections of 1 mg/kg every 12 hours until hospital discharge).[93] The composite endpoint of 30-day mortality, in-hospital reinfarction, or in-hospital refractory ischemia was reduced from 15.4 percent with unfractionated heparin to 11.4 percent with enoxaparin (RR, 0.74; 95 percent CI, 0.63-0.87). The rate of intracranial hemorrhage was similar with unfractionated heparin versus enoxaparin (0.93 percent versus 0.88 percent; $p = 0.98$).

The ASSENT-3 PLUS study compared the same unfractionated heparin and enoxaparin regimens but initiated therapy in the prehospital setting.[120] The composite endpoint of 30-day mortality, in-hospital reinfarction, or in-hospital refractory ischemia was reduced from 17.4 percent with unfractionated heparin to 14.2 percent with enoxaparin ($p = 0.08$). Of concern, however, was the increased rate of intracranial hemorrhage observed in ASSENT-3 PLUS: 1.0 percent with unfractionated heparin versus 2.2 percent with enoxaparin ($p = 0.05$). The increase in intracranial hemorrhage in ASSENT-3 PLUS was seen predominantly in patients older than 75 years of age: 0.8 percent with unfractionated heparin versus 6.7 percent with enoxaparin ($p = 0.01$). The ongoing ExTRACT-TIMI 25 trial is testing the hypothesis that enoxaparin is superior to unfractionated heparin when administered as an adjunct to fibrinolytic therapy with respect to the primary composite endpoint of death or nonfatal recurrent myocardial infarction through 30 days. Because of the observations noted earlier regarding the excess risk of intracranial hemorrhage in elderly patients receiving enoxaparin, a dose modification has been introduced so that elderly patients do not receive an initial 30 mg intravenous bolus and receive 0.75 mg/kg subcutaneously every 12 hours throughout the index hospitalization; this represents 75 percent of the maintenance dose administered to patients younger than 75 years of age.

Recommendations for Antithrombin Therapy

Given the pivotal role thrombin plays in the pathogenesis of STEMI, antithrombotic therapy remains an important intervention (see Fig. 47–17). Patients undergoing percutaneous or surgical revascularization should receive unfractionated heparin (see Chaps. 48 and 76). Patients undergoing reperfusion therapy with alteplase, reteplase, or tenecteplase should receive unfractionated heparin as a weight-based bolus of 60 U/kg (maximum 4000 U) followed by an initial infusion of 12 U/kg/hr (maximum 1000 U/hr) adjusted to maintain an aPTT at one and a half to two times control.[7] Unfractionated heparin should also be given intravenously to patients treated with nonselective fibrinolytic agents (e.g., streptokinase) who are at high risk for systemic emboli (large or anterior myocardial infarction, atrial fibrillation, previous embolus, or known left ventricular thrombus). It is not unreasonable to also consider administration of unfractionated heparin intravenously to all patients undergoing reperfusion therapy with streptokinase.

Low-molecular-weight-heparin can be considered an acceptable alternative to unfractionated heparin as ancillary therapy for patients younger than 75 years of age who are receiving fibrinolytic therapy if significant renal dysfunction (serum creatinine > 2.5 mg/dl in men or > 2.0 mg/dl in women) is not present. Enoxaparin (30-mg intravenous bolus followed by 1.0 mg/kg subcutaneously every 12 hours until hospital discharge) used in combination with full-dose tenecteplase is the most comprehensively studied regimen in patients younger than 75 years of age. Low-molecular-weight heparin should not be used as an alternative to unfractionated heparin as ancillary therapy in patients older than 75 years of age who are receiving fibrinolytic therapy until a safe dosing regimen for elderly patients is established from clinical trials.

In patients with known heparin-induced thrombocytopenia, it is reasonable to consider bivalirudin as a useful alternative to heparin to be used in conjunction with streptokinase. Dosing according to the HERO 2 regimen (a bolus of 0.25 mg/kg followed by an intravenous infusion of 0.5 mg/kg/hr for the first 12 hours and 0.25 mg/kg/hr for the subsequent 36 hours) is recommended but with a reduction in the infusion rate if the aPTT is greater than 75 seconds within the first 12 hours.[116] (Bivalirudin is currently indicated only for anticoagulation in patients with unstable angina who are undergoing percutaneous coronary angioplasty, but in view of the limited alternatives available to clinicians when treating patients with heparin-induced thrombocytopenia, the recommendation noted above should be considered.)

Antiplatelet Therapy

Platelets play a major role in the thrombotic response to disruption of a coronary artery plaque (see Fig. 46–1).[121] Platelets are activated in response to fibrinolysis, and platelet-rich thrombi are also more resistant to fibrinolysis than are fibrin and erythrocyte-rich thrombi (Fig. 47–17).[122] Thus, there is a sound scientific basis for inhibiting platelet aggregation in *all* STEMI patients, regardless of whether a thrombolytic agent is prescribed. Comprehensive overviews of randomized trials of antiplatelet therapy have summarized the overwhelming evidence of benefit of antiplatelet therapy for a wide range of vascular disorders.[123] In patients at risk for STEMI, patients with a documented prior STEMI, and patients in the acute phase of STEMI, there is a 22 percent reduction in the odds of the composite endpoint of death, nonfatal recurrent infarction, and nonfatal stroke with antiplatelet therapy (Fig. 47–18). Not unexpectedly, the absolute benefits are greatest in those patients at highest baseline risk. Although several antiplatelet regimens have been evaluated, the agent most extensively tested has been aspirin, and this also is the drug for which the most compelling evidence of benefit exists.

The ISIS-2 study was the largest trial of aspirin in STEMI patients; it provides the single strongest piece of evidence that aspirin reduces mortality in STEMI patients.[109] In contrast to the observations of a time-dependent mortality effect of fibrinolytic therapy, the mortality reduction with aspirin was similar in patients treated within 4 hours (25 percent reduction in mortality), between 5 and 12 hours (21 percent reduction), and between 13 and 24 hours (21 percent reduction). There was an overall 23 percent reduction in mortality from aspirin in ISIS-2 that was largely additive to the 25 percent reduction in mortality from streptokinase, so that patients receiving both therapies experienced a 42 percent reduction in mortality.[109] The mortality reduction was as high as 53 percent in those patients who received both aspirin and streptokinase within 6 hours of symptoms. Of particular interest was the finding that the combination of streptokinase and aspirin reduced mortality *without* increasing the risk of stroke or hemorrhage.

Obstructive arterial thrombi that are platelet rich are resistant to fibrinolysis and have an increased tendency to produce reocclusion after initial successful reperfusion in patients with STEMI.[124] Despite the inhibition of cyclooxygenase by aspirin, platelet activation continues to occur through thromboxane A_2-independent pathways, leading to platelet aggregation and increased thrombin formation. Activation of platelets by a variety of agonists results in the expression of functional receptors for fibrinogen and other ligands on the platelet surface—the glycoprotein (GP) IIb/IIIa receptor.[125] GP IIb/IIIa inhibition accelerates fibrinolysis and prevents reocclusion of successfully recanalized infarct arteries.[126] Potential mechanistic explanations for the beneficial of the effects of GP IIb/IIIa inhibition when combined with fibrinolytics center around important interactions between fibrinolytics and platelets (see Fig. 47–17). Platelets can be stimulated by fibrinolytics—for example, by the exposure of clot-bound thrombin. A narrowed lumen and a highly stenosed infarct-related artery generates high shear forces, a potent stimulus to platelet activation. Activated platelets may inhibit thrombolysis through the release of substances such as plasminogen activator inhibitor-1, alpha-2 plasminogen inhibitor, and factor XIII, which stabilize the clot and also

Category of trial	No. of trials with data	No. (%) of vascular events: Allocated antiplatelet	No. (%) of vascular events: Adjusted control	Observed-expected	Variance	% Odds reduction (SE)
Previous myocardial infarction	12	1345/9984 (13.5)	1708/10022 (17.0)	−159.8	567.6	25 (4)
Acute myocardial infarction	15	1007/9658 (10.4)	1370/9644 (14.2)	−181.5	519.2	30 (4)
Previous stroke/transient ischemic attack	21	2045/11493 (17.8)	2464/11527 (21.4)	−152.1	625.8	22 (4)
Acute stroke	7	1670/20418 (8.2)	1858/20403 (9.1)	−94.6	795.3	11 (3)
Other high risk	140	1638/20359 (8.0)	2102/20543 (10.2)	−222.3	737.0	26 (3)
Subtotal: all except acute stroke	188	6035/51494 (11.7)	7644/51736 (14.8)	−715.7	2449.6	25 (2)
All trials	**195**	**7705/71912 (10.7)**	**9502/72139 (13.2)**	**−810.3**	**3244.9**	**22 (2)**

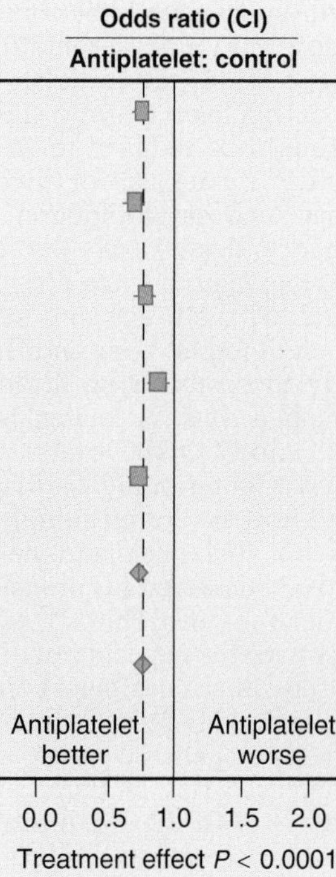

Odds ratio (CI) Antiplatelet: control; Antiplatelet better | Antiplatelet worse; 0.0 0.5 1.0 1.5 2.0; Treatment effect $P < 0.0001$

Heterogeneity of odds reductions between:
5 categories of trial: $\chi^2 = 21.4$, df = 4; $P = 0.0003$
Acute stroke vs. other: $\chi^2 = 18.0$, df = 1; $P = 0.00002$

FIGURE 47–18 Proportional effects of antiplatelet therapy on vascular events (myocardial infarction, stroke, or vascular death) in the main high-risk categories. Stratified ratio of odds of an event in treatment groups to that in control groups is plotted for each group of trials (square) along with its 99 percent confidence interval (horizontal line). Meta-analysis of results for all trials (and 95 percent confidence interval) is represented by a diamond. (From Antithromboitc Trialists' Collaboration: Collaborative meta-analysis of randomised trials of antiplatelet therapy for prevention of death, myocardial infarction, and stroke in high-risk patients. BMJ 324:71, 2002.)

enhance clot retraction—all features that make the clot more resistant to thrombolysis. Observations such as those noted earlier served as the foundation for testing the hypothesis that GP IIb/IIIa inhibition is a potent and safe addition to thrombolytic regimens and introduced the concept of *combination reperfusion* for patients with STEMI.

Aspirin only partially inhibits platelet aggregation by inhibiting the thromboxane A_2 pathway. Thienopyridines such as ticlopidine and clopidogrel inhibit binding to the adenosine diphosphate receptor and also block adenosine diphosphate-dependent pathways for platelet activation. Platelet inhibition by aspirin and the thienopyridines block only a limited number of the pathways of platelet activation. Irrespective of the stimulus for platelet activation, the final common pathway is expression of the GP IIb/IIIa receptor on the platelet surface. Therefore, direct inhibition of the GP IIb/IIIa receptor with intravenous agents such as abciximab, tirofiban, and eptifibatide has been studied in patients with STEMI.[34]

COMBINATION PHARMACOLOGICAL REPERFUSION. Several studies evaluated the combination of GP IIb/IIIa inhibitors and fibrinolytics.[127] The first series of trials combined full doses of thrombolytic agents with IIb/IIIa inhibitors.[128-131] Although these initial trials provided proof of the concept that the addition of an intravenous GP IIb/IIIa inhibitor enhanced the efficacy of a full dose of a fibrinolytic agent, unacceptably high rates of major bleeding were observed.

The combination of a reduced dose of a fibrinolytic agent and IIb/IIIa inhibitor was tested in a subsequent series of trials.[62,132-135] The rates of TIMI grade 3 flow at 60 and 90 minutes were only slightly higher with combination reperfusion compared with full-dose fibrinolytic monotherapy. A generally consistent observation across the trials was evidence of improved myocardial perfusion reflected in enhanced ST segment resolution and faster angiographic frame counts.[132,134-136]

GLYCOPROTEIN IIB/IIIA INHIBITION. The GUSTO V trial tested half-dose reteplase (5 U and 5 U) and full-dose abciximab compared with full-dose reteplase (10 U and 10 U) in 16,588 patients in the first 6 hours of STEMI.[137] Thirty-day mortality rates were similar in the two treatment groups (5.9 percent versus 5.6 percent). However, nonfatal reinfarction and other complications of myocardial infarction were reduced in the group receiving combination reperfusion therapy. Although the rates of intracranial hemorrhage were the same in the two treatment groups (0.6 percent), moderate to severe bleeding was significantly increased from 2.3 percent to 4.6 percent with combination reperfusion therapy ($p < 0.001$). This excess bleeding risk appeared to be limited to patients older than 75 years of age. The greatest mortality benefit was observed in those patients who presented with anterior myocardial infarction.

The ASSENT-3 trial randomized 6095 patients with STEMI to full-dose tenecteplase with unfractionated heparin versus full-dose tenecteplase with enoxaparin or half-dose tenecteplase plus abciximab (with weight-adjusted reduced-dose unfractionated heparin).[93] Similar to the GUSTO V trial, combination reperfusion therapy with half-dose tenecteplase and abciximab was not associated with a reduction in 30-day mortality; however, in-hospital reinfarction and refractory ischemia were reduced with combination reperfusion therapy. Of note, the major bleeding rate other than intracranial hemorrhage was increased from 2.2 percent to 4.3 percent with combination reperfusion therapy ($p < 0.0005$). The elderly were at greatest risk for excess bleeding, experiencing a threefold increase in the rate of that complication.

Nonenteric-coated aspirin should be chewed by patients who have not taken aspirin prior to presentation with STEMI. The dose should be 162 to 325 mg initially. During the maintenance phase of antiplatelet therapy following STEMI, the dose of aspirin should be reduced to 75 to 162 mg to minimize bleeding risk.[138] If true aspirin allergy is present, other antiplatelet agents such as clopidogrel (loading dose 300-600 mg; maintenance dose 75 mg per day) or ticlopidine (loading dose 500 mg; maintenance dose 250 mg twice daily) can be substituted. The efficacy and safety of the routine combination of clopidogrel plus aspirin in patients with STEMI, especially those receiving fibrinolytic therapy, has not been established but is being investigated in the CLARITY-TIMI 28 and COMMIT trials.

In selected patients (anterior myocardial infarction, age less than 75 years, and low risk for bleeding), combination reperfusion therapy with abciximab and half-dose reteplase or tenecteplase can be considered for prevention of reinfarction and other complications of STEMI,[137] although this should not be undertaken with the expectation of a reduction in mortality. Combination pharmacological reperfusion therapy with abciximab and half-dose reteplase or tenecteplase should not be given to patients older than 75 years of age because of an increased risk of intracranial hemorrhage. A discussion of the use of GP IIb/IIIa inhibitors either alone or in combination with reduced dose fibrinolytic as a preparatory regimen in patients for whom PCI is planned (i.e., facilitated PCI) is found in Chapter 48.

Hospital Management

Coronary Care Units

Deaths from primary ventricular fibrillation in patients with STEMI have been prevented because the coronary care unit (CCU) allows continuous monitoring of cardiac rhythm by highly trained nurses with the authority to initiate immediate treatment of arrhythmias in the absence of physicians, and because of the specialized equipment (defibrillators, pacemakers) and drugs available. Although all of these benefits can be achieved for patients scattered throughout the hospital, the clustering of patients with STEMI in the CCU has greatly improved the efficient use of the trained personnel, facilities, and equipment. With increasing emphasis on hemodynamic monitoring and treatment of the serious complications of STEMI with such modalities as pharmacological or catheter-based reperfusion therapy, afterload reduction, and intraaortic balloon counterpulsation, the presence of a CCU and experienced teams of physicians has assumed even greater importance. Improvements in the 30-day survival rate of elderly patients with STEMI can be traced to advances in therapy delivered in CCUs.[139] As reperfusion strategies including fibrinolytic therapy and PCI are used more routinely in STEMI patients, facilities in which patients can undergo diagnostic and therapeutic angiographic procedures are being integrated into an expanded structure of a coronary care team.[140]

At the same time, the value of CCUs for patients with uncomplicated STEMI has been questioned and restudied.[7] With increasing attention directed to the limitations of resources and to the economic impact of intensive care, efforts have been made to select patients likely to benefit from hospitalization in a CCU. The ECG reading, on presentation, particularly in conjunction with previous tracings and an immediate general clinical assessment, can be useful both for predicting which patients will have the diagnosis of acute myocardial infarction confirmed and for identifying low-risk patients who may require less intensive care. Analysis of the quality of pain can help identify low-risk patients. Patients without a history of angina pectoris or myocardial infarction presenting with pain that is sharp or stabbing and pleuritic, positional, or reproduced by palpation of the chest wall are extremely unlikely to be experiencing STEMI.[25] Computer-guided decision protocols are being developed to aid clinicians in identifying those STEMI patients who require admission to the CCU as opposed to a less intensive hospital ward.[141]

Contemporary CCUs typically have equipment available for noninvasive monitoring of single or multiple ECG leads, cardiac rhythm, ST segment deviation, arterial pressure, and arterial oxygen saturation. Computer algorithms for detection and analysis of arrhythmias are superior to visual surveillance by skilled CCU staff. However, even the most sophisticated ECG monitoring systems are susceptible to artifacts due to patient movement or noise on the signal from poor skin preparation when monitoring electrodes are applied. Noninvasive monitoring of arterial blood pressure using a sphygmomanometric cuff that undergoes cycles of inflation and deflation at programmed intervals is suitable for the majority of patients admitted to a CCU. Invasive arterial monitoring is preferred in patients with a low output syndrome under circumstances in which inotropic therapy is initiated for severe left ventricular failure.

The CCU remains the appropriate hospital unit for patients with complicated infarctions (e.g., hemodynamic instability, recurrent arrhythmias) and those patients requiring intensive nursing care for devices such as an intraaortic balloon pump. STEMI patients with an uncomplicated status, such as those without a history of previous infarction, persistent ischemic-type discomfort, congestive heart failure, hypotension, heart block, or hemodynamically compromising ventricular arrhythmias, can be safely transferred out of the CCU within 24 to 36 hours. In patients with a complicated STEMI, the duration of the CCU stay should be dictated by the need for "intensive" care; that is, hemodynamic monitoring, close nursing supervision, intravenous vasoactive drugs, and frequent changes in the medical regimen.

For patients with a low risk of mortality from STEMI, the clinician should consider admission to an intermediate care facility (see later) equipped with simple ECG monitoring and resuscitation equipment.[7] This strategy has been shown to be cost-effective and may reduce CCU use by one-third, shorten hospital stays, and have no deleterious effect on patients' recovery. Intermediate care units for low-risk STEMI patients can also be appealing to patients who stand to gain little benefit from the high staffing, intense activity, and elaborate technology available in current CCUs (with their attendant high costs) and who may be disturbed by that activity and equipment.

General Measures

The CCU staff must be sensitive to patient concerns about mortality, prognosis, and future productivity. A calm, quiet atmosphere and the "laying on of hands" with a gentle but confident touch help allay anxiety and reduce sympathetic tone, ultimately leading to a reduction in hypertension, tachycardia, and arrhythmias.[7] To reduce the risk of nausea and vomiting early after infarction and to reduce the risk of aspiration, during the first 4 to 12 hours after admission patients should receive either nothing by mouth or a clear liquid diet (see Table 47–5). Subsequently, a diet with 50 to 55 percent of calories from complex carbohydrates and up to 30 percent from mono- and unsaturated fats should be given. The diet should be enriched in foods that are high in

TABLE 47–5 Sample Admitting Orders for the STEMI patient

1. Condition: Serious
2. IV: NS on D_5W to keep vein open. Start a second IV if IV medication is being given. This may be a saline lock.
3. Vital signs: every 1.5 hours until stable, then every 4 hours and as needed. Notify physician if HR is less than 60 beats/min or greater than 100 beats/min, BP is less than 100 mm Hg systolic or greater than 150 mm Hg systolic, respiratory rate is less than 8 or greater than 22.
4. Monitor: Continuous ECG monitoring for dysrhythmia and ST segment deviation
5. Diet: NPO except for sips of water until stable. Then start 2 gm sodium/day, low saturated fat (less than 7% of total calories/day), low cholesterol (less than 200 mg/day) diet, such as Total Lifestyle Change (TLC) diet
6. Activity: Bedside commode and light activity when stable
7. Oxygen: Continuous oximetry monitoring. Nasal cannula at 2 liters/min when stable for 6 hr, reassess for oxygen need (i.e., O_2 saturation of less than 90%) and consider discontinuing oxygen.
8. Medications:
   a. Nitroglycerin (NTG)
      1. Use sublingual NTG 0.4 mg every 5 min as needed for chest discomfort.
      2. Intravenous NTG for CHF, hypertension, or persistent ischemia.
   b. ASA
      1. If ASA not given in the emergency department (ED), chew nonenteric-coated ASA* 162-325 mg.
      2. If ASA has been given, start daily maintenance of 75-162 mg daily; may use enteric coated for gastrointestinal protection.
   c. Beta blocker
      1. If not given in the ED, assess for contraindications, i.e., bradycardia and hypotension; continue daily assessment to ascertain eligibility for beta blocker.
      2. If given in the ED, continue daily dose and optimize as dictated by heart rate and blood pressure.
   d. ACE inhibitor
      1. Start ACE inhibitor orally in patients with pulmonary congestion or LVEF less than 40 percent if the following are absent: hypotension (SBP less than 100 mm Hg or less than 30 mm Hg below baseline) or known contraindications to this class of medications.
   e. Angiotensin receptor blocker (ARB)
      1. Start ARB orally in patients who are intolerant of ACE inhibitors and with either clinical or radiological signs of heart failure or LVEF less than 40 percent.
   f. Pain medications
      1. IV morphine sulfate 2-4 mg with increments of 2-8 mg IV at 5- to 15-min intervals as needed to control pain.
   g. Anxiolytics (based on a nursing assessment)
   h. Daily stool softener

Modified from Ryan TJ, Antman EM, Brooks NH, et al: 1999 update: ACC/AHA guidelines for the management of patients with acute myocardial infarction. A report of the American College of Cardiology/American Heart Association Task Force on Practice Guidelines (Committee on Management of Acute Myocardial Infarction). J Am Coll Cardiol 34:890, 1999.

*Although some trials have used enteric-coated ASA for initial dosing, more rapid buccal absorption occurs with nonenteric-coated formulations.

potassium, magnesium, and fiber but low in sodium (Table 47–5).

The results of laboratory tests obtained in the CCU should be scrutinized for any derangements potentially contributing to arrhythmias, such as hypoxemia, hypovolemia, disturbances of acid-base balance or of electrolytes, and drug toxicity. Oxazepam, 15 to 30 mg orally four times a day, is useful to allay the anxiety that is common in the first 24 to 48 hours (see Table 47–5). Delirium can be provoked by medications frequently used in the CCU, including antiarrhythmic drugs, H_2 blockers, narcotics, and beta blockers. Potentially offending agents should be discontinued in patients with an abnormal mental status. Haloperidol, a butyrophenone, can be used safely in patients with STEMI beginning with a dose of 2 mg intravenously for mildly agitated patients and 5 to 10 mg for progressively more agitated patients. Hypnotics, such as temazepam, 15 to 30 mg or an equivalent, should be provided as needed for sleep. Dioctyl sodium sulfosuccinate, 200 mg daily, or another stool softener should be used to prevent constipation and straining (see Table 47–5).

"Coronary precautions" that do *not* appear to be supported by evidence from clinical research include the avoidance of iced fluids, hot beverages, caffeinated beverages, rectal examinations, and back rubs.[7]

PHYSICAL ACTIVITY. In the absence of complications, patients with STEMI need not be confined to bed for more than 12 hours and, unless they are hemodynamically compromised, they may use a bedside commode shortly after admission (see Table 47–5). Progression of activity should be individualized depending on the patient's clinical status, age, and physical capacity.

In patients without hemodynamic compromise, early ambulation, including dangling the feet on the side of the bed, sitting in a chair, standing, and walking around the bed, does not cause important changes in heart rate, blood pressure, or pulmonary wedge pressure. Although heart rate increases slightly (usually by less than 10 percent), pulmonary wedge pressures fall slightly as the patient assumes the upright posture for activities. Early ambulatory activities are rarely associated with any symptoms, and when symptoms do occur, they generally are related to hypotension. Thus, when Levine and Lown proposed the "armchair" treatment of STEMI in the 1950s, they were undoubtedly correct that stress to the myocardium is less in the upright position. As long as blood pressure and heart rate are monitored, early ambulation offers considerable psychological and physical benefit without any clear medical risk.

The Intermediate Coronary Care Unit

Patients with STEMI are at risk for late in-hospital mortality from recurrent ischemia or infarction, hemodynamically significant ventricular arrhythmias, and severe congestive heart failure after discharge from the CCU. Therefore, continued surveillance in intermediate CCUs (also called step-down units) is justifiable. Risk factors for mortality in the hospital after discharge from the coronary care unit include significant congestive heart failure evidenced by persistent sinus tachycardia for more than 2 days and rales greater than one-third of the lung fields; recurrent ventricular tachycardia and ventricular fibrillation; atrial fibrillation or flutter while in the CCU; intraventricular conduction delays or heart block; anterior location of infarction; and recurrent episodes of angina with marked electrocardiographic ST-segment abnormalities at low activity levels.

The availability of intermediate care units may also be helpful in identifying those patients who remain free of complications and are suitable candidates for early discharge from the hospital. Aggressive reperfusion protocols with angioplasty or thrombolytics can reduce the length of hospital stay.[142] In patients who are believed to have undergone successful reperfusion, the *absence* of early sustained ventricular tachyarrhythmias, hypotension, or heart failure, coupled with a well-preserved left ventricular ejection fraction, predicts a low risk of late complications in-hospital.[143] Such patients are suitable candidates for discharge from the hospital in less than 5 days from the onset of symptoms.

Following STEMI, patients are often eager for information, in need of reassurance, confused by misinformation and prior impressions, capable of counterproductive denial, and simply frightened. Intermediate care facilities provide ideal settings and ample opportunities to begin the rehabilitation process.[144] The capacity for the early detection of problems following STEMI and the social and educational benefits of grouping such patients together strongly argue for continued utilization of intermediate CCUs. Furthermore, the economic advantage of grouping such patients together for sharing of skilled personnel and resources outweighs any questions raised by the lack of a clear consensus regarding reduced mortality. An additional potential advantage is the facilitation of patient education in a group setting with lectures and audiovisual programs.

Pharmacological Therapy

Beta Blockers (see Chaps. 49 and 50)

The effects of beta blockers in the treatment of patients with STEMI can be divided into those that are immediate (when the drug is given very early in the course of infarction) and those that are long-term (secondary prevention), when the drug is initiated sometime after infarction. The immediate intravenous administration of beta-adrenoceptor blockers reduces cardiac index, heart rate, and blood pressure.[50] The net effect is a reduction in myocardial oxygen consumption per minute and per beat. Favorable effects of acute intravenous administration of beta-adrenoceptor blockers on the balance of myocardial oxygen supply and demand are reflected in reductions in chest pain, in the proportion of patients with threatened infarction who actually evolve STEMI, and in the development of ventricular arrhythmias.[145] Because beta-adrenoceptor blockade diminishes circulating levels of free fatty acids by antagonizing the lipolytic effects of catecholamines and because elevated levels of fatty acids augment myocardial oxygen consumption and probably increase the incidence of arrhythmias, these metabolic actions of beta-blocking agents may also be beneficial to the ischemic heart.

Objective evidence of beneficial effects of beta blockers in acute myocardial ischemia has been reported using the precordial ST segment mapping technique. Acute beta blockade probably reduces infarct size in patients with STEMI. Reduction in release of serum cardiac biomarkers with beta blockade is suggestive of a smaller infarct, as is the preservation of R waves and reduction in the development of Q waves.

At least 30 randomized beta blocker trials involving more than 29,000 patients have been undertaken. Intravenous followed by oral beta blocker therapy is associated with about a 13 percent relative reduction in the risk of mortality (Fig. 47–19). Although antagonism of sympathetic stimulation to the heart might be expected to exacerbate pulmonary edema in patients with occult heart failure, usually only small changes in pulmonary capillary wedge pressure occur when the drug is used in patients with STEMI. Thus, in appropriately selected patients (Table 47–6), the benefits occur at a cost of about a 3 percent incidence of provocation of congestive heart failure or complete heart block and a 2 percent incidence of the development of cardiogenic shock.

Because reduction of infarct size in STEMI patients treated with beta blockers is likely to occur only with early treatment (<4 hours from the onset of pain), investigators have sought other explanations for the reduction in the mortality in the acute phase that has been observed. Intriguing observations from the ISIS-1 trial raise the possibility that a reduction in the development of cardiac rupture or electromechanical dissociation during the first day is achieved with early beta blockade.[146]

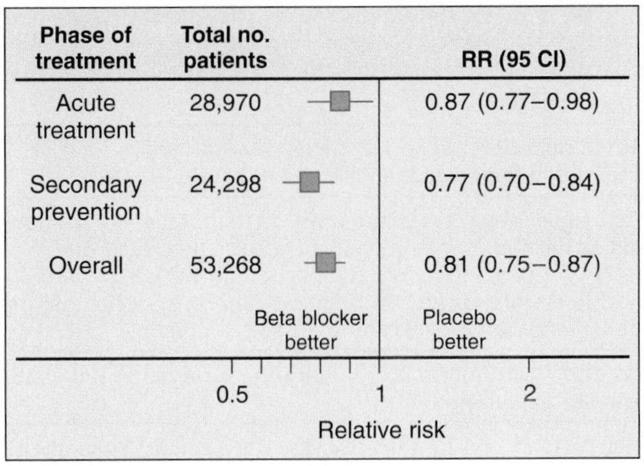

Phase of treatment	Total no. patients	RR (95 CI)
Acute treatment	28,970	0.87 (0.77–0.98)
Secondary prevention	24,298	0.77 (0.70–0.84)
Overall	53,268	0.81 (0.75–0.87)

FIGURE 47–19 Effect of beta blockers on mortality rate in patients with myocardial infarction. The relative risk of mortality is reduced with beta blockers both during the acute phase of treatment and when prescribed as secondary prevention after acute myocardial infarction. (Data from Chae CU, Hennekens CH: Beta blockers. *In* Hennekens CH [ed]: Clinical Trials in Cardiovascular Disease: A Companion to Braunwald's Heart Disease. Philadelphia, WB Saunders, 1999, p 84.)

TABLE 47–6 Contraindications to Beta-Adrenoceptor Blocker Therapy in Acute Myocardial Infarction
Heart rate < 60 beats/min
Systolic arterial pressure < 100 mm Hg
Moderate or severe left ventricular failure
Signs of peripheral hypoperfusion
PR interval > 0.24 second
Second- or third-degree atrioventricular block
Severe chronic obstructive pulmonary disease
History of asthma
Severe peripheral vascular disease
Insulin-dependent diabetes mellitus

In the TIMI-II trial, the addition of a beta blocker (metoprolol) to fibrinolytic therapy was studied.[147] Although recurrent ischemia and reinfarction were reduced by immediate intravenous versus delayed use of metoprolol, mortality was not reduced, nor was ventricular function improved. Thus, immediate intravenous beta blockade, although clinically beneficial, may not enhance salvage of myocardium in the setting of early reperfusion but may confer clinical benefit by means of its antiischemic effect.[148]

Substantial proportions of elderly patients who are hospitalized with STEMI and are ideal candidates for early beta blocker therapy do not receive this treatment.[50] Compared with elderly patients who receive early beta blockade in STEMI, those who do not receive beta blockade are older, more likely to be women, and less likely to be white. Elderly patients who receive early beta blocker therapy have significantly lower in-hospital mortality rates than those who do not receive beta blockers.

RECOMMENDATIONS. Given the overwhelming evidence of benefits of early blockade in STEMI, patients without a contraindication who can be treated within 12 hours of the onset of infarction, irrespective of administration of concomitant thrombolytic therapy or performance of primary PCI, should receive beta blockers. A regimen that we like to use is metoprolol 5 mg intravenously every 2 to 5 minutes for three doses provided the heart rate does not fall below 60 beats/min and the systolic blood pressure does not drop below 100 mm Hg. Oral maintenance dosing is initiated with metoprolol 50 mg every 6 hours for 2 days and then 100 mg twice daily.

Beta blockers are especially helpful in patients in whom STEMI is complicated by persistent or recurrent ischemic pain, progressive or repetitive serum enzyme elevations suggestive of infarct extension, or tachyarrhythmias early after the onset of infarction. If adverse effects of beta blockers develop or if patients present with complications of infarction that are contraindications to beta blockade such as heart failure or heart block, the beta blocker should be withheld. Unless there are contraindications (Table 47–6), beta blockade probably should be continued in patients who develop STEMI.

Selection of Beta Blocker. Favorable effects have been reported with metoprolol, atenolol, timolol, and alprenolol; these benefits probably occur with propranolol and with esmolol, an ultra-short-acting agent, as well. In the absence of any favorable evidence supporting the benefit of agents with intrinsic sympathomimetic activity, such as pindolol and oxprenolol, and with some unfavorable evidence for these agents in secondary prevention, beta blockers with intrinsic sympathomimetic activity probably should not be chosen for treatment of STEMI. The CAPRICORN trial randomized 1959 patients with myocardial infarction and systolic dysfunction (ejection fraction < 40 percent) to carvedilol or placebo in addition to contemporary pharmacotherapy, including ACE inhibitors in 98 percent of patients.[149] All-cause mortality was reduced from 15.3 percent in the placebo group to 11.9 percent in the carvedilol group (23 percent relative risk reduction; $p = 0.031$). Thus, CAPRICORN confirms the benefit of beta blockade in addition to ACE inhibitor therapy in patients with transient or sustained left ventricular dysfunction after myocardial infarction. An algorithm for the use of beta blockers in the STEMI patients is shown in Figure 47–20.

Occasionally, the clinician may wish to proceed with beta blocker therapy even in the presence of relative contraindications, such as a history of mild asthma, mild bradycardia, mild heart failure, or first-degree heart block. In this situation, a trial of esmolol may help determine whether the patient can tolerate beta blockade. Because the hemodynamic effects of this drug, with a half-life of 9 minutes, disappear in less than 30 minutes, it offers considerable advantage over

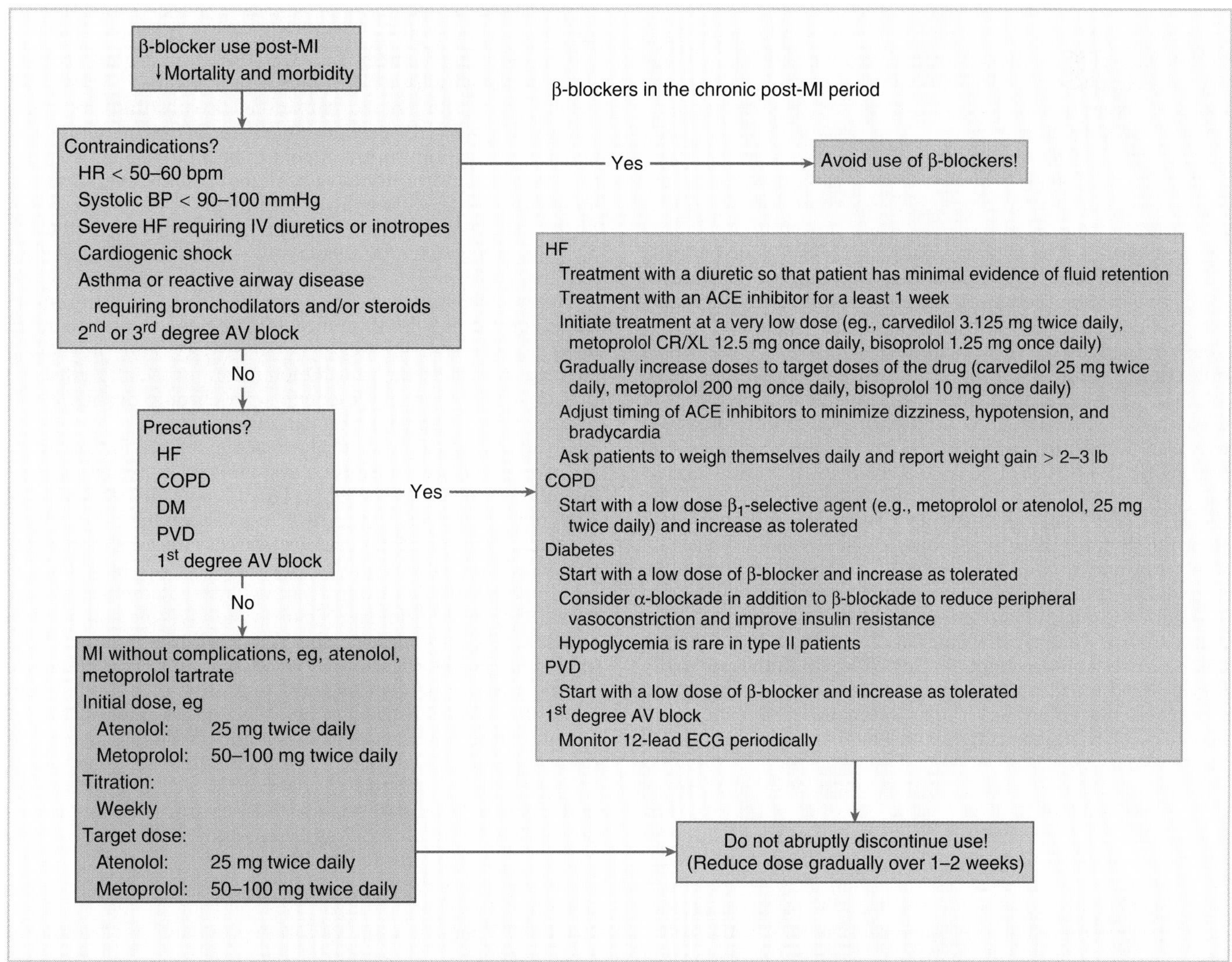

FIGURE 47–20 Algorithm for use of beta blockers in the treatment of patients with ST segment elevation myocardial infarction. COPD = chronic obstructive pulmonary disease; DM = diabetes mellitus; HF = heart failure; PVD = peripheral vascular disease. (From Gheorghiade M, Goldstein S: Beta-blockers in the post-myocardial infarction patient. Circulation 106:394, 2002.)

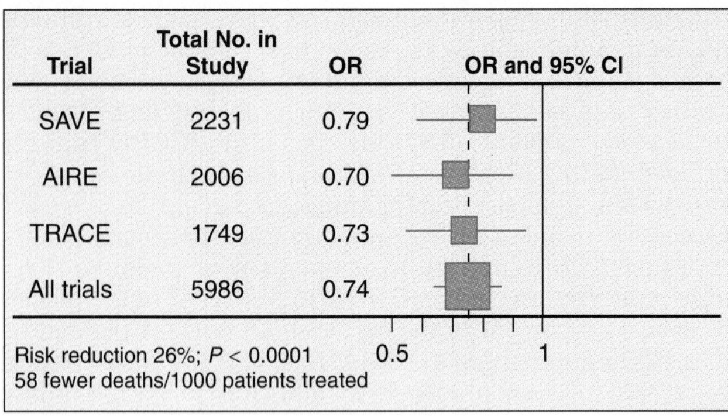

Trial
Total No. in Study
OR
OR and 95% CI
SAVE 2231 0.79
AIRE 2006 0.70
TRACE 1749 0.73
All trials 5986 0.74
Risk reduction 26%; P < 0.0001
58 fewer deaths/1000 patients treated
0.5
1

FIGURE 47–21 Effect of angiotensin-converting enzyme inhibitors on mortality after myocardial infarction: results from the long-term trials. (From Flather MD, Pfeffer MA: Angiotensin-converting enzyme inhibitors. *In* Hennekens CH [ed]: Clinical Trials in Cardiovascular Disease: A Companion to Braunwald's Heart Disease. Philadelphia, WB Saunders, 1999, p 97.)

Trial	Total No. in Study	OR	OR and 95% CI
CONSENSUS-II	6090	1.1	
GISSI-3	19394	0.88	
SMILE	1556	0.67	
ISIS-4	58050	0.94	
CCS-1	13634	0.94	
All trials	98724	0.93	

Risk reduction 6.7%; $P < 0.006$
4.9 fewer deaths/1000 patients treated
0.5 1

FIGURE 47–22 Effects of angiotensin-converting enzyme inhibitors on mortality after myocardial infarction: results from the short-term trials. (From Flather MD, Pfeffer MA: Angiotensin-converting enzyme inhibitors. *In* Hennekens CH [ed]: Clinical Trials in Cardiovascular Disease: A Companion to Braunwald's Heart Disease. Philadelphia, WB Saunders, 1999, p 101.)

longer acting agents when the risk of a beta blocker complication is relatively high.

Inhibition of the Renin-Angiotensin-Aldosterone System

In 1992, with the publication of the SAVE trial, ACE inhibitors were established as an important addition to the list of treatments for STEMI. The rationale for their use includes experimental and clinical evidence of a favorable impact on ventricular remodeling, improvement in hemodynamics, and reductions in congestive heart failure.[150] There is now unequivocal evidence from randomized, placebo-controlled mortality trials that ACE inhibitors reduce the rate of mortality from STEMI. These trials can be grouped into two categories. The first consisted of *selected* myocardial infarction patients for randomization, based on features indicative of increased mortality such as left ventricular ejection fraction less than 40 percent, clinical signs and symptoms of congestive heart failure,[151] anterior location of infarction,[152] and abnormal wall motion score index (Fig. 47–21).[153] The second group were *unselective* trials that randomized all patients with myocardial infarction provided they had a minimum systolic pressure of approximately 100 mm Hg (ISIS-4,[154] GISSI-3,[155] CONSENSUS II,[156] and Chinese Captopril Study) (Fig. 47–22). With the exception of the SMILE trial,[152] all of the selective trials initiated ACE inhibitor therapy between 3 and 16 days after myocardial infarction and maintained it for 1 to 4 years, whereas the unselective trials all initiated treatment within the first 24 to 36 hours and maintained it for only 4 to 6 weeks.

A consistent survival benefit was observed in all of the trials already noted, except for CONSENSUS II, the one study that utilized an intravenous preparation early in the course of myocardial infarction.[156] An estimate of the mortality benefit of ACE inhibitors in the unselective, short duration of therapy trials was 5 per 1000 patients treated.[157,158] Analysis of these unselective short-term trials indicates that approximately one-third of the lives saved occurred within the first 1 to 2 days. Certain subgroups, such as patients with anterior infarction, showed proportionately greater benefit from early administration (11 lives saved per 1000) of ACE inhibitors. Not unexpectedly, greater survival benefits of 42 to 76 lives saved per 1000 patients treated were obtained in the *selective*, long duration of therapy trials. Of note, there was generally a 20 percent reduction in the risk of death attributable to ACE inhibitor treatment in the selective trials. The mortality reduction with ACE inhibitors is accompanied by significant reductions in the development of congestive heart failure, supporting the underlying pathophysiological rationale for administering this class of drugs in patients with STEMI.[151,153,155] In addition, some data suggest that ischemic events, including recurrent infarction and the need for coronary revascularization, can also be reduced by chronic administration of ACE inhibitors after a STEMI.[159]

The mortality benefits of ACE inhibitors are additive to those achieved with aspirin and beta blockers.[155] Thus, ACE inhibitors should not be considered a substitute for these other therapies with proven benefit in STEMI patients. The benefits of ACE inhibition appear to be a class effect because mortality and morbidity have been reduced by several agents. To replicate these benefits in clinical practice, however, physicians should select a specific agent and prescribe the drug according to the protocols utilized in the successful clinical trials reported to date.

The major *contraindications* to the use of ACE inhibitors in patients with STEMI include hypotension in the setting of adequate preload, known hypersensitivity, and pregnancy. Adverse reactions include hypotension, especially after the first dose, and intolerable cough with chronic dosing; much less commonly, angioedema can occur (see Chap. 38).

An alternative method of pharmacological inhibition of the renin-angiotensin-aldosterone system is by administration of angiotensin-2 receptor blockers (ARBs). The OPTIMAAL trial evaluated the effects of the ARB losartan versus captopril on survival and other major cardiovascular outcomes in myocardial infarction patients with clinical evidence of heart failure. Although losartan was significantly better tolerated than captopril, there was a nonsignificant trend favoring captopril in terms of total mortality.[160] The VALIANT trial compared the effects of the ARB valsartan versus captopril alone and in combination with captopril on mortality in patients with acute myocardial infarction complicated by left ventricular systolic dysfunction and/or heart failure.[161] Patients were randomized within 10 days of myocardial infarction to valsartan (20 mg initially, titrated to 160 mg twice daily), valsartan added to captopril (20 mg and 6.25 mg initially, titrated to 80 mg twice daily and 50 mg three times daily), or captopril (6.25 mg initially, titrated to 50 mg three times daily), added to conventional therapy. Rates of mortality were similar in the three treatment groups: 19.9 percent in the valsartan group, 19.3 percent in the valsartan plus captopril group, and 19.5 percent in the captopril alone group (Fig. 47–23). Permanent discontinuation of study medication was more frequent in the groups receiving captopril (valsartan, 20.5 percent; valsartan plus captopril 23.4 percent; captopril alone

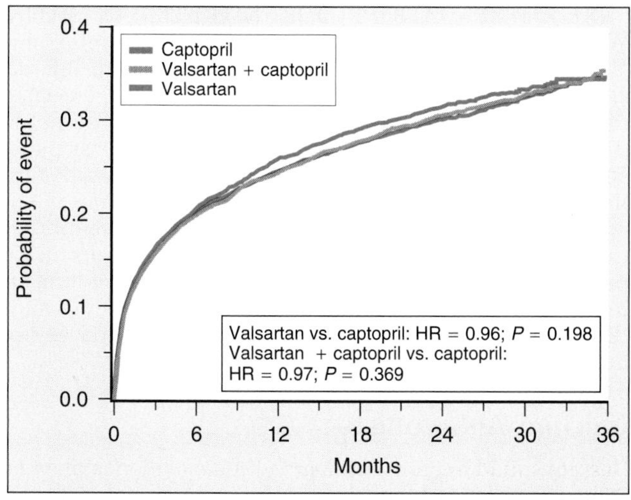

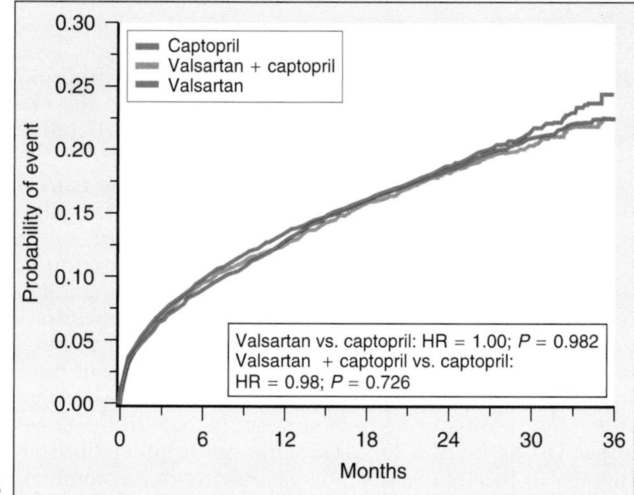

FIGURE 47–23 Effects of an angiotensin-converting enzyme inhibitor (captopril), angiotensin receptor blocker (valsartan), or the combination after myocardial infarction. The Kaplan-Meier estimates of **(A)** mortality and **(B)** cardiovascular death, reinfarction, or hospitalization for heart failure, by treatment in the VALIANT trial are depicted. (From Pfeffer M, McMurray JJ, Velasquez EJ, et al: Effects of valsartan relative to captopril in patients with myocardial infarction complicated by heart failure and or left ventricular dysfunction. N Engl J Med 349:1893, 2003.)

21.6 percent; $p = 0.129$ for valsartan compared to captopril and $p = 0.021$ for valsartan plus captopril versus captopril alone).

Aldosterone blockade is the last pharmacological strategy for inhibition the renin-angiotensin-aldosterone system. The EPHESUS trial randomized 6642 patients with acute myocardial infarction complicated by left ventricular dysfunction and heart failure to the selective aldosterone blocker eplerenone or placebo in conjunction with contemporary postinfarction pharmacotherapy.[162] During a mean follow-up period of 16 months, there was a 15 percent reduction in the relative risk of mortality favoring eplerenone (Fig. 47–24). Cardiovascular mortality or hospitalization for cardiovascular events was also reduced by eplerenone. Serious hyperkalemia (serum potassium concentration ≥ 6.0 mmol/liter) occurred in 5.5 percent of patients in the eplerenone group compared with 3.9 percent of patients in the placebo group ($p = 0.002$).

RECOMMENDATIONS. After administration of aspirin and initiation of reperfusion strategies and, where appropriate, beta blockade, *all* STEMI patients should be considered for inhibition of the renin-angiotensin-aldosterone system.

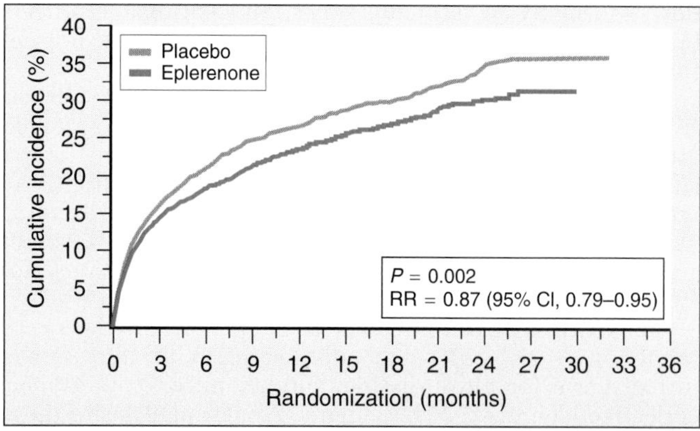

FIGURE 47–24 Effect of a selective aldosterone receptor blocker (eplerenone) after myocardial infarction. The Kaplan-Meier estimates of the rate of death from cardiovascular causes or hospitalization for cardiovascular events in the EPHESUS trial are depicted. (From Pitt B, Remme W, Zannad F, et al: Eplerenone, a selective aldosterone blocker, in patients with left ventricular dysfunction after myocardial infarction (abstract). N Engl J Med 348:14, 2003.)

Although there is little disagreement that high-risk STEMI patients (elderly, anterior infarction, prior infarction, Killip class II or greater, and asymptomatic patients with evidence of depressed global ventricular function on an imaging study) should receive life-long treatment with ACE inhibitors,[163] short-term (4-6 weeks) therapy to a broader group of patients has also been proposed based on the pooled results of the unselective mortality trials.[154]

Considering all the available data, we favor a strategy of an initial trial of oral ACE inhibitors in all STEMI patients with congestive heart failure as well as in hemodynamically stable patients with ST segment elevation or left bundle branch block, commencing within the first 24 hours.[158,164] ACE inhibition therapy should be continued indefinitely in patients with congestive heart failure, evidence of a reduction in global function, or a large regional wall motion abnormality. In patients without these findings at discharge, ACE inhibitors can be discontinued.

The results of the VALIANT trial expand the range of options available to clinicians treating patients with STEMI. Since the ARB was at least as effective as the ACE inhibitor in reducing mortality and other adverse cardiovascular outcomes following myocardial infarction, it should be considered as a clinically effective alternative to captopril. The choice between ACE inhibition and angiotensin receptor blockade following STEMI should be based on physician experience with the agents, patient tolerability, safety, convenience, and cost. Finally, based on experience from the EPHESUS study, long-term aldosterone blockade with eplerenone 25 mg/day initially and then titrated to 50 mg/day for high-risk patients following STEMI (ejection fraction ≤ 40 percent, clinical heart failure, diabetes mellitus) should be considered. Given the small but definite increase in the risk of serious hypokalemia when aldosterone blockade is prescribed, particularly when other measures for inhibition of the renin-angiotensin-aldosterone system are used concurrently, periodic monitoring of the serum potassium level should be undertaken.[165]

Nitrates (see Chap. 50)

Sublingual nitroglycerin very rarely opens occluded coronary arteries. However, in patients with STEMI, the potential for reductions in ventricular filling pressures, wall tension, and cardiac work coupled with improvement in coronary blood flow, especially in ischemic zones, and antiplatelet effects make nitrates a logical and attractive pharmacological intervention.[7]

In patients with STEMI, the administration of nitrates reduces pulmonary capillary wedge pressure and systemic arterial pressure, left ventricular chamber volume, infarct size, and the incidence of mechanical complications. As with other interventions to spare ischemic myocardium in cases of STEMI, intravenous nitroglycerin appears to be of greatest benefit in patients treated earliest after the onset of symptoms.

CLINICAL TRIAL RESULTS. In the prefibrinolytic era, 10 randomized trials of acute administration of intravenous nitroglycerin (or nitroprusside, another nitric oxide donor) collectively enrolled 2042 patients. A meta-analysis of these trial results showed a reduction in mortality of 35 percent associated with nitrate therapy.

In the fibrinolytic era, two megatrials of nitrate therapy have been conducted: GISSI-3[155] and ISIS-4.[154] In GISSI-3, there was no independent effect of nitrates on short-term mortality.[155] Similarly, in ISIS-4, no effect of a mononitrate on 35-day mortality was observed. A pooled analysis of more than 80,000 patients treated with nitrate-like preparations intravenously or orally in 22 trials revealed a mortality rate of 7.7 per cent in the control group, which was reduced to 7.4 percent in the nitrate group. These data are consistent with a small treatment effect of nitrates on mortality such that 3 to 4 fewer deaths would occur for every 1000 patients treated.[154]

NITRATE PREPARATIONS AND MODE OF ADMINISTRATION. Intravenous nitroglycerin can be administered safely to patients with evolving STEMI as long as the dose is titrated to avoid induction of reflex tachycardia or systemic arterial hypotension. Patients with inferior wall infarction are particularly sensitive to an excessive fall in preload, particularly if concurrent right ventricular infarction is present.[166] In such cases, nitrate-induced venodilation could impair cardiac output and reduce coronary block flow, thus worsening myocardial oxygenation rather than improving it.

A useful regimen employs an initial infusion rate of 5 to 10 mg/min with increases of 5 to 20 mg/min until the mean arterial blood pressure is reduced by 10 percent of its baseline level in normotensive patients and by 30 percent for hypertensive patients, but in no case below a systolic pressure of 90 mm Hg. Alternatively, nitroglycerin can be administered as a sustained-release oral preparation (30-60 mg/day) or as an ointment (1 to 3 inches every 6 to 8 hours for patients with a systolic pressure greater than 120 mm Hg). Nitroglycerin can also be given sublingually at doses of 0.3 to 0.6 mg. This route can be more hazardous because the rate of absorption is difficult to control and arterial pressure may decline precipitously.

ADVERSE EFFECTS. Clinically significant methemoglobinemia has been reported to occur during administration of intravenous nitroglycerin. Although uncommon, this problem is seen when unusually large doses of nitrates are administered. It is important not only for its potential to cause symptoms of lethargy and headache but also because elevated methemoglobin levels can impair the oxygen-carrying capacity of blood, potentially exacerbating ischemia. Dilation of the pulmonary vasculature supplying poorly ventilated lung segments may produce a ventilation-perfusion mismatch.

Tolerance to intravenous nitroglycerin (as manifested by increasing nitrate requirements) develops in many patients, often as soon as 12 hours after the infusion is started. Despite the theoretical and demonstrated benefit of sulfhydryl agents in diminishing tolerance, their use has not become widespread.

RECOMMENDATIONS FOR NITRATES IN PATIENT WITH STEMI. Nitroglycerin is indicated for the relief of persistent pain and as a vasodilator in patients with infarction associated with left ventricular failure. In the absence of recurrent angina or congestive heart failure, we do not routinely prescribe them for STEMI patients. Higher risk patients such as those with large transmural infarctions, especially of the anterior wall, have the most to gain from nitrates in terms of reduction of ventricular remodeling, and we therefore routinely use intravenous nitrates for 24 to 48 hours in such patients. There is no clear benefit to empirical long-term cutaneous or oral nitrates in the asymptomatic patient, and we therefore do not prescribe nitrates beyond the first 48 hours unless angina or ventricular failure is present.

Calcium Antagonists (see Chap. 50)

Despite sound experimental and clinical evidence of an anti-ischemic effect, calcium antagonists have *not* been found to be helpful in the acute phase of STEMI, and concern has been raised in several systematic overviews about an increased risk of mortality when they are prescribed on a routine basis. A distinction should be made between the dihydropyridine type of calcium antagonists (e.g., nifedipine) and the nondihydropyridine calcium antagonists (e.g., verapamil and diltiazem).

NIFEDIPINE. In multiple trials involving more than 5000 patients, the immediate-release preparation of nifedipine has not resulted in any reduction in infarct size, prevention of progression to infarction, control of recurrent ischemia, or lowering of mortality rate. When trials of the immediate-release form of nifedipine are pooled in a meta-analysis, evidence suggests a dose-related increased risk of in-hospital mortality (especially at a dose higher than 80 mg of nifedipine), although posthospital mortality does not appear to be increased in nifedipine-treated patients. Nifedipine does not appear to be helpful in conjunction with either fibrinolytic therapy or beta blockade.[167] Thus, we do not recommend the use of immediate-release nifedipine early in the treatment of STEMI. No trials of the sustained-release preparations of nifedipine in patients with acute myocardial infarction have been reported to date.

VERAPAMIL AND DILTIAZEM. When administered during the acute phase of STEMI, these drugs have not had any demonstrated favorable effect on infarct size or other important endpoints in patients with STEMI, with the exception of control of supraventricular arrhythmias.[168] The INTERCEPT trial compared 300 mg of diltiazem with placebo in patients who received fibrinolytic therapy for STEMI.[169] Diltiazem did not reduce the cumulative occurrence of cardiac death, nonfatal reinfarction, or refractory ischemia during a 6-month follow-up.

Based on the available data, we do *not* recommend the routine use of either verapamil or diltiazem in patients with STEMI. Verapamil and diltiazem can be given for relief of ongoing ischemia or slowing of a rapid ventricular response in atrial fibrillation in patients for whom beta blockers are ineffective or contraindicated.[7] Their use should be avoided in patients with Killip class II or greater hemodynamic findings.

OTHER THERAPIES

MAGNESIUM. Patients with STEMI may have a total body deficit of magnesium because of a low dietary intake, advanced age, or prior diuretic use. They may also acquire a functional deficit of available magnesium due to trapping of free magnesium in adipocytes, as soaps are formed when free fatty acids are released by catecholamine-induced lipolysis with the onset of infarction.

The ISIS-4 investigators enrolled 58,050 patients, 29,011 to magnesium and 29,039 to control. The control group mortality was 7.2 percent in ISIS-4 compared with 7.6 percent in the magnesium group.[154] The MAGIC trial investigated the benefits of early administration of intravenous magnesium to high-risk patients with STEMI.[48] At 30 days, the mortality rate was 15.3 percent in the magnesium group and 15.2 percent in the placebo group (OR, 1.0; 95 percent CI, 0.9-1.2; $p = 0.96$).

RECOMMENDATIONS. Because of the risk of cardiac arrhythmias when electrolyte deficits are present in the early phase of infarction, all patients with STEMI should have a serum magnesium measurement on admission. We advocate repleting magnesium deficits to maintain a serum magnesium level of 2.0 mEq/liter or more. In the presence of hypokalemia (<4.0 mEq/liter) during the course of treatment of STEMI, the serum magnesium level should be rechecked and repleted if necessary because it is often difficult to correct a potassium deficit in the presence of a concurrent magnesium deficit. Episodes of torsades de pointes should be treated with 1 to 2 gm of magnesium delivered as a bolus over about 5 minutes. Between 1980 and 2002, 68,684 patients were studied in a series of 14 randomized trials. Based on the totality of available evidence and current coronary care practice, there is no indication for the routine administration of intravenous magnesium to patients with STEMI at any level of risk.

GLUCOSE-INSULIN-POTASSIUM. Administration of a solution of glucose-insulin-potassium (GIK) lowers the concentration of plasma free fatty acids and improves ventricular performance, as reflected in systolic arterial pressure, cardiac output, and stroke work at any level of left ventricular filling pressure; also, the frequency of ventricular premature beats decreases. Fath-Ordoubadi and colleagues reported in a meta-analysis of nine studies conducted between 1965 and 1987 enrolling a cumulative total of 1932 patients that the mortality rate was reduced from 21 percent in the placebo group to 16.1 percent in the GIK group (OR, 0.72; 95 percent CI, 0.57-0.90; $p = 0.004$).[170] Subsequently, the ECLA group performed a randomized trial of STEMI patients treated within 24 hours of the onset of symptoms.[171] The mortality rate was reduced from 15.2 percent in the control group to 5.2 percent in the GIK group for the subset of patients who received thrombolysis (OR, 0.34; 95 percent CI, 0.15-0.77; $p = 0.01$).

The DIGAMI (Diabetes Mellitus Insulin-Glucose Infusion in Acute Myocardial Infarction) Study reported a significant 30 percent relative decrease in mortality at 1 year in diabetic patients with myocardial infarction who received a strict regimen of an insulin-glucose infusion for 24 hours, followed by 3 months of subcutaneous injections of insulin four times daily as compared with standard therapy. Thus, infusions of GIK may provide necessary metabolic support for the ischemic myocardium; this could be particularly important in patients with large anterior infarcts and cardiogenic shock.

The most contemporary of the studies of GIK treatment in cases of STEMI was conducted by Dutch investigators who randomized 940 patients treated with PCI to either a GIK infusion (3 ml/kg/hr over 8 to 12 hours) or no infusion.[49] The 30-day mortality rate was 4.8 percent in patients receiving GIK compared with 5.8 percent in the control group (RR, 0.82; 95 percent CI, 0.46-1.46). Among the 91 percent of patients who presented without heart failure (Killip class I), the 30-day mortality rate was 1.2 percent in the GIK group versus 4.2 percent in the control group (RR, 0.28; 95 percent CI, 0.1-0.75). Among the 8.9 percent of patients with Killip class ≥ II, the 30-day mortality rate was 36 percent in the GIK group versus 26.5 percent in the control group (RR, 1.44; 95 percent CI, 0.65-3.22). As pointed out by Apstein, the rate of the GIK infusion in the Dutch study (3.8 ml/kg/hr) was twice as high as that used in the ECLA study (1.5 ml/kg/hr). For example, in the Dutch study, an 80 kg patient with heart failure received approximately 2 liters of fluid in the first 8 hours—a volume load that may have not been tolerated and was associated with an increased mortality risk.[172]

Thus, the benefits of routine administration of GIK to patients with STEMI, although intriguing, remain controversial. Additional studies are required to define the optimal dose and rate of infusion of GIK as well as the cohort of STEMI patients for whom GIK is efficacious and safe.

INTRAAORTIC BALLOON COUNTERPULSATION (see also Chap. 25). From a theoretical standpoint, intraaortic balloon counterpulsation might be expected to limit infarct size for several reasons. In experimental animals, intraaortic balloon counterpulsation decreases preload, increases coronary blood flow, and improves cardiac performance. No definitive information is available indicating that intraaortic balloon counterpulsation alters the prognosis in patients with relatively uncomplicated STEMI, especially in the context of other proven mortality-reducing therapies used in contemporary clinical practice. Intraaortic balloon pumping should be reserved for hemodynamically compromised patients and for those with refractory ischemia. Although noninvasive external forms of counterpulsation have been developed, these approaches have not been rigorously studied in patients with STEMI.

OTHER AGENTS. Several adjunctive pharmacotherapies have been investigated to prevent inflammatory damage in the infarct zone.[173] Trials with antibodies against the CD11/CD18 receptor on white blood cells failed to show a reduction in infarct size.[44,45]

Pexelizumab, a monoclonal antibody against the C5 component of complement had no effect on infarct size in STEMI patients treated either with fibrinolytics or PCI.[31,47] However, the rate of mortality was lower in the pexelizumab group compared with the placebo group in patients treated with PCI, prompting further clinical trials with this agent.

The AMISTAD II trial was a dose-ranging study of adenosine in patients with anterior STEMI.[174] Although high-dose adenosine (70 μg/kg/min infusion for 3 hours) was associated with a reduction in infarct size, neither high- nor low-dose adenosine reduced the primary composite clinical endpoint of death or the development of heart failure at 6 months compared with placebo.

Contrary to earlier beliefs that the heart is a terminally differentiated organ without the capacity to regenerate, evidence now exists that human cardiac myocytes divide after STEMI, and stem cells can promote regeneration of cardiac tissue.[175,176] These observations open up the possibility of myocardial replacement therapy after STEMI.[177]

Hemodynamic Disturbances

Hemodynamic Assessment

In patients with clinically uncomplicated STEMI, invasive hemodynamic monitoring is not necessary because the status of the circulation can be assessed by clinical evaluation. This ordinarily consists of monitoring of heart rate and rhythm, repeated measurement of systemic arterial pressure by cuff, obtaining chest radiographs to detect heart failure, repeated auscultation of the lung fields for pulmonary congestion, measurement of urine flow, examination of the skin and mucous membranes for evidence of the adequacy of perfusion, and arterial sampling for P_{O_2}, P_{CO_2}, and pH when hypoxemia or metabolic acidosis is suspected.

In contrast, in patients with STEMI whose ventricular contractile performance is not normal, as evidenced by clinical signs and symptoms of heart failure, it is important to assess the degree of hemodynamic compromise to initiate therapy with drugs such as vasodilators and diuretics. In the past, central venous or right atrial pressure was used to gauge the degree of left ventricular failure in patients with STEMI. However, this technique is fraught with error because central venous pressure actually reflects right rather than left ventricular function. Right ventricular function and therefore systemic venous pressure may be normal or nearly so in patients with significant left ventricular failure. Conversely, patients with right ventricular failure due to right ventricular infarction or pulmonary embolism may exhibit elevated right atrial and central venous pressures despite normal left ventricular function. Low values for right atrial and central venous pressures imply hypovolemia, whereas elevated right atrial pressures usually result from right ventricular failure secondary to left ventricular failure, pulmonary hypertension, or right ventricular infarction, or less commonly from tricuspid regurgitation or pericardial tamponade.

Major advances in the management of STEMI have resulted from the hemodynamic monitoring that has become widespread in CCUs (Table 47-7). This often consists of both an intraarterial catheter and a pulmonary artery catheter for measurement of pulmonary artery, pulmonary artery occlusive (equivalent to pulmonary wedge), and right atrial

TABLE 47–7 Indications for Hemodynamic Monitoring in Patients with STEMI

Management of complicated acute myocardial infarction Hypovolemia vs. cardiogenic shock Ventricular septal rupture vs. acute mitral regurgitation Severe left ventricular failure Right ventricular failure
Refractory ventricular tachycardia
Differentiating severe pulmonary disease from left ventricular failure
Assessment of cardiac tamponade
Assessment of therapy in *selected* individuals Afterload reduction in patients with severe left ventricular failure Inotropic agent therapy Beta blocker therapy Temporary pacing (ventricular vs. atrioventricular) Intraaortic balloon counterpulsation Mechanical ventilation

From Gore JM, Zwernet PL: Hemodynamic monitoring of acute myocardial infarction. *In* Francis GS, Alpert JS (eds): Modern Coronary Care, Boston, Little, Brown. 1990, p 138.

pressures, and cardiac output by thermodilution. In patients with hypotension, a Foley catheter provides accurate and continuous measurement of urine output.

NEED FOR INVASIVE MONITORING. The use of invasive hemodynamic monitoring is based on the following principal factors:

1. Difficulty in interpreting clinical and radiographic findings of pulmonary congestion because of phase lags, such as those occurring after diuretic therapy. Severe depression of cardiac index and/or elevation of left ventricular filling pressure may be unsuspected in as many as 15 percent of patients when estimates are based exclusively on clinical criteria.
2. Need for identifying noncardiac causes of arterial hypotension, particularly hypovolemia.
3. Possible contribution of reduced ventricular compliance to impaired hemodynamics, requiring judicious adjustment of intravascular volume to optimize left ventricular filling pressure.
4. Difficulty in assessing the severity and sometimes even determining the presence of lesions such as mitral regurgitation and ventricular septal defect when the cardiac output or the systemic pressures are depressed.
5. Establishing a baseline of hemodynamic measurements and guiding therapy in patients with clinically apparent pulmonary edema or cardiogenic shock.
6. Underestimation of systemic arterial pressure by the cuff method in patients with intense vasoconstriction.

The prognosis and the clinical status are related to both the cardiac output and the pulmonary artery wedge pressure. Patients with normal cardiac output after STEMI have an extremely low expected chance of mortality; prognosis worsens as cardiac output declines. Patients with intraventricular conduction defects, atrioventricular (AV) block, or both after anterior infarction have lower cardiac indices and higher pulmonary capillary wedge pressures than do patients without these conduction disturbances. On the other hand, patients with these conduction defects and inferior STEMI usually do not demonstrate such hemodynamic abnormalities.

PULMONARY ARTERY PRESSURE MONITORING. Patients most likely to benefit from pulmonary artery catheter monitoring include those whose STEMI is complicated by (1) hypotension that is not easily corrected by fluid administration; (2) hypotension in the presence of congestive heart failure; (3) hemodynamic compromise severe enough to require intravenous vasopressors or vasodilators or intraaortic balloon counterpulsation; (4) mechanical lesions (or suspected ones) such as cardiac tamponade, severe mitral regurgitation, and a ruptured ventricular septum; and (5) right ventricular infarction.[26] Other indications for hemodynamic monitoring include assessment of the effects of mechanical ventilation, differentiating pulmonary disease from left ventricular failure as the cause of hypoxemia, and management of septic shock (see Table 47–7).[7]

Before inserting a pulmonary artery catheter into a patient with STEMI, the physician must weigh that the potential benefit of the information to be obtained outweighs any potential risks. Major complications from pulmonary artery catheters are relatively rare (about 3 to 5 percent of cases), but severe problems can occur, including sepsis, pulmonary infarction, and pulmonary artery rupture. By minimizing the duration of catheterization and by strict adherence to aseptic techniques, risk can be diminished. Catheter-related bloodstream infections can also be reduced by using antiseptic-impregnated catheters.[178]

Accurate determination of hemodynamics by clinical assessment is difficult in critically ill patients. The use of a pulmonary artery catheter often leads to important changes in therapy that would not have occurred if the hemodynamic information had not been available. Of note, reports exist that rates of complications and mortality may be higher in patients who undergo pulmonary artery catheterization, although such patients are often at higher risk initially. These observations emphasize the importance of patient selection, meticulous technique, and correct interpretation of the data obtained.

Hemodynamic Abnormalities

In 1976, Swan, Forrester, and their associates measured the cardiac output and wedge pressure simultaneously in a large series of patients with acute myocardial infarction and identified four major hemodynamic subsets of patients (Table 47–8): (1) patients with normal perfusion and without pulmonary congestion (normal cardiac output and normal wedge pressure); (2) patients with normal perfusion and pulmonary congestion (normal cardiac output and elevated wedge pressure); (3) patients with decreased perfusion but without pulmonary congestion (reduced cardiac output and normal wedge pressure); and (4) patients with decreased perfusion and pulmonary congestion (reduced cardiac output and elevated wedge pressure). This classification, which overlaps with a crude clinical classification proposed earlier by Killip and Kimball (Table 47–9), has proved to be quite useful, but it should be noted that patients frequently pass from one category to another with therapy and sometimes apparently even spontaneously.

HEMODYNAMIC SUBSETS. These are usually reflected in the patient's clinical status. Hypoperfusion usually becomes evident clinically when the cardiac index falls below approximately 2.2 liters/min/m^2, whereas pulmonary congestion is noted when the wedge pressure exceeds approximately 20 mm Hg. However, approximately 25 percent of patients with cardiac indices less than 2.2 liters/min/m^2 and 15 percent of patients with elevated pulmonary capillary wedge pressures are not recognized clinically. Discrepancies in hemodynamic and clinical classification of patients with STEMI arise for a variety of reasons.

Patients may exhibit "phase lags" as clinical pulmonary congestion develops or resolves, symptoms secondary to chronic obstructive pulmonary disease may be confused with those resulting from pulmonary congestion, or longstanding left ventricular dysfunction may mask signs of hypoperfusion secondary to compensatory vasoconstriction.

The hemodynamic findings shown in Tables 47–8 and 47–9 allow for rational approaches to therapy. The goals of hemodynamic therapy are to maintain ventricular performance, support blood pressure, and protect jeopardized myocardium. Because these goals occasionally may be at cross purposes, recognition of the hemodynamic profile, as assessed clinically or as available from hemodynamic monitoring, is required before optimal therapeutic interventions can be designed along the lines discussed later.

HYPOTENSION IN THE PREHOSPITAL PHASE. During the prehospital phase of STEMI, invasive hemodynamic monitoring is not feasible, and during this period, therapy should be guided by frequent clinical assessment and measurement of arterial pressure by cuff, with the recognition that intense vasoconstriction can provide a falsely low pressure measured by this method. Hypotension associated with bradycardia often reflects excessive vagotonia. Relative or absolute hypovolemia is often present when hypotension occurs with a normal or rapid heart rate, particularly among patients receiving diuretics just prior to the occurrence of infarction. Marked diaphoresis, reduction of fluid intake, or vomiting during the period preceding and accompanying the onset of STEMI may all contribute to the development of hypovolemia. Even if the effective vascular volume is normal, relative hypovolemia may be present because ventricular compliance is reduced in cases of STEMI and a left ventricular filling pressure as high as 20 mm Hg may be needed to provide an optimal preload.

MANAGEMENT. In the absence of rales involving more than one-third of the lung fields, the patient should be put in the reverse Trendelenburg position, and in patients with sinus bradycardia and hypotension, atropine should be administered (0.3-0.6 mg IV repeated at 3- to 10-minute intervals up to 2.0 mg). If these measures do not correct the hypotension, normal saline should be administered intravenously, beginning with a bolus of 100 ml followed by 50 ml increments every 5 minutes. The patient should be observed and the infusion stopped when the systolic pressure returns to approximately 100 mm Hg, if the patient becomes dyspneic, or if pulmonary rales develop or increase. Because of the poor correlation between left ventricular filling pressure and mean right atrial pressure, assessment of systemic (even central) venous pressure is of limited value as a guide to fluid therapy.

Administration of cardiotonic agents is indicated during the prehospital phase if systemic hypotension persists despite correction of hypovolemia and excessive vagotonia. In the absence of invasive hemodynamic monitoring, assessment of peripheral vascular resistance must be based on clinical observations. If cutaneous vasoconstriction is present, therapy with dobutamine, which stimulates cardiac contractility without unduly accelerating heart rate and which does not increase the impedance to ventricular outflow, may be helpful. In hypotensive patients with STEMI with clinical evidence of vasodilation, an uncommon circumstance, phenylephrine hydrochloride is preferable, although this agent, which increases coronary as well as peripheral vascular tone, should be used with caution.

HYPOVOLEMIC HYPOTENSION. Recognition of hypovolemia is of particular importance in hypotensive patients with STEMI because of the hazard it poses and because of the improvement in circulatory dynamics that can be achieved so readily and safely by augmentation of vascular volume. Because hypovolemia is often occult, it is frequently over-

TABLE 47–8 Hemodynamic Classifications of Patients with Acute Myocardial Infarction

A. Based on Clinical Examination		B. Based on Invasive Monitoring	
Class	*Definition*	*Subset*	*Definition*
A	Rales and S_3 absent	I	Normal hemodynamics PCWP < 18, CI > 2.2
B	Rales over >50% of lung	II	Pulmonary congestion PCWP > 18, CI > 2.2
C	Rales over <50% of lung fields (pulmonary edema)	III	Peripheral hypoperfusion PCWP < 18, CI < 2.2
D	Shock	IV	Pulmonary congestion and peripheral hypoperfusion PCWP > 18, CI < 2.2

A, Modified from Killip T, Kimball J: Treatment of myocardial infarction in a coronary care unit. A two year experience with 250 patients. Am J Cardiol *20*:457, 1967; and **B,** From Forrester J, Diamond G, Chatterjee K, et al: Medical therapy of acute myocardial infarction by the application of hemodynamic subsets. N Engl J Med 295:1356, 1976.
PCWP = pulmonary capillary wedge pressure; CI = cardiac index.

TABLE 47–9 Hemodynamic Patterns for Common Clinical Conditions

	Chamber Pressure (mm Hg)				
Cardiac Condition	*RA*	*RV*	*PA*	*PCW*	*CI*
Normal	0-6	25/0-6	25/0-12	6-12	≥2.5
AMI without LVF	0-6	25/0-6	30/12-18	≤18	≥2.5
AMI with LVF	0-6	30-40/0-6	30-40/18-25	>18	>2.0
Biventricular failure	>6	50-60/>6	50-60/25	18-25	>2.0
RVMI	12-20	30/12-20	30/12	≤12	<2.0
Cardiac tamponade	12-16	25/12-16	25/12-16	12-16	<2.0
Pulmonary embolism	12-20	50-60/12-20	50-60/12	<12	<2.0

AMI = acute myocardial infarction; CI = cardiac index; LVF = left ventricular failure; PA = pulmonary artery; PCW = pulmonary capillary wedge; RA = right atrium; RV = right ventricle; RVMI = right ventricular myocardial infarction.
From Gore JM, Zwerner PL: Hemodynamic monitoring of acute myocardial infarction. *In* Francis GS, Alpert JS (eds): Modern Coronary Care, 1990, pp 139-164.

looked in the absence of invasive hemodynamic monitoring. Hypovolemia may be absolute, with low left ventricular filling pressure (8 mm Hg), or relative, with normal (8 to 12 mm Hg) or even modestly increased (13 to 18 mm Hg) left ventricular filling pressures. Because of the reduction of left ventricular compliance that occurs with acute ischemia and infarction, left ventricular filling pressures between 13 and 18 mm Hg, although above the upper limits of normal, may actually be suboptimal.

Exclusion of hypovolemia as the cause of hypotension requires the documentation of a reduced cardiac output despite left ventricular filling pressure exceeding 18 mm Hg. If, in a hypotensive patient, the pulmonary capillary wedge pressure (ordinarily measured as the pulmonary artery occlusive pressure) is below this level, fluid challenge should be carried out as described earlier. If hypovolemia is documented or suspected, the fluid replaced should resemble the fluid lost. Thus, when a low hematocrit complicates STEMI, infusion of packed red blood cells or whole blood is the treatment of choice.[179] On the other hand, crystalloid or colloid solutions should be administered when the hematocrit is normal or elevated.

Hypotension caused by right ventricular infarction may be confused with that caused by hypovolemia because both are associated with a low, normal, or minimally elevated left ventricular filling pressure. The findings and management of right ventricular infarction are discussed elsewhere in this chapter.

THE HYPERDYNAMIC STATE. When infarction is not complicated by hemodynamic impairment, no therapy other than general supportive measures and treatment of arrhythmias is necessary. However, if the hemodynamic profile is of the hyperdynamic state, that is, elevation of sinus rate, arterial pressure, and cardiac index, occurring singly or together in the presence of a normal or low left ventricular filling pressure, and if other causes of tachycardia such as fever, infection, and pericarditis can be excluded, treatment with beta-adrenoceptor blockers is indicated. Presumably, the increased heart rate and blood pressure are the result of inappropriate activation of the sympathetic nervous system, possibly secondary to augmented release of catecholamines, pain and anxiety, or some combination of these.

Left Ventricular Failure

Left ventricular dysfunction is the single most important predictor of mortality following STEMI (Fig. 47–25).[79,85] In patients with STEMI, heart failure is characterized either by systolic dysfunction alone or by both systolic and diastolic dysfunction. Left ventricular diastolic dysfunction leads to pulmonary venous hypertension and pulmonary congestion, whereas systolic dysfunction is principally responsible for a depression of cardiac output and of the ejection fraction. Clinical manifestations of left ventricular failure become more common as the extent of the injury to the left ventricle increases.[180] In addition to infarct size, other important predictors of the development of symptomatic left ventricular dysfunction include advanced age and diabetes.[180] Mortality increases in association with the severity of the hemodynamic deficit.

THERAPEUTIC IMPLICATIONS. Classification of patients with STEMI by hemodynamic subsets has therapeutic relevance. As already noted, patients with normal wedge pressures and hypoperfusion often benefit from infusion of fluids, because the peak value of stroke volume is usually not attained until left ventricular filling pressure reaches 18 to 24 mm Hg. However, a low level of left ventricular filling pressure does not imply that left ventricular damage is necessarily slight. Such patients may be relatively hypovolemic

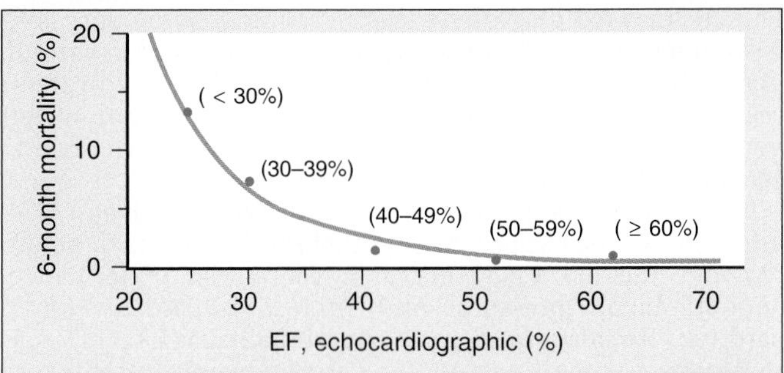

FIGURE 47–25 Impact of left ventricular function on survival following myocardial infarction. The curvilinear relationship between left ventricular ejection fraction (LVEF) for patients treated in the fibrinolytic era is shown. Among patients with an LVEF below 40 percent, the rate of mortality is markedly increased at 6 months. Thus, interventions such as thrombolysis, aspirin, and angiotensin-converting enzyme inhibitors should be of considerable benefit in patients with acute myocardial infarction to minimize the amount of left ventricular damage and interrupt the neurohumoral activation seen with congestive heart failure. (Adapted from Volpi A, De VC, Franzosi MG, et al: Determinants of 6-month mortality in survivors of myocardial infarction after thrombolysis. Results of the GISSI-2 data base. The Ad Hoc Working Group of the Gruppo Italiano per lo Studio della Sopravvivenza nell'Infarto Miocardico (GISSI)-2 Data Base. Circulation 88:416, 1993.)

and/or may have suffered a right ventricular infarct with or without severe left ventricular damage.

The relationship between ventricular filling pressure and cardiac index when preload is increased by an infusion of saline or dextran can provide valuable hemodynamic information, in addition to that obtained from baseline measurements. For example, the ventricular function curve rises steeply (marked increase in cardiac index, small increase in filling pressure) in patients with normal left ventricular function and hypovolemia, whereas the curve rises gradually or remains flat in those patients with a combination of hypovolemia and depressed cardiac function.

Invasive hemodynamic monitoring is essential to guide therapy of patients with severe left ventricular failure (pulmonary capillary wedge pressure > 18 mm Hg *and* cardiac index < 2.5 liters/min/m^2).

AVOIDANCE OF HYPOXEMIA. Patients whose STEMI is complicated by congestive heart failure characteristically develop hypoxemia due to a combination of pulmonary vascular engorgement (and in some cases pulmonary interstitial edema), diminished vital capacity, and respiratory depression from narcotic analgesics. Hypoxemia can impair the function of ischemic tissue at the margin of the infarct and thereby contribute to establishing or perpetuating the vicious circle (see Fig. 46–10). The ventilation-perfusion mismatch that results in hypoxemia requires careful attention to ventilatory support. Increasing fractions of inspired oxygen (FIO_2) via face mask should be used initially, but if the oxygen saturation of the patient's blood cannot be maintained above 85 to 90 percent on 100 percent FIO_2, strong consideration should be given to endotracheal intubation with positive-pressure ventilation. The improvement of arterial oxygenation and hence myocardial oxygen supply may help to restore ventricular performance. Positive end-expiratory pressure may diminish systemic venous return and reduce effective left ventricular filling pressure. This may require reduction in the amount of positive end-expiratory pressure, normal saline infusions to maintain left ventricular filling pressure, adjustment of the rate of infusion of vasodilators such as nitroglycerin, or some combination of these. Because myocardial ischemia frequently occurs during the return to unsupported spontaneous breathing, the weaning process should be accompanied by observation for signs of ischemia and is potentially facilitated by a period of intermittent mandatory ventilation or pressure support ventilation before extubation.

Although positive inotropic agents can be useful, they do not represent the initial therapy of choice in patients with STEMI. Instead, heart failure is managed most effectively first by reduction of ventricular preload, and then, if possible, by lowering of afterload. Arrhythmias can contribute to hemodynamic compromise and should be treated promptly in patients with left ventricular failure.

DIURETICS (see Chaps. 23 and 38). Mild heart failure in patients with STEMI frequently responds well to diuretics such as furosemide, administered intravenously in doses of 10 to 40 mg, repeated at 3- to 4-hour intervals if necessary. The resultant reduction of pulmonary capillary pressure reduces dyspnea, and the lowering of left ventricular wall tension that accompanies the reduction of left ventricular diastolic volume diminishes myocardial oxygen requirements and may lead to improvement of contractility and augmentation of the ejection fraction, stroke volume, and cardiac output. The reduction of elevated left ventricular filling pressure may also enhance myocardial oxygen delivery by diminishing the impedance to coronary perfusion attributable to elevated ventricular wall tension. It may also improve arterial oxygenation by reducing pulmonary vascular congestion.

The intravenous administration of furosemide reduces pulmonary vascular congestion and pulmonary venous pressure within 15 minutes, before renal excretion of sodium and water has occurred; presumably this action results from a direct dilating effect of this drug on the systemic arterial bed. It is important not to reduce left ventricular filling pressure much below 18 mm Hg, the lower range associated with optimal left ventricular performance in STEMI, because this may reduce cardiac output further and cause arterial hypotension. Excessive diuresis may also result in hypokalemia, with its attendant risk of digitalis intoxication.

AFTERLOAD REDUCTION. Myocardial oxygen requirements depend on left ventricular wall stress, which in turn is proportional to the product of peak developed left ventricular pressure, volume, and wall thickness. Vasodilator therapy is recommended in patients with STEMI complicated by (1) heart failure unresponsive to treatment with diuretics, (2) hypertension, (3) mitral regurgitation, or (4) ventricular septal defect. In these patients, treatment with vasodilator agents increases stroke volume and may reduce myocardial oxygen requirements and thereby lessen ischemia. Hemodynamic monitoring of systemic arterial and, in many cases, pulmonary capillary wedge (or at least pulmonary artery) pressure and cardiac output in patients treated with these agents is important. Improvement of cardiac performance and energetics requires three simultaneous effects: (1) reduction of left ventricular afterload, (2) avoidance of excessive systemic arterial hypotension to maintain effective coronary perfusion pressure, and (3) avoidance of excessive reduction of ventricular filling pressure with consequent diminution of cardiac output. In general, pulmonary capillary wedge pressure should be maintained at approximately 20 mm Hg and arterial pressure above 90/60 mm Hg in patients who were normotensive before developing the STEMI.

Vasodilator therapy is particularly useful when STEMI is complicated by mitral regurgitation or rupture of the ventricular septum. In such patients, vasodilators alone or in combination with intraaortic balloon counterpulsation can sometimes serve as a "holding maneuver" and provide hemodynamic stabilization to permit definitive catheterization and angiographic studies to be carried out and to prepare the patient for early surgical intervention. Because of the precarious state of patients with complicated infarction and the need for meticulous adjustment of dosage, therapy is best initiated with agents that can be administered intravenously and that have a short duration of action, such as nitroprusside, nitroglycerin, or isosorbide dinitrate. After initial stabilization, the medication of choice is generally an ACE inhibitor, but long-acting nitrates given by mouth, sublingually, or by ointment can also be useful.

Nitroglycerin. This drug has been shown in animal experiments to be less likely than nitroprusside to produce a "coronary steal"—that is, to divert blood flow from the ischemic to the nonischemic zone. Therefore, apart from consideration of its routine use in STEMI patients discussed earlier, it may be a particularly useful vasodilator in patients with STEMI complicated by left ventricular failure. Ten to 15 mg/min is infused and the dose is increased by 10 mg/min every 5 minutes until (1) the desired effect (improvement of hemodynamics or relief of ischemic chest pain) is achieved or (2) a decline in systolic arterial pressure to 90 mm Hg, or by more than 15 mm Hg, has occurred. Although both nitroglycerin and nitroprusside lower systemic arterial pressure, systemic vascular resistance, and the heart rate-systolic blood pressure product, the reduction of left ventricular filling pressure is more prominent with nitroglycerin because of its relatively greater effect than nitroprusside on venous capacitance vessels. Nevertheless, in patients with severe left ventricular failure, cardiac output often increases despite the reduction in left ventricular filling pressure produced by nitroglycerin.

Oral Vasodilators. The use of oral vasodilators in the treatment of chronic congestive heart failure is discussed in Chapter 23. In patients with STEMI and persistent heart failure, long-term inhibition of the renin-angiotensin-aldosterone system should be carried out. This reduced ventricular load decreases the remodeling of the left ventricle that occurs commonly in the period after STEMI and thereby reduces the development of heart failure and risk of death.[181]

DIGITALIS (see Chap. 23). Although digitalis increases the contractility and the oxygen consumption of normal hearts, when heart failure is present the diminution of heart size and wall tension frequently results in a net reduction of myocardial oxygen requirements. In animal experiments, it fails to improve ventricular performance immediately following experimental coronary occlusion, but salutary effects are elicited when it is administered several days later. The absence of early beneficial effects may be due to the inability of ischemic tissue to respond to digitalis or the already maximal stimulation of contractility of the normal heart by circulating and neuronally released catecholamines.

Although the issue is still controversial, arrhythmias can be increased by digitalis glycosides when they are given to patients in the first few hours after the onset of STEMI, particularly in the absence of hypokalemia. Also, undesirable peripheral systemic and coronary vasoconstriction can result from the rapid intravenous administration of rapidly acting glycosides such as ouabain.

Administration of digitalis to patients with STEMI in the hospital phase should generally be reserved for the management of supraventricular tachyarrhythmias such as atrial flutter and fibrillation and of heart failure that persists despite treatment with diuretics, vasodilators, and beta-adrenoceptor agonists. There is no indication for its use as an inotropic agent in patients without clinical evidence of left ventricular dysfunction, and it is too weak an inotropic agent to be relied upon as the principal cardiac stimulant in patients with overt pulmonary edema or cardiogenic shock. It may, however, be useful as a supplement to agents that inhibit the renin-angiotensin-aldosterone system and in the maintenance phase of treatment for persistent or recurrent left ventricular failure.[182]

BETA-ADRENOCEPTOR AGONISTS. When left ventricular failure is severe, as manifested by marked reduction of cardiac index (<2 liters/min/m^2), and pulmonary capillary wedge pressure is at optimal (18-24 mm Hg) or excessive (>24 mm Hg) levels despite therapy with diuretics, beta-adrenoceptor agonists are indicated. Although isoproterenol is a potent cardiac stimulant and improves ventricular performance, it should be avoided in STEMI patients. It also causes tachycardia and augments myocardial oxygen consumption and lactate production; in addition, it reduces coronary perfusion pressure by causing systemic vasodilation and in animal experiments it increases the extent of experimentally induced infarction. Norepinephrine also increases myocardial oxygen consumption because of its peripheral vasoconstrictor as well as positive inotropic actions.

Dopamine and dobutamine (see Chap. 23) can be particularly useful in patients with STEMI and reduced cardiac output, increased left ventricular filling pressure, pulmonary vascular congestion, and hypotension. Fortunately, the potentially deleterious alpha-adrenergic vasoconstrictor effects exerted by dopamine occur only at higher doses than those required to increase contractility. The vasodilating actions of dopamine on renal and splanchnic vessels and its positive inotropic effects generally improve hemodynamics and renal function. In patients with STEMI and severe left ventricular failure, this drug should be administered at a dose of 3 μg/kg/min while pulmonary capillary wedge and systemic arterial pressures as well as cardiac output are monitored. The dose can be increased stepwise to 20 μg/kg/min to reduce pulmonary capillary wedge pressure to approximately 20 mm Hg and elevate cardiac index to exceed 2 liters/min/m^2. It must be recognized, however, that doses exceeding 5 μg/kg/min activate peripheral alpha receptors and cause vasoconstriction.

Dobutamine has a positive inotropic action comparable to that of dopamine but a slightly less positive chronotropic effect and less vasoconstrictor activity. In patients with STEMI, dobutamine improves left ventricular performance without augmenting enzymatically estimated infarct size. It can be administered in a starting dose of 2.5 μg/kg/min and increased stepwise to a maximum of 30 μg/kg/min. Both dopamine and dobutamine must be given carefully and with constant monitoring of the electrocardiogram, systemic arterial pressure, and pulmonary artery or pulmonary artery occlusive pressure and, if possible, with frequent measurements of cardiac output. The dose must be reduced if the heart rate exceeds 100 to 110 beats/min, if supraventricular or ventricular tachyarrhythmias are precipitated, or if ST segment changes increase.

OTHER POSITIVE INOTROPIC AGENTS. Milrinone is a noncatecholamine, nonglycoside, phosphodiesterase inhibitor with inotropic and vasodilating actions. It is useful in selected patients whose heart failure persists despite treatment with diuretics, who are not hypotensive, and who are likely to benefit from both an enhancement in contractility and afterload reduction. Milrinone should be given as a loading dose of 0.5 μg/kg/min over 10 minutes, followed by a maintenance infusion of 0.375 to 0.75 μg/kg/min.

Cardiogenic Shock

Cardiogenic shock is the most severe clinical expression of left ventricular failure and is associated with extensive damage to the left ventricular myocardium in more than 80 percent of STEMI patients in whom it occurs; the remainder have a mechanical defect such as ventricular septal or papillary muscle rupture or predominant right ventricular infarction.[27] In the past, cardiogenic shock has been reported to occur in up to 20 percent of patients with STEMI, but estimates from recent large randomized trials of fibrinolytic therapy and observational databases report an incidence rate in the range of 7 percent.[27] About 10 percent of patients with cardiogenic shock present with this condition at the time of admission, whereas 90 percent develop it during hospitalization. This low-output state is characterized by elevated ventricular filling pressures, low cardiac output, systemic hypotension, and evidence of vital organ hypoperfusion (e.g., clouded sensorium, cool extremities, oliguria, acidosis). Patients with cardiogenic shock due to STEMI are more likely to be older, to have a history of a prior myocardial infarction or congestive heart failure, and to have sustained an anterior infarction at the time of development of shock. Of note, although the incidence of cardiogenic shock in patients with STEMI has been relatively stable since the mid-1970s, the short-term mortality rate has decreased from 70 to 80 percent in the 1970s to 50 to 60 percent in the 1990s.[183] Cardiogenic shock is the cause of death in about 60 percent of patients dying after fibrinolysis for STEMI.[27]

PATHOLOGICAL FINDINGS. At autopsy, more than two-thirds of patients with cardiogenic shock demonstrate stenosis of 75 percent or more of the luminal diameter of all three major coronary vessels, usually including the left anterior descending coronary artery.[184] Almost all patients with cardiogenic shock are found to have thrombotic occlusion of the artery supplying the major region of recent infarction, with loss of about 40 percent of the left ventricular mass.[27] In addition to culprit vessel location, correlates of 1-year survival in patients with shock complicating STEMI include age, the initial TIMI flow grade, and extent of left ventricular dysfunction.[185] Other causes of cardiogenic shock in patients with STEMI include mechanical defects such as rupture of the ventricular septum, a papillary muscle, or free wall with tamponade; right ventricular infarction; or marked reduction of preload due to conditions such as hypovolemia.[27]

Patients who die as a consequence of cardiogenic shock often have "piecemeal" necrosis, that is, progressive myocardial necrosis from marginal extension of their infarct into an ischemic zone bordering on the infarction. This is generally associated with persistent elevation of creatine kinase-MB (CK-MB). Early deterioration in left ventricular function secondary to apparent extension of infarction may, in some cases, result from expansion of the necrotic zone of myocardium without actual extension of the necrotic process. Shear forces that develop during ventricular systole can disrupt necrotic myocardial muscle bundles, with resultant expansion and thinning of the akinetic zone of myocardium, which in turn results in deterioration of overall left ventricular function.

At autopsy, patients with cardiogenic shock consistently demonstrate marginal extension of recent areas of infarction. Additionally, focal areas of necrosis are frequently found in regions of the left and right ventricles that are not adjacent to the major area of recent infarction. Such extensions and focal lesions are probably in part the result of the shock state itself, because they can also be found in the hearts of patients dying of noncardiogenic shock. Infarction of the ischemic periinfarction zone can be precipitated by a number of factors that adversely affect the supply of oxygen or the metabolic demand in this zone of myocardium. These include a reduction of coronary perfusion pressure causing impaired myocardial perfusion in the presence of atherosclerotic obstructions of the nonculprit artery. An augmentation of myocardial oxygen demand resulting from the local release of catecholamines from ischemic adrenergic nerve endings in the heart as well as from circulating endogenous or infused catecholamines may also play a role. Patients with shock due to a mechanical defect often have smaller infarcts than do those with cardiogenic shock secondary to ventricular failure without a mechanical lesion. The prognosis is better in such patients because the smaller infarct allows their left ventricle to support the circulation if the mechanical defect has been corrected surgically.

PATHOPHYSIOLOGY. The shock state in patients with STEMI appears to be the result of a vicious circle, demonstrated in Figure 46–10.

DIAGNOSIS. Cardiogenic shock is characterized by marked and persistent (>30 min) hypotension with systolic arterial pressure less than 80 mm Hg and a marked reduction of cardiac index (generally <1.8 liters/mm/m^2) in the face of elevated left ventricular filling pressure (pulmonary capillary wedge pressure > 18 mm Hg). Spurious estimates of left ventricular filling pressure based on measurements of the pulmonary artery wedge pressure can occur in the presence of marked mitral regurgitation, in which the tall *v* wave in the left atrial (and pulmonary artery wedge) pressure tracing elevates the mean pressure above left ventricular end-diastolic pressure. Accordingly, mitral regurgitation and other mechanical lesions such as ventricular septal defect, ventricular aneurysm, and pseudoaneurysm must be excluded before the diagnosis of cardiogenic shock due to impairment of left ventricular function can be established. Mechanical complications should be suspected in any patient with acute myocardial infarction in whom circulatory collapse occurs.[27] Immediate hemodynamic, angiographic, and echocardiographic evaluations are necessary in patients with cardiogenic shock. It is important to exclude mechanical complications, because primary therapy of such lesions usually requires immediate operative treatment with intervening support of the circulation by intraaortic balloon counterpulsation.

Medical Management

When the aforementioned mechanical complications are not present, cardiogenic shock is due to impairment of left ventricular function. Although dopamine or dobutamine usually improves the hemodynamics in these patients, unfortunately neither appears to improve hospital survival significantly. Similarly, vasodilators have been used in an effort to elevate cardiac output and to reduce left ventricular filling pressure. However, by lowering the already markedly reduced coronary perfusion pressure, myocardial perfusion can be compromised further, accelerating the vicious circle illustrated in Figure 46–10. Vasodilators may nonetheless be used in conjunction with intraaortic balloon counterpulsation and inotropic agents in an effort to increase cardiac output while sustaining or elevating coronary perfusion pressure.

The systemic vascular resistance is usually elevated in patients with cardiogenic shock, but occasionally resistance is normal and in a few cases vasodilation actually predominates.[186] When systemic vascular resistance is not elevated (i.e., <1800 dynes/sec/cm^5) in patients with cardiogenic shock, norepinephrine, which has both alpha- and beta-adrenoceptor agonist properties (in doses ranging from 2 to 10 μg/min), can be employed to increase diastolic arterial pressure, maintain coronary perfusion, and improve contractility. Norepinephrine should be used only when other means, including balloon counterpulsation, fail to maintain arterial diastolic pressure above 50 to 60 mm Hg in a previously normotensive patient. The use of alpha-adrenoceptor agents such as phenylephrine and methoxamine is contraindicated in patients with cardiogenic shock (unless systemic vascular resistance is inordinately low). Inspired by the observation that many patients with shock have a low systemic vascular resistance, Cotter and associates evaluated the benefit of the nitric oxide synthase inhibitor L-NMMA in patients in refractory shock.[187] The favorable impact of L-NMMA on the hemodynamics and clinical outcomes in this pilot study serves as the foundation for further investigation of nitric oxide synthase inhibition of cardiogenic shock.[186]

Intraaortic Balloon Counterpulsation (see Chap. 25)

Intraaortic balloon counterpulsation is used in the treatment of STEMI in three groups of patients: (1) those whose conditions are hemodynamically unstable and in whom support of the circulation is required for the performance of cardiac catheterization and angiography carried out to assess lesions that are potentially correctable surgically or by angioplasty; (2) those with cardiogenic shock that is unresponsive to medical management; and (3) rarely, those with persistent ischemic pain that is unresponsive to treatment with inhalation of 100 percent oxygen, beta-adrenoceptor blockade, and nitrates. Unfortunately, among patients with cardiogenic shock, improvement is often only temporary, and "balloon dependence" commonly develops. Patients with cardiogenic shock treated with this modality can be successfully weaned from the supporting system only occasionally. Counterpulsation alone does not improve overall survival in patients either with or without a surgically remediable mechanical lesion.

COMPLICATIONS. Complications occur infrequently but include damage to or perforation of the aortic wall, ischemia distal to the site of insertion of the balloon in the femoral artery, thrombocytopenia, hemolysis, renal emboli, and mechanical failure such as rupture of the balloon. Patients at highest risk include those with peripheral vascular disease, the elderly, and women, particularly if they are small. These factors should be taken into consideration before an attempt is made to institute intraaortic balloon counterpulsation. Because of the potential for vascular bleeding complications, there has been a reluctance to use intraaortic pumps in patients who have undergone fibrinolytic therapy. However, despite the increased bleeding risk, because of the poor outcome among patients with shock following thrombolysis (usually ineffective thrombolysis), this modality should be considered in selected patients who are candidates for an aggressive approach to revascularization.

Revascularization

Of the five therapies frequently used to treat patients with cardiogenic shock (vasopressors, intraaortic balloon counterpulsation, fibrinolysis, PCI, and coronary artery bypass surgery), the first two are useful temporizing maneuvers. Surgical treatment in patients with cardiogenic shock (aside from correcting mechanical abnormalities) may involve bypassing occluded as well as severely obstructed nonoccluded vessels. Occlusion of one major vessel can cause left ventricular dysfunction and hypotension, which can then lead to hypoperfusion and ischemia of myocardium subserved by the other diseased vessels. Left ventricular function can be improved by relief of this ischemia with revascularization.

The SHOCK study evaluated early revascularization for the treatment of patients with acute myocardial infarction complicated by cardiogenic shock. Patients with shock due to left ventricular failure complicating STEMI were randomized to emergency revascularization (n = 152), accomplished by either coronary artery bypass grafting or angioplasty, or initial medical stabilization (n = 150). In 86 percent of patients in both groups, intraaortic balloon counterpulsation was performed. The primary endpoint was all-cause mortality at 30 days; a secondary endpoint was mortality at 6 months. At 30 days, the overall mortality rate was 46.7 percent in the revascularization group, not significantly different from the 56.0 percent mortality rate observed in the medical therapy group (p = 0.11). Subgroups of patients in the SHOCK trial that showed particular benefit from the early revascularization strategy (i.e., reduced 6-month mortality) were those who were younger than 75 years of age, had a prior myocardial infarction, and were randomized less than 6 hours from onset of infarction.[188] The 1-year survival rate was significantly higher in the revascularization group than in the medical therapy group, with rates of 46.7 percent versus 33.6 percent, respectively ($p = 0.027$).

RECOMMENDATIONS. We recommend assessment of patients on an individualized basis to determine their desire for aggressive care and overall candidacy for further treatment (e.g., age, mental status, comorbidities). Patients who are potential candidates for revascularization should then rapidly receive intraaortic balloon counterpulsation and be referred for coronary arteriography. Those with suitable anatomy should be revascularized as completely as possible with PCI and/or coronary artery bypass surgery.[189] Encouraging initial experience has been reported with a percutaneous left ventricular assist device as a bridge to a revascularization procedure.[190] In appropriately selected patients, emergency cardiac transplantation has also been used successfully to manage cardiogenic shock.

Right Ventricular Infarction

A characteristic hemodynamic pattern (Table 47–10) has been observed in patients with right ventricular infarction, which frequently accompanies inferior left ventricular infarction or rarely occurs in isolated form. Right-heart filling pressures (central venous, right atrial, and right ventricular end-diastolic pressures) are elevated, whereas left ventricular filling pressure is normal or only slightly raised; right ventricular systolic and pulse pressures are decreased, and cardiac output is often markedly depressed. Rarely, this disproportionate elevation of right-sided filling pressure causes right-to-left shunting through a patent foramen ovale. This possibility should be considered in patients with right ventricular infarction who have unexplained systemic hypoxemia. The finding of an elevation in atrial natriuretic factor level in patients with this condition has led to the suggestion that abnormally high levels of this peptide might be in part responsible for the hypotension seen in patients with right ventricular infarction. Of note, the same protective effect of ischemic preconditioning that has been described in cases of infarction of the left ventricle has also been reported in patients with infarction of the right ventricle.[191]

TABLE 47–10 Features of Right Ventricular Myocardial Infarction

Clinical Findings
Normal or depressed right ventricular function
Shock
Tricuspid regurgitation
Ruptured ventricular septum
Hemodynamic Measurements
Abnormally elevated right atrial pressure
Normal right ventricular and pulmonary artery systolic pressures
Increased ratio of right ventricular to left ventricular filling presure
Depressed right ventricular function curve
Scintigraphy
Uptake in right ventricular free wall
Increased right ventricular dimensions and decreased wall motion
Echocardiography
Increased right ventricular dimension
Absence of pericardial effusion
Cardiac Biomarkers
Increased magnitude of biomarker values relative to degree of left ventricular dysfunction
Cardiac Catheterization
Involvement of right (usually) or left (rarely) circumflex coronary arteries
Right ventricular akinesis
Differential Diagnosis
Hypotension with acute myocardial infarction
Pericardial tamponade
Constrictive pericarditis
Pulmonary embolus

Modified from Rackley CE, Russell RO Jr, Mantle JA, et al: Right ventricular infarction and function. Am Heart J 101:215, 1981.

Diagnosis

Many patients with the combination of normal left ventricular filling pressure and depressed cardiac index have right ventricular infarcts (with accompanying inferior left ventricular infarcts). The hemodynamic picture may superficially resemble that seen in patients with pericardial disease (see Chap. 64). It includes elevated right ventricular filling pressure; steep, right atrial *y* descent; and an early diastolic drop and plateau (resembling the square root sign) in the right ventricular pressure tracing. Moreover, the Kussmaul sign (an increase in jugular venous pressure with inspiration) and pulsus paradoxus (a fall in systolic pressure of greater than 10 mm Hg with inspiration) may be present in patients with right ventricular infarction.[26] In fact, Kussmaul sign in the setting of inferior STEMI is highly predictive of right ventricular involvement.

The electrocardiogram can provide the first clue that right ventricular involvement is present in the patient with inferior STEMI. Most patients with right ventricular infarction have ST segment elevation in lead V_4R (right precordial lead in V_4 position).[192] Transient elevation of the ST segment in any of the right precordial leads can occur with right ventricular myocardial infarction, and the presence of ST segment elevation of 0.1 mV or more in any one or combination of leads V_4R, V_5R, and V_6R in patients with the clinical picture of acute myocardial infarction is highly sensitive and specific for the diagnosis of right ventricular myocardial infarction. Wellens has emphasized that in addition to noting the presence or absence of convex upward ST elevation in V_4R, clinicians should determine whether the T wave is positive or negative—such distinctions help distinguish proximal versus distal occlusion of the right coronary artery versus occlusion of the left circumflex artery.[193] Elevation of the ST segments in leads V_1 through V_4 due to right ventricular infarction can be confused with elevation due to anteroseptal infarction. Although the elevated ST segments are oriented anteriorly in both cases, it is the frontal plane that provides important clues—the ST segments are oriented to the right in right ventricular infarction (e.g., +120 degrees) whereas they are oriented to the left in anteroseptal infarction (e.g., −30 degrees).[194]

ECHOCARDIOGRAPHY AND RADIONUCLIDE ANGIOGRAPHY. Echocardiography is helpful in the differential diagnosis because in right ventricular infarction, in contrast to pericardial tamponade, no significant quantities of pericardial fluid are seen. On two-dimensional echocardiography, abnormal wall motion of the right ventricle as well as right ventricular dilation and depression of right ventricular ejection fraction are noted.[26] Gated equilibrium radionuclide angiography is also useful for recognizing right ventricular infarction. Serial studies have shown that some degree of recovery of an initially depressed right ventricular ejection fraction is the rule with right ventricular infarction, whereas this is less apparent in cases of left ventricular ejection fraction.[26]

HEMODYNAMICS. Loss of atrial transport in patients with right ventricular infarction can result in marked reductions in stroke volume and arterial blood pressure. As already noted, disproportionate elevation of the right-sided filling pressure is the hemodynamic hallmark of right ventricular infarction. Therefore, ventricular pacing may fail to increase cardiac output, and atrioventricular sequential pacing may be required.

Treatment

Because of their ability to reduce preload, medications routinely prescribed for left ventricular infarction may produce profound hypotension in patients with right ventricular infarction.[26] In patients with hypotension due to right ventricular myocardial infarction, hemodynamics can be improved by a combination of expanding plasma volume to augment right ventricular preload and cardiac output and, when left ventricular failure is present, arterial vasodilators. The initial therapy for hypotension in patients with right ventricular infarction should almost always be volume expansion. If hypotension has not been corrected after 1 or more liters of fluid have been administered briskly, however, consideration should be given to hemodynamic monitoring with a pulmonary artery catheter, because further volume infusion may be of little use and may produce pulmonary congestion. Vasodilators reduce the impedance to left ventricular outflow and in turn left ventricular diastolic, left atrial, and pulmonary (arterial) pressures, thereby lowering the impedance to right ventricular outflow and enhancing right ventricular output.

Right ventricular infarction is common among patients with inferior left ventricular infarction. Therefore, otherwise unexplained systemic arterial hypotension or diminished cardiac output, or marked hypotension in response to small doses of nitroglycerin in patients with inferior infarction, should lead to the prompt consideration of this diagnosis. In view of the importance of atrial transport, patients requiring pacing should have atrial or atrioventricular sequential pacing.[195] Successful reperfusion of the right coronary artery significantly improves right ventricular mechanical function and lowers in-hospital mortality in patients with right ventricular infarction. Replacement of the tricuspid valve and repair of the valve with annuloplasty rings have been carried out in the treatment of severe tricuspid regurgitation secondary to right ventricular infarction.

Mechanical Causes of Heart Failure

Free Wall Rupture

The most dramatic complications of STEMI are those that involve tearing or rupture of acutely infarcted tissue (Fig. 47–26).[7] The clinical characteristics of these lesions vary considerably and depend on the site of rupture, which may involve the papillary muscles, the interventricular septum, or the free wall of either ventricle. The overall incidence of these complications is hard to assess because clinical and autopsy series differ considerably.[196] The comparative clinical profile of these complications, as gathered from different studies, is shown in Table 47–11. The incidence of myocardial rupture has increased since the late 1960s. The prior use of corticosteroids or nonsteroidal antiinflammatory agents has been implicated as predisposing to rupture as a result of impaired healing. Controversy remains about the actual relationship between the use of such agents and the frequency of rupture, with several series suggesting a correlation of rupture with their use and others not. Conversely, the early use of fibrinolytic therapy appears to reduce the incidence of cardiac rupture, an effect that is responsible in part for improved survival with effective fibrinolysis. Late fibrinolytic therapy may actually *increase* the risk of cardiac rupture despite improving overall survival.

Rupture of the free wall of the infarcted ventricle (see Fig. 47–26) occurs in up to 10 percent of patients dying in the hospital of STEMI.[197] Thinness of the apical wall, marked intensity of necrosis at the terminal end of the blood supply, poor collateral flow, the shearing effect of muscular contraction against an inert and stiffened necrotic area, and aging of the myocardium with laceration of the myocardial microstructure have all been proposed as the local factors that lead to rupture (Fig. 47–27).[198]

CLINICAL CHARACTERISTICS. The following are some features that characterize this serious complication of STEMI[199]:

1. Occurs more frequently in elderly patients and possibly more frequently in women than in men with infarction.[197]
2. Appears to be more common in hypertensive than in normotensive patients.

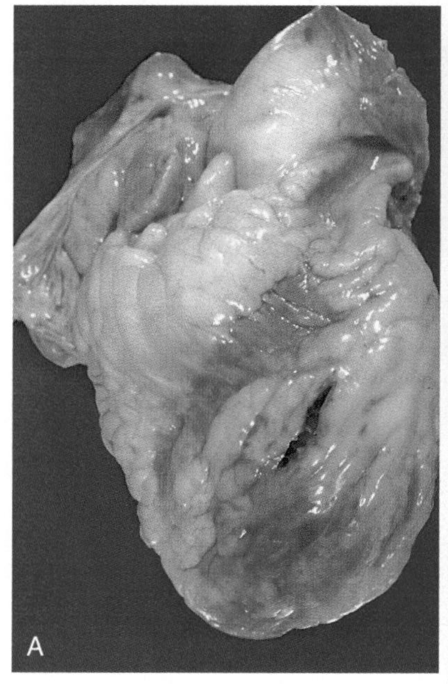

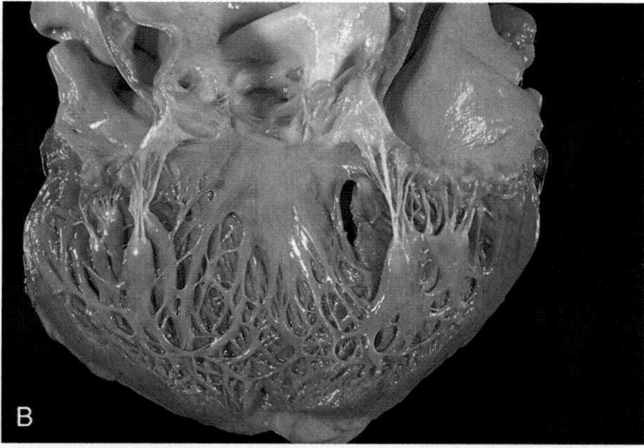

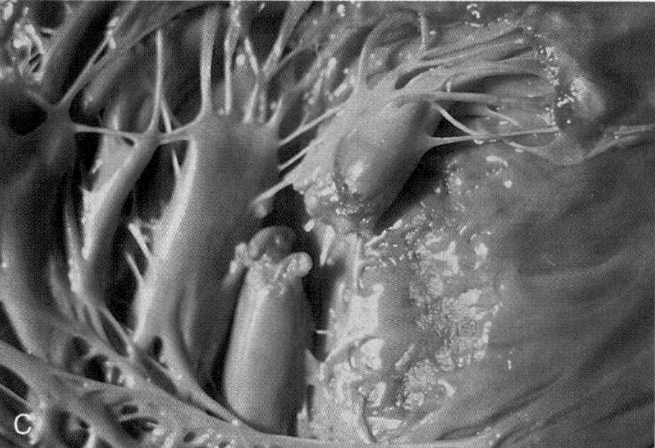

FIGURE 47–26 Cardiac rupture syndromes complicating STEMI. **A,** Anterior myocardial rupture in an acute infarct (arrow). **B,** Rupture of the ventricular septum (arrow). **C,** Complete rupture of a necrotic papillary muscle. (From Schoen FJ: The heart. *In* Cotran RS, Kumar V, Collins T [eds]: Pathologic Basis of Disease. 6th ed. Philadelphia, WB Saunders Company, 1999, p 562.)

TABLE 47–11 Clinical Profile of Mechanical Complications of Myocardial Infarction

Variable	Ventricular Septal Defect	Free Wall Rupture	Papillary Muscle Rupture
Age (mean, yr)	63	69	65
Days post-MI	3-5	3-6	3-5
Anterior MI	66%	50%	25%
New murmur	90%	25%	50%
Palpable thrill	Yes	No	Rare
Previous MI	25%	25%	30%
Echocardiographic findings			
Two-dimensional	Visualize defect	May have pericardial effusion	Flail or prolapsing leaflet
Doppler	Detect shunt		Regurgitant jet in LA
PA catheterization	Oxygen step-up in RV	Equalization of diastolic pressure	Prominent *c-v* wave in PCW tracing
Mortality			
Medical	90%	90%	90%
Surgical	50%	Case reports	40-90%

MI = myocardial infarction; LA = left atrium; PA = pulmonary artery; RV = right ventricle; PCW = pulmonary capillary wedge.
Modified from Labovitz AJ, et al: Mechanical complications of acute myocardial infarction. Cardiovasc Rev Rep 5:948, 1984.

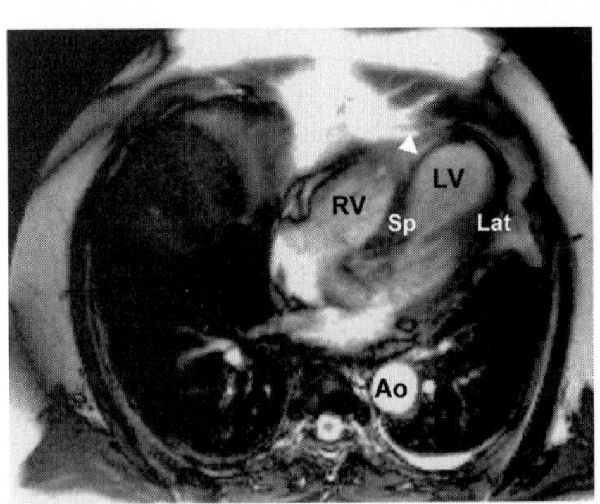

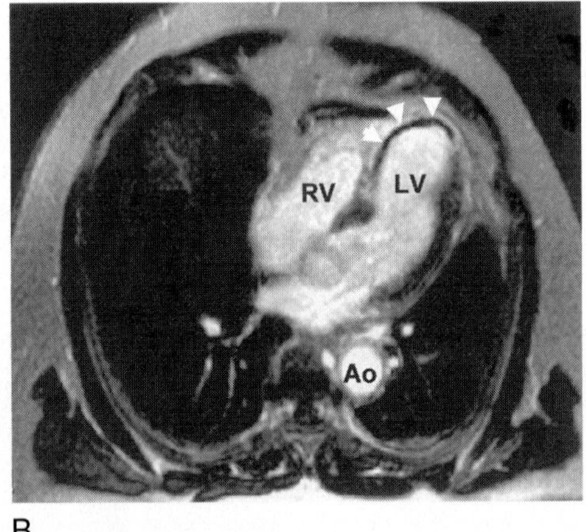

FIGURE 47–27 **A,** Gadolinium-enhanced cardiac magnetic resonance horizontal long-axis image at end diastole. The white arrowhead indicates a very dark region in the mid- to distal septum and true apical regions. The lack of gadolinium perfusion represents microvascular obstruction. **B,** Cine images show dyskinetic systolic wall motion in the regions with microvascular obstruction (as in part A). Marked wall thinning is again visible. Ao = aorta; Lat = lateral left wall; LV = left ventricular cavity; RV = right ventricular cavity; Sp = interventricular septum. (From Lesser JR, Johnson K, Lindberg JL, et al: Myocardial rupture, microvascular obstruction, and infarct expansion: Elucidation by cardiac magnetic resonance. Circulation 108:116, 2003.

3. Occurs more frequently in the left than in the right ventricle and seldom occurs in the atria.
4. Usually involves the anterior or lateral walls[197] of the ventricle in the area of the terminal distribution of the left anterior descending coronary artery.
5. Is usually associated with a relatively large transmural infarction involving at least 20 percent of the left ventricle.
6. Occurs between 1 day and 3 weeks, but most commonly 1 to 4 days, after infarction.
7. Is usually preceded by infarct expansion, that is, thinning and a disproportionate dilation within the softened necrotic zone (see Fig. 47–27).
8. Most commonly results from a distinct tear in the myocardial wall or a dissecting hematoma that perforates a necrotic area of myocardium (see Fig. 47–26).
9. Usually occurs near the junction of the infarct and the normal muscle.
10. Occurs less frequently in the center of the infarct, but when rupture occurs here, it is usually during the second rather than the first week after the infarct.
11. Rarely occurs in a greatly thickened ventricle or in an area of extensive collateral vessels.
12. Most often occurs in patients *without* previous infarction.
13. There is no evidence that the intensity of anticoagulation influences the occurrence of rupture.[200]
14. Occurs more commonly in patients who received reperfusion therapy with a fibrinolytic versus PCI.[197]

Rupture of the free wall of the left ventricle usually leads to hemopericardium and death from cardiac tamponade. Occasionally, rupture of the free wall of the ventricle occurs as the first clinical manifestation in patients with undetected or silent myocardial infarction, and then it may be considered a form of "sudden cardiac death" (see Chap. 33).

The course of rupture varies from catastrophic, with an acute tear leading to immediate death, to subacute, with nausea, hypotension, and pericardial type of discomfort being the major clinical clues to its presence.[198] Survival depends on the recognition of this complication, hemodynamic stabilization of the patient—usually with inotropic agents and/or intraaortic balloon pump—and most importantly on prompt surgical repair.

PSEUDOANEURYSM. Incomplete rupture of the heart may occur when organizing thrombus and hematoma, together with pericardium, seal a rupture of the left ventricle and thus prevent the development of hemopericardium (Fig. 47–28). With time, this area of organized thrombus and pericardium can become a pseudoaneurysm (false aneurysm) that maintains communication with the cavity of the left

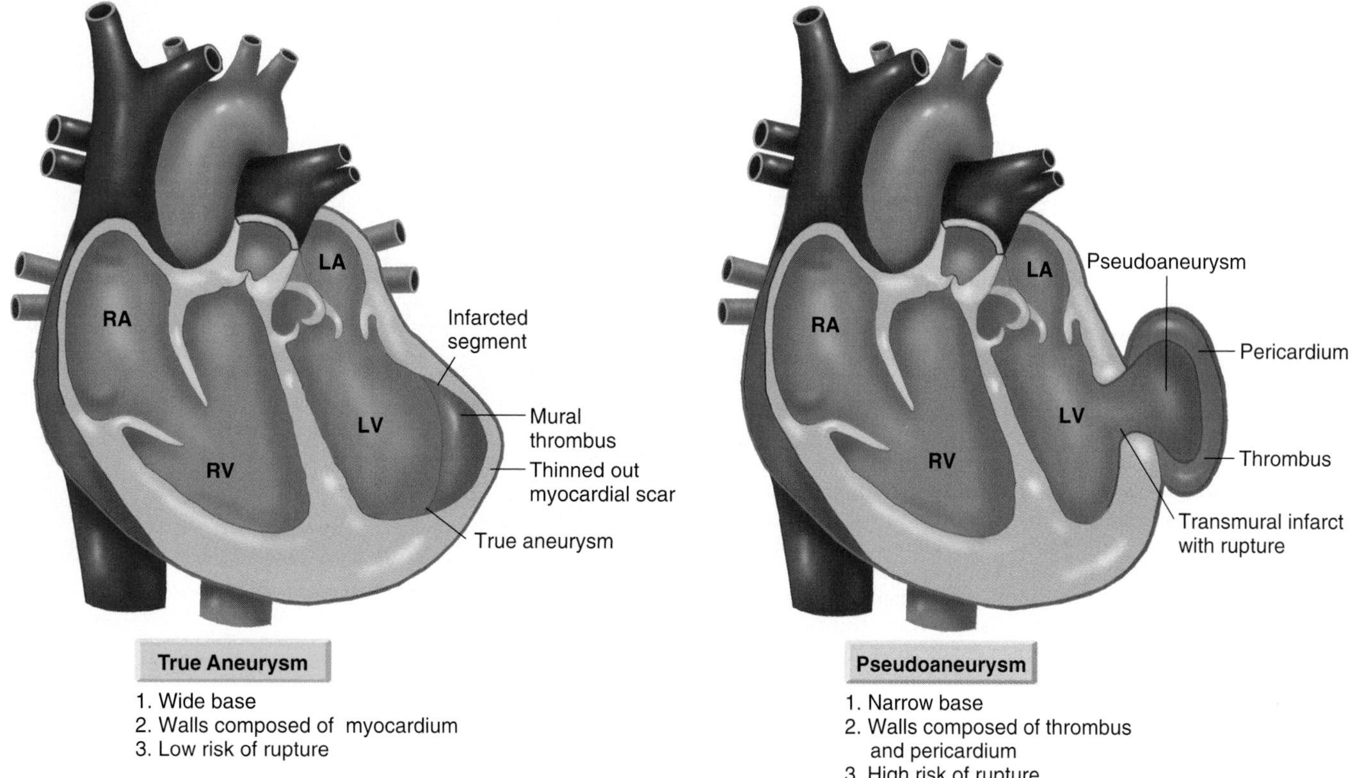

FIGURE 47–28 Differences between a pseudoaneurysm and a true aneurysm. (From Shah PK: Complications of acute myocardial infarction. *In* Parmley W, Chatterjee K [eds]: Cardiology. Philadelphia, JB Lippincott, 1987.)

ventricle. In contrast to true aneurysms, which always contain some myocardial elements in their walls, the walls of pseudoaneurysms are composed of organized hematoma and pericardium and lack any elements of the original myocardial wall. Pseudoaneurysms can become quite large, even equaling the true ventricular cavity in size, and they communicate with the left ventricular cavity through a narrow neck. Frequently, pseudoaneurysms contain significant quantities of old and recent thrombi, superficial portions of which can cause arterial emboli. Pseudoaneurysms can drain off a portion of each ventricular stroke volume exactly as do true aneurysms. The diagnosis of pseudoaneurysm can usually be made by two-dimensional echocardiography and contrast angiography, although at times differentiation between true aneurysm and pseudoaneurysm can be difficult by any imaging technique.[201]

DIAGNOSIS. The rupture usually is first suggested by the development of sudden profound shock, often rapidly leading to electromechanical dissociation due to pericardial tamponade. Immediate pericardiocentesis confirms the diagnosis and relieves the pericardial tamponade, at least momentarily. If the patient's condition is relatively stable, echocardiography may help in establishing the diagnosis of tamponade.[7] Under the most favorable conditions, cardiac catheterization can be carried out, not necessarily to confirm the diagnosis of rupture but to delineate the coronary anatomy. This is helpful so that, in addition to ventricular repair, coronary artery bypass surgery can be performed in patients in whom high-grade obstructive lesions are present. In patients in whom hemodynamics are critically compromised, establishment of the diagnosis should be followed immediately by surgical resection of the necrotic and ruptured myocardium with primary reconstruction (Fig. 47–29). When rupture is subacute and a pseudoaneurysm is suspected or present, prompt elective surgery is indicated

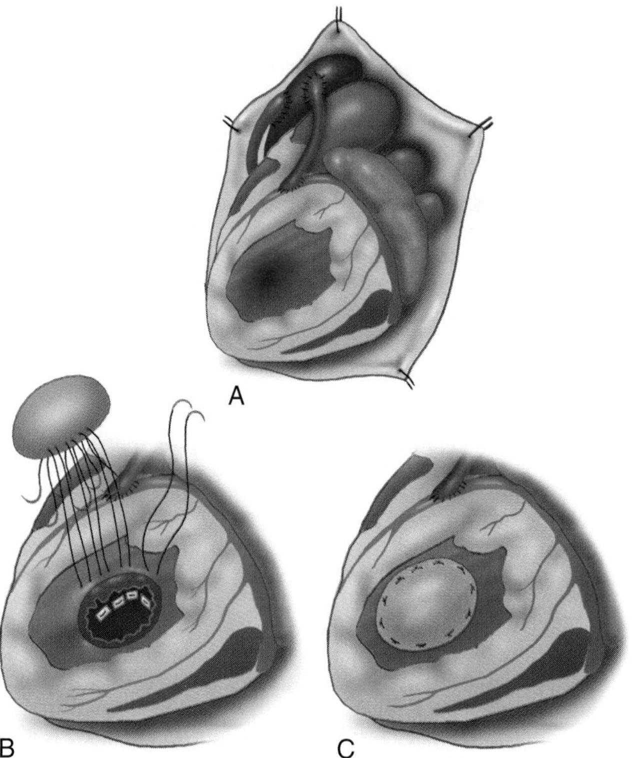

FIGURE 47–29 Management of free wall rupture. **A,** Typically, the rupture site is within a larger area of necrotic muscle. **B,** After debridement, pledgeted sutures are placed inside the ventricle and through a tailored prosthetic patch. **C,** The patch is then secured to the free wall. (Courtesy of Dr. David Adams, Mt. Sinai Hospital, New York.)

because rupture of the pseudoaneurysm occurs relatively frequently.

Rupture of the Interventricular Septum

Although rupture of the interventricular septum previously was reported in up to 11 percent of autopsied cases and 2 percent of acute myocardial infarction patients in the prefibrinolytic era, it occurs in only 0.2 percent of patients in contemporary fibrinolytic trials.[196] Clinical features associated with an increased risk of rupture of the interventricular septum include lack of development of a collateral network, advanced age, hypertension, anterior location of infarction, and possibly thrombolysis.[196] Patients who develop a rupture of the interventricular septum after STEMI have a much higher 30-day mortality rate (74 percent) than patients who do not develop this complication (7 percent).[202]

The perforation can range in length from one to several centimeters (see Fig. 47–26). It can be a direct through-and-through opening or more irregular and serpiginous. The size of the defect determines the magnitude of the left-to-right shunt and the extent of hemodynamic deterioration, which in turn affects the likelihood of survival.[196] As in rupture of the free wall of the ventricle, transmural infarction underlies rupture of the ventricular septum. Rupture of the septum with an anterior infarction tends to be apical in location, whereas inferior infarctions are associated with perforation of the basal septum and with a worse prognosis than those in an anterior location. In contrast with rupture of the free wall, rupture of the ventricular septum is more likely (20-30 percent of cases) to be associated with complete heart block, right bundle branch block, and atrial fibrillation.[203] Virtually all patients have multivessel coronary artery disease, with the majority exhibiting lesions in all of the major vessels. The likelihood of survival depends on the degree of impairment of ventricular function and the size of the defect.[196]

A ruptured interventricular septum is characterized by the appearance of a new harsh, loud holosystolic murmur that is heard best at the lower left sternal border and that is usually accompanied by a thrill.[7] Biventricular failure generally ensues within hours to days. The defect can also be recognized by two-dimensional echocardiography with color flow Doppler imaging or insertion of a pulmonary artery balloon catheter to document the left-to-right shunt. Catheter placement of an umbrella-shaped device within the ruptured septum has been reported to stabilize the conditions of critically ill patients with acute septal rupture after STEMI.

Rupture of a Papillary Muscle

Partial or total rupture of a papillary muscle is a rare but often fatal complication of transmural myocardial infarction (see Fig. 47–26).[204] Inferior wall infarction can lead to rupture of the posteromedial papillary muscle, which occurs more commonly than rupture of the anterolateral muscle, a consequence of anterolateral myocardial infarction. Rupture of a right ventricular papillary muscle is rare but can cause massive tricuspid regurgitation and right ventricular failure. Complete transection of a left ventricular papillary muscle is incompatible with life because the sudden massive mitral regurgitation that develops cannot be tolerated. Rupture of a portion of a papillary muscle, usually the tip or head of the muscle, resulting in severe, although not necessarily overwhelming, mitral regurgitation, is much more frequent and is not immediately fatal (Fig. 47–30). Unlike rupture of the ventricular septum, which occurs with large infarcts, papillary muscle rupture occurs with a relatively small infarction in approximately one-half of the cases seen. The extent of coronary artery disease in these patients sometimes is modest as well.

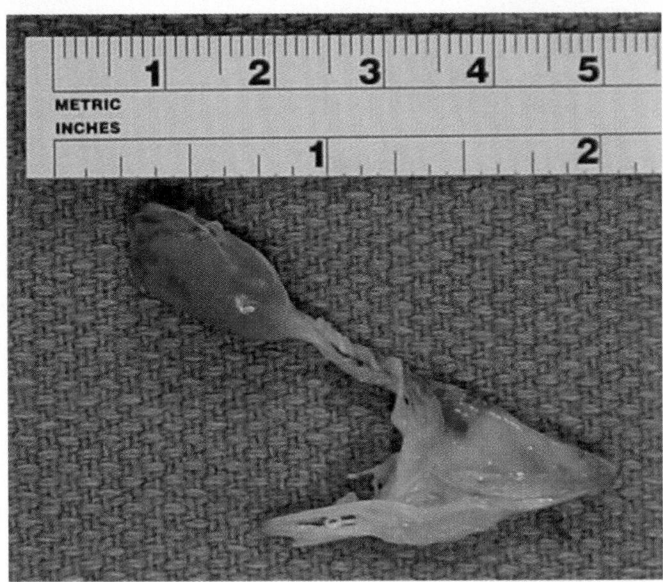

FIGURE 47–30 Surgical specimen showing papillary muscle (top left), chordae, and anterior mitral leaflet (bottom right) from a patient who had partial rupture of the papillary muscle and underwent mitral valve replacement for severe mitral regurgitation after ST elevation myocardial infarction. (Courtesy of John Byrne, MD, Brigham and Women's Hospital, Boston.)

In a small number of patients, rupture of more than one cardiac structure is noted clinically or at postmortem examination; all possible combinations of rupture of the free left ventricular wall, the interventricular septum, and papillary muscles have been described.[203]

As with patients who have a ruptured ventricular septal defect, those with papillary muscle rupture manifest a new holosystolic murmur and develop increasingly severe heart failure. In both conditions, the murmur may become softer or disappear as arterial pressure falls. Mitral regurgitation due to partial or complete rupture of a papillary muscle can be promptly recognized echocardiographically.[205] Color flow Doppler imaging is particularly helpful in distinguishing acute mitral regurgitation from a ventricular septal defect in the setting of STEMI (see Table 47–11).[7] Therefore, an echocardiogram should be obtained immediately on any patient in whom the diagnosis is suspected, because hemodynamic deterioration can ensue rapidly. Echocardiography also often permits differentiation of papillary muscle rupture from other, generally less severe forms of mitral regurgitation that occur with STEMI.

Differentiation Between Ventricular Septal Rupture and Mitral Regurgitation

It may be difficult, on clinical grounds, to distinguish between acute mitral regurgitation and rupture of the ventricular septum in patients with STEMI who suddenly develop a loud systolic murmur. This differentiation can be made most readily by color flow Doppler echocardiography. In addition, a right-heart catheterization with a balloon-tipped catheter can readily distinguish between these two complications. Patients with ventricular septal rupture demonstrate a "step-up" in oxygen saturation in blood samples from the right ventricle and pulmonary artery compared with those from the right atrium. Patients with acute mitral regurgitation lack this step-up; they may demonstrate tall *c-v* waves in both the pulmonary capillary and pulmonary arterial pressure tracings.

Invasive monitoring, which is essential in these patients, also allows for the critically important assessment of ventricular function.[7] Right and left ventricular filling pressures (right atrial pressure and pulmonary capillary wedge pressure) dictate fluid administration or the use of diuretics, whereas measurements of cardiac output and mean arterial pressure are obtained for calculation of systemic vascular resistance as a guide for vasodilator therapy. Unless systolic pressure is below 90 mm Hg, this therapy, generally using nitroglycerin or nitroprusside, should be instituted as soon as possible once hemodynamic monitoring is available. This may be critically important for stabilizing the patient's condition in preparation for further diagnostic studies and surgical repair. If vasodilator therapy is not tolerated or if it fails to achieve hemodynamic stability, intraaortic balloon counterpulsation should be rapidly instituted.

Surgical Treatment

Operative intervention is most successful in patients with STEMI and circulatory collapse when a surgically correctable mechanical lesion such as ventricular septal defect or mitral regurgitation can be identified and repaired. In such patients, the circulation should at first be supported by intraaortic balloon pulsation and a positive inotropic agent such as dopamine or dobutamine in combination with a vasodilator, unless the patient is hypotensive. Surgery should not be delayed in patients with a correctable lesion who agree to an aggressive management strategy and require pharmacological and/or mechanical (counterpulsation) support. Such patients frequently develop a serious complication—infection, adult respiratory distress syndrome, extension of the infarct, or renal failure—if surgery is delayed. Surgical survival is predicted by early operation, short duration of shock, and mild degrees of right and left ventricular impairment. When the hemodynamic status of a patient with one of these mechanical lesions complicating STEMI remains stable after the patient has been weaned from pharmacological and/or mechanical support, it may be possible to postpone the operation for 2 to 4 weeks to allow some healing of the infarct to occur. Surgical repair involves correction of mitral regurgitation, insertion of a prosthetic mitral valve repair, or closure of a ventricular septal defect, usually accompanied by coronary revascularization (Figs. 47–31 and 47–32).[7]

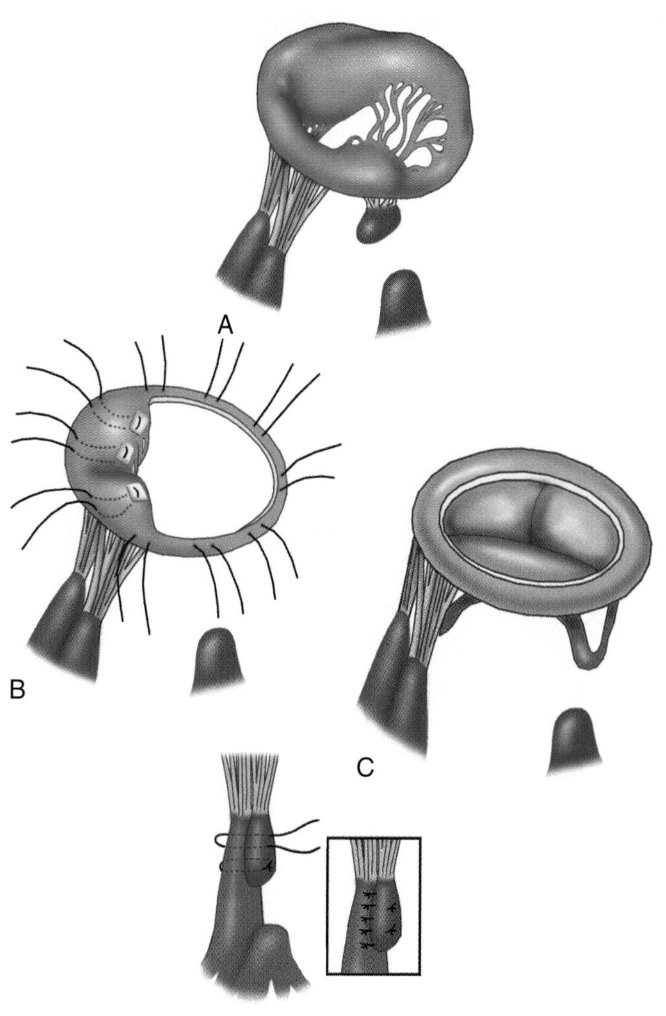

FIGURE 47–31 Surgical management of mitral regurgitation due to ruptured papillary muscle. **A,** Acute papillary muscle rupture results in severe mitral regurgitation due to leaflet and commissural prolapse. Mitral valve replacement is usually necessary. **B,** Mitral debridement with retention of the unruptured commissural and leaflet segment is performed to preserve partial annular papillary continuity. **C,** Mitral valve replacement is then performed. **D,** Occasionally, mitral valve repair can be performed by transfer of a papillary head to a nonrupture segment. (Courtesy of Dr. David Adams, Mt. Sinai Hospital, New York.)

Arrhythmias

The genesis and diagnosis of arrhythmias are presented in Chapters 27 and 29 and their treatment in Chapters 30 and 31. The role of arrhythmias in complicating the course of patients with STEMI and the prevention and treatment of these arrhythmias in this setting are discussed here and summarized in Table 47–12.

The incidence of arrhythmias is higher in patients the earlier they are seen after the onset of symptoms. Many serious arrhythmias develop before hospitalization, even before the patient is monitored. Some abnormality of cardiac rhythm also occurs in the majority of patients with STEMI treated in CCUs. When patients are seen very early during the course of STEMI, they almost invariably exhibit evidence of increased activity of the autonomic nervous system. Thus, sinus bradycardia, sometimes associated with AV block, and hypotension reflect augmented vagal activity.

MECHANISM OF ARRHYTHMIAS. A leading hypothesis for a major mechanism of arrhythmias in the acute phase of coronary occlusion is reentry due to inhomogeneity of the electrical characteristics of ischemic myocardium.[206] The cellular electrophysiological mechanisms for reperfusion arrhythmias appear to include washout of various ions such as lactate and potassium and toxic metabolic substances that have accumulated in the ischemic zone.

HEMODYNAMIC CONSEQUENCES. Patients with significant left ventricular dysfunction have a relatively fixed stroke volume and depend on changes in heart rate to alter cardiac output. However, there is a narrow range of heart rate over which the cardiac output is maximal, with significant reductions occurring at both faster and slower rates. Thus, all forms of bradycardia and tachycardia can depress the cardiac output in patients with STEMI. Although the optimal rate insofar as cardiac output is concerned may exceed 100 beats/min, it is important to consider that heart rate is one of the major determinants of myocardial oxygen consumption and that at more rapid heart rates, myocardial energy needs can be elevated to levels that adversely affect ischemic myocardium. Therefore, in patients with STEMI, the optimal rate is usually lower, in the range of 60 to 80 beats/min.

A second factor to consider in assessing the hemodynamic consequences of a particular arrhythmia is the loss of the atrial contribution to ventricular preload. Studies in patients without STEMI have demonstrated that loss of atrial transport decreases left ventricular output by 15 to 20 percent. In patients with reduced diastolic left ventricular compliance of any cause (including STEMI), however, atrial systole is of greater importance for left ventricular filling. In patients with STEMI, atrial systole boosts end-diastolic volume by 15 percent, end-diastolic pressure by 29 percent, and stroke volume by 35 percent.

TABLE 47–12 Cardiac Arrhythmias and Their Management During Acute Myocardial Infarction

Category	Arrhythmia	Objective of Treatment	Therapeutic Options
1. Electrical instability	Ventricular premature beats	Correction of electrolyte deficits and increased sympathetic tone	Potassium and magnesium solutions, beta blocker
	Ventricular tachycardia	Prophylaxis against ventricular fibrillation, restoration of hemodynamic stability	Antiarrhythmic agents; cardioversion/defibrillation
	Ventricular fibrillation	Urgent reversion to sinus rhythm	Defibrillation; bretylium tosylate
	Accelerated idioventricular rhythm	Observation unless hemodynamic function is compromised	Increase sinus rate (atropine, atrial pacing); antiarrhythmic agents
	Nonparoxysmal atrioventricular junctional tachycardia	Search for precipitating causes (e.g., digitalis intoxication); suppress arrhythmia only if hemodynamic function is compromised	Atrial overdrive pacing; antiarrhythmic agents; cardioversion relatively contraindicated if digitalis intoxication present
2. Pump failure/ excessive sympathetic stimulation	Sinus tachycardia	Reduce heart rate to diminish myocardial oxygen demands	Antipyretics; analgesics; consider beta blocker unless congestive heart failure present; treat latter if present with anticongestive measures (diuretics, afterload reduction)
	Atrial fibrillation and/or atrial flutter	Reduce ventricular rate; restore sinus rhythm	Verapamil, digitalis glycosides; anticongestive measures (diuretics, afterload reduction); cardioversion; rapid atrial pacing (for atrial flutter)
	Paroxysmal supraventricular tachycardia	Reduce ventricular rate; restore sinus rhythm	Vagal maneuvers; verapamil, cardiac glycosides, beta-adrenergic blockers; cardioversion; rapid atrial pacing
3. Bradyarrhythmias and conduction disturbances	Sinus bradycardia	Acceleration of heart rate only if hemodynamic function is compromised	Atropine; atrial pacing
	Junctional escape rhythm	Acceleration of sinus rate only if loss of atrial "kick" causes hemodynamic compromise	Atropine; atrial pacing
	Atrioventricular block and intraventricular block		Insertion of pacemaker

Modified from Antman EM, Rutherford JD (eds): Coronary Care Medicine: A Practical Approach. Boston, Martinus Nijhoff Publishing, 1986, p 78.

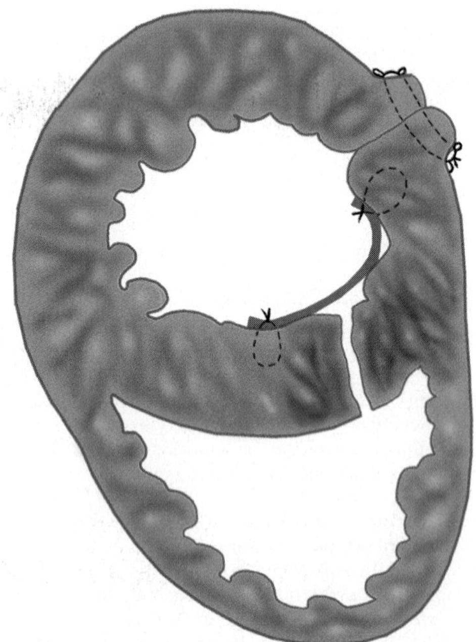

FIGURE 47–32 Repair of ischemic ventricular septal defect. The infarct typically involves a free wall and septum. Repair of the defect is performed through an incision in the ventricular wall infarct. The septal defect is closed with a prosthetic patch and a second patch is used to close the incision in the free wall. (Courtesy of Dr. David Adams, Mt. Sinai Hospital, New York.)

VENTRICULAR ARRHYTHMIAS (see Chap. 29)

Ventricular Premature Complexes

Prior to the widespread use of reperfusion therapy, aspirin, beta blockers, and intravenous nitrates in the management of STEMI, it was believed that frequent ventricular premature complexes (more than 5 per minute), ventricular premature complexes with multiform configuration, early coupling (the "R-on-T" phenomenon), and repetitive patterns in the form of couplets or salvos presaged ventricular fibrillation. It is now clear, however, that such "warning arrhythmias" are present in as many patients who do not develop fibrillation as those who do. Several reports have shown that primary ventricular fibrillation (see later) occurs without antecedent warning arrhythmias and may even develop in spite of suppression of warning arrhythmias.[207] Both primary ventricular fibrillation and ventricular premature complexes, especially R-on-T beats, occur during the early phase of STEMI, when considerable heterogeneity of electrical activity is present. Although R-on-T beats expose this heterogeneity and can precipitate ventricular fibrillation in a small minority of patients, the ubiquitous nature of VPCs in patients with STEMI and the extremely infrequent nature of ventricular fibrillation in the current era of STEMI management produces unacceptably low sensitivity and specificity of ECG patterns observed on monitoring systems for identifying patients at risk of ventricular fibrillation.

MANAGEMENT. Since the incidence of ventricular fibrillation in patients with STEMI seen in CCUs over the last three decades appears to be declining, the prior practice of prophylactic suppression of ventricular premature beats with antiarrhythmic drugs no longer is necessary and there is the possibility that its use may actually be associated with an increased risk of fatal bradycardic and asystolic events.[208] Therefore, we pursue a conservative course when ventricular premature complexes are observed in STEMI patients and do not routinely prescribe

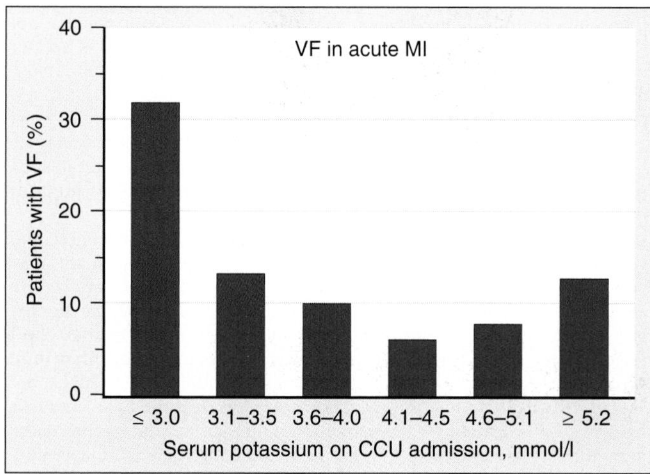

FIGURE 47–33 Importance of electrolyte deficits, as shown in this study in which the risk for ventricular fibrillation (VF) was strikingly increased in patients who presented to the critical care unit (CCU) with hypokalemia. MI = myocardial infarction. (From Nordrehaug JE, van der Lippe G: Hypokalemia and ventricular fibrillation in acute myocardial infarction. Br Heart J 50:525, 1983.)

antiarrhythmic drugs but instead determine whether recurrent ischemia or electrolyte (Fig. 47-33) or metabolic disturbances are present.[207,209]

When, at the very inception of an infarction, ventricular premature complexes are encountered in the presence of sinus tachycardia, augmented sympathoadrenal stimulation is often a contributing factor and can be treated by beta-adrenoceptor blockade. In fact, early administration of an intravenous beta blocker is effective in reducing the incidence of ventricular fibrillation in cases of evolving myocardial infarction.

ACCELERATED IDIOVENTRICULAR RHYTHM. This arrhythmia is seen in up to 20 percent of patients with STEMI. It occurs frequently during the first 2 days, with about equal frequency in anterior and inferior infarctions. Most episodes are of short duration. Accelerated idioventricular rhythm is often observed shortly after successful reperfusion has been established. However, the frequent occurrence of this rhythm in patients without reperfusion limits their reliability as markers of restoration of patency of the infarct-related coronary artery.[7] In contrast to rapid ventricular tachycardia, accelerated idioventricular rhythm is thought not to affect prognosis, and we do not routinely treat accelerated idioventricular rhythms.

Ventricular Tachycardia

Nonsustained runs of ventricular tachycardia do not appear to be associated with an increased mortality risk, either during hospitalization or over the first year. Ventricular tachycardia occurring late in the course of STEMI is more common in patients with transmural infarction and left ventricular dysfunction, is likely to be sustained, usually induces marked hemodynamic deterioration, and is associated with increased rates of both hospital mortality and long-term mortality.

MANAGEMENT. Since hypokalemia can increase the risk of developing ventricular tachycardia, low serum potassium levels should be identified quickly after a patient's admission for STEMI and should be treated promptly. We strive to maintain the serum potassium level above 4.5 mEq/liter and serum magnesium level above 2 mEq/liter. Rapid abolition of sustained ventricular tachycardia in patients with STEMI is mandatory because of its deleterious effect on pump function and because it frequently deteriorates into ventricular fibrillation. After reversion to sinus rhythm, every effort should be made to correct underlying abnormalities such as hypoxia, hypotension, acid-base or electrolyte disturbances, and digitalis excess. Although no definitive data are available, it is a common clinical practice to continue maintenance infusions of antiarrhythmic drugs for several days after an index episode of ventricular tachycardia and to discontinue the drug and either observe the patient for recurrence or perform a diagnostic electrophysiology study. Patients with recurrent or refractory ventricular tachycardia should be considered for specialized procedures such as implantation of antitachycardia devices or surgery. Occasionally, urgent attempts at revascularization with angioplasty or coronary artery bypass graft surgery help control refractory ventricular tachycardia.

Ventricular Fibrillation

Ventricular fibrillation can occur in three settings in hospitalized patients with STEMI. (Its occurrence as a mechanism of sudden death is discussed in Chapter 33.) *Primary* ventricular fibrillation occurs suddenly and unexpectedly in patients with no or few signs or symptoms of left ventricular failure. Although primary ventricular fibrillation occurred in up to 10 percent of patients hospitalized with STEMI several decades ago, analyses suggest that its incidence has declined. *Secondary* ventricular fibrillation is often the final event of a progressive downhill course with left ventricular failure and cardiogenic shock. So-called *late* ventricular fibrillation develops more than 48 hours after STEMI and frequently but not exclusively occurs in patients with large infarcts and ventricular dysfunction. Patients with intraventricular conduction defects and anterior wall infarction, patients with persistent sinus tachycardia, atrial flutter, or fibrillation early in the clinical course, and patients with right ventricular infarction who require ventricular pacing are at higher risk for suffering late in-hospital ventricular fibrillation than are patients without these features.

PROGNOSIS. The effect of primary ventricular fibrillation on prognosis continues to be debated.[208] The MILIS study, conducted in the prethrombolytic era, suggested that it does not have an adverse effect on hospital mortality, whereas the GISSI investigators reporting observations in large cohorts of thrombolytic-treated patients, suggested there was an excess mortality due to primary ventricular fibrillation during the hospital phase but not thereafter.[210] Now, with the availability of amiodarone and implantable cardioverter-defibrillators, the prognosis of late ventricular fibrillation is improving and is probably driven more by residual ventricular function and recurrent ischemia than by the arrhythmic risk per se.

PROPHYLAXIS. Lidocaine prophylaxis to prevent primary ventricular fibrillation is no longer advised. There is an association between hypokalemia and the risk of ventricular fibrillation in the CCU (see Fig. 47-33). Although it has not been conclusively shown that correction of hypokalemia to a level of 4.5 mEq/liter actually reduces the incidence of ventricular fibrillation, our experience suggests that this probably is protective and of little risk. Despite the fact that no consistent relationship between hypomagnesemia and ventricular fibrillation has been observed, magnesium deficits may still be involved in the risk of ventricular fibrillation because intracellular magnesium levels are reduced in patients with STEMI and are not adequately reflected by serum measurements. For these reasons, plus the fact that it is often difficult to repair a potassium deficit without administering supplemental magnesium, we routinely replete magnesium to a level of 2 mEq/liter.

The only situation in which we might consider prophylactic lidocaine (bolus of 1.5 mg/kg followed by 20-50 μg/kg/min) would be the unusual circumstance in which a patient within the first 12 hours of a STEMI must be managed in a facility where cardiac monitoring is not available and equipment for prompt defibrillation is not readily accessible.

MANAGEMENT (see Chaps. 32 and 33). Treatment for ventricular fibrillation consists of an unsynchronized electrical countershock with at least 200 to 300 joules, implemented as rapidly as possible.[7] When ventricular fibrillation occurs outside an intensive care unit, resuscitative efforts are much less likely to be successful, primarily because the time interval between the onset of the episode and institution of definitive therapy tends to be prolonged. Failure of electrical countershock to restore an effective cardiac rhythm is almost always due to rapidly recurrent ventricular tachycardia or ventricular fibrillation, to electromechanical dissociation, or, very rarely, to electrical asystole.

Successful interruption of ventricular fibrillation or prevention of refractory recurrent episodes can also be facilitated by administration of intravenous amiodarone. When synchronous cardiac electrical activity is restored by countershock but contraction is ineffective—that is, during electromechanical dissociation—the usual underlying cause is very extensive myocardial ischemia or necrosis or rupture of the ventricular free wall or septum. If rupture has not occurred, intracardiac administration of calcium gluconate or epinephrine may promote restoration of an effective heartbeat. We do *not* usually administer bicarbonate injections to correct acidosis because of the high osmotic load they impose and the fact that hyperventilation of the patient is probably a more suitable means of clearing the acidosis.

BRADYARRHYTHMIAS (see Chap. 29)

Sinus Bradycardia

Sinus bradycardia is a common arrhythmia occurring during the early phases of STEMI, and it is particularly frequent in patients with inferior and posterior infarction.[7,211] On the basis of data obtained in experimental infarction and from some clinical observations, it appears that the increased vagal tone that produces sinus bradycardia during the early phase of STEMI may actually be protective, perhaps because it reduces myocardial oxygen demands.[212] Thus, the acute mortality rate appears to be as low in patients with sinus bradycardia as in patients without this arrhythmia.

MANAGEMENT. Isolated sinus bradycardia, unaccompanied by hypotension or ventricular ectopy, should be observed rather than treated initially. In the first 4 to 6 hours after infarction, if the sinus rate is extremely slow (less than 40 to 50 beats/min) and associated with hypotension, intravenous atropine in aliquots of 0.3 to 0.6 mg every 3 to 10 minutes (with a total dose not exceeding 2 mg) can be administered to bring the heart rate up to approximately 60 beats/min.

Atrioventricular and Intraventricular Block

Ischemic injury can produce conduction block at any level of the AV or intraventricular conduction system. Such blocks can occur in the atrioventricular node and the bundle of His, producing various grades of AV block; in either main bundle branch, producing right or left bundle branch block; and in the anterior and posterior divisions of the left bundle, producing left anterior or left posterior (fascicular) divisional blocks. Disturbances of conduction can, of course, occur in various combinations. Clinical features of proximal and distal AV conduction disturbances in patients with STEMI are summarized in Table 47-13.

FIRST-DEGREE ATRIOVENTRICULAR BLOCK. First-degree AV block generally does not require specific treatment. Beta blockers and calcium antagonists (other than nifedipine) prolong AV conduction and may be responsible for first-degree AV block as well. However, discontinuation of these drugs in the setting of STEMI has the potential of increasing ischemia and ischemic injury. Therefore, it is our practice not to decrease the dosage of these drugs unless the PR interval is greater than 0.24 second. Only if higher degree block or hemodynamic impairment occurs should these agents be stopped. If the block is a manifestation of excessive vagotonia and is associated with sinus bradycardia and hypotension, administration of atropine, as already outlined, may be helpful. Continued electrocardiographic monitoring is important in such patients in view of the possibility of progression to higher degrees of block.

SECOND-DEGREE ATRIOVENTRICULAR BLOCK. First-degree and type I second-degree AV blocks do not appear to affect survival, are most commonly associated with occlusion of the right coronary artery, and are caused by ischemia of the AV node (see Table 47-13). Specific therapy is not required in patients with second-degree AV block of the type I variety when the ventricular rate exceeds 50 beats/min and premature ventricular contractions, heart failure, and bundle branch block are absent. However, if these complications develop or if the heart rate falls below approximately 50 beats/min and the patient is symptomatic, immediate treatment with atropine (0.3 to 0.6 mg) is indicated; temporary pacing systems are almost never needed in the management of this arrhythmia.

Type II second-degree block usually originates from a lesion in the conduction system below the bundle of His (see Table 47-13). Because of its potential for progression to complete heart block, type II second-degree AV block should be treated with a temporary external or transvenous demand pacemaker with the rate set at approximately 60 beats/min.[7]

COMPLETE (THIRD-DEGREE) ATRIOVENTRICULAR BLOCK. Complete AV block can occur in patients with either anterior or inferior

TABLE 47-13 Atrioventricular (AV) Conduction Disturbances in Acute Myocardial Infarction

	Location of AV Conduction Disturbance	
	Proximal	***Distal***
Site of block	Intranodal	Infranodal
Site of infarction	Inferoposterior	Anteroseptal
Compromised arterial supply	RCA (90%), LCX (10%)	Septal perforators of LAD
Pathogenesis	Ischemia, necrosis, hydropic cell swelling, excess parasympathetic activity	Ischemia, necrosis, hydropic cell swelling
Predominant type of AV nodal block	First-degree (PR > 200 msec) Mobitz type I second-degree	Mobitz type II second-degree Third-degree
Common premonitory features of third-degree AV block	(a) First–second-degree AV block (b) Mobitz I pattern	(a) Intraventricular conduction block (b) Mobitz II pattern
Features of escape rhythm following third-degree block (a) Location (b) QRS width (c) Rate (d) Stability of escape rhythm	 (a) Proximal conduction system (His bundle) (b) <0.12/sec* (c) 45-60/min but may be as low as 30/min (d) Rate usually stable; asystole uncommon	 (a) Distal conduction system (bundle branches) (b) >0.12/sec (c) Often <30/min (d) Rate often unstable with moderate to high risk of ventricular asystole
Duration of high-grade AV block	Usually transient (2-3 days)	Usually transient but some form of AV conduction disturbance and/or intraventricular defect may persist
Associated mortality rate	Low unless associated with hypotension and/or congestive heart failure	High because of extensive infarction associated with power failure or ventricular arrhythmias
Pacemaker therapy (a) Temporary (b) Permanent	 (a) Rarely required; may be considered for bradycardia associated with left ventricular power failure, syncope, or angina (b) Almost never indicated because conduction defect is usually transient	 (a) Should be considered in patients with anteroseptal infarction and acute bifascicular block (b) Indicated for patients with high-grade AV block with block in His-Purkinje system and those with transient advanced AV block and associated bundle branch block

LAD = left anterior descending coronary artery. LCX = left circumflex coronary artery; RCA = right coronary artery.

Modified from Antman EM, Rutherford JD: Coronary Care Medicine: A Practical Approach. Boston, Martinus Nijhoff, 1986; and Dreifus LS, et al: Guidelines for implantation of cardiac pacemakers and antiarrhythmia devices. J Am Coll Cardiol 18:1, 1991. Reprinted with permission from the American College of Cardiology.

*Some studies suggest that a wide QRS escape rhythm (>0.12 sec) following high-grade AV block in inferior infarction is associated with a worse prognosis.

infarction. Complete heart block in patients with inferior infarction usually results from an intranodal or supranodal lesion and develops gradually, often progressing from first-degree or type I second-degree block. The escape rhythm is usually stable without asystole and often junctional, with a rate exceeding 40 beats/min and a narrow QRS complex in 70 percent of cases and a slower rate and wide QRS in the others. This form of complete AV block is often transient, may be responsive to pharmacological antagonism of adenosine with methylxanthines,[213] and resolves in the majority of patients within a few days (see Table 47-13).

In patients with anterior infarction, third-degree AV block often occurs suddenly, 12 to 24 hours after the onset of infarction, although it is usually preceded by intraventricular block and often type II (not first-degree or type I) AV block. Such patients have unstable escape rhythms with wide QRS complexes and rates less than 40 beats/min; ventricular systole may occur quite suddenly. In patients with anterior infarction, AV block usually develops as a result of extensive septal necrosis that involves the bundle branches. The high rate of mortality in this group of patients with slow idioventricular rhythm and wide QRS complexes is the consequence of extensive myocardial necrosis resulting in severe left ventricular failure and often shock (see Table 47-13).

Patients with inferior infarction often have concomitant ischemia or infarction of the AV node secondary to hypoperfusion of the AV node artery. However, the His-Purkinje system usually escapes injury in such individuals. Patients with inferior STEMI who develop AV block usually have lesions in both right and left anterior descending coronary arteries. Likewise, patients with inferior STEMI and AV block have larger infarcts and more depressed right ventricular and left ventricular function than do patients with inferior infarct and no AV block. As already noted, junctional escape rhythms with narrow QRS complexes occur commonly in this setting.

Although data suggest that complete AV block is *not* an independent risk factor for mortality, whether temporary transvenous pacing per se improves survival of patients with anterior STEMI remains controversial. Some investigators contend that ventricular pacing is useless when employed to correct complete AV block in patients with anterior infarction in view of the poor prognosis in this group regardless of therapy. However, pacing may protect against transient hypotension with its attendant risks of extending infarction and precipitating malignant ventricular tachyarrhythmias. Also, pacing protects against asystole (see Chap. 31), a particular hazard in patients with anterior infarction and infranodal block. Improved survival with pacing probably occurs in only a small fraction of patients with complete AV block and anterior wall infarcts, because the extensive destruction of the myocardium that almost invariably accompanies this condition results in a very high mortality rate, even in paced patients. Given these considerations, an extremely large series of patients would be required to demonstrate the small reduction of mortality that might be achieved by pacing. The absence of data supporting such an effect, however, by no means excludes the possibility that it may be present.

Pacing is not usually needed in patients with inferior wall infarction and complete AV block that is often transient in nature, but it is indicated if the ventricular rate is very slow (<40 to 50 beats/min), if ventricular arrhythmias or hypotension is present, or if pump failure develops; atropine is only rarely of value in these patients. Only when complete heart block develops in less than 6 hours after the onset of symptoms is atropine likely to abolish the AV block or cause acceleration of the escape rhythm. In such cases, the AV block is more likely to be transient and related to increases in vagal tone, rather than the more persistent block seen later in the course of STEMI, which generally requires cardiac pacing.

Intraventricular Block

The right bundle branch and the left posterior division have a dual blood supply from the left anterior descending and right coronary arteries, whereas the left anterior division is supplied by septal perforators originating from the left anterior descending coronary artery. Not all conduction blocks observed in patients with STEMI can be considered to be complications of infarcts, because almost half are already present at the time the first electrocardiogram is recorded, and they may represent antecedent disease of the conduction system.[214] Compared with patients without conduction defects, STEMI patients with bundle branch blocks have more comorbid conditions, are less likely to receive therapies such as thrombolytics, aspirin, and beta blockers, and have an increased in-hospital mortality rate.[215] In the prefibrinolytic era, studies of intraventricular conduction disturbances—that is, block within one or more of the three subdivisions (fascicles) of the His-Purkinje system (the anterior and posterior divisions of the left bundle and the right bundle)—had been reported to occur in 5 to 10 percent of patients with STEMI. More recent series in the fibrinolytic era suggest that intraventricular blocks occur in about 2 to 5 percent of patients with myocardial infarction.[216]

ISOLATED FASCICULAR BLOCKS. Isolated left anterior divisional block is unlikely to progress to complete AV block. Mortality is increased in these patients, although not as much as in patients with other forms of conduction block. The posterior fascicle is larger than the anterior fascicle, and, in general, a larger infarct is required to block it. As a consequence, mortality is markedly increased. Complete AV block is not a frequent complication of either form of isolated divisional block.

RIGHT BUNDLE BRANCH BLOCK. This conduction defect alone can lead to AV block because it is often a new lesion, associated with anteroseptal infarction. Isolated right bundle branch block is associated with an increased mortality risk in patients with anterior STEMI even if complete AV block does not occur, but this appears to be the case only if it is accompanied by congestive heart failure.

BIFASCICULAR BLOCK. The combination of right bundle branch block with either left anterior or posterior divisional block or the combination of left anterior and posterior divisional blocks (i.e., left bundle branch block) is known as bidivisional or bifascicular block. If new block occurs in two of the three divisions of the conduction system, the risk of developing complete AV block is quite high. Mortality is also high because of the occurrence of severe pump failure secondary to the extensive myocardial necrosis required to produce such an extensive intraventricular block.[216] Patients with intraventricular conduction defects, particularly right bundle branch block, account for the majority of patients who develop ventricular fibrillation late in their hospital stay. However, the high rate of mortality in these patients occurs even in the absence of high-grade AV block and appears to be related to cardiac failure and massive infarction rather than to the conduction disturbance.[215]

Preexisting bundle branch block or divisional block is less often associated with the development of complete heart block in patients with STEMI than are conduction defects acquired during the course of the infarct. Bidivisional block in the presence of prolongation of the P-R interval (first-degree AV block) may indicate disease of the third subdivision rather than of the AV node and is associated with a greater risk of complete heart block than if first-degree AV block is absent.

Complete bundle branch block (either left or right), the combination of right bundle branch block and left anterior divisional (fascicular) block, and any of the various forms of trifascicular block are all more often associated with anterior than with inferoposterior infarction. All these forms are more frequent with large infarcts and in older patients and have a higher incidence of other accompanying arrhythmias than is seen in patients without bundle branch block.

Use of Pacemakers in Patients with Acute Myocardial Infarction (see Chap. 31)

TEMPORARY PACING. Just as is the case for complete AV block, transvenous ventricular pacing has not resulted in statistically demonstrable improvement in prognosis among patients with acute myocardial infarction who develop intraventricular conductions defects. However, temporary pacing is advisable in some of these patients because of the high risk of developing complete AV block. This includes patients with new bilateral (bifascicular) bundle branch block—that is, right bundle branch block with left anterior or posterior divisional block and alternating right and left bundle branch block; first-degree AV block adds to this risk. Isolated new block in only one of the three fascicles even with P-R prolongation and preexisting bifascicular block and normal P-R interval poses somewhat less risk; these patients should be monitored closely, with insertion of a temporary pacemaker deferred unless higher degree AV block occurs.

Noninvasive external temporary cardiac pacing is possible routinely in conscious patients and is acceptable to many but not all patients despite the discomfort. Used in a standby mode, it is virtually free of complications and contraindications and provides an important alternative to transvenous endocardial pacing.[7] Once it is clinically evident that continuous pacing is required, external pacing, which is generally not well tolerated for more than minutes to hours, should be replaced by a temporary transvenous pacemaker.

ASYSTOLE. The presence of apparent ventricular asystole on monitor displays of continuously recorded electrocardiograms may be misleading, because the mechanism may in fact be fine ventricular fibrillation. Because of the predominance of ventricular fibrillation as the cause of cardiac arrest in this setting, initial therapy should include electrical countershock, even if definitive electrocardiographic documentation of this arrhythmia is not available. In the rare instance in which asystole can be documented to be the responsible electrophysiological disturbance, immediate transcutaneous pacing (or stimulation with a transvenous pacemaker if one is already in place) is indicated.[7]

PERMANENT PACING. The question of the advisability of permanent pacemaker insertion is complicated by the fact that not all sudden deaths in STEMI patients with conduction defects are due to high-grade AV block. A high incidence of late ventricular fibrillation occurs in CCU survivors with anterior STEMI complicated by either right or left bundle branch block. Therefore, ventricular fibrillation rather than asystole due to failure of AV conduction and infranodal pacemakers could be responsible for late sudden death.

Long-term pacing is often helpful when complete heart block persists throughout the hospital phase in a patient with STEMI, when sinus node function is markedly impaired, or when type II second- or third-degree block occurs intermittently.[7] When high-grade AV block is associated with newly acquired bundle branch block or other criteria of impairment of conduction system function, prophylactic long-term pacing may be justified as well. Additional considerations that drive a decision to insert a permanent pacemaker include whether the patient is a candidate for an implantable cardioverter-defibrillator or has severe heart failure that might be improved with biventricular pacing (see Chap. 24).

SUPRAVENTRICULAR TACHYARRHYTHMIAS (see Chap. 29)

SINUS TACHYCARDIA. This arrhythmia is typically associated with augmented sympathetic activity and may provoke transient hypertension or hypotension. Common causes are anxiety, persistent pain, left ventricular failure, fever, pericarditis, hypovolemia, pulmonary embolism, and the administration of cardioaccelerator drugs such as atropine, epinephrine, or dopamine; rarely, it occurs in patients with atrial infarction. Sinus tachycardia is particularly common in patients with anterior infarction, especially if there is significant accompanying left ventricular dysfunction. It is an undesirable rhythm in patients with STEMI because it results in an augmentation of myocardial oxygen consumption, as well as a reduction in the time available for coronary perfusion, thereby intensifying myocardial ischemia and/or external myocardial necrosis. Persistent sinus tachycardia can signify persistent heart failure and under these circumstances is a poor prognostic sign associated with an excess mortality. An underlying cause should be sought and appropriate treatment instituted, such as analgesics for pain; diuretics for heart failure; oxygen, beta blockers, and nitroglycerin for ischemia; and aspirin for fever or pericarditis.

Administration of beta-adrenoceptor blocking agents, in the dosage and manner described elsewhere in this chapter, may be helpful in the treatment of sinus tachycardia, particularly when this arrhythmia is a manifestation of a hyperdynamic circulation, which is seen particularly in young patients with an initial STEMI without extensive cardiac damage. Beta blockade is contraindicated, however, in patients in whom the sinus tachycardia is a manifestation of hypovolemia or of pump failure, the latter reflected by a systolic arterial pressure below 100 mm Hg, rales involving more than one-third of the lung fields, a pulmonary capillary wedge pressure exceeding 20 to 25 mm Hg, or a cardiac index below approximately 2.2 liters/min/m^2. A possible exception to this is a patient in whom persistent ischemia is believed to be the cause or the result of tachycardia-cautious administration of an ultra-short-acting beta-adrenoceptor blocker such as esmolol (25 to 200 μg/kg/min) can be tried to ascertain the patient's response to slowing of the heart rate.

ATRIAL FLUTTER AND FIBRILLATION. Atrial flutter is usually transient, and in patients with STEMI it is typically a consequence of augmented sympathetic stimulation of the atria, often occurring in patients with left ventricular failure or pulmonary emboli in whom the arrhythmia intensifies hemodynamic deterioration (see Table 47-12).

As with atrial premature complexes and atrial flutter, fibrillation is usually transient and tends to occur in patients with left ventricular failure but is also observed in patients with pericarditis and ischemic injury to the atria and right ventricular infarction.[26] The increased ventricular rate and the loss of the atrial contribution to left ventricular filling result in a significant reduction in cardiac output. Atrial fibrillation during STEMI is associated with increased mortality and stroke, particularly in patients with anterior wall infarction.[217] However, because it is more common in patients with clinical and hemodynamic manifestations of extensive infarction and a poor prognosis, atrial fibrillation is probably a marker of poor prognosis, with only a small independent contribution to increased mortality.

Management. Atrial flutter and fibrillation in patients with STEMI are treated in a manner similar to these conditions in other settings (see Chap. 29). Patients with recurrent episodes of atrial fibrillation should be treated with oral anticoagulants (to reduce the risk of stroke), even if sinus rhythm is present at the time of hospital discharge, because no antiarrhythmic regimen can be relied upon to be completely effective in suppressing atrial fibrillation. In the absence of contraindications, patients should receive a beta blocker after STEMI; in addition to their several other beneficial effects, these agents are helpful in slowing the ventricular rate, should atrial fibrillation recur.

Other Complications

Recurrent Chest Discomfort

Evaluation of postinfarction chest discomfort is sometimes complicated by previous abnormalities on the electrocardiogram and a vague description of the discomfort by the patient, who either may be exquisitely sensitive to fleeting discomfort or may deny a potential recrudescence of symptoms. The critical task for clinicians is to distinguish recurrent angina or infarction from nonischemic causes of discomfort that might be caused by infarct expansion, pericarditis, pulmonary embolism, and noncardiac conditions. Important diagnostic maneuvers include a repeat physical examination, repeat ECG reading, and assessment of the response to sublingual nitroglycerin, 0.4 mg. (The use of noninvasive diagnostic evaluation for recurrent ischemia in patients whose symptoms appear only with moderate levels of exertion is discussed elsewhere in this chapter.)

RECURRENT ISCHEMIA AND INFARCTION. The incidence of postinfarction angina without reinfarction is 20 percent in patients treated with fibrinolytics and is significantly reduced to 6 percent in patients undergoing primary PCI for STEMI.[99] It does not appear to be reduced by the use of thrombolytic therapy as the management strategy during the acute phase[218] but has been reported to be lower in patients who undergo primary percutaneous transluminal coronary angioplasty for acute myocardial infarction, especially if stents are used.[219] When accompanied by ST and T wave changes in the same leads where Q waves have appeared, it may be due to occlusion of an initially patent vessel, reocclusion of an initially recanalized or stented vessel, or coronary spasm.

DIAGNOSIS. *Extension* of the original zone of necrosis or *reinfarction* in a separate myocardial zone can be a difficult diagnosis, especially within the first 24 hours after the index event. It is more convenient to refer to both extension and reinfarction collectively under the more general term *recurrent infarction.* Serum cardiac markers may still be elevated from the initial infarction, and it may not be possible to distinguish the ECG changes that are part of the normal evolution after the index infarction from those due to recurrent infarction. Because the levels of cardiac-specific troponins remain elevated for more than 1 week following the index event, they are of less value for diagnosing recurrent infarction than are more rapidly rising and falling markers, such as CK-MB. Within the first 18 to 24 hours following the initial infarction, when serum cardiac markers may not have returned to the normal range, recurrent infarction should be strongly considered when there is repeat ST segment elevation on the electrocardiogram. Although pericarditis remains a possibility in such patients, the two can usually be distinguished by the presence of a rub and lack of responsiveness to nitroglycerin in patients with pericardial discomfort.

Beyond the first 24 hours, when serum cardiac markers such as CK-MB have usually returned to the normal range, recurrent infarction can be diagnosed either by re-elevation of the CK-MB level above the upper limit of normal and increased by at least 50 percent of the previous value or the appearance of new Q waves on the ECG reading.[7] Because of variations in patient populations and definitions of recurrent infarction, estimates of the incidence of this complication vary; large fibrinolytic trials report 30-day reinfarction rates of about 5 to 6 percent as compared with about 20 percent in patients undergoing primary PCI.[79,85,99,220] Reinfarction is more common in patients with diabetes mellitus and those with a previous myocardial infarction. In patients treated with fibrinolytics, the rate of reinfarction is lower if a low-molecular-weight heparin or direct thrombin inhibitor is used instead of unfractionated heparin as adjunctive antithrombin therapy.[67] The predominant angiographic predictors of reinfarction in patients undergoing primary PCI include a final coronary stenosis greater than 30 percent, post-PCI coronary dissection, and post-PCI intracoronary thrombus.[220]

PROGNOSIS. Regardless of whether postinfarction angina is persistent or limited, its presence is important because the short-term morbidity rate is higher among such patients; mortality is increased if the recurrent ischemia is accompanied by ECG changes and hemodynamic compromise.[7] Recurrent infarction (due in many cases to reocclusion of the infarct-related coronary artery) carries serious adverse prognostic information because it is associated with two- to fourfold higher rates of in-hospital complications (congestive heart failure, heart block) and early and long-term mortality.[221] Presumably, the higher mortality rate is related to the larger mass of myocardium whose function becomes compromised.

Of the standard therapies that are routinely prescribed during the acute phase of STEMI, aspirin and beta blockers have been associated with a reduction in the incidence of recurrent infarction.[147,166]

Management. As with the acute phase of treatment of STEMI, algorithms for management of patients with recurrent ischemic discomfort at rest center on the 12-lead electrocardiogram (Fig. 47–34). Patients with ST segment re-elevation should be referred for urgent catheterization and PCI; repeat fibrinolysis can be considered if PCI is not available. Insertion of an intraaortic balloon pump may help stabilize the patient while other procedures are being arranged. For patients believed to have recurrent ischemia who do not have evidence of hemodynamic compromise, an attempt should be made to control symptoms with sublingual or intravenous nitroglycerin and intravenous beta blockade to slow the heart rate to 60 beats/min. When hypotension, congestive heart failure, or ventricular arrhythmias develop during recurrent ischemia, urgent catheterization and revascularization are indicated.

Prior studies failed to show any benefit of a strategy of *routine* referral for catheterization and revascularization, either early or after a delay of 1 or 2 days. It should be realized, however, that those studies were conducted in an era in which the catheterization equipment was less technologically advanced than it is today and glycoprotein IIb/IIIa inhibitors and stents were not part of the interventionist's armamentarium. The de facto practice in many centers currently is to pursue a routine invasive strategy after fibrinolysis for STEMI. Although no large-scale randomized trials have been conducted in the contemporary era to support such a practice, we find it quite persuasive. Investigators in Germany reported lower rates of the composite endpoint of death/recurrent myocardial infarction/target vessel revascularization/ischemic events in patients treated with routine PCI as compared to a conservative strategy of medical therapy with referral for PCI when symptoms recurred.[222,223] The expanded use of PCI beyond rescue PCI, referred to by Dauerman and Sobel as "pharmacoinvasive recanalization," is in need of more vigorous testing but holds considerable promise for reducing rates of mortality and morbidity after STEMI.[224-227]

Pericardial Effusion and Pericarditis (see Chap. 64)

PERICARDIAL EFFUSION. Effusions are generally detected echocardiographically, and their incidence varies with technique, criteria, and laboratory expertise.[228] Effusions are more common in patients with anterior STEMI and with larger infarcts and when congestive failure is present. The majority of pericardial effusions that are seen following STEMI do not cause hemodynamic compromise; when

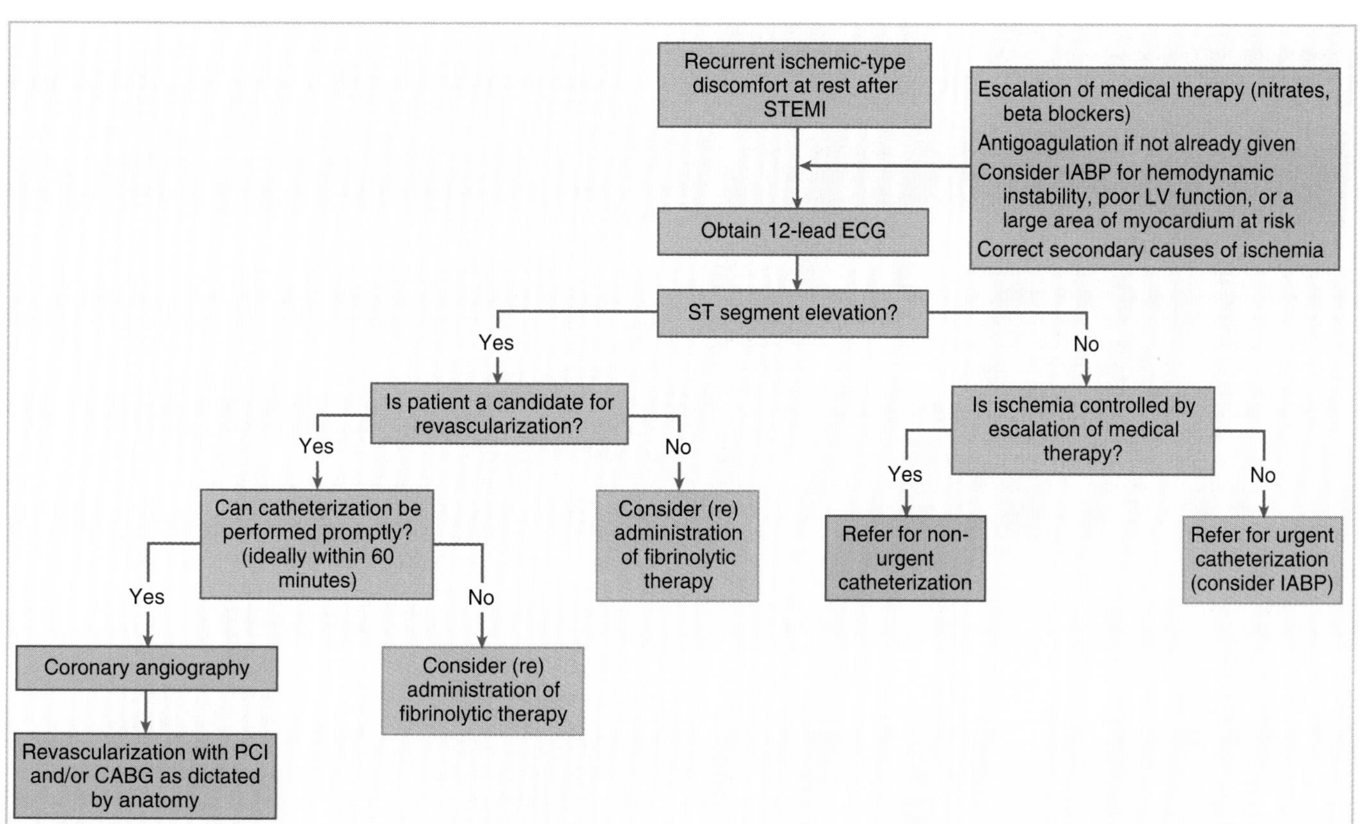

FIGURE 47–34 Algorithm for management of ischemia/infarction after ST segment elevation myocardial infarction (STEMI). CABG = coronary artery bypass grafting; ECG = electrocardiogram; IABP = intraaortic balloon pump; PCI = percutaneous coronary intervention. (Modified from Braunwald E, Zipes D, Libby P: Heart Disease: A Textbook of Cardiovascular Medicine. 6th ed. Philadelphia, WB Saunders, 2001, p 1195.)

tamponade occurs, it is usually due to ventricular rupture or hemorrhagic pericarditis.

The reabsorption rate of a postinfarction pericardial effusion is slow, with resolution often taking several months. The presence of an effusion does not indicate that pericarditis is present; although they may occur together, the majority of effusions occur without other evidence of pericarditis.

PERICARDITIS. Pericarditis can produce pain as early as the first day and as late as 6 weeks after STEMI. The pain of pericarditis may be confused with that resulting from postinfarction angina, recurrent infarction, or both. An important distinguishing feature is the radiation of the pain to either trapezius ridge, a finding that is nearly pathognomonic of pericarditis and rarely seen with ischemic discomfort. Transmural myocardial infarction, by definition, extends to the epicardial surface and is responsible for local pericardial inflammation. An acute fibrinous pericarditis (pericarditis epistenocardica) occurs commonly after transmural infarction, but the majority of patients do not report any symptoms from this process. Although transient pericardial friction rubs are relatively common among patients with transmural infarction within the first 48 hours, pain or electrocardiographic changes occur much less often. However, the development of a pericardial rub appears to be correlated with a larger infarct and greater hemodynamic compromise. The discomfort of pericarditis usually becomes worse during a deep inspiration, but it can be relieved or diminished when the patient sits up and leans forward.

Although anticoagulation clearly increases the risk for hemorrhagic pericarditis early after STEMI, this complication has not been reported with sufficient frequency during heparinization or following fibrinolytic therapy to warrant absolute prohibition of such agents when a rub is present. Nevertheless, the detection of a pericardial effusion on echocardiogram is usually an indication for discontinuation of anticoagulation. In patients in whom continuation or initiation of anticoagulant therapy is strongly indicated (such as during cardiac catheterization or following coronary angioplasty), heightened monitoring of clotting parameters and observation for clinical signs of possible tamponade are needed. Late pericardial constriction due to anticoagulant-induced hemopericardium has been reported.

Treatment of pericardial discomfort consists of aspirin, but usually in higher doses than prescribed routinely following infarction—doses of 650 mg orally every 4 to 6 hours may be needed. Nonsteroidal anti-inflammatory agents and steroids should be avoided because they may interfere with myocardial scar formation.[7]

DRESSLER SYNDROME. Also known as the *postmyocardial infarction syndrome*, Dressler syndrome usually occurs 1 to 8 weeks after infarction. Dressler cited an incidence of 3 to 4 percent of all myocardial infarction patients in 1957, but the incidence has decreased dramatically since that time. Clinically, patients with Dressler syndrome present with malaise, fever, pericardial discomfort, leukocytosis, an elevated sedimentation rate, and a pericardial effusion. At autopsy, patients with this syndrome usually demonstrate localized fibrinous pericarditis containing polymorphonuclear leukocytes. The cause of this syndrome is not clearly established, although the detection of antibodies to cardiac tissue has raised the notion of an immunopathological process. Treatment is with aspirin, 650 mg, as often as every 4 hours. Glucocorticosteroids and nonsteroidal antiinflammatory agents are best avoided in patients with Dressler syndrome within 4 weeks of STEMI because of their potential to impair infarct healing, to cause ventricular rupture,[229] and to increase coronary vascular resistance. Aspirin in large doses is effective.

Venous Thrombosis and Pulmonary Embolism

Almost all pulmonary emboli originate from thrombi in the veins of the lower extremities; much less commonly, they originate from mural thrombi overlying an area of right ventricular infarction. Bed rest and heart failure predispose to venous thrombosis and subsequent pulmonary embolism, and both of these factors occur commonly in patients with STEMI, particularly those with large infarcts. At a time when patients with STEMI were routinely subjected to prolonged periods of bed rest, significant pulmonary embolism was found in more than 20 percent of patients with STEMI coming to autopsy, and massive pulmonary embolism accounted for 10 percent of deaths from myocardial infarction. In contemporary practice, with early mobilization and the widespread use of low-dose anticoagulant prophylaxis, especially using low-molecular-weight heparins, pulmonary embolism has become an uncommon cause of death in patients with STEMI. When pulmonary embolism does occur in patients with STEMI, management is generally along the lines described for noninfarction patients (see Chap. 66).

Left Ventricular Aneurysm

The term *left ventricular aneurysm* (often termed *true aneurysm*) is generally reserved for a discrete, dyskinetic area of the left ventricular wall with a broad neck (to differentiate it from pseudoaneurysm due to a contained myocardial rupture). Dyskinetic or akinetic areas of the left ventricle are far more common than true aneurysms after STEMI; such poorly contracting segments are referred to as *regional wall motion abnormalities*.[228] True left ventricular aneurysms probably develop in less than 5 percent of all patients with STEMI and perhaps somewhat more frequently in patients with transmural infarction (especially anterior).[41] The wall of the true aneurysm is thinner than the wall of the rest of the left ventricle (see Fig. 47–28), and it is usually composed of fibrous tissue as well as necrotic muscle, occasionally mixed with viable myocardium.

PATHOGENESIS. Aneurysm formation presumably occurs when intraventricular tension stretches the noncontracting infarcted heart muscle, thus producing infarct expansion, a relatively weak, thin layer of necrotic muscle, and fibrous tissue that bulges with each cardiac contraction. With the passage of time, the wall of the aneurysm becomes more densely fibrotic, but it continues to bulge with systole, causing some of the left ventricular stroke volume during each systole to be ineffective.

When an aneurysm is present after anterior STEMI, there is generally a total occlusion of a poorly collateralized left anterior descending coronary artery. An aneurysm is rarely seen with multivessel disease when there are either extensive collaterals or a nonoccluded left anterior descending artery. Aneurysms usually range from 1 to 8 cm in diameter. They occur approximately four times more often at the apex and in the anterior wall than in the inferoposterior wall. The overlying pericardium is usually densely adherent to the wall of the aneurysm, which may even become partially calcified after several years. True left ventricular aneurysms (in contrast to pseudoaneurysms) rarely rupture soon after development. Late rupture, when the true aneurysm has become stabilized by the formation of dense fibrous tissue in its wall, almost never occurs.

The rate of mortality in patients with a left ventricular aneurysm is up to six times higher than in patients without aneurysms, even when compared with that in patients with comparable left ventricular ejection fraction. Death in these patients is often sudden and presumably related to the high incidence of ventricular tachyarrhythmias that occur with aneurysms.[207]

DIAGNOSIS. The presence of persistent ST segment elevation in an electrocardiographic area of infarction, classically thought to suggest aneurysm formation, actually indicates a large infarct with a regional wall motion abnormality but does not necessarily imply an aneurysm. The diagnosis of aneurysm is best made noninvasively by an echocardiographic study by radionuclide ventriculography, or at the time of cardiac catheterization by left ventriculography. With the loss of shortening from the area of the aneurysm, the remainder of the ventricle must be hyper-

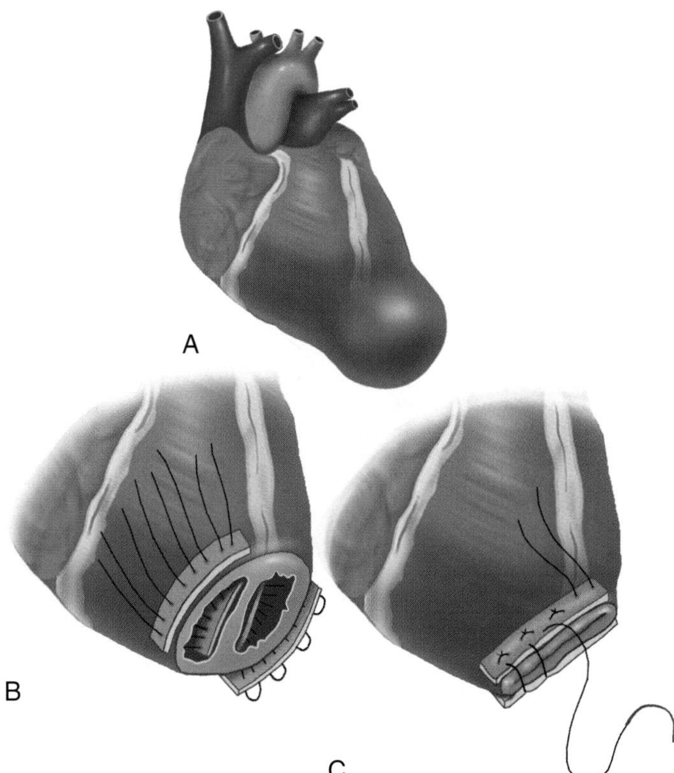

FIGURE 47–35 Surgical management of ventricular aneurysm. **A,** In this case, the aneurysm is located at the apex. **B,** The aneurysmal segment is resected and felt pledget strips are used to reinforce interrupted suture closure of the apex. **C,** Completed repair partially restores apical geometry. (Courtesy of Dr. David Adams, Division of Cardiac Surgery, Mt. Sinai Hospital, New York.)

kinetic in order to compensate. With relatively large aneurysms, complete compensation is impossible. The stroke volume falls, or, if it is maintained, it is at the expense of an increase in end-diastolic volume, which in turn leads to increased wall tension and myocardial oxygen demand. Heart failure may ensue, and angina may appear or worsen.

TREATMENT. Aggressive management of STEMI, including prompt reperfusion, may diminish the incidence of ventricular aneurysms. Surgical aneurysmectomy generally is successful only if there is relative preservation of contractile performance in the nonaneurysmal portion of the left ventricle (Fig. 47–35). In such circumstances, when the operation is performed for worsening heart failure or angina, operative mortality is relatively low and clinical improvement can be expected.[230] Aneurysmectomy and special procedures carried out to control ventricular tachyarrhythmias occurring with left ventricular aneurysms are described elsewhere in this chapter. Because of the risk of mural thrombosis and systemic embolization, we favor long-term oral anticoagulation with warfarin in patients with a left ventricular aneurysm after STEMI.

LEFT VENTRICULAR THROMBUS AND ARTERIAL EMBOLISM

The most convenient and accurate method for diagnosing left ventricular thrombosis is two-dimensional echocardiography.[228] It is hypothesized that endocardial inflammation during the acute phase of infarction provides a thrombogenic surface for clots to form in the left ventricle. With extensive transmural infarction of the septum, however, mural thrombi may overlie infarcted myocardium in both ventricles. Prospective studies have suggested that patients who develop a mural thrombus early (within 48 to 72 hours of infarction) have an extremely poor early prognosis,[231] with a high rate of mortality from the complications of a large infarction (shock, reinfarction, rupture, and ventricular tachyarrhythmia), rather than emboli from the left ventricular thrombus.

Although a mural thrombus adheres to the endocardium overlying the infarcted myocardium, superficial portions of it can become detached and produce systemic arterial emboli. Although estimates vary based on patient selection, about 10 percent of mural thrombi result in systemic embolization.[231] Echocardiographically detectable features that suggest that a given thrombus is more likely to embolize include increased mobility and protrusion into the ventricular chamber, visualization in multiple views, and contiguous zones of akinesis and hyperkinesis.

MANAGEMENT. Data from previous trials with limited sample size suggested that anticoagulation (intravenous heparin or high-dose subcutaneous heparin) reduced the development of left ventricular *thrombi* by 50 percent, but, because of the low event rate, it was not possible to demonstrate a reduction in the incidence of *systemic embolism.* Fibrinolysis reduces the rate of thrombus formation and the character of the thrombi so that they are less protuberant. Of note, however, the data from fibrinolytic trials are difficult to interpret because of the confounding effect of antithrombotic therapy with heparin. Recommendations for anticoagulation vary considerably, and fibrinolysis has precipitated fatal embolization. Nevertheless, anticoagulation for 3 to 6 months with warfarin is advocated for many patients with demonstrable mural thrombi.[7,232]

Based on the available data, it is our practice to recommend anticoagulation (intravenous heparin to elevate the aPTT to one and a half to two times that of control, followed by a minimum of 3 to 6 months of warfarin) in the following clinical situations: (1) an embolic event has already occurred, or (2) the patient has a large anterior infarction whether or not a thrombus is visualized echocardiographically. We are also inclined to follow the same anticoagulation practice in patients with infarctions other than in the anterior distribution if a thrombus or large wall motion abnormality is detected.

Aspirin, although probably not capable of affecting thrombus size in most patients, may prevent further platelet deposition on existing thrombi and also is protective against recurrent ischemic events. It should be prescribed in conjunction with warfarin to patients who are candidates for long-term anticoagulation therapy based on the indications discussed earlier.

Convalescence, Discharge, and Post-Myocardial Infarction Care

TIMING OF HOSPITAL DISCHARGE. The timing of discharge from the hospital is variable. As noted earlier, patients who have undergone aggressive reperfusion protocols and have no significant ventricular arrhythmias, recurrent ischemia, or congestive heart failure have been safely discharged in less than 5 days. More commonly, discharge occurs 5 or 6 days after admission for patients who experience no complications, who can be followed readily at home, and whose family setting is conducive to convalescence. Most complications that would preclude early discharge occur within the first day or two of admission; therefore, patients suitable for early discharge can be identified early during the hospitalization.[233] Several controlled trials and many uncontrolled trials of early discharge after STEMI have failed to show any increase in risk in patients appropriately selected for early discharge. The decision regarding timing of discharge in the patients with uncomplicated STEMI should take into account the patient's psychological state after STEMI, the adequacy of the dose titration for essential drugs such as beta blockers and inhibitors of the renin-angiotensin-aldosterone system, and the availability and timing of follow-up with visiting nurses and the patient's primary care physician.[144]

For patients who have experienced a complication, discharge is deferred until their condition has been stable for several days and it is clear that they are responding appropriately to necessary medications such as antiarrhythmic agents, vasodilators, or positive inotropic agents or that they have undergone the appropriate work-up for recurrent ischemia.

COUNSELING. Before discharge from the hospital, all patients should receive detailed instruction concerning physical activity. Initially, this should consist of ambulation at home but avoidance of isometric exercise such as lifting; several rest periods should be taken daily. In addition, the patient should be given fresh nitroglycerin tablets and instructed in their use and should receive careful instructions about the use of any other medications prescribed. As convalescence progresses, graded resumption of activity should be encouraged. Many approaches have been utilized, ranging from formal rigid guidelines to general advice advocating moderation and avoidance of any activity that evokes symptoms. Sexual counseling is often overlooked during recovery from STEMI and should also be included as part of the educational process. Such counseling should begin early after STEMI and should include the recommendation that sexual activity be resumed after successful completion of either early submaximal or later symptom-limited exercise stress testing.[7]

Some evidence indicates that behavioral alteration is possible after recovery from STEMI and that this may improve prognosis. A cardiac rehabilitation program with supervised physical exercise and an educational component has been recommended for most STEMI patients after discharge. Although the overall clinical benefit of such programs continues to be debated, there is little question that most people derive considerable knowledge and psychological security from such interventions, and they continue to be endorsed by experienced clinicians.[7] Meta-analyses of randomized trials of medically supervised rehabilitation programs versus usual care that were conducted in an era before widespread use of beta-adrenoceptor blockers and aggressive reperfusion strategies have shown a reduction in cardiovascular death but no change in the incidence of nonfatal reinfarction. Given the relationship between depression and STEMI, interest has arisen in psychosocial intervention programs in the convalescent phase of STEMI.[234] Psychosocial intervention programs have been shown to be helpful for decreasing symptoms of depression and are a useful adjunct to standard cardiac rehabilitation programs after STEMI; however, they do not have a significant impact on the risk of mortality or recurrent myocardial infarction after STEMI.[234] More detailed information on physical and psychological aspects of rehabilitation of patients convalescing from STEMI is given in Chapter 43.

Risk Stratification After STEMI

The process of risk stratification following STEMI occurs in several stages: initial presentation, in-hospital course (CCU, intermediate care unit), and at the time of hospital discharge. The tools used to form an integrated assessment of the patient consist of baseline demographic information, serial electrocardiograms and serum cardiac marker measurements, hemodynamic monitoring data, a variety of noninvasive tests, and, if performed, the findings at cardiac catheterization (Fig. 47–36).[7]

INITIAL PRESENTATION. Certain demographic and historical factors are associated with a poor prognosis in patients with STEMI, including female gender, age greater than 70 years, a history of diabetes mellitus, prior angina pectoris, and previous myocardial infarction (see Fig. 47–10).[143] Diabetes mellitus, in particular, appears to confer a three- to fourfold increase in risk. Whether this is due to accelerated atherosclerosis or some other characteristic induced by the diabetic state (such as a larger infarct size) is unclear. (Surviving diabetic patients also experience a more complicated post-myocardial infarction course, including a greater incidence of postinfarction angina, infarct extension, and heart failure.[7])

In addition to playing a central role in the decision pathway for management of patients with STEMI based on the presence or absence of ST segment elevation, the 12-lead electrocardiogram carries important prognostic information. Mortality is greater in patients experiencing anterior wall myocardial infarction than after inferior myocardial infarction, even when corrected for infarct size. Patients with right ventricular infarction complicating inferior infarction, as suggested by ST segment elevation in V_4R, have a greater mortality rate than patients sustaining an inferior infarction without right ventricular involvement.[26,235] Patients with multiple leads showing ST elevation and a high sum of ST segment elevation have an increased mortality rate, especially if their infarct is anterior in location.[235] Patients whose electrocardiogram demonstrates persistent advanced heart block (e.g., type II, second-degree, or third-degree AV block) or new intraventricular conduction abnormalities (bifascicular or trifascicular) in the course of a STEMI have a worse prognosis than do patients without these abnormalities. The influence of high degrees of heart block is particularly important in patients with right ventricular infarction, because such patients have a markedly increased mortality risk. Other electrocardiographic findings that augur poorly are persistent horizontal or downsloping ST segment depression, Q waves in multiple leads, evidence of right ventricular infarction accompanying inferior infarction,[26] ST segment depressions in anterior leads in patients with inferior infarction,[235] and atrial arrhythmias (especially atrial fibrillation).

HOSPITAL COURSE. Soon after CCUs were instituted, it became apparent that left ventricular function is an important early determinant of survival. Hospital mortality from acute myocardial infarction depends directly on the severity of left ventricular dysfunction.[143] Risk stratification via clinical findings, estimation of infarct size, and, in appropriate patients, invasive hemodynamic monitoring in the CCU provide an assessment of the likelihood of a complicated hospital course and may also identify important abnormalities, such as hemodynamically significant mitral regurgitation, that convey an adverse long-term prognosis (see Table 47–8).

Recurrent ischemia and infarction following STEMI, either in the same location as the index infarction or "at a distance," influence prognosis adversely.[221] Poor prognosis comes from the loss of viable myocardium, with the resulting larger area of infarction creating a greater compromise in ventricular function. Postinfarction angina generally connotes a less favorable prognosis because it indicates the presence of jeopardized myocardium. In the current era of aggressive revascularization, early postinfarction angina often leads to early interventions that tend to improve outcome, diminishing the long-term impact and significance of angina early after STEMI.[220]

Assessment at Hospital Discharge

Both short-term and long-term survival after STEMI depend on three factors: resting left ventricular function, residual potentially ischemic myocardium, and susceptibility to serious ventricular arrhythmias. The most important of these factors is the state of left ventricular function (see Fig. 47–25).[7] The second most important factor is how the severity and extent of the obstructive lesions in the coronary vascular bed perfusing residual viable myocardium affect the risk of recurrent infarction, additional myocardial damage, and serious ventricular arrhythmias.[7] Thus, survival relates to the quantity of myocardium that has become necrotic and the quantity at risk of becoming necrotic.

At one end of the spectrum, the prognosis is best for the patient with normal intrinsic coronary vessels whose completed infarction constitutes a small fraction (5 percent) of the left ventricle as a consequence of a coronary embolus and who has no jeopardized myocardium. At the other extreme is the patient with a massive infarct with left ventricular failure whose residual viable myocardium is perfused by markedly obstructed vessels. Progression of atherosclerosis or lowering of perfusion pressure in these vessels impairs the function and viability of the residual myocardium on which left ventricular function depends. The situation may not be hopeless even in such a patient, however, because revascularization may reduce the threat to the jeopardized myocardium. The third risk factor, the susceptibility to serious arrhythmias, is reflected in ventricular ectopic activ-

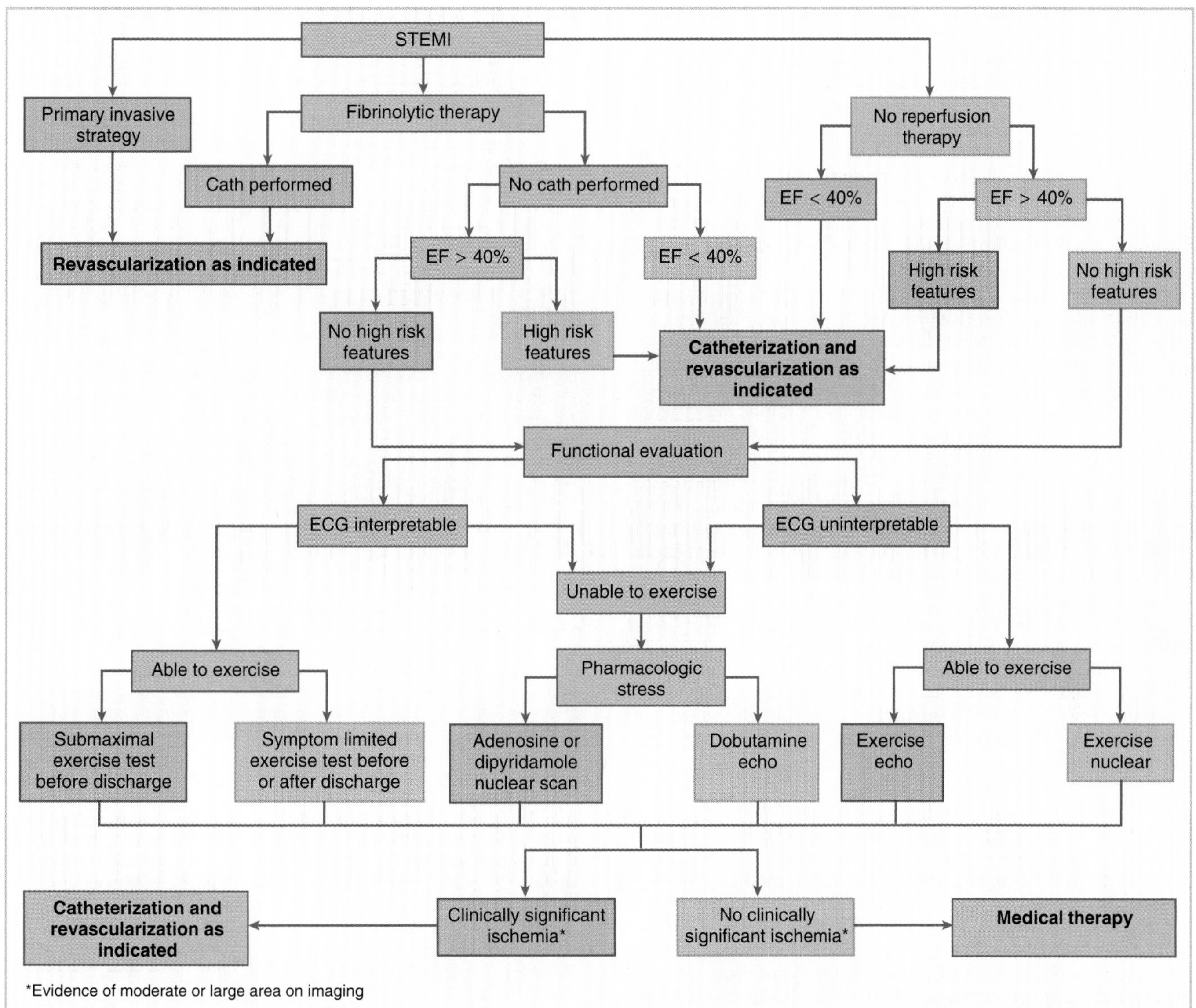

FIGURE 47–36 Algorithm for catheterization and revascularization after ST segment elevation myocardial infarction (STEMI). The algorithm shows the treatment paths for patients who initially undergo a primary invasive strategy, receive fibrinolytic therapy, or do not undergo reperfusion therapy for STEMI. Patients who have not undergone a primary invasive strategy and have no high-risk features should undergo functional evaluation using one of the noninvasive tests shown. When clinically significant ischemia (evidence of moderate or large area of ischemia by imaging) is detected, patients should undergo catheterization and revascularization as indicated; if no clinically significant ischemia is detected, medical therapy is prescribed post-STEMI. (From Antman EM, et al: ACC/AHA Guidelines for the Management of Patients with ST-Elevation Myocardial Infarction. 2004 [http://www.acc.org/clinical/guidelines/stemi/index.htm].)

ity and other indicators of electrical instability, such as reduced heart rate variability or baroreflex sensitivity and an abnormal signal-averaged electrocardiogram. All of these identify patients at increased risk of death.

In addition, patients with an occluded infarct-related artery late (e.g., 1 to 2 weeks) after STEMI have a higher long-term mortality rate.[29] Persistent occlusion of the culprit artery is associated with an increased incidence of abnormal late potentials on the electrocardiogram and appears to have an adverse prognostic effect independent of the level of ventricular function.

ASSESSMENT OF LEFT VENTRICULAR FUNCTION. Left ventricular ejection fraction may be the most easily assessed measurement of left ventricular function and is extremely useful for risk stratification (see Fig. 47–25). However, imaging of the left ventricle at rest may not distinguish adequately between infarcted, irreversibly damaged, and stunned or hibernating myocardium. To circumvent this difficulty, a variety of techniques has been investigated to assess the extent of residual viable myocardium, including exercise and pharmacological stress echocardiography, stress radionuclide ventricular angiography, perfusion imaging in conjunction with pharmacological stress, and positron emission tomography.[236] All of these techniques can be performed safely in postinfarction patients. Since no study has clearly shown one imaging modality to be superior to others, clinicians should be guided in their selection of ventricular imaging technique by the availability and level of expertise with a given modality at their local institution.[143,228,237]

In patients with low left ventricular ejection fraction, the measurement of exercise capacity is useful for further identifying those patients at particularly high risk and also for establishing safe exercise limits after discharge.[238] Patients with a good exercise capacity despite a reduced ejection fraction have a better long-term outcome than those who cannot perform more than modest exercise.

ASSESSMENT OF MYOCARDIAL ISCHEMIA. Because of the potent adverse consequences of recurrent myocardial infarction after STEMI, it is important to assess a patient's risk for future ischemia and infarction. Given the increasing array of pharmacological, interventional catheterization, and surgical options available to modify the likelihood of developing recurrent episodes of myocardial ischemia, most clinicians find it helpful to identify patients at risk for provocable myocardial ischemia prior to discharge. A predischarge evaluation for ischemia allows clinicians to select patients who might benefit from catheterization and revascularization following STEMI and to assess the adequacy of medical therapy for those patients who are suitable for a more conservative management strategy (see Fig. 47–36).

Exercise Testing. An exercise test also offers the clinician an opportunity to formulate a more precise exercise prescription and is helpful in boosting patients' confidence in their ability to conduct their daily activities after discharge. Patients who are unable to exercise can be evaluated by the use of a pharmacological stress protocol, such as an infusion of dobutamine or dipyridamole with echocardiography or perfusion imaging (see Fig. 47–36).

Treadmill exercise testing after STEMI has traditionally utilized a submaximal protocol that requires the patient to exercise until symptoms of angina appear, electrocardiographic evidence of ischemia is seen, or a target workload (approximately 5 metabolic equivalents) has been reached (see Chap. 10). It has been proposed that symptom-limited exercise tests can be safely performed before discharge in patients with an uncomplicated postinfarction course in-hospital.[238] Variables derived from exercise tests after STEMI that have been evaluated for their ability to predict the occurrence of death or recurrent nonfatal infarction include the development and magnitude of ST segment depression, the development of angina, exercise capacity, and the systolic blood pressure response during exercise.

The DANAMI (Danish Acute Myocardial Infarction) investigators reported that when patients with provocable ischemia after infarction were randomized to catheterization and revascularization versus conservative medical therapy, they experienced a lower requirement for antianginal medications, less unstable angina, and fewer nonfatal infarctions.[239] These observations, coupled with emerging data on the potential benefits of PCI after fibrinolysis, lend support for the increasingly common practice of routine referral for catheterization after lytic therapy.

ASSESSMENT FOR ELECTRICAL INSTABILITY. After STEMI, patients are at greatest risk for the development of sudden cardiac death due to malignant ventricular arrhythmias over the course of the first 1 to 2 years.[240] Several techniques have been devised to stratify patients into those who are at increased risk of sudden death following STEMI: measurement of Q-T dispersion (variability of Q-T intervals between ECG leads), ambulatory ECG recordings for detection of ventricular arrhythmias (Holter monitoring), invasive electrophysiological testing, recording a signal-averaged electrocardiogram (a measure of delayed, fragmented conduction in the infarct zone), and measuring heart rate variability (beat-to-beat variability in R-R intervals) or baroreflex sensitivity (slope of a line relating beat-to-beat change in sinus rate in response to alteration of blood pressure).[207]

Despite the increased risk of arrhythmic events following acute myocardial infarction in patients who are found to have abnormal results on one or more of the noninvasive tests described earlier, several points should be emphasized. The low positive predictive value (<30 percent) for the noninvasive screening tests limits their usefulness when viewed in isolation. Although the predictive value of screening tests can be improved by combining several of them together, the therapeutic implications of an increased risk profile for arrhythmic events have not been established. The mortality reductions achievable with the general use of beta blockers, ACE inhibitors, aspirin, and revascularization when appropriate after infarction, coupled with concerns about the efficacy and safety of antiarrhythmic drugs and the cost of implanted defibrillators, leave considerable uncertainty about the therapeutic implications of an abnormal noninvasive test for electrical instability in an asymptomatic patient. Additional data on patient outcomes when clinicians act on the results of an abnormal finding are required before definitive recommendations can be made for asymptomatic patients.[166] The management of patients with sustained, hemodynamically compromising arrhythmias is discussed in Chapters 30 and 31.

PROPHYLACTIC ANTIARRHYTHMIC THERAPY. Although it has been recognized for decades that antiarrhythmic therapy can control atrial and ventricular arrhythmias effectively in many patients, reviews of clinical trials following STEMI have reported an increased risk of mortality with type I drugs. The most notable postinfarction trial in this area was the Cardiac Arrhythmia Suppression Trial (CAST), which tested whether encainide, flecainide, or moricizine for suppression of ventricular arrhythmias detected on ambulatory electrocardiographic monitoring would reduce the risk of cardiac arrest and death over the long term. Both the first phase of the trial (encainide or flecainide versus placebo) and the second phase of the trial (moricizine versus placebo) were stopped prematurely because of increased mortality in the active treatment groups. The mechanism of the increased risk after STEMI remains a subject of investigation, but one hypothesis that has been put forth is an adverse interaction between recurrent ischemia and the presence of an antiarrhythmic drug because the risk of death or cardiac arrest was greater in patients with a non-Q-wave acute myocardial infarction than with Q-wave myocardial infarction. Sodium channel blockade by antiarrhythmics may exacerbate electrophysiological differences between subepicardial and subendocardial zones of myocardium, rendering the latter more susceptible to ischemic injury.

Subsequent to CAST, another postinfarction prophylactic antiarrhythmic drug trial was undertaken with oral D-sotalol (Survival With ORal D-sotalol, or SWORD). This trial was designed to test the hypothesis that prophylactic administration of D-sotalol to patients with depressed left ventricular function (ejection fraction < 40 percent) and either a recent (6 to 42 days) or remote (42 days) acute myocardial infarction would reduce total mortality. SWORD also was stopped prematurely after enrollment of only 3121 of a planned 6400 patients because statistical evidence of increased mortality emerged in the active treatment group.

The Canadian Amiodarone Myocardial Infarction Trial (CAMIAT) showed that amiodarone reduced the frequency of ventricular premature depolarization in patients with recent myocardial infarction; this correlated with a reduction in arrhythmic death or resuscitation from ventricular fibrillation.[241] However, 42 percent of patients discontinued amiodarone during maintenance therapy in CAMIAT because of intolerable side effects. The European Amiodarone Myocardial Infarction Trial (EMIAT) showed a reduction in arrhythmic death after myocardial infarction in patients with depressed left ventricular function, but there was no reduction in total mortality or other cardiovascular-related mortality.[242]

RECOMMENDATIONS. At this time, the *routine* use of antiarrhythmic agents (including amiodarone) cannot be recommended. Given the data cited earlier on the protective effects of beta-adrenoceptor blockers against sudden death and the ability of aspirin to reduce the risk of reinfarction, it is unclear that additional mortality reductions would be achieved by the empirical addition of amiodarone in the patient who is convalescing from a STEMI and is free of symptomatic sustained ventricular arrhythmias.

Several trials that included post-STEMI patients in the study population have shown significant mortality reductions in patients randomized to ICD implantation versus conventional medical therapy (see Chap. 31). At present, the selection of STEMI patients who are candidates for ICD implantation is based on the left ventricular ejection fraction and the time since the acute STEMI event. An algorithm incorporating these factors is given in Figure 47–37.

Secondary Prevention of Acute Myocardial Infarction (see Chap. 42)

The concept of secondary prevention of reinfarction and death after recovery from a STEMI has been investigated actively for several decades. Problems in proving the efficacy of various interventions have been related both to the ineffectiveness of certain strategies and to the difficulty in proving a benefit as mortality and morbidity have improved after STEMI. Nevertheless, patients who survive the initial course of STEMI are at increased risk because of coronary artery disease and its complications; therefore, it is imperative that efforts be made to reduce this risk. Although secondary prevention drug trials generally have tested one form of therapy against placebo in an attempt to demonstrate a benefit of that therapy, the physician must remember that disciplined clinical care of the individual patient is far more important than rote use of an agent found beneficial in the latest drug trial.

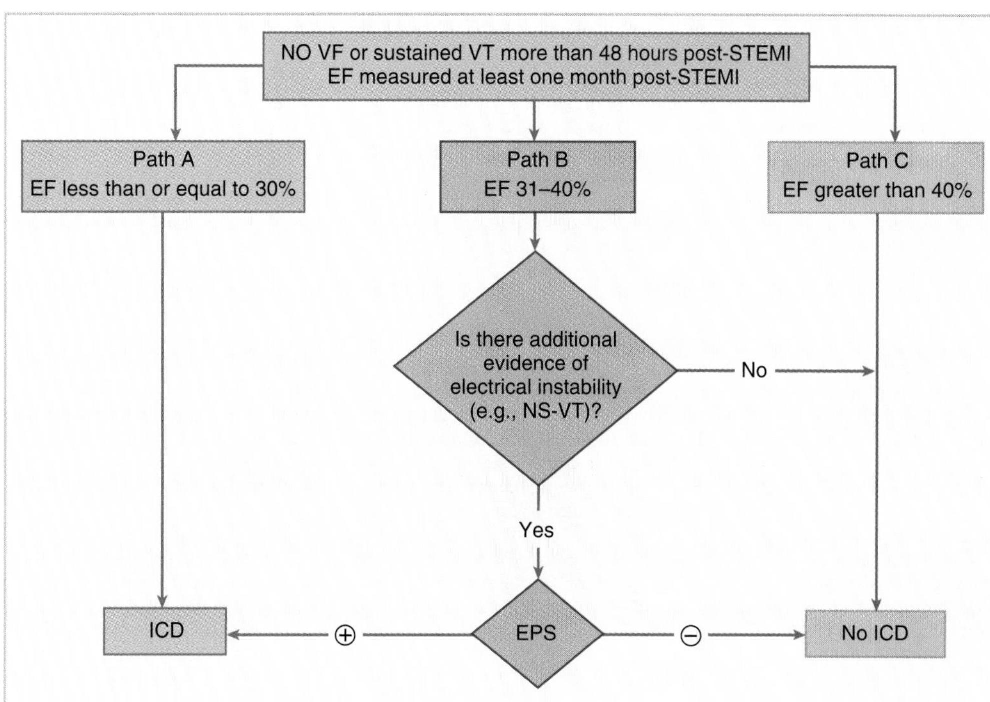

FIGURE 47–37 Algorithm for assessment of need for electrophysiological study and implantation of an implantable cardioverter-defibrillator (ICD) in ST segment elevation myocardial infarction (STEMI) patients without ventricular fibrillation (VF) or sustained ventricular tachycardia (VT) more than 72 hours after STEMI. The appropriate management path is selected based on the timing and measurement of left ventricular ejection fraction (EF) (see table at top of figure). EF measurements obtained 3 days or less after STEMI should be repeated before proceeding with the algorithm. In path A, patients with markedly depressed left ventricular function at least 1 month post-STEMI are referred for insertion of an ICD. Path B illustrates the management of patients in an intermediate-risk category who require further evaluation with an electrophysiology study (EPS). If the EPS reveals inducible ventricular tachycardia/ventricular fibrillation, an ICD is implanted; if the EPS is negative, no ICD is implanted and the patient receives medical therapy post-STEMI. Path C illustrates the management of patients with preserved left ventricular function who do not receive an ICD and are treated with medical therapy post-STEMI. LOE = level of evidence; NS-VT = nonsustained ventricular tachycardia. (From Antman EM, et al: ACC/AHA Guidelines for the Management of Patients with ST-Elevation Myocardial Infarction. 2004 [http://www.acc.org/clinical/guidelines/stemi/index.htm].)

LIFE-STYLE MODIFICATION. Efforts to improve survival and the quality of life after myocardial infarction that relate to life-style modification of known risk factors are considered in Chapter 42. Of these, cessation of smoking and control of hypertension are probably most important. It has been shown that within 2 years of quitting smoking, the risk of a nonfatal myocardial infarction in former smokers falls to a level similar to that in patients who never smoked. Being hospitalized for a STEMI is a powerful motivation for patients to cease cigarette smoking, and this is an ideal time to encourage that clearly beneficial and highly cost-effective life-style change. It is also an ideal time to begin to treat hypertension, to counsel patients to achieve optimal body weight, and to consider various strategies to improve the patient's lipid profile.[7]

DEPRESSION. Physicians caring for patients following a STEMI need to be sensitive to the fact that some patients experience major depression after infarction, and the development of this problem is an independent risk factor for mortality. In addition, lack of an emotionally supportive network in the patient's environment after discharge is associated with an increased risk of mortality and recurrent cardiac events.[7] The precise mechanisms relating depression and lack of social support to worse prognosis after STEMI are not clear, but one possibility is lack of adherence to prescribed treatments, a behavior that has been shown to be associated with increased risk of mortality after infarction.[7] Evidence exists that a comprehensive rehabilitation program utilizing primary health care personnel who counsel patients and make home visits favorably impacts the clinical course of patients after infarction and reduces the rate of rehospitalization for recurrent ischemia and infarction. A supportive physician attitude can also have a positive impact on the rate of return to work after STEMI.

MODIFICATION OF LIPID PROFILE. Compelling evidence now exists that an increased cholesterol level, and most importantly an increased low-density lipoprotein (LDL) cholesterol level, is associated with an increased risk of coronary heart disease (see Chap. 39). Based on this observation and the finding that lowering cholesterol reduces the risk of coronary heart disease, a target LDL cholesterol level of less than 100 mg/dl has been recommended in patients with clinically evident coronary heart disease.[243] This recommendation clearly applies to patients with STEMI, and it is therefore important to obtain a lipid profile on admission in all patients admitted with acute infarction. (It should be recalled that cholesterol levels may fall 24 to 48 hours after infarction.) In addition to lowering LDL cholesterol, therapy with statins reduces levels of C-reactive protein, suggesting an antiinflammatory effect.[244]

Surveys of physician practice in the past have revealed a disappointingly low rate of treatment of hypercholesterolemia in patients with proven coronary artery disease, indicating considerable room for improvement in this aspect of secondary prevention after STEMI.

Recommendations. The dietary prescription after STEMI should be low saturated fat (<7 percent of total calories) and low cholesterol (<200 mg/day). Patients with an LDL cholesterol level greater than 100 mg/dl should be discharged on statin therapy with the goal of reducing the LDL level to less than 70 mg/dl (see Chap. 49). It is also reasonable to prescribe statin therapy to patients recovering from STEMI whose LDL cholesterol level is either unknown or is less than 100 mg/dl.[7] For many patients recovering from an acute myocardial infarction, a low high-density lipoprotein cholesterol level is their primary lipid abnormality. Gemfibrozil (1200 mg/day) reduces the risk of death, reinfarction, and stroke in such patients.[7]

ANTIPLATELET AGENTS. On the basis of the compelling data from the Antiplatelet Trialists' Collaboration of a 22 percent reduction in the risk of recurrent infarction, stroke, or vascular death in high-risk vascular patients receiving prolonged antiplatelet therapy in the absence of a true aspirin allergy, all STEMI patients should receive 75 to 162 mg of aspirin daily indefinitely.[123,138] Additional benefits of long-term aspirin that can accrue in the STEMI patient are an increased likelihood of patency of the infarct artery and smaller infarcts if recurrent myocardial infarction does take place. Patients with true aspirin allergy can be treated with clopidogrel (75 mg once daily), based on experience from patients with unstable angina/non-ST segment elevation myocardial infarction (see Chap. 49).

INHIBITION OF THE RENIN-ANGIOTENSIN-ALDOSTERONE SYSTEM. The rationale for inhibition of this neurohormonal axis after STEMI was discussed earlier. To prevent late remodeling of the left ventricle and also to decrease the likelihood of recurrent ischemic events, we advocate indefinite therapy with an ACE inhibitor to all patients with clinically evident congestive heart failure, a moderate decrease in global ejection fraction, or a large regional wall-motion abnormality, even in the face of a normal global ejection fraction. Once the STEMI patient is discharged from the hospital, the evidence base on long-term management of patients with chronic coronary artery disease is the most relevant for long-term decision-making. Based on the results of the HOPE and EUROPA trials, we advocate indefinite treatment with an ACE inhibitor in all STEMI patients, provided no contraindications exist.[245,246] As discussed earlier, the VALIANT trial results suggest that valsartan may be used as an alternative to an ACE inhibitor for long-term management of patients with left ventricular dysfunction after STEMI.[161]

BETA-ADRENOCEPTOR BLOCKERS. Meta-analyses of trials from the prethrombolytic era involving more than 24,000 patients who received beta-adrenoceptor blockers in the convalescent phase of STEMI have shown a 23 percent reduction in long-term mortality (see Fig. 47-19). When beta blockade is initiated early (6 hours) in the acute phase of infarction and continued in the chronic phase of treatment, some of the benefit may result from a reduction in infarct size. In the majority of patients who have beta blockade initiated during the convalescent phase of STEMI, however, reduction in long-term mortality is probably due to a combination of an antiarrhythmic effect (prevention of sudden death) and prevention of reinfarction. Beta blockade over the long term is also effective for reducing the rate of mortality in patients who have undergone revascularization.[247]

Given the well-documented benefits of beta-adrenoceptor blockade, it is disturbing that this form of therapy continues to be underutilized, especially in high-risk groups such as the elderly.[7] Patients with a relative contraindication to beta blockade (moderate heart failure, bradyarrhythmias) should undergo a monitored trial of therapy in the hospital. The dosage should be sufficient to blunt the heart rate response to stress or exercise. Much of the impact of beta blockers in preventing mortality occurs in the first weeks; treatment should commence as soon as possible. Evidence exists that programs providing physician feedback improve adherence to guidelines such as those noted earlier for prescription of beta-adrenoceptor blockers after acute myocardial infarction.[1]

Some controversy exists as to how long patients should be treated. The collective data from five trials providing information on long-term follow-up of beta-adrenoceptor blockers after infarction suggest that therapy should be continued for at least 2 to 3 years (see Fig. 47-19). At that time, if the beta blocker is well tolerated and if there is no reason to discontinue therapy, such therapy probably should be continued in most patients.

Not all patients derive the same benefit from beta blocker therapy. The cost-effectiveness of treatment in medium- or high-risk persons compares very favorably with that of many other accepted interventions, such as coronary bypass surgery, angioplasty, and lipid-lowering therapy. In patients with an extremely good prognosis (first acute myocardial infarction, good ventricular function, no angina, negative stress test result, and no complex ventricular ectopy) among whom a mortality rate of

TABLE 47-14 Aspirin vs. Warfarin Therapy after ST-Elevation Myocardial Infarction (STEMI)

Study	Study Design	Drugs Used	ASA	Second Arm	Third Arm
STEMI-Specific Trials					
WARIS II*	Randomized Open label N = 3630 FU = Mean 4 yr	ASA monotherapy vs. warfarin monotherapy vs. warfarin + ASA	160 mg daily	Dosed to target INR 2.8-4.2	Dosed to target INR 2.0-2.5 + ASA 75 mg daily
APRICOT II†	Randomized Open label N = 308 FU = 3 mo	ASA monotherapy vs. warfarin + ASA	If TIMI grade 3 post 48 hr UFH then 160 mg initially and then 80 mg daily	Dosed to target INR 2-3 if TIMI 3 post 48 hr UFH + 160 mg initially and then 80 mg daily	N/A
Trials not Specific to STEMI					
ASPECT II‡	Randomized Open label N = 999 FU = 26 mo	ASA monotherapy vs. warfarin monotherapy vs.warfarin + ASA	80 mg daily	Dosed to target INR 3-4	Dosed to target INR 2-2.5 + ASA 80 mg daily
CHAMP§	Randomized Open label N = 5059 FU = median 2.7 yr	ASA monotherapy vs. warfarin +ASA	162 mg daily	Dosed to target INR 1.5-2.5 + 81 mg ASA daily	N/A
CARS¶	Randomized Blinded N = 8803 FU = 33 mo Median = 14 mo	ASA monotherapy vs. warfarin 1 mg + ASA	160 mg daily (avg INR @ wk 4 = 1.02	1 mg + 80 mg ASA (avg INR @ wk 4 = 1.05)	N/A

N/A = not applicable; ASA = acetylsalicylic acid (aspirin); FU = follow-up; INR = international normalized ratio; MI = myocardial infarction; STEMI = ST-elevation myocardial infarction; Tx = treatment; UA = unstable angina; UFH = unfractionated heparin.

*Hurlen M, et al: N Engl J Med 347:969, 2002.

†Brouwer MA, et al: Circulation 106:659, 2002.

‡Van Es RF, et al: Lancet 360:109, 2002.

approximately 1 percent per year can be anticipated, beta blockers would have a smaller impact on survival. However, it is our preference to prescribe beta blockers to such patients for whatever postinfarction benefit is achieved and also to have them as part of the patient's usual regimen should acute myocardial infarction recur at an unpredictable time in the future.

NITRATES. Although these agents are suitable for management of specific conditions after STEMI, such as recurrent angina or as part of a treatment regimen for congestive heart failure, little evidence indicates that they reduce mortality over the long term when prescribed on a routine basis to all patients with infarction.[7]

ANTICOAGULANTS. At least three theoretical reasons exist for anticipating that anticoagulants might be beneficial in the long-term management of patients after STEMI. (1) Because the coronary occlusion responsible for the STEMI is often due to a thrombus, anticoagulants might be expected to halt progression, slow progression, or prevent the development of new thrombi elsewhere in the coronary arterial tree. (2) Anticoagulants might be expected to diminish the formation of mural thrombi and resultant systemic embolization. (3) Anticoagulants might be expected to reduce the incidence of venous thrombosis and pulmonary embolization.

After several decades of evaluation, the weight of evidence now suggests that anticoagulants have a favorable effect on late mortality, stroke, and reinfarction among patients hospitalized with STEMI (Table 47-14). Given the complexities of combining long-term therapy with warfarin alone with antiplatelet therapy, clinicians must weigh the need for warfarin based on established indications for anticoagulation and the risk of bleeding. An algorithm to guide decision-making is given in Figure 47-38.

CALCIUM ANTAGONISTS. At present, we do not recommend the routine use of calcium antagonists for secondary prevention of infarction. A possible exception is a patient who cannot tolerate a beta-adrenoceptor blocker because of adverse effects on bronchospastic lung disease but who has well-preserved left ventricular function; such patients may be candidates for a rate-slowing calcium antagonist such as diltiazem or verapamil.

HORMONE THERAPY. The decision to prescribe hormone therapy is often a complex one that involves the desire to suppress postmenopausal symptoms versus the risks of breast and endometrial cancer and vascular events. Despite improvement in lipid profiles, hormone therapy with estrogen plus progestin to postmenopausal women with established coronary heart disease does not prevent recurrent coronary events and is associated with significantly increased risk of coronary heart disease and venous thromboembolic events.[7] At present, we recommend not starting hormone therapy with estrogen plus progestin after STEMI and discontinuing it in postmenopausal women after STEMI.

ANTIOXIDANTS. Dietary supplementation with omega-3 polyunsaturated fatty acids has been associated with a reduction in congestive heart disease death and nonfatal reinfarction in patients within 3 months of a myocardial infarction.[248] Vitamin E (300 mg/day) was not associated with any significant clinical benefit, however.[248]

		Results		
Patients	**Endpoints**	***ASA Alone***	***Warfarin Alone***	***ASA + Warfarin***
Age < 75 yr Hospitalized for acute MI **% STEMI = 71.8**	Death, nonfatal reinfarction, or thromboembolic stroke Major, nonfatal bleeding ($p < 0.001$)	20% 0.17%	16.7% ($p = 0.03$ vs. ASA) 0.68%	15% ($p = 0.001$ vs. ASA) 0.57%
Age ≤ 76 yr Acute ST MI ≤ 6 hr prior to thrombolytic Tx **% STEMI = 100**	Reooclusion (TIMI ≤ 2) ($p < 0.02$) Total occlusion (TIMI 0-1) ($p < 0.02$) Revascularization ($p < 0.01$) Reinfarction ($p < 0.05$) Event-free survival rate* ($p < 0.01$) Bleeding (TIMI major and minor ($p = $ NS)	28% 20% 31% 8% 66% 3%	N/A	15% 9% 13% 2% 86% 5%
Acute MI or UA within preceding 8 wk	Death, MI, or stroke ($p = 0.0479$) Major bleeding Minor bleeding ($p < 0.0001$) Almost 20% of the warfarin and combined group discontinued therapy; 40% in therapeutic range	9% 1% 5%	5% 1% 8%	5% 2% 15%
Acute MI within preceding 14 days prior to enrollment	Death ($p = 0.76$) Recurrent MI ($p = 0.78$) Stroke ($p = 0.52$) Major bleeding ($p = 0.001$)	17.3% 13.1% 3.5% 0.72**	N/A	17.6% 13.3% 3.1% 1.2**
Age 21-85 yr (82% < 70 yr) MI 3-21 days (mean 9.6 days) prior to enrollment	Ischemic stroke ($p = 0.0534$)	0.6%	N/A	1.1%

§Fiore LD, et al: Circulation 105:557, 2002.
¶O'Connor CM, et al: Am J Cardiol 88:541, 2001.
**Reported as number of events per 100 person-years of follow-up.
Adapted from Antman EM, et al: ACC/AHA Guidelines for the Management of Patients with ST-Elevation Myocardial Infarction. 2004 (http://www.acc.org/clinical/guidelines/stemi/index.htm).

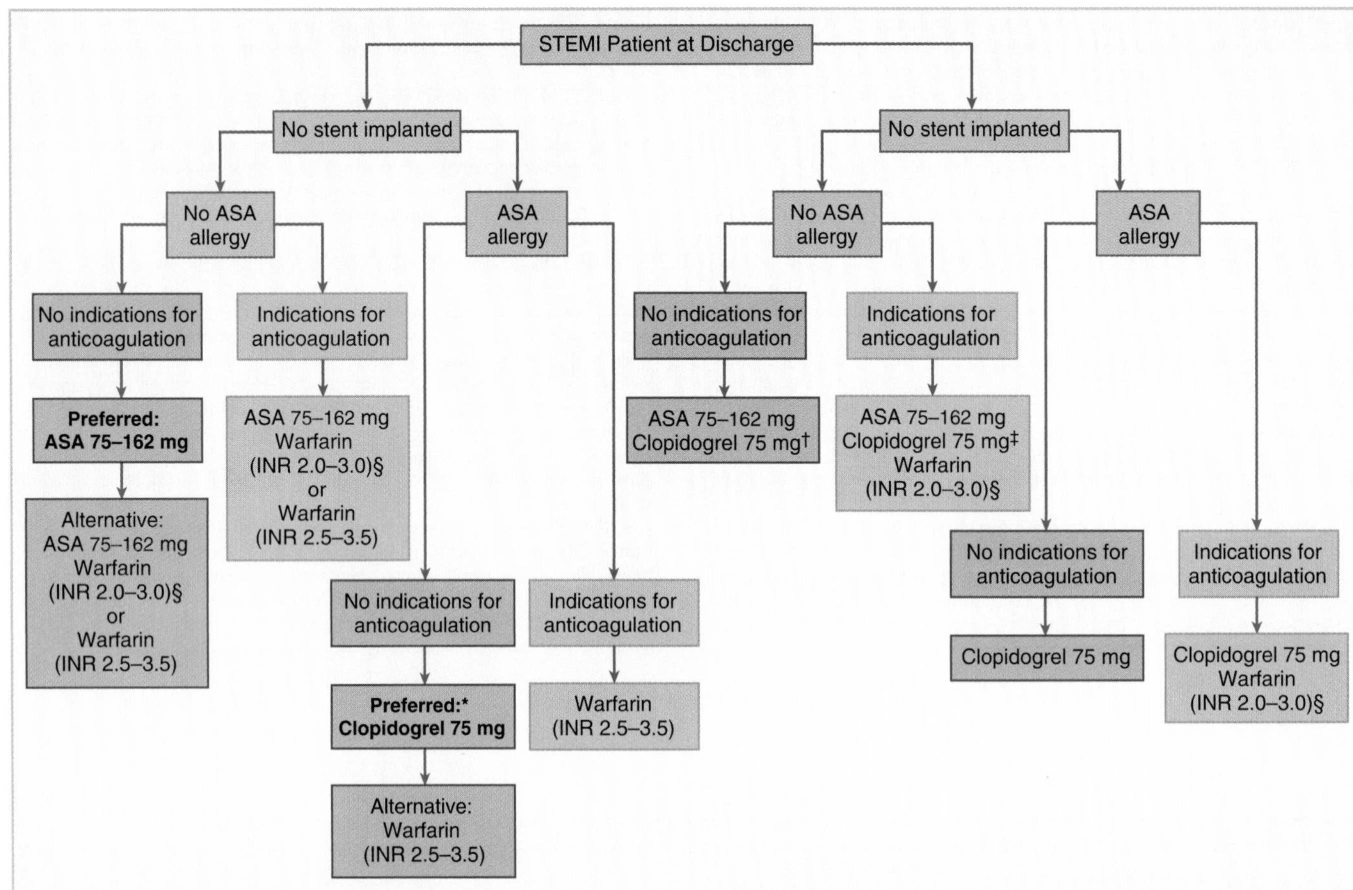

FIGURE 47–38 Algorithm for antithrombotic therapy at hospital discharge after ST segment elevation myocardial ischemia (STEMI). *Clopidogrel is preferred over warfarin due to increased risk of bleeding and low patient compliance in warfarin trials. †For 12 months. ‡Discontinue clopidogrel 1 month after implantation of a bare metal stent or several months after implantation of a drug-eluting stent (3 months after sirolimus and 6 months after paclitaxel) because of the potential increased risk of bleeding with warfarin and two antiplatelet agents. Continue ASA and warfarin long term if warfarin is indicated for other reasons such as atrial fibrillation, LV thrombus, cerebral emboli, or extensive regional wall motion abnormality. §An INR of 2.0–3.0 is acceptable with tight control, but the lower end of this range is preferable. The combination of antiplatelet therapy and warfarin may be considered in patients aged less than 75 years, with low bleeding risk, who can be monitored reliably. ASA = acetylsalicyclic acid; INR = international normalized ratio; LV = left ventricular. (From Antman EM, et al: ACC/AHA Guidelines for the Management of Patients with ST-Elevation Myocardial Infarction. 2004 [http://www.acc.org/clinical/guidelines/stemi/index.htm].)

REFERENCES

1. Mehta RH, Montoye CK, Gallogly M, et al: Improving quality of care for acute myocardial infarction: The Guidelines Applied in Practice (GAP) Initiative. JAMA 287:1269, 2002.
2. Jencks SF, Huff ED, Cuerdon T: Change in the quality of care delivered to Medicare beneficiaries, 1998-1999 to 2000-2001. JAMA 289:305, 2003.
3. National Committee for Quality Assurance: The State of Health Care Quality. Washington, DC, NCQA, 2003.
4. Schneider EC, Zaslavsky AM, Epstein AM: Racial disparities in the quality of care for enrollees in medicare managed care. JAMA 287:1288, 2002.
5. Faxon D, Lenfant C: Timing is everything: Motivating patients to call 9-1-1 at onset of acute myocardial infarction. Circulation 104:1210, 2001.

Prehospital Care

6. Luepker RV, Raczynski JM, Osganian S, et al: Effect of a community intervention on patient delay and emergency medical service use in acute coronary heart disease: The Rapid Early Action for Coronary Treatment (REACT) Trial. JAMA 284:60, 2000.
7. Antman EM, et al: ACC/AHA Guidelines for the Management of Patients with ST-Elevation Myocardial Infarction. 2004 (http://www.acc.org/clinical/guidelines/stemi/index.htm).
8. Ornato JP, Hand MM: Warning signs of a heart attack. Circulation 104:1212, 2001.
9. Canto JG, Zalenski RJ, Ornato JP, et al: Use of emergency medical services in acute myocardial infarction and subsequent quality of care: Observations from the National Registry of Myocardial Infarction 2. Circulation 106:3018, 2002.
10. National Heart Lung and Blood Institute: Act in time to heart attack signs. Accessed 10/6/03. (www.nhlbi.nih.gov/actintime)
11. American Heart Association. Accessed 10/6/03. (www.americanheart.org.)
12. Caffrey SL, Willoughby PJ, Pepe PE, et al: Public use of automated external defibrillators. N Engl J Med 347:1242, 2002.
13. Gibson CM: Time is myocardium and time is outcomes. Circulation 104:2632, 2001.
14. Morrow DA, Antman EM, Giugliano RP, et al: A simple risk index for rapid initial triage of patients with ST-elevation myocardial infarction: An InTIME II substudy. Lancet 358:1571, 2001.
15. Morrison LJ, Verbeek PR, McDonald AC, et al: Mortality and prehospital thrombolysis for acute myocardial infarction: A meta-analysis. JAMA 283:2686, 2000.
16. Bonnefoy E, Lapostolle F, Leizorovicz A, et al: Primary angioplasty versus prehospital fibrinolysis in acute myocardial infarction: A randomised study. Lancet 360:825, 2002.
17. Steg G, Bonnefoy E, Chabaud S, et al: Impact of time to treatment on mortality after prehospital fibrinolysis or primary angioplasty: Data from the CAPTIM randomized clinical trial. Circulation 108:2851, 2003.
18. Hanamia G, Sauval P, LaBlanche JM, et al: Impact of prehospital thrombolysis on 1-month outcome after ST-elevation myocardial infarction: Data from the nationwide French USIC 2000 survey. Abstract 2703. Vienna, European Society of Cardiology, 2003.
19. Fibrinolytic Therapy Trialists (FTT) Collaborative Group: Indications for fibrinolytic therapy in suspected acute myocardial infarction: Collaborative overview of early mortality and major morbidity results from all randomised trials of more than 1000 patients. Lancet 343:311, 1994.
20. Pedley DK, Bissett K, Connolly EM, et al: Prospective observational cohort study of time saved by prehospital thrombolysis for ST elevation myocardial infarction delivered by paramedics. BMJ 327:22, 2003.

Care in the Emergency Department

21. Hamm CW, Bertrand M, Braunwald E: Acute coronary syndrome without ST elevation: Implementation of new guidelines. Lancet 358:1533, 2001.
22. Van de Werf F, Ardissino D, Betriu A, et al: Management of acute myocardial infarction in patients presenting with ST-segment elevation. The Task Force on the Management of Acute Myocardial Infarction of the European Society of Cardiology. Eur Heart J 24:28, 2003.
23. Califf RM, Faxon DP: Need for centers to care for patients with acute coronary syndromes. Circulation 107:1467, 2003.
24. Willerson JT: Editor's commentary: Centers of excellence. Circulation 107:1471, 2003.
25. Braunwald E, Antman EM, Beasley JW, et al: ACC/AHA 2002 guideline update for the management of patients with unstable angina and non-ST-segment elevation myocardial infarction—Summary article: A report of the American College of Cardiology/

American Heart Association task force on practice guidelines (Committee on the Management of Patients With Unstable Angina). J Am Coll Cardiol 40:1366, 2002.
26. Pfisterer M: Right ventricular involvement in myocardial infarction and cardiogenic shock. Lancet 362:392, 2003.
27. Holmes DR Jr: Cardiogenic shock: A lethal complication of acute myocardial infarction. Rev Cardiovasc Med 4:131, 2003.
28. Schomig A, Ndrepepa G, Mehilli J, et al: Therapy-dependent influence of time-to-treatment interval on myocardial salvage in patients with acute myocardial infarction treated with coronary artery stenting or thrombolysis. Circulation 108:1084, 2003.
29. Sadanandan S, Buller CE, Menon V, et al: The late open artery hypothesis—A decade later. Am Heart J 142:411, 2001.
30. Gibson CM: Has my patient achieved adequate myocardial reperfusion? Circulation 108:504, 2003.
31. Granger CB, Mahaffey KW, Weaver WD, et al: Pexelizumab, an anti-C5 complement antibody, as adjunctive therapy to primary percutaneous coronary intervention in acute myocardial infarction: The COMplement inhibition in Myocardial infarction treated with Angioplasty (COMMA) trial. Circulation 108:1184, 2003.
32. Kopecky SL, Aviles RJ, Bell MR, et al: A randomized, double-blinded, placebo-controlled, dose-ranging study measuring the effect of an adenosine agonist on infarct size reduction in patients undergoing primary percutaneous transluminal coronary angioplasty: The ADMIRE (AmP579 Delivery for Myocardial Infarction REduction) study. Am Heart J 146:146, 2003.
33. Przyklenk K, Bauer B, Ovize M, et al: Regional ischemic 'preconditioning' protects remote virgin myocardium from subsequent sustained coronary occlusion. Circulation 87:893, 1993.
34. Katritsis D, Karvouni E, Webb-Peploe MM: Reperfusion in acute myocardial infarction: Current concepts. Prog Cardiovasc Dis 45:481, 2003.
35. De Luca G, Suryapranata H, Zijlstra F, et al: Symptom-onset-to-balloon time and mortality in patients with acute myocardial infarction treated by primary angioplasty. J Am Coll Cardiol 42:991, 2003.
36. De Luca G, Suryapranata H, Ottervanger JP, et al: Time-delay to treatment and mortality in primary angioplasty for acute myocardial infarction: every minute counts. Circulation 109:1223, 2004.
37. Fujita M, Nakae I, Kihara Y, et al: Determinants of collateral development in patients with acute myocardial infarction. Clin Cardiol 22:595, 1999.
38. Bolli R, Marban E: Molecular and cellular mechanisms of myocardial stunning. Physiol Rev 79:609, 1999.
39. Gerber BL, Wijns W, Vanoverschelde JL, et al: Myocardial perfusion and oxygen consumption in reperfused noninfarcted dysfunctional myocardium after unstable angina: Direct evidence for myocardial stunning in humans. J Am Coll Cardiol 34:1939, 1999.
40. Davies CH, Ormerod OJ: Failed coronary thrombolysis. Lancet 351:1191, 1998.
41. Vargas SO, Sampson BA, Schoen FJ: Pathologic detection of early myocardial infarction: A critical review of the evolution and usefulness of modern techniques. Mod Pathol 12:635, 1999.
42. de Lemos JA, Gibson CM, Antman EM, et al: Abciximab and early adjunctive percutaneous coronary intervention are associated with improved ST-segment resolution after thrombolysis: Observations from the TIMI 14 Trial. Am Heart J 141:592, 2001.
43. Antman EM, Cooper HA, Gibson CM, et al: Determinants of improvement in epicardial flow and myocardial perfusion for ST elevation myocardial infarction: Insights from TIMI 14 and InTIME-II. Eur Heart J 23:928, 2002.
44. Baran KW, Nguyen M, McKendall GR, et al: Double-blind, randomized trial of an anti-CD18 antibody in conjunction with recombinant tissue plasminogen activator for acute myocardial infarction: Limitation of myocardial infarction following thrombolysis in acute myocardial infarction (LIMIT AMI) study. Circulation 104:2778, 2001.
45. Faxon DP, Gibbons RJ, Chronos NA, et al: The effect of blockade of the CD11/CD18 integrin receptor on infarct size in patients with acute myocardial infarction treated with direct angioplasty: The results of the HALT-MI study. J Am Coll Cardiol 40:1199, 2002.
46. Wang K, Zhou X, Zhou Z, et al: Recombinant soluble P-selectin glycoprotein ligand-Ig (rPSGL-Ig) attenuates infarct size and myeloperoxidase activity in a canine model of ischemia-reperfusion. Thromb Haemost 88:149, 2002.
47. Mahaffey KW, Granger CB, Nicolau JC, et al: Effect of pexelizumab, an anti-C5 complement antibody, as adjunctive therapy to fibrinolysis in acute myocardial infarction: The COMPlement inhibition in myocardial infarction treated with thromboLYtics (COMPLY) trial. Circulation 108:1176, 2003.
48. Magnesium in Coronaries (MAGIC) Trial Investigators: Early administration of intravenous magnesium to high-risk patients with acute myocardial infarction in the Magnesium in Coronaries (MAGIC) Trial: A randomised controlled trial. Lancet 360:1189, 2002.
49. van der Horst IC, Zijlstra F, van't Hof AW, et al: Glucose-insulin-potassium infusion inpatients treated with primary angioplasty for acute myocardial infarction: The glucose-insulin-potassium study: A randomized trial. J Am Coll Cardiol 42:784, 2003.
50. Gheorghiade M, Goldstein S: Beta-blockers in the post-myocardial infarction patient. Circulation 106:394, 2002.
51. Chiladakis JA, Patsouras N, Manolis AS: The Bezold-Jarisch reflex in acute inferior myocardial infarction: Clinical and sympathovagal spectral correlates. Clin Cardiol 26:323, 2003.
52. Hochman JS, Califf RM: Acute myocardial infarction. *In* Antman E (ed): Cardiovascular Therapeutics: A Companion to Braunwald's Heart Disease. 2nd ed. Philadelphia, WB Saunders, 2002, pp 233-291.
53. Sadanandan S, Hochman JS: Early reperfusion, late reperfusion, and the open artery hypothesis: An overview. Prog Cardiovasc Dis 42:397, 2000.
54. Kloner RA, Jennings RB: Consequences of brief ischemia: Stunning, preconditioning, and their clinical implications: Part 2. Circulation 104:3158, 2001.
55. Yousef ZR, Redwood SR, Bucknall CA, et al: Late intervention after anterior myocardial infarction: Effects on left ventricular size, function, quality of life, and exercise tolerance: Results of the Open Artery Trial (TOAT Study). J Am Coll Cardiol 40:869, 2002.
56. Van De Werf F, Baim DS: Reperfusion for ST-segment elevation myocardial infarction: An overview of current treatment options. Circulation 105:2813, 2002.
57. Nakatani D, Sato H, Kinjo K, et al: Effect of successful late reperfusion by primary coronary angioplasty on mechanical complications of acute myocardial infarction. Am J Cardiol 92:785, 2003.

Coronary Fibrinolysis

58. Boersma E, Mercado N, Poldermans D, et al: Acute myocardial infarction. Lancet 361:847, 2003.
59. Franzosi MG, Santoro E, De Vita C, et al: Ten-year follow-up of the first megatrial testing thrombolytic therapy in patients with acute myocardial infarction: Results of the Gruppo Italiano per lo Studio della Sopravvivenza nell'Infarto-1 study. The GISSI Investigators. Circulation 98:2659, 1998.
60. TIMI Study Group: The Thrombolysis in Myocardial Infarction (TIMI) Trial; Phase I findings. N Engl J Med 312:932, 1985.
61. Chesebro JH, Knatterud G, Roberts R, et al: Thrombolysis in Myocardial Infarction (TIMI) Trial, Phase 1: A comparison between intravenous tissue plasminogen activator and intravenous streptokinase. Circulation 76:142, 1987.
62. Antman EM, Giugliano RP, Gibson CM, et al: Abciximab facilitates the rate and extent of thrombolysis: Results of the thrombolysis in myocardial infarction (TIMI) 14 trial. The TIMI 14 Investigators. Circulation 99:2720, 1999.
63. Gibson CM, Murphy SA, Rizzo JM, et al: Relationship between TIMI frame count and clinical outcomes after thrombolytic administration. Thrombolysis In Myocardial Infarction (TIMI) Study Group. Circulation 99:1945, 1999.
64. Gibson CM, Murphy S, Menown IB, et al: Determinants of coronary blood flow after thrombolytic administration. TIMI Study Group. Thrombolysis in Myocardial Infarction. J Am Coll Cardiol 34:1403, 1999.
65. Schroder R: ST segment resolution on 12-lead ECG. Circulation 2004, in press.
66. Krucoff MW, Johanson P, Crater SW, et al: The clinical utility of serial and continuous ST-segment recovery in patients with acute ST elevation myocardial infarction: Assessing the dynamics of epicardial and myocardial reperfusion. Circulation 2004, in press.
67. Armstrong PW, Collen D, Antman E: Fibrinolysis for acute myocardial infarction: The future is here and now. Circulation 107:2533, 2003.
68. Angeja BG, Gunda M, Murphy SA, et al: TIMI myocardial perfusion grade and ST segment resolution: Association with infarct size as assessed by single photon emission computed tomography imaging. Circulation 105:282, 2002.
69. Boersma E, Maas AC, Deckers JW, et al: Early thrombolytic treatment in acute myocardial infarction: Reappraisal of the golden hour. Lancet 348:771, 1996.
70. Thiemann DR, Coresh J, Schulman SP, et al: Lack of benefit for intravenous thrombolysis in patients with myocardial infarction who are older than 75 years. Circulation 101:2239, 2000.
71. Berger AK, Radford MJ, Wang Y, et al: Thrombolytic therapy in older patients. J Am Coll Cardiol 36:366, 2000.
72. Stenestrand U, Wallentin L: Fibrinolytic therapy in patients 75 years and older with ST-segment-elevation myocardial infarction: One-year follow-up of a large prospective cohort. Arch Intern Med 163:965, 2003.
73. White HD: Thrombolytic therapy in the elderly. Lancet 356:2028, 2000.
74. Morrow DA, Antman EM, Charlesworth A, et al: TIMI risk score for ST-elevation myocardial infarction: A convenient, bedside, clinical score for risk assessment at presentation: An intravenous nPA for treatment of infarcting myocardium early II trial substudy. Circulation 102:2031, 2000.
75. Morrow DA, Antman EM, Parsons L, et al: Application of the TIMI risk score for ST-elevation MI in the National Registry of Myocardial Infarction 3. JAMA 286:1356, 2001.
76. Brouwer MA, van den Bergh PJ, Aengevaeren WR, et al: Aspirin plus coumarin versus aspirin alone in the prevention of reocclusion after fibrinolysis for acute myocardial infarction: Results of the Antithrombotics in the Prevention of Reocclusion In Coronary Thrombolysis (APRICOT)-2 Trial. Circulation 106:659, 2002.
77. Aversano T, Aversano LT, Passamani E, et al: Thrombolytic therapy vs primary percutaneous coronary intervention for myocardial infarction in patients presenting to hospitals without on-site cardiac surgery: A randomized controlled trial. JAMA 287:1943, 2002.
78. Llevadot J, Giugliano RP, Antman EM: Bolus fibrinolytic therapy in acute myocardial infarction. JAMA 286:442, 2001.
79. The Global Use of Strategies to Open Occluded Coronary Arteries (GUSTO III) Investigators: A comparison of reteplase with alteplase for acute myocardial infarction. N Engl J Med 337:1118, 1997.
80. Ware JH, Antman EM: Equivalence trials. N Engl J Med 337:1159, 1997.
81. White HD: Thrombolytic therapy and equivalence trials. J Am Coll Cardiol 31:494, 1998.
82. Cannon CP, McCabe CH, Gibson CM, et al: TNK-tissue plasminogen activator in acute myocardial infarction. Results of the Thrombolysis in Myocardial Infarction (TIMI) 10A dose-ranging trial. Circulation 95:351, 1997.
83. Cannon CP, Gibson CM, McCabe CH, et al: TNK-tissue plasminogen activator compared with front-loaded alteplase in acute myocardial infarction: Results of the TIMI 10B trial. Thrombolysis in Myocardial Infarction (TIMI) 10B Investigators. Circulation 98:2805, 1998.
84. Van de Werf F, Cannon CP, Luyten A, et al: Safety assessment of single-bolus administration of TNK tissue-plasminogen activator in acute myocardial infarction: The ASSENT-1 trial. The ASSENT-1 Investigators. Am Heart J 137:786, 1999.
85. Assessment of the Safety and Efficacy of a New Thrombolytic (ASSENT-2) Investigators: Single-bolus tenecteplase compared with front-loaded alteplase in acute myocardial infarction: The ASSENT-2 double-blind randomised trial. Assessment of the Safety and Efficacy of a New Thrombolytic Investigators. Lancet 354:716, 1999.
86. The InTIME-II Investigators: Intravenous NPA for the treatment of infarcting myocardium early; InTIME-II, a double-blind comparison of single-bolus lanoteplase

vs accelerated alteplase for the treatment of patients with acute myocardial infarction. Eur Heart J 21:2005, 2000.

87. Armstrong PW, Burton J, Pakola S, et al: Collaborative Angiographic Patency Trial Of Recombinant Staphylokinase (CAPTORS II). Am Heart J 146:484, 2003.
88. The GUSTO Angiographic Investigators: The comparative effects of tissue plasminogen activator, streptokinase, or both on coronary artery patency, ventricular function and survival after acute myocardial infarction. N Engl J Med 329:1615, 1993.
89. Dubois CL, Belmans A, Granger CB, et al: Outcome of urgent and elective percutaneous coronary interventions after pharmacologic reperfusion with tenecteplase combined with unfractionated heparin, enoxaparin, or abciximab. J Am Coll Cardiol 42:1178, 2003.
90. Gore JM, Granger CB, Simoons ML, et al: Stroke after thrombolysis: Mortality and functional outcomes in the GUSTO-I Trial. Circulation 92:2811, 1995.
91. Kleiman NS, Terrin M, Mueller H, et al: Mechanisms of early death despite thrombolytic therapy: Experience from the Thrombolysis in Myocardial Infarction Investigation Phase II (TIMI II) Study. J Am Coll Cardiol 19:1129, 1992.
92. Eagle KA, Goodman SG, Avezum A, et al: Practice variation and missed opportunities for reperfusion in ST-segment-elevation myocardial infarction: Findings from the Global Registry of Acute Coronary Events (GRACE). Lancet 359:373, 2002.
93. Assessment of the Safety and Efficacy of a New Thrombolytic Regimen (ASSENT)-3 Investigators: Efficacy and safety of tenecteplase in combination with enoxaparin, abciximab, or unfractionated heparin: The ASSENT-3 randomised trial in acute myocardial infarction. Lancet 358:605, 2001.
94. Van de Werf F, Barron HV, Armstrong PW, et al: Incidence and predictors of bleeding events after fibrinolytic therapy with fibrin-specific agents: A comparison of TNK-tPA and rt-PA. Eur Heart J 22:2253, 2001.
95. Giugliano RP, Antman EM: Caeteris paribus—All things being equal. Eur Heart J 22:2221, 2001.
96. Lee DC, Oz MC, Weinberg AD, et al: Optimal timing of revascularization: Transmural versus nontransmural acute myocardial infarction. Ann Thorac Surg 71:1197, discussion 1202, 2001.
97. Hasdai D, Behar S, Wallentin L, et al: A prospective survey of the characteristics, treatments and outcomes of patients with acute coronary syndromes in Europe and the Mediterranean basin: The Euro Heart Survey of Acute Coronary Syndromes (Euro Heart Survey ACS). Eur Heart J 23:1190, 2002.
98. Weaver WD: All hospitals are not equal for treatment of patients with acute myocardial infarction. Circulation 108:1768, 2003.
99. Keeley EC, Boura JA, Grines CL: Primary angioplasty versus intravenous thrombolytic therapy for acute myocardial infarction: A quantitative review of 23 randomised trials. Lancet 361:13, 2003.
100. Hochman JS, Sleeper LA, White HD, et al: One-year survival following early revascularization for cardiogenic shock. JAMA 285:190, 2001.
101. Wu AH, Parsons L, Every NR, et al: Hospital outcomes in patients presenting with congestive heart failure complicating acute myocardial infarction: A report from the Second National Registry of Myocardial Infarction (NRMI-2). J Am Coll Cardiol 40:1389, 2002.
102. Kent DM, Schmid CH, Lau J, et al: Is primary angioplasty for some as good as primary angioplasty for all? J Gen Intern Med 17:887, 2002.
103. Grzybowski M, Clements EA, Parsons L, et al: Mortality benefit of immediate revascularization of acute ST-segment elevation myocardial infarction in patients with contraindications to thrombolytic therapy: A propensity analysis. JAMA 290:1891, 2003.
104. Herrmann HC: Optimizing outcomes in ST-segment elevation myocardial infarction. J Am Coll Cardiol 42:1357, 2003.
105. Widimsky P, Budesinsky T, Vorac D, et al: Long distance transport for primary angioplasty vs immediate thrombolysis in acute myocardial infarction: Final results of the randomized national multicentre trial—PRAGUE-2. Eur Heart J 24:94, 2003.
106. Andersen HR, Nielsen TT, Rasmussen K, et al: A comparison of coronary angioplasty with fibrinolytic therapy in acute myocardial infarction. N Engl J Med 349:733, 2003.
107. Dalby M, Lechat P, Montalescot G: Transfer for primary angioplasty versus immediate thrombolysis in acute myocardial infarction. Circulation 108:1809, 2003.
108. Nallamothu BK, Bates ER: Percutaneous coronary intervention versus fibrinolytic therapy in acute myocardial infarction: Is timing (almost) everything? Am J Cardiol 92:824, 2003.

Antithrombin and Antiplatelet Therapy

109. ISIS-2 (Second International Study of Infarct Survival) Collaborative Group: Randomised trial of intravenous streptokinase, oral aspirin, both, or neither among 17,187 cases of suspected acute myocardial infarction: ISIS-2. Lancet 2:349, 1988.
110. Baigent C, Collins R: Aspirin and heparin. *In* Hennekens CH (ed): Clinical Trials in Cardiovascular Disease: Companion to Braunwald's Health Disease. Philadelphia, WB Saunders, 1999, p 60.
111. The Global Use of Strategies to Open Occluded Coronary Arteries (GUSTO) IIb Investigators: A comparison of recombinant hirudin with heparin for the treatment of acute coronary syndromes. N Engl J Med 335:775, 1996.
112. Menon V, Berkowitz SD, Antman EM, et al: New heparin dosing recommendations for patients with acute coronary syndromes. Am J Med 110:641, 2001.
113. Hirsh J, Anand SS, Halperin JL, et al: Guide to anticoagulant therapy: Heparin: A statement for healthcare professionals from the American Heart Association. Circulation 103:2994, 2001.
114. Antman EM: The search for replacements for unfractionated heparin. Circulation 103:2310, 2001.
115. Direct Thrombin Inhibitor Trialists' Collaborative Group: Direct thrombin inhibitors in acute coronary syndromes: Principal results of a meta-analysis based on individual patients' data. Lancet 359:294, 2002.
116. White H: Thrombin-specific anticoagulation with bivalirudin versus heparin in patients receiving fibrinolytic therapy for acute myocardial infarction: The HERO-2 randomised trial. Lancet 358:1855, 2001.
117. Ross AM, Molhoek P, Lundergan C, et al: Randomized comparison of enoxaparin, a low-molecular-weight heparin, with unfractionated heparin adjunctive to recombinant tissue plasminogen activator thrombolysis and aspirin: Second trial of Heparin and Aspirin Reperfusion Therapy (HART II). Circulation 104:648, 2001.
118. Simoons M, Krzeminska-Pakula M, Alonso A, et al: Improved reperfusion and clinical outcome with enoxaparin as an adjunct to streptokinase thrombolysis in acute myocardial infarction. The AMI-SK study. Eur Heart J 23:1282, 2002.
119. Antman EM, Louwerenburg HW, Baars HF, et al: Enoxaparin as adjunctive antithrombin therapy for ST-elevation myocardial infarction: Results of the ENTIRE-Thrombolysis in Myocardial Infarction (TIMI) 23 Trial. Circulation 105:1642, 2002.
120. Wallentin L, Goldstein P, Armstrong PW, et al: Efficacy and safety of tenecteplase in combination with the low-molecular-weight heparin enoxaparin or unfractionated heparin in the prehospital setting: The Assessment of the Safety and Efficacy of a New Thrombolytic Regimen (ASSENT)-3 PLUS randomized trial in acute myocardial infarction. Circulation 108:135, 2003.
121. Naghavi M, Libby P, Falk E, et al: From vulnerable plaque to vulnerable patient: A call for new definitions and risk assessment strategies: Part I. Circulation 108:1664, 2003.
122. Serebruany VL, Malinin AI, Callahan KP, et al: Effect of tenecteplase versus alteplase on platelets during the first 3 hours of treatment for acute myocardial infarction: The Assessment of the Safety and Efficacy of a New Thrombolytic Agent (ASSENT-2) platelet substudy. Am Heart J 145:636, 2003.
123. Antithrombotic Trialists' Collaboration: Collaborative meta-analysis of randomised trials of antiplatelet therapy for prevention of death, myocardial infarction, and stroke in high risk patients. BMJ 324:71, 2002.
124. Gawaz M, Neumann FJ, Schomig A: Evaluation of platelet membrane glycoproteins in coronary artery disease: Consequences for diagnosis and therapy. Circulation 99:E1, 1999.
125. Moliterno DJ, Chan AW: Glycoprotein IIb/IIIa inhibition in early intent-to-stent treatment of acute coronary syndromes: EPISTENT, ADMIRAL, CADILLAC, and TARGET. J Am Coll Cardiol 41:49S, 2003.
126. Vivekananthan DP, Patel VB, Moliterno DJ: Glycoprotein IIb/IIIa antagonism and fibrinolytic therapy for acute myocardial infarction. J Interv Cardiol 15:131, 2002.
127. Eisenberg MJ, Jamal S: Glycoprotein IIb/IIIa inhibition in the setting of acute ST-segment elevation myocardial infarction. J Am Coll Cardiol 42:1, 2003.
128. Kleiman N, Ohman EM, Califf RM, et al: Profound inhibition of platelet aggregation with monoclonal antibody 7E3 Fab after thrombolytic therapy: Results of the Thrombolysis and Angioplasty in Myocardial Infarction (TAMI) 8 pilot study. J Am Coll Cardiol 22:381, 1993.
129. Ohman EM, Kleiman NS, Gacioch G, et al: Combined accelerated tissue-plasminogen activator and platelet glycoprotein IIb/IIIa integrin receptor blockade with Integrilin in acute myocardial infarction. Results of a randomized, placebo-controlled, dose-ranging trial. IMPACT-AMI Investigators. Circulation 95:846, 1997.
130. Ronner E, van Kesteren HA, Zijnen P, et al: Safety and efficacy of eptifibatide vs placebo in patients receiving thrombolytic therapy with streptokinase for acute myocardial infarction: A phase II dose escalation, randomized, double-blind study. Eur Heart J 21:1530, 2000.
131. The PARADIGM Investigators: Combining thrombolysis with the platelet glycoprotein IIb/IIIa inhibitor lamifiban: Results of the Platelet Aggregation Receptor Antagonist Dose Investigation and Reperfusion Gain in Myocardial Infarction (PARADIGM) trial. J Am Coll Cardiol 32:2003, 1998.
132. Strategies for Patency Enhancement in the Emergency Department (SPEED) Group: Trial of abciximab with and without low-dose reteplase for acute myocardial infarction. Circulation 101:2788, 2000.
133. Brener SJ, Zeymer U, Adgey AA, et al: Eptifibatide and low-dose tissue plasminogen activator in acute myocardial infarction: The integrilin and low-dose thrombolysis in acute myocardial infarction (INTRO AMI) trial. J Am Coll Cardiol 39:377, 2002.
134. Giugliano RP, Roe MT, Harrington RA, et al: Combination reperfusion therapy with eptifibatide and reduced-dose tenecteplase for ST-elevation myocardial infarction: Results of the integrilin and tenecteplase in acute myocardial infarction (INTEGRITI) Phase II Angiographic Trial. J Am Coll Cardiol 41:1251, 2003.
135. Ohman EM, Oliverio RM, Harrelson L: Results of the Fibrinolytics and Aggrastat in ST Elevation Resolution (FASTER, TIMI 24) randomized trial. 2004, in press.
136. de Lemos JA, Antman EM, Gibson CM, et al: Abciximab improves both epicardial flow and myocardial reperfusion in ST-elevation myocardial infarction: Observations from the TIMI 14 trial. Circulation 101:239, 2000.
137. Topol EJ: Reperfusion therapy for acute myocardial infarction with fibrinolytic therapy or combination reduced fibrinolytic therapy and platelet glycoprotein IIb/IIIa inhibition: The GUSTO V randomised trial. Lancet 357:1905, 2001.
138. Peters RJ, Mehta SR, Fox KA, et al: Effects of aspirin dose when used alone or in combination with clopidogrel in patients with acute coronary syndromes: Observations from the Clopidogrel in Unstable angina to prevent Recurrent Events (CURE) Study. Circulation 108:1682, 2003.
139. Reikvam A, Kvan E, Aursnes I: Use of cardiovascular drugs after acute myocardial infarction: A marked shift towards evidence-based drug therapy. Cardiovasc Drugs Ther 16:451, 2002.
140. Fonarow GC, Gawlinski A, Moughrabi S, et al: Improved treatment of coronary heart disease by implementation of a Cardiac Hospitalization Atherosclerosis Management Program (CHAMP). Am J Cardiol 87:819, 2001.
141. Pope JH, Selker HP: Diagnosis of acute cardiac ischemia. Emerg Med Clin North Am 21:27, 2003.
142. Bartholomew BA, Harjai KJ, Grines CL, et al: Variation in hospital length of stay in patients with acute myocardial infarction undergoing primary angioplasty and the need to change the diagnostic-related group system. Am J Cardiol 92:830, 2003.
143. Peterson ED, Shaw LJ, Califf RM: Risk stratification after myocardial infarction. Ann Intern Med 126:561, 1997.
144. Antman EM, Kuntz KM: The length of the hospital stay after myocardial infarction. N Engl J Med 342:808, 2000.

Pharmacological Therapy

145. Freemantle N, Cleland J, Young P, et al: Beta blockade after myocardial infarction: Systematic review and meta regression analysis. BMJ 318:1730, 1999.
146. ISIS-1 (First International Study of Infarct Survival) Collaborative Group: Mechanisms for the early mortality reduction produced by beta-blockade started early in acute myocardial infarction: ISIS-1. Lancet 1:921, 1988.
147. The TIMI Study Group: Comparison of invasive and conservative strategies after treatment with intravenous tissue plasminogen activator in acute myocardial infarction: Results of the Thrombolysis in Myocardial Infarction (TIMI) Phase II Trial. N Engl J Med 320:618, 1989.
148. Roberts R, Rogers WJ, Mueller HS, et al: Immediate versus deferred B-blockade following thrombolytic therapy in patients with acute myocardial infarction: Results of the Thrombolysis in Myocardial Infarction (TIMI) II-B Study. Circulation 83:422, 1991.
149. Dargie HJ: Effect of carvedilol on outcome after myocardial infarction in patients with left-ventricular dysfunction: The CAPRICORN randomised trial. Lancet 357:1385, 2001.
150. Pfeffer MA: Left ventricular remodeling after acute myocardial infarction. Ann Rev Med 46:455, 1995.
151. The Acute Infarction Ramipril Efficacy (AIRE) Study Investigators: Effect of ramipril on mortality and morbidity of survivors of acute myocardial infarction with clinical evidence of heart failure. Lancet 342:821, 1993.
152. Ambrosioni E, Borghi C, Magnani B, et al: Effects of the early administration of zofenopril on mortality and morbidity in patients with anterior myocardial infarction: Results of the Survival of Myocardial Infarction Long-Term Evaluation Trial. N Engl J Med 332:280, 1995.
153. Kobler L, Torp-Pedersen C, Carlsen JE, et al: A clinical trial of the angiotensin-converting-enzyme inhibitor trandolapril in patients with left ventricular dysfunction after myocardial infarction. N Engl J Med 333:1670, 1995.
154. ISIS-4 Collaborative Group: ISIS-4: A randomized factorial trial assessing early oral captopril, oral mononitrate, and intravenous magnesium sulphate in 58,050 patients with suspected acute myocardial infarction. Lancet 345:669, 1995.
155. Gruppo Italiano per lo Studio della Sopravvivenza nell'Infarto Miocardico: GISSI-3: Effects of lisinopril and transdermal glyceryl trinitrate singly and together on 6-week mortality and ventricular function after acute myocardial infarction. Lancet 343:1115, 1994.
156. Swedberg K, Held P, Kjekshus J, et al: Effects of early administration of enalapril on mortality in patients with acute myocardial infarction. Results of the Cooperative North Scandinavian Enalapril Survival Study II (CONSENSUS II). N Engl J Med 327:678, 1992.
157. ACE Inhibitor Myocardial Infarction Collaborative Group: Indications for ACE inhibitors in the early treatment of acute myocardial infarction: Systematic overview of individual data from 100,000 patients in randomized trials. Circulation 97:2202, 1998.
158. Pfeffer MA: ACE inhibitors in acute myocardial infarction: Patient selection and timing. Circulation 97:2192, 1998.
159. Rutherford JD, Pfeffer MA, Moye LA, et al: Effects of captopril on ischemic events after myocardial infarction. Results of the Survival and Ventricular Enlargement Trial. Circulation 90:1731, 1994.
160. Dickstein K, Kjekshus J: Effects of losartan and captopril on mortality and morbidity in high-risk patients after acute myocardial infarction: The OPTIMAAL randomised trial. Optimal Trial in Myocardial Infarction with Angiotensin II Antagonist Losartan. Lancet 360:752, 2002.
161. Pfeffer MA: Effects of valsartan relative to captopril in patients with myocardial infarction complicated by heart failure and/or left ventricular dysfunction. N Engl J Med 349:1843, 2003.
162. Pitt B, Remme W, Zannad F, et al: Eplerenone, a selective aldosterone blocker, in patients with left ventricular dysfunction after myocardial infarction. N Engl J Med 348:1309, 2003.
163. Lindsay HSJ, Zaman AG, Cowan JC: ACE inhibitors after myocardial infarction: Patient selection or treatment for all? Br Heart J 73:397, 1995.
164. Pfeffer MA, Greaves SC, Arnold JM, et al: Early versus delayed angiotensin-converting enzyme inhibition therapy in acute myocardial infarction: The healing and early afterload reducing therapy trial. Circulation 95:2643, 1997.
165. Pitt B: Aldosterone blockade in patients with systolic left ventricular dysfunction. Circulation 108:1790, 2003.
166. Ryan TJ, Antman EM, Brooks NH, et al: 1999 update: ACC/AHA Guidelines for the Management of Patients with Acute Myocardial Infarction: Executive Summary and Recommendations: A report of the American College of Cardiology/American Heart Association Task Force on Practice Guidelines (Committee on Management of Acute Myocardial Infarction). Circulation 100:1016, 1999.
167. Report of the Holland Interuniversity Nifedipine/Metoprolol Trial Research Group: Early treatment of unstable angina in the coronary care unit: A randomised, double-blind, placebo-controlled comparison of recurrent ischaemia and thrombolytic therapy in patients treated with nifedipine or metoprolol or both. Br Heart J 56:400, 1986.
168. The Danish Study Group on Verapamil in Myocardial Infarction: Verapamil in acute myocardial infarction. Eur Heart J 54:516, 1984.
169. Boden WE, van Gilst WH, Scheldewaert RG, et al: Diltiazem in acute myocardial infarction treated with thrombolytic agents: A randomised placebo-controlled trial. Incomplete Infarction Trial of European Research Collaborators Evaluating Prognosis post-Thrombolysis (INTERCEPT). Lancet 355:1751, 2000.
170. Fath-Ordoubadi F, Beatt KJ: Glucose-insulin-potassium therapy for treatment of acute myocardial infarction: An overview of randomized placebo-controlled trials. Circulation 96:1152, 1997.
171. Diaz R, Paolasso EA, Piegas LS, et al: Metabolic modulation of acute myocardial infarction. The ECLA (Estudios Cardiologicos Latinoamerica) Collaborative Group. Circulation 98:2227, 1998.
172. Apstein CS: The benefits of glucose-insulin-potassium for acute myocardial infarction (and some concerns). J Am Coll Cardiol 42:792, 2003.
173. Falati S, Liu Q, Gross P, et al: Accumulation of tissue factor into developing thrombi in vivo is dependent upon microparticle P-selectin glycoprotein ligand 1 and platelet P-selectin. J Exp Med 197:1585, 2003.
174. Ross A, Gibbons R, Kloner RA, et al: Acute Myocardial Infarction Study of Adenosine (AMISTAD II). J Am Coll Cardiol 39:883, 2002.
175. Beltrami AP, Urbanek K, Kajstura J, et al: Evidence that human cardiac myocytes divide after myocardial infarction. N Engl J Med 344:1750, 2001.
176. Quaini F, Urbanek K, Beltrami AP, et al: Chimerism of the transplanted heart. N Engl J Med 346:5, 2002.
177. Siminiak T, Kurpisz M: Myocardial replacement therapy. Circulation 108:1167, 2003.

Hemodynamic Disturbances

178. Veenstra DL, Saint S, Saha S, et al: Efficacy of antiseptic-impregnated central venous catheters in preventing catheter-related bloodstream infection: A meta-analysis. JAMA 281:261, 1999.
179. Wu WC, Rathore SS, Wang Y, et al: Blood transfusion in elderly patients with acute myocardial infarction. N Engl J Med 345:1230, 2001.
180. Lewis EF, Moye LA, Rouleau JL, et al: Predictors of late development of heart failure in stable survivors of myocardial infarction: The CARE study. J Am Coll Cardiol 42:1446, 2003.
181. Udelson JE, Patten RD, Konstam MA: New concepts in post-infarction ventricular remodeling. Rev Cardiovasc Med 4(Suppl 3):S3, 2003.
182. Eichhorn EJ, Gheorghiade M: Digoxin—New perspective on an old drug. N Engl J Med 347:1394, 2002.
183. Goldberg RJ, Samad NA, Yarzebski J, et al: Temporal trends in cardiogenic shock complicating acute myocardial infarction. N Engl J Med 340:1162, 1999.
184. Webb JG, Lowe AM, Sanborn TA, et al: Percutaneous shock intervention for cardiogenic shock in the SHOCK Trial. J Am Coll Cardiol 42:1380, 2003.
185. Sanborn TA, Sleeper LA, Webb JG, et al: Correlates of one-year survival in patients with cardiogenic shock complicating acute myocardial infarction: Angiographic findings from the SHOCK trial. J Am Coll Cardiol 42:1373, 2003.
186. Hochman JS: Cardiogenic shock complicating acute myocardial infarction: Expanding the paradigm. Circulation 107:2998, 2003.
187. Cotter G, Kaluski E, Milo O, et al: LINCS: L-NAME (a NO synthase inhibitor) in the treatment of refractory cardiogenic shock: A prospective randomized study. Eur Heart J 24:1287, 2003.
188. Hochman JS, Sleeper LA, Webb JG, et al: Early revascularization in acute myocardial infarction complicated by cardiogenic shock. SHOCK Investigators: Should we emergently revascularize occluded coronaries for cardiogenic shock? N Engl J Med 341:625, 1999.
189. Bertrand M, McFadden E: Cardiogenic shock: Is there light at the end of the tunnel? J Am Coll Cardiol 42:1387, 2003.
190. Lemos PA, Cummins P, Lee CH, et al: Usefulness of percutaneous left ventricular assistance to support high-risk percutaneous coronary interventions. Am J Cardiol 91:479, 2003.
191. Inoue K, Ito H, Kitakaze M, et al: Antecedent angina pectoris as a predictor of better functional and clinical outcomes in patients with an inferior wall acute myocardial infarction. Am J Cardiol 83:159, 1999.
192. Zimetbaum PJ, Josephson ME: Use of the electrocardiogram in acute myocardial infarction. N Engl J Med 348:933, 2003.
193. Wellens HJ: The value of the right precordial leads of the electrocardiogram. N Engl J Med 340:381, 1999.
194. Hurst JW: Comments about the electrocardiographic signs of right ventricular infarction. Clin Cardiol 21:289, 1998.
195. Jacobs AK, Leopold JA, Bates E, et al: Cardiogenic shock caused by right ventricular infarction: A report from the SHOCK registry. J Am Coll Cardiol 41:1273, 2003.
196. Birnbaum Y, Fishbein MC, Blanche C, et al: Ventricular septal rupture after acute myocardial infarction. N Engl J Med 347:1426, 2002.
197. Sugiura T, Nagahama Y, Nakamura S, et al: Left ventricular free wall rupture after reperfusion therapy for acute myocardial infarction. Am J Cardiol 92:282, 2003.
198. Birnbaum Y, Chamoun AJ, Anzuini A, et al: Ventricular free wall rupture following acute myocardial infarction. Coron Artery Dis 14:463, 2003.
199. Figueras J, Cortadellas J, Calvo F, et al: Relevance of delayed hospital admission on development of cardiac rupture during acute myocardial infarction: Study in 225 patients with free wall, septal or papillary muscle rupture. J Am Coll Cardiol 32:135, 1998.
200. Becker RC, Hochman JS, Cannon CP, et al: Fatal cardiac rupture among patients treated with thrombolytic agents and adjunctive thrombin antagonists: Observations from the Thrombolysis and Thrombin Inhibition in Myocardial Infarction 9 Study. J Am Coll Cardiol 33:479, 1999.
201. Reynen K, Strasser RH: Images in clinical medicine. Impending rupture of the myocardial wall. N Engl J Med 348:e3, 2003.
202. Crenshaw BS, Granger CB, Birnbaum Y, et al: Risk factors, angiographic patterns, and outcomes in patients with ventricular septal defect complicating acute myocardial infarction. Circulation 101:27, 2000.
203. Figueras J, Cortadellas J, Soler-Soler J: Comparison of ventricular septal and left ventricular free wall rupture in acute myocardial infarction. Am J Cardiol 81:495, 1998.
204. Birnbaum Y, Chamoun AJ, Conti VR, et al: Mitral regurgitation following acute myocardial infarction. Coron Artery Dis 13:337, 2002.
205. Dias B, Graba J, Siu S, et al: Papillary muscle rupture complicating an acute myocardial infarction. Can J Cardiol 17:722, 2001.

206. Carmeliet E: Cardiac ionic currents and acute ischemia: From channels to arrhythmias. Physiol Rev 79:917, 1999.
207. Cannom DS, Prystowsky EN: Management of ventricular arrhythmias: Detection, drugs, and devices. JAMA 281:172, 1999.
208. Tan HL, Lie KI: Prophylactic lidocaine use in acute myocardial infarction revisited in the thrombolytic era. Am Heart J 137:770, 1999.
209. Thompson CA, Yarzebski J, Goldberg RJ, et al: Changes over time in the incidence and case-fatality rates of primary ventricular fibrillation complicating acute myocardial infarction: Perspectives from the Worcester Heart Attack Study. Am Heart J 139:1014, 2000.
210. Volpi A, Cavalli A, Santoro L, et al: Incidence and prognosis of early primary ventricular fibrillation in acute myocardial infarction—Results of the Gruppo Italiano per lo Studio della Sopravvivenza nell'Infarto Miocardico (GISSI-2) database. Am J Cardiol 82:265, 1998.
211. Brady WJ Jr, Harrigan RA: Diagnosis and management of bradycardia and atrioventricular block associated with acute coronary ischemia. Emerg Med Clin North Am 19:371, xi, 2001.
212. Zuanetti G, Mantini L, Hernandez-Bernal F, et al: Relevance of heart rate as a prognostic factor in patients with acute myocardial infarction: Insights from the GISSI-2 study. Eur Heart J 19(Suppl F):F19, 1998.
213. Altun A, Kirdar C, Ozbay G: Effect of aminophylline in patients with atropine-resistant late advanced atrioventricular block during acute inferior myocardial infarction. Clin Cardiol 21:759, 1998.
214. Herlitz J, Karlson BW, Bang A, et al: Mortality and risk indicators for death during five years after acute myocardial infarction among patients with and without ST elevation on admission electrocardiogram. Cardiology 89:33, 1998.
215. Go AS, Barron HV, Rundle AC, et al: Bundle-branch block and in-hospital mortality in acute myocardial infarction. National Registry of Myocardial Infarction 2 Investigators. Ann Intern Med 129:690, 1998.
216. Sgarbossa EB, Pinski SL, Topol EJ, et al: Acute myocardial infarction and complete bundle branch block at hospital admission: Clinical characteristics and outcome in the thrombolytic era. GUSTO-I Investigators. Global Utilization of Streptokinase and t-PA [tissue-type plasminogen activator] for Occluded Coronary Arteries. J Am Coll Cardiol 31:105, 1998.
217. Pedersen OD, Bagger H, Kober L, et al: The occurrence and prognostic significance of atrial fibrillation/flutter following acute myocardial infarction. TRACE Study group. TRAndolapril Cardiac Evalution. Eur Heart J 20:748, 1999.
218. The GUSTO Investigators: An international randomized trial comparing four thrombolytic strategies for acute myocardial infarction. N Engl J Med 329:673, 1993.
219. Grines CL, Cox DA, Stone GW, et al: Coronary angioplasty with or without stent implantation for acute myocardial infarction. N Engl J Med 341:1949, 1999.
220. Kernis SJ, Harjai KJ, Stone GW, et al: The incidence, predictors, and outcomes of early reinfarction after primary angioplasty for acute myocardial infarction. J Am Coll Cardiol 42:1173, 2003.
221. Gibson CM, Karha J, Murphy SA, et al: Early and long-term clinical outcomes associated with reinfarction following fibrinolytic administration in the Thrombolysis in Myocardial Infarction trials. J Am Coll Cardiol 42:7, 2003.
222. Scheller B, Hennen B, Hammer B, et al: Beneficial effects of immediate stenting after thrombolysis in acute myocardial infarction. J Am Coll Cardiol 42:634, 2003.
223. Zeymer U, Uebis R, Vogt A, et al: Randomized comparison of percutaneous transluminal coronary angioplasty and medical therapy in stable survivors of acute myocardial infarction with single vessel disease: A study of the Arbeitsgemeinschaft Leitende Kardiologische Krankenhausarzte. Circulation 108:1324, 2003.
224. Dauerman HL, Sobel BE: Synergistic treatment of ST-segment elevation myocardial infarction with pharmacoinvasive recanalization. J Am Coll Cardiol 42:646, 2003.
225. O'Neill WW: "Watchful waiting" after thrombolysis: It's time for a re-evaluation. J Am Coll Cardiol 42:17, 2003.
226. Dauerman HL: The early days after ST-segment elevation acute myocardial infarction: Reconsidering the delayed invasive approach. J Am Coll Cardiol 42:420, 2003.
227. McKay RG: Evolving strategies in the treatment of acute myocardial infarction in the community hospital setting. J Am Coll Cardiol 42:642, 2003.
228. Cheitlin MD, Armstrong WF, Aurigemma GP, et al: ACC/AHA/ASE 2003 guideline update for the clinical application of echocardiography: A report of the American College of Cardiology/American Heart Association Task Force on Practice Guidelines (ACC/AHA/ASE Committee to Update the 1997 Guidelines on the Clinical Application of Echocardiography). American College of Cardiology, 2003 (http://www.acc.org/clinical/guidelines/echocardiography/dirIndex.htm. 2003).
229. Reinecke H, Wichter T, Weyand M: Left ventricular pseudoaneurysm in a patient with Dressler's syndrome after myocardial infarction. Heart 80:98, 1998.
230. Ohara K: Current surgical strategy for post-infarction left ventricular aneurysm—From linear aneurysmectomy to Dor's operation. Ann Thorac Cardiovasc Surg 6:289, 2000.
231. Barbera S, Hillis LD: Echocardiographic recognition of left ventricular mural thrombus. Echocardiography 16:289, 1999.
232. Hirsh J, Fuster V, Ansell J, et al: American Heart Association/American College of Cardiology Foundation guide to warfarin therapy. Circulation 107:1692, 2003.

Post-Myocardial Infarction Care

233. Newby LK, Califf RM, Guerci A, et al: Early discharge in the thrombolytic era: An analysis of criteria for uncomplicated infarction from the Global Utilization of Streptokinase and t-PA for Occluded Coronary Arteries (GUSTO) trial. J Am Coll Cardiol 27:625, 1996.
234. Berkman LF, Blumenthal J, Burg M, et al: Effects of treating depression and low perceived social support on clinical events after myocardial infarction: The Enhancing Recovery in Coronary Heart Disease Patients (ENRICHD) Randomized Trial. JAMA 289:3106, 2003.
235. Birnbaum Y, Drew BJ: The electrocardiogram in ST elevation acute myocardial infarction: Correlation with coronary anatomy and prognosis. Postgrad Med J 79:490, 2003.
236. Agati L, De Majo F, Madonna MP, et al: Assessment of myocardial viability in patients with postischemic left ventricular dysfunction: Role of myocardial contrast echocardiography. Echocardiography 20(Suppl 1):S19, 2003.
237. Klocke FJ, Baird MG, Bateman TM, et al: ACC/AHA/ASNC guidelines for the clinical use of cardiac radionuclide imaging: A report of the American College of Cardiology/American Heart Association Task Force on Practice Guidelines (ACC/AHA/ASNC Committee to Revise the 1995 Guidelines for the Clinical Use of Radionuclide Imaging). American College of Cardiology, 2003. (http://www.acc.org/clinical/guidelines/radio/dirIndex.htm. 2003).
238. Gibbons RJ, Balady GJ, Bridker JT, et al: ACC/AHA 2002 guideline update for exercise testing: A report of the American College of Cardiology/American Heart Association Task Force on Practice Guidelines (Committee on Exercise Testing). 2002. American College of Cardiology, 2002 (http://www.acc.org/clinical/guidelines/exercise/dirIndex.htm. 2002).
239. Madsen JK, Grande P, Saunamaki K, et al: Danish multicenter randomized study of invasive versus conservative treatment in patients with inducible ischemia after thrombolysis in acute myocardial infarction (DANAMI). DANish trial in Acute Myocardial Infarction. Circulation 96:748, 1997.
240. Moss AJ, Zareba W, Hall WJ, et al: Prophylactic implantation of a defibrillator in patients with myocardial infarction and reduced ejection fraction. N Engl J Med 346:877, 2002.
241. Cairns JA, Connolly SJ, Roberts R, et al: Randomised trial of outcome after myocardial infarction in patients with frequent or repetitive ventricular premature depolarisations: CAMIAT. Canadian Amiodarone Myocardial Infarction Arrhythmia Trial Investigators. Lancet 349:675, 1997.
242. Julian DG, Camm AJ, Frangin G, et al: Randomised trial of effect of amiodarone on mortality in patients with left-ventricular dysfunction after recent myocardial infarction: EMIAT. European Myocardial Infarct Amiodarone Trial Investigators. Lancet 349:667, 1997.
243. Expert Panel on Detection, Evaluation, and Treatment of High Blood Cholesterol in Adults: Executive Summary of The Third Report of The National Cholesterol Education Program (NCEP) Expert Panel on Detection, Evaluation, And Treatment of High Blood Cholesterol In Adults (Adult Treatment Panel III). JAMA 285:2486, 2001.
244. Libby P, Ridker PM, Maseri A: Inflammation and atherosclerosis. Circulation 105:1135, 2002.
245. Yusuf S, Sleight P, Pogue J, et al: Effects of an angiotensin-converting-enzyme inhibitor, ramipril, on cardiovascular events in high-risk patients. The Heart Outcomes Prevention Evaluation Study Investigators. N Engl J Med 342:145, 2000.
246. Fox KM: Efficacy of perindopril in reduction of cardiovascular events among patients with stable coronary artery disease: Randomised, double-blind, placebo-controlled, multicentre trial (the EUROPA study). Lancet 362:782, 2003.
247. Chen J, Radford MJ, Wang Y, et al: Are beta-blockers effective in elderly patients who undergo coronary revascularization after acute myocardial infarction? Arch Intern Med 160:947, 2000.
248. Gruppo Italiano per lo Studio della Sopravvivenza nell'Infarto Miocardico: Dietary supplementation with n-3 polyunsaturated fatty acids and vitamin E after myocardial infarction: Results of the GISSI-Prevenzione trial. Lancet 354:447, 1999.

CHAPTER 48

Primary Percutaneous Coronary Intervention in the Management of Acute Myocardial Infarction

Gary E. Lane • David R. Holmes, Jr.

The restoration of blood flow to ischemic myocardium is established as the preeminent objective for treatment of patients with acute myocardial infarction. Primary angioplasty or percutaneous coronary intervention (PCI) has evolved through continued innovation of the method and dissemination to an expanding proportion of patients. This chapter examines the evidence favoring a primary angioplasty (PCI) strategy, modern application of the technique, and emerging innovations in reperfusion science.

OBSERVATIONAL DATA

Multiple centers have described their experience with primary angioplasty over the past 20 years. These series have frequently included patients with contraindications to thrombolysis and cardiogenic shock. For example, O'Keefe and colleagues[1] reported a large consecutive series (1980 to 1993) of 1000 patients (7.9 percent with cardiogenic shock). The infarct artery was recanalized in 94 percent and the overall mortality was 7.8 percent (44 percent with cardiogenic shock). Historically, these reports may be compromised by selection bias, but they established primary angioplasty as an alternative reperfusion modality.

Several large registries have been reported comparing primary angioplasty with thrombolysis. Although these registries evaluate reperfusion treatment in contemporary practice, their importance is limited by significant drawbacks including nonuniform availability of primary angioplasty, unidentified imbalance of patients' characteristics, and the influence of clinical opinions concerning treatment. Nevertheless, they provide information regarding the applicability of lessons learned from randomized trials.

The Myocardial Infarction Triage and Intervention (MITI) registry ($n = 3145$) (1988 to 1994) did not identify differences in mortality (hospital or at 3 years) or reinfarction, although 26 percent of patients in the thrombolytic group underwent "rescue" revascularization.[2] In the Second National Registry of Myocardial Infarction (NRMI-2) ($n = 29{,}644$) (1994 to 1995) total strokes were less (0.7 percent versus 1.6 percent, $p < 0.0001$) with primary angioplasty but the combined endpoint of death and nonfatal stroke was equivalent (5.6 percent for angioplasty and 6.2 percent for thrombolysis).[3]

In contrast, logistic regression multivariate analysis of the combined German Maximal Individual Therapy in Acute Myocardial Infarction–Myocardial Infarction Registry (MITRA-MIR) registries ($n = 9906$) (1994 to 1998) found a significantly reduced risk of hospital mortality for patients undergoing primary angioplasty compared with thrombolysis (6.4. percent versus 11.3 percent; odds ratio [OR] 0.54, confidence interval [CI] 0.43 to 0.67).[4] This effect was persistent across almost all preidentified subgroups of patients analyzed, including those related to gender, age, and infarct location. Furthermore, as mortality in the groups of patients increased, presumably reflecting higher risk patients, there was an increase in the absolute benefit of primary angioplasty compared with thrombolysis. The advantage noted in this analysis may reflect the improving methodology of catheter-based reperfusion. A separate examination of this registry revealed an improving hospital mortality from 1994 to 1998 with primary angioplasty but not with thrombolytic therapy.[5] From registry data, it appears that interventional advances have led to continued separation in the relative benefits of the two reperfusion strategies.

Randomized Trials Comparing Primary Angioplasty with Thrombolysis

The foundation of evidence-based medicine rests on the data obtained from carefully conducted randomized trials. On the question of reperfusion strategy, significant information has accumulated, yet even randomized trials may have inherent limitations including the inability to "blind" treatment groups and the common crossover to revascularization in patients allocated to thrombolysis.

Three randomized trials published simultaneously in 1993 provided a stimulus for expanded application and investigation of the primary angioplasty strategy. The largest ($n = 395$) of these trials, the Primary Angioplasty in Myocardial Infarction (PAMI) trial, achieved reperfusion success in 97 percent (94 percent Thrombolysis in Myocardial Infarction [TIMI] 3 flow) within 60 minutes in the angioplasty group.[6] Although there was no significant improvement in left ventricular function during rest or exercise at 6-week follow-up, there was a trend for a reduction of in-hospital mortality (2.6 percent versus 6.5 percent, $p = 0.06$) in the angioplasty group in comparison with the group treated with tissue plasminogen activator (t-PA). There was a significant reduction in combined death or reinfarction (5.1 percent versus 12 percent, $p = 0.02$) and intracranial hemorrhage (0 percent versus 2.0 percent, $p = 0.05$) with angioplasty. Patients classified as "not low risk" (older than 70 years, anterior infarction or heart rate >100) had a lower mortality rate (2.0 percent versus 10.4 percent, $p = 0.01$) with angioplasty.

The Mayo Clinic trial ($n = 108$, primary angioplasty versus t-PA) assessed myocardial salvage by technetium-99m sestamibi tomographic imaging in 108 patients.[7] No significant difference in salvage was detected. The Netherlands (Zwolle) trial compared primary angioplasty with streptokinase in 142 patients and found a significant reduction in reinfarction with angioplasty (0 percent versus 13 percent, $p = 0.003$) and a higher predischarge left ventricular ejection fraction (0.51 versus 0.45, $p = 0.004$).[8]

The Global Use of Strategies to Open Occluded Coronary Arteries in Acute Coronary Syndromes (GUSTO-IIb) angioplasty substudy was the largest trial comparing primary balloon angioplasty with thrombolysis (t-PA).[9] Although the incidence of the primary endpoint (death, nonfatal reinfarction, or disabling stroke at 30 days) was significantly reduced in the angioplasty group (9.6 percent versus 13.7 percent, $p = 0.033$), there was no significant advantage evident at 6 months (14.1 percent versus 16.1 percent, p = not significant). In comparison of this trial with other trials, it has been noted that only 81 percent of patients assigned to angioplasty underwent the procedure and TIMI-3 flow was achieved in only 73 percent. This finding may reflect the number of relatively inexperienced centers in this trial.

Evidence favoring the primary angioplasty strategy was derived from the Primary Coronary Angioplasty Trialists (PCAT) meta-analysis of 10 randomized trials (conducted 1989 to 1996).[10] The details of these trials are highlighted in Table 48–1. Primary balloon angioplasty resulted in a significant reduction in 30-day mortality (4.4 percent versus 6.5 percent, $p = 0.02$; 34 percent risk reduction) and the combination of death plus reinfarction (7.2 percent versus 11.9 percent, $p < 0.001$; 40 percent risk reduction). These effects were not significantly affected by the thrombolytic regimen. Primary angioplasty was also associated with a reduction in total stroke (0.7 percent versus 2.0 percent, $p = 0.007$) and a marked decrease in hemorrhagic stroke (0.1 percent versus 1.1 percent, $p < 0.001$).

A follow-up study from the PCAT investigators revealed that 26 lives were saved per 1000 patients treated with a primary angioplasty strategy.[11] This beneficial effect persisted at 6 months (Fig. 48–1). A similar reduction in estimated relative risk of death or reinfarction was noted across each of the major clinical subgroups analyzed, but the absolute benefits were greater in proportion to baseline risk. A 5-year follow-up from the Zwolle investigators has demonstrated the durability of primary angioplasty results with a persistent attenuation of mortality (13 percent versus 24 percent, $p < 0.01$) and reinfarction (6 percent versus 22 percent, $p < 0.001$).[12]

These studies occurred before adoption of more advanced angioplasty techniques. More recent trials have compared thrombolysis with catheter-based reperfusion utilizing stents and glycoprotein (GP) IIb/IIIa receptor inhibitors. For example, the Stent versus Thrombolysis for Occluded Coronary Arteries in Patients with Acute Myocardial Infarction (STOPAMI) trial compared patients reperfused with a stent plus abciximab with patients receiving t-PA.[13] Scintigraphic infarct size was significantly reduced in the stent group because of a larger salvage index. In addition, the composite endpoint of death, reinfarction, and stroke was lower in the stent group (8.5 percent versus 23.2 percent at 6 months, $p = 0.02$). Conversely, primary angioplasty was compared with

TABLE 48–1 Randomized Trials Comparing Primary Angioplasty with Thrombolysis*

Reference	*N*	Population of Patients	Symptom Duration (hr)	Thrombolytic Regimen	Treatment Interval (min) *PTCA*	*Thrombolysis*	Primary Follow-Up Duration (d)	Trial Period	Stents	IIb/IIIa
Dewood[†25]	90	<75 yr; ↑ST	<12	Duteplase (4 hr)	126	84	30	—	No	No
PAMI-1[†6]	395	↑ST	<12	t-PA (3 hr)	60	32	D/C	90-92	No	No
Zijlstra[†8]	294	<75 yr; ↑ST	<6	Streptokinase	68	30	30	90-92	No	No
Mayo[†7]	103	<80 yr; ↑ST	<12	Duteplase (4 hr)	45	20	D/C	89-91	No	No
Zijlstra[†22]	95	Low risk; ↑ST	<6	Streptokinase	68	30	30	93-95	No	No
Ribeiro[†23]	100	<75 yr; ↑ST	<6	Streptokinase	238	179	D/C	89	No	No
Grinfeld[†24]	112	↑ST	<12	Streptokinase	63	18	30	96[‡]	No	No
Ribichini[†26]	83	<80 yr: IWMI	<6	t-PA (90 min)	40	43	D/C	93-96	Yes	No
Garcia[†27]	189	AWMI	5	t-PA (90 min)	84	69	30	91-96	No	No
GUSTO IIB[†9]	1138	↑ST, LBBB	<12	t-PA (90 min)	114	72	30	94-96	No	No
Akhras[28]	87	↑ST	<12	Streptokinase	—	—	240	97[‡]	No	No
de Boer[29]	87	>75 yr; ↑ST	<6	Streptokinase	59	31	30	96-99	Yes	No
STOPAMI[13]	140	↑ST	<12	t-PA (90 min)	65	30	180	97-99	Yes	Yes
STAT[30]	133	↑ST, LBBB	<12	t-PA (90 min)	77	15	180	97-99	Yes	Yes
Kastrati[31]	162	↑ST, LBBB	<12	t-PA (90 min)	75	35	180	99-01	Yes	Yes
PRAGUE-1[15]	200	↑ST, LBBB	<6	Streptokinase	93	10	30	97-99	Yes	No
PRAGUE-2[16]	850	↑ST	<12	Streptokinase	94	12	30	99-02	Yes	No
LIMI[32]	150	<80 yr; ↑ST	<6	t-PA (90 min)	100	45	42	95-97	Yes	No
Air-PAMI[17]	137	↑ST; high risk	<12	t-PA/streptokinase	155	155	55	—	Yes	Yes
DANAMI-2[18]	1129	↑ST	<12	t-PA (90 min)	100	40	30	—	Yes	NA
C-PORT[20]	451	↑ST	<12	t-PA (90 min)	101	46	42/180	96-99	Yes	Yes
CAPTIM[14]	840	↑ST	<6	t-PA (90 min)	190	130	30	97-00	Yes	Yes
SHOCK[§33]	302	Cardiogenic shock	<36	t-PA (90 min)	152	150	30	93-98	Yes	Yes

AW = anterior wall; D/C = hospital discharge; IW = inferior wall; LBBB = left bundle branch block; MI = myocardial infarction; NA = not available; t-PA = tissue plasminogen activator. Trials: Air-PAMI = Air Primary Angioplasty in Myocardial Infarction; CAPTIM = Comparison of Angioplasty and Prehospital Thrombolysis In acute Myocardial infarction; C-PORT = Atlantic Cardiovascular Patient Outcomes Research Team; DANAMI = DANish trial in Acute Myocardial Infarction; GUSTO = Global Use of Strategies to Open Occluded Coronary Arteries in Acute Coronary Syndromes; PAMI = Primary Angioplasty in Myocardial Infarction; PRAGUE = PRimary Angioplasty in patients transferred from General community hospitals to specialized PTCA Units without Emergency thrombolysis; SHOCK = SHould we emergently revascularize Occluded coronaries for Cardiogenic shocK; STAT = Stenting versus Thrombolysis in Acute myocardial infarction Trial; STOPAMI = Stent versus Thrombolysis for Occluded Coronary Arteries in Patients with Acute Myocardial Infarction.

*The first 10 trials (above the horizontal line) were included in the PCAT analysis conducted in 1989-1996. The other 13 trials (below the horizontal line) were conducted in 1997-2002.

†Initial PCAT analysis trials.

‡Publication date.

§In the SHOCK trial patients were randomly assigned to revascularization or medical treatment (see text).

Data from Keeley EC, Boura JA, Grines CL: Primary angioplasty versus intravenous thrombolytic therapy for acute myocardial infarction: A quantitative review of 23 randomised trials. Lancet 361:13-20, 2003.

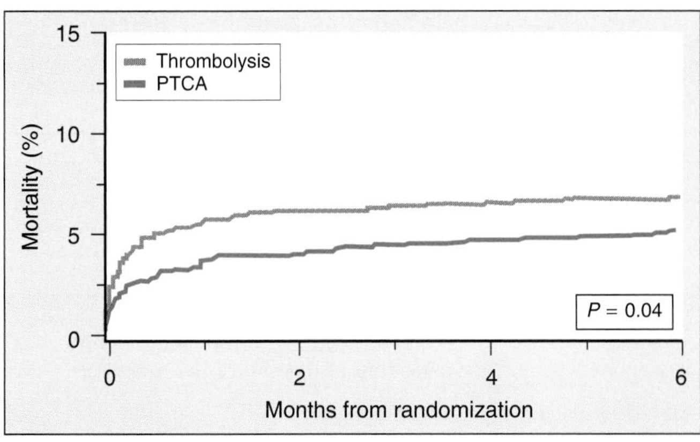

FIGURE 48–1 Mortality over 6 months from Primary Coronary Angioplasty Trialists analysis of 11 randomized trials.[11] PTCA = percutaneous transluminal coronary angioplasty.

prehospital thrombolysis in the Comparison of Angioplasty and Prehospital Thrombolysis In acute Myocardial infarction (CAPTIM) trial.[14] Although the trial was discontinued prematurely because of lack of funding, there was no significant difference in the primary endpoint of death, reinfarction, or stroke at 30 days. Rescue angioplasty was performed in 26 percent of the prehospital thrombolysis group, and a physician was part of the ambulance team. Notably, the incidence of cardiogenic shock on admission was significantly reduced in the thrombolysis group.

Additional data from randomized trials comparing primary angioplasty and thrombolysis have accumulated from trials examining logistical constraints to the application of catheter-based reperfusion. Several trials have compared a protocol of on-site thrombolysis with interhospital transport for primary angioplasty (Table 48–2). The PRimary Angioplasty in patients transferred from General community hospitals to specialized PTCA Units without Emergency thrombolysis (PRAGUE) 1 and 2,[15,16] Air Primary Angioplasty in Myocardial Infarction (Air PAMI),[17] and Danish multicenter randomized on thrombolytic treatment versus acute coronary angioplasty (DANAMI-2)[18] trials all demonstrated more favorable outcomes for patients treated with primary angioplasty despite the intrinsic transportation delay. Pooled analysis of comparative interhospital transportation trials ($n = 1242$) revealed a significant reduction in 30-day mortality (6.8 percent versus 9.6 percent, $p = 0.01$).[19] The Atlantic Cardiovascular Outcomes Research Team (C-PORT) trial compared thrombolysis (t-PA) with primary angioplasty at hospitals without on-site cardiac surgery.[20] The composite endpoint (death, reinfarction, stoke) was lower with primary angioplasty at 6 weeks (10.7 percent versus 17.7 percent, $p = 0.03$) and 6 months (12.4 percent versus 19.9 percent, $p = 0.03$).

A comprehensive review by Keeley and colleagues[21] combined the previous trials from the PCAT analysis[6-9,22-27] with 13 (conducted 1997 to 2002) more recent investigations[13-18,20,28-33] (see Table 48–1) in which stents were utilized in 12 of 13 and GP IIb/IIIa inhibitors in 7 of 13. The summary results (Fig. 48–2) ($n = 7437$) delineated a significant reduction in death, reinfarction, stroke, and hemorrhagic stroke.[21] Major hemorrhage (5 percent versus 7 percent, $p = 0.032$) was increased in the angioplasty patients. The benefit was similar irrespective of the thrombolytic regimen. Long-term (6 months) outcomes in several trials were persistently favorable for the angioplasty patients.

As with registry observations, the increasing advantage of catheter-based reperfusion strategies over thrombolysis in the more recently conducted (1996 to 2002) trials may represent increased institutional experience and advancing technology.

Advantages of the Primary Angioplasty (Percutaneous Coronary Intervention) Strategy

SUPERIOR RESTORATION OF FLOW. The GUSTO-I trial confirmed the critical link between early establishment of TIMI-3 flow and myocardial salvage and subsequent survival (Table 48–3).[34] A relationship between TIMI-3 flow and survival has also been verified for primary angioplasty.[35] Catheter-based reperfusion techniques attain TIMI-3 flow in 93 to 98 percent of patients.[6,7,36,37] In contrast, only 54 percent of patients achieve this reperfusion benchmark with accelerated t-PA.[34] This discrepancy provides a theoretical basis for

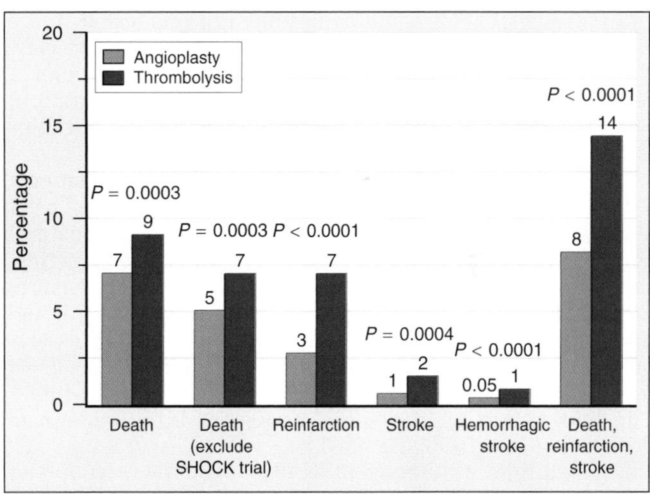

FIGURE 48–2 Short-term clinical outcomes of patients in 23 randomized trials of primary angioplasty versus thrombolysis.[21]

TABLE 48–2 Trials of Thrombolysis versus Transfer for Primary Angioplasty

			Treatment Interval (min)		% Death, Reinfarction, Stroke at 30 days		
Trial	*n*	Lytic Agent	*PTCA*	*Thrombolysis*	*PTCA*	*Thrombolysis*	*p*
PRAGUE-1[15]	200	SK	93	10	8	23	<0.02
PRAGUE-2[16]	850	SK	94	12	8.4	15.2	<0.003
Air-PAMI[17]	138	t-PA/SK	155	51	8.4	13.6	0.33
DANAMI-2[18]	1129	t-PA	100	40	8.5	14.2	0.002

Air-PAMI = Air Primary Angioplasty in Myocardial Infarction; DANAMI = DANish trial in Acute Myocardial Infarction; PRAGUE = PRimary Angioplasty in patients transferred from General community hospitals to specialized PTCA Units without Emergency thrombolysis; SK = streptokinase; t-PA = tissue plasminogen activator.

TABLE 48–3 TIMI Flow Grade Classification Scheme[42]

Flow Grade	Definition
Grade 0	No perfusion. No antegrade flow beyond the point of occlusion.
Grade 1	Penetration without perfusion. Contrast material passes beyond the area of obstruction but fails to opacify the entire coronary bed distal to the obstruction for the duration of the cineangiographic filming sequence.
Grade 2	Partial perfusion. Contrast material passes across the obstruction and opacifies the coronary distal to the obstruction. However, the rate of entry of contrast material into the vessel distal to the obstruction or its rate of clearance form the distal bed (or both) is perceptibly slower than its flow into or clearance from comparable areas not perfused by the previously occluded vessel.
Grade 3	Complete perfusion. Antegrade flow into the bed distal to the obstruction occurs as promptly as antegrade flow into the bed proximal to the obstruction, and clearance of contast material from the involved bed is as rapid as clearance from an uninvolved bed in the same vessel or the opposite artery.

TIMI: Thrombolysis In Myocardial Infarction.

TABLE 48–4 TIMI Myocardial Perfusion Grades[43]

Perfusion Grade	Definition
Grade 0	Minimal or no myocardial blush.
Grade 1	Dye stains the myocardium and this stain persists on the next injection.
Grade 2	Dye enters the myocardium but washes out slowly so that dye is strongly persistent at the end of the injection.
Grade 3	There is normal entrance and exit of dye in the myocardium so that dye is mildly persistent at the end of the injection.

TIMI = Thrombolysis In Myocardial Infarction.

the incremental improvement in outcomes with primary angioplasty.

Modification of pharmacological reperfusion utilizing a reduced-dose lytic agent and addition of a GP IIb/IIIa inhibitor resulted in TIMI-3 flow rates as high as 76 percent at 90 minutes.[38] This combination therapy was tested in the GUSTO-V and Assessment of the Safety and Efficacy of a New Thrombolytic Regimen (ASSENT)-3 trials.[39,40] Although a reduction in early ischemic events (including reinfarction) was seen, there was no reduction in 30-day[39,40] or 1-year mortality[40] compared with standard lytic therapy.

Despite restoration of epicardial flow, many patients exhibit suboptimal tissue level perfusion. This has been demonstrated by several techniques including myocardial contrast echocardiography, magnetic resonance imaging, scintigraphic methods, and Doppler flow wire measurements.[41] Epicardial flow has been more precisely quantitated utilizing the TIMI frame count,[42] and angiographic assessments of perfusion have been introduced including the TIMI myocardial perfusion grade (Table 48–4)[43] and blush score.[44] The implication of inadequate perfusion despite adequate flow is depicted in Figure 48–3.[43]

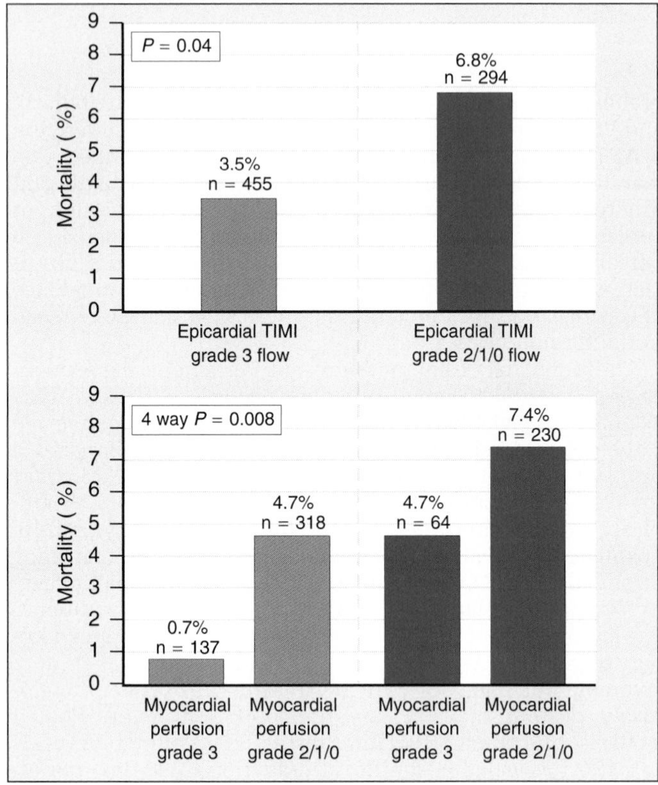

FIGURE 48–3 Relationship of both the Thrombolysis in Myocardial Infarction (TIMI) flow grade and TIMI myocardial perfusion grade at 90 minutes in the TIMI 10B trial (randomized comparison of TNK and tissue plasminogen activator). Even among patients with TIMI-3 flow, 30-day mortality was increased as myocardial perfusion decreased.[43]

Blended into this concept is the phenomenon of "no reflow" indicating impaired function of the microvasculature within the distribution of the infarct.[45] The impaired perfusion is associated with adverse left ventricular remodeling, heart failure, and reduced survival.[41,45] A multitude of factors contribute to microvascular dysfunction including platelet embolization and obstruction, vasoconstriction, and reperfusion injury processes leading to neutrophil adhesion or infiltration, endothelial cell damage, and edema.[41,45,46]

Although a significant proportion of patients exhibit impaired perfusion (30 to 70 percent)[43,44,47] after successful restoration of infarct artery flow, there appears to be more preserved microvascular perfusion among patients undergoing primary angioplasty. In a study of patients with TIMI-3 flow, 72 percent of patients treated with t-PA exhibited persistent microvascular dysfunction (myocardial echo contrast defects) at 1 month compared with 31 percent of patients treated by primary angioplasty.[47] Analysis of ST segment resolution during infarction provides a simple surrogate for monitoring myocardial perfusion. In a retrospective study of thrombolytic ($n = 851$) and primary angioplasty ($n = 528$) reperfusion, ST resolution was accelerated in the latter group and this correlated with an improved outcome.[48]

Modern objectives for reperfusion therapy should include the maintenance of microvascular integrity. Continued investigation into methods to prevent embolization, modify distal vascular tone, and enhance the microcirculatory environment may augment the results of reperfusion therapy.[41,45]

TREATMENT OF THE INCITING PATHOBIOLOGY IN ACUTE MYOCARDIAL INFARCTION. Although reperfusion therapy is based upon thrombotic coronary occlusion, thrombus may not play the predominant role in a significant proportion of acute myocardial infarctions. One study found that intracoronary aspiration thrombectomy successfully resolved coronary occlusion in 58 percent of patients, whereas thrombectomy alone or followed by primary angioplasty was successful in more than 90 percent.[49] The thrombectomy success is similar to that seen with optimal thrombolysis. Dynamic occlusive events apart from thrombus, including plaque rupture, intramural hemorrhage, dissection, and spasm, may explain at least part of the advantage of primary angioplasty over thrombolysis.

After successful thrombolysis, a significant residual stenosis remains in the majority of patients (Fig. 48–4).[50] Among patients in the TIMI trials the composite of death, reinfarction, and congestive heart failure was higher with a residual stenosis greater than 50 percent (7.8 percent versus 2.8 percent, $p = 0.03$). Treatment of the stenosis during primary angioplasty appears to lower the risk of recurrent ischemic events. In the meta-analysis of randomized trials, reinfarction was reduced to 3 percent with primary angioplasty compared with 7 percent for thrombolytic therapy ($p < 0.0001$).[21]

Late reocclusion rates (5 to 14 percent) compare favorably with those reported after thrombolysis (25 to 30 percent).[51,52] Restenosis after primary balloon angioplasty has been reported in 28 to 47 percent of patients.[51-53] Stenting further reduces the risk of reocclusion (5.1 percent versus 9.3 percent with percutaneous transluminal coronary angioplasty [PTCA], $p = 0.04$ in Stent Primary Angioplasty in Myocardial Infarction [Stent-PAMI]) and restenosis (20.3 percent versus 33.5 percent, $p < 0.001$).[36,53]

ANATOMICAL DEFINITION AND RISK STRATIFICATION. The angiographic and hemodynamic data obtained at the time of emergency catheterization impart valuable decision-facilitating information and more precise risk stratification. Definition of the coronary pathology is confirmed in patients with equivocal or uninterpretable electrocardiographic changes. After urgent coronary angiography, approximately 5 percent of patients require emergent coronary bypass surgery for severe multivessel or left main coronary artery disease.[54] Mechanical complications can also be identified during cardiac catheterization. An additional 5 percent of patients exhibit spontaneous reperfusion without a significant residual stenosis.

Stratification of patients into a low-risk group (age ≤ 70 years, left ventricular ejection fraction > 0.45, one- or two-vessel disease, successful angioplasty, no persistent arrhythmias) at the time of the procedure facilitates rapid safe recovery. It may allow omission of intensive care and noninvasive testing with early (day 3) hospital discharge.[55]

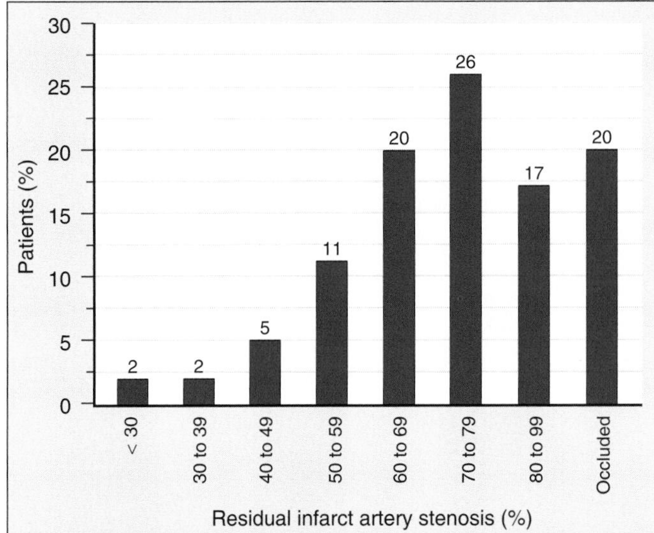

FIGURE 48–4 Distribution of residual stenosis in the infarct-related artery at 90 minutes after thrombolysis in 2119 patients in the TIMI 4, 10A, 10B, and 14 trials. (Modified from Llevadot J, Giugliano RP, McCabe CH, et al: Degree of residual stenosis in the culprit coronary artery after thrombolytic administration (Thrombolysis in Myocardial Infarction [TIMI] trials). Am J Cardiol 85:1409, 2000.)

REDUCTION IN COMPLICATIONS. Treatment with primary angioplasty appears to reduce the complications of myocardial infarct rupture. In a combined meta-analysis of the GUSTO-I and PAMI-I/II trials, primary angioplasty resulted in an 86 percent reduction in the risk of mechanical complications compared with that of patients undergoing thrombolysis.[56] There was a significant reduction in acute mitral regurgitation (0.31 percent versus 1.73 percent, $p < 0.001$) and ventricular septal defects (0.0 percent versus 0.47 percent, $p < 0.001$). In a multivariate analysis of 1375 patients, treatment with primary angioplasty was independently associated with a lower risk of free wall rupture.[57]

Intracranial hemorrhage remains a serious complication of thrombolysis. In the NRMI-2 registry the overall risk after t-PA therapy was 1.0 percent.[3] A primary angioplasty strategy nearly eliminated the peril of this complication.[21] One-third of the mortality reduction with primary angioplasty compared with thrombolysis has been attributed to curtailment of intracranial hemorrhage.[10]

Challenging Groups of Patients

ELDERLY PATIENTS. The population of elderly patients (older than 65 years) accounts for 85 percent of deaths from myocardial infarction.[58] Senescent transformation of the cardiovascular system limits cardiac reserve and complicates the management of myocardial injury.

Although the relative benefit of thrombolytic therapy is diminished in elderly patients, an analysis of the Fibrinolytic Trialists' data demonstrated a 15 percent reduction in mortality for eligible patients older than 75 years[59] compared with conservative therapy. Despite this evidence, reperfusion therapy is applied to less than half of eligible elderly patients.[60] Apprehension regarding the risk of intracranial hemorrhage significantly contributes to this diminished treatment.

Observations from the Cooperative Cardiovascular Project (CCP) Medicare data base identified a 38 percent statistically significant relative increase in mortality for thrombolysis-treated patients 76 to 84 years of age compared with conservative management.[61] The risk of intracranial hemorrhage was 2.5 percent among those older than 75 years in the NRMI-2 registry.[3] Trials of thrombolytic therapy including more aged patients have demonstrated a 2 to 3 percent risk of intracranial hemorrhage in this group. Attempts to enhance the results of thrombolysis with combination regimens in the ASSENT-3 and GUSTO-V trials did not improve overall efficacy and increased bleeding risk in patients older than 75 years.[39,40]

In contrast, the CCP patients undergoing primary angioplasty ($n = 2038$) exhibited lower 30-day (8.7 percent versus 11.9 percent, $p = 0.001$) and 1-year (14.4 percent versus 17.6 percent, $p = 0.001$) mortality compared with those undergoing thrombolysis ($n = 18{,}645$).[60] For patients older than 75 years in the NRMI-2 registry, the combined endpoint of death and nonfatal stroke was significantly higher in patients treated with t-PA compared with primary angioplasty (18.4 percent versus 14.6 percent, $p = 0.001$).[3]

Pooled analysis of the PAMI, Zwolle, and Mayo Clinic randomized trials revealed a significant mortality reduction for the elderly (older than 70 years) subgroup treated with angioplasty (3.5 percent versus 16 percent, $p = 0.02$) but not for younger patients.[62] A small randomized trial demonstrated no advantage for primary balloon angioplasty over conservative therapy in 120 patients older than 80 years.[63] However a trial ($n = 87$) comparing streptokinase (perhaps the preferred lytic agent in elderly patients) with angioplasty (stents in 51 percent) demonstrated a striking reduction (9 percent versus 29 percent, $p = 0.01$) in the primary endpoint (death, reinfarction, or stroke) and considerable reduction in 30-day (7 percent versus 22 percent, $p = 0.04$) and 1-year mortality (11 percent versus 29 percent, $p = 0.03$) with angioplasty in patients older than 75 years.[29]

Despite a shortage of randomized trial data, the advantage of primary angioplasty may be magnified in the elderly population. Clearly, further investigation is needed emphasizing the selection of patients who can safely benefit from reperfusion therapy.

PRIOR CORONARY BYPASS SURGERY. Mortality is increased in patients with prior coronary bypass surgery and acute myocardial infarction.[64,65] The increased risk of mortality and infarct complications may be attributed to more frequent coexistent factors such as advanced age, prior infarction, multivessel disease, diabetes, and impaired ventricular function. However, prior bypass surgery remains an independent risk factor for mortality.[66] No randomized controlled trials specifically address reperfusion therapy in this cohort.

In the NRMI-2 registry, 2544 patients with previous bypass surgery were treated with t-PA and 375 underwent primary angioplasty.[65] There was no significant difference in the mortality rate. The large thrombus burden often present in vein grafts may be more resistant to the action of lytic agents. In the GUSTO-I trial of thrombolysis, TIMI-3 flow in bypass grafts was achieved in only 32 percent compared with 49.2 percent without previous surgery.[64]

Primary balloon angioplasty of vein grafts has been associated with higher rates of TIMI-3 flow compared with thrombolysis (83 percent in the PAMI trials, $n = 93$) but reduced rates compared with native vessel reperfusion.[66,67] In addition to more extensive thrombus, vein graft angioplasty is often complicated by graft ectasia, limited runoff, atherosclerotic debris, and increased risk of distal embolization. Reperfusion of the infarct artery through the native circulation should be attempted if feasible.

In a retrospective series of 158 patients with acute vein graft occlusion, primary stenting ($n = 74$) resulted in more frequent TIMI-3 flow than balloon angioplasty ($n = 84$) (96 percent versus 72 percent, $p = 0.0001$) but without a difference in clinical outcome.[68] The role of GP IIb/IIIa inhibitors is unclear, although they appear to be of little value during vein graft intervention in other settings. Alternative methodology (thrombectomy, distal protection devices, ultrasound thrombolysis) requires investigation to optimize reperfusion within bypass grafts.

PATIENTS WITH THROMBOLYTIC CONTRAINDICATIONS. A significant proportion (25 to 30 percent) of patients presenting with ST elevation (or left bundle branch block) infarction who are eligible do not receive reperfusion therapy. In the Global Registry of Acute Coronary Events (GRACE) registry, 2084 patients presented within 12 hours of the onset of ST elevation infarction.[69] Thrombolytic contraindications were present in 15 percent, and overall 30 percent of eligible patients did not receive reperfusion therapy. Correlates of the latter group included prior bypass surgery, diabetes, history of congestive failure, and age older than 75 years. There remains a bias against thrombolysis particularly for elderly patients. Patients with clear-cut and relative contraindications to thrombolysis are at higher risk for death.

Patients with thrombolytic contraindications who underwent primary angioplasty in the MITRA registry had significantly lower mortality than conservatively managed patients (2.2 percent versus 24.7 percent, $p = 0.001$).[70] Juliard and colleagues[71] reported that reperfusion therapy with thrombolysis or angioplasty, or both, could be accomplished in 98 percent of 500 consecutive patients. Primary angioplasty can be applied in most higher risk patients who are not ideal candidates for thrombolytic therapy. The contraindications to primary angioplasty are limited to patients who cannot receive heparin or aspirin-thienopyridines, patients with documented life-threatening contrast allergy, or those with lack of vascular access.

CARDIOGENIC SHOCK. Infarct artery patency correlates with improved survival in cardiogenic shock secondary to left ventricular damage. Multiple observational series of patients undergoing angioplasty in cardiogenic shock have demonstrated an improved hemodynamic status and suggested enhanced survival.[72]

In contrast, thrombolysis appears to be less effective when administered to patients in shock. Limited trial data suggest an equivocal or marginal benefit in cardiogenic shock.[72] Intraaortic balloon counterpulsation may improve the results of thrombolytic therapy in cardiogenic shock.[73]

The SHould we emergently revascularize Occluded Coronaries for cardiogenic shocK (SHOCK) trial[33] verified a role for revascularization in cardiogenic shock. Patients ($n = 302$) were randomly assigned to an early (within 6 hours) revascularization strategy (angioplasty [55 percent] or bypass surgery [38 percent]) or medical stabilization (thrombolysis 63 percent) with delayed revascularization if appropriate. Intraaortic balloon support was recommended (86 percent in both groups). A significant survival advantage for revascularization was noted at 6 months and 1 year but not at the 30-day primary endpoint (Fig. 48–5).[74] The 30-day mortality was significantly lower with early revascularization for patients younger than 75 years (41 percent versus 57 percent, $p < 0.05$). These data strongly support the utilization of early revascularization in patients with shock younger than 75 years. The approach in elderly patients is less clear, although a survival advantage was seen for those older than 75 years who were clinically selected for early revascularization in the SHOCK registry.[75] Clearly, rapid reperfusion is critical to success in patients with cardiogenic shock (Fig. 48–6).[76]

Multivessel or left main disease is found in 60 to 90 percent of patients with cardiogenic shock.[72] In the SHOCK trial angioplasty was recommended for patients with one- or two-vessel disease and bypass surgery for those with left main or three-vessel disease. The role for multivessel angioplasty in cardiogenic shock remains to be defined, but stenting may allow safer application of this strategy.

THE LOGISTIC CHALLENGE OF EFFECTIVE REPERFUSION THERAPY

Rapid reperfusion of the infarct artery leading to myocardial salvage has remained the basis for the reperfusion paradigm. The survival benefit of

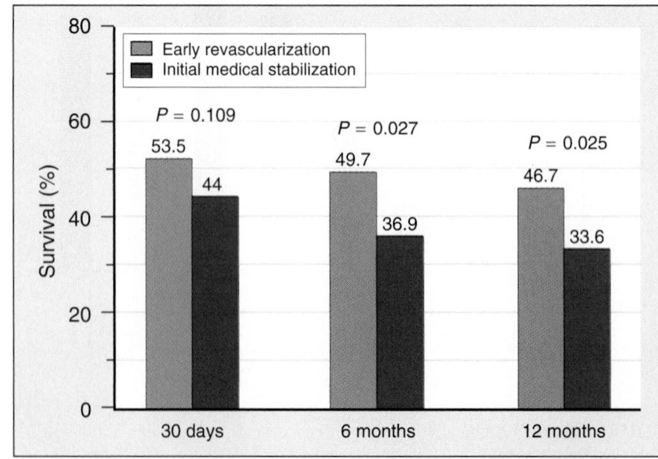

FIGURE 48–5 The temporal relation to survival for patients randomized in the SHould we emergently revascularize Occluded Coronaries for cardiogenic shocK (SHOCK) trial by treatment strategy.[74]

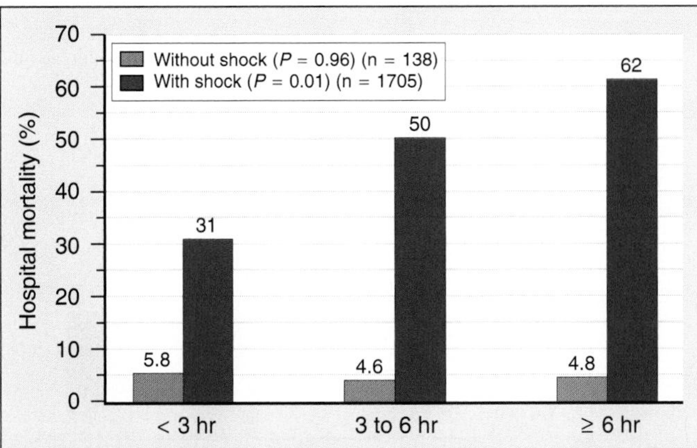

FIGURE 48–6 In-hospital mortality by time to reperfusion (symptom onset) in patients with and without shock. In this study after adjustment for baseline variables, reperfusion time was a significant predictor of mortality in patients with shock but not in patients without shock.[76]

reperfusion with thrombolytic therapy decreases with increasing delay in treatment.[77] A similar time-dependent relationship has been assumed for primary angioplasty.

There is an inherent delay in application of primary angioplasty compared with thrombolysis. The results of early randomized trials demonstrating an advantage for primary angioplasty over thrombolysis were not reproduced when some community-based registries were examined. These differences were attributed to the prolonged treatment interval to effect catheter-based reperfusion compared with thrombolysis seen in some of these registries. In the PCAT randomized trials, the mean primary angioplasty treatment delay was 26 minutes longer than the thrombolysis delay, compared with about 45 minutes relative delay in MITI and NRMI-2 registries.[2,3,10] This relative delay is an impediment to widespread application of a mechanical reperfusion strategy.

A relationship between increased mortality and prolonged treatment intervals (especially "door-to-balloon" times > 2 hours) was demonstrated in the GUSTO-IIB trial and the NRMI-2 registry.[35,78] Yet, in the same populations no survival relationship was found between time from symptom onset and reperfusion. In a series ($n = 1352$) reported by Brodie and colleagues,[79] mortality was lower when patients were reperfused early (<2 hours) but thereafter remained constant (2 to 12 hours after symptom onset). The investigators in PCAT ($n = 2635$) demonstrated increasing major adverse cardiac event rates with increasing presentation delay for thrombolysis but relatively stable event rates for primary angioplasty.[80]

An expanded concept of the mechanism of reperfusion benefit should be considered. Clearly, the earliest possible restoration of blood flow into the infarct artery is desirable. The occurrence of the most favorable outcomes with early (<2 hour) reperfusion is evident in most catheter-based reperfusion studies. This timely gain correlates with enhanced salvage of myocardium as measured by sestamibi perfusion and preservation of left ventricular function.[1,81] Myocardial salvage beyond the 2- to 3-hour window is probably modest. However, less than 20 percent of patients present early enough to achieve reperfusion in less than 2 hours.[78] Attainment of reperfusion in this early time period is more critical for patients with cardiogenic shock.[33] Moreover, in an analysis of primary PCI in 1843 patients again reported by Brodie and colleagues,[76] reperfusion time (from symptom onset) was important for the survival of patients with shock but independent of mortality in patients without shock (see Fig. 48–6).

The benefit of primary angioplasty may be less dependent on the treatment interval because of several possibilities. A consistent and high reperfusion efficacy is attained with primary angioplasty, but achievement of TIMI-3 flow decreases as treatment is delayed with thrombolysis.[82] In patients receiving thrombolysis, the complications of intracranial hemorrhage and myocardial rupture occur more frequently with longer treatment delays.[56,77] Myocardial rupture is reduced and intracranial hemorrhage is nearly eliminated with a primary angioplasty strategy.[56,57,77] Despite limited gains in myocardial salvage from primary angioplasty with later treatment, the improved patency may enhance survival by stabilizing myocardium at risk for rupture, having positive effects on ventricular remodeling, augmenting electrical stability, and providing a conduit for collateral flow.[79] The intrinsic value of infarct artery patency may be more than previously realized.

Expanding the Population for Catheter-Based Reperfusion

Only a minority of hospitals have catheterization laboratories, and even fewer offer coronary bypass surgery. The improving results of primary angioplasty (PCI) provide momentum to extend this advantage to more patients.

The prolonged temporal margin of benefit seen with a primary angioplasty strategy has created a foundation for expanding catheter-based reperfusion by transfer to capable centers. Summary evidence favoring this concept from several randomized trials (see Table 48–2) indicates a reduction in 30-day mortality (6.8 percent versus 9.6 percent, $p = 0.01$; 33 lives saved per 1000 patients treated) and adverse events (death, stroke, or reinfarction) (8.5 percent versus 15.5 percent, $p < 0.001$; 70 fewer events per 1000 treated).[19] Individually, there was a statistically insignificant reduction in mortality for each trial. In the PRAGUE-2 trial the survival benefit appeared to be limited to patients presenting more than 3 hours after symptom onset, consistent with the delayed temporal advantage of primary angioplasty.[16] In these trials, interhospital transport appeared to be safe without increasing the patient's risk. Because of rapid transport and concurrent preparation for primary angioplasty in the DANAMI-2 trial, the treatment delay for transferred patients was minimal (<15 minutes) compared with that for a group presenting at the interventional centers.[18]

An alternative approach involves increasing the number of hospitals offering primary angioplasty. Experienced operators have performed primary angioplasty at hospitals without cardiac surgery with high procedural success even in patients with cardiogenic shock. A randomized trial (C-PORT) ($n = 451$) compared primary angioplasty (70 percent stents) with thrombolysis at 11 hospitals without on-site cardiac surgery.[20] A formal development program was completed prior to the trial at all hospitals and included American College of Cardiology/American Heart Association (ACC/AHA) guidelines.[83] The composite primary endpoint (death, reinfarction, stroke) was significantly reduced at 6 weeks and 6 months (12.4 percent versus 19.9 percent, $p = 0.03$) in the angioplasty group. No patient experienced a complication from attempted angioplasty that required emergency surgery.

The risk of an interventional complication requiring surgery (dissection or closure, side branch occlusion, perforation) in the setting of infarct artery angioplasty is low in the current era of stents and GP IIb/IIIa inhibitors.[54] However, a small percentage of patients require emergency surgery because of left main or complex multivessel disease and mechanical complications of infarction. In addition, institutional and operator expertise has been shown to affect the results of primary angioplasty procedures. Analysis of data from the NRMI data base indicates that mortality is lower among patients treated with primary angioplasty compared with thrombolysis at hospitals performing at intermediate (17 to 48 per year; 4.5 percent versus 5.9 percent, $p < 0.001$) and high volumes (>49 per year; 3.4 percent versus 5.4 percent, $p < 00.1$). At low-volume (<17 per year) hospitals, there was no mortality reduction for patients undergoing angioplasty (6.2 percent versus 5.9 percent, $p = 0.58$).[84] In-hospital mortality was reduced 57 percent when angioplasty was performed by high-volume operators (defined as >10 primary angioplasty procedures per year) in an analysis of the New York State registry.[85] These and other factors must be considered if primary angioplasty is considered at an institution without on-site cardiac surgery.[83]

The optimal reperfusion strategy for patients with acute myocardial infarction continues to evolve. Many regional factors may influence decisions regarding local protocols. Increasing utilization of prehospital diagnostic and risk assessment strategies should allow appropriate triage and initiation of timely reperfusion therapy for all eligible patients.

Modern Catheter-Based Reperfusion Techniques

Glycoprotein IIb/IIIa Inhibition

There is a strong theoretical basis for utilization of GP IIb/IIIa inhibition during catheter-based reperfusion therapy. Antagonism of platelet aggregation may "passivate" the unstable mechanically injured atherosclerotic arterial wall, avert thrombus formation on acutely deployed stents, and prevent microembolization with subsequent no reflow. Abciximab was shown to improve recovery of microvascular perfusion and to enhance contractile function after stenting in a randomized study of 200 patients with acute myocardial infarction.[86]

The ReoPro in AMI Primary PTCA Organization Randomized Trial (RAPPORT) randomly assigned 483 patients to placebo or abciximab while undergoing primary balloon angioplasty.[87] The incidence of death, reinfarction, or urgent target vessel revascularization (TVR) was significantly reduced at 30 days (5.8 percent versus 11.2 percent, $p = 0.03$) and 6 months (11.6 percent versus 17.8, $p = 0.05$) with abciximab. However the primary 6-month endpoint of death, reinfarction, and any TVR was equivalent (28.1 percent versus 28.2 percent).

Despite the apparent benefits of stenting in myocardial infarction, there was concern regarding the reduced rate of TIMI-3 flow achieved by stenting compared with balloon angioplasty (89.5 percent versus 92.7 percent, $p = 0.046$) in the Stent-PAMI trial.[36] This concern was amplified by the strong trend for higher mortality in the stent group at 1 year (5.4 percent versus 3 percent, $p = 0.054$).[53] It was postulated that this phenomenon may be due to thrombus embolization by stent devices during deployment. Thus, IIb/IIIa inhibition could be an important adjunct to stenting in acute myocardial infarction.

Two trials have examined the combination of primary infarct stenting and GP IIb/IIIa inhibition. The Abciximab before Direct angioplasty and stenting in Myocardial Infarction Regarding Acute and Long-term results (ADMIRAL) trial randomly assigned 300 patients undergoing primary stenting to abciximab given before angiography or placebo.[88] Patients receiving abciximab attained a greater frequency of TIMI-3 flow before stenting (16.8 percent versus 5.4 percent, $p = 0.01$), immediately after stenting (95.1 percent versus 86.7 percent, $p = 0.04$), and at 6 months (94.3 percent versus 82.8 percent, $p = 0.04$). The primary endpoint of death, reinfarction, or urgent TVR was also significantly reduced with abciximab treatment at 30 days (6 percent versus 14.6 percent, $p = 0.01$) and 6 months (7.4 percent versus 15.9 percent, $p = 0.02$). At 6 months, abciximab therapy was associated with less reocclusion (2.9 percent versus 12.1 percent, $p = 0.04$) and enhanced left ventricular function.

The risk of subacute thrombosis (stent and PTCA) at 30 days was reduced (0.4 percent versus 1.4 percent, $p < 0.001$) by abciximab in the Controlled Abciximab and Device Investigation to Lower Late Angioplasty Complications (CADILLAC) trial.[37] However, no significant advantage for abciximab treatment was evident at 6 months although a nonsignificant reduction in ischemic TVR was seen in patients with PTCA. In addition, abciximab did not significantly affect TIMI-3 flow rates or left ventricular function.

The discrepant results of these trials may be explained by differences in inclusion criteria (8 percent with shock in ADMIRAL), different stent designs, or, perhaps more important, the timing of abciximab administration. In CADILLAC, abciximab was given after angiography, whereas patients in ADMIRAL received drug before sheath insertion. In fact, in the ADMIRAL trial 26 percent of patients had abciximab administered in the emergency room or ambulance. A large benefit was identified for an early administration strategy (Fig. 48–7).[88] It must be remembered that abciximab has been associated with a small increase in minor bleeding (nonintracranial) and thrombocytopenia.

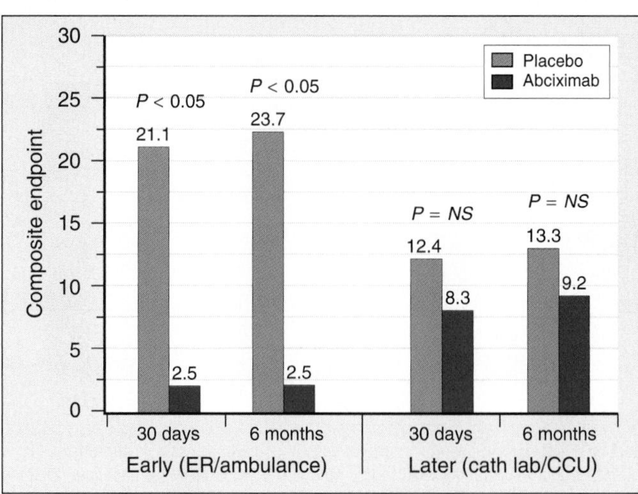

FIGURE 48–7 The incidence of the primary composite endpoint (death, reinfarction, or urgent target vessel revascularization) in the Abciximab before Direct angioplasty and stenting in Myocardial Infarction Regarding Acute and Long-term results (ADMIRAL) trial stratified by randomization and study drug administration time.[88] CCU = cardiac care unit; ER = emergency room.

Although the incremental benefits of adjunctive GP IIb/IIIa inhibition remain controversial, there is evidence supporting administration, especially early in the reperfusion process.

Primary Stent Implantation

Stents have ascended to an essential role in interventional practice. Early concerns regarding the safety of stent implantation in the presence of intracoronary thrombus have abated. High-pressure stent deployment techniques and additive antiplatelet therapy mitigated the risk of stent thrombosis and allowed utilization in acute coronary syndromes.

Suboptimal results after primary angioplasty are predictive of recurrent ischemia or reocclusion.[89] Initial use of stents was restricted to "bailout" indications, but several studies demonstrated the feasibility and safety of stents in acute myocardial infarction.[90]

Several randomized trials (Table 48–5)[36,37,91-97] have been conducted comparing primary stenting with primary balloon angioplasty. The Stent-PAMI trial reported a reduction in the 6-month combined endpoint of death, recurrent infarction, and TVR related entirely to diminished TVR in the stent group (7.7 percent versus 17 percent, $p < 0.001$).[36] Stenting also reduced recurrent ischemia (9 percent versus 28 percent, $p = 0.003$) and restenosis or reocclusion (17 percent versus 43 percent, $p = 0.001$). Despite a favorable influence on the combined endpoint, concern was raised regarding a trend toward increased late mortality in the stent group, possibly related to decreased TIMI-3 flow after stenting.[53] In the CADILLAC trial primary balloon angioplasty or primary stenting (newer generation device) without abciximab was compared in 1030 patients.[37] There was no significant difference in TIMI-3 flow rates (94.7 percent versus 94.5 percent) and 30-day mortality (2.5 percent versus 2.2 percent), but the 30-day TVR was significantly lower with stenting (6.0 percent versus 3.4 percent, $p < 0.05$). At 6 months the combined endpoint of death, reinfarction, stroke, and ischemic TVR was significantly lower in the stent group (11.5 percent versus 20 percent, $p < 0.001$), driven by lower rates of ischemic TVR with stenting (8.3 percent versus 15.7 percent, $p < .001$). The 6-month mortality was insignificantly lower with stenting (3 percent versus 4.5 percent).

TABLE 48–5 Randomized Trials of Primary Stenting Versus Primary Angioplasty in Acute Myocardial Infarction

				MACE			Death		
Reference	n	PTCA → Stent Crossover (%)	F/U time (mo)	*Stent*	*PTCA*	*P* value	*Stent*	*PTCA*	*P* value
Zwolle[92]	227	13	6	5	20	0.0012	2	3	1
FRESCO[91]	150	0	6	9	28	0.003	0	0	—
PASTA[93]	136	10	12	22	49	0.0011	5	9	0.32
GRAMI[94]	104	25	0.2	17.3	34.6	0.002	3.8	7.7	NS
STENTIM-2[95]	211	36	6	19.8	28.2	0.14	3	1.9	NS
Stent PAMI[36]	900	15	12	17	25	<0.01	5.8	3.1	0.07
PSAAMI[97]	88	27	12	23	43	0.03	9	18	0.18
PRISAM[96]	222	1	6	—	—	—	0	0.9	—
CADILLACa*[37]	1030	18	6	11.5	20	<0.001	3	4.5	0.23
CADILLACb†[37]	1054	14	6	10.2	16.5	0.004	4.2	2.5	0.23

CADILLAC = Controlled Abciximab and Device Investigation to Lower Late Angioplasty Complications; FRESCO = Florence Randomized Elective Stenting in Acute Coronary Occlusions; F/U = follow-up; GRAMI = Gianturco-Roubin in Acute Myocardial Infarction; MACE = major adverse cardiac events—death, reinfarction, target vessel revascularization (stroke included in CADILLAC and Stent-PAMI); PAMI = Primary Angioplasty in Myocardial Infarction; PASTA = Primary Angioplasty versus STent implantation in Acute myocardial infarction; PRISAM = PRImary Stenting for Acute Myocardial infarction; PSAAMI = Primary Stenting vs. Angioplasty in Acute Myocardial Infarction; PTCA = percutaneous transluminal coronary angioplasty; STENTIM = STENT In acute Myocardial infarction.

*CADILLACa, stent alone and balloon angioplasty alone arms.

†CADILLACb, stent plus abciximab and balloon angioplasty plus abciximab arms.

A meta-analysis of the reported trials confirms the advantage of stent deployment.[98] The composite incidence of major adverse events at 6 to 12 months is significantly reduced (OR 0.52, 95 percent CI 0.44 to 0.62) without a significant difference in mortality again principally secondary to a reduction in TVR (OR 0.43, 95 percent CI 0.36 to 0.52) (Fig. 48–8). As with other PCI indications, stents should be routinely applied in acute myocardial infarction.

ADVANCES IN THE PROCESS OF REPERFUSION

There is considerable interest in developing the science of reperfusion beyond ensuring prompt and stable coronary patency. Methods for protection of microvascular integrity and preservation of the injured myocyte are evolving.

The importance of optimal myocardial perfusion and hazards of the no-reflow phenomenon have already been highlighted. Distal embolization identified by angiography during primary angioplasty was noted in 15.2 percent of patients in the Zwolle trial.[99] Procedural success (TIMI-3 flow) and perfusion (blush score) were reduced with embolization and associated with larger infarct size, lower ejection fraction, and higher 5-year mortality (44 percent versus 9 percent, $p < 0.001$).

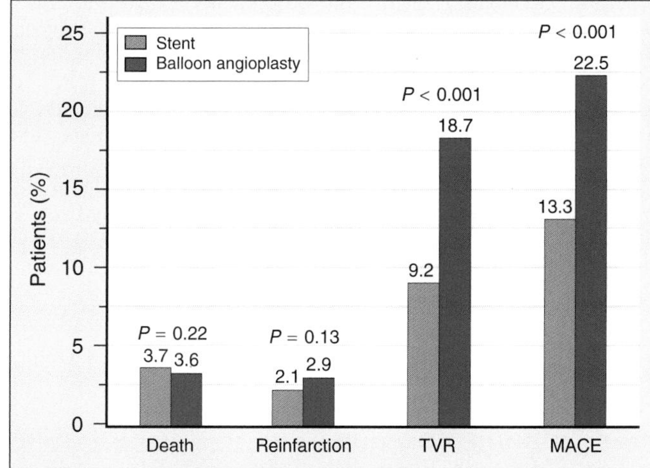

FIGURE 48–8 Results of meta-analysis comparing primary stenting with primary balloon angioplasty.[98] MACE = major adverse cardiac events including death, reinfarction, and target vessel revascularization (TVR) (stroke in Controlled Abciximab and Device Investigation to Lower Late Angioplasty Complications [CADILLAC] and Stent Primary Angioplasty in Myocardial Infarction [Stent-PAMI] trials).

In addition to pharmacological protection of the microvasculature with GP IIb/IIIa inhibition, several mechanical techniques employing thrombus removal have been reported. Kaplan and coworkers[100] reported utilization of the transluminal extraction catheter device in acute infarction with a 94 percent procedural success rate in 100 patients. However, restenosis occurred in 68 percent and this technique is limited by the large profile and complexity. Ultrasound thrombolysis has also been utilized successfully to induce patency (94 percent) in a small series.[101]

Several small series reported successful application of the AngioJet rheolytic thrombectomy catheter. This device utilizes high-velocity saline jets to create a low-pressure zone at the catheter tip through a Bernoulli effect, allowing fragmentation and aspiration of thrombus. For example, Silva and associates[102] reported a series of 79 patients with acute infarction and angiographic evidence for thrombus. Procedural success occurred in 94 percent with greater success in native arteries than venous bypass grafts. Angioplasty or stenting, or both, followed in most patients. Complications included distal embolization (10 percent) or perforation (3 percent). Beside the obvious application to patients with a large thrombus burden, utilization of this device has been reported to achieve superior outcomes in cardiogenic shock[103] and stent thrombosis,[104] in which usual catheter-based revascularization has been less successful. A randomized trial examining routine application of AngioJet thrombectomy during catheter-based reperfusion is in progress.

The X-sizer device employs helical thrombectomy and vacuum aspiration. It has been reported in a randomized trial ($n = 92$) to attain normal myocardial blush scores in a greater proportion of patients than primary stenting alone (72 percent versus 37 percent, $p = 0.006$).[105] Other thrombus removal devices using vacuum-assisted aspiration through specialized catheters have also been successfully utilized in myocardial infarction.[49,106]

Protection can also be accomplished with systems designed to prevent embolization through distal balloon occlusion and aspiration or filters designed to trap debris. The former mechanism in the form of the PercuSurge device has been reported with successful removal of thrombus and effective reperfusion in a few cases.[107] A current randomized trial is testing routine use of this device during acute infarct angioplasty. Other distal protection devices are under development and will be investigated in this setting.

Many pharmacological interventions have been proposed and investigated as methods of myocardial preservation. Considerable effort has been focused on reperfusion injury, which has been described to consist of several processes including oxygen free radical production, contraction band necrosis related to calcium overload, activation of inflammatory mediators, endothelial dysfunction, and microvascular injury contributing to no reflow.[46] Despite promising experimental data, clinical trials including those targeting neutrophil migration, free radical formation, and metabolic stabilization have failed to affect infarct size or outcomes significantly.[46,108,109]

In contrast, more favorable effects have been observed with the vasodilator adenosine, which may also work through cardioprotective mechanisms including replenishment of high-energy phosphate stores, ischemic preconditioning, free radical suppression, and platelet and neutrophil inhibition. Intracoronary adenosine reduced no reflow and improved ventricular function during primary angioplasty.[110] In the Acute Myocardial Infarction Study of Adenosine (AMISTAD) I and II trials, infarct size was significantly reduced (27 to 33 percent) by adenosine with a trend toward reduced death and heart failure in AMISTAD II.[111,112] Nicorandil, another agent with multiple effects (adenosine triphosphate-sensitive K^+ channel opener with nitrate properties) reduced no reflow and was associated with better clinical outcomes in a randomized trial involving 81 patients undergoing primary angioplasty.[113] In the COMplement inhibition in Myocardial infarction treated with Angioplasty (COMMA) trial a monoclonal antibody to the C5 terminal component of the complement cascade (pexelizumab) was tested in 814 patients undergoing primary angioplasty. Although there was no effect on the primary endpoint of infarct size, 6-month mortality was significantly lower in the antibody-treated group (3.2 percent vs, 7.4 percent, $p = 0.018$).[114]

Preliminary evidence suggests that infusion of aqueous hyperoxemic blood (oxygen partial pressure 600 to 800 mm Hg) for 60 to 90 minutes after primary angioplasty may attenuate microvascular injury and enhance myocardial salvage.[115] Induction of moderate systemic hypothermia through a heat exchange catheter in the vena cava may also reduce infarct size.[116] These and other interventions for myocardial protection during reperfusion are being tested in randomized trials.

Combining Thrombolysis and Angioplasty as Reperfusion Therapy

RESCUE ANGIOPLASTY. Despite growth in the proportion of patients undergoing primary angioplasty, in most countries the majority of patients with infarction receive thrombolytic reperfusion therapy. There remains a paucity of investigational data regarding the value of rescue angioplasty in patients who do not achieve reperfusion after thrombolysis. Observational data and early trials suggested little benefit and high mortality (>30 percent) among patients in whom attempted rescue angioplasty fails.[117] This finding is reflective of the higher risk profile in patients with failed thrombolysis and the complex management related to the uncertainty of lytic success and possible need for transfer to enable rescue procedures.

An analysis of four small randomized trials of rescue angioplasty ($n = 368$) identified a significant reduction in early severe heart failure (3.8 percent versus 11.7 percent, $p = 0.04$) and a trend toward reduced early mortality (8.5 percent versus 12.2 percent, $p = 0.26$).[118] Aggregate 1-year follow-up data from two of these trials revealed a significant survival benefit.[118] More contemporary data indicate that patients undergoing rescue intervention benefit from GP IIb/IIIa inhibition and stenting with improved procedural success and enhanced clinical outcomes.[119,120]

The difficulty of noninvasive determination of the status of infarct artery perfusion remains an important limitation of this approach. Utilization of clinical features, baseline/60-minute biomarkers, and ST segment resolution in combination as a predictive instrument may improve accuracy.[121] The role of rescue angioplasty will continue to be investigated as the concept of facilitated intervention evolves.

THE CONCEPT OF FACILITATED ANGIOPLASTY. The parallel nascent development of thrombolytic reperfusion therapy and transluminal revascularization within the catheterization laboratory invited combined application in acute myocardial infarction in an effort to optimize the arterial lumen and reduce the risk of recurrent ischemia and reocclusion. However, several trials conducted more than a decade ago demonstrated an adverse outcome for early compared with delayed angioplasty after thrombolysis with more complications (bypass surgery and bleeding), a trend for higher mortality, and no difference in left ventricular function.[83] This hazard was presumed to originate from enhanced platelet activation or extensive intramural hemorrhage, or both. Yet, advanced angioplasty techniques have improved the safety of the procedure in this setting. In a multivariate analysis of the patients in the TIMI-10B (tenecteplase [TNK] versus t-PA) and TIMI-14 (reduced dose t-PA and/or abciximab) trials, those undergoing adjunctive or delayed intervention (>60 percent stents) had a lower risk of 30-day mortality or reinfarction than patients with successful (TIMI-3 flow at 90 minutes) thrombolysis without intervention.[122]

A further impetus for revisiting a combined pharmacological and mechanical approach to reperfusion comes from an analysis of the four PAMI trials ($n = 2507$).[123] Patients (16 percent) with spontaneous reperfusion (TIMI-3 flow) on initial angiography prior to intervention had improved left ventricular function with less heart failure, hypotension, and hospital mortality. Procedural success was improved and, by multivariate analysis, TIMI-3 flow before angioplasty was an independent determinant of survival.

This information has stimulated further development of the synergistic concept of facilitated angioplasty achieving the speed advantage of pharmacological reperfusion while allowing the security of mechanical bailout and "definitive" treatment of the arterial lumen. In the Plasminogen-activator Angioplasty Compatibility Trial (PACT), patients receiving half-dose t-PA had a higher TIMI-3 flow rate (33 percent versus 15 percent with placebo) prior to angioplasty.[124] The benefits of early initiation of abciximab before primary stenting were noted in the ADMIRAL trial (see Fig. 48–7). Administration of abciximab alone before angiography resulted in 90-minute TIMI-3 flow rates of about 30 percent.[38,125] When abciximab was combined with reduced-dose (usually half) thrombolysis, the 90-minute TIMI-3 flow rates were 62 to 77 percent[38] with no increased risk of major bleeding or intracranial hemorrhage over full-dose thrombolysis. In the SPEED (Strategies for Patency Enhancement in the Emergency Department) (GUSTO IV pilot) trial, 323 patients who underwent PCI in the setting of prior combined reteplase and abciximab therapy were compared with 162 patients without intervention.[125] The patients with early PCI experienced a reduction in the composite endpoint of death, reinfarction, or urgent revascularization (5.6 percent versus 16 percent, $p = 0.001$). The risk of ischemic events or bleeding complications was also reduced with early PCI (15 percent versus 30 percent, $p = 0.001$).

Facilitated angioplasty (PCI) may augment the results of catheter-based reperfusion by enhancing myocardial salvage, the stability of the procedure, and the safety of transfer of patients. However, these benefits need to be counterbalanced by the hemorrhagic risk of combined pharmacological reperfusion therapy, especially in the elderly population.[39,40] Several trials are now in progress that will elucidate further the role of a facilitated angioplasty strategy.

The Conduct of the Primary Angioplasty (Percutaneous Coronary Intervention) Procedure

A primary interventional strategy for reperfusion in myocardial infarction is a multidisciplinary institutional commitment. Precise protocols and standards should be imposed, including mechanisms for urgent transfer to the interventional center preferably after prehospital triage utilizing

12-lead electrocardiograms. This will allow mobilization of the reperfusion team. Upon hospital arrival, evaluation should proceed in a swift and thorough manner while infarct care is begun (including aspirin, heparin, and beta blockade or nitrates as appropriate). In the PAMI trials, patients treated with precatheterization beta blockade had fewer procedural complications and lower hospital mortality (1.8 percent versus 3.7 percent, $p = 0.0035$).[126] Assessment must include acknowledgment of factors that may influence the procedure (e.g., peripheral vascular disease, renal function) with early involvement of the interventional operator in this process.

ACC/AHA guidelines for performance of primary angioplasty at hospitals without cardiac surgery have been published.[83] The importance of a formalized transfer arrangement for urgent cardiac surgery and ongoing outcomes analysis should not be underestimated.[20] Operator experience in ongoing interventional practice at a surgery center is critical to program success. Efforts to minimize the treatment interval should be diligently pursued.

In the catheterization laboratory, ongoing intensive medical care must be provided. Comprehensive protocols provide a dedicated environment where events and complications are anticipated. In most circumstances, primary angioplasty is more complicated than an elective procedure. The operator must tailor the approach to the environment of acute infarction

Preparation of both femoral access sites is a facile precautionary step. Primary angioplasty can usually be performed utilizing 6 French (6F) guide catheters and familiar guidewires, but larger guide catheters may be needed to utilize thrombectomy or distal protection devices. Attention should be paid to collateral flow during initial angiography to guide intervention in the infarct artery. Angiography of the infarct vessel can be performed with the guide catheter. Care should be taken to maintain the guidewire in the main vessel with advancement through the occlusion. An appropriately sized balloon catheter should be positioned efficiently and inflated to allow early reperfusion. In most cases, stenting should follow balloon angioplasty of the culprit lesion. Although direct stenting without predilation has been proposed as a method to minimize embolization, this practice did not reduce no reflow in one study compared with conventional stenting techniques.[127]

Heparin anticoagulation should be monitored during the procedure and adjustments made reflecting the use of GP IIb/IIIa inhibition. Thienopyridines are necessary adjuncts to stent implantation, and in the PAMI trials administration of ticlopidine prior to angiography (in addition to standard heparin and aspirin) was associated with higher preintervention TIMI-3 flow rates (20.7 percent versus 11.4 percent, $p < 0.001$).[123] The role of direct thrombin inhibitors and primary angioplasty awaits further study

Thrombectomy and distal protection devices are being tested as routine adjuncts to catheter-based reperfusion in randomized trials. The current utilization of these devices is largely based upon the operator's judgment and experience. Angiographic morphology predictive of slow or no reflow includes "cutoff" occlusion, reference diameter greater than 4 mm, floating thrombus, persistent dye stasis distal to the obstruction, thrombus more than 5 mm proximal to the occlusion, or accumulated linear thrombus more than three times the reference diameter.[128] These findings might be utilized to define circumstances for effective use of thromboembolic protective devices.

Discovery of these predictors of impaired flow should promote the use of GP IIb/IIIa inhibition and consideration of other prophylactic pharmacological measures. Giri and colleagues[129] reported less no reflow with abciximab in a consecutive case series ($n = 650$). In patients who develop angiographic evidence of no reflow (TIMI flow grade ≤2) (see Table 48–4) after primary angioplasty, epicardial vessel complications such as dissection, a suboptimal result, or spasm must be excluded. Both intracoronary adenosine[110] and intravenous nicorandil[113] reduce no reflow when given before and after intervention. Intracoronary calcium channel blockers have been reported to be effective in attenuating microvascular dysfunction during myocardial infarction.[45] Intracoronary nitroprusside resulted in improved flow compared with verapamil in a review of 68 patients with no reflow.[130] In some cases, the onset of no reflow can result in profound hemodynamic deterioration. Intracoronary epinephrine has been utilized to improve flow significantly in patients with refractory no reflow and may be appropriate treatment in patients who are hypotensive.[131] These agents are preferably administered distally in the epicardial vessels. Despite favorable effects, no agent has clearly improved clinical outcomes.[130]

Multivessel disease is encountered in 40 to 75 percent of patients undergoing reperfusion therapy.[36,37,132] The conventional approach to the patient with multivessel disease has incorporated either urgent surgery, staged angioplasty, late surgery, or noninvasive evaluation after reperfusion. The advent of modern angioplasty technology has allowed consideration of multivessel revascularization at the time of the primary angioplasty procedure. This strategy seems a logical approach in the patient with cardiogenic shock, but it should be tested against emergency bypass surgery. In the hemodynamically stable patient, multivessel disease impairs recovery of left ventricular function.[133] Multiple complex coronary lesions have been identified in approximately 40 percent of patients with acute infarction and may reflect a systemic process (inflammation, deranged lipid metabolism) affecting widespread vulnerable plaques.[132] The presence of multiple complex plaques is associated with more recurrent ischemic events. Investigation examining multivessel angioplasty during the primary procedure is lacking. Small reports suggest mixed results, and randomized trials are needed to determine the optimal revascularization strategy for patients with multivessel disease.[134,135]

The benefits of rapid reperfusion are amplified in cardiogenic shock.[33,76] If prompt reperfusion is accomplished and the patient does not improve, mechanical complications should be considered utilizing hemodynamic, ventriculographic, or echocardiographic assessment.

Intraaortic balloon counterpulsation is a necessary adjunct during reperfusion therapy of the patient with cardiogenic shock.[33] Brodie and colleagues[136] reported a reduction of adverse catheterization laboratory events in high-risk infarct patients with cardiogenic shock, heart failure, or a low (<0.30) ejection fraction. Early studies of routine counterpulsation after primary angioplasty reported reduced reocclusion and improved ventricular function. However the PAMI-2 trial identified no reduction in the risk of reocclusion, reinfarction, or death or improved ventricular function with balloon pump support of hemodynamically stable high-risk patients.[137]

The interventional team is obligated to review outcomes and modify processes continually, incorporating advances derived from investigation in the dynamic field of reperfusion therapy.

Synopsis of the Primary Angioplasty Strategy

- In comparison with thrombolysis, a primary angioplasty strategy provides a greater chance for restoring blood flow and stabilization of the infarct artery. This method increases the population that can gain effective and safe reperfusion.
- The expanded latitude of temporal benefit for primary angioplasty may mitigate the logistical constraints of this approach.

- Stents enhance the durability of the procedure. Early administration of GP IIb/IIIa inhibitors may augment the results of primary stenting.
- There is considerable promise for evolution of the science of microcirculatory and myocardial protection during infarction.

The challenge ahead is to focus on early entry of the infarct patient into a triage process that can accelerate reperfusion. Local factors are likely to influence whether a primary, facilitated, or transfer procedure is the optimal strategy.

REFERENCES

1. O'Keefe JH Jr, Bailey WL, Rutherford BD, Hartzler GO: Primary angioplasty for acute myocardial infarction in 1,000 consecutive patients. Results in an unselected population and high-risk subgroups. Am J Cardiol 72:107G, 1993.
2. Every NR, Parsons LS, Hlatky M, et al: A comparison of thrombolytic therapy with primary coronary angioplasty for acute myocardial infarction. Myocardial Infarction Triage and Intervention Investigators. N Engl J Med 335:1253, 1996.
3. Tiefenbrunn AJ, Chandra NC, French WJ, et al: Clinical experience with primary percutaneous transluminal coronary angioplasty compared with alteplase (recombinant tissue-type plasminogen activator) in patients with acute myocardial infarction: A report from the Second National Registry of Myocardial Infarction (NRMI-2). J Am Coll Cardiol 31:1240, 1998.
4. Zahn R, Schiele R, Schneider S, et al: Primary angioplasty versus intravenous thrombolysis in acute myocardial infarction: Can we define subgroups of patients benefiting most from primary angioplasty? Results from the pooled data of the Maximal Individual Therapy in Acute Myocardial Infarction Registry and the Myocardial Infarction Registry. J Am Coll Cardiol 37:1827, 2001.
5. Zahn R, Schiele R, Schneider S, et al: Decreasing hospital mortality between 1994 and 1998 in patients with acute myocardial infarction treated with primary angioplasty but not in patients treated with intravenous thrombolysis. Results from the pooled data of the Maximal Individual Therapy in Acute Myocardial Infarction (MITRA) Registry and the Myocardial Infarction Registry (MIR). J Am Coll Cardiol 36:2064, 2000.

Randomized Trials Comparing Primary Angioplasty with Thrombolysis

6. Grines CL, Browne KF, Marco J, et al: A comparison of immediate angioplasty with thrombolytic therapy for acute myocardial infarction. The Primary Angioplasty in Myocardial Infarction Study Group. N Engl J Med 328:673, 1993.
7. Gibbons RJ, Holmes DR, Reeder GS, et al: Immediate angioplasty compared with the administration of a thrombolytic agent followed by conservative treatment for myocardial infarction. The Mayo Coronary Care Unit and Catheterization Laboratory Groups. N Engl J Med 328:685, 1993.
8. Zijlstra F, de Boer MJ, Hoorntje JC, et al: A comparison of immediate coronary angioplasty with intravenous streptokinase in acute myocardial infarction. N Engl J Med 328:680, 1993.
9. GUSTO IIb Angioplasty Substudy Investigators: A clinical trial comparing primary coronary angioplasty with tissue plasminogen activator for acute myocardial infarction. The Global Use of Strategies to Open Occluded Coronary Arteries in Acute Coronary Syndromes (GUSTO IIb) Angioplasty Substudy Investigators. N Engl J Med 336:1621, 1997.
10. Weaver WD, Simes RJ, Betriu A, et al: Comparison of primary coronary angioplasty and intravenous thrombolytic therapy for acute myocardial infarction: A quantitative review. JAMA 278:2093, 1997.
11. Grines C, Patel A, Zijlstra F, et al: Primary coronary angioplasty compared with intravenous thrombolytic therapy for acute myocardial infarction: Six-month follow up and analysis of individual patient data from randomized trials. Am Heart J 145:47, 2003.
12. Zijlstra F, Hoorntje JC, de Boer MJ, et al:. Long-term benefit of primary angioplasty as compared with thrombolytic therapy for acute myocardial infarction. N Engl J Med 341:1413, 1999.
13. Schomig A, Kastrati A, Dirschinger J, et al: Coronary stenting plus platelet glycoprotein IIb/IIIa blockade compared with tissue plasminogen activator in acute myocardial infarction. Stent versus Thrombolysis for Occluded Coronary Arteries in Patients with Acute Myocardial Infarction Study Investigators. N Engl J Med 343:385, 2000.
14. Bonnefoy E, Lapostolle F, Leizorovicz A, et al: Primary angioplasty versus prehospital fibrinolysis in acute myocardial infarction: A randomised study. Lancet 360:825, 2002.
15. Widimsky P, Groch L, Zelizko M, et al: Multicentre randomized trial comparing transport to primary angioplasty vs immediate thrombolysis vs combined strategy for patients with acute myocardial infarction presenting to a community hospital without a catheterization laboratory. The PRAGUE study. Eur Heart J 21:823, 2000.
16. Widimsky P, Budesinsky T, Vorac D, et al: Long distance transport for primary angioplasty vs immediate thrombolysis in acute myocardial infarction. Final results of the randomized national multicentre trial—PRAGUE-2. Eur Heart J 24:94, 2003.
17. Grines CL, Westerhausen DR Jr, Grines LL, et al: A randomized trial of transfer for primary angioplasty versus on-site thrombolysis in patients with high-risk myocardial infarction: The Air Primary Angioplasty in Myocardial Infarction study. J Am Coll Cardiol 39:1713, 2002.
18. Moon JC, Kalra PR, Coats AJ: DANAMI-2: Is primary angioplasty superior to thrombolysis in acute MI when the patient has to be transferred to an invasive centre? Int J Cardiol 85:199, 2002.
19. Zijlstra F: Angioplasty vs thrombolysis for acute myocardial infarction: A quantitative overview of the effects of interhospital transportation. Eur Heart J 24:21, 2003.
20. Aversano T, Aversano LT, Passamani E, et al: Thrombolytic therapy vs primary percutaneous coronary intervention for myocardial infarction in patients presenting to hospitals without on-site cardiac surgery: A randomized controlled trial. JAMA 287:1943, 2002.
21. Keeley EC, Boura JA, Grines CL: Primary angioplasty versus intravenous thrombolytic therapy for acute myocardial infarction: A quantitative review of 23 randomised trials. Lancet 361:13, 2003.
22. Zijlstra F, Beukema WP, van't Hof AW, et al: Randomized comparison of primary coronary angioplasty with thrombolytic therapy in low risk patients with acute myocardial infarction. J Am Coll Cardiol 29:908, 1997.
23. Ribeiro EE, Silva LA, Carneiro R, et al: Randomized trial of direct coronary angioplasty versus intravenous streptokinase in acute myocardial infarction. J Am Coll Cardiol 22:376, 1993.
24. Grinfeld L, Berrocal D, Belardi J, et al: Fibrinolytics vs. primary angioplasty in acute myocardial infarction (FAP). J Am Coll Cardiol 27:222A, 1996.
25. Dewood MA: Direct PTCA vs. intravenous t-Pa in acute myocardial infarction: Results from a prospective randomized trial. *In* The Thrombolysis and Interventional Therapy in Acute Myocardial Infarction Symposium VI. Washington, DC, George Washington University, 1990, pp 28-29.
26. Ribichini F, Steffenino G, Dellavalle A, et al: Comparison of thrombolytic therapy and primary coronary angioplasty with liberal stenting for inferior myocardial infarction with precordial ST-segment depression: Immediate and long-term results of a randomized study. J Am Coll Cardiol 32:1687, 1998.
27. Garcia E, Elizaga J, Perez-Castellano N, et al: Primary angioplasty versus systemic thrombolysis in anterior myocardial infarction. J Am Coll Cardiol 33:605, 1999.
28. Akhras F, Abu Ousa A, Swann G: Primary coronary angioplasty or intravenous thrombolysis for patients with acute myocardial infarction? Acute and late follow-up results in a new cardiac unit. J Am Coll Cardiol 29:A235, 1997.
29. de Boer MJ, Ottervanger JP, van't Hof AW, et al: Reperfusion therapy in elderly patients with acute myocardial infarction: A randomized comparison of primary angioplasty and thrombolytic therapy. J Am Coll Cardiol 39:1723, 2002.
30. Le May MR, Labinaz M, Davies RF, et al: Stenting versus thrombolysis in acute myocardial infarction trial (STAT). J Am Coll Cardiol 37:985, 2001.
31. Kastrati A, Mehilli J, Dirschinger J, et al: Myocardial salvage after coronary stenting plus abciximab versus fibrinolysis plus abciximab in patients with acute myocardial infarction: A randomised trial. Lancet 359:920, 2002.
32. Vermeer F, Oude Ophuis AJ, vd Berg EJ, et al: Prospective randomised comparison between thrombolysis, rescue PTCA, and primary PTCA in patients with extensive myocardial infarction admitted to a hospital without PTCA facilities: A safety and feasibility study. Heart 82:426, 1999.
33. Hochman JS, Sleeper LA, Webb JG, et al: Early revascularization in acute myocardial infarction complicated by cardiogenic shock. SHOCK Investigators. Should We Emergently Revascularize Occluded Coronaries for Cardiogenic Shock. N Engl J Med 341:625, 1999.
34. GUSTO Angiographic Investigators: The effects of tissue plasminogen activator, streptokinase, or both on coronary artery patency, ventricular function, and survival after acute myocardial infarction. N Engl J Med 329:1615, 1993.
35. Berger PB, Ellis SG, Holmes DR Jr, et al: Relationship between delay in performing direct coronary angioplasty and early clinical outcome in patients with acute myocardial infarction: Results from the global use of strategies to open occluded arteries in Acute Coronary Syndromes (GUSTO-IIb) trial. Circulation 100:14, 1999.
36. Grines CL, Cox DA, Stone GW, et al: Coronary angioplasty with or without stent implantation for acute myocardial infarction. Stent Primary Angioplasty in Myocardial Infarction Study Group. N Engl J Med 341:1949, 1999.
37. Stone GW, Grines CL, Cox DA, et al: Comparison of angioplasty with stenting, with or without abciximab, in acute myocardial infarction. N Engl J Med 346:957, 2002.
38. Antman EM, Giugliano RP, Gibson CM, et al: Abciximab facilitates the rate and extent of thrombolysis: Results of the thrombolysis in myocardial infarction (TIMI) 14 trial. The TIMI 14 Investigators. Circulation 99:2720, 1999.
39. ASSENT-3 Investigators: Efficacy and safety of tenecteplase in combination with enoxaparin, abciximab, or unfractionated heparin: The ASSENT-3 randomised trial in acute myocardial infarction. Lancet 358:605, 2001.
40. Lincoff AM, Califf RM, Van de Werf F, et al: Mortality at 1 year with combination platelet glycoprotein IIb/IIIa inhibition and reduced-dose fibrinolytic therapy vs conventional fibrinolytic therapy for acute myocardial infarction: GUSTO V randomized trial. JAMA 288:2130, 2002.
41. Roe MT, Ohman EM, Maas AC, et al: Shifting the open-artery hypothesis downstream: The quest for optimal reperfusion. J Am Coll Cardiol 37:9, 2001.
42. Gibson CM, Cannon CP, Daley WL, et al: TIMI frame count: A quantitative method of assessing coronary artery flow. Circulation 93:879, 1996.
43. Gibson CM, Cannon CP, Murphy SA, et al: Relationship of TIMI myocardial perfusion grade to mortality after administration of thrombolytic drugs. Circulation 101:125, 2000.
44. van 't Hof AW, Liem A, Suryapranata H, et al: Angiographic assessment of myocardial reperfusion in patients treated with primary angioplasty for acute myocardial infarction: Myocardial blush grade. Zwolle Myocardial Infarction Study Group. Circulation 97:2302, 1998.
45. Rezkalla SH, Kloner RA: No-reflow phenomenon. Circulation 105:656, 2002.
46. Verma S, Fedak PW, Weisel RD, et al: Fundamentals of reperfusion injury for the clinical cardiologist. Circulation 105:2332, 2002.
47. Agati L, Voci P, Hickle P, et al: Tissue-type plasminogen activator therapy versus primary coronary angioplasty: Impact on myocardial tissue perfusion and regional function 1 month after uncomplicated myocardial infarction. J Am Coll Cardiol 31:338, 1998.
48. Zeymer U, Schroder R, Neuhaus K: Primary PTCA accelerates myocardial reperfusion compared to thrombolysis in patients with acute myocardial infarction. Circulation 104:II-466, 2001.

49. Murakami T, Mizuno S, Takahashi Y, et al: Intracoronary aspiration thrombectomy for acute myocardial infarction. Am J Cardiol 82:839, 1998.
50. Llevadot J, Giugliano RP, McCabe CH, et al: Degree of residual stenosis in the culprit coronary artery after thrombolytic administration (Thrombolysis In Myocardial Infarction [TIMI] trials). Am J Cardiol 85:1409, 2000.
51. Veen G, de Boer MJ, Zijlstra F, Verheugt FW: Improvement in three-month angiographic outcome suggested after primary angioplasty for acute myocardial infarction (Zwolle trial) compared with successful thrombolysis (APRICOT trial). Antithrombotics in the Prevention of Reocclusion In COronary Thrombolysis. Am J Cardiol 84:763, 1999.
52. Brodie BR, Grines CL, Ivanhoe R, et al: Six-month clinical and angiographic follow-up after direct angioplasty for acute myocardial infarction. Final results from the Primary Angioplasty Registry. Circulation 90:156, 1994.
53. Grines CL, Cox DA, Stone GW, et al: Stent PAMI: 12 month results and predictors of mortality. J Am Coll Cardiol 35:402A, 2000.
54. Stone GW, Brodie BR, Griffin JJ, et al: Role of cardiac surgery in the hospital phase management of patients treated with primary angioplasty for acute myocardial infarction. Am J Cardiol 85:1292, 2000.
55. Grines CL, Marsalese DL, Brodie B, et al: Safety and cost-effectiveness of early discharge after primary angioplasty in low risk patients with acute myocardial infarction. PAMI-II Investigators. Primary Angioplasty in Myocardial Infarction. J Am Coll Cardiol 31:967, 1998.
56. Kinn JW, O'Neill WW, Benzuly KH, et al: Primary angioplasty reduces risk of myocardial rupture compared to thrombolysis for acute myocardial infarction. Cathet Cardiovasc Diagn 42:151, 1997.
57. Moreno R, Lopez-Sendon J, Garcia E, et al: Primary angioplasty reduces the risk of left ventricular free wall rupture compared with thrombolysis in patients with acute myocardial infarction. J Am Coll Cardiol 39:598, 2002.
58. Biostatistical Fact Sheet: Older Americans and Cardiovascular Diseases. Chicago, American Heart Association, 1998.
59. White HD: Thrombolytic therapy in the elderly. Lancet 356:2028, 2000.
60. Berger AK, Schulman KA, Gersh BJ, et al: Primary coronary angioplasty vs thrombolysis for the management of acute myocardial infarction in elderly patients. JAMA 282:341, 1999.
61. Thiemann DR, Coresh J, Schulman SP, et al: Lack of benefit for intravenous thrombolysis in patients with myocardial infarction who are older than 75 years. Circulation 101:2239, 2000.
62. O'Neill WW, De Boer MJ, Gibbons RJ, et al: Lessons from the pooled outcome of the PAMI, ZWOLLE, and Mayo Clinic randomized trials of primary angioplasty versus thrombolytic therapy of acute myocardial infarction. J Invasive Cardiol 10(Suppl A):4A, 1998.
63. Minai K, Horie H, Takahashi M, et al: Long-term outcome of primary percutaneous transluminal coronary angioplasty for low-risk acute myocardial infarction in patients older than 80 years: A single-center, open, randomized trial. Am Heart J 143:497, 2002.
64. Labinaz M, Sketch MH Jr, Ellis SG, et al: Outcome of acute ST-segment elevation myocardial infarction in patients with prior coronary artery bypass surgery receiving thrombolytic therapy. Am Heart J 141:469, 2001.
65. Peterson LR, Chandra NC, French WJ, et al: Reperfusion therapy in patients with acute myocardial infarction and prior coronary artery bypass graft surgery (National Registry of Myocardial Infarction-2). Am J Cardiol 84:1287, 1999.
66. Al Suwaidi J, Velianou JL, Berger PB, et al: Primary percutaneous coronary interventions in patients with acute myocardial infarction and prior coronary artery bypass grafting. Am Heart J 142:452, 2001.
67. Nguyen TT, O'Neill WW, Dixon SR, et al: Poor one year prognosis in acute myocardial infarction patients with saphenous vein grafts as the infarct related vessel treated by primary balloon angioplasty. J Am Coll Cardiol 39:309A, 2002.
68. Mattos L, Sousa A, Neto CC, et al: Primary stenting versus balloon PTCA for the treatment of acute vein graft occlusion in myocardial infarction: In-hospital results from the Brazilian Coronary Interventional Registry (CENIC). J Am Coll Cardiol 35:39A, 2000.
69. Eagle KA, Goodman SG, Avezum A, et al: Practice variation and missed opportunities for reperfusion in ST-segment-elevation myocardial infarction: Findings from the Global Registry of Acute Coronary Events (GRACE). Lancet 359:373, 2002.
70. Zahn R, Schuster S, Schiele R, et al: Comparison of primary angioplasty with conservative therapy in patients with acute myocardial infarction and contraindications for thrombolytic therapy. Maximal Individual Therapy in Acute Myocardial Infarction (MITRA) Study Group. Catheter Cardiovasc Interv 46:127, 1999.
71. Juliard JM, Himbert D, Golmard JL, et al: Can we provide reperfusion therapy to all unselected patients admitted with acute myocardial infarction? J Am Coll Cardiol 30:157, 1997.
72. Lane GE, Holmes DR: The modern strategy for cardiogenic shock. *In* Cannon CP (ed): Management of Acute Coronary Syndromes. Totowa, NJ, Humana Press, 2003, pp 603-52.
73. Barron HV, Every NR, Parsons LS, et al: The use of intra-aortic balloon counterpulsation in patients with cardiogenic shock complicating acute myocardial infarction: Data from the National Registry of Myocardial Infarction 2. Am Heart J 141:933, 2001.
74. Hochman JS, Sleeper LA, White HD, et al: One-year survival following early revascularization for cardiogenic shock. JAMA 285:190, 2001.
75. Dzavik V, Sleeper LA, Hosat S, et al: Effect of age on treatment and outcome of patients in cardiogenic shock. Eur Heart J 19:28, 1998.
76. Brodie BR, Stuckey TD, Muncy DB, et al: Importance of time-to-reperfusion in patients with acute myocardial infarction with and without cardiogenic shock treated with primary percutaneous coronary intervention. Am Heart J 145:708, 2003.
77. Newby LK, Rutsch WR, Califf RM, et al: Time from symptom onset to treatment and outcomes after thrombolytic therapy. GUSTO-1 Investigators. J Am Coll Cardiol 27:1646, 1996.
78. Cannon CP, Gibson CM, Lambrew CT, et al: Relationship of symptom-onset-to-balloon time and door-to-balloon time with mortality in patients undergoing angioplasty for acute myocardial infarction. JAMA 283:2941, 2000.
79. Brodie BR, Stuckey TD, Wall TC, et al: Importance of time to reperfusion for 30-day and late survival and recovery of left ventricular function after primary angioplasty for acute myocardial infarction. J Am Coll Cardiol 32:1312, 1998.
80. Zijlstra F, Patel A, Jones M, et al: Clinical characteristics and outcome of patients with early (<2 h), intermediate (2-4 h) and late (>4 h) presentation treated by primary coronary angioplasty or thrombolytic therapy for acute myocardial infarction. Eur Heart J 23:550, 2002.
81. Milavetz JJ, Giebel DW, Christian TF, et al: Time to therapy and salvage in myocardial infarction. J Am Coll Cardiol 31:1246, 1998.
82. Bode C, Smalling RW, Berg G, et al: Randomized comparison of coronary thrombolysis achieved with double-bolus reteplase (recombinant plasminogen activator) and front-loaded, accelerated alteplase (recombinant tissue plasminogen activator) in patients with acute myocardial infarction. The RAPID II Investigators. Circulation 94:891, 1996.
83. Smith SC Jr, Dove JT, Jacobs AK, et al: ACC/AHA guidelines of percutaneous coronary interventions (revision of the 1993 PTCA guidelines)—Executive summary. A report of the American College of Cardiology/American Heart Association Task Force on Practice Guidelines (committee to revise the 1993 guidelines for percutaneous transluminal coronary angioplasty). J Am Coll Cardiol 37:2215, 2001.
84. Magid DJ, Calonge BN, Rumsfeld JS, et al: Relation between hospital primary angioplasty volume and mortality for patients with acute MI treated with primary angioplasty vs thrombolytic therapy. JAMA 284:3131, 2000.
85. Vakili BA, Kaplan R, Brown DL: Volume-outcome relation for physicians and hospitals performing angioplasty for acute myocardial infarction in New York state. Circulation 104:2171, 2001.

Modern Catheter-Based Reperfusion Techniques

86. Neumann FJ, Blasini R, Schmitt C, et al: Effect of glycoprotein IIb/IIIa receptor blockade on recovery of coronary flow and left ventricular function after the placement of coronary-artery stents in acute myocardial infarction. Circulation 98:2695, 1998.
87. Brener SJ, Barr LA, Burchenal JE, et al: Randomized, placebo-controlled trial of platelet glycoprotein IIb/IIIa blockade with primary angioplasty for acute myocardial infarction. ReoPro and Primary PTCA Organization and Randomized Trial (RAPPORT) Investigators. Circulation 98:734, 1998.
88. Montalescot G, Barragan P, Wittenberg O, et al: Platelet glycoprotein IIb/IIIa inhibition with coronary stenting for acute myocardial infarction. N Engl J Med 344:1895, 2001.
89. Grines CL, Brodie BR, Griffin J, et al: Which primary PTCA patients may benefit form new technologies? Circulation 92:I-146, 1995.
90. Stone GW, Brodie BR, Griffin JJ, et al: Prospective, multicenter study of the safety and feasibility of primary stenting in acute myocardial infarction: In-hospital and 30-day results of the PAMI stent pilot trial. Primary Angioplasty in Myocardial Infarction Stent Pilot Trial Investigators. J Am Coll Cardiol 31:23, 1998.
91. Antoniucci D, Santoro GM, Bolognese L, et al: A clinical trial comparing primary stenting of the infarct-related artery with optimal primary angioplasty for acute myocardial infarction: Results from the Florence Randomized Elective Stenting in Acute Coronary Occlusions (FRESCO) trial. J Am Coll Cardiol 31:1234, 1998.
92. Suryapranata H, van't Hof AW, Hoorntje JC, et al: Randomized comparison of coronary stenting with balloon angioplasty in selected patients with acute myocardial infarction. Circulation 97:2502, 1998.
93. Saito S, Hosokawa G, Tanaka S, Nakamura S: Primary stent implantation is superior to balloon angioplasty in acute myocardial infarction: Final results of the primary angioplasty versus stent implantation in acute myocardial infarction (PASTA) trial. PASTA Trial Investigators. Catheter Cardiovasc Interv 48:262, 1999.
94. Rodriguez A, Bernardi V, Fernandez M, et al: In-hospital and late results of coronary stents versus conventional balloon angioplasty in acute myocardial infarction (GRAMI trial). Gianturco-Roubin in Acute Myocardial Infarction. Am J Cardiol 81:1286, 1998.
95. Maillard L, Hamon M, Khalife K, et al: A comparison of systematic stenting and conventional balloon angioplasty during primary percutaneous transluminal coronary angioplasty for acute myocardial infarction. STENTIM-2 Investigators. J Am Coll Cardiol 35:1729, 2000.
96. Kawashima A, Ueda K, Nishida Y, et al: Quantitative angiographic analysis of restenosis of primary stenting using the Wiktor stent for acute myocardial infarction: Results of the multicenter randomized PRISAM study. Circulation 100:I-856, 1999.
97. Scheller B, Hennen B, Severin-Kneib S, et al: Long-term follow-up of a randomized study of primary stenting versus angioplasty in acute myocardial infarction. Am J Med 110:1, 2001.
98. Zhu MM, Feit A, Chadow H, et al: Primary stent implantation compared with primary balloon angioplasty for acute myocardial infarction: A meta-analysis of randomized clinical trials. Am J Cardiol 88:297, 2001.
99. Henriques JP, Zijlstra F, Ottervanger JP, et al: Incidence and clinical significance of distal embolization during primary angioplasty for acute myocardial infarction. Eur Heart J 23:1112, 2002.
100. Kaplan BM, Larkin T, Safian RD, et al: Prospective study of extraction atherectomy in patients with acute myocardial infarction. Am J Cardiol 78:383, 1996.
101. Rosenschein H, Hertz I, Tenebaum-Koren E, et al: Coronary ultrasound thrombolysis in acute myocardial infarction: Results from the acute study. J Am Coll Cardiol 31:192A, 1998.
102. Silva JA, Ramee SR, Cohen DJ, et al: Rheolytic thrombectomy during percutaneous revascularization for acute myocardial infarction: Experience with the AngioJet catheter. Am Heart J 141:353, 2001.
103. Taghizadeh B, Chiu JA, Papaleo R, et al: AngioJet thrombectomy and stenting for reperfusion in acute MI complicated with cardiogenic shock. Catheter Cardiovasc Interv 57:79, 2002.
104. Silva JA, White CJ, Ramee SR, et al: Treatment of coronary stent thrombosis with rheolytic thrombectomy: Results from a multicenter experience. Catheter Cardiovasc Interv 58:11, 2003.

105. Napodano M, Reimers B, Pasquetto G, et al: Intracoronary thrombectomy improves myocardial perfusion in patients undergoing direct angioplasty: A single center randomized study. J Am Coll Cardiol 41:357A, 2003.
106. van Ommen V, Michels R, Heymen E, et al: Usefulness of the rescue PT catheter to remove fresh thrombus from coronary arteries and bypass grafts in acute myocardial infarction. Am J Cardiol 88:306, 2001.
107. Belli G, Pezzano A, De Biase AM, et al: Adjunctive thrombus aspiration and mechanical protection from distal embolization in primary percutaneous intervention for acute myocardial infarction. Catheter Cardiovasc Interv 50:362, 2000.
108. Zeymer U, Suryapranata H, Monassier JP, et al: The Na(+)/H(+) exchange inhibitor eniporide as an adjunct to early reperfusion therapy for acute myocardial infarction. Results of the evaluation of the safety and cardioprotective effects of eniporide in acute myocardial infarction (ESCAMI) trial. J Am Coll Cardiol 38:1644, 2001.
109. Faxon DP, Gibbons RJ, Chronos NA, et al: The effect of blockade of the CD11/CD18 integrin receptor on infarct size in patients with acute myocardial infarction treated with direct angioplasty: The results of the HALT-MI study. J Am Coll Cardiol 40:1199, 2002.
110. Marzilli M, Orsini E, Marraccini P, Testa R: Beneficial effects of intracoronary adenosine as an adjunct to primary angioplasty in acute myocardial infarction. Circulation 101:2154, 2000.
111. Ross AM, Gibbons RJ, Kloner RA, et al: Acute myocardial infarction study of adenosine (AMISTAD II). J Am Coll Cardiol 39:338A, 2002.
112. Mahaffey KW, Puma JA, Barbagelata NA, et al: Adenosine as an adjunct to thrombolytic therapy for acute myocardial infarction: Results of a multicenter, randomized, placebo-controlled trial: The Acute Myocardial Infarction STudy of ADenosine (AMISTAD) trial. J Am Coll Cardiol 34:1711, 1999.
113. Ito H, Taniyama Y, Iwakura K, et al: Intravenous nicorandil can preserve microvascular integrity and myocardial viability in patients with reperfused anterior wall myocardial infarction. J Am Coll Cardiol 33:654, 1999.
114. Granger C: Complement and Reduction of Infarct Size after Angioplasty or Lytics (CARDINAL) Trials. Chicago, American Heart Association, 2002.
115. Dixon SR, Bartorelli AL, Marcovitz PA, et al: Initial experience with hyperoxemic reperfusion after primary angioplasty for acute myocardial infarction: Results of a pilot study utilizing intracoronary aqueous oxygen therapy. J Am Coll Cardiol 39:387, 2002.
116. Dixon SR, Whitbourn RJ, Dae MW, et al: Induction of mild systemic hypothermia with endovascular cooling during primary percutaneous coronary intervention for acute myocardial infarction. J Am Coll Cardiol 40:1928, 2002.
117. Gibson CM, Cannon CP, Greene RM, et al: Rescue angioplasty in the thrombolysis in myocardial infarction (TIMI) 4 trial. Am J Cardiol 80:21, 1997.
118. Ellis SG, Da Silva ER, Spaulding CM, et al: Review of immediate angioplasty after fibrinolytic therapy for acute myocardial infarction: Insights from the RESCUE I, RESCUE II, and other contemporary clinical experiences. Am Heart J 139:1046, 2000.
119. Dauerman HL, Prpic R, Andreou C, et al: Angiographic and clinical outcomes after rescue coronary stenting. Catheter Cardiovasc Interv 50:269, 2000.
120. Petronio AS, Musumeci G, Limbruno U, et al: Abciximab improves 6-month clinical outcome after rescue coronary angioplasty. Am Heart J 143:334, 2002.
121. French JK, Ramanathan K, Stewart JT, et al: A score predicts failure of reperfusion after fibrinolytic therapy for acute myocardial infarction. Am Heart J 145:508, 2003.
122. Schweiger MJ, Cannon CP, Murphy SA, et al: Early coronary intervention following pharmacologic therapy for acute myocardial infarction (the combined TIMI 10B-TIMI 14 experience). Am J Cardiol 88:831, 2001.
123. Stone GW, Cox D, Garcia E, et al: Normal flow (TIMI-3) before mechanical reperfusion therapy is an independent determinant of survival in acute myocardial infarction: Analysis from the primary angioplasty in myocardial infarction trials. Circulation 104:636, 2001.
124. Ross AM, Coyne KS, Reiner JS, et al: A randomized trial comparing primary angioplasty with a strategy of short-acting thrombolysis and immediate planned rescue angioplasty in acute myocardial infarction: The PACT trial. PACT investigators. Plasminogen-activator Angioplasty Compatibility Trial. J Am Coll Cardiol 34:1954, 1999.
125. Herrmann HC, Moliterno DJ, Ohman EM, et al: Facilitation of early percutaneous coronary intervention after reteplase with or without abciximab in acute myocardial infarction: Results from the SPEED (GUSTO-4 Pilot) Trial. J Am Coll Cardiol 36:1489, 2000.
126. Harjai KJ, Stone GW, Boura J, et al: Effects of prior beta-blocker therapy on clinical outcomes after primary coronary angioplasty for acute myocardial infarction. Am J Cardiol 91:655, 2002.
127. Sabatier R, Hamon M, Zhao QM, et al: Could direct stenting reduce no-reflow in acute coronary syndromes? A randomized pilot study. Am Heart J 143:1027, 2002.
128. Yip HK, Chen MC, Chang HW, et al: Angiographic morphologic features of infarct-related arteries and timely reperfusion in acute myocardial infarction: Predictors of slow-flow and no-reflow phenomenon. Chest 122:1322, 2002.
129. Giri S, Mitchel JF, Hirst JA, et al: Synergy between intracoronary stenting and abciximab in improving angiographic and clinical outcomes of primary angioplasty in acute myocardial infarction. Am J Cardiol 86:269, 2000.
130. Resnic FS, Wainstein M, Lee MK, et al: No-reflow is an independent predictor of death and myocardial infarction after percutaneous coronary intervention. Am Heart J 145:42 2003.
131. Skelding KA, Goldstein JA, Mehta L, et al: Resolution of refractory no-reflow with intracoronary epinephrine. Catheter Cardiovasc Interv 57:305, 2002.
132. Goldstein JA, Demetriou D, Grines CL, et al: Multiple complex coronary plaques in patients with acute myocardial infarction. N Engl J Med 343:915, 2000.
133. Dambrink JE, van der Schaaf RJ, Hoorntje JC, et al: Impact of multivessel disease on recovery of left ventricular function after primary angioplasty for acute myocardial infarction. J Am Coll Cardiol 41:389A, 2003.
134. Denklas AE, Orford JL, Fasseas P, et al: Multivessel percutaneous intervention for ST-segment elevation myocardial infarction: The Mayo Clinic experience. J Am Coll Cardiol 41:324A, 2003.
135. Roe MT, Cura FA, Joski PS, et al: Initial experience with multivessel percutaneous coronary intervention during mechanical reperfusion for acute myocardial infarction. Am J Cardiol 88:170, 2001.
136. Brodie BR, Stuckey TD, Hansen C, Muncy D: Intra-aortic balloon counterpulsation before primary percutaneous transluminal coronary angioplasty reduces catheterization laboratory events in high-risk patients with acute myocardial infarction. Am J Cardiol 84:18, 1999.
137. Stone GW, Marsalese D, Brodie BR, et al: A prospective, randomized evaluation of prophylactic intraaortic balloon counterpulsation in high risk patients with acute myocardial infarction treated with primary angioplasty. Second Primary Angioplasty in Myocardial Infarction (PAMI-II) Trial Investigators. J Am Coll Cardiol 29:1459, 1997.

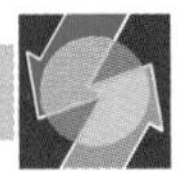

GUIDELINES *Thomas H. Lee*

Primary Percutaneous Coronary Intervention in Acute Myocardial Infarction

The American College of Cardiology and American Heart Association (ACC/AHA) updated comprehensive guidelines on percutaneous coronary interventions (PCIs) in 2001.[1] These guidelines included recommendations regarding several specific issues relevant to primary PCI. These issues were also addressed in prior ACC/AHA guidelines on acute myocardial infarction[2] and unstable angina.[3,4] The PCI guidelines use the ACC/AHA classification system for the indications (class I for generally accepted indications, class IIa when indications are controversial but the weight of evidence is supportive, class IIb when usefulness or efficacy is less well established, and class III when there is a consensus against the usefulness of the intervention). The updated guidelines use a convention for rating levels of evidence upon which recommendations have been based. *Level A* recommendations were derived from data from multiple randomized clinical trials, *level B* recommendations were derived from a single randomized trial or nonrandomized studies, and *level C* recommendations were based upon the consensus opinion of experts.

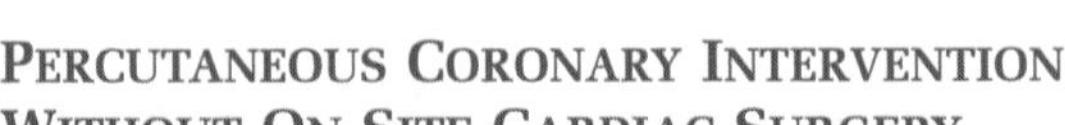

Percutaneous Coronary Intervention Without On-Site Cardiac Surgery

The guidelines note that the use of cardiac surgical backup for PCI has become less formal because of low rates of use and that some institutions use "off-site surgical backup." However, the guidelines note the greater risk associated with emergent PCI and describe specific volume thresholds for hospitals providing this service without cardiac surgical backup. The guidelines stipulate that the operators must be experienced interventionalists who regularly perform at least 75 elective PCI cases per year at a surgical center and that the institution must perform a minimum of 36 primary PCI procedures per year. The guidelines also stipulate that the procedure should be limited to patients with ST segment elevation myocardial infarction (MI) or new left bundle branch block on electrocardiography and done in a timely fashion (balloon inflation within 90 ± 30 minutes of admission). The laboratory must have written protocols in place for immediate (within 1 hour) transfer of patients to the nearest cardiac surgical facility.

Primary Percutaneous Coronary Intervention Versus Thrombolysis for Acute Transmural Myocardial Infarction

The ACC/AHA guidelines support use of PCI as an alternative to thrombolysis for acute MI (AMI) with ST segment elevation or new or presumed left bundle branch block within the first 12 hours after the onset of symptoms and afterward if such symptoms continue. As already noted, the guidelines define a performance standard for the average time from admission to balloon inflation of 90 ± 30 minutes and stipulate that the PCI should be performed by experienced operators and high-volume facilities (Table 48G–1). PCI is endorsed for a longer period (up to 36 hours after the onset of infarction) for patients who present in cardiogenic shock if the patients are younger than 75 years and the procedure can be performed within 18 hours of the onset of shock.

The guidelines do not support use of PCI for non-infarct-related arteries at the time of AMI and for patients who are asymptomatic after receiving fibrinolytic therapy within 12 hours.

Percutaneous Coronary Intervention After Thrombolysis

Coronary angiography and PCI are commonly performed after thrombolysis even though this strategy has not been studied extensively in clinical trials. Therefore, the ACC/AHA guidelines support relatively conservative use of angiography and PCI for patients after thrombolysis (Table 48G–2). PCI is considered appropriate for patients with objective evidence of recurrent infarction or ischemia and is also given support for patients with cardiogenic shock or hemodynamic instability. However, PCI is not considered routinely appropriate for patients who have successful or unsuccessful thrombolysis.

TABLE 48G–1 ACC/AHA Guidelines for Primary Percutaneous Coronary Intervention for Patients with Acute Transmural Myocardial Infarction as an Alternative to Thrombolysis

Class	Indication	Level of Evidence
Class I (indicated)	As an alternative to thrombolytic therapy in patients with AMI and ST segment elevation or new or presumed new left bundle branch block who can undergo angioplasty of the infarct artery <12 hr from the onset of ischemic symptoms or >12 hr if symptoms persist, if performed in a timely fashion (performance standard: balloon inflation within 90 ± 30 min of hospital admission) by individuals skilled in the procedure* and supported by experienced personnel in an appropriate laboratory environment.†	A
	In patients who are within 36 hr of an acute ST elevation/Q wave or new left bundle branch block MI who develop cardiogenic shock, are younger than 75 yr, and revascularization can be performed within 18 hr of the onset of shock by individuals skilled in the procedure* and supported by experienced personnel in an appropriate laboratory environment.†	A
Class IIa (good supportive evidence)	As a reperfusion strategy in candidates who have a contraindication to thrombolytic therapy.	C
Class IIb (weak supportive evidence)		
Class III (not indicated)	Elective PCI of a non–infarct-related artery at the time of acute MI (*level of evidence: C*).	C
	In patients with acute MI who Have received fibrinolytic therapy within 12 hr and have no symptoms of myocardial ischemia. Are eligible for thrombolytic therapy and are undergoing primary angioplasty by an inexperienced operator (individual who performs <75 PCI procedures per year). Are beyond 12 hr after onset of symptoms and have no evidence of myocardial ischemia.	C

ACC/AHA = American College of Cardiology/American Heart Association; AMI = acute myocardial infarction; MI = myocardial infarction; PCI = percutaneous coronary intervention.
*Individuals who perform at least 75 PCI procedures per year.
†Centers that perform at least 200 PCI procedures per year and have cardiac surgical capability.

TABLE 48G–2 ACC/AHA Guidelines for Percutaneous Coronary Intervention After Thrombolysis

Class	Indication	Level of Evidence
Class I (indicated)	Objective evidence for recurrent infarction or ischemia (rescue PCI)	B
Class IIa (good supportive evidence)	Cardiogenic shock or hemodynamic instability	B
Class IIb (weak supportive evidence)	Recurrent angina without objective evidence of ischemia or infarction (*level of evidence: C*)	C
	Angioplasty of the infarct-related artery stenosis within hours to days (48 hr) following successful thrombolytic therapy in asymptomatic patients without clinical and/or inducible evidence of ischemia	B
Class III (not indicated)	Routine PCI within 48 hr following failed thrombolysis	B
	Routine PCI of the infarct artery stenosis immediately after thrombolytic therapy	A

ACC/AHA = American College of Cardiology /American Heart Association; PCI = percutaneous coronary intervention.

TABLE 48G–3 ACC/AHA Guidelines for Percutaneous Coronary Intervention (PCI) During Subsequent Hospital Management After Acute Therapy for Acute Myocardial Infarction Including Primary PCI

Class	Indication	Level of Evidence
Class I (indicated)	Spontaneous or provocable myocardial ischemia during recovery from infarction	C
	Persistent hemodynamic instability	C
Class IIa (good supportive evidence)	Patients with LV ejection fraction <0.4, CHF, or serious ventricular arrhythmias	C
Class IIb (weak supportive evidence)	Coronary angiography and angioplasty for an occluded infarct-related artery in an otherwise stable patient to revascularize that artery (open artery hypothesis)	C
	All patients after a non-Q-wave MI	C
	Clinical HF during the acute episode but subsequent demonstration of preserved LV function (LV ejection fraction >0.4)	C
Class III (not indicated)	PCI of the infarct-related artery within 48 to 72 hr after thrombolytic therapy without evidence of spontaneous or provocable ischemia	C

ACC/AHA = American College of Cardiology/American Heart Association; CHF = congestive heart failure; HF = heart failure; LV = left ventricular; MI = myocardial infarction.

Percutaneous Coronary Intervention Later During Hospitalization

The guidelines support use of PCI after the immediate treatment of AMI in reaction to clinical evidence of ischemia and for persistent hemodynamic instability (Table 48G–3). The ACC/AHA task force did not provide much support for use of PCI for routine care of patients who were clinically stable. However, the Treat Angina with Aggrastat and determine Cost of Therapy with an Invasive or Conservative Strategy–Thrombolysis in Myocardial Infarction 18 (TACTICS-TIMI 18) trial, which demonstrated clinical benefit from an early invasive strategy for patients with unstable angina or AMI without ST segment elevation,[5] had been presented only as an abstract at the time the guidelines were written. Thus, future revisions of these guidelines may support a lower threshold for use of PCI after AMI.

References

1. Smith SC Jr, Dove JT, Jacobs AK, et al: ACC/AHA guidelines for percutaneous coronary intervention: A report of the American College of Cardiology/American Heart Association Task Force on Practice Guidelines (Committee to Revise the 1993 Guidelines for Percutaneous Transluminal Coronary Angioplasty). J Am Coll Cardiol 37:2239i, 2001.
2. Ryan TJ, Antman EM, Brooks NH, et al: 1999 update: ACC/AHA guidelines for the management of patients with acute myocardial infarction: Executive summary and recommendations: A report of the American College of Cardiology/American Heart Association Task Force on Practice Guidelines (Committee on Management of Acute Myocardial Infarction). J Am Coll Cardiol 34:890, 1999.
3. Braunwald E, Antman EM, Beasley JW, et al: ACC/AHA guidelines for the management of patients with unstable angina and non-ST-segment elevation myocardial infarction: A report of the American College of Cardiology/American Heart Association Task Force on Practice Guidelines (Committee on the Management of Patients With Unstable Angina). J Am Coll Cardiol 36:970, 2000.
4. Braunwald E, Antman EM, Beasley JW, et al: ACC/AHA 2002 guideline update for the management of patients with unstable angina and non-ST-segment elevation myocardial infarction: Summary article: A report of the American College of Cardiology/American Heart Association Task Force on Practice Guidelines (Committee on the Management of Patients With Unstable Angina). Circulation 106:1893, 2002.
5. Cannon CP, Weinstraub WS, Demopoulos LA, et al: Comparison of early invasive and conservative strategies in patients with unstable coronary syndromes treated with the glycoprotein IIb/IIIa inhibitor tirofiban. N Engl J Med 344:1879, 2001.

CHAPTER 49

Unstable Angina and Non-ST Elevation Myocardial Infarction

Christopher P. Cannon • Eugene Braunwald

Current estimates are that 1.7 million patients with acute coronary syndromes (ACSs) are admitted each year to hospitals in the United States (see Fig. 46–1).[1] Of these, only one-quarter present with acute myocardial infarction (MI) associated with electrocardiographic ST segment elevation (Chaps. 46 and 47); three-quarters, or approximately 1.4 million patients, have unstable angina or non-ST elevation myocardial infarction (UA/NSTEMI).[1] The former is most commonly caused by acute total thrombotic occlusion of a coronary artery and urgent reperfusion is the mainstay of therapy, whereas UA/NSTEMI is usually associated with severe coronary obstruction but not total occlusion of the culprit coronary artery.[2] Among patients with UA/NSTEMI, between 40 and 60 percent have evidence of myocardial necrosis with elevated troponin.[3]

Definition and Classification

DEFINITION. The definition of unstable angina is largely based on the clinical presentation (see Chap. 45). *Stable* angina pectoris is characterized by a deep, poorly localized chest or arm discomfort (rarely described as pain) that is reproducibly associated with physical exertion or emotional stress and relieved within 5 to 15 minutes by rest or sublingual nitroglycerin, or both. In contrast, *unstable* angina is defined as angina pectoris (or equivalent type of ischemic discomfort) with at least one of three features: (1) occurring at rest (or with minimal exertion) and usually lasting more than 20 minutes (if not interrupted by nitroglycerin), (2) being severe and described as frank pain and of new onset (i.e., within 1 month), and (3) occurring with a crescendo pattern (i.e., more severe, prolonged, or frequent than previously).[4] Some patients with this pattern of ischemic discomfort, especially those with prolonged rest pain, develop evidence of myocardial necrosis on the basis of cardiac serum markers (such as creatine kinase muscle-brain fraction [CK-MB] or troponin T or I, or both) and thus have a diagnosis of NSTEMI.

CLASSIFICATION. Because UA/NSTEMI comprises such a heterogeneous group of patients, classification schemes based on clinical features are useful. A clinical classification of UA/NSTEMI (Table 49–1)[5,6] has been found to be a useful means of stratifying risk.[7] Patients are divided into three groups according to the clinical circumstances of the acute ischemic episode: primary unstable angina, secondary angina (e.g., with angina related to obvious precipitating factors such as anemia, infection, or cardiac arrhythmias), and post-MI angina. Patients are also classified according to the severity of the ischemia (acute rest pain, subacute rest pain, or new-onset severe angina). This classification has been shown to be predictive of coronary thrombus at angiography or in atherectomy specimens and in determination of prognosis.[6,7]

Because UA/NSTEMI is a clinical syndrome rather than a specific disease (much like hypertension rather than pneumococcal pneumonia), an etiological approach has been proposed.[8] There are five pathophysiological processes that may contribute to the development of UA/NSTEMI (Fig. 49–1). These are (1) plaque rupture or erosion with superimposed nonocclusive thrombus (by far the most common cause of UA/NSTEMI), (2) dynamic obstruction (i.e., coronary spasm of an epicardial artery, as in Prinzmetal angina [see Prinzmetal (Variant) Angina] or constriction of the small muscular coronary arteries), (3) progressive mechanical obstruction, (4) inflammation or infection or both, and (5) secondary unstable angina, related to increased myocardial oxygen demand or decreased supply (e.g., anemia). Individual patients may have several of these processes coexisting as the cause of their episode of UA/NSTEMI. Use of this etiological approach may help refine the diagnostic approach and help target therapeutic strategies to treat the underlying disease that precipitated the episode of UA/NSTEMI. As noted later (see Risk Stratification), several new serum markers have been shown to be effective tools in identifying these pathophysiological processes and in predicting outcome; this approach is evolving into a "multimarker strategy" for evaluation and risk stratification (Fig. 49–2; see Fig. 49–10).[9]

Pathophysiology

The pathophysiology of UA/NSTEMI involves a broad time line with three phases rather than an isolated ischemic event. Traditionally, focus had been only on the acute phase of UA/NSTEMI, whereas the true pathophysiology actually spans two or more decades before the acute clinical event and then may span more than 20 years afterward. The acute event, which usually involves thrombus formation at the site of a ruptured or eroded atherosclerotic plaque, is the clinical manifestation of a generalized and progressive disease, currently referred to as *atherothrombosis* (see Chap. 35). This new term has emerged in place of atherosclerosis because it more fully describes the pathophysiology of the disease, in which there is both progression of the atheroma (e.g., cholesterol plaque development) and disruption of the plaque with superimposed thrombosis. Thus, the full pathophysiology of an ACS event can be divided into three phases: (1) the development of the unstable plaque that ruptures, (2) the acute ischemic event, and (3) the long-term risk of recurrent coronary events that remains after the acute event. As noted in Chapter 35, inflammation can play a major role in causing plaque instability, with inflammatory cells

TABLE 49–1 Braunwald Clinical Classification of Unstable Angina or Non-ST Elevation Myocardial Infarction

Class	Definition	Death or Myocardial Infarction 1 Year* (%)
Severity		
Class I	New onset of severe angina or accelerated angina; no rest pain	7.3
Class II	Angina at rest within past month but not within preceding 48 hr (angina at rest, subacute)	10.3
Class III	Angina at rest within 48 hr (angina at rest, subacute)	10.8†
Clinical circumstances		
A (secondary angina)	Develops in the presence of extracardiac condition that intensifies myocardial ischemia	14.1
B (primary angina)	Develops in the absence of extracardiac condition	8.5
C (postinfarction angina)	Develops within 2 wks after acute myocardial infarction	18.5‡
Intensity of treatment	Patients with unstable angina may also be divided into three groups depending on whether unstable angina occurs (1) in the absence of treatment for chronic stable angina, (2) during treatment for chronic stable angina, or (3) despite maximal antiischemic drug therapy. The three groups may be designated by subscripts 1, 2, and 3, respectively.	
Electrocardiographic changes	Patients with unstable angina may be further divided into those with or without transient ST-T wave changes during pain.	

*Data from TIMI III Registry: Scirica BM, Cannon CP, McCabe CH, et al, for the Thrombolysis In Myocardial Ischemia III Registry Investigators: Prognosis in the Thrombolysis in Myocardial Ischemia III Registry according to the Braunwald unstable angina pectoris classification. Am J Cardiol 90:821, 2002.
†$p = 0.057$.
‡$p < 0.001$.
From Braunwald E: Unstable angina: A classification. Circulation 80:410, 1989.

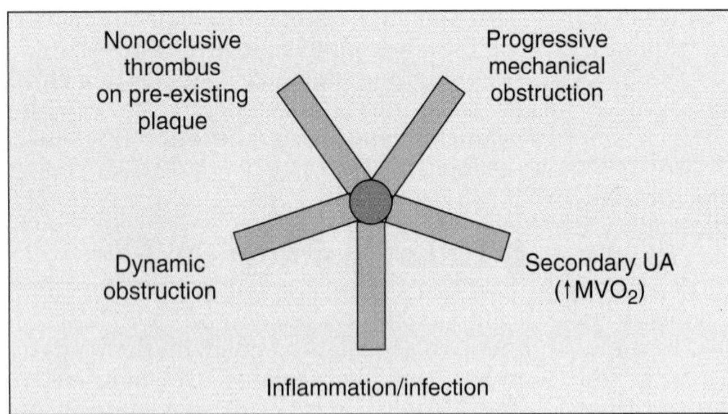

FIGURE 49–1 Schematic representation of the causes of unstable angina (UA). MVO_2 = myocardial O_2 consumption. (From Braunwald E: Unstable angina: An etiologic approach to management [editorial]. Circulation 98:2219, 1998.)

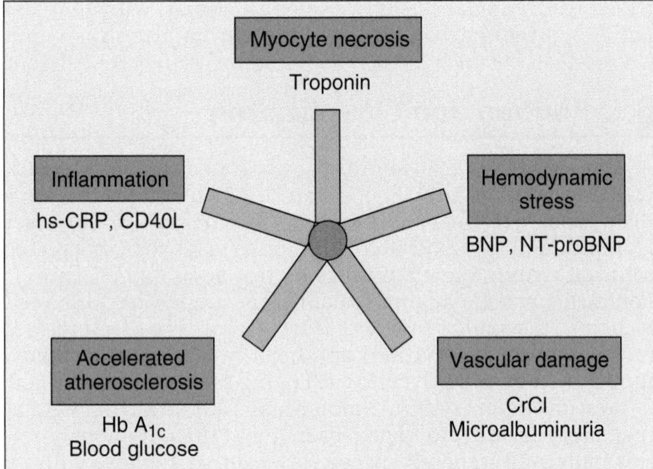

FIGURE 49–2 A multimarker strategy for evaluation of the etiology and prognosis of unstable angina or non-ST elevation myocardial infarction. Many new markers have been shown to be independent markers of an adverse prognosis. Troponin is a marker for myocyte necrosis; high-sensitivity C-reactive protein (hs-CRP) and CD40 ligand (CD40L) are markers of vascular inflammation; creatinine clearance (CrCl) and microalbuminuria are markers of vascular damage; hemoglobin (Hb) A_{1c} and blood glucose are markers of diabetes and accelerated atherosclerosis. (Adapted from Morrow DA, Braunwald E: Future of biomarkers in acute coronary syndromes: Moving toward a multimarker strategy. Circulation 108:250, 2003.)

releasing cytokines, which in turn increase the release of matrix metalloproteinases, which then make the fibrous cap thinner and more likely to rupture or erode. In parallel, inflammation can decrease the synthesis of collagen, thus further weakening the plaque and increasing the likelihood of rupture.

The acute ischemia in UA/NSTEMI can be caused by an increase in myocardial oxygen demand (e.g., precipitated by tachycardia or hypertension), more commonly by a reduction in supply (e.g., related to reduction in coronary lumen diameter by platelet-rich thrombi or vasospasm), or both. Rapid progression of the underlying coronary artery disease (CAD) has also been documented in some patients. A sequence of events can be documented in UA/NSTEMI, in which there is first a reduction in coronary sinus oxygen saturation (signifying a reduction in coronary blood flow), then ST segment depression, followed by chest discomfort.[10] Elevations in blood pressure or heart rate sometimes ensue. A patient may have a small increase in myocardial oxygen demand in conjunction with a reduction in coronary blood flow, leading to the episode of ischemia. The five major contributing causes of UA/NSTEMI are reviewed next.

THROMBOSIS (see also Chap. 80). The central role of coronary artery thrombosis in the pathogenesis of UA/NSTEMI is supported by six sets of observations:

1. At autopsy, thrombi can usually be identified at the site of a ruptured or eroded coronary plaque.[11]
2. Coronary atherectomy specimens obtained from patients with UA/NSTEMI demonstrate a high inci-

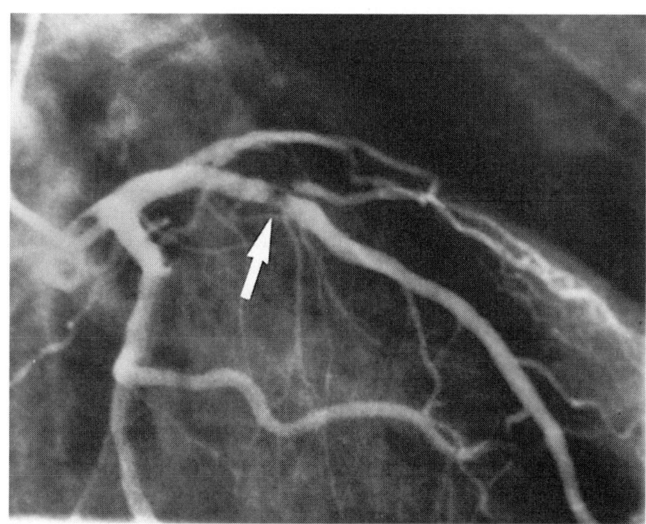

FIGURE 49–3 Coronary artery thrombus in a patient with unstable angina. A 60-year-old man presented with prolonged rest pain and transient anterior ST elevations. Coronary angiography shows an irregular hazy filling defect in the left anterior descending artery at the level of the second diagonal branch (arrow). Contrast medium surrounds the globular thrombus, which extends into the diagonal branch.

dence of thrombotic lesions compared with those obtained from patients with stable angina.[12]

3. Coronary angioscopic observations in UA/NSTEMI indicate that thrombus is frequently present.[13]
4. Coronary angiography has demonstrated ulceration or irregularities suggesting a ruptured plaque and/or thrombus in many patients (Fig. 49–3).[2] In the Thrombolysis in Myocardial Ischemia (TIMI) IIIA trial involving patients with UA/NSTEMI, 35 percent of patients had definite thrombus and an additional 40 percent had possible thrombus at angiography.[2]
5. Evidence of ongoing thrombosis has been noted with elevation of several markers of platelet activity and fibrin formation.[14,15]
6. The clinical outcome of patients with ACSs has been improved by antithrombotic therapy with aspirin,[16] unfractionated heparin (UFH) or low-molecular-weight heparin (LMWH),[17-19] platelet glycoprotein (GP) IIb/IIIa inhibitors,[20-22] or clopidogrel.[23]

PLATELET ACTIVATION AND AGGREGATION (see also Chap. 80). Platelets play a key role in the transformation of a stable atherosclerotic plaque to an unstable lesion (Fig. 49–4). With rupture or ulceration of an atherosclerotic plaque, the subendothelial matrix (e.g., collagen and tissue factor) is exposed to the circulating blood. The first step is *platelet adhesion* through the platelet GP Ib receptor by its interaction with von Willebrand factor. This is followed by *platelet activation*, which leads to (1) a shape change in the platelet (from a smooth discoid shape to a spiculated form, which increases the surface area upon which thrombin generation can occur); (2) degranulation of the alpha and dense granules, thereby releasing thromboxane A_2, serotonin, and other platelet aggregatory and chemoattractant agents; and (3) expression of GP IIb/IIIa receptors on the platelet surface with activation of the receptor, such that it can bind fibrinogen. The final step is *platelet aggregation*, i.e., the formation of the platelet plug. Fibrinogen (or von Willebrand factor) binds to the activated GP IIb/IIIa receptors of two platelets, thereby creating a growing platelet aggregate. Antiplatelet therapy is one of the cornerstones of therapy in UA/NSTEMI (see Medical Therapy) and is directed at decreasing the formation of thromboxane A_2 (aspirin), inhibiting the P2Y12 component of the adenosine diphosphate (ADP) receptor pathway of platelet activation (ticlopidine and clopidogrel),[24] and directly inhibiting platelet aggregation (GP IIb/IIIa inhibitors) (see Fig. 49–4).

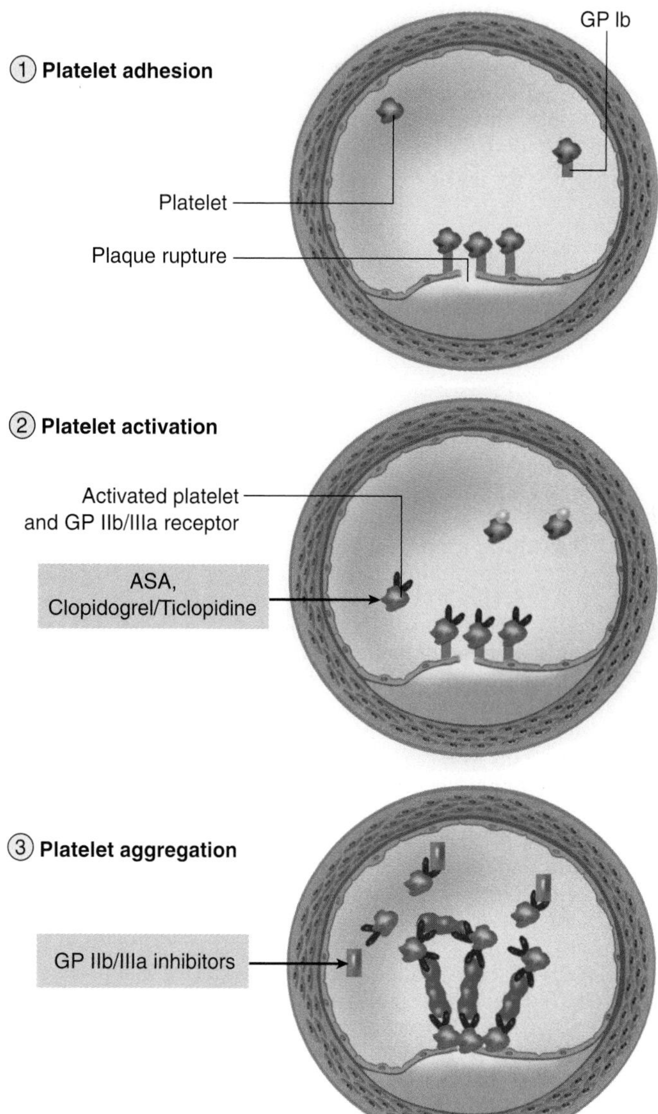

FIGURE 49–4 Primary hemostasis—process of platelet adhesion (1), activation (2), and aggregation (3) and the site of action of antiplatelet drugs. Platelets initiate thrombosis at the site of a ruptured plaque; the first step is *platelet adhesion* (1) through the glycoprotein (GP) Ib receptor in conjunction with von Willebrand factor. This is followed by *platelet activation* (2), which leads to a shape change in the platelet, degranulation of the alpha and dense granules, and expression of GP IIb/IIIa receptors on the platelet surface with activation of the receptor so that it can bind fibrinogen. The final step is *platelet aggregation* (3), in which fibrinogen (or von Willebrand factor) binds to the activated GP IIb/IIIa receptors of two platelets. Aspirin (acetylsalicylic acid [ASA]) and clopidogrel act to decrease platelet activation (see text for details), whereas the GP IIb/IIIa inhibitors inhibit the final step of platelet aggregation.

SECONDARY HEMOSTASIS. Simultaneously with formation of the platelet plug, the plasma coagulation system is activated. Release of tissue factor appears to be the predominant mechanism of initiating hemostasis following plaque rupture (see Chap. 80).[25] Ultimately, factor X is activated to factor Xa, which leads to generation of thrombin (Factor IIa), which plays a central role in arterial thrombosis: (1) thrombin converts fibrinogen to fibrin in the final common pathway for clot formation, (2) it is a powerful stimulus for platelet aggregation, and (3) it activates factor XIII, which leads to cross-linking and stabilization of the fibrin clot. Thrombin molecules are incorporated into coronary thrombi and can form the nidus of rethrombosis (i.e., reocclusion or reinfarction) as the thrombus undergoes spontaneous or pharmacologically induced fibrinolysis. Accordingly, effective inhibition of thrombin and factor Xa plays an important part in the therapy of UA/NSTEMI.

CORONARY VASOCONSTRICTION. There are three settings in which the process of dynamic coronary obstruction is identified:

1. Prinzmetal variant angina, with intense focal spasm of a segment of an epicardial coronary artery, is the prototypic example.[26] It can occur in patients without coronary atherosclerosis or in patients with one or more atheromatous plaques.
2. Coronary vasoconstriction causing "microcirculatory angina," which results from constriction of the small intramural coronary resistance vessels,[27] is the second setting. Although there are no epicardial coronary artery stenoses, coronary flow is usually slowed (see Chap. 44).
3. The third and probably most common setting in which vasoconstriction occurs is that of coronary atherosclerotic plaques.[28] Vasoconstriction can occur as the result of local vasoconstrictors released from platelets, serotonin and thromboxane A_2, as well as those present within the thrombus, such as thrombin. A dysfunctional coronary endothelium, with reduced production of nitric oxide and increased release of endothelin, can also lead to vasoconstriction. Adrenergic stimuli, cold immersion, cocaine,[29] or mental stress[30] can also cause coronary vasoconstriction.

PROGRESSIVE MECHANICAL OBSTRUCTION. The fourth etiology of UA/NSTEMI is that of progressive luminal narrowing. This narrowing was most commonly seen in the setting of restenosis following percutaneous coronary intervention (PCI) in the absence of drug-eluting stents (see Chap. 52). Angiographic and atherectomy studies have demonstrated that many patients without previous intracoronary procedures have shown progressive luminal narrowing of the culprit vessel in the period preceding the onset of UA/NSTEMI that is related to rapid cellular proliferation.[31]

SECONDARY UNSTABLE ANGINA. This form of unstable angina is precipitated by an imbalance in myocardial oxygen supply and demand caused by conditions extrinsic to the coronary arteries in patients with prior coronary stenosis and chronic stable angina.[5-7] It can result from either an increase in myocardial oxygen demand, a decrease in coronary flow, or both. Conditions that increase oxygen demand include tachycardia (e.g., supraventricular tachycardia or new-onset atrial fibrillation with rapid ventricular response), fever, thyrotoxicosis, hyperadrenergic states, and elevations of left ventricular afterload such as in hypertension or aortic stenosis. Secondary unstable angina can also be due to impaired oxygen delivery, as occurs in anemia, hypoxemia (e.g., related to pneumonia or congestive heart failure), and hyperviscosity states, or hypotension. Secondary angina appears to have a worse prognosis than primary unstable angina (see Table 49–1).[7]

Clinical Presentation

The clinical profile of patients presenting with UA/NSTEMI differs from that of patients with STEMI. Women present more often with unstable angina, constituting 30 to 45 percent of patients with unstable angina in several studies,[32-34] compared with 25 to 30 percent of patients with NSTEMI and approximately 20 percent of patients with STEMI.[32,33] In comparison with the latter, patients with unstable angina also have higher rates of prior MI, angina, previous coronary revascularization, and extracardiac vascular disease.[33,35] Indeed, approximately 80 percent of patients with UA/NSTEMI have a prior history of cardiovascular disease and most have evidence of prior coronary risk factors.[36]

CLINICAL EXAMINATION. A description of "ischemic pain" is the hallmark of UA/NSTEMI (see Chap. 45). The physical examination may be unremarkable or may support the diagnosis of cardiac ischemia (see Chap. 8). Signs that suggest that the culprit artery perfuses a larger fraction of the left ventricle include diaphoresis, pale cool skin, sinus tachycardia, a third or fourth heart sound, and basilar rales on lung examination. Rarely, in UA/NSTEMI the severity of left ventricular dysfunction causes hypotension (i.e., cardiogenic shock).

ELECTROCARDIOGRAM. In UA/NSTEMI, ST depression (or transient ST elevation) and T wave changes occur in up to 50 percent of patients.[3,22,37] New (or presumably new) ST segment deviation is a specific and important measure of ischemia and prognosis. Traditionally, ST depression has been considered significant only if it was greater than 0.1 mV, which occurs in 20 to 25 percent of patients. However, an additional 20 percent of patients present with 0.05 mV ST depression,[3,37] and they have been observed to have an adverse prognosis approaching that of patients with 0.1 mV ST depression.[37,38] The worst prognosis occurs among patients with transient (i.e., <20 minutes) ST elevation, which occurs in approximately 10 percent of patients with UA/NSTEMI. T wave changes are sensitive but not as specific measures of acute ischemia unless they are marked (≥0.3 mV).[22]

CONTINUOUS ELECTROCARDIOGRAPHIC MONITORING. Continuous monitoring of the electrocardiogram (ECG) can be used for two purposes in UA/NSTEMI: to monitor for arrhythmias or for recurrent ST segment deviation indicative of ischemia. For the former, telemetry of patients admitted to monitored beds can detect arrhythmias in association with the acute episode; although life-threatening arrhythmias are rare in unstable angina, they may be more common among patients with NSTEMI. For the latter goal, high-fidelity Holter monitors have been used in clinical trials to detect ST segment deviation as evidence of recurrent ischemia. In several studies, the ST segment monitoring appeared to be more sensitive than patients' symptoms and identified up to 25 percent of patients with evidence of ischemia during the first 24 hours after admission.[39,40] In addition, the presence of ST deviation is a strong marker of adverse short- and long-term outcome,[39,40] even when used in conjunction with troponins and clinical variables.[41] As with recurrent cardiac events of symptomatic ischemia or recurrent MI, silent ischemia is more frequent and prolonged in patients with NSTEMI than those with unstable angina.

CARDIAC NECROSIS MARKERS FOR DIAGNOSIS OF NSTEMI. Among patients presenting with symptoms consistent with UA/NSTEMI, elevations of markers of myocardial necrosis (i.e., CK-MB, troponin T or I) are used to identify patients with the diagnosis of NSTEMI (as opposed to UA).[42] With the use of troponins, which are both more sensitive and more specific than CK-MB, a greater percentage of patients are classified as having NSTEMI. Despite worries about the consequences of the apparent change in definition of MI, several studies have lent support to the use of these more sensitive markers, which are helpful in the assessment of prognosis.[43]

The issue of the appropriate "cut point" to define an elevated troponin level has been controversial. An important aspect is that the assay clearly discriminates truly elevated levels of troponin from false-positive results related to poor analytical performance of the assay. It has been proposed that the upper limit of normal for each specific assay be defined as the 99th percentile of a normal population of subjects[44] and meet acceptable criteria for precision of the assay at that concentration (defined as a 10 percent coefficient of variation, a measure of reproducibility from repeated testing on the same sample). Clinicians and laboratorians have debated the clinical relevance of very low-level elevation of cardiac troponin. However, studies have found that low-level elevation of cardiac troponin is associated with a higher risk of death or recurrent ischemic events[45,46] and thus support the European Society of Cardiology/American College of Cardiology proposal to ensure high accuracy at the low troponin levels.[47]

Because each assay is different, each hospital needs to review the specific cut points defined by that assay.[48] Point-of-care tests can have a positive versus negative result or provide a quantitative result, although the sensitivity and diagnostic accuracy of these tests have only recently been able to match those of current generation laboratory-based assays.

Despite increasingly accurate assays, apparent false-positive troponin elevations have been found in patients later found at coronary angiography not to have epicardial stenoses.[49] These elevations may be due to an alternative diagnosis, such as congestive heart failure, in which elevations have been observed in the absence of CAD and were associated with an adverse prognosis.[50] An analysis from the Treat Angina with Aggrastat and determine Cost of Therapy with an Invasive or Conservative Strategy (TACTICS)-TIMI 18 trial also raised a cautionary note that these troponin elevations should not be discarded as simply false positive. Patients presenting with UA/NSTEMI who had elevations of troponin but no apparent CAD on angiography were found to have a significantly worse prognosis than those who were troponin negative without coronary disease, with a 6-month rate of death or MI of 5.3 versus 0 percent, respectively.[51] This group had a prognosis similar to that of patients with documented coronary disease who were troponin negative at presentation. These data suggest that the elevations in troponin may be signs of alternative diagnoses such as heart failure that are associated with adverse outcomes.

CORONARY ARTERIOGRAPHIC FINDINGS. Patients with UA/NSTEMI enrolled in the invasive arm of TACTICS-TIMI 18 systematically underwent angiography. Thirty-four percent had critical obstruction (>50 percent luminal diameter stenosis) of three vessels, 28 percent had two-vessel disease, 26 percent had single-vessel disease, and 13 percent had no coronary stenosis greater than 50 percent.[3] Approximately 5 to 10 percent had left main stem stenosis greater than 50 percent.[3] Similar findings have been reported from registries of unselected UA/NSTEMI patients.[37,52] Women and nonwhites with UA/NSTEMI have less extensive coronary disease than their counterparts,[32,33,52,53] and patients with NSTEMI have more extensive disease than those who present with unstable angina.[33]

Approximately 15 percent of patients who present with symptoms of UA/NSTEMI have no significant coronary stenosis on coronary angiography.[32,33,37,52,53] Women and nonwhites constitute a larger proportion of such patients without epicardial coronary disease, suggesting either a difficulty in making a firm diagnosis of UA/NSTEMI in these groups or a different pathophysiological mechanism for their clinical presentation.[32-34,37,52,53] Approximately one-third of patients with UA/NSTEMI without a critical epicardial obstruction exhibit impaired coronary flow assessed angiographically, suggesting a pathophysiological role for coronary microvascular dysfunction.[54] The short-term prognosis is excellent in this group of patients.[55]

The culprit lesion in UA/NSTEMI typically exhibits an eccentric stenosis with scalloped or overhanging edges and a narrow neck.[2] These angiographic findings may represent disrupted atherosclerotic plaque, thrombus, or a combination. Features suggesting thrombus include globular intraluminal masses with a rounded or polypoid shape (see Fig. 49–3).[2] "Haziness" of a lesion has been used as an angiographic marker of possible thrombus, but this finding is less specific. Patients with angiographically visualized thrombus have impaired coronary flow and worse clinical outcomes than those without thrombus.[56]

Coronary flow as measured by the TIMI flow grade or frame count and TIMI myocardial perfusion grade have also been found to be impaired in patients with UA/NSTEMI, especially those with an elevated troponin.[56,57] Furthermore, as has been observed in patients with STEMI, abnormal tissue level perfusion is also associated with adverse outcomes in patients with UA/NSTEMI, independent of the presence of thrombus and abnormal flow in the epicardial artery.

ANGIOSCOPY AND INTRAVASCULAR ULTRASONOGRAPHY. Greater definition of the culprit lesion has been possible using angioscopy, where "white" (platelet-rich) thrombi are frequently observed, as opposed to "red" thrombi, more often seen in patients with acute ST elevation MI (Fig. 49–5).[13] Intravascular ultrasound examination identified more soft "echolucent" plaques and fewer calcified lesions among patients with unstable versus stable angina.[58]

OTHER LABORATORY TESTS. A chest roentgenogram may be useful in identifying pulmonary congestion or edema, which is more frequent in patients with NSTEMI involving a significant proportion of the left ventricle or in those with prior known left ventricular dysfunction. The presence of congestion has been shown to confer an adverse prognosis.[59]

Obtaining a serum cholesterol level and levels of its principal fractions, low-density lipoprotein (LDL) and high-density lipoprotein cholesterol, is useful in identifying an important, treatable risk factor for coronary atherothombosis. Because serum cholesterol falls 24 hours following STEMI or UA/NSTEMI, it should be measured at the time of initial presentation. If only a later sample is obtained but the value falls into a range that warrants long-term treatment (see Chap. 39), appropriate therapy can be initiated. Other circulating markers of increased risk are discussed later. Evaluation for other secondary causes of UA/NSTEMI[5] may also be appropriate in selected patients (e.g., assessing thyroid function in patients who present with UA/NSTEMI and a persistent tachycardia).

Risk Stratification

PATHOPHYSIOLOGY OF LONG-TERM RISK FOLLOWING ACUTE CORONARY SYNDROME. An important concept that has emerged regarding the long-term risk following an ACS event is that the observed high risk of recurrent ischemic events is linked to multifocal lesions other than the culprit lesion responsible for the ACS event. Studies of coronary anatomy using angiography,[60-62] intravascular coronary ultrasonography,[63] or angioscopy[64] have shown multiple active plaques in addition to the culprit lesion (see Fig. 49–5). Thus, as aggressive interventional approaches are used successfully to treat the culprit lesion, the remaining plaques, which frequently have unstable features on angiographic or angioscopic examination, are responsible for recurrent events. The link to inflammation was also seen in one of these studies (Fig. 49–6): Multiple active plaques on angiography occurred more frequently with an increasing C-reactive protein (CRP) level.[63] This provides an important pathophysiological link between inflammation, more diffuse active coronary disease, and recurrent cardiac events in the months to years following a clinical ACS event.

NATURAL HISTORY. The short-term mortality of patients with unstable angina has been shown to be lower (1.7 percent at 30 days) than that of patients with NSTEMI or STEMI, whereas the mortality risk with the two types of MI is similar (5.1 percent for each type).[38] The early mortality risk in ACS is related to the extent of myocardial damage and resulting hemodynamic compromise.[65] In contrast, long-term outcomes—for both mortality and nonfatal events—are actually *worse* for patients with either unstable angina or NSTEMI compared with STEMI (Fig. 49–7).[38] This is probably due to

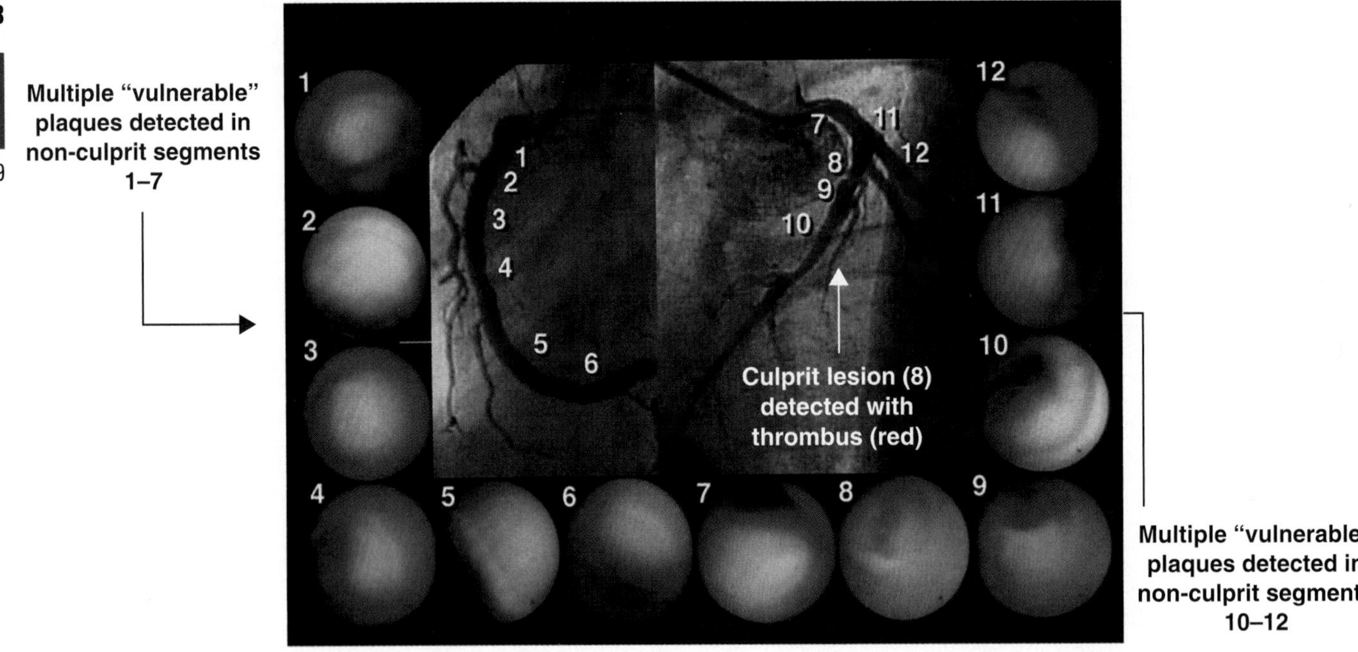

FIGURE 49–5 Evidence of multiple vulnerable plaques in a patient with acute coronary syndrome. Angiographic and angioscopic images of a 58-year-old male with anterior myocardial infarction are shown. The culprit lesion is seen in the proximal left anterior descending artery at site 8. However, other segments of the artery, which appear normal on the coronary angiogram, at angioscopy demonstrate the presence of vulnerable plaques (sites 10 to 12 and 1, 3, 4, 7). (Adapted from Asakura M, Ueda Y, Yamaguchi O, et al: Extensive development of vulnerable plaques as a pan-coronary process in patients with myocardial infarction: An angioscopic study. J Am Coll Cardiol 37:1284, 2001.)

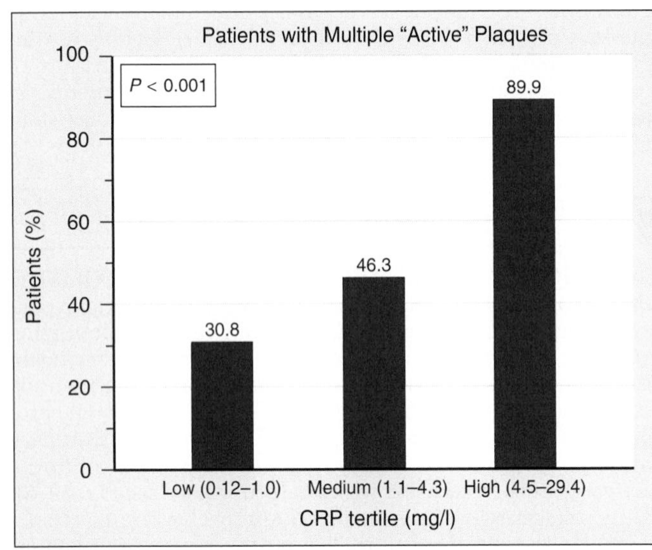

FIGURE 49–6 The level of C-reactive protein (CRP) correlated with the prevalence of multiple thrombus–containing coronary plaques in 228 patients with unstable angina or non-ST elevation myocardial infarction. (Data from Zairis MN, Papadaki OA, Manousakis SJ, et al: C-reactive protein and multiple complex coronary artery plaques in patients with primary unstable angina. Atherosclerosis 164:355, 2002.)

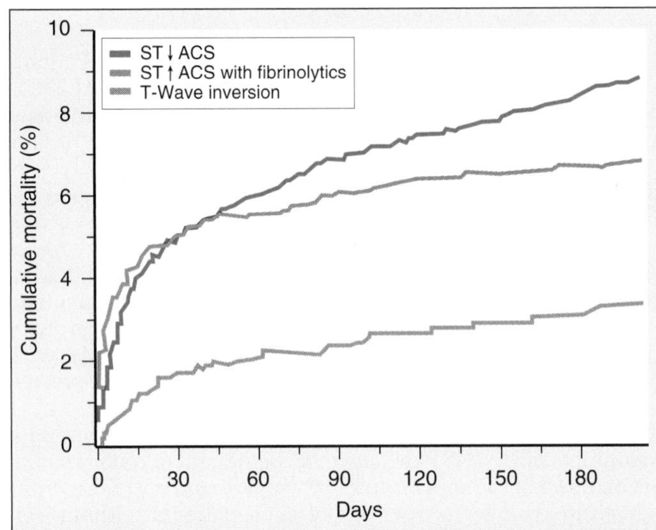

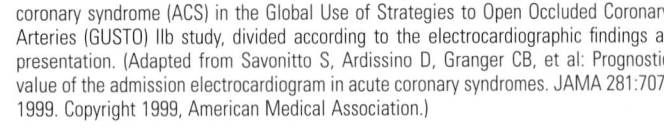

FIGURE 49–7 Kaplan-Meier curves showing mortality in patients with acute coronary syndrome (ACS) in the Global Use of Strategies to Open Occluded Coronary Arteries (GUSTO) IIb study, divided according to the electrocardiographic findings at presentation. (Adapted from Savonitto S, Ardissino D, Granger CB, et al: Prognostic value of the admission electrocardiogram in acute coronary syndromes. JAMA 281:707, 1999. Copyright 1999, American Medical Association.)

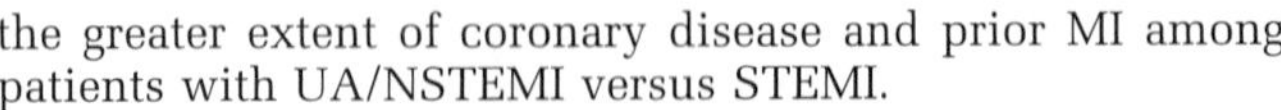

the greater extent of coronary disease and prior MI among patients with UA/NSTEMI versus STEMI.

Methods of Risk Stratification

Patients with UA/NSTEMI are a heterogeneous group, with a prognosis that ranges from an excellent outcome with modest adjustments in therapeutic regimen to one in which the risk of death or MI is high and intensive treatment is needed. Accordingly, risk stratification now plays a central role in the evaluation and management of this condition. Specific subgroups of patients, identified by clinical features, electrocardiographic findings, or cardiac (or vascular) markers are at higher risk for adverse outcomes (Table 49–2). Furthermore, these groups appear to derive greater benefit from more aggressive antithrombotic or interventional therapy, or both (see later). Clinical predictors can also be used to assist in triage of patients with unstable angina to the coronary care unit or a monitored bed. Patients determined to be at highest risk should be admitted to the coronary care unit, whereas those with intermediate or lower risk could be admitted to a monitored bed on a cardiac step-down unit. Patients sometimes referred to as at "low risk," but who are best characterized by their "low likelihood" of having an ACS, are

TABLE 49–2 Clinical Indicators of Increased Risk in Unstable Angina or Non-ST Elevation Myocardial Infarction

History
Advanced age (>70 yr)
Diabetes mellitus
Post-myocardial infarction angina
Prior peripheral vascular disease
Prior cerebrovascular disease

Clinical Presentation
Braunwald class II or III (acute or subacute rest pain)
Braunwald class B (secondary unstable angina)
Heart failure or hypotension; ventricular arrhythmias

Electrocardiogram
ST segment deviation ≥0.05 mV
T wave inversion ≥0.3 mV
Left bundle branch block

Cardiac Markers
Increased troponin T or I or creatine kinase muscle-brain (MB) fraction
Increased C-reactive protein or white blood cell count
Increased B-type natriuretic peptide
Elevated CD40 ligand
Elevated glucose or hemoglobin A_{1c}; elevated creatinine

Angiogram
Thrombus; three vessel disease; reduced ejection fraction

evaluated and managed in emergency department observation units or chest pain centers (see Chap. 45).

Clinical Variables

The aforementioned classification of unstable angina[5] (see Table 49–1) has been shown in several studies to be useful clinically in identifying high-risk patients. In the TIMI III Registry, which included 3318 consecutive patients with UA/NSTEMI, this classification was an important predictor of rate of death or MI to 1 year.[7] High-risk groups of patients with unstable angina are those with acute rest pain, those with post-MI unstable angina, and those with secondary unstable angina.

HIGH-RISK CLINICAL SUBGROUPS. Increasing age has been shown to be associated with a significant increase in adverse outcomes in patients with UA/NSTEMI.[66-68] Diabetic patients with UA/NSTEMI are at approximately 50 percent higher risk than nondiabetics.[69] Patients with extracardiac vascular disease, i.e., those with either cerebrovascular disease or peripheral arterial vascular disease, also appear to have approximately 50 percent higher rates of death or recurrent ischemic events compared with patients without previous peripheral or cerebrovascular disease, even after controlling for other differences in baseline characteristics.[70]

As with STEMI, patients with UA/NSTEMI who present with evidence of congestive heart failure (Killip Class > II) have an increased risk of death.[71] In addition, patients who develop recurrent ischemia after initial presentation have been found to be at increased risk.[72]

Risk Assessment by Electrocardiography

The admission ECG is very useful in predicting long-term adverse outcomes. In the TIMI III Registry of patients with UA/NSTEMI, independent predictors of 1-year death or MI included left bundle branch block (risk ratio 2.8), ST segment deviation greater than 0.05 mV (risk ratio 2.45), both p less than 0.001.[37] There appears to be a gradient of risk based on the degree of ST segment deviation.[73,74] In contrast, the presence of T wave changes greater than 0.1 mV was associated with a modest[73] or no increase in subsequent death or MI.[37,38]

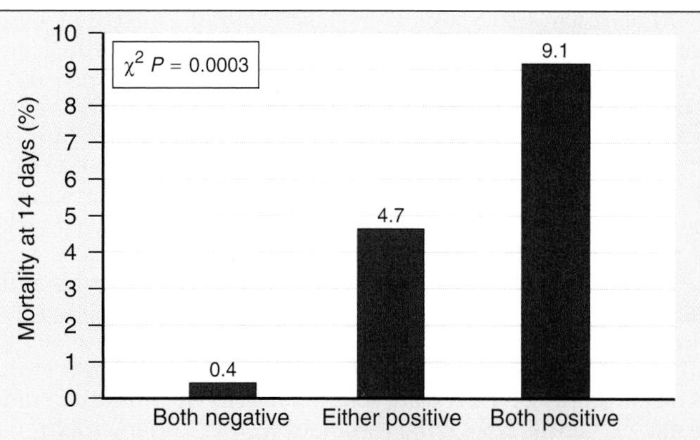

FIGURE 49–8 Use of both troponin T and C-reactive protein (CRP) to predict mortality. These data demonstrate that an elevated high-sensitivity CRP (>15.5 mg/liter in this study) and an "early positive" rapid bedside troponin T assay (defined as positive < 10 minutes) are independent predictors of increased mortality. (From Morrow DA, Rifai N, Antman EM, et al: C-reactive protein is a potent predictor of mortality independently and in combination with troponin T in acute coronary syndromes: A TIMI 11A substudy. J Am Coll Cardiol 31:1460, 1998.)

Risk Assessment by Cardiac Markers

CREATINE KINASE-MB AND THE TROPONINS. Patients with NSTEMI, defined as those with an elevated biomarker of necrosis, CK-MB, or troponin, have a worse long-term prognosis than those with unstable angina.[45,75-79] Beyond just a positive versus negative test result, there is a linear relationship between the level of troponin T or I in the blood and subsequent risk of death—the higher the troponin, the higher the mortality risk.[75] On the other hand, a higher risk of MI was observed with *lower* levels of troponin in several studies, and thus the overall rate of death or MI is equally high among patients with low or higher troponin values.[45,80] Similar results have been obtained using a bedside rapid assay for troponin T, in which time to positivity is a semiquantitative measure of serum troponin T, and related to increased mortality.[81] Thus, troponin T and troponin I are useful not only in diagnosing infarction but also in risk assessment and in targeting therapies to high-risk patients.

C-REACTIVE PROTEIN. Among the growing list of markers that appear to be useful in assessing patients with UA/NSTEMI, CRP is very promising. Elevated CRP has been related to increased risk of death, MI, or need for urgent revascularization.[80,82-84] Of note, because CRP is an acute phase reactant, it is known to be elevated by an ACS. Thus, elevated levels of CRP in patients with ACS are approximately five times higher than those of stable patients.[82,85] Among patients with negative troponin I at baseline, who overall had a 14-day mortality of only 1.5 percent, CRP was able to discriminate a high- and a low-risk group; mortality for patients with an elevated CRP was 5.8 percent versus 0.4 percent for patients without elevated CRP.[82] When using both CRP and troponin T, mortality could be stratified from 0.4 percent for patients with both markers negative to 4.7 percent if either CRP or troponin was positive to 9.1 percent if both were positive (Fig. 49–8).[82] Similar results have been seen in other studies.[80,83,84,86-89] Of note, however, in contrast to troponin, which is extremely useful in selecting patients for more aggressive treatment, CRP has not been shown in the setting of UA/NSTEMI to predict a differential benefit of a therapy.[90] CRP measured at the time of hospital discharge has been found to be a strong predictor of outcome to 3 to 12 months.[91]

Other inflammatory markers have offered consistent evidence of an association between systemic inflammation and recurrent adverse events, including serum amyloid A,[92] monocyte chemoattractant protein-1 (MCP-1),[93] and interleukin-6.[94] In addition, some of these markers of inflammation may be potential therapeutic targets, as may be the case for MCP-1.[93] Thus, these studies indicate that inflammation is related to the instability of patients and an increased risk of recurrent cardiac events.

WHITE BLOOD CELL COUNT. Another, even simpler and universally available marker of inflammation is the white blood cell (WBC) count. Several studies of patients with acute MI[95,96] and UA/NSTEMI[96-98] have observed that patients with elevated WBC counts were at higher risk of mortality and recurrent acute MI. This association was independent of CRP,[87,97] suggesting that not all the information about the influence of inflammation on outcomes is captured in one marker such as CRP.

CD40 LIGAND. Another emerging and important marker is CD40 ligand (CD40L), a member of the tumor necrosis factor-alpha family of proteins. CD40L is expressed on the platelet surface when platelets are activated and is subsequently cleaved, generating a soluble hydrolytic fragment termed sCD40L. It has been found to be both prothrombotic[99] and proinflammatory and to have a role in atherosclerotic lesion progression.[100] CD40L has been correlated with the degree of platelet activation, as measured by platelet-monocyte aggregates, and thus is a novel marker of platelet activation.[101] Studies have found that increasing levels of CD40L are associated with increased risk of death, MI, and recurrent ischemic events, independent of troponin and CRP, in patients with ACS[101,102] as well as in more stable populations of patients,[103] suggesting that this is a useful new marker of risk.

B-TYPE NATRIURETIC PEPTIDE. B-type natriuretic peptide (BNP) is a neurohormone that is synthesized in ventricular myocardium and released in response to increased wall stress.[104] It has many actions including natriuresis, vasodilation, inhibition of sympathetic nerve activity, and inhibition of the renin-angiotensin-aldosterone system. BNP has been show to be a diagnostic and prognostic marker in patients with congestive heart failure[105] and patients with acute MI.[106] BNP has now been seen to have prognostic value across the full spectrum of patients with ACS, including those with UA/NSTEMI: patients with elevated levels of BNP (>80 pg/ml) had a two- to threefold higher risk of death by 10 months.[107] This finding was confirmed in the TIMI 11 and TACTICS-TIMI 18 trials.[108,109] Together, these data suggest that measurement of BNP in patients presenting with UA/NSTEMI adds importantly to our current tools for risk stratification (see Fig. 49–2).

MYELOPEROXIDASE. Myeloperoxidase (MPO) is a hemoprotein expressed by polymorphonuclear neutrophils that possesses potent proinflammatory properties and that promotes oxidation of lipoproteins in vascular atheroma. One case-control study found an association of MPO levels with the presence of angiographically documented CAD, independent of other cardiovascular risk factors and of WBC count.[110] In patients with UA/NSTEMI, MPO serum levels were associated with increased risk for subsequent death or MI, independent of other risk factors and other cardiac markers.[111] Elevations of MPO have been seen throughout the coronary vasculature in patients with UA/NSTEMI.[112] Thus, MPO may be both a marker of inflammation, and its presence also suggests a direct role of neutrophil activation in the pathophysiology of vascular inflammation and ACS.

CREATININE. Another simple tool for risk stratification is the use of creatinine or calculation of creatinine clearance, or both. Several studies have found elevated creatinine to be associated with an adverse prognosis (see Fig. 49–2).[113-116] The risk appears to be independent of other standard risk factors, such as troponin elevation. This factor may also play a role in decreased drug clearance, in which dosages of medications such as LMWH need to be adjusted.[117]

GLUCOSE. Adverse outcomes have been seen among diabetic patients with acute MI with elevated admission glucose values compared with patients without hyperglycemia.[118] Studies have found that this association is present even among patients without a prior diagnosis of diabetes. In addition, this association was seen in patients with both STEMI and UA/NSTEMI and was independent of other baseline risk factors.[119,120] A similar association of poor glycemic control, as measured by hemoglobin A_{1c}, has been seen in other studies.[121] Thus, in patients with UA/NSTEMI, a higher baseline glucose level at the time of presentation is associated with significantly higher long-term mortality, independent of a history of diabetes, a risk factor that may be modifiable with aggressive treatment.[122]

Combined Risk Assessment Scores

Integrating all of the preceding factors, several groups have developed comprehensive risk scores that use clinical variables, findings from the ECG, and findings from serum cardiac markers.[67,68] From the Platelet Glycoprotein IIb/IIIa in Unstable Angina: Receptor Suppression Using Integrilin Therapy (PURSUIT) trial, Boersma and colleagues identified factors that were independently associated with increased mortality and with death or MI. The most important baseline determinants of higher mortality were increasing age, increasing heart rate, lower systolic blood pressure, ST segment depression, signs of heart failure, and elevated cardiac marker enzymes. The TIMI risk score identified seven independent risk factors: age older than 65 years, more than three risk factors for CAD, documented CAD at catheterization, ST deviation greater than 0.5 mm, more than two episodes of angina in the last 24 hours, aspirin within the prior week, and elevated cardiac markers. This scoring system was used to stratify the risk for patients across a 10-fold gradient of risk, from 4.7 to 40.9 percent ($p < 0.001$) (Fig. 49–9A).[67] More important, this risk score has been found to predict the response to several of the therapies used in UA/NSTEMI: patients with higher TIMI risk scores had significant reductions in events when treated with enoxaparin compared with UFH,[67] with a GP IIb/IIIa inhibitor compared with placebo,[123] and with an invasive versus conservative strategy (Fig. 49–9B).[3] With the ever-growing number of new cardiac markers (see earlier), it is expected that these comprehensive risk scores can be expanded to include these new markers as they become more widely available in clinical practice, as shown in one study using three markers in a "multimarker strategy for evaluation" (Fig. 49–10; see Fig. 49–2).

Medical Therapy

TREATMENT GOALS. The treatment objectives for patients with UA/NSTEMI are to stabilize and "passivate" the acute coronary lesion, to treat residual ischemia, and to employ long-term secondary prevention. Antithrombotic therapy (e.g., aspirin, clopidogrel, UFH or LMWH, and GP IIb/IIIa inhibitors) is used to prevent further thrombosis and allow endogenous fibrinolysis to dissolve the thrombus and reduce the degree of coronary stenosis. Antithrombotic therapy is continued in the long term to reduce the risk of developing future events or to prevent progression to complete occlusion of the coronary artery, or both. Antiischemic therapies (e.g., beta blockers, nitrates, and calcium antagonists) are used primarily to reduce myocardial oxygen demand but also appear to have effects in preventing plaque rupture, as shown in prevention of clinical events with beta

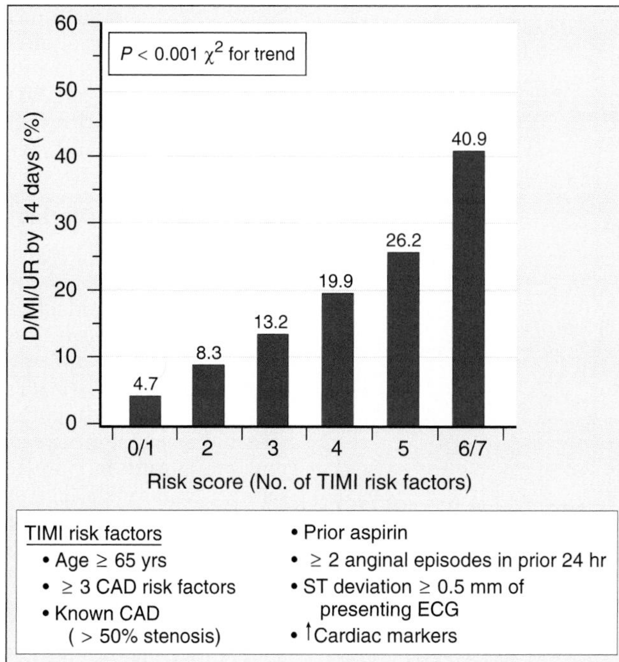

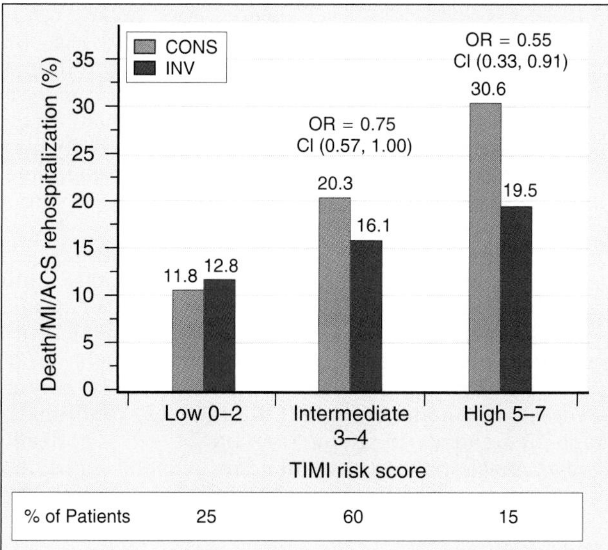

FIGURE 49–9 **A,** Thrombolysis in Myocardial Ischemia (TIMI) risk score for unstable angina or non-ST elevation myocardial infarction (UA/NSTEMI). The risk factors are shown on the right and the risk of death (D), myocardial infarction (MI), or urgent revascularization (UR) is shown along the vertical axis. **B,** Use of the TIMI risk score for UA/NSTEMI to predict the benefit of an early invasive strategy. In a prospectively defined analysis, the TIMI risk score was applied in the Treat Angina with Aggrastat and determine Cost of Therapy with an Invasive or Conservative Strategy (TACTICS)-TIMI 18 trial. As shown, 75 percent of patients had a risk score of 3 or higher, and in these patients a significant benefit of an invasive strategy was observed. ACS = acute coronary syndrome; CAD = coronary artery disease; CI = confidence interval; CONS = conservative; ECG = electrocardiogram; INV = invasive; OR = odds ratio. (**A,** Adapted from Antman EM, Cohen M, Bernink PJLM, et al: The TIMI risk score for unstable angina/non-ST elevation MI: A method for prognostication and therapeutic decision making. JAMA 284:835, 2000; **B,** data from Cannon CP, Weintraub WS, Demopoulos LA, et al: Comparison of early invasive and conservative strategies in patients with unstable coronary syndromes treated with the glycoprotein IIb/IIIa inhibitor tirofiban. N Engl J Med 344:1879, 2001.)

blockers and angiotensin-converting enzyme (ACE) inhibition. Coronary revascularization is frequently used to treat the severe stenosis of a culprit lesion, thereby preventing the thrombus from progressing and causing recurrent ischemia. After the acute event is stabilized, the many factors that led up to the event need to be reversed, i.e., treatment of atherosclerotic risk factors such as hypercholesterolemia, hypertension, and cessation of smoking, each of which contributes to stabilization of the cholesterol-laden plaque and healing of the endothelium.

General Measures

Patients with UA/NSTEMI should be admitted to a monitored bed. Continuous ECG monitoring (i.e., telemetry) is used to detect cardiac arrhythmias. Higher fidelity continuous ECG tracings can be obtained with a Holter monitor and can assess asymptomatic ST deviations as markers for ischemia. This approach has been shown to be useful in clinical trials in risk stratification with core laboratory analysis of the tracings,[41] but its usefulness "on line" in clinical practice has not been well established and deserves further study.

Bed rest is usually prescribed initially for patients with UA/NSTEMI. Ambulation as tolerated is permitted if the patient has been stable without recurrent chest discomfort for at least 12 to 24 hours or following revascularization. Means of improving the physical and emotional surroundings for the patient, such as placing the patient in a quiet atmosphere away from any emotionally taxing arguments and offering the physician's reassurance or mild sedation, may act to reduce sympathetic drive and thereby reduce ischemia. It is advisable to provide supplemental oxygen only to patients with cyanosis, extensive rales, or documented hypoxemia. Oxygen saturation determined by oxymetry is useful with supplemental oxygen administered when the arterial O_2 saturation declines below 92 percent.

Relief of chest pain is an initial goal of treatment. In patients with persistent pain despite therapy with nitrates and beta blockers (see later), morphine sulfate 1 to 5 mg intravenously is recommended. Contraindications include hypotension or prior allergy; meperidine hydrochloride can be substituted in the latter patients. With careful blood pressure monitoring, repeated doses can be administered every 5 to 30 minutes. Morphine may act as both an analgesic and anxiolytic, but its venodilatory effects may produce beneficial hemodynamic effects by reducing preload. The latter is especially useful in the setting of acute pulmonary edema. If hypotension develops after administration of morphine, supine positioning or intravenous saline should restore blood pressure, and pressors are rarely needed. If respiratory depression develops, naloxone (0.4 to 2.0 mg) may be given.

Nitrates (see also Chap. 50)

Nitrates are endothelium-independent vasodilators that both increase myocardial blood flow by coronary vasodilation and reduce myocardial oxygen demand. The latter effect is produced by venodilation, which leads to reduced myocardial preload, reduction in ventricular wall stress, and thereby reduced myocardial oxygen demand. Nitrates should initially be given sublingually or by buccal spray (0.3 to 0.6 mg) if the patient is experiencing ischemic pain. If pain persists after three sublingual tablets (or buccal sprays) given 5 minutes apart and initiation of beta blockade (see later), intravenous nitroglycerin (5 to 10 μg/min using nonabsorbing tubing) is recommended. The rate of the infusion may be increased by 10 μg/min every 3 to 5 minutes until symptoms are relieved or systolic blood pressure falls to below 100 mm Hg. Although there is no absolute maximum dose, a dose of 200 μg/min is generally used as a ceiling. Contraindications to use of nitrates are hypotension or the use of sildenafil (Viagra) or related compounds within the previous 24 to 48 hours.[124] Topical or oral nitrates can be used if the episode of pain has resolved, or they may replace intravenous nitroglycerin if the patient has been pain free for 12 to 24 hours. Dosing of nitrates depends on the formulation, but one

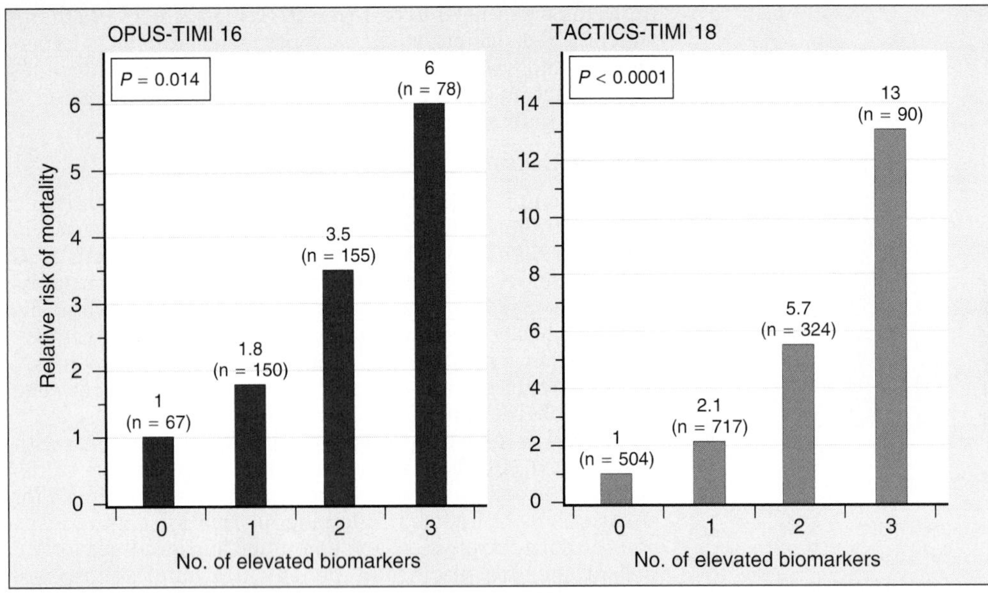

FIGURE 49–10 A multimarker strategy to predict mortality in acute coronary syndrome. Troponin I, C-reactive protein, and B-type natriuretic peptide as determinants of 30-day mortality in unstable angina or non-ST elevation myocardial infarction. Mortality is a function of the number of elevated biomarkers in two separate trials. OPUS-TIMI = Orbofiban in Patients with Unstable Coronary Syndromes–Thrombolysis in Myocardial Infarction; TACTICS-TIMI = Treat Angina with aggrastat and determine Cost of Therapy with an Invasive or Conservative Strategy–TIMI. (Adapted from Sabatine MS, Morrow DA, de Lemos JA, et al: Multimarker approach to risk stratification in non-ST elevation acute coronary syndromes: Simultaneous assessment of troponin I, C-reactive protein, and B-type natriuretic peptide. Circulation 105:1760, 2002.)

should attempt to have an 8- to 10-hour nitrate-free interval to avoid the development of tolerance.

The effect of nitrates on mortality was evaluated in the Gruppo Italiano per lo Studio della Sopravvivenza nell'Infarto Miocardico (GISSI)-3 and Fourth International Study of Infarct Survival (ISIS-4) trials for patients with suspected MI (both ST elevation and NSTEMI).[125,126] No beneficial effect on mortality was observed in the overall population or in the subgroup of patients with NSTEMI. Consequently, the goal of nitrate therapy is relief of pain; chronic nitrate therapy can frequently be tapered off in the long-term management of patients, with primary therapy being aspirin, clopidogrel, beta blockers, and so forth with sublingual or buccal nitroglycerin given as needed for new episodes of pain.

Beta Blockers (see also Chap. 50)

Several placebo-controlled trials in UA/NSTEMI have shown benefit of beta blockers in reducing subsequent MI or recurrent ischemia, or both.[127-129] Subgroup analyses of patients with non-Q-wave MI in several trials demonstrated the benefits of beta blockers (intravenous followed by oral).[130] Thus, beta blockers are recommended for patients with UA/NSTEMI who do not have contraindications to beta blockade (bradycardia, advanced atrioventricular [AV] block, persistent hypotension, known systolic dysfunction with acute pulmonary edema, history of bronchospasm). If ischemia and chest pain are ongoing, early intravenous beta blockade should be used, followed by oral beta blockade. A reduced ejection fraction, which was formerly a contraindication, has now become an *indication* for chronic beta blockade (see Chap. 23), but the dose must be escalated slowly in patients with left ventricular dysfunction, and intravenous administration should be avoided.[131]

The choice of beta blocker can be made individually on the basis of the drug's pharmacokinetics and cost and the physician's familiarity with it. However, those with intrinsic sympathomimetic activity, such as pindolol, should not be selected. Examples of doses tested in large trials include atenolol (5- to 10-mg intravenous bolus followed by 100 mg orally daily) and metoprolol (5-mg intravenous boluses, three given 2 to 5 minutes apart, followed by 50 mg orally twice daily titrated up to 100 mg twice daily).[132]

Calcium Channel Blockers (see also Chap. 50)

Calcium channel blockers have vasodilatory effects and lower blood pressure, and some (verapamil and diltiazem) also slow heart rate. They may be used in patients who have persistent or recurrent symptoms but are currently recommended only for patients who have persistent ischemia after treatment with full-dose nitrates and beta blockers or patients with contraindications to beta blockade. Such patients should be treated with heart rate–slowing calcium channel blockers (e.g., diltiazem or verapamil). Oral doses of diltiazem and verapamil range from 30 mg three times daily for the former and 80 mg three times daily for the latter to 480 mg once daily of the long-acting preparation.

In the Diltiazem Reinfarction Study, involving 576 patients with non-Q-wave MI, diltiazem reduced recurrent MI from 9.3 percent with placebo to 5.2 percent with diltiazem.[133] A pilot study using intravenous diltiazem and a larger clinical trial using long-acting diltiazem[134] in patients following thrombolytic therapy found trends toward benefit of diltiazem versus placebo. In the Danish Verapamil Infarction Trial II (DAVIT II) involving patients with suspected MI or unstable angina, of whom nearly half did not have confirmed MI, verapamil tended to reduce recurrent MI or death.[135] However, meta-analyses have found no beneficial effect of the calcium antagonist drugs as a class in reducing mortality or subsequent infarction.[136] One overview did suggest benefit of verapamil alone.[137]

In patients with acute MI with left ventricular dysfunction or congestive heart failure, a harmful effect of diltiazem was observed.[138] Nifedipine, which does not lower heart rate, has been shown to be harmful in patients with acute MI when not coadministered with a beta blocker. In contrast, no harm was observed in one study with verapamil in patients with congestive heart failure, all of whom were treated with ACE inhibitors.[139] Similarly, no harm with long-term treatment with amlodipine or felodipine[140] was observed in patients with documented left ventricular dysfunction and CAD, indicating that these vasoselective calcium antagonists may be safely used in patients with UA/NSTEMI with left ventricular dysfunction.

In summary, calcium antagonists should be used in patients with UA/NSTEMI if needed for recurrent ischemia despite beta blockade or in patients in whom beta blockade is contraindicated (e.g., bronchospasm); diltiazem should be avoided in patients with left ventricular dysfunction or congestive heart failure, or both.

Angiotensin-Converting Enzyme Inhibitors

For acute treatment, three large trials showed a 0.5 percent absolute mortality benefit of early (initiated within 24 hours)

ACE inhibition in patients with acute MI.[125,126,141] However, in the ISIS-4 study, no benefit was observed in patients without ST elevation. Thus, short-term ACE inhibition does not appear to confer any benefit for patients with UA/NSTEMI.

On the other hand, *long-term* use of ACE inhibition is beneficial in preventing recurrent ischemic events and mortality in a broad population of patients now including those with any evidence of CAD (see also Chap. 50).[142,143] It is of note that recurrent MI and the need for revascularization were reduced with captopril and enalapril in the Survival and Ventricular Enlargement (SAVE) and Studies of Left Ventricular Dysfunction (SOLVD) trials,[144,145] which has now been confirmed using ramipril and perindopril in the Heart Outcomes Prevention Evaluation (HOPE) and EURopean trial On reduction of cardiac events with Perindopril in stable coronary Artery disease (EUROPA),[142,143] suggesting an antiischemic effect of this entire class of agents.

Lipid-Lowering Therapy (see also Chap. 39)

When compared to placebo, long-term treatment with lipid-lowering therapy, especially with statins, has been shown to be beneficial in patients following acute MI and unstable angina.[146-149] In the Scandinavian Simvastatin Survival Study (4S), carried out in hypercholesterolemic patients with a history of MI *or* unstable angina, mortality was reduced by 30 percent ($p = 0.0003$) and coronary deaths were significantly reduced by 42 percent.[146] In addition, recurrent MI was significantly reduced by 37 percent ($p < 0.001$), coronary revascularization by 37 percent ($p < 0.0001$), and rehospitalization for acute cardiovascular disease by 26 percent ($p < 0.001$).[146,150] In the Long-term Intervention with Pravastatin in Ischemic Disease (LIPID) trial, involving a prespecified subgroup of more than 3200 patients with unstable angina, pravastatin therapy led to a significant 26 percent reduction in total mortality ($p = 0.004$).[151]

The National Cholesterol Education Program recommends treatment with diet and drug therapy if the LDL is greater than 100 mg/dl, with a target of reducing LDL to less than 100 mg/dl.[152] The timing of the blood sample is ideally in the first 24 hours after admission because cholesterol levels fall with acute illness. However, cholesterol should be measured at some time during admission because if it is high, therapy is warranted. Because treatment with statin drugs was associated with the benefits for mortality and cardiovascular morbidity cited earlier, these are the current first-line drugs. Additional or alternative therapy is also warranted according to the National Cholesterol Education Program (see also Chap. 39).[153]

Several pilot studies and observational studies have sought to determine whether there is an early clinical benefit of early initiation of statin therapy in ACS.[154-157] The larger, randomized Myocardial Ischaemia Reduction with Aggressive Cholesterol Lowering (MIRACL) trial found that short-term (4 months) treatment with high-dose atorvastatin (80 mg/d) reduced the primary composite endpoint of cardiac death, nonfatal MI, resuscitated sudden cardiac death, or urgent rehospitalization for recurrent ischemia by 16 percent ($p = 0.048$). The potential benefits of early aggressive statin therapy compared to placebo are also being studied in the Aggrastat to Zocor (A to Z; TIMI 21) trial.[158]

The Pravastatin or Atorvastatin Evaluation and Infection Therapy—Thrombolysis in Myocardial Infarction (PROVE IT-TIMI) 22 trial evaluated the role of intensive lipid lowering as compared with standard lipid lowering in 4162 patients within 10 days of admission for an acute coronary syndrome.[158a] Treatment with standard therapy (pravastatin, 40 mg) achieved a median LDL of 95 mg/dl (range, 79 to 113 mg/dl), while intensive therapy (atorvastatin, 80 mg) achieved a median LDL of 62 mg/dl (interquartile range, 50 to 79 mg/dl) ($p < 0.001$). The risk of death, nonfatal myocar-

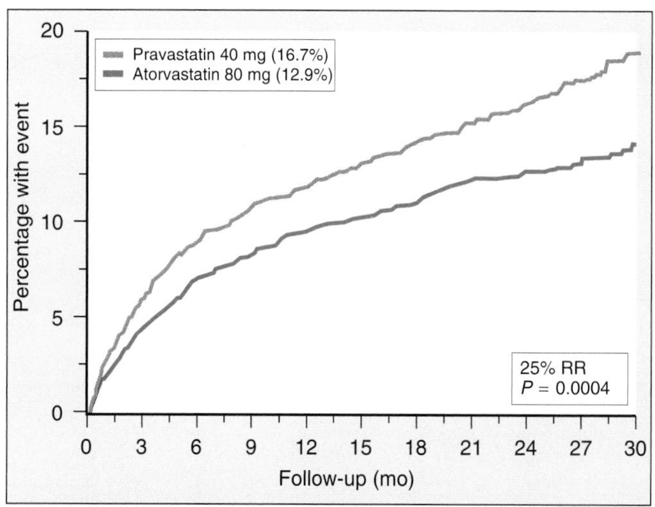

FIGURE 49–11 Results of the PROVE-IT TIMI 22 Trial showing reduction of adverse outcomes (death, nonfatal MI, or urgent revascularization) with intensive lipid lowering with atorvastatin 80 mg/day, compared to standard lipid lowering with pravastatin 40 mg/day. Rates in parentheses are at 2 years.

dial infarction, documented unstable angina, revascularization, or stroke was reduced by 16% ($p = 0.005$), with rates at 2 years (mean time of follow-up) falling from 26.3 percent to 22.4 percent in the standard versus intensive therapy groups. The risk of death, nonfatal myocardial infarction, or revascularization was reduced by 25 percent ($p = 0.0004$) (Fig. 49–11). In addition, all-cause mortality was reduced by 28 percent ($p = 0.07$), with 2-year mortality rates of 32 percent for standard statin therapy versus 2.2 percent for intensive therapy. Benefit emerged within 30 days postrandomization and continued throughout the 2.5 years of follow-up. Thus, this study demonstrated that (1) early use of high-dose statins following acute coronary syndrome is beneficial in reducing death or recurrent cardiac events, and (2) more intensive lipid-lowering therapy that achieved LDL cholesterol concentrations substantially below current target levels is beneficial.

Beyond the issue of whether an early clinical benefit is achieved and the optimal degree of lipid lowering, studies have found that early initiation of therapy after ACS can improve long-term compliance. One study used standardized orders to ensure that all the patients are receiving appropriate guideline-recommended therapies and found an increase in the use of statins at the time of discharge and at 1-year follow-up, with 91 percent of appropriate patients receiving therapy.[159] Others have also found improved long-term treatment rates with institution of in-hospital quality improvement programs.[160]

Antithrombotic Therapy

Aspirin (see also Chap. 80)

Aspirin permanently acetylates cyclooxygenase 1, thereby blocking the synthesis of thromboxane A_2 by the platelet (Fig. 49–12). By reducing the amount of thromboxane A_2 released, which would act to stimulate other platelets, this effect decreases overall platelet aggregation at the site of the thrombus. This inhibition of cyclooxygenase is permanent, and thus the antiplatelet effects last for the lifetime of the platelets, on the order of 7 to 10 days. Several trials have demonstrated clear beneficial effects of aspirin, with a more than 50 percent reduction in the risk of death or MI in patients presenting with UA/NSTEMI (Fig. 49–13).[16,161] The benefit emerges within the first day of treatment.[161] Thus, aspirin has a dramatic effect in reducing adverse clinical

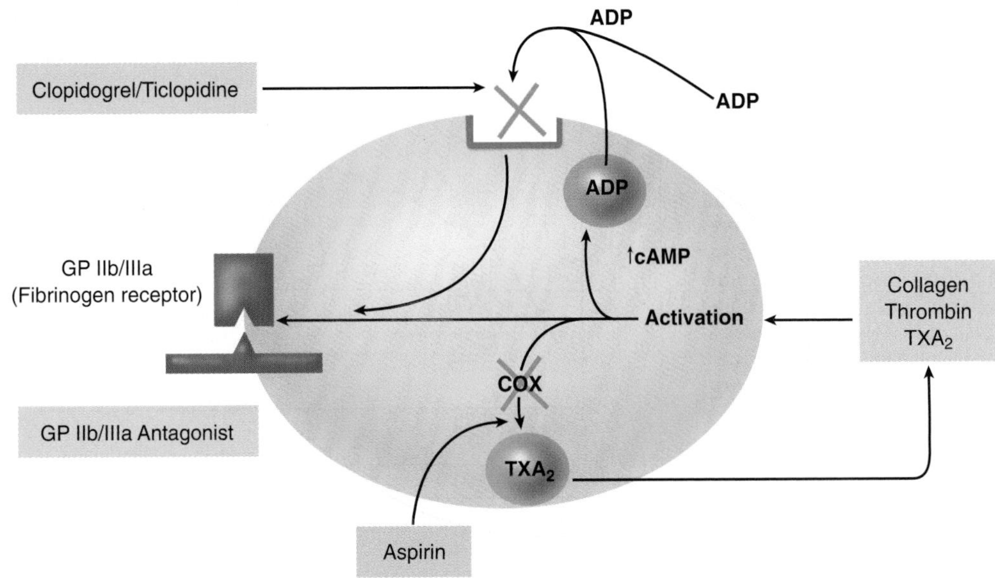

FIGURE 49–12 Mechanisms of action of antiplatelet therapies. See text and Chapter 80 for details. ADP = adenosine diphosphate; cAMP = cyclic adenosine monophosphate; COX = cyclooxygenase; GP = glycoprotein; TXA_2 = thromboxane A_2. (Adapted from Schafer AI: Antiplatelet therapy. Am J Med 101:199, 1996.)

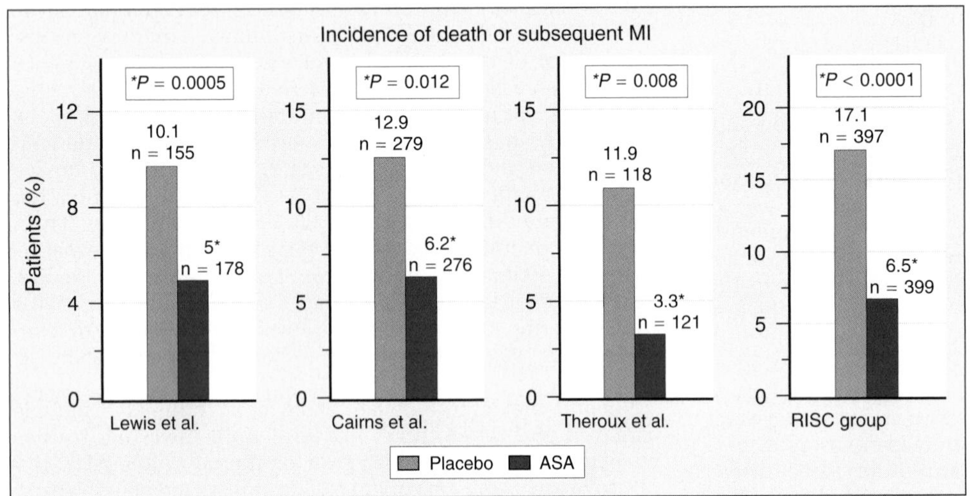

FIGURE 49–13 Four randomized trials showing the benefit of aspirin in unstable angina or non-ST elevation myocardial infarction (UA/NSTEMI). In UA/NSTEMI, the incidence of death or myocardial infarction (MI) was reduced by more than 50 percent in each of the four trials. The doses of aspirin in the four trials were 325, 1300, 650, and 75 mg/d, respectively, indicating no difference in efficacy for aspirin across these doses. ASA = acetylsalicylic acid (aspirin). (Data from Lewis HD, et al: N Engl J Med 309:396, 1983; Cairns, et al: N Engl J Med 313:1499, 1985; Theroux P, et al: N Engl J Med 319:1105, 1988; RISC Group: Lancet 349:827, 1990.)

events early in the course of treatment of UA/NSTEMI and thus is primary therapy for these patients.

The dose of aspirin in the four randomized trials ranged from 75 to 1300 mg/d, and each trial showed a roughly 50 percent reduction in death or MI.[16,161-163] In the large overview of all short- and long-term trials, there does not appear to be a dose-response effect in efficacy of aspirin.[164] In ISIS-2, a dose of 160 mg/d was shown to have a mortality benefit, and this dose is the minimum initial dose recommended.[165] In terms of safety (e.g., gastrointestinal bleeding), two observational studies have found that the rate of bleeding appears to be lower with low-dose aspirin than with medium-dose aspirin (i.e., 325 mg/d) (Table 49–3).[166,167] This was seen among patients treated with medical therapy, PCI, or coronary artery bypass graft (CABG) surgery. Thus, after an initial loading dose of 162 to 325 mg, a dose of 75 to 81 mg/d appears be appropriate for both early and long-term therapy.

During chronic therapy, aspirin resistance has been reported.[168,169] Small studies have identified 5 to 8 percent of patients who have minimal inhibition of platelet aggregation when treated with aspirin. These patients tend to have a greater risk of recurrent cardiac events.[169] No dose response has been seen with this measure of aspirin resistance. A larger study correlated outcomes at 5 years with the amount of thromboxane metabolites in the urine.[168] When patients were divided into quartiles according to the amount of thromboxane in the urine, which could be viewed as a measure of thromboxane "breakthrough" despite aspirin therapy, higher event rates were seen as the amount of thromboxane metabolites rose.[168]

Absolute contraindications for aspirin therapy are few but include documented aspirin allergy (e.g., asthma), active bleeding, or a known platelet disorder. In patients who report dyspepsia or other gastrointestinal symptoms with long-term aspirin therapy (i.e., intolerance), this would not be expected to be an acute problem for in-hospital treatment, and aspirin therapy may be considered for such patients, at least for the short term. In patients who have an allergy or who cannot tolerate aspirin, use of clopidogrel is recommended.[4]

Clopidogrel and Ticlopidine

(see also Chap. 80)

Clopidogrel and ticlopidine are thienopyridine derivatives that inhibit platelet aggregation, increase bleeding time, and reduce blood viscosity by inhibiting adenosine diphosphate (ADP) action on platelet receptors.[24] They achieve their antiaggregatory action by inhibiting the binding of ADP to its platelet receptors, specifically the P_2Y_{12} component of the ADP receptor (see Fig. 49–12).[24] Blockade of this receptor not

TABLE 49–3 Major Bleeding by Aspirin Dose

Aspirin Dose (mg)	Aspirin + Placebo	Aspirin + Clopidogrel
75-100	1.9%	3.0%
100-199	2.8%	3.4%
200-325	3.7%	4.9%

Data from Peters RJ, Mehta SR, Fox KA, et al: Circulation 108:1682, 2003.

only inhibits the ADP-induced platelet activation and subsequent aggregation but also appears to decrease platelet activation by other outside stimuli (e.g., von Willebrand factor).[170] Thus, because the P_2Y_{12} receptor is part of the overall amplification of platelet activation within the platelet, inhibition of this receptor appears to have a broader effect in decreasing platelet activation than just inhibition ADP-induced aggregation.

Ticlopidine was compared with placebo (without aspirin) in a randomized trial involving 652 patients with UA/NSTEMI and was found to produce a significant 46 percent reduction in vascular death or nonfatal MI.[171] Ticlopidine has also been demonstrated to be effective in combination with aspirin for prevention of thrombosis and recurrent ischemic events in patients undergoing coronary stent implantation, a portion of whom have recently suffered UA/NSTEMI (see also Chap. 80).[172] However, ticlopidine is associated with neutropenia and thrombocytopenia in approximately 1 percent of patients and quite rarely with thrombotic thrombocytopenic purpura, which can be fatal in 25 to 40 percent of cases.[173] Thus, if ticlopidine is used, short courses (2 to 3 weeks) and biweekly monitoring of complete blood count are generally recommended.

Clopidogrel was developed to avoid these hematological complications and in clinical trials to date has not been associated with an increased incidence of neutropenia or thrombotic thrombocytopenic purpura compared with aspirin alone.[23,174,175] When added to aspirin, clopidogrel appears to be as effective as ticlopidine in preventing stent thrombosis.[176]

THE CURE TRIAL. The addition of clopidogrel to aspirin was studied in the large Clopidogrel in Unstable angina to prevent Recurrent Events (CURE) trial, in which patients were treated with aspirin (75 to 325 mg), heparin or LMWH, and other standard therapies and were randomly assigned to receive a 300-mg loading dose of clopidogrel followed by 75 mg/d.The combination of clopidogrel plus aspirin conferred a 20 percent reduction in cardiovascular death, MI, or stroke compared with aspirin alone in both low- and high-risk patients with UA/NSTEMI (Fig. 49-14).[23] Benefit was seen as early as 24 hours, with the Kaplan-Meier curves diverging after just 2 hours, indicating a very early antithrombotic and clinical effect (Fig. 49-15).[177] Moreover, the benefit continued throughout the trial's 1-year treatment period, consistent with data from the Clopidogrel for Recurrent Events During Observation (CREDO) and Clopidogrel versus Aspirin in Patients at Risk of Ischaemic Events (CAPRIE) trials showing benefit of clopidogrel through 1 and 3 years, respectively, of follow-up in patients with prior atherothrombotic disease.[174,178]

In PCI-CURE, benefit of early treatment with clopidogrel prior to PCI was also seen with a 31 percent reduction in cardiac events at 30 days and 1 year in patients.[179]

THE CREDO TRIAL. In the CREDO trial involving patients undergoing planned or likely PCI (which included approximately two-thirds of patients with ACS), patients were randomly assigned to receive a loading dose of clopidogrel (300 mg) or placebo between 3 and 24 hours before PCI. Following stenting, all patients received open-label clopidogrel for 28 days; after 28 days, patients in the pretreatment group continued on clopidogrel for 1 year, whereas the nonpretreatment group was treated with matching placebo.This study found a small but not statistically significant increase in bleeding in patients receiving clopidogrel versus placebo in addition to aspirin, heparin, and GP IIb/IIIa inhibition. Similar safety observations have been made in other studies.[179-181]

The efficacy results from CREDO also lend further support to both early and long-term use of clopidogrel in patients with UA/NSTEMI. Pretreatment with clopidogrel led to a nonsignificant 19 percent risk reduction in events; however, those given clopidogrel at least 6 hours before PCI had a 38.6 percent relative risk reduction in major events at 28 days ($p = 0.05$) compared with no reduction with treatment less than 6 hours before PCI. This emphasizes the need to initiate clopidogrel as soon as possible on admission for UA/NSTEMI, prior to any planned catheterization and possible PCI. Overall, treatment for 1 year with clopidogrel plus aspirin led to a 26.9 percent relative reduction in death, MI, or stroke compared with post-PCI clopidogrel therapy for 1 month (8.5 versus 11.5 percent [placebo], $p = 0.02$). This included an additional 37.4 percent relative reduction in major events from day 29 to 1 year with clopidogrel ($p = 0.04$). In summary, the results of PCI-CURE and CREDO support preprocedural loading and long-term therapy with clopidogrel in those scheduled or expected to undergo PCI. The significant benefits were seen with or without the concomitant use of GP IIb/IIIa inhibitors.

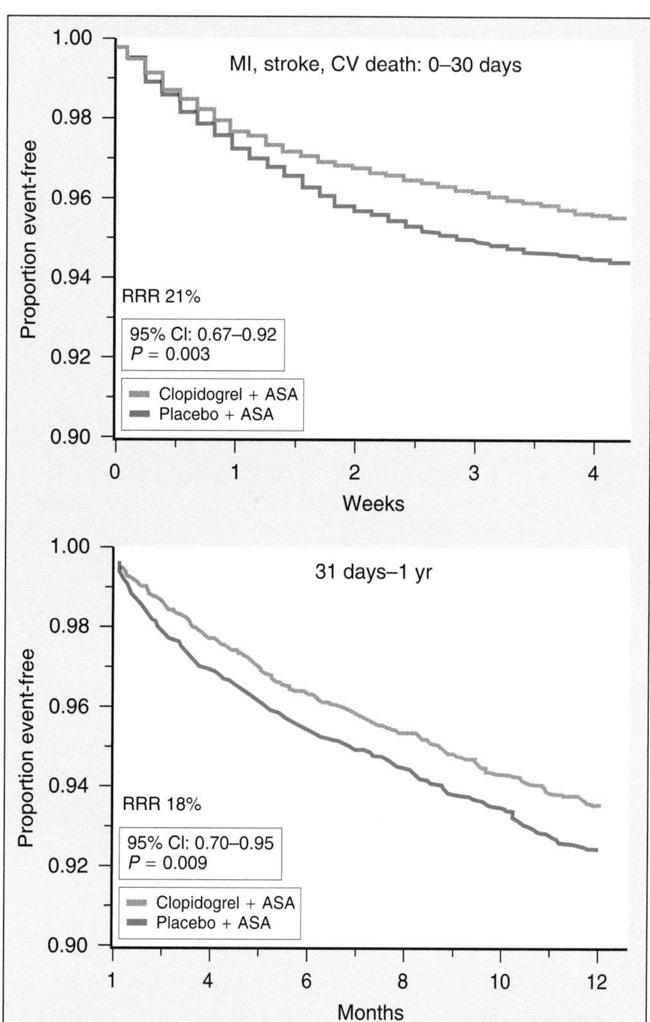

FIGURE 49–14 Benefit of the addition of clopidogrel to aspirin compared with placebo and aspirin during the first 30 days **(top)** and between 31 days and 1 year **(bottom)**. The second analysis was restricted to patients who did not experience an event during the first 31 days. ASA = acetylsalicylic acid (aspirin); CI = confidence interval; CV = cardiovascular; MI = myocardial infarction. (From Yusuf S, Mehta SR, Zhao F, et al: Early and late effects of clopidogrel in patients with acute coronary syndromes. Circulation 107:966, 2003.)

In UA/NSTEMI, the dose of clopidogrel should be an initial loading dose of 300 mg, followed by 75 mg/d. Initiation of only 75 mg/d achieves the target level of platelet inhibition after 3 to 5 days, whereas the loading dose of 300 mg achieves effective platelet inhibition within 4 to 6 hours.[182] Use of a 600-mg loading dose has been shown to achieve a steady-state level of platelet inhibition after just 2 hours.[183] This dose has been utilized in two large clinical studies and been well tolerated.[184,185] In one study, all 2159 patients received a 600-mg loading dose at least 2 hours prior to PCI and were randomly assigned to abciximab and reduced-dose heparin versus placebo and standard-dose heparin. There was no difference in outcomes between the groups at 30 days.[185] This is in contrast to 35 to 50 percent reductions seen with abciximab in other placebo-controlled trials conducted before widespread pretreatment with thienopyridines,[186-188] suggesting that the achievement of effective levels of platelet inhibition with clopidogrel before PCI is effective in reducing events. More studies are ongoing to evaluate the 600-mg loading dose.

As with aspirin, "low responders" to clopidogrel have been identified in several studies.[189,190] As with the aspirin resistance issue, defining what a low response is and determi-

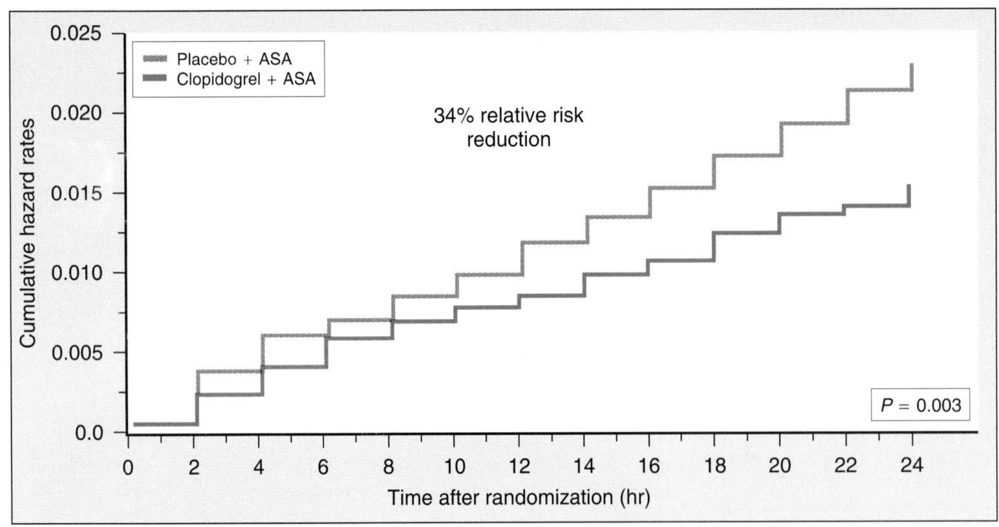

FIGURE 49–15 Effects of clopidogrel in the first 24 hours of the Clopidogrel in Unstable angina to prevent Recurrent Events (CURE) trial. ASA = acetylsalicylic acid (aspirin). (From Yusuf S, Mehta SR, Zhao F, et al: Early and late effects of clopidogrel in patients with acute coronary syndromes. Circulation 107:966, 2003.)

whether it reflects variability in the state of platelet aggregation in the patient or variability in the platelet response to the drug has been difficult using current assays. These findings have fueled interest in development of newer drugs in this class that might achieve higher levels of platelet inhibition.[24] The balance of the efficacy and safety of higher levels of inhibition with this class of drugs needs to be defined in prospective clinical trials.

Heparin (see also Chap. 80)

Anticoagulation with UFH has been a cornerstone of therapy for patients with UA/NSTEMI for over a decade on the basis of several randomized trials that found lower rates of death or MI with UFH plus aspirin compared with aspirin alone.[16,161,191,192] A meta-analysis showed a 33 percent reduction in death or MI at 2 to 12 weeks follow-up with UFH plus aspirin versus aspirin alone, although this reduction was of borderline statistical significance.[17]

Variability in the anticoagulant effects of UFH, so-called heparin resistance, is thought to be due to the heterogeneity of heparin and to the neutralization of heparin by circulating plasma factors and by proteins released by activated platelets.[193] Clinically, frequent monitoring of the anticoagulant response using the activated partial thromboplastin time (aPTT) is recommended with titrations carried out using a standardized nomogram (Table 49–4). The latter minimizes the variability in the dosing adjustments given by various physicians and has been shown to improve the achievement of a target aPTT.[194]

The level of anticoagulation that constitutes the therapeutic range is not yet firmly established. Small studies have suggested that lower aPTT values may be related to recurrent ischemic events,[195,196] suggesting that the lower limit of the target range of aPTT is at least 1.5 times the control value. On the upper boundary of the target range, higher aPTT values are associated with an increased risk of hemorrhage.[196] The lowest rate of bleeding (and mortality) in patients with STEMI treated with thrombolytic therapy was observed when the 12-hour aPTT was between 50 and 70 seconds.[196] Furthermore, in TIMI IIIB, there appeared to be no advantage in reducing ischemic events with higher levels of anticoagulation.[197]

DOSING. On the basis of available data,[198] the current optimal regimen appears to consist of weight-adjusted dosing of UFH (60 units/kg bolus and 12 units/kg/hr infusion), frequent monitoring of aPTT (every 6 hours until in the target range and every 12 to 24 hours thereafter), and titration of UFH using a standardized nomogram (see Table 49–4) with a target range of aPTT between 1.5 to 2 times the control value or approximately 50 and 70 seconds.

Low-Molecular-Weight Heparin (see also Chap. 80)

LMWHs have been widely tested as a means of improving on anticoagulation with UFH. These agents *combine* factor IIa and factor Xa inhibition and thus inhibit both the action and generation of thrombin.[199] LMWHs are obtained by depolymerization of standard UFHs and selection of those with lower molecular weight. Compared with UFH that has nearly equal anti-IIa (thrombin) and anti-Xa activity, LMWHs have increased ratios of anti-IIa to anti-Xa activity of either 2:1 (e.g., dalteparin) or 3.8:1 (e.g., enoxaparin).

LMWH has several potential advantages over UFH. First, its greater anti-factor Xa activity inhibits thrombin generation more effectively. LMWH also induces a greater release of tissue factor pathway inhibitor than UFH, and it is not neutralized by platelet factor 4.[199] LMWH has been found to induce thrombocytopenia at a lower rate than UFH.[200] Its high bioavailability allows subcutaneous administration, which provides a long duration of systemic anticoagulation so that dosing can be administered twice daily. Also, LMWH has less binding to plasma proteins (including acute phase reactant proteins) and thus has a more consistent anticoagulant effect in relation to the dose administered. Accordingly, monitoring of the level of anticoagulation (which is necessary using aPTT for UFH) is not necessary. These last two differences make LMWH a much simpler anticoagulant to administer

TABLE 49–4 Standardized Nomogram for Titration of Heparin

Initial dose: 60 U/kg bolus and 12 U/kg/hr infusion
The activated partial thromboplastin time (aPTT) should be checked and infusion adjusted at 6, 12, and 24 hr after initiation of heparin, daily thereafter, and 4 to 6 hr after any adjustment in dose.

aPTT (sec)	Change	Intravenous Infusion (U/kg/hr)
<35	60 U/kg bolus	+3
35-49	30 U/kg bolus	+2
50-70	0	0
71-90	0	−2
>100	Hold infusion for 30 min	−3

Adapted from Becker RC, Ball SP, Eisenberg P, et al: A randomized, multicenter trial of weight-adjusted intravenous heparin dose titration and point-of-care coagulation monitoring in hospitalized patients with active thromboembolic disease. Antithrombotic Therapy Consortium Investigators. Am Heart J 137:59, 1999.

than UFH. However, it should be noted that LMWHs are more affected by renal dysfunction than UFH, and a reduced dose should be considered in patients with creatinine clearance less than 30 ml/min.

CLINICAL TRIALS

There have been more than 12 randomized trials comparing LMWH with placebo[201] or UFH[18,202,203] and one comparing two different LMWHs. LMWH (plus aspirin) has been found to be effective compared with aspirin alone, leading to a 66 percent reduction in the odds of death or MI.[201,204]

In comparisons between LMWHs and UFH, heterogeneity has been seen between the LMWHs. To date, no difference was observed between dalteparin[202] or nadroparin compared with UFH.[202,203]

On the other hand, three of four trials with enoxaparin have found a significant improvement in clinical outcomes. In the Evaluation of the Safety and Efficacy of Enoxaparin in Non-ST elevation Coronary Events (ESSENCE)[18] and TIMI 11B,[19] enoxaparin conferred a significant approximately 20 percent reduction in death, MI, or recurrent ischemia compared with UFH. In both trials, patients with ST segment deviation exhibited a significant reduction in cardiac events with enoxaparin compared with UFH, whereas those without ST deviation did not.[18,19] Similarly, in the TIMI 11B troponin substudy, among patients who were CK-MB negative, those with elevations of troponin I derived a significantly greater benefit from enoxaparin versus UFH than those with negative troponins.[205] Using the TIMI risk score (see Fig. 49-9A), the benefit of enoxaparin over UFH was seen among patients with a score of 3 or higher (in both ESSENCE and TIMI 11B).[67] Thus, the clinical benefit of enoxaparin is seen among higher risk patients.

In a formal pharmacoeconomic analysis, use of enoxaparin was found to be cost effective: There was a small increase in the cost of the drug (enoxaparin versus UFH with aPTT measurements), but it was balanced by significantly lower rates of catheterization and revascularization, and thus treatment with enoxaparin led to *savings* of $1172 per patient treated.[206] Thus, both improved outcomes and lower costs were observed with in-hospital treatment with enoxaparin versus UFH. No additional benefit of continuing enoxaparin beyond hospital discharge was observed.[19] On the other hand, a more dramatic benefit of enoxaparin was seen among patients undergoing PCI.[207]

Three studies evaluated the merit of enoxaparin versus UFH among patients receiving aspirin and a GP IIb/IIIa inhibitor.[40,158,208] In one study, in which enoxaparin was administered for approximately 4 days prior to any revascularization procedure, if performed, enoxaparin led to a significant reduction in death or MI and of recurrent ischemia documented by ST segment depression on Holter monitoring.[40] In the A to Z trial, a nonsignificant trend toward improved outcomes was seen.[208] A third study (Superior Yield of the New strategy of Enoxaparin, Revascularization, GlYcoprotein IIb/IIIa inhibitors [SYNERGY]) of approximately 10,000 found no significant difference in death or myocardial infarction between enoxaparin and UFH but an increase in bleeding with enoxaparin.[208a] of the two agents in the setting of an early invasive strategy and GP IIb/IIIa inhibition. Figure 49-16 summarizes data on enoxaparin in UA/NSTEMI: a significant approximately 15 to 20 percent relative risk reduction in death or MI and of the combined endpoint of death, MI, or recurrent ischemia at 7 days.[208]

Finally, one study of 438 patients with UA/NSTEMI directly compared two LMWHs—enoxaparin and tinzaparin. The primary composite endpoint, death, MI, or recurrent angina at 7 days, was significantly lower in the enoxaparin group (12.3 percent versus 21.1 percent in the tinzaparin group, $p = 0.015$).[209] These data, combined with the multiple studies of enoxaparin versus UFH, suggest that enoxaparin has a particular benefit in UA/NSTEMI, and unless new trials with other LMWHs demonstrate a benefit over UFH, enoxaparin appears to be the LWMH (and antithrombin) of choice in UA/NSTEMI.

Because one of the purported advantages of LMWH over UFH is the greater factor Xa inhibition, research is progressing with testing of pure factor Xa inhibitors. One agent is a synthetic pentasaccharide, which has been found to be more effective than enoxaparin in prevention of deep vein thrombosis[210]; it is currently being tested in UA/NSTEMI and STEMI.

Direct Thrombin Inhibitors (see also Chap. 80)

Direct thrombin (factor IIa) inhibitors have also undergone extensive evaluation. The prototypic agent is hirudin, a naturally occurring anticoagulant from the medicinal leech. Hirudin, which is manufactured by a recombinant DNA technique, is a 65-amino-acid polypeptide that binds directly to

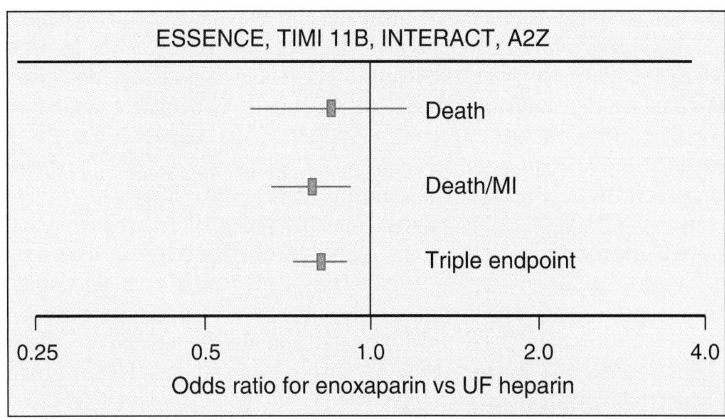

FIGURE 49–16 Meta-analysis of Thrombolysis in Myocardial Infarction (TIMI 11B), Evaluation of the Safety and Efficacy of Enoxaparin in Non-ST elevation Coronary Events (ESSENCE), Interact, and Aggrastat to Zocor (A to Z) trials comparing enoxaparin with unfractionated (UF) heparin. There is a significant reduction in the rate of death or myocardial infarction (MI) in patients treated with enoxaparin. (From Blazing MA: The A-to-Z Trial: Results of the A-Phase, investigating combined use of low-molecular-weight heparin with the glycoprotein IIb/IIIa inhibitor tirofiban. Presented at the American College of Cardiology Scientific Sessions, New Orleans, LA, March 2003.)

thrombin, independent of antithrombin. The hirudin desirudin was tested in the Global Use of Strategies to Open Occluded Coronary Arteries (GUSTO) IIb trial involving 12,142 patients with UA/NSTEMI and STEMI. In the entire cohort, the 30-day rate of death or MI tended to be lower, 8.9 versus 9.8 percent ($p = 0.06$),[35] with no difference in mortality and a modest reduction in reinfarction (5.4 versus 6.3 percent for heparin, $p = 0.04$). In the 8011 patients with UA/NSTEMI, 30-day death or MI was not significantly reduced (8.3 versus 9.1 percent, $p = 0.22$).[35]

The Organisation to Assess Strategies for Ischemic Syndromes (OASIS-2) trial[211] compared lepirudin, another form of hirudin, and UFH; cardiovascular death or MI at 7 days tended to be lower with lepirudin (3.6 versus 4.2 percent, respectively, $p = 0.08$). Major bleeding requiring transfusion was rare but more frequent with lepirudin (1.2 versus 0.7 percent for heparin, $p = 0.01$). A meta-analysis of all hirudin trials showed a modest 10 percent benefit favoring hirudin, which was not statistically significant for patients with UA/NSTEMI. Other synthetic direct thrombin inhibitors have also been tested in small trials to date (e.g., argatroban and bivalirudin), with trends toward lower rates of recurrent cardiac events and lower rates of bleeding.[212-214]

BIVALIRUDIN. This directly acting antithrombin has been tested during PCI and found to have a trend toward superior outcomes compared with UFH[215] and outcomes similar to those with the combination of UFH plus a GP IIb/IIIa inhibitor.[216] In the latter trial, only 40 percent of patients were characterized as having UA/NSTEMI, and the difference in recurrent cardiac events was numerically higher but not statistically different among this high-risk subgroup. Thus, the efficacy of bivalirudin has not been fully studied in UA/NSTEMI, but a large trial is underway. The direct thrombin inhibitors have been observed to provide a stable level of anticoagulation, as measured by aPTT,[35,217] and no episodes of thrombocytopenia have been reported for the hirudin class. Of note, lepirudin and argatroban are approved by the Food and Drug Administration for use as anticoagulants in patients with heparin-induced thrombocytopenia and associated thromboembolic disease.

Oral Anticoagulation (see also Chap. 80)

Oral anticoagulation with warfarin following ACSs has been examined in several trials, with the rationale that prolonged treatment might extend the benefit of early anticoagulation with an antithrombin agent (e.g., heparin, LMWH). Three of the initial large trials have failed to show a significant benefit of long-term warfarin plus aspirin over aspirin alone. In the OASIS-2 trial involving patients with UA/NSTEMI, the rate of cardiovascular death, MI, or stroke to 5 months was 7.6 percent for those receiving warfarin plus aspirin and 8.3 percent for those receiving aspirin alone ($p = NS$).[218] Similarly, in the Combination Hemotherapy and Mortality Prevention (CHAMP) trial involving survivors of MI, there was no difference in the rate of all-cause mortality over an average 2.7 years of follow-up between the combination of warfarin plus aspirin and aspirin alone, but there was a higher rate of major bleeding.[219] In addition, fixed-dose warfarin plus aspirin was not better than aspirin alone in the Coumadin Aspirin Reinfarction Study (CARS).[220]

However, three subsequent trials, in addition to a post hoc analysis of OASIS-2, suggested that if a sufficient degree of anticoagulation is achieved, a benefit can be observed with the combination of aspirin plus warfarin compared with aspirin alone.[221-224] In each of these studies, the International Normalized Ratio (INR) for the warfarin (plus aspirin) treatment arm had a mean of 2.3 to 2.4, indicating a full degree of anticoagulation, compared with 1.9 in the CHAMP study, which did not find a benefit of warfarin. In the largest study,[223] 4930 patients with ACS within the prior 8 weeks were randomly assigned to warfarin alone (target INR of 2.8 to 4.2), aspirin (160 mg/d), or aspirin (75 mg/d) combined with warfarin (target INR of 2.0 to 2.5). During an average of 4 years of follow-up, death, MI, or thromboembolic cerebral stroke occurred in 20.0 percent of patients receiving aspirin, 16.7 percent of patients receiving warfarin ($p = 0.03$), and 15.0 percent of patients receiving warfarin and aspirin ($p = 0.001$). Rates of major bleeding were 0.62 percent per treatment year in both groups receiving warfarin and 0.17 percent in patients receiving aspirin ($p < 0.001$). Thus, the combination of aspirin plus warfarin is more effective than aspirin alone for long-term secondary prevention.

However, given the similar benefit seen with clopidogrel plus aspirin, the lack of need for monitoring the INR, and the frequent use of PCI and stenting in the population of patients in which clopidogrel is well established, the clinical use of aspirin plus warfarin is limited. However, among patients with another indication for warfarin, such as chronic atrial fibrillation or severe left ventricular dysfunction, who are at high risk for systemic embolization, the combination of aspirin plus warfarin would be preferable as the long-term antithrombotic strategy.[225] The combination of all three agents has not been tested to date but might portend a higher bleeding risk during long-term therapy. Use of all three agents together is sometimes needed among patients with atrial fibrillation or other strong indications for warfarin who undergo stenting. In such patients, one approach is to use aspirin (75 to 81 mg/d) and warfarin (INR 2.0 to 2.5) and to use clopidogrel for only 1 month (the period during which the risk of stent thrombosis is highest).

Research is ongoing to identify alternative oral anticoagulants. One agent, ximelagatran, an oral direct thrombin inhibitor, has been tested in patients following ACS in a dose-ranging study. Overall, the combination of ximelagatran plus aspirin reduced the rate of death, MI, or severe recurrent ischemia by 24 percent compared with aspirin, from 16.3 to 12.7 percent ($p = 0.049$).[226] Although this agent was associated with elevations of liver function tests, it is administered at a fixed dose and does not require monitoring of the level of anticoagulation, but it does require monitoring of liver function tests. Oral factor Xa inhibitors are also in early stages of development.

Glycoprotein IIb/IIIa Inhibitors (see also Chap. 80)

The GP IIb/IIIa receptor inhibitors are a potent class of antiplatelet drugs that act by preventing the final common pathway of platelet aggregation, i.e., fibrinogen-mediated cross-linkage of platelets through the GP IIb/IIIa receptor (see Fig. 49–4). These agents are potent inhibitors of platelet aggregation caused by all types of stimuli (e.g., thrombin, ADP, collagen, serotonin). Three agents are now available for use in UA/NSTEMI, abciximab, eptifibatide, and tirofiban, with the former currently approved only in patients undergoing PCI. *Abciximab* is an Fab fragment of a monoclonal antibody directed at the GP IIb/IIIa receptor. *Eptifibatide*, a synthetic heptapeptide, and *tirofiban*, a nonpeptide molecule, are antagonists of the GP IIb/IIIa receptor whose structure mimics the arginine-glycine-aspartic acid (abbreviated RGD) amino acid sequence by which fibrinogen binds to the GP IIb/IIIa receptor.

Several trials have shown benefit of IIb/IIIa inhibition in UA/NSTEMI in patients receiving predominantly medical management,[21] early interventional management,[227] or both.[20,22,228] In Platelet Receptor Inhibition for Ischemic Syndrome Management in Patients Limited by Unstable Signs and Symptoms (PRISM-PLUS), tirofiban plus heparin and aspirin significantly reduced the rate of death, MI, or refractory ischemia at 7 days compared with heparin plus aspirin.[22] Death or MI at 30 days was also significantly reduced by 30 percent, from 11.9 to 8.7 percent. In the PURSUIT trial, involving 10,948 patients, eptifibatide also significantly reduced the rate of death or MI at 30 days.[20]

There appeared to be a greater benefit of treatment when administered earlier in relation to the onset of pain, i.e., within the first 6 to 12 hours.[229] This benefit may be related in part to reduction in the amount of myocardial necrosis with early treatment.[230] In addition, GP IIb/IIIa inhibitors have been observed to lead to greater resolution of thrombus and improved coronary flow compared with aspirin and heparin alone.[56,231] Together, these data establish the pathophysiological link between the potent platelet inhibition achieved by GP IIb/IIIa inhibition, a reduction in thrombus, improvement in coronary blood flow, and consequent improvement in clinical outcome for patients.

However, the most recent trial, GUSTO-IV ACS, found no benefit and higher early mortality with the use of abciximab in high-risk UA/NSTEMI patients for whom an early conservative strategy (initial medical management) was planned.[232] The higher mortality in the 48-hour infusion group has been proposed to be due to low levels of inhibition of platelet aggregation during the infusion of abciximab at the dose tested. This proposal is in part based on data from other studies showing that during the 12-hour infusion, the level of platelet inhibition falls steadily.[233] Low levels of platelet inhibition have been found to lead to shedding of CD40L, a prothrombotic and proinflammatory protein. Thus, the failure of this agent to improve outcomes in the setting of medically managed UA/NSTEMI may have related to the pharmacodynamics of the agent at the dose tested. In meta-analyses not including GUSTO-IV ACS, largely evaluating the "small molecule" GPIIb/IIIa inhibitors, a 20 percent reduction in death or MI was observed at 30 days.[234] However, when GUSTO-IV ACS was included, the benefit of IIb/IIIa inhibition was only a 9 percent reduction in death or MI at 30 days ($p = 0.015$).

RISK STRATIFICATION TO TARGET GLYCOPROTEIN IIB/IIIA INHIBITORS. GP IIb/IIIa inhibition appears to be a treatment than can be targeted to higher risk patients. In the initial trials, it was observed that the subgroup of patients with ST segment depression or transient ST elevation had a two to three times greater absolute benefit than patients without ST changes.[22] Diabetic patients with UA/NSTEMI were found to have a 26 percent reduction in mortality with GP IIb/IIIa inhibition compared with no reduction in nondiabetics.[69]

Substudies using baseline troponin (and now other cardiac markers) have found that the benefit of GP IIb/IIIa inhibition appears to be greatest in these high-risk patients. This was first seen in the Chimeric c7E3 AntiPlatelet Therapy in Unstable angina REfractory to standard treatment (CAPTURE) trial: among patients who were troponin T positive at baseline, treatment with abciximab before PCI led to a 68 percent reduction in death or MI at 6 months compared with no significant benefit for those who were troponin T negative ($p < 0.001$).[78] These findings have been essentially duplicated with tirofiban versus heparin in the PRISM trial (Fig. 49–17)[79] and two other trials.[235,236] Similar findings were seen using the TIMI risk score to identify high-risk patients who benefit from GP IIb/IIIa inhibition.[123] These subgroups have been seen to have more thrombus at coronary angiography[57,237] and thus be at risk for microvascular embolization[238] and are subgroups in which this potent class of antithrombotic drugs would be of great benefit.

Other cardiac markers have also been able to identify patients at high risk, who derive benefit from GP IIb/IIIa inhibition. CD40L appeared to add information in addition to that provided by troponin in identifying patients who benefit; among troponin-positive patients, those with low levels of CD40L had no benefit from abciximab. Conversely, among troponin-negative patients, who overall had no benefit from abciximab in the original study,[78] those with elevated levels of CD40L had a significant reduction in events with the addition of abciximab. These data suggest that more careful identification of coronary thrombosis and platelet activation with these new cardiac markers may help identify patients in whom GP IIb/IIIa inhibitors will be of greater benefit.

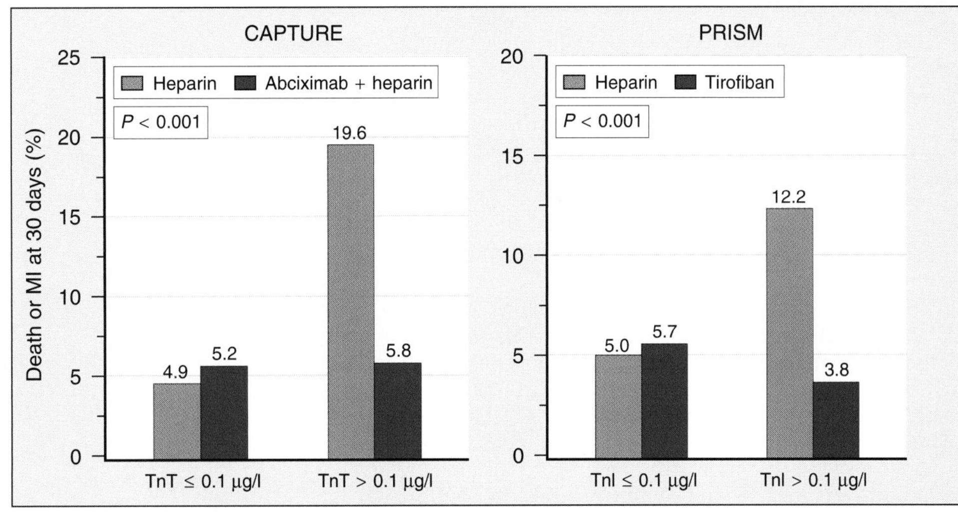

FIGURE 49–17 **Left,** Benefit of abciximab in the CAPTURE trial involving patients with refractory unstable angina treated with angioplasty in those with positive versus negative troponin T (TnT) values at study entry. **Right,** Greater benefit of tirofiban versus heparin in patients with unstable angina or non-ST elevation myocardial infarction was also seen in those with positive troponin I (TnI) values in the PRISM trial, with a nearly 70 percent reduction in death or myocardial infarction (MI) at 30 days with the IIb/IIIa inhibitor. (**Left,** Data from Hamm CW, Heeschen C, Goldmann B, et al: Benefit of abciximab in patients with refractory unstable angina in relation to serum troponin T levels. C7E3 Fab antiplatelet therapy in unstable refractory angina [CAPTURE] study investigators. N Engl J Med 340:1623, 1999; **right,** from Heeschen C, Hamm CW, Goldmann B, et al: Troponin concentrations for stratification of patients with acute coronary syndromes in relation to therapeutic efficacy of tirofiban. PRISM study investigators. Platelet Receptor Inhibition in Ischemic Syndrome Management. Lancet 354:1757, 1999.)

GLYCOPROTEIN IIB/IIIA INHIBITION AND PERCUTANEOUS CORONARY INTERVENTION. With the greater relative benefit of GP IIb/IIIa inhibitors seen in trials of patients undergoing PCI,[186,188] compared with the 9 percent overall benefit in UA/NSTEMI, many have felt that this class of drugs can be reserved for those who undergo PCI. Two meta-analyses found that the majority of the benefit in the UA/NSTEMI trials was seen in those who had early PCI (or CABG).[239] However, one aspect not accounted for in these analyses was the proportion of benefit that was achieved before the PCI procedure. In a pooled analysis of three trials, PRISM-PLUS, PURSUIT, and CAPTURE, involving 12,296 patients, there was a 34 percent relative reduction in death or MI during a period of 24 hours of medical management only (3.8 versus 2.5 percent, $p = 0.001$), with that benefit continuing up through the time of PCI.[240] Furthermore, there is evidence that initial medical treatment with a small-molecule GP IIb/IIIa inhibitor leads to clinical benefit; in the PRISM trial a significant 32 percent reduction in death, MI, or refractory ischemia at 48 hours was found, suggesting a significant clinical benefit during medical treatment alone.[21]

CORONARY ARTERY BYPASS GRAFTING. Patients who undergo CABG also appear to derive particular benefit from early treatment with GP IIb/IIIa inhibition.[241] This benefit of early GP IIb/IIIa inhibition was also seen in the meta-analysis for patients who underwent CABG within 5 days of randomization.[228] As is the case for patients undergoing PCI, the benefit of GP IIb/IIIa inhibition is observed both prior to the CABG and in the early post-CABG phase. The hypothesis is that the early antiplatelet therapy reduces the thrombus and stabilizes the patient preoperatively, thereby reducing perioperative complications.

Thus, it appears that there is benefit of GP IIb/IIIa inhibition during the phase of medical treatment as well as in patients undergoing PCI and CABG. Because patients with UA/NSTEMI are such a high-risk group, the benefit of GP IIb/IIIa inhibition has been quite dramatic, with reductions of death or MI ranging from 30 to 70 percent.[242] Thus, patients who undergo PCI should have been treated with a GP IIb/IIIa inhibitor at the time of presentation or, if not, should receive it during the procedure.

RISK-BASED VERSUS STRATEGY-BASED TARGETING OF THERAPY. The relative merits of targeting GP IIb/IIIa inhibition to the patients' risk versus the treatment strategy have been addressed in several studies. In the PRISM trial, the benefit of GP IIb/IIIa inhibition in patients with positive troponin was seen with or without revascularization,[79] suggesting that risk-based rather than intervention-based targeting of these agents may be optimal. Similar results were seen in PRISM-PLUS, using the risk score; among higher risk patients, the degree of benefit of GP IIb/IIIa inhibition was similar in those who had PCI and those who did not.[123,243] Because it is not clear at the time of presentation whether a patient will be managed with PCI, CABG, or medical therapy alone, the targeting of GP IIb/IIIa inhibition to high-risk patients appears warranted.

New data from two large observational studies provide additional support for early treatment. The National Registry of Myocardial Infarction (NRMI) included 60,770 patients with NSTEMI. Patients who received GP IIb/IIIa inhibition within 24 hours after presentation were compared with those who did not, with 10 percent of the latter group receiving GP IIb/IIIa inhibition for PCI later during the hospital course.[244] Only 25 percent of eligible patients received early GP IIb/IIIa therapy. Patients treated with early GP IIb/IIIa inhibition had 12 percent lower adjusted mortality. In addition, patients treated at hospitals with greater use of early GP IIb/IIIa inhibition also had lower adjusted mortality rates than those treated at hospitals in which GP IIb/IIIa inhibition was used less frequently.[244] A nearly identical finding has been seen in a similar analysis of the CRUSADE (Can Rapid Risk Stratification of Unstable Angina Patients Suppress Adverse Outcomes with Early Implementation of the ACC/AHA Guidelines) registry, with greater benefit in patients with positive troponin at the time of presentation.[245] These data provide support for the early use of GP IIb/IIIa inhibition in high-risk patients with NSTEMI. Currently, randomized trials are underway to study further the question of appropriate timing of GP IIb/IIIa inhibition.

SAFETY. The rate of major hemorrhage was slightly higher for patients treated with GP IIb/IIIa inhibitors than for those receiving aspirin and heparin alone. In a meta-analysis of the large placebo-controlled trials, major bleeding occurred in 2.4 percent of patients treated with GP IIb/IIIa inhibition versus 1.4 percent for placebo, p less than 0.0001.[228] Thrombocytopenia is an uncommon but important complication of GP IIb/IIIa inhibitors. For tirofiban in PRISM-PLUS, the rate of severe thrombocytopenia (<50,000 cells/mm^3) was 0.5 versus 0.3 percent for heparin (p = not significant)[22]; in the PURSUIT trial, thrombocytopenia (<20,000 cells/mm^3) occurred in 0.2 percent compared with less than 0.1 percent for heparin.[20] Thrombocytopenia is associated with increased bleeding and, in a smaller proportion of patients, recurrent thrombotic events.[246] This syndrome bears resemblance to heparin-induced thrombocytopenia and indicates a need to monitor platelet count daily during GP IIb/IIIa infusion.

ORAL IIB/IIIA INHIBITION. Because the benefit of intravenous GP IIb/IIIa inhibitors occurs only during the infusion, it was hypothesized that prolonged IIb/IIIa inhibition, using oral agents, might further improve outcomes. Unfortunately, five large trials failed to show any benefit of this approach.[166,247-250] In addition, a 35 percent increase in mortality was seen across all of the trials.

THROMBOLYTIC THERAPY. Because thrombolytic therapy is beneficial in the treatment of patients with acute MI presenting with ST elevation, it was thought that it might also play a role in the other ACSs in which thrombosis is involved. In TIMI IIIB, 1473 patients with UA/NSTEMI were treated with aspirin, UFH, and antiischemic therapy and were randomly assigned to receive either tissue plasminogen activator or its placebo. No differences were observed in the incidence of death, postrandomization MI, or recurrent, objectively documented ischemia through 6 weeks.[251] The proposed mechanism for an adverse effect of thrombolysis in UA/NSTEMI is a prothrombotic effect of thrombolysis.

Invasive Versus Conservative Strategies

Two general approaches to the use of cardiac catheterization and revascularization in UA/NSTEMI exist. The first is an "early invasive" strategy, involving routine early cardiac catheterization and revascularization with PCI or bypass surgery, depending on the coronary anatomy. The other is a more "conservative" approach with initial medical management with catheterization and revascularization only for recurrent ischemia either at rest or in a noninvasive stress test.

CLINICAL TRIALS

To date, nine randomized trials have studied the relative merits of an invasive strategy, involving routine cardiac catheterization with revascularization if feasible, compared with a conservative strategy in which angiography and revascularization are reserved for patients who have evidence of recurrent ischemia either at rest or on provocative testing. The first three trials failed to demonstrate a significant benefit,[251] but the subsequent six have all shown a significant benefit, including the FRagmin and Fast Revascularisation during InStability in Coronary artery disease (FRISC) II and TACTICS-TIMI 18 trials and the Randomized Intervention Trial of unstable Angina (RITA) (Fig. 49–18).[3,252,253]

In FRISC II, 2457 patients with UA/NSTEMI were randomly assigned to an invasive strategy involving coronary angiography carried out on average 4 days after randomization, thus a "delayed" invasive strategy, or a conservative strategy. The latter had strict criteria for catheterization requiring refractory angina despite maximal medical treatment or a positive ECG exercise test with greater than 0.3 mV ST depression. Accordingly, with these strict criteria in the conservative strategy, only 9 percent of patients underwent revascularization during the first 7 days. This trial found that the rate of death or MI at 6 months was significantly lower in the invasive than in the conservative group, 9.4 versus 12.1 percent, p = 0.031. At 1 year there was a significant reduction in mortality in the invasive compared with the conservative group (2.2 versus 3.9 percent, respectively, p = 0.016).[252]

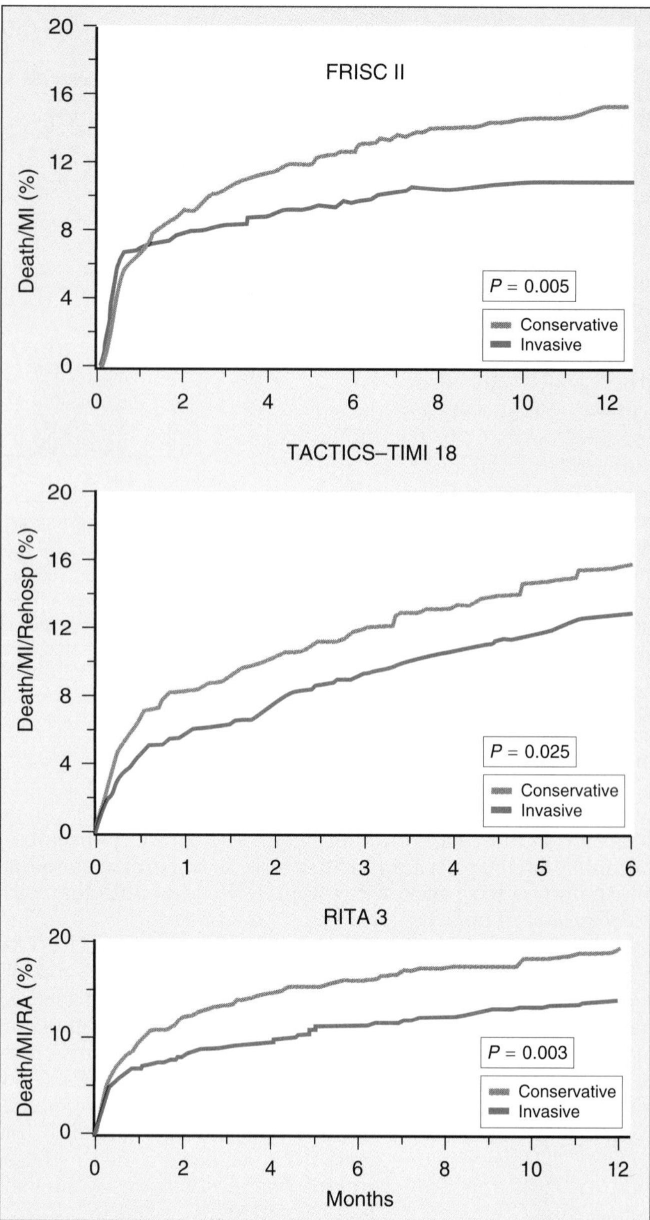

FIGURE 49–18 Kaplan-Meier event curves of three trials comparing invasive versus conservative strategies in ACA. **Top,** Probability of death or myocardial infarction (MI) according to assignment to the invasive or noninvasive strategies in the FRagmin and Fast Revascularisation during InStability in Coronary artery disease (FRISC) II trial. **Middle,** Adverse outcomes (death, MI, or rehospitalization) of both treatment groups in the Treat Angina with aggrastat and determine Cost of Therapy with an Invasive or Conservative Strategy–Thrombolysis in Myocardial Infarction (TACTICS-TIMI) 18 trial. **Bottom,** Death, MI, or refractory angina (RA) in the Randomized Intervention Trial of unstable Angina (RITA) 3 trial. (**Top,** Adapted from Wallentin L, Lagerqvist B, Husted S, et al: Outcome at 1 year after an invasive compared with a non-invasive strategy in unstable coronary artery disease: The FRISC II invasive randomized trial. Lancet 356:9, 2000; **middle,** from Cannon CP, Weintraub WS, Demopoulos LA, et al: Comparison of early invasive and conservative strategies in patients with unstable coronary syndromes treated with the glycoprotein IIb/IIIa inhibitor tirofiban. N Engl J Med 344:1879, 2001; **bottom,** adapted from Fox KAA, Poole-Wilson PA, Henderson RA, et al: Interventional versus conservative treatment for patients with unstable angina or non-ST-elevation myocardial infarction: The British Heart Foundation RITA 3 randomised trial. Lancet 360:743, 2002.)

In TACTICS-TIMI 18, all patients received aspirin, heparin, and the GP IIb/IIIa inhibitor tirofiban at the time of randomization for at least 48 hours, including more than 12 hours following PCI. The rate of death, MI, or rehospitalization for ACS at 6 months was reduced with the early invasive strategy, from 19.4 percent in the conservative group to 15.9 percent in the early invasive group, $p = 0.025$.[3] At 30 days the event rates were 10.5 percent for conservative and 7.4 percent for invasive, $p = 0.009$. Death or nonfatal MI was significantly reduced at 30 days (7.0 to 4.7 percent, respectively, $p = 0.02$) and at 6 months ($p = 0.0498$). In a prospective analysis of costs, the estimated cost per year of life gained for the invasive strategy, based on projected life expectancy, was $12,739, indicating that an early invasive strategy is very cost effective relative to other cardiac medications and interventions.[254]

RISK STRATIFICATION. The benefits of the early invasive strategy have been observed in higher risk patients, especially in those with ST segment changes who had positive troponin on admission.[3,45,252] In TACTICS-TIMI 18, a prespecified hypothesis was that there would be a significantly greater benefit in patients with positive troponin values than in those with negative values.[3] In patients with a troponin T greater than 0.01 ng/ml, there was a relative 39 percent risk reduction in the primary endpoint with the invasive versus the conservative strategy ($p < 0.001$), whereas patients with negative troponin had similar outcomes with either strategy. Death or nonfatal MI was also significantly reduced with the invasive strategy in patients with troponin T greater than 0.01 ng/ml. Similar results were obtained using a troponin T cut point of 0.1 ng/ml and with troponin I.[45]

The same findings of benefit were seen in patients with ST segment changes on admission, with a 10 percent absolute benefit in the primary endpoint in TACTICS-TIMI 18[3] compared with no benefit in those without ST segment changes on admission. Similar findings were observed in FRISC II.[252]

Using the TIMI risk score in TACTICS, there was significant benefit of the early invasive strategy in intermediate-risk (score 3 to 4) and high-risk patients (5 to 7), whereas low-risk (0 to 2) patients had similar outcomes when managed with either strategy (see Fig. 49-9B).[3] The intermediate- and high-risk groups constituted 75 percent of the total population in the trial.

TIMING OF AN INVASIVE STRATEGY. With the benefit of an early invasive strategy now well established, research has turned to the optimal timing. The Intracoronary Stenting with Antithrombotic Regimen Cooling-Off (ISAR-COOL) study found a benefit of an immediate invasive strategy with an average time to catheterization of 2 hours, compared with a delayed invasive strategy (average time to catheterization 4 days).[184] An analysis of the timing of angiography within the early invasive arm of TACTICS-TIMI failed to find any major differences in outcomes among patients who underwent protocol-mandated catheterization within the first 12 hours versus 12 to 24 hours and 24 to 48 hours.[255] Additional trials are ongoing to evaluate the optimal timing of an invasive approach, but on the basis of available data the optimal timing appears to be within the first 48 hours of presentation.

Summary: Indications for Invasive Versus Conservative Management Strategies

On the basis of multiple randomized trials, an early invasive strategy is now strongly recommended for high-risk patients with UA/NSTEMI with ST segment changes or a positive troponin (on admission or that evolves over the next 24 hours), or both. In addition, other high-risk indicators, such as recurrent ischemia and evidence of congestive heart failure, are indications for an early invasive strategy.[4] An early invasive approach appears warranted in those with cardiogenic shock on the basis of studies in acute MI.[256] In addition, an early invasive strategy in those who present with UA/NSTEMI within 6 months of a prior PCI or in patients with prior CABG is indicated.[257]

CURRENT UTILIZATION. The use of cardiac procedures varies by region around the world, although management of patients with UA/NSTEMI is shifting toward a more invasive approach worldwide. In the United States in 2003, in the CRUSADE registry of patients with high-risk UA/NSTEMI, 62 percent underwent cardiac catheterization during hospitalization, 37 percent underwent PCI, and 11 percent underwent coronary bypass surgery.[258] In the 2002 Euro Heart Survey of ACS, involving 10,484 patients admitted to 103 hospitals in 25 countries, the corresponding rates of these procedures were 52.0, 25.4, and 5.4 percent in UA/NSTEMI patients. Cardiac procedures are used more frequently in lower risk patients, not higher risk patients, as recommended in the guidelines.[259]

Noninvasive Testing

In the management of UA/NSTEMI, noninvasive testing is used (1) at presentation, usually in the emergency department to diagnose the presence or absence of CAD (in patients with a low likelihood of coronary disease) (see Chap. 45); (2) to guide further therapy as part of an early conservative strategy; (3) after medical therapy has been carried out, to evaluate the extent of residual ischemia; (4) to evaluate left ventricular function; and (5) to estimate prognosis (i.e., risk stratification).

The results from noninvasive tests that portend high risk of future cardiac events are shown in Table 49–5 (see also Chaps. 10, 16, and 50). These results are derived from studies involving patients with unstable angina, MI, and stable CAD. The marker of high risk is either evidence of ischemia on stress testing or left ventricular dysfunction (either at rest or

TABLE 49–5 Noninvasive Test Results Predicting High Risk for Adverse Outcomes

Exercise Electrocardiographic Testing
Abnormal horizontal or downsloping ST segment depression with
Onset at heart rate <120 beats/min or ≤6.5 METs
Magnitude ≥2.0 mm
Postexercise duration of ≥6 min
Depression in multiple leads
Abnormal systolic blood pressure response
With sustained decrease of >10 mm Hg or flat blood pressure response ≤130 mm Hg, associated with abnormal electrocardiogram
Other
Exercise-induced ST segment elevation
Ventricular tachycardia
Radionuclide Myocardial Perfusion Imaging
Abnormal myocardial tracer distribution in more than one coronary artery region at rest or with stress or an anterior defect that reperfuses
Abnormal myocardial distribution with increased lung uptake
Cardiac enlargement
Left Ventricular Imaging
Stress radionuclide ventriculography
Exercise EF ≤50%
Rest EF ≤35%
Fall in EF ≥10%
Stress echocardiography
Rest EF ≤35%
Wall motion score index >1

EF = ejection fraction; METs = metabolic equivalents.

Adapted from Schlant RC, Blomqvist CG, Brandenburg RO, et al: Guidelines for exercise testing. Circulation 74:653A, 1986; Guidelines for Clinical Use of Cardiac Radionuclide Imaging, December 1986. J Am Coll Cardiol 8:1471, 1986; Cheitlin MD, Alpert JS, Armstrong WF, et al: ACC/AHA Guidelines for the Clinical Application of Echocardiography. Circulation 95:1686, 1997.

stress induced). The use of angiography and revascularization for patients who had a positive stress test (i.e., evidence of ischemia) has long been assumed to be necessary and has been included in the "conservative" arms of most randomized trials.[3,251,260] A benefit of revascularization for provocable ischemia has been documented in patients with a positive ECG stress test following thrombolytic therapy for STEMI.[261]

The safety of early stress testing in patients with UA/NSTEMI has been debated, but evidence from several trials has suggested that pharmacological[262] or symptom-limited stress testing[263] is safe after a period of at least 24 to 48 hours of stabilization in patients with UA/NSTEMI.[264] A contraindication to stress testing is a recent recurrence of rest pain, especially if associated with ECG changes or other signs of instability (hemodynamic or significant arrhythmias).

The merits of various modalities of stress testing have been compared directly in relatively small series of patients (see also Chaps. 10 and 16). For most patients ECG exercise stress testing is recommended if the ECG is without significant ST segment abnormalities. If ST abnormalities exist, perfusion or echo imaging is recommended. Exercise testing is generally recommended unless the patient cannot walk sufficiently to achieve a significant workload, in which case pharmacological stress testing is recommended.

Revascularization

PERCUTANEOUS CORONARY INTERVENTION (see also Chap. 52). PCI is an effective means of reducing coronary obstruction, improving acute ischemia, and improving regional and global left ventricular function in patients with UA/NSTEMI. Current angiographic success rates are high, generally greater than 95 percent, although the presence of UA/NSTEMI or visualized thrombus is associated with an increased risk of acute complications such as abrupt closure or MI (as compared with patients with stable angina or those without visualized thrombus).[56,265] Thus, use of IIb/IIIa inhibitors, clopidogrel, bivalirudin, or other antithrombotic drugs in such patients is associated with improved acute and long-term outcomes following PCI. Use of drug-eluting stents has been shown to reduce the risk of restenosis,[266] further enhancing the overall clinical benefit of an invasive approach.

PERCUTANEOUS CORONARY INTERVENTION VERSUS CORONARY ARTERY BYPASS GRAFTING. When revascularization is required in patients with UA/NSTEMI, the choice is between PCI and CABG. More than eight trials have compared PCI and CABG in patients with ischemic heart disease, many of whom had UA/NSTEMI.[267,268] The results of these trials are reviewed in Chapter 50. On the basis of the results of these trials, CABG is recommended for patients with disease of the left main coronary artery, multivessel disease, and impaired left ventricular function. For other patients, either PCI or CABG may be suitable. PCI is associated with a slightly lower initial morbidity and mortality than CABG but a higher rate of repeated procedures; CABG is associated with more effective relief from angina.

INTRAAORTIC BALLOON COUNTERPULSATION. Intraaortic balloon counterpulsation (IABP) is an effective means of increasing diastolic coronary blood flow and reducing left ventricular afterload, which act in concert to reduce ischemia (see Chap. 25). IABP is usually reserved for patients with UA/NSTEMI who are refractory to maximal medical therapy, those with hemodynamic compromise who are awaiting cardiac catheterization, or those with very high risk coronary anatomy (e.g., left main stenosis) as a bridge to PCI or CABG. Although no randomized trials have documented the benefit of IABP, this method is effective in stabilizing patients with refractory ischemia.

Summary: Acute Management of Unstable Angina or Non-ST Elevation Myocardial Infarction

The evaluation of patients with UA/NSTEMI begins with the clinical history, ECG, and measurement of cardiac biomarkers to assess (1) the likelihood of coronary disease and (2) the patient's risk of death or recurrent cardiac events (Fig. 49–19). Patients with a low likelihood of having UA/NSTEMI should undergo a "diagnostic pathway" evaluation through serial ECGs, cardiac biomarkers, and early stress testing to evaluate for coronary disease (Fig. 49–20). This evaluation can frequently be accomplished in an emergency department observation–chest pain unit. For patients with a clinical history strongly consistent with UA/NSTEMI, those at low risk should be treated with antithrombotic therapy with aspirin, clopidogrel, either heparin or LMWH, beta blockers, and nitrates. An early conservative strategy is adequate in low-risk patients, although an invasive strategy is equally clinically beneficial. For high-risk patients (e.g., those with positive troponin, ST segment changes, TIMI risk score > 3), GP IIb/IIIa inhibition should be added to the preceding medications, and an early invasive strategy is preferred (Fig. 49–21).

Long-Term Secondary Prevention Following Unstable Angina or Non-ST Elevation Myocardial Infarction

The time of hospital discharge following UA/NSTEMI has been noted to be a "teachable moment" for the patient,[269] when the physician and staff can review and optimize the medical regimen for long-term treatment. Risk factor modification is critical and includes discussions with the patient (as appropriate to the patient's risk factors) concerning the importance of smoking cessation, achieving optimal weight, daily exercise, following an appropriate diet, good blood pressure control, tight control of hyperglycemia in diabetics, and lipid management (Table 49–6).

Five classes of drugs that have been shown in large randomized trials to improve outcomes following UA/NSTEMI are now recommended for long-term treatment. Each agent

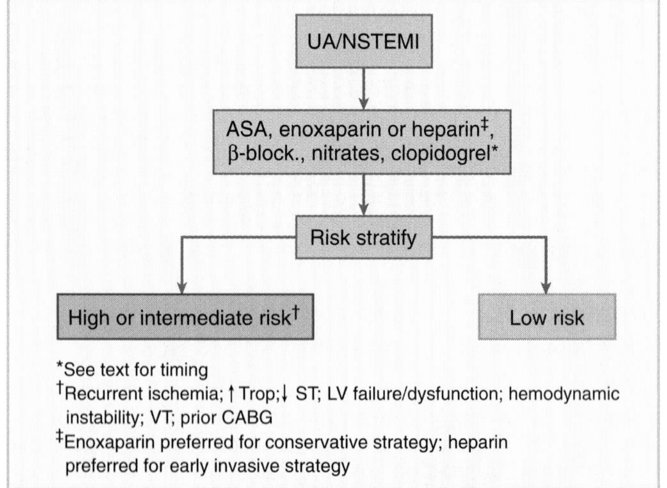

FIGURE 49–19 Algorithm for the management of patients with unstable angina or non-ST elevation myocardial infarction (UA/NSTEMI). Patients in whom the diagnosis is confirmed or suspected are treated with aspirin (ASA), heparin (enoxaparin preferred to unfractionated heparin), beta blockade, nitrates, and clopidogrel. Risk stratification is then performed, and their subsequent management is dictated by their risk category. CABG = coronary artery bypass graft; LV = left ventricular; VT = ventricular tachyarrhythmia. (From Braunwald E: Application of current guidelines to the management of unstable angina and non-ST elevation myocardial infarction. Circulation 108:III-28, 2003.)

may contribute to long-term clinical stability in different ways. Statins[149,270] and ACE inhibitors[143,144,271] are recommended for long-term treatment that may facilitate plaque stabilization. Beta blockers are indicated for antiischemic therapy[130,272] and may help decrease "triggers" for MI during follow-up. For antiplatelet therapy, the combination of aspirin and clopidogrel for at least a year has been shown to be beneficial[175,177] and would prevent or decrease the severity of any thrombosis if a plaque rupture does occur. Thus, a multifactorial approach to long-term medical therapy is directed toward preventing the various components of atherothrombosis.

Registry Experience

A major problem identified in clinical practice is that a large proportion of patients do not receive guideline-recommended therapies. Five large registries, in the United States and worldwide, have documented that only 80 to 85 percent of patients received aspirin.[34,66,253,273,274] In addition to guideline development and education, there is a need for specific tools to ensure that the guideline recommendations are implemented on a patient-by-patient basis. Adherence to practice guidelines has been found to be associated with improved outcomes.[269] This was first observed in UA/NSTEMI, by Giugliano and colleagues, who observed in a single-center study that patients who were treated according

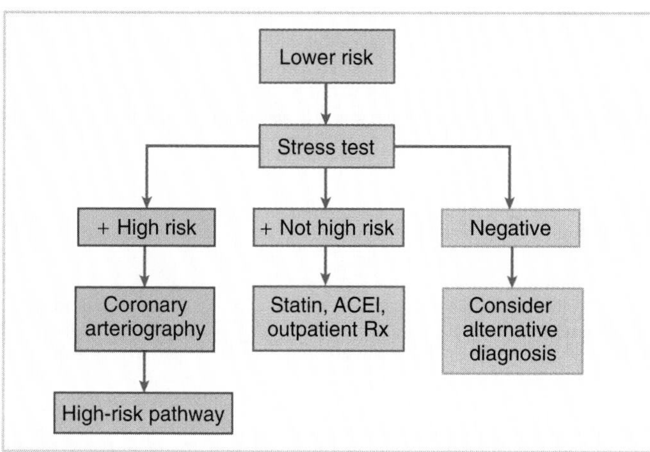

FIGURE 49–20 Management of lower risk patients with unstable angina or non-ST elevation myocardial infarction. ACEI = angiotensin-converting enzyme inhibitor. (From Braunwald E: Application of current guidelines to the management of unstable angina and non-ST elevation myocardial infarction. Circulation 108:III-28, 2003.)

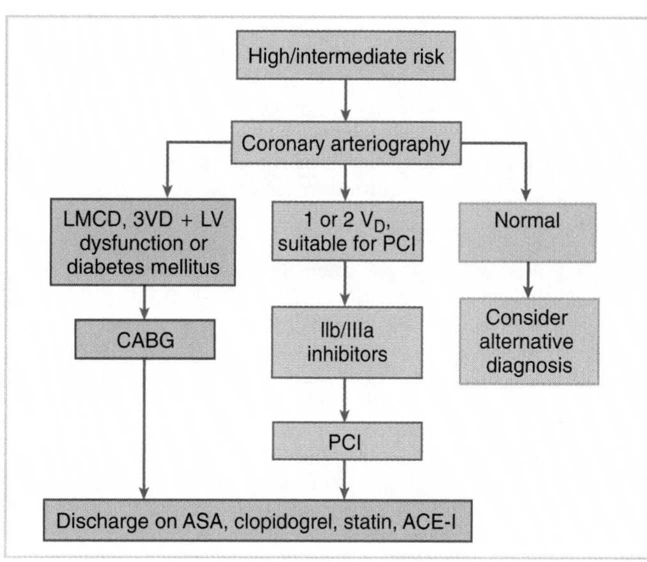

FIGURE 49–21 Management of high- and medium-risk patients with unstable angina or non-ST elevation myocardial infarction. ACE-I = angiotensin-converting enzyme inhibitor; ASA = aspirin; LMCD = left main coronary disease; LV dys = left ventricular dysfunction; VD = vessel disease. (From Braunwald E: Application of current guidelines to the management of unstable angina and non-ST elevation myocardial infarction. Circulation 108:III-28, 2003.)

TABLE 49–6 Cardiac Checklist for Unstable Angina or Non-ST Elevation Myocardial Infarction*

Cardiac Checklist—Admission		Cardiac Checklist—Discharge	
Patient Name: ______ (First Name) (Middle Initial) (Last Name)	**Admit Date:** ______	**Patient Name:** ______ (First Name) (Middle Initial) (Last Name)	**Admit Date:** ______
Brief History: ______		**Brief History:** ______	
Medications		**Medications**	
1. Aspirin	□	1. Aspirin	□
2. Clopidogrel	□	2. Clopidogrel	□
3. Heparin (or LMWH)	□	3. Statin	□
4. GP IIb/IIIa inhibitor	□	4. ACE inhibitor	□
5. Beta blocker	□	5. Beta blocker	□
6. Nitrate	□	**Interventions**	
7. ACE inhibitor	□	6. LDL controlled to goal	□
Interventions		7. Blood pressure controlled	□
8. Cath/revascularization for recurrent ischemia or in intermediate and high-risk patients	□	8. Diabetes controlled	□
Risk Factor Modification		9. Smoking cessation counseling (if applicable)	□
9. Cholesterol—check and treat as needed	□	10. Cardiac rehab/life-style change	□
10. Treat other risk factors (e.g., smoking)	□		

*These simple lists serve as reminders of guideline-recommended therapies, such as aspirin, clopidogrel, heparin, or low-molecular-weight heparin. This "cardiac checklist" could be used in two ways: physicians could keep a copy on a small index card in their pocket or in their personal digital assistant (PDA) and run down the list when writing admission orders for patients, or it could be used in developing standard orders for unstable angina or non-ST elevation myocardial infarction—either printed order sheets or computerized orders. See text for details of specific indications and contraindications for medications.
ACE = angiotensin-converting enzyme; GP = glycoprotein; LDL = low-density lipoprotein; LMWH = low-molecular-weight heparin.

to the guidelines had an adjusted 1-year survival that was significantly improved compared with those who had lower compliance with guideline recommendations.[275]

Critical Pathways and Continuous Quality Improvement

Critical pathways and the process of continuous quality improvement (CQI) are means of trying to improve care.[276,277] Critical pathways are standardized protocols for the management of specific diseases (e.g., ACS) that aim to optimize and streamline care of patients.[276,278] In general, these pathways involve having standardized order sets (or computerized ones), simple pocket cards, reminders, or checklists of the appropriate therapies (see Table 49–6). The process of implementation of pathways generally involves physician and nursing education, including presentations at grand rounds, inservices, and other educational meetings throughout the institution involving the relevant caretakers. Another key part of an overall CQI effort is to monitor data on performance, i.e., utilization of guideline-recommended therapies.

Critical Pathways Improve Outcomes

There are now several well-conducted studies showing that use of critical pathways can lead to improved quality of care. The Cardiac Hospitalization Atherosclerosis Management Program (CHAMP) involved staff who assisted the physicians to ensure that all the patients were treated with appropriate guideline-recommended therapies.[269] They were able to improve the use of therapies, such as aspirin, from 78 percent before the program up to 92 percent at the time of hospital discharge. Notably, at 1-year follow-up the CHAMP program had further increased utilization, up to 94 percent of patients, whereas prior to the program compliance had actually fallen to 68 percent.[159] The same was seen for beta blocker, ACE inhibitor, and statin use.

The American College of Cardiology–sponsored Guideline Applied in Practice (GAP) Program provided important multicenter data supporting the efficacy of critical pathways.[279] They found improvement in the use of guideline-recommended therapies and procedures following implementation of their pathways: early use of aspirin and beta blockers and measurement of LDL cholesterol were all improved after implementation of the GAP quality improvement effort.[279] Most interestingly, patients for whom there was evidence in the medical records that the pathways and tools had been used had the highest rates of treatment with the recommended therapies. This finding demonstrated that having tools available for clinicians to use as reminders really can lead to improvements in the use of various therapies.

Thus, critical pathways have now been shown to lead to improvements in the quality of care and to be associated with improved outcomes. Monitoring of performance is key to ensuring that the efforts in education on guideline implementation and changes in the system actually translate into improved care.

Prinzmetal (Variant) Angina

In 1959, Prinzmetal and associates described an unusual syndrome of cardiac pain secondary to myocardial ischemia that occurs almost exclusively at rest, is not usually precipitated by physical exertion or emotional stress, and is associated with ST segment elevations on the ECG (Fig. 49–22).[280] This syndrome, now known as *Prinzmetal,* or *variant, angina* (the terms are interchangeable), may be associated with acute MI and severe cardiac arrhythmias, including ventricular tachycardia and fibrillation, as well as sudden death. A prevailing clinical impression is that Prinzmetal angina has become less frequent in North America for reasons that are unclear, but it appears to remain common in Japan.

Mechanisms

The original hypothesis of Prinzmetal and colleagues, that variant angina is the result of transient increases in coronary vasomotor tone or vasospasm, has been convincingly demonstrated by coronary angiography. Vasospasm causes a transient, abrupt, marked decrease in the diameter of an epicardial (or large septal) coronary artery resulting in severe myocardial ischemia. This event occurs in the absence of any preceding increases in myocardial O_2 demand, as reflected in an increased heart rate or blood pressure. The decrease in luminal diameter can usually be reversed by nitroglycerin, sometimes requiring large doses. Although the sites of vasospasm may correspond to areas of severe focal stenosis, in some patients with apparently normal vessels at angiography the vasospastic segments appear to occur at sites of at least minimal atherosclerotic change, as detected by intravascular ultrasonography.[281] This severe focal vasospasm should not be confused with vasoconstriction of both the large and small coronary vessels, a *normal* response to stimuli such as cold exposure. The latter response is much less intense and occurs diffusely throughout the coronary vascular bed.

Although responses to various vasoconstrictor substances, including catecholamines, thromboxane A_2, serotonin, endothelin, and arginine vasopressin, are greater in spastic segments of the coronary arteries, hypersensitivity to vasoconstrictor stimuli also occurs throughout the entire coronary tree in patients with Prinzmetal angina,[282] perhaps as a manifestation of a more generalized response to vasoactive stimuli. The precise mechanisms have not been established, but a systemic alteration in NO production or an imbalance between endothelium-derived relaxing and contracting factors has been suggested.[282,283] Impaired endothelium-dependent vasodilation in the brachial artery has been demonstrated in Prinzmetal angina,[284] and diurnal fluctuations in flow-mediated endothelium-dependent dilation in this vessel are associated with variations in the frequency of ischemic episodes.[285] Cultured skin fibroblasts obtained from patients with Prinzmetal angina have demonstrated enhanced phospholipase C (PLC) activity. Because PLC (through activating the inositol triphosphate pathway) mobilizes Ca^{2+} from intracellular stores, it may enhance contraction of smooth muscle cells.[286]

The sites of spasm in Prinzmetal angina may be adjacent to atheromatous plaque. It has been suggested that in this subgroup of patients, the basic abnormality may be hypercontractility of the arterial wall associated with the atherosclerotic process itself. Other suggested mechanisms include endothelial injury (which reverses the dilator response to a variety of stimuli, e.g., acetylcholine [see Chap. 44]) and hypercontractility of vascular smooth muscle as a result of vasoconstrictor mitogens, leukotrienes, serotonin, endothelin, angiotensin II, histamine,[287] and higher local concentrations of blood-borne vasoconstrictors in areas adjacent to neovascularized atherosclerotic plaque.

The sequelae of coronary spasm may accelerate atherosclerosis and predispose to further spasm. One mechanism may involve the release of potent vasoconstrictor substances, such as platelet-derived growth factors, in addition to activation of the coagulation system.[288] The combination of a reduction in blood flow and an increase in platelet activation and local thrombosis may accelerate atherosclerosis.[288] Histological findings in patients undergoing coronary atherectomy suggest that repetitive coronary vasospasm may provoke vascular injury and lead to the formation of neointimal hyperplasia at the initial site of spasm. In this respect, coronary spasm may have a key role in the rapid progression of coronary stenosis in some patients.[289]

Imaging with iodine-123-labeled metaiodobenzylguanidine (^{123}I-MIBG) has demonstrated regional myocardial sympathetic denervation in the area of distribution of the vessel in which vasospasm developed.[290]

Coronary spasm in patients with variant angina may induce stasis and result in the conversion of fibrinogen to fibrin in the coronary vessels, with elevated levels of both plasma fibrinogen[291] and fibrinopeptide A, an index of fibrin formation.[292] It has been reported that hypomagnesemia predisposes to variant angina,[293] and magnesium sulfate has been shown to terminate and to suppress attacks.

Clinical and Laboratory Findings

Patients with variant angina tend to be younger than patients with chronic stable angina or unstable angina secondary to coronary atherosclerosis, and many do not exhibit classical coronary risk factors except that they are often heavy cigarette smokers.[294] The anginal discomfort is often extremely severe and may be accompanied by syncope. Features associated with syncope include inferior ST segment elevation and serious arrhythmias, either AV block and asystole or ventricular tachyarrhythmias.[295-297]

Attacks of Prinzmetal angina tend to be clustered between midnight and 8 AM[292] and sometimes occur in clusters of two or three within 30 to 60 minutes. Patients studied by means of ambulatory ECG, even those without clinically apparent angina pectoris, show more frequent abnormalities in the morning. Although exercise capacity is generally well preserved in patients with Prinzmetal angina, some patients experience typical pain and ST segment elevations not only at rest but during or after exertion as well. Exertion of angina usually signifies exertion-induced vasospasm or associated fixed obstruction.

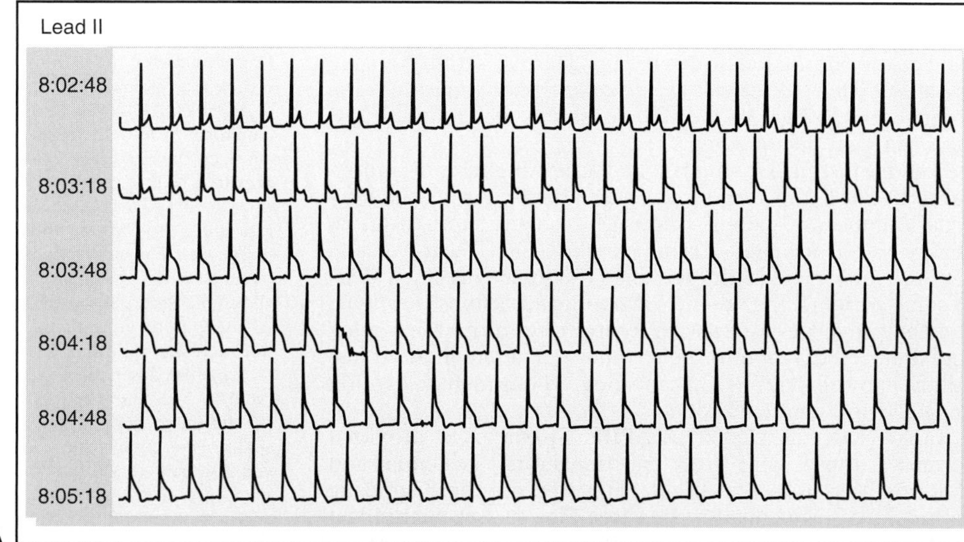

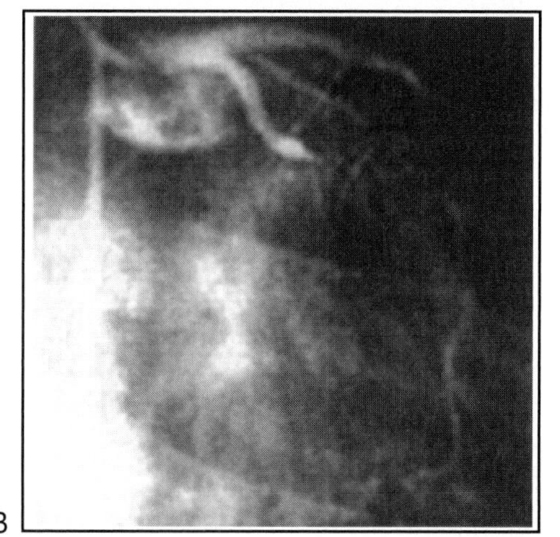

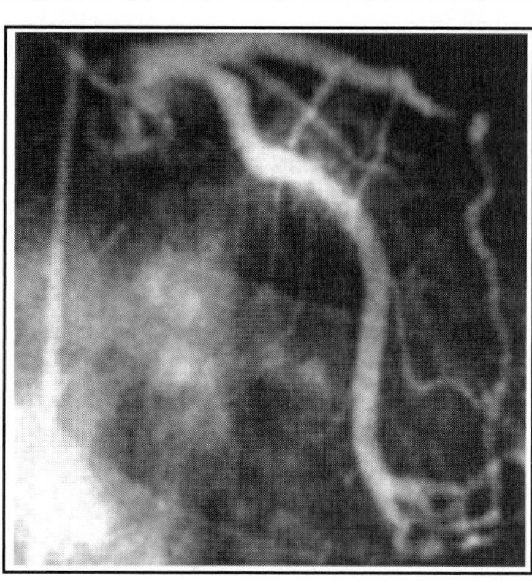

FIGURE 49–22 Findings in a 39-year-old man with Prinzmetal angina. **A,** During an episode of angina, transient ST segment elevation (in lead II) was noted on continuous telemetry. Continuous telemetric recording demonstrating dynamic ST segment elevation. **B,** Hyperventilation-induced total occlusion of the proximal left circumflex artery (visible on angiography from the right anterior oblique caudal view). **C,** Spasm that resolved with the administration of intracoronary nitroglycerine and diltiazem. The patient's symptoms were controlled with oral nitrates and calcium channel blockade during a follow-up of 2 years. (From Chen HSV, Pinto DS: Prinzmetal's angina. N Engl J Med 349:e1, 2003.)

Patients with Prinzmetal angina and severe fixed coronary obstruction may have a combination of fixed-threshold, exertion-induced angina with ST segment depression and episodes of angina at rest with ST segment elevation. Some patients appear to demonstrate a distinct relationship between emotional distress and episodes of coronary vasospasm, which is consistent with studies suggesting that a sympathovagal imbalance may precipitate spasm in patients with variant angina. In rare cases, Prinzmetal angina develops after coronary artery bypass surgery, and occasionally it appears to be a manifestation of a generalized vasospastic disorder associated with migraine and Raynaud phenomenon; it has also been reported in association with aspirin-induced asthma[298] and has been reported to be provoked by 5-fluorouracil and by cyclophosphamide (see Chaps. 62 and 83). Alcohol withdrawal may precipitate variant angina and, conversely, alcohol ingestion may prevent coronary spasm.[299]

ELECTROCARDIOGRAPHY. The key to the diagnosis of variant angina lies in the detection of episodic ST segment elevation with pain (see Fig. 49–22). In one series of patients with variant angina and normal coronary arteries monitored with a computerized 24-hour, 12-lead ECG recording and analysis system, approximately 90 percent of episodes were associated with ST segment elevation, with accompanying arrhythmias in 19 percent, but no arrhythmias were noted in the small proportion of patients with ST segment depression.[295] In some patients, episodes of ST segment depression follow episodes of ST segment elevation and are associated with T wave changes. ST segment and T wave alternans and increased QT dispersion are the result of ischemic conduction delay and may be associated with potentially lethal ventricular arrhythmias. Many patients exhibit multiple episodes of asymptomatic ST segment elevation (silent ischemia). ST segment deviations may be present in any leads.

Transient conduction disturbances may occur during episodes of ischemia.[296] Ventricular ectopic activity is more frequent during longer episodes of ischemia, is often associated with ST segment and T wave alternans, and is of ominous prognostic import. In survivors of out-of-hospital cardiac arrest without flow-limiting coronary stenoses, spontaneous or induced focal coronary spasm has been found to be associated with life-threatening ventricular arrhythmias. In some patients, reperfusion rather than ischemia itself correlates with the onset of the arrhythmias.[300] Myocardial cell damage, as reflected in the release of small quantities of CK-MB, may occur in the absence of persistent ECG changes in patients with prolonged attacks of variant angina; transient Q waves have been observed, which may be explained by a transient loss of normal cell membrane electrical activity during spasm. Q wave MI caused by coronary artery spasm in the absence of angiographically demonstrable obstructive CAD has been well documented.[301]

Exercise testing in patients with variant angina is of limited value because the response is so variable. Approximately equal numbers of patients show ST segment depression, no change in ST segments during exercise, or ST segment elevation, which reflects the presence of underlying fixed CAD in some patients, the absence of significant lesions in others, and the provocation of spasm by exercise in the remainder. Ambulatory ECG monitoring or the use of a telephone transmitter may be helpful in capturing ST segment elevation during symptomatic episodes.[302]

CORONARY ARTERIOGRAPHY. Spasm of a proximal coronary artery with resultant transmural ischemia and abnormalities in left ventricular function are the diagnostic hallmarks of Prinzmetal angina (see Fig. 49–22). Significant fixed proximal coronary obstruction of at least one major artery occurs in the majority of patients, and in them spasm usually occurs within 1 cm of this obstruction. The remainder have normal coronary arteries in the absence of ischemia. Patients with no or mild fixed coronary obstruction tend to experience a more benign course than patients with associated severe obstructive lesions.[303] The vasospastic process almost always involves large segments of the epicardial vessels at a single site, but at different times other sites may be involved. The right coronary artery is the most frequent site, followed by the left anterior descending coronary artery.[302]

PROVOCATIVE TESTS

THE ERGONOVINE TEST. Several provocative tests for coronary spasm have been developed. Of these, the ergonovine test is the most sensitive. Ergonovine maleate, an ergot alkaloid that stimulates both alpha-adrenergic and serotonergic receptors and therefore exerts a direct constrictive effect on vascular smooth muscle,[304] has been used to induce coronary artery spasm, which results in chest pain and ST segment elevation in patients with Prinzmetal angina. Occasionally, ergonovine may produce a similar response in patients with more typical effort-related anginal symptoms.[302] When administered intravenously in doses ranging from 0.05 to 0.40 mg, ergonovine provides a sensitive and specific test for provoking coronary artery spasm. The majority of patients who have a response to ergonovine do so at a dose of less than 0.20 mg.[302]

In low doses and in carefully controlled clinical situations, ergonovine is a relatively safe drug, but prolonged coronary artery spasm precipitated by ergonovine may cause MI. Occasionally, conduction disturbances develop (heart block, asystole, or severe tachyarrhythmias). Because of these hazards, it is recommended that ergonovine be administered only to patients in whom coronary arteriography has demonstrated normal or nearly normal coronary arteries and in gradually increasing doses, beginning with a very low dose. Nitrates and calcium antagonists are usually effective in providing prompt relief from drug-induced spasm, and the intracoronary route for these drugs is usually the most expeditious in patients already undergoing angiography.

The ergonovine test should be conducted only in a setting where appropriate resuscitative equipment, drugs, and personnel are readily available, usually in the cardiac catheterization laboratory, and with a catheter poised to enter the coronary arteries, so that the angiographic diagnosis of spasm can be made and intracoronary nitroglycerin administered to abolish the spasm. Absolute contraindications to ergonovine testing include pregnancy, severe hypertension, severe left ventricular dysfunction, moderate to severe aortic stenosis, and high-grade left main coronary artery stenosis. Relative contraindications include uncontrolled or unstable angina, uncontrolled ventricular arrhythmias, recent MI, and advanced CAD. Although the provocative test with ergonovine is a useful test, the drug is no longer readily available in the United States.

HYPERVENTILATION. This stimulus has also been demonstrated to provoke episodes of intense angina,[305] ST segment elevations on the ECG, angiographic evidence of coronary artery spasm, and ventricular arrhythmias. A large series documented the relative specificity of the hyperventilation test in patients with vasospastic angina.[306] Patients with positive tests had a statistically significantly greater frequency of high disease activity (five or more attacks per week), severe arrhythmias during attacks, and multivessel spasm.

ACETYLCHOLINE. Stimulation of acetylcholine receptors produces a uniform endothelium-dependent dilation of normal coronary vessels of all sizes but leads to vasoconstriction when endothelial function is impaired.[307] In patients with variant angina, intracoronary injections of acetylcholine have been shown to induce severe coronary spasm and reproduce the clinical syndrome.[308] This focal spasm should not be confused with the mild diffuse constriction that acetylcholine induces in patients with abnormal coronary endothelium. Because this method allows induction of spasm separately in the left and right coronary arteries, it is useful in patients with known multivessel disease or spasm. Acetylcholine is infused over a 1-minute period into a coronary artery in incremental doses of 10, 25, 50, and 100 μg, and doses should be separated by 5-minute intervals.

Histamine, dopamine, and serotonin can also induce coronary artery spasm. Like ergonovine and acetylcholine, these agents are capable of causing marked coronary artery spasm in patients with variant angina who have severe underlying arteriosclerotic coronary artery narrowing and in those without such fixed stenoses. Exercise, the cold pressor test, and induced alkalosis can all cause coronary spasm in patients with variant angina, but none of these tests is as sensitive as ergonovine or acetylcholine.

Management

Patients with variant angina should be urged strongly to stop smoking. The mainstay of therapy for vasospastic angina is a calcium antagonist alone or in combination with long-acting nitrates. There are several important differences between the optimal management of Prinzmetal angina and that of classical (stable and unstable) angina.

1. Patients with both variant and classical angina usually respond well to nitrates; sublingual or intravenous nitroglycerin often abolishes attacks of variant angina promptly, and long-acting nitrates are useful in preventing attacks.[309] However, the mechanisms of action of the drugs may differ in the two types of angina. As discussed in Chapter 50, in chronic (effort-induced) stable angina as well as in unstable angina, one important action of nitrates is to reduce myocardial O_2 need and another is to cause coronary vasodilation. In Prinzmetal angina, nitrates abolish or prevent myocardial ischemia *exclusively* by exerting a direct vasodilating effect on the spastic coronary arteries.
2. In patients with classical angina (stable and unstable), beta blockade is usually beneficial, but the response to these agents in patients with Prinzmetal angina is variable.[310] Some, particularly those with associated fixed lesions, exhibit a reduction in the frequency of exertion-induced angina caused primarily by augmentation of myocardial O_2 requirements. In others, however, nonselective beta adrenoreceptor blockers may actually be detrimental because blockade of $beta_2$ receptors, which subserve coronary dilation, allows unopposed alpha receptor–mediated coronary vasoconstriction to occur; in these patients, the duration of episodes of vasotonic angina may be prolonged by propranolol.
3. In contrast to the variable effectiveness of beta blockers, calcium antagonists are extremely effective in preventing the coronary artery spasm of variant angina,[311] and they should ordinarily be prescribed in maximally tolerated doses on a long-term basis. These drugs, along with long- and short-acting nitrates, are the mainstay of therapy. Because calcium antagonists act through a different mechanism than nitrates, the vasodilatory actions of these two classes of drugs may be additive. All first- and second-generation calcium antagonists have similar (approximately 90 percent) efficacy in

producing relief of symptoms,[282,312-314] and they also suppress asymptomatic ischemia. In rare instances, a patient responds to only one of these agents, and even less commonly, the simultaneous administration of two or even three calcium antagonists is required. Some patients need extremely high doses, although side effects are increased. Reports have suggested a rebound of symptoms when calcium antagonist therapy is discontinued.[314] Prolonged, in some instances life-long, treatment may be required.

4. *Prazosin*, a selective alpha adrenoreceptor blocker, has also been found to be of value in patients with Prinzmetal angina.[315] *Nicorandil*,* a vasodilator that influences coronary arterial tone by acting through potassium channel activation, appears to be effective for the treatment of vasospastic angina.[316] *Aspirin*, helpful in unstable angina, may actually *increase* the severity of ischemic episodes in patients with Prinzmetal angina because it inhibits biosynthesis of the naturally occurring coronary vasodilator prostacyclin. *ACE inhibition* has been shown to be ineffective.[317] Other novel but promising approaches to the management of vasospastic angina include troglitazone, an insulin sensitizer,[318] and in a small study of patients in whom vasospastic angina was induced by hyperventilation, the infusion of B-type (brain) natriuretic peptide was highly effective.[319] Estradiol supplementation has been reported to suppress hyperventilation-induced coronary vasospasm in women with variant angina.[320]
5. PCI and occasionally CABG may be helpful in patients with variant angina and discrete, proximal fixed obstructive lesions.[321,322] However, spasm may develop at a site different from the initial stenosis; therefore, calcium antagonists should be continued for at least 6 months following successful revascularization. PCI and coronary artery bypass surgery are *contraindicated* in patients with isolated coronary artery spasm without accompanying fixed obstructive disease.
6. Patients who have experienced ischemia-associated ventricular fibrillation who continue to manifest ischemia despite treatment should receive an implantable cardioverter-defibrillator.[323]

Prognosis

Many patients with Prinzmetal angina pass through an acute, active phase, with frequent episodes of angina and cardiac events during the first 6 months after diagnosis. In a series of 277 patients with a median follow-up of 7.5 years, recurrent angina was common (39 percent), but cardiac death and MI were relatively infrequent and occurred in 3.5 and 6.5 percent of patients, respectively.[324] The extent and severity of the underlying CAD and the activity or the tempo of the syndrome have a major effect on the incidence of late mortality and MI. Patients with variant angina in whom serious arrhythmias (ventricular tachycardia, ventricular fibrillation, high-degree AV block, or asystole) develop during spontaneous episodes of pain have a higher risk of sudden death.[325]

In most patients who survive an infarction or the initial 3- to 6-month period of frequent episodes, the condition stabilizes and symptoms and cardiac events tend to diminish with time. In patients who experience such remissions, cautious tapering of calcium antagonists may be attempted. In one series, 16 percent of patients had spontaneous remission for 3 months after withdrawal of therapy, 44 percent continued to have symptoms despite treatment with calcium antagonists and nitrates, and the other 40 percent were free of angina but receiving treatment. Remission occurred more frequently in patients without significant coronary artery stenoses and in those who stopped smoking.[326]

For reasons that are not clear, some patients, after a relatively quiescent period of months or even years, experience a recrudescence of vasospastic activity with frequent and severe episodes of ischemia. Fortunately, these patients respond to retreatment with calcium antagonists and nitrates.

*Nicorandil is not available in the United States at the time of this writing.

REFERENCES

1. American Heart Association: 2004 Heart and Stroke Statistical Update (www.americanheart.org).
2. The TIMI IIIA Investigators: Early effects of tissue-type plasminogen activator added to conventional therapy on the culprit lesion in patients presenting with ischemic cardiac pain at rest. Results of the Thrombolysis in Myocardial Ischemia (TIMI IIIA) Trial. Circulation 87:38, 1993.
3. Cannon CP, Weintraub WS, Demopoulos LA, et al: Comparison of early invasive and conservative strategies in patients with unstable coronary syndromes treated with the glycoprotein IIb/IIIa inhibitor tirofiban. N Engl J Med 344:1879, 2001.
4. Braunwald E, Antman EM, Beasley JW, et al: ACC/AHA guideline update for the management of patients with unstable angina and non-ST-segment elevation myocardial infarction-2002: Summary article: A report of the American College of Cardiology/American Heart Association Task Force on Practice Guidelines (Committee on the Management of Patients With Unstable Angina). Circulation 106:1893, 2002.
5. Braunwald E: Unstable angina: A classification. Circulation 80:410, 1989.
6. Hamm CW, Braunwald E: A classification of unstable angina—Revisited. Circulation 102:118, 2000.
7. Scirica BM, Cannon CP, McCabe CH, et al, for the Thrombolysis In Myocardial Ischemia III Registry Investigators: Prognosis in the Thrombolysis in Myocardial Ischemia III Registry according to the Braunwald unstable angina pectoris classification. Am J Cardiol 90:821, 2002.
8. Braunwald E: Unstable angina: An etiologic approach to management. Circulation 98:2219, 1998.
9. Morrow DA, Braunwald E: Future of biomarkers in acute coronary syndromes: Moving toward a multimarker strategy. Circulation 108:250, 2003.

Pathophysiology

10. Maseri A: Ischemic Heart Disease: A Rational Basis for Clinical Practice and Clinical Research. New York, Churchill Livingstone, 1995.
11. Davies MJ: The composition of coronary-artery plaques. N Engl J Med 336:1312, 1997.
12. Harrington RA, Califf RM, Holmes DR Jr, et al, for the CAVEAT Investigators: Is all unstable angina the same? Insights from the Coronary Angioplasty Versus Excisional Atherectomy Trial (CAVEAT-I). Am Heart J 137:227, 1999.
13. Nesto RW, Waxman S, Mittleman MA, et al: Angioscopy of culprit coronary lesions in unstable angina pectoris and correlation of clinical presentation with plaque morphology. Am J Cardiol 81:225, 1998.
14. Kennon S, Price CP, Mills PG, et al: The central role of platelet activation in determining the severity of acute coronary syndromes. Heart 89:1253, 2003.
15. Serebruany VL, Glassman AH, Malinin AI, et al: Enhanced platelet/endothelial activation in depressed patients with acute coronary syndromes: Evidence from recent clinical trials. Blood Coagul Fibrinolysis 14:563, 2003.
16. Theroux P, Ouimet H, McCans J, et al: Aspirin, heparin or both to treat unstable angina. N Engl J Med 319:1105, 1988.
17. Oler A, Whooley MA, Oler J, Grady D: Adding heparin to aspirin reduces the incidence of myocardial infarction and death in patients with unstable angina. A meta-analysis. JAMA 276:811, 1996.
18. Cohen M, Demers C, Gurfinkel EP, et al, for the Efficacy and Safety of Subcutaneous Enoxaparin in Non-Q-Wave Coronary Events Study Group: A comparison of low-molecular-weight heparin with unfractionated heparin for unstable coronary artery disease. N Engl J Med 337:447, 1997.
19. Antman EM, McCabe CH, Gurfinkel EP, et al: Enoxaparin prevents death and cardiac ischemic events in unstable angina/non-Q-wave myocardial infarction: Results of the Thrombolysis In Myocardial Infarction (TIMI) 11B trial. Circulation 100:1593, 1999.
20. The PURSUIT Trial Investigators: Inhibition of platelet glycoprotein IIb/IIIa with eptifibatide in patients with acute coronary syndromes. N Engl J Med 339:436, 1998.
21. The Platelet Receptor Inhibition for Ischemic Syndrome Management (PRISM) Study Investigators: A comparison of aspirin plus tirofiban with aspirin plus heparin for unstable angina. N Engl J Med 338:1498, 1998.
22. The Platelet Receptor Inhibition for Ischemic Syndrome Management in Patients Limited by Unstable Signs and Symptoms (PRISM-PLUS) Trial Investigators: Inhibition of the platelet glycoprotein IIb/IIIa receptor with tirofiban in unstable angina and non-Q-wave myocardial infarction. N Engl J Med 338:1488, 1998.
23. Clopidogrel in Unstable Angina to Prevent Recurrent Events Trial Investigators: Effects of clopidogrel in addition to aspirin in patients with acute coronary syndromes without ST-segment elevation. N Engl J Med 345:494, 2001.
24. Storey RF, Newby LJ, Heptinstall S: Effects of P2Y(1) and P2Y(12) receptor antagonists on platelet aggregation induced by different agonists in human whole blood. Platelets 12:443, 2001.
25. Badimon JJ, Lettino M, Toschi V, et al: Local inhibition of tissue factor reduces the thrombogenicity of disrupted human atherosclerotic plaques: Effects of tissue factor

pathway inhibitor on plaque thrombogenicity under flow conditions. Circulation 99:1780, 1999.
26. Prinzmetal M, Kennamer R, Merliss R, et al: A variant form of angina pectoris. Am J Med 27:375, 1959.
27. Bottcher M, Botker HE, Sonne H, et al: Endothelium-dependent and -independent perfusion reserve and the effect of L-arginine on myocardial perfusion in patients with syndrome X. Circulation 99:1795, 1999.
28. Marzilli M, Sambuceti G, Fedele S, L'Abbate A: Coronary microcirculatory vasoconstriction during ischemia in patients with unstable angina. J Am Coll Cardiol 35:327, 2000.
29. Pitts WR, Lange RA, Cigarroa JE, Hillis LD: Cocaine-induced myocardial ischemia and infarction: Pathophysiology, recognition, and management. Prog Cardiovasc Dis 40:65, 1997.
30. Strike PC, Steptoe A: Systematic review of mental stress–induced myocardial ischaemia. Eur Heart J 24:690, 2003.
31. Kaski JC: Rapid coronary artery disease progression and angiographic stenosis morphology. Ital Heart J 1:21, 2000.

Clinical Presentation

32. Hochman JS, McCabe CH, Stone PH, et al, for the TIMI Investigators: Outcome and profile of women and men presenting with acute coronary syndromes: A report from TIMI IIIB. J Am Coll Cardiol 30:141, 1997.
33. Hochman JS, Tamis JE, Thompson TD, et al: Sex, clinical presentation, and outcome in patients with acute coronary syndromes. Global Use of Strategies to Open Occluded Coronary Arteries in Acute Coronary Syndromes IIb Investigators. N Engl J Med 341:226, 1999.
34. Scirica BM, Moliterno DJ, Every NR, et al, and the GUARANTEE Investigators: Differences between men and women in the management of unstable angina pectoris (the GUARANTEE Registry). Am J Cardiol 84:1145, 1999.
35. The Global Use of Strategies to Open Occluded Coronary Arteries (GUSTO) IIb Investigators: A comparison of recombinant hirudin with heparin for the treatment of acute coronary syndromes. N Engl J Med 335:775, 1996.
36. Khot UN, Khot MB, Bajzer CT, et al: Prevalence of conventional risk factors in patients with coronary heart disease. JAMA 290:898, 2003.
37. Cannon CP, McCabe CH, Stone PH, et al, for the TIMI III Registry ECG Ancillary Study Investigators: The electrocardiogram predicts one-year outcome of patients with unstable angina and non-Q wave myocardial infarction: Results of the TIMI III Registry ECG Ancillary Study. J Am Coll Cardiol 30:133, 1997.
38. Savonitto S, Ardissino D, Granger CB, et al: Prognostic value of the admission electrocardiogram in acute coronary syndromes. JAMA 281:707, 1999.
39. Akkerhuis KM, Klootwijk PA, Lindeboom W, et al: Recurrent ischaemia during continuous multilead ST-segment monitoring identifies patients with acute coronary syndromes at high risk of adverse cardiac events; meta-analysis of three studies involving 995 patients. Eur Heart J 22:1997, 2001.
40. Goodman SG, Fitchett D, Armstrong PW, et al: Randomized evaluation of the safety and efficacy of enoxaparin versus unfractionated heparin in high-risk patients with non-ST-segment elevation acute coronary syndromes receiving the glycoprotein IIb/IIIa inhibitor eptifibatide. Circulation 107:238, 2003.
41. Jernberg T, Lindahl B, Wallentin L: ST-segment monitoring with continuous 12-lead ECG improves early risk stratification in patients with chest pain and ECG nondiagnostic of acute myocardial infarction. J Am Coll Cardiol 34:1413, 1999.
42. The Joint European Society of Cardiology/American College of Cardiology committee: Myocardial infarction redefined—A consensus document of The Joint European Society of Cardiology/American College of Cardiology committee for the redefinition of myocardial infarction. J Am Coll Cardiol 36:959, 2000.
43. Meier MA, Al-Badr WH, Cooper JV, et al: The new definition of myocardial infarction: Diagnostic and prognostic implications in patients with acute coronary syndromes. Arch Intern Med 162:1585, 2002.
44. Panteghini M, Apple FS, Christenson RH, et al: Use of biochemical markers in acute coronary syndromes. IFCC Scientific Division, Committee on Standardization of Markers of Cardiac Damage. International Federation of Clinical Chemistry. Clin Chem Lab Med 37:687, 1999.
45. Morrow DA, Cannon CP, Rifai N, et al, for the TACTICS-TIMI 18 Investigators: Ability of minor elevations of troponin I and T to predict benefit from an early invasive strategy in patients with unstable angina and non-ST elevation myocardial infarction: Results from a randomized trial. JAMA 286:2405, 2001.
46. Diderholm E, Andren B, Frostfeldt G, et al: The prognostic and therapeutic implications of increased troponin T levels and ST depression in unstable coronary artery disease: The FRISC II invasive troponin T electrocardiogram substudy. Am Heart J 143:760, 2002.
47. The Joint European Society of Cardiology/American College of Cardiology committee: Myocardial infarction redefined—A consensus document of The Joint European Society of Cardiology/American College of Cardiology committee for the redefinition of myocardial infarction. Eur Heart J 21:1502, 2000.
48. Morrow DA, Rifai N, Sabatine MS, et al: Evaluation of the AccuTnI assay for cardiac troponin I for risk assessment in acute coronary syndromes. Clin Chem 49:1396, 2003.
49. Wright SA, Sawyer DB, Sacks DB, et al: Elevation of troponin I levels in patients without evidence of myocardial injury. JAMA 278:2144, 1997.
50. Horwich TB, Patel J, MacLellan WR, Fonarow GC: Cardiac troponin I is associated with impaired hemodynamics, progressive left ventricular dysfunction, and increased mortality rates in advanced heart failure. Circulation 108:833, 2003.
51. Dokainish H, Pillai M, Murphy S, et al, for the TACTICS -TIMI 18 Investigators: Prognostic implications of elevated troponin in patients with suspected acute coronary syndromes but no epicardial coronary disease. J Am Coll Cardiol (in press).
52. Cannon CP, Johnson EB, Cermignani M, et al: Emergency department thrombolysis critical pathway reduces door-to-drug times in acute myocardial infarction. Clin Cardiol 22:17, 1999.
53. Scirica BM, Moliterno DJ, Every NR, et al, and the GUARANTEE Investigators: Racial differences in the management of unstable angina: Results from the GUARANTEE Registry. Am Heart J 138:1065, 1999.
54. Diver DJ, Bier JD, Ferreira PE, et al, for the TIMI-IIIA Investigators. Clinical and arteriographic characterization of patients with unstable angina without critical coronary arterial narrowing (from the TIMI-IIIA trial). Am J Cardiol 74:531, 1994.
55. Roe MT, Harrington RA, Prosper DM, et al: Clinical and therapeutic profile of patients presenting with acute coronary syndromes who do not have significant coronary artery disease. The Platelet Glycoprotein IIb/IIIa in Unstable Angina: Receptor Suppression Using Integrilin Therapy (PURSUIT) Trial Investigators. Circulation 102:1101, 2000.
56. Zhao X-Q, Theroux P, Snapinn SM, Sax FL, for the PRISM-PLUS Investigators: Intracoronary thrombus and platelet glycoprotein IIb/IIIa receptor blockade with tirofiban in unstable angina or non-Q-wave myocardial infarction. Angiographic results from the PRISM-PLUS trial (Platelet Receptor Inhibition for Ischemic Syndrome Management in Patients Limited by Unstable Signs and Symptoms). Circulation 100:1609, 1999.
57. Wong GC, Morrow DA, Murphy S, et al, for the TACTICS-TIMI 18 Study Group: Elevations in troponin T and I are associated with abnormal tissue level perfusion: A TACTICS-TIMI 18 substudy. Circulation 106:202, 2002.
58. De Servi S, Arbustini E, Marsico F, et al: Correlation between clinical and morphologic findings in unstable angina. Am J Cardiol 77:128, 1996.
59. Jaber WA, Prior DL, Marso SP, et al: CHF on presentation is associated with markedly worse outcomes among patients with acute coronary syndromes: PURSUIT trial findings. Circulation 100(Suppl I):I-433, 1999.

Risk Stratification

60. Kerensky RA, Wade M, Deedwania P, et al: Revisiting the culprit lesion in non-Q-wave myocardial infarction. Results from the VANQWISH trial angiographic core laboratory. J Am Coll Cardiol 39:1456, 2002.
61. Goldstein JA, Demetriou D, Grines CL, et al: Multiple complex coronary plaques in patients with acute myocardial infarction. N Engl J Med 343:915, 2000.
62. Rioufol G, Finet G, Ginon I, et al: Multiple atherosclerotic plaque rupture in acute coronary syndrome: A three-vessel intravascular ultrasound study. Circulation 106:804, 2002.
63. Zairis MN, Papadaki OA, Manousakis SJ, et al: C-reactive protein and multiple complex coronary artery plaques in patients with primary unstable angina. Atherosclerosis 164:355, 2002.
64. Asakura M, Ueda Y, Yamaguchi O, et al: Extensive development of vulnerable plaques as a pan-coronary process in patients with myocardial infarction: An angioscopic study. J Am Coll Cardiol 37:1284, 2001.
65. Lindahl B, Diderholm E, Lagerqvist B, et al: Mechanisms behind the prognostic value of troponin T in unstable coronary artery disease: A FRISC II substudy. J Am Coll Cardiol 38:979, 2001.
66. Stone PH, Thompson B, Anderson HV, et al, for the TIMI III Registry Study Group: Influence of race, sex, and age on management of unstable angina and non-Q-wave myocardial infarction: The TIMI III Registry. JAMA 275:1104, 1996.
67. Antman EM, Cohen M, Bernink PJ, et al: The TIMI risk score for unstable angina/non-ST elevation MI: A method for prognostication and therapeutic decision making. JAMA 284:835, 2000.
68. Boersma E, Pieper KS, Steyerberg EW, et al, for the PURSUIT Investigators: Predictors of outcome in patients with acute coronary syndromes without persistent ST-segment elevation. Results from an international trial of 9461 patients. Circulation 101:2557, 2000.
69. Roffi M, Chew DP, Mukherjee D, et al: Platelet glycoprotein IIb/IIIa inhibitors reduce mortality in diabetic patients with non-ST-segment-elevation acute coronary syndromes. Circulation 104:2767, 2001.
70. Cotter G, Cannon CP, McCabe CH, et al: Prior peripheral arterial disease and cerebrovascular disease are independent predictors of adverse outcome in patients with acute coronary syndromes: Are we doing enough? Results from the Orbofiban in Patients with Unstable Coronary Syndromes-Thrombolysis In Myocardial Infarction (OPUS-TIMI) 16 study. Am Heart J 145:622, 2003.
71. Khot UN, Jia G, Moliterno DJ, et al: Prognostic importance of physical examination for heart failure in non-ST-elevation acute coronary syndromes: The enduring value of Killip classification. JAMA 290:2174, 2003.
72. Klootwijk P, Meij S, Melkert R, et al: Reduction of recurrent ischemia with abciximab during continuous ECG-ischemia monitoring in patients with unstable angina refractory to standard treatment (CAPTURE). Circulation 98:1358, 1998.
73. Hyde TA, French JK, Wong CK, et al: Four-year survival of patients with acute coronary syndromes without ST-segment elevation and prognostic significance of 0.5-mm ST-segment depression. Am J Cardiol 84:379, 1999.
74. Holmvang L, Clemmensen P, Lindahl B, et al: Quantitative analysis of the admission electrocardiogram identifies patients with unstable coronary artery disease who benefit the most from early invasive treatment. J Am Coll Cardiol 41:905, 2003.
75. Antman EM, Tanasijevic MJ, Thompson B, et al: Cardiac-specific troponin I levels to predict the risk of mortality in patients with acute coronary syndromes. N Engl J Med 335:1342, 1996.
76. Kleiman N, Lakkis N, Cannon C, et al: Prospective analysis of creatine kinase muscle-brain fraction and comparison with troponin T to predict cardiac risk and benefit of an invasive strategy in patients with non-ST-elevation acute coronary syndromes. J Am Coll Cardiol 40:1044, 2002.
77. Newby LK, Christenson RH, Ohman EM, et al: Value of serial troponin T measures for early and late risk stratification in patients with acute coronary syndromes. The GUSTO-IIa Investigators. Circulation 98:1853, 1998.
78. Hamm CW, Heeschen C, Goldmann B, et al, for the c7E3 Fab Antiplatelet Therapy in Unstable Refractory Angina (CAPTURE) Study Investigators: Benefit of abciximab in patients with refractory unstable angina in relation to serum troponin T levels. N Engl J Med 340:1623, 1999.

79. Heeschen C, Hamm CW, Goldmann B, et al, for the PRISM Study Investigators: Troponin concentrations for stratification of patients with acute coronary syndromes in relation to therapeutic efficacy of tirofiban. Lancet 354:1757, 1999.
80. James SK, Armstrong P, Barnathan E, et al: Troponin and C-reactive protein have different relations to subsequent mortality and myocardial infarction after acute coronary syndrome: A GUSTO-IV substudy. J Am Coll Cardiol 41:916, 2003.
81. Antman EM, Sacks DB, Rifai N, et al: Time to positivity of a rapid bedside assay for cardiac-specific troponin T predicts prognosis in acute coronary syndromes: A Thrombolysis in Myocardial Infarction (TIMI) 11A substudy. J Am Coll Cardiol 31:326, 1998.
82. Morrow DA, Rifai N, Antman EM, et al: C-reactive protein is a potent predictor of mortality independently and in combination with troponin T in acute coronary syndromes: A TIMI 11A substudy. J Am Coll Cardiol 31:1460, 1998.
83. Rebuzzi AG, Quaranta G, Liuzzo G, et al: Incremental prognostic value of serum levels of troponin T and C-reactive protein on admission in patients with unstable angina pectoris. Am J Cardiol 82:715, 1998.
84. de Winter RJ, Bholasingh R, Lijmer JG, et al: Independent prognostic value of C-reactive protein and troponin I in patients with unstable angina or non-Q-wave myocardial infarction. Cardiovasc Res 42:240, 1999.
85. Ridker PM, Rifai N, Rose L, et al: Comparison of C-reactive protein and low-density lipoprotein cholesterol levels in the prediction of first cardiovascular events. N Engl J Med 347:1557, 2002.
86. Lindahl B, Toss H, Siegbahn A, et al, for the FRISC Study Group: Fragmin during Instability in Coronary Artery Disease. Markers of myocardial damage and inflammation in relation to long-term mortality in unstable coronary artery disease. N Engl J Med 343:1139, 2000.
87. Cannon CP, McCabe CH, Wilcox RG, et al: High-sensitivity C-reactive protein is a potent predictor of long-term mortality in 3225 patients with acute coronary syndromes: Results from OPUS-TIMI 16. Circulation 102(Suppl II):II-499, 2000.
88. Lenderink T, Boersma E, Heeschen C, et al: Elevated troponin T and C-reactive protein predict impaired outcome for 4 years in patients with refractory unstable angina, and troponin T predicts benefit of treatment with abciximab in combination with PTCA. Eur Heart J 24:77, 2003.
89. Sabatine MS, Morrow DA, de Lemos JA, et al: Multimarker approach to risk stratification in non-ST elevation acute coronary syndromes: Simultaneous assessment of troponin I, C-reactive protein, and B-type natriuretic peptide. Circulation 105:1760, 2002.
90. Heeschen C, Hamm CW, Bruemmer J, Simoons ML, for the Chimeric c7E3 AntiPlatelet Therapy in Unstable angina REfractory to standard treatment trial (CAPTURE) Investigators: Predictive value of C-reactive protein and troponin T in patients with unstable angina: A comparative analysis. J Am Coll Cardiol 35:1535, 2000.
91. Biasucci LM, Liuzzo G, Grillo RL, et al: Elevated levels of C-reactive protein at discharge in patients with unstable angina predict recurrent instability. Circulation 99:855, 1999.
92. Morrow DA, Rifai N, Antman EM, et al: Serum amyloid A predicts early mortality in acute coronary syndromes: A TIMI 11A substudy. J Am Coll Cardiol 35:358, 2000.
93. de Lemos JA, Morrow DA, Sabatine MS, et al: Association between plasma levels of monocyte chemoattractant protein-1 and long-term clinical outcomes in patients with acute coronary syndromes. Circulation 107:690, 2003.
94. Lindmark E, Diderholm E, Wallentin L, Siegbahn A: Relationship between interleukin 6 and mortality in patients with unstable coronary artery disease: Effects of an early invasive or noninvasive strategy. JAMA 286:2107, 2001.
95. Barron HV, Cannon CP, Murphy SA, et al: Association between white blood cell count, epicardial blood flow, myocardial perfusion, and clinical outcomes in the setting of acute myocardial infarction: A Thrombolysis In Myocardial Infarction 10 substudy. Circulation 102:2329, 2000.
96. Cannon CP, McCabe CH, Wilcox RG, et al, for the OPUS-TIMI 16 Investigators: Association of white blood cell count with increased mortality in acute myocardial infarction and unstable angina pectoris. Am J Cardiol 87:636, 2001.
97. Sabatine MS, Morrow DA, Cannon CP, et al: Relationship between baseline white blood cell count and degree of coronary artery disease and mortality in patients with acute coronary syndromes: A TACTICS-TIMI 18 (Treat Angina with Aggrastat and determine Cost of Therapy with an Invasive or Conservative Strategy –Thrombolysis in Myocardial Infarction 18 trial) substudy. J Am Coll Cardiol 40:1761, 2002.
98. Mueller C, Neumann FJ, Roskamm H, et al: Women do have an improved long-term outcome after non-ST-elevation acute coronary syndromes treated very early and predominantly with percutaneous coronary intervention: A prospective study in 1,450 consecutive patients. J Am Coll Cardiol 40:245, 2002.
99. Andre P, Prasad KS, Denis CV, et al: CD40L stabilizes arterial thrombi by a beta3 integrin–dependent mechanism. Nat Med 8:247, 2002.
100. Schonbeck U, Sukhova GK, Shimizu K, et al: Inhibition of CD40 signaling limits evolution of established atherosclerosis in mice. Proc Natl Acad Sci USA 97:7458, 2000.
101. Heeschen C, Dimmeler S, Hamm CW, et al: Soluble CD40 ligand in acute coronary syndromes. N Engl J Med 348:1104, 2003.
102. Varo N, de Lemos JA, Libby P, et al: Soluble CD40L: Risk prediction after acute coronary syndromes. Circulation 108:1049, 2003.
103. Schonbeck U, Varo N, Libby P, et al: Soluble CD40L and cardiovascular risk in women. Circulation 104:2266, 2001.
104. Wiese S, Breyer T, Dragu A, et al: Gene expression of brain natriuretic peptide in isolated atrial and ventricular human myocardium: Influence of angiotensin II and diastolic fiber length. Circulation 102:3074, 2000.
105. Dao Q, Krishnaswamy P, Kazanegra R, et al: Utility of B-type natriuretic peptide in the diagnosis of congestive heart failure in an urgent-care setting. J Am Coll Cardiol 37:379, 2001.
106. Richards AM, Nicholls MG, Yandle TG, et al: Plasma N-terminal pro-brain natriuretic peptide and adrenomedullin: New neurohormonal predictors of left ventricular function and prognosis after myocardial infarction. Circulation 97:1921, 1998.
107. de Lemos JA, Morrow DA, Bentley JH, et al: The prognostic value of B-type natriuretic peptide in patients with acute coronary syndromes. N Engl J Med 345:1014, 2001.
108. Morrow DA, de Lemos JA, Sabatine MS, et al: Evaluation of B-type natriuretic peptide for risk assessment in unstable angina/non-ST-elevation myocardial infarction: B-type natriuretic peptide and prognosis in TACTICS-TIMI 18. J Am Coll Cardiol 41:1264, 2003.
109. Omland T, de Lemos JA, Morrow DA, et al: Prognostic value of N-terminal pro-atrial and pro-brain natriuretic peptide in patients with acute coronary syndromes. Am J Cardiol 89:463, 2002.
110. Zhang R, Brennan ML, Fu X, et al: Association between myeloperoxidase levels and risk of coronary artery disease. JAMA 286:2136, 2001.
111. Baldus S, Heeschen C, Meinertz T, et al: Myeloperoxidase serum levels predict risk in patients with acute coronary syndromes. Circulation 108:1440, 2003.
112. Buffon A, Biasucci LM, Liuzzo G, et al: Widespread coronary inflammation in unstable angina. N Engl J Med 347:5, 2002.
113. Januzzi JL, Cannon CP, DiBattiste PM, et al: Effects of renal insufficiency on early invasive management in patients with acute coronary syndromes (the TACTICS-TIMI 18 trial). Am J Cardiol 90:1246, 2002.
114. Januzzi JL Jr, Snapinn SM, DiBattiste PM, et al: Benefits and safety of tirofiban among acute coronary syndrome patients with mild to moderate renal insufficiency: Results from the Platelet Receptor Inhibition in Ischemic Syndrome Management in Patients Limited by Unstable Signs and Symptoms (PRISM-PLUS) trial. Circulation 105:2361, 2002.
115. Aviles RJ, Askari AT, Lindahl B, et al: Troponin T levels in patients with acute coronary syndromes, with or without renal dysfunction. N Engl J Med 346:2047, 2002.
116. Gibson CM, Pinto DS, Murphy SA, et al: Association of creatinine and creatinine clearance on presentation in acute myocardial infarction with subsequent mortality. J Am Coll Cardiol 42:1535, 2003.
117. Becker RC, Spencer FA, Gibson M, et al: Influence of patient characteristics and renal function on factor Xa inhibition pharmacokinetics and pharmacodynamics after enoxaparin administration in non-ST-segment elevation acute coronary syndromes. Am Heart J 143:753, 2002.
118. Malmberg K, Norhammar A, Wedel H, Ryden L: Glycometabolic state at admission: Important risk marker of mortality in conventionally treated patients with diabetes mellitus and acute myocardial infarction: Long-term results from the Diabetes and Insulin-Glucose Infusion in Acute Myocardial Infarction (DIGAMI) study. Circulation 99:2626, 1999.
119. Bhadriraju S, Cannon CP, DeFranco AC, et al: Association between blood glucose and long term mortality in patients with acute coronary syndromes in the OPUS-TIMI 16 trial. Circulation 108(Suppl 1):1475, 2003.
120. Foo K, Cooper J, Deaner A, et al: A single serum glucose measurement predicts adverse outcomes across the whole range of acute coronary syndromes. Heart 89:512, 2003.
121. Tenerz A, Nilsson G, Forberg R, et al: Basal glucometabolic status has an impact on long-term prognosis following an acute myocardial infarction in non-diabetic patients. J Intern Med 254:494, 2003.
122. Malmberg K, Ryden L, Hamsten A, et al, for the Diabetes Insulin-Glucose in Acute Myocardial Infarction (DIGAMI) Study Group. Effects of insulin treatment on cause-specific one-year mortality and morbidity in diabetic patients with acute myocardial infarction. Eur Heart J 17:1337, 1996.
123. Morrow DA, Antman EM, Snapinn SM, et al: An integrated clinical approach to predicting the benefit of tirofiban in non-ST elevation acute coronary syndromes: Application of the TIMI risk score for UA/NSTEMI in PRISM-PLUS. Eur Heart J 23:223, 2002.

Medical Therapy

124. Cheitlin MD, Hutter AM Jr, Brindis RG, et al: ACC/AHA expert consensus document. Use of sildenafil (Viagra) in patients with cardiovascular disease. American College of Cardiology/American Heart Association. J Am Coll Cardiol 33:273, 1999.
125. Gruppo Italiano per lo Studio della Sopravvivenza nell'Infarto Miocardico: GISSI-3: Effect of lisinopril and transdermal glyceryl trinitrate singly and together on 6-week mortality and ventricular function after acute myocardial infarction. Lancet 343:1115, 1994.
126. ISIS-4 Collaborative Group: ISIS-4: Randomized factorial trial assessing early oral captopril, oral mononitrate, and intravenous magnesium sulphate in 58,050 patients with suspected acute myocardial infarction. Lancet 345:669, 1995.
127. Gottlieb SO, Weisfeldt ML, Ouyang P, et al: Effect of the addition of propranolol to therapy with nifedipine for unstable angina: A randomized, double-blind, placebo-controlled trial. Circulation 73:331, 1986.
128. The Holland Interuniversity Nifedipine/Metoprolol Trial (HINT) Research Group: Early treatment of unstable angina in the coronary care unit: A randomised, double blind, placebo controlled comparison of recurrent ischaemia in patients treated with nifedipine or metoprolol or both. Br Heart J 56:400, 1986.
129. Theroux P, Taeymans Y, Morissette D, et al: A randomized study comparing propranolol and diltiazem in the treatment of unstable angina. J Am Coll Cardiol 5:717, 1985.
130. Yusuf S, Peto R, Lewis J, et al: Beta-blockade during and after myocardial infarction: An overview of the randomized trials. Prog Cardiovasc Dis 27:335, 1985.
131. Foody JM, Farrell MH, Krumholz HM: Beta-blocker therapy in heart failure: Scientific review. JAMA 287:883, 2002.
132. TIMI Study Group: Comparison of invasive and conservative strategies after treatment with intravenous tissue plasminogen activator in acute myocardial infarction. Results of the Thrombolysis in Myocardial Infarction (TIMI) Phase II Trial. N Engl J Med 320:618, 1989.
133. Gibson RS, Boden WE, Theroux P, et al, and the Diltiazem Re-Infarction Study (DRS) Group: Diltiazem and reinfarction in patients with non-Q wave myocardial infarction. Results of a double-blind, randomized, multicenter trial. N Engl J Med 315:423, 1986.
134. Boden WE, van Gilst WH, Scheldewaert RG, et al: Diltiazem in acute myocardial infarction treated with thrombolytic agents: A randomised placebo-controlled trial. Incomplete Infarction Trial of European Research Collaborators Evaluating Prognosis post-Thrombolysis (INTERCEPT). Lancet 355:1751, 2000.

135. The Danish Study Group on Verapamil in Myocardial Infarction: Effect of verapamil on mortality and major events after acute infarction (the Danish Verapamil Infarction Trial II—DAVIT II). Am J Cardiol 66:779, 1990.
136. Hennekens CH, Albert CM, Godfried SL, et al: Adjunctive drug therapy of acute myocardial infarction—Evidence from clinical trials. N Engl J Med 335:1660, 1996.
137. Pepine CJ, Faich G, Makuch R: Verapamil use in patients with cardiovascular disease: An overview of randomized trials. Clin Cardiol 21:633, 1998.
138. The Multicenter Diltiazem Postinfarction Trial Research Group: The effect of diltiazem on mortality and reinfarction after myocardial infarction. N Engl J Med 319:385, 1988.
139. Hansen JF, Hagerup L, Sigurd B, et al, for the Danish Verapamil Infarction Trial (DAVIT) Study Group. Cardiac event rates after acute myocardial infarction in patients treated with verapamil and trandolapril versus trandolapril alone. Am J Cardiol 79:738, 1997.
140. Cohn JN, Ziesche S, Smith R, et al: Effect of the calcium antagonist felodipine as supplementary vasodilator therapy in patients with chronic heart failure treated with enalapril: V-HeFT III. Vasodilator-Heart Failure Trial (V-HeFT) Study Group. Circulation 96:856, 1997.
141. Chinese Cardiac Study Collaborative Group: Oral captopril versus placebo among 13,634 patients with suspected myocardial infarction: Interim report from the Chinese Cardiac Study (CCS-1). Lancet 345:686, 1995.
142. Yusuf S, Sleight P, Pogue J, et al, for the Heart Outcomes Prevention Evaluation Study Investigators. Effects of an angiotensin-converting-enzyme inhibitor, ramipril, on cardiovascular events in high-risk patients. N Engl J Med 342:145, 2000 [published erratum appears in N Engl J Med 342:748, 2000].
143. Fox KM: Efficacy of perindopril in reduction of cardiovascular events among patients with stable coronary artery disease: Randomised, double-blind, placebo-controlled, multicentre trial (the EUROPA study). Lancet 362:782, 2003.
144. Rutherford JD, Pfeffer MA, Moye LA, et al, on behalf of the SAVE Investigators. Effects of captopril on ischemic events after myocardial infarction. Results of the Survival and Ventricular Enlargement Trial. Circulation 90:1731, 1994.
145. The SOLVD Investigators: Effect of enalapril on survival in patients with reduced left ventricular ejection fractions and congestive heart failure. N Engl J Med 325:293, 1991.
146. Scandinavian Simvastatin Survival Study Group: Randomised trial of cholesterol lowering in 4444 patients with coronary heart disease: The Scandinavian Simvastatin Survival Study (4S). Lancet 344:1383, 1994.
147. Sacks RM, Pfeffer MA, Moye LA, et al, for the Cholesterol and Recurrent Events Trial Investigators. The effect of pravastatin on coronary events after myocardial infarction in patients with average cholesterol levels. N Engl J Med 335:1001, 1996.
148. The Long-Term Intervention with Pravastatin in Ischaemic Disease (LIPID) Study Group: Prevention of cardiovascular events and death with pravastatin in patients with coronary heart disease and a broad range of initial cholesterol levels. N Engl J Med 339:1349, 1998.
149. Heart Protection Study Collaborative Group: MRC/BHF Heart Protection Study of cholesterol lowering with simvastatin in 20,536 high-risk individuals: A randomised placebo controlled trial. Lancet 360:7, 2002.
150. Pedersen TR, Kjekshus J, Berg K, et al, for the Scandinavian Simvastatin Survival Study Group: Cholesterol lowering and the use of healthcare resources. Results of the Scandinavian Simvastatin Survival Study. Circulation 93:1796, 1996.
151. Tonkin AM, Colquhoun D, Emberson J, et al: Effects of pravastatin in 3260 patients with unstable angina: Results from the LIPID study. Lancet 356:1871, 2000.
152. Executive Summary of The Third Report of The National Cholesterol Education Program (NCEP) Expert Panel on Detection, Evaluation, and Treatment of High Blood Cholesterol in Adults (Adult Treatment Panel III). JAMA 285:2486, 2001.
153. Expert Panel on Detection, Evaluation, and Treatment of High Blood Cholesterol in Adults: Summary of the second report of the National Cholesterol Education Program (NCEP) expert panel on detection, evaluation, and treatment of high blood cholesterol in adults (Adult Treatment Panel II). JAMA 269:3015, 1993.
154. Arntz HR, Agrawal R, Wunderlich W, et al: Beneficial effects of pravastatin (+/− cholestyramine/niacin) initiated immediately after a coronary event (the randomized Lipid-Coronary Artery Disease [L-CAD] Study). Am J Cardiol 86:1293, 2000.
155. Liem AH, van Boven AJ, Veeger NJ, et al: Effect of fluvastatin on ischaemia following acute myocardial infarction: A randomized trial. Eur Heart J 23:1931, 2002.
156. Aronow HD, Topol EJ, Roe MT, et al: Effect of lipid-lowering therapy on early mortality after acute coronary syndromes: An observational study. Lancet 357:1063, 2001.
157. Stenestrand U, Wallentin L: Early statin treatment following acute myocardial infarction and 1-year survival. JAMA 285:430, 2001.
158. Blazing MA, De Lemos JA, Dyke CK, et al: The A-to-Z Trial: Methods and rationale for a single trial investigating combined use of low-molecular-weight heparin with the glycoprotein IIb/IIIa inhibitor tirofiban and defining the efficacy of early aggressive simvastatin therapy. Am Heart J 142:211, 2001.
158a. Cannon CP, Braunwald E, McCabe CH, et al: Intensive versus moderate lipid lowering with statins after acute coronary syndromes. N Engl J Med 350:1495, 2004.
159. Fonarow GC, Gawlinski A, Moughrabi S, Tillisch JH: Improved treatment of coronary heart disease by implementation of a Cardiac Hospitalization Atherosclerosis Management Program (CHAMP). Am J Cardiol 87:819, 2001.
160. Jha AK, Perlin JB, Kizer KW, Dudley RA: Effect of the transformation of the Veterans Affairs Health Care System on the quality of care. N Engl J Med 348:2218, 2003.
161. The RISC Group: Risk of myocardial infarction and death during treatment with low dose aspirin and intravenous heparin in men with unstable coronary artery disease. Lancet 336:827, 1990.
162. Lewis HD, Davis JW, Archibald DG, et al: Protective effects of aspirin against acute myocardial infarction and death in men with unstable angina. N Engl J Med 309:396, 1983.
163. Cairns JA, Gent M, Singer J, et al: Aspirin, sulfinpyrazone, or both in unstable angina. N Engl J Med 313:1369, 1985.
164. Antithrombotic Trialists' Collaboration: Collaborative meta-analysis of randomised trials of antiplatelet therapy for prevention of death, myocardial infarction, and stroke in high risk patients. BMJ 324:71, 2002.
165. ISIS-2 (Second International Study of Infarct Survival) Collaborative Group: Randomised trial of intravenous streptokinase, oral aspirin, both, or neither among 17,187 cases of suspected acute myocardial infarction: ISIS-2. Lancet 2:349, 1988.
166. Topol EJ, Easton D, Harrington RA, et al: Randomized, double-blind, placebo-controlled, international trial of the oral IIb/IIIa antagonist lotrafiban in coronary and cerebrovascular disease. Circulation 108:399, 2003.
167. Peters RJ, Mehta SR, Fox KA, et al: Effects of aspirin dose when used alone or in combination with clopidogrel in patients with acute coronary syndromes: Observations from the Clopidogrel in Unstable angina to prevent Recurrent Events (CURE) study. Circulation 108:1682, 2003.
168. Eikelboom JW, Hirsh J, Weitz JI, et al: Aspirin-resistant thromboxane biosynthesis and the risk of myocardial infarction, stroke, or cardiovascular death in patients at high risk for cardiovascular events. Circulation 105:1650, 2002.
169. Gum PA, Kottke-Marchant K, Welsh PA, et al: A prospective, blinded determination of the natural history of aspirin resistance among stable patients with cardiovascular disease. J Am Coll Cardiol 41:961, 2003.
170. Goto S, Tamura N, Eto K, et al: Functional significance of adenosine 5'-diphosphate receptor (P2Y(12)) in platelet activation initiated by binding of von Willebrand factor to platelet GP Ibalpha induced by conditions of high shear rate. Circulation 105:2531, 2002.
171. Balsano F, Rizzon P, Violi F, et al, the Studio della Ticlopidina nell'Angina Instabile Group: Antiplatelet treatment with ticlopidine in unstable angina: A controlled multicenter clinical trial. Circulation 82:17, 1990.
172. Leon MB, Baim DS, Popma JJ, et al: A clinical trial comparing three antithrombotic-drug regimens after coronary-artery stenting. Stent Anticoagulation Restenosis Study Investigators. N Engl J Med 339:1665, 1998.
173. Steinhubl SR, Tan WA, Foody JM, Topol EJ, for the EPISTENT Investigators: Incidence and clinical course of thrombotic thrombocytopenic purpura due to ticlopidine following coronary stenting. JAMA 281:806, 1999.
174. CAPRIE Steering Committee: A randomised, blinded, trial of clopidogrel versus aspirin in patients at risk of ischaemic events (CAPRIE). Lancet 348:1329, 1996.
175. Steinhubl SR, Berger PB, Mann JT 3rd, et al: Early and sustained dual oral antiplatelet therapy following percutaneous coronary intervention: A randomized controlled trial. JAMA 288:2411, 2002.
176. Bhatt DL, Bertrand ME, Berger PB, et al: Meta-analysis of randomized and registry comparisons of ticlopidine with clopidogrel after stenting. J Am Coll Cardiol 39:9, 2002.
177. Yusuf S, Mehta SR, Zhao F, et al: Early and late effects of clopidogrel in patients with acute coronary syndromes. Circulation 107:966, 2003.
178. Cannon CP, on behalf of the CAPRIE Investigators: Effectiveness of clopidogrel versus aspirin in preventing acute myocardial infarction in patients with symptomatic atherothrombosis (CAPRIE trial). Am J Cardiol 90:960, 2002.
179. Mehta SR, Yusuf S, Peters RJ, et al: Effects of pretreatment with clopidogrel and aspirin followed by long-term therapy in patients undergoing percutaneous coronary intervention: The PCI-CURE study. Lancet 358:527, 2001.
180. Topol EJ, Moliterno DJ, Herrmann HC, et al: Comparison of two platelet glycoprotein IIb/IIIa inhibitors, tirofiban and abciximab, for the prevention of ischemic events with percutaneous coronary revascularization. N Engl J Med 344:1888, 2001.
181. Bonz AW, Lengenfelder B, Strotmann J, et al: Effect of additional temporary glycoprotein IIb/IIIa receptor inhibition on troponin release in elective percutaneous coronary interventions after pretreatment with aspirin and clopidogrel (TOPSTAR trial). J Am Coll Cardiol 40:662, 2002.
182. Helft G, Osende JI, Worthley SG, et al: Acute antithrombotic effect of a front-loaded regimen of clopidogrel in patients with atherosclerosis on aspirin. Arterioscler Thromb Vasc Biol 20:2316, 2000.
183. Muller I, Seyfarth M, Rudiger S, et al: Effect of a high loading dose of clopidogrel on platelet function in patients undergoing coronary stent placement. Heart 85:92, 2001.
184. Neumann FJ, Kastrati A, Pogatsa-Murray G, et al: Evaluation of prolonged antithrombotic pretreatment ("cooling-off" strategy) before intervention in patients with unstable coronary syndromes: A randomized controlled trial. JAMA 290:1593, 2003.
185. Neumann F: Intracoronary Stenting and Antithrombotic Regimen Rapid Early Action for Coronary Treatment (ISAR REACT). In: American College of Cardiology Scientific Sessions; 2003.
186. The EPISTENT Investigators: Randomised placebo-controlled and balloon-angioplasty-controlled trail to assess the safety of coronary stenting with use of platelet glycoprotein-IIb/IIIa blockade. Lancet 352:87, 1998.
187. The EPILOG Investigators: Platelet glycoprotein IIb/IIIa receptor blockade and low-dose heparin during percutaneous coronary revascularization. N Engl J Med 336:1689, 1997.
188. The ESPRIT Investigators: Novel dosing regimen of eptifibatide in planned coronary stent implantation (ESPRIT): A randomised, placebo-controlled trial. Lancet 356:2037, 2000.
189. Muller I, Besta F, Schulz C, et al: Prevalence of clopidogrel non-responders among patients with stable angina pectoris scheduled for elective coronary stent placement. Thromb Haemost 89:783, 2003.
190. Gurbel PA, Bliden KP, Hiatt BL, O'Connor CM: Clopidogrel for coronary stenting: Response variability, drug resistance, and the effect of pretreatment platelet reactivity. Circulation 107:2908, 2003.
191. Theroux P, Waters D, Qiu S, et al: Aspirin versus heparin to prevent myocardial infarction during the acute phase of unstable angina. Circulation 88:2045, 1993.
192. Cohen M, Adams PC, Parry G, et al, and the Antithrombotic Therapy in Acute Coronary Syndromes Research Group: Combination antithrombotic therapy in unstable rest angina and non-Q-wave infarction in nonprior aspirin users. Primary end points analysis from the ATACS trial. Circulation 89:81, 1994.

193. Hirsh J, Anand SS, Halperin JL, Fuster V: Guide to anticoagulant therapy: Heparin: A statement for healthcare professionals from the American Heart Association. Circulation 103:2994, 2001.
194. Flaker GC, Bartolozzi J, Davis V, et al: Use of a standardized nomogram to achieve therapeutic anticoagulation after thrombolytic therapy in myocardial infarction. Arch Intern Med 154:1492, 1994.
195. Anand SS, Yusuf S, Pogue J, et al: Relationship of activated partial thromboplastin time to coronary events and bleeding in patients with acute coronary syndromes who receive heparin. Circulation 107:2884, 2003.
196. Granger CB, Hirsh J, Califf RM, et al, for the GUSTO-I Investigators: Activated partial thromboplastin time and outcome after thrombolytic therapy for acute myocardial infarction: Results from the GUSTO-I Trial. Circulation 93:870, 1996.
197. Becker RC, Cannon CP, Tracy RP, et al, for the Thrombolysis in Myocardial Ischemia IIIB Investigators: Relationship between systemic anticoagulation as determined by activated partial thromboplastin time and heparin measurements and in-hospital clinical events in unstable angina and non-Q wave myocardial infarction. Am Heart J 131:421, 1996.
198. Hochman JS, Wali AU, Gavrila D, et al: A new regimen for heparin use in acute coronary syndromes. Am Heart J 138:313, 1999.
199. Hirsh J, Warkentin TE, Shaughnessy SG, et al: Heparin and low-molecular-weight heparin: Mechanisms of action, pharmacokinetics, dosing, monitoring, efficacy, and safety. Chest 119:64S, 2001.
200. Warkentin TE, Levine MN, Hirsh J, et al: Heparin-induced thrombocytopenia in patients treated with low-molecular-weight heparin or unfractionated heparin. N Engl J Med 332:1330, 1995.
201. Fragmin during Instability in Coronary Artery Disease (FRISC) Study Group: Low-molecular-weight heparin during instability in coronary artery disease. Lancet 347:561, 1996.
202. Klein W, Buchwald A, Hillis SE, et al, for the FRIC Investigators: Comparison of low-molecular-weight heparin with unfractionated heparin acutely and with placebo for 6 weeks in the management of unstable coronary artery disease. Fragmin in Unstable Coronary Artery Disease Study (FRIC). Circulation 96:61, 1997.
203. The FRAX.I.S Study Group: Comparison of two treatment durations (6 days and 14 days) of a low molecular weight heparin with a 6-day treatment of unfractionated heparin in the initial management of unstable angina or non-Q wave myocardial infarction: FRAX.I.S. (FRAXiparine in Ischaemic Syndrome). Eur Heart J 20:1553, 1999.
204. Eikelboom JW, Anand SS, Malmberg K, et al: Unfractionated heparin and low-molecular-weight heparin in acute coronary syndrome without ST elevation: A meta-analysis. Lancet 355:1936, 2000.
205. Morrow DA, Antman EM, Tanasijevic M, et al: Cardiac troponin I for stratification of early outcomes and the efficacy of enoxaparin in unstable angina: A TIMI 11B sub-study. J Am Coll Cardiol 36:1812, 2000.
206. Mark DB, Cowper PA, Berkowitz SD, et al: Economic assessment of low-molecular-weight heparin (enoxaparin) versus unfractionated heparin in acute coronary syndrome patients: Results from the ESSENCE randomized trial. Circulation 97:1702, 1998.
207. Fox KA, Antman EM, Cohen M, Bigonzi F: Comparison of enoxaparin versus unfractionated heparin in patients with unstable angina pectoris/non-ST-segment elevation acute myocardial infarction having subsequent percutaneous coronary intervention. Am J Cardiol 90:477, 2002.
208. Blazing MA: The A-to-Z Trial: Results of the A-Phase, investigating combined use of low-molecular-weight heparin with the glycoprotein IIb/IIIa inhibitor tirofiban. Presented at the American College of Cardiology Scientific Sessions, New Orleans, LA, March 2003.
208a. SYNERGY Steering Committee: Superior yield of the New strategy of Enoxaparin, Revascularization and GlYcoprotein IIb/IIIa inhibitors (SYNERGY): Primary results. JAMA 2004 (in press).
209. Michalis LK, Katsouras CS, Papamichael N, et al: Enoxaparin versus tinzaparin in non-ST-segment elevation acute coronary syndromes: The EVET trial. Am Heart J 146:304, 2003.
210. Eriksson BI, Bauer KA, Lassen MR, Turpie AG: Fondaparinux compared with enoxaparin for the prevention of venous thromboembolism after hip-fracture surgery. N Engl J Med 345:1298, 2001.
211. Organisation to Assess Strategies for Ischemic Syndromes (OASIS-2) Investigators: Effects of recombinant hirudin (lepirudin) compared with heparin on death, myocardial infarction, refractory angina, and revascularisation procedures in patients with acute myocardial ischaemia without ST elevation: A randomised trial. Lancet 353:429, 1999.
212. Antman EM, McCabe CH, Braunwald E: Bivalirudin as a replacement for unfractionated heparin in unstable angina/non-ST-elevation myocardial infarction: Observations from the TIMI 8 trial. Am Heart J 143:229, 2002.
213. Kong DF, Topol EJ, Bittl JA, et al: Clinical outcomes of bivalirudin for ischemic heart disease. Circulation 100:2049, 1999.
214. Direct Thrombin Inhibitor Trialists' Collaborative Group: Direct thrombin inhibitors in acute coronary syndromes and during percutaneous coronary intervention: Design of a meta-analysis based on individual patient data. Am Heart J 141:E2, 2001.
215. Bittl JA, Strony J, Brinker JA, et al, for the Hirulog Angioplasty Study Investigators: Treatment with bivalirudin (Hirulog) as compared with heparin during coronary angioplasty for unstable or post-infarction angina. N Engl J Med 333:764, 1995.
216. Lincoff AM, Bittl JA, Harrington RA, et al: Bivalirudin and provisional glycoprotein IIb/IIIa blockade compared with heparin and planned glycoprotein IIb/IIIa blockade during percutaneous coronary intervention: REPLACE-2 randomized trial. JAMA 289:853, 2003.
217. Fuchs J, Cannon CP, and the TIMI 7 Investigators: Hirulog in the treatment of unstable angina: Results of the Thrombin Inhibition in Myocardial Ischemia (TIMI) 7 trial. Circulation 92:727, 1995.
218. The Organization to Assess Strategies for Ischemic Syndromes (OASIS) Investigators: Effects of long-term, moderate-intensity oral anticoagulation in addition to aspirin in unstable angina. J Am Coll Cardiol 37:475, 2001.
219. Fiore LD, Ezekowitz MD, Brophy MT, et al: Department of Veterans Affairs Cooperative Studies Program clinical trial comparing combined warfarin and aspirin with aspirin alone in survivors of acute myocardial infarction: Primary results of the CHAMP Study. Circulation 105:557, 2002.
220. Coumadin Aspirin Reinfarction Study (CARS) Investigators: Randomised double-blind trial of fixed low-dose warfarin with aspirin after myocardial infarction. Lancet 350:389, 1997.
221. Anand SS, Yusuf S, for the OASIS Investigators: Randomized trial of oral anticoagulation therapy in patient with acute ischemic syndromes without ST elevation: Importance of good compliance. J Am Coll Cardiol 33(Suppl A):396A, 1999.
222. van Es RF, Jonker JJ, Verheugt FW, et al: Aspirin and Coumadin after acute coronary syndromes (the ASPECT-2 study): A randomised controlled trial. Lancet 360:109, 2002.
223. Hurlen M, Abdelnoor M, Smith P, et al: Warfarin, aspirin, or both after myocardial infarction. N Engl J Med 347:969, 2002.
224. Brouwer MA, van den Bergh PJ, Aengevaeren WR, et al: Aspirin plus coumarin versus aspirin alone in the prevention of reocclusion after fibrinolysis for acute myocardial infarction: Results of the Antithrombotics in the Prevention of Reocclusion In Coronary Thrombolysis (APRICOT)-2 Trial. Circulation 106:659, 2002.
225. Loh E, Sutton MS, Wun CC, et al: Ventricular dysfunction and the risk of stroke after myocardial infarction. N Engl J Med 336:251, 1997.
226. Wallentin L, Wilcox RG, Weaver WD, et al: Oral ximelagatran for secondary prophylaxis after myocardial infarction: The ESTEEM randomised controlled trial. Lancet 362:789, 2003.

Glycoprotein IIb/IIIa Inhibitors

227. The CAPTURE Investigators: Randomised placebo-controlled trial of abciximab before and during coronary intervention in refractory unstable angina: The CAPTURE study. Lancet 349:1429, 1997 [published erratum appears in Lancet 350:744, 1997].
228. Boersma E, Harrington RA, Moliterno DJ, et al: Platelet glycoprotein IIb/IIIa inhibitors in acute coronary syndromes: A meta-analysis of all major randomised clinical trials. Lancet 359:189, 2002.
229. Bhatt DL, Topol EJ: Current role of platelet glycoprotein IIb/IIIa inhibitors in acute coronary syndromes. JAMA 284:1549, 2000.
230. Januzzi JL, Hahn SS, Chae CU, et al: Effects of tirofiban plus heparin versus heparin alone on troponin I levels in patients with acute coronary syndromes. Am J Cardiol 86:713, 2000.
231. van den Brand M, Laarman GJ, Steg PG, et al: Assessment of coronary angiograms prior to and after treatment with abciximab, and the outcome of angioplasty in refractory unstable angina patients. Angiographic results from the CAPTURE trial. Eur Heart J 20:1572, 1999.
232. The GUSTO IV-ACS Investigators: Effect of glycoprotein IIb/IIIa receptor blocker abciximab on outcome in patients with acute coronary syndromes without early coronary revascularisation: The GUSTO IV-ACS randomised trial. Lancet 357:1915, 2001.
233. Steinhubl SR, Talley JD, Braden GA, et al: Point-of-care measured platelet inhibition correlates with a reduced risk of an adverse cardiac event after percutaneous coronary intervention: Results of the GOLD (AU-Assessing Ultegra) multicenter study. Circulation 103:2572, 2001.
234. Kong DF, Califf RM, Miller DP, et al: Clinical outcomes of therapeutic agents that block the platelet glycoprotein IIb/IIIa integrin in ischemic heart disease. Circulation 98:2829, 1998.
235. Newby LK, Ohman EM, Christenson RH, et al: Benefit of glycoprotein IIb/IIIa inhibition in patients with acute coronary syndromes and troponin t-positive status: The PARAGON-B troponin T substudy. Circulation 103:2891, 2001.
236. Januzzi JL, Chai CU, Sabatine MS, Jang IK: Elevation in serum troponin I predicts the benefit of tirofiban. J Thromb Thrombolysis 11:211, 2001.
237. Heeschen C, van Den Brand MJ, Hamm CW, Simoons ML: Angiographic findings in patients with refractory unstable angina according to troponin T status. Circulation 100:1509, 1999.
238. Topol EJ, Yadav JS: Recognition of the importance of embolization in atherosclerotic vascular disease. Circulation 101:570, 2000.
239. Roffi M, Chew D, Mukherjee D, et al: Platelet glycoprotein IIb/IIIa inhibition in acute coronary syndromes. Gradient of benefit related to the revascularization strategy. Eur Heart J 23:1441, 2002.
240. Boersma E, Akkerhuis KM, Theroux P, et al: Platelet glycoprotein IIb/IIIa receptor inhibition in non-ST-elevation acute coronary syndromes: Early benefit during medical treatment only, with additional protection during percutaneous coronary intervention. Circulation 100:2045, 1999.
241. Marso SP, Bhatt DL, Roe MT, et al: Enhanced efficacy of eptifibatide administration in patients with acute coronary syndrome requiring in-hospital coronary artery bypass grafting. Circulation 102:2952, 2000.
242. Braunwald E, Antman EM, Beasley JW, et al: ACC/AHA guidelines for the management of patients with unstable angina and non-ST-segment elevation myocardial infarction: Executive summary and recommendations: A report of the American College of Cardiology/American Heart Association task force on practice guidelines (Committee on the management of patients with unstable angina). Circulation 102:1193, 2000.
243. Morrow DA, Sabatine MS, Cannon CP, Theroux P: Benefit of tirofiban among patients treated without coronary intervention: Application of the TIMI Risk Score for Unstable Angina and Non-ST Elevation MI in PRISM-PLUS. Circulation 104(Suppl II):II-782, 2001.
244. Peterson ED, Pollack CV Jr, Roe MT, et al: Early use of glycoprotein IIb/IIIa inhibitors in non-ST-elevation acute myocardial infarction: Observations from the National Registry of Myocardial Infarction 4. J Am Coll Cardiol 42:45, 2003.

245. Peterson ED: Early glycoprotein IIb/IIIa inhibition is associated with improved outcomes: A CRUSADE registry substudy. Presented at the First International Quality Improvement Summit on Acute Coronary Syndromes, Orlando, Fla, 2003.
246. Mahaffey KW, Harrington RA, Simoons ML, et al, for the PURSUIT Investigators: Stroke in patients with acute coronary syndromes: Incidence and outcomes in the Platelet glycoprotein IIb/IIIa in Unstable angina Receptor suppression using Integrilin therapy (PURSUIT) trial. Circulation 99:2371, 1999.
247. O'Neill WW, Serruys P, Knudtson M, et al, for the EXCITE Trial Investigators: Long-term treatment with a platelet glycoprotein-receptor antagonist after pecutaneous coronary revascularization. N Engl J Med 342:1316, 2000.
248. Cannon CP, McCabe CH, Wilcox RG, et al, for the OPUS-TIMI 16 Investigators: Oral glycoprotein IIb/IIIa inhibition with Orbofiban in patients with unstable coronary syndromes (OPUS-TIMI 16) trial. Circulation 102:149, 2000.
249. The SYMPHONY Investigators: Comparison of sibrafiban with aspirin for prevention of cardiovascular events after acute coronary syndromes: A randomised trial. Lancet 355:337, 2000.
250. Second Symphony Investigators: Randomized trial of aspirin, sibrafiban, or both for secondary prevention after acute coronary syndromes. Circulation 103:1727, 2001.
251. The TIMI IIIB Investigators: Effects of tissue plasminogen activator and a comparison of early invasive and conservative strategies in unstable angina and non-Q-wave myocardial infarction: Results of the TIMI IIIB Trial. Circulation 89:1545, 1994.

Invasive Versus Conservative Strategies

252. FRagmin and Fast Revascularisation during InStability in Coronary artery disease Investigators: Invasive compared with non-invasive treatment in unstable coronary-artery disease: FRISC II prospective randomised multicentre study. Lancet 354:708, 1999.
253. Fox KA, Goodman SG, Klein W, et al: Management of acute coronary syndromes. Variations in practice and outcome; findings from the Global Registry of Acute Coronary Events (GRACE). Eur Heart J 23:1177, 2002.
254. Mahoney EM, Jurkovitz CT, Chu H, et al, for the "Treat Angina with Aggrastat and Determine Cost of Therapy with an Invasive or Conservative Strategy (TACTICS)-TIMI 18" Investigators: Cost and cost-effectiveness of an early invasive versus conservative strategy for the treatment of unstable angina and non-ST elevation myocardial infarction. JAMA 288:1851, 2002.
255. McCullough PA, Gibson CM, DiBattiste PM, et al, for the TACTICS TIMI-18 Investigators: Timing of angiography and revascularization in acute coronary syndromes: An analysis from the TACTICS-TIMI 18 trial. J Interv Cardiol 17:81, 2004.
256. Hochman JS, Sleeper LA, Webb JG, et al, for the SHOCK Investigators: Early revascularization in acute myocardial infarction complicated by cardiogenic shock. N Engl J Med 341:625, 1999.
257. Kugelmass AD, Sadanandan S, Cannon CP, et al, for the TACTICS-TIMI 18 Investigators: Early invasive strategy improves outcomes in acute coronary syndrome patients with prior CABG: Results from TACTICS-TIMI 18. Circulation 104(Suppl II):II-548, 2001.
258. Bhatt DL, Greenbaum A, Roe MT, et al: An early invasive approach to acute coronary syndromes in CRUSADE: Dissociation between clinical guidelines and current practice. Circulation 106(Suppl II):II-494, 2002.
259. Sharis PJ, Cannon CP, Rogers WJ, et al: Predictors of mortality, coronary angiography, and revascularization in unstable angina pectoris and acute non-ST elevation myocardial infarction (the TIMI III Registry). Am J Cardiol 90:1154, 2002.
260. Boden WE, O'Rourke RA, Crawford MH, et al, for the Veterans Affairs Non-Q-Wave Infarction Strategies in Hospital (VANQWISH) Trial Investigators: Outcomes in patients with acute non-Q-wave myocardial infarction randomly assigned to an invasive as compared with a conservative strategy. N Engl J Med 338:1785, 1998.
261. Madsen JK, Grande P, Saunamaki K, et al, on behalf of the DANAMI Study Group: Danish multicenter randomized study of invasive versus conservative treatment in patients with inducible ischemia after thrombolysis in acute myocardial infarction (DANAMI). Circulation 96:748, 1997.
262. Heller GV, Brown KA, Landin RJ, Haber SB: Safety of early intravenous dipyridamole technetium 99m sestamibi SPECT myocardial perfusion imaging after uncomplicated first myocardial infarction. Early Post MI IV Dipyridamole Study (EPIDS). Am Heart J 134:105, 1997.
263. Larsson H, Areskog M, Areskog NH, et al: Should the exercise test (ET) be performed at discharge or one month later after an episode of unstable angina or non-Q-wave myocardial infarction? Int J Card Imaging 7:7, 1991.
264. Karha J, Cannon CP, for the TIMI Study Group: Safety of stress testing following an acute coronary syndrome. J Am Coll Cardiol (in press).
265. Kamp O, Beatt KJ, De Feyter PJ, et al: Short-, medium-, and long-term follow-up after percutaneous transluminal coronary angioplasty for stable and unstable angina pectoris. Am Heart J 117:991, 1989.
266. Moses JW, Leon MB, Popma JJ, et al: Sirolimus-eluting stents versus standard stents in patients with stenosis in a native coronary artery. N Engl J Med 349:1315, 2003.
267. The Bypass Angioplasty Revascularization Investigation (BARI) Investigators: Comparison of coronary bypass surgery with angioplasty in patients with multivessel disease. N Engl J Med 335:217, 1996.
268. Morrison DA, Sethi G, Sacks J, et al: Percutaneous coronary intervention versus coronary bypass graft surgery for patients with medically refractory myocardial ischemia and risk factors for adverse outcomes with bypass: The VA AWESOME multicenter registry: Comparison with the randomized clinical trial. J Am Coll Cardiol 39:266, 2002.
269. Fonarow GC: In-hospital initiation of statins: Taking advantage of the 'teachable moment'. Cleve Clin J Med 70:502, 504, 2003.
270. Schwartz GG, Olsson AG, Ezekowitz MD, et al: Effects of atorvastatin on early recurrent ischemic events in acute coronary syndromes: The MIRACL study: A randomized controlled trial. JAMA 285:1711, 2001.
271. Heart Outcomes Prevention Evaluation Study Investigators: Effects of ramipril on cardiovascular and microvascular outcomes in people with diabetes mellitus: Results of the HOPE study and MICRO-HOPE substudy. Lancet 355:253, 2000.
272. Shivkumar K, Schultz L, Goldstein S, Gheorghiade M: Effects of propranolol in patients entered in the Beta-Blocker Heart Attack Trial with their first myocardial infarction and persistent electrocardiographic ST-segment depression. Am Heart J 135:261, 1998.
273. Hasdai D, Behar S, Wallentin L, et al: A prospective survey of the characteristics, treatments and outcomes of patients with acute coronary syndromes in Europe and the Mediterranean basin; the Euro Heart Survey of Acute Coronary Syndromes (Euro Heart Survey ACS). Eur Heart J 23:1190, 2002.
274. Hoekstra JW, Pollack CV Jr, Roe MT, et al: Improving the care of patients with non-ST-elevation acute coronary syndromes in the emergency department: The CRUSADE initiative. Acad Emerg Med 9:1146, 2002.
275. Giugliano RP, Lloyd-Jones DM, Camargo CA Jr, et al: Association of unstable angina guideline care with improved survival. Arch Intern Med 160:1775, 2000.
276. Cannon CP, O'Gara PT: Goals, design and implementation of critical pathways in cardiology. *In* Cannon CP, O'Gara PT (eds): Critical Pathways in Cardiology. Philadelphia, Lippincott Williams & Wilkins, 2001, pp 3-6.
277. Califf RM, Peterson ED, Gibbons RJ, et al: Integrating quality into the cycle of therapeutic development. J Am Coll Cardiol 40:1895, 2002.
278. Cannon CP, Hand MH, Bahr R, et al: Critical pathways for management of patients with acute coronary syndromes: An assessment by the National Heart Attack Alert Program. Am Heart J 143:777, 2002.
279. Mehta RH, Montoye CK, Gallogly M, et al, on behalf of the GAP Steering Committee of the American College of Cardiology: Improving quality of care of acute myocardial infarction: The Guideline Applied in Practice (GAP) initiative in southeast Michigan. JAMA 287:1269, 2002.

Prinzmetal (Variant) Angina

280. Prinzmetal M, Kennamer R, Merliss R, et al: Angina pectoris. I. A variant form of angina pectoris: Preliminary report. Am J Med 27:375, 1959.
281. Yamagishi M, Miyatake K, Tamai J, et al: Intravascular ultrasound detection of atherosclerosis at the site of focal vasospasm in angiographically normal or minimally narrowed coronary segments. J Am Coll Cardiol 23:352, 1994.
282. Mayer S, Hillis LD: Prinzmetal's variant angina. Clin Cardiol 21:243, 1998.
283. Cox ID, Kaski JC, Clague JR: Endothelial dysfunction in the absence of coronary atheroma causing Prinzmetal's angina. Heart 77:584, 1997.
284. Hamabe A, Takase B, Uehata A, et al: Impaired endothelium-dependent vasodilation in the brachial artery in variant angina pectoris and the effect of intravenous administration of vitamin C. Am J Cardiol 87:1154, 2001.
285. Kawano H, Motoyama T, Yasue H, et al: Endothelial function fluctuates with diurnal variation in the frequency of ischemic episodes in patients with variant angina. J Am Coll Cardiol 40:266, 2002.
286. Okumura K, Osanai T, Kosugi T, et al: Enhanced phospholipase C activity in the cultured skin fibroblast obtained from patients with coronary spastic angina: Possible role for enhanced vasoconstrictor response. J Am Coll Cardiol 36:1847, 2000.
287. Sakata Y, Komamura K, Hirayama A, et al: Elevation of the plasma histamine concentration in the coronary circulation in patients with variant angina. Am J Cardiol 77:1121, 1996.
288. Vandergoten P, Benit E, Dendale P: Prinzmetal's variant angina: Three case reports and a review of the literature. Acta Cardiol 54:71, 1999.
289. Suzuki H, Kawai S, Aizawa T, et al: Histological evaluation of coronary plaque in patients with variant angina: Relationship between vasospasm and neointimal hyperplasia in primary coronary lesions. J Am Coll Cardiol 33:198, 1999.
290. Sakata K, Miura F, Sugino H, et al: Assessment of regional sympathetic nerve activity in vasospastic angina: Analysis of iodine 123-labeled metaiodobenzylguanidine scintigraphy. Am Heart J 133:484, 1997.
291. Umemoto S, Suzuki N, Fujii K, et al: Eosinophil counts and plasma fibrinogen in patients with vasospastic angina pectoris. Am J Cardiol 85:715, 2000.
292. Ogawa H, Yasue H, Oshima S, et al: Circadian variation of plasma fibrinopeptide A level in patients with variant angina. Circulation 80:1617, 1989.
293. Igawa A, Miwa K, Miyagi Y, et al: Comparison of frequency of magnesium deficiency in patients with vasospastic angina and fixed coronary artery disease. Am J Cardiol 75:728, 1995.
294. Kim HS, Lee MM, Oh BH, et al: Variant angina is not associated with angiotensin I converting enzyme gene polymorphism but rather with smoking. Coron Artery Dis 10:227, 1999.
295. Onaka H, Hirota Y, Shimada S, et al: Clinical observation of spontaneous anginal attacks and multivessel spasm in variant angina pectoris with normal coronary arteries: Evaluation by 24-hour 12-lead electrocardiography with computer analysis. J Am Coll Cardiol 27:38, 1996.
296. Unverdorben M, Haag M, Fuerste T, et al: Vasospasm in smooth coronary arteries as a cause of asystole and syncope. Cathet Cardiovasc Diagn 41:430, 1997.
297. Tsurukawa T, Kawabata K, Miyahara K, et al: Sudden death during Holter electrocardiogram monitoring in a patient with variant angina. Intern Med 35:966, 1996.
298. Waters DD, Theroux P, Crittin J, et al: Previously undiagnosed variant angina as a cause of chest pain after coronary artery bypass surgery. Circulation 61:1159, 1980.
299. Matsuguchi T, Araki H, Nakamura N, et al: Prevention of vasospastic angina by alcohol ingestion: Report of 2 cases. Angiology 39:394, 1988.
300. Myerburg RJ, Kessler KM, Mallon SM, et al: Life-threatening ventricular arrhythmias in patients with silent myocardial ischemia due to coronary-artery spasm. N Engl J Med 326:1451, 1992.
301. Lip GY, Gupta J, Khan MM, et al: Recurrent myocardial infarction with angina and normal coronary arteries. Int J Cardiol 51:65, 1995.
302. Pepine CJ, el-Tamimi H, Lambert CR: Prinzmetal's angina (variant angina). Heart Dis Stroke 1:281, 1992.
303. Crea F: Variant angina in patients without obstructive coronary atherosclerosis: A benign form of spasm (editorial). Eur Heart J 17:980, 1996.

304. Tatineni S, Kern MJ, Deligonul U, et al: The effects of ionic and nonionic radiographic contrast media on coronary hyperemia in patients during coronary angiography. Am Heart J 123:621, 1992.
305. Minoda K, Yasue H, Kugiyama K, et al: Comparison of the distribution of myocardial blood flow between exercise-induced and hyperventilation-induced attacks of coronary spasm: A study with thallium-201 myocardial scintigraphy. Am Heart J 127:1474, 1994.
306. Nakao K, Ohgushi M, Yoshimura M, et al: Hyperventilation as a specific test for diagnosis of coronary artery spasm. Am J Cardiol 80:545, 1997.
307. Marcus ML, Chilian WM, Kanatsuka H, et al: Understanding the coronary circulation through studies at the microvascular level. Circulation 82:1, 1990.
308. Kugiyama K, Ohgushi M, Motoyama T, et al: Enhancement of constrictor response of spastic coronary arteries to acetylcholine but not to phenylephrine in patients with coronary spastic angina. J Cardiovasc Pharmacol 33:414, 1999.
309. Lombardi M, Morales MA, Michelassi C, et al: Efficacy of isosorbide-5-mononitrate versus nifedipine in preventing spontaneous and ergonovine-induced myocardial ischaemia. A double-blind, placebo-controlled study. Eur Heart J 14:845, 1993.
310. De Cesare N, Cozzi S, Apostolo A, et al: Facilitation of coronary spasm by propranolol in Prinzmetal's angina: Fact or unproven extrapolation? Coron Artery Dis 5:323, 1994.
311. Antman E, Muller J, Goldberg S, et al: Nifedipine therapy for coronary-artery spasm. Experience in 127 patients. N Engl J Med 302:1269, 1980.
312. Ginsburg R, Lamb IH, Schroeder JS, et al: Randomized double-blind comparison of nifedipine and isosorbide dinitrate therapy in variant angina pectoris due to coronary artery spasm. Am Heart J 103:44, 1982.
313. Morikami Y, Yasue H: Efficacy of slow-release nifedipine on myocardial ischemic episodes in variant angina pectoris. Am J Cardiol 68:580, 1991.
314. Winniford MD, Johnson SM, Mauritson DR, et al: Verapamil therapy for Prinzmetal's variant angina: Comparison with placebo and nifedipine. Am J Cardiol 50:913, 1982.
315. Tzivoni D, Keren A, Benhorin J, et al: Prazosin therapy for refractory variant angina. Am Heart J 105:262, 1983.
316. Kaski JC: Management of vasospastic angina—Role of nicorandil. Cardiovasc Drugs Ther 9(Suppl 2):221, 1995.
317. Guazzi M, Agostoni P, Loaldi A: Ineffectiveness of angiotensin converting enzyme inhibition (enalapril) on overt and silent myocardial ischemia in vasospastic angina and comparison with verapamil. Clin Pharmacol Ther 59:476, 1996.
318. Murakami T, Mizuno S, Ohsato K, et al: Effects of troglitazone on frequency of coronary vasospastic-induced angina pectoris in patients with diabetes mellitus. Am J Cardiol 84:92, 1999.
319. Kato H, Yasue H, Yoshimura M, et al: Suppression of hyperventilation-induced attacks with infusion of B-type (brain) natriuretic peptide in patients with variant angina. Am Heart J 128:1098, 1994.
320. Kawano H, Motoyama T, Hirai N, et al: Estradiol supplementation suppresses hyperventilation-induced attacks in postmenopausal women with variant angina. J Am Coll Cardiol 37:735, 2001.
321. Gaspardone A, Tomai F, Versaci F, et al: Coronary artery stent placement in patients with variant angina refractory to medical treatment. Am J Cardiol 84:96, 1999.
322. Tanabe Y, Itoh E, Suzuki K, et al: Limited role of coronary angioplasty and stenting in coronary spastic angina with organic stenosis. J Am Coll Cardiol 39:1120, 2002.
323. Meisel SR, Mazur A, Chetboun I, et al: Usefulness of implantable cardioverter-defibrillators in refractory variant angina pectoris complicated by ventricular fibrillation in patients with angiographically normal coronary arteries. Am J Cardiol 89:1114, 2002.
324. Bory M, Pierron F, Panagides D, et al: Coronary artery spasm in patients with normal or near normal coronary arteries. Long-term follow-up of 277 patients. Eur Heart J 17:1015, 1996.
325. Shimokawa H, Nagasawa K, Irie T, et al: Clinical characteristics and long-term prognosis of patients with variant angina. A comparative study between western and Japanese populations. Int J Cardiol 18:331, 1988.
326. Tashiro H, Shimokawa H, Koyanagi S, et al: Clinical characteristics of patients with spontaneous remission of variant angina. Jpn Circ J 57:117, 1993.

GUIDELINES *Thomas H. Lee*

Unstable Angina

American College of Cardiology/American Heart Association (ACC/AHA) guidelines for the management of unstable angina and non-ST-segment elevation myocardial infarction (UA/NSTEMI) were published in 2000[1] and updated just 2 years later because of rapid progress in clinical research in this area.[2] The full text of the updated guidelines incorporating the changes is available on the Internet (www.acc.org or www.americanheart.org). Recommendations contained within these guidelines that are relevant to the initial evaluation of the patient with acute chest pain are included in the text of Chapter 45. Other recommendations relevant to this topic have been published in the guidelines for use of percutaneous coronary interventions (PCIs), summarized in the appendix to Chapter 52, and in the guidelines for management of acute myocardial infarction, summarized in the appendix to Chapter 48.

These guidelines continue to use the ACC/AHA classification system for the indications (class I for generally accepted indications, class IIa when indications are controversial but the weight of evidence is supportive, class IIb when usefulness or efficacy is less well established, and class III when there is a consensus against the usefulness of the intervention). The guidelines also use a convention for rating levels of evidence upon which recommendations have been based. *Level A* recommendations were derived from data from multiple randomized clinical trials, *level B* recommendations were derived from a single randomized trial or nonrandomized studies, and *level C* recommendations were based upon the consensus opinion of experts.

Early Risk Stratification and Management

The ACC/AHA guidelines describe a framework for classification of patients into groups at high, intermediate, and low risk for complications on the basis of early clinical data (Table 49G–1). (Details of the components of the initial clinical evaluation and management of the patient with possible acute ischemic heart disease are given in Chapter 45.) Of note is the recommendation that a cardiac-specific troponin is the preferred biomarker of myocardial injury and that biomarkers of injury should be sampled within 6 hours and then again at 6 to 12 hours from the onset of symptoms (Table 49G–2). The guidelines considered evidence to be somewhat favorable (class IIa) for use of an early marker of cardiac injury such as myoglobin or creatine kinase muscle and brain (CK-MB) subforms in patients who present early after the onset of symptoms but were less encouraging of other tests.

The ACC/AHA guidelines recommend admission to hospital for patients with definite acute coronary syndromes and any of the following:

- Ongoing pain
- Positive cardiac markers
- New ST segment deviations
- New deep T wave inversions
- Hemodynamic abnormalities
- Positive stress test

For patients with possible acute coronary syndrome and negative cardiac markers, early stress testing is recommended; this testing can be performed on an outpatient basis for lower risk patients.

Hospital Care

The guidelines recommend that patients admitted for acute coronary syndromes with continuing discomfort or hemodynamic instability, or both, be hospitalized for at least 24 hours in a coronary care unit characterized by a nurse-to-patient ratio sufficient to provide continuous rhythm monitoring and rapid resuscitation and defibrillation should it be necessary. Patients who do not have continuing discomfort or hemodynamic instability can be admitted to a step-down unit.

When a patient with high-risk acute coronary syndrome is admitted, treatment should be initiated with aspirin, a beta blocker, antithrombin therapy, and a glycoprotein IIb/IIIa inhibitor unless contraindications exist (Fig. 49G–1). Clinicians should choose between an early invasive strategy, including prompt angiography and revascularization if appropriate, and an early conservative strategy, in which patients are stabilized with medical therapy and angiography is performed if patients have recurrent symptoms or ischemia, heart failure, or serious arrhythmias. Patients managed according to the early conservative strategy should undergo an assessment of left ventricular function and a stress test; they should also undergo angiography if they are found to have an ejection fraction below 40 percent or if they have an intermediate- or high-risk exercise test.

TABLE 49G–1 American College of Cardiology/American Heart Association System for Risk Stratification of Patients with Unstable Angina

Feature	High Risk *At Least One of the Following Features*	Intermediate Risk *No High-Risk Feature but Must Have One of the Following*	Low Risk *No High- or Intermediate-Risk Feature but May Have Any of the Following Features*
History	Accelerating tempo of ischemic symptoms in preceding 48 hr	Prior MI, peripheral or cerebrovascular disease, or CABG, prior aspirin use	
Character of pain	Prolonged ongoing (>20 min) rest pain	Prolonged rest angina, now resolved, with moderate or high likelihood of CAD Rest angina <20 min or relieved with rest or sublingual NTG	New-onset or progressive CCS Class III or IV angina the past 2 wk without prolonged rest pain but with moderate or high likelihood of CAD
Clinical findings	Pulmonary edema, most likely due to ischemia New or worsening MR murmur S_3 or new worsening rales Hypotension, bradycardia, tachycardia Age >75 yr	Age >70 yr	
ECG	Angina at rest with transient ST segment changes >0.05 mV Bundle branch block, new or presumed new Sustained ventricular tachycardia	T wave inversions >0.2 mV Pathological Q waves	Normal or unchanged ECG during an episode of chest discomfort
Cardiac markers	Elevated	Slightly elevated	Normal

CABG = coronary artery bypass graft; CAD = coronary artery disease; CCS = Canadian Cardiovascular Society; ECG = electrocardiogram; MI = myocardial infarction; MR = mitral regurgitation; NTG = nitroglycerin.

TABLE 49G–2 American College of Cardiology/American Heart Association Guidelines for Data Collection for Early Risk Stratification

Class	Indication	Level of Evidence
Class I (indicated)	A determination should be made in all patients with chest discomfort of the likelihood of acute ischemia caused by CAD as high, intermediate, or low.	C
	Patients who present with chest discomfort should undergo early risk stratification that focuses on anginal symptoms, physical findings, ECG findings, and biomarkers of cardiac injury.	B
	A 12-lead ECG should be obtained immediately (within 10 min) in patients with ongoing chest discomfort and as rapidly as possible in patients who have a history of chest discomfort consistent with ACS but whose discomfort has resolved by the time of evaluation.	C
	Biomarkers of cardiac injury should be measured in all patients who present with chest discomfort consistent with ACS. A cardiac-specific troponin is the preferred marker, and, if available, it should be measured in patients with negative cardiac markers within 6 hr of the onset of pain; another sample should be drawn in the 6- to 12-hr time frame (e.g., at 9 hr after the onset of symptoms).	C
Class IIa (good supportive evidence)	For patients who present within 6 hr of the onset of symptoms, an early marker of cardiac injury (e.g., myoglobin or CK-MB subforms) should be considered in addition to a cardiac troponin.	C
Class IIb (weak supportive evidence)	C-reactive protein (CRP) and other markers of inflammation should be measured.	B
Class III (not indicated)	Total CK (without MB), aspartate aminotransferase (AST, SGOT), beta-hydroxybutyric dehydrogenase, and/or lactate dehydrogenase should be the markers for the detection of myocardial injury in patients with chest discomfort suggestive of ACS.	C

ACS = acute coronary syndrome; AST = aspartate aminotransferase; CAD = coronary artery disease; CK-MB = creatine kinase muscle and brain fraction; ECG = electrocardiogram; SGOT = serum glutamic-oxaloacetic transaminase.

Patients admitted with acute coronary syndromes should be placed at bed rest with electrocardiographic monitoring (Table 49G–3). Supplemental oxygen is not recommended for routine use by the guidelines because of lack of evidence for benefit; instead, it should be used when patients have cyanosis or respiratory distress. Medical therapy should include nitrates and, in the absence of contraindications, beta blockers. If contraindications to beta blockers exist, patients with recurrent ischemia can be treated with a nondihydropyridine calcium antagonist (e.g., verapamil or diltiazem). Morphine sulfate should be used for patients whose condition is not controlled with nitrates or when patients have pulmonary congestion or severe agitation, or both. An angiotensin-converting enzyme (ACE) inhibitor should be started if hypertension persists despite antiischemic therapy or if patients have left ventricular systolic dysfunction or diabetes. The guidelines consider use of immediate-release dihydropyridine calcium antagonists in the absence of a beta blocker inappropriate (class III).

Recommendations for use of antithrombotic therapy were revised considerably to reflect more recent research in the 2002 update to the guidelines, leading to an expanded role for clopidogrel and more complex tactics for use of platelet glycoprotein IIb/IIIa inhibitors.[2] Aspirin continues to be recommended for initial therapy, but the 2002 guidelines describe class I indications for clopidogrel for patients who are unable to take aspirin, for patients in whom an early noninterventional approach is planned, and for patients in whom percutaneous coronary intervention (PCI) is planned (Table 49G–4). Clopidogrel should be withheld for 5 to 7 days before elective coronary artery bypass graft (CABG) surgery. The guidelines also recommend anticoagulation with low-molecular-weight or unfractionated heparin in addition to antiplatelet therapy.

Glycoprotein IIb/IIIa inhibitors are considered in the 2002 guidelines to be clearly indicated (class I) when PCI is planned for patients receiving aspirin and heparin. If such patients are already receiving heparin, aspirin, *and clopidogrel,* the ACC/AHA task force considered evidence less conclusive but still generally supportive for addition of a glycoprotein IIb/IIIa inhibitor (class IIa indication) (see Table 49G–4). These agents also received some support for use in high-risk subsets of patients with acute coronary syndromes even if an invasive strategy is not planned (Class IIa), but the task force thought evidence was generally not favorable for their use in patients without continuing ischemia or other high-risk features. Abciximab was considered inappropriate in patients for whom PCI is not planned.

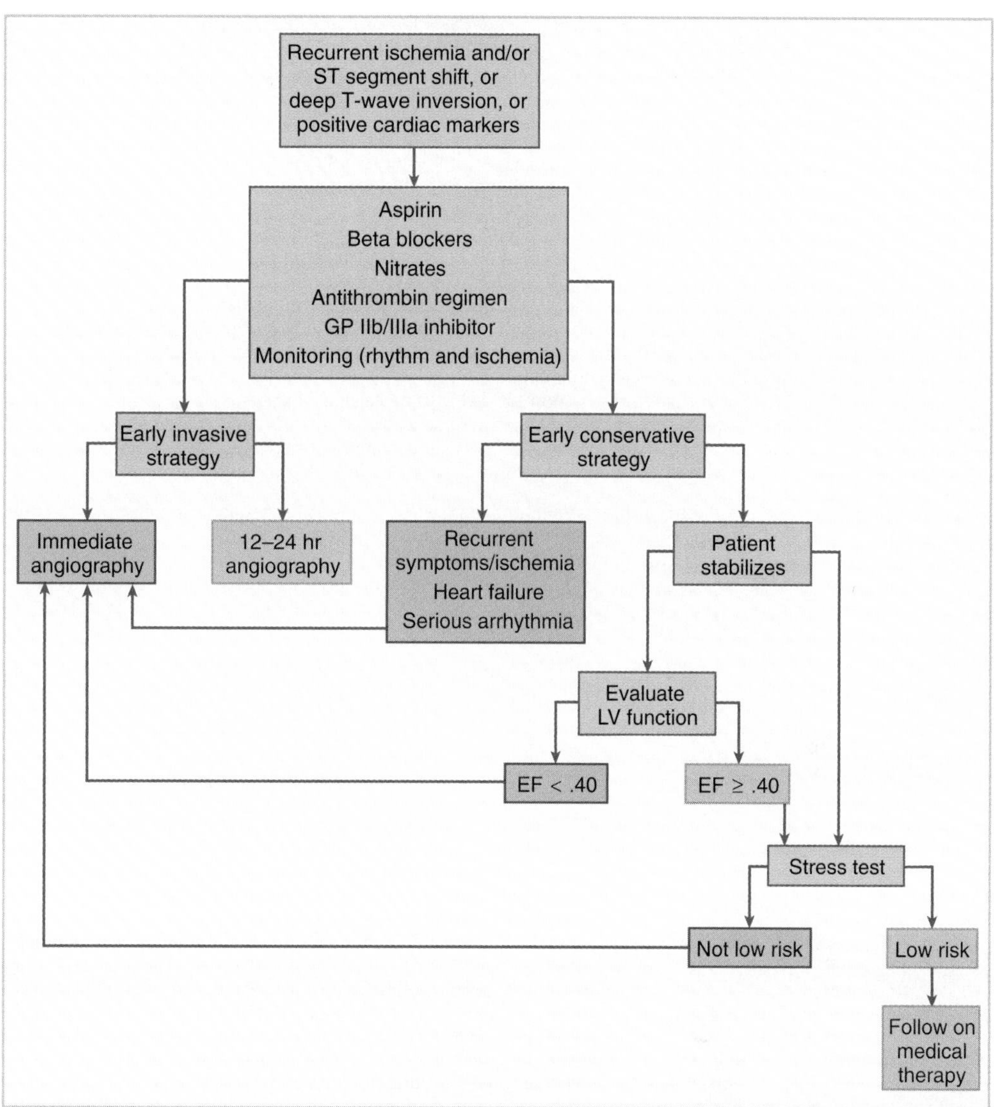

FIGURE 49G–1 Acute ischemia pathway. EF = ejection fraction; GP = glycoprotein. (From Braunwald E, Antman EM, Beasley JW, et al: ACC/AHA 2002 guideline update for the management of patients with unstable angina and non-ST-segment elevation myocardial infarction: Summary article: A report of the American College of Cardiology/American Heart Association Task Force on Practice Guidelines (Committee on the Management of Patients with Unstable Angina). J Am Coll Cardiol 36:970, 2000.

Later Risk Stratification and Management

The ACC/AHA guidelines support early stress testing in low-risk patients (see Table 49G–1 for risk category definition); for intermediate-risk patients, stress testing can be performed after they have been free of ischemia and heart failure for a minimum of 2 to 3 days (Table 49G–5). The first choice in noninvasive tests is exercise electrocardiography; imaging technologies and pharmacological stress tests should be used for subsets of patients for whom exercise electrocardiography would be expected to have a high likelihood of providing inadequate data. Data from noninvasive tests can be used to stratify patients into high-, intermediate-, and low-risk groups (Table 49G–6). The guidelines endorse prompt angiography without noninvasive risk stratification for patients who are not readily stabilized by intensive medical therapy.

The guidelines recommend an early invasive strategy for patients with acute coronary syndromes and high-risk indicators from their clinical data or noninvasive testing (Table 49G–7). In the absence of such high-risk indicators, the guidelines consider either an early conservative or early invasive strategy to be reasonable. The guidelines also provided some support for use of an early invasive strategy in patients with repeated episodes of suspected acute coronary syndrome without clear evidence for ischemia.

For patients who require coronary revascularization, the principles for choosing between CABG and PCI are similar to those used for patients with chronic stable angina. The guidelines recommend CABG over PCI for patients with significant left main coronary artery disease and for patients with multivessel disease and diminished ejection fraction or diabetes (Tables 49G–8 and 49G–9). CABG and PCI were both considered appropriate for patients with one- or two-vessel disease without proximal left anterior descending (LAD) coronary artery disease but who had large areas of myocardium in jeopardy (see Table 49G–9). The guidelines provided some support for revascularization with either CABG or PCI for patients with proximal LAD disease alone (class IIa) but did not recommend revascularization for patients without proximal LAD disease or those who had only small amounts of ischemia detected by noninvasive testing.

TABLE 49G–3 American College of Cardiology/American Heart Association Recommendations for Antiischemic Therapy

Class	Indication	Level of Evidence
Class I (indicated)	Bed rest with continuous ECG monitoring for ischemia and arrhythmia detection in patients with ongoing rest pain.	C
	NTG, sublingual tablet or spray, followed by intravenous administration, for the immediate relief of ischemia and associated symptoms.	C
	Supplemental oxygen for patients with cyanosis or respiratory distress; finger pulse oximetry or arterial blood gas determination to confirm adequate arterial oxygen saturation (SaO_2 greater than 90%) and continued need for supplemental oxygen in the presence of hypoxemia.	C
	Morphine sulfate intravenously when symptoms are not immediately relieved with NTG or when acute pulmonary congestion and/or severe agitation is present.	C
	A beta blocker, with the first dose administered intravenously if there is ongoing chest pain, followed by oral administration, in the absence of contraindications.	B
	In patients with continuing or frequently recurring ischemia when beta blockers are contraindicated, a nondihydropyridine calcium antagonist (e.g., verapamil or diltiazem) as initial therapy in the absence of severe LV dysfunction or other contraindications.	B
	An ACEI when hypertension persists despite treatment with NTG and a beta blocker in patients with LV systolic dysfunction or CHF and in ACS patients with diabetes.	B
Class IIa (good supportive evidence)	Oral long-acting calcium antagonists for recurrent ischemia in the absence of contraindications and when beta blockers and nitrates are fully used.	C
	An ACEI for all post-ACS patients.	B
	Intraaortic balloon pump (IABP) counterpulsation for severe ischemia that is continuing or recurs frequently despite intensive medical therapy or for hemodynamic instability in patients before or after coronary angiography.	C
Class IIb (weak supportive evidence)	Extended-release form of nondihydropyridine calcium antagonists instead of a beta blocker.	B
	Immediate-release dihydropyridine calcium antagonists in the presence of a beta blocker.	B
Class III (not indicated)	NTG or other nitrate within 24 hr of sildenafil (Viagra) use.	C
	Immediate-release dihydropyridine calcium antagonists in the absence of a beta blocker.	A

ACEI = angiotensin-converting enzyme inhibitor; ACS = acute coronary syndrome; CHF = congestive heart failure; ECG = electrocardiographic, LV = left ventricular; NTG = nitroglycerin; SaO_2 = oxygen saturation in arterial blood.

TABLE 49G–4 American College of Cardiology/American Heart Association Guidelines for Antiplatelet and Anticoagulation Therapy

Class	Indication	Level of Evidence
Class I (indicated)	Antiplatelet therapy should be initiated promptly. ASA should be administered as soon as possible after presentation and continued indefinitely.	A
	Clopidogrel should be administered to hospitalized patients who are unable to take ASA because of hypersensitivity or major gastrointestinal intolerance.	A
	In hospitalized patients in whom an early noninterventional approach is planned, clopidogrel should be added to ASA as soon as possible on admission and administered for at least 1 mo and for up to 9 mo.	B
	In patients for whom a PCI is planned, clopidogrel should be started and continued for at least 1 mo and up to 9 mo in patients who are not at high risk for bleeding.	B
	In patients taking clopidogrel in whom elective CABG is planned, the drug should be withheld for 5 to 7 d.	B
	Anticoagulation with subcutaneous LMWH or intravenous UFH should be added to antiplatelet therapy with ASA and/or clopidogrel.	A
	A platelet GP IIb/IIIa antagonist should be administered, in addition to ASA and heparin, to patients in whom catheterization and PCI are planned. The GP IIb/IIIa antagonist may also be administered just prior to PCI.	A
Class IIa (good supportive evidence)	Eptifibatide or tirofiban should be administered, in addition to ASA and LMWH or UFH, to patients *with* continuing ischemia, elevated troponin, or other high-risk features in whom an invasive management strategy is *not* planned.	A
	Enoxaparin is preferable to UFH as an anticoagulant in patients with UA/NSTEMI, unless CABG is planned within 24 hr.	A
	A platelet GP IIb/IIIa antagonist should be administered to patients already receiving heparin, ASA, *and clopidogrel* in whom catheterization and PCI are planned. The GP IIb/IIIa antagonist may also be administered just prior to PCI.	B
Class IIb (weak supportive evidence)	Eptifibatide or tirofiban, in addition to ASA and LMWH or UFH, to patients *without* continuing ischemia who have no other high-risk features and in whom PCI is *not* planned.	A
Class III (not indicated)	Intravenous fibrinolytic therapy in patients without acute ST segment elevation, a true posterior MI, or a presumed new left bundle branch block.	A
	Abciximab administration in patients in whom PCI is not planned.	A

ASA = acetylsalicylic acid (aspirin); CABG = coronary artery bypass graft; GP = glycoprotein; LMWH = low-molecular-weight heparin; MI = myocardial infarction; PCI = percutaneous coronary intervention; UA/NSTEMI = unstable angina or non-ST elevation myocardial infarction; UFH = unfractionated heparin.

TABLE 49G–5 American College of Cardiology/American Heart Association Guidelines for Risk Stratification in Patients with Acute Coronary Syndromes

Class	Indication	Level of Evidence
Class I (indicated)	Noninvasive stress testing in low-risk patients (see Table 49G–1) who have been free of ischemia at rest or with low-level activity and of CHF for a minimum of 12 to 24 hr.	C
	Noninvasive stress testing in patients at intermediate risk who have been free of ischemia at rest or with low-level activity and of CHF for a minimum of 2 or 3 d.	C
	Choice of stress test is based on the resting ECG, ability to perform exercise, local expertise, and technologies available. Treadmill exercise is suitable in patients able to exercise in whom the ECG is free of baseline ST segment abnormalities, bundle branch block, LV hypertrophy, intraventricular conduction defect, paced rhythm, preexcitation, and digoxin effect.	C
	An imaging modality is added in patients with resting ST segment depression (greater than or equal to 0.10 mV), LV hypertrophy, bundle branch block, intraventricular conduction defect, preexcitation, or digoxin who are able to exercise. In patients undergoing a low-level exercise test, imaging modality may add sensitivity.	B
	Pharmacological stress testing with imaging when physical limitations (e.g., arthritis, amputation, severe peripheral vascular disease, severe COPD, general debility) preclude adequate exercise stress.	B
	Prompt angiography without noninvasive risk stratification for failure of stabilization with intensive medical treatment.	B
Class IIa (good supportive evidence)	A noninvasive test (echocardiogram or radionuclide angiogram) to evaluate LV function in patients with definite ACS who are not scheduled for coronary arteriography and left ventriculography.	C
Class IIb (weak supportive evidence)	None	
Class III (not indicated)	None	

ACS = acute coronary syndrome; CHF = congestive heart failure; COPD = chronic obstructive pulmonary disease; ECG = electrocardiogram; LV = left ventricular.

TABLE 49G–6 American College of Cardiology/American Heart Association Noninvasive Risk Stratification

High Risk (>3% Annual Mortality Rate)

1. Severe resting LV dysfunction (LVEF <0.35)
2. High-risk treadmill score (score ≤–11)
3. Severe exercise LV dysfunction (exercise LVEF <0.35)
4. Stress-induced large perfusion defect (particularly if anterior)
5. Stress-induced multiple perfusion defects of moderate size
6. Large, fixed perfusion defect with LV dilation or increased lung uptake (thallium-201)
7. Stress-induced moderate perfusion defect with LV dilation or increased lung uptake (thallium-201)
8. Echocardiographic wall motion abnormality (involving > two segments) developing at a low dose of dobutamine (≤10 mg/kg/min) or at a low heart rate (<120 beats/min)
9. Stress echocardiographic evidence of extensive ischemia

Intermediate Risk (1–3% Annual Mortality Rate)

1. Mild/moderate resting LV dysfunction (LVEF 0.35–0.49)
2. Intermediate-risk treadmill score (–11 < score <5)
3. Stress-induced moderate perfusion defect without LV dilation or increased lung intake (thallium-201)
4. Limited stress echocardiographic ischemia with a wall motion abnormality only at higher doses of dobutamine involving ≤ two segments

Low Risk (<1% Annual Mortality Rate)

1. Low-risk treadmill score (score ≥5)
2. Normal or small myocardial perfusion defect at rest or with stress
3. Normal stress echocardiographic wall motion or no change of limited resting wall motion abnormalities during stress

LV = left ventricular; LVEF = left ventricular ejection fraction.

From Table 23 in Gibbons RJ, Chatterjee K, Daley J, et al: ACC/AHA/ACP-ASIM guidelines for the management of patients with chronic stable angina. J Am Coll Cardiol 33:2092, 1999.

TABLE 49G–7 American College of Cardiology/American Heart Association Guidelines for Early Conservative Versus Invasive Strategies

Class	Indication	Level of Evidence
Class I (indicated)	An early invasive strategy in patients with UA/NSTEMI and any of the following high-risk indicators: Recurrent angina or ischemia at rest or with low-level activities despite intensive antiischemic therapy Elevated TnT or TnI New or presumably new ST segment depression Recurrent angina or ischemia with CHF symptoms, an S_3 gallop, pulmonary edema, worsening rales, or new or worsening MR High-risk findings on noninvasive stress testing Depressed LV systolic function (e.g., EF less than 0.40 on noninvasive study) Hemodynamic instability Sustained ventricular tachycardia PCI within 6 mo Prior CABG	A
	In the absence of these findings, either an early conservative or an early invasive strategy in hospitalized patients without contraindications for revascularization.	B
Class IIa (good supportive evidence	An early invasive strategy in patients with repeated presentations for ACS despite therapy and without evidence for ongoing ischemia or high risk.	C
Class IIb (weak supportive evidence)		
Class III (not indicated)	Coronary angiography in patients with extensive comorbidities (e.g., liver or pulmonary failure, cancer) in whom the risks of revascularization are not likely to outweigh the benefits.	C
	Coronary angiography in patients with acute chest pain and a low likelihood of ACS.	C
	Coronary angiography in patients who do not consent to revascularization regardless of the findings.	C

ACS = acute coronary syndrome; CABG = coronary artery bypass graft; CHF = congestive heart failure; EF = ejection fraction; LV = left ventricular; MR = mitral regurgitation; PCI = percutaneous coronary intervention; TnI = troponin I; TnT = troponin T; UA/NSTEMI = unstable angina or non-ST elevation myocardial infarction.

TABLE 49G–8 American College of Cardiology/American Heart Association Guidelines for Revascularization with Percutaneous Coronary Intervention and Coronary Artery Bypass Graft in Patients with Unstable Angina or Non-ST Elevation Myocardial Infarction

Class	Indication	Level of Evidence
Class I (indicated)	CABG for patients with significant left main CAD.	A
	CABG for patients with three-vessel disease; the survival benefit is greater in patients with abnormal LV function (EF less than 0.50).	A
	CABG for patients with two-vessel disease with significant proximal left anterior descending CAD and either abnormal LV function (EF less than 0.50) or demonstrable ischemia on noninvasive testing.	A
	PCI or CABG for patients with one- or two-vessel CAD without significant proximal left anterior descending CAD but with a large area of viable myocardium and high-risk criteria on noninvasive testing.	B
	PCI for patients with multivessel coronary disease with suitable coronary anatomy, with normal LV function and without diabetes.	A
	Intravenous platelet GP IIb/IIIa inhibitor in patients with UA/NSTEMI undergoing PCI.	A
Class IIa (good supportive evidence)	Repeat CABG for patients with multiple saphenous vein graft (SVG) stenoses, especially when there is significant stenosis of a graft that supplies the LAD.	C
	PCI for focal SVG lesions or multiple stenoses in poor candidates for reoperative surgery.	C
	PCI or CABG for patients with one- or two-vessel CAD without significant proximal left anterior descending CAD but with a moderate area of viable myocardium and ischemia on noninvasive testing.	B
	PCI or CABG for patients with one-vessel disease with significant proximal left anterior descending CAD.	B
	CABG with the internal mammary artery for patients with multivessel disease and treated diabetes mellitus.	B
Class IIb (weak supportive evidence)	PCI for patients with two- or three-vessel disease with significant proximal left anterior descending CAD, with treated diabetes or abnormal LV function, and with anatomy suitable for catheter-based therapy.	B
Class III (not indicated)	PCI or CABG for patients with one- or two-vessel CAD without significant proximal left anterior descending CAD or with mild symptoms or symptoms that are unlikely to be due to myocardial ischemia or who have not received an adequate trial of medical therapy and who have no demonstrable ischemia on noninvasive testing.	C
	PCI or CABG for patients with insignificant coronary stenosis (less than 50% diameter).	C
	PCI in patients with significant left main coronary artery disease who are candidates for CABG.	B

CABG = coronary artery bypass graft; CAD = coronary artery disease; EF = ejection fraction; GP = glycoprotein; LAD = left anterior descending; LV = left ventricular; PCI = percutaneous coronary intervention; UA/NSTEMI = unstable angina or non-ST elevation myocardial infarction.

TABLE 49G–9 American College of Cardiology/American Heart Association Guidelines for Mode of Coronary Revascularization for Unstable Angina or Non-ST Elevation Myocardial Infarction

Extent of Disease	Treatment	Appropriateness Class	Level of Evidence
Left main disease (≥50% stenosis), candidate for CABG	CABG PCI	I III	A C
Left main disease, not candidate for CABG	PCI	IIb	C
Three-vessel disease with EF<0.50	CABG	I	A
Multivessel disease including proximal LAD with EF<0.50 or treated diabetes	CABG PCI	I IIb	A B
Multivessel disease with EF>0.50 and without diabetes	PCI	I	A
One- or two-vessel disease without proximal LAD but with large areas of myocardial ischemia or high-risk criteria on noninvasive testing	CABG or PCI	I	B
One-vessel disease with proximal LAD	CABG or PCI	IIa	B
One- or two-vessel disease without proximal LAD with small area of ischemia or no ischemia on noninvasive testing	CABG or PCI	III*	C
Insignificant coronary stenosis	CABG	CABG or PCI	IIIC

*Class = I if severe angina persists despite medical therapy.
CABG = coronary artery bypass graft; EF = ejection fraction; LAD = left anterior descending; PCI = percutaneous coronary intervention.

Hospital Discharge and Post-Hospital Discharge Care

The ACC/AHA guidelines emphasize the importance of aggressive risk factor modification and teaching of patients about management of ischemic episodes. Class I indications for pharmacological therapy include:

Aspirin 75 to 325 mg/d in the absence of contraindications
Clopidogrel 75 mg/d in the absence of contraindications when aspirin is not tolerated
The combination of aspirin and clopidogrel for 9 months after UA/NSTEMI
Beta blockers in the absence of contraindications
Lipid-lowering agents and diet with low-density lipoprotein (LDL) cholesterol greater than 130 mg/dl
Lipid-lowering agents if the LDL cholesterol level after diet is greater than 100 mg/dl
ACE inhibitors for patients with heart failure, left ventricular dysfunction, hypertension, or diabetes

Special Groups

The guidelines indicate that women with acute coronary syndromes should be managed according to the same principles as men, using the same indications for noninvasive tests and treatments. For elderly patients, the guidelines recommend that physicians weigh the patients' overall health, comorbidities, cognitive status, and life expectancy as choices are made regarding aggressiveness of management.

For patients with diabetes, the guidelines recommend CABG with internal mammary artery grafts over PCI for diabetic patients with multivessel disease who require revascularization; otherwise, management decisions should be similar to those made for nondiabetics. The task force noted that the use of stents, particularly with abciximab, may provide more favorable results in diabetics but that further data are needed before this approach can be routinely recommended.

For patients with acute coronary syndromes who have previously undergone CABG, the guidelines recommend a lower threshold for angiography because of the many potential causes of ischemia. The guidelines support use of imaging with stress testing in patients who have previously had CABG (class IIa indication).

Calcium antagonists and nitrates are recommended for patients with chest pain after cocaine use and for patients with clinical syndromes consistent with coronary spasm. In patients who have used cocaine, coronary angiography is recommended for patients whose ST segments remain elevated after such medical treatment.

References

1. Braunwald E, Antman EM, Beasley JW, et al: ACC/AHA guidelines for the management of patients with unstable angina and non-ST-segment elevation myocardial infarction: A report of the American College of Cardiology/American Heart Association Task Force on Practice Guidelines (Committee on the Management of Patients with Unstable Angina). J Am Coll Cardiol 36:970, 2000.
2. Braunwald E, Antman EM, Beasley JW, et al: ACC/AHA 2002 guideline update for the management of patients with unstable angina and non-ST-segment elevation myocardial infarction: Summary article: A report of the American College of Cardiology/American Heart Association Task Force on Practice Guidelines (Committee on the Management of Patients with Unstable Angina). Circulation 106:1893, 2002.
3. Smith SC Jr, Dove JT, Jacobs AK, et al: ACC/AHA guidelines for percutaneous coronary intervention: A report of the American College of Cardiology/American Heart Association Task Force on Practice Guidelines (Committee to Revise the 1993 Guidelines for Percutaneous Transluminal Coronary Angioplasty). J Am Coll Cardiol 37:2239i, 2001.

CHAPTER 50

Chronic Coronary Artery Disease

David A. Morrow • Bernard J. Gersh • Eugene Braunwald

Chronic coronary artery disease (CAD) is most commonly due to obstruction of the coronary arteries by atheromatous plaque (the pathogenesis of atherosclerosis is described in Chap. 35).[1] Factors that predispose to this condition are discussed in Chapter 36, the control of coronary blood flow in Chapter 44, acute myocardial infarction in Chapter 46, and unstable angina in Chapter 49; sudden cardiac death, another significant consequence of CAD, is presented in Chapter 33.

No uniform syndrome of signs and symptoms is initially seen in patients with CAD. Chest discomfort is usually the predominant symptom in chronic (stable) angina, unstable angina, Prinzmetal (variant) angina (see Chap. 49), microvascular angina, and acute myocardial infarction. However, syndromes of CAD also occur in which ischemic chest discomfort is absent or not prominent, such as asymptomatic (silent) myocardial ischemia, congestive heart failure, cardiac arrhythmias, and sudden death. Obstructive CAD also has many nonatherosclerotic causes, including congenital abnormalities of the coronary artery, myocardial bridging, coronary arteritis in association with the systemic vasculitides, and radiation-induced coronary disease.[2] Myocardial ischemia and angina pectoris may also occur in the *absence* of obstructive CAD, as in the case of aortic valve disease (see Chap. 57), hypertrophic cardiomyopathy, and idiopathic dilated cardiomyopathy (see Chap. 59). Moreover, CAD may coexist with these other forms of heart disease.

The Magnitude of the Problem

The importance of CAD in contemporary society is attested to by the almost epidemic number of persons afflicted (see Chap. 1). It is estimated that 13,200,000 Americans have CAD, 6,800,00 of whom have angina pectoris and 7,800,000 have had myocardial infarction.[3] Based on data from the Framingham Heart Study, the lifetime risk of developing symptomatic CAD after age 40 is 49 percent for men and 32 percent for women.[3] In 2001, CAD accounted for 54 percent of all deaths due to cardiovascular disease and was the single most frequent cause of death in American men and women, resulting in more than 1 in 5 of deaths in the United States.[3] The economic cost of CAD in the United States in 2003 is estimated at $133.2 billion.[3] Ischemic heart disease is now the leading cause of death worldwide,[4] and it is expected that the rate of CAD will only accelerate in the next decade, contributed to by aging of the population, alarming increases in the worldwide prevalence of obesity, type 2 diabetes, and the metabolic syndrome, as well as a rise in cardiovascular risk factors among younger generations.[5] The World Health Organization estimates that by 2020 the global number of deaths from CAD will have risen from 7.1 in 2002 to 11.1 million.[6]

Stable Angina Pectoris

Clinical Manifestations

CHARACTERISTICS OF ANGINA (see Chap. 7). Angina pectoris is a discomfort in the chest or adjacent areas caused by myocardial ischemia. It is usually brought on by exertion and is associated with a disturbance in myocardial function, but without myocardial necrosis. Heberden's initial description of the chest discomfort as conveying a sense of "strangling and anxiety" is still remarkably pertinent, although adjectives frequently used to describe this distress include "viselike," "constricting," "suffocating," "crushing," "heavy," and "squeezing." In other patients, the quality of the sensation is more vague and described as a mild pressure-like discomfort, an uncomfortable numb sensation, or a burning sensation. The site of the discomfort is usually retrosternal, but radiation is common and usually occurs down the ulnar surface of the left arm; the right arm and the outer surfaces of both arms may also be involved (see Fig. 7–2). Epigastric discomfort alone or in association with chest pressure is not uncommon. Anginal discomfort above the mandible or below the epigastrium is rare. Anginal "equivalents" (i.e., symptoms of myocardial ischemia other than angina), such as dyspnea, faintness, fatigue, and eructations, are common, particularly in the elderly.[7] A history of abnormal exertional dyspnea may be an early indicator of CAD even when angina is absent or no electrocardiographic (ECG) evidence of ischemic heart disease can be found. Dyspnea at rest or with exertion may be a manifestation of severe ischemia, leading to increases in left ventricular filling pressure. Nocturnal angina should raise the suspicion of sleep apnea.

The typical episode of angina pectoris usually begins gradually and reaches its maximum intensity over a period of minutes before dissipating. It is unusual for angina pectoris to reach its maximum severity within seconds, and it is characteristic that patients with angina usually prefer to rest, sit, or stop walking during episodes.

Chest discomfort while walking in the cold, uphill, or after a meal is suggestive of angina. Features suggesting the *absence* of angina pectoris include pleuritic pain, pain localized to the tip of one finger, pain reproduced by movement or palpation of the chest wall or arms, and constant pain lasting many hours or, alternatively, very brief episodes of pain lasting seconds. Pain radiating into the lower extremities is also a highly unusual manifestation of angina pectoris.

Typical angina pectoris is relieved within minutes by rest or by the use of nitroglycerin. The response to the latter is often a useful diagnostic tool, although it should be remembered that esophageal pain and other syndromes may also respond to nitroglycerin. A delay of more than 5 to 10 minutes before relief is obtained by rest and nitroglycerin suggests that the symptoms are either not due to ischemia or, alternatively, are due to severe ischemia, as with acute myocardial infarction or unstable angina. The phenomenon of "first-effort" or "warm-up" angina is used to describe the ability of some patients in whom angina develops with exertion to subsequently continue at the same or even greater level of exertion without symptoms after an intervening period of rest. This attenuation of myocardial ischemia observed with repeated exertion has been postulated to be due to ischemic preconditioning[8] and may require preceding ischemia of at least moderate intensity to induce the warm-up phenomenon.[9]

GRADING OF ANGINA PECTORIS. A system of grading the severity of angina pectoris proposed by the Canadian Cardiovascular Society has gained widespread acceptance (see Table 7–7).[10] The system is a modification of the New York Heart Association (NYHA) functional classification but allows patients to be categorized in more specific terms. Other grading systems include a specific activity scale developed by Goldman and associates[11] and an anginal "score" developed by Califf and colleagues.[12] The Goldman scale is based on the metabolic cost of specific activities and appears to be valid when used by both physicians and nonphysicians. The anginal score of Califf and coworkers integrates the clinical features and "tempo" of angina together with ECG ST and T wave changes and offers independent prognostic information above that provided by age, gender, left ventricular function, and coronary angiographic anatomy. A limitation of all of these grading systems is their dependence on accurate patient observation and patients' widely varying tolerance for symptoms. Functional estimates based on the Canadian Cardiovascular Society criteria showed a reproducibility of only 73 percent and still did not correlate well with objective measures of exercise performance.[11]

MECHANISMS. The mechanisms of cardiac pain and the neural pathways involved are poorly understood.[1] It is presumed that angina pectoris results from ischemic episodes that excite chemosensitive and mechanoreceptive receptors in the heart. Stimulation of these receptors results in the release of adenosine, bradykinin, and other substances that excite the sensory ends of the sympathetic and vagal afferent fibers. The afferent fibers traverse the nerves that connect to the upper five thoracic sympathetic ganglia and upper five distal thoracic roots of the spinal cord. Impulses are transmitted by the spinal cord to the thalamus and hence to the neocortex. Within the spinal cord, cardiac sympathetic afferent impulses may converge with impulses from somatic thoracic structures, which may be the basis for referred cardiac pain, for example, to the chest. In comparison, cardiac vagal afferent fibers synapse in the nucleus tractus solitarius of the medulla and then descend to excite the upper cervical spinothalamic tract cells, which may contribute to the anginal pain experienced in the neck and jaw.[13] Positron-emission tomographic (PET) imaging of the brain in subjects with silent ischemia suggests that failed transmission of signals from the thalamus to the frontal cortex may contribute to this phenomenon, along with impaired afferent signaling, such as that due to autonomic neuropathy.[14]

Differential Diagnosis of Chest Pain (see Table 7–3 and Fig. 7–2)

ESOPHAGEAL DISORDERS. Common disorders that may simulate or coexist with angina pectoris are gastroesophageal reflux and disorders of esophageal motility, including diffuse spasm as well as "nutcracker" esophagus, which is characterized by high-amplitude peristaltic contractions and vigorous achalasia. To compound the difficulty in distinguishing between angina and esophageal pain, both may be relieved by nitroglycerin. However, esophageal pain is often relieved by milk, antacids, foods, or, occasionally, warm liquids.

ESOPHAGEAL MOTILITY DISORDERS. Esophageal motility disorders are not uncommon in patients with retrosternal chest pain of unclear cause and should be specifically excluded or confirmed, if possible. In addition to chest pain, most such patients have dysphagia. Although barium studies may reveal motility problems, esophageal manometry may show diffuse esophageal spasm, increased pressure at the lower esophageal sphincter, and other motility disorders. Provocative pharmacological agents such as methacholine may provoke esophageal pain and manometric signs of spasm.

Both CAD and esophageal disease are common clinical entities that may coexist. Diagnostic evaluation for an esophageal disorder may be indicated in patients with CAD who have a poor symptomatic response to antianginal therapy in the absence of documentation of severe ischemia or in patients with persistent symptoms despite adequate coronary revascularization.

BILIARY COLIC. Although visceral symptoms are a common association of myocardial ischemia (particularly acute inferior myocardial infarction [see Chap. 46]), cholecystitis and related hepatobiliary disorders may also mimic ischemia and should always be considered in patients with atypical chest discomfort, particularly those with diabetes. The pain is steady, usually lasts 2 to 4 hours, and subsides spontaneously without any symptoms between attacks. It is generally most intense in the right upper abdominal area but may also be felt in the epigastrium or precordium. This discomfort is often referred to the scapula, may radiate around the costal margin to the back, or may in rare cases be felt in the shoulder and suggest diaphragmatic irritation. Ultrasonography is accurate in diagnosing gallstones and allows determination of gallbladder size and thickness and whether the bile ducts are dilated.

COSTOSTERNAL SYNDROME. In 1921, Tietze first described a syndrome of local pain and tenderness, usually limited to the anterior chest wall and associated with swelling of costal cartilage. This condition causes pain that can resemble angina pectoris. The full-blown Tietze syndrome (i.e., pain associated with tender *swelling* of the costochondral junctions) is uncommon, whereas costochondritis causing tenderness of the costochondral junctions (without swelling) is relatively common. Pain on palpation of these joints is a useful clinical sign. Local pressure should be applied routinely to the anterior chest wall during examination of a patient with suspected angina pectoris. In addition, costochondritis is usually well localized. Although palpation of the chest wall often reproduces pain in patients with various musculoskeletal conditions, it should be appreciated that chest wall tenderness may also be associated with and does not exclude symptomatic CAD.[15]

OTHER MUSCULOSKELETAL DISORDERS. Cervical radiculitis may be confused with angina. This condition may occur as a constant ache, sometimes resulting in a sensory deficit. The pain may be related to motion of the neck, just as motion of the shoulder triggers attacks of pain from bursitis. A hyperalgesic area noted by running the finger down the back and exerting pressure may lead to a suspicion of thoracic root pain. Occasionally, pain mimicking angina can be due to compression of the brachial plexus by the cervical ribs, and tendinitis or bursitis involving the left shoulder may also cause angina-like pain. Physical examination may also detect pain brought about by movement of an arthritic shoulder or a calcified shoulder tendon.

OTHER CAUSES OF ANGINA-LIKE PAIN. *Acute myocardial infarction* is usually associated with prolonged (>30 minutes), severe pain occurring at rest that, apart from duration and intensity, may be similar to angina pectoris. It is associated with characteristic ECG changes and the release of cardiac markers (see Chap. 46). Unstable angina is a severe form of angina that may also occur at rest and may not be relieved by nitroglycerin (see Chap. 49). The classic symptom of *aortic dissection* is a severe, often sharp pain that radiates to the back (see Chap. 53).

Severe pulmonary hypertension may be associated with exertional chest pain with the characteristics of angina pectoris, and indeed, this pain is thought to be due to right ventricular ischemia that develops during exertion (see Chap. 67). Other associated symptoms include exertional dyspnea, dizziness, and syncope. Associated findings on physical examination, such as parasternal lift, a palpable and loud pulmonary component of the second sound, and right ventricular hypertrophy on the ECG, are usually readily recognized.

Pulmonary embolism is initially characterized by dyspnea as the cardinal symptom, but chest pain may also be present (see Chap. 66). Pleuritic pain suggests pulmonary infarction, and a history of exacerbation of the pain with inspiration, along with a pleural friction rub, usually helps distinguish it from angina pectoris.

The pain of *acute pericarditis* (see Chap. 64) may at times be difficult to distinguish from angina pectoris. However, pericarditis tends to occur in younger patients than angina does, and the diagnosis depends on the combination of chest pain not relieved by rest or nitroglycerin; exacerbation by movement, deep breathing, and lying flat; a pericardial friction rub; and ECG changes.

Physical Examination

Many patients with chronic CAD present with normal physical findings. Nonetheless, careful examination may reveal the presence of risk factors for coronary atherosclerosis or the consequences of myocardial ischemia.

GENERAL EXAMINATION. Inspection of the eyes may reveal a *corneal arcus*, and examination of the skin may show xanthomas. Among patients with heterozygous familial hypercholesterolemia (in whom CAD is common), the presence of a corneal arcus increases with age and, in some studies, correlates positively with levels of cholesterol and low-density lipoprotein (LDL) as well as with the prognosis. *Xanthelasma*, in which lipid deposits are intracellular, appears to be promoted by increased levels of triglycerides and a relative deficiency of high-density lipoprotein (HDL). The presence of xanthelasma is a strong marker of dyslipidemia and, often, a family history of cardiovascular disease and should provide a strong impetus for performing a comprehensive lipid profile. Retinal arteriolar changes are common in patients with CAD and diabetes mellitus or hypertension.[16] A unilateral diagonal earlobe crease is often present in younger persons with CAD and becomes bilateral with advancing age.

Blood pressure may be chronically elevated or may rise acutely (along with the heart rate) during an angina attack. Changes in blood pressure may precede (and precipitate) or follow (and be caused by) angina.

The association between peripheral vascular disease and CAD is strong and well documented.[17] This association is not confined to patients with symptomatic or clinically overt peripheral vascular disease or CAD but is also seen in asymptomatic subjects with a reduced ankle-brachial blood pressure index or evidence of early carotid disease on ultrasonography. The presence of carotid and peripheral arterial disease on palpation and auscultation increases the likelihood that chest discomfort of unclear origin is caused by CAD.

CARDIAC EXAMINATION. The physical findings of hypertrophic cardiomyopathy (see Chap. 59) or aortic valve disease (Chap. 57) suggest that angina may be due to conditions other than (or in addition to) CAD. It is often helpful to examine the heart *during* an episode of pain because ischemia may produce transient left ventricular dysfunction with a third heart sound and pulmonary rales detectable on physical examination.[18] If massage of the carotid sinus produces pain relief, the pain is probably anginal. Paradoxical splitting of the second heart sound (see Chap. 8) may occur transiently during angina and appears to be related to asynergy and prolongation of left ventricular contraction, which results in delayed closure of the aortic valve. If other obvious cardiac diseases are absent, a third or loud fourth heart sound suggests ischemia as the basis for the chest pain. A displaced ventricular impulse, particularly if dyskinetic, is a sign of significant left ventricular systolic dysfunction.

Transient apical systolic murmurs are quite common in CAD and have been attributed to reversible papillary muscle dysfunction secondary to transient myocardial ischemia. These murmurs are more prevalent in patients with extensive CAD, especially those with prior myocardial infarction and left ventricular dysfunction, and may indicate an adverse prognosis. Systolic murmurs may assume a variety of configurations (early, late, or holosystolic) and may be accentuated by exertion or during angina. A midsystolic click, often followed by a late systolic murmur produced by mitral valve prolapse (see Chap. 57), also occurs in patients with CAD. A diastolic murmur or a continuous murmur is a rare finding in CAD and has been attributed to turbulent flow across a proximal coronary artery stenosis.

Pathophysiology

Angina pectoris results from myocardial ischemia, which is caused by an imbalance between myocardial O_2 requirements and myocardial O_2 supply.[1] The former may be elevated by increases in heart rate, left ventricular wall stress, and contractility (see Chap. 19); the latter is determined by coronary blood flow and coronary arterial O_2 content (Fig. 50–1).

ANGINA CAUSED BY INCREASED MYOCARDIAL O_2 REQUIREMENTS. In this condition, sometimes termed *demand angina*, the myocardial O_2 requirement increases in the face of a constant and usually restricted O_2 supply. The increased requirement commonly stems from norepinephrine release by adrenergic nerve endings in the heart and vascular bed, a physiological response to exertion, emotion, or mental stress. Of great importance to the myocardial O_2 requirement is the *rate* at which any task is carried out. Hurrying is particularly likely to precipitate angina, as are efforts involving motion of the hands over the head. Mental stress may also precipitate angina, presumably by increased hemodynamic and catecholamine responses to stress, increased adrenergic tone, and reduced vagal activity.[19,20] The combination of physical exertion and emotion in association with sexual activity commonly precipitates angina pectoris. Anger may produce constriction of coronary arteries with preexisting narrowing without necessarily affecting O_2 demand. Other precipitants of angina include physical exertion after a heavy meal and the excessive metabolic demands imposed by chills, fever, thyrotoxicosis, tachycardia from any cause, and hypoglycemia.

ANGINA CAUSED BY TRANSIENTLY DECREASED O_2 SUPPLY. Increasing evidence suggests that not only unstable angina but also chronic stable angina may be caused by transient reductions in O_2 supply as a consequence of coronary vasoconstriction,[21] a condition that is sometimes termed *supply angina* and due to the entity of *dynamic stenosis*.[22] In the presence of organic stenoses, platelet thrombi and leukocytes may elaborate vasoconstrictor substances such as serotonin and thromboxane A_2. Also, endothelial damage in atherosclerotic coronary arteries may result in decreased production of vasodilator substances and an abnormal vasoconstrictor response to exercise and other stimuli. A variable threshold of myocardial ischemia in patients with chronic stable angina may be due to dynamic changes in peristenotic smooth muscle tone and also to constriction of arteries distal to the stenosis.[23]

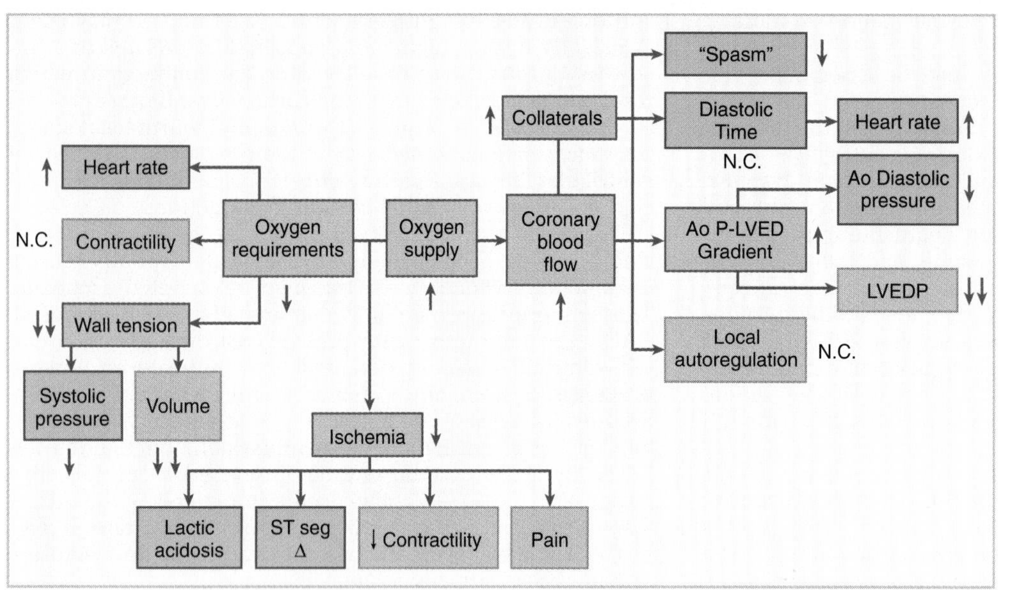

FIGURE 50–1 Factors influencing the balance between myocardial O_2 requirement **(left)** and supply **(right).** Arrows indicate effects of nitrates. In relieving angina pectoris, nitrates exert favorable effects by reducing O_2 requirements and increasing supply. Although a reflex increase in heart rate would tend to reduce the time for coronary flow, dilation of collaterals and enhancement of the pressure gradient for flow to occur as the left ventricular end-diastolic pressure (LVEDP) falls tend to increase coronary flow. Ao P-LVED = aortic pressure–left ventricular end-diastolic; LVEDP = left ventricular end-diastolic pressure; N.C. = no change. (From Frishman WH: Pharmacology of the nitrates in angina pectoris. Am J Cardiol 56:8I, 1985.)

In rare patients without organic obstructing lesions, severe dynamic obstruction occurring at rest alone can cause myocardial ischemia and result in angina (see Prinzmetal [Variant] Angina, Chap. 49). On the other hand, in patients with severe fixed obstruction to coronary blood flow, only a minor increase in dynamic obstruction is necessary for blood flow to fall below a critical level and cause myocardial ischemia.

FIXED COMPARED WITH VARIABLE-THRESHOLD ANGINA. In patients with fixed-threshold angina precipitated by increased O_2 demands with few if any dynamic (vasoconstrictor) components, the level of physical activity required to precipitate angina is relatively constant. Characteristically, these patients can predict the amount of physical activity that will precipitate angina, for example, walking up exactly two flights of stairs at a customary pace. When tested on a treadmill or bicycle, the pressure-rate product (the so-called double product, a correlate of the myocardial O_2 requirement) that elicits angina and/or ECG evidence of ischemia is relatively constant. As the activity of the left ventricle (and therefore its O_2 requirement) increases in patients with fixed-threshold, demand angina, a point is reached at which perfusion distal to a critical coronary arterial obstruction cannot supply sufficient O_2 to myocardium perfused by the obstructed artery; ischemia and angina ensue.

Most patients with variable-threshold angina have atherosclerotic coronary arterial narrowing, but dynamic obstruction caused by vasoconstriction plays an important role in causing myocardial ischemia. These patients typically have "good days," when they are capable of substantial physical activity, as well as "bad days," when even minimal activity can cause clinical and/or ECG evidence of myocardial ischemia or angina at rest. They often complain of a circadian variation in angina that is more common in the morning. Angina on exertion and sometimes even at rest may be precipitated by cold temperature,[24] emotion, and mental stress. A cold environment has been shown to increase peripheral resistance, both at rest and during exercise. The rise in arterial pressure, by augmenting myocardial O_2 requirements, lowers the threshold for the development of angina.

Postprandial angina may be a marker of severe multivessel CAD. The mechanism has not been explained, but it may be due to redistribution of coronary blood flow away from the territory supplied by severely stenosed vessels.[25] Some evidence indicates that this phenomenon is more prominent after high-carbohydrate than high-fat meals.

MIXED ANGINA. The term *mixed angina* has been proposed by Maseri and colleagues to describe the many patients who fall between the two extremes of fixed-threshold and variable-threshold angina.[26]

The pathophysiological and clinical correlations of ischemia in patients with stable CAD may have important implications for the selection of antiischemic agents, as well as for their timing. The greater the contribution from increased myocardial O_2 requirements to the imbalance between supply and demand, the greater the likelihood that beta-blocking agents will be effective, whereas nitrates and calcium-channel blocking agents, at least on theoretical grounds, are likely to be especially effective in episodes caused primarily by coronary vasoconstriction. The finding that in most patients with chronic stable angina an increase in myocardial O_2 requirement precedes episodes of ischemia, that is, that they have demand angina, argues in favor of beta blockers as essential therapeutic agents.

Noninvasive Testing

Biochemical Tests

In patients with chronic stable angina, metabolic abnormalities that are risk factors for the development of CAD are frequently detected. These abnormalities include hypercholesterolemia and other dyslipidemias (see Chap. 39), carbohydrate intolerance, and insulin resistance. All patients with established or suspected CAD warrant biochemical evaluation of total cholesterol, LDL cholesterol, HDL cholesterol, triglycerides, and fasting blood glucose.[27]

Several other biochemical markers have been shown to be associated with higher risk of future cardiovascular events (see Chap. 36). Measurement of lipoprotein Lp(a) and other lipid elements that are particularly atherogenic, such as apoprotein B and small dense LDL, appear to add to measurement of total cholesterol and LDL, but no consensus has been reached regarding routine measurement.[28] Homocysteine has also been linked to atherogenesis and to correlate with the risk of CAD; however, in aggregate, prospective studies have supported at most a modest increase in risk associated with elevated homocyst(e)ine, and have not consistently demonstrated a relationship that is independent of traditional risk factors or other biochemical markers.[29] Therefore, general screening for elevated homocyst(e)ine levels is not recommended.[30] Advances in understanding regarding the pathobiology of atherothrombosis (see Chap. 35) have generated intense interest in inflammatory biomarkers as noninvasive indicators of underlying atherosclerosis and cardiovascular risk. High-sensitivity measurement of the acute-phase protein C-reactive protein (hs-CRP) has shown a strong and consistent relationship to the risk of incident cardiovascular events.[31] The prognostic value of hs-CRP is additive to traditional risk factors, including lipid screening.[32] Measurement of hs-CRP in patients judged at intermediate risk by global risk assessment (10 to 20 percent risk of CHD/10 years) may help direct further evaluation and therapy in the primary prevention of CHD (see Chap. 36) and may be useful as an independent marker of prognosis in patients with established CAD.[33]

Blood levels of cardiac markers of necrosis (e.g., cardiac troponin) are normal in patients with chronic stable angina, which serves to differentiate them from patients with acute myocardial infarction. Novel biomarkers of myocardial ischemia are currently under study and may ultimately prove valuable in the noninvasive detection of ischemia in patients with stable CAD.[34]

Resting Electrocardiogram (see Chap. 9)

The resting ECG is normal in approximately half of patients with chronic stable angina pectoris, and even patients with severe CAD may have a normal tracing at rest. A normal resting ECG suggests the presence of normal resting left ventricular function and is an unusual finding in a patient with an extensive previous infarction. The most common ECG abnormalities in patients with chronic CAD are nonspecific ST-T wave changes with or without abnormal Q waves. Numerous pitfalls must be avoided when using the *resting* ECG for the diagnosis of myocardial ischemia. In addition to myocardial ischemia, other conditions that can produce ST-T wave abnormalities include left ventricular hypertrophy and dilation, electrolyte abnormalities, neurogenic effects, and antiarrhythmic drugs. In patients with *known* CAD, however, the occurrence of ST-T wave abnormalities on the resting ECG may correlate with the severity of the underlying heart disease. This association may explain the adverse association of ST-T wave changes with prognosis in these patients. In contrast, a normal resting ECG is a more favorable long-term prognostic sign in patients with suspected or definite CAD.[35]

Interval ECGs may reveal the development of Q wave infarctions that have gone unrecognized clinically. Various conduction disturbances, most frequently left bundle branch block and left anterior fascicular block, may occur in patients with chronic stable angina, and they are often associated with impairment of left ventricular function and reflect multivessel disease and previous myocardial damage. Hence, such conduction disturbances are an indicator of a relatively poor prognosis.[18] Abnormal Q waves are relatively specific but insensitive indicators of previous myocardial infarction. Various arrhythmias, especially ventricular premature beats, may be present on the ECG, but they too have low sensitivity and specificity for CAD. Left ventricular hypertrophy on the ECG suggests a poor prognosis in patients with chronic stable angina. This finding suggests the presence of underlying hypertension, aortic stenosis, or hypertrophic cardiomyopathy and warrants further evaluation, such as echocardiography to assess left ventricular size, wall thickness, and function.

During an episode of angina pectoris, the ECG becomes abnormal in 50 percent or more of patients with normal resting ECGs. The most common finding is ST segment depression, although ST segment elevation and normalization of previous resting ST-T wave depression or inversion ("pseudonormalization") may develop. Ambulatory ECG monitoring has shown that many patients with symptomatic myocardial ischemia also have episodes of silent ischemia that would otherwise go unrecognized during normal daily activities. Although this form of ECG testing provides a quantitative estimate of the frequency and duration of ischemic episodes during routine activities, its sensitivity for detecting CAD is less than that of exercise ECG.

Noninvasive Stress Testing (see Chap. 10)

Noninvasive stress testing can provide useful and often indispensable information to establish the diagnosis and estimate the prognosis in patients with chronic stable angina.[36] However, the indiscriminate use of such tests may provide limited *incremental* information over and above that provided by the physician's detailed and thoughtful clinical assessment.[37] Appropriate application of noninvasive tests requires consideration of Bayesian principles. These principles state that the reliability and predictive accuracy of any test are defined not only by its sensitivity and specificity but also by the prevalence of disease (or pretest probability) in the population under study. A reasonable estimate of the pretest probability of CAD may be made on clinical grounds (Table 50–1).

Noninvasive testing should be performed only if the *incremental* amount of information provided by a test is likely to alter the planned management strategy. The value of noninvasive stress testing is greatest when the pretest likelihood is intermediate because the test result is likely to have the greatest effect on the posttest probability of CAD and, hence, on clinical decision making.

Exercise Electrocardiography (see Chap. 10)

DIAGNOSIS OF CORONARY ARTERY DISEASE. The exercise ECG is particularly helpful in patients with chest pain syndromes who are considered to have a moderate probability of CAD and in whom the resting ECG is normal, provided that they are capable of achieving an adequate workload.[36] Although the incremental diagnostic value of exercise testing is limited in patients in whom the estimated prevalence of CAD is either high or low, the test provides useful additional information about the degree of functional limitation in both groups of patients and about the severity of ischemia and prognosis in patients with a high pretest probability of CAD.[36] Interpretation of the exercise test should include consideration of the exercise capacity (duration and metabolic equivalents) and clinical, hemodynamic, and ECG response.[36]

The predictive value for the detection of CAD is 90 percent if typical chest discomfort occurs during exercise along with horizontal or downward-sloping ST segment depression of 1 mm or more. ST segment depression of 2 mm or more

TABLE 50–1 Pretest Likelihood of Coronary Artery Disease in Symptomatic Patients According to Age and Sex*

Age (years)	Nonanginal Chest Pain		Atypical Angina		Typical Angina	
	Men	*Women*	*Men*	*Women*	*Men*	*Women*
30-39	4	2	34	12	76	26
40-49	13	3	51	22	87	55
50-59	20	7	65	31	93	73
60-69	27	14	72	51	94	86

From Gibbons RJ, Abrams J, Chatterjee K, et al: ACC/AHA 2002 guideline update for the management of patients with chronic stable angina: A report of the American College of Cardiology/American Heart Association Task Force on Practice Guidelines (Committee to update the 1999 guidelines for the management of patients with chronic stable angina). © 2002 American College of Cardiology and American Heart Association (Available at www.acc.org/clinical/guidelines/stable/stable.pdf).

*Each value represents the percentage with significant coronary artery disease at coronary angiography.

accompanied by typical chest discomfort is virtually diagnostic of significant CAD. In the absence of typical angina pectoris, downsloping or horizontal ST segment depression of 1 mm or more has a predictive value of 70 percent for the detection of significant coronary stenosis, but the predictive value increases to 90 percent with ST segment depression of 2 mm or more. The early onset of ST segment depression during exercise, its long persistence following discontinuation of exercise, a downsloping or horizontal depression, and a low work capacity or exercise duration all are strongly associated with multivessel disease and an adverse prognosis. Exercise-induced QRS prolongation also appears to be a function of exercise-induced ischemia and is related to the extent of exercise-induced segmental contraction abnormalities.

A meta-analysis of 147 published studies involving more than 24,000 patients was performed in the process of establishing the American College of Cardiology (ACC)/American Heart Association (AHA) Guidelines on Exercise Testing (Table 50–2).[36] Wide variability in sensitivity and specificity was reported, with a mean sensitivity of 68 percent and mean specificity of 77 percent. The results of stress testing often influence the subsequent decision for angiography and create a posttest referral bias that tends to inflate sensitivity and decrease specificity. When meta-analysis is restricted to studies designed to avoid such work-up bias, the sensitivity is only 45 to 50 percent but the specificity is 85 to 90 percent.[36,38] Clinical scores (e.g., Duke Treadmill Score)[39] or more complex equations that include variables in addition to the ST segment response may improve the discrimination of angiographically significant CAD compared to the ST-segment response alone.[36,39]

A major factor contributing to the low sensitivity of exercise ECG is that many patients are incapable of reaching the level of exercise required for near-maximal effort (≥85 percent of the maximal predicted heart rate), particularly those receiving beta-adrenergic blockers; those in whom fatigue, leg cramps, or dyspnea develops; and those with musculoskeletal symptoms. ST segment changes have low specificity in patients taking digitalis and those with left ventricular hypertrophy and repolarization abnormalities. In these subsets of patients, noninvasive *imaging* with exercise or pharmacological stress testing or diagnostic coronary angiography may be indicated.

INFLUENCE OF ANTIANGINAL THERAPY. Antianginal pharmacological therapy reduces the sensitivity of exercise testing as a screening tool. Beta blockade increases the exercise duration and suppresses, diminishes, or delays the appearance of ST segment depression, and thus obscures the diagnostic interpretation of exercise testing. A negative exercise test in patients receiving antianginal drugs does not exclude significant and possibly severe CAD. Therefore if the purpose of the exercise test is to diagnose ischemia, it should be performed, if possible, in the absence of antianginal medications. Two or 3 days is required for patients receiving long-acting beta blockers. Unless the patient has severe angina, sublingual nitroglycerin for 1 or 2 days is likely to be sufficient to control symptoms if other therapy is withdrawn. For long-acting nitrates, calcium antagonists, and short-acting beta blockers, discontinuing use of the medications the day before testing usually suffices. If the purpose of the exercise test is to identify safe levels of daily activity or the extent of functional disability, or as a guide to prognosis, the test should be performed while patients are taking their usual medications.

Nuclear Cardiology Techniques (see Chap. 13)

STRESS MYOCARDIAL PERFUSION IMAGING. Exercise perfusion imaging with simultaneous ECG is superior to exercise ECG alone in detecting CAD, in identifying multivessel disease, in localizing diseased vessels, and in determining the magnitude of ischemic and infarcted myocardium. The published results of exercise single-photon emission computed tomographic (SPECT) imaging involving more than 5200 patients with angiographic documentation of the presence or absence of CAD yield an average sensitivity and specificity of 88 and 72 percent, respectively (range, 71 to 98 percent and 36 to 92 percent, respectively) (Table 50–3).[18] Referral bias may account, in part, for the low specificity of many studies, and the few studies that adjusted for referral bias report a specificity higher than 90 percent.[18] The results with thallium-201 are comparable to those obtained with ^{99m}Tc-sestamibi or ^{99m}Tc-tetrofosmin, so these agents can in general be used interchangeably for the diagnosis of CAD.[40] Perfusion imaging is also valuable for detecting myocardial viability in patients with regional or global left ventricular dysfunction, with or without Q waves.[41] Stress perfusion imaging also provides important information in regard to prognosis.[40,42]

Stress myocardial scintigraphy is particularly helpful in the diagnosis of CAD in patients with abnormal resting ECGs and those in whom ST segment responses cannot be interpreted accurately, such as patients with left ventricular hypertrophy and repolarization abnormalities, those with left bundle branch block, and those receiving digitalis. Because stress myocardial perfusion imaging is a relatively expensive test (three to four times the cost of an exercise ECG), certain issues should be considered: (1) a regular exercise ECG should always be considered first in patients with chest pain and a normal resting ECG for screening and detection of CAD[18]; (2) stress myocardial perfusion scintigraphy should *not* be used as a screening test in patients in whom the prevalence of CAD is low because the majority of abnormal tests will yield false-positive results; (3) stress perfusion imaging

TABLE 50–2 Predictive Accuracy of Exercise Electrocardiography

Grouping	Number of Studies	Total Number of Patients	Sensitivity (%)	Specificity (%)	Predictive Accuracy (%)
Meta-analysis of standard exercise test	147	24,047	68	77	73
Meta-analysis without MI	58	11,691	67	72	69
Meta-analysis without workup bias	3	>1,000	50	90	69
Meta-analysis with ST depression	22	9,153	69	70	69
Meta-analysis without ST depression	3	840	67	84	75
Meta-analysis with digoxin	15	6,338	68	74	71
Meta-analysis without digoxin	9	3,548	72	69	70
Meta-analysis with LVH	15	8,016	68	69	68
Meta-analysis without LVH	10	1,977	72	77	74

MI = myocardial infarction; LVH = left ventricular hypertrophy.

From Gibbons RJ, Balady GJ, Bricker JT, et al: ACC/AHA 2002 guideline update for exercise testing: A report of the American College of Cardiology/American Heart Association Task Force on Practice Guidelines (Committee on exercise testing). © 2002 American College of Cardiology and American Heart Association. (Available at www.acc.org/clinical/guidelines/exercise/dirIndex.htm).

TABLE 50–3 Sensitivity and Specificity of Stress Imaging*

Modality	Total Patients	Sensitivity†	Specificity†
Exercise SPECT	5272	0.88	0.72
Adenosine SPECT	2137	0.90	0.82
Exercise echocardiography	2788	0.85	0.81
Dobutamine echocardiography	2582	0.81	0.79

SPECT = single-photon emission computed tomography.

Data from Gibbons RJ, Abrams J, Chatterjee K, et al: ACC/AHA 2002 guideline update for the management of patients with chronic stable angina: A report of the American College of Cardiology/American Heart Association Task Force on Practice Guidelines (Committee to update the 1999 guidelines for the management of patients with chronic stable angina). © 2002 American College of Cardiology and American Heart Association. (Available at www.acc.org/clinical/guidelines/stable/stable.pdf).

*Without correction for referral bias.

†Weighted average pooled across individual trials.

is more sensitive in detecting CAD, especially in patients with single-vessel CAD, than is exercise ECG[43]; (4) perfusion imaging is more accurate in patients with resting ECG abnormalities and those receiving digitalis; and (5) perfusion imaging is more accurate in localizing and quantifying regions of myocardial ischemia, which is of particular importance in patients who previously had revascularization, and in determining the extent of viable myocardium in patients with left ventricular dysfunction.[18]

PHARMACOLOGICAL NUCLEAR STRESS TESTING. For patients unable to exercise adequately, especially the elderly and patients with peripheral vascular disease, pulmonary disease, arthritis, or a previous stroke, pharmacological vasodilator stress with dipyridamole or adenosine may be used.[18] In most nuclear cardiology laboratories, such patients account for approximately 40 percent of those referred for perfusion imaging. Although the diagnostic accuracy of pharmacological vasodilator stress perfusion imaging is comparable to that achieved with exercise perfusion imaging (see Table 50-3),[18] treadmill testing is preferred for patients who are capable of exercising because the exercise component of the test provides additional diagnostic and prognostic information, including ST segment changes, effort tolerance and symptomatic response, and heart rate and blood pressure response.

POSITRON EMISSION TOMOGRAPHY (see Chap. 13). PET is considered by many to be the gold standard for evaluation of myocardial viability among patients with ischemic heart disease.[40] Most commonly PET uses ^{18}F-fluorodeoxyglucose (FDG) as the metabolic marker and ^{13}N-labeled ammonia as the perfusion tracer to evaluate for mismatch between myocardial perfusion and metabolic activity. In addition to assessment of myocardial viability, PET may be used to noninvasively measure coronary flow reserve.[44]

EXERCISE RADIONUCLIDE ANGIOGRAPHY. The use of radionuclide angiography for detecting and estimating prognosis in CAD has been supplanted largely by exercise echocardiography and is now performed infrequently.[18] Echocardiography provides a more accurate assessment of exercise-induced changes in regional wall motion and systolic wall thickening, which are more specific markers of reversible ischemia than are changes in ejection fraction.

Stress Echocardiography (see Chap. 11)

EXERCISE ECHOCARDIOGRAPHY. Two-dimensional echocardiography is useful in the evaluation of patients with chronic CAD because it can assess global and regional left ventricular function in the absence and presence of ischemia, as well as detect left ventricular hypertrophy and associated valve disease. Stress echocardiography allows the detection of regional ischemia by identifying new areas of wall motion disorders. Adequate images can be obtained in more than 85 percent of patients, and the test is highly reproducible. Detection of ischemic myocardium has been enhanced with the development of systems that allow simultaneous side-by-side display of rest and postexercise images. Numerous studies have shown that exercise echocardiography can detect the presence of CAD with an accuracy that is similar to that of stress myocardial perfusion imaging and superior to exercise ECG alone (see Table 50-3).[45] Stress echocardiography is also valuable in localizing and quantifying ischemic myocardium. As with perfusion imaging, stress echocardiography also provides important prognostic information in patients with known or suspected CAD.

Indications for stress echocardiography are similar to those discussed earlier for stress myocardial perfusion imaging. Stress echocardiography is an excellent alternative to nuclear cardiology procedures. Although less expensive than nuclear perfusion imaging, stress echocardiography is more expensive and less available than exercise ECG.

PHARMACOLOGICAL STRESS ECHOCARDIOGRAPHY. In patients unable to exercise, those unable to achieve adequate heart rates with exercise, and those in whom the quality of the echocardiographic images during or immediately after exercise is poor, alternative approaches are available. The most well studied and clinically available method is dobutamine stress echocardiography. Dobutamine increases both the heart rate and contractility and produces diagnostic changes in regional wall motion and systolic wall thickening as ischemia develops. Low-dose dobutamine infusion (5 to 10 μg/kg/min) is also valuable for assessing contractile reserve in regions with hypokinetic or akinetic wall motion at rest as a means of identifying viable myocardium that may improve in function after revascularization.[46] Atropine increases the accuracy of dobutamine stress echocardiography in patients with inadequate heart rate responses, especially those taking beta blockers and those in whom second-degree heart block develops at higher atrial rates. Dobutamine stress imaging achieves diagnostic accuracy comparable to that of exercise echocardiography.

Transesophageal dobutamine stress echocardiography has been shown to be feasible, safe, and accurate for the detection of myocardial ischemia. Although not readily available for large numbers of patients, it may allow extension of dobutamine stress testing to patients with inadequate transthoracic echocardiographic imaging.[18] Poor visualization of endocardial borders in a sizable subset of patients has been a limitation of stress echocardiography. However, two developments, contrast echocardiography and harmonic imaging, have significantly improved endocardial border definition, with the potential for enhanced detection of ischemic myocardium.[47,48] Doppler tissue imaging, which allows quantification of intramural myocardial velocities, provides a more direct measure of myocardial function during stress and may provide objective, quantitative evidence of induced ischemia during stress echocardiography.[49]

STRESS ECHOCARDIOGRAPHY VERSUS STRESS NUCLEAR PERFUSION IMAGING. See Chapter 16.

Clinical Application of Noninvasive Testing

GENDER DIFFERENCES IN THE DIAGNOSIS OF CAD (see Chap. 73). On the basis of earlier studies that indicated a much higher frequency of false-positive stress test results in women than in men, it is generally accepted that ECG stress testing is not as reliable in women. However, the prevalence of CAD among women in the patient populations under study was low, and the lower positive predictive value of exercise ECG in women can be accounted for, in large part, on the basis of Bayesian principles (see Table 50-1).[36] Once men and women are stratified appropriately according to the pretest prevalence of disease, the results of stress testing are similar, although the specificity is probably slightly less in women.[36]

Exercise imaging modalities have greater diagnostic accuracy than exercise ECG in both men and women.[36] Although soft tissue attenuation artifacts, especially those caused by breast tissue, may reduce the specificity of myocardial perfusion imaging in women, these artifacts can usually be identified by experienced observers without a substantial reduction in diagnostic accuracy, and risk assessment by nuclear perfusion imaging is not diminished in women versus men.[50] In addition, the use of gated SPECT imaging has greatly improved identification of these artifacts by demonstrating that regions with apparently irreversible perfusion defects have normal wall motion, thereby enhancing diagnostic accuracy.[51]

IDENTIFICATION OF PATIENTS AT HIGH RISK. When applying noninvasive tests to the diagnosis and management of CAD, it is useful to grade the results as "negative"; "indeterminate"; "positive, not high risk"; and "positive, high risk." The criteria for high-risk findings on stress ECG, myocardial perfusion imaging, and stress echocardiography are listed in Table 50–4.

TABLE 50–4 Risk Stratification Based on Noninvasive Testing

High Risk (>3% annual mortality rate)

1. Severe resting left ventricular dysfunction (LVEF < 0.35)
2. High-risk treadmill score (score ≤ –11)
3. Severe exercise left ventricular dysfunction (exercise LVEF < 0.35)
4. Stress-induced large perfusion defect (particularly if anterior)
5. Stress-induced multiple perfusion defects of moderate size
6. Large, fixed perfusion defect with LV dilation or increased lung uptake (thallium-201)
7. Stress-induced moderate perfusion defect with LV dilation or increased lung uptake (thallium-201)
8. Echocardiographic wall motion abnormality (involving > two segments) developing at low dose of dobutamine (≤10 mg/kg/min) or at a low heart rate (<120 beats/min)
9. Stress echocardiographic evidence of extensive ischemia

Intermediate Risk (1-3% annual mortality rate)

1. Mild/moderate resting left ventricular dysfunction (LVEF = 0.35-0.49)
2. Intermediate-risk treadmill score (–11 < score < 5)
3. Stress-induced moderate perfusion defect without LV dilation or increased lung intake (thallium-201)
4. Limited stress echocardiographic ischemia with a wall motion abnormality only at higher doses of dobutamine involving ≤ two segments

Low Risk (<1% annual mortality rate)

1. Low-risk treadmill score (score ≥ 5)
2. Normal or small myocardial perfusion defect at rest or with stress*
3. Normal stress echocardiographic wall motion or no change of limited resting wall motion abnormalities during stress*

LV = left ventricular; LVEF = LV ejection fraction.

From Gibbons RJ, Abrams J, Chatterjee K, et al: ACC/AHA 2002 guideline update for the management of patients with chronic stable angina: A report of the American College of Cardiology/American Heart Association Task Force on Practice Guidelines (Committee to update the 1999 guidelines for the management of patients with chronic stable angina). © 2002 American College of Cardiology and American Heart Association. (Available at www.acc.org/clinical/guidelines/stable/stable.pdf).

*Although the published data are limited, patients with these findings will probably not be at low risk in the presence of either a high-risk treadmill score or severe resting left ventricular dysfunction (LVEF < 0.35).

Regardless of the severity of symptoms, patients with high-risk noninvasive test results have a high likelihood of CAD and, if they have no obvious contraindications to revascularization, should undergo coronary arteriography. Such patients, even if asymptomatic, are at risk for left main or triple-vessel CAD, and many have impaired left ventricular function. Hence, they are at high risk for experiencing coronary events and may be candidates for coronary revascularization. In contrast, patients with clearly negative exercise tests, regardless of symptoms, have an excellent prognosis that cannot usually be improved by revascularization. If they do not have serious symptoms, coronary arteriography is generally not indicated.

The Duke Treadmill Score (see Fig. 10–15) is an integrative tool that incorporates exercise duration, the magnitude of ST segment deviation, and exercise-induced angina, and it effectively identifies patients with a high probability of severe CAD (triple-vessel or left main CAD) at angiography and with higher mortality risk. Among groups defined by low-, moderate-, and high-risk Duke Treadmill Scores, mortality at 5 years is 3 percent, 10 percent, and 35 percent, respectively.[39]

ASYMPTOMATIC PERSONS. Exercise testing in asymptomatic individuals without known CAD is generally not recommended.[36] Exercise testing may be appropriate for asymptomatic individuals with diabetes mellitus who plan to begin vigorous exercise,[36] for those with evidence of myocardial ischemia on ambulatory ECG monitoring, or for those with severe coronary calcifications on electron-beam CT.[18]

In asymptomatic persons or in those with chest pain not likely to be angina, the pretest likelihood of CAD is low (<15 percent). In such patients, a negative exercise ECG, for practical purposes, excludes ischemic heart disease. However, if such a patient has an abnormal exercise ST segment response, several alternatives exist. If the ST segment is abnormal but not high risk (<2-mm depression) and the patient demonstrates excellent exercise capacity (i.e., to stage IV of a Bruce protocol or the equivalent), the likelihood of left main CAD or multivessel CAD is low, the prognosis is favorable, and the patient may usually be observed without further testing, although an imaging study may provide further clarification and assurance. If, however, such a patient has a high-risk positive exercise ECG, coronary angiography is usually indicated to determine whether left main CAD or severe multivessel disease with left ventricular dysfunction is present. If the patient falls into an intermediate category (a positive but not high-risk exercise test result), a stress imaging study (echocardiography or perfusion scintigraphy) may provide further information. If both studies are abnormal but not high risk, the likelihood of CAD approaches 90 percent.

PATIENTS WITH ATYPICAL ANGINA. In these patients, the pretest probability of CAD is approximately 50 percent. If two noninvasive tests are abnormal, the likelihood of CAD exceeds 95 percent; if both tests are normal, it falls below 5 percent. When test results are discordant, they should be evaluated in light of the exercise level achieved, the presence of accompanying symptoms, and whether one of the tests is positive with high risk. Thus, for example, a patient who has atypical angina and a normal exercise ECG with multiple large perfusion defects on a stress thallium-201 scintigram at a heart rate of 130 beats/min has a much greater likelihood of having CAD than one who has a normal exercise ECG and a single small perfusion defect without chest pain at a heart rate of 185 beats/min. Although the indications for performing a stress imaging test directly in such a patient without an initial exercise ECG are controversial, such an approach is reasonable if the patient with atypical angina also has multiple cardiovascular risk factors, such as smoking, hypercholesterolemia, or a positive family history of premature CAD.

PATIENTS WITH TYPICAL ANGINA. In patients with a high pretest likelihood of disease of approximately 90 percent, noninvasive testing is most valuable for estimating the extent and severity of CAD and thereby the prognosis. The development of a high-risk positive stress test points to multivessel disease and a high risk of subsequent coronary events, and unless the patient has contraindications to revascularization, coronary angiography is indicated.

Chest Roentgenogram (see Chap. 12)

The chest roentgenogram is usually within normal limits in patients with chronic stable angina, particularly if they have a normal resting ECG and have not experienced a myocardial infarction. If cardiomegaly is present, it is indicative of severe CAD with previous myocardial infarction, preexisting hypertension, or an associated nonischemic condition such as concomitant valvular heart disease or cardiomyopathy.

Computed Tomography (see Chap. 15)

Noninvasive detection of coronary artery calcification has long been possible with fluoroscopy. Such calcific deposits are diagnostic of coronary atherosclerosis.[52] Electron-beam, and now multislice cardiac, CT has emerged as a highly sensitive method for detecting coronary calcification and is being used at some centers as a screening technique for CAD. CT quantification of coronary calcium has also been proposed as a method for assessing the response to treatment of risk factors such as dyslipidemia or hypertension among individuals with suspected or established CAD.[53] The calcium score is a quantitative index of total coronary artery calcium detected by CT, and this score has been shown to be a good marker of the total coronary atherosclerotic burden.[54] However, the relationship of the coronary calcium score to subsequent cardiac events in asymptomatic persons has not been fully established.[55,56] Several other uncertainties persist as well, including (1) the value of coronary calcium screening in comparison to multiple risk factor assessment; (2) whether coronary calcium scores add incremental value beyond the standard risk factors; and (3) whether coronary calcium screening is more accurate and cost-effective in asymptomatic persons than are other established noninvasive tests or other new methods that assess atherosclerotic burden, such as inflammatory biomarkers (see Chap. 36), the ankle-brachial index, and ultrasonic carotid intimal-medial thickening.[57]

The *absence* of calcium on CT imaging is predictive of the absence of significant atherosclerotic disease in older persons, but it is possible for young people (men younger than 45 years, women younger than 55) to have obstructive CAD and, hence, a risk for future cardiac events in the absence of detectable calcification or with a low calcium score.[58] Although coronary calcification is a highly sensitive (~90 percent) finding in patients who have CAD and the presence of coronary calcification is an accurate marker of coronary atherosclerosis, the specificity of this finding for identifying patients with obstructive CAD is low (~50 percent).[57,59] In light of the poor specificity and the potential consequences of expensive and unnecessary testing as the result of false-positive results, CT is currently *not* recommended as a routine approach toward screening for obstructive CAD.[18,57] Moreover, in patients with known or suspected CAD, exercise testing is preferable to CT imaging for determining the extent of CAD and the indication for coronary angiography.[57] Selective screening of individuals at intermediate risk of CAD may be appropriate.[57] The results of ongoing investigation will guide future recommendations regarding the role of this technique in the assessment and management of CAD.

In addition to application for detection of coronary calcification, CT technology may also evolve to enable reliable noninvasive coronary angiography. In particular, the emergence of new generations of multislice spiral CT scanners has reduced the motion artifact that constitutes a critical barrier to CT becoming a viable method for coronary angiography. Preliminary data with this technology in conjunction with aggressive beta blockade to reduce heart rate during imaging show promise for detection of obstructive CAD in the major epicardial arteries.[60]

Magnetic Resonance Imaging (see Chap. 14)

Magnetic resonance imaging (MRI) is established as a valuable clinical tool for imaging the aorta and the cerebral and peripheral arterial vasculature and is emerging as a versatile noninvasive cardiac imaging modality that has multiple applications for patients with CAD.[61] At present, the clinical use of MRI for myocardial viability assessment is growing based on data demonstrating its ability to predict functional recovery after percutaneous or surgical revascularization[62] and its very good correlation with PET.[63] Specifically, delayed hyperenhancement with gadolinium identifies areas of myocardial scar, and the transmural extent of hyperenhancement is strongly inversely associated with the probability of recovery after revascularization[62] and may be useful in assessing the probability of regaining contractile function after myocardial infarction.[64] Pharmacological stress perfusion imaging with MRI also compares favorably to other methods and is being employed clinically in some centers, particularly for individuals who present limitations for other imaging modalities.[65] In these patients, MRI also offers accurate characterization of left ventricular function. New techniques are likely to lead to further improvements in MRI as a tool for stress testing.[66,67]

By virtue of its ability to visualize arteries in three dimensions and differentiate tissue constituents, MRI has received intense interest as a potential, but as yet unproven, method to characterize arterial atheroma and assess vulnerability to rupture on the basis of compositional analysis.[61,68] Characterization of arterial plaque has been achieved in the aorta and carotid arteries[69] in humans and has been shown to be predictive of subsequent vascular events.[70] Initial studies evaluating MRI coronary angiography in humans demonstrate the ability to detect stenoses in the proximal and middle of major epicardial vessels[71] or surgical bypass grafts,[72] as well as to characterize congenital coronary anomalies.[73] Analogous to CT, new MRI technology is also likely to improve myocardial definition, enhance discrimination of wall motion, and also present new methods for ischemia detection based on assessment of regional oxygen content or detection of molecular changes (e.g., phosphocreatinine and adenosine triphosphate [ATP]) during ischemia.[61] However, routine clinical use of MRI scanning of coronary plaque will require substantial additional technical developments.[61]

Catheterization, Angiography, and Coronary Arteriography

The clinical examination and noninvasive techniques described earlier are extremely valuable in establishing the diagnosis of CAD and are indispensable to an overall assessment of patients with this condition. However, currently, definitive diagnosis of CAD and precise assessment of its anatomical severity still require cardiac catheterization and coronary arteriography (see Chaps. 17 and 18). Among patients with chronic stable angina pectoris referred for coronary arteriography, approximately 25 percent each have single-, double-, or triple-vessel disease (i.e., >70 percent luminal diameter narrowing). Five to 10 percent have obstruction of the left main coronary artery, and in approximately 15 percent no critical obstruction is detectable. Newer invasive techniques such as intravascular ultrasonography (IVUS) provide a cross-sectional view of the coronary artery and have substantially enhanced the detection and quantification of coronary atherosclerosis (see Chap. 52).[74] Studies incorporating both coronary angiography and IVUS demonstrate that the severity of CAD may be underestimated by angiography alone. In addition, IVUS images provide insight regarding plaque composition, discriminating lipid-laden versus fibrous or calcified elements based on echo-density.[75] In clinical practice, IVUS is a valuable tool to assess the cross-sectional lumen dimensions and to detect coronary artery stucture and pathology. Although IVUS is used in fewer than 10 percent of percutaneous interventions, it is particularly useful when angiography provides equivocal findings, such as occult left main or ostial CAD, or when there is haziness within the vessel after coronary stent implantation.

Coronary angiographic findings differ between patients presenting with acute myocardial infarction and those with chronic stable angina. Patients with unheralded myocardial infarction have fewer diseased vessels, fewer stenoses and chronic occlusions, and less diffuse disease than do chronic stable angina patients, thus suggesting that the pathophysiological substrate and the propensity for thrombosis differ between these two groups of patients.[76] In patients with chronic angina who have a history of prior infarction, total occlusion of at least one major coronary artery is more common than in those without such a history.

CORONARY ARTERY ECTASIA AND ANEURYSMS. Patulous, aneurysmal dilation involving most of the length of a major epicardial coronary artery is present in approximately 1 to 3 percent of patients with obstructive CAD at autopsy or angiography. This angiographic lesion does not appear to affect symptoms, survival, or incidence of myocardial infarction. Most coronary artery ectasia and/or aneurysms are due to coronary atherosclerosis (50 percent), and the rest are due to congenital anomalies and inflammatory diseases such as Kawasaki disease. Despite the absence of overt obstruction, 70 percent of patients with multivessel fusiform coronary artery ectasia/aneurysms demonstrated evidence of cardiac ischemia based on cardiac lactate levels during ergometry and atrial pacing. Moreover, nitroglycerin was of no benefit.[77]

Coronary ectasia should be distinguished from discrete *coronary artery aneurysms*, which are almost never found in arteries without severe stenosis, are most common in the left anterior descending coronary artery, and are usually associated with extensive CAD.[78] These discrete atherosclerotic coronary artery aneurysms do not appear to rupture, and resection of them is not warranted.

CORONARY COLLATERAL VESSELS (see Chap. 18). Provided that they are of adequate size, collaterals may protect against myocardial infarction when total occlusion occurs. In patients with abundant collateral vessels, myocardial infarct size is smaller than in patients without collaterals, and total occlusion of a major epicardial artery may not lead to left ventricular dysfunction. In patients with chronic occlusion of a major coronary artery but without infarction, collateral-dependent myocardial segments show nearly normal baseline blood flow and O_2 consumption but severely limited flow reserve. This finding provides an explanation for the ability of collaterals to protect against resting ischemia but not exercise-induced angina.[79]

MYOCARDIAL BRIDGING. Bridging of coronary arteries (see Chap. 18) is observed at coronary angiography at a rate of less than 5 percent in otherwise angiographically normal coronary arteries and ordinarily does not constitute a hazard.[80] Occasionally, compression of a portion of a coronary artery by a myocardial bridge can be associated with clinical manifestations of myocardial ischemia during strenuous physical activity and may even result in myocardial infarction or initiate malignant ventricular arrhythmias.[80] The functional consequences of myocardial bridging may be better characterized with the use of IVUS and intracoronary Doppler measurements.[80]

LEFT VENTRICULAR FUNCTION. Left ventricular function can be assessed by means of biplane contrast ventriculography (see also Chap. 20). Global abnormalities of left ventricular systolic function are reflected by elevations in left ventricular end-diastolic and end-systolic volume and depression of the ejection fraction. These changes are, however, quite nonspecific and can occur in many forms of heart disease. Abnormalities of *regional* wall motion (hypokinesis, akinesia, or dyskinesia) are more characteristic of CAD because the latter is usually regional in distribution. Also, hyperkinetic contraction of nonischemic myocardium may compensate for hypokinetic or akinetic ischemic or necrotic myocardium, thereby maintaining normal or nearly normal global left ventricular function despite marked depression of function in one region of the ventricle.

Ventricular relaxation, as reflected in the early diastolic ventricular filling rate, may be impaired at rest in patients with chronic CAD. Diastolic filling becomes even more abnormal (slowed) during exercise, when ischemia intensifies. In patients with chronic stable angina, the frequency of elevated left ventricular end-diastolic pressure and reduced cardiac output at rest, generally attributed to abnormal left ventricular dynamics, increases with the number of vessels exhibiting critical narrowing and with the number of prior infarctions. Left ventricular end-diastolic pressure may be elevated secondary to reduced ventricular compliance, left ventricular systolic failure, or a combination of these two processes.[81] Left ventricular function (global or regional) may be normal at rest in patients with chronic CAD without previous myocardial infarction but may become abnormal during or after stress. Abnormalities of left ventricular function detected angiographically may signify irreversible damage (i.e., prior infarction) or they may indicate acute ischemia or chronic hypoperfusion sufficient to maintain viability, but not contractility of the myocardium (i.e., "myocardial hibernation") (see Chap. 19).[82] Reversibility of this form of left ventricular dysfunction in patients with CAD and chronic stable angina is reflected by improved contraction assessed angiographically after an inotropic stimulus (postextrasystolic potentiation or the infusion of a sympathomimetic amine) and is accompanied by long-term improvement after myocardial revascularization.

Left ventriculography may also show mitral valve prolapse, which occurs in up to 20 percent of patients with obstructive CAD[83] and probably results from impaired contractility of the ventricular myocardium and papillary muscles. Mitral regurgitation secondary to left ventricular dilation may be observed in patients with chronic stable angina and ischemic cardiomyopathy.

CORONARY BLOOD FLOW AND MYOCARDIAL METABOLISM. Cardiac catheterization can also document abnormal myocardial metabolism in patients with chronic stable angina. With a catheter in the coronary sinus, arterial and coronary venous lactate measurements are obtained at rest and after suitable stress, such as the infusion of isoproterenol or pacing-induced tachycardia.[84] Because lactate is a byproduct of anaerobic glycolysis, its production by the heart and subsequent appearance in coronary sinus blood is a reliable sign of myocardial ischemia.

Studies of coronary flow reserve (maximum flow divided by resting flow) and endothelial function are frequently abnormal in patients with CAD and chronic stable angina. These techniques are discussed in Chapter 44.

Natural History, Prognosis, and Risk Stratification

Data from the Framingham Study, obtained before the widespread use of aspirin, beta blockers, and aggressive modification of risk factors, showed that the average annual mortality rate of patients with chronic stable angina was 4 percent. The combination of these treatments has improved prognosis. More recent data among middle-aged men with prevalent CAD indicate an annual mortality rate of 1.7 to 3 percent and an annual rate of major ischemic events of 1.4 to 2.4 percent.[85] Clinical, noninvasive, and invasive tools

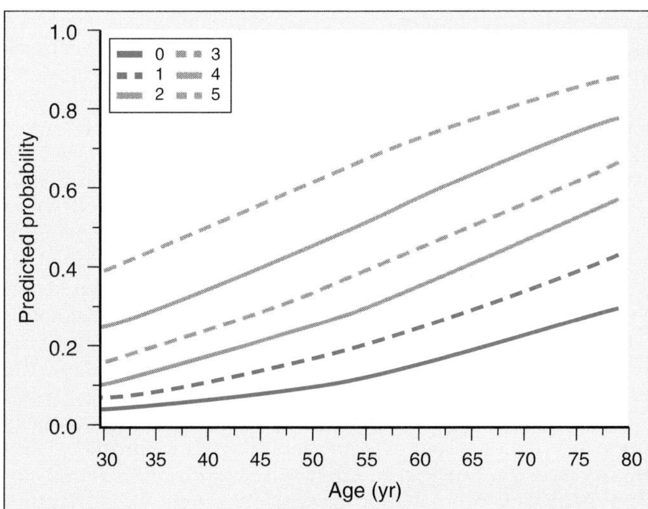

FIGURE 50–2 Nomogram showing the probability of severe (triple-vessel or left main) coronary artery disease based on a five-point clinical score assigned on the basis of the clinical variables: male gender, typical angina, history and electrocardiographic evidence of myocardial infarction, and diabetes. (Adapted from Hubbard BL, Gibbons RJ, Lapyre AC, et al: Identification of severe coronary artery disease using simple clinical parameters. Arch Intern Med 152:309-312, 1992.)

are useful in refining the estimate of risk for the individual patient with stable angina. Moreover, noninvasively acquired information is valuable in identifying patients who are candidates for invasive evaluation with cardiac catheterization.

CLINICAL AND ELECTROCARDIOGRAPHIC CRITERIA. A composite risk score based on multiple clinical variables (e.g., age, sex, diabetes, previous myocardial infarction, and the nature of the chest pain) may be quite strongly predictive of the presence of severe CAD (triple-vessel or left main CAD) and thus provide a strong indication for angiography (Fig. 50–2). Numerous studies attest to the adverse prognostic effect of congestive heart failure (based on a clinical history and/or the presence of cardiomegaly on chest radiography), previous myocardial infarction, hypertension, and advanced age in patients with stable angina pectoris.[18] A third heart sound is a useful clinical predictor of an abnormal left ventricular ejection fraction and an adverse prognosis in patients with CAD. The severity of angina, especially the tempo of intensification, is also an important predictor of outcome. On the other hand, a normal resting ECG in patients with stable angina pectoris speaks in favor of well-preserved left ventricular function and a favorable long-term prognosis.

NONINVASIVE TESTING

Exercise Electrocardiography. The prognostic importance of the treadmill exercise test was determined by several observational studies in the 1980s and early 1990s. One of the most important and consistent predictors is the maximal exercise capacity, regardless of whether it is measured by exercise duration or workload achieved or whether the test was terminated because of dyspnea, fatigue, or angina. After adjustment for age, the peak exercise capacity measured in metabolic equivalents is among the strongest predictors of mortality among men with cardiovascular disease.[86] Other factors with a poor prognosis identified in individual series of patients with chronic stable angina are described in Table 50–4 .

Stress Nuclear Myocardial Perfusion Imaging (see Chaps. 13 and 16). Although myocardial perfusion imaging was developed as a diagnostic tool for determining the presence or absence of CAD, its prognostic value is now well established.[87] In particular, the ability of myocardial perfusion SPECT to identify patients at low (<1 percent), intermediate (1 to 5 percent), or high (>5 percent) risk for future cardiac events is essential to patient management decisions. The prognostic data obtained from myocardial perfusion SPECT are incremental over the clinical and treadmill exercise data for predicting future cardiac events. Among patients with normal SPECT imaging the annual risk of death or myocardial infarction is less than 1 percent.

Echocardiography. Echocardiographic assessment of left ventricular function is one of the most valuable aspects of noninvasive imaging. Such testing is not necessary for all patients with angina pectoris, and among patients with a normal ECG and no previous history of myocardial infarction, the likelihood of preserved left ventricular systolic function is high. In contrast, among patients with a history of myocardial infarction, ST-T wave changes, or conduction defects or Q waves on the ECG, left ventricular function should be measured with echocardiography or an equivalent technique.

Evidence is increasingly demonstrating that echocardiography with exercise or pharmacological stress (dobutamine, arbutamine, or dipyridamole) is both sensitive and specific for the identification of myocardial ischemia and for risk stratification in patients with chronic stable angina.[88] The presence or absence of inducible regional wall motion abnormalities and the response of the ejection fraction to exercise appear to provide incremental prognostic information in addition to the assessment of cardiac structure and function provided by the resting echocardiogram. Moreover, a negative stress test portends a low risk for future events (<1 percent per person-year).

ANGIOGRAPHIC CRITERIA. The independent impact of multivessel disease and left ventricular dysfunction and their interaction on the prognosis of patients with CAD is well established (Fig. 50–3). The adverse effects of impaired ventricular function on prognosis are more pronounced as the number of stenotic vessels increases.[18]

Although several indices have been used to quantify the extent of severity of CAD, the simple classification of disease into single-, double-, triple-vessel, or left main CAD is the most widely used and is effective. Additional prognostic information is provided by the severity of obstruction and the location, whether proximal or distal. The concept of the gradient of risk is illustrated in Figure 50–4. Studies of treated symptomatic patients have revealed that if only one of the three major coronary arteries has more than 50 percent stenosis, the annual mortality rate is approximately 2 percent. The importance to survival of the quantity of myocardium that is jeopardized is reflected in the observation that an obstructive lesion proximal to the first septal perforating branch of the left anterior descending coronary artery was associated with a 5-year survival rate of 90 percent in comparison with 98 percent for patients with more distal lesions.[89] The survival rate of patients with isolated right CAD at 5 years appeared to be higher (96 percent) than for patients with disease of the left anterior descending coronary artery (92 percent). The overall survival of medically treated patients with left anterior descending and left circumflex CAD was not significantly different, but both were less than the survival of patients with isolated right CAD.

High-grade lesions of the left main coronary artery or its "equivalent," as defined by severe proximal left anterior descending and proximal left circumflex CAD, are particularly life threatening.[90] Mortality among medically treated patients has been reported to be 29 percent at 18 months and 43 percent at 5 years. Survival is better for patients with 50 to 70 percent stenosis (1- and 3-year survival rates of 91 and 66 percent, respectively) than for patients with a left main coronary artery stenosis greater than 70 percent (1- and 3-year survival rates of 72 and 41 percent). Furthermore, a number of characteristics found at catheterization or on noninvasive examination are predictors of an adverse prognosis in

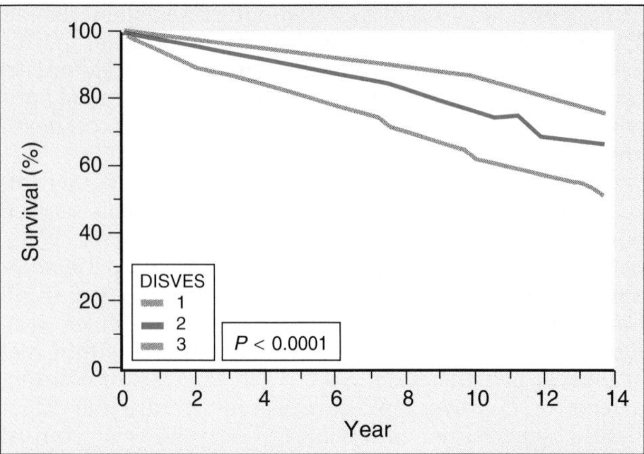

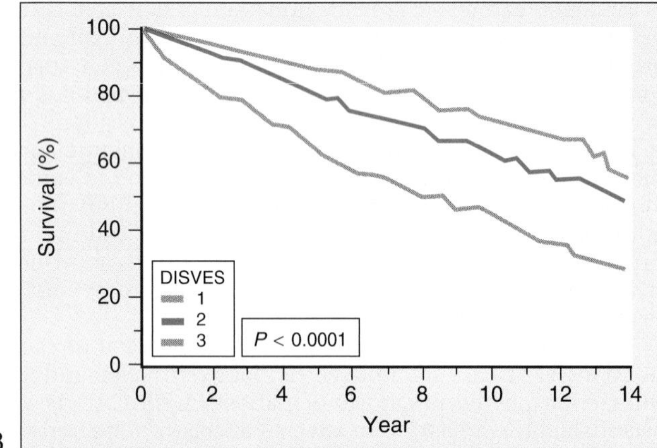

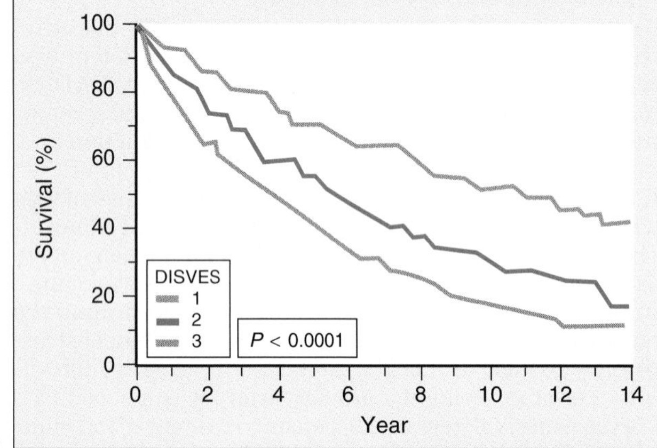

FIGURE 50–3 Graphs showing survival for medically treated CASS patients. **A,** Patients with single-, double-, or triple-vessel disease and an ejection fraction of 0.50 to 1.00 stratified by the number of diseased vessels (DISVES). **B,** Patients with single-, double-, or triple-vessel disease and an ejection fraction of 0.35 to 0.49 stratified by the number of diseased vessels. **C,** Patients with single-, double-, or triple-vessel disease and an ejection fraction of ≤0.34 stratified by the number of diseased vessels. (**A** to **C,** From Emond M, Mock MB, Davis KB, et al: Long-term survival of medically treated patients in the Coronary Artery Surgery Study [CASS] Registry. Circulation 90:2645, 1994.)

patients with 70 percent or greater left main coronary artery stenosis, including chest pain at rest, ST-T wave changes on resting ECG, cardiomegaly on chest radiography, a history of congestive heart failure, and the presence of left ventricular dysfunction at catheterization.

Limitations of Angiography. The pathophysiological significance of coronary stenoses lies in their impact on resting and exercise-induced blood flow, *and* in their potential for plaque rupture with superimposed thrombotic occlusion. It is generally accepted that a stenosis of greater than 60 percent of the luminal diameter is hemodynamically significant in that it may be responsible for a reduction in exercise-induced myocardial blood flow and cause angina and ischemia. The immediate functional significance of obstruction of "intermediate" severity (~50 percent diameter stenosis) is less well established. Coronary angiography is not a reliable indicator of the functional significance of stenosis, nor is it sensitive to the presence of thrombus. Moreover, the coronary angiographic determinants of the severity of stenosis are based on a decrease in the caliber of the lumen at the site of the lesion *relative* to adjacent reference segments, which are considered, often erroneously, to be relatively free of disease. This approach may lead to significant underestimation of the severity and extent of atherosclerosis.[74]

The most serious limitation to the routine use of coronary angiography for prognosis in patients with chronic stable angina is its inability to identify which coronary lesions can be considered to be at high risk, or "vulnerable," for future events, such as myocardial infarction or sudden death. Although it is widely accepted that myocardial infarction is the result of thrombotic occlusion at the site of plaque rupture or erosion (see Chap. 46), it is clear that it is not necessarily the plaque causing the most severe stenosis that subsequently ruptures. Lesions causing mild obstructions can rupture, thrombose, and occlude, thereby leading to myocardial infarction and sudden death. Approaches to quantifying the extent of coronary disease, inclusive of nonobstructive lesions, appear to offer additional prognostic information.[91] In contrast, arteries with severe preexisting stenoses may proceed to clinically silent complete occlusion, often without infarction, presumably because of the formation of collaterals as ischemia gradually becomes more severe.

In summary, angiographic documentation of the extent of CAD provides useful information toward assessment of the patient's risk of death and future ischemic events and is an indispensable step in the selection of patients for coronary revascularization, particularly if the interaction between the anatomical extent of disease, left ventricular function, and the severity of ischemia is taken into account. However, angiography is *not* helpful in predicting the site of subsequent plaque rupture or erosion that can precipitate myocardial infarction or sudden cardiac death. Additional tools that improve the imaging of coronary atheroma (e.g., IVUS), or the functional assessment of a stenosis (Doppler determination of coronary flow reserve) may be helpful in deciding on the flow-limiting significance of a specific lesion and the need for coronary revascularization.

Medical Management

Comprehensive management of chronic stable angina has five aspects: (1) identification and treatment of associated diseases that can precipitate or worsen angina; (2) reduction of coronary risk factors; (3) application of general and nonpharmacological methods, with particular attention toward adjustments in life style; (4) pharmacological management; and (5) revascularization by percutaneous catheter-based techniques or by coronary bypass surgery. Although discussed individually in this chapter, all five of these approaches must be considered, often simultaneously, in each patient. Among the medical therapies, three (aspirin, angiotensin-converting enzyme [ACE] inhibition, and effective lipid lowering) have been convincingly shown to reduce mortality and morbidity in patients with chronic stable angina and preserved left ventricular function. Other therapies such as nitrates, beta blockers, and calcium antagonists have been shown to improve symptomatology and exercise performance, but their effect, if any, on survival in patients with stable angina has not been demonstrated.

In stable patients with left ventricular dysfunction following myocardial infarction, data consistently indicate that ACE inhibitors and beta blockers reduce both mortality and the risk of repeat infarction, and these agents are recommended in such patients, with or without chronic angina, along with aspirin and lipid-lowering drugs.

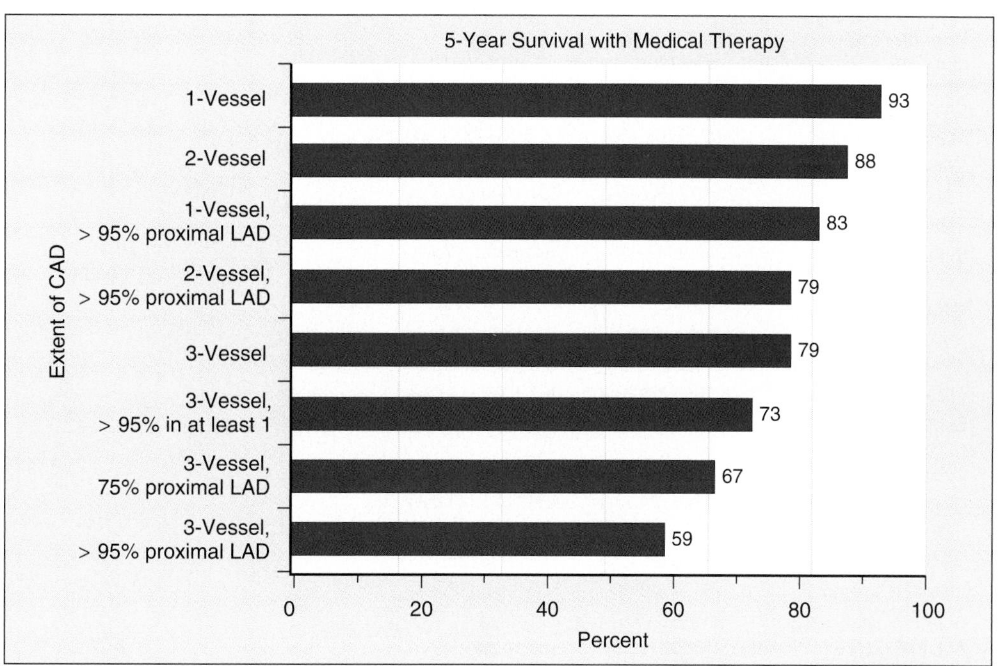

FIGURE 50–4 Angiographic extent of coronary artery disease (CAD) and subsequent survival with medical therapy. A gradient of mortality risk is established based on the number of diseased vessels and the presence and severity of disease of the proximal left anterior descending (LAD) artery. (Data from Califf RM, Armstrong PW, Carver, JR, et al: Task Force 5: Stratification of patients into high-, medium-, and low-risk subgroups for purposes of risk factor management. J Am Coll Cardiol 27:964-1047, 1996.)

TREATMENT OF ASSOCIATED DISEASES. Several common medical conditions that can increase myocardial O_2 demand or reduce O_2 delivery may contribute to the onset of new angina pectoris or the exacerbation of previously stable angina. These conditions include anemia, marked weight gain, occult thyrotoxicosis, fever, infections, and tachycardia. Drugs such as amphetamines and isoproterenol increase myocardial O_2 demand, as do other agents that stimulate the sympathetic nervous system. Cocaine, which can cause acute coronary spasm and myocardial infarction, is discussed in Chapter 62. In patients with CAD, heart failure, by causing cardiac dilation, mitral regurgitation, or tachyarrhythmias (including sinus tachycardia), can increase myocardial O_2 need, along with an increase in the frequency and severity of angina. Identification and treatment of these conditions are critical to the management of chronic stable angina.

Reduction of Coronary Risk Factors

HYPERTENSION (see Chaps. 37, 38, and 42). Epidemiological links between increased blood pressure and CAD severity and mortality are well established.[92] For individuals aged 40 to 70 years, the risk of ischemic heart disease doubles for each 20 mm Hg increment in systolic blood pressure across the entire range of 115 to 185 mm Hg.[93] Hypertension predisposes to vascular injury, accelerates the development of atherosclerosis, increases myocardial O_2 demand, and intensifies ischemia in patients with preexisting obstructive coronary vascular disease. Although the relationship between hypertension and CAD is linear,[93] left ventricular hypertrophy is a stronger predictor of myocardial infarction and CAD death than is the actual degree of increase in blood pressure.[94] A meta-analysis of clinical trials of treatment of mild to moderate hypertension showed a statistically significant 16 percent reduction in CAD events and mortality in patients receiving antihypertensive therapy.[95] This treatment effect is nearly twice as great in older compared with younger persons. It is logical to extend these observations on the benefits of antihypertensive therapy to patients with established CAD.[96] Moreover, the number of individuals treated to avoid one death is lower in subjects with established cardiovascular disease.[97] Therefore, blood pressure control is an essential aspect of the management of patients with chronic stable angina.

CIGARETTE SMOKING. This remains one of the most powerful risk factors for the development of CAD in all age groups (see Chap. 36). Among patients with angiographically documented CAD, cigarette smokers have a higher 5-year risk of sudden death, myocardial infarction, and all-cause mortality than do those who have stopped smoking. Moreover, smoking cessation lessens the risk of adverse coronary events in patients with established CAD.[98] Cigarette smoking may be responsible for aggravating angina pectoris other than through the progression of atherosclerosis. It may increase myocardial O_2 demand and reduce coronary blood flow by means of an alpha-adrenergically mediated increase in coronary artery tone and thereby cause acute ischemia.[99] Cigarette smoking also appears to reduce the efficacy of antianginal drugs. Smoking cessation is one of the most effective and certainly the least expensive approach to the prevention of disease progression in native vessels and bypass grafts. Strategies for smoking cessation are discussed in Chapter 43.

MANAGEMENT OF DYSLIPIDEMIA (see Chap. 39). Clinical trials in patients with established atherosclerotic vascular disease have demonstrated a significant reduction in subsequent cardiovascular events in patients with a wide range of serum cholesterol and LDL cholesterol levels who are treated with 3-hydroxy-3-methylglutaryl coenzyme A (HMG-CoA) reductase inhibitors (statins).[100-104] Angiographic trials of cholesterol lowering in patients with chronic CAD, many of whom had chronic stable angina, have shown that the effects on coronary obstruction are modest, in contrast with the substantive reduction in cardiovascular events. Several, but not all, studies have shown that statins significantly improve endothelium-mediated responses in the coronary and systemic arteries of patients with hypercholesterolemia or known atherosclerosis.[105]

Lipid-lowering with statins has been shown to reduce circulating levels of C-reactive protein[106,107] decrease thrombogenicity,[108] and favorably alter the collagen and inflammatory components of arterial atheroma;[109] these effects do not appear to correlate well with the change in serum LDL cholesterol and suggest antiatherothrombotic properties of statins.[110] These findings may explain the improvement in

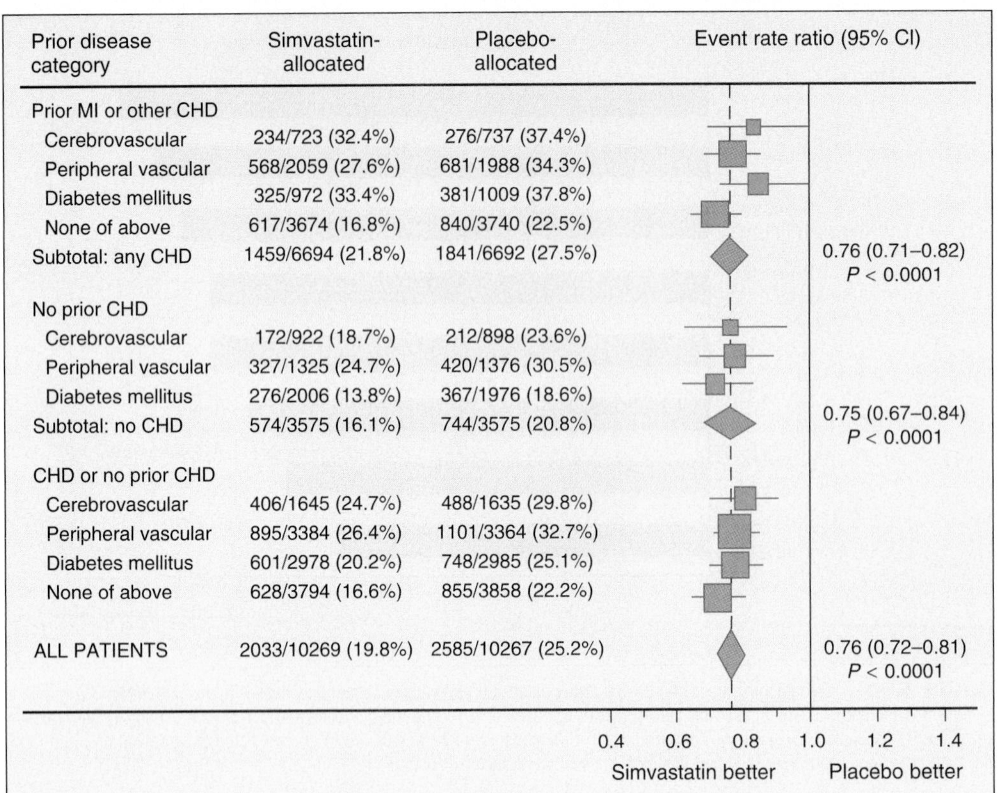

Prior disease category
Simvastatin-allocated
Placebo-allocated
Event rate ratio (95% CI)
Prior MI or other CHD
Cerebrovascular 234/723 (32.4%) 276/737 (37.4%)
Peripheral vascular 568/2059 (27.6%) 681/1988 (34.3%)
Diabetes mellitus 325/972 (33.4%) 381/1009 (37.8%)
None of above 617/3674 (16.8%) 840/3740 (22.5%)
Subtotal: any CHD 1459/6694 (21.8%) 1841/6692 (27.5%)
0.76 (0.71–0.82)
P < 0.0001
No prior CHD
Cerebrovascular 172/922 (18.7%) 212/898 (23.6%)
Peripheral vascular 327/1325 (24.7%) 420/1376 (30.5%)
Diabetes mellitus 276/2006 (13.8%) 367/1976 (18.6%)
Subtotal: no CHD 574/3575 (16.1%) 744/3575 (20.8%)
0.75 (0.67–0.84)
P < 0.0001
CHD or no prior CHD
Cerebrovascular 406/1645 (24.7%) 488/1635 (29.8%)
Peripheral vascular 895/3384 (26.4%) 1101/3364 (32.7%)
Diabetes mellitus 601/2978 (20.2%) 748/2985 (25.1%)
None of above 628/3794 (16.6%) 855/3858 (22.2%)
ALL PATIENTS 2033/10269 (19.8%) 2585/10267 (25.2%)
0.76 (0.72–0.81)
P < 0.0001
0.4 0.6 0.8 1.0 1.2 1.4
Simvastatin better
Placebo better

FIGURE 50–5 Effect of simvastatin on cardiovascular events among patients with and without coronary heart disease (CHD) in the Heart Protection Study. Among 13,386 patients with CHD enrolled in the Heart Protection Study, simvastatin (40 mg daily) reduced the risk of major vascular events (cardiovascular death, myocardial infarction [MI], stroke, or arterial revascularization) by 24 percent. CI = confidence interval. (From the Heart Protection Study Collaborative Group: MRC/BHF Heart Protection Study of cholesterol lowering with simvastatin in 20536 high risk individuals: A randomized placebo-controlled trial. Lancet 360:7-22, 2002.)

blood flow, the reduction in inducible myocardial ischemia, and the disproportionate reduction in coronary events in patients treated with statins despite small degrees of anatomical regression of atherosclerotic stenoses.

Results from secondary prevention trials of patients with a history of chronic stable angina, unstable angina, or previous myocardial infarction provide convincing evidence that effective lipid-lowering therapy significantly improves overall survival and reduces cardiovascular mortality in patients with coronary heart disease (see Chap. 39).[100-102] These effects have been demonstrated in both men and women and in the elderly[111,112] and provide a cost-effective approach to the management of large numbers of patients with chronic CAD.[113]

The National Cholesterol Education Program Guidelines (see Chap. 39)[27] advocate cholesterol-lowering therapy for all patients with coronary heart disease or extracardiac atherosclerosis to LDL levels below 100 mg/dl, and these guidelines have been adopted in recommendations from the ACC/AHA.[18] Moreover, the Heart Protection Study demonstrated an improvement in survival and reduction in future coronary events with statin therapy among individuals with diabetes, or cerebrovascular or peripheral vascular disease, as well as those with established CAD regardless of their baseline levels of cholesterol (Fig. 50–5).[104] In addition, results from the Pravastatin or Atorvastatin Evaluation and Infection Therapy (PROVE-IT)-TIMI 22 Trial demonstrated that among patients with a recent acute coronary syndrome, more aggressive lipid-lowering therapy, achieving LDL concentrations well below 100 mg/dl, provided greater protection against death or major cardiovascular events (see Fig. 49–11).[113a] These data provide additional support for aggressive cholesterol-lowering therapy among patients with established CAD.

Low HDL Cholesterol. Patients with established CAD and low levels of HDL cholesterol represent a subgroup with considerable risk for future coronary events.[114] Low HDL levels are often associated with obesity, hypertriglyceridemia, and insulin resistance and often signify the presence of small lipoprotein remnants and small dense LDL particles that are thought to be particularly atherogenic.[115] Therapy has focused on diet and exercise, as well as LDL cholesterol reduction in patients with a concomitant increase in LDL cholesterol.[27] The Veterans Affairs High-Density Lipoprotein Cholesterol Intervention Trial (VA-HIT) Study Group has demonstrated the efficacy of gemfibrozil treatment in patients with low HDL cholesterol (≤40 mg/dl) without elevations in LDL cholesterol (≤140 mg/dl) or triglycerides (mean, 160 mg/dl).[116] Gemfibrozil resulted in a 6 percent increase in HDL cholesterol and a 31 percent decrease in triglycerides, and these changes were associated with a 24 percent reduction in death, nonfatal myocardial infarction, and stroke ($p = 0.006$). The 22 percent reduction in cardiac death achieved only borderline statistical significance ($p = 0.07$).

Dyslipidemia after Myocardial Revascularization. In patients who have undergone coronary artery bypass grafting (CABG), elevation of LDL cholesterol is a risk factor for the development of saphenous vein graft occlusive disease, as well as progression of atherosclerosis in the native coronary arteries. Lipid-lowering therapy reduces mortality and acute coronary events in patients who have undergone either surgical or percutaneous revascularization,[117,118] and therapy for dyslipidemia should be given to these patients, as to all patients with chronic CAD.

ESTROGEN REPLACEMENT. A large data base derived from observational studies suggested a protective effect of hormone replacement therapy for postmenopausal women, with a 30 to 50 percent reduction in overall mortality from cardiovascular disease observed in these studies.[119] However, the major randomized, controlled secondary prevention trials have shown no cardiovascular benefit from hormone replacement therapy. Specifically, in the Heart and Estrogen/Progestin Replacement Study (HERS),[120] which randomly assigned postmenopausal women (mean age, 68 years) with established CAD to receive conjugated estrogen plus medroxyprogesterone or placebo, with a follow-up period of 4 years, no difference was seen in cumulative cardiac mortality or total cardiovascular events between the two groups despite a greater decrease in LDL cholesterol and increase in HDL cholesterol in the treatment group. The HERS-II study, which continued follow-up on unblinded therapy for an additional 2.7 years, also showed no difference between the treatment groups after 6.8 years.[121] Subsequent secondary prevention trials have added to the data indicating either no cardiovascular benefit or suggesting an increase in risk of coronary events with hormone replacement.[122-125] The increased risk of coronary heart disease among subjects treated with combined estrogen and progestin for primary prevention in the Women's Health Initiative bolsters these findings.[126] Thus, in light of the collective data from randomized clinical trials, it is *not* advised that hormone replacement therapy be initiated or continued for the purpose of secondary cardiovascular prevention in women with CAD.[18,127]

EXERCISE (see Chap. 43). The conditioning effect of exercise on skeletal muscles allows a greater workload at any level of total-body O_2 consumption. By decreasing the heart rate at any level of exertion, a higher cardiac output can be achieved at any level of myocardial O_2 consumption. The combination of these two effects of exercise conditioning permits patients with chronic stable angina to increase physical performance substantially following institution of a continuing exercise program.[128]

Most of the information about the physiological effects of exercise and their effect on prognosis in patients with CAD comes from studies on patients entered into cardiac rehabilitation programs, many of whom previously sustained a myocardial infarction.[129] Less information is available on the benefits of exercise in patients with chronic stable CAD, but nine small, randomized studies with a total of 980 patients have consistently demonstrated improved effort tolerance, O_2 consumption, and quality of life in patients undergoing exercise training.[18] Randomized trials evaluating symptom reduction and objective measures of ischemia in patients with stable CAD are few, with most supporting a reduction in symptoms or evidence of ischemia, such as with myocardial perfusion imaging.[18,128] Others have demonstrated a striking and direct relationship between the intensity of exercise and favorable changes in the morphology of obstructive lesions on angiography,[130] as well as favorable effects on vascular endothelial function thought to be mediated through expression and phosphorylation of endothelial nitric oxide synthase.[131] The question of whether exercise accelerates the development of collateral vessels in patients with chronic CAD remains unsettled.[132]

Exercise is safe if begun under supervision and increased gradually,[128,133] and if survivors of myocardial infarction can be used as a yardstick, it is probably cost-effective.[134] The psychological benefits of exercise are difficult to evaluate. However, a single nonrandomized study demonstrated significant improvement in well-being scores and positive-affect scores, as well as a reduction in disability scores, in patients in a structured exercise program.[18] In addition, exercise conditioning programs may be quite helpful in increasing the self-confidence of patients with chronic CAD. Patients who are involved in exercise programs are also more likely to be health conscious, to pay attention to diet and weight, and to discontinue cigarette smoking. For all the aforementioned reasons, patients should be urged to participate in regular exercise programs—usually walking—in conjunction with their drug therapy.[18,128]

INFLAMMATION (see Chaps. 35 and 42). Atherothrombosis has been identified as an inflammatory disease. Moreover, markers of systemic inflammation, including high-sensitivity C-reactive protein in particular, identify patients with established vascular disease who are at higher risk for death and future ischemic events.[135] Inflammation has now been identified as a potential target for therapeutic intervention in patients with CAD. Laboratory and clinical studies have provided evidence for antiinflammatory effects of established treatments aimed at other risk factors for atherogenesis (e.g., aspirin, statins, and ACE inhibitors); effects that may contribute, at least in part, to the proven clinical efficacy of these therapies.[136] For example, additional analyses from the Cholesterol and Recurrent Events (CARE) trial and the Air Force/Texas Coronary Atherosclerosis Prevention Study (AFCAPS/TexCAPS) are among the numerous studies that have demonstrated lowering of circulating levels of hs-CRP after treatment with statins.[136a] These findings lend support to the hypothesis that statins are effective in modifying the risk associated with evidence of systemic inflammation.[135,136] Other established preventive interventions, as well as novel therapeutic strategies, may also have antiinflammatory effects that could target inflammation as a risk factor in patients with CAD. ACE inhibitors, thiazolidinediones, thienopyridines, and fibric acid derivatives are among those agents that have been shown to exert antiinflammatory or immunoregulatory actions in animal models and/or in human studies.[136] Additional research is needed to clarify whether inflammation is a viable target for risk reduction in patients with stable CAD.

Additional Pharmacotherapy for Secondary Prevention

ASPIRIN (see Chaps. 42 and 80). A meta-analysis of 140,000 patients in 300 studies confirmed the prophylactic benefit of aspirin in both men and women with angina pectoris, previous myocardial infarction, or previous stroke and after bypass surgery.[137] In a Swedish trial of men and women with chronic stable angina, 75 mg of aspirin in conjunction with the beta blocker sotalol conferred a 34 percent reduction in acute myocardial infarction and sudden death.[138] In a smaller study confined to men with chronic stable angina but without a history of myocardial infarction, 325 mg of aspirin on alternate days reduced the risk of myocardial infarction during 5 years of follow-up by 87 percent.[139] Therefore, 75 to 325 mg of aspirin daily is advisable in patients with chronic stable angina but without contraindications to this drug.[18,140] Dosing at 75 to 150 mg daily appears to have comparable effects for secondary prevention to dosing at 160 to 325 mg daily[141] and may be associated with lower bleeding risk.[142]

Aspirin reduces the risk of subsequent myocardial infarction in healthy men with increased levels of C-reactive protein.[143] However, direct evidence that aspirin, administered in doses routinely used for secondary prevention, exerts antiinflammatory effects is mixed. In patients with established CAD and inducible myocardial ischemia, aspirin (300 mg/day) reduces circulating levels of C-reactive protein, macrophage colony–stimulating factor, and interleukin 6.[144] In contrast, aspirin (81 mg/day or 325 mg every third day) administered to healthy volunteers reduced measures of platelet activation but not C-reactive protein.[145] Aspirin also improves endothelial function in patients with atherosclerosis through a mechanism that may involve blockade of cyclooxygenase-dependent release of endothelium-derived constricting factors.[146]

Although warfarin has proved beneficial in patients after MI, no data support the use of chronic anticoagulation in patients with stable angina. However, a single large, randomized trial in patients with risk factors for atherosclerosis but without symptoms of angina has shown that low doses of warfarin (achieving a mean international normalized ratio [INR] of 1.47) combined with aspirin decrease the risk of coronary death and myocardial infarction when used for primary prevention in high-risk groups.[147] Any benefit of this combination must be balanced against the potential for increased bleeding, which was also noted in this study.

ASPIRIN INTERACTION WITH ACE INHIBITORS. With the increasing use of ACE inhibitors in patients with cardiovascular disease, concern has arisen about a possible adverse interaction between aspirin and these drugs. Aspirin has the potential to inhibit prostaglandin-mediated pathways of ACE inhibition, and evidence of such antagonism has been demonstrated in patients with hypertension and heart failure.[148] However, no evidence for an adverse interaction between aspirin and ACE inhibition (with ramipril) was observed in the substantially larger Heart Outcomes Prevention Evaluation (HOPE) trial.[149] Thus, current evidence supports aspirin therapy for all patients with CAD, including those taking ACE inhibitors. Ongoing clinical trials in this area will provide additional information.

CLOPIDOGREL. Another orally acting class of agents that block platelet aggregation are the thienopyridine derivatives, including clopidogrel.[150] Clopidogrel may be substituted for aspirin in patients with aspirin hypersensitivity or those who cannot tolerate aspirin (see Chap. 49). In a randomized comparison between clopidogrel and aspirin among patients with established atherosclerotic vascular disease (the Clopidogrel versus Aspirin in Patients at Risk of Ischaemic Events [CAPRIE] trial) treatment with clopidogrel resulted in a modest 8.7 percent relative reduction in the risk of vascular death, ischemic stroke, or myocardial infarction ($p = 0.043$) over 2 years.[151] Subsequent studies evaluating the addition of clopidogrel to aspirin among patients with non-ST elevation acute coronary syndromes[152] or after percutaneous coronary intervention[153] have indicated more robust risk reductions in these patient populations with CAD. Ongoing investigation will clarify the role of chronic treatment with clopidogrel for secondary prevention in patients with chronic stable angina.

BETA BLOCKERS. The value of beta blockers in reducing death and recurrent myocardial infarction in patients who have experienced a myocardial infarction is well established (see Chap. 46),[154] as is their usefulness in the treatment of angina. Whether these drugs are also of value in preventing infarction and sudden death in patients with chronic stable angina without previous infarction is uncertain, and there have been no controlled trials against placebo. However, there is no reason to assume that the favorable effects of beta blockers on ischemia and perhaps on arrhythmias should not apply to patients with chronic stable angina pectoris. Therefore, it is sensible to use these drugs when angina, hypertension, or both are present in patients with chronic CAD and when these drugs are well tolerated.

ACE INHIBITORS. Although ACE inhibitors are not indicated for the treatment of angina, these drugs appear to have important benefits in reducing the risk of future ischemic events. An unexpected and far-reaching finding from randomized trials of ACE inhibitors in postinfarct and other patients with ischemic and nonischemic causes of left ventricular dysfunction is the striking reduction in incidence of subsequent ischemic events such as myocardial infarction, unstable angina, and the need for coronary revascularization procedures.[155,156] Data from four trials including approximately 11,000 patients demonstrated a statistically significant risk reduction in myocardial infarction of 21 percent and in subsequent unstable angina of 15 percent.[156] The potentially beneficial effects of ACE inhibitors include a reduction in left ventricular hypertrophy, vascular hypertrophy, progression of atherosclerosis, plaque rupture, and thrombosis, in addition to a potentially favorable influence on myocardial O_2 supply/demand relationships and cardiac hemodynamics and a reduction in sympathetic activity.[156] Recent evidence also indicates that ACE inhibitors enhance coronary endothelial vasomotor function in patients with CAD,[157] which may contribute to enhanced myocardial blood flow during increases in myocardial demand.[158] In addition, in vitro experiments show that angiotensin II induces inflammatory changes in human vascular smooth muscle cells,[159] and treatment with ACE inhibitors can reduce signs of inflammation in animal models of atherosclerosis.[160]

These beneficial effects of ACE inhibitors on vascular structure and function should in theory extend beyond patients with left ventricular dysfunction to a much wider range of patients with CAD, including those with normal left ventricular function. This is the subject of several randomized, multicenter trials. The first of these trials to be completed provided strong evidence supporting the therapeutic benefit of ACE inhibitors. The HOPE study enrolled 9297 patients with atherosclerotic vascular disease or diabetes and at least one other CAD risk factor and randomly assigned them to receive ramipril (10 mg daily) or placebo; the mean follow-up was 5 years.[149] Eighty percent of patients had CAD, only 12 percent of whom had a myocardial infarction within 1 year after enrollment. No patient had heart failure symptoms on study entry, and echocardiograms (available for 5183 patients) demonstrated preserved left ventricular function (ejection fraction ≥0.40) in 92 percent of patients. Ramipril significantly decreased the risk of the primary composite endpoint of cardiovascular death, myocardial infarction, and stroke from 17.7 to 14.1 percent (relative risk reduction of 22 percent, $p < 0.001$). The relative decreases in cardiovascular death, myocardial infarction, and stroke were 25, 20, and 31 percent, respectively. The European Trial on Reduction of Cardiac Events with Perindopril in stable CAD (EUROPA) provided additional convincing support for the benefit of ACE inhibitors with respect to future cardiovascular events in patients with stable CAD in the absence of heart failure (Fig. 50–6).[160a] In both HOPE and EUROPA, the results were similar when examined in patient subsets defined by age, sex, known CAD, hypertension, diabetes, left ventricular function, or previous myocardial infarction. Beneficial effects were also similar in patients who were or were not taking aspirin in the HOPE trial.

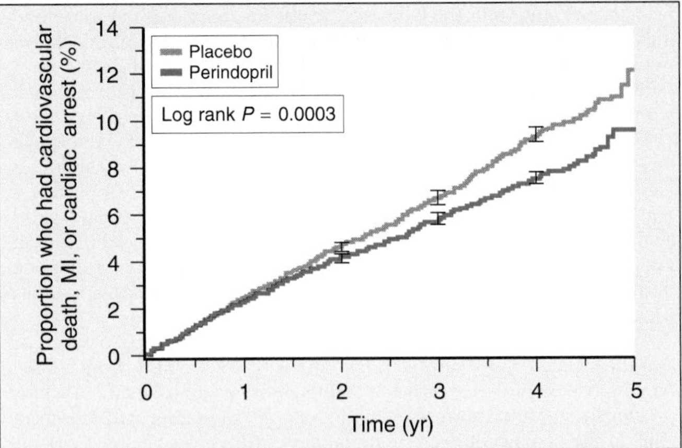

FIGURE 50–6 Kaplan-Meier time-to-event curves for the primary endpoint (cardiovascular death, myocardial infarction [MI], or cardiac arrest) with perindopril versus placebo among patients with stable coronary artery disease without apparent heart failure enrolled in the European Trial on the Reduction of Cardiac Events with Perindopril in Stable Coronary Artery Disease (EUROPA Trial). The angiotensin-converting enzyme inhibitor perindopril conferred a 20 percent relative reduction in the risk of the primary endpoint ($p = 0.0003$). (From EUROPA Investigators: Efficacy of perindopril in reduction of cardiovascular events among patients with stable coronary artery disease: Randomized double-blind, placebo-controlled, multicenter trial [the EUROPA study]. Lancet 363:782-788, 2003.)

In the 2002 AHA/ACC Guideline Update for management of patients with chronic stable angina, ACE inhibitors are recommended for all patients with CAD in conjunction with diabetes and/or left ventricular dysfunction.[18] The EUROPA study was reported after development of these guidelines. Considered together, the results of the HOPE and EUROPA studies have wide-reaching implications and suggest that patients with stable CAD, such as those enrolled in HOPE and EUROPA, should receive ACE inhibitor therapy. The role of ACE inhibition in lower risk patients with CAD is being studied in the PEACE trial.[160b]

ANTIOXIDANTS (see Chap. 42). Oxidized LDL particles are strongly linked to the pathophysiology of atherogenesis, and descriptive, prospective cohort, and case-control studies suggest that a high dietary intake of antioxidant vitamins (A, C, and beta-carotene) and flavonoids (polyphenolic antioxidants), naturally present in vegetables, fruits, tea, and wine, is associated with a decrease in coronary heart disease events.[161]

Despite this evidence for a beneficial effect of high dietary intake of antioxidant vitamins, randomized trials have not detected an advantage to treatment with supplemental beta-carotene, vitamin C, or vitamin E with respect to cardiovascular risk. Although the Cambridge Heart Antioxidant Study (CHAOS) reported a 77 percent reduction in myocardial infarction and a 47 percent reduction in all cardiovascular events among 2002 patients with angiographic CAD randomized to alpha-tocopherol compared with placebo,[162] two subsequent large, randomized, placebo-controlled trials have detected no benefit among individuals at high risk for or with established CAD.[163,164] The Heart Protection Study Collaborative Group enrolled more than 20,000 individuals with established atherosclerotic vascular disease or diabetes mellitus and found no reduction in all-cause mortality, myocardial infarction, or other vascular events with supplementation of vitamin E, vitamin C, and beta-carotene versus matched placebo during 5 years of follow-up.[164] Thus, based on present evidence, there is no basis for recommending that individuals take supplemental vitamin E, vitamin C, or beta-carotene for the purpose of treating CAD.[18]

Counseling and Changes in Life Style

The psychosocial issues faced by a patient who develops chronic stable angina for the first time are similar to, although usually less intense than, those experienced by a patient with an acute myocardial infarction. Recent data have reinforced that depressive symptoms are strongly associated with health status as reported by the patient, including the burden of symptoms and overall quality of life, independently of left ventricular function and the presence of provokable ischemia.[165] In conjunction with counseling, treatment with a selective serotonin reuptake inhibitor appears to be safe and effective in managing depression among patients with acute coronary syndromes and may be expected to be safe among patients with stable CAD.[166] Thus, efforts to evaluate and treat depression among patients with CAD is an important element of their overall management.

An important aspect of the physician's role is to counsel patients in the kinds of work they can do and in their leisure activities, eating habits, vacation plans, and the like.[167] Certain changes in life style may be helpful, such as modifying strenuous activities if they constantly and repeatedly produce angina. These changes may be minor in many instances. For example, golfing could be modified to include the use of a golf cart instead of walking. A history of CAD and stable angina is not inconsistent with the ability to continue to perform exertion, which is important not only in regard to recreational activities and life style but also for patients in whom some physical exertion is required in their employment. However, isometric activities such as weight lifting and other activities such as snow shoveling, which involves an energy expenditure between 60 and 65 percent of peak oxygen consumption, and cross-country or downhill skiing are undesirable. In addition, some activities expose the individual to the detrimental effects of cold on the O_2 demand/supply relationship, and these activities should also be avoided whenever possible.

Eliminating or reducing the factors that precipitate anginal episodes is of obvious importance. Patients learn their usual threshold by trial and error. Patients should avoid *sudden* bursts of activity, particularly after long periods of rest or after meals and in cold weather. Both chronic angina and unstable angina exhibit a circadian rhythm characterized by a lower angina threshold shortly after arising.[168] Therefore, morning activities such as showering, shaving, and dressing should be done at a slower pace and, if necessary, with the use of prophylactic nitroglycerin. The stress of sexual intercourse is approximately equal to that of climbing one flight of stairs at a normal pace or any activity that induces a heart rate of approximately 120 beats/min. With proper precautions (i.e., commencing more than 2 hours postprandially and taking an additional dose of a short-acting beta blocker 1 hour before and nitroglycerin 15 minutes before), most patients with chronic stable angina are able to continue satisfactory sexual activity. Although it is desirable to minimize the number of bouts of angina, an occasional episode is not to be feared. Indeed, unless patients occasionally reach their angina threshold, they may not appreciate the extent of their exercise capacity. Patients with stable CAD may use sildenafil but not in conjunction with nitrates.

Marked restriction in activity or even complete bed rest, in addition to drug therapy, may occasionally be necessary to control symptoms. In less critical situations, merely reducing the amount of time spent working or increasing the rest periods has a beneficial effect. For example, a long lunch break that includes a short nap may be beneficial. It may be helpful for the patient to use a face mask or scarf to cover the mouth or nose in cold weather. A hot, humid environment may also precipitate angina, and air conditioning may be a necessity rather than a luxury for patients with chronic angina. Large meals can have a similar effect if they are followed by exertion. An effort should be made to minimize emotional outbursts because they too increase myocardial O_2 requirements and sometimes induce coronary vasoconstriction. Occasionally, antianxiety drugs and sedatives or relaxation techniques using biofeedback mechanisms may be helpful.

Pharmacological Management of Angina Pectoris

Nitrates

MECHANISM OF ACTION. Even though the clinical effectiveness of amyl nitrite in angina pectoris was first described in 1867 by Brunton, organic nitrates are still the drugs most commonly used in the treatment of patients with this condition. The action of these agents is to relax vascular smooth muscle.[169] The vasodilator effects of nitrates are evident in both systemic (including coronary) arteries and veins in normal subjects and in patients with ischemic heart disease, but they appear to be predominant in the venous circulation. The venodilator effect reduces ventricular preload, which in turn reduces myocardial wall tension and O_2 requirements. The action of nitrates in reducing both preload and afterload makes them useful in the treatment of heart failure (see Fig. 50-1), as well as angina pectoris. By reducing the heart's mechanical activity, volume, and O_2 consumption, nitrates increase exercise capacity in patients with ischemic heart disease, thereby allowing a greater total-body workload to be achieved before the angina threshold is reached. In patients with stable angina, nitrates improve exercise tolerance and time to ST segment depression during treadmill exercise tests. When used in combination with calcium-channel blockers and/or beta blockers, the antianginal effects appear greater.[18]

EFFECTS ON THE CORONARY CIRCULATION (Table 50–5). Quantitative, computer-assisted measurements of coronary arterial diameter have been used to show that nitroglycerin causes dilation of epicardial stenoses. These stenoses are often eccentric lesions, and nitroglycerin causes relaxation of the smooth muscle in the wall of the coronary artery that is not encompassed by plaque. Even a small increase in a narrowed arterial lumen can produce a significant reduction in resistance to blood flow across obstructed regions.[170] Nitrates may also exert a beneficial effect in patients with impaired coronary flow reserve by alleviating the vasoconstriction caused by endothelial dysfunction.[171]

REDISTRIBUTION OF BLOOD FLOW. Studies in experimental animals with coronary obstruction have shown that nitroglycerin causes redistribution of blood flow from normally perfused to ischemic areas, particularly in the subendocardium.[172] This redistribution may be mediated in part by an increase in collateral blood flow and in part by lowering of ventricular diastolic pressure, thereby reducing subendocardial compression. Nitroglycerin appears to preferentially reduce coronary vascular resistance in viable myocardium with ischemia as detected by SPECT imaging.[173] In patients with chronic stable angina responsive to nitroglycerin, topical nitroglycerin under resting conditions alters myocardial perfusion by preferentially increasing flow to areas of reduced perfusion with little or no change in global myocardial perfusion.[174]

ANTITHROMBOTIC EFFECTS. Stimulation of guanylate cyclase by nitric oxide (NO) results in inhibitory action on platelets in addition to vasodilation. Although the antithrombotic effects of intravenous nitroglycerin have been demonstrated both in patients with unstable angina and in those with chronic stable angina, the clinical significance of these actions is not clear.[175]

CELLULAR MECHANISM OF ACTION. Nitrates have the ability to cause vasodilation regardless of whether the endothelium is intact. After entering the vascular smooth muscle cell, nitrates are converted to

TABLE 50–5 Effects of Antianginal Agents on Indices of Myocardial Oxygen Supply and Demand*

		Beta-Adrenoceptor Blockers						
		ISA		*Cardioselective*		Calcium Antagonists		
Index	**Nitrates**	***No***	***Yes***	***No***	***Yes***	***Nifedipine***	***Verapamil***	***Diltiazem***
Supply								
Coronary resistance								
Vascular tone	↓↓	↑	0	↑	0↑	↓↓↓	↓↓↓	↓↓↓
Intramyocardial diastolic tension	↓↓↓	↑	0	↑	↑	↓↓	0↑	0
Coronary collateral circulation	↑	0	0	0	0	↑	0	↑
Duration of diastole	0(↓)	↑↑↑	0↓	↑↑↑	↑↑↑	0↑(↓↓)	↑↑↑(↓)	↑↑(↓)
Demand								
Intramyocardial systolic tension								
Preload	↓↓↓	↑	0	↑	↑	↓0	↑0↓	0↓
Afterload (peripheral vascular resistance)	↓	↑	↑	↑↑	↑	↓↓	↓	↓
Contractility	0(↑)	↓↓↓	↓	↓↓↓	↓↓↓	↓(↑↑)†	↓↓(↑)†	↓(↑)†
Heart rate	0(↑)	↓↓↓	0↓	↓↓↓	↓↓↓	0(↑↑)	↓↓(↑)	↓↓(↑)

ISA = intrinsic sympathomimetic activity.
From Shub C, Vlietstra RE, McGoon MD: Selection of optimal drug therapy for the patient with angina pectoris. Mayo Clin Proc 60:539, 1985.
*↑ = Increase; ↓ = decrease; 0 = little or no definite effect. The number of arrows represents the relative intensity of effect. Symbols in parentheses indicate reflex-mediated effects.
†Effect of calcium entry on left ventricular *contractility*, as assessed in the intact animal model. The net effect on *left ventricular performance* is variable since it is influenced by alterations in afterload, reflex cardiac stimulation, and the underlying state of the myocardium.

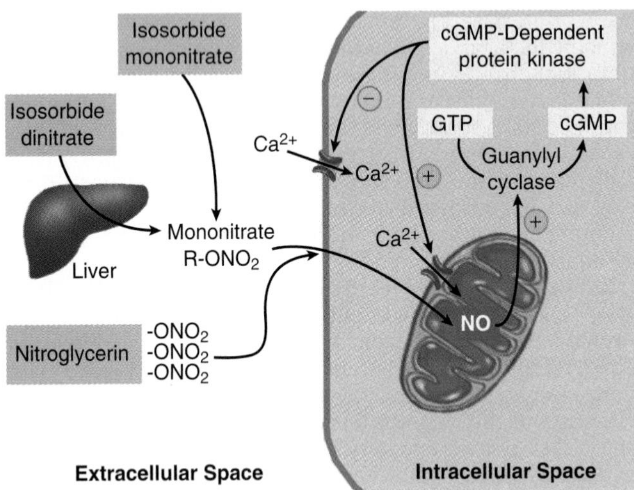

FIGURE 50–7 Mechanism of action of nitrates. Evidence exists that biotransformation of mononitrates occurs through action of mitochondrial aldehyde reductase producing nitric oxide (NO). NO activates soluble guanylyl cyclase, resulting in increased production of cyclic guanosine monophosphate (cGMP). The second messenger cGMP reduces cytoplasmic calcium (Ca^{2+}) by inhibiting inflow and stimulating mitochondrial uptake of calcium, thus mediating relaxation of smooth muscle cells and causing vasodilation. Isosorbide dinitrate is metabolized by the liver, whereas the liver is bypassed by mononitrates. GTP = guanosine triphosphate. R-ONO_2 = mononitrate. (Adapted from Gori T, Parker JD: Nitrate tolerance: A unifying hypothesis. Circulation 106:2510-2513, 2002; and Opie LH: Drugs for the Heart. 4th ed. Philadelphia, WB Saunders, 1995, p 33.)

reactive (NO) or *S*-nitrosothiols, which activate intracellular guanylate cyclase to produce cyclic guanosine monophosphate,[176] which in turn triggers smooth muscle relaxation and antiplatelet aggregatory effects (Fig. 50-7). Evidence now exists that the biotransformation of nitroglycerin occurs via mitochondrial aldehyde dehydrogenase and that inhibition of this enzyme may contribute to the development of tolerance.[177] Sulfhydryl (SH) groups appear to be required, at least as a cofactor, for both formation of NO and stimulation of guanylate cyclase, and nitroglycerin-induced vasodilation can be enhanced by prior administration of *N*-acetylcysteine, an agent that increases the availability of SH groups.[169] This action of *N*-acetylcysteine potentiates peripheral hemodynamic responses and the coronary vasodilator effect of nitroglycerin[178] and reverses the partial tolerance to the coronary vasodilator effect of nitroglycerin.

TABLE 50–6 Recommended Dosing Regimens for Long-Term Nitrate Therapy

Preparation of Agent	Dose	Schedule
Nitroglycerin*		
Ointment	0.5-2 inches	2 or 3 times daily
Buccal or transmucosal	1-3 mg	3 times daily
Transdermal patch	0.2-0.8 mg/hr	q 24 hr; remove at bedtime for 12-14 hr
Sublingual tablet	0.3-0.6 mg	As needed up to 3 doses 5 min apart
Spray	1-2 sprays	As needed up to 3 doses 5 min apart
Oral sustained release	2.5-6.5 mg	2 or 3 times daily†
Isosorbide Dinitrate*		
Oral	10-40 mg	2 or 3 times daily
Oral sustained release	80-120 mg	1 or 2 times daily (eccentric schedule)
Isosorbide 5-Mononitrate		
Oral	20 mg	2 times daily (given 7-8 hr apart)
Oral sustained release	30-240 mg	Once daily

*A 10- to 12-hour nitrate-free interval is recommended.
†Very limited data available on efficacy.

Types of Preparations and Routes of Administration (Table 50–6)

Nitroglycerin administered sublingually remains the drug of choice for the treatment of acute angina episodes and for the prevention of angina. Because sublingual administration avoids first-pass hepatic metabolism, a transient but effective concentration of the drug rapidly appears in the circulation. The half-life of nitroglycerin itself is brief, and it is rapidly converted to two inactive metabolites, both of which are found in the urine. Within 30 to 60 minutes, hepatic breakdown has abolished the hemodynamic and clinical effects. The usual sublingual dose is 0.3 to 0.6 mg, and most patients respond within 5 minutes to one or two 0.3-mg tablets. If symptoms are not relieved by a single dose, additional doses of 0.3 mg may be taken at 5-minute intervals, but no more than 1.2 mg should be used within a 15-minute period. The development of tolerance (see later) is rarely a problem with intermittent use. Sublingual nitroglycerin is especially useful when it is taken prophylactically shortly before undertaking physical activities that are likely to cause angina. When used for this purpose, it may prevent angina for up to 40 minutes.

ADVERSE REACTIONS. Adverse reactions are common and include headache, flushing, and hypotension. The last is rarely severe, but in some patients with volume depletion and in an upright posture, nitrate-induced hypotension is accompanied by a paradoxical bradycardia, consistent with a vasovagal or vasodepressor response. This reaction is more common in the elderly, who are less able to tolerate hypovolemia. Administration of nitrates before or soon after a meal, particularly in patients with a tendency toward postprandial hypotension, may augment venous pooling, preload reduction, and the extent of the fall in blood pressure after the meal. In addition, the partial pressure of O_2 in arterial blood may fall after large doses of nitroglycerin because of a ventilation-perfusion imbalance caused by inability of the pulmonary vascular bed to constrict in areas of alveolar hypoxia, thereby leading to perfusion of less hypoxic tissues. Methemoglobinemia is a rare complication of very large doses of nitrates; commonly used doses of nitrates cause small elevations of methemoglobin that are probably not of clinical significance.

PREPARATIONS (see Table 50–6)

Nitroglycerin Tablets. Nitroglycerin tablets tend to lose their potency, especially if exposed to light, and should thus be kept in dark containers. Other nitrate preparations are available in sublingual, buccal, oral, spray, and ointment forms. An oral nitroglycerin spray that dispenses metered, aerosolized doses of 0.4 mg may be better absorbed than the sublingual form in patients with dry mucosal membranes.[179] It can also be quickly sprayed onto or under the tongue. For prophylaxis, the spray should be used 5 to 10 minutes before angina-provoking activities.

Isosorbide Dinitrate. This drug is an effective antianginal agent but has low bioavailability after oral administration. It undergoes hepatic metabolism rapidly, and marked variation in plasma concentrations may be seen after oral administration. It has two metabolites (one has potent vasodilator action) that are cleared less rapidly than the parent drug and excreted unchanged in the urine. It is available in tablets for sublingual use, in chewable form, in tablets for oral use, and in sustained-release capsules.

Partial or complete nitrate tolerance (see later) develops with regimens of isosorbide dinitrate when it is administered as 30 mg three or four times daily.[180] A dosage schedule should be adopted that allows a 10- to 12-hour nitrate-free interval. If the drug is administered on a three-times-daily schedule (e.g., at 8 AM, 1 PM, and 6 PM), the antianginal benefit lasts for approximately 6 hours, and the magnitude of the antianginal benefit decreases with each successive dose.[180]

Isosorbide 5-Mononitrate. This active metabolite of the dinitrate is completely bioavailable with oral administration because it does not undergo first-pass hepatic metabolism, and it is efficacious in the treatment of chronic stable angina.[181] Plasma levels of isosorbide 5-mononitrate reach their peak between 30 minutes and 2 hours after ingestion, and the drug has a plasma half-life of 4 to 6 hours. A single 20-mg tablet still exhibits activity 8 hours after administration. Tolerance has not been demonstrated with once-a-day or eccentric dosing intervals but does occur with a twice-daily dosing regimen at 12-hour intervals. The only sustained-release preparation of isosorbide 5-mononitrate is Imdur, which is given once daily in a dose of 30 to 240 mg. Presumably, this preparation avoids tolerance by either providing a sufficiently low nitrate level or a duration of activity of 12 hours or less.

TOPICAL NITROGLYCERIN

Ointment. Nitroglycerin ointment (15 mg/inch) is efficacious when applied (most commonly to the chest) in strips of 0.5 to 2.0 inches. The delay in onset of action is approximately 30 minutes. Because this form of the drug is effective for 4 to 6 hours, it is particularly useful in patients with severe angina or unstable angina who are confined to bed and chair. Nitroglycerin ointment may also be used prophylactically after retiring by patients with nocturnal angina. Skin permeability increases with increased hydration, and absorption is also enhanced if the paste is covered with plastic whose edges are taped to the skin.

Transdermal Patches. Application of silicone gel or polymer matrix impregnated with nitroglycerin results in absorption for 24 to 48 hours at a rate determined by various methods of preparation of the patch, including a semipermeable membrane placed between the drug reservoir and the skin. The release rate of the patches varies from 0.1 to 0.8 mg per hour. Relatively low doses (0.1 to 0.2 mg/hr) may not produce sufficient plasma and tissue concentrations to sustain consistent, effective antianginal effects. Transdermal nitroglycerin therapy has been shown to increase exercise duration and maintain antiischemic effects for 12 hours after patch application throughout 30 days of therapy without significant evidence of nitrate tolerance or rebound phenomena,[182] provided that the patch is not applied for more than 12 out of 24 hours.

NITRATE TOLERANCE

A major problem with the use of nitrates is the development of nitrate tolerance, which has been demonstrated with all forms of nitrate administration delivering continuous, relatively stable blood levels of the drug.[169,180,182] Although nitrate tolerance is rapid in onset, renewed responsiveness is easily established after a short nitrate-free interval. The problem of tolerance applies to all nitrate preparations and is particularly important in patients with chronic stable angina pectoris, as opposed to those receiving short-acting courses of nitrates (e.g., unstable angina and myocardial infarction). Nitrate tolerance appears to be limited to the capacitance and resistance vessels and has not been noted in the large conductance vessels, including the epicardial coronary arteries and radial arteries, despite continuous administration of nitroglycerin for 48 hours.[183]

MECHANISMS. Several mechanisms of nitrate tolerance have been proposed.[169] Accumulating data support the hypothesis that increased generation of vascular superoxide anion ($\cdot O_2^-$) is central to the process.[184] There are multiple possible contributors to generation of oxygen free radicals, including effects of nitroglycerin on endothelial oxide synthase ("NOS uncoupling") and counterregulatory neurohormonal activation. The consequences of increased superoxide anion formation are also multiple and include plausible links to many of the proposed mechanisms of nitrate tolerance: (1) plasma volume expansion and neurohormonal activation; (2) impaired biotransformation of nitrates to NO; and (3) decreased end-organ responsiveness to NO.[184] A secondary implication of these emerging findings is that extended treatment with organic nitrates may have unfavorable consequences (free radical generation, endothelial dysfunction, and sympathetic activation) that could adversely affect long-term clinical outcomes.[184] Such data raise a cautionary note that warrants additional investigation.

MANAGEMENT. The only practical strategy to manage nitrate tolerance is to prevent it by providing a "nitrate-free" interval. The optimal interval is unknown, but with patches or ointment of nitroglycerin or preparations of isosorbide dinitrate or isosorbide 5-mononitrate, a 12-hour off period is recommended. The timing of administration should be adapted to the pattern of nitroglycerin administered by the sublingual route, which does not ordinarily result in tolerance, and even after 2 weeks of therapy, efficacy is not reduced when sublingual nitroglycerin is administered two or three times daily.[185]

NITRATE WITHDRAWAL. A common form of nitrate withdrawal (rebound) is observed in patients whose angina is intensified after discontinuation of large doses of long-acting nitrates.[186] In this situation, patients may also have heightened sensitivity to constrictor stimuli.[187] The potential for rebound can be modified by adjusting the dose and timing of administration in addition to the use of other antianginal drugs.

INTERACTION WITH SILDENAFIL. The combination of nitrates and sildenafil may cause serious, prolonged, and potentially life-threatening hypotension.[188] Nitrate therapy is an absolute contraindication to the use of sildenafil and vice versa. Patients who wish to take sildenafil should be aware of the serious nature of this adverse drug interaction and be warned about taking sildenafil within 24 hours of any nitrate preparation, including short-acting sublingual nitroglycerin tablets.

Beta-adrenoceptor blocking drugs (beta blockers) constitute a cornerstone of therapy for angina pectoris. In addition to their antiischemic properties, beta blockers are effective antihypertensives (see Chap. 38) and antiarrhythmics (see Chap. 30). They have also been shown to reduce mortality and reinfarction in patients after myocardial infarction (see Chap. 47) and to reduce mortality in patients with heart failure (see Chap. 23). This combination of actions makes them extremely useful in the management of chronic stable angina. A number of studies have shown that beta blockers, in doses that are generally well tolerated, reduce the frequency of anginal episodes and raise the anginal threshold, both when given alone and when added to other antianginal agents.

The salutary action of these drugs (which have a chemical structure resembling that of beta-adrenoceptor agonists) depends on their ability to cause competitive inhibition of the effects of neuronally released and circulating catecholamines on beta adrenoceptors (Table 50–7).[189] Beta blockade reduces myocardial O_2 requirements, primarily by slowing the heart rate; the slower heart rate in turn increases the fraction of the cardiac cycle occupied by diastole, with a corresponding increase in the time available for coronary perfusion (Fig. 50–8; see also Table 50–5). These drugs also reduce exercise-induced increases in blood pressure and limit exercise-induced increases in contractility. Thus, beta blockers reduce myocardial O_2 demand primarily during activity or excitement, when surges of increased sympathetic activity occur. In the face of impaired myocardial perfusion, the effects of beta blockers on myocardial O_2 demand may critically and favorably alter the imbalance between supply and demand, thereby resulting in the elimination of ischemia.

Beta blockers may reduce blood flow to most organs by means of the combination of unopposed alpha-adrenergic vasoconstriction and beta$_2$ receptor blockade. Complications are relatively minor, but in patients with peripheral vascular disease, the reduction in blood flow to skeletal muscles with the use of nonselective beta blockers may reduce maximal exercise capacity. In patients with preexisting left ventricular dysfunction, beta blockade may increase ventricular volume and thereby enhance O_2 demand.

Characteristics of Different Beta Blockers (Table 50–8)

SELECTIVITY. Two major subtypes of beta receptors, designated *beta$_1$* and *beta$_2$*, are present in different proportions in different tissues. Beta$_1$ receptors predominate in the heart, and stimulation of these receptors leads to an increase in heart rate, atrioventricular (AV) conduction, and contractility; release of renin from juxtaglomerular cells in the kidneys; and lipolysis in adipocytes. Beta$_2$ stimulation causes bronchodilation, vasodilation, and glycogenolysis. Nonselective beta-blocking drugs (propranolol, nadolol, penbutolol, pindolol, sotalol, timolol, carteolol) block both beta$_1$ and beta$_2$ receptors, whereas cardioselective beta blockers (acebutolol, atenolol, betaxolol, bisoprolol, esmolol, and metoprolol) block beta$_1$ receptors while having less effect on beta$_2$ receptors. Thus, cardioselective beta blockers reduce myocardial O_2 requirements while tending to not block bronchodilation, vasodilation, or glycogenolysis. However, as the doses of these drugs are increased, this cardioselectivity diminishes. Because cardioselectivity is only relative, the use of cardioselective beta blockers in doses sufficient to control angina may still cause bronchoconstriction in some susceptible patients.

Some beta blockers also cause vasodilation. Such drugs include labetalol (an alpha-adrenergic blocking agent and beta$_2$ agonist; see Chap. 38), carvedilol (with alpha- and beta$_1$-blocking activity), and bucindolol (a nonselective beta blocker that causes direct [non-alpha-adrenergic-mediated] vasodilation).[190]

ANTIARRHYTHMIC ACTIONS (see Chap. 30). Beta blockers have antiarrhythmic properties as a direct effect of their ability to block sym-

TABLE 50–7 Physiological Actions of Beta-Adrenergic Receptors

Organ	Receptor Type	Response to Stimulus
Heart		
SA node	Beta$_1$	Increased heart rate
Atria	Beta$_1$	Increased contractility and conduction velocity
AV node	Beta$_1$	Increased automaticity and conduction velocity
His-Purkinje system	Beta$_1$	Increased automaticity and conduction velocity
Ventricles	Beta$_1$	Increased automaticity, contractility, and conduction velocity
Arteries		
Peripheral	Beta$_2$	Dilation
Coronary	Beta$_2$	Dilation
Carotid	Beta$_2$	Dilation
Other	Beta$_1$	Increased insulin release Increased liver and muscle glycogenolysis
Lungs	Beta$_2$	Dilation of bronchi
Uterus	Beta$_2$	Smooth muscle relaxation

AV = atrioventricular; SA = sinoatrial.
From Abrams J: Medical therapy of stable angina pectoris. *In* Beller G, Braunwald E (eds): Chronic Ischemic Heart Disease. Atlas of Heart Disease. Vol 5. Philadelphia, WB Saunders 1995, p 7.19.

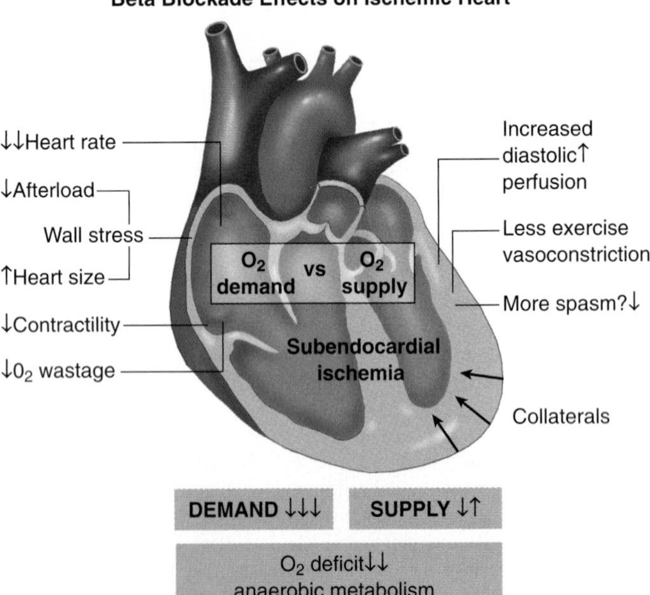

FIGURE 50–8 Effects of beta blockade on the ischemic heart. Beta blockade has a beneficial effect on ischemic myocardium unless (1) the preload rises substantially as in left-sided heart failure or (2) vasospastic angina is present, in which case spasm may be promoted in some patients. Note the proposal that beta blockade diminishes exercise-induced vasoconstriction. (Redrawn from Opie LH: Drugs for the Heart. 4th ed. Philadelphia, WB Saunders, 1995.)

pathoadrenal myocardial stimulation, which in certain situations may be arrhythmogenic.[191] Sotalol has combined class II (beta-blocking) and class III antiarrhythmic activities; it is a potentially attractive drug when it is desired to treat angina and suppress ventricular tachyarrhythmias[192] but should be used with caution in patients with left ventricular dysfunction and left ventricular hypertrophy, and it does have proarrhythmic effects.

INTRINSIC SYMPATHOMIMETIC ACTIVITY. Beta blockers with intrinsic sympathomimetic activity (ISA), such as acebutolol, bucindolol, carteolol, celiprolol, penbutolol, and pindolol, are partial beta agonists that also produce blockade by shielding beta receptors from more potent beta agonists. Pindolol and acebutolol produce low-grade beta stimulation when sympathetic activity is low (at rest), whereas these partial agonists behave more like conventional beta blockers when sympathetic activity is high. Agents with ISA may not be as effective as those without this property in reducing the heart rate or the frequency, duration, and magnitude of ambulatory ST segment changes or in increasing the duration of exercise in patients with severe angina.

POTENCY. Potency can be measured by the ability of beta blockers to inhibit the tachycardia produced by isoproterenol. All drugs are considered in reference to propranolol, which is given a value of 1.0 (see Table 50-8). Timolol and pindolol are the most potent agents, and acebutolol and labetalol are the least potent.

LIPID SOLUBILITY. The hydrophilicity or lipid solubility of beta blockers is a major determination of their absorption and metabolism. The lipid-soluble (lipophilic) beta blockers propranolol, metoprolol, and pindolol are readily absorbed from the gastrointestinal tract, are metabolized predominantly by the liver, have a relatively short half-life, and usually require administration twice or more daily to achieve continuing pharmacological effects. If either metoprolol or propranolol is administered intravenously, a much higher concentration reaches the bloodstream, and therefore intravenous dosing has much greater potency than oral dosing does. The water-soluble (hydrophilic) beta blockers (atenolol, sotalol, and nadolol) are not as readily absorbed from the gastrointestinal tract, are not as extensively metabolized, have relatively long plasma half-lives, and can be administered once daily. Water-soluble beta blockers are generally eliminated unchanged by the kidneys. Lipid-soluble agents are often preferable in patients with significant renal dysfunction for whom clearance of water-soluble agents is reduced. Greater lipid solubility is associated with greater penetration to the central nervous system and may contribute to side effects (e.g., lethargy, depression, and hallucinations) that are not clearly related to beta-blocking activity.

ALPHA-ADRENOCEPTOR BLOCKING ACTIVITY. The alpha-blocking potency of labetalol (approximately one-tenth that of phentolamine) is approximately 20 percent of its beta-blocking potency (see Table 50-8). Labetalol's combined alpha- and beta-blocking effects make it a particularly useful antihypertensive agent (see Chap. 38), and it is especially so in patients with hypertension and angina. The major side effects of labetalol are postural hypotension and retrograde ejaculation. Carvedilol is a newer beta blocker that also possesses alpha-adrenergic blocking activity with an $alpha_1$ to beta-blocking ratio of approximately 1 : 10.[190]

OXIDATION PHENOTYPE. The metabolism of metoprolol, carvedilol, and propranolol may be influenced by genetic polymorphisms or other medications.[193] The oxidative metabolism of metoprolol occurs primarily through the cytochrome P450 enzyme CYP2D6 and exhibits the debrisoquin type of genetic polymorphism; poor hydroxylators or metabolizers ($\leq$10 percent of whites) have significant prolongation of the elimination half-life of the drug in comparison to extensive hydroxylators or metabolizers. Thus, angina might be controlled by a single daily dose of metoprolol in poor metabolizers, whereas extensive metabolizers require the same dose two or three times a day.[194] If a patient exhibits an exaggerated clinical response (e.g., extreme bradycardia) following the administration of metoprolol, propranolol, or other lipid-soluble beta blockers, it may be the result of prolongation of the elimination half-life because of slow oxidative metabolism. Metabolism of metoprolol may also be altered by drugs that interact with CYP2D6.[193,195]

EFFECTS ON SERUM LIPIDS. Beta-blocker therapy (with agents lacking ISA) usually causes no significant changes in total or LDL cholesterol but increases triglycerides and reduces HDL cholesterol.[196] The most commonly studied drug has been propranolol, which can increase plasma triglyceride concentrations by 20 to 50 percent and reduce HDL cholesterol by 10 to 20 percent. Increasing $beta_1$ selectivity is associated with lesser effects on lipids. Adverse effects on the lipid profile may be more frequent with nonselective than with $beta_1$-selective blockers. The effects of these changes in serum lipids by long-term administration of beta blockers must be considered when this therapy is begun or maintained for either hypertension or angina.

DOSAGE. For optimal results, the dosage of a beta blocker should be carefully adjusted. In the case of atenolol, it is useful to start with a dose of 50 mg once daily. The usual effective dose is 50 to 100 mg daily; however, some patients benefit from up to 200 mg daily. In the case of metoprolol, it is often preferable from a perspective of the patient's compliance to use an extended-release formulation, which may be started at a dose of 100 mg once daily. Other beta blockers should be started at comparable doses. Efficacy is determined by the effect on the heart rate and symptoms, and when these are unclear, the effect on exercise performance can be evaluated by treadmill exercise testing. The resting heart rate should be reduced to between 50 and 60 beats/min, and an increase of less than 20 beats/min should occur with modest exercise (e.g., climbing one flight of stairs). Therapy with beta blockers needs to be individualized and requires repeated clinical evaluation during the initial period of drug administration.

ADVERSE EFFECTS AND CONTRAINDICATIONS. Most of the adverse effects of beta blockers occur as a consequence of the known properties of these drugs and include cardiac effects (severe sinus bradycardia, sinus arrest, AV block, reduced left ventricular contractility), bronchoconstriction, fatigue, mental depression, nightmares, gastrointestinal upset, sexual dysfunction, intensification of insulin-induced hypoglycemia, and cutaneous reactions (Table 50–9; see also Table 50–7). Lethargy, weakness, and fatigue may be caused by reduced cardiac output or may arise from a direct effect on the central nervous system.[197] Bronchoconstriction results from blockade of $beta_2$ receptors in the tracheobronchial tree. As a consequence, asthma and chronic obstructive lung disease are relative contraindications to beta blockers, even to $beta_1$-selective agents.

In patients who already have impaired left ventricular function, congestive heart failure may be intensified, an effect that can be counteracted in part by the use of digitalis or diuretics. Beginning therapy with a very low dose (e.g., metoprolol XL, 25 mg daily, for 2 weeks in patients with NYHA functional Class II) and then gradually increasing the dose over the course of several weeks has been shown to be well tolerated and beneficial in patients with idiopathic dilated cardiomyopathy and those with heart failure caused by ischemic heart disease (see Chap. 23).[198] This approach is recommended when using beta blockers in patients with angina and heart failure.

Beta blockers should be prescribed with caution in patients with cardiac conduction disease involving either the sinus node or the AV conduction system. In patients with symptomatic conduction disease, beta blockers are contraindicated unless a pacemaker is in place. In patients with asymptomatic sinus node dysfunction or first-degree AV block, beta blockers may be tolerated, but their administration requires careful observation. Pindolol, because of its ISA activity, may be preferable in this situation. Blockade of noncardiac $beta_2$ receptors inhibits catecholamine-induced glycogenolysis, so noncardioselective beta blockers can impair the defense to insulin-induced hypoglycemia. Blockade of $beta_2$ receptors also inhibits the vasodilating effects of catecholamines in peripheral blood vessels and leaves the constrictor (alpha-adrenergic) receptors unopposed, thereby enhancing vasoconstriction. Noncardioselective beta blockers may precipitate episodes of Raynaud phenomenon in patients with this condition and may cause uncomfortable coldness in the distal extremities. Reduced flow to the limbs may occur in patients with peripheral vascular disease.

Abrupt withdrawal of beta-adrenoceptor blocking agents after prolonged administration can result in increased total ischemic activity in patients with chronic stable angina. This increased ischemia may be caused by a return to the previously high levels of myocardial O_2 demand while the under-

TABLE 50–8 Pharmacokinetics and Pharmacology of Some Beta-Adrenoceptor Blockers

Characteristic	Atenolol	Metoprolol/XL	Nadolol	Pindolol	Propranolol/LA	Timolol
Extent of absorption (%)	~50	>95	~30	>90	>90	>90
Extent of bioavailability (% of dose)	~40	~50/77	~30	~90	~30/20	75
Beta-blocking plasma concentration	0.2-0.5 μg/ml	50-100 ng/ml	50-100 ng/ml	50-100 ng/ml	50-100 ng/ml	50-100 ng/ml
Protein binding (%)	<5	12	~30	57	93	~10
Lipophilicity*	Low	Moderate	Low	Moderate	High	Low
Elimination half-life (hr)	6-9	3-7	14-25	3-4	3.5 to 6/8-11	3-4
Drug accumulation in renal disease	Yes	No	Yes	No	No	No
Route of elimination	RE (mostly unchanged)	HM	RE	RE (40% unchanged and HM)	HM	RE (20% unchanged and HM)
Beta-blocker potency ratio (propranolol = 1)	1.0	1	1.0	6.0	1	6.0
Adrenergic-receptor blocking activity	β_1¶	β_1¶	β_1/β_2	β_1/β_2	β_1/β_2	β_1/β_2
Intrinsic sympathetic activity	0	0	0	+	0	0
Membrane-stabilizing activity	0	0	0	+	++	0
Usual maintenance dose	50-100 mg/d	50-100 mg b.i.d.–q.i.d./50-400 mg/d	40-80 mg/d	10-40 mg/d (b.i.d.–t.i.d.)	80-320 mg/d (b.i.d.–t.i.d.)/ 80-160 mg/d	10-30 mg b.i.d.
FDA-approved indications						
Hypertension	Yes	Yes/Yes	Yes	Yes	Yes/Yes	Yes
Angina	Yes	Yes/Yes	Yes	No	Yes/Yes	No
Post MI	Yes	Yes/No	No	No	Yes/No	Yes
Heart failure	No	Yes/Yes	No	No	No/No	No

FDA = Food and Drug Administration; HM = hepatic metabolism; ND = no data; RE = renal excretion; MI = myocardial infarction.
*Determined by the distribution ratio between octanol and water.
†Half-life of the active metabolite, diacetolol, is 12 to 15 hours.
‡Acebutolol is mainly eliminated by the liver, but its major metabolite, diacetolol, is excreted by the kidney.
§Rapid metabolism by esterases in the cytosol of red blood cells.
¶Beta$_1$ selectivity is maintained at lower doses, but beta$_2$ receptors are inhibited at higher doses.

lying atherosclerotic process has progressed,[199] but a rebound phenomenon resulting in increased beta-adrenergic sensitivity probably occurs in some patients. Occasionally, such withdrawal can precipitate unstable angina and may in rare cases even provoke myocardial infarction. Chronic beta-blocker therapy can be safely discontinued by slowly withdrawing the drug in a stepwise manner over the course of 2 to 3 weeks. If abrupt withdrawal of beta blockers is required, patients should be instructed to reduce exertion and manage angina episodes with sublingual nitroglycerin and/or substitute a calcium antagonist.

Calcium Antagonists (see Chap. 38)

The critical role of calcium ions in the normal contraction of cardiac and vascular smooth muscle is discussed in Chapter 19. Calcium antagonists are a heterogeneous group of compounds that inhibit calcium ion movement through slow channels in cardiac and smooth muscle membranes by noncompetitive blockade of voltage-sensitive L-type calcium channels (see Fig. 19–8).[200,201] The three major classes of calcium antagonists are the dihydropyridines (nifedipine is the prototype), the phenylalkylamines (verapamil is the prototype), and the modified benzothiazepines (diltiazem is the prototype). Amlodipine and felodipine are additional dihydropyridines that are among the most commonly used calcium antagonists in the United States. The two predominant effects of calcium antagonists result from blocking the entry of calcium ions and slowing recovery of the channel. Phenylalkylamines have a marked effect on recovery of the channel and thereby exert depressant effects on cardiac pacemakers and conduction, whereas dihydropyridines, which do not impair channel recovery, have little effect on the conduction system.

MECHANISM OF ACTION. The efficacy of calcium antagonists in patients with angina pectoris is related to the reduction in myocardial O_2 demand and the increase in O_2 supply that they induce (see Table 50–5).[200] The latter effect is particularly important in patients with conditions in which a prominent vasospastic or vasoconstrictor component may be present, such as Prinzmetal (variant) angina (see Chap. 49), variable-threshold angina, and angina related to impaired

Acebutolol	Labetalol	Bisoprolol	Betaxolol	Carteolol	Penbutolol	Carvedilol	Esmolol (IV)	Sotalol
~70	>90	>90	>90	>90	100	ND	ND	ND
~50	~25	80	90	85	100	~30	100	>90
0.2-2.0 μg/ml	0.7-3.0 μg/ml	0.01-0.1 μg/ml	20-50 ng/ml	40-160 ng/ml	ND	ND	0.15-2.0 μg/ml	ND
30-40	~50	30	50-60	23-30	80-98	95-98	55	0
Low	Low	Moderate	Moderate	Low	High	High	Low	Low
3-4[†]	~6	7-15	12-22	5-7	17-26	6-10	4.5 min	12
Yes[‡]	No	Yes	Yes	Yes	Yes	No	No	Yes
HM[‡]	HM	HM 50% RE 50%	HM	RE	HM	HM	[§]	RE
0.3	0.3	10	4	10	1	10	0.02	0.3
β_1[¶]	$\beta_1/\beta_2/\alpha_1$	β_1[¶]	β_1[¶]	β_1/β_2	β_1/β_2	$\beta_1/\beta_2/\alpha_1$	β_1[¶]	β_1/β_2
+	0	0	0	+	+	0	0	0
+	0	0	0	0	0	+	0	0
200-600 mg b.i.d.	100-400 mg b.i.d.	5-20 mg/d	5-20 mg/d	2.5-10 mg/d	10-40 mg/d	3.125-50 mg/ b.i.d.	Bolus of 500 μg/kg; infusion at 50-200 μg/kg/min	80-160 mg b.i.d.
Yes	Yes	Yes	Yes	Yes	Yes	Yes	Yes	No
No	No	No	No	No	No	No	No	No
No	No	No	No	No	No	No	Yes	No
No	No	No	No	No	No	Yes	No	No

vasodilator reserve of small coronary arteries.[202] Calcium antagonists may be effective on their own or in combination with beta-adrenoceptor blockers and nitrates in patients with chronic stable angina.[200] Several calcium antagonists are effective for the treatment of angina pectoris (Table 50–10). Each relaxes vascular smooth muscle in both the systemic arterial and coronary arterial beds. In addition, blockade of the entry of calcium into myocytes results in a negative inotropic effect, which is counteracted to some extent by peripheral vascular dilation and by activation of the sympathetic nervous system in response to drug-induced hypotension.[203] However, the negative inotropic effect must be taken into consideration in patients with significant left ventricular dysfunction.

With a rapid onset of action and metabolism by the liver, calcium antagonists have a limited bioavailability of between 13 and 52 percent and a half-life of between 3 and 12 hours. Amlodipine and felodipine are exceptions in that both drugs have long half-lives and may be administered once daily. In the case of some of the other calcium antagonists (e.g., nifedipine and diltiazem), sustained-release preparations have been shown to be effective.

ANTIATHEROGENIC ACTION. Hyperlipidemia-induced changes in the permeability of smooth muscle cells to calcium may play a role in atherogenesis; thus, the hypothesis that calcium antagonists might inhibit atherogenesis has been explored since the 1970s but not yet achieved consensus.[204] Studies of first-generation calcium antagonists showed mixed results with respect to lesion progression. Subsequent experimental work with more lipophilic second-generation calcium-channel blockers such as amlodipine have demonstrated inhibition of smooth muscle cell proliferation, migration, and ameliorated unfavorable membrane alterations.[205] In a randomized trial among patients with established CAD, treatment with amlodipine, compared with placebo, was associated with less progression of carotid atherosclerosis measured by intimal-medial thickness; however, no difference was detected in the progression of coronary atherosclerosis.[206] The role of calcium antagonists in atheroprotection is the subject of ongoing study.

First-Generation Calcium Antagonists

NIFEDIPINE. This dihydropyridine is a particularly effective dilator of vascular smooth muscle and is a more potent vasodilator than either diltiazem or verapamil. Although its in vitro actions on myocardium and specialized cardiac tissue are similar to those of other agents, the concentration required to reproduce effects on these tissues is not reached in vivo because of the early appearance of its powerful vasodilating effects. Thus, in clinical practice, the potential negative chronotropic, inotropic, and dromotropic (on AV conduction) effects of nifedipine are seldom a problem, with the exception that nifedipine has been reported to worsen heart failure in patients with preexisting chronic congestive heart failure.[207]

TABLE 50–9 Candidates for Use of Beta-Blocking Agents for Angina

Ideal Candidates
Prominent relationship of physical activity to attacks of angina
Coexistent hypertension
History of supraventricular or ventricular arrhythmias
Previous myocardial infarction
Left ventricular systolic dysfunction
Mild to moderate heart failure symptoms (NYHA functional Classes II, III)
Prominent anxiety state

Poor Candidates
Asthma or reversible airway component in chronic lung disease patients
Severe left ventricular dysfunction with severe heart failure symptoms (NYHA functional Class IV)
History of severe depression
Raynaud phenomenon
Symptomatic peripheral vascular disease
Severe bradycardia or heart block
Brittle diabetes

NYHA = New York Heart Association.
Modified from Abrams JA: Medical therapy of stable angina pectoris. *In* Beller G: Chronic Ischemic Heart Disease. *In* Braunwald E (ed): Atlas of Heart Disease. Vol 5. Philadelphia, WB Saunders, 1995, p 7.22.

The beneficial effects of nifedipine in the treatment of angina result from its capacity to reduce myocardial O_2 requirements because of its afterload-reducing effect and to increase myocardial O_2 delivery as a result of its dilating action on the coronary vascular bed (see Table 50–5). Oral nifedipine in capsule form exerts hypotensive effects within 20 minutes of administration. This immediate-release formulation is no longer recommended because of concerns regarding adverse events.[208] An extended-release formulation using the gastrointestinal therapeutic system of drug delivery (see Table 50–10) is designed to deliver 30, 60, or 90 mg of nifedipine in a single daily dose at a relatively constant rate over a 24-hour period and is useful for the treatment of chronic stable angina, Prinzmetal angina, and hypertension. Steady-state plasma levels are typically achieved within 48 hours of initiation. The efficacy of the extended-release preparation, either alone or in conjunction with beta blockers, in reducing episodes of angina and ischemia on ambulatory monitoring has been documented.[209]

Adverse Effects. These occur in 15 to 20 percent of patients and require discontinuation of medication in about 5 percent. Most adverse effects are related to systemic vasodilation and include headache, dizziness, palpitations, flushing, hypotension, and leg edema (unrelated to heart failure). Gastrointestinal side effects, including nausea, epigastric pressure, and vomiting, are noted in approximately 5 percent of patients. In rare instances, in patients with extremely severe, fixed coronary obstructions, nifedipine aggravates angina, presumably by lowering arterial pressure excessively, with subsequent reflex tachycardia. For this reason, combined treatment of angina with nifedipine and a beta blocker is particularly effective and superior to nifedipine alone.[209] Most of the adverse effects are reduced by the use of extended-release preparations.

TABLE 50–10 Pharmacokinetics of Calcium Antagonists Used Commonly for Angina Pectoris

Characteristic	Diltiazem/SR		Nicardipine	Nifedipine/SR	
Usual adult dose	IV: 0.25 mg/kg bolus, then 5-15 mg/hr Oral: 30-90 mg t.i.d.–q.i.d. SR: 60-180 mg b.i.d. CD: 120-480 mg/d		IV: 3-15 mg/hr Oral: 20-40 mg t.i.d. SR: 30-60 mg b.i.d.	Oral: 10-30 mg t.i.d. SR: 90 mg/d	
Extent of absorption (%)	80-90		100	90	
Extent of bioavailability (%)	40-70		30	65-75/86	
Onset of action	IV: 3 min Oral: 30-60 min		IV: 1 min Oral: 20 min	20 min	
Time to peak serum concentration (hr)	2-3/6-11		0.5-2.0	0.5/6	
Therapeutic serum levels (ng/ml)	50-200		30-50	25-100	
Elimination half-life (hr)	3.5/5-7		2.0-4.0	2.0-5.0	
Elimination	60% metabolized by liver; remainder excreted by kidneys		High first-pass hepatic metabolism	High first-pass hepatic metabolism	
Heart rate	↓		↑	↑↑	
Peripheral vascular resistance	↓		↓↓↓	↓↓↓	
FDA-approved indications	IR	SR		IR	SR
Hypertension	No	Yes	Yes†	No	Yes
Angina	Yes	Yes	Yes	Yes	Yes
Coronary spasm	Yes	No	No	Yes	Yes

CD = combination drug; CR = controlled release; FDA = Food and Drug Administration; IR = immediate release; ND = no data; SR = sustained release.
*Half-life of 4.5 to 12 hours with multiple dosing; may be prolonged in the elderly.
†The sustained-release formulation may preferred for hypertension.

Several clinical case-control studies of hypertension and associated reviews have suggested that *short-acting nifedipine* may cause an increase in mortality.[208] No firm data indicate that this risk applies to extended-release nifedipine or to other calcium antagonists. Although insufficient data are available to assess the long-term risks (if any) of calcium antagonists in chronic CAD, *long-acting nifedipine* should be considered an effective and safe antianginal drug for the treatment of symptomatic patients with chronic CAD who are already receiving beta blockers, with or without nitrates. Short-acting nifedipine should ordinarily be avoided.

Because of its potent vasodilator effects, nifedipine is contraindicated in patients who are hypotensive or have severe aortic valve stenosis and in patients with unstable angina who are not simultaneously receiving a beta blocker and in whom reflex-mediated increases in the heart rate may be harmful. Nifedipine (or one of the second-generation dihydropyridines) is the calcium antagonist of choice in patients with sinus bradycardia, sick sinus syndrome, or AV block (particularly if a beta-adrenoceptor blocking agent is administered concurrently and additional drug therapy for angina is indicated). This recommendation is based on the observation that in doses used clinically, nifedipine has fewer negative effects on myocardial contractility, heart rate, and AV conduction than verapamil or diltiazem.[207]

Nifedipine interacts significantly with prazosin (resulting in excessive hypotension), cimetidine, and phenytoin (resulting in increased bioavailability of nifedipine). In patients with Prinzmetal angina, abrupt cessation of nifedipine therapy may result in a rebound increase in the frequency and duration of attacks (see Chap. 49).

VERAPAMIL. Verapamil dilates systemic and coronary resistance vessels and large coronary conductance vessels. It slows the heart rate and reduces myocardial contractility. This combination of actions results in a reduction in myocardial O_2 requirement, which is the basis for the drug's efficacy in the management of chronic stable angina.

Verapamil reduces the frequency of angina and prolongs exercise tolerance in patients with symptomatic chronic CAD, and the combination of verapamil and a beta blocker provides clinical benefit that is additive.[210] When evaluated in the International Verapamil-Trandolapril Study (INVEST), a strategy combining sustained-release verapamil and trandolapril compared to atenolol and a diuretic for the treatment of patients with hypertension and CAD showed equivalent outcomes with respect to death, MI, or stroke.[210a] Despite the marked negative inotropic effects of verapamil in isolated cardiac muscle preparations, changes in contractility are modest in patients with normal cardiac function. However, in patients with cardiac dysfunction, verapamil may reduce cardiac output, increase left ventricular filling pressure, and cause clinical heart failure. In clinically useful doses, verapamil inhibits calcium influx into specialized cardiac cells, sometimes causing slowing of the heart rate and AV conduction. Therefore, it is contraindicated in patients with preexisting AV nodal disease or sick sinus syndrome, congestive heart failure, and suspected digitalis or quinidine toxicity.

The usual starting dose of verapamil for oral administration is 40 to 80 mg three times daily to a maximal dose of 480 mg daily (see Table 50-10). Sustained-release preparations of verapamil are available, and starting doses are 120 to 240 mg twice daily with a usual optimal dose range of 240 to 360 mg daily.

Verapamil interacts significantly with several other drugs. *Intravenous* verapamil should generally not be used together with a beta blocker (given intravenously or orally), nor should a beta blocker be administered *intravenously* in patients receiving oral verapamil. Both drugs can be administered orally but with caution in view of the potential for bradyarrhythmias and negative inotropic effects. The

Verapamil/SR		Amlodipine	Felodipine	Isradipine	Nisoldipine
IV: 0.075-0.15 mg/kg Oral: 80-120 mg t.i.d.–q.i.d. SR: 180-480 mg/d		Oral 2.5-10 mg/d	Oral SR: 2.5-10 mg/d	Oral CR: 2.5-10 mg b.i.d.	Oral SR: 10-40 mg/d
90		>90	>90	>90	ND
20-35		60-90	20	25	5
IV: 2-5 min Oral: 30 min		0.5-1.0 hr	2 hr	20 min	1-3 hr
IV: 3-5 min Oral: 1-2 SR: 7-9		6-12	2-5	1.5	6-12
80-300		5-20	1-5	2-10	ND
3.0-7.0*		30-50	11-16	8	7-12
85% eliminated by first-pass hepatic metabolism		Hepatic	High first-pass hepatic metabolism	High first-pass hepatic metabolism	Hepatic
↓		0	↑	0	0
↓↓		↓↓↓	↓↓↓	↓↓↓	↓↓↓
IR	SR				
Yes	Yes	Yes	Yes	Yes	Yes
Yes	No	Yes	No	No	Yes
Yes	No	Yes	No	No	No

bioavailability of verapamil is increased by cimetidine and carbamazepine, whereas verapamil may increase plasma levels of cyclosporine and digoxin and may be associated with excessive hypotension in patients receiving quinidine or prazosin. Hepatic enzyme inducers such as phenobarbital may reduce the effects of verapamil. Verapamil should not be administered in conjunction with the antiarrhythmic drug dofetilide.

Adverse effects of verapamil are noted in approximately 10 percent of patients and relate to systemic vasodilation (hypotension and facial flushing), gastrointestinal symptoms (constipation and nausea), and central nervous system reactions such as headache and dizziness. A rare side effect is gingival hyperplasia, which appears after 1 to 9 months of therapy.

DILTIAZEM. Diltiazem's actions are intermediate between those of nifedipine and verapamil. In clinically useful doses, its vasodilator effects are less profound than those of nifedipine, and its cardiac depressant action (on the sinoatrial and AV nodes and myocardium) is less than that of verapamil. This profile may explain the remarkably low incidence of adverse effects of diltiazem. Diltiazem is a systemic vasodilator that lowers arterial pressure at rest and during exertion and increases the workload required to produce myocardial ischemia, but it may also increase myocardial O_2 delivery. Although this drug causes little vasodilation of epicardial coronary arteries under basal conditions, it may enhance perfusion of the subendocardium distal to a flow-limiting coronary stenosis; it also blocks exercise-induced coronary vasoconstriction. In patients with chronic stable angina receiving maximally tolerated doses of diltiazem, the heart rate is significantly reduced at rest, but no effect on peak blood pressure is achieved during exercise, and the duration of symptom-limited treadmill exercise is prolonged.

Several sustained-release formulations of diltiazem are available for once-daily treatment of systemic hypertension and angina pectoris.[211] The usual starting dose of sustained-release formulations is 120 mg once daily up to a typical maintenance dose of 180 to 360 mg once daily. The maximum effect on blood pressure may not be observed until 14 days after starting therapy.

Diltiazem is a highly effective antianginal agent. Atenolol and diltiazem have similar efficacy in increasing nonischemic exercise duration in patients with variable-threshold angina and act primarily by slowing the resting heart rate.[212] High doses (mean dose, 340 mg) have been shown to be a relatively safe addition to maximally tolerated doses of isosorbide dinitrate and a beta blocker and cause increases in exercise tolerance and resting and exercise left ventricular ejection fraction.[211] Major side effects are similar to those of the other calcium channel blockers and are related to vasodilation, but they are relatively infrequent, particularly if the dose does not exceed 240 mg daily. As is the case with verapamil, diltiazem should be prescribed with caution for patients with sick sinus syndrome or AV block. In patients with preexisting left ventricular dysfunction, diltiazem may exacerbate or precipitate heart failure.

Diltiazem interacts with other drugs, including beta-adrenergic blocking agents (causing enhanced negative inotropic, chronotropic, and dromotropic effects), flecainide, and cimetidine (which increases the bioavailability of diltiazem), and diltiazem has been associated with increased plasma levels of cyclosporine, carbamazepine, and lithium carbonate. Diltiazem may cause excessive sinus node depression if administered with disopyramide and may reduce digoxin clearance, especially in patients with renal failure.

Second-Generation Calcium Antagonists

The second-generation calcium antagonists (nicardipine, isradipine, amlodipine, and felodipine) are mainly dihydropyridine derivatives, with nifedipine being the prototypical agent. Considerable experience has also accumulated with nimodipine, nisoldipine, and nitrendipine. These agents differ in potency, tissue specificity, and pharmacokinetics and, in general, are potent vasodilators because of greater vascular selectivity than seen with the first-generation antagonists (i.e., verapamil, nifedipine, and diltiazem).

AMLODIPINE. This agent, which is less lipid soluble than nifedipine, has a slow, smooth onset and ultra-long duration of action (plasma half-life of 36 hours). It causes marked coronary and peripheral dilation and may be useful in the treatment of patients with angina accompanied by hypertension. It may be used as a once-daily hypotensive or antianginal agent.[213] In a series of randomized, placebo-controlled studies in patients with stable exercise-induced angina pectoris, amlodipine was shown to be effective and well tolerated.[214] In two trials among patients with established CAD, amlodipine reduced the risk of major cardiovascular events.[206,214a] Amlodipine has little, if any, negative inotropic action and may be especially useful in patients with chronic angina and left ventricular dysfunction.[215]

The usual dose of amlodipine is 5 to 10 mg once daily. Downward adjustment of the starting dose is appropriate among patients with liver disease and the elderly. Significant changes in blood pressure are typically not evident until 24 to 48 hours after initiation. Steady-state serum levels are achieved at 7 to 8 days.

NICARDIPINE. This drug has a half-life similar to that of nifedipine (2 to 4 hours), but it appears to have greater vascular selectivity. Nicardipine may be used as an antianginal and antihypertensive agent and requires three-times-daily administration, although a sustained-release formulation is available for twice-daily dosing in hypertension. For chronic stable angina pectoris, it appears to be as effective as verapamil or diltiazem, and its efficacy is enhanced when combined with a beta blocker.

FELODIPINE AND ISRADIPINE. In the United States, both drugs are approved by the U.S. Food and Drug Administration (FDA) for the treatment of hypertension but not for angina pectoris. A recent study documented similar efficacy between felodipine and nifedipine in patients with chronic stable angina.[216] Felodipine has also been reported to be more vascular selective than nifedipine and to have a mild positive inotropic effect as a result of calcium-channel agonist properties. Isradipine has a longer half-life than nifedipine and demonstrates greater vascular sensitivity.

OTHER PHARMACOLOGICAL AGENTS

NICORANDIL.* Nicorandil is a nicotinamide ester that dilates peripheral and coronary resistance vessels via action on ATP-sensitive potassium channels and possesses a nitrate moiety that promotes systemic venous and coronary vasodilation. As a result of these dual actions, nicorandil reduces preload and afterload and results in an increase in coronary blood flow. In addition to these effects, nicorandil may have cardioprotective actions mediated through activation of potassium channels.[217]

Nicorandil has antianginal efficacy similar to beta blockers, nitrates, and calcium-channel blockers. In a recent randomized clinical trial (N = 5126), nicorandil reduced the risk of cardiac death, myocardial infarction, or hospital admission for angina (hazard ratio 0.83; $p = 0.014$) compared with placebo when added to standard antianginal therapy.[218]

METABOLIC AGENTS.† Agents aimed at increasing the metabolic efficiency of cardiac myocytes have also been studied in patients with chronic stable angina. Partial inhibitors of fatty acid oxidation appear to shift myocardial metabolism to more oxygen-efficient pathways.[219] Trimetazidine and ranolazine are agents that have been shown to inhibit fatty acid oxidation and to reduce the frequency of angina without hemodynamic effects among patients with chronic stable angina. When eval-

*This drug has not been approved by the FDA at the time of this writing.

†These agents have not been approved by the FDA at the time of this writing.

uated in patients with chronic stable angina ($N = 823$) taking standard doses of atenolol, amlodipine, or diltiazem, the addition of ranolazine administered twice daily increased exericise duration on treadmill testing and reduced the frequency of angina and use of nitroglycerin.[219a]

Selection of Pharmacologic Therapy for Angina Pectoris

RELATIVE ADVANTAGES OF BETA BLOCKERS AND CALCIUM ANTAGONISTS (Table 50–11). The choice between a beta blocker and a calcium-channel antagonist as initial therapy in patients with chronic stable angina is controversial because both classes of agents are effective in relieving symptoms and reducing ischemia.[18] Trials comparing beta blockers and calcium antagonists have not shown any difference in the rate of death or myocardial infarction,[18] although in some studies beta blockers appeared to have greater clinical efficacy,[220-222] and less frequent discontinuation due to side effects.[223] Because long-term administration of beta blockers has been demonstrated to prolong life in patients after acute myocardial infarction and in the treatment of hypertension, it is reasonable to consider beta blockers over calcium antagonists as the agents of choice in treating patients with chronic stable angina.[18] However, it must be recognized that beta blockers (without ISA) increase serum triglycerides and decrease HDL cholesterol with uncertain long-term consequences. In addition, these drugs may produce fatigue, depression, and sexual dysfunction. In contrast, although calcium antagonists do not show these adverse effects, their long-term administration has *not* been shown to improve long-term survival after acute myocardial infarction.[224] However, diltiazem is apparently effective in preventing severe angina and early reinfarction after non-Q-wave infarction.[225] Verapamil reduces reinfarction rates in patients post-MI[266] and, when combined with trandolapril, achieves similar outcomes to atenolol together with a diuretic for the treatment of patients with hypertension and CAD.[210a]

TABLE 50–11 Recommended Drug Therapy* (Calcium Antagonist vs. Beta Blocker) in Patients Who Have Angina in Conjunction with Other Medical Conditions

Clinical Condition	Recommended Drug
Cardiac Arrhythmia or Conduction Disturbance	
Sinus bradycardia	Nifedipine or amlodipine
Sinus tachycardia (not caused by cardiac failure)	Beta blocker
Supraventricular tachycardia	Beta blocker (verapamil)
Atrioventricular block	Nifedipine or amlodipine
Rapid atrial fibrillation	Verapamil or beta blocker
Ventricular arrhythmia	Beta blocker
Left Ventricular Dysfunction	
Heart failure	Beta blocker
Miscellaneous Medical Conditions	
Systemic hypertension	Beta blocker (calcium antagonist)
Severe preexisting headaches	Beta blocker (verapamil or diltiazem)
COPD with bronchospasm or asthma	Nifedipine, amlodipine, verapamil, or diltiazem
Hyperthyroidism	Beta blocker
Raynaud syndrome	Nifedipine or amlodipine
Claudication	Calcium antagonist
Severe depression	Calcium antagonist

COPD = chronic obstructive pulmonary disease.
*Alternatives in parentheses.

The choice of drug with which to initiate therapy is influenced by a number of clinical factors (see Table 50-11),[18] as discussed in the following:

1. Calcium antagonists are the preferred agents in patients with a history of asthma, chronic obstructive lung disease, and/or wheezing on clinical examination, in whom beta blockers, even relatively selective agents, are contraindicated.
2. Nifedipine (long acting), amlodipine, and nicardipine are the calcium antagonists of choice in patients with chronic stable angina and sick sinus syndrome, sinus bradycardia, or significant AV conduction disturbances, whereas beta blockers and verapamil should be used only with great caution in such patients. In patients with symptomatic conduction disease, neither a beta blocker nor a calcium-channel blocker should be used unless a pacemaker is in place. If a beta blocker is required in patients with asymptomatic evidence of conduction disease, pindolol, which has the greatest ISA, is useful. In the case of calcium-channel blockers in patients with conduction system disease, nifedipine or nicardipine is preferable to verapamil and diltiazem, but careful observation for deterioration of conduction is mandatory.
3. Calcium antagonists are clearly preferred in patients with suspected Prinzmetal (variant) angina (see Chap. 49); beta blockers may even aggravate angina under these circumstances.
4. Calcium antagonists may be preferred over beta blockers in patients with significant, symptomatic peripheral arterial disease because the latter may cause peripheral vasoconstriction.
5. Beta blockers should usually be avoided in patients with a history of significant depressive illness and should be prescribed cautiously for patients with sexual dysfunction, sleep disturbance, nightmares, fatigue, or lethargy.
6. The presence of moderate to severe left ventricular dysfunction in patients with angina limits the therapeutic options. The beneficial effects of beta blockers on survival in patients with left ventricular dysfunction after myocardial infarction,[154] coupled with their beneficial effects on survival and left ventricular performance in patients with heart failure,[227] has established beta blockers as the drug class of choice for the treatment of angina in patients with left ventricular dysfunction, with or without symptoms of heart failure, together with ACE inhibitors, diuretics, and digitalis. If angina persists despite beta blockade and nitrates, amlodipine can be administered.[215] Verapamil, nifedipine, and diltiazem should be avoided.
7. Short-acting nifedipine should not be used because the reflex-mediated tachycardia may aggravate ischemia.
8. Hypertensive patients with angina pectoris do well with either beta blockers or calcium antagonists because both agents have antihypertensive effects. However, beta blockers are the preferred initial agent for treating angina in such patients, as noted earlier, and an ACE inhibitor should be strongly considered for all patients with CAD with hypertension.[149]

COMBINATION THERAPY. The combination of a beta blocker, calcium antagonist, and long-acting nitrate is widely used in the management of chronic stable angina.[222] When adrenergic blockers and calcium antagonists are used together in the treatment of angina pectoris, several issues should be considered, as follows:

1. The addition of a beta blocker enhances the clinical effect of nifedipine and other dihydropyridines.
2. In patients with moderate or severe left ventricular dysfunction, sinus bradycardia, or AV conduction

disturbances, combination therapy with calcium antagonists and beta blockers either should be avoided or should be initiated with caution. In patients with AV conduction system disease, the preferred combination is a long-acting dihydropyridine and a beta blocker. The negative inotropic effects of calcium antagonists are not usually a problem in combined therapy with low doses of beta blockers but can become significant with higher doses. With such doses, amlodipine is the calcium antagonist of choice, but it should be used cautiously.

3. The combination of a dihydropyridine and a long-acting nitrate (without a beta blocker) is not an optimal combination because both are vasodilators.

Approach to Patients with Chronic Stable Angina

1. Identify and treat precipitating factors, such as anemia, uncontrolled hypertension, thyrotoxicosis, tachyarrhythmias, uncontrolled congestive heart failure, and concomitant valvular heart disease.
2. Initiate risk factor modification, physical exercise, diet, and life-style counseling. Initiate therapy with an HMG-CoA reductase inhibitor, as needed, to reduce LDL cholesterol to at least below 100 mg/dl.
3. Initiate pharmacotherapy with aspirin and a beta blocker. Strongly consider an ACE inhibitor as first-line therapy in all patients with chronic CAD.
4. Use sublingual nitroglycerin for alleviation of symptoms and for prophylaxis.
5. If angina occurs more than two or three times per week, the next step is addition of a calcium antagonist or a long-acting nitrate via dosing schedules to prevent nitrate tolerance. The decision to add a calcium antagonist or a long-acting nitrate is not based entirely on the frequency and severity of symptoms. The need to treat concomitant hypertension or the presence of left ventricular dysfunction and symptoms of heart failure may be an indication for the use of one of these agents, even in patients in whom episodes of symptomatic angina are infrequent.
6. If angina persists despite two antianginal agents (a beta blocker with either a long-acting nitrate preparation or a calcium antagonist), add the third antianginal agent.
7. Coronary angiography, with a view to considering coronary revascularization, is indicated in patients with refractory symptoms or ischemia despite optimal medical therapy; it should also be carried out in patients with "high-risk" noninvasive test results (see Table 50–4) and in those with occupations or life styles that require a more aggressive approach.

OTHER THERAPIES

SPINAL CORD STIMULATION. An option for patients with refractory angina who are not candidates for coronary revascularization is spinal cord stimulation using a specially designed electrode inserted into the epidural space. The beneficial effects of neuromodulation via this technique on pain are based on the gate theory, in which stimulation of axons in the spinal cord that do not transmit pain to the brain will reduce input to the brain from axons that do so. Irrespective of the mechanism, several observational studies have reported success rates of up to 80 percent in terms of reducing the frequency and severity of angina.[228] What is less easily explained is an apparent antiischemic effect of this technique. In a small randomized trial among patients with angina and with CAD not amenable to percutaneous coronary intervention (PCI), spinal cord stimulation was associated with similar symptom relief and long-term quality of life compared to CABG.[228,229] Mortality was lower after 6 months among those treated with spinal stimulation and comparable at 5 years between the two groups. Exercise capacity was better in the CABG group.[228] Randomized, placebo-controlled trials are impossible to perform, and this approach should be reserved for patients in whom all other treatment options have been exhausted.[230]

ENHANCED EXTERNAL COUNTERPULSATION. The use of enhanced external counterpulsation (EECP) is another promising alternative treatment of refractory angina.[231,232] EECP is generally administered as 35 1-hour treatments over 7 weeks. Observational data suggest that EECP reduces the frequency of angina and the use of nitroglycerin and improves exercise tolerance and quality of life.[232] In a randomized, double-blind, sham-controlled study of EECP for patients with chronic stable angina, active counterpulsation was associated with an increase in time to ST segment depression during exercise testing and a reduction in angina, as well as an improvement in health-related quality of life that extends to at least 1 year.[233] EECP also reduces the extent of ischemia detected with myocardial perfusion imaging.[234]

The mechanisms underlying the effects of EECP are poorly understood. Possible mechanisms include (1) durable hemodynamic changes that reduce myocardial O_2 demand; (2) improvement in myocardial perfusion due to the capacity of increased transmyocardial pressure to open collaterals; and (3) the elaboration of various substances that improve endothelial function and vascular remodeling due to augmented flow through the arterial vascular bed.[232] Lastly, the possibility of placebo effects should be recognized; most of the evidence demonstrating favorable effects of EECP are from uncontrolled studies, and data from sham-controlled studies are few.

CHELATION. Randomized trials have shown no benefit and these agents may be harmful. They have no place in the management of acute or chronic CAD.[235]

Percutaneous Coronary Intervention (see Chap. 52)

PCI, which includes percutaneous transluminal coronary angioplasty (PTCA), stenting, and related techniques, represents an important therapeutic option in the management of chronic stable angina. The practice of interventional cardiology has changed radically with increased operator experience; improved adjunctive pharmacotherapy; and advances in technology, including drug-eluting stents, distal protection devices, and devices directed at specific technical issues (e.g., thrombectomy and atherectomy catheters).[236] In line with more frequent use of percutaneous intervention for complex and/or multivessel CAD, the number of coronary interventions increased by 266 percent from 1987 to 2001.[3] Despite these advances, it must be appreciated that a dilatable lesion represents an isolated target, whereas atherosclerosis is a frequently a diffuse or multifocal process. Thus, PCI is but one aspect of a comprehensive therapeutic strategy that should vigorously address the risk factors for CAD.

PATIENT SELECTION. Improved technology and increasing operator experience have continued to expand the pool of patients with both single-vessel and multivessel disease who are candidates for PCI (and other catheter-based techniques for revascularization).[236] Factors that need to be considered in patient selection include the following:

1. The need for mechanical revascularization (surgical or catheter based) as opposed to intensification of medical therapy, including stringent risk factor modification.
2. The likelihood of successful catheter-based revascularization based on the angiographic characteristics of the lesion. Equally important are factors such as vessel size, extent of calcification, tortuosity, and relationships to side branches
3. The risk and potential consequences of acute failure of PCI, which are a function, in part, of the coronary artery anatomy (multivessel and/or diffuse disease), the percentage of viable myocardium at risk, and underlying left ventricular function.
4. The likelihood of restenosis, which has been associated with clinical (e.g., diabetes, prior restenosis) and

angiographic factors (small-vessel diameter, long-lesion length, total occlusion, and saphenous vein graft disease).

5. The need for complete revascularization based on the extent of CAD, the volume of myocardium in the distribution of the narrowed artery(ies), the severity of ischemia, and the presence or absence of left ventricular dysfunction.
6. The presence of comorbid conditions and the suitability of the patient for surgery.
7. Patient preference.

Patients with chronic stable angina who are ideal for PCI are those with significant symptoms despite intensive medical therapy, who are at low risk for complications, and in whom the likelihood of technical success is high (e.g., the patient who is younger than 70 years and has single-vessel and single-lesion CAD), the anatomical characteristics of a low risk lesion with less than 90 percent stenosis, no history of congestive heart failure, and an ejection fraction greater than 0.40. Although these characteristics define the ideal candidate, excellent technical and clinical results can still be obtained in many patients who do not fulfill these ideal criteria; newer technologies have substantially expanded the pool of suitable candidates and during the last 5 years, the majority of revascularization procedures in the United States and the United Kingdom were PCI as opposed to CABG.[3]

Features associated with an increased risk for PCI failure include advanced age, female gender, unstable angina, congestive heart failure, left main coronary artery–equivalent disease, and multivessel CAD. Diabetes mellitus in patients with multivessel disease has been associated with increased periprocedural ischemic complications and late mortality in comparison with patients without diabetes. Patients with impaired renal function, particularly those with diabetes, are also at increased risk for periprocedural morbidity and, in particular, contrast agent nephropathy.[237,238]

The ACC/AHA lesion classification criteria have been revised to reflect low, moderate, and high risk in the stent era (Table 50–12).[239,240] Factors associated with increased risk of procedural failure include the presence of total occlusion for more than 3 months old, excessive vessel tortuosity, bifurcation lesions, the presence of thrombus, the inability to protect a side branch, and degenerative vein graft lesions. The presence of the aforementioned features should be considered in weighing the risks and potential benefits of PCI.

TABLE 50–12 American College of Cardiology/American Heart Association Coronary Lesion Classification*

Low Risk
Discrete (length <10 mm)
Concentric
Readily accessible
Nonangulated segment (<45 degrees)
Smooth contour
Little or no calcification
Less than totally occlusive
Not ostial in location
No major side branch involvement
Absence of thrombus
Moderate Risk
Tubular (length 10-20 mm)
Eccentric
Moderate tortuosity of proximal segment
Moderately angulated segment (>45, <90 degrees)
Irregular contour
Moderate or heavy calcification
Total occlusions <3 mo old
Ostial in location
Bifurcation lesions requiring double guidewires
Some thrombus present
High Risk
Diffuse (length >20 mm)
Excessive tortuosity of proximal segment
Extremely angulated segments >90 degrees
Total occlusions >3 mo old and/or bridging collaterals
Inability to protect major side branches
Degenerated vein grafts with friable lesions

From Smith SC Jr, Dove JT, Jacobs AK, et al: ACC/AHA guidelines of percutaneous coronary interventions (revision of the 1993 PTCA guidelines)–executive summary. A report of the American College of Cardiology/American Heart Association Task Force on Practice Guidelines (Committee to Revise the 1993 Guidelines for Percutaneous Transluminal Coronary Angioplasty). J Am Coll Cardiol 37:2215-2239, 2001.

*Anatomic risk groups.

EARLY OUTCOME. Continued improvement in the technical aspects of PCI (predominantly coronary stenting), as well as increasing operator experience, has had a favorable impact on the rate of primary success (defined angiographically as a final stenosis diameter <20 percent in the presence of Thrombosis in Myocardial Infarction [TIMI] grade 3 flow) and the rate of reductions in complications (i.e., death, myocardial infarction, and emergency coronary bypass surgery).[241] These improvements have occurred despite broadening of the selection criteria for PCI to include higher risk patients with more complex anatomy. Current expectations for PCI, particularly with the widespread use of coronary stents, are an overall procedural success rate of at least 90 percent with a mortality of less than 1 percent, rate of Q wave myocardial infarction of less than 1.5 percent, and rate of emergency bypass surgery of 1 to 2 percent.

LONG-TERM OUTCOME. Long-term outcome after PCI is well characterized, with left ventricular function, extent of coronary disease, diabetes, and the patient's age being the major determinants of mortality risk, and restenosis at the site of intervention being a major contributor to recurrent ischemia and the need for subsequent procedures. The incidence of restenosis following balloon angioplasty is 30 to 40 percent and appears higher in certain clinical and angiographic subsets, accounting in large part for the high frequency of repeat revascularization procedures (up to 40 percent at 1 to 2 years) after angioplasty. However, contemporary datasets reflecting the widespread use of intracoronary stenting document significantly lower rates of repeat revascularization procedures at 1 year (CABG 8.6 percent and PCI 12.4 percent) than observed in the era of balloon angioplasty.[241]

STENTS (see Chap. 52). Since their entry into clinical practice in the early 1990s, stents have improved both the early and late results of PCI. In regard to the former, stents have produced a marked reduction in the need for emergency bypass surgery, and in comparison with PTCA, stents have been associated with a significant reduction in the incidence of major cardiac events after discharge.[242] These favorable results have occurred primarily through reduction in clinical restenosis and the need for repeat revascularization without translating into a reduction in death or myocardial infarction.[243] Despite the significant reduction in restenosis achieved with bare-metal stents compared with balloon angioplasty, restenosis within the stent (in-stent restenosis), occurring in 15 to 30 percent of stented lesions, has remained a limitation to long-term outcomes with PCI.[242] Drug-eluting stents (coated stents that release single or multiple bioactive agents into the surrounding tissue) have shown dramatic reductions in restenosis in patients selected for clinical trials (binary restenosis 0 to 10 percent) compared to bare-metal stents.[244] This advantage may translate into an additional decline in the need for repeat revascularization procedures after PCI, including multivessel interventions, and in patients, such as those with diabetes mellitus, who are at high risk for restenosis with bare-metal stents.[236]

CHRONIC TOTAL OCCLUSION. Chronic total occlusions are present in 20 to 40 percent of patients with angiographic documentation of CAD and are particularly frequent in patients with multivessel disease and left ventricular dysfunction, in whom a total occlusion is often a barrier to complete revascularization. The availability of newer devices, particularly guidewires dedicated to treatment of chronic total occlusions, has increased the probability of initial technical success. Nevertheless, the rate of primary success is lower (51 to 74 percent) and the rate of restenosis higher during PCI for chronic total occlusions compared with nonoccluded vessels.[245] Long-term survival appears greater and anginal symptoms are less frequent among patients with chronic total occlusions who undergo successful PCI compared with those who have failed procedures even after adjusting for differences in their baseline risk profile.[245]

RESTENOSIS. See Chapter 52.

Comparisons Between PCI and Medical Therapy

Randomized clinical trials comparing PCI to medical therapy are few in number, have involved fewer than 2000 patients (in total) with predominantly single-vessel disease, and were completed prior to routine use of coronary stenting and enhanced adjunctive pharmacotherapy.[246] In aggregate, the results of these trials have supported superior control of angina and improved exercise capacity in patients treated with angioplasty compared with medical therapy (Fig. 50–9). In addition, results from long-term follow-up in the second Randomized Intervention Treatment of Angina (RITA-2) trial indicated improved quality of life among those treated with angioplasty through 1 year of follow-up, although this benefit was attenuated by 3 years.[247] No randomized trial to date has demonstrated a reduction in death or myocardial infarction with PCI compared with medical therapy for patients with chronic stable angina. To the contrary, the RITA-2 investigators observed an excess of death and periprocedural myocardial infarction with angioplasty compared to medical therapy (6.3 percent vs. 3.3 percent; $p = 0.02$); it is worthy of note that 62 percent of the patients enrolled in RITA-2 had multivessel CAD. Among patients with stable single- or double-vessel CAD and mild symptoms (asymptomatic or Canadian Cardiovascular Society class I or II angina) and preserved left ventricular function, medical therapy, including aggressive lipid lowering, provided similar results to angioplasty with respect to a composite of cardiovascular death, need for (repeat) revascularization, myocardial infarction, or worsening angina resulting in hospitalization.[103]

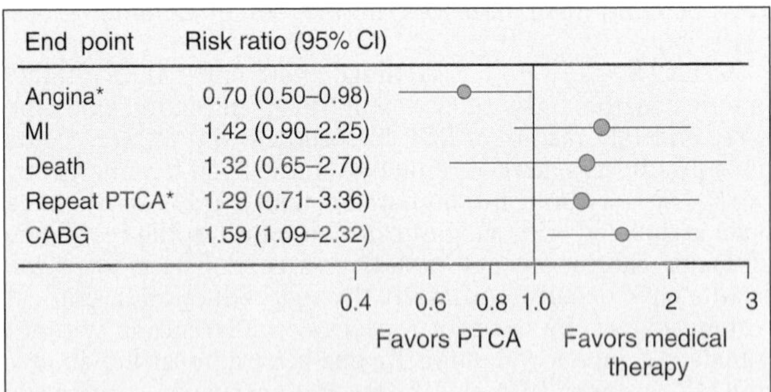

End point
Risk ratio (95% CI)
Angina*
0.70 (0.50–0.98)
MI
1.42 (0.90–2.25)
Death
1.32 (0.65–2.70)
Repeat PTCA*
1.29 (0.71–3.36)
CABG
1.59 (1.09–2.32)
0.4
0.6
0.8
1.0
2
3
Favors PTCA
Favors medical therapy

FIGURE 50–9 Relative risk of recurrent cardiac events with percutaneous transluminal coronary angioplasty (PTCA) versus medical therapy from meta-analysis of six randomized trials ($N = 1904$). Compared with medical therapy, angioplasty reduced the relative risk of recurrent angina by 30 percent. Randomized trials have not included sufficient numbers of patients for informative estimates of the effect of angioplasty on myocardial infarction (MI), death, or subsequent revascularization; however, trends in the available data do not favor angioplasty. These trials do not reflect the widespread use of coronary stenting. *Test for heterogeneity, $p < 0.0001$. CABG = coronary artery bypass grafting; CI = confidence interval. (From Bucher HC, Hengstler P, Schindler C, et al: Percutaneous transluminal coronary angioplasty versus medical therapy for treatment of non-acute coronary heart disease: A meta-analysis of randomised controlled trials. BMJ 321:73-77, 2000.)

Based on these best available data from randomized trials, it appears reasonable to pursue a strategy of initial medical therapy for most patients with chronic stable angina and Canadian Cardiovascular Society class I or II symptoms and reserve revascularization for those with persistent and/or more severe symptoms despite optimal medical therapy, or those with high-risk criteria on noninvasive testing, such as inducible ischemia involving a moderate or large territory of myocardium.[18] The ongoing Clinical Outcomes Utilization Revascularization and Aggressive drug Evaluation (COURAGE) trial will provide additional insight regarding the comparison of intensive medical therapy versus revascularization using contemporary technology.

PCI in Specific Subgroups of Patients with Chronic Stable Angina

LEFT VENTRICULAR DYSFUNCTION. Studies of balloon angioplasty in patients with chronic stable angina and left ventricular dysfunction have documented high rates of initial procedural success[248] but less complete revascularization and less favorable long-term outcomes (including survival) than in patients with normal left ventricular function. Despite advances in interventional cardiology, left ventricular dysfunction remains associated with higher in-hospital and long-term mortality after PCI.[248] Specifically, among patients with stable CAD and estimated ejection fractions of 0.40 percent or less, 0.41 to 0.49, and 0.50 or higher in the National Heart, Lung, and Blood Institute (NHLBI) Dynamic Registry, mortality at 1 year after PCI was 11.0 percent, 4.5 percent, and 1.9 percent, respectively.[248] Patients with left ventricular dysfunction are more likely to have other important factors associated with increased risk, including advanced age, diabetes mellitus, and more extensive epicardial disease. However, systolic dysfunction remains an independent predictor of mortality after PCI in the stent era.

WOMEN. Compared with men, women undergoing PCI tend to be older and to have more comorbid disease, a higher prevalence of diabetes mellitus, and more severe angina.[249] However, the extent of epicardial coronary disease is typically similar or less among women. The apparent discordance between the number of risk factors and severity of symptoms with the angiographic extent of disease has been attributed to greater abnormalities of vasomotor function and micovascular and endothelial dysfunction among women.[249] Although reports in the early 1990s demonstrated worrisome higher mortality among women undergoing PCI, subsequent studies have documented consistent reduction in the risk of early complications, despite persistent high-risk characteristics, and similar long-term outcomes compared to men.[250]

THE ELDERLY. Catheter-based revascularization is particularly attractive in the elderly because of age-related changes in cognitive function and cerebrovascular events after CABG and because of the adverse effect of coexisting disease (which is frequent in the elderly) on perioperative outcome. Nonetheless, the increased prevalence of multivessel and diffuse disease and left ventricular dysfunction in the elderly diminishes the proportion of patients likely to have significant long-term benefits in comparison to CABG. The more unfavorable coronary artery anatomy in the elderly population together with left ventricular dysfunction is reflected by the twofold to fourfold higher mortality and periprocedural complication rates in the elderly undergoing PCI,[251] in addition to greater recurrence of angina in hospital survivors.[252] In elderly patients without ventricular dysfunction or renal insufficiency, outcomes are comparable to those in younger patients. Moreover, despite a persistently high burden of comorbidities, the rate of periprocedural complications for the elderly have decreased.[251]

The Trial of Invasive versus Medical therapy in the Eldery (TIME), a randomized trial of invasive versus medical management of chronic stable angina in patients 75 years of age and older, demonstrated a trend toward an early hazard with respect to the risk of death or myocardial infarction but improved functional outcomes among survivors of invasive management.[252a] In long-term follow-up, both of these outcomes converged between the arms so that no difference in quality of life, functional outcomes, or death/myocardial infarction was detected (Fig 50–10). Elderly patients who were managed medically had a significantly higher risk of major adverse cardiac events, when rehospitalization and the need for subsequent revascularization were included (49.3 percent vs. 19.0 percent; $p < 0.001$), but no difference in death/myocardial infarction.[252a] Nonrandomized data from at least one observational study that included a propensity analysis indicate that absolute benefit of treatment with PCI compared with medical therapy may increase with age.[253]

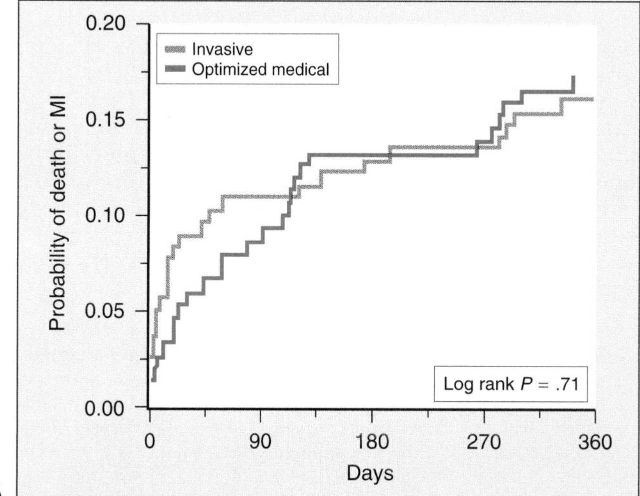

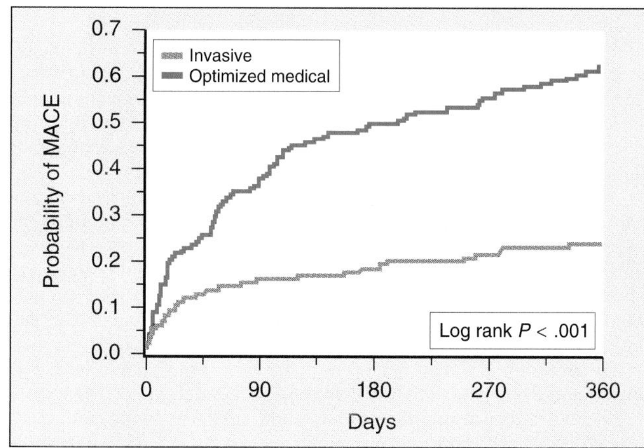

FIGURE 50–10 Results of a randomized trial of invasive versus medical management for patients ($N = 282$) aged 75 years or older with chronic coronary artery disease (Trial of Invasive vs. Medical therapy in the Eldery [TIME] Trial). **A,** After 1 year, rates of death or nonfatal myocardial infarction were not significantly different between the two treatment strategies. **B,** However, the rate of major adverse cardiac events (MACE; death, nonfatal myocardial infarction [MI], or hospitalization for uncontrolled symptoms or acute coronary syndrome) was significantly higher in patients randomized to a strategy of medical therapy. (**A** and **B,** From Pfisterer M, Buser P, Osswald S, et al: Outcome of elderly patients with chronic symptomatic coronary artery disease with an invasive vs. optimized medical treatment strategy: One-year results of the randomized TIME trial. JAMA 289:1117-1123, 2003.)

DIABETES MELLITUS. Patients with diabetes are at substantially higher risk for complications after PCI. Possible explanations for the higher rate of adverse outcomes include an altered vascular biological response in diabetic patients to balloon injury and rapid progression of disease in nondilated segments. The diabetic atherosclerotic milieu is characterized by a procoagulant state, decreased fibrinolytic activity, increased proliferation, and inflammation.[254]

Restenosis is more frequent in diabetic patients, as is disease progression. In a study of patients referred for diagnostic angiography 1 month or more after successful PTCA, the number of new narrowings in the arteries of diabetic patients was 22 percent higher, particularly at other sites in the artery that initially underwent PTCA. For this reason, CABG, which bypasses the majority of the vessel instead of a specific lesion, may offer a better intermediate- to long-term outcome.[255] The optimal revascularization strategy (CABG vs. PCI) for patients with diabetes and multivessel disease bears further study in the era of drug-eluting stents that have been shown to substantially reduce restenosis, including among patients with diabetes.[256,257]

PREVIOUS CORONARY BYPASS GRAFTING. CABG and PCI are often considered competitive procedures, but it is more appropriate to view them as complementary. An increasing number of patients who have had CABG and later have recurrent ischemia undergo revascularization with PCI. At the Mayo Clinic, approximately 20 percent of all PCIs are in patients who have had previous CABG.[258]

With advances in technology, the rates of initial success with PCI in venous bypass grafts have approximated those encountered for intervention in native coronaries.[259] Specifically, studies indicate procedural success in more than 90 percent of lesions and mortality rates less than 2 percent. However, the incidence of periprocedural myocardial infarction due to distal embolization remains higher with PCI in venous grafts compared with native coronary arteries. Restenosis in saphenous vein grafts has been reduced with the introduction of elective stenting but remains more frequent than in native arteries. The age of the bypass graft should be taken into consideration, because patients with older and severely diseased venous grafts may benefit from repeat CABG as an alternative to PCI.[258]

Innovative approaches to the PCI in vein graft atherosclerosis include catheter-based aspiration systems, in which the techniques of aspiration and filters are combined to prevent distal emboli.[260] These have provided important reductions in the risk of periprocedural myocardial infarction. Platelet glycoprotein IIb/IIIa antagonists and other newer devices, such as coronary ultrasound thrombolysis, have not yet been shown to improve outcomes.

OTHER CATHETER-BASED TECHNIQUES. Directional coronary atherectomy, rotational atherectomy, transluminal extraction catheters, thrombectomy, Excimer laser atherectomy, distal protection devices, and other newer catheter-based techniques are discussed in Chapter 52.

Coronary Artery Bypass Surgery

In 1964, Garrett, Dennis, and DeBakey first used CABG as a "bailout" procedure. Widespread use of the technique by Favoloro and Johnson and their respective collaborators followed in the late 1960s. Use of the internal mammary artery

(IMA) graft was pioneered by Kolessov in 1967 and by Green and colleagues in 1970.[261]

The annual number of coronary bypass operations in the United States rose steadily between 1979 and 1997, increasing by 227 percent over that period. In 2001, approximately 305,000 patients underwent coronary bypass surgery; a decline of 16 percent since 1997 that may be attributed in part to the growth of PCI.[3] Nevertheless, CABG remains one of the most frequently performed operations in the United States, resulting in the expenditure of almost $50 billion annually. CABG provides excellent short- and intermediate-term results in the management of stable CAD; its long-term results are affected by failure of venous grafts. Long-term data with totally arterial surgical revascularization are few.

Technical Considerations

When a decision has been reached to proceed with CABG, administration of beta blockers, nitrates, and calcium antagonists is continued until surgery. It is crucial to minimize perioperative damage and protect the myocardium. The most commonly used method involves a single period of aortic cross-clamping with intermittent infusion of cold cardioplegia solution. Technical modifications of traditional CABG, either using more limited incisions or eliminating cardiopulmonary bypass (CPB), or both, have been aimed at reducing the morbidity associated with this major surgery.[261] It is estimated that in 2002 approximately 20 percent of CABG was performed off-pump[262] and that this proportion is increasing. Other technical factors include the selection and method of preparation of bypass conduits, use of sutureless anastomotic devices, and the method of cardioplegia, if utilized.

MINIMALLY INVASIVE CABG. "Less invasive" or "minimally invasive" approaches may be divided into four major categories based on the approach and use of CPB. Port-access CABG is performed using limited incisions with femoral-femoral CPB and cardioplegic arrest. Port-access technology has also now enabled totally endoscopic robotically assisted CABG (TECAB) to be performed on the arrested heart.[263] Off-pump CABG is performed using a standard median sternotomy, with generally small skin incisions, and stabilization devices to reduce motion of the target vessels while anastomoses are performed without CPB. Finally, minimally invasive direct coronary artery bypass (MIDCAB) is performed through a left anterior thoracotomy without CPB.[261] Thus, off-pump approaches to CABG include both off-pump CAB (OPCAB) and MIDCAB techniques (Fig 50–11).

The potential advantages of the minimally invasive approaches include reduced postoperative patient discomfort, minimized risk of wound infection, and shorter recovery times. The avoidance of CPB may mitigate the risk of bleeding, systemic thromboembolism, renal insufficiency, myocardial stunning, stroke, and damaging neurological effects of bypass, particularly in the elderly and in patients with heavily calcified aortas.[262] Amelioration of the systemic inflammatory response that occurs after CABG using CPB is viewed as an additional advantage that may affect these clinical outcomes.[262] The "learning curve" of minimally invasive CABG has led to reports of early graft failure. In many centers, intraoperative or early postoperative angiography has been performed to assess the quality of the anastomosis. It should be emphasized that with conventional surgical techniques, the *early* patency rates of an IMA graft are excellent (98.7 percent in one large series), and less than 50 percent stenosis was noted in 91 percent of grafts.[264] Short-term clinical and angiographic outcomes suggest that the less invasive techniques can be used to achieve results comparable to traditional CABG.[265] The ultimate success of these "nontraditional" approaches to CABG will depend on long-term graft patency and the continued development of new techniques that will increase exposure to allow for more complete revascularization.

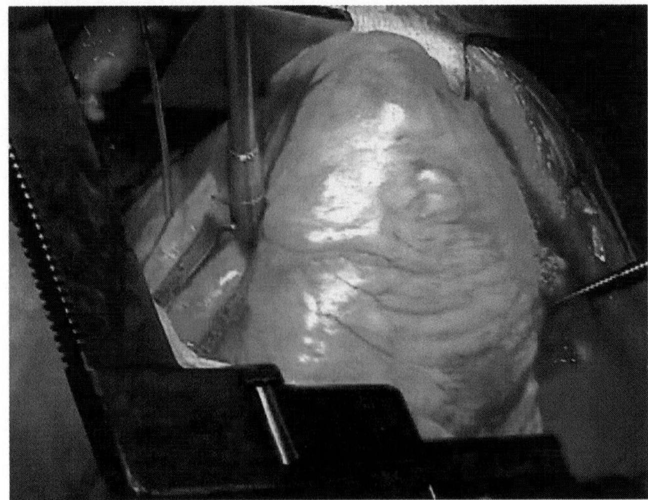

FIGURE 50–11 Off-pump coronary artery bypass grafting performed using a standard median sternotomy and a stabilization device to reduce motion of the target vessel while the anastomosis is performed without cardiopulmonary bypass. (Courtesy of Dr. Tomislav Mihaljevic.)

In addition, novel approaches to coronary revascularization may also include CABG with PCI by combining a minimally invasive coronary bypass surgical procedure on the left anterior descending coronary artery with PCI on the remaining vessels. Further experience is needed to clarify appropriate selection criteria and whether this strategy offers important advantages over multivessel bypass surgery alone.[266]

PORT-ACCESS CABG. An innovative approach to coronary revascularization is the *port-access method*, which uses small thoracotomy ports for cardiac manipulation; CPB is established by groin cannulation and an intraaortic balloon clamp for occlusion of the aorta. The two largest single-center series and the first report of the Port-Access International Registry, which documented the results of 555 bypass procedures, were encouraging.[267] Data comparing port-access to traditional CABG are few but indicate similar short-term outcomes.[268] Limitations to the use of this technique include atherosclerotic involvement of the aortic arch, high cost, long operating times due to technically very demanding surgery, and the risk of aortic dissection.[268] As a result, the port-access approach is now not widely used. However, port-access technology has enabled robotically enhanced totally endoscopic CABG to be performed and may increase in use if this new approach becomes more widely adopted.[263]

MINIMALLY INVASIVE DIRECT CABG. MIDCAB is performed through a limited left thoracotomy on the beating heart (off-pump), most commonly with grafting of the left internal thoracic artery to the left anterior descending artery. Studies of early angiographic patency have shown rates (98 percent) comparable to traditional CABG.[269] In a randomized trial comparing MIDCAB to stenting for treatment of isolated left anterior descending (LAD) artery disease, the rate of death or myocardial infarction was similar between the two groups (3 percent with stenting vs. 6 percent with MIDCAB; $p = 0.5$, $n = 220$). The need for repeated revascularization during the following 6 months was significantly higher in patients treated with coronary stenting (29 percent vs. 8 percent; $p = 0.003$).[270] In this trial, early reoperation for graft failure was necessary in 3 percent of patients and conversion to a full sternotomy was necessary in 5 percent. All grafts were patent at 6 months.[270] Outcomes were favorable (major cardiac events 7.8 percent, mortality 2.5 percent) at 1 year among 274 patients who underwent MIDCAB in an experienced center. Accumulation of operator experience appears to reduce perioperative adverse events.[271]

Limitations include the requirement that the patient can tolerate single-lung ventilation and that the operation is generally limited to revascularization of the LAD territory due to lesser accessibility of the left circumflex and right coronary arteries. The latter limitation may be successfully addressed by combined MIDCAB of the LAD with revascularization of other diseased arteries by PCI.[266] This approach has been evaluated predominantly in small observational studies; the benefit of so-called integrated coronary revascularization compared to established strategies remains to be adequately studied.

OFF-PUMP CABG. An alternative approach to revascularization on the beating heart is OPCAB, entailing a conventional median sternotomy and mechanical suction stabilizing systems. This combination enhances surgical exposure compared with MIDCAB and is particularly useful if multivessel bypass grafting is contemplated. Most surgeons consider only hemodynamic instability or severe cardiomegaly as contraindications.[262] In studies of small numbers of patients, angiographic patency rates have been documented as 99 percent at hospital discharge and 1 month and as 95 percent at 6 months.[262]

Observational data among 2223 patients who underwent OPCAB in the United Kingdom suggest better survival in analysis adjusted for baseline risk (odds ratio for CPB vs. OPCAB 1.85; 95 percent confidence interval (CI), 1.19 to 2.92).[272] The number of patients studied in randomized, controlled trials are few. A meta-analysis of nine randomized trials (<600 randomized to off-pump procedures, including MIDCAB), performed primarily in younger patients at lower risk, showed a trend toward lower risk of a composite of death, stroke, or myocardial infarction (odds ratio, 0.48; 95 percent CI, 0.21 to 1.09).[273] Generally consistent findings across randomized and observational data sets include comparable completeness of revascularization, reductions in blood loss and/or transfusion requirements, fewer wound infections, lower indices of myocardial injury, shorter duration of mechanical ventilation, and earlier hospital discharge with OPCAB.[262,274] Although trends toward neurocognitive benefits are evident, important reductions in stroke or long-term cognitive impairment with OPCAB versus traditional CABG have not yet been demonstrated.[275] Moreover, a randomized trial of OPCAB versus traditional CABG suggests that the former provides similar long-term outcomes (death, myocardial infarction, stroke, or need for reintervention) and is more cost-effective in low-risk patients,[276] but additional data regarding optimal patient selection for OPCAB are needed.

CARDIOPLEGIA

Favorable outcomes with respect to postoperative ventricular function are in large part dependent on optimal intraoperative myocardial protection.[277] Early cardioplegic techniques relied on cold crystalloid to initiate and maintain intraoperative cardiac arrest. However, blood cardioplegia facilitates myocardial aerobic metabolism, preserves myocardial high-energy phosphate stores, and reduces lactate production compared with crystalloid cardioplegia.[277] Enhancement of cardioplegia using metabolic substrates such as glutamate has also been shown to improve metabolic recovery. Other alternatives include retrograde and/or antegrade delivery, continuous versus intermittent cardioplegia, and the use of "warm" (37° C) or "tepid" (29° C) induction of cardioplegic arrest[278] and/or a terminal infusion of warm blood cardioplegia to facilitate a return to aerobic metabolism. Retrograde cardioplegia through the coronary sinus provides more uniform distribution of cardioplegic solution; many surgeons now use a combination of antegrade and retrograde perfusion. Intermittent delivery facilitates visualization of the distal anastomosis. Novel approaches with separate administration or additional additives such as sodium/hydrogen exchange inhibitors, L-arginine, insulin, or adenosine as additional myocardial protectants are under study.[277] Future advances may stem from ongoing investigation of the mediators of myocardial injury during cardioplegia and the impact of cardioplegic alternatives.[279]

Among patients with satisfactory preoperative cardiac function, a wide range of techniques have produced excellent results. For example, both cold crystalloid and warm blood cardioplegia in elective bypass surgery in patients with well-preserved preoperative ventricular function have been associated with low mortality and morbidity. This success is probably a reflection of the extent of myocardial functional reserve in those with well-preserved systolic function. In contrast, among patients with depressed left ventricular function (both acutely and chronically), it is easier to demonstrate a benefit with more specialized protocols, including the use of sanguineous cardioplegic techniques, with or without substrate enhancement, and blood cardioplegia.[277]

VENOUS CONDUITS. The saphenous vein is used mainly for distal branches of the right and circumflex coronary arteries and for sequential grafts to these vessels and diagonal branches (Figs. 50–12 and 50–13). In emergency situations, many surgeons prefer the saphenous vein to the IMA, because

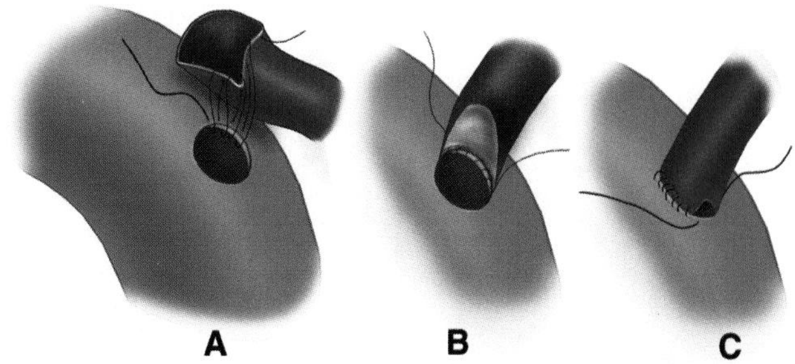

FIGURE 50–12 Aorticovenous anastomosis in a coronary artery–saphenous vein bypass graft. **A,** The technique of single cross-clamp is demonstrated. An aortotomy is created with a knife and punch Appropriate conduit length and orientation are established and a fine polypropylene suture is used in a running fashion toward and around the anastomotic heel. **B,** The conduit is carefully parachuted down onto the aorta. **C,** The suture is continued toward and around the anastomotic toe. (**A** to **C,** From Woo YJ, Gardner TJ: Myocardial revascularization with cardiopulmonary bypass. *In* Cohn LC, Edmunds LH [eds]: Cardiac Surgery in the Adult. New York, McGraw-Hill, 2003, p 597.)

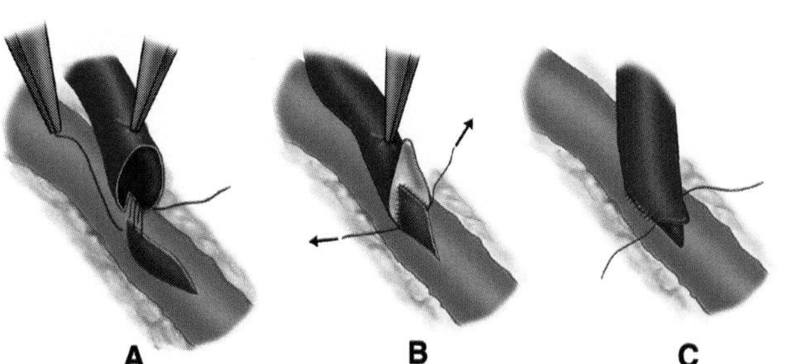

FIGURE 50–13 Venocoronary anastomosis. **A,** An initial arteriotomy is created with a knife and then extended with angled fine scissors. A fine polypropylene suture is used in a running fashion toward and around the anastomotic heel. **B,** After several throws of the suture, the conduit is carefully parachuted down onto the coronary artery. **C,** The suture is continued toward and around the anastomotic toe until the other end of the suture is reached. (From Woo YJ, Gardner TJ: Myocardia revascularization with cardiopulmonary bypass. *In* Cohn LC, Edmunds LH (eds): Cardiac Surgery in the Adult. New York: McGraw Hill, 2003, p 593.)

the saphenous vein can be harvested and grafted more rapidly. When the greater saphenous vein is not available, the lesser saphenous vein and the upper extremity veins (typically the cephalic or basilic) may be used. However, arm vein grafts are not as effective as either IMA or saphenous vein grafts. Endoscopic harvesting of saphenous vein provides improved cosmetic results and may reduce morbidity compared with open harvesting.[280] Cryopreserved homologous saphenous vein grafts and glutaraldehyde-treated umbilical veins have been used, but the patency rates are not optimal and thus these veins should be used only when there are no other alternatives.[261]

Trauma to the vein during surgical preparation can denude the endothelium, impair the intrinsic fibrinolytic activity of the saphenous vein, and damage the vessel wall, thereby predisposing to early thrombosis. Careful harvesting of the graft, with particular attention to avoidance of overdistention and the use of modified storage solutions, and inclusion of surrounding tissue to minimize manipulation of the graft have been shown to improve patency and preserve the integrity of the graft in both animal models and the clinical setting.[281-283]

Recently developed aortic-saphenous vein graft connectors enable surgeons to create the proximal anastomosis without the use of side-biting aortic clamps that may contribute to aortic injury and perioperative stroke. Early experience with sutureless connectors suggests high rates of stenosis during the first 6 months after placement; thus, although these devices have potential for substantial expansion of use in

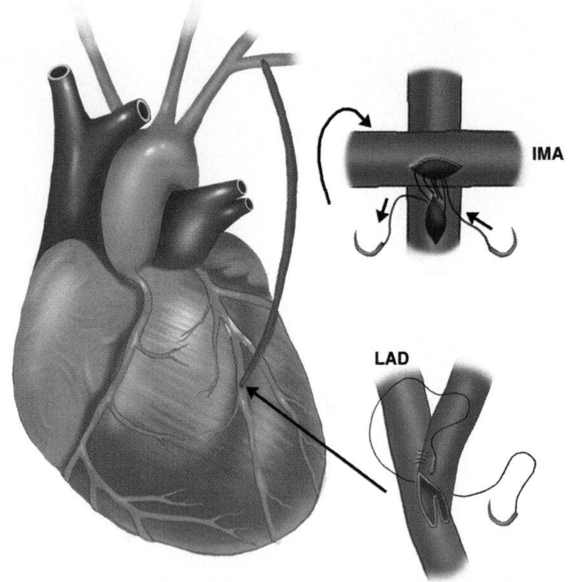

FIGURE 50–14 Internal mammary grafting consisting of an in situ left internal mammary artery (IMA) graft to the left anterior descending (LAD) artery (end to side) and diagonal branch (side to side), with the diamond anastomotic technique used for the latter. The details show the IMA pedicle rolled up over the diagonal coronary artery to facilitate exposure and the use of continuous suture. (From Jones EL: Extended use of the internal mammary–coronary artery bypass. J Card Surg 1:13, 1986.)

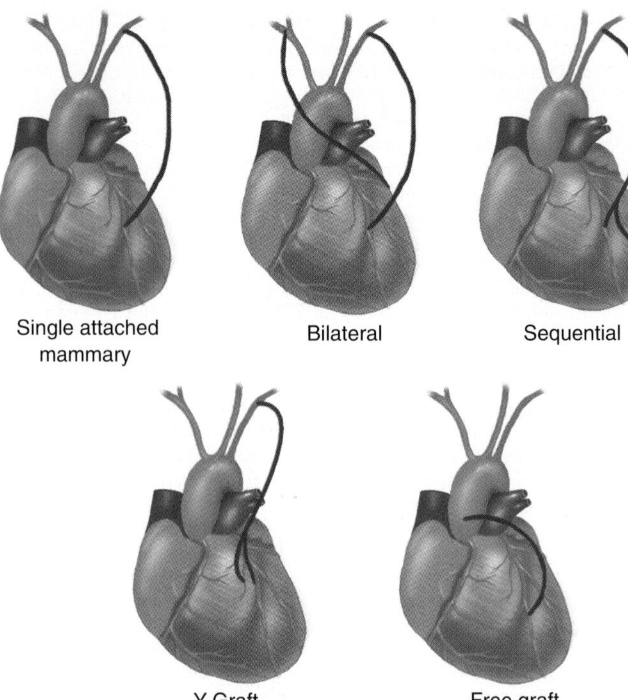

FIGURE 50–15 Different types of internal mammary artery grafts. A single attached internal mammary artery graft (either the right or left) remains attached proximally to the subclavian artery and is connected to the coronary arteries. Bilateral internal mammary artery grafts (right and left) are joined end to side to coronary arteries. Sequential internal mammary artery grafts consist of an attached or free internal mammary artery with one or more side-to-side anastomoses and one end-to-side anastomosis. The internal mammary artery Y graft has two terminal branches of either the attached or free internal mammary artery sutured to two coronary arteries. A free internal mammary graft is placed by transecting the right or left internal mammary artery near its origin in the subclavian artery and anastomosing the proximal portion of the artery to the aorta and the distal end to the coronary artery. (From Tector AJ, Schmahl TM, Canino VR: Expanding the use of the internal mammary artery to improve patency in coronary artery bypass grafting. J Thorac Cardiovasc Surg 91:9, 1986.)

conjunction with minimally invasive CABG, additional experience and long-term data are needed to clarify their role.[284]

Flow Rates. When measured at the time of surgery, flow rates through saphenous vein grafts average nearly 70 ml/min. Flow rates less than 45 ml/min—and especially less than 25 ml/min—are more frequently associated with graft closure than are higher flow rates.[285] The usefulness of measuring flow rates is enhanced by taking into account the type of conduit used and the size of the distal vasculature. If flow rates are lower than expected, reassessment of the anastomosis with a probe may be helpful. Possible causes of reduced flow include (1) subcritical obstruction of the coronary artery; (2) a technically poor anastomosis with narrowing of the lumen from kinking of the vessel or pinching at the site of anastomosis; (3) a small myocardial mass perfused by the graft; and (4) a diseased distal vascular bed.

INTERNAL MAMMARY ARTERY BYPASS GRAFTS. The IMA, also known as the internal thoracic artery, is usually remarkably free of atheroma, especially in patients younger than 65 years. When it is grafted to a coronary artery (Figs. 50–14 and 50–15), it appears to be virtually immune to the development of intimal hyperplasia, which is almost universally seen in aortocoronary vein grafts,[286] and the functional (endothelium-dependent vasodilatory) capacity of the artery remains intact.[287] The diameter of the IMA graft is usually a closer match to that of the recipient coronary artery than is the diameter of a saphenous vein.

The current standard for bypass grafting advocates routine use of the left IMA for grafting the left anterior descending coronary artery, with supplemental saphenous vein grafts to other vessels.[261] Limitations to this approach are few; the primary consideration is that the procedure is time consuming; thus, the IMA is not often used for emergency surgery.

Although the benefits of a single IMA graft over a saphenous vein graft alone are not in dispute,[288] the superiority of bilateral IMA grafts over a single IMA graft and one saphenous vein graft is less well accepted.[289] Initial enthusiasm for the use of bilateral IMA grafts was tempered by a higher rate of postoperative complications, including bleeding, wound infection, and prolonged ventilatory support. Wound infection, which has been of particular concern, remains modest in frequency (<3 percent), except among patients who are obese or diabetic or those who require prolonged ventilatory support. Subsequent series have shown that bilateral versus single IMA grafting is associated with lower rates of recurrent angina pectoris, reoperation, and myocardial infarction and improved survival in nonrandomized studies.[289] The increased technical demands and longer operative times of bilateral IMA grafting have also been a barrier to more widespread adoption but may be overcome if data supporting a survival advantage continue to accumulate.

Complications. Inadequate flow rates with evidence of myocardial ischemia in the perioperative period are rare after IMA grafts to the LAD coronary artery or its diagonal branches. Perioperative spasm is the presumed cause and can be managed by the administration of sodium nitroprusside or a combination of glyceryl trinitrate and verapamil. Other complications include an increased incidence of sternal wound infections, which is more frequent in obese patients and diabetics and after bilateral IMA implants.

OTHER CONDUITS. The success of IMA grafts has stimulated interest in the use of other arterial conduits, particularly in patients who are younger, diabetic, or hyperlipidemic or in whom the saphenous veins are unsuitable or unavailable.[261] Options for arterial grafts include the radial, right gastroepiploic, inferior epigastric, and very rarely the subscapular, intercostal, splenic, left gastric, and gastroduodenal arteries. Initial enthusiasm for use of the radial artery was blunted by reports of high reocclusion rates. More recent experience, in which attention has been paid to avoiding spasm by minimizing manipulation and the use of calcium-channel blockers, has been favorable. Early rates of patency are as high as 95 percent with mid-term patency comparable to that for IMA grafts (~85 percent at 5 years). Radial arterial grafts may be associated with fewer perioperative complications and thus preferable to the right IMA as a second arterial graft.[290] Total arterial revascularization using both IMAs and free radial or alternative arterial grafts has also gained interest. A randomized trial comparing grafting using the left IMA plus additional venous grafts versus total arterial revascularization detected no differences in the number of vessels grafted, time on CPB, or postoperative complications. At a mean follow-up of 12 months, patients managed with total arterial revascularization were less likely to have recurrent angina or to require additional revascularization.[291]

The right gastroepiploic artery can be harvested by extending the median sternotomy incision toward the umbilicus.[292] It is frequently placed as a graft to the right coronary artery, but both the circumflex and the left anterior descending coronary arteries can be grafted with this conduit. Early results demonstrated excellent patency rates, but there is a paucity of data on long-term results. Similarly, the inferior epigastric artery has been used as a free graft for coronary revascularization, with good short-term patency rates but without long-term data. Bovine IMA, Dacron, and polytetrafluoroethylene (PTFE) grafts have also been used with lower patency (~50 to 60 percent) over the mid-term. These grafts should only be used as a last resort.[261]

THE DISTAL VASCULATURE. The state of the distal coronary vasculature is important for the fate of bypass grafts. Late patency of grafts is related to coronary arterial runoff as determined by the diameter of the coronary artery into which the graft is inserted, the size of the distal vascular bed, and the severity of coronary atherosclerosis distal to the site of insertion of the graft. The highest graft patency rates are found when the lumina of the vessels distal to the graft insertion are greater than 1.5 mm in diameter, perfuse a large vascular bed, and are free of atheroma obstructing more than 25 percent of the vessel lumen. For saphenous veins, optimal patency rates are achieved with a lumen of 2.0 mm or greater.

Surgical Outcomes

The patient population undergoing CABG has been changing over time, particularly with the wider use of PCI. In comparison with the 1970s, patients undergoing CABG today are older, include a higher percentage of women, and are "sicker" in that a greater proportion have unstable angina, triple-vessel disease, previous coronary revascularization with either CABG or PCI, left ventricular dysfunction, and comorbid conditions, including hypertension, diabetes, and peripheral vascular disease. Despite the increasing risk profile of this population, outcomes with CABG have generally remained stable or improved.

OPERATIVE MORTALITY. Risk factors for death following coronary artery surgery may be separated into five categories: (1) preoperative factors related to CAD, including recent acute myocardial infarction, hemodynamic instability, left ventricular dysfunction, extensive CAD, the presence of left main CAD, and severe or unstable angina; (2) preoperative factors related to the aggressiveness of the arteriosclerotic process, as reflected in associated carotid or peripheral vascular disease; (3) preoperative biological factors (older age at surgery, diabetes mellitus, comorbidities, including pulmonary and renal disease, and perhaps female gender); (4) intraoperative factors (intraoperative ischemic damage and failure to use IMA grafts); and (5) environmental or institutional factors, including the specific surgeon and treatment protocols used. Of these factors, several variables have consistently emerged as the most potent predictors of mortality after CABG: (1) age; (2) urgency of operation; (3) prior cardiac surgery; (4) left ventricular function; (5) percent stenosis of the left main coronary artery; and (6) number of epicardial vessels with significant disease.[261]

In-hospital mortality after isolated CABG was characterized by a steady decline from 1967 to the 1980s. Despite a shift toward higher risk demographics with an older population of patients with more comorbidities being referred for CABG, early mortality continued to decline in the 1990s.[293] Specifically, during the period from 1990 to 1999, crude mortality through 30 days after CABG in the United States fell by 0.9 percent, (23.1 percent relative decrease; $p < 0.0001$). Mortality among the 503,478 CABG-only operations recorded in the Society of Thoracic Surgeons data base between 1997 and 1999 was 3.05 percent.[294] Moreover, with increasingly wide scrutiny of procedural results, it has become recognized that *absolute* rates of morbidity and mortality might not provide a fair basis for comparing institutions and individuals, unless the characteristics of the patients are considered. Several models have been developed and refined with the objective of predicting perioperative mortality.[294] Application of such models demonstrate even greater declines in CABG mortality over the past decade when adjusted for changes in risk profile.[293]

A useful perspective of long-term survival after CABG during an earlier phase in the evaluation of this therapy is provided by the most recent follow-up data (mean, 15 years) from the Coronary Artery Surgery Study (CASS) Registry. Ninety percent of patients were alive at 5 years, 74 percent at 10 years, and 56 percent at 15 years. The hazard function for death decreases rapidly after surgery to its nadir at 9 to 12 months,[295] followed by a steady increase with a doubling of the hazard ratio at 15 years in comparison to that at 5 years.

PERIOPERATIVE COMPLICATIONS

Perioperative morbidity (see Chap. 76) has increased because of a larger fraction of higher risk patients. Major morbidity (death, stroke, renal failure, reoperation, prolonged ventilation, and sternal infection) occurred in 13.4 percent through 30 days among the 503,478 CABG-only operations recorded in the Society of Thoracic Surgeons data base between 1997 and 1999.[294]

MYOCARDIAL INFARCTION. Perioperative myocardial infarction, particularly if it is associated with hemodynamic or arrhythmic complications or preexisting left ventricular dysfunction, has a major adverse effect on early and late prognosis. The reported incidence varies widely (0 to >10 percent), in large part due to heterogeneous diagnostic criteria, with an average of 3.9 percent (median 2.9 percent).[296] The cardiac troponins and myocardial creatine phosphokinase-MB (CK-MB) may be useful as markers of perioperative infarction.[297] Elevation of CK-MB more than five times the upper limit of normal is commonly considered diagnostic of myocardial infarction in this setting. Predictors of perioperative myocardial infarction in CASS were female gender, severe perioperative angina pectoris, severe stenosis of the left main coronary artery, and triple-vessel disease. Preconditioning the myocardium with short periods of ischemic stress interspersed with reperfusion increases the resistance to infarction and appears to reduce myocardial damage during cardiac surgery, but the appropriateness of this technique as a routine clinical tool has not been determined.

RESPIRATORY COMPLICATIONS. Most patients are extubated within 6 to 8 hours after undergoing CABG. Prolonged mechanical ventilation (>24 hours) is necessary in 5 to 6 percent of first-time CABGs and 10 to 11 percent of reoperations.[298] The etiology is multifactorial and includes the presence of preexisting pulmonary disease and numerous perioperative factors related directly to anesthesia, level of consciousness, CPB, incisional pain, chest tube placement, and occasionally phrenic nerve damage.[299] Severe chronic obstructive pulmonary disease, as defined by a forced expiratory volume in 1 second (FEV_1) of less than 50 percent or an FEV_1/forced vital capacity (FVC) ratio less than 0.70, is associated with a high incidence of postoperative pulmonary complications (29 percent). The left ventricular ejection fraction is also an important determinant of prolonged ventilation.[300]

Postoperative changes in pulmonary function after CABG are frequent and troublesome, but rarely serious, except in patients with preexisting chronic lung disease or the elderly.[299] A potentially serious complication is phrenic nerve injury, which may be related to cold-induced damage during myocardial protection strategies or possibly to mechanical injury while harvesting the IMA. The pulmonary consequences vary and range from an asymptomatic radiographic abnormality to severe pulmonary dysfunction requiring prolonged ventilation.[261]

BLEEDING. Impaired hemostasis and bleeding complications are an inherent risk of CABG. Reoperation for bleeding is required in 2 to 6 percent of patients and is associated with nearly threefold higher in-hospital mortality.[301] CPB causes derangement of the intrinsic coagulation and fibrinolytic systems in addition to impairing platelet function. The risk of bleeding is increased with age, a smaller body surface area, duration of CPB, reoperation, bilateral internal thoracic artery grafts, and the preoperative use of heparin, aspirin, and fibrinolytic agents. Bleeding may be reduced with aprotinin and lysine analogs such as aminocaproic acid and tranexamic acid.[302]

WOUND INFECTIONS. Major perioperative wound complications, especially mediastinitis and/or wound dehiscence, occur in 1 to 4 percent of patients and are associated with significant morbidity as well as higher mortality. This risk is substantially increased in those undergoing reoperation and by the use of double IMA grafts, particularly in diabetic patients, and it is markedly increased in obese patients. Preventive measures include careful skin preparation, increased attention to sterility in the perioperative environment, and preoperative use of antimicrobial agents. Other factors that may decrease perioperative infection include strict control of glucose in patients with diabetes and the avoidance of unnecessary blood transfusion in view of the immunosuppressive effect of the latter.[261] Successful management of deep sternal wound infection involves prompt recognition and aggressive débridement with muscle flap closure.

POSTOPERATIVE HYPERTENSION. Hypertension can occur in up to one-third of patients postoperatively. The mechanisms are unclear but may be related to increased levels of circulating catecholamines and other humoral factors in addition to vasoconstriction secondary to activation of the renin-angiotensin system. Control of postoperative hypertension is important to prevent myocardial ischemia, cardiac failure, and perioperative bleeding. Regardless of the cause, sodium nitroprusside is an effective approach to afterload reduction, and other drugs such as calcium antagonists, nitrates, and beta blockers, including short-acting esmolol, are helpful.[261]

CEREBROVASCULAR COMPLICATIONS. Neurological abnormalities following cardiac surgery are dreaded complications. Postulated mechanisms include emboli from atherosclerosis of the aorta or other large arteries, emboli possibly from the CPB machine circuit and its tubing, and intraoperative hypotension, particularly in patients with preexisting hypertension.[303] Type I injury is associated with major neurological deficits, stupor, and coma, and type II is characterized by a deterioration in intellectual function and memory.[261] The incidence of neurological abnormalities is variably estimated depending on how the deficits are defined. The incidence of stroke reported in the Society of Thoracic Surgeons data base between 1997 to 1999 was 1.63 percent and has been documented as higher in prospective studies (1.5 to 5 percent). Studies aimed at careful evaluation of neurological deficits report more frequent neurological sequelae; type I deficits have been documented in 6 percent of patients early after CABG, with short-term cognitive decline in 33 to 83 percent.[304] A prospective long-term study employing sophisticated neurocognitive testing revealed cognitive decline in 53 percent of patients at the time of hospital discharge, 36 percent at 6 weeks, and 24 percent at 6 months.[305] In regard to the neurological sequelae of CPB (including stroke, delirium, and neurocognitive dysfunction), older age in addition to other comorbid conditions (particularly diabetes) associated with atherosclerosis and intraoperative manipulation of the aorta are the more powerful predictors. In most studies, atherosclerosis of the proximal aorta has also been a strong predictor of stroke, as has the use of an intraaortic balloon pump.

ATRIAL FIBRILLATION. This arrhythmia is one of the most frequent complications of CABG. It occurs in up to 40 percent of patients, primarily within 2 to 3 days.[306] In the early postoperative period, rapid ventricular rates and loss of atrial transport may compromise systemic hemodynamics, increase the risk of embolization, and lead to a significant increase in the duration and cost of the hospital stay, and it is associated with a twofold to threefold increase in postoperative stroke. Older age, hypertension, prior atrial fibrillation, and congestive heart failure are associated with higher risk of developing atrial fibrillation after cardiac surgery.

Prophylactic use of beta blockers reduces the frequency of postoperative atrial fibrillation and should be administered routinely before and after CABG to patients without contraindications. Amiodarone is also effective in prophylaxis against postoperative atrial fibrillation and may be considered in patients at high risk for developing this dysrhythmia (see Chap. 76). Up to 80 percent of patients spontaneously revert to sinus rhythm within 24 hours without treatment other than digoxin or other agents used for controlling the ventricular rate. Most patients return to sinus rhythm by 6 weeks after surgery.

BRADYARRHYTHMIAS AND CONDUCTION DISTURBANCES. The incidence of postoperative bradyarrhythmias requiring permanent pacemaker implantation was 0.8 percent in a series of 1614 consecutive patients discharged from the hospital after coronary bypass surgery. Predictive factors were preoperative left bundle branch block, concomitant left ventricular aneurysmectomy, and older age. Most patients continued to require permanent pacemaker support during follow-up.

RENAL DYSFUNCTION. The incidence of renal failure requiring dialysis after CABG remains low (0.5 to 1.0 percent) but is associated with significantly greater morbidity and mortality.[296] A decline in renal function defined by a postoperative serum creatinine higher than 2.0 mg/dl or an increase of more than 0.7 mg/dl is more frequent (7 to 8 percent). Predictors of postoperative renal dysfunction include advanced age, diabetes, preexisting renal dysfunction, and heart failure.[307] Patients with preoperative renal dysfunction and serum creatinine higher than 2.5 mg/dl appear to be at increased risk of the need for hemodialysis and may be candidates for alternative approaches to revascularization or prophylactic dialysis.[308]

SYMPTOMATIC RESULTS. CABG is highly effective in the relief of angina and results in improved quality of life. Approximately 80 percent of patients are free of angina at 5 years and 63 percent at 10 years, but by 15 years only about 15 percent are alive and free of an ischemic event.[261] Recurrent angina is associated with a higher risk of myocardial infarction and more frequent coronary reintervention but does not appear to affect survival. The acceleration in adverse events after 5 to 15 years is due to gradual occlusion of vein grafts in addition to progressive disease in the native coronary vessels. Independent predictors of recurrence of angina are female gender, obesity, preoperative hypertension, and lack of use of the IMA as a conduit.[261] In patients with triple-vessel disease undergoing coronary bypass surgery, the completeness of revascularization was a significant determinant of the relief of symptoms at 1 year and over a 5-year period.[309] In the bypass surgery arms of recent randomized trials of PCI and CABG, recurrent angina pectoris was reported in 21.5 to 34 percent of patients at a follow-up ranging from 2 to 3 years, but (Canadian classification) grade III or IV angina was present in only 6 percent at 2.5 years.[261]

RETURN TO EMPLOYMENT. Return to full employment has been variable (35 to 80 percent) but is as high as 80 percent among those who were employed prior to undergoing CABG.[310] Patients who undergo CABG take approximately 6 weeks longer to return to work than those who are treated with PCI; however, long-term employment is similar (>80 percent) among patients treated with CABG or PCI.[310] Factors that adversely affect the prospects of patients for returning to work include advanced age, postoperative angina, job satisfaction prior to surgery, and a period of either unemployment or disability before surgery.[311]

PATENCY OF VENOUS GRAFTS. Experimental studies and observations in patients suggest that the development of disease in *venous* aortocoronary artery bypass grafts occurs in several phases. The occlusion rate, which is high in the first year, decreases substantially between the first and sixth years. Between 6 and 10 years after surgery, the attrition rate for grafts increases again. Early occlusion (before hospital discharge) occurs in 8 to 12 percent of venous grafts, and by 1 year, 15 to 30 percent of vein grafts have become occluded.[261] After the first year, the annual occlusion rate is 2 percent and rises to approximately 4 percent annually between years 6 and 10. At 10 years, approximately 50 percent of vein grafts have become occluded, and significant atherosclerosis is present in the substantial proportion of grafts remaining patent, with significant stenoses in 20 to 40 percent.[261] Patency rates with IMA grafts are superior. Predictors of graft occlusion include small target-vessel diameter and patient risk factors such as high LDL cholesterol, low HDL cholesterol, prior myocardial infarction, male gender, and active smoking.[312]

EARLY PHASE (FIRST MONTH). Technical factors that may cause thrombotic closure at the proximal or distal anastomoses include kinking because of excessive length, tension from insufficient length, poor graft flow, and inadequate distal runoff. Surgical manipulation of the saphenous vein during harvesting and preparation prior to grafting play key roles in initiating the sequence of endothelial damage with subsequent platelet and fibrin deposition leading to thrombosis.

INTERMEDIATE PHASE (1 MONTH TO 1 YEAR). Vein grafts that have been implanted in the arterial circulation for 1 month to 1 year are subject to substantial endothelial denudation and proliferation and to migration of medial cells to the intima. Migration of vascular smooth muscle cells through the internal elastic lamina into the intima may also occur.[313] This initial phase of rapid proliferation is followed after several months by a marked increase in the connective tissue matrix, which further increases intimal and medial thickness. This accelerated process of intimal hyperplasia and thickening is an early stage of atherosclerotic plaque formation and is believed to occur because of interaction between platelets and macrophages and endothelial damage. If the proliferation is severe and localized, as may occur at the site of anastomosis between the grafts and the recipient artery, total occlusion can occur within 1 year.

LATE PHASE (BEYOND 1 YEAR). Some investigators believe that the development of atherosclerosis in vein grafts, as in native arteries, is a continuum starting from platelet deposition and advancing to smooth muscle cell proliferation and finally to lipid incorporation into the plaque. By 10 years, nearly half of venous grafts patent at 5 years have become occluded.[314] Beyond the first year, particularly after 3 to 5 years, the histological appearance of occluded or obstructed coronary bypass grafts is consistent with atherosclerosis. There is clear evidence of mature lipid-laden plaque, foam cells, cholesterol clefts, ulceration, and areas of calcification with disruption of the medial layer. Late graft atherosclerosis is often characterized by an extensive thrombotic burden and marked friability of the lesions; the resultant intermittent distal embolization in turn complicates repeat revascularization procedures either by percutaneous coronary reintervention or reoperation.[315]

DETERMINATION OF GRAFT PATENCY. Although angiography is the most frequently used method for the determination of vein graft patency, the diffuseness of the atherosclerotic process, which in many patients decreases the luminal diameter of the entire vessel, may lead to an underestimation of the severity of a more focal lesion. Alternative approaches to the evaluation of vein graft patency that are being investigated include contrast-enhanced CT (see Chap. 15),[316] phase-contrast magnetic resonance angiography (see Chap. 14),[317] and transcutaneous ultrasonographic[318] and magnetic resonance measurements of angiographic flow.[72]

ARTERIAL GRAFT PATENCY. Comparative morphological and angiographic studies of IMA and saphenous vein bypass grafts that have been implanted long-term show that accelerated atherosclerosis occurs commonly in saphenous vein grafts but is extremely rare in IMA grafts. Several potential explanations may be offered for the superiority of the IMA graft. The media of the artery may derive nourishment from the lumen as well as from the vasa vasorum, and the internal elastic lamina of the IMA is uniform. Moreover, the finding that the endothelium of the IMA produces significantly more prostacyclin than that of the saphenous vein may explain the more pronounced endothelium-dependent relaxation and may allow flow-dependent autoregulation to occur. Fibrointimal proliferation occasionally develops in IMA grafts, and the resultant narrowing may be a factor in late graft closure.[261]

Clinical and angiographic outcomes are superior when IMA grafts are used compared with venous grafts. In one series, IMA grafts had patency rates of 95, 88, and 83 percent at 1, 5, and 10 years, respectively. Although comparable at 1 year, these rates are significantly higher than those observed for venous grafts at 5 and 10 years. Excellent long-term results have also been achieved with use of the right IMA as a free or sequential graft. Consistent with these angiographic findings, patients receiving an IMA graft have a decreased risk of short-term and long-term major cardiac events, including death, myocardial infarction, and reoperations, and this clinical advantage persists for up to 20 years.[261,288]

PROGRESSION OF DISEASE IN NONGRAFTED ARTERIES. Disease progression, defined as worsening of a preexisting lesion or the appearance of a new diameter narrowing of 50 percent or greater, can occur at a rate of 20 to 40 percent over 5 to 10 years in nongrafted native vessels.[319] The rate of disease progression appears highest in arterial segments already showing evidence of disease, and it is between three and six times higher in grafted native coronary arteries than in ungrafted native vessels. Disease progression is also greater in arteries with patent grafts than in arteries with occluded grafts[320] and usually occurs proximal to the site of graft insertion. These data suggest that bypassing an artery with minimal disease, even if initially successful, may ultimately be harmful to patients, who incur both the risk of graft closure and the increased risk of accelerated obstruction of native vessels. Lesions in the native vessel that are long (>10 mm) and more than 70 percent in diameter are at increased risk of progressing to total occlusion.[321]

EFFECTS OF THERAPY ON VEIN GRAFT OCCLUSION AND NATIVE VESSEL PROGRESSION

Measures aimed at enhancing long-term patency are generally directed at delaying the overall process of atherosclerosis, and thus they may have several additional benefits.[315] Secondary preventive therapy, in particular lipid-lowering treatment, is important to reducing the risk of failure of venous grafts.[282] Chronic anticoagulant therapy has *not* been shown convincingly to alter outcomes.[282] Other novel approaches, such as pretreatment of venous grafts to increase resistance to atherothrombosis, are in early stages of evaluation.[283]

ANTIPLATELET THERAPY. Several trials have demonstrated the efficacy of aspirin therapy when started 1, 7, or 24 hours preoperatively, but the benefit is lost when aspirin is started more than 48 hours postoperatively.[322] Aspirin, 80 to 325 mg daily, should be continued indefinitely. The addition of dipyridamole or warfarin in conventional doses has not been shown definitively to provide added benefit.[282] Although the effects of clopidogrel on graft patency have not been studied specifically, it is likely to be at least as effective as aspirin.

LIPID-LOWERING THERAPY. The rationale for lowering lipid levels in patients with CAD was extended to postoperative patients with at least one patent vein graft and LDL cholesterol concentrations between 130 and 175 mg/dl in the Post-Coronary Artery Bypass Graft Trial.[282] Patients who received aggressive treatment with lovastatin and, if needed, cholestyramine to decrease LDL cholesterol to less than 100 mg/dl, in comparison with "moderate" therapy resulting in an LDL cholesterol level of 134 mg/dl, had a lower rate of progressive atherosclerosis in grafts (27 vs. 39 percent; $p < 0.001$) and a lower rate of repeat revascularization procedures over a 4-year period. Similar benefits are achieved with other lipid-lowering therapies, including colestipol and niacin, and gemfibrozil. Moreover, the favorable effects of lipid-lowering on the progression of graft disease appear similar in women and men, the elderly and young, and those with and without diabetes.

SMOKING CESSATION. Strong evidence from the CASS randomized trial and other series indicates that continued smoking after bypass surgery increases mortality, the recurrence rate of angina, the need for repeat hospitalization, and repeat revascularization procedures. Not unexpectedly, continued smoking has been associated with angiographic progression of graft disease.[312]

Patient Selection

Indications for CABG consist of the need for improvement in the quality or duration of life. Patients whose angina is not adequately controlled by medical management or who have unacceptable side effects with such management should be considered for coronary revascularization. The decision to perform PCI or CABG is based partly on coronary anatomy, left ventricular function, other medical comorbidities that may affect the patient's risk for either procedure, and patient preference. Recent technological developments have enlarged the pool of patients with single-vessel or multivessel disease amenable to PCI. For patients who are suitable for

PCI and who do not fulfill the criteria of anatomy requiring surgery (e.g., left main CAD or severe triple-vessel disease and left ventricular dysfunction), PCI is generally the procedure of choice. However, if medical therapy has failed (i.e., the symptoms are severe or sufficient to impair quality of life), and the patient is not a good candidate for initial or repeat PCI, CABG should be strongly considered. This procedure is also indicated for patients with CAD, regardless of symptoms, in whom survival is likely to be prolonged, and for patients in whom noninvasive testing suggests "high risk."[261]

In making the decision about revascularization, it is important to assess the patient's prognosis (Tables 50–13 and 50–14) and how it may be affected by surgery. The key initial step is to stratify patients into categories of risk with continued medical therapy based on an analysis of clinical, noninvasive, and, in some patients, angiographic variables. This process defines the *indications* for revascularization over medical therapy and, by implication, the indications for coronary angiography in patients with chronic stable angina, as well as which *modality* of revascularization (PCI or surgery) is preferable.[18]

The four major determinants of risk in CAD are the extent of ischemia, the number of vessels diseased, left ventricular function, and the electrical substrate. The major effect of coronary revascularization is on ischemia, and the magnitude of the benefit compared with that of medical therapy is enhanced with left ventricular dysfunction, particularly in the presence of reversibly ischemic jeopardized myocardium. In this context, patients can be risk stratified according to the expected benefit of revascularization versus medical therapy. Patients with more extensive and severe CAD have an increasing magnitude of benefit from CABG over medical therapy (Figs. 50–16 and 50–17 and Table 50–15). Selection of patients for surgery is based on clinical, angiographic, and noninvasive testing characteristics that may be considered markers or, in some cases, surrogates of the three major predictors—ischemia, left ventricular function, and, to a lesser extent, arrhythmia. Other factors that must always be considered in the decision are general health and noncoronary comorbid conditions.

The appropriate use of invasive cardiovascular procedures is undergoing increasing scrutiny. It is therefore reassuring to note that in studies of coronary angiography and bypass surgery less than 4 percent of bypass procedures are

TABLE 50–13 Determinants of Adverse Prognosis in Patients with Coronary Artery Disease

Cardiac Determinants
Left ventricular dysfunction
Extent of myocardium in jeopardy
Abnormal arrhythmic substrate

Clinical and Electrocardiographic Modifying Factors
Advanced age
History of congestive heart failure
Diabetes
Rapidly accelerating angina
Resting electrocardiographic abnormalities
Left ventricular hypertrophy and hypertension
Peripheral vascular disease
Hyperlipidemia
Increased C-reactive protein (inflammation)

TABLE 50–14 Impact of Coronary Bypass Surgery on Survival in Subsets of Patients Studied in the Coronary Artery Surgery Study (CASS) Randomized Trial and Registry Studies

Category of Risk	Number of Vessels Diseased	Severity of Ischemia	Ejection Fraction	Results of Surgery on Survival
Mild	2	Mild	>0.50	Unchanged*
	3			Unchanged*
Moderate	2	Moderate to severe	>0.50	Unchanged*
	3			Improved†
	2	Mild	<0.50	Unchanged*
	3			Improved†
Severe	2	Moderate to severe	<0.50	Improved†
	3			Improved†

*Randomized trial.
†Survival improved with surgery versus medicine. In the European Coronary Surgery Trial, patients with double-vessel disease and involvement of the proximal left anterior descending coronary artery had improved survival with surgery irrespective of left ventricular function.

TABLE 50–15 Effects of Coronary Artery Bypass Grafting on Survival*

Subgroup	Medical Treatment Mortality Rate (%)	*p* Value for CABG Surgery vs. Medical Treatment
Vessel Disease		
One vessel	9.9	0.18
Two vessels	11.7	0.45
Three vessels	17.6	<0.001
Left main artery	36.5	0.004
No LAD Disease		
One or two vessels	8.3	0.88
Three vessels	14.5	0.02
Left main artery	45.8	0.03
Overall	12.3	0.05
LAD Disease Present		
One or two vessels	14.6	0.05
Three vessels	19.1	0.009
Left main artery	32.7	0.02
Overall	18.3	0.001
LV Function		
Normal	13.3	<0.001
Abnormal	25.2	0.02
Exercise Test Status		
Missing	17.4	0.10
Normal	11.6	0.38
Abnormal	16.8	<0.001
Severity of Angina		
Class 0, I, II	12.5	0.005
Class III, IV	22.4	0.001

LAD = left anterior descending artery; LV = left ventricular.
From Yusuf S, Zucker D, Peduzzi P, et al: Effect of coronary artery bypass surgery on survival: Overview of 10-year results from randomized trials by the Coronary Artery Bypass Surgery Trialists Collaboration. Lancet 344:563, 1994.
*Systematic overview of the effect of coronary artery bypass grafting (CABG) vs. medical therapy on survival based on data from the seven randomized trials comparing a strategy of initial CABG surgery with one of initial medical therapy. Subgroup results at 5 years are shown.

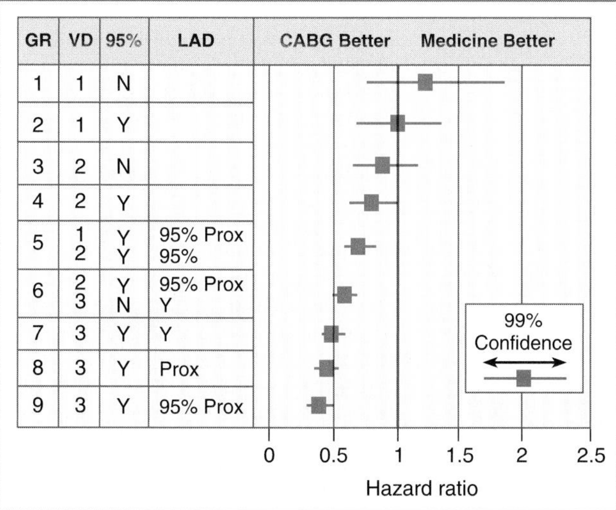

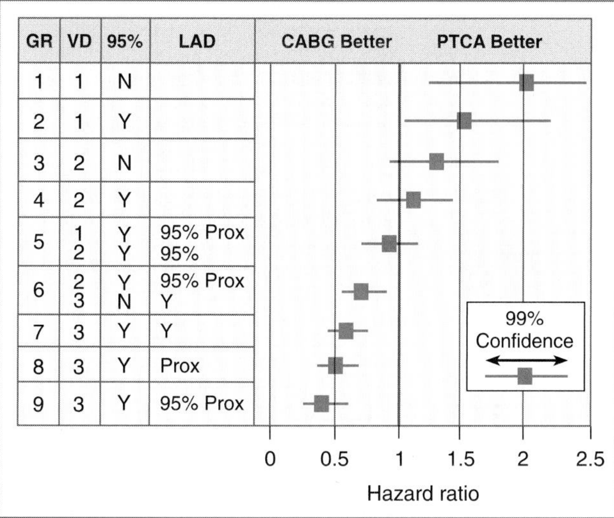

FIGURE 50–16 **A,** Adjusted hazard (mortality) ratios comparing coronary artery bypass grafting (CABG) and medical therapy for nine coronary anatomy severity groups (GR) according to the number of vessels diseased (VD), the presence or absence of a 95 percent proximal stenosis (95 percent), and involvement of the left anterior descending coronary artery (LAD). **B,** Adjusted hazard (mortality) ratios comparing CABG and percutaneous transluminal angioplasty (PTCA) for nine coronary anatomy groups according to the number of vessels diseased, the presence or absence of a 95 percent proximal stenosis, and LAD involvement. Among patients with the least severe categories of disease, 5-year survival appears to be better with PTCA (single-vessel disease without proximal stenosis and without LAD involvement), whereas for patients with triple-vessel disease and higher grade, more complex double-vessel disease, a survival benefit is noted with surgery. For other subsets of patients with double-vessel disease, no difference in survival was seen in those treated with CABG or PTCA, and many of these patients are probably similar to those included in the randomized trials. (Data from the Duke University data base. **A** and **B,** From Jones RH, Kesler K, Phillips HR III, et al: Long-term survival benefits of coronary artery bypass grafting and percutaneous transluminal angioplasty in patients with coronary artery disease. J Thorac Cardiovasc Surg 111:1013, 1996.)

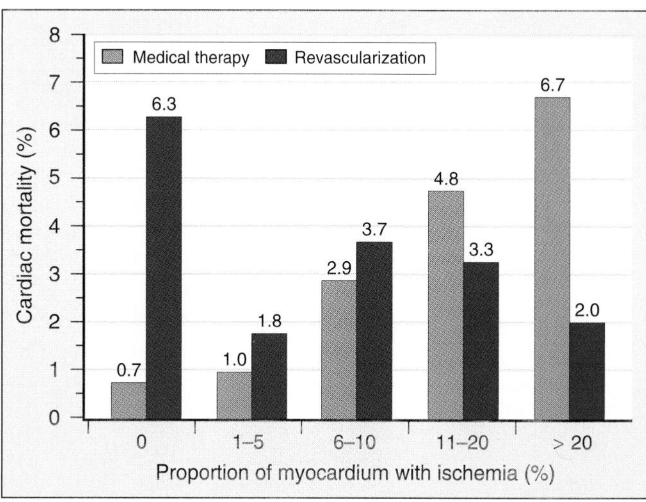

FIGURE 50–17 Rate of cardiac death among patients treated with medical therapy versus revascularization, stratified by the proportion of ischemic myocardium on stress nuclear imaging. A total of 10,627 consecutive patients without prior myocardial infarction or revascularization were followed for a mean of 1.6 years after exercise or adenosine myocardial perfusion imaging. Patients with moderate to severe ischemia who underwent percutaneous or surgical coronary revascularization within 60 days of stress imaging had lower mortality than those treated with medical therapy ($p < 0.0001$). However, those patients with no or mild ischemia had no survival advantage with revascularization. (From Hachamovitch R, Hayes SW, Friedman JD, et al: Comparison of the short-term survival benefit associated with revascularization compared with medical therapy in patients with no prior coronary artery disease undergoing stress myocardial perfusion single photon emission computed tomography. Circulation 107:2900-2906, 2003.)

considered inappropriate using criteria from an international panel.[323]

Results

In 1972, a committee of the AHA indicated that the most widely accepted indication for surgical revascularization was "significant disability from moderate to severe angina pectoris, unresponsive to optimal medical care." More than three decades later, with the development of PCI and improvements both in medical therapy of CAD and in CABG, the realization that CABG prolongs survival in subgroups of patients with either minimal or mild to moderate symptoms has shifted the emphasis toward *ischemia* instead of *symptoms alone* as the target for coronary revascularization. Consequently and appropriately, CABG is currently performed in an increasing number of patients with multivessel disease and/or left ventricular dysfunction (particularly in the face of viable jeopardized dysfunctioning myocardium). Severe ischemia and/or reversible left ventricular dysfunction provides a window of opportunity for improving survival (in comparison to medical therapy) that has resulted in an increase in the frequency of CABG in patients with unstable angina and in survivors of acute myocardial infarction. Left ventricular dysfunction, initially a relative contraindication for surgery, has become a major indication. Nonetheless, severe symptoms or even moderate symptoms that interfere with the quality of life despite adequate medical therapy remain as firm an indication for coronary revascularization (PCI or CABG) as they were for CABG three decades ago.

RELIEF OF ANGINA. CABG is highly effective in providing complete relief from angina in some patients and improvement in the severity of symptoms in most of the remainder. For example, in a series of patients who received saphenous vein grafts alone, approximately 90 percent were free of angina at 1 year. In the following 4 years, the recurrence rate was approximately 3 percent per year and 5 percent per year thereafter. Approximate rates of freedom from angina were 78 percent at 5 years, which decreased to 52 and 23 percent at 10 and 15 years, respectively.[324] Trials in which the contemporary practice of using one or more arterial grafts was prevalent demonstrate similar to superior rates of freedom from angina during short-term and mid-term follow-up.[325] The major randomized trials all have demonstrated greater relief of angina, better exercise performance, and a lower requirement for antianginal medications for surgically versus medically treated patients 5 years postoperatively.[261] Beyond 5 years, differences in symptoms between

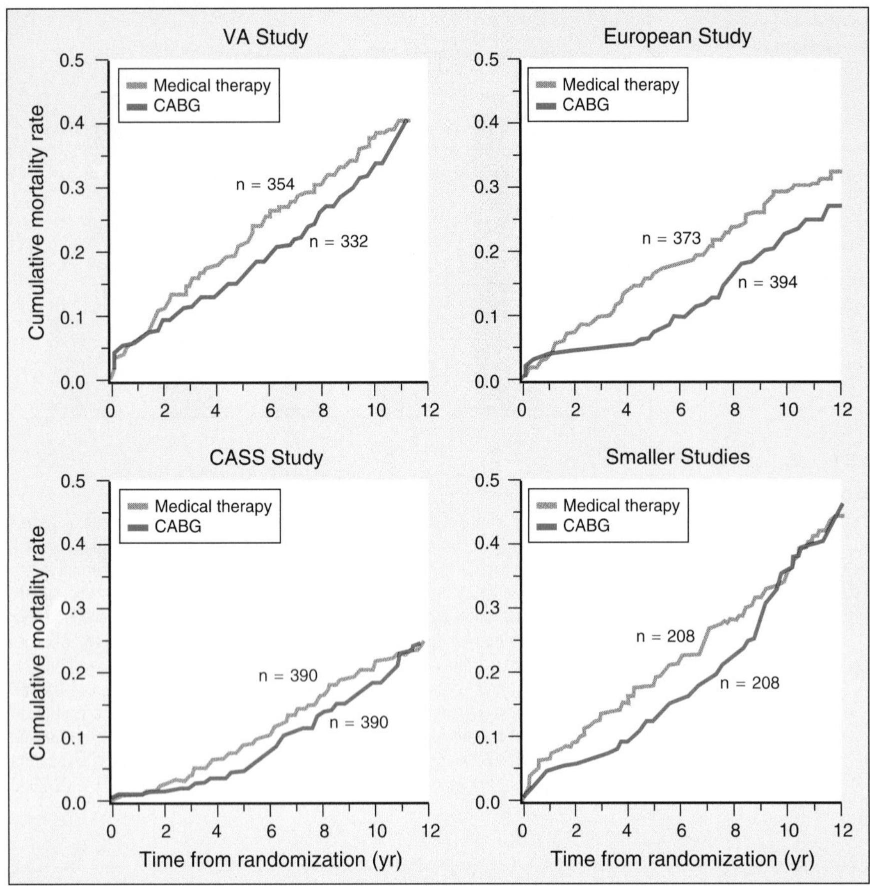

FIGURE 50–18 Survival curves of the three large randomized trials and four smaller studies combined. (From Eagle KA, Guyton RA, Davidoff R, et al: ACC/AHA guidelines for coronary artery bypass graft surgery: A report of the American College of Cardiology/American Heart Association Task Force on Practice Guidelines [Committee to Revise the 1991 Guidelines for Coronary Artery Bypass Graft Surgery]. American College of Cardiology/American Heart Association. J Am Coll Cardiol 34:1262-1347, 1999.)

patients initially treated medically and surgically are diminished, in part because of the high crossover rate from medical to surgical therapy in patients with continued symptoms and progression of disease in vein grafts and in nonbypassed vessels in the surgical group.[326] The reoperation rate for recurrence of symptoms has been reported to be in the range of 6 to 8 percent per year.

For patients with persistent angina despite adequate medical therapy or for patients who do not tolerate medications and who are not suitable candidates for PCI, CABG provides excellent symptomatic relief.[261] With increasing use of IMA grafts, long-term relief from angina and freedom from subsequent cardiac events are improved in comparison to previous patient populations who received vein grafts alone.

In summary, after 5 years, approximately three-fourths of surgically treated patients can be predicted to be free of an ischemic event, sudden death, occurrence of myocardial infarction, or the recurrence of angina; about half remain free for approximately 10 years and about 15 percent for 15 or more years. Symptomatic improvement is best maintained in patients with the most complete revascularization.

EFFECTS ON SURVIVAL. Current clinical practice has been shaped by three major randomized trials of CABG compared to medical therapy that enrolled patients between 1972 and 1984: the Veterans Affairs (VA) Trial, the European Cardiac Society Study (ECSS), and the National Institutes of Health–supported CASS (Fig. 50–18).[261] The evidence base comprised data from 2649 patients participating in these and several smaller trials.[327] It has provided a wealth of important information but has several important limitations with respect to application to current practice as the risk profile of patients referred for surgery, as well as the available surgical and medical interventions have evolved substantially. In particular, these trials antedated the widespread use of one or two IMAs. As a result, the extent of the completeness of coronary revascularization, graft patency rates, and perioperative mortality in the VA trial fall far short of current expectations and reflect, in part, the initial learning experience of coronary bypass surgery. Moreover, although the patients allocated to initial CABG had a significantly lower mortality at 5, 7, and 10 years, 41 percent of the patients assigned to medical treatment had undergone CABG by 10 years (so-called crossovers).

The results of the trials of surgical versus medical therapy were generally highly consistent, and thus the major points guiding clinical practice may still be drawn from a meta-analysis of the results.[327] In each of the trials, a survival benefit of CABG emerged during mid-term follow-up (2 to 6 years), but this advantage eroded during long-term follow-up and remained statistically significant only in the ECSS. Considered together, the results of these trials support a 4.1 percent absolute reduction in long-term mortality (10 years) with CABG ($p = 0.03$). Subgroup analyses reveal several high-risk criteria that identify patients who are likely to sustain a more substantial survival benefit: (1) left main CAD; (2) single- or double-vessel disease with proximal LAD disease; (3) left ventricular systolic dysfunction; (4) a composite evaluation that indicates high risk, including severity of symptoms, high-risk exercise tolerance test, history of prior myocardial infarction, and the presence of ST depression on the resting ECG.

The only randomized data comparing CABG with medical therapy in the current era are from the Asymptomatic Cardiac Ischemia Pilot (ACIP) Study of 558 patients (Fig. 50–19).[328] This trial of angina-guided versus angina plus ischemia-guided medical therapy (using ambulatory monitoring) in comparison to revascularization by either PTCA (92 patients) or CABG (79 patients) enrolled relatively low-risk patients. After 2 years of follow-up, mortality was significantly lower among the patients assigned to routine revascularization (1.1 vs. 6.6 and 4.4 percent for the two medical groups [$p < 0.02$]), and rates of death or myocardial infarction were 12.1 percent (angina-guided medical therapy), 8.9 percent (ischemia-guided medical therapy), and 4.7 percent (coronary revascularization) ($p < 0.04$). Although this trial was designed as a pilot study and the number of patients was relatively small, the observed risk reductions were statistically significant and suggest that the benefits of revascularization in the context of current revascularization technique may be greater than previously appreciated. The trial was not designed to assess differences between PTCA and bypass surgery but does point to the need for larger, more definitive randomized trials testing current strategies of revascularization with optimal medical therapy and risk factor reduction.

Taken together, the results of all the trials and registries indicate that the "sicker" the patient (based on the severity of symptoms or ischemia, age, the number of vessels diseased, and the presence of left ventricular dysfunction), the greater the benefit of surgical over medical therapy on survival (see Figs. 50-16 and 50-17 and Table 50-15). CABG prolongs survival in patients with significant left main CAD irrespective of symptoms, in patients with multivessel disease and impaired left ventricular function, and in patients with triple-vessel disease that includes the proximal LAD coronary artery (irrespective of left ventricular function).[261] Surgical therapy has also been demonstrated to prolong life in patients with *double-vessel disease* and left ventricular dysfunction, particularly those with proximal narrowing of one or more coronary arteries and in the presence of severe angina. Although no study has documented a survival

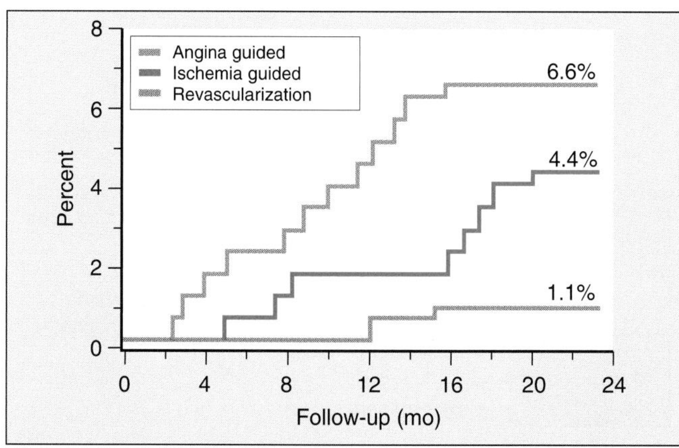

FIGURE 50–19 Two-year cumulative mortality rates for the three treatment strategies in the Asymptomatic Cardiac Ischemia Pilot (ACIP) study. Significant differences were seen between revascularization and angina-guided strategies ($p \leq 0.005$) and between revascularization and ischemia-guided strategies ($p \leq 0.05$). Angina-guided and ischemia-guided strategies were not significantly different from each other ($p = 0.34$). Similar results were noted for the endpoints of cumulative rates of death, myocardial infarction, or cardiac hospitalization. (From Davies RF, Goldberg AD, Forman S, et al: Asymptomatic Cardiac Ischemia Pilot [ACIP] study two-year follow-up: Outcomes of patients randomized to initial strategies of medical therapy versus revascularization. Circulation 95:2037, 1997.)

benefit with surgical treatment in patients with *single-vessel disease*, some evidence indicates that such patients who have impaired left ventricular function have a poor long-term survival with medical therapy. Such patients with angina or evidence of ischemia at a low or moderate level of exercise, especially those with obstruction of the proximal left anterior descending coronary artery, may benefit from coronary revascularization by either PCI or bypass surgery.

LEFT MAIN CORONARY ARTERY STENOSIS. It is widely agreed that surgical treatment improves survival in patients with left main coronary artery obstruction or its "equivalent."[261] The CASS Registry demonstrated that the superiority of revascularization was equivalent in both symptomatic and asymptomatic patients with disease affecting the left main coronary artery.

Whether a "left main–equivalent" anatomy exists that has a natural history similar to that of left main CAD is uncertain. The condition in question may consist of disease in the proximal portions of both the LAD and left circumflex coronary arteries. It is likely that significant left main coronary disease has an ominous nature because a single event (rupture of a single plaque) can cause infarction of a very large quantity of myocardium. Consequently, although combined disease of the proximal left anterior descending and circumflex coronary arteries does identify a subgroup of high-risk patients, the prognosis is not as poor as it is for patients with left main CAD.[329] Nevertheless, patients with combined stenoses of 70 percent or greater in the LAD coronary artery, before the first septal perforating branch, and in the proximal circumflex coronary artery, before the first obtuse marginal branch, who have impaired ventricular function also have improved survival and less angina following surgical revascularization than if they are treated medically, particularly in the face of left ventricular dysfunction. The median survival of surgically treated patients with left main–equivalent disease is 13.1 years versus 6.2 years for those medically treated.[261]

EFFECT ON SUBSEQUENT MYOCARDIAL INFARCTION. The major randomized trials of patients with mild to moderate angina suggested that the likelihood of occurrence of myocardial infarction after 5 to 10 years of follow-up was similar in medically and surgically treated patients. In both the VA study and the CASS, the major benefit of surgery on myocardial infarction does not appear to be mediated by a decrease in the frequency of myocardial infarction but by a decrease in the case fatality rate of patients who subsequently have infarction.[330] Potential explanations are that previous bypass surgery results in smaller infarcts caused by distal occlusions and that the bypass may enhance myocardial perfusion distal to the obstructing lesion.

Patients with Depressed Left Ventricular Function

Depressed left ventricular function is one of the most powerful predictors of perioperative and late mortality.[294] In the Society of Thoracic Surgeons data base, the mean ejection fraction among approximately 136,330 patients undergoing initial coronary bypass in 1999 was approximately 0.51, and approximately 25 percent had an ejection fraction of less than 0.45.[293] Moreover, as the population ages and the proportion undergoing reoperation increases, the number of patients with preoperative left ventricular dysfunction and clinical heart failure will increase. In the CABG Patch trial confined to patients with an ejection fraction of 0.35 or less, perioperative mortality was 3.5 percent for patients without clinical signs of heart failure versus 7.7 percent for those with NYHA Class I to IV heart failure.[331] The latter was a powerful independent predictor of increased operative mortality in patients with ventricular dysfunction and a positive signal-averaged ECG (odds ratio, 2.4; $p = 0.01$).

Although the effect of a reduced ejection fraction on operative mortality cannot be eliminated, careful attention to intraoperative metabolic, inotropic, and mechanical support, including preoperative intraaortic balloon counterpulsation in some patients, may decrease perioperative mortality in comparison with the mortality rates expected from prediction models. In addition to advances in myocardial protection for those undergoing CABG with CPB, off-pump approaches to CABG may also lead to improved surgical outcomes in this high-risk population.[332] Thus, in experienced centers, the in-hospital mortality for patients with severe left ventricular dysfunction is less than 4 percent.[333]

The powerful effect of the preoperative ejection fraction on late survival emphasizes that in the current era, the presence of left ventricular dysfunction, in association with viable myocardium, has changed from a relative contraindication to coronary bypass to a strong indication.[18] This shift in focus has been due to the realization that viable dysfunctioning myocardium may improve after coronary revascularization.[334] Indeed, the most striking survival benefits of CABG, as well as symptomatic and functional improvement, are shown by patients with seriously impaired left ventricular function in whom the prognosis of medical therapy is poor.[333] In patients with a history of congestive heart failure and multivessel (particularly triple-vessel) disease, coronary bypass surgery may also reduce the incidence of sudden cardiac death.[335] Although preoperative left ventricular dysfunction creates the potential for significant benefit, the perioperative risk should not be underestimated, particularly in the setting of clinical congestive heart failure. Selection of patients with viable myocardium supplied by a reasonable target vessel(s) for grafting appears critical in considering CABG for patients with severe left ventricular dysfunction.[336]

MYOCARDIAL HIBERNATION (see Chap. 19). Improvement in survival and left ventricular function following CABG depends on successful reperfusion of viable but noncontractile or poorly contracting myocardium.[337] Two related pathophysiological conditions have been described to explain reversible ischemic contractile dysfunction[338]: (1) myocardial stunning (prolonged but temporary postischemic ventricular dysfunction without myocardial necrosis) and (2) myocardial hibernation (persistent left ventricular dysfunction when myocardial perfusion is chronically reduced (or repetitively stunned) but sufficient to maintain the viability

TABLE 50–16 Markers of Viable Myocardium

Clinical Indicator	Diagnostic Test	Alternative Test
Diastolic wall thickness	Echo	CT, MRI
Systolic wall thickening	Echo	CT, MRI, gated SPECT
Regional wall motion	Echo	CT, MRI, gated SPECT
Regional blood flow	SPECT	PET, MRI
Myocardial metabolism	PET	SPECT
Cell membrane integrity	SPECT	PET
Contractile reserve	Dobutamine, Echo	Angiography, CT, MRI

CT = computed tomography; Echo = echocardiography; MRI = magnetic resonance imaging; PET = positron-emission tomography; SPECT = single-photon emission computed tomography.

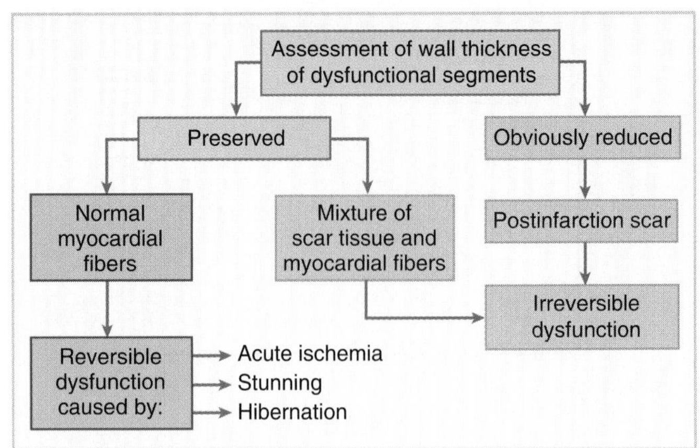

FIGURE 50–20 Flow diagram for the practical assessment of noncontractile segments of myocardial wall potentially recoverable by revascularization procedures. An obviously reduced wall thickness is indicative of a postinfarction scar. Absence of contractile function in segments of the ventricular wall with preserved wall thickness may be caused by different mechanisms. An acute ischemic cause can be excluded by the administration of sublingual nitrates. Stunning can be excluded by repeating the ventricular wall motion study several days after the last ischemic episode. Hibernating myocardium should be distinguished from a mixture of scar tissue and viable myocardial cells. (From Maseri A: Ischemic Heart Disease: A Rational Basis for Clinical Practice and Clinical Research. New York, Churchill Livingstone, 1995.)

of tissue. The reduction in myocardial contractility in hibernating myocardium conserves metabolic demands and may be protective, but more prolonged and severe hibernation may lead to severe ultrastructural abnormalities, irreversible loss of contractile units, and apoptosis.

Hibernating myocardium can cause abnormal systolic or diastolic ventricular function or both. The predominant clinical feature of myocardial ischemia in these patients may not be angina but dyspnea secondary to increased left ventricular diastolic pressure. Symptoms of heart failure resulting from chronic left ventricular dysfunction may be inappropriately ascribed to myocardial necrosis and scarring when the symptoms may, in fact, be reversed after the chronic ischemia is relieved by coronary revascularization.[334]

Detection of Hibernating Myocardium. Several clinical markers may be used to determine the likelihood that a dysfunctional myocardial segment is viable or nonviable (Table 50–16). The presence of angina and the absence of Q waves on the ECG or a history of prior myocardial infarction are useful clues. A severe reduction in the diastolic wall thickness of dysfunctional left ventricular segments is indicative of scarring. On the other hand, akinetic or dyskinetic segments with preserved diastolic wall thickness may represent a mixture of scarred and viable myocardium. A useful strategy for the assessment of dysfunctional segments has been developed by Maseri (Fig. 50–20). Although a number of imaging tools may be used for this assessment (see Chap. 16), the most readily available in most settings is low-dose dobutamine echocardiography.[339]

The term *contractile reserve* describes the ability of hibernating myocardium to exhibit augmented contractility to a suitable temporary stimulus, often causing transient improvement in the global ejection fraction. Contractile reserve underscores the fact that many hypokinetic (and even akinetic) areas of the ventricular wall are composed entirely or in part of viable, hibernating myocardium or a mixture of the latter and fibrous scar. Viable muscle is capable of responding to a sympathomimetic agent. In contrast, necrotic tissue obviously cannot be stimulated to contract by any pharmacological or hemodynamic intervention or by improved perfusion. The most common method of identifying contractile reserve is echocardiographic imaging during infusion of a low dose of dobutamine.[339] Numerous studies have demonstrated that the finding of contractile reserve by low-dose dobutamine echocardiography identifies dysfunctional but viable myocardium with the potential to improve in function after myocardial revascularization.[337]

PET (see Chap. 13) has emerged as an excellent method for demonstrating viable myocardium in patients with impaired left ventricular function. In comparative studies, PET has yielded the highest predictive accuracy of all imaging modalities in detecting dysfunctional myocardium that will improve after revascularization.[340] However, the high cost, technical difficulty, and need for a cyclotron continue to limit this technique's widespread applicability. MRI is emerging as a valuable alternative technique for assessment of myocardial viability.[63] MRI has been shown to have very good correlation with PET [63] and to predict functional recovery after percutaneous or surgical revascularization.[62] Specifically, delayed hyperenhancement with gadolinium identifies areas of myocardial scar, and the transmural extent of hyperenhancement is strongly inversely associated with the probability of recovery after revascularization[62] and may be useful in assessing the probability of regaining contractile function after myocardial infarction.[64]

Thallium-201 rest-redistribution imaging may also be used to determine whether regions with hypoperfusion at rest manifest uptake in the resting defect with time, and stress-redistribution-reinjection imaging, in which a second injection of thallium is administered, may be used to determine whether defects that do not redistribute after exercise represent fibrotic myocardium or myocardium that is severely ischemic (see Chap. 13).[40]

Prognostic Implications of Identifying Viable Myocardium. A growing body of evidence indicates that the detection of viable myocardium in patients with CAD and left ventricular dysfunction not only identifies those in whom improvement in cardiac function is likely after revascularization but also identifies a group of high-risk patients in whom revascularization improves survival (Fig 50–21).[337] Studies with PET, thallium-201, and dobutamine echocardiography have uniformly demonstrated that patients with left ventricular dysfunction and evidence of hibernating myocardium have a high mortality rate during medical therapy and appear to have a better outcome with revascularization. All these studies have limitations, including a small number of patients, the retrospective nature of the analysis, and lack of a randomized control group.[341] However, the consistency of the findings has been striking. Recent data point out that viability assessment is also helpful in the selection of patients for revascularization because patients

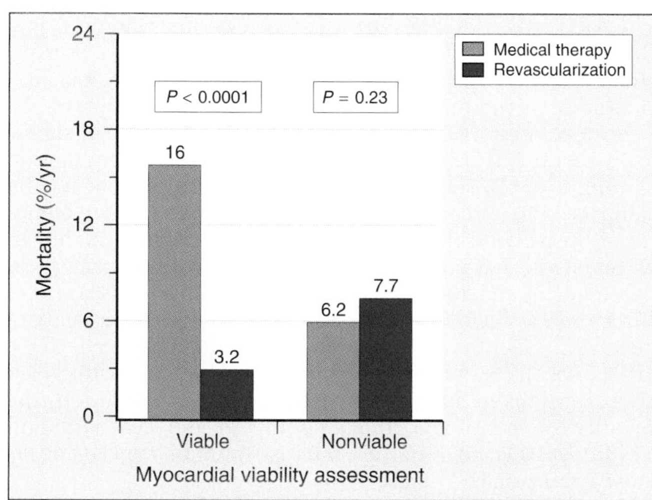

FIGURE 50–21 Meta-analysis of observational studies examining late survival with revascularization versus medical therapy for patients with coronary artery disease and left ventricular dysfunction. Analysis of results from 24 studies ($n = 3088$) demonstrated that revascularization was associated with a significant reduction in annual mortality compared with medical therapy among patients with myocardial viability. No advantage of revascularization was detected in patients without myocardial viability. (Adapted from Allman KC, Shaw LJ, Hachamovitch R, et al: Mycoardial viability testing and impact of revascularization on prognosis in patients with coronary artery disease and left-ventricular dysfunction: A meta-analysis. J Am Coll Cardiol 39:1151-1158, 2002.)

selected for revascularization on the basis of an imaging study demonstrating myocardial viability have lower operative mortality and a higher long-term survival rate than do those who have no evidence of important myocardial viability or those in whom a viability assessment is not performed.[342] Perioperative mortality in the latter patients approaches 10 percent.

The mechanisms for improved survival after revascularization in patients with hibernating myocardium may be related to improvement in left ventricular function, but it is likely that other factors are also operative, including the reduction of left ventricular remodeling, the propensity for serious arrhythmias, and the likelihood of a future fatal acute ischemic event. What remains to be established is the relationship among the extent of viability and the severity of left ventricular dysfunction and the prognostic impact of revascularization.

Surgical Treatment in Special Groups

WOMEN (see Chap. 73). Women are less likely than men to be referred for coronary angiography and subsequent revascularization.[343] In some studies, sex-based differences in referral for revascularization are explained fully by clinical factors.[344] Moreover, it has not been established whether sex-based differences represent underutilization in women, overutilization in men, or both.[343] In comparison with men, women who undergo CABG are "sicker," as defined by age, comorbid conditions, the severity of angina, and history of congestive heart failure.[249] In-hospital mortality and perioperative morbidity after CABG has remained, on average, two times higher in women compared with men. However, when adjusted for the greater risk profile of women referred for CABG, short-term mortality rates as well as long-term outcomes are similar to those for men in most, but not all studies.[345] The independent predictors of long-term prognosis in women are similar to those in men and include older age, previous coronary bypass surgery, previous myocardial infarction, and diabetes.

An excess risk of short-term mortality recently reported in younger women undergoing CABG in one study has not been well explained.[346] Smaller vessel size (as a function of smaller body surface area), a higher incidence of left ventricular hypertrophy, and hypertensive heart disease have been raised as potential contributors to higher surgical risk in women. However, these differences are reasonably expected to be more important in elderly women; the pathophysiological bases for the observed difference in younger women compared with men require further exploration.[249]

With generally similar long-term outcomes after surgical revascularization, sex should not be a significant factor in decisions regarding whether to offer CABG.[249] Newer technical approaches such as OPCAB may be particularly advantageous to women.[347]

YOUNGER PATIENTS. Patients 35 years of age or younger who undergo CABG usually have hyperlipidemia and other major risk factors for CAD. Despite the severity of the underlying disease and the rapidity of the atherosclerotic process, CABG is associated with excellent actuarial survival rates of 94 percent at 5 years and 85 percent at 10 years.[348] Nonetheless, in the CASS Registry, patients younger than 35 years had markedly impaired survival over a 15-year period in comparison with an age- and sex-matched U.S. population. This impaired survival is probably the result of progression of premature atherosclerotic disease, the presence of multiple risk factors, and the development of progressive vein graft disease. The latter underlies the current trend for the use of bilateral IMA grafts and other arterial conduits in younger patients.

THE ELDERLY. A demographic tide in combination with marked improvement in perioperative care and in the outcomes of CABG has resulted in a burgeoning population of elderly patients with extensive disease undergoing such surgery. The number of individuals older than 75 years of age in the United States is expected to quadruple in the next 50 years, with cardiovascular disease being the leading cause of morbidity and mortality in this population.[349] Many such individuals are likely to become candidates for CABG.

Older patients are sicker than their younger counterparts in that they have a greater frequency of comorbid conditions, including peripheral vascular and cerebrovascular disease, more extensive triple-vessel and left main CAD, and a higher frequency of left ventricular dysfunction and history of congestive heart failure. Not unexpectedly, these differences are translated into higher perioperative mortality and complication rates, with a sharp increase in the slope of the curve relating mortality to age seen in patients older than 70 years.[261] Despite these differences, in-hospital mortality for the elderly has declined over time to 7 to 9 percent among those undergoing CABG only and has been reported to be as low as 3 to 4 percent among the subgroup of octogenarians without significant medical comorbidities. Perioperative morbidity is greater in the elderly, with high rates of low-output syndrome, stroke, gastrointestinal complications, wound infection, and postoperative atrial fibrillation.

RENAL DISEASE. Cardiovascular disease is the major cause of mortality in patients with end-stage renal disease (ESRD) and accounts for 54 percent of deaths (see Chap. 86). Patients with ESRD, as well as those with less severe renal insufficiency, have numerous risk factors that not only accelerate the development of CAD but also complicate its medical management. These risk factors include diabetes, hypertension with left ventricular hypertrophy, both systolic and diastolic dysfunction, abnormal lipid metabolism, anemia, and increased homocysteine levels.[350] Coronary revascularization with PCI or CABG is feasible and well documented in patients with ESRD, but the mortality and complication rates are increased.[350,351] Patients with renal insufficiency (serum creatinine >2.0 mg/dl) who are not dependent on dialysis are also at higher risk of major perioperative complications, longer recovery times, and lower rates of short and mid-term survival. Observational data suggest that in patients on chronic dialysis, CABG is the preferred strategy for revascularization over PCI. However, randomized data are very few, and 30-day mortality in patients with ESRD undergoing CABG ranges from 9 to as high as 20 percent.[238]

In summary, coronary bypass surgery can be performed with an acceptable risk and a reasonable expectation of long-term benefit in carefully selected patients with ESRD. As for all high-risk situations, careful attention to patient selection is essential.

PATIENTS WITH DIABETES. In comparison with age-matched nondiabetic patients, diabetic patients with angiographically proven CAD are more likely to be women with evidence of peripheral vascular disease and a higher number of coronary occlusions. Diabetes is an important independent predictor of mortality among patients undergoing surgical revascularization. However, the benefit of CABG versus medical therapy is maintained in patients with diabetes, with a significant 44 percent relative reduction in mortality provided by surgery.[261] Patients with diabetes have smaller distal vessels judged to be poorer targets for bypass grafting. Nevertheless, the patency of arterial and venous grafts appears similar in diabetics and nondiabetic patients.[352] In the absence of new data to the contrary, patients with diabetes and multivessel disease, who are at acceptable surgical risk, should be considered as candidates for surgical revascularization.[353]

CORONARY BYPASS SURGERY IN PATIENTS WITH ASSOCIATED VASCULAR DISEASE

Management of patients with combined CAD and peripheral vascular disease involving the carotid arteries, the abdominal aorta, or the vessels of the lower extremities presents many challenges. Combined disease is becoming increasingly frequent as the population of patients under consideration for CABG ages and as technical improvements allow the application of coronary revascularization to ever more complex cases.

IMPACT OF COMBINED CAD AND PERIPHERAL VASCULAR DISEASE. Clinically apparent CAD occurs frequently in patients with peripheral vascular disease. Among patients undergoing peripheral vascular surgery, late outcomes are dominated by cardiac causes of morbidity and mortality. Conversely, in patients with CAD, the presence of peripheral vascular disease, even if asymptomatic, is associated with an adverse prognosis, presumably because of the greater total atherosclerotic burden borne by these patients.

Because patients with CAD and peripheral atherosclerosis tend to be older and have more widespread vascular disease and end-organ damage than do patients without peripheral atherosclerosis, the perioperative mortality and morbidity consequent to CABG are high and the late outcome is not as favorable.[354] In the Northern New England Cardiovascular data base, in-hospital mortality after CABG was 2.4-fold greater in patients with peripheral vascular disease than in those without it, particularly for patients with lower extremity disease.[355] In the BARI trial, approximately one-third of patients had peripheral vascular disease, among whom the risk of major complications after both bypass surgery and PTCA was markedly increased in comparison to those without peripheral vascular disease, even after controlling for baseline differences.[354] Diffuse *atheroembolism* is a particularly serious complication of CABG in patients with peripheral vascular disease and aortic atherosclerosis. It is a major cause of perioperative death, stroke, neurocognitive dysfunction, and multiorgan dysfunction after CABG.

Peripheral vascular disease is also a strong marker of an adverse long-term outcome. At any point during a 10-year period, patients in either the medical or surgical group in the CASS Registry who had peripheral vascular disease had a 25 percent greater likelihood of mortality than did those without this condition. Similarly, in the Northern New England Cardiovascular data base, the 5-year mortality remained approximately twofold greater in patients with peripheral vascular disease than in those without it, even after adjusting for other comorbid conditions, which are more frequent in patients with peripheral vascular disease.[355] In the BARI trial, patients with asymptomatic lower extremity disease, as defined by the ankle-arm index, had an almost fivefold greater mortality than did those without lower extremity arterial disease. Indeed, mortality was similar for patients with symptomatic and patients with asymptomatic lower extremity disease.

CAROTID ARTERY DISEASE. In patients with stable CAD and *carotid artery disease* in whom coronary endarterectomy is planned, exercise stress testing and consideration of coronary revascularization can ordinarily be performed after the carotid surgery. The prevalence of significant carotid disease in an increasingly elderly population coming to CABG is high—approximately 20 percent have a stenosis of 50 percent or greater, 6 to 12 percent have a stenosis of 80 percent or greater, and the percentage is higher in patients with left main CAD.[356] In patients for whom surgical treatment is considered for both carotid artery disease and CAD, the merits of a combined versus a staged approach are debated.[357] Neither strategy has been demonstrated to be unequivocally superior to the other, and an individualized approach, depending on the patient's initial condition, the severity of symptoms, the anatomy of the coronary and carotid vessels, and individual institutional experience, is most appropriate.[358]

MANAGEMENT OF PATIENTS WITH ASSOCIATED VASCULAR DISEASE. Patients with severe or unstable CAD requiring revascularization can be categorized into two groups according to the severity and instability of the accompanying vascular disease.[358] When the noncoronary vascular procedures are elective, they can generally be postponed until the cardiac symptoms have stabilized, either by intensive medical therapy or by revascularization. A combined procedure is necessary in patients with both unstable CAD and an unstable vascular condition such as frequent recurrent transient ischemic attacks or a rapidly expanding abdominal aortic aneurysm.[359] In some patients in this category, PCI offers the potential for stabilizing the patient's cardiac condition before proceeding with a definitive vascular repair. A problem is posed by the use of clopidogrel after stenting that will increase bleeding, unless surgery is performed at least 5 days after discontinuation of clopidogrel.

PATIENTS REQUIRING REOPERATION. Currently, approximately 12 percent of coronary artery procedures are reoperations, and in some centers, particularly tertiary care centers, the proportion is increasing rapidly and accounts for 20 percent of all CABG operations.[261] The major indication for reoperation is late disease of saphenous vein grafts. An added factor underlying recurrent symptoms is progression of disease in native vessels between the first and second operations.[360] Several series have emphasized the sicker preoperative status of patients undergoing reoperation, including older age, more serious comorbidity, associated valvular heart disease, and a greater prevalence of left ventricular dysfunction and greater extent of ischemic jeopardized myocardium.[361]

Not unexpectedly, the mortality associated with reoperation is significantly higher than that of initial bypass procedures. In the 1997 data base of the Society of Thoracic Surgeons, the mortality among 99,810 patients undergoing an elective first CABG procedure was 1.7 percent versus 5.2 percent for elective reoperations. For patients undergoing first operations, mortality was 2.6 percent for urgent and 6 percent for emergency procedures in comparison with 7.4 and 13.5 percent, respectively, among patients undergoing repeat bypass surgery. Indications for reoperation have not been defined by randomized trials, but in general, the same principles that apply to patients with initial disease should be followed.

Summary of Indications for Coronary Revascularization

1. Certain anatomical subsets of patients are candidates for CABG, regardless of the severity of symptoms or left ventricular dysfunction. Such patients include those with significant left main CAD and most patients with triple-vessel disease that includes the proximal LAD coronary artery, especially those with left ventricular dysfunction (ejection fraction < 0.50). Patients with chronic stable angina and double-vessel CAD with

significant proximal disease of the LAD, and either left ventricular dysfunction or high-risk findings on noninvasive testing should also be considered for CABG.[18]

2. The benefits of CABG are well documented in patients with left ventricular dysfunction and multivessel disease, regardless of symptoms. In patients whose dominant symptom is heart failure without severe angina, the benefits of coronary revascularization are less well defined, but this approach should be considered in patients who also have evidence of severe ischemia (regardless of angina symptoms), particularly in the presence of a significant extent of potentially viable dysfunctioning (hibernating) myocardium.
3. The primary objective of coronary revascularization in patients with single-vessel disease is relief of significant symptoms or objective evidence of severe ischemia. For most of these patients, PCI is the revascularization modality of choice.
4. In patients with angina who are *not* considered to be at high risk, survival is similar for surgery, PCI, and medical management.
5. All the indications discussed earlier relate to the potential benefits of surgery over medical therapy on *survival.* Coronary revascularization with PCI *or* CABG is highly efficacious in relieving symptoms and may be considered for patients with moderate to severe ischemic symptoms who are not controlled by and/or are dissatisfied with medical therapy, even if they are not in a high-risk subset. For such patients, the optimal method of revascularization is selected on the basis of left ventricular function and arteriographic findings and the likelihood of technical success.

Comparisons Between PCI and CABG

OBSERVATIONAL STUDIES. Since the catheter-based revascularizations in these comparative studies were limited largely to PTCA, this term instead of PCI is used in this section. The findings from observational studies have been largely consistent. Over a period of 1 to 5 years, the rates of mortality and nonfatal infarction were not significantly different between patients revascularized with CABG versus PTCA, but recurrent events, including angina pectoris and the need for repeat revascularization procedures, were significantly more frequent in the PTCA than the CABG group, largely as a consequence of incomplete revascularization and restenosis. Specifically, 1 year after PTCA, the recurrence of symptoms and/or the need for repeat revascularization procedures is frequent (~40 percent), and approximately 20 percent of patients are referred for CABG.

When the overall population is considered, observational data show no differences in survival. However, several subgroups of patients who may derive a survival benefit from CABG compared to PTCA are identified. These include patients with left ventricular dysfunction, probably because of the ability to achieve more complete revascularization with the CABG. In addition, CABG provided a survival benefit compared with PTCA when proximal LAD stenosis (>70 percent) was present. This finding was most evident in an analysis of 3-year survival in approximately 30,000 patients enrolled in the New York State PTCA registry.[362] In this data set, patients with single-, double-, or triple-vessel disease involving the proximal LAD had lower mortality when treated with CABG.

RANDOMIZED TRIALS

PCI VERSUS CABG IN PATIENTS WITH SINGLE-VESSEL DISEASE. Both the Lausanne trial and the Medicine, Angioplasty, or Surgery Study (MASS) trial from Brazil, which included a medical arm, were limited to patients with isolated disease of the proximal LAD coronary artery. The RITA investigators also published results for the subset of patients (45 percent) who had single-vessel disease. The results of these small trials were consistent in that over 2 to 3 years the rates of mortality and myocardial infarction were similar in the two treatment arms, as was improvement in symptoms, but at the cost of more frequent reintervention in patients treated with PTCA. At 5 years in the Lausanne trial, mortality rates and functional status were similar for the two groups; however, an excess incidence of non-Q-wave myocardial infarction was noted in patients treated with PTCA, but this complication did not affect vital status or symptomatic outcome.[363] At least one trial has now compared minimally invasive direct CABG to stenting for patients with isolated stenosis in the proximal LAD.[270] Results from this small study (N = 220) were similar to prior trials. Although patients treated with CABG were less likely to have recurrent symptoms or undergo repeat revascularization, there was no detectable difference in the risk of death or myocardial infarction with PCI versus CABG (3 percent vs. 6 percent; $p = 0.5$).

These results suggest that PCI and CABG are both highly effective in preventing symptoms in patients with single-vessel disease, with similar long-term survival. Moreover, technological advances in PCI since PTCA (the use of stents, first bare metal and more recently drug eluting) have achieved reductions in the frequency of reintervention among patients undergoing these procedures.

MULTIVESSEL DISEASE. At least nine published studies have compared PCI with CABG in patients with multivessel disease. Despite the heterogeneity of the trials in regard to design, methods, and the patient population enrolled, the results are generally comparable and provide a consistent perspective of CABG and PCI in selected patients with multivessel disease. A major limitation is that these trials, except for the Arterial Revascularization Therapy Study (ARTS) and the Argentine randomized trial of PTCA versus CAB surgery in multivessel disease (ERACI II) trial, were conducted before the widespread use of stents and other advances in PCI technology, as well as newer adjunctive therapy, such as clopidogrel and glycoprotein IIb/IIIa platelet inhibition. Also, these trials lacked an aggressive approach to lipid lowering in both groups of patients. In RITA, the Argentine randomized stent study (ERACI), ARTS, and the French Monocentric trials, the ability to achieve "equivalent" degrees of revascularization in the two groups was an inclusion criterion. Moreover, the majority of patients entered into the trials had well-preserved left ventricular function with a mean ejection fraction exceeding 0.50. Therefore, patients enrolled in these trials were at relatively low risk, with predominantly double-vessel disease and well-preserved left ventricular function, that is, a high proportion of patients in whom CABG surgery had *not* been previously shown to be superior to medical therapy in regard to survival. Thus, one would not expect a significant mortality difference between PCI and CABG, particularly with the relatively small sample size of the trials.[18]

The Bypass Angioplasty Revascularization Investigation (BARI) trial, conducted by the NHLBI, enrolled 1829 patients with multivessel disease in the United States and Canada. This trial is the largest of the completed randomized trials of PTCA and bypass surgery and the only trial with sufficient statistical power to detect a substantial mortality difference. At 5 years, overall survival rates were not different between the two groups (89.3 percent with CABG and 86.3 percent with PTCA; $p = 0.19$), nor was any difference noted in the incidence of Q wave myocardial infarction. An initially unexpected finding—but one that has subsequently been reinforced by ARTS[364] and observational data[365]—was that patients with previously treated diabetes who underwent PTCA had a 5-year mortality of 34.5 percent versus 19.4 percent for those who underwent CABG ($p = 0.003$) (Fig. 50-22). This advantage of CABG over PTCA among patients with diabetes became more robust by 7 years of follow-up, at which time no survival advantage was evident for patients without diabetes.[353] More rapid progression of atherosclerosis and high rates of restenosis in patients undergoing percutaneous revascularization are largely responsible for this difference. It is possible that the introduction of drug-eluting stents and more aggressive medical therapy of diabetes will reduce or eliminate this advantage of CABG over PCI in patients with diabetes.

NONFATAL OUTCOMES. Review of the nonfatal outcomes in the randomized trials reveals some differences between CABG and PCI. In each of the studies, CABG was initially associated with greater improvement in angina, which appears to be proportional to the more complete revascularization in patients with multivessel disease. Moreover, as anticipated from the observational data, repeat revascularization procedures were more frequent after PCI. This difference was less in the ARTS trial in which repeat revascularization through 1 year was performed in only 16.9 percent of patients in the stented group (Fig 50-23), contrasting

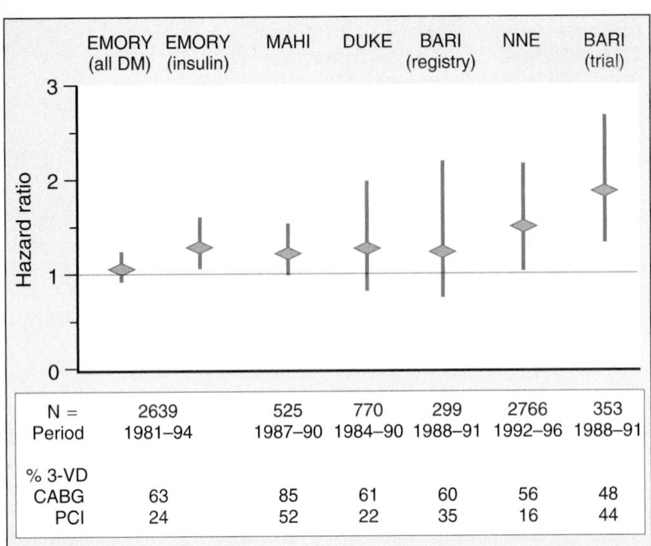

FIGURE 50–22 Five- to six-year survival after coronary artery bypass grafting (CABG) versus percutaneous coronary intervention (PCI) among patients with diabetes mellitus (DM) and multivessel coronary artery disease. Data from both observational and randomized studies show either trends toward or superior survival with CABG. All hazard ratios are adjusted with the exception of the data from the Mid America Heart Institute (MAHI). BARI = Bypass-Angioplasty Revascularization Investigation; NNE = Northern New England data base study; 3-VD = triple-vessel coronary artery disease. (Adapted from Niles NW, McGrath PD, Malenka D, et al: Survival of patients with diabetes and multivessel coronary artery disease after surgical or percutaneous revascularization: Results of a large regional prospective study. J Am Coll Cardiol 37:1008-1015, 2001.)

with 38 percent within 2 years after angioplasty in RITA-1. In the ERACI II study, results were similar to those in the ARTS trial, with only 16.8 percent of patients who had PCI with stenting requiring repeat revascularization in follow-up versus 4.8 percent of bypass surgical patients.[366] However, in the BARI trial, other measures of procedural success, including indices of the quality of life, cognitive function, and return to employment, were similar between PTCA and CABG.

Another consistent but not unexpected finding was the lower in-hospital cost for patients undergoing PCI. This initial cost advantage was sustained at 1 year in ARTS. However, the need for recurrent hospitalization and repeat revascularization procedures over the long term contributed to an increase in postdischarge cost in the PCI arms, resulting in similar overall cost over 3 to 5 years in BARI and a diminished cost advantage at 3 years in ARTS.[367,367a] A major determinant of lower cost is the presence of double-vessel disease; in comparison, patients with congestive heart failure, comorbid conditions, or diabetes are likely to accrue higher cost regardless of the procedure.[367]

The Choice Between PCI and CABG

(Figs. 50–22, 50–23, and 50–24 and Table 50–17)

Medical management of chronic CAD involves a reduction in reversible risk factors, counseling in life-style alteration, treatment of conditions that intensify angina, and pharmacological management of ischemia. When an unacceptable level of angina persists despite medical management, the patient has troubling side effects from the antiischemic drugs, and/or exhibits a "high-risk" result on noninvasive testing, the coronary anatomy should be defined to allow selection of the appropriate technique for revascularization. After elucidation of the coronary anatomy, selection of the technique of revascularization is made as follows:

SINGLE-VESSEL DISEASE. Among patients with single-vessel disease in whom revascularization is deemed necessary and the lesion is anatomically suitable, PCI is generally preferred over bypass surgery.

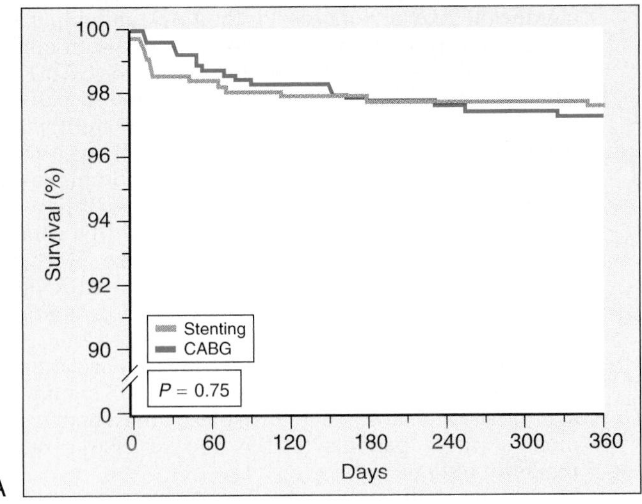

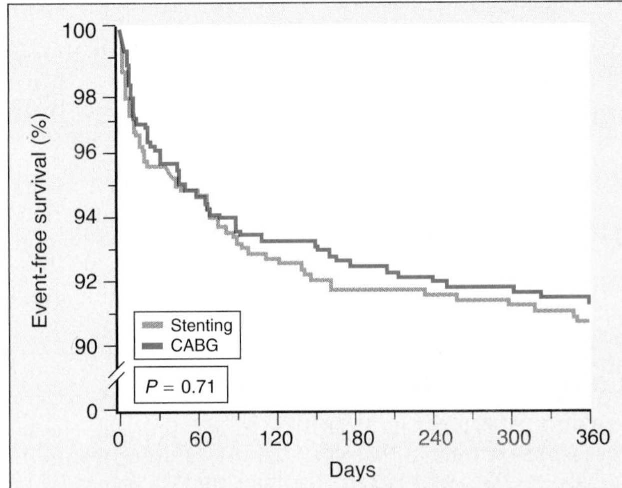

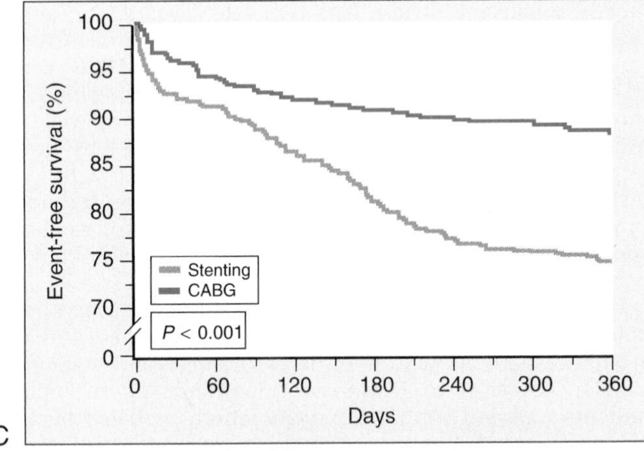

FIGURE 50–23 Outcomes among 1205 patients with multivessel coronary artery disease randomly assigned to undergo percutaneous revascularization with coronary stenting or coronary artery bypass grafting (CABG) in the Arterial Revascularization Therapies Study (ARTS). One year after the revascularization procedure, rates of death, myocardial infarction, and cerebrovascular events were not statistically different between the two revascularization strategies. However, patients undergoing initial stenting were more likely to require repeat revascularization. **A,** Actuarial survival in the stenting versus CABG groups. **B,** Kaplan-Meier estimates of survival free of myocardial infarction or cerebrovascular events. **C,** Kaplan-Meier estimates of survival free of myocardial infarction, cerebrovascular events, or repeated revascularization. (**A** to **C,** From Serruys PW, Unger F, Sousa JE, et al: Comparison of coronary artery bypass surgery and stenting for the treatment of multivessel disease. N Engl J Med 344:1117-1124, 2001.)

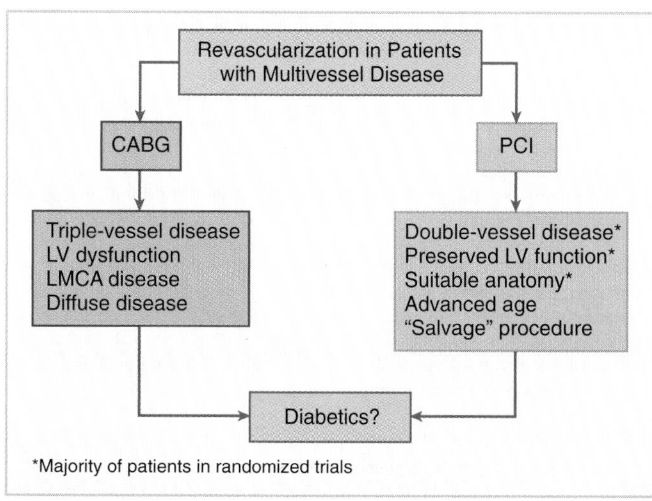

FIGURE 50–24 Indications for coronary revascularization with bypass surgery (CABG) or percutaneous coronary intervention (PCI) in patients with multivessel disease. The combination of triple-vessel disease and left ventricular (LV) dysfunction and/or left main coronary artery (LMCA) disease is primarily surgical, whereas the majority of the patients entered into the randomized trials were suitable for angioplasty on the basis of double-vessel disease, preserved LV dysfunction, and suitable anatomy. Diabetics should be treated individually.

TABLE 50–17 Comparison of Revascularization Strategies in Multivessel Disease

Advantages	Disadvantages
Percutaneous Coronary Intervention	
Less invasive	Restenosis
Shorter hospital stay	High incidence of incomplete revascularization
Lower initial cost	Relative inefficacy in patients with severe left ventricular dysfunction
Easily repeated	Less favorable outcome in diabetics
Effective in relieving symptoms	Limited to specific anatomical subsets
Coronary Artery Bypass Graft Surgery	
Effective in relieving symptoms	Cost
Improved survival in certain subsets	Morbidity
Ability to achieve complete revascularization	
Wider applicability (anatomical subsets)	

Modified from Faxon DP: Coronary angioplasty for stable angina pectoris. *In* Beller G (ed): Chronic Ischemic Heart Disease. *In* Braunwald E (ed): Atlas of Heart Disease. Vol 5. Philadelphia, WB Saunders, 1995.

MULTIVESSEL DISEASE. The first step is to decide whether a patient falls into the category of those who were included in randomized trials comparing PCI and CABG. Most of the patients included in these trials were at lower risk, as defined by double-vessel disease and well-preserved ventricular function. Moreover, several trials required that equivalent degrees of revascularization be achievable by both techniques. Most patients with chronically occluded coronary arteries were excluded, and of those who were clinically eligible, approximately two-thirds were excluded for angiographic reasons. The lack of any difference in late mortality and myocardial infarction between the two treatment arms in such patients indicates that PCI is a reasonable *initial* strategy, provided that the patient accepts the distinct possibility of symptom recurrence and need for repeat revascularization. Patients with a single localized lesion in each affected vessel and preserved left ventricular function fare best with PCI. Additional anatomical factors, such as the presence of severe proximal LAD disease, should also be considered and weigh in favor of surgery (see Fig. 50–16).

NEED FOR COMPLETE REVASCULARIZATION. Complete revascularization is an important goal in patients with left ventricular dysfunction and/or multivessel disease. The major advantage of CABG surgery over PCI is its greater ability to achieve complete revascularization, particularly in patients with triple-vessel disease. In the majority of such patients, particularly those with chronic total coronary occlusion, left ventricular dysfunction, or left main CAD, CABG is the procedure of choice. Among patients with borderline left ventricular function (ejection fraction between 0.40 and 0.50) and milder degrees of ischemia, PCI may provide adequate revascularization, even if it is not complete anatomically.

In many patients, either method of revascularization is suitable. Other factors that come into consideration include the following:

1. Access to a high-quality team and operator (surgeon or interventional cardiologist) with an excellent record of success
2. Patient preference—some patients are made anxious by the idea that after PCI they remain at risk for symptom recurrence and may require reintervention; such patients are better candidates for surgical treatment. Other patients are attracted by the less invasive nature and much more rapid recovery from PCI; these patients prefer to have PCI as their initial revascularization with the idea of "falling back" on CABG if symptoms persist and/or an excellent revascularization has not been achieved
3. Advanced patient age and comorbidity—frail, very elderly patients and those with comorbid conditions, such as cancer or serious liver disease with a limited life expectancy, but who have disabling angina, are often better candidates for PCI
4. Younger patient age—PCI is also often preferable in younger patients (<50 years of age) with the expectation that they may require CABG at some time in the future and that PCI will postpone the need for surgery; this sequence may be preferable to two operations. Patient preference is a pivotal aspect of the decision to perform PCI or CABG in these patient groups

PCI AND CABG IN DIABETIC PATIENTS (see Chap. 51). The poorer outcomes after PCI than after CABG in treated diabetic patients in the BARI trial, together with similar findings in the ARTS trial, have raised concern about whether all diabetic patients with multivessel disease should be treated surgically. This important issue has significant economic implications. Further analysis suggests that treatment of diabetic patients can be individualized, as in nondiabetic patients.

One point of debate is related to the patient selection criteria for enrollment into the trials. In the BARI Registry, in which patients were treated according to the preference of the individual physician, and in two large data base studies, poorer outcomes were noted for both CABG and PTCA in diabetics versus nondiabetics, but *among diabetics*, no survival difference was noted between PTCA and CABG.[368] Similar trends were noted in two large community studies.[369] Diabetic patients as a group in the BARI trial had a greater prevalence of triple-vessel disease, left ventricular dysfunction, and a history of congestive heart failure. It is noteworthy that in the Emory University study of diabetic patients, approximately 85 percent of those with triple-vessel disease underwent bypass surgery, whereas the use of PTCA and CABG was similar among those with double-vessel disease. A plausible explanation for the differences in results in the registry and data base studies compared to the randomized trials is that in the latter, sicker diabetic patients with triple-vessel disease and left ventricular dysfunction, by design, were treated equally with bypass surgery and PTCA, whereas in clinical practice, such patients are referred appropriately for surgery. Consistent with this notion, earlier data base studies suggest that 3- to 5-year survival after CABG in the higher-risk subgroups is superior to that obtained with PCI.

The therapeutic implications of these observations are evident. The revascularization strategy in diabetic patients should be based on the number of vessels diseased, lesion-related technical factors, the caliber of the distal vessels, and the presence or absence of left ventricular dysfunction. Most of the earlier-described comparisons between PCI and CABG involved balloon angioplasty or bare-metal stents. No comparisons between PCI using drug-eluting stents and CABG are available at this time. Since the major disadvantage of PCI prior to the development of drug-eluting stents has been the high rate of restenosis, which has now been substantially reduced, the fraction of patients referred for PCI is increasing, with a corresponding reduction in those referred for CABG. The choice between PCI with drug-eluting stents and CABG will likely revolve around the ability of each procedure to achieve complete revascularization in any given patient.

Other Surgical Procedures for Ischemic Heart Disease

CABG may be combined with surgical procedures aimed at correction of atherosclerotic disease elsewhere in the cardiovascular system, correction of mechanical complications of myocardial infarction (mitral regurgitation or ventricular septal defect), left ventricular aneurysms, and concomitant valvular heart disease. Not unexpectedly, morbidity and mortality are correspondingly increased because of the added complexity of the procedure and, in many patients who require these other procedures, the presence of underlying left ventricular dysfunction (see later).

TRANSMYOCARDIAL LASER REVASCULARIZATION. Transmyocardial laser revascularization is performed by placing a laser on the epicardial surface of the left ventricle, exposed through a lateral thoracotomy, and creating small channels from the epicardial to the endocardial surfaces. This innovative approach to the treatment of ischemic heart disease appears to improve symptoms in patients with refractory angina; however, the mechanism and magnitude of benefit remain uncertain.[370] The initial assumption was that laser-mediated channels would provide a network of functional connections between the left ventricular cavity and the ischemic myocardium. Subsequent observations demonstrating closure of the channels within hours or days despite apparent relief of symptoms have led to alternative explanations for the apparent clinical success of the procedure. These explanations include improved perfusion by stimulation of angiogenesis, a placebo effect, and an anesthetic effect mediated by the destruction of sympathetic nerves carrying pain-sensitive afferent fibers or periprocedural infarction.[371] One study evaluated sympathetic innervation with [^{11}C]hydroxyephedrine and demonstrated decreased myocardial uptake of this substance in most patients, without significant change in resting or stress myocardial perfusion, which suggests that the improvement in angina after the procedure may be partly due to sympathetic denervation.

Initial clinical studies in patients with severe CAD not amenable to a bypass procedure were promising in that most demonstrated a reduction in anginal severity and improved exercise tolerance. Several small randomized trials of transmyocardial laser revascularization resulted in improvement in comparison with maximal medical therapy. The results of one trial suggested improvement in perfusion as assessed by PET, but such improvement was not shown with thallium scintigraphy in another trial. In contrast to the positive studies, Schofield and associates reported no significant improvement in exercise time and 12-minute walking distance up to 1 year after translaser myocardial revascularization with a carbon dioxide laser, although the laser-treated patients had a modest reduction in the frequency of angina.[372] The subjective improvement in the severity of angina found in this study, in the absence of any measurable effect on myocardial perfusion or exercise tolerance, argues for a placebo effect or denervation.[371] Subsequent trials have provided mixed results with respect to the durability of symptom improvement after surgical transmyocardial laser revascularization.[373] Moreover, the failure of two sham-controlled trials of percutaneous laser myocardial revascularization to show any benefit has highlighted the impact of placebo effect in response to laser myocardial revascularization.[370] On the basis of data from the randomized trials, it would appear that the widespread use of translaser myocardial revascularization as a stand-alone method cannot be justified, but it may still have a role as an adjunctive procedure during CABG in patients who have some vessels suitable for bypass but others that are unsuitable. Because of the perioperative morbidity associated with surgical transmyocardial laser revascularization, careful selection of patients is necessary.[374] Larger sham-controlled studies of percutaneous laser myocardial revascularization are ongoing. Whether this technique will fulfill its potential as a vehicle for the delivery of angiogenic factors and other forms of gene therapy remains to be determined.

Other Manifestations of Coronary Artery Disease

Prinzmetal (Variant) Angina

See Chapter 49.

Chest Pain with Normal Coronary Arteriogram

The syndrome of angina or angina-like chest pain with a normal coronary arteriogram, often referred to as *syndrome X* (to be distinguished from the metabolic syndrome X characterized by abdominal obesity, hypertriglyceridemia, low HDL cholesterol, insulin resistance, hyperinsulinemia, and hypertension), is an important clinical entity that should be differentiated from classic ischemic heart disease caused by CAD. In this condition, the prognosis is usually excellent,[375] in contrast to the variable outcome in patients with angina caused by coronary atherosclerosis. Patients with chest pain and normal coronary arteriograms may represent as many as 10 to 20 percent of those undergoing coronary arteriography because of clinical suspicion of angina. The cause(s) of the syndrome is not conclusively defined. However, microvascular dysfunction and myocardial metabolic abnormalities have been implicated.[376] True myocardial ischemia, reflected in the production of lactate by the myocardium during exercise or pacing, is present in some of these patients; however, others have no metabolic evidence for ischemia as the cause of their discomfort. The incidence of coronary calcification on multislice CT scanning is significantly higher than that of normal controls (53 vs. 20 percent) but lower than that in patients with angina secondary to obstructive CAD (96 percent).[377]

It is postulated that the syndrome of angina pectoris with normal coronary arteries reflects a number of conditions. Included in syndrome X are patients with endothelial dysfunction or microvascular dysfunction or spasm in whom angina may be the result of ischemia.[376] This condition is frequently referred to as *microvascular angina*. In others, chest discomfort without ischemia may be due to abnormal pain perception or sensitivity.[378] Also, IVUS studies have demonstrated anatomical and physiological heterogeneity of syndrome X, with a spectrum ranging from normal coronary arteries to vessels with intimal thickening and atheromatous plaque but without critical obstructions. It is likely that some patients with syndrome X have a combination of pathobiological contributors. In addition, it is difficult to distinguish patients with syndrome X in whom chest pain is caused by ischemia from patients with noncardiac pain. Behavioral or psychiatric disorders may be evident.[379]

MICROVASCULAR DYSFUNCTION (INADEQUATE VASODILATOR RESERVE). Patients with chest pain, angiographically normal coronary arteries, and no evidence of large-vessel spasm even after an acetylcholine challenge may demonstrate an abnormally decreased capacity to reduce coronary resistance and increase coronary flow in response to stimuli such as exercise, adenosine, dipyridamole, and atrial pacing. These patients also have an exaggerated response of small coronary vessels to vasoconstrictor stimuli and an impaired response to intracoronary papaverine. In some patients, this abnormality appears to affect the smaller resistance vessels that are not visible angiographically, while the large proximal conductance vessels are normal.[380] Abnormal endothelium-dependent vasoreactivity has been associated with regional myocardial perfusion defects on SPECT and PET imaging.[381] It has been reported that patients with syndrome X also have impaired vasodilator reserve in forearm vessels and airway hyperresponsiveness, which suggests that the smooth muscle of systemic arteries and other organs may be affected in addition to that of the coronary circulation.

Endothelial dysfunction and endothelial cell activation, reported in patients with syndrome X, may participate in the release of cellular adhesion molecules, proinflammatory cytokines, and constricting mediators that induce changes in the arterial wall, resulting in microvascular dysfunction. Patients with syndrome X have been observed to have higher levels of circulating intercellular adhesion molecule-1, the vasoconstrictor endothelin-1, and the inflammatory marker hs-CRP; moreover, the level of hs-CRP appears to correlate with the severity of symptoms and burden of ischemic ECG changes.[382]

EVIDENCE FOR ISCHEMIA. Despite general acceptance that microvascular and/or endothelial dysfunction is present in many patients with syndrome X, whether ischemia is in fact the putative cause of the symptoms in these patients is not clear.[383] Studies of transmyocardial production of lactate have generated mixed results.[376,382] The development of left ventricular dysfunction and ECG or scintigraphic abnormalities during exercise in some of these patients supports an ischemic cause. However, stress echocardiography with dobutamine has failed to detect regional contraction abnormalities consistent with ischemia.[384] More sensitive techniques, such as perfusion analysis with MRI, have demonstrated that subendocardial perfusion abnormalities, in particular, may be associated with syndrome X.[385]

ABNORMAL PAIN PERCEPTION. The lack of definitive evidence of ischemia in some patients with syndrome X has focused attention on alternative nonischemic causes of cardiac-related pain, including a decreased threshold for pain perception—the so-called sensitive heart syndrome.[385] This hypersensitivity may result in an awareness of chest pain in response to stimuli such as arterial stretch or changes in heart rate, rhythm, or contractility. A sympathovagal imbalance with sympathetic predominance in some of these patients has also been postulated. At the time of cardiac catheterization, some patients with syndrome X are unusually sensitive to intracardiac instrumentation, with typical chest pain being consistently produced by direct right atrial stimulation and saline infusion.[386] Measurements of regional cerebral blood flow at rest and during chest pain suggest differential handling of afferent stimuli between patients with syndrome X and those with obstructive CAD.[378]

Clinical Features

The syndrome of angina or angina-like chest pain with normal epicardial arteries occurs more frequently in women,[385] many of whom are premenopausal, whereas obstructive CAD is found more commonly in men and postmenopausal women. Fewer than half of patients with syndrome X have typical angina pectoris; most have a variety of forms of atypical chest pain. Although the features are frequently atypical, the chest pain may nonetheless be severe and disabling. The condition may be benign in regard to survival, but it may have markedly adverse effects on the quality of life, employment, and use of health care resources.

In some patients with minimal or no CAD, an exaggerated preoccupation with personal health is associated with the chest pain, and panic disorder may be responsible in a proportion of such patients. Potts and Bass found that two-thirds of patients with chest pain and normal coronary arteries have psychiatric disorders.[379] Others have reported that the incidence of obstructive CAD is extremely low in patients with atypical chest pain who are anxious and/or depressed. The association between syndrome X and insulin resistance warrants further study.

PHYSICAL AND LABORATORY EXAMINATION. Abnormal physical findings reflecting ischemia, such as a precordial bulge, gallop sound, and the murmur of mitral regurgitation, are uncommon in syndrome X. The resting ECG may be normal, but nonspecific ST-T wave abnormalities are often observed, sometimes occurring in association with the chest pain. Approximately 20 percent of patients with chest pain and normal coronary arteriograms have positive exercise tests. However, many patients with this syndrome do not complete the exercise test because of fatigue or mild chest discomfort. Left ventricular function is usually normal at rest and during stress, unlike the situation in obstructive CAD, in which function often becomes impaired during stress.[384]

PROGNOSIS. Important prognostic information on patients with angina and either normal or nearly normal coronary arteriograms has been obtained from the CASS Registry.[387] In patients with an ejection fraction of 0.50 or more, the 7-year survival rate was 96 percent for patients with a normal arteriogram and 92 percent for those whose arteriographic study revealed mild disease (50 percent luminal stenosis). In such patients, an ischemic response to exercise was not associated with increased mortality, although a history of smoking or hypertension was. Thus, long-term survival of patients with anginal chest pain and normal coronary angiograms is excellent, markedly better than in patients with obstructive CAD and no different from that in an age-matched general population. Nonetheless, the symptoms are persistent, and most patients continue to experience chest pain that leads to repeated cardiac catheterization and hospital admission.[388]

MANAGEMENT. In patients with angina-like chest pain syndrome and normal epicardial coronary arteries, noncardiac etiologies, such as esophageal abnormalities, should be considered. In patients with syndrome X in whom ischemia can be demonstrated by noninvasive stress testing, a trial of antiischemic therapy with nitrates, calcium-channel blockers and beta blockers is logical, but the response to this therapy is variable.[388] Perhaps because of the heterogeneity of this population, studies testing these antianginal therapies have provided conflicting results. For example, beta blockers may be most effective in patients with syndrome X who also have evidence of increased sympathetic nervous activity (e.g., tachycardia and reduced heart rate variability). Calcium antagonists are effective in reducing the frequency and severity of angina and improving exercise tolerance in some patients. Sublingual nitroglycerin has shown paradoxical effects on blood flow and exercise tolerance in some studies and beneficial effects in others.[388] Alpha blockers have been demonstrated to be ineffective.

ACE inhibitors have favorable effects on endothelial function, vascular remodeling, and sympathetic tone that may be relevant to the pathophysiology of syndrome X. Preliminary data studying ACE inhibitors in this population are promising.[388] Similarly, estrogen has been shown to attenuate normal coronary vasomotor responses to acetylcholine, increase coronary blood flow, and potentiate endothelium-dependent vasodilation in postmenopausal women. Studies of estrogen replacement in postmenopausal women with syndrome X have shown improvement in symptoms and/or exercise performance; however, the role of exogenous estrogen in treatment of this group remains in question. Aimed at the altered somatic and visceral pain perception in many patients with syndrome X, imipramine (50 mg) and structured psychological intervention have been reported to be helpful in some.[389]

Oral aminophylline (an adenosine receptor blocker) may have a favorable effect on the exercise-induced chest pain threshold without any effect on exercise-induced ST segment changes.

Silent Myocardial Ischemia

The prognostic importance and the mechanisms of silent ischemia have been the subject of considerable interest for almost 30 years.[390] Patients with silent ischemia have been stratified into three categories by Cohn. The first and least common form, type I silent ischemia, occurs in totally asymptomatic patients with obstructive CAD (which may be severe). These patients *do not experience angina at any time*; indeed, some type I patients do not even experience pain in the course of myocardial infarction. Epidemiological studies of sudden death (see Chap. 33), as well as clinical and postmortem studies of patients with silent myocardial infarction and studies of patients with chronic angina pectoris, suggest that many patients with extensive coronary artery obstruction never experience angina pectoris in any of its recognized forms (stable, unstable, or variant). These patients with type I silent ischemia may be considered to have a *defective anginal warning system.* Type II silent ischemia is the form that occurs in patients with documented previous myocardial infarction.

The third and much more frequent form, designated *type III silent ischemia,* occurs in patients with the usual forms of chronic stable angina, unstable angina, and Prinzmetal angina. When monitored, patients with this form of silent ischemia exhibit some episodes of ischemia that are associated with chest discomfort and other episodes that are not—that is, episodes of silent (asymptomatic) ischemia. The *total ischemic burden* in these patients refers to the total period of ischemia, both symptomatic and asymptomatic.

AMBULATORY ELECTROCARDIOGRAPHY. The extensive use of ambulatory ECG monitoring has led to a greater appreciation of the high frequency of type III silent ischemia, occurring in up to one-third of patients with stable angina treated with appropriate therapy (Fig. 50–25).[390] It has become apparent that anginal pain is a poor indicator and underestimates the frequency of significant cardiac ischemia. Exercise-induced hemodynamic changes indicative of myocardial ischemia (increasing left ventricular end-diastolic pressure and decreasing left ventricular ejection fraction) occur in patients with CAD, regardless of the development of ischemic discomfort.

The role of myocardial O_2 demand in the genesis of myocardial ischemia has been evaluated by measuring the heart rate and blood pressure changes preceding silent ischemic events during ambulatory studies. In one series, 92 percent of all episodes were silent, and 60 to 70 percent were preceded by significant increases in heart rate or blood pressure. The circadian variations in heart rate and blood pressure also paralleled the increase in silent ischemic events. This and other studies have suggested that increases in myocardial O_2 demand have a significant role in the genesis of silent ischemia, but in other patients reductions in myocardial O_2 supply may make an important contribution to the initiation of both symptomatic and asymptomatic episodes. The mechanisms underlying the development of ischemia, as detected by ambulatory ECG and exercise testing, may be different, and in patients in the ACIP study, concordance between the ambulatory ECG and SPECT was only 50 percent. For identification of silent ischemia, the two techniques probably complement each other.

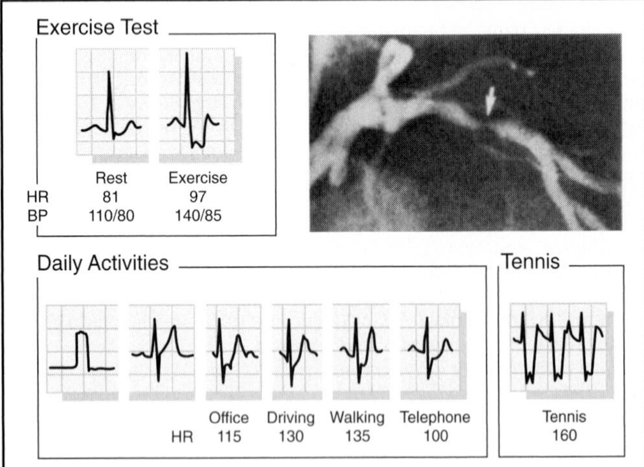

FIGURE 50–25 Ambulatory electrocardiograms and coronary angiogram of a severe left anterior descending stenosis in a patient with fatigue (but not angina) during a tennis match. In stage II of a treadmill exercise test (Bruce protocol), 4 mm of ST segment depression was seen in lead V_5. Ambulatory Holter monitoring of lead V_5 demonstrates ischemic ST segment depressions during a number of ordinary activities, such as walking and telephoning. During a game of tennis, marked ST segment depression was recorded when the patient was asymptomatic. HR = heart rate; BP = blood pressure. (From Nabel EG, Rocco MB, Selwyn AB: Characteristics and significance of ischemia detected by ambulatory electrocardiographic monitoring. Circulation 75[Suppl 5]:74, 1987.)

Transient ST segment depression of 0.1 mV or more that lasts longer than 30 seconds is a rare finding in normal subjects. Patients with known CAD show a strong correlation between such transient ST segment depression and independent measurements of impaired regional myocardial perfusion and ischemia determined by rubidium-82 uptake as measured by PET. In patients with type III silent ischemia, perfusion defects occur in the same myocardial regions during symptomatic and asymptomatic episodes of ST segment depression. Other methods of detecting silent ischemia include measurement of the left ventricular ejection fraction with a "nuclear vest," the presence of regional wall motion abnormalities, and perfusion defects on echocardiography or radionuclide scintigraphy.

Type III silent ischemia is extremely common. Analysis of ambulatory ECG recordings among patients with CAD who had both symptomatic and silent myocardial ischemia found that 85 percent of ambulant ischemic episodes occur without chest pain and 66 percent of angina reports were unaccompanied by ST segment depression.[391] Their frequency is such that it has been suggested that overt angina pectoris is merely the "tip of the ischemic iceberg." Among patients with stable CAD enrolled 1 to 6 months after hospitalization for an acute ischemic event, only 15 percent had angina with exercise, yet 28 percent had ST segment depression and 41 percent had reversible myocardial perfusion defects on thallium scintigraphy.[392] Episodes of silent ischemia have been estimated to be present in approximately one-third of all treated patients with angina, although a higher prevalence has been reported in diabetics. Episodes of ST segment depression, both symptomatic and asymptomatic, exhibit a circadian rhythm and are more common in the morning. Asymptomatic nocturnal ST segment changes are almost invariably an indicator of double- or triple-vessel CAD or left main coronary artery stenosis.

Pharmacological agents that reduce or abolish episodes of symptomatic ischemia (i.e., nitrates, beta blockers, and calcium antagonists) also reduce or abolish episodes of silent ischemia.[390]

MECHANISMS OF SILENT ISCHEMIA. It is not clear why some patients with unequivocal evidence of ischemia do not experience chest pain whereas others are symptomatic. Differences in both peripheral and central neural processing of pain have been proposed as important factors underlying silent ischemia. PET imaging of cerebral blood flow during painful versus silent ischemia has pointed toward differences in handling of afferent signals by the central nervous system.[378] Specifically, "overactive" gating of afferent signals in the thalamus may reduce the cortical activation necessary for perception of pain from the heart. Autonomic neuropathy has also been implicated as a reason for reduced sensation of pain during ischemia. Although increased release of endorphins may play a role in some patients with silent ischemia, the results of clinical studies are mixed.[390] Some researchers have suggested that antiinflammatory cytokines are at play in reducing inflammatory processes that may participate in the genesis of cardiac pain.[393]

PROGNOSIS. Although some controversy remains, ample evidence supports the view that episodes of myocardial ischemia, regardless of whether they are symptomatic or asymptomatic, are of prognostic importance in patients with CAD.[390] In asymptomatic patients (type I), the presence of exercise-induced ST segment depression has been shown to predict a fourfold to fivefold increase in cardiac mortality in comparison with patients without this finding.[394] Similarly, in patients with stable angina or prior myocardial infarction, the presence of inducible ischemia evident by ST depression or perfusion abnormalities during exercise testing is associated with unfavorable outcomes, regardless of whether symptoms are present.[395] The strength of this association is greatest when the ischemia is found to occur at a low workload. Several studies evaluating the prognostic implications of silent ischemia on ambulatory monitoring in patients with stable angina (type III) have demonstrated that the presence of myocardial ischemia on ambulatory ECG, whether silent or symptomatic, is also associated with an adverse cardiac outcome.[220,221,396] Moreover, in the ACIP study, among patients treated medically, myocardial ischemia detected by ambulatory ECG and by an abnormal exercise treadmill test were each *independently* associated with adverse cardiac outcomes.[397] However, revascularization and/or intensification of medical therapy were included as subjective elements of the composite endpoints for these studies along with death and myocardial infarction. In addition, other studies have not detected a relationship between silent ischemia on ambulatory monitoring and subsequent hard outcomes.[398]

Nevertheless, when the subgroup of patients with ischemia on stress testing is considered, silent ischemia on Holter monitoring is also a significant predictor of subsequent death or myocardial infarction. In addition, patients with ischemia on ambulatory ECG are more likely to have multivessel CAD, severe proximal stenoses, and a greater frequency of complex lesion morphology, including intracoronary thrombus, ulceration, and eccentric lesions, than are patients without evidence of ischemia on ambulatory monitoring. The presence of severe and complex CAD may partly explain the apparent independent effect of silent ischemia during ambulatory monitoring on prognosis.[399]

Whether the incremental prognostic information provided by adding an ambulatory ECG to a standard stress test justifies the cost of using this modality as a tool for widespread screening remains to be determined, but it is unlikely. Exercise ECG can identify most of the patients likely to have significant ischemia during their daily activities and remains the most important screening test for significant CAD. Many patients with type I silent ischemia have been identified because of an asymptomatic positive exercise ECG obtained following myocardial infarction. In such patients with a defective anginal warning system, it is reasonable to assume that asymptomatic ischemia has a significance similar to that of symptomatic ischemia and that their management with respect to coronary angiography and revascularization should be similar.

MANAGEMENT. Drugs that are effective in preventing episodes of symptomatic ischemia (nitrates, calcium antagonists, and beta blockers) are also effective in reducing or eliminating episodes of silent ischemia (Fig. 50–26).[390] Multiple studies have shown beta blockers to reduce the frequency, duration, and severity of silent ischemia in a dose-dependent fashion.[400] For example, in the Atenolol Silent Ischemia Study Trial (ASIST), 4 weeks of atenolol therapy decreased the number of ischemic episodes detected on ambulatory ECG (from 3.6 to 1.7; $p < 0.001$) and also the average duration (from 30 to 16.4 minutes per 48 hours; $p < 0.001$).[220] In a randomized study comparing beta blockade versus calcium-channel antagonism, metoprolol was shown to be superior to diltiazem in decreasing the mean number of ischemic episodes and the mean duration of ischemia.[401] Beta blockers may also blunt the circadian increase in ischemic events in the early morning. A combination of a beta blocker and a calcium antagonist is superior to either class of drug alone in suppressing ischemia detected by ambulatory ECG. Coronary revascularization is also effective in reducing the rate of both angina and ambulatory ischemia. In the ACIP pilot study, 57 percent of patients treated with revascularization were free of ischemia at 1 year, compared with 31 and 36 percent in the "ischemia-" and "angina-guided" strategies, respectively ($p < 0.0001$).[402] Aggressive secondary prevention with lipid-lowering therapy has also been shown to reduce ischemia on ambulatory monitoring.[403]

Although suppression of ischemia in patients with asymptomatic ischemia appears a worthwhile objective, whether treatment should be guided by symptoms or by ischemia as reflected by the ambulatory ECG has not been established. In a study of bisoprolol, nifedipine, and the combination, patients achieving complete eradication of ischemia, symptomatic and asymptomatic, were less likely to suffer death, myocardial infarction, or angina requiring revascularization. Similarly, amelioration of all symptomatic and asymptomatic ischemia in the ASIST trial conferred an advantage with respect to the primary endpoint of death, resuscitated ventricular tachycardia or ventricular fibrillation, myocardial infarction, unstable angina, revascularization, or worsening angina.[220] However, in the ACIP trial, no differences in outcome were detected between the groups allocated to ischemia-guided versus angina-guided therapy. In contrast, the early benefits of revascularization on ischemia were associated with improved clinical outcomes. Specifically, the rate of death or myocardial infarction was 12.1 percent in the angina-guided strategy, 8.8 percent in the ischemia-guided strategy, and 4.7 percent in the revascularization strategy, and a strong reduction was also seen in recurrent hospitalizations and the revascularization strategies.[328] Patients who continue to suffer silent ischemia after revascularization may be at increased risk for recurrent cardiac events compared to those who are free of any ischemia.[404]

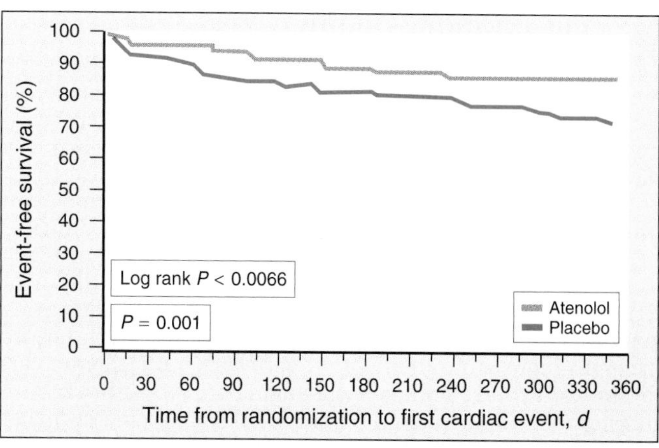

FIGURE 50–26 The Atenolol in Silent Ischemia Trial (ASIST) is the first controlled trial to demonstrate modification of cardiac risk through treatment of silent myocardial ischemia (SMI). A total of 306 asymptomatic or minimally symptomatic patients with coronary artery disease, positive exercise tests, and ambulatory electrocardiographic (ECG) episodes of SMI were randomized to receive atenolol or placebo. Ambulatory ECG monitoring was repeated at 4 weeks, and outcome was assessed after 1 year. At 4 weeks, atenolol was associated with a significant reduction in SMI. After 1 year, a significant (56 percent) relative reduction in adverse events (death, resuscitated ventricular tachycardia and fibrillation, nonfatal myocardial infarction, and unstable or worsening angina) was found when patients given atenolol were compared with those given placebo. The presence of ischemia at 4 weeks was the most important independent factor associated with adverse outcomes after 1 year. (From Bertolet BD, Pepine CJ: Silent myocardial ischemia. *In* Beller GA [ed]: Chronic Ischemic Heart Disease. *In* Braunwald E [ed]: Atlas of Heart Diseases. Vol 5. Philadelphia, WB Saunders, 1995, p 8.9.)

Heart Failure in Ischemic Heart Disease

In the current era, the leading cause of heart failure in developed countries is CAD.[405] In the United States, CAD and its complications account for two-thirds to three-fourths of all cases of heart failure. In many patients, the progressive nature of heart failure reflects the progressive nature of the underlying CAD. The term *ischemic cardiomyopathy* is used for the clinical syndrome in which one or more of the pathophysiological features just discussed result in left ventricular dysfunction and heart failure symptoms.[406] This condition is the predominant form of heart failure related to CAD. Additional complications of CAD that may become superimposed on ischemic cardiomyopathy and precipitate heart failure are the development of left ventricular aneurysm and mitral regurgitation caused by papillary muscle dysfunction.

Ischemic Cardiomyopathy

In 1970, Burch and colleagues first used the term *ischemic cardiomyopathy* to describe the condition in which CAD results in severe myocardial dysfunction, with clinical manifestations often indistinguishable from those of primary dilated cardiomyopathy (see Chap. 59). Symptoms of heart failure caused by ischemic myocardial dysfunction and hibernation, diffuse fibrosis, or multiple infarctions, alone or in combination, may dominate the clinical picture of CAD. In some patients with chronic CAD, angina may be the principal clinical manifestation at one time, but later this symptom diminishes or even disappears as heart failure becomes more prominent. Other patients with ischemic cardiomyopathy have no history of angina or myocardial infarction (type I silent ischemia), and it is in this subgroup that ischemic cardiomyopathy is most often confused with dilated cardiomyopathy.

It is important to recognize hibernating myocardium in patients with ischemic cardiomyopathy because symptoms resulting from chronic left ventricular dysfunction may be incorrectly thought to result from necrotic and scarred myocardium rather than from a reversible ischemic process. Hibernating myocardium may be present in patients with known or suspected CAD with a degree of cardiac dysfunction or heart failure not readily accounted for by previous myocardial infarctions.[407]

The outlook for patients with ischemic cardiomyopathy treated medically is quite poor, and revascularization or cardiac transplantation may be considered.[333,408] The prognosis is particularly poor for patients in whom ischemic cardiomyopathy is due to multiple myocardial infarctions, in those with associated ventricular arrhythmias, and in those with extensive amounts of hibernating myocardium. However, this last group of patients, whose heart failure, even if severe, is due to large segments of reversibly dysfunctional but viable myocardium, has a significantly better prognosis after revascularization.[333] Revascularization in this group also significantly improves heart failure symptoms. Thus, the key to management of patients with ischemic cardiomyopathy is to assess the extent of residual viable myocardium with a view to coronary revascularization of viable myocardium (see Chap. 16). Patients with little or no viable myocardium in whom heart failure is secondary to extensive myocardial infarction and/or fibrosis should be managed in a manner similar to those with dilated cardiomyopathy (see Chaps. 24 and 59). Their prognosis is poor.

Left Ventricular Aneurysm

Left ventricular aneurysm is usually defined as a segment of the ventricular wall that exhibits paradoxical (dyskinetic) systolic expansion. Chronic fibrous aneurysms interfere with ventricular performance principally through loss of contractile tissue. Aneurysms made up largely of a mixture of scar tissue and viable myocardium or of thin scar tissue also impair left ventricular function by a combination of paradoxical expansion and loss of effective contraction.[409] *False aneurysms* (pseudoaneurysms) represent localized myocardial rupture in which the hemorrhage is limited by pericardial adhesions, and they have a mouth that is considerably smaller than the maximal diameter (Fig. 50–27). True and false aneurysms may coexist, although the combination is extremely rare.

The frequency of ventricular aneurysms depends on the incidence of transmural myocardial infarction and congestive heart failure in the population studied. Left ventricular aneurysms and the need for aneurysmectomy have declined dramatically during the last 5 to 10 years in concert with the expanded use of acute reperfusion therapy in evolving myocardial infarction. More than 80 percent of left ventricular aneurysms are located anterolaterally near the apex. They

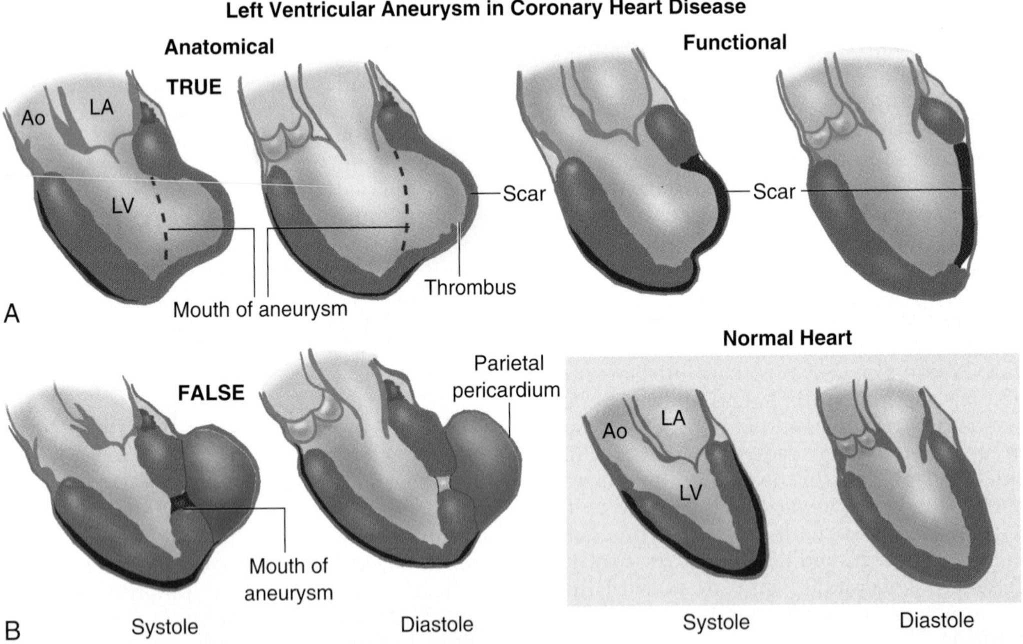

FIGURE 50–27 Hearts in systole and diastole with true and false anatomical and functional left ventricular (LV) aneurysms and healed myocardial infarction. A normal heart in systole and diastole is shown for comparison **(inset)**. A true anatomical left ventricular aneurysm **(A)** protrudes during both systole and diastole, has a mouth that is as wide as or wider than the maximal diameter, has a wall that was formerly the wall of the left ventricle, and is composed of fibrous tissue with or without residual myocardial fibers. A true aneurysm may or may not contain thrombus and almost never ruptures once the wall is healed. A false anatomical left ventricular aneurysm **(B)** protrudes during both systole and diastole, has a mouth that is considerably smaller than the maximal diameter of the aneurysm and represents a myocardial rupture site, has a wall made up of parietal pericardium, virtually always contains thrombus, and often ruptures. A functional left ventricular aneurysm protrudes during ventricular systole but not during diastole and consists of fibrous tissue with or without myocardial fibers. Ao = aorta; LA = left atrium. (From Cabin HS, Roberts WC: Left ventricular aneurysm, intraaneurysmal thrombus, and systemic embolus in coronary heart disease. Chest 77:586, 1980.)

are often associated with total occlusion of the LAD coronary artery and a poor collateral blood supply. Approximately 5 to 10 percent of aneurysms are located posteriorly. Three-fourths of patients with aneurysms have multivessel CAD.

Almost 50 percent of patients with moderate or large aneurysms have symptoms of heart failure (with or without associated angina), approximately 33 percent have severe angina alone, and approximately 15 percent have symptomatic ventricular arrhythmias that may be intractable and life threatening. Mural thrombi are found in almost half of patients with chronic left ventricular aneurysms and can be detected by angiography and two-dimensional echocardiography (see Chap. 11). Systemic embolic events in patients with thrombi and left ventricular aneurysm tend to occur early after myocardial infarction. In the Mayo Clinic series of patients with chronic left ventricular aneurysm (documented at least 1 month after infarction), subsequent systemic emboli were extremely uncommon (0.35 per 100 patient-years in patients not receiving anticoagulants).

DETECTION. Clues to the presence of aneurysm include persistent ST segment elevations on the resting ECG (in the absence of chest pain)[410] and a characteristic bulge of the silhouette of the left ventricle on a chest roentgenogram. Marked calcification of the left ventricular silhouette may be present. These findings, when clear-cut, are relatively specific, but they have limited sensitivity. Radionuclide ventriculography and two-dimensional echocardiography can demonstrate ventricular aneurysm more readily; the latter is also helpful in distinguishing between true and false aneurysms based on the demonstration of a narrow neck in relation to cavity size in the latter.[411] Color-flow echocardiographic imaging is useful in establishing the diagnosis because flow "in and out" of the aneurysm as well as abnormal flow within the aneurysm can be detected, and subsequent pulsed Doppler imaging can reveal a "to-and-fro" pattern with characteristic respiratory variation in the peak systolic velocity. MRI may be emerging as the preferred noninvasive technique for the preoperative assessment of ventricular shape, thinning, and resectability.[409]

LEFT VENTRICULAR ANEURYSMECTOMY. True ventricular aneurysms do not rupture, and operative excision is carried out to improve the clinical manifestations, most often heart failure but sometimes also angina, embolization, and life-threatening tachyarrhythmias.[409] Coronary revascularization is frequently performed along with aneurysmectomy, especially in patients in whom angina accompanies heart failure.

A large left ventricular aneurysm in a patient with symptoms of heart failure, particularly if angina pectoris is also present, is an indication for surgery. The operative mortality rate for left ventricular aneurysmectomy is approximately 8 percent (ranging from 2 to 19 percent),[412] with rates as low as 3 percent reported in more recent series.[413] Risk factors for early death include poor left ventricular function, triple-vessel disease, recent myocardial infarction, the presence of mitral regurgitation, and intractable ventricular arrhythmias.[413] The presence of angina pectoris instead of dyspnea as the dominant preoperative symptom is associated with lower operative mortality.[414] Surgery carries a particularly high risk in patients with severe heart failure, a low-output state, and akinesis of the interventricular septum, as assessed echocardiographically. Akinesis or dyskinesia of the posterior basal segment of the left ventricle and significant right coronary artery stenoses are additional risk factors.

Risk factors for late mortality following survival from surgery include incomplete revascularization, impaired systolic function of the basal segments of the ventricle and septum not involved by the aneurysm, the presence of a large aneurysm with a small quantity of residual viable myocardium, and the presence of severe cardiac failure as the initial feature.[415]

Improvement in left ventricular function has been reported in survivors of resection of left ventricular aneurysms.[416] Anterior ventricular restoration has the potential to reverse adverse remodeling, realign contractile fibers, and decrease ventricular wall stress.[417-419] By removing the abnormal mechanical burden, left ventricular aneurysmectomy has been associated with late improvement in overall systolic function and improvement in the performance of regional nonischemic myocardium in zones remote from the left ventricular aneurysm, in addition to improvement in measures of ventricular relaxation and cardiovascular neuroregulatory mechanisms.[416] A concomitant improvement in exercise performance and clinical symptoms may also occur, particularly in patients who have undergone complete revascularization. In one series, 78 percent of patients undergoing ventricular reconstruction had an improvement in symptoms, with survival of 84 percent at 5 years.[409]

New surgical approaches to the repair of left ventricular aneurysms are designed to restore normal left ventricular geometry by using an alternative method of epicardial closure and/or an endocardial patch to divide the area of the aneurysm from the remainder of the ventricular cavity (Fig. 50–28). Favorable clinical and hemodynamic results following the use of these newer techniques have been reported, with 5-year survival rates ranging from 73 to 87.5 percent and a corresponding improvement in hemodynamics and clinical symptoms.[413] In one series, 88 percent of patients treated with the endoaneurysmorrhaphy technique were in NYHA Class I or II after a mean follow-up of approximately 3.5 years.[420]

Mitral Regurgitation Secondary To Coronary Artery Disease (see Chap. 57)

Mitral regurgitation is an important cause of heart failure in some patients with CAD. Rupture of a papillary muscle or the head of a papillary muscle usually causes severe acute mitral

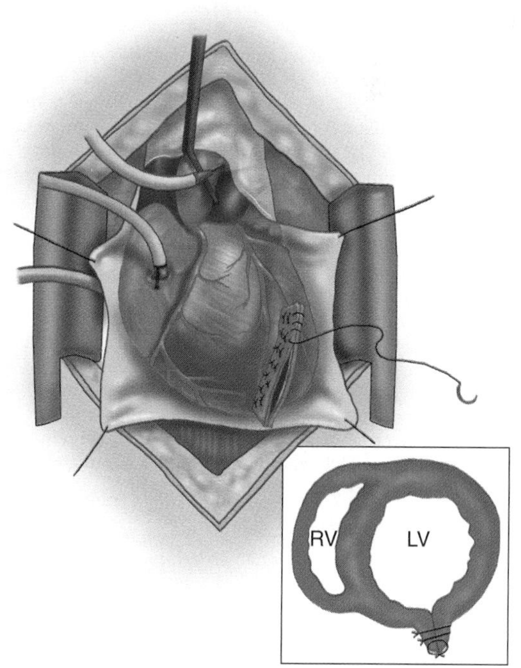

FIGURE 50–28 Linear repair technique used in left ventricular (LV) aneurysm repair. The aneurysm walls are closed in a vertical line between two layers of Teflon felt. Two layers of interrupted horizontal mattress sutures are reinforced with two layers of running sutures. RV = right ventricle. (From Glower DD, Lowe JE: Left ventricular aneurysm. *In* Cohn LC, Edmunds LH [eds]: Cardiac Surgery in the Adult. New York, McGraw-Hill, 2003, p 597.)

regurgitation in the course of acute myocardial infarction (see Chap. 57). The cause of chronic mitral regurgitation in patients with CAD is multifactorial, and the geometrical determinants are complex and include papillary muscle dysfunction from ischemia and fibrosis in conjunction with a wall motion abnormality and changes in ventricular shape in the region of the papillary muscle and/or dilation of the mitral annulus.[421,422] Enlargement of the mitral annulus at end-systole is asymmetrical, with lengthening primarily involving the posterior annular segments and leading to prolapse of leaflet tissue tethered by the posterior papillary muscle and restriction of leaflet tissue attached to the anterior leaflet. Most patients with chronic CAD and mitral regurgitation have suffered a previous myocardial infarction. Clinical features that help identify mitral regurgitation secondary to papillary muscle dysfunction as the cause of acute pulmonary edema or the cause of milder symptoms of left-sided failure include a loud systolic murmur and demonstration of a flail mitral valve leaflet on echocardiography.

In some patients with severe mitral regurgitation into a small "unprepared" left atrium, the murmur may be unimpressive or inaudible. Doppler echocardiography is helpful in assessing the severity of the regurgitation (see Chap. 11). As in mitral regurgitation of other causes, the left atrium is not usually greatly enlarged unless mitral regurgitation has been present for more than 6 months. The ECG is nonspecific, and most patients have angiographic evidence of multivessel CAD.

MANAGEMENT. In patients with severe mitral regurgitation, the indications for surgical correction, usually in association with CABG, are fairly clear-cut. Mitral valve repair, as opposed to mitral replacement, is the procedure of choice, but the decision is based on the anatomical characteristics of the structures forming the mitral valve apparatus, the urgency of the need for surgery, and the severity of left ventricular dysfunction.[423] A more complex and frequently encountered problem involves the indications for mitral valve surgery in patients undergoing coronary bypass surgery in whom the severity of mitral regurgitation is moderate.[424] The decision is based partly on the presence or absence of structural abnormalities of the mitral apparatus and the amenability of the valve to repair. Intraoperative transesophageal echocardiography is invaluable in assessing the severity of regurgitation, the reparability of the valve, and the success of the integrity of the repair after discontinuation of CPB.

The mortality associated with combined coronary bypass surgery and mitral valve placement in the 2002 Society of Thoracic Surgeons data base was 12 percent. For bypass surgery and mitral valve repair, mortality was 7 percent overall including emergency and reoperative procedures.[425] Predictors of early mortality include the need for replacement versus repair (in some but not all series) but, in addition, may include other variables such as age, comorbid conditions, the urgency of surgery, and left ventricular function.[426] Late results are strongly influenced by the pathophysiological mechanisms underlying mitral regurgitation and are poorer in patients with regurgitation resulting from annular dilation or restrictive leaflet motion than in patients with chordal or papillary muscle rupture. It is encouraging that despite the relatively high operative mortality, late survival of hospital survivors is excellent. In patients with very poor left ventricular function and dilation of the mitral annulus, mitral regurgitation can intensify the severity of left ventricular failure. In such patients, the risk of surgery is high and the benefits are less obvious, and a trial of intensive medical therapy, including afterload reduction to decrease left ventricular volume and the diameter of the annulus, may be worthwhile.

CARDIAC ARRHYTHMIAS

In some patients with CAD, cardiac arrhythmias are the dominant clinical manifestation of the disease. Various degrees and forms of ventricular ectopic activity are the most common arrhythmias in patients with CAD, but serious ventricular arrhythmias may be a major component of the clinical findings in other subgroups. The clinical presentation of arrhythmias and their management in patients with CAD are discussed in Chapter 29.

NONATHEROMATOUS CORONARY ARTERY DISEASE

Although atherosclerosis is by far the most important cause of CAD, other conditions may also be responsible. The most common causes of nonatheromatous CAD resulting in myocardial ischemia are the syndrome of angina-like pain with normal coronary arteriograms (i.e., so-called syndrome X) and Prinzmetal angina (see Chap. 49).

Nonatheromatous CAD may result from other diverse abnormalities, including congenital abnormalities in the origin or distribution of the coronary arteries (see Chap. 56). The most important of these abnormalities are anomalous origin of a coronary artery (usually the left) from the pulmonary artery, origin of both coronary arteries from either the right or the left sinus of Valsalva, and coronary arteriovenous fistula. An anomalous origin of either the left main coronary artery or right coronary artery from the aorta with subsequent coursing between the aorta and pulmonary trunk is a rare and sometimes fatal coronary arterial anomaly.[427] Coronary anomalies are reported to cause between 12 and 19 percent of sports-related deaths in U.S. high school and college athletes.[427]

MYOCARDIAL BRIDGING. This cause of systolic compression of the LAD coronary artery is a well-recognized angiographic phenomenon of questionable clinical significance.

CONNECTIVE TISSUE DISORDERS. Several inherited connective tissue disorders are associated with myocardial ischemia (see Chap. 70), including Marfan syndrome (causing aortic and coronary artery dissection), Hurler syndrome (causing coronary obstruction), homocystinuria (causing coronary artery thrombosis), Ehlers-Danlos syndrome (causing coronary artery dissection), and pseudoxanthoma elasticum (causing accelerated CAD). Kawasaki disease (the mucocutaneous lymph node syndrome) may cause coronary artery aneurysms and ischemic heart disease in children.

SPONTANEOUS CORONARY DISSECTION. This is a rare cause of myocardial infarction and sudden cardiac death.[428] Chronic dissection manifested as congestive heart failure has been described. In one series, approximately 75 percent of cases were diagnosed at autopsy, and 75 percent occurred in women, half of which were associated with a postpartum state. Some cases are associated with atherosclerosis. Hypertension has been postulated as a cause of multivessel spontaneous coronary dissection in some patients, and in others, no obvious cause has been identified. In the acute phase, thrombolytic therapy may be dangerous, but early angiography may identify patients who could benefit from stenting or bypass surgery.[429] In survivors of spontaneous coronary artery dissection, the subsequent 3-year mortality was 20 percent, but complete healing as defined angiographically may lead to a favorable outcome without intervention.[430]

CORONARY VASCULITIS. This condition resulting from connective tissue diseases or autoimmune forms of vasculitis, including polyarteritis nodosa, giant cell (temporal) arteritis, and scleroderma, is well described (see Chap. 82). Coronary arteritis is seen at autopsy in about 20 percent of patients with rheumatoid arthritis but is rarely associated with clinical manifestations. The incidence of CAD is increased in women with systemic lupus erythematosus. In patients with systemic lupus erythematosus, CAD has been attributed to a vasculitis, immune complex–mediated endothelial damage, and coronary thrombosis from antiphospholipid antibodies, as well as accelerated atherosclerosis. Giant coronary artery aneurysm associated with systemic lupus erythematosus is an unusual manifestation that has been associated with the development of acute myocardial infarction despite therapy. The antiphospholipid syndrome, which is characterized by arterial and venous thrombosis and is associated with the presence of antiphospholipid antibodies, may be associated with myocardial infarction, angina, and diffuse left ventricular dysfunction.

TAKAYASU ARTERITIS. In rare cases, (see Chap. 82) this condition is associated with angina, myocardial infarction, and cardiac failure in patients younger than 40 years of age. Coronary blood flow may be decreased by involvement of the ostia or proximal segments of the coronary arteries, but disease in distal coronary segments is rare.[431] The average age at the onset of symptoms is 24 years, and the event-free survival rate 10 years after diagnosis is approximately 60 percent. Luetic aortitis may also produce myocardial ischemia by causing coronary ostial obstruction.

POSTMEDIASTINAL IRRADIATION. The occurrence of CAD and morbid cardiac events in young persons after mediastinal irradiation is highly suggestive of a cause-and-effect relationship.[432] Pathological changes include adventitial scarring and medial hypertrophy with severe intimal atherosclerotic disease. Radiation injury may be latent and may not be manifested clinically for many years after therapy. Contributory factors include higher doses than currently administered and the presence of cardiac risk factors. Among patients without risk factors who receive an intermediate total dose of 30 and 40 Gy, the risk of cardiac death and myocardial infarction is low.

Myocardial ischemia not caused by coronary atherosclerosis can also result from embolism from infective endocarditis (see Chap. 58), implanted prosthetic cardiac valves (see Chap. 57), calcified aortic valves, mural thrombi, and primary cardiac tumors (see Chap. 63).

COCAINE (see Chap. 62). Because of its widespread use, cocaine has become a well-documented cause of chest pain, myocardial infarction, and sudden cardiac death.[433] In a population-based study of sudden death among persons 20 to 40 years old in Olmsted County over a 30-year period, a high prevalence of cocaine abuse was observed in the more recent cohort of young adults who died suddenly. The principal effects of cocaine are mediated by alpha-adrenergic stimulation, which causes an increase in myocardial O_2 demand and a reduction in O_2 supply because of coronary vasoconstriction.

Cardiac Transplant–Associated Coronary Arteriopathy

See Chapters 26 and 35.

REFERENCES

1. Maseri A: Ischemic heart disease. *In* A Rational Basis for Clinical Practice and Clinical Research. New York, Churchill Livingstone, 1995.
2. Virmani R, Forman MB: Nonatherosclerotic Ischemic Heart Disease. New York, Raven, 1989.
3. American Heart Association: Heart Disease and Stroke Statistics—2004 Update. Dallas, American Heart Association, 2004.
4. Murray CJ, Lopez AD: Mortality by cause for eight regions of the world: Global Burden of Disease Study. Lancet 349:1269-1276, 1997.
5. Bonow RO, Smaha LA, Smith SC Jr, et al: World Heart Day 2002: The international burden of cardiovascular disease—responding to the emerging global epidemic. Circulation 106:1602-1605, 2002.
6. American Heart Association: International Cardiovascular Disease Statistics. Dallas, American Heart Association, 2004.
7. Duprez DA: Angina in the elderly. Eur Heart J 17(Suppl G):8-13, 1996.
8. Bogaty P, Kingma JG Jr, Robitaille NM, et al: Attenuation of myocardial ischemia with repeated exercise in subjects with chronic stable angina: Relation to myocardial contractility, intensity of exercise, and the adenosine triphosphate–sensitive potassium channel. J Am Coll Cardiol 32:1665-1671, 1998.
9. Bogaty P, Poirier P, Boyer L, et al: What induces the warm-up ischemia/angina phenomenon: Exercise or myocardial ischemia? Circulation 107:1858-1863, 2003.
10. Campeau L: Grading of angina pectoris [letter]. Circulation 54:522-523, 1976.
11. Goldman L, Hashimoto B, Cook EF, et al: Comparative reproducibility and validity of systems for assessing cardiovascular functional class: Advantages of a new specific activity scale. Circulation 64:1227-1234, 1981.
12. Califf RM, Mark DB, Harrell FE Jr, et al: Importance of clinical measures of ischemia in the prognosis of patients with documented coronary artery disease. J Am Coll Cardiol 11:20-26, 1988.
13. Foreman RD: Mechanisms of cardiac pain. Annu Rev Physiol 61:143-167, 1999.
14. Rosen SD, Camici PG: The brain-heart axis in the perception of cardiac pain: The elusive link between ischaemia and pain. Ann Med 32:350-364, 2000.
15. Wise CM, Semble EL, Dalton CB: Musculoskeletal chest wall syndromes in patients with noncardiac chest pain: A study of 100 patients. Arch Phys Med Rehabil 73:147-149, 1992.
16. Klein R, Klein BE, Moss SE, et al: Association of ocular disease and mortality in a diabetic population. Arch Ophthalmol 117:1487-1495, 1999.
17. Eagle KA, Rihal CS, Foster ED, et al: Long-term survival in patients with coronary artery disease: Importance of peripheral vascular disease. The Coronary Artery Surgery Study (CASS) Investigators. J Am Coll Cardiol 23:1091-1095, 1994.
18. Gibbons RJ, Abrams J, Chatterjee K, et al: ACC/AHA 2002 guideline update for the management of patients with chronic stable angina—summary article: A report of the American College of Cardiology/American Heart Association Task Force on Practice Guidelines (Committee on the Management of Patients with Chronic Stable Angina). J Am Coll Cardiol 41:159-168, 2003.
19. Freedman SB, Wong CK: Triggers of daily life ischaemia. Heart 80:489-492, 1998.
20. Gullette EC, Blumenthal JA, Babyak M, et al: Effects of mental stress on myocardial ischemia during daily life. JAMA 277:1521-1526, 1997.
21. Hillis LD, Braunwald E: Coronary artery spasm. N Engl J Med 299:695-702, 1978.
22. Opie LH: The Heart: Physiology, From Cell to Circulation. 3rd ed. Philadelphia, Lippincott-Raven, 1998.
23. Maseri A, Crea F, Lanza GA: Coronary vasoconstriction: Where do we stand in 1999? An important, multifaceted but elusive role. Cardiologia 44:115-118, 1999.
24. Benhorin J, Banai S, Moriel M, et al: Circadian variations in ischemic threshold and their relation to the occurrence of ischemic episodes. Circulation 87:808-814, 1993.
25. Baliga RR, Rosen SD, Camici PG, et al: Regional myocardial blood flow redistribution as a cause of postprandial angina pectoris. Circulation 97:1144-1149, 1998.
26. Maseri A, Chierchia S, Kaski JC: Mixed angina pectoris. Am J Cardiol 56:30E-33E, 1985.

Noninvasive Testing

27. Expert Panel on Detection, Evaluation, and Treatment of High Blood Cholesterol in Adults: Executive Summary of the Third Report of the National Cholesterol Education Program (NCEP) Expert Panel on Detection, Evaluation, and Treatment of High Blood Cholesterol in Adults (Adult Treatment Panel III). JAMA 285:2486-2497, 2001.
28. Lamarche B, Tchernof A, Mauriege P, et al: Fasting insulin and apolipoprotein B levels and low-density lipoprotein particle size as risk factors for ischemic heart disease. JAMA 279:1955-1961, 1998.
29. The Homocysteine Studies Collaboration: Homocysteine and risk of ischemic heart disease and stroke: A meta-analysis. JAMA 288:2015-2022, 2002.
30. Malinow MR, Bostom AG, Krauss RM: Homocyst(e)ine, diet, and cardiovascular diseases: A statement for healthcare professionals from the Nutrition Committee, American Heart Association. Circulation 99:178-182, 1999.
31. Ridker PM: Clinical application of C-reactive protein for cardiovascular disease detection and prevention. Circulation 107:363-369, 2003.
32. Ridker PM, Rifai N, Rose L, et al: Comparison of C-reactive protein and low-density lipoprotein cholesterol levels in the prediction of first cardiovascular events. N Engl J Med 347:1557-1565, 2002.
33. Pearson TA, Mensah GA, Alexander RW, et al: Markers of inflammation and cardiovascular disease—application to clinical and public health practice: A statement for healthcare professionals from the Centers for Disease Control and Prevention and the American Heart Association. Circulation 107:499-511, 2003.
34. Morrow DA, de Lemos JA, Sabatine MS, et al: The search for a biomarker of cardiac ischemia. Clin Chem 49:537-539, 2003.
35. Crenshaw JH, Mirvis DM, el-Zeky F, et al: Interactive effects of ST-T wave abnormalities on survival of patients with coronary artery disease. J Am Coll Cardiol 18:413-420, 1991.
36. Gibbons RJ, Balady GJ, Bricker JT, et al: ACC/AHA 2002 guideline update for exercise testing—summary article: A report of the American College of Cardiology/American Heart Association Task Force on Practice Guidelines (Committee to Update the 1997 Exercise Testing Guidelines). Circulation 106:1883-1892, 2002.
37. Shaw LJ, Hachamovitch R, Berman DS, et al: The economic consequences of available diagnostic and prognostic strategies for the evaluation of stable angina patients: An observational assessment of the value of precatheterization ischemia. Economics of Noninvasive Diagnosis (END) Multicenter Study Group. J Am Coll Cardiol 33:661-669, 1999.
38. Froelicher VF, Lehmann KG, Thomas R, et al: The electrocardiographic exercise test in a population with reduced workup bias: Diagnostic performance, computerized interpretation, and multivariable prediction. Veterans Affairs Cooperative Study in Health Services 016 (QUEXTA) Study Group. Quantitative Exercise Testing and Angiography. Ann Intern Med 128:965-974, 1998.
39. Shaw LJ, Peterson ED, Shaw LK, et al: Use of a prognostic treadmill score in identifying diagnostic coronary disease subgroups. Circulation 98:1622-1630, 1998.
40. Beller GA, Zaret BL: Contributions of nuclear cardiology to diagnosis and prognosis of patients with coronary artery disease. Circulation 101:1465-1478, 2000.
41. Pagley PR, Beller GA, Watson DD, et al: Improved outcome after coronary bypass surgery in patients with ischemic cardiomyopathy and residual myocardial viability. Circulation 96:793-800, 1997.
42. Gibbons RJ, Hodge DO, Berman DS, et al: Long-term outcome of patients with intermediate-risk exercise electrocardiograms who do not have myocardial perfusion defects on radionuclide imaging. Circulation 100:2140-2145, 1999.
43. Ritchie J, Bateman TM, Bonow RO, et al: Guidelines for clinical use of cardiac radionuclide imaging: A report of the American Heart Association/American College of Cardiology Task Force on Assessment of Diagnostic and Therapeutic Cardiovascular Procedures, Committee on Radionuclide Imaging, developed in collaboration with the American Society of Nuclear Cardiology. Circulation 91:1278-1303, 1995.
44. Ibrahim T, Nekolla SG, Schreiber K, et al: Assessment of coronary flow reserve: Comparison between contrast-enhanced magnetic resonance imaging and positron emission tomography. J Am Coll Cardiol 39:864-870, 2002.
45. Fleischmann KE, Hunink MG, Kuntz KM, et al: Exercise echocardiography or exercise SPECT imaging? A meta-analysis of diagnostic test performance. JAMA 280:913-920, 1998.
46. Bax JJ, Poldermans D, Elhendy A, et al: Improvement of left ventricular ejection fraction, heart failure symptoms, and prognosis after revascularization in patients with chronic coronary artery disease and viable myocardium detected by dobutamine stress echocardiography. J Am Coll Cardiol 34:163-169, 1999.
47. Finkelhor RS, Pajouh M, Kett A, et al: Clinical impact of second harmonic imaging and left heart contrast in echocardiographic stress testing. Am J Cardiol 85:740-743, 2000.
48. Vlassak I, Rubin DN, Odabashian JA, et al: Contrast and harmonic imaging improves accuracy and efficiency of novice readers for dobutamine stress echocardiography. Echocardiography 19:483-488, 2002.
49. Voigt JU, Exner B, Schmiedehausen K, et al: Strain-rate imaging during dobutamine stress echocardiography provides objective evidence of inducible ischemia. Circulation 107:2120-2126, 2003.
50. Hachamovitch R, Berman DS, Kiat H, et al: Effective risk stratification using exercise myocardial perfusion SPECT in women: Gender-related differences in prognostic nuclear testing. J Am Coll Cardiol 28:34-44, 1996.
51. Taillefer R, DePuey EG, Udelson JE, et al: Comparative diagnostic accuracy of Tl-201 and Tc-99m sestamibi SPECT imaging (perfusion and ECG-gated SPECT) in detecting coronary artery disease in women. J Am Coll Cardiol 29:69-77, 1997.
52. Loecker TH, Schwartz RS, Cotta CW, et al: Fluoroscopic coronary artery calcification and associated coronary disease in asymptomatic young men. J Am Coll Cardiol 19:1167-1172, 1992.
53. Callister TQ, Raggi P, Cooil B, et al: Effect of HMG-CoA reductase inhibitors on coronary artery disease as assessed by electron-beam computed tomography. N Engl J Med 339:1972-1978, 1998.

54. Budoff MJ, Diamond GA, Raggi P, et al: Continuous probabilistic prediction of angiographically significant coronary artery disease using electron beam tomography. Circulation 105:1791-1796, 2002.
55. Detrano RC, Wong ND, Doherty TM, et al: Coronary calcium does not accurately predict near-term future coronary events in high-risk adults. Circulation 99:2633-2638, 1999.
56. Kondos GT, Hoff JA, Sevrukov A, et al: Electron-beam tomography coronary artery calcium and cardiac events: A 37-month follow-up of 5635 initially asymptomatic low- to intermediate-risk adults. Circulation 107:2571-2576, 2003.
57. O'Rourke RA, Brundage BH, Froelicher VF, et al: American College of Cardiology/ American Heart Association Expert Consensus document on electron-beam computed tomography for the diagnosis and prognosis of coronary artery disease. Circulation 102:126-140, 2000.
58. Budoff MJ, Georgiou D, Brody A, et al: Ultrafast computed tomography as a diagnostic modality in the detection of coronary artery disease: A multicenter study. Circulation 93:898-904, 1996.
59. Nallamothu BK, Saint S, Bielak LF, et al. Electron-beam computed tomography in the diagnosis of coronary artery disease: A meta-analysis. Arch Intern Med 161:833-838, 2001.
60. Ropers D, Baum U, Pohle K, et al: Detection of coronary artery stenoses with thin-slice multi-detector row spiral computed tomography and multiplanar reconstruction. Circulation 107:664-666, 2003.
61. Forder JR, Pohost GM: Cardiovascular nuclear magnetic resonance: Basic and clinical applications. J Clin Invest 111:1630-1639, 2003.
62. Kim RJ, Wu E, Rafael A, et al: The use of contrast-enhanced magnetic resonance imaging to identify reversible myocardial dysfunction. N Engl J Med 343:1445-1453, 2000.
63. Klein C, Nekolla SG, Bengel FM, et al: Assessment of myocardial viability with contrast-enhanced magnetic resonance imaging: Comparison with positron emission tomography. Circulation 105:162-167, 2002.
64. Gerber BL, Garot J, Bluemke DA, et al: Accuracy of contrast-enhanced magnetic resonance imaging in predicting improvement of regional myocardial function in patients after acute myocardial infarction. Circulation 106:1083-1089, 2002.
65. Schwitter J, Nanz D, Kneifel S, et al: Assessment of myocardial perfusion in coronary artery disease by magnetic resonance: A comparison with positron emission tomography and coronary angiography. Circulation 103:2230-2235, 2001.
66. Kuijpers D, Ho KY, van Dijkman PR, et al: Dobutamine cardiovascular magnetic resonance for the detection of myocardial ischemia with the use of myocardial tagging. Circulation 107:1592-1597, 2003.
67. Kraitchman DL, Sampath S, Castillo E, et al: Quantitative ischemia detection during cardiac magnetic resonance stress testing by use of FastHARP. Circulation 107:2025-2030, 2003.
68. Fuster V, Corti R, Fayad ZA, et al: Integration of vascular biology and magnetic resonance imaging in the understanding of atherothrombosis and acute coronary syndromes. J Thromb Haemost 1:1410-1421, 2003.
69. Hatsukami TS, Ross R, Polissar NL, et al: Visualization of fibrous cap thickness and rupture in human atherosclerotic carotid plaque in vivo with high-resolution magnetic resonance imaging. Circulation 102:959-964, 2000.
70. Moody AR, Murphy RE, Morgan PS, et al: Characterization of complicated carotid plaque with magnetic resonance direct thrombus imaging in patients with cerebral ischemia. Circulation 107:3047-3052, 2003.
71. Kim WY, Danias PG, Stuber M, et al: Coronary magnetic resonance angiography for the detection of coronary stenoses. N Engl J Med 345:1863-1869, 2001.
72. Langerak SE, Vliegen HW, Jukema JW, et al: Value of magnetic resonance imaging for the noninvasive detection of stenosis in coronary artery bypass grafts and recipient coronary arteries. Circulation 107:1502-1508, 2003.
73. Taylor AM, Thorne SA, Rubens MB, et al: Coronary artery imaging in grown up congenital heart disease: Complementary role of magnetic resonance and x-ray coronary angiography. Circulation 101:1670-1678, 2000.

Catheterization, Angiography, and Coronary Arteriography

74. Schoenhagen P, Nissen S: Understanding coronary artery disease: Tomographic imaging with intravascular ultrasound. Heart 88:91-96, 2002.
75. Nair A, Kuban BD, Tuzcu EM, et al: Coronary plaque classification with intravascular ultrasound radiofrequency data analysis. Circulation 106:2200-2206, 2002.
76. Bogaty P, Brecker SJ, White SE, et al: Comparison of coronary angiographic findings in acute and chronic first presentation of ischemic heart disease. Circulation 87:1938-1946, 1993.
77. Kruger D, Stierle U, Herrmann G, et al: Exercise-induced myocardial ischemia in isolated coronary artery ectasias and aneurysms ("dilated coronopathy"). J Am Coll Cardiol 34:1461-1470, 1999.
78. Tunick PA, Slater J, Kronzon I, et al: Discrete atherosclerotic coronary artery aneurysms: A study of 20 patients. J Am Coll Cardiol 15:279-282, 1990.
79. Vanoverschelde JL, Wijns W, Depre C, et al: Mechanisms of chronic regional postischemic dysfunction in humans: New insights from the study of noninfarcted collateral-dependent myocardium. Circulation 87:1513-1523, 1993.
80. Mohlenkamp S, Hort W, Ge J, et al: Update on myocardial bridging. Circulation 106:2616-2622, 2002.
81. Mann T, Brodie BR, Grossman W, et al: Effect of angina on the left ventricular diastolic pressure-volume relationship. Circulation 55:761-766, 1977.
82. Braunwald E, Rutherford JD: Reversible ischemic left ventricular dysfunction: Evidence for the "hibernating myocardium." J Am Coll Cardiol 8:1467-1470, 1986.
83. Verani MS, Carroll RJ, Falsetti HL: Mitral valve prolapse in coronary artery disease. Am J Cardiol 37:1-6, 1976.
84. Gertz EW, Wisneski JA, Neese R, et al: Myocardial lactate metabolism: Evidence of lactate release during net chemical extraction in man. Circulation 63:1273-1279, 1981.
85. Lampe FC, Whincup PH, Wannamethee SG, et al: The natural history of prevalent ischaemic heart disease in middle-aged men. Eur Heart J 21:1052-1062, 2000.
86. Myers J, Prakash M, Froelicher V, et al: Exercise capacity and mortality among men referred for exercise testing. N Engl J Med 346:793-801, 2002.
87. Yao SS, Rozanski A: Principal uses of myocardial perfusion scintigraphy in the management of patients with known or suspected coronary artery disease. Prog Cardiovasc Dis 43:281-302, 2001.
88. Lee TH, Boucher CA: Clinical practice: Noninvasive tests in patients with stable coronary artery disease. N Engl J Med 344:1840-1845, 2001.
89. Califf RM, Tomabechi Y, Lee KL, et al: Outcome in one-vessel coronary artery disease. Circulation 67:283-290, 1983.
90. Caracciolo EA, Davis KB, Sopko G, et al: Comparison of surgical and medical group survival in patients with left main coronary artery disease: Long-term CASS experience. Circulation 91:2325-2334, 1995.
91. Bigi R, Cortigiani L, Colombo P, et al: Prognostic and clinical correlates of angiographically diffuse non-obstructive coronary lesions. Heart 89:1009-1013, 2003.

Medical Management

92. Jousilahti P, Vartiainen E, Tuomilehto J, et al: Sex, age, cardiovascular risk factors, and coronary heart disease: A prospective follow-up study of 14 786 middle-aged men and women in Finland. Circulation 99:1165-1172, 1999.
93. Lewington S, Clarke R, Qizilbash N, et al: Age-specific relevance of usual blood pressure to vascular mortality: A meta-analysis of individual data for one million adults in 61 prospective studies. Lancet 360:1903-1913, 2002.
94. Devereux RB, Roman MJ: Inter-relationships between hypertension, left ventricular hypertrophy, and coronary heart disease. J Hypertens 11(Suppl):S3-S9, 1993.
95. Hebert PR, Moser M, Mayer J, et al: Recent evidence on drug therapy of mild to moderate hypertension and decreased risk of coronary heart disease. Arch Intern Med 153:578-581, 1993.
96. Psaty BM, Lumley T, Furberg CD, et al: Health outcomes associated with various antihypertensive therapies used as first-line agents: A network meta-analysis. JAMA 289:2534-2544, 2003.
97. Ogden LG, He J, Lydick E, et al: Long-term absolute benefit of lowering blood pressure in hypertensive patients according to the JNC VI risk stratification. Hypertension 35:539-543, 2000.
98. Critchley JA, Capewell S: Mortality risk reduction associated with smoking cessation in patients with coronary heart disease: A systematic review. JAMA 290:86-97, 2003.
99. Czernin J, Sun K, Brunken R, et al: Effect of acute and long-term smoking on myocardial blood flow and flow reserve. Circulation 91:2891-2897, 1995.
100. Scandinavian Simvastatin Survival Study Group: Randomised trial of cholesterol lowering in 4444 patients with coronary heart disease: The Scandinavian Simvastatin Survival Study (4S). Lancet 344:1383-1389, 1994.
101. Sacks FM, Pfeffer MA, Moye LA, et al: The effect of pravastatin on coronary events after myocardial infarction in patients with average cholesterol levels. Cholesterol and Recurrent Events Trial investigators. N Engl J Med 335:1001-1009, 1996.
102. Long-Term Intervention with Pravastatin in Ischaemic Disease (LIPID) Study Group: Prevention of cardiovascular events and death with pravastatin in patients with coronary heart disease and a broad range of initial cholesterol levels. N Engl J Med 339:1349-1357, 1998.
103. Pitt B, Waters D, Brown WV, et al: Aggressive lipid-lowering therapy compared with angioplasty in stable coronary artery disease. Atorvastatin versus Revascularization Treatment Investigators. N Engl J Med 341:70-76, 1999.
104. Heart Protection Study Collaborative Group: MRC/BHF Heart Protection Study of cholesterol lowering with simvastatin in 20,536 high-risk individuals: A randomised placebo-controlled trial. Lancet 360:7-22, 2002.
105. Dupuis J, Tardif JC, Cernacek P, et al: Cholesterol reduction rapidly improves endothelial function after acute coronary syndromes. The RECIFE (Reduction of Cholesterol in Ischemia and Function of the Endothelium) trial. Circulation 99:3227-3233, 1999.
106. Ridker PM, Rifai N, Pfeffer MA, et al: Long-term effects of pravastatin on plasma concentration of C-reactive protein. Circulation 100:230-235, 1999.
107. Albert MA, Danielson E, Rifai N, et al: Effect of statin therapy on C-reactive protein levels: The pravastatin inflammation/CRP evaluation (PRINCE)—a randomized trial and cohort study. JAMA 286:64-70, 2001.
108. Dangas G, Badimon JJ, Smith DA, et al: Pravastatin therapy in hyperlipidemia: Effects on thrombus formation and the systemic hemostatic profile. J Am Coll Cardiol 33:1294-1304, 1999.
109. Crisby M, Nordin-Fredriksson G, Shah PK, et al: Pravastatin treatment increases collagen content and decreases lipid content, inflammation, metalloproteinases, and cell death in human carotid plaques: Implications for plaque stabilization. Circulation 103:926-933, 2001.
110. Rosenson RS, Tangney CC: Antiatherothrombotic properties of statins: Implications for cardiovascular event reduction. JAMA 279:1643-1650, 1998.
111. Lewis SJ, Sacks FM, Mitchell JS, et al: Effect of pravastatin on cardiovascular events in women after myocardial infarction: The Cholesterol and Recurrent Events (CARE) trial. J Am Coll Cardiol 32:140-146, 1998.
112. Shepherd J, Blauw GJ, Murphy MB, et al: Pravastatin in elderly individuals at risk of vascular disease (PROSPER): A randomised controlled trial. Lancet 360:1623-1630, 2002.
113. Tsevat J, Kuntz KM, Orav EJ, et al: Cost-effectiveness of pravastatin therapy for survivors of myocardial infarction with average cholesterol levels. Am Heart J 141:727-734, 2001.
113a. Cannon CP, Braunwald E, McCabe CH, et al: Pravastatin or Atorvastatin Evaluation and Infection Therapy (PROVE-IT)-TIMI 22 Investigators. Intensive versus moderate lipid lowering with statins after acute coronary syndromes. N Engl J Med 350:1495-1504, 2004.
114. Gotto AM Jr: Low high-density lipoprotein cholesterol as a risk factor in coronary heart disease: A working group report. Circulation 103:2213-2218, 2001.

115. Lamarche B, Tchernof A, Moorjani S, et al: Small, dense low-density lipoprotein particles as a predictor of the risk of ischemic heart disease in men: Prospective results from the Quebec Cardiovascular Study. Circulation 95:69-75, 1997.
116. Rubins HB, Robins SJ, Collins D, et al: Gemfibrozil for the secondary prevention of coronary heart disease in men with low levels of high-density lipoprotein cholesterol. Veterans Affairs High-Density Lipoprotein Cholesterol Intervention Trial Study Group. N Engl J Med 341:410-418, 1999.
117. Flaker GC, Warnica JW, Sacks FM, et al: Pravastatin prevents clinical events in revascularized patients with average cholesterol concentrations. Cholesterol and Recurrent Events CARE Investigators. J Am Coll Cardiol 34:106-112, 1999.
118. Serruys PW, de Feyter P, Macaya C, et al: Fluvastatin for prevention of cardiac events following successful first percutaneous coronary intervention: A randomized controlled trial. JAMA 287:3215-3222, 2002.
119. Grodstein F, Stampfer MJ, Colditz GA, et al: Postmenopausal hormone therapy and mortality. N Engl J Med 336:1769-1775, 1997.
120. Hulley S, Grady D, Bush T, et al: Randomized trial of estrogen plus progestin for secondary prevention of coronary heart disease in postmenopausal women. Heart and Estrogen/progestin Replacement Study (HERS) Research Group. JAMA 280:605-613, 1998.
121. Grady D, Herrington D, Bittner V, et al: Cardiovascular disease outcomes during 6.8 years of hormone therapy: Heart and Estrogen/progestin Replacement Study follow-up (HERS II). JAMA 288:49-57, 2002.
122. Clarke SC, Kelleher J, Lloyd-Jones H, et al: A study of hormone replacement therapy in postmenopausal women with ischaemic heart disease: The Papworth HRT atherosclerosis study. Br J Obstet Gynaecol 109:1056-1062, 2002.
123. Herrington DM, Reboussin DM, Brosnihan KB, et al: Effects of estrogen replacement on the progression of coronary-artery atherosclerosis. N Engl J Med 343:522-529, 2000.
124. Waters DD, Alderman EL, Hsia J, et al: Effects of hormone replacement therapy and antioxidant vitamin supplements on coronary atherosclerosis in postmenopausal women: A randomized controlled trial. JAMA 288:2432-2440, 2002.
125. Cherry N, Gilmour K, Hannaford P, et al: Oestrogen therapy for prevention of reinfarction in postmenopausal women: A randomised placebo-controlled trial. Lancet 360:2001-2008, 2002.
126. Rossouw JE, Anderson GL, Prentice RL, et al: Risks and benefits of estrogen plus progestin in healthy postmenopausal women: Principal results from the Women's Health Initiative randomized controlled trial. JAMA 288:321-333, 2002.
127. Mosca L, Collins P, Herrington DM, et al: Hormone replacement therapy and cardiovascular disease: A statement for healthcare professionals from the American Heart Association. Circulation 104:499-503, 2001.
128. Thompson PD, Buchner D, Pina IL, et al: Exercise and physical activity in the prevention and treatment of atherosclerotic cardiovascular disease. Circulation 107:3109-3116, 2003.
129. Jolliffe JA, Rees K, Taylor RS, et al: Exercise-based rehabilitation for coronary heart disease. Cochrane Database Syst Rev CD001800, 2004.
130. Hambrecht R, Niebauer J, Marburger C, et al: Various intensities of leisure time physical activity in patients with coronary artery disease: Effects on cardiorespiratory fitness and progression of coronary atherosclerotic lesions. J Am Coll Cardiol 22:468-477, 1993.
131. Hambrecht R, Adams V, Erbs S, et al: Regular physical activity improves endothelial function in patients with coronary artery disease by increasing phosphorylation of endothelial nitric oxide synthase. Circulation 107:3152-3158, 2003.
132. Hambrecht R, Wolf A, Gielen S, et al: Effect of exercise on coronary endothelial function in patients with coronary artery disease. N Engl J Med 342:454-460, 2000.
133. Fletcher GF, Balady GJ, Amsterdam EA, et al: Exercise standards for testing and training: A statement for healthcare professionals from the American Heart Association. Circulation 104:1694-1740, 2001.
134. Oldridge N, Furlong W, Feeny D, et al: Economic evaluation of cardiac rehabilitation soon after acute myocardial infarction. Am J Cardiol 72:154-161, 1993.
135. Ridker PM, Rifai N, Pfeffer MA, et al: Inflammation, pravastatin, and the risk of coronary events after myocardial infarction in patients with average cholesterol levels. Cholesterol and Recurrent Events (CARE) Investigators. Circulation 98:839-844, 1998.
136. Libby P, Aikawa M: Stabilization of atherosclerotic plaques: New mechanisms and clinical targets. Nat Med 8:1257-1262, 2002.
136a. Ridker PM, Rifai N, Clearfield M, et al: Air Force/Texas Coronary Atherosclerosis Prevention Study Investigators. Measurement of C-reactive protein for the targeting of statin therapy in the primary prevention of acute coronary events. N Engl J Med 344:1959-1965, 2001.
137. Antiplatelet Trialists' Collaboration: Collaborative overview of randomised trials of antiplatelet therapy: I. Prevention of death, myocardial infarction, and stroke by prolonged antiplatelet therapy in various categories of patients. BMJ 308:81-106, 1994.
138. Juul-Moller S, Edvardsson N, Jahnmatz B, et al: Double-blind trial of aspirin in primary prevention of myocardial infarction in patients with stable chronic angina pectoris. The Swedish Angina Pectoris Aspirin Trial (SAPAT) Group. Lancet 340:1421-1425, 1992.
139. Ridker PM, Manson JE, Gaziano JM, et al: Low-dose aspirin therapy for chronic stable angina: A randomized, placebo-controlled clinical trial. Ann Intern Med 114:835-839, 1991.
140. Hennekens CH, Dyken ML, Fuster V: Aspirin as a therapeutic agent in cardiovascular disease: A statement for healthcare professionals from the American Heart Association. Circulation 96:2751-2753, 1997.
141. Antithrombotic Trialists' Collaboration: Collaborative meta-analysis of randomised trials of antiplatelet therapy for prevention of death, myocardial infarction, and stroke in high-risk patients. BMJ 324:71-86, 2002.
142. Peters RJ, Mehta SR, Fox KA, et al: Effects of aspirin dose when used alone or in combination with clopidogrel in patients with acute coronary syndromes: Observations from the Clopidogrel in Unstable angina to prevent Recurrent Events (CURE) study. Circulation 108:1682-1687, 2003.
143. Ridker PM, Cushman M, Stampfer MJ, et al: Inflammation, aspirin, and the risk of cardiovascular disease in apparently healthy men. N Engl J Med 336:973-979, 1997.
144. Ikonomidis I, Andreotti F, Economou E, et al: Increased proinflammatory cytokines in patients with chronic stable angina and their reduction by aspirin. Circulation 100:793-798, 1999.
145. Feldman M, Jialal I, Devaraj S, et al: Effects of low-dose aspirin on serum C-reactive protein and thromboxane B_2 concentrations: A placebo-controlled study using a highly sensitive C-reactive protein assay. J Am Coll Cardiol 37:2036-2041, 2001.
146. Husain S, Andrews NP, Mulcahy D, et al: Aspirin improves endothelial dysfunction in atherosclerosis. Circulation 97:716-720, 1998.
147. The Medical Research Council's General Practice Research Framework. Thrombosis Prevention Trial: Randomised trial of low-intensity oral anticoagulation with warfarin and low-dose aspirin in the primary prevention of ischaemic heart disease in men at increased risk. Lancet 351:233-241, 1998.
148. Nguyen KN, Aursnes I, Kjekshus J: Interaction between enalapril and aspirin on mortality after acute myocardial infarction: Subgroup analysis of the Cooperative New Scandinavian Enalapril Survival Study II (CONSENSUS II). Am J Cardiol 79:115-119, 1997.
149. Yusuf S, Sleight P, Pogue J, et al: Effects of an angiotensin-converting-enzyme inhibitor, ramipril, on cardiovascular events in high-risk patients. The Heart Outcomes Prevention Evaluation Study Investigators. N Engl J Med 342:145-153, 2000.
150. Quinn MJ, Fitzgerald DJ: Ticlopidine and clopidogrel. Circulation 100:1667-1672, 1999.
151. CAPRIE Steering Committee: A randomised, blinded, trial of clopidogrel versus aspirin in patients at risk of ischaemic events (CAPRIE). Lancet 348:1329-1339, 1996.
152. Yusuf S, Zhao F, Mehta SR, et al: Effects of clopidogrel in addition to aspirin in patients with acute coronary syndromes without ST-segment elevation. N Engl J Med 345:494-502, 2001.
153. Steinhubl SR, Berger PB, Mann JT III, et al: Early and sustained dual oral antiplatelet therapy following percutaneous coronary intervention: A randomized controlled trial. JAMA 288:2411-2420, 2002.
154. Gottlieb SS, McCarter RJ, Vogel RA: Effect of beta-blockade on mortality among high-risk and low-risk patients after myocardial infarction. N Engl J Med 339:489-497, 1998.
155. Pfeffer MA, Braunwald E, Moye LA, et al: Effect of captopril on mortality and morbidity in patients with left ventricular dysfunction after myocardial infarction: Results of the survival and ventricular enlargement trial. The SAVE Investigators. N Engl J Med 327:669-677, 1992.
156. Lonn EM, Yusuf S, Jha P, et al: Emerging role of angiotensin-converting enzyme inhibitors in cardiac and vascular protection. Circulation 90:2056-2069, 1994.
157. Prasad A, Husain S, Quyyumi AA: Abnormal flow-mediated epicardial vasomotion in human coronary arteries is improved by angiotensin-converting enzyme inhibition: A potential role of bradykinin. J Am Coll Cardiol 33:796-804, 1999.
158. Schneider CA, Voth E, Moka D, et al: Improvement of myocardial blood flow to ischemic regions by angiotensin-converting enzyme inhibition with quinaprilat IV: A study using [15O] water dobutamine stress positron emission tomography. J Am Coll Cardiol 34:1005-1011, 1999.
159. Kranzhofer R, Schmidt J, Pfeiffer CA, et al: Angiotensin induces inflammatory activation of human vascular smooth muscle cells. Arterioscler Thromb Vasc Biol 19:1623-1629, 1999.
160. Tummala PE, Chen XL, Sundell CL, et al: Angiotensin II induces vascular cell adhesion molecule-1 expression in rat vasculature: A potential link between the renin-angiotensin system and atherosclerosis. Circulation 100:1223-1229, 1999.
160a. Fox KM: EURopean trial On reduction of cardiac events with Perindopril in stable coronary Artery disease Investigators. Efficacy of perindopril in reduction of cardiovascular events among patients with stable coronary artery disease: Randomised, double-blind, placebo-controlled, multicentre trial (the EUROPA study). Lancet 362:782-788, 2003.
160b. Pfeffer MA, Domanski M, Verter J, et al: The continuation of the Prevention of Events with Angiotensin-Converting Enzyme Inhibition (PEACE) trial. Am Heart J 142:375-377, 2001.
161. Kushi LH, Folsom AR, Prineas RJ, et al: Dietary antioxidant vitamins and death from coronary heart disease in postmenopausal women. N Engl J Med 334:1156-1162, 1996.
162. Stephens NG, Parsons A, Schofield PM, et al: Randomised controlled trial of vitamin E in patients with coronary disease: Cambridge Heart Antioxidant Study (CHAOS). Lancet 347:781-786, 1996.
163. Yusuf S, Dagenais G, Pogue J, et al: Vitamin E supplementation and cardiovascular events in high-risk patients. The Heart Outcomes Prevention Evaluation Study Investigators. N Engl J Med 342:154-160, 2000.
164. Heart Protection Study Collaborative Group. MRC/BHF Heart Protection Study of antioxidant vitamin supplementation in 20,536 high-risk individuals: A randomised placebo-controlled trial. Lancet 360:23-33, 2002.
165. Ruo B, Rumsfeld JS, Hlatky MA, et al: Depressive symptoms and health-related quality of life: The Heart and Soul Study. JAMA 290:215-221, 2003.
166. Glassman AH, O'Connor CM, Califf RM, et al: Sertraline treatment of major depression in patients with acute MI or unstable angina. JAMA 288:701-709, 2002.
167. Larson CO, Nelson EC, Gustafson D, et al: The relationship between meeting patients' information needs and their satisfaction with hospital care and general health status outcomes. Int J Qual Health Care 8:447-456, 1996.
168. Figueras J, Lidon RM: Early morning reduction in ischemic threshold in patients with unstable angina and significant coronary disease. Circulation 92:1737-1742, 1995.

Pharmacological Management of Angina Pectoris

169. Parker JD, Parker JO: Nitrate therapy for stable angina pectoris. N Engl J Med 38:520-531, 1998.
170. Brown BG, Bolson E, Petersen RB, et al: The mechanisms of nitroglycerin action: Stenosis vasodilatation as a major component of the drug response. Circulation 64:1089-1097, 1981.

171. Parker JO: Nitrates and angina pectoris. Am J Cardiol 72:3C-6C, 1993.
172. Bottcher M, Madsen MM, Randsbaek F, et al: Effect of oral nitroglycerin and cold stress on myocardial perfusion in areas subtended by stenosed and nonstenosed coronary arteries. Am J Cardiol 89:1019-1024, 2002.
173. Tadamura E, Mamede M, Kubo S, et al: The effect of nitroglycerin on myocardial blood flow in various segments characterized by rest-redistribution thallium SPECT. J Nucl Med 44:745-751, 2003.
174. Fallen EL, Nahmias C, Scheffel A, et al: Redistribution of myocardial blood flow with topical nitroglycerin in patients with coronary artery disease. Circulation 91:1381-1388, 1995.
175. Munzel T, Mulsch A, Kleschyov A: Mechanisms underlying nitroglycerin-induced superoxide production in platelets: Some insight, more questions. Circulation 106:170-172, 2002.
176. Anderson TJ, Meredith IT, Ganz P, et al: Nitric oxide and nitrovasodilators: Similarities, differences, and potential interactions. J Am Coll Cardiol 24:555-566, 1994.
177. Chen Z, Zhang J, Stamler JS: Identification of the enzymatic mechanism of nitroglycerin bioactivation. Proc Natl Acad Sci U S A 99:8306-8311, 2002.
178. Winniford MD, Kennedy PL, Wells PJ, et al: Potentiation of nitroglycerin-induced coronary dilatation by *N*-acetylcysteine. Circulation 73:138-142, 1986.
179. Parker JO, Vankoughnett KA, Farrell B: Nitroglycerin lingual spray: Clinical efficacy and dose-response relation. Am J Cardiol 57:1-5, 1986.
180. Bassan MM: The day-long pattern of the antianginal effect of long-term three times daily administered isosorbide dinitrate. J Am Coll Cardiol 16:936-940, 1990.
181. Nordlander R, Walter M: Once- versus twice-daily administration of controlled-release isosorbide-5-mononitrate 60 mg in the treatment of stable angina pectoris: A randomized, double-blind, cross-over study. The Swedish Multicentre Group. Eur Heart J 15:108-113, 1994.
182. Parker JO, Amies MH, Hawkinson RW, et al: Intermittent transdermal nitroglycerin therapy in angina pectoris. Clinically effective without tolerance or rebound. Minitran Efficacy Study Group. Circulation 91:1368-1374, 1995.
183. Jeserich M, Munzel T, Pape L, et al: Absence of vascular tolerance in conductance vessels after 48 hours of intravenous nitroglycerin in patients with coronary artery disease. J Am Coll Cardiol 26:50-56, 1995.
184. Gori T, Parker JD: Nitrate tolerance: A unifying hypothesis. Circulation 106:2510-2513, 2002.
185. May DC, Popma JJ, Black WH, et al: In vivo induction and reversal of nitroglycerin tolerance in human coronary arteries. N Engl J Med 317:805-809, 1987.
186. Przybojewski JZ, Heyns MH: Acute coronary vasospasm secondary to industrial nitroglycerin withdrawal: A case presentation and review. S Afr Med J 63:158-165, 1983.
187. Caramori PR, Adelman AG, Azevedo ER, et al: Therapy with nitroglycerin increases coronary vasoconstriction in response to acetylcholine. J Am Coll Cardiol 32:1969-1974, 1998.
188. Cheitlin MD, Hutter AM Jr, Brindis RG, et al: ACC/AHA expert consensus document: Use of sildenafil (Viagra) in patients with cardiovascular disease. American College of Cardiology/American Heart Association. J Am Coll Cardiol 33:273-282, 1999.
189. Hoffman BB: Catecholamines, sympathomimetic drugs, and adrenergic receptor antagonists. *In* Hardman JG, Limbird LE, Goodman A (eds): Goodman & Gilman's The Pharmacological Basis of Therapeutics. 10th ed. New York, McGraw-Hill, 2001, pp 215-268.
190. Frishman WH: Carvedilol. N Engl J Med 339:1759-1765, 1998.
191. Steinbeck G, Andresen D, Bach P, et al: A comparison of electrophysiologically guided antiarrhythmic drug therapy with beta-blocker therapy in patients with symptomatic, sustained ventricular tachyarrhythmias. N Engl J Med 327:987-992, 1992.
192. Hohnloser SH, Meinertz T, Stubbs P, et al: Efficacy and safety of *d*-sotalol, a pure class III antiarrhythmic compound, in patients with symptomatic complex ventricular ectopy: Results of a multicenter, randomized, double-blind, placebo-controlled dose-finding study. The *d*-Sotalol PVC Study Group. Circulation 92:1517-1525, 1995.
193. Flockhart DA, Tanus-Santos JE: Implications of cytochrome P450 interactions when prescribing medication for hypertension. Arch Intern Med 162:405-412, 2002.
194. Lennard MS: The polymorphic oxidation of beta-adrenoceptor antagonists. Pharmacol Ther 41:461-477, 1989.
195. Werner U, Werner D, Rau T, et al: Celecoxib inhibits metabolism of cytochrome P450 2D6 substrate metoprolol in humans. Clin Pharmacol Ther 74:130-137, 2003.
196. Weir MR, Moser M: Diuretics and beta-blockers: Is there a risk for dyslipidemia? Am Heart J 139:174-183, 2000.
197. Ko DT, Hebert PR, Coffey CS, et al: Beta-blocker therapy and symptoms of depression, fatigue, and sexual dysfunction. JAMA 288:351-357, 2002.
198. Gottlieb SS, Fisher ML, Kjekshus J, et al: Tolerability of beta-blocker initiation and titration in the Metoprolol CR/XL Randomized Intervention Trial in Congestive Heart Failure (MERIT-HF). Circulation 105:1182-1188, 2002.
199. Miller RR, Olson HG, Amsterdam EA, et al: Propranolol-withdrawal rebound phenomenon: Exacerbation of coronary events after abrupt cessation of antianginal therapy. N Engl J Med 293:416-418, 1975.
200. Braunwald E: Mechanism of action of calcium-channel-blocking agents. N Engl J Med 307:1618-1627, 1982.
201. Abernethy DR, Schwartz JB: Calcium-antagonist drugs. N Engl J Med 341:1447-1457, 1999.
202. Cannon RO III, Watson RM, Rosing DR, et al: Efficacy of calcium channel blocker therapy for angina pectoris resulting from small-vessel coronary artery disease and abnormal vasodilator reserve. Am J Cardiol 56:242-246, 1985.
203. Freher M, Challapalli S, Pinto JV, et al: Current status of calcium channel blockers in patients with cardiovascular disease. Curr Probl Cardiol 24:236-340, 1999.
204. Mason RP: Mechanisms of atherosclerotic plaque stabilization for a lipophilic calcium antagonist amlodipine. Am J Cardiol 88:2M-6M, 2001.
205. Tulenko TN, Sumner AE, Chen M, et al: The smooth muscle cell membrane during atherogenesis: A potential target for amlodipine in atheroprotection. Am Heart J 141:S1-S11, 2001.
206. Pitt B, Byington RP, Furberg CD, et al: Effect of amlodipine on the progression of atherosclerosis and the occurrence of clinical events. PREVENT Investigators. Circulation 102:1503-1510, 2000.
207. Elkayam U, Amin J, Mehra A, et al: A prospective, randomized, double-blind, crossover study to compare the efficacy and safety of chronic nifedipine therapy with that of isosorbide dinitrate and their combination in the treatment of chronic congestive heart failure. Circulation 82:1954-1961, 1990.
208. Alderman MH, Cohen H, Roque R, et al: Effect of long-acting and short-acting calcium antagonists on cardiovascular outcomes in hypertensive patients. Lancet 349:594-598, 1997.
209. Parmley WW, Nesto RW, Singh BN, et al: Attenuation of the circadian patterns of myocardial ischemia with nifedipine GITS in patients with chronic stable angina. N-CAP Study Group. J Am Coll Cardiol 19:1380-1389, 1992.
210. Leon MB, Rosing DR, Bonow RO, et al: Clinical efficacy of verapamil alone and combined with propranolol in treating patients with chronic stable angina pectoris. Am J Cardiol 48:131-139, 1981.
210a. Pepine CJ, Handberg EM, Cooper-DeHoff RM, et al: A calcium antagonist vs a non-calcium antagonist hypertension treatment strategy for patients with coronary artery disease. The International Verapamil-Trandolapril Study (INVEST): A randomized controlled trial. JAMA 290:2805-2816, 2003.
211. Klinke WP, Baird M, Juneau M, et al: Antianginal efficacy and safety of controlled-delivery diltiazem QD versus an equivalent dose of immediate-release diltiazem TID. Cardiovasc Drugs Ther 9:319-330, 1995.
212. Nadazdin A, Davies GJ: Investigation of therapeutic mechanisms of atenolol and diltiazem in patients with variable-threshold angina. Am Heart J 127:312-317, 1994.
213. Deanfield JE, Detry JM, Lichtlen PR, et al: Amlodipine reduces transient myocardial ischemia in patients with coronary artery disease: Double-blind Circadian Anti-Ischemia Program in Europe (CAPE Trial). J Am Coll Cardiol 24:1460-1467, 1994.
214. Ezekowitz MD, Hossack K, Mehta JL, et al: Amlodipine in chronic stable angina: Results of a multicenter double-blind crossover trial. Am Heart J 129:527-535, 1995.
214a. Jorgensen B, Simonsen S, Endresen K, et al: Restenosis and clinical outcome in patients treated with amlodipine after angioplasty: Results from the Coronary Angio-Plasty Amlodipine REStenosis Study (CAPARES). J Am Coll Cardiol 35:592-599, 2000.
215. Packer M, O'Connor CM, Ghali JK, et al: Effect of amlodipine on morbidity and mortality in severe chronic heart failure. Prospective Randomized Amlodipine Survival Evaluation Study Group. N Engl J Med 335:1107-1114, 1996.
216. Ekelund LG, Ulvenstam G, Walldius G, et al: Effects of felodipine versus nifedipine on exercise tolerance in stable angina pectoris. Am J Cardiol 73:658-660, 1994.
217. Sato T, Sasaki N, O'Rourke B, et al: Nicorandil, a potent cardioprotective agent, acts by opening mitochondrial ATP-dependent potassium channels. J Am Coll Cardiol 35:514-518, 2000.
218. The IONA Study Group: Effect of nicorandil on coronary events in patients with stable angina: The Impact of Nicorandil in Angina (IONA) randomised trial. Lancet 359:1269-1275, 2002.
219. Rupp H, Zarain-Herzberg A, Maisch B: The use of partial fatty acid oxidation inhibitors for metabolic therapy of angina pectoris and heart failure. Herz 27:621-636, 2002.
219a. Chaitman BR, Pepine CJ, Parker JO, et al: Combination Assessment of Ranolazine In Stable Angina (CARISA) Investigators. Effects of ranolazine with atenolol, amlodipine, or diltiazem on exercise tolerance and angina frequency in patients with severe chronic angina: A randomized controlled trial. JAMA 291:309-316, 2004.
220. Pepine CJ, Cohn PF, Deedwania PC, et al: Effects of treatment on outcome in mildly symptomatic patients with ischemia during daily life. The Atenolol Silent Ischemia Study (ASIST). Circulation 90:762-768, 1994.
221. von Arnim T: Medical treatment to reduce total ischemic burden: Total ischemic burden bisoprolol study (TIBBS), a multicenter trial comparing bisoprolol and nifedipine. The TIBBS Investigators. J Am Coll Cardiol 25:231-238, 1995.
222. Savonitto S, Ardissiono D, Egstrup K, et al: Combination therapy with metoprolol and nifedipine versus monotherapy in patients with stable angina pectoris: Results of the International Multicenter Angina Exercise (IMAGE) Study. J Am Coll Cardiol 27:311-316, 1996.
223. Heidenreich PA, McDonald KM, Hastie T, et al: Meta-analysis of trials comparing beta-blockers, calcium antagonists, and nitrates for stable angina. JAMA 281:1927-1936, 1999.
224. Ishikawa K, Nakai S, Takenaka T, et al: Short-acting nifedipine and diltiazem do not reduce the incidence of cardiac events in patients with healed myocardial infarction. Secondary Prevention Group. Circulation 95:2368-2373, 1997.
225. The Multicenter Diltiazem Postinfarction Trial Research Group: The effect of diltiazem on mortality and reinfarction after myocardial infarction. N Engl J Med 319:385-392, 1988.
226. The DAVIT II Investigators: Effect of verapamil on mortality and major events after acute myocardial infarction (the Danish Verapamil Infarction Trial II—DAVIT II). Am J Cardiol 66:779-785, 1990.
227. Gheorghiade M, Colucci WS, Swedberg K: Beta-blockers in chronic heart failure. Circulation 107:1570-1575, 2003.
228. Mannheimer C, Eliasson T, Augustinsson LE, et al: Electrical stimulation versus coronary artery bypass surgery in severe angina pectoris: The ESBY study. Circulation 97:1157-1163, 1998.
229. Ekre O, Eliasson T, Norrsell H, et al: Long-term effects of spinal cord stimulation and coronary artery bypass grafting on quality of life and survival in the ESBY study. Eur Heart J 23:1938-1945, 2002.
230. Brodison A, Chauhan A: Spinal-cord stimulation in management of angina. Lancet 354:1748-1749, 1999.
231. Sinvhal RM, Gowda RM, Khan IA: Enhanced external counterpulsation for refractory angina pectoris. Heart 89:830-833, 2003.
232. Bonetti PO, Holmes DR Jr, Lerman A, et al: Enhanced external counterpulsation for ischemic heart disease: What's behind the curtain? J Am Coll Cardiol 41:1918-1925, 2003.

233. Arora RR, Chou TM, Jain D, et al: The multicenter study of enhanced external counterpulsation (MUST-EECP): Effect of EECP on exercise-induced myocardial ischemia and anginal episodes. J Am Coll Cardiol 33:1833-1840, 1999.
234. Stys TP, Lawson WE, Hui JC, et al: Effects of enhanced external counterpulsation on stress radionuclide coronary perfusion and exercise capacity in chronic stable angina pectoris. Am J Cardiol 89:822-824, 2002.
235. Ernst E: Chelation therapy for coronary heart disease: An overview of all clinical investigations. Am Heart J 140:139-141, 2000.

Percutaneous Coronary Interventions

236. Popma JJ, Kuntz RE, Baim DS: A decade of improvement in the clinical outcomes of percutaneous coronary intervention for multivessel coronary artery disease. Circulation 106:1592-1594, 2002.
237. Herzog CA, Ma JZ, Collins AJ: Comparative survival of dialysis patients in the United States after coronary angioplasty, coronary artery stenting, and coronary artery bypass surgery and impact of diabetes. Circulation 106:2207-2211, 2002.
238. Szczech LA, Best PJ, Crowley E, et al: Outcomes of patients with chronic renal insufficiency in the bypass angioplasty revascularization investigation. Circulation 105:2253-2258, 2002.
239. Kastrati A, Schomig A, Elezi S, et al: Prognostic value of the modified American College of Cardiology/American Heart Association stenosis morphology classification for long-term angiographic and clinical outcome after coronary stent placement. Circulation 100:1285-1290, 1999.
240. Krone RJ, Shaw RE, Klein LW, et al: Evaluation of the American College of Cardiology/American Heart Association and the Society for Coronary Angiography and Interventions lesion classification system in the current "stent era" of coronary interventions (from the ACC-National Cardiovascular Data Registry). Am J Cardiol 92:389-394, 2003.
241. Srinivas VS, Brooks MM, Detre KM, et al: Contemporary percutaneous coronary intervention versus balloon angioplasty for multivessel coronary artery disease: A comparison of the National Heart, Lung and Blood Institute Dynamic Registry and the Bypass Angioplasty Revascularization Investigation (BARI) study. Circulation 106:1627-1633, 2002.
242. Al Suwaidi J, Berger PB, Holmes DR Jr: Coronary artery stents. JAMA 284:1828-1836, 2000.
243. Brophy JM, Belisle P, Joseph L: Evidence for use of coronary stents: A hierarchical bayesian meta-analysis. Ann Intern Med 138:777-786, 2003.
244. Sousa JE, Serruys PW, Costa MA: New frontiers in cardiology: Drug-eluting stents: I. Circulation 107:2274-2279, 2003.
245. Olivari Z, Rubartelli P, Piscione F, et al: Immediate results and one-year clinical outcome after percutaneous coronary interventions in chronic total occlusions: Data from a multicenter, prospective, observational study (TOAST-GISE). J Am Coll Cardiol 41:1672-1678, 2003.
246. Bucher HC, Hengstler P, Schindler C, et al: Percutaneous transluminal coronary angioplasty versus medical treatment for non-acute coronary heart disease: Meta-analysis of randomised controlled trials. BMJ 321:73-77, 2000.
247. Pocock SJ, Henderson RA, Clayton T, et al: Quality of life after coronary angioplasty or continued medical treatment for angina: Three-year follow-up in the RITA-2 trial. Randomized Intervention Treatment of Angina. J Am Coll Cardiol 35:907-914, 2000.
248. Keelan PC, Johnston JM, Koru-Sengul T, et al: Comparison of in-hospital and one-year outcomes in patients with left ventricular ejection fractions ≤40%, 41% to 49%, and ≥50% having percutaneous coronary revascularization. Am J Cardiol 91:1168-1172, 2003.
249. Jacobs AK: Coronary revascularization in women in 2003: Sex revisited. Circulation 107:375-377, 2003.
250. Malenka DJ, Wennberg DE, Quinton HA, et al: Gender-related changes in the practice and outcomes of percutaneous coronary interventions in Northern New England from 1994 to 1999. J Am Coll Cardiol 40:2092-2101, 2002.
251. Batchelor WB, Anstrom KJ, Muhlbaier LH, et al: Contemporary outcome trends in the elderly undergoing percutaneous coronary interventions: Results in 7,472 octogenarians. National Cardiovascular Network Collaboration. J Am Coll Cardiol 36:723-730, 2000.
252. Taddei CF, Weintraub WS, Douglas JS Jr, et al: Influence of age on outcome after percutaneous transluminal angioplasty. Am J Cardiol 84:245-251, 1999.
252a. Pfisterer M, Buser P, Osswald S, et al: Outcome of elderly patients with chronic symptomatic coronary artery disease with an invasive vs. optimized medical treatment strategy: One-year results of the randomized TIME trial. JAMA 289:1117-1123, 2003.
253. Graham MM, Ghali WA, Faris PD, et al: Survival after coronary revascularization in the elderly. Circulation 105:2378-2384, 2002.
254. Beckman JA, Creager MA, Libby P: Diabetes and atherosclerosis: Epidemiology, pathophysiology, and management. JAMA 287:2570-2581, 2002.
255. Kuntz RE: Importance of considering atherosclerosis progression when choosing a coronary revascularization strategy: The diabetes–percutaneous transluminal coronary angioplasty dilemma. Circulation 99:847-851, 1999.
256. Park SJ, Shim WH, Ho DS, et al: A paclitaxel-eluting stent for the prevention of coronary restenosis. N Engl J Med 348:1537-1545, 2003.
257. Moses JW, Leon MB, Popma JJ, et al: Sirolimus-eluting stents versus standard stents in patients with stenosis in a native coronary artery. N Engl J Med 349:1315-1323, 2003.
258. Mathew V, Clavell AL, Lennon RJ, et al: Percutaneous coronary interventions in patients with prior coronary artery bypass surgery: Changes in patient characteristics and outcome during two decades. Am J Med 108:127-135, 2000.
259. Hong MK, Mehran R, Dangas G, et al: Are we making progress with percutaneous saphenous vein graft treatment? A comparison of 1990 to 1994 and 1995 to 1998 results. J Am Coll Cardiol 38:150-154, 2001.
260. Stone GW, Rogers C, Hermiller J, et al: Randomized comparison of distal protection with a filter-based catheter and a balloon occlusion and aspiration system during percutaneous intervention of diseased saphenous vein aorto-coronary bypass grafts. Circulation 108:548-553, 2003.

Coronary Artery Bypass Surgery

261. Eagle KA, Guyton RA, Davidoff R, et al: ACC/AHA Guidelines for Coronary Artery Bypass Graft Surgery: A Report of the American College of Cardiology/American Heart Association Task Force on Practice Guidelines (Committee to Revise the 1991 Guidelines for Coronary Artery Bypass Graft Surgery). American College of Cardiology/American Heart Association. J Am Coll Cardiol 34:1262-1347, 1999.
262. Abu-Omar Y, Taggart DP: Off-pump coronary artery bypass grafting. Lancet 360:327-330, 2002.
263. Dogan S, Aybek T, Andressen E, et al: Totally endoscopic coronary artery bypass grafting on cardiopulmonary bypass with robotically enhanced telemanipulation: Report of forty-five cases. J Thorac Cardiovasc Surg 123:1125-1131, 2002.
264. Berger PB, Alderman EL, Nadel A, et al: Frequency of early occlusion and stenosis in a left internal mammary artery to left anterior descending artery bypass graft after surgery through a median sternotomy on conventional bypass: Benchmark for minimally invasive direct coronary artery bypass. Circulation 100:2353-2358, 1999.
265. de Jaegere PP, Suyker WJ: Off-pump coronary artery bypass surgery. Heart 88:313-318, 2002.
266. Cisowski M, Morawski W, Drzewiecki J, et al: Integrated minimally invasive direct coronary artery bypass grafting and angioplasty for coronary artery revascularization. Eur J Cardiothorac Surg 22:261-265, 2002.
267. Galloway AC, Shemin RJ, Glower DD, et al: First report of the Port-Access International Registry. Ann Thorac Surg 67:51-56, 1999.
268. Dogan S, Graubitz K, Aybek T, et al: How safe is the port-access technique in minimally invasive coronary artery bypass grafting? Ann Thorac Surg 74:1537-1543, 2002.
269. Oliveira SA, Lisboa LA, Dallan LA, et al: Minimally invasive single-vessel coronary artery bypass with the internal thoracic artery and early postoperative angiography: Midterm results of a prospective study in 120 consecutive patients. Ann Thorac Surg 73:505-510, 2002.
270. Diegeler A, Thiele H, Falk V, et al: Comparison of stenting with minimally invasive bypass surgery for stenosis of the left anterior descending coronary artery. N Engl J Med 347:561-566, 2002.
271. Mehran R, Dangas G, Stamou SC, et al: One-year clinical outcome after minimally invasive direct coronary artery bypass. Circulation 102:2799-2802, 2000.
272. Al-Ruzzeh S, Ambler G, Asimakopoulos G, et al: Off-pump coronary artery bypass (OPCAB) surgery reduces risk-stratified morbidity and mortality: A United Kingdom multicenter comparative analysis of early clinical outcome. Circulation 108:II1-II8, 2003.
273. Parolari A, Alamanni F, Cannata A, et al: Off-pump versus on-pump coronary artery bypass: Meta-analysis of currently available randomized trials. Ann Thorac Surg 76:37-40, 2003.
274. Puskas JD, Williams WH, Duke PG, et al: Off-pump coronary artery bypass grafting provides complete revascularization with reduced myocardial injury, transfusion requirements, and length of stay: A prospective randomized comparison of two hundred unselected patients undergoing off-pump versus conventional coronary artery bypass grafting. J Thorac Cardiovasc Surg 125:797-808, 2003.
275. Van Dijk D, Jansen EW, Hijman R, et al: Cognitive outcome after off-pump and on-pump coronary artery bypass graft surgery: A randomized trial. JAMA 287:1405-1412, 2002.
276. Nathoe HM, van Dijk D, Jansen EW, et al: A comparison of on-pump and off-pump coronary bypass surgery in low-risk patients. N Engl J Med 348:394-402, 2003.
277. Cohen G, Borger MA, Weisel RD, et al: Intraoperative myocardial protection: Current trends and future perspectives. Ann Thorac Surg 68:1995-2001, 1999.
278. Mallidi HR, Sever J, Tamariz M, et al: The short-term and long-term effects of warm or tepid cardioplegia. J Thorac Cardiovasc Surg 125:711-720, 2003.
279. Kalawski R, Majewski M, Kaszkowiak E, et al: Transcardiac release of soluble adhesion molecules during coronary artery bypass grafting: Effects of crystalloid and blood cardioplegia. Chest 123:1355-1360, 2003.
280. Kiaii B, Moon BC, Massel D, et al: A prospective randomized trial of endoscopic versus conventional harvesting of the saphenous vein in coronary artery bypass surgery. J Thorac Cardiovasc Surg 123:204-212, 2002.
281. Souza DS, Dashwood MR, Tsui JC, et al: Improved patency in vein grafts harvested with surrounding tissue: Results of a randomized study using three harvesting techniques. Ann Thorac Surg 73:1189-1195, 2002.
282. Knatterud GL, Rosenberg Y, Campeau L, et al: Long-term effects on clinical outcomes of aggressive lowering of low-density lipoprotein cholesterol levels and low-dose anticoagulation in the post coronary artery bypass graft trial. Post CABG Investigators. Circulation 102:157-165, 2000.
283. West NE, Qian H, Guzik TJ, et al: Nitric oxide synthase (nNOS) gene transfer modifies venous bypass graft remodeling: Effects on vascular smooth muscle cell differentiation and superoxide production. Circulation 104:1526-1532, 2001.
284. Traverse JH, Mooney MR, Pedersen WR, et al: Clinical, angiographic, and interventional follow-up of patients with aortic-saphenous vein graft connectors. Circulation 108:452-456, 2003.
285. Grondin CM, Lepage G, Castonguay YR, et al: Aortocoronary bypass graft: Initial blood flow through the graft, and early postoperative patency. Circulation 44:815-819, 1971.
286. Loop FD: Internal thoracic artery grafts: Biologically better coronary arteries. N Engl J Med 334:263-265, 1996.
287. Amoroso G, Tio RA, Mariani MA, et al: Functional integrity and aging of the left internal thoracic artery after coronary artery bypass surgery. J Thorac Cardiovasc Surg 120:313-318, 2000.
288. Dabal RJ, Goss JR, Maynard C, et al: The effect of left internal mammary artery utilization on short-term outcomes after coronary revascularization. Ann Thorac Surg 76:464-470, 2003.

289. Taggart DP, D'Amico R, Altman DG: Effect of arterial revascularisation on survival: A systematic review of studies comparing bilateral and single internal mammary arteries. Lancet 358:870-875, 2001.
290. Caputo M, Reeves B, Marchetto G, et al: Radial versus right internal thoracic artery as a second arterial conduit for coronary surgery: early and midterm outcomes. J Thorac Cardiovasc Surg 126:39-47, 2003.
291. Muneretto C, Negri A, Manfredi J, et al: Safety and usefulness of composite grafts for total arterial myocardial revascularization: A prospective randomized evaluation. J Thorac Cardiovasc Surg 125:826-835, 2003.
292. Chavanon O, Durand M, Hacini R, et al: Coronary artery bypass grafting with left internal mammary artery and right gastroepiploic artery, with and without bypass. Ann Thorac Surg 73:499-504, 2002.
293. Ferguson TB Jr, Hammill BG, Peterson ED, et al: A decade of change—risk profiles and outcomes for isolated coronary artery bypass grafting procedures, 1990-1999: A Report from the STS National Database Committee and the Duke Clinical Research Institute. Society of Thoracic Surgeons. Ann Thorac Surg 73:480-489, 2002.
294. Shroyer AL, Coombs LP, Peterson ED, et al: The Society of Thoracic Surgeons: 30-day operative mortality and morbidity risk models. Ann Thorac Surg 75:1856-1864, 2003.
295. Gao D, Grunwald GK, Rumsfeld JS, et al: Variation in mortality risk factors with time after coronary artery bypass graft operation. Ann Thorac Surg 75:74-81, 2003.
296. Nalysnyk L, Fahrbach K, Reynolds MW, et al: Adverse events in coronary artery bypass graft (CABG) trials: A systematic review and analysis. Heart 89:767-772, 2003.
297. Holmvang L, Jurlander B, Rasmussen C, et al: Use of biochemical markers of infarction for diagnosing perioperative myocardial infarction and early graft occlusion after coronary artery bypass surgery. Chest 121:103-111, 2002.
298. Yende S, Wunderink R: Causes of prolonged mechanical ventilation after coronary artery bypass surgery. Chest 122:245-252, 2002.
299. Canver CC, Chanda J: Intraoperative and postoperative risk factors for respiratory failure after coronary bypass. Ann Thorac Surg 75:853-857, 2003.
300. Branca P, McGaw P, Light R: Factors associated with prolonged mechanical ventilation following coronary artery bypass surgery. Chest 119:537-546, 2001.
301. Dacey LJ, Munoz JJ, Baribeau YR, et al: Reexploration for hemorrhage following coronary artery bypass grafting: Incidence and risk factors. Northern New England Cardiovascular Disease Study Group. Arch Surg 133:442-447, 1998.
302. Pleym H, Stenseth R, Wahba A, et al: Single-dose tranexamic acid reduces postoperative bleeding after coronary surgery in patients treated with aspirin until surgery. Anesth Analg 96:923-928, 2003.
303. Taggart DP, Westaby S: Neurological and cognitive disorders after coronary artery bypass grafting. Curr Opin Cardiol 16:271-276, 2001.
304. Selnes OA, McKhann GM: Coronary artery bypass surgery and the brain. N Engl J Med 344:451-452, 2001.
305. Newman MF, Kirchner JL, Phillips-Bute B, et al: Longitudinal assessment of neurocognitive function after coronary artery bypass surgery. N Engl J Med 344:395-402, 2001.
306. Maisel WH, Rawn JD, Stevenson WG: Atrial fibrillation after cardiac surgery. Ann Intern Med 135:1061-1073, 2001.
307. Eriksen BO, Hoff KR, Solberg S: Prediction of acute renal failure after cardiac surgery: Retrospective cross-validation of a clinical algorithm. Nephrol Dial Transplant 18:77-81, 2003.
308. Durmaz I, Yagdi T, Calkavur T, et al: Prophylactic dialysis in patients with renal dysfunction undergoing on-pump coronary artery bypass surgery. Ann Thorac Surg 75:859-864, 2003.
309. Bell MR, Gersh BJ, Schaff HV, et al: Effect of completeness of revascularization on long-term outcome of patients with three-vessel disease undergoing coronary artery bypass surgery: A report from the Coronary Artery Surgery Study (CASS) Registry. Circulation 86:446-457, 1992.
310. Hlatky MA, Boothroyd D, Horine S, et al: Employment after coronary angioplasty or coronary bypass surgery in patients employed at the time of revascularization. Ann Intern Med 129:543-547, 1998.
311. Mittag O, Kolenda KD, Nordman KJ, et al: Return to work after myocardial infarction/coronary artery bypass grafting: Patients' and physicians' initial viewpoints and outcome 12 months later. Soc Sci Med 52:1441-1450, 2001.
312. Domanski MJ, Borkowf CB, Campeau L, et al: Prognostic factors for atherosclerosis progression in saphenous vein grafts: The Postcoronary Artery Bypass Graft (Post-CABG) trial. Post-CABG Trial Investigators. J Am Coll Cardiol 36:1877-1883, 2000.
313. Tsui JC, Dashwood MR: Recent strategies to reduce vein graft occlusion: A need to limit the effect of vascular damage. Eur J Vasc Endovasc Surg 23:202-208, 2002.
314. FitzGibbon GM, Leach AJ, Kafka HP, et al: Coronary bypass graft fate: Long-term angiographic study. J Am Coll Cardiol 17:1075-1080, 1991.
315. Motwani JG, Topol EJ: Aortocoronary saphenous vein graft disease: Pathogenesis, predisposition, and prevention. Circulation 97:916-931, 1998.
316. Lu B, Dai RP, Zhuang N, et al: Noninvasive assessment of coronary artery bypass graft patency and flow characteristics by electron-beam tomography. J Invasive Cardiol 14:19-24, 2002.
317. Bunce NH, Lorenz CH, John AS, et al: Coronary artery bypass graft patency: Assessment with true AST imaging with steady-state precession versus gadolinium-enhanced MR angiography. Radiology 227:440-446, 2003.
318. Chirillo F, Bruni A, Balestra G, et al: Assessment of internal mammary artery and saphenous vein graft patency and flow reserve using transthoracic Doppler echocardiography. Heart 86:424-431, 2001.
319. Hwang MH, Meadows WR, Palac RT, et al: Progression of native coronary artery disease at 10 years: Insights from a randomized study of medical versus surgical therapy for angina. J Am Coll Cardiol 16:1066-1070, 1990.
320. Kroncke GM, Kosolcharoen P, Clayman JA, et al: Five-year changes in coronary arteries of medical and surgical patients of the Veterans Administration Randomized Study of Bypass Surgery. Circulation 78:I144-I1450, 1988.
321. Pond KK, Martin GV, Every N, et al: Predictors of progression of native coronary narrowing to total occlusion after coronary artery bypass grafting. Am J Cardiol 91:971-974, A4, 2003.
322. Mangano DT: Aspirin and mortality from coronary bypass surgery. N Engl J Med 347:1309-1317, 2002.
323. Bernstein SJ, Lazaro P, Fitch K, et al: Appropriateness of coronary revascularization for patients with chronic stable angina or following an acute myocardial infarction: Multinational versus Dutch criteria. Int J Qual Health Care 14:103-109, 2002.
324. van Brussel BL, Plokker HW, Ernst SM, et al: Venous coronary artery bypass surgery: A 15-year follow-up study. Circulation 88:II87-I192, 1993.
325. Unger F, Serruys PW, Yacoub MH, et al: Revascularization in multivessel disease: Comparison between two-year outcomes of coronary bypass surgery and stenting. J Thorac Cardiovasc Surg 125:809-820, 2003.
326. Peduzzi P, Kamina A, Detre K: Twenty-two-year follow-up in the VA Cooperative Study of Coronary Artery Bypass Surgery for Stable Angina. Am J Cardiol 81:1393-1399, 1998.
327. Yusuf S, Zucker D, Peduzzi P, et al: Effect of coronary artery bypass graft surgery on survival: Overview of 10-year results from randomised trials by the Coronary Artery Bypass Graft Surgery Trialists Collaboration. Lancet 344:563-570, 1994.
328. Davies RF, Goldberg AD, Forman S, et al: Asymptomatic Cardiac Ischemia Pilot (ACIP) study two-year follow-up: Outcomes of patients randomized to initial strategies of medical therapy versus revascularization. Circulation 95:2037-2043, 1997.
329. Califf RM, Conley MJ, Behar VS, et al: "Left main equivalent" coronary artery disease: Its clinical presentation and prognostic significance with nonsurgical therapy. Am J Cardiol 53:1489, 1984.
330. Davis KB, Alderman EL, Kosinski AS, et al: Early mortality of acute myocardial infarction in patients with and without prior coronary revascularization surgery. A Coronary Artery Surgery Study Registry Study. Circulation 85:2100-2109, 1992.
331. Argenziano M, Spotnitz HM, Whang W, et al: Risk stratification for coronary bypass surgery in patients with left ventricular dysfunction: Analysis of the coronary artery bypass grafting patch trial database. Circulation. 100:II119-II124, 1999.
332. Antunes PE, de Oliveira JM, Antunes MJ: Coronary surgery with non-cardioplegic methods in patients with advanced left ventricular dysfunction: Immediate and long term results. Heart 89:427-431, 2003.
333. Lytle BW: The role of coronary revascularization in the treatment of ischemic cardiomyopathy. Ann Thorac Surg 75:S2-S5, 2003.
334. Carr JA, Haithcock BE, Paone G, et al: Long-term outcome after coronary artery bypass grafting in patients with severe left ventricular dysfunction. Ann Thorac Surg 74:1531-1536, 2002.
335. Veenhuyzen GD, Singh SN, McAreavey D, et al: Prior coronary artery bypass surgery and risk of death among patients with ischemic left ventricular dysfunction. Circulation 104:1489-1493, 2001.
336. Kleikamp G, Maleszka A, Reiss N, et al: Determinants of mid- and long-term results in patients after surgical revascularization for ischemic cardiomyopathy. Ann Thorac Surg 75:1406-1412, 2003.
337. Allman KC, Shaw LJ, Hachamovitch R, et al: Myocardial viability testing and impact of revascularization on prognosis in patients with coronary artery disease and left ventricular dysfunction: A meta-analysis. J Am Coll Cardiol 39:1151-1158, 2002.
338. Wijns W, Vatner SF, Camici PG: Hibernating myocardium. N Engl J Med 339:173-181, 1998.
339. Pasquet A, Lauer MS, Williams MJ, et al: Prediction of global left ventricular function after bypass surgery in patients with severe left ventricular dysfunction: Impact of preoperative myocardial function, perfusion, and metabolism. Eur Heart J 21:125-136, 2000.
340. Bax JJ, Wijns W, Cornel JH, et al: Accuracy of currently available techniques for prediction of functional recovery after revascularization in patients with left ventricular dysfunction due to chronic coronary artery disease: Comparison of pooled data. J Am Coll Cardiol 30:1451-1460, 1997.
341. Bonow RO: Myocardial viability and prognosis in patients with ischemic left ventricular dysfunction. J Am Coll Cardiol 39:1159-1162, 2002.
342. Kleikamp G, Maleszka A, Reiss N, et al: Determinants of mid- and long-term results in patients after surgical revascularization for ischemic cardiomyopathy. Ann Thorac Surg 75:1406-1412, 2003.
343. Schulman KA, Berlin JA, Harless W, et al: The effect of race and sex on physicians' recommendations for cardiac catheterization. N Engl J Med 340:618-626, 1999.
344. Ghali WA, Faris PD, Galbraith PD, et al: Sex differences in access to coronary revascularization after cardiac catheterization: Importance of detailed clinical data. Ann Intern Med 136:723-732, 2002.
345. Jacobs AK, Kelsey SF, Brooks MM, et al: Better outcome for women compared with men undergoing coronary revascularization: A report from the Bypass Angioplasty Revascularization Investigation (BARI). Circulation 98:1279-1285, 1998.
346. Vaccarino V, Abramson JL, Veledar E, et al: Sex differences in hospital mortality after coronary artery bypass surgery: Evidence for a higher mortality in younger women. Circulation 105:1176-1181, 2002.
347. Brown PP, Mack MJ, Simon AW, et al: Outcomes experience with off-pump coronary artery bypass surgery in women. Ann Thorac Surg 74:2113-2119, 2002.
348. Myers WO, Blackstone EH, Davis K, et al: CASS Registry long-term surgical survival. Coronary Artery Surgery Study. J Am Coll Cardiol 33:488-498, 1999.
349. Kurlansky PA, Williams DB, Traad EA, et al: Arterial grafting results in reduced operative mortality and enhanced long-term quality of life in octogenarians. Ann Thorac Surg 76:418-426, 2003.
350. Khaitan L, Sutter FP, Goldman SM: Coronary artery bypass grafting in patients who require long-term dialysis. Ann Thorac Surg 69:1135-1139, 2000.
351. Nakayama Y, Sakata R, Ura M, et al: Long-term results of coronary artery bypass grafting in patients with renal insufficiency. Ann Thorac Surg 75:496-500, 2003.
352. Schwartz L, Kip KE, Frye RL, et al: Coronary bypass graft patency in patients with diabetes in the Bypass Angioplasty Revascularization Investigation (BARI). Circulation 106:2652-2658, 2002.

353. The BARI Investigators: Seven-year outcome in the Bypass Angioplasty Revascularization Investigation (BARI) by treatment and diabetic status. J Am Coll Cardiol 35:1122-1129, 2000.
354. Rihal CS, Sutton-Tyrrell K, Guo P, et al: Increased incidence of periprocedural complications among patients with peripheral vascular disease undergoing myocardial revascularization in the bypass angioplasty revascularization investigation. Circulation 100:171-177, 1999.
355. Birkmeyer JD, Quinton HB, O'Connor NJ, et al: The effect of peripheral vascular disease on long-term mortality after coronary artery bypass surgery. Northern New England Cardiovascular Disease Study Group. Arch Surg 131:316-321, 1996.
356. Naylor AR, Mehta Z, Rothwell PM, et al: Carotid artery disease and stroke during coronary artery bypass: A critical review of the literature. Eur J Vasc Endovasc Surg 23:283-294, 2002.
357. Gansera B, Angelis I, Weingartner J, et al: Simultaneous carotid endarterectomy and cardiac surgery—additional risk factor or safety procedure? Thorac Cardiovasc Surg 51:22-27, 2003.
358. Borger MA, Fremes SE: Management of patients with concomitant coronary and carotid vascular disease. Semin Thorac Cardiovasc Surg 13:192-198, 2001.
359. Zacharias A, Schwann TA, Riordan CJ, et al: Operative and 5-year outcomes of combined carotid and coronary revascularization: Review of a large contemporary experience. Ann Thorac Surg 73:491-497, 2002.
360. Yamamuro M, Lytle BW, Sapp SK, et al: Risk factors and outcomes after coronary reoperation in 739 elderly patients. Ann Thorac Surg 69:464-474, 2000.
361. van Eck FM, Noyez L, Verheugt FW, et al: Changing profile of patients undergoing redo-coronary artery surgery. Eur J Cardiothorac Surg 21:205-211, 2002.
362. Hannan EL, Racz MJ, McCallister BD, et al: A comparison of three-year survival after coronary artery bypass graft surgery and percutaneous transluminal coronary angioplasty. J Am Coll Cardiol 33:63-72, 1999.
363. Goy JJ, Eeckhout E, Moret C, et al: Five-year outcome in patients with isolated proximal left anterior descending coronary artery stenosis treated by angioplasty or left internal mammary artery grafting: A prospective trial. Circulation 99:3255-3259, 1999.
364. Abizaid A, Costa MA, Centemero M, et al: Clinical and economic impact of diabetes mellitus on percutaneous and surgical treatment of multivessel coronary disease patients: Insights from the Arterial Revascularization Therapy Study (ARTS) trial. Circulation 104:533-538, 2001.
365. Niles NW, McGrath PD, Malenka D, et al: Survival of patients with diabetes and multivessel coronary artery disease after surgical or percutaneous coronary revascularization: Results of a large regional prospective study. Northern New England Cardiovascular Disease Study Group. J Am Coll Cardiol 37:1008-1015, 2001.
366. Rodriguez A, Bernardi V, Navia J, et al: Argentine Randomized Study: Coronary Angioplasty with Stenting versus Coronary Bypass Surgery in patients with Multiple-Vessel Disease (ERACI II): 30-day and one-year follow-up results. ERACI II Investigators. J Am Coll Cardiol 37:51-58, 2001.
367. Hlatky MA, Rogers WJ, Johnstone I, et al: Medical care costs and quality of life after randomization to coronary angioplasty or coronary bypass surgery. Bypass Angioplasty Revascularization Investigation (BARI) Investigators. N Engl J Med 336:92-99, 1997.
367a. Legrand VM, Serruys PW, Unger F, et al: Arterial Revascularization Therapy Study (ARTS) Investigators. Three-year outcome after coronary stenting versus bypass surgery for the treatment of multivessel disease. Circulation 109:1114-1120, 2004.
368. Detre KM, Guo P, Holubkov R, et al: Coronary revascularization in diabetic patients: A comparison of the randomized and observational components of the Bypass Angioplasty Revascularization Investigation (BARI). Circulation 99:633-640, 1999.
369. Weintraub WS, Stein B, Kosinski A, et al: Outcome of coronary bypass surgery versus coronary angioplasty in diabetic patients with multivessel coronary artery disease. J Am Coll Cardiol 31:10-19, 1998.
370. Saririan M, Eisenberg MJ: Myocardial laser revascularization for the treatment of end-stage coronary artery disease. J Am Coll Cardiol 41:173-183, 2003.
371. Lange RA, Hillis LD: Transmyocardial laser revascularization. N Engl J Med 341:1075-1076, 1999.
372. Schofield PM, Sharples LD, Caine N, et al: Transmyocardial laser revascularisation in patients with refractory angina: A randomised controlled trial. Lancet 353:519-524, 1999.
373. Horvath KA, Aranki SF, Cohn LH, et al: Sustained angina relief 5 years after transmyocardial laser revascularization with a CO_2 laser. Circulation 104:I81-I84, 2001.
374. Hughes GC, Landolfo KP, Lowe JE, et al: Perioperative morbidity and mortality after transmyocardial laser revascularization: Incidence and risk factors for adverse events. J Am Coll Cardiol 33:1021-1026, 1999.

Chest Pain with Normal Coronary Arteriogram

375. Lichtlen PR, Bargheer K, Wenzlaff P: Long-term prognosis of patients with angina-like chest pain and normal coronary angiographic findings. J Am Coll Cardiol 25:1013-1018, 1995.
376. Panting JR, Gatehouse PD, Yang GZ, et al: Abnormal subendocardial perfusion in cardiac syndrome X detected by cardiovascular magnetic resonance imaging. N Engl J Med 346:1948-1953, 2002.
377. Chen LC, Chen JW, Wu MH, et al: Differential coronary calcification on electron-beam CT between syndrome X and coronary artery disease in patients with chronic stable angina pectoris. Chest 120:1525-1533, 2001.
378. Rosen SD, Paulesu E, Wise RJ, et al: Central neural contribution to the perception of chest pain in cardiac syndrome X. Heart 87:513-519, 2002.
379. Potts SG, Bass CM: Psychological morbidity in patients with chest pain and normal or near-normal coronary arteries: A long-term follow-up study. Psychol Med 25:339-347, 1995.
380. Sun H, Mohri M, Shimokawa H, et al: Coronary microvascular spasm causes myocardial ischemia in patients with vasospastic angina. J Am Coll Cardiol 39:847-851, 2002.
381. Schindler TH, Nitzsche E, Magosaki N, et al: Regional myocardial perfusion defects during exercise, as assessed by three dimensional integration of morphology and function, in relation to abnormal endothelium-dependent vasoreactivity of the coronary microcirculation. Heart 89:517-526, 2003.
382. Cosin-Sales J, Pizzi C, Brown S, et al: C-reactive protein, clinical presentation, and ischemic activity in patients with chest pain and normal coronary angiograms. J Am Coll Cardiol 41:1468-1474, 2003.
383. Panza JA: Myocardial ischemia and the pains of the heart. N Engl J Med 346:1934-1935, 2002.
384. Zouridakis EG, Cox ID, Garcia-Moll X, et al: Negative stress echocardiographic responses in normotensive and hypertensive patients with angina pectoris, positive exercise stress testing, and normal coronary arteriograms. Heart 83:141-146, 2000.
385. Cannon RO III: Chest pain and the sensitive heart. Eur J Gastroenterol Hepatol 7:1161-1171, 1995.
386. Rosen SD: The pathophysiology of cardiac syndrome X—a tale of paradigm shifts. Cardiovasc Res 52:174-177, 2001.
387. Kemp HG, Kronmal RA, Vlietstra RE, et al: Seven-year survival of patients with normal or near-normal coronary arteriograms: A CASS registry study. J Am Coll Cardiol 7:479-483, 1986.
388. Kaski JC, Valenzuela Garcia LF: Therapeutic options for the management of patients with cardiac syndrome X. Eur Heart J 22:283-293, 2001.
389. Cannon RO III, Quyyumi AA, Mincemoyer R, et al: Imipramine in patients with chest pain despite normal coronary angiograms. N Engl J Med 330:1411-1417, 1994.

Silent Myocardial Ischemia

390. Cohn PF, Fox KM, Daly C: Silent myocardial ischemia. Circulation 108:1263-1277, 2003.
391. Krantz DS, Hedges SM, Gabbay FH, et al: Triggers of angina and ST-segment depression in ambulatory patients with coronary artery disease: Evidence for an uncoupling of angina and ischemia. Am Heart J 128:703-712, 1994.
392. Krone RJ, Gregory JJ, Freedland KE, et al: Limited usefulness of exercise testing and thallium scintigraphy in evaluation of ambulatory patients several months after recovery from an acute coronary event: Implications for management of stable coronary heart disease. Multicenter Myocardial Ischemia Research Group. J Am Coll Cardiol 24:1274-1281, 1994.
393. Mazzone A, Cusa C, Mazzucchelli I, et al: Increased production of inflammatory cytokines in patients with silent myocardial ischemia. J Am Coll Cardiol 38:1895-1901, 2001.
394. Laukkanen JA, Kurl S, Lakka TA, et al: Exercise-induced silent myocardial ischemia and coronary morbidity and mortality in middle-aged men. J Am Coll Cardiol 38:72-79, 2001.
395. Elhendy A, Schinkel AF, van Domburg RT, et al: Comparison of late outcome in patients with versus without angina pectoris having reversible perfusion abnormalities during dobutamine stress technetium-99m sestamibi single-photon emission computed tomography. Am J Cardiol 91:264-268, 2003.
396. Pepine CJ, Sharaf B, Andrews TC, et al: Relation between clinical, angiographic and ischemic findings at baseline and ischemia-related adverse outcomes at 1 year in the Asymptomatic Cardiac Ischemia Pilot study. ACIP Study Group. J Am Coll Cardiol 29:1483-1489, 1997.
397. Stone PH, Chaitman BR, Forman S, et al: Prognostic significance of myocardial ischemia detected by ambulatory electrocardiography, exercise treadmill testing, and electrocardiogram at rest to predict cardiac events by one year (the Asymptomatic Cardiac Ischemia Pilot [ACIP] study). Am J Cardiol 80:1395-1401, 1997.
398. Dargie HJ, Ford I, Fox KM: Total Ischaemic Burden European Trial (TIBET): Effects of ischaemia and treatment with atenolol, nifedipine SR, and their combination on outcome in patients with chronic stable angina. The TIBET Study Group. Eur Heart J 17:104-112, 1996.
399. Sharaf BL, Williams DO, Miele NJ, et al: A detailed angiographic analysis of patients with ambulatory electrocardiographic ischemia: Results from the Asymptomatic Cardiac Ischemia Pilot (ACIP) study angiographic core laboratory. J Am Coll Cardiol 29:78-84, 1997.
400. Tzivoni D, Medina A, David D, et al: Comparison between metoprolol orally osmotic once daily and metoprolol two or three times daily in suppressing exercise-induced and daily myocardial ischemia. Am J Cardiol 78:1362-1368, 1996.
401. Portegies MC, Sijbring P, Gobel EJ, et al: Efficacy of metoprolol and diltiazem in treating silent myocardial ischemia. Am J Cardiol 74:1095-1098, 1994.
402. Rogers WJ, Bourassa MG, Andrews TC, et al: Asymptomatic Cardiac Ischemia Pilot (ACIP) study: Outcome at 1 year for patients with asymptomatic cardiac ischemia randomized to medical therapy or revascularization. The ACIP Investigators. J Am Coll Cardiol 26:594-605, 1995.
403. Andrews TC, Raby K, Barry J, et al: Effect of cholesterol reduction on myocardial ischemia in patients with coronary disease. Circulation 95:324-328, 1997.
404. Zellweger MJ, Weinbacher M, Zutter AW, et al: Long-term outcome of patients with silent versus symptomatic ischemia six months after percutaneous coronary intervention and stenting. J Am Coll Cardiol 42:33-40, 2003.

Heart Failure in Ischemic Heart Disease

405. Gheorghiade M, Bonow RO: Chronic heart failure in the United States: A manifestation of coronary artery disease. Circulation 97:282-289, 1998.
406. Felker GM, Shaw LK, O'Connor CM: A standardized definition of ischemic cardiomyopathy for use in clinical research. J Am Coll Cardiol 39:210-218, 2002.
407. Schinkel AF, Bax JJ, Sozzi FB, et al: Prevalence of myocardial viability assessed by single photon emission computed tomography in patients with chronic ischaemic left ventricular dysfunction. Heart 88:125-130, 2002.
408. Baker DW, Jones R, Hodges J, et al: Management of heart failure: III. The role of revascularization in the treatment of patients with moderate or severe left ventricular systolic dysfunction. JAMA 272:1528-1534, 1994.
409. Mickleborough LL, Merchant N, Provost Y, et al: Ventricular reconstruction for ischemic cardiomyopathy. Ann Thorac Surg 75:S6-S12, 2003.

410. Candell-Riera J, Santana-Boado C, Armadans-Gil L, et al: Comparison of patients with anterior wall healed myocardial infarction with and without exercise-induced ST-segment elevation. Am J Cardiol 81:12-16, 1998.
411. Buck T, Hunold P, Wentz KU, et al: Tomographic three-dimensional echocardiographic determination of chamber size and systolic function in patients with left ventricular aneurysm: Comparison to magnetic resonance imaging, cineventriculography, and two-dimensional echocardiography. Circulation 96:4286-4297, 1997.
412. Jones RH: Is it time for a randomized trial of surgical treatment of ischemic heart failure? J Am Coll Cardiol 37:1210-1213, 2001.
413. Lundblad R, Abdelnoor M, Svennevig JL: Repair of left ventricular aneurysm: Surgical risk and long-term survival. Ann Thorac Surg 76:719-725, 2003.
414. Vural KM, Sener E, Ozatik MA, et al: Left ventricular aneurysm repair: An assessment of surgical treatment modalities. Eur J Cardiothorac Surg 13:49-56, 1998.
415. Di Mattia DG, Di Biasi P, Salati M, et al: Surgical treatment of left ventricular post-infarction aneurysm with endoventriculoplasty: Late clinical and functional results. Eur J Cardiothorac Surg 15:413-418, 1999.
416. Athanasuleas CL, Stanley AW, Buckberg GD, et al: Surgical anterior ventricular endocardial restoration (SAVER) for dilated ischemic cardiomyopathy. Semin Thorac Cardiovasc Surg 13:448-458, 2001.
417. Stanley AW Jr, Athanasuleas CL, Buckberg GD: Left ventricular remodeling and functional mitral regurgitation: Mechanisms and therapy. Semin Thorac Cardiovasc Surg 13:486-495, 2001.
418. Athanasuleas CL, Stanley AW Jr, Buckberg GD, et al: Surgical anterior ventricular endocardial restoration (SAVER) in the dilated remodeled ventricle after anterior myocardial infarction. RESTORE group. Reconstructive Endoventricular Surgery, returning Torsion Original Radius Elliptical Shape to the LV. J Am Coll Cardiol 37:1199-1209, 2001.
419. Di Donato M, Sabatier M, Dor V, et al: Effects of the Dor procedure on left ventricular dimension and shape and geometric correlates of mitral regurgitation one year after surgery. J Thorac Cardiovasc Surg 121:91-96, 2001.
420. Shapira OM, Davidoff R, Hilkert RJ, et al: Repair of left ventricular aneurysm: Long-term results of linear repair versus endoaneurysmorrhaphy. Ann Thorac Surg 63:701-705, 1997.
421. Tibayan FA, Rodriguez F, Zasio MK, et al: Geometric distortions of the mitral valvular-ventricular complex in chronic ischemic mitral regurgitation. Circulation 108(Suppl 1):II116-II121, 2003.
422. Kwan J, Shiota T, Agler DA, et al: Geometric differences of the mitral apparatus between ischemic and dilated cardiomyopathy with significant mitral regurgitation: Real-time three-dimensional echocardiography study. Circulation 107:1135-1140, 2003.
423. Gillinov AM, Wierup PN, Blackstone EH, et al: Is repair preferable to replacement for ischemic mitral regurgitation? J Thorac Cardiovasc Surg 122:1125-1141, 2001.
424. Paparella D, Mickleborough LL, Carson S, et al: Mild to moderate mitral regurgitation in patients undergoing coronary bypass grafting: Effects on operative mortality and long-term significance. Ann Thorac Surg 76:1094-1100, 2003.
425. Society of Thoracic Surgeons Database, 2002 (www.ctsnet.org).
426. Cohn LH, Rizzo RJ, Adams DH, et al: The effect of pathophysiology on the surgical treatment of ischemic mitral regurgitation: Operative and late risks of repair versus replacement. Eur J Cardiothorac Surg 9:568-574, 1995.
427. Angelini P, Velasco JA, Flamm S: Coronary anomalies: Incidence, pathophysiology, and clinical relevance. Circulation 105:2449-2454, 2002.
428. Maehara A, Mintz GS, Castagna MT, et al: Intravascular ultrasound assessment of spontaneous coronary artery dissection. Am J Cardiol 89:466-468, 2002.
429. Lane JE, Cartledge RG, Johnson JH: Successful surgical treatment of spontaneous coronary artery dissection. Curr Surg 58:316-318, 2001.
430. Longheval G, Badot V, Cosyns B, et al: Spontaneous coronary artery dissection: Favorable outcome illustrated by angiographic data. Clin Cardiol 22:374-375, 1999.
431. Endo M, Tomizawa Y, Nishida H, et al: Angiographic findings and surgical treatments of coronary artery involvement in Takayasu arteritis. J Thorac Cardiovasc Surg 125:570-577, 2003.
432. Byrd BF III, Mendes LA: Cardiac complications of mediastinal radiotherapy: The other side of the coin. J Am Coll Cardiol 42:750-751, 2003.
433. Lange RA, Hillis LD: Cardiovascular complications of cocaine use. N Engl J Med 345:351-358, 2001.

GUIDELINES *Thomas H. Lee*

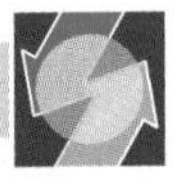

Chronic Stable Angina

The American College of Cardiology and the American Heart Association (ACC/AHA) updated guidelines for management of patients with stable chest pain syndromes and known or suspected ischemic heart disease in 2002.[1] Populations addressed by these guidelines include patients with "ischemic equivalents" such as dyspnea or arm pain with exertion, and patients with ischemic heart disease who have become asymptomatic, including those who have undergone revascularization procedures. Patients with unstable ischemic syndromes are not included in these guidelines but are instead addressed in guidelines summarized in appendices to Chapter 49. As with other ACC/AHA guidelines, indications for interventions are classified into the following four groups:

- Class I—for generally accepted indications
- Class IIa—when indications are controversial, but the weight of evidence is supportive
- Class IIb—when usefulness or efficacy is less well established
- Class III—when there is consensus against the usefulness of the intervention

The guidelines use a convention for rating levels of evidence on which recommendations have been based, as follows:

- Level A—derived from data from multiple randomized clinical trials
- Level B—derived from a single randomized trial or nonrandomized studies
- Level C—based on the consensus opinion of experts

Overview

The ACC/AHA guidelines emphasize the importance of detailed symptom history, focused physical examination, and directed risk-factor assessment for patients presenting with chest pain. These data are to be used by the clinician to estimate the probability of significant coronary artery disease as low, intermediate, or high. For patients with a low probability of coronary disease (e.g., ≤5 percent), cardiovascular interventions should be limited, while noncardiac causes of chest pain should be evaluated (Fig. 50G–1). Recommended initial tests are summarized in Table 50G–1. Routine use of chest radiographs or electron-beam computed tomography (CT) is not recommended.[2]

For patients with an intermediate or high probability of coronary disease, the clinician should exclude unstable ischemic syndromes and conditions that might exacerbate or cause angina. If these are not present, then noninvasive testing should be considered to refine the diagnostic assessment of patients with an intermediate probability of coronary disease and to perform risk stratification for patients with a high probability of coronary disease (Fig. 50G–2).

The ACC/AHA guidelines do not mandate exercise testing in all such patients. Pharmacological imaging studies are recommended for patients who are unable to exercise. Exercise imaging studies are recommended for patients who have had previous coronary revascularization or whose resting electrocardiograms (ECGs) are uninterpretable. Imaging studies are also supported when the clinical evaluation and exercise ECGs have not provided sufficient information to guide management. If the results of noninvasive studies suggest a high risk for complications of coronary heart disease, then coronary angiography and revascularization should be considered.

The treatment algorithm recommended by the ACC/AHA guidelines emphasizes the importance of patient education about coronary disease; prevention of ischemia through use of nitrates, beta blockers, and calcium blockers; and prevention of progression of atherosclerosis through risk factor management (Fig. 50G–3).

The ACC/AHA guidelines require clarity from the clinician in defining the critical issues for the individual patient. For patients with a chest pain complaint of uncertain etiology, the dominant question may be whether coronary artery disease is present or absent (diagnosis). For patients with known or strongly suspected coronary disease, the focus is likely to be on the patient's risk. In these guidelines, a specific test

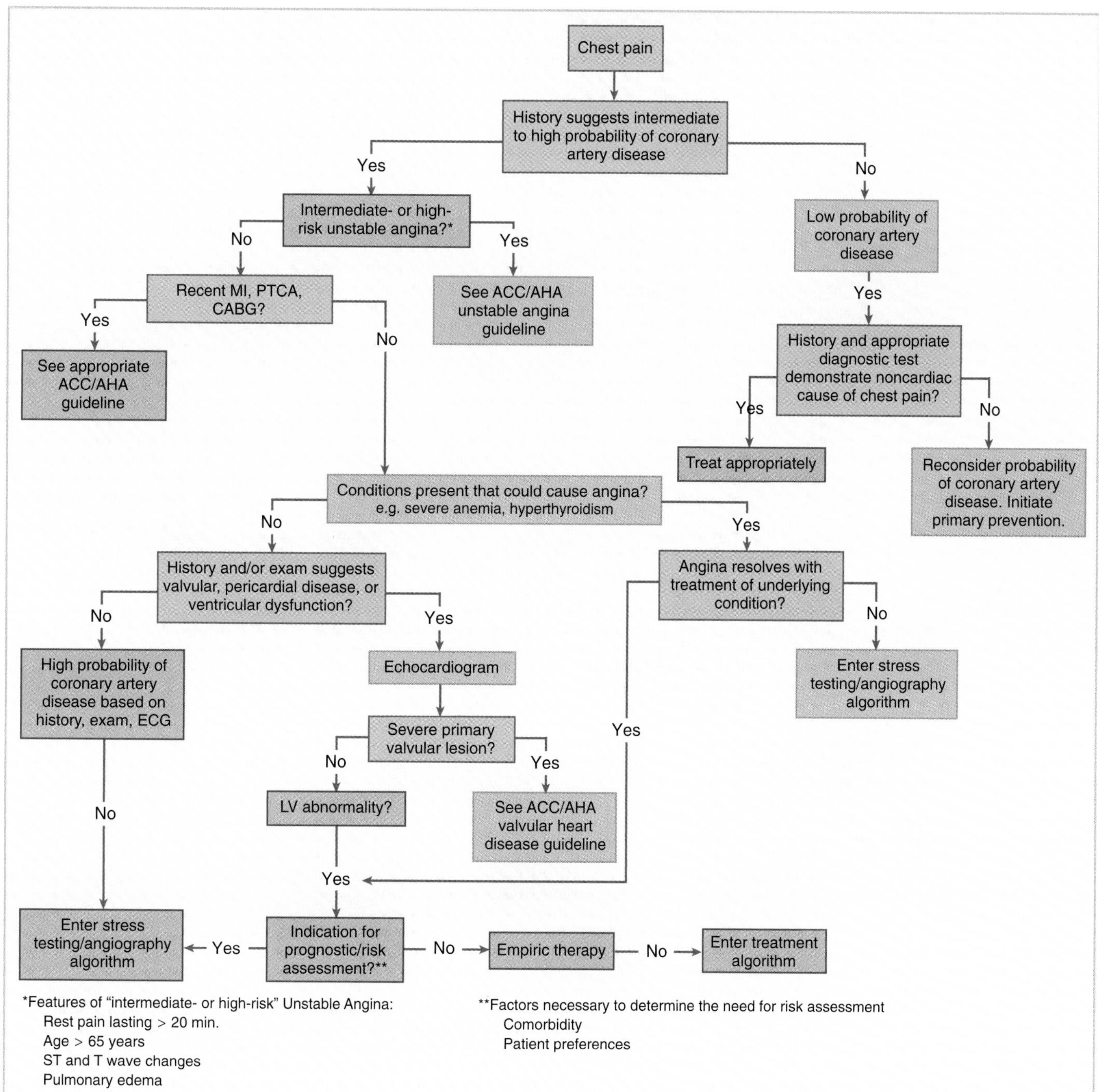

FIGURE 50G–1 Approach to the clinical assessment of chest pain. ACC = American College of Cardiology; AHA = American Heart Association; CABG = coronary artery bypass grafting; ECG = electrocardiogram; LV = left ventricular; MI = myocardial infarction; PTCA = percutaneous transluminal coronary angioplasty. (From ACC/AHA 2002 guideline update for the management of patients with chronic stable angina: A report of the American College of Cardiology/American Heart Association Task Force on Practice Guidelines [Committee to Update the 1999 Guidelines for the Management of Patients with Chronic Stable Angina]. ©2002, American College of Cardiology Foundation and the American Heart Association, p 8 [www.acc.org/clinical/guidelines/stable/stable.pdf]).

may be considered an appropriate option for addressing one or the other of these issues.

The guidelines clearly differentiate between indications for the same tests for the purpose of diagnosis and risk stratification. For example, exercise ECGs are discouraged for establishing diagnosis in patients with a high clinical probability of coronary artery disease based on age, gender, and symptoms (class IIb indication). However, exercise ECGs are strongly supported as a class I indication when used to assess prognosis in this same patient population. Thus, interpretation of these guidelines demands rigorous definition of the clinical question at hand.

Diagnosis

Noninvasive Studies

Exercise Electrocardiography. Exercise testing is considered most valuable for diagnosis when the patient's other clinical data suggest an intermediate probability of coronary disease. The ACC/AHA guidelines support the use of exercise ECGs for such patients unless their baseline ECGs show abnormalities likely to render the exercise tracing uninterpretable (Table 50G–2). However, exercise ECGs were considered appropriate for patients with complete right

TABLE 50G–1 ACC/AHA Guidelines for Routine Clinical Testing in Patients with Chronic Stable Angina

Class	Indication	Evidence*
I (indicated)	1. Rest ECG in patients without an obvious noncardiac cause of chest pain	B
	2. Rest ECG during an episode of chest pain	B
	3. Chest radiograph in patients with signs or symptoms of congestive heart failure, valvular heart disease, pericardial disease, or aortic dissection/aneurysm	B
	4. Hemoglobin	C
	5. Fasting glucose	C
	6. Fasting lipid panel	C
IIa (good supportive evidence)	Chest radiograph in patients with signs or symptoms of pulmonary disease	B
IIb (weak supportive evidence)	1. Chest radiograph in other patients	C
	2. Electron-beam CT	B
III (not indicated)	none	

ACC = American College of Cardiology; AHA = American Heart Association; ECG = electrocardiogram.
*See guidelines text for definitions of level of evidence.

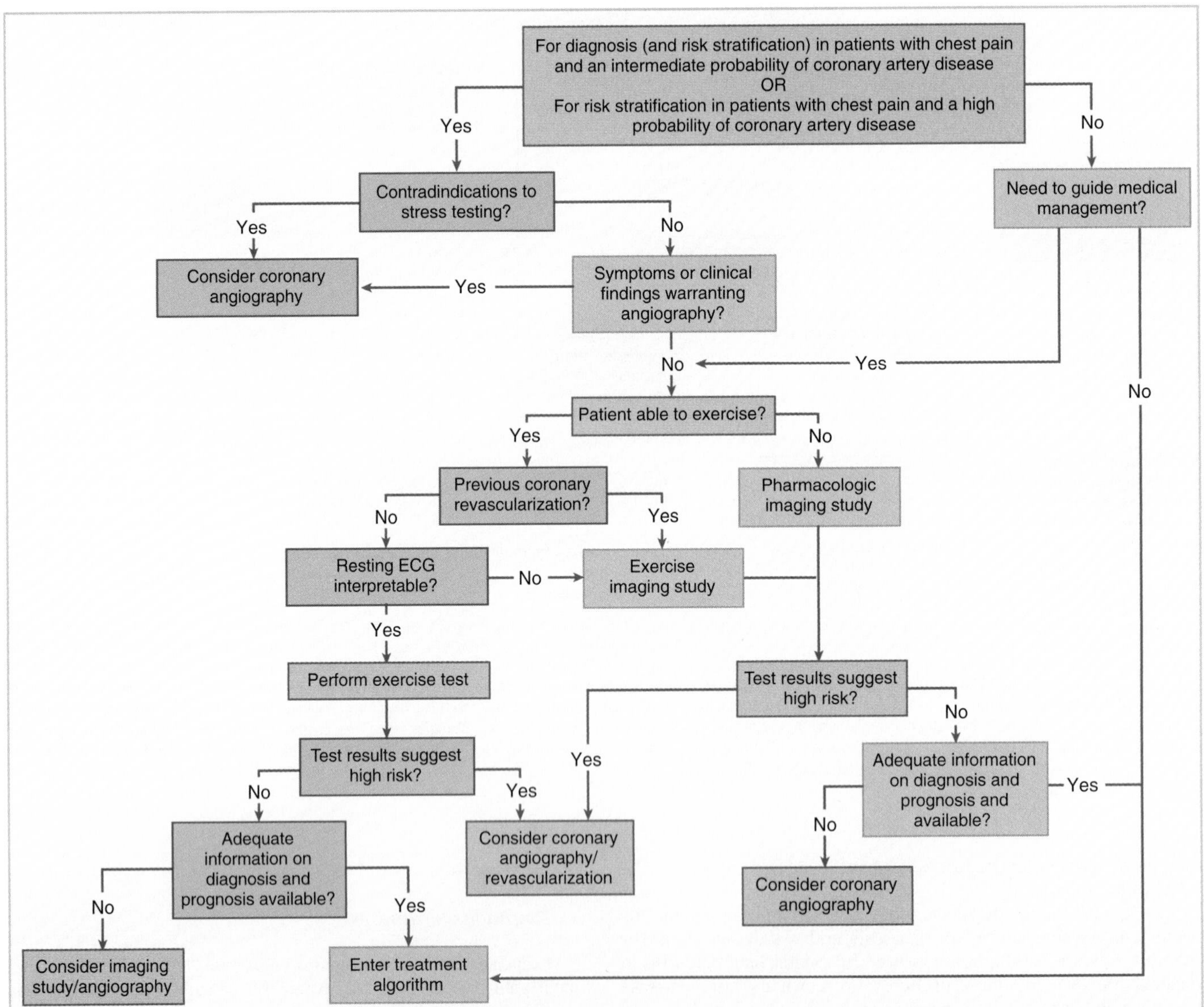

FIGURE 50G–2 Stress testing and angiography in patients with chest pain. ECG = electrocardiogram. (From ACC/AHA 2002 guideline update for the management of patients with chronic stable angina: A report of the American College of Cardiology/American Heart Association Task Force on Practice Guildeines [Committee to Update the 1999 Guidelines for the Management of Patients with Chronic Stable Angina]. ©2002, American College of Cardiology Foundation and the American Heart Association, p 9 [www.acc.org/clinical/guidelines/stable/stable.pdf]).

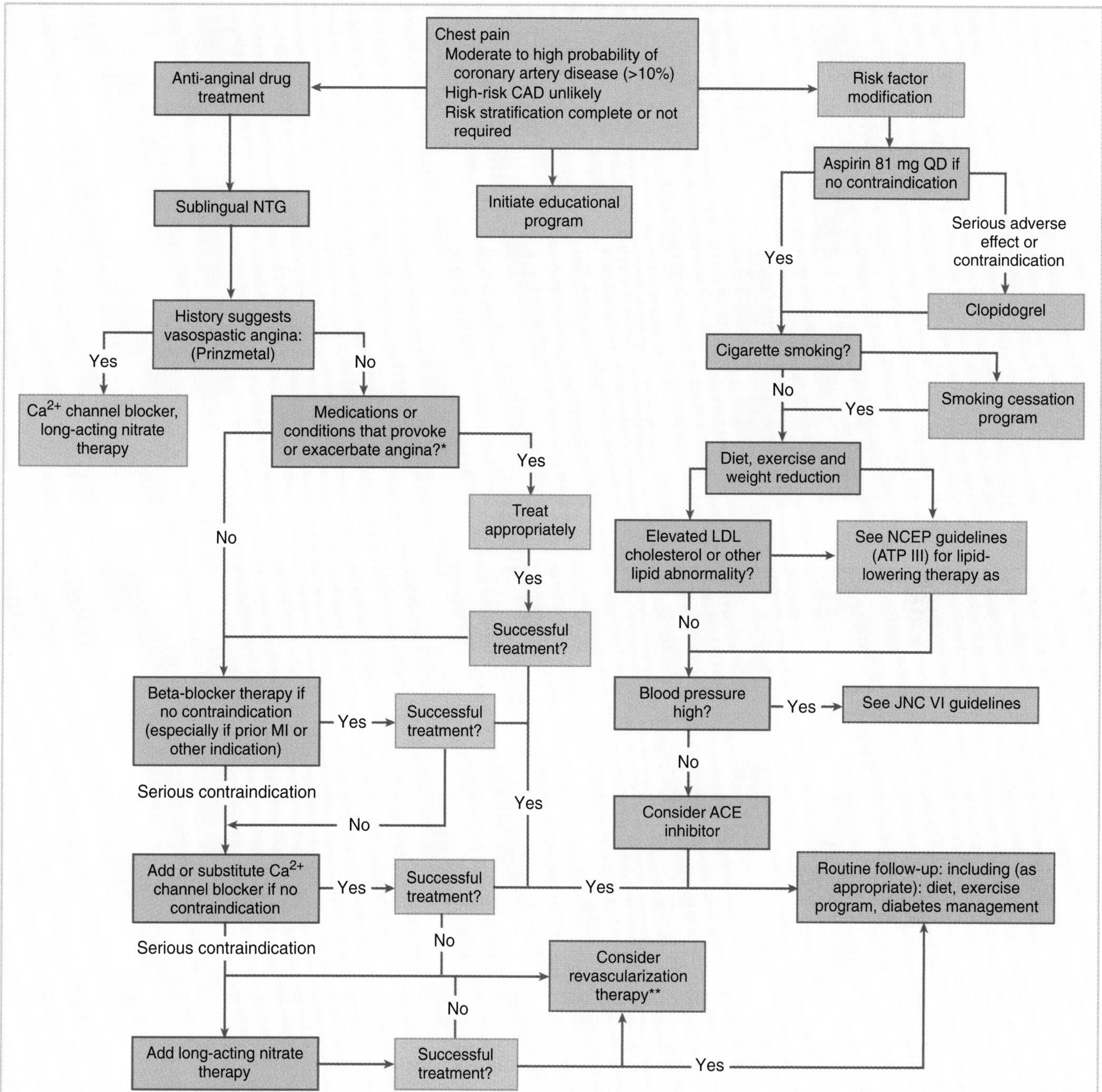

FIGURE 50G–3 Approach to the treatment of chest pain. CAD = coronary artery disease; JNC = Joint National Committee; MI = myocardial infarction; NCEP = National Cholesterol Education Program; NTG = nitroglycerin. *Conditions that exacerbate or provoke angina are medications (vasodilators, excessive thyroid replacement, and vasoconstrictors), other cardiac problems (tachyarrhythmias, bradyarrhythmias, valvular heart disease, especially aortic stenosis), and other medical problems (hypertrophic cardiomyopathy, profound anemia, uncontrolled hypertension, hyperthyroidism, hypoxemia). **At any point in this process, based on coronary anatomy, severity of anginal symptoms, and patient preferences, it is reasonable to consider evaluation for coronary revascularization. Unless a patient is documented to have left main, triple-vessel, or double-vessel coronary artery disease with significant stenosis of the proximal left anterior descending coronary artery, there is no demonstrated survival advantage associated with revascularization in low-risk patients with chronic stable angina; thus, medical therapy should be attempted in most patients before considering percutaneous coronary intervention or coronary artery bypass grafting. (From ACC/AHA 2002 guideline update for the management of patients with chronic stable angina: A report of the American College of Cardiology/American Heart Association Task Force on Practice Guidelines [Committee to Update the 1999 Guidelines for the Management of Patients with Chronic Stable Angina]. ©2002, American College of Cardiology Foundation and the American Heart Association, p 10 [www.acc.org/clinical/guidelines/stable/stable.pdf]).

bundle branch block or less than 1 mm of ST depression at rest. Use of the exercise test was considered of uncertain value (class IIb) for patients with high or low pretest probability of coronary disease; or who had less than 1 mm of ST depression and were either using digoxin or had ECG evidence of left ventricular hypertrophy.

Echocardiography. The ACC/AHA guidelines state that "most patients undergoing a diagnostic evaluation for angina do not need an echocardiogram." Echocardiograms are supported to evaluate systolic murmurs suggestive of aortic stenosis or hypertrophic cardiomyopathy and for evaluation of the extent of ischemia when the study can be obtained within 30 minutes after the end of an ischemic episode (Table 50G–3). However, routine use of echocardiography for patients with a normal ECG, no history of myocardial infarction, and no evidence of structural heart disease is considered inappropriate (class III).

Stress Imaging Studies. The ACC/AHA guidelines recommend stress imaging as opposed to exercise ECG when patients have (1)

TABLE 50G–2 ACC/AHA Guidelines for Diagnosis of Obstructive CAD With Exercise ECG Testing Without an Imaging Modality

Class	Indication	Evidence*
I (indicated)	Patients with an intermediate pretest probability of CAD based on age, gender, and symptoms, including those with complete right bundle branch block or <1 mm of ST depression at rest (exceptions are listed in classes II and III)	B
IIa (good supportive evidence)	Patients with suspected vasospastic angina	C
IIb (weak supportive evidence)	1. Patients with a high pretest probability of CAD by age, gender, and symptoms	B
	2. Patients with a low pretest probability of CAD by age, gender, and symptoms	B
	3. Patients taking digoxin whose ECG has <1 mm of baseline ST segment depression	B
	4. Patients with ECG criteria for LVH and <1 mm of baseline ST segment depression	B
III (not indicated)	1. Patients with the following baseline ECG abnormalities:	
	a. Preexcitation (Wolff-Parkinson-White) syndrome	B
	b. Electronically paced ventricular rhythm	B
	c. More than 1 mm of ST depression at rest	B
	d. Complete left bundle branch block	B
	2. Patients with an established diagnosis of CAD owing to prior myocardial infarction or coronary angiography; however, testing can assess functional capacity and prognosis	

ACC = American College of Cardiology; AHA = American Heart Association; CAD = coronary artery disease; ECG = electrocardiogram; LVH = left ventricular hypertrophy.
*See guidelines text for definitions of level of evidence.

TABLE 50G–3 ACC/AHA Guidelines for Echocardiography for Diagnosis of Cause of Chest Pain in Patients with Suspected Chronic Stable Angina Pectoris

Class	Indication	Evidence*
I (indicated)	1. Patients with systolic murmur suggestive of aortic stenosis or hypertrophic cardiomyopathy	C
	2. Evaluation of extent (severity) of ischemia (e.g., LV segmental wall motion abnormality) when the echocardiogram can be obtained during pain or within 30 min after its abatement	C
IIa (good supportive evidence)		
IIb (weak supportive evidence)	Patients with a click or murmur to diagnose mitral valve prolapse	C
III (not indicated)	Patients with a normal ECG, no history of myocardial infarction, and no signs or symptoms suggestive of heart failure, valvular heart disease, or hypertrophic cardiomyopathy	C

ACC = American College of Cardiology; AHA = American Heart Association; ECG = electrocardiograph; LV = left ventricular.
*See guidelines text for definitions of level of evidence.

complete left bundle branch block, electronically paced ventricular rhythm, preexcitation (Wolff-Parkinson-White) syndrome, and other such ECG conduction abnormalities; (2) patients who have more than 1 mm of ST segment depression at rest, including those with left ventricular hypertrophy or taking drugs such as digitalis; (3) patients who are unable to exercise to a level high enough to give meaningful results on exercise ECGs; and (4) patients with coronary disease who have undergone prior revascularization, in whom localization of ischemia and establishing the significance of lesions is important.

The guidelines specify that exercise stress testing is preferable to pharmacological stress testing when the patient can exercise to develop an appropriate level of cardiovascular stress (e.g., 6 to 12 minutes). Tables 50G–4 and 50G–5 summarize the appropriate indications for stress imaging in patients who are and who are not able to exercise, respectively. As is the case with exercise ECGs, these tests are considered most useful for diagnosis in patients with an intermediate probability of disease.

The guidelines comment on the choice among stress imaging technologies. They conclude that dobutamine perfusion imaging has significant limitations compared with dipyridamole or adenosine perfusion imaging because it does not provoke as great an increase in coronary flow. Therefore, the guidelines recommend that dobutamine be used to provoke ischemia for perfusion imaging only when patients have contraindications to the other agents. In contrast, dobutamine is the agent of choice for pharmacological stress echocardiography because it enhances myocardial contractile performance and wall motion, which can be directly observed by echocardiography.

Specific Patient Subsets. Although treadmill ECG testing is less accurate for diagnosis in women than in men, the guidelines note that the diagnostic performance of imaging technologies is also compromised by technical issues (e.g., breast tissue) in women. Therefore, the guidelines conclude that "there currently are insufficient data to justify replacing standard exercise testing with stress imaging in the initial evaluation of women."

The ACC/AHA guidelines discourage use of noninvasive testing for coronary disease with and without imaging for asymptomatic patients. There are no class I and class IIa indications for exercise testing of asymptomatic patients, and there is just one class IIb indication (weak support): asymptomatic patients with possible myocardial ischemia on ambulatory ECG monitoring or with severe coronary calcification on electron-beam CT scanning. Myocardial perfusion imaging testing also receives only weak support (class IIb) for asymptomatic patients who, despite the recommendations of guidelines, had undergone exercise ECGs and who had an intermediate-risk or high-risk Duke treadmill score or an inadequate exercise ECG.

Coronary Angiography

Coronary angiography is a necessary step in the management of patients for whom revascularization with percutaneous coronary

TABLE 50G–4 ACC/AHA Guidelines for Cardiac Stress Imaging as the Initial Test for Diagnosis in Patients with Chronic Stable Angina Who Are Able to Exercise

Class	Indication	Evidence*
I (indicated)	1. Exercise myocardial perfusion imaging or exercise echocardiography in patients with an intermediate pretest probability of CAD who have one of the following baseline ECG abnormalities: a. Preexcitation (Wolff-Parkinson-White) syndrome b. More than 1 mm of ST depression at rest 2. Exercise myocardial perfusion imaging or exercise echocardiography in patients with prior revascularization (either PCI or CABG) 3. Adenosine or dipyridamole myocardial perfusion imaging in patients with an intermediate pretest probability of CAD and one of the following baseline ECG abnormalities: a. Electronically paced ventricular rhythm b. Left bundle branch block	B B B C B
IIa (good supportive evidence)		
IIb (weak supportive evidence)	1. Exercise myocardial perfusion imaging or exercise echocardiography in patients with a low or high probability of CAD who have one of the following baseline ECG abnormalities: a. EPreexcitation (Wolff-Parkinson-White) syndrome b. EMore than 1 mm of ST depression 2. Adenosine or dipyridamole myocardial perfusion imaging in patients with a low or high probability of CAD and one of the following baseline ECG abnormalities: a. EElectronically paced ventricular rhythm b. ELeft bundle branch block 3. Exercise myocardial perfusion imaging or exercise echocardiography in patients with an intermediate probability of CAD who have one of the following: a. EDigoxin use with <1 mm ST depression on the baseline ECG b. LVH with <1 mm ST depression on the baseline ECG 4. Exercise myocardial perfusion imaging, exercise echocardiography, adenosine or dipyridamole myocardial perfusion imaging, or dobutamine echocardiography as the initial stress test in a patient with a normal rest ECG who is not taking digoxin 5. Exercise or dobutamine echocardiography in patients with left bundle branch block	B B C B B B B C
III (not indicated)		

ACC = American College of Cardiology; AHA = American Heart Association; CABG = coronary artery bypass grafting; CAD = coronary artery disease; ECG = electrocardiograph; LVH = left ventricular hypertrophy; PCI = percutaneous coronary intervention.
*See guidelines text for definitions of level of evidence.

TABLE 50G–5 ACC/AHA Guidelines for Cardiac Stress Imaging as the Initial Test for Diagnosis in Patients with Chronic Stable Angina Who Are Unable to Exercise

Class	Indication	Evidence*
I (indicated)	1. Adenosine or dipyridamole myocardial perfusion imaging or dobutamine echocardiography in patients with an intermediate pretest probability of CAD 2. Adenosine or dipyridamole stress myocardial perfusion imaging or dobutamine echocardiography in patients with prior revascularization (either PCI or CABG)	B B
IIa (good supportive evidence)		
IIb (weak supportive evidence)	1. Adenosine or dipyridamole stress myocardial perfusion imaging or dobutamine echocardiography in patients with a low or high probability of CAD in the absence of electronically paced ventricular rhythm or left bundle branch block 2. Adenosine or dipyridamole myocardial perfusion imaging in patients with a low or a high probability of CAD and one of the following baseline ECG abnormalities: a. Electronically paced ventricular rhythm b. Left bundle branch block 3. Dobutamine echocardiography in patients with left bundle branch block	B C B C
III (not indicated)		

ACC = American College of Cardiology; AHA = American Heart Association; CAD = coronary artery disease; PCI = percutaneous coronary intervention; CABG = coronary artery bypass grafting; ECG = electrocardiograph.
*See guidelines text for definitions of level of evidence.

intervention (PCI) or coronary artery bypass grafting (CABG) is likely to be beneficial because of a high risk for complications with medical therapy alone. Thus, the ACC/AHA guidelines support coronary angiography for diagnosis in patients with angina who have survived sudden death (Table 50G–6). The guidelines consider coronary angiography to be possibly indicated (class IIa) when patients with chest pain have contraindications to noninvasive testing or such testing is inadequate or likely to be inadequate to guide management.

The committee thought that noninvasive and clinical data are usually sufficient to establish or exclude the diagnosis of coronary disease and that coronary angiography should rarely be used for this purpose. The guidelines assert that coronary angiography is "generally not indicated" for diagnosis in asymptomatic patients. They offer

TABLE 50G–6 ACC/AHA Guidelines for Coronary Angiography to Establish a Diagnosis in Patients With Suspected Angina, Including Those With Known CAD Who Have a Significant Change in Anginal Symptoms

Class	Indication	Evidence*
I (indicated)	Patients with known or possible angina pectoris who have survived sudden cardiac death	B
IIa (good supportive evidence)	1. Patients with an uncertain diagnosis after noninvasive testing in whom the benefit of a more certain diagnosis outweighs the risk and cost of coronary angiography 2. Patients who cannot undergo noninvasive testing because of disability, illness, or morbid obesity 3. Patients with an occupational requirement for a definitive diagnosis 4. Patients who by virtue of young age at onset of symptoms, noninvasive imaging, or other clinical parameters are suspected of having a nonatherosclerotic cause for myocardial ischemia (coronary artery anomaly, Kawasaki disease, primary coronary artery dissection, radiation-induced vasculopathy) 5. Patients in whom coronary artery spasm is suspected and provocative testing may be necessary 6. Patients with a high pretest probability of left main or triple-vessel CAD	C C C C C C
IIb (weak supportive evidence)	1. Patients with recurrent hospitalization for chest pain in whom a definite diagnosis is judged necessary 2. Patients with an overriding desire for a definitive diagnosis and a > low probability of CAD	C C
III (not indicated)	1. Patients with significant comorbidity in whom the risk of coronary arteriography outweighs the benefit of the procedure 2. Patients with an overriding personal desire for a definitive diagnosis and a low probability of CAD	C C

ACC = American College of Cardiology; AHA = American Heart Association; CAD = coronary artery disease.
*See guidelines text for definitions of level of evidence.

TABLE 50G–7 ACC/AHA Guidelines for Exercise Testing Risk Assessment and Prognosis in Patients with an Intermediate or High Probability of CAD

Class	Indication	Evidence*
I (indicated)	1. Patients undergoing initial evaluation (exceptions are listed below in classes IIb and III) 2. Patients after a significant change in cardiac symptoms	B C
IIa (good supportive evidence)		
IIb (weak supportive evidence)	1. Patients with the following ECG abnormalities: a. Preexcitation (Wolff-Parkinson-White) syndrome b. Electronically paced ventricular rhythm c. More than 1 mm of ST depression at rest d. Complete left bundle branch block 2. Patients who have undergone cardiac catheterization to identify ischemia in the distribution of coronary lesion of borderline severity 3. Postrevascularization patients who have a significant change in anginal pattern suggestive of ischemia	B B B B C C
III (not indicated)	Patients with severe comorbidity likely to limit life expectancy or prevent revascularization	C

ACC = American College of Cardiology; AHA = American Heart Association; ECG = electrocardiograph.
*See guidelines text for definitions of level of evidence.

only weak support (class IIb) for coronary angiography to establish a definitive diagnosis for patients with recurrent hospitalization for chest pain.

Risk Stratification

The ACC/AHA guidelines emphasize the following four factors that predict survival for patients with coronary artery disease: (1) left ventricular function; (2) anatomical extent and severity of coronary atherosclerosis; (3) presence of recent plaque rupture; and (4) the patient's general health and noncoronary comorbidity.

Assessment of Left Ventricular Function

The guidelines consider assessment of left ventricular function with either echocardiography or radionuclide angiography appropriate (class I) in patients with symptoms or signs of heart failure, a history of prior myocardial infarction, or pathological Q waves on ECG. Echocardiography is also considered appropriate for patients with mitral regurgitation to assess its severity and etiology and for patients with complex ventricular arrhythmias to assess left ventricular function. However, the guidelines note that a normal ECG correlates strongly with normal left ventricular function at rest and therefore do not endorse echocardiography as a routine test for patients with a normal ECG, no history of myocardial infarction, and no symptoms or signs of congestive heart failure. They also do not support routine periodic echocardiography for stable patients in whom no new change in therapy is contemplated.

Noninvasive Tests for Ischemia

Exercise testing is recommended for assessment of prognosis for all patients with an intermediate or high probability of coronary artery disease, except those with ECG abnormalities that compromise interpretation of the exercise tracing and those in which the information is unlikely to alter management (Table 50G–7). The committee directly addressed the issue of whether the additional information provided by imaging technologies might make them preferable tests for risk stratification but concluded the greater costs of these tests could not be justified for most patients. Therefore, the guidelines endorse a stepwise approach in which the exercise ECG is used as the initial test in

TABLE 50G–8 ACC/AHA Guidelines for Cardiac Stress Imaging as the Initial Test for Risk Stratification of Patients with Chronic Stable Angina Who Are Able to Exercise

Class	Indication	Evidence*
I (indicated)	1. Exercise myocardial perfusion imaging or exercise echocardiography to identify the extent, severity, and location of ischemia in patients who do not have left bundle-branch block or an electronically paced ventricular rhythm and who either have an abnormal rest ECG or are using digoxin.	B
	2. Dipyridamole or adenosine myocardial perfusion imaging in patients with left bundle-branch block or electronically paced ventricular rhythm.	B
	3. Exericse myocardial perfusion imaging or exercise echocardiography to assess the functional significance of coronary lesions (if not already known) in planning PCI.	B
IIa (good supportive evidence)		
IIb (weak supportive evidence)	1. Exercise or dobutamine echocardiography in patients with left bundle-branch block.	C
	2. Exercise, dipyridamole, or adenosine myocardial perfusion imaging, or exercise or dobutamine echocardiography as the initial test in patients who have a normal rest ECG and who are not taking digoxin.	B
III (not indicated)	1. Exercise myocardial perfusion imaging in patients with left bundle-branch block.	C
	2. Exercise, dipyridamole, or adenosine myocardial perfusion imaging, or exercise or dobutamine echocardiography in patients with severe comorbidity likely to limit life expectation or prevent revascularization.	C

ACC = American College of Cardiology; AHA = American Heart Association; ECG = electrocardiograph; PCI = percutaneous coronary intervention.
*See guidelines text for definitions of level of evidence.

TABLE 50G–9 ACC/AHA Guidelines for Cardiac Stress Imaging as the Initial Test for Risk Stratification of Patients with Chronic Stable Angina Who Are Unable to Exercise

Class	Indication	Evidence*
I (indicated)	1. Dipyridamole or adenosine myocardial perfusion imaging or dobutamine echocardiography to identify the extent, severity, and location of ischemia in patients who do not have left bundle branch block or electronically paced ventricular rhythm	B
	2. Dipyridamole or adenosine myocardial perfusion imaging in patients with left bundle branch block or electronically paced ventricular rhythm	B
	3. Dipyridamole or adenosine myocardial perfusion imaging or dobutamine echocardiography to assess the functional significance of coronary lesions (if not already known) in planning PCI	B
IIa (good supportive evidence)		
IIb (weak supportive evidence)	Dobutamine echocardiography in patients with left bundle branch block	C
III (not indicated)	Dipyridamole or adenosine myocardial perfusion imaging or dobutamine echocardiography in patients with severe comorbidity likely to limit life expectation or prevent revascularization	C

ACC = American College of Cardiology; AHA = American Heart Association; PCI = percutaneous coronary intervention.
*See guidelines text for definitions of level of evidence.

patients who are not taking digoxin, have a normal rest ECG, and are able to exercise.

The ACC/AHA guidelines support use of stress testing with either echocardiographic or radionuclide imaging to identify the severity of ischemia in patients who have ECG abnormalities precluding interpretation of the exercise tracing and for patients in whom the functional significance of coronary lesions will guide management (Tables 50G–8 and 50G–9). Dipyridamole or adenosine myocardial perfusion imaging is recommended for patients with left bundle branch block or electronically paced ventricular rhythms because of higher rates of false-positive septal perfusion defects with exercise than with either dipryridamole or adenosine. There are relatively few data on the performance of dobutamine echocardiography in this setting, so this approach is not endorsed by the guidelines for patients with left bundle branch block or electronically paced ventricular rhythms. Stress imaging studies are also supported for assessment of the functional significance of coronary lesions in planning PCI.

The guidelines discourage use of noninvasive testing for risk stratification of patients who have no symptoms of coronary disease. There were no class I or class IIa indications for use of cardiac stress imaging as an initial test for risk stratification. Supporting evidence is considered weak for use of cardiac stress imaging for asymptomatic patients with severe coronary calcification on electron-beam CT or who had undergone an exercise ECG and had inadequate tests or intermediate- or high-risk Duke treadmill scores.

Coronary Angiography

In the ACC/AHA guidelines, the decision to proceed to coronary angiography should be based on symptomatic status and risk stratification derived from clinical data and noninvasive test results. The guidelines define noninvasive findings that predict a high (>3 percent), intermediate (1 to 3 percent) and low (<1 percent) expected annual mortality rate (Table 50G–10). Coronary angiography for risk stratification and as a prelude to intervention is endorsed for patients with high-risk criteria, as well as those with disabling chronic stable angina despite medical therapy or other clinical characteristics suggesting high risk (Table 50G–11). The committee considered evidence to be generally supportive (class IIa) for coronary angiography for patients with milder angina in the setting of left ventricular dysfunction even if they do not have high-risk criteria on noninvasive testing; for

TABLE 50G–10 ACC/AHA Guideline Criteria for Noninvasive Risk Stratification

High Risk (>3% annual mortality rate)

1. Severe resting left ventricular dysfunction (LVEF <0.35)
2. High-risk treadmill score (score ≤–11)
3. Severe exercise LV dysfunction (exercise LVEF <0.35)
4. Stress-induced large perfusion defect (particularly if anterior)
5. Stress-induced multiple perfusion defects of moderate size
6. Large, fixed perfusion defect with LV dilation or increased lung uptake (thallium-201)
7. Stress-induced moderate perfusion defect with LV dilation or increased lung uptake (thallium-201)
8. Echocardiographic wall motion abnormality (involving > two segments) developing at low dose of dobutamine (≤10 mg/kg/min) or at a low heart rate (<120 beats/min)
9. Stress echocardiographic evidence of extensive ischemia

Intermediate Risk (1-3% annual mortality rate)

1. Mild/moderate resting LV dysfunction (LVEF =0.35-0.49)
2. Intermediate-risk treadmill score (–11 < score < 5)
3. Stress-induced moderate perfusion defect without LV dilation or increased lung intake (thallium-201)
4. Limited stress echocardiographic ischemia with a wall motion abnormality only at higher doses of dobutamine involving ≥ two segments

Low Risk (<1% annual mortality rate)

1. Low-risk treadmill score (score ≥5)
2. Normal or small myocardial perfusion defect at rest or with stress*
3. Normal stress echocardiographic wall motion or no change of limited resting wall motion abnormalities during stress*

ACC = American College of Cardiology; AHA = American Heart Association; LV = left ventricular; LVEF = LV ejection fraction.

From ACC/AHA 2002 guideline update for the management of patients with chronic stable angina: A report of the American College of Cardiology/American Heart Association Task Force on Practice Guidelines (Committee to Update the 1999 Guidelines for the Management of Patients with Chronic Stable Angina). ©2002, American College of Cardiology Foundation and the American Heart Association (www.acc.org/clinical/guidelines/stable/stable.pdf).

*Although the published data are limited, patients with these findings will probably not be at low risk in the presence of either a high-risk treadmill score or severe resting left ventricular dysfunction (LVEF <0.35).

TABLE 50G–11 ACC/AHA Guidelines for Coronary Angiography for Risk Stratification in Patients with Chronic Stable Angina

Class	Indication	Evidence*
I (indicated)	1. Patients with disabling (Canadian Cardiovascular Society [CCS] classes III and IV) chronic stable angina despite medical therapy	B
	2. Patients with high-risk criteria on noninvasive testing regardless of anginal severity	B
	3. Patients with angina who have survived sudden cardiac death or serious ventricular arrhythmia	B
	4. Patients with angina and symptoms and signs of CHF	C
	5. Patients with clinical characteristics that indicate a high likelihood of severe CAD	C
IIa (good supportive evidence)	1. Patients with significant LV dysfunction (ejection fraction <0.45), CCS class I or II angina, and demonstrable ischemia but < high-risk criteria on noninvasive testing	C
	2. Patients with inadequate prognostic information after noninvasive testing	C
	3. Patients with high-risk criteria suggesting ischemia on noninvasive testing	C
IIb (weak supportive evidence)	1. Patients with CCS class I or II angina, preserved LV function (ejection fraction >0.45), and < high-risk criteria on noninvasive testing	C
	2. Patients with CCS class III (not indicated) or IV angina, which with medical therapy improves to class I or II	C
	3. Patients with CCS class I or II angina but intolerance (unacceptable side effects) to adequate medical therapy	C
III (not indicated)	1. Patients with CCS class I or II angina who respond to medical therapy and who have no evidence of ischemia on noninvasive testing	C
	2. Patients who prefer to avoid revascularization	C

ACC = American College of Cardiology; AHA = American Heart Association; CHF = congestive heart failure; CAD = coronary artery disease; LV = left ventricular.
*See guidelines text for definitions of level of evidence.

asymptomatic patients with high-risk criteria; and for patients whose risk status is uncertain despite noninvasive testing.

Conversely, coronary angiography is discouraged (class III) for patients who have mild angina and no evidence of ischemia on noninvasive testing or would not undergo revascularization. There is only weak support (class IIb) for coronary angiography for patients with mild angina and good left ventricular function in the absence of high-risk criteria on noninvasive testing, for patients with severe angina whose symptoms were controlled with medical therapy, or for patients with mild angina but unacceptable side effects to adequate medical therapy.

Treatment

ACC/AHA guidelines for medical therapy of patients with chronic stable angina are oriented toward preventing myocardial infarction and death and reducing symptoms. When coronary revascularization has been shown to extend life, it is the recommended approach, but in many settings there are a variety of reasonable options, including medical therapy, PCI, and CABG. Cost-effectiveness and patient preference are considered important components of the decision-making process.

The guidelines assert that the goal of treatment of patients with chronic stable angina should be the complete or nearly complete

TABLE 50G–12 ACC/AHA Guidelines for Pharmacotherapy for Chronic Stable Angina

Class	Indication	Evidence*
I (indicated)	1. Aspirin in the absence of contraindications	A
	2. Beta-blockers as initial therapy in the absence of contraindications in patients with prior myocardial infarction or without prior myocardial infarction	A,B
	3. ACE inhibitor in all patients with CAD who also have diabetes and/or LV systolic dysfunction	A
	4. LDL-lowering therapy in patients with documented or suspected CAD and LDL cholesterol >130 mg/dl, with a target LDL of <100 mg/dl	A
	5. Sublingual nitroglycerin or nitroglycerin spray for the immediate relief of angina	B
	6. Calcium antagonists† or long-acting nitrates as initial therapy for reduction of symptoms when beta blockers are contraindicated	B
	7. Calcium antagonists† or long-acting nitrates in combination with beta blockers when initial treatment with beta blockers is not successful	B
	8. Calcium antagonists† and long-acting nitrates as a substitute for beta blockers if initial treatment with beta blockers leads to unacceptable side effects	C
IIa (good supportive evidence)	1. Clopidogrel when aspirin is absolutely contraindicated	B
	2. Long-acting nondihydropyridine calcium antagonists† instead of beta blockers as initial therapy	B
	3. In patients with documented or suspected CAD and LDL cholesterol 100-129 mg/dl, several therapeutic options are available: a. Lifestyle and/or drug therapies to lower LDL to <100 mg/dl b. Weight reduction and increased physical activity in persons with the metabolic syndrome c. Institution of treatment of other lipid or nonlipid risk factors; consider use of nicotinic acid or fibric acid for elevated triglycerides or low HDL cholesterol	B
	4. ACE inhibitor in patients with CAD or other vascular disease	B
IIb (weak supportive evidence)	Low-intensity anticoagulation with warfarin in addition to aspirin	B
III (not indicated)	1. Dipyridamole	B
	2. Chelation therapy	B

ACC = American College of Cardiology; AHA = American Heart Association; ACE = angiotensin-converting enzyme; CAD = coronary artery disease; LDL = low-density lipoprotein; LV = left ventricular.
*See guidelines text for definitions of level of evidence.
†Short-acting dihydropyridine calcium antagonists should be avoided.

elimination of anginal chest pain and return to normal activities, with minimal side effects. They recommend that the initial treatment of the patient should include all the elements in the following menomic:

A = Aspirin and Antianginal therapy
B = Beta blocker and Blood pressure
C = Cigarette smoking and Cholesterol
D = Diet and Diabetes
E = Education and Exercise

Pharmacological Therapy

The guidelines emphasize the importance of aspirin and beta blockers for patients with coronary disease in the absence of contraindications (Table 50G–12). Absolute contraindications to beta blockers include severe bradycardia, preexisting high degree of atrioventricular block, sick sinus syndrome, and severe, unstable left ventricular failure. Relative contraindications to beta blockers include asthma and bronchospastic disease, severe depression, and peripheral vascular disease. The guidelines note that most patients with diabetes tolerate beta blockers, although these drugs should be used with caution in patients who require insulin.

Angiotensin-converting enzyme (ACE) inhibitors are recommended (class I indication) for patients with diabetes and/or left ventricular systolic dysfunction, and evidence is considered good for their use in other patients with coronary disease (class IIa). The guidelines recommende that nitrates and calcium antagonists and nitrates should be used for symptom control but indicate that short-acting dihydropyridine calcium antagonists should be avoided. Low-density lipoprotein (LDL) cholesterol should be controlled with a target of less than 100 mg/dl (see Risk Reduction).

Several of the recommendations about pharmacological therapy may be altered in future revisions of these guidelines owing to subsequent research providing insight into the effects of these agents. For example, the guidelines give some support to use of clopidogrel only when aspirin is contraindicated (class IIa), but research on this and other antiplatelet agents is advancing rapidly so that insights into their optimal use can be expected to change in the next several years. Evidence is considered weak for anticoagulation with warfarin in addition to aspirin; since these guidelines were published, a randomized trial has shown that the combination of warfarin and aspirin were superior to aspirin alone in preventing future events but at the price of a higher rate of bleeding complications.[3] Use of dipyridamole or chelation therapy is discouraged.

For asymptomatic patients with known coronary disease (e.g., patients with prior myocardial infarction), the guidelines recommend aspirin and beta blockers in the absence of contraindications and the use of lipid-lowering therapies and ACE inhibitors as described earlier.

Risk Reduction

For patients with chronic stable angina, the ACC/AHA guidelines support intensive management of risk factors including hypertension, cigarette smoking, diabetes, LDL cholesterol, and obesity (Table 50G–13). The guidelines support use of pharmacological therapy for patients with LDL levels greater than 130 mg/dl, with a target of 100 mg/dL. For patients with coronary disease who have an LDL of 100 to 129 mg/dl, the guidelines consider several options reasonable (class IIa), including life-style modifications or drug therapies.

In changes from prior guidelines, initiation of hormone therapy for the purpose of reducing cardiovascular risk is considered inappropriate (class III), as is use of vitamins C and E supplementation, chelation therapy, garlic, acupuncture, and coenzyme Q for this purpose. Evidence to support interventions based on lipoprotein(a) and homocysteine levels are considered inconclusive.

Specific goals for key risk reduction interventions are summarized in Table 50G–14.

TABLE 50G–13 ACC/AHA Guidelines for Treatment of Risk Factors

Class	Indication	Evidence*
I (indicated)	1. Treatment of hypertension according to Joint National Conference VI guidelines	A
	2. Smoking cessation therapy	B
	3. Management of diabetes	C
	4. Comprehensive cardiac rehabilitation program (including exercise)	B
	5. LDL-lowering therapy in patients with documented or suspected CAD and LDL cholesterol ≥130 mg/dl, with a target LDL of <100 mg/dl	A
	6. Weight reduction in obese patients in the presence of hypertension, hyperlipidemia, or diabetes mellitus	C
IIa (good supportive evidence)	1. In patients with documented or suspected CAD and LDL cholesterol 100-129 mg/dl, several therapeutic options are available:	B
	a. Lifestyle and/or drug therapies to lower LDL to <100 mg/dl	B
	b. Weight reduction and increased physical activity in persons with the metabolic syndrome	B
	c. Institution of treatment of other lipid or nonlipid risk factors; consider use of nicotinic acid or fibric acid for elevated triglycerides or low HDL cholesterol	B
	2. Therapy to lower non-HDL cholesterol in patients with documented or suspected CAD and triglycerides >200 mg/dl, with a target non-HDL cholesterol <130 mg/dl	B
	3. Weight reduction in obese patients in the absence of hypertension, hyperlipidemia, or diabetes mellitus	C
IIb (weak supportive evidence)	1. Folate therapy in patients with elevated homocysteine levels	C
	2. Identification and appropriate treatment of clinical depression to improve CAD outcomes	C
	3. Intervention directed at psychosocial stress reduction	C
III (not indicated)	1. Initiation of hormone replacement therapy in postmenopausal women for the purpose of reducing cardiovascular risk	A
	2. Vitamins C and E supplementation	A
	3. Chelation therapy	C
	4. GarlicC	
	5. Acupuncture	C
	6. Coenzyme Q	C

ACC = American College of Cardiology; AHA = American Heart Association; CAD = coronary artery disease; HDL = high-density lipoprotein; LDL = low-density lipoprotein.
*See guidelines text for definitions of level of evidence.

TABLE 50G–14 Specific Goals for Risk Reduction Strategies in Patients with Chronic Stable Angina

Risk Factor/Strategy	Goal
Smoking	Complete cessation
Blood pressure	<140/90 or 130/85 mm Hg if heart failure or renal insufficiency; <130/85 mm Hg if diabetes
Lipid management	Primary goal: LDL <100 mg/dl Secondary goal: If triglycerides ≥200 mg/dl, then non-HDL should be <130 mg/dl
Physical activity	Minimum goal: 30 min 3 or 4 d/w Optimal goal: daily
Weight management	BMI 18.5-24.9 kg/m^2
Diabetes management	HbA1c <7%
Antiplatelet agents/anticoagulants	All patients: indefinite use of aspirin 75-325 mg per day if not contraindicated. Consider clopidogrel as an alternative if aspirin is contraindicated. Manage warfarin to international normalized ratio = 2.0 to 3.0 in patients after myocardial infarction when clinically indicated or for those not able to take aspirin or clopidogrel
ACE inhibitors	Treat all patients indefinitely after myocardial infarction; start early in stable high-risk patients (anterior myocardial infarction, previous myocardial infarction, Killip class II [S_3 gallop, rales, radiographic CHF]). Consider chronic therapy for all other patients with coronary or other vascular disease unless contraindicated. Use as needed to manage blood pressure or symptoms in all other patients
Beta blockers	Start in all post-myocardial infarction and acute patients (arrhythmia, LV dysfunction, inducible ischemia) at 5-28 days. Continue 6 mo minimum. Observe usual contraindications. Use as needed to manage angina, rhythm, or blood pressure in all patients

ACE = angiotensin-converting enzyme; LDL = low-density lipoprotein; BMI = body mass index; HbA1c = hemoglobin A1c; CHF = congestive heart failure; LV = left ventricular.

Revascularization

ACC/AHA guidelines for revascularization with PCI or CABG for patients with chronic stable angina focus on improvement of survival for patients with high clinical risk of mortality on medical therapy and on controlling symptoms in patients who have an inadequate quality of life on medical therapy. Recommendations include the use of CABG for patients with significant left main coronary artery disease and in patients with triple-vessel disease, particularly in those with abnormal left ventricular function (Table 50G–15). PCI and CABG are supported for patients with double- and triple-vessel coronary disease and who do not have treated diabetes. Revascularization is also supported for

TABLE 50G–15 ACC/AHA Guidelines for Revascularization with PCI and CABG in Patients with Stable Angina

Class	Indication	Evidence*
I (indicated)	1. CABG for patients with significant left main coronary disease	A
	2. CABG for patients with triple-vessel disease. The survival benefit is greater in patients with abnormal LV function (ejection fraction <0.50)	A
	3. CABG for patients with double-vessel disease with significant proximal LAD CAD and either abnormal LV function (ejection fraction less than 50%) or demonstrable ischemia on noninvasive testing	A
	4. Percutaneous coronary intervention for patients with double-or triple-vessel disease with significant proximal LAD CAD, who have anatomy suitable for catheter-based therapy and normal LV function and who do not have treated diabetes	B
	5. PCI or CABG for patients with single- or double-vessel CAD without significant proximal LAD CAD but with a large area of viable myocardium and high-risk criteria on noninvasive testing	B
	6. CABG for patients with single- or double-vessel CAD without significant proximal LAD CAD who have survived sudden cardiac death or sustained ventricular tachycardia	C
	7. In patients with prior PCI, CABG or PCI for recurrent stenosis associated with a large area of viable myocardium or high-risk criteria on noninvasive testing	C
	8. PCI or CABG for patients who have not been successfully treated by medical therapy and can undergo revascularization with acceptable risk	B
IIa (good supportive evidence)	1. Repeat CABG for patients with multiple saphenous vein graft stenoses, especially when there is significant stenosis of a graft supplying the LAD; it may be appropriate to use PCI for focal saphenous vein graft lesions or multiple stenoses in poor candidates for reoperative surgery	C
	2. Use of PCI or CABG for patients with single- or double-vessel CAD without significant proximal LAD disease but with a moderate area of viable myocardium and demonstrable ischemia on noninvasive testing	B
	3. Use of PCI or CABG for patients with single-vessel disease with significant proximal LAD disease	B
IIb (weak supportive evidence)	1. Compared with CABG, PCI for patients with double- or triple-vessel disease with significant proximal LAD CAD, who have anatomy suitable for catheter-based therapy, and who have treated diabetes or abnormal LV function	B
	2. Use of PCI for patients with significant left main coronary disease who are not candidates for CABG	C
	3. PCI for patients with single- or double-vessel CAD without significant proximal LAD CAD who have survived sudden cardiac death or sustained ventricular tachycardia	C
III (not indicated)	1. Use of PCI or CABG for patients with single- or double-vessel CAD without significant proximal LAD CAD, who have mild symptoms that are unlikely due to myocardial ischemia, or who have not received an adequate trial of medical therapy and a. have only a small area of viable myocardium *or* b. have no demonstrable ischemia on noninvasive testing	C
	2. Use of PCI or CABG for patients with borderline coronary stenoses (50-60% diameter in locations other than the left main coronary artery) and no demonstrable ischemia on noninvasive testing	C
	3. Use of PCI or CABG for patients with insignificant coronary stenosis (<50% diameter)	C
	4. Use of PCI in patients with significant left main coronary artery disease who are candidates for CABG	B

ACC = American College of Cardiology; AHA = American Heart Association; CAD = coronary artery disease; CABG = coronary artery bypass grafting; LAD = left anterior descending [coronary artery]; LV = left ventricular; PCI = percutaneous coronary intervention.
*See guidelines text for definitions of level of evidence.

patients with single- or double-vessel coronary disease who have a large area of viable myocardium and high-risk criteria on noninvasive testing.

The guidelines discourage use of PCI or CABG for single- or double-vessel coronary disease without significant proximal left anterior descending (LAD) coronary artery disease if they have mild symptoms or have not received an adequate trial of medical therapy, particularly if noninvasive testing data indicate either that they have only a small area of viable myocardium or have no demonstrable ischemia on noninvasive testing. PCI for patients with diabetes is considered a second-choice strategy compared with CABG.

For asymptomatic patients, the guidelines for revascularization with PCI or CABG are identical to those for other patients with chronic stable angina (see Table 50G-15), except that the following indications that were considered class IIa are regarded as weaker (class IIb) in asymptomatic patients:

Use of PCI or CABG for patients with single- or double-vessel CAD without significant proximal LAD disease but with a moderate area of viable myocardium and demonstrable ischemia on noninvasive testing

Use of PCI or CABG for patients with single-vessel disease with significant proximal LAD disease

Alternative Therapies

The guidelines do not consider alternative therapies to be sufficiently supported by evidence to warrant a class I indication for patients with chronic stable angina. Surgical laser transmyocardial revascularization is given a class IIa indication, and enhanced external counterpulsation and spinal cord stimulation are given class IIb indications.

PATIENT FOLLOW-UP

The ACC/AHA guidelines recommend that patients with chronic stable angina should have follow-up evaluations every 4 to 12 months during the first year of therapy; subsequently, annual evaluations are recommended if the patient is stable and reliable enough to call when angina symptoms become worse or other symptoms occur. The guidelines urge restraint in the use of routine testing in follow-up of patients with chronic stable angina if they have not had a change in clinical status (Table 50G-16). All of the class I indications for testing are for patients who have had a significant change in clinical status, except for the use of coronary angiography for patients with marked limitations of ordinary activity despite maximal medical therapy.

TABLE 50G–16 ACC/AHA Guidelines for Echocardiography, Treadmill Exercise Testing, Stress Radionuclide Imaging, Stress Echocardiography Studies, and Coronary Angiography During Patient Follow-Up

Class	Indication	Evidence*
I (indicated)	1. Chest radiograph for patients with evidence of new or worsening CHF	C
	2. Assessment of LV ejection fraction and segmental wall motion by echocardiography or radionuclide imaging in patients with new or worsening CHF or evidence of intervening myocardial infarction by history or ECG	C
	3. Echocardiography for evidence of new or worsening valvular heart disease	C
	4. Treadmill exercise test for patients without prior revascularization who have a significant change in clinical status, are able to exercise, and do not have any of the ECG abnormalities listed in No. 5	C
	5. Stress radionuclide imaging or stress echocardiography procedures for patients without prior revascularization who have a significant change in clinical status and are unable to exercise or have one of the following ECG abnormalities: a. Preexcitation (Wolff-Parkinson-White) syndrome b. Electronically paced ventricular rhythm c. More than 1 mm of rest ST depression d. Complete left bundle branch block	C
	6. Stress radionuclide imaging or stress echocardiography procedures for patients who have a significant change in clinical status and required a stress imaging procedure on their initial evaluation because of equivocal or intermediate-risk treadmill results	C
	7. Stress radionuclide imaging or stress echocardiography procedures for patients with prior revascularization who have a significant change in clinical status	C
	8. Coronary angiography in patients with marked limitation of ordinary activity (CCS class III) despite maximal medical therapy	C
IIa (good supportive evidence)		
IIb (weak supportive evidence)	Annual treadmill exercise testing in patients who have no change in clinical status, can exercise, have none of the ECG abnormalities listed in No. 5, and have an estimated annual mortality rate >1%	C
III (not indicated)	1. Echocardiography or radionuclide imaging for assessment of LV ejection fraction and segmental wall motion in patients with a normal ECG, no history of myocardial infarction, and no evidence of CHF	C
	2. Repeat treadmill exercise testing in <3 yr in patients who have no change in clinical status and an estimated annual mortality rate <1% on their initial evaluation, as demonstrated by one of the following: a. Low-risk Duke treadmill score (without imaging) b. Low-risk Duke treadmill score with negative imaging c. Normal LV function and a normal coronary angiogram d. Normal LV function and insignificant CAD	C
	3. Stress imaging or echocardiograph procedures for patients who have no change in clinical status and a normal rest ECG, are not taking digoxin, are able to exercise, and did not require a stress imaging or echocardiographic procedure on their initial evaluation because of equivocal or intermediate-risk treadmill results	C
	4. Repeat coronary angiography in patients with no change in clinical status, no change on repeat exercise testing or stress imaging, and insignificant CAD on initial evaluation	C

ACC = American College of Cardiology; AHA = American Heart Association; CAD = coronary artery disease; CCS = Canadian Cardiovascular Society; CHF = congestive heart failure; ECG = electrocardiograph; LV = left ventricular.

*See guidelines text for definitions of level of evidence.

References

1. Gibbons RJ, Abrams J, Chatterjee K, et al: ACC/AHA 2002 guideline update for the management of patients with chronic stable angina: A report of the American College of Cardiology/American Heart Association Task Force on Practice Guidelines (Committee to Update the 1999 Guidelines for the Management of Patients with Chronic Stable Angina). 2002 (Available at www.acc.org/clinical/guidelines/stable/stable.pdf).
2. O'Rourke RA, Brundage BH, Froelicher VF, et al: American College of Cardiology/American Heart Association Expert Consensus Document on electron-beam computed tomography for the diagnosis and prognosis of coronary artery disease. Circulation 102:126-140, 2000.
3. Hurlen M, Abdelnoor M, Smith P, et al: Warfarin, aspirin, or both after myocardial infarction. N Engl J Med 347:969-974, 2002.

CHAPTER 51

Diabetes and Heart Disease

Richard W. Nesto

Scope of the Problem

People with diabetes have an increased prevalence of atherosclerosis and coronary heart disease (CHD) (see Chap. 40) and experience higher morbidity and mortality after acute coronary syndrome and myocardial infarction (MI) than people without diabetes. Diabetes has dramatic impact on outcomes following unstable angina or MI. Analyzing data collected for the Organization to Assess Strategies for Ischemic Syndromes (OASIS) Registry, Malmberg and colleagues showed that diabetes significantly increased all-cause death and the incidence of new MI, stroke, and heart failure during a 2-year mean follow-up in patients who were hospitalized for unstable angina or non-Q-wave MI.[1] In a similar study of patients hospitalized with a confirmed MI, Mukamal and colleagues found that diabetes was associated with an adjusted hazard ratio for mortality of 1.7 (95 percent confidence interval [CI] 1.2 to 2.3) compared with patients without diabetes and no previous MI.[2] In general, diabetes confers as much additional risk as having had a previous MI.

Diabetes also increases the risk of heart failure. Patients with diabetes are two to five times more likely to develop heart failure than those without diabetes,[3] and following development of heart failure, diabetic patients have higher mortality and heart failure–related morbidity.[4] The fundamental causes of heart failure are similar in diabetic and nondiabetic subjects: previous MI and the resultant loss of contracting myocardium cause most chronic congestive heart failure (CHF). Other contributors to CHF in diabetic patients include hypertension, left ventricular hypertrophy, and valvular heart disease. Although diabetes is an important risk factor for CHF, it rarely occurs independently and in fact appears to act synergistically with other risk factors.

Traditional CHD risk factors such as hypertension, dyslipidemia, and overweight and obesity cluster in patients with impaired glucose tolerance or diabetes (see discussion of metabolic syndrome in Chap. 40), but this clustering cannot account for all of the increased risk in these patients. In addition to the traditional risk factors associated with CHD and heart failure, a number of diabetes-specific risk factors contribute to the increased morbidity and mortality of coronary artery disease (CAD) in diabetes. For example, patients with diabetes have lipid-rich atherosclerotic plaque that is more vulnerable to rupture than plaque found in patients without diabetes.[5] Diabetes is associated with the presence of multiple vulnerable coronary plaques in patients undergoing catheterization for acute coronary syndromes, which may account for the increased risk of reinfarction in these patients. Platelets harvested from patients with diabetes exhibit enhanced aggregation and increased expression of activation-dependent adhesion molecules, such as glycoprotein (GP) IIb/IIIa, which contributes to thrombus formation.[6]

Changes in vascular function may also contribute to the poorer outcomes in diabetes. No reflow following successful percutaneous recanalization of an infarct-related coronary artery occurs more commonly in the presence of diabetes and/or hyperglycemia and may contribute to left ventricular dysfunction. No reflow in this circumstance probably results from platelet–endothelial cell interactions that impair microvascular function and decrease myocardial blood flow. Patients with diabetes have increased levels of plasminogen activator inhibitor type 1 (PAI-1) in plasma and in atheromas.[7,8] Elevated tissue PAI-1 could decrease fibrinolysis, increase thrombus formation, and accelerate plaque formation. Other vascular changes, including increased endothelin activity and reduced prostacyclin and nitric oxide activity, lead to abnormal control of blood flow.[9,10] The emerging recognition that CHD is part of a proinflammatory state suggests that the increased plasma C-reactive protein levels seen in people with diabetes may contribute to the increased risk.[11] Other diabetes-specific changes that occur include diabetic cardiomyopathy, which impairs myocardial performance and renders the myocardium more susceptible to and less able to recover from ischemia, and diabetic autonomic neuropathy, which results in sympathovagal imbalance and contributes to cardiovascular mortality.[12] Advanced glycation end products (AGEs) are thought to contribute to many of these diabetes-specific changes (see Chap. 40).

Medical Therapy of Acute Coronary Syndromes

A history of diabetes is important in determining the treatment of patients during and following an acute MI. However, patients with acute coronary syndromes commonly have undiagnosed diabetes and impaired glucose metabolism. In a study of 3266 patients scheduled for coronary angiography, Taubert and colleagues reported that the prevalence of previously undiagnosed diabetes was nearly 18 percent.[13] Patients with acute MI have an even higher percentage (25 to 31 percent) of previously undiagnosed diabetes.[14]

The negative interaction between diabetes and the prognosis after MI extends to patients with elevated blood glucose at the time of admission. Several studies have shown this relationship. For example, 1664 consecutively hospitalized patients with an acute MI were categorized by history of diabetes and by whether they had a blood glucose concentration greater than 198 mg/dl.[15] The patients who had a history of diabetes or who were hyperglycemic had a significantly elevated risk of in-hospital mortality compared with those without either condition. In a similar study, admission blood glucose level in nondiabetic patients independently predicted nonfatal reinfarction ($p = 0.006$), hospitalization for heart failure ($p = 0.0034$), and a major cardiovascular event ($p = 0.0042$) during the 1.5- to 2.5-year follow-up period.[16]

Antiplatelet Drugs

Studies have consistently shown that patients with either type 1 or type 2 diabetes have enhanced platelet aggregation in response to a variety of agonists.[6] This enhanced aggregability results in part from increased production of thromboxane, altered calcium and magnesium homeostasis, and increased expression of activation-dependent adhesion molecules. Endothelial dysfunction, characterized by decreased production of nitric oxide and prostacyclin, is common in diabetic individuals and enhances platelet aggregation and adhesiveness in vivo.[6] Thus, agents directed at inhibiting platelet aggregation in vivo consistently reduce the incidence of thrombotic events in nondiabetic and diabetic individuals.

Aspirin

In the Early Treatment of Diabetic Retinopathy Study (ETDRS), patients with type 1 or type 2 diabetes randomly assigned to aspirin 650 mg/day had a significantly lowered risk of MI without incurring an increase in the risk of vitreous or retinal bleeding, even in patients with retinopathy.[17] The Hypertension Optimal Treatment (HOT) trial confirmed this benefit in 1501 diabetic subjects who experienced a significant 15 percent reduction in cardiovascular events and a 36 percent reduction in MI while being treated with aspirin 75 mg/day.[17] This cardiovascular benefit resembled that seen in the nondiabetic cohort. The American Diabetes Association currently recommends enteric-coated aspirin (81 to 325 mg/day) for (1) secondary prevention in men and women with diabetes and evidence of macrovascular disease and (2) primary prevention in persons with type 1 or type 2 diabetes and additional coronary risk factors.[17]

Adenosine Diphosphate Receptor Antagonists

Ticlopidine and clopidogrel irreversibly block platelet adenosine diphosphate (ADP) receptors, preventing activation of the GP IIb/IIIa receptor and thereby inhibiting binding of fibrinogen. In the Clopidogrel versus Aspirin in Patients at Risk of Ischemic Events (CAPRIE) trial, patients who had suffered a recent MI, stroke, or had established peripheral arterial disease were randomly assigned to receive aspirin 325 mg/day or clopidogrel 75 mg/day.[18,19] During the 1.9-year follow-up, the incidence of the combined primary endpoint, stroke, MI, or vascular death, was 8.7 percent lower in the clopidogrel group than in the aspirin group. Although the incidence of the primary endpoint was higher in the nearly 4000 diabetic participants, the benefit of clopidogrel over aspirin extended to this subgroup.[19] The Clopidogrel in Unstable Angina to Prevent Recurrent Events (CURE) study tested clopidogrel plus aspirin against aspirin alone in patients with unstable angina or non-Q-wave MI. After 9 months the incidence of the primary composite endpoint (cardiovascular death, nonfatal MI, or stroke) was reduced in the clopidogrel plus aspirin group by 20 percent.[20] Subgroup analysis showed that this effect extended to the patients with diabetes.

Glycoprotein IIb/IIIa Blockers

These potent antiplatelet agents have improved outcomes in patients with unstable angina and non-Q-wave infarction and have reduced the incidence of acute ischemic events by 35 to 50 percent in patients undergoing percutaneous coronary intervention (PCI).[21] At least one of the GP IIb/IIIa inhibitors, abciximab, positively influenced long-term mortality.[21] In general, these agents appear to have equal or better efficacy in diabetic than nondiabetic patients, although most studies have not been sufficiently powered to evaluate this interaction fully. However, meta-analyses clearly show a major benefit in the diabetic population.

Four placebo-controlled trials of the use of GP IIb/IIIa blockade during PCI included detailed outcome data for the diabetic subgroups.[21] Three studies (the Evaluation of c7E3 for Prevention of Ischemic Complications [EPIC], Evaluation in PTCA to Improve Long-term Outcome with abciximab GP IIb/IIIa blockade [EPILOG], and Evaluation of Platelet Inhibition in STENTing [EPISTENT]) evaluated abciximab, and the fourth (Enhanced Suppression of the Platelet IIb/IIIa Receptor with Integrilin Therapy [ESPRIT]) tested eptifibatide. The magnitude of the reduction in acute ischemic events (death, MI, or urgent revascularization occurring within 30 days) in the active treatment group compared with the placebo group was similar in both diabetic (21 to 67 percent reduction) and nondiabetic patients (30 to 51 percent reduction). This treatment effect was durable, as indicated by the similar reductions in death or MI at 6 months in both the diabetic and nondiabetic groups. The incidence of target vessel revascularization at 6 months, a surrogate for restenosis, varied considerably between treatment groups and among trials. Thus, whether GP IIb/IIIa treatment reduces the incidence of restenosis in diabetic or nondiabetic patients remains an open issue. Long-term mortality is also reduced by abciximab in the general population, and multivariate analysis has shown that diabetes is an important factor in predicting this survival benefit.[22]

The survival benefit of GP IIb/IIIa blockade may be greater in diabetic patients treated with stents. In EPISTENT, 1-year mortality was reduced from 4.1 to 1.2 percent in stented, diabetic patients, a larger benefit than seen in the nondiabetic group (1.9 to 1.0 percent).[23] A similar reduction in 1-year mortality was found in stented, diabetic patients treated with eptifibatide in the ESPRIT trial.[24] Although these differences did not achieve statistical significance because of the studies' limited power, the results suggest that GP IIb/IIIa blockade neutralizes the mortality risk usually seen in diabetic patients following PCI. GP IIb/IIIa blockers also confer a survival benefit on diabetic patients treated for non-ST-segment elevation acute coronary syndromes. A meta-analysis of six major studies involving 6458 diabetic patients showed a reduction in 30-day mortality from 6.2 percent in the placebo group to 4.8 percent in the treated group ($p = 0.007$).[25] No benefit was seen in the 23,072 nondiabetic patients.

Part of the increased risk of thrombotic events in diabetic patients stems from their altered platelet function, including altered arachidonic acid metabolism and increased expression of activation-dependent adhesion molecules such as GP IIb/IIIa, resulting in enhanced platelet aggregation.[6] This diabetic thrombocytopathy may explain in part the greater effect of GP IIb/IIIa blockers in diabetic patients compared with nondiabetic patients. GP IIb/IIIa blockade may also improve microvascular dysfunction in acute coronary syndrome patients,[26] although the mechanism of this platelet-endothelial interaction has not yet been elucidated.

Beta-Adrenergic Blocking Agents

Overwhelming evidence exists that beta-adrenergic blocking agents (beta blockers) reduce mortality and reinfarction in patients with MI. However, the use of beta blockers in the diabetic population has been controversial because of their potential to reduce hypoglycemic symptoms, precipitate glucose intolerance, inhibit the release of insulin, and affect adversely the plasma lipid profile. Despite these concerns, treatment of diabetic patients with beta blockers following MI has reduced mortality, and the benefit in several studies exceeded that seen in the nondiabetic counterparts. Although these data derive from retrospective subgroup analyses of trials in the prethrombolytic era, they concur with more recent results. The National Cooperative Cardiovascular Project reviewed records of more than 45,000 patients who had experienced an acute MI, 26 percent of whom had diabetes. After adjusting for confounding variables, beta blocker use was associated with a lower 1-year mortality in diabetic patients without an increase in diabetes-related complications.[27]

The greater relative benefit of beta blockers in diabetic patients may derive from several factors. Beta blockers can help restore sympathovagal balance in diabetic patients with autonomic neuropathy and may decrease fatty acid utilization within the myocardium, thus reducing oxygen demand. However, despite the continuing growth of evidence regarding their efficacy and safety in the diabetic patient, beta blockers continue to be underprescribed in this group. Physicians have concerns that beta blockers can mask the warning signs of hypoglycemia, suppress glycogenolysis, interfere with insulin release, and further impair glucose tolerance in patients with diabetes. Some are also concerned that beta blockers may elevate serum triglycerides, reduce high-density lipoprotein, and increase low-density lipoprotein and thereby potentially counteract some of the widely accepted cardioprotective benefits of these drugs. However, much of the concern surrounding the use of these drugs in diabetes stems from earlier experience with noncardioselective agents in higher doses. The risk of hypoglycemia in diabetic hypertensive patients taking cardioselective beta blockers was no different from that of patients taking placebo.[28] Cardioselective agents have less tendency to worsen glycemic control than nonselective agents do, although diabetes may develop in over 20 percent of nondiabetic hypertensive patients given beta blockers.[29]

Angiotensin-Converting Enzyme Inhibitors

Angiotensin-converting enzyme (ACE) inhibitors reduce infarct size, limit ventricular remodeling, improve survival after myocardial infarction, and may be of particular benefit in patients with diabetes.[30] A post hoc analysis of one thrombolytic trial (Grupo Italiano per lo Studio della Sopravivenza nell'Infarto Miocardico-3 [GISSI-3]) revealed that early administration of lisinopril in the setting of acute MI reduced 6-week and 6-month mortality comparatively more in diabetic versus nondiabetic patients (30 versus 5 percent reduction at 6 weeks and 20 versus 0 percent at 6 months, respectively).[31] Lisinopril administration resulted in some 37 lives saved per 1000 treated diabetic patients. Another retrospective analysis, the Trandolapril Cardiac Evaluation (TRACE) study, compared the effect of oral trandolapril versus placebo in anterior MI in patients with and without diabetes.[32] Patients with diabetes experienced a greater relative improvement in survival over 5 years of follow-up than the nondiabetic cohort. Furthermore, ACE inhibition reduced by nearly 50 percent the risk of sudden death, reinfarction, and progression of CHF in patients with diabetes, whereas subjects without diabetes experienced only trends in protection against these secondary outcomes.

Many factors may explain the particular benefits of ACE inhibitors in diabetic patients with acute MI. These agents can prevent or limit remodeling of the ventricle, particularly when administered early in the course of acute MI; reduce recurrent ischemic events; and restore sympathovagal imbalance. ACE inhibitors may also improve endothelial function in diabetes, counteract reduced fibrinolysis by suppression of PAI-1 expression, and decrease insulin resistance.[33] In the Heart Outcomes Prevention Evaluation (HOPE) study, ramipril significantly reduced the rates of MI, stroke, and cardiovascular death in diabetic subjects with or without a prior history of CAD or CHF over a 5-year period when compared with placebo.[34]

Insulin

Studies have evaluated the role of strict glycemic control in diabetic patients during the acute phase of MI. The blood glucose level may increase in proportion to infarct size and hemodynamic stress in nondiabetic patients with MI as catecholamines, cortisol, and growth hormone are released. These hormones may create "transient" insulin resistance, with serum glucose returning to normal at discharge. In some cases, a very high admission glucose level out of proportion to infarct size indicates previously undiagnosed diabetes. Nevertheless, substantial evidence points to the admission glucose level as an independent predictor of early and late mortality after MI in patients with and without diabetes mellitus.[35]

Aggressive control of plasma glucose levels during the treatment of myocardial ischemia in diabetic patients can improve outcomes. In the Diabetes and Insulin-Glucose Infusion in Acute Myocardial Infarction (DIGAMI) study, 620 diabetic patients with acute MI were randomly assigned to either intensive insulin therapy (insulin-glucose infusion for 24 hours, followed by subcutaneous insulin injection for at least 3 months) or a standard glycemic control strategy.[36] Those receiving the intensive insulin regimen had a lower blood glucose level during the first hour (9.6 versus 11.7 mmol/liter, $p < 0.01$) and at discharge (8.2 versus 9.0 mmol/liter, $p < 0.01$) than the control group. During the first year of follow-up, a significant reduction in mortality was seen in the intensive insulin group compared with the conventionally treated group (19 versus 26 percent, $p = 0.027$). Mortality remained lower in the intensive control group through 3.4 years than in the conventional care group (33 versus 44 percent, $p = 0.011$).[37] Predictors of mortality were age, history of CHF, diabetes duration, admission glucose, and admission hemoglobin (Hb) A_{1c} level. The subgroup whose diabetes had been managed with diet or oral hypoglycemic drugs before infarction enjoyed the greatest survival benefit. A study of diabetic patients undergoing coronary artery bypass graft (CABG) surgery showed that continuous insulin infusion compared with subcutaneous insulin treatment reduced mortality (2.5 versus 5.3 percent, $p < 0.0001$.[38] Although no placebo group was reported, mortality in the insulin infusion group was significantly less than predicted by Society of Thoracic Surgeons risk model.

Several mechanisms may explain the findings of the DIGAMI trial. Insulin-glucose infusion may (1) increase the availability of glucose as a substrate for adenosine triphosphate (ATP) generation in cardiac muscle; (2) reduce lipolysis and decrease the generation of free fatty acids, which can impair myocardial contractility and trigger ventricular arrhythmia; and (3) shift cardiac metabolism from free fatty acid oxidation to glycolysis. In addition, tight glycemic control can reverse hyperglycemia-induced platelet reactivity and reduce the typically elevated PAI-1 activity in patients with diabetes. Part of the benefit derived from the use of insulin in the tight control arm may have resulted from the removal of any potential cardiac risk associated with the use of sulfonylureas (see later).

Infusion of glucose-insulin-potassium (GIK) solution, originally used in the 1960s and 1970s as a polarizing agent to maintain electrical stability, is regaining favor as a method to influence myocardial metabolism positively during treatment of MI, coronary revascularization procedures, and CABG surgery. A meta-analysis of nine studies including 1932 patients conducted between 1965 and 1987 concluded that GIK infusion reduced in-hospital mortality from 21 to 16.1 percent.[39] However, only two of the studies were double blind, and no information about diabetic patients was provided. In a prospective, randomized, open-label study of GIK infusion in 940 patients undergoing percutaneous transluminal coronary angioplasty (PTCA) for an acute MI, no mortality benefit was seen in the GIK group compared with the placebo group.[40] Although there seemed to be a benefit in the diabetic subgroup, in which GIK infusion reduced mortality from 12.2 to 4 percent, the small size of the subgroup and the small number of deaths prevented this effect from reaching statistical significance. In diabetic patients undergoing elective CABG surgery, GIK infusion beneficially influenced metabolism, as indicated by an elimination of myocardial extraction of nonesterified fatty acids and an increase in myocardial uptake of lactate and glucose.[41] Patients treated with GIK infusion during CABG may have a reduced prevalence of atrial fibrillation, enhanced cardiac function, and faster recovery than those who do not receive this treatment.[42] Further prospective studies are necessary to determine the long-term effect of GIK infusion in diabetic patients treated for MI or acute coronary syndromes.

Heart Failure

Heart failure, the pathophysiological state in which the heart is unable to maintain cardiac output sufficient to meet the metabolic needs of the body, and its attendant morbidity and mortality continue to be a growing problem in the United States. Although MI and hypertension are the most common risk factors associated with CHF, diabetes mellitus is also a strong and independent risk factor. In the Framingham Heart Study (Fig. 51–1), men with diabetes had an age- and risk factor–adjusted hazard ratio for CHF of 1.82 (95 percent CI = 1.28 to 2.58) compared with men without diabetes.[43] The hazard ratio in diabetic women was even larger, 3.73 (CI = 1.49 to 3.21). Patients with diabetes account for more than 33 percent of hospital admissions for heart failure, clearly a disproportionately high fraction.[44]

Not only are diabetic patients at higher risk for CHF, but the diabetic patients who develop CHF have a worse prognosis than those without diabetes. In the Studies of Left Ventricular Dysfunction (SOLVD) trials and registry, diabetic patients with symptomatic heart failure or asymptomatic left ventricular dysfunction had an increased risk of all-cause mortality (risk ratio = 1.29, CI = 1.10 to 1.50) and hospitalization for CHF (risk ratio = 1.55, CI = 1.32 to 1.82) during the average 37 months of follow-up.[4] The increased mortality was seen primarily in the diabetic patients with ischemic cardiomyopathy.[45]

Factors Responsible for the Increased Incidence of Heart Failure in Diabetic Patients

Coronary Heart Disease

As already noted, diabetes is a major risk factor for acute MI. Following an acute MI, the presence of diabetes increases the risk of developing new CHF.[1] Using the OASIS registry, which provided long-term data on 8013 patients with unstable coronary syndromes, Malmberg and colleagues showed that diabetes increases the risk of developing new CHF after hospitalization for unstable angina or non-Q-wave MI by 82 percent ($p < 0.001$; Fig. 51–2).[1] In diabetic patients with a history of previous CHD, the risk was considerably higher. The reasons for the increased incidence of CHF following an acute MI are not fully understood, but several factors may contribute. Diabetic patients may have a decreased awareness of pain or an atypical presentation of symptoms during an acute MI (Fig. 51–3).[30] These patients often delay seeking and receiving treatment, leading to more extensive and severe ischemic myocardial damage. In some cases, these patients suffer unrecognized or silent MI, creating a myocardial substrate predisposed to develop heart failure. However, the increased incidence of heart failure in diabetes cannot be accounted for solely by more extensive or severe myocardial infarctions. When the data are adjusted to account for differences in infarct size and baseline risk factors, CHF still occurs much more often in patients with diabetes than in those without the disease.

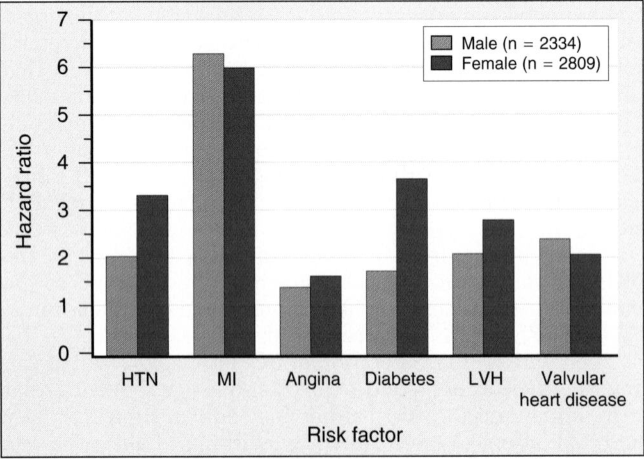

FIGURE 51–1 Risk factors for the development of heart failure in the Framingham Heart Study. In this study diabetes was defined as fasting blood glucose greater than 200 mg/dl or the use of insulin or an oral hypoglycemic agent. HTN = hypertension; LVH = left ventricular hypertrophy; MI = myocardial infarction. (From Levy D, Larson MG, Vasan RS, et al: The progression from hypertension to congestive heart failure. JAMA 275:1557, 1996.)

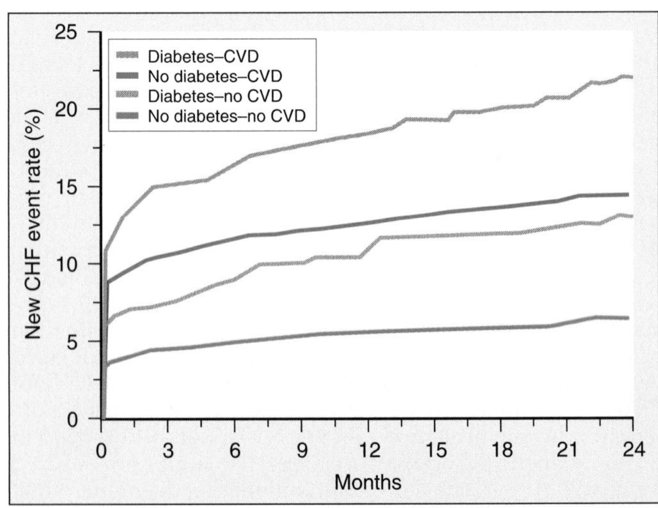

FIGURE 51–2 Heart failure is more prevalent in patients with type 2 diabetes than in those without diabetes after acute coronary syndrome. CHF = congestive heart failure; CVD = cardiovascular disease. (From Malmberg K, Yusuf S, Gerstein HC, et al: Impact of diabetes on long-term prognosis in patients with unstable angina and non-Q-wave myocardial infarction: Results of the OASIS [Organization to Assess Strategies for Ischemic Syndromes] Registry. Circulation 102:1014, 2000.)

Remodeling Following Myocardial Infarction
(see also Chap. 46)

Following a MI, the heart undergoes short- and long-term adaptation in response to the loss of contractile function, a process accentuated in diabetes. In the hours immediately after an acute MI, diabetic patients show less compensatory increase in contractility of noninfarcted myocardium than nondiabetic patients. This deficit persists over time, and thus the diabetic heart may be less capable of adapting to compensate for the loss of stroke volume than the nondiabetic heart. For example, Solomon and colleagues showed that left ventricular size increased less in diabetic patients than in nondiabetic patients in the 2 years following a MI, a difference associated with a twofold higher incidence of heart failure in the diabetic cohort.[46] The failure of the diabetic myocardium to remodel appropriately is probably due to a combination of factors associated with diabetic cardiomyopathy, including heart muscle metabolism, insufficient glucose transport, endothelial dysfunction and impaired control of myocardial blood flow, left ventricular fibrosis leading to impaired filling, and diabetic autonomic dysfunction.[30,47]

Diabetic Cardiomyopathy

The increased incidence of CHF and its poorer prognosis in diabetic patients compared with those without diabetes suggest alterations in the underlying myocardium in the diabetic patient, rendering it more susceptible to ischemia and less able to recover after an ischemic insult. Over the years, substantial evidence has accumulated that a specific, "true" diabetic cardiomyopathy distinct from ischemic injury does indeed exist. The exact prevalence, nature, and cause of cardiac dysfunction directly attributable to diabetes have given rise to considerable debate because other factors common in diabetes, such as hypertension, coronary atherosclerosis, and microvascular dysfunction, can independently impair myocardial performance (Fig. 51–4).

Epidemiological Evidence

Epidemiological studies using case-control analyses have confirmed the association between diabetes and idiopathic cardiomyopathy in men and in women, and have emphasized a possible interaction between diabetes and a history of hypertension. In men screened for the Multiple Risk Factor Intervention Trial (MRFIT) who had cardiomyopathy, diabetes was a risk factor for mortality. By combining the original Framingham Study cohort and the Framingham Offspring Study, gender-specific linear regression analysis probed the contribution of diabetes and glucose intolerance to age-adjusted echocardiographic parameters in more than 4500 men and women.[48] Diabetic individuals, particularly women, had higher heart rates, greater left ventricular wall thicknesses, and greater cardiac mass than unaffected subjects. In a reexamination of 2623 participants in the Framingham Offspring Study who had no history of myocardial infarction or heart failure, worsening glucose intolerance was associated with increasing left ventricular mass, a finding that was more significant ($p < 0.001$) in women than in men ($p = 0.054$).[48]

PATHOLOGICAL FINDINGS

Autopsy and biopsy specimens from diabetic patients with heart failure have revealed a number of morphological changes, including myocardial hypertrophy, myocyte hypertrophy, myofibril depletion, interstitial fibrosis, increased microvascular basement membrane thickness, increased matrix and basement membrane within arteriolar walls, and intramyocardial microangiopathy.[49] None of these lesions is specific to diabetes, and all can be found to some degree in cardiomyopathy of other etiologies. However, the coexistence of diabetes and other risk factors for cardiomyopathy can amplify the pathology. For example,

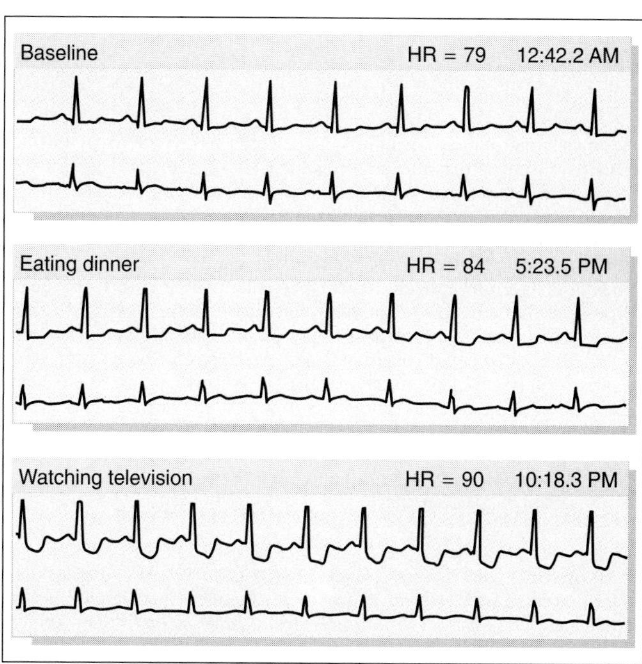

FIGURE 51–3 Holter ST segment monitoring shows no ST changes at baseline in the tracing **(top)**. Two episodes of ST depression **(middle, bottom)** are identified, demonstrating asymptomatic ischemia at rest. The lack of angina is due to cardiac autonomic neuropathy in diabetes. HR = heart rate.

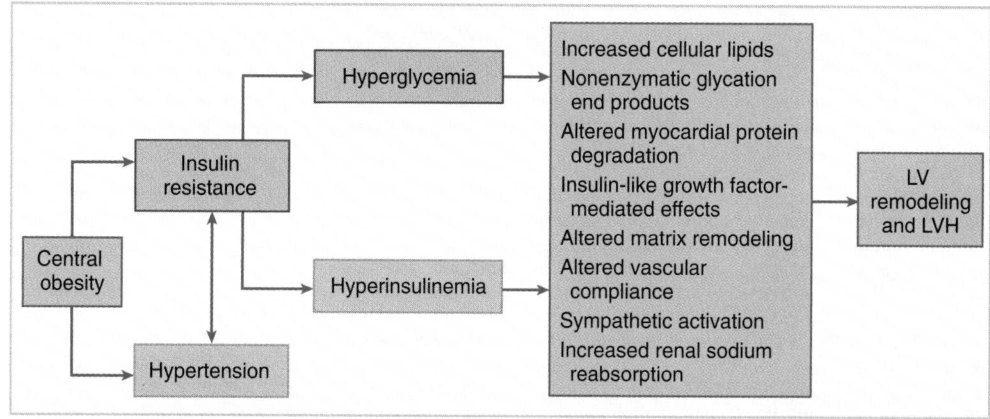

FIGURE 51–4 Central obesity is related to insulin resistance, hyperglycemia, and hyperinsulinemia and results in numerous mechanisms that may lead to remodeling of the left ventricle (LV) and left ventricular hypertrophy (LVH). Such mechanisms may also render the heart more vulnerable to maladaptive remodeling after myocardial injury. (From Rutter MK, Parise H, Benjamin EJ, et al: Impact of glucose intolerance and insulin resistance on cardiac structure and function: Sex-related differences in the Framingham Heart Study. Circulation 107:448, 2003.)

TABLE 51–1 Possible Contributors to Diabetic Cardiomyopathy
Collagen accumulation leading to decreased myocardial compliance
Accumulation of advanced glycosylation end product–modified extracellular matrix proteins causing diastolic dysfunction
Direct effects of altered energy substrate supply and utilization
Abnormal myocardial calcium handling leading to abnormal cardiac mechanics
Endothelial dysfunction characterized by decreased bioavailability of nitric oxide
Deposition of intramyocardial fat secondary to increased circulating free fatty acids
Cardiac autonomic neuropathy
Genetic abnormalities

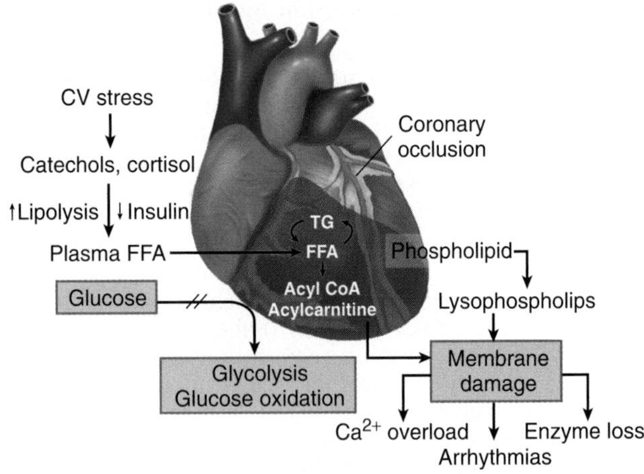

FIGURE 51–5 In the setting of insulin resistance, there is a release of free fatty acids (FFAs) from adipose tissue into the plasma. FFA becomes the dominant fuel for myocardial energy in the form of free fatty acid oxidation within cardiac myocytes. In addition, the rise in plasma free fatty acids leads to a decrease in glycolysis and glucose oxidation in these cells. Free fatty acid oxidation is a less efficient means of generating adenosine triphosphate than glucose oxidation (see text for details). CoA = coenzyme A; CV = cardiovascular; TG = triglyceride. (Adapted from Oliver MF, Opie LH: Effects of glucose and fatty acids on myocardial ischaemia and arrhythmias. Lancet 343:155, 1994.)

endomyocardial biopsy or autopsy specimens from patients with diabetes have shown that the ultrastructural changes, including capillary basement membrane thickening and interstitial and myocardial fibrosis, are accentuated by coexisting hypertension.[50]

Noninvasive methods have confirmed fibrosis as a key feature of the heart in diabetic patients without evident cardiac disease. Increased levels of collagen have been detected in patients with type 1 or type 2 diabetes, as have changes in left ventricular diastolic function.[51] Changes in left ventricular function can occur even in patients with well-controlled type 2 diabetes. One study used magnetic resonance imaging to measure left ventricular function in 12 asymptomatic normotensive newly diagnosed type 2 diabetic patients compared with 12 control subjects. The diabetic patients had normal left ventricular mass and systolic function, but all measures of left ventricular diastolic function were reduced compared with those in the control group.[52]

MECHANISMS OF DIABETIC CARDIOMYOPATHY
(Table 51-1)

ADVANCED GLYCATION END PRODUCTS. Because the lesions described earlier occur together in diabetes, the metabolic derangements of diabetes account for the morphological changes seen in the diabetic heart. AGEs accumulate in tissue exposed to hyperglycemia and are implicated in the morphological changes that occur in the diabetic heart. Accumulation of AGE-modified extracellular matrix results in inelasticity of the vessel wall and could interfere with myocardial function as well. Serum levels of AGEs correlate with microvascular and renal complications in type 1 diabetes. In 52 patients with type 1 diabetes, prolongation of the isovolumic relaxation time as assessed by Doppler echocardiography correlated with serum levels of AGEs after adjustment for age, diabetes duration, renal function, blood pressure, and autonomic function parameters.[53] Experimental studies in diabetic dogs have also shown decreased left ventricular compliance associated with intramyocardial deposition of collagen in the absence of hypertrophy.[54] These data help explain the clinical observation that diabetic patients can have CHF as a result of diastolic dysfunction in the absence of hypertension or increased wall thickness, or both.

MYOCARDIAL CALCIUM HANDLING. Abnormalities in myocardial calcium handling may also contribute to abnormal cardiac mechanics in the diabetic heart. Insulin-dependent diabetes impairs sarcoplasmic reticular Ca^{2+} pump activities, which reduces the rate of calcium removal from the cytoplasm in diastole.[55] Such alterations may contribute to the increased diastolic stiffness characteristic of diabetic cardiomyopathy. Diabetes-related changes in troponin T, the contractile regulatory protein of the thin myofilament, may also contribute to both diastolic and systolic dysfunction.

MYOCARDIAL METABOLISM (Fig. 51-5). The direct effects of hyperglycemia and insulin resistance on myocardial cellular metabolism may contribute to chronic left ventricular dysfunction (cardiomyopathy) in diabetes. Altered energy substrate supply and utilization may explain some of the morphological changes seen in the diabetic heart.[56,57] Type 2 diabetes has complex effects on the energy metabolism of the heart. Normally, the heart uses nonesterified (or "free") fatty acids as its primary energy source during aerobic perfusion at normal workloads and increasingly relies on glycolysis and pyruvate oxidation during periods of ischemia or increased work. Because of reduced glucose transport into cardiac myocytes, the diabetic heart can have an exaggerated impairment in ATP generation by glycolysis during ischemia. Accumulated free fatty acids and their oxidation products may also be directly toxic to the myocardial cells and thus contribute to the development of diabetic cardiomyopathy.[57]

CORONARY MICROCIRCULATION. Not only do diabetic patients suffer more severe and diffuse CAD,[58] but also, as noted previously, the structure and function of the coronary microcirculation may be abnormal in diabetes and contribute to the development of CHF. Endothelial dysfunction, characterized by reduced synthesis or bioavailability of the potent vasodilator nitric oxide, commonly occurs in the diabetic coronary vasculature and may lead to abnormal control of blood flow (see also Chap. 40). Despite endothelial dysfunction, resting coronary blood flow in diabetic subjects is normal or even slightly elevated.[59] However, diabetic patients have reduced capacity of the myocardial circulation to vasodilate. When maximal coronary blood flow is measured during intracoronary infusion of a non-endothelium-dependent vasodilator (e.g., papaverine, dipyridamole, adenosine), diabetic subjects exhibit a smaller increase, or coronary reserve, than nondiabetic subjects.[59,60]

The angiogenic response to ischemia also appears to be impaired in diabetes. In a study of 205 diabetic and 205 nondiabetic patients undergoing coronary angiography, Abaci and coworkers[61] determined functional collateral blood vessel formation. Collateral formation was significantly less in the diabetic cohort than in the normal subjects, and the authors speculated that this observation might explain why diabetic patients have such a poor prognosis following myocardial infarction. Others have reported substantially lower capillary density in diabetic patients who had experienced a MI than in patients without diabetes (with or without a previous MI) or in diabetic patients who had not had a prior MI.[62] This failure of the diabetic heart to mount an appropriate angiogenic response following a MI may contribute to diabetic cardiomyopathy.

FAILURE OF ISCHEMIC PRECONDITIONING. Ischemic preconditioning describes the observation that short periods of transient ischemia protect the myocardium against subsequent, longer ischemic insults. Evidence of this protective effect has been shown in animal experiments[63] and in human myocardial biopsy samples.[64] Diabetes appears to eliminate ischemic preconditioning in human myocardium.[64,65] The opening of myocardial adenosine triphosphate (ATP)-sensitive potassium (K_{ATP}) channels is an essential factor in ischemic preconditioning, and the clinical use of sulfonylureas, which block K_{ATP} channels, by type 2 diabetic patients has engendered controversy, as discussed in more detail in a later section.

Reducing the Risk of Heart Failure in Diabetes

Glycemic Control

Poor glycemic control increases the risk of developing heart failure in diabetes.[66] Two studies clearly illustrate the relationship between glycemic control and the incidence of heart failure in diabetes. Iribarren and colleagues observed a group of 48,858 diabetic subjects with no history of heart failure for a median period of 2.2 years after measurement of Hb A_{1c} levels.[66] The incidence of hospitalizations for heart failure or death related to heart failure depended on baseline Hb A_{1c} in the diabetic cohort. The association was stronger in men than in women. In men, each absolute 1 percent increase in Hb A_{1c} was associated with a 12 percent increase (CI = 7 to 18 percent) in heart failure after adjustment for other factors, including use of ACE inhibitors, beta blockers, and incidence of MI during the follow-up period. In women, each absolute 1 percent increase in Hb A_{1c} was associated with a 4 percent increase (CI = −2 to 9 percent) in heart failure. A similar, although steeper, relationship was found in the United Kingdom Prospective Diabetes Study (UKPDS)[67] among 4585 participants with type 2 diabetes. During the 7.5- to 12.5-year follow-up period, each absolute 1 percent increase in average Hb A_{1c} was associated with a 16 percent increase in the incidence of heart failure ($p = 0.021$). These studies suggest that tight glycemic control might reduce the incidence of heart failure, and because no threshold was identified, the target Hb A_{1c} levels should be as close to normal as possible.

Control of Blood Pressure

Diabetes and hypertension often occur together, and this combination amplifies the morphological changes seen in diabetic cardiomyopathy. In UKPDS, systolic blood pressure was associated strongly with the incidence of nonfatal heart failure.[68] For each 10 mm Hg increase in systolic blood pressure, a 12 percent increase in the risk of heart failure ($p = 0.0028$) was observed. In the treatment phase of the study, 1148 hypertensive type 2 diabetic patients received either tight control (target blood pressure <150/85 mm Hg using either captopril or atenolol as the primary drug) or less tight control of blood pressure (target blood pressure <180/105 mm Hg avoiding the use of ACE inhibitors or beta blockers), and follow-up was for a median of 8.4 years.[69] The average blood pressure achieved in the two treatment groups was 144/82 mm Hg in the tight control group and 154/87 mm Hg in the less tight group. This small difference in average blood pressure was associated with a large difference in the incidence of heart failure—the incidence of heart failure fell by 56 percent in the tight control group compared with the less tight control group (2.77 versus 6.15 percent, $p = 0.0043$). In the tight control group, those treated with captopril or those treated with atenolol showed no difference in the incidence of heart failure (3.00 versus 2.51 percent, $p = 0.66$).[70]

The Antihypertensive and Lipid-Lowering Treatment to Prevent Heart Attack Trial (ALLHAT) addressed the issue of whether a certain class of antihypertensive drugs might more effectively reduce the incidence of heart failure in hypertensive diabetic patients.[71] In ALLHAT, a calcium channel blocker (amlodipine) or an ACE inhibitor (lisinopril) was compared with a thiazide diuretic (chlorthalidone) as first-line therapy for their ability to prevent cardiovascular events in 33,357 hypertensive subjects, 36 percent of whom were diabetic at baseline. During the average 4.9-year follow-up, the incidence of new-onset heart failure in the diabetic patients was significantly lower in the thiazide diuretic group than in either of the other treatment groups. The Second Australian National Blood Pressure Study had few diabetic patients and showed no treatment-dependent difference in the incidence of heart failure.[72]

Medical Therapy to Treat or Prevent Heart Failure in Diabetic Patients

The goals of treatment of left ventricular dysfunction and heart failure in diabetic patients are the same as those in nondiabetic patients: relief of pulmonary congestion, slowing the progression of the disease, and prolonging survival. In general, drug therapies for heart failure have similar if not better efficacy in diabetic patients than in those without the disease.

Beta-Adrenergic Blocking Agents

As noted earlier, beta blockers reduce mortality and reinfarction in diabetic patients after a MI. These benefits also extend to diabetic patients with heart failure of various severities.[73-79] The mortality benefit in patients with heart failure has been seen with nonselective beta blockers (e.g., bucindolol[73,79]), with cardioselective beta blockers (e.g., metoprolol[75]), and with a nonselective beta blocker that also blocks $alpha_1$-adrenergic receptors (carvedilol[77,80]). Beta blockers with intrinsic sympathomimetic activity, such as pindolol, may be contraindicated in patients with heart failure, particularly in diabetic patients with heart failure. Carvedilol may offer advantages in the diabetic patients because of its favorable effects on insulin sensitivity and plasma lipid profile as well as its peripheral vasodilating activity. In the Carvedilol Or Metoprolol European Trial (COMET), patients with New York Heart Association (NYHA) Class II to IV heart failure were randomly assigned to either carvedilol or metoprolol and observed for a mean of 5 years.[80] All-cause mortality was reduced by 17 percent in the carvedilol group compared with the metoprolol group. A similar benefit of carvedilol was seen in the 24 percent of the study population who were diabetic at baseline.

Angiotensin-Converting Enzyme Inhibitors

ACE inhibitors clearly and convincingly reduce the morbidity and mortality associated with left ventricular dysfunction, but the early studies lacked sufficient power to address rigorously the question of whether ACE inhibitors could influence the morbidity and mortality associated with diabetes and heart failure. Several more recent studies have addressed these questions and have shown that, indeed, ACE inhibitors are effective in diabetic patients.

In GISSI-3, lisinopril reduced 6-week and 6-month mortality in the diabetic subgroup when started within 24 hours of an acute MI but did not affect the incidence of heart failure or other signs of left ventricular dysfunction.[31] In the TRACE study,[32] patients with an enzyme-confirmed acute MI and left ventricular dysfunction (left ventricular ejection fraction ≤35 percent) present 2 to 6 days after the MI were randomly assigned to receive either the ACE inhibitor trandolapril or matching placebo. In the diabetic group, trandolapril reduced the rate of progression to severe heart failure by 62 percent ($p < 0.001$), a beneficial effect not seen in those without diabetes (Fig. 51–6).

Angiotensin II Receptor Blockers

In three major studies involving patients with chronic heart failure, angiotensin II receptor blockers (ARBs) have demonstrated rough equivalence to ACE inhibitors in preventing morbidity and mortality associated with heart failure.[81-83] However, this benefit may be smaller in the diabetic cohort.[82,83] Two studies of the ARB losartan suggest that this

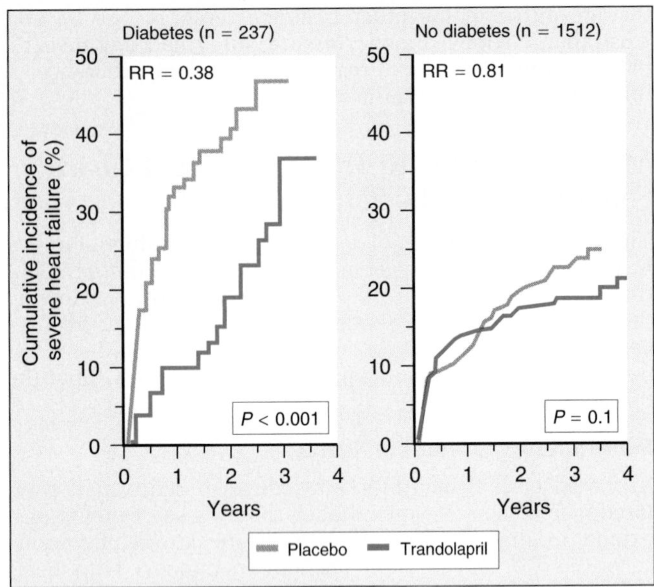

FIGURE 51–6 The Trandolapril Cardiac Evaluation (TRACE) study was carried out in patients with myocardial infarction with congestive heart failure (CHF), depressed ejection fraction, and anterior infarction. The diabetic cohort demonstrated the benefit of trandolapril in a reduction of the high incidence of early and late CHF in patients with diabetes. RR = relative risk. (From Gustafsson I, Torp-Pedersen C, Kober L, et al: Effect of the angiotensin-converting enzyme inhibitor trandolapril on mortality and morbidity in diabetic patients with left ventricular dysfunction after acute myocardial infarction. TRACE Study Group. J Am Coll Cardiol 34:83, 1999%.)

pharmacological class may prevent heart failure in type 2 diabetes. In the Reduction in Endpoints in NIDDM with the Angiotensin II Antagonist Losartan (RENAAL) study,[84] type 2 diabetic patients with nephropathy and no history of heart failure received either losartan or placebo in addition to conventional antihypertensive therapy. In addition to slowing of the progression of kidney failure over the 4-year study, the incidence of heart failure was reduced by 32 percent in the losartan group ($p = 0.005$). In the Losartan Intervention For Endpoint Reduction (LIFE) study, 1195 diabetic patients with hypertension and signs of left ventricular hypertrophy were randomly assigned either losartan or atenolol as the primary antihypertensive agent and were observed for an average of 4.7 years.[85] Not only was the incidence of the primary composite endpoint (cardiovascular death, MI, or stroke) reduced but hospitalizations for heart failure also fell by 41 percent ($p = 0.013$).

ARBs are well tolerated and have an excellent safety record. With ARBs, unlike ACE inhibitors, the incidence of cough is no higher than in patients treated with placebo and angioedema occurs rarely. However, despite these advantages, until results of clinical studies clearly demonstrate superiority or equivalence to ACE inhibitors in the treatment of heart failure, ARBs should probably be reserved for patients who are unable to tolerate ACE inhibition. Currently, only valsartan is approved for this indication

Aldosterone Antagonists

Aldosterone was traditionally thought to contribute to the pathophysiology of heart failure only through its action to increase sodium retention and potassium excretion. However, aldosterone may stimulate directly the production of inflammatory mediators, cause myocardial fibrosis, and promote endothelial dysfunction and vascular stiffening.[86,87] Evidence of the benefit of blocking aldosterone receptors was presented in the results of the Eplerenone Post-Acute Myocardial Infarction Heart Failure Efficacy and Survival Study (EPHESUS).[88] In EPHESUS, the mineralocorticoid-selective aldosterone antagonist eplerenone was added to optimal therapy (usually ACE inhibition 87 percent, beta blockade 75 percent, diuretics 60 percent, and aspirin 88 percent) in patients who had suffered a recent myocardial infarction with documented reduction in left ventricular ejection fraction and symptoms of heart failure. With this treatment, compared with placebo, the risk of death from cardiovascular causes or hospitalizations for cardiovascular causes was reduced by 13 percent ($p = 0.002$). This benefit was similar in diabetic patients, who were 32 percent of the total population of patients, but the study was not powered to evaluate the effect fully in this subgroup.

Treating Diabetes in Patients with Coronary Heart Disease, Acute Coronary Syndromes, or Heart Failure

Sulfonylureas

In the 1970s, evidence emerged that suggested that the sulfonylurea tolbutamide increased cardiovascular mortality and CAD compared with results for patients with type 2 diabetes treated with insulin. The sulfonylureas induce insulin release through a mechanism involving the blocking of K_{ATP} channels in pancreatic beta cells. The discovery that K_{ATP} channels also exist in the myocardium and that blocking them with sulfonylureas prevented ischemic preconditioning, a cardioprotective mechanism, and attenuated coronary vasodilation in animal models[63] suggested a mechanism by which these drugs might promote ischemic injury in diabetic patients. However, the results reported in the UKPDS argue strongly against a proischemic class effect of sulfonylureas. That prospective, randomized study reported the impact of tight glycemic control using a variety of treatment strategies on the incidence and severity of microvascular and macrovascular complications in newly diagnosed diabetes.[89] Patients treated with chlorpropamide or glibenclamide had a rate of myocardial infarction and sudden death over the 10-year follow-up similar to that of patients treated with insulin.

Ischemic preconditioning can be demonstrated with human myocardial biopsy samples[64] and in patients undergoing angioplasty.[90] The presence of diabetes itself appears to attenuate or eliminate ischemic preconditioning in the human heart,[64,65] and certain sulfonylureas may further inhibit this phenomenon. The discovery that cardiac and vascular K_{ATP} channels are structurally distinct from those in the pancreatic beta cells[91] stimulated studies that describe differences in specificity that sulfonylureas may exhibit toward these receptor subtypes. Although clinical extrapolation of these observations is complex, functional differences among the sulfonylureas exist that may have important implications in the treatment of diabetes in patients with CHD. For example, in a double-blind, placebo-controlled study, glibenclamide, but not glimepiride, prevented electrocardiographic evidence of ischemic preconditioning in nondiabetic patients undergoing elective balloon angioplasty of high-grade coronary artery stenoses.[90] A similar difference in response to ischemia has been reported in diabetic patients chronically treated with either glimepiride or glibenclamide.[92] Sulfonylureas may be either proarrhythmic or antiarrhythmic, depending on the presence or absence of ischemia, as a result of the role of the K_{ATP} channel in regulating the duration of the cardiac action potential.[63]

Despite these controversies, this class of hypoglycemic drugs is widely used, given the well-established benefits of improved glycemic control in preventing diabetes-related microvascular complications. However, the choice of specific sulfonylureas for patients with diabetes on the basis of the presence or absence of coronary disease remains unclear at this time.

Thiazolidinediones

Thiazolidinediones (TZDs) decrease glucose levels in type 2 diabetes by increasing the sensitivity to insulin in target tissues.[93] TZDs can increase the incidence of edema, raising concern about the use of these drugs in heart failure.[94] In addition to their glucose lowering ability, these agents induce a wide variety of effects mediated through activation of the PPAR gamma nuclear receptor on liquids, thrombosis, inflammation, and endothelial function that may benefit the cardiovascular system.[94a] An increase in the incidence of heart failure or exacerbation of symptoms has been reported for both rosiglitazone and pioglitazone, particularly when administered concomitantly with insulin.[95] Neither drug is recommended for use in patients with NYHA Class III or IV heart failure.

Metformin

Metformin (dimethylbiguanide) lowers blood glucose both by increasing insulin sensitivity and by decreasing hepatic glucose output.[96] Although epidemiological studies had suggested that the addition of metformin to sulfonylurea therapy was associated with increased mortality, a population-based cohort study involving 12,272 subjects with newly diagnosed type 2 diabetes reported significantly reduced mortality in those treated with metformin monotherapy or metformin combined with a sulfonylurea compared with the patients treated with sulfonylurea monotherapy during the average 5.1-year follow-up.[97]

Lactic acidosis is a rare but potentially life-threatening complication of metformin use, with a reported incidence of about 0.03 cases per 1000 patient-years of use and with a fatality rate of about 50 percent.[98] It occurs more commonly in patients with renal insufficiency or with tissue hypoperfusion and hypoxemia. Because patients with heart failure are at higher risk for hypoperfusion or hypoxemia, the use of metformin is contraindicated in those with CHF who require pharmacological treatment.[98]

Coronary Revascularization

Percutaneous Transluminal Coronary Angioplasty

(see also Chap. 52)

Large-scale trials generally have not shown a benefit of aggressive revascularization after thrombolytic therapy for acute myocardial infarction. Similar considerations apply to diabetic patients. Although diabetic and nondiabetic patients have similar rates of initial angioplasty success, diabetic patients have higher restenosis rates after PTCA[99] and worse long-term outcomes.[100,101]

Diabetic patients also have a higher risk of in-hospital mortality, restenosis, and long-term mortality after coronary artery stenting and atherectomy.[102] Although stenting has reduced restenosis rates in both diabetic and nondiabetic patients, diabetic patients have smaller lumina in the stented vessels and a significantly higher restenosis rate (55 versus 20 percent, $p = 0.001$) within 4 months of the procedure despite similar baseline and procedural characteristics. The mechanism underlying the increased restenosis rate in diabetes after coronary intervention is unclear. Serial intravascular ultrasonography has suggested that exaggerated intimal hyperplasia develops in diabetic patients after intervention.[103] A histological study found increased collagen-rich fibrous tissue in atherectomy specimens from diabetic patients.[104] Clinical trials of paclitaxel- and sirolimus-eluting stents have shown dramatic reductions in the restenosis rates in the general population of patients.[105,106] Although similar benefit has been observed in diabetic patients, the total number of diabetic patients studied has been small, and the studies excluded patients with multivessel disease.[107]

Coronary Artery Bypass Graft Surgery

Most studies comparing outcomes in diabetic and nondiabetic patients undergoing CABG surgery show an increased risk of postoperative death, 30-day and long-term mortality, and an increased need for subsequent reoperation in the diabetic population.[108] Although diabetic patients have a worse risk profile, tend to be older, and have more extensive CAD and poorer left ventricular function than nondiabetic patients,[109] their higher long-term mortality does not depend entirely on these factors and continues to diverge from that in nondiabetic patients during long-term follow-up. The difference probably reflects accelerated disease progression in both the nonbypassed and the bypassed native coronary vessels.

The Bypass Angioplasty Revascularization Investigation (BARI) trial, which included 641 patients with and 2962 patients without diabetes, evaluated the role of CABG in diabetic patients.[110] Five-year mortality was higher in diabetic patients. Q wave myocardial infarction occurred more frequently in diabetic patients (8 versus 4 percent). CABG significantly reduced the mortality after a myocardial infarction when compared with angioplasty, whereas no such protective effect of surgery was noted in nondiabetic patients experiencing a myocardial infarction. After 7 years, CABG showed an even more pronounced benefit over PTCA in patients with treated diabetes.[111]

Coronary Artery Bypass Graft Versus Percutaneous Transluminal Coronary Angioplasty

In general, randomized trials comparing PTCA with CABG have reported similar outcomes. However, in patients with diabetes CABG may provide better outcomes than classical PTCA, especially in patients with three-vessel disease.[112,113] The BARI trial, which randomly assigned patients with multivessel disease to CABG or PTCA, reported that bypass surgery in treated diabetic patients yielded a higher survival rate at 5 years than PTCA (81 versus 66 percent, $p = 0.003$).[113] The benefit of CABG accrued primarily in patients receiving internal mammary artery conduits. Cardiac mortality was 2.9 percent when an internal mammary artery graft was used compared with 18.2 percent when only saphenous vein grafts were used, a mortality similar to that observed with PTCA.[113] Diabetic patients undergoing stenting for multivessel disease may also have a worse outcome than those undergoing CABG. In the Arterial Revascularization Therapy Study (ARTS), the 208 patients with diabetes who underwent percutaneous revascularization had a lower 1-year survival (63 percent) than those undergoing CABG (84 percent).[114] In contrast, no difference was detected in the Veterans Affairs Angina With Extremely Serious Operative Mortality Evaluation (AWESOME) study between diabetic patients who underwent PTCA (54 percent with stents) and those who underwent CABG.[115] Survival was similar in the two groups at 30 days, 6 months, and 36 months.

Cardiovascular Autonomic Neuropathy

(see also Chap. 87)

Cardiovascular autonomic neuropathy (CAN) probably contributes to the poor prognosis of CHD and CHF in both type 1 and type 2 diabetes mellitus. The majority of patients with CAN come to clinical attention with complaints of postural hypotension, resting tachycardia, exercise intolerance, or painless myocardial ischemia or infarction. The risk for CAN depends on the duration of diabetes and the degree of glycemic control and tends to parallel the development of other end-organ disease related to diabetes such as retinopathy, nephropathy, and vasculopathy.[116] Symptoms and signs of CAN often occur relatively late in the natural history of this complication. Because reliable and quantitative noninvasive methods to assess autonomic function have become available, the diagnosis of CAN may now precede the development of symptoms. Most clinicians regard CAN as a major complication of type 1 diabetes because the challenge of managing this complication often dominates the care of these patients. CAN tends to be less fully expressed in patients with type 2 diabetes, who are typically older and have a wider variety of comorbid conditions.

DIAGNOSIS. A variety of tests can assess parasympathetic and sympathetic function in diabetes. A series of bedside maneuvers can aid in the diagnosis of CAN and differentiate the relative contribution of parasympathetic and sympathetic dysfunction in CAN. These tests use the electrocardiogram to measure beat-to-beat heart rate variation during deep breathing, at assumption of an upright posture, and during the Valsalva maneuver.[12] Tests that can detect the presence of CAN before symptoms develop include methods that assess heart rate variability during 24-hour recordings and thereby permit detection of subtle disorders in autonomic balance. Cardiac radionuclide imaging with the norepinephrine analog metaiodobenzylguanidine (MIBG) can directly image the sympathetic nerve activity of the myocardium. Diabetic individuals generally have less myocardial MIBG uptake with more pronounced regional differences from base to apex than patients without diabetes. In addition, positron-emission tomographic scanning with the sympathetic neurotransmitter analog ^{11}C-labeled hydroxyephedrine can evaluate myocardial sympathetic innervation. These noninvasive methods, alone or in combination with the standard bedside examination, can establish the presence and severity of CAN and can be used to evaluate the effects of interventions.

PREVALENCE. The reported prevalence of CAN varies with the populations studied and methods used. Regardless of this variation, CAN appears to be common in diabetes. A summary of 15 reports on CAN suggests that the prevalence is between 2.6 and 90 percent in the diabetic population, with an average prevalence of about 30 percent.[12]

PROGNOSIS. Numerous studies have documented increased mortality in diabetic patients with CAN. Maser and colleagues[117] have reviewed 15 studies involving a total of 2900 diabetic patients with and without evidence of CAN. During the follow-up period, which ranged from 0.5 to 16 years, mortality was consistently higher in the patients with CAN (30 percent) than in those without CAN at baseline (13 percent). A pooled estimate of the hazard ratio for CAN in these studies was 3.45 (CI 2.66 to 4.47, $p < 0.001$) for studies using two or more indicators of CAN and 1.20 (CI 1.02 to 1.41, $p = 0.03$) for studies using only one measure to define CAN.

The mechanisms by which CAN increases mortality remain uncertain (Table 51–2). Part of this association may derive from the high prevalence of other complications and risk factors in diabetic patients with CAN. For example, the progression of microvascular complications, such as diabetic nephropathy, appears to parallel that of CAN and can result in an increase in cardiovascular risk related to hypertension and dyslipidemia.[12] CAN may also decrease the perception of myocardial ischemia. Clinicians have long recognized that diabetic patients often experience fewer ischemic symptoms such as angina than do nondiabetic patients. Thus, compared with nondiabetic individuals with exercise-limited ischemia, diabetic individuals with CAN are less likely to be limited by angina at the time of ST segment depression.[118] Resting tachycardia, an early manifestation of parasympathetic denervation of CAN, increases myocardial oxygen demand and can place the diabetic patient with CAN closer to the ischemic threshold. In addition, CAN can cause abnormal coronary blood flow regulation. Thus, CAN may provoke ischemic episodes by upsetting the balance between myocardial supply and demand.[118]

Sudden cardiovascular death may be related to CAN in diabetic individuals. Prolongation of the QT interval in diabetic patients correlates with the degree of autonomic neuropathy and may predispose these individuals to serious arrhythmias and sudden death.[12,118] The presence of QT dispersion on the 12-lead electrocardiogram reflects dispersion of ventricular refractoriness and an increased risk for arrhythmia. In a study of 471 patients with type 2 diabetes, both QT dispersion and prolongation of the QT interval independently predicted cardiovascular and coronary mortality during the median 5.7-year follow-up.[119]

TABLE 51–2 Cardiovascular Autonomic Neuropathy and Increased Cardiovascular Morbidity and Mortality in Diabetes Mellitus—Possible Mechanisms

Impaired angina recognition Silent ischemia and infarction
Decreased threshold for ischemia Increased resting heart rate and blunted chronotropic response to exercise Impaired coronary vasomotor regulation
Prolonged QT interval Increased lethal arrhythmias and sudden death (with or without myocardial ischemia)
Abnormal diastolic and systolic function Contributes to diabetic cardiomyopathy Increased cardiac mass Adversely affects the natural history of congestive heart failure
Increased perioperative risk Increased need for hemodynamic support Reduced hypoxia-induced respiratory drive
Alteration of normal circadian variation of sympathovagal activity Lack of normal nighttime decrease in blood pressure Loss of nighttime protection against myocardial infarction
Increased prevalence of other cardiovascular risk factors and other complications Increased microvascular complications Increased rate of progression of glomerulopathy Increased prevalence of hypertension and dyslipidemias

REFERENCES

Scope of the Problem

1. Malmberg K, Yusuf S, Gerstein HC, et al: Impact of diabetes on long-term prognosis in patients with unstable angina and non-Q-wave myocardial infarction: Results of the OASIS (Organization to Assess Strategies for Ischemic Syndromes) Registry. Circulation 102:1014, 2000.
2. Mukamal KJ, Nesto RW, Cohen MC, et al: Impact of diabetes on long-term survival after acute myocardial infarction: Comparability of risk with prior myocardial infarction. Diabetes Care 24:1422, 2001.
3. Nichols GA, Hillier TA, Erbey JR, et al: Congestive heart failure in type 2 diabetes: Prevalence, incidence, and risk factors. Diabetes Care 24:1614, 2001.
4. Shindler DM, Kostis JB, Yusuf S, et al: Diabetes mellitus, a predictor of morbidity and mortality in the Studies of Left Ventricular Dysfunction (SOLVD) Trials and Registry. Am J Cardiol 77:1017, 1996.
5. Moreno PR, Murcia AM, Palacios IF, et al: Coronary composition and macrophage infiltration in atherectomy specimens from patients with diabetes mellitus. Circulation 102:2180, 2000.
6. Colwell JA, Nesto RW: The platelet in diabetes: Focus on prevention of ischemic events. Diabetes Care 26:2181, 2003.
7. Sobel BE, Woodcock-Mitchell J, Schneider DJ, et al: Increased plasminogen activator inhibitor type 1 in coronary artery atherectomy specimens from type 2 diabetic compared with nondiabetic patients: A potential factor predisposing to thrombosis and its persistence. Circulation 97:2213, 1998.
8. Pandolfi A, Cetrullo D, Polishuck R, et al: Plasminogen activator inhibitor type 1 is increased in the arterial wall of type II diabetic subjects. Arterioscler Thromb Vasc Biol 21:1378, 2001.
9. Cosentino F, Eto M, De Paolis P, et al: High glucose causes upregulation of cyclooxygenase-2 and alters prostanoid profile in human endothelial cells: Role of protein kinase C and reactive oxygen species. Circulation 107:1017, 2003.
10. Cardillo C, Campia U, Bryant MB, et al: Increased activity of endogenous endothelin in patients with type II diabetes mellitus. Circulation 106:1783, 2002.
11. Ford ES: Body mass index, diabetes, and C-reactive protein among U.S. adults. Diabetes Care 22:1971, 1999.
12. Vinik AI, Maser RE, Mitchell BD, et al: Diabetic autonomic neuropathy. Diabetes Care 26:1553, 2003.

Medical Therapy of Acute Coronary Syndromes

13. Taubert G, Winkelmann BR, Schleiffer T, et al: Prevalence, predictors, and consequences of unrecognized diabetes mellitus in 3266 patients scheduled for coronary angiography. Am Heart J 145:285, 2003.
14. Norhammar A, Tenerz A, Nilsson G, et al: Glucose metabolism in patients with acute myocardial infarction and no previous diagnosis of diabetes mellitus: A prospective study. Lancet 359:2140, 2002.

15. Wahab NN, Cowden EA, Pearce NJ, et al: Is blood glucose an independent predictor of mortality in acute myocardial infarction in the thrombolytic era? J Am Coll Cardiol 40:1748, 2002.
16. Norhammar AM, Ryden L, Malmberg K: Admission plasma glucose. Independent risk factor for long-term prognosis after myocardial infarction even in nondiabetic patients. Diabetes Care 22:1827, 1999.
17. Colwell JA: Aspirin therapy in diabetes. Diabetes Care 26:S87, 2003.
18. A randomised, blinded, trial of clopidogrel versus aspirin in patients at risk of ischaemic events (CAPRIE). CAPRIE Steering Committee. Lancet 348:1329, 1996.
19. Bhatt DL, Marso SP, Hirsch AT, et al: Amplified benefit of clopidogrel versus aspirin in patients with diabetes mellitus. Am J Cardiol 90:625, 2002.
20. Yusuf S, Zhao F, Mehta SR, et al: Effects of clopidogrel in addition to aspirin in patients with acute coronary syndromes without ST-segment elevation. N Engl J Med 345:494, 2001.
21. Lincoff AM: Important triad in cardiovascular medicine: Diabetes, coronary intervention, and platelet glycoprotein IIb/IIIa receptor blockade. Circulation 107:1556, 2003.
22. Kereiakes DJ, Lincoff AM, Anderson KM, et al: Abciximab survival advantage following percutaneous coronary intervention is predicted by clinical risk profile. Am J Cardiol 90:628, 2002.
23. Topol EJ, Mark DB, Lincoff AM, et al: Outcomes at 1 year and economic implications of platelet glycoprotein IIb/IIIa blockade in patients undergoing coronary stenting: Results from a multicentre randomised trial. EPISTENT Investigators. Evaluation of Platelet IIb/IIIa Inhibitor for Stenting. Lancet 354:2019, 1999.
24. Labinaz M, Madan M, O'Shea JO, et al: Comparison of one-year outcomes following coronary artery stenting in diabetic versus nondiabetic patients (from the Enhanced Suppression of the Platelet IIb/IIIa Receptor With Integrilin Therapy [ESPRIT] trial). Am J Cardiol 90:585, 2002.
25. Roffi M, Chew DP, Mukherjee D, et al: Platelet glycoprotein IIb/IIIa inhibitors reduce mortality in diabetic patients with non-ST-segment-elevation acute coronary syndromes. Circulation 104:2767, 2001.
26. Heitzer T, Ollmann I, Koke K, et al: Platelet glycoprotein IIb/IIIa receptor blockade improves vascular nitric oxide bioavailability in patients with coronary artery disease. Circulation 108:536, 2003.
27. Chen J, Marciniak TA, Radford MJ, et al: Beta-blocker therapy for secondary prevention of myocardial infarction in elderly diabetic patients. Results from the National Cooperative Cardiovascular Project. J Am Coll Cardiol 34:1388, 1999.
28. Shorr RI, Ray WA, Daugherty JR, et al: Antihypertensives and the risk of serious hypoglycemia in older persons using insulin or sulfonylureas. JAMA 278:40, 1997.
29. Gress TW, Nieto FJ, Shahar E, et al: Hypertension and antihypertensive therapy as risk factors for type 2 diabetes mellitus. N Engl J Med 342:905, 2000.
30. Nesto RW, Zarich S: Acute myocardial infarction in diabetes mellitus: Lessons learned from ACE inhibition. Circulation 97:12, 1998.
31. Zuanetti G, Latini R, Maggioni AP, et al: Effect of the ACE inhibitor lisinopril on mortality in diabetic patients with acute myocardial infarction: Data from the GISSI-3 study. Circulation 96:4239, 1997.
32. Gustafsson I, Torp-Pedersen C, Køber L, et al: Effect of the angiotensin-converting enzyme inhibitor trandolapril on mortality and morbidity in diabetic patients with left ventricular dysfunction after acute myocardial infarction. Trace Study Group. J Am Coll Cardiol 34:83, 1999.
33. McFarlane SI, Kumar A, Sowers JR: Mechanisms by which angiotensin-converting enzyme inhibitors prevent diabetes and cardiovascular disease. Am J Cardiol 91:30H, 2003.
34. Effects of ramipril on cardiovascular and microvascular outcomes in people with diabetes mellitus: Results of the HOPE study and MICRO-HOPE substudy. Lancet 355:253, 2000.
35. Capes SE, Hunt D, Malmberg K, et al: Stress hyperglycaemia and increased risk of death after myocardial infarction in patients with and without diabetes: A systematic overview. Lancet 355:773, 2000.
36. Malmberg K, Ryden L, Efendic S, et al: Randomized trial of insulin-glucose infusion followed by subcutaneous insulin treatment in diabetic patients with acute myocardial infarction (DIGAMI study): Effects on mortality at 1 year. J Am Coll Cardiol 26:57, 1995.
37. Malmberg K, Norhammar A, Wedel H, et al: Glycometabolic state at admission: Important risk marker of mortality in conventionally treated patients with diabetes mellitus and acute myocardial infarction: Long-term results from the Diabetes and Insulin-Glucose Infusion in Acute Myocardial Infarction (DIGAMI) study. Circulation 99:2626, 1999.
38. Furnary AP, Gao G, Grunkemeier GL, et al: Continuous insulin infusion reduces mortality in patients with diabetes undergoing coronary artery bypass grafting. J Thorac Cardiovasc Surg 125:1007, 2003.
39. Fath-Ordoubadi F, Beatt KJ: Glucose-insulin-potassium therapy for treatment of acute myocardial infarction: An overview of randomized placebo-controlled trials. Circulation 96:1152, 1997.
40. van der Horst IC, Zijlstra F, van't Hof AW, et al: Glucose-insulin-potassium infusion inpatients treated with primary angioplasty for acute myocardial infarction: The glucose-insulin-potassium study: A randomized trial. J Am Coll Cardiol 42:784, 2003.
41. Szabo Z, Arnqvist H, Hakanson E, et al: Effects of high-dose glucose-insulin-potassium on myocardial metabolism after coronary surgery in patients with type II diabetes. Clin Sci (Lond) 101:37, 2001.
42. Lazar HL, Chipkin S, Philippides G, et al: Glucose-insulin-potassium solutions improve outcomes in diabetics who have coronary artery operations. Ann Thorac Surg 70:145, 2000.

Heart Failure

43. Levy D, Larson MG, Vasan RS, et al: The progression from hypertension to congestive heart failure. JAMA 275:1557, 1996.
44. Reis SE, Holubkov R, Edmundowicz D, et al: Treatment of patients admitted to the hospital with congestive heart failure: Specialty-related disparities in practice patterns and outcomes. J Am Coll Cardiol 30:733, 1997.
45. Dries DL, Sweitzer NK, Drazner MH, et al: Prognostic impact of diabetes mellitus in patients with heart failure according to the etiology of left ventricular systolic dysfunction. J Am Coll Cardiol 38:421, 2001.
46. Solomon SD, St John Sutton M, Lamas GA, et al: Ventricular remodeling does not accompany the development of heart failure in diabetic patients after myocardial infarction. Circulation 106:1251, 2002.
47. Standl E, Schnell O: A new look at the heart in diabetes mellitus: From ailing to failing. Diabetologia 43:1455, 2000.

Diabetic Cardiomyopathy

48. Rutter MK, Parise H, Benjamin EJ, et al: Impact of glucose intolerance and insulin resistance on cardiac structure and function: Sex-related differences in the Framingham Heart Study. Circulation 107:448, 2003.
49. Zarich SW, Nesto RW: Diabetic cardiomyopathy. Am Heart J 118:1000, 1989.
50. Kawaguchi M, Techigawara M, Ishihata T, et al: A comparison of ultrastructural changes on endomyocardial biopsy specimens obtained from patients with diabetes mellitus with and without hypertension. Heart Vessels 12:267, 1997.
51. Picano E: Diabetic cardiomyopathy. The importance of being earliest. J Am Coll Cardiol 42:454, 2003.
52. Diamant M, Lamb HJ, Groeneveld Y, et al: Diastolic dysfunction is associated with altered myocardial metabolism in asymptomatic normotensive patients with well-controlled type 2 diabetes mellitus. J Am Coll Cardiol 42:328, 2003.
53. Berg TJ, Snorgaard O, Faber J, et al: Serum levels of advanced glycation end products are associated with left ventricular diastolic function in patients with type 1 diabetes. Diabetes Care 22:1186, 1999.
54. Avendano GF, Agarwal RK, Bashey RI, et al: Effects of glucose intolerance on myocardial function and collagen-linked glycation. Diabetes 48:1443, 1999.
55. Pierce GN, Russell JC: Regulation of intracellular Ca^{2+} in the heart during diabetes. Cardiovasc Res 34:41, 1997.
56. Taegtmeyer H, McNulty P, Young ME: Adaptation and maladaptation of the heart in diabetes: Part I. Circulation 105:1727, 2002.
57. Young ME, McNulty P, Taegtmeyer H: Adaptation and maladaptation of the heart in diabetes: Part II. Circulation 105:1861, 2002.
58. Ledru F, Ducimetiere P, Battaglia S, et al: New diagnostic criteria for diabetes and coronary artery disease: Insights from an angiographic study. J Am Coll Cardiol 37:1543, 2001.
59. McDonagh PF, Hokama JY: Microvascular perfusion and transport in the diabetic heart. Microcirculation 7:163, 2000.
60. Pitkanen OP, Nuutila P, Raitakari OT, et al: Coronary flow reserve is reduced in young men with IDDM. Diabetes 47:248, 1998.
61. Abaci A, Oguzhan A, Kahraman S, et al: Effect of diabetes mellitus on formation of coronary collateral vessels. Circulation 99:2239, 1999.
62. Yarom R, Zirkin H, Stammler G, et al: Human coronary microvessels in diabetes and ischaemia. Morphometric study of autopsy material. J Pathol 166:265, 1992.
63. Grover GJ, Garlid KD: ATP-sensitive potassium channels: A review of their cardioprotective pharmacology. J Mol Cell Cardiol 32:677, 2000.
64. Ghosh S, Standen NB, Galinianes M: Failure to precondition pathological human myocardium. J Am Coll Cardiol 37:711, 2001.
65. Ishihara M, Inoue I, Kawagoe T, et al: Diabetes mellitus prevents ischemic preconditioning in patients with a first acute anterior wall myocardial infarction. J Am Coll Cardiol 38:1007, 2001.

Reducing the Risk of Heart Failure in Diabetes

66. Iribarren C, Karter AJ, Go AS, et al: Glycemic control and heart failure among adult patients with diabetes. Circulation 103:2668, 2001.
67. Stratton IM, Adler AI, Neil HA, et al: Association of glycaemia with macrovascular and microvascular complications of type 2 diabetes (UKPDS 35): Prospective observational study. BMJ 321:405, 2000.
68. Adler AI, Stratton IM, Neil HA, et al: Association of systolic blood pressure with macrovascular and microvascular complications of type 2 diabetes (UKPDS 36): Prospective observational study. BMJ 321:412, 2000.
69. Tight blood pressure control and risk of macrovascular and microvascular complications in type 2 diabetes: UKPDS 38. BMJ 317:703, 1998.
70. Efficacy of atenolol and captopril in reducing risk of macrovascular and microvascular complications in type 2 diabetes: UKPDS 39. UK Prospective Diabetes Study Group. BMJ 317:713, 1998.
71. Major outcomes in high-risk hypertensive patients randomized to angiotensin-converting enzyme inhibitor or calcium channel blocker vs diuretic: The Antihypertensive and Lipid-Lowering Treatment to Prevent Heart Attack Trial (ALLHAT). JAMA 288:2981, 2002.
72. Wing LM, Reid CM, Ryan P, et al: A comparison of outcomes with angiotensin-converting-enzyme inhibitors and diuretics for hypertension in the elderly. N Engl J Med 348:583, 2003.
73. A trial of the beta-blocker bucindolol in patients with advanced chronic heart failure. N Engl J Med 344:1659, 2001.
74. The cardiac insufficiency bisoprolol study II (CIBIS-II): A randomised trial. Lancet 353:9, 1999.
75. Hjalmarson A, Goldstein S, Fagerberg B, et al: Effects of controlled-release metoprolol on total mortality, hospitalizations, and well-being in patients with heart failure: The Metoprolol CR/XL Randomized Intervention Trial in congestive heart failure (MERIT-HF). JAMA 283:1295, 2000.
76. Packer M, Bristow MR, Cohn JN, et al: The effect of carvedilol on morbidity and mortality in patients with chronic heart failure. N Engl J Med 334:1349, 1996.

77. Packer M, Coats AJ, Fowler MB, et al: Effect of carvedilol on survival in severe chronic heart failure. N Engl J Med 344:1651, 2001.
78. Packer M, Fowler MB, Roecker EB, et al: Effect of carvedilol on the morbidity of patients with severe chronic heart failure: Results of the carvedilol prospective randomized cumulative survival (COPERNICUS) study. Circulation 106:2194, 2002.
79. Domanski M, Krause-Steinrauf H, Deedwania P, et al: The effect of diabetes on outcomes of patients with advanced heart failure in the BEST trial. J Am Coll Cardiol 42:914, 2003.
80. Poole-Wilson PA, Swedberg K, Cleland JG, et al: Comparison of carvedilol and metoprolol on clinical outcomes in patients with chronic heart failure in the Carvedilol Or Metoprolol European Trial (COMET): Randomised controlled trial. Lancet 362:7, 2003.
81. Pitt B, Poole-Wilson PA, Segal R, et al: Effect of losartan compared with captopril on mortality in patients with symptomatic heart failure: Randomised trial—The Losartan Heart Failure Survival Study ELITE II. Lancet 355:1582, 2000.
82. Cohn JN, Tognoni G: A randomized trial of the angiotensin-receptor blocker valsartan in chronic heart failure. N Engl J Med 345:1667, 2001.
83. Pfeffer MA, Swedberg K, Granger CB, et al: Effects of candesartan on mortality and morbidity in patients with chronic heart failure: The CHARM-Overall programme. Lancet 362:759, 2003.
84. Brenner BM, Cooper ME, de Zeeuw D, et al: Effects of losartan on renal and cardiovascular outcomes in patients with type 2 diabetes and nephropathy. N Engl J Med 345:861, 2001.
85. Lindholm LH, Ibsen H, Dahlof B, et al: Cardiovascular morbidity and mortality in patients with diabetes in the Losartan Intervention For Endpoint reduction in hypertension study (LIFE): A randomised trial against atenolol. Lancet 359:1004, 2002.
86. Stier CT Jr, Chander PN, Rocha R: Aldosterone as a mediator in cardiovascular injury. Cardiol Rev 10:97, 2002.
87. Weber KT: Aldosterone in congestive heart failure. N Engl J Med 345:1689, 2001.
88. Pitt B, Remme W, Zannad F, et al: Eplerenone, a selective aldosterone blocker, in patients with left ventricular dysfunction after myocardial infarction. N Engl J Med 348:1309, 2003.

Treating Diabetes in Patients with Coronary Heart Disease, Acute Coronary Syndromes, or Heart Failure

89. Intensive blood-glucose control with sulphonylureas or insulin compared with conventional treatment and risk of complications in patients with type 2 diabetes (UKPDS 33). Lancet 352:837, 1998.
90. Klepzig H, Kober G, Matter C, et al: Sulfonylureas and ischaemic preconditioning; a double-blind, placebo-controlled evaluation of glimepiride and glibenclamide. Eur Heart J 20:439, 1999.
91. Brady PA, Terzic A: The sulfonylurea controversy: More questions from the heart. J Am Coll Cardiol 31:950, 1998.
92. Lee TM, Chou TF: Impairment of myocardial protection in type 2 diabetic patients. J Clin Endocrinol Metab 88:531, 2003.
93. Goldstein BJ: Differentiating members of the thiazolidinedione class: A focus on efficacy. Diabetes Metab Res Rev 18(Suppl 2):S16, 2002.
94. Lebovitz HE: Differentiating members of the thiazolidinedione class: A focus on safety. Diabetes Metab Res Rev 18(Suppl 2):S23, 2002.\
94a. Nesto RW, Bell D, Bonow RO, et al: Thiazolidinedione use, fluid retention, and congestive heart failure: A consensus statement from the American Heart Association and American Diabetes Associaiton. Circulation 108:2941, 2003.
95. Wooltorton E: Rosiglitazone (Avandia) and pioglitazone (Actos) and heart failure. Can Med Assoc J 166:219, 2002.
96. Libby P: Metformin and vascular protection: A cardiologist's view. Diabetes Metab 29:6S117, 2003.
97. Johnson JA, Majumdar SR, Simpson SH, et al: Decreased mortality associated with the use of metformin compared with sulfonylurea monotherapy in type 2 diabetes. Diabetes Care 25:2244, 2002.
98. Bailey CJ, Turner RC: Metformin. N Engl J Med 334:574, 1996.
99. Van Belle E, Bauters C, Hubert E, et al: Restenosis rates in diabetic patients: A comparison of coronary stenting and balloon angioplasty in native coronary vessels. Circulation 96:1454, 1997.
100. Kip KE, Alderman EL, Bourassa MG, et al: Differential influence of diabetes mellitus on increased jeopardized myocardium after initial angioplasty or bypass surgery: Bypass angioplasty revascularization investigation. Circulation 105:1914, 2002.
101. Kip KE, Faxon DP, Detre KM, et al: Coronary angioplasty in diabetic patients. The National Heart, Lung, and Blood Institute Percutaneous Transluminal Coronary Angioplasty Registry. Circulation 94:1818, 1996.
102. Reginelli JP, Bhatt DL: Why diabetics are at risk in percutaneous coronary intervention and the appropriate management of diabetics in interventional cardiology. J Invasive Cardiol 14(Suppl E):2E, 2002.
103. Kornowski R, Mintz GS, Kent KM, et al: Increased restenosis in diabetes mellitus after coronary interventions is due to exaggerated intimal hyperplasia. A serial intravascular ultrasound study. Circulation 95:1366, 1997.
104. Moreno PR, Fallon JT, Murcia AM, et al: Tissue characteristics of restenosis after percutaneous transluminal coronary angioplasty in diabetic patients. J Am Coll Cardiol 34:1045, 1999.
105. Chevalier B, DeScheerder I, Gershlick A: Effect on restenosis with a paclitaxel eluting stent: Factors associated with inhibition in the ELUTES clinical study [abstract]. J Am Coll Cardiol 39:59A, 2002.
106. Serruys PW, Degertekin M, Tanabe K, et al: Intravascular ultrasound findings in the multicenter, randomized, double-blind RAVEL (RAndomized study with the sirolimus-eluting VElocity balloon-expandable stent in the treatment of patients with de novo native coronary artery Lesions) trial. Circulation 106:798, 2002.
107. Lepor NE, Madyoon H, Kereiakes D: Effective and efficient strategies for coronary revascularization in the drug-eluting stent era. Rev Cardiovasc Med 3:S38, 2002.
108. Carson JL, Scholz PM, Chen AY, et al: Diabetes mellitus increases short-term mortality and morbidity in patients undergoing coronary artery bypass graft surgery. J Am Coll Cardiol 40:418, 2002.
109. Cohen Y, Raz I, Merin G, et al: Comparison of factors associated with 30-day mortality after coronary artery bypass grafting in patients with versus without diabetes mellitus. Israeli Coronary Artery Bypass (ISCAB) Study Consortium. Am J Cardiol 81:7, 1998.
110. Detre KM, Lombardero MS, Brooks MM, et al: The effect of previous coronary-artery bypass surgery on the prognosis of patients with diabetes who have acute myocardial infarction. Bypass Angioplasty Revascularization Investigation Investigators. N Engl J Med 342:989, 2000.
111. Seven-year outcome in the Bypass Angioplasty Revascularization Investigation (BARI) by treatment and diabetic status. J Am Coll Cardiol 35:1122, 2000.
112. Niles NW, McGrath PD, Malenka D, et al: Survival of patients with diabetes and multivessel coronary artery disease after surgical or percutaneous coronary revascularization: Results of a large regional prospective study. Northern New England Cardiovascular Disease Study Group. J Am Coll Cardiol 37:1008, 2001.
113. Influence of diabetes on 5-year mortality and morbidity in a randomized trial comparing CABG and PTCA in patients with multivessel disease: The Bypass Angioplasty Revascularization Investigation (BARI). Circulation 96:1761, 1997.
114. Abizaid A, Costa MA, Centemero M, et al: Clinical and economic impact of diabetes mellitus on percutaneous and surgical treatment of multivessel coronary disease patients: Insights from the Arterial Revascularization Therapy Study (ARTS) trial. Circulation 104:533, 2001.
115. Sedlis SP, Morrison DA, Lorin JD, et al: Percutaneous coronary intervention versus coronary bypass graft surgery for diabetic patients with unstable angina and risk factors for adverse outcomes with bypass: Outcome of diabetic patients in the AWESOME randomized trial and registry. J Am Coll Cardiol 40:1555, 2002.
116. Valensi P, Huard JP, Giroux C, et al: Factors involved in cardiac autonomic neuropathy in diabetic patients. J Diabetes Complications 11:180, 1997.
117. Maser RE, Mitchell BD, Vinik AI, et al: The association between cardiovascular autonomic neuropathy and mortality in individuals with diabetes: A meta-analysis. Diabetes Care 26:1895, 2003.
118. Nesto RW, Libby P: Diabetes mellitus and the cardiovascular system. *In* Braunwald E, Zipes DP, Libby P (eds): Heart Disease. A Textbook of Cardiovascular Medicine. 6th ed. Philadelphia, WB Saunders, 2001, p 2133.
119. Cardoso CR, Salles GF, Deccache W: Prognostic value of QT interval parameters in type 2 diabetes mellitus: Results of a long-term follow-up prospective study. J Diabetes Complications 17:169, 2003.

CHAPTER 52

Percutaneous Coronary and Valvular Intervention

Jeffrey J. Popma • Richard E. Kuntz • Donald S. Baim

The use of percutaneous coronary intervention (PCI) to treat ischemic coronary artery disease (CAD) has expanded dramatically over the past two decades. From its beginning as a therapeutic novelty, PCI was performed in more than 900,000 patients in 2003 in the United States, far exceeding the number of patients undergoing coronary artery bypass graft (CABG) surgery, which peaked at 500,000 yearly and has been falling by 10 percent per year. At the same time, the procedural success, safety, and durability of PCI have improved dramatically because of continual technological improvements (e.g., drug stents, distal protection devices), refinements in periprocedural adjunctive pharmacology (e.g., glycoprotein IIb/IIIa [GP IIb/IIIa] inhibitors, alternative thrombin inhibitors), and a better understanding of early and late outcomes. These improvements support the expanded use of PCI as definitive therapy for many patients with ischemia-producing CAD.

This chapter reviews (1) the historical and current methods used for PCI, including conventional balloon angioplasty and new coronary devices; (2) the procedural outcomes and complication rates obtained with contemporary PCI methods; (3) the periprocedural pharmacological strategies to reduce acute complications and restenosis after PCI; (4) the use of drug-eluting stents and radiation brachytherapy for the prevention of restenosis; and (5) recommendations for coronary revascularization in patients with ischemic CAD, with consideration of the alternatives of medical therapy, PCI, and CABG. A discussion of the current issues in selection of patients, technical performance, and outcomes associated with percutaneous mitral and aortic valvuloplasty is also included. Primary PCI for acute coronary syndromes is the subject of Chapter 48.

HISTORICAL PERSPECTIVE

Balloon angioplasty, or percutaneous transluminal coronary angioplasty (PTCA), was first performed by Andreas Gruentzig in 1977 using a prototype, fixed-wire balloon catheter. The procedure was initially limited to the less than 10 percent of patients with symptomatic CAD who had focal noncalcified lesions of a single, proximal coronary vessel, where it was used as an alternative to CABG. As equipment design and operator experience evolved rapidly over the next decade, PCI was expanded to a broader spectrum of patients, such as those with multivessel disease, more challenging anatomy, reduced left ventricular function, and other serious comorbid medical conditions. Despite these improvements, two major complications limited the widespread use of balloon PTCA. The first was abrupt closure of the treated vessel, which occurred in 5 to 8 percent of cases and required emergency CABG for correction in 3 to 5 percent of cases. The second was the development of symptom recurrence because of restenosis of the treated segment in 15 to 30 percent of patients within 6 to 9 months after the initial procedure.

A series of new coronary devices were developed in the early 1990s that sought to improve upon the procedural outcomes achieved with balloon PTCA. Although these novel methods removed (e.g., directional, rotational, or extraction atherectomy) (Fig. 52–1), ablated (e.g., excimer laser angioplasty), or scaffolded (e.g., stents) atherosclerotic plaque, only coronary stenting consistently improved the procedural safety and late clinical outcomes compared with balloon angioplasty in the routine patients undergoing what is now referred to more broadly as PCI. Stents are currently used in more than 80 percent of PCI procedures, whereas atherectomy is used in less than 10 percent of PCI, relegated to "niche use" in patients with certain complex coronary lesions. As a result of these advances, the procedural outcome of PCI has improved substantially in the past two decades (Table 52–1).[1-7]

Balloon Percutaneous Transluminal Coronary Angioplasty

Balloon angioplasty expands the coronary lumen by stretching and tearing the atherosclerotic plaque and vessel wall and, to a lesser extent, by redistributing atherosclerotic plaque along its longitudinal axis ("footprints in the sand"). Although ischemia was generally (>90 percent) improved after balloon angioplasty alone in early series, elastic recoil of the stretched vessel wall left an average residual stenosis of 30 to 35 percent, with higher residual stenoses correlated with higher subsequent recurrence rates. Before the availability of

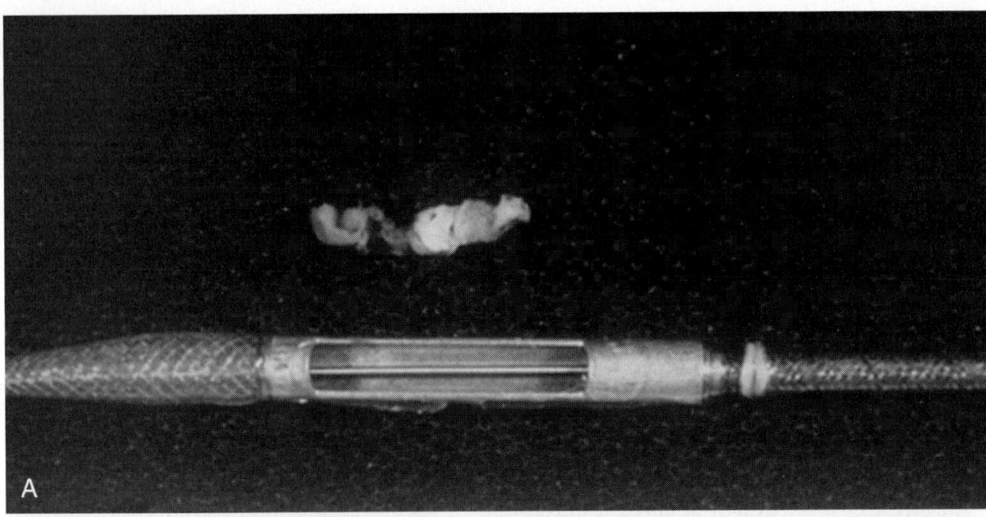

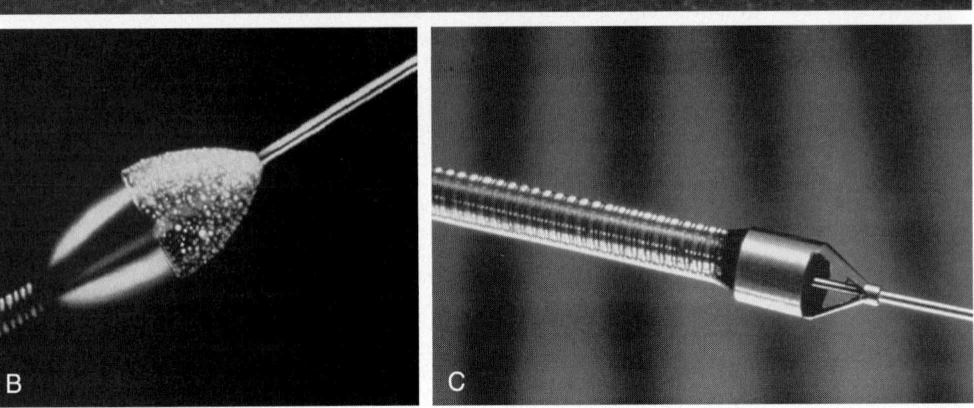

FIGURE 52–1 Atherectomy devices. **A,** Directional coronary atherectomy device alongside tissue resected. **B,** Rotational atherectomy device. **C,** Transluminal extraction catheter.

TABLE 52–1 In-Hospital Outcomes Associated with Perctaneous Intervention over Time

Variable	NHLBI-I[1]	NHLBI-II[1]	MAPS[2]	MAPS[2]	BOAT PTCA Arm[3]	STRESS PTCA Arm[4]	Benestent II PTCA Arm[5]	Cutting Balloon PTCA Arm[6]	Dynamic Registry All PCI[7]
Years of entry	1977-1981	1985-1986	1986-1987	1991	1994-1995	1991-1993	1995-1996	1994-1996	1997-1998
Number of patients	1155	1802	400	200	492	203	413	621	1559
New device use	No	No	No	Yes	"Bailout"	"Bailout"	"Bailout"	"Bailout"	64% stent
Baseline factors									
Mean age, yr	54	58	58	62	58	60	50	58	62
Women, %	25	26	29	30	24	27	23	23	32
Diabetes mellitus	9	14	19	25	14	16	13	12	26
Unstable angina, %	37	49	48	51	NA	48	45	64	43
Multivessel disease, %	25	53	100	100	NA	32	NA	NR	54
Angiographic success, %	68	91	NR	92	NA	92.6	99	NR	94
Procedure success, %	61	78	83.5	90	87	89.6	96	94.7	92
Early complications					3.3[1]	7.9[1]	7.0	2.7	4.9
Death, %	1.2	1.0	1.0	1.0	0.4	1.5	0	0	1.9
Q wave infarction, %	4.9	4.3	2.0	1.5	1.2	3.0	1.2	1.0	NR
Emergency CABG, %	5.8	3.4	5.5	1.0	2.0	4.0	0.7	1.0	1.5
Late clinical outcome	5 yr	5 yr	1 yr	1 yr	1 yr	240 d	12 mo	6 mo	NA
Any Event					31.1	23.8	23.2	15.1	NA
Death, %	4.9	8.3	NA	NA	1.6	0	1.0	0.3	NA
Q wave MI	9.7	9.1	NA	NA	1.6	0.5	1.9	1.1	NA
Revascularization, %	32.1	38.8			19.7	15.4	18.9	14.8	NA
Repeat PTCA	22.5	30.9	16.2	13.2	NA	11.4	9.4	NA	NA
CABG	15.5	13.4	13.4	8.1	NA	4.5	1.9	NA	NA

BOAT = Balloon vs Optimal Atherectomy Trial; CABG = coronary artery bypass graft; MAPS = Multivessel Angioplasty Prognosis Study; MI = myocardial infarction; NA = not applicable; NHLBI = National Heart, Lung, and Blood Institute; NR = not reported; PCI = percutaneous coronary intervention; PTCA = percutaneous transluminal coronary angioplasty; STRESS = Stent Restenosis Study.

Modified from Hirshfeld J, Ellis S, Faxon D: Recommendations for the assessment and maintenance of proficiency in coronary interventional procedures: Statement of the American College of Cardiology. J Am Coll Cardiol 31:722, 1998.

stents, the stretching process left propagating coronary dissections that resulted in abrupt vessel closure in 5 to 8 percent of patients.

Balloon angioplasty has remained an integral component of PCI, whether to dilate the vessel prior to stent placement, deploy a coronary stent, or further expand the stent after deployment. But "stand-alone" balloon angioplasty is now reserved for cases such as smaller (<2.5-mm) vessels, long (>25-mm) lesions, anastomotic stenosis in saphenous vein grafts (SVGs) in which the long-term benefits of coronary stenting are limited, or the treatment of in-stent restenosis before brachytherapy. A "provisional" stent strategy may still be used for these complex lesions, with coronary stent placement reserved for lesions with abrupt or threatened closure or suboptimal (>40 percent) residual stenosis after attempts at adequate vessel expansion with balloon angioplasty have failed. The availability of "bailout" coronary stents to treat angioplasty-induced dissection reduced the emergency CABG rate to less than 1 percent in most institutions.

Two modifications of balloon PTCA have been developed as niche devices for patients undergoing PCI. The cutting balloon (Boston Scientific, Natick, MA) is a conventional balloon that contains either three or four longitudinal microtome blades that incise the atherosclerotic plaque during balloon dilation. The cutting balloon does not reduce restenosis compared with conventional balloon angioplasty but has been approved in the United States by the Food and Drug Administration (FDA) for use in undilatable lesions.[6] The cutting balloon is also useful in patients with in-stent restenosis because the longitudinal blades prevent slippage of the balloon along the axial length of the vessel (Fig. 52-2), particularly when radiation brachytherapy is used as an adjunct. The Fx Minirail (Guidant, Santa Clara, CA) employs a similar concept by adding an additional guidewire that runs outside the balloon dilation catheter in order to score the plaque and prevent balloon slippage. These devices are used in about 10 percent of interventional procedures.

Coronary Atherectomy

Atherectomy assists with PCI by removing the obstructing atherosclerotic plaque and improving lesion wall compliance by fracturing and scoring the remaining plaque. The primary advantage of atherectomy-assisted angioplasty over balloon alone is that a larger final minimal lumen diameter can be achieved. Atherectomy use reached its peak (30 percent of interventional procedures) between 1992 and 1994 but fell dramatically after the clinical availability of coronary stents. It is estimated that 5 to 10 percent of cases currently involve the use of atherectomy devices, alone or in combination with coronary stenting.

DIRECTIONAL CORONARY ATHERECTOMY

Directional coronary atherectomy (DCA) (Guidant, Santa Clara, CA) uses a directional cutting device to remove 18 to 20 mg of tissue, with the remaining lumen gain provided by mechanical dilation by the DCA catheter and balloon angioplasty and changes in radial compliance produced by the vessel by excision of deep wall elastic components. Intravascular ultrasound studies show that a substantial amount (43 to 55 percent cross-sectional narrowing) of atherosclerotic plaque remains even after aggressive DCA.

An "optimal" DCA result is defined as a final diameter stenosis less than 10 percent, tissue removal, and the avoidance of major clinical complications (death, Q wave myocardial infarction [MI], or emergency CABG). The lowest angiographic restenosis rates are obtained in patients with discrete, native vessel lesions who undergo optimal DCA (31.4 percent) as compared with balloon PTCA (39.8 percent; $p < 0.05$) (Table 52-2).[3,8-12] More "conservative" atherectomy using smaller DCA devices and no adjunct balloon PTCA results in higher (>25 percent) residual stenosis and more complications and has no benefit over balloon PTCA. Arterial constrictive remodeling is the major cause of restenosis after DCA and can be avoided when DCA is used before stent placement. Although the strategy of debulking before stenting may lessen the chance of late restenosis, the Atherectomy before Multilink Stent Improves Lumen Gain and Clinical Outcomes Study (AMIGO) trial compared DCA followed by stent implantation with stent implantation alone in more than 800 patients and showed benefit for DCA only when very aggressive atherectomy was performed or there was a significant bifurcation stenosis involving both the parent vessel and the side branch. Accordingly, routine use of DCA before stent placement to remove atherosclerotic plaque is not recommended.

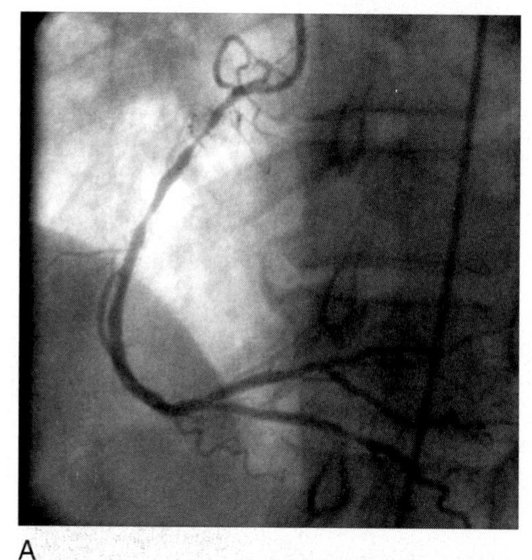
A

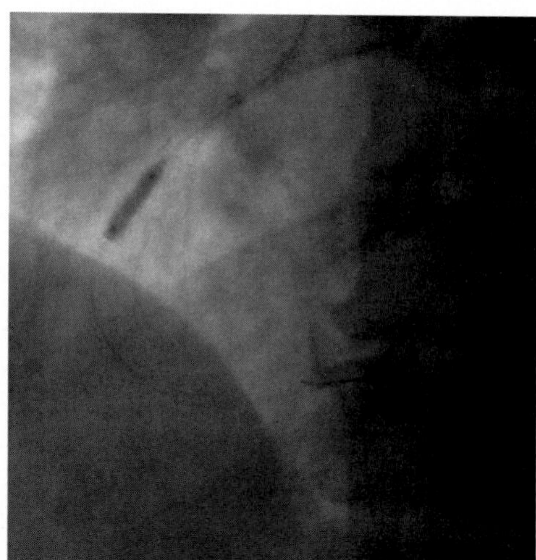
B

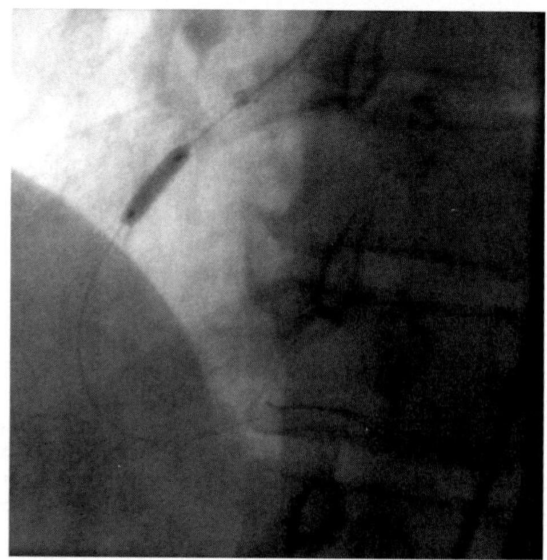
C

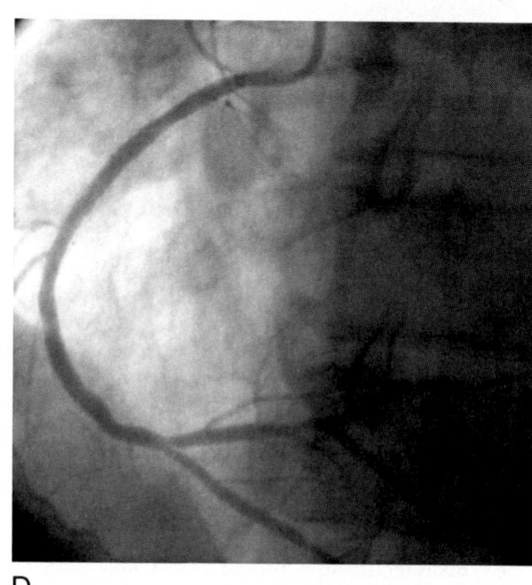
D

FIGURE 52–2 **A,** Sequential restenoses within a long stent within the right coronary artery. **B,** A 3.5-mm × 15-mm cutting balloon is advanced across the in-stent restenosis and inflated. **C,** The cutting balloon is positioned more proximally and a repeated inflation is performed. **D,** At the end of the cutting balloon inflation, there is a 10 percent residual stenosis. The cutting balloon limits slippage of the balloon within the stent because of the longitudinal cutting blades that score the plaque while inflating the balloon.

TABLE 52–2 Early and Late Outcome After Directional Coronary Atherectomy in Native Coronary Arteries

	CAVEAT[8]		C-CAT[9]		ABACUS[10]		BOAT[3]		START[11]		SOLD[12]
Method	*PTCA*	*DCA*	*PTCA*	*DCA*	*DCA*	*DCA + PTCA*	*PTCA*	*DCA*	*Stent*	*DCA*	*DCA + Stent*
Years of entry	1991-1992		1991-1992		1994-1995		1994-1995		1995-1997		1996-1997
Number of patients	500	512	136	138	106	108	492	497	62	60	71
Baseline factors											
Mean age, yr	59	59	55	58	62	60	58	58	62	64	57
Diabetes mellitus, %	19	19	15	17	19	21	14	14	29	22	14
Unstable angina, %	70	66	52	39	30	22	NA	NA	NR	NR	33
Procedure success, %	76	82+	88	94		99.5	87	93‡	NR	NR	96
RVD, mm	2.9	2.9	3.13	3.23	3.24	3.21	3.20	3.25	3.23	3.29	3.27
Final MLD, mm											
Baseline MLD	NR	NR	0.89	0.94	1.04	1.03	1.04	1.07	1.00	1.01	0.87
Final MLD, mm	1.80	2.02§	2.10	2.34§	2.60	2.88†	2.33	2.82§	2.80	2.89	3.47
Follow-up MLD, mm	NR	NR	1.55	1.61	1.80	1.85	1.68	1.86‡	1.89	2.18	2.57
% Diameter stenosis											
Baseline	73	71	71.5	70.6	68.7	68.0	NR	NR			74
Final	36	29	33	26§	15.0	10.8†	28.1	14.7§	14.7	12.7	0.4
Follow-up	NR	NR	48.4	48.7	32.3	33.4	45.6	40.1‡	40.1	32.1	21
Restenosis rate, %	57	50	43	46	19.6	23.6	39.8	31.4*	32.8	15.8	11
Early complications	5	11§	6	5							
Death, %	0.4	0	0	0	0	0	0.4	0	NR	NR	1.4
Q wave MI, %	2	2	0	0.7	0.9	0	1.2	2.0	NR	NR	2.8
Emergency CABG, %	2	3	4.4	1.4	0	0	2.0	1.0	NR	NR	1.4
Follow-up time	1 yr		6 mo		1 yr		1 yr		1 yr		NR
Late clinical events	42.4	38.7	29	29	18.1	21.9	24.8	21.1¶	33.9	18.3¶	NR
Death, %	0.6	2.2+	0	0.7	0	0	0.6	0.6	1.6	0	NR
Q-wave MI	1.2	2.9	1.6	0	0.9	0	1.6	2.0	NR	NR	NR
TLR, %			27.9	28.7	15.2	21.9			29	15	NR
Repeat PCI	25.9	24.4	23.3	23.5	NR	NR	NR	NR	NR	NR	NR
CABG	9.1	9.3	4.6	5.2	NR	NR	NR	NR	3.2	0	NR

ABACUS = Adjunctive Balloon Angioplasty After Coronary Atherectomy Study; BOAT = Balloon vs Optimal Atherectomy Trial; CABG = coronary artery bypass graft; CAVEAT = Coronary Angioplasty Versus Excisional Atherectomy Trial; C-CAT = Canadian Coronary Atherectomy Trial; DCA = directional coronary atherectomy; MLD = minimum lumen diameter; MI = myocardial infarction; NR = not reported; PCI = percutaneous coronary intervention; PTCA = percutaneous transluminal coronary angioplasty; RVD = reference vessel diameter; SOLD = stenting after optimal lesion debulking; START = Stent versus directional coronary Atherectomy Randomized Trial; TLR = target lesion revascularization.

*$p < 0.05$.

†$p < 0.01$.

‡$p < 0.005$.

§$p < 0.001$.

¶Target vessel failure (death, Q wave myocardial infarction, or target vessel revascularization).

In current practice, DCA is reserved for patients with noncalcified bifurcation lesions involving a large branch or in the ostium of the left anterior descending artery, particularly when there is an acute angle with the origin of the left circumflex. DCA may also be useful for the treatment of in-stent restenosis in larger vessels.

ROTATIONAL ATHERECTOMY

The rotational atherectomy (RA) device or Rotablator (Boston Scientific, Natick, MA) removes the atheromatous plaque by the differential abrasion of inelastic tissue (i.e., calcified plaque) while elastic tissue (i.e., arterial wall) is deflected away from the microscopic diamond chips on the rotating atherectomy burr. The device consists of an olive-shaped, stainless steel burr coated with diamond chips measuring 20 to 50 microns with burr diameters ranging from 1.25 to 2.50-mm. A burr about 0.7 the diameter of the reference vessel adjacent to the target lesion is spun at roughly 160,000 rpm and advanced slowly across that lesion to abrade plaque elements that intrude into the coronary lumen. This abrasion process generates 2- to 5-µm microparticles that pass through the coronary microcirculation for removal by the reticuloendothelial system. Correct technique is important to avoid slowing of rotational speed by excessive contact force between burr and lesion. Deceleration by more than 5000 rpm can lead to inadvertent stalling, burr entrapment, dissection, or vessel occlusion.[13] Two to four passes are made with each burr, with 30 to 60 seconds between passes to allow coronary perfusion. Aggressive RA (using burr-to-artery ratios of >0.7) techniques do not provide a restenosis advantage over more conservative (burr-to-artery ratio of approximately 0.7) methods and tend to increase acute procedural complications.[13] Adjunctive balloon PTCA is used in most (82 to 88 percent) cases to reduce residual percent diameter stenosis or to treat coronary dissections. RA does not appear to reduce restenosis compared with balloon angioplasty in noncalcified vessels.[14] Current RA procedures generally conclude by placement of a coronary stent within the treated segment.

RA registries have reported high (88 to 98.6 percent) procedural success rates in complex lesions. Major complications are uncommon after RA, but transient bradycardia and atrioventricular block are occasionally seen during RA, particularly during RA of the right coronary artery. In the Excimer, Rotablator, or Balloon Angioplasty for Complex Lesions (ERBAC) Study, angiographic restenosis at 6 months was similar in patients treated with RA (57 percent), excimer laser angioplasty (59 percent), or balloon PTCA (47 percent).[15] No advantage of RA over balloon angioplasty was found in noncalcified lesions.[14]

RA is currently reserved for lesions not suitable for balloon PTCA because of excess procedural risk, such as ostial and heavily calcified lesions, selected bifurcation lesions, and lesions that are undilatable with balloon PTCA (Fig. 52-3). RA may also be useful for the treatment of in-stent restenosis but should be avoided in the presence of focal or extensive dissection after balloon PTCA, visible thrombus, or extremely eccentric lesions located on the outer surface of a severe bend.

ABLATIVE LASER-ASSISTED ANGIOPLASTY

Delivery of laser energy through optical fibers can also be used to ablate atherosclerotic obstructions. Two laser systems have been used in coronary arteries: the XeCl excimer laser coronary angioplasty (ELCA) system and the holmium:yttrium aluminum garnet (Ho:YAG) laser system. The ELCA system uses laser light at 308 nm, and the Ho:YAG system uses light at a wavelength of 2100 nm. This light is delivered during a single slow (0.5 to 1.0-mm/sec) pass of the laser catheter through the lesion under fluoroscopic guidance. A concurrent saline flush through the guiding catheter removes blood and contrast medium from the coronary artery to minimize the degree of photoacoustic injury to the surrounding vessel. After successful laser passage, adjunctive balloon PTCA is needed in most (90 percent) cases to reduce the residual stenosis to below 30 percent.

Randomized trials have failed to show a reduction in restenosis associated with the use of the Ho:YAG or excimer laser system compared with balloon angioplasty in either simple or complex lesions. As a result, laser angioplasty has a limited role in PCI and is reserved for patients with in-stent restenosis, particularly those in SVGs, aortoostial SVG lesions, undilatable total occlusions, and, potentially, lesions located in friable SVGs. Laser angioplasty should be used with caution in patients with thrombus or in the presence of severe calcification.

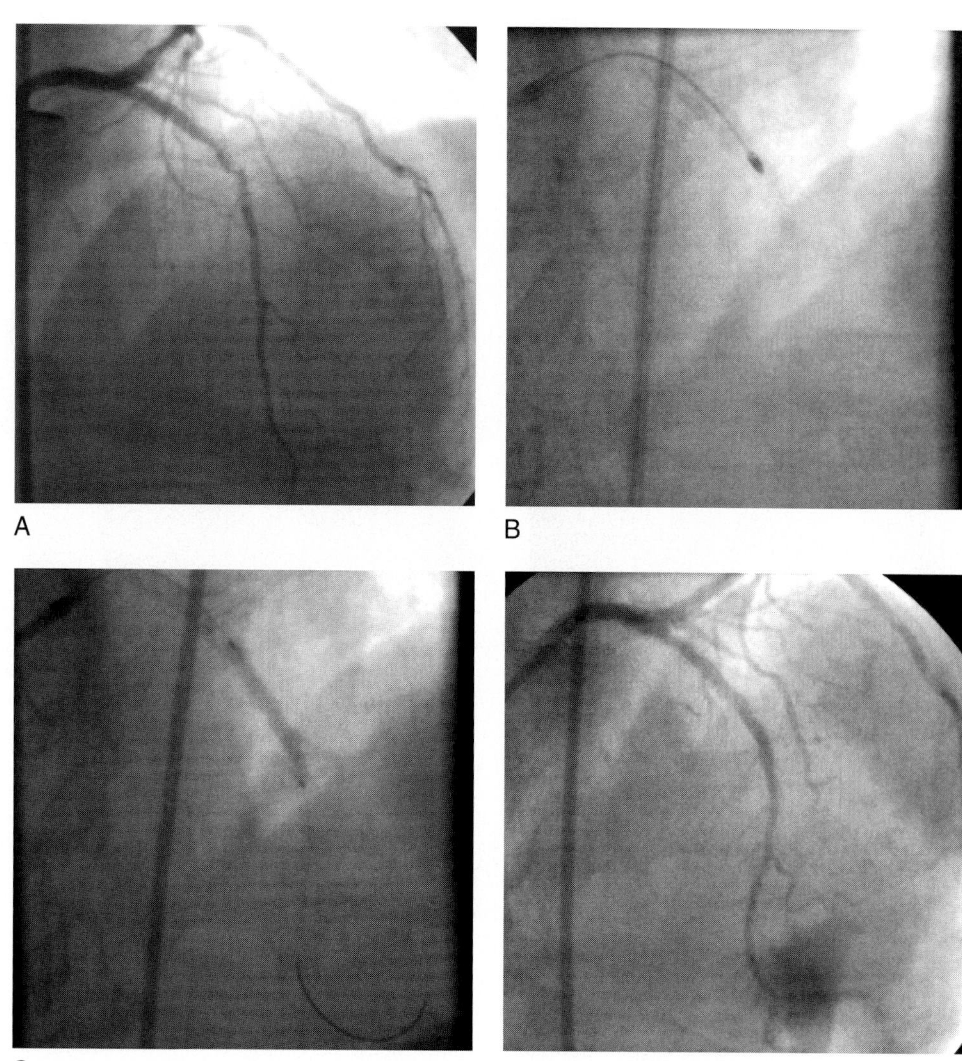

FIGURE 52–3 **A,** A heavily calcified diffuse lesion in the left anterior descending artery is generally considered undilatable with conventional balloon techniques. **B,** A 1.5-mm rotational atherectomy burr revolving at 160,000 rpm is advanced to ablate the calcified lesion. **C,** A 3.0-mm × 28-mm stent can then be advanced across the blockage and inflated to 16 atm of pressure. It is unlikely that full stent expansion could have occurred without pretreatment with rotational atherectomy. **D,** The final angiographic result shows no residual stenosis and normal flow into the distal vessel.

Catheter-Based Thrombolysis and Mechanical Thrombectomy

The presence of thrombus within the native vessel or SVG imparts a substantial risk for distal embolization, "no reflow," or other embolic complications during PCI (Fig. 52–4). Early experience with the Transluminal Extraction Catheter (TEC) (Boston Scientific, Natick, MA) showed moderate success in removing intraluminal clot, but its commercial use was limited by the need for large diameter (9 French [9F]) guiding catheters and stiffness of the device. In the mid-1990s, the Angiojet (Possis Medical, Minneapolis, MN) was introduced as a dedicated device for thrombus removal. A 4F catheter contains a high-pressure hypotube through which saline is injected through a distal tip. These high-speed saline jets are directed toward the proximal end of the catheter lumen and create intense local suction by the Venturi effect, pulling surrounding blood, thrombus, and saline into the lumen of the catheter opening and propelling the debris proximally through the catheter lumen. Repeated passes of the Angiojet may be performed until angiography shows no further evidence of thrombus (Fig. 52–5).

The Vein Graft AngioJet Study 2 (VEGAS-2) trial randomly assigned 349 patients with angiographic thrombus to treatment with the Angiojet or prolonged intraluminal urokinase consisting of a 250,000-unit bolus over a 30-minute period followed by intravenous urokinase for 6 to 30 hours.[16] The procedure success rate was higher and the complication rate was lower in patients treated with the Angiojet device.[16] The Angiojet is currently indicated in patients with moderate to large thrombus-containing native vessels or SVGs prior to definitive therapy with balloon PTCA and stents. The Angiojet should not be used in small (<2.0-mm) vessels because of the risk of perforation.

Distal Embolic Protection Devices

Although distal embolization of atherosclerotic debris was thought not to be a problem during the early years of catheter-based intervention, it is now recognized as a potential cause of distal myocardial necrosis after PCI. The first demonstration of atheroembolization was in diseased SVGs, where such embolization is now seen as the primary etiology for post-procedural cardiac enzyme elevation (17 percent of cases)

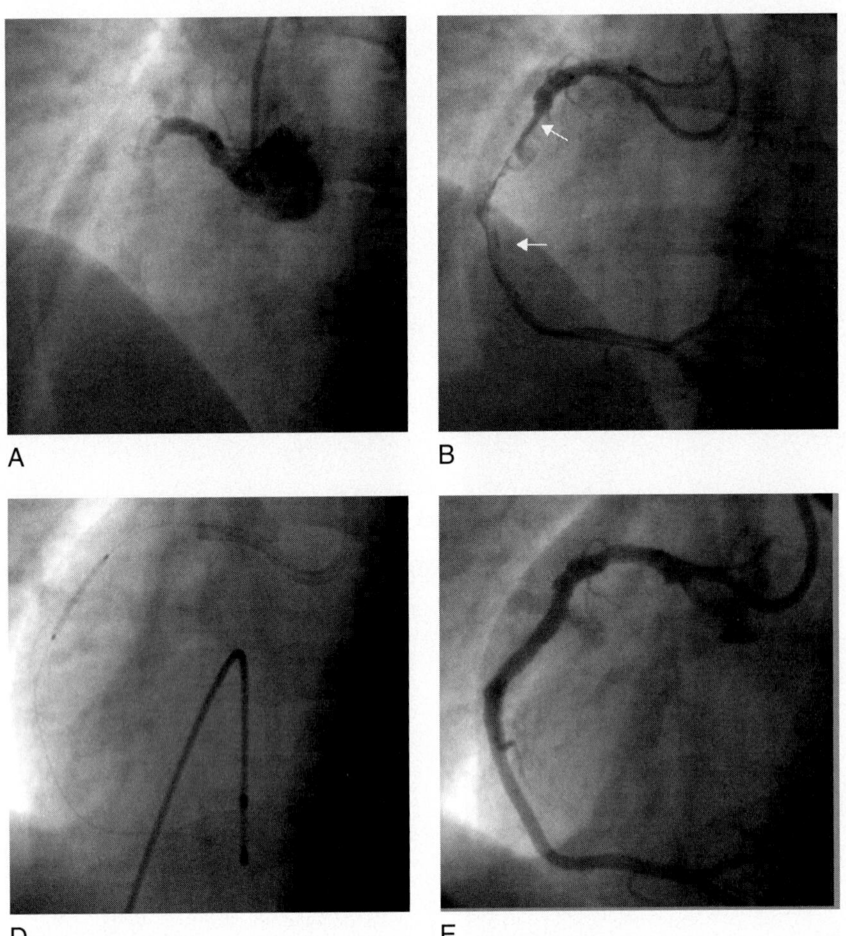

FIGURE 52–4 **A,** A thrombotic occlusion of the proximal right coronary artery persists after thrombolytic therapy. **B,** Following recanalization with a wire, there is a long thrombotic occlusion (arrows). **C,** Following Angiojet thrombectomy (not shown), there is resolution of the thrombus and Thrombolysis in Myocardial Infarction (TIMI) 3 flow into the distal vessel. **D,** A 4.0-mm stent is positioned and then deployed at the site of the infarction. **E,** After stent deployment, there is return of TIMI 3 flow to the distal vessel.

and the no-reflow phenomenon (8 percent of cases) manifest as reduced myocardial perfusion despite a patent epicardial vessel. Microvascular (arteriolar) spasm and platelet aggregation are contributory mechanisms, but only protection against distal atherosclerotic embolization has been shown to reduce the incidence of these complications.

Three classes of embolic protection devices are being evaluated. The first involves distal occlusion using a low-pressure balloon mounted on a hollow guidewire shaft. The Percusurge Guardwire (Medtronic Vascular, Santa Rosa, CA) device is passed across the target lesion and inflated to occlude flow so that any debris liberated by intervention remains trapped in the stagnant column of blood and can be aspirated before the occlusion balloon is deflated to restore antegrade flow[17] (Fig. 52–6). Preliminary data showed that embolic debris (size range between 25 μm and 2 mm) was recovered in more than 95 percent of such procedures, that the histology of the debris (cholesterol clefts, foam cells) resembled that of the treated lesion, and that the incidence of cardiac enzyme elevation was much lower (4 percent) than expected.[18] This benefit was confirmed in the 801-patient Saphenous vein graft Angioplasty Free of Emboli Randomized (SAFER) trial, in which patients undergoing SVG intervention were randomly assigned to stenting over the occlusion wire or a conventional guidewire, showing substantial reductions in 30-day major adverse clinical events (from 16.9 to 9.6 percent) and no reflow (from 8.3 to 3.3 percent) (Fig. 52–7).[17]

The second class of embolic protection devices consists of distal filters that are passed across the target lesion in their smaller collapsed state, opened to approximate the edges of the filter material against the vessel wall, and remain in place to catch any liberated embolic material larger than the filter pore size (usually 100 to 150 μm), until they are collapsed after stent deployment, thereby removing the captured embolic material from the body (Fig. 52–8).[19] This type of device has the advantages of maintaining antegrade flow during the procedure and allowing intermittent injection of contrast material to visualize underlying anatomy but the inherent disadvantage of allowing the component of debris with a diameter less than the filter pore size to pass. The first such filter to complete a pivotal clinical trial is the Embolic Protection Incorporated FilterWire (Boston Scientific, Natick, MA), which was evaluated against the Guardwire distal occlusion device in a 656-patient randomized trial (Fig. 52–9).[19] That trial showed that the distal filter was noninferior (equivalent or better) compared with the distal occlusion device in 30-day major adverse cardiac events.

The third type of embolic protection device involves proximal occlusion of the treated vessel with balloon on the tip of or just beyond the tip of the guiding catheter. With such inflow occlusion, retrograde flow generated by distal collaterals or infusion through a "rinsing" catheter can propel any liberated debris back into the lumen of the guiding catheter. Although devices of this type have thus far undergone only limited clinical testing, they have the advantage of providing protection even before the first wire is advanced across the target lesion.

Devices of all three types are also being evaluated for other anatomical and clinical situations. In native coronaries of patients experiencing acute MI, liberation of thrombus and underlying atherosclerotic debris may contribute to limited myocardial reperfusion and impaired resolution of ST

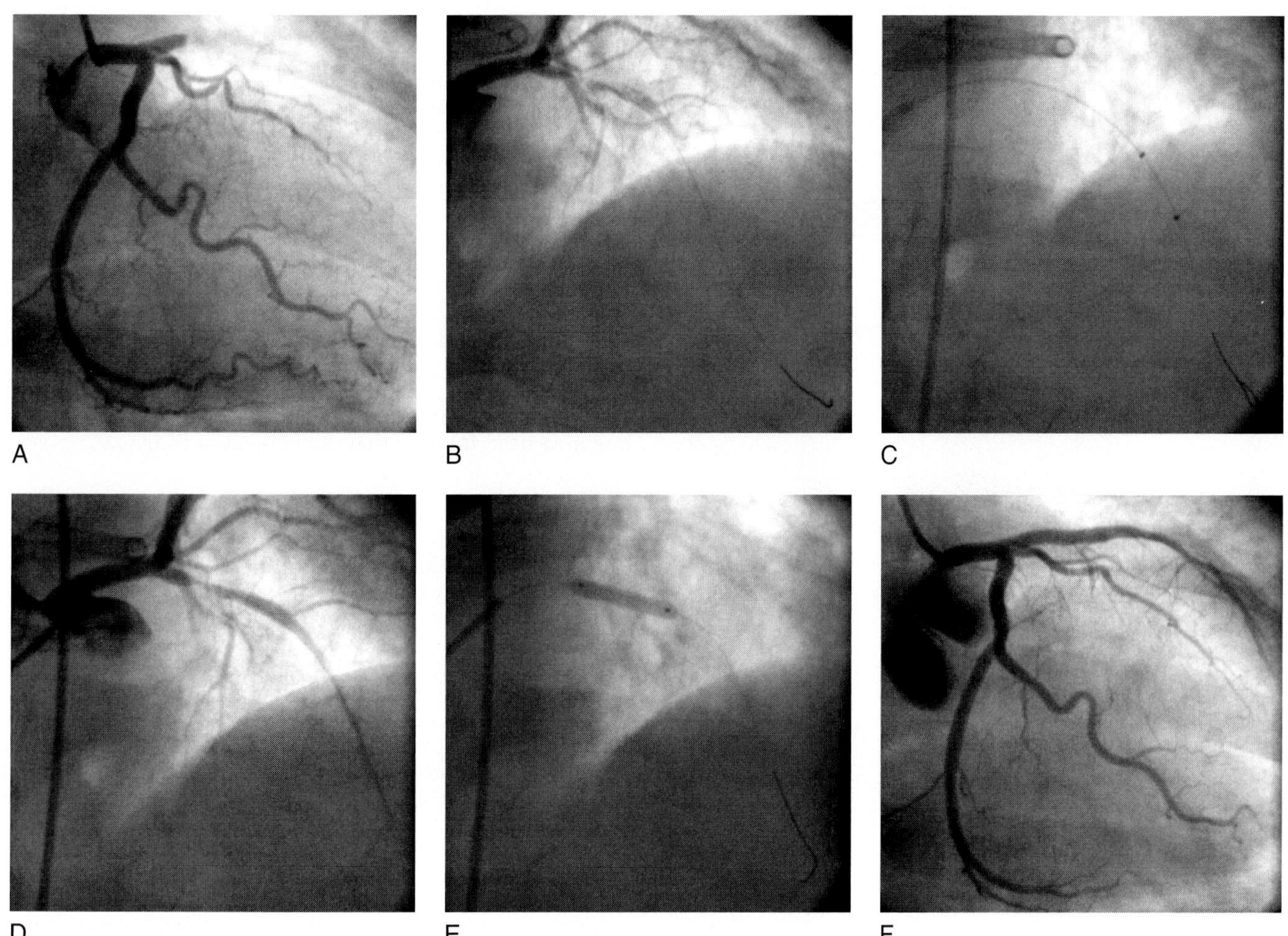

FIGURE 52–5 **A,** A thrombotic occlusion of the proximal segment of the left anterior descending artery is shown. **B,** The vessel is recanalized with a coronary guidewire. **C,** A 4F Angiojet is advanced across the lesion and multiple passes are made to relieve the stenosis. **D,** The thrombus is removed (residual stenosis shown, panels **E, A**), and a 3.5-mm stent is placed at the site of plaque rupture. **F,** There is no residual stenosis and flow is re-established into the distal left anterior descending artery.

segment elevation.[18] The Enhanced Myocardial Efficacy and Recovery by Aspiration of Liberalized Debris (EMERALD) study is a large randomized trial involving patients with acute MI in native vessels, with patients assigned to the distal occlusion device or no distal protection and nuclear imaging assessment of myocardial infarct size as the primary endpoint (Fig. 52–10). Although carotid artery stenting is still investigational, there is ample evidence from transcranial Doppler studies that stent placement is associated with cerebral embolization that probably contributes to the 3 to 5 percent incidence of postprocedural stroke. Embolic protection devices of all three types have been effective in recovering emboli and reducing the neurological complication rate, making them part of all ongoing carotid stenting protocols (see also Chap. 55).

Thus, mounting evidence indicates that distal atherosclerotic debris commonly embolizes from lesions in many vascular territories during percutaneous intervention, that it can be recovered using any of the three types of embolic protection device, and that use of those devices reduces the incidence of end-organ injury.

Total Occlusion–Crossing Devices

Many patients presenting with chronic angina have one or more coronary arteries that are completely occluded rather than just severely stenotic. The distal myocardium may still be viable as the result of inter- or intracoronary collaterals, but such collaterals are generally unable to meet increased oxygen demands during exercise or stress. Restoration of blood flow to such territories is thus an important part of any revascularization strategy. Conventional angioplasty guidewires are only 60 to 70 percent effective in crossing such occlusions, giving this anatomical subgroup the lowest success with PCI and making the presence of one or more chronic total occlusions the leading reason why patients are referred to bypass surgery instead of PCI. Slightly better results in crossing chronic total occlusions are possible with the use of stiffer and hydrophilic-coated guidewires, albeit with a concomitant increase in vessel dissection or perforation.

Considerable effort is thus being made to develop new devices for crossing total occlusions that are steerable and potent enough to make headway through the fibrous caps at either end of the occlusion (and fibrocalcific islands in between) but selective enough to minimize injury to the vessel wall. Two devices are currently approved by the FDA for this indication.

The Lumend Front Runner (Lumend, Santa Clara, CA) has a pair of mechanically openable jaws at its tip that can perform blunt microdissection to cross the total occlusion. This device can cross more than half of the total occlusions in which conventional guidewires have failed, although

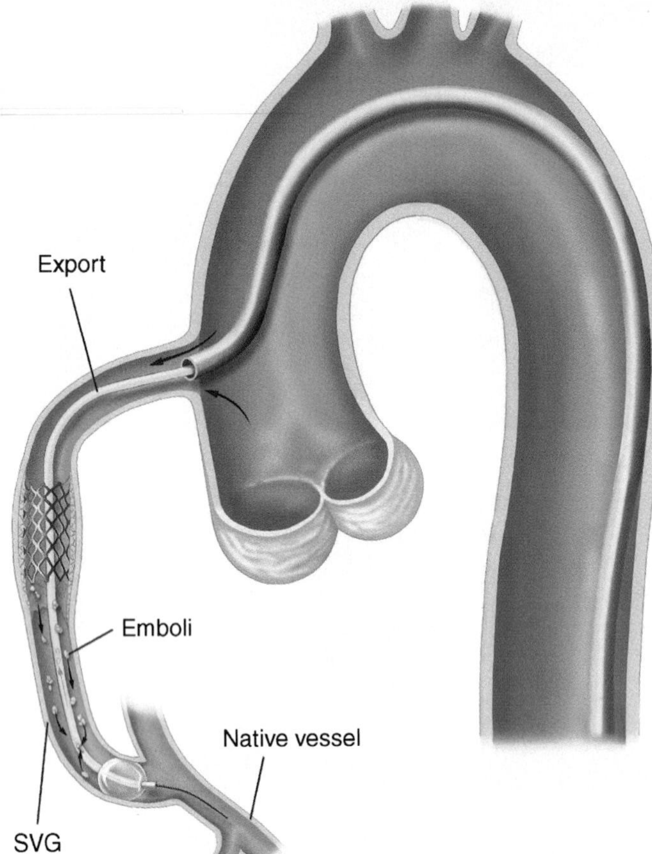

FIGURE 52–6 Key components of the Guardwire Distal Protection Balloon. The Guardwire device is advanced through the saphenous vein graft (SVG) to a distal portion of the SVG that is free of significant stenosis. The occlusion balloon is inflated and, after demonstration of occlusion, stent placement is performed within the SVG. At the end of stent deployment, an Export catheter is advanced and approximately 40 ml of blood and particulate material are removed. (From Baim D, Wahr D, George B, et al: Randomized trial of a distal embolic protection device during percutaneous intervention of saphenous vein aorto-coronary bypass grafts. Circulation 105:1285, 2002. Reproduced with permission.)

it often passes the occlusion in a subintimal dissection plane that requires guidewire use to reenter the distal true lumen.

The IntraLuminal Therapeutics SafeCross (Intraluminal Therapeutics, Kansas City, MO) guidewire is a standard size (0.014-inch) guidewire that contains a single optical fiber. This fiber carries a beam of low-coherence light to the plaque at the tip of the wire and collects the reflected light. When only amorphous plaque is ahead of the wire, that reflection falls off rapidly with increasing distance, but if the tip of the wire is near the vessel wall there is a secondary increase in reflection by the organized collagen fibers therein (i.e., a specular reflector). The system monitors the reflected signal for the presence of the vessel wall signature and alerts the operator to change directions if it is seen. If the fiber detects only plaque and mechanical advancement force is insufficient, it can be supplemented by a brief radiofrequency electrical discharge to help penetrate more fibrocalcific elements of the occlusion. This approach results in successful passage of roughly half of the total occlusions where a conventional guidewire has failed. Once the first wire has crossed the total occluded segment and entered the true lumen beyond, treatment with conventional angioplasty balloons and stents can generally be performed.

Coronary Stents

More than any other of the new devices, coronary stents have revolutionized the practice of interventional cardiology by both reducing early complications and improving late clinical outcomes in a broad array of patients. The concept of a temporary endoluminal splint to scaffold an occluded peripheral vessel was introduced by Charles Dotter nearly 40 years ago but was not practical until the first human coronary implantation was performed in 1986. Self-expanding wire mesh stents were initially used but never attained broad clinical use because of high thrombosis rates. In contrast, a series of balloon-expandable stents has been available in the United States since 1994, and because of improving designs and a large number of randomized trials demonstrating clear benefits in specific lesion subsets (Table 52–3),[4,5,20-23] these devices are now used in more than 80 percent of PCIs.

Indications

DE NOVO OR RESTENOTIC LESIONS. Randomized trials have shown that coronary stenting in relatively large (>3.0-mm), de novo native coronary vessels improves short- and long-term outcomes compared with conventional balloon PTCA. The Stent Restenosis Study (STRESS) and the Belgium Netherlands Stent (BENESTENT) trials showed that Palmaz-Schatz stent placement resulted in a 26 to 31 percent reduction in angiographic restenosis and a 27 to 31 percent lowering of 1-year clinical events compared with balloon PTCA.[4,20] The Restenosis Stent (REST) Study, a randomized trial of 383 patients with prior restenosis after balloon PTCA who were assigned to Palmaz-Schatz stenting or repeated balloon PTCA, showed that angiographic restenosis was lower in stent-treated patients than in balloon PTCA-treated patients (18 versus 32 percent, $p = 0.03$); target lesion revascularization (TLR) also occurred less often in patients treated with coronary stents (10 percent) than in patients treated with balloon PTCA alone (27 percent, $p = 0.001$).[21]

ABRUPT OR THREATENED CLOSURE AFTER BALLOON PTCA. Self-expanding and balloon-expandable coiled and slotted tube stents have been used to scaffold coronary dissections in patients with balloon PTCA–induced complications. The clinical use of coronary stents to treat procedural complications has reduced the emergency CABG rates to less than 1 percent, although clinical trials that attempted to compare prolonged balloon inflations with stent placement for abrupt closure were inconclusive because of difficulties in recruitment of patients (Fig. 52–11). Because stents are used primarily in a broad array of patients, use of stents for bailout purposes alone is uncommon and useful for suboptimal results in smaller vessels or with the development of guiding catheter or guidewire dissections.

SAPHENOUS VEIN GRAFTS. Although balloon PTCA of SVG lesions is associated with reasonably high (88 percent) procedural success rates, clinical recurrence related to restenosis or progression of disease at other SVG sites is common. The Saphenous Vein Graft De Novo (SAVED) Trial randomly assigned 220 patients with de novo SVG lesions to treatment with Palmaz-Schatz stent placement or balloon PTCA alone.[22] Stenting was associated with higher procedural success rates (92 versus 69 percent in balloon-treated patients; $p < 0.001$) at the expense of more bleeding events (17 versus 5 percent in balloon PTCA-treated patients; $p < 0.01$) because of the aggressive anticoagulation regimen used in this study. Although restenosis was not significantly lower in stent-treated patients (37 percent) than in balloon PTCA-treated patients (46 percent), freedom from significant cardiac events was better in the stent group (73 versus 58 percent in balloon PTCA-treated patients; $p = 0.03$). Stents are the pre-

TABLE 52–3 Early and Late Outcome in Randomized Trials of Coronary Stent Placement Versus Balloon Percutaneous Transluminal Coronary Angioplasty

	STRESS[4]		Benestent[20]		Benestent II[5]		REST[21]		SAVED[22]		TOSCA[23]	
Variable	*PTCA*	*Stent*	*PTCA*	*Stent*	*PTCA*	*Stent*	*PTCA*	*Stent*	*PTCA*	*Stent*	*PTCA*	*Stent*
Lesion type	De novo, native		De novo, native		De novo, native		Restenotic, native		SVGs		Chronic occlusion	
Years of entry	1991-1993		1991-1993		1995-1996		1991-1996		1993-1995		1996-1997	
Number of patients	202	205	257	259	410	413	176	178	107	108	208	202
Baseline factors												
Mean age, yr	60	60	58	57	59	50	60	59	66	66	58	58
Women, %	27	17	18	20	20	23	18	20	21	18	20	16
Diabetes mellitus	16	15	6	7	11	13	15	20	36	23	18	15
Unstable angina, %	48	47	NA	NA	40	45	22	17	77	82	25	24
Multivessel disease, %	32	36	NA	NA	NA	NA	32	33	NA	NA	NA	NA
Angiographic success, %	92.6	99.5	98.1	96.9	99	99	93.2	98.9	86	97	NA	NA
Clinical success, %s	89.6	96.1	91.1	92.7	95	96	100	100	69	92	87.9	94.6
Reference diameter, mm	2.99	3.03	3.01	2.99	2.93	2.96	3.04	3.01	3.19	3.18	3.53	3.61
Final % stenosis	35	19	33	22	8	7	30	6	32	12	38	27
Stent use, %	6.9	96.1	5.1	94.6	13.4	96.6	6.8	98.9	7.0	97	9.6	96
Early complications	0-14 d		In hospital		1 mo		In hospital		In hospital		In hospital	
Death, %	1.5	0	0	0	0.2	0	0.6	1.1	2	2	0	0
Q wave Infarction, %	3.0	2.9	0.8	1.9	1.0	1.2	0.6	2.8	1	2	NR	NR
Emergency CABG, %	4.0	2.4	1.6	1.9	0.5	0.7	0.6	1.1	4	2	0	0.5
CK-MB elevation > 3x												
Late clinical outcome	15-240 d		7 mo		12 mo		6 mo		240 d		180 d	
Death, %	0	1.5	0.4	0.8	1.0	1.0	1.1	1.1	9	7	0	0
Q wave MI	0.5	1.0	1.6	2.7	1.5	1.9	0.6	2.8	4	5	NR	NR
Revascularization, %	15.4	10.2	NA	NA	NA	NA	NA	NA	NA	NA	15.4	8.4*
Repeat PTCA	11.4	9.8	20.6	10.0	15.6	9.4	26.6	10.3	16	13	14.4	6.9
CABG	4.5	2.4	2.3	3.1	1.5	1.9	0.6	2.2	12	7	1.4	1.5
Follow-up angiography												
Restenosis, %	42.1	31.6	32	22	31	16	32	18	47	36	70	55†
Follow-up MLD	1.56	1.74	1.73	1.82	1.66	1.89	1.85	2.04	1.49	1.73	1.23	1.49
Follow-up % stenosis	49	42	43	38	17	17	47	30	51	46	61	53
Any bleeding complication	4.0	7.3	3.1	13.5	1.0	1.2	1.1	11.2	5	17	NR	NR

*$p < 0.05$.
†$p < 0.005$.
CABG = coronary artery bypass graft; CK-MB = creatine kinase with muscle and brain subunits; MLD = minimum lumen diameter; MI = myocardial infarction; NA = not applicable; NR = not reported; SAVED = Saphenous for Vein Graft Lesions de novo trial; PTCA = percutaneous transluminal coronary angioplasty; REST = Restenosis Stent Study; STRESS = Stent Restenosis Study; TOSCA = Total Occlusion Study of Canada.

ferred therapy in patients with ostial or body SVG lesions. The risk of no reflow or distal embolization is higher in patients with severe SVG friability and in those with SVG thrombus, although it is improved by the use of thrombectomy and distal embolic protection devices.

TOTAL CORONARY OCCLUSIONS. Balloon PTCA of chronic coronary occlusions is associated with reduced (47 to 69 percent) procedural success, primarily because of failure to cross with a guidewire (see Total Occlusion–Crossing Devices). Even when crossed successfully, total occlusions have a high (45 to 55 percent) incidence of restenotic recurrence, often (19 percent) as recurrent total coronary occlusion. There appears to be no significant benefit of plaque debulking for the treatment of chronic total occlusions. A number of randomized trials have shown the benefit of stent placement over balloon PTCA alone in patients with chronic occlusions. The Total Occlusion Study of Canada (TOSCA) trial randomly assigned 410 patients with native coronary occlusions to balloon PTCA or primary stenting with the heparin-coated Palmaz-Schatz stent. A reduced binary restenosis rate was found in patients treated with the heparin-coated stent (55 percent) compared with the bare metal stent (70 percent; $p < 0.0.01$).[23] In the Stenting in Chronic Coronary Occlusion (SICCO) Study, 119 patients with successful balloon PTCA of a chronic coronary occlusion were assigned to no further intervention or to Palmaz-Schatz stent placement.[24] Angiographic restenosis occurred less often in stent-treated patients (32 percent) than in patients receiving no further therapy (74 percent) ($p < 0.001$). TLR was also needed less often in stent-treated patients (22 percent) than in balloon PTCA–treated patients (42 percent) ($p = 0.025$). This benefit was sustained at late follow-up.[24]

ST SEGMENT ELEVATION MYOCARDIAL INFARCTION. When compared with thrombolytic therapy, primary balloon PTCA improves thrombolysis in myocardial infarction (TIMI) 3 flow rates and reduces the frequency of mortality, reinfarction, and stroke in patients with ST segment elevation myocardial infarction (STEMI) (see also Chap. 48). Primary balloon PTCA may be limited in this setting by recurrent in-hospital ischemia or reinfarction (10 to 15 percent), restenosis (37 to 49 percent), or late reocclusion (9 to 14 percent). Primary stenting confers advantages over balloon

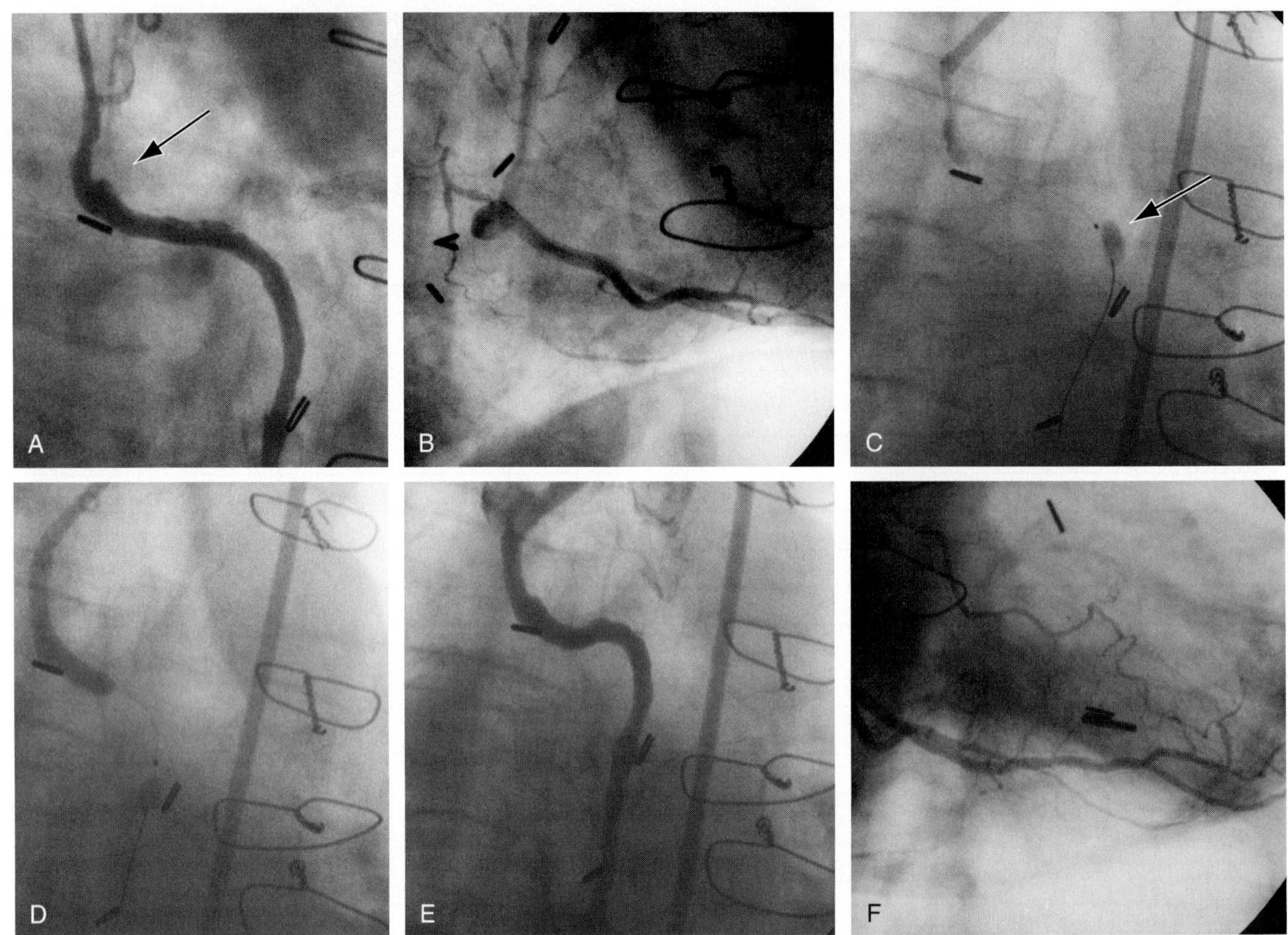

FIGURE 52–7 **A,** Degenerated saphenous vein graft (SVG) to the posterior descending artery with a diffuse stenosis in the proximal segment of the SVG (arrow). **B,** Normal distal perfusion of the SVG with demonstration of secondary and tertiary branches. Positioning of the PercuSurge balloon in the distal portion of the SVG (**C,** arrow) and a 4.0-mm stent in the proximal SVG **(D)** resulted in minimal residual stenosis **(E)** and no evidence of distal embolization **(F)**.

PTCA in patients with STEMI by scaffolding the ruptured plaque and preventing the arterial remodeling that occurs with balloon angioplasty. The Primary Angioplasty in Myocardial Infarction (PAMI) stent trial randomly assigned 900 patients with acute MI to treatment with primary balloon PTCA or placement of the Palmaz-Schatz heparin-coated stent.[25] After 6 months, fewer patients in the stent group had angina (11.3 versus 16.9 percent in the balloon group; $p = 0.02$) or needed TLR (7.7 versus 17.0 percent in the balloon group; $p < 0.001$). Angiographic restenosis also occurred less often in stent-treated patients (20.3 versus 33.5 percent in balloon-treated patients; $p < 0.001$).[25]

Another study, the Controlled Abciximab and Device Investigation to Lower Late Angioplasty Complications (CADILLAC) trial, evaluated the use of abciximab and stents in a 2 × 2 factorial design in 2082 patients with STEMI.[26] At 6 months, the primary endpoint—a composite of death, reinfarction, disabling stroke, and ischemia-driven revascularization of the target vessel—had occurred in 20.0 percent of patients after PTCA, 16.5 percent after PTCA plus abciximab, 11.5 percent after stenting, and 10.2 percent after stenting plus abciximab ($p < 0.001$).[26] There was little incremental benefit associated with routine abciximab use in patients with STEMI, although another study suggested that abciximab may be useful in reducing events in high-risk patients undergoing stent placement.[27] The CADILLAC trial also found that angiographic restenosis occurred in 40.8 percent after PTCA and 22.2 percent after stenting ($p < 0.001$), and the respective rates of reocclusion of the infarct-related artery were 11.3 percent and 5.7 percent ($p = 0.01$), both independent of abciximab use.[26]

STENT DESIGNS

A number of balloon-expandable and self-expanding stents have become available for clinical use. Each stent varies with respect to its metallic composition, strut design, stent length, delivery and deployment system, and arterial surface coverage, among other factors. Although there may be differences in flexibility, ease of delivery, and side branch access among the different stent designs, randomized stent-versus-stent trials comparing various second-generation stent designs with the benchmark Palmaz-Schatz stent have generally failed to show significant differences in subacute stent thrombosis or subsequent restenosis behavior (Table 52–4).[28-32]

Because of the inherent limitations of 316L stainless steel as the major filament component of most commercially available stents, including limited radiopacity and lack of flexibility with thicker filaments, alternative alloys have been considered. Cobalt chromium appears to have better radiopacity and deliverability than stainless steel for comparable strut thicknesses. The Guidant Vision stent (Guidant, Santa Clara, CA), the Medtronic Driver stent (Medtronic Vascular, Santa Rosa, CA), and the Cordis Steeplechaser stent (Cordis, Warren, NJ) all use cobalt chromium alloys and the new generation of balloon-expandable stent and will be the platform for drug elution.

Thromboresistant stents have also been developed to reduce the occurrence of subacute thrombosis, and potentially restenosis, after PCI. The most frequently used is a heparin-coated Bx Velocity stent (Hepa-

TABLE 52–4 Early and Late Outcome in Randomized Trials of Stent Versus Stent Equivalence Trials in Native Vessels

	ASCENT[30]		Paragon[28]		NIRVANA[29]		SCORES[31]		GR-II[32]	
Variable	***PS 153***	***ML***	***Paragon***	***PS 153***	***PS 153***	***NIR***	***PS 153***	***Radius***	***PS 153***	***GR-II***
Number of patients	522	518	349	339	430	418	551	545	375	380
Lesion type	Focal, <25-mm De novo lesion 3.00-3.75-mm		Focal, <25-mm De novo or RS 3.00-4.00-mm		Focal, <25-mm De novo or RS 3.00-3.75-mm		Focal, <25-mm De novo or RS 2.75-4.35-mm		Focal, <25-mm De novo or RS 3.00-4.00-mm	
Baseline factors										
Mean age, yr	61	61	62	62	62	62	62	62	61	61
Women, %	31	33	32	32	32	30	32	30	28.5	31.3
Diabetes mellitus	20	19	21	21	22	23	19	22	22.4	23.2
Unstable angina	70	69	81	82	73	75	65	65	NR	NR
LAD location, %	44	42	41	45	40	42	38	40	43.4	39.7
Lesion length, mm	11.0	10.9	12.4	12.2	13.3	13.3	13.0	12.8	14.0	14.3
ACC/AHA B_2 or C	59	63	63	69	65	69	NR	NR	NR	NR
Maximum inflation pressure	17.1	16.7	16.7	17.1	16.6	15.5	16.8	13.3	NR	NR
Reference diameter, mm	2.94	2.95	2.97*	3.05	2.97	3.03	3.05	3.06	3.08	3.08
MLD, mm										
Baseline	1.05	1.05	1.05	1.07	1.09	1.04	0.99	1.01	1.06	1.08
Final	2.72	2.77	2.83	2.83	2.73	2.74	2.80	2.86	2.83	2.64
Follow-up	1.92	1.96	1.78	1.93	1.90	2.00	1.88	1.88	1.90	1.48
% Diameter stenosis										
Baseline	64	64	64	65	63	65	66.5	67.3	65.2	64.7
Final	10	8	6.3	8.8*	8	8	11.8	12.2	9.8	15.6
Follow-up	32	35	39.8	37.9			36.1	36.3	36.4	50.6§
Restenosis rate	22.1	16.0	29.1	23.7	22.4	19.3	18.7	24.2	20.6	47.3§
Device success, %	96.9	98.8	NR	NR	97.9	99.5	95.3	98.3‡	NR	NR
Procedural success, %s	93.9	95.7	91.9	95.5	94.3	95.4	93.5	97.0	NR	NR
30-d event rates	6.5	5.0	8.3‖	4.4	4.4	4.3	3.1	2.9	1.3	4.2
Death, %	1.1	0*	0.3	0	0.2	0	0.4	0.4	0.5	0.3
Q wave infarction, %	1.0	0.6	0.9	0.3	0.9	0.5	0.4	0.2	0.5	1.3
Emergency CABG, %	0.8	0.6	0.3	0.3	0	0.2	0.7	0.9	0.3	1.9
Subacute thrombosis, %	1.8	0.6	0.6	0.3	0.5	0.5	0.4	0.2	0.3	3.9‡
Follow-up period, mo	9 mo		6 mo		6 mo		9 mo			
TLR, %	9.8	7.7	12.0	5.9*	13.4	12.2	10.7	9.5	15.3	27.4§
Late clinical events, %	19.5	17.8	19.8	11.2†	15.3	14.1	NR	NR	17.8	29.8§
Death	2.5	1.4	2.0	1.2	0.9	1.0	1.1	1.5	2.7	2.7
Q wave MI	1.0	0.6	2.0	0.3	0.9	0.7	0.5	0.7	0.8	1.4
CABG, %	2.9	2.3	2.9	2.4	3.0	2.4	5.3	5.1	4.4	5.1
Repeat PCI, %	6.9	5.4	9.7	4.1†	8.6	7.2	11.1	10.3	10.9	22.8§

ACC/AHA = American College of Cardiology/American Heart Association; ASCENT = ACS Stent Clinical Equivalence in De Novo Lesions trial; CABG = coronary artery bypass graft; GR-II = Gianturco-Roubin stent; MI = myocardial infarction; MLD = minimal lumen diameter; NIRVANA = The NIR Vascular Advanced North American trial; NR = not reported; PS = Palmaz-Schatz stent; RS = restenotic lesion; SCORES = the Stent Comparative Restenosis Trial; TLR = target lesion revascularization.

*$p < 0.05$.

†$p < 0.01$.

‡$p < 0.005$.

§$p < 0.001$.

‖In-hospital events.

¶Balloon PTCA with "bailout" stenting.

coat, Cordis, Warren, NJ) that has been shown to have a low thrombosis rate in a number of complex subsets.[5,23,25] Silicon carbide–coated stents have also been developed with low subacute thrombosis rates.

Clinical Outcomes and Complications of Percutaneous Coronary Intervention

Anatomical (or angiographic) success after PCI is defined as the attainment of residual diameter stenosis less than 50 percent and normal TIMI 3 flow (see Chap. 18). Procedural success is defined as angiographic success without the occurrence of major complications (death, MI, or CABG) within 30 days of the procedure. Clinical success is defined as procedural success without the need for urgent repeated PCI or surgical revascularization within the first 30 days of the procedure.[33]

With stenting to control dissection and abrupt closure (and thereby to avert emergency CABG), the most common complication of current PCI is periprocedural MI. The incidence of Q wave MI remains 1 to 2 percent, and the most common events are non-Q-wave MIs as diagnosed by postprocedure

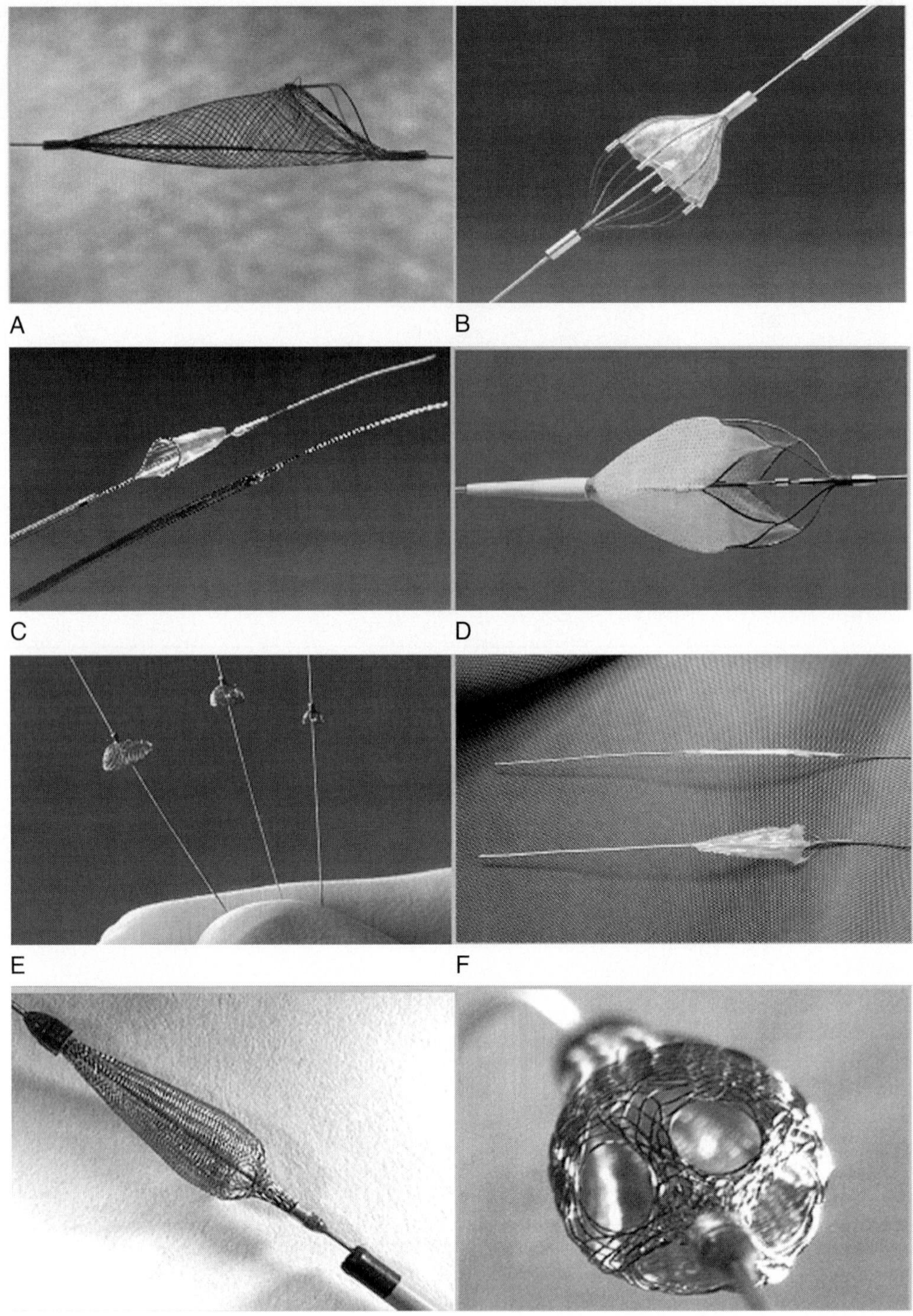

FIGURE 52–8 Filters for distal protection. **A,** The Spider filter (ev3, Minneapolis, MN). **B,** Angioguard device (Cordis, Warren, NJ). **C,** EPI Filterwire (Boston Scientific, Natick, MA). **D,** Accunet device (Guidant, Santa Clara, CA). **E,** MedNova (Abbott, Chicago, IL). **F,** Rubicon filter (Rubicon). **G** and **H,** The Interceptor filter (Medtronic Vascular, Santa Rosa, CA), in longitudinal view **(G)** and axial view **(H)**.

elevation of cardiac enzymes. Two classification systems are in use: (1) the World Health Organization (WHO) classification system, which includes a total creatine phosphokinase (CPK) isoenzyme elevation more than two times normal in association with elevation of the CPK-MB isoform and occurs after 1 to 2 percent of PCI procedures, and (2) the FDA classification system, which includes an elevation in CPK-MB of three times normal or higher after the procedure and occurs after 5 to 10 percent of procedures.[34] The incidence of such events may be significantly higher when atherectomy devices are used or in high-risk lesion subgroups, such as SVGs. Although several studies have shown that CK or CK-MB elevations over five to eight times the upper limit of normal adversely affect subsequent survival, the causal relationship of small (one to eight times normal CPK-MB) elevations to late mortality is unclear. Some studies have suggested worse long-term outcomes with even one to three times elevations of cardiac enzymes, but it is not clear whether this is a cause-and-effect relationship or just a reflection of the ability of more diffuse atherosclerotic involvement to cause both

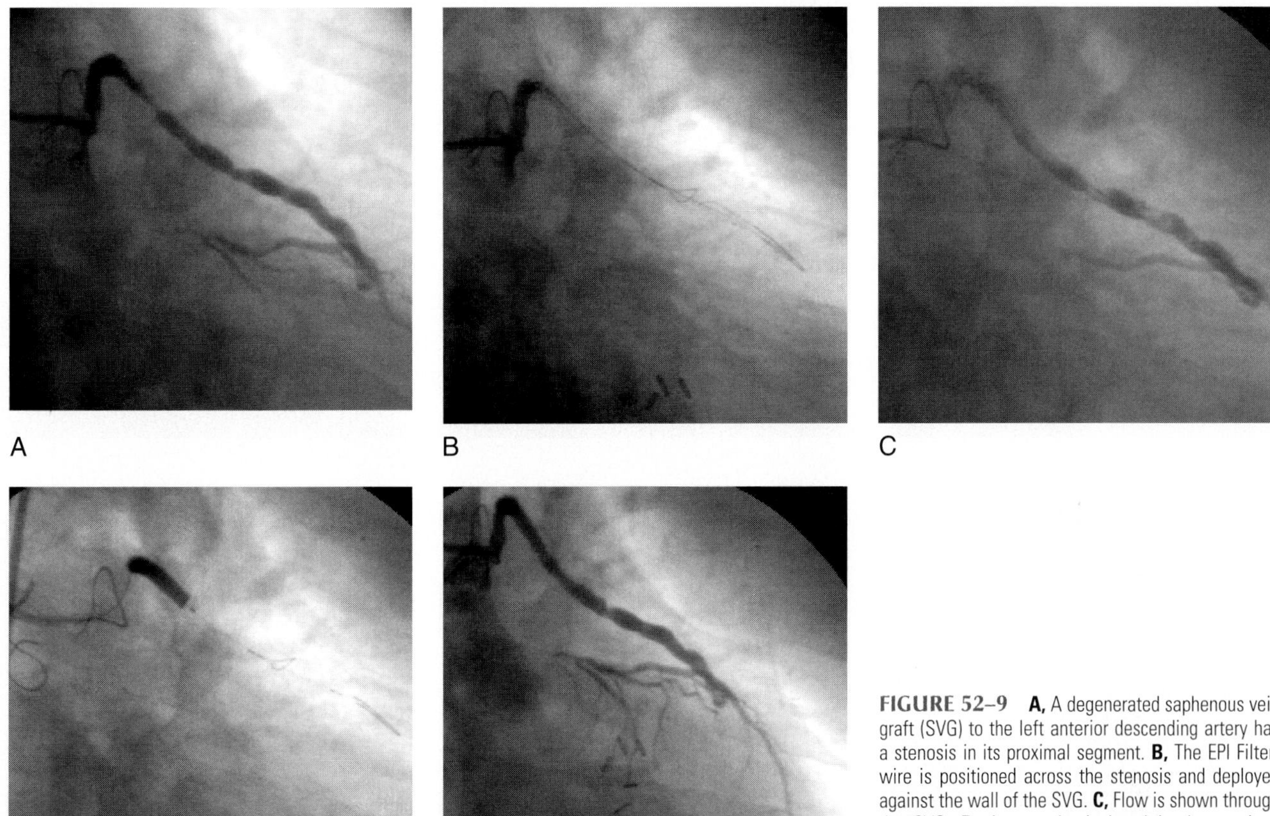

FIGURE 52–9 **A,** A degenerated saphenous vein graft (SVG) to the left anterior descending artery has a stenosis in its proximal segment. **B,** The EPI Filterwire is positioned across the stenosis and deployed against the wall of the SVG. **C,** Flow is shown through the SVG. **D,** A stent is deployed in the proximal segment of the SVG. **E,** The Filterwire is removed, and there is excellent flow into the distal SVG without evidence of distal embolization.

greater periprocedural CK elevation and worse long-term outcome.

Early procedural outcome after PCI is correlated with clinical factors, including age, unstable and Canadian Cardiovascular Society (CCS) class IV angina, congestive heart failure, cardiogenic shock, renal insufficiency, and preprocedural instability requiring intraaortic balloon pump support, among other factors. Anatomical risk variables include multivessel CAD, presence of thrombus, SVG intervention, and American College of Cardiology/American Heart Association (ACC/AHA) type C lesion morphology, including chronic total coronary occlusion. Procedural factors also affect procedure outcomes, including a higher final percent diameter stenosis, smaller minimal lumen diameter, and the presence of a residual dissection or transstenotic pressure gradient (see Chap. 18 for definitions of ACC/AHA lesion types). Procedural mortality is associated with balloon PTCA of arteries subtending 50 percent or more of the myocardium, a left ventricular ejection fraction less than 25 percent, a more severe preprocedural percent diameter stenosis, multivessel CAD, and female gender, among other factors.[35,36] The latter factors indicate a greater risk for cardiovascular collapse should abrupt vessel closure occur.

The early use of coronary stents was limited by high (3.5 to 8.6 percent) subacute thrombosis rates despite aggressive antithrombotic therapy with aspirin (>325 mg daily), dipyridamole (225 mg daily), periprocedural low-molecular-weight dextran, and an uninterrupted transition from intravenous heparin to oral warfarin. Clinical events associated with subacute thrombosis were profound, resulting in an untoward outcome (e.g., death, MI, or emergency revascularization) in virtually every such patient. Patients at high risk for subacute thrombosis included those with unstable angina, residual proximal or distal dissection, angiographic thrombus or a filling defect, in-laboratory transient or sustained abrupt closure, multiple (more than three) stent implants, smaller (<3.0-mm) vessels, total occlusions, or stent placement for failed balloon PTCA. Anatomical factors were also important contributors to subacute thrombosis after stent deployment (e.g., underdilation of the stent, proximal and distal dissections, poor inflow or outflow obstruction, <3-mm vessel diameter). Lower frequencies of subacute stent thrombosis (roughly 0.5 percent) are now achieved with optimal stent deployment and with a modern drug regimen including aspirin and a thienopyridine (ticlopidine or clopidogrel) started just after stent placement.[37]

Side branch occlusion may also occur in some patients after stent placement (6 to 14 percent), particularly in bifurcation lesions involving the origin of the side branch. The clinical importance of the side branch occlusion is related to the size of the side branch and extent of myocardium that the side branch supplies. Open-cell and coiled stent designs may provide better access to side branches than afforded by the closed-cell, tubular slotted stent designs. Stent dislodgment from the delivery catheter is an uncommon occurrence with second- and third-generation stents, but it occurred more often in the era when stents were "hand crimped" onto a balloon catheter, although generally without serious complication. Stent margin dissections can occur during stent deployment or during postdeployment stent dilation, particularly when stent dilation strategies are directed at maximizing the internal stent diameter. The availability of shorter (15-mm), noncompliant balloons allows more precise stent dilation when using high (>16 atm) pressure, thereby

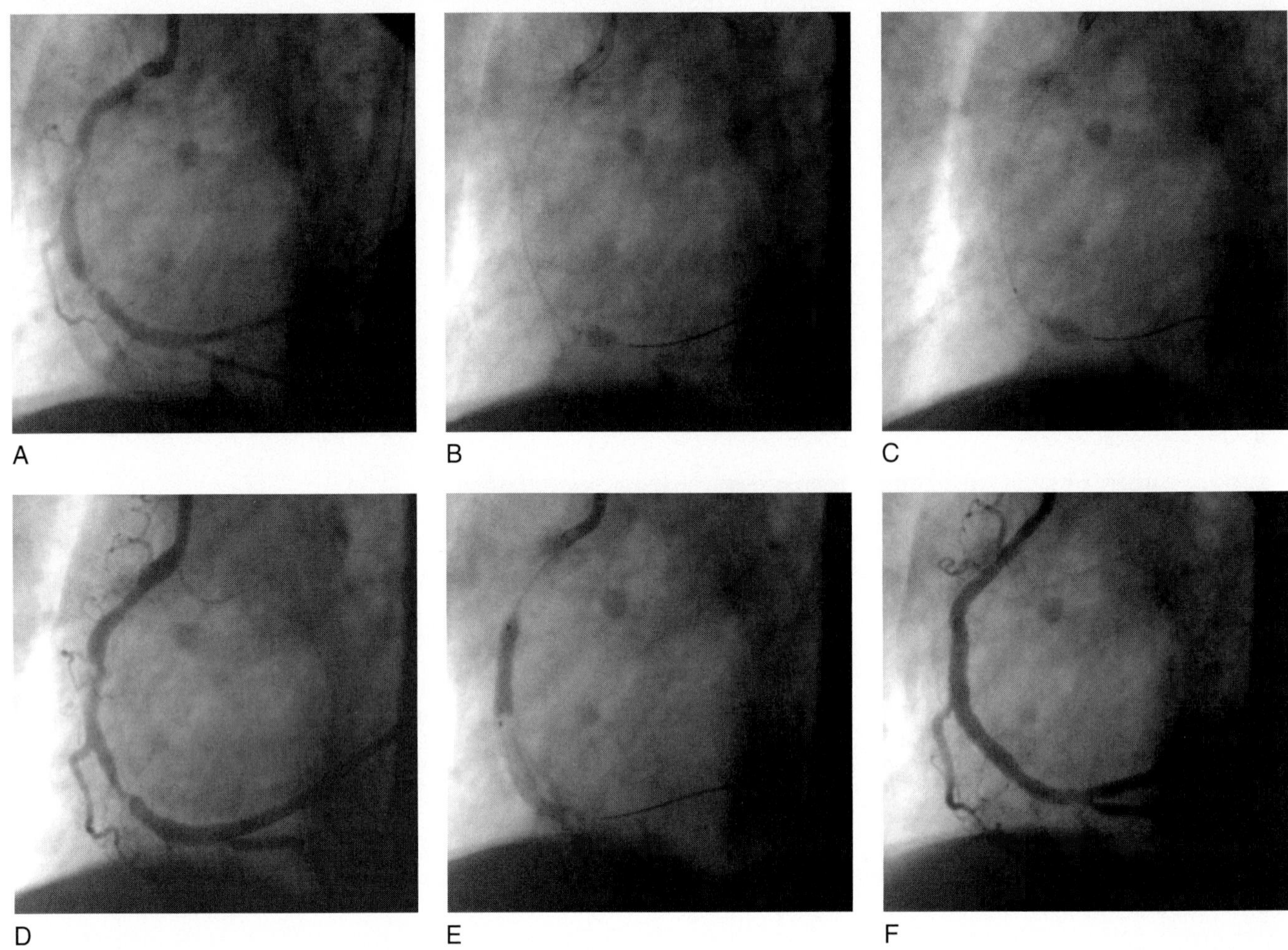

FIGURE 52–10 **A,** A thrombotic lesion causing occlusion of the middle right coronary artery (RCA) is demonstrated in a patient who experienced reperfusion after thrombolytic therapy. The vessel was at high risk for distal embolization because of the underlying thrombus burden. **B,** The Percusurge Guardwire was positioned in the distal RCA (arrow). **C,** The Export catheter (arrow) was advanced and 20 ml of blood and clot was removed before stent placement. **D,** The export catheter removed a substantial amount of thrombus. **E,** A 4.0-mm stent was placed with distal protection, and the Export catheter was again used to remove the residual thrombus. **F,** The final angiographic result demonstrated no evidence of distal embolization.

reducing the frequency of edge dissections. Coronary perforation is also an uncommon occurrence after stent deployment, but it may occur during poststent deployment dilation with an oversized balloon inflated to high pressure. No evidence indicates that higher balloon inflation pressures predispose to higher rates of stent restenosis.

Late Clinical Outcome

Clinical events after PCI are attributable to arterial renarrowing at the PTCA site, intimal hyperplasia in the region of coronary stenting, progression or instability of atherosclerotic disease at remote sites, or a combination of these events. These processes can be partially distinguished by the time of occurrence of the event, with angiographic and clinical restenosis generally developing within 6 to 9 months after balloon PTCA and death, MI, and progression of atherosclerosis occurring as a low but constant hazard (1 to 2 percent risk per year) indefinitely after the procedure. Predictors of higher risk of all-cause late mortality include advanced age, reduced left ventricular function or congestive heart failure, presence of diabetes mellitus, number of diseased vessels, inoperable disease, and severe comorbid conditions. A 95 percent 10-year survival rate can be expected in patients with single-vessel CAD and an 80 percent survival rate after PCI can be achieved in those with multivessel CAD.

The risk of restenosis after balloon PTCA depends on clinical factors, such as diabetes mellitus, unstable angina, acute MI, and prior restenosis; anatomical factors, such as total occlusions, proximal left anterior descending artery lesions, smaller vessel size, long lesions, and lesions involving an SVG; and procedural factors, such as the final minimal lumen diameter or percent diameter stenosis. Exposure to infectious agents may also predispose to the development of restenosis. Risk factors for restenosis after coronary stent placement include age, a history of diabetes, a longer lesion or total stent length, small postprocedural minimal lumen diameters, and the left anterior descending lesion location.

In-Stent Restenosis

Accumulation of neointimal tissue within the axial stent length accounts for virtually all cases of in-stent restenosis. Recurrence of symptoms may occur in 10 to 20 percent of patients within 12 months after stent implantation; after 6 to 12 months, improvements of the lumen dimensions related to scar retraction have been noted. Although some patients with multivessel CAD or multiple stent restenoses are best served by referral for CABG, the majority of patients with in-stent restenosis can be safety and effectively treated with repeated PCI, with the mechanism of benefit related to both expansion of the stent and extrusion of the tissue through the

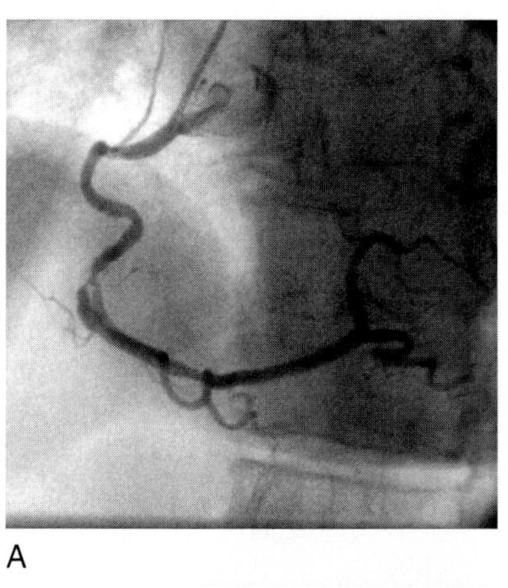
A

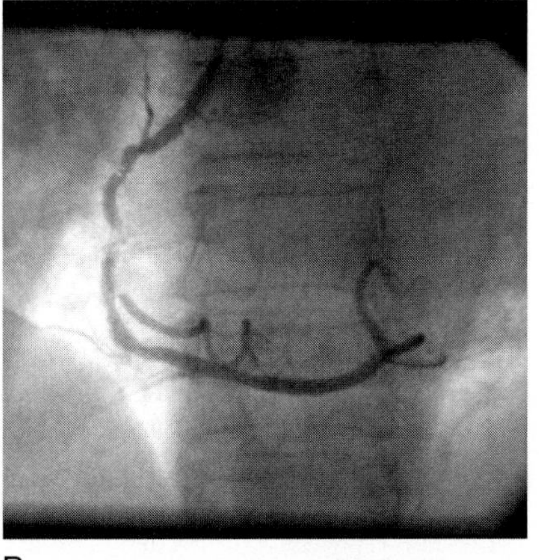
B

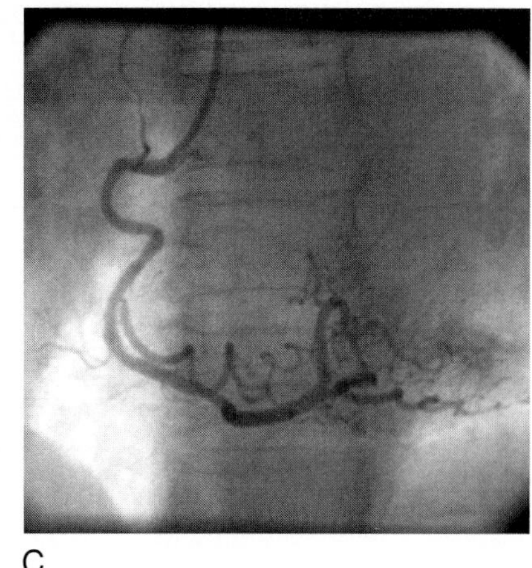
C

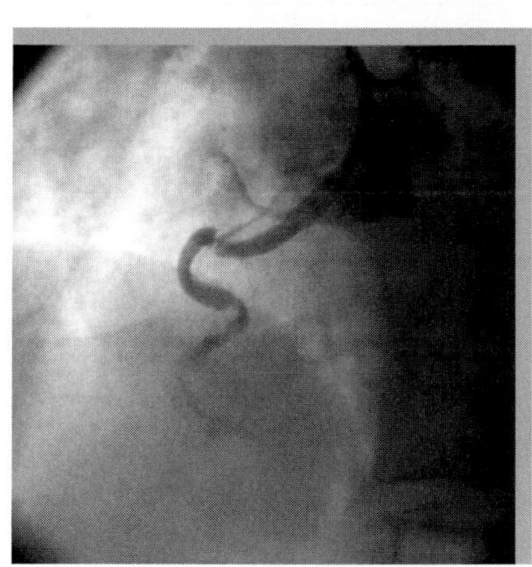
D

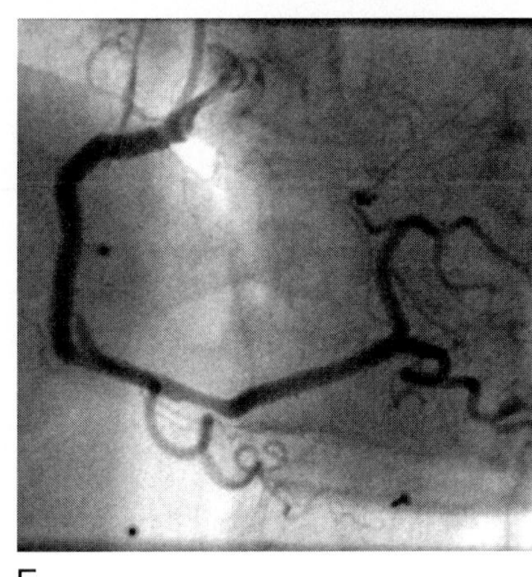
E

FIGURE 52–11 **A,** An extremely tortuous right coronary artery has a stenosis in its midportion. **B,** After crossing with a coronary guidewire, there is marked straightening of the vessel. **C,** After a stent is placed and the guidewire is removed, there is an excellent initial result. **D,** Abrupt closure develops because of a guide catheter dissection, resulting in typical chest pain and ST segment elevation. **E,** Coronary stents are placed to "bail out" the severe coronary dissection that developed, and normal flow is reestablished to the vessel. Without the availability of coronary stents, it is highly likely that coronary bypass surgery would have been needed to reverse the abrupt closure event.

stent struts and along its length. Early tissue recoil may also occur immediately after PCI in those with in-stent restenosis. Recurrence rates after balloon PTCA for stent restenosis ranged from 10 to 20 percent, although higher (up to 80 percent) recurrence rates have been reported depending on vessel size, pattern of restenosis (e.g., intrastent, stent margin, or remote disease), and the time to presentation.

Atheroablation by DCA, RA, or ELCA has been used in patients at "high risk" for recurrence after PCI for in-stent restenosis, but an advantage over conventional balloon PTCA alone has not been demonstrated in a prospective, randomized study. The Angioplasty versus Rotational Atherectomy for Treatment of Diffuse In-Stent Restenosis Trial (ARTIST) study was a multicenter, randomized, prospective trial with 298 patients with in-stent restenosis who were assigned to treatment with balloon angioplasty or rotablation performed using a stepped-burr approach followed by adjunctive balloon angioplasty.[38] Although restenosis rates were lower (51 percent) in the balloon angioplasty arm than in the RA arm (65 percent; $p = 0.039$),[38] these differences were related to the use of low-pressure inflations after RA that resulted in incomplete stent expansion.

"Very late" (>1 year) restenosis occurs rarely after coronary stenting in native coronary arteries. Three-year angiographic and clinical follow-up was obtained for 143 patients (147 lesions) who underwent Palmaz-Schatz stent placement in native coronaries.[39] After 14 months, TLR was necessary in only 2.1 percent of patients, whereas balloon PTCA of a new lesion was required in 7.7 percent of patients. Follow-up coronary angiography showed no further decrease in minimal lumen diameter between 6 months and 1 year (1.95-mm in both groups), as well as a significant ($p < 0.001$) improvement in minimal lumen diameter between 6 months (1.94-mm) and 3 years (2.09-mm).[39]

Radiation Brachytherapy for In-Stent Restenosis

Because in-stent restenosis is solely due to excessive neointimal proliferation within the stent, it is reasonable that local radiation therapy could retard such proliferation and reduce the chance of recurrence when an in-stent restenotic lesion is treated (Table 52–5).[40-44] Three studies have shown the value of gamma irradiation with iridium-192 (^{192}Ir) in reducing the frequency of angiographic and clinical recurrence in patients undergoing treatment for in-stent restenosis.[40-42] In the largest of these studies, the multicenter Gamma-1 trial randomly assigned 252 patients with in-stent restenosis to either ^{192}Ir intracoronary radiation or placebo after treatment of in-stent restenosis.[42] Six-month angiographic follow-up demonstrated a significant reduction of in-stent restenosis in the radiation group compared with placebo (21 percent in the gamma radiation group versus 49.5 percent in the placebo group, $p < 0.001$).[42] The beneficial effects of gamma radiation have been sustained for up to 5 years after the procedure. Gamma brachytherapy has also been shown to be particularly useful in long lesions, total occlusions, and in patients with SVG stenoses and diabetes mellitus. Its limitations are prolonged treatment times and the need for extensive shielding within the procedure room.

TABLE 52–5 Late Outcome in Randomized Trials of Radiation Brachytherapy for the Prevention of In-Stent Restenosis

	Scripps[40]		WRIST[41]		Gamma-1[42]		START[44]		INHIBIT[43]	
Variable	*Ir-192*	*PL*	*Ir-192*	*PL*	*Ir-192*	*PL*	*Sr-90*	*PL*	*P-32*	*PL*
Number of patients	26	29	65	65	131	121	244	232	166	166
Baseline factors										
Mean age, yr	70	69	63	62	58	61	61	61	62	61
Women, %	27	24	34	28	25.2	26.6	32	37	30	27
Diabetes mellitus	27	41	39	45	31.3	31.4	31	32	33	27
Lesion length, mm	12.9	11.9	28.8	26.7	19	20.3	16.3	16.0	16.9	17.9
Reference diameter, mm	2.88	2.78	2.71	2.72	2.69	2.73	2.76	2.77	2.68	2.71
MLD, mm										
Baseline	1.10	1.03	0.94	0.81	0.98	0.96	0.98	0.98	1.01	0.95
Final	2.82	2.88	2.23	2.25	2.09	2.12	1.94	1.94	1.92	1.96
Follow-up	2.43*	1.85	2.03§	1.24	1.47	1.31	1.65§	1.41	1.54*	1.38
% Diameter stenosis										
Baseline	62	62	65	70	63.3	64.6	64.2	64.2	61.9	65.2
Final	7	5	19	20	23.9	24.5	31.4	30.7	29.6	28.5
Follow-up	17*	54	30§	57	45.6	53.2	41.7§	50.1	43.3‡	51.3
Restenosis rate, %	17*	54	22§	60	32.4*	55.3	28.8§	45.2	26§	52
Stent thrombosis, %	1	0	9.2	3.5	6.3	1.6	0	0.4	3	1
Follow-up period, mo	6 mo		12 mo		9 mo		8 mo		290 d	
TLR, %	12*	45	23.0§	63.1	24.4†	42.1	13.9§	24.9	8§	26
Late clinical events, %	19*	62	35.3§	67.6	28.2*	43.8	19.1*	28.7	12§	28
Death	0	3	6.2	6.2	3.1	0.8	1.3	0.5	3	2
Q wave MI	4	0	0	0	4.6	2.5	0	0	2	0

INHIBIT = Intimal Hyperplasia Inhibition with Beta In-Stent trial; MLD = minimal lumen diameter; MI = myocardial infarction; PL = placebo; START = Stents and Radiation Therapy trial; TLR = target lesion revascularization; WRIST = Washington Radiation for In-Stent Restenosis Trial.

*$p < 0.05$.
†$p < 0.01$.
‡$p < 0.005$.
§$p < 0.001$.

Beta radiation therapy also reduces the recurrence rates in patients undergoing treatment for in-stent restenosis (Fig. 52-12).[43,44] In a multicenter, "blinded," and randomized trial 476 patients with in-stent restenosis treated with either intracoronary radiation using a $^{90}Sr/^{90}Y$ beta source or placebo for in-stent restenosis, the primary endpoint, 8-month clinically driven target vessel revascularization, was reduced from 26.8 percent in the patients assigned to placebo to 17.0 percent in patients assigned to radiation ($p = 0.015$).[44] The binary 8-month angiographic restenosis (more than 50 percent diameter stenosis) within the entire segment treated with radiation was reduced from 45.2 percent in the placebo-treated patients to 28.8 percent in the $^{90}Sr/^{90}Y$-treated patients ($p = 0.001$).[44] In another study of 332 patients with in-stent restenosis who underwent successful coronary intervention, random assignment was made to intracoronary beta radiation with a phosphorus-32 source or placebo delivered into a centering balloon catheter through an automatic afterloader.[43] The binary angiographic restenosis rate was significantly lower in the radiated group than the placebo group for the entire analyzed segment.[43] Similar results have been demonstrated with a ^{32}P beta balloon source.[45] Beta radiation is more convenient than gamma radiation, requiring shorter treatment times and less shielding in the laboratory. Its limitation is that it may have limited use in larger (>4.0-mm) vessels. Beta radiation has not proved beneficial in patients undergoing primary balloon angioplasty or provisional stenting.

Two limitations of brachytherapy were identified from these studies. Some patients developed restenosis at the margin of the treatment zone, attributable to vessel injury with incomplete radiation coverage. This limitation has been lessened by the use of longer radiation sources with a 5- to 10-mm margin proximal and distal to the regions of balloon dilation. The second limitation was the occurrence of late (>30 day) subacute stent thrombosis in patients receiving a new stent.[42] The occurrence of late vessel occlusion has been substantially reduced with the use of long-term (up to 12 months) clopidogrel administration. Indications for brachytherapy for the treatment of in-stent restenosis include early (<3 month) restenosis, recurrent restenosis, diabetes, SVG restenosis, and longer lesions.

Vascular Closure Devices

Most (90 percent) coronary interventional procedures are performed from the femoral artery using the Seldinger technique, although there is increasing use of the radial approach in obese patients, patients with a bleeding diathesis, or patients with peripheral vascular disease. At the end of the procedure, the standard approach has been to discontinue further unfractionated heparin use and allow the activated clotting time (ACT) to fall below 150 to 180 seconds. The vascular sheath was then removed and manual or mechanical external compression was applied for 10 to 30 minutes until a hemostatic plug formed over the arterial entry site. Patients were then kept at bed rest for 4 to 6 hours before ambulation and discharge. Complications at the catheter entry site occurred in 5 to 7 percent of patients and included free rebleeding, local hematoma, femoral arterial pseudoaneurysm, retroperitoneal bleeding, and femoral arteriovenous fistulas. Discomfort, prolonged hospitalization, transfusion, or even surgical repair of the femoral artery was occasionally (3 to 10 percent) required. This motivated the search for devices that could achieve immediate hemostasis at the puncture site regardless of ongoing anticoagulation, reduce subsequent complications, and allow immediate ambulation.

Several classes of approach to puncture site management have been attempted. The suture-based approach (e.g., Perclose, Sutura) is to deliver surgical suture remotely through the margins of the puncture site, knot the ends of the suture together, and slide the resulting knot down to the arterial surface to duplicate surgical closure. Initial trials showed rapid hemostasis and ambulation but with some residual complications related to incorrect placement of sutures,

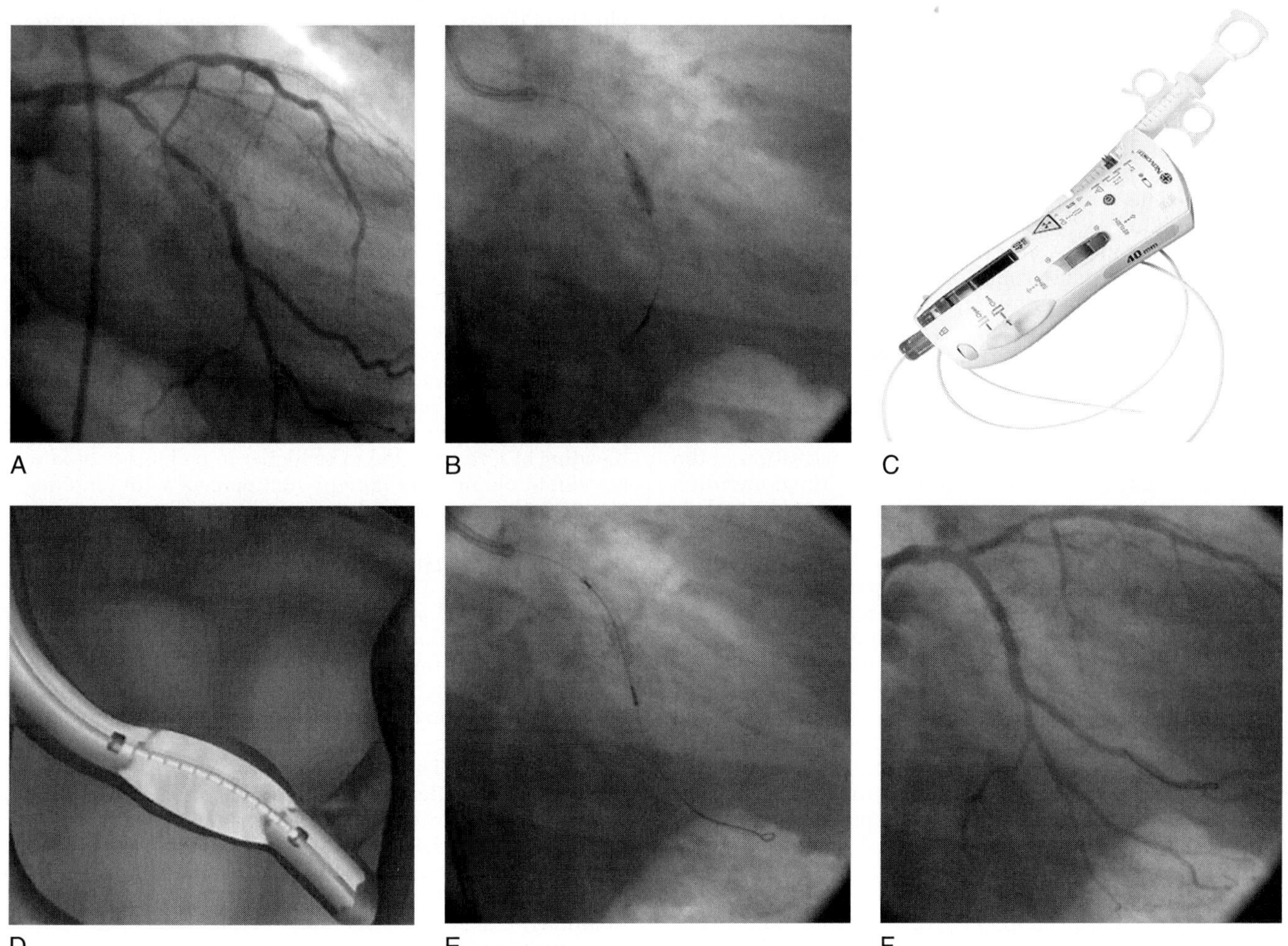

FIGURE 52–12 **A,** Restenosis after coronary stent placement in the midportion of the left circumflex coronary artery. **B,** A 3.5-mm cutting balloon was used to dilate the lesion proximally and distally. **C,** The Novoste Transfer Device uses a saline-filled syringe to advance the radiation seeds to the treatment site. The same device is used to remove the seeds at the end of the brachytherapy treatment. **D,** The Novoste delivery catheter advances $^{90}Sr/^{90}Y$ seeds to the site of angioplasty. **E,** The fluoroscopic position of the catheter is positioned to provide a 5- to 10-mm proximal and distal margin at the region of injury. **F,** The final angiographic result after radiation brachytherapy is shown.

mechanical breakage, or infection caused by the foreign body. Subsequent generations of devices have reduced the size and complexity of placement, and meticulous attention to aseptic technique or even use of prophylactic antibiotics has controlled the infection risk.

Collagen-based approaches seek to apply a small pack of purified bovine collagen to the external surface of the artery. This can be done just externally (VasoSeal, Datascope) or in conjunction with an intraarterial absorbable anchor and suture (AngioSeal, Kensey-Nash). These devices are generally easier to employ than the suture approach,[46] although correct technical placement is essential to efficacy and minimizing complications.

Procoagulant-based approaches (Vascular Solutions Duett) seek to achieve internal mechanical hemostasis temporarily with a miniature balloon-tip catheter while a liquid procoagulant (thrombin and collagen) is deposited in the soft tissue just outside the artery. Once this material is in place, the balloon can be deflated and removed, with rapid formation of the hemostatic plug following contact of the blood with the procoagulant. Incorrect deposition can lead to poor hemostasis or procoagulant deposition within the arterial lumen with production of distal limb ischemic complications.

The balance of the patient's comfort related to elimination of manual or mechanical compression and prolonged bed rest, greater staff efficiencies in not having to supervise delayed sheath removal, and the ability to facilitate outpatient procedures have made the use of one or more of the groin closure devices described previously fairly routine in catheter-based interventional procedures. Still, failure to eliminate the standard groin complications compared with manual compression and the potential for introducing unique complications such as infection and intraarterial administration of procoagulants have led other laboratories to continue to favor manual or mechanical groin compression following catheter-based intervention.

Anticoagulation During Percutaneous Coronary Intervention

(see also Chaps. 48 and 80)

PCI requires the use of one or more antiplatelet agents (e.g., aspirin, clopidogrel, and GP IIb/IIIa inhibitors) combined with some level of thrombin inhibition (e.g., intravenous heparin, low-molecular-weight heparin [LMWH], or bivalirudin) in order to prevent thrombus formation on the denuded endothelium, balloons, stents, and wires that are used to perform the PCI.

Aspirin

Aspirin is an irreversible inhibitor of the enzyme cyclooxygenase that blocks the synthesis of thromboxane A_2, a vasoconstricting agent that promotes platelet aggregation. Compared with placebo, aspirin substantially reduced periprocedural MI related to thrombotic occlusions and has been established as a standard for all patients undergoing PCI. Although the minimum effective aspirin dosage in the setting of PCI has not been established, oral or intravenous doses greater than 75 mg given at least 2 hours before the procedure appear to be effective. The inhibitory effect of aspirin occurs within 60 minutes, and its effect on platelet inhibition lasts for up to 7 days after aspirin discontinuation. It is now recognized that a substantial number of patients have aspirin resistance with standard doses of aspirin therapy.

Thienopyridine Derivatives

Thienopyridine derivatives cause irreversible platelet inhibition related to their effects on the P2Y12 adenosine diphosphate (ADP) receptor that is responsible for activation of the GP IIb/IIIa complex. Because aspirin and thienopyridine derivatives have synergistic mechanisms of action, their combination may inhibit platelet aggregation to a greater extent than either agent alone. Clopidogrel, 300 mg loading followed by 75 mg daily, or, less preferred, ticlopidine, 500 mg loading followed by 250 mg twice daily, may also be used as an alternative in aspirin-sensitive patients undergoing balloon angioplasty or coronary atherectomy.

Subacute vessel closure is a recognized complication of stent placement and occurred in 3 to 5 percent of cases in the initial stent series,[4,20] and this risk was substantially reduced with the addition of a thienopyridine derivate in addition to aspirin.[37,47] In a study of 517 high-risk patients treated with Palmaz-Schatz stents for acute MI, suboptimal angioplasty, or other high-risk clinical and anatomical features, random assignment to aspirin plus ticlopidine or anticoagulant therapy was performed after successful stent placement.[47] The primary composite endpoint of cardiac death, MI, CABG, or repeated angioplasty occurred in 6.2 percent of patients assigned to anticoagulant therapy and 1.5 percent of patients assigned to antiplatelet therapy ($p = 0.01$).[47] Subacute stent thrombosis developed in 5.4 percent of patients assigned to anticoagulant therapy and in 0.8 percent of the antiplatelet therapy group. A second study was performed in 1653 lower risk patients undergoing successful Palmaz-Schatz stent placement.[37] The Stent Anticoagulation Restenosis Study (STARS) compared the effect of aspirin, 325 mg daily; the combination of aspirin, 325 mg daily, plus ticlopidine, 500 mg daily, for 1 month; and aspirin, 325 mg daily, plus warfarin on 30-day ischemic endpoints.[37] The composite of death, TLR, angiographic thrombosis, or MI was reduced from 3.6 percent of patients assigned to aspirin only and 2.7 percent assigned to aspirin plus warfarin to 0.5 percent of those assigned to aspirin plus ticlopidine ($p < 0.001$).[37]

Ticlopidine use has been virtually abandoned because of frequent side effects and hematological toxicities with the availability of the safer thienopyridine derivative clopidogrel. Rare hematological complications have been reported with clopidogrel, including hemolytic-uremic syndrome and thrombotic thrombocytopenic purpura, but it is still considered much safer than ticlopidine. Randomized trials have shown no difference in clinical efficacy between clopidogrel and ticlopidine, with fewer side effects in patients treated with clopidogrel. Although higher (450 to 600 mg) doses of clopidogrel prior to PCI may provide additional benefit compared with conventional loading doses, additional study is needed before this is routinely recommended.

Prolonged (up to 10 days) pretreatment with clopidogrel before PCI in patients with acute coronary syndromes was associated with improved 30-day outcomes compared with patients who were not pretreated with clopidogrel,[48] although the incremental benefit of clopidogrel given just before elective PCI has not been clearly established. The combination of aspirin and clopidogrel may also be useful in preventing ischemic complications for up to 9 months after PCI in patients with acute coronary syndromes[48] and after elective angioplasty.[49] The Clopidogrel for the Reduction of Events During Observation (CREDO) trial was a randomized, double-blind, placebo-controlled trial involving 2116 patients who were to undergo elective PCI who were randomly assigned to receive a 300-mg clopidogrel loading dose or placebo 3 to 24 hours before PCI. Thereafter, all patients received clopidogrel, 75 mg/d, through day 28. From day 29 through 12 months, patients in the loading-dose group received clopidogrel, 75 mg/d, and those in the control group received placebo. Both groups received aspirin throughout the study. The 12-month incidence of the composite of death, MI, or stroke in the intent-to-treat population was reduced by 26.9 percent in patients treated with clopidogrel ($p = 0.02$).[49] Risk of major bleeding at 1 year tended to be higher in patients treated with combined clopidogrel therapy (8.8 percent with clopidogrel versus 6.7 percent with placebo; $p = 0.07$).[49]

Glycoprotein IIb/IIIa Inhibitors

Thrombin and collagen are potent platelet agonists that can cause ADP and serotonin release and activate GP IIb/IIIa fibrinogen receptors on the platelet surface. Functionally active GP IIb/IIIa activation serves as the final common pathway of platelet aggregation by binding fibrinogen and other adhesive proteins that bridge adjacent platelets.

ABCIXIMAB. The safety and efficacy of abciximab were first evaluated in the Evaluation of 7E3 for the Prevention of Ischemic Complications (EPIC) trial, a clinical study of 2099 patients at high risk for complications after PCI.[50] Patients also received aspirin 325 mg and a non-weight-adjusted, 10,000- to 12,000-IU heparin bolus prior to PCI and were then randomly assigned to treatment with placebo, a bolus of abciximab 0.25 mg/kg, or the same bolus of abciximab followed by a 12-hour abciximab infusion at 10 μg/min. Bolus and infusion abciximab was associated with a 35 percent reduction in frequency of the composite clinical endpoint, defined as death, nonfatal MI, repeated revascularization, or procedural failure (8.3 versus 12.8 percent in placebo-treated patients; $p = 0.008$).[50] Bleeding complications occurred twice as often in patients receiving abciximab, attributable to the high dose of heparin used with the procedure.

The Evaluation of PTCA to Improve Long-Term Outcome by Abciximab GP IIb/IIIa Blockade (EPILOG) trial randomly assigned 2792 "low-risk" patients who were treated with aspirin to standard-dose, weight-adjusted (100 units/kg) heparin and placebo; standard-dose, weight-adjusted heparin and abciximab; or low-dose, weight-adjusted (70 units/kg) heparin.[51] The 30-day composite event rate was significantly ($p < 0.001$) lower in patients treated with abciximab and low-dose (5.2 percent) or standard-dose (5.4 percent) heparin than in patients treated with standard-dose heparin and placebo (11.7 percent).[51] Abciximab does not reduce complication rates associated with SVG intervention. Bailout abciximab is often given during or just after PCI for the presence of residual dissection, thrombus, or suboptimal results, although its value has not been demonstrated in prospective studies.

The Evaluation of Platelet IIb/IIIa Inhibitor for Stenting Trial (EPISTENT) randomly assigned 2399 patients with ischemic CAD to stenting plus placebo, stenting plus abciximab, or balloon PTCA plus abciximab.[52] The primary 30-day endpoint, a combination of death, MI, or need for urgent revascularization, occurred in 10.8 percent of patients in the stent-plus-placebo group, 5.3 percent of patients in the stent-plus-abciximab group (hazard ratio 0.48; $p < 0.001$), and 6.9 percent of patients in the balloon-plus-abciximab group (hazard ratio 0.63; $p = 0.007$).[52] No significant differences in bleeding complications were noted among the groups. A pooled analysis also suggests that abciximab may reduce mortality in diabetic patients.

EPTIFIBATIDE. The Integrilin to Minimise Platelet Aggregation and Coronary Thrombosis-II (IMPACT-II) trial enrolled 4010 patients undergoing PCI who were randomly assigned to treatment with a single, low-dose bolus of eptifibatide (135 μg/kg) followed by a low-dose infusion (0.5 μg/kg/min for 20 to 24 hours) or the same eptifibatide bolus and a modestly higher dose infusion of 0.75 μg/kg/min for 20 to 24 hours.[53] The primary endpoint was the 30-day composite occurrence of death, MI, unplanned CABG or repeated PCI, or coronary stenting for abrupt closure. Such events occurred in 11.4 percent of patients in the placebo group versus 9.2 percent in the eptifibatide135/0.5 group ($p = 0.063$) and 9.9 percent in the eptifibatide 135/0.75 group ($p = 0.22$).[53] It is now recognized that the eptifibatide infusion dosage in the IMPACT-II trial was insufficient to provide adequate platelet inhibition during PCI.

The Enhanced Suppression of the Platelet IIb/IIIa Receptor with Integrilin Therapy (ESPRIT) study evaluated a larger double eptifibatide bolus (180 μg/kg boluses 10 minutes apart) and infusion dose (2.0 μg/kg/min for 18 to 24 hours) or placebo in a randomized study of 2064 patients undergoing stent implantation in a native coronary artery.[54] The primary endpoint was the composite of death, MI, urgent target vessel revascularization, and thrombotic bailout GP IIb/IIIa inhibitor therapy within 48 hours after randomization, and it occurred in 10.5 percent of 1024 patients receiving placebo and in 6.6 percent of patients treated with eptifibatide ($p = 0.0015$). The key 30-day secondary endpoint was also reduced, from 10.5 percent to 6.8 percent ($p = 0.0034$). Major bleeding was infrequent but arose more often with eptifibatide than placebo (1.3 percent versus 0.4 percent in placebo-treated patients; $p = 0.027$). These effects were sustained 1 year after the procedure and were effective in high-risk diabetic patients.

TIROFIBAN. Tirofiban, a nonpeptidyl tyrosine derivative, has also been evaluated for its adjunctive benefit during PCI. In the Randomized Efficacy Study of Tirofiban for Outcomes and Restenosis (RESTORE) trial that included 2139 patients undergoing PCI within 72 hours of an acute coronary syndrome, the primary 30-day composite endpoint was 16 percent lower with tirofiban treatment ($p = 0.160$), although a 38 percent relative reduction in the composite endpoint was noted at 48 hours ($p = 0.005$) and a 27 percent relative reduction at 7 days ($p = 0.022$).[55] In a larger study using the same bolus and infusion dose of tirofiban, 4809 patients were randomly assigned to receive either tirofiban or abciximab before PCI with the intent to perform stenting.[56] The primary endpoint, a composite of death, nonfatal MI, and urgent target vessel revascularization at 30 days, occurred more frequently among the patients in the tirofiban group than among patients in the abciximab group (7.6 percent versus 6.0 percent; $p = 0.038$). Subsequent studies have suggested that the tirofiban bolus dose given in this study may have been insufficient to obtain optimal anticoagulation during PCI, and larger bolus doses have been shown to improve the inhibition of platelet aggregation but have not been tested in clinical studies.

Unfractionated Heparin (see also Chap. 80)

Unfractionated heparin is the thrombin inhibitor most commonly used during PCI. "Near-patient" ACT monitoring has facilitated heparin dose titration during PCI, as the required level of anticoagulation activity is beyond the range of the activated partial thromboplastin time. Retrospective studies have related the ACT value to clinical outcome after PCI, and an analysis of 5216 patients undergoing PCI in which unfractionated heparin was used showed that an ACT in the range of 350 to 375 seconds provided the lowest composite ischemic event rate of 6.6 percent, or a 34 percent relative risk reduction in 7-day ischemic events compared with rates observed between 171 and 295 seconds by quartile analysis ($p = 0.001$).[57] Any level of ACT greater than 200 seconds was associated with no further reductions in ischemic complications with concomitant use of GP IIb/IIIa inhibitors, but bleeding complications increased incrementally at all ACTs greater than 200 seconds.[57]

Although randomized trials that have evaluated empirical and weight-adjusted heparin dosing have shown comparable results, weight-adjusted heparin dosing regimens of 50 to 70 IU/kg are now used in an attempt to avoid "overshooting" the ACT. It is generally recommended that sufficient unfractionated heparin be administered during PCI to achieve an ACT around 300 seconds if no GP IIb/IIIa inhibitor is given and more than 200 seconds if GP IIb/IIIa inhibitors are given. Routine use of intravenous heparin after PCI is no longer indicated because several randomized studies showed no benefit in reducing ischemic complications and higher access site bleeding complication rates. Early sheath removal is encouraged when the ACT falls to less than 150 to 180 seconds.

Low-Molecular-Weight Heparin

(see also Chap. 80)

An increasing number of patients with unstable angina are treated with LMWH prior to PCI, but because of difficulties monitoring anticoagulation levels with LMWH during PCI, empirical dose algorithms have been designed to guide additional anticoagulation therapy during PCI. If the last dose of enoxaparin was given less than 8 hours before PCI, no additional antithrombin is needed. If the last dose of enoxaparin was given between 8 and 12 hours, a 0.3-mg/kg bolus of intravenous enoxaparin should be given.[58] If the dose was administrated more than 12 hours before PCI, conventional anticoagulation therapy is indicated. A near-patient assay for estimating the anticoagulant activity (by estimating anti-Xa activity) with enoxaparin has been developed and is available for clinical use. The use of enoxaparin appears safe and effective when it is given in combination with tirofiban or eptifibatide during PCI.

Direct Thrombin Inhibitors

Three direct thrombin inhibitors, hirudin, bivalirudin, and argatroban, have been evaluated as alternatives to heparin during PCI. In the Hirudin in a European Trial Versus Heparin in the Prevention of Restenosis after PTCA (HELVETICA) study,[59] 1141 patients with unstable angina undergoing PCI were treated with aspirin and randomly assigned to receive a heparin bolus of 10,000 units plus infusion at 15 units/kg/hr for 24 hours; a hirudin bolus of 40 mg plus intravenous infusion at 0.2 mg/kg/hr for 24 hours; or a hirudin bolus of 40 mg, intravenous infusion at 0.2 mg/kg/hr for 24 hours, and subcutaneous infusion of 40 mg twice daily for an additional 3 days. Hirudin use was associated with a 39 percent reduction in early cardiac events ($p = 0.023$), although clinical outcomes were similar 7 months later in the three groups. A recombinant hirudin (lepirudin) bolus of 0.4 mg/kg and infusion at 0.15 mg/kg/hr are approved for use in the United States in patients with heparin-induced thrombocytopenia.

Bivalirudin (Angiomax) was compared with unfractionated heparin in a randomized trial involving 4098 patients with postinfarction or unstable angina undergoing PCI. Patients were assigned to treatment with a high-dose (175 units/kg) heparin bolus and an infusion of 15 units/kg/hr for 18 to 24 hours or to a bivalirudin bolus (1.0 mg/kg) and an infusion of 2.5 mg/kg/hr for 4 hours, followed by 0.2 mg/kg/hr for 14 to 20 hours.[60] Bivalirudin did not reduce the likelihood of in-hospital death, Q wave or non-Q-wave MI, or emergency CABG but did reduce the likelihood of bleeding complications (odds ratio of 0.4; $p < 0.001$).[60] In patients with post-MI angina, bivalirudin resulted in lower rates of major ischemic complications (9.1 versus 14.2 percent in heparin-treated patients; $p = 0.04$) and lower rates of bleeding (3.0 versus 11.1 percent in heparin-treated patients; $p < 0.001$).[60]

The Randomized Evaluation in PCI Linking Angiomax to Reduced Clinical Events (REPLACE)-2 trial randomly assigned 6010 patients undergoing PCI to receive intravenous bivalirudin (0.75 mg/kg bolus plus 1.75 mg/kg per hour for the duration of PCI), with provisional GP IIb/IIIa inhibition, or heparin (65 U/kg bolus) with planned GP IIb/IIIa inhibition (abciximab or eptifibatide).[61] The primary composite endpoint was the 30-day incidence of death, MI, urgent repeated revascularization, or in-hospital major bleeding and occurred among 9.2 percent of patients in the bivalirudin group and 10.0 percent of patients in the heparin-plus-GP IIb/IIIa group ($p = 0.32$). Bivalirudin with provisional GP IIb/IIIa blockade was statistically not inferior to heparin plus planned GP IIb/IIIa blockade during contemporary PCI with regard to suppression of acute ischemic endpoints and was associated with less bleeding. Bivalirudin may be particularly useful in patients with heparin-induced thrombocytopenia, those with excessive bleeding risk, elderly patients, and patients with renal insufficiency.

Pharmacological Approaches to Restenosis

A number of systemic agents have been used to prevent restenosis after balloon angioplasty and directional atherectomy, but none has had a consistent effect on restenosis prevention. Detailed review of the multiple trials is beyond the scope of this chapter, but a summary of ongoing evaluation of newer potential therapies may be found in Table 52–6.[62-76]

Studies that have evaluated aspirin in preventing restenosis after PCI have provided conflicting results, potentially owing to the varied dosage, timing, and duration of aspirin therapy; limited sample sizes; and incomplete angiographic follow-up. Aspirin therapy (75 to 325 mg/d) should be continued indefinitely after PCI for the secondary prevention of cardiovascular events (death, MI, or stroke) rather than for the prevention of late restenosis.

Cilostazol selectively inhibits 3′,5′-cyclic nucleotide phosphodiesterase III and has antiplatelet and vasodilating effects. Smaller studies suggest a benefit of cilostazol in preventing restenosis after coronary stenting, but one larger study failed to demonstrate a restenosis benefit of cilostazol after elective stent placement.[63] The Cilostazol for Restenosis (CREST) trial is an ongoing evaluation of 600 patients undergoing elective treatment with stent implantation treated with either aspirin and clopidogrel or aspirin, clopidogrel, and cilostazol (William Weintraub, personal communication).

Although a subgroup analysis of diabetic patients undergoing stent implantation in EPISTENT demonstrated a reduction in revascularization in diabetic patients assigned to stenting plus abciximab (8.1 percent) compared with patients receiving stenting plus placebo (16.6 percent),[77] a larger subgroup analysis in another prospective trial failed to demonstrate a difference in late outcomes in diabetic patients treated with periprocedural abciximab and tirofiban.[78] GP IIb/IIIa inhibitors are no longer recommended for the prevention of restenosis in diabetic patients undergoing stent implantation.

C-reactive protein (CRP) rises and remains elevated for up to 36 hours after stent implantation, and preprocedural elevation of CRP is an important predictor of restenosis. Although a single bolus of systemic corticosteroids does not reduce restenosis, sustained oral prednisone therapy reduced restenosis in a series of 83 patients with persistent elevation of CRP after successful stent placement,[67] reducing 6-month restenosis rates from 33 percent in placebo-treated patients to 7 percent in prednisone-treated patients.

Probucol is an antioxidant that has been shown to reduce intimal hyperplasia. Although one smaller study failed to demonstrate a reduction in angiographic restenosis after stent placement, a larger study randomly assigned 317 patients 1 month before angioplasty to treatment with placebo, probucol (500 mg), multivitamins (30,000 IU of beta carotene, 500 mg of vitamin C, and 700 IU of vitamin E), or both probucol and multivitamins—all given twice daily.[79] Restenosis rates per segment were 20.7 percent in the probucol group, 28.9 percent in the combined treatment group, 40.3 percent in the multivitamin group, and 38.9 percent in the placebo group ($p = 0.003$ for probucol versus no probucol).[79] In a subgroup of 189 patients with small (<3.0-mm) vessels in the MultiVitamins and Probucol (MVP) trial, restenosis was lower in patients treated with probucol. Although probucol has potential benefit in restenosis prevention, the prolonged pretreatment time, prolongation of the QTc interval, and unfavorable effect on high-density lipoprotein limit its clinical use. AGI-1067, a metabolically stable modification of probucol with an equipotent antioxidant effect, also has a potential beneficial effect on restenosis after stent placement.[68]

Oral rapamycin, 6 mg loading dose and 2 mg per day for 4 weeks, was given to 22 patients at high risk for restenosis after stent placement.[80] Nearly 50 percent of patients discontinued therapy because of side effects, and no reduction in the occurrence of clinical or angiographic restenosis was found.[80]

A number of studies have evaluated lipid-lowering therapy for the prevention of restenosis after coronary intervention, but none has shown a consistent reduction in restenosis. The Fluvastatin Angioplasty Restenosis (FLARE) trial found no difference in angiographic restenosis with high-dose fluvastatin use, although there was a significantly lower incidence of total death and MI was observed in 6 patients (1.4 percent) in the fluvastatin group and 17 (4.0 percent) in the placebo group (log rank $p = 0.025$).[81] A larger clinical study, the Lescol Intervention Prevention Study (LIPS), assigned patients to receive fluvastatin, 80 mg/d, or matching placebo at hospital discharge for 3 to 4 years.[82] At least one major adverse cardiac event (MACE) event occurred in 21.4 percent of patients in the fluvastatin group and 26.7 percent of patients in the placebo group ($p = 0.01$).[82] In aggregate, these findings suggest that lipid-lowering agents play a limited role in the reduction of restenosis after coronary stent placement, but their use is highly beneficial for the progression of coronary atherosclerosis and clinical events attributable to sites remote from stent placement.

Drug-Eluting Stents

In sharp contradistinction to the failed attempts to prevent restenosis with systemic drug therapy, sustained local delivery of several agents from a stent coating system (termed *drug-eluting stent system*) has been very effective at suppressing the local neointimal proliferation that causes angiographic and clinical restenosis (Table 52–7). Some drug-eluting stent systems have prevented restenosis (e.g., sirolimus, everolimus, polymer-delivered paclitaxel), whereas others have had no or a limited effect (e.g., batimastat, dexamethasone, stent-based paclitaxel) or were clinically detrimental (e.g., actinomycin D, 7-hexanoyltaxol [QP2], a taxane derivative). These studies have demonstrated the important interaction between the stent design, the presence (or absence) of a polymeric coating that is used to deliver the drug, and the types of agents that are delivered to the vessel wall.

Sirolimus

The CYPHER (Cordis, Warren, NJ) stent contains sirolimus, which is a naturally occurring antimicrobial and immunosuppressive agent that causes cytostatic inhibition of growth factor– and cytokine-stimulated cell proliferation in the G1 phase. The polymeric (Topcoat) coating on the Bx Velocity stent provides sustained release of sirolimus over a 30- to 45-day period. The CYPHER stent received CE Mark approval in Europe in April 2002 and approval by the FDA in the United States in May 2003.

TABLE 52–6 Trials of the Use of Oral Agents for the Prevention of Restenosis After Percutaneous Coronary Intervention

Author	Year	Total patients	Angio FU	Stent Use	Treatment	Pretreatment Duration	Duration of Therapy	Restenosis Rates# (%)
Cilostazol								
Tsuchikane et al[62]	1999	211	193	No	Cilostazol 200 mg qd	None	3 mo	18*
					Aspirin 250 mg qd			40
Park et al[63]	2000	409	380	Yes	Cilostazol 100 mg b.i.d.	48 hr	6 mo	23
					Ticlopidine	48 hr	1 mo	27
Kamishirado et al[64]	2002	130	111	Yes	Cilostazol 200 mg qd	48 hr	6 mo	13†
					Ticlopidine			31
Coumadin								
Garachemani et al[65]	2002	191	172	35%	Warfarin (INR = 2.5-4.0)	None	6 mo	30
					Aspirin			33
ten Berg et al[66]	2003	531	480	34%	Coumarin (INR = 2.1-4.8)	7 d	6 mo	38.9§
					Placebo			39.1
Steroids								
Versaci et al[67]	2002	83	83	Yes	Prednisolone orally with taper	None	45 d	7†
					Placebo			33
Antiinflammatory agents								
Tardif et al[68]	2003	305	NR	Yes	AGI-1067, 70 mg	14 d	4 wk	23.6
					AGI-1067, 140 mg			23.6
					AGI-1067, 280 mg			23.6
					Probucol			25.9
					Placebo			37.7
Tranilast								
Holmes et al[69]	2002	11,484		Yes	Tranilast 300 mg b.i.d.	None	1 mo	35
					Tranilast 450 mg b.i.d.		1 mo	33
					Tranilast 300 mg b.i.d.		3 mo	35
					Tranilast 450 mg b.i.d.		3 mo	32
					Placebo			33
Trapidil								
Serruys et al[70]	2001	303	269	Wallstent	Trapidil 200 mg qd	>1 hr	6 mo	31
					Placebo			24
ACE inhibitors								
Meurice et al[71]	2001	91	79	No	Quinapril 40 mg qd	None	6 mo	37
					Placebo			24
Kondo et al[72]	2001	100	99	Yes	Quinapril 10-20 mg qd	None	6 mo	12†
					Placebo			24
Angiotensin receptor blockers								
Peters et al[73]	2001	250	200	Yes	Valsartan 80 mg qd	NR	6 mo	19.2‡
					Placebo			38.6
Calcium channel antagonists								
Dens et al[74]	2001	826	646	No	Nisoldipine 40 mg qd	None	6 mo	49‖
					Placebo			55
Jorgensen et al[75]	2000	585	451	16%	Amlodipine 10 mg qd	2 wk	4 mo	28
					Placebo			28
Carvedilol								
Serruys et al[76]	2000	324	292	No	Carvedilol 12.5 mg b.i.d.	>24 hr	5 mo	23.4
					Placebo			23.9

ACE = angiotensin-converting enzyme; Angio = angiographic; FU = follow-up; INR = international normalized ratio; NR = not reported.
* $p < 0.001$.
† $p < 0.05$.
‡ $p < 0.005$.
§ Mean follow-up percent stenosis.
‖ Restenosis defined as a loss of 50% of initial gain.
\# Restenosis defined as more than 50% follow-up diameter strenosis unless indicated otherwise.

FIRST IN-HUMAN STUDIES. Sirolimus-eluting Bx Velocity stents were first implanted in 45 patients with focal native vessel disease.[83-85] In-stent minimal lumen diameter and percent diameter stenosis were essentially unchanged from the postprocedural study to the 18- to 24-month follow-up study.[86] Intravascular ultrasound–detected neointimal hyperplasia was virtually absent at 12 months in both groups (Fig. 52–13).

RAVEL. The Randomized Study with the Sirolimus-Eluting Bx Velocity Balloon-Expandable Stent (RAVEL) trial randomly assigned 238 patients with single, primary lesions located in native coronary arteries to treatment with the sirolimus stent or the bare metal stent (Table 52–8).[87] The degree of late lumen loss at 6 months was significantly lower in the sirolimus stent group (−0.01 ± 0.33-mm) than in the standard stent group (0.80 ± 0.53-mm) ($p < 0.001$). None of

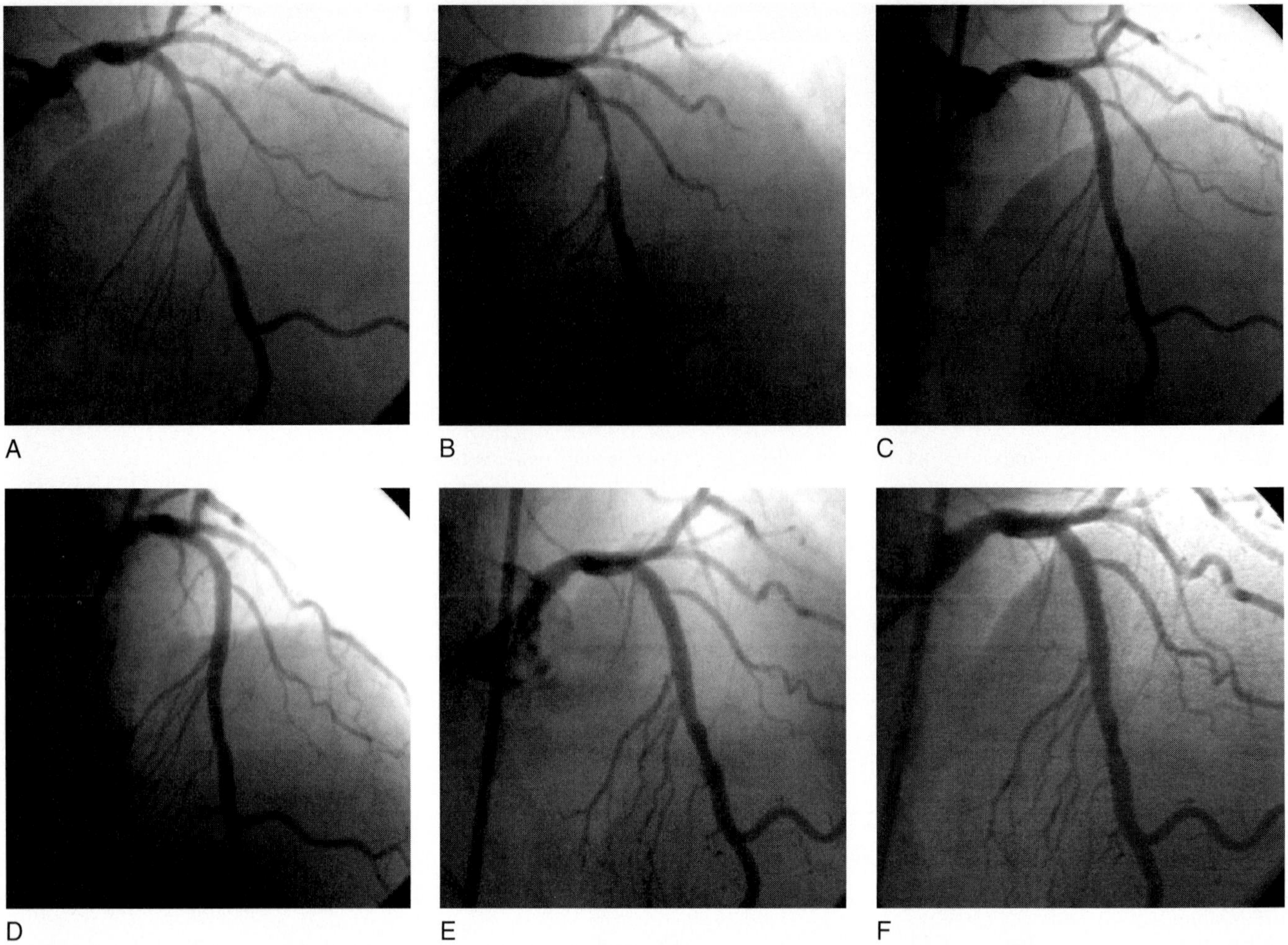

A B C

D E F

FIGURE 52–13 First in-human CYPHER stent implantation. **A,** A focal stenosis is shown in the middle left anterior descending artery. **B,** A CYPHER sirolimus-eluting stent is positioned across the stenosis. **C,** There is an excellent initial angiographic result and no residual stenosis. Follow-up angiography was performed at 4 months **(D)**, 1 year **(E)**, and 2 years after the procedure **(F)** without evidence of lumen renarrowing. This pattern of markedly reduced intimal hyperplasia was found in virtually all patients in the first in-human study. (Courtesy of Dr. Eduardo Sousa, São Paulo, Brazil.)

TABLE 52–7 Angiographic and Clinical Endpoints for Restenosis Percutaneous Coronary Intervention

Angiographic	Clinical
Binary	**Binary**
>50% follow-up diameter stenosis	Death
>0.72-mm loss in lumen diameter	Nonfatal myocardial infarction
>20% loss in gain achieved	Revascularization
Continuous	Target vessel failure
Follow-up minimal lumen diameter	Target vessel revascularization
Follow-up % diameter stenosis	Target lesion revascularization
Late lumen loss	Recurrence of angina
Loss index	**Continuous**
	Exercise test duration

the patients in the sirolimus stent group had restenosis, compared with 26.6 percent of those in the standard stent group ($p < 0.001$).[87] There were no episodes of stent thrombosis. During a follow-up period of up to 1 year, the overall rate of major cardiac events was 5.8 percent in the sirolimus stent group and 28.8 percent in the standard stent group ($p < 0.001$).[87] Volumetric intravascular ultrasound analysis also demonstrated a 90 percent reduction in intimal hyperplasia associated with the use of the CYPHER stent.[88]

SIRIUS. The Sirolimus-Eluting Stent in de novo Coronary Artery Lesions (SIRIUS) trial included 1058 patients with a lesion length between 15 and 30-mm and a reference diameter between 2.5 and 3.5-mm and randomly assigned them to treatment with a sirolimus-eluting stent or a bare metal stent.[89] The primary clinical endpoint in the SIRIUS trial was 8-month target vessel failure, defined as target vessel revascularization, death, or MI, and it was reduced from 21.0 percent in patients treated with bare metal stents to 8.6 percent in patients with sirolimus-eluting stents ($p < 0.001$). Target vessel revascularization was reduced from 16.6 percent with bare metal stents to 4.1 percent in patients treated with sirolimus-eluting stents ($p < 0.001$).[89] Compared with patients treated with bare metal stents, patients treated with sirolimus-eluting stents had lower rates of binary angiographic restenosis within the treated segment (36.3 percent with bare metal stents versus 8.9 percent with sirolimus-eluting stents; $p < 0.001$) and within the stent (35.4 percent with bare metal stents versus 3.2 percent with sirolimus-eluting stents; $p < 0.001$).[89]

OTHER INDICATIONS. The CYPHER stent may also be useful in patients with in-stent restenosis. Twenty-five patients with in-stent restenosis were successfully treated with the implantation of one or two sirolimus-eluting Bx Velocity stents.[90] Angiographic late loss averaged 0.07 ±

TABLE 52–8 Late Outcome in Randomized Trials of Sirolimus Eluting Stents for the Prevention of Restenosis

	RAVEL[87]		SIRIUS[89]	
Variable	***Sirolimus***	***Bare***		
Number of patients	120	118	533	525
Baseline factors				
Mean age, yr	61.8	59.7	62.1	62.4
Women, %	30	29	27	30
Diabetes mellitus	16	21	24.6	28.2
Lesion length, mm	9.6	9.6	14.4	14.4
Reference diameter, mm	2.56	2.64	2.79	2.82
MLD, mm				
Baseline	0.94	0.95	0.97	0.98
Final	2.43	2.41	2.39	2.40
Follow-up	2.42*	1.64	2.15	1.60
Late lumen loss, mm	−0.01	0.80	0.24	0.81
% Diameter stenosis				
Baseline	63.6	64.0	65.6	65.3
Final	11.9	14.0	15.8	16.1
Follow-up	14.7	36.7	23.6	43.2
Restenosis rate, %	0	26.6	8.9	36.3
Stent thrombosis, %	0	0		
Follow-up period	12 mo		9 mo	
TLR, %	0	27	4.1	16.6
Late clinical events, %	5.8	28.8	8.6	21.0
Death	2	2	0.9	0.6
Q wave MI	0	0	0.8	0.4

*$p < 0.001$.

MI = myocardial infarction; MLD = minimum lumen diameter; RAVEL = Randomized Study with the Sirolimus-Eluting Bx Velocity Balloon-Expandable Stent; SIRIUS = Sirolimus-Eluting Stent in de novo Coronary Artery Lesions; TLR = target lesion revascularization.

0.2-mm within the stent and −0.05 ± 0.3-mm within the lesion at 4 months and 0.36 ± 0.46-mm within the stent and 0.16 ± 0.42-mm within the lesion 12 months later. Only one patient had in-stent restenosis at 1-year follow-up. A second series of 16 patients with more complex recurrent in-stent restenosis in native coronary arteries (average lesion length 18.4-mm) were treated with one or more 18-mm Bx Velocity sirolimus-eluting stents.[91] Four patients had recurrent restenosis following brachytherapy, and three patients had totally occluded vessels before the procedure.[91] At 4-month follow-up, one patient had died and three patients had angiographic evidence of restenosis (one in stent and two in lesion).[91] Although there was a minimal amount of in-stent late lumen loss (averaging 0.21-mm), three patients had experienced four major adverse cardiac events by 9 months (two deaths and one acute MI necessitating repeated target vessel angioplasty).[91] One randomized trial comparing brachytherapy and the CYPHER stent in patients with in-stent restenosis is ongoing.

Paclitaxel

Paclitaxel stabilizes microtubules and prevents cell division at the M phase. In lower doses this agent may also have cytostatic effects on cell proliferation, and in higher doses it may have cytotoxic effects. Paclitaxel has been delivered to the vessel wall in two formulations—one with a polymeric coating that elutes the drug to the vessel wall over a period of 30 to 45 days (TAXUS programs, Boston Scientific, Natick, MA) and one with a spray coating of the drug on the stent that provides more rapid release (Cook, Bloomington, IN, and Guidant, Santa Clara, CA).

POLYMERIC-COATED, PACLITAXEL-ELUTING STENT: THE TAXUS STUDIES. The TAXUS I trial was a prospective, double-blind, three-center study randomly assigning 61 patients with de novo or restenotic lesions to receive an NIR stent with a polymeric coating that eluted paclitaxel or a bare metal stent (Table 52–9).[92-95] There were no cases of angiographic restenosis 6 months after the procedure, compared with 10 percent in patients treated with control stents, and these beneficial effects persisted up to 1 year after the procedure.[92] The TAXUS II study was a larger randomized trial involving 536 patients with native vessel CAD who were randomly assigned to treatment with a bare NIR Express stent, an NIR Express stent containing a slow-release vascularly compatible Translute polymeric coating that released paclitaxel, or a bare NIR Express or an NIR Express containing a moderate-release Translute polymer that released paclitaxel over a more sustained period. There was a significant reduction in the clinical and angiographic restenosis rate in patients treated with both the slow- and moderate-release formulations.[93]

Twenty-eight patients with in-stent restenosis were treated with a paclitaxel-eluting NIR stent in the TAXUS III study.[96] No subacute stent thrombosis occurred up to 12 months, but there was one late chronic total occlusion and three additional patients showed angiographic restenosis.[96] The major adverse cardiac event rate was 29 percent (eight patients; one non-Q-wave MI, one coronary artery bypass grafting, and six TLR).[96] Of the patients with TLR, one had restenosis in a bare stent implanted for edge dissection and two had restenosis in a gap between two paclitaxel-eluting stents.[96]

The TAXUS IV trial randomized 1314 patients to treatment with a bare metal or paclitaxel-coated stent. Target lesion

TABLE 52–9 Late Outcome in Randomized Trials, Patients Treated with Paclitaxel-Eluting Stents for the Prevention of Restenosis

	TAXUS-I[92]		TAXUS-II[93]				TAXUS-IV[94]		ASPECT[95]	
Variable	*SL*	*Bare*	*SL*	*Bare*	*MR*	*Bare*	*SL*	*Bare*	*High Dose*	*Placebo*
Number of patients	31	30	131	136	135	134	662	652	60	59
Baseline factors										
Mean Age, yr	66	64	62	60	59	59	63	62	58	58
Women, %	6	17	30	21	24	23	28	28	20	24
Diabetes mellitus	23	13	11	16	17	14	31	33	18	17
Lesion length, mm	10.7	11.9	10.6	10.5	10.2	10.7	14.4	14.4		
Reference diameter, mm	2.99	2.94	2.78	2.77	2.72	2.73	2.75	2.75	2.94	2.88
MLD, mm										
Baseline	1.30	1.23	1.02	1.03	0.95	0.91	0.92	0.95	0.64	0.54
Final	2.95	2.87	2.53	2.58	2.53	2.52	2.26	2.29	2.85	2.82
Follow-up	2.60	1.19	2.23	1.79	2.24	1.76	2.03	1.68	2.53*	1.79
Late lumen loss	0.36	0.71	0.31	0.79	0.30	0.77	0.23	0.61	0.29*	1.04
% Diameter stenosis										
Baseline	57	58	63.3	62.8	64.9	66.6	66.5	65.6	79.4	80.9
Final	6	10	10.9	10.2	11.0	12.0	19.1	19.1	1.8	3.8
Follow-up	14	27	19.5	31.8	18.2	33.9	26.3	39.8	14*	39
Restenosis rate, %	0	10	5.5	20.1	8.6	23.8	7.9	26.6	4*	27
Stent thrombosis, number	0	0	1	0	1	0	0.6%	0.8%	3	0
Follow-up period	12 mo		12 mo				9 mo		6 mo	
TLR, %	0	10	4.7†	12.9	3.8‡	16.0	11.3	3.0	2	2
Late clinical events, %	3	10	10.9†	22.0	9.9†	21.4	8.5	15.0	10%	5%
Death	0	0	0	1.5	0	0	1.4	1.1	0	0
Q wave MI	0	0	0.8	1.5	1.5	0.8	0.8	0.3	0	0

*$p < 0.001$.
†$p < 0.05$.
‡$p < 0.005$.
ASPECT = Asian Paclitaxel-Eluting Stent Clinical Trial; MI = myocardial infarction; MLD = minimum lumen diameter; MR = moderate release; SL = slow release; TLR = target lesion revascularization.

revascularization and angiographic restenosis were significantly reduced in patients treated with the TAXUS stent.[94]

PACLITAXEL-COATED STENTS. Another method of delivering paclitaxel by means of a spray coating was evaluated in a randomized study of 177 patients with discrete coronary lesions using low-dose paclitaxel (1.3 μg/mm^2), high dose paclitaxel (3.1 μg/mm^2), or control stents.[95] At follow-up, the high-dose paclitaxel group had significantly lower binary restenosis rates than control-treated patients (4 percent versus 27 percent; $p < 0.001$).[95] Intravascular ultrasonography showed a stepwise reduction in intimal hyperplasia accumulation within the stented segment in patients treated with high-dose paclitaxel .[97] The DELIVER trial was a large randomized trial that evaluated the Penta stent with paclitaxel coating and failed to demonstrate a significant benefit with a drug-eluting stent.

PACLITAXEL DERIVATIVE–ELUTING POLYMERIC SLEEVE. The Study to COmpare REstenosis rate between QueST and QuaDS-QP2 (SCORE) trial was a randomized, multicenter trial that compared QP2-eluting stents with bare metal stents in the treatment of de novo coronary lesions. This system was associated with a high (10 percent) subacute thrombosis rate, although restenosis was reduced.[98] At 6 months, three patients had TLR (20 percent). Two patients had restenosis (13.3 percent) with a minimal amount of intimal hyperplasia observed in all the segments covered by drug-eluting stents.[98] At 12 months, one patient suffered from non-Q-wave MI and 61.5 percent had angiographic restenosis.[98] Five patients with restenosis underwent DCA for recurrent in-stent restenosis.[99] Restenotic lesions from QuaDS-QP2-eluting stents at 12 months showed persistent fibrin deposition with varying degrees of inflammation.[99] These pathological changes, representing delayed healing, are usually observed up to only 3 months in human coronary arteries with stainless steel balloon-expandable stents.[99] The nonreabsorbable polymer alone may have induced chronic inflammation.[99]

Other Drug Elution Programs

Everolimus (Novartis) is another rapamycin analog that has both immunosuppressive and antiproliferative effects, and it has been submitted for FDA regulatory approval for patients with renal transplantation. Like sirolimus, everolimus inhibits the cytoplasmic phase (G1) of cell replication by inhibiting mammalian target of rapamycin (mTOR). Two programs have been proposed for the evaluation of everolimus-eluting stents. The first involves the use of a bioresorbable polymeric coating for everolimus delivery (Biosensors). The FUTURE-1 trial involving 27 patients treated with the Biosensors stent eluting everolimus and 15 patients treated with bare metal stents demonstrated no cases of restenosis in everolimus-treated patients and 9.1 percent restenosis in those treated with control metal stents with an in-stent late lumen loss of 0.10-mm. The second proposed program involves use of the Vision cobalt chromium stent (Guidant, Santa Clara, CA) with a TrueCoat polymeric coating for the elution of everolimus to the vessel wall. A randomized efficacy trial called SPIRIT FIRST is planned in Europe.

ABT-578, another rapamycin analog, has been tested in pilot studies in Australia on both the phosphylcholine (PC)-coated biodivYsio stent (Abbott Vascular, Chicago, IL) and the PC-coated cobalt chromium Driver stent (Medtronic Vascular, Santa Rosa, CA). The ENDEAVOR-II trial is the pivotal trial evaluating the Medtronic Program in Europe, commencing in the summer of 2003.

Tacrolimus elution from a ceramic coating on the Jomed was evaluated in the Endovascular Investigation Determining the Safety of a New Tacrolimus-Eluting Stent Graft (EVIDENT) and Preliminary Safety Evaluation of Nanoporous Tacrolimus-Eluting Stents (PRESENT) studies with limited results because of underdosing of the tacrolimus. The STRIDE Registry evaluated the use of dexamethasone elution from a phosphorylcholine coating in a 70-patient pilot series and reported a 13.3 percent binary restenosis rate. Although the angiographic restenosis rate was higher than expected given the noncomplex patients included in the study, the Dexamet stent received CE Mark approval in late 2002.

The value of actinomycin D elution from a polymeric coated balloon expandable stent was evaluated in the Actinomycin Eluting Stent Improves Outcomes by Reducing Neointimal Hyperplasia (ACTION) trial, but actinomycin in two doses failed to show benefit in preventing restenosis. Other agents that have been tried include Resten-NG, estrogen, and batimastat, but their effect on reducing restenosis after stent placement has not been convincing.

Indications for Percutaneous Coronary Interventions

The major value of percutaneous or surgical coronary revascularization is the relief of symptoms and signs of ischemic CAD.[33] PCI may reduce mortality and subsequent MI risk compared with medical therapy in unstable patients,[100,101] but these events are better treated with systemic therapies aimed at reducing the extent of atherosclerosis, such as lipid-lowering therapy, hypertension control, and smoking cessation.[102] In contrast, CABG prolongs life in patients in certain anatomical subsets, such as patients with left main disease, three-vessel CAD, or left anterior descending artery disease with involvement of one or two additional vessels, irrespective of left ventricular function.[103] The risks and benefits of coronary revascularization must be carefully reviewed with the patient and family members, and relative to the options of surgical bypass or continued medical therapy, before these procedures are performed. Guidelines for the performance of PCI and CABG have been published by a joint task force of the American College of Cardiology and American Heart Association.[33,103]

Asymptomatic Patients or Those with Mild Angina

Patients who are asymptomatic or have only mild symptoms are generally best treated with medical therapy unless one or more significant lesions subtend a moderate to large area of viable myocardium, the patient prefers to maintain an aggressive life style or has a high-risk occupation, and the procedure can be performed with a high chance of success and low likelihood of complications.[33] Coronary revascularization should not be performed in patients with absent or mild symptoms if only a small area of myocardium is at risk, if no objective evidence of ischemia can be found, or if the likelihood of success is low or the chance of complications is high.[33] There is no evidence that preemptive PCI of a hemodynamically insignificant "vulnerable" plaque prevents a subsequent MI.

Patients with Moderate to Severe Angina

(see Chap. 50)

Patients with CCS class II to IV angina, particularly those who are refractory to medical therapy, are suitable candidates for coronary revascularization provided that the lesion subtends a moderate to large area of viable myocardium as determined by noninvasive testing.[33] Patients who have recurrent symptoms while receiving medical therapy are candidates for revascularization even if they have a higher risk for an adverse outcome with revascularization.[33] Patients with class II to IV symptoms should not undergo revascularization without noninvasive evidence of myocardial ischemia or a trial of medical therapy, particularly if only a small region of myocardium is at risk, the likelihood of success is low, or the chance of complications is high.

Patients with Unstable Angina or Non-ST-Segment Myocardial Infarction (see Chap. 49)

Cardiac catheterization and coronary revascularization in moderate- to high-risk patients who present with unstable angina or non-ST-segment elevation MI (NSTEMI) may improve the prognosis and reduce the rate of reinfarction,[104] although two earlier studies failed to demonstrate a benefit for death or MI with the routine revascularization.[105,106] These studies were performed before the availability of GP IIb/IIIa inhibitors and coronary stents.[107]

Three subsequent trials have demonstrated benefit of routine revascularization in patients with acute coronary syndromes. The Fragmin and Fast Revascularization During Instability in Coronary Artery Disease (FRISC II) study demonstrated a 22 percent reduction ($p = 0.031$) in death or MI at 6 months in patients assigned to routine catheterization and revascularization (9.4 percent) versus those assigned to a conservative approach (12.1 percent).[108] The Treat Angina with Aggrastat and determine Cost of Therapy with an Invasive or Conservative Strategy– Thrombolysis in Myocardial Infarction 18 (TACTICS-TIMI 18) trial treated 2200 patients with NSTEMI or unstable angina with aspirin, unfractionated heparin, and intravenous tirofiban and randomly assigned patients to an early aggressive strategy with coronary arteriography and coronary revascularization within 4 to 48 hours after presentation or to a conservative strategy whereby coronary arteriography was performed only for recurrent ischemia or exercise stress testing demonstrating reversible ischemia.[100] The rate of the 6-month primary composite endpoint of death, recurrent MI, or urgent revascularization was reduced by 22 percent in patients assigned to the invasive strategy compared with the conservative strategy (15.9 percent versus 19.4 percent, respectively; $p = 0.025$).[100] The rate of death or MI at 6 months was reduced by 26 percent (7.3 percent versus 9.5 percent, respectively; $p < 0.05$).[100] These benefits were highest in patients presenting with unfavorable prognostic factors, such as rest pain, cardiac enzyme elevation, or electrocardiographic changes.[100]

The British Heart Foundation Randomized Intervention Trial of unstable Angina (RITA-3) randomly assigned 1810 patients with NSTEMI to an early intervention or conservative revascularization strategy.[101] At 4 months, 9.6 percent of patients in the intervention group had died or had MI or refractory angina, compared with 14.5 percent of patients in the conservative group (risk ratio 0.66; $p = 0.001$).[101] This difference was mainly due to a halving of refractory angina in the intervention group, as the frequency of death or MI was similar in both treatment groups.[101] Symptoms of angina were improved and use of antianginal medications significantly reduced with the interventional strategy ($p < 0.0001$).[101]

Patients with acute coronary syndromes are also excellent candidates for drug-eluting stents. The Rapamycin-Eluting Stent Evaluated At Rotterdam Cardiology Hospital (RESEARCH) registry compared 198 patients with acute coronary syndromes treated exclusively with drug-eluting stents with 301 patients with acute coronary syndromes treated with bare stents in the same time period immediately before the study.[109] The 30-day major adverse cardiac event rate was similar in both groups, with stent thrombosis occurring in 0.5 percent of patients treated with drug-eluting stents and 1.7 percent of patients treated with bare metal stents ($p = 0.4$).[109]

Options for Medical Therapy or Coronary Revascularization (see also Chap. 50)

For patients with symptomatic CAD, the clinician must decide whether medical therapy or referral for coronary revascularization by PCI or CABG would provide the better prognosis for the individual patient. A number of factors ultimately affect the decision to undertake one strategy over another, including (1) the patient's general vigor, comorbid conditions, initial symptoms, and personal preferences; (2) the coronary anatomy, number of lesions, and their location and morphology, including the presence of total occlusions; (3) left ventricular function; and (4) whether CABG has already been performed.

Percutaneous Coronary Intervention Versus Medical Therapy (see Chap. 50)

Two trials have compared medical therapy with PCI in patients with single-vessel CAD. The Veterans Administration Angioplasty Compared to Medicine (ACME) trial randomly assigned 212 patients with single-vessel coronary disease and stable angina to treatment with medical therapy or balloon PTCA. Death and MI rates were similar in both groups, but superior symptom control and a better exercise duration were shown in patients treated with balloon PTCA. The Atorvastatin Versus Revascularization Therapy (AVERT) trial compared the effect of aggressive lipid lowering with atorvastatin at 80 mg/d and coronary angioplasty in 341 patients with asymptomatic or mildly symptomatic (class I or II) CAD.[110] At an 18-month follow-up, 13 percent of medically treated patients had experienced an ischemic event compared with 21 percent of patients treated with PCI ($p = 0.048$), although more improvement in angina was shown in patients treated with PCI.

Two other trials have evaluated medical therapy with PCI in patients with more extensive CAD. The RITA-2 trial randomly assigned 1018 patients with single-vessel or multivessel disease to medical therapy or PCI. Death or definite MI occurred significantly ($p = 0.02$) more often in PCI-treated patients (6.3 percent) than in medically treated patients (3.3 percent), attributable to the occurrence of periprocedural MI. Angina improvement and exercise durations were better in the PCI group. The Asymptomatic Cardiac Ischemia Pilot (ACIP) study randomly assigned 558 patients with asymptomatic ischemia determined by stress testing and ambulatory ischemia monitoring and randomly assigned them to angina-guided therapy, angina plus ischemia–guided therapy, or revascularization using PCI or CABG. The incidence of death or MI at 2 years was significantly lower ($p < 0.01$) in patients treated with revascularization (4.7 percent) than in patients assigned to angina-guided (12.1 percent) or ischemia-guided (8.8 percent) therapy.

In aggregate, these studies suggest that patients with mild class I or II angina have a favorable prognosis whether treated with medical therapy or PCI. Angina relief is generally greater in patients treated with PCI than those receiving medical therapy. Patients with moderate to severe angina, particularly those who have not responded to medical therapy, should be considered candidates for PCI. The availability of durable treatment with drug-eluting stents may alter these paradigms in patients with documented ischemia, given that symptom recurrence is markedly reduced with these new therapies.

Percutaneous Coronary Intervention Versus Coronary Artery Bypass Graft (see Chap. 50)

At least nine randomized trials have evaluated the relative value of balloon angioplasty and CABG in patients with multivessel CAD.[103,111,112] These trials were performed before the availability of improved anticoagulation during PCI (e.g., GP IIb/IIIa inhibitors, direct thrombin inhibitors) and before the widespread use of coronary stents (i.e., bare metal or drug-eluting stents). These randomized trials had certain unavoidable design limitations, including relatively small sample sizes (127 to 1792 patients), low screened-to-recruitment ratios (limiting the generalizability of the study), and limited (1 to 5 years) follow-up. Despite these limitations, one of these studies led to a significant debate about the role of CABG in diabetic patients. The Bypass And Revascularization Investigation (BARI) found that diabetic patients assigned to PCI had a significantly ($p = 0.003$) worse survival rate (65.5 percent) than diabetic patients assigned to CABG (80.6 percent), primarily because of a reduced cardiac mortality rate (20.6 percent in PCI patients versus 5.8 percent in CABG patients; $p = 0.003$) from subsequent Q wave MI.[113] Placement of a left internal mammary artery to the left anterior descending artery appears responsible for the majority of this benefit.

With the improved outcomes associated with PCI over the past decade, a number of studies subsequently compared CABG with single-vessel or multivessel stent placement and showed that death and MI are similar in patients treated with CABG or multivessel stenting,[114-116] although one study suggested the persistence of a surgical 2-year mortality benefit in diabetic patients.[117,118] Restenosis has remained the major limitation after bare metal stenting, but with the availability of drug-eluting stents and aggressive risk factor modification after PCI, further studies are needed to evaluate the long-term outcomes of patients treated with these two therapies, particularly diabetic patients.

The ultimate choice of the method of revascularization should be made after a frank discussion with the patient about the options of revascularization. In patients with diffuse involvement of three coronary vessels, particularly in the setting of complex anatomy, including total occlusions, CABG may provide a more definitive long-term benefit, especially if one or more arterial conduits are used. In contrast, in a patient with focal lesions involving two or three large epicardial vessels, multivessel coronary stent placement may be the preferred approach as it is associated with a lower risk of Q wave MI and a shorter hospital stay than CABG. Diabetic patients with diffuse two- or three-vessel CAD may be best served with CABG.

Patients Without Options for Revascularization

Patients who suffer from substantial angina but are poor candidates for conventional revascularization have limited therapeutic options. These patients generally have a single, proximal vessel occlusion that subtends a large amount of myocardium or have undergone one or more prior CABG surgeries with stenoses of the SVGs poorly suited for conventional repeated revascularization. Patients with limited options make up approximately 4 to 12 percent of those undergoing coronary angiography; a larger percentage of patients (20 to 30 percent) have incomplete revascularization because of unsuitable coronary anatomy with surgery or percutaneous techniques.

Creation of new blood vessels in the ischemic tissue, also known as therapeutic angiogenesis, may provide symptom relief in these patients. Both surgical and percutaneous approaches have been used to improve regional blood flow to the ischemic myocardium in these patients, although these strategies vary with respect to the depth of myocardial injury, the laser-tissue interactions, the presence or absence of guidance, and the number of channels created. No such therapy has yet been proved effective in blinded clinical trials.

Percutaneous approaches to myocardial revascularization vary in the laser source, delivery catheter types, and use of guidance to direct placement of the laser channels. These techniques provide partial-thickness myocardial channels, ranging from 3 to 5-mm in depth, in contrast to the full-thickness myocardial channel produced with surgical methods. Although studies with several of the laser systems reported dramatic clinical improvement in angina severity and exercise time in open-label studies, the few placebo-controlled randomized studies performed with this group of devices have shown much of the improvement to be due to a placebo effect.[119] No such percutaneous laser myocardial revascularization systems are currently approved for use in the United States.

LOCALIZED MYOCARDIAL GENE TRANSFER. Using electromechanical localization with the Biosense system, direct intramyocardial administration of the naked plasmid VEGF-165 has been used in an attempt to stimulate angiogenesis.[120] In small series of 13 consecutive patients treated with a direct intramyocardial injection of VEGF-165, partial or complete resolution of perfusion defects seen on the sestamibi scan was observed 60 days after the procedure.[120] A multicenter placebo-controlled study evaluating this approach is ongoing.

Percutaneous Valvuloplasty

In parallel with the development of percutaneous treatments for coronary and peripheral vascular lesions, there has been an ongoing effort to provide percutaneous treatments for valvular heart disease. Percutaneous valve dilation has been used as an alternative to definitive surgical repair or replacement in selected patients with symptomatic valvular stenosis, particularly of the mitral valve. Mitral valvuloplasty is a safe and effective alternative to surgical repair in selected patients with mitral stenosis, whereas aortic valvuloplasty provides only short-term palliation and should be reserved for inoperable cases with degenerative calcific aortic stenosis. The indications and contraindications for mitral and aortic valvuloplasty are reviewed in detail elsewhere (see Chap. 57). This chapter focuses on the technical issues, selection of patients, and outcomes associated with mitral and aortic valvuloplasty.

Mitral Valvuloplasty (see also Chap. 57)

Percutaneous mitral valvuloplasty (PMV) was first performed in 1984 as an alternative to surgical mitral valve commissurotomy; subsequent reports confirmed the immediate and long-term benefits of this procedure. Although the majority of PMV procedures are performed in developing countries where rheumatic fever and valvular heart disease continue to be endemic, a few specialized centers in Western countries have developed technical expertise in PMV (Fig. 52–14).

TECHNICAL ISSUES. Several approaches for PMV have been described. The most common is transvenous or anterograde, using a transseptal puncture to gain access to the left atrium. A balloon catheter is then floated across the mitral valve into the left ventricle. A retrograde, transarterial approach can be used to avoid the creation of a large atrial septal defect but is uncommon in clinical practice, and experience with this method is limited except for a few specialized centers.

There are several variants of the anterograde approach. With the double-balloon method, a transseptal puncture is performed and a balloon catheter is advanced across the mitral valve into the left ventricle. Two long exchange wires are then positioned in the left ventricle, and the interatrial septum is dilated with a 6- to 8-mm peripheral dilation balloon. Two mitral valvuloplasty balloons of appropriate size are advanced across the mitral valve and inflated simultaneously to split the sclerosed mitral commissures. The second technique uses the special Inoue balloon, which is a self-positioning, pressure-distensible, dumbbell-shaped balloon that locks itself into the stenotic mitral orifice and progressively dilates the orifice as the inflation pressure is increased. A stepwise dilation technique is performed to minimize the risk of mitral valve rupture and mitral regurgitation. Selection of balloon size is generally based on the patient's height, body surface area, and diameter of the mitral annulus. A mechanical valve dilator has also been used percutaneously and has the advantage of resterilization and reuse in developing countries.

Comparative studies of these two techniques have shown similar clinical success rates but shorter procedure times and higher disposable costs with the Inoue technique. The Inoue balloon has also been used in patients with severe mitral valve calcification and subvalvular fibrosis.

HEMODYNAMIC ASSESSMENT. Serial hemodynamic measurements, alone or in combination with echocardiography, may be used to evaluate the result achieved with PMV.[121] An immediate improvement in left atrial mean pressure (and reduction of the transmittal gradient) should be seen, with a gradual decrease in pulmonary artery pressure and an increase in cardiac output. Criteria for termination of the procedure include (1) a mitral valve area larger than 1 cm^2 per square meter of body surface area, (2) complete opening of at least one commissure, or (3) the appearance of an increment in mitral regurgitation. Transesophageal echocardiography may also be performed during the procedure and, in particular, may guide the transseptal puncture in patients with obscure cardiac landmarks or skeletal deformity.

PROCEDURAL OUTCOME. A favorable procedural outcome has been related to institutional volume (>25 cases per year), baseline mitral valve area (>0.5 cm^2), and the age of the patient (younger than 70 years). Procedural mortality associated with mitral valvuloplasty ranges from 0 to 3 percent in most series and is primarily related to left ventricular perforation resulting from the transseptal technique or advancement of the guidewire or balloon catheter into the left ventricle or to general comorbidity in the patient. Cerebral or coronary emboli occur in 0.5 to 5.0 percent of patients and are related to dislodgment of thromboembolic material from the left atrium or air within the dilatation apparatus, underscoring the importance of transesophageal echocardiography for detection of atrial thrombi. Severe mitral regurgitation resulting from rupture of the chordae tendineae or papillary muscle rupture may also occur. Atrial septal defects are commonly (80 percent) seen after PMV, but the magnitude of the left-to-right shunt is generally insignificant. The atrial septal defect also closes in the majority (90 to 100 percent) of cases within 3 months after PMV. Emergency surgery may be required in a minority of cases after PMV. When surgery is required for mitral regurgitation, left ven-

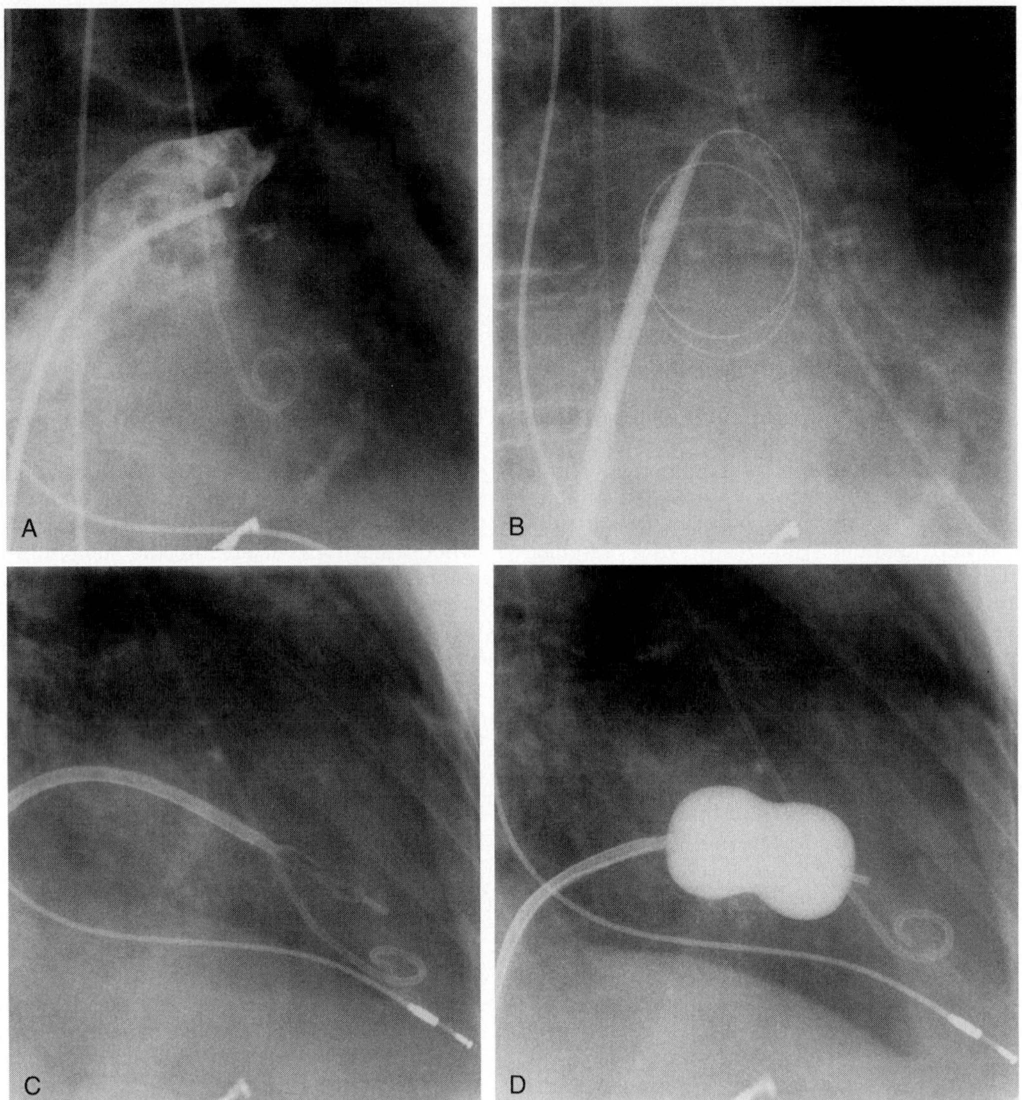

FIGURE 52–14 Mitral valvuloplasty. After transseptal puncture, a Mullins sheath is advanced into the left atrium, as demonstrated by injection of contrast medium **(A)**. An Inoue guidewire is coiled in the left atrium and an Inoue dilator is advanced across the intraatrial septum **(B)**. Advancement of the Inoue balloon dilation catheter into the left ventricle **(C)** and inflation **(D)** resulted in a successful procedure. (Courtesy of Dr. Andrew Eisenhauer.)

tricular rupture, or the development of a left-to-right shunt or as a result of a failed procedure, the mortality rate rises substantially.

LATE OUTCOME. Transthoracic echocardiography may be useful to assess the prognosis after PMV by semiquantitatively scoring leaflet mobility, valvular and subvalvular thickening, and valvular calcification. In one series of 136 patients undergoing successful PMV, the estimated 5-year mortality rate was 24 percent and the 5-year event rate (i.e., mitral valve replacement, repeated valvuloplasty, or death from cardiac causes) was 49 percent.[122] Multivariable predictors of late events after PMV were a high mitral valve echocardiographic score, an elevated left ventricular end-diastolic pressure, and a worse New York Heart Association (NYHA) functional class ($p = 0.04$).[122] Patients with fewer than two risk factors for early restenosis (echocardiographic score >8, left ventricular end-diastolic pressure >10-mm Hg, or NYHA functional Class IV) had a predicted 5-year event-free survival rate of 60 to 84 percent, whereas patients with two or three risk factors had a predicted 5-year event-free survival rate of only 13 to 41 percent.[122]

Aortic Valvuloplasty (see also Chap. 57)

The most frequent cause of acquired valvular heart disease in Western countries is degenerative calcific aortic stenosis.[121] Whereas in mitral stenosis the problem is commissural fusion, in acquired calcific stenosis the problem is rigid valve leaflets. Percutaneous aortic valvuloplasty (PAV) fractures the calcified aortic leaflets, thereby increasing their flexibility, and somewhat dilates the surrounding aortic annulus. When the annulus recoils and the leaflets recalcify, even the modest hemodynamic improvements abate (days to weeks). The long-term clinical benefit associated with PAV for calcific aortic stenosis is thus limited.

PAV is generally reserved for adult patients with severe calcific aortic stenosis who have severe comorbidities that preclude aortic valve replacement, such as patients with cardiogenic shock or other significant comorbid conditions; for patients as a "bridge" to definitive surgical correction; or for patients with severe left ventricular dysfunction (i.e., low flow, low gradient) in whom the hemodynamic response to aortic valve replacement cannot be determined (Fig. 52–15).

In the absence of these indications, definitive aortic valve replacement rather than PAV should be performed, even in elderly patients. PAV in patients with congenital aortic stenosis is discussed in Chapter 56. New percutaneous procedures are being developed to stent the calcified valve open and allow a new pericardial valve sewn with the stent to open and close with the cardiac cycle, which may allow more durable percutaneous correction of calcific aortic stenosis.[123]

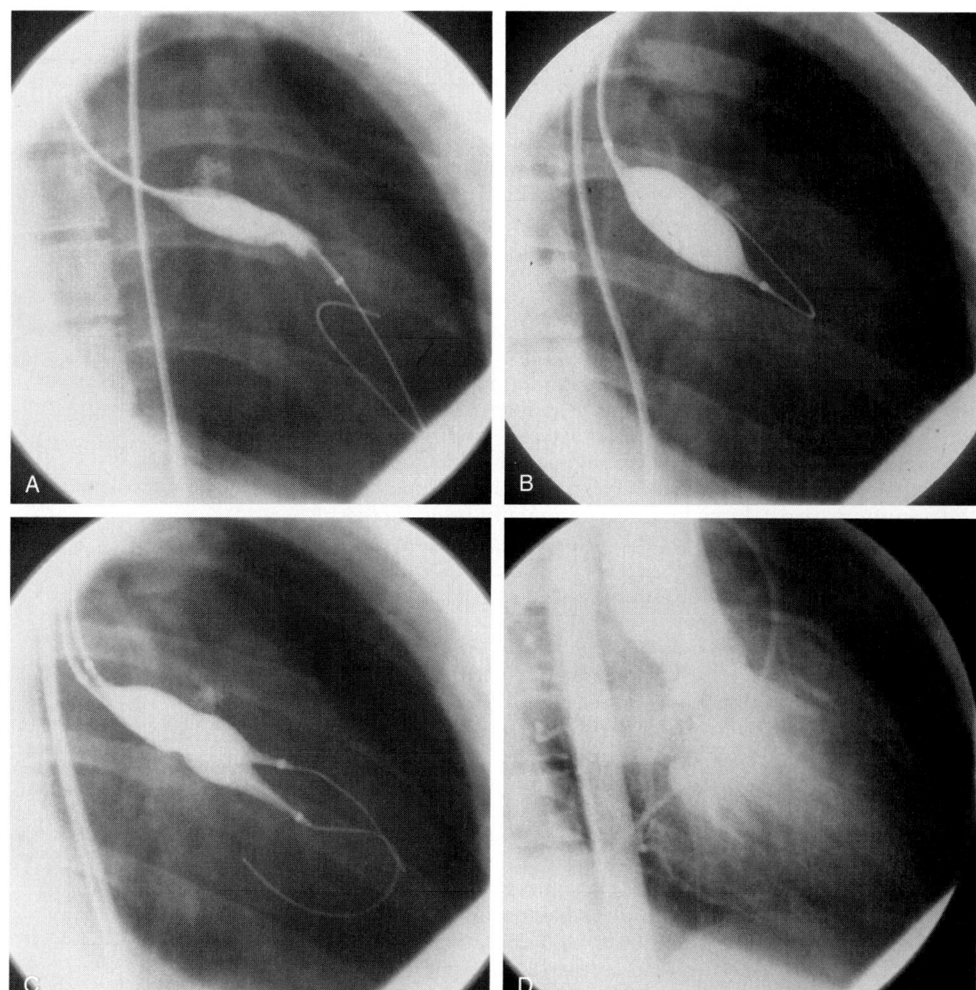

FIGURE 52–15 Aortic valvuloplasty. A 16-mm aortic valvuloplasty balloon is inflated across the aortic valve **(A)** and exchanged for a 24-mm balloon **(B)** because of a persistent gradient. To improve the aortic gradient further, two 16-mm valvuloplasty balloons are advanced across the aortic valve **(C)**. Because of the relative oversizing of the balloons to the aortic ring, aortic regurgitation results **(D)**. (Courtesy of Dr. Andrew Eisenhauer.)

TECHNICAL ISSUES. The femoral approach is most frequently used for PAV. After crossing the aortic valve with a guidewire, an extra-stiff 0.038-inch wire is inserted into the apex of the left ventricle to stabilize the balloon during inflation. In patients with severe peripheral vascular disease, a brachial approach or antero-grade approach with a transseptal puncture can be used to pass a long wire through the left ventricle, across the aortic valve, and into the descending aorta. The interatrium septum is dilated with a peripheral balloon, and the PAV balloon is then advanced across the aortic valve. PAV balloons ranging in diameter between 15 and 25-mm and in length between 3 and 5 cm have variable shapes, including conventional, bifoil, trifoil, and double-sized configurations, with the proximal portion measuring 20 to 23-mm and the distal portion 15 to 18-mm.[121] The size of the balloon should not exceed 1.2 to 1.3 times the diameter of the aortic ring.

HEMODYNAMIC ASSESSMENT. The transaortic valve gradient should be reduced immediately after the procedure, although little change may be noted in cardiac output. After successful dilation, 25 to 47 percent of patients obtain a final valve area larger than 1 cm^2 and 22 to 39 percent of patients achieve a valve area less than 0.7 cm^2.

PROCEDURAL SUCCESS AND COMPLICATION RATES. The clinical success rate for patients undergoing PAV ranges from 68 to 75 percent. Hospital mortality after PAV varies from 3.5 to 13.5 percent, and 20 to 25 percent of patients experience at least one complication during their hospitalization. Complications include a need for vascular access repair, embolic cerebrovascular events, aortic regurgitation, and, with the use of oversized balloons, rupture of the aortic ring. Predictors of procedural mortality include the patient's age, NYHA class, concomitant CAD, congestive heart failure, lower initial left ventricular systolic pressure, smaller final aortic valve area, lower baseline cardiac output, and the development of procedural complications. Predictors of morbidity are depressed left ventricular function, low cardiac output, diffuse coronary disease, and final valve area smaller than 0.7 cm^2.

The major limitation of PAV is the early recurrence of symptoms in most patients. The estimated incidence of late restenosis is 36 to 80 percent in the first year. Determinants of late outcomes after PAV were studied in 205 patients undergoing this procedure. The event-free survival rate, defined as survival without recurrent symptoms, repeated valvuloplasty, or aortic valve replacement, was 18 percent over the 24-month follow-up (range, 1 to 47 months). Significant predictors of event-free survival included the left ventricular ejection fraction, left ventricular and aortic systolic pressure before PAV, and percent reduction in the aortic valve pressure gradient; the pulmonary capillary wedge pressure was inversely associated with event-free survival. Although the predicted event-free survival rate for the entire group of patients was 50 percent at 1 year and 25 percent at 2 years, the probability of event-free survival at 1 year varied between 23 and 65 percent when patients were stratified according to three independent predictors: aortic systolic pressure, pulmonary capillary wedge pressure, and percent reduction in the peak aortic valve gradient. The best long-term results after valvuloplasty were observed in patients who would also have been expected to have excellent long-term results after aortic valve replacement. Repeated PAV for symptom recurrence may also be useful.

Training Standards and Proficiency in Interventional Cardiology

As the number of devices, procedures, and associated pharmacology has grown, interventional cardiology has evolved into a separate discipline in medicine. Standards for core curriculum development and procedural proficiency for interventional cardiology training programs have been established by the American College of Cardiology and by the Society for Cardiac Angiography and Intervention.[124-126] These criteria form the basis for an additional 12-month dedicated training program established under the guidelines of the American Board of Internal Medicine Accreditation Council for Graduate Medical Education. Successful completion of this training program is a prerequisite for new graduates prior to sitting for the Certification Examination for Added Qualification in Interventional Cardiology. Proficiency requirements for interventional training have become more rigorous over time, with the minimum case volume for interventional training increasing from 125 to 250 cases as the primary operator; maintenance of proficiency now requires more than 75 cases per year as the primary operator unless special circumstances are identified.[126]

Operator- and hospital-specific procedural outcomes after PCI are also collected by hospital, governmental, and managed care organizations and should be monitored to ensure quality in care of patients provided by the interventional operators. The focus on minimum volume criteria is based on studies that relate procedural outcome after PCI to both hospital and individual operator volumes. PCI complication rates are higher when the hospital procedural volume is less than 200 to 400 cases per year or individual operator volume is less than 75 to 100 coronary interventions per year. The American College of Cardiology has recommended that hospitals perform more than 200 to 400 cases per year and individual operators perform more than 75 cases per year.[33,125] Accordingly, individual institutions need to establish valid methods for peer review, including documentation of procedural success and failure rates of individual operators, minimum volume performance for the hospital and individual operators, quality of the laboratory facility, and training of the support staff. Establishment of an outcomes data base is strongly encouraged for all institutions as part of an ongoing quality assurance program.[127,128]

REFERENCES

Outcomes After Percutaneous Coronary Intervention

1. Detre K, Holubkov R, Kelsey S, et al: Percutaneous transluminal coronary angioplasty in 1985-1986 and 1977-1981. The National Heart, Lung, and Blood Institute Registry. N Engl J Med 318:265, 1988.
2. Ellis SG, Cowley MJ, Whitlow PL, et al: Prospective case-control comparison of percutaneous transluminal coronary revascularization in patients with multivessel disease treated in 1986-1987 versus 1991: Improved in-hospital and 12-month results. Multivessel Angioplasty Prognosis Study (MAPS) Group. J Am Coll Cardiol 25:1137, 1995.
3. Baim DS, Cutlip DE, Sharma SK, et al: Final results of the Balloon vs Optimal Atherectomy Trial (BOAT). Circulation 97:322, 1998.
4. Fischman DL, Leon MB, Baim DS, et al: A randomized comparison of coronary-stent placement and balloon angioplasty in the treatment of coronary artery disease. Stent Restenosis Study Investigators. N Engl J Med 331:496, 1994.
5. Serruys PW, van Hout B, Bonnier H, et al: Randomised comparison of implantation of heparin-coated stents with balloon angioplasty in selected patients with coronary artery disease (Benestent II). Lancet 352:673, 1998.
6. Mauri L, Bonan R, Weiner B, et al: Cutting balloon angioplasty for the prevention of restenosis: Results of the Cutting Balloon Global Randomized Trial. Am J Cardiol 90:1079, 2002.
7. Williams D, Holubkov R, Yeh W, et al: Percutaneous coronary intervention in the current era compared with 1985-1986: The National Heart, Lung, and Blood Institute Registries. Circulation 102:2945, 2000.

Coronary Atherectomy and Thrombectomy

8. Topol EJ, Leya F, Pinkerton CA, et al: A comparison of directional atherectomy with coronary angioplasty in patients with coronary artery disease. The CAVEAT Study Group. N Engl J Med 329:221, 1993.
9. Adelman AG, Cohen EA, Kimball BP, et al: A comparison of directional atherectomy with balloon angioplasty for lesions of the left anterior descending coronary artery. N Engl J Med 329:228, 1993.
10. Suzuki T, Hosokawa H, Katoh O, et al: Effects of adjunctive balloon angioplasty after intravascular ultrasound-guided optimal directional coronary atherectomy: The result of Adjunctive Balloon Angioplasty After Coronary Atherectomy Study (ABACAS). J Am Coll Cardiol 34:1028, 1999.
11. Tsuchikane E, Sumitsuji S, Awata N, et al: Final results of the STent versus directional coronary Atherectomy Randomized Trial (START). J Am Coll Cardiol 34:1050, 1999.
12. Moussa I, Moses J, Di Mario C, et al: Stenting after optimal lesion debulking (sold) registry. Angiographic and clinical outcome. Circulation 98:1604, 1998.
13. Whitlow PL, Bass TA, Kipperman RM, et al: Results of the study to determine rotablator and transluminal angioplasty strategy (STRATAS). Am J Cardiol 87:699, 2001.
14. Mauri L, Reisman M, Buchbinder M, et al: Comparison of rotational atherectomy with conventional balloon angioplasty in the prevention of restenosis of small coronary arteries: Results of the Dilatation vs Ablation Revascularization Trial Targeting Restenosis (DART). Am Heart J 145:847, 2003.
15. Reifart N, Vandormael M, Krajcar M, et al: Randomized comparison of angioplasty of complex coronary lesions at a single center. Excimer Laser, Rotational Atherectomy, and Balloon Angioplasty Comparison (ERBAC) Study. Circulation 96:91, 1997.
16. Kuntz R, Baim D, Cohen D, et al: A trial comparing rheolytic thrombectomy with intracoronary urokinase for coronary and vein graft thrombus (the Vein Graft AngioJet Study [VeGAS 2]). Am J Cardiol 89:326, 2002.
17. Baim D, Wahr D, George B, et al: Randomized trial of a distal embolic protection device during percutaneous intervention of saphenous vein aorto-coronary bypass grafts. Circulation 105:1285, 2002.
18. Webb J, Carere R, Virmani R, et al: Retrieval and analysis of particulate debris after saphenous vein graft intervention. J Am Coll Cardiol 34:468, 1999.
19. Stone GW, Rogers C, Hermiller J, et al: Randomized comparison of distal protection with a filter-based catheter and a balloon occlusion and aspiration system during percutaneous intervention of a diseased saphenous vein aorto-coronary bypass graft. Circulation 108:548, 2003.

Coronary Stenting

20. Serruys P, de Jaegere P, Kiemeneij F, et al: A comparison of balloon expandable stent implantation with balloon angioplasty in patients with coronary artery disease. N Engl J Med 8:489, 1994.
21. Erbel R, Haude M, Hopp H, et al: Coronary-artery stenting compared with balloon angioplasty for restenosis after initial balloon angioplasty. N Engl J Med 339:1672, 1998.
22. Savage MP, Douglas JS Jr, Fischman DL, et al: Stent placement compared with balloon angioplasty for obstructed coronary bypass grafts. Saphenous Vein De Novo Trial Investigators. N Engl J Med 337:740, 1997.
23. Buller C, Dzavik V, Carere R, et al: Primary stenting versus balloon angioplasty in occluded coronary arteries: The Total Occlusion Study of Canada (TOSCA). Circulation 100:236, 1999.
24. Sirnes PA, Golf S, Myreng Y, et al: Stenting in Chronic Coronary Occlusion (SICCO): A randomized, controlled trial of adding stent implantation after successful angioplasty. J Am Coll Cardiol 28:1444, 1996.
25. Grines C, Cox D, Stone G, et al: Coronary angioplasty with or without stent implantation for acute myocardial infarction. Stent Primary Angioplasty in Myocardial Infarction Study Group. N Engl J Med 341:1949, 1999.
26. Stone G, Grines C, Cox D, et al: Comparison of angioplasty with stenting, with or without abciximab, in acute myocardial infarction. N Engl J Med 346:957, 2002.
27. Neumann F-J, Kastrati A, Schmitt C, et al: Effect of glycoprotein IIb-IIa receptor blockade with abciximab on clinical and angiographic restenosis rates after the placement of coronary stents following acute myocardial infarction. J Am Coll Cardiol 35:915, 2000.
28. Holmes D, Lansky A, Kuntz R, et al: The PARAGON stent study: A randomized trial of a new martensitic nitinol stent versus the Palmaz-Schatz stent for treatment of complex native coronary arterial lesions. Am J Cardiol 86:1073, 2000.
29. Baim D, Cutlip D, O'Shaughnessy C, et al: Final results of a randomized trial comparing the NIR stent to the Palmaz-Schatz stent for narrowings in native coronary arteries. Am J Cardiol 87:152, 2001.
30. Baim D, Cutlip D, Midei M, et al: Final results of a randomized trial comparing the MULTI-LINK stent with the Palmaz-Schatz stent for narrowings in native coronary arteries. Am J Cardiol 87:157, 2001.
31. Han R, Schwartz R, Kobayashi Y, et al: Comparison of self-expanding and balloon-expandable stents for the reduction of restenosis. Am J Cardiol 88:253, 2001.
32. Lansky A, Roubin G, O'Shaughnessy C, et al: Randomized comparison of GR-II stent and Palmaz-Schatz stent for elective treatment of coronary stenoses. Circulation 102:1364, 2000.

Clinical Results After Percutaneous Coronary Intervention

33. Smith S, Dove J, Jacobs A, et al: ACC/AHA guidelines of percutaneous coronary interventions (revision of the 1993 PTCA guidelines)—Executive summary. A report of the American College of Cardiology/American Heart Association Task Force on Practice Guidelines (committee to revise the 1993 guidelines for percutaneous transluminal coronary angioplasty). J Am Coll Cardiol 37:2215, 2001.
34. Califf RM, Abdelmeguid AE, Kuntz RE, et al: Myonecrosis after revascularization procedures. J Am Coll Cardiol 31:241, 1998.
35. O'Conner G, Malenka D, Quiton H, et al: Multivariate prediction of in-hospital mortality after percutaneous coronary interventions in 1994-1996. J Am Coll Cardiol 34:681, 1999.
36. Moscucci M, O'Connor G, Ellis S, et al: Validation of risk adjustment models for in-hospital percutaneous transluminal coronary angioplasty on an independent data set. J Am Coll Cardiol 34:692, 1999.

37. Leon M, Baim D, Popma J, et al: A clinical trial comparing three antithrombotic-drug regimens after coronary-artery stenting. N Engl J Med 339:1665, 1998.

Treatment of In-Stent Restenosis

38. vom Dahl J, Dietz U, Haager P, et al: Rotational atherectomy does not reduce recurrent in-stent restenosis: Results of the angioplasty versus rotational atherectomy for treatment of diffuse in-stent restenosis trial (ARTIST). Circulation 105:583, 2002.
39. Kimura T, Yokoi H, Nakagawa T, et al: Three-year follow-up after implantation of metallic coronary artery stents. N Engl J Med 334:561, 1996.
40. Teirstein PS, Massullo V, Jani S, et al: Catheter-based radiotherapy to inhibit restenosis after coronary stenting. N Engl J Med 336:1697, 1997.
41. Waksman R, White R, Chan R, et al: Intracoronary gamma-radiation therapy after angioplasty inhibits recurrence in patients with in-stent restenosis. Circulation 101:2130, 2000.
42. Leon M, Teirstein P, Moses J, et al: Localized intracoronary gamma radiation therapy to inhibit the recurrence of restenosis after stenting. N Engl J Med 344:250, 2001.
43. Waksman R, Raizner A, Yeung A, et al: Use of localised intracoronary beta radiation in treatment of in-stent restenosis: The INHIBIT randomised controlled trial. Lancet 359:551, 2002.
44. Popma J, Suntharalingam M, Lansky A, et al: Randomized trial of ^{90}Sr/^{90}Y beta-radiation versus placebo control for treatment of in-stent restenosis. Circulation 106:1090, 2002.
45. Waksman R, Buchbinder M, Reisman M, et al: Balloon-based radiation therapy for treatment of in-stent restenosis in human coronary arteries: Results from the BRITE I study. Catheter Cardiovasc Interv 57:286, 2002.
46. Duffin D, Muhlestein J, Allisson S, et al: Femoral arterial puncture management after percutaneous coronary procedures: A comparison of clinical outcomes and patient satisfaction between manual compression and two different vascular closure devices. J Invasive Cardiol 13:354, 2001.

Anticoagulation During Percutaneous Coronary Intervention

47. Schomig A, Neumann FJ, Kastrati A, et al: A randomized comparison of antiplatelet and anticoagulant therapy after the placement of coronary-artery stents. N Engl J Med 334:1084, 1996.
48. Mehta S, Yusuf S, Peters R, et al: Effects of pretreatment with clopidogrel and aspirin followed by long-term therapy in patients undergoing percutaneous coronary intervention: The PCI-CURE study. Lancet 358:527, 2001.
49. Steinhubl S, Berger P, Mann J, et al: Early and sustained dual oral antiplatelet therapy following percutaneous coronary intervention: A randomized controlled trial. JAMA 288:2411, 2002.
50. The EPIC Investigators: Use of a monoclonal antibody directed against the platelet glycoprotein IIb/IIIa receptor in high-risk coronary angioplasty. The EPIC Investigation. N Engl J Med 330:956, 1994.
51. The EPILOG Investigators: Platelet glycoprotein IIb/IIIa receptor blockade and low-dose heparin during percutaneous coronary revascularization. The EPILOG Investigators. N Engl J Med 336:1689, 1997.
52. The EPISTENT Investigators: Randomised placebo-controlled and balloon-angioplasty-controlled trial to assess safety of coronary stenting with use of platelet glycoprotein-IIb/IIIa blockade. Evaluation of Platelet IIb/IIIa Inhibitor for Stenting. Lancet 352:87, 1998.
53. The IMPACT-II Investigators: Randomised placebo-controlled trial of effect of eptifibatide on complications of percutaneous coronary intervention: IMPACT-II. Integrilin to Minimise Platelet Aggregation and Coronary Thrombosis-II. Lancet 349:1422, 1997.
54. The ESPRIT Investigators: Novel dosing regimen of eptifibatide in planned coronary stent implantation (ESPRIT): A randomised, placebo-controlled trial. Lancet 356:2037, 2000.
55. The RESTORE Investigators: Effects of platelet glycoprotein IIb/IIIa blockade with tirofiban on adverse cardiac events in patients with unstable angina or acute myocardial infarction undergoing coronary angioplasty. The RESTORE Investigators. Randomized Efficacy Study of Tirofiban for Outcomes and REstenosis. Circulation 96:1445, 1997.
56. Topol E, Moliterno D, Herrmann H, et al: Comparison of two platelet glycoprotein IIb/IIIa inhibitors, tirofiban and abciximab, for the prevention of ischemic events with percutaneous coronary revascularization. N Engl J Med 344:1888, 2001.
57. Chew D, Bhatt D, Lincoff A, et al: Defining the optimal activated clotting time during percutaneous coronary intervention: Aggregate results from 6 randomized, controlled trials. Circulation 103:961, 2001.
58. Levine GN, Ferguson JJ: Low-molecular-weight heparin during percutaneous coronary interventions: Rationale, results, and recommendations. Cathet Cardiovasc Interv 60:185, 2003.
59. Serruys PW, Herrman JP, Simon R, et al: A comparison of hirudin with heparin in the prevention of restenosis after coronary angioplasty. Helvetica Investigators. N Engl J Med 333:757, 1995;.
60. Bittl JA, Strony J, Brinker JA, et al: Treatment with bivalirudin (Hirulog) as compared with heparin during coronary angioplasty for unstable or postinfarction angina. Hirulog Angioplasty Study Investigators. N Engl J Med 333:764, 1995.
61. Lincoff A, Bittl J, Harrington R, et al: Bivalirudin and provisional glycoprotein IIb/IIIa blockade compared with heparin and planned glycoprotein IIb/IIIa blockade during percutaneous coronary intervention: REPLACE-2 randomized trial. JAMA 289:853, 2003.

Systemic Approaches to Restenosis

62. Tsuchikane E, Fukuhara A, Kobayashi T, et al: Impact of cilostazol on restenosis after percutaneous coronary balloon angioplasty. Circulation 100:21, 1999.
63. Park S, Lee C, Kim H, et al: Effects of cilostazol on angiographic restenosis after coronary stent placement. Am J Cardiol 86:499, 2000.
64. Kamishirado H, Inoue T, Mizoguchi K, et al: Randomized comparison of cilostazol versus ticlopidine hydrochloride for antiplatelet therapy after coronary stent implantation for prevention of late restenosis. Am Heart J 144:303, 2002.
65. Garachemani A, Fleisch M, Windecker S, et al: Heparin and Coumadin versus acetylsalicylic acid for prevention of restenosis after coronary angioplasty. Catheter Cardiovasc Interv 55:315, 2002.
66. ten Berg J, Kelder J, Suttorp M, et al: A randomized trial assessing the effect of coumarins started before coronary angioplasty on restenosis: Results of the 6-month angiographic substudy of the Balloon Angioplasty and Anticoagulation Study (BAAS). Am Heart J 145:58, 2003.
67. Versaci F, Gaspardone A, Tomai F, et al: Immunosuppressive Therapy for the Prevention of Restenosis after Coronary Artery Stent Implantation (IMPRESS Study). J Am Coll Cardiol 40:1935, 2002.
68. Tardif J, Gregoire J, Schwartz L, et al: Effects of AGI-1067 and probucol after percutaneous coronary interventions. Circulation 107:552, 2003.
69. Holmes D, Savage M, La Blanche J, et al: Results of Prevention of REStenosis with Tranilast and its Outcomes (PRESTO) trial. Circulation 106:1243, 2002.
70. Serruys P, Foley D, Pieper M, et al: The TRAPIST Study. A multicentre randomized placebo controlled clinical trial of trapidil for prevention of restenosis after coronary stenting, measured by 3-D intravascular ultrasound. Eur Heart J 22:1938, 2001.
71. Meurice T, Bauters C, Hermant X, et al: Effect of ACE inhibitors on angiographic restenosis after coronary stenting (PARIS): A randomised, double-blind, placebo-controlled trial. Lancet 357:1321, 2001.
72. Kondo J, Sone T, Tsuboi H, et al: Effect of quinapril on intimal hyperplasia after coronary stenting as assessed by intravascular ultrasound. Am J Cardiol 87:443, 2001.
73. Peters S, Gotting B, Trummel M, et al: Valsartan for prevention of restenosis after stenting of type B2/C lesions: The VAL-PREST trial. J Invasive Cardiol 13:93, 2001.
74. Dens J, Desmet W, Coussement P, et al: Usefulness of Nisoldipine for prevention of restenosis after percutaneous transluminal coronary angioplasty (results of the NICOLE study). NIsoldipine in COronary artery disease in LEuven. Am J Cardiol 87:28, 2001.
75. Jorgensen B, Simonsen S, Endresen K, et al: Restenosis and clinical outcome in patients treated with amlodipine after angioplasty: Results from the Coronary AngioPlasty Amlodipine REStenosis Study (CAPARES). J Am Coll Cardiol 35:592, 2000.
76. Serruys P, Foley D, Hofling B, et al: Carvedilol for prevention of restenosis after directional coronary atherectomy: Final results of the European carvedilol atherectomy restenosis (EUROCARE) trial. Circulation 101:1512, 2000.
77. Lincoff A, Califf RM, Moliterno D, et al: Complementary clinical benefits of coronary artery stenting and blockade of platelet glycoprotein IIb-IIIa receptors. N Engl J Med 341:319, 1999.
78. Roffi M, Moliterno D, Meier B, et al: Impact of different platelet glycoprotein IIb/IIIa receptor inhibitors among diabetic patients undergoing percutaneous coronary intervention: Do Tirofiban and ReoPro Give Similar Efficacy Outcomes Trial (TARGET) 1-year follow-up. Circulation 105:2730, 2002.
79. Tardif JC, Cote G, Lesperance J, et al: Probucol and multivitamins in the prevention of restenosis after coronary angioplasty. Multivitamins and Probucol Study Group. N Engl J Med 337:365, 1997.
80. Brara P, Moussavian M, Grise M, et al: Pilot trial of oral rapamycin for recalcitrant restenosis. Circulation 107:1722, 2003.
81. Serruys P, Foley D, Jackson G, et al: A randomized placebo-controlled trial of fluvastatin for prevention of restenosis after successful coronary balloon angioplasty; final results of the fluvastatin angiographic restenosis (FLARE) trial. Eur Heart J 20:58, 1999.
82. Serruys P, de Feyter P, Macaya C, et al: Fluvastatin for prevention of cardiac events following successful first percutaneous coronary intervention: A randomized controlled trial. JAMA 287:3215, 2002.

Drug-Eluting Stents

83. Sousa JE, Costa MA, Abizaid AC, et al: Sustained suppression of neointimal proliferation by sirolimus-eluting stents: One-year angiographic and intravascular ultrasound follow-up. Circulation 104:2007, 2001.
84. Degertekin M, Serruys P, Foley D, et al: Persistent inhibition of neointimal hyperplasia after sirolimus-eluting stent implantation: Long-term (up to 2 years) clinical, angiographic, and intravascular ultrasound follow-up. Circulation 106:1610, 2002.
85. Rensing B, Vos J, Smits P, et al: Coronary restenosis elimination with a sirolimus eluting stent: First European human experience with 6-month angiographic and intravascular ultrasonic follow-up. Eur Heart J 22:2125, 2001.
86. Sousa J, Costa M, Sousa A, et al: Two-year angiographic and intravascular ultrasound follow-up after implantation of sirolimus-eluting stents in human coronary arteries Circulation 107:381, 2003.
87. Morice M, Serruys P, Sousa J, et al: A randomized comparison of a sirolimus-eluting stent with a standard stent for coronary revascularization. N Engl J Med 346:1773, 2002.
88. Serruys P, Degertekin M, Tanabe K, et al: Intravascular ultrasound findings in the multicenter, randomized, double-blind RAVEL (RAndomized study with the sirolimus-eluting VElocity balloon-expandable stent in the treatment of patients with de novo native coronary artery Lesions) trial. Circulation 106:798, 2002.
89. Moses J, Leon M, Popma J, et al: Angiographic and clinical outcomes after a sirolimus-eluting stent compared to a standard stent in patients with complex coronary stenoses. N Engl J Med 349:1315, 2003.
90. Sousa J, Costa M, Abizaid A, et al: Sirolimus-eluting stent for the treatment of in-stent restenosis: A quantitative coronary angiography and three-dimensional intravascular ultrasound study. Circulation 107:24, 2003.
91. Degertekin M, Regar E, Tanabe K, et al: Sirolimus-eluting stent for treatment of complex in-stent restenosis. The first clinical experience. J Am Coll Cardiol 41:184, 2003.

92. Grube E, Silber S, Hauptmann K, et al: TAXUS I: Six- and twelve-month results from a randomized, double-blind trial on a slow-release paclitaxel-eluting stent for de novo coronary lesions. Circulation 107:38, 2003.
93. Colombo A, Drzewiecki J, Banning A, et al: Randomized study to assess the effectiveness of slow- and moderate-release polymer-based paclitaxel-eluting stents for coronary artery lesions Circulation 108:788, 2003.
94. Stone C, Ellis SG, Cox DA, et al: A polymer-based, paclitaxel-eluting stent in patients with coronary artery disease. N Engl J Med 350:221, 2004.
95. Park S, Shim W, Ho D, et al: A paclitaxel-eluting stent for the prevention of coronary restenosis. N Engl J Med 348:1537, 2003.
96. Tanabe K, Serruys P, Grube E, et al: TAXUS III trial: In-stent restenosis treated with stent-based delivery of paclitaxel incorporated in a slow-release polymer formulation. Circulation 107:559, 2003.
97. Hong M, Mintz G, Lee C, et al: Paclitaxel coating reduces in-stent intimal hyperplasia in human coronary arteries: A serial volumetric intravascular ultrasound analysis from the Asian Paclitaxel-Eluting Stent Clinical Trial (ASPECT). Circulation 107:517, 2003.
98. Liistro F, Stankovic G, Di Mario C, et al: First clinical experience with a paclitaxel derivate-eluting polymer stent system implantation for in-stent restenosis: Immediate and long-term clinical and angiographic outcome. Circulation 105:1883, 2002.
99. Virmani R, Liistro F, Stankovic G, et al: Mechanism of late in-stent restenosis after implantation of a paclitaxel derivate-eluting polymer stent system in humans. Circulation 106:2649, 2002.

Indications for Coronary Revascularization

100. Cannon C, Weintraub W, Demopoulos L, et al: Comparison of early invasive and conservative strategies in patients with unstable coronary syndromes treated with the glycoprotein IIb/IIIa inhibitor tirofiban. N Engl J Med 344:1879, 2001.
101. Fox K, Poole-Wilson P, Henderson R, et al: Interventional versus conservative treatment for patients with unstable angina or non-ST-elevation myocardial infarction: The British Heart Foundation RITA 3 randomised trial. Randomized Intervention Trial of unstable Angina. Lancet 360:743, 2002.
102. Popma J, Sawyer M, Selwyn A, et al: Lipid-lowering therapy after coronary revascularization. Am J Cardiol 86(4 Suppl 2):18H, 2000.
103. Eagle K, Guyton R, Davidoff R, et al: ACC/AHA Guidelines for Coronary Artery Bypass Surgery. J Am Coll Cardiol 34:1262, 1999.
104. Braunwald E, Antman E, Beasley J, et al: ACC/AHA 2002 guideline update for the management of patients with unstable angina and non-ST-segment elevation myocardial infarction—Summary article: A report of the American College of Cardiology/American Heart Association task force on practice guidelines (Committee on the Management of Patients With Unstable Angina). J Am Coll Cardiol 40:1366, 2002.
105. Anderson H, Cannon C, Stone P, et al: One year results of the Thrombolysis In Myocardial Infarction (TIMI) IIIB clinical trial: A randomized comparison of tissue-type plasminogen activator versus placebo and early invasive versus early conservative strategies in unstable angina and non-Q-wave myocardial infarction. J Am Coll Cardiol 26:1643, 1995.
106. Boden WE, O'Rourke RA, Crawford MH, et al: Outcomes in patients with acute non-Q-wave myocardial infarction randomly assigned to an invasive as compared with a conservative management strategy. Veterans Affairs Non-Q-Wave Infarction Strategies in Hospital (VANQWISH) Trial Investigators. N Engl J Med 338:1785, 1998.
107. Boden W: "Routine invasive" versus "selective invasive" approaches to non-ST-segment elevation acute coronary syndromes management in the post-stent/platelet inhibition era. J Am Coll Cardiol 41(4 Suppl S):113S, 2003.
108. The FRISC-II Investigators: Invasive compared with non-invasive treatment in unstable coronary artery disease: FRISC II prospective randomised multcentre study. Lancet 354:708, 1999.
109. Lemos P, Lee C, Degertekin M, et al: Early outcome after sirolimus-eluting stent implantation in patients with acute coronary syndromes. Insights from the Rapamycin-Eluting Stent Evaluated At Rotterdam Cardiology Hospital (RESEARCH) registry. J Am Coll Cardiol 41:2093, 2003
110. Pitt B, Waters D, Brown W: Aggressive lipid lowering compared with angioplasty in stable coronary artery disease. N Engl J Med 341:70, 1999.

Coronary Artery Bypass Surgery Versus Percutaneous Coronary Intervention

111. Solomon AJ, Gersh BJ: Management of chronic stable angina: medical therapy, percutaneous transluminal coronary angioplasty, and coronary artery bypass graft surgery. Lessons from the randomized trials. Ann Intern Med 128:216, 1998.
112. Pocock S, Henderson R, Rickards A, et al: Meta-analysis of randomized trials comparing coronary angioplasty with bypass surgery. Lancet 346:1184, 1995.
113. Detre KM, Lombardero MS, Brooks MM, et al: The effect of previous coronary-artery bypass surgery on the prognosis of patients with diabetes who have acute myocardial infarction. Bypass Angioplasty Revascularization Investigation Investigators. N Engl J Med 342:989, 2000.
114. Diegeler A, Thiele H, Falk V, et al: Comparison of stenting with minimally invasive bypass surgery for stenosis of the left anterior descending coronary artery. N Engl J Med 347:561, 2002.
115. de Feyter P, Serruys P, Unger F, et al: Bypass surgery versus stenting for the treatment of multivessel disease in patients with unstable angina compared with stable angina. Circulation 105:2367, 2002.
116. Serruys PW, Unger F, Sousa JE, et al: Comparison of coronary-artery bypass surgery and stenting for the treatment of multivessel disease. N Engl J Med 344:1117, 2001.
117. The SOS Investigators: Coronary artery bypass surgery versus percutaneous coronary intervention with stent implantation in patients with multivessel coronary artery disease (the Stent or Surgery trial): A randomised controlled trial. Lancet 360:965, 2002;.
118. Unger F, Serruys P, Yacoub M, et al: Revascularization in multivessel disease: Comparison between two-year outcomes of coronary bypass surgery and stenting. J Thorac Cardiovasc Surg 125:809, 2003.
119. Stone G, St Goar F, Taussig A, et al: First experience with hybrid percutaneous transmyocardial laser revascularization and angioplasty in patients with lesions at high risk for restenosis: Results of a phase I feasibility study. Am Heart J 142:679, 2001.
120. Vale PR, Losordo D, Milliken CE, et al: Left ventricular electromechanical mapping to assess efficacy of phVEGF165 gene transfer for therapeutic angiogenesis in chronic myocardial ischemia. Circulation 102:965, 2000.

Aortic and Mitral Valvuloplasty

121. Vahanian A: Valvuloplasty. *In* Topol E (ed): Textbook of Cardiovascular Medicine. Philadelphia, Lippincott-Raven, 1998, pp 2155-2175.
122. Cohen DJ, Kuntz RE, Gordon SP, et al: Predictors of long-term outcome after percutaneous balloon mitral valvuloplasty. N Engl J Med 327:1329, 1992.
123. Cribier A, Eltchaninoff H, Bash A, et al: Percutaneous transcatheter implantation of an aortic valve prosthesis for calcific aortic stenosis: First human case description. Circulation 106:3006, 2002.

Institutional and Operator Proficiency

124. Pepine C, Babb J, Brinker J, et al: Guidelines for training in adult cardiovascular medicine. Core Cardiology Training Symposium (COCATS). Task Force 3: Training in cardiac catheterization and interventional cardiology. J Am Coll Cardiol 25:14, 1995.
125. Hirshfeld J, Banas J, Brundage B, et al: American College of Cardiology training statement on recommendations for the structure of an optimal adult interventional cardiology training program: A report of the American College of Cardiology task force on clinical expert consensus documents. J Am Coll Cardiol 34:2141, 1999.
126. Hirshfeld J, Ellis S, Faxon D: Recommendations for the assessment and maintenance of proficiency in coronary interventional procedures: Statement of the American College of Cardiology. J Am Coll Cardiol 31:722, 1998.
127. Shaw R, Anderson H, Brindis R, et al: Development of a risk adjustment mortality model using the American College of Cardiology-National Cardiovascular Data Registry (ACC-NCDR) experience: 1998-2000. J Am Coll Cardiol 39:1104, 2002.
128. Bashore T, Bates E, Berger P, et al: American College of Cardiology/Society for Cardiac Angiography and Interventions Clinical Expert Consensus Document on cardiac catheterization laboratory standards. A report of the American College of Cardiology Task Force on Clinical Expert Consensus Documents. J Am Coll Cardiol 37:2170, 2001.

GUIDELINES *Thomas H. Lee*

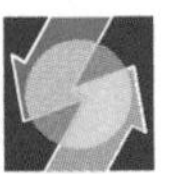

Percutaneous Coronary and Valvular Intervention

The American College of Cardiology/American Heart Association (ACC/AHA) updated guidelines for percutaneous coronary interventions (PCIs) in 2001.[1] Recommendations from these guidelines for use of PCI in the setting of acute myocardial infarction are summarized in the appendix to Chapter 48. Guidelines for use of percutaneous valvular interventions were published by the ACC/AHA in 1998[2] and are summarized in the appendix to Chapter 57. Therefore, this appendix focuses on recommendations relevant to use of PCI for stable ischemic heart disease and for unstable angina without acute myocardial infarction.

These guidelines use the ACC/AHA classification system for the indications (class I for generally accepted indications, class IIa when indications are controversial but the weight of evidence is supportive, class IIb when usefulness or efficacy is less well established, and class III when there is consensus against the usefulness of the intervention). The guidelines also use a convention for rating levels of evidence upon which recommendations have been based. *Level A* recommendations were derived from data from multiple randomized clinical trials, *level B* recommendations were derived from a single randomized trial or nonrandomized studies, and *level C* recommendations were based upon the consensus opinion of experts.

The guidelines acknowledged variability in outcomes of PCI in different populations, with particular attention to poorer outcomes in patients with diabetes mellitus. The committee concluded that much of the increase in adverse outcomes in women and elderly people was due to comorbidities; thus, with rare exception, separate recommendations for subgroups defined by gender and age were not developed.

Institutional and Operator Competence

These guidelines gave considerable attention to institutional and physician-specific factors associated with better outcomes and lower complication rates, such as higher procedure volume. Citing an ACC Training Statement,[3] the guidelines recommend that physicians undergo a 3-year comprehensive cardiac training program with 12 months of training in diagnostic catheterization during which the trainee performs 300 diagnostic catheterizations, including 200 as the primary operator. Interventional training requires a fourth year of training including more than 250 interventional procedures, a volume level that is also required for physicians to be eligible for the American Board of Internal Medicine certifying examination in interventional cardiology.

Institutions must have a system for quality measurement and improvement that includes valid peer review. The guidelines recommend that credentials committees should evaluate physician outcomes and cite benchmarks for unadjusted mortality (0.9 percent) and need for emergency coronary artery bypass surgery (<3.0 percent). The guidelines favor performance of PCI by higher volume operators (>75 cases per year) with advanced technical skills (e.g., subspecialty certification) at high-volume centers (>400 cases per year) associated with an on-site cardiovascular surgical program, except in underserved areas that are geographically far removed from major centers (Table 52G–1).

Despite technical improvements that have decreased the intensity of surgical "backup" coverage for PCI at many institutions, the guidelines continue to recommend that elective PCI should not be performed in facilities without on-site cardiac surgery.

Indications

The most recent guidelines for PCI differ from previous versions in that they no longer make recommendations based upon the number of diseased vessels. The guidelines assume that the operator can perform either single-vessel or multivessel PCI with a high likelihood of initial success and low risk. Therefore, recommendations are based upon the patient's clinical condition, specific coronary lesion morphology and anatomy, left ventricular function, and associated medical conditions.

The guidelines assert that the majority of patients with coronary disease who are asymptomatic or have mild angina should be treated medically. However, for patients with moderate or severe ischemia and few symptoms, revascularization with PCI or coronary artery bypass graft (CABG) surgery is considered reasonable and considered class I

TABLE 52G–1 Recommendations for Percutaneous Coronary Intervention Institutional and Operator Volumes at Centers with On-Site Cardiac Surgery

Operator Volume	Minimal Institutional Volume (200-400 Procedures Annually)	Optimal Institutional Volume (>400 Procedures Annually)
Low (<75 procedures annually)	Class IIb (an institution with a volume of <200 procedures per year, unless in a region that is underserved because of geography, should carefully consider whether it should continue to offer the service)	Class IIa (ideally, operators with annual procedure volume <75 should work only at institutions with an activity level of >600 procedures per year)
Acceptable (≥75 procedures annually)	Class IIa	Class I

TABLE 52G–2 ACC/AHA Recommendations for Percutaneous Coronary Intervention in Asymptomatic Patients or Patients with Class I Angina

Class	Indication	Level of Evidence
Class I (indicated)	Patients who do not have treated diabetes with asymptomatic ischemia or mild angina with one or more significant lesions in one or two coronary arteries suitable for PCI with a high likelihood of success and a low risk of morbidity and mortality. The vessels to be dilated must subtend a large area of viable myocardium.	B
Class IIa (good supportive evidence)	The same clinical and anatomical requirements as for class I, except the myocardial area at risk is of moderate size or the patient has treated diabetes.	B
Class IIb (weak supportive evidence)	Patients with asymptomatic ischemia or mild angina with > three coronary arteries suitable for PCI with a high likelihood of success and a low risk of morbidity and mortality. The vessels to be dilated must subtend at least a moderate area of viable myocardium. In the physician's judgment, there should be evidence of myocardial ischemia by ECG exercise testing, stress nuclear imaging, stress echocardiography or ambulatory ECG monitoring, or intracoronary physiological measurements.	B
Class III (not indicated)	Patients with asymptomatic ischemia or mild angina who do not meet the criteria as listed under class I or class II and who have: Only a small area of viable myocardium at risk. No objective evidence of ischemia. Lesions that have a low likelihood of successful dilation. Mild symptoms that are unlikely to be due to myocardial ischemia. Factors associated with increased risk of morbidity or mortality. Left main disease. Insignificant disease <50%.	C

ACC/AHA = American College of Cardiology/American Heart Association; ECG = electrocardiographic; PCI = percutaneous coronary intervention.

or II in appropriateness (Table 52G–2). PCI is considered inappropriate when the amount of viable myocardium at risk is small, when symptoms are unlikely to be due to ischemia, or when there is a high risk of complications.

For patients with more severe angina, the threshold for performing PCI is lower (Table 52G–3). PCI is considered appropriate in patients with single-vessel or multivessel disease if a moderate or large area of viable myocardium is at risk, the procedure has a high likelihood of success, and the risk of complications is low. PCI is considered inappropriate if patients have minimal myocardium at risk or a high risk of complications or if they have significant left main disease and are candidates for CABG.

For patients who have had CABG, the guidelines are supportive of an aggressive approach to detecting and addressing ischemia detected soon after surgery (Table 52G–4). Usually, such ischemia represents graft failure, often related to thrombosis, which can be corrected with PCI. When ischemia occurs 1 to 12 months after surgery, the etiology is usually perianastomotic graft stenosis, which also responds well to PCI. In contrast, PCI for chronic vein occlusions is characterized by lower success and higher complication rates, and thresholds for PCI are therefore higher when patients have ischemia more than 1 year after CABG.

Adjunctive Technologies

Intravascular ultrasonography can be used to facilitate deployment of coronary stents, but the guidelines do not consider it necessary for all stent procedures (Table 52G–5). The guidelines recommend that it be considered for use (class IIa) in high-risk procedures, such as those with multiple stents, impaired Thrombolysis in Myocardial Infarction (TIMI) grade flow or coronary flow reserve, and marginal angiographic appearance.

The guidelines similarly recommend a narrow role for assessment of coronary flow velocity and coronary vasodilator reserve. This tool might have a role in assessment of the physiological effects of intermediate coronary stenosis (30 to 70 percent luminal narrowing in patients with angina symptoms, class IIa), but the guidelines were dubious about its value in patients who had undergone successful PCI (Table 52G–6).

Management Issues

Recommendations for use of medications in patients undergoing PCI electively and with acute myocardial infarction are summarized in Table 52G–7. Antiplatelet therapy with aspirin and clopidogrel are considered class I indications for all patients, whereas warfarin is inappropriate except in patients with other indications for this medication. Glycoprotein IIb/IIIa inhibitors were considered clearly appropriate for patients undergoing PCI for severe or unstable angina but less clearly so (class II) for patients with class I angina. Unfractionated heparin was considered appropriate during PCI; the role of low-molecular-weight heparin was considered unresolved.

During long-term follow-up of patients after PCI, the guidelines do not endorse routine exercise testing of asymptomatic patients. If patients are symptomatic, the guidelines recommend that they undergo stress imaging studies in order to localize disease.

TABLE 52G–3 ACC/AHA Recommendations for Patients with Moderate or Severe Symptoms (Angina Class II to IV, Unstable Angina or Non-ST-Elevation Myocardial Infarction) with Single- or Multivessel Coronary Disease Receiving Medical Therapy

Class	Indication	Level of Evidence
Class I (indicated)	Patients with one or more significant lesions in one or more coronary arteries suitable for PCI with a high likelihood of success and low risk of morbidity or mortality. The vessel(s) to be dilated must subtend a moderate or large area of viable myocardium and have high risk.	B
Class IIa (good supportive evidence)	Patients with focal saphenous vein graft lesions or multiple stenoses who are poor candidates for reoperative surgery.	C
Class IIb (weak supportive evidence)	Patient has one or more lesions to be dilated with reduced likelihood of success or the vessel(s) subtends a less than moderate area of viable myocardium. Patients with two- or three-vessel disease, with significant proximal LAD CAD and treated diabetes or abnormal LV function.	C
Class III (not indicated)	Patient has no evidence of myocardial injury or ischemia on objective testing and has not had a trial of medical therapy or has Only a small area of myocardium at risk. All lesions or the culprit lesion to be dilated with morphology with a low likelihood of success. A high risk of procedure-related morbidity or mortality.	C
	Patients with insignificant coronary stenosis (e.g., <50% diameter).	C
	Patients with significant left main CAD who are candidates for CABG.	B

ACC/AHA = American College of Cardiology/American Heart Association; CABG = coronary artery bypass graft; CAD = coronary artery disease; LAD = left anterior descending; LV = left ventricular; PCA = percutaneous coronary intervention.

TABLE 52G–4 ACC/AHA Recommendations for Percutaneous Coronary Intervention with Prior Coronary Artery Bypass Graft

Class	Indication	Level of Evidence
Class I (indicated)	Patients with early ischemia (usually within 30 d) after CABG.	B
Class IIa (good supportive evidence)	Patients with ischemia occurring 1 to 3 yr postoperatively and preserved LV function with discrete lesions in graft conduits.	B
	Disabling angina secondary to new disease in a native coronary circulation. (If angina is not typical, the objective evidence of ischemia should be obtained.)	B
	Patients with diseased vein grafts >3 yr following CABG.	B
Class IIb (weak supportive evidence)		
Class III (not indicated)	PCI to chronic total vein graft occlusions.	B
	Patients with multivessel disease, failure or multiple SVGs, and impaired LV function.	B

ACC/AHA = American College of Cardiology/American Heart Association; CABG = coronary artery bypass graft; LV = left ventricular; SVG = saphenous vein graft.

TABLE 52G–5 ACC/AHA Recommendations for Coronary Intravascular Ultrasonography

Class	Indication	Level of Evidence
Class I (indicated)		
Class IIa (good supportive evidence)	Assessment of the adequacy of deployment of coronary stents, including the extent of stent apposition and determination of the minimum luminal diameter within the stent.	B
	Determination of the mechanism of stent restenosis (inadequate expansion versus neointimal proliferation) and to enable selection of appropriate therapy (plaque ablation versus repeated balloon expansion).	B
	Evaluation of coronary obstruction at a location difficult to image by angiography in a patient with a suspected flow-limiting stenosis.	C
	Assessment of a suboptimal angiographic result following PCI.	C
	Diagnosis and management of coronary disease following cardiac transplantation.	C
	Establishing presence and distribution of coronary calcium in patients for whom adjunctive rotational atherectomy is contemplated.	C
	Determination of plaque location and circumferential distribution for guidance of directional coronary atherectomy.	B
Class IIb (weak supportive evidence)	Determining extent of atherosclerosis in patients with characteristic anginal symptoms and a positive functional study with no focal stenoses or mild CAD on angiography.	C
	Preinterventional assessment of lesional characteristics and vessel dimensions as a means to select an optimal revascularization device.	C
Class III (not indicated)	When angiographic diagnosis is clear and no interventional treatment is planned.	C

ACC/AHA = American College of Cardiology/American Heart Association; CAD = coronary artery disease; PCI = percutaneous coronary intervention.

TABLE 52G–6 Recommendations for Intracoronary Physiological Measurements

Class	Indication	Level of Evidence
Class I (indicated)		
Class IIa (good supportive evidence)	Assessment of the physiological effects of intermediate coronary stenoses (30% to 70% luminal narrowing) in patients with anginal symptoms. Coronary pressure or Doppler velocimetry may also be useful as an alternative to performing noninvasive functional testing (e.g., when the functional study is absent or ambiguous) to determine whether an intervention is warranted.	B
Class IIb (weak supportive evidence)	Evaluation of the success of percutaneous coronary revascularization in restoring flow reserve and to predict the risk of restenosis.	C
	Evaluation of patients with anginal symptoms without an apparent angiographic culprit lesion.	C
Class III (not indicated)	Routine assessment of the severity of angiographic disease in patients with a positive, unequivocal noninvasive functional study.	C

TABLE 52G–7 ACC/AHA Recommendations for Pharmacological Management of Patients Undergoing Percutaneous Coronary Intervention*

Drugs	Clinical Status				
			Transmural MI		
	Class I Angina	*Class II-IV Angina, Unstable Angina, NSTEMI*	*Acute Phase MI*	*After Thrombolysis*	*Hospital Management Phase*
Aspirin	I	I	I	I	I
Ticlopidine, clopidogrel (in conjunction with stenting)	I (to be given 24-48 hours before planned stenting, if possible)	I	I	I	I (2-4 weeks after stent placement)
Warfarin	III (in patients without atrial fibrillation or other pre-existing clinical indications)	III	III	II	I (patients with anterior myocardial wall motion abnormalities or left ventricular thrombus)
Glycoprotein IIb/IIIa inhibitors	II	I	II	I	III
Unfractionated heparin	I	I	I	II	III

ACC/AHA = American College of Cardiology/American Heart Association; MI = myocardial infarction; NSTEMI = non–ST-segment elevation myocardial infarction.

*Roman numerals indicate ACC/AHA class indication.

References

1. Smith SC Jr, Dove JT, Jacobs AK, et al: ACC/AHA guidelines for percutaneous coronary intervention: A report of the American College of Cardiology/American Heart Association Task Force on Practice Guidelines (Committee to Revise the 1993 Guidelines for Percutaneous Transluminal Coronary Angioplasty). J Am Coll Cardiol 37:2239i, 2001.
2. Bonow RO, Carabello B, de Leon AC Jr, et al: ACC/AHA guidelines for the management of patients with valvular heart disease: Executive summary: A report of the American College of Cardiology/American Heart Association Task Force on Practice Guidelines (Committee on Management of Patients with Valvular Heart Disease). Circulation 98:1949, 1998.
3. Hirshfeld JW Jr, Banas JS Jr, Brudage BH, et al: American College of Cardiology training statement on recommendations for the structure of an optimal adult interventional cardiology training program: A report of the American College of Cardiology Task Force on Clinical Expert Consensus Documents. J Am Coll Cardiol 34:2141, 1999.

CHAPTER 53

Diseases of the Aorta

Eric M. Isselbacher

The Normal Aorta

Function

The aorta is the largest and strongest artery in the body, carrying roughly 200 million liters of blood through the body in an average lifetime. Three layers comprise the aorta: the thin inner layer, or *intima;* a thick middle layer, or *media;* and a rather thin outer layer, the *adventitia* (see Chap. 35). The strength of the aorta lies in the media, which is composed of laminated but intertwining sheets of elastic tissue arranged in a spiral manner that affords maximum tensile strength. Indeed, as thin as it is, experimentally the aortic wall can withstand the pressure of thousands of millimeters of mercury without bursting. In contrast to smaller muscular arteries, the aortic media contains multiple layers of elastic laminae (see Chap. 35). It is this tremendous accretion of elastic tissue that gives the aorta not only tensile strength but also distensibility and elasticity, which serve a vital circulatory role. The endothelium-lined aortic intima is a thin, delicate layer and is easily traumatized. The adventitia contains mainly collagen and carries the important vasa vasorum, which nourish the outer half of the aortic wall, including much of the media.

Ventricular systole distends the aorta by the force of the blood ejected from the left ventricle. In this manner, part of the kinetic energy generated by the contracting left ventricle is converted into potential energy stored in the aortic wall. Then, during diastole, this potential energy is transformed back into kinetic energy as the aortic walls recoil and propel the blood in the aortic lumen distally into the arterial bed. Thus, the aorta plays an essential role in maintaining forward circulation of the blood in diastole after it is delivered into the aorta by the left ventricle during systole. The pulse wave itself, with its milking effect, is transmitted along the aorta to the periphery at a speed of about 5 m/sec. This speed is much faster than the velocity of the intraluminal blood itself, which travels at only 40 to 50 cm/sec.

The systolic pressure developing within the aorta is a function of the volume of blood ejected into the aorta, the compliance or distensibility of the aorta, and resistance to blood flow. This resistance depends primarily on the tone of the peripheral muscular arteries and arterioles and, to a slight extent, on the inertia of the column of blood in the aorta when systole commences.

In addition to its conductance and pumping functions, the aorta also plays a role in indirectly controlling systemic vascular resistance and heart rate. Pressure-responsive receptors, analogous to those in the carotid sinus, lie in the ascending aorta and aortic arch and send afferent signals to the vasomotor center in the brain stem by way of the vagus nerves. An increase in intraaortic pressure causes reflex bradycardia and a reduction in systemic vascular resistance, whereas a decrease in intraaortic pressure increases the heart rate and vascular resistance.

Anatomical Considerations

The aorta is divided anatomically into thoracic and abdominal components. The thoracic aorta is further divided into the *ascending, arch,* and *descending* segments, and the abdominal aorta consists of *suprarenal* and *infrarenal* segments.

The ascending aorta is some 5 cm long and has two distinct segments. The lower segment is the *aortic root,* which begins at the level of the aortic valve and extends to the sinotubular junction. This portion of the ascending aorta is the widest and measures about 3.5 cm. The bases of the aortic leaflets are supported by the aortic root, from which the three sinuses of Valsalva bulge outward to allow for full excursion of the aortic valve leaflets during systole. In addition, the two coronary artery trunks arise from these sinuses of Valsalva. The upper tubular segment of the ascending aorta begins at the sinotubular junction and rises to join the aortic arch. Normally, the ascending aorta sits just to the right of midline, with its proximal portion lying within the pericardial cavity.

The arch of the aorta gives rise to all the brachiocephalic arteries. From the ascending aorta, the arch courses slightly leftward in front of the trachea and then proceeds posteriorly to the left of the trachea and esophagus. The pulmonary artery bifurcation and right pulmonary artery lie inferior to the arch, as does the left lung.

The descending thoracic aorta begins in the posterior mediastinum to the left of the vertebral column and gradually courses in front of the vertebral column as it descends, where it occupies a position immediately behind the esophagus. Distally, it passes through the diaphragm, usually at the level of the 12th thoracic vertebra.

The point at which the aortic arch joins the descending aorta is called the *aortic isthmus.* The aorta is especially vulnerable to trauma at this site because it is here that the relatively mobile portion of the aorta—the ascending aorta and arch—becomes relatively fixed to the thoracic cage by the pleural reflections, the paired intercostal arteries, and the left subclavian artery. Coarctations of the aorta also localize to this region.

The abdominal aorta continues from the thoracic aorta, gives rise to the mesenteric and renal arteries, and ends at its bifurcation into common iliac arteries at the level of the fourth lumbar vertebra.

Aging of the Aorta

As discussed, the elastic properties of the aorta contribute crucially to its normal function. However, the elasticity and distensibility of the aorta decline with age. Such changes occur even in normal healthy adults. The loss of elasticity and aortic compliance probably accounts for the increase in pulse pressure commonly seen in elderly persons and is accompanied by slow but progressive dilatation of the aorta.[1] This loss of aortic elasticity with aging is accelerated among persons with hypertension, hypercholesterolemia, or coronary artery disease, as compared with control subjects. Conversely, among healthy athletes, aortic elasticity is higher than in their age-matched controls.

Histologically, the aging aortic wall exhibits fragmentation of elastin with a concomitant increase in collagen that results in an increased collagen-to-elastin ratio, which contributes to the loss of aortic distensibility observed physiologically. Experimental animal data suggest that impairment of vasa vasorum flow to the aortic wall results in stiffening of the aorta with similar histological changes and may therefore be one cause of the degenerative changes seen with age.[2]

In animals, loss of aortic distensibility directly affects the mechanical performance of the left ventricle, with increases noted in left ventricular systolic pressure and wall tension and in end-diastolic pressure and volume. Furthermore, reduced aortic compliance causes a 20 to 40 percent increase in myocardial oxygen consumption to maintain a given stroke volume.[3] Over time, the changes in aortic compliance seen with age may cause clinically important alternations in cardiac function.

Examination of the Aorta

Unless the aorta is abnormally enlarged, the only location in which it can be palpated is the abdomen. The ease with which it can be felt depends largely on body habitus and pulse pressure: It is readily felt in thin individuals. It may be quite sensitive to palpation. Auscultation is usually unrevealing in patients with aortic diseases, except for occasional bruits at sites of narrowing of the aorta or its arterial branches. Diseases of the aortic root and proximal ascending aorta sometimes involve the aortic valve, with resultant aortic regurgitation that may be detectable on auscultation. Regurgitant murmurs secondary to root dilatation rather than primary valvular disease are often loudest along the right rather than the left sternal border.

Chest radiography and fluoroscopy are valuable and simple procedures for assessing the aorta. Normally, the ascending aorta is not visible on the direct anteroposterior chest radiograph. The aorta appears as a "knob" in the superior mediastinum just to the left of the vertebral column. The lateral border of the descending thoracic aorta can often be found to the left of the spine. On the lateral chest radiograph, the aortic root and proximal ascending aorta are visible as an indistinct shadow in the middle of the mediastinum arising from the base of the heart. The left anterior oblique projection best demonstrates the ascending aorta and arch.

A number of imaging modalities are available for diagnostic examination of the aorta, including aortography, computed tomography (CT), magnetic resonance imaging (MRI), and both transthoracic echocardiography (TTE) and transesophageal echocardiography (TEE). The respective utility of these imaging modalities is discussed here in the context of specific aortic diseases.

Aortic Aneurysms

The term *aortic aneurysm* refers to a pathological dilatation of the normal aortic lumen involving one or several segments. One useful criterion defines aortic aneurysm as a permanent localized dilation of the aorta having a diameter at least 1.5 times that of the expected normal diameter of that given aortic segment, although no definition is universally accepted. Aneurysms are usually described in terms of their location, size, morphologic appearance, and origin. The morphology of an aortic aneurysm is typically either *fusiform,* which is the more common shape, or *saccular.* A fusiform aneurysm has a fairly uniform shape, with symmetrical dilation that involves the full circumference of the aortic wall. Saccular aneurysms, on the other hand, have more localized dilation that appears as an outpouching of only a portion of the aortic wall. In addition, the aorta may have a *pseudoaneurysm* or *false aneurysm,* which is not actually an aneurysm at all, but rather a well-defined collection of blood and connective tissue outside the vessel wall. This defect may result from a contained rupture of the aortic wall.

The presence of an aortic aneurysm may be a marker of more diffuse aortic disease. Overall, up to 13 percent of all patients in whom an aortic aneurysm is diagnosed have multiple aneurysms, with 25 to 28 percent of those with thoracic aortic aneurysms having concomitant abdominal aortic aneurysms. For this reason, a patient in whom an aortic aneurysm is discovered should undergo examination of the entire aorta for the possible presence of other aneurysms.

Abdominal Aortic Aneurysms

Abdominal aortic aneurysms are much more common than thoracic aortic aneurysms. Age is an important risk factor. The incidence of abdominal aortic aneurysm rises rapidly after 55 years of age in men and 70 years of age in women, and abdominal aortic aneurysms occur 5 to 10 times more frequently in men than women. Men 65 years of age and older screened by ultrasonography have a prevalence of abdominal aortic aneurysms of 4 to 9 percent. The true prevalence of abdominal aortic aneurysms is difficult to determine, as there may be as much as a 10-fold variation depending on the diagnostic criteria, the imaging modality used, and the age, gender distribution, and baseline risk of the population examined.[4] Nevertheless, the incidence of abdominal aneurysms appears to have increased two- to threefold in recent decades. Some of the increase may reflect more widespread screening than in the past and more frequent use of abdominal CT scanning, which may reveal aortic aneurysms as incidental findings, for other diagnostic purposes. However, these data likely reflect, at least in part, a true increase in disease incidence.

The large majority of abdominal aortic aneurysms arise below the renal arteries and are known as *infrarenal* aneurysms. Only a small minority, known as *suprarenal aneurysms,* arise between the level of the diaphragm and the renal arteries. As a result of flow disturbance through the aneurysmal aortic segment, blood may stagnate along the walls and thus allow the formation of mural thrombus. Such thrombus, as well as atherosclerotic debris, may embolize and compromise the circulation of distal arteries. However, rupture poses the major risk of abdominal aortic aneurysms. When rupture does occur, 80 percent rupture into the left retroperitoneum, which may contain the rupture, whereas most of the remainder rupture into the peritoneal cavity and cause uncontrolled hemorrhage and rapid circulatory collapse.

ETIOLOGY AND PATHOGENESIS (see also Chap. 35). A number of risk factors favor the development of aneurysms. Smoking is most strongly associated with abdominal aortic aneurysms, followed by age, hypertension, hyperlipidemia, and atherosclerosis.[5] Gender and genes also influence aneurysm formation. Men are 10 times more likely than women to have an abdominal aortic aneurysm of 4.0 cm or greater.[6] However, women with aneurysms have a risk of rupture significantly higher than men. Those with a family history (first-degree relative) of abdominal aortic aneurysm have an increased risk of 13 to 32 percent compared with the 2 to 5 percent risk in the general population. In addition, those with familial aneurysms tend to be younger and have higher rates of rupture than those with sporadic aneurysms. Given the results of pedigree analysis and the fact that single gene defects have not yet been identified, the increased risk is probably polygenic.[7]

The aortic wall resists expansion because of the strength of its extracellular matrix, notably elastin and collagen. Degradation of these structural proteins, due to any of a number of factors, in turn weakens the aortic wall and allows aneurysms to develop. As the aorta then widens, tension in the vessel wall rises in accordance with Laplace law, which states that tension is proportional to the product of pressure and radius. Further widening results in even greater wall tension, which in turn leads to acceleration of aneurysm enlargement. A vicious cycle ensues in which the dilatation often progresses rapidly.

Classically, atherosclerosis has been considered the underlying cause of abdominal aortic aneurysms. The infrarenal abdominal aorta is most affected by the atherosclerotic process and is similarly the most common site of abdominal aneurysm formation; only a fraction of abdominal aortic aneurysms are suprarenal, and these tend to arise as an extension of a thoracic (thoracoabdominal) aneurysm. The atherosclerotic process less often involves the thoracic aorta. Atherosclerotic disease of the aorta may produce either stenotic obstruction, a process that tends to be confined to the infrarenal abdominal aorta, or aneurysmal dilatation; why one process should predominate over the other in any given individual, however, is unknown.

Although aortic atherosclerosis clearly contributes to the process, ongoing research supports a multifactorial pathogenesis of abdominal aortic aneurysms. Genetic, environmental, hemodynamic, and immunological factors all appear to play a role in the development and progressive growth of aneurysms. Moreover, although it was once thought that atherosclerotic and inflammatory abdominal aortic aneurysms were distinct conditions, it now appears that their underlying pathophysiology is actually similar, with inflammatory aneurysms simply representing an extreme of atherosclerotic aneurysms.

Inflammation within the aortic wall has been implicated in the degradation of the extracellular matrix. There is histological evidence of inflammatory infiltrates—in particular macrophages and T lymphocytes—within the media and adventitia of aneurysms. This may represent a primary inflammatory response whose target antigens within the aortic wall are unknown. Infection is one possible causal factor, with a number of studies identifying viral or bacterial antigens within aneurysm wall tissue. For example, a large proportion of men with abdominal aortic aneurysms have evidence of infection with *Chlamydia pneumoniae*. Moreover, the titer of IgA and the titer of IgG both have been found to correlate with more rapid expansion of aneurysms.[8] The infiltration with macrophages and T lymphocytes in turn results in local production of proteolytic enzymes that degrade aortic elastin, collagen, and other matrix proteins. It should be noted, however, that there is also some competing protein synthesis, so ultimately the process is one of a dynamic balance between protein degradation and synthesis that leads to remodeling of the aortic wall. T lymphocytes may induce smooth muscle cell apoptosis within the aneurysm wall. Since smooth muscle cells produce elastin and collagen, the loss of cellularity may lead to impaired maintenance and repair of the extracellular matrix in the face of ongoing degradation.[9]

Matrix metalloproteinases are zinc- and calcium-dependent enzymes that are produced by smooth muscle and inflammatory cells, and several of these proteinases may participate in abdominal aortic aneurysm formation. Indeed, certain matrix metalloproteinases can degrade elastin and collagen, primary components of the aortic extracellular matrix. The levels of some matrix metalloproteinases (e.g., MMP-9, MMP-2, MMP-14) are significantly elevated in the walls of aneurysms compared with control aortas. Moreover, in one study, the levels of MMP-9 messenger RNA expression was fourfold higher in large (5.0 to 6.9 cm) than in small (3.0-4.9 cm) aneurysms.[10] Circulating levels of MMP-9 are elevated in at least 50 percent of patients with abdominal aortic aneurysms, and levels decrease after open or endovascular aneurysm repair. The evidence linking the matrix metalloproteinases to aneurysm formation is, however, more than just circumstantial. In fact, in an experimental mouse model of aneurysm formation in which MMP-2 and MMP-9 levels are increased, both MMP-2 and MMP-9 knockout mice resisted aneurysm formation.[11] Reduced levels of metalloproteinases inhibitors, known as TIMPs (tissue inhibitors of metalloproteinases), in the walls of aneurysms may promote matrix breakdown by MMPs as well.

Pharmacological inhibition of proteolysis may slow the growth of aneurysms. The tetracyclines inhibit matrix metalloproteinases through a mechanism unrelated to their antibiotic activity. In animal models of abdominal aortic aneurysms, treatment with either doxycycline or tetracycline derivatives without antibiotic activity has reduced aortic wall production of MMP-9, led to preservation of medial elastin, and reduced aneurysmal expansion. In one murine model, doxycycline administration reduced aneurysm growth by 33 to 66 percent at circulating doxycycline levels similar to those achieved in humans at standard doses.[12] The early data in human trials is encouraging. Curci and colleagues found that preoperative treatment with oral doxycycline resulted in a fivefold reduction in the amount of MMP-9 expressed within aneurysm wall tissue resected at surgery.[13] A multicenter group led by Robert Thompson has reported a phase II trial demonstrating the safety of prolonged 6-month administration of doxycycline (100 mg bid) to subjects with abdominal aortic aneurysms. Their findings also showed that therapy is associated with a gradual reduction in plasma MMP-9 levels.[14] In a relatively small trial of 92 subjects, roxithromycin therapy for 28 days reduced the rate of aneurysm expansion by 44 percent in the first year, although by only 5 percent in the second year of follow-up.[15] As discussed earlier, *C. pneumoniae* may contribute to the inflammatory process underlying aneurysm formation. Because doxycycline is effective in the treatment of *C. pneumoniae* infection as well, this may provide another mechanism by which the drug might slow aneurysm expansion.

In addition to the matrix metalloproteinases, several other proteinases, including plasminogen activators, serine elastases, and cathepsins, may contribute to the formation of aneurysms. Cathepsins S and K are potent elastases overexpressed in human atheromas. Increased levels of cathepsin S have been demonstrated in both atherosclerotic plaques and aneurysms. On the other hand, patients with wider aortas have lower levels of cystatin C, an endogenous cathepsin S inhibitor, compared with control subjects.[16]

CLINICAL MANIFESTATIONS. The majority of abdominal aortic aneurysms are asymptomatic and discovered incidentally on routine physical examination or on imaging studies ordered for other indications. Younger patients (50 years old or younger), however, are several times more likely to be symptomatic at the time of diagnosis.[17] Among these patients, pain is the most frequent complaint and is usually located in the hypogastrium or lower part of the back. The pain is usually steady, has a gnawing quality, and may last for hours to days at a time. In contrast to musculoskeletal back pain, movement does not affect aneurysm pain, although patients may be more comfortable in certain positions, such as with the legs drawn up.

RUPTURED ANEURYSM. The development of new or worsening pain, often of sudden onset, may herald expansion or impending rupture of an aneurysm. This pain is characteristically constant, severe, and located in the back or lower part of the abdomen, sometimes with radiation into the groin, buttocks, or legs. Actual rupture is associated with abrupt

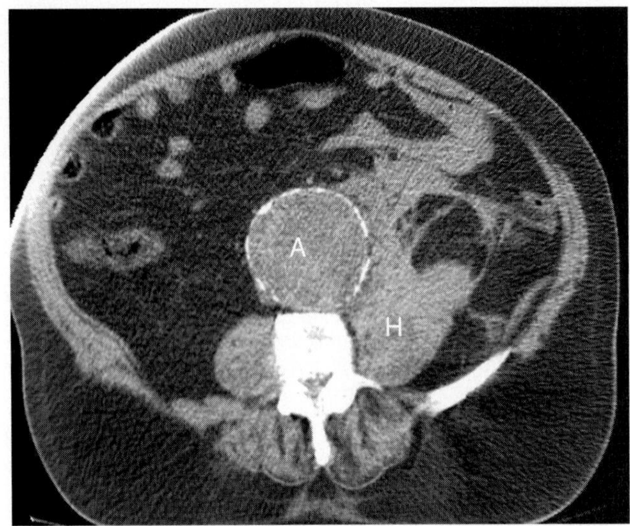

FIGURE 53–1 A non-contrast-enhanced computed tomography scan of the abdomen revealing a ruptured infrarenal abdominal aortic aneurysm. The aneurysm (A) is large, measuring 8.7 cm in greatest diameter, and its wall is well defined by the intimal calcification. The high-attenuation material (approximately 50 Hounsfield units) extending from the aneurysm into the left perirenal space is consistent with hemorrhage (H).

onset of back pain along with abdominal pain and tenderness. Most patients have a palpable, pulsatile abdominal mass, and many are hypotensive when initially seen. However, this familiar triad of abdominal/back pain, a pulsatile abdominal mass, and hypotension—recognized as pathognomonic of a ruptured abdominal aortic aneurysm—is seen in as few as one-third of cases.[18] Moreover, a ruptured aneurysm may mimic other acute abdominal conditions, such as renal colic, diverticulitis, or a gastrointestinal hemorrhage, and may therefore be initially misdiagnosed in as many as 30 percent of cases.

Patients who suffer rupture of an abdominal aortic aneurysm (Fig. 53–1) are critically ill. Hemorrhagic shock and its complications may ensue rapidly. Retroperitoneal hemorrhage may be signaled by hematomas in the flanks and groin. Rupture into the abdominal cavity may result in abdominal distention, whereas rupture into the duodenum is manifested as massive gastrointestinal hemorrhage.

PHYSICAL EXAMINATION. Many aneurysms can be detected on physical examination, although even large aneurysms may be difficult or impossible to detect in obese individuals.[19] When palpable, a pulsatile mass extending variably from the xiphoid process to the umbilicus may be appreciated. Because of difficulty distinguishing the abdominal aorta from surrounding structures by palpation, the size of an aneurysm tends to be overestimated on physical examination. Moreover, it may be difficult to differentiate a tortuous, ectatic aorta from true aneurysmal dilatation. Aneurysms are often sensitive to palpation and may be quite tender if rapidly expanding or about to rupture. Although tender aneurysms should be examined cautiously, no risk is known to be associated with palpation of the abdominal aorta.[20]

Associated occlusive arterial disease is sometimes present in the femoral pulses and distal pulses in the legs and feet. Bruits arising from associated narrowed arteries can be heard over the aneurysm. Occasionally, an arteriovenous fistula is formed by spontaneous rupture into the inferior vena cava, iliac vein, or renal vein and can cause a syndrome of hemodynamic collapse and acute high-output cardiac failure.

DIAGNOSIS AND SIZING. Several diagnostic imaging modalities are currently used for detecting, sizing, and serially monitoring abdominal aortic aneurysms, as well as for precise definition of the aortic anatomy preoperatively. Abdominal ultrasonography is perhaps the most practical way to screen for abdominal aortic aneurysms. It can visualize an aneurysm in the transverse and longitudinal planes, has a sensitivity of 87 to 99 percent (depending on the segment involved),[21] and can accurately define aneurysm size to within ±0.3 cm, but it is limited by less reliable measurements of the suprarenal aorta and significant interobserver variability. Its major advantages are that it is relatively inexpensive, is noninvasive, and does not require the use of a contrast agent. However, because ultrasonography is limited in its ability to visualize the cephalic or pelvic extent of disease or define the associated mesenteric and renal arterial anatomy, it is insufficient for planning operative repair.

Computed tomography is an extremely accurate method for both diagnosing aortic aneurysms (Fig. 53–2A) and sizing them to within ±0.2 cm. CT has an advantage over ultrasonography in that it can better define the shape and extent of the aneurysm as well as the local anatomical relationships of the visceral and renal vessels. Its disadvantages are that the procedure is more expensive and less widely available than ultrasonography, and it also requires the use of ionizing radiation and intravenous contrast. Although CT may therefore be less practical than ultrasonography as a screening tool, its high accuracy in sizing aneurysms makes it an excellent modality for serially monitoring changes in aneurysm size. It is important to note that CT measurements of aneurysm size tend to be larger than ultrasonographic measurements by an average of 0.27 cm.[22] Spiral (helical) CT, which permits three-dimensional display of the aorta and its branches, provides more comprehensive evaluation of the anatomy of an abdominal aortic aneurysm and information regarding renal, mesenteric, or iliac arterial occlusive disease and thus may be sufficient for preoperative evaluation of abdominal aneurysms (see Fig. 53–2B).

Magnetic resonance angiography (MRA) is also an alternative for the preoperative evaluation of aortic aneurysms. On conventional spin-echo MRI, flowing blood appears as a signal void, but with the use of MRA, blood has a bright appearance and vessels can be visualized in a projective fashion, similar to traditional angiography. Moreover, because tomographic images are reconstructed to create a three-dimensional image, the aorta can be visualized from a series of projections to facilitate appreciation of anatomical relationships. MRA is extremely accurate in determining aneurysm size, and it correctly defines the proximal extent of disease and iliofemoral involvement in more than 80 percent of cases.[23]

Aortography may underestimate aneurysm size in the presence of nonopacified mural thrombus lining the aneurysm walls, but it nevertheless remains an excellent technique for defining the suprarenal extent of the aneurysm and any associated renal, mesenteric, or iliofemoral arterial disease. Its disadvantages are that it is expensive, it is an invasive procedure with inherent risks, and it requires the use of intraarterial contrast and ionizing radiation. Preoperative aortography is now used only in selected cases, as CT and MRA provide sufficient information in most cases.

Many practitioners currently recommend the use of screening ultrasonography only for patients at high risk, in particular those with a family history of abdominal aortic aneurysm or those older than 60 years who have a history of smoking or hypertension. However, an important, but not fully resolved, issue is the potential utility of routine screening of asymptomatic patients for the presence of abdominal aneurysms. The largest and most definitive trial to date is the recent report of the Multicentre Aneurysm Screening Study Group, which provides a 4-year cost-effective analysis based on the results of a controlled trial in which a population-based sample of 67,800 men (aged 65-74 years) were randomized to an invitation to ultrasonography screening or to a control group not offered screening.[24] Eighty percent accepted the invitation for screening. Men found to have an abdominal aortic aneurysm of 3 cm or greater were followed with serial ultrasonographic scans for a mean of 4 years. Surgery was considered when the diameter reached 5.5 cm or greater, grew more than 1 cm per year, or became tender. There were 65 deaths related to the aneurysm in the invited

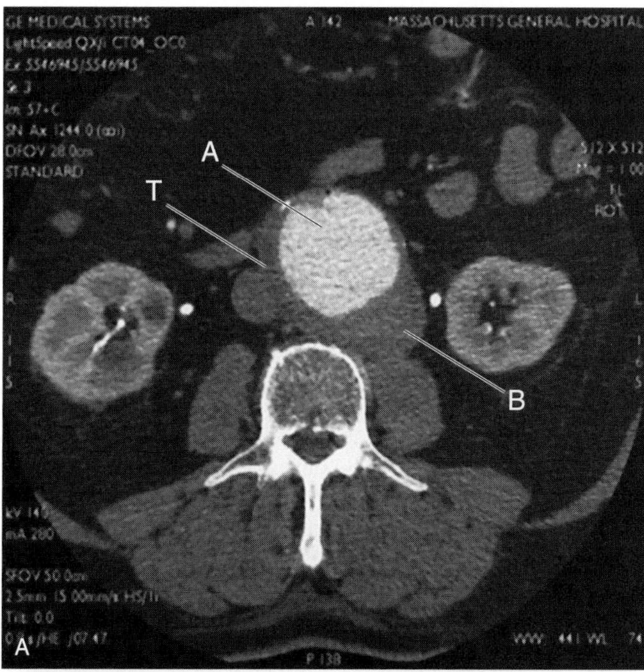

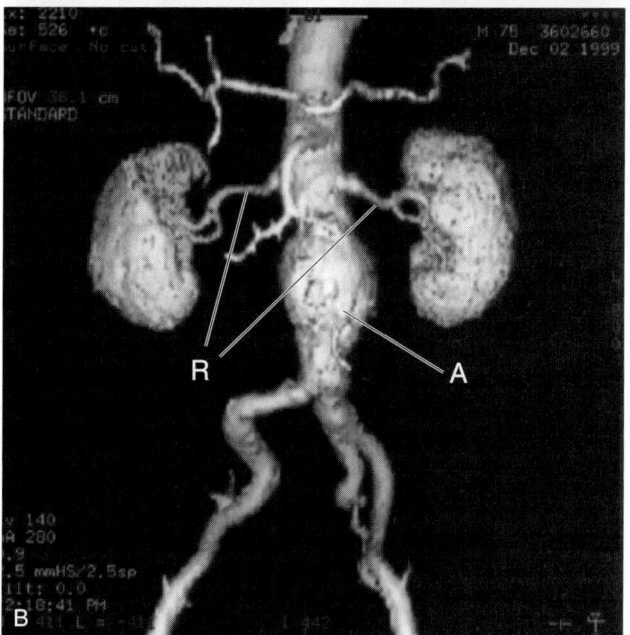

FIGURE 53–2 A, Axial contrast-enhanced computed tomography (CT) scan showing a 6.6-cm abdominal aortic aneurysm (A) lined with mural thrombus (T). Blistering of the aneurysm (B) is indicative of a weakened aortic wall and suggests impending rupture. **B,** Three-dimensional shaded-surface display of the same CT scan. This anteroposterior projection demonstrates that the aneurysm (A) is infrarenal and displays its anatomical relationship to surrounding structures, including the renal arteries (R) proximally and the aortic bifurcation distally. (Courtesy of John A. Kaufman, M.D., Division of Vascular Radiology, Massachusetts General Hospital, Boston.)

group, compared with 113 in the control group, yielding an estimated risk reduction of 42 percent. After 4 years, the cost was estimated to be $57,000 per quality-adjusted life year gained; it was expected to fall to $14,200 at 10 years. Screening of 710 subjects was required to prevent one death. The authors conclude that at 4 years, the cost-effectiveness of screening for abdominal aortic aneurysm is acceptable and is likely to become increasingly favorable over time. However, one important question left unanswered by this study is the cost-effectiveness of screening women for abdominal aneurysms. Another British study addressed the potential utility of repeated screening for abdominal aneurysms.[25] The investigators followed 223 65-year-old men who had abdominal aortic diameters of less than 2.6 cm at baseline with repeated ultrasonographic evaluations at 5 and 12 years. None of those who survived the 12-year interval had any clinically significant increase in the mean aortic diameter, and none of those who died did so from a ruptured abdominal aneurysm. The authors conclude that a normal ultrasonogram at age 65 effectively excludes the risk of a clinically significant aneurysm for life.

NATURAL HISTORY. The paramount concern in managing abdominal aortic aneurysms is their tendency to rupture. Mortality from rupture is quite high: Among the participants in the United Kingdom Small Aneurysm Trial who suffered a ruptured abdominal aneurysm, 25 percent died before reaching a hospital and 51 percent died in the hospital without undergoing surgery. The operative mortality rate for the 13 percent undergoing surgery was 46 percent (compared with 4 to 6 percent for elective surgery), yielding an overall 30-day survival of just 11 percent.[26] To prevent the associated mortality, surgical repair is the therapy of choice for aneurysms considered to be at significant risk of rupture.

It is well established that the risk of rupture increases with aneurysm size. The United Kingdom Small Aneurysm Trial found that aneurysms smaller than 4.0 cm have a 0.3 percent annual risk of rupture, those 4.0 to 4.9 cm have a 1.5 percent annual risk of rupture, and those 5.0 to 5.9 cm have a 6.5 percent annual risk of rupture.[26] For aneurysms 6.0 cm or larger, the risk of rupture rises sharply, although an exact risk cannot be estimated. Although abdominal aneurysms are less prevalent among women than men, when present they rupture three times more frequently among women and at a smaller aortic diameter (mean diameter of 5.0 cm among women versus 6.0 cm among men). Rupture is also more common among current smokers and those with hypertension.[26]

Because 80 percent of abdominal aortic aneurysms expand over time, with as many as 15 to 20 percent expanding rapidly (>0.5 cm/yr), the risk of rupture may concomitantly increase with time. Accordingly, the ability to predict rates of aortic aneurysm expansion would be useful in estimating the risk of future rupture. Although the mean rate of abdominal aortic aneurysm expansion is thought to approximate 0.4 cm per year, the rates of expansion within a population are extremely variable. Expansion rates even vary within one individual over time, as would be expected given the "vicious cycle" of aneurysm growth explained earlier. Baseline aneurysm size is perhaps the best predictor of aneurysm expansion rate, with larger aneurysms expanding more rapidly than small ones, probably as a consequence of the Laplace law. A rapid rate of expansion apparently also predicts aneurysm rupture, especially abdominal aneurysms 5.0 cm or greater in diameter. Many surgeons therefore consider both large size and rapid expansion to be indications for repair.

Management

SURGICAL TREATMENT. The goal of treating abdominal aortic aneurysms is to prolong life by preventing rupture. The decision to operate must weigh the natural history of the aneurysm and life expectancy of the patient against the anticipated morbidity and mortality of the proposed surgical procedure. Operative mortality is 4 to 6 percent overall for elective aneurysm repair and as low as 2 percent in low-risk patients. However, operative mortality rises to 19 percent for urgent aortic repair and reaches 50 percent for repair of a ruptured aneurysm. Aneurysm size remains the primary indicator for repair of asymptomatic aneurysms, and for many years there has been debate on the minimum aneurysm diameter that necessitates surgery. Recently, two large-scale clinical trials investigating this very question have been completed.

The United Kingdom Small Aneurysm Trial[27] randomized 1090 patients aged 60 to 76 years with small aortic aneurysms (diameter 4.0 to 5.5 cm) to either early elective surgery or regular ultrasonographic surveillance. They found no long-term difference in survival between the early-surgery group and the surveillance group, although after 8 years, total mortality was slightly lower in the early-surgery group. However, since the operative mortality rate in this trial was 5.8 percent, some practitioners have questioned whether there may have been a survival benefit from early surgery had the operative mortality rate been lower. However, a similar trial known as the Aneurysm Detection and Management (ADAM) Veterans Affairs Cooperative Study[28] has suggested otherwise. In ADAM 1136, patients with small asymptomatic aneurysms (diameter 4.0 to 5.4 cm) were randomized to undergo immediate surgical repair or surveillance at 6-month intervals by ultrasonography or CT scanning. Despite a remarkably low operative mortality rate of 2.1 percent, after a mean follow-up of 5 years there was no difference in survival between the two groups. Collectively, these trials suggest that surgery is not indicated in most instances for patients with asymptomatic aneurysms less than 5.5 cm in size. However, it should be recognized that the subjects randomized to the surveillance arms of these trials have careful clinical follow-up with both medical management and regular surveillance imaging to monitor the aneurysm. Such careful follow-up does not always take place in general practice settings outside a trial. Another important limitation is that these two study populations consisted almost entirely of men (United Kingdom Aneurysm Trial, 78 percent; ADAM, 99 percent), and since the risk of aneurysm rupture is greater and occurs at smaller diameters in women than in men, these results may well not be equally applicable to women.[29]

Surgical repair of abdominal aortic aneurysms consists of opening of the aneurysm and insertion of a synthetic prosthesis, usually fabricated of Dacron or expanded polytetrafluoroethylene (Gore-Tex). Sometimes, a simple tube graft is all that is necessary, although frequently the operation must be carried distally into one or both of the iliac arteries to excise the aneurysm completely. In the case of large aneurysms, much of the aneurysm wall may be left in situ ("intrasaccular approach of Creech"), thereby reducing the need for extensive dissection and thus decreasing aortic cross-clamping time.

A less invasive alternative to open surgery for repair of abdominal aortic aneurysms is the use of percutaneously implanted, expanding endovascular stent-grafts (see Chap. 55 and Figs. 53–3 and 53–4). The device consists of a collapsible prosthetic tube graft that is inserted remotely (e.g., via the femoral artery), advanced transluminally across the aneurysm under fluoroscopic guidance, and then secured at both its proximal and distal ends with an expandable stent attachment system. For aortic aneurysm repair, the stent-graft serves to bridge the region of the aneurysm, thereby excluding it from the circulation while allowing aortic blood flow to continue distally through the prosthetic stent-graft lumen. In some cases, stent-grafts are bifurcated, with two arms on the distal end designed to extend into the common iliac arteries when these vessels are aneurysmal as well. The rate of successful stent-graft implantation in several recent series ranged from 78 to 94 percent,[30-32] with some outcome variability resulting from differing definitions of procedural success. Despite these promising results, only 30 to 60 percent of patients

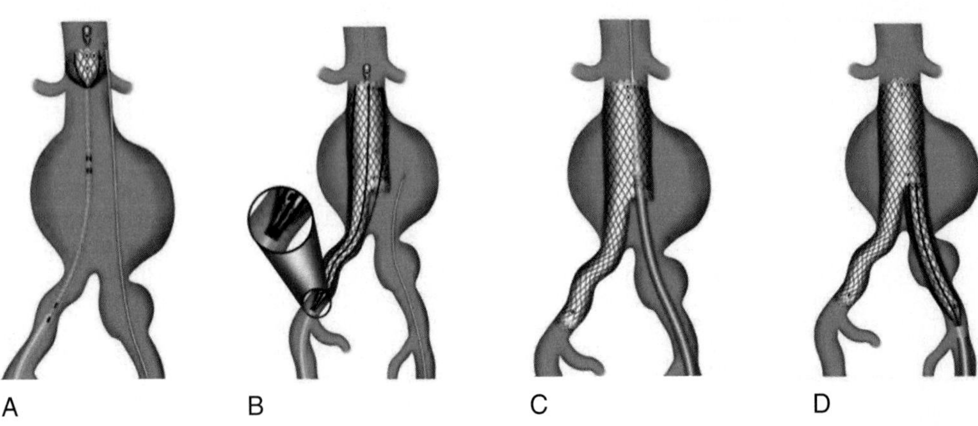

FIGURE 53–3 Diagram of deployment of an aortic stent graft. **A,** The catheter placement and proximal stabilization are achieved via right femoral access. **B,** The body and right limb of the stent graft are positioned and deployed. **C,** The cannula for deployment of the left limb of the graft is placed via left femoral access. **D,** The left limb of the graft is deployed, completing the endovascular repair of the aortic aneurysm with left iliac involvement. (Courtesy of Medtronics Corporation.)

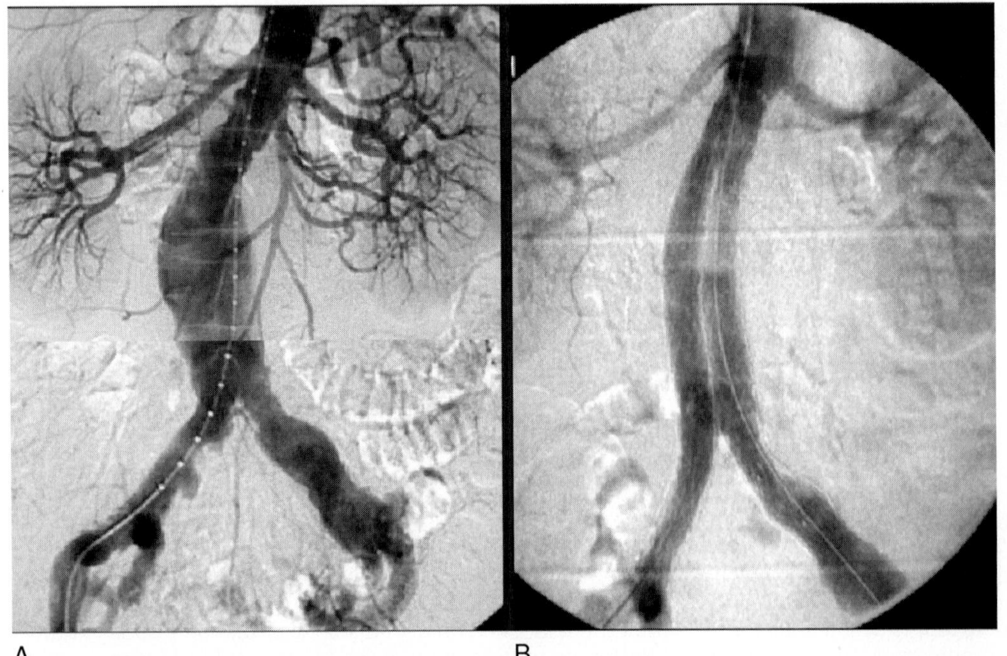

FIGURE 53–4 Angiographic views of an infrarenal abdominal aortic aneurysm with bi-iliac involvement treated by stent grafting before **(A)** and following **(B)** deployment of the aortic stent graft. (Courtesy of Dr. Edwin Graveraux, Brigham and Women's Hospital, Boston.)

with abdominal aortic aneurysms have aneurysm anatomy suitable for endovascular repair. Moreover, the long-term outcomes of endovascular repair versus conventional surgical repair are not yet known. One of the major technical difficulties associated with the stent-graft technique that has yet to be overcome is the frequent occurrence of *endoleaks,* which are seen angiographically as persistent contrast flow into the aneurysm sac because of failure to completely exclude the aneurysm from the aortic circulation. Such endoleaks, if left untreated, may leave the patient at continued risk for aneurysm expansion or rupture.[33] Therefore, at present, the use of stent-grafts for endovascular repair of abdominal aortic aneurysms has generally been limited to a subset of patients, typically older patients or those at high operative risk.

ASSESSING OPERATIVE RISK (see Chap. 77). Because patients with abdominal aortic aneurysms in almost all cases have atherosclerosis, their high likelihood of concomitant coronary, renal, and cerebrovascular arterial disease significantly increases the risk of major vascular surgery. Indeed, half of all perioperative deaths from aneurysm repair result from myocardial infarction. In addition, in one study, routine coronary arteriography in patients undergoing aneurysm repair revealed severe revascularizable coronary artery disease in 18 percent of all patients, including an 8 percent incidence in patients without prior symptoms of coronary ischemia.[34] Moreover, among those with angiographically significant coronary artery disease, about half have multivessel disease.

Several studies have demonstrated that cardiac scintigraphy is an effective means of identifying patients at highest risk for perioperative ischemic events (see Chaps. 9, 13, and 77). Patients with reversible perfusion defects in multiple segments of myocardium are at highest risk, and it is in this subgroup that coronary angiography is likely to be most helpful. The safety of nuclear imaging with pharmacological stress in such patients has been well established. Although exercise scintigraphy is also a useful screening method, many patients with vascular disease fail to achieve an adequate heart rate because of limited exercise capacity. Other useful techniques for preoperative evaluation of myocardial ischemia include dobutamine stress echocardiography and electrocardiographic exercise testing in patients with a normal baseline electrocardiogram and adequate exercise tolerance.

Selective preoperative evaluation to identify the presence and severity of coronary artery disease in patients with clinical markers of coronary artery disease has been widely advocated, and some investigators further suggest screening those with strong cardiac risk factors despite the absence of clinical evidence of coronary artery disease. Although patients found to have significant revascularizable coronary artery disease are presumed to benefit from preoperative coronary revascularization with selective coronary artery bypass surgery or angioplasty, at present this conclusion remains unproven. Data available from nonrandomized studies of patients with significant coronary artery disease undergoing vascular surgery do demonstrate lower mortality for those who have undergone coronary bypass surgery. Furthermore, a randomized study has demonstrated that the long-term outcome of patients with combined peripheral vascular disease and high-risk coronary artery disease is improved by coronary artery revascularization in patients with three-vessel coronary disease.[35] As is the case for coronary artery bypass surgery, no data are yet available to confirm that preoperative percutaneous coronary revascularization for significant coronary stenoses decreases the risk from major vascular surgery.

In addition to such preoperative screening and potential coronary revascularization, the use of perioperative invasive hemodynamic monitoring and careful perioperative surveillance for evidence of ischemia may further reduce operative risk secondary to cardiac ischemic events. Furthermore, myocardial ischemia and perhaps myocardial infarction may be prevented by using beta-adrenergic blockers perioperatively (see Chap. 77).

Late Survival. A review of late survival following abdominal aortic aneurysm repair among almost 2500 patients revealed 1-, 5-, and 10-year survival rates of 93, 63, and 40 percent, respectively.[18]

MEDICAL MANAGEMENT. Risk factor modification is fundamental in the medical management of abdominal aortic aneurysms. Hypercholesterolemia and hypertension should be carefully controlled. Most patients with abdominal aortic aneurysms are cigarette smokers, and given the increased risk of aneurysm rupture among active smokers, the habit must be discontinued. Beta blockers have long been considered an important therapy for reducing the risk of aneurysm expansion and rupture, and both animal and human studies support such a role. Brophy and coworkers demonstrated that propranolol delays the development of aneurysms in a mouse model prone to spontaneous aortic aneurysms.[36] Interestingly, it appears that the drug's efficacy in this model may have been independent of reductions in blood pressure or diminution of the rate of left ventricular ejection (dP/dt) and, instead, may have resulted from changes in connective tissue metabolism and the structure of the aortic wall. In humans, the data are mixed. Several trials have shown that treatment with propranolol has no significant impact on the rate of growth of smaller aneurysms (less than 4 cm in diameter), but decreases the rate of growth of larger aneurysms (4.0 to 5.0 cm in diameter, or larger) by 50 percent or more.[37] Therefore beta blockers should be recommended for patients with larger aneurysms managed medically.

When following an abdominal aortic aneurysm 4.0 cm in size or larger, careful routine follow-up is indicated to detect either rapid expansion (≥0.5 cm/yr) or an increase in size to 5.5 cm or larger, either of which is an indication for surgery. CT scanning every 6 months, perhaps as frequently as every 3 months for those at higher risk, has been advocated as an effective method of follow-up in such patients. CT scanning is preferable to ultrasonography for monitoring aneurysm growth because CT measurements of aneurysm size are more accurate.

Thoracic Aortic Aneurysms

Thoracic aortic aneurysms are much less common than aneurysms of the abdominal aorta. Thoracic aneurysms are classified by the portion of aorta involved, i.e., the ascending, arch, or descending thoracic aorta. This anatomical distinction is important because the etiology, natural history, and treatment of thoracic aneurysms differ for each of these segments. In modern series aneurysms of the ascending aorta occur most commonly (60 percent), followed by aneurysms of the descending aorta (40 percent), whereas arch aneurysms (10 percent) and thoracoabdominal aneurysms (10 percent) occur less often. *Thoracoabdominal aortic aneurysm* refers to descending thoracic aneurysms that extend distally to involve the abdominal aorta. Sometimes, the entire aorta may be ectatic, with localized aneurysms seen at sites in both the thoracic and abdominal aorta.

ETIOLOGY AND PATHOGENESIS. Aneurysms of the ascending thoracic aorta most often result from cystic medial degeneration (or cystic medial necrosis). Histologically, cystic medial degeneration has the appearance of smooth muscle cell drop-out and elastic fiber degeneration, with the presence in the media of cystic spaces filled with mucoid material. Although these changes occur most frequently in the ascending aorta, some cases may involve the entire aorta.

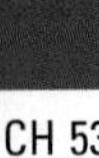

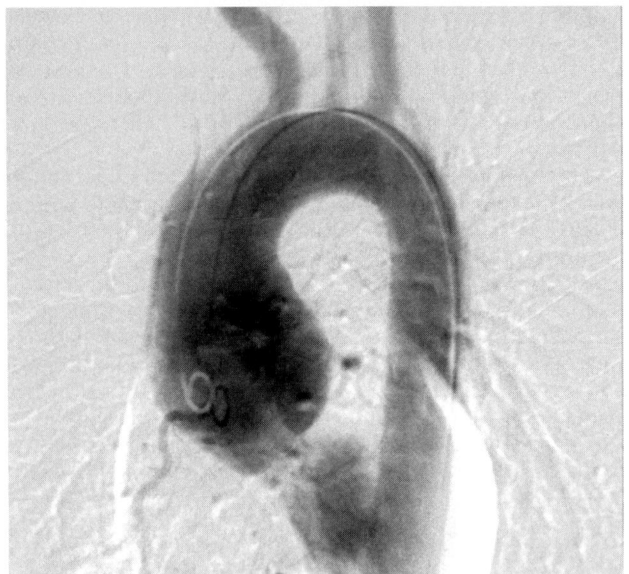

FIGURE 53–5 Left anterior oblique digital-subtraction aortogram in a man with annuloaortic ectasia and aneurysmal dilatation of the ascending thoracic aorta. The bulbous, pear-shaped aortic root can easily be seen. The aorta tapers to a normal diameter before the aortic arch, which is normal in size. Also of note, some contrast material is seen within the left ventricle, signifying the presence of aortic regurgitation.

The histological changes lead to weakening of the aortic wall, which in turn results in the formation of a fusiform aneurysm. Such aneurysms often involve the aortic root and may consequently result in aortic regurgitation: The term *annuloaortic ectasia* (Fig. 53–5) is often used to describe this condition (see later).

Cystic medial necrosis occurs to some extent with aging and is accelerated by hypertension.[38] At younger ages, cystic medial degeneration is classically associated with Marfan syndrome and can be associated with other connective tissue disorders as well, such as the Ehlers-Danlos syndrome. The Marfan syndrome (see Chap. 70) is an autosomal dominant heritable disorder of connective tissue that has been discovered to be due to mutations in one of the genes for fibrillin-1, a structural protein that is the major component of microfibrils of elastin. These mutations result in a decrease in the amount of elastin in the aortic wall, together with a loss of elastin's normally highly organized structure. As a consequence, from an early age a marfanoid aorta exhibits markedly abnormal elastic properties and increased systemic pulse wave velocities, and over time the aorta exhibits progressively increasing degrees of stiffness and dilatation.

But cystic medial degeneration is also seen in patients with ascending thoracic aortic aneurysms who do not have overt connective tissue disorders. It has long been suspected that some patients who have annuloaortic ectasia and proven cystic medial degeneration without the classic phenotypic manifestations of the Marfan syndrome may, in fact, have a variation, or *forme fruste,* of the Marfan syndrome. Indeed, increasing evidence suggests that many of these patients also have a genetic mutation that may account for cystic medial degeneration. Moreover, it is now recognized that although cases of thoracic aortic aneurysms in the absence of overt connective tissue disorders may be sporadic, they are often familial in nature and are now referred to as the *familial thoracic aortic aneurysm syndrome*.

In an analysis using the large database of patients treated at Yale, Coady and colleagues identified those with a familial pattern of thoracic aortic aneurysms and compared them with both sporadic cases and those with the Marfan syndrome. At least 19 percent of patients had a family history of a thoracic aortic aneurysm. The mean age of presentation for patients with familial syndromes was 57 years, which was significantly younger than sporadic cases (64 years) but older than the Marfan syndrome cases (25 years). Most pedigrees suggested an autosomal dominant mode of inheritance, but some suggested a recessive mode and possibly X-linked inheritance as well.[39] Biddinger and colleagues investigated the families of 158 patients referred for surgical repair or thoracic aortic aneurysms or dissections and found that first-degree relatives of probands had a higher risk (risk ratio [RR] 1.8 for fathers and sisters, RR 10.9 for brothers) of thoracic aortic aneurysms or sudden death compared with control subjects.[40]

Milewicz and colleagues have identified a mutation on 3p24.2-25 that can cause both isolated and familial thoracic aortic aneurysms. Although there appears to be dominant inheritance, there is marked variability in the expression and penetrance of the disorder, such that some inherit and pass on the gene but show no manifestation. Pathological evaluation of the aorta and these families reveals cystic medial degeneration.[41] Recently, two studies of familial thoracic aortic aneurysm syndromes have successfully mapped the mutations to at least two different chromosomal loci, but some families mapped to neither of these, suggesting at least a third locus.[38,42] As more families are studied, the extent of genetic heterogeneity is likely to become more evident. Indeed, the fact that there is such variable expression and penetrance suggests that this may be a polygenic condition.

Some cases of ascending thoracic aortic aneurysms are associated with an underlying bicuspid aortic valve (see Chap. 57). In fact, the risks of aortic dilatation, aneurysm, and dissection are significantly increased among those with a bicuspid aortic valve. Historical teaching attributed such aneurysms to "poststenotic dilatation" of the ascending aorta, but the data suggest otherwise. Nistri and colleagues found that 52 percent of young people with normally functioning bicuspid aortic valves have echocardiographic evidence of aortic dilatation. Dilatation occurred most frequently at the level of the tubular portion of the ascending aorta (44 percent), but the 20 percent had dilatation at the level of sinuses.[43] In a community sample, Nkomo and colleagues demonstrated that bicuspid aortic valve is associated with a dilated aorta regardless of the presence or absence of hemodynamically significant valve dysfunction.[44]

Cystic medial degeneration appears to be the underlying cause of the aortic aneurysms associated with bicuspid aortic valve. Indeed, 75 percent of patients with bicuspid aortic valve undergoing aortic valve replacement surgery have biopsy-proven significant cystic medial necrosis of the ascending aorta, compared with only 14 percent of patients with tricuspid aortic valves undergoing similar surgery.[45] Inadequate production of fibrillin-1 during embryogenesis may result in both the bicuspid aortic valve and a weakened aortic wall.[46] In addition, among those with bicuspid aortic valve, deficient microfibrillar elements within the aortic wall may cause smooth muscle cell detachment, matrix metalloproteinase release, matrix disruption, and cell death.[47] No single gene responsible for bicuspid aortic valve has yet been identified, and it is likely genetically heterogeneous. Moreover, in the study by Nistri and colleagues, 48 percent of patients with bicuspid valves had aortic dimensions equal to those of control subjects, so it appears that not all are at increased risk.[43]

ATHEROSCLEROSIS. Atherosclerotic aneurysms infrequently occur in the ascending aorta and, when they do, tend to be associated with diffuse aortic atherosclerosis. Aneurysms in the aortic arch are often contiguous with aneurysms of the ascending or descending aorta. They may be due to atherosclerotic disease, cystic medial degeneration, and syphilis or other infections. The predominant cause of aneurysms of the descending thoracic aorta is atherosclerosis. These aneurysms tend to originate just distal to the origin of the left subclavian artery and may be either fusiform or saccular. The pathogenesis of such atherosclerotic aneurysms in the thoracic aorta may resemble that of abdominal aneurysms but has not been extensively examined.

SYPHILIS. Syphilis was once a common cause of ascending thoracic aortic aneurysm, but today it has become a rarity in most major medical centers as a result of aggressive antibiotic treatment of the disease in its early stages. The latent period from initial spirochetal infection to aortic complications may range from 5 to 40 years but is most commonly 10 to 25 years. During the secondary phase of the disease, spirochetes directly infect the aortic media, most commonly involving the ascending aorta. The infection and attendant inflammatory response destroys the muscular and elastic medial elements, which undergo replacement by fibrous tissue that frequently calcifies. Weakening of the aortic wall from medial destruction results in progressive aneurysmal dilatation. In addition, the infection may spread into the aortic root, and the subsequent root dilation may result in aortic regurgitation.

INFECTIOUS AORTITIS. Infectious aortitis is a rare cause of aortic aneurysm that can result from a primary infection of the aortic wall causing aortic dilation with the formation of fusiform or saccular aneurysms. More commonly, infected, or mycotic, aneurysms arise secondarily from an infection occurring in a preexisting aneurysm of another cause. When an infected aneurysm involves the ascending aorta, it is often the consequence of direct spread from aortic valve bacterial endocarditis.

Several other causes of thoracic aortic aneurysms are discussed in detail elsewhere in this or other chapters, including giant cell arteritis (see Chap. 82), aortic trauma (see Chap. 65), and aortic dissection (see below). Note that the clinical features, natural history, and treatment of thoracic aneurysms discussed here apply specifically to nondissecting thoracic aortic aneurysms.

CLINICAL MANIFESTATIONS. At least half the patients with thoracic aortic aneurysms are asymptomatic at the time of diagnosis, with such aneurysms typically discovered as incidental findings on a routine physical examination, chest radiograph, or CT scan. When patients do experience symptoms, the symptoms tend to reflect either a vascular consequence of the aneurysm or a local mass effect. Vascular consequences include aortic regurgitation from dilatation of the aortic root, often associated with secondary congestive heart failure, or thromboembolism causing stroke, lower extremity ischemia, renal infarction, or mesenteric ischemia. A local mass effect from an ascending or arch aneurysm may cause superior vena cava syndrome as a result of obstruction of venous return via compression of the superior vena cava or innominate vein. Aneurysms of the arch or descending aorta may compress the trachea (Fig. 53–6) or main stem bronchus and produce tracheal deviation, wheezing, cough, dyspnea (with symptoms that may be positional), hemoptysis, or recurrent pneumonitis. Compression of the esophagus can produce dysphagia, and compression of the recurrent laryngeal nerve can cause hoarseness. Chest pain or back pain occur in one-quarter of cases of nondissecting aneurysms and result from direct compression of other intrathoracic structures or the chest wall, or from erosion into adjacent bone. Typically, such pain is steady, deep, boring, and at times severe.

As with abdominal aortic aneurysms, the most worrisome consequence of thoracic aneurysms is leakage or rupture. Rupture is accompanied by the dramatic onset of excruciating pain, often in the region where less severe pain had previously existed. Rupture occurs most commonly into the left intrapleural space or the mediastinum and is manifested as hypotension. Less often, an aneurysm of the descending thoracic aorta ruptures into the adjacent esophagus (an aortoesophageal fistula), which causes life-threatening hematemesis. Acute aneurysm expansion, which may herald rupture, can cause similar pain. Thoracic aneurysms can also be accompanied by aortic dissection, as discussed in detail later in this chapter.

DIAGNOSIS AND SIZING. Many thoracic aneurysms are readily visible on chest radiographs (Fig. 53–7) and are characterized by widening of the mediastinal silhouette, enlargement of the aortic knob, or displacement of the trachea from the midline. Unfortunately, smaller aneurysms, especially saccular ones, may not be evident on the chest radiograph; therefore, this technique cannot exclude the diagnosis of aortic aneurysm.

Aortography had long been the preferred modality for the preoperative evaluation of thoracic aortic aneurysms and for precise definition of the anatomy of the aneurysm and great vessels (see Fig. 53–5). However, as is the case for abdominal aortic aneurysms, CT and MRA are now often sufficient in most cases to define both aortic and branch vessel anatomy. Both contrast-enhanced CT scanning (Fig. 53–8) and MRI very accurately detect and size thoracic aortic aneurysms. When aneurysms involve the aortic root, MRA is preferable to CT scanning, as CT images the root less well and is less accurate in sizing its diameter. When patients have a tortuous thoracic aorta, which is often the case among the elderly, one should use caution in using axial images to measure the aortic diameter. The axial images often cut through the descending aorta off-axis, resulting in a falsely large aortic diameter. When the axial data are reconstructed into three-dimensional images (i.e., CT angiography), one can measure the tortuous aorta in true cross section and obtain an accurate diameter. Such three-dimensional imaging should then always be used to follow such patients over time.

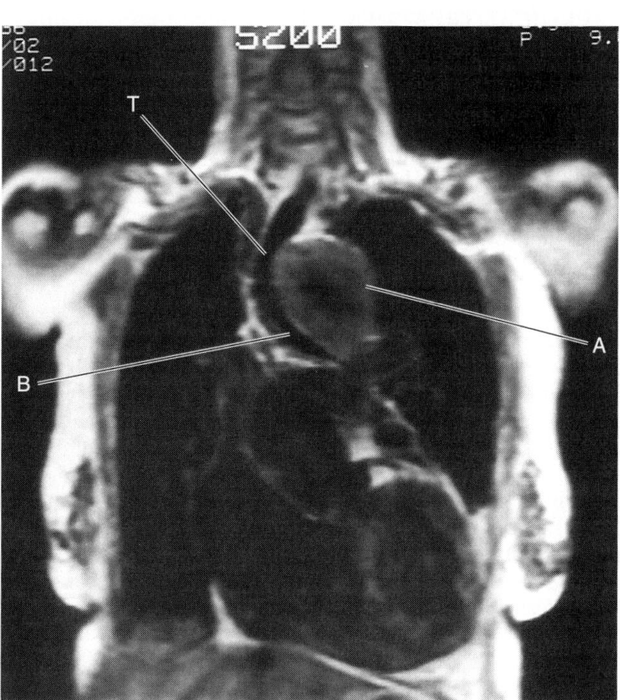

FIGURE 53–6 Magnetic resonance imaging scan in the coronal projection of a large thoracic aortic aneurysm in an elderly woman with dyspnea and cough. In this view, the markedly dilated aortic arch (A) is compressing the trachea (T) and causing rightward tracheal deviation. The aneurysm is also compressing the left main stem bronchus (B). In addition, all four cardiac chambers are dilated, consistent with the patient's known idiopathic dilated cardiomyopathy

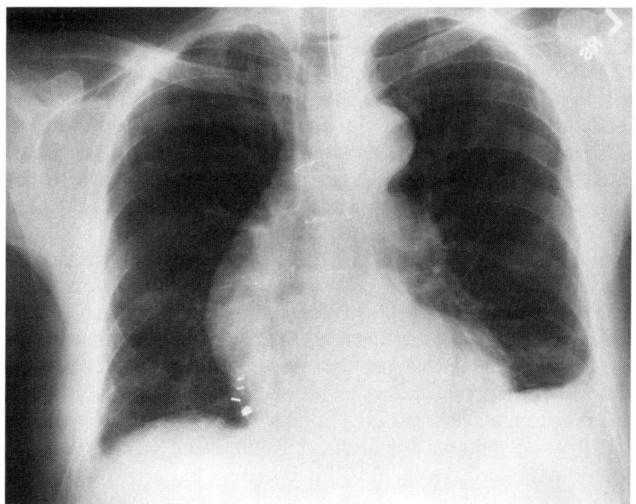

FIGURE 53–7 Chest radiograph of a patient with a very large aneurysm of the ascending thoracic aorta. Evident are both marked widening of the mediastinum and an abnormal aortic contour.

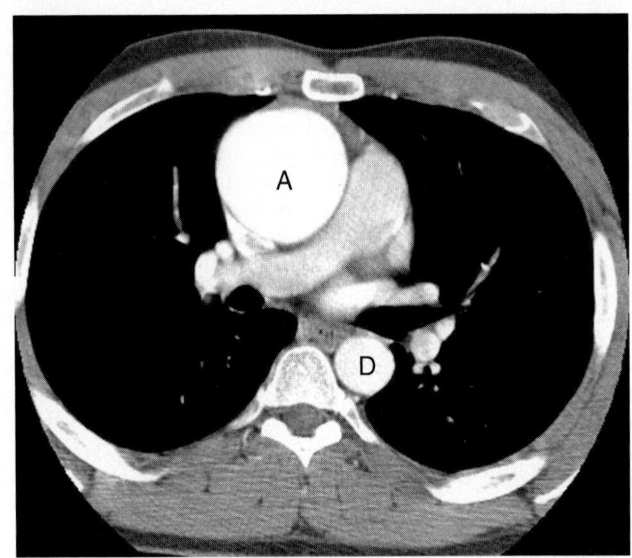

FIGURE 53–8 Contrast-enhanced computed tomography scan of the chest at the level of the right pulmonary artery demonstrating a 6.5-cm ascending thoracic aortic aneurysm (A).The descending aorta (D) is normal in caliber.

TTE is an excellent modality for imaging the aortic root, which is important for patients with the Marfan syndrome, but it is not able to visualize the middle or distal ascending aorta well in many cases and is particularly limited in its ability to examine the descending thoracic aorta. Therefore, among patients other than those with the Marfan syndrome, TTE should not be used for diagnosing thoracic aneurysms. TEE, on the other hand, can visualize the entire thoracic aorta quite well and therefore has become widely used for detection of aortic dissection. However, given that TEE is a semi-invasive procedure, CT and MR are usually preferred imaging techniques in the evaluation of nondissecting thoracic aneurysms. (The advantages and disadvantage of each imaging modality are discussed later in greater detail.)

NATURAL HISTORY. Defining the natural history of thoracic aortic aneurysms has been challenging for a number of reasons. Both the origin and the location of a thoracic aneurysm can affect its rate of growth and propensity for dissection or rupture. The presence or absence of aneurysm symptoms is another important predictor inasmuch as symptomatic patients have a much poorer prognosis than do those without symptoms, in large part because the onset of new symptoms is frequently a harbinger of rupture or death. Finally, during the recent decades in which it has been routine to image aneurysms serially to document growth and size, surgery has typically been performed when aneurysms have been large enough to be considered at high risk for rupture. Those patients whose large aneurysms have been managed without surgery are often elderly or have important comorbidities, thus increasing their mortality irrespective of the aneurysm.

Perhaps the best data currently available on the natural history of thoracic aortic aneurysms come from a longitudinal study recent reported by Davies and colleagues from the Yale group in which 304 patients with thoracic aortic aneurysms at least 3.5 cm in size were followed for a mean of more than 31 months.[48] The mean rate of growth for all thoracic aneurysms was 0.1 cm/yr. The rate of growth was significantly greater for aneurysms of the descending aorta (0.19 cm/yr), however, than for those of the ascending aorta (0.07 cm/yr). In addition, dissected thoracic aneurysms grew significantly more rapidly (0.14 cm/yr) than did nondissected ones (0.09 cm/yr), and patients with Marfan syndrome also had higher growth rates. The mean rate of rupture or dissection was only 2 percent per year for aneurysms less than 5 cm in diameter, rose slightly to 3 percent per year for aneurysms 5.0 to 5.9 cm, but increased sharply to 7 percent per year for aneurysms 6.0 cm or larger. In a multivariate logistic regression analysis of the predictors of dissection or rupture, the relative risk associated with an aneurysm diameter of 5.0 to 5.9 cm was 2.5; with an aneurysm diameter of 6.0 cm or larger, 5.2; with Marfan syndrome, 3.7; and with female gender, 2.9. In addition, concomitant vascular disease or abdominal aortic aneurysm were univariate predictors of both dissection/rupture and mortality. Other natural history studies focused on thoracic and thoracoabdominal aneurysms have found that the odds of rupture are increased by chronic obstructive pulmonary disease (COPD) (RR, 3.6), advanced age (RR, 2.6/decade), and aneurysm-related pain (RR, 2.3).[49]

As with abdominal aneurysms, initial size is an important predictor of the rate of thoracic aneurysm growth. Dapunt and colleagues[50] monitored 67 patients with thoracic aortic aneurysms by serial CT scanning and found that the only independent predictor of rapid expansion (>0.5 cm/yr) was an initial aortic diameter larger than 5.0 cm. Aneurysms that were 5.0 cm or smaller grew more slowly than did those larger than 5.0 cm. Unfortunately, even when controlling for initial aneurysm size, substantial variation was still seen in individual aneurysm growth rates, thus rendering such mean growth rates of little value in predicting aneurysm growth for a given patient. More helpful, however, was the finding that growth rates among small aneurysms were more consistent, with only 1 of 25 aneurysms 4.0 cm or smaller at baseline showing rapid growth.

Rupture or acute dissection are the major complications of thoracic aortic aneurysms and can be fatal. Fewer than half of patients with rupture may arrive at the hospital alive; mortality at 6 hours is 54 percent and at 24 hours reaches 76 percent.[51]

Management

SURGICAL TREATMENT. The optimal timing of surgical repair of thoracic aortic aneurysms remains uncertain for several reasons. First, as noted earlier, the data available on the natural history of thoracic aneurysms are limited, especially with respect to the outcomes of surgical intervention. Second, with the high incidence of coexisting cardiovascular disease in this population, many patients die of other cardiovascular diseases before their aneurysms ever rupture. Finally, significant risks are associated with thoracic aortic surgery, particularly in the arch and descending aorta, which in many cases may outweigh the potential benefits of aortic repair.

We currently recommend surgery when aneurysms of the ascending thoracic aorta reach 5.5 cm or larger and those of the descending thoracic aorta reach 6.0 cm or larger, or perhaps 6.0 and 7.0 cm or larger, respectively, in patients at high operative risk. Indications for surgery in patients with smaller aneurysms include a rapid rate of expansion, associated significant aortic regurgitation, or the presence of aneurysm-related symptoms. In patients with the Marfan syndrome, bicuspid aortic valve, or a familial thoracic aortic aneurysm syndrome, given their higher risk of dissection and rupture, we often recommend repair of ascending thoracic aneurysms when they reach only 5.0 cm in size. Surgery can be considered even sooner (e.g., 4.5 cm) in Marfan syndrome patients at especially high risk, such as those with rapid and progressive aortic dilatation, those with a family history of the Marfan syndrome plus aortic dissection, or women planning pregnancy.[52] Finally, if patients require aortic valve replacement for a dysfunctional bicuspid valve, we recommend replacement of the ascending aorta if its diameter is 4 cm or larger, given that they are now recognized to be at high risk for postoperative aortic dissection.[53,54] Of course, the aggressiveness with which surgical repair is undertaken in any case should be appropriately influenced by the general condition of the individual patient.

Thoracic aortic aneurysms are generally resected and replaced with a prosthetic sleeve of appropriate size. Cardiopulmonary bypass is necessary for the removal of ascending aortic aneurysms, and partial bypass to support the circulation distal to the aneurysm while the aortic site being repaired is cross-clamped is often advisable when resecting descending thoracic aortic aneurysms. The use of such adjuncts is less important, however, than the nature and extent of the aneurysm in determining the incidence of postoperative complications.

The use of a composite graft consisting of a Dacron tube with a prosthetic aortic valve sewn into one end (known as a *composite aortic repair* or the *Bentall procedure*) is generally the method of choice in treating ascending thoracic aneurysms involving the root and associated with significant aortic regurgitation. The valve and graft are sewn directly into the aortic annulus, and the coronary arteries are then reimplanted into the Dacron aortic graft (Fig. 53–9). The operative risk for mortality is about 5 percent.[55] For patients with structurally normal aortic valve leaflets whose aortic regurgitation is secondary to dilatation of the root, David and colleagues have successfully repaired the native valve either by reimplanting it within a Dacron graft or by remodeling of the aortic root. By avoiding valve replacement, it is expected that this procedure, when successful, will eliminate the long-term risks associated with a prosthetic valve and reduce the risk for repeat valve surgery. In a series of 151 patients with aortic root aneurysms who underwent valve-sparing surgery, 67 percent had mild or no aortic regurgitation during the first 8 years of follow-up, with only 2 percent developing severe aortic regurgitation.[56]

Aneurysms of the aortic arch can be successfully excised surgically, but the procedure remains particularly challenging. Neurological damage is a major cause of morbidity and mortality from aortic arch repair and typically results from embolization of atherosclerotic debris or as a consequence of global ischemic injury during antegrade circulatory arrest. The brachiocephalic vessels must be removed from the aortic arch before its resection and then reimplanted into the prosthetic tube graft arch after its interposition. Traditionally, the surgical procedure involves removing and then reimplanting the brachiocephalic vessels en bloc (i.e., as an island of native aortic tissue containing the three branch-vessels), after which normal cerebral perfusion is restored. Recently, however, several novel surgical techniques have been introduced to reduce the hypothermic circulatory arrest times and embolic events by placing a multilimbed prosthetic arch graft, to which each arch vessel is in turn anastomosed individually (Fig. 53–10).

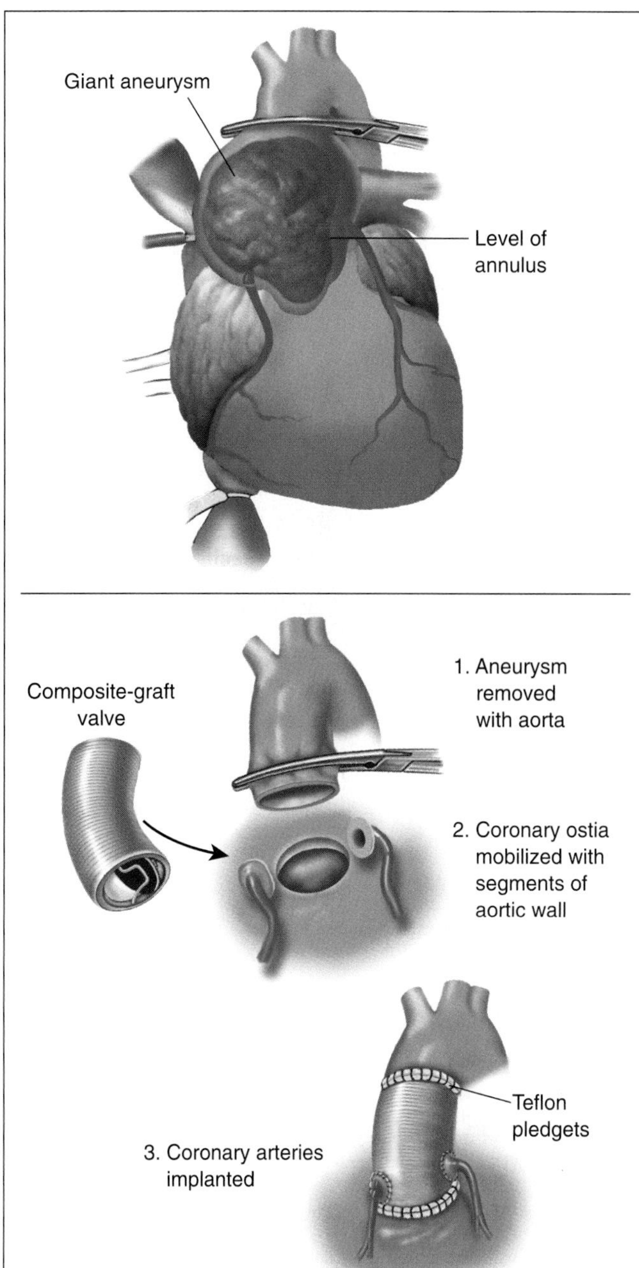

FIGURE 53–9 Technique for the composite graft replacement of an aneurysm of the ascending aorta. **Top,** The aneurysm is shown involving the sinuses of Valsalva. The patient is maintained on total cardiopulmonary bypass. **Bottom,** The composite graft is shown, with a low-profile, tilting disc aortic prosthesis attached to its inferior end. (1) The aneurysm is resected with the native aortic valve. (2) The coronary ostia have been excised and mobilized with a button of aortic wall. (3) The composite graft has been secured in place with Teflon felt reinforcement for the suture line. The coronary artery ostia are then reimplanted directly into the graft.

Three methods of cerebral protection have been used for aortic arch surgery. The traditional method has been the use of profound hypothermic circulatory arrest with arrest of cerebral perfusion. The hypothermia is intended to reduce the cerebral metabolic rate by cooling to 10°C to 13°C. The simplicity of the technique, however, is offset by the high incidence of stroke and temporary neurological dysfunction. In 1990, the use of retrograde cerebral perfusion via a superior vena cava cannula was introduced as an adjunct for cerebral protection during hypothermic arrest. It was originally suggested that this technique would improve outcomes by providing nutrients and oxygen to the brain and to flush out both air and particulate matter from the cerebral and carotid arteries that would otherwise embolize. More extensive studies have shown that there is, in fact, no metabolic benefit to the brain from retrograde cerebral perfusion and several studies have shown no improvement in outcomes.[57,58] More recently, the technique of selective antegrade cerebral perfusion has been introduced, in which perfusion cannulae inserted directly into the cerebral vessels allows perfusion of the brain through all but brief periods during the procedure. Indeed, the use of the multilimbed prosthetic aortic graft makes selective antegrade cerebral perfusion easier and more effective. This technique allows for a longer time of safe circulatory arrest, which is of greater importance in more complex arch procedures. The available data suggest that selective antegrade cerebral perfusion does not reduce the risk of stroke but does significantly reduce the incidence of temporary neurological dysfunction.[58] Historically, for aortic arch repair, the rates of mortality and stroke were as high as 6 to 20 percent and 4 to 11 percent, respectively, but with the use of these modern techniques in experienced hands, the rates are as low as 4 percent and 2 percent, respectively.[59]

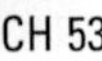

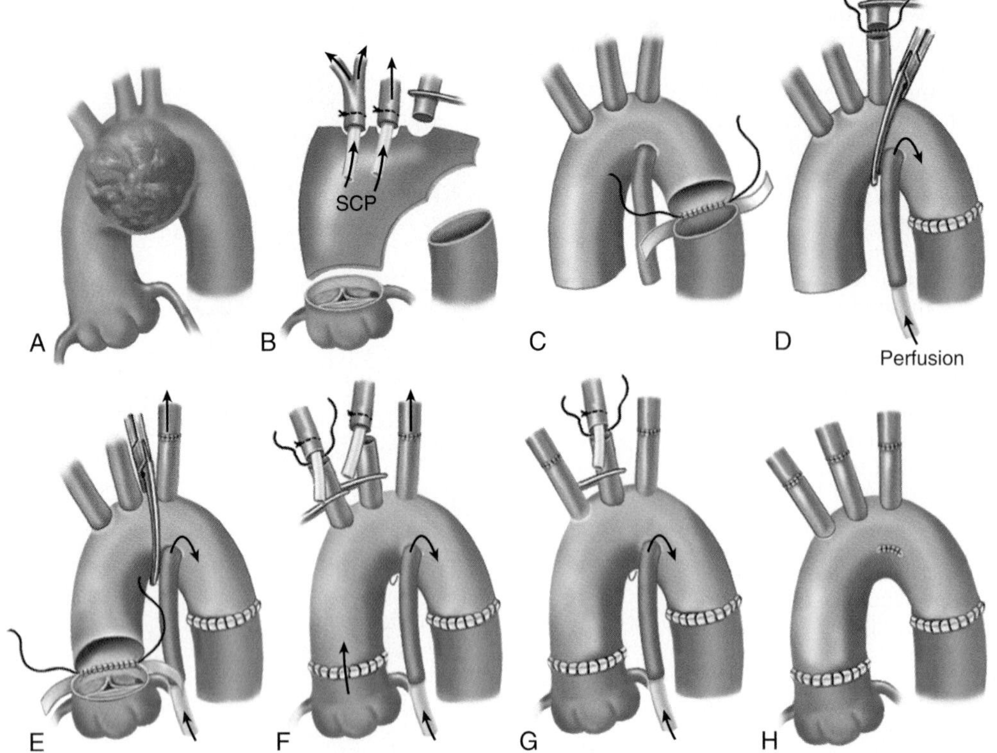

FIGURE 53–10 **A-H,** Surgical technique for total arch replacement with a branched aortic graft. Following initiation of circulatory arrest, the aneurysm is transected in the ascending aorta and where it meets the proximal descending aorta. The branched graft is anastomosed at its distal end. The graft proximal to the fourth limb is clamped and perfusion is restored through this limb to the distal circulation. The third limb is anastomosed to the left subclavian artery and flow to this vessel is restored. Then, the proximal end of the graft is anastomosed to the stump of the ascending aorta, flow is restored to the remaining arch vessels, and the fourth branch is then resected. (Adapted from Kazui T, Washiyama N, Muhammad BAH, et al: Improved results of atherosclerotic arch aneurysm operations with a refined technique. J Thorac Cardiovasc Surg 121:491, 2001.)

Many of the patients undergoing surgical repair of a thoracic aortic aneurysm have multiple aortic segments involved. Such widespread aneurysmal dilatation of the aorta presents a particular challenge to the surgeon and often precludes surgery. Although it is possible to successfully replace virtually the entire diseased thoracic aorta, attempts to replace the ascending, arch, and descending thoracic aorta in one surgery carry increased risks. An alternative strategy is the use of a staged procedure, known as the "elephant trunk" technique, in which the ascending aorta and arch are replaced initially, whereas the descending aorta is replaced at a later date. Use of the elephant trunk technique has been shown to facilitate such extensive surgical procedures and reduce the associated risks.[60]

Elective surgical repair of ascending and descending thoracic aortic aneurysms in large centers is associated with mortality rates of 3 to 10 percent and 5 to 14 percent, respectively. Major complications include stroke and hemorrhage. A catastrophic complication of resection of descending thoracic aortic aneurysms is postoperative paraplegia secondary to interruption of the blood supply to the spinal cord. The incidence of paraplegia has been as high as 13 to 17 percent, but in most modern series is 5 to 6 percent. A number of methods have been proposed to reduce the likelihood of paraplegia, although none has proved to be consistently safe and effective. One of the more promising techniques involves regional hypothermic protection of the spinal cord with epidural cooling during surgical repair of the aorta, which has reduced the frequency of spinal cord complications to 3 percent (compared with a historical control of 20 percent) in one large series by Cambria and colleagues.[61] The use of cerebrospinal fluid drainage was similarly shown to reduce the rate of paraplegia to 3 percent in a recent randomized trial by Coselli and colleagues.[62] Other important techniques that may also reduce the risk of spinal cord injury include the reimplantation of patent critical intercostal arteries, the use of intraoperative somatosensory-evoked potential monitoring, and maintenance of distal aortic perfusion during surgery with the use of atriofemoral (left heart) bypass to the distal aorta during the proximal anastomosis.[63] Controlled trials might better clarify the efficacy of such techniques.

An alternative approach to the surgical management of descending thoracic aneurysms is the use of a transluminally placed endovascular stent-graft (see Chap. 55). This technique has the advantage of being far less invasive than surgery with potentially fewer postoperative complications and a lower morbidity rate. Dake and coworkers reported the results of a large series in which "first-generation" endovascular stentgrafts were implanted in 103 patients with thoracic aortic aneurysms, only 62 (60 percent) of whom were judged to be reasonable candidates for traditional surgical aortic repair.[64] Complete thrombosis of the aortic aneurysm was achieved in 83 percent of patients, but rates of early stroke and paraplegia were 3 and 7 percent, respectively. The authors suggest that with newer and more refined devices together with more precise stent-graft deployment, the overall success rates should rise and complication rates fall. Although still experimental at present, such a device may in the future have an important role in the management of patients who are at risk for aortic rupture but are otherwise poor surgical candidates. Unfortunately, the curvilinear nature of the ascending aorta and arch makes application of similar techniques to aneurysms of these proximal aortic segments far more challenging.

Complications of associated atherosclerosis, such as myocardial infarction, cerebrovascular accidents, and renal failure, often arise under the massive physiological stress of aortic surgery. The most frequent causes of early postoperative death are myocardial infarction, congestive heart failure, stroke, renal failure, hemorrhage, respiratory failure, and sepsis. Advanced age, emergency surgery, prolonged aortic cross-clamp time, extent of the aneurysm, diabetes, prior aortic surgery, aneurysm symptoms, and intraoperative hypotension are the most important factors determining perioperative morbidity and mortality. Many patients with atherosclerotic aneurysms are heavy smokers, and pulmonary complications following surgery are common. The left lung may be severely traumatized by compression during resection of large aneurysms of the descending thoracic aorta, a complication that can seriously jeopardize the patient's survival, particularly in the setting of underlying pulmonary disease.

MEDICAL MANAGEMENT. The long-term impact of medical therapy on aneurysm growth and survival in patients with typical atherosclerotic thoracic aneurysms has not been examined. However, Shores and colleagues examined the efficacy of beta blockers in adult patients with the Marfan syndrome[65] (see Chap. 70). They randomized 70 patients to treatment with propranolol versus no beta blocker therapy and monitored them over a 10-year period. The treated group showed a significantly slower rate of aortic dilatation, fewer adverse clinical endpoints (death, aortic dissection, aortic regurgitation, aortic root larger than 6 cm), and significantly lower mortality from the 4-year point onward. Although this study examined only the effect of beta blockade in patients with the Marfan syndrome, it follows logically that medical therapy to reduce dP/dt and control blood pressure is essential to the treatment of thoracic aortic aneurysms, both for patients with smaller aneurysms being monitored serially and for patients who have undergone aortic aneurysm repair.

Aortic Dissection

Acute aortic dissection is an uncommon but potentially catastrophic illness that occurs with an incidence of approximately 2.9/100,000/yr with at least 7000 cases per year in the United States.[66] Early mortality is as high as 1 percent per hour if untreated,[66] but survival may be significantly improved by the timely institution of appropriate medical and/or surgical therapy. Prompt clinical recognition and definitive diagnostic testing are therefore essential in the management of patients with aortic dissection.

Aortic dissection is believed to begin with the formation of a tear in the aortic intima that directly exposes an underlying diseased medial layer to the driving force (or pulse pressure) of intraluminal blood (Fig. 53–11A). This blood penetrates the diseased medial layer and cleaves the media longitudinally, thereby dissecting the aortic wall. Driven by persistent intraluminal pressure, the dissection process extends a variable length along the aortic wall, typically antegrade (driven by the forward force of aortic blood flow) but sometimes retrograde from the site of the intimal tear. The blood-filled space between the dissected layers of the aortic wall becomes the false lumen. Shear forces may lead to further tears in the intimal flap (the inner portion of the dissected aortic wall) and produce exit sites or additional entry sites for blood flow into the false lumen. Distention of the false lumen with blood may cause the intimal flap to bow into the true lumen and thereby narrow its caliber and distort its shape.

Alternatively, aortic dissection may begin with rupture of the vasa vasorum within the aortic media; that is, with the development of an intramural hematoma (see Fig. 53–11B). Local hemorrhage then secondarily ruptures through the intimal layer and creates the intimal tear and aortic dissection. Since in autopsy series as many as 13 percent of aortic dissections do not have an identifiable intimal tear, at least in a minority of cases independent medial hemorrhage does appear to be the primary cause of dissection. On the other hand, one might argue that the lack of an intimal tear in these patients indicates they do not, in fact, have classic aortic dissection but rather have intramural hematoma of the aorta, a closely related condition (see later).

CLASSIFICATION. Most classification schemes for aortic dissection are based on the fact that the vast majority of aortic dissections originate in one of two locations: (1) the ascending aorta, within several centimeters of the aortic valve, and (2) the descending aorta, just distal to the origin of the left subclavian artery at the site of the ligamentum arteriosum. Sixty-five percent of intimal tears occur in the ascending aorta, 20 percent in the descending aorta, 10 percent in the aortic arch, and 5 percent in the abdominal aorta.

Three major classification systems are used to define the location and extent of aortic involvement, as defined in Table 53–1 and depicted in Figure 53–12: (1) DeBakey types I, II, and III; (2) Stanford types A and B; and (3) the anatomical categories "proximal" and "distal." All three schemes share the same basic principle of distinguishing aortic dissections with and without ascending aortic involvement for prognostic and therapeutic reasons; in general, surgery is indicated for dissections involving the ascending aorta, whereas medical management is reserved for dissections without ascending aortic involvement. Accordingly, because both DeBakey types I and II involve the ascending aorta, they are grouped together for simplicity in the Stanford (type A) and anatomical (proximal) classification systems, irrespective of the site of intimal tear. Less experienced clinicians will sometimes misclassify as type A dissections that begin in the aortic arch and progress distally, but since the ascending aorta is not involved, such cases should, in fact, be classified as type B. Aortic dissections confined to the abdominal aorta, although quite uncommon, are best categorized as type B or distal dissections. Proximal or type A dissections occur in about two-thirds of cases, with distal dissections comprising the remaining one-third.

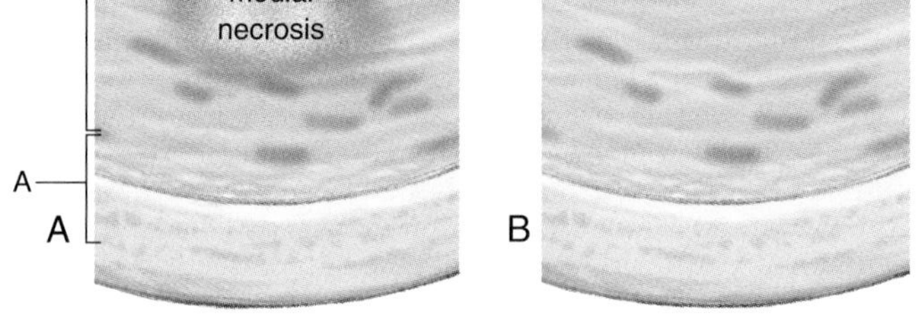

FIGURE 53–11 Proposed mechanisms of initiation of aortic dissection. A = adventitia; I = intima; M = media.

TABLE 53–1 Commonly Used Classification Systems to Describe Aortic Dissection

Type	Site of Origin and Extent of Aortic Involvement
DeBakey	
Type I	Originates in the ascending aorta, propagates at least to the aortic arch and often beyond it distally
Type II	Originates in and is confined to the ascending aorta
Type III	Originates in the descending aorta and extends distally down the aorta or, rarely, retrograde into the aortic arch and ascending aorta
Stanford	
Type A	All dissections involving the ascending aorta, regardless of the site of origin
Type B	All dissections not involving the ascending aorta
Descriptive	
Proximal	Includes DeBakey types I and II or Stanford type A
Distal	Includes DeBakey type III or Stanford type B

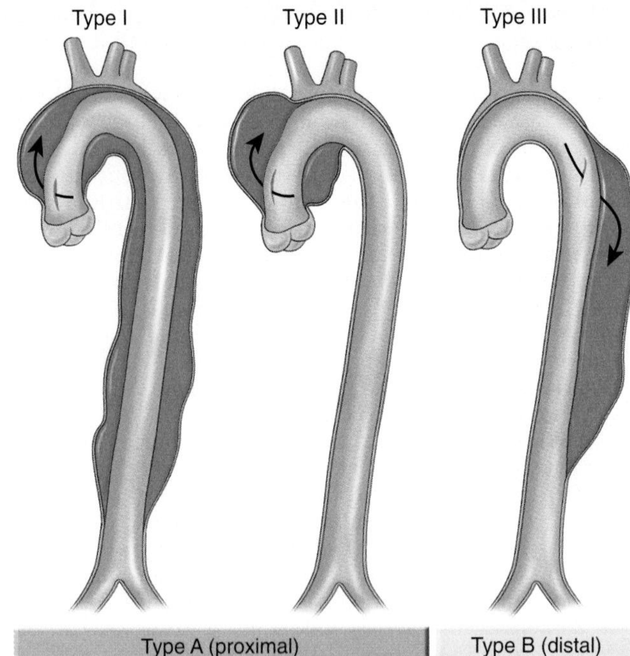

FIGURE 53–12 Commonly used classification systems for aortic dissection. (Refer to Table 53–1 for definitions.)

In addition to its location, aortic dissection is also classified according to its duration, defined as the length of time from symptom onset to medical evaluation. The mortality from dissection and its risk of progression decrease progressively over time, which makes therapeutic strategies for longstanding aortic dissections quite different from those seen acutely. A dissection present less than 2 weeks is defined as "acute," whereas those present 2 weeks or more are defined as "chronic" because the mortality curve for untreated aortic dissections begins to level off at 75 to 80 percent at this time. At diagnosis, the large majority of aortic dissections are acute.

ETIOLOGY AND PATHOGENESIS. Cystic medial degeneration, as described earlier, is the chief predisposing factor in aortic dissection. Therefore, any disease process or other condition that undermines the integrity of the elastic or muscular components of the media predisposes the aorta to dissection. Cystic medial degeneration is an intrinsic feature of several hereditary defects of connective tissue, most notably the Marfan and Ehlers-Danlos (see Chap. 70) syndromes, and is also common among patients with bicuspid aortic valve. In addition to their propensity for thoracic aortic aneurysms, patients with the Marfan syndrome are indeed at high risk for aortic dissection, especially proximal dissection, at a relatively young age. In fact, the Marfan syndrome accounts for 5 percent of all aortic dissections.[67]

In the absence of the Marfan syndrome, only a minority of cases of aortic dissection have histologically classic cystic medial degeneration. Nevertheless, the degree of medial degeneration found in most other cases of aortic dissection still tends to be qualitatively and quantitatively much greater than expected as part of the aging process. Although the cause of such medial degeneration remains unclear, advanced age and hypertension appear to be two of the most important factors.

The peak incidence of aortic dissection is in the sixth and seventh decades of life, with men affected twice as often as women. About three-quarters of patients with aortic dissection have a history of hypertension. [67] A bicuspid aortic valve is a well-established risk factor for proximal aortic dissection and occurs in 5 to 7 percent of aortic dissections. As is the case with ascending thoracic aortic aneurysms, the risk of aortic dissection appears to be independent of the severity of the bicuspid valve stenosis. Certain other congenital cardiovascular abnormalities predispose the aorta to dissection, including coarctation of the aorta. Rarely, aortic dissection complicates arteritis involving the aorta (see Chap. 82), particularly giant cell arteritis. A number of reports describe aortic dissection in association with cocaine abuse, typically among young, black, and hypertensive men. However, cocaine likely accounts for less than 1 percent of cases of aortic dissection and the mechanisms by which it causes dissection remain speculative.[68]

An unexplained relationship exists between pregnancy and aortic dissection (see Chap. 74). About half of all aortic dissections in women younger than 40 years occur during pregnancy, typically in the third trimester and also occasionally in the early postpartum period. The increases in blood volume, cardiac output, and blood pressure seen in late pregnancy may contribute to the risk, although this explanation cannot account for postpartum occurrence. Women with the Marfan syndrome and a dilated aortic root are at particular risk for acute aortic dissection during pregnancy,[69] and in some cases, diagnosis of the Marfan syndrome is first made when such women are evaluated for peripartum aortic dissection.

Direct trauma to the aorta may also cause aortic dissection. Blunt trauma tends to cause localized tears, hematomas, or frank aortic transection (see Chap. 65) and only rarely causes classic aortic dissection. Iatrogenic trauma, on the other hand, is associated with true aortic dissection and accounts for 5 percent of cases.[70] Both intraarterial catheterization and the insertion of intraaortic balloon pumps may induce aortic dissection, probably from direct trauma to the aortic intima. Cardiac surgery also entails a very small risk (0.12 to 0.16 percent) of acute aortic dissection. The majority of these dissections are discovered intraoperatively and repaired at that time, although 20 percent are detected only after a delay. In addition, aortic dissection sometimes occurs late (months to years) after cardiac surgery; in fact, as many as 18 percent of those with acute aortic dissection have a history of prior cardiac surgery. Of cardiac surgical patients, those undergoing aortic valve replacement have the highest risk for aortic dissection as a late complication. The association with aortic valve surgery may occur because many such patients had surgery to replace dysfunctional bicuspid aortic valves. As discussed earlier, cystic medial degeneration often accompanies this condition and can predispose them to subsequent dissection. Von Kodolitsch and colleagues have found that patients with a dilated ascending aorta together with aortic regurgitation or a thinned aortic wall at the time of aortic valve replacement are most likely to have such a late aortic dissection.[71] This association argues for an aggressive approach in replacing even a mildly dilated ascending aorta at the time of bicuspid aortic valve replacement, as discussed earlier.

Clinical Manifestations

SYMPTOMS. Much of the data presented regarding the clinical manifestations of aortic dissection are from the older clinical series of Slater and DeSanctis[72] and Spittel and colleagues,[73] as well as from a more recent series from the International Registry of Acute Aortic Dissection (IRAD), which studied 464 consecutive patients with acute aortic dissection from 12 international referral centers.[67] By far the most common initial symptom of acute aortic dissection is pain, which is found in up to 96 percent of cases, whereas the large majority of those without pain are found to have chronic dissections. The pain is typically severe and of sudden onset and is as severe at its inception as it ever becomes, in contrast to the pain of myocardial infarction, which usually has a crescendo-like onset and is not as intense. In fact, the pain of aortic dissection may be all but unbearable in some instances and force the patient to writhe in agony, fall to the ground, or pace restlessly in an attempt to gain relief. Several features of the pain should arouse suspicion of aortic dissection. The quality of the pain as described by the patient is often morbidly appropriate to the actual event, with adjectives such as "tearing," "ripping," "sharp," and "stabbing" frequently used in more than half the cases. In fact, it is not uncommon to hear descriptors that are collectively almost diagnostic of aortic dissection, but quite unlike the symptoms of myocardial ischemia or infarction, such as someone "stabbed me in the chest with a knife" or "hit me in the back with an ax."

Another important characteristic of the pain of aortic dissection is its tendency to migrate from its point of origin to other sites, generally following the path of the dissection as it extends through the aorta. However, such migratory pain is described in as few as 17 percent of cases. The location of pain may be quite helpful in suggesting the location of the aortic dissection because localized symptoms tend to reflect involvement of the underlying aorta. Spittell and colleagues found that when the location of chest pain was anterior only (or if the most severe pain was anterior), more than 90 percent of patients had involvement of the ascending aorta. Conversely, when the chest pain was interscapular only (or when the most severe pain was interscapular), more than 90 percent of patients had involvement of the descending thoracic aorta (i.e., DeBakey type I or III). The presence of any pain in the neck, throat, jaw, or face strongly predicted involvement of the ascending aorta, whereas pain anywhere in the back, abdomen, or lower extremities strongly predicted involvement of the descending aorta.[73] In rare cases, the presenting pain is only pleuritic in nature, owing to acute pericarditis that results from hemorrhage into the pericardial space from the dissected ascending aorta. In such cases, the underlying diagnosis may be overlooked if one does not search for other symptoms or signs that might suggest the presence of aortic dissection.

Less common symptoms at initial evaluation, occurring with or without associated chest pain, include congestive heart failure (7 percent), syncope (13 percent), cerebrovascular accident (6 percent), ischemic peripheral neuropathy, paraplegia, and cardiac arrest or sudden death. The presence of acute congestive heart failure in this setting is almost invariably due to severe aortic regurgitation induced by a proximal aortic dissection (discussed later). Patients with syncope have been found to have a higher rate of mortality than those without syncope and are more likely to have cardiac tamponade or stroke. However, when the complications of cardiac tamponade and stroke are excluded, syncope alone does not increase mortality.[74] On occasion, a patient presents with acute chest pain, and the initial imaging study reveals hemopericardium yet fails to demonstrate an aortic dissection. In such a scenario, unless another diagnosis, such as tumor metastatic to the pericardium, is evident, one must still suspect the presence of acute aortic dissection (or contained aortic rupture). Ideally, such a patient would be taken presumptively to the operating room or, at the very least, immediately undergo additional imaging with other modalities to confirm the diagnosis.[75]

PHYSICAL FINDINGS. Although extremely variable, findings on physical examination generally reflect the location of aortic dissection and the extent of associated cardiovascular involvement. In some cases, physical findings alone may be sufficient to suggest the diagnosis, whereas in other cases, such pertinent physical findings may be subtle or absent, even in the presence of extensive aortic dissection. Hypertension is seen in 70 percent of patients with distal aortic dissection but in only 36 percent with proximal dissection. Hypotension, on the other hand, occurs much more commonly among those with proximal than with distal aortic dissection (25 and 4 percent, respectively). True hypotension is usually the result of cardiac tamponade, acute severe aortic regurgitation, intrapleural rupture, or intraperitoneal rupture. Dissection involving the brachiocephalic vessels may result in "pseudohypotension," an inaccurate measurement of blood pressure caused by compromise or occlusion of the brachial arteries.

The physical findings most typically associated with aortic dissection—pulse deficits, the murmur of aortic regurgitation, and neurological manifestations—are more characteristic of proximal than distal dissection. Reduced or absent pulses in patients with acute chest pain strongly suggest the presence of aortic dissection. Such pulse abnormalities are present in about 30 percent of proximal aortic dissections and occur throughout the arterial tree, but they are seen in only 15 percent of distal dissections, where they usually involve the femoral or left subclavian artery. The presence of pulse deficits predicts an increased risk for adverse outcomes.[76] Impaired pulses, and similarly, visceral ischemia, result from extension of the dissection flap into a branch artery with compression of the true lumen by the false channel (Fig. 53–13), which diminishes blood flow in the aortic true lumen because of narrowing or obliteration by the distended false lumen (occurring most commonly in the descending or abdominal aorta); impaired pulses may also result from proximal obstruction of flow caused by a mobile portion of the intimal flap overlying the branch vessel's orifice. Whichever the cause, the pulse deficits in aortic dissection may be transient, secondary to decompression of the false lumen by distal reentry into the true lumen or secondary to movement of the intimal flap away from the occluded orifice.

Aortic regurgitation is an important feature of proximal aortic dissection, with the murmur of aortic regurgitation detected in one-third of cases. When present in patients with distal dissection, aortic regurgitation generally antedates the dissection and may be the result of preexisting dilation of the aortic root from the underlying aortic pathologic condition, such as cystic medial degeneration. The murmur of aortic regurgitation may wax and wane, the intensity varying directly with the height of the arterial blood pressure. Depending on the severity of the regurgitation, other peripheral signs of aortic incompetence may be present, such as collapsing pulses and a wide pulse pressure. In some cases, however, congestive heart failure secondary to severe acute aortic regurgitation may occur with little or no murmur and no peripheral signs of aortic runoff.

The acute aortic regurgitation associated with proximal aortic dissection, which occurs in one-half to two-thirds of such cases, may result from any of several mechanisms (Fig. 53–14). First, the dissection may dilate the aortic root, thereby widening the sinotubular junction from which the aortic leaflets hang so that the leaflets are unable to coapt properly in diastole (incomplete closure). Second, the dissection may extend into the aortic root and detach one or more aortic leaflets from their commissural attachments at the sinotubular junction, thereby resulting in diastolic leaflet prolapse. Not infrequently, both incomplete closure and leaflet prolapse are present at the same time. Finally, in the setting of an extensive or circumferential intimal tear the unsupported intimal flap may prolapse into the left ventricular outflow tract, occasionally appearing as frank intimal intussusception, and produce severe aortic regurgitation.

Neurological manifestations occur in as many as 6 to 19 percent of all aortic dissections and accompany proximal dissection more frequently. Cerebrovascular accidents may occur in 3 to 6 percent when the innominate or left common

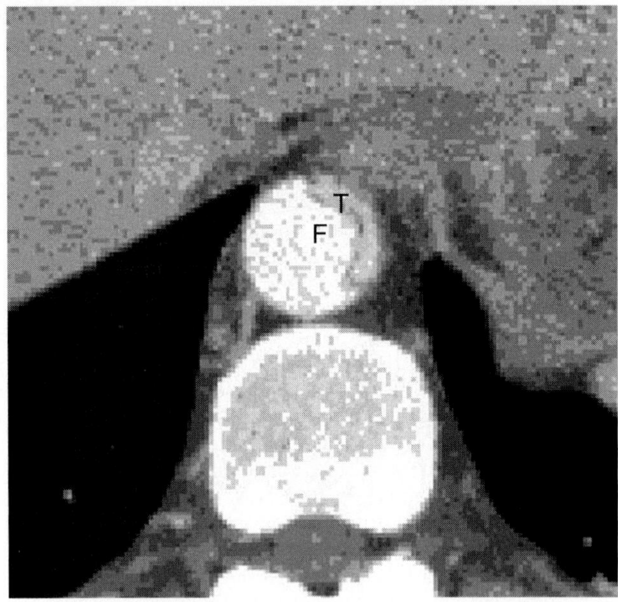

A

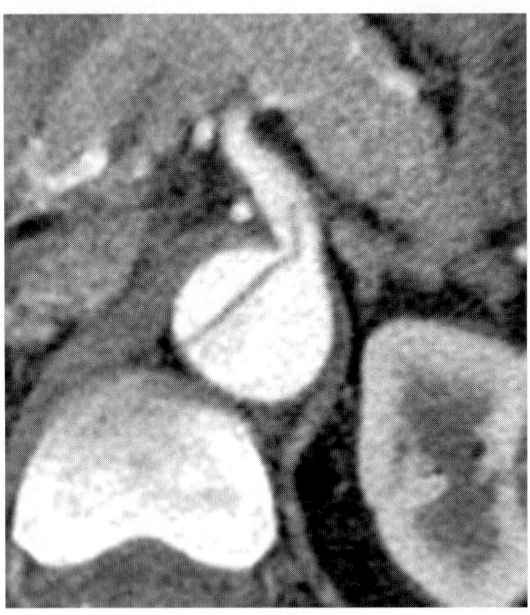

B

FIGURE 53–13 Mechanisms of compromised perfusion of branch arteries due to aortic dissection. **A,** The branch artery still originates from the true lumen, but the true lumen (T) is markedly compressed by the false lumen (F) throughout the cardiac cycle, resulting in low pressure and reduced flow within the true lumen and its branches. **B,** The intimal flap of the aortic dissection extends into the ostium of a branch artery, potentially narrowing or obstructing it.

carotid arteries are directly involved. Less often, patients may have altered consciousness or even coma. When spinal artery perfusion is compromised, ischemic spinal cord damage may produce paraparesis or paraplegia.

In a small minority, about 1 to 2 percent, of cases, a proximal dissection flap may involve the ostium of a coronary artery and cause acute myocardial infarction. Because most proximal dissections arise above the right sinus of Valsalva, retrograde extension into the aortic root more often affects the right coronary artery than the left, which explains why these myocardial infarctions tend to be inferior in location. Unfortunately, when secondary myocardial infarction does occur, its symptoms may complicate the clinical picture by obscuring symptoms of the primary aortic dissection. Most worrisome is the possibility that in the setting of electrocardiographic evidence of myocardial infarction, the underlying aortic dissection may go unrecognized. Moreover, the consequences of such a misdiagnosis in the era of thrombolytic therapy can be catastrophic. In a review of the literature, Kamp and colleagues described an early mortality rate of 71 percent (many from cardiac tamponade) among 21 patients with aortic dissection treated with thrombolysis.[77] It thus remains essential that when evaluating patients with acute myocardial infarction, particularly inferior infarctions, one carefully consider the possibility of an underlying aortic dissection before thrombolytic or anticoagulant therapy is instituted. Although some physicians feel reassured that performing a chest radiograph before the institution of thrombolysis is adequate to exclude the diagnosis of dissection, studies have shown it is not sufficient.

Extension of aortic dissection into the abdominal aorta can cause other vascular complications. Compromise of one or both renal arteries occurs in about 5 to 8 percent and can lead to renal ischemia or frank infarction and, eventually, severe hypertension and acute renal failure. Mesenteric ischemia and infarction are also occasional and potentially lethal complications of abdominal dissection seen in 3 to 5 percent of cases. In addition, aortic dissection may extend into the iliac arteries and cause diminished femoral pulses (12 percent) and acute lower extremity ischemia. If in such cases, the associated chest pain is minimal or absent, the pulse deficit and ischemic peripheral neuropathy may be mistaken for a peripheral embolic event.

Additional clinical manifestations of aortic dissection include the presence of small pleural effusions, seen more commonly on the left side. The effusion typically arises secondary to an inflammatory reaction around the involved aorta, but in some cases larger effusions may result from hemothorax caused by a transient rupture or leak from a descending dissection. Several rarely encountered clinical manifestations of aortic dissection include hoarseness, upper airway obstruction, rupture into the tracheobronchial tree with hemoptysis, dysphagia, hematemesis from rupture into the esophagus, superior vena cava syndrome, pulsating neck masses, Horner syndrome, and unexplained fever. Other rare findings associated with the presence of a continuous murmur include rupture of the aortic dissection into the right atrium, into the right ventricle, or into the left atrium with secondary congestive heart failure.

A variety of conditions can mimic aortic dissection, including myocardial infarction or ischemia, pericarditis, pulmonary embolism, acute aortic regurgitation without dissection, nondissecting thoracic or abdominal aortic aneurysms, or mediastinal tumors.

LABORATORY FINDINGS. Chest radiography is included in the discussion of clinical manifestations of aortic dissection rather than the discussion of diagnostic techniques because an abnormal incidental finding on a routine chest radiograph may first raise clinical suspicion of aortic dissection (Fig. 53–15). Moreover, although chest radiography may help support a diagnosis of suspected aortic dissection, the findings are nonspecific and rarely diagnostic. The results of chest radiography therefore add to the other available clinical data used in deciding whether suspicion of aortic dissection warrants proceeding to a more definitive diagnostic study.

The most common abnormality seen on a chest radiograph in cases of aortic dissection is widening of the aortic silhouette, which appears in 81 to 90 percent of cases. Less often, nonspecific widening of the superior mediastinum is seen. If calcification of the aortic knob is present, separation of the intimal calcification from the outer aortic soft tissue border by more than 1.0 cm—the "calcium sign"—is suggestive, although not diagnostic, of aortic dissection. Comparison of the current chest radiograph with a previous study may reveal acute changes in the aortic or mediastinal silhouettes that would otherwise have gone unrecognized. Pleural effusions are common, typically occur on the left side, and are more often associated with dissection involving the descending aorta. Although the majority of patients with aortic dissection have one or more of these radiographic abnormalities, the remainder, up to 12 percent, have chest radiographs that appear unremarkable. Therefore, a normal chest radiograph can never exclude the presence of aortic dissection.

Electrocardiographic findings in patients with aortic dissection are nonspecific. One-third of electrocardiograms show changes consistent with left ventricular hypertrophy, whereas another third are normal. Nevertheless, obtaining an electrocardiogram is diagnostically important for two reasons: (1) in cases of aortic dissection, nonspecific chest pain and the absence of ischemic ST segment and T wave changes on electrocardiogram may argue against the diagnosis of myocardial ischemia and thereby prompt consideration of other chest pain syndromes, including aortic dissection, and (2) in patients with proximal dissection, the electrocardiogram may reveal acute myocardial infarction when the dissection flap has involved a coronary artery.

Because of the variable extent of aortic, branch vessel, and cardiac involvement occurring with aortic dissection, the signs and symptoms associated with the condition occur sporadically. Consequently, the presence or absence of aortic dissection cannot be diagnosed accurately in most cases on the basis of symptoms and clinical findings alone. In the series of Spittell and associates,[73] of all aortic dissections (without a known diagnosis), the initial clinical diagnosis was aortic dissection in only 62 percent, and the other 38 percent of patients were initially thought to have myocardial ischemia, congestive heart failure, nondissecting aneurysms of the thoracic or abdominal aorta, symptomatic aortic stenosis, pulmonary embolism, and so forth. Among this 38 percent in whom aortic dissection went undiagnosed at initial evaluation, nearly two-thirds of patients had their aortic dissection detected incidentally while undergoing a diagnostic procedure for other clinical questions, and in

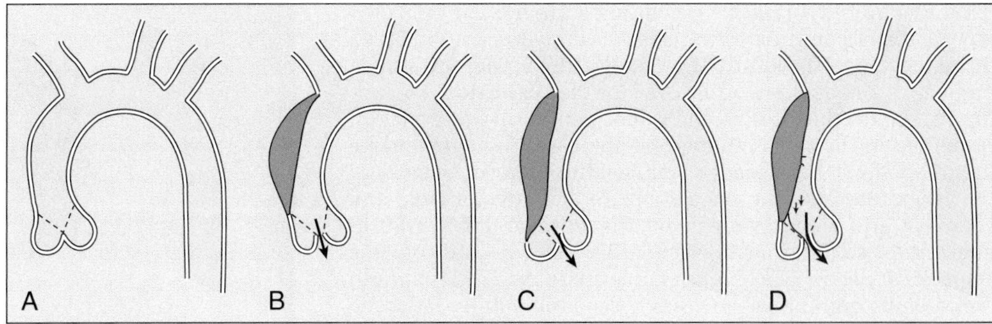

FIGURE 53–14 Mechanisms of aortic regurgitation in proximal aortic dissection. **A,** Normal aortic valve anatomy, with the leaflets suspended (dotted lines) from the sinotubular junction. **B,** A type A dissection dilates the ascending aorta, which in turn widens the sinotubular junction from which the aortic leaflets hang so that the leaflets are unable to coapt properly in diastole (incomplete closure). Aortic regurgitation (arrow) results. **C,** A type A dissection extends into the aortic root and detaches an aortic leaflet from its commissural attachment to the sinotubular junction. Diastolic leaflet prolapse results. **D,** In the setting of an extensive or circumferential intimal tear, the unsupported intimal flap may prolapse across the aortic valve and into the left ventricular outflow tract and prevent normal leaflet coaptation.

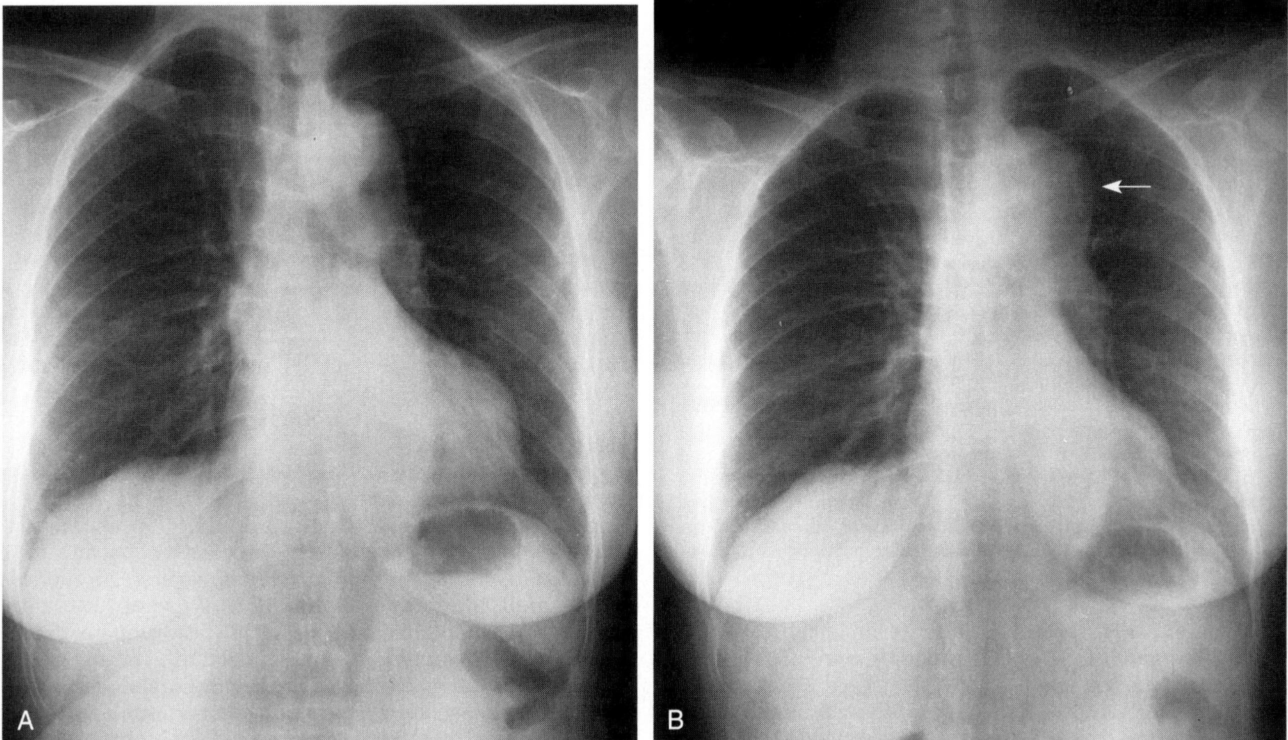

FIGURE 53–15 Chest radiograph of a patient with aortic dissection. **A,** The patient's baseline study from 3 years prior to admission, with a normal-appearing aorta. **B,** The chest radiograph upon admission, which is remarkable for the interval enlargement of the aortic knob (arrow). The patient was found to have a proximal aortic dissection. (From Isselbacher EM: Aortic dissection. *In* Creager, MA [ed]: Atlas of Vascular Disease. 2nd ed. Philadelphia, Current Medicine, 2003.)

nearly one-third, the aortic dissection remained undiagnosed until necropsy. Given the clinical challenge that detection of aortic dissection presents, physicians should remain vigilant for any risk factors, symptoms, and signs consistent with aortic dissection if a timely diagnosis is to be made.

DIAGNOSTIC TECHNIQUES. Once the diagnosis of aortic dissection is suspected on clinical grounds, it is essential to confirm the diagnosis both promptly and accurately. The diagnostic modalities currently available for this purpose include aortography, contrast-enhanced CT, MRI, and TTE or TEE. Each modality has certain advantages and disadvantages with respect to diagnostic accuracy, speed, convenience, risk, and cost, but none is appropriate in all situations.

When comparing the four imaging modalities, one must begin by considering what diagnostic information is needed. First and foremost, the study must confirm or refute the diagnosis of aortic dissection. Second, it must determine whether the dissection involves the ascending aorta (i.e., proximal or type A) or is confined to the descending aorta or arch (i.e., distal or type B). Third, if possible, it should identify a number of the anatomical features of the dissection, including its extent, the sites of entry and reentry, the presence of thrombus in the false lumen, branch vessel involvement by the dissection, the presence and severity of aortic regurgitation, the presence or absence of pericardial effusion, and any coronary artery involvement by the intimal flap. Unfortunately, no single imaging modality provides all of this anatomical detail. The choice of diagnostic modalities should therefore be guided by the clinical scenario and by targeting information that will best assist patient management.

Aortography. Retrograde aortography was the first accurate diagnostic technique for evaluating suspected aortic dissection. The diagnosis of aortic dissection is based on direct angiographic signs, including visualization of two lumina or an intimal flap (considered diagnostic), as in Figure 53–16, or on indirect signs (considered suggestive), such as deformity of the aortic lumen, thickening of the aortic walls, branch vessel abnormalities, and aortic regurgitation.

Aortography had long been considered the diagnostic standard for the evaluation of aortic dissection because for several decades it was the only accurate method of diagnosing aortic dissection antemortem, although its true sensitivity could not be defined. However, the more recent introduction of alternative diagnostic modalities has shown that aortography is not as sensitive as previously thought. Prospective studies have found that for the diagnosis of aortic dissection, the sensitivity of aortography is 88 percent and falls to only 77 percent when the definition of aortic dissection included intramural hematoma with noncommunicating dissection.[78] The specificity of aortography is 94 percent. False-negative aortograms occur because of thrombosis of the false lumen, equal and simultaneous opacification of both the true and false lumina, or the presence of an intramural hematoma.

Important advantages of aortography include its ability to delineate the extent of the aortic dissection, including branch vessel involvement (Fig. 53–17). It is also useful in detecting some of the major complications of aortic dissection, such as the presence of aortic regurgitation, and is often useful in revealing patency of the coronary arteries. In addition to the limited sensitivity of aortography, other disadvantages are the inherent risks of the invasive procedure, the risks associated with the use of contrast material, and the time needed to complete the study, both in assembling an angiography team and the long duration of the procedure. Finally, aortography requires that potentially unstable patients travel to the angiography suite.

Computed Tomography. In contrast-enhanced CT scanning, aortic dissection is diagnosed by the presence of two distinct aortic lumina, either visibly separated by an intimal flap (Fig. 53–18) or distinguished by a differential rate of contrast opacification. Spiral (helical) CT scanning, which is now used routinely, permits three-dimensional display of the aorta and its branches (Fig. 53–19), has improved the accuracy of CT in diagnosing aortic dissection, as well as in

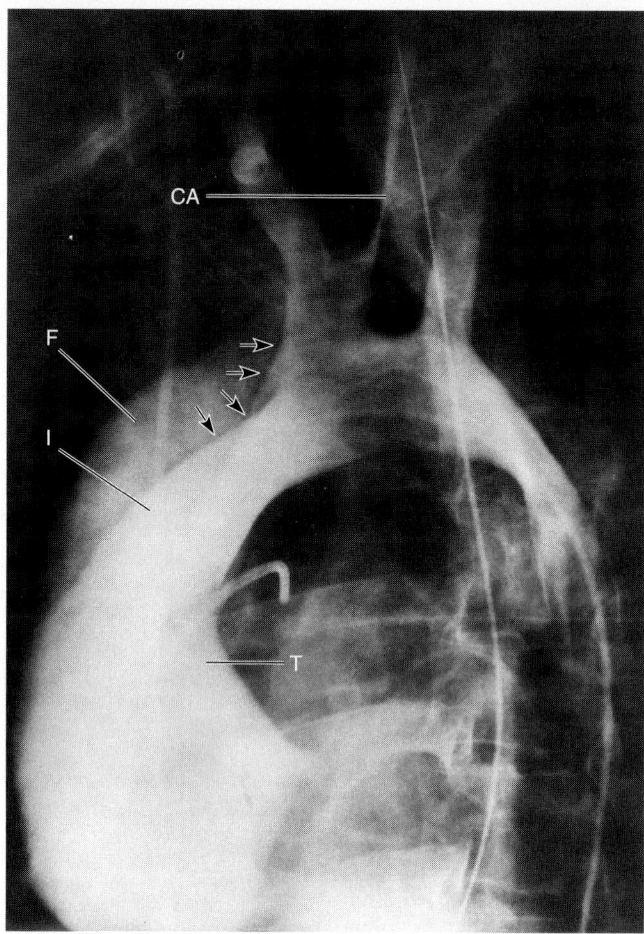

FIGURE 53–16 Aortogram in the left oblique view demonstrating proximal aortic dissection and its associated cardiovascular complications. The true lumen (T) and false lumen (F) are separated by the intimal flap (I), which is faintly visible as a radiolucent line following the contour of the pigtail catheter. The true lumen is better opacified than the false lumen, and two planes of the intimal flap can be distinguished (arrows). The branch vessels are opacified, along with marked narrowing of the right carotid artery (CA), which suggests that its lumen is compromised by the dissection. (From Isselbacher EM: Aortic dissection. *In* Creager MA [ed.]: Atlas of Vascular Disease. 2nd ed. Philadelphia, Current Medicine, 2003.)

defining anatomical features. Several series have found that spiral CT scanning has both a sensitivity and specificity for acute aortic dissection of 96 to 100 percent (see Chap. 14).

Computed tomography scanning has the advantage that, unlike aortography, it is noninvasive. However, it does require the use of an intravenous contrast agent. Most hospitals are equipped with a readily accessible CT scanner available on an emergency basis. CT is also helpful in identifying the presence of thrombus in the false lumen and in detecting pericardial effusion. The use of CT angiography (three-dimensional reconstruction of axial CT data) permits assessment of branch vessel compromise in both the thoracic and abdominal segments. A disadvantage of CT scanning is that the site of intimal tear is rarely identified. CT scanning also cannot reliably detect the presence of aortic regurgitation.

Magnetic Resonance Imaging. The use of MRI has particular appeal for diagnosing aortic dissection in that it is entirely noninvasive and does not require the use of intravenous contrast material or ionizing radiation. Furthermore, MRI produces high-quality images in the transverse, sagittal, and coronal planes, as well as in a left anterior oblique view that displays the entire thoracic aorta in one plane (see Chap. 14). The availability of these multiple views facilitates the diagnosis of aortic dissection and determination of its extent

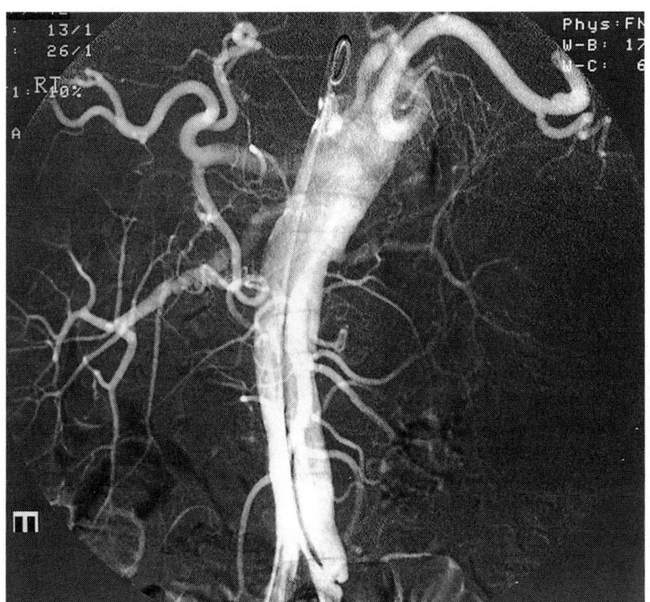

FIGURE 53–17 Digital subtraction angiogram of the abdominal aorta, in a patient with a distal thoracic aortic dissection, to assess the status of renal perfusion. This study confirmed the presence of an intimal flap extending down into the left common iliac artery. The celiac axis, superior mesenteric artery, and right renal artery are widely patent and fill from the true lumen. The left renal artery fills from the false lumen, with the intimal flap involving the ostium of the artery and impairing distal flow. As a consequence, there is minimal contrast excretion by the left kidney compared to the right.

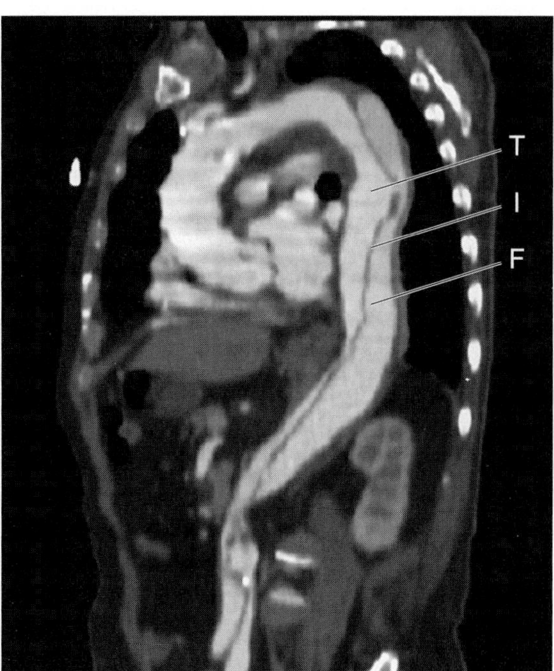

FIGURE 53–19 Computed tomography (CT) for diagnosing aortic dissection. Shown is a contrast-enhanced spiral CT scan of the chest at the level of the pulmonary artery showing an intimal flap (I) in the descending thoracic aorta separating the two lumina in a type B aortic dissection. F = false lumen; T = true lumen.

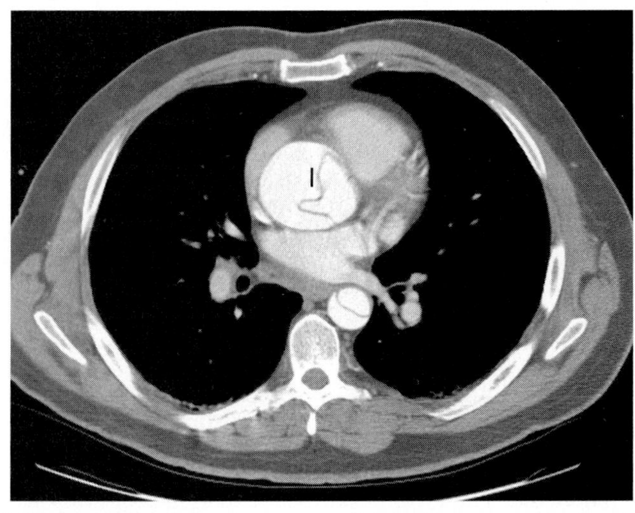

FIGURE 53–18 Computed tomography (CT) for diagnosing aortic dissection. Shown is a contrast-enhanced spiral CT scan of the chest at the level of the right pulmonary artery showing an intimal flap (I) in both the ascending and descending thoracic aorta separating the two lumina in a type B aortic dissection. (Reprinted with permission from Isselbacher EM: Aortic dissection. *In* Creager MA [ed]: Atlas of Vascular Disease. 2nd ed. Philadelphia, Current Medicine, 2003.)

and in many cases reveals the presence of branch vessel involvement.

Magnetic resonance imaging has been found to have both a sensitivity and a specificity of approximately 98 percent. Furthermore, use of the cine-MRI technique in a subset of these patients showed 85 percent sensitivity for detecting aortic regurgitation. Intravenous administration of gadolinium yields a magnetic resonance angiogram, which can be used to define the patency of aortic branch vessels. Still, MRI does have a number of disadvantages. It is contraindicated in patients with pacemakers or implantable defibrillators and certain types of vascular clips. MRI provides only limited images of branch vessels (unless gadolinium is used) and does not consistently identify the presence of aortic regurgitation. In most hospitals, magnetic resonance scanners are not readily available on an emergency basis. Many patients with aortic dissection are hemodynamically unstable, often intubated or receiving intravenous antihypertensive medications with arterial pressure monitoring, but magnetic resonance scanners limit the presence of many monitoring and support devices in the imaging suite and also limit patient accessibility during the lengthy study. Understandably, concern for the safety of unstable patients has led many physicians to conclude that the use of MRI is relatively contraindicated for unstable patients.

Echocardiography. Echocardiography is well suited for the evaluation of patients with suspected aortic dissection because it is readily available in most hospitals, it is noninvasive and quick to perform, and the full examination can be completed at the bedside. The echocardiographic finding considered diagnostic of an aortic dissection is the presence of an undulating intimal flap within the aortic lumen that separates the true and false channels. Reverberations and other artifacts can cause linear echodensities within the aortic lumen that mimic aortic dissection; to distinguish an intimal flap definitively from such artifacts, the flap should be identified in more than one view, it should have motion independent of that of the aortic walls or other cardiac structures, and a differential in color Doppler flow patterns should be noted between the two lumina. In cases in which the false lumen is thrombosed, displacement of intimal calcification or thickening of the aortic wall may suggest aortic dissection.

TRANSTHORACIC ECHOCARDIOGRAPHY. TTE has a sensitivity of 59 to 85 percent and a specificity of 63 to 96 percent for the diagnosis of aortic dissection. Such poor sensitivity significantly limits the general utility of this technique. Furthermore, image quality is often adversely affected by obesity,

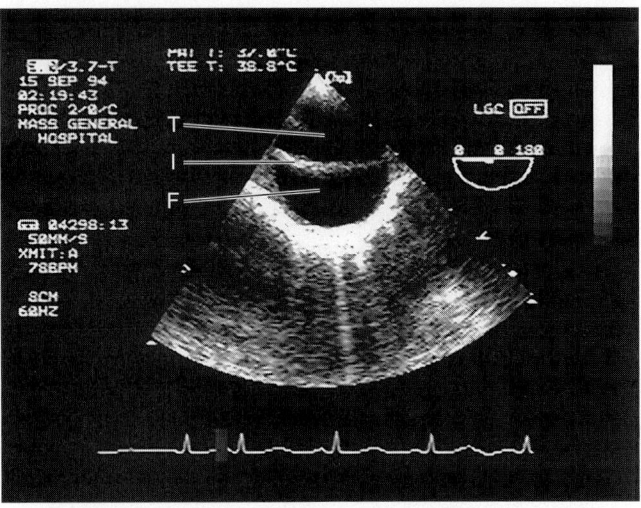

FIGURE 53–20 Cross-sectional transesophageal echocardiogram of the descending thoracic aorta demonstrating aortic dissection. The aorta is dilated. Evident is an intimal flap (I) dividing the true lumen (T) anteriorly and the false lumen (F) posteriorly. The true lumen fills during systole and is therefore seen bowing slightly into the false lumen in this systolic image.

emphysema, mechanical ventilation, or small intercostal spaces.

TRANSESOPHAGEAL ECHOCARDIOGRAPHY. The proximity of the esophagus to the aorta enables TEE to overcome many of the limitations of transthoracic imaging and permits the use of higher frequency ultrasonography, which provides better anatomical detail (Figs. 53–20 and 53–21). The examination is generally performed at the bedside with the patient under sedation or light general anesthesia and typically requires 10 to 15 minutes to complete. The procedure does not require arterial access nor intravenous contrast or ionizing radiation. Relative contraindications include known esophageal disease such as strictures or tumors. The incidence of important side effects (such as hypertension, bradycardia, bronchospasm, or rarely, esophageal perforation) is much less than 1 percent. One important disadvantage of TEE is its limited ability to visualize the distal ascending aorta and proximal arch because of interposition of the air-filled trachea and main stem bronchus.

The results of large prospective studies have demonstrated that the sensitivity of TEE for aortic dissection is 98 to 99 percent, whereas the sensitivity for detecting an intimal tear (Fig. 53–22) is 73 percent. Furthermore, TEE detects both aortic regurgitation and pericardial effusion in 100 percent of cases. The specificity of TEE for the diagnosis of aortic dissection is less well defined but is likely in the range of 94 to 97 percent.

In addition to its high sensitivity for detecting aortic dissection, TEE can provide other important information useful to the surgeon. Some surgeons want to know preoperatively whether the intimal flap involves the ostia of the coronary arteries, but this determination has traditionally required the performance of coronary angiography. Ballal and colleagues performed TEE on 34 patients with aortic dissection, 7 of whom had coronary artery involvement confirmed at surgery.[79] In six of these seven patients, TEE identified the intimal flap extending into the coronary ostia. However, TEE delineates only the very proximal portions of the coronary arteries, so when assessment of coronary atherosclerosis is necessary, coronary angiography is still required (see later).

Among patients with suspected aortic dissection, the diagnosis is excluded in as many as two-thirds of cases, which yields a group of patients with a chest pain syndrome of unknown origin. Among patients determined not to have aortic dissection, TEE identifies alternative cardiovascular diagnoses (e.g., other aortic abnormalities or evidence of acute myocardial infarction or ischemia) in 66 to 73 percent.[80]

Selecting an Imaging Modality. Each of the four imaging modalities has particular advantages and disadvantages. In selecting among them, one must consider the accuracy as well as the safety and availability of each test. Given their extremely high sensitivity and specificity and ability to provide three-dimensional images, CT angiography and MRA are considered the current standards for evaluating aortic dissection. The four imaging modalities described earlier differ in their ability to detect complications associated with dissection, so the specific diagnostic information sought by the treating physician and/or surgeon should have a bearing on the procedure chosen.

Both the accessibility of imaging studies and the time required to complete them are key considerations given the high rate of early mortality associated with unoperated proximal aortic dissection. Aortography can only rarely be performed on an emergency basis, because it often requires assembly of an angiography team and is subject to the risks associated with an invasive procedure and use of a contrast agent. MRI is also generally unavailable on an emergency basis and poses the risk of limited patient monitoring and accessibility during the lengthy procedure. CT scanning is more readily available in most emergency departments and is quickly completed. TEE is also readily available in most larger centers and can be completed quickly at the bedside, which makes it ideal for evaluating unstable patients. Among the centers in the IRAD, CT was used most often (63 percent) as the imaging study of first choice, with TEE performed first about half as often (32 percent).[81] Aortography and MRI were rarely used as the initial imaging modality (4 percent and 1 percent, respectively).

In a setting in which all these imaging modalities are available, CT should be considered first in the evaluation of suspected aortic dissection in light of its accuracy, safety, speed, and convenience. When CT identifies a type A aortic dissection, the patient may be taken directly to the operating room, where TEE can then be performed to assess the anatomy and competence of the aortic valve without unduly delaying surgery. However, in cases of suspected aortic dissection in which aortic valve disease is suspected or the patient is unstable, TEE may be the initial procedure of choice.

Despite its relative disadvantages, aortography still plays an important role when clear definition of the anatomy of the branch vessels is essential for management. Performance of aortography should also be considered when a definitive diagnosis is not made by one or more of the other imaging modalities.

In the final analysis, each institution must determine its own best diagnostic approach to the evaluation of suspected aortic dissection and base it on available human and material resources and the speed with which such resources can be mobilized. The level of skill and experience of those who carry out each diagnostic procedure should also enter into the choice of diagnostic modality.

The Role of Coronary Angiography. The importance of assessing the status of coronary artery patency before surgical repair of acute aortic dissection continues to be controversial. Some surgeons believe that obtaining this information before surgery is essential, whereas others are content to assess the coronary arteries intraoperatively. Two types of coronary artery involvement must be considered in the setting of aortic dissection. The first is acute proximal coronary narrowing or occlusion as a result of the dissection itself, often caused by occlusion of the coronary ostia by the intimal flap. The second is the possible presence of chronic atherosclerotic coronary artery disease, which, although generally independent of the dissection process, may complicate its surgical management.

In some cases, coronary involvement by the intimal flap is self-evident if the electrocardiogram shows evidence of acute myocardial ischemia or infarction. Should this acute process not be clinically evident, however, TEE can effectively define the patency of the proximal coronary arteries in a majority of cases. Aortography may also reveal such coronary artery involvement. More comprehensive evaluation requires the performance of coronary angiography; however, this study may be risky in patients with aortic dissection and often prolongs the time to aortic repair by several hours. Moreover, catheterization of the coronary arteries is sometimes unsuccessful in patients with proximal dissection and a dilated root, in which case the added procedural delay offers no potential benefit. In addition, such proximal coronary obstructions can usually be readily identified at the time of surgery.

Chronic coronary artery disease is seen in about one-quarter of patients with aortic dissection. Identifying the presence of this underlying coronary disease is beyond the capability of any of the four imaging modalities discussed earlier. Furthermore, accurately defining such atherosclerotic disease intraoperatively is challenging, although Rizzo and coworkers have suggested probing of the proximal coronary arteries, epicardial palpation, and angioscopy as possible means to identify coronary stenoses.[82]

The impact of unrecognized coronary artery disease on outcome is not certain. In a 10-year review examining 54 patients undergoing urgent aortic repair, Kern and colleagues found that only 1 of 27 patients with a proximal dissection had a perioperative myocardial infarction; this patient had a prior history of coronary artery disease.[83] In addition, Rizzo and associates observed that among patients in whom unrecognized coronary artery disease was discovered at autopsy, none died of coronary ischemia but several died of aortic rupture.[82] Lastly, Penn and colleagues studied 122 consecutive patients undergoing emergency aortic repair and found no difference in in-hospital mortality between patients who had preoperative angiography and those who did not.[84] Accordingly, we and others recommend avoiding preoperative coronary angiography unless a specific indication exists, such as a known history of coronary artery disease, prior coronary artery bypass grafting, or the presence of ischemic electrocardiographic changes. Conversely, Creswell and coauthors reported good outcomes when performing combined aortic repair and coronary artery bypass grafting in patients with underlying coronary artery disease and therefore argue that all stable patients with acute proximal dissec-

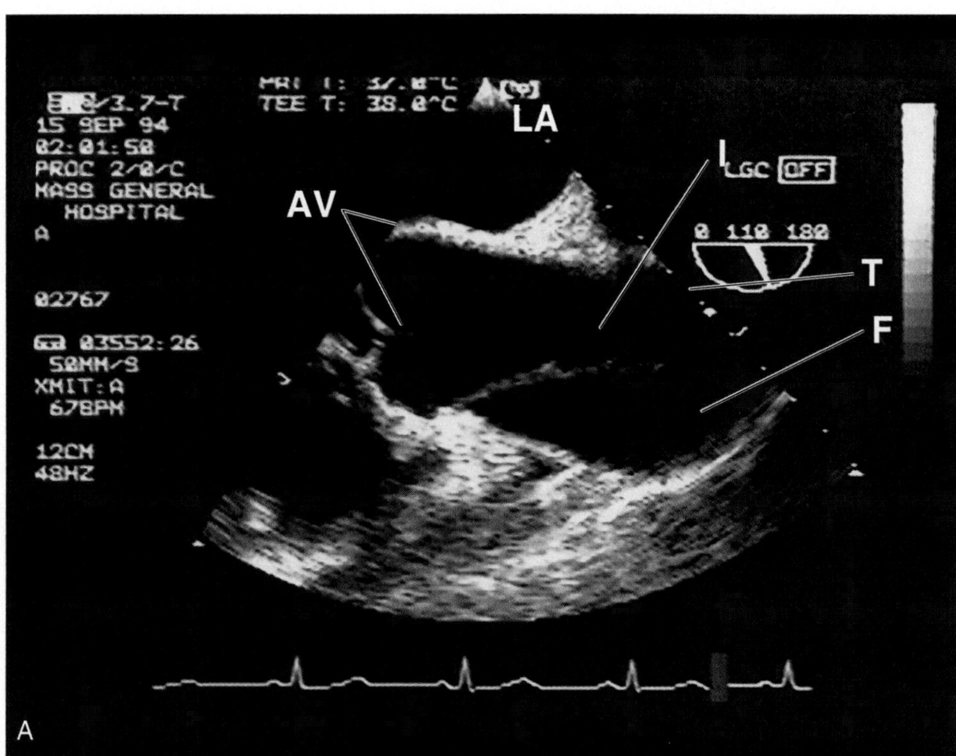

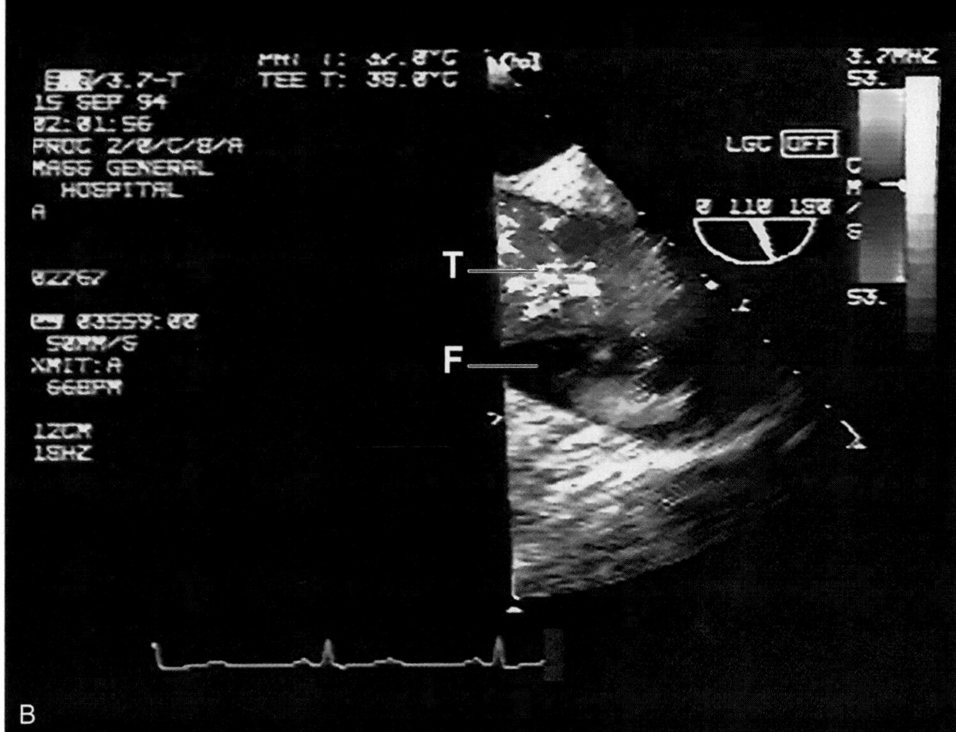

FIGURE 53–21 Transesophageal echocardiogram of the proximal ascending aorta in long-axis view in a patient with proximal aortic dissection. **A,** The left atrium (LA) is closest to the transducer. The aortic valve (AV) is seen on the left in this view, with the ascending aorta extending to the right. Within the proximal aorta is an intimal flap (I) that originates just at the level of the sinotubular junction above the right sinus of Valsalva. The true lumen (T) and the false lumen (F) are separated by the intimal flap. **B,** The addition of color flow Doppler in the same view confirms the presence of two distinct lumina. The true lumen (T) fills completely with brisk blood flow (bright blue color), while at the same time minimal retrograde flow (dark orange) is seen in the false lumen (F).

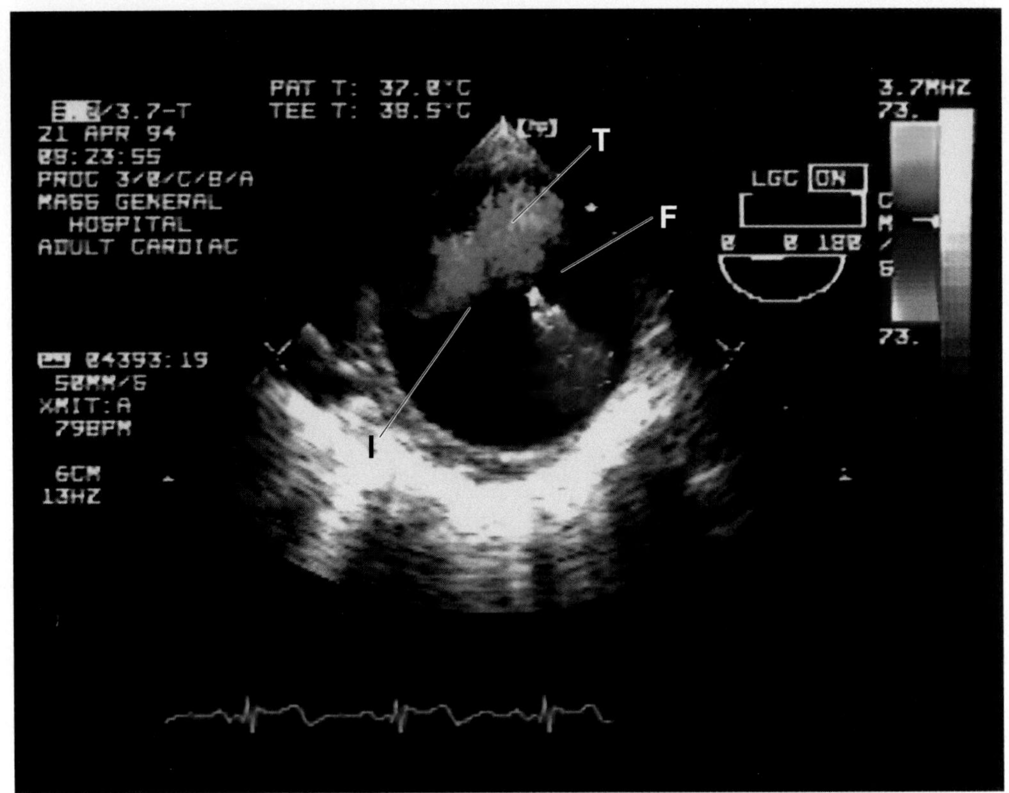

FIGURE 53–22 Cross-sectional transesophageal echocardiogram of a descending aortic dissection demonstrating a site of intimal tear. Blood flow (in orange) is evident in the true lumen (T) during systole, while a narrow jet of high-velocity blood (in blue) crosses into the false lumen (F) through a tear in the intimal flap (I).

tion should undergo preoperative coronary angiography.[85] While the debate continues unresolved, the trend in the literature has been a retreat from the routine performance of coronary angiography in cases of acute aortic dissection.

Management

Therapy for aortic dissection aims to halt progression of the dissecting hematoma because lethal complications arise not from the intimal tear itself but rather from the subsequent course taken by the dissecting aorta, such as vascular compromise or aortic rupture. Without treatment, aortic dissection has a high mortality rate. In a collective review of long-term survival in patients with untreated aortic dissection, more than 25 percent of all patients died within the first 24 hours after the onset of dissection, more than 50 percent died within the first week, more than 75 percent died within 1 month, and more than 90 percent died within 1 year.

The first surgical approach to aortic dissection was a fenestration procedure in which the dissected aorta was incised and a distal communication created between the true and false channels, thereby decompressing the false lumen. This procedure is, in fact, still used by some surgeons in selected cases of dissection involving the descending aorta to relieve limb, renal, or mesenteric ischemia. Definitive surgical therapy was pioneered by DeBakey and colleagues in the early 1950s. Its purpose is to excise the intimal tear, obliterate the false channel by oversewing the aortic edges, reconstitute the aorta directly or with the interposition of a synthetic graft, and in the case of proximal dissection, restore aortic valve competence either by resuspension of the displaced aortic leaflets or by prosthetic aortic valve replacement.

Aggressive medical treatment of aortic dissection was first advocated by Wheat and colleagues in the 1960s. The authors established reduction of systolic blood pressure and diminution of the rate of left ventricular ejection (dP/dt) as the two primary goals of pharmacological therapy. Originally introduced for patients too ill to withstand surgery, medical therapy is now the initial treatment for virtually all patients with aortic dissection before definitive diagnosis and furthermore serves as the primary long-term therapy in a subset of patients, particularly those with distal dissections.

IMMEDIATE MEDICAL MANAGEMENT. All patients in whom acute aortic dissection is strongly suspected should immediately be placed in an acute care setting for hemodynamic stabilization and monitoring of blood pressure, cardiac rhythm, and urine output. Two large-bore intravenous catheters should be inserted for intravenous medications and fluid resuscitation if necessary. An arterial line should be placed, preferably in the right arm so that it remains functional during surgery when the aorta is cross-clamped. However, in cases in which the blood pressure is significantly greater on the left than on the right, the arterial line should be placed on the left. In patients with a lower likelihood of dissection who are hemodynamically stable, an automatic blood pressure cuff should suffice.

A central venous or pulmonary arterial line to monitor central venous or pulmonary artery wedge pressure and cardiac output should be considered in patients with hypotension or congestive heart failure. Femoral lines and blood gas studies should be avoided if possible to conserve these sites for bypass cannulation during potential aortic repair. If a femoral line must be placed urgently, the opposite groin site should be protected from needle puncture.

BLOOD PRESSURE REDUCTION. Initial therapeutic goals include the elimination of pain and reduction of systolic blood pressure to 100 to 120 mm Hg (mean of 60 to 75 mm Hg) or the lowest level commensurate with adequate vital organ (cardiac, cerebral, renal) perfusion. Simultaneously, beta-blocking agents should be administered as well, regardless of whether pain or systolic hypertension is present. The use of long-acting medications should be avoided in patients who are surgical candidates because they may complicate intraoperative arterial pressure management. Pain, which may itself exacerbate hypertension and tachycardia, should be promptly treated with intravenous morphine sulfate.

For the acute reduction of arterial pressure, the potent vasodilator sodium nitroprusside is very effective. It is initially infused at 20 μg/min with the dosage titrated upward, as high as 800 μg/min, according to the blood pressure response. When used alone, however, sodium nitroprusside can actually cause an increase in dP/dt, which in turn may potentially contribute to propagation of the dissection. Therefore, concomitant beta-blocking treatment is essential. For those patients with acute or chronic renal insufficiency, intravenous fenoldopam may be preferable to sodium nitroprusside.[86]

To reduce dP/dt acutely, an intravenous beta blocker should be administered in incremental doses until evidence of satisfactory beta blockade is noted, usually indicated by a heart rate of 60 to 80 beats/min in the acute setting. Because propranolol was the first generally available beta blocker, it has been used most widely in treating aortic dissection. However, it is believed that other noncardioselective beta blockers are equally effective. Propranolol should be administered in intravenous doses of 1 mg every 3 to 5 minutes until the desired effect is achieved, although the maximum initial dose should not exceed 0.15 mg/kg (or approximately 10 mg). To maintain adequate beta blockade, as evidenced by the heart rate, additional propranolol should be given intravenously every 4 to 6 hours, or administered as a continuous infusion.

Labetalol, which acts as both an alpha- and a beta-adrenergic receptor blocker, can be especially useful in the setting of aortic dissection because it effectively lowers both dP/dt and arterial pressure. The initial dose of labetalol is 20 mg, administered intravenously over a 2-minute period, followed by additional doses of 40 to 80 mg every 10 to 15 minutes (up to a maximum total dose of 300 mg) until the heart rate and blood pressure have been controlled. Maintenance dosing can then be achieved with a continuous intravenous infusion starting at 2 mg/min and titrating up to 5 to 10 mg/min.

The ultra-short-acting beta blocker esmolol may be particularly useful in patients with labile arterial pressure, especially if surgery is planned, because use of this drug can be abruptly discontinued if necessary. It is administered as a 500 μg/kg intravenous bolus followed by continuous infusion at 50 μg/kg/min and titrated up to 200 μg/kg/min. Esmolol can also be useful as a means to test beta blocker safety and tolerance in patients with a history of obstructive pulmonary disease who may be at uncertain risk for bronchospasm from beta blockade. In such patients, a cardioselective beta blocker, such as atenolol or metoprolol, can be considered.

When contraindications exist to the use of beta blockers—including sinus bradycardia, second- or third-degree atrioventricular block, congestive heart failure, or bronchospasm—other agents to reduce arterial pressure and dP/dt should be considered. Calcium channel antagonists, which are effective in managing hypertensive crisis, are used on occasion in the treatment of aortic dissection. The combined vasodilator and negative inotropic effects of both diltiazem and verapamil make these agents well suited for the treatment of aortic dissection. Moreover, these agents may be administered intravenously. Nifedipine has the advantage that it can be given immediately by the sublingual route while other medications are being prepared. A key limitation of nifedipine, however, is that it has little negative chronotropic or inotropic effect.

Refractory hypertension may result when a dissection flap compromises one or both of the renal arteries, thereby causing the release of large amounts of renin. In this situation, the most efficacious antihypertensive may be the intravenous angiotensin-converting enzyme (ACE) inhibitor enalaprilat, which is administered initially in doses of 0.625 to 1.25 mg every 6 hours and then titrated upward if necessary to a maximum of 5 mg every 6 hours.

In the event that a patient with suspected aortic dissection has significant hypotension, rapid volume expansion should be considered given the possible presence of cardiac tamponade or aortic rupture. Before initiating aggressive treatment of such hypotension, however, the possibility of *pseudohypotension*, which occurs when arterial pressure is being measured in an extremity where the circulation is selectively compromised by the dissection, should be carefully excluded. If vasopressors are absolutely required for refractory hypotension, norepinephrine (Levophed) or phenylephrine (Neo-Synephrine) is preferred. Dopamine should be reserved for improving renal perfusion and used only at very low doses, given that it may raise dP/dt.

Once appropriate medical therapy has been initiated and the patient sufficiently stabilized, a definitive diagnostic study should be promptly undertaken. If a patient remains unstable, TEE is preferred because it can be performed at the bedside in the emergency department or intensive care unit, thereby allowing both monitoring and therapeutic intervention to continue uninterrupted. When a patient with a strongly suspected dissection becomes extremely unstable, aortic rupture or cardiac tamponade is likely and the patient should go directly to the operating room rather than delaying surgery for diagnostic imaging. In such situations, intraoperative TEE can be used both to confirm the diagnosis and to guide surgical repair.

MANAGEMENT OF CARDIAC TAMPONADE. Cardiac tamponade frequently complicates acute proximal aortic dissection and is one of the most common mechanisms of death in these patients. It is often the cause of hypotension when patients have aortic dissection, and pericardiocentesis is commonly performed in this setting in an effort to stabilize patients while they await definitive surgical repair. In a retrospective series, however, we found that pericardiocentesis may be harmful rather than beneficial in this setting because it can precipitate hemodynamic collapse and death rather than stabilize the patient as intended.[87] Seven patients in this series were relatively stable initially (six hypotensive, one normotensive). Three of four who underwent successful pericardiocentesis died suddenly between 5 and 40 minutes after the procedure due to acute pulseless electrical activity. In contrast, none of the three patients without pericardiocentesis died before surgery. It may be that in such patients, the increase in intraaortic pressure that follows pericardiocentesis causes a closed communication between the false lumen and pericardial space to reopen, thereby leading to recurrent hemorrhage and lethal cardiac tamponade.

Therefore, when a patient with acute aortic dissection complicated by cardiac tamponade is relatively stable, the risks of pericardiocentesis probably outweigh the benefits and *every effort should be made to proceed as urgently as possible to the operating room for direct surgical repair of the aorta with intraoperative drainage of the hemopericardium.* However, when patients have pulseless electrical activity or marked hypotension, an attempt to resuscitate the patient with pericardiocentesis is warranted and may indeed be successful. A prudent strategy in such cases is to aspirate only enough pericardial fluid to raise blood pressure to the lowest acceptable level.

Definitive Therapy

Despite minor variations from center to center, a reasonable consensus regarding definitive therapy for aortic dissection has evolved over the past several decades. All practitioners agree that surgical therapy is superior to medical therapy for acute proximal dissection. With even limited progression of a proximal dissection, patients may suffer the potentially devastating consequences of aortic rupture or cardiac tamponade, acute aortic regurgitation, or neurological compromise. Thus, by controlling this risk, immediate surgical repair promises a better outcome. Occasional patients with proximal dissection who refuse surgery or for whom surgery is contraindicated (e.g., by age or prior debilitating illness) may

TABLE 53–2 Indications for Definitive Surgical and Medical Therapy in Aortic Dissection

Surgical
Treatment of choice for acute proximal dissection
Treatment for acute distal dissection complicated by the following:
- Progression with vital organ compromise
- Rupture or impending rupture (e.g., saccular aneurysm formation)
- Retrograde extension into the ascending aorta
- Dissection in the Marfan syndrome

Medical
Treatment of choice for uncomplicated distal dissection
Treatment for stable, isolated arch dissection
Treatment of choice for stable chronic dissection (uncomplicated dissection presenting 2 weeks or later after onset)

be treated successfully with medical therapy with a 30-day survival rate of up to 42 percent.[67]

Patients suffering acute distal aortic dissection, on the other hand, are at significantly lower risk of early death from complications of the dissection than are those with proximal dissection. Furthermore, because patients with distal dissection tend to be older and have a relatively increased prevalence of advanced atherosclerosis or cardiopulmonary disease, their surgical risk is often considerably higher. A large retrospective series involving patients from both Duke and Stanford universities has, by multivariate analysis, shown that medical therapy provides an outcome equivalent to that of surgical therapy in patients with uncomplicated distal dissection. As a consequence, medical therapy for such patients is favored. An important exception is that when distal dissection is complicated by vital organ or limb ischemia, uncontrolled pain, rapid expansion, medical therapy yields poor results and surgery is therefore recommended.

Patients with chronic aortic dissection have, through self-selection, survived the early period of highest mortality, and whether treated medically or surgically, their subsequent hospital survival rate is approximately 90 percent. Accordingly, medical therapy is recommended for the management of all stable patients with chronic proximal and distal dissection, again unless complicated by rupture, aneurysm formation, aortic regurgitation, arterial occlusion, or extension or recurrence of dissection.

SURGICAL MANAGEMENT. Generally advocated indications for definitive surgical therapy are summarized in Table 53–2. Surgical candidacy should be determined whenever possible at the start of the patient's evaluation because this option guides the selection of diagnostic studies. Surgical risk for all patients is increased by age, comorbid disease (especially pulmonary emphysema), aneurysm leakage, cardiac tamponade, shock, or vital organ compromise as a result of such conditions as myocardial infarction, cerebrovascular accident, and in particular, preexisting renal failure.

Preoperative mortality in patients with acute dissection ranges from 3 percent when surgery is expedited to as high as 20 percent when the preoperative evaluation is more prolonged. These data reinforce the need for prompt diagnosis and repair to prevent even minimal progression of the dissection, which might lead to further complications.

The usual objectives of definitive surgical therapy include resection of the most severely damaged segment of aorta, excision of the intimal tear when possible, and obliteration of entry into the false lumen by suturing of the edges of the dissected aorta both proximally and distally. After the diseased segment containing the intimal tear is resected, typically a segment of the ascending aorta in proximal dissections or the proximal descending aorta in distal dissections, aortic continuity is then reestablished by interposing a prosthetic sleeve graft between the two ends of the aorta (Fig. 53–23).

Importantly, several studies have demonstrated that the immediate and long-term survival of patients treated surgically was not significantly affected by failure to excise the intimal tear. Some patients with proxi-

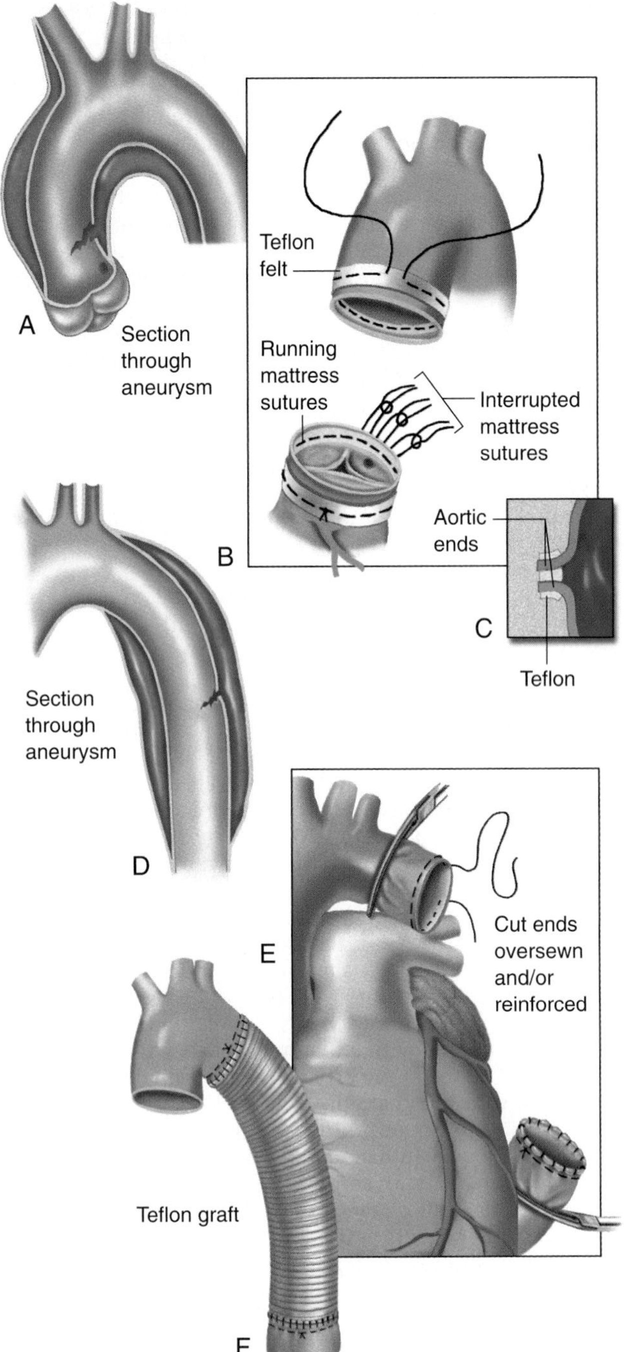

FIGURE 53–23 Several steps in the surgical repair of proximal **(A, B,** and **C)** and distal **(D, E,** and **F)** aortic dissections. **A** and **D,** Dissections and intimal tears. **B,** The aorta has been transected, and the ends of the aorta have been oversewn to obliterate the false lumen and buttressed with Teflon felt to prevent the sutures from tearing through the fragile tissue. **C,** The aortic ends are brought together in such a way that the Teflon is again used to reinforce the suture line between the two ends of the aorta and between the aorta and a sleeve graft, if such a graft is necessary for reconstitution of the aorta. **E,** Resection of a distal dissection, with a Teflon graft interposed in **F.** (**D, E,** and **F** from Austen WG, DeSanctis RW: Surgical treatment of dissecting aneurysm of the thoracic aorta. N Engl J Med 272:1314, 1965.)

mal dissection have an intimal tear located in the aortic arch. Because surgical repair of the arch may increase the morbidity and mortality associated with the procedure and because resection of the tear may not necessarily improve mortality,[88] many surgeons elect not to repair the arch if the sole purpose of surgery is resection of the intimal tear. However, with improvements in surgical technique during the last decade, several groups suggest that even these challenging lesions can be resected with favorable results.[89]

When aortic regurgitation complicates aortic dissection, simple decompression of the false lumen is sometimes all that is required to allow resuspension of the aortic leaflets and restoration of valvular competence. More often, however, preservation of the aortic valve requires approximation of the two layers of dissected aortic wall and resuspension of the commissures with pledgeted sutures. In this setting, the use of intraoperative TEE may be particularly helpful to the surgeon in guiding aortic valve repair.[90] This resuspension technique has had favorable results with a fairly low incidence of recurrent aortic regurgitation in long-term follow-up. Preserving the aortic valve in this fashion may avoid the complications associated with prosthetic valve replacement, especially the requirement for oral anticoagulation, which may pose an added risk in patients prone to future aortic rupture.

Prosthetic aortic valve replacement is sometimes necessary, however, either because attempts at valve repair are unsuccessful or in the setting of preexisting valvular disease or Marfan syndrome. Many surgeons are aggressive about replacing the aortic valve if it appears that even moderate aortic regurgitation will remain after the leaflets are resuspended and choose to avoid the risk of having to replace the aortic valve at some later date in a second operation through a diseased aorta. When the proximal aorta is fragile or badly torn, most surgeons use a composite prosthetic graft (described earlier) for replacement of both the ascending aorta and the aortic valve together. The operative procedure for aortic dissection is technically demanding. The wall of the diseased aorta is often friable, and the repair must be performed with meticulous care. Use of Teflon felt to buttress the wall and prevent sutures from tearing through the fragile aorta is essential (see Fig. 53-23). Determining the sources of vital organ perfusion distal to the surgical site by diagnostic imaging studies may be of critical importance. For example, if one or both renal arteries are supplied by the false lumen and are not going to be directly corrected surgically, the surgeon may leave communication between the true and false channels distal to the site of aortic repair so that renal perfusion is not jeopardized.

Complications. Bleeding, infection, pulmonary failure, and renal insufficiency constitute the most common early complications of surgical therapy. Spinal cord ischemia with paraplegia caused by inadvertent interruption of the blood supply from the anterior spinal or intercostal arteries is an uncommon but dreaded consequence of descending thoracic aortic repair. Late complications include progressive aortic regurgitation if the aortic valve has not been replaced, localized aneurysm formation, and recurrent dissection at the original site or at a secondary site. With modern operative techniques, 30-day surgical survival rates for proximal and distal dissections are 74 and 69 percent, respectively.[67]

Newer Surgical Techniques. As a modification of more standard operative techniques, many surgeons now use tissue glues to appose permanently the dissected aortic layers to both eliminate the false lumen and to strengthen friable aortic tissue in order to improve the anastomoses. After resection of the diseased aortic segment, this glue is used in place of pledgeted sutures to seal the false lumen of the aortic stumps, before implantation of the Dacron prosthesis. The glue not only hardens and reinforces the fragile dissected aortic tissue but may also simplify the operation, facilitate resuspension of the aortic valve, and potentially reduce the incidence of late aortic root aneurysm formation.[91] Although some reports have shown favorable morbidity and mortality with the use of these new techniques, others suggest that glue use may result in late complications of tissue necrosis,[92] particularly if the glue is used improperly. Before the use of tissue glue can be widely adopted, a direct comparison with standard operative techniques is needed.

Endovascular Techniques. One of the more promising avenues of investigation is the use of endovascular techniques for treating high-risk patients with aortic dissection. For example, because patients with renal or visceral artery compromise from dissection have had operative mortality rates exceeding 50 percent, alternative management strategies are desirable. Two endovascular techniques have been used in many centers to manage patients with acute vascular complications secondary to aortic dissection. The first is balloon fenestration of the intimal flap, which involves crossing an intact intimal flap with a wire, passing a balloon-tipped catheter over the wire, and then expanding the balloon to tear a hole in the intimal flap. The hole acts as a site of reentry to allow blood to flow from the false into the true lumen, thereby decompressing the distended false lumen. The second technique involves percutaneous stenting of an affected arterial branch whose flow has been compromised by the dissection process. Slonim and coauthors reported the use of percutaneous management of ischemic complications of aortic dissection in a series of 22 patients.[93] Sixteen patients were treated with endovascular stents, three with balloon fenestration of the intimal flap, and three with fenestration in combination with stenting of the aorta or its branches; revascularization with clinical success was achieved in all 22 patients, with excellent long-term outcomes. In comparing our recent 10-year experience with a previously reported 30-year experience, we found that current methods of peripheral vascular intervention have reduced the overall mortality of dissection-associated branch vessel occlusion from 51 percent to 23 percent.[94] In the large IRAD series of acute aortic dissection, 3.2 percent of patients were treated with percutaneous fenestration procedures.[67]

More recently, intraluminal stent-grafts placed percutaneously by the transfemoral catheter technique have been introduced as a potential alternative to aortic repair. This procedure aims to close the site of entry into the false lumen (intimal tear), decompress and promote thrombosis of the false lumen, and relieve any obstruction of branch vessels that may accompany the dissection. It is hoped that this approach will reduce the morbidity and mortality of aortic dissection and reduce the risk of subsequent aneurysm formation. Nienaber and colleagues compared the use of stent-graft placement with standard surgical repair in a group of 24 patients with subacute or chronic type B aortic dissection and a patent false lumen.[95] No procedural complications occurred among the 12 patients undergoing stent-graft treatment, and when compared with the surgical group, the stent-graft group had a significantly shorter hospital stay, lower rate of morbidity, and lower 1-year postprocedural mortality rate. Dake and colleagues inserted stent-grafts in the descending thoracic aortas of 19 patients with acute aortic dissection and a patent false lumen who suffered from obstruction of branch vessels, acute aortic rupture, or persistent back pain.[96] Endovascular stent-graft deployment was successful in all cases, with complete thrombosis of the false lumen in 79 percent and partial thrombosis in the remaining 21 percent. Restoration of flow to ischemic arterial branches with relief of corresponding symptoms occurred in 76 percent of obstructed branches. The results of these two series are extremely promising, but larger studies with more patients and longer follow-up will be required before stent-graft therapy becomes an accepted therapy for aortic dissection.

DEFINITIVE MEDICAL MANAGEMENT. As discussed earlier, we prefer medical therapy for stable patients with uncomplicated acute distal dissection (see Table 53-2) given that the 30-day survival rate for those with distal dissection treated medically is 92 percent.[67] However, surgery (or percutaneous intervention) clearly must be performed in cases of medical management failure, such as in the presence of rupture or impending rupture, progression of the dissection with vital organ compromise, an inability to control pain with medicines, or retrograde progression of a type B dissection into the ascending aorta. Because of the extreme difficulty of surgery to repair the aortic arch when it is involved by the dissection, medical therapy is also usually advocated for type B dissections that either originate in the arch or extend retrograde into the arch. Operative therapy is again reserved for patients with serious complications. Medical therapy is also generally recommended for patients with chronic aortic dissection, whether proximal or distal, unless late complications of the dissection, such as aortic regurgitation or localized aneurysm formation, necessitate surgery.

Severe hypertension is relatively common during the period of hospitalization after acute aortic dissection and may occur even in patients without a history of significant hypertension. In the past, some practitioners have argued that such refractory hypertension should be considered an indication for aortic repair, as it might increase the risk of early complications. In a retrospective analysis, however, we found that although almost two-thirds of our patients with distal dissections required the administration of four or more antihypertensive medications to control refractory hypertension early in their hospitalization, there was no increase in adverse events as compared with patients without such hypertension, and surgery is generally not necessary in this setting.[97] The etiology for this hypertensive response is unclear but it may reflect a marked increase in sympathetic tone triggered by the severe inflammation of the aortic wall that accompanies dissection. In our experience, renal ischemia rarely caused hypertension, so in the absence of a fall in urine output or a rise in serum creatinine, renal artery imaging is typically not necessary. Furthermore, the severe hypertension usually improves 5 to 7 days after onset of the aortic dissection, allowing a reduction in antihypertensive therapy.

When patients with type B aortic dissection are managed medically, in addition to the reduction in dP/dt and heart rate, a second goal is to monitor the patient vigilantly for any evidence of branch arterial compromise, with the most lethal consequence being mesenteric ischemia. Unfortunately, the clinical features of mesenteric ischemia may be subtle initially and therefore go unrecognized, and by the time they have become clinically obvious, organ damage may be irreversible. Adding to the challenge of this condition is the fact that in as many as half such cases,[98] imaging studies such as urgent CT scanning may show patent mesenteric vessels arising from the true lumen with no evidence of the dissection flap extending into the branches. However, often a large false lumen is distended with blood and compresses a small true lumen throughout most of the cardiac cycle, markedly reducing antegrade flow through the true lumen to the mesenteric vessels and resulting in nonobstructive ischemia (see Fig. 53–13). In this setting, a strong clinical suspicion and a low threshold for surgical or percutaneous intervention are the keys to preventing a catastrophic outcome.

Long-Term Therapy and Late Follow-Up

Late follow-up of patients leaving the hospital with treated aortic dissection shows an actuarial survival rate not much worse than that of individuals of comparable age without dissection. No significant differences are seen among discharged patients when comparing proximal versus distal dissection, acute versus chronic dissection, or medical versus surgical treatment.[99] Five-year survival rates for all these groups (among discharged patients) are typically 75 to 82 percent. Thus, the initial success of surgical or medical therapy is usually sustained on long-term follow-up. Late complications include aortic regurgitation, recurrent dissection, and aneurysm formation or rupture. The presence of a persistently patent false lumen is one of the strongest predictors of adverse late outcomes, including more rapid aortic dilatation, a greater likelihood of requiring subsequent aortic surgery, and late mortality.[100,101]

Long-term medical therapy to control hypertension and reduce dP/dt is indicated for all patients who have sustained an aortic dissection, regardless of whether their in-hospital definitive treatment was surgical or medical. Indeed, one study found that late aneurysm rupture after aortic dissection was 10 times more common in patients with poorly controlled hypertension than in those with controlled blood pressure,[102] which dramatically demonstrates the importance of aggressive lifelong antihypertensive therapy. Systolic blood pressure should be maintained at or below 130 mm Hg. The preferred agents are beta blockers or, if contraindicated, other agents with a negative inotropic as well as a hypotensive effect, such as verapamil or diltiazem. Pure vasodilators, such as dihydropyridine calcium channel antagonists or hydralazine, may cause an increase in dP/dt and should therefore be used only in conjunction with adequate beta blockade. ACE inhibitors are attractive antihypertensive agents for treating aortic dissection and may be of particular benefit in patients with some degree of renal ischemia as a consequence of the dissection.

Up to 29 percent of late deaths following surgery result from rupture of either the dissecting aneurysm or another aneurysm at a remote site. Moreover, the incidence of subsequent aneurysm formation at a site remote from the surgical repair is 17 to 25 percent, with these remote aneurysms accounting for many of the rupture-related deaths. The mean time interval from primary aortic dissection to the appearance of subsequent aneurysms is 18 months, with the majority appearing within 2 years. Many such aneurysms occur from dilatation of the residual false lumen in the more distal aortic segments not resected at the time of surgery. Because the dissected aneurysm wall is relatively thin and consists of only the outer half of the original aortic wall, these aneurysms rupture more frequently than do typical atherosclerotic thoracic aneurysms. Thus, an aggressive approach to treating such late-appearing aneurysms may be indicated.

The high incidence of late aneurysm formation and rupture emphasizes both the diffuse nature of the aortic disease process in this population and the tremendous importance of careful follow-up. The primary goal of long-term surveillance is the early detection of aortic lesions that might require subsequent surgical intervention, such as the appearance of new aneurysms or rapid aneurysm expansion, progression or recurrence of dissection, aortic regurgitation, or peripheral vascular compromise.

Follow-up evaluation of patients after aortic dissection should include careful and repeated physical examinations, periodic chest radiographs, and serial aortic imaging with CT, MRI, or TEE. We generally prefer CT for serially monitoring of these patients because it is completely noninvasive and provides excellent anatomical detail that may be exceedingly helpful in evaluating interval changes. Patients are at highest risk immediately after hospitalization and during the first 2 years, with the risk progressively declining thereafter. It is therefore important to have more frequent early follow-up; for example, patients can be seen and imaged at 3 and 6 months initially and then return every 6 months for 2 years, after which time they can be reevaluated at 6- to 12-month intervals, depending on the given patient's risk.

Atypical Aortic Dissection

In aortic dissection as classically described, two other diseases of the aorta are closely related, *intramural hematoma* of the aorta and *penetrating atherosclerotic ulcer* of the aorta. These two conditions share with aortic dissection many of the predisposing risk factors and initial symptoms, and indeed, both may lead to either classic aortic dissection or aortic rupture. In light of their clinical similarities, it is appropriate to consider classic aortic dissection and its variants collectively among the "acute thoracic aortic syndromes," a category that also includes traumatic aortic transection and rupture, contained rupture (pseudoaneurysm), or acute expansion of thoracic aortic aneurysms.

INTRAMURAL HEMATOMA. Intramural hematoma is an acute aortic syndrome that is essentially a hemorrhage contained within the medial layer of the aortic wall but—unlike classic aortic dissection—without an evident tear in the intima or active communication between the hematoma and the aortic lumen. Hence, some practitioners have termed it *aortic dissection without intimal rupture.* The actual causes of intramural hematoma remain debatable. Historically, it has been presumed that intramural hematoma results from rupture of the vasa vasorum within the aortic wall. Others have argued, however, that the hematoma results from a tear in the intima (too small to visualize) that permits transient blood flow from the lumen into the aortic wall, which then thromboses to form a hematoma rather than a false lumen. The hematoma can be localized or discrete, but more often the hemorrhage extends for a variable distance by dissecting along the outer media beneath the adventitia.

Clinically, intramural hematoma can be indistinguishable from true aortic dissection. The risk factors, signs, and symptoms associated with intramural hematoma resemble those seen in classic aortic dissection, and it is therefore impossible to predict on clinical grounds (without an imaging study) whether a patient with suspected aortic dissection has a classic aortic dissection or intramural hematoma. Indeed, a significant minority—historically 10 percent to 17 percent—of apparent aortic dissection cases are diagnosed as intramural hematoma. Furthermore, many of the acute complications of aortic dissection such as aortic insufficiency, rupture into the pericardium, pleural and pericardial effusions, and branch vessel occlusion also occur with intramural hematoma, raising the question of whether intramural hematoma is just a morphological variant of aortic dissection or a distinct clinical entity with a different course and prognosis.

On axial imaging studies (i.e., CT, MRI, and TEE) intramural hematoma appears as a crescentic or sometimes circumferential thickening of the aortic wall, with no evidence of flow within the hematoma. The appearance of the thickened wall, especially in the ascending aorta, is often subtle on TEE, so the reader must be vigilant when clinical suspicion is high. CT scanning is the modality that best demonstrates the intramural hematoma. On a non-contrast-enhanced CT scan (see Fig. 53–24A) it appears as a continuous, crescentic, high-attenuation area along the aortic wall without evidence of an intimal tear, false lumen, or associated intimal atherosclerotic ulcer. This first examination is followed by a contrast-enhanced CT scan (see Fig. 53–24B), which demonstrates failure of the intramural hematoma to enhance (appearing as a darker crescentic thickening of the aortic wall), thereby excluding communication with the aortic lumen. In some cases, it may be challenging to distinguish intramural hematoma from aortic dissection with thrombosis of the false lumen or from mural thrombus within an aortic aneurysm. With an intramural hematoma, however, the aortic lumen retains its overall size and round shape, unlike the case with aortic dissection or a thrombus-lined aneurysm.

Conversely, intramural hematoma is often not detected by catheter-based contrast aortography, because this technique images the aortic lumen itself—which, in this case, appears normal—and not the aortic wall where the abnormality lies. During the years that contrast aortography was the standard imaging technique for suspected aortic dissection, intramural hematomas often went clinically unrecognized. In fact, the sensitivity of aortography for detecting intramural hematoma is as low as 19 percent[103]; therefore, although a negative aortogram can exclude the presence of classic aortic dissection, it does not reliably exclude the important variant of intramural hematoma.

Although intramural hematoma is now recognized as pathoanatomically distinct from classic aortic dissection, its natural history is still debated. When followed with serial imaging studies, it can have four possible courses: the hematoma may persist (although its thickness may change); it may be reabsorbed, so that the appearance of the aortic wall

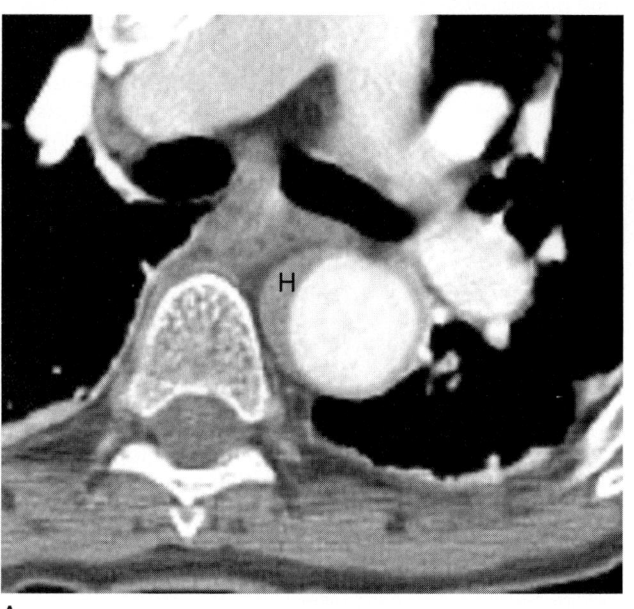

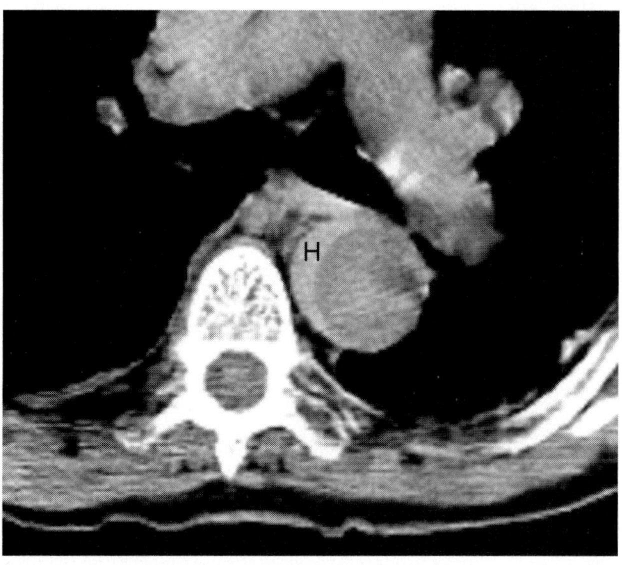

FIGURE 53–24 Intramural hematoma of the descending thoracic aorta. **A,** An axial contrast-enhanced computed tomography (CT) scan at the level of the pulmonary artery demonstrating crescentic dark thickening of the aortic wall (H) that does not enhance, confirming the presence of an intramural hematoma. Note that neither the size nor the shape of the aortic lumen is distorted the way it would typically be in the presence of a classic aortic dissection. **B,** On a non-contrast-enhanced CT scan there is crescentic thickening of the aortic wall that is of increased density (H) compared with blood in the lumen, consistent with an intramural hematoma of the aorta.

returns to normal; it may lead to an aortic aneurysm; or it may convert to a classic aortic dissection, with the development of a typical intimal flap and flow in a false lumen.

In the 1990s, several retrospective reports described the outcomes of intramural hematoma, but the study samples were small. More recently, Sawhney and colleagues[104] performed a review of 160 patients from 11 studies reporting outcomes of aortic intramural hematoma and found that proximal intramural hematoma was associated with a mortality rate of 47 percent when managed medically compared with 24 percent when managed surgically. On the other hand, distal intramural hematoma was associated with a mortality rate of 13 percent with medical management compared with 15 percent with surgical repair. These rates are similar to those for classic aortic dissection as reported by the IRAD[67]: 58 percent for proximal aortic dissection when managed medically compared with 26 percent when managed surgically, and 11 percent for distal aortic dissection with medical management compared with 31 percent with surgical repair. Consequently, most treatment centers currently accept a general management strategy for aortic intramural hematoma similar to that used for classic aortic dissection: proximal aortic involvement is treated surgically[105] and distal aortic involvement is managed medically. Physicians should have a low threshold for proceeding to surgery in patients with distal disease if symptoms persist or evidence of progression is seen, however. Medical management should therefore include serial imaging studies to monitor progression or regression of the intramural hematoma.

It should be noted that several recent reports have suggested that the outcomes associated with proximal intramural hematoma may be more benign than with classic aortic dissection, with a large proportion of patients surviving with medical therapy alone. For example, Song and coworkers[106] reported in-hospital mortality rates for medically managed proximal and distal intramural hematoma of only 7 percent and 1 percent, respectively, both of which are substantially lower than the rates of 47 percent and 13 percent, respectively, reported by Sawhney and coworkers.

How can such dramatic differences be reconciled? It may be that the samples studied were not comparable. In fact, in Song's series, 29 percent of apparent aortic dissection cases were diagnosed as intramural hematoma, a proportion about double what other investigators have reported. It is therefore possible that in this series, more "subtle" cases of intramural hematoma, which would go undetected in other hospitals and which are likely to be associated with a lower risk of progression or rupture, were identified and included. There may in fact be a continuum of risk for intramural hematoma rather than an absolute risk. The morphological features that distinguish intramural hematoma from classic aortic dissection, such as the absence of a patent false lumen, suggest that intramural hematomas are somewhat less likely to rupture. However, factors that increase aortic wall stress, such as large aortic diameters and thick hematomas, could increase the risk of rupture or dissection. Indeed, one recent study of acute intramural hematoma[107] found that a maximum aortic diameter 50 mm or larger was an independent predictor of progression, whereas in another study of patients with distal intramural hematoma managed medically,[108] both a maximum aortic diameter of 40 mm or larger and a maximum aortic wall thickness of 10 mm or larger were independent predictors of progression. These findings confirm that some patients with intramural hematoma may be at considerably lower risk than others, suggesting that baseline differences in patient characteristics could substantially influence outcomes. However, until further studies help to better define those patients at very low risk, we still recommend the strategy of routine aortic surgery for proximal intramural hematoma.[109]

PENETRATING ATHEROSCLEROTIC ULCER. Penetrating atherosclerotic ulcer, first defined in the modern literature in 1986, is an ulceration of an atherosclerotic lesion of the aorta that penetrates the internal elastic lamina and allows hematoma formation within the media of the aortic wall (Fig. 53–25). Although such ulcerations usually occur in the descending thoracic aorta, they may also localize in the arch or rarely in the ascending aorta. The hematoma that results from a penetrating atherosclerotic ulcer usually remains localized or extends several centimeters in length, but a classic false lumen typically does not develop. However, some cases of intramural hematoma of the aorta may in fact result from small penetrating atherosclerotic ulcers that have escaped detection on imaging studies but are later identified at the time of surgery.[110]

Atherosclerotic aortic ulcers penetrate through the media in one-quarter of cases to cause aortic pseudoaneurysms or less often through the adventitia to cause transmural aortic rupture. Rarely, a penetrating atherosclerotic ulcer may progress to an extensive classic aortic dissection. Over time, penetrating atherosclerotic ulcers frequently lead to the late formation of saccular or fusiform aortic aneurysms.

Patients in whom penetrating atherosclerotic ulcers develop tend to be elderly with a history of hypertension and smoking. The majority have evidence of other atherosclerotic cardiovascular disease and as many as half also have a history of a preexisting abdominal or thoracic aortic aneurysm. Initial symptoms include chest and back pain similar to that of aortic dissection, and the majority are hypertensive

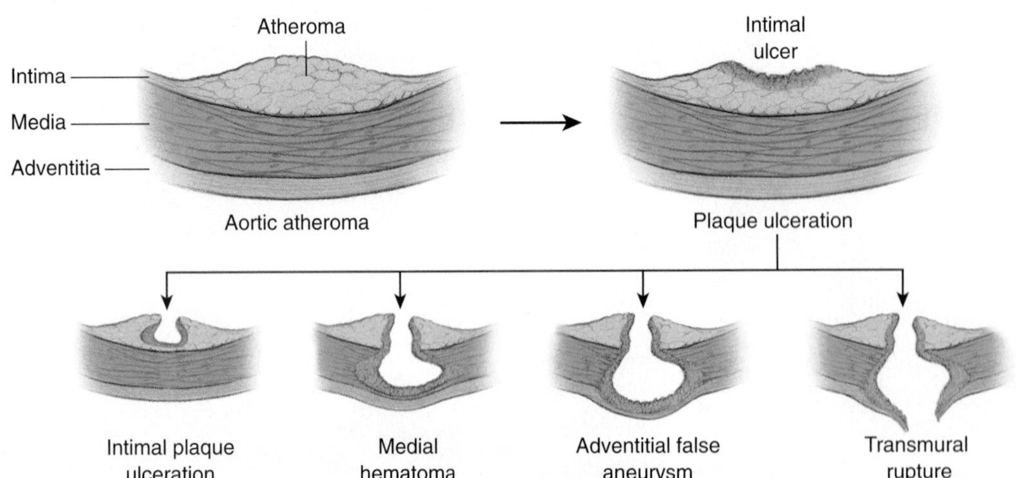

FIGURE 53–25 Evolution of a penetrating atherosclerotic ulcer of the aorta. Once an intimal ulcer has formed, it may then progress to a variable depth. Penetration through the intima causes a medial hematoma, while penetration through the media leads to the formation of a pseudoaneurysm, and perforation through the adventitial layer results in aortic rupture. (From Stanson AW, Kazmier FJ, Hollier LH, et al: Penetrating atherosclerotic ulcers of the thoracic aorta: Natural history and clinicopathological correlations. Ann Vasc Surg 1:15, 1986.)

at initial evaluation. However, since penetrating atherosclerotic ulcers tend to be localized, the vascular compromise or aortic regurgitation that often complicates aortic dissection does not develop.

Chest radiographs often demonstrate a dilated descending thoracic aorta as well as left-sided or bilateral pleural effusions. Aortography had been the diagnostic standard for detecting a penetrating atherosclerotic ulcer, with the lesion appearing as a contrast-filled outpouching in the descending aorta in the absence of an intimal flap or false lumen. However, penetrating atherosclerotic ulcers are now particularly well visualized with the use of CT or MRA (Fig. 53–26), in which the lesion appears as a focal ulceration with thickening of the aortic wall and consistent with an associated intramural hematoma. TEE may identify the presence of a culprit atherosclerotic ulcer in the setting of a visible intramural hematoma, but making the diagnosis is more difficult than with the above mentioned imaging modalities.

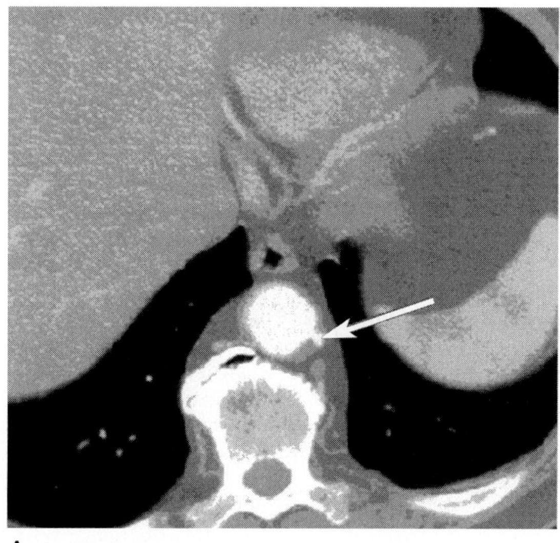

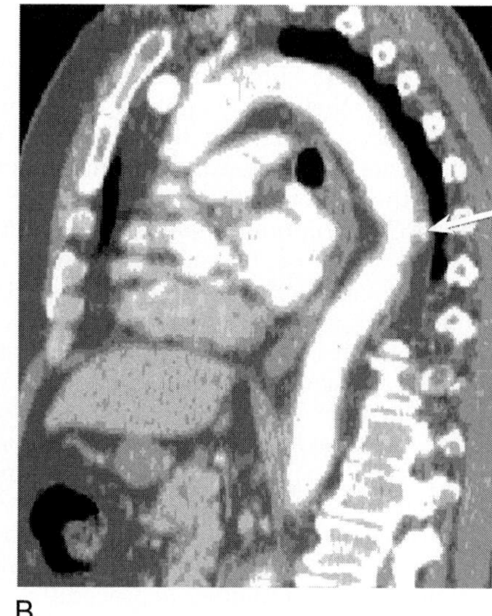

FIGURE 53–26 Contrast-enhanced CT scan through the distal descending aorta demonstrating the presence of a penetrating atherosclerotic ulcer. **A,** An axial image showing a small discrete ulcer (arrow) penetrating the aortic intima and producing a very localized hematoma within the aortic wall. **B,** Computed tomography angiogram in the same patient showing how the ulcer (arrow) projects out from the lumen of the distal descending aorta.

The natural history of a penetrating atherosclerotic ulcer remains largely unclear, and likely differs significantly between patients presenting with symptoms (i.e., acute aortic syndrome) versus without symptoms (i.e., an incidental finding). Coady and colleagues found that the risk of rupture and 1-year mortality are greater among patients with penetrating atherosclerotic ulcer than among those with aortic dissection.[111] At present, no definitive treatment strategy has been agreed upon. Certainly, patients who are hemodynamically unstable or who have evidence of pseudoaneurysm formation or transmural rupture should undergo urgent surgical repair. Continued or recurrent pain, distal embolization, and progressive aneurysmal dilation are also indications for surgery. However, it remains unclear if otherwise stable patients with distal penetrating atherosclerotic ulcers should undergo surgery or can be safely managed medically, as in the case of classic aortic dissection. In a study by Tittle and colleagues[112] of 26 patients with penetrating atherosclerotic ulcer, there was no difference in the 1- or 5-year survival between surgical and medical management strategies, suggesting that surgery may not improve the otherwise poor prognosis. On the other hand, there is growing optimism that transluminal placement of an endovascular stent-graft may become a lower risk alternative to surgery in such patients.

Ganaha and coworkers[113] recently examined the outcomes of 31 patients with penetrating atherosclerotic ulcers, of whom 17 were managed medically, whereas 8 underwent surgical repair and the other 6 underwent stent-grafting for evidence of aortic rupture or impending rupture. Importantly, there was no significant difference in early survival among the three strategies. The authors compared patients with a progressive in-hospital course—defined as aortic rupture, hematoma expansion, or appearance of a distinct false lumen—to those with a stable course. Uncontrolled pain and an enlarging pleural effusion were both highly predictive of a progressive course. CT findings associated with a progressive rather than a stable course included maximum diameter of the ulcer (21 mm versus 12 mm, respectively), maximum depth of the ulcer (14 mm versus 7 mm, respectively), and an ulcer located in the proximal third of the descending aorta rather than more distal. Using these various markers, about half of the patients in their study would have been considered low-risk for a progressive course. We recommend treating patients with such uncomplicated conditions with antihypertensive medications and close monitoring with serial imaging studies, similar to the management of a patient with a distal aortic dissection.

Aortic Trauma

See Chapter 65.

Aortic Atheroembolic Disease

See Chapter 54.

Acute Aortic Occlusion

Acute aortic occlusion is an infrequent, but potentially catastrophic, condition with an early mortality rate of 31 to 52 percent. It is caused by either embolic occlusion of the infrarenal aorta at the bifurcation, known as a "saddle embolus," or acute thrombosis of the abdominal aorta. At least 95 percent of aortic emboli originate from the left side of the heart, typically as a thrombus from the left atrium secondary to atrial fibrillation, particularly in the setting of rheumatic mitral stenosis, or from the left ventricle secondary to myocardial infarction, aneurysm, or dilated cardiomyopathy. Less common cardiac sources of emboli include atrial myxoma, prosthetic valve thrombus, and acute bacterial or fungal endocarditis. Primary thrombosis accounts for the remaining 35 to 92 percent of acute aortic occlusions. Seventy-five to 80 percent of thrombotic aortic occlusions occur in the setting of underlying severe aortoiliac occlusive disease and are frequently precipitated by a low-flow state secondary to heart failure or dehydration. In patients without aortoiliac occlusive disease, a hypercoagulable state may precipitate thrombosis of an abdominal aortic aneurysm and lead to aortic occlusion.[114]

Acute aortic occlusion is in most cases heralded by the sudden onset of excruciating bilateral lower extremity pain, usually radiating from the midportion of the thigh distally and associated with weakness, numbness, and paresthesias. Nonclassic manifestations include sudden onset of bilateral lower extremity weakness, severe hypertension from renal artery involvement, and abdominal pain from mesenteric ischemia. Persistent ischemia may lead to myonecrosis with secondary hypotension, hyperkalemia, myoglobinuria, and acute tubular necrosis. If perfusion is not reestablished within hours, death is almost inevitable.

DIAGNOSIS. Physical examination reveals cold pale extremities that are cyanotic and often exhibit a mottled, reticulated, and reddish blue appearance that may progress to the blue-black color of gangrene. Pulses are notably absent below the abdominal aorta, and capillary refill is absent. Signs of ischemic neuropathy are present and include symmetrical weakness, loss of all modalities of sensation (usually with demarcation at the level of the midthigh), and diminished or absent deep tendon reflexes. When neurological symptoms predominate, patients are often mistakenly thought to have spinal cord infarction or compression and their ischemic symptoms may initially be overlooked. In fact, as many as 11 to 17 percent of such patients first undergo neurological or neurosurgical evaluation before the vascular cause is recognized.

The diagnosis of acute aortic occlusion is confirmed by aortography. While some practitioners suggest that all stable patients should undergo the procedure, others advise prompt surgical intervention without angiography if the diagnosis is strongly suspected, since added delays increase the likelihood of irreversible ischemic damage to the limbs. Aortography is desirable in the presence of concomitant abdominal pain, hypertension, or anuria to evaluate the possibility of renal and mesenteric arterial involvement.

MANAGEMENT. Once a clinical diagnosis of acute aortic occlusion is made, intravenous heparin therapy should be initiated while the patient awaits immediate surgery. A saddle embolus can be removed by using Fogarty balloon-tipped catheters inserted through a transfemoral arterial approach under local anesthesia. If the embolus cannot be retrieved with Fogarty catheters, removal by direct transabdominal aortotomy is undertaken. Patients with thrombotic occlusion generally undergo either direct aortic reconstruction or revascularization with aortofemoral or axillofemoral bypass. The operative mortality rate for acute aortic occlusion is 31 to 40 percent and as high as 85 percent among patients with severe left ventricular dysfunction or a hypercoagulable state. Limb salvage rates are as high as 98 percent. Lifelong anticoagulant therapy is necessary after surgery in almost all cases to prevent recurrent emboli.

Aortoarteritis Syndromes

See Chapters 54 and 82.

Bacterial Infections of the Aorta

Infected aortic aneurysms are rare, with as few as one case per year reported from large medical centers. In an effort to avoid confusion with infections truly of fungal origin, the term *infected aneurysm* has gradually replaced the original designation, *mycotic aneurysm*, used by Osler to define localized dilation in the wall of the aorta caused by sepsis. Although saccular aneurysms are seen most commonly, infections can also cause fusiform and false aneurysms. In a minority of cases, infection may arise in a preexistent aortic aneurysm, typically atherosclerotic ones. Rarely, one may encounter nonaneurysmal bacterial aortitis.

PATHOGENESIS. Aortic infection can arise by several mechanisms. A septic embolus from bacterial endocarditis was once the most common cause but has become rare in the era of efficacious antibiotic treatment of septicemia. Contiguous spread of infection from adjacent sites is also infrequently seen. The most common cause of an infected aneurysm is direct deposition of circulating bacteria in a diseased, atherosclerotic, or traumatized aortic intima, after which organisms penetrate the aortic wall through breeches in intimal integrity to cause microbial arteritis. In some cases, aortic infections occur in patients with impaired immunity as a consequence of chronic disease, immunosuppressive therapy, or immune deficiency, whereas in other cases, the infection is introduced from distant surgical sites or via intraaortic catheterization procedures.[115]

MICROBIOLOGY. Although virtually any organism can infect the aorta, certain bacteria seem to have a proclivity for this site. *Staphylococcus aureus* and *Salmonella* species are consistently the most frequently identified organisms.[115,116] *Salmonella* commonly infects atherosclerotic arteries but can also adhere to a normal aortic wall and directly penetrate an intact intima. Other gram-positive organisms, particularly *Pneumococcus*, and gram-negative organisms can also cause infected aortic aneurysms. *Pseudomonas*, *Bacteroides fragilis*, *Campylobacter fetus*, *Neisseria gonorrhoeae*, and fungal infections are seen less often. Aortic infections with unusual organisms now occur with increasing frequency in the overtly immunocompromised population.

CLINICAL MANIFESTATIONS. Most patients with infected aortic aneurysm are febrile, with extremely high fevers and rigors being common. Symptoms can arise from localized expansion of an infected aneurysm, which is palpable in as many as 50 percent of patients and almost always tender. A tender and pulsatile abdominal mass in a febrile patient should therefore be considered an infected aneurysm until proved otherwise.

Leukocytosis and an elevated erythrocyte sedimentation rate are present in most cases. When positive, blood cultures are helpful in suggesting the diagnosis and identifying the pathogen. In any patient with fever of unknown origin and documented *Salmonella* bacteremia, an arterial source of infection should be considered. The absence of positive blood cultures, however, does not exclude the diagnosis of infected aortic aneurysm, because cultures have been found to be negative in 25 percent of cases.

Although abdominal ultrasonography may identify the presence of an aortic aneurysm, CT scanning is superior in demonstrating associated pathological findings suggestive of an infectious cause. Sometimes the aorta is normal in size when bacterial aortitis is first evaluated, however, so lack of aneurysmal dilation does not exclude the diagnosis. In such cases, if a patient's fever, leukocytosis, and pain persist, follow-up imaging should be performed because the aorta can rapidly dilate during the course of the infection. Aortography can also be used to make the diagnosis and is sometimes performed preoperatively to assist in surgical planning.

The natural history of infected aortic aneurysms is that of expansion and eventual rupture, with extremely rapid progression. *Salmonella* and other gram-negative infections have a greater tendency to early rupture and death. Overall mortality from infected aortic aneurysms is more than 50 percent, despite advances in therapy.

MANAGEMENT. Infected aortic aneurysms require treatment with intravenous antibiotics and most often surgical excision. The standard surgical approach involves resection of the infected aneurysm and infected retroperitoneal tissue, oversewing of the native aorta as stumps, and restoration of distal perfusion by placement of an extraanatomical bypass graft tunneled through unaffected tissue planes to avoid placing a graft in a contaminated region. Antibiotic therapy must be continued postoperatively for at least 6 weeks. Several reports suggest that in selected patients with localized infection and no gross pus, an effective and simpler surgical approach is in situ reconstruction of the aorta with a prosthetic graft[117] or cryopreserved arterial allograft.[118]

Primary Tumors of the Aorta

Primary tumors of the aorta are quite rare, although as a result of improvements in noninvasive imaging techniques, the frequency of reports of such tumors has increased significantly over the past two decades. Most are diagnosed in the seventh to eighth decades of life. The thoracic aorta and abdominal aorta are involved with equal frequency. In several cases, aortic tumors have appeared in association with previously inserted Dacron aortic grafts. Histologically, the majority of primary aortic tumors are classified as sarcomas, with the malignant fibrous histiocytoma subtype especially common.

The majority of primary aortic tumors arise in the intima and grow along the intimal surface and into the aortic lumen to form polypoid masses (often with superimposed thrombus), but they tend to not invade the aortic wall.[119] Intimal tumors may be characterized by symptoms of vascular obstruction from narrowing of the aortic lumen or, more typically, by signs and symptoms of peripheral embolization identical to those of atherothrombotic emboli. Emboli are commonly a mixture of tumor and thrombus, and the correct diagnosis may remain obscure until histological analysis of an embolectomy specimen is completed. Less commonly, aortic tumors arise in the medial or adventitial layers of the aortic wall. Such tumors tend to not invade the aortic lumen but, instead, behave as aggressive mass lesions and cause constitutional symptoms or back pain.

Since primary aortic tumors are so uncommon and their features nonspecific, the diagnosis is rarely considered before surgical exploration or necropsy. However, several imaging modalities can be helpful in suggesting the diagnosis. Aortography demonstrates narrowing of the lumen or an intraluminal filling defect in the presence of an intimal tumor, but it may be negative if the tumor is adventitial. Intraaortic biopsy of an intraluminal aortic mass with intravascular biopsy forceps guided by aortography has been reported.[120] CT scanning can detect intimal tumors but may not easily differentiate these masses from protruding atheromas. MRI may better define both the tumor anatomy and the extent of invasion. Finally, the ability of TEE to image the aortic intima may make it especially useful in the detection of intimal tumors of the thoracic aorta (Fig. 53–27).

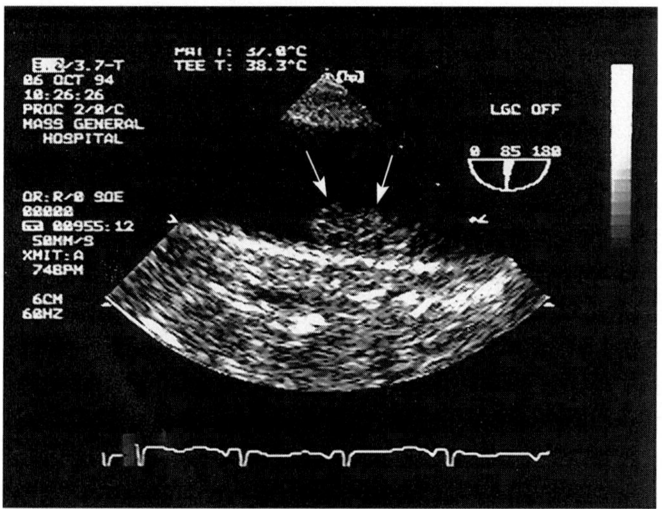

FIGURE 53–27 Transesophageal echocardiogram in a long-axis view of the descending thoracic aorta demonstrating a primary tumor of the aorta (arrows) protruding into the lumen. The tumor, 3.5 cm in length, involves the intimal layer but does not appear to be invading any farther into the aortic wall.

Treatment of primary aortic tumors has met with little success. Because the majority of patients initially have metastatic disease, surgical approaches are often only palliative, to prevent further embolization. Many patients die secondary to the consequences of multiple emboli to vital organs. Of those undergoing surgical therapy, the large majority die within days to months postoperatively.

Acknowledgment

The author wishes to gratefully acknowledge the contributions of Drs. Kim A. Eagle, Roman W. DeSanctis, and Eve E. Slater to previous versions of this chapter in earlier editions of this text.

REFERENCES

1. Fleishmann D, Hastie TJ, Dannegger FC, et al: Quantitative determination of age-related geometric changes in the normal abdominal aorta. J Vasc Surg 33:97, 2001.
2. Stefanadis C, Vlachopoulos C, Karayannacos P, et al: Effect of vasa vasorum flow on structure and function of the aorta in experimental animals. Circulation 91:2669, 1995.
3. Kelly RP, Tunin R, Kass DA: Effect of reduced aortic compliance on cardiac efficiency and contractile function of in situ canine left ventricle. Circ Res 71:490, 1992.
4. Wanhainen A, Bjork M, Boman K, et al: Influence of diagnostic criteria on the prevalence of abdominal aortic aneurysm. J Vasc Surg 34:229, 2001.
5. Lederle FA, Johnson GR, Wilson SE, et al: Prevalence and associations of abdominal aortic aneurysm detected through screening. Aneurysm Detection and Management (ADAM) Veterans Affairs Cooperative Study Group. Ann Intern Med 126:441, 1997.
6. Lederle FA, Johnson GR, Wilson SE, et al: Abdominal aortic aneurysm in women. J Vasc Surg 34:122, 2001.
7. Davies MJ: Aortic aneurysm formation: Lessons from human studies and experimental models. Circulation 98:193, 1998.
8. Lindholt JS, Juul S, Ashton HA, Scott RAP: Indicators of infection *Chlamydia pneumoniae* are associated with expansion of abdominal aortic aneurysm. J Vasc Surg 34:212, 2001.
9. Henderson EL, Geng Y-J, Sukhova GK, et al: Death of smooth muscle cells and expression of mediators of apoptosis by T lymphocytes in human abdominal aortic aneurysms. Circulation 99:96, 1999.
10. McMillan WD, Tamarina NA, Cipollone M, et al: Size matters: The relationship between MMP-9 expression and aortic diameter. Circulation 96:2228, 1997.
11. Longo GM, Xiong W, Greiner TC, et al: Matrix metalloproteinases 2 and 9 work in concert to produce aortic aneurysms. J Clin Invest 110:625, 2002.
12. Prall AK, Longo M, Mayhan WG, et al: Doxycycline in patients with abdominal aortic aneurysms and in mice: Comparison of serum levels and effect on aneurysm growth in mice. J Vasc Surg 35:923, 2002.
13. Curci JA, Mao D, Bohner DG, et al: Preoperative treatment with doxycycline reduces aortic wall expression and activation of matrix metalloproteinases in patients with abdominal aortic aneurysms. J Vasc Surg 31:325, 2000.
14. Baxter BT, Pearce WH, Waltke EA, et al: Prolonged administration of doxycycline in patients with small asymptomatic abdominal aortic aneurysms: Report of a prospective (phase II) multicenter study. J Vasc Surg 36:1, 2002.
15. Vammen S, Lindholt JS, Ostergaard L, et al: Randomized double-blind trial of roxithromycin for prevention of abdominal aortic aneurysm expansion. Br J Surg 88:1066, 2001.
16. Shi G-P, Sukhova GK, Grubb A: Cystatin C deficiency in human atherosclerosis and aortic aneurysms. J Clin Invest 104:1191, 1999.
17. Muluk SC, Gertler JP, Brewster DC, et al: Presentation and patterns of aortic aneurysms in young patients. J Vasc Surg 20:880, 1994.
18. Kiell CS, Ernst CB: Advances in the management of abdominal aortic aneurysm. Adv Surg 26:73, 1993.
19. Lederle FA, Simel DL: Does this patient have abdominal aortic aneurysm? JAMA 281:77, 1999.
20. Fink HA, Lederle FA, Roth CS, et al: The accuracy of physical examination to detect aortic aneurysms. Arch Intern Med 160:833, 2000.
21. Lindholt JS, Vammen S, Juul S, et al: The validity of ultrasonographic scanning as screening method for abdominal aortic aneurysm. Eur J Vasc Endovasc Surg 17:472, 1999.
22. Lederle FA, Wilson SE, Johnson GR, et al: Variability in measurement of abdominal aortic aneurysms. J Vasc Surg 21:945, 1995.
23. Petersen MJ, Cambria RP, Kaufman JA, et al: Magnetic resonance angiography in the preoperative evaluation of abdominal aortic aneurysms. J Vasc Surg 21:891, 1995.
24. Multicentre Aneurysm Screening Study Group: Multicentre aneurysm screening study (MASS): Cost-effectiveness analysis of screening for abdominal aortic aneurysms based on four year results from a randomised controlled trial. BMJ 325:1135, 2002.
25. Crow P, Shaw E, Earnshaw JJ, et al: A single normal ultrasonographic scanning at age 65 years rules out significant aneurysm disease for life in men. Br J Surg 88:941, 2001.
26. Brown LC, Powell JT: Risk factors for aneurysm rupture in patients kept under ultrasound surveillance. UK Small Aneurysm Trial Participants. Ann Surg 230:289, 1999.

27. The United Kingdom Small Aneurysm Trial Participants: Long-term outcomes of immediate repair compared with surveillance of small abdominal aortic aneurysms. N Engl J Med 346:1445, 2002.
28. Lederle FA, Wilson ES, Johnson GR, et al: Immediate repair compared with surveillance of small abdominal aortic aneurysms. N Engl J Med 346:1437, 2002.
29. Thompson RW: Detection and management of small aortic aneurysms. N Engl J Med 346:1484, 2002.
30. Brewster DC, Geller SC, Kaufman JA, et al: Initial experience with endovascular aneurysm repair: Comparison of early results with outcome of conventional open repair. J Vasc Surg 27:992, 1998.
31. Blum U, Voshage G, Lammer J, et al: Endoluminal stent-grafts for infrarenal abdominal aortic aneurysms. N Engl J Med 336:13, 1997.
32. Zarins CK, White RA, Schwarten D, et al: AneuRx stent graft versus open surgical repair of abdominal aortic aneurysms: Multicenter prospective clinical trial. J Vasc Surg 29:292, 1999.
33. Finlayson SR, Birkmeyer JD, Fillinger MF, et al: Should endovascular surgery lower the threshold for repair of abdominal aortic aneurysms? J Vasc Surg 29:973, 1999.
34. Kioka Y, Tanabe A, Kotani Y, et al: Review of coronary artery disease in patients with infrarenal abdominal aortic aneurysm. Circulation 66:1110, 2002.
35. Rihal CS, Eagle KA, Mickel MC, et al: Surgical therapy for coronary artery disease among patients with combined coronary artery and peripheral vascular disease. Circulation 91:46, 1995.
36. Brophy C, Tilson JE, Tilson MD: Propranolol delays the formation of aneurysms in the male blotchy mouse. J Surg Res 44:687, 1988.
37. The Propranolol Aneurysm Trial Investigators: The propranolol for small abdominal aortic aneurysms: Results of a randomized trial. J Vasc Surg 35:72, 2002.
38. Guo D, Hasham S, Kuang S-Q, et al: Familial thoracic aortic aneurysms and dissections. Circulation 103:2461, 2001.
39. Coady MA, Davis RR, Roberts M, et al: Familial patterns of thoracic aortic aneurysms. Arch Surg 134:361, 1999.
40. Biddinger A, Rocklin M, Coselli J, Milewicz DM: Familial thoracic aortic dilatations and dissections: A case control study. J Vasc Surg 25:506, 1997.
41. Milewicz DM, Chen H, Park E-S, et al: Reduced penetrance and variable expressivity of familial thoracic aneurysms/dissections. Am J Cardiol 82:474, 1998.
42. Vaughan CJ, Casey M, He J, et al: Identification of a chromosome 11q23.2-q24 locus for familial aortic aneurysm disease, a genetically heterogeneous disorder. Circulation 103:2469, 2001.
43. Nistri S, Sorbo MD, Marin M, et al: Aortic root dilatation in young men with normally functioning bicuspid aortic valves. Heart 82:19, 1999.
44. Nkomo VT, Enriquez-Sarano M, Ammash NM, et al: Bicuspid aortic valve associated with aortic dilatation: A community-based study. Arterioscler Thromb Vasc Biol 23:351, 2003.
45. DeSa M, Moshkovitz Y, Butany J, David TE: Histologic abnormalities of the ascending aorta and pulmonary trunk in patients with bicuspid aortic valve disease: Clinical relevance to the Ross procedure. J Thorac Cardiovasc Surg 118:588, 1999.
46. Huntington K, Hunter AGW, Chan K-L: A prospective study to assess the frequency of familial clustering of congential bicuspid aortic valve. J Am Coll Cardiol 30:1809, 1997.
47. Fedak PWM, Verma S, David T, et al: Clinical and pathophysiological implications of a bicuspid aortic valve. Circulation 106:900, 2002.
48. Davies RR, Goldstein LJ, Coady MA, et al: Yearly rupture or dissection rates for thoracic aortic aneurysms: Simple prediction based on size. Ann Thorac Surg 73:17, 2002.
49. Griepp RB, Ergin A, Gall JD, et al: Natural history of descending thoracic and thoracoabdominal aneurysms. Ann Thorac Surg 67:1927, 1999.
50. Dapunt OE, Galla JD, Sadeghi AM, et al: The natural history of thoracic aortic aneurysms. J Thorac Cardiovasc Surg 107:1323, 1994.
51. Johansson G, Markström U, Swedenborg J: Ruptured thoracic aortic aneurysms: A study of incidence and mortality rates. J Vasc Surg 21:985, 1995.
52. Devereux RB, Roman MJ: Aortic disease in Marfan's syndrome. N Engl J Med 340:1358, 1999.
53. Sundt TM, Mora BN, Moon MR, et al: Options for repair of a bicuspid aortic valve and ascending aortic aneurysm. Ann Thorac Surg 69;1333, 2000.
54. Russo CF, Massett S, Garatti A, et al: Aortic complications after bicuspid aortic valve replacement: Long-term results. Ann Thorac Surg 74:S1773, 2002.
55. Gott VL, Gillinov AM, Pyeritz RE, et al: Aortic root replacement: Risk factor analysis of a seventeen-year experience with 270 patients. J Thorac Cardiovasc Surg 109:536, 1995.
56. David TE, Ivanov J, Armstrong S, et al: Aortic valve-sparing operations in patients with aneurysms of the aortic root or ascending aorta. Ann Thorac Surg 74:S1758, 2002.
57. Moon MR, Sundt TM: Influence of retrograde cerebral perfu-sion during aortic arch procedures. Ann Thorac Surg 74:426, 2002.
58. Hagl C, Ergin MA, Galla JD, et al: Neurologic outcome after ascending aorta-aortic arch operations: Effect of brain protection technique in high-risk patients. J Thorac Cardiovasc Surg 121:1107, 2001.
59. Kazui T, Washiyama N, Muhammad BAH, et al: Improved results of atherosclerotic arch aneurysm operations with a refined technique. J Thorac Cardiovasc Surg 121:491, 2001.
60. Estera AL, Miller CC, Porat EE, et al: Staged repair of extensive aortic aneurysms. Ann Thorac Surg 74:S1803, 2002.
61. Cambria RP, Davison JK, Zannetti S, et al: Clinical experience with epidural cooling for spinal cord protection during thoracic and thoracoabdominal aneurysm repair. J Vasc Surg 25:234, 1997.
62. Coselli JS, LeMaire SA, Koksoy C, et al: Cerebrospinal fluid drainage reduces paraplegia following thoracoabdominal aortic aneurysm repair: Results of a randomized clinical trial. J Vasc Surg 35:635, 2002.
63. Coselli JS, Conkin LD, LeMaire SA: Thoracoabdominal aortic aneurysm repair: Review and update of current strategies. Ann Thorac Surg 74:S1881, 2002.
64. Dake MD, Miller DC, Mitchell RS, et al: The "first generation" of endovascular stent-grafts for patients with aneurysms of the descending thoracic aorta. J Thorac Cardiovasc Surg 116:689, 1998.
65. Shores J, Berger KR, Murphy EA, Pyeritz RE: Progression of aortic dilatation and the benefit of long-term β-adrenergic blockade in Marfan's syndrome. N Engl J Med 330:1335, 1994.
66. Meszaros I, Morocz J, Szlavi J, et al: Epidemiology and clinicopathology of aortic dissection: A population-based longitudinal study over 27 years. Chest 117:1271, 2000.
67. Hagan PG, Nienaber CA, Isselbacher EM, et al: International Registry of Acute Aortic Dissection (IRAD): New insights into an old disease. JAMA 283:897, 2000.
68. Eagle KA, Isselbacher EM, DeSanctis W: Cocaine-related aortic dissection in perspective. Circulation 105:1529, 2002.
69. Elkayam U, Ostzega E, Shotan A, Mehra A: Cardiovascular problems in pregnant women with the Marfan syndrome. Ann Intern Med 123:117, 1995.
70. Januzzi JL, Sabatine MS, Eagle KA, et al: Iatrogenic aortic dissection. Am J Cardiol 89:623, 2002.
71. von Kodolitsch Y, Simic O, Schwartz A, et al: Predictors of proximal aortic dissection at the time of aortic valve replacement. Circulation 100(Suppl 2):287, 1999.
72. Slater EE, DeSanctis RW: The clinical recognition of dissecting aortic aneurysm. Am J Med 60:625, 1976.
73. Spittell PC, Spittell JA Jr, Joyce JW, et al: Clinical features and differential diagnosis of aortic dissection: Experience with 236 cases (1980 through 1990). Mayo Clin Proc 68:642, 1993.
74. Nallamothu BK, Mahta RH, Saint S, et al: Syncope in acute aortic dissection: Diagnostic, prognostic, and clinical implications. Am J Med 133:468, 2002.
75. Kim MH, Eagle KA, Isselbacher EM: Bayesian persuasion. Circulation 100:e68, 1999.
76. Bossone E, Rampoldi V, Nienaber CA, et al: Usefulness of pulse deficits to predict in-hospital complications and mortality in patients with acute type A aortic dissection. Am J Cardiol 89:851, 2002.
77. Kamp TJ, Goldschmidt-Clermont PJ, Brinker JA, Resar JR: Myocardial infarction, aortic dissection, and thrombolytic therapy. Am Heart J 128:1234, 1994.
78. Bansal RC, Chandrasekaran K, Ayala K, Smith D: Frequency and explanation of false negative diagnosis of aortic dissection by aortography and transesophageal echocardiography. J Am Coll Cardiol 25:1393, 1995.
79. Ballal RS, Nanda NC, Gatewood R, et al: Usefulness of transesophageal echocardiography in assessment of aortic dissection. Circulation 84:1903, 1991.
80. Armstrong WF, Bach DS, Carey LM, et al: Clinical and echocardiographic findings in patients with suspected acute aortic dissection. Am Heart J 136:1051, 1998.
81. Moore AG, Eagle KA, Bruckman D, et al: Choice of computed tomography, transesophageal echocardiography, magnetic resonance imaging, and aortography in acute aortic dissection: International Registry of Acute Aortic Dissection (IRAD). Am J Cardiol 89:1235, 2002.
82. Rizzo RJ, Aranki SF, Aklog L, et al: Rapid noninvasive diagnosis and surgical repair of acute ascending aortic dissection. J Thorac Cardiovasc Surg 108:567, 1994.
83. Kern MJ, Serota H, Callicoat P, et al: Use of coronary arteriography in the preoperative management of patients undergoing urgent repair of the thoracic aorta. Am Heart J 119:143, 1990.
84. Penn MS, Smedira N, Lytle B, Brener SJ: Does coronary angiography before emergency aortic surgery affect in-hospital mortality? J Am Coll Cardiol 35:889, 2000.
85. Creswell LL, Kouchoukos NT, Cox JL, Rosenbloom M: Coronary artery disease in patients with type A aortic dissection. Ann Thorac Surg 59:585, 1995.
86. Murphy MB, Murray C, Shorten GD: Fenoldopam: A selective peripheral dopamine-receptor agonist for the treatment of hypertension. N Engl J Med 345:1548, 2001.
87. Isselbacher EM, Cigarroa JE, Eagle KA: Cardiac tamponade complicating proximal aortic dissection: Is pericardiocentesis harmful? Circulation 90:2375, 1994.
88. Sabik JF, Lytle BW, Blackstone EH, et al: Long-term effectiveness of operations for ascending aortic dissections. J Thorac Cardiovasc Surg 119:946, 2000.
89. Hirotani T, Kameda T, Kumamoto T, Shirota S: Results of a total aortic arch replacement of an acute aortic arch dissection. J Thorac Cardiovasc Surg 120:686, 2000.
90. Movsowitz HD, Levine RA, Hilgenberg AD, Isselbacher EM: Transesophageal echocardiographic description of the mechanisms of aortic regurgitation in acute type A aortic dissection: Implications for aortic valve repair. J Am Coll Cardiol 36:884, 2000.
91. Bavaria JE, Brinster DR, Gorman RC, et al: Advances in the treatment of acute type a dissection: An integrated approach, Ann Thorac Surg 74:S1848, 2002.
92. Kazui T, Washiyama N, Bashar AHM, et al: Role of biologic glue repair of proximal aortic dissection in the development of early and midterm redissection of the aortic root. Ann Thorac Surg 72:509, 2001.
93. Slonim SM, Nyman U, Semba CP, et al: Aortic dissection: Percutaneous management of ischemic complications with endovascular stents and balloon fenestration. J Vasc Surg 23:241, 1996.
94. Lauterbach SE, Cambria RP, Brewster DC, et al: Contemporary management of aortic branch compromise resulting from acute aortic dissection. J Vasc Surg 33:1185, 2001.
95. Nienaber CA, Fattori R, Lund G, et al: Nonsurgical reconstruction of thoracic aortic dissection by stent-graft placement. N Engl J Med 340:1539, 1999.
96. Dake MD, Kato N, Mitchell RS, et al: Endovascular stent-graft placement for the treatment of acute aortic dissection. N Engl J Med 340:1546, 1999.
97. Januzzi JL, Sabatine MS, Choi JC, et al: Refractory systemic hypertension following type B aortic dissection. Am J Cardiol 88:686, 2001.
98. Neri E, Sassi S, Massetti M, et al: Nonocclusive intestinal ischemia in patients with acute aortic dissection. J Vasc Surg 36:738, 2002.
99. Doroghazi RM, Slater EE, DeSanctis RW, et al: Long-term survival of patients with treated aortic dissection. J Am Coll Cardiol 3:1026, 1984.

100. Fattori R, Bacchi-Reggiani L, Bertaccini P, et al: Evolution of aortic dissection after surgical repair. Am J Cardiol 86:868, 2000.
101. Bernard Y, Zimmermann H, Chocron S, et al: False lumen patency as a predictor of late outcome in aortic dissection. Am J Cardiol 87:1378, 2001.
102. Neya K, Omoto R, Kyo S, et al: Outcome of Stanford type B acute aortic dissection. Circulation 86(Suppl 2):1, 1992.
103. Vilacosta I, San Roman JA, Ferreiros J, et al: Natural history and serial morphology of aortic intramural hematoma: A novel variant of aortic dissection. Am Heart J 134:495, 1997.
104. Sawhney NS, DeMaria AN, Blanchard DG: Aortic intramural hematoma: An increasingly recognized and potentially fatal entity. Chest 120:1340, 2001.
105. von Kodolitsch Y, Csosz SK, Koschyk DH, et al: Intramural hematoma of the aorta: Predictors of progression to dissection and rupture. Circulation 107:1158, 2003.
106. Song J-K, Kim H-S, Song JM, et al: Outcomes of medically treated patients with aortic intramural hematoma. Am J Med 113:244, 2002.
107. Kaji S, Nishigami K, Akasaka T, et al: Prediction of progression or regression of type A aortic intramural hematoma by computed tomography. Circulation 100(suppl II):II281, 1999.
108. Sueyoshi E, Imada T, Sakamoto I, et al: Analysis of predictive factors for progression of type B aortic intramural hematoma with computed tomography. J Vasc Surg 35:1179, 2002.
109. Isselbacher EM: Intramural hematoma of the aorta: Should we let down our guard? Am J Med 113:181, 2002.
110. Muluk SC, Kaufman JA, Torchiana DF, et al: Diagnosis and treatment of thoracic aortic intramural hematoma. J Vasc Surg 24:1022, 1996.
111. Coady MA, Rizzo JA, Hammond GL, et al: Penetrating ulcer of the thoracic aorta: How do we recognize it? How do we manage it? J Vasc Surg 27:1006, 1998.
112. Tittle SL, Lynch RJ, Cole PE, et al: Midterm follow-up of penetrating ulcer and intramural hematoma of the aorta. J Thorac Cardiovasc Surg 123:1051, 2002.
113. Ganaha F, Miller DC, Sugimoto K, et al: Prognosis of aortic intramural hematoma with and without penetrating atherosclerotic ulcer: A clinical and radiological analysis. Circulation 106:342, 2002.
114. Babu SC, Shah PM, Nitahara J: Acute aortic occlusion: Factors that influence outcome. J Vasc Surg 21:567, 1995.
115. Muller BT, Wegener OR, Grabitz K, et al: Mycotic aneurysms of the thoracic and abdominal aorta and iliac arteries: Experience with anatomic and extra-anatomic repair in 33 cases. J Vasc Surg 33:106, 2001.
116. Williamson WK, Keller FS: SCVIR annual meeting film panel session: Diagnosis and discussion of Case 4. J Vasc Interv Radiol 12:544, 2001.
117. Oderich GS, Panneton JM, Bower TC, et al: Infected aortic aneurysms: Aggressive presentation, complicated early outcome, and durable results. J Vasc Surg 34:900, 2001.
118. Leseche G, Castier Y, Petit M-D, et al: Long-term results of cryopreserved arterial allograft reconstruction in infected prosthetic grafts and mycotic aneurysms of the abdominal aorta. J Vasc Surg 34:616, 2001.
119. Khan A, Jilani F, Kaye S, Greenberg BR: Aortic wall sarcoma with tumor emboli and peripheral ischemia: Case report with review of literature. Am J Clin Oncol 20:73, 1997.
120. Ronaghi AH, Roberts AC, Rosenkrantz H: Intraaortic biopsy of a primary aortic tumor. J Vasc Interv Radiol 5:777, 1994.

CHAPTER 54

Peripheral Arterial Diseases

Mark A. Creager • Peter Libby

The term *peripheral arterial disease* (PAD) generally refers to atherosclerosis that obstructs the blood supply to the lower or upper extremities. The term *peripheral vascular disease* has less specificity because it encompasses a group of diseases affecting blood vessels, including not only PAD but also vasculitis, vasospasm, venous thrombosis, venous insufficiency, and lymphatic disorders.

Traditionally, cardiologists have devoted most of their efforts to the diagnosis and treatment of arterial disease of the coronary tree. Although cardiology training and practice often accord a place to diseases of the aorta, focus on the disease of the peripheral arteries has lagged. PAD strongly correlates with risk of major cardiovascular events, since it frequently associates with coronary and cerebral atherosclerosis. Moreover, symptoms of PAD, including intermittent claudication, jeopardize quality of life and independence for many patients. In contrast to coronary artery afflictions, PAD is commonly underdiagnosed and undertreated. Thus, practitioners of cardiology have increasing interest in the diagnosis and management of PAD. This chapter provides a framework for the approach to the diagnosis and management of the patient with PAD.

Epidemiology

The prevalence of PAD varies depending on the population studied, the diagnostic method used, and whether symptoms are included to derive estimates. Most epidemiological studies have used a noninvasive measurement, the ankle/brachial index (ABI), to diagnose PAD. The ABI is the ratio of the ankle to brachial systolic blood pressure and is described in greater detail later in this chapter. In relatively large population-based studies conducted in the United States, Europe, and the Middle East, the prevalence of PAD based on abnormal ABI ranged from 4.6 to 29 percent (Table 54–1).[1-5] In a free-living population, PAD was detected in less than 3 percent of persons younger than 60 years of age, but in more than 20 percent of those 75 years and older and 27 percent greater in men than in women.[6] In other studies, however, women had similar or greater prevalence of PAD. These aggregate data indicate that some 8 to 10 million individuals in the United States have PAD.

Questionnaires specifically designed to elicit symptoms of intermittent claudication can assess the prevalence of symptomatic disease in these populations. Estimates have varied depending on the age and gender of the population but generally indicate that only one-third to one-half of patients with PAD have symptoms of claudication. Overall, the estimated prevalence of claudication ranges from 1.0 to 4.5 percent of a population typically older than 40 years of age.[1,2] The prevalence and incidence of claudication increase with age and are greater in men than in women in most but not all studies (Fig. 54–1).[1,2,6]

There is less information regarding the incidence of critical limb ischemia, but it is estimated at 400 to 450 per million population per year.[1] The incidence of amputation ranges from 112 to 250 per million population per year.

Contribution of Risk Factors (see Chap. 36)

The well-known modifiable risk factors associated with coronary atherosclerosis also contribute to atherosclerosis of the peripheral circulation. Cigarette smoking, diabetes mellitus, dyslipidemia, hypertension, and hyperhomocysteinemia increase the risk of PAD (Table 54–2). Data derived from several observational studies (including the Edinburgh Artery Study, the Framingham Heart Study, and the Cardiovascular Health Study, among others) indicates a two- to fivefold increase in the risk of developing PAD in smokers.[1,2,7] Approximately 84 to 90 percent of patients with claudication are current or ex-smokers.[8] Progression of disease to critical limb ischemia and limb loss is more likely to occur in patients who continue to smoke than in those who stop.[9] Smoking can even increase the risk of developing PAD more than it does coronary artery disease. Patients with diabetes mellitus often have extensive and severe PAD and a greater propensity for vascular calcification.[10] Involvement of the femoral and popliteal arteries resembles that of nondiabetic persons, but distal disease affecting the tibial and peroneal arteries occurs more fre-

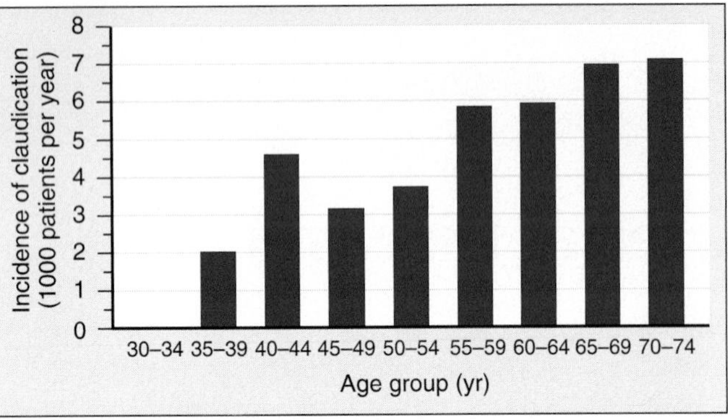

FIGURE 54–1 Age-related incidence of intermittent claudication derived from large population-based studies. (From Dormandy JA, Rutherford RB: Management of peripheral arterial disease (PAD), TASC Working Group. J Vasc Surg 31:51, 2000.)

TABLE 54–1 The Prevalence of Peripheral Arterial Disease

Study/Location	Population (No.)	Age (years)	Prevalence (%)
San Diego	613	38-82	11.7
The Jerusalem Lipid Research Clinic Prevalence Study	1592	≥35	4.6
The Edinburgh Artery Study	1592	55-74	9.0
The Cardiovascular Health Study	5084	≥65	12.4
The Rotterdam Study	7715	≥55	19.1
The Limburg PAOD Study	3650	40-78	12.4
The Strong Heart Study	4549	45-74	5.3
The PARTNERS Program	6979	50-69*; ≥70	29
The Framingham Offspring Study	3313	≥40	3.6

*Age 50-69 plus diabetes or cigarette smoking.

quently.[11] The risk of developing PAD increases two- to fourfold in patients with diabetes mellitus.[7] Among patients with PAD, diabetic patients are more likely to have an amputation than nondiabetic patients.

Abnormalities in lipid metabolism also are associated with an increased prevalence of PAD. Elevations in total or low-density lipoprotein (LDL) cholesterol increase the risk of developing PAD and claudication in some studies but not in others.[7,12,13] The odds ratio for developing claudication in the Framingham Heart Study was 1.2 for each 40 mg/dl increase in total cholesterol.[14] In a cohort of patients participating in a Lipid Research Clinic protocol, however, no association was found between LDL cholesterol and PAD based on a multiple logistic regression analysis that included cigarette smoking, blood pressure, glucose, and obesity.[6] Hypertriglyceridemia independently predicts risk for PAD.[7] Increased levels of lipoprotein(a) impart a twofold increased risk of developing PAD, with higher levels associated with a greater risk for critical limb ischemia.[15]

Hypertension increased the risk of claudication in the Framingham and the Framingham Offspring Studies, and the risk increased proportionally with the severity of hypertension.[5,16] Similarly, in the Edinburgh Artery Study, elevations in systolic blood pressure correlated with PAD. In the Limburg study, diastolic hypertension was associated with PAD.[17] However, not all epidemiological studies have found a link between hypertension and PAD.

TABLE 54–2 Risk of Peripheral Arterial Disease in Persons with Modifiable Risk Factors

Risk Factor	Estimated Relative Risk
Cigarette smoking	2.0-5.0
Diabetes mellitus	3.0-4.0
Hypertension	1.1-2.2
Hypercholesterolemia (per 40-50 mg/dl increase in total cholesterol)	1.2-1.4
Fibrinogen (per 0.7 g/liter increase in fibrinogen)	1.35
C-reactive protein	2.1
Hyperhomocysteinemia	2.0-3.2

Hyperhomocysteinemia increases the risk of developing atherosclerosis (see Chap. 36). In a meta-analysis of studies relating homocysteine level to atherosclerotic disease, the odds ratio for PAD in patients with increased homocysteine levels was 6.8.[18] Some 30 to 40 percent of patients with PAD have high levels of homocysteine. The plasma levels of B complex vitamins, including folate, cobalamin, and pyridoxal 5′ phosphate, all inversely relate to plasma homocysteine concentration, and patients taking B vitamin supplements have a lower risk of vascular disease.[19]

Fibrinogen levels also correlate with risk of developing PAD.[5,20] In the Edinburgh Artery Study, the risk for developing PAD increased 35 percent over 5 years for each 0.70 g/liter increase in fibrinogen.[21] Patients with PAD have elevated levels of C-reactive protein, a serological marker of systemic inflammation. In the Physicians' Health Study, the relative risk of developing PAD among men in the highest quartile for C-reactive protein concentrations was 2.5 (see Chap. 36).[13,22]

The risk of developing PAD and intermittent claudication increases progressively with the burden of contributing factors. In the Framingham study, the probability of claudication in a 70-year-old man whose only risk factor was smoking versus nonsmoking was 2.5 percent versus 0.8 percent per 4 years. In a 70-year-old male smoker who was also hypertensive, hypercholesterolemic, and diabetic, the risk increased to 24 percent per 4 years (Fig. 54–2).[14] Similar observations apply to women.

Pathobiology

Heterogeneity of Blood Vessels in Different Circulatory Beds

Atherosclerosis preferentially affects certain locations in the circulation. As discussed in Chapter 35, atheromatous lesions tend to form at flow dividers and branch points in arteries and usually spare veins. Recent progress has increased the understanding of the link between hydrodynamics of the circulation and the cellular and molecular mechanisms of atherosclerosis, and the atheroprotective functions of vascular wall cells. Chapter 35 discusses the focality of atherosclerosis in terms of local hemodynamic differences. Other questions remain, however: Are blood vessels intrinsically different in particular regions of the circulation? Do regional variations in the propensity for atherosclerosis merely depend on the external hemodynamic forces that impinge upon them? Indeed, vessels in different beds have distinct

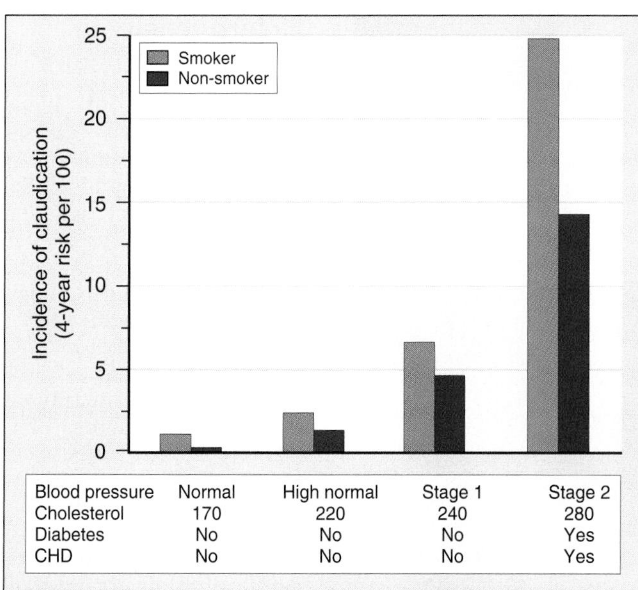

Blood pressure	Normal	High normal	Stage 1	Stage 2
Cholesterol	170	220	240	280
Diabetes	No	No	No	Yes
CHD	No	No	No	Yes

FIGURE 54–2 The incidence of intermittent claudication in the Framingham Heart Study in smokers and nonsmokers is compounded by an increased burden of risk factors. (From Murabito JM, D'Agostino RB, Silbershatz H, Wilson WF: Intermittent claudication: A risk profile from the Framingham Heart Study. Circulation 96:44, 1997.)

morphological, physiological, and pharmacological features, indicating intrinsic heterogeneity. Recent advances help us to understand the biological basis of differences among blood vessels. This section considers, in turn, new information regarding the development of blood vessels related to arterial heterogeneity, differences in functions of blood vessels depending on the circulatory bed, and finally, whether the mechanisms leading to clinical manifestations of arterial disease vary from one circulatory bed (e.g., the coronary circulation) and other arteries (e.g., the carotid, the aorta, or the femoral).

Developmental Biology of the Heterogeneity Among Blood Vessels

Endothelial cells have a common origin but acquire bed-specific characteristics during development.[23] The endothelial cells that form the inner lining of all blood vessels arise during embryogenesis from regions known as the blood islands, located on the embryo's periphery. Angioblasts, the predecessors of the endothelial cells, share this site with the precursors of blood cells. Despite arising from the same site, cells display considerable heterogeneity even during embryological and early postnatal development. Although endothelial cells presumably derive from a common precursor, the signals they encounter during vessel development differ. As rudimentary blood vessels begin to form, endothelial precursors interact with surrounding cells. The interchange permits spatial and temporal gradients of various stimuli and their receptors on the endothelial cells, leading to this cell type's heterogeneity in the adult.

Recent evidence has indicated that the cells that make up various compartments of the arterial wall can originate from bone marrow during postnatal life as well as from their traditional embryological sources. In particular, peripheral blood appears to contain endothelial precursor cells that may help the repair of areas of endothelial desquamation. Moreover, in injured or transplanted arteries, smooth muscle cells of apparent bone marrow origin can take up residence in the intima or media.[24,25] The endothelial progenitor cells bear characteristic markers such as CD133, CD34, and vascular endothelial growth factor receptor-2.[26]

Differential expression of endothelial genes in various types of blood vessels depends on transcriptional regulation by the local environment. For example, the promoter region of the gene that encodes von Willebrand factor directs expression in the endothelium of brain and heart microvessels but not in larger arteries. Indeed, co-culture of endothelial cells with cardiac myocytes, but not other cell types, could selectively activate a von Willebrand factor gene promoter construct.[27] Likewise, endothelial nitric oxide synthase gene activity in the heart shows bed-specific regulation.[28] Members of the EPH family of tyrosine kinase receptors and their ligands, known as ephrins, display heterogeneous expressions in arterial versus venous endothelial cells during development.[29] In the adult, arterial endothelial and smooth muscle cells, but not venous vascular cells, express EphrinB2.[30] This finding supports a stable lineage difference between cells that make up arteries and veins. These examples illustrate the molecular diversity of cells' location in the circulation. Phage display techniques have begun to substantiate the in vivo significance of vascular cell heterogeneity in atherogenesis.[31,32]

Smooth Muscle Cells Derive from Several Local Sources During Development

In contrast to endothelial cells thought to derive from a common precursor, smooth muscle cells can arise from many sources.[33] After endothelial cells form tubes, the rudimentary precursor of blood vessels, they recruit the cells that will become smooth muscle, or pericytes (smooth muscle-like cells associated with microvessels). In the descending aorta and arteries of the lower body, the regional mesoderm serves as the source of smooth muscle precursors. The mesodermal cells in somites give rise to the smooth muscle cells that invest much of the distal aorta and its branches. In arteries of the upper body, however, smooth muscle cells can actually derive from a completely different germ layer, neurectoderm rather than mesoderm. Before the neural tube closes, neurectodermal cells migrate and become the precursors of smooth muscle cells in the ascending aorta and some of its branches, including the carotid arteries (Fig. 54–3).[34] Smooth muscle cells in the coronary arteries derive from mesoderm, but in a special way. The precursors of coronary artery smooth muscle cells arise from yet another embryological source, a structure known as the *proepicardial organ*.[35]

As in the case of endothelial cells, smooth muscle cells show molecular heterogeneity early during development.[36] For example, the promoter of a characteristic smooth muscle gene, known as SM22, drives gene expression in venous but not arterial smooth muscle cells during embryogenesis.[37] A specific transcription factor known as dHAND signals the recruitment of mesenchyme by endothelial cells in an anatomically heterogeneous manner during development. In particular, dHAND regulation participates selectively in recruitment of mesenchyme in upper body blood vessels versus those of the more caudal portions of the embryo.[38] A CArG box-dependent enhancer within the regulatory regions of the cysteine-rich protein 1 gene directs this protein's expression in arterial but not venous or visceral smooth muscle cells.[39] These findings also point to molecular distinctions between the cells that compose different types of vessels.

Clinical Implications of Vascular Developmental Biology

Far from being of mere theoretical concern, the developmental biology of the arterial tree has important clinical implications in terms of issues that arise in daily practice. The distinct embryonic origins of smooth muscle cells in various arteries can help explain why some regions of the arterial tree have particular predilection to atherogenesis. Although local hydrodynamics doubtless control the expression of genes that protect against or promote atherogenesis (see Chap. 35), the cellular substrate acted on by biomechanical forces varies, as described earlier.

Curiously, certain regions of the arterial tree develop intimal "cushions" early in life. These cushions consist of regions of intimal expansion populated by smooth muscle cells and extracellular matrix (Fig. 54–4). Two regions of intimal cushion formation of particular consequence for cardiologists include the proximal left anterior descending coronary artery and the carotid siphon.[40,41] The intimal cushion in the proximal left anterior descending coronary artery begins to form even during intrauterine life. It progresses rapidly in early postnatal life, leading to intimal cushions in the proximal left anterior coronary artery in all humans by 2 years of age. It remains unclear to what extent lineage

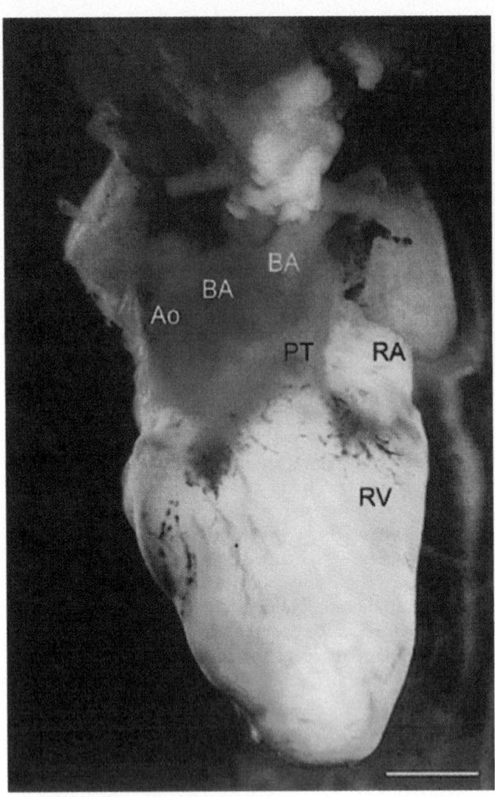

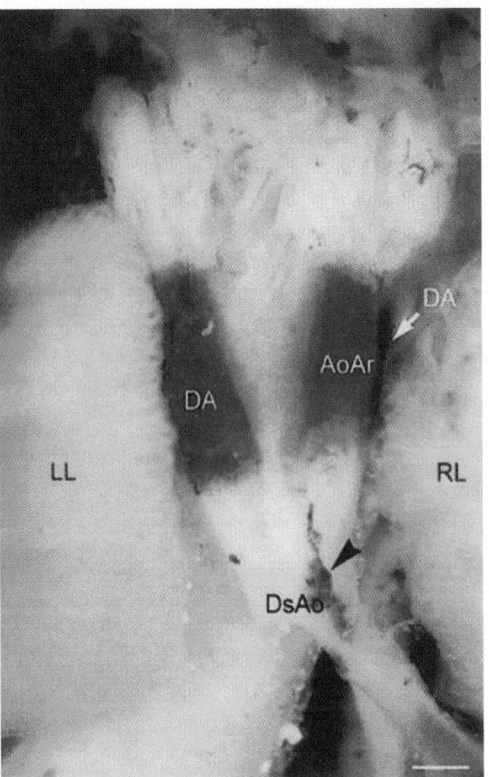

FIGURE 54–3 **Left,** Anterior view of an embryonic chick heart in which cells of neural crest origin stain blue. Note the focal localization of cells derived from neural crest in the great arteries as well as the cardiac innervation plexus spread over the ventricles. Ao = aorta; BA = brachiocephalic artery; PT = pulmonary trunk; RA = right atrium; RV = right ventricle. Bar = 750 μm. **Right,** Posterior view of a chicken embryo heart-lung whole-mount similarly tagged. Note the sharp demarcation in the localization of the blue neural crest-derived cells in the aortic arch (AoAr) and dorsal aorta (DA) before they unite to form the descending aorta (DsAo). The arrowhead indicates neural crest–derived neural tissue. LL and RL indicate left and right lung, respectively. Bar = 250 μm. (From Bergwerff M, Verberne ME, DeRuiter MC, et al: Neural crest cell contribution to the developing circulatory system. Circ Res 82:221, 1998.)

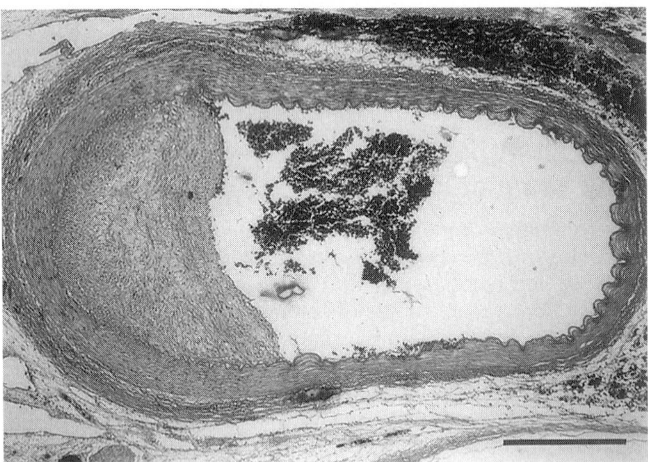

FIGURE 54–4 An intimal cushion shown in a cross-section through the internal carotid artery of a 10-week-old male infant. Areas where intimal cushions form in early life tend to develop atheroma more commonly in later years. The bar shows 0.5 mm. (From Weniger WJ, Muller GB, Reiter C, et al: Intimal hyperplasia of the infant parasellar carotid artery: A potential developmental factor in atherosclerosis and SIDS. Circ Res 85:970, 1999.)

differences versus local hemodynamic forces contribute to the formation of these intimal cushions in arteries prone to develop atherosclerosis. These cushions of smooth muscle and connective tissue form the "soil" in which atheromatous lesions can grow in later life.[42]

Heterogeneity in Vascular Functions

The functions of blood vessels differ in various regions of the circulation, as evidenced by preferential effects on select vascular beds of many vasoactive drugs commonly used in the practice of cardiology. Nitrates dilate both arteries and veins, whereas other vasodilators, such as hydralazine, act primarily as arterial vasodilators. The well-recognized differences in the clinical outcomes of saphenous vein and internal mammary artery bypass grafts furnish another example of clinically relevant heterogeneity among vessels. Internal mammary arteries release more nitric oxide than do saphenous veins. In addition, saphenous veins produce more vasoconstrictor endothelial-derived cyclooxygenase products than do internal mammary arteries. Such differences can help to explain the superior clinical outcomes with internal mammary grafts versus autologous venous bypass grafts.

Indeed, the reactions of blood vessels or vascular cells from various regions of the circulation sometimes differ directionally. The pulmonary vasoconstrictive versus systemic vasodilator response to hypoxia, or the disparate response of the cerebral versus systemic arterial circulation to carbon dioxide furnish commonly encountered examples. Neurectoderm-derived smooth muscle cells in upper body blood vessels grow in response to transforming growth factor-beta, but mesenchymal-derived smooth muscle cells from lower body arteries may actually show growth inhibition when exposed to this mediator. Perhaps the different embryonic origins of smooth muscle cells in the ascending versus descending aorta explain why certain gene defects express themselves primarily in the ascending aorta. In cases of Marfan syndrome, for example, the fibrillin mutation characteristically involves the ascending aorta first (see Chap. 70). Likewise, in cases of Williams syndrome, the genetic defect affects elastin throughout the body, yet the vascular phenotype of these patients manifests primarily in the supravalvular portion of the ascending aorta just where smooth muscle cells of neurectodermal origin reside (see Fig. 54–3).

Heterogeneity of the Clinical Manifestations of Arterial Disease

The Pathobiological Determinants of Atherosclerosis in Youth (PDAY) study collected arterial specimens from Americans younger than 35 years of age who died of noncardiac causes. This study found that fatty streaks and raised arterial lesions localize initially in the dorsal portion of the abdominal aorta. Involvement of the thoracic aorta with fatty streaks or early atheroma follows lesion formation in the abdominal aorta (see Chap. 35). The PDAY data suggest that the formation of coronary atheroma actually lags behind the development of fatty lesions in the aorta.[43,44] Interventions that lower lipids, however, benefit the coronary, carotid, and femoral arteries, although intimal changes in one bed do not necessarily track well with changes in another in a given individual.[45,46]

The most dreaded clinical consequences of atherosclerosis include thrombosis, the cause of most myocardial infarctions and many strokes. A physical disruption of the atherosclerotic plaque causes most fatal coronary events. The role of plaque disruption as a cause of thrombosis in other arterial beds has received less attention. The above discussion has highlighted the developmental and anatomical reasons that coronary arteries differ from peripheral arteries. In addition, the hemodynamic stresses impinging on lesions in the coronary versus the peripheral arterial tree differ. Notably, most coronary artery flow occurs during diastole, whereas the peak pressure and flow in peripheral arteries occurs during systole. Thus, the underlying mechanism of the thrombotic complications of atheroma might well differ in the coronary versus peripheral arteries. Yet, commonalties also exist that link the fundamental mechanisms of stenosis formation, plaque instability, and thrombosis in the coronary and peripheral arteries. Constrictive remodeling, or a failure of compensatory enlargement, appears to cause stenosis in the femoral as well as coronary arteries.[47] Intravascular ultrasound elastography shows that both femoral and coronary arteries harbor atheromata of the fibro-fatty or fibrous variety.[48] Importantly, inflammation appears to occur in disrupted plaques in the carotid as it does in the coronary circulations.[49] These pathoanatomical findings agree well with studies of serum markers of inflammation that show greater incidence of PAD in individuals with higher levels of biomarkers of inflammation, such as C-reactive protein or soluble intercellular adhesion molecule-1.[22,50]

In the aorta, mural thrombi seldom develop into occlusive clots because of the high flow. Nonetheless, aortic plaques frequently rupture, and aortic thrombi are recognized as a clinically important source of embolic disease (Fig. 54–5). Plaques in the aorta encounter high "hoop" (circumferential) stress, due to the large radius, according to the Laplace relationship. This difference may account for the common finding of multiple disrupted plaques in the atherosclerotic aorta (see Fig. 54–5). Recent evidence suggests that plaque rupture also underlies symptoms of carotid artery disease. Features associated with vulnerability of coronary plaques, such as ulcerated plaque with superimposed thrombus, occur frequently in carotid plaques as detected by magnetic resonance imaging.[51] Features such as abundance of foam cells and thinned fibrous caps can help distinguish symptomatic from asymptomatic carotid plaques. As in the unstable coronary plaque, there is infiltration with inflammatory cells and activation of these cells (determined by expression of the histocompatibility antigen HLA-DR). The proportion of active inflammatory cells is consistently higher in the ruptured plaque than in the asymptomatic plaques of similar degree of stenosis.[49]

An independent line of clinical evidence supports a commonality in the mechanisms of complication shared by carotid and coronary arteries. One large study dichotomized patients with symptomatic carotid artery lesions into those with or without irregularity of the carotid lesion by angiography. Over 10 years of follow-up, patients with irregular carotid lesions had a greater than twofold higher cumulative incidence of non-stroke vascular death (mostly due to coronary events) than did those presenting with smooth lesions.[52] Nonvascular deaths and the risk factors assessed in this study did not differ between groups. Similar mechanisms are likely to account for acute thromboses in peripheral arteries, although detailed investigations are not available. Despite the considerable biological and functional heterogeneity among arterial beds, the mechanisms causing the most important clinical manifestations appear similar.

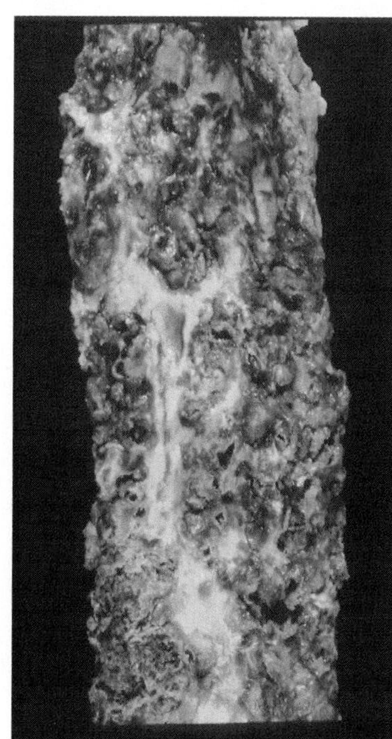

FIGURE 54–5 Atherosclerotic aorta of a patient with atheroemboli. There are multiple, protruding, shaggy atheromas with superimposed mural thrombi. (Courtesy of R.N. Mitchell, MD, PhD, Department of Pathology, Brigham and Women's Hospital, Boston, MA.)

Pathophysiology of Limb Ischemia

Pathophysiological considerations in patients with PAD must take into account the balance of circulatory supply of nutrients to the skeletal muscle and the oxygen and nutrient demand of the skeletal muscle (Table 54–3).

Factors Regulating Blood Supply (see Chap. 44)

The primary determinant of inadequate blood supply to the extremity is a flow-limiting lesion of a conduit artery. Flow through an artery is directly proportional to perfusion pressure and inversely proportional to

TABLE 54–3 Pathophysiological Considerations in Peripheral Arterial Disease
Factors regulating blood supply to limb
Flow-limiting lesion (stenosis severity, inadequate collateral vessels)
Impaired vasodilation (decreased nitric oxide and reduced responsiveness to vasodilators)
Accentuated vasoconstriction (thromboxane, serotonin, angiotensin II, endothelin, norepinephrine)
Abnormal rheology (reduced red blood cell deformability, increased leukocyte adhesivity, platelet aggregation, microthombosis, increased fibrinogen)
Altered skeletal muscle structure and function
Axonal denervation of skeletal muscle
Loss of type II, glycolytic fast twist fibers
Impaired mitochondrial enzymatic activity

the vascular resistance. If atherosclerosis causes a stenosis, flow through the artery is reduced, as described in the Poiseuille equation, in which

$$Q = \frac{\Delta P \pi r^4}{8 \eta l},$$

where ΔP is the pressure gradient across the stenosis, r is the radius of the residual lumen, η is blood viscosity, and l is the length of the vessel affected by the stenosis. As the severity of a stenotic lesion increases, flow becomes progressively reduced. The pressure gradient across the stenosis increases in a nonlinear manner, emphasizing the importance of a stenosis at high blood flow rates. Usually, a blood pressure gradient exists at rest if the stenosis reduces the lumen diameter by more than 50 percent, because as distorted flow develops there is loss of kinetic energy. A stenosis that does not cause a pressure gradient at rest may cause a gradient during exercise, when blood flow rises consequent to higher cardiac output and decreased vascular resistance. Thus, as flow through a stenosis increases, distal perfusion pressure is not maintained. Also, as the metabolic demand of exercising muscle outstrips its blood supply, local metabolites, including adenosine, nitric oxide, potassium, and hydrogen ion, accumulate and peripheral resistance vessels dilate. This results in a further drop of perfusion pressure, since the stenosis limits flow. In addition, intramuscular pressure rises during exercise and may exceed the arterial pressure distal to an occlusion, causing blood flow to cease. Flow through collateral blood vessels is usually adequate to meet the resting metabolic needs of the skeletal muscle tissue but is not enough during exercise.

Functional abnormalities in vasomotor reactivity also may interfere with blood flow. Vasodilator capability of both conduit and resistance vessels is reduced in patients with peripheral atherosclerosis. Normally, arteries dilate in response to pharmacological and biochemical stimuli, such as acetylcholine, serotonin, thrombin, or bradykinin, as well as to shear stress induced by increases in blood flow. This vasodilator response results from the release of biologically active substances from the endothelium, particularly nitric oxide. The vascular relaxation of a conduit vessel that occurs after a flow stimulus, such as that induced by exercise, may facilitate the delivery of blood to exercising muscles in healthy persons. Endothelium-dependent vasodilation subsequent to flow or pharmacological stimuli is impaired in the atherosclerotic femoral arteries and calf resistance vessels of patients with PAD. This failure of vasodilation might prevent an increase in nutritive blood supply to exercising muscle, since endothelium-derived nitric oxide can contribute to hyperemic blood volume after an ischemic stimulus.[53] Several studies have suggested that L-arginine, the precursor for endothelium-derived nitric oxide, increases muscle blood flow and improves claudication distance in patients with PAD, further supporting the contention that endothelium-dependent vasodilation is abnormal in these individuals.[54-56] No large trials have as yet established the clinical benefits of L-arginine, however. It is not known whether vasodilator function with respect to prostacyclin, adenosine, or ion-channels is abnormal in atherosclerotic peripheral arteries. Endogenous vasoconstrictor substances such as prostanoids and other lipid mediators, thrombin, serotonin, angiotensin II, endothelin, and norepinephrine may interfere with vasodilation.

Skeletal Muscle Structure and Metabolic Function

Electrophysiological and histopathological examination has found evidence of partial axonal denervation of the skeletal muscle in legs affected by PAD. There is preservation of type I, oxidative slow twitch fibers, but a loss of type II, or glycolytic, fast twitch fibers in the skeletal muscle of patients with PAD.[57] The loss of type II fibers correlates with decreased muscle strength and reduced exercise capacity. In skeletal muscle distal to PAD, there is a shift to anaerobic metabolism earlier during exercise and it persists longer after cessation of exercise. Patients with claudication have increased lactate release and accumulation of acylcarnitines during exercise, indicative of ineffective oxidative metabolism.[57] Moreover, mitochondrial respiratory activity and phosphocreatine and adenosine triphosphate recovery time decrease in the calf muscles of PAD patients as assessed after submaximal exercise by ^{31}P magnetic resonance spectroscopy.[58]

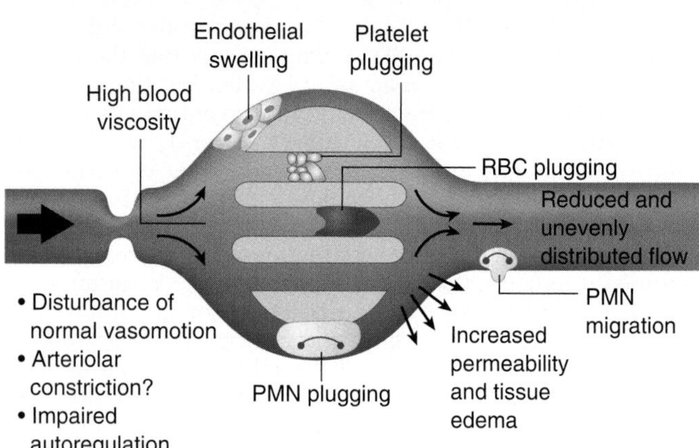

FIGURE 54–6 Schematic representation of potential pathophysiological mechanisms that lead to microvascular obstruction in patients with critical limb ischemia. (From Brevetti G, Corrado S, Marone VD, et al: Microcirculation and tissue metabolism in peripheral arterial disease. Clin Hemorheol Microcirc 21:245, 1999.)

Pathophysiology of Critical Limb Ischemia

Abnormalities in the microcirculation contribute to the pathophysiology of critical limb ischemia. Patients with severe limb ischemia have a reduced number of perfused skin capillaries.[59] Other potential causes of decreased capillary perfusion in this condition include reduced red blood cell deformability, increased leukocyte adhesivity, platelet aggregates, fibrinogen, microthrombosis, excessive vasoconstriction, and interstitial edema (Fig. 54–6). Intravascular pressure may also decrease because of precapillary arteriolar dilation due to locally released vasoactive metabolites.[60]

Clinical Presentation

Symptoms

The cardinal symptoms of PAD include intermittent claudication and rest pain. The term *claudication* is derived from the Latin word *claudicare*, "to limp." Intermittent claudication is characterized by a pain, ache, sense of fatigue, or other discomfort that occurs in the affected muscle group with exercise, particularly walking, and resolves with rest. Claudication occurs when skeletal muscle oxygen demand during effort exceeds blood oxygen supply and results from activation of local sensory receptors by accumulation of lactate or other metabolites. The location of the symptom often relates to the site of the most proximal stenosis. Buttock, hip or thigh claudication typically occurs in patients with obstruction of the aorta and iliac arteries. Calf claudication characterizes femoral and popliteal artery stenoses. The gastrocnemius muscle consumes more oxygen during walking than other muscle groups in the leg and hence causes the most frequent symptom reported by patients. Ankle or pedal claudication occurs in patients with tibial and peroneal artery disease. Similarly, stenoses of the subclavian, axillary, or brachial arteries may cause shoulder, biceps, or forearm claudication, respectively. Symptoms should resolve several minutes after cessation of effort. Calf and thigh pain that occurs at rest, such as nocturnal cramps, should not be confused with claudication and is not a symptom of PAD. The history obtained from persons reporting claudication should note the walking distance, speed, and incline that precipitate claudication. This baseline assessment evaluates disability and provides an initial qualitative measure with which to determine stability, improvement, or deterioration during subsequent encounters with the patient. Symptoms other than claudication can limit functional capacity.[61] Patients with PAD walk more slowly and have less walking endurance than patients who do not have PAD.[62,63]

Several questionnaires have been developed to assess the presence and severity of claudication. The Rose Questionnaire was developed initially to diagnose both angina and intermittent claudication in epidemiological surveys. It questions whether the patient develops pain in either calf with walking and whether the pain occurs at rest, while walking at an ordinary or hurried pace, or when walking uphill. There have been several modifications in this questionnaire, including the Edinburgh Claudication Questionnaire and the San Diego Claudication Questionnaire,[64,65] both of which are more sensitive and specific in comparison to a physician's diagnosis of intermittent claudication based on walking distance, walking speed, and nature of symptoms. A more recently validated instrument, the Walking Impairment Questionnaire, asks a series of questions and develops a point score based on walking distance, walking speed, and nature of symptoms.[66]

Limb claudication occasionally results from nonatherosclerotic causes of arterial occlusive disease (Table 54–4). Several of these are discussed later in the chapter and include arterial embolism, vasculitides such as thromboangiitis obliterans, Takayasu arteritis, giant cell arteritis, aortic coarctation, fibromuscular dysplasia, irradiation, or extravascular compression due to arterial entrapment or adventitial cyst (see Chap. 82).

Several nonvascular causes of exertional leg pain should be considered in patients who present with symptoms suggestive of intermittent claudication (see Table 54–4). Lumbosacral radiculopathy resulting from degenerative joint disease, spinal stenosis, and herniated disks can cause pain in the buttock, hip, thigh, calf, and/or foot with walking, often after very short distances, or even with standing. The term *neurogenic pseudoclaudication* has been used to describe this symptom. Lumbosacral spine disease and PAD both preferentially affect the elderly, and hence may coexist in the same individual. Arthritis of the hips and knees also provokes leg pain with walking. Typically, the pain localizes to the affected joint and can be elicited on physical examination through palpation and range of motion maneuvers. Rarely, skeletal muscle disorders such as myositis can cause exertional leg pain. Muscle tenderness, an abnormal neuromuscular examination finding, elevated skeletal muscle enzyme levels, and a normal pulse examination finding should distinguish myositis from PAD. McArdle syndrome, in which there is a deficiency of skeletal muscle phosphorylase, can cause symptoms mimicking the claudication of PAD. Patients with chronic venous insufficiency sometimes report leg discomfort with exertion, which is designated *venous claudication*. Venous hypertension during exercise increases arterial resistance in the affected limb and limits blood flow. In the case of venous insufficiency, elevated extravascular pressure caused by interstitial edema further diminishes capillary perfusion. A physical examination demonstrating peripheral edema, venous stasis pigmentation, and occasionally venous varicosities will identify this unusual cause of exertional leg pain.

TABLE 54–4 Differential Diagnosis of Exertional Leg Pain

Vascular causes
- Atherosclerosis
- Thrombosis
- Embolism
- Vasculitis
  - Thromboangiitis obliterans
  - Takayasu arteritis
  - Giant cell arteritis
- Aortic coarctation
- Fibromuscular dysplasia
- Irradiation
- Extravascular compression
  - Arterial entrapment (e.g., popliteal artery entrapment, thoracic outlet syndrome)
  - Adventitial cysts

Nonvascular causes
- Lumbosacral radiculopathy
  - Degenerative arthritis
  - Spinal stenosis
  - Herniated disc
- Arthritis
  - Hips, knees
- Venous insufficiency
- Myositis
- McArdle syndrome

Rest pain occurs in patients with critical limb ischemia in whom the available blood supply does not adequately meet the resting metabolic needs of the tissue. Typically, patients complain of pain or paresthesias in the foot or toes of the affected extremity. This discomfort worsens upon leg elevation and improves with leg dependency, as might be anticipated by the respective effects of gravity on perfusion pressure. The pain can be particularly severe at sites of skin fissuring, ulceration, or necrosis. Often the skin is very sensitive and even the weight of bedclothes or sheets elicits pain. Patients may sit on the edge of the bed and dangle their legs to alleviate the discomfort. Patients with ischemic or diabetic neuropathy can experience little or no pain despite the presence of severe ischemia.

Critical limb and digital ischemia can result from arterial occlusions other than those caused by atherosclerosis. These include vasculitides, such as thromboangiitis obliterans, connective tissue disorders such as systemic lupus erythematosus and scleroderma, vasospasm, atheromatous embolism, and acute arterial occlusion caused by thrombosis or embolism (see later). Acute gouty arthritis, trauma, and sensory neuropathies such as that caused by diabetes mellitus, lumbosacral radiculopathies, and reflex sympathetic dystrophy can cause foot pain. Leg ulcers also occur in patients with venous insufficiency and sensory neuropathies, particularly that related to diabetes. These ulcers are easily distinguished from arterial ulcers. The venous ulcer usually localizes near the medial malleolus and has an irregular border and a pink base with granulation tissue. Venous ulcers produce milder pain than arterial ulcers. Neurotrophic ulcers occur where there is pressure or trauma, usually on the sole of the foot. These ulcers are deep, frequently infected, and usually not painful because of the loss of sensation (Fig. 54–7, right panel).

Physical Findings

A careful vascular examination includes palpation of pulses and auscultation of accessible arteries for bruits. Pulses that are readily palpable in healthy individuals include the brachial, radial, and ulnar arteries of the upper extremity and the femoral, popliteal, dorsalis pedis, and posterior tibial arteries of the lower extremities. The aorta also can be palpated in asthenic persons. A decreased or absent pulse provides insight into the location of arterial stenoses. For example, a normal right femoral pulse but absent left femoral

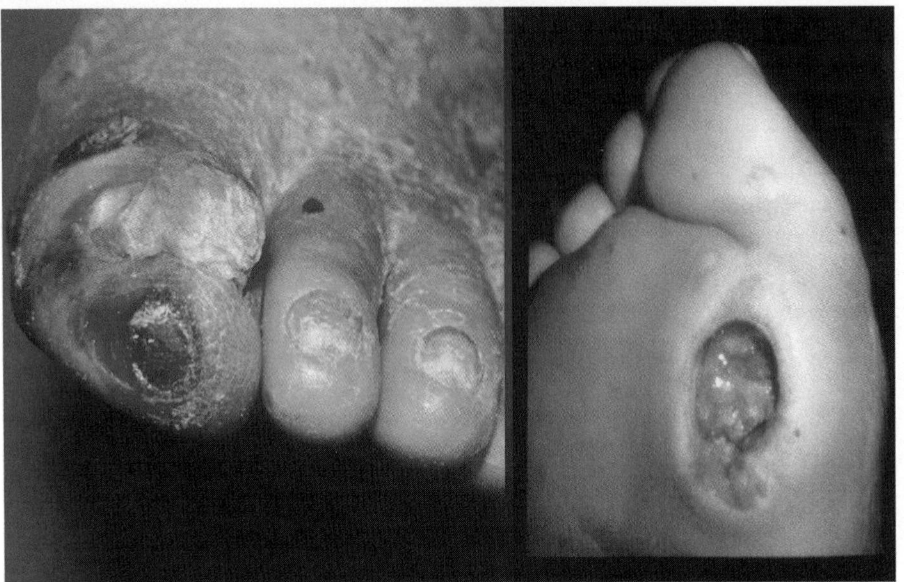

FIGURE 54–7 **Left,** A typical arterial ulcer. It is a discrete, circumscribed, necrotic ulcer located on the great toe. **Right,** A trophic ulcer in a patient with diabetes mellitus. It is located on the volar surface of the foot beneath the head of the first metatarsal bone, a typical area of pressure; its base has granulation tissue.

pulse suggests the presence of left iliofemoral arterial stenosis. A normal femoral artery pulse but absent popliteal artery pulse would indicate a stenosis in the superficial femoral artery or proximal popliteal artery. Similarly, disease of the anterior and posterior tibial arteries can be inferred when the popliteal artery pulse is present but the dorsalis pedis and posterior tibial pulses, respectively, are not palpable. Bruits are often indicative of accelerated blood flow velocity and flow disturbance at sites of stenosis. A stethoscope should be used to auscultate the supraclavicular and infraclavicular fossae for evidence of subclavian artery stenosis, the abdomen, flank, and pelvis for evidence of stenoses in the aorta and its branch vessels, and each groin for evidence of femoral artery stenoses. Pallor can be elicited on the soles of the feet of some patients with PAD by performing a maneuver in which the feet are elevated above the level of the heart and the calf muscles are exercised by repeated dorsiflexion and plantar flexion of the ankle. The legs are then placed in the dependent position and the time to the onset of hyperemia and venous distention is measured. Each of these variables depends on the rate of blood flow, which in turn reflects the severity of stenosis and adequacy of collateral vessels.

The legs of patients with chronic aortoiliac disease may show muscle atrophy. Additional signs of chronic low-grade ischemia include hair loss, thickened and brittle toenails, smooth and shiny skin, and subcutaneous fat atrophy of the digital pads. Patients with severe limb ischemia have cool skin and may also have petechiae, persistent cyanosis or pallor, dependent rubor, pedal edema resulting from prolonged dependency, skin fissures, ulceration, or gangrene. Arterial ulcers typically have a pale base with irregular borders and usually involve the tips of the toes or the heel of the foot, or develop at sites of pressure (see Fig. 54–7, left panel). These ulcers vary in size and may be as small as 3 to 5 mm.

Categorization

Classification of patients with PAD depends on the severity of the symptoms and abnormalities detected on physical examination. Categorization of the clinical manifestations of PAD improves communication among professionals caring for these patients and provides a structure for defining guidelines for therapeutic interventions. Fontaine described one widely used scheme that classified patients in one of four stages progressing from asymptomatic to critical limb ischemia (Table 54–5). Several professional vascular societies have adopted a contemporary, more descriptive classification that includes asymptomatic patients, three grades of claudication, and three grades of critical limb ischemia ranging from rest pain alone to minor and major tissue loss (Table 54–6).[67]

Testing

Segmental Pressure Measurement and Ankle/Brachial Indices

The measurement of systolic blood pressure along selected segments of each extremity furnishes one of the most useful and simplest noninvasive tests to evaluate the presence and severity of stenoses in the peripheral arteries. In the lower extremities, pneumatic cuffs are placed on the upper and lower portions of the thigh, the calf, above the ankle, and often over the metatarsal area of the foot. Likewise, in the upper extremity, pneumatic cuffs

TABLE 54–5 Fontaine Classification of Peripheral Arterial Disease

Stage	Symptoms
I	Asymptomatic
II	Intermittent claudication
IIa	Pain-free, claudication walking >200 m
IIb	Pain-free, claudication walking <200 m
III	Rest and nocturnal pain
IV	Necrosis, gangrene

TABLE 54–6 Clinical Categories of Chronic Limb Ischemia

Grade	Category	Clinical Description
	0	Asymptomatic, not hemodynamically correct
I	1 2 3	Mild claudication Moderate claudication Severe claudication
II	4 5	Ischemic rest pain Minor tissue loss: nonhealing ulcer, focal gangrene with diffuse pedal ulcer
III	6	Major tissue loss extending above transmetatarsal level, functional foot no longer salvageable

Adapted from Rutherford RB, Baker JD, Ernst C, et al. Recommended standards for reports dealing with lower extremity ischemia: Revised version. J Vasc Surg 26:517, 1997.

TABLE 54–7 Leg Segmental Pressure Measurements in a Patient with Bilateral Calf Claudication

	152/84	
Brachial Artery	*Right leg*	*Left leg*
Upper thigh	160	162
Lower thigh	110	140
Calf	108	100
Ankle	64	78
Ankle/brachial index	0.42	0.51

are placed on the upper arm over the biceps, on the forearm below the elbow, and at the wrist. Systolic blood pressure at each respective limb segment can be measured by first inflating the pneumatic cuff to suprasystolic pressure and then determining the pressure at which blood flow occurs during cuff deflation. The onset of flow can be assessed by placing a Doppler ultrasound flow probe over an artery distal to the cuff. In the lower extremities, it is most convenient to place the Doppler probe on the foot over the posterior tibial artery as it courses inferior and posterior to the medial malleolus or over the dorsalis pedis artery on the dorsum of the metatarsal arch. In the upper extremities, the Doppler probe can be placed over the brachial artery in the antecubital fossa or over the radial and ulnar arteries at the wrist.

Left ventricular contraction imparts kinetic energy to blood, which is maintained throughout the large and medium-sized vessels. Systolic blood pressure in the more distal vessels may be higher than in the aorta and proximal vessels because of reflection of blood pressure waves.[68] A stenosis can cause loss of pressure energy as a result of increased frictional forces and flow disturbance at the site of the stenosis. Approximately 90 percent of the cross-sectional area of the aorta must be narrowed before a pressure gradient develops. In smaller vessels, such as the iliac and femoral arteries, a 70 to 90 percent decrease in cross-sectional area will cause a resting pressure gradient sufficient to decrease systolic blood pressure distal to the stenosis. Taking into consideration the precision of this noninvasive method and the variability in blood pressure over even short periods of time, a blood pressure gradient in excess of 20 mm Hg between successive cuffs is generally used as evidence of arterial stenosis in the lower extremity, whereas a 10 mm Hg gradient is indicative of a stenosis between sequential cuffs in the upper extremity. Systolic blood pressure in the toes and fingers approximates 60 percent of the systolic blood pressure at the ankle and wrist, respectively, as pressure diminishes further in the smaller distal vessels.

Table 54–7 gives examples of leg segmental pressure measurements in a patient with bilateral calf claudication. In the right leg, there are pressure gradients between upper and lower thigh and between the calf and ankle. These are indicative of stenoses in the superficial femoral artery and in the tibioperoneal arteries. In the left leg, there are pressure gradients between the upper and lower thigh, between the lower thigh and calf, and between the calf and ankle. These are indicative of stenoses in the superficial femoral and popliteal arteries and in the tibioperoneal arteries.

Ankle/Brachial Index

Determination of the ABI furnishes a simplified application of leg segmental blood pressure measurements readily used at the bedside. This index is the ratio of the systolic blood pressure measured at the ankle to the systolic blood pressure measured at the brachial artery. A pneumatic cuff placed around the ankle is inflated to suprasystolic pressure and subsequently deflated, while the onset of flow is detected with a Doppler ultrasound probe placed over the dorsalis pedis and posterior tibial arteries, thus denoting ankle systolic blood pressure. Brachial artery systolic pressure can be assessed in a routine manner, using either a stethoscope to listen for the first Korotkoff sound or a Doppler probe to listen for the onset of flow during cuff deflation. The normal ABI should be 1.0 or greater. However, recognizing the variability intrinsic to sequential blood pressure measurements, an ABI of less than 0.90 is considered abnormal and is 95 percent sensitive for angiographically verified peripheral arterial stenosis.[1] The ABI is often used to gauge the severity of PAD. Patients with symptoms of leg claudication often have ABIs ranging from 0.5 to 0.8, and patients with critical limb ischemia usually have an ABI of less than 0.5. The ABI correlates inversely with walking distance and speed. Fewer than 40 percent of patients whose ABI is less than 0.40 can complete a 6-minute walk.[69] In patients with skin ulcerations, an ankle pressure of less than 55 mm Hg would predict poor ulcer healing.

One limitation of leg blood pressure recordings is that they cannot be used reliably in patients with calcified vessels, as might occur in persons with diabetes mellitus or renal insufficiency. The calcified vessel cannot be compressed during inflation of the pneumatic cuff and therefore the Doppler probe indicates continuous blood flow, even when the mercury manometer records pressure in excess of 250 mm Hg.

Treadmill Exercise Testing

Treadmill exercise testing serves to evaluate the clinical significance of peripheral arterial stenoses and to provide objective evidence of the patient's walking capacity. The initial claudication distance is defined as the point at which symptoms of claudication first develop and the absolute claudication distance is when the patient is no longer able to continue walking because of severe leg discomfort. This standardized and more objective measurement of walking capacity supplements the patient's history and thus provides a quantitative assessment of the patient's disability as well as a metric that can be monitored after therapeutic interventions.

Treadmill exercise protocols use a motorized treadmill that incorporates fixed or progressive speeds and angles of incline. A fixed workload test usually maintains a constant grade of 12 percent and speed of 1.5 to 2.0 miles per hour. A progressive, or graded, treadmill protocol typically maintains a constant speed of 2 miles per hour while the grade is gradually increased by 2 percent every 2 to 3 minutes. Reproducibility of repeated treadmill test results is reportedly better with progressive than with constant grade protocols.[70]

Treadmill testing provides a means to determine whether arterial stenoses contribute to the patient's symptoms of exertional leg pain. During exercise, blood flow through a stenosis increases as vascular resistance falls in the exercising muscle. According to Poiseuille's Law, described previously, the pressure gradient across the stenosis increases in direct proportion to flow. Thus, ankle and brachial systolic blood pressures are measured under resting conditions before treadmill exercise, within 1 minute after exercise, and repeatedly until baseline values are reestablished. Normally, the blood pressure increase that occurs during exercise should be the same in both upper and lower extremities, maintaining a constant ABI of 1.0 or greater. In the presence of peripheral arterial stenoses, the ABI decreases, because the increase in blood pressure that is observed in the arm is not matched by a comparable increase in ankle blood pressure. A 25 percent or greater decrease in ABI after exercise in a patient whose walking capacity is limited by claudication is considered diagnostic, implicating PAD as a cause of the patient's symptoms.

Many patients with PAD also have coronary atherosclerosis. The addition of cardiac monitoring to the exercise protocol may provide adjunctive information regarding the presence of myocardial ischemia. A workload sufficient to increase myocardial oxygen demand and provoke myocardial ischemia may not be achieved in patients whose exercise capacity is limited by claudication. Nonetheless, electrocardiographic changes, particularly during low levels of treadmill exercise, may provide evidence of severe coronary artery disease.

Pulse Volume Recording

The pulse volume recording graphically illustrates the volumetric change in a segment of the limb that occurs with each pulse. Plethysmographic instruments, typically utilizing strain gauges or pneumatic cuffs, are used to transduce volumetric changes in the limb, which can be displayed on a graphic recorder. These transducers are strategically placed along the limb to record the pulse volume in its different segments, such as the thigh, calf, ankle, metatarsal region, and toes or the upper arm, forearm, and fingers. The normal pulse volume contour is influenced by both local arterial pressure and vascular wall distensibility and resembles a blood pressure waveform. It consists of a sharp systolic upstroke, rising rapidly to a peak, a dicrotic notch, and a concave downslope that drops off gradually toward the baseline.[71] The contour of the pulse wave changes distal to a stenosis. There is loss of the dicrotic notch, a slower rate of rise, a more rounded peak, and a slower descent. The amplitude becomes lower with increasing severity of disease, and the pulse wave may not be recordable at all in the critically ischemic limb. Segmental analysis of the pulse wave may indicate the location of an arterial stenosis, which is likely to be sited in the artery between a normal and an abnormal pulse volume recording. The pulse volume wave also provides information regarding the integrity of blood flow when blood pressure measurements cannot be accurately obtained because of noncompressible vessels.

Doppler Ultrasonography

Continuous wave and pulsed wave Doppler systems transmit and receive high-frequency ultrasound signals. The Doppler frequency shift caused by moving red blood cells varies directly with the velocity of blood flow. Typically, the perceived frequency shift is between 1 and 20 kHz and is within the audible range of the human ear. Therefore, placement of a Doppler probe along an artery enables the examiner to hear whether blood flow is present and the vessel is patent. Processing and graphically recording the Doppler signal permits a more detailed analysis of the frequency components.

Doppler instruments can be used without or with gray scale imaging to evaluate an artery for the presence of stenoses. The Doppler probe is positioned at approximately a 60-degree angle over the common femoral, superficial femoral, popliteal, dorsalis pedis, and posterior tibial arteries. The normal Doppler waveform has three components: a rapid forward flow component during systole, a transient flow reversal during early diastole, and a slow antegrade component during late diastole. The Doppler waveform becomes altered if the probe is placed distal to an arterial stenosis and is characterized by deceleration of systolic flow, loss of the early diastolic reversal, and diminished peak frequencies. Arteries in a limb with critical ischemia may not show any Doppler frequency shift. As with pulse volume recordings, a change from a normal to an abnormal Doppler waveform as the artery is interrogated more distally provides inferential evidence of the location of a stenosis.[71,72]

Duplex Ultrasound Imaging

Duplex ultrasound imaging provides a direct, noninvasive means of assessing both the anatomic characteristics of peripheral arteries and the functional significance of arterial stenoses. The methodology incorporates gray scale B-mode ultrasound imaging, pulsed Doppler velocity measurements, and color coding of the Doppler-shift information (Fig. 54–8). Real-time ultrasonography scanners emit and receive high-frequency sound waves, typically ranging from 2 to 10 mHz, to construct an image. The acoustic properties of the vascular wall differ from those of the surrounding tissue, enabling them

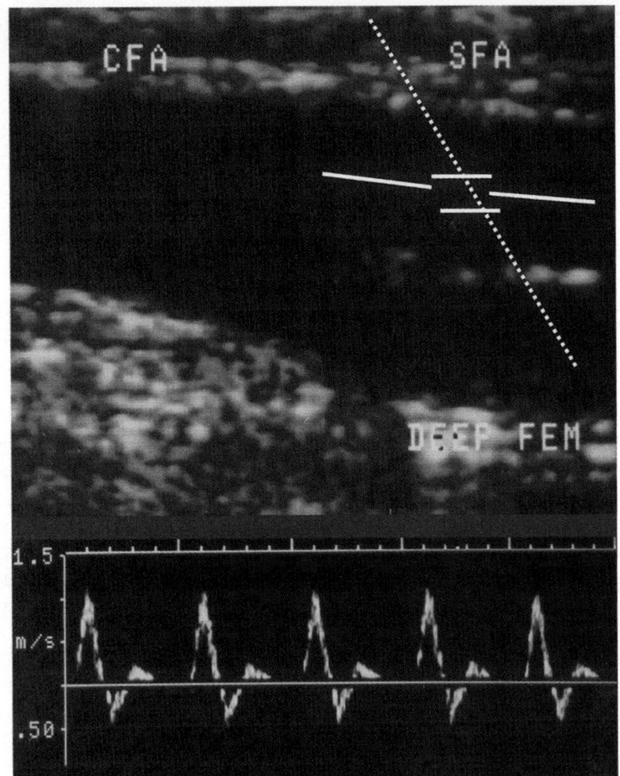

FIGURE 54–8 Duplex ultrasonogram of the common femoral artery bifurcation into the superficial and deep femoral arteries. The **upper image** shows a normal gray scale image of the artery in which the intima is not thickened and the lumen is widely patent. The **lower image** is a recording of the pulse Doppler velocity sampled from the superficial femoral artery. The triphasic profile is apparent, the envelope is thin, and the peak systolic velocity is within normal limits.

to be imaged easily. Atherosclerotic plaque may be present and visible on gray scale images. Pulsed wave Doppler systems emit ultrasound beams at precise times and can therefore sample the reflected ultrasound waves at specific depths, enabling the examiner to determine the blood cell velocity within the lumen of the artery. By positioning the pulsed Doppler beam at a known angle, the examiner can calculate blood flow velocity according to the following equation:

$$Df = 2VF\cos\theta/C,$$

where *Df* is the frequency shift, *V* is the velocity, *F* is the frequency of the transmitted sound, θ is the angle between the transmitted sound and the velocity vector, and *C* is the velocity of sound and tissue. For optimal measurements, the angle of the pulsed Doppler beam should be less than 60 degrees. With color Doppler, the frequency shift information within the entire field sampled by the ultrasound beam can be superimposed on the gray scale image. This provides a composite real-time display of flow velocity within the vessel.

Color-assisted duplex ultrasound imaging is an effective means of localizing peripheral arterial stenoses (Fig. 54–9). Normal arteries have laminar flow, with the highest velocity at the center of the artery. The corresponding color image is usually homogeneous, with relatively constant hue and intensity. In the presence of an arterial stenosis, blood flow velocity increases through the narrowed lumen. As the velocity increases, there is progressive desaturation of the color display, and flow disturbance distal to the stenosis causes changes in hue and color. Pulsed Doppler velocity measurements can be made along the length of the artery and particularly at areas of flow abnormalities suggested by the color images. A twofold or greater increase in peak systolic velocity at the site of an atherosclerotic plaque indicates a 50 percent or greater diameter stenosis (see Fig. 54–9). A threefold increase in velocity suggests 75 percent or greater stenosis. An occluded artery generates no Doppler signal. Using contrast angiography as a reference standard, duplex ultrasound imaging for identifying sites of arterial stenoses has approximately a 95 percent specificity and an 80 to 90 percent sensitivity.[73,74]

Magnetic Resonance Angiography

Magnetic resonance angiography (MRA) can noninvasively visualize the aorta and the peripheral arteries (see Chaps. 14 and 53). A detailed description of the instrumentation and technique is beyond the scope of this chapter. The resolution of the vascular anatomy with gadolinium-enhanced MRA approaches that of conventional contrast digital subtraction angiography (Fig. 54–10). Comparative studies have reported sensitivities of 93 to 100 percent and specificity of 96 to 100 percent for the aorta, iliac, femoropopliteal, and tibioperoneal arteries.[74-79] MRA currently has greatest utility for the evaluation of symptomatic patients to assist decision-making before endovascular and surgical intervention or in patients at risk for renal, allergic, or other complications during conventional angiography.

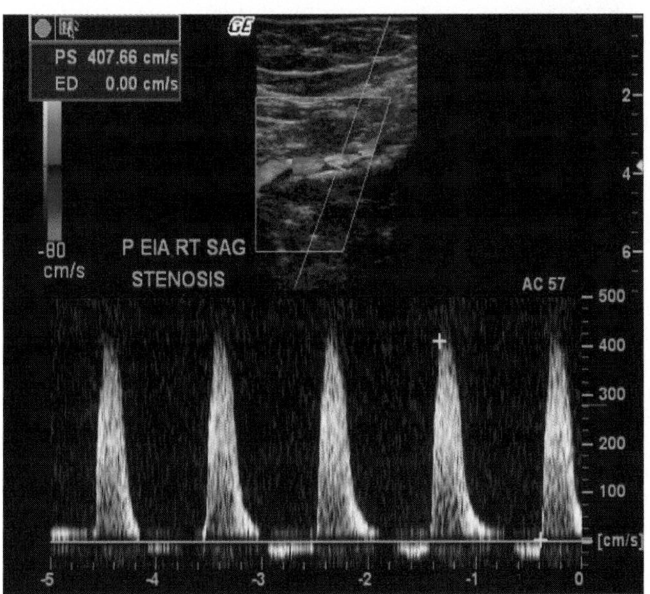

FIGURE 54–9 Duplex ultrasonogram of the external iliac artery. The **upper image** shows a color image of the artery in which there is heterogeneity and desaturation of color indicative of high-velocity flow through a stenosis. The **lower image** is a recording of the pulse Doppler velocity sampled from the right external iliac artery. The peak velocity of 350 cm/sec is elevated. These features are consistent with a significant stenosis.

Computed Tomographic Angiography

Computed tomographic angiography (CTA) utilizes intravenous administration of radiocontrast material to opacify and visualize the aorta and peripheral arteries (see Chap. 15). New computed tomography scanners using multidetector technology can acquire up to 16 simultaneous cross-sectional images displayed with maximal intensity projection. This advance permits imaging of peripheral arteries with excellent spatial resolution over a relatively short period of time and using reduced amount of radiocontrast (Fig. 54–11).[80] Images can be displayed in three dimensions and rotated to optimize visualization of arterial stenoses. Compared to conventional contrast angiography, the sensitivity and specificity for occlusions reported for CTA using single detector technology are 94 to 100 percent and 98 to 100 percent, respectively. For stenoses greater than 75 percent, the sensitivity is 73 to 88 percent and the specificity is 94 to 100 percent.[81] The use of newer generation multidetector scanners improves this accuracy.[80,82]

Experience with CTA is still relatively limited compared to that of MRA and conventional intraarterial angiography. CTA offers an advantage over MRA in that it can be used in patients with stents, metal clips, and pacemakers, although it also has the disadvantage of requiring radiocontrast and ionizing radiation.

Contrast Angiography (see Chap. 18)

Conventional angiography, using a radioiodinated or other contrast agent, is indicated for evaluation of the arterial anatomy prior to a revascularization procedure. It still has occasional utility when the diagnosis is in doubt. Most contemporary angiography laboratories use digital subtraction techniques following intraarterial administration of contrast

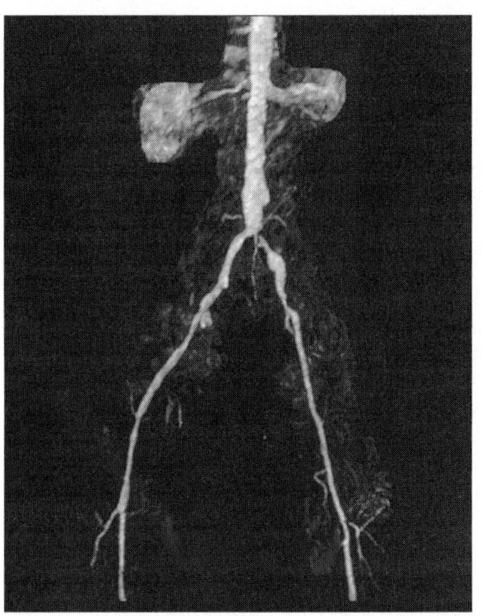
A

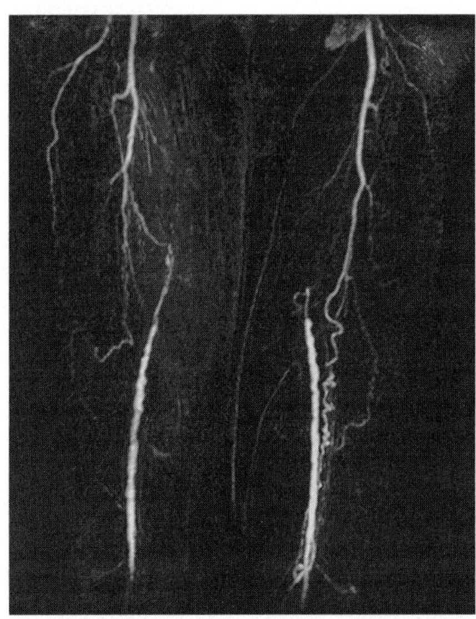
B

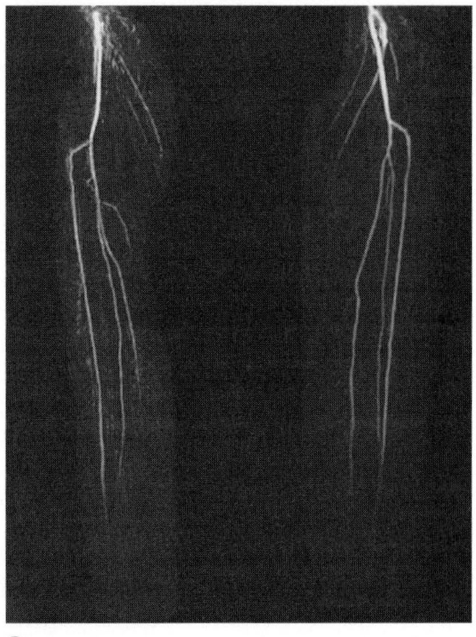
C

FIGURE 54–10 Gadolinium-enhanced two-dimensional magnetic resonance angiogram of the aorta and both legs, extending from the thighs to above the ankle. **A,** Aortoiliac atherosclerosis with stenosed left common iliac artery. **B,** Bilateral superficial femoral artery occlusion with reconstitution of the distal portion of the right and left superficial femoral arteries. **C,** The anterior tibial, posterior tibial, and peroneal arteries, which are patent in each leg.

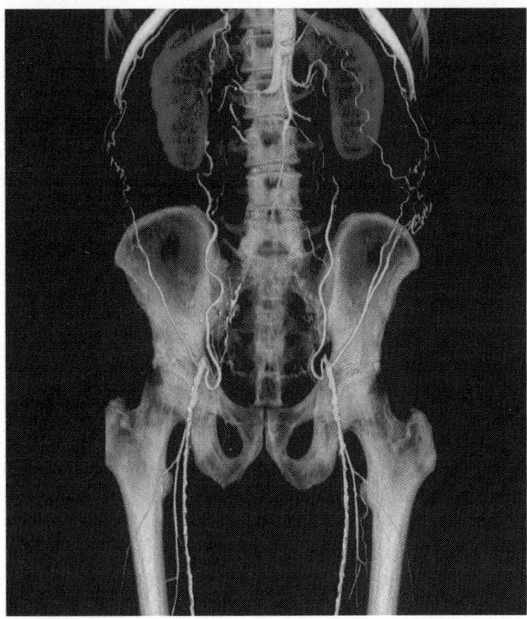

FIGURE 54–11 Computed tomographic angiogram of a patient with complete occlusion of the aorta and both iliac arteries. There is reconstitution of the common femoral arteries. (Courtesy of the 3D and Image Processing Center of Brigham and Women's Hospital, Boston, MA.)

material to enhance resolution. Evaluation of the aorta and the peripheral arteries generally uses retrograde transfemoral catheterization. Injection of the radiocontrast material into the aorta permits visualization of the aorta and iliac arteries, and injection of contrast material into the iliofemoral segment of the involved leg permits optimal visualization of the femoral, popliteal, tibial, and peroneal arteries (Fig. 54–12). In patients with aortic occlusion, catheterization of the femoral arteries is not feasible. The aorta can be approached by brachial or axillary artery cannulation or, if necessary, directly by a translumbar approach.

Prognosis

Patients with PAD have an increased risk for adverse cardiovascular events as well as the risk of limb loss and impaired quality of life.[2,12,83,84] Patients with PAD frequently have concomitant coronary artery disease and cerebrovascular disease.[1,85,86] The relative prevalence of each of these manifestations of atherosclerosis depends, in part, on the diagnostic criteria used to establish their diagnosis. In the Clopidogrel vs. Aspirin in Patients at Risk of Ischemic Events (CAPRIE) trial, 21 percent of the patients with PAD had a history of myocardial infarction and 26 percent had angina.[85] Patients with abnormal ABIs are twice as likely as those with normal ABIs to have a history of myocardial infarction, angina, congestive heart failure, or cerebrovascular ischemia.[1] Approximately 15 to 25 percent of patients with peripheral artery disease have significant carotid artery stenoses as detected by duplex ultrasonography. The risk of death from cardiovascular causes increases 2.5- to sixfold in patients with PAD, and their annual mortality rate is 4.3 to 4.9 percent.[1,87] The risk of death is greatest in those with the most severe PAD, and mortality correlates with decreasing ABI (Fig. 54–13). Approximately 25 percent of patients with critical limb ischemia die within 1 year, and the 1-year mortality rate among patients who have undergone amputation for PAD may be as high as 45 percent.[1,88]

Approximately 25 percent of patients with claudication develop worsening symptoms. Clinical progression to critical limb ischemia occurs in 7.5 to 8.0 percent of patients with claudication in the first year after diagnosis and in approximately 2.2 percent each year thereafter.[89] Both smoking and diabetes mellitus independently predict progression of disease.[1] Of patients with PAD, the risk of amputation in those with diabetes mellitus is at least 12-fold higher than in nondiabetic persons.[90]

Treatment

The goals of treatment for PAD include reduction in cardiovascular morbidity and mortality as well as improvement in quality of life by decreasing symptoms of claudication, eliminating rest pain, and preserving limb viability.[5] Therapeutic considerations, therefore, include risk factor modification by lifestyle measures and pharmacological therapy to reduce the risk of adverse cardiovascular events, such as myocardial infarction, stroke, and death. Symptoms of claudication can improve with pharmacotherapy or exercise rehabilitation, whereas optimal management of critical limb ischemia often includes endovascular interventions or surgical reconstruction to improve blood supply and maintain limb viability.[1,2,91]

Risk Factor Modification (see Chaps. 39 and 42)

Lipid-lowering therapy reduces the risk of adverse cardiovascular events in patients with coronary artery disease. Secondary prevention trials with statins documented reduced risk of nonfatal myocardial infarction or death from coronary artery disease by 24 to 34 percent (see Chap. 39). The recent Heart Protection Study found that lipid-lowering therapy with simvastatin reduced the risk of adverse cardiovascular outcomes by 25 percent in patients with atherosclerosis, including more than 6700 patients with PAD (Fig. 54–14).[92] The National Cholesterol Education Program Adult Treatment Panel III designated PAD a "coronary risk equivalent," hence the current recommendations for lipid-lowering therapy in patients with PAD. Such patients should receive diet and drug therapy to achieve a target LDL cholesterol level of 100 mg/dl or less.[93]

Several clinical trials have found that lipid-lowering therapy with diet, niacin, binding resins, or clofibrate reduces the progression of femoral artery atherosclerosis. In one study, the addition of probucol to cholestyramine did not affect femoral atherosclerosis.[94] Lipid-lowering therapy may also reduce the incidence or severity of claudication. The Program on the Surgical Control of the Hyperlipidemia (POSCH) found that partial ileal bypass surgery, a surgical procedure that lowers cholesterol levels, reduced the incidence of intermittent claudication or critical limb ischemia by 34 percent and reduced the risk for developing an abnormal ABI by 44 percent.[95] A post hoc analysis of the Scandinavian Simvastatin Survival Study (4S) found that simvastatin, as compared with placebo, reduced the risk of developing new or worsening claudication by 38 percent.[96]

Prospective trials have found that statins improve walking distance in patients with PAD.[97-99] In the Treatment of Peripheral Atherosclerotic Disease with Moderate or Intensive Lipid Lowering (TREADMILL) trial, atorvastatin (80 mg) increased pain-free walking distance by more than 60 percent as compared with 38 percent increase with placebo (Fig. 54-15).[98] Also, patients treated with statins have superior leg functioning as assessed by walking speed and distance compared to those not so treated.[100]

Smoking Cessation

Prospective trials examining the benefits of smoking cessation are lacking. However, observational evidence unequivocally supports the notion that cigarette smoking increases the risk of atherosclerosis and its clinical sequelae. Nonsmokers with PAD have lower rates of myocardial infarction and mortality than those who have smoked or continue to smoke, and

PAD patients who discontinue smoking have approximately twice the 5-year survival rate of those who continue to smoke.[8] Smoking cessation also lowers the risk of developing critical limb ischemia.

Treatment of Diabetes

(see Chaps. 40 and 51)

Aggressive treatment of diabetes decreases the risk for microangiopathic events such as nephropathy and retinopathy; however, only limited data support the benefit of aggressive treatment of diabetes on the clinical manifestations of atherosclerosis (see Chap. 40). In the Diabetes Control and Complications Trial (DCCT), which involved patients with type 1 diabetes mellitus, a post-hoc analysis found that intensive insulin therapy, as compared with usual care, caused a nonsignificant 42 percent reduction in cardiovascular events, including a 22 percent reduction in events related to PAD.[101] Also, after 6 years, the rate of growth of carotid intima–media thickness was less in the intensive treatment group, indicating a favorable effect on atherosclerosis progression.[102] The United Kingdom Prospective Diabetes Study (UKPDS) of patients with type 2 diabetes mellitus found that intensive treatment with sulfonylureas or insulin was associated with a 16 percent reduction in myocardial infarction, a finding of borderline statistical significance, and a trend for a decrease in the incidence of death or amputation from PAD.[103]

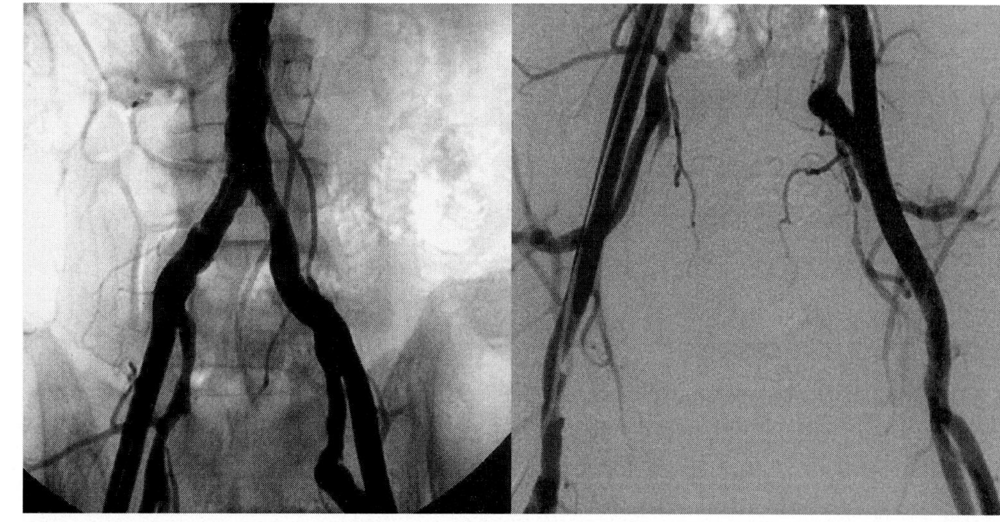

A

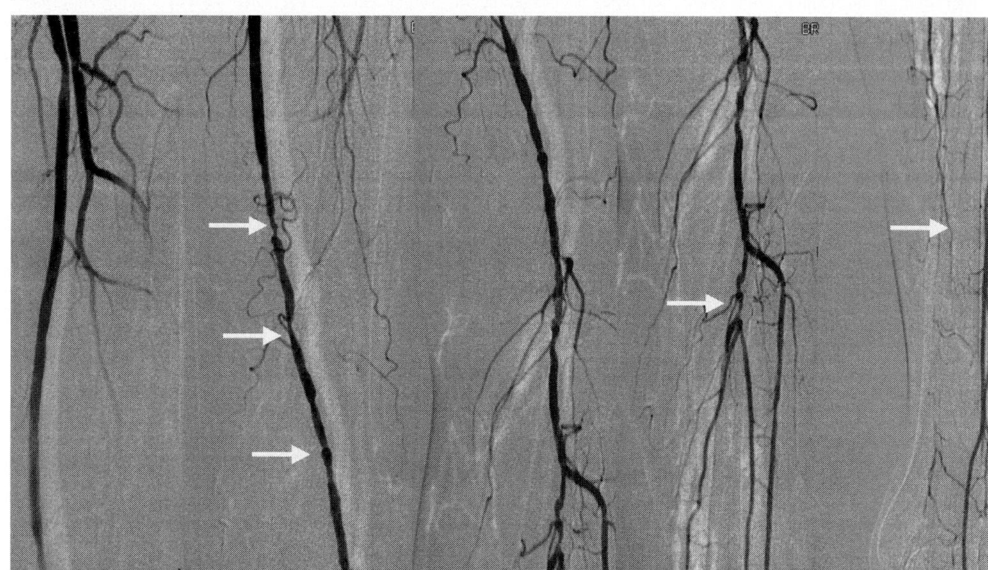

B

FIGURE 54–12 Angiogram of a patient with disabling left calf claudication. **A,** The aorta and bilateral common iliac arteries are patent. **B,** The left superficial femoral artery has multiple stenotic lesions (arrows). There is a significant stenosis of the left tibioperoneal trunk and left posterior tibial artery (arrows).

Blood Pressure Control

Antihypertensive therapy reduces the risk of stroke, coronary artery disease, and vascular death. In the Appropriate Blood Pressure Control in Diabetes (ABCD) trial, intensive blood pressure control to levels approximating 128/75 mm Hg substantially reduced cardiovascular events as compared with moderate blood pressure control in patients with PAD.[104] It is not known whether antihypertensive therapy prevents the progression of PAD. Treatment of hypertension might decrease perfusion pressure to extremities already compromised by peripheral arterial stenoses. In addition, concern has been raised regarding the potential adverse affects of beta-adrenergic receptor blockers on peripheral blood flow and symptoms of claudication or critical limb ischemia. Beta-adrenergic blocking agents worsen claudication in some trials but not in others. A meta-analysis that included 11 studies of beta-blocker therapy, as compared with placebo, in patients with intermittent claudication found no significant impairment on walking capacity.[105] Beta-blocking drugs reduce the risk of myocardial infarction and death in patients with coronary artery disease, a problem affecting many patients with PAD.[106] Thus, if clinically indicated for other conditions, these drugs should not be withheld in patients with PAD. The balance of evidence supports treatment of hypertension in patients with PAD according to established clinical guidelines (see Chap. 38).[107]

Angiotensin-converting enzyme inhibitors reduce cardiovascular events in patients with atherosclerosis. In the Heart Outcomes Prevention Evaluation study (HOPE), the angiotensin-converting enzyme inhibitor ramipril decreased the risk for vascular death, myocardial infarction, or stroke by 22 percent. Forty-four percent of the patients enrolled in the HOPE trial had evidence of PAD as manifested by an ABI less than 0.9. Ramipril reduced cardiovascular events in the patients with PAD to a comparable degree as in those without PAD (Fig. 54–16).[108]

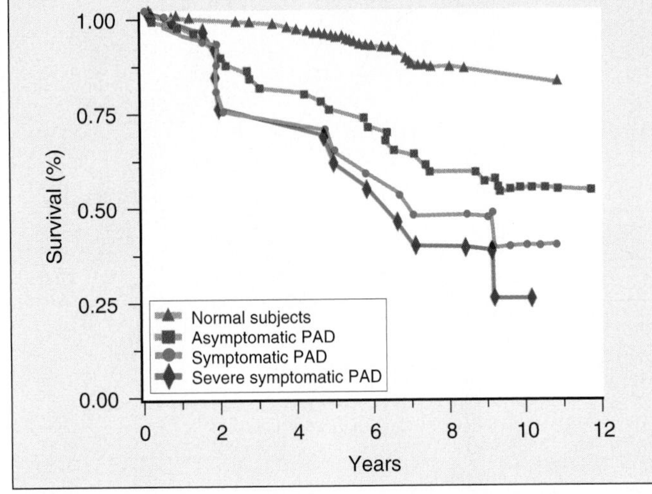

FIGURE 54–13 Survival rates of patients with peripheral arterial disease (PAD) derived from a population-based study. PAD was diagnosed by measuring the ankle/brachial index. Just the presence of PAD, even in the absence of symptoms, was associated with decreased survival. Survival was poorest in patients with symptoms. (From Criqui M, Langer RD, Fronek A, et al: Mortality over a period of 10 years in patients with peripheral arterial disease. N Engl J Med 326:381, 1992.)

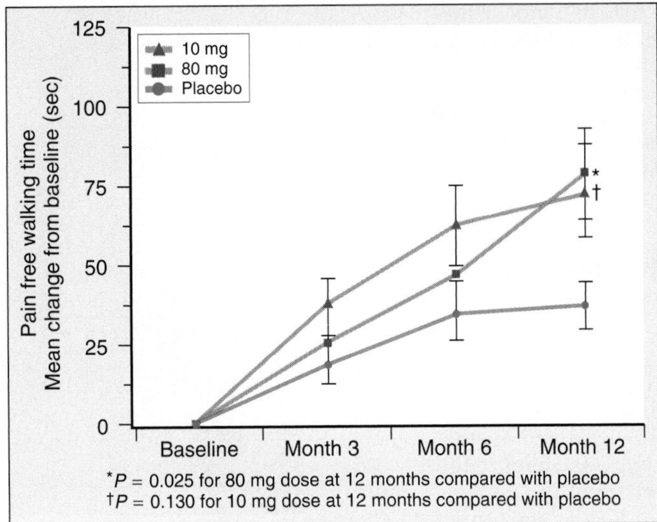

FIGURE 54–15 In the TREADMILL Study, lipid-lowering therapy with atorvastatin improved pain-free walking time in patients with intermittent claudication. (From Mohler ER 3rd, Hiatt Wr, Creager MA: Cholesterol reduction with atorvastatin improves walking distance in patients with arterial artery disease. Circulation 108:1481, 2003.)

Antiplatelet Therapy

Substantial evidence supports the use of antiplatelet agents to reduce adverse cardiovascular outcome in patients with atherosclerosis. A meta-analysis that included approximately 135,000 high-risk patients with atherosclerosis, including those with acute and prior myocardial infarction, stroke, and transient cerebrovascular ischemia, and other high-risk groups, including those with PAD, found that antiplatelet therapy yielded a 22 percent odds reduction for subsequent vascular death, myocardial infarction, or stroke (see Chap. 80).[109] Among the 9214 patients with PAD included in this analysis, antiplatelet therapy reduced the risk of myocardial infarction, stroke, or death by 22 percent (Fig. 54–17).[109] The CAPRIE trial compared clopidogrel with aspirin in terms of efficacy in preventing ischemic events in patients with recent myocardial infarction, recent ischemic stroke, or PAD. Overall, there was 8.7 percent relative risk reduction for

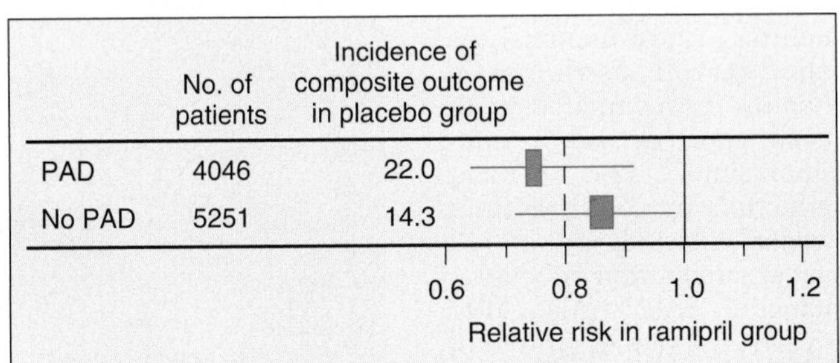

FIGURE 54–16 The relative risk of adverse cardiovascular events in the patients with and without peripheral arterial disease (PAD) according to treatment with the angiotensin-converting enzyme inhibitor ramipril in the Heart Outcomes Prevention Evaluation (HOPE) study. (Modified from Yusuf S, Sleight P, Pogue J, et al: Effects of an angiotensin-converting enzyme inhibitor, ramipril, on cardiovascular events in high-risk patients. The Heart Outcomes Prevention Evaluation Study Investigators [published erratum appears in N Engl J Med 342:748, 2000]. N Engl J Med 342:145, 2000.)

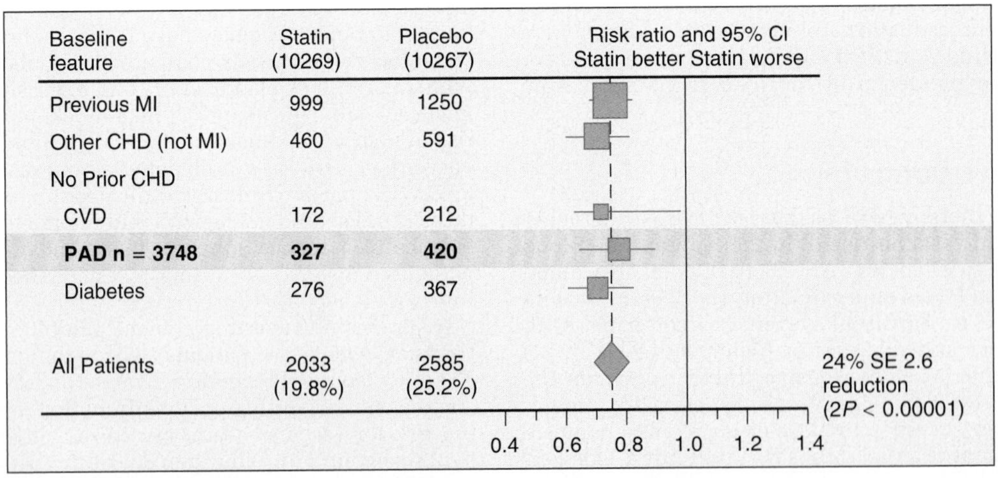

Baseline feature	Statin (10269)	Placebo (10267)	Risk ratio and 95% CI Statin better Statin worse
Previous MI	999	1250	
Other CHD (not MI)	460	591	
No Prior CHD			
CVD	172	212	
PAD n = 3748	**327**	**420**	
Diabetes	276	367	
All Patients	2033 (19.8%)	2585 (25.2%)	24% SE 2.6 reduction ($2P < 0.00001$)

0.4 0.6 0.8 1.0 1.2 1.4

FIGURE 54–14 Relative risk of adverse cardiovascular events in participants in the Heart Protection Study based on treatment with statin or placebo. Included in this study were 6700 patients with peripheral arterial disease (PAD), including 3748 patients who had no prior coronary heart disease, in whom there was an approximate 24 percent risk reduction of vascular events. CHD = congestive heart disease; MI = myocardial infarction. (From MRC/BHF: Heart Protection Study of cholesterol lowering with simvastatin in 20,536 high-risk individuals: A randomized placebo-controlled trial. Lancet 360:7, 2002.)

myocardial infarction, ischemic stroke, or vascular death in the group treated with clopidogrel.[85] Notably, among the 6452 patients in the PAD subgroup, clopidogrel treatment reduced adverse cardiovascular events by 23.8 percent (Fig. 54–18).

Antiplatelet therapy also prevents occlusion in the peripheral circulation after revascularization procdures. Of approximately 3000 patients with peripheral arterial procedures previously analyzed by the Antiplatelet Trialists Collaboration, the odds reduction for arterial or graft occlusion by antiplatelet therapy, primarily aspirin or aspirin plus dipyridamole, was 43 percent. Ticlopidine improved long-term patency of peripheral saphenous vein bypass grafts.[110] Several studies suggested that ticlopidine improves claudication or reduces the need for reconstructive vascular surgery, but these observations will require confirmation in additional clinical trials.

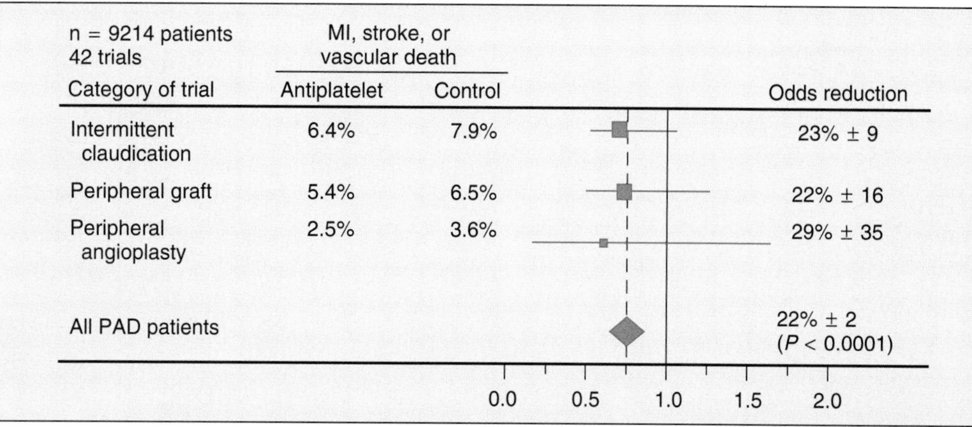

n = 9214 patients
42 trials
MI, stroke, or vascular death
Category of trial
Antiplatelet
Control
Odds reduction
Intermittent claudication
6.4%
7.9%
23% ± 9
Peripheral graft
5.4%
6.5%
22% ± 16
Peripheral angioplasty
2.5%
3.6%
29% ± 35
All PAD patients
22% ± 2
(P < 0.0001)
0.0
0.5
1.0
1.5
2.0

FIGURE 54–17 The effect of antiplatelet therapy on cardiovascular events in patients with peripheral arterial disease (PAD) based on the Antiplatelet Trialists' Collaboration. The odds ratios are shown for patients with claudication, infrainguinal bypass grafts, and percutaneous transluminal angioplasty. MI = myocardial infarction. (From Antithrombotic Trialists' Collaboration: Collaborative meta-analysis of randomised trials of antiplatelet therapy for prevention of death, myocardial infarction, and stroke in high risk patients. BMJ 324:71, 2002.)

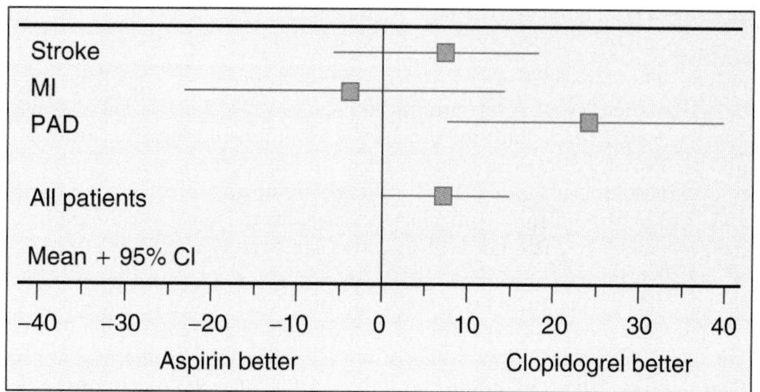

FIGURE 54–18 The relative risk reduction in adverse cardiovascular events in the Clopidogrel vs. Aspirin in Patients at Risk for Ischemic Events (CAPRIE) study. Patients with peripheral arterial disease (PAD) who received placebo had a 24 percent risk reduction compared with those receiving aspirin. (From CAPRIE Steering Committee: A randomised, blinded trial of clopidogrel versus aspirin in patients at risk of ischaemic events (CAPRIE). Lancet 348:1329, 1996.)

Pharmacotherapy

The development of effective pharmacotherapy for treating symptoms of PAD has lagged substantially behind pharmacotherapy for treating coronary artery disease. Published consensus guidelines for conducting clinical trials of pharmacological agents for treatment of patients with PAD should provide common ground for the objective evaluation of new drugs.[111] Most studies of vasodilator therapy have failed to demonstrate any efficacy in patients with intermittent claudication. Several pathophysiological explanations may account for the failure of vasodilator therapy in patients with PAD. During exercise, resistance vessels distal to a stenosis dilate in response to ischemia. Vasodilators would have minimal, if any, effect on these endogenously dilated vessels but would decrease resistance in other vessels and create a relative steal phenomenon, reducing blood flow and perfusion pressure to the affected leg. Moreover, in contrast to their effects on myocardial oxygen consumption in patients with coronary artery disease (due to afterload reduction), vasodilators do not reduce skeletal muscle oxygen demand.

In the United States, the Food and Drug Administration has approved two drugs, pentoxifylline (Trental) and cilostazol (Pletal), for treating claudication in patients with PAD. Additional drugs have been approved by licensing bodies in Europe, Asia, and South America. Pentoxifylline is a xanthine derivative used to treat patients with intermittent claudication. Its action is thought to be mediated via its hemorheological properties, including its ability to decrease blood viscosity and improve erythrocyte flexibility. It may have antiinflammatory and antiproliferative effects.[112,113] Two meta-analyses of randomized placebo-controlled trials of pentoxifylline found that it increased initial claudication distance by approximately 20 to 30 meters and absolute claudication distance by approximately 45 to 50 meters.[114,115]

Cilostazol is a quinolinone derivative that inhibits phosphodiesterase III, thereby decreasing cyclic adenosine monophosphate degradation and increasing its concentration in platelets and blood vessels. Although cilostazol inhibits platelet aggregation and causes vasodilation in experimental animals, its mechanism of action in patients with PAD is not known.[116] Several trials have reported that cilostazol improves absolute claudication distance by 40 to 50 percent as compared with placebo (Fig. 54–19).[117-119] Quality of life measures, assessed by the Medical Outcomes Scale (SF-36) and Walking Impairment Questionnaire, also demonstrated improvement. One study also found that absolute walking distance improves more with cilostazol than with either pentoxifylline or placebo, with the latter two having equivalent efficacy.[120] An advisory from the Food and Drug Administration stated that cilostazol should not be used in patients with congestive heart failure, since other phosphodiesterase III inhibitors have been shown to decrease survival in these patients.[121] The effect of cilostazol on cardiac morbidity and mortality is not known.

Other classes of drugs have been studied or are currently under investigation for treatment of either claudication or critical limb ischemia. These include serotonin (5HT-2) antagonists, calcium channel blockers, L-arginine, carnitine derivatives, vasodilator prostaglandins, and angiogenic growth factors. Naftidrofuryl, a serotonin-antagonist, has been reported to have improved symptoms of claudication in some trials and is currently available for use in Europe.[122] L-Arginine, the precursor for endothelium-derived nitric oxide, was found to have improved claudication distance after 3 weeks of intravenous therapy.[54] A nutritional bar enriched with L-arginine improved claudication time in a small study, but a large clinical trial did not confirm this observation.[56] Propionyl L-carnitine, a cofactor for fatty acid metabolism, has been reported to improve claudication, particularly in patients whose baseline maximum walking distance is less than 250 meters.[123,124]

Therapy with vasodilator prostaglandins has been investigated in patients with intermittent claudication and in those with critical limb ischemia. Intravenous administration of prostaglandin E_1 (PGE_1) or its precursor and oral administration of prostacyclin analogs improved claudication distance in preliminary trials.[125-127] A phase III study with the oral

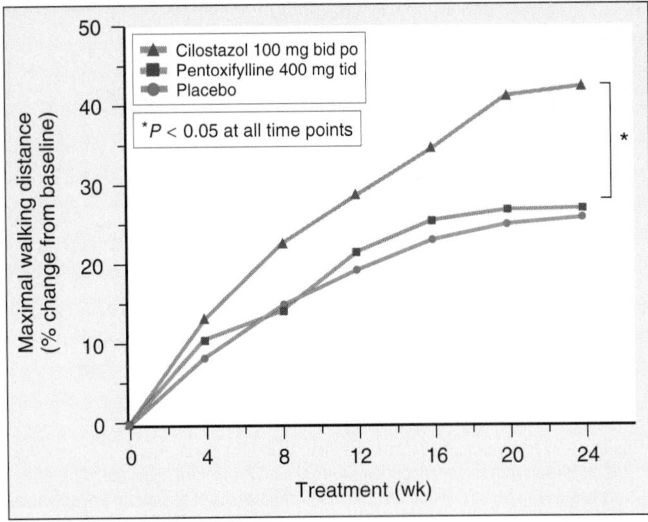

FIGURE 54–19 The effect of cilostazol, compared with pentoxifylline and placebo, on maximal walking distance. (From Dawson DL, Cutler BS, Hiatt WR, et al: A comparison of cilostazol and pentoxifylline for treating intermittent claudication. Am J Med 109:523, 2000.)

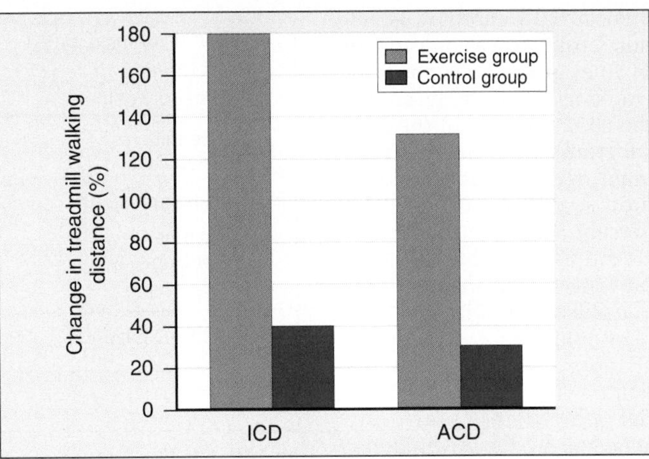

FIGURE 54–20 The effect of supervised exercise training on peak treadmill exercise time in patients with intermittent claudication. ACD = absolute claudication difference; ICD = initial claudication distance. (Adapted from Gardner AW, Poehlman ET: Exercise rehabilitation programs for the treatment of claudication pain. A meta-analysis. JAMA 274:975, 1995.)

prostacyclin derivative beraprost found no improvement in walking distance in patients with intermittent claudication.[128] In a large trial of 1560 patients with critical limb ischemia, PGE_1 administered intravenously for up to 28 days reduced the composite endpoint of death, major amputation, persistence of critical limb ischemia, acute myocardial infarction, and stroke at the time of hospital discharge from 73 to 64 percent, but its effect on this outcome did not differ significantly from the effect of placebo at the 6-month timepoint.[129] Most of the benefit of PGE_1 in this trial was related to recovery from leg ischemia.

The therapeutic use of angiogenic growth factors has engendered considerable enthusiasm. Administration of basic fibroblast growth factor and vascular endothelial growth factor as protein or gene therapy increases collateral blood vessel development, capillary number, and blood flow in experimental models of hindlimb ischemia. Gene transfer of human plasmid phVEGF165 by intraarterial catheter-based technique or by intramuscular injection into the ischemic extremity improved collateral blood vessel development in small case series.[130] Also, one recent study found that intramuscular administration of bone marrow–derived mononuclear cells to induce angiogenesis improved ABI, rest pain, and pain-free walking time in patients with chronic limb ischemia.[131] To date, few placebo-controlled clinical trials have evaluated angiogenic growth factors in patients with either claudication or critical limb ischemia. Intramuscular delivery of $AdVEGF_{121}$, an adenovirus encoding the 121 isoform of vascular endothelial growth factor, did not improve walking time or ABI in patients with claudication.[132] Intrafemoral artery administration of recombinant fibroblast growth factor-2 modestly improved maximal walking time but not ABI in patients with claudication.[133] Other studies are in progress.

Exercise Rehabilitation

Supervised exercise rehabilitation programs improve symptoms of claudication in patients with PAD. Meta-analyses of controlled studies of exercise rehabilitation found that supervised exercise programs increase the average distance walked to the onset of claudication by 180 percent and the maximal distance walked by 120 to 150 percent (Fig. 54–20).[134,135] The greatest benefit occurred when sessions were at least 30 minutes in duration, sessions occurred at least three times per week for 6 months, and walking was used as the mode of exercise. Postulated mechanisms through which exercise training improves claudication include formation of collateral vessels and improvement in endothelium-dependent vasodilation, hemorheology, muscle metabolism, and walking efficiency.[136] Studies in experimental models of hindlimb ischemia have suggested that regular exercise increases the development of collateral blood vessels.[136] Expression of angiogenic factors is increased by exercise, particularly in hypoxic tissue.[137,138] Exercise training may improve endothelium-dependent vasodilation in patients with PAD, as it does in patients with coronary atherosclerosis and in the peripheral circulation of patients with congestive heart failure.[139-141] Improvement in calf blood flow has not been demonstrated consistently in patients with claudication after exercise training, although one study found that maximal calf blood flow increased commensurate with improvement in walking distance.[136,142] To date, no imaging studies have demonstrated increased collateral blood vessels after exercise training in patients with PAD.

The benefits of exercise training in patients with PAD may result from changes in skeletal muscle function, such as increased muscle mitochondrial enzyme activity, ATP production rate, and lactate production. In patients with PAD, improvement in exercise performance is associated with a decrease in plasma and skeletal muscle short chain acylcarnitine concentrations, which indicate improvement in oxidative metabolism, and increased peak oxygen consumption.[57] Training may also enhance biomechanical performance, enabling patients to walk more efficiently with less energy expenditure.

Percutaneous Transluminal Angioplasty and Stents (see Chap. 55)

Peripheral Arterial Surgery

Surgical revascularization is generally indicated to improve quality of life in patients with disabling claudication on maximal medical therapy and to relieve rest pain and preserve limb viability in patients with critical limb ischemia not amenable to percutaneous interventions. The specific operation must take into account the anatomic location of the arterial lesions and the presence of comorbid conditions. The surgical procedure is planned after identification of the arterial obstruction by imaging, ensuring that there is sufficient arterial inflow to and outflow from the graft to maintain patency. A preoperative evaluation to assess the risk of vascular surgery should be performed, since many of these patients have coexisting coronary artery disease. Guidelines for this evaluation have been established and are beyond the scope of this chapter (see Chap. 77).[143]

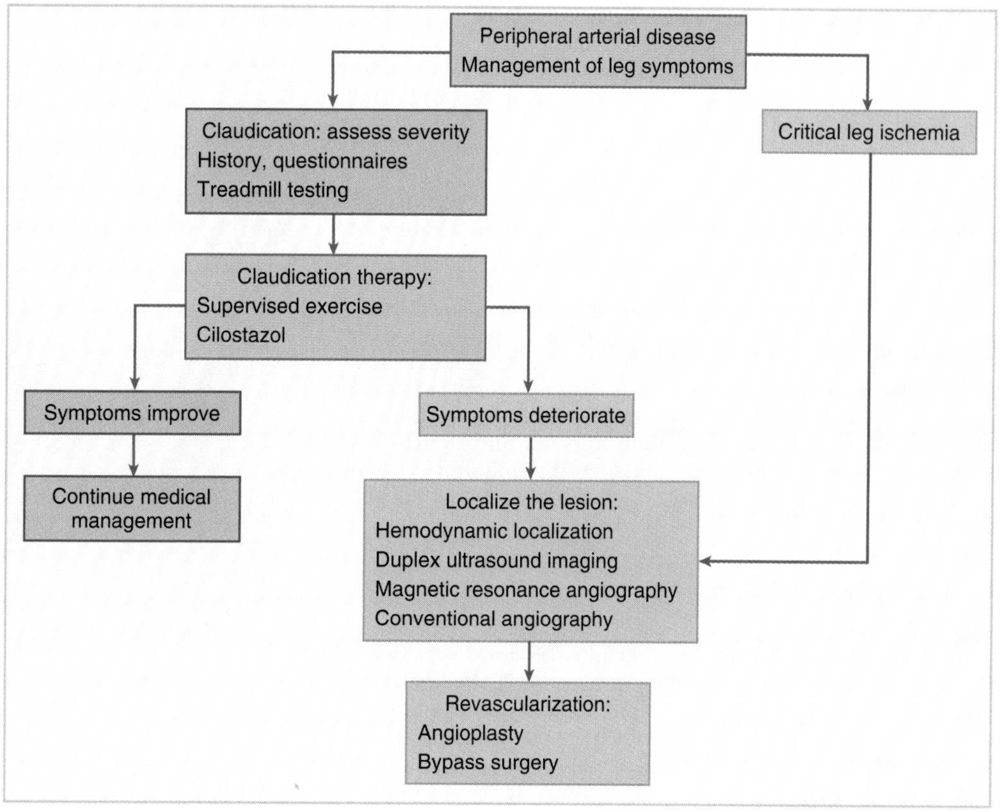

Aorta–bifemoral bypass is the most frequent operation for patients with aortoiliac disease. Typically, a knitted or woven prosthesis made of Dacron or polytetrafluoroethylene (PTFE) is anastomosed proximally to the aorta and distally to each common femoral artery. Occasionally, the iliac artery is used for the distal anastomosis, to maintain antegrade flow into at least one hypogastric artery. A meta-analysis of aortic bifurcation grafts based on 23 studies reported from 1970 to 1996 noted that 5 and 10-year limb patency rates were 91 percent and 87 percent for patients with claudication, respectively, and were 88 percent and 82 percent for patients with critical limb ischemia, respectively.[144] Patency rates appear to be lower in younger than in older patients, and this may result from more aggressive atherosclerosis in the aorta and outflow vessels in these younger patients.[145] Among the more recent series in the meta-analysis, operative morbidity and mortality rates were 8.3 percent and 3.3 percent, respectively.[144]

Peripheral arterial disease
Management of leg symptoms

Claudication: assess severity
History, questionnaires
Treadmill testing

Critical leg ischemia

Claudication therapy:
Supervised exercise
Cilostazol

Symptoms improve

Symptoms deteriorate

Continue medical management

Localize the lesion:
Hemodynamic localization
Duplex ultrasound imaging
Magnetic resonance angiography
Conventional angiography

Revascularization:
Angioplasty
Bypass surgery

FIGURE 54–21 Management algorithm for the treatment of symptomatic peripheral arterial disease (PAD). (From Hiatt WR: Medical treatment of peripheral arterial disease and claudication. N Engl J Med 344:1608, 2001.) See also Fig. 55–1 for an aggressive scheme for life-style limiting claudication.

Extra-anatomic surgical reconstructive procedures for aortoiliac disease include axillo-bifemoral bypass, ilio-bifemoral bypass, and femoral-femoral bypass. These bypass grafts, made of Dacron or PTFE, circumvent the aorta and iliac arteries and are generally utilized in high-risk patients with critical limb ischemia.[146] Long-term patency rates are inferior to those of aorto-bifemoral bypass procedures. Five-year patency rates for axillo-bifemoral bypass operations range from 50 to 70 percent, and for femoral-femoral bypass grafts from 70 to 80 percent. The operative mortality rate for extra-anatomic bypass procedures is 3 to 5 percent, reflecting, in part, the serious comorbid conditions and advanced atherosclerosis of many of the patients who undergo these procedures.

Reconstructive surgery for infrainguinal arterial disease includes femoral-popliteal and femoral-tibial or femoral-peroneal artery bypass. In situ or reversed autologous saphenous veins or synthetic grafts made of PTFE are used for the infrainguinal bypass. Patency rates for autologous saphenous vein bypass grafts exceed those with PTFE grafts.[1,2,147,148] Also, patency rates are better for grafts in which the distal anastomosis is placed in the popliteal artery above the knee as compared with below the knee.[1] Five-year primary patency rates for femoral-popliteal reconstruction in patients with claudication are approximately 80 percent and 75 percent for autogenous vein grafts or PTFE grafts, respectively, and in patients with critical limb ischemia are approximately 65 percent and 45 percent, respectively. For femoral-below knee bypass, including tibioperoneal artery reconstruction, the 5-year patency rates for saphenous vein grafts in patients with claudication or critical limb ischemia are comparable to those for femoral-popliteal above knee grafts and range from 60 to 80 percent. The 5-year patency rate for PTFE grafts in the infrapopliteal position is considerably inferior, approximating 65 percent in patients with claudication and 33 percent in patients with critical limb ischemia. The operative mortality rate for infrainguinal bypass operations is 1 to 2 percent.

Graft stenoses can result from technical errors at the time of surgery, such as retained valve cuffs or intimal flap or valvotome injury; from fibrous intimal hyperplasia, usually within 6 months of surgery; or from atherosclerosis, usually occurring within the vein graft at least 1 to 2 years after surgery. Institution of graft surveillance protocols using color-assisted duplex ultrasonography has enabled the identification of graft stenoses, prompting graft revision and avoiding complete graft failure.[2] Graft outcome is improved as a result of routine ultrasonographic surveillance. Also, antithrombotic agents, including antiplatelet drugs and coumarin derivatives, improve graft patency. Several studies have suggested that antiplatelet drugs may be more effective in preserving synthetic grafts, whereas coumarin derivates may be more effective for vein bypass grafts.[149,150]

A management algorithm for treating symptomatic PAD is illustrated in Figure 54–21.

Vasculitis

See Chapter 82.

Thromboangiitis Obliterans

Thromboangiitis obliterans (TAO) is a segmental vasculitis that affects the distal arteries, veins, and nerves of the upper and lower extremities. It typically occurs in young persons who smoke. A patient with characteristics of TAO was described initially by von Winiwater in 1879.[151] Leo Buerger coined the term *thromboangiitis obliterans* and described its pathology in 11 amputated limbs.[152]

Pathology and Pathogenesis

Thromboangiitis obliterans primarily affects the medium and small vessels of the arms, including the radial, ulnar, palmar, and digital arteries, and their counterparts in the legs, including the tibial, peroneal, plantar, and digital arteries. Involvement can extend to the cerebral, coronary, renal, mesenteric, aortoiliac, and pulmonary arteries.[153-155] The pathological findings include an occlusive, highly cellular thrombus incorporating polymorphonuclear leukocytes, microabscesses, and occasionally multinucleated giant cells.[156] The inflammatory infiltrate can also affect the vascular wall, but the internal elastic membrane remains intact. In the chronic phase of the disease, the thrombus becomes organized and the vascular wall becomes fibrotic.

The precise cause of TAO is not known. Tobacco use or exposure is present in virtually every patient. Potential immunological mechanisms include increased cellular sensitivity to type I and type III collagen or the presence of antiendothelial cell antibodies. CD4 T cells have been identified in cellular infiltrates of vessels of patients with TAO.[157,158] The prevalence of anticardiolipin antibodies may be increased, particularly among the more severely affected patients.[159] Decreased endothelium-dependent vasodilation to acetylcholine can occur in both affected and unaffected limbs of patients with TAO, raising the possibility that reduced bioavailability of nitric oxide contributes to the disorder.[160]

Clinical Presentation

The prevalence of TAO is greater in Asia than in North America or Western Europe. In the United States, TAO occurs in approximately 13 per 100,000 population.[156] Most patients with TAO develop symptoms before 45 years of age, and 75 to 90 percent are men. Patients can have claudication of the hands, forearms, feet, or calves. The majority of patients with TAO present with rest pain and digital ulcerations. Often more than one extremity is affected. Raynaud phenomenon occurs in approximately 45 percent of patients, and superficial thrombophlebitis, which may be migratory, occurs in approximately 40 percent of patients.

The radial, ulnar, dorsalis pedis, and posterior tibial pulses may be absent if the corresponding vessel is involved. The clinical characteristics of critical limb ischemia and ischemic digital ulcerations are described earlier in this chapter. The Allen test result is abnormal in two-thirds of patients.[156] To perform the Allen test, both radial and ulnar arteries are compressed while the hand is clenched and then opened. This maneuver causes palmar blanching. Release of compression from either pulse should normally produce palmar erythema if the palmar arches are patent. If these are occluded, pallor persists on the side where compression is maintained. The distal aspects of the extremities may have discrete, tender, erythematous subcutaneous cords, indicating a superficial thrombophlebitis .

Diagnosis

No specific laboratory tests other than biopsy can diagnose TAO. Most tests, therefore, require exclusion of other diseases that might have similar clinical presentations, including autoimmune diseases, such as scleroderma or systemic lupus erythematosus, hypercoagulable states, diabetes, or acute arterial occlusion due to embolism. Acute phase indicators, such as the erythrocyte sedimentation rate or C-reactive protein, are usually normal. Serum immunological markers, including antinuclear antibodies and rheumatoid factor, should not be present, and serum complement levels should be normal. If clinically indicated, a proximal source of embolism should be excluded by cardiac and vascular ultrasonography or by arteriography. Arteriography of an affected limb supports the diagnosis of TAO if there is segmental occlusion of small and medium-size arteries, absence of atherosclerosis, and corkscrew collateral vessels circumventing the occlusion (Fig. 54–22). These same findings, however, can occur in patients with scleroderma, systemic lupus erythematosus, mixed connective tissue disease, and antiphospholipid antibody syndrome. The pathognomonic test is a biopsy showing the classic pathological findings. This procedure is rarely indicated, and biopsy sites may fail to heal because of severe ischemia. The diagnosis, therefore, usually depends on an age of onset younger than 45 years, a history of tobacco use, physical examination demonstrating distal limb ischemia, exclusion of other diseases, and, if necessary, angiographic demonstration of typical lesions.[161]

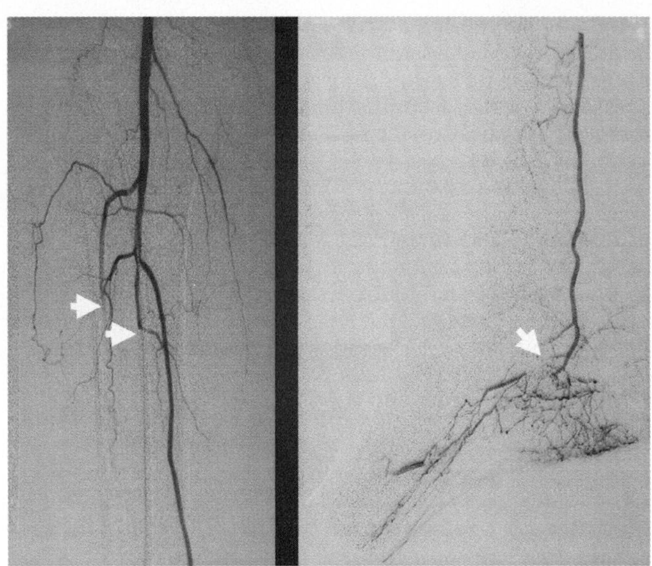

FIGURE 54–22 Angiogram of a young woman with thromboangiitis obliterans. The **left panel** demonstrates occlusion of the anterior tibial and peroneal arteries (arrows). The **right panel** demonstrates an occlusion of the distal portion of the posterior tibial artery (arrow) with bridging collateral vessels.

Treatment

The cornerstone of treatment is cessation of tobacco use.[162] Patients without gangrene who stop smoking rarely require amputation.[163,164] In contrast, one or more amputations may ultimately be required in 40 to 45 percent of those patients with TAO who continue to smoke.

Several drugs can benefit patients with TAO. The prostacyclin analogue iloprost, administered 6 hours per day for 28 days, was more effective than aspirin in relieving rest pain and healing ulcers.[165] In a multicenter trial, however, oral iloprost administered for 8 weeks had no greater effect than placebo in healing ulcers, although there was somewhat more effective relief of pain at low doses.[166] Cyclophosphamide improved symptoms but not the angiographic appearance of TAO in one study.[167] A naked plasmid DNA-encoding vascular endothelial growth factor (phVEGF 165) was administered intramuscularly into seven limbs of six patients with TAO, with subsequent healing of ulcers in three to five limbs and relief of rest pain in two others.[168]

Vascular reconstructive surgery is usually not a viable option because of the segmental nature of this disease and involvement of distal vessels. An autogenous saphenous vein bypass graft can be considered if a target vessel for the distal anastomosis is available. Long-term patency rates are better in ex-smokers than in smokers.[169]

Takayasu Arteritis and Giant Cell Arteritis

See Chapter 82.

Acute Limb Ischemia

Acute limb ischemia occurs when an arterial occlusion suddenly reduces blood flow to the arm or leg. The metabolic needs of the tissue outstrip perfusion, placing limb viability in jeopardy. The clinical presentation of patients with acute limb ischemia relates to the location of the arterial occlusion and the resulting decrease in blood flow. Depending on the severity of ischemia, patients may note disabling claudication or pain at rest. Pain may develop over a short period and is manifest in the affected extremity distal to the site of obstruction. It is not necessarily confined to the foot or toes, or hand or fingers, as is usually the case in chronic limb ischemia. Concurrent ischemia of peripheral nerves causes sensory loss and motor dysfunction.

The physical findings can include absence of pulses distal to the occlusion, cool skin, pallor, delayed capillary return and venous filling, diminished or absent sensory perception, and muscular weakness or paralysis. This constellation of symptoms and signs is often recalled as the five Ps, *p*ain, *p*ulselessness, *p*allor, *p*aresthesias, and *p*aralysis.

Prognosis

Comorbid cardiovascular disorders are usually found in patients who present with acute limb ischemia and may even be responsible for the event. Therefore, long-term prognosis is limited in this population.[170] The 5-year survival rate after acute limb ischemia caused by thrombosis approximates 45 percent and after embolism is less than 20 percent.[171] The 1-month survival rate in persons older than 75 years of age with acute limb ischemia approximates 40 percent.[172] The risk of limb loss depends on the severity of the ischemia and the elapsed time before a revascularization procedure is undertaken.

A classification scheme that takes into consideration the severity of ischemia and the viability of the limb, along with related neurological findings and Doppler signals, has been developed by the Society for Vascular Surgery and the International Society for Cardiovascular Surgery (Table 54–8).[67] A viable limb, category 1, is not immediately threatened, has neither sensory nor motor abnormalities, and has blood flow detectable by Doppler. Threatened viability, category 2, indicates that the severity of ischemia will cause limb loss unless the blood supply is restored promptly. The category is subdivided into marginally and immediately threatened limbs, the latter characterized by pain, sensory deficits, and muscular weakness. Arterial blood flow cannot be detected by Doppler. Irreversible limb ischemia leading to tissue loss and requiring amputation, category 3, is characterized by loss of sensation, paralysis, and the absence of Doppler-detected blood flow in both arteries and veins distal to the occlusion.

Pathogenesis

The causes of acute limb ischemia include arterial embolism, thrombosis in situ, dissection, and trauma. Most arterial emboli arise from thrombotic sources in the heart. Atrial fibrillation complicating valvular heart disease, congestive heart failure, coronary artery disease, and hypertension accounts for approximately 50 percent of cardiac emboli to the limbs. Other sources include rheumatic or prosthetic cardiac valves, ventricular thrombus resulting from myocardial infarction or left ventricular aneurysm, paradoxical embolism of venous thrombi through the intraatrial or intraventricular communications, and cardiac tumors such as left atrial myxomas. Aneurysms of the aorta or peripheral arteries may harbor thrombi, which subsequently embolize to more distal arterial sites, usually lodging at branch points where the artery decreases in size.

Thrombosis in situ occurs in atherosclerotic peripheral arteries, infrainguinal bypass grafts, peripheral artery aneurysms, and normal arteries of patients with hypercoagulable states. In patients with peripheral atherosclerosis, thrombosis in situ may complicate plaque rupture, causing acute arterial occlusion and limb ischemia, in a manner analogous to that which occurs in coronary arteries in patients with acute myocardial infarction. Thrombosis complicating popliteal artery aneurysms is a much more common complication than rupture and may account for 10 percent of cases of acute limb ischemia in elderly men.[1,173] Acute thrombotic occlusion of a normal artery is unusual but may occur in patients with procoagulant disorders such as antiphospholipid antibody syndrome, activated protein C resistance (Factor V Leiden), deficiency of protein C or S, heparin-induced thrombocytopenia, essential thrombocythemia, and hyperhomocysteinemia. One of the most common causes of acute limb ischemia is thrombotic occlusion of an infrainguinal bypass graft, as discussed previously.

Diagnostic Tests

The history and physical examination usually establish the diagnosis of acute limb ischemia. Time available for diagnostic tests is often limited, and diagnostic tests should not delay urgent revascularization procedures if limb viability is immediately threatened. The pressure in the affected limb and corresponding ABI can be measured if flow is detectable by Doppler ultrasonography. A Doppler probe can be used to

TABLE 54–8 Clinical Categories of Acute Limb Ischemia (Modified from the SVS/ISCVS Classification)

		Findings		Doppler Signals	
Category	Description/Prognosis	*Sensory loss*	*Muscle weakness*	*Arterial*	*Venous*
I. Viable	Not immediately threatened	None	None	audible	Audible
II. Threatened					
a. Marginally	Salvageable if promptly treated	Minimal (toes) or none	None	(Often) inaudible	Audible
b. Immediately	Salvageable with immediate revascularization	More than toes, rest pain	Mild, moderate	(Usually) inaudible	Audible
III. Irreversible	Major tissue loss or permanent nerve damage inevitable	Profound, anesthetic	Profound, paralysis (rigor)	Inaudible	Inaudible

Adapted from Rutherford RB, Baker JD, Ernst C, et al. Recommended standards for reports dealing with lower extremity ischemia: revised version. J Vasc Surg 26:517, 1997.

detect the presence of blood flow in peripheral arteries, particularly when pulses are not palpable. Color-assisted duplex ultrasonography can be used to determine the site of occlusion. It is particularly applicable to evaluate the patency of infrainguinal bypass grafts. Contrast arteriography demonstrates the site of occlusion and provides an anatomic guide for revascularization.

Treatment

Analgesic medications should be administered to reduce pain. For patients with acute leg ischemia, the bed should be positioned such that the feet are lower than chest level, thereby increasing limb perfusion pressure via gravitational effects. This can be accomplished by putting blocks under the posts at the head of the bed. Efforts should be made to reduce pressure on the heels, on bony prominences, and between the toes by appropriate placement of soft material on the bed, such as sheep skin, and between the toes, such as lamb's wool. The room should be kept warm to prevent cold-induced cutaneous vasoconstriction.

Heparin is administered intravenously as soon as the diagnosis of acute limb ischemia is made. The dose should be sufficient to increase the partial thromboplastin time by 1.5 to 2.5 times control values to prevent thrombus propagation or recurrent embolism. It is not known whether low-molecular-weight heparin would be as effective as unfractionated heparin in patients with acute limb ischemia.

Catheter-directed intraarterial thrombolysis is an initial treatment option for patients presenting with category I and IIA acute limb ischemia, if there is no contraindication to thrombolysis.[174-176] Catheter-based thrombolysis can also be considered for patients with more severe limb ischemia who are considered a high risk for surgical intervention. Long-term patency after thrombolysis is greater in patients with category I and II critical limb ischemia than in those with category III, in native arteries than in grafts, and in vein grafts than in prosthetic grafts.[176] Identification and repair of a graft stenosis after successful thrombolysis improves long-term graft patency.[176,177] Thrombolytic regimens have employed streptokinase, urokinase, recombinant tissue plasminogen activator, and reteplase. The duration of catheter-based thrombolytic therapy should generally not exceed 48 hours to achieve optimal benefit and limit the risk of bleeding. Percutaneous, catheter-based, mechanical thrombectomy can be used alone or in addition to pharmacological thrombolysis to treat patients with acute limb ischemia.[175,178]

Urgent revascularization is indicated for patients presenting with category IIB and early category III acute limb ischemia. The procedure depends on the nature and location of the arterial occlusion. Thromboembolectomy can be attempted in patients whose acute limb ischemia is caused by systemic embolism.[179] If thromboembolectomy is neither feasible nor successful, then surgical reconstruction, bypassing the occluded area, should be performed. These techniques were discussed previously in this chapter.

Five prospective randomized trials, comprising 1283 patients, have compared the benefits and risks of thrombolysis and surgical reconstruction in patients presenting with acute limb ischemia (Table 54-9).[180] The Surgery versus Thrombolysis for Ischemia of the Lower Extremity (STILE) trial compared thrombolysis with either recombinant tissue plasminogen activator or urokinase to surgery after native artery or graft occlusion in patients with limb ischemia of less than 6 months' duration. The trial was stopped prematurely after enrollment of 393 patients. The composite outcome of death, ongoing or recurrent ischemia, major amputation, and major morbidity occurred in 62 percent of the group randomized to thrombolysis compared with 36 percent of those randomized to surgery. Of those patients who had symptoms for less than 14 days, however, amputation-free survival at 6 months was greater in the patients treated with thrombolysis than in those treated with surgery.[181] In the Thrombolysis or Peripheral Arterial Study (TOPAS), intraarterial thrombolysis with urokinase was compared to surgery in 554 patients with acute limb ischemia of less than 14 days. Amputation-free survival at 6 and 12 months was 72 and 65 percent, respectively, in the thrombolysis group and 75 and 70 percent, respectively, in the surgery group.[182] Taken together, the findings from these trials would suggest that catheter-based thrombolysis is an appropriate initial option in patients with category I and IIA acute limb ischemia of less than 7 days' duration, whereas surgical revascularization would be more appropriate for those with category IIB and early III acute limb ischemia and in those whose symptoms have been present for more than 7 days (Fig. 54-23).

Atheroembolism

Atheroembolism refers to the occlusion of arteries resulting from detachment and embolization of atheromatous debris, including fibrin, platelets, cholesterol crystals, and calcium fragments. Other terms include *atherogenic embolism* and *cholesterol embolism*. Atheroemboli originate most frequently from shaggy protruding atheromas of the aorta and less frequently from atherosclerotic branch arteries. The atheroemboli typically occlude small downstream arteries and arterioles of the extremities, brain, eye, kidneys, or mesentery.[183,184]

The prevalence of atheroembolism in the general population is not known. Most affected individuals are males who are older than 60 years of age with clinical evidence of atherosclerosis. The Dutch National Pathology Information System reported an incidence of atheroemboli in 6.2 patients per million per year, and atheroemboli were present in 0.3 percent of autopsy cases.[185] In autopsy series of persons over the age of 60, the incidence of atheroembolism has ranged from 0.8 to 2.4 percent.

Pathogenesis

The risk of atheroembolism is greatest in patients with aortic atherosclerosis characterized by large protruding atheromas (see Fig. 54–5). There is a strong association between large

TABLE 54–9 Comparison of Catheter-Directed Thrombolysis and Surgical Revascularization in Treatment of Limb Ischemia

		Catheter Directed Thrombolysis			Surgical Revascularization		
Study	Results at	*Patients*	*Limb Salvage (%)*	*Mortality (%)*	*Patients*	*Limb Salvage (%)*	*Mortality (%)*
Rochester	12 mo	57	82	16	57	82	42
STILE[181]	6 mo	248	88	6	144	89	8
TOPAS[182]	12 mo	272	85	20	272	86	17

Adapted from Dormandy JA, Rutherford RB: Management of peripheral arterial disease (PAD), TASC Working Group. J Vasc Surg 31:S1, 2000.

aortic plaques identified by ultrasonography and previous embolic disease.[186-188] Similarly, identification of large protruding atheromas by transesophageal echocardiography predicts future embolic events.[186,189,190] Approximately 50 percent of atheroemboli involve vessels in the lower extremities.

Catheter manipulation causes a large proportion of atheroemboli.[191] Similarly, surgical manipulation of the aorta during cardiac or vascular operations precipitates atheroembolism in 2 to 3 percent of patients.[192] Controversy remains as to whether anticoagulants or thrombolytic drugs contribute to atheroembolism.[183,184,190,193,194] In the Stroke Prevention and Atrial Fibrillation (SPAF) study, atheroembolism occurred in 0.7 percent per patient-year in those patients assigned to adjusted-dose warfarin.[195] In the French Study of Aortic Plaques in Stroke Group, no patient receiving warfarin developed clinical evidence of atheroembolism.[189] Muscle biopsies at the time of coronary artery bypass surgery in patients with recent myocardial infarction detected atheroemboli in 14 percent of patients who received thrombolysis and 10 percent of those who did not.[196]

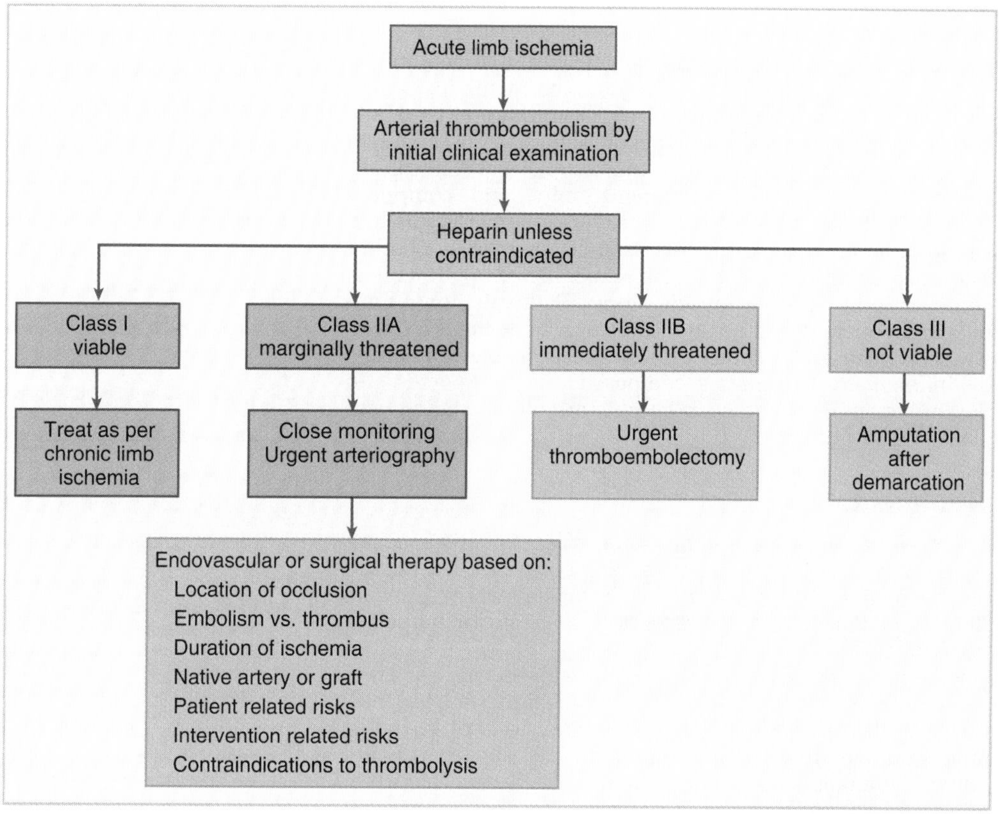

Acute limb ischemia
Arterial thromboembolism by initial clinical examination
Heparin unless contraindicated
Class I viable
Class IIA marginally threatened
Class IIB immediately threatened
Class III not viable
Treat as per chronic limb ischemia
Close monitoring Urgent arteriography
Urgent thromboembolectomy
Amputation after demarcation
Endovascular or surgical therapy based on:
Location of occlusion
Embolism vs. thrombus
Duration of ischemia
Native artery or graft
Patient related risks
Intervention related risks
Contraindications to thrombolysis

FIGURE 54–23 Management algorithm for the treatment of acute limb ischemia. (Adapted from Dormandy JA, Rutherford RB: Management of peripheral arterial disease (PAD). TASC Working Group. J Vasc Surg 31:S1, 2000.)

Clinical Presentation

The most notable clinical features of atheroembolism to the extremities includes painful cyanotic toes, resulting in the appellation *blue-toe syndrome* (Fig. 54–24). Livedo reticularis occurs in approximately 50 percent of patients. Local areas of erythematous or violaceous discoloration may be present on the lateral aspects of the feet and the soles and also on the calves. Other findings include digital and foot ulcerations, nodules, purpura, and petechiae. Pedal pulses are typically present, since the emboli tend to lodge in the more distal digital arteries and arterioles. Symptoms and signs indicating additional organ involvement with atheroemboli should be sought. Fundoscopy can visualize Hollenhorst plaques in patients with visual loss secondary to retinal ischemia or infarction. Renal involvement manifested by increased blood pressure and azotemia commonly occurs in patients with peripheral atheroemboli. Patients also sometimes have evidence of mesenteric or bladder ischemia and splenic infarction.

The clinical setting and findings are usually sufficient to diagnose atheroembolism. However, some of the manifestations of atheroemboli may be present with other diseases. As discussed previously, critical limb ischemia occurs in patients with severe peripheral atherosclerosis, and acute limb ischemia is a consequence of thromboembolism, each of which would be characterized by an abnormal pulse examination. Hypersensitivity vasculitides secondary to connective tissue diseases, infections, drugs, polyarteritis nodosa, or

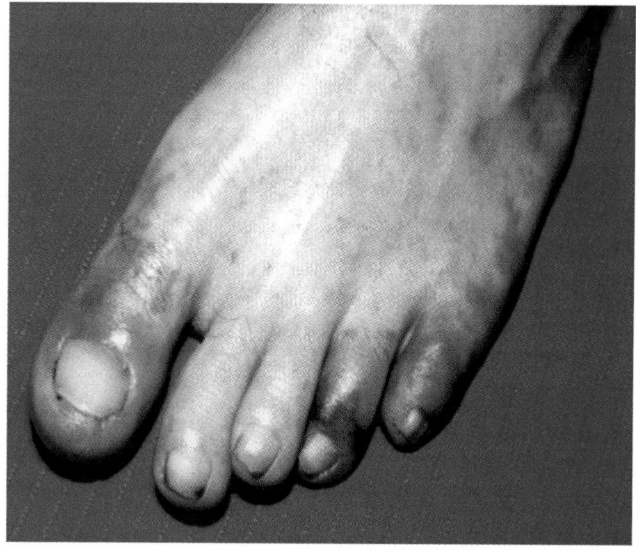

FIGURE 54–24 Atheroemboli to the foot, or "blue toe syndrome." There is cyanotic discoloration of the first, fourth, and fifth toes, as well as localized areas of violaceous discoloration along the lateral aspect of the foot.

cryoglobulinemia, for example, may manifest with multisystem organ damage and cutaneous findings of purpura, ulcers, and digital ischemia similar to those findings that result from atheroemboli (see Chap. 82). Procoagulant disorders such as antiphospholipid antibody syndrome, heparin-induced thrombocytopenia, and myeloproliferative disorders such as essential thrombocythemia can cause digital artery thrombosis with resultant digital ischemia, cyanosis, and ulceration.

Diagnostic Tests

Laboratory studies that are consistent with atheroembolism include an elevated erythrocyte sedimentation rate, eosinophilia, and eosinophiluria. Other findings may include anemia, thrombocytopenia, hypocomplementemia, and azotemia. Imaging of the aorta with transesophageal echocardiography, magnetic resonance angiography, and computed tomography may identify sites of severe atherosclerosis and shaggy atheroma indicative of a source for atheroemboli.[197] The only definitive test for atheroembolism is pathological confirmation by skin or muscle biopsy. Pathognomonic findings include elongated needle-shaped clefts in small arteries, which are caused by cholesterol crystals, often accompanied by inflammatory infiltrates composed of lymphocytes and possibly giant cells and eosinophils, intimal thickening, and perivascular fibrosis.

Treatment

There is no definitive treatment for atheroembolism. Analgesics should be administered for pain. Local foot care should be provided as described previously for patients with acute limb ischemia. It may be necessary to excise or amputate necrotic areas.

Patients with this condition are subject to recurrent atheroembolic events. Risk factor modification, such as lipid-lowering therapy and smoking cessation, can have favorable effects on overall outcome from atherosclerosis, but it is not known whether such intervention will prevent recurrent atheroembolism. The use of antiplatelet drugs to prevent recurrent atheroembolism remains controversial.[184,188] It is reasonable, however, to administer antiplatelet agents even in the absence of strong clinical evidence of efficacy, since the agents will prevent other adverse cardiovascular events in patients with atherosclerosis. The use of warfarin also engenders controversy, and some investigators have even suggested that anticoagulants precipitate atheroemboli.[183,184,186,193] Others have found that warfarin reduces atheroembolic events, particularly in patients with mobile aortic atheroma.[190,194] The use of corticosteroids to treat atheroembolism also remains controversial.[184]

Surgical removal of the source should be considered in patients with atheroembolism, particularly in those in whom it recurs. Surgical procedures include excision and replacement of affected portions of the aorta, endarterectomy, and bypass operations. Operative intervention is targeted to the site of the aorta, iliac, or femoral arteries where there is aneurysm formation or obvious shaggy friable atherosclerotic plaque. Often, the aorta is diffusely affected by severe atherosclerosis and it is not possible to identify the precise segment that is responsible for atheroembolism. In addition, many of these patients are elderly and have coexisting coronary artery disease, which increases the risk of major vascular operations.

REFERENCES

General Considerations and Epidemiology

1. Dormandy JA, Rutherford RB: Management of peripheral arterial disease (PAD). TASC Working Group. J Vasc Surg 31:S1, 2000.
2. ACC/AHA Guidelines for the Management of Peripheral Arterial Disease. J Am Coll Cardiol. In press. Available at http://www.acc.org/xxx.
3. Meijer WT, Hoes AW, Rutgers D, et al: Peripheral arterial disease in the elderly: The Rotterdam Study. Arterioscler Thromb Vasc Biol 18:185, 1998.
4. Hirsch AT, Criqui MH, Treat-Jacobson D, et al: Peripheral arterial disease detection, awareness, and treatment in primary care. JAMA 286:1317, 2001.
5. Murabito JM, Evans JC, Nieto K, et al: Prevalence and clinical correlates of peripheral arterial disease in the Framingham Offspring Study. Am Heart J 143:961, 2002.
6. Criqui MH: Peripheral arterial disease—epidemiological aspects. Vasc Med 6(Suppl 1):3, 2001.
7. Beckman J, Creager M: Risk factors. *In* Creager M (ed): Management of Peripheral Arterial Disease. London, ReMEDICA Publishing, 2000, pp 19-42.
8. Lu J, Creager MA: The relationship of cigarette smoking to peripheral arterial disease. Rev Cardiovasc Med. In press.
9. Doyle J, Creager MA: Pharmacotherapy and behavioral intervention for peripheral arterial disease. Rev Cardiovasc Med 4:18, 2003.
10. Beckman JA, Creager MA, Libby P: Diabetes and atherosclerosis: Epidemiology, pathophysiology, and management. JAMA 287:2570, 2002.
11. Jude EB, Oyibo SO, Chalmers N, Boulton AJ: Peripheral arterial disease in diabetic and nondiabetic patients: A comparison of severity and outcome. Diabetes Care 24:1433, 2001.
12. Criqui MH, Denenberg JO, Langer RD, Fronek A: The epidemiology of peripheral arterial disease: Importance of identifying the population at risk. Vasc Med 2:221, 1997.
13. Ridker PM, Stampfer MJ, Rifai N: Novel risk factors for systemic atherosclerosis: A comparison of C-reactive protein, fibrinogen, homocysteine, lipoprotein(a), and standard cholesterol screening as predictors of peripheral arterial disease. JAMA 285:2481, 2001.
14. Murabito JM, D'Agostino RB, Silbershatz H, Wilson WF: Intermittent claudication: A risk profile from The Framingham Heart Study. Circulation 96:44, 1997.
15. Cheng SW, Ting AC, Wong J: Lipoprotein (a) and its relationship to risk factors and severity of atherosclerotic peripheral vascular disease. Eur J Vasc Endovasc Surg 14:17, 1997.
16. Kannel WB: The demographics of claudication and the aging of the American population. Vasc Med 1:60, 1996.
17. Hooi JD, Kester AD, Stoffers HE, et al: Incidence of and risk factors for asymptomatic peripheral arterial occlusive disease: A longitudinal study. Am J Epidemiol 153:666, 2001.
18. Boushey CJ, Beresford SA, Omenn GS, Motulsky AG: A quantitative assessment of plasma homocysteine as a risk factor for vascular disease. Probable benefits of increasing folic acid intakes. JAMA 274:1049, 1995.
19. Graham IM, Daly LE, Refsum HM, et al: Plasma homocysteine as a risk factor for vascular disease. The European Concerted Action Project. JAMA 277:1775, 1997.
20. Smith FB, Lowe GD, Lee AJ, et al: Smoking, hemorheologic factors, and progression of peripheral arterial disease in patients with claudication. J Vasc Surg 28:129, 1998.
21. Smith FB, Lee AJ, Hau CM, et al: Plasma fibrinogen, haemostatic factors and prediction of peripheral arterial disease in the Edinburgh Artery Study. Blood Coagul Fibrinolysis 11:43, 2000.
22. Ridker PM, Cushman M, Stampfer MJ, et al: Plasma concentration of C-reactive protein and risk of developing peripheral vascular disease. Circulation 97:425, 1998.

Pathophysiology of PAD

23. Aird WC: Endothelial cell heterogeneity. Crit Care Med 31:S221, 2003.
24. Shimizu K, Sugiyama S, Aikawa M, et al: Host bone-marrow cells are a source of donor intimal smooth-muscle-like cells in murine aortic transplant arteriopathy. Nat Med 7:738, 2001.
25. Saiura A, Sata M, Hirata Y, et al: Circulating smooth muscle progenitor cells contribute to atherosclerosis. Nat Med 7:382, 2001.
26. Hristov M, Erl W, Weber PC: Endothelial progenitor cells: Mobilization, differentiation, and homing. Arterioscler Thromb Vasc Biol 23:1185, 2003.
27. Aird WC, Edelberg JM, Weiler-Guettler H, et al: Vascular bed-specific expression of an endothelial cell gene is programmed by the tissue microenvironment. J Cell Biol 138:1117, 1997.
28. Guillot PV, Guan J, Liu L, et al: A vascular bed-specific pathway. J Clin Invest 103:799, 1999.
29. Adams RH, Wilkinson GA, Weiss C, et al: Roles of ephrinB ligands and EphB receptors in cardiovascular development: Demarcation of arterial/venous domains, vascular morphogenesis, and sprouting angiogenesis. Genes Develop 13:295, 1999.
30. Shin D, Garcia-Cardena G, Hayashi S, et al: Expression of ephrinB2 identifies a stable genetic difference between arterial and venous vascular smooth muscle as well as endothelial cells, and marks subsets of microvessels at sites of adult neovascularization. Dev Biol 230:139, 2001.
31. Tomlinson JE, Topper JN: New insights into endothelial diversity. Curr Atheroscler Rep 5:223, 2003.
32. Liu C, Bhattacharjee G, Boisvert W, et al: In vivo interrogation of the molecular display of atherosclerotic lesion surfaces. Am J Pathol 163:1859, 2003.
33. Majesky MW: Vascular smooth muscle diversity: Insights from developmental biology. Curr Atheroscler Rep 5:208, 2003.
34. Bergwerff M, Gittenberger-de Groot AC, Wisse LJ, et al: Loss of function of the Prx1 and Prx2 homeobox genes alters architecture of the great elastic arteries and ductus arteriosus. Virchows Arch 436:12, 2000.
35. Lu J, Landerholm TE, Wei JS, et al: Coronary smooth muscle differentiation from proepicardial cells requires rhoA-mediated actin reorganization and p160 rho-kinase activity. Dev Biol 240:404, 2001.
36. Miano JM: Mammalian smooth muscle differentiation: Origins, markers and transcriptional control. Results Probl Cell Differ 38:39, 2002.
37. Li L, Liu Z, Mercer B, et al: Evidence for serum response factor-mediated regulatory networks governing SM22alpha transcription in smooth, skeletal, and cardiac muscle cells. Dev Biol 187:311, 1997.
38. Yamagishi H, Olson EN, Srivastava D: The basic helix-loop-helix transcription factor, dHAND, is required for vascular development [review]. J Clin Invest 105:261, 2000.
39. Lilly B, Olson EN, Beckerle MC: Identification of a CArG box–dependent enhancer within the cysteine-rich protein 1 gene that directs expression in arterial but not venous or visceral smooth muscle cells. Dev Biol 240:531, 2001.
40. Ikari Y, McManus BM, Kenyon J, Schwartz SM: Neonatal intima formation in the human coronary artery. Arterioscler Thromb Vasc Biol 19:2036, 1999.
41. Weninger WJ, Muller GB, Reiter C, et al: Intimal hyperplasia of the infant parasellar carotid artery: A potential developmental factor in atherosclerosis and SIDS. Circ Res 85:970, 1999.
42. Schwartz SM: The intima: A new soil. Circ Res 85:877, 1999.

43. Rainwater DL, McMahan CA, Malcom GT, et al: Lipid and apolipoprotein predictors of atherosclerosis in youth: Apolipoprotein concentrations do not materially improve prediction of arterial lesions in PDAY subjects. The PDAY Research Group. Arterioscler Thromb Vasc Biol 19:753, 1999.
44. Strong JP, Malcom GT, Oalmann MC, Wissler RW: The PDAY Study: Natural history, risk factors, and pathobiology. Pathobiological Determinants of Atherosclerosis in Youth. Ann N Y Acad Sci 811:226, 1997.
45. de Groot E, Jukema JW, Montauban van Swijndregt AD, et al: B-mode ultrasound assessment of pravastatin treatment effect on carotid and femoral artery walls and its correlations with coronary arteriographic findings: A report of the Regression Growth Evaluation Statin Study (REGRESS). J Am Coll Cardiol 31:1561, 1998.
46. Zhao XQ, Yuan C, Hatsukami TS, et al: Effects of prolonged intensive lipid-lowering therapy on the characteristics of carotid atherosclerotic plaques in vivo by MRI: A case-control study. Arterioscler Thromb Vasc Biol 21:1623, 2001.
47. Vink A, Schoneveld AH, Borst C, Pasterkamp G: The contribution of plaque and arterial remodeling to de novo atherosclerotic luminal narrowing in the femoral artery. J Vasc Surg 36:1194, 2002.
48. de Korte CL, Pasterkamp G, van der Steen AF, et al: Characterization of plaque components with intravascular ultrasound elastography in human femoral and coronary arteries in vitro. Circulation 102:617, 2000.
49. Carr SC, Farb A, Pearce WH, et al: Activated inflammatory cells are associated with plaque rupture in carotid artery stenosis. Surgery 122:757, discussion 763, 1997.
50. Pradhan AD, Rifai N, Ridker PM: Soluble intercellular adhesion molecule–1, soluble vascular adhesion molecule-1, and the development of symptomatic peripheral arterial disease in men. Circulation 106:820, 2002.
51. Yuan C, Zhang SX, Polissar NL, et al: Identification of fibrous cap rupture with magnetic resonance imaging is highly associated with recent transient ischemic attack or stroke. Circulation 105:181, 2002.
52. Rothwell PM, Villagra R, Gibson R, et al: Evidence of a chronic systemic cause of instability of atherosclerotic plaques. Lancet 355:19, 2000.

Pathophysiology of Limb Ischemia

53. Meredith IT, Currie KE, Anderson TJ, et al: Postischemic vasodilation in human forearm is dependent on endothelium-derived nitric oxide. Am J Physiol 270:H1435, 1996.
54. Böger RH, Bode-Böger SM, Thiele W, et al: Restoring vascular nitric oxide formation by L-arginine improves the symptoms of intermittent claudication in patients with peripheral arterial occlusive disease. J Am Coll Cardiol 32:1336, 1998.
55. Schellong SM, Boger RH, Burchert W, et al: Dose-related effect of intravenous L-arginine on muscular blood flow of the calf in patients with peripheral vascular disease: A H215O positron emission tomography study. Clin Sci (Colch) 93:159, 1997.
56. Maxwell AJ, Anderson BE, Cooke JP: Nutritional therapy for peripheral arterial disease: A double-blind, placebo-controlled, randomized trial of HeartBar. Vasc Med 5:11, 2000.
57. Hiatt WR: Pathophysiology. *In* Creager M (ed): Management of Peripheral Arterial Disease. London, ReMEDICA Publishing Limited, 2000, pp 43-56.
58. Pipinos II, Shepard AD, Anagnostopoulos PV, et al: Phosphorus 31 nuclear magnetic resonance spectroscopy suggests a mitochondrial defect in claudicating skeletal muscle. J Vasc Surg 31:944, 2000.
59. Bollinger A, Hoffmann U, Franzeck UK: Microvascular changes in arterial occlusive disease: Target for pharmacotherapy. Vasc Med 1:50, 1996.
60. Brevetti G, Corrado S, Martone VD, et al: Microcirculation and tissue metabolism in peripheral arterial disease. Clin Hemorheol Microcirc 21:245, 1999.
61. McDermott MM, Mehta S, Greenland P: Exertional leg symptoms other than intermittent claudication are common in peripheral arterial disease. Arch Intern Med 159:387, 1999.
62. McDermott MM, Fried L, Simonsick E, et al: Asymptomatic peripheral arterial disease is independently associated with impaired lower extremity functioning: The women's health and aging study. Circulation 101:1007, 2000.

Testing for PAD

63. McDermott MM, Liu K, Guralnik JM, et al: The ankle brachial index independently predicts walking velocity and walking endurance in peripheral arterial disease. J Am Geriatr Soc 46:1355, 1998.
64. Leng GC, Fowkes FG: The Edinburgh Claudication Questionnaire: An improved version of the WHO/Rose Questionnaire for use in epidemiological surveys. J Clin Epidemiol 45:1101, 1992.
65. Criqui MH, Denenberg JO, Bird CE, et al: The correlation between symptoms and non-invasive test results in patients referred for peripheral arterial disease testing. Vasc Med 1:65, 1996.
66. Coyne KS, Margolis MK, Gilchrist KA, et al: Evaluating effects of method of administration on Walking Impairment Questionnaire. J Vasc Surg 38:296, 2003.
67. Rutherford RB, Baker JD, Ernst C, et al: Recommended standards for reports dealing with lower extremity ischemia: Revised version. J Vasc Surg 26:517, 1997.
68. Nichols WW, O'Rourke MF: Wave reflections. *In* Nichols WW, O'Rourke MF (eds): McDonald's Blood Flow in Arteries. 4th ed. London, Arnold, 1998, pp 201-222.
69. McDermott MM, Greenland P, Liu K, et al: The ankle brachial index is associated with leg function and physical activity: The Walking and Leg Circulation Study. Ann Intern Med 136:873, 2002.
70. Chaudhry H, Holland A, Dormandy J: Comparison of graded versus constant treadmill test protocols for quantifying intermittent claudication. Vasc Med 2:93, 1997.
71. Creager MA: Clinical assessment of the patient with claudication: The role of the vascular laboratory. Vasc Med 2:231, 1997.
72. Gale SS, Scissons RP, Salles-Cunha SX, et al: Lower extremity arterial evaluation: Are segmental arterial blood pressures worthwhile? J Vasc Surg 27:831, discussion 838, 1998.
73. Pemberton M, London NJ: Colour flow duplex imaging of occlusive arterial disease of the lower limb. Br J Surg 84:912, 1997.
74. Visser K, Hunink MG: Peripheral arterial disease: Gadolinium-enhanced MR angiography versus color-guided duplex US—a meta-analysis. Radiology 216:67, 2000.
75. Poon E, Yucel EK, Pagan-Marin H, Kayne H: Iliac artery stenosis measurements: Comparison of two-dimensional time-of-flight and three-dimensional dynamic gadolinium-enhanced MR angiography. AJR Am J Roentgenol 169:1139, 1997.
76. Ho KY, de Haan MW, Kessels AG, et al: Peripheral vascular tree stenoses: Detection with subtracted and nonsubtracted MR angiography. Radiology 206:673, 1998.
77. Quinn SF, Sheley RC, Semonsen KG, et al: Aortic and lower-extremity arterial disease: Evaluation with MR angiography versus conventional angiography. Radiology 206:693, 1998.
78. Rofsky NM, Johnson G, Adelman MA, et al: Peripheral vascular disease evaluated with reduced-dose gadolinium-enhanced MR angiography. Radiology 205:163, 1997.
79. Nelemans PJ, Leiner T, de Vet HC, van Engelshoven JM: Peripheral arterial disease: Meta-analysis of the diagnostic performance of MR angiography. Radiology 217:105, 2000.
80. Rubin GD, Schmidt AJ, Logan LJ, Sofilos MC: Multi-detector row CT angiography of lower extremity arterial inflow and runoff: Initial experience. Radiology 221:146, 2001.
81. Rieker O, Duber C, Schmiedt W, et al: Prospective comparison of CT angiography of the legs with intraarterial digital subtraction angiography. AJR Am J Roentgenol 166:269, 1996.
82. Rubin GD: MDCT imaging of the aorta and peripheral vessels. Eur J Radiol 45(Suppl 1):S42, 2003.

Prognosis of PAD

83. Belch JJ, Topol EJ, Agnelli G, et al: Critical issues in peripheral arterial disease detection and management: A call to action. Arch Intern Med 163:884, 2003.
84. Ouriel K: Peripheral arterial disease. Lancet 358:1257, 2001.
85. A randomised, blinded, trial of clopidogrel versus aspirin in patients at risk of ischaemic events (CAPRIE). CAPRIE Steering Committee. Lancet 348:1329, 1996.
86. Ness J, Aronow WS: Prevalence of coexistence of coronary artery disease, ischemic stroke, and peripheral arterial disease in older persons, mean age 80 years, in an academic hospital-based geriatrics practice. J Am Geriatr Soc 47:1255, 1999.
87. Criqui MH, Denenberg JO: The generalized nature of atherosclerosis: How peripheral arterial disease may predict adverse events from coronary artery disease. Vasc Med 3:241, 1998.
88. Criqui M, Langer RD, Fronek A, et al: Mortality over a period of 10 years in patients with peripheral arterial disease. N Engl J Med 326:381, 1992.
89. Leng GC, Lee AJ, Fowkes FG, et al: Incidence, natural history and cardiovascular events in symptomatic and asymptomatic peripheral arterial disease in the general population. Int J Epidemiol 25:1172, 1996.
90. Diabetes-related amputations of lower extremities in the Medicare population—Minnesota, 1993-1995. MMWR Morb Mortal Wkly Rep 47:649, 1998.

Management of PAD

91. Hiatt WR: Medical treatment of peripheral arterial disease and claudication. N Engl J Med 344:1608, 2001.
92. MRC/BHF Heart Protection Study of cholesterol lowering with simvastatin in 20,536 high-risk individuals: A randomised placebo-controlled trial. Lancet 360:7, 2002.
93. Executive Summary of the Third Report of the National Cholesterol Education Program (NCEP) Expert Panel on Detection, Evaluation, and Treatment of High Blood Cholesterol in Adults (Adult Treatment Panel III). JAMA 285:2486, 2001.
94. Walldius G, Erikson U, Olsson AG, et al: The effect of probucol on femoral atherosclerosis: The Probucol Quantitative Regression Swedish Trial (PQRST). Am J Cardiol 74:875, 1994.
95. Buchwald H, Bourdages HR, Campos CT, et al: Impact of cholesterol reduction on peripheral arterial disease in the Program on the Surgical Control of the Hyperlipidemias (POSCH). Surgery 120:672, 1996.
96. Pedersen TR, Kjekshus J, Pyorala K, et al: Effect of simvastatin on ischemic signs and symptoms in the Scandinavian simvastatin survival study (4S). Am J Cardiol 81:333, 1998.
97. Aronow WS, Nayak D, Woodworth S, Ahn C: Effect of simvastatin versus placebo on treadmill exercise time until the onset of intermittent claudication in older patients with peripheral arterial disease at six months and at one year after treatment. Am J Cardiol 92:711, 2003.
98. Mohler ER 3rd, Hiatt WR, Creager MA: Cholesterol reduction with atorvastatin improves walking distance in patients with peripheral arterial disease. Circulation 108:1481, 2003.
99. Mondillo S, Ballo P, Barbati R, et al: Effects of simvastatin on walking performance and symptoms of intermittent claudication in hypercholesterolemic patients with peripheral vascular disease. Am J Med 114:359, 2003.
100. McDermott MM, Guralnik JM, Greenland P, et al: Statin use and leg functioning in patients with and without lower-extremity peripheral arterial disease. Circulation 107:757, 2003.
101. Effect of intensive diabetes management on macrovascular events and risk factors in the Diabetes Control and Complications Trial. Am J Cardiol 75:894, 1995.
102. Nathan DM, Lachin J, Cleary P, et al: Intensive diabetes therapy and carotid intima-media thickness in type 1 diabetes mellitus. N Engl J Med 348:2294, 2003.
103. Intensive blood-glucose control with sulphonylureas or insulin compared with conventional treatment and risk of complications in patients with type 2 diabetes (UKPDS 33). UK Prospective Diabetes Study (UKPDS) Group [published erratum appears in Lancet 354:602, 1999]. Lancet 352:837, 1998.
104. Mehler PS, Coll JR, Estacio R, et al: Intensive blood pressure control reduces the risk of cardiovascular events in patients with peripheral arterial disease and type 2 diabetes. Circulation 107:753, 2003.

105. Radack K, Deck C: Beta-adrenergic blocker therapy does not worsen intermittent claudication in subjects with peripheral arterial disease: A meta-analysis of randomized controlled trials. Arch Intern Med 151:1769, 1991.
106. Freemantle N, Cleland J, Young P, et al: Beta blockade after myocardial infarction: Systematic review and meta regression analysis. BMJ 318:1730, 1999.
107. Chobanian AV, Bakris GL, Black HR, et al: The Seventh Report of the Joint National Committee on Prevention, Detection, Evaluation, and Treatment of High Blood Pressure: The JNC 7 Report. JAMA 289:2560, 2003.
108. Yusuf S, Sleight P, Pogue J, et al: Effects of an angiotensin-converting-enzyme inhibitor, ramipril, on cardiovascular events in high-risk patients. The Heart Outcomes Prevention Evaluation Study Investigators [published erratum appears in N Engl J Med 342:748, 2000]. N Engl J Med 342:145, 2000.
109. Antithrombotic Trialists' Collaboration: Collaborative meta-analysis of randomised trials of antiplatelet therapy for prevention of death, myocardial infarction, and stroke in high risk patients. BMJ 324:71, 2002.
110. Becquemin JP: Effect of ticlopidine on the long-term patency of saphenous-vein bypass grafts in the legs. Etude de la Ticlopidine apres Pontage Femoro-Poplite and the Association Universitaire de Recherche en Chirurgie. N Engl J Med 337:1726, 1997.
111. Labs KH, Dormandy JA, Jaeger KA, et al: Transatlantic Conference on Clinical Trial Guidelines in Peripheral Arterial Disease: Clinical trial methodology. Basel PAD Clinical Trial Methodology Group. Circulation 100:e75, 1999.
112. Hansen PR, Holm AM, Qi JH, et al: Pentoxifylline inhibits neointimal formation and stimulates constrictive vascular remodeling after arterial injury. J Cardiovasc Pharmacol 34:683, 1999.
113. Chen YM, Wu KD, Tsai TJ, Hsieh BS: Pentoxifylline inhibits PDGF-induced proliferation of and TGF-beta-stimulated collagen synthesis by vascular smooth muscle cells. J Mol Cell Cardiol 31:773, 1999.
114. Hood SC, Moher D, Barber GG: Management of intermittent claudication with pentoxifylline: Meta-analysis of randomized controlled trials. CMAJ 155:1053, 1996.
115. Girolami B, Bernardi E, Prins MH, et al: Treatment of intermittent claudication with physical training, smoking cessation, pentoxifylline, or nafronyl: A meta-analysis. Arch Intern Med 159:337, 1999.
116. Ikeda Y: Antiplatelet therapy using cilostazol, a specific PDE3 inhibitor. Thromb Haemost 82:435, 1999.
117. Money SR, Herd JA, Isaacsohn JL, et al: Effect of cilostazol on walking distances in patients with intermittent claudication caused by peripheral vascular disease. J Vasc Surg 27:267, discussion 274, 1998.
118. Beebe HG, Dawson DL, Cutler BS, et al: A new pharmacological treatment for intermittent claudication: Results of a randomized, multicenter trial. Arch Intern Med 159:2041, 1999.
119. Regensteiner JG, Ware JE Jr, McCarthy WJ, et al: Effect of cilostazol on treadmill walking, community-based walking ability, and health-related quality of life in patients with intermittent claudication due to peripheral arterial disease: Meta-analysis of six randomized controlled trials. J Am Geriatr Soc 50:1939, 2002.
120. Dawson DL, Cutler BS, Hiatt WR, et al: A comparison of cilostazol and pentoxifylline for treating intermittent claudication. Am J Med 109:523, 2000.
121. Cohn JN, Goldstein SO, Greenberg BH, et al: A dose-dependent increase in mortality with vesnarinone among patients with severe heart failure. Vesnarinone Trial Investigators. N Engl J Med 339:1810, 1998.
122. Barradell LB, Brogden RN: Oral naftidrofuryl: A review of its pharmacology and therapeutic use in the management of peripheral occlusive arterial disease. Drugs Aging 8:299, 1996.
123. Brevetti G, Diehm C, Lambert D: European multicenter study on propionyl-L-carnitine in intermittent claudication. J Am Coll Cardiol 34:1618, 1999.
124. Hiatt WR, Regensteiner JG, Creager MA, et al: Propionyl-L-carnitine improves exercise performance and functional status in patients with claudication. Am J Med 110:616, 2001.
125. Belch JJ, Bell PR, Creissen D, et al: Randomized, double-blind, placebo-controlled study evaluating the efficacy and safety of AS-013, a prostaglandin E1 prodrug, in patients with intermittent claudication. Circulation 95:2298, 1997.
126. Boger RH, Bode-Boger SM, Thiele W, et al: Restoring vascular nitric oxide formation by L-arginine improves the symptoms of intermittent claudication in patients with peripheral arterial occlusive disease. J Am Coll Cardiol 32:1336, 1998.
127. Lievre M, Morand S, Besse B, et al: Oral Beraprost sodium, a prostaglandin I(2) analogue, for intermittent claudication: A double-blind, randomized, multicenter controlled trial. Beraprost et Claudication Intermittente (BERCI) Research Group. Circulation 102:426, 2000.
128. Mohler ER 3rd, Hiatt WR, Olin JW, et al: Treatment of intermittent claudication with beraprost sodium, an orally active prostaglandin I2 analogue: A double-blinded, randomized, controlled trial. J Am Coll Cardiol 41:1679, 2003.
129. ICAI Study Group: Prostanoids for chronic critical leg ischemia: A randomized, controlled, open-label trial with prostaglandin E1. Ischemia Cronica degli Arti Inferiori. Ann Intern Med 130:412, 1999.
130. Baumgartner I, Pieczek A, Manor O, et al: Constitutive expression of phVEGF165 after intramuscular gene transfer promotes collateral vessel development in patients with critical limb ischemia. Circulation 97:1114, 1998.
131. Tateishi-Yuyama E, Matsubara H, Murohara T, et al: Therapeutic angiogenesis for patients with limb ischaemia by autologous transplantation of bone-marrow cells: A pilot study and a randomised controlled trial. Lancet 360:427, 2002.
132. Rajagopalan S, Mohler ER 3rd, Lederman RJ, et al: Regional angiogenesis with vascular endothelial growth factor in peripheral arterial disease: A phase II randomized, double-blind, controlled study of adenoviral delivery of vascular endothelial growth factor 121 in patients with disabling intermittent claudication. Circulation 108:1933, 2003.
133. Lederman RJ, Mendelsohn FO, Anderson RD, et al: Therapeutic angiogenesis with recombinant fibroblast growth factor-2 for intermittent claudication (the TRAFFIC study): A randomised trial. Lancet 359:2053, 2002.
134. Gardner AW, Poehlman ET: Exercise rehabilitation programs for the treatment of claudication pain: A meta-analysis. JAMA 274:975, 1995.
135. Leng GC, Fowler B, Ernst E: Exercise for intermittent claudication. Cochrane Database Syst Rev CD000990, 2000.
136. Stewart KJ, Hiatt WR, Regensteiner JG, Hirsch AT: Exercise training for claudication. N Engl J Med 347:1941, 2002.
137. Hoppeler H: Vascular growth in hypoxic skeletal muscle. Adv Exp Med Biol 474:277, 1999.
138. Gustafsson T, Puntschart A, Kaijser L, et al: Exercise-induced expression of angiogenesis-related transcription and growth factors in human skeletal muscle. Am J Physiol 276:H679, 1999.
139. Hambrecht R, Wolf A, Gielen S, et al: Effect of exercise on coronary endothelial function in patients with coronary artery disease. N Engl J Med 342:454, 2000.
140. Hambrecht R, Fiehn E, Weigl C, et al: Regular physical exercise corrects endothelial dysfunction and improves exercise capacity in patients with chronic heart failure. Circulation 98:2709, 1998.
141. Brendle DC, Joseph LJ, Corretti MC, et al: Effects of exercise rehabilitation on endothelial reactivity in older patients with peripheral arterial disease. Am J Cardiol 87:324, 2001.
142. Gardner AW, Katzel LI, Sorkin JD, et al: Exercise rehabilitation improves functional outcomes and peripheral circulation in patients with intermittent claudication: A randomized controlled trial. J Am Geriatr Soc 49:755, 2001.
143. Eagle KA, Berger PB, Calkins H, et al: ACC/AHA guideline update for perioperative cardiovascular evaluation for noncardiac surgery—executive summary a report of the American College of Cardiology/American Heart Association Task Force on Practice Guidelines (Committee to Update the 1996 Guidelines on Perioperative Cardiovascular Evaluation for Noncardiac Surgery). Circulation 105:1257, 2002.
144. de Vries SO, Hunink MG: Results of aortic bifurcation grafts for aortoiliac occlusive disease: A meta-analysis. J Vasc Surg 26:558, 1997.
145. Reed AB, Conte MS, Donaldson MC, et al: The impact of patient age and aortic size on the results of aortobifemoral bypass grafting. J Vasc Surg 37:1219, 2003.
146. Biancari F, Lepantalo M: Extra-anatomic bypass surgery for critical leg ischemia: A review. J Cardiovasc Surg (Torino) 39:295, 1998.
147. Abbott WM, Green RM, Matsumoto T, et al: Prosthetic above-knee femoropopliteal bypass grafting: Results of a multicenter randomized prospective trial. Above-Knee Femoropopliteal Study Group. J Vasc Surg 25:19, 1997.
148. Illig KA, Green RM: Prosthetic above-knee femoropopliteal bypass. Semin Vasc Surg 12:38, 1999.
149. Dorffler-Melly J, Koopman MM, Adam DJ, et al: Antiplatelet agents for preventing thrombosis after peripheral arterial bypass surgery. Cochrane Database Syst Rev CD000535, 2003.
150. Dorffler-Melly J, Buller H, Koopman M, Prins M: Antithrombotic agents for preventing thrombosis after infrainguinal arterial bypass surgery. Cochrane Database Syst Rev 4:CD000536, 2003.

Thromboangiitis Obliterans

151. von Winiwater F: Ueber eine eighenthumliche Form von Endarteritis und Endophlebitis mit Gangran des Fusses. Arch Klin Chir 23:202, 1879.
152. Buerger L: Thromboangiitis obliterans: A study of the vascular lesions leading to presenile spontaneous gangrene. Am J Med Sci 136:567, 1908.
153. Donatelli F, Triggiani M, Nascimbene S, et al: Thromboangiitis obliterans of coronary and internal thoracic arteries in a young woman. J Thorac Cardiovasc Surg 113:800, 1997.
154. Lie JT: Visceral intestinal Buerger's disease. Int J Cardiol 66(Suppl 1):S249, 1998.
155. Michail PO, Filis KA, Delladetsima JK, et al: Thromboangiitis obliterans (Buerger's disease) in visceral vessels confirmed by angiographic and histological findings. Eur J Vasc Endovasc Surg 16:445, 1998.
156. Olin JW: Thromboangiitis obliterans (Buerger's disease). N Engl J Med 343:864, 2000.
157. Lee T, Seo JW, Sumpio BE, Kim SJ: Immunobiologic analysis of arterial tissue in Buerger's disease. Eur J Vasc Endovasc Surg 25:451, 2003.
158. Eichhorn J, Sima D, Lindschau C, et al: Antiendothelial cell antibodies in thromboangiitis obliterans. Am J Med Sci 315:17, 1998.
159. Maslowski L, McBane R, Alexewicz P, Wysokinski WE: Antiphospholipid antibodies in thromboangiitis obliterans. Vasc Med 7:259, 2002.
160. Makita S, Nakamura M, Murakami H, et al: Impaired endothelium-dependent vasorelaxation in peripheral vasculature of patients with thromboangiitis obliterans (Buerger's disease). Circulation 94:II211, 1996.
161. Shionoya S: Diagnostic criteria of Buerger's disease. Int J Cardiol 66(Suppl 1):S243, 1998.
162. Jaff MR: Thromboangiitis Obliterans (Buerger's Disease). Curr Treat Options Cardiovasc Med 2:205, 2000.
163. Olin JW: Thromboangiitis obliterans (Buerger's disease). *In* Rutherford RB (ed): Vascular Surgery. 4th ed. Philadelphia, WB Saunders, 2000, pp 350-364.
164. Shigematsu H, Shigematsu K: Factors affecting the long-term outcome of Buerger's disease (thromboangiitis obliterans). Int Angiol 18:58, 1999.
165. Fiessinger JN, Schafer M: Trial of iloprost versus aspirin treatment for critical limb ischaemia of thromboangiitis obliterans. The TAO Study. Lancet 335:555, 1990.
166. Oral iloprost in the treatment of thromboangiitis obliterans (Buerger's disease): A double-blind, randomised, placebo-controlled trial. The European TAO Study Group [published erratum appears in Eur J Vasc Endovasc Surg 16]:456, 1998]. Eur J Vasc Endovasc Surg 15:300, 1998.
167. Saha K, Chabra N, Gulati SM: Treatment of patients with thromboangiitis obliterans with cyclophosphamide. Angiology 52:399, 2001.
168. Isner JM, Baumgartner I, Rauh G, et al: Treatment of thromboangiitis obliterans (Buerger's disease) by intramuscular gene transfer of vascular endothelial growth factor: Preliminary clinical results. J Vasc Surg 28:964, 1998.

169. Sasajima T, Kubo Y, Inaba M, et al: Role of infrainguinal bypass in Buerger's disease: An eighteen-year experience. Eur J Vasc Endovasc Surg 13:186, 1997.

Acute Limb Ischemia

170. Dormandy J, Heeck L, Vig S: The fate of patients with critical leg ischemia. Semin Vasc Surg 12:142, 1999.
171. Aune S, Trippestad A: Operative mortality and long-term survival of patients operated on for acute lower limb ischaemia. Eur J Vasc Endovasc Surg 15:143, 1998.
172. Braithwaite BD, Davies B, Birch PA, et al: Management of acute leg ischaemia in the elderly. Br J Surg 85:217, 1998.
173. Ascher E, Markevich N, Schutzer RW, et al: Small popliteal artery aneurysms: Are they clinically significant? J Vasc Surg 37:755, 2003.
174. Working Party on Thrombolysis in the Management of Limb Ischemia: Thrombolysis in the management of lower limb peripheral arterial occlusion—a consensus document. Am J Cardiol 81:207, 1998.
175. Ouriel K: Acute arterial occlusion. Curr Treat Options Cardiovasc Med 2:255, 2000.
176. Thrombolysis in the management of lower limb peripheral arterial occlusion—a consensus document. J Vasc Interv Radiol 14:S337, 2003.
177. Semba CP, Murphy TP, Bakal CW, et al: Thrombolytic therapy with use of alteplase (rt-PA) in peripheral arterial occlusive disease: Review of the clinical literature. The Advisory Panel. J Vasc Interv Radiol 11:149, 2000.
178. Kasirajan K, Gray B, Beavers FP, et al: Rheolytic thrombectomy in the management of acute and subacute limb-threatening ischemia. J Vasc Interv Radiol 12:413, 2001.
179. Dormandy J, Heeck L, Vig S: Acute limb ischemia. Semin Vasc Surg 12:148, 1999.
180. Berridge DC, Kessel D, Robertson I: Surgery versus thrombolysis for acute limb ischaemia: Initial management. Cochrane Database Syst Rev CD002784, 2002.
181. Results of a prospective randomized trial evaluating surgery versus thrombolysis for ischemia of the lower extremity. The STILE trial. Ann Surg 220:251, 1994.
182. Ouriel K, Veith FJ, Sasahara AA: A comparison of recombinant urokinase with vascular surgery as initial treatment for acute arterial occlusion of the legs. Thrombolysis or Peripheral Arterial Surgery (TOPAS) Investigators. N Engl J Med 338:1105, 1998.

Atheroembolism

183. Tunick PA, Kronzon I: Embolism from the aorta: Atheroemboli and thromboemboli. Curr Treat Options Cardiovasc Med 3:181, 2001.
184. Smyth JS, Scoble JE: Atheroembolism. Curr Treat Options Cardiovasc Med 4:255, 2002.
185. Moolenaar W, Lamers CB: Cholesterol crystal embolization in the Netherlands. Arch Intern Med 156:653, 1996.
186. Kronzon I, Tunick PA: Atheromatous disease of the thoracic aorta: Pathologic and clinical implications. Ann Intern Med 126:629, 1997.
187. Spittell PC, Seward JB, Hallett JW Jr: Mobile thrombi in the abdominal aorta in cases of lower extremity embolic arterial occlusion: Value of extended transthoracic echocardiography. Am Heart J 139:241, 2000.
188. Tunick PA, Kronzon I: Atheromas of the thoracic aorta: Clinical and therapeutic update. J Am Coll Cardiol 35:545, 2000.
189. The French Study of Aortic Plaques in Stroke Group: Atherosclerotic disease of the aortic arch as a risk factor for recurrent ischemic stroke. N Engl J Med 334:1216, 1996.
190. Ferrari E, Vidal R, Chevallier T, Baudouy M: Atherosclerosis of the thoracic aorta and aortic debris as a marker of poor prognosis: benefit of oral anticoagulants. J Am Coll Cardiol 33:1317, 1999.
191. Fukumoto Y, Tsutsui H, Tsuchihashi M, et al: The incidence and risk factors of cholesterol embolization syndrome, a complication of cardiac catheterization: A prospective study. J Am Coll Cardiol 42:211, 2003.
192. Kolh PH, Torchiana DF, Buckley MJ: Atheroembolization in cardiac surgery: The need for preoperative diagnosis. J Cardiovasc Surg (Torino) 40:77, 1999.
193. Bols A, Nevelsteen A, Verhaeghe R: Atheromatous embolization precipitated by oral anticoagulants. Int Angiol 13:271, 1994.
194. Dressler FA, Craig WR, Castello R, Labovitz AJ: Mobile aortic atheroma and systemic emboli: Efficacy of anticoagulation and influence of plaque morphology on recurrent stroke. J Am Coll Cardiol 31:134, 1998.
195. Blackshear JL, Zabalgoitia M, Pennock G, et al: Warfarin safety and efficacy in patients with thoracic aortic plaque and atrial fibrillation. SPAF TEE Investigators. Stroke Prevention and Atrial Fibrillation. Transesophageal echocardiography. Am J Cardiol 83:453, A9, 1999.
196. Blankenship JC, Butler M, Garbes A: Prospective assessment of cholesterol embolization in patients with acute myocardial infarction treated with thrombolytic vs conservative therapy. Chest 107:662, 1995.
197. Vaduganathan P, Ewton A, Nagueh SF, et al: Pathologic correlates of aortic plaques, thrombi and mobile "aortic debris" imaged in vivo with transesophageal echocardiography. J Am Coll Cardiol 30:357, 1997.

CHAPTER 55

Endovascular Treatment of Noncoronary Obstructive Vascular Disease

Andrew C. Eisenhauer • Kenneth Rosenfield

Noncoronary arterial disease, otherwise known as peripheral artery disease (PAD), is increasingly recognized for its high prevalence and clinical importance (see Chap. 54). As the population ages and the number of people with both symptomatic and asymptomatic PAD grows, physicians and patients alike are developing more awareness of the ramifications of PAD, including its associated morbidity and power to predict mortality. Percutaneous transluminal angioplasty (PTA) was initially developed as treatment for PAD, although it is the explosion of its use for treatment of coronary artery disease (CAD) that has fueled the commercial development and academic interest in catheter-based techniques in general. The resulting major improvements in technology and results, combined with patient demand for less invasive therapies, has provided impetus for their extended use in PAD. The widespread availability of high-resolution noninvasive diagnostic imaging, capable of accurately identifying disease and distinguishing lesions amenable to less invasive treatment, has further lowered the threshold for considering treatment for symptomatic PAD.

Although surgery has been the historical mainstay of revascularization therapy for PAD, percutaneous vascular intervention now provides patients with a less invasive, effective modality for the treatment of atheromatous disease over a wide spectrum of anatomical and clinical situations. Catheter-based intervention can provide symptomatic relief of claudication and amelioration of limb ischemia. It can be used for definitive therapy of stenosis in the renal, brachiocephalic, and carotid arteries. In addition, effective methods have been developed to treat aneurysmal disease and venous conditions percutaneously. Nonetheless, establishing recommendations for therapy in PAD can be more complex than in CAD, owing to the wide range of available options (surgical, endovascular, medical, or combination therapy), the involvement of multiple different end-organs, and the relative paucity of definitive data in this rapidly evolving field. Given these complexities, the clinician, whose focus is on providing the optimal treatment strategy, must be knowledgeable about the disease state and aware of the full range of options. In complicated cases, the patient may benefit from the input of physicians from multiple specialties.

Interventions for Atherosclerotic Disease

For Lower Extremity Claudication or Limb Salvage

Intermittent claudication involving the lower extremities is commonly caused by stenosis or occlusion of the iliac, femoral, or infrapopliteal vessels (see Chap. 54). Although first-line therapy has included aggressive risk factor modification and exercise training, life-style–limiting claudication, rest pain, or tissue loss can dictate more aggressive investigation and therapy. The goals of therapy for lower extremity obstructive disease are symptomatic relief of claudication and, in more advanced cases, limb salvage. Although surgical therapy has been reserved historically for patients with limb-threatening ischemia and rest pain, the availability of endovascular therapies has lowered the threshold for intervention. Because most percutaneous interventions have low procedural risk, patients with life-style–limiting claudication are now often considered for angiographic investigation and intervention. In addition, percutaneous treatment usually preserves the surgical option, should it be needed subsequently. An increasingly informed patient population will, given the choice, often opt for less invasive therapies, accepting results that may be less durable or even less effective than those associated with a more invasive approach. For the clinician treating patients with lower extremity vascular disease, improvement in functional capacity and quality of life, as well as long-term results, are important in weighing the value of potential treatments. Evaluation of a patient with lower extremity symptoms requires awareness of the variable manifestations of PAD. In some instances, patients and even physicians misconstrue hip discomfort and other symptoms of claudication as those of "arthritis," or as a normal component of aging. Some patients unintentionally self-restrict their activities to avoid ischemic pain: their symptoms abate because they no longer exercise. These patients are akin to the patient with exertional angina who limits his or her activity to below the angina threshold.

Though progression from claudication to limb-threatening ischemia is relatively uncommon—occurring in only 10 to 20 percent of claudicants—even asymptomatic PAD is associated with significant morbidity (see Chap. 54). The U.S. National Institutes of Health suggest that peripheral arterial disease results in more than 60,000 hospitalizations annually, with an average length of stay greater than 11 days.[1] Approximately 1 to 2 percent of people aged 45 to 69 years have clinical evidence of intermittent claudication, and risk factors for lower extremity disease include tobacco use, diabetes mellitus, hyperlipidemia, and systolic hypertension (see Chap. 54). Smoking appears to be the greatest modifiable risk factor and one of the most potent—perhaps even more so than in association with coronary atherosclerosis.

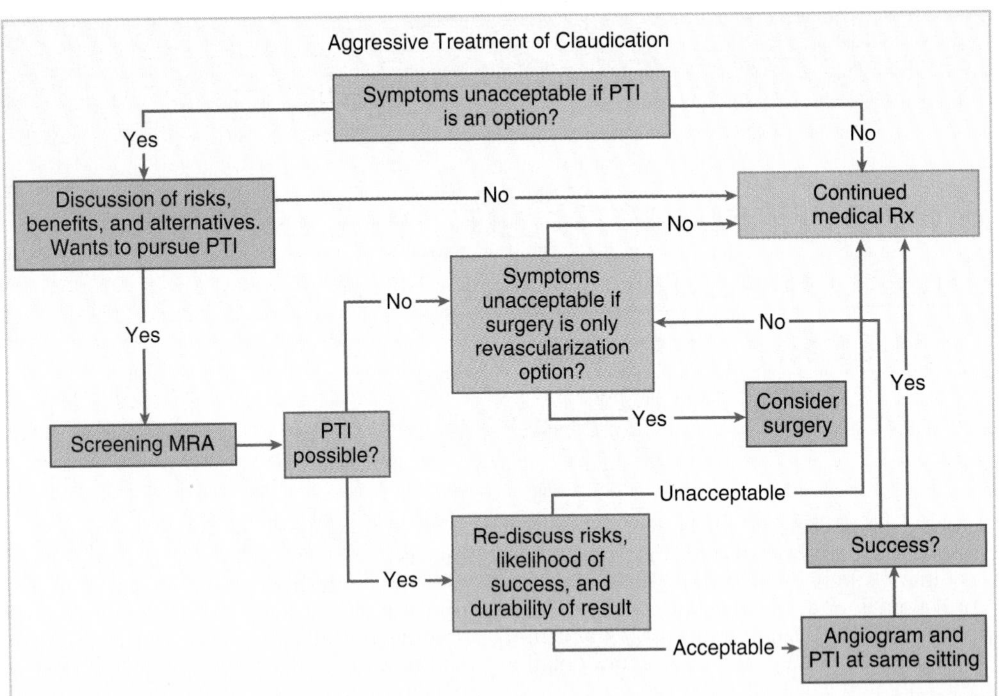

FIGURE 55–1 A strategy for aggressive treatment of claudication. The strategy is based on assessment of symptoms and frank discussion with patients about the risks and benefits of available therapies. In the current era, noninvasive diagnostic imaging is used not to make a diagnosis but to ascertain the anatomical suitability for intervention and to assess the patient's procedural risk profile. MRA = magnetic resonance angiography; PTI = percutaneous transluminal intervention; Rx = treatment. See also Figure 54–21 for a management scheme for less life-style limiting claudication.

Noninvasive functional testing, such as pulse volume recordings and segmental Doppler pressures (ankle-brachial index) with or without exercise, is helpful in confirming the presence of obstructive disease and estimating its level and severity. The broad indications for lower extremity angiography of any kind, noninvasive or invasive, include symptoms of PAD where, if the angiogram demonstrates a suitable anatomic situation, surgery or PTA would be undertaken. Recent advances in axial imaging techniques (both magnetic resonance [MR] angiography and computed tomography [CT] angiography) now enable remarkable definition of the vascular anatomy. These studies are now frequently obtained to confirm the diagnosis and to help formulate a strategy and approach to revascularization. Invasive angiography is necessary when the results from axial imaging are ambiguous. For critical limb ischemia, anatomical definition is required to plan therapy in nearly all cases. In the case of claudication, imaging should be performed as outlined in Figure 55–1.

The goals of revascularization include not only limb salvage and wound healing but also relief of exertional symptoms. The likelihood of clinical success, the durability, and the technical approach vary according to anatomical site. These aspects are best considered separately for aortoiliac, femoropopliteal, and infrapopliteal segments.

Aortoiliac Obstruction

Obstructive disease in the aorta and iliac vessels is usually atherosclerotic in origin, and treatment for both sites, typically labeled *inflow vessels* to the leg, is similar. Many patients with aortoiliac disease have concomitant femoral and tibial obstructive disease. In these patients with multilevel disease, correction of hemodynamically significant inflow lesions is usually undertaken as the first stage in revascularization. In some cases, aortoiliac treatment alone may result in symptomatic improvement by increasing the proximal pressure head and thus collateral blood flow to the distal extremity.

Perhaps more so than for any other vascular territory in the body, the preferred mode of revascularization of the aortoiliac vessels has shifted over the past 15 years from predominantly surgical to nearly all percutaneous. This change in strategy is based on both the less invasive nature of PTA and its short- and long-term success, which are comparable to that of more high-risk surgical bypass.[2,3] Furthermore, the primary use of stents, as opposed to balloon angioplasty alone, has gained enormous popularity in the aortoiliac (and other) vessels, due to generally superior angiographic and hemodynamic results and the paucity of complications associated with stents. Insufficient data exist to support or reject the strategy of primary stenting. One trial did suggest that patency rates (~70 percent) and clinical success rates (~78 percent) at 2 years are similar to stenting when excellent angiographic and hemodynamic results are obtained from balloon angioplasty alone.[4] This has led some to favor a strategy of "provisional stenting," wherein stents are reserved for cases of failed balloon angioplasty. However, in the single trial comparing the two strategies, nearly half of the patients (43 percent) randomized to receive balloon alone crossed over to receive stents. Moreover, a meta-analysis of all trials published after 1990 suggests that both immediate success rate (96 vs. 91 percent) and 4-year patency (77 vs. 65 percent for stenoses) are superior for stenting versus balloon alone.[2] These data support the strategy of primary stenting when treating aortoiliac lesions. Long lesions, diffuse disease, and occlusions, in particular, benefit from primary stenting. Since stented segments that restenose can be treated successfully with repeat angioplasty, long-term patency may be even greater when one includes secondary procedures. Finally, with regard to type of stent selected (balloon-expandable vs. self-expanding; stainless steel vs. nitinol), there are insufficient data to recommend one over another; however, recent experience suggests that nitinol may offer advantages in placement accuracy and long-term patency for self-expanding stents over that achieved with stainless steel in the past.[5]

Although endovascular therapy is the preferred initial therapy for focal aortoiliac stenosis, the approach to diffusely diseased vessels and total occlusions is more controversial. Early studies demonstrated poor technical results and high complication rates. However, the advent of hydrophilic guidewires and other technical advances have enabled recanalization of occluded iliac segments with a greater than 80 percent rate of primary success, independent of location (external, internal, or common iliac artery); secondary patency rates at 6 years are as high as 80 percent. There is general agreement that stents should be used primarily (not provisionally) when treating occlusions. The same is true of a subset of patients with stenotic or occlusive disease that involves the terminal aorta, extends into its bifurcation, and compromises the origins of the common iliac arteries. These patients do well with reconstruction of the bifurcation using stents.

The most serious complications of endovascular aortoiliac repair remain distal embolization, with rates ranging from 4 to 7 percent,[6] and arterial perforation or rupture, which is rare. Routine treatment with covered stents is now possible for the latter. Based on these improved outcomes, percutaneous treatment is generally attempted for short occlusions and for longer iliac stenosis or occlusions that are technically suitable (Fig. 55–2). Total occlusions of the abdominal aorta are more often treated surgically, though thrombolysis followed by PTA remains an option.

Pretreatment before PTA with therapies that dissolve or remove thrombus, such as thrombolytic therapy, rheolytic thrombectomy, and suction thrombectomy, can reduce embolic complications in thrombus-containing lesions. Distal embolic protection devices have also been used for the same purpose. Although individual reports and small series show favorable outcomes in selected cases, further delineation of the specific indications is required for these adjunct therapies. Finally, covered stents are now used for iliac artery lesions with associated aneurysm or anatomical complexities, further extending the applicability of percutaneous therapy.

In summary, PTA and stenting represent appropriate first-line therapy for aortoiliac obstructive disease. They offer durability similar to that of surgical reconstruction, with less risk and at reduced cost. In the small percentage of patients in whom patency cannot be maintained, surgery remains an option. The availability of these effective and less invasive techniques has lowered the threshold at which intervention can be offered to patients with aortoiliac disease who are disabled by claudication or limb ischemia (Table 55–1).

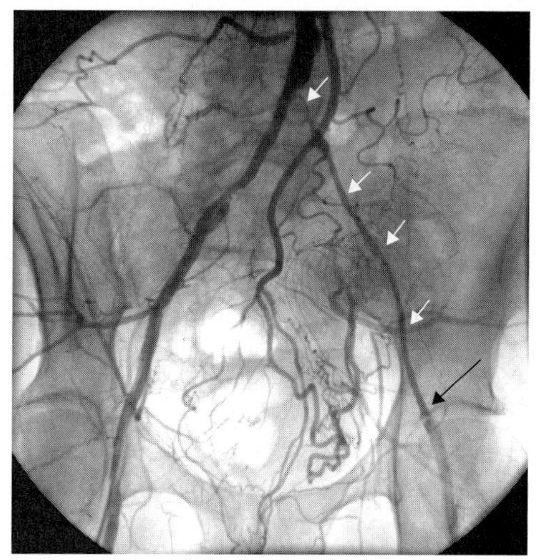

A

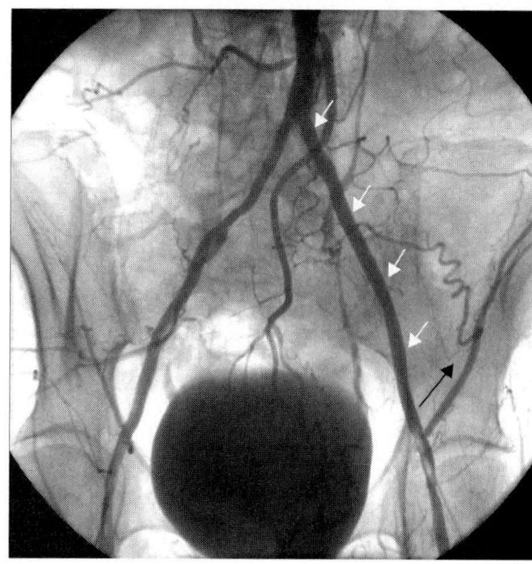

B

FIGURE 55–2 Iliac stenting. **A** shows a severe long segment disease of the left common and external iliac arteries (white arrows). The black arrow shows the level of collateral inflow and the resulting mixing opacified and unopacified blood. This patient was treated with predilation and a single balloon-expandable stent placed at the origin of the left common iliac artery (white arrows). This was followed by implantation of a self-expanding stent in the remainder of the vessel. **B** shows wide patency of that vessel and reversal of flow to antegrade in the collateral vessel (black arrow). This patient's claudication was abolished.

TABLE 55–1 Recent Results of Iliac Artery Stent Placement*

Lead Author	Reference	Year	No. of Patients	Lesions Treated	Percent with Occlusions	Technical Success (%)	Ankle-Brachial Index *Before*	Ankle-Brachial Index *After*	Mean Lesion Length (cm)	Stent Used	Primary Patency at 2 Years (%)	Cumulative Patency at 2 Years (%)
Reyes	16	1997	59	61	100	92	0.51	0.9	10	SES	73	88
Dyet	17	1997	72	72	100	93	NA	NA	6.7	BES, SES	85	85
Murphy	15	1998	65	90	31	97	0.62	0.9	5.6	BES, SES	69	80
Tetleroo	4	1998	143	187	9	NA	0.78	NA	NA	BES	NA	71.3
Powell	14	2000	87	210	NA	97	0.56	0.75	NA	Various	43	72
Saha	12	2001	50	61	4	97	NA	NA	NA	BES, SES	97	100
Timaran	13	2001	189	247	NA	97	NA	NA	NA	BES, SES	NA	
Haulon	7	2002	106	212	NA	100	NA	NA	NA	BES/SES	79.4	97.7
Siskin	8	2002	42	59	8.5	95	0.68	0.99	NA	BES/SES	72	88
Mohamed	9	2002	24	48	42	100	NA	NA	5.2	BES/SES	58	84
Reekers	10	2002	126	143	10	100	0.67	0.92	3.3	BES	84†	89†
Funovics	11	2002	78	94	100	96	NA	NA	6.2	Various	74.5	88.8

BES = balloon-expandable stainless steel; SES = self-expanding stainless steel; SEN = self-expanding nitinol; SESG = self-expanding stent graft; NA = not assessed or reported.

*Historical and contemporary results of iliac artery stent placement. The difficulty in determining the literature is that these reports of experience include patients with widely varying degrees of disease and incorporate a variety of stent types and techniques. Nevertheless, cumulative 2-year patency is approximately 90% in most series.

†At 12 months.

Prior experience has shown little difference between the results of endovascular therapy for the superficial femoral (SFA) and popliteal arteries. Accordingly, these two vessels traditionally are considered together with respect to indications and results. The SFA, particularly within the adductor canal of the thigh, has a tremendous propensity to accumulate atherosclerotic plaque. Whether this is due to the inherent physical stresses and flow patterns specific to this vessel (low flow vessel, high resistance bed), the presence of a natural collateral (the profunda femoris artery), or other undefined factors is not known. In the current era, procedural success for femoropopliteal recanalization exceeds 90 percent. The advent of hydrophilic guidewires and catheters has greatly enhanced the ability to traverse femoropopliteal occlusions, which now can be treated successfully in 80 to 90 percent of cases. Even though hydrophilic wires and other technological advances have improved acute success, the rate of restenosis remains more than twofold that of iliac disease and far exceeds what would be expected considering the size (mean lumen diameter, 5 to 6 mm) of the SFA.

A variety of adjunct technologies has been used in an attempt to improve long-term patency. Debulking devices, such as directional atherectomy, excimer laser, and rotational atherectomy, although sometimes enhancing acute success and providing a better angiographic result, have failed to demonstrate a reduction in restenosis. Newer debulking devices, which are more aggressive and "thorough" in their tissue removal, have not been evaluated yet for long-term efficacy.

Though it had been hoped that stent placement would offer advantages over balloon angioplasty, as it does in the coronary circulation, initial reports of long-term results were disappointing. Restenosis rates after 6 months were in the 30 to 70 percent range, with poorer results associated with longer lesions, total occlusions, and more distal disease. However, following recanalization, there was little evidence to support the superiority of endovascular stents over balloon angioplasty alone in this anatomical locale.

However, the advent of flexible thin-strutted nitinol self-expanding stents improved the clinically perceived rates of restenosis following long-segment SFA recanalization and stenting have improved. Given the past moderate rates of procedural success with femoropopliteal intervention, percutaneous treatment has been relatively neglected in the treatment of claudication, and many believed it was unsatisfactory for the treatment of limb-threatening ischemia. Traditionally, it has been reserved for claudicants with isolated short-segment disease and those with limb-threatening ischemia believed to be at high risk for surgical therapy.

Recognition is increasing that a great potential advantage of endovascular therapy is that restenosis or occlusion of previously successfully treated limbs seldom results in greater clinical deterioration than simply a return to the preprocedure state. In contrast, occlusion of surgical bypasses can worsen ischemia. Thus, the use of endovascular approaches to recanalize and stent diffuse SFA disease is reemerging.

In addition, the development of stent coatings containing drugs such as rapamycin may further reduce the incidence of renarrowing to that approaching the patency of surgical bypass. In a randomized series of long-segment SFA disease patients, those receiving rapamycin-coated nitinol self-expanding stents developed much less intimal thickening and no restenosis at 6 months.[18] Of additional interest, the control group that received identical but noncoated stents had only 23 percent restenosis—suggesting that stent design may also influence the success of the treatment of long-segment SFA disease. Although it is likely that longer follow-up and additional studies will demonstrate that drug-eluting stents do not abolish restenosis completely, these initial findings have engendered tremendous interest in the development of recanalization technologies to treat the long-segment chronic total occlusion.

Because it is the rule rather than the exception for lower extremity arterial disease of the SFA to present with chronic total occlusion, there is renewed interest in both the treatment of long-segment disease and the recanalization of chronic total occlusions, especially with the excimer laser. Scheinert and colleagues have reported 411 lesions in 318 patients successfully recanalized with the excimer laser. The success achieved in this group was remarkable when one considers the mean lesion length was 19.4 cm.[19,20] Table 55–2 summarizes recently reported femoropoliteal interventional studies.

How is one to decide on the best treatment for his or her patient today? Unfortunately, there is scant evidence on which to base this decision. Surgical revascularization and its initial technologies were developed long before balloon angioplasty and other catheter-based technologies emerged, and surgery thus became the traditional or gold standard. However, "traditional" does not necessarily mean "superior," and "new" does not necessarily mean "better." We lack prospective, randomized series or surgery versus catheter-based intervention to permit valid comparisons.

Adherents of surgical technique particularly point to the superior durability and primary patency of autologous saphenous vein bypass as well as poorer technical success and long-term patency of endovascular recanalization and/or stenting. They note that salvage of critically ischemic limbs probably requires reconstitution of unobstructed "straight-line" flow to the foot (i.e., through revascularized native arteries or bypass grafts and not via collaterals).

Interventionalists remark that their ability to recanalize the long-segment chronic total occlusion has improved rival surgical technical success rates and that if straight-line perfusion can be achieved with endovascular technique, the results can be hemodynamically equivalent. They further note that interventional procedure-related cardiac mortality is rare and interventional therapy, because of its minimally invasive nature, should be considered a *course* of treatment and not judged by the surgical primary patency standard. In addition, angiographic restenosis may play a less critical role in the follow-up of *endovascular* treatment of critical limb ischemia—when applied properly, there is little or no surgical dissection and disruption of native anatomy. Thus, slowly developing restenosis may afford time for the continued development of collaterals and, after giving the distal tissues time to heal, closure of the revascularized segment may be less consequential than the original occlusion.

Those who advocate the medical treatment of claudication point to the success of exercise programs, ongoing research into new palliative drugs, the increasingly documented benefits of aggressive risk factor modification, and the complete lack of "procedure-related mortality" with medical treatment alone as a demonstration of the need for conservatism in the treatment of claudicants (see Chap. 54). In many instances, either surgery or interventional techniques can ameliorate the patient's symptoms. The decision regarding the most appropriate therapy can be made by the patient and the physician, taking into account the risks and discomforts of the proposed procedure, its probable durability and reproducibility, the degree to which a procedure closes the door to other therapies, the magnitude of life-style limitation, and the individual patient's tolerance for risk.

The treatment of femoropopliteal disease now stands at a new threshold. The advent of new stent design, better recanalization techniques, and the promise of drug-eluting

TABLE 55–2 Recent Results of Femoropopliteal Interventions*

Lead Author	Reference	Year	No. of Patients	Lesions Treated	Percent with Occlusions	Technical Success (%)	Ankle-Brachial Index		Mean Lesion Length (cm)	Devices Used Primarily	Primary Success[†] (%)	Duration (mo)	Cumulative Success[†] (%)	Duration (mo)
							Before	After						
Gray	21	1997	55	58	NA	NA	0.48	0.71	16.5	SES, BES	22	24	46	24
Martin	22	1999	68	NA	6	100	NA	NA	NA	PTA	NA	—	57	24
Kessel	23	2000	20	NA	—	95	0.6	1	17	SG	29	12	64	12
Conroy	24	2000	48	61	100	100	NA	NA[¶]	13.5	SES, Some BES	47	12	79	12
Cheng	25	2001	55	69	NA	92	NA	NA	13.8	SEN, SES	53.8	24	72.1	24
Gordon	26	2001	57	71	100	NA	0.59	0.86	14.4	SES	38.2	24	76.2	24
Scheinert	19	2001	318	411	100	83	0.62	NA	19.4	LPTA, some SEN	33.6[†]	12	75.9	12
Lofberg	27	2001	92	121	47	88	NA	NA	NA	PTA	27	60	34	60
Bauermeister	28	2001	35	NA	100	100	0.25	0.87	22	SG[§]	73.2	12	82.6	12
Duda	18	2002	36	36	57	100	NA	NA	8.5	DEN vs. SEN	100/77	6	NA	—
Steinkamp	29	2002	312	312	100	91.7	0.56	0.88	7.5	LPTA, some SEN	61.5	24	90.2	24
Gray	30	2002	23	NA	84	88	0.54	0.84	6.2	LPTA	33	24	75	24
Jamsen	31	2002	173	218	NA	83.5	NA	NA	NA	PTA	25	60	4.1	60
Cho	5	2003	40	40	100	100	0.61	0.93	NA	SEN	NA	—	NA	—
Becquemin	32	2003	251	277	NA	90	0.52	NA	2.5	BES vs. PTA	65/67[‡]	12	NA	—
Jahnke	33	2003	52	63	83	100	0.54	0.89	10.9	SG	74.1	24	83.2	24

BES = balloon-expandable stainless steel; SES = self-expanding stainless steel; SEN = self-expanding nitinol; DEN = drug-eluting nitinol; PTA = percutaneous transluminal (balloon) angioplasty; LPTA = excimer laser-assisted PTA; SG = stent graft; NA = not assessed or reported.

*Summary of reports of femoropopliteal interventions from the literature. A wide variety of anatomical situations are represented here, including many with chronic long-segment total occlusions. Of note is that primary patency of 2 years, when reported, is considerably lower than that for iliac interventions yet cumulative patency ranges from approximately 75% to 90%. This emphasizes the need for both postprocedure surveillance and consideration of the performance of a femoral intervention when embarking on a course of therapy.

†Clinical or objective patency.

‡Angiographic patency (<50% stenosis) in mandatory stent group vs. PTA with selective stenting group.

§Devices placed surgically.

¶Average increase of 0.26.

stents will provide many more effective treatment options for patients (Figs. 55–3 through 55–6).

Infrapopliteal Obstruction

PAD is typically a diffuse process involving multiple arterial levels and segments. Thus, when disease is seen in the proximal vessels, significant occlusive disease is often seen in the three infrapopliteal arteries (anterior tibial, peroneal, and posterior tibial). Similarly, when infrapopliteal narrowing is present, one is likely to find coexisting proximal disease. Rarely, stenosis may be isolated to one or more vessels below the knee. Revascularization considerations below the knee must take into account the extent, severity, and distribution of disease in more proximal vessels. Indeed, for patients with claudication and compromised outflow, correction of coexisting disease in a proximal vessel is often sufficient in and of itself to achieve symptomatic relief. This differs from patients with critical limb ischemia, in whom lesion healing generally requires restoration of uninterrupted patency of at least one vessel to the foot. In the absence of severe and flow-limiting proximal disease, significant disease of all three crural vessels is usually required to provoke symptomatic calf claudication or higher grades of ischemia (rest pain or tissue loss).

Traditionally, revascularization for vessels below the knee has been reserved for patients with rest pain; limbs threatened by ulcers, infection, or gangrene; or symptoms at very low levels of exertion. Until recently, the preferred mode of treatment has been surgical bypass. However, paradigms that challenge the traditional approach are emerging with respect to both indications and mode of revascularization. Dramatic technological advances and incremental experience now allow for routine and uncomplicated access to vessels in the infrapopliteal distribution. Although the relative advantages of catheter-based arterial revascularization have been more clearly established for lesions in more proximal vessels, numerous studies have now confirmed the feasibility, safety, and efficacy of tibial PTA. Infrapopliteal PTA was initially limited to patients with critical limb ischemia who were at high risk for bypass graft surgery; those who had no saphenous vein available for bypass conduit; or those with more proximal interventions in whom improving distal runoff might help maintain overall vessel patency. In these patients, the less invasive approach is now preferred routinely over higher risk surgical intervention. Primary success rates are generally 80 to 95 percent, and cumulative 2-year patency rates can approximate 75 percent (Table 55–3). More important, limb salvage rates of percutaneous intervention have now been demonstrated to rival those of surgical reconstruction.[36,38,39] Even in diabetic patients, in whom skepticism regarding small-vessel intervention previously prevailed, balloon angioplasty can effectively salvage ischemic limbs.[41,42]

The safe and effective reconstruction achieved with the percutaneous approach in this higher-risk cohort has caused a shift in the management of patients who have critical limb ischemia due to infrapopliteal disease. When anatomically feasible, an initial attempt at PTA is now considered a reasonable and appropriate strategy for revascularization in *all* patients, even those who are suitable candidates for infrapopliteal bypass (Figs. 55–7 and 55–8). The exception to this may be in patients with more extensive disease, in whom long-term outcomes may be hampered by restenosis rates as high as 40 to 60 percent. Rotational atherectomy or excimer laser angioplasty can be useful as adjunctive therapy in lesions that have unfavorable morphology, such as total occlusion, heavy calcification, and/or ostial location. Previous studies with rotational atherectomy have shown it to be useful acutely, though data on long-term follow-up are no more favorable than balloon angioplasty alone. Though wide-ranging use may not be appropriate, selected patients (particularly those with limited surgical options) clearly benefit from these "niche" devices.[30]

Strategies for revascularization must reflect the limitations of technology but also must be considered in the context of the patient's overall clinical condition. Selection of a higher-risk open surgical procedure based on anticipation of better long-term patency should be tempered by the knowledge that shorter-term patency established by less risky percutaneous means is often adequate to salvage the extremity. In many instances, critical limb ischemia does not recur once the extremity has healed, even in the face of restenosis or reocclusion. The optimal strategy is one that is safest and most likely to provide both acute improvement and—to the greatest extent possible—long-term benefit.

The changing paradigm for revascularization also relates to the indications for intervention in patients with symptomatic but less critical infrapopliteal disease. The traditionally high threshold for intervention was maintained largely due to the associated risk and invasive nature of the surgical approach. Currently, however, a lower threshold for intervention may be considered. Specifically, in the subset of patients who claudicate solely due to infrapopliteal disease, favorable acute and intermediate term patency and clinical results have been achieved using PTA.[39] Such a strategy should be limited to patients with severe symptoms (Rutherford category 3) and straightforward anatomy. Infrapopliteal PTA may also be useful in claudicants undergoing proximal revascularization (either with surgery or PTA), in whom the runoff is severely impaired. When tibial outflow is a major

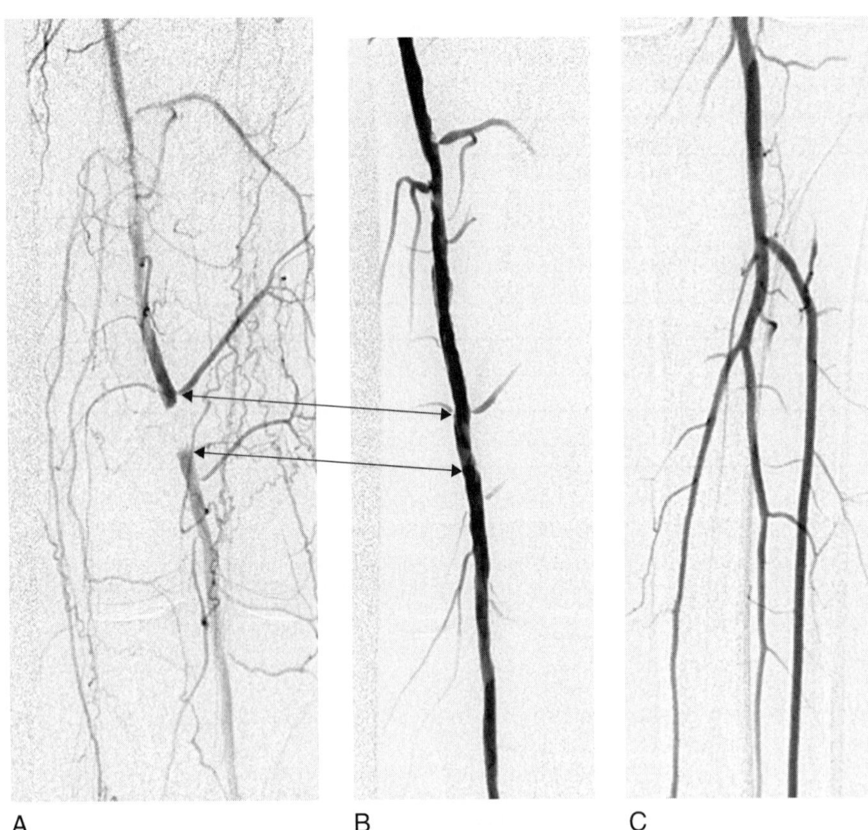

FIGURE 55–3 The result of recanalization and balloon dilation of a short-segment femoropopliteal occlusion. In **A,** a digital subtraction angiogram illustrates the area of total occlusion and compares it to that in **B,** showing the results of balloon dilation only. Both areas are indicated by the double-ended black arrows. **C** shows an intact three-vessel runoff without evidence of distal embolization.

TABLE 55–3 Results of Tibial Artery Interventions*

Lead Author	Reference	Year	No. of Patients	Lesions Treated	Percent with Occlusions	Technical Success (%)	Ankle-Brachial Index	
							Before	*After*
Sivananthan	34	1994	38	73	24	96	NA	NA
Varty	35	1995	38	40	17	98	0.55	0.84
Dorros	36	1998	312	657	27	98	NA	NA
Desgranges	37	2000	33	NA	NA	82	NA	NA
Soder	38	2000	60	72	35	84/61†	NA	NA
Dorros	39	2001	235	529	28.9	92	NA	NA
Tsetis	40	2002	12	13	100	92.3	0.35	0.68

PTA = percultaneous transluminal (balloon) angioplasty; VPTA = vibrational PTA; NA = not assessed or reported.
*Summary of recent literature on tibial artery interventions. Most reports are those of review of single-center experience and procedural results. The 2001 report of Dorros and associates deserves special mention: It is of long-term follow-up of event-free survival and limb salvage.
†Stenosis/occlusion.

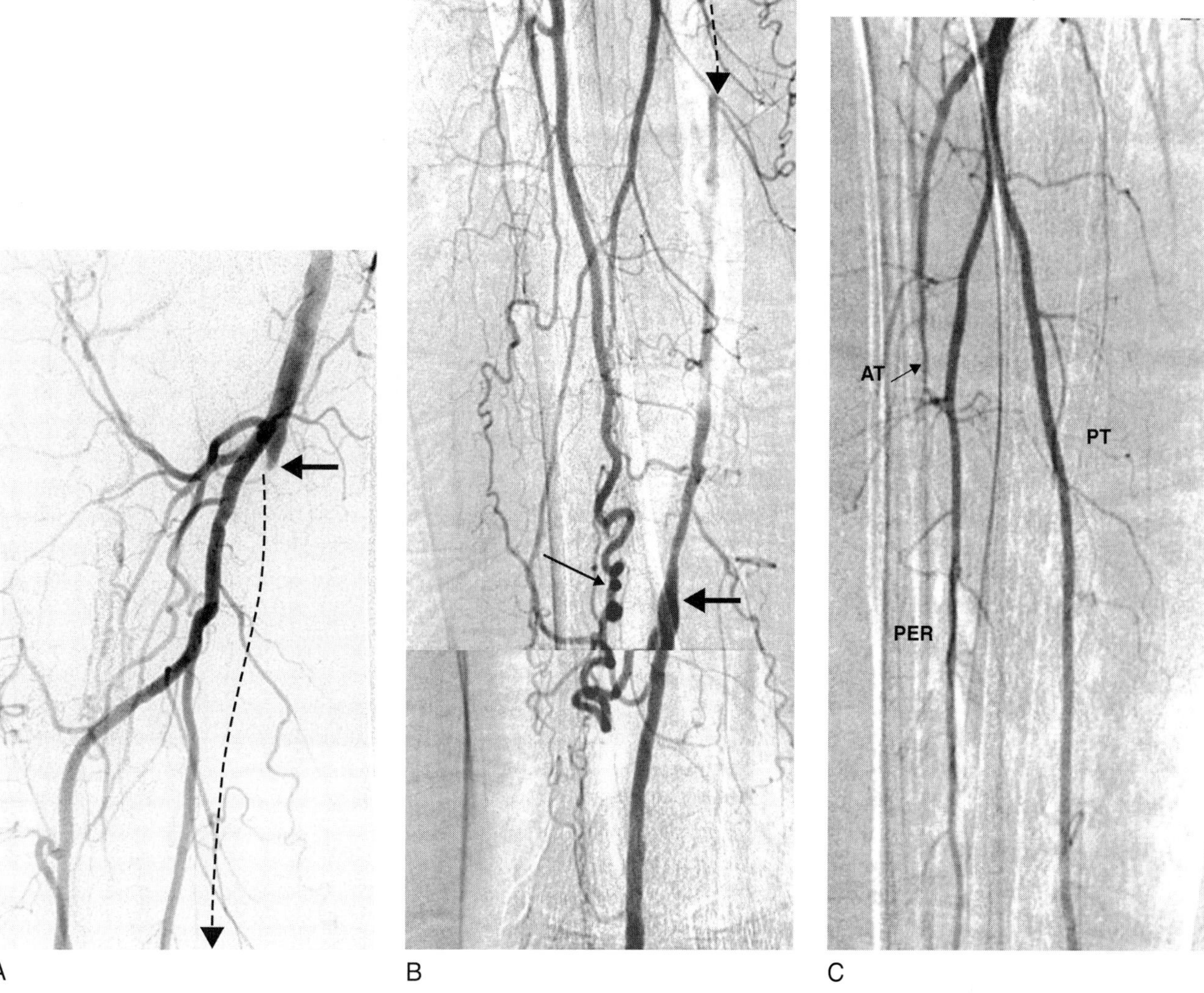

FIGURE 55–4 A long-segment chronic total occlusion. In contrast to the short-segment disease in Figure 55-3, this requires recanalization from the origin of the superficial femoral artery (SFA) (**A,** thick arrow) along the path of the SFA (dashed arrow) continuing to the level of the most significant collateral inflow and reconstitution of the vessel (**B**). **C** shows the crural vessels and demonstrates occlusion of the anterior tibial (AT) with patent peroneal (PER) and posterior tibial (PT) runoff.

Mean Lesion Length (cm)	Primary Device	Primary Patency		Cumulative Patency		Event-Free Survival		Limb Salvage	
		Percent	*Duration (mo)*	*Percent*	*Duration (mo)*	*Percent*	*Duration (mo)*	*Percent*	*Duration (mo)*
NA	PTA	NA	—	NA	—	NA	—	NA	—
1	PTA	59	24	68	24	NA	—	77	12
NA	PTA	NA	—	NA	—	NA	—	NA	—
NA	PTA	66	12	77	12	94	12	91	12
NA	PTA	68/48†	10	56	18	NA	—	80	18
NA	PTA	NA	—	NA	—	31	60	91	60
7	VPTA	NA	—	NA	—	NA	—	NA	—

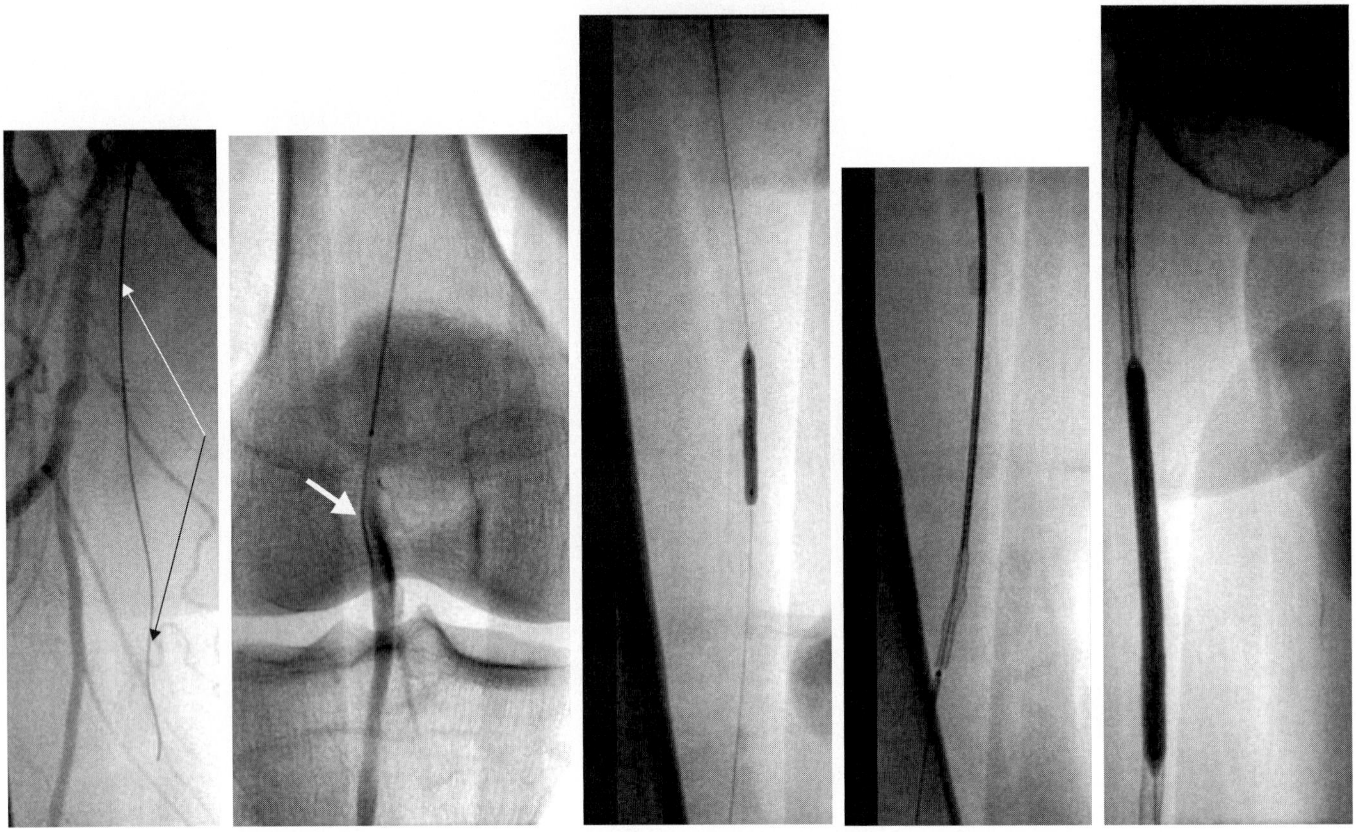

A B C D E

FIGURE 55–5 Recanalization of this lesion was accomplished from the contralateral approach using a hydrophilic guidewire advanced into the occluded segment **(A)**. Once the guidewire is free in the distal vessel, a small catheter is passed over the wire and a contrast agent injection is made to confirm the intravascular position **(B)**. This is followed by "pre"-dilation **(C)**, self-expanding stent placement from distal to proximal **(D)**, and, finally, "post"-dilation to the appropriate size **(E)**

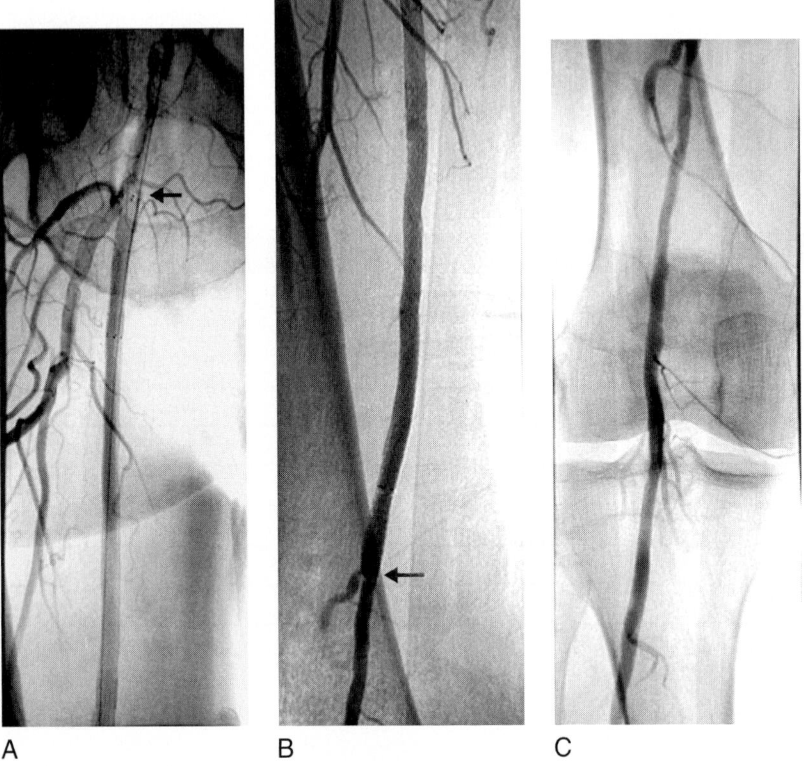

FIGURE 55–6 Recanalization of this long-segment occlusion and stenting from the origin of the superficial femoral artery (SFA) in **A** (arrow) to the level of collateral reconstitution in **B** (arrow) resulted in reconstitution of the normal anatomy, return of pedal pulses, and healing of digital ulcers. Care was taken to preserve the collateral vessel ostia so that, in the event of restenosis, collateral pathways are reestablished. This anatomy should be contrasted with total occlusion of the SFA but short-segment disease shown in Figure 55-3. These cases illustrate the anatomical variations that commonly occur and emphasize the difficulty in characterizing the true extent of disease in patients with total occlusions of this vessel.

determinant of long-term patency, recanalizing the runoff vessels may provide a benefit. In any case, when performing PTA for critical limb ischemia or claudication, particular care must be taken not to compromise subsequent surgical options. For example, disruption of a distal, previously uncompromised vessel may prohibit subsequent bypass to that site. Although this is a rare occurrence, a thoughtful strategy is required to avoid "burning a bridge" to a subsequent surgical intervention.

In summary, optimal management of patients with lower extremity arterial occlusive disease and associated symptoms

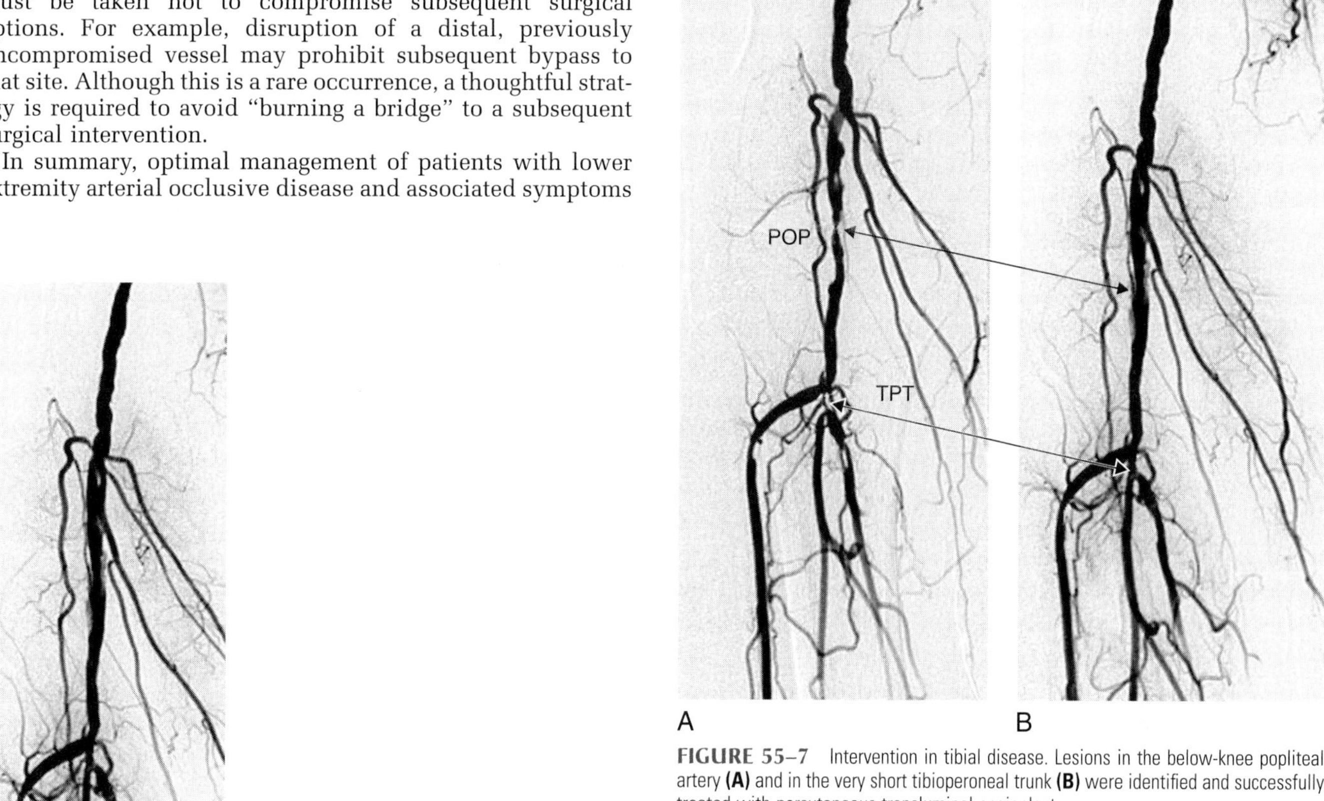

FIGURE 55–7 Intervention in tibial disease. Lesions in the below-knee popliteal artery **(A)** and in the very short tibioperoneal trunk **(B)** were identified and successfully treated with percutaneous transluminal angioplasty.

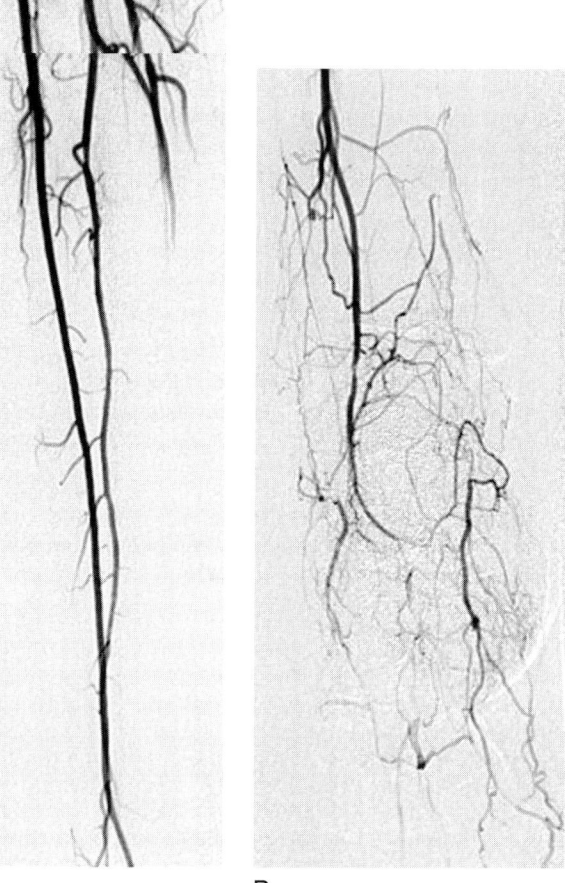

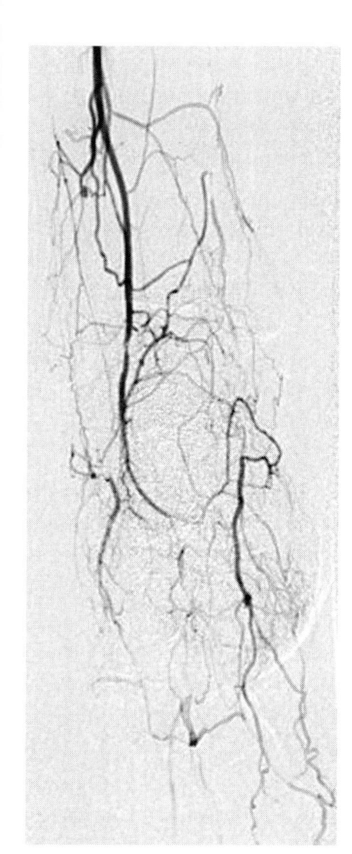

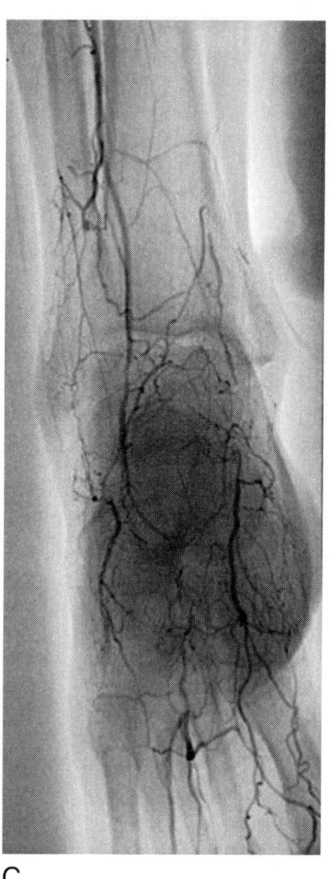

FIGURE 55–8 **A** shows a composite angiogram from the patient in Figure 55-7 demonstrating the intact anterior tibial runoff in the calf. The peroneal normally attenuates by the level of the malleoli and, in this case, the posterior tibial is also occluded. **B** and **C** show the pedal circulation in both digital subtraction angiography and native views. Though "straight-line" flow to the foot was reconstituted and the patient's ulcers healed, the evident diffuse small-vessel disease in the pedal vessels still places the foot in long-term jeopardy. Careful surveillance and compulsive continuing medical management are critical in this group of patients, even in the context of technical procedural success.

requires the input of practitioners knowledgeable of the capabilities of both percutaneous and surgical revascularization. If their disease is anatomically suitable, patients should be considered for percutaneous endovascular treatment. The physician must provide a frank discussion of the risks, potential symptomatic benefit, and durability of the proposed intervention. For patients with claudication, there is little evidence to suggest that an early and aggressive revascularization alters the natural history of lower extremity occlusive disease. Thus, treatment should be guided by the patient's degree of impairment and personal wishes. Limb-threatening ischemia, in contrast, should be treated promptly, utilizing the modality that will provide the most complete revascularization with the lowest procedural risk. For example, endovascular treatment of isolated iliac occlusive disease is often equivalent hemodynamically and may be preferable to surgery. Infrainguinal disease that is diffuse or associated with long-segment femoral obstruction has traditionally been addressed with saphenous vein bypass. However, given the coexistence of coronary disease with peripheral vascular disease, a less invasive endovascular approach may be a preferable first step in a given patient. Generally, the greater the patient's comorbidity, the more likely one is to turn to a percutaneous approach.

Determination of optimal strategy in the future will likely be based on accumulating evidence and data, wherein patient and lesion characteristics, functional outcome measures, and cost analyses will be standardized to enable comparison among pure endovascular, pure surgical, and combined percutaneous and surgical approaches.[43] As the short- and long-term outcomes of catheter-based interventions continue to improve, it is likely that these techniques will be used in an increasing number of patients presenting with either claudication or critical limb ischemia.

Regardless of initial treatment strategy, a key determinant of the long-term outcome is the requirement for intensive follow-up surveillance. Although surveillance strategies for surgical bypass grafts have been developed, no formal guidelines exist for monitoring patients following percutaneous therapy. However, there is general agreement that these individuals should be subjected to regular evaluation, examination of the affected limb, and noninvasive testing. Early and prompt reintervention is indicated for restenosis to maximize the chances of long-term symptom relief, wound healing, and integrity of the limb.

For Visceral Ischemia

Renal Artery Obstructive Disease

Renovascular disease is an important and often unrecognized contributor to renal insufficiency, refractory hypertension, and overall cardiovascular mortality. However, because not all patients with angiographic evidence of renovascular disease are hypertensive or have renal dysfunction, patient selection for more invasive therapy requires careful consideration. Additionally, since the clinical syndrome associated with this anatomical diagnosis can resemble that of more common clinical diagnoses, such as isolated essential hypertension, a renovascular cause may not be considered. The onset of diastolic hypertension after the age of 55 years, refractory or malignant hypertension, resistant hypertension in a previously well-controlled patient, and/or an increasing serum creatinine level should alert the clinician and prompt further diagnostic testing. Unfortunately, modalities such as angiotensin-converting enzyme (ACE) inhibitor–induced venous plasma renin sampling and intravenous urography have insufficient sensitivity and specificity to provide a reliable screening and diagnostic tool.[44] Although post-ACE renal scintigraphy has high levels of sensitivity and specificity in some patient subsets, its utility is limited by lower sensitivity and specificity in patients with bilateral disease or abnormal renal function.[45] Duplex renal artery ultrasound,[46] spiral CT,[47] and more recently, MR angiography[46] all have been used in the noninvasive assessment of the renal vasculature with high degrees of accuracy. Although these modalities vary in their sensitivity and specificity, ultimately one's clinical conviction regarding the diagnosis must weigh heavily in the decision to pursue angiographic evaluation, because none of the techniques allows assessment of the functional significance of a renovascular lesion. Furthermore, even the traditional reference standard, contrast angiography, has considerable intraobserver and interobserver variability.[48,49] Determining the functional significance of an anatomical finding remains one of the greatest challenges of renal intervention. Nevertheless, significant renal artery obstruction is associated with an adverse prognosis in patients with atherosclerosis.[50]

After establishing the anatomical diagnosis of renal artery stenosis, one must consider the most appropriate management. The goals of treatment, both surgical and percutaneous, for renal artery stenosis include preservation of renal function, improved control of hypertension, and prevention of hemodialysis. Improvement in blood pressure control and reduction in the number of antihypertensive medications is common, but complete resolution of hypertension is unusual because concomitant essential hypertension often coexists. To the extent that severe renal artery disease can cause renal dysfunction, the identification and treatment of functionally significant renal artery stenosis could have major health benefits.[51] A major question remaining is whether percutaneous renal revascularization can slow, delay, or prevent deterioration in renal function and subsequent hemodialysis.

Historical data from the surgical literature support treatment of patients with both unilateral and bilateral renal artery stenosis. Although anatomical revascularization may allow improved antihypertensive management and preserve renal parenchymal function, how does percutaneous therapy compare to surgery? This question has particular importance, given the advanced age of many patients with atherosclerotic disease and the significant perioperative morbidity and operative mortality rates of up to 6 percent associated with surgical therapy. Only one randomized, controlled study has compared surgical therapy versus balloon angioplasty for unilateral atherosclerotic renal artery stenosis.[52] The authors reported slightly lower primary patency rates in the balloon angioplasty group, as one may expect in the prestent era. However, secondary patency was 90 percent in the PTA group and 97 percent in the surgical group, with comparable improvement in blood pressure and similar likelihood of improvement or stabilization in renal function after intervention. Even in the prestent era, the results of percutaneous intervention compared favorably to those of surgery.[53,54]

The availability of stents and the associated technological improvements that facilitate secure delivery of devices to the target site have led to more predictable and hemodynamically favorable results in renal revascularization. In spite of technical success rates in excess of 95 percent using stents, not all patients undergoing this procedure enjoy a clinical benefit. Thus, the presence of arterial stenosis does not guarantee a causal relationship to the patient's coexisting hypertension or renal insufficiency. In addition, patients with renovascular disease are commonly afflicted by other nephrotoxic conditions, including diabetes, essential hypertension, atheroemboli, and medication-related insults. Thus, the outcome of intervention in patients with isolated renovascular disease differs from that in candidates with renal artery stenosis and concomitant renal parenchymal disease. For this reason, it is likely that the desired clinical outcome of

TABLE 55–4 Clinical and/or Historical Factors Influencing the Degree of Suspicion of Renal Artery Stenosis*

Type of Influence	Effects	
Indication	Hypertension of recent onset or newly refractory Mildly elevated creatinine level (≤2.5) without diabetes Increasing creatinine on ACE inhibitor Disparate renal size (1 normal, 1 small) Pulmonary edema not explained by cardiac dysfunction	*The presence of any two is indication for determining renovascular anatomy*
Increases	Coronary atherosclerosis Claudication Known aortic branch vessel (brachiocephalic/mesenteric) atherosclerosis Abdominal bruit Known atherosclerotic abdominal aortic aneurysm Mild proteinuria without diabetes	
Decreases	Normal creatinine Severely elevated creatinine level (>3.5 mg/dl) Diabetes *with* evidence of nephropathy/retinopathy Severe (nephrotic range) proteinuria Longstanding stable hypertension Bilateral atrophic kidneys	

ACE = angiotensin-converting enzyme.

*Current potential indications for investigating the anatomical presence of renal artery stenosis and intervening if it is found. In our laboratories, the presence of any two with the indications in concert is cause for anatomical definition of the renal arteries. The intensity of this set of indications is augmented by the presence of the factors causing increases and is reduced in the presence of mitigating factors causing decreases.

improved blood pressure, with concomitant reduction in requirement for antihypertensive medications, is seen in only two-thirds of patients treated with stenting for renovascular disease.

This discrepancy between anatomical result and clinical outcome remains a challenge for the clinician who must assess the potential efficacy of a proposed renal artery intervention. How can one determine if revascularizing one of two kidneys will achieve the intended goals? The Dutch Renal Artery Stenosis Intervention Cooperative Study Group performed a study to determine whether an aggressive approach with invasive therapy is superior to that of "provisional" angioplasty. The group, consisting of some 26 centers, prospectively studied 106 patients with difficult-to-control hypertension, unilateral atherosclerotic renal artery stenosis (>50 percent decrease in luminal diameter), and a serum creatinine of less than 2.3 mg/dl, randomizing between angioplasty and best medical therapy.[55] The results suggested little advantage of angioplasty over medical therapy in the control of hypertension based on an intention-to-treat analysis. However, several issues severely limited the utility of this investigation, including the small sample size; inclusion of patients with only moderate renal artery stenoses; failure to use vascular stents; high percentage (44 percent) of cross-over to balloon angioplasty among patients in the control arm; and the authors' focus on the effect of therapy on blood pressure control to the exclusion of effect on renal function.

Many investigators and clinicians believe the routine use of vascular stents improves the results. Harden and associates studied patients with both bilateral and unilateral renal artery stenosis. Although the number of patients investigated was small, evidence suggested a slowing of renal impairment after stenting.[56] Additionally, when the entire renal mass is involved ("global renal ischemia"), the response is more dramatic: Renal intervention in patients with severe (>75 percent) bilateral disease or unilateral disease in a solitary kidney uniformly improves or stabilizes renal function and preserves kidney size.[57]

In summary, percutaneous treatment of renovascular disease offers a safe, flexible, and effective therapy that is preferable to open surgical revascularization. Renal artery stenting can ameliorate hypertension, can improve or stabilize renal function, and may delay the need for hemodialysis in appropriately selected patients. Controversy remains regarding the appropriate threshold for intervention in patients with severe unilateral renal artery stenosis, associated with normal renal function and only modest hypertension that is reasonably controlled. Future randomized trials and the adoption of uniform reporting standards will hopefully shed light on this issue.[58,59] Lastly, the advent of distal protection devices to limit atheroembolic complications may further improve safety and renal parenchymal preservation. The current recommended systematic approach to the investigation and treatment of this condition is outlined in Table 55–4 and Figures 55–9 and 55–10, and examples of complex renal intervention are shown in Figures 55–11 through 55–13.

Mesenteric Ischemia

The clinical syndrome of mesenteric ischemia is surprisingly uncommon, given the high frequency of atherosclerotic disease of the aorta and the common finding of aorto-ostial stenosis of the visceral vessels. It is likely that the rarity of the clinical syndrome reflects the good collateralization and redundancy of the visceral circulation with multiple pathways from the superior mesenteric artery and the inferior mesenteric artery. In addition, there are clearly lesser degrees of ischemia, often misdiagnosed, that manifest with moderate postprandial discomfort, bloating, or gas rather than the full-blown syndrome of delayed postprandial pain, vomiting, food avoidance, and weight loss. Even in advanced cases, multiple other etiologies for the manifest of weight loss and abdominal pain are often entertained before "intestinal angina" comes into focus as the diagnosis of exclusion. Evidence of significant obstruction of two or more of these vessels is often found when classic symptoms and endoscopy suggest bowel ischemia.[60] With the advent of MR angiography imaging, it is now possible to make the "anatomical" diagnosis without resorting to invasive angiography.[61] When the symptoms are classic, the anatomical findings severe, and the alternative pathological explanations few, the diagnosis is confirmed and revascularization is in order. As might be expected, however, this patient group has a high incidence of CAD, and surgical mortality and morbidity ranges from 5 to 8 percent,[62-65] with the highest incidence of complications

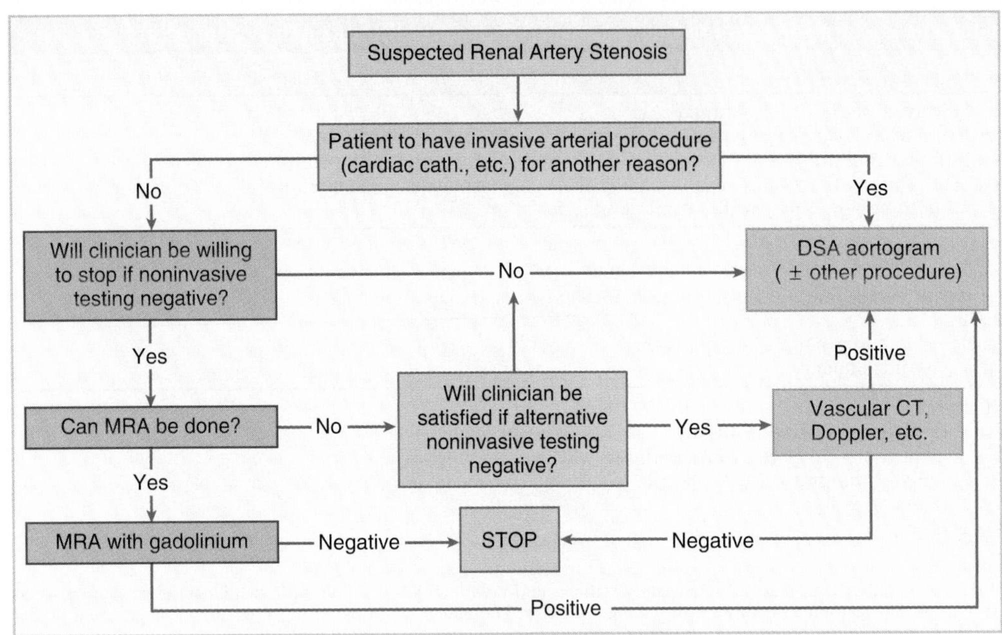

FIGURE 55–9 The approach to the anatomical evaluation of renal artery stenosis. Once stenosis is suspected, if the patient is to have another invasive arterial procedure, noninvasive imaging is deferred and a low-volume digital subtraction aortogram (DSA) is done at the time of that procedure. In other cases, the clinician should assess whether a negative noninvasive test would be sufficient evidence to acquit the renal arteries. If so, noninvasive testing should be performed. If not, consideration should be given to DSA and selective angiography. cath = catheterization; MRA = magnetic resonance angiography.

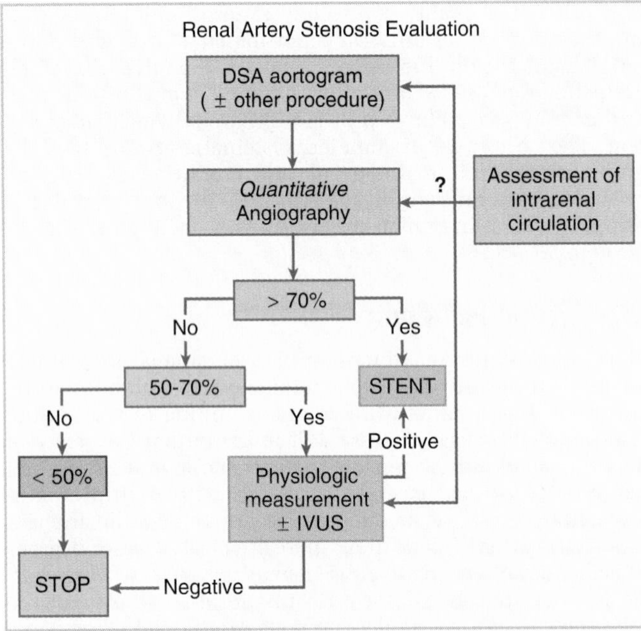

FIGURE 55–10 The approach to the angiographic evaluation and treatment of renal artery stenosis. Once a digital subtraction aortogram (DSA) is performed confirming the presence of renovascular disease, quantitative angiography and objective evaluation of the severity of stenosis should be performed. Very severe (>70 percent diameter stenosis) lesions are subjected to revascularization and mild lesions (<50 percent diameter stenosis) are not. We believe that the intermediate lesion should be assessed with physiological evaluation and/or an additional anatomical documentation of severity such as intravascular ultrasound (IVUS). The absence of translesional flow acceleration or a pressure gradient should mitigate the desire to intervene.

occurring in patients older than 70 years of age.[64] Mortality for operation on *acute* mesenteric ischemia is an order of magnitude higher.[66] In view of these risks, the clinician must have a high degree of diagnostic certainty before commending the patient to surgery for chronic mesenteric ischemia.

Obstructions of the visceral vessels are similar to those of the renal arteries, and the technical considerations for PTA and stent placement are similar to those for renal artery intervention. The endovascular approach circumvents the need for general anesthesia, and the operative trauma associated with open surgery and, it is believed, will result in a lower acute mortality and morbidity.[67-69]

As is true for the evaluation of alternative therapies in most other peripheral vascular beds, there is no side-by-side comparison of surgery versus endovascular treatment for chronic mesenteric ischemia. Interpretation of the literature, which reports successful case series of both surgical and interventional treatment, is confounded by the obvious case selection and other inherent biases. Interventional treatment offers a clear alternative for the management of chronic visceral ischemia that may have advantages over surgery, especially in those patients with advanced age or additional increased risk of morbidity and mortality (Figs. 55–14 and 55–15).

For Cerebral Ischemia

Brachiocephalic and Subclavian Obstructive Disease

Once considered rare, brachiocephalic and subclavian artery obstructions have received increased attention due to the use of internal mammary conduits for coronary bypass surgery. Subclavian steal syndrome arises due to reversal of flow in the vertebral artery as blood is shunted into the brachial circulation. Symptoms of dizziness, syncope, and vertigo are most common along with extremity claudication in the ipsilateral limb. In coronary-subclavian steal, there is reversal of flow within the left internal mammary artery because of proximal subclavian stenosis. These patients often come to clinical attention with myocardial ischemia. Although some clinical improvement may be seen with conservative therapy, relief of the anatomical obstruction is usually necessary.[70]

Balloon angioplasty for subclavian artery stenosis was described in the early 1980s, with subsequent reports showing that acute success and patency rates at follow-up were comparable to surgery. Furthermore, there was a low rate of complications and infrequent mortality.[71,72] There was initial concern about the potential for distal embolization and stroke, uncertain long-term patency, and difficulty in treating total occlusions. This concern, in conjunction with continued improvements in anesthetic and operative technique, short hospital stays, and early discharge, has led many practitioners to continue to regard surgery as the standard therapy against which endovascular methods must be compared.

Vascular stents have become the endovascular treatment of choice for atherosclerotic obstructive disease of branches of

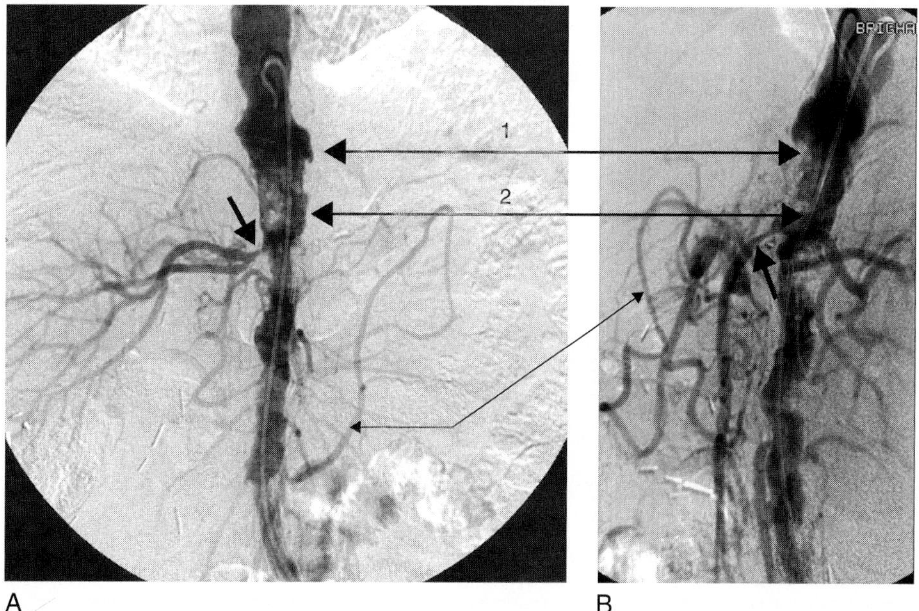

FIGURE 55–11 The anatomical complexity in treatment of advanced renovascular disease. **A** shows an anteroposterior aortogram in a patient with refractory hypertension and monthly hospitalizations for hypertensive crises and pulmonary edema. Initially, this patient was to have aortic and renovascular surgery, but on exploration, the aorta was so calcified that no operative approach was deemed feasible. Medical therapy was elected, but after continued refractory hypertension, aortography and intervention were performed. Between levels 1 and 2, shown by the double-headed arrows, an eccentric atherosclerotic excrescence produced a pressure gradient of between 30 and 50 mm Hg. In addition, there was an intrinsic ostial renal artery stenosis indicated by the single thick arrow in **A.** In **B** the thick arrow shows an origin stenosis of the superior mesenteric artery, and the thin arrow projecting into both panels identifies the marginal artery collaterals filling the mesenteric circulation.

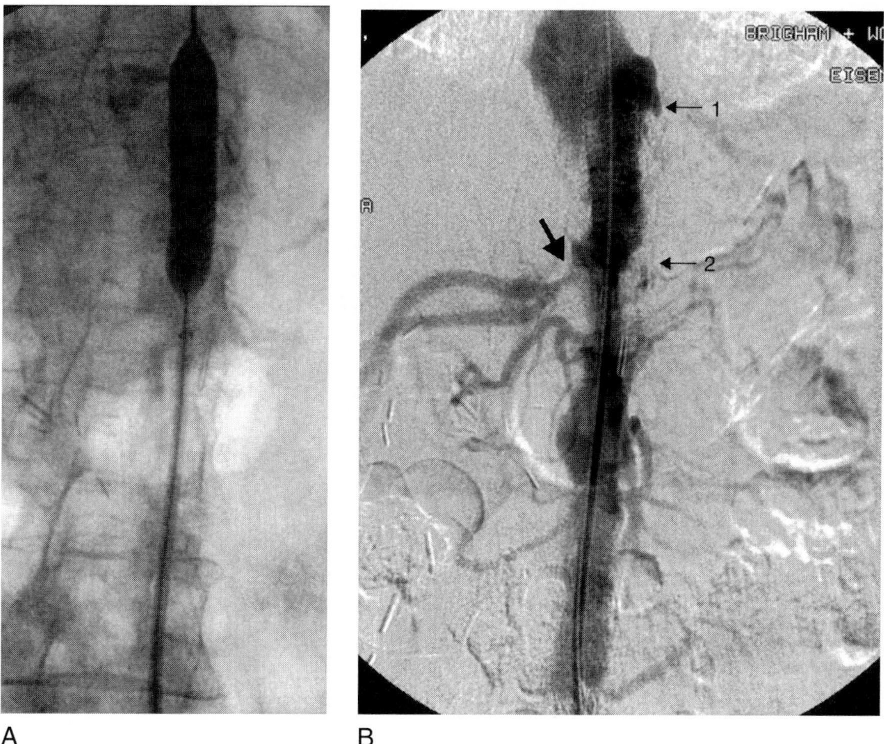

FIGURE 55–12 **A,** Balloon postdilation of a 14-mm self-expanding stent. **B,** This stent obliterated the translesional gradient from position 1 to position 2, yet the intrinsic renal artery stenosis remained (thick arrow).

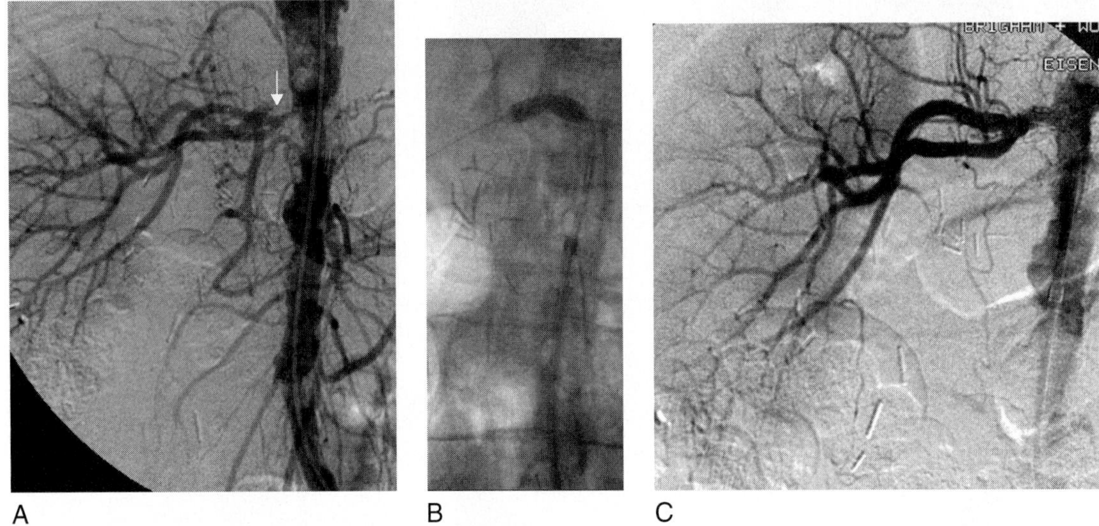

FIGURE 55–13 Selective balloon and stent placement in this vessel. **A,** The initial stenosis. **B,** Balloon-expandable stent placement. **C,** Selective angiography demonstrating resolution of the stenosis. Final hemodynamic measurements showed no pressure gradient from the thoracic aorta and downstream of the renal stent. This patient tolerated the procedure well, had mild improvement in the serum creatinine level, but most significantly was no longer refractory to antihypertensive medications, and her blood pressure control prevented further hospitalizations for hypertensive crises and pulmonary edema.

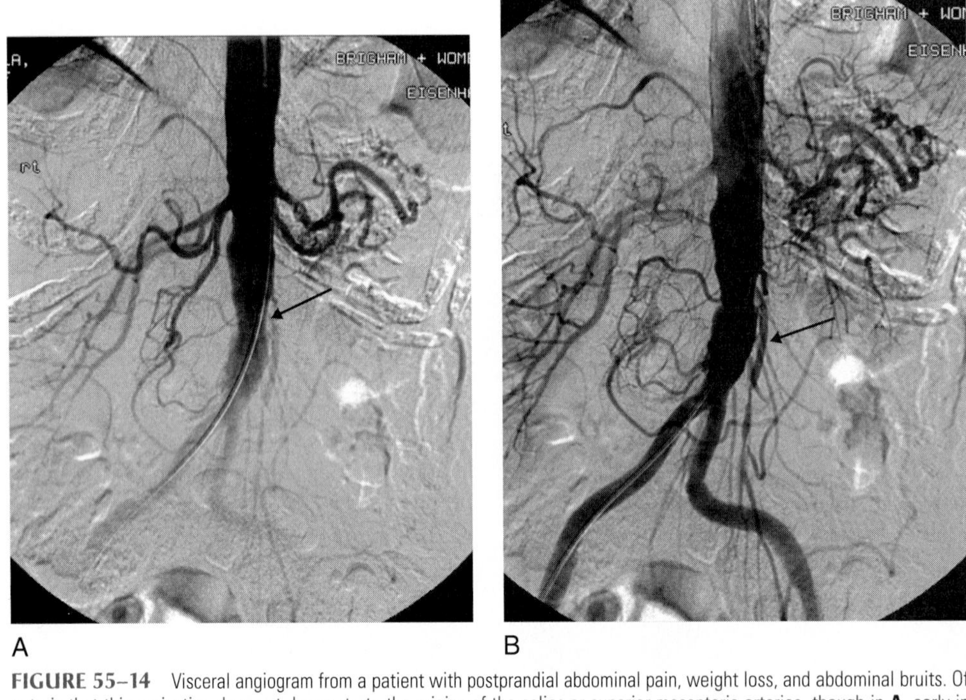

FIGURE 55–14 Visceral angiogram from a patient with postprandial abdominal pain, weight loss, and abdominal bruits. Of note is that this projection does not demonstrate the origins of the celiac or superior mesenteric arteries, though in **A,** early in the run, the thin arrow indicates a stenosis at the origin of the inferior mesenteric artery. Then, from a later frame, **B** shows the origins of the renal arteries; though potentially not seen in absolute profile, they appear unobstructed.

the aorta, including the subclavian and carotid arteries. However, long-term patency and clinical data for percutaneous treatment of the subclavian/brachiocephalic vessels are limited. An evaluation of the reports of surgery versus angioplasty/stenting of this condition has been published, compiling technical success (the ability to perform the planned procedure yielding target lesion revascularization and survival to discharge), patient death, stroke, and patency of the treated segment.[73] There was no uniformity or standardization for evaluation or reporting of complications in the studies in which stenting was performed; however, adverse events were reported in approximately 6 percent of patients.[73] Similarly, the overall incidence of postprocedure complications such as vascular access difficulty, hemorrhage, pseudoaneurysm, transfusion, or contrast-mediated transient renal insufficiency is not known. Of the patients represented in the reports, technical success was achieved in 97 percent. No strokes or deaths occurred. Follow-up data were available in about two-thirds of technically successful cases at a mean duration of 16.8 months. Occlusion or restenosis was reported in 6 percent. Following publication of this review, there were editorials from interventionalists suggesting broadening the horizons of interventional therapy[74] and from surgeons advising to proceed with caution.[75]

The reports of vascular stenting continue to suggest that perioperative strokes are quite uncommon. Al-Mubarak and colleagues reported no strokes in their series of 38 patients,[71] and strokes occurred in only 0.9 percent of subclavian procedures described by Henry and coworkers.[72] In addition, treatment failures, when they occurred, were limited to totally occluded arteries. Primary patency ranged from 94 percent at 20 months to 75 percent at 8 years; with overall patency of 100 percent at 20 months to 90 percent at 8 years.[71]

There have been some conflicting reports regarding the efficacy of stent implantation. There are concerns about not only long-term patency but also durability of the stent owing to wire fracture at the site of flexion and compression.[76] Motarjeme reported disappointing patency rates for

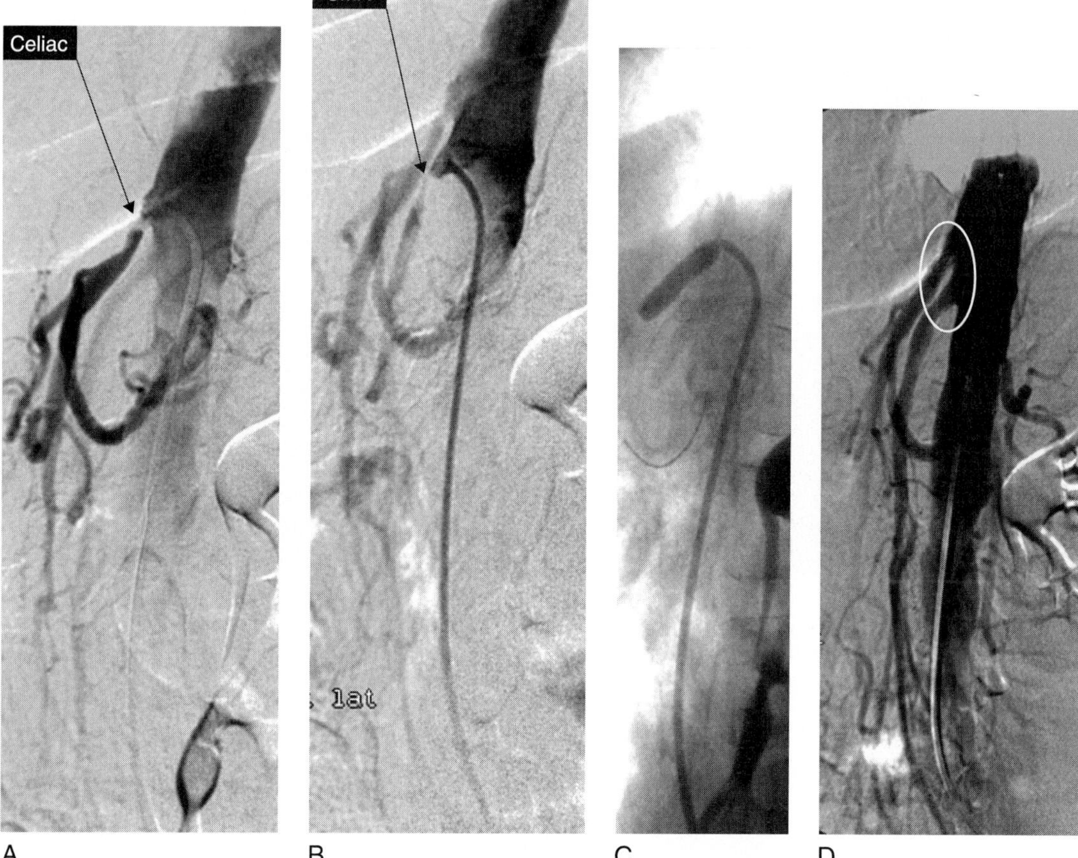

FIGURE 55–15 The selective evaluation of the celiac and superior mesenteric arteries (SMA) in the lateral projection of the patient in Figure 55–21. Both these vessels proved to be critically stenosed (**A** and **B**) and were treated interventionally (**C**), restoring wide patency to both as outlined in **D**. The patient's symptoms abated, and she began to gain weight.

balloon angioplasty alone in a group of patients with total occlusions of the subclavian,[77] whereas Henry and associates reported good short and intermediate results in both those who underwent angioplasty alone and those who had angioplasty and stenting.[72] A European series reviewed 115 patients with subclavian disease who were treated percutaneously.[78] The procedures were performed between 1984 and 1998, and all patients after January 1, 1996, routinely received balloon-expandable stents. Successful revascularization was achieved in 98 patients. There were no periprocedural deaths, 1 patient had a transient ischemic attack (TIA) from the left vertebral artery, and 2 patients had emboli (one to the renal artery and 1 to the mesenteric artery). All 3 patients recovered completely from these events. Although patency rates were significantly higher at 1 year in the stented group compared with those treated only with angioplasty (95 vs. 76 percent), by 4 years of follow-up there was more restenosis in the stented patients.[78] Furthermore, in a multivariate model, predictors of restenosis in this study included lesion length, residual stenosis after angioplasty, and stent implantation.[78] However, this analysis was limited by the large difference in patient numbers in the two groups (26 in the stented group vs. 72 in the angioplasty group) and because stents were placed only in patients treated after 1996. By that time technological advances had made it easier to open totally occluded vessels that were previously rarely successfully treated percutaneously. Thus, many of these lesions in the stent group had other factors increasing their risk of restenosis and would not have been successfully treated percutaneously before the introduction of stents.

It remains unlikely that the near future will produce a large well-designed trial comparing surgical and interventional treatment of patients with brachiocephalic and subclavian disease. At present, experience and examination of the literature support the consideration of a primary percutaneous approach in most patients with symptomatic obstructive disease (Fig. 55–16; also see Fig. 55–22).

Carotid Disease

Stroke and its associated debilitation is one of the most dreaded threats to health. As a result, prophylactic surgical therapy for significant carotid stenosis was embraced by both patients and physicians, and carotid endarterectomy became one of the most commonly performed procedures by vascular surgeons. Now, developing endovascular technology has allowed the expansion of available treatment modalities for cerebrovascular disease. Although catheter-based therapy may offer a less invasive alternative to carotid endarterectomy, controversy still exists regarding where and when the endovascular treatment of cerebrovascular disease should be applied.

The goals of treating carotid artery disease are to prevent disabling stroke and to prolong life. All therapies should be judged ultimately on their ability to achieve these endpoints rather than surrogate ones. Planning mechanical treatment for cerebrovascular disease requires knowledge of the natural history of the problem. In the Dutch TIA trial, 3000 patients with a history of recent TIA were randomized to treatment with low or moderate dose aspirin.[79] After 36 months, the risk of nonfatal stroke was 5.7 percent in the low-dose group and 6.9 percent in the high-dose group. Thus the risk of stroke in unselected aspirin-treated patients is 3 percent per year after an index event. Given the concerning natural history of cerebrovascular disease and the unknown effects of carotid endarterectomy, several randomized trials were organized to determine whether endarterectomy had benefits over medical therapy for both symptomatic and asymptomatic disease. In the early 1990s, European Carotid Endarterectomy Surgery

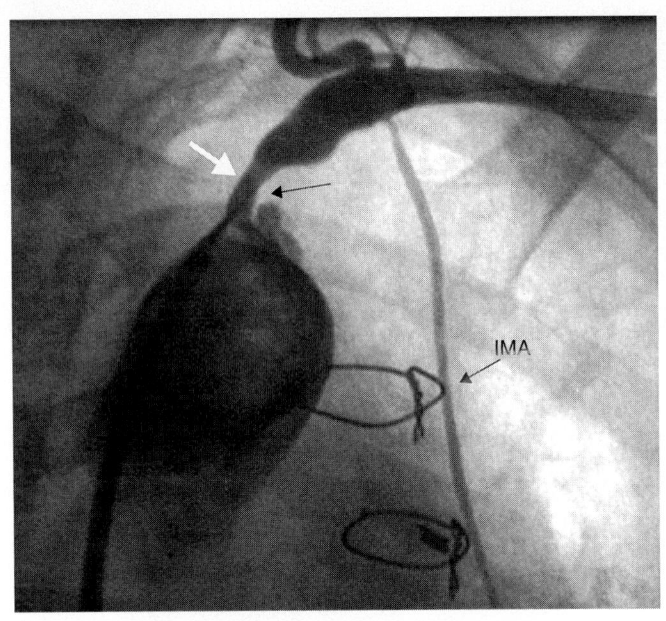

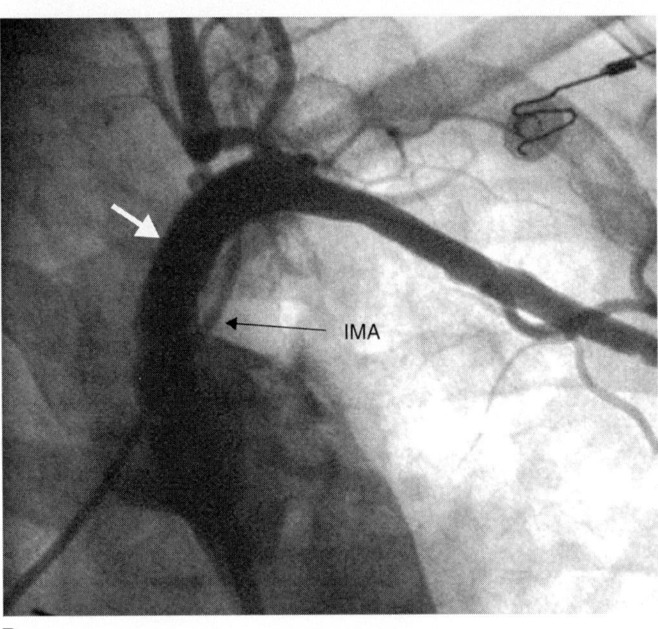

A B

FIGURE 55–16 The treatment of proximal subclavian disease. In **A,** a severe stenosis at the origin of the left subclavian artery is identified (thick white arrow). This is in association with an atherosclerotic ulcer (thin black arrow). The internal mammary artery (IMA) is indicated. Following balloon dilation and stent placement **(B),** the subclavian artery is widely patent and the IMA is preserved.

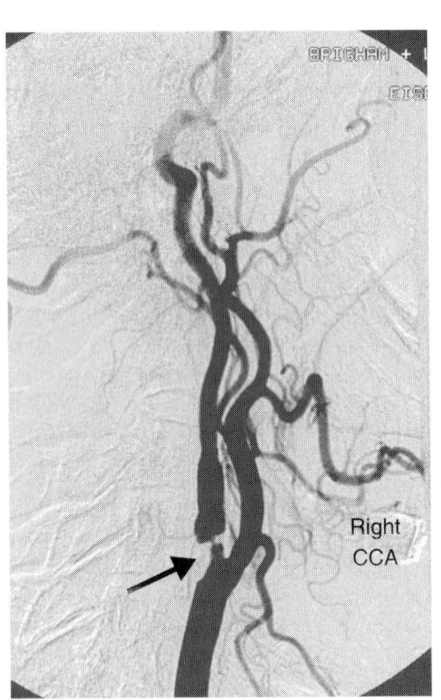

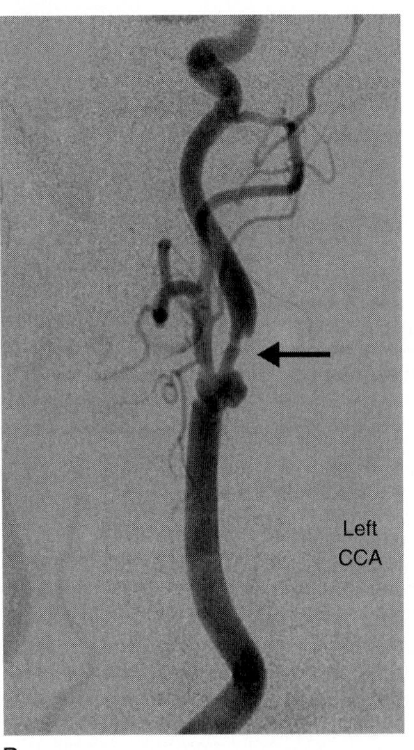

A B

FIGURE 55–17 Selective digital subtraction angiograms of the cervical carotid artery (CCA) in a patient with disseminated atherosclerosis and severe bilateral internal carotid obstruction. This patient had a recent right hemisphere transient ischemic attack, and the stenosis at the origin of the right internal carotid artery (**A,** arrow) is extremely severe. In **B,** the left carotid angiogram demonstrates a severe stenosis (arrow), but one with a lesser degree of obstruction than the contralateral artery.

Trialists (ECST)[80] enrolled patients with 70 to 99 percent carotid stenosis within 180 days of an ipsilateral TIA. Patients were randomized to medical versus surgical therapy, yielding a 21.9 percent risk of stroke at 36 months for the medically treated group and a 12.3 percent risk in the surgically treated group. The North American Symptomatic Carotid Endarterectomy Trial (NASCET) randomized patients with 70 to 99 percent stenosis and ipsilateral TIA symptoms within 120 days of randomization to medical or surgical therapy.[81] The 30-day follow-up favored medical therapy with a 5.8 percent rate of all stroke and death in the surgical group and a 3.6 percent risk in the medical group. Similarly, the major stroke rate was increased more than twofold to 2.1 percent in the surgical group. As in the ECST data, the 36-month death rate did not differ significantly between groups in the NASCET study (12.7 vs. 9.9 percent, surgical vs. medical), with most of these deaths related to cardiovascular causes. However, the 36-month total stroke rate (9 vs. 26 percent) and major stroke rate (2.5 vs. 13.1 percent, surgical vs. medical) were significantly less in the surgical group. The results of this study have served as the gold standard for treatment of symptomatic carotid disease and clearly suggest that surgical endarterectomy stabilizes the index lesion. Similar data have been developed for severe asymptomatic stenoses,[82] albeit with results that are less compelling compared to those in patients with symptomatic disease.

Although these randomized trials suggest that high-quality carotid endarterectomy, despite procedural risk, decreases long-term incidence of ipsilateral stroke in patients with severe carotid stenoses, endarterectomy has not been shown to prolong life. The patients in these studies were carefully selected to avoid confounding conditions, and many with significant comorbidities were excluded—such as those with atrial fibrillation, severe symptomatic coronary disease, recent myocardial

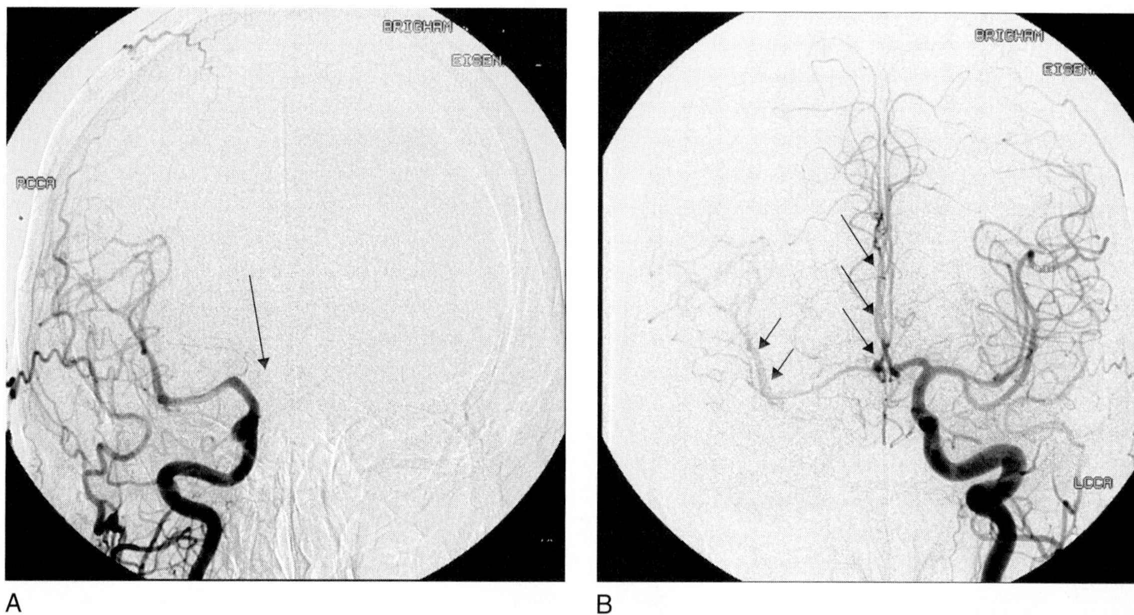

FIGURE 55–18 The corresponding anteroposterior (Townes) view of the right and left carotid angiograms (**A** and **B,** respectively). **A** shows perfusion of the right middle cerebral territory only, and no flow is seen into the anterior cerebral vessel, the expected location of which is delineated by the arrow. In contrast, **B** shows the injection of the left carotid artery and demonstrates filling of both hemispheres, including the right anterior cerebral (three long arrows) and middle cerebral (two short arrows) territories.

infarction, past ipsilateral carotid endarterectomy, ipsilateral disabling stroke, age older than 79 years, or life expectancy less than 5 years. To participate, institutions and surgeons had to demonstrate acceptably low rates of complications and stroke in their surgical patients.

Clearly, for endarterectomy to have achieved those benefits in the populations studied, the strokes *prevented* by the operation must significantly exceed the strokes *caused* by the operation. Similarly, operative mortality could obliterate any benefit of surgery. In NASCET, carotid endarterectomy was associated with a 6.5 percent complication rate of combined stroke and death, with about 0.9 percent of death not related to stroke. Most strokes in NASCET resulted from thromboembolism within 6 hours of the procedure. These perioperative strokes were mostly ipsilateral to the carotid endarterectomy and were attributed to thrombus formation at a denuded arterial site. The longer term results of NASCET showed that although there was no mortality benefit, the reduction in stroke ipsilateral to the endarterectomy during the operative and 3-year follow-up period favored endarterectomy. After the perioperative period, the risk of ipsilateral major stroke was almost zero,

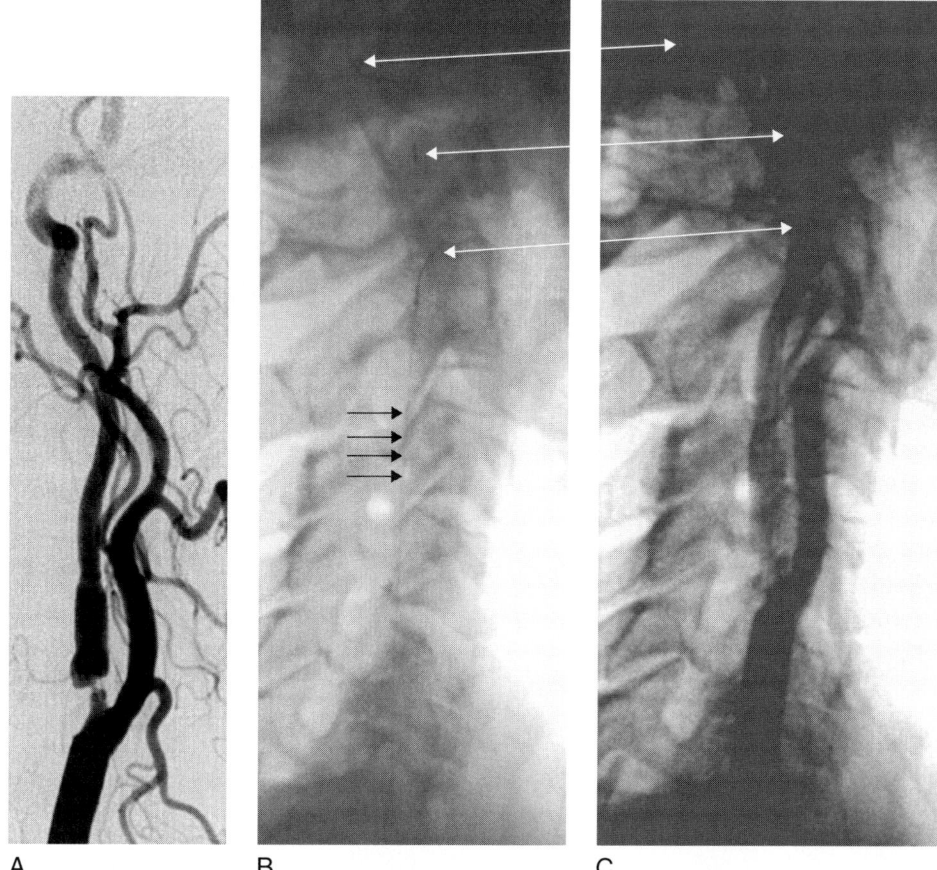

FIGURE 55–19 **A,** The prestenting angiogram; the right carotid is repeated. **B** and **C** illustrate the Filterwire distal protection device in place. In **B,** the four short arrows indicate the body of the guidewire, with the uppermost horizontal arrow indicating the distal portion of the guidewire; the middle horizontal arrow showing the end of the cone of the distal protection device; and the lowermost horizontal arrow showing the hoop supporting the entry into the conically shaped microporous membrane of the distal protection device. **C** is an unsubtracted angiogram with the device in place, demonstrating distal perfusion through the membrane of this device.

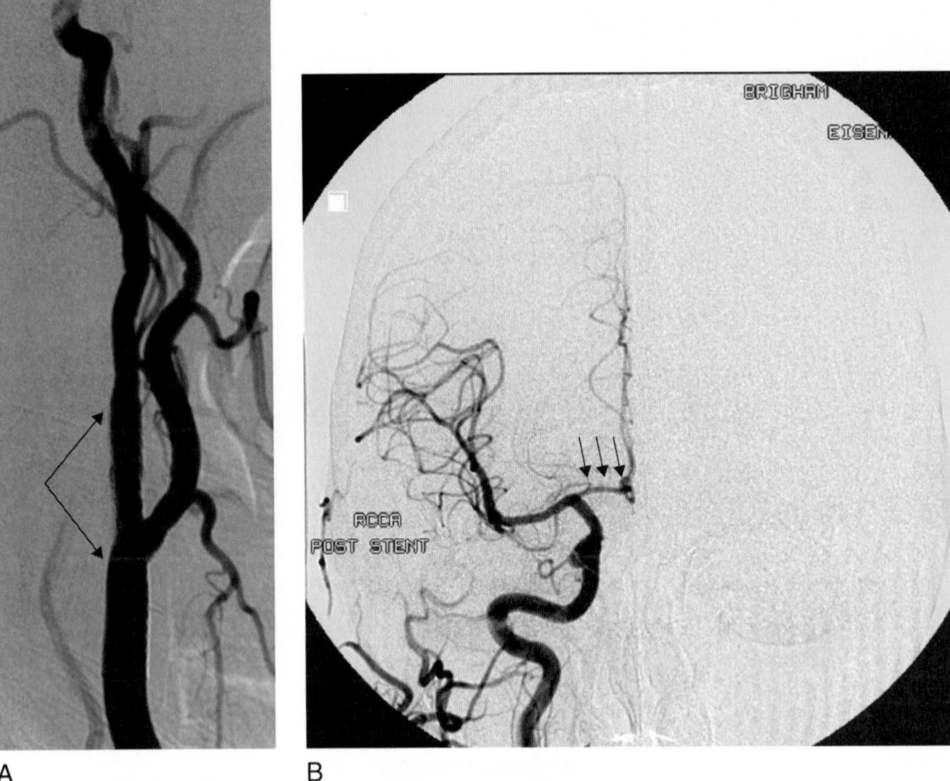

FIGURE 55–20 **A** illustrates the results of stent placement; the extent of the stent is indicated by the arrows, and wide patency of the carotid has been restored. **B** shows a poststenting right carotid angiogram illustrating renewed vigorous flow into the anterior cerebral artery in this hemisphere (three arrows).

implying that strokes occurring outside the perioperative period are *not* under the influence of the operation or surgical technique.[83,84] The large size of the trial and the relatively low adverse event rates indicated that small absolute differences in these rates could have obliterated the statistical benefit of endarterectomy. Indeed, subsequent analysis of operative stroke rates in the general population at the NASCET-participating hospitals suggested the reported rates were unusually low.[85] On balance, however, the randomized surgical data demonstrate that once a perioperative stroke is avoided, endarterectomy is a durable prophylaxis against ipsilateral stroke.

Endovascular Carotid Treatment

It was a logical evolution of endovascular technique to consider its potential in extracranial cerebrovascular disease. Given the results of the randomized surgical trials, this extension encountered a number of conceptual and ethical hurdles. First, was it ethical to extend a new and untested therapy to a clinical situation in which there was already another therapy shown to be superior to medical treatment alone? Because of this consideration, early endovascular efforts were not extended to every patient whose clinical characteristics matched those in the NASCET, the European Carotid Endarterectomy Surgery Trial (ECST), or the Asymptomatic Carotid Atherosclerosis Study (ACAS). Instead, stenting was first offered to patients who were at high risk. They would have been ineligible for the surgical trials but had carotid *lesions* similar to those benefiting from surgical revascularization. Results were encouraging, but the rate of periprocedure central nervous system events did not appear to be *identical* to those in the NASCET population. Alternative possibilities advanced to explain these results were that the endovascular technique was responsible or that the incongruent outcomes were the result of the inclusion of high-risk patients not studied in the surgical trials.

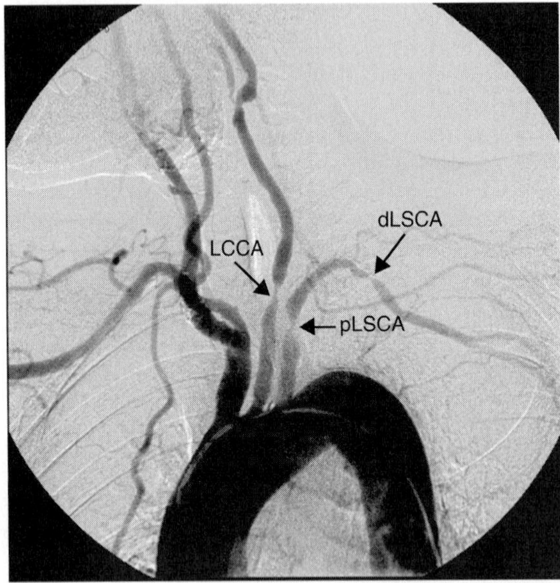

FIGURE 55–21 A digital subtraction aortic arch angiogram, in the left anterior oblique projection, of an elderly patient with severe aortic arch disease. This patient had evidence of both left hemisphere transient ischemic attacks and left arm claudication. This case illustrates the ability to treat complex aortic arch vessel disease with interventional technique. dLSCA = distal left subcavian artery; LCCA = left common carotid artery; pLSCA = proximal left subclavian artery.

Currently, experience with carotid stenting is accumulating. Some early publications suggested a high rate of procedural complications. However, Roubin and associates reported the complications of TIA, stroke, myocardial infarction, and death in their first series of patients treated with carotid stenting.[86] The 5.7 percent procedural stroke incidence corresponds to an overall stroke and death rate at 30 days of 5.8 percent in the surgically treated group in NASCET—certainly suggesting clinical equipoise. Five-year follow-up results of 528 patients[87] undergoing carotid stenting showed a 1.6 percent fatal stroke and nonstroke death rate at 30 days. The major stroke rate was 1 percent and the minor stroke rate was 4.8 percent. The overall 30-day stroke and death rate was 7.4 percent ($n = 43$). Over the course of follow-up there was a 3-year freedom from stroke rate of 92 ± 1 percent. Of particular note is the learning curve that is appar-

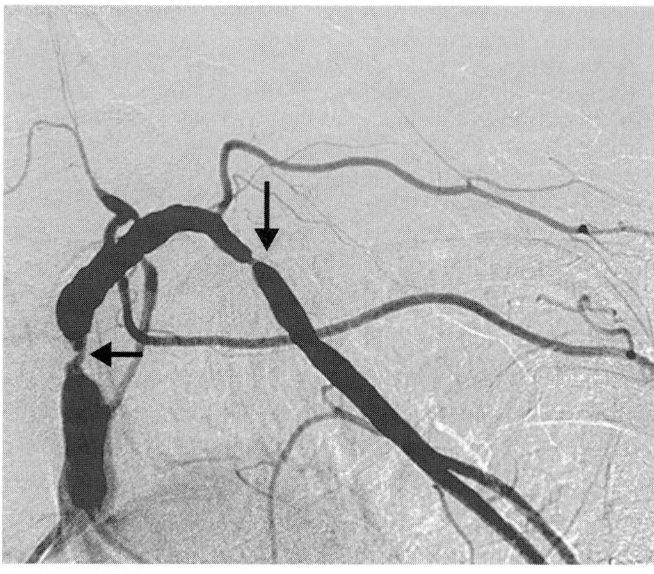

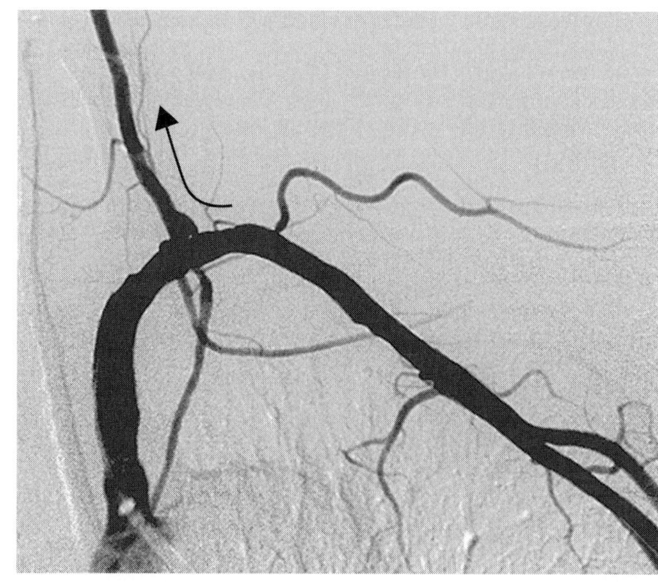

FIGURE 55–22 **A,** A selective digital subtraction angiogram of the left subclavian. This study shows a stenosis proximal to the origin of the left vertebral and left internal mammary artery (horizontal black arrow) and a severe stenosis distal to the left vertebral, internal mammary, and thyrocervical trunk. Treatment of the distal lesion without relief of the proximal obstruction would potentially exacerbate the subclavian steal, and thus both lesions require treatment. **B,** A repeat subclavian angiogram after placement of proximal and distal stents. In **A** and **B,** the injection technique was similar, yet **B** shows antegrade flow in the left vertebral, indicated by the curved black arrow in **B**. Because of the potential for external compression, a self-expanding stent with appropriate postdilation was used to treat the more distal subclavian lesion.

ent in the application of this technology—over the 5-year study period, the 30-day minor stroke rate significantly improved from 7.1 percent for the first year to 3.1 percent for the fifth year.

The International Society for Carotid Artery Treatment has compiled an ongoing voluntary, self-reported registry of procedures performed outside of formal trials.[88,89] This registry also discloses a learning, or experience, curve, with the highest rates of major stroke and death (~3 percent each) occurring in centers that have performed procedures on fewer than 50 patients. Overall, however, in this patient group, the reported rates of TIA and minor stroke in 1999 were less than 3 percent, major stroke 1.35 percent, and death less than 1 percent. An additional report[90] of 8612 procedures describes 2.3 percent TIA, 2.5 percent minor stroke, and 1.32 percent major stroke, for a summed ischemic complication rate of 6.12 percent. The overall procedural mortality was 0.72 percent. Of course, these are self-reported registry data and not independently collected or adjudicated, as would be the case in prospective, randomized studies. However, these data suggest the rate of complications that is likely to be encountered in practice.

The Carotid and Vertebral Artery Transluminal Angioplasty Study (CAVATAS) provided the first prospective, randomized comparative data on patients with cerebrovascular disease randomized to endovascular or surgical treatment.[91] In this study, the mortality was equivalent in both arms and the neurovascular event rates were statistically similar. The major stroke and death rate was 5.9 percent among the surgical patients and 6.4 percent among the angioplasty patients (10 percent and 9.9 percent for any stroke lasting >7days within 30 days of treatment). All deaths in the endovascular group were due to fatal strokes, but there was only one fatal stroke in the surgical arm. The high event rate in both arms of CAVATAS led to criticism of both carotid endarterectomy and endovascular intervention in this trial.[92] In a small randomized series comparing carotid stenting and endarterectomy, there were no strokes in either the surgical or the endovascular stent groups, and only one death in the surgical group.[93] Though the rate of adverse events did not differ between the groups, the small size of this study raises the question of whether it had sufficient power to prove equivalence of the techniques. As of this writing, these are the only peer-reviewed reports of direct comparisons of carotid endarterectomy with endovascular technique. However, the results of the high-risk randomized trial of Stenting and Angioplasty with (embolic) Protection in Patients at High Risk for Endarterectomy (SAPPHIRE) trial, comparing stenting to endarterectomy in high-risk patients, have been presented in abstract form. This trial, although designed as an equivalency study, surprisingly indicated an advantage of endovascular therapy over carotid endarterectomy with regards to the primary endpoint of stroke, death, or myocardial infarctin at 30 days. One-year data, recently reported but not peer reviewed, indicate a persistent advantage to stenting at 1 year, with favorable rates of combined ipsilateral stroke and death compared to the surgical approach.

Carotid Intervention and Embolic Debris

The key to the overall benefit of any carotid procedure is the *avoidance of the periprocedural stroke.* Both stenting and endarterectomy appear to stabilize the area of the lesion effectively. The trade-off versus medical therapy alone is the exchange of procedure-related strokes in the short term with spontaneous lesion–related strokes in the follow-up period.

The recognition that the avoidance of periprocedure stroke is critical and that distal emboli are potentially disastrous, combined with the desire to improve percutaneous methods of treating obstructive carotid atherosclerosis, has underscored the need to identify risk factors to optimize patient selection. Neurological deficits can be predicted by the presence of symptomatic lesion, a lesion length greater than 11.2 mm, and the absence of hypercholesterolemia.[94] The lesion length was thought to predict stroke because the treatment of long stenoses required more manipulations, longer stents, and multiple postdilations after stent placement. It was postulated that the postdilation surface provided a prothrombotic area immediately following intervention; thromboembolic stroke was an implicated outcome. In addition, neurological complications of endovascular treatment were found in one study to be predicted by advanced age (>80 years) and long (>10 mm) or multiple (>1 lesion separated by normal vessel wall) stenoses.[95] The incidence of stroke in patients younger than 80 years was 5.6 percent, whereas in those 80 years or older, the incidence was 19.2 percent.

However, thrombotic debris is not the only cause of embolic stroke. Evidence of carotid plaque embolization as a result of stenting and PTA was reported by Manninen and colleagues.[96,97] The results of stenting, including postdilation when necessary ($n = 9$) and PTA ($n = 10$), were compared in situ in human cadavers, and embolic debris was detected in equal amounts for both types of interventions. Histological analysis of the debris determined that it was composed primarily of atherosclerotic plaque constituents. Observations of the postintervention surfaces with intravascular ultrasound and MR imaging led the investigators to postulate that the smoother stent surface could be preferable to the post-PTA surface. Additional ex vivo studies have confirmed that embolic debris is commonly released during endovascular plaque manipulation at many stages.[98] Ohki,[99] Rapp,[100] and their associates found that embolic debris was released from all specimens.

Clinically, Doppler evidence of emboli is found in 30 to 40 percent of symptomatic patients and 4 to 20 percent of asymptomatic patients, and it has been said that microembolization is universal. The clinical consequences of embolic showers likely depend on the size and number of emboli and the nature of the distal vascular bed.[101] Thus, the major concern associated with balloon angioplasty and stenting of carotid lesions has been the periprocedural complications that arise due to embolic debris and not the long-term outcome.[102]

Distal Embolization Protection (see also Chap. 52)

The determination that distal embolization is both dire and common during endovascular carotid procedures has prompted a search for devices and techniques to limit its occurrence. Devices that employ distal balloon occlusion, the distal positioning of a porous filter, and proximal occlusion with aspiration all have been developed.[103] Henry and coworkers[104] were first to report use of balloon occlusion and aspiration for carotid applications in high-risk patients. Carotid occlusion was well tolerated in all but 1 of the 48 patients; intolerance was due to the presence of multiple severe carotid lesions and poor collateralization. Analysis of debris retrieved in a similar patient population[105] revealed particle sizes ranging from 50 to 2500 μm in diameter composed of atherothrombotic material—fresh thrombus, old thrombus, lipoid masses, fibrous particles, and calcified particles.

Technical reports of experience with distal embolic protection devices report aggregate rates of periprocedural stroke and death from 2 to 5 percent.[106-110] The use of the devices can be associated with difficult placement distal to the lesion, distal carotid spasm, or difficulty in protection device retrieval through stents. Debris is often grossly visible, and histological analysis of the particulate routinely demonstrates typical components of atherosclerotic plaque. Although occlusion balloons currently have a more favorable, lower crossing profile, they do not allow flow and are not tolerated by all patients. Filters provide distal perfusion and, in doing so, not only benefit the target organ but also allow better visualization for stent placement. Although there are no randomized studies and the technology continues to evolve rapidly, carotid stenting distal cerebral protection appears safe, and further investigation with such devices is warranted. Recent peer-reviewed procedural results of carotid intervention are outlined in Table 55–5.

Though it is an evolving technology, carotid stenting offers an appealing, less invasive modality with benefits comparable to surgical endarterectomy. With increasing operator experience and use of increasingly effective distal embolization protection devices and antiplatelet therapy, endovascular techniques will undoubtedly advance rapidly. Large-scale randomized, controlled trials and registries, some currently ongoing, will ultimately determine relative advantages of surgical and endovascular approaches to carotid disease. For the present, endarterectomy remains the reference standard. Refinements of endovascular technique will be led by devices that mitigate distal embolization; reports suggest that these devices are clearly effective in reducing the incidence of

TABLE 55–5 Recent Carotid Intervention Series*

Lead Author	Reference	Year	Protected (P), Unprotected (U), or Mixed (M)	*N*	TIA (%)	Minor Stroke (%)	Major Stroke %	All Stroke (%)	Death (%)	MACE (%)
Wholey	90	2000	M	8612	2.3	2.5	1.32	—	—	6.12
Shawl	112	2000	U	170	—	—	—	2.9	0	2.9‡
Roubin	86	2001	U	528	—	4.8	1	—	1.6	7.4
Spence	92	2001	U	—	—	—	—	—	—	9.9
Brooks	93	2001	U	53	1.9	—	—	—	0	1.9
Dietz	107	2001	P	43	—	—	—	—	—	5
Reimers	110	2001	P	86	—	1.2	—	—	—	2.3
Henry	104	2002	M	315	1.3	1.3	1.6	4.2	0.3	4.5
Schluter	108	2002	P	93	2.1	—	—	3.1	—	5.2
Al-Mubarak	109	2002	P	162	—	1	—	—	1	2
Mean†										**4.72**
Range										**1.9–9.9%**

MACE = major adverse cardiac event; TIA = transient ischemic attack.

*A recent published series of carotid artery interventions. Of note is that the mean MACE rate is <5%, ranging from 1.9% to 9.9%. Major stroke appears rare in the series in which embolic protection is used.

†Mean of all studies, not weighted by patient numbers.

‡Excludes death.

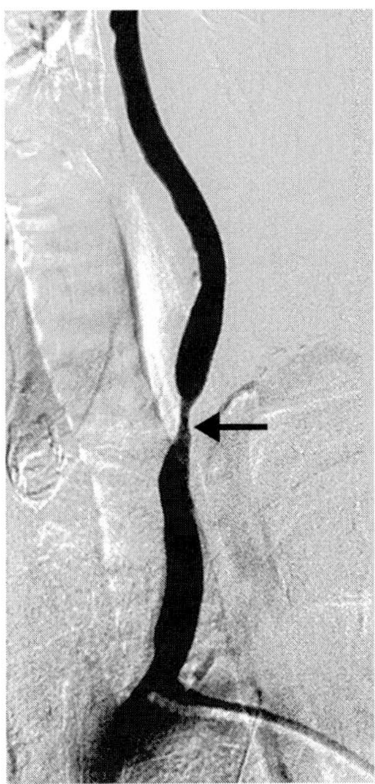
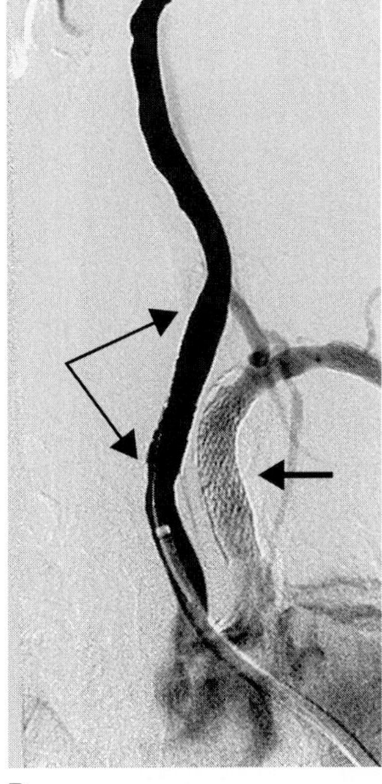

A B

FIGURE 55–23 **A**, A selective digital subtraction angiogram of the left common carotid. This reveals a severe stenosis of the intrathoracic portion of the left common carotid, which was treated with a single-balloon expandable stent. The stented segment is between the two long arrows. Wide patency was restored. The large horizontal arrow in **B** shows the previously stented left subclavian. The patient's arm claudication and transient ischemic attacks were successfully treated by this procedure.

symptomatic embolization. However, the reduction in risk is likely influenced by the overall risk of the patients being studied. Elderly patients, for example, have an excess risk of distal embolization, whereas those who are younger are at lesser risk. Thus the immediate effectiveness of carotid stenting with embolic protection depends on the risk profile of the patients for whom it is employed. The risk of adverse outcomes of carotid stenting in the current literature is from 2 to 10 percent, and future stent systems and embolic protection devices should be expected to perform within that range as we work to improve the results of carotid revascularization. At present, the global experience with carotid stenting, both with and without distal protection, suggests clinical equivalence to carotid endarterectomy as neurovascular interventions to prevent stroke in the several years after the procedure.[111] The very long-term effects on prevention of stroke and death and the more subtle influences on cognitive function will require further investigation. However, the clinical practice of carotid intervention will likely advance in light of the accumulating experience in support of its safety and efficacy (Figs. 55–17 through 55–23).

Interventions for Venous Disease

For Extremity Venous Thrombosis

Unlike atherosclerotic arterial obstructive disease, the major presenting obstructive element in venous obstruction is thrombus. Thus, dissolution or removal of the offending thrombus is the most evident goal of interventions for extremity venous thrombosis. Yet underlying the thrombus is almost always a predisposing factor such as a hypercoagulable state, external obstruction, venous stricture, scarring, or an indwelling foreign body. As a result, the treatment of venous thrombosis comprises not only the removal of thrombus but also attempt to correct the underlying predisposition(s). For most patients, anticoagulation and/or thrombolytic therapy are the mainstays of therapy (see Chap. 66). Both systemic and catheter-directed thrombolysis have achieved some success. Mechanical thrombectomy, balloon venoplasty, and stenting all have been reported, yet compelling data supporting the use of catheter-directed therapy are limited.

Despite the reports of experience, the data do not support the *routine* use of catheter-directed thrombolysis in the treatment of lower extremity deep venous thrombosis. Because of the suggestion of a reduction in the incidence of postthrombotic syndrome with lysis compared to anticoagulation alone and because of the suggestion of reduced major bleeding, catheter-directed therapy seems reasonable to apply in patients at higher risk for the complications of systemic lysis and in those who have a large thrombus burden and/or a high risk of developing a postthrombotic syndrome. In addition, more interventional concepts are emerging. There are reports of experience with rheolytic thrombectomy[113] or mechanical clot disruption. Additional experience with stents suggests that in cases where there is residual venous obstruction from scarring or external compression, relief of that obstruction with self-expanding stents may be important to maintain venous patency and prevent recurrent thrombosis. This is particularly true when the initial insult, such as an indwelling port infusion catheter, has been removed. Balloon venoplasty is also increasingly used to provide temporary relief of venous obstruction to facilitate the placement of transvenous pacing and/or defibrillator leads. Thus, the selective application of catheter-based thrombolysis, thrombectomy, and venous stenting is appropriate based on individual circumstances.

For Central Venous Obstruction

Superior vena cava (SVC) syndrome results from the obstruction of the blood flow in the SVC (see Chap. 83). Pathological processes from contiguous structures can compress or directly invade the SVC. Superimposed venous thrombosis may contribute to the development of SVC syndrome in up to 50 percent of patients. Historically, SVC syndrome was most frequently caused by direct tumor compression. Currently, the use of indwelling venous access catheters, coupled with the improved survival of chemotherapy patients, is increasing the occurrence of "nonmalignant" SVC syndrome in patients whose cancers have been cured. The explosion in the use of the automatic implantable cardioverter-defibrillator and sophisticated multilead pacing systems has increased the incidence and recognition of this condition.

Percutaneous Treatment

Medical and surgical options for the treatment of SVC obstruction are well established (see Chap. 83). Since the initial description of successful percutaneous treatment of SVC syndrome in the adult, the use of angioplasty alone was limited by a high rate of initial failure and early restenosis due to recoil of highly elastic SVC wall. Stenting therefore quickly gained acceptance in this area of vascular intervention after it was first reported in the 1980s.

Stenting in malignant SVC syndrome rapidly improves symptoms. Patients report almost immediate resolution of headache, visual disturbances, and other central nervous system symptoms. Dyspnea, cough, and edema usually resolve within 1 to 3 days but occasionally may take up to 1 week. Stenting results in complete resolution of symptoms in 68 to 100 percent of patients with malignant SVC syndrome.[114] In the largest series, 76 consecutive patients with

SVC syndrome were treated with stents and compared with historical control of patients treated with radiation. Procedural success was 100 percent, and all patients had improvement of symptoms within 48 hours. Ninety percent of patients treated with a stent had no symptoms of SVC obstruction at the time of death compared with 12 percent of patients treated with radiation.[114] The recurrence rate of SVC syndrome after percutaneous intervention has been reported between 0 and 45 percent.[115,116] Many pathophysiological mechanisms of recurrence have been documented. Acute stent thrombosis can develop shortly after stent placement in patients on insufficient anticoagulation or antiplatelet therapy; tumor ingrowth through stent struts had been reported; and intimal hyperplasia or fibrous scarring can occur. Stent length oversizing may prevent recurrence of SVC syndrome due to stent edge overgrowth; however, it may increase risk of SVC stent thrombosis or restenosis. The highest recurrence rate of SVC syndrome has been reported in patients with total SVC occlusion, but repeated procedures in these patients are uniformly successful, with additional stent placement, angioplasty, and/or thrombolysis used alone or in combination

Superior Vena Cava Syndrome of Nonmalignant Etiology

In the developed world, SVC syndrome of nonmalignant etiology ("benign" SVC syndrome) is usually iatrogenic in origin and it is most frequently due to indwelling intravenous catheters and pacing leads. Complications of pacemaker lead placement such as venous thrombosis or stenosis occurs in up to 30 percent of patients. Only a few patients, however, become symptomatic, but the presence of multiple leads, retention of severed lead(s), and previous lead infection may increase the risk of SVC syndrome. The largest series of percutaneous therapy in benign SVC syndrome included 16 patients. Ten patients had SVC syndrome due to the indwelling catheter, 2 due to the pacemaker wire, and 1 each due to goiter, fibrous mediastinitis, heart-lung transplant, and spontaneous thrombosis. The patency rate in 13 patients who were followed for a mean of 17 months was 85 percent.[117] Similar results can be expected in patients with SVC syndrome associated with central venous infusion catheters. Ideally, interventional treatment should also include removal of the inciting lead or catheter.

SVC stenting is a low-risk procedure that provides fast and durable symptomatic relief in malignant caval obstruction, often in combination with chemotherapy or radiation to provide patients with benefit of life prolongation together with effective symptom control. In patients with SVC syndrome of nonmalignant etiology, based on mid-term follow-up results, stenting is the treatment of choice. Surgical therapy should be reserved for patients with benign SVC syndrome refractory to percutaneous therapy. Only a few patients are likely to become truly refractory because most patients with recurrent SVC syndrome can be treated successfully with repeated percutaneous intervention (Figs. 55–24 through 55–26).

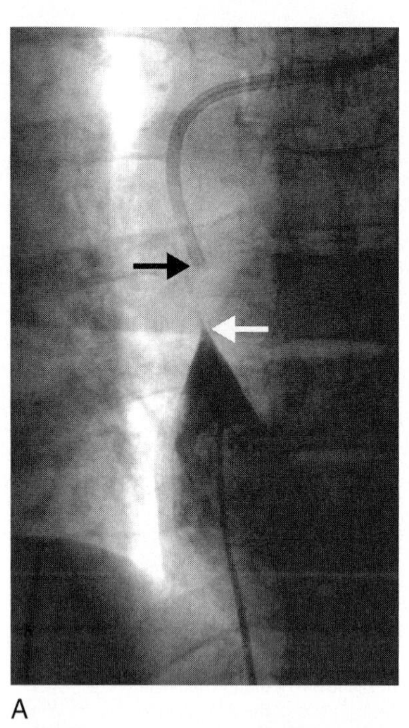

A

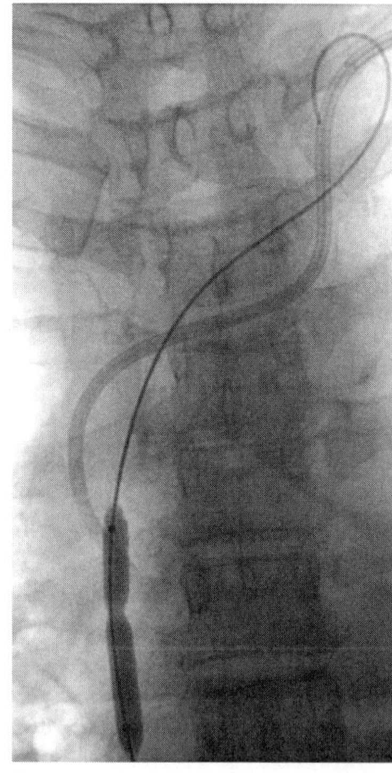

B

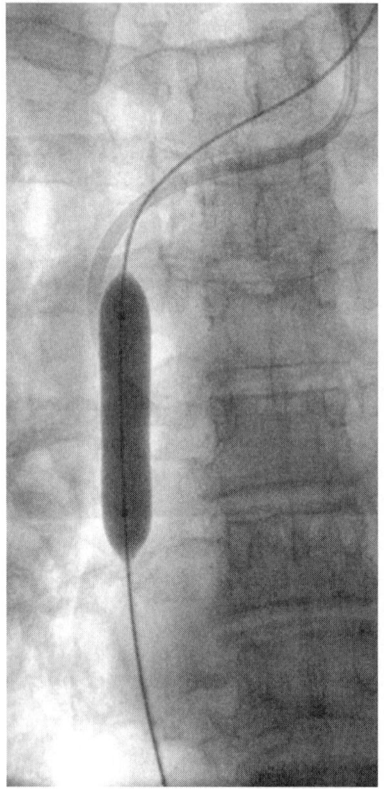

C

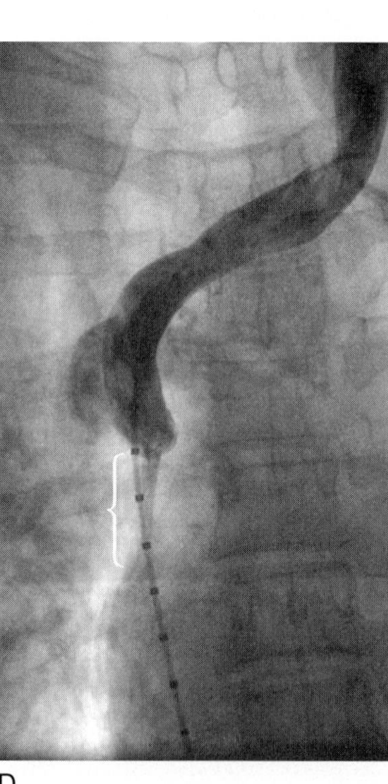

D

FIGURE 55–24 Superior vena cava (SVC) syndrome and its treatment in a middle-aged woman with an indwelling port access catheter who had received chemotherapy for breast cancer. Though these catheters allow potentially sclerosing agents to be given into the central circulation, the position of the catheter tip along the wall of the SVC likely induces an inflammatory reaction and fibrous scarring. In this case the catheter tip, identified by the black arrow in **A,** ends at an area of complete occlusion of the superior vena cava. Injection of contrast agent into the right atrial–SVC junction shows the SVC to be completely occluded at that point (horizontal white arrow, **A**). This total occlusion was pierced with a hydrophilic guidewire, and a series of balloon dilations were performed. **B** shows the first dilation with a small balloon indicating an indentation in that balloon. This was likely the nidus of the complete occlusion. Successive dilations with up to a 10-mm balloon **(C)** were successful, but given the fibrous and elastic nature of these venous obstructions, there is severe elastic recoil. **D** demonstrates a venogram performed with a catheter across the total occlusion and shows the reestablishment of a small channel (bracket) between the SVC and the right atrium. Stenting is required to ensure wide and durable patency; however, the indwelling port access catheter may be entrapped by the placement of a stent.

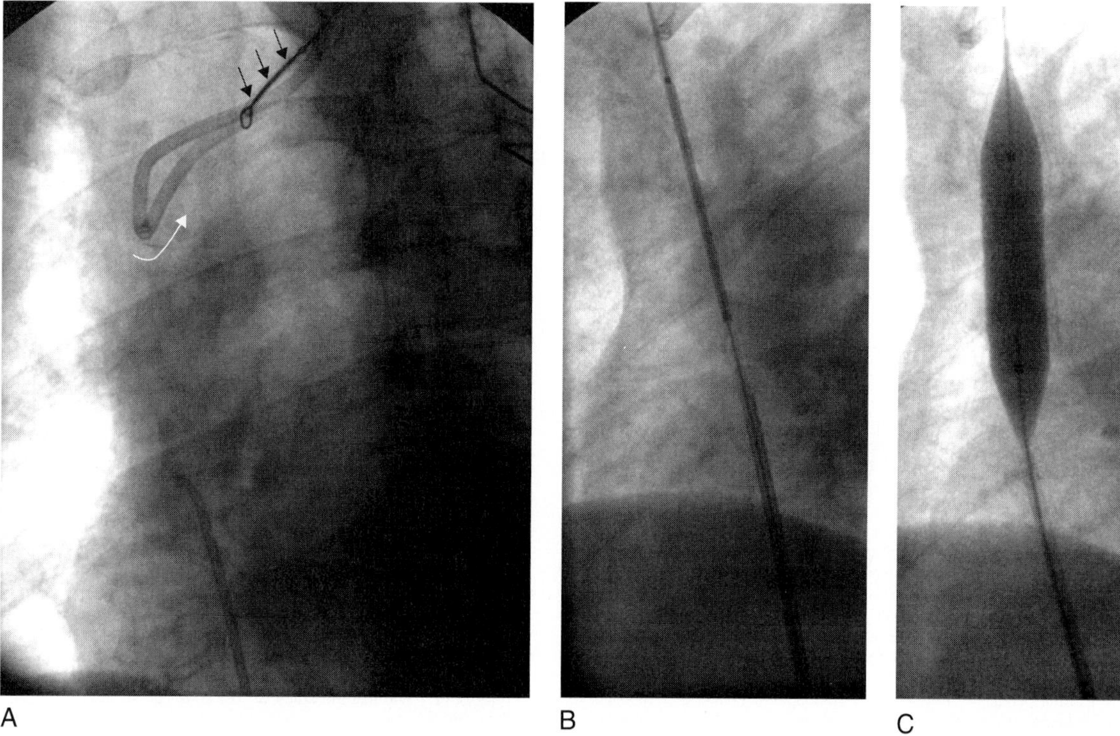

FIGURE 55–25 An option for stenting in the presence of an indwelling port access catheter. When indwelling pacing or implantable cardioverter-defibrillator leads traverse the cavoatrial junction, these leads must be removed before being trapped between stents and the vascular wall. In this case, the end of the port access catheter was snared from the left brachial approach (**A,** three short arrows) and the tip withdrawn by doubling it over in the superior vena cava (white arrow). From below, a large self-expanding nitinol stent **(B)** was positioned in the area of residual stenosis, deployed, and postdilated with a 14-mm balloon **(C)**.

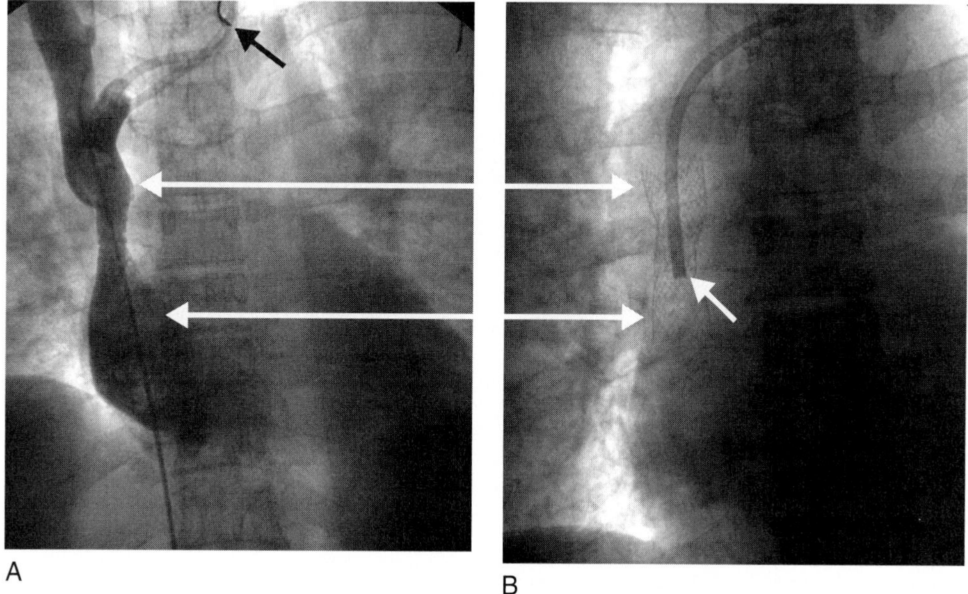

FIGURE 55–26 Final result from stent placement. In **A,** an injection into the superior vena cava shows free flow of contrast agent into the right atrium via the stented segment (delineated by the uppermost and lowermost horizontal arrows). The end of the indwelling port access catheter can still be seen trapped by the snare in **A** (black arrow). The tip of this catheter was repositioned within the stented segment (**B,** white arrow). The patient's symptoms were completely resolved, and the use of the port access catheter was preserved.

Conclusion

Though the specific tools and techniques vary, the theme of endovascular intervention is similar across many vascular territories. In general, vascular stenting has become the mainstay of percutaneous revascularization for relief of symptoms. The challenge for the future will be to continue to improve the long-term durability of endovascular therapy and to explore its potential for preventing the complications of progressive vascular disease.

1. U.S. Department of Health and Human Services: Chartbook on Cardiovascular, Lung and Blood Diseases: Morbidity and Mortality. Bethesda, National Heart, Blood, and Lung Institute, National Institutes of Health, 1994.

Aortoiliac Obstruction

2. Bosch JL, Hunink MG: Meta-analysis of the results of percutaneous transluminal angioplasty and stent placement for aortoiliac occlusive disease. Radiology 204:87-96, 1997.
3. Wilson SE, Wolf GL, Cross AP: Percutaneous transluminal angioplasty versus operation for peripheral arteriosclerosis: Report of a prospective randomized trial in a selected group of patients. J Vasc Surg 9:1-9, 1989.
4. Tetteroo E, van der Graaf Y, Bosch JL, et al: Randomised /comparison of primary stent placement versus primary angioplasty followed by selective stent placement in patients with iliac artery occlusive disease. Dutch Iliac Stent Trial study group. Lancet 351:1153-1159, 1998.
5. Cho L, Roffi M, Mukherjee D, et al: Superficial femoral artery occlusion: Nitinol stents achieve better flow and reduce the need for medications than balloon angioplasty alone. J Invasive Cardiol 15:198-200, 2003.
6. Henry M, Amor M, Ethevenot G, et al: Percutaneous endoluminal treatment of iliac occlusions: Long-term follow-up of 105 patients. J Endovasc Surg 5:228-235, 1998.
7. Haulon S, Mounier-Vehier C, Gaxotte V, et al: Percutaneous reconstruction of the aortoiliac bifurcation with the "kissing stents" technique: Long-term follow-up in 106 patients. J Endovasc Ther 9:363-368, 2002.
8. Siskin GP, Englander M, Roddy S, et al: Results of iliac artery stent placement in patients younger than 50 years of age. J Vasc Interv Radiol 13:785-790, 2002.
9. Mohamed F, Sarkar B, Timmons G, et al: Outcome of "kissing stents" for aortoiliac atherosclerotic disease, including the effect on the non-diseased contralateral iliac limb. Cardiovasc Intervent Radiol 25:472-475, 2002.
10. Reekers JA, Vorwerk D, Rousseau H, et al: Results of a European multicentre iliac stent trial with a flexible balloon expandable stent. Eur J Vasc Endovasc Surg 24:511-515, 2002.
11. Funovics MA, Lackner B, Cejna M, et al: Predictors of long-term results after treatment of iliac artery obliteration by transluminal angioplasty and stent deployment. Cardiovasc Intervent Radiol 25:397-402, 2002.
12. Saha S, Gibson M, Torrie EP, et al: Stenting for localised arterial stenoses in the aorto-iliac segment. Eur J Vasc Endovasc Surg 22:37-40, 2001.
13. Timaran CH, Stevens SL, Freeman MB, Goldman MH: External iliac and common iliac artery angioplasty and stenting in men and women. J Vasc Surg 34:440-446, 2001.
14. Powell RJ, Fillinger M, Bettmann M, et al: The durability of endovascular treatment of multisegment iliac occlusive disease. J Vasc Surg 31:1178-1184, 2000.
15. Murphy TP, Khwaja AA, Webb MS: Aortoiliac stent placement in patients treated for intermittent claudication. J Vasc Interv Radiol 9:421-428, 1998.
16. Reyes R, Maynar M, Lopera J, et al: Treatment of chronic iliac artery occlusions with guide wire recanalization and primary stent placement. J Vasc Interv Radiol 8:1049-1055, 1997.
17. Dyet JF, Gaines PA, Nicholson AA, et al: Treatment of chronic iliac artery occlusions by means of percutaneous endovascular stent placement. J Vasc Interv Radiol 8:349-353, 1997.

Femoropopliteal Obstruction

18. Duda SH, Pusich B, Richter G, et al: Sirolimus-eluting stents for the treatment of obstructive superficial femoral artery disease: Six-month results. Circulation 106:1505-1509, 2002.
19. Scheinert D, Biamino G: Femoropopliteal occlusions: Experience with peripheral excimer laser angioplasty. Curr Interv Cardiol Rep 3:130-138, 2001.
20. Scheinert D, Laird JR Jr., Schroder M, et al: Excimer laser-assisted recanalization of long, chronic superficial femoral artery occlusions. J Endovasc Ther 8:156-166, 2001.
21. Gray BH, Sullivan TM, Childs MB, et al: High incidence of restenosis/reocclusion of stents in the percutaneous treatment of long-segment superficial femoral artery disease after suboptimal angioplasty. J Vasc Surg 25:74-83, 1997.
22. Martin DR, Katz SG, Kohl RD, Qian D: Percutaneous transluminal angioplasty of infrainguinal vessels. Ann Vasc Surg 13:184-187, 1999.
23. Kessel DO, Wijesinghe LD, Robertson I, et al: Endovascular stent-grafts for superficial femoral artery disease: Results of 1-year follow-up. J Vasc Interv Radiol 10:289-296, 1999.
24. Conroy RM, Gordon IL, Tobis JM, et al: Angioplasty and stent placement in chronic occlusion of the superficial femoral artery: Technique and results. J Vasc Interv Radiol 11:1009-1020, 2000.
25. Cheng SW, Ting AC, Wong J: Endovascular stenting of superficial femoral artery stenosis and occlusions: Results and risk factor analysis. Cardiovasc Surg 9:133-140, 2001.
26. Gordon IL, Conroy RM, Arefi M, et al: Three-year outcome of endovascular treatment of superficial femoral artery occlusion. Arch Surg 136:221-228, 2001.
27. Lofberg AM, Karacagil S, Ljungman C, et al: Percutaneous transluminal angioplasty of the femoropopliteal arteries in limbs with chronic critical lower limb ischemia. J Vasc Surg 34:114-121, 2001.
28. Bauermeister G: Endovascular stent-grafting in the treatment of superficial femoral artery occlusive disease. J Endovasc Ther 8:315-320, 2001.
29. Steinkamp HJ, Wissgott C, Rademaker J, et al: Short (1–10 cm) superficial femoral artery occlusions: Results of treatment with excimer laser angioplasty. Cardiovasc Intervent Radiol 25:388-396, 2002.
30. Gray BH, Laird JR, Ansel GM, Shuck JW: Complex endovascular treatment for critical limb ischemia in poor surgical candidates: A pilot study. J Endovasc Ther 9:599-604, 2002.
31. Jamsen TS, Manninen HI, Jaakkola PA, Matsi PJ: Long-term outcome of patients with claudication after balloon angioplasty of the femoropopliteal arteries. Radiology 225:345-352, 2002.
32. Becquemin JP, Favre JP, Marzelle J, et al: Systematic versus selective stent placement after superficial femoral artery balloon angioplasty: A multicenter prospective randomized study. J Vasc Surg 37: 487-494, 2003.
33. Jahnke T, Andresen R, Muller-Hulsbeck S, et al: Hemobahn stent-grafts for treatment of femoropopliteal arterial obstructions: Midterm results of a prospective trial. J Vasc Interv Radiol 14:41-51, 2003.

Infrapopliteal Obstruction

34. Sivananthan UM, Browne TF, Thorley PJ, Rees MR: Percutaneous transluminal angioplasty of the tibial arteries. Br J Surg 81:1282-1285, 1994.
35. Varty K, Bolia A, Naylor AR, et al: Infrapopliteal percutaneous transluminal angioplasty: A safe and successful procedure. Eur J Vasc Endovasc Surg 9:341-345, 1995.
36. Dorros G, Jaff MR, Murphy KJ, Mathiak L: The acute outcome of tibioperoneal vessel angioplasty in 417 cases with claudication and critical limb ischemia. Cathet Cardiovasc Diagn 45:251-256, 1998.
37. Desgranges P, Kobeiter K, d'Audiffret A, et al: Acute occlusion of popliteal and/or tibial arteries: The value of percutaneous treatment. Eur J Vasc Endovasc Surg 20:138-145, 2000.
38. Soder HK, Manninen HI, Jaakkola P, et al: Prospective trial of infrapopliteal artery balloon angioplasty for critical limb ischemia: Angiographic and clinical results. J Vasc Interv Radiol 11:1021-1031, 2000.
39. Dorros G, Jaff MR, Dorros AM, et al: Tibioperoneal (outflow lesion) angioplasty can be used as primary treatment in 235 patients with critical limb ischemia: Five-year follow-up. Circulation 104:2057-2062, 2001.
40. Tsetis DK, Michalis LK, Rees MR, et al: Vibrational angioplasty in the treatment of chronic infrapopliteal arterial occlusions: Preliminary experience. J Endovasc Ther 9:889-895, 2002.
41. Hanna GP, Fujise K, Kjellgren O, et al: Infrapopliteal transcatheter interventions for limb salvage in diabetic patients: Importance of aggressive interventional approach and role of transcutaneous oximetry. J Am Coll Cardiol 30:664-669, 1997.
42. Faglia E, Mantero M, Caminiti M, et al: Extensive use of peripheral angioplasty, particularly infrapopliteal, in the treatment of ischaemic diabetic foot ulcers: Clinical results of a multicentric study of 221 consecutive diabetic subjects. J Intern Med 252:225-232, 2002.
43. Bakal CW, Cynamon J, Sprayregen S: Infrapopliteal percutaneous transluminal angioplasty: What we know. Radiology 200:36-43, 1996.

Renal Artery Obstructive Disease

44. Lenz T, Kia T, Rupprecht G, et al: Captopril test: Time over? J Hum Hypertens 13:431-435, 1999.
45. Olin JW, Novick AC: Renovascular disease. *In* Young JR, et al (eds): Peripheral Vascular Diseases. St. Louis, CV Mosby, 1996, pp 321-342.
46. Leung DA, Hoffman U, Pfammatter T, et al: Magnetic resonance angiography versus duplex sonography for diagnosis renovascular disease. Hypertension 33:726-731, 1999.
47. Johnson PT, Halpern EJ, Kuszyk BS, et al: Renal artery stenosis: CT angiography—comparison of real-time volume-rendering and maximal intensity projection algorithms. Radiology 211:337-343, 1999.
48. van Jaarsveld BC, Pieterman H, vanDijk LC, et al: Inter-observer variability in the angiographic assessment of renal artery stenosis. J Hypertens 17:1731-1736, 1999.
49. Schreij G, deHaan MW, Oei TK, et al: Interpretation of renal angiography by radiologists. J Hypertens 17:1737-1741, 1999.
50. Conlon PJ, Little MA, Pieper K, Mark DB: Severity of renal vascular disease predicts mortality in patients undergoing coronary angiography. Kidney Int 60:1490-1497, 2001.
51. Caps MT, Erissinotto C, Zierler RE, et al: Prospective study of atherosclerotic disease progression in the renal artery. Circulation 98:2866-2872, 1998.
52. Weibull H, Bergquist P, Bergentz SE, et al: Percutaneous transluminal renal angioplasty versus surgical reconstruction of atherosclerotic renal artery stenosis: A prospective randomized study. J Vasc Surg 18:841-852, 1993.
53. Eisenhauer AC: Atherosclerotic renovascular disease: Diagnosis and treatment. Curr Opin Nephrol Hypertens 9:659-668, 2000.
54. Safian RD, Textor SC: Renal artery stenosis. N Engl J Med 344:431-442, 2001.
55. van Jaarsveld BC, Krijnen P, Pieterman H, et al: The effect of balloon angioplasty on hypertension in atherosclerotic renal artery stenosis. N Engl J Med 342:1007-1014, 2000.
56. Harden PN, Macleod MJ, Rodger RSC, et al: Effect of renal artery stenting on progression of renovascular renal failure. Lancet 349:1133-1136, 1997.
57. Watson PS, Hadjipetrou P, Cox SV, et al: Effect of renal artery stenting on renal function and size in patients with atherosclerotic renovascular disease. Circulation 102:1671-1677, 2000.
58. Rundback JH, Murphy TP, Cooper C, Weintraub JL: Chronic renal ischemia: Pathophysiologic mechanisms of cardiovascular and renal disease. J Vasc Interv Radiol 13:1085-1092, 2002.
59. Rundback, JH, Sacks D, Kent KC, et al: Guidelines for the reporting of renal artery revascularization in clinical trials. J Vasc Interv Radiol 13:959-974, 2002.

Mesenteric Ischemia

60. Matsumoto AH, Tegtmeyer CJ, Fitzcharles EK, et al: Percutaneous transluminal angioplasty of visceral arterial stenoses: Results and long-term clinical follow-up. J Vasc Interv Radiol 6:165-174, 1995.
61. Chow LC, Chan FP, Li KC: A comprehensive approach to MR imaging of mesenteric ischemia. Abdom Imaging 27:507-516, 2002.
62. Mateo RB, O'Hara PJ, Hertzer NR, et al: Elective surgical treatment of symptomatic chronic mesenteric occlusive disease: Early results and late outcomes. J Vasc Surg 29:821-831, 1999; discussion 832.
63. Kihara TK, Blebea J, Anderson KM, et al: Risk factors and outcomes following revascularization for chronic mesenteric ischemia. Ann Vasc Surg 13:37-44, 1999.

64. Park WM, Cherry KJ Jr., Chua HK, et al: Current results of open revascularization for chronic mesenteric ischemia: A standard for comparison. J Vasc Surg 35:853-859, 2002.
65. Leke MA, Hood DB, Rowe VL, et al: Technical consideration in the management of chronic mesenteric ischemia. Am Surg 68:1088-1092, 2002.
66. Park WM, Gloviczki P, Cherry KJ Jr., et al: Contemporary management of acute mesenteric ischemia: Factors associated with survival. J Vasc Surg 35:445-452, 2002.
67. Maspes F, Mazzetti di Pietralata G, Gandini R, et al: Percutaneous transluminal angioplasty in the treatment of chronic mesenteric ischemia: Results and 3 years of follow-up in 23 patients. Abdom Imaging 23:358-363, 1998.
68. Cognet F, Bensalem D, Dranssart M, et al: Chronic mesenteric ischemia: Imaging and percutaneous treatment. Radiographics 22:863-879, 2002; discussion 879-880.
69. Matsumoto AH, Angle JF, Spinosa DJ, et al: Percutaneous transluminal angioplasty and stenting in the treatment of chronic mesenteric ischemia: Results and long-term followup. J Am Coll Surg 194(1 Suppl): S22-S31, 2002.

Brachiocephalic and Subclavian Obstructive Disease

70. Eisenhauer AC: Subclavian and innominate revascularization: Surgical therapy versus catheter-based intervention. Curr Interv Cardiol Rep 2:101-110, 2000.
71. Al-Mubarak N, Liu MW, Dean LS, et al: Immediate and late outcomes of subclavian artery stenting. Cathet Cardiovasc Intervent 46:169-172, 1999.
72. Henry M, Amor M, Henry I, et al: Percutaneous transluminal angioplasty of the subclavian arteries. J Endovasc Surg 6:33-41, 1999.
73. Hadjipetrou P, Cox S, Piemonte T, Eisenhauer A: Percutaneous revascularization of atherosclerotic obstruction of aortic arch vessels. J Am Coll Cardiol 33:1238-1245, 1999.
74. White CJ: The times they are a-changin'. J Am Coll Cardiol 33:1246-1247, 1999.
75. Hollier LH: Combining endovascular and surgical techniques: The best of both worlds. J Endovasc Surg 5:333-334, 1998.
76. Phipp LH, Scott DJ, Kessel D, Robertson I: Subclavian stents and stent-grafts: Cause for concern? J Endovasc Surg 6: 223-226, 1999.
77. Motarjeme A: Percutaneous transluminal angioplasty of supra-aortic vessels. J Endovasc Surg 3:171-181, 1996.
78. Schillinger M, Haumer M, Schillinger S, et al: Risk stratification for subclavian artery angioplasty: Is there an increased rate of restenosis after stent implantation? J Endovasc Ther 8:550-557, 2001.

Carotid and Distal Embolic Protection

79. The Dutch TIA Trial Study Group: A comparison of two doses of aspirin (30 mg vs. 283 mg a day) in patients after a transient ischemic attack or minor stroke. N Engl J Med 325:1261-1266, 1991.
80. Randomised trial of endarterectomy for recently symptomatic carotid stenosis: Final results of the MRC European Carotid Surgery Trial (ECST). Lancet 351:1379-1387, 1998.
81. NASCET Collaborators: Beneficial effect of carotid endarterectomy in symptomatic patients with high-grade carotid stenosis. N Engl J Med 325:445-453, 1991.
82. Endarterectomy for asymptomatic carotid artery stenosis. Executive Committee for the Asymptomatic Carotid Atherosclerosis Study. JAMA 273:1421-1428, 1995.
83. Barnett HJ, Taylor DW, Eliasziw M, et al: Benefit of carotid endarterectomy in patients with symptomatic moderate or severe stenosis. North American Symptomatic Carotid Endarterectomy Trial Collaborators. N Engl J Med 339:1415-1425, 1998.
84. Ferguson GG, Eliasziw M, Barr HW, et al: The North American Symptomatic Carotid Endarterectomy Trial : Surgical results in 1415 patients. Stroke 30:1751-1758, 1999.
85. Wennberg DE, Lucas FL, Birkmeyer JD, et al: Variation in carotid endarterectomy mortality in the Medicare Population: Trial hospitals, volume and patient characteristics. JAMA 279:1278-1281, 1998.
86. Roubin GS, Iyer SS, Vitek J: Carotid artery stenting: rationale, indications, technique. *In* Heuser R (ed): Peripheral Vascular Stenting for Cardiologists. New York, Martin Dunitz, 1999, pp 67-117.
87. Roubin GS, New G, Iyer SS, et al: Immediate and late clinical outcomes of carotid artery stenting in patients with symptomatic and asymptomatic carotid artery stenosis: A 5-year prospective analysis. Circulation 103:532-537, 2001.
88. Wholey MH, Wholey M, Bergeron P, et al: Current global status of carotid artery stent placement. Cathet Cardiovasc Diagn 44:1-6, 1998.
89. Wholey MH, Wholey MH, Eles G: Clinical experience in cervical carotid artery stent placement: Carotid and neurovascular intervention. 1:2-9, 1998.
90. Wholey MH, Wholey M, Mathias K, et al: Global experience in cervical carotid artery stent placement. Cathet Cardiovasc Interv 50:160-167, 2000.
91. Veith FJ, Amor M, Ohki T, et al: Current status of carotid bifurcation angioplasty and stenting based on a consensus of opinion leaders. J Vasc Surg 33:S111, 2001.
92. Spence D, Eliasziw M: Endarterectomy or angioplasty for treatment of carotid stenosis? Lancet 357:1722-1723, 2001.
93. Brooks WH, McClure RR, Jones MR, et al: Carotid angioplasty and stenting versus carotid endarterectomy: Randomized trial in a community hospital. J Am Coll Cardiol 38:1589-1595, 2001.
94. Qureshi AI, Luft AR, Janardhan V, et al: Identification of patients at risk for periprocedural neurological deficits associated with carotid angioplasty and stenting. Stroke 31:376-382, 2000.
95. Mathur A, Roubin GS, Iyer SS, et al: Predictors of stroke complicating carotid artery stenting. Circulation 97: 1239-1245, 1998.
96. Manninen HI, Rasanen H, Vanninen RL, et al: Human carotid arteries: Correlation of intravascular US with angiographic and histopathologic findings. Radiology 206:65-74, 1998.
97. Manninen HI, Rasanen HT, Vanninen RL, et al: Stent placement versus percutaneous transluminal angioplasty of human carotid arteries in cadavers in situ: Distal embolization and findings at intravascular US, MR imaging, and histopathologic analysis. Radiology 212:483-492, 1999.
98. Coggia M, Goeau-Brissonniere O, Duval JL, et al: Embolic risk of the different stages of carotid bifurcation balloon angioplasty: An experimental study. J Vasc Surg 31:550-557, 2000.
99. Ohki T, Marin ML, Lyon RT, et al: Ex vivo human carotid artery bifurcation stenting: Correlation of lesion characteristics with embolic potential. J Vasc Surg 27:463-471, 1998.
100. Rapp JH, Pan XM, Sharp FR, et al: Atheroemboli to the brain: size threshold for causing acute neuronal cell death. J Vasc Surg 32:68-76, 2000.
101. Markus H: Monitoring embolism in real time. Circulation 102:826-828, 2000.
102. Ohki T, Veith FJ: Carotid stenting with and without protection devices: Should protection be used in all patients? Semin Vasc Surg 13:144-152, 2000.
103. Macdonald S, Gaines PA: Current concepts of mechanical cerebral protection during precutaneous carotid intervention. Vasc Med 8:25-32, 2003.
104. Henry M, Amor M, Henry I, et al: Carotid stenting with cerebral protection: First clinical experience using the PercuSurge GuardWire system. J Endovasc Surg 6:321-331, 1999.
105. Kowntor S, et al: Relationship between the structure of the plaque and the importance of embolization during carotid angioplasty. J Am Coll Cardiol 35(Suppl A):67, 2000.
106. Henry M, Henry I, Klonaris C, et al: Benefits of cerebral protection during carotid stenting with the PercuSurge GuardWire system: Midterm results. J Endovasc Ther 9:1-13, 2002.
107. Dietz A, Berkefeld J, Theron JG, et al: Endovascular treatment of symptomatic carotid stenosis using stent placement: Long-term follow-up of patients with a balanced surgical risk/benefit ratio. Stroke 32:1855-1859, 2001.
108. Schluter M, Tubler T, Mathey DG, Schofer J: Feasibility and efficacy of balloon-based neuroprotection during carotid artery stenting in a single-center setting. J Am Coll Cardiol 40:890-895, 2002.
109. Al-Mubarak N, Colombo A, Gaines PA, et al: Multicenter evaluation of carotid artery stenting with a filter protection system. J Am Coll Cardiol 39:841-846, 2002.
110. Reimers B, Corvaja N, Moshiri S, et al: Cerebral protection with filter devices during carotid artery stenting. Circulation 104:12-15, 2001.
111. Wholey MH, Al-Mubarak N, Wholey M: Fifth-year update of carotid artery stenting global registry: What have we learned? J Am Coll Cardiol 30H, 2002.
112. Shawl F, Kadro W, Domanski MJ, et al: Safety and efficacy of elective carotid artery stenting in high-risk patients. J Am Coll Cardiol 35:1721-1728, 2000.

Peripheral Venous Disease and Superior Vena Cava Syndrome

113. Kasirajan K, Gray B, Ouriel K: Percutaneous AngioJet thrombectomy in the management of extensive deep venous thrombosis. J Vasc Interv Radiol 12:179-185, 2001.
114. Nicholson AA, Ettles DF, Arnold A, et al: Treatment of malignant superior vena cava obstruction: Metal stents or radiation therapy. J Vasc Interv Radiol 8:781-788, 1997.
115. Crowe MT, Davies CH, Gaines PA: Percutaneous management of superior vena cava occlusions. Cardiovasc Intervent Radiol 18:367-372, 1995.
116. Gross CM, Kramer J, Waigand J, et al: Stent implantation in patients with superior vena cava syndrome. AJR Am J Roentgenol 169:429-432, 1997.
117. Kee ST, Kinoshita L, Razavi MK, et al: Superior vena cava syndrome: Treatment with catheter-directed thrombolysis and endovascular stent placement. Radiology 206:187-193, 1998.

PART VII

Diseases of the Heart, Pericardium, and Pulmonary Vasculature Bed

CHAPTER 56

Congenital Heart Disease

Gary D. Webb • Jeffrey F. Smallhorn • Judith Therrien • Andrew N. Redington

This chapter has been written for the practicing cardiologist and is compatible with the existing expert management recommendations[1-3] for the care of adult patients with congenital cardiac defects. These guidelines are available on the Internet at www.cachnet.org, at www.achd-library.com, and at www.isaccd.org. For the occasions when more detailed information is needed, the reader is referred to other sources.[4-9]

Congenital cardiovascular disease is defined as an abnormality in cardiocirculatory structure or function that is present at birth, even if it is discovered much later. Congenital cardiovascular malformations usually result from altered embryonic development of a normal structure or failure of such a structure to progress beyond an early stage of embryonic or fetal development. The aberrant patterns of flow created by an anatomical defect may, in turn, significantly influence the structural and functional development of the remainder of the circulation. For instance, the presence in utero of mitral atresia may prohibit normal development of the left ventricle, aortic valve, and ascending aorta. Similarly, constriction of the fetal ductus arteriosus may result in right ventricular dilation and tricuspid regurgitation in the fetus and newborn, or it may contribute importantly to the development of pulmonary arterial aneurysms in the presence of a ventricular septal defect (VSD) and absent pulmonary valve, or it may result in an alteration in the number and caliber of fetal and newborn pulmonary vascular resistance vessels.

Postnatal events can markedly influence the clinical presentation of a specific "isolated" malformation. Infants with Ebstein malformation of the tricuspid valve may improve dramatically as the magnitude of tricuspid regurgitation diminishes with the normal fall in pulmonary vascular resistance after birth; and infants with pulmonary atresia or severe stenosis may not become cyanotic until normal spontaneous closure of a patent ductus arteriosus (PDA) occurs. Ductal constriction many days after birth also may be a central factor in some infants in the development of coarctation of the aorta. Still later in life, patients with a VSD may experience spontaneous closure of the abnormal communication or may develop right ventricular outflow tract obstruction and/or aortic regurgitation or pulmonary vascular obstructive disease. These selected examples serve to emphasize that anatomical and physiological changes in the heart and circulation can continue indefinitely from prenatal life in association with any specific congenital cardiocirculatory lesion.

INCIDENCE. The true incidence of congenital cardiovascular malformations is difficult to determine accurately, partly because of difficulties in definition. About 0.8 percent of live births are complicated by a cardiovascular malformation. This figure does not take into account what may be the two most common cardiac anomalies: the congenital, functionally normal bicuspid aortic valve and prolapse of the mitral valve.

Specific defects can show a definite gender preponderance: PDA, Ebstein anomaly of the tricuspid valve, and atrial septal defect (ASD) are more common in females, whereas aortic valve stenosis, coarctation of the aorta, hypoplastic left heart, pulmonary and tricuspid atresia, and transposition of the great arteries (TGA) are more common in males.

Extracardiac anomalies occur in about 25 percent of infants with significant cardiac disease, and their presence may significantly increase mortality. The extracardiac anomalies are often multiple. One-third of infants with both cardiac and extracardiac anomalies have some established syndrome.

ADULT PATIENT. Thanks to the great successes of pediatric cardiac care, the overall number of adult patients with congenital heart disease (CHD) is now greater than the number of pediatric cases. In 2000, there were about 485,000 American adults with moderately complex to very complex CHD. There were another 300,000 patients with simple forms of CHD, for a total population of 785,000 adult CHD patients in the United States. The 485,000 moderately to very complex patients are at significant risk of premature mortality, reoperation, or future complications of their conditions and their treatments. Many patients, especially those with moderately to very complex conditions, should see a specialist. At present, there are not enough such practitioners or facilities to always make this possible. Adult patients should have been taught in adolescence about their condition, their future outlook, and the possibility of further surgery and complications if appropriate, and they also should have been advised about their responsibilities in ensuring self-care and professional surveillance. Copies of operative reports should accompany patients being transferred for adult care and other key documents from the pediatric file.

Table 56–1 shows a listing of the types of patients who should be considered "simple" and suitable for community care. Tables 56–2 and 56–3 show the diagnoses for "moderately complex" and "very complex" patients. The moderately and very complex patients should be monitored throughout their life.

CHD in the adult is not simply a continuation of the childhood experience. The patterns of many lesions change in adult life. Arrhythmias are more frequent and of a different character. Cardiac chambers often enlarge, and ventricles tend to develop systolic dysfunction. Bioprosthetic valves, prone to early failure in childhood, last longer when implanted at an older age. The comorbidities that tend to develop in adult life often become important factors needing attention. As a result, the needs of these adult CHD patients are often best met by a physician or a team familiar with both pediatric and adult cardiology issues. Congenital heart surgery and interventional catheterization procedures should be performed at centers with adequate surgical and institu-

TABLE 56–1 Types of Adult Patients with Simple Congenital Heart Disease*

Native disease Isolated congenital aortic valve disease Isolated congenital mitral valve disease (except parachute valve, cleft leaflet) Isolated patent foramen ovale or small atrial septal defect Isolated small ventricular septal defect (no associated lesions) Mild pulmonic stenosis
Repaired conditions Previously ligated or occluded ductus arteriosus Repaired secundum or sinus venosus atrial septal defect without residua Repaired ventricular septal defect without residua

From Webb G, Williams R, Alpert J, et al: 32nd Bethesda Conference: Care of the Adult with Congenital Heart Disease, October 2-3, 2000. J Am Coll Cardiol 37:1161-1198, 2001.

*These patients can usually be cared for in the general medical community.

TABLE 56–2 Types of Adult Patients with Congenital Heart Disease of Moderate Severity*

Aorto–left ventricular fistulas
Anomalous pulmonary venous drainage, partial or total
Atrioventricular septal defects (partial or complete)
Coarctation of the aorta
Ebstein anomaly
Infundibular right ventricular outflow obstruction of significance
Ostium primum atrial septal defect
Patent ductus arteriosus (not closed)
Pulmonary valve regurgitation (moderate to severe)
Pulmonic valve stenosis (moderate to severe)
Sinus of Valsalva fistula/aneurysm
Sinus venosus atrial septal defect
Subvalvular or supravalvular aortic stenosis (except HOCM)
Tetralogy of Fallot
Ventricular septal defect with Absent valve or valves Aortic regurgitation Coarctation of the aorta Mitral disease Right ventricular outflow tract obstruction Straddling tricuspid/mitral valve Subaortic stenosis

HOCM = hypertrophic obstructive cardiomyopathy.

From Webb G, Williams R, Alpert J, et al: 32nd Bethesda Conference: Care of the Adult with Congenital Heart Disease, October 2-3, 2000. J Am Coll Cardiol 37:1161-1198, 2001.

*These patients should be seen periodically at regional adult congenital heart disease centers.

TABLE 56–3 Types of Adult Patients with Congenital Heart Disease of Great Complexity*

Conduits, valved or nonvalved
Cyanotic congenital heart (all forms)
Double-outlet ventricle
Eisenmenger syndrome
Fontan procedure
Mitral atresia
Single ventricle (also called *double inlet* or *outlet*, *common* or *primitive*)
Pulmonary atresia (all forms)
Pulmonary vascular obstructive diseases
Transposition of the great arteries
Tricuspid atresia
Truncus arteriosus/hemitruncus
Other abnormalities of atrioventricular or ventriculoarterial connection not included above (i.e., crisscross heart, isomerism, heterotaxy syndromes, ventricular inversion)

From Webb G, Williams R, Alpert J, et al: 32nd Bethesda Conference: Care of the Adult with Congenital Heart Disease, October 2-3, 2000. J Am Coll Cardiol 37:1161-1198, 2001.

*These patients should be seen regularly at adult congenital heart disease centers.

tional volumes of congenital heart cases at any age. Echocardiographic studies, diagnostic heart catheterizations, electrophysiological studies, and magnetic resonance imaging (MRI) and other imaging of complex cases are best done where qualified staff have relevant training, experience, and equipment. Patient care ideally should be multidisciplinary. Special cardiology and echocardiography skills are essential, but individuals with other special training, experience, and interest should also be accessible. These include congenital heart surgeons and their teams, nurses, reproductive health staff, mental health professionals, medical imaging technicians, respiratory consultants, and others.

Etiology

Congenital cardiac malformations can occur with mendelian inheritance directly as a result of a genetic abnormality, be strongly associated with an underlying genetic disorder (e.g., trisomy), be related directly to the effect of an environmental toxin (e.g., alcohol), or result from an interaction between multifactorial genetic and environmental systems too complex to allow a single specification of cause (e.g., CHARGE syndrome [see Syndromes in Congenital Heart Disease]). The latter group is shrinking as new genetic research identifies new genetic abnormalities underlying many conditions.

GENETIC. A single gene mutation can be causative in the familial forms of ASD with prolonged atrioventricular (AV) conduction, mitral valve prolapse, VSD, congenital heart block, situs inversus, pulmonary hypertension, and the syndromes of Noonan, LEOPARD, Ellis-van Creveld, and Kartagener (see Syndromes in Congenital Heart Disease). The genes responsible for several defects have either been mapped (e.g., long-QT syndrome, Holt-Oram syndrome) or identified (e.g., Marfan syndrome, hypertrophic cardiomyopathy, supravalvular aortic stenosis). Contiguous gene defects on the long arm of chromosome 22 likely underlie the conotruncal malformations of DiGeorge and velocardiofacial syndromes. At present, fewer than 15 percent of all cardiac malformations can be accounted for by chromosomal aberrations or genetic mutations or transmission (see Chap. 69).

The finding that, with some exceptions, only one of a pair of monozygotic twins is affected by CHD indicates that most cardiovascular malformations are not inherited in a simple manner. However, this observation may have led, in the past, to an underestimation of genetic contribution, because most recent twin studies reveal more than double the incidence of heart defects in monozygotic twins but usually in only one of the pair. Family studies indicate a 2-fold to 10-fold increase in the incidence of CHD in siblings of affected patients or in the offspring of an affected parent. Malformations often are concordant or partially concordant within families. Routine fetal cardiac screening seems a worthwhile investigation in such circumstances.

ENVIRONMENTAL. Maternal rubella, ingestion of thalidomide and isotretinoin early during gestation, and chronic maternal alcohol abuse are environmental insults known to interfere with normal cardiogenesis in humans. Rubella syndrome consists of cataracts, deafness, microcephaly, and, either singly or in combination, PDA, pulmonary valve and/or arterial stenosis, and ASD. Thalidomide exposure is associated with major limb deformities and, occasionally, with cardiac malformations without a predilection for a specific lesion. Tricuspid valve anomalies are associated with ingestion of lithium during pregnancy. The fetal alcohol syndrome consists of microcephaly, micrognathia, microphthalmia, prenatal growth retardation, developmental delay, and cardiac defects (often defects of the ventricular septum) occur in about 45 percent of affected infants.

Prevention

Physicians who deal with pregnant women should be aware of known teratogens as well as drugs that may have a functional rather than a structural damaging influence on the fetal and newborn heart and circulation, and they should recognize that for many drugs, information about their teratogenic potential is inadequate. Similarly, appropriate radiological equipment and techniques for reducing gonadal and fetal radiation exposure should always be used to reduce the potential hazards of this likely cause of birth defects.

Detection of genetic abnormalities is becoming an increasing reality for many problems. Fetal cells are obtained from amniotic fluid or chorionic villus biopsy. Many fetuses in whom CHD is detected will undergo genetic testing, and fetal echo is frequently indicated when a chromosomal abnormality is diagnosed for other reasons. Many social, religious, and legal considerations influence whether termination of pregnancy is performed under these circumstances, but the improved outcomes for even the most complex CHDs frequently mandate against the cardiac condition being used as the sole reason. Immunization of children with rubella vaccine has been one of the most effective preventive strategies against fetal rubella syndrome and its associated congenital cardiac abnormalities.

Anatomy and Embryology

Embryology

NORMAL CARDIAC DEVELOPMENT. During the first month of gestation, the primitive, straight cardiac tube is formed, comprising the sinuatrium (most cephalad), the primitive ventricle, the bulbus cordis, and the truncus arteriosus (most caudad) in series. In the second month of gestation, this tube doubles over on itself to form two parallel pumping systems, each with two chambers and a great artery. The two atria develop from the sinuatrium, the AV canal is divided by the endocardial cushions into tricuspid and mitral orifices, and the right and left ventricles develop from the primitive ventricle and bulbus cordis. Differential growth of myocardial cells causes the straight cardiac tube to bear to the right, and the bulboventricular portion of the tube doubles over on itself, bringing the ventricles side by side. Migration of the AV canal to the right and of the ventricular septum to the left serves to align each ventricle with its appropriate AV valve. At the distal end of the cardiac tube, the bulbus cordis divides into a subaortic muscular conus and a subpulmonary muscular conus; the subpulmonary conus elongates and the subaortic conus resorbs, allowing the aorta to move posteriorly and connect with the left ventricle.

ABNORMAL DEVELOPMENT. A host of anomalies can result from defects in this basic developmental pattern. Double-inlet left ventricle is observed if the tricuspid orifice does not align over the right ventricle. The various types of persistent truncus arteriosus result from failure of the truncus to divide into main pulmonary artery and aorta. Double-outlet anomalies of the right ventricle are produced by failure of either the subpulmonary or subaortic conus to resorb, whereas resorption of the subpulmonary instead of the subaortic conus may lead to TGA.

ATRIA. The primitive sinuatrium is separated into right and left atria by the downgrowth from its roof of the septum primum toward the AV canal, thereby creating an inferior interatrial ostium primum opening. Numerous perforations form in the anterosuperior portion of the septum primum as the septum secundum begins to develop to the right of the former. The coalescence of these perforations forms the ostium secundum. The septum secundum completely separates the atrial chambers except for a central opening—the fossa ovalis—that is covered by tissue of the septum primum, forming the valve of the foramen ovale.

Fusion of the endocardial cushions anteriorly and posteriorly divides the AV canal into tricuspid and mitral inlets. The inferior portion of the atrial septum, the superior portion of the ventricular septum, and portions of the septal leaflets of both the tricuspid and mitral valves are formed from the endocardial cushions. The integrity of the atrial septum depends on growth of the septum primum and septum secundum and proper fusion of the endocardial cushions. ASDs and various degrees of AV defect are the result of developmental deficiencies of this process.

VENTRICLES. Partitioning of the ventricles occurs as cephalic growth of the main ventricular septum results in its fusion with the endocardial cushions and the infundibular or conus septum. Defects in the ventricular septum may occur owing to a deficiency of septal substance; malalignment of septal components in different planes preventing their fusion; or an overly long conus, keeping the septal components apart. Isolated defects probably result from the first mechanism, whereas the latter two appear to generate the VSDs in tetralogy of Fallot and transposition complexes.

PULMONARY VEINS. These structures arise from the primitive foregut and are drained early in embryogenesis by channels from the splanchnic plexus to the cardinal and umbilicovitelline veins. An outpouching from the posterior left atrium forms the common pulmonary vein, which communicates with the splanchnic plexus establishing pulmonary venous drainage to the left atrium. The umbilicovitelline and anterior cardinal vein communications atrophy as the common pulmonary vein is incorporated into the left atrium. Anomalous pulmonary venous connections to the umbilicovitelline (portal) venous system or to the cardinal system (superior vena cava) result from failure of the common pulmonary vein to develop or establish communications to the splanchnic plexus. Cor triatriatum results from a narrowing of the common pulmonary vein to left atrial junction.

GREAT ARTERIES. The truncus arteriosus is connected to the dorsal aorta in the embryo by six pairs of aortic arches. Partition of the truncus arteriosus into two great arteries is a result of the fusion of tissue arising from the back wall of the vessel and the truncus septum. Rotation of the truncus coils the aortopulmonary septum and creates the normal spiral relation between aorta and pulmonary artery. Semilunar valves and their related sinuses are created by absorption and hollowing out of tissue at the distal side of the truncus ridges. Aortopulmonary septal defect and persistent truncus arteriosus represent various degrees of partitioning failure.

Although the six aortic arches appear sequentially, portions of the arch system and dorsal aorta disappear at different times during embryogenesis. The first, second, and fifth sets of paired arches regress completely. The proximal portions of the sixth arches become the right and left pulmonary arteries, and the distal left sixth arch becomes the ductus arteriosus. The third aortic arch forms the connection between internal and external carotid arteries, and the left fourth arch becomes the arterial segment between left carotid and subclavian arteries. The proximal portion of the right subclavian artery forms from the right fourth arch. An abnormality in regression of the arch system in a number of sites can produce a wide variety of arch anomalies, whereas a failure of regression usually results in a double aortic arch malformation.

Normal Cardiac Anatomy

The key to understanding CHD is an appreciation of the segmental approach to the diagnosis of both simple and complex lesions.

CARDIAC SITUS. This refers to the status of the atrial appendages. The normal left atrial appendage is a finger-like structure with a narrow base and no guarding crista. On the other hand, the right atrial appendage is broad based and has a guarding crista and pectinate muscles. *Situs solitus* or *inversus* refers to hearts with both a morphological left and right atrium. *Situs ambiguous* refers to hearts with two morphological left or right atrial appendages. These are dealt with in the section on isomerism and have implications with regard to associated intracardiac and extracardiac abnormalities.

ATRIOVENTRICULAR CONNECTIONS. This refers to the connections between the atria and ventricles. The AV connections are said to be concordant if the morphological left atrium is connected to a morphological left ventricle via the mitral valve, with the morphological right atrium connecting to the morphological right ventricle via a tricuspid valve. They are said to be discordant in other circumstances, such as in congenitally corrected TGA (cc-TGA).

VENTRICULOARTERIAL CONNECTIONS. This refers to the connections between the semilunar valve and the ventricles. Ventriculoarterial concordance occurs when the morphological left ventricle is connected to the aorta, while the morphological right ventricle is connected to the pulmonary artery. Ventriculoarterial discordance is when the morphological left ventricle is connected to the pulmonary artery, with the aorta being connected to the morphological right ventricle. Double-outlet right ventricle is where more than 50 percent of both great arteries are connected to the morphological right ventricle. A single-outlet heart is where there is only one great artery that is connected to the heart.

ATRIA. The assignment of either a morphological left or right atrium is determined by the morphology of the atrial appendages and not by the status of the systemic or pulmonary venous drainage. Although the pulmonary veins usually drain to a morphological left atrium, and the systemic veins drain into a morphological right atrium, this is not always the case.

ATRIOVENTRICULAR VALVES. The morphological mitral valve is a bileaflet valve with the anterior leaflet in fibrous continuity with the noncoronary cusp of the aortic valve. The mitral valve leaflets are supported by two papillary muscle groups located in the anterolateral and posteromedial positions. Each papillary muscle supports the adjacent part of both valve leaflets, with considerable variation in the morphology of the papillary muscles.

The tricuspid valve is a trileaflet valve, although it can frequently be difficult to identify all three leaflets. With close inspection, the commissural chordae that arise from the papillary muscles may permit the identification of the three leaflets. The three leaflets occupy a septal anterior, superior, and inferior position. The commissures between the leaflets are the anterior septal, anterior inferior, and inferior. The papillary muscles supporting the valve leaflets arise mostly from the trabeculoseptomarginalis and its apical ramifications.

MORPHOLOGICAL RIGHT VENTRICLE. The morphological right ventricle is a triangular-shaped structure with an inlet, trabecular, and outlet component. The inlet component of the right ventricle has attachments from the septal leaflet of the tricuspid valve. Inferior to this is the moderator band, which arises at the base of the trabeculoseptomarginalis, with extensive trabeculations toward the apex of the right ventricle. The outlet component of the right ventricle consists of a fusion of three structures, that is, the infundibular septum separating the aortic from the pulmonary valve, the ventriculoinfundibular fold separating the tricuspid valve from the pulmonary valve, and finally the anterior and posterior limbs of the trabeculoseptomarginalis.

MORPHOLOGICAL LEFT VENTRICLE. The morphological left ventricle is an elliptical-shaped structure with a fine trabecular pattern, with absent septal attachments of the mitral valve in the normal heart. It consists of an inlet portion containing the mitral valve and a tension apparatus, with an apical trabecular zone that is characterized by fine trabeculations and an outlet zone that supports the aortic valve.

SEMILUNAR VALVES. The aortic valve is a trileaflet valve with the left and right cusps giving rise to the left and right coronary arteries, respectively, with the noncoronary cusp lacking a coronary artery connection. Of note, the noncoronary cusp is in fibrous continuity with the anterior leaflet of the mitral valve. The aortic valve has a semilunar attachment to the junction of the ventricular outlet and its great arteries. The aortic cusps have a main core of fibrous tissue with endocardial linings on each surface. The cusps are thickened at the midpoint to form a nodule. The characteristics of the pulmonary valve are similar to its aortic counterpart, noting the absence of the coronary ostia arising at the superior portion of the sinuses.

AORTIC ARCH AND PULMONARY ARTERIES. In the normal heart the aortic arch usually points to the left with the first branch, the innominate artery, giving rise to the right carotid and subclavian artery. In general, the left carotid and left subclavian arteries arise separately from the aortic arch. By definition the ascending aorta is proximal to the origin of the innominate artery, with the transverse aortic arch being from the innominate artery to the origin of the left subclavian artery. The aortic isthmus is the area between the left subclavian artery and a PDA or ligamentum arteriosum.

SYSTEMIC VENOUS CONNECTIONS. In the normal heart the left and right innominate veins form the superior vena cava, which connects to the roof of the right atrium. The inferior vena cava connects to the inferior portion of the morphological right atrium, with hepatic veins joining the inferior vena cava prior to its insertion into the atrium. The coronary veins drain into the flow of the coronary sinus, with the latter running in the posterior AV groove and terminating in the right atrium. The inferior vena cava is guarded by the eustachian valve, which may vary in size between different hearts.

PULMONARY VENOUS DRAINAGE IN THE NORMAL HEART. The pulmonary veins drain to the left-sided atrium. There are usually three pulmonary veins arising from the trilobed right lung and two pulmonary veins from the bilobed left lung. The pulmonary veins drain into the left atrium in superior and inferior locations. There is a short segment of extraparenchymal pulmonary vein prior to it disappearing into the adjacent hila of the lungs.

Fetal and Transitional Circulations

(Fig. 56–1)

CHD is being diagnosed with increasing frequency during fetal life. Our ability to modify the evolution of structural (by fetal intervention) and physiological (by drug therapy) heart disease is increasing. Knowledge of the changes in cardiocirculatory structure, function, and metabolism that occur during fetal development is more important today than at any time in the past.

FETAL CIRCULATORY PATHWAYS. Dynamic alterations occur in the circulation during the transition from fetal to neonatal life when the lungs take over the function of gas exchange from the placenta. The fetal circulation consists of parallel pulmonary and systemic pathways in contrast to the "in series" circuit of the normal postnatal circulation. Oxygenated blood returns from the placenta through the

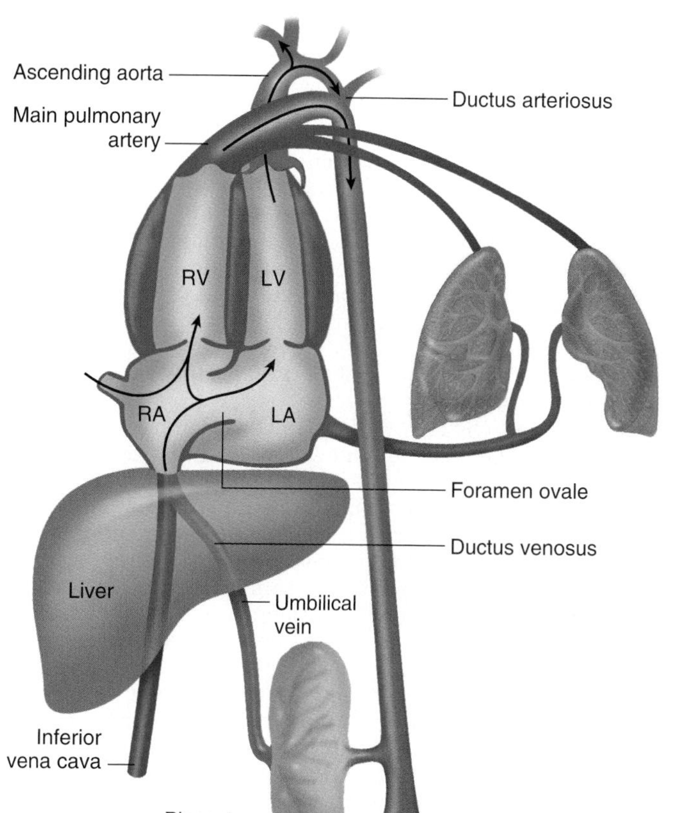

FIGURE 56–1 The fetal circulation, with arrows indicating the directions of flow. A fraction of umbilical venous blood enters the ductus venosus and bypasses the liver. This relatively highly oxygenated blood flows across the foramen ovale to the left side of the heart, preferentially perfusing the coronary arteries, head, and upper trunk. The output of the right ventricle flows preferentially across the ductus arteriosus and circulates to the placenta, as well as to the abdominal viscera and lower trunk. (Courtesy of Dr. David Teitel.)

umbilical vein and enters the portal venous system. A variable amount of this stream bypasses the hepatic microcirculation and enters the inferior vena cava by way of the ductus venosus. Inferior vena caval blood is from the ductus venosus, hepatic veins, and lower body venous drainage and is partly deflected across the foramen ovale into the left atrium. Almost all superior vena caval blood passes directly through the tricuspid valve, entering the right ventricle. Most of the blood that reaches the right ventricle bypasses the high-resistance, unexpanded lungs and passes through the ductus arteriosus into the descending aorta. The right ventricle contributes about 55 percent and the left 45 percent to the total fetal cardiac output. The major portion of blood ejected from the left ventricle supplies the brain and upper body, with lesser flow to the coronary arteries; the balance passes across the aortic isthmus to the descending aorta, where it joins with the large stream from the ductus arteriosus before flowing to the lower body and back to the placenta.

FETAL PULMONARY CIRCULATION. In fetal life, the alveoli are fluid filled, and the pulmonary arteries and arterioles have relatively thick walls and a small lumen, similar to arteries in the systemic circulation. The low pulmonary blood flow in the fetus (7 to 10 percent of the total cardiac output) is the result of high pulmonary vascular resistance. Fetal pulmonary vessels are highly reactive to changes in oxygen tension or in the pH of blood perfusing them as well as to a number of other physiological and pharmacological influences.

EFFECTS OF CARDIAC MALFORMATIONS ON THE FETUS. Although fetal somatic growth may be unimpaired, the hemodynamic effects of many cardiac malformations can alter the development and structure of the fetal heart and circulation. For example, while lesions associated with left-to-right shunts in postnatal life rarely influence fetal cardiac development directly, regurgitant AV valves can lead to chamber dilation, hydrops, and fetal death. Ventricular obstructive lesions (e.g., aortic valve stenosis) may variably lead to hypertrophy, dilation, and failure. The secondary effects of congenital lesions are also important. Reduced flow through the left heart can result in aortic hypoplasia and coarctation. Reduced antegrade pulmonary blood flow is associated with pulmonary artery hypoplasia. These effects rarely affect the fetal circulation overtly, however, and often only become exposed as problems after birth as the ductus arteriosus closes.

FUNCTION OF THE FETAL HEART. Compared with the adult heart, the fetal and newborn heart is unique with respect to its ultrastructural appearance, its mechanical and biochemical properties, and its autonomic innervation. During late fetal and early neonatal development there is maturation of the excitation-contraction coupling process and changes in the biochemical composition of the heart's energy-utilizing myofibrillar proteins and of adenosine triphosphate and creatine phosphate energy-producing proteins. Moreover, fetal and neonatal myocardial cells are small in diameter and reduced in density, so that the young heart contains relatively more noncontractile mass (primarily mitochondria, nuclei, and surface membranes) than later in postnatal life. As a result, force generation and the extent and velocity of shortening are decreased, and stiffness and water content of ventricular myocardium are increased in the fetal and early newborn periods. The fetal heart is surrounded by fluid-filled rather than air-filled lungs. As a result, the fetal and neonatal heart has limited ability to increase cardiac output in the presence of either a volume load or a lesion that increases resistance to emptying. Ultimately cardiac output is much more dependent on changes in heart rate, explaining why bradycardia is so poorly tolerated by the fetal circulation. Tachycardia can also rapidly lead to heart failure in the fetus, whether due to the hemodynamic issues discussed earlier or a manifestation of energy-substrate utilization.

CHANGES AT BIRTH. Inflation of the lungs at the first inspiration produces a marked reduction in pulmonary vascular resistance. The reduced extravascular pressure and increased alveolar oxygen content, as fluid is removed from the lungs and replaced by air, leads to pulmonary vasodilation and recruitment. As a result, pulmonary artery pressure falls, and pulmonary blood flow increases greatly, raising left atrial pressure and closing the flap valve of the foramen ovale. Conversely, systemic vascular resistance rises. This is related to loss of the low-resistance placental circulation and gradual closure of the ductus arteriosus. It is also related to a sudden increase in arterial blood oxygen tension, consequent to the lack of mixing of oxygenated and deoxygenated blood that characterizes the fetal milieu. In healthy, mature infants, the ductus arteriosus is profoundly constricted at 10 to 15 hours and is closed functionally by 72 hours, with total anatomical closure following within a few weeks by a process of thrombosis, intimal proliferation, and fibrosis. Preterm infants have a high incidence of persistent patency of the ductus arteriosus because of an immaturity of those mechanisms responsible for constriction.

The ductus venosus, ductus arteriosus, and foramen ovale remain potential channels for blood flow after birth. Thus, persistent patency of the ductus venosus is capitalized on during balloon atrial septostomy performed via the umbilical vein. Lesions producing right or left atrial volume or pressure overload can stretch the foramen ovale and render incompetent the flap valve mechanism for its closure. Anomalies that depend on patency of the ductus arteriosus for preserving pulmonary or systemic blood flow remain latent until the ductus arteriosus constricts. A common example is the rapid intensification of cyanosis observed in infants with tetralogy of Fallot when the magnitude of pulmonary hypoperfusion is unmasked by spontaneous closure of the ductus arteriosus. Moreover, increasing evidence shows that ductal constriction is a key factor in the postnatal development of coarctation of the aorta and is clearly the most important factor governing the presentation in babies with a duct-dependent systemic circulation. The management of these conditions is discussed in the appropriate sections.

NEONATE AND INFANT. Most management decisions in patients with significant CHD occur during the first few months of life. An increase in the prenatal diagnosis of major congenital heart defects has resulted in earlier admission and intervention in the neonate with CHD. These neonates are, in general, healthier than in the past owing to the administration of prostaglandins at the time of delivery, thus maintaining hemodynamic stability. With improved surgery and interventional catheterization techniques, many of these neonates undergo early intervention. There has been a trend toward complete repair in the neonate and young infant due to an improvement in myocardial preservation and surgical techniques. In most major cardiac centers, the surgical mortality for this age group is in the range of 2 to 4 percent, which is an improvement on the results of the past, where a palliative procedure often preceded a complete repair.

With increasing experience in this age group, the focus has now shifted from mortality to morbidity. Because the expectation is that most of these neonates and young infants will survive into their adult years, their neurodevelopmental outcome has become as important as the results of the cardiac intervention. Ongoing research in this age group will provide increasing data as to the benefit of early intervention in neonates and infants with CHD.

CHILD AND ADOLESCENT. The rapid somatic growth rates of infancy and adolescence are periods of rapid hemodynamic change. Stenotic lesions that may be relatively slowly progressive throughout early childhood need more frequent surveillance during adolescence. Childhood and adolescence is a time to begin educating the patient, not just the parents, about their heart disease, and the responsibilities that go with it. Issues such as the need for compliance with medications, avoidance of smoking and illicit drug use, and pregnancy and contraception counseling are by no means exclusively issues of the adult with CHD, and increasingly require discussion in the pediatric cardiac clinic.

Indeed, the early teenage years should be regarded as part of the transition process prior to transfer to adult follow-up. The whole area of the follow-up of adults with newly discovered or previously treated CHD is a burgeoning new subspecialty that will require careful planning to ensure adequate resources for the increasing number of adult "graduates" of pediatric programs. A coordinated approach with specialists in an affiliated adult congenital clinic is clearly desirable.

ADULT. Patients and often family members should understand their cardiac condition[10] both in terms of what has been done so far and what could happen in the future. This is important for a young patient graduating into the adult world. Patients need information and should become partners in their own care.

Potential long-term complications in adults with CHD (such as arrhythmias, ventricular failure, conduit obstruction and endocarditis) should be explained to patients who are at relatively high risk. The possible need for future therapy—medical (antiarrhythmics, anticoagulation, heart failure therapy), catheter based (valve dilation, stents, arrhythmia ablation), or surgical (redo surgery, transplantation)—should be discussed if the patient may require them in the short or intermediate future. Day-to-day issues of concern for these young adults need to be addressed, such as exercise prescriptions,[11,12] driving restrictions, and traveling limitations. Many young people with CHD need advice regarding career choices, entering the work force, insurability, and life expectancy.

Many will want to start a family, and reproductive issues will need to be addressed. Discussion of appropriate contraception methods for any given patient should be offered. Counseling prior to conception as to the risk to the mother and the fetus for any given pregnancy should be done by specialized physicians. They will take into account the maternal cardiac anatomy, maternal functional status, maternal life expectancy, risk of CHD transmission to the offspring, and risk of premature birth. High-risk patients (e.g., Marfan with aortic root dilation, severe pulmonary hypertension, New York Heart Association [NYHA] Class III or IV, and severe aortic stenosis) must be advised against pregnancy. Intermediate-risk patients (e.g., cyanotic, mechanical valve and other warfarin [Coumadin]-requiring patients, left ventricular outflow tract obstruction, moderate-to-severe left ventricular dysfunction) need to know that pregnancy, although possible, may be complicated and that they will require careful follow-up.[13,14]

Last but not least, comorbidities such as obesity, smoking, high blood pressure, diabetes, and high cholesterol level add new levels of complexity to these adults as they age and must be part of the mandate of the patient's cardiologist.

Pathological Consequences of Congenital Cardiac Lesions

Congestive Heart Failure

Although the basic mechanisms of cardiac failure are similar for all ages, the common causes, time of onset, and often the approach to treatment vary with age (see Chaps. 20 to 25). The development of fetal echocardiography has allowed the diagnosis of intrauterine cardiac failure. The cardinal findings of *fetal heart failure* are scalp edema, ascites, pericardial effusion, and decreased fetal movements. In *preterm infants*, especially of less than 1500 gm birth weight, persistent patency of the ductus arteriosus is the most common cause of cardiac decompensation, and other forms of structural heart disease are rare. In *full-term newborns*, the earliest important causes of heart failure are the hypoplastic left heart and aortic coarctation syndromes, sustained tachyarrhythmia, cerebral or hepatic arteriovenous fistula, and myocarditis. Among the lesions commonly producing heart failure *beyond age 1 to 2 weeks*, when diminished pulmonary vascular resistance allows substantial left-to-right shunting, are VSDs and AV septal defects, TGA, truncus arteriosus, and total anomalous pulmonary venous connection. *Infants younger than 1 year* who have cardiac malformations account for 80 to 90 percent of pediatric patients who develop congestive failure. In *older children*, heart failure often is due to acquired disease or is a complication of open-heart surgical procedures. In the acquired category are rheumatic and endomyocardial diseases, infective endocarditis, hematological and nutritional disorders, and severe cardiac arrhythmias.

The distinction between left and right heart failure is less obvious in infants than in the older children or adults. Conversely, augmented filling or elevated pressure of the right ventricle in infants reduces left ventricular compliance disproportionately when compared with older children or adults and gives rise to signs of both systemic and pulmonary venous congestion.

Care of infants with heart failure must include careful consideration of the underlying structural or functional disturbance. The general aims of treatment are to achieve an increase in cardiac performance, augment peripheral perfusion, and decrease pulmonary and systemic venous congestion. In many conditions, medical management cannot control the effects of the abnormal loads imposed by a host of congenital cardiac lesions. Under these circumstances, cardiac diagnosis and interventional catheter or operative intervention may be urgently required.

Congestive heart failure is not common in adult congenital heart practice, although prevention of myocardial dysfunction is a common concern. The adult patient with CHD develops heart failure in the presence of a substrate (e.g., myocardial dysfunction, valvular regurgitation) and a precipitant (e.g., sustained arrhythmia, pregnancy, hyperthyroidism). Patients prone to congestive failure include those with long-standing volume loads (e.g., valvular regurgitation and left-to-right shunts), those with a primary depression of myocardial function (e.g., systemic right ventricles, ventricles damaged during surgery or because of late treatment of ventricular overload). Treatment depends on a clear understanding of the elements contributing to decompensation and addressing each of the treatable components. The greatest success is achieved when the main elements can be eliminated. When this is not possible, standard palliative adult heart failure regimens are applied and may include angiotensin-converting enzyme (ACE) inhibitors,[15,16] angiotensin receptor blockers, beta blockers,[17] diuretics, resynchronization pacing,[18] transplantation,[19,20] and other novel therapies.

Cyanosis

DEFINITION. *Central cyanosis* refers to arterial oxygen desaturation resulting from the shunting or mixing of systemic venous blood into the arterial circulation. The magnitude of shunting/mixing and the amount of pulmonary blood flow determine the severity of desaturation.

MORPHOLOGY. Cardiac defects that result in central cyanosis can be divided into two categories: (1) those with increased pulmonary blood flow or (2) those with decreased pulmonary blood flow (Table 56–4).[21]

PATHOPHYSIOLOGY. Hypoxemia increases renal production of erythropoietin, which in turn stimulates bone marrow production of circulating red blood cells, enhancing oxygen-carrying capacity. Secondary erythrocytosis should be present in all cyanotic patients since it is a physiological response to tissue hypoxia. The improved tissue oxygenation that results from this adaptation may be sufficient to reach a new equilibrium at a higher hematocrit. However, adaptive failure can occur if the increased whole blood viscosity rises so much that it impairs oxygen delivery.

TABLE 56–4 Cardiac Defects Causing Central Cyanosis

Transposition of the great arteries	Ebstein's anomaly
Tetralogy of Fallot	Eisenmenger physiology
Tricuspid atresia	Critical pulmonary stenosis or atresia
Truncus arteriosus	Functionally single ventricle
Total anomalous pulmonary venous return	

Note 5 Ts and 2 Es.

CLINICAL FEATURES

Hyperviscosity Syndrome. Erythrocytosis, by virtue of increasing whole blood viscosity, may cause hyperviscosity symptoms, including headaches, faintness, dizziness, fatigue, altered mentation, visual disturbances, paresthesias, tinnitus and myalgias. Iron deficiency, a common finding in cyanotic adult patients if repeated phlebotomies or excessive bleeding occurs, may cause hyperviscosity symptoms at hematocrit levels well below 65 percent. The patient usually experiences the same hyperviscosity symptoms each time (e.g., headache, visual disturbances, fatigue), and they must be relieved by phlebotomy to qualify as hyperviscosity symptoms.

Hematological. Hemostatic abnormalities have been documented in cyanotic patients with erythrocytosis and can occur in up to 20 percent of patients. A bleeding tendency can be mild and superficial, leading to easy bruising, skin petechiae, and mucosal bleeding, or it can be moderate or life-threatening with hemoptysis or intracranial, gastrointestinal, or postoperative bleeding. An elevated prothrombin and partial thromboplastin time; decreased levels of factors V, VII, VIII, and IX; qualitative and quantitative platelet disorders; and increased fibrinolysis all have been implicated.[22]

Central Nervous System. Neurological complications including cerebral hemorrhage can occur secondary to hemostatic defects and can be seen in patients taking anticoagulants. Patients with right-to-left shunts may be at risk for paradoxical cerebral emboli, especially if they are iron deficient. A brain abscess should be suspected in a cyanotic patient with a new or different headache or new neurological symptoms. Air filters should be used in peripheral/central venous lines in cyanotic patients to avoid paradoxical emboli through a right-to-left shunt.

Renal. Renal dysfunction can manifest itself as proteinuria, hyperuricemia, or renal failure. Pathological studies at the level of the glomeruli show evidence of vascular abnormalities as well as increased cellularity and fibrosis.[23] Hyperuricemia is common and is thought to be due mainly to the decreased reabsorption of uric acid rather than to overproduction with erythrocytosis. Urate nephropathy, uric acid nephrolithiasis, and gouty arthritis may occur.

Arthritic. Rheumatological complications include gout and especially hypertrophic osteoarthropathy, which is thought to be responsible for the arthralgias and bone pain affecting up to one-third of patients. In patients with right-to-left shunting, megakaryocytes released from the bone marrow can bypass the lung. The entrapment of megakaryocytes in the systemic arterioles and capillaries induces the release of platelet-derived growth factor, promoting local cell proliferation. New osseous formation with periostitis ensues and gives rise to arthralgia and bony pain.

INTERVENTIONAL OPTIONS AND OUTCOMES

Physiological Repair. Physiological repair results in total or near-total anatomical and physiological separation of the pulmonary and systemic circulations in complex cyanotic lesions that leads to relief of cyanosis. Such procedures should be performed whenever feasible.

Palliative Surgical Intervention. Palliative surgical interventions can be performed in patients with cyanotic lesions to increase pulmonary blood flow while allowing cyanosis to persist. Palliative surgical shunts are summarized in Table 56–5. Blalock-Taussig, central, and Glenn (also called *cavopulmonary*) shunts are still in use today. Blalock-Taussig shunts seldom caused pulmonary hypertension and were less prone to causing pulmonary artery distortion. Glenn shunts have the advantage of increasing pulmonary flow without imposing a volume load on the systemic ventricle. Glenn shunts require low pulmonary artery pressures to work, and they are associated with the development over time of pulmonary arteriovenous fistulas, which can worsen cyanosis.

TABLE 56–5 Palliative Systemic-to-Pulmonary Shunts

Arterial
Blalock-Taussig shunt (subclavian artery to PA)
Classic—end-to-side, no or reduced ipsilateral arm pulses
Current—side-to-side tubular grafts, preserved arm pulses
Central shunt (side-to-side tubular graft, aorta to PA)
Potts shunt (descending aorta to LPA)
Waterston shunt (ascending aorta to RPA)
Venous
Glenn shunt (SVC to ipsilateral PA without cardiac or other PA connection)
Bidirectional cavopulmonary (Glenn) shunt (end-to-side SVC to LPA and RPA shunt)

PA = pulmonary artery; LPA = left PA; RPA = right PA; SVC = superior vena cava.

Transplantation (see Chap. 26). Transplantation of heart, one or both lungs with surgical cardiac repair, and heart-lung transplantation have been performed in cyanotic patients with or without palliation who were no longer candidates for other forms of intervention. Pulmonary vascular obstructive disease precludes isolated heart transplantation. An increasing number of CHD patients with previous palliation and ventricular failure are successfully undergoing cardiac transplantation.[24] Timing of transplantation in these patients remains difficult.

OTHER MANAGEMENT

Phlebotomy. The goal of phlebotomy is symptom control. When patients have troubling symptoms of hyperviscosity, are iron replete, and are not dehydrated, removal of 250 to 500 ml of blood over 30 to 45 minutes should be performed with concomitant quantitative volume replacement. The procedure may be repeated every 24 hours until symptomatic improvement occurs or the hemoglobin level has fallen too far.[25] Phlebotomy is not indicated for asymptomatic patients. The only indication for prophylactic phlebotomy is in the preoperative patient when the hematocrit is higher than 65 percent to reduce the chances of perioperative bleeding.

Iron Replacement. If iron deficiency anemia is found or anticipated, iron supplements should be prescribed. Cyanotic patients should be helped to avoid iron deficiency, which can cause functional deterioration and is associated with an increased risk of stroke.

Bleeding Diathesis. Platelet transfusions, fresh frozen plasma, vitamin K, cryoprecipitate, and desmopressin can be used to treat severe bleeding. Given the inherent tendency to bleed, aspirin, heparin, and warfarin should be avoided unless the risks of treatment are outweighed by the risks of nontreatment. Likewise, nonsteroidal antiinflammatory drugs should be avoided to prevent bleeding.

Gouty Arthritis. Symptomatic hyperuricemia and gouty arthritis can be treated as necessary with colchicine, probenecid, antiinflammatory drugs, or allopurinol.

REPRODUCTIVE ISSUES. Pregnancy in cyanotic CHD (excluding Eisenmenger syndrome) results in a 32 percent incidence of maternal cardiovascular complications and a 37 percent incidence of fetal prematurity. Pregnant women with a resting oxygen saturation greater than 85 percent fare better than women with an oxygen saturation less than 85 percent.[13]

FOLLOW-UP ISSUES. All cyanotic patients should be followed by a CHD cardiologist, and particular attention should be paid to the underlying heart condition; symptoms of hyperviscosity; systemic complications of cyanosis; change in exercise tolerance; change in saturation levels; and prophylaxis against endocarditis, influenza, and pneumococcal infections. In stable cyanotic patients, yearly follow-up is recommended and should include annual flu shots, periodic pneumococcal vaccination, yearly blood work (complete blood count, ferritin, clotting profile, renal function, uric acid), and regular echo Doppler studies.

Pulmonary Hypertension

Pulmonary hypertension is a common accompaniment of many congenital cardiac lesions, and the status of the pulmonary vascular bed is often the principal determinant of the clinical manifestations, the course, and whether corrective treatment is feasible (see Chap. 67). Increases in pulmonary arterial pressure result from elevations of pulmonary blood flow and/or resistance, the latter sometimes caused by an increase in vascular tone but usually the result of underdevelopment and/or obstructive/obliterative structural changes within the pulmonary vascular bed. Although pulmonary hypertension usually affects the entire pulmonary vascular bed, it may occur focally. For example, unilateral pulmonary hypertension may occur in an overshunted lung (the other lung perhaps protected and fed by a cavopulmonary Glenn shunt), or in lung segments supplied by aortopulmonary collateral flow.

Pulmonary vascular resistance normally falls rapidly immediately after birth, owing to the onset of ventilation and subsequent release of hypoxic pulmonary vasoconstriction. Subsequently, the medial smooth muscle of pulmonary arterial resistance vessels thins gradually. This latter process often is delayed by several months in infants with large aortopulmonary or ventricular communications, at which time levels of pulmonary vascular resistance are still somewhat elevated. In patients with high pulmonary arterial pressures from birth, failure of normal growth of the pulmonary circulation may occur, and anatomical changes in the pulmonary vessels in the form of proliferation of intimal cells and intimal and medial thickening often progress, so that in an older child or adult vascular resistance ultimately may become relatively fixed by obliterative changes in the pulmonary vascular bed. The causes of pulmonary vascular obstructive disease remain unknown, although increased pulmonary arterial blood pressure, elevated pulmonary venous pressure, erythrocytosis, systemic hypoxia, acidemia, and the nature of the bronchial circulation all have been implicated. Quite likely, injury to pulmonary vascular endothelial cells initiates a cascade of events that involve the release or activation of factors that alter the extracellular matrix, induce hypertrophy, cause proliferation of vascular smooth muscle cells, and promote connective tissue protein synthesis. Considered together, these may permanently alter vessel structure and function.

MECHANISMS OF DEVELOPMENT. Intimal damage appears to be related to shear stresses because endothelial cell damage occurs at high shear rates. A reduction in pulmonary arteriolar lumen size due to either thickened medial muscle or vasoconstriction increases the velocity of flow. Shear stress also increases as blood viscosity rises; therefore, infants with hypoxemia and high hematocrit levels as well as increased pulmonary blood flow are at increased risk of developing pulmonary vascular disease. In patients with left-to-right shunts, pulmonary arterial hypertension, if not present in infancy or childhood, may never occur or may not develop until the third or fourth decade or later. Once developed, intimal proliferative changes with hyalinization and fibrosis are not reversible by repair of the underlying cardiac defect. In severe pulmonary vascular obstructive disease, arteriovenous malformations may develop and predispose to massive hemoptysis.

Most vexing is the variability among patients with the same or similar cardiac lesions in both the time of appearance and the rate of progression of their pulmonary vascular obstructive process. Although genetic influences may be operative (an example is the apparent acceleration of pulmonary vascular disease in patients with CHD and trisomy 21), evidence is now accumulating for important prenatal and postnatal modifiers of the pulmonary vascular bed that appear, at least in part, to be lesion dependent. Thus, a quantitative variability exists in the pulmonary vascular bed related to the number, not just the size and wall structure, of arterial vessels within the pulmonary circulation.

Modeling of the blood vessels occurs proximal to and within terminal bronchioles (preacinar and intraacinar vessels, respectively) continuously from before birth. The intraacinar vessels, in particular, increase in size and number from late fetal life throughout childhood, with minimal muscularization of their walls. The ensuing increase in the cross-sectional area of the pulmonary arterial circulation allows the cardiac output to rise substantially without an increase in pulmonary arterial pressure. If, however, the presence of a cardiac lesion interferes with the normal growth and multiplication of these peripheral arteries, the resulting elevation of pulmonary vascular resistance may first be related to failure of the intraacinar pulmonary circulation to develop fully, and then secondarily to the morphological changes of obliterative vascular disease—medial thickening, intimal proliferation, hyalinization and fibrosis, angiomatoid and plexiform lesions, and ultimately, arterial necrosis.

Eisenmenger Syndrome

DEFINITION. *Eisenmenger syndrome*, a term coined by Paul Wood, is defined as pulmonary vascular obstructive disease that develops as a consequence of a large preexisting left-to-right shunt such that pulmonary artery pressures approach systemic levels and the direction of the flow becomes bidirectional or right-to-left. Congenital heart defects that can result in Eisenmenger syndrome include "simple" defects such as ASD, VSD, and PDA as well as more "complex" defects such as AV septal defect, truncus arteriosus, aortopulmonary window, and univentricular heart. The high pulmonary vascular resistance is usually established in infancy (by age 2 years, except in ASD) and is present sometimes from birth.

NATURAL HISTORY OF THE UNOPERATED PATIENT. Patients with defects that allow free communication between the pulmonary and systemic circuits at the aortic or ventricular levels usually have a fairly healthy childhood and gradually become overtly cyanotic during their second or third decade. Exercise intolerance (dyspnea and fatigue) is proportional to the degree of hypoxemia or cyanosis. In the absence of complications, these patients generally have an excellent to good functional capacity up to their third decade[26,27] and thereafter usually experience a slowly progressive decline in their physical abilities. Most patients survive to adulthood,[27-29] with a reported 77 percent and 42 percent survival rate at 15 and 25 years of age, respectively.[27]

Congestive heart failure in patients with Eisenmenger syndrome usually occurs after 40 years of age.[26] The most common modes of death are sudden death (~30 percent), congestive heart failure (~25 percent), and hemoptysis (~15 percent). Pregnancy, perioperative mortality after noncardiac surgery, and infectious causes (brain abscesses and endocarditis) account for most of the remainder.[26,27,29]

CLINICAL MANIFESTATIONS. Patients can present with the following complications: those related to their cyanotic state; palpitations in nearly half the patients (atrial fibrillation/flutter in 35 percent, ventricular tachycardia in up to 10 percent); hemoptysis in about 20 percent; pulmonary thromboembolism, angina, syncope, and endocarditis in about 10 percent each; and congestive heart failure.[26] Hemoptysis is usually due to bleeding bronchial vessels or pulmonary infarction. Physical examination reveals central cyanosis and clubbing of the nail beds. Patients with Eisenmenger PDA can have pink nail beds on the right (> left) hand and cyanosis and clubbing of both feet, so-called differential cyanosis. This occurs because venous blood shunts through the ductus and enters the aorta distal to the subclavian arteries. The jugular venous pressure in patients with Eisenmenger syndrome can be normal or elevated, especially with prominent v waves when tricuspid regurgitation is present. Signs of pulmonary hypertension—a right ventricular heave, palpable and loud P_2, and a right-sided S_4—are typically present. In many patients, a pulmonary ejection click and a soft and scratchy systolic ejection murmur, attributable to dilation of the pulmonary trunk, and a high-pitched decrescendo diastolic murmur of pulmonary regurgitation (Graham Steell) are audible. Peripheral edema is absent until right-sided heart failure ensues.

LABORATORY INVESTIGATIONS

Electrocardiography (ECG). Peaked P waves consistent with right atrial overload and evidence of right ventricular hypertrophy with right axis deviation are the rule. Atrial arrhythmias can be present.

Chest Radiography. Dilated central pulmonary arteries with rapid tapering of the peripheral pulmonary vasculature are the radiographic hallmarks of Eisenmenger syndrome. Pulmonary artery calcification may be seen and is diagnostic of long-standing pulmonary hypertension. Eisenmenger syndrome due to VSD or PDA usually has a normal or slightly increased cardiothoracic ratio. Eisenmenger syndrome due to an ASD typically has a large cardiothoracic ratio due to right atrial and ventricular dilation, along with an inconspicuous aorta. Calcification of the duct may be seen in Eisenmenger PDA.

Echocardiography. The intracardiac defect should be seen readily along with bidirectional shunting. A pulmonary hypertensive PDA is not easily seen. Evidence of pulmonary hypertension is found. Assessment of pulmonary right ventricular function adds prognostic value.

Cardiac Catheterization. Cardiac catheterization not only provides direct measurement of the pulmonary artery pressure, documenting the existence of severe pulmonary hypertension, but also can allow assessment of reactivity of the pulmonary vasculature. Administration of pulmonary arterial vasodilators (O_2, nitric oxide, prostaglandin I_2 [epoprostenol]) can discriminate between patients in whom surgical repair is contraindicated and those with reversible pulmonary hypertension who may benefit from surgical repair. Radiographic contrast material may cause hypotension and worsening cyanosis and should be used cautiously.

Open-Lung Biopsy. Open-lung biopsy should be considered only when the reversibility of the pulmonary hypertension is uncertain from the hemodynamic data. An expert opinion will determine the severity of the changes, often using the Heath-Edwards classification.

INDICATIONS FOR INTERVENTION. The underlying principle of clinical management in patients with Eisenmenger syndrome is to avoid any factors that may destabilize the delicately balanced physiology. In general, an approach of nonintervention has been traditionally recommended, although research in the treatment of pulmonary hypertension may alter this approach in the future. The main interventions, therefore, are directed toward preventing complications (e.g., flu shots to reduce the morbidity of respiratory infections) or to restore the physiological balance (e.g., iron replacement for iron deficiency, antiarrhythmic management of atrial arrhythmias, diuretics for right-sided heart failure). As a general rule, the first episode of hemoptysis should be considered an indication for investigation. Bed rest is usually recommended; and, although usually self-limiting, each such episode should be regarded as potentially life threatening, and a treatable cause should be sought. When patients are severely incapacitated from severe hypoxemia or congestive heart failure, the main intervention available is lung (plus repair of the cardiac defect) or, with somewhat better results, heart-lung transplantation. This is generally reserved for individuals without contraindications who are thought to have a 1-year survival of less than 50 percent. Such assessment is fraught with difficulty because of the unpredictability of the time course of the disease and the risk of sudden death.

Noncardiac surgery should be performed only when absolutely necessary because of its high associated mortality.[30] Eisenmenger syndrome patients are particularly vulnerable to alterations in hemodynamics induced by anesthesia or surgery, such as a minor decrease in systemic vascular resistance that can increase right-to-left shunting and possibly potentiate cardiovascular collapse. Local anesthesia should be used whenever possible. Avoidance of prolonged fasting and especially dehydration, the use of antibiotic prophylaxis when appropriate, and careful intraoperative monitoring are recommended. The choice of general versus epidural-spinal anesthesia is controversial.[31] An experienced cardiac anesthetist with an understanding of Eisenmenger syndrome physiology should administer anesthesia. Additional risks of surgery include excessive bleeding, postoperative arrhythmias, and deep venous thrombosis with paradoxical emboli. An "air filter" or "bubble trap" should be used for most intravenous lines in cyanotic patients. Early ambulation is recommended. Postoperative care in an intensive care unit setting is optimal.

INTERVENTIONAL OPTIONS AND OUTCOMES

Oxygen. Supplemental nocturnal oxygen has recently been shown to have no impact on exercise capacity or on survival in adult patients with Eisenmenger syndrome.[32] Supplemental oxygen during commercial air travel is often recommended, but the scientific basis for this recommendation is lacking.[33]

Transplantation. Lung transplant may be undertaken in association with repair of existing cardiovascular defect(s). Alternatively, heart-lung transplantation may be required if the intracardiac anatomy is not correctable. The 1-year survival rate for adults undergoing lung transplantation with primary intracardiac repair is 55 percent. The 1-year survival rate after heart-lung transplantation is 70 percent.[34] These procedures offer the best hope to individuals with end-stage CHD who are confronting death and have an intolerable quality of life.

INVESTIGATIONAL OPTIONS[35,36]

Calcium-Channel Blockers. The chronic use of nifedipine in a small group of patients with Eisenmenger syndrome demonstrated a small but significant increase in exercise tolerance and a decrease in pulmonary vascular resistance, especially in children. This therapy is still considered investigational and should be prescribed only in a clinical research setting. Indeed with the advent of newer therapies that may have a more direct role on the pulmonary vasculature, there are fewer proponents for their use.

ACE Inhibitors. Data available[37] on a highly selected group of 10 patients with cyanotic CHD showed no change in oxygen saturation despite a subjective improvement in functional capacity. Proponents of the use of ACE inhibitors in these patients argue that, by decreasing systemic vascular resistance, one improves the cardiac output and thus oxygen delivery.[37] The counterargument is that these agents are potentially dangerous because they lower systemic vascular resistance without changing pulmonary vascular resistance and lead to an increase in right-to-left shunting. The use of this medication remains highly experimental and again should be administered only within the boundaries of a study trial guided by rigorous monitoring.

Prostacyclin. There are two reports of the use of long-term prostacyclin therapy for patients with Eisenmenger syndrome. In 20 patients (9 ASDs, 7 VSDs, 4 TGAs, 3 PDAs, 3 partial anomalous pulmonary venous drainage, and 1 aortopulmonary window), the chronic infusion of prostacyclin led to an improvement in hemodynamics after a 1-year period of therapy.[38] Pulmonary arterial pressure was reduced from 77 ± 20 to 61 ± 5 mm Hg ($p < 0.01$), and pulmonary vascular resistance decreased from 25 ± 13 to 12 ± 7 units ($p < 0.01$). Exercise capacity also improved from 408 ± 149 meters to 460 ± 99 meters during a 6-minute walk. Eight of the 12 patients listed for transplantation were removed from the active transplant list because of persistent clinical and hemodynamic improvement. One patient with an ASD initially believed to be inoperable improved enough that her ASD was closed with a device. A subsequent study of McLaughlin and associates evaluated 33 patients with secondary forms of pulmonary hypertension, 7 of whom had CHD. In these patients mean pulmonary arterial pressure decreased by 18 percent over a mean 1-year follow-up.[39]

Endothelin Receptor Antagonists. A large randomized North American trial of a nonselective endothelin receptor antagonist (Bosentan) has been recently completed in patients with pulmonary hypertension. There was a statistically significant increase in exercise tolerance in the entire cohort.[40] Fourteen patients in that study had congenital cardiac disease (11 in the Bosentan group and 3 in the placebo group). In this subgroup there was an increase of 46 meters traveled in a 6-minute walk test compared with 7.7 meters in the placebo group (personal communication, 2003). The results of two small studies of Bosentan in patients with Eisenmenger syndrome are pending. Given the high levels of endothelin in patients with congenital cardiac disease, it would seem logical to evaluate this therapy more rigorously in a larger prospective trial.

Sildenafil (Viagra) is another promising agent. Despite biological plausibility and early reports of benefit of sildenafil in pulmonary hypertension, at present there are little data to warrant its use outside a clinical trial. The results of a large multicenter trial of sildenafil in primary and secondary forms of pulmonary artery hypertension is anticipated.

FOLLOW-UP. Patient education is critical. Avoidance of over-the-counter medications, dehydration, smoking, high-altitude exposure, and excessive physical activity should be stressed. Avoidance of pregnancy is of paramount importance. Annual flu shots and use of endocarditis prophylaxis together with proper skin hygiene (avoidance of nail biting) are recommended. A yearly assessment of complete blood cell count and uric acid, creatinine, and ferritin levels should be done to monitor treatable causes of deterioration.

Cardiac Arrhythmias

In teenagers and young adults, most arrhythmias (see Chap. 32) encountered are in association with previously operated CHD. Arrhythmias can be a major clinical challenge in adolescent and adult congenital heart patients. They are the most frequent reason for emergency department visits and hospital admissions, and they are usually recurrent and may worsen or become less responsive to treatment with time. Treatment may be challenging.

ATRIAL ARRHYTHMIAS. Atrial flutter and, to a lesser degree, atrial fibrillation are most common. Atrial flutter tends to reflect right atrial, and atrial fibrillation left atrial abnormalities. Atrial flutter in such patients is often atypical in appearance and behavior and is better called intraatrial reentrant tachycardia. Recognition of atrial flutter can be difficult, and the observer will need to be vigilant in recognizing 2:1 conduction masquerading as sinus rhythm. Recurrence is likely and should not necessarily be assumed to represent failure of the management strategy. The conditions in which atrial flutter is most likely are Mustard/Senning repairs of TGA,[41-43] repaired or unrepaired ASDs,[44-46] repaired tetralogy of Fallot,[47] Ebstein anomaly of the tricuspid valve,[48-50] and after a Fontan operation.[51-53] Atrial flutter may reflect hemodynamic deterioration in patients who have had Mustard, Senning, tetralogy of Fallot, or Fontan repairs. Its arrival is usually associated with more symptoms and functional limitation.

The pharmaceutical agents most commonly used in therapy are warfarin, beta blockers, amiodarone, sotalol, propafenone, and digoxin. As a rule, patients with good ventricular function can receive sotalol or propafenone, whereas those with depressed ventricular function should receive amiodarone. Other therapies, including pacemakers, ablative procedures,[47,54,55] and innovative surgery,[56-59] are being both applied and refined. Sustained ventricular tachycardia[47,60-62] or ventricular fibrillation occurs less often, usually in the setting of ventricular dilation, dysfunction, and scarring. Although sudden death is common in several conditions,[63,64] the mechanism is poorly understood.

VENTRICULAR TACHYCARDIA. This arrhythmia can be seen as a manifestation of proarrhythmic effects of various agents; in patients with acute myocardial injury or infarction; and in CHD patients with severe ventricular dysfunction. In particular, sustained VT has been seen in patients with repaired tetralogy of Fallot, where it is seen as a manifestation of hemodynamic problems requiring repair; as a reflection of right ventricular dilation and dysfunction[61,62]; and in relation to ventricular scarring.

SUDDEN DEATH. In contrast to adults, children seldom die suddenly and unexpectedly of cardiovascular disease. Nonetheless, sudden death has been reported with arrhythmias, aortic stenosis, hypertrophic obstructive cardiomyopathy, primary pulmonary hypertension, Eisenmenger syndrome, myocarditis, congenital complete heart block, primary endocardial fibroelastosis, and when there are undiagnosed anomalies of the coronary arteries. Sudden death is more frequent in older patients with postoperative heart disease,[63-65] particularly after atrial switch procedures,[65] and repair of tetralogy of Fallot.[63,64]

ATRIOVENTRICULAR BLOCK. First-degree AV block is commonly seen in patients with AV septal defects, the older ASD patient, Ebstein, and complete TGA (D-TGA).[41-43] Complete heart block may develop in patients with cc-TGA[66] and may develop postoperatively in other patients. When pacing is required, epicardial leads are usually placed in cyanotic patients. Many adult patients with CHD are prone to problems of vascular access because of prior surgeries and pacing leads.

INFECTIVE ENDOCARDITIS

Infective endocarditis complicating CHD is uncommon before 2 years of age, except in the immediate postoperative period. The list of those conditions not requiring antibiotic prophylaxis is shorter than for those requiring it and is limited to patients before and after closure of a secundum ASD, after closure of a PDA, after spontaneous closure of a muscular and sometimes a perimembranous VSD, and in those with unoperated or operated anomalous pulmonary venous drainage in whom there is no residual hemodynamic abnormality.

CHEST PAIN

Angina pectoris is an uncommon symptom of cardiac disease in young infants and children, although it probably explains the irritability and crying during or after feeding in babies with coronary ischemia resulting from anomalous origin of the coronary artery from the pulmonary artery. In older children and young adults with severe left or right ventricular outflow tract obstruction and pulmonary hypertension, chest pain commonly follows effort and may be identical to effort angina of coronary artery disease in older adults. A sensation of chest discomfort or cardiac awareness is frequently interpreted as pain by the parents of children with cardiac arrhythmias. Careful questioning serves to identify palpitations rather than pain as the symptom and often elicits an additional history of anxiety, pallor, and sweating. Pain caused by pericarditis is commonly of acute onset and associated with fever, and can be identified by specific physical, radiographic, and echocardiographic findings. Most commonly, late postoperative chest pain is musculoskeletal in origin and may be reproduced on upper extremity movement or by palpation. Finally, children and adults may suffer chest pain of nonspecific form owing to anxiety, with or without hyperventilation.

SYNDROMES IN CONGENITAL HEART DISEASE[67]

ALCAPA SYNDROME. The acronym stands for *a*nomalous *l*eft *c*oronary *a*rtery arising from the *p*ulmonary *a*rtery. It is also called *Bland-White-Garland syndrome*.

ALAGILLE SYNDROME. This is a hereditary syndrome consisting of intrahepatic cholestasis, characteristic facies, butterfly-like vertebral anomalies, and varying degrees of peripheral pulmonary artery stenoses or diffuse hypoplasia of the pulmonary artery and its branches. It is associated with deletion in chromosome 20p.

CATCH-22. This is a syndrome that is due to microdeletion at chromosome 22q11 resulting in a wide clinical spectrum. CATCH stands for *c*ardiac defect, *a*bnormal facies, *t*hymic hypoplasia, cleft palate, and *h*ypocalcemia. Cardiac defects include conotruncal defects such as interrupted aortic arch, tetralogy of Fallot, truncus arteriosus, and double-outlet right ventricle. It is also known as *DiGeorge syndrome* and *velocardiofacial syndrome*.

CHARGE ASSOCIATION. This anomaly is characterized by the presence of coloboma or choanal atresia and three of the following defects: CHD, nervous system anomaly or mental retardation, genital abnormalities, ear abnormality, or deafness. Congenital heart defects seen in the CHARGE association are tetralogy of Fallot with or without other cardiac defects, AV septal defect, double-outlet right ventricle, double-inlet left ventricle, TGA, interrupted aortic arch, and others.

DOWN SYNDROME. This is the most common malformation caused by trisomy 21. Most of the patients (95 percent) have complete trisomy of chromosome 21; some have translocation or mosaic forms. The phenotype is diagnostic (short stature, characteristic facial appearance, mental retardation, brachydactyly, atlantoaxial instability, and thyroid and white blood cell disorders). Congenital heart defects are frequent, AV septal defect and VSD being the most common. Mitral valve prolapse and aortic regurgitation may be present. Patients with Down syndrome are prone to earlier and more severe pulmonary vascular disease than otherwise expected as a result of the lesions identified.

ELLIS–VAN CREVELD SYNDROME. This is an autosomal recessive syndrome in which common atrium, primum ASD, and partial AV septal defect are the most common cardiac lesions.

HOLT-ORAM SYNDROME. This is an autosomal dominant syndrome consisting of radial abnormalities of the forearm and hand associated with secundum ASD (most common), VSD, or, rarely, other cardiac malformations.

LEOPARD SYNDROME. This autosomal dominant condition includes *l*entigines, *E*CG abnormalities, ocular hypertelorism, *p*ulmonary stenosis, *a*bnormal genitalia, *r*etardation of growth, and *d*eafness. Rarely, cardiomyopathy or complex CHD may be present.

NOONAN SYNDROME. This is an autosomal dominant syndrome, phenotypically somewhat similar to Turner syndrome but with a normal chromosomal complement. It is associated with congenital cardiac anomalies, especially dysplastic pulmonary valve stenosis, pulmonary artery stenosis, and ASD. Hypertrophic cardiomyopathy is less common. Congenital lymphedema is a commonly associated anomaly that may be unrecognized.

RUBELLA SYNDROME. This is a wide spectrum of malformations caused by rubella infection early in pregnancy, including cataracts, retinopathy, deafness, CHD, bone lesions, and mental retardation. The spectrum of congenital heart lesions is wide and includes pulmonary artery stenosis, PDA, tetralogy of Fallot, and VSD.

SCIMITAR SYNDROME. This is a constellation of anomalies including total or partial anomalous pulmonary venous connection (PAPVC) of the right lung to the inferior vena cava, often associated with hypoplasia of the right lung and right pulmonary artery. The lower portion of the right lung (sequestered lobe) tends to receive its arterial supply from the abdominal aorta. The name of the syndrome derives from the appearance on posteroanterior chest radiograph of the shadow formed by the anomalous pulmonary venous connection that resembles a Turkish sword, or scimitar.

SHONE COMPLEX (SYNDROME). This is an association of multiple levels of left ventricular inflow and outflow obstruction (subvalvular and valvular left ventricular outflow tract obstruction, coarctation of the aorta, and mitral stenosis [parachute mitral valve and supramitral ring]).

TURNER SYNDROME. This is a clinical syndrome due to the 45 XO karyotype in about 50 percent of cases, with various other X chromosome abnormalities comprising the remainder. There is a characteristic but variable phenotype, an association with congenital cardiac anomalies, especially postductal coarctation of the aorta and other left-sided obstructive lesions, as well as PAPVC without ASD. The female phenotype varies with the age of presentation and is somewhat similar to that of Noonan syndrome.

WILLIAMS SYNDROME. This is a congenital syndrome of heterogeneous cause, often sporadic, occasionally autosomal dominant, associated with infantile hypercalcemia, characteristic phenotype, and CHD, especially supravalvular aortic stenosis and multiple peripheral pulmonary stenoses.

Evaluation of the Patient with Congenital Heart Disease

Physical Examination

Although the advances in technology have profoundly improved our diagnostic abilities, there is still a role for detailed clinical examination in the assessment and follow-up of unoperated, palliated, and repaired CHD. The relevant findings pertaining to specific abnormalities are outlined in the appropriate sections that follow, but some general principles bear consideration (see Chap. 8).

PHYSICAL ASSESSMENT. One should assess both cardiac and visceral situs and not assume the heart will be left sided. The presence of characteristic facial or somatic features of an underlying syndrome may be a strong clue to the type of heart disease (e.g., Williams, Noonan, Down) at any age. Central cyanosis can be difficult to diagnose clinically when mild but should be actively excluded by oximetry in any patient with suspected CHD. It is also important to perform careful surveillance of the chest wall for scars in older patients and adults, who do not always know or report the type and sequence of their surgical interventions. The thin chest wall of children and many young adults with CHD facilitates the detection of chamber enlargement by palpation, as well as the detection of systolic or diastolic thrills.

The infant or child with hemodynamically significant heart disease may show signs of failure to thrive. Simply put, the infant or child is underweight, small, or both. The weight and height should therefore be plotted sequentially against normal growth curves appropriate to race, sex, and underlying syndrome (e.g., Down syndrome growth chart). The manifestations of "heart failure" vary with age and underlying problem. In children, peripheral edema is rare, but intercostal recession, nasal flaring, and grunting with respiration are signs of congestive heart failure. In small children, liver size and pulsatility are an excellent barometer of cardiac function, reflecting right atrial pressure, right ventricular filling time, and diastolic dysfunction or tricuspid regurgitation. The jugular venous pressure is difficult to assess in young children but is a fundamental part of the examination of the older child, teenager, and adult.

Examination of the upper and lower limb peripheral pulses is important at any age. Delay, absence, or reduction of a pulse is an important clue to the presence of arterial obstruction and its site. The left brachial pulse is often compromised by surgery for coarctation, and blood pressure measurements should not be taken in only the left arm. Similarly, other palliative procedures (Blalock-Taussig shunt, interposition grafts) may affect either or both upper limb pulses. It is always important to assess the femoral and carotid pulses in addition to the upper limb pulses in such patients. The pulse volume and character also provide important information regarding severity of obstructive or regurgitant left heart disease. A low-volume pulse (usually with a narrow pulse pressure) reflects a low cardiac output. Pulsus alternans signifies severe systemic ventricular dysfunction. Pulsus paradoxus points to cardiac tamponade.

In adolescents and adults, the jugular venous pressure examination is often very important. It may give indication of cardiac decompensation, cardiac chamber hypertrophy or noncompliance, valvular regurgitation or stenosis, arrhythmia or conduction disturbance, cardiac tamponade, pericardial constriction, and other phenomena.

AUSCULTATION. The rules of auscultation follow those developed for acquired heart disease. However, cardiac and vascular malposition may significantly affect the appreciation of heart sounds and murmurs. For example, in TGA treated by an atrial switch procedure, the aorta remains anterior to the pulmonary artery. Consequently the aortic component of the second sound can be exceptionally loud, and the pulmonary component may be virtually inaudible, making it difficult to assess the pulmonary artery pressure under such circumstances. Conversely, when there is a valved conduit between the right ventricle and pulmonary artery, the pulmonary closure sound may be extremely loud, even though the pulmonary artery diastolic pressure is low. This is because the conduit is frequently "stuck" to the chest wall, facilitating sound transmission to the stethoscope placed just above it. Calcification of semilunar valves is relatively unusual in childhood and early adult life, making the differentiation of valve stenosis from subvalve or supravalve narrowing, by the presence of an ejection click, more precise in these patients. The differentiation of multiple murmurs is sometimes a challenge. There may be several causes of systolic and/or diastolic murmurs in an individual, and supplementary clinical information may be required to establish their significance in some cases. It is important to auscultate over the entire anterior and posterior chest wall. The continuous murmurs of aorto-aortic collateral arteries in coarctation may be audible only between the shoulder blades posteriorly, for example, and similarly the presence of a localized distal pulmonary artery stenosis or the presence of an aortopulmonary collateral artery may be detected only in a very localized area of the chest wall, particularly in adults.

Electrocardiogram

The ECG remains an important tool in the assessment of CHD (see Chap. 9). Heart rhythm and rate as well as AV conduction can be evaluated. The dominant theme that runs through ECGs in CHD is the prevalence of right heart disease. This often takes the form of right axis deviation along with right atrial and right ventricular hypertrophy. Right ventricular hypertrophy may reflect pulmonary hypertension, right ventricular outflow tract obstruction, or a subaortic right ventricle. Incomplete right bundle branch block often indicates right ventricular hypertrophy due to pressure (e.g., pulmonary hypertension or pulmonary stenosis) or volume (e.g., ASD) overload. Right ventricular volume overload is likely when the r′ in V_1 is less than 7 mm. Very wide QRS complexes should be seen as possible manifestations of very dilated and dysfunctional ventricles, most specifically in patients with repaired tetralogy, complete right bundle branch block, and severe pulmonary regurgitation. The ECG may be uninterpretable in patients with abnormal cardiac or visceral situs unless it is clear where the leads were placed.

Atrial flutter (often in an atypical form—so-called intra-atrial reentrant tachycardia) is much more common in young patients than is atrial fibrillation. First-degree block is often seen in AV septal defects, cc-TGA, and Ebstein anomaly. Complete heart block is most often seen in patients with cc-TGA, as well those with older VSD repairs.

Left atrial overload may reflect increased pulmonary blood flow as well as AV valve dysfunction and myocardial failure. Left axis deviation should make one think of AV septal defect, a univentricular heart, and a hypoplastic right ventricle. Deep q waves in the left chest leads can be caused by left ventricular volume overload in a young person with aortic or mitral regurgitation. Pathological Q waves can be evidence of the anomalous origin of the left coronary from the pulmonary artery.

Chest Radiograph

The chest radiograph is another valuable tool for the discerning physician caring for patients with congenital heart defects (see Chap. 12). Although more recent technologies have rightly attracted much attention, there is value in learning how to interpret the chest radiograph. Some teaching points can be made that may anchor the interpretation of chest radiographs of some CHD patients. In the following sections are provided a number of clinical and radiographic differential diagnoses.

CRITERIA FOR SHUNT VASCULARITY. These include (1) uniformly distributed vascular markings with absence of the normal lower lobe vascular predominance; (2) right descending pulmonary artery diameter that exceeds 17 mm; and (3) a pulmonary artery branch that is larger than its accompanying bronchus (best noted in the right parahilar area). Prominent vascularity is apparent only if the pulmonary-to-systemic flow ratio is greater than 1.5 to 1.0. As a rule, cardiac enlargement usually implies a shunt greater than 2.5 to 1.0. Anemia, pregnancy, thyrotoxicosis, and a pulmonary AV fistula may mimic shunt vascularity.

CYANOTIC PATIENTS WITH SHUNT VASCULARITY. This group includes single ventricle with transposition, persistent truncus arteriosus, tricuspid atresia without significant pulmonary outflow obstruction, total anomalous pulmonary venous connection, double-outlet right ventricle, and a common atrium.

CYANOTIC PATIENTS WITH A VSD AND NORMAL OR DECREASED PULMONARY VASCULARITY. This group includes tetralogy of Fallot; tricuspid atresia with pulmonary stenosis; single ventricle and pulmonary stenosis; D-TGA with pulmonary stenosis; cc-TGA with pulmonary stenosis; double-outlet right ventricle with pulmonary stenosis; pulmonary atresia; and asplenia syndrome.

CAUSES OF RETROSTERNAL FILLING ON LATERAL CHEST RADIOGRAPH. These include right ventricular dilation, TGA, ascending aortic aneurysm, and noncardiovascular masses (e.g., lymphoma, thymoma, teratoma, and thyroid).

CAUSES OF A STRAIGHT LEFT HEART BORDER. These include right ventricular dilation, left atrial dilation, cc-TGA, pericardial effusion, Ebstein anomaly, and congenital absence of the left pericardium.

CARDIOVASCULAR DISEASES ASSOCIATED WITH SCOLIOSIS. These include cyanotic CHD, Eisenmenger syndrome, Marfan syndrome, and occasionally mitral prolapse.

CAUSES OF LARGE CENTRAL PULMONARY ARTERIES. These include increased pulmonary flow (main pulmonary artery and branches), increased pulmonary pressure (main pulmonary artery and branches), pulmonary stenosis (main and left pulmonary artery), and idiopathic dilation of the pulmonary artery (main pulmonary artery).

SITUS SOLITUS WITH CARDIAC DEXTROVERSION. Situs solitus with cardiac dextroversion is associated with CHD in more than 90 percent of cases. Up to 80 percent have a congenitally corrected transposition with a high incidence of associated VSD, pulmonary stenosis, and tricuspid atresia. *Situs inversus with dextrocardia* carries a low incidence of CHD, whereas *situs inversus with levocardia* is virtually always associated with severe CHD.

Cardiovascular MRI

Cardiac MRI in adolescents and adults with CHD has become of ever-increasing importance in the past decade (see Chap. 14). MRI is able to circumvent the echocardiographic problem of suboptimal visualization of the heart in adult patients, especially those who have had surgery. This technique can now generate information never previously available and also more easily or more accurately than by other means. New MRI image acquisition methods are faster and provide improved temporal and spatial resolution. Major advances in hardware design, new pulse sequences, and faster image reconstruction techniques now permit rapid high-resolution imaging of complex cardiovascular anatomy. MRI can produce quantitative measures of ventricular volumes, mass, and ejection fraction. MRI can quantify blood flow in any vessel.

Cardiac MRI is of particular value when transthoracic echocardiography cannot provide the needed diagnostic information; as an alternative to diagnostic cardiac catheterization; and for MRI's unique capabilities such as tissue imaging, myocardial tagging, and vessel-specific flow quantification. The value of MRI over echocardiography in the evaluation of the right ventricle is becoming increasingly appreciated. The capability of MRI to assess the right ventricle is of great importance since the right ventricle is a key component of many of the more complex CHD lesions. In addition, MRI can evaluate valve regurgitation, postoperative systemic and pulmonary venous pathways, Fontan pathways, and the great vessels. MRI should be considered the main imaging modality in adolescents and adults with repaired tetralogy of Fallot, TGA, Fontan procedure, and diseases of the aorta. In the near future, we will see real-time MRI to allow MR-guided interventional procedures, and molecular imaging that will further expand MRI's capabilities.

Transthoracic Echocardiography (see Chap. 11)

FETAL ECHOCARDIOGRAPHY

General Considerations. Fetal echocardiography has graduated from being a special area of interest to some pediatric cardiologists to one of standard care. As early as 16 weeks' gestation excellent images of the fetal cardiac structures can be obtained by the transabdominal route, along with an appreciation of cardiac and placental physiology through the use of Doppler technology. Transvaginal ultrasound is a newer approach that permits the echocardiographer to obtain images at around 13 to 14 weeks' gestation. Although it has some application for cases with a higher risk of recurrent CHD (e.g., obstructive left-sided lesions), its accuracy has yet to be determined. This is in part due to the limited number of views that are possible due to a relatively fixed position of the transducer. Although there are specific indications for fetal echocardiographic scanning, the highest number of cases arise from anatomical or functional abnormalities detected at routine obstetrical screening. A routine anatomical screen has become a standard of care in many obstetrical practices throughout the world. As a result there has been a tremendous push by pediatric fetal echocardiographers to improve the standard of routine screening of the prenatal heart. There has been a rapid rise in the number of abnormalities that are detected by general obstetrical ultrasonographers that are subsequently referred in a timely manner to the pediatric cardiologist and echocardiographer.

Impact of Fetal Echocardiography. Most major structural congenital heart defects are now accurately categorized through fetal echocardiography. Once the abnormalities are identified families and obstetrical caregivers can be counseled as to the impact of the abnormality to the fetus and the family. Decisions appropriate to the individual family and fetus can then be made. Although termination of pregnancy is one of the consequences of prenatal diagnosis, it is not the main objective.[68] In fact data are starting to appear in the literature indicating that prenatal diagnosis of some major cardiac malformations has a direct impact on outcome, from a survival, morbidity, and cost outcome.[69] This is in part due to the fact that when a prenatal diagnosis is made, subsequent caregivers are prepared for the immediate postnatal effects of the defect. For example, in hypoplastic left heart syndrome and other duct-dependent lesions prostaglandin E_1 can be started immediately after birth, hopefully in a hospital within or attached to a pediatric cardiology facility.

Fetal echocardiography has also permitted us to understand more about the evolution of certain congenital cardiac malformations. For example, although the fetal heart is fully formed by the time a prenatal scan is performed, there is a tremendous growth of the cardiac structures that still has to occur. Therefore, in some circumstances a cardiac chamber that may appear only mildly hypoplastic at 16 weeks' gestation may be profoundly affected at the time of birth. This has a major impact on the management of the newborn as well as the counseling process at 16 weeks' gestation.

Direct Fetal Intervention. The next step is direct intervention for specific cardiac lesions. This has initially involved obstructive lesions, thus far mainly being limited to the left ventricle. The rationale behind this therapy is based on the notion that the relief of obstructive outflow tract lesions will permit growth of the affected ventricle, potentially changing a neonatal pathway from univentricular to biventricular. Cardiac surgery to the fetus is also a future option, and indeed there is already a considerable amount of research on the impact of this in fetal animal models.

SEGMENTAL APPROACH[70,71] TO ECHOCARDIOGRAPHY IN CONGENITAL HEART DISEASE. The following four echocardiographic steps of segmental analysis are crucial in any patient with CHD. Starting from a standard subcostal view, one should determine the position of the apex, the situs of the atria, as well as the AV and ventriculoarterial relationships.

1. Apex Position. From a standard subcostal view, determine if the apex of the heart is pointing to the right (dextrocardia), to the left (levocardia), or to the middle (mesocardia).

2. Situs of the Atria (Fig. 56–2). The right and left atria differ morphologically with regard to their appendages. A morphological right atrium has a broad right atrial appendage, whereas a morphological left atrium has a narrow left atrial appendage. Right and left atrial appendages, however, are difficult to visualize by transthoracic echocardiography, and one often has to rely on abdominal situs to determine the atrial situs. Atrial situs follows abdominal situs in about 70 to 80 percent of the cases. From a standard subcostal view with the probe pointing at a right angle to the spine, one can visualize the abdominal aorta as well as the inferior vena cava and the spine at the back. When the aorta is to the left of the spine and the inferior vena cava to the right of the spine, there is abdominal situs solitus and, in all probability, corresponding atrial situs solitus (meaning the morphological right atrium is on the right side and the morphological left atrium is on the left side). When the aorta is to the right of the spine and the inferior vena cava is to the left of the spine, there is abdominal situs inversus and, in all probability, corresponding atrial situs inversus (morphological right atrium on the left side and morphological left atrium on the right side). When both the aorta and inferior vena cava are to the left of the spine, there is abdominal as well as atrial left isomerism (two morphological left atria). When both the aorta and inferior vena cava are to the right of the spine, there is abdominal as well as atrial right isomerism (two morphological right atria).

3. Atrioventricular Relationship. Once the situs of the atria is determined, one has to assess the position of the ventricles in relation to the atria. The morphological right ventricle has four characteristic features that distinguish it from the morphological left ventricle: (1) a trabeculated apex, (2) a moderator band, (3) septal attachment of the tricuspid valve, and (4) lower (apical) insertion of the tricuspid valve. The tricuspid valve is always "attached" to the morphological right ventricle. The morphological left ventricle has the following characteristics: (1) a smooth apex, (2) no moderator band, (3) no septal attachment of the mitral valve, and (4) higher (basal) insertion of the mitral valve. The mitral valve is always "attached" to the morphological left ventricle. Once the position of the ventricles is determined, one can then establish the AV relationship. When the morphological right atrium empties into to the morphological right ventricle, and the morphological left atrium empties into to the morphological left ventricle, there is AV concordance. When the morphological right atrium empties into to the morphological left ventricle, and the morphological left atrium empties into to the morphological right ventricle, there is AV discordance. When both atria empty into one ventricle (right or left), it is called a *double-inlet* (right or left) *ventricle*.

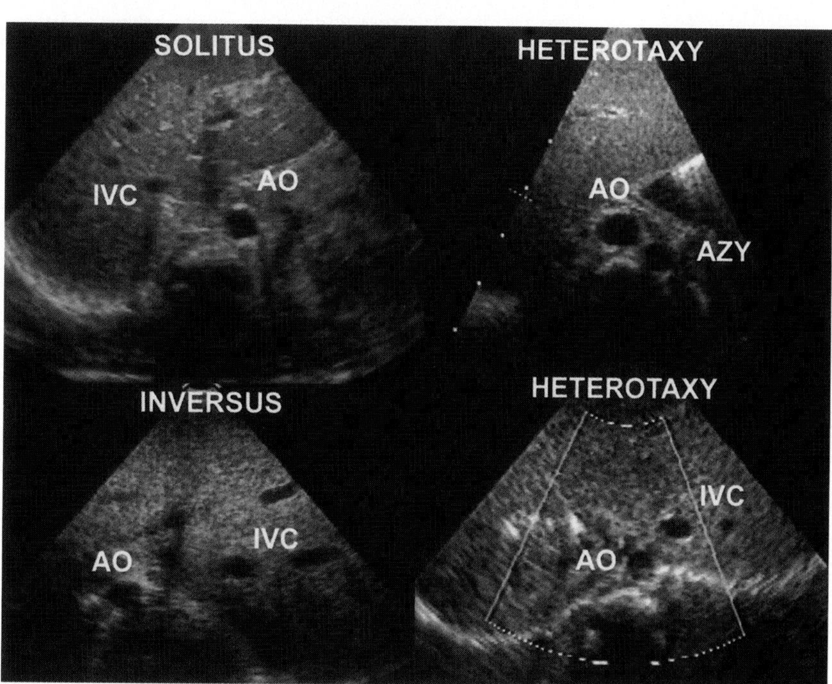

FIGURE 56–2 Montage of the different types of situs as seen by a subcostal echocardiographic scan. Note that situs solitus and inversus are just the mirror image of each other. The upper right picture is in the setting of heterotaxy with an interrupted intrahepatic inferior vena cava, with azygos continuation on the left. This is seen more frequently in left atrial isomerism. The lower right picture is also in the setting of heterotaxy with an intrahepatic inferior vena cava that is positioned closer to the aorta that in solitus or inversus. Note also the midline liver. This pattern is seen more commonly in right atrial isomerism. AO = aorta; AZY = azygos; IVC = inferior vena cava.

4. Ventriculoarterial Relationship. Once the AV relationship has been determined, one should assess the position of the great arteries in relation to the ventricles. The pulmonary artery can be distinguished by: its early branching pattern into the left and right pulmonary arteries; the pulmonary valve is always "attached" to the pulmonary artery. Similarly, the aorta can be distinguished by its "candy cane" shape and the take-off of its three head and neck vessels (innominate, carotid, and subclavian arteries). The aortic valve is always "attached" to the aorta. Once the position of the great arteries is determined, one can then establish the ventriculoarterial relationship. When the morphological right ventricle ejects into to the pulmonary artery, and the morphological left ventricle ejects into to the aorta, there is ventriculoarterial concordance. When the morphological right ventricle ejects into to the aorta, and the morphological left ventricle ejects into to the pulmonary artery, there is ventriculoarterial discordance. When both great arteries are exiting from one ventricle (right or left), it is called *double-outlet* (right or left) *ventricle*.

Once segmental analysis has been completed, one can then proceed to the usual echocardiographic windows to determine the nature of the specific lesions as well as their hemodynamic relevance.

ECHOCARDIOGRAPHY IN THE NEONATE AND INFANT. Echocardiography is of immense value in differentiating between heart disease and lung disease in newborns. Indeed, it has become the standard for the diagnosis of virtually all cardiovascular malformations. Most neonates and infants are now referred directly after ultrasound study for operative repair, without intervening cardiac catheterization. It is simpler to list those lesions where it cannot be used as the sole mode of investigation prior to making a management decision.[72] For example, in pulmonary atresia and VSD with multiple aortopulmonary collaterals, echocardiography is used as an adjunct to angiocardiography. Echocardiography provides details about the intracardiac pathology, whereas angiocardiography is necessary to delineate the sources of pulmonary blood supply. In pulmonary atresia with intact ventricular septum, the presence or absence of a right ventricular dependent coronary circulation is best assessed by angiocardiography. Apart from these two lesions, there are few other preoperative decisions that cannot be made by echocardiography alone in the newborn and infant. Postoperative management is different, particularly for those defects that are on Fontan track where precise hemodynamic measurements are of key importance in the decision process.

Transesophageal echocardiography (TEE) is usually unnecessary for the preoperative evaluation of the neonate or infant with heart disease. This technique has now become a standard in the immediate postoperative period for the evaluation of residual anatomical or functional abnormalities. Newer techniques such as tissue Doppler and three-dimensional (3D) echocardiography are starting to be applied to this age group and will add important additional information in the future.

ECHOCARDIOGRAPHY IN THE OLDER CHILD AND ADOLESCENT. This technique still plays a key role in the diagnosis and follow-up of the older child and adolescent with congenital or acquired heart disease. As many of the patients underwent surgery in the neonatal or infant periods they often have suboptimal ultrasound windows that necessitate other modes of investigation, especially magnetic resonance angiography (MRA). The application of newer technologies such as tissue Doppler and 3D echocardiography are already possible in this population and provide additional information that has thus far not been obtainable from standard techniques. For example, force-frequency relationships have been obtained in postoperative patients to try and predict the optimal heart rates to maintain maximum cardiac efficiency. On the other hand 3D echocardiography can provide new insights into AV valve function[73] that have not been possible from standard 2D techniques. In the future, 3D echocardiography may replace some TEE procedures.

ECHOCARDIOGRAPHY IN THE ADULT. Advances in cardiac ultrasonography now allow comprehensive noninvasive assessment of cardiovascular structure and function in adults with CHD. Because of its widespread availability, easy use, and quick interpretation, transthoracic echocardiography remains the technique of choice for the initial diagnosis and for follow-up in adults with CHD. The general initial approach to the diagnosis of CHD by transthoracic echocardiography starts with a segmental approach to ascertain the relative position of the various cardiac chambers. Once the segmental approach has been completed, a more lesion-specific approach can then be carried out, as discussed in the individual lesion sections.

Transesophageal Echocardiography

DIAGNOSTIC ASSESSMENT. TEE offers a better 2D resolution than transthoracic echocardiography. This is especially important in adult patients with multiple previous cardiac operations, when adequate transthoracic windows are often difficult to obtain.

TEE should be used whenever transthoracic echo does not provide adequate 2D, color, or Doppler information. TEE should be considered in the setting of the conditions discussed in the following sections.

Secundum Atrial Septal Defect. Use TEE for assessment of device closure feasibility, measuring ASD size, assessing adequacy of margins for device anchoring, and ruling out anomalous pulmonary venous connection.

Mitral Regurgitation. Use TEE for preoperative evaluation of mitral valve leaflet morphology and suitability for mitral valve repair versus replacement.

Ebstein Anomaly. Use TEE for preoperative assessment of tricuspid valve morphology and the potential for tricuspid valve repair.[74]

Fontan. Use TEE when right atrial clot is suspected on clinical grounds or by transthoracic echocardiography, or when circuit obstruction is suspected.

Precardioversion. For any patient who is not anticoagulated, presenting with atrial flutter or fibrillation longer than 24 hours, TEE should be performed prior to chemical or electrical cardioversion. Patients with a Fontan circuit should undergo TEE irrespective of the duration of atrial tachyarrhythmia to rule out a right or left atrial thrombus.

GUIDANCE OF THERAPEUTIC INTERVENTION. TEE can be instrumental in helping guide therapy at the time of transcatheter or surgical procedures. TEE is particularly helpful in the following situations.

Percutaneous Device Closure. TEE is performed at the time of transcatheter ASD closure to assist ASD-stretched balloon sizing and device deployment, unless intracardiac echocardiography (ICE) (see later) is available.

Intraoperative and Postoperative Assessment. TEE is often required for the intraoperative and postoperative assessment of the adult patient undergoing congenital cardiac surgery. It has a particular role in the intraoperative assessment of adequacy of valve repair. A TEE service by an experienced echocardiographer is an essential requirement for centers performing adult congenital cardiac surgery.

Three-Dimensional Echocardiography

DIAGNOSTIC ASSESSMENT. Presently, 3D echocardiography is not being widely used for the adult with CHD. However, with the expected improvement in technology that will permit real-time 3D echocardiography, its clinical applications will widen. By providing unique imaging planes and projections of the septa and AV and semilunar valves, 3D echocardiography offers the potential to enhance the understanding of complex cardiac anatomy.[75] It will also permit volumetric analyses independent of geometric assumptions, which will make it a particularly useful method for the assessment of the irregularly shaped, and thus problematic, right ventricle.[76]

Intracardiac Echocardiography

Intracardiac echocardiography (ICE) uses lower frequency transducers that have been miniaturized and mounted into catheters capable of percutaneous insertion into the heart. ICE not only provides high-resolution 2D and hemodynamic data with full Doppler capabilities but also eliminates the need for general anesthesia, which is often required for TEE.

CURRENT APPLICATIONS

Percutaneous ASD Device Closure. ICE supports percutaneous ASD device closure by adequately sizing the defect and by assisting device positioning[77] while avoiding the need for general anesthesia.

Electrophysiological Studies. ICE facilitates electrophysiological procedures by guiding transseptal puncture, enabling endocardial visualization, and ensuring electrode/tissue contact at the time of ablative procedures.[78]

Cardiac Catheterization

With the development of cross-sectional echocardiography, and the subsequent introduction of MRI and fast computed tomographic (CT) methods, truly diagnostic cardiac catheterization is a thing of the past for both children and adults. "Diagnostic" catheterization is reserved for resolving unanswered questions from the less-invasive techniques and measuring hemodynamics. A good example of this is the assessment of major aortopulmonary collateral arteries in tetralogy with pulmonary atresia, where their presence and distribution may be shown beautifully by MRA, but cardiac catheterization is required to demonstrate the presence of communications with the central pulmonary arteries and measure the pressure within them. There is no adequate substitute for cardiac catheterization to measure ventricular end-diastolic pressures or pulmonary artery pressures and resistance with the precision required to plan for, or to assess, the Fontan circulation. Such diagnostic testing may also be needed to evaluate possible coronary artery disease, especially prior to heart surgery.

THERAPEUTIC CATHETERIZATION. Balloon atrial septostomy was the first catheter intervention that proved useful in treating CHD, and it remains the standard initial palliation in many infants with D-TGA unless the arterial switch operation is performed immediately. Many transcatheter techniques are now used successfully to treat CHD: blade atrial septostomy; device or coil closure of PDA; closure of ASD and patent foramen ovale; transluminal balloon dilation of pulmonary and aortic valve stenosis; radiofrequency perforation of pulmonary valve atresia; balloon-expandable intravascular stents for right ventricular outflow tract, pulmonary artery, aortic coarctation, and other vascular stenoses; and device occlusion of unwanted collateral vessels and AV fistulas. These have all become treatments of choice in some centers with these capabilities. Some are universally accepted as standard of care (e.g., balloon pulmonary valvuloplasty), whereas debate continues for other interventions (e.g., unoperated coarctation).[79,80] Going along with the extraordinary expansion of interventional techniques for the treatment of structural abnormalities, ablative techniques for the treatment of tachycardias are now performed routinely in centers with congenital heart electrophysiology programs and are crucial to the management of the adult with operated and unoperated CHD, where arrhythmias are such a burden in terms of their morbidity, as well as a significant cause of late mortality. The indications, outcomes, and current status of each of these techniques are discussed in detail in the sections concerning specific lesions that follow.

Specific Cardiac Defects

Left-to-Right Shunts

Atrial Septal Defect

MORPHOLOGY. There are four types of ASDs or interatrial communications: ostium primum, ostium secundum, sinus venosus, and coronary sinus defects (Fig. 56–3A and D). (Ostium primum is discussed in the section on AV septal defect.) Ostium secundum defects occur from either excessive resorption of the septum primum or from deficient growth of the septum secundum and are occasionally associated with anomalous pulmonary venous connection (<10 percent). Sinus venosus defect of the superior vena cava type occurs at the cardiac junction of the superior vena cava, giving rise to a superior vena cava connected to both atria, and almost always associated with anomalous pulmonary venous connection (right >> left). Sinus venosus–inferior vena cava-type defects are very uncommon, and abut the junction of the inferior vena cava, inferior to the fossa ovalis. Coronary sinus septal defects are rare and arise from an opening of its wall with the left atrium, allowing left-to-right atrial shunting.

PATHOPHYSIOLOGY. In any type of ASD, the degree of left-to-right atrial shunting depends on the size of the defect and the relative diastolic filling properties of the two ventricles. Any condition causing reduced left ventricular compliance (e.g., systemic hypertension, cardiomyopathy, or myocardial infarction) or increased left atrial pressure (mitral stenosis and/or regurgitation) tends to increase the left-to-right shunt. If similar forces are present in the right heart, this will diminish the left-to-right shunt and promote right-to-left shunting.

NATURAL HISTORY. A large ASD (pulmonary artery blood flow relative to systemic blood flow [Qp/Qs] > 2.0/1.0) may cause congestive heart failure and failure to thrive in an infant or child. An undetected ASD with a significant shunt (Qp/Qs > 1.5/1.0) probably causes symptoms over time in adolescence or adulthood, and symptomatic patients usually become progressively more limited as they age. Effort dyspnea is seen in about 30 percent of patients by the third decade and more than 75 percent of patients by the fifth decade.[81] Supraventricular arrhythmias (atrial fibrillation or flutter) and right-sided heart failure develop by 40 years of age in about 10 percent of patients and become more prevalent with aging.[82] Paradoxical embolism resulting in a transient ischemic attack or stroke can call the diagnosis to attention. The development of pulmonary hypertension, although probably not as common as originally thought,[82] can occur at an early age. If pulmonary hypertension is severe, a second causative diagnosis should be sought. Life expectancy is clearly reduced, although not as severely as was quoted in earlier papers, since only patients with large ASDs were reported.

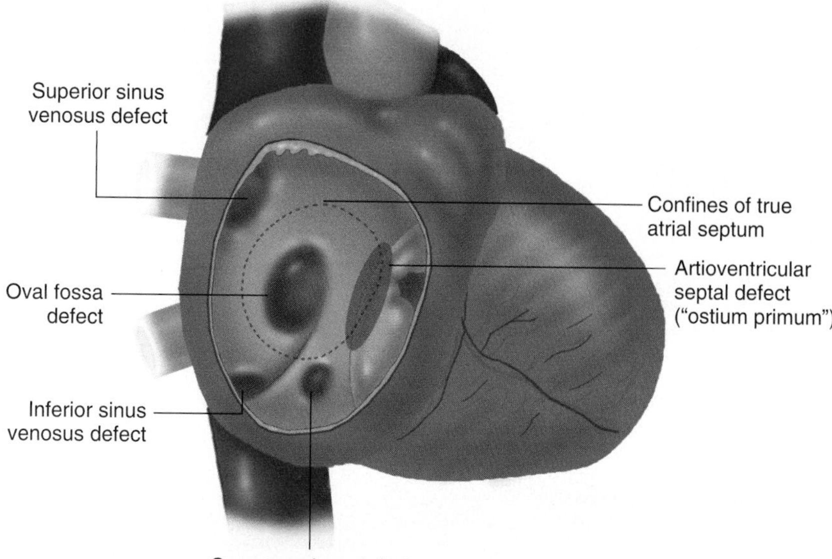

A

SVC
LA
*
RA
SVC
right atrial appendage
ASD
IVC
CS
Tric valve
Eust valve

B

FIGURE 56–3 **A,** Schematic diagram outlining the different types of interatrial shunting that can be encountered. Note that only the central defect is suitable for device closure. **B,** Subcostal right anterior oblique view of a secundum atrial septal defect (asterisk) that is suitable for device closure. The right panel is a specimen as seen in a similar view, outlining the landmarks of the defect. *Continued*

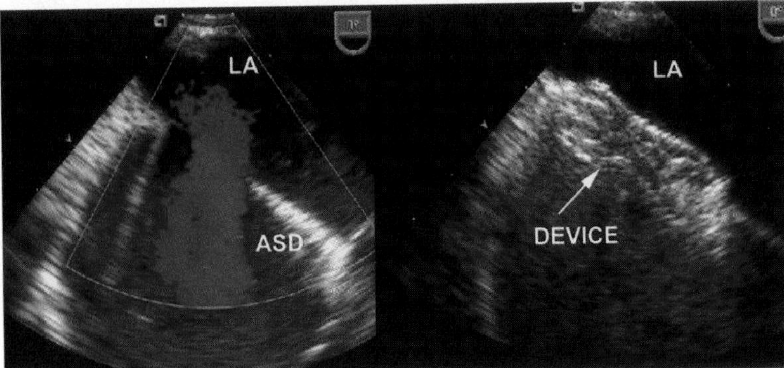

C

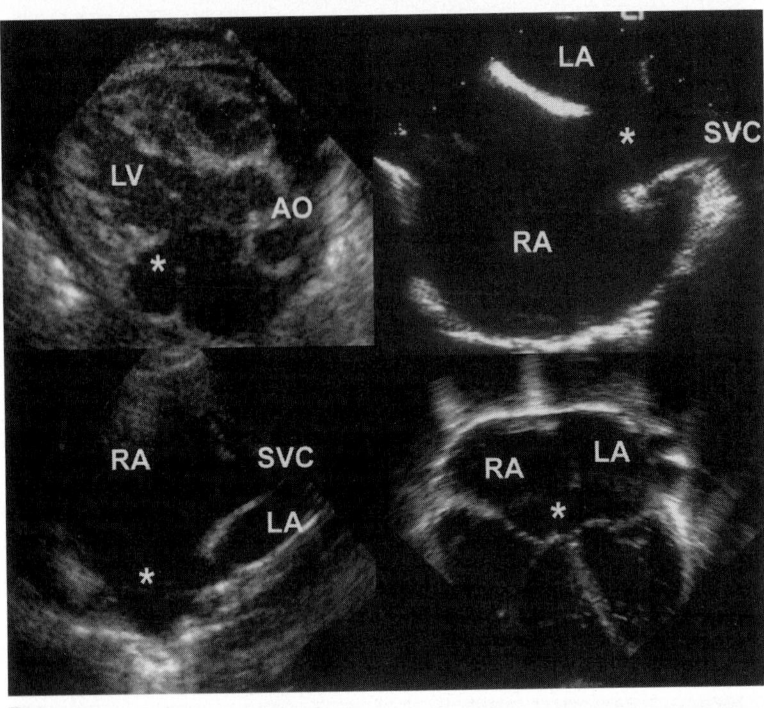

D

FIGURE 56–3, cont'd **C,** The left image is a transesophageal echocardiogram with color flow before device closure, whereas the right side shows postrelease of an Amplatzer device. **D,** Montage of interatrial communications that are not atrial septal defects (asterisks) and therefore not suitable for device closure. The upper left is a coronary sinus defect, due to unroofing; the top right is a superior sinus venosus defect; the bottom left is an inferior sinus venosus defect; and the bottom right is an atrial septal defect in the setting of an atrioventricular septal defect. AO = aorta; ASD = atrial septal defect; CS = coronary sinus; Eust = eustachian; IVC = inferior vena cava; LA = left atrium; LV = left ventricle; RA = right atrium; SVC = superior vena cava; Tric = tricuspid.

CLINICAL FEATURES

Pediatrics. Most children are asymptomatic, and the diagnosis is made following the discovery of a murmur. Occasionally, increased pulmonary blood flow may be so great that congestive heart failure, recurrent chest infections, chronic wheeze, or even pulmonary hypertension may necessitate closure in infancy. Spontaneous closure of an ASD may occur within the first year of life. Even quite substantial defects diagnosed in the neonatal period (<7 mm) may reduce in size and not require later intervention. Thus, in asymptomatic children with isolated secundum ASD, intervention is usually deferred so that elective device closure becomes an option if indicated.

Adults. The most common presenting symptoms in adults are exercise intolerance (exertional dyspnea and fatigue) and palpitations (typically from atrial flutter, atrial fibrillation, or sick sinus syndrome). Right ventricular failure can be the presenting symptom in older patients. The presence of cyanosis should alert one to the possibility of shunt reversal and Eisenmenger syndrome or, alternatively, to a prominent eustachian valve directing inferior vena cava flow to the left atrium via a secundum ASD or sinus venosus ASD of the inferior vena cava type.

On examination, there is "left atrialization" of the jugular venous pressure (A wave = V wave). A hyperdynamic right ventricular impulse may be felt at the left sternal border at the end of expiration or in the subxyphoid area on deep inspiration. A dilated pulmonary artery trunk may be palpated in the second left intercostal space. A wide and fixed split of S_2 is the auscultatory hallmark of ASD, although not always present. A systolic ejection murmur, usually grade 2 and often scratchy, is best heard at the second left intercostal space and a mid-diastolic rumble, from increased flow through the tricuspid valve, may be present at the left lower sternal border. When right ventricular failure occurs, a pansystolic murmur of tricuspid regurgitation is usual.

LABORATORY INVESTIGATIONS

ECG. Sinus rhythm or atrial fibrillation or flutter may be present. The QRS axis is typically rightward in secundum ASD. Negative P waves in the inferior leads indicate a low atrial pacemaker often seen in sinus venosus–superior vena cava-type defects, which are located in the area of the sinoatrial node and render it deficient. Complete right bundle branch block appears as a function of age. Tall R or R′ waves in V_1 often indicate pulmonary hypertension.

Chest Radiography. The classic radiographic features are of cardiomegaly (from right atrial and ventricular enlargement), dilated central pulmonary arteries with pulmonary plethora indicating increased pulmonary flow, and a small aortic knuckle (reflecting a chronic low cardiac output state).

Echocardiography. Transthoracic echocardiography documents the type(s) and size (defect diameter) of the ASD(s), the direction(s) of the shunt (see Fig. 56–3B) and sometimes the presence of anomalous pulmonary venous return. The functional importance of the defect can be estimated by the size of the right ventricle, the presence or absence of right ventricular volume overload (paradoxical septal motion), and the calculation of Qp/Qs. Indirect measurement of the pulmonary artery pressure can be obtained from the Doppler velocity of the tricuspid regurgitation jet. TEE permits better visualization of the interatrial septum and is usually required when device closure is contemplated, partly to ensure that pulmonary venous drainage is normal.

INDICATIONS FOR INTERVENTION. In asymptomatic children, the decision to intervene is based on the presence of right-sided heart dilation and a significant ASD (>5 mm) that shows no sign of spontaneous closure. Shunt fractions are now rarely measured and are reserved for "borderline" cases. Hemodynamically insignificant ASDs (Qp/Qs < 1.5) do not require closure, with the possible exception of trying to prevent paradoxical emboli in older patients after a stroke. "Significant" ASDs (Qp/Qs > 1.5, or ASDs associated with right ventricular volume overload) should be closed, especially if device closure is available and appropriate.[83,84] For patients with pulmonary hypertension (pulmonary artery pressure > ⅔ systemic arterial blood pressure, or pulmonary arteriolar resistance > ⅔ systemic arteriolar resistance), closure can be recommended if there is a net left-to-right shunt of at least 1.5:1, evidence of pulmonary artery reactivity when challenged with a pulmonary vasodilator (e.g., oxygen or nitric oxide), or evidence on lung biopsy (rarely required) that pulmonary arterial changes are potentially reversible.

INTERVENTIONAL OPTIONS AND OUTCOMES

Device Closure. Device closure of secundum ASDs percutaneously under fluoroscopy and TEE or with intracardiac echo guidance[83] is the therapy of choice when appropriate (see Fig. 56–3C).[85] Indications for device closure are the same as for surgical closure, but the selection criteria are stricter. Depending on the device, this technique is available only for patients with a secundum ASD with a stretched diameter of less than 36 mm and with adequate rims to enable secure deployment of the device. Anomalous pulmonary venous connection or proximity of the defect to the AV valves or coronary sinus or systemic venous drainage usually precludes the use of this technique. It is a safe and effective procedure in experienced hands, with major complications (e.g., device embolization, atrial perforation) occurring in less than 1 percent of patients, and clinical closure achieved in more than 80 percent of patients. Device closure of an ASD improves functional status in symptomatic patients and exercise capacity in asymptomatic and symptomatic patients,[86] but long-term follow-up data are not available.

Surgery. Device closure is not an option for those with sinus venosus or ostium primum defects or with secundum defects with unsuitable anatomy. Surgical closure of ASDs can be performed by primary suture closure or using a pericardial or synthetic patch. The procedure is usually performed via a midline sternotomy, but the availability of an inframammary or minithoracotomy approach to a typical secundum ASD should be made known to cosmetically sensitive patients. Surgical mortality in the adult without pulmonary hypertension should be less than 1 percent. Surgical closure of an ASD improves functional status and exercise capacity in symptomatic patients[87] and improves (but usually does not normalize) survival and improves or eliminates congestive heart failure, especially when patients are operated on at an earlier age. However, surgical closure of ASD in adult life does not prevent atrial fibrillation/flutter or stroke, especially when patients are operated on after the age of 40 years.[88] The role of a concomitant Cox/maze procedure in patients with a prior history of atrial flutter/fibrillation is unclear (see Chap. 30).[89]

REPRODUCTIVE ISSUES. Pregnancy is well tolerated in patients after ASD closure. Pregnancy is also well tolerated in women with unrepaired ASDs, but the risk of paradoxical embolism is increased (still only to a very low risk) during pregnancy as well as in the postpartum period. Pregnancy is contraindicated in Eisenmenger syndrome because of the high maternal (≤50 percent) and fetal (≤60 percent) mortality.

FOLLOW-UP ISSUES. Most children with isolated secundum defect can be discharged to the care of their family physician 6 months after complete closure is confirmed, no matter whether surgical or by device. They do not require any special precautions or endocarditis prophylaxis. Patients with sinus venosus defect are at risk of developing caval and/or pulmonary vein stenosis and should be kept under intermittent review. Patients who have had surgical or device repair as adults, patients with atrial arrhythmias preoperatively or postoperatively, and patients with ventricular dysfunction should remain under long-term cardiology surveillance.

Atrioventricular Septal Defect

TERMINOLOGY. The terms *atrioventricular septal defect, atrioventricular canal defect,* and *endocardial cushion defect* can be used interchangeably to describe this group of defects. The variable components of these lesions are explained in the following sections.

MORPHOLOGY. The basic morphology of AV septal defect is common to all types and is independent of the presence or absence of an ASD or VSD.[72,90-92] These common features (Figs. 56–4 and 56–5) are absence of the muscular AV septum (resulting in the AV valves being at the same level on echo); inlet/outlet disproportion (resulting in an elongated left ventricular outflow tract, the so-called goose-neck deformity); abnormal lateral rotation of the posteromedial papillary muscle; and abnormal configuration of the AV valves. The left AV valve is a trileaflet valve made of superior and inferior bridging leaflets separated by a mural leaflet. The space between the superior and inferior leaflets as they bridge the interventricular septum is called the *cleft* in the left AV valve. The bridging leaflets may be completely adherent to the crest of the interventricular septum, free floating, or attached by chordal apparatus.

PARTITIONED VERSUS COMPLETE ATRIOVENTRICULAR SEPTAL DEFECTS. A *partitioned* orifice is one where the superior and inferior leaflets are joined together by a connecting tongue of tissue as they bridge the interventricular septum. This partitions the valve into a separate left and right orifice. A *common* AV valve orifice is one where there is no such connecting tongue, resulting in one large orifice that encompasses the left- and right-sided components. Interatrial (ostium primum) and interventricular defects are common in AV septal defect.

The left ventricular outflow tract is elongated and predisposes to subaortic stenosis. The papillary muscles are closer together than normal. The term *unbalanced AV septal defect* refers to cases where one ventricle is hypoplastic. This is seen

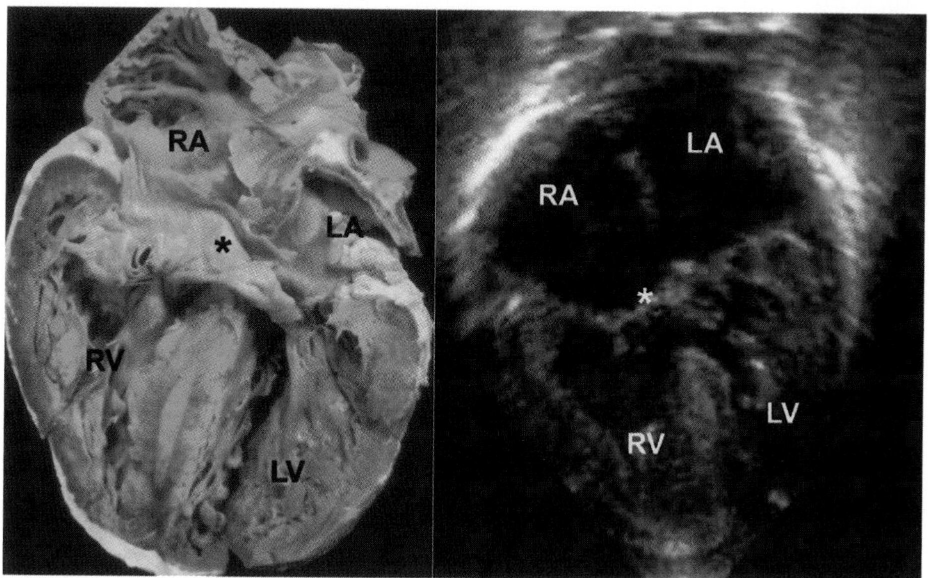

FIGURE 56–4 Apical four-chamber view in a complete atrioventricular septal defect with a common atrioventricular valve orifice (*). Note the large interatrial and interventricular communications and the large free-floating superior bridging leaflet. LA = left atrium; LV = left ventricle; RA = right atrium; RV = right ventricle.

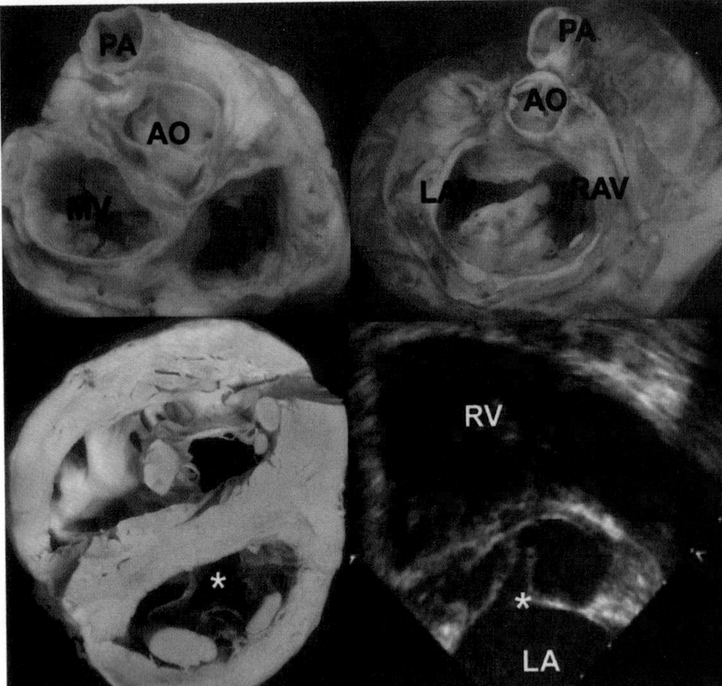

FIGURE 56–5 Montage comparing the normal atrioventricular junction to that seen in an atrioventricular septal defect. The upper left picture is the normal atrioventricular junction as seen from above. Note the normal morphology of the mitral and tricuspid valve, with the aorta wedged between them. The upper right picture is a similar view in an atrioventricular septal defect. Note the unwedged aorta, the trileaflet left atrioventricular valve, and the cleft between the superior and inferior bridging leaflets. The lower left picture is a specimen of an atrioventricular septal defect demonstrating the cleft. The lower right picture is an echo showing the cleft. AO = aorta; LA = left atrium; LAV = left atrioventricular valve; MV = mitral valve; PA = pulmonary artery; RAV = right atrioventricular valve; RV = right ventricle; TV = tricuspid valve.

more commonly in patients with heterotaxy and those with left-sided obstructive defects.

PATHOPHYSIOLOGY

Native. The pathophysiology of those with an isolated shunt at atrial level (commonly referred to as a *primum ASD*) is similar to that of a large secundum ASD, with unrestricted left-to-right shunting through the primum ASD, leading to right-sided atrial and ventricular volume overload. Chronic left AV valve regurgitation may produce left-sided ventricular and atrial volume overload. Complete AV septal defect has a greater degree of left-to-right shunting from the primum ASD as well as the nonrestrictive VSD, which triggers earlier left ventricular dilation as well as a greater degree of pulmonary hypertension.

After Correction. Residual significant left AV valve regurgitation may occur and cause significant left atrial as well as left ventricular dilation. Left AV valve stenosis from overzealous repair of the valve may also occur. The long, narrow left ventricular outflow tract of AV septal defect promotes left ventricular outflow tract obstruction and leads to subaortic stenosis in about 5 percent of patients.

NATURAL HISTORY. Patients with an isolated primum ASD have a course similar to that of those with large secundum ASDs, although symptoms may appear sooner when significant left AV valve regurgitation is present. Patients are usually asymptomatic until their third or fourth decade, but progressive symptoms related to congestive heart failure, atrial arrhythmias, complete heart block, and variable degrees of pulmonary hypertension develop in virtually all of them by the fifth decade.[93,94]

Most patients with complete AV septal defect have had surgical repair in infancy. Infants present with dyspnea, congestive heart failure, and failure to thrive. When presenting unrepaired, most adults have established pulmonary vascular disease. Patients with Down syndrome have a propensity to develop pulmonary hypertension at an even earlier age than do other patients with AV septal defect.

CLINICAL ISSUES

Down Syndrome. Down syndrome occurs in 35 percent of patients with AV septal defect. These patients more commonly have a complete AV septal defect with a common AV valve orifice and a large associated VSD. They often present in infancy with pulmonary hypertension. Clinical features are cardiomegaly, a right ventricular heave, and a pulmonary outflow tract murmur. If there is associated AV valve regurgitation, there is a pansystolic murmur.

Non-Down Syndrome. Clinical presentation depends on the presence and size of the ASD and the VSD and on the competence of the left AV valve. A large left-to-right shunt gives rise to symptoms of heart failure (exertional dyspnea or fatigue) or pulmonary vascular disease (exertional syncope, cyanosis). In adulthood, palpitations from atrial arrhythmias are common. Cardiac findings on physical examination for patients with an isolated shunt at atrial level are similar to those of patients with secundum ASD, with the important addition of a prominent left ventricular apex and pansystolic murmur when significant left AV valve regurgitation is present. Cases with a primum ASD and a restrictive VSD have similar findings, but with the addition of a pansystolic VSD murmur heard best at the left sternal border. Complete AV septal defects have a single S_1 (common AV valve), a mid-diastolic murmur from augmented AV valve inflow, and findings of pulmonary hypertension and/or a right-to-left shunt.

LABORATORY INVESTIGATIONS

ECG. Most patients have first-degree AV block and left axis deviation. Complete AV block and/or atrial fibrillation/flutter can be present in older patients. Partial or complete right bundle branch block is usually associated with right ventricular dilation or prior surgery.

Chest Radiography. If unrepaired, this demonstrates cardiomegaly with right atrial and right ventricular prominence with increased pulmonary vascular markings. In those cases with a small interatrial communication and left AV valve regurgitation, there is cardiomegaly due to left ventricular enlargement and normal pulmonary vascular markings. Findings of Eisenmenger syndrome are also possible. When repaired, the study may be normal with sternal wires.

Echocardiography. This has replaced angiography in assessing virtually all cases with AV septal defect.[72,90,91] The cardinal and common features discussed in the morphology section are readily recognized by echocardiography. In the four-chamber view the AV valve(s) appear at the same level, irrespective of the presence or absence of a VSD. The typical inferior ASD and the posteriorly positioned VSD will be sought. The degree of associated AV valve regurgitation, the left-to-right shunt from left ventricle to right atrium, and the estimated right ventricular systolic pressure should be assessed. When using the right AV valve to assess right ventricular pressure, care must be taken to ensure that the jet is not contaminated by an obligatory left ventricle-right atrial shunt.

Cardiac Catheterization. In general this technique has been replaced by echocardiography for the evaluation of patients with an AV septal defect. The one role it still has is in the evaluation of the patient who presents late and may have associated pulmonary vascular disease.

Open-Lung Biopsy. This should be considered only when the reversibility of pulmonary hypertension is uncertain from the hemodynamic data.

INDICATIONS FOR INTERVENTION. The patient with an unoperated or newly diagnosed AV septal defect and significant hemodynamic defects requires surgical repair. Equally, patients with persistent left AV valve regurgitation (or stenosis from previous repair) causing symptoms, atrial arrhythmia or deterioration in ventricular function, or patients with significant subaortic obstruction (a gradient ≥50 mm Hg at rest) require surgical intervention.[83]

In the presence of severe pulmonary hypertension (pulmonary artery pressure > ⅔ systemic blood pressure or pulmonary arteriolar resistance > ⅔ systemic arteriolar resistance), there must be a net left-to-right shunt of at least 1.5:1.0, evidence of pulmonary artery reactivity when challenged with a pulmonary vasodilator (e.g., oxygen, nitric oxide, and/or prostaglandins), or lung biopsy evidence that pulmonary arterial changes are potentially reversible (Heath-Edwards grade ≤ II-III) before surgical intervention can be carried out.

INTERVENTIONAL OPTIONS AND OUTCOMES

Isolated Shunt at Atrial Level (Primum Atrial Septal Defect). Pericardial patch closure of the primum ASD with concomitant suture (with or without annuloplasty) of the "cleft" left AV valve is usually performed. When left AV valve repair is not possible, replacement may be necessary. In the short term, the results of repair of partial AV septal defect are similar to those following closure of secundum ASD,[95-97] but sequelae of left AV ("mitral") valve regurgitation,[96-101] subaortic stenosis[102,103] and AV block may develop or progress.

Complete Atrial Septal Defect. The "staged approach" (pulmonary artery banding followed by intracardiac repair) has been supplanted by primary intracardiac repair in infancy. The goals of intracardiac repair are ventricular and atrial septation with adequate mitral and tricuspid reconstruction. Both single- and double-patch techniques[104] to close ASDs and VSDs have been described with comparable results. Occasionally, left AV valve replacement is necessary when valve repair is not possible. The long-term results of repair of complete AV septal defect are not well known, but similar problems as with partial AV septal defect are likely.

REPRODUCTIVE ISSUES. Pregnancy is well tolerated in patients with complete repair and no significant residual lesions. Women in NYHA Classes I and II with unoperated isolated primum ASD usually tolerate pregnancy very well. Pregnancy is contraindicated in Eisenmenger syndrome because of the high maternal (≤50 percent) and fetal (≤60 percent) mortality.

FOLLOW-UP ISSUES. All patients require periodic follow-up by an expert cardiologist because of the possibility of the postoperative complications, which include patch dehiscence or residual septal defects (1 percent), the development of complete heart block (3 percent), late atrial fibrillation/flutter, left AV valve dysfunction,[96-101] and subaortic stenosis.[102,103] Left AV valve regurgitation requires reoperation in at least 10 percent of patients.[105] Subaortic stenosis develops or progresses in 5 to 10 percent of patients after repair, particularly in patients with primum ASD, especially if the left AV ("mitral") valve has been replaced. Particular attention should be paid to those patients with pulmonary hypertension preoperatively.[106] Antibiotic prophylaxis is needed in most patients after repair, given the common occurrence of residual "mitral" regurgitation.

Isolated Ventricular Septal Defect

MORPHOLOGY. The ventricular septum can be divided into three major components—inlet, trabecular, and outlet—all abutting on a small membranous septum lying just underneath the aortic valve. VSDs (Fig. 56–6) are classified into three main categories according to their location and margins (Fig. 56–7). *Muscular* VSDs are bordered entirely by myocardium and can be trabecular, inlet, or outlet in location. *Membranous* VSDs often have inlet, outlet, or trabecular extension and are bordered in part by fibrous continuity between the leaflets of an AV valve and an arterial valve. *Doubly committed* subarterial VSDs are more common in Asian patients, are situated in the outlet septum, and are bordered by fibrous continuity of the aortic and pulmonary valves.[107] This section deals with VSDs occurring in isolation from major associated cardiac anomalies.

PATHOPHYSIOLOGY. A *restrictive* VSD is a defect that produces a significant pressure gradient between the left ventricle and the right ventricle (pulmonary/aortic systolic pressure ratio < 0.3) and is accompanied by a small (<1.4/1.0) shunt. A *moderately restrictive* VSD is accompanied by a moderate shunt (Qp/Qs = 1.4 to 2.2/1.0) with a pulmonary/aortic systolic pressure ratio less than 0.66. A large or *nonrestrictive* VSD is accompanied by a large shunt (Qp/Qs > 2.2) and a pulmonary/aortic systolic pressure ratio greater than

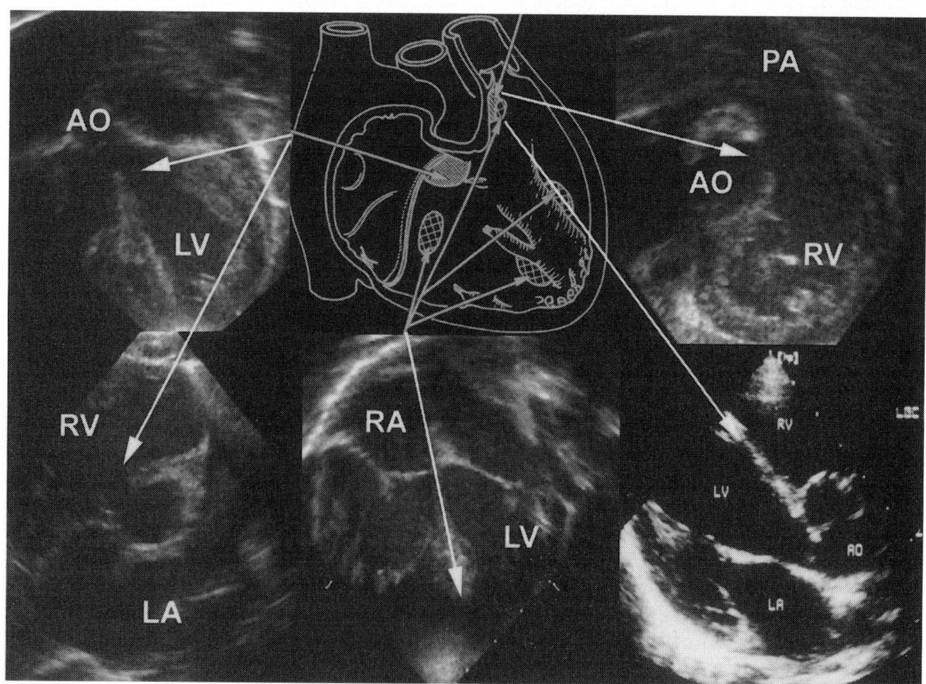

FIGURE 56–6 Montage of the different types of ventricular septal defects. The central diagram outlines the location of the various types of defects as seen from the right ventricle. The two left images show a perimembranous ventricular septal defect as seen in the five-chamber and short-axis views. Note the defect is roofed by the aorta and is next to the tricuspid valve. The bottom middle echocardiogram is a muscular apical defect. The upper right image is a right anterior oblique view in a doubly committed ventricular septal defect. The lower right is a short-axis view showing an outlet ventricular septal defect with prolapse of the right coronary cusp. AO = aorta; LV = left ventricle; PA = pulmonary artery; RA = right atrium; RV = right ventricle.

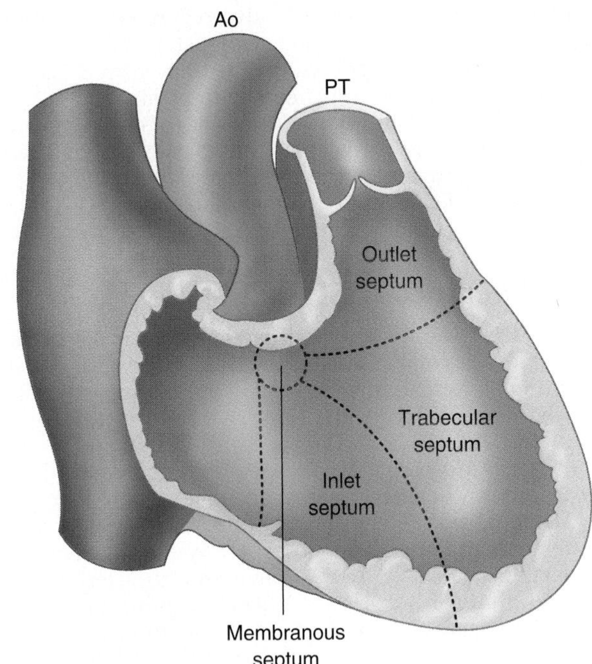

FIGURE 56–7 Four components of the ventricular septum shown here from the right ventricular aspect are now described by Anderson and associates as inlet and outlet components of the right ventricle because these areas do not correspond to septal structures as initially suggested. Ao = aorta; PT = pulmonary trunk. (Modified from Anderson RH, Becker AE, Lucchese E, et al: Morphology of Congenital Heart Disease. Baltimore, University Park Press, 1983.)

0.66. An *Eisenmenger VSD* has a systolic pressure ratio of 1.0 and Qp/Qs less than 1:1, a net right-to-left shunt.[83]

NATURAL HISTORY. A *restrictive* VSD does not cause significant hemodynamic derangement[108] and may close spontaneously during childhood and sometimes in adult life. Small VSDs pose an ongoing and relatively high risk of endocarditis. A perimembranous defect in an immediately subaortic position, or any doubly committed VSD, may be associated with progressive aortic regurgitation.[109] Late development of subaortic and subpulmonary stenosis (see double-chambered right ventricle) as well as the formation of a left ventricular to right atrial shunt all are well described and should be excluded at follow-up.[110] A *moderately restrictive* VSD imposes a hemodynamic burden on the left ventricle, which leads to left atrial and ventricular dilation and dysfunction as well as a variable increase in pulmonary vascular resistance. A large or nonrestrictive VSD features left ventricular volume overload early in life with a progressive rise in pulmonary artery pressure and a fall in left-to-right shunting. In turn, this leads to higher pulmonary vascular resistance and to Eisenmenger syndrome.

CLINICAL FEATURES

Pediatrics. Neonatal presentation with a murmur is increasingly frequent. Most of these patients have a restrictive defect, the murmur becoming apparent only as the pulmonary vascular resistance falls. Paradoxically, those infants with large nonrestrictive defects tend to present later. This is because equalization of pressures across the defect obviates the generation of a pansystolic murmur. Instead, pulmonary blood flow increases progressively as the pulmonary vascular resistance falls. Presentation with breathlessness, congestive heart failure, and failure to thrive in the 2nd and 3rd months of life is usual. At that time a pulmonary ejection murmur and a mitral rumble may be heard, reflecting increased pulmonary flow and pulmonary venous return. Cyanosis is rare in early childhood, and if present, other causes of a raised pulmonary vascular resistance should be excluded (e.g., mitral stenosis or coexisting lung pathology).

Medical management of the symptomatic infant is directed at improving symptoms prior to surgery, or "buying time" while spontaneous closure, or diminution in size, occurs. Treatment with diuretics is universally accepted, and increasingly, the successful use of ACE inhibition is being reported.

Adults. Most adult patients with a small *restrictive* VSD are asymptomatic. Physical examination reveals a harsh or high frequency pansystolic murmur, usually grade 3 to 4/6, heard with maximal intensity at the left sternal border in the 3rd or 4th intercostal space. Patients with a *moderately restrictive* VSD often present with dyspnea in adult life perhaps triggered by atrial fibrillation. Physical examination typically reveals a displaced cardiac apex with a similar pansystolic murmur as well as an apical diastolic rumble and third heart sound at the apex from the increased flow through the mitral valve. Patients with large *nonrestrictive* Eisenmenger VSDs present with central cyanosis and clubbing of the nail beds. Signs of pulmonary hypertension—a right ventricular heave, palpable and loud P_2, and a right-sided S_4—are typically present. A pulmonary ejection click, a soft and scratchy systolic ejection murmur, and a high-pitched decrescendo diastolic murmur of pulmonary regurgitation (Graham Steell) may be audible. Peripheral edema usually reflects right-sided heart failure.

LABORATORY INVESTIGATIONS

ECG. The ECG mirrors the size of the shunt and the degree of pulmonary hypertension. Small, *restrictive* VSDs usually produce a normal tracing. *Moderate*-sized VSDs produce a broad notched P wave characteristic of left atrial overload as well as evidence of left ventricular volume overload, namely deep Q and tall R waves with tall T waves in leads V_5 and V_6, and perhaps eventually atrial fibrillation. Following repair, the ECG is usually normal with right bundle branch block.

Chest Radiography. The chest radiograph reflects the magnitude of the shunt as well as the degree of pulmonary hypertension. A *moderate*-sized shunt causes signs of left ventricular dilation with some pulmonary plethora.

Echocardiography. Transthoracic echocardiography can identify the location, size, and hemodynamic consequences of the VSD as well as any associated lesions (aortic regurgitation, right ventricular outflow tract obstruction, or left ventricular outflow tract obstruction).

Cardiac Catheterization. Cardiac catheterization may be required when the hemodynamic significance of a VSD is questioned or when assessment of pulmonary artery pressures and resistances is needed. In some centers therapeutic catheterization is performed for percutaneous closure (see later).

INDICATIONS FOR INTERVENTION. The presence of a significant VSD (the symptomatic patient shows a Qp/Qs > 1.5/1.0; pulmonary artery systolic pressure > 50 mm Hg; increased LV and LA size, or deteriorating left ventricular function) in the absence of irreversible pulmonary hypertension warrants surgical closure. If severe pulmonary hypertension (see ASD section) is present, closure is seldom feasible. Other relative indications for VSD closure include the presence of a perimembranous or outlet VSD with more than mild aortic regurgitation[111] and a history of recurrent endocarditis.

In children, the presence of a nonrestrictive VSD, or a smaller VSD with significant symptoms failing to respond to medication, are indications for surgical or device closure. Elective surgery is usually performed between 3 and 9 months of age. Some patients have pulmonary hypertension. If pulmonary arteriolar resistance is less than 7 Wood units, closure can be safely undertaken if there is a net left-to-right shunt of at least 1.5/1.0, strong evidence of pulmonary reactivity when challenged with a pulmonary vasodilator (oxygen, nitric oxide), or lung biopsy evidence that pulmonary artery changes are reversible (rarely required).

INTERVENTIONAL OPTIONS AND OUTCOMES

Surgery. Surgical closure by direct suture or with a patch has been used for more than 50 years with a low perioperative mortality—even in adults—and a very high closure rate. VSDs should be closed by congenital heart surgeons. Patch leaks are not uncommon but seldom need reoperation.

Device Closure. Successful transcatheter device closure of trabecular (muscular) and perimembranous VSDs has recently been reported. Trabecular VSDs have proven more amenable to this technique because of their relatively straightforward anatomy and muscular rim to which the device attaches well. The closure of perimembranous VSDs is technically more challenging due to its proximity to valve structures and requires careful patient selection.[112] It should be performed only in centers with appropriate expertise. No long-term follow-up is available.

REPRODUCTIVE ISSUES. Pregnancy is well tolerated in women with small or moderate VSD and in women with repaired VSDs. Pregnancy is contraindicated in Eisenmenger syndrome because of high maternal (≤50 percent) and fetal (≤60 percent) mortality.

FOLLOW-UP ISSUES. For patients with good to excellent functional class and good left ventricular function prior to surgical closure, life expectancy after surgical correction is close to normal. The risk of progressive aortic regurgitation is reduced after surgery, as is the risk of endocarditis, unless a residual VSD persists. Yearly cardiac evaluation is suggested for patients with right ventricular outflow tract obstruction, left ventricular outflow tract obstruction, and aortic regurgitation not undergoing surgical repair; patients with Eisenmenger syndrome; and adults with significant atrial or ventricular arrhythmias. Cardiac surveillance is also recommended for patients who had late repair of moderate or large defects, which are often associated with left ventricular impairment and elevated pulmonary artery pressure at the time of surgery.

Patent Ductus Arteriosus

MORPHOLOGY. The ductus arteriosus derives from the left sixth primitive aortic arch and connects the proximal left pulmonary artery to the descending aorta, just distal to the left subclavian artery.[113]

PATHOPHYSIOLOGY. The ductus is widely patent in the normal fetus, carrying unoxygenated blood from the right ventricle through the descending aorta to the placenta, where the blood is oxygenated. Functional closure of the ductus from vasoconstriction occurs shortly after a term birth, whereas anatomical closure from intimal proliferation and fibrosis takes several weeks to complete. Some patients have "ductus-dependent" physiology as neonates. This means their circulation is dependent on the ductus for pulmonary blood flow such as in severe aortic coarctation, hypoplastic left heart syndrome, and sometimes D-TGA. If spontaneous closure of the ductus occurs in such neonates, clinical deterioration and death usually follow.

Isolated PDAs, the subject of this section, are often categorized according to the degree of left-to-right shunting, which is determined by both the size and length of the duct and the difference between systemic and pulmonary vascular resistances, as follows:

- Silent: tiny PDA detected only by nonclinical means (usually echo)
- Small: continuous murmur common; Qp/Qs < 1.5:1.0
- Moderate: continuous murmur common; Qp/Qs = 1.5 to 2.2:1.0
- Large: Qp/Qs > 2.2:1.0
- Eisenmenger: continuous murmur absent; substantial pulmonary hypertension, differential hypoxemia, and differential cyanosis

NATURAL HISTORY

Premature Infants. Patency of a ductus arteriosus is common in a preterm infant who lacks the normal mechanisms for postnatal ductal closure because of immaturity. A PDA is thus an expected finding in a premature infant, and delayed spontaneous closure of the ductus may be anticipated if the infant does not succumb to other problems.

Full-Term Infant. In a full-term newborn, patency of a ductus is a true congenital malformation. Occasionally, some full-term newborns have persistent patency of the ductus arteriosus because their relative hypoxemia contributes to vasodilation of the channel. This includes infants born at high altitude; those with congenital malformations causing hypoxemia; or malformations in which ductal flow supplies the systemic circulation, such as hypoplastic left heart syndrome, interrupted aortic arch, or aortic coarctation.

Children and Adults. Children and adults with *silent* PDAs are detected by nonclinical means, usually echocardiography, and face virtually no long-term complications. An exception occurs if the patient's murmur is inaudible because of obesity or other somatic factors. A *small* ductus accompanied by a small shunt does not cause a significant hemodynamic derangement but may predispose to endarteritis, especially when a murmur is present. A *moderate-sized* duct and shunt pose a volume load on the left atrium and ventricle with resultant left ventricular dilation and dysfunction and perhaps eventual atrial fibrillation. A *large* duct results initially in left ventricular volume overload but develops a progressive rise in pulmonary artery pressures and eventually irreversible pulmonary vascular changes by 2 years of age (Eisenmenger syndrome).

CLINICAL FEATURES

Premature Infants. Most preterm infants with a birth weight less than 1500 gm have a PDA, and about one-third have a large enough shunt to cause significant cardiopulmonary deterioration. Clinical findings in these patients include bounding peripheral pulses, an infraclavicular and interscapular systolic murmur (occasionally a continuous murmur), precordial hyperactivity, hepatomegaly, and either multiple episodes of apnea and bradycardia or ventilator dependence.

Full-Term Infants, Children, and Adults. A *small* audible duct usually causes no symptoms but may rarely present as an endovascular infection. Physical examination may reveal a grade 1 or 2 continuous murmur peaking in late systole and best heard in the 1st or 2nd left intercostal space. Patients with a *moderate-sized* duct may present with dyspnea or palpitations from atrial arrhythmias. A louder continuous or "machinery" murmur in the 1st or 2nd left intercostal space is typically accompanied by a wide systemic pulse pressure from aortic diastolic runoff into the pulmonary trunk and signs of left ventricular volume overload, such as a displaced left ventricular apex and sometimes a left-sided S_3 (meaningful in adults only). With a moderate degree of pulmonary hypertension, the diastolic component of the murmur disappears, leaving a systolic murmur. Adults with a *large* uncorrected PDA eventually present with a short systolic ejection murmur, hypoxemia in the feet more than the hands (differential cyanosis), and Eisenmenger physiology.

LABORATORY INVESTIGATIONS IN PREMATURE INFANTS

ECG. This may be normal or demonstrate right or left ventricular hypertrophy or both, depending on the amount of left-to-right shunting and the degree of associated pulmonary hypertension.

Chest Radiography. This may demonstrate cardiomegaly and increased pulmonary vascular markings that may be difficult to interpret in the setting of hyaline membrane disease.

Echocardiography. This is the key to diagnosis. The ductus arteriosus can be imaged in its entirety and its size estimated. Doppler demonstrates the shunt and permits an accurate assessment of mean pulmonary artery pressure. This is achieved from calculating the mean left-to-right spectral trace and subtracting it from the mean blood pressure. Measurements of the left atrial and left ventricular size provide indirect evidence of the magnitude of left-to-right shunting.

LABORATORY INVESTIGATIONS IN FULL-TERM INFANTS, CHILDREN, AND ADULTS

ECG. The ECG reflects the size and degree of shunting occurring through the duct. A *small* duct produces a normal ECG. A *moderate* duct may show left ventricular volume overload with broad, notched P waves together with deep Q waves, tall R waves, and peaked T waves in V_5 and V_6. A *large* duct produces findings of right ventricular hypertrophy.

Chest Radiography. A *small* duct produces a normal chest radiograph. A *moderate*-sized duct causes moderate cardiomegaly with left-sided heart enlargement, a prominent aortic knuckle, and increased pulmonary perfusion. Ring calcification of the ductus may be seen through the soft tissue density of the aortic arch or pulmonary trunk in older adults. The large PDA produces an Eisenmenger appearance with a prominent aortic knuckle.

Echocardiography. This determines the presence, size, and degree of shunting and the physiological consequences of the shunt. The PDA is seen with difficulty in an Eisenmenger context. A bubble study shows the communication.

INDICATIONS FOR INTERVENTION

Premature Infants. Treatment of preterm infants with a PDA varies with the magnitude of shunting and the severity of hyaline membrane disease because the ductus may contribute importantly to mortality in infants with respiratory distress syndrome. Intervention in an asymptomatic infant with a small left-to-right shunt is unnecessary because the PDA almost invariably undergoes spontaneous closure. Those infants who demonstrate unmistakable signs of a significant ductal left-to-right shunt during the course of the respiratory distress syndrome are often unresponsive to medical measures to control congestive heart failure and require closure of the PDA to survive. These infants are best treated by pharmacological inhibition of prostaglandin synthesis with indomethacin or ibuprofen to constrict and close the ductus.[114] Surgical ligation is required in the estimated 10 percent of infants who are unresponsive to indomethacin.

Full-Term Infants. In the clinical settings in which the ductus preserves pulmonary blood flow, the inevitable spontaneous closure of the vessel is associated with profound clinical deterioration and often death. Undesirable ductal closure may be reversed medically within the first 4 or 5 days of life by an infusion of prostaglandin E_1. By dilating the constricted ductus arteriosus, a temporary increase should occur in arterial blood oxygen tension and saturation and correction of acidemia.

Children and Adults. Closure of an isolated, clinically detectable PDA, in the absence of irreversible pulmonary hypertension, is often recommended. There is no debate about the desirability of closing a hemodynamically important PDA. There is debate about closing a PDA strictly to reduce the risk of endarteritis. The risk of endarteritis in a patient with a silent PDA is considered negligible, and closure of such ducts is seldom recommended for that reason. In the presence of severe pulmonary hypertension (see ASD section), closure is seldom indicated. Contraindications to ductal closure include irreversible pulmonary hypertension or active endarteritis.[83]

INTERVENTIONAL OPTIONS AND OUTCOMES

Transcatheter Treatment (Fig. 56–8). Over the past 20 years, the efficacy and safety of transcatheter device closure for ducts smaller than 8 mm have been established with complete ductal closure achieved in more than 85 percent of patients by 1 year following device placement at a mortality rate of less than 1 percent.[115] In centers with appropriate resources and experience, transcatheter device occlusion should be the method of choice for ductal closure.[115,116]

Surgical Treatment. Surgical closure, by ductal ligation and/or division, has been performed for more than 50 years with a marginally greater closure rate than device closure but somewhat greater morbidity and mortality. Immediate clinical closure (no shunt audible on physical examination) is achieved in more than 95 percent of patients. Surgical closure is a low-risk procedure in children. Surgical mortality in adults is 1.0 to 3.5 percent and relates to the presence of pulmonary arterial hypertension and difficult ductal morphology (calcified or aneurysmal) often seen in adults. Surgical closure should be reserved for those in whom the PDA is too large for device closure or at centers without access to device closure.

REPRODUCTIVE ISSUES. Pregnancy is well tolerated in women with silent and small PDA or in patients who were asymptomatic prior to pregnancy. In the woman with a hemodynamically important PDA, pregnancy may precipitate or worsen heart failure. Pregnancy is contraindicated in Eisenmenger syndrome because of the high maternal (≤50 percent) and fetal (≤60 percent) mortality.

FOLLOW-UP ISSUES. Patients with device occlusion or after surgical closure should be examined periodically for possible recanalization. Silent residual shunts may be found by transthoracic echocardiography.[117] The risk of late endarteritis from a clinically silent residual shunt after device implantation or surgical closure is low, and the need for endocarditis prophylaxis in such patients is uncertain. Endocarditis prophylaxis is recommended for 6 months following PDA device closure or for life if any residual defect persists.

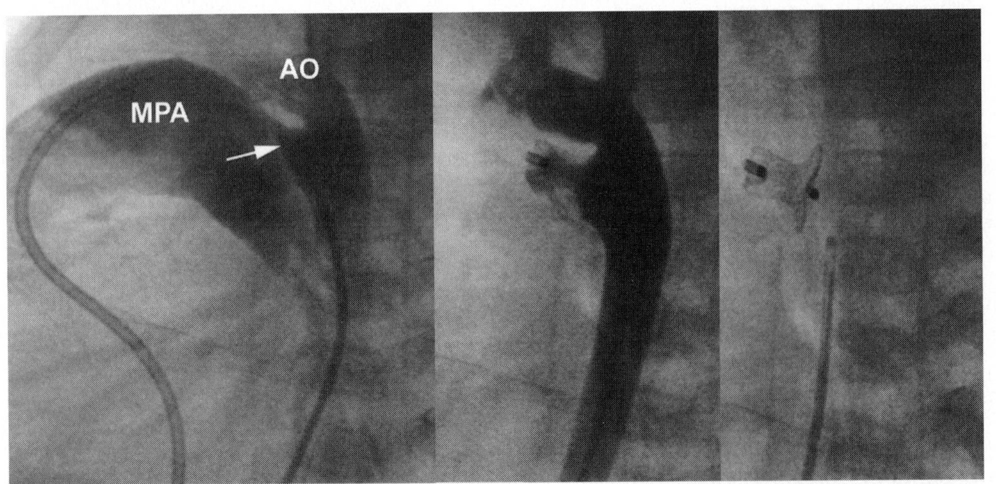

FIGURE 56–8 Montage of a patent arterial duct, before and after device occlusion. AO = aorta; MPA = main pulmonary artery.

Patients with a silent PDA probably do not require endocarditis prophylaxis or follow-up.

Persistent Truncus Arteriosus

MORPHOLOGY. Persistent truncus arteriosus is an anomaly in which a single vessel forms the outlet of both ventricles and gives rise to the systemic, pulmonary, and coronary arteries. It is always accompanied by a VSD, and frequently with a right-sided aortic arch. The truncal valve is usually tricuspid but is quadricuspid in about one-third of patients. Truncal valve regurgitation and truncal valve stenosis are each seen in 10 to 15 percent of patients. There can be a single coronary artery.

Truncus malformations can be classified either anatomically according to the mode of origin of pulmonary vessels from the common trunk or from a functional point of view, based on the magnitude of blood flow to the lungs. In the common type (type I) of truncus arteriosus, a partially separate pulmonary trunk of variable length exists and gives rise to left and right pulmonary arteries. In type II, each pulmonary artery arises separately but close to the other from the posterior aspect of the truncus. In type III, each pulmonary artery arises from the lateral aspect of the truncus. Less commonly, one pulmonary artery branch may be absent, with aortopulmonary collateral arteries supplying the lung that does not receive a pulmonary artery branch from the truncus.

PATHOPHYSIOLOGY. Pulmonary blood flow is governed by the size of the pulmonary arteries and the pulmonary vascular resistance. In infancy, pulmonary blood flow is usually excessive because pulmonary vascular resistance is not greatly increased. Thus, in the neonate, only minimal cyanosis is present. With time, pulmonary vascular resistance increases, relieving the left ventricular volume load but at the price of increasing cyanosis. When pulmonary vascular resistance reaches systemic levels, Eisenmenger physiology and bidirectional shunting occur. Significant truncal valve regurgitation produces a volume load on both right and left ventricles because of the biventricular origin of the truncal artery.

NATURAL HISTORY. Most deaths from congestive heart failure occur before 1 year of age. Unoperated patients who survive past 1 year most likely present with established pulmonary hypertension. The prevalence of truncal valve regurgitation increases with age, causing biventricular heart failure and increasing susceptibility to endocarditis.

CLINICAL FEATURES

Pediatrics. Infants with truncus arteriosus usually present with mild cyanosis coexisting with the cardiac findings of a large left-to-right shunt. This is the result of excessive pulmonary blood flow due to a low pulmonary vascular resistance. Symptoms of heart failure and poor physical development usually appear in the first weeks or months of life. The most frequent physical findings include cardiomegaly, collapsing peripheral pulses, a loud single second heart sound, a harsh systolic murmur preceded by an ejection click, and a low-pitched mid-diastolic rumbling murmur and bounding pulses. A decrescendo diastolic murmur suggests associated truncal valve regurgitation.

DiGeorge syndrome may be seen with truncus arteriosus. Facial dysmorphism, a high incidence of extracardiac malformations (particularly of the limbs, kidneys, and intestine), atrophy or absence of the thymus gland, T-lymphocyte deficiency, and a predilection to infection also may be features of the clinical presentation.

The physical findings are different if pulmonary blood flow is restricted by a high pulmonary vascular resistance: Cyanosis is prominent, and only a short systolic murmur may be heard in association with an ejection click. Pulmonary vascular obstruction usually does not restrict pulmonary blood flow before 1 year of age.

Adults. Adults presenting with an unrepaired truncus arteriosus have Eisenmenger syndrome and its typical findings.

LABORATORY INVESTIGATIONS (UNREPAIRED)

ECG. This demonstrates biventricular hypertrophy with strain as the pulmonary resistance rises.

Chest Radiography. This demonstrates cardiomegaly with prominent pulmonary arterial markings and by unusually high hilar areas. A right aortic arch occurs in 50 percent of cases.

Echocardiography (Fig. 56–9). In most cases, 2D echocardiography provides a complete diagnosis. The study should demonstrate the overriding truncal root, the origin of the pulmonary arteries, the number of truncal cusps, the origin of the coronary arteries, the functional status of the truncal valve, and VSD size.

Cardiac Catheterization and Angiography. This is rarely necessary and in fact carries a risk of both morbidity and mortality. In general, significant arterial desaturation in the absence of branch pulmonary artery stenosis indicates that the lesion cannot be repaired.

INDICATIONS FOR INTERVENTION. Early surgical intervention is indicated in all cases within the first 2 months of life. In the presence of severe pulmonary hypertension (see ASD section), surgical intervention is usually not performed.

INTERVENTIONAL OPTIONS AND OUTCOMES. Operation consists of closure of the VSD, leaving the aorta arising from the left ventricle; excision of the pulmonary arteries from their truncus origin; and a valve-containing prosthetic conduit or aortic homograft valve conduit between the right ventricle and the pulmonary arteries to establish circulatory continuity.[118] Truncal valve insufficiency is a challenging problem and may require valve replacement or repair.[119]

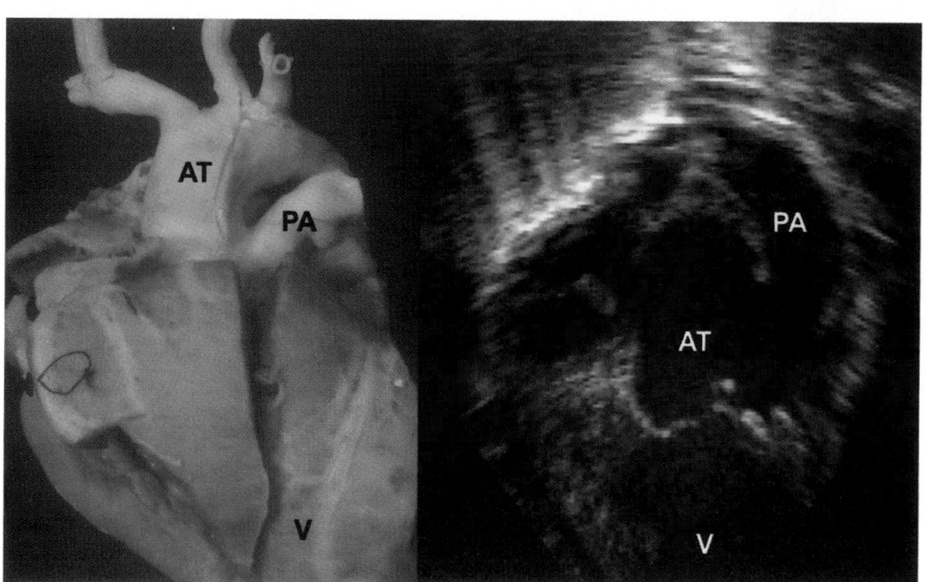

FIGURE 56–9 View of the origin of the pulmonary artery in truncus arteriosus. Note the lateral origin of the pulmonary artery. AT = ascending trunk; PA = pulmonary artery; V = ventricle.

Important risk factors for perioperative death are severe truncal valve regurgitation, interrupted aortic arch, coronary artery anomalies, and age at operation older than 100 days. Patients with only one pulmonary artery are especially prone to early development of severe pulmonary vascular disease.

REPRODUCTIVE ISSUES. Patients with a repaired truncus arteriosus and no hemodynamically important residual lesions should tolerate pregnancy well. Patients with significant conduit obstruction and/or important truncal valve regurgitation need prepregnancy counseling, with correction of the lesions prior to pregnancy and/or careful follow-up throughout pregnancy. Pregnancy is contraindicated in patients with Eisenmenger syndrome, given its 50 percent maternal mortality.

FOLLOW-UP ISSUES. Patients operated on early (<1 year of age) generally do well. However, conduit change is often indicated within the first few years after repair as the patient outgrows its size.[118] Those cases with significant truncal valve stenosis and/or regurgitation may eventually require truncal valve replacement. Patients operated on late (>1 year of age) require careful follow-up for any signs of pulmonary hypertension progression. Endocarditis prophylaxis is required in all patients.

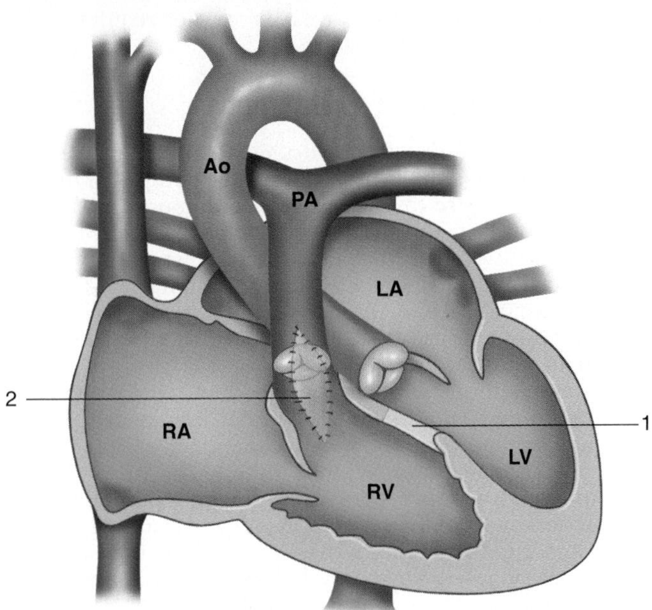

FIGURE 56–11 Diagrammatic representation of the surgical repair of tetralogy of Fallot. 1, Patch closure of ventricular septal defect; 2, right ventricular outflow/main pulmonary artery outflow patch (transannular patch). RA = right atrium; RV = right ventricle; LA = left atrium; LV = left ventricle; Ao = aorta; PA = pulmonary artery. (From Mullins CE, Mayer DC: Congenital Heart Disease: A Diagrammatic Atlas. New York, Wiley-Liss, 1988.)

Cyanotic Heart Disease

Tetralogy of Fallot (Including Tetralogy with Pulmonary Atresia)

MORPHOLOGY (Figs. 56–10 and 56–11). The four components of tetralogy of Fallot are an outlet VSD, obstruction to right ventricular outflow, overriding of the aorta (< 50 percent), and right ventricular hypertrophy. The fundamental abnormality contributing to each of these features is anterior and cephalad deviation of the outlet septum, which is malaligned with respect to the trabecular septum. Tetralogy may also coexist with an AV septal defect. Right ventricular outflow tract obstruction is variable. There is often a stenotic, bicuspid pulmonary valve with supravalvular hypoplasia. The dominant site of obstruction is usually at the subvalve level. In some cases the outflow tract is atretic, and the heart can be diagnosed as having tetralogy of Fallot with pulmonary atresia (also known as *complex pulmonary atresia* when major aortopulmonary collateral arteries are present). The management and outcome for patients with major aortopulmonary collateral arteries are significantly different from those with less extreme forms of tetralogy and are discussed separately at the end of this section.

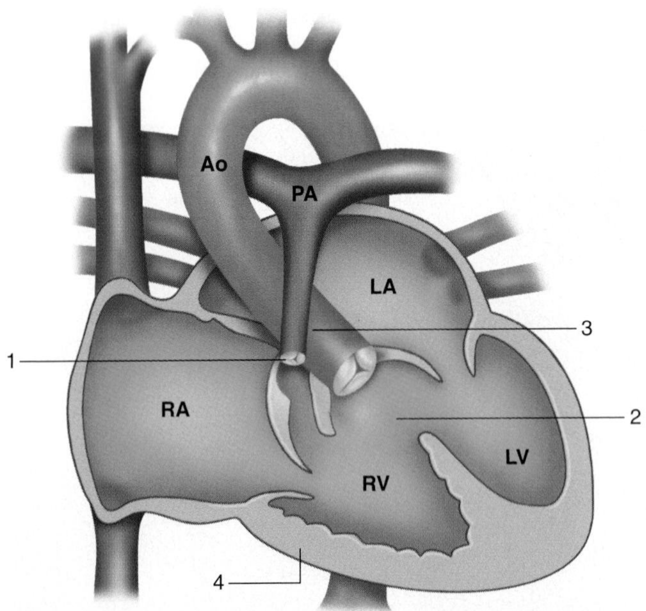

FIGURE 56–10 Diagrammatic representation of tetralogy of Fallot. 1, Pulmonary stenosis; 2, ventricular septal defect; 3, overriding aorta; 4, right ventricle hypertrophy. RA = right atrium; RV = right ventricle; LA = left atrium; LV = left ventricle; Ao = aorta; PA = pulmonary artery. (From Mullins CE, Mayer DC: Congenital Heart Disease: A Diagrammatic Atlas. New York, Wiley-Liss, 1988.)

Associated Anomalies. A right aortic arch occurs in about 25 percent of patients, and abnormalities of the course of the coronary arteries occur in approximately 5 percent. The most common anomaly is when the anterior descending artery originates from the right coronary artery and may course anteriorly to cross the infundibulum of the right ventricle. Absent pulmonary valve syndrome is a rare form of tetralogy in which stenosis and regurgitation of the right ventricular outflow tract is due to a markedly stenotic pulmonary valve ring with poorly formed or absent valve leaflets. The pulmonary arteries are markedly dilated or aneurysmal. This may produce airway compression at birth, a poor prognostic feature.

PATHOPHYSIOLOGY. In the absence of alternative sources of pulmonary blood flow, the degree of cyanosis reflects the severity of right ventricular outflow tract obstruction and the level of systemic vascular resistance. There is right-to-left shunting across the VSD. A tetralogy "spell" is an acute fall in arterial saturation and it may be life threatening. Its treatment is aimed at relieving obstruction and increasing (e.g., with norepinephrine) systemic resistance. Relief of hypoxic pain with morphine, intravenous propranolol, and systemic vasoconstriction (e.g., squatting) usually reverses the cyanosis.

NATURAL HISTORY. Progressive hypoxemia in the first years of life is expected. Survival to adult life is rare without palliation or correction. The presence of additional sources of blood supply (see later) modifies the rate of progression of cyanosis and its complications.

CLINICAL FEATURES

Unoperated Patients. There is variable cyanosis. A right ventricular impulse and systolic thrill are often palpable along the left sternal border. An early systolic ejection sound that is aortic in origin may be heard at the lower left sternal border and apex; the second heart sound is usually single. The intensity and duration of the systolic ejection murmur vary inversely with the severity of obstruction—the opposite of the relation that exists in patients with pulmonary stenosis and an intact ventricular septum. With extreme outflow tract stenosis or pulmonary atresia and during an attack of paroxysmal hypoxemia, no murmur or only a very short, faint murmur may be detected. A continuous murmur faintly audible over the anterior or posterior chest reflects flow through enlarged bronchial collateral vessels.

After Surgery, Palliated. Progressive cyanosis with its complications can result from worsening right ventricular outflow tract obstruction, gradual stenosis and occlusion of palliative aortopulmonary shunts, or the development of pulmonary hypertension (sometimes seen after Waterston or Potts shunts). Progressive aortic dilation and aortic regurgitation are becoming increasingly recognized. Central cyanosis and clubbing are invariably present.

After Surgery, Repaired. After intracardiac repair more than 85 percent of patients are asymptomatic on follow-up,[120] although objective testing may demonstrate a marked reduction in maximal performance.[121] Palpitations from atrial and ventricular arrhythmias and exertional dyspnea from progressive right ventricular dilation secondary to chronic pulmonary regurgitation or severe residual right ventricular outflow tract obstruction occur in 10 to 15 percent of patients at 20 years after initial repair. An ascending aortic aneurysm and progressive aortic regurgitation from a dilated aortic root can also be present.[122] There may be a parasternal right ventricular lift and a soft and delayed P_2 with a low-pitched diastolic murmur from pulmonary regurgitation. A systolic ejection murmur from right ventricular outflow tract obstruction, a high-pitched diastolic murmur from aortic regurgitation, and a pansystolic murmur from a VSD patch leak can also be heard.

Tetralogy of Fallot with Pulmonary Atresia and Major Aortopulmonary Collateral Arteries. This subgroup represents one of the greatest challenges in CHD. The aim of unifocalization surgery is to amalgamate all the sources of pulmonary blood flow and to establish unobstructed right ventricular-to-pulmonary artery continuity while achieving a normal pulmonary artery pressure and a closed ventricular septum.[123] If an adequate number of segments can be unifocalized in an unobstructed fashion, then coincident intracardiac repair can be contemplated. When this is not possible, a combined interventional catheterization and surgical approach is required.[124] Balloon dilation and stenting of stenosed arteries and anastomoses can "rehabilitate" segmental supply and allow subsequent VSD closure, or if already closed, reduce right ventricular pressure.

LABORATORY INVESTIGATIONS

ECG. Right axis deviation with right ventricular and right atrial hypertrophy is common. In adults with repaired tetralogy of Fallot, a complete right bundle branch block following repair has been the rule. QRS width may reflect the degree of right ventricular dilation.[61,125] A QRS duration 180 milliseconds or longer is a risk factor for sustained ventricular tachycardia and sudden death.

Chest Radiography. Characteristically, there is a normal-sized boot-shaped heart (*coeur en sabot*) with prominence of the right ventricle and a concavity in the region of the underdeveloped right ventricular outflow tract and main pulmonary artery. The pulmonary vascular markings are typically diminished, and the aortic arch may be on the right side (25 percent). The ascending aorta is often prominent.

Echocardiography (Fig. 56–12). A complete diagnosis can usually be established by echo-Doppler alone. The study should identify the malaligned and nonrestrictive VSD and overriding aorta (<50 percent override) and the presence and degree of right ventricular outflow tract obstruction (infundibular, valvular, and/or pulmonary arterial stenosis). It is rare that any other investigations are required prior to corrective surgery. The exception to this rule is when there are additional sources of pulmonary blood flow. In patients with *repaired* tetralogy of Fallot, residual pulmonary stenosis and regurgitation, residual VSD, right and left ventricular sizes and function, aortic root size, and the degree of aortic regurgitation should be assessed.

Cardiac Catheterization and Angiocardiography. Although echocardiography, MRA, and fast CT may delineate the presence and proximal course of the pulmonary blood vessels, the preoperative assessment of tetralogy with pulmonary atresia with major aortopulmonary collateral arteries must include delineation of the arterial supply to both lungs by selective catheterization and angiography to show the course and segmental supply from the collateral arteries and central pulmonary arteries. Major aortopulmonary collateral arteries usually arise from the descending aorta at the level of the tracheal bifurcation.

MRI. The goals of MRI examination after tetralogy of Fallot repair include the quantitative assessment of left and particularly right ventricular volumes, stroke volumes and ejection fraction; imaging of the anatomy of the right ventricular outflow tract, the pulmonary arteries, the aorta and

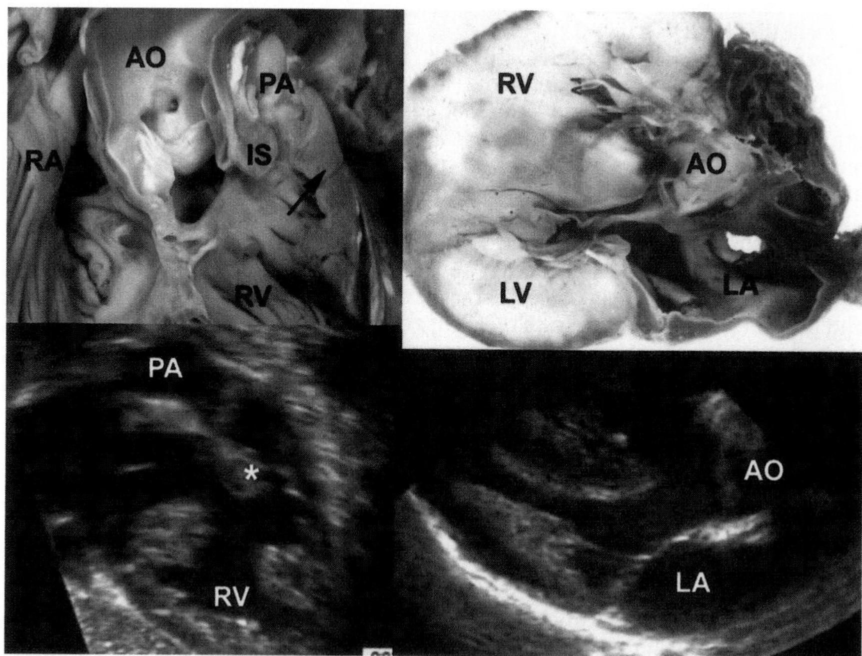

FIGURE 56–12 Montage of tetralogy of Fallot. The two left images are in the right anterior oblique view that demonstrates the anteriorly deviated infundibular septum and the ventricular septal defect. The arrow on the specimen points to the hypertrophied septoparietal trabeculations. The right images demonstrate the overriding aorta and the ventricular septal defect. AO = aorta; IS = infundibular septum; LA = left atrium; PA = pulmonary artery; RA = right atrium; RV = right ventricle.

aortopulmonary collaterals; and quantifying pulmonary, aortic, and tricuspid regurgitation.

INDICATIONS FOR INTERVENTION

Children. Symptomatic infants are now repaired at any age, and elective repair in asymptomatic infants during the first 6 months is advocated by many.[126,127] This is often at the expense of a transannular patch enlargement of the right ventricular outflow tract, which may be a risk factor for later failure. Marked hypoplasia of the pulmonary arteries, small body size, and prematurity are relative contraindications for early corrective operation, and these patients may be successfully palliated by balloon dilation of the right ventricular outflow tract and pulmonary arteries.

Adults, Unoperated. For unoperated adults, surgical repair is still recommended because the results are gratifying and the operative risk is comparable to pediatric series provided there is no serious coexisting morbidity.[128]

Palliated. Palliation was seldom intended as a permanent treatment strategy, and most of these patients should undergo surgical repair. In particular, palliated patients with increasing cyanosis and erythrocytosis (from gradual shunt stenosis or development of pulmonary hypertension), left ventricular dilation, or aneurysm formation in the shunt should undergo intracardiac repair with takedown of the shunt unless irreversible pulmonary hypertension has developed.

Repaired. The following situations *may* warrant intervention after repair: a residual VSD with a shunt greater than 1.5/1.0; residual pulmonary stenosis (either the native right ventricular outflow or valved conduit if one is present) with right ventricular pressure ⅔ or more of systemic pressure; or severe pulmonary regurgitation associated with substantial right ventricular dilation/dysfunction, exercise intolerance, or sustained arrhythmias.[83] The development of major cardiac arrhythmias, most commonly atrial flutter/fibrillation or sustained ventricular tachycardia, usually reflects hemodynamic deterioration and should be treated accordingly. Surgery is occasionally necessary for significant aortic regurgitation associated with symptoms and/or progressive left ventricular dilation and for aortic root enlargement of 55 mm or more. Rapid enlargement of a right ventricular outflow tract aneurysm needs surgical attention.

INTERVENTIONAL OPTIONS

Surgery. Reparative surgery involves closing the VSD with a Dacron patch and relieving the right ventricular outflow tract obstruction. The latter may involve resection of infundibular muscle, and insertion of a right ventricular outflow tract or transannular patch—a patch across the pulmonary valve annulus that disrupts the integrity of the pulmonary valve and causes important pulmonary regurgitation. When an anomalous coronary artery crosses the right ventricular outflow tract and precludes transection of the latter, an extracardiac conduit is placed between the right ventricle and pulmonary artery, bypassing the right ventricular outflow tract obstruction. A patent foramen ovale or secundum ASD is closed. Additional treatable lesions such as muscular VSDs, PDA, and aortopulmonary collaterals should also be addressed at the time of surgery.

Reoperation is necessary in 10 to 15 percent of patients after reparative surgery over a 20-year follow-up.[47] For persistent right ventricular outflow tract obstruction, resection of residual infundibular stenosis or placement of a right ventricular outflow or transannular patch, with or without pulmonary arterioplasty, can be performed. Occasionally, an extracardiac valved conduit may be necessary. Pulmonary valve replacement (either homograft or xenograft) is used to treat severe pulmonary regurgitation. Concomitant tricuspid valve annuloplasty may be performed for moderate or severe tricuspid regurgitation. Concomitant cryoablation should often be performed at the time of surgery for patients with either preexisting atrial or ventricular arrhythmias.[129]

Interventional. Significant branch pulmonary artery stenosis can be managed with balloon dilation and usually stent insertion. A catheter-delivered pulmonary bioprosthesis is being developed.

INTERVENTIONAL OUTCOMES. The overall survival of patients who have had initial operative repair is excellent, provided the VSD has been closed and the right ventricular outflow tract obstruction has been relieved. A 25-year survival of 94 percent has been reported.[130] Pulmonary valve replacement for chronic pulmonary regurgitation or right ventricular outflow tract obstruction after initial intracardiac repair can be done safely with a mortality rate of 1 percent.[131] Pulmonary valve replacement, when performed for significant pulmonary regurgitation, leads to an improvement in exercise tolerance as well as right ventricular dimension and function.[132] Sudden death can occur. Ventricular tachycardia can arise at the site of the right ventriculotomy, from VSD patch sutures, or from the right ventricular outflow tract. Patients at high risk for sudden death include those with right ventricular dilation and a QRS duration of 180 milliseconds or more on their ECG.[61] Moderate to severe left ventricular dysfunction is another risk factor for sudden death.[133] The reported incidence of sudden death is approximately 5 percent, which accounts for approximately one-third of late deaths over the first 20 years of follow-up.

FOLLOW-UP. All patients should have expert cardiology follow-up every 1 to 2 years.

Fontan Procedure–Requiring Lesions

The next four sections describe lesions usually or often treated with a Fontan procedure. These include tricuspid atresia, hypoplastic left heart syndrome, double-inlet ventricle, and isomerism. *Fontan procedure* has become a generic term to describe a palliative surgical procedure that redirects the systemic venous return directly to the pulmonary arteries without passing through a subpulmonary ventricle. It is performed in patients having a "functionally single" ventricle or when an intracardiac repair is not possible even though there are two good-sized ventricles. Although undoubtedly imperfect, the Fontan circuit restores an in-series pulmonary-to-systemic circulation, removing the chronic volume load of the systemic ventricle previously supporting a parallel circuit of pulmonary and systemic circulations. The earliest iteration of the Fontan procedure was a simple "atriopulmonary" connection, whereby the right atrium or its appendage was anastomosed to the pulmonary arteries. Because of the long-term problems of atrial dilation, arrhythmia, and thrombosis, this procedure has been abandoned in favor of hemodynamically superior versions. In the early 1990s the total cavopulmonary anastomosis was introduced. This consisted of a direct, end-to-side superior cavopulmonary anastomosis (bidirectional Glenn operation) in combination with an intraatrial baffle or tube connection of the inferior vena cava to the underside of the confluent pulmonary arteries. More recently the inferior vena cava has been directed to the pulmonary arteries via an extracardiac conduit, completely excluding the atrium from the circuit. It remains to be seen whether these modifications will have the desired effect of reducing late morbidity, and all patients will require regular and careful review in special centers.

Tricuspid Atresia (Absent Right Atrioventricular Connection)

MORPHOLOGY. *Classic tricuspid atresia* is best described as absence of the right AV connection (Figs. 56–13 and 56–14). Consequently, there must be an ASD. There is usually hypoplasia of the morphological right ventricle, which communicates to the dominant ventricle via a VSD. Patients may be subdivided into those with concordant ventriculoarterial connections and normally related great arteries (70 to 80 percent of cases) and those with discordant connections, where the aorta arises from the small right ventricle and is fed via the VSD. Associated lesions in the latter group include subaortic stenosis and aortic arch anomalies.

PATHOPHYSIOLOGY. The clinical picture and management are dominated by issues related to the ventriculoarterial connections. All patients have "mixing" of atrial blood, and their degree of cyanosis is governed by the amount of pulmonary blood flow. Patients with concordant ventriculoarterial connections tend to be more cyanosed (depending on the size of the VSD), whereas those with discordant connections are pinker and tend to develop heart failure (because the unobstructed pulmonary circulation arises directly from the left ventricle). Some present with a critical reduction of systemic blood flow, because of obstruction at the VSD and/or associated aortic arch anomalies, and behave much like hypoplastic left heart syndrome.

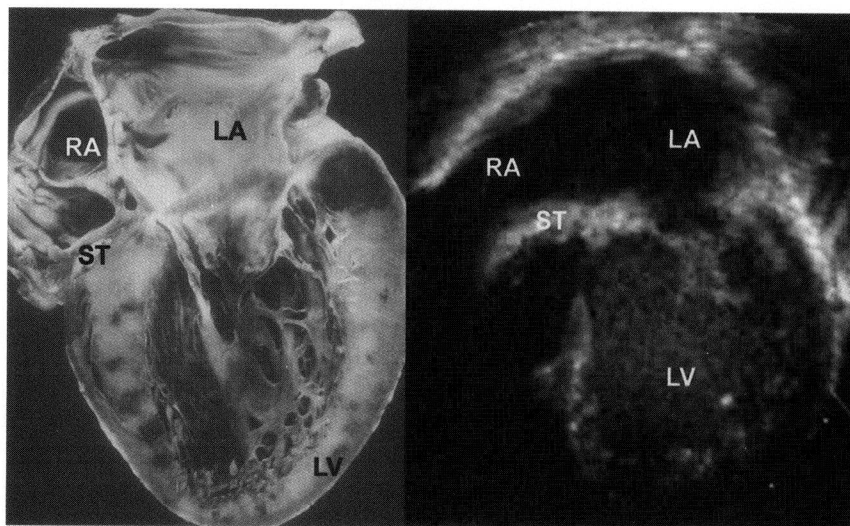

FIGURE 56–13 Apical four-chamber view in univentricular connection of left ventricular type with absent right connection (tricuspid atresia). Note the wedge of sulcus tissue in the floor of the right atrium. LA = left atrium; LV = left ventricle; RA = right atrium; ST = sulcus tissue.

LABORATORY INVESTIGATIONS

ECG. There is often left axis deviation, right atrial enlargement, and left ventricular hypertrophy. Left atrial enlargement may be present if pulmonary flow is high.

Chest Radiography. There is usually situs solitus, levocardia, and a left-sided aortic arch. The heart size and pulmonary vascular markings vary with the amount of pulmonary blood flow. The main pulmonary trunk is inapparent. There is a right aortic arch in 25 percent.

Echocardiogram. This establishes the full segmental diagnosis. The size of the ASD, VSD, and aortic arch all must be carefully assessed.

Cardiac Catheterization. This is rarely required for initial diagnosis or management. It can be useful to assess the degree of subaortic stenosis (by assessing the change in left ventricle-to-aortic pressure gradient while performing a dobutamine challenge) and is mandatory to measure the pulmonary artery pressure and resistance prior to venopulmonary connections.

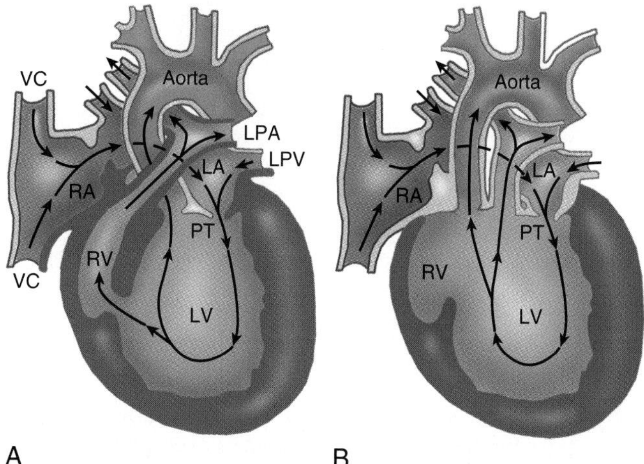

FIGURE 56–14 **A,** Tricuspid atresia with normally related great arteries, a small ventricular septal defect, diminutive right ventricular chamber, and narrowed outflow tract. **B,** An example of tricuspid atresia and complete transposition of the great arteries in which the left ventricular chamber is essentially a common ventricle, with the aorta arising from an infundibular component (RV) of the common ventricle. VC = vena cava; RA = right atrium; LA = left atrium; RV = right ventricle; LV = left ventricle; LPV = left pulmonary vein; LPA = left pulmonary artery; PT = pulmonary trunk. (**A** and **B,** Modified from Edwards JE, Burchell HB: Congenital tricuspid atresia: Classification. Med Clin North Am 33:1177, 1949.)

MANAGEMENT OPTIONS. In those with concordant ventriculoarterial connections and severe cyanosis, a systemic-to-pulmonary shunt is performed in the first 6 to 8 weeks of life, and in older children, a primary bidirectional Glenn procedure can be considered. In infants with discordant arterial connections, early palliation ranges from pulmonary artery banding to reduce pulmonary blood flow when there is no subaortic narrowing, to a full Norwood stage 1 procedure in those presenting with severe stenosis and a hypoplastic ascending aorta and arch.

The aim of early palliation is to prepare for a Fontan procedure. This should be performed only when there is good ventricular function, unobstructed systemic blood flow, and minimal AV valve regurgitation. Candidates for these corrective procedures must also have normal pulmonary vascular resistance and a low pulmonary resistance, a mean pulmonary artery pressure less than 15 mm Hg, and pulmonary arteries of adequate size.

Hypoplastic Left Heart Syndrome

DEFINITION. *Hypoplastic left heart syndrome* is a generic term used to describe a group of closely related cardiac anomalies characterized by underdevelopment of the left cardiac chambers, in association with atresia or stenosis of the aortic and/or the mitral orifices, and hypoplasia of the aorta. The term should be restricted to those with normally connected hearts with concordant AV and ventriculoarterial connections. Hypoplastic left heart syndrome (Fig. 56–15) is characterized by duct-dependent systemic blood flow and so tends to present with severe symptoms within the first week of life, as ductal constriction occurs. Untreated, the disease is almost uniformly fatal in infancy. In the past, many infants would present with severe acidemic circulatory collapse, but this is becoming less frequent as fetal ultrasound screening for cardiac anomalies becomes more generally available and successful. Fetal diagnosis allows for a planned delivery and institution of prostaglandin therapy from birth and has now been proven to reduce subsequent preoperative morbidity

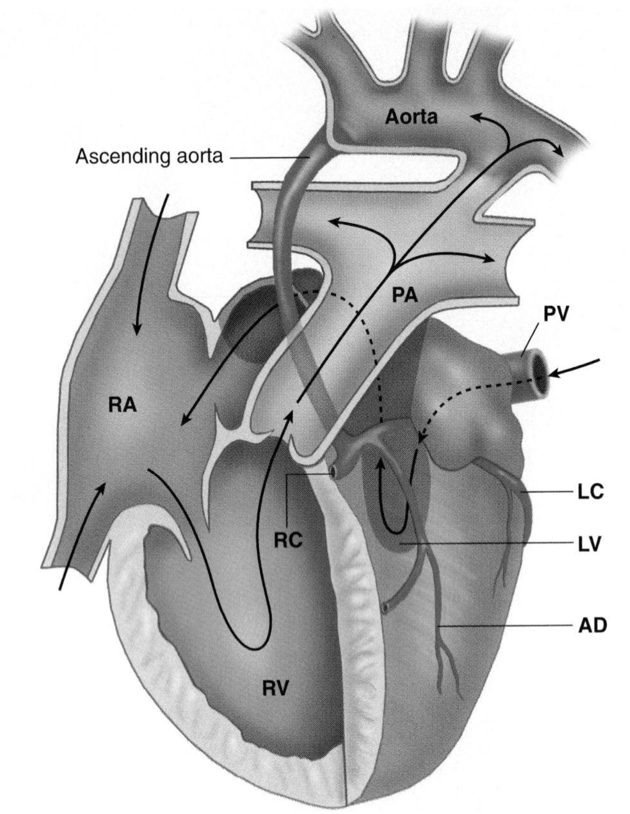

FIGURE 56–15 Hypoplastic left heart with aortic hypoplasia, aortic valve atresia, and a hypoplastic mitral valve and left ventricle. AD = anterior descending; RA = right atrium; RV = right ventricle; RC = right coronary artery; PA = pulmonary artery; PV = pulmonary vein; LC = left circumflex. (From Neufeld HN, Adams P Jr, Edwards JE, et al: Diagnosis of aortic atresia by retrograde aortography. Circulation 25:278, 1962.)

and perioperative mortality during the first stage of surgical repair.

PATHOPHYSIOLOGY. It remains uncertain whether hypoplastic left heart syndrome reflects a primary myocardial disease or is a consequence of a structural or hemodynamic abnormality. There is no doubt that in some patients, an apparently isolated dilated cardiomyopathy in early fetal life may evolve (as a result of a subsequent lack of left ventricular growth) into hypoplastic left heart syndrome later in gestation. Congenital structural abnormalities clearly play a significant role as well. This is exemplified by the effect of isolated valvular stenosis to produce a continuum of hypoplastic left heart syndrome to critical aortic stenosis with a normal-sized left ventricle. It is likely therefore that hypoplastic left heart syndrome is multifactorial in origin.

CLINICAL FEATURES. The diagnosis should be considered in any infant with the sudden onset of circulatory collapse and severe lactic acidosis. As such, it must be distinguished from neonatal sepsis and metabolic disorders. Until excluded, any child presenting in this way should be treated with prostaglandin, which may have a dramatic positive effect if there is an underlying cardiac abnormality and little effect if there is not.

LABORATORY INVESTIGATIONS

ECG. This frequently shows right axis deviation, right atrial and ventricular enlargement, and ST and T wave abnormalities in the left precordial leads.

Chest Radiography. This usually shows some cardiac enlargement shortly after birth, but with clinical deterioration there may be marked cardiomegaly and increased pulmonary venous and arterial vascular markings.

Echocardiography (Fig. 56–16). Cross-sectional echocardiography provides a full segmental diagnosis. In its classic form, the left ventricular cavity is small, with a diminutive mitral valve. The myocardium may be thinned or be of normal thickness, but the endocardium is usually thickened, consistent with endocardial fibroelastosis. There may be fistulous communications between the left ventricular cavity and the coronary arteries, a feature much more likely when the mitral valve is patent rather than atretic. The aortic root is usually diminutive, less than 4 to 5 mm in diameter at the level of the sinuses of Valsalva and narrowed in its ascending portion. The aortic arch is usually larger, but there is often a juxtaductal coarctation. The duct varies in size according to treatment, and assessment of this and the size of the interatrial communication are crucial to management. There may be profound desaturation and rapid demise (because of a combination of reduced pulmonary blood flow and pulmonary edema) in children with an intact atrial septum or restrictive patent foramen ovale.

MANAGEMENT OPTIONS. Early treatment with prostaglandin is mandatory. Those presenting in shock require paralysis, mechanical ventilation, and inotropic support. Crucial to managing these patients is maintenance of a balanced pulmonary and systemic blood flow. The cardiac output is fixed and is distributed according to the relative magnitude of the systemic and pulmonary vascular resistance. Thus, measures to elevate the pulmonary resistance (by imposing hypercapnia or by alveolar hypoxia) and reduce the systemic resistance (using vasodilators) are frequently required.

Surgical Treatment. Staged surgical management now provides long-term palliation to most patients with hypoplastic left heart syndrome. The first stage, often referred to as the *Norwood procedure*, now has many versions, but its essence is the creation of an unobstructed communication between the right ventricle and an unobstructed aorta. The right ventricular to aortic connection is accomplished by direct connection between the transected proximal pulmonary trunk and ascending aorta, usually with a patch extending around the augmented aortic arch. Pulmonary blood flow is established via a systemic-to-pulmonary shunt, or the more recently introduced right ventricle-to-pulmonary artery conduit. The

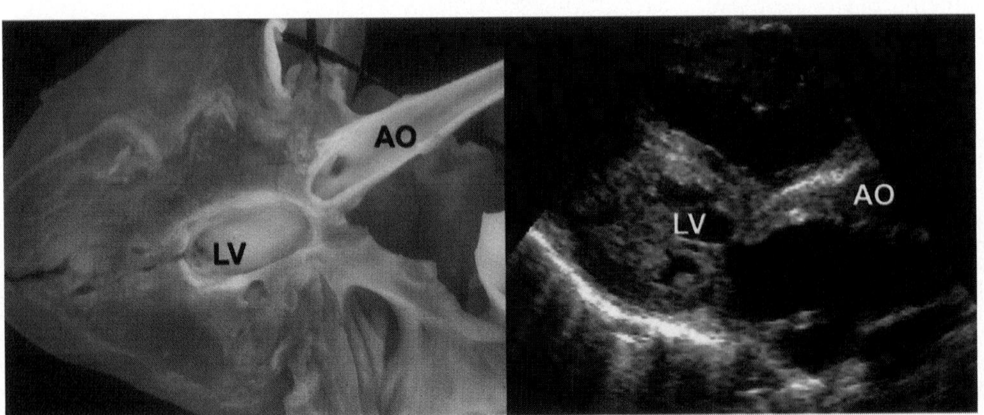

FIGURE 56–16 Long-axis view of the left ventricle and aorta in hypoplastic left heart syndrome. Note the associated endocardial fibroelastosis in the specimen. AO = aorta, LV = left ventricle.

PDA is ligated and a large interatrial communication is created. Early results of this procedure were poor, but survival rates higher than 85 percent have recently been published. Institutional variations, the interval mortality, and those unsuitable to progress to stage 2 must also be taken into account, however, and in some centers, the preferred operation is cardiac transplantation.

Stage 2 consists of an end-to-side superior vena cava-to-pulmonary artery connection (bidirectional Glenn procedure) or a hemi-Fontan (incorporating the roof of the atrium into the pulmonary artery anastomosis. This is performed at approximately 6 months of age as an intermediate step before stage 3, a Fontan operation.

ADULT ISSUES. The survivors of the earliest attempts at staged Norwood palliation are just now entering adult life. Their issues are likely to be common to all late survivors of Fontan palliation.[134]

Double-Inlet Ventricle

DEFINITION. Double-inlet connection falls under the umbrella of univentricular AV connections. These hearts are defined by having more than 50 percent of both AV connections connected to a dominant ventricle. In practice this usually means the whole of one and greater than 50 percent of the alternative junction is connected to either a left or right ventricle. When there is a common junction, then more than 75 percent of the junction must be connected to the dominant ventricle.

MORPHOLOGY. In about 75 percent of patients, the dominant ventricle is a left ventricle that is separated from the right ventricle by a VSD. In 20 percent the dominant ventricle is a right ventricle and the small, incomplete ventricle is of left ventricular apical morphology. In only 5 percent of cases is there truly only one ventricle in the ventricular mass. In double-inlet left ventricle the most common ventriculoarterial connection is discordant. Thus the aorta arises from the small right ventricle and is fed via the VSD, and the generally unobstructed pulmonary artery arises from the left ventricle. Aortic and aortic arch anomalies are frequent in these patients.

PATHOPHYSIOLOGY. The basic circulatory physiology of *double-inlet left ventricle* is identical to that of tricuspid atresia. There is common mixing of systemic and pulmonary venous blood, which is then ejected from the left ventricle into the pulmonary artery (with discordant connections) or aorta (with concordant connections). In the former, the blood must pass through the VSD to gain egress to the aorta. Subaortic stenosis, aortic hypoplasia, and arch anomalies are therefore common. In *double-inlet right ventricle,* it is those patients with concordant ventriculoarterial connections who are at particular risk of systemic outflow obstruction. One or the other or both of the two AV valves (when present) may be stenotic, atretic, or regurgitant. Under these circumstances the integrity of the atrial septum becomes important. If there is left or right atrial outflow obstruction, then a septectomy or septostomy will be required.

CLINICAL FEATURES. When there is critical reduction of systemic outflow, infants may be duct dependent and present with acidemic shock. Conversely, when pulmonary blood flow is reduced, presentation may be with severe cyanosis or with duct-dependent pulmonary blood flow. Other patients may not present in the neonatal period and will develop heart failure because of increased pulmonary blood flow. Patients undergo the same surgical algorithms as those with tricuspid atresia and so ultimately will undergo a Fontan operation. Their clinical issues are typical of any patient after this procedure.

LABORATORY INVESTIGATIONS

ECG. This is highly variable. Ventricular hypertrophy appropriate to the dominant ventricle is expected.

Chest Radiography. This is similarly variable and rarely diagnostic.

Echocardiography (Fig. 56–17). A full segmental diagnosis should be possible in all patients. Particular attention should be paid to defining AV valve anomalies and the presence and anatomy of any subaortic obstruction. This may develop, even if not present at birth, and should be part of the routine surveillance of these patients.

INDICATIONS AND OPTIONS FOR INTERVENTION. Survival without intervention may be prolonged, but at the expense of increasing cyanosis (when there is restriction to pulmonary blood flow) or pulmonary vascular disease (when there is unrestricted pulmonary blood flow). Those born with restricted systemic blood flow require urgent surgical intervention, usually undergoing a Norwood-type repair to establish the pulmonary valve as the unobstructed systemic outflow tract. Pulmonary artery banding is only offered to those infants with pulmonary overcirculation, heart failure, and unobstructed systemic outflow. Subsequently, and sometimes as the primary procedure, a bidirectional Glenn anastomosis is performed as a prelude to a Fontan procedure.

FOLLOW-UP. These patients should be reviewed frequently and in a center conversant with the issues of the Fontan operation.

Isomerism

DEFINITION. For the purposes of describing the cardiac manifestations, isomerism describes the situation where both atrial appendages have either left or right anatomical features (i.e., bilateral right or bilateral left atrial appendages).

MORPHOLOGY. There have been many attempts to describe hearts with complex abnormalities of visceral and atrial situs, whereby normal lateralization is lost. Terms such as *heterotaxy, asplenia,* and *polysplenia* fail to adequately describe either the visceral or cardiac manifestations with enough precision. The left atrial appendage is characterized by its tubular shape and pectinate muscles confined to the

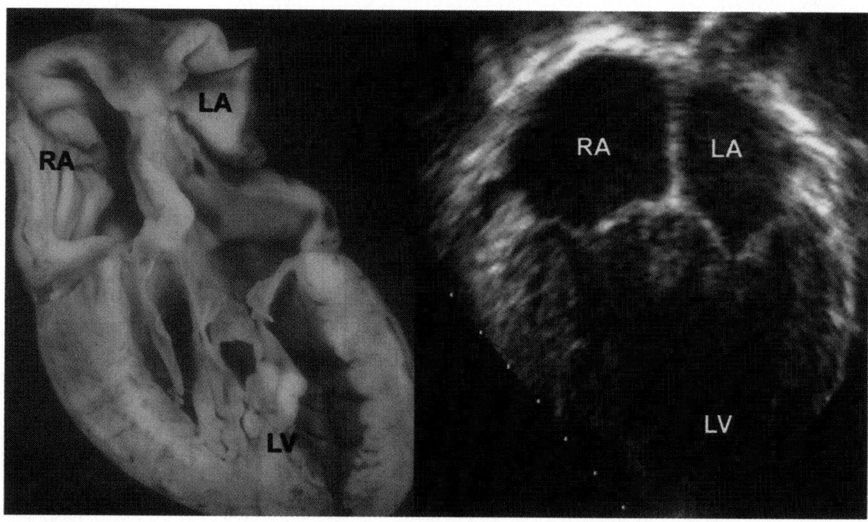

FIGURE 56–17 Apical four-chamber view in a double-inlet univentricular connection of left ventricular type with two atrioventricular valves. LA = left atrium; LV = left ventricle; RA = right atrium.

appendage. The pectinate muscles of the triangular right atrial appendage extend from its broad junction with the atrium, to extend around the vestibule or AV junction. Thus the arrangement of the atria (be it usual, mirror image, right or left isomerism) can be defined independent of the venous anatomy.

In left isomerism it is not unusual to have a biventricular AV connection, with separate AV junctions. A common junction (with an AV septal defect) is seen in approximately 30 percent of cases of left isomerism and more than 90 percent of hearts with isomerism of the right atrial appendages. Concordant ventriculoarterial connections predominate in left isomerism, and a double-outlet right ventricle with an anterior aorta is most frequently seen when there is right isomerism. The venous connections are very variable. These variations significantly affect the clinical and interventional management of these patients.

Isomerism of the Right Atrial Appendages

CLINICAL FEATURES. Bilateral "right-sidedness" results in a pattern of visceral abnormalities sometimes described as asplenia syndrome. The liver is midline, both lungs are trilobed with symmetrically short bronchi on the chest radiograph, and the spleen is hypoplastic or absent. The latter mandates immunization against pneumococcal infection and continuous penicillin prophylaxis against gram-positive sepsis. The diagnosis can be inferred from the bronchial pattern on the chest radiograph but most often is established by cross-sectional echocardiography because of early presentation with severe CHD. Abdominal scanning shows ipsilateral arrangement of the aorta and an anterior inferior vena cava. The intracardiac anatomy is most often that of an AV septal defect with varying degrees of right ventricular dominance, and frequently there is associated double-outlet right ventricle with an anterior aorta and subpulmonary stenosis or atresia. Thus cyanosis is the most common presentation. The inferior vena cava may connect to either right atrium, and superior vena cavae are often lateralized and separate. It is the pulmonary venous drainage that is crucial to the presentation and outcome of these children. By definition, the pulmonary veins are draining anomalously to one or other right atrium, but frequently this is indirect and/or obstructed. Adequate repair of the latter is fundamental to the outcome of these children, who almost uniformly ultimately require a Fontan procedure.

MANAGEMENT OPTIONS AND OUTCOMES. Initial palliation is usually directed toward regulating pulmonary blood flow and dealing with anomalies of pulmonary venous connection. Subsequently these patients (even when there are equal-sized ventricles) are treated along a Fontan algorithm. This is because repair of complete AV septal defect in the setting of abnormal ventriculoarterial connections is technically difficult or impossible. Thus a unilateral, or bilateral superior cavopulmonary anastomosis is performed at approximately 6 months of age, followed when possible by a Fontan procedure when aged 2 to 4 years.

The long-term outcome of surgery for right isomerism, however, has been poor. Improved early palliation and a staged approach toward the Fontan procedure have led to improved results. The prognosis for these infants, particularly when there is obstruction to pulmonary venous return, must remain guarded.

Isomerism of the Left Atrial Appendages

CLINICAL FEATURES. These patients have bilateral "left-sidedness." Hence they have two left lungs and bronchi, tend to have polysplenia, and frequently have malrotation of the gut. The cardiac abnormalities tend to be less severe than those of right isomerism. These patients are particularly prone to develop atrial arrhythmias, since the normal sinoatrial node is a right atrial structure and is usually absent in these patients. The ECG often shows an abnormal P wave axis, or wandering pacemaker. The anatomical diagnosis is usually established by echocardiography. The abdominal great vessels are both to the right or left of the spine, as with right isomerism, but in left isomerism the vein is a posterior azygos vein that continues to connect to a left- or right-sided superior vena cava. The intrahepatic inferior vena cava is absent in 90 percent, and under these circumstances the hepatic veins drain directly to the atria. The pulmonary venous connection needs to be defined precisely prior to any surgical intervention. Pulmonary arteriovenous malformations are not infrequently seen in patients with left isomerism. These can lead to cyanosis in unoperated or operated patients. The intracardiac anatomy varies from essentially normal to very complex. Again, AV septal defect (partial and complete) is overrepresented but with less frequent ventricular imbalance and abnormalities of ventriculoarterial connection.

MANAGEMENT OPTIONS. A biventricular repair is achieved in many more of these patients, albeit with the need for complex atrial baffle surgery to separate the systemic and pulmonary venous returns. The long-term outcome for patients with left isomerism is therefore much better than for those with right isomerism. The issues are very much those related to the type of surgery, but monitoring for arrhythmia needs to be even more intense than usual.

The Fontan Patient (Fig. 56–18)

BACKGROUND. As stated in the introduction to this section, such is the uncertain nature of the Fontan circulation, and the frequency of its failure,[135,136] that all patients should be followed regularly in a specialized center for CHD, and new symptoms should prompt early re-evaluation in such a center.

Since its description for the surgical management of tricuspid atresia in 1971, the Fontan procedure has become the definitive palliative surgical treatment when a biventricular repair is not possible. The principle is diversion of the systemic venous return directly to the pulmonary arteries without passing through a subpulmonary ventricle. Over the years, many modifications of the original procedure have been described and performed, namely, direct atriopulmonary connection, total cavopulmonary connection, and extracardiac conduit. Fenestration (5-mm diameter) of the Fontan circuit into the left atrium is sometimes performed at the time of surgery in high-risk patients, permitting right-to-left shunting and decompression of the Fontan circuit.

PATHOPHYSIOLOGY. Elevation of the central venous pressure and a reduced cardiac output (sometimes at rest[137] but always on exercise[138]) are inevitable consequences of the Fontan procedure. Small adverse changes in ventricular function (particularly diastolic), circuit efficiency (elevated pulmonary resistance, obstruction, thrombosis), or the onset of arrhythmia, all potentially lead to major symptomatic deterioration.

Although it is reasonable to describe patients after the Fontan procedure as existing in a form of chronic heart failure (since their right atrial pressure must be high), this is seldom due to marked systolic dysfunction.[139] Indeed, a small elevation in ventricular diastolic pressure may be much more harmful. Thus it may be incorrect to treat these patients with traditional heart failure medications. In a randomized, blinded placebo-controlled study, ACE inhibition failed to improve functional performance, and some indices worsened.[140]

The more "steamlined" Fontan circulations (total cavopulmonary anastomosis, extracardiac conduit) that exclude the right atrium from the circulation have demonstrably better fluid dynamic properties and improved functional performance.[138] Physical obstruction at surgical anastomoses, the distal pulmonary arteries, or pulmonary veins (often due to compression by a dilated right atrium) all reduce circulatory efficiency, however. Similarly, elevated pulmonary arteriolar resistances have adverse effects. This is because the pulmonary vascular resistance is the single biggest contributor to impairment of venous return and elevation of venous pressure. Relatively little is known about pulmonary vascular resistance late after the procedure, but it has recently been shown to be elevated in a significant number of patients and to be reactive to inhaled nitric oxide, suggesting pulmonary endothelial dysfunction.[141]

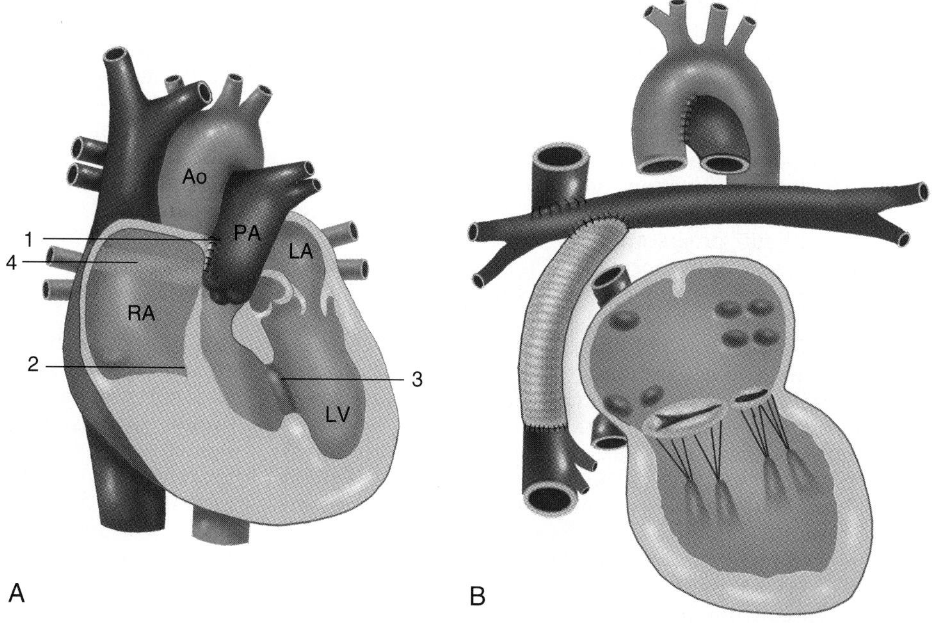

FIGURE 56–18 Modification of the Fontan operation. **A,** Direct atriopulmonary connection (1) for tricuspid valve atresia (2); ventricular septal defect, oversewn (3); patch closure of atrial septal defect (4). **B,** Extracardiac conduit made of a Dacron graft bypassing the right atrium, connecting the inferior vena cava to the inferior aspect of the right pulmonary artery. Superior vena cava is anastomosed to the superior aspect of the right pulmonary artery. RA = right atrium; LA = left atrium; LV = left ventricle; Ao = aorta; PA = pulmonary artery. (**A,** From Mullins CE, Mayer DC: Congenital Heart Disease: A Diagrammatic Atlas. New York, Wiley-Liss, 1988; and **B,** From Marcelletti C: Inferior vena cava–pulmonary artery extracardiac conduit: A new form of right heart bypass. J Thorac Cardiovasc Surg 100:228-232, 1990.)

CLINICAL FEATURES. The majority of patients (~90 percent) present with functional Class I to II at 5 years' follow-up after a Fontan procedure.[136,142,143] Progressive deterioration of functional status with time is the rule.[136,142-144] Supraventricular arrhythmias such as atrial tachycardia, flutter, and fibrillation are common. Physical examination in an otherwise uncomplicated patient reveals an elevated, usually nonpulsatile jugular venous pulse (10 cm above the sternal angle and needed to provide the hydrostatic pressure to drive cardiac output through the pulmonary circulation), a quiet apex, a normal S_1, and a single S_2 (the pulmonary artery having been tied off). A heart murmur should not be present, and its identification suggests the presence of systemic AV valve regurgitation or subaortic obstruction. Generalized edema may be a sign of protein-losing enteropathy.

COMPLICATIONS AND SEQUELAE

Arrhythmia. Although often associated with marked symptomatic decline, atrial arrhythmias tend to reflect the consequences of the abnormalities of ventricular function and circulatory efficiency described earlier. The massively dilated right atrium after an atriopulmonary connection is commonly associated with atrial flutter and fibrillation. With new-onset arrhythmia, hemodynamic abnormalities and atrial/venous thrombosis—which may develop within 2 hours of arrhythmia onset—should be actively excluded prior to therapy. Atrial flutter/fibrillation is common (15 to 20 percent at 5 years' follow-up)[51,52,145,146] and increases with duration of follow-up.[51-53] Atrial flutter/fibrillation carries significant morbidity, can be associated with profound hemodynamic deterioration, and needs prompt medical attention. The combination of atrial incisions and multiple suture lines at the time of Fontan surgery combined with increased right atrial pressure and size probably explains the high incidence of atrial arrhythmias in such patients. Patients at greater risk for atrial tachyarrhythmias are those who were operated on at an older age, with poor ventricular function, systemic AV valve regurgitation, or increased pulmonary artery pressure. It has been suggested that the exclusion of the right atrium from elevated systemic venous pressure (as in total cavopulmonary connection or extracardiac conduit) leads to a decrease in the incidence of atrial arrhythmias. This apparent benefit may, however, be due exclusively to the shorter length of follow-up in this group of patients. Sinus node dysfunction and complete heart block can occur and require pacemaker insertion.

Thrombosis and Stroke. The reported incidence of thromboembolic complications in the Fontan circuit varies from 6 to 25 percent, depending on the diagnostic method used and the length of follow-up.[147-149] Thrombus formation may relate to the presence of supraventricular arrhythmias, right atrial dilation, right atrial "smoke," and the presence of artificial material used to construct the Fontan circuit.[147-149] Accordingly, a similar incidence of thrombus formation had been reported for all types of Fontan circuits. Systemic arterial embolism in patients with and without a fenestrated Fontan has also been reported. Protein C deficiency has been reported in these patients and may explain in part their propensity to thromboembolism.

Protein-Losing Enteropathy. Protein-losing enteropathy, defined as severe loss of serum protein into the intestine, occurs in 4 to 13 percent of patients after a Fontan procedure.[145,150,151] Patients present with generalized edema, ascites, pleural effusion, and/or chronic diarrhea. Protein-losing enteropathy is thought to result principally from chronically elevated systemic venous pressure causing intestinal lymphangiectasia with consequent loss of albumin, protein, lymphocytes, and immunoglobulin into the gastrointestinal tract. The diagnosis is confirmed by finding low serum albumin and protein, low plasma $alpha_1$-antitrypsin level and lymphocyte counts, and, most important, a high $alpha_1$-antitrypsin stool clearance. It carries a dismal prognosis, with a 5-year survival of 46 to 59 percent.[150,151]

Right Pulmonary Vein Compression/Obstruction. Right pulmonary vein obstruction/compression can occur from the enlarged right atrium or atrial baffle bulging into the left atrium and can lead to increased pulmonary artery pressure with further dilation of the right atrium. It should be sought.

Pulmonary thromboembolism is increasingly recognized[147-149,152] and will elevate central venous pressure. There is continuing debate as to the role of anticoagulation, antiplatelet therapy, or both in the long-term management of these patients, but most receive some form of therapy,[153-155]

Fontan Obstruction. Stenosis or partial obstruction of the Fontan connection leads to exercise intolerance, atrial tachyarrhythmias, and right-sided heart failure. Sudden total obstruction can present as sudden death.

Ventricular Dysfunction and Valvular Regurgitation. Progressive deterioration of systemic ventricular function, with or without progressive AV valve regurgitation, is common. Patients with morphological systemic right ventricles may fare less well than those with morphological left ventricles.

Hepatic Dysfunction. Mildly raised hepatic transaminase levels from hepatic congestion are frequent but seldom clinically important. Cirrhosis apparently due to chronic venous hypertension has been described.

Cyanosis. Worsening cyanosis may relate to worsening of ventricular function, the development of venous collateral channels draining to the left atrium, or the development of pulmonary arteriovenous malformations (especially if a classic Glenn procedure remains as part of the Fontan circulation).

LABORATORY INVESTIGATIONS

ECG. Sinus rhythm, atrial flutter, junctional rhythm, or complete heart block may be present. The QRS complex reflects the basic underlying cardiac anomaly. In patients with tricuspid atresia, left axis deviation is the norm. In patients with univentricular hearts, the conduction pattern varies widely and depends on the morphology and relative position of the rudimentary chamber.

Chest Radiography. Mild bulging of the right lower heart border from a dilated right atrium is often seen in patients with an atriopulmonary connection.

Echocardiography. The presence or absence of right atrial stasis, thrombus, patency of a fenestration, and Fontan circuit obstruction should be sought. Superior and inferior vena cavae biphasic and pulmonary artery triphasic flow patterns suggest unobstructed flow in the Fontan circuit, whereas a mean gradient between the Fontan circuit and the pulmonary artery of 2 mm Hg or more may represent significant obstruction. Assessment of the pulmonary venous flow pattern is important in detecting pulmonary vein obstruction (right pulmonary vein > left pulmonary vein) sometimes caused by an enlarged right atrium (often ~ 80 × 60 mm in adults with atriopulmonary connections). Concomitant assessment of systemic ventricular function and AV valve regurgitation can be readily accomplished. TEE may be required if there is inadequate visualization of the Fontan anastomosis or to exclude thrombus in the right atrium.

Diagnostic Catheterization. Complete heart catheterization is advised if surgical reintervention is planned or if adequate assessment of the hemodynamics is not obtained by noninvasive means.

MRI. The objectives of MRI in Fontan patients include assessment of the pathways from the systemic veins to the pulmonary arteries for obstruction and thrombus; detection of Fontan baffle fenestration or leaks; evaluation of the pulmonary veins for compression; assessing systemic ventricular volume, mass, and ejection fraction; imaging of the systemic ventricular outflow tract for obstruction; and quantitative assessment of the AV and semilunar valve(s) for regurgitation, the aorta for obstruction or an aneurysm, and for aortopulmonary, systemic venous, or systemic-to-pulmonary venous collateral vessels.

MANAGEMENT OPTIONS AND OUTCOMES. Patient selection is of utmost importance and has a major impact on clinical outcome. Long-term survival in "ideal" candidates is 81 percent at 10 years,[142] compared with 60 to 71 percent in "all comers."[144] Death occurs mostly from congestive heart failure and atrial arrhythmias. The Fontan procedure remains a palliative, not curative, procedure. A more radical approach to the failing Fontan circulation including surgical revision of the circuit to an extracardiac conduit, in combination with a Cox/maze procedure and, frequently, simultaneous epicardial pacemaker insertion, has recently been shown to provide good early palliation.[59,59,156-159] Ultimately cardiac transplantation is likely to be required by many of these patients.[150]

Arrhythmias. Atrial tachyarrhythmias are quite difficult to manage and should quickly raise the thought of long-term warfarin therapy. When atrial flutter/fibrillation are present, an underlying hemodynamic cause should always be sought, and, in particular, evidence for obstruction of the Fontan circuit needs to be sought. Prompt attempts should be made to restore sinus rhythm. Antiarrhythmic medications, alone or combined with an epicardial antitachycardia pacing device, and radiofrequency catheter ablation techniques have had limited success. Surgical conversion from an atriopulmonary Fontan to a total cavopulmonary connection with concomitant atrial cryoablation therapy at the time of surgery has been reported with good short-term success.[59,158,159] Epicardial pacemaker insertion for sinus node dysfunction and/or complete heart block may be necessary. Epicardial AV sequential pacing should be employed whenever possible.

Anticoagulant Therapy. The use of prophylactic long-term anticoagulation is contentious. It is recommended that patients with a history of documented arrhythmias, fenestration in the Fontan connection, or spontaneous contrast (smoke) in the right atrium on echocardiography be anticoagulated.[153,154] For established thrombus, thrombolytic therapy versus surgical removal of the clot and conversion of the Fontan circuit have been described, both with high mortality rates.

Protein-Losing Enteropathy. Treatment modalities include a low-fat, high-protein, medium-chain triglyceride diet to reduce intestinal lymphatic production; albumin infusions to increase intravascular osmotic pressure; and/or the introduction of diuretics, afterload-reducing agents, and positive inotropic agents to lower central venous pressure. Most often these therapies are ineffective and should not be continued if indeed tried at all. Catheter-based interventions such as balloon dilation of pathway obstruction or creation of an atrial fenestration as well as surgical interventions from conversion or takedown of the Fontan circuit to cardiac transplantation have also been advocated. Other reportedly effective treatment modalities include subcutaneous heparin, octreotide treatment, and prednisone therapy. All therapies have a similar approximately 50 percent failure rate.[151,160]

Right Pulmonary Vein Compression/Obstruction. When hemodynamically significant, Fontan conversion to a total cavopulmonary connection or extracardiac conduit may be recommended.

Fontan Obstruction. Surgical revision of obstructed right atrium to pulmonary artery or superior and inferior vena cavae to pulmonary artery connections is recommended, usually to an extracardiac Fontan. Alternatively, balloon angioplasty with or without stenting may be used when appropriate and feasible.

Ventricular Failure and Valvular Regurgitation. ACE inhibitors are of unproven benefit, do not appear to enhance exercise capacity, and may cause clinical deterioration. Patients with systemic AV valve regurgitation may require AV valve repair or replacement. Cardiac transplantation should also be considered.

Cyanosis. In the setting of a fenestrated Fontan, surgical or preferably transcatheter closure of the fenestration can be attempted. Pulmonary arteriovenous fistulas from a classic Glenn may be improved by surgical conversion to a bidirectional Glenn connection.

FOLLOW-UP ISSUES. Close and expert follow-up is recommended with particular attention to ventricular function and systemic AV valve regurgitation. The development of atrial tachyarrhythmia should instigate a search for possible obstruction at the Fontan anastomosis, right pulmonary vein obstruction, or thrombus within the right atrium.

Total Anomalous Pulmonary Venous Connection

DEFINITION. This describes the situation where all pulmonary veins fail to drain directly to the left atrium. As a result, all of the systemic and pulmonary venous return drains to the right atrium, albeit using varied routes.

MORPHOLOGY (Fig. 56–19). The anatomical varieties of total anomalous pulmonary venous connection may be subdivided, depending on the level of the abnormal drainage. The anomalous connection is most often supradiaphragmatic, connecting via a vertical vein to the left brachiocephalic vein, direct to the right atrium, to the coronary sinus, or directly to the superior vena cava. In about 10 to 15 percent the site of connection is below the diaphragm. The anomalous trunk then connects into the portal vein or one of its tributaries, the ductus venosus, or, rarely, to the hepatic or other abdominal veins.

PATHOPHYSIOLOGY. The physiological consequences and, accordingly, the clinical picture depend on the size of the interatrial communication and on the magnitude of the pulmonary vascular resistance. When the interatrial communication is small, systemic blood flow is severely limited with right-sided heart failure. Obstruction to pulmonary venous return and pulmonary venous hypertension are invariably present in patients with infradiaphragmatic anomalous pulmonary venous connection.

NATURAL HISTORY. Most patients with total anomalous pulmonary venous connection have symptoms during the first year of life, and 80 percent die before 1 year of age if not treated. The presence of obstruction in the pulmonary venous pathway or at the atrial septum leads to earlier presentation. When the obstruction is severe, neonatal presentation with severe cyanosis and cardiovascular collapse may occur. This is incompatible with survival without urgent surgical intervention.

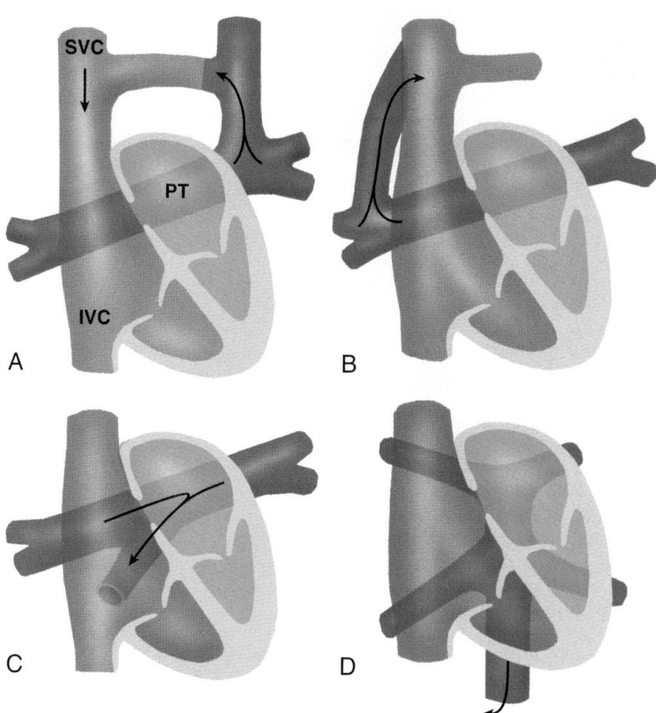

FIGURE 56–19 Anatomical types of total anomalous pulmonary venous return: supracardiac, in which the pulmonary veins drain either via the vertical vein to the anomalous vein **(A)** or directly to the superior vena cava (SVC) with the orifice close to the orifice of the azygos vein **(B)**. **C,** Drainage into the right atrium via the coronary sinus. **D,** Infracardiac drainage via a vertical vein into the portal vein or the inferior vena cava (IVC). PT = pulmonary trunk. (**A** to **D,** From Stark J, deLeval M: Surgery for Congenital Heart Defects. 2nd ed. Philadelphia, WB Saunders, 1994, p 330.)

CLINICAL FEATURES. Symptomatic infants with total anomalous pulmonary venous connection present with signs of heart failure and/or cyanosis. Infants with pulmonary venous obstruction present with the early onset of severe dyspnea, pulmonary edema, cyanosis, and right-sided heart failure. When unobstructed, cyanosis may be minimal and go undetected. On auscultation there is usually a fixed, widely split second heart sound with an accentuated pulmonic component.

LABORATORY INVESTIGATIONS

ECG. This usually shows right axis deviation and right atrial and right ventricular hypertrophy.

Chest Radiography. In the unrepaired patient, this usually shows cardiomegaly with increased pulmonary blood flow. The right atrium and ventricle are dilated and hypertrophied, and the pulmonary artery segment is enlarged. The so-called "figure-of-8" or "snowman" heart is due to enlargement of the heart and the presence of a dilated right superior vena cava, innominate vein, and left vertical vein.

Echocardiography (Fig. 56–20). This will usually show marked enlargement of the right ventricle and a small left atrium. It is usually possible to demonstrate the entire pathway of pulmonary venous drainage, and cardiac catheterization (which may be hazardous) is almost never performed now. An echo-free space representing the pulmonary venous confluence can usually be seen behind the left atrium. The drainage of all four pulmonary veins and their connections must be identified.

MRI. Although not often used, especially in infants, MRI may be helpful to delineate the site of connections of total anomalous pulmonary venous return, when there are multiple mixed sites, in older children, and to detect stenosis in postoperative patients.

INDICATIONS FOR INTERVENTION. Medical therapy, other than mechanical ventilation, has a limited role in the symptomatic infant, and corrective surgery should be performed as soon as possible. In asymptomatic children without pulmonary hypertension, surgery can be deferred to 3 to 6 months of age.

INTERVENTIONAL OPTIONS AND OUTCOMES. Occasionally an urgent balloon atrial septostomy is required to increase systemic blood flow prior to surgery. Otherwise, interventional catheterization is restricted to attempts at relieving postoperative pulmonary venous stenosis, although this is often unrewarding. Historically, surgical repair of restenosis was also disappointing. However, the sutureless technique, whereby the pulmonary veins are opened widely into the retroatrial space, has markedly improved the results of such surgery. Adult patients have almost always had surgical repair in childhood. As a rule, they function normally and are not too prone to arrhythmias or other problems. They are seen as low- to moderate-risk adults.

FOLLOW-UP. Early follow-up should be frequent and aimed at early detection of stenosis of the pulmonary veins or the surgical anastomosis. If not present within the first year, stenosis is rare, but annual follow-up during childhood is required.

Transposition Complexes

The key anatomical feature that characterizes this group of diagnoses is ventriculoarterial discordance. This is most commonly seen in the context of AV concordance, also known as

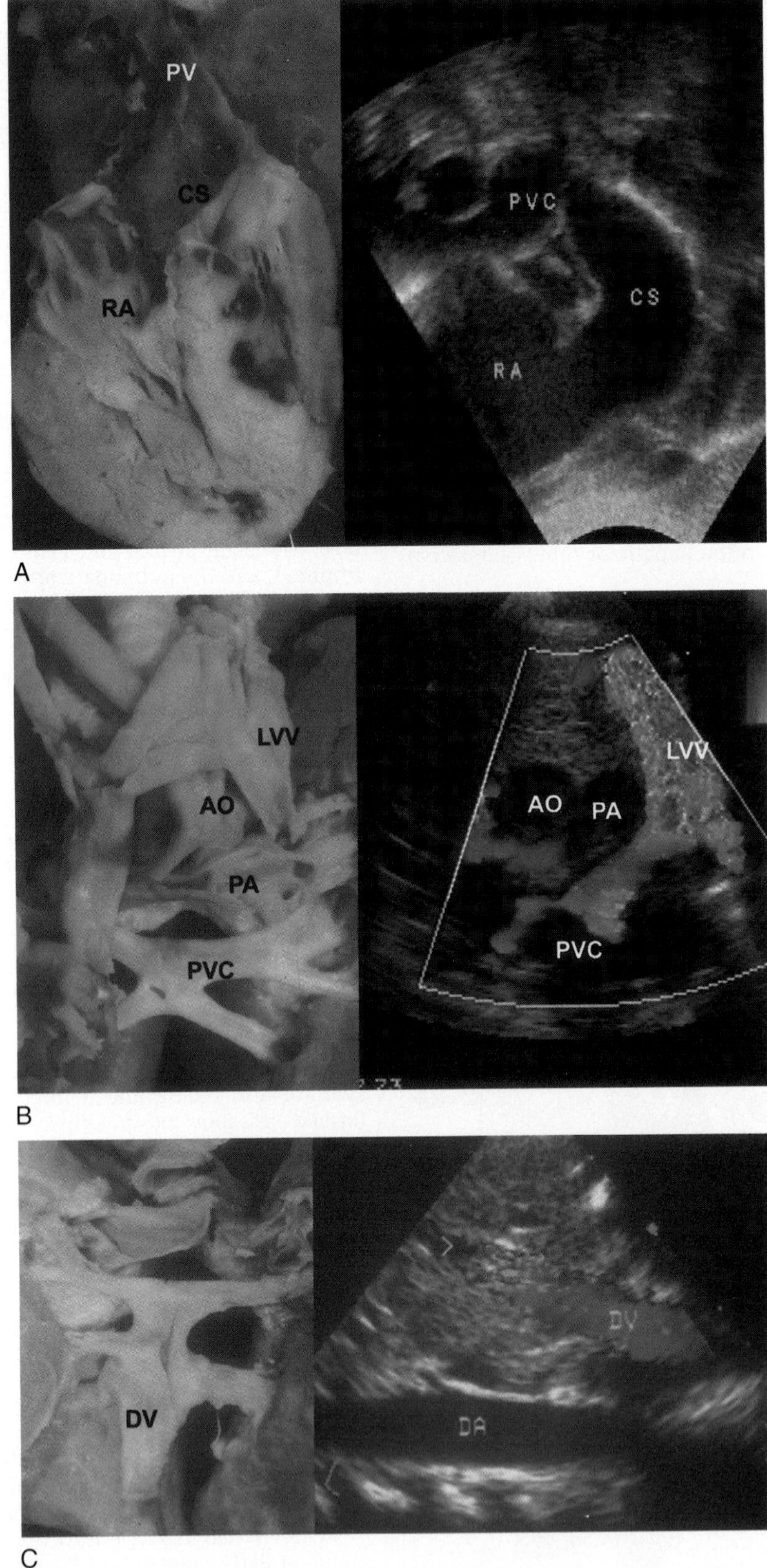

FIGURE 56–20 **A,** Subcostal view demonstrating total anomalous pulmonary drainage to the coronary sinus. Note the dilated coronary sinus in both images. The echocardiogram also demonstrates an associated confluence that connects to the coronary sinus. **B,** Suprasternal view demonstrating total anomalous pulmonary venous drainage to a left vertical vein. Note the direction of flow in the vertical vein that differentiates it from a left superior vena cava. **C,** Total anomalous pulmonary venous drainage below the diaphragm. The specimen shows the pulmonary veins as they enter the confluence, whereas the echocardiogram demonstrates the descending veins as it enters the liver. Note the direction of flow is away from the heart. CS = coronary sinus; PVC = pulmonary venous confluence; RA = right atrium; DA = descending aorta; DV = descending vein; AO = aorta; LVV = left vertical vein; PA = pulmonary artery.

complete transposition or *D-TGA*. The second condition that is discussed in this section is the combination of ventriculoarterial discordance with AV discordance, commonly referred to as *congenitally corrected TGA* or *L-TGA*. More complex arrangements are not considered here.

Complete Transposition of the Great Arteries

DEFINITION AND NATURAL HISTORY. This is a common and potentially lethal form of heart disease in newborns and infants. The malformation consists of the origin of the aorta from the morphological right ventricle and that of the pulmonary artery from the morphological left ventricle. Consequently, the pulmonary and systemic circulations are connected in parallel rather than the normal in-series connection. In one circuit, systemic venous blood passes to the right atrium, the right ventricle, and then to the aorta. In the other, pulmonary venous blood passes through the left atrium and ventricle to the pulmonary artery. This situation is incompatible with life unless mixing of the two circuits occurs.

Approximately two-thirds of patients have no major associated abnormalities (*"simple" transposition*) and one-third have associated abnormalities (*"complex" transposition*). The most common associated abnormalities are VSD and pulmonary/subpulmonary stenosis. It is increasingly being diagnosed in utero.[161] Without treatment, about 30 percent of these infants die within the first week of life, and 90 percent die within the first year.

MORPHOLOGY. Some communication between the two circulations must exist after birth to sustain life; otherwise, unoxygenated systemic venous blood is directed inappropriately to the systemic circulation and oxygenated pulmonary venous blood is directed to the pulmonary circulation. Almost all patients have an interatrial communication, blood flow across which governs the amount of desaturation. Two-thirds have a PDA, and about one-third have an associated VSD.

PATHOPHYSIOLOGY. The degree of tissue hypoxia, the nature of the associated cardiovascular anomalies, and the anatomical and functional status of the pulmonary vascular bed determine the clinical course.

The anatomical arrangement results in two separate and parallel circulations. The systemic arterial oxygen saturation is governed by the amount of blood exchanged between the two circulations. Infants with D-TGA are particularly susceptible to the early development of pulmonary vascular obstructive disease even in the absence of a PDA and with an intact ventricular septum.

CLINICAL FEATURES

Pediatric. Average birth weight and size of infants born with complete transposition of the great arteries are greater than normal. The usual clinical manifestations are dyspnea and cyanosis from birth, progressive hypoxemia, and congestive heart failure. The most severe cyanosis and hypoxemia are observed in infants who have only a small patent foramen ovale or ductus arteriosus and an intact ventricular septum, or in those infants with relatively reduced pulmonary blood flow because of left ventricular outflow tract obstruction. With a large PDA or a large VSD, cyanosis can be minimal, and heart failure is usually the dominant problem after the first few weeks of life. Cardiac murmurs are of little diagnostic significance.

The 2D echocardiogram should establish the complete diagnosis, including the coronary artery pattern. Prenatal detection is possible and favorably modifies neonatal morbidity and mortality. Ultrasound imaging has become a standard procedure to guide catheter placement and manipulation during balloon atrial septostomy and to assess the anatomical adequacy of the septostomy.

MANAGEMENT OPTIONS. Dilation of the duct by prostaglandin E_1 in the early neonatal period improves the arterial saturation by enhancing mixing. There is a frequent misconception that significant mixing occurs at ductal level. This is incorrect; the effect of prostaglandin is to increase pulmonary blood flow, and by so doing to increase left atrial pressure, and increase mixing at atrial level. This is usually as a prelude to the creation or enlargement of an interatrial communication by a balloon or blade atrial septostomy. Surgical atrial septectomy is seldom required now.

Surgery. Although balloon atrial septostomy is often life saving, it is palliative prior to "corrective" surgery. Atrial redirection procedures were developed in the 1950s and 1960s but were replaced by the arterial switch operation, which became widely adopted in the 1980s.[162]

Atrial Switch (Fig. 56–21). The most common surgical procedure in patients who are currently adults is the atrial switch operation. Patients will have had either a Mustard or a Senning procedure. Blood is redirected at the atrial level using a baffle made of Dacron or pericardium (Mustard operation) or atrial flaps (Senning operation), achieving physiological correction. Systemic venous return is diverted through the mitral valve into the subpulmonary left ventricle, and the pulmonary venous return is rerouted through the tricuspid valve into the subaortic right ventricle. By virtue of this repair, the morphological right ventricle is left to support the systemic circulation.

Palliative Atrial Switch. Uncommonly, in patients with a large VSD and established pulmonary vascular disease, a palliative atrial switch operation is done to improve oxygenation. The VSD is left open or enlarged at the time of atrial baffle surgery. These patients resemble patients with Eisenmenger VSDs and should be managed as such.

Arterial Switch Operation (Fig. 56–22). In this operation, the arterial trunks are transected and reanastomosed to the contralateral root. If present, a VSD is closed. The coronary arteries must be transposed to the neoaorta. This is the most

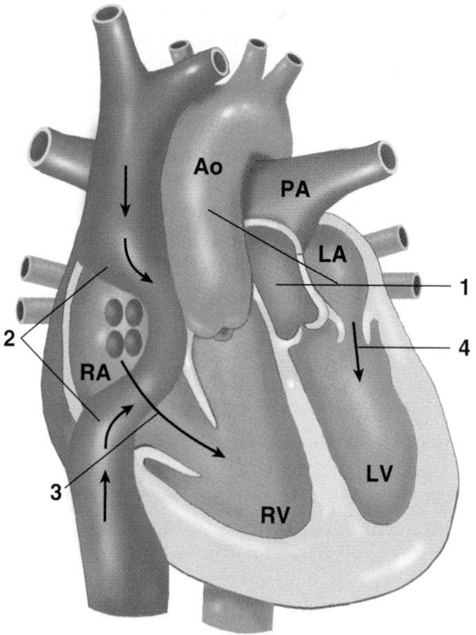

FIGURE 56–21 Diagrammatic representation of atrial switch surgery (Mustard/Senning procedure). Superior vena cava (SVC) and inferior vena cava (IVC) blood is redirected into the morphological left ventricle (LV), which pumps blood into the pulmonary artery (PA), whereas the pulmonary venous blood flow is rerouted to the morphological right ventricle (RV), which empties into the aorta (Ao). RA = right atrium; LA = left atrium; 1 = transposition of the great arteries; 2 = atrial baffles; 3 = pulmonary vein blood flow through tricuspid valve to RV; 4 = IVC and SVC blood flow through mitral valve to LV. (From Mullins CE, Mayer DC: Congenital Heart Disease: A Diagrammatic Atlas. New York, Wiley-Liss, 1988.)

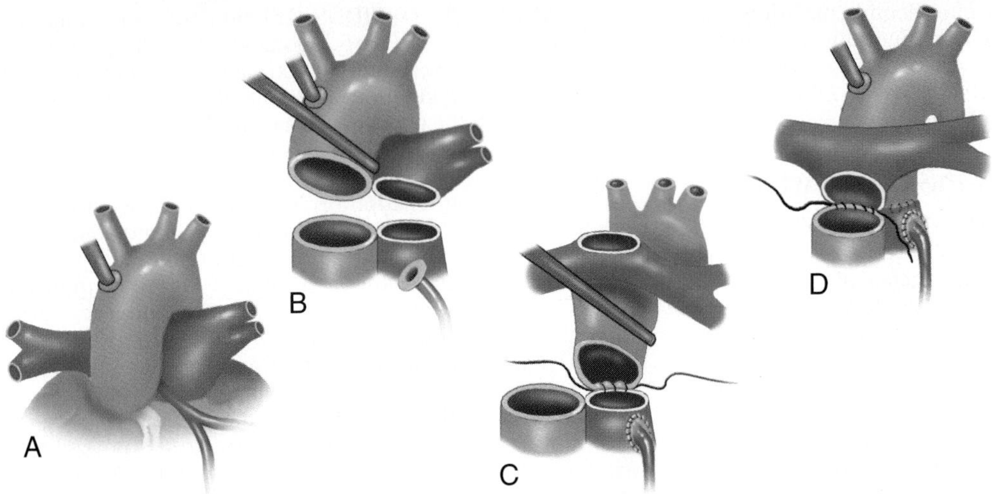

FIGURE 56–22 Complete transposition of the great arteries, corrected by a modified arterial switch operation **(A)**. The aorta and pulmonary artery are transected, and the orifices of the coronary arteries are excised with a rim of adjacent aortic wall **(B)**. The aorta is brought under the bifurcation of the pulmonary artery, and the pulmonary artery and the aorta are anastomosed without necessitating graft interposition. The coronary arteries are transferred to the pulmonary artery **(C)**. The mobilized pulmonary artery is directly anastomosed to the proximal aortic stump **(D)**. (**A** to **D**, From Stark J, deLaval M: Surgery for Congenital Heart Defects. New York, Grune & Stratton, 1983, p 379.)

challenging part of the procedure and accounts for most of the mortality. Nonetheless, this rate has fallen to less than 2 percent in most large centers.[162,163] The major advantages of the arterial switch procedure, when compared with the atrial switch procedure, are restoration of the left ventricle as the systemic pump and the potential for long-term maintenance of sinus rhythm.

Follow-up studies after the arterial switch operation have demonstrated good left ventricular function and normal exercise capacity.[163,164] Potential sequelae of the operation include coronary occlusion, supravalvular pulmonary stenosis (which may be treated by either reoperation or balloon angioplasty), supravalvular aortic stenosis, and neoaortic regurgitation, usually mild.[165-167] Long-term patency and growth of the coronary arteries appear satisfactory.

Rastelli Procedure. Infants with TGA plus a VSD and left ventricular outflow tract obstruction may require an early systemic-to-pulmonary artery anastomosis when a pronounced diminution in pulmonary blood flow exists. A later corrective procedure for these patients bypasses the left ventricular outflow obstruction with an extracardiac prosthetic conduit between the right ventricle and the distal end of a divided pulmonary artery and uses an intracardiac ventricular baffle to tunnel the left ventricle to the aorta.

MANAGEMENT OUTCOMES

Atrial Switch. After atrial baffle surgery, most patients who reach adulthood are in NYHA Classes I and II,[41,168,169] but abnormalities of ventricular filling, due to the abnormal atrial pathways, may be of more direct importance to functional capacity than right ventricular performance issues in many.[170] Some present with symptoms of congestive heart failure (2 to 15 percent). Echocardiographic evidence of moderate or severe systemic right ventricular dysfunction is present in up to 40 percent of patients. Relative right ventricular ischemia (supply-demand mismatch) is thought to perhaps play a role in systemic right ventricular dysfunction.[171-173] More than mild systemic tricuspid regurgitation is present in 10 to 40 percent, both reflecting and exacerbating right ventricular dysfunction. Palpitations and near-syncope/syncope from rhythm disturbances is fairly common. Atrial flutter occurs in 20 percent of patients by 20 years of age, and sinus node dysfunction is seen in half of the patients by that time.[42,174-176] These rhythm disturbances are a consequence of direct and indirect atrial and sinus node damage at the time of atrial baffle surgery.[177]

A shortened life expectancy is the rule, with 70 to 80 percent survival at 20 to 30 years' follow-up.[41] Patients with "complex" TGA in general fare much worse than those with "simple" TGA. Sudden cardiac death occurs in about 5 percent of these patients and may relate to systemic right ventricular dysfunction, the presence of atrial flutter, and pulmonary hypertension. Significant pulmonary vascular disease can develop over time and relates to older age at the time of atrial switch operation, particularly in patients with a substantial VSD, as well as in those with long-standing left-to-right shunts through a baffle leak. Superior vena cava or inferior vena cava baffle obstruction often goes undetected because collateral drainage through the azygos vein prevents systemic venous congestion. Pulmonary venous baffle obstruction causes elevated pulmonary artery pressure, and patients can present with dyspnea and pulmonary venous congestive features.

Physical examination of a patient whose condition is otherwise uncomplicated reveals a right ventricular parasternal lift, a normal S_1, a single S_2 (P_2 is not heard because of its posterior location), a pansystolic murmur from tricuspid regurgitation if present (best heard at the left lower sternal border, but not increasing with inspiration), and a right-sided S_3 when severe systemic ventricular dysfunction is present.

Arterial Switch. Data on clinical presentation in adults who have undergone the arterial switch procedure are lacking, because most patients have not yet reached adulthood. Clinical arrhythmia promises to be less of a problem in this group of patients.[165,178] Concerns about the development of supra-neopulmonary artery stenosis, ostial coronary artery disease, and progressive neoaortic valve regurgitation remain to be addressed over the long-term. Cardiac examination in uncomplicated patients is normal.

Rastelli. Progressive right ventricular-to-pulmonary artery conduit obstruction can cause exercise intolerance or right ventricular angina. Left ventricular tunnel obstruction can present as dyspnea or syncope. Conduit replacement is inevitably required in surviving patients. Physical examination in uncomplicated patients reveals, in contrast to atrial switches, no right ventricular lift, an ejection systolic murmur from the conduit, and two components to the S_2.

LABORATORY INVESTIGATIONS

ECG. Sinus bradycardia or junctional rhythm (without a right atrial overload pattern) with evidence of marked right ventricular hypertrophy is characteristically present in patients after the atrial switch procedure. The ECG is typically normal in patients after the arterial switch procedure. The ECG typically shows right bundle branch block after a Rastelli procedure.

Chest Radiography. On the posteroanterior film, a narrow vascular pedicle with an oblong cardiac silhouette ("egg on side") is typically seen in patients after the atrial switch procedure. On the lateral view, the anterior aorta is seen to fill the retrosternal space. For the arterial switch, normal mediastinal borders are present despite the Lecompte maneuver. After the Rastelli procedure, the chest radiograph is normal unless the conduit becomes calcified or a nonhomograft prosthesis is employed.

Echocardiography. After the atrial switch procedure, parallel great arteries are the hallmark of TGA (Fig. 56–23). They are best visualized from a parasternal long-axis view (running side by side) or from a parasternal short-axis view (seen *en face*, with the aorta anterior and rightward).[179] Qualitative assessment of systemic right ventricular function, the degree of tricuspid regurgitation, and the presence or absence of subpulmonary left ventricular obstruction (dynamic or fixed) is possible. Assessment of baffle leak or obstruction (Fig. 56–24) is best done using color and Doppler flow imaging. Normal baffle flow should be phasic in nature and vary with respiration, with a peak velocity less than 1 meter per second. After arterial switch, neoaortic valve regurgitation, supra-neopulmonary valve stenosis, and segmental wall motion abnormality from ischemia due to coronary ostial stenosis should be sought. In patients who have undergone the Rastelli operation, left ventricular-to-aorta tunnel obstruction as well as right ventricular-to-pulmonary artery conduit degeneration (stenosis/regurgitation) must be sought.

MRI. The major role of MRI in patients with atrial switch is to evaluate the baffles and systemic right ventricular volume and ejection fraction. As a rule, MRI reports better right ventricular size and function than does echo. For patients who are claustrophobic or have a pacemaker, a high-quality radionuclide angiogram with volume estimates will serve as a substitute. MRI can evaluate issues in arterial switch and Rastelli patients as well.

Cardiac Catheterization. Diagnostic cardiac catheterization may be required for assessing the presence or severity of systemic/pulmonary baffle obstruction, baffle leak, and pulmonary hypertension; coronary ostial stenosis; or tunnel or conduit obstruction when not diagnosed by noninvasive means.

INDICATIONS FOR REINTERVENTION. After the *atrial switch procedure*, severe symptomatic right ventricular dysfunction may warrant surgical treatment in the form of a *two-stage arterial switch* procedure[180-184] or cardiac transplantation. Tricuspid valve replacement is rarely performed for severe systemic (tricuspid) AV valve regurgitation if due to a flail leaflet or cusp perforation providing right ventricular function is adequate. A baffle leak resulting in a significant left-to-right shunt (>1.5/1.0), any right-to-left shunt, or attributable symptoms requires surgical or transcatheter closure. Superior vena cava or inferior vena cava pathway obstruction may require intervention. Superior vena cava stenosis is usually benign, whereas inferior vena cava stenosis may be life threatening. Balloon dilation of superior vena cava or inferior vena cava stenosis is an option in expert hands. Stenting usually relieves the stenosis completely.

Pathway obstruction after the Senning operation is usually more amenable to balloon dilation and stenting. Pulmonary venous obstruction, although usually seen early and reoperated on in childhood, may present in adulthood. Symptomatic bradycardia warrants permanent pacemaker implantation, whereas tachyarrhythmias may require catheter ablation, an antitachycardia pacemaker device, or medical therapy. After an atrial switch, transvenous pacing leads must traverse the upper limb of the baffle to enter the morphological left ventricle. Active fixation is required because coarse trabeculation is absent in the morphological left ventricle. Transvenous pacing should be avoided in patients with residual intracardiac communications because paradoxical emboli can occur.

After an *arterial switch procedure*, significant right ventricular outflow tract obstruction at any level (gradient > 50 mm Hg or right-to-left ventricular pressure ratio > 0.6) may require surgical or catheter augmentation of the right ventricular outflow tract.[21] Myocardial ischemia from coronary artery obstruction may require coronary artery bypass grafting, preferably with arterial conduits. Significant neoaortic valve regurgitation may warrant aortic valve replacement.

In patients who have had the *Rastelli procedure*, significant right ventricle-to-pulmonary artery conduit stenosis (>50 mm Hg withdrawal gradient or mean echo gradient) or significant regurgitation necessitates conduit replacement.

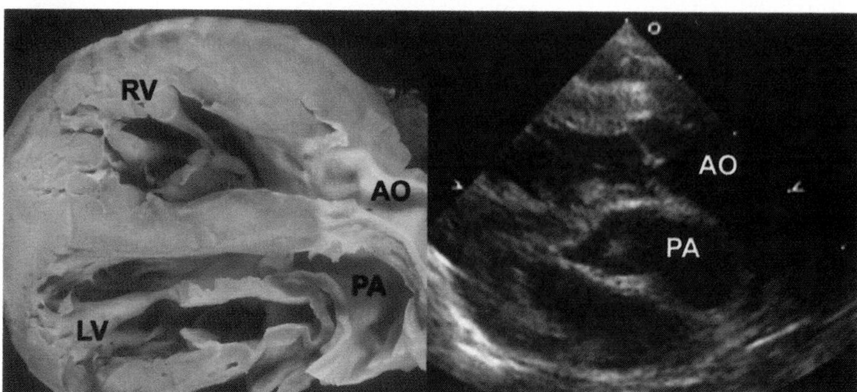

FIGURE 56–23 Parasternal long-axis view in transposition of the great arteries. Note the parallel nature of the aorta and pulmonary artery. AO = aorta; LV = left ventricle; PA = pulmonary artery; RV = right ventricle.

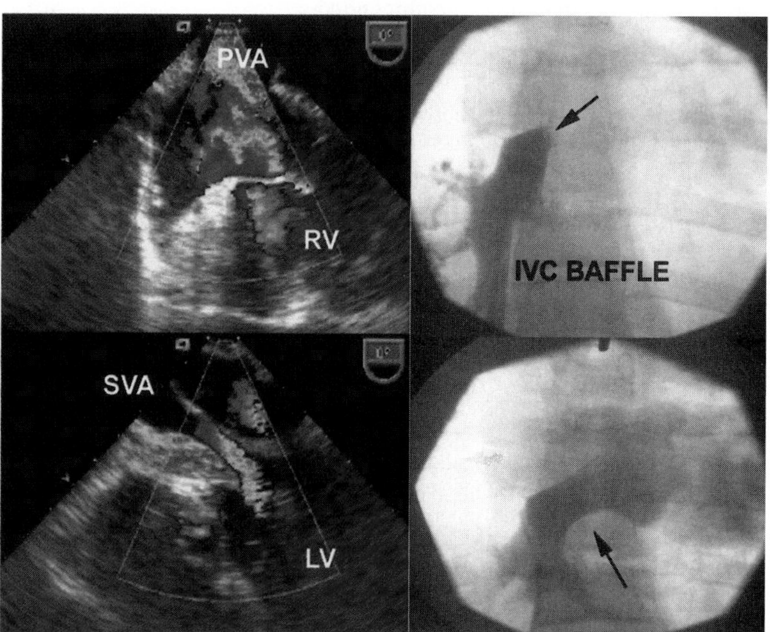

FIGURE 56–24 Montage of post-Mustard cases. The angiogram on the right upper panel shows complete obstruction of the inferior limb of the systemic venous baffle, whereas the lower right panel is the same case after stenting. The upper left image is a transesophageal echocardiogram showing the pulmonary venous baffle with some mild flow acceleration in its midpoint. The lower left panel shows the systemic venous baffle at its left ventricular end. LV = left ventricle; PVA = pulmonary venous atrium; RV = right ventricle; SVA = systemic venous atrium; IVC = inferior vena cava.

Subaortic obstruction across the left ventricle-to-aorta tunnel necessitates left ventricle-to-aorta baffle reconstruction. A significant residual VSD (shunt > 1.5/1.0) may require surgical closure.

Patients with clinical deterioration and a palliative atrial switch should be considered for lung or heart-lung transplantation.

REINTERVENTION OPTIONS

Medical Therapy. The role of afterload reduction with ACE inhibitors to preserve systemic right ventricular function is unknown. In light of the effects of these drugs on dysfunctional systemic left ventricles, it seems logical to assume that similar beneficial effects on systemic right ventricles may occur.[15,16]

Two-Stage Arterial Switch. Patients with symptomatic, severe systemic (right) ventricular dysfunction with or without severe systemic (tricuspid) AV valve regurgitation, following an atrial switch procedure, may require consideration of a conversion procedure to an arterial switch (two-stage arterial switch)[181-183] or heart transplantation. The two-stage arterial switch, or switch-conversion procedure, consists of banding the pulmonary artery in the first stage to induce subpulmonary left ventricular hypertrophy and "train" the left ventricle to support systemic pressure. Once left ventricular systolic pressure is more than 75 percent of systemic pressure and the left ventricular mass is considered adequate, in the second stage the atrial baffles and the pulmonary band are taken down, the atrial septum is reconstructed, and the great arteries are switched, leaving the morphological left ventricle as the systemic ventricle. This procedure is still experimental in adults, with little data available to assess its short- and long-term efficacy.

Cardiac Transplantation. Heart transplantation should be considered as an alternative, given its relatively good 5- to 10-year survival.

REPRODUCTIVE ISSUES. Severe systemic ventricular dysfunction or intractable arrhythmias may be a contraindication to pregnancy, and baffle obstruction should, ideally, be relieved before childbearing.

FOLLOW-UP. Regular follow-up by physicians with special expertise in CHD is recommended.

Atrial Switch. Serial follow-up of systemic right ventricular function is warranted. MRI is best, followed by radionuclide angiography and perhaps by echocardiography. Asymptomatic baffle obstruction should be sought with echocardiography or MRI. Regular Holter monitoring is recommended to diagnose unacceptable bradyarrhythmias or tachyarrhythmias.

Arterial Switch. Regular follow-up with echocardiography is recommended.

Rastelli. Regular follow-up with echocardiography is warranted given the inevitability of conduit degeneration over time.

Congenitally Corrected Transposition of the Great Arteries

DEFINITION. This term describes hearts in which there are discordant AV connections in combination with discordant ventriculoarterial connections.[185]

MORPHOLOGY (Fig. 56–25). cc-TGA is a rare condition, accounting for less than 1 percent of all CHD. When there is the usual atrial arrangement, systemic venous blood passes from the right atrium through a mitral valve to a left ventricle and then to the posteriorly located pulmonary artery. Pulmonary venous blood passes from the left atrium through a tricuspid valve to a left-sided right ventricle and then to an anterior, left-sided aorta. The circulation is thus "physiologically" corrected, but the morphological right ventricle supports the systemic circulation. Associated anomalies occur in up to 95 percent of patients and consist of VSD (75 percent), pulmonary or subpulmonary stenosis (75 percent), and left-sided (tricuspid and often "Ebstein-like") valve anomalies (>75 percent).

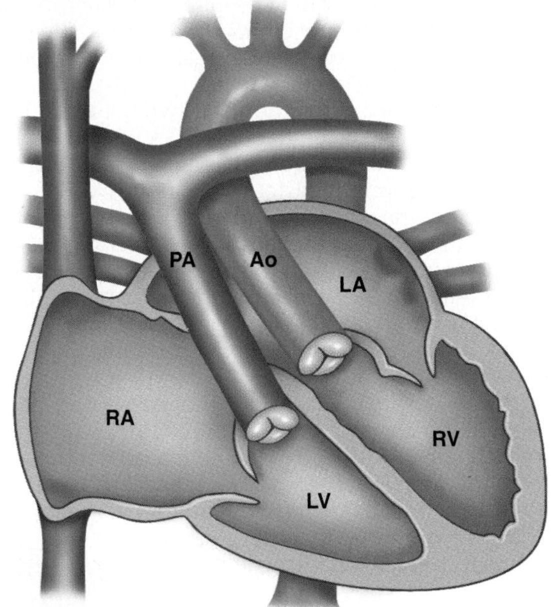

FIGURE 56–25 Diagrammatic representation of congenitally corrected transposition of the great arteries. RA = right atrium; RV = right ventricle; LA = left atrium; LV = left ventricle; Ao = aorta; PA = pulmonary artery. (From Mullins CE, Mayer DC: Congenital Heart Disease: A Diagrammatic Atlas. New York, Wiley-Liss, 1988.)

Because of the inherently abnormal conduction system, 5 percent of patients with cc-TGA are born with congenital complete heart block.

PATHOPHYSIOLOGY. Patients with no associated abnormalities ("isolated" cc-TGA) can exceptionally survive until the seventh or eighth decade.[186] Progressive systemic (tricuspid) AV valve regurgitation and systemic (right) ventricular dysfunction tend to occur from the fourth decade onward, whereas atrial tachyarrhythmias are more common from the fifth decade onward.[187] In addition to those born with congenital complete heart block, acquired complete AV block continues to develop at a rate of 2 percent per year, concentrated mainly at the time of cardiac surgery. Patients with associated anomalies (VSD, pulmonary stenosis, left-sided [tricuspid] valve anomaly) often have undergone surgical palliation (systemic-to-pulmonary artery shunt for cyanosis) or repair of the associated anomalies (see surgical procedures), but a significant number of patients are naturally balanced by a combination of their VSD and subpulmonary left ventricular outflow tract obstruction. While cyanosed they often remain well, with no intervention for many years.[188]

CLINICAL FEATURES

Unoperated. Patients with no associated defects (≤5 percent) can be asymptomatic until late adulthood. Dyspnea, exercise intolerance from developing congestive heart failure, and palpitations from supraventricular arrhythmias most often arise in the fifth or sixth decade.[189] Patients with well-balanced VSD and pulmonary stenosis can present with paradoxical emboli or cyanosis, especially if pulmonary stenosis is severe. Physical examination of a patient whose condition is otherwise uncomplicated reveals a somewhat more medial apex due to the side-by-side orientation of the two ventricles. The A_2 is often palpable in the 2nd left intercostal space due to the anterior location of the aorta. A single S_2 (A_2) is heard, with P_2 often being silent due to its variably posterior location. The murmur of an associated VSD or of left AV valve regurgitation may be heard. The murmur of pulmonary stenosis radiates upward and to the right, given the rightward direction of the main pulmonary artery. If there is complete heart block, cannon "*a* waves" with an S_1 of variable intensity are present.

VSD Patch and Left Ventricular-to-Pulmonary Artery Conduit Repair. Most patients are in functional Class I at 5 to 10 years after surgery despite the common development of tricuspid regurgitation and systemic right ventricular dysfunction after surgical repair. Dyspnea, exercise intolerance, and palpitations from supraventricular arrhythmia often occur in the fourth decade. Complete heart block may complicate surgery in an additional 25 percent. Physical examination reflects the basic cardiac malformation with or without residual coexisting anomalies.

LABORATORY INVESTIGATIONS

ECG. An abnormal direction of initial (septal) depolarization from right to left causes reversal of the precordial Q wave pattern (Q waves are often present in the right precordial leads and absent in the left). First-degree AV block occurs in about 50 percent, and complete AV block occurs in up to 25 percent of patients. Atrial arrhythmias may be seen.

Chest Radiography. Characteristically reveals absence of the normal pulmonary artery segment in favor of a smooth convexity of the left supracardiac border produced by the left-sided ascending aorta. The main pulmonary trunk is medially displaced and absent from the cardiac silhouette; the right pulmonary hilum is often prominent and elevated compared with the left, producing a right-sided "waterfall" appearance.

Echocardiography (Fig. 56–26). Echocardiography permits the identification of the basic malformation as well as any associated anomalies. The morphological left ventricle is characterized by its smooth endocardial surface and is guarded by a bileaflet AV (mitral) valve with no direct septal attachment. The morphological right ventricle is recognized by its apical trabeculation and moderator band and is guarded by a trileaflet apically displaced AV valve (tricuspid valve) with direct attachment to the septum. The AV valves therefore show reversed offsetting, a strong clue to the diagnosis. Ebstein-like malformation of the left (tricuspid) AV valve is defined by excessive (>8 mm/m^2 BSA) apical displacement of the left (tricuspid) AV valve, with or without dysplastic features.

MRI. The major role of MRI in cc-TGA patients is to evaluate the systemic right ventricular volume and ejection fraction. It does so better than echocardiography can at present. For claustrophobic or pacemaker patients, a high-quality radionuclide angiogram with volume estimates serves as a substitute. MRI can evaluate other issues as well, including conduit function and AV valve regurgitation.

Cardiac Catheterization. This is rarely required for diagnosis but may be indicated prior to surgical repair, to demonstrate the coronary artery anatomy as well as ventricular end-diastolic and pulmonary artery pressures.

INDICATIONS FOR INTERVENTION AND REINTERVENTION. If moderate or severe systemic (tricuspid, left) AV valve regurgitation develops, valve replacement should be considered. Left AV valve replacement should be performed before systemic right ventricular function deteriorates, namely at an ejection fraction of 45 percent or more.[190,191] When tricuspid regurgitation is associated with poor systemic (right) ventricular function, the double-switch procedure should perhaps be considered.[192-195] Patients with end-stage symptomatic heart failure should be referred for cardiac transplantation. The presence of a hemodynamically significant VSD (Qp/Qs > 1.5:1.0) or residual VSD with significant native or postsurgical (conduit) pulmonary outflow tract stenosis (echo mean or catheter gradient > 50 mm Hg) may require surgical correction. Left AV valve replacement at the time of VSD and pulmonary stenosis surgery should be considered if concomitant left AV valve regurgitation is present. Pacemaker implantation is usual when complete AV block is present. The optimal pacing modality is DDD. Active fixation electrodes are required, owing to the lack of apical trabeculation in the morphological left ventricle. Transvenous pacing should be avoided if there are intracardiac shunts because paradoxical emboli may occur. Epicardial leads are preferred under these circumstances.

INTERVENTIONAL OPTIONS

Medical Therapy. ACE inhibitor or beta-blocker therapy for patients with systemic ventricular dysfunction may be intuitive, but the role of such agents has not yet been demonstrated.

Conduit Replacement. This is inevitably required in survivors of this type of initial surgery.

Tricuspid Valve Replacement. For significant regurgitation, this is preferable to tricuspid valve repair.[190] Valve repair is usually unsuccessful because of the abnormal, often Ebstein-like anatomy of the valve.

Double-Switch Procedure. This procedure has been successfully performed in children. It should be considered for patients with severe tricuspid regurgitation and systemic ventricular dysfunction.[192] Its purpose is to relocate the left ventricle into the systemic circulation and the right ventricle into the pulmonary circulation, achieving physiological correction. An atrial switch procedure (Mustard or Senning), together with either an arterial switch procedure (when pulmonary stenosis is not present) or a Rastelli-type repair, the so-called Ilbawi procedure[196] (left ventricle tunneled to aorta and right ventricle-to-pulmonary artery valved conduit when VSD and pulmonary stenosis are present), can be performed after adequate left ventricular retraining, leaving the regurgitant tricuspid valve and failing right ventricle on the pulmonary side.

Cardiac Transplantation. Patients with deteriorating systemic (right) ventricular function should be treated aggressively with medical therapy but may need to be considered for transplantation.

INTERVENTIONAL OUTCOMES. After conduit repair and VSD patching, the median survival of patients reaching adulthood is 40 years.[197] The usual causes of death are sudden (presumed arrhythmic) or, more commonly, progressive systemic right ventricular dysfunction with systemic (tricuspid) AV valve regurgitation. The major predictor of poor outcome

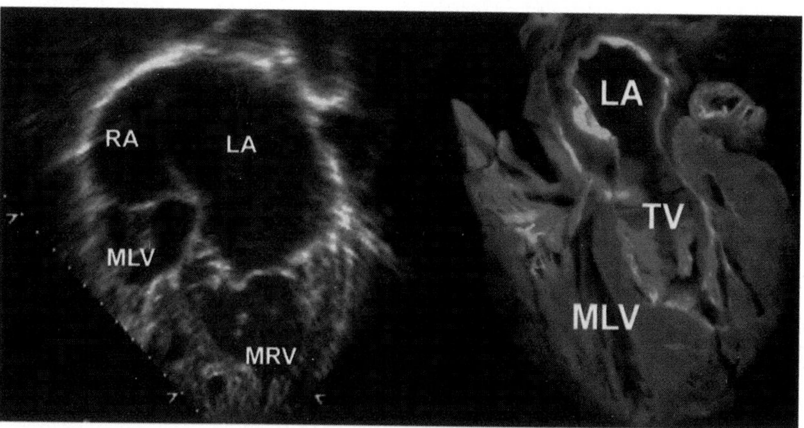

FIGURE 56–26 Four-chamber view in congenitally corrected transposition with dysplasia and displacement of the morphological left-sided tricuspid valve. LA = left atrium; MLV = morphological left ventricle; MRV = morphological right ventricle; RA = right atrium; TV = tricuspid valve.

is the presence of left AV (tricuspid) valve regurgitation.[197] Reoperation is common (15 to 25 percent), with left AV valve replacement usually being the primary reason. Data in adults using the double-switch procedure are lacking, and this procedure should be considered experimental in this patient population.

FOLLOW-UP. All patients should have at least annual cardiology follow-up with an expert in the care of patients with congenital cardiac defects. Regular assessment of systemic (tricuspid) AV valve regurgitation by serial echocardiographic studies and systemic ventricular function by MRI or radionuclide angiography should be done. Holter recording can be useful if paroxysmal atrial arrhythmias or transient complete AV block is suspected.

Double-Outlet Right Ventricle

DEFINITION. The term *double-outlet right ventricle* describes hearts in which more than 50 percent of both semilunar valves arise from the morphological right ventricle. It may coexist with any form of atrial arrangement or AV connection and is independent of infundibular (conal) anatomy.

MORPHOLOGY (Fig. 56–27). There are few morphological descriptors that have invoked more discussion and controversy than double-outlet right ventricle. The definition given earlier is flawed but pragmatic.[198] To some extent this anatomical definition is less important than the understanding of the relationship between the great vessels and the VSD, and the anatomy of the outlets to the great vessels, both of which are crucial determinants of clinical presentation and management.

CLINICAL FEATURES. There are three main categories of double-outlet right ventricle: (1) double-outlet right ventricle with a subaortic VSD, (2) double-outlet right ventricle with a subpulmonary VSD, and (3) double-outlet right ventricle with a noncommitted VSD.

When present, the anatomy of the infundibular septum further modifies the hemodynamics. Taking double-outlet right ventricle with a *subaortic VSD* as an example, where the aorta and its semilunar valve is closest to, or overriding, the trabecular septum, anterior deviation of the outlet septum causes subpulmonary stenosis, and the clinical scenario and management algorithm are similar or identical to that of tetralogy of Fallot. Conversely, if the outlet septum is deviated posteriorly, there will be subaortic stenosis, often with a coexisting abnormality of the aortic arch. The presentation and management of this variation are therefore entirely different. If there is no deviation of the outlet septum, and no outlet obstruction, the clinical scenario will be that of a simple VSD. Double-outlet right ventricle with a *subpulmonary VSD* (Taussig-Bing anomaly) can be considered along with TGA. This is because the usual position of the pulmonary artery (posterior and leftward to the aorta) means that the streaming of deoxygenated and oxygenated blood is similar to that of transposition, even though most of the pulmonary valve is connected to the right ventricle. Anterior deviation of the outlet septum causes subaortic stenosis and aortic anomalies, and posterior deviation causes subpulmonary stenosis and limits pulmonary blood flow. It is also important to recognize double-outlet right ventricle with a *noncommitted VSD*. This defines hearts in which the VSD is remote from the outlets. Surgical management may be particularly difficult.

ASSOCIATED LESIONS. More than half of patients with double-outlet right ventricle have associated anomalies of the AV valves. Mitral valve atresia associated with a hypoplastic left ventricle is common. Ebstein anomaly of the tricuspid valve, complete AV septal defect, and overriding or straddling of either AV valve may occur.[199]

LABORATORY INVESTIGATIONS. Because of the diversity of underlying anatomies, discussion of the ECG and radiographic features is not included here.

Echocardiography. This is the mainstay of diagnosis. The commitment of the semilunar valves to the ventricles is ascertained. When present, deviation of the outlet septum beneath a semilunar valve likely has implications for downstream development. For example, when there is subaortic stenosis, the echocardiographic examination is incomplete until abnormalities of the aorta and arch have been excluded. Preoperative evaluation must also take account of potential AV valve anomalies and straddling in particular.

INDICATIONS FOR INTERVENTION. The goals of operative treatment are to establish left ventricle-to-aorta continuity, create adequate right ventricle-to-pulmonary continuity, and repair associated lesions. Palliative surgery is reserved for those in whom biventricular repair is not possible and in those with markedly reduced pulmonary blood flow. In the latter, an aortopulmonary shunt may be placed to temporize prior to complete correction. For the remainder, complete repair is now performed as a primary procedure in the majority.[200] In double-outlet right ventricle with a subaortic VSD, repair is accomplished by creating an intraventricular baffle that conducts left ventricular blood to the aorta. If there is coexisting subpulmonary stenosis, the repair is similar to that of tetralogy of Fallot. When the VSD is subpulmonary, but without subpulmonary stenosis, repair is accomplished by closure of the VSD and arterial switch. Subpulmonary stenosis frequently is present in double-outlet right ventricle with a subpulmonary VSD. In these cases the aorta is connected to the left ventricle using an intraventricular baffle, and a

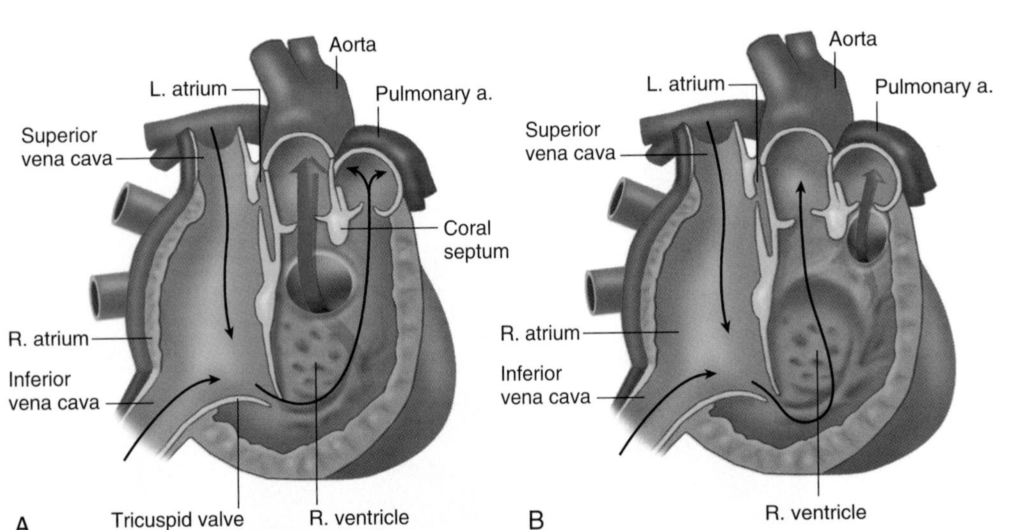

FIGURE 56–27 Double-outlet right ventricle with side-by-side relation of great arteries is illustrated in both panels. **A,** A subaortic ventricular septal defect below the crista supraventricularis favors delivery of left ventricular blood to the aorta. **B,** Subpulmonary location of the ventricular septal defect above the crista favors streaming to the pulmonary trunk. (**A** and **B,** From Castañeda A, Jonas RA, Mayer JE, et al: Cardiac Surgery of the Neonate and Infant. Philadelphia, WB Saunders, 1994, p 446.)

right ventricle-to-pulmonary artery conduit is placed to complete the repair (Rastelli procedure). Classic surgical approaches cannot be used when the VSD is remote and uncommitted to either semilunar orifice.[201] Occasionally the VSD can be baffled toward the aorta, but when this is not possible, the right ventricle may be used as the systemic ventricle. This requires a Mustard or Senning atrial redirection procedure, closure of the VSD, and placement of a conduit between the left ventricle and the pulmonary trunk.

INTERVENTIONAL OPTIONS AND OUTCOMES. The late follow-up of the surgical procedures described earlier (e.g., tetralogy of Fallot repair, arterial switch, Rastelli) tend to be less satisfactory when there is double-outlet right ventricle than when performed for more classic indications.[200,202,203] The development of subaortic stenosis is more likely because of the abnormal geometry of the left ventricular outflow tract that often results after correction.[204] Similarly, right ventricle-to-pulmonary conduit obstruction is more likely because of the spatial difficulties imposed on placement of the conduit, with respect to the position on the right ventricle and the sternum. Because of these considerations, the options for catheter interventions are often fairly limited. However, recurrent arch obstruction and distal pulmonary artery obstruction are amenable to balloon dilation with or without stenting.

FOLLOW-UP. All of these patients require at least annual review by a congenital heart cardiologist.

Ebstein Anomaly

MORPHOLOGY (Fig. 56–28). The common feature in all cases of Ebstein anomaly is apical displacement of the septal tricuspid leaflet in conjunction with leaflet dysplasia. Many, but not all, have associated displacement of the posterior mural leaflet, with the anterior leaflet never being displaced. Although the anterior leaflet is never displaced apically, it may be adherent to the free wall of the right ventricle, causing right ventricular outflow tract obstruction. The displacement of the tricuspid valve results in "atrialization" (functioning as an atrial chamber) of the inflow tract of the right ventricle

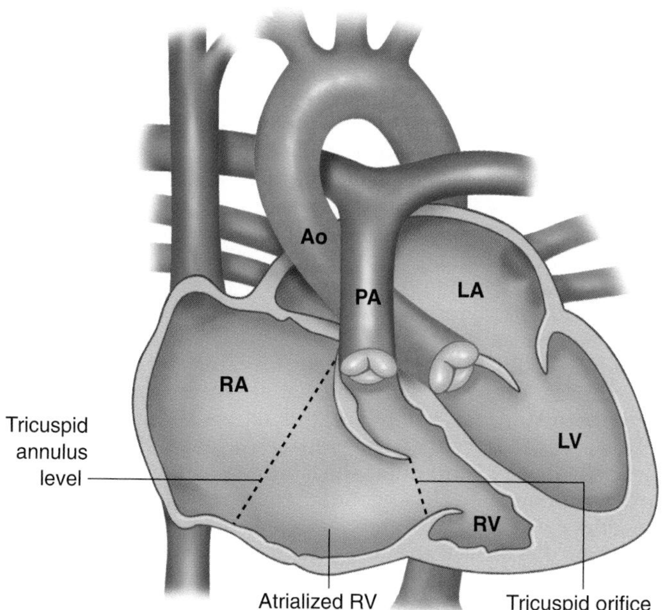

FIGURE 56–28 Diagrammatic representation of Ebstein anomaly. RA = right atrium; RV = right ventricle; LA = left atrium; LV = left ventricle; Ao = aorta; PA = pulmonary artery. (From Mullins CE, Mayer DC: Congenital Heart Disease: A Diagrammatic Atlas. New York, Wiley-Liss, 1988.)

and consequently produces a variably small, functional right ventricle. Associated anomalies include patent foramen ovale or ASD in approximately 50 percent of patients, accessory conduction pathways in 25 percent (usually right sided), and, occasionally, varying degrees of right ventricular outflow tract obstruction, VSD, aortic coarctation, PDA, or mitral valve disease.

PATHOPHYSIOLOGY. Varying degrees of tricuspid regurgitation (or exceptionally tricuspid stenosis) result from the abnormal tricuspid leaflet morphology with consequent further right atrial enlargement. Right ventricular volume overload from significant tricuspid regurgitation and infundibular dilation can also be present. Right-to-left shunting through a patent foramen ovale or ASD occurs if the right atrial pressure exceeds the left atrial pressure (which is often the case when severe tricuspid regurgitation is present).

NATURAL HISTORY. The natural history of patients with Ebstein anomaly depends on its severity.[205] When the tricuspid valve deformity and dysfunction are extreme, death in utero from hydrops fetalis is the norm. When the tricuspid valve deformity is severe, symptoms usually develop in newborn infants. Patients with moderate tricuspid valve deformity and dysfunction usually develop symptoms during late adolescence or young adult life. Adults with Ebstein anomaly can occasionally remain asymptomatic throughout their life if the anomaly is mild—exceptional survival to the ninth decade has been reported.

CLINICAL ISSUES

Pediatrics. With severe tricuspid valve deformity, newborns and infants present with failure to thrive and right-sided congestive heart failure. Most other pediatric patients who present after the neonatal period remain asymptomatic until late adolescence or early adult life.

Adults. Most adult patients present with exercise intolerance (exertional dyspnea and fatigue), palpitations of supraventricular origin, or cyanosis from a right-to-left shunt at atrial level. Occasionally, a paradoxical embolus resulting in a transient ischemic attack or stroke can call attention to the diagnosis. Right-sided cardiac failure from severe tricuspid regurgitation and right ventricular dysfunction is possible. Sudden death (presumed to be arrhythmic in nature) is described. Physical examination typically reveals an unimpressive jugular venous pressure because of the large and compliant right atrium and atrialized right ventricle; a widely split S_1 with a loud tricuspid component (the "sail sound"); a widely split S_2 from the right bundle branch block; and a right-sided third heart sound. A pansystolic murmur increasing on inspiration from tricuspid regurgitation is best heard at the lower left sternal border. Cyanosis from a right-to-left shunt at the atrial level may or may not be present.

LABORATORY INVESTIGATIONS

ECG. The ECG presentation of Ebstein anomaly varies widely. Low voltage is typical. Peaked P waves in leads II and V_1 reflect right atrial enlargement. The PR interval is usually prolonged, but a short PR interval and a delta wave from early activation through an accessory pathway can be present. An rsr′ pattern consistent with right ventricular conduction delay is typically seen in lead V_1, and right bundle branch block is common in adults. Atrial flutter and fibrillation are common. The ECG may be normal.

Chest Radiography. A rightward convexity from an enlarged right atrium and atrialized right ventricle coupled with a leftward convexity from a dilated infundibulum give the heart a "water bottle" appearance on chest radiograph. Cardiomegaly, highly variable in degree, is the rule. The aorta and the pulmonary trunk are inconspicuous. The pulmonary vasculature is usually normal to reduced.

Echocardiography (Fig. 56–29). The diagnosis of Ebstein anomaly is usually made by echocardiography. Apical displacement of the septal leaflet of the tricuspid valve by

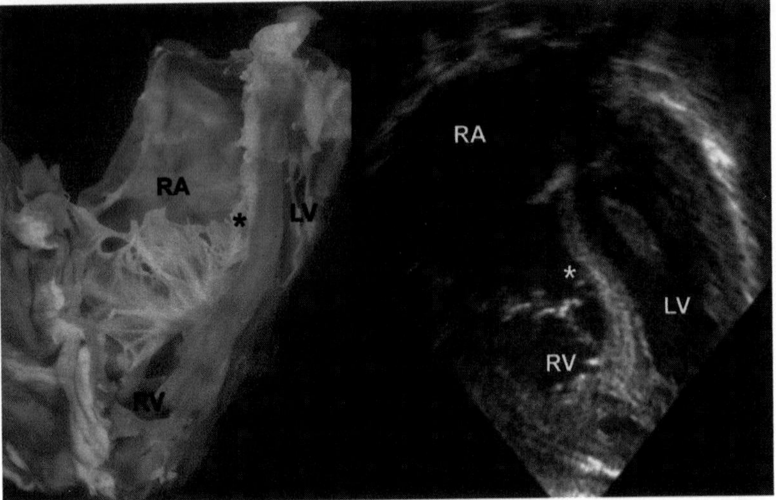

FIGURE 56–29 Apical four-chamber view in Ebstein malformation of the tricuspid valve. Note the significant displacement of the septal tricuspid valve leaflet (asterisk), with associated valve dysplasia. LV = left ventricle; RA = right atrium; RV = right ventricle.

8 mm/m^2 or more, combined with an elongated sail-like appearance of the anterior leaflet, confirms the diagnosis. The size of the atrialized portion of the right ventricle (identified between the tricuspid annulus and the ventricular attachment of the tricuspid valve leaflets) and the systolic performance of the functional right ventricle can be estimated. The degree of tricuspid regurgitation (and more rarely stenosis) can be assessed. Associated defects such as ASDs as well as the presence and direction of shunting can also be identified.

Angiography. Cardiac catheterization is required mainly when concomitant coronary artery disease is suspected and to determine if pulmonary artery pressures are elevated. When performed, selective right ventricular angiography shows the extent of tricuspid valve displacement, the size of the functional right ventricle, and configuration of its outflow tract.

MRI. This investigation can offer insights into functional right ventricular volume and function.

INDICATIONS FOR INTERVENTION. Indications for intervention include substantial cyanosis, right-sided heart failure, deteriorating functional capacity (NYHA ≥ class III), and perhaps the occurrence of paradoxical emboli. Recurrent supraventricular arrhythmias not controlled by medical or ablation therapy, and asymptomatic substantial cardiomegaly (cardiothoracic ratio >65 percent) are relative indications.[206]

INTERVENTIONAL OPTIONS. Tricuspid valve repair when feasible is preferable to tricuspid valve replacement. The feasibility of tricuspid valve repair depends primarily on the experience and skill of the surgeon, as well as on the adequacy of the anterior leaflet of the tricuspid valve to form a monocusp valve. Tricuspid valve repair is possible when the edges of the anterior leaflet of the tricuspid valve are not severely tethered down to the myocardium and when the functional right ventricle is of adequate size (>35 percent of the total right ventricle).[74] If the tricuspid valve is not repairable, valve replacement will be necessary, usually with a bioprosthetic tricuspid valve. For “high-risk” patients (those with severe tricuspid regurgitation, an inadequate functional right ventricle [because of size or function], and/or chronic supraventricular arrhythmias), a bidirectional cavopulmonary connection can be added to reduce right ventricular preload if pulmonary artery pressures are low.[207] Occasionally a Fontan operation may be the best option in patients with tricuspid stenosis and/or a hypoplastic right ventricle. A concomitant right atrial or biatrial maze procedure at the time of surgery should be considered in patients with chronic atrial flutter/fibrillation.[58] If an accessory pathway is present, this should be mapped and obliterated either at the time of surgical repair or preoperatively in the catheter laboratory. An atrial communication, if present, should be closed.

With satisfactory valve repair, with or without plication of the atrialized right ventricle or bidirectional cavopulmonary connection, the medium-term prognosis is excellent.[50,208] Late arrhythmias can occur.[209] With valve replacement, results are less satisfactory. Valve replacement may be necessary because of a failing bioprosthesis or a thrombosed mechanical valve.

REPRODUCTIVE ISSUES. In the absence of maternal cyanosis, right-sided heart failure, or arrhythmias, pregnancy is usually well tolerated.[210]

FOLLOW-UP ISSUES. All patients with Ebstein anomaly should have regular follow-up, the frequency being dictated by the severity of their disease. Particular attention should be paid to patients with cyanosis, substantial cardiomegaly, poor right ventricular function, and recurrent atrial arrhythmias. Patients with substantial tricuspid regurgitation following tricuspid valve repair need close follow-up, as do patients with recurrent atrial arrhythmias, degenerating bioprostheses, or dysfunctional mechanical valves.

Valvular and Vascular Conditions

Left Ventricular Outflow Tract Lesions (Fig. 56–30)

COARCTATION OF THE AORTA

Aortic arch obstruction may be divided into (1) localized coarctation in close proximity to a PDA or ligamentum, (2) tubular hypoplasia of some part of the aortic arch system, and (3) aortic arch interruption.

Localized Aortic Coarctation

MORPHOLOGY. This lesion consists of a localized shelf in the posterolateral aortic wall opposite the ductus arteriosus. A neonatal presentation is more often associated with a shelf plus transverse aortic arch and isthmic hypoplasia, whereas with a later presentation these areas are larger.[211,212]

CLINICAL FEATURES. Coarctation occurs two to five times more commonly in males, and there is a high degree of association with gonadal dysgenesis (Turner syndrome) and bicuspid aortic valve. Other common associated anomalies include VSD and mitral stenosis or regurgitation. Additional lesions have an impact on outcome.[213]

NEONATES. Rapid, severe obstruction in infancy is a prominent cause of left ventricular failure and systemic hypoperfusion. Heart failure in this setting is due to a sudden increase in left ventricular wall stress after closure of the arterial duct. Substantial left-to-right shunting across a patent foramen ovale and pulmonary venous hypertension secondary to heart failure cause pulmonary arterial hypertension. Because little or no aortic obstruction existed during fetal life, the collateral circulation in the newborn period is often poorly developed. In these infants, peripheral pulses characteristically are weak throughout the body until left ventricular function is improved with medical management; a significant pressure difference then develops between the arms and the legs, allowing detection of a pulse discrepancy. Cardiac murmurs are nonspecific in infancy and commonly are derived from associated lesions.

ECG. This shows right axis deviation and right ventricular hypertrophy.

Chest Radiography. This shows generalized cardiomegaly and pulmonary arterial and venous engorgement.

Echocardiography (Fig. 56–31A). This demonstrates the posterior shelf and the degree of associated isthmic and/or transverse arch hypoplasia. Doppler echocardiography is helpful if the ductus is closed or partially restrictive and demonstrates a high-velocity jet during systole and diastole. On the other hand, if the ductus is widely patent, then the usual right-to-left shunting makes the Doppler assessment invalid, because the distal pressure then reflects the high pulmonary artery pressure. With associated tubular hypoplasia, Doppler-derived gradients provide higher and less reliable values compared with those obtained by blood pressure or catheterization measurements.[214,215]

MRA. Although this is the gold standard for evaluation of the aortic arch in the older child and adult, it is usually unnecessary in the neonate and infant.[216]

Management usually involves prostaglandin therapy in an attempt to reopen or maintain patency of a ductus arteriosus. After prostaglandin E_1 infusion to dilate the ductus arteriosus, the pressure difference may be obliterated across the site of coarctation because the fetal flow pattern is reestablished. This has the additional benefit of improving renal perfusion, which in turn helps reverse the frequently associated metabolic acidosis.

Intervention in this age group usually involves surgical relief of the obstruction with excision of the area of coarctation and extended end-to-end repair or end-to-side anastomosis with absorbable sutures to allow remodeling of the aorta with time.[217] Subclavian flap aortoplasty, which was employed extensively in the past, is now less popular than the earlier-mentioned procedures. It is generally believed that balloon dilation does not play a role in management in this age group. Early surgery is associated with a lower incidence of long-term hypertension.[217]

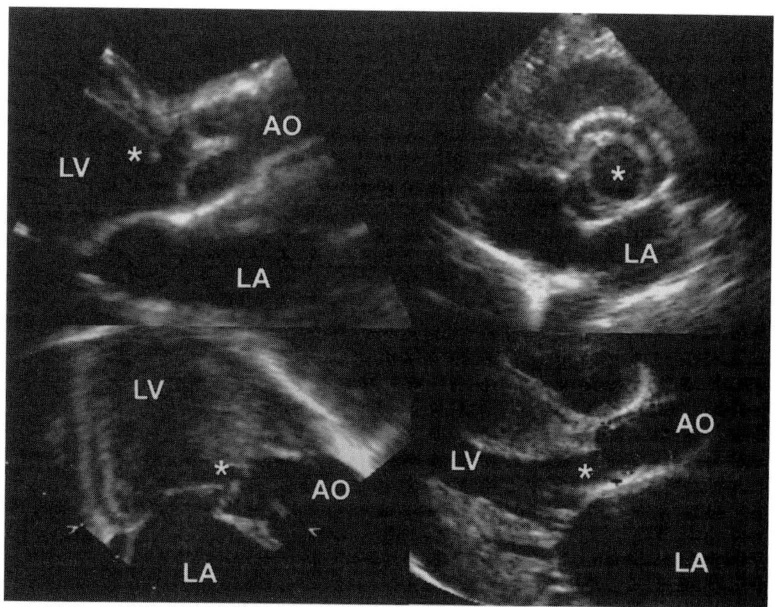

FIGURE 56–30 Montage demonstrating the different types of left ventricular outflow tract obstruction (asterisks). The upper left image shows isolated fibromuscular obstruction, the upper right stenosis due to a bicuspid aortic valve, the lower left due to chordal apparatus from the anterior mitral leaflet, and the lower right due to tunnel narrowing at the valve, annular, and subvalve level. AO = aorta; LA = left atrium; LV = left ventricle.

INFANTS AND CHILDREN

Presentation. Most infants and children with isolated coarctation are asymptomatic, with the findings of reduced femoral pulses and/or hypertension being detected during routine medical care of the pediatric patient. Heart failure is uncommon because the left ventricle has a chance to become hypertrophied, thus maintaining a normal wall stress. Complaints of headache, cold extremities, and claudication with exercise may be noted in the older child and adolescent.

A midsystolic murmur over the anterior chest, back, and spinous processes is most frequent, becoming continuous if the lumen is sufficiently narrowed to result in a high-velocity jet across the lesion throughout the cardiac cycle. Additional systolic and continuous murmurs over the lateral thoracic wall may reflect increased flow through dilated and tortuous collateral vessels, which are commonly not heard until later childhood.

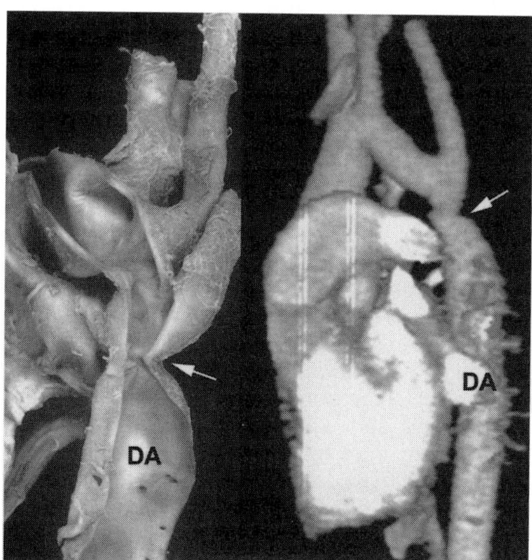

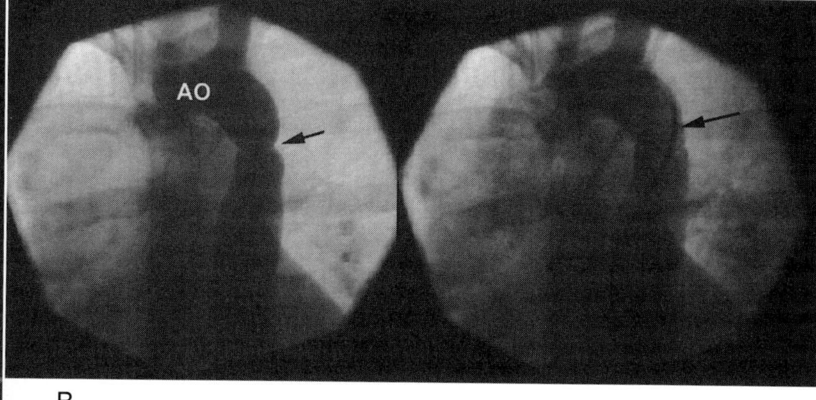

FIGURE 56–31 **A,** Montage of a coarctation of the aorta. The left image is a specimen that shows the site of the posterior shelf, as outlined by the arrow. The right image is from an MRI and shows the posterior shelf and some associated transverse arch hypoplasia. **B,** Angiogram of a coarctation of the aorta, before and after stenting. AO = aorta; DA = descending aorta.

ECG. This reveals left ventricular hypertrophy of various degrees, depending on the height of arterial pressure above the obstruction and the patient's age. Coexisting right ventricular hypertrophy usually implies a complicated lesion.

Chest Radiography. The characteristic posteroanterior film feature is the so-called figure-3 configuration of the proximal descending thoracic aorta due to both prestenotic and poststenotic dilation. Rib notching (unilateral or bilateral, second to ninth ribs) is present in 50 percent of cases. Rib notching is unilateral if the right or left subclavian arteries arise from the aorta distal to the coarctation. Rib notching is noted as an erosion of the undersurface of a posterior rib, usually at its outer third, with a sclerotic margin.

Echocardiography. This demonstrates a posterior shelf, a well-expanded isthmus and transverse aortic arch (in most cases), and a high-velocity continuous jet through the coarctation site. Of interest there is a slow upstroke on the abdominal aortic velocity profile when compared to that seen in the ascending aorta.

MRI. This provides detailed information in this age group and may be performed prior to intervention, particularly if balloon dilation is the treatment of choice. This is the best tool for post-intervention imaging and has become routine in many centers.[216]

Angiocardiography. This is reserved for delineating the coarctation at the time of balloon dilation.

Primary management in those cases with a well-expanded isthmus and transverse aortic arch invariably involves balloon dilation.[218] Surgery is usually reserved for cases where there is associated arch hypoplasia that requires a patch, as well as coarctation resection.

Paradoxical hypertension of short duration is often noted in the immediate postoperative period, a phenomenon much less common after balloon angioplasty. A resetting of carotid baroreceptors and increased catecholamine secretion appears to be responsible for the initial phase of postoperative systemic hypertension, with a later, second phase of prolonged elevation of systolic and particularly diastolic blood pressure related to activation of the renin-angiotensin system. A necrotizing panarteritis of the small vessels of the gastrointestinal tract of uncertain cause occasionally complicates the course of recovery.

Recoarctation. The risk of recurrent narrowing after repair of coarctation in infancy is 5 to 10 percent. Such narrowing is best screened for with Doppler ultrasonography, with MRI being the gold standard for imaging. Clinical decisions to intervene are usually based on a cuff blood pressure difference between the right arm and leg (for a left aortic arch and normal innominate artery). Although there are no hard and fast rules for absolute blood pressure difference, it has been common practice to reintervene when the blood pressure difference is more than 25 to 30 mm Hg, in the presence of systemic hypertension. Although Doppler measurements can detect the presence of a recurrent obstruction, this technique provides an overestimation of the blood pressure–measured gradients due to the phenomenon of pressure recovery.[214] Recoarctation is usually addressed with balloon dilation if the obstruction is relatively localized. In the presence of long-segment narrowings, surgical intervention may be necessary, with the use of patch augmentation of the hypoplastic segment. More recently in the adolescent or adult, balloon-expandable stents have been employed with good success.[219] This has the advantage of avoiding the risk of potential neurological damage in post-intervention cases that invariably have poorly developed collaterals.

Long-Term Complications. In those patients who survive the first 2 years of life, complications of juxtaductal coarctation are uncommon before the second or third decade.[220-222] The chief hazards to patients with coarctation result from severe hypertension and include the development of cerebral aneurysms and hemorrhage, hypertensive encephalopathy, rupture of the aorta, left ventricular failure, and infective endocarditis. Systemic hypertension in the absence of residual coarctation has been observed in resting or exercise-stressed patients postoperatively and appears to be related to the duration of preoperative hypertension.[11,223] Life-long observation is desirable because of the late onset of hypertension in some postoperative patients.

ADULTS. Although much of the previous material is also relevant in the adult, there are some differences in the issues faced by adult patients. *Complex coarctation* is used to describe coarctation in the presence of other important intracardiac anomalies (e.g., VSD, left ventricular outflow tract obstruction, and mitral stenosis) and is usually detected in infancy. *Simple coarctation* refers to coarctation in the absence of such lesions. It is the most common form detected de novo in adults. Associated abnormalities include bicuspid aortic valve in most cases; intracranial aneurysms (most commonly of the circle of Willis) in up to 10 percent; and acquired intercostal artery aneurysms. One definition of *significant coarctation* requires a gradient greater than 20 mm Hg across the coarctation site at angiography with or without proximal systemic hypertension. A second definition of significant coarctation requires the presence of proximal hypertension in the company of echocardiographic or angiographic evidence of aortic coarctation. If there is an extensive collateral circulation, there may be minimal or no pressure gradient and acquired aortic atresia.

Death in patients who do not undergo repair is usually due to heart failure (usually > 30 years of age), coronary artery disease, aortic rupture/dissection, concomitant aortic valve disease, infective endarteritis/endocarditis, or cerebral hemorrhage.[224,225] Of Turner syndrome patients, 35 percent have aortic coarctation.

Clinical Features. Patients can be asymptomatic, or they can present with minimal symptoms of epistaxis, headache, and leg weakness on exertion or more serious symptoms of congestive heart failure, angina, aortic stenosis, aortic dissection, or unexplained intracerebral hemorrhage. Leg claudication (pain) is rare unless there is concomitant abdominal aortic coarctation (Somerville J, personal communication, 1998). A thorough clinical examination reveals upper limb systemic hypertension as well as a differential systolic blood pressure of at least 10 mm Hg (brachial > popliteal artery pressure). Radial-femoral pulse delay is evident unless significant aortic regurgitation coexists. Auscultation may reveal an interscapular systolic murmur emanating from the coarctation site and a widespread crescendo-decrescendo systolic murmur throughout the chest wall from intercostal collateral arteries. Fundoscopic examination can reveal "corkscrew" tortuosity of retinal arterioles.

INTERVENTIONAL OUTCOMES

Surgical. After surgical repair of simple coarctation, the obstruction is usually relieved with minimal mortality (1 percent). Paraplegia due to spinal cord ischemia is uncommon (0.4 percent) and may occur in patients who do not have well-developed collateral circulation. The prevalence of recoarctation reported in the literature varies widely, from 7 to 60 percent depending on the definition used, the length of follow-up, and the age at surgery. The appropriateness of the surgical repair for a given anatomy is probably the main factor dictating the chance of recoarctation rather than the type of surgical repair itself.[226] True aneurysm formation at the site of coarctation repair is also a well-recognized entity, with a reported incidence between 2 and 27 percent.[227-229] Aneurysms are particularly common after Dacron patch aortoplasty and usually occur in the native aorta opposite the patch. Late dissection at the repair site is rare, but false aneurysms, usually at the suture line, can occur. Long-term follow-up after surgical correction of coarctation of the aorta still reveals an increased incidence of premature cardiovascular disease and death.[230,231]

Transcatheter. After balloon dilation (Fig. 56–31B), aortic dissection, restenosis, and aneurysm formation at the site of coarctation all have been documented.[232-236] These complications may well be reduced if stents are used.[219] The significance of aneurysm formation is often unknown, and longer-term data are needed.[237]

Prior hypertension resolves in up to 50 percent of patients but may recur later in life, especially if the intervention is performed at an older age.[230,231] In some of these patients this may be essential hypertension, but a hemodynamic basis should be sought and blood pressure control should be attained. Systolic hypertension is also common with exercise and is not a surrogate marker for recoarctation of the aorta.[11] It may be related to residual arch hypoplasia or to increased renin and catecholamine activity from residual functional abnormalities of the precoarctation vessels. The criteria for and significance of exertional systolic hypertension are controversial.[11] Late cerebrovascular events occur, notably in those patients undergoing repair as adults and in those with residual hypertension. Endocarditis or endarteritis can occur at the coarctation site or on intracardiac lesions; and if this occurs at the coarctation site, embolic manifestations are restricted to the legs.

FOLLOW-UP. All patients should have follow-up examination every 1 to 3 years. Particular attention should be directed toward residual hypertension; heart failure; intracardiac disease, such as an associated bicuspid aortic valve, which can become stenotic or regurgitant later in life; or an ascending aortopathy sometimes seen in the presence of bicuspid aortic valve. Complications at the site of repair such as restenosis and aneurysm formation should also be sought using clinical examination, chest radiography, echocardiography, and periodic MRI or CT scanning. Patients with Dacron patch repair should probably undergo an MRI[238] or spiral CT examination every 3 to 5 years or so to detect subclinical aneurysm formation. Hemoptysis from a leaking or ruptured aneurysm is a serious complication requiring immediate investigation and surgery. New or unusual headaches raise the possibility of berry aneurysms. Endocarditis prophylaxis is recommended for any residual turbulent flow.

AORTIC ARCH HYPOPLASIA

MORPHOLOGY. The aortic isthmus, the portion of the aorta between the left subclavian artery and the ductus arteriosus, should be narrowed in the fetus and newborn. The lumen of the aortic isthmus is about two-thirds that of the ascending and descending portions of the aorta until age 6 to 9 months, when the physiological narrowing disappears. Pathological tubular hypoplasia of the aortic arch usually is noted in the aortic isthmus and is most commonly associated with presentation of aortic coarctation in the newborn period. Despite this, there is a small group of cases where the arch obstruction is due primarily to tubular hypoplasia, usually involving both the aortic isthmus and transverse aortic arch (between the innominate and subclavian artery). These cases usually present early on in life with similar findings to those with a severe coarctation of the aorta. As with the latter, they are duct dependent and may also be associated with other left-sided obstructive lesions.

MANAGEMENT OPTIONS. Provided the other left-sided structures are formed well enough to sustain life, the management involves arch reconstruction with a patch, in a similar fashion to those cases undergoing a Norwood procedure for hypoplastic left heart syndrome. If the left-sided structures are hypoplastic, then palliative surgery with a Norwood procedure or cardiac transplantation are the two treatments of choice.

Complex Coarctation. In some instances the coarctation of the aorta is part of a more complex spectrum of lesions. This can be seen in cases with double-outlet right ventricle, cc-TGA, D-TGA, functionally single ventricle, truncus arteriosus, and AV septal defect. In these cases the decision process involves not only the coarctation repair but the management of the associated lesion(s). In the current era, the general trend is to complete repair of the intracardiac lesion at the same time as the arch repair.

SINUS OF VALSALVA ANEURYSM AND FISTULA

MORPHOLOGY. The malformation consists of a separation, or lack of fusion, between the media of the aorta and the annulus fibrosus of the aortic valve. The receiving chamber of a right aortic sinus aortocardiac fistula is usually the right ventricle, but occasionally, when the noncoronary cusp is involved, the fistula drains into the right atrium. Five to 15 percent of aneurysms originate in the posterior or noncoronary sinus. The left aortic sinus is seldom involved. Associated anomalies are common and include a VSD, bicuspid aortic valve, and aortic coarctation.

CLINICAL FEATURES. The deficiency in the aortic media appears to be congenital. Reports in infants are exceedingly rare and are infrequent in children, because progressive aneurysmal dilation of the weakened area develops but may not be recognized until the third or fourth decade of life, when rupture into a cardiac chamber occurs.[239-241] A congenital aneurysm of an aortic sinus of Valsalva, particularly the right coronary sinus, is an uncommon anomaly that occurs three times more often in males. An unruptured aneurysm usually does not produce a hemodynamic abnormality. Rarely, myocardial ischemia may be caused by coronary arterial compression. Rupture is often of abrupt onset, causes chest pain, and creates continuous arteriovenous shunting and acute volume loading of both right and left heart chambers, which promptly results in heart failure. An additional complication is infective endocarditis, which may originate either on the edges of the aneurysm or on those areas in the right side of the heart that are traumatized by the jetlike stream of blood flowing through the fistula.

The presence of this anomaly should be suspected in a patient with a combination of chest pain of sudden onset, resting or exertional dyspnea, bounding pulses, and a loud, superficial, continuous murmur accentuated in diastole when the fistula opens into the right ventricle, as well as a thrill along the right or left lower sternal border. The physical findings can be difficult to distinguish from those produced by a coronary arteriovenous fistula.

LABORATORY INVESTIGATIONS

ECG. This may show biventricular hypertrophy, or it may be normal.

Chest Radiography. This may demonstrate generalized cardiomegaly and usually heart failure.

Echocardiography. Studies based on 2D and pulsed Doppler echocardiography may detect the walls of the aneurysm and disturbed flow within the aneurysm or at the site of perforation, respectively. TEE may provide more precise information than the transthoracic approach.[242,243]

Cardiac Catheterization. This reveals a left-to-right shunt at the ventricular or, less commonly, the atrial level; the diagnosis may be established definitively by retrograde thoracic aortography.

MANAGEMENT OPTIONS AND OUTCOMES. Preoperative medical management consists of measures to relieve cardiac failure and to treat coexistent arrhythmias or endocarditis, if present. At operation, the aneurysm is closed and amputated, and the aortic wall is reunited with the heart, either by direct suture or with a prosthesis. Every effort should be made to preserve the aortic valve in children because patch closure of the defect combined with prosthetic valve replacement greatly enhances the risk of operation in small patients. Rarely, device closure of the ruptured aneurysm has been attempted.[244]

VASCULAR RINGS

MORPHOLOGY. The term *vascular ring* is used for those aortic arch or pulmonary artery malformations that exhibit an abnormal relation with the esophagus and trachea, often causing dysphagia and/or respiratory symptoms.[245]

DOUBLE AORTIC ARCH (Fig. 56–32). The most common vascular ring is produced by a double aortic arch in which both the right and left fourth embryonic aortic arches persist. In the most common type of double aortic arch, there is a left ligamentum arteriosum or occasionally a ductus arteriosus. Although both arches may be patent at the time of diagnosis, invariably the left arch distal to the left subclavian artery is atretic and is connected to the descending aorta by a fibrous remnant that completes the ring. In the setting where both arches are patent, the right arch is usually larger than the left. This usually occurs as an isolated lesion, with the respiratory symptoms being caused by tracheal compression and frequently associated laryngomalacia, usually in the neonate and young infant.

RIGHT AORTIC ARCH. A right aortic arch with a left ductus or ligamentum arteriosum connecting the left pulmonary artery and the upper part of the descending aorta is the next most important vascular ring seen. Although all with this lesion have a vascular ring, not all cases are symptomatic. Indeed those patients who are symptomatic usually have an associated diverticulum of Kommerrell.[246] This is a large outpouching at the distal takeoff of the left subclavian artery from the descending aorta. It is the combination of the diverticulum and the ring that causes the airway compression.

ANOMALOUS ORIGIN OF A RIGHT SUBCLAVIAN ARTERY. This is one of the most common abnormalities of the aortic arch that is encountered. Although the aberrant right subclavian artery runs posterior to the esophagus it does not form a vascular ring unless there is an associated right-sided ductus or ligamentum to complete the ring. During adulthood about 5 percent of patients with an aberrant right subclavian artery (and a left ductus) develop symptoms due to rigidity of the aberrant vessel.

RETROESOPHAGEAL DESCENDING AORTA. This is a rarer but more problematic type of vascular ring. In this setting there may be either an ascending left and descending right, or an ascending right and descending left, aorta. The retroesophageal component of the descending aorta causes the tracheal compression, in conjunction with the left- or right-sided ligamentum.[247,248]

PULMONARY ARTERY SLING. This is usually made up of the left pulmonary artery arising from the right pulmonary artery and runs posterior to the trachea but anterior to the esophagus. This is usually seen in isolation and is associated with significant hypoplasia of the bronchial tree, which is the predominant cause of the airway symptoms.

CLINICAL FEATURES. The symptoms produced by vascular rings depend on the tightness of anatomical constriction of the trachea and esophagus and consist principally of respiratory difficulties including stridor, cyanosis (especially with feeding), and dysphagia. Not all patients with a vascular ring are symptomatic, and cases with an aberrant left subclavian artery are frequently detected at the time of evaluation for associated CHD. Although most patients with a true ring and some airway compression present early on in life, others present later on with dysphagia, with others escaping diagnosis forever.

LABORATORY INVESTIGATIONS

ECG. This appears normal unless associated cardiovascular anomalies are present.

Chest Radiography. If there is evidence of a right aortic arch in a symptomatic patient, then a vascular ring should be suspected. In some instances there is evidence of some airway narrowing. The barium esophagogram is a useful screening procedure. Prominent posterior indentation of the esophagus is observed in many of the common vascular ring arrangements, although the pulmonary artery vascular sling produces an anterior indentation.

Echocardiography. This is a very sensitive tool for evaluating the laterality of the aortic arch, including a detailed assessment of the associated brachiocephalic vessels.[249] In general if there is normal branching of the innominate artery, to the right for a left aortic arch and to the left for a right, along with the correct "sidedness" of the descending aorta, then a vascular ring can be excluded. *Most cases with a double aortic arch* have a dominant right arch, with the descending aorta appearing to dip posteriorly as it runs behind the esophagus. A patent ductus or ligamentum can usually be identified by echocardiography. When both arches are patent, a frontal plane sweep from inferior to superior demonstrates both patent arches, as well as their brachiocephalic vessels. *A right aortic arch with an aberrant left subclavian artery* is suspected when it is not possible to identify normal branching of the left-sided innominate artery. *A retroesophageal descending aorta* should be suspected when the ascending aorta and its brachiocephalic arteries are readily identified but there is difficulty in identifying the descending aorta as it traverses behind the esophagus. *A left pulmonary artery sling* is suspected when the normal branching pattern of pulmonary arteries cannot be identified. In this setting color Doppler permits the identification of the left pulmonary artery as it arises from the right pulmonary artery and runs in a posterior and leftward direction.

MRI and CT. MRI and CT play a major role in the evaluation of patients with a vascular ring. In fact MRA has become the gold standard for the evaluation of the aorta and its branches. The only disadvantage for infants is that it often requires general anesthesia to achieve a successful examination. On the other hand, spiral CT is a technique that is fast and provides better definition of the affected airways. This latter technique is particularly valuable for patients with a pulmonary artery sling, where the vascular ring plays a secondary role to the airway abnormalities. The advantages of these techniques are that, unlike echocardiog-

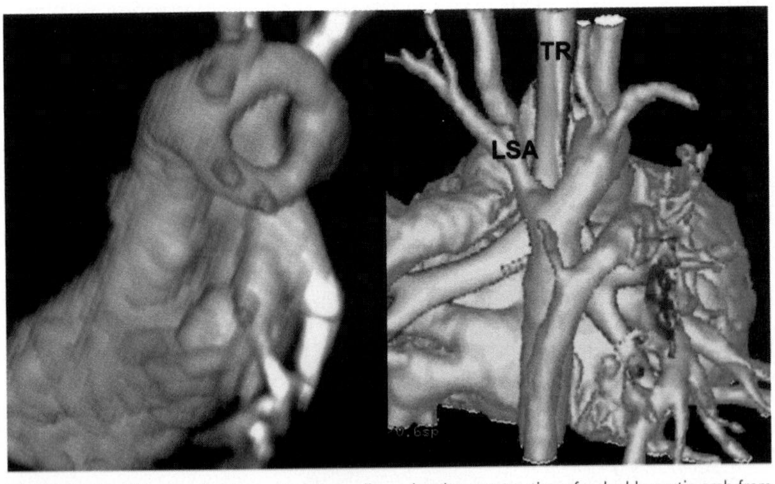

FIGURE 56–32 The left image is a three-dimensional reconstruction of a double aortic arch from an MRI, whereas the right image is from an aberrant left subclavian artery as seen by spiral CT. LSA = left subclavian artery; TR = trachea.

raphy, they permit a precise assessment of the more posterior vascular structures and their relationships to the esophagus and airways. These techniques are particularly valuable in the more complex forms, such as a retroesophageal descending aorta.

Management Options and Outcomes. The severity of symptoms and the anatomy of the malformation are the most important factors in determining treatment. Patients, particularly infants, with respiratory obstruction require prompt surgical intervention.[250] A left thoracotomy is the surgical approach in most patients with a vascular ring. For the most common vascular rings such as a double aortic arch or aberrant left subclavian artery, the combination of a chest radiograph, barium swallow, and echocardiogram is all that is necessary prior to surgical intervention.

Operative repair of the double aortic arch requires division of the minor arch (usually the left) and the ligamentum. Patients with a right aortic arch and a left ductus or ligamentum arteriosum require division of the ductus or ligamentum and/or ligation and division of the left subclavian artery, which is the posterior component of the ring. Video-assisted thoracoscopy holds promise as an alternative to open thoracotomy for management.[251,252] In patients with a pulmonary artery vascular sling, operation consists of detachment of the left pulmonary artery at its origin and anastomosis to the main pulmonary artery directly or by way of a conduit with its proximal end brought anterior to the trachea.

CONGENITAL AORTIC VALVE STENOSIS

GENERAL CONSIDERATIONS. We deal here only with this condition in newborns and children, since the adult presentation is dealt with in Chapter 52. Congenital aortic valve stenosis is a relatively common anomaly. Congenital aortic valve stenosis occurs much more frequently in males, with a gender ratio of 4:1. Associated cardiovascular anomalies have been noted in as many as 20 percent of patients. PDA and coarctation of the aorta occur most frequently with aortic valve stenosis; all three of these lesions may coexist.

MORPHOLOGY. The basic malformation consists of thickening of valve tissue with various degrees of commissural fusion. The valve most commonly is bicuspid. In some patients, the stenotic aortic valve is unicuspid and dome shaped, with no or one lateral attachment to the aorta at the level of the orifice. In infants and young children with severe aortic stenosis, the aortic valve annulus may be relatively underdeveloped. This lesion forms a continuum with the hypoplastic left heart syndrome and the aortic atresia and hypoplasia complexes. Secondary calcification of the valve is rare in childhood. When the obstruction is hemodynamically significant, concentric hypertrophy of the left ventricular wall and dilation of the ascending aorta occur.

NEONATAL PRESENTATION. The newborn presentation is often similar to that seen with other obstructive left-sided lesions, such as coarctation of the aorta or interrupted aortic arch. They present with heart failure and are dependent on ductal patency for survival. There is a frequent association with varying degrees of left ventricular hypoplasia, mitral valve abnormalities, and endocardial fibroelastosis. With the advent of good prenatal screening, many are detected before birth, with deliveries being performed in a high-risk obstetrical unit attached to a congenital heart facility. The decision process around single versus biventricular repair is a complex one and beyond the scope of this chapter. Suffice it to say there are formulas that have been derived to assist the pediatric cardiologist in the decision process.[253]

Clinical Findings. The newborns generally have weak pulses throughout, signs of heart failure, and often little in the way of murmurs, despite the severe left ventricular outflow tract obstruction.

ECG. This usually shows right ventricular dominance with evidence of diffuse ST wave changes due to left ventricular strain.

Chest Radiography. This usually shows cardiomegaly due to a large right ventricle and varying degrees of pulmonary edema.

Echocardiography. This is currently the diagnostic test of choice. It usually shows a poorly contracting left ventricle with varying degrees of endocardial fibroelastosis and frequently hypoplasia of the left ventricle and aortic root. Doppler assessment of gradients are often unreliable due to poor left ventricular function. The presence of right ventricular hypertension and tricuspid valve regurgitation are common associated findings.

Management. Prostaglandin therapy is instituted in this patient population to maintain the fetal circulation with retrograde ductal flow that permits coronary and cerebral perfusion. The nature of further treatment depends on whether the left ventricle and aortic root are believed to be of a sufficient size to support a biventricular repair. If so, balloon dilation is rapidly becoming the treatment of choice,[254] though surgical intervention is still preferred by some.[255] If the left heart structures are believed to be too small to sustain life, then either cardiac transplantation or a Norwood procedure can be undertaken.[253]

PRESENTATION BEYOND THE NEWBORN PERIOD. The diagnosis is invariably made following the detection of a murmur. Occasionally heart failure ensues, usually in the first 1 to 2 months of life when there is a rapid progression of the obstruction and lack of left ventricular mass to maintain a normal wall stress. The natural history studies performed several years ago demonstrated that more rapid progression of aortic valve stenosis is more likely to happen within the first 2 years of life, following which the rate of progressive obstruction is more uniform.[256,257]

Clinical Findings. In general the children are asymptomatic, having normal peripheral pulses if the stenosis is less severe and low-volume, slow-rising pulses when it progresses. Exercise fatigue and chest pain are rare complaints and occur only when the stenosis is severe. With severe stenosis there is systolic thrill in the same area that can also be felt in the suprasternal notch and carotid arteries. Beyond the newborn period there is usually an ejection click at the apex that precedes the murmur. The second heart sound is usually normal in children. There is an ejection systolic murmur heard along the left sternal border, with radiation into the right infraclavicular area. Associated aortic regurgitation may be heard.

ECG. Left ventricular hypertrophy with or without strain are the hallmark features.

Chest Radiography. Overall heart size is normal, or the degree of enlargement is slight in most children with congenital aortic valve stenosis.

Echocardiography. 2D echocardiography provides detailed information about the morphology of the valve, the left ventricular function, and the presence of associated left-sided lesions. Doppler echocardiography can be used to determine the severity of stenosis and the presence or absence of associated aortic regurgitation. Doppler provides peak instantaneous gradients that are higher than the peak-to-peak gradients determined from cardiac catheterization.[258,259] The importance of this lies in the fact that the natural history studies and clinical decision-making have thus far been based on peak-to-peak catheterization gradients in the infant, child, and adolescent. Valve areas are usually not calculated in this age group because there are no good data to support their use in pediatric patients. Mean gradients as derived from Doppler and catheterization correlate closely, but again there is lack of data to support their use in clinical decision-making. Some data exist that convert the Doppler-derived mean gradients to peak to peak, with the addition of the pulse pressure as obtained from blood pressure measurements. Whatever absolute number is chosen to work with, the additional finding of left ventricular hypertrophy on ECG and echocardiography provide supportive data regarding timing for intervention. There is general agreement in the pediatric population that a peak-to-peak gradient of 60 mm Hg or more probably warrants intervention.

Diagnostic Cardiac Catheterization. Cardiac catheterization is now rarely used to establish the site and severity of obstruction to left ventricular outflow. Instead, catheterization is undertaken when therapeutic interventional balloon aortic valvuloplasty is indicated.

Management Options. In this current era balloon dilation has almost completely replaced primary surgical valvotomy in children.

FOLLOW-UP. Follow-up studies indicate that aortic valvotomy is a safe and effective means of palliative treatment with excellent relief of symptoms. Aortic insufficiency can occasionally be progressive and require valve replacement.[260-262] Moreover, after commissurotomy, the valve leaflets remain somewhat deformed, and it is likely that further degenerative changes, including calcification, will lead to significant stenosis in later years. Thus, prosthetic aortic valve replacement is required in approximately 35 percent of patients within 15 to 20 years of the original operation. For those children and adolescents requiring aortic valve replacement, the surgical options include replacement with a mechanical aortic valve, an aortic homograft, or a pulmonary autograft in the aortic position. Accumulating evidence shows that the pulmonary autograft may ultimately be preferable to the aortic homograft. In the pulmonary autograft, called the *Ross procedure*, the patient's pulmonary valve is removed and used to replace the diseased aortic valve, and the right ventricular outflow tract is reconstructed with a pulmonary valve homograft.[262,263] We consider it likely that the Ross procedure will emerge as the approach of choice in the future,[263] although caution is needed when applied to patients with bicuspid aortic valve and aortic regurgitation.[264] This surgical approach can be applied from neonatal through to adult life. Neither homografts nor autografts require anticoagulation.

SUBAORTIC STENOSIS

MORPHOLOGY

Discrete Fibromuscular. This lesion consists of a ridge or fibrous ring encircling the left ventricular outflow tract at varying distances from the aortic valve.[265] The subvalvular fibrous process usually extends onto the aortic valve cusps and almost always makes contact with the ventricular aspect of the anterior mitral leaflet at its base. In other cases with fibrous discontinuity between the mitral and aortic valves, it forms more of a tunnel obstruction.

Focal Muscular. Rarely there is no fibrous element, but rather a focal muscular obstruction on the crest of the interventricular septum, which differs from cases with hypertrophic cardiomyopathy.

Hypoplasia of the Left Ventricular Outflow Tract. In some cases, valvular and subvalvular aortic stenoses coexist with hypoplasia of the aortic valve annulus and thickened valve leaflets, producing a tunnel-like narrowing of the left ventricular outflow tract. Additional findings often include a small ascending aorta.

Discrete Subaortic Stenosis and VSD. This combination is frequently encountered in the pediatric age group, with the fibromuscular component often being absent at the initial echocardiographic evaluation. The association should be suspected in those VSDs with some associated anterior malalignment of the aorta and a more acute aortoseptal angle.[266] These hearts frequently develop subpulmonary stenosis. In a different subset of patients with aortic arch interruption and a VSD, there is muscular subaortic stenosis due to posterior deviation of the infundibular septum.

Complex Subaortic Stenosis. Various anatomical lesions other than a discrete ridge may produce subaortic stenosis. Among these are abnormal adherence of the anterior leaflet of the mitral valve to the septum and the presence in the left ventricular outflow tract of accessory endocardial cushion tissue.[267,268] These are frequently associated with a "cleft in the anterior mitral valve leaflet," which is to be differentiated from that seen in an AV septal defect. These types of obstruction are seen more commonly in those cases with abnormalities of the ventriculoarterial connection in association with a VSD (e.g., double-outlet right ventricle, transposition, and VSD).

CLINICAL FEATURES. These types of obstruction are usually identified as secondary lesions in those cases with associated VSDs, with or without abnormalities of the ventriculoarterial connections or aortic arch obstruction. In general the substrate for left ventricular outflow tract obstruction is present, though in some cases actual physiological obstruction is absent. In other cases the patients are referred with a systolic murmur for evaluation. In the those cases with a gradient across their left ventricular outflow tract, there is an ejection systolic murmur heard along the lower left sternal border with the absence of an ejection click.

LABORATORY INVESTIGATIONS

ECG. In those with associated defects the ECG reflects the major abnormality rather than the associated left ventricular outflow tract obstruction. With isolated forms of left ventricular outflow tract obstruction, there may be left ventricular hypertrophy when the obstruction is significant.

Chest Radiography. This is usually unhelpful in these cases.

Echocardiography. Echocardiography is the current standard diagnostic tool in this lesion.[269] Not only can it permit an accurate delineation of the mechanisms of obstruction but it provides detailed data regarding associated lesions. In all forms the parasternal long-axis view is key to providing an accurate diagnosis. The presence of mitral aortic discontinuity, the relationship of a fibromuscular ridge to the aortic valve, the presence of accessory obstructive tissue, and the dimensions of the aortic annulus and root all are well imaged in this view. As well, color-flow mapping permits the identification of associated aortic valve regurgitation and provides hemodynamic evidence of the site of onset of obstruction. The extension of a fibromuscular ridge onto the anterior mitral leaflet is best appreciated in the apical five-chamber view. As well, this provides the best site for pulsed or continuous-wave Doppler assessment of the maximum gradient across the left ventricular outflow tract. In the older patient TEE plays an important role in delineating the pathology.[270]

Cardiac Catheterization. This technique is no longer of importance in evaluating this lesion. Although balloon dilation has been attempted, it is generally believed that this is a surgical lesion.

MRI. In general, MRI is unnecessary unless there are problems obtaining the needed information by echocardiography.

INTERVENTIONAL OPTIONS. Surgical intervention is indicated either at the time of the repair of the underlying primary lesion or in those cases with discrete obstruction when the obstruction is severe enough to raise concerns.

Discrete Subaortic Stenosis (Fibrous and Muscular). The rate of progression is varied and may be slow.[271] In general the approach to the latter group has been to intervene when there is a mean gradient across the left ventricular outflow tract of greater than 30 mm Hg to avoid future aortic leaflet damage.[272] Surgery involves a fibromectomy, with care to avoid damage to the aortic valve or to create a traumatic VSD.[273] There is a recurrence rate of subaortic stenosis requiring reoperation in up to 20 percent of cases. In some the recurrence is in the form of a fibrous ridge, whereas in others there is acquired pathology of the aortic valve in the form of stenosis as well as regurgitation. Reoperation may involve just repeat resection of a recurrent fibrous ridge, or it may involve surgery for the aortic valve in those cases with significant aortic regurgitation.

Complex Forms of Left Ventricular Outflow Tract Obstruction and an Intact Ventricular Septum. In cases with an intact ventricular septum the indications for intervention are similar to those cases with discrete obstruction. The difference lies in the fact that the surgical approach has to be modified according to the underlying pathology. Resection of any fibromuscular component or accessory tissue (provided it is not a primary support mechanism for the mitral valve), a valve-sparing Konno operation, and, in those cases with a hypoplastic aortic annulus, a classic Konno procedure with aortic valve replacement, are the potential surgical options.[274,275]

Left Ventricular Outflow Tract Obstruction and Complex Forms of CHD. In general, surgery to the left ventricular outflow tract is part of the general repair of the lesion and is not dependent on the precise degree of obstruction across this site.

OUTCOMES. Immediate complications related to surgery include complete AV block, creation of a VSD, or mitral regurgitation from intraoperative damage to the mitral valve apparatus. Long-term complications include recurrence of fibromuscular subvalvular left ventricular outflow tract obstruction (up to 20 percent). Clinically important aortic regurgitation is not uncommon (up to 25 percent of patients). In some cases with predominant acquired aortic valve stenosis, balloon dilation has been the treatment of choice.

FOLLOW-UP. Particular attention should be paid to patients with residual or recurrent subaortic stenosis or those with an associated bicuspid aortic valve or important aortic regurgitation because they are most likely to require surgery eventually. Patients with bioprosthetic aortic valves in the aortic position (following the Konno procedure) or the pulmonary position (following the Ross-Konno procedure) need close follow-up. Endocarditis prophylaxis should be used for prosthetic valves or in the presence of any residual lesions.

SUPRAVALVULAR AORTIC STENOSIS

MORPHOLOGY. Three anatomical types of supravalvular aortic stenosis are recognized, although some patients may have findings of more than one type. Most common is the hourglass type, in which marked thickening and disorganization of the aortic media produce a constricting annular ridge at the superior margin of the sinuses of Valsalva. The membranous type is the result of a fibrous or fibromuscular semicircular diaphragm with a small central opening stretched across the lumen of the aorta. Diffuse hypoplasia of the ascending aorta characterizes the third type.

Because the coronary arteries arise proximal to the site of outflow obstruction in supravalvular aortic stenosis, they are subjected to the elevated pressure that exists within the left ventricle. These vessels often are dilated and tortuous, and premature coronary arteriosclerosis has been described. Moreover, if the free edges of some or all of the aortic cusps adhere to the site of supravalvular stenosis, coronary artery inflow may be compromised. The left ventricle may have a "ballerina foot" configuration, which can result in muscular left ventricular outflow tract obstruction, particularly when associated with significant supravalvular obstruction.

CLINICAL FEATURES. The clinical picture of supravalvular obstruction differs in major respects from that observed in the other forms of aortic stenosis. Chief among these differences is the association of supravalvular aortic stenosis with idiopathic infantile hypercalcemia, a disease that occurs in the first years of life and can be associated with deranged vitamin D metabolism.

WILLIAMS SYNDROME. The designation *supravalvular aortic stenosis syndrome, Williams syndrome,* or *Williams-Beuren syndrome* has been applied to the distinctive picture produced by coexistence of the cardiac and a multisystem disorder.[276] Beyond infancy in these patients, a challenge with vitamin D- or calcium-loading tests unmasks abnormalities in the regulation of circulating 25-hydroxyvitamin D. Infants with Williams syndrome often exhibit feeding difficulties, failure to thrive, and gastrointestinal problems in the form of vomiting, constipation, and colic. The entire spectrum of clinical manifestations includes auditory hyperacusis, inguinal hernia, a hoarse voice, and a typical personality that is outgoing and engaging. Other manifestations of this syndrome include intellectual impairment, "elfin facies", narrowing of peripheral systemic and pulmonary arteries, strabismus, and abnormalities of dental development consisting of microdontia, enamel hypoplasia, and malocclusion.

Many medical conditions can complicate the course of Williams syndrome, including systemic hypertension, gastrointestinal problems, and urinary tract abnormalities. In an older child or adult, progressive joint limitation and hypertonia may become a problem. Adult patients are usually handicapped by their developmental disabilities.

Williams syndrome was previously considered to be nonfamilial; however, a number of families in which parent-to-child transmission of Williams syndrome has occurred have now been identified. All of these families show a parent and child to be affected with Williams syndrome, including one instance of male-to-male transmission. This supports autosomal dominant inheritance as the likely pattern, with most cases of Williams syndrome probably occurring as the result of a new mutation. New information indicates that a genetic defect for supravalvular aortic stenosis is located in the same chromosomal subunit as elastin on chromosome 7q11.23.[277] Elastin is an important component of the arterial wall, but precisely how mutations in elastin genes cause the phenotypes of supravalvular aortic stenosis is not known.

FAMILIAL AUTOSOMAL DOMINANT PRESENTATION. Occasionally the aortic anomaly and peripheral pulmonary arterial stenosis are also found in familial and sporadic forms not associated with the other features of the syndrome.[278] Affected patients have normal intelligence and are normal in facial appearance. Genetic studies suggest that when the anomaly is familial, it is transmitted as autosomal dominant with variable expression. Some family members may have peripheral pulmonary stenosis either as an isolated lesion or in combination with the supravalvular aortic anomaly.

CLINICAL FEATURES. Patients with Williams syndrome are intellectually challenged (Fig. 56–33). The typical appearance is similar to that of the elfin facies observed in the severe form of idiopathic infantile hypercalcemia and is characterized by a high prominent forehead, stellate or lacy iris patterns, epicanthal folds, underdeveloped bridge of the nose and mandible, overhanging upper lip, strabismus, and anomalies of dentition. Recognition of this distinctive appearance, even in infancy, should alert the physician to the possibility of underlying multisystem disease. In addition, a positive family history in a patient with a normal appearance and clinical signs suggesting left ventricular outflow obstruction should lead to the suspicion of either supravalvular aortic stenosis or hypertrophic obstructive cardiomyopathy.

Studies of the natural history of the principal vascular lesions in these patients—supravalvular aortic stenosis and peripheral pulmonary artery stenosis[279]—indicate that the aortic lesion is usually progressive, with an increase in the

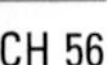

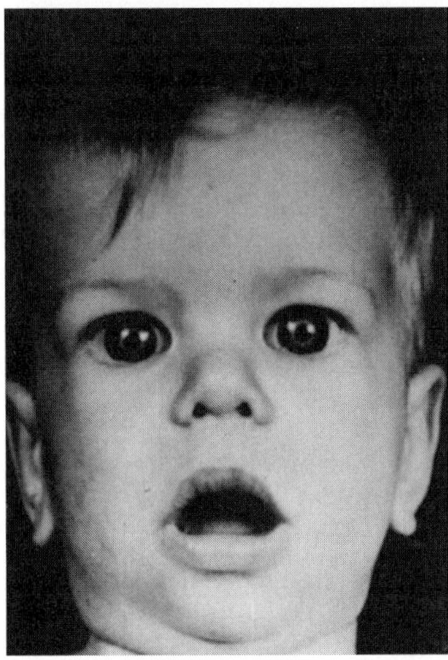

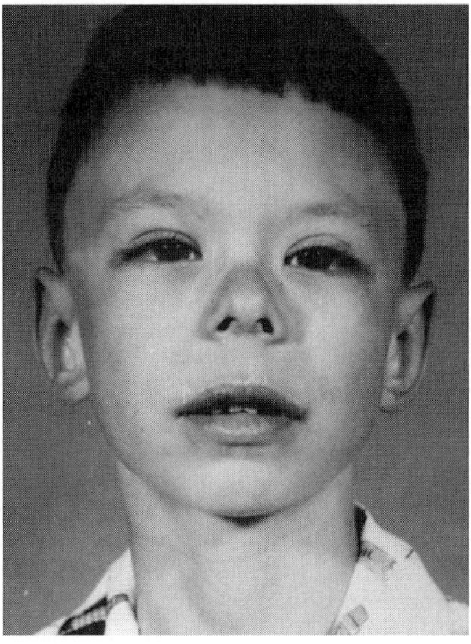

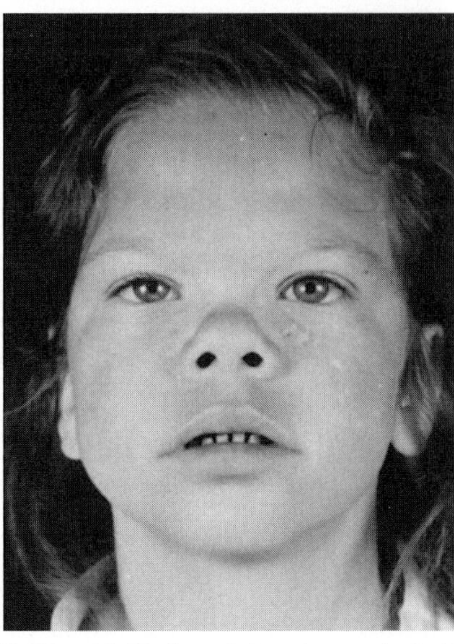

FIGURE 56–33 Typical elfin facies in three patients with supravalvular aortic stenosis. (From Friedman WF, Kirkpatrick SE: Congenital aortic stenosis. *In* Adams FH, Emmanouilides GC, Riemenschneider TA, et al [eds]: Moss' Heart Disease in Infants, Children, and Adolescents. 4th ed. Baltimore, Williams & Wilkins, 1989.)

intensity of obstruction related often to poor growth of the ascending aorta. In contrast, the patients with pulmonary branch stenosis, whether associated with the aortic lesion or not, tend to show no change or a reduction in right ventricular pressure with time.[280,281]

With few exceptions, the major *physical findings* resemble those observed in patients with aortic valve stenosis. Among these exceptions are accentuation of aortic valve closure due to elevated pressure in the aorta proximal to the stenosis, an absent ejection click, and the especially prominent transmission of a thrill and murmur into the jugular notch and along the carotid vessels. The narrowing of the peripheral pulmonary arteries may produce a late systolic or continuous murmur heard best in the lung fields and usually are accentuated by inspiration. Another hallmark of supravalvular aortic stenosis is that the systolic pressure in the right arm is usually higher than in the left arm. This pulse disparity may relate to the tendency of a jet stream to adhere to a vessel wall (Coanda effect) and selective streaming of blood into the innominate artery.

LABORATORY INVESTIGATIONS

ECG. This usually reveals left ventricular hypertrophy when obstruction is severe. Biventricular or even right ventricular hypertrophy may be found if there is significant narrowing of peripheral pulmonary arteries.

Chest Radiography. In contrast to valvular and discrete subvalvular aortic stenosis, poststenotic dilation of the ascending aorta is absent.

Echocardiography. This is a valuable technique for localizing the site of obstruction to the supravalvular area.[282] Most often the sinuses of Valsalva are dilated, and the ascending aorta and arch appear small or of normal size. The diameter of the aortic annulus is always greater than that of the sinotubular junction. Doppler examination determines the location of obstruction but usually overestimates the gradient compared with that obtained at cardiac catheterization. This results from the obstruction being lengthy, and the Doppler gradient is overestimated due to the phenomena of pressure recovery.

Angiocardiography. In most cases, this is necessary to define an accurate hemodynamic gradient across the left ventricular outflow tract, as well as to determine the status of the coronary arteries. Usually it also involves an assessment of the branch pulmonary arteries as well as the brachiocephalic, renal, and mesenteric arteries, all of which can be stenotic. Because of the nature of the anatomical defect, transcatheter balloon angioplasty, with or without stenting, is not an effective treatment option.

INTERVENTIONAL OPTIONS AND OUTCOMES. Surgical intervention for the supravalvular aortic stenosis has been successful in most cases with good medium and long-term results.[283,284] A variety of surgical procedures may be performed, all of which are tailored to the type of pathology. The use of a Y patch, resection with end-to-end anastomosis, or a Ross procedure are the main techniques employed. Additional lesions, including coronary ostial stenosis, aortic valvuloplasty, and subaortic resection, may be necessary in some cases.

The cardiac prognosis is very good, with some patients requiring further surgery for recurrent supravalvular stenosis.[279,285] As peripheral pulmonary artery stenosis tends to improve with time, there is a reluctance to attempt intervention, either surgical or via balloon angioplasty. Long-term behavioral and intellectual problems persist.[285]

Congenital Mitral Valve Anomalies

CONGENITAL MITRAL STENOSIS

MORPHOLOGY. Anatomical types of mitral stenosis include the parachute deformity of the valve, in which shortened chordae tendineae converge and insert into a single large papillary muscle; thickened leaflets with shortening and fusion of the chordae tendineae; an anomalous arcade of obstructing papillary muscles; accessory mitral valve tissue; and a supravalvar circumferential ridge or "ring" of connective tissue arising at the base of the atrial aspect of the mitral leaflets.[286] Associated cardiac defects are common, including endocardial fibroelastosis, coarctation of the aorta, PDA, and left ventricular outflow tract obstruction. There is also an association between persistence of the left superior vena cava and obstructive left-sided lesions.[287]

CLINICAL FEATURES. In most cases the findings are incidental at the time of evaluation of another left-sided obstructive lesion, such as coarctation of the aorta or aortic valve stenosis. The classic auscultatory findings seen with rheumatic mitral valve stenosis are often absent in the congenital form. Typical findings include a normal S_1, a mid-diastolic murmur with or without some presystolic accentuation, and no opening snap.

LABORATORY INVESTIGATIONS

ECG. In milder forms this is usually normal, or there may be left atrial overload, with or without right ventricular hypertrophy due to associated pulmonary hypertension.

Chest Radiography. This is normal in milder forms, with evidence of pulmonary edema in those cases with more severe obstruction.

Echocardiography. The 2D echocardiography, combined with Doppler studies, usually provides a complete analysis of the anatomy and function of congenital mitral stenosis.[288] The status of the papillary muscles is best appreciated in the precordial short-axis view. In patients with two papillary muscles, they are usually closer together than is seen in the normal heart. The precordial long-axis view permits identification of a supravalvular mitral ring as well as the degree of mobility of the valve leaflets. Color flow Doppler allows identification of the level of the obstruction, as well as the presence of mitral valve regurgitation. Pulsed or continuous-wave Doppler provides an accurate assessment of the mean gradient across the mitral valve. The advantage of the pressure half-time lies in the fact that it is independent of cardiac output, unlike the mean gradient across the mitral valve. Due to more rapid heart rates in children, the pressure half-time is of less value.

INTERVENTIONAL OPTIONS AND OUTCOMES. In asymptomatic cases clinical and echocardiographic follow-up is all that is necessary. If the patient starts to develop pulmonary hypertension or symptoms, surgical intervention is usually indicated. Mitral valve balloon dilation[289] is not as successful as it is in rheumatic mitral valve stenosis. Surgery usually involves removing a supramitral ring if present, splitting papillary muscles and fused chordal apparatus in those cases with more common forms of congenital mitral stenosis. In general, surgical intervention provides temporary relief, with many operated cases requiring valve replacement later in life.[290,291]

CONGENITAL MITRAL REGURGITATION

MORPHOLOGY

Isolated Congenital Mitral Valve Regurgitation. This is usually due to either an isolated cleft of the anterior mitral valve leaflet[292] or as the result of leaflet dysplasia. In these cases there is evidence of shortened chordae in conjunction with dysplastic valve leaflets. In those with an isolated mitral valve *cleft*, the deficiency in the anterior mitral leaflet points toward the left ventricular outflow tract, unlike those cases with an AV septal defect. In general, the larger the cleft in the anterior mitral leaflet, the greater the degree of regurgitation.

In cases with a *dysplastic* mitral valve the chordal apparatus is shortened with varying degrees of dysplasia of the leaflets. Other anatomical lesions such as mitral valve arcade resulting in regurgitation are usually part of a more generalized abnormality of the left side of the heart.

Complex Congenital Mitral Valve Regurgitation. This is seen more frequently in association with abnormalities of the ventriculoarterial connection, such as double-outlet right ventricle, transposition and VSD, and corrected transposition. In the first two it is frequent to have a cleft in the anterior mitral valve leaflet with some chordal support apparatus that renders the valve less regurgitant than in those cases with an isolated cleft. In cc-TGA the morphological mitral valve may have an associated cleft, be dysplastic, or have multiple papillary muscles, all of which increase the tendency for it to be regurgitant.

CLINICAL FEATURES. The presence of symptoms relates to the severity of the regurgitation in those cases where the pathology is isolated to the valve. Exercise intolerance, combined with a pansystolic murmur at the apex, with or without a mid-diastolic murmur, are the cardinal clinical features.

LABORATORY INVESTIGATIONS

ECG. This is either normal or demonstrates left atrial and left ventricular hypertrophy.

Chest Radiography. This demonstrates cardiomegaly predominantly involving the left ventricle and atrium.

Echocardiography. Doppler and 2D echocardiography provide an accurate evaluation of the mechanisms and degree of valvular regurgitation.[288,292] The cleft in the anterior mitral valve leaflet is best seen in the precordial short-axis view, pointing toward the left ventricular outflow tract. Patients with a dysplastic mitral valve lack mobility of the valve leaflets and have shortened chordae. Color Doppler interrogation helps in locating the site of regurgitation. The severity of regurgitation is assessed in the standard fashion. The 3D echocardiography permits a comprehensive evaluation of the mechanisms of regurgitation, with additional information being obtained regarding commissural length, leaflet area, and sites of regurgitation from color flow Doppler.

Angiocardiography and MRI. These procedures are seldom helpful in management planning.

INTERVENTIONAL OPTIONS AND OUTCOMES. This depends on the severity of regurgitation and its impact on left ventricular function. Surgery should not be delayed until the patients become symptomatic. Surgery involves suture of an isolated cleft, with or without associated commissuroplasties. In those cases with a dysplastic mitral valve, leaflet extension in conjunction with an annuloplasty and commissuroplasty usually results in effective control of the regurgitation in the short and medium term.[293] Despite this, many of these patients most likely end up with a mitral valve replacement at some stage in the future. Attempted surgical repair, rather than replacement, is important in the pediatric age group, because it permits temporary relief that allows the child to grow such that future surgery can be done into a larger mitral annulus. When required, mitral valve replacement has had a good short- and medium-term outcome in those cases where repair is not possible.[294]

Right Ventricular Outflow Tract Lesions

PERIPHERAL PULMONARY ARTERY STENOSIS (Fig. 56–34)

Right ventricular outflow tract is a term that applies to those patients with both peripheral pulmonary artery stenosis and an intact ventricular septum. It excludes those with an associated VSD, which is dealt with in the sections on tetralogy

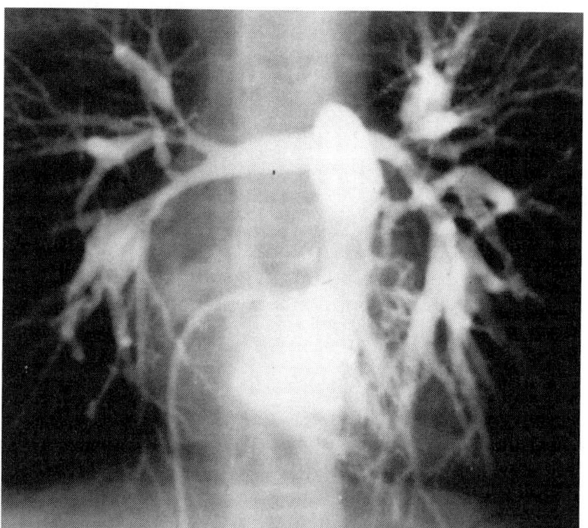

FIGURE 56–34 Right ventricular angiocardiogram showing numerous sites of peripheral pulmonic stenosis and poststenotic dilation of the peripheral pulmonic arteries.

of Fallot and pulmonary atresia with a ventricular septal defect. Also excluded is Noonan syndrome, which is dealt with in the subsequent section on pulmonary valve stenosis.

ETIOLOGY

Rubella Syndrome. The most important cause of significant pulmonary artery stenoses producing symptoms in newborns used to be intrauterine rubella infection. Other cardiovascular malformations commonly found in association with congenital rubella include PDA, pulmonary valve stenosis, and ASD. Generalized systemic arterial stenotic lesions also may be a feature of the rubella embryopathy, which may involve large and medium-sized vessels such as the aorta and coronary, cerebral, mesenteric, and renal arteries. Cardiovascular lesions are but one manifestation of intrauterine rubella infection because cataracts, microphthalmia, deafness, thrombocytopenia, hepatitis, and blood dyscrasias are also common. The clinical picture in infants with rubella syndrome depends on the severity of the cardiovascular lesions and the associated abnormalities.

Williams Syndrome. Peripheral pulmonary artery stenosis is also associated with supravalvular aortic stenosis in patients with Williams syndrome, which is discussed in the section on supravalvular aortic stenosis.[295]

Alagille Syndrome. Peripheral pulmonary artery stenosis is a component of this syndrome, with some cases having a *JAG1* mutation.[296]

Isolated Branch Pulmonary Artery Stenosis. This is encountered mainly in the proximal left pulmonary artery and is invariably related to a sling of ductal tissue that causes stenosis when the ductus arteriosus closes after birth. In most cases this is fairly mild, but a significant obstruction resulting in failure of distal growth of the left pulmonary artery may also be seen.

MORPHOLOGY. Apart from the isolated form mentioned earlier, the stenoses are usually diffuse and bilateral and extend into the mediastinal, hilar, and intraparenchymal pulmonary arteries.

CLINICAL FEATURES. The degree of obstruction is the principal determinant of clinical severity. The type of obstruction determines the feasibility of intervention. Most patients are asymptomatic. An ejection systolic murmur heard at the upper left sternal border and well transmitted to the axillae and back is most common. There is no pulmonary ejection click. The pulmonic component of the second heart sound may be accentuated and is loud only if there is proximal pulmonary hypertension. A continuous murmur is often audible in patients with significant branch stenosis. The murmurs in the lung fields are typically increased by inspiration.

LABORATORY INVESTIGATIONS

ECG. Right ventricular hypertrophy is seen when obstruction is severe. Left axis deviation with counterclockwise orientation of the frontal QRS vector is common in rubella syndrome and when there is also supravalvular aortic stenosis.

Chest Radiography. Mild or moderate stenosis usually produces normal findings. Detectable differences in vascularity between regions of the lungs or dilated pulmonary artery segments are uncommon. When obstruction is bilateral and severe, right atrial and ventricular enlargement may be seen.

Echocardiography. Echocardiography is helpful in making the diagnosis and excluding associated lesions; however, it is limited in its ability to image the distal pulmonary arteries beyond the hilum of the lung. Right ventricular pressure assessment may be predicted if there is associated tricuspid valve regurgitation.

MRI and Spiral CT. These are valuable diagnostic tests because they permit a more distal evaluation of the branch pulmonary arteries. The advantage of spiral CT in young children is that it can be performed without the need for heavy sedation or even general anesthesia. Although most patients require cardiac catheterization and angiography, these other techniques are excellent for the initial evaluation and for following the progress of the lesions.

Radionuclide Quantitative Lung Perfusion Scan. This is valuable in those cases with unilateral stenosis to determine whether intervention is necessary. Similar flow estimates can now be obtained by MRI.

Cardiac Catheterization and Angiocardiography. This permits the assessment of right ventricular pressure and the pressures in the pulmonary arterial tree. Angiocardiography is the key to precisely assessing the extent and severity of the stenoses.

INTERVENTIONAL OPTIONS AND OUTCOMES. For those cases with isolated left pulmonary artery stenosis where there is less than 30 percent of flow to the lung, balloon dilation with or without stent insertion is effective in relieving the obstruction. In those cases with more diffuse bilateral stenoses, the indications for intervention depend on the right ventricular pressure. As the natural history of diffuse peripheral pulmonary artery stenosis in Williams syndrome is one of potential regression over time, intervention is in general reserved for those cases with systemic or suprasystemic right ventricular pressure. Intervention is also dependent in part on the extent of the stenosis and the dilation capability of the lesions, with or without stenting.[297-299] In some cases, several attempts at dilation are required to achieve any improvement in vessel caliber. High-pressure balloons are usually needed, but some lesions cannot be dilated even with such balloons. Recently, improved results have been reported using "cutting" balloons, which may facilitate dilation in an otherwise undilatable stenosis. As a rule, surgery has little to offer those patients with diffuse peripheral pulmonary artery stenoses and can indeed make the situation worse.

SUPRAVALVULAR RIGHT VENTRICULAR OUTFLOW TRACT OBSTRUCTION

Supravalvular right ventricular outflow tract obstruction seldom occurs in isolation. It can occur in tetralogy of Fallot, Williams syndrome, Noonan syndrome, VSD, or arteriohepatic dysplasia (Alagille syndrome). Supravalvular right ventricular outflow tract obstruction can progress in severity and should be monitored. Dilation of the pulmonary trunk is not a feature of subvalvular and supravalvular right ventricular outflow tract obstruction. Intervention is recommended when the peak gradient across the right ventricular outflow tract is more than 50 mm Hg at rest or when the patient is symptomatic.

PULMONARY STENOSIS WITH INTACT VENTRICULAR SEPTUM (Figs. 56–35 and 56–36)

This lesion exists as a continuum, ranging from those patients with isolated valvular stenosis to others where there is complete atresia of the pulmonary outflow tract. There are two modes of presentation. The first presents in the neonatal period, usually with associated pathology of the tricuspid valve, right ventricle, and/or coronary arteries. The second mode of presentation is beyond the neonatal period, when the valvular stenosis is usually isolated. Some cases with severe stenosis diagnosed in utero can present with valvular atresia at the time of birth.

MORPHOLOGY. The pulmonary valve may vary from a well-formed trileaflet valve with varying degrees of commissural fusion to an imperforate membrane. If stenosis is present, the right ventricle is usually of normal size or only mildly hypoplastic. Those patients with an imperforate valve and a patent infundibulum invariably have a larger right ventricular volume than cases with both infundibular and valve atresia.

CLINICAL FEATURES

Neonate with Critical Pulmonary Valve Stenosis. The neonate presents with central cyanosis due to right-to-left shunting at the atrial level and depends on a prostaglandin infusion to maintain the patency of the ductus arteriosus. Auscultatory findings include a single second heart sound, no ejection click, and a murmur that, when present, is due to tricuspid valve regurgitation.

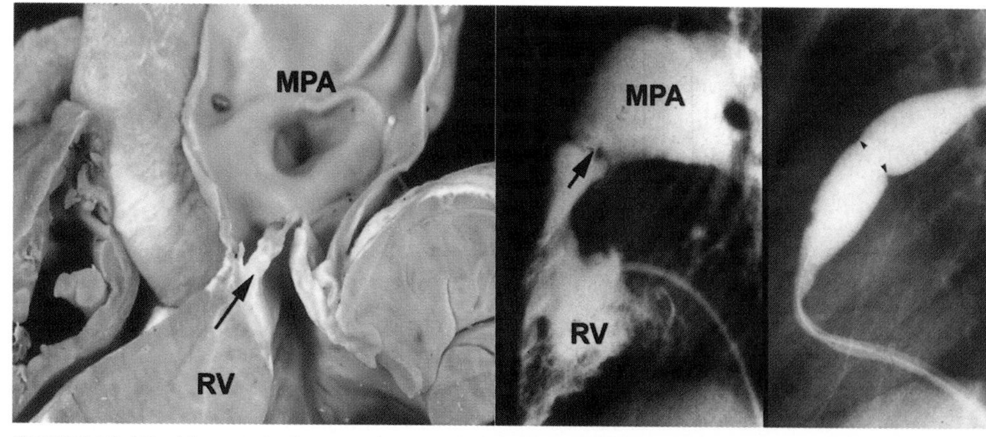

FIGURE 56–35 Montage of pulmonary valve stenosis demonstrating typical pathology (**left**, arrow) with a thickened pulmonary valve and obstruction due to commissural fusion. Note the post-stenotic dilation. The angiogram demonstrates a case before (**middle**, arrow) and during (**right**) balloon dilation. MPA = main pulmonary artery; RV = right ventricle.

Infant and Child. In cases beyond the newborn period the referral is usually for the assessment of a cardiac murmur. This may be detected within the first few weeks of life, more commonly at the routine 6-week postnatal visit or later. These patients usually have an ejection click and a second heart sound that moves with respiration but with a soft pulmonary component. There is an ejection murmur of varying intensity and duration heard best in the pulmonary area.

Adult. Adults with isolated mild to moderate right ventricular outflow tract obstruction of any type are usually asymptomatic. Patients with severe right ventricular outflow tract obstruction may present with exertional fatigue, dyspnea, lightheadedness, and chest discomfort (right ventricular angina). Physical examination may reveal a prominent jugular A wave, a right ventricular lift, and possibly a thrill in the 2nd left interspace. Auscultation reveals a normal S_1, a single or split S_2 with a diminished P_2 (unless the obstruction is supravalvular in which case the intensity of the P_2 is normal or increased) and a systolic ejection murmur best heard in the 2nd left intercostal space. When the pulmonary valve is thin and pliable, a systolic ejection click will be heard which decreases on inspiration. As the severity of the pulmonary stenosis progresses, the interval between S_1 and the systolic ejection click becomes shorter, S_2 becomes widely split, P_2 diminishes or disappears, and the systolic ejection murmur lengthens and peaks later in systole, often extending beyond A_2. An ejection click seldoms occur with dysplastic pulmonary stenosis. Cyanosis may be present when a patent foramen ovale or ASD permits right-to-left shunting.

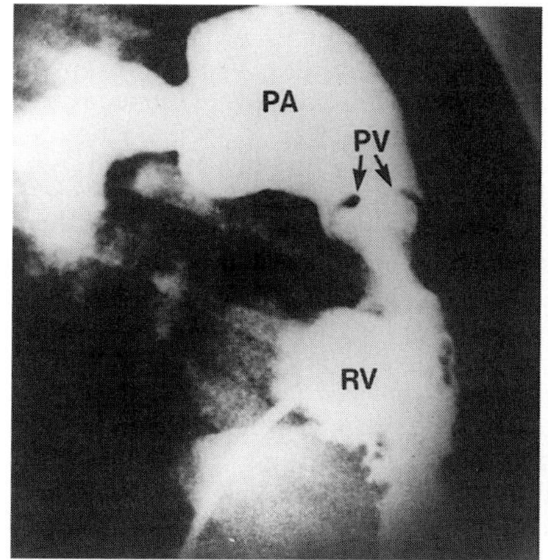

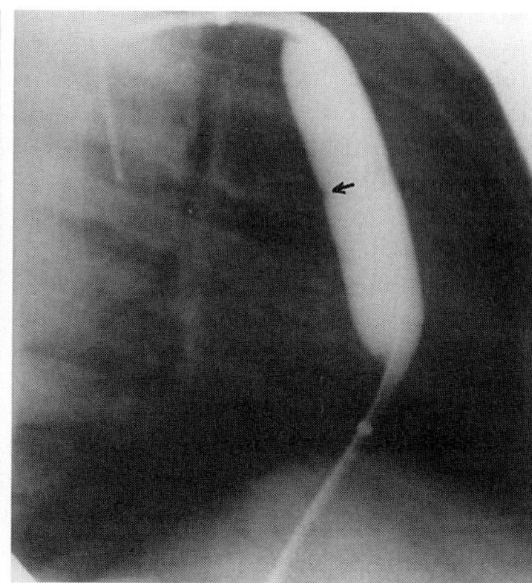

FIGURE 56–36 Right ventriculogram (RV) in the lateral projection (left) from a patient with valvular pulmonic stenosis. The pulmonary valve (PV) is thickened and domes in systole (arrows). Poststenotic dilation of the pulmonary artery (PA) is seen. At the right, successful balloon valvuloplasty shows almost complete disappearance of the stenotic waist (arrow). (Courtesy of Dr. Thomas G. DiSessa.)

Adult patients with trivial and mild valvular right ventricular outflow tract obstruction do not become worse with time. Moderate valvular right ventricular outflow tract obstruction can progress in 20 percent of unoperated patients,[300] especially in adults because of calcification of the valve, and may require intervention. Some of these patients can also become symptomatic, particularly in later life, because of atrial arrhythmias resulting from right ventricular pressure overload and tricuspid regurgitation. Patients with severe valvular right ventricular outflow tract obstruction will have had balloon or surgical valvotomy to survive to adult life. Long-term survival in patients with repaired pulmonary valve stenosis is similar to that of the general population, with excellent to good functional class at long-term follow-up in most patients. A few patients have severe pulmonary regurgitation.

LABORATORY INVESTIGATIONS

ECG. *In the newborn* period this may show left axis deviation and left ventricular dominance in those cases with significant right ventricular hypoplasia. Other patients may have a normal QRS axis. Right atrial overload is present in those with increased right atrial pressure. *In the infant, child, and adult* the findings are dependent on the severity of the stenosis. In milder cases the ECG should be normal. As the stenosis progresses, evidence of right ventricular hypertrophy appears. Severe stenosis is seen in the form of a tall R wave in lead V_4R or V_1 with a deep S wave in V_6. A tall QR wave in the right precordial leads with T wave inversion and ST segment depression (right ventricular "strain") reflects very severe stenosis. When an rSR′ pattern is observed in lead V_1 (20 percent of patients), lower right ventricular pressures are found than in patients with a pure R wave of equal amplitude. Right atrial overload is associated with moderate to severe pulmonary stenosis.

Chest Radiography. *In the neonate* this demonstrates pulmonary oligemia with a prominent right heart border in those with associated tricuspid valve regurgitation. *In the infant, child, and adult* with mild or moderate pulmonary stenosis, chest radiography often shows a heart of normal size and normal pulmonary vascularity. Poststenotic dilation of the main and left pulmonary arteries is often seen. Right atrial and right ventricular enlargement are observed in patients with severe obstruction and right ventricular failure. The pulmonary vascularity is usually normal in the absence of a right-to-left atrial shunt but may be reduced in patients with severe stenosis and right ventricular failure.

Echocardiography. Combined 2D echocardiographic and continuous-wave Doppler examination characterizes the anatomical valve abnormality and its severity and has essentially eliminated the requirement for diagnostic cardiac catheterization. Invasive studies are currently used for balloon valvuloplasty.

Right ventricular size is currently best assessed indirectly from the tricuspid annular dimension. In the absence of a VSD there is an excellent correlation between the two. Right ventricular pressure can be assessed indirectly from the tricuspid regurgitation gradient. Tricuspid valve morphology and function and the status of the interatrial septum all need to be addressed.

INTERVENTIONAL OPTIONS AND OUTCOMES

Neonate. In the neonate, prostaglandin E_1 is instituted in those cases with ductal dependency. Following this, balloon dilation is performed in those with stenosis, whereas radiofrequency perforation in conjunction with dilation may be undertaken in those with pulmonary valve atresia. If relief of the obstruction is successful, then the prostaglandins are slowly weaned to determine if the right ventricle is large enough to support the circulation. If not, a systemic-to-pulmonary artery shunt is necessary early in the management. In those cases with a normal-sized right ventricle, no further therapy is usually necessary in the future, since there is a very low recurrence rate of stenosis. Newborns with isolated pulmonary stenosis do well after relief of the stenosis.

Infant and Older Child. Balloon dilation of the pulmonary valve is the therapeutic procedure of choice with excellent short- and medium-term results.

Adults. Balloon valvuloplasty is recommended when the gradient across the right ventricular outflow tract is greater than 50 mm Hg at rest[206] or when the patient is symptomatic. Intermediate- and long-term outcomes are excellent.[301]

DYSPLASTIC PULMONARY VALVE STENOSIS

MORPHOLOGY. In pulmonary valve stenosis due to valvular dysplasia the obstruction is caused not by commissural fusion but by a combination of thickened and dysplastic pulmonary valve leaflets in combination with varying degrees of supravalvular pulmonary stenosis. The supravalvular stenosis is classically at the distal part of pulmonary valve sinuses, and there is usually no poststenotic pulmonary artery dilation. This entity is associated with Noonan syndrome, which in turn may be associated with hypertrophic cardiomyopathy.

CLINICAL FEATURES. In most cases, the diagnosis is made either during an evaluation of a systolic murmur or in a child with dysmorphic features who is undergoing clinical evaluation. Children with Noonan syndrome have short stature, webbed necks, and broad-shaped chests in a fashion similar to Turner syndrome. Although this syndrome does not have an associated chromosomal abnormality, it may be familial and affects both sexes equally. A unique association in the newborn is pulmonary lymphangiectasia. The auscultatory finding that differentiates the dysplastic valves from simple pulmonary valve stenosis is the lack of an ejection click. The other features of the murmur are similar to that described in pulmonary valve stenosis.

ECG. The ECG is helpful in that patients with dysplastic pulmonary stenosis frequently have a leftward QRS axis, particularly when associated with hypertrophic cardiomyopathy. The remainder of the ECG is similar to that seen in pulmonary valve stenosis.

Chest Radiography. The findings are similar to typical pulmonary valve stenosis, apart from the lack of post-stenotic pulmonary trunk dilation, even in the presence of severe obstruction. In those with pulmonary lymphangiectasia the chest radiograph has a ground-glass appearance, which can be difficult to differentiate from pulmonary venous obstruction.

Echocardiography. This demonstrates a thickened fleshy pulmonary valve, lack of post-stenotic dilation, and varying degrees of supravalvular pulmonary stenosis. The associated diagnosis of hypertrophic cardiomyopathy can be confirmed or excluded. If the initial echocardiogram does not demonstrate hypertrophic cardiomyopathy, then further studies should be performed throughout childhood and adolescence, particularly in those cases with left axis deviation.

INTERVENTIONAL OPTIONS AND OUTCOMES

Cardiac Catheterization and Angiography. Although the results of balloon valvuloplasty are less rewarding than those with stenosis due to commissural fusion, it is worth attempting this before considering surgical intervention. There has been varied success, with many cases having some reduction in gradient that can delay surgery.

Surgical Intervention. If balloon valvuloplasty fails, then surgical intervention is indicated. This usually involves a partial valvectomy in conjunction with patch repair of the supravalvular stenosis.

Outcomes. Adequate relief of the right ventricular outflow tract obstruction results in an excellent outlook, with the greatest long-term risk factor being the presence of hypertrophic cardiomyopathy.

SUBPULMONARY RIGHT VENTRICULAR OUTFLOW TRACT OBSTRUCTION (ANOMALOUS MUSCLE BUNDLES OR A DOUBLE-CHAMBERED RIGHT VENTRICLE)

MORPHOLOGY. A double-chambered right ventricle is formed by right ventricular obstruction due to anomalous muscle bundles.[302,303] Although this can occur in isolation, it is more frequently part of a combination of lesions that includes right ventricular muscle bundles, a perimembranous-outlet VSD, and subaortic stenosis with or without aortic valve prolapse.

CLINICAL FEATURES. Most cases are discovered as an incidental finding during the evaluation of a VSD.[304] In some cases there may be only an ejection systolic murmur. If the obstruction is isolated, then there is an ejection systolic murmur heard best in the upper left sternal border. If the VSD is the predominant lesion, the right ventricular outflow tract murmur may not be appreciated. Before the routine use of echocardiography, the diagnosis was often made during follow-up for a VSD when the pansystolic murmur decreased in intensity and a systolic ejection murmur emerged. The patients are usually pink unless there is progression of the subpulmonary stenosis in the setting of a VSD. The diagnosis may be more problematic in adults.[305,306]

LABORATORY INVESTIGATIONS

ECG. The ECG is similar to those with isolated pulmonary valve stenosis beyond the newborn period. In cases with a nonrestrictive VSD and mild subpulmonary stenosis, the ECG typically shows biventricular hypertrophy due to a left-to-right shunt and associated pulmonary hypertension. If the stenosis is more severe, right ventricular hypertrophy will be seen. Those with a restrictive VSD may have a normal ECG or left ventricular hypertrophy, the latter of which is replaced with right ventricular hypertrophy if the subpulmonary stenosis increases in severity.

Chest Radiography. This is usually normal in those with isolated subpulmonary stenosis, whereas those with a VSD may have increased or reduced pulmonary blood flow, depending on the severity of the obstruction.

Echocardiography. Doppler and 2D echocardiography usually provide a complete diagnosis.[304] The level of subpulmonary obstruction is appreciated best in a combination of subcostal right anterior oblique and precordial short-axis views. These views permit the identification of the relationship of the VSD to the muscle bundles, as well as the degree of anterior malalignment of the infundibular septum in those with a VSD. The precordial short-axis view is the best position to evaluate the presence of possible subaortic stenosis and aortic cusp prolapse. Color and pulsed or continuous-wave Doppler evaluation usually allows differentiation of the VSD flow jet from that originating from the muscle bundles. This permits an accurate assessment of the hemodynamic effect of the subpulmonary obstruction.

Cardiac Catheterization and Angiocardiography. This technique is rarely necessary.[304] In older patients where the echocardiographic images of the subpulmonary region may be suboptimal, a combination of MRA[307] and echocardiography is all that is generally needed.

MANAGEMENT OPTIONS AND OUTCOMES. Management is dictated by the severity of the subpulmonary stenosis and the presence of associated defects. In those patients with isolated subpulmonary stenosis, surgery is indicated when the right ventricular pressure is more than 60 percent of systemic. This involves resection of the muscle bundles through the right atrium. For those cases with an associated VSD, the decision is based on the size of the VSD, the degree of associated subaortic stenosis, the presence of aortic valve prolapse, and the severity of the subpulmonary stenosis. These patients tend to have a progressive disease, so many cases that are followed conservatively for several years will eventually require surgery.[306] In general, the outcome is excellent with a low rate of recurrence after surgical resection of obstructive muscle bundles.[308] Infrequently, recurrence of the subaortic obstruction may occur.

Miscellaneous Lesions

Cor Triatriatum

MORPHOLOGY. In this malformation, failure of resorption of the common pulmonary vein results in a left atrium divided by an abnormal fibromuscular diaphragm into a posterosuperior chamber receiving the pulmonary veins and an anteroinferior chamber giving rise to the left atrial appendage and leading to the mitral orifice.[309] The communication between the divided atrial chambers may be large, small, or absent, depending on the size of the opening(s) in the diaphragm, which determines the degree of obstruction to pulmonary venous return. Elevations of both pulmonary venous pressure and pulmonary vascular resistance may result in severe pulmonary artery hypertension.

CLINICAL FEATURES. Cor triatriatum may be detected as an incidental finding in a patient who has an echocardiogram for another reason. In general these represent the unobstructed form that requires no early intervention. Cases with more severe obstruction present in a fashion similar to patients with congenital pulmonary vein stenosis.

LABORATORY INVESTIGATIONS

ECG. In unobstructed cases this is normal, whereas in those with significant obstruction there is right ventricular hypertrophy due to the associated pulmonary hypertension.

Chest Radiography. This may be normal in those with mild obstruction or demonstrate pulmonary edema with significant obstruction.

Echocardiography. The diagnosis is established by 2D or TEE, with further insight from 3D reconstruction.[310] The obstructive diaphragm is visualized in the parasternal long- and short-axis and four-chamber views and can be distinguished from a supravalvular mitral ring by its position superior to the left atrial appendage, which forms part of the distal chamber. Also present is diastolic fluttering of the mitral leaflets and high-velocity flow detected by Doppler examination in the distal atrial chamber and at the mitral orifice.

Cardiac Catheterization and Angiocardiography. This technique is usually unnecessary with the advent of echocardiography and MRI.

MANAGEMENT OPTIONS AND OUTCOMES. Surgical resection of the membrane is the treatment of choice for patients with significant obstruction.[311] This results in symptom relief and a reduction of pulmonary artery pressure. In general the outcome following surgery is very good. With the advent of more routine echocardiography a subset of cases with typical but nonobstructive forms has been recognized.[312] Thus far these cases appear to remain asymptomatic, with an infrequent need for surgical intervention.

Pulmonary Vein Stenosis

Congenital pulmonary vein stenosis may occur as a focal stenosis at the atrial junction or generalized hypoplasia of one or more pulmonary veins. The incidence of associated cardiac malformations is extremely high, including VSD, ASD, tetralogy of Fallot, tricuspid and mitral atresia, and AV septal defect.[313] In other cases the pulmonary vein stenosis is acquired after surgical intervention for total anomalous pulmonary venous connection. Children frequently present with recurrent respiratory infections, whereas adults exhibit exercise intolerance. Pulmonary hypertension is one of the consequences of pulmonary vein stenosis, whether it is congenital or acquired. In those cases with unilateral pulmonary vein stenosis, clinical symptoms are frequently absent because there is pulmonary blood flow redistribution away from the affected lung.

LABORATORY INVESTIGATIONS

ECG. The ECG is usually normal unless there is evidence of pulmonary hypertension, in which case right ventricular hypertrophy may be seen.

Chest Radiography. With unilateral pulmonary vein stenosis there is oligemia of the affected lung and increased flow to the contralateral side. If the obstruction is bilateral, then pulmonary edema is seen.

Echocardiography. This can usually exclude or confirm the diagnosis of pulmonary vein stenosis. Assessment of pulmonary artery pressure from tricuspid or pulmonary valve regurgitation is possible. Doppler color flow assessment of the right- and left-sided pulmonary veins is the best screening tool.[314] If there is evidence of turbulence or aliasing in the color flow pattern, then spectral analysis with pulsed Doppler will help confirm the diagnosis. Usually pulmonary venous flow is low velocity and phasic. If the pattern is high velocity and turbulent, there is disturbed pulmonary venous flow. Absolute Doppler gradients may or may not be helpful for two reasons. First, the absolute velocity is dependent on the amount of pulmonary blood flow to that segment of lung. Second, it is often difficult to obtain a parallel line of interrogation of the pulmonary veins that will impact on gradient assessment. The absolute velocity is less important than the diagnosis of pulmonary vein stenosis and its effect on pulmonary artery pressure.

MRI (Fig. 56–37). This technique has now become the gold standard for the diagnosis of pulmonary vein stenosis. This permits a detailed assessment of the pulmonary veins. Velocity assessment is now possible, though this is in the actual veins themselves rather than at the venoatrial junction, which is the site assessed by Doppler echocardiography.

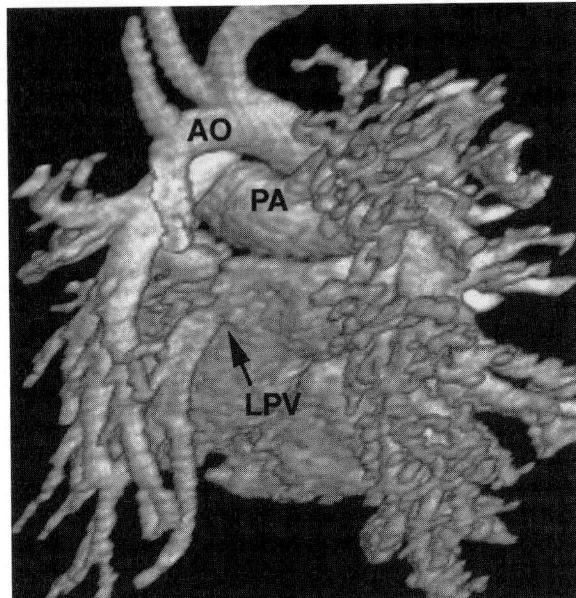

FIGURE 56–37 Three-dimensional MRI demonstrating stenosis of the left lower lobe pulmonary vein. AO = aorta; LPV = left pulmonary vein; PA = pulmonary artery.

Cardiac Catheterization and Angiography. In general a combination of echocardiography and MRI makes invasive procedures unnecessary.

MANAGEMENT OPTIONS AND OUTCOMES. If the patient has unilateral pulmonary vein stenosis and normal pulmonary artery pressure, no treatment may be necessary. Continued follow-up is important because this is often a progressive disease that can subsequently affect both sides. In cases with bilateral stenoses the outlook in the past was believed to be hopeless, with a virtually 100 percent mortality. Stents usually provided only temporary relief. More recently a pericardial reflection procedure using native tissue has resulted in some early success in this lesion. This involves using native atrial tissue to form a pocket around the surgically resected stenotic region.[201,315]

Partial Anomalous Pulmonary Venous Connection

MORPHOLOGY. This refers to those conditions where part or all of one lung drains to a site other than the left atrium. Sinus venosus defects have PAPVC typically from the right upper and middle lobe pulmonary veins to the superior vena cava.[316] PAPVC may be directed to a left vertical vein, to the superior vena cava at the level of or above the right pulmonary artery, to the azygos vein, or to the coronary sinus. PAPVC to the inferior vena cava (scimitar syndrome) may have associated hypoplasia of the right lung, pulmonary sequestration, and abnormal collateral supply to the sequestered segment. It can be seen in some patients (<10 percent) with a secundum ASD, as well as in association with many other forms of CHD. PAPVC to the right atrium has the pulmonary veins lying in the normal position; however, there is deviation of the septum primum to the left with absence of the septum secundum. This type of lesion is seen more frequently in hearts with visceral heterotaxy.

CLINICAL FEATURES. In the absence of associated anomalies, the physiological disturbance is determined by the number of anomalous veins and their site of connection, the presence and size of an ASD, and the state of the pulmonary vascular bed. In the usual patient with isolated partial pulmonary venous connection, the hemodynamic state and physical findings are similar to those in ASD.

LABORATORY INVESTIGATIONS

ECG. In isolated cases findings similar to a secundum ASD may be seen.

Chest Radiography. Isolated cases shows cardiomegaly involving the right ventricle with increased pulmonary vascular markings. In scimitar syndrome there is invariably right lung hypoplasia, with a secondary shift of the heart into the right thorax and a right-sided scimitar sign that represents the anomalous pulmonary vein.

Echocardiography. If there is a significant left-to-right shunt, then there is right ventricular volume overload with paradoxical interventricular septal motion.[317] A dilated coronary sinus is seen in PAPVC to the coronary sinus. In scimitar syndrome the abnormal pulmonary vein can be seen from the subcostal position during evaluation of the inferior vena cava.[318,319] There may be associated stenosis of the pulmonary vein. The suprasternal position permits identification of a left vertical vein, and in general it is possible in children to identify the number of connecting veins on that side. Abnormal venous drainage to the right superior vena cava may be more difficult to identify, unless a systematic approach is undertaken. The suprasternal frontal plane view allows the identification of those veins that connect just above the right pulmonary artery. Those that connect just behind the right pulmonary artery, either into the superior vena cava or the azygos, can be identified with a right anterior oblique view of the superior vena cava, whether from the subcostal position or a high right parasternal location. In adults, TEE may also be useful in detecting PAPVC.[320]

MRI. Although TEE can be used in older patients with a poorer ultrasound window with a considerable degree of accuracy,[320] it is less invasive to obtain the data using MRI.[321] This provides superb images of the connecting veins that can be seen more distally to their connections with the hilum of the lung. The pulmonary-to-systemic flow ratio can be calculated, obviating the need for hemodynamic evaluation. The pulmonary-to-systemic flow ratio can also be calculated by radionuclide techniques.

MANAGEMENT OPTIONS. In cases with a volume-loaded right ventricle, surgical intervention should be considered. Surgery is not needed when a single anomalously draining vein has not produced right ventricular volume loading. Surgery is typically performed at a similar time to an ASD at around 3 to 5 years of age. The type of surgery depends on the location of the drainage[322,323] but in general consists of reconnecting the abnormal vein(s) to the left atrium, either directly in the case of a left vertical vein or via a baffle in most other instances. In scimitar syndrome occlusion of the collateral arteries may be necessary as well as redirection of the pulmonary veins.

OUTCOMES. In general patients with repaired PAPVC have a good outcome similar to patients with an isolated ASD. What is unclear is the exact patency rate of the veins that are reconnected or baffled back to the left atrium. Patients with scimitar syndrome fare well if the lesion is relatively isolated but do poorly if there is significant associated intracardiac pathology.

Pulmonary Arteriovenous Fistula

Abnormal development of the pulmonary arteries and veins in a common vascular complex is responsible for this uncommon congenital anomaly. A variable number of pulmonary arteries communicate directly with branches of the pulmonary veins. Most patients have an associated Weber-Osler-Rendu syndrome; associated problems include bronchiectasis and other malformations of the bronchial tree, as well as absence of the right lower lobe. Pulmonary AV fistulas may also complicate classic Glenn shunts used in the palliation of cyanotic CHD and are believed to be due to the absence of "hepatic factor" in the venous blood feeding the superior vena cava–pulmonary artery connection. The amount of right-to-left shunting depends on the extent of the fistulous communications and may result in cyanosis. Paradoxical emboli or a brain abscess may cause major neurological deficits.[324,325] Patients with hereditary hemorrhagic telangiectasia often are anemic owing to repeated blood loss and may have less obvious cyanosis because of anemia. Systolic and continuous murmurs may be audible over areas of the fistula. Rounded opacities of various sizes in one or both lungs on chest radiography may suggest the presence of the lesion.

LABORATORY INVESTIGATIONS. Echocardiography is helpful in the initial diagnostic process with the use of a saline contrast injection into a systemic vein.[326] With pulmonary arteriovenous malformations there is early pulmonary venous return to the left atrium, but not as quickly as for patients with a patent foramen ovale or ASD and right-to-left atrial shunting. More recently CT and MRI techniques have provided valuable diagnostic information.[327,328] Pulmonary angiography reveals the site and extent of the abnormal communication.

MANAGEMENT OPTIONS. Unless the lesions are widespread throughout both lungs, surgical treatment aimed at removing the lesions with preservation of healthy lung tissue commonly is indicated to avoid the complications of massive hemorrhage,[324] bacterial endocarditis, and rupture of arteriovenous aneurysms. Transcatheter balloon or plug or coil occlusion embolotherapy may prove to be the therapeutic procedure of choice in some patients.[329]

Coronary Arteriovenous Fistula

MORPHOLOGY. A coronary arteriovenous fistula is a communication between one of the coronary arteries and a cardiac chamber or vein. The right coronary artery (or its branches) is the site of the fistula in about 55 percent of patients; the left coronary artery is involved in about 35 percent; and both coronary arteries are involved in a few. Connections between the coronary system and a cardiac chamber appear to represent persistence of embryonic intertrabecular spaces and sinusoids. Most of these fistulas drain into the right ventricle, right atrium, or the coronary sinus. Coronary to pulmonary artery fistulas are an occasional and usually incidental finding in the adult coronary angiography suite.

CLINICAL FEATURES. The shunt through the fistula is usually small and myocardial blood flow is not compromised. Potential complications include pulmonary hypertension and congestive heart failure if a large left-to-right shunt exists, bacterial endocarditis, rupture or thrombosis of the fistula or of an associated arterial aneurysm, and myocardial ischemia distal to the fistula due to a "myocardial steal."

Most pediatric patients are asymptomatic and are referred because of a cardiac murmur that is loud, superficial, and continuous at the lower or midsternal border. The site of maximal intensity of the murmur is related to the site of drainage and is usually away from the 2nd left intercostal space—the classic site of the continuous murmur of persistent ductus arteriosus.

LABORATORY INVESTIGATIONS

ECG. This is usually normal unless there is a large left-to-right shunt.

Chest Radiography. Radiographic findings often are normal and seldom show selective chamber enlargement.

Echocardiography. Coronary artery fistulas are now recognized with a high degree of accuracy with the advent of routine coronary artery evaluation during most pediatric echocardiography examinations. A significantly enlarged feeding coronary artery can be detected, and the entire course and site of entry of the arteriovenous fistula can be traced by Doppler color flow mapping. The shunt entry site is characterized by a continuous turbulent systolic and diastolic flow pattern. Multiplane TEE also accurately defines the origin, course, and drainage site of the fistula.

Cardiac Catheterization and Angiocardiography. If echocardiography demonstrates a significant coronary artery fistula, then hemodynamic evaluation is warranted. Standard retrograde thoracic aortography, balloon occlusion angiography of the aortic root with a 45-degree caudal tilt of the frontal camera ("laid back" aortogram), or coronary arteriography can be used reliably to identify the size and anatomical features of the fistulous tract.[330]

MANAGEMENT OPTIONS AND OUTCOMES. Small fistulas have an excellent long-term prognosis.[331] Untreated larger fistulas may predispose the individual to premature coronary artery disease in the affected vessel. Coil embolization at the time of cardiac catheterization is rapidly becoming the treatment of choice.[332] Surgical treatment is still required in some instances.[333]

REFERENCES

1. Therrien J, Somerville J, Webb G, et al: Canadian Cardiovascular Society Consensus Conference 2001 update: Recommendations for the Management of Adults with Congenital Heart Disease, Parts I, II, III. Can J Cardiol 17:940-959; 1029-1050; 1135-1158, 2001.
2. Deanfield J, Thaulow E, Warnes C, et al: Task Force on the Management of Grown-Up Congenital Heart Disease ESoC, ESC Committee for Practice Guidelines: Management of grown-up congenital heart disease. Eur Heart J 24:1035-1084, 2003.
3. Webb G, Williams R, Alpert J, et al: 32nd Bethesda Conference: Care of the Adult with Congenital Heart Disease, October 2-3, 2000. J Am Coll Cardiol 37:1161-1198, 2001.
4. Gatzoulis MA, Webb GD, Daubeney PE: Diagnosis and Management of Adult Congenital Heart Disease. Philadelphia, Churchill Livingstone, 2003.
5. Emmanouilides GC, Allen HD, Gutgesell HP, et al: Clinical Synopsis of Moss and Adams Heart Disease in Infants, Children, and Adolescents: Including the Fetus and Young Adult. Baltimore, Williams & Wilkins, 1998.
6. Anderson RH, Baker E, Macartney F, et al: Paediatric Cardiology. 2nd ed. London, Churchill Livingstone, 2002.
7. Nadas AS, Fyler DC: Pediatric Cardiology. 3rd ed. Philadelphia, WB Saunders, 1972.
8. Park MK: Pediatric Cardiology for Practitioners. 3rd ed. St. Louis, Mosby, 1996.
9. Garson A Jr, Bricker JT, Fisher DJ, et al: The Science and Practice of Pediatric Cardiology. 2nd ed. Baltimore, Williams & Wilkins, 1998.
10. Dore A, De Guise P, Mercier LA: Transition of care to adult congenital heart centres: What do patients know about their heart condition? Can J Cardiol 18:141-146, 2002.
11. Swan L, Goyal S, Hsia C, et al: Exercise systolic blood pressures are of questionable value in the assessment of the adult with a previous coarctation repair. Heart 89:189-192, 2003.
12. Graham TP Jr, Bricker JT, James FW, Strong WB: 26th Bethesda Conference: Recommendations for Determining Eligibility for Competition in Athletes with Cardiovascular Abnormalities. Task Force 1: Congenital Heart Disease. J Am Coll Cardiol 24:867-873, 1994.
13. Siu SC, Sermer M, Colman JM, et al: Cardiac Disease in Pregnancy (CARPREG) Investigators: Prospective multicenter study of pregnancy outcomes in women with heart disease. Circulation 104:515-521, 2001.
14. Siu SC, Colman JM: Heart disease and pregnancy. Heart 85:710-715, 2001.
15. Hechter SJ, Fredriksen PM, Liu P, et al: Angiotensin-converting enzyme inhibitors in adults after the Mustard procedure. Am J Cardiol 87:660-663, 2001.
16. Lester SJ, McElhinney DB, Viloria E, et al: Effects of losartan in patients with a systemically functioning morphologic right ventricle after atrial repair of transposition of the great arteries. Am J Cardiol 88:1314-1316, 2001.
17. Laer S, Mir TS, Behn F, et al: Carvedilol therapy in pediatric patients with congestive heart failure: A study investigating clinical and pharmacokinetic parameters. Am Heart J 143:916-922, 2002.
18. Rodriguez-Cruz E, Karpawich PP, Lieberman RA, Tantengco MV: Biventricular pacing as alternative therapy for dilated cardiomyopathy associated with congenital heart disease. Pacing Clin Electrophysiol 24:235-237, 2001.
19. Odim J, Laks H, Burch C, et al: Transplantation for congenital heart disease. Adv Cardiac Surg 12:59-76, 2000.
20. Pigula FA, Gandhi SK, Ristich J, et al: Cardiopulmonary transplantation for congenital heart disease in the adult. J Heart Lung Transplant 20:297-303, 2001.
21. Therrien J, Warnes C, Daliento L, et al: Canadian Cardiovascular Society Consensus Conference 2001 update: Recommendations for the Management of Adults with Congenital Heart Disease: Part III. Can J Cardiol 17:1135-1158, 2001.
22. Tempe DK, Virmani S: Coagulation abnormalities in patients with cyanotic congenital heart disease. J Cardiothorac Vasc Anesth 16:752-765, 2002.
23. Perloff JK, Latta H, Barsotti P: Pathogenesis of the glomerular abnormality in cyanotic congenital heart disease. Am J Cardiol 86:1198-1204, 2000.

24. Lamour JM, Addonizio LJ, Galantowicz ME, et al: Outcome after orthotopic cardiac transplantation in adults with congenital heart disease. Circulation 100(Suppl):5, 1999.
25. Thorne S: Management of polycythaemia in adults with cyanotic congenital heart disease. Heart 79:315-316, 1998.

Eisenmenger Syndrome

26. Daliento L, Somerville J, Presbitero P, et al: Eisenmenger syndrome: Factors relating to deterioration and death. Eur Heart J 19:1845-1855, 1998.
27. Saha A, Balakrishnan KG, Jaiswal PK, et al: Prognosis for patients with Eisenmenger syndrome of various aetiology. Int J Cardiol 45:199-207, 1994.
28. Vongpatanasin W, Brickner ME, Hillis LD, Lange RA: The Eisenmenger syndrome in adults. Ann Intern Med 128:745-755, 1998.
29. Corone S, Davido A, Lang T, Corone P: [Outcome of patients with Eisenmenger syndrome. Apropos of 62 cases followed-up for an average of 16 years]. [French]. Arch Mal Coeur Vaiss 85:521-526, 1992.
30. Ammash NM, Connolly HM, Abel MD, Warnes CA: Noncardiac surgery in Eisenmenger syndrome. J Am Coll Cardiol 33:222-227, 1999.
31. Martin JT, Tautz TJ, Antognini JF: Safety of regional anesthesia in Eisenmenger's syndrome. Reg Anesth Pain Med 27:509-513, 2002.
32. Sandoval J, Aguirre JS, Pulido T, et al: Nocturnal oxygen therapy in patients with the Eisenmenger syndrome. Am J Respir Crit Care Med 164:1682-1687, 2001.
33. Harinck E, Hutter PA, Hoorntje TM, et al: Air travel and adults with cyanotic congenital heart disease. Circulation 93:272-276, 1996.
34. Waddell TK, Bennett L, Kennedy R, et al: Heart-lung or lung transplantation for Eisenmenger syndrome. J Heart Lung Transplant 21:731-737, 2002.
35. Berman EB, Barst RJ: Eisenmenger's syndrome: Current management. Prog Cardiovasc Dis 45:129-138, 2002.
36. Granton JT, Rabinovitch M: Pulmonary arterial hypertension in congenital heart disease. Cardiol Clin 20:441-457, 2002.
37. Hopkins WE, Kelly DP: Angiotensin-converting enzyme inhibitors in adults with cyanotic congenital heart disease. Am J Cardiol 77:439-440, 1996.
38. Rosenzweig EB, Kerstein D, Barst RJ: Long-term prostacyclin for pulmonary hypertension with associated congenital heart defects. Circulation 99:1858-1865, 1999.
39. McLaughlin VV, Genthner DE, Panella MM, et al: Compassionate use of continuous prostacyclin in the management of secondary pulmonary hypertension: A case series. Ann Intern Med 130:740-743, 1999.
40. Rubin LJ, Badesch DB, Barst RJ, et al: Bosentan therapy for pulmonary arterial hypertension. N Engl J Med 346:896-903, 2002.

Cardiac Arrhythmias

41. Wilson NJ, Clarkson PM, Barratt-Boyes BG, et al: Long-term outcome after the Mustard repair for simple transposition of the great arteries: 28-year follow-up. J Am Coll Cardiol 32:758-765, 1998.
42. Puley G, Siu S, Connelly M, et al: Arrhythmia and survival in patients > 18 years of age after the Mustard procedure for complete transposition of the great arteries. Am J Cardiol 83:1080-1084, 1999.
43. Myridakis DJ, Ehlers KH, Engle MA: Late follow-up after venous switch operation (Mustard procedure) for simple and complex transposition of the great arteries. Am J Cardiol 74:1030-1036, 1994.
44. Gatzoulis MA, Freeman MA, Siu SC, et al: Atrial arrhythmia after surgical closure of atrial septal defects in adults. N Engl J Med 340:839-846, 1999.
45. Murphy JG, Gersh BJ, McGoon MD, et al: Long-term outcome after surgical repair of isolated atrial septal defect: Follow-up at 27 to 32 years. N Engl J Med 323:1645-1650, 1990.
46. Konstantinides S, Geibel A, Olschewski M, et al: A comparison of surgical and medical therapy for atrial septal defect in adults. N Engl J Med 333:469-473, 1995.
47. Oechslin EN, Harrison DA, Harris L, et al: Reoperation in adults with repair of tetralogy of Fallot: Indications and outcomes. J Thorac Cardiovasc Surg 118:245-251, 1999.
48. Gentles TL, Calder AL, Clarkson PM, Neutze JM: Predictors of long-term survival with Ebstein's anomaly of the tricuspid valve. Am J Cardiol 69:377-381, 1992.
49. Giuliani ER, Fuster V, Brandenburg RO, Mair DD: Ebstein's anomaly: The clinical features and natural history of Ebstein's anomaly of the tricuspid valve. Mayo Clin Proc 54:163-173, 1979.
50. Augustin N, Schmidt-Habelmann P, Wottke M, et al: Results after surgical repair of Ebstein's anomaly. Ann Thorac Surg 63:1650-1656, 1997.
51. Fishberger SB, Wernovsky G, Gentles TL, et al: Factors that influence the development of atrial flutter after the Fontan operation. J Thorac Cardiovasc Surg 113:80-86, 1997.
52. Gelatt M, Hamilton RM, McCrindle BW, et al: Risk factors for atrial tachyarrhythmias after the Fontan operation. J Am Coll Cardiol 24:1735-1741, 1994.
53. Peters NS, Somerville J: Arrhythmias after the Fontan procedure. Br Heart J 68:199-204, 1992.
54. Downar E, Harris L, Kimber S, et al: Ventricular tachycardia after surgical repair of tetralogy of Fallot: Results of intraoperative mapping studies. J Am Coll Cardiol 20:648-655, 1992.
55. Balaji S, Johnson TB, Sade RM, et al: Management of atrial flutter after the Fontan procedure. J Am Coll Cardiol 23:1209-1215, 1994.
56. Bonchek LI, Burlingame MW, Worley SJ, et al: Cox/maze procedure for atrial septal defect with atrial fibrillation: Management strategies. Ann Thorac Surg 55:607-610, 1993.
57. Sandoval N, Velasco VM, Orjuela H, et al: Concomitant mitral valve or atrial septal defect surgery and the modified Cox-maze procedure. Am J Cardiol 77:591-596, 1996.
58. Theodoro DA, Danielson GK, Porter CJ, Warnes CA: Right-sided maze procedure for right atrial arrhythmias in congenital heart disease. Ann Thorac Surg 65:149-153, 1998.
59. Mavroudis C, Backer CL, Deal BJ, Johnsrude CL: Fontan conversion to cavopulmonary connection and arrhythmia circuit cryoblation. J Thorac Cardiovasc Surg 115:547-556, 1998.
60. Harrison DA, Harris L, Siu SC, et al: Sustained ventricular tachycardia in adult patients late after repair of tetralogy of Fallot. J Am Coll Cardiol 30:1368–1373, 1997.
61. Gatzoulis MA, Till JA, Somerville J, Redington AN: Mechanoelectrical interaction in tetralogy of Fallot: QRS prolongation relates to right ventricular size and predicts malignant ventricular arrhythmias and sudden death. Circulation 92:231-237, 1995.
62. Berul CI, Hill SL, Geggel RL, et al: Electrocardiographic markers of late sudden death risk in postoperative tetralogy of Fallot children. J Cardiovasc Electrophysiol 8:1349-1356, 1997.
63. Murphy JG, Gersh BJ, Mair DD, et al: Long-term outcome in patients undergoing surgical repair of tetralogy of Fallot. N Engl J Med 329:593-599, 1993.
64. Nollert G, Fischlein T, Bouterwek S, et al: Long-term survival in patients with repair of tetralogy of Fallot: 36-year follow-up of 490 survivors of the first year after surgical repair. J Am Coll Cardiol 30:1374-1383, 1997.
65. Oechslin EN, Harrison DA, Connelly MS, et al: Mode of death in adults with congenital heart disease. Am J Cardiol 86:1111-1116, 2000.
66. Huhta JC, Maloney JD, Ritter DG, et al: Complete atrioventricular block in patients with atrioventricular discordance. Circulation 67:1374-1377, 1983.
67. Colman JM, Oechslin E: Adapted from Abbreviations and Glossary, Canadian Consensus Conference on Adult Congenital Heart Disease, 1996. Can J Cardiol 14:395-452, 1996.
68. Bull C: Current and potential impact of fetal diagnosis on prevalence and spectrum of serious congenital heart disease at term in the UK. British Paediatric Cardiac Association. Lancet 354:1242-1247, 1999.
69. Bonnet D, Coltri A, Butera G, et al: Detection of transposition of the great arteries in fetuses reduces neonatal morbidity and mortality. Circulation 99:916-918, 1999.
70. Van Praagh R: The segmental approach to diagnosis in congenital heart disease. *In* Bergsma D (ed): Birth Defects: Original Article Series. Baltimore, Williams & Wilkins, 1972.
71. Shinebourne EA, Macartney FJ, Anderson RH: Sequential chamber localization: Logical approach to diagnosis in congenital heart disease. Br Heart J 38:327-340, 1976.
72. Sittiwangkul R, Ma RY, McCrindle BW, et al: Echocardiographic assessment of obstructive lesions in atrioventricular septal defects. J Am Coll Cardiol 38:253-261, 2001.
73. Sugeng L, Spenser KT, Mor-Avi V, et al: Dynamic three-dimensional color-flow Doppler: An improved technique for the assessment of mitral regurgitation. Echocardiography 20:265, 2003.
74. Shiina A, Seward JB, Tajik AJ, et al: Two-dimensional echocardiographic-surgical correlation in Ebstein's anomaly: Preoperative determination of patients requiring tricuspid valve plication vs. replacement. Circulation 68:534-544, 1983.
75. Marx GR, Sherwood MC: Three-dimensional echocardiography in congenital heart disease: A continuum of unfulfilled promises? No. A presently clinically applicable technology with an important future? Yes. Pediatr Cardiol 23:266-285, 2002.
76. Heusch A, Rubo J, Krogmann ON, Bourgeois M: Volumetric analysis of the right ventricle in children with congenital heart defects: Comparison of biplane angiography and transthoracic 3-dimensional echocardiography. Cardiol Young 9:577-584, 1999.
77. Jan SL, Hwang B, Lee PC, et al: Intracardiac ultrasound assessment of atrial septal defect: Comparison with transthoracic echocardiographic, angiocardiographic, and balloon-sizing measurements. Cardiovasc Intervent Radiol 24:84-89, 2001.
78. Bruce CJ, Friedman PA: Intracardiac echocardiography. Eur J Echocardiogr 2:234-244, 2001.
79. Cowley CG, Lloyd TR: Interventional cardiac catheterization advances in nonsurgical approaches to congenital heart disease. Curr Opin Pediatr 11:425-432, 1999.
80. Hornung TS, Benson LN, McLaughlin PR: Catheter interventions in adult patients with congenital heart disease. Curr Cardiol Rep 4:54-62, 2002.

Atrial Septal Defect

81. Campbell M: Natural history of atrial septal defect. Br Heart J 32:820-826, 1970.
82. Craig RJ, Selzer A: Natural history and prognosis of atrial septal defect. Circulation 37:805-815, 1968.
83. Therrien J, Dore A, Gersony W, et al: Canadian Cardiovascular Society: CCS Consensus Conference 2001 update: Recommendations for the management of adults with congenital heart disease: Part I. Can J Cardiol 17:940-959, 2001.
84. Attie F, Rosas M Granados N, et al: Surgical treatment for secundum atrial septal defects in patients older than 40 years old: A randomized clinical trial. J Am Coll Cardiol 38:2035-2042, 2001.
85. Mullen MJ, Dias BF, Walker F, et al: Intracardiac echocardiography guided device closure of atrial septal defects. J Am Coll Cardiol 41:285-292, 2003.
86. Du ZD, Hijazi ZM, Kleinman CS, et al: Comparison between transcatheter and surgical closure of secundum atrial septal defect in children and adults: Results of a multicenter nonrandomized trial. J Am Coll Cardiol 39:1836-1844, 2002.
87. Brochu MC, Baril JF, Dore A, et al: Improvement in exercise capacity in asymptomatic and mildly symptomatic adults after atrial septal defect percutaneous closure. Circulation 106:1821-1826, 2002.
88. Helber U, Baumann R, Seboldt H, et al: Atrial septal defect in adults: Cardiopulmonary exercise capacity before and 4 months and 10 years after defect closure. J Am Coll Cardiol 29:1345-1350, 1997.
89. McCarthy PM, Gillinov AM, Castle L, et al: The Cox-maze procedure: The Cleveland Clinic experience. Semin Thorac Cardiovasc Surg 12:25-29, 2000.

Atrioventricular Septal Defect

90. Lange A, Mankad P, Walayat M, et al: Transthoracic three-dimensional echocardiography in the preoperative assessment of atrioventricular septal defect morphology. Am J Cardiol 85:630-635, 2000.
91. Smallhorn JF: Cross-sectional echocardiographic assessment of atrioventricular septal defect: Basic morphology and preoperative risk factors. Echocardiography 18:415-432, 2001.
92. Suzuki K, Ho SY, Anderson RH, Becker AE, et al: Morphometric analysis of atrioventricular septal defect with common valve orifice. J Am Coll Cardiol 31:217-223, 1998.

93. Ostium primum defect: Factors causing deterioration in the natural history. Br Heart J 27:413-419. 1965.
94. Hynes JK, Tajik AJ, Seward JB, et al: Partial atrioventricular canal defect in adults. Circulation 66:284-287, 1982.
95. Barnett MG, Chopra PS, Young WP: Long-term follow-up of partial atrioventricular septal defect repair in adults. Chest 94:321-324, 1988.
96. Burke RP, Horvath K, Landzberg M, et al: Long-term follow-up after surgical repair of ostium primum atrial septal defects in adults. J Am Coll Cardiol 27:696-699, 1996.
97. Bergin ML, Warnes CA, Tajik AJ, Danielson GK: Partial atrioventricular canal defect: Long-term follow-up after initial repair in patients ≥ 40 years old. J Am Coll Cardiol 25:1189-1194, 1995.
98. Pearl JM, Laks H: Intermediate and complete forms of atrioventricular canal. Semin Thorac Cardiovasc Surg 9:8-20, 1997.
99. Hanley FL, Fenton KN, Jonas RA, et al: Surgical repair of complete atrioventricular canal defects in infancy: Twenty-year trends. J Thorac Cardiovasc Surg 106:387-394, 1993.
100. Michielon G, Stellin G, Rizzoli G, et al: Left atrioventricular valve incompetence after repair of common atrioventricular canal defects. Ann Thorac Surg 60(Suppl):9, 1995.
101. Bando K, Turrentine MW, Sun K, et al: Surgical management of complete atrioventricular septal defects: A twenty-year experience. J Thorac Cardiovasc Surg 110:1543-1552, 1995.
102. Van Arsdell GS, Williams WG, Boutin C, et al: Subaortic stenosis in the spectrum of atrioventricular septal defects: Solutions may be complex and palliative. J Thorac Cardiovasc Surg 110:1534-1541, 1995.
103. DeLeon SY, Ilbawi MN, Wilson WR Jr, et al: Surgical options in subaortic stenosis associated with endocardial cushion defects. Ann Thorac Surg 52:1076-1082, 1991.
104. Mavroudis C, Backer CL: The two-patch technique for complete atrioventricular canal. Semin Thorac Cardiovasc Surg 9:35-43, 1997.
105. El Najdawi EK, Driscoll DJ, Puga FJ, et al: Operation for partial atrioventricular septal defect: A forty-year review. J Thorac Cardiovasc Surg 119:880-889, 2000.
106. Kameyama T, Ando F, Okamoto F, et al: Long term follow-up of atrioventricular valve function after repair of atrioventricular septal defect. Ann Thorac Cardiovasc Surg 5:101-106, 1999.

Ventricular Septal Defect

107. Perloff J: Ventricular septal defect. *In* The Clinical Recognition of Congenital Heart Disease. 4th ed. Philadelphia, WB Saunders, 1999, pp 467-489.
108. Gabriel HM, Heger M, Innerhofer P, et al: Long-term outcome of patients with ventricular septal defect considered not to require surgical closure during childhood. J Am Coll Cardiol 39:1066-1071, 2002.
109. Neumayer U, Stone S, Somerville J: Small ventricular septal defects in adults. Eur Heart J 19:1573-1582, 1998.
110. Eroglu AG, Oztunc F, Saltik L, et al: Evolution of ventricular septal defect with special reference to spontaneous closure rate, subaortic ridge and aortic valve prolapse. Pediatr Cardiol 24:31-35, 2003.
111. Eroglu AG, Oztunc F, Saltik L, et al: Aortic valve prolapse and aortic regurgitation in patients with ventricular septal defect. Pediatr Cardiol 24:36-39, 2003.
112. Arora R, Trahan V, Kumar A, et al: Transcatheter closure of congenital ventricular septal defects: Experience with various devices. J Intervent Cardiol 16:83-91, 2003.

Patent Ductus Arteriosus

113. Perloff J: Patent ductus arteriosus. *In* The Clinical Recognition of Congenital Heart Disease. 4th ed. Philadelphia, WB Saunders, 1999, pp 467-489.
114. Van Overmeire B, Smets K, Lecoutere D, et al: A comparison of ibuprofen and indomethacin for closure of patent ductus arteriosus. N Engl J Med 343:674-681, 2000.
115. Galal MO: Advantages and disadvantages of coils for transcatheter closure of patent ductus arteriosus. J Intervent Cardiol 16:157-163, 2003.
116. Landzberg MJ: Transcatheter occlusion: The treatment of choice for the adult with patent ductus arteriosus. Circulation 84(Suppl II):67, 1999.
117. Bennhagen RG, Benson LN: Silent and audible persistent ductus arteriosus: An angiographic study. Pediatr Cardiol 24:27-30, 2003.
118. Dearani JA, Danielson GK, Puga FJ, et al: Late follow-up of 1095 patients undergoing operation for complex congenital heart disease utilizing pulmonary ventricle to pulmonary artery conduits. Ann Thorac Surg 75:399-410, 2003.
119. Mavroudis C, Backer CL: Surgical management of severe truncal insufficiency: Experience with truncal valve remodeling techniques. Ann Thorac Surg 72:396-400, 2001.

Tetralogy of Fallot

120. Hokanson JS, Moller JH: Adults with tetralogy of Fallot: Long-term follow-up. Cardiol Rev 7:149-155, 1999.
121. Graham TP Jr: Management of pulmonary regurgitation after tetralogy of Fallot repair. Curr Cardiol Rep 4:63-67, 2002.
122. Niwa K, Perloff JK, Bhuta SM, et al: Structural abnormalities of great arterial walls in congenital heart disease: Light and electron microscopic analyses. Circulation 103:393-400, 2001.
123. Reddy VM, McElhinney DB, Amin Z, et al: Early and intermediate outcomes after repair of pulmonary atresia with ventricular septal defect and major aortopulmonary collateral arteries: Experience with 85 patients. Circulation 101:1826-1832, 2000.
124. Mair DD, Puga FJ: Management of pulmonary atresia with ventricular septal defect. Curr Treat Options Cardiovasc Med 5:409-415, 2003.
125. Abd El Rahman MY, Abdul-Khaliq H, Vogel M, et al: Relation between right ventricular enlargement, QRS duration, and right ventricular function in patients with tetralogy of Fallot and pulmonary regurgitation after surgical repair. Heart 84:416-420, 2000.
126. Alexiou C, Mahmoud H, Al Khaddour A, et al: Outcome after repair of tetralogy of Fallot in the first year of life. Ann Thorac Surg 71:494-500, 2001.
127. Parry AJ, McElhinney DB, Kung GC, et al: Elective primary repair of acyanotic tetralogy of Fallot in early infancy: Overall outcome and impact on the pulmonary valve. J Am Coll Cardiol 36:2279-2283, 2000.
128. Hu DC, Seward JB, Puga FJ, et al: Total correction of tetralogy of Fallot at age 40 years and older: Long-term follow-up. J Am Coll Cardiol 5:40-44, 1985.
129. Therrien J, Siu SC, Harris L, et al: Impact of pulmonary valve replacement on arrhythmia propensity late after repair of tetralogy of Fallot. Circulation 103:2489-2494, 2001.
130. Nollert G, Fischlein T, Bouterwek S, et al: Long-term results of total repair of tetralogy of Fallot in adulthood: 35 years follow-up in 104 patients corrected at the age of 18 or older. Thorac Cardiovasc Surgeon 45:178-181, 1997.
131. Yemets IM, Williams WG, Webb GD, et al: Pulmonary valve replacement late after repair of tetralogy of Fallot. Ann Thorac Surg 64:526-530, 1997.
132. Vliegen HW, van Straten A, de Roos A, et al: Magnetic resonance imaging to assess the hemodynamic effects of pulmonary valve replacement in adults late after repair of tetralogy of fallot. Circulation 106:1703-1707, 2002.
133. Ghai A, Silversides C, Harris L, et al: Left ventricular dysfunction is a risk factor for sudden cardiac death in adults late after repair of tetralogy of Fallot. J Am Coll Cardiol 40:1675-1680, 2003.
134. Mahle WT, Spray TL, Wernovsky G, et al: Survival after reconstructive surgery for hypoplastic left heart syndrome: A 15-year experience from a single institution. Circulation 102(Suppl):41, 2000.

Fontan Patient

135. Gentles TL, Mayer JE Jr, Gauvreau K, et al: Fontan operation in five hundred consecutive patients: Factors influencing early and late outcome. J Thorac Cardiovasc Surg 114:376-391, 1997.
136. Gentles TL, Gauvreau K, Mayer JE Jr, et al: Functional outcome after the Fontan operation: Factors influencing late morbidity. J Thorac Cardiovasc Surg 114:392-403, 1997.
137. Senzaki H, Masutani S, Kobayashi J, et al: Ventricular afterload and ventricular work in fontan circulation: Comparison with normal two-ventricle circulation and single-ventricle circulation with Blalock-Taussig shunts. Circulation 105:2885-2892, 2002.
138. Rosenthal M, Bush A, Deanfield J, Redington A: Comparison of cardiopulmonary adaptation during exercise in children after the atriopulmonary and total cavopulmonary connection Fontan procedures. Circulation 91:372-378, 1995.
139. Milanesi O, Stellin G, Colan SD, et al: Systolic and diastolic performance late after the Fontan procedure for a single ventricle and comparison of those undergoing operation at <12 months of age and at >12 months of age. Am J Cardiol 89:276-280, 2002.
140. Kouatli AA, Garcia JA, Zellers TM, et al: Enalapril does not enhance exercise capacity in patients after Fontan procedure. Circulation 96:1507-1512, 1997.
141. Khambadkone S, Li J, de Leval MR, et al: Basal pulmonary vascular resistance and nitric oxide responsiveness late after Fontan-type operation. Circulation 107:3204-3208, 2003.
142. Fontan F, Kirklin JW, Fernandez G, et al: Outcome after a "perfect" Fontan operation. Circulation 81:1520-1536, 1990.
143. Gates RN, Laks H, Drinkwater DC, et al: The Fontan procedure in adults. Ann Thorac Surg 63:1085-1090, 1997.
144. Driscoll DJ, Offord KP, Feldt RH, et al: Five- to fifteen-year follow up after Fontan operation. Circulation 85:469-496, 1992.
145. Durongpisitkul K, Porter CJ, Cetta F, et al: Predictors of early- and late-onset supraventricular tachyarrhythmias after Fontan operation. Circulation 98:1099-1107, 1998.
146. Gewillig M, Wyse RK, de Leval MR, Deanfield JE: Early and late arrhythmias after the Fontan operation: Predisposing factors and clinical consequences. Br Heart J 67:72-79, 1992.
147. Shirai LK, Rosenthal DN, Reitz BA, et al: Arrhythmias and thromboembolic complications after the extracardiac Fontan operation. J Thorac Cardiovasc Surg 115:499-505, 1998.
148. Balling G, Vogt M, Kaemmerer H, et al: Intracardiac thrombus formation after the Fontan operation. J Thorac Cardiovasc Surg 119:52, 2000.
149. Coon PD, Rychik J, Novello RT, et al: Thrombus formation after the Fontan operation. Ann Thorac Surg 71:1990-1994, 2001.
150. Brancaccio G, Carotti A, D'Argenio P, et al: Protein-losing enteropathy after Fontan surgery: Resolution after cardiac transplantation. J Heart Lung Transplant 22:484-486, 2003.
151. Mertens L, Hagler DJ, Sauer U, et al: Protein-losing enteropathy after the Fontan operation: An international multicenter study. PLE Study Group. J Thorac Cardiovasc Surg 115:1063-1073, 1998.
152. Varma C, Warr MR, Hendler AL, et al: Prevalence of "silent" pulmonary emboli in adults after the Fontan operation. J Am Coll Cardiol 41:2252-2258, 2003.
153. Monagle P, Cochrane A, McCrindle B, et al: Thromboembolic complications after Fontan procedures: The role of prophylactic anticoagulation. J Thorac Cardiovasc Surg 115:493-498, 1998.
154. Jacobs ML, Pourmoghadam KK, Geary EM, et al: Fontan's operation: is aspirin enough? Is Coumadin too much? Ann Thorac Surg 73:64-68, 2002.
155. Seipelt RG, Franke A, Vazquez-Jimenez JF, et al: Thromboembolic complications after Fontan procedures: Comparison of different therapeutic approaches. Ann Thorac Surg 74:556-562, 2002.
156. Deal BJ, Mavroudis C, Backer CL: Beyond Fontan conversion: Surgical therapy of arrhythmias including patients with associated complex congenital heart disease. Ann Thorac Cardiovasc Surg 76:542-553; Discussion 553-554, 2003.
157. Mavroudis C, Deal BJ, Backer CL: Arrhythmia surgery in association with complex congenital heart repairs excluding patients with Fontan conversion. Semin Thorac Cardiovasc Surg Pediatr Card Surg Annu 6:33-50, 2003.
158. Deal BJ, Mavroudis C, Backer CL, et al: Impact of arrhythmia circuit cryoablation during Fontan conversion for refractory atrial tachycardia. Am J Cardiol 83:563-568, 1999.

159. Mavroudis C, Backer CL, Deal BJ, et al: Total cavopulmonary and Maze procedure for patients with failure of the Fontan operation. Thorac Cardiovasc Surgeon 122:863-871, 2001.
160. Feldt RH, Driscoll DJ, Offord KP, et al: Protein-losing enteropathy after the Fontan operation. J Thorac Cardiovasc Surg 112:672-680, 1996.

Transposition Complexes

161. Bonnet D, Coltri A, Butera G, et al: [Prenatal diagnosis of transposition of great vessels reduces neonatal morbidity and mortality]. [French]. Arch Mal Coeur Vaiss 92:637-640, 1999.
162. Williams W, McCrindle B, Ashburn DA, et al: Congenital Heart Surgeon's Society: Outcome of 829 neonates with complete transposition of the great arteries 12-17 years after repair. Eur J Cardiothorac Surg 24:1-9, 2003.
163. Rehnstrom P, Gilljam T, Sudow G, Berggren H: Excellent survival and low complication rate in medium-term follow-up after arterial switch operation for complete transposition. Scand Cardiovasc J 37:104-106, 2003.
164. Hovels-Gurich HH, Kunz D, Seghaye M, et al: Results of exercise testing at a mean age of 10 years after neonatal arterial switch operation. Acta Paediatr 92:190-196, 2003.
165. Losay J, Touchot A, Serraf A, et al: Late outcome after arterial switch operation for transposition of the great arteries. Circulation 104(Suppl):6, 2001.
166. Yoshizumi K, Yagihara T, Uemura H: Approach to the neoaortic valve for replacement after the arterial switch procedure in patients with complete transposition. Cardiol Young 11:666-669, 2001.
167. Legendre A, Losay J, Touchot-Kone A, et al: [Prevalence and diagnosis of coronary lesions after arterial switch]. [French]. Arch Mal Coeur Vaiss 96:485-488, 2003.
168. Wells WJ, Blackstone E: Intermediate outcome after Mustard and Senning procedures: A study by the Congenital Heart Surgeons Society. Semin Thorac Cardiovasc Surg Pediatr Card Surg Annu 3:186-197, 2000.
169. Connelly M, Walters JE, McLaughlin PR, et al: Functional capacity in adult patients with Mustard operation. J Am Coll Cardiol 25:378A, 1995.
170. Derrick GP, Narang I, White PA, et al: Failure of stroke volume augmentation during exercise and dobutamine stress is unrelated to load-independent indexes of right ventricular performance after the Mustard operation. Circulation 102(Suppl):9, 2000.
171. Hauser M, Bengel FM, Kuhn A, et al: Myocardial blood flow and flow reserve after coronary reimplantation in patients after arterial switch and Ross operation. Circulation 103:1875-1880, 2001.
172. Lubiszewska B, Gosiewska E, Hoffman P, et al: Myocardial perfusion and function of the systemic right ventricle in patients after atrial switch procedure for complete transposition: Long-term follow-up. J Am Coll Cardiol 36:1365-1370, 2000.
173. Millane T, Bernard EJ, Jaeggi E, et al: Role of ischemia and infarction in late right ventricular dysfunction after atrial repair of transposition of the great arteries. J Am Coll Cardiol 35:1661-1668, 2000.
174. Gelatt M, Hamilton RM, McCrindle BW, et al: Arrhythmia and mortality after the Mustard procedure: A 30-year single-center experience. J Am Coll Cardiol 29:194-201, 1997.
175. Gewillig M, Cullen S, Mertens B, et al: Risk factors for arrhythmia and death after Mustard operation for simple transposition of the great arteries. Circulation 84(Suppl):92, 1991.
176. Rhodes LA, Wernovsky G, Keane JF, et al: Arrhythmias and intracardiac conduction after the arterial switch operation. J Thorac Cardiovasc Surg109:303-310, 1995.
177. Gatzoulis MA, Walters J, McLaughlin PR, et al: Late arrhythmia in adults with the Mustard procedure for transposition of great arteries: A surrogate marker for right ventricular dysfunction? Heart 84:409-415, 2000.
178. Haas F, Wottke M, Poppert H, Meisner H: Long-term survival and functional follow-up in patients after the arterial switch operation. Ann Thorac Surg 68:1692-1697, 1999.
179. Mahoney LT, Knoedel DL, Skorton DJ: Echocardiographic postoperative assessment of patients with transposition of the great arteries. J Cardiovasc Ultrasound Allied Tech 12:545-557, 1999.
180. Daebritz SH, Tiete AR, Sachweh JS, et al: Systemic right ventricular failure after atrial switch operation: Midterm results of conversion into an arterial switch. Ann Thorac Surg 71:1255-1259, 2001.
181. Chang AC, Wernovsky G, Wessel DL, et al: Surgical management of late right ventricular failure after Mustard or Senning repair. Circulation 86(Suppl):9, 1992.
182. Cochrane AD, Karl TR, Mee RB: Staged conversion to arterial switch for late failure of the systemic right ventricle. Ann Thorac Surg 56:854-861, 1993.
183. van Son JA, Reddy VM, Silverman NH, Hanley FL: Regression of tricuspid regurgitation after two-stage arterial switch operation for failing systemic ventricle after atrial inversion operation. J Thorac Cardiovasc Surg 111:342-347, 1996.
184. Carrel T, Pfammatter JP: Complete transposition of the great arteries: Surgical concepts for patients with systemic right ventricular failure following intraatrial repair. Thorac Cardiovasc Surgeon 48:224-227, 2000.

Congenitally Corrected Transposition of the Great Arteries

185. Webb GD, McLaughlin PR, Gow RM, et al: Transposition complexes. Cardiol Clin 11:651-664, 1993.
186. Roffi M, de Marchi SF, Seiler C: Congenitally corrected transposition of the great arteries in an 80-year-old woman. Heart 79:622-623, 1998.
187. Kafali G, Elsharshari H, Ozer S, et al: Incidence of dysrhythmias in congenitally corrected transposition of the great arteries. Turk J Pediatr 44:219-223, 2002.
188. Rutledge JM, Nihill MR, Fraser CD, et al: Outcome of 121 patients with congenitally corrected transposition of the great arteries. Pediatr Cardiol 23:137-145, 2002.
189. Presbitero P, Somerville J, Rabajoli F, et al: Corrected transposition of the great arteries without associated defects in adult patients: Clinical profile and follow up. Br Heart J 74:57-59, 1995.
190. Beauchesne LM, Warnes CA, Connolly HM, et al: Outcome of the unoperated adult who presents with congenitally corrected transposition of the great arteries. J Am Coll Cardiol 40:285-290, 2002.
191. van Son JA, Danielson GK, Huhta JC, et al: Late results of systemic atrioventricular valve replacement in corrected transposition. J Thorac Cardiovasc Surg 109:642-652, 1995.
192. Duncan BW, Mee RB, Mesia CI, et al: Results of the double-switch operation for congenitally corrected transposition of the great arteries. Eur J Cardiothorac Surg 24:11-19, 2003.
193. Imai Y: Double-switch operation for congenitally corrected transposition. Adv Cardiac Surg 9:65-86, 1997.
194. Karl TR, Weintraub RG, Brizard CP, et al: Senning plus arterial switch operation for discordant (congenitally corrected) transposition. Ann Thorac Surg 64:495-502, 1997.
195. Prieto LR, Hordof AJ, Secic M, et al: Progressive tricuspid valve disease in patients with congenitally corrected transposition of the great arteries. Circulation 98:997-1005, 1998.
196. Ilbawi MN, Ocampo CB, Allen BS, et al: Intermediate results of the anatomic repair for congenitally corrected transposition. Ann Thorac Surg 73:594-599, 2002.
197. Graham TP Jr, Bernard YD, Mellen BG, et al: Long-term outcome in congenitally corrected transposition of the great arteries: A multi-institutional study. J Am Coll Cardiol 36:255-261, 2000.

Double-Outlet Right Ventricle

198. Anderson RH: Double-outlet right ventricle. Eur J Cardiothorac Surg 22:853, 2002.
199. Anderson RH, McCarthy K, Cook AC: Continuing medical education: Double-outlet right ventricle. Cardiol Young 11:329-344, 2001.
200. Brown JW, Ruzmetov M, Okada Y, et al: Surgical results in patients with double-outlet right ventricle: A 20-year experience. Ann Thorac Surg 72:1630-1635, 2001.
201. Lacour-Gayet F, Zoghbi J, Serraf AE, et al: Surgical management of progressive pulmonary venous obstruction after repair of total anomalous pulmonary venous connection. J Thorac Cardiovasc Surg 117:679-687, 1999.
202. Belli E, Serraf A, Lacour-Gayet F, et al: Biventricular repair for double-outlet right ventricle: Results and long-term follow-up. Circulation 98(Suppl):5, 1998.
203. Aoki M, Forbess JM, Jonas RA, et al: Result of biventricular repair for double-outlet right ventricle. J Thorac Cardiovasc Surg 107:338-349, 1994.
204. Rychik J, Jacobs ML, Norwood WI: Early changes in ventricular geometry and ventricular septal defect size following Rastelli operation or intraventricular baffle repair for conotruncal anomaly: A cause for development of subaortic stenosis. Circulation 90:II13-19, 1994.
205. Celermajer DS, Bull C, Till JA, et al: Ebstein's anomaly: Presentation and outcome from fetus to adult. J Am Coll Cardiol 23:170-176, 1994.
206. Therrien J, Gatzoulis M, Graham T, et al: Canadian Cardiovascular Society Consensus Conference 2001 update: Recommendations for the Management of Adults with Congenital Heart Disease: Part II. Can J Cardiol 17:1029-1050, 2001.
207. Chauvaud S, Fuzellier JF, Berrebi A, et al: Bi-directional cavopulmonary shunt associated with ventriculo and valvuloplasty in Ebstein's anomaly: Benefits in high-risk patients. Eur J Cardiothorac Surg 13:514-519, 1998.
208. Chauvaud S: Ebstein's malformation: Surgical treatment and results. Thorac Cardiovasc Surgeon 48:220-223, 2000.
209. Chauvaud SM, Brancaccio G, Carpentier A: Cardiac arrhythmia in patients undergoing surgical repair of Ebstein's anomaly. Ann Thorac Surg 71:1547-1552, 2001.
210. Almange C: [Ebstein anomaly and pregnancy]. [French]. Arch Mal Coeur Vaiss 95:525, 2002.

Coarctation of the Aorta

211. Aluquin VP, Shutte D, Nihill MR, et al: Normal aortic arch growth and comparison with isolated coarctation of the aorta. Am J Cardiol 91:502-505, 2003.
212. Bharati S, Lev M: The surgical anatomy of the heart in tubular hypoplasia of the transverse aorta (preductal coarctation). J Thorac Cardiovasc Surg 91:79-85, 1986.
213. Levine JC, Sanders SP, Colan SD, et al: The risk of having additional obstructive lesions in neonatal coarctation of the aorta. Cardiol Young 11:44-53, 2001.
214. De Mey S, Segers P, Coomans I, et al: Limitations of Doppler echocardiography for the post-operative evaluation of aortic coarctation. J Biomechan 34:951-960, 2001.
215. Lim DS, Ralston MA: Echocardiographic indices of Doppler flow patterns compared with MRI or angiographic measurements to detect significant coarctation of the aorta. Echocardiography 19:55-60, 2002.
216. Godart F, Labrot G, Devos P, et al: Coarctation of the aorta: Comparison of aortic dimensions between conventional MR imaging, 3D MR angiography, and conventional angiography. Eur Radiol 12:2034-2039, 2002.
217. Seirafi PA, Warner KG, Geggel RL, et al: Repair of coarctation of the aorta during infancy minimizes the risk of late hypertension. Ann Thorac Surg 66:1378-1382, 1998.
218. Ovaert C, Benson LN, Nykanen D, Freedom RM: Transcatheter treatment of coarctation of the aorta: A review. Pediatr Cardiol 19:27-44, 1998.
219. Zabal C, Attie F, Rosas M, et al: The adult patient with native coarctation of the aorta: Balloon angioplasty or primary stenting? Heart 89:77-83, 2003.
220. Bouchart F, Dubar A, Tabley A, et al: Coarctation of the aorta in adults: Surgical results and long-term follow-up. Ann Thorac Surg 70:1483-1488, 2000.
221. Toro-Salazar OH, Steinberger J, Thomas W, et al: Long-term follow-up of patients after coarctation of the aorta repair. Am J Cardiol 89:541-547, 2002.
222. von Kodolitsch Y, Aydin MA, Koschyk DH, et al: Predictors of aneurysmal formation after surgical correction of aortic coarctation. J Am Coll Cardiol 39:617-624, 2002.
223. O'Sullivan JJ, Derrick G, Darnell R: Prevalence of hypertension in children after early repair of coarctation of the aorta: A cohort study using casual and 24-hour blood pressure measurement. Heart (British Cardiac Society) 88:163-166, 2002.
224. Jenkins NP, Ward C: Coarctation of the aorta: Natural history and outcome after surgical treatment. QJM 92:365-371, 1999.
225. Campbell M: Natural history of coarctation of the aorta. Br Heart J 32:633-640, 1970
226. Messmer BJ, Minale C, Muhler E, von Bernuth G: Surgical correction of coarctation in early infancy: Does surgical technique influence the result? Ann Thorac Surg 52:594-600, 1991.

227. Ala-Kulju K, Jarvinen A, Maamies T, et al: Late aneurysms after patch aortoplasty for coarctation of the aorta in adults. Thorac Cardiovasc Surg 31:301-306, 1983.
228. Hehrlein FW, Mulch J, Rautenburg HW, et al: Incidence and pathogenesis of late aneurysms after patch graft aortoplasty for coarctation. J Thorac Cardiovasc Surg 92:226-230, 1986.
229. Maron BJ, Humphries JO, Rowe RD, Mellits ED: Prognosis of surgically corrected coarctation of the aorta: A 20-year postoperative appraisal. Circulation 47:119-126, 1973.
230. Bergdahl L, Bjork VO, Jonasson R: Surgical correction of coarctation of the aorta: Influence of age on late results. J Thorac Cardiovasc Surg 85:532-536, 1983.
231. Clarkson PM, Nicholson MR, Barratt-Boyes BG, et al: Results after repair of coarctation of the aorta beyond infancy: A 10- to 28-year follow-up with particular reference to late systemic hypertension. Am J Cardiol 51:1481-1488, 1983.
232. Siblini G, Rao PS, Nouri S, et al: Long-term follow-up results of balloon angioplasty of postoperative aortic recoarctation. Am J Cardiol 81:61-67, 1998.
233. Ebeid MR, Prieto LR, Latson LA: Use of balloon-expandable stents for coarctation of the aorta: Initial results and intermediate-term follow-up. J Am Coll Cardiol 30:1847-1852, 1997.
234. Yetman AT, Nykanen D, McCrindle BW, et al: Balloon angioplasty of recurrent coarctation: A 12-year review. J Am Coll Cardiol 30:811-816, 1997.
235. McCrindle BW, Jones TK, Morrow WR, et al: Acute results of balloon angioplasty of native coarctation versus recurrent aortic obstruction are equivalent. Valvuloplasty and Angioplasty of Congenital Anomalies (VACA) Registry Investigators. J Am Coll Cardiol 28:1810-1817, 1996.
236. Rothman A: Interventional therapy for coarctation of the aorta. Curr Opin Cardiol 13:66-72, 1998.
237. Harrison DA, McLaughlin PR, Lazzam C, et al: Endovascular stents in the management of coarctation of the aorta in the adolescent and adult: One-year follow-up. Heart 85:561-566, 2001.
238. Therrien J, Thorne SA, Wright A, et al: Repaired coarctation: A "cost-effective" approach to identify complications in adults. J Am Coll Cardiol 35:997-1002, 2000.

Sinus of Valsalva Aneurysm and Fistula

239. Barragry TP, Ring WS, Moller JH, Lillehei CW: 15- to 30-year follow-up of patients undergoing repair of ruptured congenital aneurysms of the sinus of Valsalva. Ann Thorac Surg 46:515-519, 1988.
240. Dong C, Wu QY, Tang Y: Ruptured sinus of Valsalva aneurysm: A Beijing experience. Ann Thorac Surg 74:1621-1624, 2002.
241. Perry LW, Martin GR, Galioto FM Jr, Midgley FM: Rupture of congenital sinus of Valsalva aneurysm in a newborn. Am J Cardiol 68:1255-1256, 1991.
242. Pasteuning WH, Roukema JA, van Straten AH, et al: Rapid hemodynamic deterioration because of acute rupture of an aneurysm of the sinus of Valsalva: The importance of echocardiography in early diagnosis. J Am Soc Echocardiogr 15:1108-1110, 2002.
243 Shah RP, Ding ZP, Ng AS, Quek SS: A ten-year review of ruptured sinus of Valsalva: Clinicopathological and echo-Doppler features. Singapore Med J 42:473-476, 2001.
244. Fedson S, Jolly N, Lang RM, Hijazi ZM: Percutaneous closure of a ruptured sinus of Valsalva aneurysm using the Amplatzer Duct Occluder. Cathet Cardiovasc Intervent 58:406-411, 2003.
245. Edwards JE: Anomalies of the derivatives of the aortic arch system. Med Clin North Am 32:925, 1948.
246. van Son JA, Konstantinov IE: Burckhard F: Kommerell and Kommerell's diverticulum. Tex Heart Instit J 29:109-112, 2002.
247. Edwards JE: Retro-esophageal segment of the left aortic arch, right ligamentum arteriosum and right descending aorta causing a congenital vascular ring about the trachea and esophagus. Proc Mayo Clin 23:108, 1948.
248. Philip S, Chen SY, Wu MH, et al: Retroesophageal aortic arch: Diagnostic and therapeutic implications of a rare vascular ring. Int J Cardiol 79:133-141, 2001.
249. Parikh SR, Ensing GJ, Darragh RK, Caldwell RL: Rings, slings and such things: Diagnosis and management with special emphasis on the role of echocardiography. J Am Soc Echocardiogr 6:1-11, 1993.
250. Sebening C, Jakob H, Tochtermann U, et al: Vascular tracheobronchial compression syndromes: Experience in surgical treatment and literature review. Thorac Cardiovasc Surgeon 48:164-174, 2000.
251. Mihaljevic T, Cannon JW, del Nido PJ: Robotically assisted division of a vascular ring in children. J Thorac Cardiovasc Surg 125:1163, 2003.
252. Decampli WM: Video-assisted thoracic surgical procedures in children. Semin Thorac Cardiovasc Surg Pediatr Card Surg Annu 1:61, 1998.

Congenital Aortic Valve Stenosis

253. Lofland GK, McCrindle BW, Williams WG, et al: Critical aortic stenosis in the neonate: A multi-institutional study of management, outcomes, and risk factors. Congenital Heart Surgeons Society. J Thorac Cardiovasc Surg 121:10-27, 2001.
254. McCrindle BW, Blackstone EH, Williams WG, et al: Are outcomes of surgical versus transcatheter balloon valvotomy equivalent in neonatal critical aortic stenosis? Circulation 104(Suppl):8, 2001.
255. Weber HS, Mart CR, Myers JL: Transcarotid balloon valvuloplasty for critical aortic valve stenosis at the bedside via continuous transesophageal echocardiographic guidance. Cathet Cardiovasc Intervent 50:326-329, 2000.
256. Lakier JB, Lewis AB, Heymann MA, et al: Isolated aortic stenosis in the neonate: Natural history and hemodynamic considerations. Circulation 50:801-808, 1974.
257. Nishimura RA, Pieroni DR, Bierman FZ, et al: Second natural history study of congenital heart defects: Pulmonary stenosis—echocardiography. Circulation 87(Suppl):9, 1993.
258. Barker PC, Ensing G, Ludomirsky A, et al: Comparison of simultaneous invasive and noninvasive measurements of pressure gradients in congenital aortic valve stenosis. J Am Soc Echocardiogr 15:1496-1502, 2002.
259. Lemler MS, Valdes-Cruz LM, Shandas RS, Cape EG: Insights into catheter/Doppler discrepancies in congenital aortic stenosis. Am J Cardiol 83:1447-1450, 1999.
260. Alexiou C, McDonald A, Langley SM, et al: Aortic valve replacement in children: Are mechanical prostheses a good option? Eur J Cardiothorac Surg 17:125-133, 2000.
261. Bacha EA, Satou GM, Moran AM, et al: Valve-sparing operation for balloon-induced aortic regurgitation in congenital aortic stenosis. J Thorac Cardiovasc Surg 122:162-168, 2001.
262. Ohye RG, Gomez CA, Ohye BJ, et al: The Ross/Konno procedure in neonates and infants: Intermediate-term survival and autograft function. Ann Thorac Surg 72:823-830, 2001.
263. Al Halees Z, Pieters F, Qadoura F, et al: The Ross procedure is the procedure of choice for congenital aortic valve disease. J Thorac Cardiovasc Surg 123:437-441, 2002.
264. Favaloro R, Stutzbach P, Gomez C, et al: Feasibility of the Ross procedure: Its relationship with the bicuspid aortic valve. J Heart Valve Dis 11:375-382, 2002.
265. Tentolouris K, Kontozoglou T, Trikas A, et al: Fixed subaortic stenosis revisited: Congenital abnormalities in 72 new cases and review of the literature. Cardiology 92:4-10, 1999.
266. Bezold LI, Smith EO, Kelly K, et al: Development and validation of an echocardiographic model for predicting progression of discrete subaortic stenosis in children. Am J Cardiol 81:314-320, 1998.
267. Cohen L, Bennani R, Hulin S, et al: Mitral valvar anomalies and discrete subaortic stenosis. Cardiol Young 12:138-146, 2002.
268. McElhinney DB, Reddy VM, Silverman NH, Hanley FL: Accessory and anomalous atrioventricular valvar tissue causing outflow tract obstruction: Surgical implications of a heterogeneous and complex problem. J Am Coll Cardiol 32:1741-1748, 1998.
269. Sigfusson G, Tacy TA, Vanauker MD, Cape EG: Abnormalities of the left ventricular outflow tract associated with discrete subaortic stenosis in children: An echocardiographic study. J Am Coll Cardiol 30:255-259, 1997.
270. Sharma S, Stamper T, Dhar P: The usefulness of transesophageal echocardiography in the surgical management of older children with subaortic stenosis. Echocardiography 13:653, 1996.
271. Oliver JM, Gonzalez A, Gallego P, et al: Discrete subaortic stenosis in adults: Increased prevalence and slow rate of progression of the obstruction and aortic regurgitation. J Am Coll Cardiol 38:835-842, 2001.
272. Coleman DM, Smallhorn JF, McCrindle BW, et al: Postoperative follow-up of fibromuscular subaortic stenosis. J Am Coll Cardiol 24:1558-1564, 1994.
273. Serraf A, Zoghby J, Lacour-Gayet F, et al: Surgical treatment of subaortic stenosis: A seventeen-year experience. J Thorac Cardiovasc Surg 117:669-678, 1999.
274. Jahangiri M, Nicholson IA, del Nido PJ, et al: Surgical management of complex and tunnel-like subaortic stenosis. Eur J Cardiothorac Surg 17:637-642, 2000.
275. Caldarone CA: Left ventricular outflow tract obstruction: The role of the modified Konno procedure. Semin Thorac Cardiovasc Surg Pediatr Card Surg Annu 6:98, 2003.
276. Garcia RC, Friedman WF, Kaback MM, Rowe RD: Idiopathic hypercalcemia and supravalvular aortic stenosis: Documentation of a new syndrome. N Engl J Med 271:117, 1964.
277. Metcalfe K, Rucka AK, Smoot L, et al: Elastin: mutational spectrum in supravalvular aortic stenosis. Eur J Hum Genet 8:955-963, 2000.
278. Vaideeswar P, Shankar V, Deshpande JR, et al: Pathology of the diffuse variant of supravalvar aortic stenosis. Cardiovasc Pathol 10:33-37, 2001.
279. Eronen M, Peippo M, Hiippala A, et al: Cardiovascular manifestations in 75 patients with Williams syndrome. J Med Genet 39:554-558, 2002.
280. Giddins NG, Finley JP, Nanton MA, Roy DL: The natural course of supravalvar aortic stenosis and peripheral pulmonary artery stenosis in Williams's syndrome. Br Heart J 62:315-319, 1989.
281. Wren C, Oslizlok P, Bull C: Natural history of supravalvular aortic stenosis and pulmonary artery stenosis. J Am Coll Cardiol 15:1625-1630, 1990.
282. Brand A, Keren A, Reifen RM, et al: Echocardiographic and Doppler findings in the Williams syndrome. Am J Cardiol 63:633-635, 1989.
283. McElhinney DB, Petrossian E, Tworetzky W, et al: Issues and outcomes in the management of supravalvar aortic stenosis. Ann Thorac Surg 69:562-567, 2000.
284. Stamm C, Kreutzer C, Zurakowski D, et al: Forty-one years of surgical experience with congenital supravalvular aortic stenosis. J Thorac Cardiovasc Surg 118:874-885, 1999.
285. Einfeld SL, Tonge BJ, Rees VW: Longitudinal course of behavioral and emotional problems in Williams syndrome. Am J Ment Retard 106:73-81, 2001.

Congenital Mitral Valve Anomalies

286. Ruckman RN, Van Praagh R: Anatomic types of congenital mitral stenosis: Report of 49 autopsy cases with consideration of diagnosis and surgical implications. Am J Cardiol 42:592-601, 1978.
287. Agnoleti G, Annecchino F, Preda L, Borghi A: Persistence of the left superior caval vein: Can it potentiate obstructive lesions of the left ventricle? Cardiol Young 9:285-290, 1999.
288. Banerjee A, Kohl T, Silverman NH: Echocardiographic evaluation of congenital mitral valve anomalies in children. Am J Cardiol 76:1284-1291, 1995.
289. Patel JJ, Munclinger MJ, Mitha AS, Patel N: Percutaneous balloon dilatation of the mitral valve in critically ill young patients with intractable heart failure. Br Heart J 73:555-558, 1995.
290. Serraf A, Zoghbi J, Belli E, et al: Congenital mitral stenosis with or without associated defects: An evolving surgical strategy. Circulation 102(Suppl):71, 2000.
291. Agarwal S, Airan B, Chowdhury UK, et al: Ventricular septal defect with congenital mitral valve disease: Long-term results of corrective surgery. Indian Heart J 54:67-73, 2002.
292. Tamura M, Menahem S, Brizard C: Clinical features and management of isolated cleft mitral valve in childhood. J Am Coll Cardiol 35:764-770, 2000.
293. Zias EA, Mavroudis C, Backer CL, et al: Surgical repair of the congenitally malformed mitral valve in infants and children. Ann Thorac Surg 66:1551-1559, 1998.
294. Erez E, Kanter KR, Isom E, et al: Mitral valve replacement in children. J Heart Valve Dis 12:25-29, 2003.

295. Kim YM, Yoo SJ, Choi JY, et al: Natural course of supravalvar aortic stenosis and peripheral pulmonary arterial stenosis in Williams' syndrome. Cardiol Young 9:37-41, 1999.
296. McElhinney DB, Krantz ID, Bason L, et al: Analysis of cardiovascular phenotype and genotype-phenotype correlation in individuals with a *JAG1* mutation and/or Alagille syndrome. Circulation 106:2567-2574, 2002.
297. Trivedi KR, Benson LN: Interventional strategies in the management of peripheral pulmonary artery stenosis. J Intervent Cardiol 16:171-188, 2003.
298. Rothman A, Levy DJ, Sklansky MS, et al: Balloon angioplasty and stenting of multiple intralobar pulmonary arterial stenoses in adult patients. Cathet Cardiovasc Intervent 58:252-260, 2003.
299. Rosales AM, Lock JE, Perry SB, Geggel RL: Interventional catheterization management of perioperative peripheral pulmonary stenosis: Balloon angioplasty or endovascular stenting. Cathet Cardiovasc Intervent 56:272-277, 2002.
300. Hayes CJ, Gersony WM, Driscoll DJ, et al: Second natural history study of congenital heart defects. Results of treatment of patients with pulmonary valvar stenosis. Circulation 87(Suppl):37, 1993.
301. Chen CR, Cheng TO, Huang T, et al: Percutaneous balloon valvuloplasty for pulmonic stenosis in adolescents and adults. N Engl J Med 335:21-25, 1996.
302. Alva C, Ortegon J, Herrera F, et al: Types of obstructions in double-chambered right ventricle: Mid-term results. Arch Med Res 33:261-264, 2002.
303. Alva C, Ho SY, Lincoln CR, et al: The nature of the obstructive muscular bundles in double-chambered right ventricle. J Thorac Cardiovasc Surg 117:1180-1189, 1999.
304. Singh M, Agarwala MK, Grover A, et al: Clinical, echocardiographic, and angiographic profile of patients with double-chambered right ventricle: Experience with 48 cases. Angiology 50:223-231, 1999.
305. Lascano ME, Schaad MS, Moodie DS, Murphy D Jr: Difficulty in diagnosing double-chambered right ventricle in adults. Am J Cardiol 88:816-819, 2001.
306. McElhinney DB, Chatterjee KM, Reddy VM: Double-chambered right ventricle presenting in adulthood. Ann Thorac Surg 70:124-127, 2000.
307. Kilner PJ, Sievers B, Meyer GP, Ho SY: Double-chambered right ventricle or sub-infundibular stenosis assessed by cardiovascular magnetic resonance. J Cardiovasc MR 4:373-379, 2002.
308. Hachiro Y, Takagi N, Koyanagi T, et al: Repair of double-chambered right ventricle: Surgical results and long-term follow-up. Ann Thorac Surg 72:1520-1522, 2001.

Cor Triatriatum

309. Marin-Garcia J, Tandon R, Lucas RV Jr, Edwards JE: Cor triatriatum: Study of 20 cases. Am J Cardiol 35:59-66, 1975.
310. Roldan FJ, Vargas-Barron J, Espinola-Zavaleta N, et al: Cor triatriatum dexter: Transesophageal echocardiographic diagnosis and 3-dimensional reconstruction. J Am Soc Echocardiogr 14:634-636, 2001.
311. Oglietti J, Cooley DA, Izquierdo JP, et al: Cor triatriatum: Operative results in 25 patients. Ann Thorac Surg 35:415-420, 1983.
312. Dauphin C, Lusson JR, Motreff P, et al: Left intra-atrial membrane without pulmonary vein obstruction: Benign condition of progressive evolution? Apropos of 7 cases. [French]. Arch Mal Coeur Vaiss 91:615-621, 1998.
313. Breinholt JP, Hawkins JA, Minich LA, et al: Pulmonary vein stenosis with normal connection: Associated cardiac abnormalities and variable outcome. Ann Thorac Surg 68:164-168, 1999.
314. Ha JW, Chung N, Yoon J, et al: Pulsed wave and color Doppler echocardiography and cardiac catheterization findings in bilateral pulmonary vein stenosis. J Am Soc Echocardiogr 11:393-396, 1998.
315. Caldarone CA, Najm HK, Kadletz M, et al: Relentless pulmonary vein stenosis after repair of total anomalous pulmonary venous drainage. Ann Thorac Surg 66:1514-1520, 1998.
316. Oliver JM, Gallego P, Gonzalez A, et al: Sinus venosus syndrome: Atrial septal defect or anomalous venous connection? A multiplane transoesophageal approach. Heart 88:634-638, 2002.
317. Wong ML, McCrindle BW, Mota C, Smallhorn JF: Echocardiographic evaluation of partial anomalous pulmonary venous drainage. J Am Coll Cardiol 26:503-507, 1995.
318. Gao YA, Burrows PE, Benson LN, et al: Scimitar syndrome in infancy. J Am Coll Cardiol 22:873-882, 1993.
319. Shibuya K, Smallhorn JE, McCrindle BW: Echocardiographic clues and accuracy in the diagnosis of scimitar syndrome. J Am Soc Echocardiogr 9:174-181, 1996.
320. Ammash NM, Seward JB, Warnes CA, et al: Partial anomalous pulmonary venous connection: Diagnosis by transesophageal echocardiography. J Am Coll Cardiol 29:1351-1358, 1997.
321. Ferrari VA, Scott CH, Holland GA, et al: Ultrafast three-dimensional contrast-enhanced magnetic resonance angiography and imaging in the diagnosis of partial anomalous pulmonary venous drainage. J Am Coll Cardiol 37:1120-1128, 2001.
322. Hijii T, Fukushige J, Hara T: Diagnosis and management of partial anomalous pulmonary venous connection: A review of 28 pediatric cases. Cardiology 89:148-151, 1998.
323. Brown JW, Ruzmetov M, Minnich DJ, et al: Surgical management of scimitar syndrome: An alternative approach. J Thorac Cardiovasc Surg 125:238-245, 2003.
324. Swanson KL, Prakash UB, Stanson AW: Pulmonary arteriovenous fistulas: Mayo Clinic experience, 1982-1997. Mayo Clin Proc 74:671-680, 1999.
325. Gonzalez VR: Pulmonary arteriovenous fistula in childhood. Z Kinderchir 40:101, 1985.
326. Gudavalli A, Kalaria VG, et al: Intrapulmonary arteriovenous shunt: Diagnosis by saline contrast bubbles in the pulmonary veins. J Am Soc Echocardiogr 15:1012-1014, 2002.
327. Tsunezuka Y, Sato H, Tsukioka T: Strategy for 3-D computed tomography diagnosis and treatment of small pulmonary arteriovenous fistula. Scand Cardiovasc J 34:90-91, 2000.
328. Berthezene Y, Howarth NR, Revel D: Pulmonary arteriovenous fistula: Detection with magnetic resonance angiography. Eur Radiol 8:1403-1404, 1998.
329. Grady RM, Sharkey AM, Bridges ND: Transcatheter coil embolisation of a pulmonary arteriovenous malformation in a neonate. Br Heart J 71:370-371, 1994.

Coronary Arteriovenous Fistula

330. Hofbeck M, Wild F, Singer H: Improved visualisation of a coronary artery fistula by the "laid-back" aortogram. Br Heart J 70:272-273, 1993.
331. Sherwood MC, Rockenmacher S, Colan SD, Geva T: Prognostic significance of clinically silent coronary artery fistulas. Am J Cardiol 83:407-411, 1999.
332. Okubo M: Outcomes of transcatheter embolization in the treatment of coronary artery fistulas. Cathet Cardiovasc Intervent 52:510, 2001.
333. Kamiya H, Yasuda T, Nagamine H, et al: Surgical treatment of congenital coronary artery fistulas: 27 years' experience and a review of the literature. J Cardiac Surg 17:173-177, 2002.

CHAPTER 57

Valvular Heart Disease

Robert O. Bonow • Eugene Braunwald

During the last quarter century, remarkable changes in the evaluation and management of patients with valvular heart disease have resulted in improvement in patient outcomes that would have been unfathomable to earlier generations of physicians. Advances in surgical approaches and interventional cardiology procedures, coupled with innovation in noninvasive imaging and understanding of the natural history of these conditions, have resulted in enhanced diagnosis and more scientific selection of patients for therapeutic interventions, which are now performed at relatively low risk. Despite the continually expanding information base and the development of clinical practice guidelines,[1,2] many aspects of the diagnostic evaluation and indications for intervention remain uncertain or controversial. Hence, clinical knowledge, experience, and judgment on the part of the practitioner remain the key components of the management of patients with cardiac valvular disease.

Mitral Stenosis

Etiology and Pathology

The predominant cause of mitral stenosis (MS) is rheumatic fever (see Chap. 81),[1,3] and rheumatic involvement is present in 99 percent of stenotic mitral valves excised at the time of mitral valve replacement (MVR). Approximately 25 percent of all patients with rheumatic heart disease have pure MS, and an additional 40 percent have combined MS and mitral regurgitation (MR).[4] Two-thirds of all patients with rheumatic MS are women.[1]

Rheumatic fever results in four forms of fusion of the mitral valve apparatus leading to stenosis: (1) commissural, (2) cuspal, (3) chordal, and (4) combined.[5] Thickening of the commissures alone occurs in 30 percent of patients, of the cusps alone in 15 percent, and of the chordae tendineae alone in 10 percent; in the remaining patients, thickening of more than one of these structures is involved. Characteristically, mitral valve cusps fuse at their edges, and fusion of the chordae tendineae results in thickening and shortening of these structures. The leaflets exhibit fibrous obliteration and revascularization. The stenotic mitral valve is typically funnel shaped (Fig. 57–1), and the orifice is frequently shaped like a "fish mouth" or buttonhole, with calcium deposits in the valve leaflets sometimes extending to involve the valve ring, which may become severely thickened. The thickened leaflets may be so adherent and rigid that they cannot open or shut, reducing or rarely even abolishing the first heart sound (S_1) and leading to combined MS and MR. When rheumatic fever results exclusively or predominantly in contraction and fusion of the chordae tendineae, with little fusion of the valvular commissures, dominant MR results.[5]

A debate continues about whether the anatomical changes in severe MS result from a smoldering rheumatic process or whether, once the valve has been deformed by the initial episode, the constant trauma produced by the turbulent blood flow leads to progressive fibrosis, thickening, and calcification of the valve apparatus.[6] Probably both processes are involved. Enlargement of the left atrium and resultant elevation of the left main stem bronchus, calcification of the left atrial wall, development of mural thrombi, and obliterative changes in the pulmonary vascular bed (see Chap. 67) all may result from chronic rheumatic MS.

Far less frequently, MS is congenital in etiology, and this form is observed almost exclusively in infants and young children (see Chap. 56). Rarely, MS is a complication of malignant carcinoid, systemic lupus erythematosus, rheumatoid arthritis, the mucopolysaccharidoses of the Hunter-Hurler phenotype, Fabry disease, and Whipple disease. Amyloid deposits may occur on rheumatic valves and contribute to the obstruction to left atrial emptying. Methysergide therapy is an unusual but documented cause of MS. Atrial septal defect is associated with MS, generally of rheumatic origin, in Lutembacher syndrome (see Chap. 56). A number of conditions may simulate MS: obstruction to left atrial outflow may be caused by a left atrial tumor, particularly myxoma (see Chap. 63); ball-valve thrombus in the left atrium (usually associated with MS); infective endocarditis with large vegetations; and a congenital membrane in the left atrium, i.e., cor triatriatum (see Chap. 56). These conditions may simulate MS. Although calcification of the mitral annulus usually causes MR, MS may result when subvalvular or intravalvular extension is extensive.

Pathophysiology

In normal adults, the cross-sectional area of the mitral valve orifice is 4 to 6 cm^2.

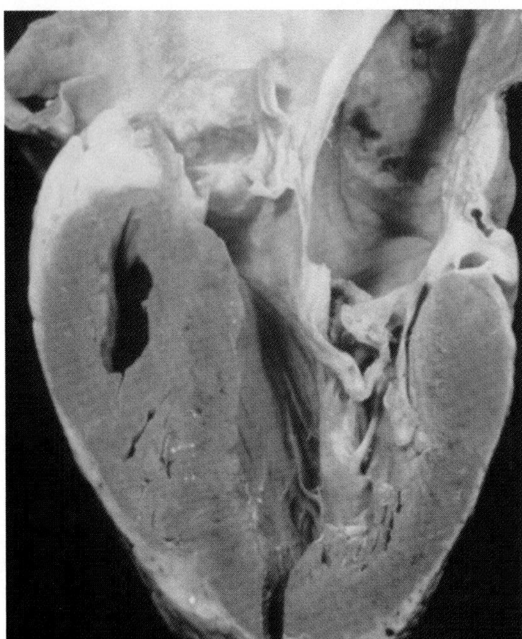

FIGURE 57–1 Rheumatic mitral stenosis. There are severe valvular changes, including marked fibrosis and calcification of the mitral valve leaflets and severe chordal thickening and fusion into pillars of fibrous tissue. (From Becker AE, Anderson RH [eds]: Cardiac Pathology: An Integrated Text and Colour Atlas. New York, Raven Press, 1983, p 4.3.)

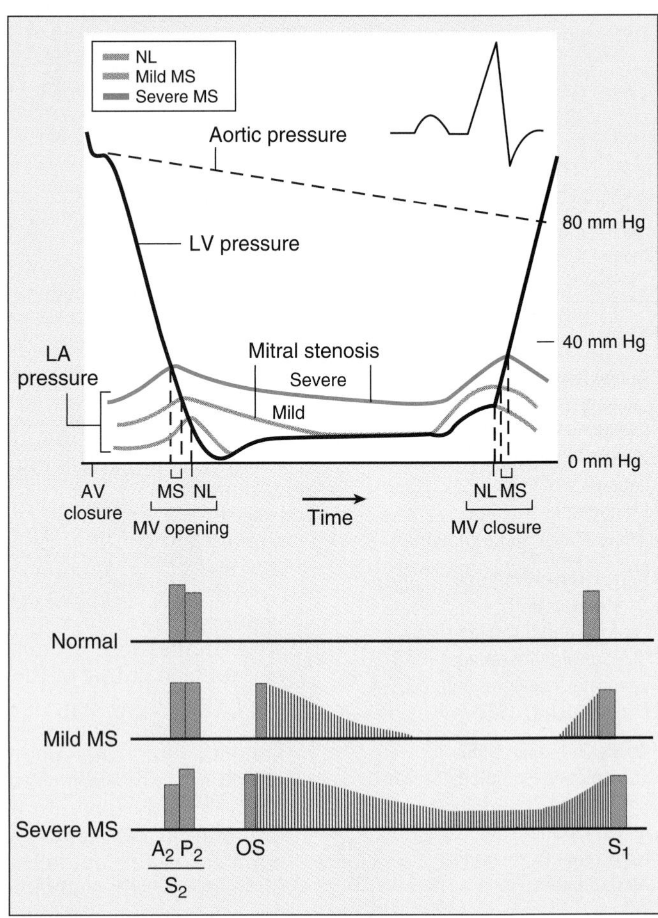

FIGURE 57–2 Schematic representation of left ventricular (LV), aortic, and left atrial (LA) pressures, showing normal relationships and alterations with mild and severe mitral stenosis (MS). Corresponding classic auscultatory signs of MS are shown at the bottom. Compared with mild MS, with severe MS the higher left atrial *v* wave causes earlier pressure crossover and earlier mitral valve (MV) opening, leading to a shorter time interval between aortic valve (AV) closure and the opening snap (OS). The higher left atrial end-diastolic pressure with severe MS also results in later closure of the mitral valve. With severe MS, the diastolic rumble becomes longer and there is accentuation of the pulmonic component (P_2) of the second heart sound (S_2) in relation to the aortic component (A_2).

When the orifice is reduced to approximately 2 cm^2, which is considered to represent *mild* MS, blood can flow from the left atrium to the left ventricle only if propelled by a small, although abnormal, pressure gradient. When the mitral valve opening is reduced to 1 cm^2, which is considered to represent *critical* MS,[3] a left atrioventricular pressure gradient of approximately 20 mm Hg (and, therefore, in the presence of a normal left ventricular diastolic pressure, a mean left atrial pressure of ≈25 mm Hg) is required to maintain normal cardiac output at rest (Fig. 57–2; see also Fig. 17–14). The elevated left atrial pressure, in turn, raises pulmonary venous and capillary pressures, resulting in exertional dyspnea. The first bouts of dyspnea in patients with MS are usually precipitated by tachycardia resulting from exercise, emotional stress, sexual intercourse, infection, or atrial fibrillation, all of which increase the rate of blood flow across the mitral orifice and result in further elevation of the left atrial pressure.[1,3,7]

To assess the severity of obstruction of the mitral valve (and, for that matter, of any valve), both the transvalvular pressure gradient and the transvalvular flow rate must be measured (see Chap. 17).[8] The latter is a function not only of the cardiac output but also of the heart rate. An increase in heart rate shortens diastole proportionately more than systole and diminishes the time available for flow across the mitral valve. Therefore, at any given level of cardiac output, tachycardia augments the transmitral valvular pressure gradient and elevates left atrial pressures further.[1] This explains the sudden occurrence of dyspnea and pulmonary edema in previously asymptomatic patients with MS who develop atrial fibrillation with a rapid ventricular rate. It also accounts for the equally rapid improvement in these patients when the ventricular rate is slowed by cardiac glycosides, beta-blocking agents, and/or heart rate–slowing calcium antagonists, even when the transvalvular flow rate per minute remains constant. Hydraulic considerations dictate that at any given orifice size the transvalvular pressure gradient is a function of the square of the transvalvular flow rate.[9] Thus, a doubling of flow rate quadruples the pressure gradient, so that a stress such as exercise in patients with moderate or severe MS causes a marked elevation of left atrial pressure.[10] Pregnancy, hypervolemia, and hyperthyroidism all increase mitral valve flow and thereby the transvalvular pressure gradient. Hence, it is common for the first clinical manifestation of MS in young women to occur during pregnancy.

Atrial contraction augments the presystolic transmitral valvular gradient by approximately 30 percent in patients with MS. Withdrawal of atrial transport when atrial fibrillation develops reduces cardiac output by about 20 percent.

Although the Gorlin formula has been the benchmark for evaluating stenotic valvular orifices since 1951,[9] there is increasing evidence that valvular orifices are not rigid and that, in fact, as transvalvular flow increases, the orifice becomes distended (see Chap. 17). Accordingly, it has been proposed that stenosis can also be expressed as valvular resistance, the quotient of the mean transvalvular pressure gradient, and the mean transvalvular flow.

INTRACARDIAC AND INTRAVASCULAR PRESSURES

Left Atrial and Right Heart Pressures. In patients with MS and sinus rhythm, mean left atrial pressure is elevated, and the left atrial pressure pulse generally exhibits a prominent atrial contraction (*a*) wave and a gradual pressure decline after mitral valve opening (*y* descent). In patients with mild to moderate MS without elevated pulmonary vascular resistance, pulmonary arterial pressure may be normal or only minimally elevated at rest but rises during exercise. However, in patients with severe MS and those in whom the pulmonary vascular resistance is significantly increased, pulmonary arterial pressure is elevated when the patient is at rest. In rare patients with extremely elevated pulmonary vascular resistance, pulmonary arterial pressure may exceed systemic arterial pressure. Further elevations of left atrial and pulmonary vascular pressures occur during exercise and/or tachycardia. With moderately elevated pulmonary arterial pressure (systolic pressure 30 to 60 mm Hg), right ventricular performance is usually maintained. However, a greater elevation of pulmonary arterial pressure represents a serious impedance to emptying of the right ventricle. Hence, patients with MS and severe pulmonary hypertension commonly fail to exhibit normal elevation of the right ventricular ejection fraction during exercise and ultimately may develop right ventricular dysfunction and dilation at rest, with accompanying tricuspid regurgitation (TR).

Left Ventricular Diastolic Pressure. This pressure is normal in patients with isolated MS; however, coexisting MR, aortic valve lesions, systemic hypertension, ischemic heart disease, and cardiomyopathy all may be responsible for elevations of left ventricular diastolic pressure. In approximately 85 percent of patients with isolated MS, the left ventricular end-diastolic volume is within the normal range, whereas it is reduced in the remaining patients. In approximately 25 percent of patients with isolated MS, the ejection fraction and other ejection indices of systolic performance (see Chap. 20) are below normal,[11] most likely resulting in part from chronic reduction in preload and elevated afterload. Regional hypokinesis is common, perhaps caused by extension of the scarring process from the mitral valve into the adjacent posterior basal myocardium or by associated ischemic heart disease. Leftward displacement of the interventricular septum secondary to more rapid early filling of the right ventricle may be responsible for a reduction of left ventricular compliance (left ventricular stiffening).[7] The left ventricular mass is usually normal but may be slightly reduced.[12]

The bulk of available evidence suggests that other than the posterior basal myocardium, left ventricular contractility is normal or only slightly impaired in the majority of patients with isolated MS. Most patients with MS have a normal elevation of ejection fraction and a reduction of end-systolic volume during exercise,[11] although ejection fraction does not increase normally with exercise in a subset of patients. In these latter patients, the normal increase in left ventricular diastolic volume during exercise fails to occur, resulting in reduced stroke volume and ejection fraction responses to exercise.[11] Associated ischemic heart disease is not common but may occur[1,13] and contribute to myocardial dysfunction in some patients.

Pulmonary Hypertension. Pulmonary hypertension in patients with MS results from (1) passive backward transmission of the elevated left atrial pressure; (2) pulmonary arteriolar constriction, which presumably is triggered by left atrial and pulmonary venous hypertension (reactive pulmonary hypertension); and (3) organic obliterative changes in the pulmonary vascular bed, which may be considered to be a complication of longstanding and severe MS (see Chap. 67).[6,7] In time, severe pulmonary hypertension results in right-sided heart failure, with dilation of the right ventricle and its annulus and secondary tricuspid and sometimes pulmonic regurgitation (PR). These changes in the pulmonary vascular bed may also exert a protective effect; the elevated precapillary resistance makes the development of symptoms of pulmonary congestion less likely by tending to prevent blood from surging into the pulmonary capillary bed and damming up behind the stenotic mitral valve, although this protection occurs at the expense of a reduced cardiac output. In patients with severe MS, pulmonary vein-bronchial vein shunts occur. Their rupture may cause hemoptysis. Patients with severe MS manifest a reduction in pulmonary compliance, an increase in the work of breathing, and a redistribution of pulmonary blood flow from the base to the apex.

Clinical and Hemodynamic Features. At any given severity of stenosis, the clinical picture is dictated largely by the levels of cardiac output and pulmonary vascular resistance. The response to a given degree of mitral obstruction may be characterized at one end of the hemodynamic spectrum by a normal cardiac output and a high left atrioventricular pressure gradient or, at the opposite end of the spectrum, by a markedly reduced cardiac output and low transvalvular pressure gradient. Thus, in some patients with moderately severe MS (mitral valve area = 1.0 to 1.5 cm^2), cardiac output at rest may be normal and rises normally during exertion. In these patients, the high transvalvular pressure gradient with exertion causes marked elevation of left atrial and pulmonary capillary pressures. This leads to severe pulmonary congestion during exertion. In contrast, in most patients with severe MS, cardiac output rises subnormally during exertion, thus reducing the pulmonary venous pressure and the severity of symptoms of pulmonary congestion more than would be the case if the cardiac output rose normally. In patients with severe MS (mitral valve area $\leq$ 1.0 cm^2), particularly when pulmonary vascular resistance is elevated, cardiac output is usually depressed at rest and may fail to rise at all during exertion. These patients frequently have severe weakness and fatigue secondary to a low cardiac output.

Left Atrial Changes. The combination of mitral valve disease and atrial inflammation secondary to rheumatic carditis causes (1) left atrial dilation, (2) fibrosis of the atrial wall, and (3) disorganization of the atrial muscle bundles. The last leads to disparate conduction velocities and inhomogeneous refractory periods. Premature atrial activation, due either to an automatic focus or to reentry, may stimulate the left atrium during the vulnerable period and thereby precipitate atrial fibrillation. The development of this arrhythmia correlates independently with the severity of the MS, the degree of left atrial dilation, and the height of the left atrial pressure.[14] Atrial fibrillation is often episodic at first but then becomes more persistent. Atrial fibrillation per se causes diffuse atrophy of atrial muscle, further atrial enlargement, and further inhomogeneity of refractoriness and conduction. These changes, in turn, lead to irreversible atrial fibrillation.

Clinical Manifestations

History

The principal symptom of MS is exertional dyspnea, largely the result of reduced pulmonary compliance. Dyspnea may be accompanied by cough and wheezing. Vital capacity is reduced, presumably owing to the presence of engorged pulmonary vessels and interstitial edema. Patients who have critical obstruction to left atrial emptying and dyspnea with ordinary activity (New York Heart Association [NYHA] Class III) generally have orthopnea as well and are at risk of experiencing attacks of frank pulmonary edema. The latter may be precipitated by effort, emotional stress, respiratory infection, fever, sexual intercourse, pregnancy, or atrial fibrillation with a rapid ventricular rate or other tachyarrhythmia. Indeed, pulmonary edema may be caused by any condition that increases flow across the stenotic mitral valve, either by increasing total cardiac output or by reducing the time available for blood flow across the mitral orifice to occur. In patients with a markedly elevated pulmonary vascular resistance, right ventricular function is often impaired.[7,15]

MS is a slowly progressive disease, and many patients remain seemingly asymptomatic merely by readjusting their life styles to a more sedentary level. Exercise testing may be useful in selected asymptomatic patients to determine functional status in an objective manner and may be combined with Doppler echocardiography (see later) to assess exercise hemodynamics.

HEMOPTYSIS. In his seminal paper 50 years ago, Wood differentiated between several kinds of *hemoptysis* complicating MS, as follows[16]:

1. Sudden hemorrhage. Although the hemorrhage is often profuse, it is only rarely life threatening. It results from the rupture of thin-walled, dilated bronchial veins, usually as a consequence of a sudden rise in left atrial pressure. With persistence of pulmonary venous hypertension, the walls of these veins thicken appreciably. This form of hemoptysis tends to disappear as MS progresses.
2. Blood-stained sputum associated with attacks of paroxysmal nocturnal dyspnea.
3. Pink, frothy sputum characteristic of acute pulmonary edema with rupture of alveolar capillaries.
4. Pulmonary infarction, a late complication of MS associated with heart failure.
5. Blood-stained sputum complicating chronic bronchitis. The edematous bronchial mucosa in patients with chronic MS increases the likelihood of chronic

bronchitis, which is a common complication of MS, particularly in Great Britain.

CHEST PAIN. A small percentage, perhaps 15 percent, of patients with MS experience chest discomfort that is indistinguishable from angina pectoris. This symptom may be caused by severe right ventricular hypertension secondary to the pulmonary vascular disease or by concomitant coronary atherosclerosis.[1,13] Rarely, chest pain may be secondary to coronary obstruction caused by coronary embolization. In many patients, however, a satisfactory explanation for the chest pain cannot be uncovered even after complete hemodynamic and angiographic studies.

SYSTEMIC EMBOLISM. Before the advent of surgical treatment, this serious complication of MS developed in at least 20 percent of patients at some time during the course of their disease.[17] Before the era of anticoagulant therapy and surgical treatment, approximately 25 percent of all fatalities in patients with mitral valve disease were secondary to systemic embolism. The tendency for development of systemic embolization correlates directly with the patient's age and the size of the left atrial appendage and inversely with the cardiac output[17,18]; 80 percent of patients with MS in whom systemic emboli develop are in atrial fibrillation. When embolization occurs in patients in sinus rhythm, the possibility of transient atrial fibrillation or underlying infective endocarditis should be considered. There is no simple correlation between the incidence of embolism on the one hand and the size of the mitral orifice on the other. Indeed, embolism may be the first symptom of MS and may occur in patients with mild MS even before the development of dyspnea.

Because thrombi are found in the left atrium at operation in only a few patients with a history of recent embolism, it is likely that only fresh clots are discharged. Approximately half of all clinically apparent emboli are found in the cerebral vessels. Coronary embolism may lead to myocardial infarction and/or angina pectoris, and renal emboli may be responsible for the development of systemic hypertension. Emboli are recurrent and multiple in approximately 25 percent of patients who develop this complication. Rarely, massive thrombosis develops in the left atrium, resulting in a pedunculated ball-valve thrombus, which may suddenly aggravate obstruction to left atrial outflow when a specific body position is assumed or may cause sudden death. Similar consequences occur in patients with free-floating thrombi in the left atrium. These two conditions are usually characterized by variability in the physical findings, often on a positional basis. They are extremely hazardous and require surgical treatment, often as an emergency.

INFECTIVE ENDOCARDITIS (see Chap. 58). This complication tends to occur *less frequently* on rigid, thickened, calcified valves and is therefore more common in patients with mild MS than those with severe MS.

OTHER SYMPTOMS. Compression of the left recurrent laryngeal nerve by a greatly dilated left atrium, enlarged tracheobronchial lymph nodes, and a dilated pulmonary artery may cause hoarseness (Ortner syndrome). A history of repeated hemoptysis is common in patients with pulmonary hemosiderosis. Systemic venous hypertension, hepatomegaly, edema, ascites, and hydrothorax all are signs of severe MS with elevated pulmonary vascular resistance and right-sided heart failure.

Physical Examination

Patients with severe MS, a low cardiac output, and systemic vasoconstriction may exhibit the so-called mitral facies, characterized by pinkish-purple patches on the cheeks. The *arterial pulse* is usually normal, but in patients with a reduced stroke volume, the pulse may be small in volume. The *jugular venous pulse* usually exhibits a prominent *a* wave in patients with sinus rhythm and elevated pulmonary vascular resistance. In patients with atrial fibrillation, the *x* descent of the jugular venous pulse disappears, and there is only one crest, a prominent *v* or *c-v* wave, per cardiac cycle. *Palpation* of the cardiac apex usually reveals an inconspicuous left ventricle; the presence of either a palpable presystolic expansion wave or an early diastolic rapid filling wave speaks strongly against serious MS. A readily palpable, tapping S_1 suggests that the anterior mitral valve leaflet is pliable. When the patient is in the left lateral recumbent position, a diastolic thrill of MS may be palpable at the apex. Often a right ventricular lift is felt in the left parasternal region in patients with pulmonary hypertension. A markedly enlarged right ventricle may displace the left ventricle posteriorly and produce a prominent apex beat that can be confused with a left ventricular lift. A loud pulmonic closure sound (P_2) may be palpable in the second left intercostal space in patients with MS and pulmonary hypertension.

AUSCULTATION

The auscultatory features of MS (see Fig. 57–2) include an accentuated first heart sound (S_1) with prolongation of the Q-S_1 interval, correlating with the level of the left atrial pressure. Accentuation of S_1 occurs when the mitral valve leaflets are flexible. It is caused, in part, by the rapidity with which left ventricular pressure rises at the time of mitral valve closure as well as by the wide closing excursion of the leaflets. Marked calcification and/or thickening of the mitral valve leaflets reduces the amplitude of S_1, probably because of diminished motion of the leaflets. As pulmonary arterial pressure rises, closure of the pulmonic valve (P_2) at first becomes accentuated and widely transmitted and can often be readily heard at both the mitral and the aortic areas. With further elevation of pulmonary arterial pressure, splitting of the second heart sound (S_2) narrows because of reduced compliance of the pulmonary vascular bed, and this shortens the "hangout interval." Finally, S_2 becomes single and accentuated. Other signs of severe pulmonary hypertension include a nonvalvular pulmonic ejection sound that diminishes during inspiration, owing to dilation of the pulmonary artery; a systolic murmur of TR; a Graham Steell murmur of PR; and a fourth heart sound (S_4) originating from the right ventricle. A third heart sound (S_3) originating from the left ventricle is absent in patients with MS unless significant MR or aortic regurgitation (AR) coexists.

The *opening snap* (OS) of the mitral valve is caused by a sudden tensing of the valve leaflets after the valve cusps have completed their opening excursion. The OS occurs when the movement of the mitral dome into the left ventricle suddenly stops. It is most readily audible at the apex, using the diaphragm of the stethoscope. The OS can usually be differentiated from P_2 because the OS occurs later, unless right bundle branch block is present. The mitral valve cannot be totally rigid if it produces an OS, which is usually accompanied by an accentuated S_1. Calcification confined to the tip of the mitral valve leaflets does not preclude an OS, although calcification of both the body and the tip does. The mitral OS follows A_2 by 0.04 to 0.12 second; this interval varies inversely with the left atrial pressure. A short A_2-OS interval is a reliable indicator of severe MS.

THE DIASTOLIC MURMUR OF MS. This murmur is a low-pitched, rumbling murmur, best heard at the apex, with the bell of the stethoscope and with the patient in the left lateral recumbent position. When this murmur is soft, it is limited to the apex, but when louder, it may radiate to the left axilla or the lower left sternal area. Although the intensity of the diastolic murmur is not closely related to the severity of stenosis, the *duration* of the murmur is a guide to the severity of mitral valve narrowing. The murmur persists for as long as the left atrioventricular pressure gradient exceeds approximately 3 mm Hg. The murmur usually commences immediately after the OS. In mild MS, the early diastolic murmur is brief, but in the presence of sinus rhythm it resumes in presystole (see Fig. 57–2). In severe MS, the murmur is holodiastolic, with presystolic accentuation while sinus rhythm is maintained.

The *diastolic rumbling murmur* of MS is heard best with the patient lying in the left lateral decubitus position. It may be masked by the presence of a thick chest wall, pulmonary emphysema, and a low cardiac output with a low flow rate across the mitral valve. This murmur may be sharply localized and thus missed unless palpation is used to detect the apex of the left ventricle and to pinpoint the area at which auscultation should be carried out. In so-called silent MS, there is usually marked right ventricular enlargement. Consequently, the right ventricle occupies the cardiac apex, the left ventricle is rotated posteriorly, and cardiac output is reduced, so that the murmur either is not audible at all or can be heard only in the mid or posterior axillary line. In addition to placing the patient in the left lateral position, auscultation of the murmur is facilitated during expiration after having the patient do a few sit-ups, walk up a flight of stairs, or other maneuvers described later.

Dynamic Auscultation (see Chap. 8). The diastolic murmur and OS of MS are often reduced during inspiration and augmented during expiration, which is the opposite of what occurs when these findings are secondary to tricuspid stenosis. During inspiration, the A_2-OS interval widens, and three sequential sounds (A_2, P_2, and OS) may be audible. Sudden standing and the resultant reduction of venous return lower the left atrial pressure and widen the A_2-OS interval; this maneuver is useful in distinguishing an A_2-OS combination from a split S_2, which narrows on standing. In contrast, the A_2-OS interval is significantly narrowed during exercise as left atrial pressure rises. The diastolic rumbling murmur of MS is reduced during the strain of a Valsalva maneuver and in any condition in which transmitral valve flow rate declines. Amyl nitrite inhalation, coughing, isometric or isotonic exercise, and sudden squatting all are useful in accentuating a faint or equivocal murmur of MS.

Differential Diagnosis. The *Carey Coombs murmur* of acute rheumatic fever is a sign of active mitral valvulitis and can be confused with the murmur of MS. The Carey Coombs murmur is a soft early diastolic murmur, usually varies from day to day, and is higher pitched than the diastolic rumbling murmur of established MS. In pure, severe MR—indeed, in any condition in which flow across a nonstenotic mitral valve is increased (e.g., a ventricular septal defect)—there may also be a short diastolic murmur following an S_3. *Left atrial myxoma* may produce auscultatory findings similar to those in rheumatic valvular MS (see Chap. 63). A diastolic rumble may also be present in some patients with hypertrophic cardiomyopathy, caused by early diastolic flow into the hypertrophied, nondistensible left ventricle.

A high-frequency early systolic murmur is audible along the lower left sternal border in one-third of patients with MS. This should be distinguished from the apical (often holosystolic or late systolic) murmur of MR. In addition, a *pansystolic murmur of TR* and an S_3 originating from the right ventricle may be audible in the 4th intercostal space in the left parasternal region in patients with severe MS. These signs, which are secondary to pulmonary hypertension, may be confused with the findings of MR. However, the inspiratory augmentation of the murmur and of the S_3 and the prominent *v* wave in the jugular venous pulse aid in establishing that the murmur originates from the tricuspid valve. A high-pitched decrescendo diastolic murmur along the left sternal border in patients with MS and pulmonary hypertension is usually due to concomitant AR but occasionally represents a Graham Steell murmur of pulmonary regurgitation. The latter, when present, characteristically increases during inspiration.

Laboratory Examination

ELECTROCARDIOGRAPHY (see Chap. 9). The electrocardiogram (ECG) is relatively insensitive for detecting mild MS, but it does show characteristic changes in moderate or severe obstruction. Left atrial enlargement (P wave duration in lead II ≥ 0.12 second and/or a P wave axis between +45 and −30 degrees) is a principal ECG feature of MS and is found in 90 percent of patients with significant MS and sinus rhythm. The ECG signs of left atrial enlargement correlate more closely with left atrial volume than with left atrial pressure and often regress following successful valvotomy. Atrial fibrillation usually develops in the presence of preexisting ECG evidence of left atrial enlargement and is related to the size of the chamber, the extent of fibrosis of the left atrial myocardium, the duration of atriomegaly, and the age of the patient.

Whether or not there is ECG evidence of right ventricular hypertrophy depends largely on the height of right ventricular systolic pressure. Approximately half of all patients with right ventricular systolic pressures between 70 and 100 mm Hg manifest the ECG criteria for right ventricular hypertrophy, including both a mean QRS axis greater than 80 degrees in the frontal plane and an R:S ratio greater than 1.0 in lead V_1. Other patients with this degree of pulmonary hypertension have no frank evidence of right ventricular hypertrophy, but the R:S ratio fails to increase from the right to the mid-precordial leads. When right ventricular systolic pressure is higher than 100 mm Hg in patients with isolated or predominant MS, ECG evidence of right ventricular hypertrophy is found quite consistently.

The *QRS axis in the frontal plane* correlates roughly with the severity of valve obstruction and with the level of pulmonary vascular resistance in patients with pure MS. Thus, a mean frontal axis between 0 and +60 degrees suggests that the mitral valve area is greater than 1.3 cm^2, whereas an axis of more than 60 degrees suggests that the valve area is less than 1.3 cm^2. In patients in whom pulmonary vascular resistance exceeds 650 $dyne \cdot sec^{-1} \cdot cm^{-5}$, the mean axis is usually greater than +110 degrees. In patients whose pulmonary artery systolic pressure approaches systemic levels, the mean axis averages +150 degrees.

RADIOLOGICAL FINDINGS (see Figs. 12–17 and 12–19). Although their cardiac silhouette may be normal in the frontal projection, patients with hemodynamically significant MS almost invariably have evidence of left atrial enlargement on the lateral and left anterior oblique views. Extreme left atrial enlargement rarely occurs in pure MS; when it is present, MR is usually severe. Enlargement of the pulmonary artery, right ventricle, and right atrium (as well as the left atrium) is commonly seen in patients with severe MS. Occasionally, calcification of the mitral valve is evident on the chest roentgenogram, but, more commonly, fluoroscopy is required to detect valvular calcification.

Radiological changes in the lung fields indirectly reflect the severity of MS. Interstitial edema, an indication of severe obstruction, is manifested as Kerley B lines (dense, short, horizontal lines most commonly seen in the costophrenic angles). This finding is present in 30 percent of patients with resting pulmonary arterial wedge pressures lower than 20 mm Hg and in 70 percent of patients with pressures higher than 20 mm Hg. Severe, longstanding mitral obstruction often results in Kerley A lines (straight, dense lines ≤ 4 cm in length running toward the hilum) as well as the findings of pulmonary hemosiderosis and rarely of parenchymal ossification. Pulmonary edema is seldom evident.

ANGIOGRAPHY. Angiograms exposed in the right and left anterior oblique projections afford the best views of the mitral valve. Although contrast material should ideally be injected into the left atrium, it is often possible to achieve good visualization of the left side of the heart by injecting a large volume of contrast material into the main pulmonary artery. Such angiograms provide an assessment of left atrial size, may demonstrate thickening and reduced motion of the valve leaflets, and outline large intraluminal thrombi. Left ventriculography makes possible simultaneous assessment of left ventricular contractile function and of the subvalvular mitral apparatus. However, echocardiography has largely superseded angiography in the evaluation of patients with MS or suspected MS.

ECHOCARDIOGRAPHY (see Chap. 11). Echocardiography is now the cornerstone of the diagnostic assessment of patients with MS. Two-dimensional transthoracic or transesophageal echocardiograms of a thickened, calcified, stenotic rheumatic valve demonstrate increased acoustic impedance and fusion of the mitral valve leaflets and poor leaflet separation in diastole (Fig. 57–3; see also Figs. 11–50 to 11–52). In mild MS, in which some leaflet mobility is preserved, the anterior leaflet may demonstrate diastolic doming. The leaflets fail to close normally in mid-diastole and may not reopen widely during atrial contraction when sinus rhythm is present. The left atrium is usually enlarged, and in isolated MS the left ventricular cavity is normal or reduced in size. Two-dimensional echocardiography may be helpful in recognizing left atrial thrombus preoperatively and in assessing mitral valve calcification and left ventricular contractility.[19] With progressive thickening and fibrosis of the

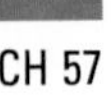

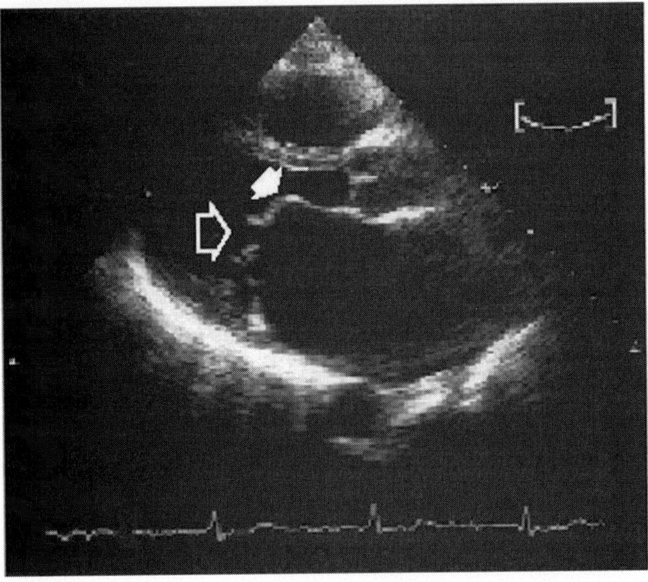

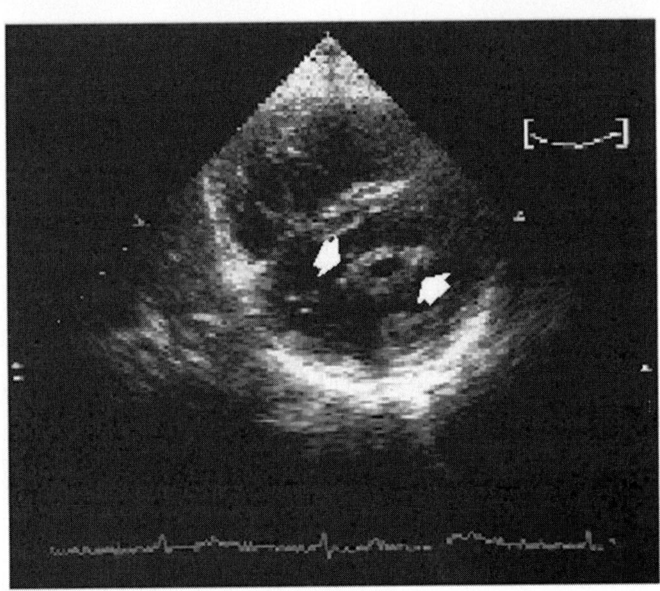

A B

FIGURE 57–3 Two-dimensional transthoracic parasternal long-axis **(A)** and short-axis **(B)** views of the mitral valve and its orifice during diastole, demonstrating leaflet thickening, the "fish mouth" appearance of the valve in the short axis (white arrows), and doming of the anterior leaflet in the long axis (white arrow). The subvalvular apparatus is not severely thickened. The open arrow indicates narrowed mitral valve orifice. (From Bach DS: Rheumatic mitral stenosis. N Engl J Med 337:31, 1997.)

leaflets, the orifice becomes fixed and can then often be imaged directly and measured. Two-dimensional echocardiography also provides information on the pliability of the leaflets, the extent of valvular calcification, thickening of the subvalvular apparatus, and fusion and retraction of the chordae tendineae, as well as calcification of the mitral annulus. This technique allows determination of left ventricular size and function and can also evaluate the aortic valve. The two-dimensional echocardiogram is helpful in determining whether the patient with MS is a suitable candidate for balloon mitral valvuloplasty (see Figs. 11–50 and 11–51). Transesophageal two-dimensional echocardiography provides images of the mitral valve that are superior to those obtained by transthoracic imaging and is more sensitive in detecting left atrial thrombus. Pedunculated and free-floating thrombi are also usually readily detected by this technique, as are atrial myxomas. Transesophageal echocardiography is necessary when the transthoracic signal is inadequate.

Doppler echocardiography is the most accurate noninvasive technique available for quantifying the severity of MS (see Fig. 11–54).[19] The pulmonary arterial pressure also can be estimated from the TR velocity signal.[20,21] Color-flow Doppler imaging can enhance the accuracy of the Doppler data by determining whether MR, AR, and other valvular abnormalities coexist.

In most patients with MS, a detailed echocardiographic examination, including two-dimensional echocardiography (transthoracic or transesophageal), a Doppler study, and color-flow Doppler imaging, can usually provide sufficient information to develop a therapeutic plan without the need for cardiac catheterization (see later).[22]

Exercise Testing with Doppler Echocardiography. Exercise testing is useful in many patients with MS to ascertain the level of physical conditioning and to elicit covert cardiac symptoms. The exercise test can be combined with Doppler echocardiography to assess exercise hemodynamics,[1] usually with the Doppler examination performed at rest after termination of exercise (see Fig. 11–54). Exercise Doppler testing is helpful in the following situations: (1) to confirm that the asymptomatic patient has satisfactory effort tolerance and has no symptoms during workloads equivalent to activities of normal living; (2) to assess pulmonary artery systolic pressure during exercise; and (3) to evaluate exercise hemodynamics in symptomatic patients who appear to have only mild MS on resting measurements.

Management

Medical Treatment

Patients with MS due to rheumatic heart disease should receive penicillin prophylaxis for beta-hemolytic streptococcal infections and prophylaxis for infective endocarditis (see Chaps. 58 and 81). Anemia and infections should be treated promptly and aggressively in patients with valvular heart disease. Adolescents and young adults with severe MS should be advised to avoid entering occupations requiring strenuous exertion. Asymptomatic patients with moderate MS should be reevaluated yearly.[1] Heavy exertion is contraindicated in symptomatic patients.

In symptomatic patients with mitral valve disease, considerable improvement occurs with the administration of oral diuretics and the restriction of sodium intake. Digitalis glycosides do not alter the hemodynamics and usually do not benefit patients with MS and sinus rhythm, but these drugs are of value in slowing the ventricular rate in patients with atrial fibrillation and in treating patients with right-sided heart failure. Hemoptysis is managed by measures designed to reduce pulmonary venous pressure, including sedation, assumption of the upright position, and aggressive diuresis. Beta-blocking agents and rate-slowing calcium antagonists may increase exercise capacity by reducing heart rate in patients with sinus rhythm and especially in patients with atrial fibrillation.[1]

Anticoagulant therapy is helpful in preventing venous thrombosis and pulmonary embolism in patients who have experienced one or more previous pulmonary embolic episodes; in patients who are at high risk of systemic embolization, i.e., with persistent or transient atrial fibrillation (especially elderly patients > 70 years of age); and in those with previous systemic emboli. Treatment with warfarin, to maintain the international normalized ratio

(INR) between 2.0 and 3.0, is indicated in such patients.[23,24] However, no firm evidence exists that anticoagulant therapy reduces the incidence of pulmonary or systemic embolism in patients in sinus rhythm in whom such episodes have not previously occurred. Although current guidelines do not recommend anticoagulation in patients in sinus rhythm, this may be considered in patients with extreme left atrial enlargement (>50 to 55 mm).[1,25]

TREATMENT OF ARRHYTHMIAS. Frequent premature atrial contractions often presage atrial fibrillation. The administration of antiarrhythmic agents (see Chap. 30) may be effective in preventing this complication. However, once atrial fibrillation has developed, these agents may be ineffective in restoring sinus rhythm because of the pathological changes that predispose to atrial fibrillation and that develop in the atrium secondary to the arrhythmia itself. After electrical cardioversion, sinus rhythm can often be maintained with antiarrhythmic agents, especially in young patients with mild MS but without marked left atrial enlargement who have been in atrial fibrillation less than 6 months.

Immediate treatment of atrial fibrillation should include intravenous heparin followed by oral warfarin. The ventricular rate should be slowed with intravenous digoxin and a beta-blocking agent or rate-slowing calcium antagonist. An effort should be made to reestablish sinus rhythm by a combination of pharmacological treatment and cardioversion. If cardioversion is planned in a patient who has had atrial fibrillation for more than 24 hours before the procedure, anticoagulation with warfarin for more than 3 weeks is indicated. Alternatively, if a transesophageal echocardiogram shows no atrial thrombus, immediate cardioversion can be carried out using intravenous heparin.[26] Paroxysmal atrial fibrillation and repeated conversions, spontaneous or induced, carry the risk of embolization. In patients who cannot be converted or maintained in sinus rhythm, digitalis should be used to maintain the ventricular rate at rest at approximately 60 beats/min. If this is not possible, small doses of a beta-blocking agent, such as atenolol (25 mg daily) or metoprolol (50 to 100 mg daily), may be added. Beta blockers are particularly helpful in preventing rapid ventricular responses that develop during exertion. Multiple repeat cardioversions are *not* indicated if the patient fails to sustain sinus rhythm while on adequate doses of an antiarrhythmic.

Patients with chronic atrial fibrillation who undergo open mitral valve repair or replacement may undergo the maze procedure (atrial compartment operation). More than 80 percent of patients undergoing this procedure can be maintained in sinus rhythm postoperatively and can regain normal atrial function,[27-29] including a satisfactory success rate in those with massive left atrial enlargement (>65 mm).[28]

NEED FOR CATHETERIZATION. There has been considerable debate concerning the need for routine cardiac catheterization in determining whether valvotomy is indicated.[1] A careful clinical evaluation and noninvasive assessment, particularly using two-dimensional and Doppler echocardiography, can provide sufficient information to permit an informed decision in the majority of patients. Preoperative catheterization is recommended for the following patients with MS: (1) patients who have a discrepancy between clinical and echocardiographic findings; hemodynamic measurements during exercise are often useful in these patients; (2) patients who have associated chronic obstructive pulmonary disease in whom it is important to determine the contribution of MS to the symptoms; (3) patients in whom left atrial myxoma should be excluded; (4) patients who have angina pectoris or angina-like chest pain in whom associated coronary artery disease must be excluded; and (5) men older than 40 years of age and women older than 50 years of age who have risk factors for coronary artery disease or a positive stress test and in whom surgery is planned; it is important to ascertain whether or not bypass grafting is indicated for those patients at risk of having coexisting coronary artery disease. Critical narrowing of one or more coronary vessels occurs in approximately 25 percent of all adults with severe MS.[1] This finding is more common in men older than 45 years of age who have angina and risk factors for coronary artery disease.

Natural History

The development of effective surgical treatment has obscured our understanding of the natural history of MS and, for that matter, of all valvular lesions. Although few meaningful data are available, it appears that in temperate zones, such as the United States and Western Europe, patients who develop acute rheumatic fever have an asymptomatic period of approximately 15 to 20 years before symptoms of MS develop. It then takes approximately 5 to 10 years for most patients to progress from mild disability (i.e., early NYHA Class II) to severe disability (i.e., NYHA Class III or IV). The progression is much more rapid in patients in tropical and subtropical areas, in Polynesians, and in Alaskan Inuit. Both economic and genetic conditions may play a role. In India, critical MS may be present in children as young as 6 to 12 years of age. In North America and Western Europe, however, symptoms develop more slowly and occur most commonly between 45 and 65 years of age.[1] Serial echocardiographic data regarding hemodynamic progression in patients with MS who have not undergone surgery demonstrate considerable interpatient variability, but on average the mitral valve area decreases by 0.09 cm^2 per year.[30]

Natural history data obtained In the *presurgical era* indicate that symptomatic patients with MS have a poor outlook. Olesen reported 5-year survival rates of 62 percent among patients with MS in NYHA Class III but only 15 percent among those in Class IV.[31] Recent data confirm these results in the current era; Horstkotte and associates[32] reported a 5-year survival rate of 44 percent in patients with symptomatic MS who refused valvotomy (Fig. 57–4).

Valvotomy

Indications

Patients with MS who are asymptomatic or minimally symptomatic frequently remain so for years. However, once moderate symptoms develop (NYHA Class II), if the stenosis is not relieved mechanically, the disease may progress relatively rapidly, as already discussed (see Fig. 57–4). Valvotomy (percutaneous balloon mitral valvuloplasty [BMV] or

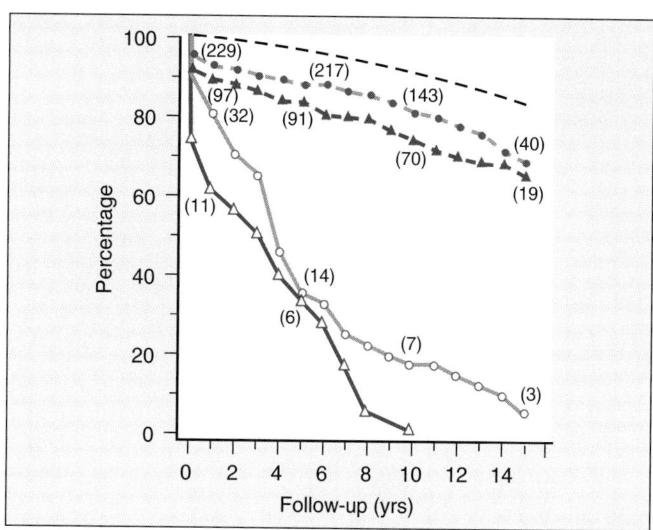

FIGURE 57–4 Natural history of 159 patients with isolated mitral stenosis (solid blue line) or mitral regurgitation (solid purple line) who were not operated on (even though the operation was indicated) compared with patients treated with valve replacement for mitral stenosis (dashed blue line) or mitral regurgitation (dashed purple line). The expected survival rate in the absence of mitral valve disease is indicated by the upper curve (dashed black line). (From Horstkotte D, Niehues R, Strauer BE: Pathomorphological aspects, aetiology, and natural history of acquired mitral valve stenosis. Eur Heart J 12[Suppl]:55-60, 1991.)

surgical valvotomy) should therefore be carried out in symptomatic patients with moderate to severe MS (i.e., a mitral valve orifice area < ≈1.0 cm²/m² body surface area [BSA] or < 1.5 to 1.7 cm² in normal-sized adults). It is also indicated in patients with mild stenosis (orifice area 1.0 to 1.5 cm²/m² BSA) who are symptomatic during ordinary activity and who develop pulmonary arterial systolic pressures exceeding 60 mm Hg or mean pulmonary capillary wedge pressures exceeding 25 mm Hg during exercise.[1,2]

Treatment must be individualized. For instance, mechanical relief of obstruction might well be deferred in a retired, mildly symptomatic, sedentary septuagenarian with a mitral valve orifice area of 0.8 cm²/m² BSA. On the other hand, a 30-year-old laborer whose family's economic well-being depends on his continued physical exertion might be an excellent candidate for mechanical relief of obstruction, although his mitral valve orifice size is 1.2 cm²/m² BSA. However, there is no evidence that valvotomy improves the prognosis of patients with no or only slight functional impairment. Therefore, valvotomy is *not* ordinarily indicated in patients who are entirely asymptomatic. Because of the high rate of recurrence, mechanical relief of obstruction is also indicated in patients with MS who have had a previous systemic embolism,[2] even if they are otherwise asymptomatic and even though there is no *definitive* evidence that the incidence of recurrent emboli will be significantly reduced. Anticoagulants should be administered to such patients up to the time of the procedure.

BALLOON MITRAL VALVOTOMY (see Chap. 52)
This percutaneous technique consists of advancing a small balloon flotation catheter across the interatrial septum (after transseptal puncture), enlarging the opening, advancing a large (23- to 25-mm) hourglass-shaped balloon (the Inoue balloon), and inflating it within the orifice (Fig. 57–5).[33-36] Alternatively, two smaller (15- to 20-mm) balloons may be employed.[33,35,36] A third technique involves retrograde, nontransseptal dilation of the mitral valve in which the balloon is positioned across the mitral valve using a steerable guide wire.[37] Commissural separation and fracture of nodular calcium appear to be the mechanisms responsible for improvement in valvular function. In several series, the hemodynamic results of BMV have been quite favorable (Fig. 57–6), with reduction of the transmitral pressure gradient from an average of approximately 18 to 6 mm Hg, a small (average 20 percent) increase in cardiac output, and an average doubling of the calculated mitral valve area from 1.0 to 2.0 cm². Although the double-balloon technique may result in a slightly greater valve opening, the clinical outcomes of the two approaches are similar.[33,35,36] Improvement in exercise tolerance has paralleled the favorable hemodynamic changes.

Results are especially impressive in younger patients without severe valvular thickening or calcification (see Fig. 57–3).[38] Elevated pulmonary vascular resistance declines rapidly, although usually not completely.[39] The reported mortality rate has ranged from 1 to 2 percent. Complications include cerebral emboli and cardiac perforation, each in approximately 1 percent of patients, and the development of MR severe enough to require operation in another 2 percent (≈15 percent develop lesser, but still undesirable, degrees of MR).

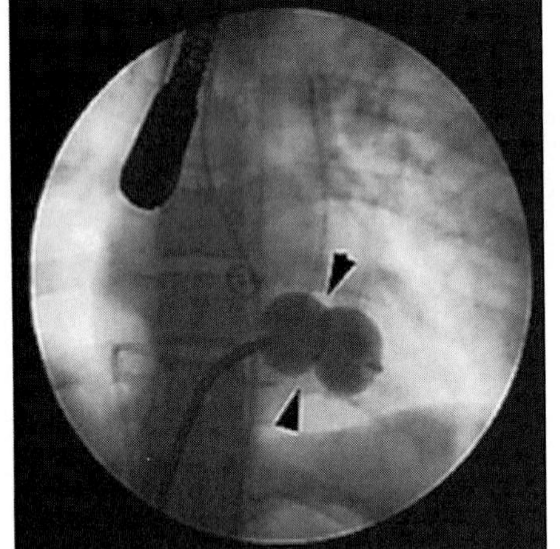

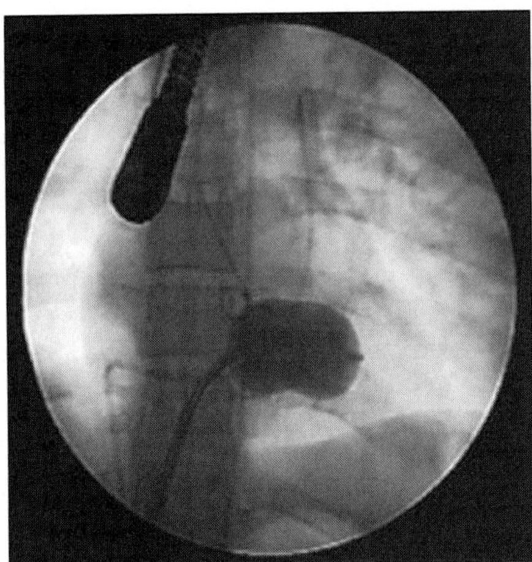

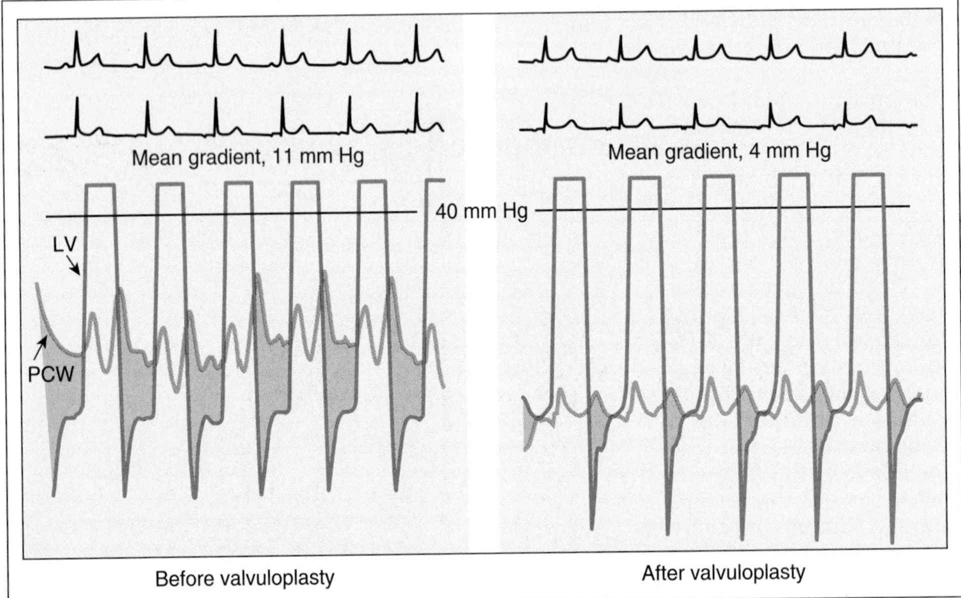

FIGURE 57–5 Percutaneous balloon mitral valvotomy (BMV) for mitral stenosis using the Inoue technique. **A,** The catheter is advanced into the left atrium via the transseptal technique and guided antegrade across the mitral orifice. As the balloon is inflated, its distal portion expands first and is pulled back so that it fits snugly against the orifice. With further inflation, the proximal portion of the balloon expands to center the balloon within the stenotic orifice (left panel). Further inflation expands the central "waist" portion of the balloon (right panel), resulting in commissural splitting and enlargement of the orifice. **B,** Successful BMV results in significant increase in mitral valve area, as reflected by reduction in the diastolic pressure gradient between left ventricle (magenta) and pulmonary capillary wedge (blue) pressure, as indicated by the shaded area. (From Delabays A, Goy JJ: Images in clinical medicine: Percutaneous mitral valvuloplasty. N Engl J Med 345:e4, 2001.)

Approximately 5 percent of patients are left with a small residual atrial septal defect, but this closes or decreases in size in the majority. Rarely, the defect is large enough to cause right-sided heart failure. Results are surgeon dependent and patients should be referred to experienced teams.

The indications for BMV are the same as those for surgical valvotomy (discussed later). A combination of significant symptoms and documented MS generally serves as the indication. Detailed two-dimensional and Doppler echocardiographic studies are indicated before a decision is made. Left atrial thrombus must be excluded by echocardiography.

An echocardiographic scoring system has been found to be particularly valuable in patient selection and has been widely adopted.[34,38,40,41] Leaflet rigidity, leaflet thickening, valvular calcification, and subvalvular disease are each scored from 0 to 4 (Table 57–1). Rigid, thickened valves with extensive subvalvular fibrosis and calcification lead to suboptimal results. A score of 8 or less is usually associated with an excellent immediate and long-term result, whereas scores exceeding 8 are associated with less impressive results (Fig. 57–7), including the risk of development of MR.[40] Significant valvular calcification[38] and coexisting MR[41,42] are additional important predictors of an adverse outcome. Transesophageal echocardiography provides a precise assessment of mitral valve structure and function and evaluation of accompanying MR and left atrial thrombus (a contraindication to BMV).[43] It also

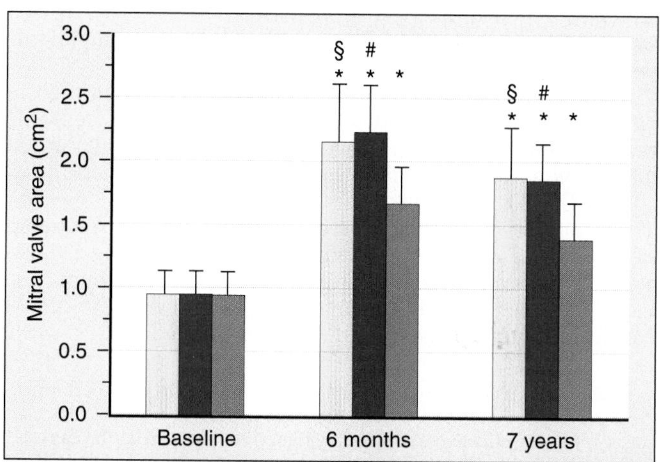

FIGURE 57–6 Mitral valve area before and 6 months and 7 years after valvotomy in a prospective, randomized trial of balloon mitral valvotomy (BMV, yellow bars), open surgical mitral commissurotomy (OMC, purple bars) and closed mitral commissurotomy (CMC, blue bars). At 6 months and 7 years, the results of BMV were equivalent to those of OMC, and superior to those of CMC. (From Farhat MB, Ayari M, Maatouk F, et al: Percutaneous balloon versus surgical closed and open mitral commissurotomy: Seven-year follow-up results of a randomized trial. Circulation 97:245, 1998.)

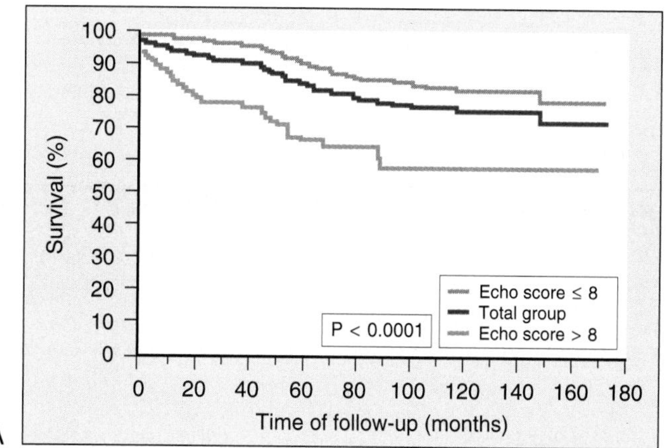

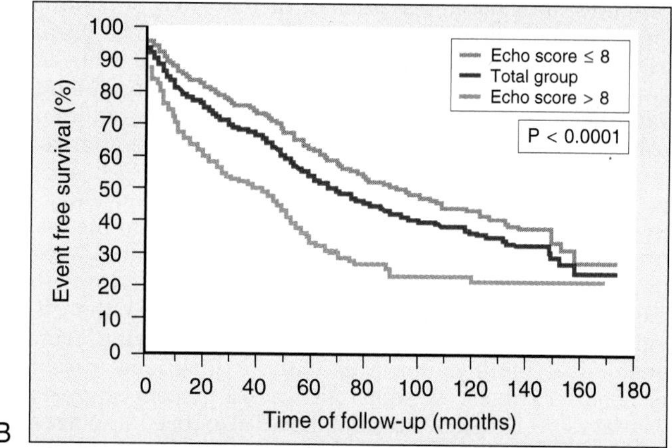

FIGURE 57–7 Long-term survival **(A)** and event-free survival **(B)** after balloon mitral valvotomy for 879 patients who were stratified by baseline echocardiographic morphology score: ≤ 8 (blue line) or > 8 (gold line). Patients with the lower echo score had a significantly better outcome initially and over the next 12 to 13 years. (From Palacios IF, Sanchez PL, Harrell LC, et al: Which patients benefit from percutaneous mitral balloon valvuloplasty? Prevalvuloplasy and postvalvuloplasty variables that predict long-term outcome. Circulation 105:1465, 2002.)

TABLE 57–1 Determinants of the Echocardiographic Mitral Valve Score

Grade	Mobility	Subvalvular Thickening	Thickening	Calcification
1	Highly mobile valve with only leaflet tips restricted	Minimal thickening just below the mitral leaflets	Leaflets near normal in thickness (4-5 mm)	A single area of increased echo brightness
2	Leaflet mid and base portions have normal mobility	Thickening of chordal structures extending up to one third of the chordal length	Midleaflets normal, considerable thickening of margins (5-8 mm)	Scattered areas of brightness confined to leaflet margins
3	Valve continues to move forward in diastole, mainly from the base	Thickening extending to the distal third of the chords	Thickening extending through the entire leaflet (5-8 mm)	Brightness extending into the midportion of the leaflets
4	No or minimal forward movement of the leaflets in diastole	Extensive thickening and shortening of all chordal structures extending down to the papillary muscles	Considerable thickening of all leaflet tissue (>8-10 mm)	Extensive brightness throughout much of the leaflet tissue

From Wilkens GT, Wyeman AL, Abscal VM, et al: Percutaneous balloon dilatation of the mitral valve: An analysis of echocardiographic variables related to outcome and the mechanism of dilatation. Br Heart J 60:299, 1988.

TABLE 57–2 Approaches to Mechanical Relief of Mitral Stenosis

Approach	Advantages	Disadvantages
Closed surgical valvotomy	Inexpensive Relatively simple Good hemodynamic results in selected patients Good long-term outcome	No direct visualization of valve Only feasible with flexible, noncalcified valves Contraindicated if MR > 2+ Surgical procedure with general anesthesia
Open surgical valvotomy	Visualization of valve allows directed valvotomy Concurrent annuloplasty for MR is feasible	Best results with flexible, noncalcified valves Surgical procedure with general anesthesia
Valve replacement	Feasible in all patients regardless of extent of valve calcification or severity of MR	Surgical procedure with general anesthesia Effect of loss of annular-papillary muscle continuity on LV function Prosthetic valve Chronic anticoagulation
Balloon mitral valvotomy	Percutaneous approach Local anesthesia Good hemodynamic results in selected patients Good long-term outcome	No direct visualization of valve Only feasible with flexible, noncalcified valves Contraindicated if MR > 2+

LV = left ventricular; MR = mitral regurgitation.
From Otto CM: Valvular Heart Disease. 2nd ed. Philadelphia, WB Saunders, 2004, p 296.

provides an accurate assessment of outcome. Three-dimensional echocardiography has also been found to be useful in assessing indications for BMV.[44] The findings on echocardiography affect the outcome of both open and closed surgical valvotomy in a similar manner. A prospective randomized trial in which patients with severe MS were randomized to undergo BMV, closed surgical valvotomy, or open surgical valvotomy resulted in similar clinical results from BMV and the open surgical technique that were superior to the results of the closed surgical valvotomy.[37] Indeed, after 7 years, mitral valve area was equivalent in the BMV and open surgical groups, both significantly greater than in the closed valvotomy group (see Fig. 57–6).[37] In patients with favorable anatomical findings, survival without functional disability or need for surgery or repeat BMV is 75 percent or greater at 7 years.[33-37] Excellent results have also been reported in children[45,46] and adolescents[47] in developing nations, where patients tend to be younger. These young patients usually have quite pliable valves, which are ideal for BMV.

Percutaneous BMV is the procedure of choice in patients who have symptomatic, hemodynamically severe stenosis with an echocardiographic score of 8 or less and without left atrial thrombus.[34,38,40,41] The lower cost and morbidity are obvious advantages. BMV can also be the initial procedure in patients with symptomatic, severe MS and less favorable valves (echocardiographic score > 8 and/or dense calcification on fluoroscopic or ultrasound examination).[34,38,41] However, the failure rate is considerable in these patients, and they may require surgical treatment, most often MVR. BMV also has acceptable results in patients with accompanying mild or moderate AR[43] and in those with mitral restenosis after surgical valvotomy.[48] It may also be used in patients with less favorable valves, including patients with restenosis after a previous BMV,[13] who are unsuitable for surgery because of very high risk. These include very elderly, frail patients; patients with associated severe ischemic heart disease; patients in whom MS is complicated by pulmonary, renal, or neoplastic disease; women of childbearing age in whom valve replacement is undesirable; and pregnant women with MS.[49,50] Patients with atrial fibrillation have a worse clinical and hemodynamic outcome with BMV than those in sinus rhythm[51]; the arrhythmia by itself does not unfavorably influence outcome, but is a marker for other clinical and morphological features associated with inferior results of BMV. BMV is contraindicated in patients with severe MR or AR and should probably not be used in patients with stenotic bioprosthetic valves.

Because the cost of the balloon catheter is deemed high in countries with restricted financial resources, a reusable metallic valvulotome has been devised. Early results are at least as good as those achieved with balloon catheters.[52]

SURGICAL VALVOTOMY

Three operative approaches are available for the treatment of rheumatic MS: (1) closed mitral valvotomy using a transatrial or transventricular approach[53]; (2) open valvotomy, i.e., valvotomy carried out under direct vision with the aid of cardiopulmonary bypass; and (3) MVR (Table 57–2).

CLOSED MITRAL VALVOTOMY. This procedure is performed without cardiopulmonary bypass but with the aid of a transventricular dilator. It is an effective operation, provided that MR, atrial thrombosis, or valvular calcification is not serious and that chordal fusion and shortening are not severe. Echocardiography is useful in selecting suitable candidates for this procedure by identifying patients without valvular calcification or dense fibrosis. If possible, closed mitral valvotomy should be carried out with "pump standby"; if the surgeon is unable to achieve a satisfactory result, the patient can be placed on cardiopulmonary bypass and the valvotomy carried out under direct vision or the valve replaced.

On average, the mitral valve area is increased by 1.0 cm^2, with only 20 to 30 percent of patients requiring MVR within 15 years.[54] In one large series,[53] the hospital mortality rate was 1.5 percent, and 0.3 percent of patients developed severe MR. Marked symptomatic improvement occurred in 86 percent of survivors. The actuarial survival rate was 89.5 percent after 18 years. Patients undergoing closed valvotomy for restenosis had a 6.7 percent mortality rate. Long-term follow-up has shown that the results are best if the operation is carried out before chronic atrial fibrillation and/or heart failure has occurred, but complication rates are higher when valves are calcified and/or severely thickened.

Closed mitral valvotomy is rarely used in the United States today, having been replaced by BMV, which is of greater effectiveness in patients who are candidates for closed mitral valvotomy.[37] Closed mitral valvotomy is more popular in developing nations, where the expense of open-heart surgery and even of balloon catheters for BMV is an important factor and where patients with mitral valve disease are younger and therefore have more pliable valves. But even in these nations, closed mitral valvotomy is being displaced by BMV.

OPEN VALVOTOMY. Most surgeons in North America and Western Europe now prefer to carry out *direct-vision* or *open valvotomy*. This operation is most frequently performed in patients with MS whose mitral valves are too distorted or calcified for BMV. Cardiopulmonary bypass is established, and to obtain a dry, quiet heart, body temperature is usually lowered, the heart is arrested, and the aorta is occluded intermittently.

Thrombi are removed from the left atrium and its appendage, and the latter is often amputated to remove a potential source of postoperative emboli. The commissures are incised, and, when necessary, fused chordae tendineae are separated, the underlying papillary muscle is split, and the valve leaflets are débrided of calcium. Mild or even moderate MR may be corrected. Left atrial and ventricular pressures are measured after bypass has been discontinued to confirm that the valvotomy has, in fact, been effective. When it has not been effective, another attempt can be made. When repair is not possible—most commonly owing to severe distortion and calcification of the valve and subvalvular apparatus with accompanying regurgitation that cannot be corrected—MVR should be carried out. In patients with atrial fibrillation, conversion to sinus rhythm is done at the completion of the operation. Open valvotomy is feasible and successful in more than 80 percent of patients referred for this procedure, with an operative mortality of 1 percent, a rate of reoperation for valve replacement of 0 to 16 percent at 36 to 53 months, and 10-year actuarial survival rates of 81 to 100 percent.[54]

In general, open valvotomy provides better hemodynamic relief of mitral valve obstruction than does the closed procedure, and the risk of dislodging thrombi from the atrium or calcium from the mitral valve is also less. Left atrial size, the need for mitral or tricuspid annuloplasty, and the presence of left atrial thrombus are all "risk factors" for a less than optimal outcome after open mitral valvotomy. Although a contemporary control series of medically and surgically treated patients is not available (nor is it likely ever to be), valvotomy appears to prolong survival substantially in patients with MS (see Fig. 57–4).

MITRAL RESTENOSIS. Mitral valvotomy, whether percutaneous or operative and whether open or closed, is *palliative* rather than curative, and even when successful, this procedure merely "turns the clock back." (The generally more effective open valvotomy and BMV turn the clock back further than does the closed valvotomy.) Thus, successful valvotomy does not result in a normal mitral valve but rather in one resembling the valve as it existed perhaps a decade earlier. Because the valve is not normal postoperatively, turbulent flow usually persists in the paravalvular region, and the resultant trauma may well play a role in restenosis. These changes are analogous to the gradual development of obstruction in a congenitally bicuspid aortic valve and are *not* usually the result of recurrent rheumatic fever.

On clinical grounds alone, i.e., based on the reappearance of symptoms, the incidence of "restenosis" has been estimated to range widely (from 2 to 60 percent). Recurrence of symptoms is usually *not* due to restenosis but may be due to one or more of the following conditions: (1) an inadequate first operation with residual stenosis; (2) the presence or development of MR, either at operation or as a consequence of infective endocarditis; (3) the progression of aortic valve disease; and (4) the development of coronary artery disease. True restenosis occurs in less than 20 percent of patients who are followed for 10 years.[1]

Thus, in properly selected patients, mitral valvotomy, however performed—balloon angioplasty, closed or open valvotomy—is a low-risk procedure that results in a significant increase in the size of the mitral orifice and favorably alters the clinical course of an otherwise progressive disease. Pulmonary arterial pressure falls promptly and decisively when mitral obstruction is effectively relieved. Most patients maintain clinical improvement for 10 to 15 years of follow-up. When a second procedure is required because of symptomatic deterioration, the valve is usually calcified and more seriously deformed than at the time of the first operation, and adequate reconstruction may not be possible. Accordingly, MVR is often necessary at that time.

Indications for Mitral Valve Replacement

This procedure is often required in patients with combined MS and moderate or severe MR; in those with extensive commissural calcification, severe fibrosis, and subvalvular fusion; and in those who have undergone previous valvotomy. The operative mortality rate following isolated MVR ranges from 3 to 8 percent in most centers and averaged 6.04 percent in the large data base of 16,105 such operations for patients with MS and/or MR reported in the Society of Thoracic Surgeons National Database (Table 57–3).[55] As described later, structural deterioration of bioprosthetic valves may occur. Also, the hazards of lifelong anticoagulant treatment in patients with mechanical prostheses must be considered. Therefore, the threshold for operation should be higher in patients in whom preoperative evaluation suggests that MVR may be required than in patients in whom valvotomy alone appears to be indicated.

MVR is indicated in two groups of patients with MS whose valves are not suitable for valvotomy: (1) those with a mitral valve area less than 1.5 cm^2 in NYHA Class III or IV; and (2) those with severe MS (mitral valve area < 1.0 cm^2), NYHA Class II, and severe pulmonary hypertension (pulmonary artery systolic pressure > 70 mm Hg).[1] Since the operative

TABLE 57–3 Operative Mortality Rates Following Valve Replacement and Repair

Operative Category	Number*	Operative Mortality* (%)	Number†	Operative Mortality† (%)
AVR (isolated)	26,317	4.3	32,968	4.0
MVR (isolated)	13,936	6.4	16,105	6.04
Multiple valve replacement	3,840	9.6	—	—
AVR + CAB	22,713	8.0	32,538	6.8
MVR + CAB	8,788	15.3	10,925	13.3
Multiple valve replacement + CAB	1,424	18.8		
AVR + any valve repair	938	7.4		
MVR + any valve repair	1,266	12.5		
Aortic valve repair	597	5.9		
Mitral valve repair	4,167	3.0		
Tricuspid valve repair	144	13.9		
AVR + aortic aneurysm repair	1,723	9.7		

AVR = aortic valve replacement; CAB = coronary artery bypass; MVR = mitral valve replacement.

*Modified from Jamieson WRE, Edwards FH, Schwartz M, et al: Risk stratification for cardiac valve replacement. National Cardiac Surgery Database, Ann Thorac Surg 67:943, 1999.

†Modified from Edwards FH, Peterson ED, Coombs LP, et al: Prediction of operative mortality after valve replacement surgery. J Am Coll Cardiol 37:885, 2001.

TABLE 57–4 Causes of Acute and Chronic Mitral Regurgitation

Acute	Chronic
Mitral Annulus Disorders Infective endocarditis (abscess formation) Trauma (valvular heart surgery) Paravalvular leak due to suture interruption (surgical technical problems or infective endocorditis)	**Inflammatory** Rheumatic heart disease Systemic lupus erythematosus Scleroderma
Mitral Leaflet Disorders Infective endocarditis (perforation or interfering with valve closure by vegetation) Trauma (tear during percutaneous balloon mitral valvotomy or penetrating chest injury) Tumors (atrial myxoma) Myxomatous degeneration Systemic lupus erythematosus (Libman-Sacks lesion)	**Degenerative** Myxomatous degeneration of mitral valve leaflets (Barlow click-murmur syndrome, prolapsing leaflet, mitral valve prolapse) Marfan syndrome Ehlers-Danlos syndrome Pseudoxanthoma elasticum Calcification of mitral valve annulus
Rupture of Chordae Tendineae Idiopathic, e.g., spontaneous Myxomatous degeneration (mitral valve prolapse, Marfan syndrome, Ehlers-Danlos syndrome) Infective endocarditis Acute rheumatic fever Trauma (percutaneous balloon valvotomy, blunt chest trauma)	**Infective** Infective endocarditis affecting normal, abnormal, or prosthetic mitral valves
Papillary Muscle Disorders Coronary artery disease (causing dysfunction and rarely rupture) Acute global left ventricular dysfunction Infiltrative diseases (amyloidosis, sarcoidosis) Trauma	**Structural** Ruptured chordae tendineae (spontaneous or secondary to myocardial infarction, trauma, mitral valve prolapse, endocarditis) Rupture or dysfunction of papillary muscle (ischemia or myocardial infarction) Dilation of mitral valve annulus and left ventricular cavity (congestive cardiomyopathies, aneurysmal dilation of the left ventricle) Hypertrophic cardiomyopathy Paravalvular prosthetic leak
Primary Mitral Valve Prosthetic Disorders Porcine cusp perforation (endocarditis) Porcine cusp degeneration Mechanical failure (strut fracture) Immobilized disc or ball of the mechanical prosthesis	**Congenital** Mitral valve clefts or fenestrations Parachute mitral valve abnormality in association with Endocardial cushion defects Endocardial fibroelastosis Transposition of the great arteries Anomalous origin of the left coronary artery

Data from Jutzy KR, Al-Zaibag M: Acute mitral and aortic valve regurgitation. *In* Al-Zaibag M, Duran CMG (eds): Valvular Heart Disease. New York, Marcel Dekker, 1994, pp 345-362 (left column); and Haffajee CI: Chronic mitral regurgitation. *In* Dalen JE. Alpert JS (eds): Valvular Heart Disease. 2nd ed. Boston, Little, Brown, 1987, p 112 (right column).

mortality risk may be quite high (10 to 20 percent) in patients in NYHA Class IV, operation should be carried out before patients reach this stage if possible. On the other hand, even such high-risk patients should not be denied operation unless they have comorbid conditions that preclude surgery or a satisfactory outcome.

Mitral Regurgitation

Etiology and Pathology

The mitral valve apparatus involves the mitral leaflets per se, chordae tendineae, papillary muscles, and mitral annulus. Abnormalities of any of these structures may cause MR.[56,57] The major causes of MR include mitral valve prolapse (MVP), rheumatic heart disease, infective endocarditis, annular calcification, cardiomyopathy, and ischemic heart disease (Table 57–4). Specific aspects of the MVP syndrome, the most important cause of significant MR in the United States, are discussed in a separate section. Less common causes of MR include collagen vascular diseases, trauma, the hypereosinophilic syndrome, carcinoid, and exposure to certain appetite suppressant drugs.

Abnormalities of Valve Leaflets

MR due to predominant involvement of the valve leaflets occurs in patients with chronic rheumatic heart disease. However, in contrast to MS, this lesion is more frequent in men than in women. It is a consequence of shortening, rigidity, deformity, and retraction of one or both mitral valve cusps and is associated with shortening and fusion of the chordae tendineae and papillary muscles. MVP involves both leaflets and chordae and may also affect the annulus. Infective endocarditis can cause MR by perforating valve leaflets (see Chap. 58); vegetations can prevent leaflet coaptation, and valvular retraction during the healing phase of endocarditis can cause MR. Destruction of the mitral valve leaflets can also occur in patients with penetrating and nonpenetrating trauma (see Chap. 65).

Abnormalities of the Mitral Annulus

DILATION. In a normal adult, the mitral annulus measures approximately 10 cm in circumference. It is soft and flexible, and contraction of the surrounding left ventricular muscle during systole causes the annular constriction that contributes importantly to valve closure. MR secondary to dilation of the mitral annulus can occur in any form of heart disease characterized by dilation of the left ventricle, especially dilated cardiomyopathy (Fig. 57–8; see also Fig. 11–57). Left ventricular submitral aneurysm has been reported as a cause of annular MR in sub-Saharan Africa and appears to be due to a congenital defect in the posterior portion of the annulus. Diagnosis by transesophageal echocardiography and surgical repair have been reported.

CALCIFICATION. Idiopathic (degenerative) calcification of the mitral annulus is one of the most common cardiac abnormalities found at autopsy; in most hearts it is of little functional consequence. However, when severe (see Fig. 12-21), it may be an important cause of MR,[57,58] and, in contrast to MR secondary to rheumatic fever, it is more common in women than in men. The development of degenerative calcification of the mitral annulus shares common risk factors with atherosclerosis, including systemic hypertension, hypercholesterolemia, and diabetes.[59] Hence, mitral annular calcification is associated with coronary[60] and carotid[61] atherosclerosis and identifies patients at higher risk for cardiovascular morbidity and mortality.[59] Annular calcification may also be accelerated by an intrinsic defect in the fibrous skeleton of the heart, as occurs in Marfan and Hurler syndromes. In these two latter syndromes, the mitral annulus is not only calcified but also dilated, further contributing to MR. The incidence of mitral annular calcification is also increased in patients who have chronic renal failure with secondary hyperparathyroidism. The annulus may also become thick, rigid, and calcified secondary to rheumatic involvement; when this process is severe, it also can interfere with valve closure.

With severe annular calcification, a rigid, curved bar or ring of calcium encircles the mitral orifice (see Fig. 12–21), and calcific spurs may project into the adjacent left ventricular myocardium. The calcification may immobilize the basal portion of the mitral leaflets, preventing their normal excursion in diastole and coaptation in systole, and aggravating the MR that results from loss of the normal sphincteric action of the mitral ring. Rarely, obstruction to left ventricular filling may occur when severe calcification encroaches on or protrudes into the mitral orifice. In patients with severe calcification, the conduction system may be invaded by calcium, leading to atrioventricular and/or intraventricular conduction defects. Calcification of the aortic valve cusps is an associated finding in approximately 50 percent of patients with severe mitral annular calcification, but this rarely causes aortic stenosis (AS). Occasionally, calcific deposits extend into the coronary arteries.

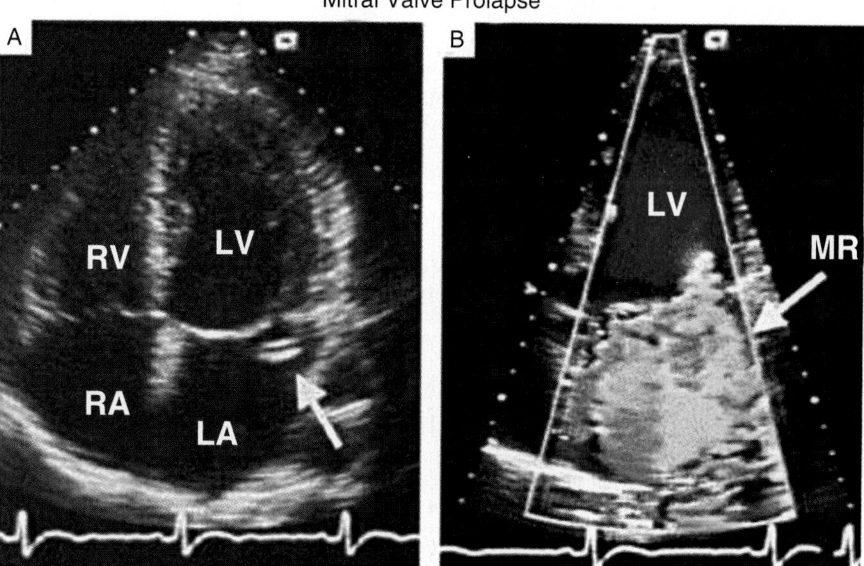

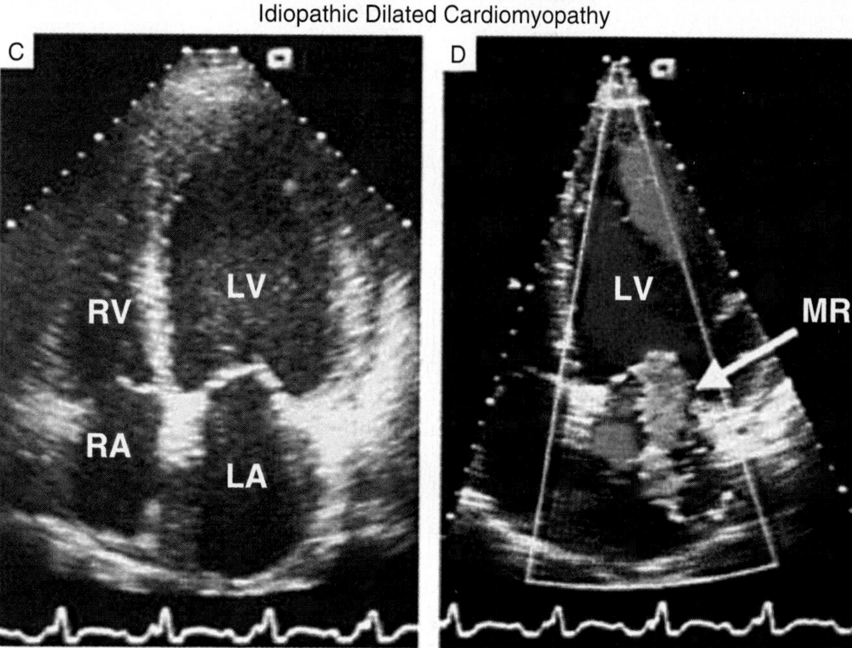

FIGURE 57–8 Echocardiographic long-axis images in two patients with mitral regurgitation **(A** and **C)** with color Doppler images of the same patients **(B** and **D)**. The top panels were obtained in a 46-year-old man with mitral valve prolapse and a partial flail posterior leaflet (arrow in **A**). The left ventricle (LV) is not dilated but the left atrium (LA) is enlarged, and there is severe mitral regurgitation (MR). The bottom images were obtained in a patient with dilated cardiomyopathy, demonstrating left ventricular dilation, normal mitral valve leaflets, and moderate MR. RA = right atrium; RV = right ventricle. (From Otto CM: Evaluation and management of chronic mitral regurgitation. N Engl J Med 345:740, 2001.)

Abnormalities of the Chordae Tendineae. Such abnormalities are important causes of MR. Lengthening and rupture of the chordae tendineae are cardinal features of the MVP syndrome (Fig. 57–8).[62] The chordae may be congenitally abnormal; rupture may be spontaneous ("primary") or may occur as a consequence of infective endocarditis, trauma, rheumatic fever, or, rarely, osteogenesis imperfecta or relapsing polychondritis. In most patients, no cause for chordal rupture is apparent other than increased mechanical strain. Chordae to the posterior leaflet rupture more frequently than those to the anterior leaflet. Patients with idiopathic rupture of mitral chordae tendineae frequently exhibit pathological fibrosis of the papillary muscles. It is possible that the dysfunction of the papillary muscles may cause stretching and ultimately rupture of the chordae tendineae. Chordal rupture may also result from acute left ventricular dilation, regardless of the cause. Depending on the number of chordae involved in rupture and the rate at which rupture occurs, the resultant MR may be mild, moderate, or severe and acute, subacute, or chronic.

Involvement of the Papillary Muscles. Diseases of the left ventricular papillary muscles are a frequent cause of MR. Because these muscles are perfused by the terminal portion of the coronary vascular bed, they are particularly vulnerable to ischemia, and any disturbance in coronary perfusion may result in papillary muscle dysfunction. When ischemia is transient, it results in temporary papillary muscle dysfunction and may cause transient episodes of MR that are sometimes associated with attacks of angina pectoris. When ischemia of papillary muscles is severe and prolonged, it causes papillary muscle dysfunction and scarring, as well as chronic MR. The posterior papillary muscle, which is supplied by the posterior descending branch of the right coronary artery, becomes ischemic and infarcted more frequently than does the anterolateral papillary muscle; the latter is supplied by diagonal branches of the left anterior descending coronary artery and often by marginal branches from the left circumflex artery as well. Ischemia of the papillary muscles is caused most commonly by coronary atherosclerosis, but it may also occur in patients with severe anemia, shock, coronary arteritis of any cause, or an anomalous left coronary artery. MR occurs frequently in patients with healed myocardial infarcts[63] and is caused by dyskinesis of the left ventricular myocardium at the base of a papillary muscle.

Left ventricular dilation of any cause, including ischemia, can alter the spatial relationships between the papillary muscles and the chordae tendineae and thereby result in MR.[64] Although *necrosis of a papillary muscle* is a frequent complication of myocardial infarction, frank rupture is far less common; the latter is usually fatal because of the extremely severe MR that it produces (see Chap. 46). However, rupture of one or two of the apical heads of a papillary muscle results in a lesser degree of MR and thus makes survival possible, usually following surgical therapy.

Some degree of MR is found in approximately 30 percent of patients with coronary artery disease who are being considered for coronary artery bypass surgery. In these patients, MR is secondary to ischemic damage to the papillary muscles and/or dilation of the mitral valve ring. In most of these patients, MR is mild; however, in the small percentage with severe MR (3 percent in one large series of patients with coronary artery disease proved by coronary arteriography), it is associated with a poor prognosis.[65,66] The incidence and severity of regurgitation vary inversely with the left ventricular ejection fraction and directly with the left ventricular end-diastolic pressure. MR occurs in approximately 20 percent of patients following acute myocardial infarction and, even when mild, is associated with a higher risk of adverse outcomes.

Various other disorders of the papillary muscles may also be responsible for the development of MR (see Table 57-4). These include congenital malposition of the muscles; absence of one papillary muscle, resulting in the so-called parachute mitral valve syndrome; and involvement or infiltration of the papillary muscles by a variety of processes, including abscesses, granulomas, neoplasms, amyloidosis, and sarcoidosis.

Other causes of MR, discussed in greater detail elsewhere, include obstructive hypertrophic cardiomyopathy (see Chap. 59), hypereosinophilic syndrome, endomyocardial fibrosis, trauma affecting the leaflets and/or papillary muscles (see Chap. 65), Kawasaki disease (see Chap. 56), left atrial myxoma (see Chap. 63), and various congenital anomalies, including cleft anterior leaflet and ostium secundum atrial septal defect (see Chap. 56).

Pathophysiology

Because the regurgitant mitral orifice is functionally in parallel with the aortic valve, the impedance to ventricular emptying is reduced in patients with MR. Consequently, MR enhances left ventricular emptying. Almost 50 percent of the regurgitant volume is ejected into the left atrium before the aortic valve opens. The volume of MR flow depends on a combination of the instantaneous size of the regurgitant orifice and the (reverse) pressure gradient between the left ventricle and the left atrium.[1,57] Both the orifice size and the pressure gradient are labile. Left ventricular systolic pressure, and therefore the left ventricular–left atrial gradient, depends on systemic vascular resistance, and in patients in whom the mitral annulus has normal flexibility, the cross-sectional area of the mitral annulus may be altered by many interventions. Thus, increase of both preload and afterload and depression of contractility increase left ventricular size and enlarge the mitral annulus and thereby the regurgitant orifice. When ventricular size is reduced by treatment with positive inotropic agents, diuretics, and particularly vasodilators, the regurgitant orifice size decreases, and the volume of regurgitant flow declines,[67,68] as reflected in the height of the *v* wave in the left atrial pressure pulse and in the intensity and duration of the systolic murmur. Conversely, left ventricular dilation, regardless of cause, may increase MR.

LEFT VENTRICULAR COMPENSATION. The left ventricle initially compensates for the development of *acute* MR in part by emptying more completely and in part by increasing preload, i.e., by use of the Frank-Starling principle. Because *acute* MR reduces both late systolic ventricular pressure and radius, left ventricular wall tension declines markedly (and proportionately to a greater extent than left ventricular pressure), permitting a reciprocal increase in both the extent and the velocity of myocardial fiber shortening, leading to a reduced end-systolic volume (Fig. 57–9). As regurgitation, particularly severe regurgitation, becomes chronic, the left ventricular end-diastolic volume increases and the end-systolic volume returns to normal. By means of the Laplace principle (which states that myocardial wall tension is related to the product of intraventricular pressure and radius), the increased ventricular end-diastolic volume increases wall tension to normal or supranormal levels in the so-called chronic compensated stage of severe MR.[57] The resultant increase in left ventricular end-diastolic volume and mitral annular diameter may create a vicious circle in which "MR begets more MR." In patients with chronic MR, both left ventricular end-diastolic volume and mass are increased; i.e., typical volume overload (eccentric) hypertrophy develops. However, the degree of hypertrophy is often not proportionate to the degree of left ventricular dilation, so that the ratio of left ventricular mass to end-diastolic volume may be less than normal.[57,69] Nonetheless, the reduced afterload permits maintenance of ejection fraction in the normal to supranormal range. The reduced left ventricular afterload allows a

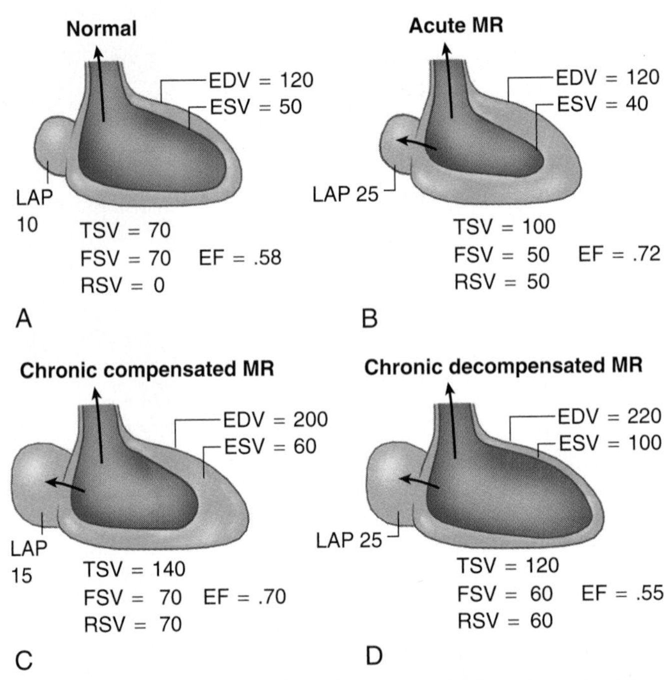

FIGURE 57–9 Three phases of mitral regurgitation (MR) are depicted and compared with normal physiology **(A)**. In acute MR **(B)**, an increase in preload and a decrease in afterload cause an increase in end-diastolic volume (EDV) and a decrease in end-systolic volume (ESV), producing an increase in total stroke volume (TSV). However, forward stroke volume (FSV) is diminished because 50 percent of the TSV regurgitates as the regurgitant stroke volume (RSV), resulting in an increase in left atrial pressure (LAP). In the chronic compensated phase **(C)**, eccentric hypertrophy has developed, and EDV is now increased substantially. Afterload has returned toward normal as the radius term of the LaPlace relationship increases with the increase in EDV. Normal muscle function and a large increase in EDV permit a substantial increase in TSV from the acute phase. This, in turn, permits a normal FSV. Left atrial enlargement now accommodates the regurgitant volume at lower LAP. Ejection fraction (EF) remains greater than normal. In the chronic decompensated phase **(D)**, muscle dysfunction has developed, impairing ejection fraction, diminishing both TSV and FSV. EF, although still "normal," has decreased to 0.55, and LAP is reelevated because less volume is ejected during systole, causing a higher ESV. (From Carabello BA: Progress in mitral and aortic regurgitation. Curr Probl Cardiol 28:553, 2003.)

greater proportion of the contractile energy of the myocardium to be expended in shortening than in tension development and explains how the left ventricle can adapt to the load imposed by MR.

The eccentric ventricular hypertrophy that accompanies the elevated end-diastolic volume of chronic MR is secondary to new sarcomeres laid down in parallel. A shift to the right (greater volume at any pressure) occurs in the left ventricular diastolic pressure-volume curve in patients with chronic MR. With decompensation, chamber stiffness increases, raising the diastolic pressure at any volume.

In most patients with severe primary MR, compensation is maintained for years, but in some patients the prolonged hemodynamic overload ultimately leads to myocardial decompensation. End-systolic volume, preload, and afterload all rise, whereas ejection fraction and stroke volume decline. In such patients, there is evidence of neurohormonal activation[70-71a] and elevation of circulating proinflammatory cytokines.[72] Plasma natriuretic peptide levels also increase in response to the volume load, more so in patients with symptomatic decompensation,[70] and a depressed ratio of phosphocreatine/adenosine triphosphate has been reported in patients with MR and severe decompensation.[73] It is not clear whether this is the cause or a marker of heart failure in these patients.

Coronary flow rates may be increased in patients with severe MR,[74] but the increases in myocardial oxygen consumption (MVO_2) are relatively modest compared to patients with AS and AR, because myocardial fiber shortening, which is elevated in patients with MR, is not one of the principal determinants of MVO_2. One of these determinants, mean left ventricular wall tension, may actually be reduced in patients with MR, whereas the other two, contractility and heart rate, may be little affected. Thus patients with MR have a low incidence of clinical manifestations of myocardial ischemia compared with the much higher incidence occurring in those with AS and AR, conditions in which MVO_2 is greatly augmented.

ASSESSMENT OF MYOCARDIAL CONTRACTILITY IN MITRAL REGURGITATION. Because the ejection phase indices of myocardial contractility are inversely correlated with afterload, patients with early MR (with reduced left ventricular afterload) often exhibit elevations in ejection phase indices of myocardial contractility, such as ejection fraction, fractional fiber shortening, and velocity of circumferential fiber shortening.[1,57] Many patients ultimately develop symptoms because of elevated left atrial and pulmonary venous pressures related to the regurgitant volume, and they may do so with no change in these ejection phase indices, which remain elevated. However, in other patients, major symptoms reflect serious contractile dysfunction, at which time ejection fraction, fiber shortening, and mean velocity of circumferential fiber shortening have declined to *low-normal* or *below-normal* levels (see Fig. 57–9). As MR persists, the reduction in afterload, which increases myocardial fiber shortening and the earlier mentioned ejection phase indices, is opposed by the impairment of myocardial function characteristic of severe chronic diastolic overload. However, even in patients with overt heart failure secondary to MR, the ejection fraction and fiber shortening may be only modestly reduced.[75] Therefore, values in the *low-normal* range for the ejection phase indices of myocardial performance in patients with chronic MR may actually reflect impaired myocardial function, whereas moderately reduced values (e.g., ejection fraction of 0.40 to 0.50) generally signify severe, often irreversible, impairment of contractility,[76,77] identifying patients who may do poorly after surgical correction of the MR (Fig. 57–10). An ejection fraction of less than 0.35 in patients with severe MR usually represents advanced myocardial dysfunction; such patients are high operative risks and may not experience satisfactory improvement following MVR.

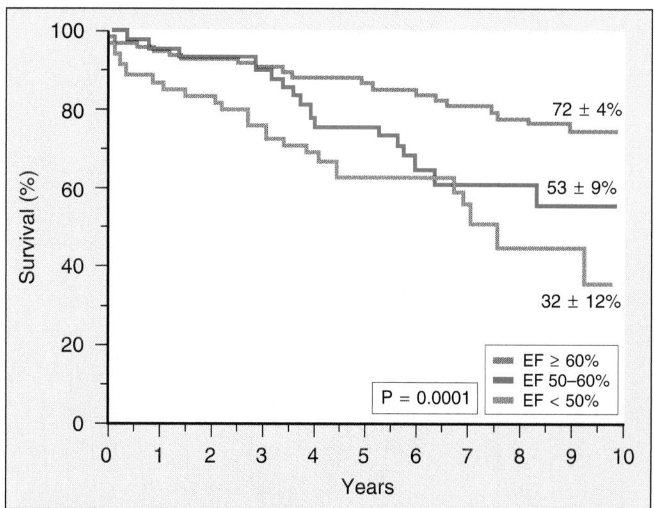

FIGURE 57–10 Graph of the late survival of patients who underwent surgical correction of mitral regurgitation as a function of the preoperative echocardiographic ejection fraction (EF). (From Enriquez-Sarano M, Tajik AJ, Schaff HV, et al: Echocardiographic prediction of survival after surgical correction of organic mitral regurgitation. Circulation 90:833, 1994.)

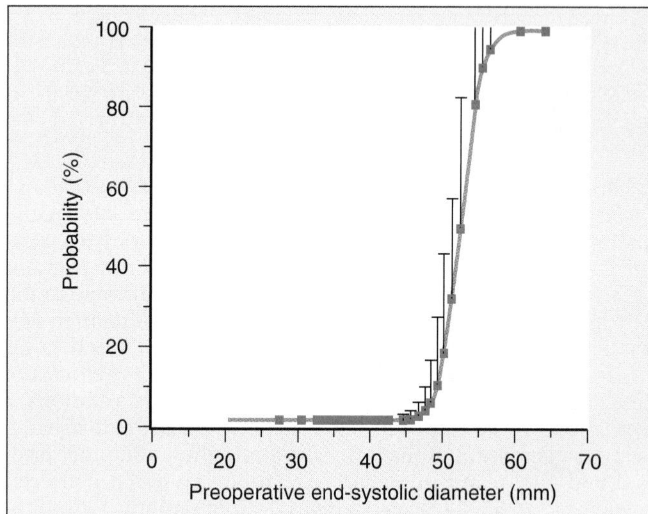

FIGURE 57–11 The probability of postoperative death or persistence of severe heart failure in patients with mitral regurgitation plotted against preoperative echocardiographic end-systolic diameter. As end-systolic diameter exceeded 45 mm, the incidence of a poor postoperative outcome increased abruptly. (From Wisenbaugh T, Skudicky D, Sareli P: Prediction of outcome after valve replacement for rheumatic mitral regurgitation in the era of chordal preservation. Circulation 89:191, 1994.)

End-Systolic Volume.. Preoperative myocardial contractility is an important determinant of the risk of operative death, of cardiac failure perioperatively, and of the level of left ventricular function postoperatively. Therefore, it is not surprising that the end-systolic pressure/volume (or stress/dimension) relation has emerged as a useful index for evaluating left ventricular function in patients with MR.[78] Indeed, the simple measurement of end-systolic volume or diameter has been found to be a useful predictor of function and survival following mitral valve surgery.[1,56,76-79] The outcome is excellent until the end-systolic diameter exceeds approximately 45 mm or 26 mm/m^2 (Fig. 57–11),[79] although even lower values of end-systolic climension have been associated with impaired postoperative ejection fraction.[76]

HEMODYNAMICS. Effective (forward) *cardiac output* is usually depressed in severely symptomatic patients with MR,

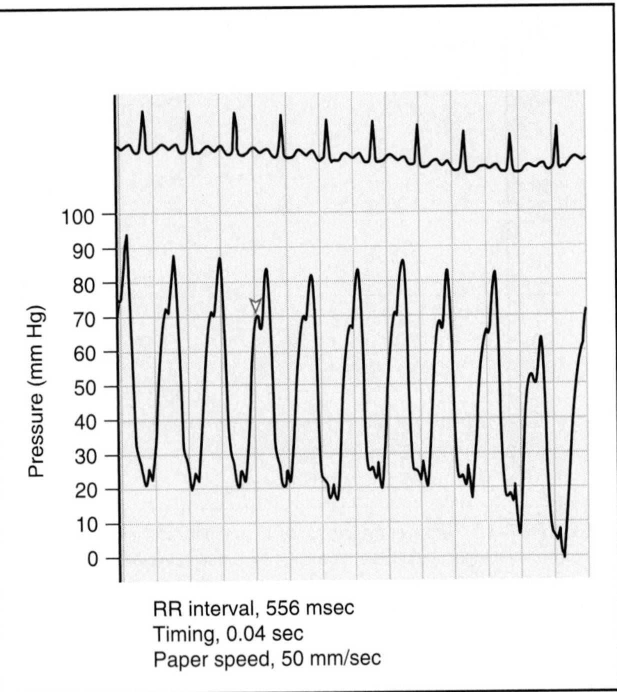

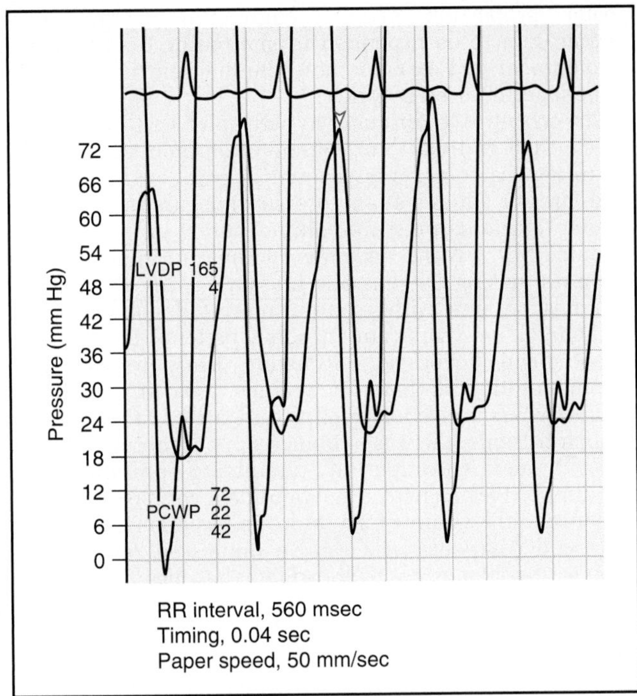

FIGURE 57–12 Hemodynamic tracings in a 45-year-old woman with acute mitral regurgitation from bacterial endocarditis. **A,** Pulmonary artery pressure. **B,** Simultaneous left ventricular diastolic pressure (LVDP) and pulmonary capillary wedge pressure (PCWP). The PCWP demonstrates a markedly elevated "v" wave (arrowhead, **B**) that transmits to the pulmonary artery pressure (arrowhead, **A**). (Adapted from Wisse B, Sniderman AD: Severe mitral regurgitation. N Engl J Med 343:1386, 2000.)

whereas *total* left ventricular output (the sum of forward and regurgitant flow) is usually elevated until quite late in the patient's course. The cardiac output achieved during exercise, not the regurgitant volume, is the principal determinant of functional capacity.[80] The atrial contraction (*a*) wave in the left atrial pressure pulse is usually not as prominent in MR as in MS, but the *v* wave is characteristically much taller because it is inscribed during ventricular systole, when the left atrium is being filled with blood from the pulmonary veins as well as from the left ventricle. Occasionally, backward transmission of the tall *v* wave into the pulmonary arterial bed may result in an early diastolic "pulmonary arterial *v* wave" (Fig. 57–12; see also Fig. 17–5). In patients with pure MR, the *y* descent in the pulmonary capillary pressure pulse is particularly rapid as the distended left atrium empties rapidly during early diastole. However, in patients with combined MS and MR, the *y* descent is gradual. Although a left atrioventricular pressure gradient persisting throughout diastole signifies the presence of significant associated MS, a brief early diastolic gradient may occur in patients with isolated, severe MR as a result of the rapid flow of blood across a normal-sized mitral orifice early in diastole, often accompanied by an early diastolic murmur at the apex.

LEFT ATRIAL COMPLIANCE

The compliance of the left atrium (and pulmonary venous bed) is an important determinant of the hemodynamic and clinical picture in patients with severe MR. Three major subgroups of patients with severe MR based on left atrial compliance have been identified and are characterized as follows:

Normal or Reduced Compliance. In this subgroup, there is little enlargement of the left atrium but marked elevation of the mean left atrial pressure (Fig. 57–13), particularly of the *v* wave, and pulmonary congestion is a prominent symptom. Severe MR usually develops acutely, as occurs with rupture of the chordae tendineae, infarction of one of the heads of a papillary muscle, or perforation of a mitral leaflet as a consequence of trauma or endocarditis. In patients with acute MR, the left atrium initially operates on the steep portion of its pressure-volume curve with a marked rise in pressure for a small increase in volume. Sinus rhythm is usually present; after the passage of weeks or a few months, the left atrial wall becomes hypertrophied, is capable of contracting vigorously, and facilitates left ventricular filling. The thicker atrium is less compliant than normal, which further increases the height of the *v* wave. Thickening of the walls of the pulmonary veins and proliferative changes in the pulmonary arteries, as well as marked elevations of pulmonary vascular resistance and pulmonary artery pressure, usually develop over the course of 6 to 12 months after the onset of acute, severe MR.

Markedly Increased Compliance. At the opposite end of the spectrum from patients in the first group are those with severe, longstanding MR with massive enlargement of the left atrium and normal or only slightly elevated left atrial pressure (see Fig. 57–13). The atrial wall contains only a small remnant of muscle surrounded by fibrous tissue. Longstanding MR in these patients has altered the physical properties of the left atrial wall and thereby displaced the atrial pressure-volume curve to the right, allowing a normal or almost-normal pressure to exist in a greatly enlarged left atrium. Pulmonary arterial pressure and pulmonary vascular resistance may be normal or only slightly elevated at rest. Atrial fibrillation and a low cardiac output are almost invariably present.

Moderately Increased Compliance. This, the most common subgroup, consists of patients between the ends of the spectrum represented by the first and second groups. These patients have severe, chronic MR and exhibit variable degrees of enlargement of the left atrium, associated with significant elevation of the left atrial pressure, and these two factors (in association with age) determine the likelihood that atrial fibrillation will ensue.

Clinical Manifestations

History

The nature and severity of symptoms in patients with chronic MR are functions of a combination of interrelated factors including the severity of MR; the rate of its progression; the level of left atrial, pulmonary venous, and pulmonary arterial pressures; the presence of episodic or chronic atrial tachyarrhythmias; and the presence of associated valvular, myocardial, or coronary artery disease. Symptoms may occur with preserved left ventricular contractile function in patients with chronic MR who have severely elevated pulmonary venous pressures or atrial fibrillation. In other

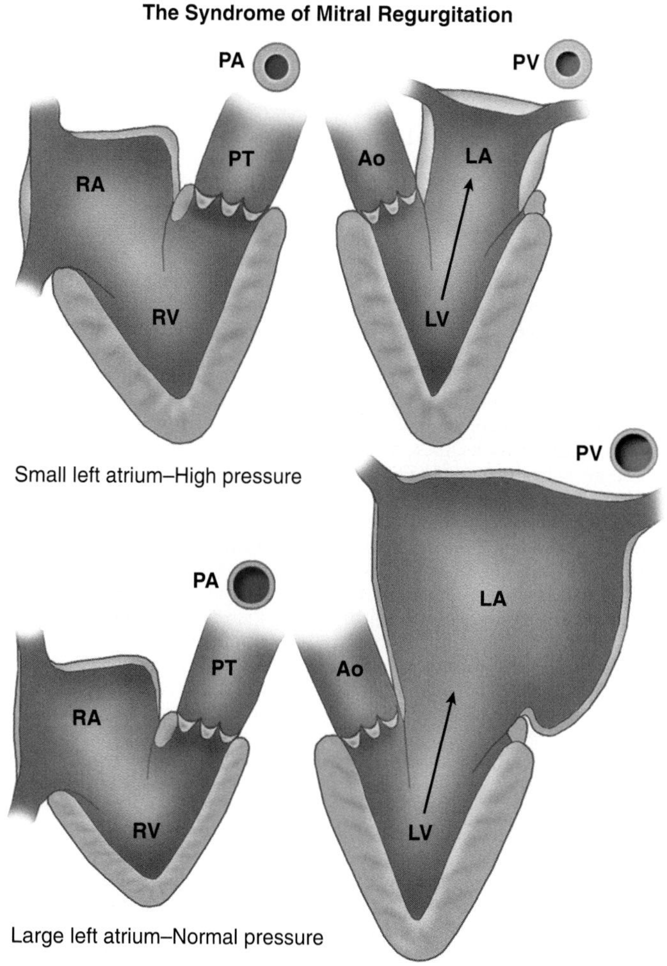

FIGURE 57–13 Diagram depicting the two extremes of the spectrum in pure mitral regurgitation. When severe mitral regurgitation appears suddenly in individuals with previously normal or near-normal hearts (top), the left atrium (LA) is relatively small and the high pressure within it is reflected back into the pulmonary vessels and right ventricle (RV). The anatomical indicator of this latter physiological event is severe hypertrophy of the LA and RV walls and marked intimal proliferation and medial hypertrophy of the pulmonary arteries (PA), arterioles, and veins (PV). At the other extreme, in patients with severe chronic mitral regurgitation (bottom), the LA cavity is of giant size and its wall is thin. It is thus able to "absorb" the left ventricular (LV) pressure without reflecting it back into the pulmonary vessels or RV. As a consequence, pulmonary vessels remain normal, and the RV wall does not thicken. PT = pulmonary trunk; RA = right atrium. (From Roberts WC, Dangel JC, Bulkley BH: Nonrheumatic valvular cardiac disease: A clinicopathologic survey of 27 different conditions causing valvular dysfunction. Cardiovasc Clin 5:403, 1973.)

patients, symptoms herald left ventricular decompensation. In patients with rheumatic MR, the time interval between the initial attack of rheumatic fever and the development of symptoms tends to be longer in patients than in those with MS and often exceeds two decades. Hemoptysis and systemic embolization are less common in patients with isolated or predominant MR than in those with MS. The development of atrial fibrillation affects the course adversely but perhaps not as dramatically as in MS. On the other hand, chronic weakness and fatigue secondary to a low cardiac output are more prominent features in MR.

Most patients with MR of rheumatic origin have only mild disability, unless regurgitation progresses as a result of chronic rheumatic activity, infective endocarditis, or rupture of the chordae tendineae. However, the indolent course of MR may be deceptive. By the time that symptoms secondary to a reduced cardiac output and/or pulmonary congestion become apparent, serious and sometimes even irreversible left ventricular dysfunction may have developed.

In patients with severe, chronic MR who have a greatly enlarged left atrium and relatively mild left atrial hypertension (patients with increased left atrial compliance [second subgroup], described earlier), pulmonary vascular resistance does not usually rise markedly. Instead, the major symptoms, fatigue and exhaustion, are related to the depressed cardiac output. Right-sided heart failure, characterized by congestive hepatomegaly, edema, and ascites, is prominent in patients with acute MR, elevated pulmonary vascular resistance, and pulmonary hypertension. Angina pectoris is rare unless coronary artery disease coexists.

NATURAL HISTORY. This is variable and depends on a combination of the volume of regurgitation, the state of the myocardium, and the cause of the underlying disorder. Asymptomatic patients with mild primary MR usually remain in a stable state for many years. Severe regurgitation develops in only a small percentage of these patients, most commonly because of intervening infective endocarditis or rupture of the chordae tendineae. In patients with mild MR related to MVP, the rate of progression in severity of MR is highly variable; in most patients progression is gradual unless a ruptured chordae or flail leaflet supervenes.[81] Regurgitation tends to progress more rapidly in patients with connective tissue diseases, such as Marfan syndrome, than in those with chronic MR of rheumatic origin. Acute rheumatic fever is a frequent cause of isolated, severe MR in adolescents in developing nations, and these patients often have a rapidly progressive course.

Because the natural history of severe MR has been altered greatly by surgical intervention, it is difficult now to predict the course of patients who receive medical therapy alone. However, Horstkotte and associates[32] reported a 5-year survival of only 30 percent in patients who were candidates for operation (presumably because of symptoms) but who declined (see Fig. 57–4). Among patients with severe MR resulting from flail leaflets, Ling and Enriquez-Sarano[82] reported an annual mortality rate of 6.3 percent; at 10 years 90 percent died or underwent surgical correction. This latter series included many patients who were initially symptomatic or had left ventricular dysfunction or atrial fibrillation and thus might be considered to be a higher risk. However, even among asymptomatic patients with initially normal left and right ventricular ejection fractions,[83] severe MR is associated with a high rate of symptoms or left ventricular dysfunction requiring surgery, and surgery is nearly unavoidable over the course of 10 years (Fig. 57–14).

Physical Examination

Palpation of the arterial pulse is helpful in differentiating AS from MR, both of which may produce a prominent systolic murmur both at the base of the heart and at the apex. The carotid arterial upstroke is sharp in severe MR and delayed in AS; the volume of the pulse may be normal or reduced in the presence of heart failure. The cardiac impulse, like the arterial pulse, is brisk and hyperdynamic. It is displaced to the left, and a prominent left ventricular filling wave is frequently palpable. Systolic expansion of the enlarged left atrium may result in a late systolic thrust in the parasternal region, which may be confused with right ventricular enlargement.

AUSCULTATION

With severe, chronic MR due to defective valve cusps, S_1, produced by mitral valve closure, is usually diminished. Wide splitting of S_2 is common and results from the shortening of left ventricular ejection and an earlier A_2 as a consequence of reduced resistance to left ventricular outflow. In patients with MR who have severe pulmonary hypertension, P_2 is louder than A_2. The abnormal increase in the flow rate across the mitral orifice during the rapid filling phase is often associated with an S_3, which should not be interpreted as a feature of heart failure in these patients, and this may be accompanied by a brief diastolic rumble.

The *systolic murmur* is the most prominent physical finding; it must be differentiated from the systolic murmur of AS, TR, and ventricular septal defect. In most patients with severe MR, the systolic murmur commences immediately after the soft S_1 and continues beyond and may obscure the A_2 because of the persisting pressure difference between the left ventricle and left atrium after aortic valve closure. The holosystolic murmur of chronic MR is usually constant in intensity, blowing, high-pitched, and loudest at the apex with radiation to the left axilla and left infrascapular area. However, radiation toward the sternum or the aortic area may occur with abnormalities of the posterior leaflet and is particularly common in patients with MVP involving this leaflet. The murmur shows little change even in the presence of large beat-to-beat variations of left ventricular stroke volume, as occur in atrial fibrillation. This contrasts with most midsystolic (ejection) murmurs, such as in AS, which vary greatly in intensity with stroke volume and therefore with the duration of diastole. There is little correlation between the intensity of the systolic murmur and the severity of MR. Indeed, in patients with severe MR due to left ventricular dilation, acute myocardial infarction, or paraprosthetic valvular regurgitation, or in those who have marked emphysema, obesity, chest deformity, or a prosthetic heart valve, the systolic murmur may be barely audible or even absent, a condition referred to as *silent MR*.

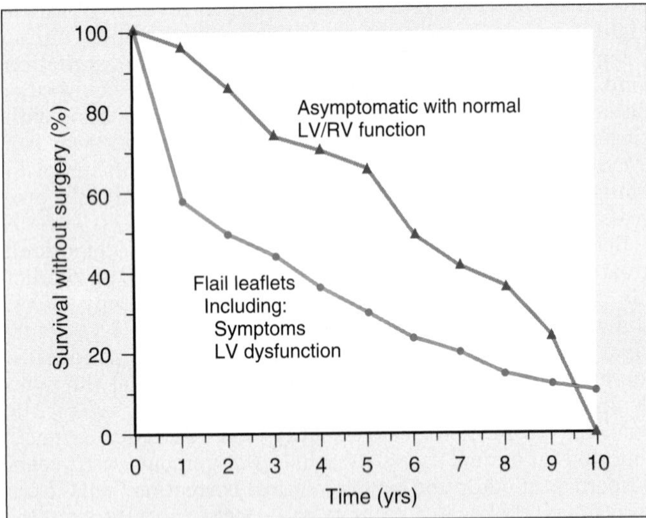

FIGURE 57–14 Two series examining the natural history of patients with severe mitral regurgitation (MR), including a series of patients with flail mitral leaflets reported by Ling and associates (magenta), many of whom were symptomatic, had atrial fibrillation, or had evidence of left ventricular (LV) dysfunction, and a second series reported by Rosen and associates (blue) who initially were asymptomatic with normal LV and right ventricular (RV) function. Although the patients with flail leaflets had a steeper initial attrition rate, both series demonstrated that patients with severe MR have a very low likelihood of remaining stable and asymptomatic over the course of 10 years. (Adapted from Ling LH, Enriquez-Sarano M, Seward JB, et al: Clinical outcome of mitral regurgitation due to flail leaflet. N Engl J Med 335:1417, 1996; and Rosen SF, Borer JS, Hochreiter C, et al: Natural history of the asymptomatic patient with severe mitral regurgitation secondary to mitral valve prolapse and normal right and left ventricular performance. Am J Cardiol 74:374, 1994.)

The murmur of MR may be holosystolic, late systolic, or early systolic. When the murmur is confined to late systole, the regurgitation is usually not severe and may be secondary to prolapse of the mitral valve or to papillary muscle dysfunction. These causes of MR are frequently associated with a normal S_1 because initial closure of the mitral valve cusps may be unimpaired. The late systolic murmur of papillary muscle dysfunction is particularly variable; it may become accentuated or holosystolic during acute myocardial ischemia and often disappears when ischemia is relieved. A midsystolic click preceding a mid to late systolic murmur and the response of that murmur to a number of maneuvers, helps establish the diagnosis of MVP. Early systolic murmurs are typical of *acute* MR. When the left atrial *v* wave is markedly elevated in acute MR, the murmur may diminish or disappear in late systole as the reverse pressure gradient declines. As noted previously, a short, low-pitched diastolic murmur following S_3 may be audible in patients with severe MR, even without accompanying MS.

Dynamic Auscultation. The holosystolic murmur of MR varies little during respiration. However, sudden standing and amyl nitrite inhalation usually diminish the murmur (Table 57–5), whereas squatting augments it. The late systolic murmur of MVP behaves in the opposite direction, decreasing in duration with squatting and increasing in duration with standing. The holosystolic MR murmur is reduced during the strain of the Valsalva maneuver and shows a left-sided response (i.e., a transient overshoot that occurs six to eight beats following release of the strain). The murmur of MR is usually intensified by isometric exercise, differentiating it from the systolic murmurs of valvular AS and hypertrophic obstructive cardiomyopathy, both of which are reduced by this intervention. The murmur of MR caused by left ventricular dilation *decreases* in intensity and duration following effective therapy with cardiac glycosides, diuretics, rest, and particularly vasodilators.

Differential Diagnosis. The holosystolic murmur of MR resembles that produced by a ventricular septal defect. However, the latter is usually loudest at the sternal border rather than the apex and is often accompanied by a parasternal, rather than an apical, thrill. The murmur of MR may also be confused with that of TR, but the latter is usually heard best along the left sternal border, is augmented during inspiration, and is accompanied by a prominent *v* wave and *y* descent in the jugular venous pulse.

When the chordae tendineae to the posterior leaflet of the mitral valve rupture, the regurgitant jet is often directed anteriorly, so that it impinges on the atrial septum adjacent to the aortic root and causes a systolic murmur that is most prominent at the base of the heart. This murmur can be confused with that of AS. On the other hand, when the chordae tendineae to the anterior leaflet rupture, the jet is usually directed to the posterior wall of the left atrium, and the murmur may be transmitted to the spine or even to the top of the head.

Patients with rheumatic disease of the mitral valve exhibit a spectrum of abnormalities, ranging from pure MS to pure MR. The presence of an S_3, a rapid left ventricular filling wave and left ventricular impulse on palpation, and a soft S_1 all favor predominant MR. In contrast, an accentuated S_1, a prominent OS with a short A_2-OS interval, and a soft, short

TABLE 57–5 Effect of Various Interventions on Systolic Murmurs

Intervention	Hypertrophic Obstructive Cardiomyopathy	Aortic Stenosis	Mitral Regurgitation	Mitral Valve Prolapse
Valsalva	↑	↓	↓	↑ or ↓
Standing	↑	↑ or unchanged	↓	↑
Handgrip or squatting	↓	↓ or unchanged	↑	↓
Supine position with legs elevated	↓	↑ or unchanged	Unchanged	↓
Exercise	↑	↑ or unchanged	↓	↑
Amyl nitrite	↑↑	↑	↓	↑
Isoproterenol	↑↑	↑	↓	↑

Modified from Paraskos JA: Combined valvular disease. *In* Dalen JE, Alpert JS, Rahimtoola SH (eds): Valvular Heart Disease. 3rd ed. Philadelphia, Lippincott Williams & Wilkins, 2000, p 332.

↑↑ = markedly increased.

systolic murmur all point to predominant MS. Elucidation of the predominant valvular lesion may be complicated by the presence of a holosystolic murmur of TR in patients with pure MS and pulmonary hypertension; this murmur may sometimes be heard at the apex when the right ventricle is greatly enlarged and may therefore be mistaken for the murmur of MR.

Laboratory Examination

ELECTROCARDIOGRAPHY. The principal ECG findings are left atrial enlargement and atrial fibrillation. ECG evidence of left ventricular enlargement occurs in about one-third of patients with severe MR. Approximately 15 percent of patients exhibit ECG evidence of right ventricular hypertrophy, a change that reflects the presence of pulmonary hypertension of sufficient severity to counterbalance the hypertrophied left ventricle of MR.

RADIOLOGICAL FINDINGS. Cardiomegaly with left ventricular enlargement, and particularly with left atrial enlargement, is a common finding in patients with chronic, severe MR (see Fig. 12–20). Although the left atrium may be severely enlarged, there is little correlation between left atrial size and pressure. Interstitial edema with Kerley B lines is frequently seen in patients with acute MR or with progressive left ventricular failure.

In patients with combined MS and MR, overall cardiac enlargement and particularly left atrial dilation are prominent findings. However, it is often difficult to determine which lesion is predominant from the plain chest roentgenogram because distinguishing between right and left ventricular enlargement may not be possible. Predominant MS is suggested by relatively mild cardiomegaly (principally straightening of the left cardiac border) and significant changes in the lung fields, whereas predominant MR is more likely when the heart is greatly enlarged and the changes in the lungs are relatively inconspicuous. Chronic MR is almost always the dominant lesion when the left atrium is aneurysmally dilated. *Calcification of the mitral annulus,* an important cause of MR in the elderly, is most prominent in the posterior third of the cardiac silhouette. The lesion is best visualized on chest films exposed in the lateral or right anterior oblique projections, in which it appears as a dense, coarse, C-shaped opacity (see Fig. 12–21).

ECHOCARDIOGRAPHY (see Chap. 11). In patients with severe MR, *two-dimensional echocardiography* shows enlargement of the left atrium and left ventricle, with increased systolic motion of both chambers. The underlying cause of the regurgitation, e.g., rupture of chordae tendineae, MVP (see Fig. 11–61), rheumatic mitral disease, a flail leaflet (see Fig. 57–8A), vegetations (see Chap. 58), and left ventricular dilation (see Fig. 57–8B; see also Fig. 11–57) can often be determined on the transthoracic echocardiogram. It may also show calcification of the mitral annulus as a band of dense echoes between the mitral apparatus and the posterior wall of the heart. This technique is also useful for estimating the hemodynamic consequences of MR; in patients with left ventricular dysfunction, end-diastolic and end-systolic volumes are increased and the ejection fraction and shortening rate may decline.

Doppler echocardiography in MR characteristically reveals a high-velocity jet in the left atrium during systole.[84] Quantitative assessment of the severity of MR has been challenging. The severity of the regurgitation is a function of the distance from the valve that the jet can be detected (see Fig. 11–56) and the size of the left atrium. Qualitative assessment using either color-flow Doppler imaging and pulsed techniques correlates reasonably well with angiographic methods in estimating the severity of MR. However, color-flow jet areas are significantly influenced by the cause of the regurgitation and jet eccentricity, thus limiting the accuracy of this approach.

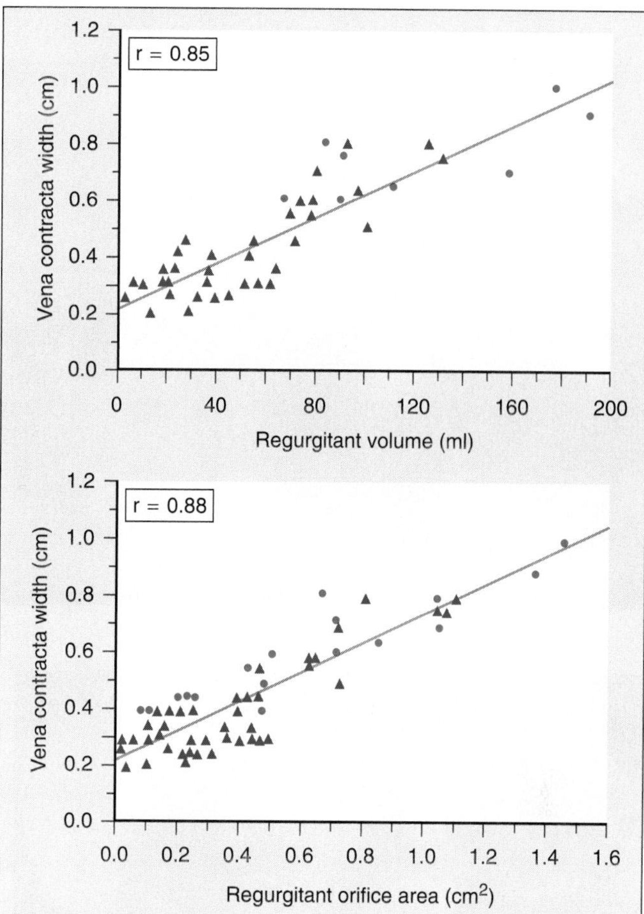

FIGURE 57–15 Linear regression plot showing good correlation between biplane vena contracta width and regurgitant volume (top) and regurgitant orifice area (bottom). Blue triangles indicate central jets and magenta circles indicate eccentric jets. (From Hall SA, Brickner E, Willen DL, et al: Assessment of mitral regurgitation severity by Doppler color-flow mapping of the vena contracta. Circulation 95:636, 1997.)

Quantitative methods to measure regurgitant fraction, regurgitant volume and regurgitant orifice area have greater accuracy in comparison with angiography (see Figs. 11–35 and 11–60),[84,85] and echocardiographic criteria to grade severity of MR have been developed (see Table 11–3).[85a] The vena contracta, defined as the narrowest cross-sectional areas of the regurgitant jet as mapped by color-flow Doppler echocardiography, also predicts the severity of MR (Fig. 57–15).[86,87] The proximal isovelocity surface area method[84] estimates MR severity with isovelocity hemispheric shells as regurgitant flow accelerates toward the mitral orifice. This latter method has not gained widespread acceptance because it is time consuming and has a number of technical limitations. Reversal of flow in the pulmonary veins during systole[88] and a high peak mitral inflow velocity[89] are also useful signs of severe MR. A mitral valve regurgitant index[90] has also been proposed to measure the severity of MR, which incorporates six variables, each graded on a scale from 0 to 3.

Doppler echocardiography is also an important tool to estimate the pulmonary artery systolic pressure and to determine the presence and severity of associated AR or TR.

Transesophageal echocardiography (see Fig. 11–58) is superior to transthoracic echocardiography in assessing the detailed anatomy of the regurgitant mitral valve and in assessing severity of MR.[91,92] Therefore, this technique is useful when the transthoracic image is suboptimal and also when determining whether mitral valve repair is feasible or whether MVR is necessary.[92a] Three-dimensional transthoracic echocardiography and three-dimensional color

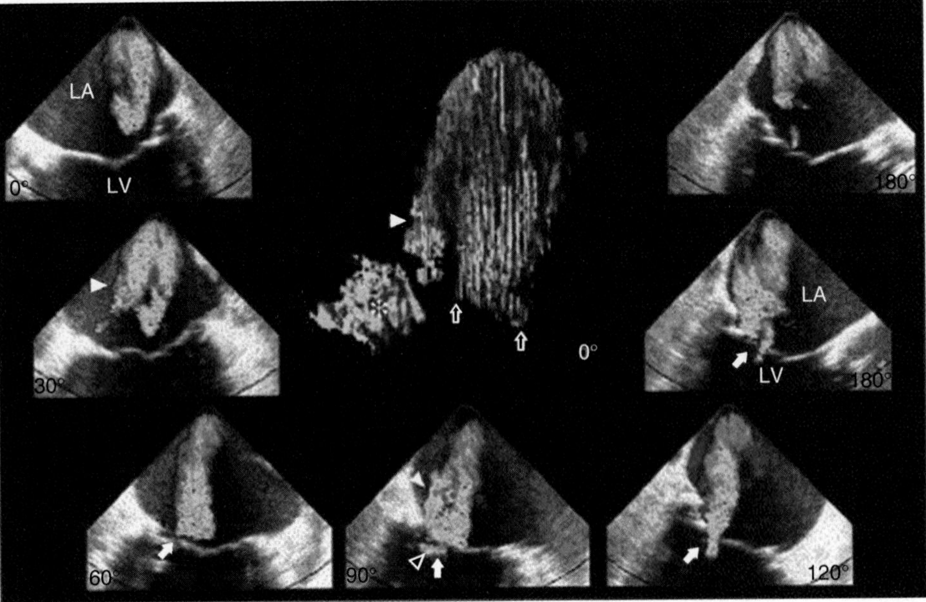

B

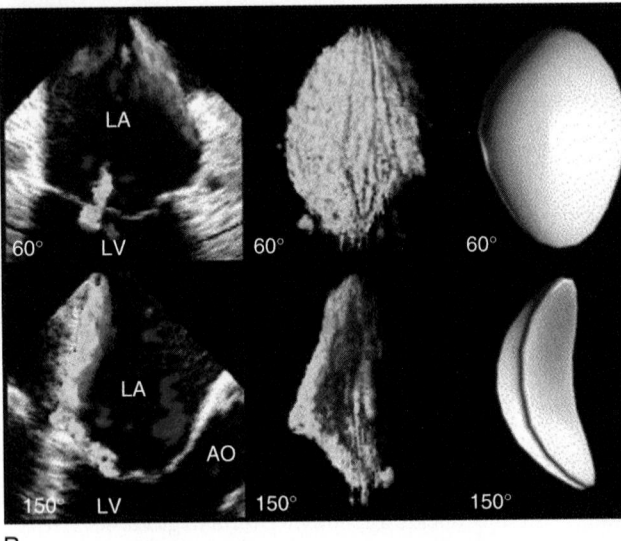

FIGURE 57–16 Three-dimensional color Doppler examination of the mitral valve. **A,** Central jet in a patient with moderate-to-severe mitral regurgitation (MR). The origin of the jet can be visualized (arrows) from multiple views from 60 to 150 degrees. The open arrows in the three-dimensional reconstruction show the extension of the regurgitant orifice, which consists of a large linear coaptation defect of the commissures. **B,** Eccentric MR jet with a "spoon" pattern in a patient with anterior leaflet prolapse. The two-dimensional view at 60 degrees can visualize only a portion of the jet at its origin. The two objects at the right represent surface reconstructions of jet geometry. LA = left atrium; LV = left ventricle. (From De Simone R, Glombitza G, Vahl CF, et al: Three-dimensional color Doppler: A clinical study in patients with mitral regurgitation. J Am Coll Cardiol 33:1646, 1999.)

Doppler[93] have also been reported to help elucidate the mechanism of MR (Fig. 57–16; see also Fig. 11–59).

Exercise echocardiography is helpful in determining severity of MR and hemodynamic abnormalities (such as pulmonary hypertension) during exercise.[94] This is a useful, objective means to evaluate symptoms in patients who appear to have only mild MR at rest and, alternatively, to determine functional status and dynamic changes in hemodynamics in patients who otherwise appear stable and asymptomatic.

Radionuclide Angiography (see Chap. 13). Although echocardiography is the imaging method most suited for routine evaluation of structure, function, and MR severity, gated blood pool nuclear imaging or first-pass angiography may be helpful in instances in which the echo images are suboptimal, there is a discrepancy between the clinical and the echocardiographic information, or there is a need for more precise measurement of left ventricular ejection fraction.[1] In addition, right ventricular function can be assessed, and the regurgitant fraction can be estimated from the ratio of left ventricular to right ventricular stroke volume. In patients with MR and impaired left ventricular function, the ejection fraction fails to rise normally during exercise. Radionuclide angiograms are useful for interval follow-up, and progressive decreases in resting ejection fraction into the low-normal range, or progressive increases in left ventricular end-diastolic and/or end-systolic volume, often suggest that surgical treatment is necessary (discussed later).

Left Ventricular Angiocardiography. The prompt appearance of contrast material in the left atrium following its injection into the left ventricle indicates the presence of MR. The injection should be rapid enough to permit left ventricular opacification but slow enough to avoid the development of premature ventricular contractions, which can induce spurious regurgitation.

The regurgitant volume can be determined from the difference between the total left ventricular stroke volume, estimated by angiocardiography, and the simultaneous measurement of the effective forward stroke volume by the Fick method. In patients with severe MR, the regurgitant volume may approach, and even exceed, the effective forward stroke volume. Qualitative but clinically useful estimates of the severity of MR may be made by cineangiographic observation of the degree of opacification of the left atrium and pulmonary veins following the injection of contrast material into the left ventricle.

The cause of the regurgitation (e.g., prolapse of the mitral valve) and a flail leaflet can often be distinguished by angiography, but this assessment has largely been superceded by echocardiography in most institutions. MR secondary to rheumatic heart disease is characterized angiographically by a central regurgitant jet and by thickened leaflets that exhibit reduced motion. In regurgitation due to other causes, particularly dilation or calcification of the mitral annulus or ruptured chordae tendineae and papillary muscles, the systolic jet may be eccentric, and the valves consist of thin filaments that display excessive motion.

Magnetic Resonance Imaging (see Chap. 14). Cardiac magnetic resonance imaging (MRI) provides accurate measurements of regurgitant flow that correlate well with quantitative Doppler imaging.[95] It is also the most accurate noninvasive technique for measuring ventricular end-diastolic volume, end-systolic volume, and mass. Detailed visualization of mitral valve structure and function is obtained more reliably with echocardiography.

Management

Medical Treatment

The role of pharmacological therapy for MR remains a subject of uncertainty and some debate. Although there is no doubt that afterload reduction therapy is indicated and, indeed, may be lifesaving, in patients with *acute* MR, the indications for such therapy in patients with *chronic* MR are much less clear. Because afterload is not excessive in most patients with chronic MR, in whom systolic shortening is facilitated by the reduced systolic wall stress, systemic vasodilator therapy to reduce afterload further may not provide additional benefit. Acute administration of nitroprusside, nifedipine, and angiotensin-converting enzyme (ACE) inhibitors to severely symptomatic patients has been demonstrated to alter hemodynamics favorably in some studies, but these effects may not pertain to asymptomatic patients with preserved systolic function. Several small studies of chronic therapy with ACE inhibitors, ranging from 4 weeks to 6 months have failed to provide evidence of hemodynamic benefit,[96] and there are no long-term studies, and no randomized trials, with which to make definitive recommendations. One study investigating oral enalapril treatment in 12 patients with MVP and chronic MR did demonstrate over the course of 6 months that ACE inhibition resulted in significant reductions in end-diastolic and end-systolic volumes and in ventricular mass, along with a significant increase in ejection fraction.[97] It is noteworthy, however, that the mean systolic blood pressure at baseline was 136 ± 15 mm Hg (which was reduced significantly by enalapril), indicating that a high proportion of these patients were hypertensive and that the improvement in left ventricular volume and function was related to blood pressure control. Currently, there is a lack of convincing data that ACE inhibitors affect left ventricular volumes or systolic function favorably in the absence of symptoms or hypertension, and current guidelines do not recommend the use of these agents for chronic therapy.[1,2] An exception would be those patients with severe chronic MR, with symptoms or left ventricular dysfunction (or both) who are not candidates for surgery because of age or other comorbidities. These patients should receive standard, aggressive management for heart failure with ACE inhibitors and beta-adrenergic blocking agents (see Chap. 23).

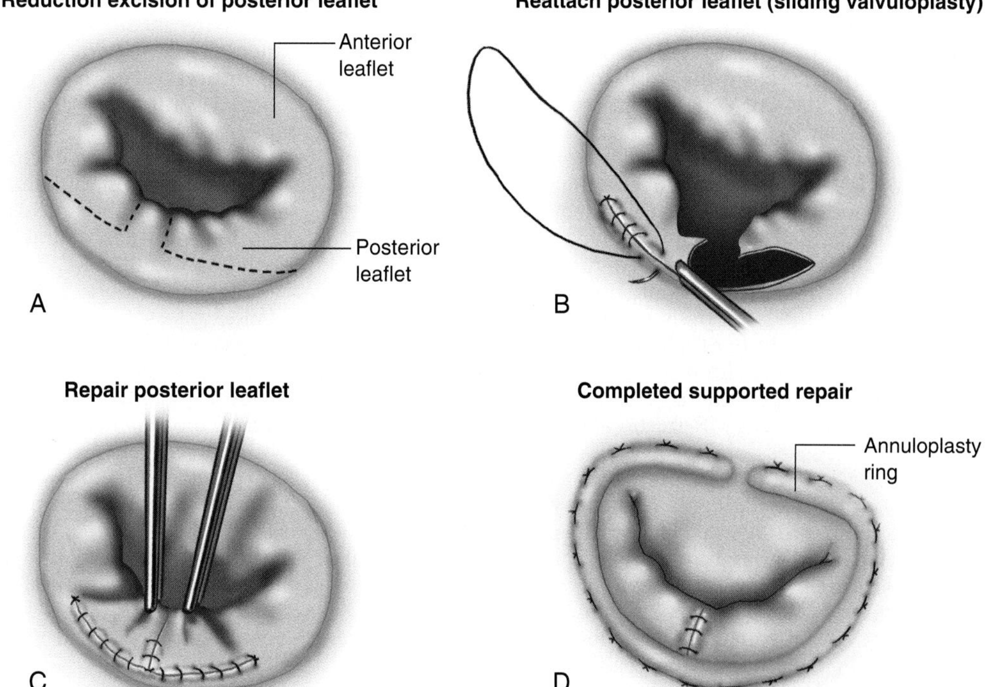

FIGURE 57–17 Mitral valve repair (**A** to **D**) employing reduction excision and reattachment of the posterior leaflet with implantation of an annuloplasty ring. (From Doty DB [ed]: Cardiac Surgery: Operative Technique. St. Louis, Mosby–Year Book, 1997, p 259.)

The accumulating experimental data suggest that beta-blocking drugs may be more beneficial than ACE inhibitors in preserving or improving left ventricular function.[57,71,98,99] Although conceptually attractive, at present there are no clinical data with which to justify chronic beta-blocker therapy.

As do all patients with valvular lesions, patients with MR require appropriate prophylaxis to prevent infective endocarditis (see Chap. 58). All patients with atrial fibrillation, paroxysmal or chronic, should receive chronic anticoagulation.

Surgical treatment should be considered for patients with functional disability and/or for patients with no symptoms or only mild symptoms but with progressively deteriorating left ventricular function or progressively increasing left ventricular dimensions as documented by noninvasive studies.[1,2] The indications for surgery are discussed subsequently.

In patients considered for surgery, two-dimensional transthoracic or transesophageal echocardiography with Doppler echocardiography and color-flow Doppler imaging provide detailed assessment of mitral valve structure and function. However, left-heart catheterization, left ventricular angiocardiography, and coronary arteriography are indicated for the following: (1) in evaluating a discrepancy between echocardiographic findings and the clinical picture; (2) in detecting and assessing the severity of any associated valvular lesions; and (3) in determining the presence and assessing the extent of coronary artery disease.

Surgical Treatment

Without surgical treatment, the prognosis for patients with MR and heart failure is poor (see Fig. 57–4). When operative treatment is being considered, the chronic and often slowly but relentlessly progressive nature of MR must be weighed against the immediate risks and long-term uncertainties attendant on surgery, especially if MVR is required. Surgical mortality depends on the patient's clinical and hemodynamic status (particularly the function of the left ventricle); on the presence of comorbid conditions such as renal, hepatic, or pulmonary disease; and on the skill and experience of the surgical team.[55] The decision to replace or to reconstruct the valve (Fig. 57–17) is of critical importance. Replacement involves the operative risk, as well as the risks of thromboembolism and anticoagulation in patients receiving mechanical prostheses; of late structural valve deterioration in patients receiving bioprostheses; and of late mortality, especially in patients with associated coronary artery disease who require coronary artery bypass grafting (see Table 57–3). Surgical mortality does not depend significantly on *which* of the currently used tissue or mechanical valve prostheses is selected.

Mitral valve repair consists of reconstruction of the valve, which usually is accompanied by an mitral annuloplasty employing a rigid or a flexible prosthetic ring (see Fig. 57–17).[100-103a] Prolapsed valves causing severe MR are usually treated with resection of the prolapsing segment with plication and reinforcement of the annulus. Replacing, reimplanting, elongating, or shortening of chordae tendineae; splitting the papillary muscles; and repairing the subvalvular apparatus have been successful in selected patients with pure or predominant MR in whom subvalvular pathology contributes to the MR.[100-104] Reconstruction of the mitral valve is most often successful in (1) children and adolescents with pliable valves; (2) adults with MR secondary to MVP; (3) annular dilation; (4) papillary muscle secondary to ischemia, dysfunction, or rupture; or (5) chordal rupture and perforation of a mitral leaflet due to infective endocarditis. These procedures are less likely to be successful in older patients with the rigid, calcified, deformed valves of rheumatic heart disease or those with severe subvalvular chordal thickening, mitral annular calcification, and major loss of leaflet substance. Many of the latter patients require MVR, which is also usually the procedure of choice for patients with badly scarred mitral valves who have previously undergone mitral valve repair. Young patients in developing countries who have severe rheumatic MR in the absence of active carditis may undergo successful repair.

Ischemic MR following rupture of a papillary muscle head during acute myocardial infarction may be managed by reattaching the papillary muscle to adjacent myocardium or by MVR. Episodic MR due to transient ischemia is often eliminated by coronary revascularization, whereas moderate to severe, chronic MR secondary ischemic heart disease usually requires MVR or repair.[105,106] Ischemic MR secondary to severe annular dilation may be treated by direct or ring annuloplasty. Annuloplasty is also successful in many patients with significant functional MR resulting from dilated cardiomyopathy.[107-109]

Although MVR with a mechanical or bioprosthesis has been used successfully in treating MR for almost four decades,[110] there has been some dissatisfaction with the results of this operation. First, left ventricular function often deteriorates following this procedure, contributing to early and late mortality and late disability. The increase in afterload consequent to abolishing the low impedance leak was first believed to be responsible, but now it is clear that the loss of annular-chordal-papillary muscle continuity (Fig. 57–18) interferes with left ventricular geometry, volume, and

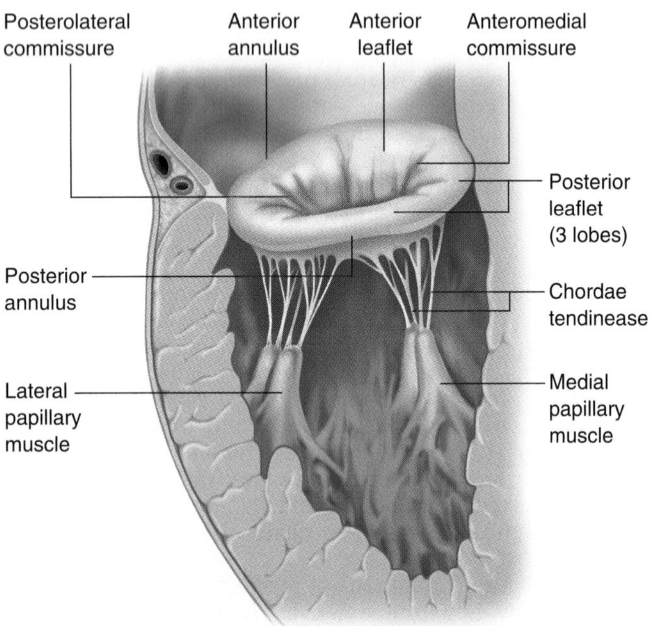

FIGURE 57–18 Continuity of the mitral apparatus and the left ventricular myocardium. Mitral regurgitation (MR) may be caused by any condition that affects the leaflets or the structure and function of the left ventricle. Similarly, a surgical procedure that disrupts the mitral apparatus in an attempt to correct MR has adverse effects on left ventricular geometry, volume, and function. (From Otto CM: Evaluation and management of chronic mitral regurgitation. N Engl J Med 345:740, 2001.)

function in patients who have undergone MVR. This does not occur after mitral valve reconstruction. Indeed, animal experiments have shown convincingly that the normal function of the mitral valve apparatus "primes" the left ventricle for normal contraction and that contraction is prevented when operation causes discontinuity of this apparatus.[57] There is evidence from animal experiments and from human patients that preservation of the papillary muscle and its chordal attachments to the mitral annulus is beneficial to postoperative left ventricular function, after both mitral valve reconstruction[76] and in MVR. Thus, preservation of these tissues, whenever possible, is now considered a critical feature of MVR.[111,112]

A second disadvantage of MVR results from the prosthesis itself. This includes thromboembolism or hemorrhage associated with mechanical prostheses, late mechanical dysfunction of bioprostheses, and the risk of infective endocarditis with all prostheses. For these reasons, increasing efforts are being made to reconstruct the mitral valve whenever possible, especially in patients with isolated or predominant MR.[100-103] The Society of Thoracic Surgeons National Database Committee reported an operative mortality rate of less than 2 percent in 3309 patients undergoing isolated mitral valve repair in 2002.[113] This compares favorably to the 6 percent operative mortality for the 4064 patients undergoing isolated MVR.

Intraoperative transesophageal color-flow Doppler mapping is extremely useful in assessing the adequacy of mitral valve repair.[114] In a few patients with persistent severe MR in whom the operative results are unsatisfactory, the problem can usually be corrected immediately, or, if necessary, the valve can be replaced. Left ventricular outflow tract obstruction due to systolic anterior motion of the mitral valve occurs in 5 to 10 percent of patients following mitral valve repair. The causes are not clear, but they may include excess valvular tissue with severe leaflet redundancy and/or an interventricular septum bulging into a small left ventricle. These complications may also be recognized intraoperatively by transesophageal echocardiography. Treatment with volume-loading and beta-blocking agents is often helpful. The obstruction usually disappears with time; if it does not, reoperation and re-repair or MVR may be necessary.

Progressive decrease in the prevalence of rheumatic heart disease (involving severely damaged valves that often are not suitable for reconstructive surgery) and a simultaneous increase in degenerative causes of MR (including MVP and rupture of chordae tendineae) as well as in ischemic MR are increasing the number of patients in whom reconstruction is carried out.[76,114a] In many centers in the United States, approximately two-thirds of all patients requiring operation for pure or predominant MR now receive reconstructive procedures, and the remainder undergo MVR. However, at the current time, the Society of Thoracic Surgeons National Cardiac Surgery Database indicates that most patients in the United States undergoing mitral valve surgery receive MVR rather than repair.[113,114a] Mitral valve repair is technically a more demanding procedure than is MVR, with a distinct learning curve for the surgeon. Furthermore, some regurgitant valves, particularly those that are thickened, severely deformed, calcified, and partly stenotic, are not suitable for reconstruction, and patients with these valves require MVR.[65,66,110,115] In addition, MR recurs after valve repair in a subset of patient with degenerative valve disease.[116]

Minimally invasive surgical techniques utilizing a small, low, asymmetrical sternotomy or anterior thoracotomy[117,118] and percutaneous cardiopulmonary bypass,[119] although quite demanding technically, have been found to be less traumatic and can be employed for both valve repair and replacement. This approach has been reported to reduce cost, improve cosmetic results, and shorten the recovery time.[120] However, it also is technically difficult and is successfully performed by only a few cardiac surgeons.

SURGICAL RESULTS. Mortality rates of 3 to 9 percent are now common in many centers for patients with pure or predominant MR (NYHA Class II or III) who undergo elective isolated MVR. The Society of Thoracic Surgeons National Database Committee reported an overall operative mortality rate of 6.04 percent in 16,105 patients undergoing isolated MVR between 1994 and 1997 (see Table 57–3); this compares with 4 percent for isolated aortic valve replacement (AVR) and 2 to 3 percent for isolated mitral valve repair.[55,113] The combination of MVR with coronary artery bypass grafting was associated with a mortality rate of 13.3 percent during this same period. The mortality rate is higher (≤25 percent) in older patients with severe left ventricular dysfunction, especially when MR is secondary to myocardial ischemia, when pulmonary or renal function is impaired, or when the operation must be carried out as an emergency. Age per se is no barrier to successful surgery; MVR can be performed in patients older than 75 years of age if their general health status is adequate; however, surgery in these patients has a higher risk than in younger patients.[76]

Surgical treatment substantially improves survival in patients with symptomatic MR. Preoperative factors such as age less than 60 years, NYHA Class II, a cardiac index exceeding 2.0 liter/min/m^2, a left ventricular end-diastolic pressure less than 12 mm Hg, and a normal ejection fraction and end-systolic volume all correlate with excellent immediate and long-term survival rates. Both preoperative ejection fraction (see Fig. 57–10) and end-systolic diameter (see Fig. 57–11) are important predictors of short-term and long-term outcomes.[76,77] Excellent survival is observed in patients with end-systolic diameters less than 45 mm and ejection fractions of 0.60 or more. Intermediate outcomes are seen in patients with end-systolic diameters between 45 and 52 mm and ejection fractions between 0.50 and 0.60. Poor outcomes are associated with values beyond these limits.

A large proportion of operative survivors have improved clinical status, quality of life, and exercise tolerance following valve replacement or repair. Severe pulmonary hypertension is reduced, left ventricular end-diastolic volume and mass decrease, and coronary flow reserve increases.[74] Depressed contractile function improves, especially if the papillary muscles and chordal attachment to the annulus remain intact.[121] However, patients with MR who have marked left ventricular dysfunction preoperatively sometimes remain symptomatic with a depressed ejection fraction despite a technically satisfactory surgical procedure.[76] Indeed, progressive left ventricular dysfunction and death from heart failure may occur in adults. Recovery of left ventricular function is much better in children.[122] Long-term survival in patients with predominant MR who undergo MVR may be poorer than in those with pure MS or with mixed stenotic and regurgitant lesions, presumably because left ventricular dysfunction may be quite advanced and largely irreversible by the time patients with pure MR develop serious symptoms. Ten-year survival was 76 percent in patients in NYHA Class I or II versus 48 percent in patients in Class III or IV.[123] Thus, every effort should be made to operate on patients before they develop serious symptoms. However, even though operating on patients with MR is clearly desirable before they develop marked left ventricular dysfunction[1,57,76] and despite the limitations of the results of surgical treatment, operation is still indicated in most patients with left ventricular dysfunction because conservative therapy has little to offer. Postoperative survival rates are lower in patients in atrial fibrillation than those in sinus rhythm.[124] As with patients with MS, the arrhythmia by itself does not unfavorably influence outcome but is a marker for older age and other clinical and hemodynamic features associated with less optimal results.

The cause of MR also plays an important role in the outcome following surgical treatment.[65,66,101-105,107,108] In patients in whom mitral dysfunction is secondary to ischemic heart disease, the 5-year survival rate is about 40 percent, whereas in patients with rheumatic MR it is approximately 75 percent. Occlusive coronary artery disease coexisting with, but not the primary cause of, mitral dysfunction requires simultaneous coronary artery bypass grafting and mitral valve repair or replacement[125] and is associated with decreased perioperative and long-term postoperative survival (Fig. 57–19). However, some improvement resulting from mitral valve repair or replacement can be expected even in patients with MR secondary to ischemic heart disease who

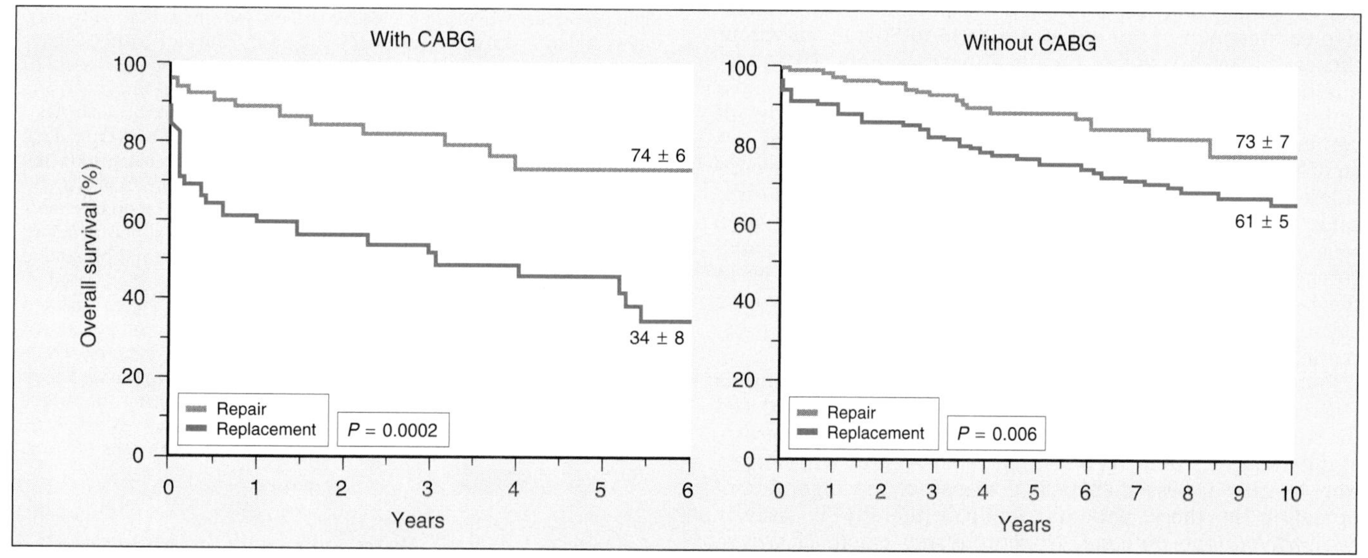

FIGURE 57–19 Plots of overall survival compared for mitral repair and replacement groups in patients who had **(left)** or did not have **(right)** associated coronary artery bypass grafting (CABG). Note that the outcome is better with repair than with replacement in both groups and that the outcome is worse in patients who underwent CABG and mitral valve replacement. (From Enriquez-Sarano M, Schaff HV, Orszulak TA, et al: Valve repair improves the outcome of surgery for mitral regurgitation: A multivariate analysis. Circulation 91:1022, 1995.)

have not responded to medical treatment and now have congestive heart failure, as long as the cardiac index exceeds 1.8 liter/min/m^2 and the ejection fraction is greater than 0.30. When left ventricular dysfunction is more severe, however, the risk of perioperative death becomes very high.[66]

INDICATIONS FOR OPERATION

The threshold for surgical treatment of MR is declining for several reasons. These include the reductions in operative mortality, the improvements in both mitral valve reconstructive procedures and procedures involving prosthetic valves, and the recognition of the poor long-term results in many patients whose MR is corrected only after a long history of symptoms, impaired left ventricular function, atrial fibrillation, or pulmonary hypertension.

A detailed echocardiographic examination should be carried out to assess the likelihood that mitral valve repair, rather than replacement, is possible. In addition, the difference in outcome between these procedures should be weighed when deciding whether or not to proceed. Asymptomatic patients (NYHA Class I) should be considered for mitral valve reconstruction only if they have left ventricular dysfunction (ejection fraction ≤ 0.60 and/or left ventricular end-systolic diameter ≤ 45 mm).[1] Class I patients with normal left ventricular function should be followed clinically and by echocardiography every 6 to 12 months. Rarely, they *may* be considered for operation if atrial fibrillation or pulmonary hypertension is present. At times, a careful history and performance of an exercise test often reveal that these patients are not truly asymptomatic.[1,94] Patients with severe MR who are asymptomatic, who perform well on an exercise test, and who have excellent ventricular function (ejection fraction > 0.70, end-systolic diameter < 40 mm, end-systolic volume < 40 ml/m^2) can be followed by echocardiography every 6 to 12 months. However, operation may be considered even in asymptomatic patients if they are younger than 70 years of age, if they are likely to be candidates for mitral valve repair, and if ventricular function (as reflected by end-systolic diameter and ejection fraction) shows *progressive* deterioration. If MVR is likely to be necessary, a higher threshold for clinical and hemodynamic impairment should be employed than if valve reconstruction is contemplated. Because of the higher operative mortality, older patients (>75 years of age) should, in general, undergo surgery only if they are symptomatic.

In asymptomatic patients with severe MR, a lower threshold for surgery may be entertained in patients with progressive enlargement of the left atrium (>45 to 50 mm) in whom successful mitral valve repair appears highly likely. A number of centers are moving toward a more aggressive surgical approach in which surgery is recommended to *all* patients with severe MR, independent of symptoms of left ventricular function. Such a recommendation should be considered *only* in centers in which the surgical experience indicates that the patient will undergo successful mitral valve repair with a high degree of certainty. Unfortunately, successful mitral valve repair cannot be guaranteed, and even in the best of circumstances, with this approach some young asymptomatic patients will be subjected to the risks of prosthetic valves prematurely and unnecessarily.

Patients with severe MR and moderate or severe symptoms (NYHA Classes II, III, and IV) should generally be considered for surgery. One exception is a patient in whom echocardiography suggests that MVR will be required and whose ejection fraction is less than 0.30. Because of the high risk of operation in these patients, medical therapy is usually advised, but the outcome is poor in any event. However, when mitral valve repair appears possible, even patients with serious left ventricular dysfunction may be considered for operation.[107-109]

ACUTE MITRAL REGURGITATION

The causes of acute MR are shown at the top of Table 57-4. They are diverse and represent acute manifestations of disease processes that may, under other circumstances, cause chronic MR. Especially important causes of acute MR are spontaneous rupture of chordae tendineae, infective endocarditis with disruption of valve leaflets or chordal rupture, ischemic dysfunction or rupture of a papillary muscle, and malfunction of a prosthetic valve.

One major hemodynamic difference between acute and chronic MR derives from the differences in left atrial compliance, as illustrated in Figure 57-13. Acute, severe MR causes a marked reduction of forward stroke volume, a slight reduction of end-systolic volume, and an increase in end-diastolic volume. Patients who develop acute, severe MR usually have a normal-sized left atrium (normal or reduced left atrial compliance [first subgroup]). The left atrial pressure rises abruptly, which often leads to pulmonary edema, marked elevation of pulmonary vascular resistance, and right-sided heart failure.

Because the *v* wave is markedly elevated in patients with acute, severe MR, the reverse pressure gradient between the left ventricle and left atrium declines at the end of systole, and the murmur may be decrescendo rather than holosystolic, ending well before A_2. It is usually lower pitched and softer than the murmur of chronic MR. A left-sided S_4 is frequently found.[130] Pulmonary hypertension, which is common in patients with acute MR, may increase the intensity of P_2 and the murmurs of pulmonary and TR may also develop along with a right-sided S_4. In patients with severe, acute MR, a *v* wave (late systolic pressure rise) in the pulmonary artery pressure pulse (see Fig. 57-12; see also Fig. 17-5) may rarely cause premature closure of the pulmonary valve, an early P_2, and paradoxical splitting of S_2. Acute MR, even if severe, often does not increase overall cardiac size, as seen on the chest roentgenogram, and may produce only mild left atrial enlargement despite marked elevation of left atrial pressure. In addition, the echocardiogram may show little increase in the internal diameter of either the left atrium or the left ventricle, but increased systolic motion of the left ventricle is prominent. Characteristic features on Doppler echocardiography are the severe jet of MR and elevation of the pulmonary artery systolic pressure.

Medical Management of Acute Mitral Regurgitation. Afterload reduction with afterload reducing agents is of particular importance in treating patients with acute MR. Intravenous nitroprusside may be lifesaving in patients with acute MR due to rupture of the head of a papillary muscle that occurs during an acute myocardial infarction. It may permit stabilization of the patient's condition and thereby allow coronary arteriography and surgery to be performed with the patient in optimal condition. In patients with acute MR who are hypotensive, an inotropic agent such as dobutamine should be administered with the nitroprusside. Intraaortic balloon counterpulsation may be necessary to stabilize the patient as preparations for surgery are made.

Surgical Treatment of Acute Mitral Regurgitation. Emergency surgical treatment may be required for patients with acute left ventricular failure caused by acute MR. Emergency surgery is associated with higher mortality rates than is elective surgery for chronic MR. However, unless patients with acute, severe MR and heart failure are treated aggressively, a fatal outcome is almost certain. If patients with MR secondary to acute myocardial infarction can be stabilized by medical treatment, it is preferable to defer operation until 4 to 6 weeks after the infarction. Vasodilator treatment may be useful during this period. However, medical management should not be prolonged if multisystem (renal and/or pulmonary) failure develops. Intraaortic balloon counterpulsation may be required to stabilize the patient preoperatively. Surgical mortality rates are also higher in patients with acute MR and refractory heart failure (NYHA Class IV), in those in whom a previously implanted prosthetic valve must be replaced because of thromboembolism or valve dysfunction, and in those with active infective endocarditis (of either a natural or a prosthetic valve). Despite the higher surgical risks, the efficacy of early operation has been established in patients with infective endocarditis complicated by medically uncontrollable congestive heart failure and/or recurrent emboli (see Chap. 58). Because fungal endocarditis responds poorly to medical management, the practice now is to recommend valve replacement in these patients *before* the onset of heart failure or embolization.

Mitral Valve Prolapse Syndrome

Etiology and Pathology

DEFINITION. The MVP syndrome has been given many names, including the *systolic click-murmur syndrome, Barlow syndrome, billowing mitral cusp syndrome, myxomatous mitral valve syndrome, floppy valve syndrome,* and *redundant cusp syndrome.*[126-129] It is a variable clinical syndrome that results from diverse pathogenic mechanisms of one or more portions of the mitral valve apparatus, valve leaflets, chordae tendineae, papillary muscle, and valve annulus. The MVP syndrome is one of the most prevalent cardiac valvular abnormalities and was previously thought to affect as much as 5 to 15 percent of the population.[130,131] It now appears likely that overdiagnosis occurred in many individuals, perhaps because of the absence of rigorous echocardiographic criteria. Using such criteria (to be discussed), a community-based study showed that MVP syndrome occurred in only 2.4 percent of the population.[131] The syndrome is twice as frequent in women as in men. However, serious MR occurs more frequently in older men (>50 years) with MVP than in young women with this disorder.

Normally, the mitral valve billows slightly into the left atrium, and an exaggerated finding should be termed *billowing mitral valve.* A "floppy valve" is regarded as an extreme form of billowing. MR occurs when the leaflet edges of the valve do not coapt. With chordal rupture, the prolapsed mitral valve is "flail," which is almost always associated with severe MR. Obviously, these conditions blend into one another, and it is often difficult to distinguish among them.

The criteria for the diagnosis of MVP have been divided into three groups (Table 57–6): (1) major criteria, the presence of one or more of which establishes the diagnosis of MVP; (2) minor criteria, the presence of which cannot be discounted and should raise the suspicion of MVP but which by themselves are not sufficient to establish the diagnosis; and (3) other findings not shown in Table 57–6, which, although often present in patients with MVP, are nonspecific. Superior displacement of the mitral valve leaflets by more than 2 mm above the plane of the annulus is an important two-dimensional echocardiographic criterion,[131,132] and systolic displacement of one or both mitral leaflets into the left atrium in the *parasternal view* improves the specificity of this finding (see Fig. 11–61). The latter criterion avoids overdiagnosis, which may occur with posterior bowing of the mitral valve on M-mode echocardiography and even in the four-chamber view on two-dimensional echocardiography.

ETIOLOGY. Most frequently, MVP occurs as a primary condition that is not associated with other diseases. However, it has also been associated with many conditions. MVP occurs quite commonly in heritable disorders of connective tissue that increase the size of the mitral leaflets and apparatus, including Marfan syndrome (see Chap. 70), Ehlers-Danlos syndrome (see Chap. 70), osteogenesis imperfecta, pseudoxanthoma elasticum, periarteritis nodosa, myotonic dystrophy, von Willebrand disease, hyperthyroidism, and congenital malformations such as Ebstein anomaly of the tricuspid valve, atrial septal defect of the ostium secundum variety, Holt-Oram syndrome, and hypertrophic cardiomyopathy. There may be a higher incidence of MVP in patients with an asthenic habitus and various congenital thoracic deformities, including "straight back" syndrome, pectus excavatum, and a shallow chest. These associations have not been proved using rigorous echocardiographic criteria, and, with the exception of connective tissue disorders, it is not clear how many of these are chance associations.

PATHOLOGY (Fig. 57–20). Findings include myxomatous proliferation of the mitral valve, in which the spongiosa component of the valve (i.e., the middle layer of the leaflet composed of loose, myxomatous material) is unusually prominent,[129,132,133] and the quantity of acid mucopolysaccharide is increased (see Fig. 57–20).[134] Electron microscopy shows a haphazard arrangement of cells with disruption and with fragmentation of collagen fibrils.

In mild cases, the valvular myxoid stroma is enlarged on histological examination, but the leaflets are grossly normal. However, with increasing quantities of myxoid stroma, the leaflets become grossly abnormal, redundant, and prolapsed. Regions of endothelial disruption are common and are possible sites of endocarditis or thrombus formation. The severity of MR depends on the extent of the prolapse. The cusps of the mitral valve, the chordae tendineae, and the annulus all may be affected by myxomatous proliferation. Degeneration of collagen and myxomatous changes within the central core of the chordae tendineae, with associated decreases in tensile strength,[62,133] are primarily responsible for chordal rupture, which often occurs and may intensify the severity of MR. Increased chordal tension resulting from the enlarged area of the valve cusps may play a contributory role. Myxomatous changes in the annulus may result in annular dilation and calcification, further contributing to the severity of MR.

Myxomatous proliferation, although most commonly affecting the mitral valve, has also been described in the tricuspid, aortic, and pulmonic valves, particularly in patients

TABLE 57–6 Diagnostic Criteria in Mitral Valve Prolapse

Criteria
Major Criteria
Auscultation
Mid to late systolic clicks and late systolic murmur or "whoop" alone or in combination at the cardiac apex
Two-dimensional echocardiogram
Marked superior systolic displacement of mitral leaflets (≥2 mm above annulus) with coaptation point at or superior to annular plane
Mild to moderate superior systolic displacement of mitral leaflets with
Chordal rupture
Doppler mitral regurgitation
Annular dilation
Echocardiogram plus auscultation
Mild to moderate superior systolic displacement of mitral leaflets with
Prominent mid to late systolic clicks at the cardiac apex
Apical late systolic or holosystolic murmur in the young patient
Late systolic "whoop"
Minor Criteria
Auscultation
Loud S_1 with an apical holosystolic murmur
Two-dimensional echocardiogram
Isolated mild to moderate superior systolic displacement of the posterior mitral leaflet
Moderate superior systolic displacement of both mitral leaflets
Echocardiogram plus history of
Mild to moderate superior systolic displacement of mitral leaflets with
Focal neurologic attacks or amaurosis fugax in the young patient
First-degree relatives with major criteria

Modified from Perloff JK, Child JS, Edwards JE: New guidelines for the clinical diagnosis of mitral valve prolapse. Am J Cardiol 57:1124, 1986.

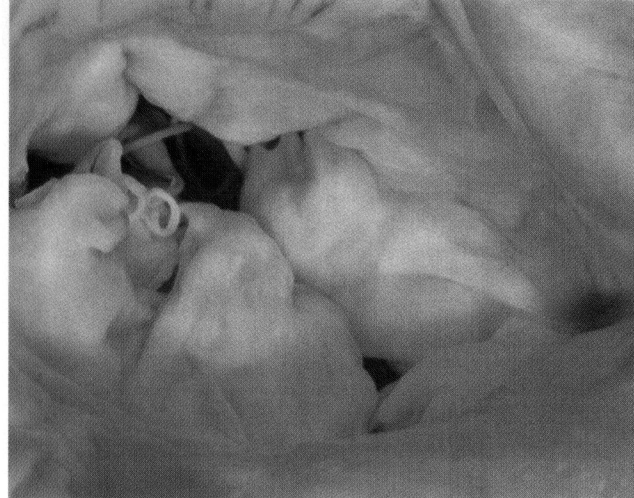

A

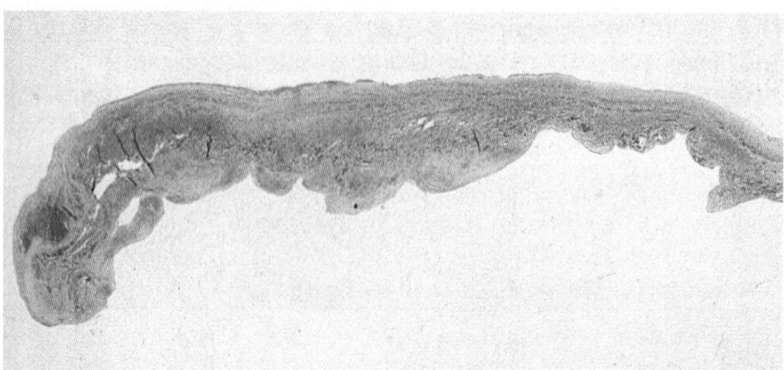

B

FIGURE 57–20 **A,** Myxomatous mitral valve in a patient with severe mitral regurgitation, viewed from the left atrium. The surface area of the valve is increased, with increased folding of the valve surface. Individual scallops of the posterior leaflet are enlarged and redundant. **B,** Histological section of posterior valve leaflet from a patient with mitral valve prolapse. The valve is thickened with marked myxomatous proliferation and interruption of the fibrosa and atrialis by the spongiosa tissue. There are extensive deposits of acid mucopolysaccharides (blue-green staining) expanding the spongiosa and extending into the fibrosa. (From Becker AE, Anderson RH [eds]: Cardiac Pathology: An Integrated Text and Colour Atlas. New York, Raven Press, 1983, pp 4.8 and 4.11.)

with Marfan syndrome, and may lead to regurgitation of these valves as well as the mitral valve.

The MVP syndrome can coexist with rheumatic MS, and it may develop following mitral valvotomy. *Ischemic heart disease* and MVP are both common disorders and sometimes coexist. MVP may also occur secondary to papillary muscle dysfunction. In some patients, MVP has been documented to develop for the first time *following* myocardial infarction. It has been proposed that MVP may *cause* myocardial ischemia by increasing tension on the base of the involved muscle, which may contribute to symptoms in some patients. During systole, the tips of the papillary muscles move basally instead of apically.

Clinical Manifestations

MVP syndrome appears to exhibit a strong hereditary component[126] and in some patients is transmitted as an autosomal dominant trait with varying penetrance. The clinical presentations of the MVP syndrome are diverse. The condition has been observed in patients of all ages and in both sexes. Despite the overestimation of the prevalence in the population referred to earlier, MVP is the most common cause of isolated MR requiring surgical treatment in the United States[128,132] and the most common cardiac condition predisposing patients to infective endocarditis (see Chap 58).[135] Echocardiographic evidence of MVP has been found in most patients with Marfan syndrome and in many of their first-degree relatives.

History

Most patients with MVP are asymptomatic and remain so throughout their lives. In many instances, otherwise asymptomatic patients with MVP suffer from undue anxiety, perhaps precipitated by their having been informed of the presence of heart disease. Although early studies called attention to an "MVP syndrome" with a characteristic systolic nonejection click and various nonspecific symptoms, such as fatigability, palpitations, postural orthostasis, and neuropsychiatric symptoms, as well as symptoms of autonomic dysfunction, these associations have not been confirmed in carefully controlled studies.[132] How, and even whether, these symptoms relate to the presence of MVP is not clear.

Patients may complain of syncope, presyncope, palpitations, chest discomfort, and, when MR is severe, symptoms of diminished cardiac reserve. Chest discomfort may be typical of angina pectoris but is more often atypical in that it is prolonged, not clearly related to exertion, and punctuated by brief attacks or severe stabbing pain at the apex. The discomfort may be secondary to abnormal tension on papillary muscles. In patients with MVP and severe MR, the symptoms of the latter (fatigue, dyspnea, and exercise limitation) are present. Patients with MVP may also develop symptomatic arrhythmias (to be discussed).

Physical Examination

The body weight is often low, and the habitus may be asthenic. Blood pressure is usually normal or low; orthostatic hypotension may be present. As already mentioned, patients with MVP have a higher than expected prevalence of straight back syndrome, scoliosis, and pectus excavatum.[129] MR ranges from nonexistent to severe.

AUSCULTATION

The auscultatory findings unique to the MVP syndrome are best elicited with the diaphragm of the stethoscope. The patient should be examined in the supine, left decubitus, and sitting positions. The most important finding is a nonejection systolic click at least 0.14 second after S_1.[136] This can be differentiated from a systolic ejection click because it occurs *after* the beginning of the carotid pulse upstroke. Occasionally, multiple mid and late systolic clicks are audible, most readily along the lower left sternal border. The clicks are believed to be produced by sudden tensing of the elongated chordae tendineae and of the prolapsing leaflets. They are often, although not invariably, followed by a mid to late crescendo systolic murmur that continues to A_2. This murmur is similar to that produced by papillary muscle dysfunction, which is readily understandable because both result from mid to late systolic MR. In general, the duration of the murmur is a function of the severity of the MR. When the murmur is confined to the latter portion of systole, MR usually is not severe. However, as MR becomes more severe, the murmur commences earlier and ultimately becomes holosystolic.

It is important to emphasize the variability of the physical findings in the MVP syndrome. Some patients exhibit both a midsystolic click and a mid to late systolic murmur; others present with only one of these two findings; still others have only a click on one occasion and only a murmur on another, both on a third examination, and no abnormality at all on a fourth. Conditions other than MVP cause midsystolic clicks; these include tricuspid valve prolapse, atrial septal aneurysms, and extracardiac causes.

Dynamic Auscultation. The auscultatory findings are exquisitely sensitive to physiological and pharmacological interventions, and recognition of the changes induced by these interventions is of great value in the diagnosis of the MVP syndrome (Fig. 57-21 and Table 57-5). The mitral valve begins to prolapse when the reduction of left ventricular volume during systole reaches a critical point at which the valve leaflets no longer coapt; at that instant, the click occurs and the murmur commences. Any maneuver that decreases left ventricular volume, such as a reduction of impedance to left ventricular outflow, a reduction in venous

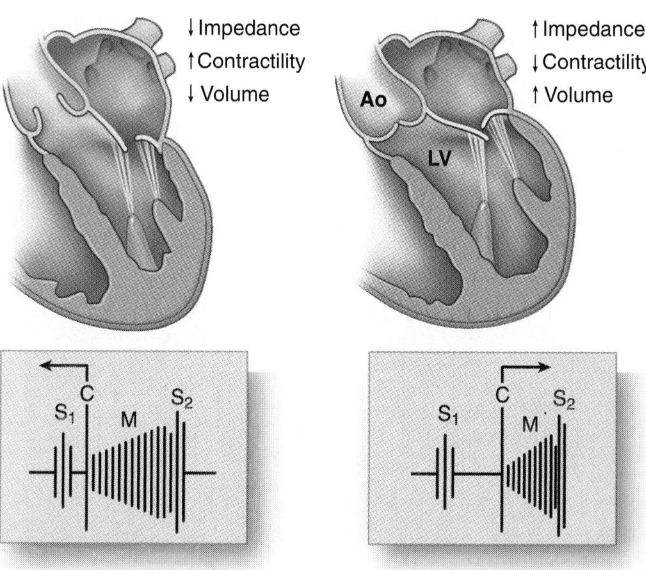

FIGURE 57–21 Dynamic auscultation in mitral valve prolapse. Any maneuver that decreases left ventricular (LV) volume (e.g., decreased venous return, tachycardia, decreased outflow impedance, increased contractility) worsens the mismatch in size between the enlarged mitral valve and LV chamber, resulting in prolapse earlier in systole and movement of the click (C) and murmur (M) toward the first heart sound (S_1). Conversely, maneuvers that increase LV volume (e.g., increased venous return, bradycardia, increased outflow impedance, decreased contractility) delay the occurrence of prolapse, resulting in movement of the click and murmur toward the second heart sound (S_2). Ao = aorta. (Adapted from O'Rourke RA, Crawford MH: The systolic click-murmur syndrome: Clinical recognition and management. Curr Probl Cardiol 1:9, 1976.)

return, tachycardia, or an augmentation of myocardial contractility, results in an earlier occurrence of prolapse during systole. As a consequence, the click and onset of the murmur move closer to S_1. When prolapse is severe and/or left ventricular size is markedly reduced, prolapse may begin with the onset of systole. As a consequence, the click may not be audible, and the murmur may be holosystolic. On the other hand, when left ventricular volume is augmented by an increase in the impedance to left ventricular emptying, an increase in venous return, a reduction of myocardial contractility, or bradycardia, both the click and the onset of the murmur will be delayed.

During the straining phase of the Valsalva maneuver, on sudden standing, and early during the inhalation of amyl nitrite, cardiac size decreases, and both the click and the onset of the murmur occur earlier in systole. In contrast, a sudden change from the standing to the supine position, leg-raising, squatting, maximal isometric exercise, and, to a lesser extent, expiration delay the click and the onset of the murmur. During the overshoot phase of the Valsalva maneuver (i.e., six to eight cycles following release) and with prolongation of the R-R interval, either following a premature contraction or in atrial fibrillation, the click and onset of the murmur are usually delayed, and the intensity of the murmur is reduced. Maneuvers that elevate arterial pressure, such as isometric exercise, increase the intensity of the click and murmur. In general, when the onset of the murmur is delayed, both its duration and intensity are diminished, reflecting a reduction in the severity of MR.

The response to several interventions may be helpful in differentiating obstructive hypertrophic cardiomyopathy from MVP (see Chap. 59). During the strain of the Valsalva maneuver, the murmur of hypertrophic cardiomyopathy increases in intensity, whereas the murmur of MVP becomes longer but usually not louder. The murmur of hypertrophic cardiomyopathy becomes louder after amyl nitrite inhalation, whereas that of MVP does not. Following a premature beat, the murmur of hypertrophic cardiomyopathy increases in intensity and duration, whereas that due to MVP usually remains unchanged or decreases.

Laboratory Examination

ELECTROCARDIOGRAPHY. The ECG is usually normal in asymptomatic patients with MVP. In a minority of asymptomatic patients and in many symptomatic patients, the ECG shows inverted or biphasic T waves and nonspecific ST segment changes in leads II, III, and aVf and occasionally in the anterolateral leads as well.

ARRHYTHMIAS. A spectrum of arrhythmias have been observed in patients with MVP. These include atrial and ventricular premature contractions and supraventricular and ventricular tachyarrhythmias,[132,137] as well as bradyarrhythmias due to sinus node dysfunction or varying degrees of atrioventricular block. The mechanism of the arrhythmias is not clear. Diastolic depolarization of muscle fibers in the anterior mitral leaflet in response to stretch has been demonstrated experimentally, and the abnormal stretch of the prolapsed leaflet may be of pathogenetic significance.

Paroxysmal supraventricular tachycardia is the most common sustained tachyarrhythmia in patients with MVP and may be related to what may be an increased incidence of left atrioventricular bypass tracts. The incidence of MVP among patients with Wolff-Parkinson-White syndrome is increased. There is also an increased association between MVP and prolongation of the QT interval, and this association may play a role in the pathogenesis of serious ventricular arrhythmias. Patients with MVP have an increased incidence of abnormal late potentials on signal-averaged ECGs, as well as reduced heart rate variability.

ECHOCARDIOGRAPHY (see Chap. 11). Echocardiography plays a key role in the diagnosis of MVP and has been most useful in the delineation of this syndrome (Fig. 57–22; see also Figs. 11–61 and 11–62).[138] The most common finding on M-mode echocardiography is abrupt posterior movement of the posterior leaflet or of both mitral leaflets in midsystole with the leaflet interface greater than 2 mm posterior to the C-D line. This movement occurs simultaneously with the systolic click. An alternate finding is pansystolic posterior prolapse of one or both leaflets, giving rise to a U- or hammock-shaped configuration 3 mm or more posterior to the C-D segment.

To establish the diagnosis, the two-dimensional echocardiogram must show that one or both mitral valve leaflets billow by at least 2 mm into the left atrium during systole in the long-axis view.[131,132,139] Thickening of the involved leaflet to greater than 5 mm supports the diagnosis. Findings of more severe myxomatous disease include increased leaflet area, leaflet redundancy, chordal elongation and annular dilation (see Fig. 57–22; see also Fig. 11–61). These findings are also helpful in identifying patients at significant risk for developing severe MR or infective endocarditis (Table 57–7). The mitral annular diameter is often abnormally increased. Transesophageal echocardiography provides additional details regarding integrity of the mitral valve apparatus, such as rupture of chordae tendineae. In MR secondary to MVP, the echocardiogram also provides valuable information regarding left ventricular size and function.

The variability in physical findings in this syndrome, already commented on, extends to the echocardiogram. Thus, some patients have a systolic click with or without a murmur and show no evidence of MVP on the echocardiogram. Conversely, the echocardiographic findings of MVP may be observed in patients without a click or murmur. Others have both the typical echocardiographic and auscultatory features. The echocardiographic findings of MVP have been reported to occur in a large number of first-degree relatives of patients with established MVP. Two-dimensional echocardiography has also revealed prolapse of the tricuspid and aortic valves in approximately 20 percent of patients with MVP.[132] Conversely, however, prolapse of the tricuspid and aortic valves occurs *uncommonly* in patients without prolapse of the mitral valve.

Doppler echocardiography frequently reveals mild MR that is not always associated with an audible murmur. Color-flow Doppler echocardiography is useful in identifying the

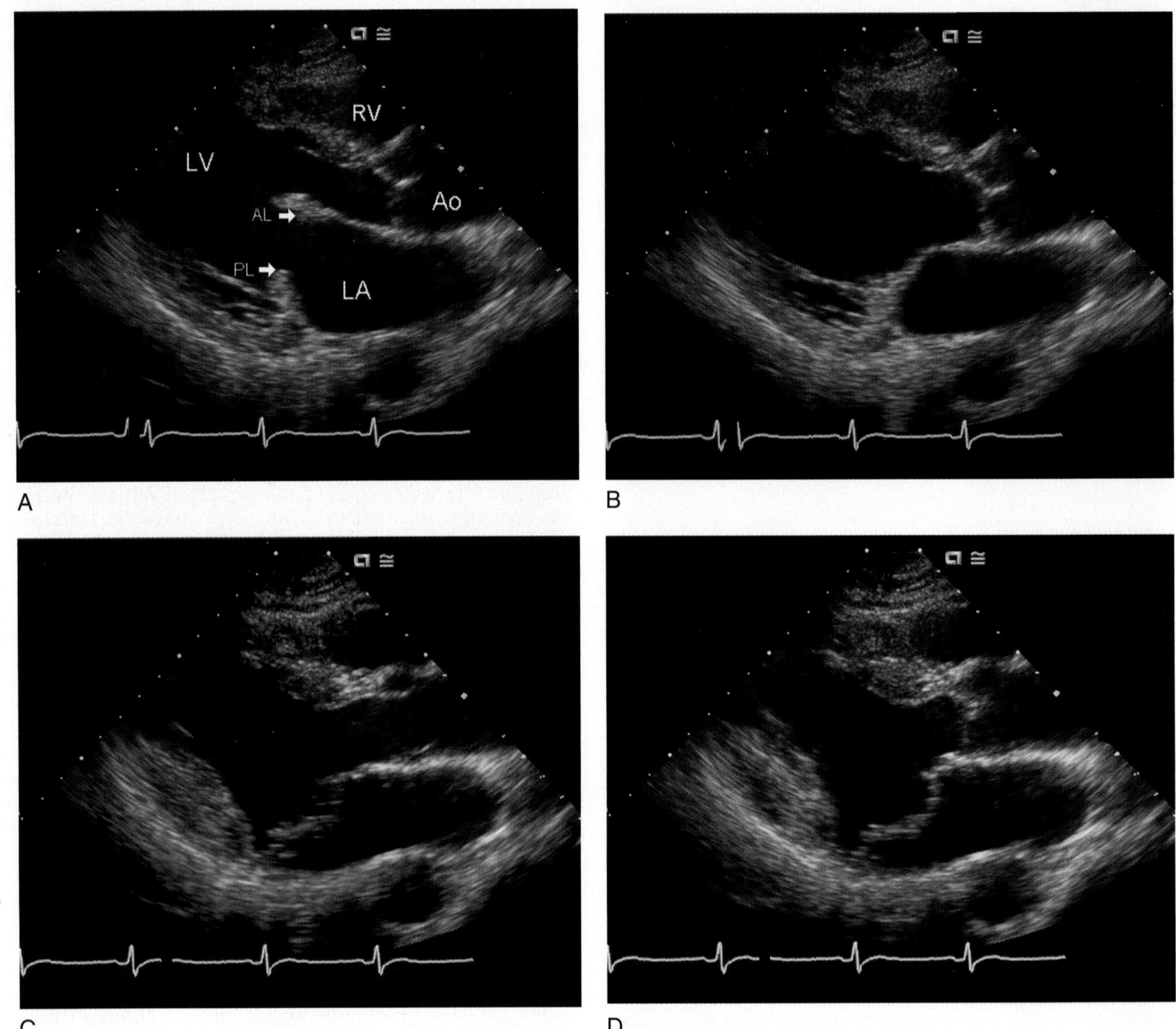

FIGURE 57–22 Parasternal long-axis two-dimensional echocardiographic images in a 41-year-old man with mitral valve prolapse and auscultatory findings of a midsystolic click and mitral regurgitation (MR). **A,** End-diastolic image. The mitral valve leaflets are severely thickened, and the anterior leaflet (AL) is elongated. **B** to **D,** Serial images from early systole to midsystole, demonstrating bileaflet prolapse, Color-flow imaging in this patient demonstrated severe MR. Patients with these findings are at increased risk of complications, such as infective endocarditis, systemic emboli, and heart failure. Ao = aorta; LA = left atrium; LV = left ventricle; PL = posterior leaflet; RV = right ventricle.

TABLE 57–7 Predictors of Clinical Outcome in Mitral Valve Prolapse

	Survival	Valve Surgery	Arrbythmias/Sudden Death	Endocarditis
Age	+++*	+++	–	–
Gender	++	++	–	–
Leaflet thickness or redundancy	+++	+++	++++	++++
Severity of mitral regurgitation	++++	++++	++++	++++
Systolic click	+	–	–	–
Left ventricular dilation	+	++++	++	–
Left atrial dilation	–	++	+	–

From Otto CM: Valvular Heart Disease. 2nd ed. Philadelphia, WB Saunders, 2004, p 376.

*The symbols indicate the relative predictive value of each variable for the listed clinical outcomes on a scale of no predictive value (–) to strongly predictive (++++).

location and severity of the regurgitant jets. MR is moderate or severe in about 10 percent of patients with MVP, most commonly in men older than 50 years of age.[140]

STRESS SCINTIGRAPHY. The differential diagnosis between two common conditions—MVP associated with atypical chest pain and ECG abnormalities and primary coronary artery disease associated with MVP—may be aided by exercise ECG. However, myocardial perfusion scintigraphy using thallium-201 or sestamibi during pharmacological exercise stress (see Chap. 13) is more specific. When findings are normal, i.e., when there is no evidence of stress-induced regional myocardial ischemia, the diagnosis of MVP unrelated to ischemic heart disease is favored.

ANGIOGRAPHY. The configuration of the left ventriculogram during systole is helpful in confirming the diagnosis of MVP. The right anterior oblique projection is most useful for defining the posterior leaflet of the mitral valve, and the left anterior oblique projection is most useful for studying the anterior leaflet. The most helpful sign is extension of the mitral leaflet tissue inferiorly and posteriorly to the point of attachment of the mitral leaflets to the mitral annulus. Angiography may also reveal scalloped edges of the leaflets, reflecting redundancy of tissue. Other abnormalities noted on angiography of some patients with MVP include dilation, decreased systolic contraction, and calcification of the mitral annulus and poor contraction of the basal portion of the left ventricle.

MAGNETIC RESONANCE IMAGING AND CARDIAC COMPUTED TOMOGRAPHY. These advanced imaging techniques can help in determining the extent of MVP and left ventricular function in patients with suboptimal echocardiographic examinations (see Fig. 15–11). MRI is also useful for evaluating the presence and severity of MR.

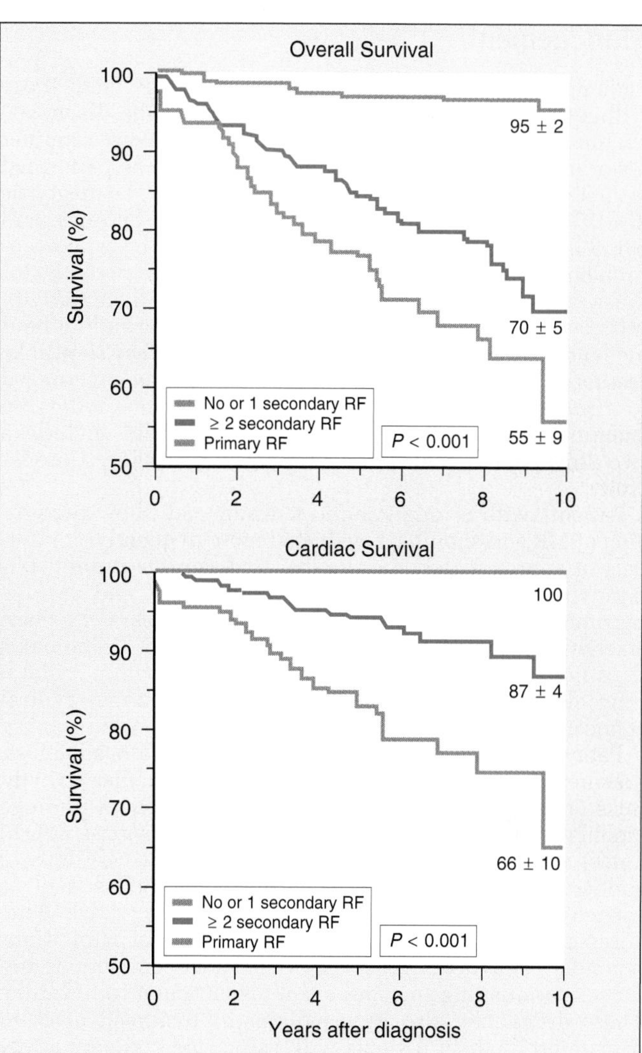

FIGURE 57–23 Survival in patients with mitral valve prolapse according to categories of baseline risk factors (RFs). Primary RFs were moderate-to-severe mitral regurgitation (MR) and ejection fraction less than 0.50. Secondary RFs were mild MR, left atrium larger than 40 mm, flail leaflet, atrial fibrillation, and age older than 50 years. (Adapted from Avierinos JF, Gersh BJ, Melton LJ, et al: Natural history of asymptomatic mitral valve prolapse in the community. Circulation 106:1355, 2002.)

NATURAL HISTORY

The outlook for patients with MVP in general is excellent; most remain asymptomatic for many years without any change in clinical or laboratory findings.[1,126,131,141,142] Zuppiroli and associates monitored 316 patients with MVP for an average of more than 8 years; 70 percent were women and 29 percent had familial MVP.[141] Serious complications (cardiac death, need for cardiac surgery, acute infective endocarditis, or cerebral embolic events) occurred at a rate of only 1 per 100 patient years, and 4 percent of patients died during the 8 years. In contrast, Avierinos and colleagues[143] observed a much more aggressive natural history in 833 patients with MVP, with a 19 percent mortality rate at 10 years and a 20 percent rate of MVP-related events, including heart failure, atrial fibrillation, cerebrovascular events, arterial thromboembolism, and endocarditis. The apparent differences between these two series can be reconciled by the finding in the latter series that patients with MVP could be risk stratified on the basis of several factors (Fig. 57-23).[143] The primary risk factors were moderate to severe MR and/or left ventricular ejection fraction less than 0.50, and secondary risk factors included mild MR, left atrial dimension greater than 40 mm, flail leaflet, and age older than 50 years. Patients with a primary risk factor had excessive mortality and morbidity, as did those with two or more secondary risk factors.[143] The data of Zuppiroli and coworkers[141] are concordant with these observations, since their patients had a high likelihood of dying or having MVP-related complications if they were men (17 percent with events), were older than 45 years of age (15 percent), or had a holosystolic murmur (67 percent) or left atrial dimension greater than 40 mm (50 percent). In keeping with these findings, other series that have reported a lower prevalence of adverse sequelae of MVP[131,144] have included relatively fewer patients with these risk factors. Variables associated with an adverse outcome are summarized in Table 57-7.

Progressive MR with gradual increase in left atrial and left ventricular size, atrial fibrillation, pulmonary hypertension, and the development of congestive heart failure is the most frequent serious complication,[1,141] occurring in about 15 percent of patients over a 10- to 15-year period. Patients with the MVP syndrome are also at risk of developing infective endocarditis.[135] Both severe MR and endocarditis develop more frequently in patients with both murmurs and clicks than in those with an isolated click, in patients with thickened (>5-mm diameter) and redundant mitral valve leaflets, and in men older than 50 years of age (see Table 57-7). In many patients, rupture of chordae tendineae is responsible for the precipitation and/or intensification of the MR.[81] Infective endocarditis often aggravates the severity of MR and therefore the need for surgical treatment.

Acute hemiplegia, transient ischemic attacks, cerebellar infarcts, amaurosis fugax, and retinal arteriolar occlusions have been reported to occur more frequently in patients with MVP syndrome, suggesting that cerebral emboli are unusually common in this condition.[132,143] It has been proposed that these neurological complications are associated with loss of endothelial continuity and tearing of the endocardium overlying the myxomatous valve, which initiates platelet aggregation and the formation of mural platelet-fibrin complexes. Although it has been proposed that embolization secondary to MVP may be a significant cause for unexplained strokes in young people without cerebrovascular disease, a large case-control study showed no association between MVP and ischemic neurological events in persons younger than 45 years of age.[144]

Mitral Valve Prolapse and Sudden Death. The relation between the MVP syndrome and sudden death is not clear. However, the best evidence suggests that MVP increases the risk of sudden death slightly,[126,129,132,145,146] especially in patients with severe MR or severe valvular deformity, and those with complex ventricular arrhythmias, QT interval prolongation, and a history of syncope and palpitations.

Management

Patients with the physical findings of MVP (and those without such findings who have been given the diagnosis) should have two-dimensional and color-flow Doppler echocardiography. This procedure should also be performed in first-degree relatives of patients with MVP.[1] The diagnosis of MVP requires definitive echocardiographic findings, and overdiagnosis and incorrect "labeling" have been a major problem with this condition. *Asymptomatic patients* (or those whose principal complaint is anxiety), with no arrhythmias evident on a routine extended ECG tracing and without evidence of MR, have an excellent prognosis. They should be reassured about the favorable prognosis and be encouraged to engage in normal life styles but should have follow-up examinations every 3 to 5 years. This should include a two-dimensional echocardiogram and a color-flow Doppler study.

Patients with a long systolic murmur may show progression of MR and should be evaluated more frequently, at intervals of approximately 12 months. *Endocarditis prophylaxis* is advisable for patients with a typical click and systolic murmur and in those with only a click who have the characteristic echocardiographic features of MVP. Prophylaxis does *not* appear to be necessary for patients with a midsystolic click without a systolic murmur or without typical echocardiographic findings (see Chap. 58).[1]

Patients with a history of palpitations, lightheadedness, dizziness, or syncope or those who have ventricular arrhythmias or QT prolongation on a routine ECG should undergo ambulatory (24-hour) ECG monitoring and/or exercise ECG to detect arrhythmias. Because of the risk, albeit very low, of sudden death, further electrophysiological studies may be carried out to characterize arrhythmias if they exist. Beta-adrenergic blockers are useful in the treatment of palpitations secondary to frequent premature ventricular contractions and for self-terminating episodes of supraventricular tachycardia. These drugs may also be useful in the treatment of chest discomfort, both in patients with associated coronary artery disease and in those with normal coronary vessels in whom the symptoms may be due to regional ischemia secondary to MVP. Radiofrequency ablation of atrioventricular bypass tracts is useful for frequent or prolonged episodes of supraventricular tachycardia.

Aspirin should be given to patients with MVP who have had a documented focal neurological event and in whom no other cause, such as a left atrial thrombus or atrial fibrillation, is apparent.

Patients with MVP and severe MR should be treated similarly to other patients with severe MR and may require mitral valve surgery. Reconstructive surgery without valve replacement is usually possible (see Fig. 57–17).[100-102,103a,104] Therefore, the threshold for surgical treatment in these patients is lower than in patients with MR in whom MVR may be necessary, providing that patients are referred to a surgical team with established success in mitral valve repair. Most mitral valve reconstructions for MR are now carried out in patients with MVP. Resection of the most deformed leaflet segment, usually the middle scallop of the posterior leaflet, and insertion of an annuloplasty ring to reduce the dilated annulus is the most commonly employed procedure. Repair or anterior leaflet prolapse is more challenging. Rupture of the chordae tendineae to the anterior leaflet can sometimes be treated by chordal transfer from the posterior leaflet. In other patients, shortening of the chordae tendineae and/or papillary muscle is necessary. The average operative mortality is 2 to 3 percent,[113] and long-term studies demonstrate excellent durability of mitral valve repair in most patients.[100-102] However, MR recurs in a subset of patients,[116,147] at which point it is usually necessary to perform MVR.

Coronary arteriography should be performed in patients with angina pectoris on effort and/or ischemic ECG changes or those with abnormalities on a stress myocardial perfusion scan. Treatment should take into account both the responsiveness of symptoms to medical management and the coronary anatomy.

Although this discussion has focused attention on complications of the MVP syndrome, it should not be forgotten that, on the whole, this is a benign condition and that the vast majority of patients with this syndrome remain asymptomatic for their entire lives and require, at most, observation every few years and reassurance.

Aortic Stenosis

Etiology and Pathology

Obstruction to left ventricular outflow is localized most commonly at the aortic valve and is discussed in this section. However, obstruction may also occur above the valve (supravalvular stenosis) or below the valve (discrete subvalvular stenosis) (see Chap. 56), or it may be caused by hypertrophic obstructive cardiomyopathy (see Chap. 59). Valvular AS has three principal causes: congenital, rheumatic, and degenerative (Fig. 57–24). Valvular AS *without accompanying mitral valve disease* is more common in men than in women, rarely occurs on a rheumatic basis, and is usually either congenital or degenerative in origin.[1,148,149]

CONGENITAL AORTIC STENOSIS (see Chap. 56). Congenital malformations of the aortic valve may be unicuspid, bicuspid, or tricuspid, or there may be a dome-shaped diaphragm. *Unicuspid valves* produce severe obstruction in infancy and are the most frequent malformations found in fatal valvular AS in children younger than 1 year of age. Congenitally *bicuspid valves* may be stenotic with commissural fusion at birth, but more often they are not responsible for serious narrowing of the aortic orifice during childhood. Their abnormal architecture induces turbulent flow, which traumatizes the leaflets and leads to fibrosis, increased rigidity, calcification of the leaflets, and narrowing of the aortic orifice in adulthood (see Fig. 57–24B).[148] With fibrosis and immobilization of the valve, in some patients a congenitally bicuspid valve may become purely or predominantly regurgitant. Infective endocarditis developing on a congenitally bicuspid valve may also lead to severe regurgitation.

Bicuspid aortic valves often have familial clustering consistent with an autosomal dominant inheritance with incomplete penetrance,[150,151] such that echocardiographic screening of first-degree relatives is justified. Bicuspid valves are also often associated with dilation of the ascending aorta[151,152] related to accelerated degeneration of the aortic media.[153] In some cases, this may progress to frank aneurysm formation. Dilation of the aortic root is another cause for development of AR in patients with bicuspid valves.

A third form of a congenitally malformed valve is *tricuspid,* with the cusps of unequal size and some commissural fusion. Although many of these valves retain normal function throughout life, it has been postulated that the turbulent flow produced by the mild congenital architectural abnormality may lead to fibrosis and ultimately to calcification and stenosis. Tricuspid stenotic aortic valves in adults may be congenital, rheumatic, or degenerative in origin.

ACQUIRED AORTIC STENOSIS. Rheumatic AS results from adhesions and fusions of the commissures and cusps and vascularization of the leaflets of the valve ring, leading

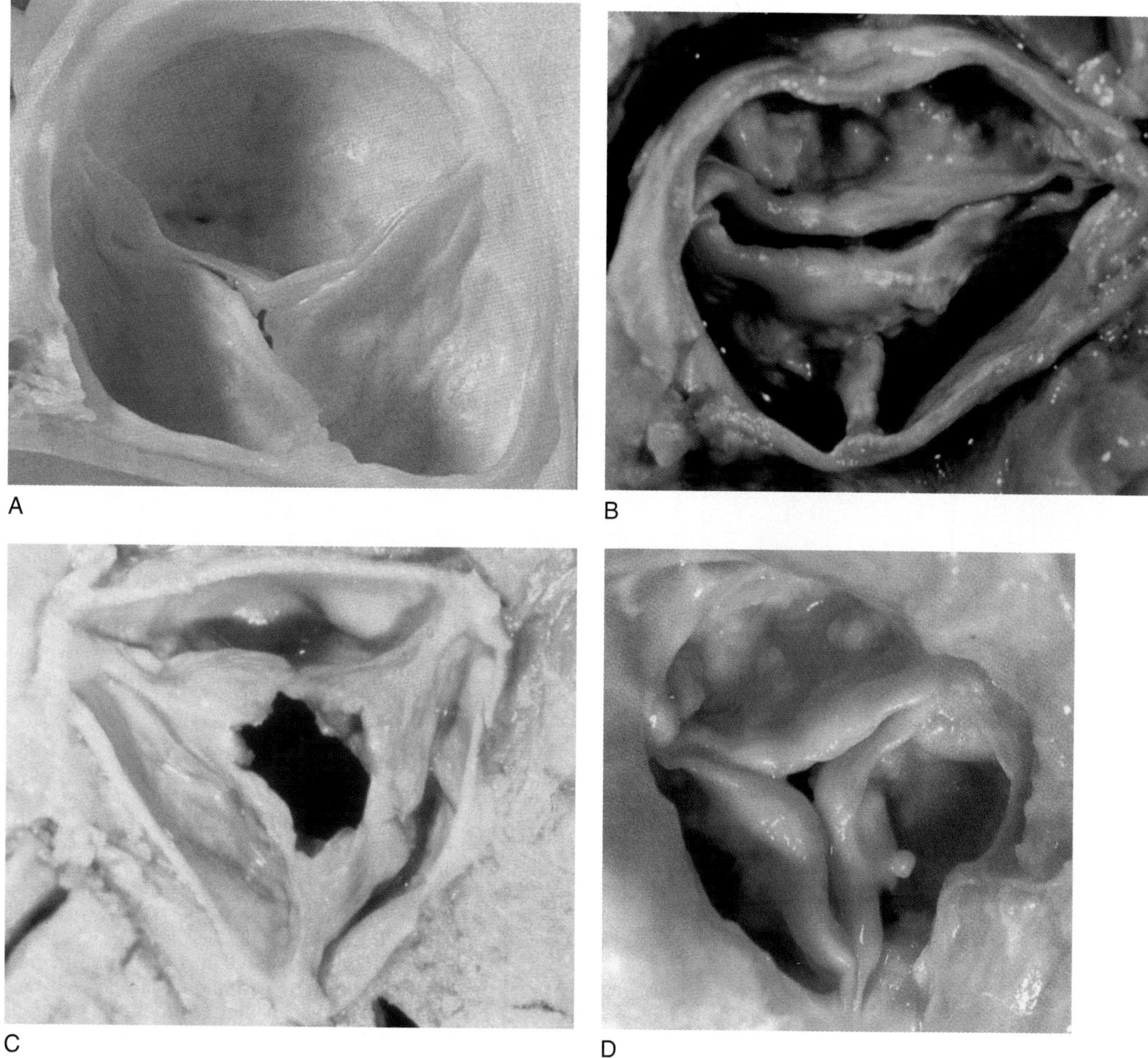

FIGURE 57–24 Major types of aortic valve stenosis. **A,** Normal aortic valve. **B,** Congenital bicuspid aortic stenosis. A false raphe is present at 6 o'clock. **C,** Rheumatic aortic stenosis. The commissures are fused with a fixed central orifice. **D,** Calcific degenerative aortic stenosis. (**A** and **D,** From Manabe H, Yutani C [eds]: Atlas of Valvular Heart Disease. Singapore, Churchill Livingstone, 1998, pp 6 and 131; **B** and **C,** Courtesy of William C. Roberts, MD.)

to retraction and stiffening of the free borders of the cusps. Calcific nodules develop on both surfaces, and the orifice is reduced to a small round or triangular opening (see Fig. 57–24C). As a consequence, the rheumatic valve is often regurgitant as well as stenotic. The heart frequently exhibits other stigmata of rheumatic disease, especially mitral valve involvement. With the decline in rheumatic fever in industrialized nations, rheumatic AS is decreasing in frequency.

Age-related degenerative calcific (formerly termed *senile*) AS is now the most common cause of AS in adults and the most frequent reason for AVR in patients with AS.[154] In a population-based echocardiographic study, 2 percent of persons 65 years of age or older had frank calcific AS, whereas 29 percent exhibited age-related aortic valve sclerosis without stenosis, defined by Otto and colleagues as irregular thickening of the aortic valve leaflets detected by echocardiography without significant obstruction and believed to represent a milder and/or earlier disease process.[155] Although once considered to represent the result of years of normal mechanical stress on an otherwise normal valve, the evolving concept is that the degenerative process represents proliferative and inflammatory changes, with lipid accumulation, upregulation of ACE activity, and infiltration of macrophages and T lymphocytes,[154,156-159] ultimately leading to bone formation[160,161] in a manner analogous to vascular calcification. Progressive calcification, initially along the flexion lines at their bases, leads to immobilization of the cusps (see Fig. 57–24D). This process rarely leads to significant AR.

Age-related AS or degenerative calcific AS shares common risk factors with mitral annular calcification,[59-61] and the two conditions often coexist. The risk factors for the development of calcific AS are similar to those for vascular atherosclerosis and include elevated serum levels of LDL cholesterol and Lp(a), diabetes, smoking, and hypertension.[162-164] Not surprisingly, age-related aortic valve sclerosis is associated with an increased risk of cardiovascular death and myocardial

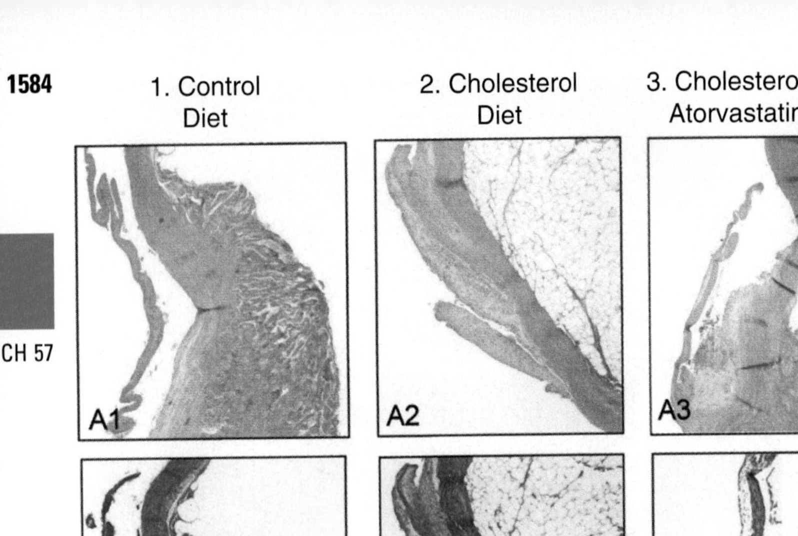

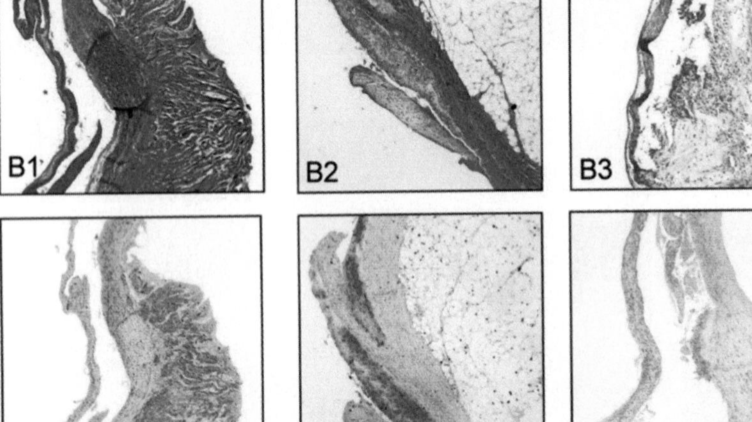

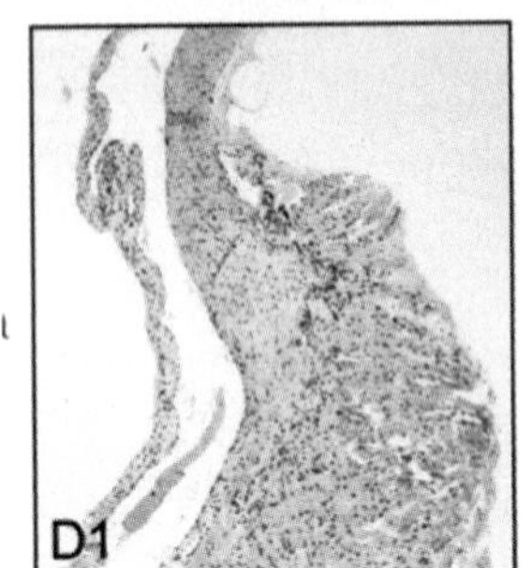

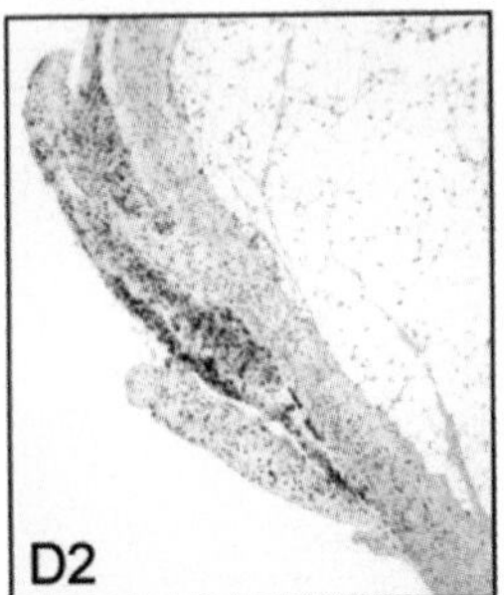

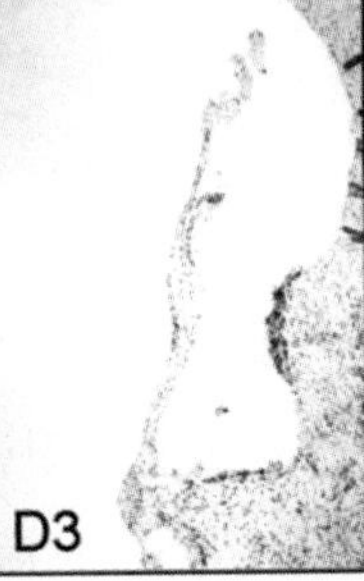

FIGURE 57–25 Light microscopy of rabbit aortic valves from a rabbit fed a conventional diet **(left column)**, one fed a high-cholesterol diet **(middle column)**, and one fed a high-cholesterol diet and treated with atorvastatin **(right column)**. In each panel, the aortic valve leaflet is positioned to the left with the aorta on the right. **A1-A3,** Hematoxylin and eosin stain. **B1-B3,** Masson trichrome stain for collagen (blue stain). **C1-C3,** Macrophage RAM-11 stain for macrophages and foam cells. **D1-D3,** Stain for proliferating cell nuclear antigen. The high-cholesterol diet results in cellular proliferation and macrophage and foam cell infiltration. These changes are prevented with atorvastatin. (From Rajamannan NM, Subramanian M, Sebo T, et al: Atorvastatin inhibits hypercholesterolemia-induced cellular proliferation and bone matrix production in the rabbit aortic valve. Circulation 105:2660, 2002.)

infarction.[155] Moreover, retrospective studies have linked treatment with HMG-CoA reductase (statin) medications with a lower rate of progression of calcific AS,[165-167] and this effect has been confirmed prospectively in an animal model of hypercholesterolemia (Fig. 57–25).[168] Hence, there is growing consensus that "degenerative" calcific AS shares many pathophysiological features with atherosclerosis and that aggressive prevention measures may retard (and perhaps even prevent) this process.[154,169,170] Whether similar preventive strategies might be used at an early age in patients with bicuspid valves to slow progressive to severe AS awaits further study.

In *atherosclerotic* aortic valve stenosis, severe atherosclerosis involves the aorta and other major arteries; this form of AS occurs most frequently in patients with severe hypercholesterolemia and is observed in children with homozygous type II hyperlipoproteinemia.[171]

Calcific AS is observed in a number of other conditions, including Paget disease of bone[172] and end-stage renal disease. *Rheumatoid involvement* of the valve is a rare cause of AS and results in nodular thickening of the valve leaflets and involvement of the proximal portion of the aorta. *Ochronosis* with alkaptonuria is another rare cause of AS.[173]

Hemodynamically significant AS leads to severe concentric left ventricular hypertrophy, with heart weights as great as 1000 gm. The interventricular septum often bulges into and encroaches on the right ventricular cavity. When left ventricular failure supervenes, the ventricle dilates, the left atrium enlarges, and changes secondary to left atrial hypertension occur in the pulmonary vascular bed, the right side of the heart, and the systemic venous bed. Isolated AS may produce significant pulmonary hypertension,[174] but this is less common than in patients with associated mitral valve disease.

Pathophysiology (Fig. 57–26)

The left ventricle responds to *sudden* severe obstruction to outflow by dilation and reduction of stroke volume. However, in adults with AS, the obstruction usually develops and increases gradually over a prolonged period. In infants and children with congenital AS, the valve orifice shows little change as the child grows, thereby intensifying the relative obstruction quite gradually. Left ventricular function can be well maintained in experimentally produced, gradually developing subcoronary AS in animals. In the experimental model, as well as in children and adults with chronic, severe AS, left ventricular output is maintained by the presence of left ventricular hypertrophy, which may sustain a large pressure gradient across the aortic valve for many years without a reduction in cardiac output, left ventricular dilation, or the development of symptoms. Critical obstruction to left ventricular outflow is usually characterized by (1) a peak systolic pressure gradient exceeding 50 mm Hg in the presence of a normal cardiac output or (2) an effective aortic orifice area (calculated by the Gorlin formula [see Chap. 17]) less than about 0.8 cm^2 in an average-sized adult, i.e., 0.5 cm^2/m^2 of BSA (less than about one-fourth of the normal aortic orifice of 3.0 to 4.0 cm^2). An aortic valve orifice of 1.0 to 1.5 cm^2 is considered moderate stenosis, and an orifice of 1.5 to 2.0 cm^2 is referred to as *mild stenosis*.

As contraction of the left ventricle becomes progressively more isometric, the left ventricular pressure pulse exhibits a rounded, rather than flattened, summit. The elevated left ventricular end-diastolic pressure, which is characteristic of severe AS, often reflects diminished compliance of the hypertrophied left ventricular wall.

In patients with severe AS, large *a* waves usually appear in the left atrial pressure pulse because of the combination of enhanced contraction of a hypertrophied left atrium and diminished left ventricular compliance. Atrial contraction plays a particularly important role in filling of the left ventricle in AS. It raises left ventricular end-diastolic pressure without causing a concomitant elevation of mean left atrial pressure. This "booster pump" function of the left atrium prevents the pulmonary venous and capillary pressures from rising to levels that would produce pulmonary congestion, while at the same time maintaining left ventricular end-diastolic pressure at the elevated level necessary for effective contraction of the hypertrophied left ventricle. Loss of appropriately timed, vigorous atrial contraction, as occurs in atrial fibrillation or atrioventricular dissociation, may result in rapid clinical deterioration in patients with severe AS.

Although the *cardiac output* at rest is within normal limits in most patients with severe AS, it often fails to rise normally during exertion. Late in the course of the disease, the cardiac output, stroke volume, and therefore the left ventricular–aortic pressure gradient all decline, whereas the mean left atrial, pulmonary capillary, pulmonary arterial, right ventricular systolic and diastolic, and right atrial pressures rise, often sequentially. As a consequence of pulmonary hypertension and/or bulging of the hypertrophied septum into the right ventricular cavity, the *a* wave in the right atrial pressure pulse becomes prominent.

Left ventricular end-diastolic volume usually remains normal until late in the course of severe AS, but left ventricular mass increases in response to the chronic pressure overload, resulting in an increase in the mass/volume ratio. However, the increase in mass may not be as great as that seen with aortic AR or combined AS and AR.

Gender differences in the response of the left ventricle to AS have been reported.[175] Women more frequently exhibit normal or even supernormal ventricular performance and a smaller, thicker walled, concentrically hypertrophied left ventricle with diastolic dysfunction (to be discussed) and normal or even subnormal systolic wall stress. Men more frequently have eccentric left ventricular hypertrophy, excessive systolic wall stress, systolic dysfunction (Fig. 57–27), and ventricular dilation.

MYOCARDIAL FUNCTION IN AORTIC STENOSIS

When the aorta is suddenly constricted in experimental animals, left ventricular pressure rises, wall stress increases significantly, and both the extent and the velocity of shortening decline. As pointed out in Chapter 21, the development of ventricular hypertrophy is one of the principal mechanisms by which the heart adapts to such an increased hemodynamic burden.[149] The increased systolic wall stress induced by AS leads to parallel replication of sarcomeres and concentric hypertrophy. The increase in left ventricular wall thickness is often sufficient to counterbalance the increased pressure, so that peak systolic wall tension returns to normal or remains normal if the obstruction develops slowly. An inverse correlation between wall stress and ejection fraction has been described in patients with AS. This suggests that the depressed ejection fraction and velocity of fiber shortening that occur in *some* patients are a consequence of inadequate wall thickening, resulting in "afterload mismatch." In others, the lower ejection fraction is secondary to a true depression of contractility; in this group, surgical treatment is less effective. Thus, both increased afterload and altered contractility are operative to varying extents in depressing left ventricular performance. To evaluate myocardial function in patients with AS, the ejection phase indices, such as ejection fraction and myocardial fiber shortening, should be related to the existing wall tension.

Diastolic Properties (see Chap. 20). Although ventricular hypertrophy is a key adaptive mechanism to the pressure load imposed by AS, it has an adverse pathophysiological consequence; i.e., it increases diastolic stiffness.[149] As a result, greater intracavitary pressure is required for ventricular filling. Some patients with AS manifest an increase in stiffness of the left ventricle (increased *chamber* stiffness) owing simply to increased muscle mass with no alteration in the diastolic properties of each unit of

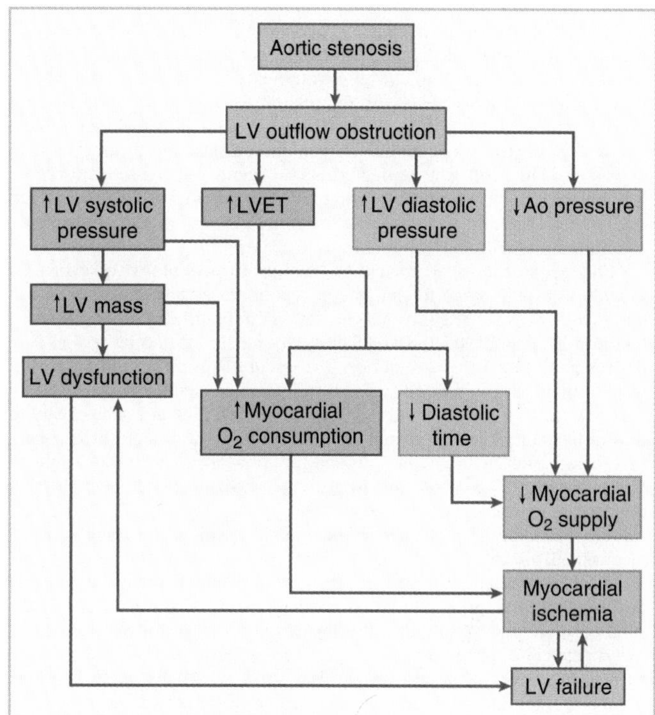

FIGURE 57–26 Pathophysiology of aortic stenosis. Left ventricular (LV) outflow obstruction results in an increased LV systolic pressure, increased LV ejection time (LVET), increased LV diastolic pressure, and decreased aortic (Ao) pressure. Increased LV systolic pressure with LV volume overload increases LV mass, which may lead to LV dysfunction and failure. Increased LV systolic pressure, LV mass, and LVET increase myocardial oxygen (O_2) consumption. Increased LVET results in a decrease of diastolic time (myocardial perfusion time). Increased LV diastolic pressure and decreased Ao diastolic pressure decrease coronary perfusion pressure. Decreased diastolic time and coronary perfusion pressure decrease myocardial O_2 supply. Increased myocardial O_2 consumption and decreased myocardial O_2 supply produce myocardial ischemia, which further deteriorates LV function. (From Boudoulas H, Gravanis MB: Valvular heart disease. *In* Gravanis MB [ed]: Cardiovascular Disorders: Pathogenesis and Pathophysiology. St. Louis, CV Mosby, 1993, p 64.)

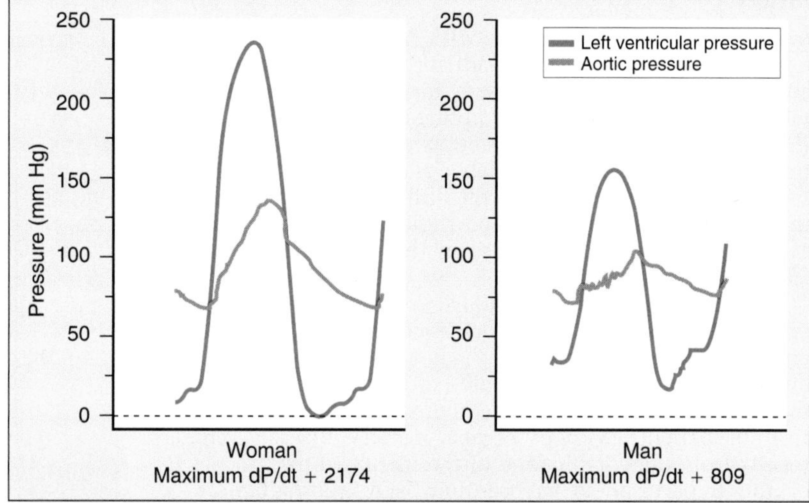

FIGURE 57–27 The difference in pressure-generating capabilities of the left ventricle in an 83-year-old woman and a 60-year-old man with a similar degree of aortic stenosis is shown. dP/dt = rate of pressure increase. (From Carroll JD, Carroll EP, Feldman T, et al: Sex-associated differences in left ventricular function in aortic stenosis of the elderly. Circulation 86:1099, 1992.)

myocardium (normal *muscle* stiffness); others exhibit increases in both chamber and muscle stiffness. This increased stiffness, however produced, contributes to the elevation of ventricular diastolic filling pressure at any level of ventricular diastolic volume and may be responsible for flash pulmonary edema in patients with AS. Diastolic dysfunction may revert toward normal with regression of hypertrophy following surgical relief of AS.

Cardiac Structure. In adults with AS, both myocardial cellular hypertrophy and relative and absolute increases in connective tissue occur. An increase in the total collagen volume of the myocardium along with increased myocardial gene expression for collagens I and III and fibronectin is related to activation of the cardiac renin-angiotensin system.[176] This likely contributes to the altered diastolic properties just discussed. The collagen and fibronectin gene expression correlate directly with the left ventricular end-diastolic pressure and inversely with the ejection fraction.[176] Reduction in renin-angiotensin activation parallels regression of hypertrophy after relief of AS.[177]

Changes in the myocardial ultrastructure in patients with severe AS include unusually large nuclei, loss of myofibrils, accumulation of mitochondria, large cytoplasmic areas devoid of contractile material, and proliferation of fibroblasts and collagen fibers in the interstitial space. The depression of myocardial function that occurs late in the course of the disease may well be related to these morphological alterations.

Ischemia. In patients with AS, coronary blood flow at rest is elevated in absolute terms but is normal when corrections are made for myocardial mass.[178] Reduced coronary blood flow reserve may produce inadequate myocardial oxygenation in patients with severe AS, even in the absence of coronary artery disease. The hypertrophied left ventricular muscle mass, the increased systolic pressure, and the prolongation of ejection all elevate myocardial oxygen consumption. The abnormally heightened pressure compressing the coronary arteries may exceed the coronary perfusion pressure, and the shortening of diastole interferes with coronary blood flow, thus leading to an imbalance between myocardial oxygen supply and demand.[179] Myocardial perfusion is also impaired by the relative decrease in myocardial capillary density as myocardial mass increases and by the elevation of left ventricular end-diastolic pressure, which lowers the aortic–left ventricular pressure gradient in diastole (i.e., the coronary perfusion pressure gradient). This underperfusion may be responsible for the development of subendocardial ischemia,[178] especially during tachycardia.

Myocardial ischemia in patients with severe AS and normal coronary arteries may also develop secondary to high systolic and diastolic stresses caused by inadequate ventricular hypertrophy and the reduced coronary flow reserve just described.[180] Metabolic evidence of myocardial ischemia, i.e., lactate production, can be demonstrated when myocardial oxygen needs are stimulated by exercise or by isoproterenol in patients with AS, even in the absence of coronary artery narrowing.[148]

Clinical Manifestations

History

In the natural history of adults with AS, a long latent period exists during which there is gradually increasing obstruction and an increase in the pressure load on the myocardium while the patient remains asymptomatic. The cardinal manifestations of acquired AS are angina pectoris, syncope, exertional dyspnea, and ultimately heart failure.[148,181] These commence most commonly in the fifth or sixth decades of life in patients with congenital or rheumatic AS and in the seventh through ninth decades in those with degenerative calcific AS.

Angina occurs in approximately two-thirds of patients with critical AS (about half of whom have associated significant coronary artery obstruction).[148] It usually resembles the angina observed in patients with coronary artery disease, in that it is commonly precipitated by exertion and relieved by rest. In patients without coronary artery disease, angina results from the combination of the increased oxygen needs of the hypertrophied myocardium and the reduction of oxygen delivery secondary to the excessive compression of coronary vessels (as discussed previously).[179] In patients with coronary artery disease, angina is caused by a combination of the epicardial coronary artery obstruction in combination with the oxygen imbalance characteristic of AS. Rarely, angina results from calcium emboli to the coronary vascular bed.

Syncope is most commonly due to the reduced cerebral perfusion that occurs during exertion when arterial pressure declines consequent to systemic vasodilation in the presence of a fixed cardiac output. Syncope has also been attributed to malfunction of the baroreceptor mechanism in severe AS, as well as to a vasodepressor response to a greatly elevated left ventricular systolic pressure during exercise. Premonitory symptoms of syncope are common. Exertional hypotension may also be manifested as "graying out" spells or dizziness on effort. Syncope at rest may be due to transient ventricular fibrillation, from which the patient recovers spontaneously; to transient atrial fibrillation with loss of the atrial contribution to left ventricular filling, which causes a precipitous decline in cardiac output; or to transient atrioventricular block due to extension of the calcification of the valve into the conduction system. Exertional dyspnea with orthopnea, paroxysmal nocturnal dyspnea, and pulmonary edema reflect varying degrees of pulmonary venous hypertension. These are relatively late symptoms in patients with AS, and their presence for more than 5 years should suggest the possibility of associated mitral valvular disease.

Because cardiac output is usually well maintained for many years in patients with severe AS, marked fatigability, debilitation, peripheral cyanosis, and other clinical manifestations of a low cardiac output are usually not prominent until quite late in the course of the disease. Other late findings in patients with isolated AS include atrial fibrillation, pulmonary hypertension, and systemic venous hypertension. Although AS may be responsible for sudden death, this usually occurs in patients who had previously been symptomatic (see Chap. 33).

In patients in whom the obstruction remains unrelieved, the prognosis is poor once these symptoms are manifested. Survival curves show that the interval from the onset of symptoms to the time of death is approximately 2 years in patients with heart failure, 3 years in those with syncope, and 5 years in those with angina (Fig. 57–28).

Gastrointestinal bleeding may develop in patients with severe AS, often associated with angiodysplasia (most commonly of the right colon) or other vascular malformations. This complication arises from shear stress–induced platelet aggregation with reduction in high-molecular-weight

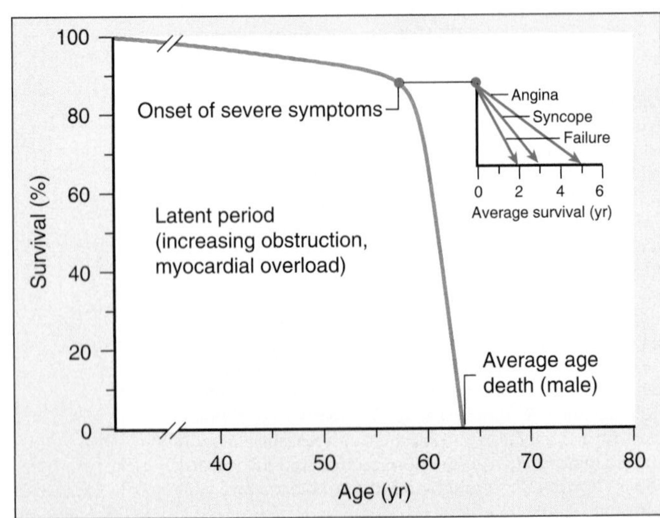

FIGURE 57–28 Natural history of aortic stenosis without operative treatment. Onset of symptoms identifies patients at high risk of death over the next 2 to 5 years. (From Ross J Jr, Braunwald E: Aortic stenosis. Circulation 38[Suppl V]:61, 1968.)

multimers of von Willebrand factor and increases in proteolytic subunit fragments. These abnormalities correlate with the severity of AS and are correctable by AVR.[182,183]

Infective endocarditis is a greater risk in younger patients with milder valvular deformity than in older patients with rock-like calcific aortic deformities. Cerebral emboli resulting in stroke or transient ischemic attacks may be due to microthrombi on thickened bicuspid valves. Calcific AS may cause embolization of calcium to various organs, including the heart, kidneys, and brain. Abrupt loss of vision has been reported when calcific emboli occlude the central retinal artery.[148]

Physical Examination (Table 57–8)

The arterial pulse characteristically rises slowly and is small and sustained (pulsus parvus et tardus). In the late stage of AS, systolic and pulse pressures are both reduced. However, in patients with mild AS with associated AR and in older patients with an inelastic arterial bed, both systolic and pulse pressures may be normal or even increased. A systolic pressure exceeding 200 mm Hg is rare in patients with critical AS. The anacrotic notch and coarse systolic vibrations are felt most readily in the carotid arterial pulse, producing the so-called carotid shudder. Simultaneous palpation of the apex and carotid arteries reveals a lag in the latter in patients with severe AS. Although left ventricular alternans occurs commonly in patients who have AS with left ventricular dysfunction, obstruction of the aortic valve may prevent its recognition in the peripheral arterial pulse. The jugular venous pulse usually shows prominent *a* waves, reflecting reduced right ventricular compliance consequent to pulmonary hypertension or hypertrophy of the ventricular septum. With pulmonary hypertension and secondary right ventricular failure and TR, *v* or *c-v* waves may become prominent.

The cardiac impulse is sustained and becomes displaced inferiorly and laterally with left ventricular failure. Presystolic distention of the left ventricle (i.e., a prominent precordial *a* wave) is often both visible and palpable. A hyperdynamic left ventricle suggests concomitant AR and/or MR. A systolic thrill is usually best appreciated when the patient leans forward during full expiration. It is palpated most readily in the second left intercostal space on either side of the sternum or in the suprasternal notch and is frequently transmitted along the carotid arteries. A systolic thrill is quite specific for severe AS.

Rarely, right ventricular failure with systemic venous congestion, hepatomegaly, and edema precedes left ventricular failure. This is probably caused by the so-called Bernheim effect, which results when the hypertrophied ventricular septum bulges into and encroaches on the right ventricular cavity and leads to impairment of right ventricular filling. In such cases, the jugular venous pressure is elevated, and the *a* wave is prominent.

AUSCULTATION (see Table 57–8)

S_1 is normal or soft and S_4 is prominent, presumably because atrial contraction is vigorous and the mitral valve is partially closed during presystole. S_2 may be single because calcification and immobility of the aortic valve make A_2 inaudible, because P_2 is buried in the prolonged aortic ejection murmur, or because prolongation of left ventricular systole makes A_2 coincide with P_2. Paradoxical splitting of S_2, which suggests associated left bundle branch block or left ventricular dysfunction, may also occur. In patients with left ventricular failure and secondary pulmonary hypertension, P_2 may become accentuated. When the aortic valve is rigid, which is the usual finding in adults with severe AS, A_2 may be inaudible, but when the valve is flexible, as may occur in patients with congenital AS, A_2 may be snapping and accentuated.

An aortic ejection sound occurs simultaneously with the halting upward movement of the aortic valve. Like an audible A_2, this sound is dependent on mobility of the valve cusps and disappears when they become severely calcified. Thus, it is common in children and young

TABLE 57–8 Differential Diagnosis of Aortic Stenosis: Physical Findings

Type of Stenosis	Maximum Murmur and Thrill	Aortic Election Sound	Aortic Component of Second Sound	Regurgitant Diastolic Murmur	Arterial Pulse
Acquired, nonrheumatic or rheumatic	Second right sternal border to neck; may be at apex in the aged	Uncommon	Decreased or absent	Common	Delayed upstroke: anacrotic notch; ± small amplitude
Hypertrophic, subaortic	Fourth left sternal border to apex (± regurgitant systolic murmur at apex)	Rare	Normal or decreased	Very rare	Brisk upstroke, sometimes bisferiens
Congenital, valvular	Second right sternal border to neck (along left sternal border in some infants)	Very common in children, disappearing with decrease in valve mobility with age	Normal or increased in children; decreased with decrease in valve mobility with age	Uncommon in children: not uncommon in adults	Delayed upstroke: anacrotic notch; ± small amplitude
Congenital, subvalvular	Discrete: like valvular; tunnel: left sternal border	Rare	Not helpful (normal, increased, decreased, or absent)	Almost all	
Congenital, supravalvular	First right sternal border to neck and sometimes to medial aspect of right arm; occasionally greater in neck than in chest	Rare	Normal or decreased	Uncommon	Rapid upstroke in right carotid, delayed in left carotid, right arm pulse pressure greater than left

From Levinson GF: Aortic stenosis. *In* Dalen JE, Alpert JS (eds): Valvular Heart Disease. 2nd ed. Boston, Little, Brown, 1987, p 202.

adults with congenital AS but is rare in adults with acquired calcific AS and rigid valves. The ejection sound occurs approximately 0.06 second after the onset of S_1.

The *systolic murmur* of AS is usually late peaking and heard best at the base of the heart but is often well transmitted both along the carotid vessels and to the apex. Cessation of the murmur before A_2 is usually helpful in differentiating it from a pansystolic mitral murmur. However, the systolic murmur may be mistaken for a pansystolic murmur because it may end with S_2, which represents pulmonic valve closure, whereas the pansystolic murmur is soft or even inaudible. In patients with calcified aortic valves, the systolic murmur is loudest at the base of the heart, but high-frequency components selectively radiate to the apex (the so-called Gallavardin phenomenon), where it may actually be more prominent and where it may be mistaken for the murmur of MR. Frequently, there is a "quiet area" between the base and apex where the murmur is diminished in intensity, supporting the erroneous impression that the apical and basal murmurs have different origins. In general, the more severe the stenosis, the longer the duration of the murmur and the more likely that it peaks later in systole. Findings on physical examination (including a delay in the carotid upstroke, a loud, long systolic murmur, and a single S_2) all correlate with severe stenosis.[184]

Patients with degenerative aortic sclerosis may have severe valvular calcification; however, obstruction may be mild or absent because the commissural fusion characteristic of congenital and rheumatic AS is not present. The nonfused, calcified cusps vibrate freely, resulting in a softer and more musical murmur that is more prominent at the apex than the murmur of congenital or rheumatic AS. High-pitched decrescendo diastolic murmurs secondary to AR are common in many patients with dominant AS.

When the left ventricle fails and the stroke volume falls, the systolic murmur of AS becomes softer; rarely, it disappears altogether. The slow rise in the arterial pulse is more difficult to recognize. Stated simply, with left ventricular failure, the clinical picture changes from typical AS to that of severe left ventricular failure with a low cardiac output. Thus, occult AS may be a cause of intractable heart failure, and critical AS should be ruled out by echocardiography in patients with severe heart failure of unknown cause because operative treatment may be life saving and may result in substantial clinical improvement.

Dynamic Auscultation (see Table 57-5). The intensity of the systolic murmur varies from beat to beat when the duration of diastolic filling varies, as in atrial fibrillation or following a premature contraction. This characteristic is helpful in differentiating AS from MR, in which the murmur is usually unaffected. The murmur of valvular AS is augmented by squatting, which increases stroke volume. It is reduced in intensity during the strain of the Valsalva maneuver and when standing, which reduce transvalvular flow.

Laboratory Examination

ELECTROCARDIOGRAPHY. The principal ECG change is left ventricular hypertrophy, which is found in approximately 85 percent of patients with severe AS. The absence of left ventricular hypertrophy does not exclude the presence of critical AS, and the correlation between the absolute ECG voltages in precordial leads and the severity of obstruction is poor in adults but is quite good in children with congenital AS. T wave inversion and ST segment depression in leads with upright QRS complexes are common. ST segment depressions greater than 0.2 mV in patients with AS (left ventricular "strain") suggest that severe ventricular hypertrophy is present. Occasionally, a "pseudoinfarction" pattern is present, characterized by a loss of R waves in the right precordial leads. There is evidence of left atrial enlargement in more than 80 percent of patients with severe, isolated AS. The principal manifestation is prominent late negativity of the P wave in lead V_1 rather than an increased duration in lead II, suggesting hypertrophy rather than dilation. Atrial fibrillation is an uncommon and late sign of pure AS, and its presence in a patient who does not appear to have end-stage aortic disease should suggest coexisting mitral valvular disease.

The extension of calcific infiltrates from the aortic valve into the conduction system may cause various forms and degrees of atrioventricular and intraventricular block in 5 percent of patients with calcific AS. Such conduction defects are more common in patients who have associated mitral annular calcification.

RADIOLOGICAL FINDINGS (see Figs. 12–8 and 12–23). Routine radiological examination may be normal in patients with critical AS. The heart is usually of normal size or slightly enlarged, with a rounding of the left ventricular border and apex, unless regurgitation or left ventricular failure is present and causes substantial cardiomegaly. Poststenotic dilation of the ascending aorta is a common finding. Marked aortic dilation suggests either a bicuspid valve or associated AR. Calcification of the aortic valve is found in almost all adults with hemodynamically significant AS, but it is more readily detected on fluoroscopy, cardiac computed tomography (see Fig. 15–11), or echocardiography than on roentgenography. The absence of calcium in the aortic valve region on careful fluoroscopic examination in a patient older than 35 years of age essentially rules out severe valvular AS. The converse is not true, however, and in patients older than 65 years of age with degenerative AS, severe calcification of the aortic valve may occur with no or only mild obstruction. The left atrium may be slightly enlarged in patients with severe AS, and there may be radiological signs of pulmonary venous hypertension. However, when left atrial enlargement is marked, the presence of associated mitral valvular disease should be suspected.

CARDIAC CATHETERIZATION AND ANGIOGRAPHY. As two-dimensional echocardiography usually defines left ventricular function, aortic valve morphology and mobility, and hemodynamic severity of AS, the principal role of the cardiac catheterization laboratory in patients with AS is to determine whether there is coexistent coronary artery disease in patients being considered for surgery. There is some hazard associated with the rapid injection of a large volume of contrast material into a high-pressure left ventricle, and therefore left ventriculography is usually not advisable in patients with AS and critical obstruction. Angiographic studies of the left ventricle and aortic valve in these patients are best performed by injecting contrast material into the pulmonary artery and filming in the 30-degree right anterior oblique and 60-degree left anterior oblique projections. These examinations often make it possible to ascertain the number of cusps of the stenotic valve and to demonstrate doming of a thickened valve and a systolic jet.

Hemodynamic assessment of AS by cardiac catheterization is not routinely necessary. However, careful hemodynamic study to determine severity of AS (see Chap. 17) is indicated when echocardiographic data are equivocal or of suboptimal quality, when there is a discrepancy between clinical information and echocardiographic findings, and when AS is associated with low cardiac output and impaired left ventricular function.[1,22] In the latter situation, hemodynamic assessment of AS severity at rest and during maneuvers to increase flow across the aortic valve (such as a dobutamine infusion) can provide information that is critical in making difficult management decisions regarding the indications for surgery (discussed subsequently).

ECHOCARDIOGRAPHY (see Chap. 11 and Figs. 11–63 to 11-68). Echocardiography has become the most important laboratory technique for evaluating and following patients with AS and selecting them for operation.

The normal range of opening of the aortic valve is 1.6 to 2.6 cm. Two-dimensional transthoracic echocardiography is helpful in detecting valvular calcification, in outlining the valve leaflets, and sometimes in determining the severity of the stenosis by imaging the orifice.[185] The orifice may be more clearly defined by transesophageal echocardiography (see Fig. 11–67), which offers a more precise short-axis view of the aortic valve.[186] Two-dimensional echocardiography is invaluable in detecting associated mitral valve disease, in assessing aortic root diameter in patients with bicuspid valves, and in assessing left ventricular systolic performance, diastolic function, dilation, and hypertrophy. Evolving three-dimensional echocardiographic methods hold promise for assessing aortic valve structure and mobility and quantifying the severity of AS.[187]

Doppler echocardiography allows calculation of the left ventricular–aortic pressure gradient from the systolic aortic valve velocity signal[188,189] using a modified Bernoulli (continuity) equation (see Figs. 11–30 and 11–65) and the continuity equation (see Figs. 11–34 and 11–68). The gradients noninvasively determined by this method correlate well with those determined by left-heart catheterization. The effective aortic valve orifice areas can also be derived from the Doppler examination.[190,191] Doppler methods can overestimate the severity of AS because of the phenomenon of pressure recovery distal to a stenosis (which has less effect on catheter-based measurements). The magnitude of this effect can be calculated and used to correct the measurements to yield accurate assessment of AS severity.[189,191,192]

Color-flow Doppler imaging is helpful in detecting and determining the severity of AR (which coexists in ≈75 percent of patients with predominant AS) and in estimating pulmonary artery pressure. Indeed, in most patients the echocardiographic examination provides the important hemodynamic information required for patient management, and under most circumstances cardiac catheterization is not essential (except to determine the status of the coronary arteries).[188-191] In patients with left ventricular dysfunction and low cardiac output, assessing the severity of AS can be enhanced by assessing hemodynamic changes during dobutamine infusion (discussed subsequently).

MAGNETIC RESONANCE IMAGING (see Chap. 14). Cardiac MRI is useful in assessing left ventricular volume, function, and mass, especially in settings in which this information cannot be obtained readily from echocardiography. MRI may also be useful in quantifying the severity of AS (see Fig. 14–13).[193,194]

NATURAL HISTORY

In contrast to MS, which leads to symptoms almost immediately after its development, patients with severe AS may be asymptomatic for many years despite the presence of severe obstruction.[1,148,181] The systolic pressure gradient may exceed 150 mm Hg, and the peak left ventricular systolic pressure may reach approximately 300 mm Hg with relatively little increase in overall heart size on radiological examination and with normal left ventricular end-diastolic and end-systolic volumes.

Patients with severe, chronic AS tend to be free of cardiovascular symptoms until relatively late in the course of the disease. Thus, there is a long latent period during which mortality and morbidity are quite low.[1,148,181] However, obstruction is progressive and often insidious, with the aortic valve area decreasing by an average of 0.12 cm^2 per year in one study,[195] associated with an average increase in aortic jet velocity of 0.32 m/sec per year and a mean gradient of 7 mm Hg per year. The rate of progression is highly variable and difficult to predict in individual patients. When symptoms develop, the valve area is, on average, 0.6 cm^2, but the severity of stenosis alone does not determine the presence or severity of symptoms. A patient may develop symptoms with a valve area of 1.0 cm^2, whereas another may remain symptom free with a valve area of 0.6 cm^2 and high systolic pressure gradients. However, the severity of AS does have predictive power regarding the likelihood that symptoms will develop with time. Most patients with peak aortic valve velocities greater than 4 m/sec experience symptom onset over the course of 3 to 4 years (Fig. 57–29),[195,197] particularly if there is evidence of severe valvular calcification or increasing severity of AS on serial examinations. Thus, the combination of high aortic jet velocity, severe valvular calcification, and increasing severity of stenosis identifies individual patients with a high likelihood of requiring surgery within a few years.

Once patients with AS develop angina pectoris or syncope, the average survival is 1 to 3 years (see Fig. 57–28).[1,148,149,196,197] Among symptomatic patients with severe AS, the outlook is poorest when the left ventricle has failed and the cardiac output and transvalvular gradient are both low.

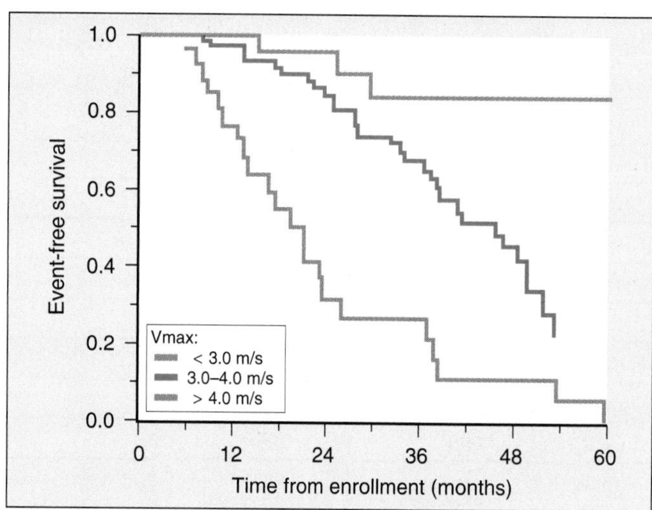

FIGURE 57–29 Natural history of asymptomatic patients with aortic stenosis. Initial aortic jet velocity (Vmax) stratifies patients according to the likelihood that symptoms requiring valve replacement will develop over time. The majority of "events" in this series were onset of symptoms warranting aortic valve replacement. (From Otto CM, Burwarsh IG, Legget ME, et al: A prospective study of asymptomatic valvular aortic stenosis: Clinical, echocardiographic, and exercise predictors of outcome. Circulation 95:2262, 1997.)

Asymptomatic patients have an excellent prognosis.[1,148,149] Sudden death, like syncope, in patients with severe AS may be due to cerebral hypoperfusion followed by arrhythmia. Although severe AS is a potentially lethal disease, death (even when sudden) usually occurs in *symptomatic* patients. A number of authors who have followed asymptomatic patients with critical AS have found that sudden death is extremely rare in this group (Table 57-9). Of 449 asymptomatic patients with critical AS, only 4 (<1 percent) died suddenly while still asymptomatic (certainly not higher than the mortality from operation).[1]

Management

Medical Treatment

Patients with known severe AS who are asymptomatic should be advised to report *promptly* the development of any symptoms possibly related to AS. Patients with critical obstruction should be cautioned to avoid vigorous athletic and physical activity. However, such restrictions do not apply to patients with mild obstruction. The need for infective endocarditis prophylaxis should be explained (see Chap 58). Because of the gradual increase in the severity of obstruction, noninvasive assessment of this finding by Doppler echocardiography should be carried out at intervals. Doppler-derived gradients have been shown to increase by 4 to 8 mm Hg per year[195] and valve areas to decrease by 0.2 to 0.3 cm^2 per year. In patients with mild obstruction, these measurements should be repeated every 2 years. In asymptomatic patients with severe obstruction, repeat echocardiography should be carried out every 6 to 12 months, with particular attention to detecting changes in left ventricular function. As patients may tailor their life styles to minimize symptoms or may ascribe fatigue and dyspnea to deconditioning or aging, they may not recognize early symptoms as important warning signals. Exercise testing may be helpful in apparently asymptomatic patients to detect covert symptoms, limited exercise capacity, and abnormal blood pressure responses.[1,195,198] Exercise stress testing should be absolutely avoided in symptomatic patients.

Symptomatic patients with severe AS are usually operative candidates, because medical therapy has little to offer. However, medical therapy may be necessary in patients who are considered to be inoperable (usually because of comorbid

TABLE 57–9 Studies of the Natural History of Asymptomatic Patients with Aortic Stenosis

Study, Year	Number of Patients	Mean Follow-up (Year)	Severity of Aortic Stenosis	Sudden Death Without Symptoms (no. of Patients)	Comments
Chizner et al, 1980	8	5.7	AVA < 1.1 cm^2	0	Retrospective study
Turina et al, 1987	17	2.0	AVA < 0.9 cm^2	0	Retrospective study
Horstkotte and Loogen, 1988	35	"years"	AVA = 0.4-0.8 cm^2	3	Retrospective study
Kelley et al, 1988	51	1.5	PV = 3.5-5.8 m/s	0	Prospective study
Pellikka et al, 1990	113	1.7	PV > 4.0 m/s	0	Prospective study
Faggiano et al, 1992	37	2.0	AVA = 0.85 ± 0.15 cm^2	0	Prospective study
Otto et al, 1997	114	2.5	PV = 3.6 ± 0.6 m/s	0	Prospective study
Rosenhek et al, 2000	106	2.3	PV > 4 m/s	1	Prospective study
Total	499	2.1		4	Average risk of sudden death ~0.4%/yr

AVA = aortic valve area; PV = peak instantaneous velocity.

Updated from Bonow RO, Carabello BA, de Leon AC, et al: ACC/AHA guidelines for the management of patients with valvular heart disease. J Am Coll Cardiol 32:1486, 1998.

conditions that preclude surgery). Digitalis glycosides are indicated if the ventricular volume is increased or the ejection fraction is reduced. Although diuretics are beneficial when there is abnormal accumulation of fluid, they must be used with caution because hypovolemia may reduce the elevated left ventricular end-diastolic pressure, lower cardiac output, and produce orthostatic hypotension. ACE inhibitors should be used with caution but are beneficial in treating patients with symptomatic left ventricular systolic dysfunction who are not candidates for surgery. They should be initiated at low doses and increased slowly to target doses, avoiding hypotension. Beta-adrenergic blockers can depress myocardial function and induce left ventricular failure and should be avoided in patients with AS.

Atrial flutter or fibrillation occurs in fewer than 10 percent of patients with severe AS, perhaps because of the late occurrence of left atrial enlargement in this condition. When such an arrhythmia is observed in a patient with AS, the possibility of associated mitral valvular disease should be considered. When atrial fibrillation occurs, the rapid ventricular rate may cause angina pectoris. The loss of the atrial contribution to ventricular filling and a sudden fall in cardiac output may cause serious hypotension. Therefore, atrial fibrillation should be treated promptly, usually with cardioversion, and a search for previously unrecognized mitral valvular disease should be undertaken. Adults with severe AS who are being considered for surgical therapy should undergo coronary arteriography. Left-heart catheterization is also indicated if there is a discrepancy between the clinical picture and the echocardiographic findings.[22]

Surgical Treatment

INDICATIONS FOR OPERATION

Children. The indications for surgery, as well as the techniques and results of operation, depend on the patient's age, the type of valvular deformity, and the function of the left ventricle. In children and adolescents with noncalcific congenital AS, who most commonly have bicuspid aortic valves, simple commissural incision under direct vision usually leads to substantial hemodynamic improvement with low risk (i.e., a mortality rate of <1 percent) (see Chap. 56). Therefore, this procedure (or now, more commonly, balloon aortic valvuloplasty [BAV]) is indicated not only in symptomatic patients but also in asymptomatic children and adolescents with severe AS,[1] which is often defined as a calculated effective orifice less than 0.8 cm^2 or 0.5 cm^2/m^2 BSA. Despite the salutary hemodynamic results following this procedure, the valve is not rendered entirely normal anatomically. The turbulent blood flow through the valve may subsequently lead to further deformation, calcification, the development of regurgitation, and restenosis after 10 to 20 years, probably requiring reoperation and valve replacement later.

Adults. In most adults with calcific AS, AVR is the surgical treatment of choice. Satisfactory long-term valvular function cannot usually be restored even by careful sculpturing procedures under direct vision, although this may be possible in a small number of selected individuals.[199] AVR should, in general, be performed in adults who have hemodynamic evidence of severe obstruction (aortic valve orifice < 1.0 cm^2 or < 0.6 cm^2/m^2 BSA) and whose symptoms are believed to result from AS. AVR should also be carried out in asymptomatic patients with *progressive* left ventricular dysfunction or a hypotensive response to exercise.[1,2,198] Although a prospective, randomized, controlled study has not been done, the long-term mortality in asymptomatic patients with critical AS and left ventricular dysfunction who undergo operation appears to be lower than that in medically treated patients who do not undergo operation.[1,2] AVR is also indicated in patients with severe stenosis who are undergoing another cardiovascular operation (e.g., coronary artery bypass grafting or surgery on the aorta or another heart valve).[1] As prosthetic valves and surgical skills continue to improve, it is likely that patients with severe AS will become candidates for operation at progressively earlier stages in the natural history of their disease,[200] and many cardiologists have already begun to lower the threshold for AVR based on severity of AS alone. Currently, however, we do *not* recommend prophylactic replacement of a critically narrow calcific aortic valve in *asymptomatic* adults unless they have progressive left ventricular dysfunction or abnormal hemodynamic responses to exercise.

Aortic Stenosis with Left Ventricular Dysfunction. Surgical risk is higher in patients with impaired left ventricular function (ejection fraction < 0.35).[201-206] However, their prognosis is poor without operation, overall survival is improved with AVR, and many patients in this group have significant clinical and functional recovery following AVR.[201-207] Hence, AVR should generally be offered to these patients. Even octogenarians with left ventricular dysfunction can have improved survival after AVR, although their operative risks are higher.[202,204,208] Exceptions are patients with advanced congestive heart failure or left ventricular dysfunction that can be related to previous myocardial infarction rather than to AS. In acutely ill patients with decompensated heart failure, nitroprusside has been reported to be safe and effective in rapidly improving hemodynamics[209] and may be used in bridging critically ill patients to AVR.

Aortic Stenosis with Low Gradient and Low Cardiac Output. Patients with critical AS, severe left ventricular dysfunction, and low cardiac output (and hence, a low transvalvular pressure gradient) often create diagnostic dilemmas for the clinician because their clinical presentation and hemodynamic data may be indistinguishable from those of patients with a dilated cardiomyopathy and a calcified valve that is not stenotic.[149,210] As aortic valve velocities and estimates of aortic valve area are dependent on flow, an important method for distinguishing between these two conditions is to reassess hemodynamics during transient increases in flow, usually by increasing cardiac output with dobutamine during Doppler echocardiography or cardiac catheterization (Fig. 56–30).[205,206,211] Patients with severe AS manifest an increase in valve gradient and no change in valve area during dobutamine, whereas those without AS manifest an increase in calculated valve area. Dobutamine echocardiography also provides evidence of myocardial contractile reserve, which is an important predictor of operative risk and improvement in left ventricular function and survival after AVR in these patients.[205,206]

RESULTS. Successful replacement of the aortic valve results in substantial clinical and hemodynamic improvement in patients with AS, AR, or combined lesions. In patients without frank left ventricular failure, the operative risk ranges from 2 to 5 percent in most centers, and in patients younger than 70 years of age, the operative risk has been reported to be as low as 1 percent. The Society of Thoracic Surgeons National Database Committee reported an overall operative mortality rate of 4 percent in 32,968 patients undergoing isolated AVR and 6.8 percent in 32,538 patients undergoing AVR and coronary artery bypass grafting (see Table 57–3).[55]

Risk factors causing a higher mortality rate include a high NYHA class, impairment of left ventricular function, advanced age, and the presence of associated coronary artery disease. The 10-year actuarial survival rate of hospital survivors in surgically treated patients is approximately 85 percent.[1,212] Risk factors for late death include higher preoperative NYHA class, advanced age, concomitant untreated coronary artery disease, preoperative impaired left ventricular function, preoperative ventricular arrhythmias, and associated significant AR.

Although age is an important determinant of risk, there is increasing experience in most surgical centers in performing AVR in symptomatic patients older than 70 or even 80 years of age with calcific AS.[208,213,214] The results of AVR are often quite satisfactory in this age group, with improved quality of life and survival, Therefore, advanced age per se, though adding to the risk, should not be considered a contraindication to operation. Particular attention must be directed to the adequacy of hepatic, renal, and pulmonary functions in these patients.

Symptoms of pulmonary congestion (exertional dyspnea) and of myocardial ischemia (angina pectoris) are relieved in almost every patient. Hemodynamic results of AVR are also impressive; elevated end-diastolic and end-systolic volumes show significant reduction. Impaired ventricular performance returns to normal more frequently in patients with AS than in those with AR or MR. However, the finding that the strongest predictor of postoperative left ventricular dysfunction is preoperative dysfunction[1,148,149] suggests that patients should, if possible, be operated on *before* left ventricular

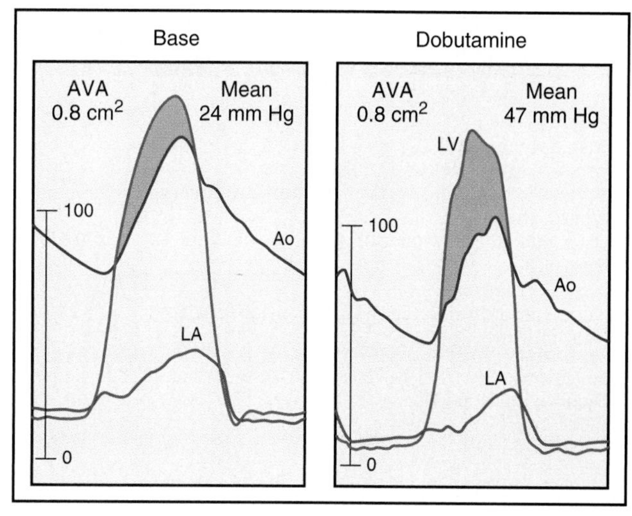

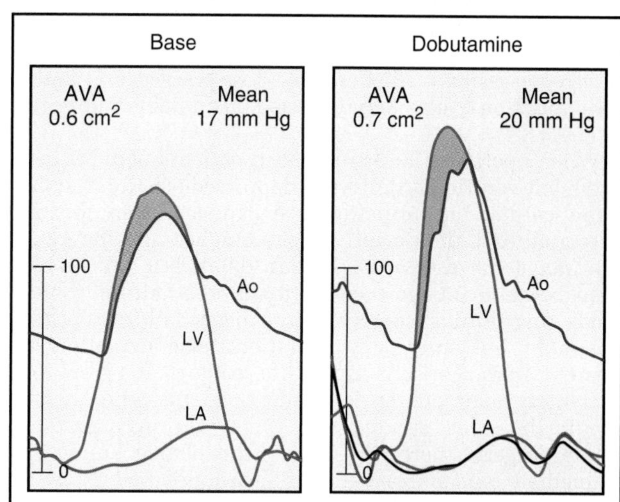

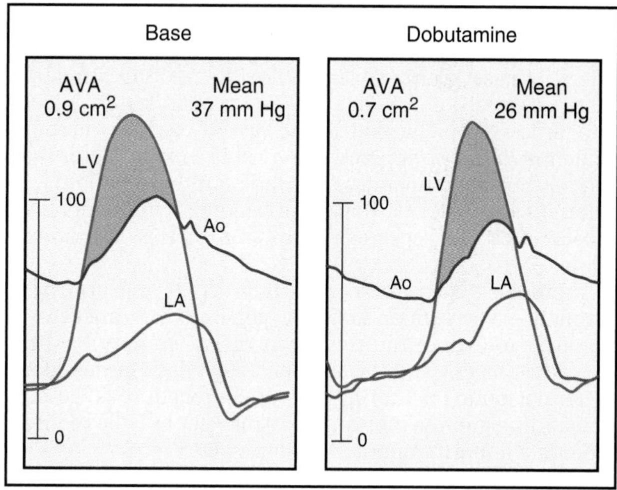

FIGURE 57–30 Hemodynamic tracings from three patients with left ventricular dysfunction, low cardiac output, and low aortic valve gradient, demonstrating three different responses to dobutamine. **A,** Increase in cardiac output and in mean aortic valve gradient from 24 to 47 mm Hg. Aortic valve area (AVA) remained 0.8 cm². This patient underwent successful valve replacement. **B,** Increase in cardiac output and minimal increase in mean pressure gradient from 17 to 20 mm Hg. The final calculated aortic valve area was 0.7 cm². The patient was found to have only minimal aortic stenosis (AS) at the time of surgery. **C,** No change in cardiac output, with decrease in mean pressure gradient from 37 to 26 mm Hg in response to dobutamine, and the test was terminated because of hypotension. The patient was found to have severe AS at the time of surgery. Ao = aortic; LA = left atrial; LV = left ventricular. (From Nishimura RA, Grantham A, Connolly HM, et al: Low-output, low-gradient aortic stenosis in patients with depressed left ventricular systolic function: The clinical utility of the dobutamine challenge in the catheterization laboratory. Circulation 106:809, 2002.)

TABLE 57–10 Predictors of Poor Outcome after Aortic Valve Replacement for Aortic Stenosis

Advanced age (>70 yr)
Female gender
Emergent surgery
Coronary artery disease
Previous coronary artery bypass grafting surgery
Hypertension
Left ventricular dysfunction (ejection fraction < 0.45 or 0.50)
Heart failure
Atrial fibrillation
Concurrent mitral valve replacement or repair
Renal failure

Adapted from Otto CM: Valvular Heart Disease. 2nd ed. Philadelphia, WB Saunders, 2004, p 227.

function becomes seriously impaired. The increased left ventricular mass is reduced toward (but not to) normal within 18 months after AVR in patients with AS,[215,216] with further reduction over the next several years.[217] Myocyte hypertrophy regresses as well. Coronary flow reserve[218,219] and diastolic function[216] also demonstrate considerable improvement after AVR.

When operation is carried out in patients with critical AS, frank left ventricular failure, a depressed ejection fraction, or a low cardiac output (and hence a reduced transaortic pressure gradient), the operative risk is higher, and the mortality rate ranges from 8 to 20 percent, depending on the skill of the surgical team and the severity of heart failure.[202-206] Obviously, performing surgery before heart failure develops is desirable, but emergency operation, even in patients with heart failure, is sometimes life saving. In view of the extremely poor prognosis of such patients who are treated medically, unless serious comorbid conditions exist that preclude surgery, there is usually little choice but to advise immediate mechanical relief of obstruction.

In patients with AS and obstructive coronary artery disease (a relatively common combination), AVR and myocardial revascularization should be performed together.[220] Although the risk of AVR is increased when accompanied by coronary artery bypass grafting (see Table 57–3),[55] the surgical risk increases even more when severe coronary artery disease is left untreated. The ability to avoid serious myocardial ischemia in the perioperative period is a major factor that has served to reduce operative mortality in these patients. Characteristics of patients that have been shown to increase the risk of AVR, as reported in different series, are shown in Table 57–10.

There has been increasing interest in performing AVR through a very small incision, generally a transverse sternotomy, so-called "minimally invasive surgery." Although the advantages (shorter hospital stay, less tissue damage, better cosmetic results) are clear, the procedure is technically demanding and the mortality rate may actually be higher than when a standard approach is employed.[221,222]

Percutaneous Treatment of Aortic Stenosis (see Chap. 52)

BAV represents an increasingly attractive alternative to aortic valvotomy in children, adolescents, and young adults with congenital noncalcific AS (see Chap. 56),[1,223] but its value is quite limited in adults with calcific AS.[1] A series of balloon dilation catheters are advanced along a guidewire positioned at the left ventricular apex. Fracture of calcified nodules, separation of fused commissures, and stretching of the aortic valve ring are responsible for the relief of obstruction. Although the response of adult patients with calcific AS varies considerably, BAV initially results in relief of obstruction in most patients, with valve areas initially increasing from approximately 0.5 to 0.8 cm^2 and the mean transvalvular gradient declining from approximately 55 to 29 mm Hg. Left ventricular ejection fraction tends to rise in patients with depressed left ventricular function who undergo BAV. In addition to the procedural mortality (3 percent), another 6 percent of patients develop serious complications such as myocardial perforation, myocardial infarction, and severe AR.

The major disadvantage of BAV in adults with critical calcified AS is restenosis due to scarring, which occurs in about 50 percent of patients within 6 months. Symptoms lessen in severity in most patients but recur in approximately 30 percent by 6 months. The 1-month and 1-year mortality rates are unacceptably high, related to the restenosis rate and the fact that the average increase in aortic valve area is slight.

Although the overall intermediate-term results (6 to 12 months) of BAV have been disappointing, the procedure does have a limited role in the management of severe calcific AS in selected patients who are not surgical candidates,[1] such as patients with cardiogenic shock due to critical AS, patients with severe heart failure who are at extremely high operative risk as a "bridge" to AVR, patients with severe comorbid conditions that preclude surgery, and patients with critical AS who refuse surgical treatment. Under most circumstances, patients with critical AS who require an urgent noncardiac operation should undergo the noncardiac operation; preoperative BAV has a very limited role in such patients. In adults with calcific AS, BAV is *not* a substitute for surgery (as BMV may be in patients with MS). In addition, nitroprusside may be a more available and effective therapy for short-term management of patients with severe heart failure,[209] but greater clinical experience with nitroprusside is needed before recommendations can be made regarding its use in this setting.[209a]

Newer percutaneous methods for implantation of prosthetic valves in seriously ill patients who are not candidates for surgery are under development.[224] Limited clinical experience has been reported to date.[225]

Aortic Regurgitation

Etiology And Pathology

AR may be caused by primary disease of the aortic valve leaflets and/or the wall of the aortic root (Fig. 57–31). Among patients with *pure* AR who undergo valve replacement, the percentage with aortic root disease has been increasing steadily during the past few decades. This now represents the most common etiology and accounts for more than 50 percent of all such patients in some series.[57,226]

Valvular Disease

Rheumatic fever is a common cause of primary disease of the aortic valve that leads to regurgitation.[57,226] The cusps become infiltrated with fibrous tissues and retract, a process that prevents cusp apposition during diastole and usually leads to regurgitation into the left ventricle through a defect in the center of the valve (see Fig. 57–24C). The associated fusion of the commissures may restrict the opening of the valve, resulting in combined AS and AR; some associated mitral valve involvement is also common. Other primary valvular causes of AR include calcific AS in the elderly, in which some degree (usually mild) of AR is present in 75 percent of patients; *infective endocarditis* (see Chap. 58), in which the infection may destroy or cause perforation of a leaflet, or the vegetations may interfere with proper coaptation of the cusps; and *trauma* that results in a tear of the ascending aorta, in which loss of commissural support can cause prolapse of an aortic cusp. Although the most common complication of a congenitally *bicuspid valve* in adults is stenosis, incomplete closure and/or prolapse of a bicuspid valve may also cause isolated regurgitation or a combination of stenosis and regurgitation.[151,227] Progressive AR may occur in patients with a large ventricular septal defect as well as in patients with membranous subaortic stenosis (see Chap. 56) and as a complication of percutaneous aortic balloon valvotomy and radiofrequency catheter ablation.[228] Progressive regurgitation may also occur in patients with myxomatous proliferation of the aortic valve. An increasingly common cause of valvular AR is structural deterioration of a bioprosthetic valve.

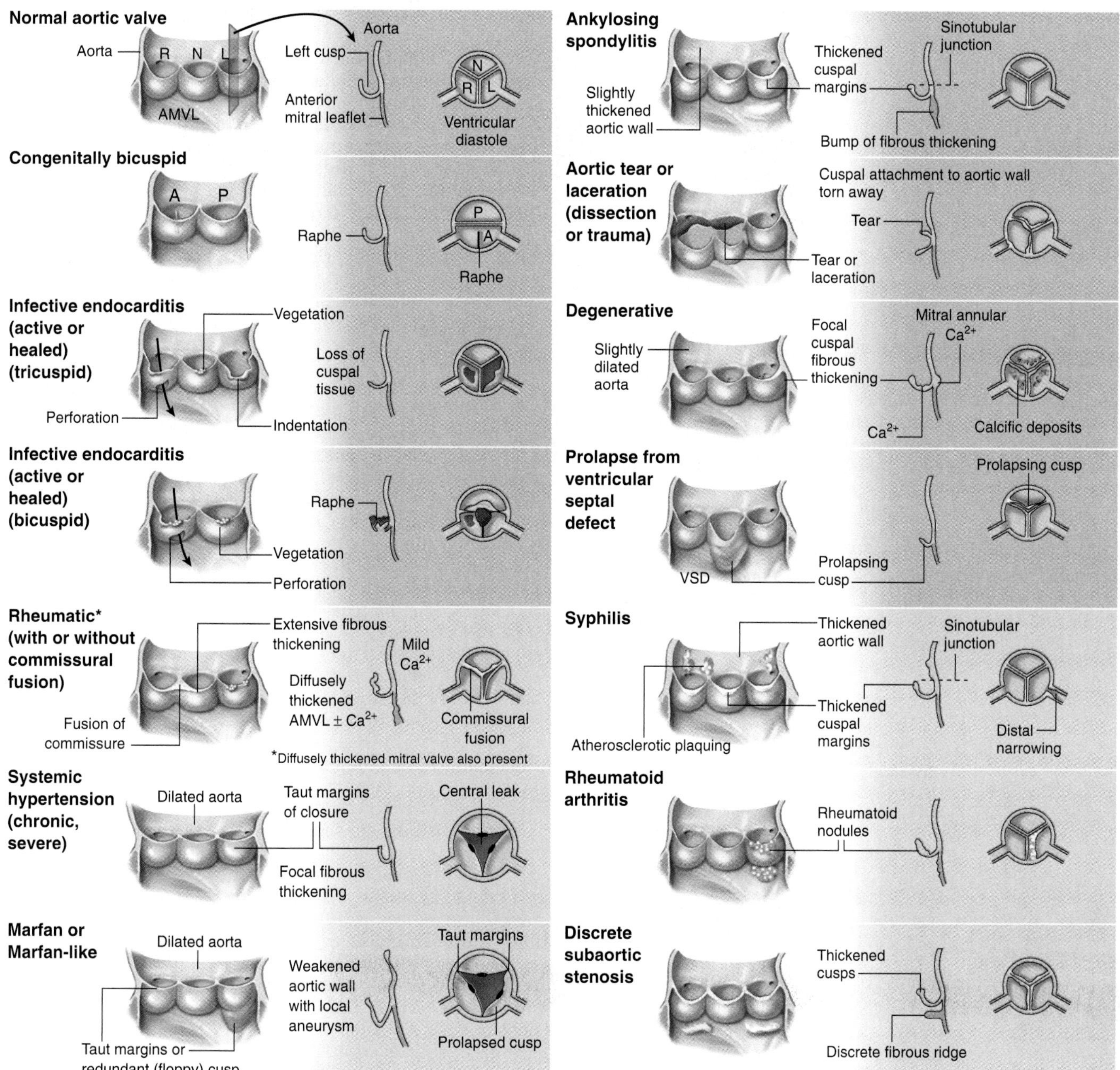

FIGURE 57–31 Diagram of various causes of pure aortic regurgitation. AMVL = anterior mitral valve leaflet; A = anterior; P = posterior; VSD = ventricular septal defect. (From Waller BF: Rheumatic and nonrheumatic conditions producing valvular heart disease. Cardiovasc Clin 16:30-31, 1986.)

Less common causes of AR include various forms of congenital AR, such as unicommissural and quadricuspid valves, or rupture of a congenitally fenestrated valve, particularly in the presence of hypertension. Other less common causes of AR occur in association with systemic lupus erythematosus, rheumatoid arthritis, ankylosing spondylitis, Jaccoud arthropathy, Takayasu disease, Whipple disease, Crohn disease, and, in the past, use of certain anorectic drugs. Isolated congenital AR is an uncommon lesion on necropsy studies, but, when present, is usually associated with a bicuspid valve.

Aortic Root Disease (see Chap. 53)

AR secondary to marked dilation of the ascending aorta is now more common than primary valve disease in patients undergoing AVR for pure AR.[57,226] The conditions responsible for aortic root disease include age-related (degenerative) aortic dilation, cystic medial necrosis of the aorta (either isolated or associated with classic Marfan syndrome), aortic dilation related to bicuspid valves, aortic dissection, osteogenesis imperfecta, syphilitic aortitis, ankylosing spondylitis, Behçet syndrome, psoriatic arthritis, arthritis associated with ulcerative colitis, relapsing polychondritis, Reiter syndrome, giant cell arteritis, and systemic hypertension, as well as exposure to some appetite-suppressant drugs.

When the aortic annulus becomes greatly dilated, the aortic leaflets separate, and AR may ensue. Dissection of the diseased aortic wall may occur and aggravate the AR. Dilation of the aortic root may also have secondary effects on the aortic valve because dilation causes tension and bowing of the individual cusps, which may thicken, retract, and become too short to close the aortic orifice. This leads to intensification of the AR, further dilating the ascending aorta and thus leading to a vicious circle in which, as is the case for MR, "regurgitation begets regurgitation."

AR, regardless of its cause, produces dilation and hypertrophy of the left ventricle, dilation of the mitral valve ring, and sometimes hypertrophy and dilation of the left atrium. Endocardial pockets frequently develop in the left ventricular cavity at sites of impact of the regurgitant jet.

Chronic Aortic Regurgitation

Pathophysiology (Fig. 57–32)

In contrast to MR, in which a fraction of the left ventricular stroke volume is ejected into the low-pressure left atrium, in AR the entire left ventricular stroke volume is ejected into a high-pressure chamber, i.e., the aorta (although the low aortic diastolic pressure does facilitate ventricular emptying during early systole). In MR, especially acute MR, the reduction of wall tension (i.e., reduced afterload) allows more complete systolic emptying; in AR, the increase in left ventricular end-diastolic volume (i.e., increased preload) provides hemodynamic compensation.[1,57,229]

Severe AR may occur with a normal effective forward stroke volume and a normal ejection fraction (forward plus regurgitant stroke volume/end-diastolic volume), together with an elevated left ventricular end-diastolic volume, pressure, and stress (Fig. 57–33).[57,230] In accord with Laplace's law (which indicates that wall tension is related to the product of the intraventricular pressure and radius divided by wall thickness), left ventricular dilation also increases the left ventricular systolic tension required to develop any level of systolic pressure. This leads to eccentric hypertrophy, with replication of sarcomeres in series and elongation of myocytes and myocardial fibers. In compensated AR, there is sufficient wall thickening so that the ratio of ventricular wall thickness to cavity radius remains normal. This maintains or returns end-diastolic wall stress to normal levels. Thus, in AR there is an increase in both preload and afterload. Left ventricular systolic function is maintained through the combination of chamber dilation and hypertrophy.[57,230] AR contrasts with AS, in which there is pressure overload (concentric) hypertrophy with replication of sarcomeres largely in parallel and an increased ratio of wall thickness to radius, but like AS there is an increase in interstitial connective tissue.[176,216,231] In AR, left ventricular mass is usually greatly increased, often to levels even higher than in isolated AS and sometimes exceeding 1000 gm (Fig. 57–34). As AR persists and increases in severity over time, wall thickening fails to keep pace with the hemodynamic load and end-systolic wall stress rises. At this point, the afterload mismatch results in a decline in systolic function, and ejection fraction falls.[57,229]

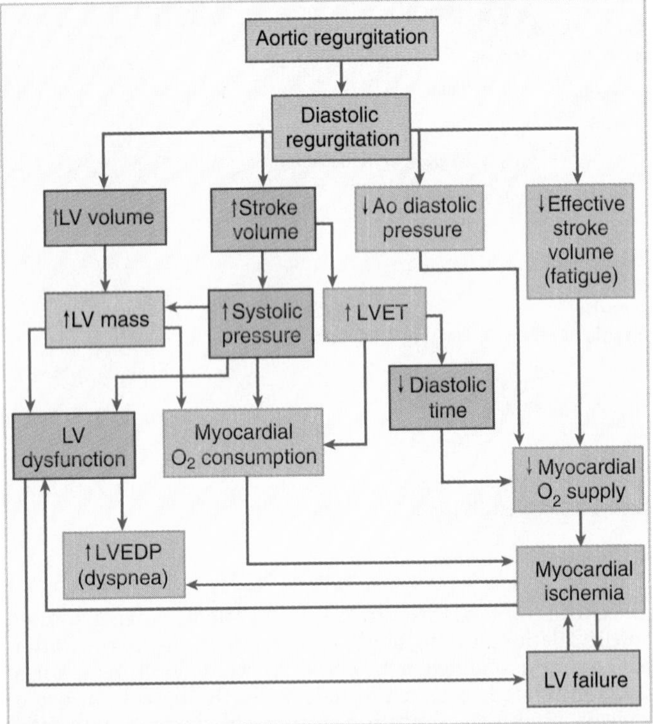

FIGURE 57–32 Pathophysiology of aortic regurgitation. Aortic regurgitation results in an increased left ventricular (LV) volume, increased stroke volume, increased aortic (Ao) systolic pressure, and decreased effective stroke volume. Increased LV volume results in an increased LV mass, which may lead to LV dysfunction and failure. Increased LV stroke volume increases systolic pressure and prolongation of LV ejection time (LVET). Increased LV systolic pressure results in a decrease in diastolic time. Decreased diastolic time (myocardial perfusion time), diastolic aortic pressure, and effective stroke volume reduce myocardial O_2 supply. Increased myocardial O_2 consumption and decreased myocardial O_2 supply produce myocardial ischemia, which further deteriorates LV function. LVEDP = LV end-diastolic pressure. (From Boudoulas H, Gravanis MB: Valvular heart disease. *In* Gravanis MB [ed]: Cardiovascular Disorders: Pathogenesis and Pathophysiology. St. Louis, CV Mosby, 1993, p 64.)

Patients with severe chronic AR have the largest end-diastolic volumes of those with any form of heart disease (resulting in so-called cor bovinum). However, end-diastolic pressure is not uniformly elevated (i.e., left ventricular compliance is often increased [see Fig. 57–33]).

In the more severe cases of AR, the regurgitant flow may exceed 20 liter/min, so that the total left ventricular output at rest approaches 25 liter/min, a level that can be achieved acutely only by a trained endurance runner during maximal exercise. Thus, the adaptive response to gradually increasing, chronic AR permits the ventricle to function as an effective high-compliance pump, handling a large stroke volume, often with little increase in filling pressure. During exercise, peripheral vascular resistance declines, and with an increase in heart rate, diastole shortens and the regurgitation per beat decreases,[1,232] facilitating an increment in effective (forward) cardiac output without substantial increases in end-diastolic volume and pressure. The ejection fraction and related ejection phase indices are often within normal limits, both at rest and during exercise, even though myocardial function, as reflected in the slope of the end-systolic pressure-volume relationship, is depressed.[233]

LEFT VENTRICULAR FUNCTION. As the left ventricle decompensates, interstitial fibrosis increases, compliance declines, and left ventricular end-diastolic pressure and volume rise (see Fig. 57–33). In advanced stages of decompensation, left atrial, pulmonary artery wedge, pulmonary arterial, right ventricular, and right atrial pressures rise and the effective (forward) cardiac output falls, at first during exercise and then at rest. The normal decline in end-systolic volume or the rise in ejection fraction fails to occur during exercise. Symptoms of heart failure, particularly those secondary to pulmonary congestion, develop.

MYOCARDIAL ISCHEMIA. When *acute* AR is induced experimentally, myocardial oxygen requirements rise substantially, secondary to an increase in wall tension. In patients with chronic, severe AR, total myocardial oxygen requirements are also augmented by the increase in left ventricular mass. Because the major portion of coronary blood flow occurs during diastole, when arterial pressure is lower than normal in AR, coronary perfusion pressure is reduced.[232] Studies in experimentally induced AR have shown a reduction in coronary flow reserve with a change in forward coronary flow from diastole to systole. The result—a combination of increased oxygen demand and reduced supply—sets the stage for the development of myocardial ischemia, especially during exercise. Thus, patients with severe AR exhibit a reduction of coronary reserve, which may be responsible for myocardial ischemia, which in turn may play a role in the deterioration of left ventricular function.

Clinical Manifestations

HISTORY

In patients with chronic, severe AR, the left ventricle gradually enlarges while the patient remains asymptomatic.[57,230] Symptoms of reduced cardiac reserve or myocardial ischemia develop, most often in the fourth or fifth decade and usually only *after* considerable cardiomegaly and myocardial dysfunction have occurred. The principal complaints of exertional dyspnea, orthopnea, and paroxysmal nocturnal dyspnea usually develop gradually. Angina pectoris is prominent late in the course; nocturnal angina may be troublesome and is often accompanied by diaphoresis that occurs when the heart rate slows and arterial diastolic pressure falls to extremely low levels. Patients with severe AR often complain of an uncomfortable awareness of the heartbeat, especially on lying down, and disagreeable thoracic pain due to pounding of the heart against the chest wall. Tachycardia, occurring with emotional stress or exertion, may cause troubling palpitations and head pounding. Premature ventricular contractions are particularly distressing because of the great heave of the volume-loaded left ventricle during the postextrasystolic beat. These complaints may be present for many years before symptoms of overt left ventricular dysfunction develop.

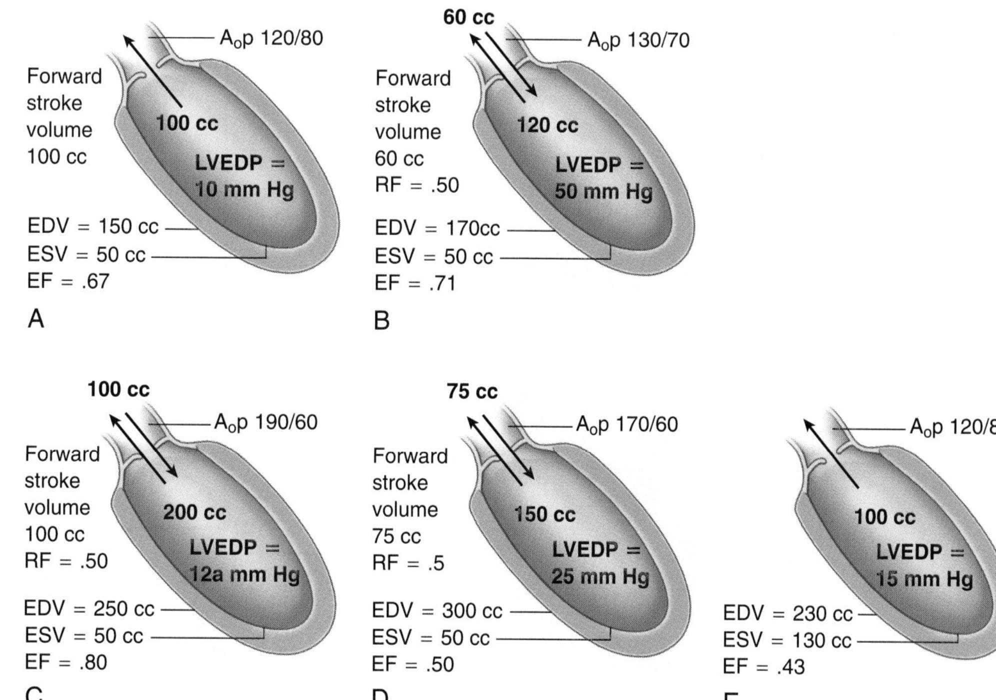

FIGURE 57–33 Hemodynamics of aortic regurgitation. **A,** Normal conditions. **B,** The hemodynamic changes that occur in severe acute aortic regurgitation. Although total stroke volume is increased, forward stroke volume is reduced. Left ventricular end-diastolic pressure (LVEDP) rises dramatically. **C,** Hemodynamic changes occurring in chronic compensated aortic regurgitation are shown. Eccentric hypertrophy produces increased end-diastolic volume (EDV), which permits an increase in total as well as forward stroke volume. The volume overload is accommodated and left ventricular filling pressure is normalized. Ventricular emptying and end-systolic volume (ESV) remain normal. **D,** In chronic decompensated aortic regurgitation, impaired left ventricular emptying produces an increase in end-systolic volume and a fall in ejection fraction (EF), total stroke volume, and forward stroke volume. There is further cardiac dilatation and reelevation of left ventricular filling pressure. **E,** Immediately following valve replacement, preload estimated by EDV decreases, as does filling pressure. ESV also is decreased, but to a lesser extent. The result is an initial fall in EF. Despite these changes, elimination of regurgitation leads to an increase in forward stroke volume. A_op = aortic pressure; RF = regurgitant fraction. (From Carabello BA: Aortic regurgitation: Hemodynamic determinants of prognosis. *In* Cohn LH, DiSesa VJ [eds]: Aortic Regurgitation: Medical and Surgical Management. New York, Marcel Dekker, 1986.)

PHYSICAL EXAMINATION (see Chap. 8)

In patients with chronic, severe AR, the head frequently bobs with each heartbeat (*de Musset sign*), and the pulses are of the "water-hammer" or collapsing type with abrupt distention and quick collapse (*Corrigan pulse*). The arterial pulse is often prominent and can be best appreciated by palpation of the radial artery with the patient's arm elevated. A *bisferiens pulse* may be present and is more readily recognized in the brachial and femoral arteries than in the carotid arteries. A variety of auscultatory findings provide confirmation of a wide pulse pressure. *Traube sign* (also known as "pistol shot sounds") refers to booming systolic and diastolic sounds heard over the femoral artery, *Müller sign* consists of systolic pulsations of the uvula, and *Duroziez sign* consists of a systolic murmur heard over the femoral artery when it is compressed proximally and a diastolic murmur when it is compressed distally. Capillary pulsations (*Quincke sign*) can be detected by pressing a glass slide on the patient's lip, by transmitting a light through the patient's fingertips, or by exerting gently pressure on the tip of a fingernail.

Systolic arterial pressure is elevated, and diastolic pressure is abnormally low. *Hill sign* refers to popliteal cuff systolic pressure exceeding brachial cuff pressure by more than 60 mm Hg. Korotkoff sounds often persist to zero even though intraarterial pressure rarely falls below 30 mm Hg.[230] The point of change in Korotkoff sounds, i.e., the muffling of these sounds in phase IV, correlates with the diastolic pressure. As heart failure develops, peripheral vasoconstriction may occur and arterial diastolic pressure may rise. This finding should not be interpreted as the presence of mild AR.

The apical impulse is diffuse and hyperdynamic and is displaced laterally and inferiorly; there may be systolic retraction over the parasternal region. A rapid ventricular filling wave is often palpable at the apex. The augmented stroke volume may create a *systolic* thrill at the base of the heart or suprasternal notch and over the carotid arteries.[230] In many patients, a carotid shudder is palpable.

AUSCULTATION

The PR interval may be prolonged, causing a soft S_1. A_2 may be normal or accentuated when AR is due to disease of the aortic root but is soft or absent when the valve is causing AR. P_2 may be obscured by the early diastolic murmur. Thus, S_2 may be absent or single or exhibit narrow or paradoxical splitting. A systolic ejection sound, presumably related to abrupt distention of the aorta by the augmented stroke volume, is frequently audible. An S_3 gallop correlates with an increased left ventricular end-diastolic volume.[230] Its development may be a sign of impaired left ventricular function, which is useful in identifying patients with severe regurgitation who are candidates for surgical treatment.

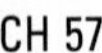

CH 57

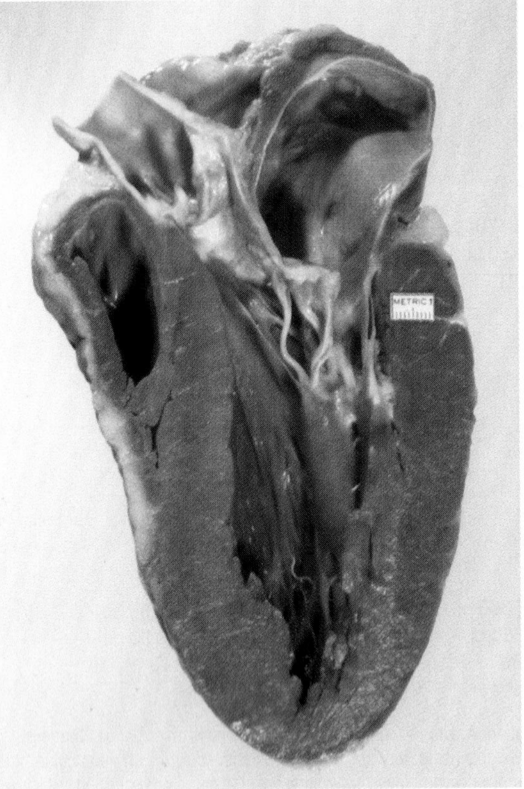

FIGURE 57–34 Heart of a young man with chronic aortic regurgitation who died suddenly, demonstrating both left ventricular dilation and marked left ventricular hypertrophy. (Courtesy of William C. Roberts, MD.)

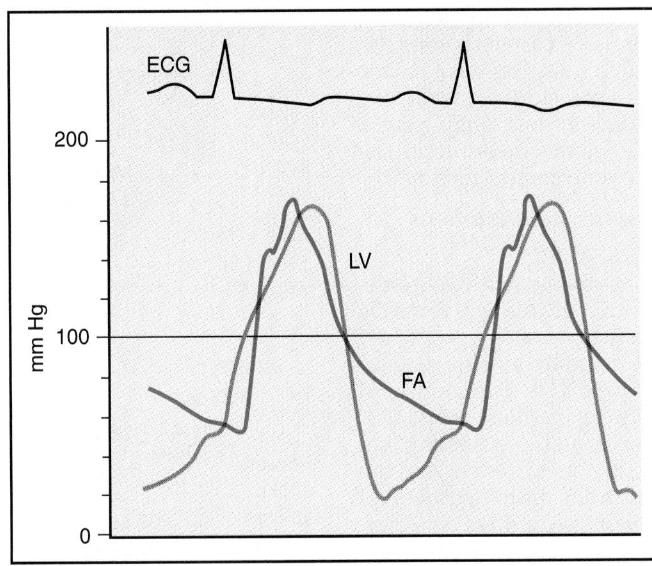

FIGURE 57–35 Pressure curves obtained from a 63-year-old man with symptoms of left ventricular (LV) failure and a loud decrescendo diastolic murmur. The femoral arterial (FA) pressure tracing demonstrates a widened pulse pressure of 115 mm Hg and equalization with LV pressure late in diastole. The LV pressure curve exhibits a steady pressure increase throughout diastole, culminating in a markedly elevated end-diastolic pressure of 45 mm Hg. These findings are indicative of severe aortic regurgitation. ECG = electrocardiogram.

The aortic regurgitant murmur, the principal physical finding of AR,[230,234] is one of high frequency that begins immediately after A_2. It may be distinguished from the murmur of PR by its earlier onset, i.e., immediately after A_2 rather than after P_2, and usually by the presence of a widened pulse pressure. The murmur is heard best with the diaphragm of the stethoscope while the patient is sitting up and leaning forward, with the breath held in deep exhalation. In severe AR, the murmur reaches an early peak and then has a dominant decrescendo pattern throughout diastole.

The severity of the regurgitation correlates better with the *duration* than with the *intensity* of the murmur. In mild AR, the murmur may be limited to early diastole and is typically high pitched and blowing. In severe AR, the murmur is holodiastolic and may have a rough quality. When the murmur is musical ("cooing dove" murmur), it usually signifies eversion or perforation of an aortic cusp. In patients with severe AR and left ventricular decompensation, equilibration of aortic and left ventricular pressures in late diastole (Fig. 57–35) abolishes the late diastolic component of the regurgitant murmur. When regurgitation is caused by primary valvular disease, the diastolic murmur is heard best along the left sternal border in the 3rd and 4th intercostal spaces. However, when it is due mainly to dilation of the ascending aorta, the murmur is often more readily audible along the right sternal border.[230]

Many patients with chronic AR have a harsh systolic outflow murmur caused by the increased total left ventricular stroke volume and ejection rate, and this often radiates to the carotid vessels.[230] The systolic murmur is often more readily audible than the diastolic murmur. It may be higher pitched and less rasping than the murmur of AS but is often accompanied by a systolic thrill. Palpation of the carotid pulses will elucidate the cause of the systolic murmur and differentiate it from the murmur of AS.

A mid and late diastolic apical rumble, the *Austin Flint murmur*, is common in severe AR and may occur in the presence of a normal mitral valve. This murmur appears to be created by rapid antegrade flow across a mitral orifice that is narrowed by the rapidly rising left ventricular diastolic pressure caused by severe aortic reflux impinging on the anterior leaflet of the mitral valve. The Austin Flint murmur may be difficult to differentiate from that due to MS, but the presence of an OS and a loud S_1 in MS and the absence of these findings in AR are helpful clues. As the left ventricular end-diastolic pressure rises, the Austin Flint murmur commences and terminates earlier.

Dynamic Auscultation. The diastolic murmur of AR may be accentuated when the patient sits up and leans forward or by interventions that raise the arterial pressure, such as squatting or isometric exercise. The intensity of the murmur is reduced by interventions that lower the systolic pressure, such as inhalation of amyl nitrite or the strain of the Valsalva maneuver. The Austin Flint murmur, like the murmur of AR, is augmented by isometric exercise and administration of vasopressors and is reduced by amyl nitrite inhalation.

Laboratory Examination

ELECTROCARDIOGRAM. *Chronic,* severe AR results in left-axis deviation and a pattern of left ventricular diastolic volume overload, characterized by an increase in initial forces (prominent Q waves in leads I, aVL, and V_3 through V_6) and a relatively small wave in lead V_1. With the passage of time, these initial forces diminish, but the total QRS amplitude increases. The T waves may be tall and upright in the left precordial leads early in the course, but, more commonly they are inverted, with ST segment depressions. A left ventricular "strain" pattern correlates with the presence of dilation and hypertrophy.[235] Left intraventricular conduction defects occur late in the course and are usually associated with left ventricular dysfunction. The ECG is not an accurate predictor of the severity of AR or cardiac weight. When AR is caused by an inflammatory process, prolongation of the PR interval may be present.[230]

RADIOLOGICAL FINDINGS (see Fig. 12–22). Cardiac size is a function of the duration and severity of regurgitation and the state of left ventricular function. In acute AR, there may be minimal cardiac enlargement, but marked enlargement is a common finding in chronic AR. Typically, the left ventricle enlarges in an inferior and leftward direction, causing a significant increase in the long axis but sometimes causing little or no increase in the transverse diameter of the heart. Calcification of the aortic valve is uncommon in patients with pure AR but is often present in patients with combined AS and AR. Distinct left atrial enlargement in the absence of heart failure suggests associated mitral valve disease. Dilation of the ascending aorta is usually more marked than in AS and may involve the entire aortic arch, including the aortic knob. Severe aneurysmal dilation of the aorta suggests that aortic root disease (e.g., Marfan syndrome, cystic medial necrosis, or annuloaortic ectasia) is responsible for the AR. Linear calcifications in the wall of the ascending aorta are seen in syphilitic aortitis but are nonspecific and are observed in degenerative disease as well.

ANGIOGRAPHY. For angiographic assessment of AR, contrast material should be injected rapidly (i.e., 25 to 35 ml/sec) into the aortic root, and filming should be carried out in the right and left anterior oblique projections. Opacification may be improved by filming during a Valsalva maneuver. In acute AR, there is only a slight increase in ventricular end-diastolic volume, but with the passage of time both the end-diastolic volume and the thickness of the ventricular wall increase, usually in parallel.

ECHOCARDIOGRAPHY (see Figs. 11–69 to 11–72 and Table 11–4). This technique is helpful in identifying the cause of AR. The echocardiogram may show thickening of the valve cusps, congenital abnormalities, prolapse of the valve, a flail leaflet, vegetations, or dilation of the aortic root. Two-dimensional studies are useful for the measurement of left ventricular end-diastolic and end-systolic dimensions, volumes, shortening fraction, ejection fraction, and mass.[232] These measurements, when made serially, are of great value in selecting the optimal time for surgical intervention. Although transthoracic imaging is usually satisfactory, transesophageal echocardiography often provides more detail.

High-frequency fluttering of the anterior leaflet of the mitral valve during diastole is an important echocardiographic finding in both acute and chronic AR (see Fig. 11–72); however, it does not develop when the mitral valve is rigid, as occurs with rheumatic involvement. This sign, which, unlike the Austin Flint murmur, occurs even in mild AR, results from the movement imparted to the anterior leaflet of the mitral valve by the jet of blood regurgitating from the aorta.

Doppler echocardiography and color-flow Doppler imaging are the most sensitive and accurate noninvasive techniques in the diagnosis and evaluation of AR. They readily detect mild degrees of AR that may be inaudible on physical examination. Both the aortic regurgitant orifice size and the aortic regurgitant flow can be estimated quantitatively (Fig. 57–36; see also Figs. 11–66 and 11–67 and Table 11–4).[236-240] Serial studies permit determination of the progression of regurgitation and its effect on the left ventricle.

RADIONUCLIDE IMAGING (see Chap. 13). In most patients, echocardiography provides the needed information regarding severity of AR and the status of the left ventricle. Radionuclide angiography is useful when the echo images are suboptimal, there is a discrepancy between the clinical and the echocardiographic information, or there is a need for more precise measurement of left ventricular ejection fraction.[1] This technique provides an accurate noninvasive assessment of the severity of AR by allowing determination of the regurgitant fraction and of the left ventricular/right ventricular stroke volume ratio. This measurement is nonspecific because the ratio is increased by the presence of associated MR and reduced by tricuspid or pulmonary regurgitation. However, in the absence of these complicating lesions, a left ventricular/right ventricular stroke volume ratio of 2.0 or more denotes severe AR. Radionuclide angiography is also of value in the assessment of left ventricular function during exercise in patients with AR.[233] Serial measurements are useful in the early detection of deterioration of left ventricular function.

MAGNETIC RESONANCE IMAGING (see Fig. 14–12B). Cardiac MRI provides accurate measurements of regurgitant volumes and the regurgitant orifice in AR. It is the most accurate noninvasive technique for assessing left ventricular end-systolic volume, diastolic volume, and mass (see Chap. 14).

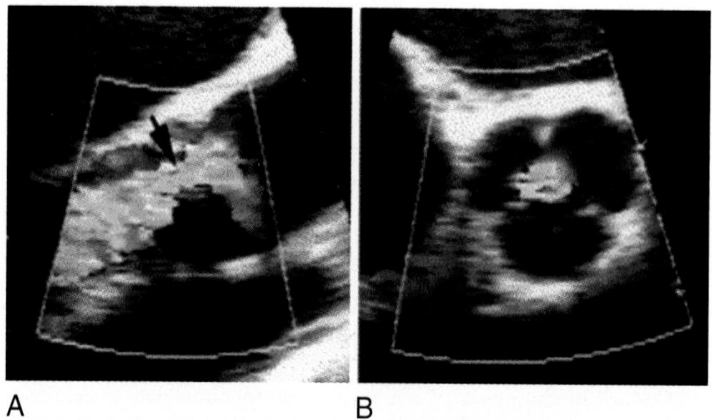

FIGURE 57–36 Transesophageal color Doppler imaging of the aortic regurgitant jet. **A,** Long-axis view. The black arrow indicates the vena contracta, the narrowest portion of the jet located at or just distal to its orifice. The width (in millimeters) of the vena contracta correlates well with volumetric measurement of regurgitant fraction and regurgitant volume. **B,** Short-axis view in the same patient. (From Willett DL, Hall SA, Jessen ME, et al: Assessment of aortic regurgitation by transesophageal color Doppler imaging of the vena contracta: Validation against an intraoperative aortic flow probe. J Am Coll Cardiol 37:1450, 2001.)

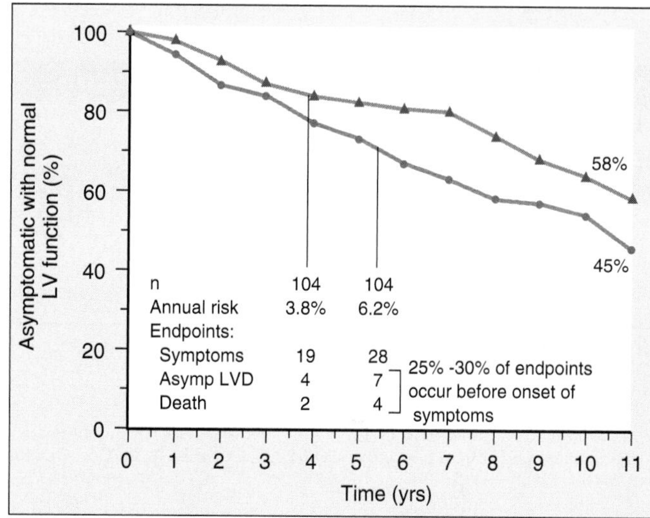

FIGURE 57–37 Natural history of chronic asymptomatic aortic regurgitation in patients with normal left ventricular (LV) ejection fraction at rest, in the series reported by Bonow and associates (blue line) and Borer and colleagues (magenta line), each enrolling 104 patients. At 11 years, 45 to 58 percent of patients remained asymptomatic with normal LV function, such that the risk of developing symptoms, LV dysfunction, or death is roughly 4 to 6 percent per year. The endpoints encountered in these series are indicated. The majority of patients who deteriorated developed symptoms leading to aortic valve replacement. However, 25 to 30 percent of the endpoints, either asymptomatic LV dysfunction (Asymp LVD) or death, occurred without warning symptoms. (Adapted from Bonow RO, Lakatos E, Maron BJ, et al: Serial long-term assessment of the natural history of asymptomatic patients with chronic aortic regurgitation and normal left ventricular systolic function. Circulation 84:1625, 1991; and Borer JS, Hochreiter C, Herrold EM, et al: Prediction of indications for valve replacement among asymptomatic and minimally symptomatic patients with chronic aortic regurgitation and normal left ventricular performance. Circulation 97:525, 1998.)

Management

NATURAL HISTORY OF CHRONIC AORTIC REGURGITATION

Moderately severe or even severe chronic AR may be associated with a generally favorable prognosis for many years. Among asymptomatic patients with severe AR and normal left ventricular ejection fractions, more than 45 percent remain asymptomatic with normal left ventricular function at 10 years (Fig. 57–37),[229,241,242] with an average rate of developing symptoms or left ventricular systolic dysfunction less than 6 percent per year (Table 57–11).[1] The likelihood of sudden death in these asymptomatic patients is less than 0.5 percent per year. However, as is the case for AS, once the patient becomes symptomatic, the downhill course becomes rapidly progressive. Congestive heart failure, punctuated by episodes of acute pulmonary edema, and sudden death may occur, usually in previously symptomatic patients who have considerable left ventricular dilation. Data compiled in the presurgical era indicate that without surgical treatment, death usually occurs within 4 years after the development of angina pectoris and within 2 years after the onset of heart failure. Dujardin and colleagues have confirmed these findings in the current era, demonstrating that 4-year survival without surgery in patients with NYHA Class III or IV symptoms is approximately 30 percent (Fig. 57–38).[244]

Gradual deterioration of left ventricular function may occur even during the asymptomatic period, and some patients may develop significant impairment of systolic function before the onset of symptoms. Numerous surgical series over the past two decades indicate that depressed left ventricular ejection fraction is among the most important determinants of mortality after AVR, particularly when ventricular dysfunction is irreversible and does not improve after operation.[1] Left ventricular dysfunction is more likely to be reversible if detected early before ejection fraction becomes severely depressed, before the left ventricle becomes markedly dilated, and before significant symptoms develop; it is therefore important to intervene surgically before these changes have become irreversible.[1,57,229,245]

TABLE 57–11 Natural History of Aortic Regurgitation

Asymptomatic Patients with Normal LV Systolic Function	
Progression to symptoms and or LV dysfunction	<6%/yr
Progression to asymptomatic LV dysfunction	<3.5%/yr
Sudden death	<0.2%/yr
Asymptomatic Patients with LV Systolic Dysfunction	
Progression to cardiac symptoms	>25%/yr
Symptomatic Patients	
Mortality rate	>10%/yr

LV = left ventricular.

From Bonow RO, Carabello B, de Leon AC Jr, et al: ACC/AHA guidelines for the management of patients with valvular heart disease. J Am Coll Cardiol 32:1486, 1988.

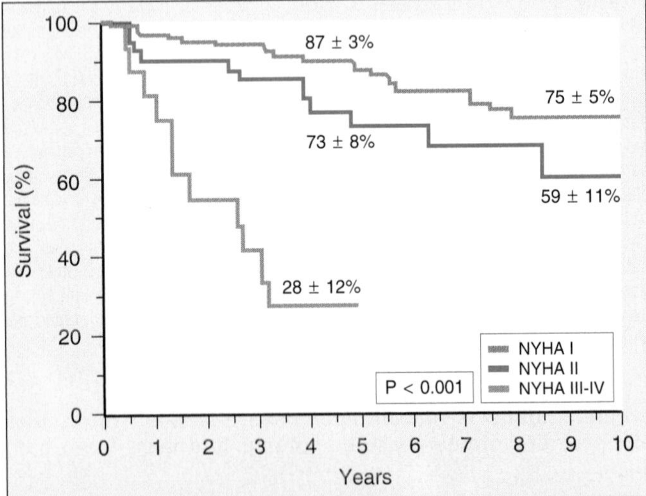

FIGURE 57–38 Survival without surgery in 242 patients with chronic aortic regurgitation, demonstrating the importance of symptoms in determining outcome. Patients with New York Heart Association (NYHA) Class III or IV symptoms had a survival of only 28 percent at 4 years. In contrast, the 10-year survival in patients in Class I was 75 percent, which was identical to that of an age-matched normal population (75 percent). (From Dujardin KS, Enriquez-Sarano M, Schaff HV, et al: Mortality and morbidity of aortic regurgitation in clinical practice: A long-term follow-up study. Circulation 99:1851, 1999.)

MEDICAL TREATMENT

All patients with AR of any severity should receive antibiotic prophylaxis for infective endocarditis (see Chap. 58). Patients with mild or moderate AR who are asymptomatic with normal or only minimally increased cardiac size require no therapy but should be followed clinically and by echocardiography every 12 or 24 months. Asymptomatic patients with chronic, severe AR and normal left ventricular function should be examined at intervals of approximately 6 months. In addition to clinical examination, serial echocardiographic assessments of left ventricular size and ejection fraction should be made. Left-heart catheterization and aortography are usually not necessary but may be useful in patients whose noninvasive test results are inconclusive or discordant with clinical findings.[1] Similarly, other noninvasive tests such as radionuclide angiography or cardiac MRI have an important role primarily when echocardiographic information is not adequate. Patients with mild to moderate AR and those with severe AR with normal ejection fractions and only mild ventricular dilation may engage in aerobic forms of exercise. However, patients with AR who have limitations of cardiac reserve and/or evidence of declining left ventricular function should not engage in vigorous sports or heavy exertion. Systemic arterial diastolic hypertension, if present, should be treated because it increases the regurgitant flow; vasodilating agents such as nifedipine or ACE inhibitors are preferred, and beta-blocking agents should be used with great caution. Atrial fibrillation and bradyarrhythmias are poorly tolerated and should be prevented if possible. If these arrhythmias occur, they must be treated promptly and vigorously.

Vasodilator Therapy. Patients with chronic AR and evidence of significant volume overload (increased end-diastolic dimension or volume) should be considered for vasodilator therapy. Short-term studies spanning 6 months to 2 years have demonstrated beneficial hemodynamic effects of oral hydralazine, nifedipine, felodipine, and ACE inhibitors.[229,246,247] One study followed asymptomatic patients with severe AR for 6 years, comparing the effects of nifedipine (69 patients) and digoxin (74 patients) on left ventricular function and symptoms.[248] Nifedipine delayed the need for operation: at 6 years, 85 percent of patients receiving nifedipine remained asymptomatic with normal left ventricular ejection fraction, compared with only 65 percent of patients receiving digoxin (Fig. 57–39).

Thus, vasodilator therapy is indicated for patients with chronic, severe AR and normal left ventricular systolic function.[1] This therapy should not be used in place of AVR in patients who fulfill the indications for surgery (discussed subsequently), except in circumstances in which AVR cannot be performed because of comorbidities or patient preference.

Symptomatic Patients. AVR is the treatment of choice in symptomatic patients. Chronic medical therapy may be necessary in some patients who refuse surgery or are considered to be inoperable because of comorbid conditions. These patients should receive an aggressive heart failure regimen (see Chap. 23) with ACE inhibitors (and perhaps other vasodilators), digoxin, diuretics, and salt restriction, but beta blockers should be avoided. Even though nitroglycerin and other nitrates are not as helpful in relieving anginal pain in patients with AR as they are in patients with coronary artery disease or AS, they are worth a trial.

In patients who are candidates for surgery but who have severely decompensated left ventricular dysfunction, vasodilator therapy may be particularly helpful in stabilizing patients while preparing for operation. Such patients also respond, at least temporarily, to treatment with digitalis glycosides, salt restriction, and diuretics.

SURGICAL TREATMENT

Indications for Operation. Because of their excellent prognosis in the short and medium term, operative correction

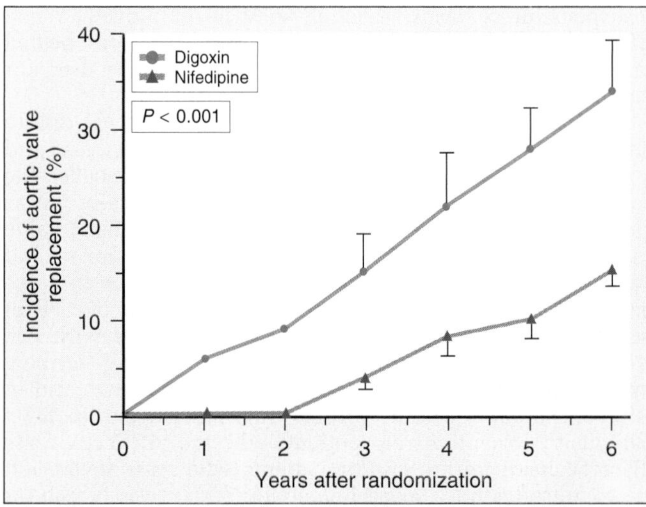

FIGURE 57–39 Randomized clinical trial of nifedipine versus digoxin in asymptomatic patients with chronic aortic regurgitation and normal left ventricular (LV) function. Data indicate the cumulative actuarial incidence of progression to aortic valve replacement because of development of symptoms or decrease in LV ejection fraction to below 50 percent. (From Scognamiglio R, Rahimtoola SH, Fasoli G, et al: Nifedipine in asymptomatic patients with severe aortic regurgitation and normal left ventricular function. N Engl J Med 331:689, 1994.)

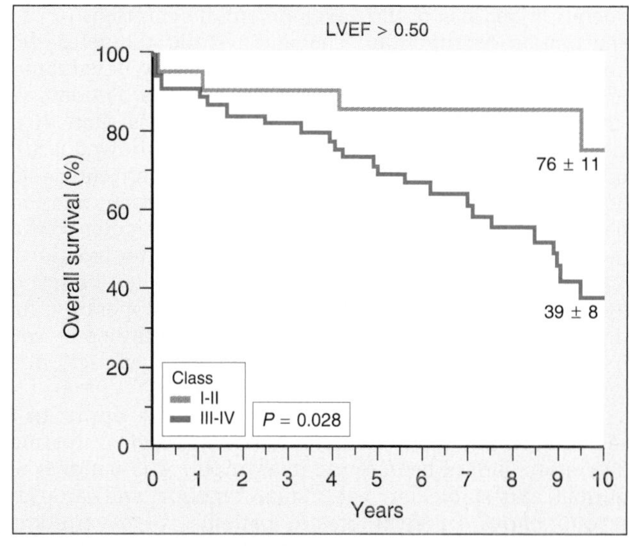

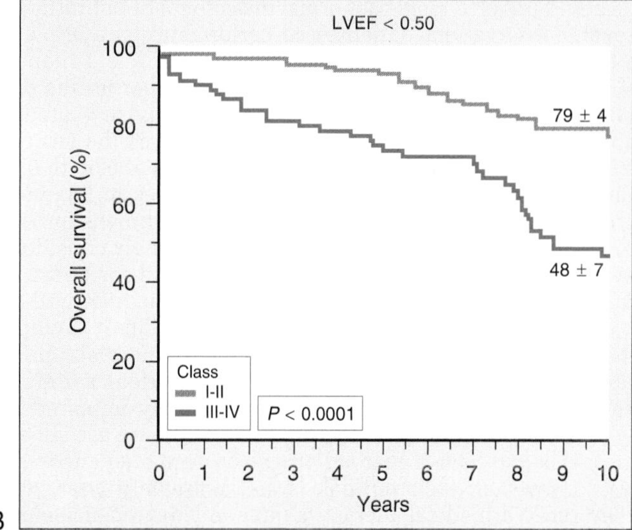

FIGURE 57–40 Long-term postoperative survival in patients with aortic regurgitation, stratified according to the severity of preoperative symptoms and preoperative left ventricular ejection fraction (LVEF). Patients with New York Heart Association (NYHA) Class III or IV symptoms experienced significantly worse survival than those with Class I or II symptoms whether the echocardiographic LVEF was higher than 0.50 **(A)** or less than 0.50 **(B)** without associated coronary artery disease. (From Klodas E, Enriquez-Sarano M, Tajik AJ, et al: Optimizing timing of surgical correction in patients with severe aortic regurgitation: Role of symptoms. J Am Coll Cardiol 30:746, 1997.)

should be deferred in patients with chronic, severe AR who are asymptomatic, have good exercise tolerance, *and* have an ejection fraction greater than 50 percent *without* severe left ventricular dilation (i.e., an end-diastolic diameter < 70 mm and an end-systolic diameter < 50 mm). Similarly, in the absence of obvious contraindications or serious comorbidity, surgical treatment is advisable for symptomatic patients with severe AR and for asymptomatic patients with an ejection fraction less than 0.50 and severe left ventricular dilation (end-diastolic diameter > 75 mm or end-systolic diameter > 55 mm).[1] Between these two ends of the clinical-hemodynamic spectrum are many patients in whom it may be quite difficult to balance the immediate risks of operation and the continuing risks of an implanted prosthetic valve on the one hand against the hazards of allowing a severe volume overload to damage the left ventricle on the other.[57,229,233,249]

Since severe symptoms (NYHA Class III or IV) and left ventricular dysfunction with an ejection fraction less than 0.50 are independent risk factors for poor postoperative survival (Fig. 57–40), surgery should be carried out in NYHA Class II patients before severe left ventricular dysfunction has developed.[1,249-252] Even after successful correction of AR, patients with severe left ventricular dysfunction may have persistent cardiomegaly and depressed left ventricular function.[229,249,251-253] Such patients often exhibit histological changes in the left ventricle, including massive fiber hypertrophy and increased interstitial fibrous tissue. Therefore, it is highly desirable to operate on patients *before* irreversible left ventricular changes have occurred.

Because AR has complex effects on both preload and afterload, the selection of appropriate indices of ventricular contractility to identify patients for operation is challenging. The relationship between end-systolic wall stress and ejection fraction or percent fractional shortening is a useful measurement,[241] as are more load-independent measures of left ventricular contractility.[254] However, in the absence of such complex measurements, *serial* changes in ventricular end-diastolic and end-systolic volumes or dimensions can be used to detect *relative* deterioration of ventricular function.[229] Although left ventricular end-diastolic volume and the ejection phase indices such as ejection fraction and ventricular fraction shortening are strongly influenced by loading conditions, they are nonetheless useful empirical predictors of postoperative function.

Serial echocardiograms or radionuclide ventriculograms should be obtained to detect changes in left ventricular size and function in asymptomatic patients with severe AR. Both techniques allow repeated evaluation of ejection fraction and end-systolic volume (or dimensions) both at rest and during exercise.[241] Impaired left ventricular function at *rest* is the basis for selecting patients for operation; normal left ventricular function at rest with failure of the ejection fraction to rise normally with *exercise* is not considered an indication for surgery per se but is an early warning sign that portends impaired function at rest.[1,233]

Asymptomatic patients with severe AR but normal left ventricular function have an excellent prognosis and do not warrant prophylactic operation (see Table 57–11).[1] On average, less than 6 percent of patients per year require operation because of the development of symptoms or of left ventricular dysfunction. The end-systolic diameter determined by two-dimensional echocardiography is valuable in predicting outcome in asymptomatic patients. Patients with severe AR and an end-systolic diameter less than 40 mm almost invariably remain stable and can be followed without immediate surgery. However, patients with an end-systolic diameter greater than 50 mm Hg have a 19 percent likelihood per year of developing symptoms of left ventricular dysfunction,[229] and those with an end-systolic diameter greater than 55 mm have an increased risk of irreversible left ventricular dysfunction if they are not operated on. Postoperative function and survival in this latter group are determined by severity of symptoms, severity of left ventricular dysfunction, and the *duration* of left ventricular dysfunction.[229]

In summary, the following considerations apply to the selection of patients with chronic AR for surgical treatment. Operation should be *deferred* in asymptomatic patients with normal and stable left ventricular function and should be *recommended* in symptomatic patients. In asymptomatic patients with left ventricular dysfunction, a decision should be based not on a single abnormal measurement but rather on several observations of depressed performance and impaired exercise tolerance, carried out at intervals of 2 to 4 months. If evidence of left ventricular dysfunction is borderline or is not consistent, continued close follow-up is indicated. If abnormalities are progressive or consistent (i.e., the left ventricular ejection fraction declines to the range of 0.50 to 0.55, the left ventricular end-systolic diameter rises to 55 mm or greater, or the left ventricular end-diastolic dimension rises to 75 mm or greater), operation should be strongly considered even in asymptomatic patients. The threshold for operation may be lower when the surgeon believes that AVR will not be necessary, but this prediction may be difficult. Symptomatic patients with severe AR who have normal, mildly depressed, or moderately depressed left ventricular function should be operated on. Patients with severely impaired left ventricular function (ejection fraction < 0.25) are at high surgical risk and have a guarded prognosis even after successful AVR. However, their outlook is also extremely poor when they receive medical therapy alone, and their management should be considered on an individual basis.

The indications for surgery in patients with severe AR secondary to aortic root disease are similar to those in patients with primary valvular disease. However, progressive expansion of the aortic root and/or a diameter greater than 50 mm by echocardiography with any degree of regurgitation is also an indication for surgery in patients with aortic root disease.[1]

As is the case for patients with other valvular lesions, adult surgical candidates who may have underlying coronary artery disease, based on symptoms, age, gender, and risk factors, should undergo preoperative coronary arteriography. Those with coronary artery stenoses should undergo revascularization at the time of AVR.

Operative Procedures. Because an increasing proportion of patients with severe, isolated AR coming to operation now have primary aortic root rather than primary valvular disease, an increasing number can be treated surgically by correcting the dilated aortic root.[103a,255,256] One of two annuloplasty procedures may be employed—an encircling suture of the aorta or a subcommissural annuloplasty. Aneurysmal dilation of the ascending aorta requires excision, replacement with a graft that includes a prosthetic valve, and reimplantation of the coronary arteries.[257]

In some patients with aortic root disease, the native valve can be spared when the aortic root is replaced or repaired (Fig. 57–41). Occasionally, when a leaflet has been torn from its attachments to the aortic annulus by trauma, surgical repair without replacement may be possible. In patients with AR secondary to prolapse of an aortic leaflet, aortic cusp resuspension or cusp resection may be employed. When AR is caused by leaflet perforation resulting from healed infective endocarditis, a pericardial patch can be used for repair.[227,258]

AVR is required for most patients with severe AR due to primary valve disease (as opposed to aortic root disease) and for many patients with combined AS and AR. Because the aortic annulus in patients with severe AR is usually not as narrow as it is in patients with AS, a larger prosthetic valve can be inserted, and mild postoperative obstruction to left ventricular outflow is less of a problem than it is in some patients with AS. In general, the risks and results of AVR in patients with AR are similar to those in patients with AS, with a large percentage of patients exhibiting striking improvement in symptoms. Reductions in heart size and in left ventricular diastolic volume and mass occur in most patients.[229] Exceptions are patients who are in NYHA Class III or IV heart failure and/or patients who have severe left ventricular dysfunction preoperatively.[215,250,252] As is true for patients with AS, the operative risk of AVR for patients with AR depends on the general condition of the patient, the state of left ventricular function, and the skill and experience of the surgical team. The mortality rate ranges from 3 to 8 percent in most medical centers (see Table 57–3). A late mortality of approximately 5 to 10 percent per year is observed in survivors who had marked cardiac enlargement and/or prolonged left ventricular dysfunction preoperatively. Follow-up studies have shown both early rapid and then slower long-term reductions of ventricular mass, ejection fraction, myocyte hypertrophy, and ventricular fibrous content following relief of AR.[216] By extending the indications for operation to symptomatic patients with normal left ventricular function as well as to asymptomatic patients with left ventricular dysfunction, both early and late results are improving.[252] With the continued improvement of surgical techniques and results, it will likely become possible to extend the recommendation for operative treatment to asymptomatic patients with severe regurgitation and normal cardiac function. However, given the risks of operation and the long-term complications of presently available prosthetic valves, we do not believe that the time for such a policy has yet arrived.

ACUTE AORTIC REGURGITATION

Acute AR is caused most commonly by infective endocarditis, aortic dissection, or trauma. The characteristic features of acute AR are tachycardia and an increase in left ventricular diastolic pressures. In contrast to the pathophysiological events in chronic AR just described, in which the left ventricle is able to adapt to the increased hemodynamic load, in acute AR the regurgitant volume fills a ventricle of normal size that cannot accommodate the combined large regurgitant volume and inflow from the left atrium. Because the ability of total stroke volume to rise acutely is limited, forward stroke volume declines. The sudden increase in left ventricular filling causes the left ventricular diastolic pressure to rise rapidly above left atrial pressure during early diastole (see Fig. 57–33),[259] causing the mitral valve to close prematurely in diastole. Premature closure of the mitral valve protects the pulmonary venous bed from backward transmission of the greatly elevated end-diastolic pressure unless it is accompanied by diastolic MR.[260] Premature closure of the mitral valve, together with tachycardia that also shortens diastole, reduces the time interval during which the mitral valve is open. The tachycardia may compensate for the reduced forward stroke volume and left ventricular and aortic *systolic* pressures may exhibit little change. However, severe acute AR may cause profound hypotension and cardiogenic shock. In light of the limited ability of the left ventricle to tolerate acute, severe AR, patients with this valvular lesion often develop clinical manifestations of sudden cardiovascular collapse, including weakness, severe dyspnea, and profound hypotension secondary to the reduced stroke volume and elevated left atrial pressure. In some patients, the aortic diastolic pressure equilibrates with the elevated left ventricular diastolic pressure.

PHYSICAL EXAMINATION. Patients with acute, severe AR appear gravely ill, with tachycardia, severe peripheral vasoconstriction and cyanosis, and sometimes pulmonary congestion and edema. The peripheral signs of AR are often not impressive and certainly not as dramatic as in patients with chronic AR. Duroziez murmur, Traube sign over the peripheral arteries, and bisferiens pulses are usually *absent* in acute AR. The normal or only slightly widened pulse pressure may lead to serious underestimation of the severity of the valvular lesion. The left ventricular impulse is normal or nearly so, and the rocking motion of the chest characteristic of chronic AR is not apparent. S_1 may be soft or absent because of premature closure of the mitral valve,[259] and the sound of mitral valve closure in mid or late diastole is occasionally audible. However, closure of the mitral valve may be incomplete, and diastolic MR may occur. Evidence of pulmonary hypertension, with an accentuated P_2, S_3, and S_4, is frequently present.

The early diastolic murmur of acute AR is lower pitched and shorter than that of chronic AR, because as left ventricular diastolic pressure rises, the (reverse) pressure gradient between the aorta and the left ventricle is rapidly reduced. A systolic murmur is common, resulting in "to and fro" sounds. The Austin Flint murmur is often present but is brief and ceases when left ventricular pressure exceeds left atrial pressure in diastole. With premature diastolic closure of the mitral valve, the presystolic portion of the Austin Flint murmur is eliminated.

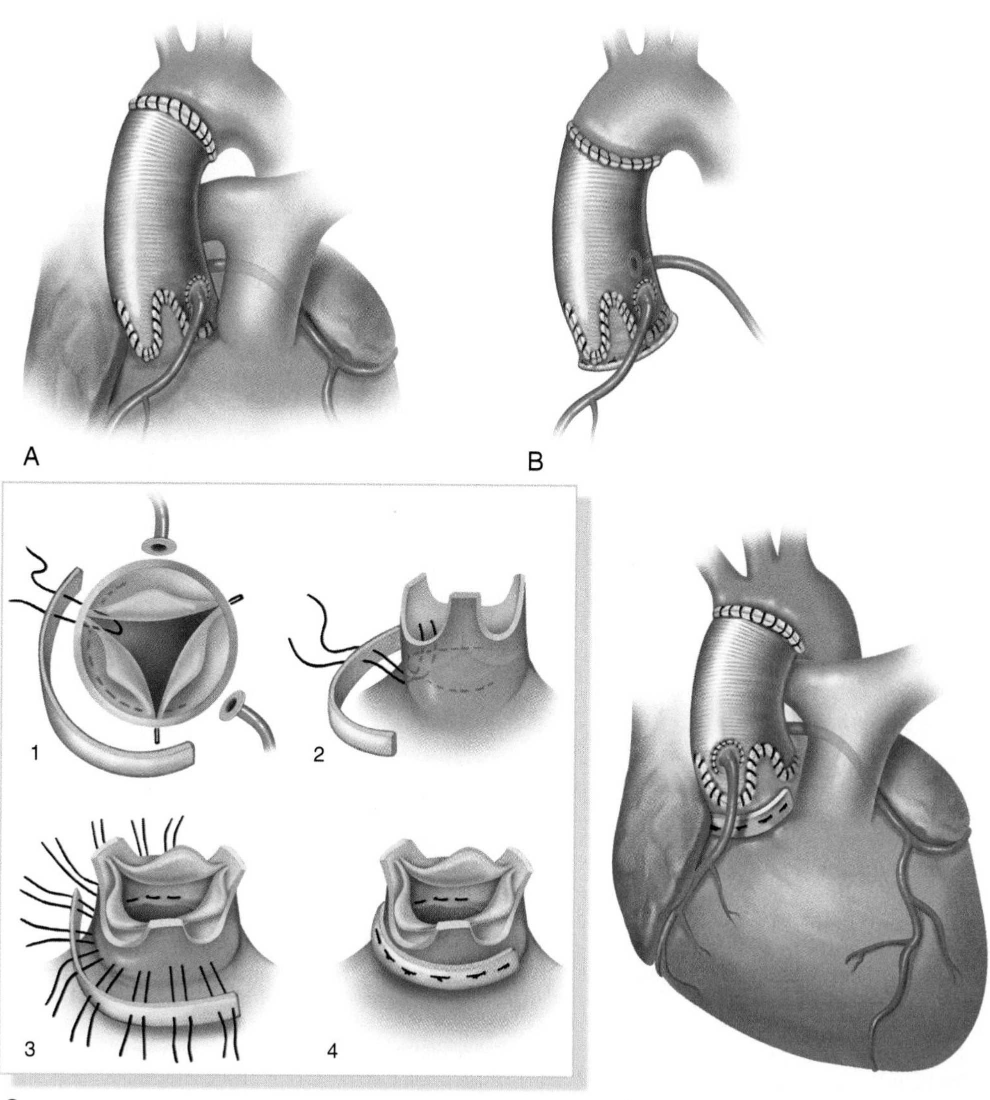

FIGURE 57–41 Repair of aortic regurgitation caused by aortic root dilation. **A,** Remodeling of the aortic root with replacement of all three aortic sinuses. **B,** Reimplantation of the aortic valve in patients with annuloaortic ectasia and aortic root aneurysm. **C** and **D,** Aortic annuloplasty in patients with annuloaortic ectasia. (From David TE: Aortic root aneurysms: Remodeling or composite replacement? Ann Thorac Surg 64:1564, 1997.)

LABORATORY EXAMINATION

Electrocardiography. In *acute* AR, the ECG may or may not show left ventricular hypertrophy, depending on the severity and duration of the regurgitation. However, nonspecific ST segment and T wave changes are common.

Radiological Findings. In acute AR, there is often evidence of marked pulmonary venous hypertension and pulmonary edema. The cardiac silhouette is usually remarkably normal, although left atrial enlargement may be present and, depending on the cause of the AR, there may be enlargement of the ascending aorta.

Echocardiography. In *acute* AR, the echocardiogram reveals a reduction in amplitude of the opening movement, premature closure, and delayed opening of the mitral valve.[259] Left ventricular end-diastolic dimensions are not markedly increased, and fractional shortening is normal. This contrasts with the findings in chronic AR, in which end-diastolic dimensions and wall motion are increased. Occasionally, with equilibration of aortic and left ventricular pressures in diastole, premature opening of the aortic valve may be detected.

MANAGEMENT OF ACUTE AORTIC REGURGITATION. Since early death due to left ventricular failure is frequent in patients with *acute, severe* AR despite intensive medical management, prompt surgical intervention is indicated. Even a normal ventricle cannot sustain the burden of acute, severe volume overload; therefore, the risk of *acute* AR is much greater than that of chronic AR.[259] While the patient is being prepared for surgery, treatment with an intravenous positive inotropic agent (dopamine or dobutamine) and/or a vasodilator (nitroprusside) is often necessary. The agent and dosage should be selected on the basis of arterial pressure (see Chap. 23). Beta-blocking agents and intraaortic balloon counterpulsation are contraindicated, because either lowering the heart rate or augmenting peripheral resistance during diastole can lead to rapid hemodynamic decompensation. In hemodynamically stable patients with acute AR secondary to active infective endocarditis, operation may be deferred to allow 5 to 7 days of intensive antibiotic therapy. However, AVR should be undertaken at the earliest sign of hemodynamic instability or if echocardiographic evidence of diastolic closure of the mitral valve develops.

Tricuspid, Pulmonic, and Multivalvular Disease

Tricuspid Stenosis

Etiology and Pathology

Tricuspid stenosis (TS) is almost always rheumatic in origin.[261] Other causes of obstruction to right atrial emptying are unusual and include congenital tricuspid atresia (see

Chap. 56); right atrial tumors, which may produce a clinical picture suggesting rapidly progressive TS (see Chap. 63)[262]; and the carcinoid syndrome (see Chap. 59),[263] which more frequently produces TR. Rarely, obstruction to right ventricular inflow can be due to endomyocardial fibrosis, tricuspid valve vegetations,[264] a pacemaker lead,[265] or extracardiac tumors.

Most patients with rheumatic tricuspid valve disease present with TR or a combination of stenosis and regurgitation. Isolated rheumatic TS is uncommon and *almost* never occurs as an isolated lesion but generally accompanies mitral valve disease.[1,261,266] In many patients with TS, the aortic valve is also involved (i.e., trivalvular stenosis is present). TS is found at autopsy in about 15 percent of patients with rheumatic heart disease but is of clinical significance in only about 5 percent.[261] Organic tricuspid valve disease is more common in India, Pakistan, and other developing nations near the equator than in North America or Western Europe. The anatomical changes of rheumatic TS resemble those of MS, with fusion and shortening of the chordae tendineae and fusion of the leaflets at their edges, producing a diaphragm with a fixed central aperture.[261] However, valvular calcification is rare. As is the case with MS, TS is more common in women. The right atrium is often greatly dilated in TS, and its walls are thickened. There may be evidence of severe passive congestion, with enlargement of the liver and spleen.

Pathophysiology

A diastolic pressure gradient between the right atrium and ventricle—the hemodynamic expression of TS—is augmented when the transvalvular blood flow increases during inspiration or exercise and is reduced when the blood flow declines during expiration. A relatively modest diastolic pressure gradient (i.e., a mean gradient of only 5 mm Hg) is usually sufficient to elevate mean right atrial pressure to a level that results in systemic venous congestion and, unless sodium intake has been restricted or diuretics have been given, is associated with jugular venous distention, ascites, and edema.

In patients with sinus rhythm, the right atrial *a* wave may be very tall and may even approach the level of the right ventricular systolic pressure. Resting cardiac output is usually markedly reduced and fails to rise during exercise. This accounts for the normal or only slightly elevated left atrial, pulmonary arterial, and right ventricular systolic pressures, despite the presence of accompanying mitral valvular disease.

A *mean* diastolic pressure gradient across the tricuspid valve as low as 2 mm Hg is sufficient to establish the diagnosis of TS. However, exercise, deep inspiration, and the rapid infusion of fluids or the administration of atropine may greatly enhance a borderline pressure gradient in a patient with TS. Therefore, when this diagnosis is suspected, right atrial and ventricular pressures should be recorded simultaneously, using two catheters or a single catheter with a double lumen, with one lumen opening on either side of the tricuspid valve. The effects of respiration on any pressure difference should be examined.

Clinical Manifestations (Table 57–12)

HISTORY. The low cardiac output characteristic of TS causes fatigue, and patients often complain of discomfort due to hepatomegaly, swelling of the abdomen, and anasarca. The severity of these symptoms, which are secondary to an elevated systemic venous pressure, is out of proportion to the degree of dyspnea. Some patients complain of a fluttering discomfort in the neck, caused by giant *a* waves in the jugular venous pulse. Despite the coexistence of MS, the symptoms characteristic of this valvular lesion (i.e., severe dyspnea, orthopnea, and paroxysmal nocturnal dyspnea) are usually mild or absent in the presence of severe TS because the latter prevents surges of blood into the pulmonary circulation behind the stenotic mitral valve. Indeed, the *absence* of symptoms of pulmonary congestion in a patient with obvious MS should suggest the possibility of TS.

TABLE 57–12 Clinical and Laboratory Features of Rheumatic Tricuspid Stenosis

History
Progressive fatigue, edema, anorexia
Minimal orthopnea, paroxysmal nocturnal dyspnea
Rheumatic fever in two-thirds of patients
Female preponderance
Pulmonary edema and hemoptysis are rare
Physical Findings
Signs of multivalvular involvement
Diastolic rumble at lower left sternal border, increasing in intensity with inspiration
Often confused with mitral stenosis
Peripheral cyanosis
Neck vein distention, with prominent *v* waves and slow *y* descent
Absent right ventricular lift
Associated murmurs of mitral and aortic valve disease
Hepatic pulsation
Ascites, peripheral edema
Laboratory Findings
Electrocardiogram: tall right atrial P waves and no right ventricular hypertrophy
Chest roentgenogram: a dilated right atrium without an enlarged pulmonary artery segment
Echocardiography: diastolic doming of tricuspid valve leaflet.

Modified from Ockene IS: Tricuspid valve disease. *In* Dalon JE. Alpert JS (eds): Valvular Heart Disease. 2nd ed. Boston, Little, Brown, 1987, pp 356, 390.

PHYSICAL EXAMINATION. Because of the high frequency with which MS occurs in patients with TS and the similarity in the physical findings between the two valvular lesions, the diagnosis of TS is commonly missed. The physical findings are mistakenly attributed to MS, which is more common and may be more obvious. Therefore, a high index of suspicion is required to detect the tricuspid valvular lesion. In the presence of sinus rhythm, the *a* wave in the jugular venous pulse is tall, and a presystolic hepatic pulsation is often palpable. The *y* descent is slow and barely appreciable. The lung fields are clear, and despite engorged neck veins and the presence of ascites and anasarca, the patient may be comfortable while lying flat. Thus, the diagnosis of TS may be suspected from inspection of the jugular venous pulse in a patient with MS but without clinical evidence of pulmonary hypertension. This suspicion is strengthened when a diastolic thrill is palpable at the lower left sternal border, particularly if the thrill appears or becomes more prominent during inspiration.

The auscultatory findings of the accompanying MS are usually prominent and often overshadow the more subtle signs of TS. A tricuspid OS may be audible but is often difficult to distinguish from a mitral OS. However, the tricuspid OS usually follows the mitral OS and is localized to the lower left sternal border, whereas the mitral OS is usually most prominent at the apex and radiates more widely. The diastolic murmur of TS is also commonly heard best along the lower left parasternal border in the 4th intercostal space and is usually softer, higher pitched, and shorter in duration than the murmur of MS. The presystolic component of the TS murmur has a scratchy quality and a crescendo-decrescendo configuration that diminishes before S_1. The diastolic murmur and OS of

TS are both augmented by maneuvers that increase transtricuspid valve flow, including inspiration, the Müller maneuver, assumption of the right lateral decubitus position, leg raising, inhalation of amyl nitrite, squatting, and isotonic exercise. They are reduced during expiration or the strain of the Valsalva maneuver and return to control levels immediately (i.e., within two or three beats) after Valsalva release.

Laboratory Examination

ELECTROCARDIOGRAM. In the absence of atrial fibrillation in a patient with valvular heart disease, TS is suggested by the presence of ECG evidence of right atrial enlargement (see Chap. 9). The P wave amplitude in leads II and V_1 exceeds 0.25 mV. Because most patients with TS have mitral valvular disease, the EGG signs of biatrial enlargement are commonly found. The amplitude of the QRS complex in lead V_1 may be reduced by the dilated right atrium.

RADIOLOGICAL FINDINGS. The key radiological finding is marked cardiomegaly with conspicuous enlargement of the right atrium (i.e., prominence of the right heart border), which extends into a dilated superior vena cava and azygos vein, but without conspicuous dilation of the pulmonary artery. The vascular changes in the lungs characteristic of mitral valvular disease may be masked, with little or no interstitial edema or vascular redistribution, but left atrial enlargement may be present.

Angiography carried out following injection of contrast material into the right atrium and filming in the 30-degree right anterior oblique projection characteristically shows thickening and decreased mobility of the leaflets, a diastolic jet through the constricted orifice, and thickening of the normal atrial wall.

ECHOCARDIOGRAM (see Chap. 11). The echocardiographic changes of the tricuspid valve in TS resemble those observed in the mitral valve in MS. Two-dimensional echocardiography characteristically shows diastolic doming of the leaflets (especially the anterior tricuspid valve leaflet), thickening and restricted motion of the other leaflets, reduced separation of the tips of the leaflets, and reduction in diameter of the tricuspid orifice. Transesophageal echocardiography allows added delineation of the details of valve structure. Doppler echocardiography shows a prolonged slope of antegrade flow and compares well with cardiac catheterization in the quantification of TS and in the assessment of associated TR.[267] Doppler evaluation of TS has largely replaced the need for catheterization to assess severity.[266]

MANAGEMENT

Although the fundamental approach to the management of severe TS is surgical treatment, intensive sodium restriction and diuretic therapy may diminish the symptoms secondary to the accumulation of excess salt and water. A preparatory period of diuresis may diminish hepatic congestion and thereby improve hepatic function sufficiently to diminish the risks of subsequent operation.

Most patients with TS have coexisting valvular disease that requires surgery. In patients with combined TS and MS, the former must *not* be corrected alone because pulmonary congestion or edema may ensue. Surgical treatment of TS should be carried out at the time of mitral valve repair or replacement in patients with TS in whom the mean diastolic pressure gradient exceeds 5 mm Hg and the tricuspid orifice is less than approximately 2.0 cm^2. The final decision concerning surgical treatment is often made at the operating table.

Because TS is almost always accompanied by some TR, simple finger fracture valvotomy may not result in significant hemodynamic improvement but may merely substitute severe regurgitation for stenosis. However, open valvotomy in which the stenotic tricuspid valve is converted into a functionally bicuspid valve may result in substantial improvement. The commissures between the anterior and septal leaflets and between the posterior and septal leaflets are opened. It is not advisable to open the commissure between the anterior and posterior leaflets for fear of producing severe regurgitation. If open valvotomy does not restore reasonably normal valve function, the tricuspid valve may have to be replaced.[268] A large porcine bioprosthesis is preferred to a mechanical prosthesis in the tricuspid position because of the high risk of thrombosis of the latter and the longer durability of bioprostheses in the tricuspid than in the mitral or aortic positions. The feasibility of tricuspid balloon valvuloplasty has been demonstrated, and this procedure may be combined with mitral balloon valvuloplasty.[269]

Tricuspid Regurgitation

Etiology and Pathology (Table 57–13)

The most common cause of TR is not intrinsic involvement of the valve itself (i.e., primary TR) but rather *dilation of the right ventricle* and of the tricuspid annulus causing secondary (functional) TR. This may be a complication of right ventricular failure of any cause. It is observed in patients with right ventricular hypertension secondary to any form of cardiac or pulmonary vascular disease, most commonly mitral valve disease.[261] In general, a systolic right ventricular systolic pressure greater than 55 mm Hg causes functional TR.[1] TR can also occur secondary to right ventricular infarction,[261] congenital heart disease (see Chap. 56) (e.g., pulmonic stenosis (PS) and pulmonary hypertension secondary to Eisenmenger syndrome), primary pulmonary hypertension, and, rarely, cor pulmonale. In infants, TR may complicate right ventricular failure secondary to neonatal pulmonary diseases and pulmonary hypertension with persistence of the

TABLE 57–13 Causes and Mechanisms of Pure Tricuspid Regurgitation

Causes

Anatomically ABNORMAL valve
- Rheumatic
- Nonrheumatic
  - Infective endocarditis
  - Ebstein anomaly
  - Floppy (prolapse)
  - Congenital (non-Ebstein)
  - Carcinoid
  - Papillary muscle dysfunction
  - Trauma
  - Connective tissue disorders (Marfan)
  - Rheumatoid arthritis
  - Radiation injury

Anatomically NORMAL valve (functional)
- Elevated right ventricular systolic pressure (dilated annulus)

Mechanisms

Condition	*Leaflet Area*	*Annular Circumference*	*Leaflet Insertion*
Floppy	↑	↑	Normal
Ebstein anomaly	↑	↑	Abnormal
Pulmonary/right ventricular systolic hypertension	Normal	↑	Normal
Papillary muscle dysfunction	Normal	Normal	Normal
Carcinoid	↓ /Normal	Normal	Normal
Rheumatic	↓ /Normal	Normal	Normal
Infective endocarditis	↓ /Normal	Normal	Normal

Modified from Waller BF: Rheumatic and nonrheumatic conditions producing valvular heart disease. *In* Frankl WS, Brest AN (eds): Cardiovascular Clinics: Valvular Heart Disease: Comprehensive Evaluation and Management. Philadelphia, FA Davis, 1989, pp 35, 95.

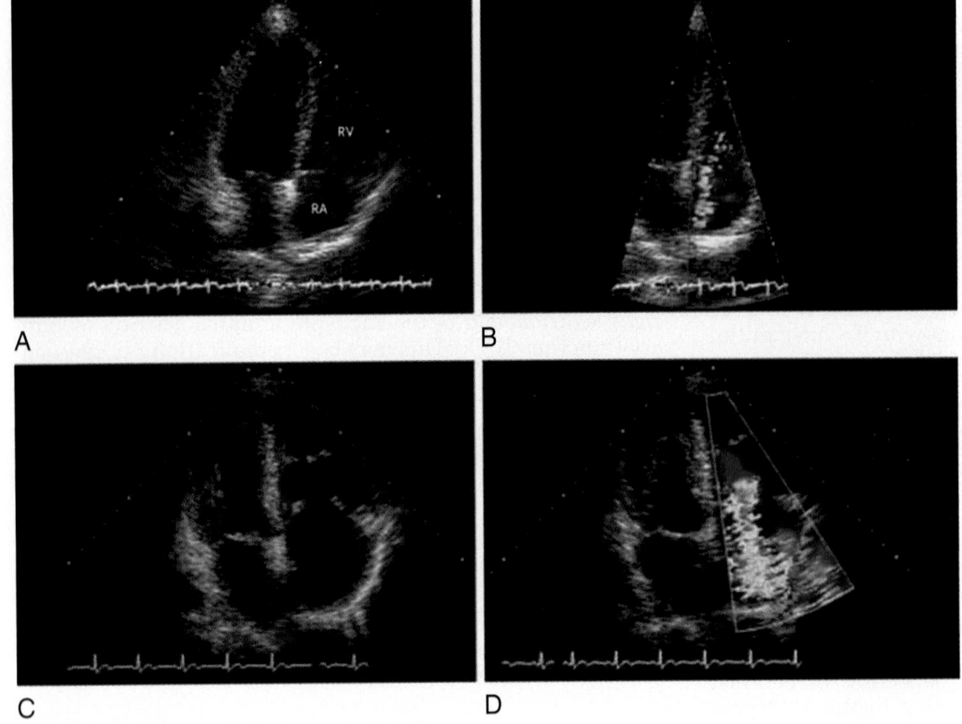

FIGURE 57–42 Tricuspid regurgitation (TR) caused by carcinoid involvement of the tricuspid valve. Serial two-dimensional echocardiograms **(A** and **C)** and color Doppler studies **(B** and **D)**, separated by 3 years are shown. After 3 years, there is severe thickening and fixation of the tricuspid leaflets **(C)**, leading to severe TR and associated right ventricular (RV) and right atrial (RA) enlargement. (From Møller JE, Connolly HM, Rubin J, et al: Factors associated with progression of carcinoid heart disease. N Engl J Med 348:1005, 2003.)

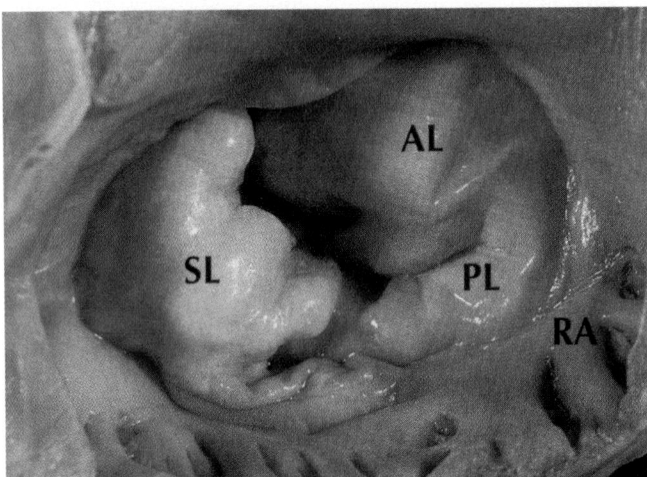

FIGURE 57–43 Tricuspid valve prolapse, viewed from the right atrium (RA). AL = anterior leaflet; PL = posterior leaflet; SL = septal leaflet. (From Virmani R, Burke AP, Farb A: Pathology of valvular heart disease. *In* Rahimtoola SH [ed]: Valvular Heart Disease. *In* Braunwald E [series ed]: Atlas of Heart Diseases. Vol 11. Philadelphia, Current Medicine, 1997, p 1.17.)

fetal pulmonary circulation. In all of these cases, TR reflects the presence of, and in turn aggravates, severe right ventricular failure. Functional TR may diminish or disappear as the right ventricle decreases in size with the treatment of heart failure. TR can also occur as a consequence of dilation of the annulus in Marfan syndrome, in which right ventricular dilation secondary to pulmonary hypertension is not present.

A variety of disease processes can affect the tricuspid valve apparatus *directly* and lead to regurgitation (primary TR). Thus, organic TR may occur on a congenital basis, as part of *Ebstein anomaly,* in atrioventricular canal, and when the tricuspid valve is involved in the formation of an aneurysm of the ventricular septum, or in corrected transposition of the great arteries,[270] or it may occur as an isolated congenital lesion. Rheumatic fever may involve the tricuspid valve directly.[266] When this occurs, it usually causes scarring of the valve leaflets and/or chordae tendineae, leading to limited leaflet mobility and either isolated TR or a combination of TR and TS. Rheumatic involvement of the mitral, and often aortic, valves coexist.

TR or the combination of TR and TS is an important feature of the *carcinoid syndrome* (Fig. 57–42), which leads to focal or diffuse deposits of fibrous tissue on the endocardium of the valvular cusps and cardiac chambers and on the intima of the great veins and coronary sinus (see Chap. 59).[263,271,272] The white, fibrous carcinoid plaques are most extensive on the right side of the heart, where they are usually deposited on the ventricular surfaces of the tricuspid valve and cause the cusps to adhere to the underlying right ventricular wall, thereby producing TR (see Fig. 57–42). Endomyocardial fibrosis with shortening of the tricuspid leaflets and chordae tendineae is an important cause of TR in tropical Africa (see Chap. 59). TR may result from prolapse of the tricuspid valve caused by myxomatous changes in the valve and chordae tendineae (Fig. 57–43); prolapse of the mitral valve is usually present in these patients as well.[261] Prolapse of the tricuspid valve occurs in about 20 percent of all patients with MVP. Tricuspid valve prolapse may also be associated with atrial septal defect. Other causes of TR include penetrating and nonpenetrating trauma, dilated cardiomyopathy, infective endocarditis (particularly staphylococcal endocarditis in narcotic addicts), and following surgical excision of the tricuspid valve in patients with infective endocarditis that is unresponsive to medical management. Less common causes of TR include cardiac tumors (particularly right atrial myxoma), transvenous pacemaker leads,[273] repeated endomyocardial biopsy in a transplanted heart,[274] endomyocardial fibrosis, methysergide-induced valvular disease, exposure to fenfluramine-phentermine,[275] and systemic lupus erythematosus involving the tricuspid valve.

Clinical Manifestations

HISTORY. In the absence of pulmonary hypertension, TR is generally well tolerated. However, when pulmonary hypertension and TR coexist, cardiac output declines and the manifestations of right-sided heart failure become intensified. Thus, the symptoms of TR result from a reduced cardiac output and from ascites, painful congestive hepatomegaly, and massive edema. Occasionally, patients have throbbing pulsations in the neck, which intensify on effort and are due to jugular venous distention, and systolic pulsations of the eyeballs have also been described. In the many patients with TR who have mitral valve disease, the symptoms of the latter usually predominate. Symptoms of pulmonary congestion may abate as TR develops, but they are replaced by weakness, fatigue, and other manifestations of a depressed cardiac output.

PHYSICAL EXAMINATION. Evidence of weight loss and cachexia, cyanosis, and jaundice are often present on inspection in patients with severe TR. Atrial fibrillation is common. There is jugular venous distention,[261] the normal *x* and *x′* descents disappear, and a prominent systolic wave, i.e., a *c-v* wave (or *s* wave), is apparent. The descent of this wave, the *y* descent, is sharp and becomes the most prominent feature of the venous pulse (unless there is coexisting TS, in which case it is slowed). A venous systolic thrill and murmur in the neck may be present in patients with severe TR. The right ventricular impulse is hyperdynamic and thrusting in quality. Systolic pulsations of an enlarged, tender liver are commonly present initially. However, in patients with chronic TR and congestive cirrhosis, the liver may become firm and nontender.[276] Ascites and edema are frequent.

Auscultation. This usually reveals an S_3 originating from the right ventricle, which is accentuated by inspiration. When TR is associated with and secondary to pulmonary hypertension, P_2 is accentuated as well. When TR occurs in the presence of pulmonary hypertension, the systolic murmur is usually high-pitched, pansystolic, and loudest in the 4th intercostal space in the parasternal region but occasionally is loudest in the subxiphoid area. When TR is mild, the murmur may be short. When TR occurs in the absence of pulmonary hypertension (e.g., in infective endocarditis or following trauma), the murmur is usually of low intensity and limited to the first half of systole. When the right ventricle is greatly dilated and occupies the anterior surface of the heart, the murmur may be prominent at the apex and difficult to distinguish from that produced by MR.

The response of the systolic murmur to respiration and other maneuvers is of considerable aid in establishing the diagnosis of TR. The murmur is characteristically augmented during inspiration (Carvallo sign). However, when the failing ventricle can no longer increase its stroke volume in the recumbent or sitting positions, the inspiratory augmentation may be elicited by standing. The murmur also increases during the Müller maneuver (forced inspiration against a closed glottis), exercise, leg-raising, and hepatic compression. It demonstrates an immediate overshoot after release of the Valsalva strain but is reduced in intensity and duration in the standing position and during the strain of the Valsalva maneuver. Increased atrioventricular flow across the tricuspid orifice in diastole may cause a short, early diastolic flow rumble in the left parasternal region following S_3. Tricuspid valve prolapse, like MVP, causes nonejection systolic clicks and late systolic murmurs. However, in tricuspid valve prolapse, these findings are more prominent at the lower left sternal border. With inspiration, the clicks occur later, and the murmurs intensify and become shorter in duration.

Laboratory Examination

ELECTROCARDIOGRAM. This is usually nonspecific and characteristic of the lesion causing TR. Incomplete right bundle branch block, Q waves in lead V_1, and atrial fibrillation are commonly found.

RADIOLOGICAL FINDINGS. In patients with functional TR, marked cardiomegaly is usually evident, and the right atrium is prominent. Evidence of elevated right atrial pressure may include distention of the azygos vein and the presence of a pleural effusion. Ascites with upward displacement of the diaphragm may be present. Systolic pulsations of the right atrium may be present on fluoroscopy.

ECHOCARDIOGRAM (see Fig. 11–73). The goal of echocardiography is to detect TR, estimate its severity, and assess pulmonary arterial pressure and right ventricular function.[267] In patients with TR secondary to dilation of the tricuspid annulus, the right atrium, right ventricle, and tricuspid annulus all are usually greatly dilated on echocardiography. There is evidence of right ventricular diastolic overload with paradoxical motion of the ventricular septum similar to that observed in atrial septal defect. Exaggerated motion and delayed closure of the tricuspid valve are evident in patients with Ebstein anomaly. Prolapse of the tricuspid valve due to myxomatous degeneration may be evident on echocardiography.[261] Echocardiographic indications of tricuspid valve abnormalities, especially TR by Doppler examination, can be detected in most patients with carcinoid heart disease.[271] In patients with TR due to endocarditis, echocardiography may reveal vegetations on the valve or a flail valve. Transesophageal echocardiography enhances detection of TR.

Doppler echocardiography is a sensitive technique for visualizing the TR jet. The magnitude of TR can be quantified using techniques similar to those used to evaluate MR (Fig. 57–44).[266,277-279] Contrast echocardiography also improves detection of TR and can trace regurgitant microbubbles into the inferior vena cava and hepatic veins.[266,278,279]

HEMODYNAMIC FINDINGS. The right atrial and right ventricular end-diastolic pressures are often elevated in TR, whether the condition is due to organic disease of the tricuspid valve or is secondary to right ventricular systolic overload. The right atrial pressure tracing usually reveals absence of the *x* descent and a prominent *v* or *c-v* wave ("ventricularization" of the atrial pressure). Absence of these findings essentially excludes moderate or severe TR.[280] As the severity of TR increases, the contour of the right atrial pressure pulse increasingly resembles that of the right ventricular pressure pulse. A rise or no change in right atrial pressure on deep inspiration, rather than the usual fall, is a characteristic finding. Determination of the pulmonary arterial (or right ventricular) systolic pressure may be helpful in deciding whether the TR is primary (i.e., due to disease of the valve or its supporting structures) or functional (i.e., secondary to right ventricular dilation). A pulmonary arterial or right ventricular systolic pressure less than 40 mm Hg favors a primary cause, whereas a pressure greater than 55 mm Hg suggests that TR is secondary.

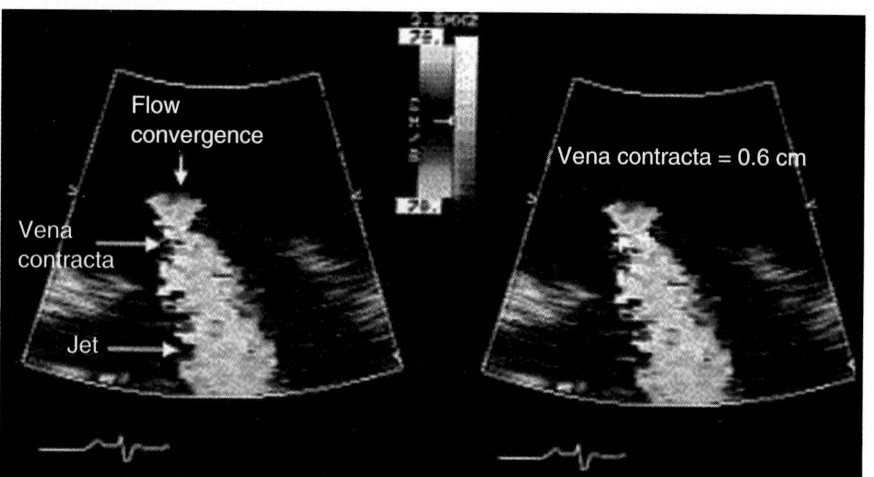

FIGURE 57–44 Tricuspid regurgitation flow visualized by color-flow Doppler echocardiography in the apical view. This defines the three components of regurgitant flow **(left)** and measurement of the width of the vena contracta **(right).** (From Tribouilloy CM, Enriquez-Sarano M, Bailey KR, et al: Quantification of tricuspid regurgitation by measuring the width of the vena contracta with Doppler color flow imaging: A clinical study. J Am Coll Cardiol 36:472, 2000.)

MANAGEMENT

TR in the absence of pulmonary hypertension usually is well tolerated and may not require surgical treatment. Indeed, both human patients and experimental animals with normal pulmonary arterial pressure may tolerate total excision of the tricuspid valve as long as right ventricular systolic pressure is normal. Dilation of the right side of the heart usually occurs months or years after tricuspid valvectomy (usually carried out for acute infective endocarditis). *Surgical treatment* of acquired regurgitation secondary to annular dilation was greatly improved with development of annuloplasty techniques, with or without an annuloplasty ring. Annuloplasty without insertion of a prosthetic ring (the so-called DeVega annuloplasty) has also been found to be effective in patients with annular dilation. This technique is now widely employed.[281,282] This reduces but does not always eliminate TR.[266]

At the time of mitral valve surgery in patients with TR secondary to pulmonary hypertension, the severity of the regurgitation should be assessed by palpation of the tricuspid valve. In addition, it should be determined whether the TR is secondary to pulmonary hypertension, in which case the valve is normal, or whether it is secondary to rheumatic fever. Patients with mild TR usually do not require surgical treatment[261]; pulmonary vascular pressures decline following successful mitral valve surgery, and the mild TR tends to disappear. Excellent results have been reported in patients with moderate TR with the use of suture annuloplasty of the posterior (unsupported) portion of the annulus. Patients with severe TR and primary rheumatic tricuspid valve disease with commissural fusion require valvotomy and ring annuloplasty. The latter is also employed for TR secondary to annular dilation. A surgical mortality rate of 13.9 percent has been reported (see Table 57–3).[283] If these procedures do not provide a good functional result at the operating table (as assessed by transesophageal echocardiography), valve replacement using a large porcine mitral heterograft may be required.

When organic disease of the tricuspid valve (Ebstein anomaly or carcinoid heart disease) causes TR severe enough to require surgery, valve replacement is usually needed. The risk of thrombosis of mechanical prostheses is greater in the tricuspid than in the mitral or aortic positions, presumably because pressure and flow rates are lower in the right side of the heart. For this reason, the artificial valve of choice for the tricuspid position in adults is a large porcine heterograft. Anticoagulants are not required, and a graft durability of more than 10 years has been established.

In treating the difficult problem of tricuspid endocarditis in heroin addicts, total excision of the tricuspid valve *without immediate replacement* can generally be tolerated by these patients, who usually do not have associated pulmonary hypertension. When antibiotic therapy is unsuccessful, valvular replacement frequently results in reinfection or continued infection. Therefore, diseased valvular tissue should be excised to eradicate the endocarditis, and antibiotic treatment can then be continued. Initially, most patients tolerate loss of the tricuspid valve without great difficulty. Later, right ventricular dysfunction usually occurs. A bioprosthetic valve may therefore be inserted 6 to 9 months after valve excision and control of the infection.

Pulmonic Valve Disease

Etiology and Pathology

PULMONIC STENOSIS. The *congenital* form is the most common cause of PS.[266] Manifestations in children and adults are discussed in Chapter 56. *Rheumatic* inflammation of the pulmonic valve is uncommon, is usually associated with involvement of other valves, and rarely leads to serious deformity. *Carcinoid* plaques, similar to those involving the tricuspid valve, are often present in the outflow tract of the right ventricle of patients with malignant carcinoid. The plaques result in constriction of the pulmonic valve ring, retraction and fusion of the valve cusps, and either PS or the combination of PS and PR (Fig. 57–45).[263,271,272] Obstruction in the region of the pulmonic valve may be extrinsic to the valve apparatus and may be produced by cardiac tumors or by aneurysm of the sinus of Valsalva.

Management of congenital PS focuses on balloon dilation (see Chaps. 52 and 56).

PULMONIC REGURGITATION. By far the most common cause of PR is dilation of the valve ring secondary to pulmonary hypertension (of any etiology) or to dilation of the pulmonary artery, either idiopathic or consequent to a connective tissue disorder such as Marfan syndrome. The second most common cause of PR is infective endocarditis. Less frequently, PR is iatrogenic and is induced at the time of surgical treatment of congenital PS or tetralogy of Fallot.[284,285] PR may also result from various lesions that directly affect the pulmonic valve. These include congenital malformations such as absent, malformed, fenestrated, or supernumerary leaflets. These anomalies may occur as isolated lesions but more often are associated with other congenital anomalies, particularly tetralogy of Fallot, ventricular septal defect, and pulmonic valvular stenosis. Less common causes include trauma, carcinoid syndrome,[263] rheumatic involvement, injury produced by a pulmonary artery flow-directed catheter, syphilis, and chest trauma.

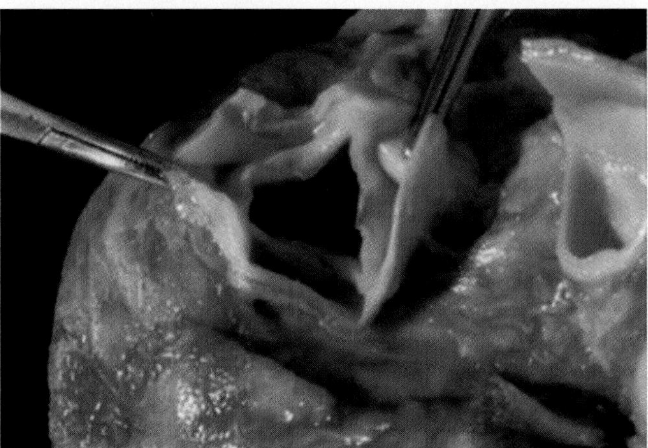

FIGURE 57–45 Carcinoid heart disease. The pulmonary valve is viewed from above. (From Kulke MH, Mayer RJ: Carcinoid tumors. N Engl J Med 340:858, 1999.)

Clinical Manifestations

Like TR, isolated PR causes right ventricular volume overload and may be tolerated for many years without difficulty unless it complicates, or is complicated by, pulmonary hypertension. In this case, PR is usually accompanied by and aggravates right ventricular failure. Patients with PR caused by infective endocarditis who develop septic pulmonary emboli and pulmonary hypertension often exhibit severe right ventricular failure. In most patients, the clinical manifestations of the primary disease are severe and usually overshadow the PR, which often results only in incidental auscultatory findings. *Physical examination* reveals a hyperdynamic right ventricle that produces palpable systolic pulsations in the left parasternal area and an enlarged pulmonary artery that often results in systolic pulsations in the 2nd left intercostal space. Sometimes systolic and diastolic thrills are felt in the same area. A tap reflecting pulmonic valve closure is usually easily palpable in the 2nd intercostal space in patients with pulmonary hypertension and secondary PR.

Auscultation. P_2 is not audible in patients with congenital absence of the pulmonic valve; however, this sound is accentuated in patients with PR secondary to pulmonary hypertension. There may be wide splitting of S_2 caused by prolongation of right ventricular ejection accompanying the augmented right ventricular stroke volume. A nonvalvular systolic ejection click due to the sudden expansion of the pulmonary artery by the augmented right ventricular stroke volume frequently initiates a midsystolic ejection murmur, most prominent in the 2nd left intercostal space. An S_3 and S_4 originating from the right ventricle are often audible, most readily in the 4th intercostal space at the left parasternal area, and are augmented by inspiration.

In the absence of pulmonary hypertension, the diastolic murmur of PR is low pitched and usually heard best at the 3rd and 4th left intercostal spaces adjacent to the sternum. The murmur commences when pressures in the pulmonary artery and right ventricle diverge, approximately 0.04 second after P_2. It is diamond shaped and brief, reaching a peak intensity when the gradient between these pressures is maximal and ending with equilibration of the pressures. The murmur becomes louder during inspiration.

When systolic pulmonary arterial pressure exceeds approximately 55 mm Hg, dilation of the pulmonic annulus results in a high-velocity regurgitant jet that is responsible for the *Graham Steell murmur* of PR. (Doppler ultrasonography reveals pulmonary regurgitation at much lower pulmonary arterial pressures.) The Graham Steell murmur is a high-pitched, blowing, decrescendo murmur beginning immediately after P_2 and is most prominent in the left parasternal region in the 2nd to 4th intercostal spaces. Thus, although it resembles the murmur of AR, it is usually accompanied by severe pulmonary hypertension, i.e., an accentuated P_2 or fused S_2, an ejection sound, and a systolic murmur of TR, and not by a widened arterial pulse pressure. Sometimes a low-frequency presystolic murmur is present, i.e., a right-sided Austin Flint murmur originating from the tricuspid valve.

The Graham Steell murmur of PR secondary to pulmonary hypertension usually increases in intensity with inspiration, exhibits little change after amyl nitrite inhalation or vasopressor administration, is diminished during the Valsalva strain, and returns to baseline intensity almost immediately after release of the Valsalva strain. This murmur resembles and may be confused with the diastolic blowing murmur of AR. However, indicator dilution studies and aortography have established that a diastolic blowing murmur along the left sternal border in patients with rheumatic heart disease and pulmonary hypertension (even in the *absence* of peripheral signs of AR) is usually due to AR rather than PR.

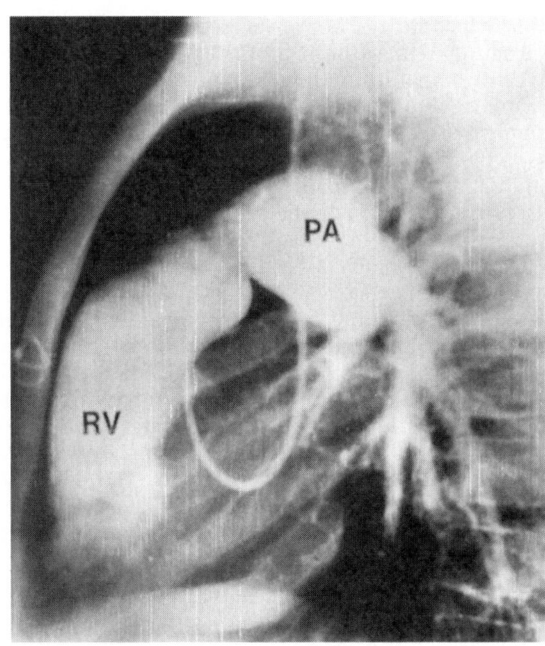

FIGURE 57–46 Pulmonic valvular regurgitation. Contrast material has been injected into the main pulmonary artery (PA) and has regurgitated back into an enlarged right ventricle (RV). (From Carlsson E, Gross R, Holt RG: The radiological diagnosis of cardiac valvular insufficiency. Circulation 55:921, 1977.)

Laboratory Examination

ELECTROCARDIOGRAM. In the absence of pulmonary hypertension, PR often results in an ECG that reflects right ventricular diastolic overload, i.e., an rSr (or rsR) configuration in the right precordial leads. PR secondary to pulmonary hypertension is usually associated with ECG evidence of right ventricular hypertrophy.

RADIOLOGICAL AND ANGIOGRAPHIC FINDINGS. Both the pulmonary artery and the right ventricle are usually enlarged, but these signs are nonspecific. Fluoroscopy may demonstrate pronounced pulsation of the main pulmonary artery. PR can be diagnosed by observing opacification of the right ventricle following injection of contrast material into the main pulmonary artery (Fig. 57–46). The diagnosis is supported by noting superimposition of the pulmonary arterial and right ventricular pressure curves during mid and late diastole. Indicator dilution studies with injections into the pulmonary artery and sampling from the right ventricle, as well as intracardiac phonocardiography, can also be helpful in establishing the diagnosis in mild cases.

ECHOCARDIOGRAM. Two-dimensional echocardiography shows right ventricular dilation and, in patients with pulmonary hypertension, right ventricular hypertrophy as well. Right ventricular function can be evaluated. Abnormal motion of the septum characteristic of volume overload of the right ventricle in diastole and/or septal flutter may be evident. The motion of the pulmonic valve may point to the cause of the PR. Absence of *a* waves and systolic notching of the posterior leaflet suggest pulmonary hypertension; large *a* waves indicate PS. PR can be detected by contrast echocardiography. The pulsed Doppler technique is also extremely accurate in detecting PR and in helping to estimate its severity. Abnormal Doppler signals in the right ventricular outflow tract with velocity sustained throughout diastole are generally observed in patients in whom PR is caused by dilation of the valve ring secondary to pulmonary hypertension. When the velocity falls during diastole, the pulmonary artery pressure is usually normal, and the regurgitation is caused by an abnormality of the valve itself.

MAGNETIC RESONANCE IMAGING. Cardiac MRI is helpful is assessing pulmonary artery dilation, imaging the regurgitant jet, and evaluating right ventricular function (see Fig. 14–12A).

MANAGEMENT

PR alone is seldom severe enough to require specific treatment. Cardiac glycosides are useful in the management of right ventricular dilation or failure. Treatment of the primary condition, such as infective endocarditis, or the lesion responsible for the pulmonary hypertension, such as surgery for mitral valvular disease, often ameliorates the PR. Surgical treatment directed specifically at the pulmonic valve (e.g., in patients in whom surgical correction of tetralogy of Fallot has caused severe PR[284,285]) is required only occasionally because of intractable right heart failure. Under such circumstances, valve replacement may be carried out, preferably with a porcine bioprosthesis or a pulmonary allograft.[286-288]

Multivalvular Disease

Multivalvular involvement is caused most frequently by rheumatic fever, and various clinical and hemodynamic syndromes can be produced by different combinations of valvular abnormalities. Marfan syndrome and other connective tissue disorders may cause multivalve prolapse and dilation, resulting in multivalvular regurgitation. Degenerative calcification of the aortic valve may be associated with degenerative mitral annular calcification and cause AS and MR. Different pathological conditions may affect two valves in the same patient, such as infective endocarditis on the aortic valve causing AR and ischemia causing MR. Development of PR and TR secondary to dilation of the pulmonic valve ring and tricuspid annulus, as a consequence of pulmonary hypertension secondary to mitral and/or aortic valvular disease, was discussed previously, as was the combination of organic rheumatic tricuspid and mitral valvular disease.

In patients with multivalvular disease, the clinical manifestations depend on the relative severities of each of the lesions. When the valvular abnormalities are of approximately equal severity, clinical manifestations produced by the more proximal (upstream) of the two valvular lesions (i.e., the mitral valve in patients with combined mitral and aortic valvular disease and the tricuspid valve in patients with combined tricuspid and mitral valvular disease) are generally more prominent than those produced by the distal lesion. Thus, the proximal lesion tends to mask the distal lesion.

It is important to recognize multivalvular involvement preoperatively because failure to correct all significant valvular disease at the time of operation increases mortality considerably. In patients with multivalvular disease, the relative severity of each lesion may be difficult to estimate by clinical examination and noninvasive techniques because one lesion may mask the manifestations of the other. For this reason, patients suspected of having multivalvular involvement and who are being considered for surgical treatment should undergo right- and left-sided cardiac catheterization and angiography. These studies are in addition to careful clinical examination and a noninvasive work-up, with emphasis on two-dimensional and Doppler echocardiography. If there is any question concerning the presence of significant AS in patients undergoing mitral valve surgery, the aortic valve should be inspected because overlooking this condition can lead to a high perioperative mortality. Similarly, it is useful to palpate the tricuspid valve at the time of mitral valve surgery.

Mitral Stenosis and Aortic Regurgitation

Approximately two-thirds of patients with severe MS have an early blowing diastolic murmur along the left sternal border with a normal pulse pressure. In about 90 percent of these patients, the murmur is due to mild or moderate AR and is usually of little clinical importance. However, approximately 10 percent of patients with MS have severe rheumatic AR,[289] which can generally be recognized by the usual signs of AR (i.e., a widened pulse pressure, left ventricular dilation and increased wall motion on echocardiography, and signs of left ventricular enlargement on radiological and ECG examinations).

In keeping with the general observation that a proximal lesion may mask a distal lesion, significant AR may be missed in patients with severe MS. The widened pulse pressure, in particular, may be absent. On the other hand, MS may be missed or, conversely, may be falsely diagnosed on clinical examination of patients with obvious AR. An accentuated S_1 and an OS in a patient with AR should suggest the possibility of mitral valvular disease. However, an Austin Flint murmur is often inappropriately considered to be the diastolic rumbling murmur of MS. These two murmurs may be distinguished at the bedside by means of amyl nitrite inhalation, which diminishes the Austin Flint murmur but augments the murmur of MS; isometric handgrip and squatting augment both the diastolic murmur of AR and the Austin Flint murmur. Echocardiography, particularly pulsed Doppler echocardiography, is of decisive value in detecting MS and MR.

Since double-valve replacement is associated with increased short-term and long-term risks,[290] balloon mitral valvotomy can be the first procedure. If this causes left ventricular dilation, AVR can follow. Alternatively, open mitral valvotomy and AVR can be performed at the same time.[1]

Mitral Stenosis and Aortic Stenosis

The left ventricle of a patient with these two lesions is usually small, stiff, and hypertrophied. When severe MS and AS coexist, the former masks many of the manifestations of the latter.[289] The cardiac output tends to be reduced more than in patients with isolated AS. The reduced cardiac output lowers both the transaortic valvular pressure gradient and the left ventricular systolic pressure, diminishes the incidence of angina pectoris, and retards the development of aortic valvular calcification and left ventricular hypertrophy. On the other hand, clinical manifestations associated with MS, such as pulmonary congestion and hemoptysis, atrial fibrillation, and systemic embolization, occur more frequently in patients with coexisting MS and AS than in those with isolated AS.

On physical examination, an S_4, (which is common in patients with pure AS) is usually not present. The midsystolic murmur characteristic of AS may be reduced in intensity and duration because the stroke volume is reduced by the MS. The ECG may fail to demonstrate left ventricular hypertrophy, but left atrial enlargement is common. The chest roentgenogram is usually typical of MS except that calcium may be present in the region of the aortic valve, and left ventricular enlargement may occur (see Fig. 12–5). The two-dimensional and Doppler echocardiograms are of the greatest value because stenosis of both valves may be evident. However, the low cardiac output characteristic of the combined lesions may reduce the transvalvular pressure gradients estimated by Doppler echocardiography.

It is vital to recognize the presence of hemodynamically significant aortic valvular disease (i.e., stenosis and/or regurgitation) preoperatively in patients who are to undergo mitral valvotomy. This procedure may be hazardous because it can impose a sudden hemodynamic load on the left ventricle that had previously been protected by the MS and may lead to acute pulmonary edema. Balloon mitral valvotomy and AVR may be the treatment of choice.

Aortic Stenosis and Mitral Regurgitation

This combination of lesions is usually caused by rheumatic heart disease, although AS may be congenital and MR may be due to MVP. The combination of severe AS and MR is a hazardous one, but fortunately it is relatively uncommon. Obstruction to left ventricular outflow augments the volume of MR flow, whereas the presence of MR diminishes the ventricular preload necessary for maintenance of the left ventricular stroke volume in patients with AS.[289] The result is a reduced forward cardiac output and marked left atrial and pulmonary venous hypertension. The development of atrial fibrillation (due to left atrial enlargement) has an adverse hemodynamic effect in the presence of AS. The physical findings may be confusing because it may be difficult to recognize two distinct systolic murmurs. On echocardiography and roentgenography, the left atrium and ventricle are usually larger than in isolated AS. In patients with severe AS and MR, both valves must usually be treated surgically by AVR and, if possible, by mitral valve repair.[290]

Aortic Regurgitation and Mitral Regurgitation

This relatively frequent combination of lesions[289] may be caused by rheumatic heart disease, by prolapse of both the aortic and the mitral valves due to myxomatous degeneration, or by dilation of both annuli in patients with connective tissue disorders. The left ventricle is usually greatly dilated. The clinical features of AR usually predominate, and it is sometimes difficult to determine whether the MR is due to organic involvement of this valve or to dilation of the mitral valve ring secondary to left ventricular enlargement. When both valvular leaks are severe, this combination of lesions is poorly tolerated. The normal mitral valve ordinarily serves as a "back-up" to the aortic valve, and premature (diastolic) closure of the mitral valve limits the volume of reflux that occurs in patients with acute AR. With severe combined regurgitant lesions, regardless of the cause of the mitral lesion, blood may reflux from the aorta through both chambers of the left side of the heart into the pulmonary veins. Physical and laboratory examinations usually show evidence of both lesions. An S_3 and a brisk arterial pulse are frequently present. The relative severity of each lesion can be assessed best by Doppler echocardiography and contrast angiography. This combination of lesions leads to severe left ventricular dilation.

MR that occurs in patients with AR secondary to left ventricular dilation often regresses following AVR alone. If severe, the MR may be corrected by annuloplasty at the time of AVR. An intrinsically normal mitral valve that is regurgitant because of a dilated annulus should not be replaced.

Surgical Treatment of Multivalvular Disease

Combined AVR and MVR is usually associated with a higher risk and poorer survival than is replacement of either of the valves alone.[291,292] The operative risk of double-valve replacement is about 70 percent higher than it is for single-valve replacement. The Society of Thoracic Surgeons National Database Committee reported an overall operative mortality rate of 9.6 percent for multiple (usually double) valve replacement in 3840 patients, compared with 4.3 percent and 6.4 percent for isolated AVR and MVR, respectively (see Table 57–3).[283] The long-term survival depends strongly on the preoperative functional status.[292] Patients operated on for combined AR and MR have poorer outcomes than patients receiving double-valve replacement for any of the other combinations of lesions, presumably because both AR and MR may produce irreversible left ventricular damage. Mitral repair or balloon valvotomy in combination with AVR is preferable to double-valve replacement and should be carried out whenever possible.[290] Risk factors that reduce long-term survival after double-valve replacement include advanced age, higher NYHA class, lower left ventricular ejection fraction, greater left ventricular enlargement, and accompanying ischemic heart disease requiring coronary artery bypass grafting.[292]

Given the higher risks, a higher threshold is required for multivalvular versus single-valve surgery. Thus, patients are generally advised not to undergo multivalvular surgery until they reach late NYHA Class II or III, unless there is evidence of declining left ventricular function. Despite a detailed noninvasive and invasive work-up, the decision to treat more than one valve is often made by palpation or by direct inspection at the operating table.

Three-Valve Disease

Hemodynamically significant disease involving the mitral, aortic, and tricuspid valves is uncommon. Patients with trivalvular disease may present in advanced heart failure with marked cardiomegaly, and surgical correction of all three valvular lesions is imperative. However, triple-valve replacement is a long and complex operation. Early in the experience with this procedure, the mortality rate was 20 percent for patients in NYHA Class III and 40 percent for patients in Class IV. More recently, the mortality rate has declined, but, nevertheless, triple-valve replacement should be avoided if possible. In many patients with trivalvular disease, it is possible to replace the aortic valve, repair the mitral valve, and perform a tricuspid annuloplasty or valvuloplasty.

Patients who survive triple-valve replacement surgery usually show substantial clinical improvement during the early postoperative period, and postoperative catheterization studies show marked reductions in pulmonary arterial and capillary pressures. However, some patients die of arrhythmias or congestive heart failure in the late postoperative period despite three normally functioning prostheses. The cause of cardiac failure in this situation is not known, but it may be related to intraoperative myocardial ischemia, microemboli from the multiple prostheses, or continued subclinical episodes of rheumatic myocarditis.

When multiple prosthetic valves must be inserted, it is logical to select either two bioprostheses or two mechanical prostheses for the left side of the heart. If the patient is to be exposed to the hazards of anticoagulants for one mechanical prosthesis, it seems unreasonable to add the potential risks of early failure of a bioprosthesis. However, if two mechanical prostheses are selected for the left side of the heart, the use of a bioprosthesis in the tricuspid position is suggested.

Prosthetic Cardiac Valves

The first successful replacements of cardiac valves in the human were accomplished by Nina Braunwald and colleagues,[293] Harken and coworkers,[294] and Starr and Edwards[295] in 1960. Two major groups of artificial (prosthetic) valves are currently available in models designed for both the atrioventricular (mitral and tricuspid) and the aortic positions: mechanical prostheses and bioprostheses (tissue valves). The major differences are related to the risk of thromboembolism (higher with mechanical valves) and the risk of structural deterioration of the prosthesis (higher with bioprostheses).

Mechanical Prostheses

Mechanical prosthetic valves are classified into three major groups: caged-ball, tilting-disc and bileaflet valves. The *Starr-Edwards* caged-ball valve, the oldest prosthetic valve in continuous use (Fig. 57–47A), has the longest record of predictable performance of any artificial valve.[296-299] The poppet is made of silicone rubber, the cage of Stellite alloy, and the sewing ring of Teflon/polypropylene cloth. A disadvantage is its bulky cage design. Therefore, the Starr-Edwards valve is not suitable for the mitral position in patients with a small left ventricular cavity or for the aortic position in those with a small aortic annulus or those requiring a valve–aortic arch composite graft. In a small number of patients, this valve induces hemolysis, which may be greatly exaggerated and become clinically important if a perivalvular leak develops. When they are small, Starr-Edwards valves may cause mild obstruction, and the incidence of thromboembolism is slightly higher than with the tilting-disc valve or bileaflet valve.[1,297,298]

The bileaflet valves are widely employed; these are less bulky, have a lower profile than the caged-ball valve, and are therefore superior hemodynamically. The *St. Jude* bileaflet valve (Fig. 57–47D), currently the most widely used prosthesis worldwide, is coated with pyrolytic carbon and has two semicircular discs that pivot between open and closed positions without the need for supporting struts.[299,300] It has favorable flow characteristics and causes a lower transvalvular pressure gradient at any outer diameter and cardiac output than the caged-ball or tilting-disc valves.[297] The St. Jude valve appears to have particularly favorable hemodynamic characteristics in the smaller sizes; therefore, it is especially useful in children. Thrombogenicity in the mitral position *may* be less than that associated with other prosthetic valves.[296,297] However, as with other mechanical prostheses, lifelong anticoagulation is needed.[1] A variation of the St. Jude valve, the *CarboMedics* prosthesis (Fig. 57–47E), is also a bileaflet valve composed of pyrolytic carbon with a titanium housing that can be rotated so as to avoid interference with disc excursion by subvalvular tissue.[301]

There are two principal tilting disc valves in current use. The *Omniscience* valve (Fig. 57–47B), the successor to the *Lillehei-Kaster* pivoting-disc valve, consists of a titanium valve housing with a polyester knit sewing ring in which a pyrolytic disc is suspended. In the open position, the disc swings to an angle of 80 degrees, providing a large central flow orifice. A closely related valve is the *Medtronic-Hall* valve (Fig. 57–47C), which has a Teflon sewing ring and titanium housing; its thin, carbon-coated pivoting disc has a central perforation that allows improved hemodynamics. Thrombogenicity appears to be quite low[296,297] (less than one episode per 100 patient-years in the mitral position), and mechanical performance is excellent over the long term. Both the bileaflet and the tilting-disc valves are associated with small (5 to 10 ml/beat) obligatory (normal) regurgitation. All have distinctive auscultatory features (Fig. 57–48).

DURABILITY AND THROMBOGENICITY. All mechanical prosthetic valves have an excellent record of durability, up to 40 years for the Starr-Edwards valve. In the mitral position, perivalvular regurgitation appears to occur more frequently with mechanical than with tissue valves.[302] Thrombosis and thromboembolism risks are greater with any mechanical valve in the mitral than in the aortic position, and higher doses of warfarin are generally recommended for mitral prostheses.[1,303] However, patients with any *mechanical* prosthesis, regardless of design or site of placement, require long-term anticoagulation and aspirin administration because of the hazard of thromboembolism, which is greatest in the first postoperative year. Without anticoagulants and aspirin, the incidence of thromboembolism is threefold to sixfold higher than when proper doses of these medications are

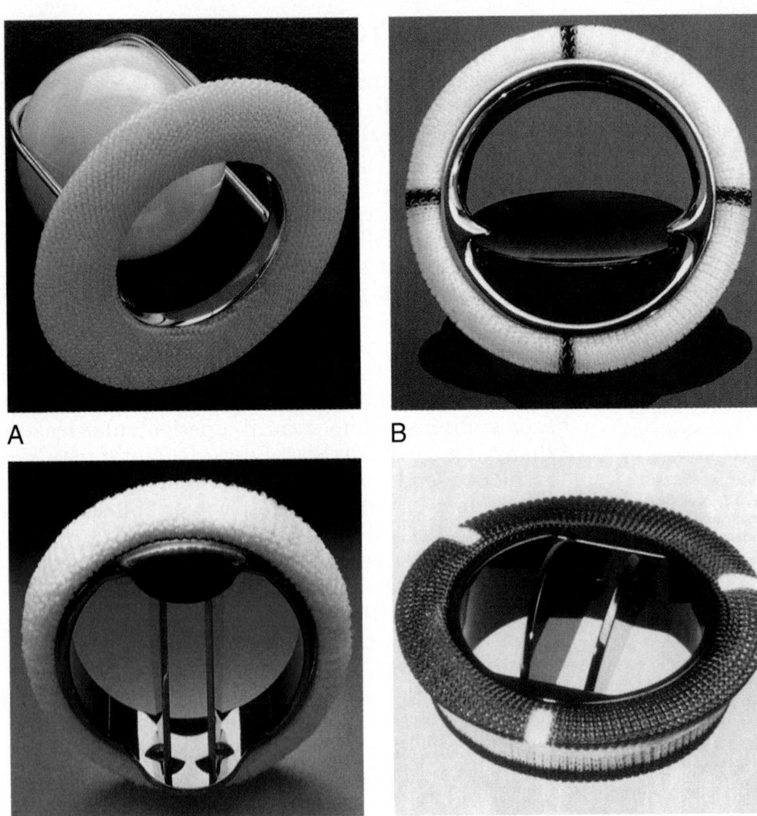

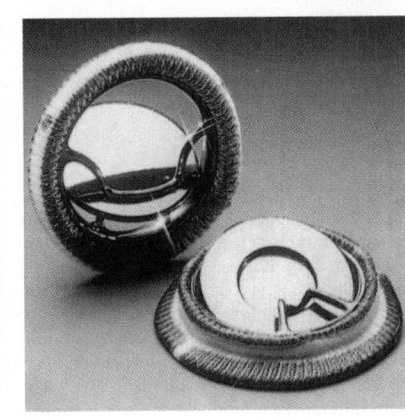

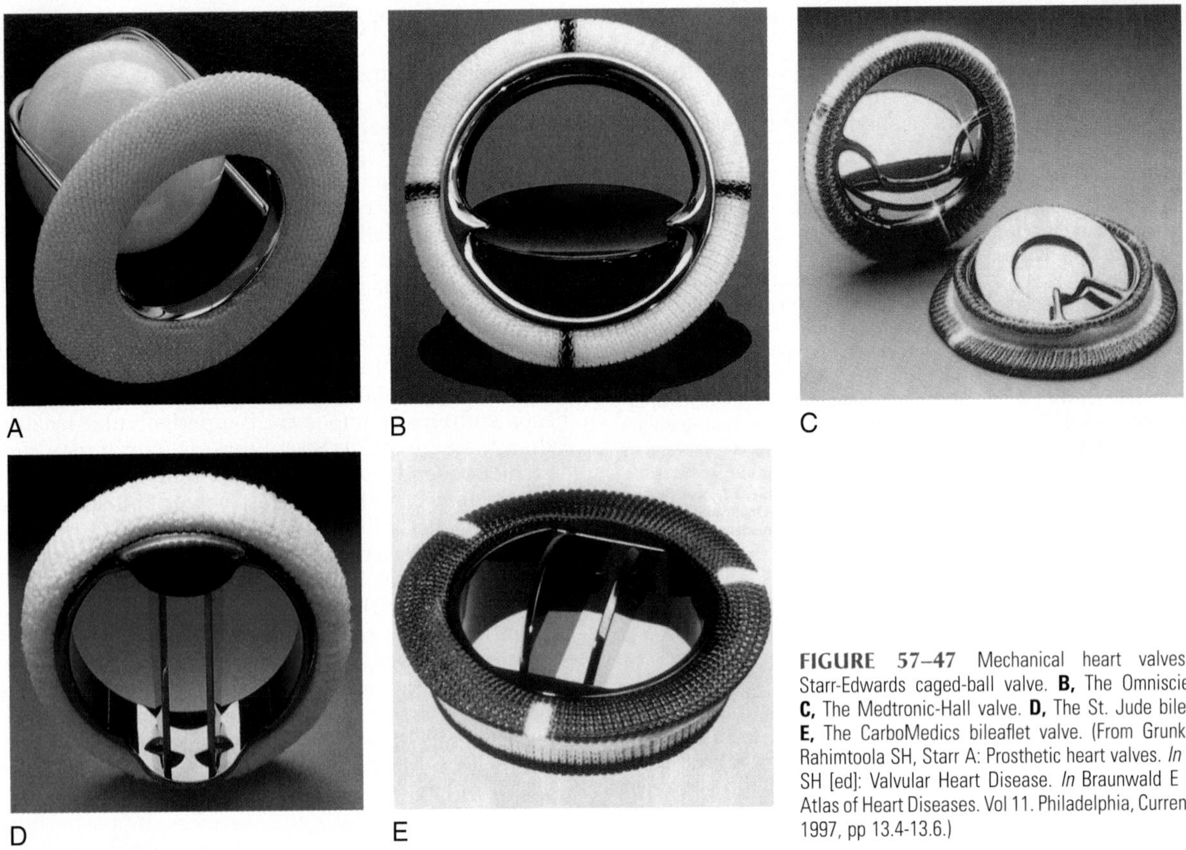

FIGURE 57–47 Mechanical heart valves. **A,** The Starr-Edwards caged-ball valve. **B,** The Omniscience valve. **C,** The Medtronic-Hall valve. **D,** The St. Jude bileaflet valve. **E,** The CarboMedics bileaflet valve. (From Grunkemeier GL, Rahimtoola SH, Starr A: Prosthetic heart valves. *In* Rahimtoola SH [ed]: Valvular Heart Disease. *In* Braunwald E [series ed]: Atlas of Heart Diseases. Vol 11. Philadelphia, Current Medicine, 1997, pp 13.4-13.6.)

Type of Valve	Aortic Prosthesis		Mitral Prosthesis	
	Normal findings	Abnormal findings	Normal findings	Abnormal findings
Caged-Ball (Starr–Edwards)	OC S_1 CC P_2 SEM	Aortic diastolic murmur Decreased intensity of opening or closing click	CC OC S_2 SEM	Low-frequency apical diastolic murmur High-frequency holosystolic murmur
Single-Tilting-Disc (Björk–Shiley or Medtronic–Hall)	OC S_1 CC P_2 SEM DM	Decreased intensity of closing click	CC OC S_2 DM	High-frequency holosystolic murmur Decreased intensity of closing click
Bileaflet-Tilting-Disc (St. Jude Medical)	OC S_1 CC P_2 SEM	Aortic diastolic murmur Decreased intensity of closing click	CC OC S_2 DM	High-frequency holosystolic murmur Decreased intensity of closing click
Heterograft Bioprosthesis (Hancock or Carpentier–Edwards)	S_1 AC P_2 SEM	Aortic diastolic murmur	MC S_2 MO SEM DM	High-frequency holosystolic murmur

FIGURE 57–48 Auscultatory characteristics of various prosthetic valves in the aortic and mitral positions, with schematic diagrams of normal findings and descriptions of abnormal findings. OC = opening click; CC = closing click; SEM = systolic ejection murmur; DM = diastolic murmur; AC = aortic closure; MC = mitral valve closure; MO = mitral opening. (From Vongpatanasin W, Hillis LD, Lange RA: Prosthetic heart valves. N Engl J Med 335:407, 1996.)

administered. Rarely, thrombosis of the mechanical valve occurs. This may be a fatal event, but when nonfatal, it interferes with prosthetic valve function.

Warfarin should begin about 2 days after operation, and the INR should be in the range of 2.0 to 3.0 for patients with the bileaflet disc and the Medtronic-Hall valve in the aortic position. The INR should be between 2.5 and 3.5 for patients at higher risk for thrombosis (e.g., atrial fibrillation, previous thromboembolism) as well as for patients with other mechanical valves in the aortic position and for *all* valves in the mitral position (see Chap. 80).[1] This relatively conservative approach reduces the risk of anticoagulant hemorrhage but does not appear to be associated with a greater frequency of thromboembolism than an INR of 3.0 to 4.0, which was used in the past.[303-305] Antiplatelet agents without anticoagulants do not provide adequate protection. However, the addition of aspirin, 80 to 150 mg daily, together with warfarin may reduce the risk of thromboembolism and should be given to all patients with prosthetic valves.[1] Although this approach does increase the risk of bleeding slightly,[306,307] there is a favorable risk-to-benefit profile.[307]

Prosthetic valve thrombosis should be suspected by the sudden appearance of dyspnea and muffled sounds or new murmurs on auscultation (see Fig. 57–48). This serious complication is diagnosed by transesophageal two-dimensional and Doppler echocardiography. Treatment consists of infusion of a thrombolytic agent for 24 to 72 hours, heparin, and aspirin. Surgery is required for nonresponders and for patients with mobile thrombi.[1,308]

It must be recognized that (1) the administration of warfarin carries its own mortality and morbidity, i.e., serious hemorrhage, estimated at 0.2 and 2.2 episodes per 100 patient-years, respectively; and (2) despite treatment with anticoagulants, the incidence of thromboembolic complications with the best mechanical prosthesis is still about 0.2 fatal complications and 1.0 to 2.0 nonfatal complications per 100 patient-years for aortic valves and 2.0 to 3.0 nonfatal complications for mitral valves. Valve thrombosis, a particularly hazardous complication, occurs at an incidence of about 0.1 percent per year in the aortic position and 0.35 percent per year in the mitral position. Thrombosis of mechanical prostheses in the tricuspid position is quite high, and for this reason bioprostheses are preferred at this site. The incidence of embolization in patients who have experienced repeated emboli from a prosthetic valve despite anticoagulants may be reduced by replacement with a tissue valve.

Mechanical prostheses regularly cause mild hemolysis, but this is not severe enough to be of clinical importance unless the patient develops periprosthetic regurgitation.

Tissue Valves

Tissue valves (bioprostheses) have been developed primarily to overcome the risk of thromboembolism that is inherent in all mechanical prosthetic valves and the attendant hazards and inconvenience of permanent anticoagulant therapy.[309] The first tissue valves to be widely used were chemically sterilized aortic homografts (allografts) obtained from cadavers. However, these had a high incidence of breakdown within 3 years, and antibiotic-treated, cryopreserved, frozen, irradiated homografts were then developed. These homografts are more durable, but, although they have many desirable properties, their use has been restricted by the problems inherent in their procurement (discussed later).

PORCINE HETEROGRAFTS. Stented porcine aortic heterografts were developed for both the mitral and the aortic positions and have been in wide clinical use since 1965.[296,297] The semirigid stents facilitate implantation and maintain the three-dimensional relationship between the leaflets. Three porcine heterografts are widely used today.[310-313] The *Hancock* valve (Fig. 57–49A) is fixed and preserved in glutaraldehyde and is mounted on a Dacron cloth–covered flexible polypropylene strut. In the smaller aortic models, the right coronary cusp is replaced by a posterior cusp from another valve to reduce obstruction resulting from the septal shelf of the valve.[310,313] The *Carpentier-Edwards* valve (Fig. 57–49B) is pressure fixed, preserved in glutaraldehyde, and mounted on a Teflon-covered strut so as to minimize the septal shelf.[311,313] The Medtronic *Intact* valve (Fig. 57–49C) is also glutaraldehyde treated but at a fixation pressure of zero and with toluidine in an attempt to inhibit calcium deposition.[312] The hemodynamic profiles of the porcine heterografts are similar to those of comparably sized low-profile mechanical prostheses.

During the first 3 postoperative months, while the sewing ring becomes endothelialized, the thromboembolic rate is high enough that anticoagulation is extremely desirable. Thereafter, anticoagulants are not required for porcine valves in the aortic position, and the thromboembolic rate is approximately one or two episodes per 100 patient-years without these drugs.[1,296,297] When these valves have been placed in the mitral position in patients who are in sinus rhythm, who do not have heart failure or thrombus in the left atrium or the left atrial appendage, and who do not have a history of embolism preoperatively, anticoagulants are not needed after the first 3 postoperative months, and the thromboembolic rate is also approximately one or two episodes per 100 patient-years. This rate is comparable to that observed in patients with the St. Jude or other mechanical valves who are receiving anticoagulants and are therefore subject to the risks of hemorrhage. It is unlikely that any MVR can be associated with a thromboembolic rate much below 0.5 episode per 100 patient-years because some of the emboli in patients with longstanding mitral disease are derived from the left atrium rather than from the valve itself. In patients undergoing MVR with a bioprosthesis who have experienced a previous embolism, in whom thrombus is found in the left atrium at operation, or who remain in atrial fibrillation postoperatively (about one-third of all patients receiving MVR), the hazard of thromboembolism and the need for anticoagulants persist. This negates the principal advantage of the tissue valves, and mechanical prostheses would appear to be preferable to bioprostheses in these patients.

Durability. The major problem with porcine bioprostheses is their limited durability (Fig. 57–50). Cuspal tears, degeneration, fibrin deposition, disruption of the fibrocollagenous structure, perforation, fibrosis, and calcification sufficiently severe to require reoperation begin to appear in some patients in the fourth or fifth postoperative year, and by 10 years the rate of primary tissue failure averages 30 percent. It then accelerates, and by 15 years postoperatively the actuarial *freedom* from bioprosthetic primary tissue failure has ranged from 30 to 60 percent in several series. Hypercholesterolemia has been shown to contribute to prosthesis calcification and degeneration,[314,315] suggesting that secondary prevention strategies may slow down this process.

Structural valve deterioration is more frequent in patients with bioprostheses in the mitral than in the aortic position,[302] presumably because of the higher closing pressure. With the passage of time, it is anticipated that many of the currently implanted valves will likely fail, especially in younger patients, and essentially all valves implanted into patients younger than 60 years of age may have to be replaced ultimately. Fortunately, however, these valves usually do not fail suddenly (as is often the case for structural failure or thrombosis of mechanical prostheses). Re-replacement of a bioprosthetic valve should be carried out when significant and/or progressive structural deterioration is evident but before operation becomes an emergency. The second operation, when carried out on an elective basis, may be associated with a surgical mortality rate of 10 to 15 percent.

Color Doppler echocardiography with two-dimensional imaging is extremely helpful in the early detection of bioprosthetic valve malfunction. Transesophageal echocardiography is more sensitive than transthoracic imaging in detecting bioprosthetic valve deterioration. Even patients without new murmurs or other physical findings of valve dysfunction should have routine echocardiographic studies to look for early bioprosthetic valve dysfunction every year for 5 to 6 years after valve replacement and every 6 months after that.

The rate of structural valve failure is age dependent and is significantly lower in patients older than 65 years than in younger patients, especially in the aortic position (Fig. 57–51A). In patients older than 65 years undergoing AVR with a porcine bioprosthesis, the rate of structural deterioration is less than 10 percent at 10 years.[1,302,310,312] Valve failure is prohibitively rapid in children and in adults younger than 35 to 40 years of age. Therefore, bioprostheses are *not* advisable in these age groups. On the other hand, degeneration is rare when these valves are implanted into patients older than 70 years of age.[1,310,312] Bioprostheses also have been reported to have extremely limited durability in patients with chronic renal failure, but recent studies have called this into question (discussed subsequently).

Prosthetic valve endocarditis is a serious, often grave illness (see Chap. 58).

STENTLESS PORCINE XENOGRAFTS. Since the stent adds to the obstruction and thereby increases stress on the leaflets, stentless valves have been developed for the aortic position (see Fig. 57–49)[316] and are now being used increasingly, especially in patients with small aortic roots.[317] These include the Toronto SPV stentless valve (St. Jude Medical valve),[318,319] the Edwards stentless valve,[320] and the Medtronic

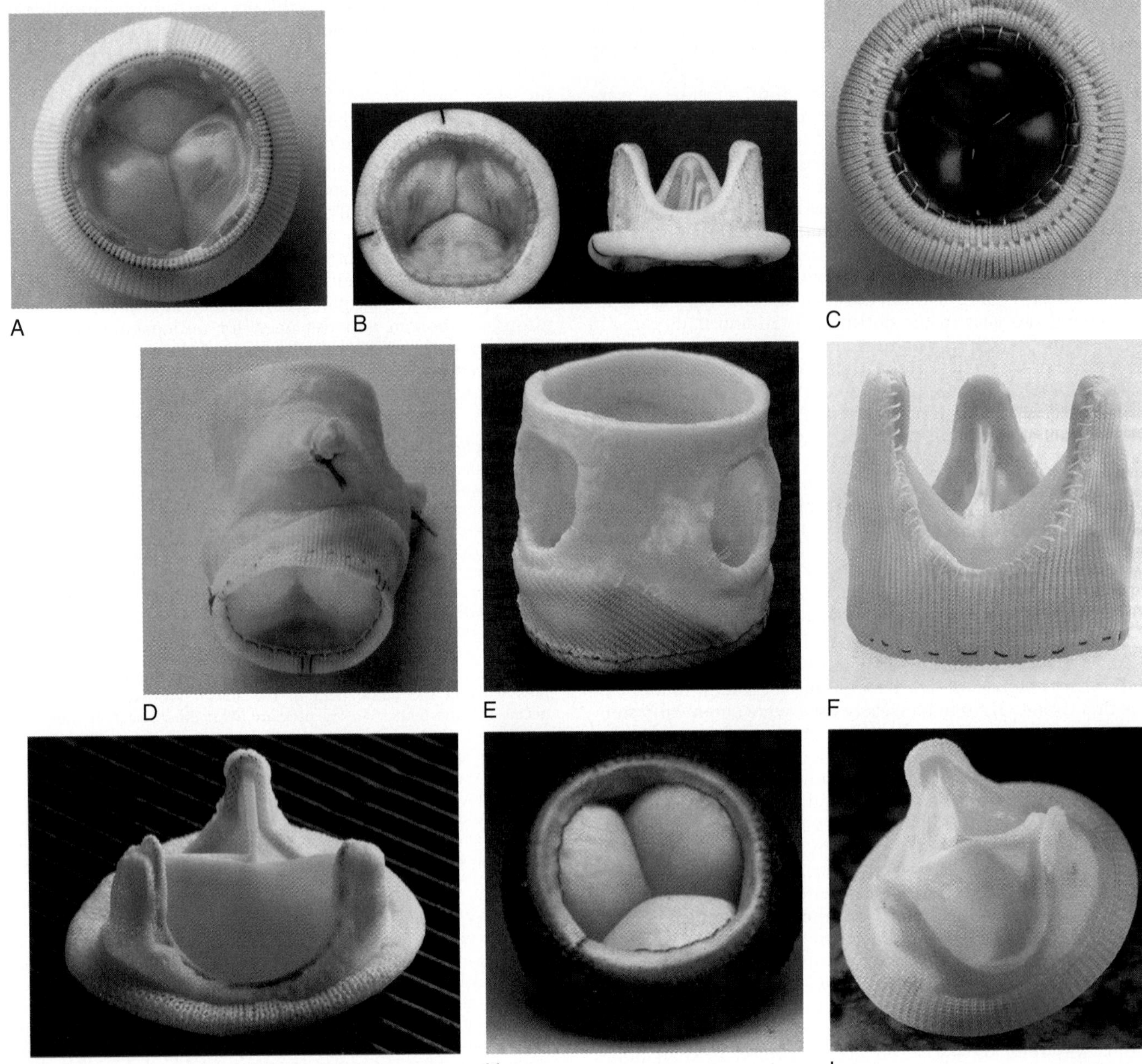

FIGURE 57–49 Bioprosthetic valves. The **top row** shows stented porcine valves: **A,** Hancock porcine valve; **B,** Carpentier-Edwards porcine valve; and **C,** Medtronic Intact porcine valve. The **middle row** shows stentless valves: **D,** Medtronic Freestyle stentless valve; **E,** Edwards Prima stentless valve; and **F,** St. Jude Medical Toronto SPV stentless valve. The **bottom row** shows pericardial valves: **G,** Carpentier-Edwards pericardial valve; **H,** Sorin Pericarbon pericardial valve; and **I,** Autologous pericardial valve. (From Grunkemeier GL, Rahimtoola SH, Starr A: Prosthetic heart valves. *In* Rahimtoola SH [ed]: Valvular Heart Disease. *In* Braunwald E [series ed]: Atlas of Heart Diseases. Vol 11. Philadelphia, Current Medicine, 1997, pp 13.9-13.13.)

Freestyle valve.[316] These valves have been reported to have more physiological flow and lower transvalvular gradients than stented porcine valves, with the potential for enhanced regression of left ventricular hypertrophy and improved left ventricular function. Although the early experience tends to confirm this,[321-323] it is yet uncertain whether this translates into improved outcomes in terms of survival and long-term prosthesis durability. It is hoped that the slightly improved hemodynamics provided by the stentless valves will translate into better valve longevity than that of valves mounted on stents.

PERICARDIAL (XENOGRAFT) AORTIC VALVES. Bovine pericardial valves, unlike porcine valves, are fabricated rather than harvested directly (see Fig. 57–49). Although the first generation of these valves had a high rate of premature structural deterioration, the current generation of stented bovine pericardial prostheses has been demonstrated to have good long-term durability that appears to be equivalent or better than that of the porcine bioprosthesis.[324,325] As with the stented porcine valves, the rate of structural deterioration is extremely low in individuals aged 70 years or older (Fig. 57–51B).[326] There is a greater risk for the development of stenosis in the mitral position.[327]

HOMOGRAFT (ALLOGRAFT) AORTIC VALVES. These are harvested from cadavers, often along with kidneys, usually within 24 hours of donor death. They are sterilized

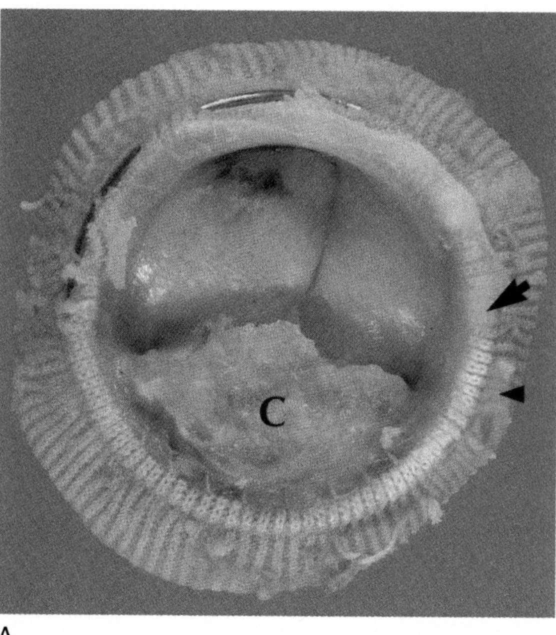

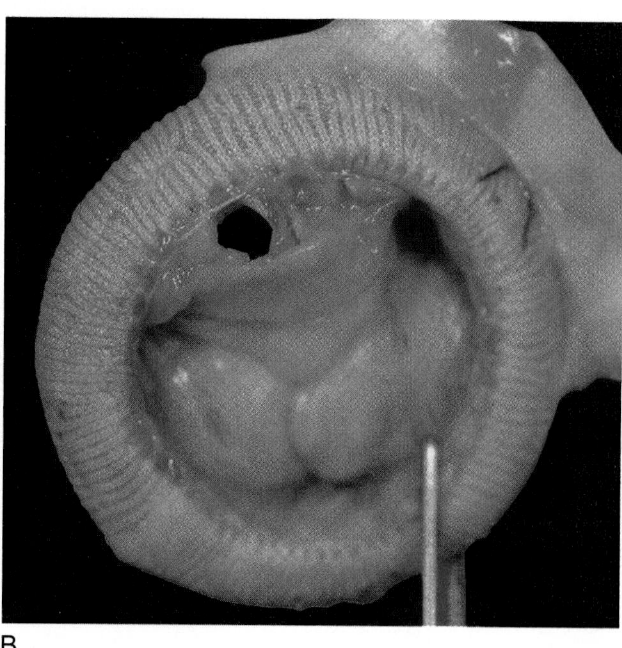

FIGURE 57–50 Structural deterioration of bioprosthetic valves. **A,** Valve failure related to mineralization and collagen degeneration. **B,** Cuspal tears and perforations. These processes may occur independently, or they may be synergistic. (**A,** From Virmani R, Burke AP, Farb A: Pathology of valvular heart disease. *In* Rahimtoola SH [ed]: Valvular Heart Disease. *In* Braunwald E [series ed]: Atlas of Heart Diseases. Vol 11. Philadelphia, Current Medicine, 1997, p 1.26; **B,** From Manabe H, Yutani C [eds]: Atlas of Valvular Heart Disease. Singapore, Churchill Livingstone, 1998, p 158.)

with antibiotics and cryopreserved for long periods at −196°C. They are inserted directly, usually in the aortic position, *without* being placed into a prosthetic stent. In the aortic position, the isolated valve is implanted in the subcoronary position, or the valve and a portion of attached aorta are implanted as a root replacement, with reimplantation of the coronary arteries into the graft. Homograft hemodynamics are superior to those of stented porcine valves and similar to those of stentless porcine valves.[328] Like porcine xenografts, their thrombogenicity is low, but cryopreserved valves appear to have similar issues with structural deterioration,[329] with evidence that this rate is reduced with the use of freshly harvested valves, approximate matching of donor's and patient's ages, and use of the root replacement technique. The subcoronary technique is associated with a higher incidence of prosthetic AR and reoperation.[329-331] Homograft aortic valves have an extremely low rate of infection and are indicated for patients with native or prosthetic valve endocarditis. They are difficult to use when the aortic root and ascending aorta are greatly enlarged, and availability is often limited.

PERICARDIAL AUTOGRAFT VALVES. The patient's own pericardium is inserted into a frame on the operating table and is inserted into either the aortic or the mitral position (see Fig. 57–49I). Long-term durability appears to be excellent; in 267 patients undergoing isolated AVR, the 14-year actuarial freedom of need for re-replacement because of structural valve dysfunction was 85 percent (94 percent in patients > 65 years of age).

PULMONARY AUTOGRAFTS. In this operation, the Ross procedure, the patient's own pulmonary valve and adjacent main pulmonary artery are removed and used to replace the diseased aortic valve and often the neighboring aorta, with reimplantation of the coronary arteries into the graft.[333] A human pulmonary or aortic homograft is then inserted into the pulmonary position. The autograft is nonthrombogenic.[334] In children and adolescents, there is evidence that the autograft grows along with the patient.[335] The risk of endocarditis is low, anticoagulants are not required, and, perhaps most important, the long-term durability appears to be excellent. A high incidence of pulmonary homograft stenosis has been reported in some series,[336,337] which may represent a postoperative inflammatory reaction. The pulmonary artery tissue adapts to the aortic pressure and usually does not dilate.[338] However, this procedure should not be performed in patients with bicuspid valves and dilated aortic roots, because the implanted pulmonary artery tissue exposed to the higher aortic pressures may also undergo degenerative changes leading to significant dilation of the autograft.[339] A subcoronary technique, in which the pulmonary autograft is inserted without a root replacement, may circumvent this problem.[340]

The pulmonary autograft is the replacement valve of choice in children, adolescents, and younger adults who have a long (>20-year) life expectancy, particularly young women who wish to become pregnant. However, its use has been limited because the operation is technically much more demanding than a simple AVR. The procedure should be carried out only by experienced surgeons.

Hemodynamics of Valve Replacements

The most commonly used prosthetic valves, i.e., mechanical prostheses and stented porcine or pericardial xenografts, have an effective in vitro orifice size that is *smaller* than the normal valve at the same site. Unstented porcine xenografts, homografts, and pulmonary autografts do not have this problem. After implantation, tissue ingrowth and endothelialization reduce the size of the effective orifice even more. Therefore, the prosthetic valves that are currently available must be considered to be mildly stenotic. However, postoperative hemodynamic measurements of the mechanical prostheses show reasonably good function, with effective mitral valve orifice areas averaging 1.7 to 2.0 cm^2 and mitral valve gradients of 4 to 8 mm Hg at rest. The cloth-covered Starr-Edwards valve appears to be intrinsically slightly more stenotic than the Medtronic-Hall or Omniscience tilting-disc valves. The bileaflet St. Jude and CarboMedics valves, in turn, may be slightly superior to the Medtronic-Hall or Omniscience valve. In hemodynamic studies, the stented porcine mitral valves

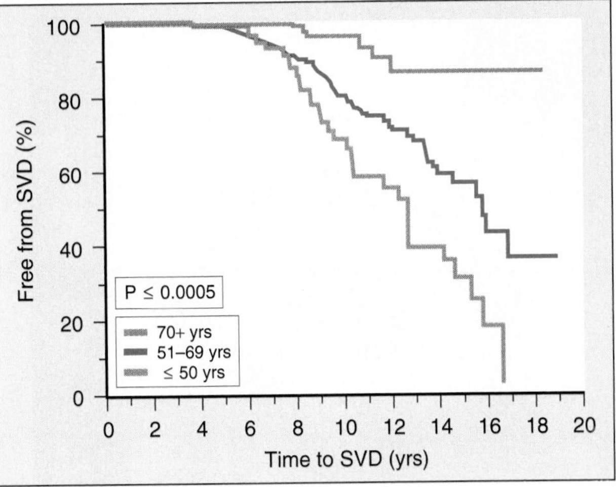

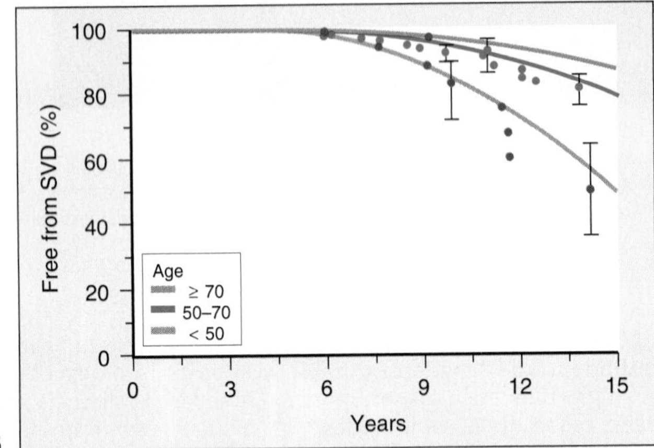

FIGURE 57–51 Estimates of freedom from structural valve deterioration (SVD) for patients undergoing porcine **(A)** and bovine pericardial **(B)** aortic valve replacement who are stratified according to age. (**A,** From Cohn LH, Collins JJ Jr, Rizzo RJ, et al: Twenty-year follow-up of the Hancock modified orifice porcine aortic valve. Ann Thorac Surg 66:S30, 1998; **B,** From Banbury MK, Cosgrove DM, White JA, et al: Age and valve size effect on the long-term durability of the Carpentier-Edwards aortic pericardial bioprosthesis. Ann Thorac Surg 72:753, 2001.)

behave in a manner similar to mechanical prosthetic valves of the same diameter. *Serious* hemodynamic obstruction of an artificial valve in the mitral position is quite uncommon, unless the valve (most commonly the Starr-Edwards valve) is placed into a small left ventricular cavity or into an unusually small mitral annulus or the prosthesis chosen is of inappropriate size.

The problem of prosthetic valve stenosis may be more serious in patients who undergo AVR for AS. The annulus into which the prosthesis is inserted in these patients is usually smaller than it is in patients with AR, and the surgeon may be forced to select an artificial valve that is relatively small. As a consequence, AVR may not abolish obstruction in patients with AS, but the "prosthesis-patient mismatch"[341] may merely convert severe to mild or moderate obstruction. When the smaller models of the stented porcine xenograft or mechanical prosthesis are placed into the aortic position, effective orifice areas of about 1.1 to 1.3 cm^2 are common. In such patients, peak transvalvular gradients as high as 40 mm Hg during exercise have been recorded. In patients with a small annulus, a stentless bioprosthesis valve has better hemodynamic performance that a stented valve.[342] The poor late results observed in a few patients undergoing replacement of stenotic aortic valves may possibly be related to the moderate stenosis of the prosthesis,[343] although the impact of prosthesis-patient mismatch on survival remains controversial.[344-344b] In patients with AS who do not exhibit clinical improvement postoperatively, it is important to evaluate the function of both the prosthetic valve and the left ventricle. Rarely, reoperation to correct a malfunctioning prosthesis may be necessary.

Selection of an Artificial Valve

Most comparisons of mechanical and bioprosthetic valves indicate similar overall results in terms of early and late mortality, prosthetic valve endocarditis and other complications, and the need for reoperation, at least for the first 5 years postoperatively. As indicated, there appear to be no significant differences insofar as hemodynamics are concerned, except that patients with an unusually small left ventricular cavity or mitral or aortic annulus may have better results with the low-profile (tilting-disc) St. Jude or Carbomedics prosthesis or a tissue valve. Patients with a small aortic annulus may be better candidates for unstented homografts, heterografts, or pulmonary autografts. In general, patient outcome after valve surgery is related more to preoperative factors, such as age, left ventricular function, associated coronary artery disease, and comorbid conditions, than to the prosthesis itself.

The major task in selecting an artificial valve is to weigh the advantage of durability and the disadvantages of the risks of thromboembolism and anticoagulant treatment inherent in mechanical prostheses on the one hand with the advantage of low thrombogenicity and the disadvantage of abbreviated durability of bioprostheses on the other. Hammermeister and associates[302] have compared the 15-year outcome in 575 men who were randomized to undergo MVR or AVR with either a mechanical or bioprosthetic valve. Patients undergoing AVR with a mechanical valve had better survival than those receiving the bioprosthesis (Fig. 57–52), principally because of the higher rate of structural deterioration of the bioprosthesis (especially in patients < 65 years of age). Much of the increased mortality in patients receiving the tissue valve was related to reoperation (which is associated with about twice the mortality of the initial procedure). The prosthetic valve did not influence survival after MVR, nor the probability of developing other valve-related complications, including endocarditis, valve thrombosis, and systemic embolism. As anticipated, anticoagulant-related bleeding was higher in patients receiving mechanical valves. Patients with mechanical valves also had a higher incidence of perivalvular regurgitation in the mitral position (see Fig. 11–79) and a trend for this complication in the aortic position. In the Edinburgh randomized trial, which also compared a mechanical with a porcine xenograft valve,[345] 20-year outcome data demonstrated no difference in overall mortality, but survival with the original prosthesis and survival without major valve-related adverse events (except bleeding) were significantly better with mechanical valves. Retrospective cohort analyses are in agreement with the results of these trials.[346,347] Therefore, mechanical prostheses, usually of the bileaflet variety, are the valves of choice in most patients younger than 65 years of age.

However, the following groups of patients should receive bioprostheses: (1) patients with coexisting disease who are prone to hemorrhage and who therefore tolerate anticoagulants poorly, such as those with bleeding disorders, intestinal polyposis, and angiodysplasia; (2) patients who are likely to be noncompliant with permanent anticoagulant treatment, who are unwilling to take anticoagulants on a regular basis, or who live in developing nations and cannot be monitored; (3) patients older than 65 years of age in whom bioprosthetic valves deteriorate slowly (see Fig. 57–51), who are unlikely to outlive their bioprostheses, and who because of their age may also be at greater risk of hemorrhage while taking anticoagulants; (4) patients with a small aortic annulus in whom an unstented (free) bioprosthetic graft may provide superior hemodynamics; and (5) younger patients (<40 years of age), especially women wishing to bear children, who require AVR and in whom a pulmonary autograft may be preferable. However, the technical difficulties associated with the last procedure must be taken into account.

Special Situations

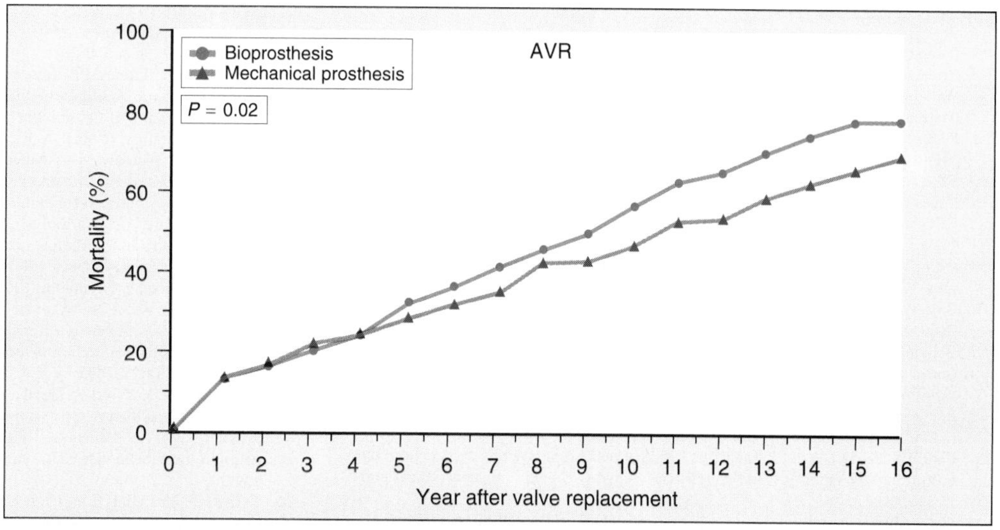

PREGNANCY (see Chap. 74). Women with artificial valves can tolerate the hemodynamic burden of pregnancy well, but the hypercoagulable state of pregnancy increases the risk of thromboembolism in pregnant patients with mechanical prostheses. Anticoagulation must not be interrupted, although an increased risk of fatal fetal hemorrhage occurs in women in whom anticoagulants are continued. There is also a risk of fetal malformation caused by the probable teratogenic effect of warfarin, but this risk is low (1.6%).[348] Although these problems represent rationales for the use of tissue valves in all women of childbearing age,[349] their limited durability in young adults makes their use unacceptable. Therefore, unless a pulmonary autograft can be employed (for patients who require AVR), every effort should be made to defer valve replacement until after childbirth. In pregnant women with critical MS or AS, balloon valvuloplasty should be considered, and, if at all possible, mitral valve repair instead of replacement should be undertaken for patients with MR. Women of childbearing potential who have a mechanical prosthesis should be counseled against pregnancy. When a woman who already has a mechanical prosthetic valve becomes pregnant, the risk to the fetus if the mother receives oral anticoagulants appears to be lower than the risk to the mother if anticoagulants are discontinued. Therefore, coumarin derivatives should be continued and the INR maintained between 2.0 and 3.0 until 2 weeks before expected delivery, at which time the patient should be switched to intravenous heparin.[1,25,350] Heparin should be discontinued at the onset of labor but may be restarted, along with coumarin, several hours after delivery. Alternatively, warfarin may be briefly interrupted at the 38th week of gestation and planned cesarean section carried out.[349] There are no data on the safety and effectiveness of low-molecular-weight heparin in pregnant patients with mechanical prosthetic valves, and this agent cannot be recommended in these patients.[348,351] Low-molecular-weight heparin is not approved for this use, and additional precautions have been added to the warning labels.

FIGURE 57–52 Mortality after aortic valve replacement (AVR) with the Björk-Shiley and porcine valves from the Department of Veterans Affairs trial. (From Hammermeister KE, Sethi GK, Henderson WG, et al: Outcomes 15 years after valve replacement with a mechanical versus a bioprosthetic valve: Final report of the Veterans Affairs randomized trial. J Am Coll Cardiol 36:1152, 2000.)

NONCARDIAC SURGERY. When noncardiac surgery is required in patients with prosthetic valves who are receiving anticoagulants, the risk is minimal when the anticoagulant is stopped 1 to 3 days preoperatively and for a similar period postoperatively. It may be desirable, however, to protect the patient with low-molecular-weight dextran during the perioperative period and to resume anticoagulation rapidly with intravenous heparin.

PATIENTS DESTINED TO RECEIVE ANTICOAGULANTS. Patients with earlier implantation of a mechanical prosthesis, chronic atrial fibrillation with an enlarged left atrium, a history of thromboembolism, or a thrombus in the left atrium at operation, and who therefore are destined to receive anticoagulants, should receive a mechanical valve prosthesis because the potential advantage of a tissue valve is negated.[1]

CHILDREN AND PATIENTS RECEIVING CHRONIC HEMODIALYSIS. The high incidence of bioprosthetic valve failure in children and adolescents virtually prohibits their use in these groups. In young adults between the ages of 25 and 35 years, the failure of bioprosthetic valves is somewhat higher than it is in older adults; this serves as a relative, but not an absolute, contraindication to their use in this age group.

In children, a mechanical prosthesis (generally the St. Jude valve) with its favorable hemodynamics and established durability is preferred despite the disadvantages inherent in the need for anticoagulants in this age group. Similarly, mechanical valve prostheses should be used in patients with chronic renal failure and/or hypercalcemia. Alternatively, if an experienced surgical team is available and the patient requires an AVR, a pulmonary autograft is an excellent alternative.

Previous studies indicated a high rate of bioprosthetic structural deterioration in patients receiving chronic renal dialysis. However, subsequent studies have reported no difference in survival of patients with a bioprosthesis or a mechanical valve, coupled with an unacceptably high rate of stroke and major bleeding in patients with the mechanical valves.[352,353] Although current guidelines recommend mechanical valves in these patients, this clearly is an area in which physician judgment is important for individual patients.

TRICUSPID POSITION. The risk of thrombosis for all valves is highest in the tricuspid position because of the lower pressures and velocity of blood flow. This complication appears to be highest for tilting-disc valves, intermediate for caged-ball valves, and lowest for bioprostheses, which are the valves of choice as tricuspid replacements. Fortunately, bioprostheses exhibit a much slower rate of mechanical deterioration in the tricuspid position than in the mitral or aortic positions.

REFERENCES

1. Bonow RO, Carabello B, de Leon AC, et al: ACC/AHA guidelines for the management of patients with valvular heart disease: A report of the American College of Cardiology/American Heart Association Task Force on Practice Guidelines (Committee on Management of Patients with Valvular Heart Disease). J Am Coll Cardiol 32:1486, 1998.
2. Iung B, Gohlke-Barwolf C, Tornos P, et al: Recommendations on the management of the asymptomatic patient with valvular heart disease. Eur Heart J 23:1253, 2002.

3. Rahimtoola SH, Durairaj A, Mehra A, et al: Current evaluation and management of patients with mitral stenosis. Circulation 106:1183, 2002.
4. Waller B, Howard J, Fess S: Pathology of mitral valve stenosis and pure mitral regurgitation: I. Clin Cardiol 17:330, 1994.
5. Filgner CL, Reichenbach DD, Otto CM: Pathology and etiology of valvular heart disease. *In* Otto CM (ed): Valvular Heart Disease. 2nd ed. Philadelphia, WB Saunders, 2004, pp 30-33.
6. Dalen JE, Fenster PE: Mitral stenosis. *In* Alpert JS, Dalen JE, Rahimtoola SH (eds): Valvular Heart Disease. 3rd ed. Philadelphia, Lippincott Williams & Wilkins, 2000, pp 75-83.
7. Otto CM: Mitral stenosis. *In* Otto CM (ed): Valvular Heart Disease. 2nd ed. Philadelphia, WB Saunders, 2004, pp 252-255.
8. Grossman W: Profiles in valvular heart disease. *In* Baim DS, Grossman W (eds): Cardiac Catheterization, Angiography and Interventions. 6th ed. Baltimore, Lippincott, Williams & Wilkins, 2000, pp 735-756.
9. Gorlin R, Gorlin SG: Hydraulic formula for calculation of the area of stenotic mitral valve, other cardiac valves, and central circulatory shunts. Am Heart J 41:1, 1951.
10. Braunwald E, Turi ZG: Pathophysiology of mitral valve disease. *In* Wells FC, Shapiro LM (eds): Mitral Valve Disease. 2nd ed. London, Butterworths, 1996, pp 28-36.
11. Choi BW, Bacharach SL, Barbour DJ, et al: Left ventricular systolic dysfunction, diastolic filling characteristics, and exercise cardiac reserve in mitral stenosis. Am J Cardiol 75:526, 1995.
12. Stefanadis C, Dernellis J, Stratos C, et al : Effects of balloon mitral valvuloplasty on left atrial function in mitral stenosis as assessed by pressure-area relation. J Am Coll Cardiol 32:159, 1998.
13. Pathan AZ, Mahdi NA, Leon MN, et al: Is redo percutaneous mitral balloon valvuloplasty (PMV) indicated in patients with post-PMV mitral restenosis? J Am Coll Cardiol 34:49, 1999.
14. Moreyra AE, Wilzon AC, Deac R, et al: Factors associated with atrial fibrillation in patients with mitral stenosis: A cardiac catheterization study. Am Heart J 135:138-145, 1998.
15. Leatham A: Assessment of mitral valve function: Clinical presentation, assessment, and prognosis. *In* Wells FC, Shapiro LM (eds): Mitral Valve Disease. 2nd ed. London, Butterworths, 1996, pp 37-46.
16. Wood P: An appreciation of mitral stenosis. BMJ 1:1051,1113, 1954.
17. Chiang CW, Lo SK, Kuo CT, et al: Noninvasive predictors of systemic embolism in mitral stenosis: An echocardiographic and clinical study of 500 patients. Chest 106:396, 1994.
18. Chiang CW, Lo SK, Ko YS, et al: Predictors of systemic embolism in patients with mitral stenosis: A prospective study. Ann Intern Med 128:885, 1998.
19. Shapiro LM: Echocardiography of the mitral valve. *In* Wells FC, Shapiro LM (eds): Mitral Valve Disease. 2nd ed. London, Butterworths, 1996, pp 47-50.
20. Sagie A, Freitas N, Chen MH, et al: Echocardiographic assessment of mitral stenosis and its associated valvular lesions in 205 patients and lack of association with mitral valve prolapse. J Am Soc Echocardiogr 10:141, 1997.
21. Faletr F, Pezzano JA, Fusc R, et al: Measurement of mitral valve area in mitral stenosis: Four echocardiographic methods compared with direct measurement of anatomic orifices. J Am Coll Cardiol 28:1190, 1996.
22. Popovic AD, Thomas JD, Neskovic AN, et al: Time-related trends in the preoperative evaluation of patients with valvular stenosis. Am J Cardiol 80:1464, 1997.
23. Prystowsky EN, Benson DW Jr, Fuster V, et al: Management of patients with atrial fibrillation: A Statement for Healthcare Professionals. From the Subcommittee on Electrocardiography and Electrophysiology. Circulation 93:1262, 1996.
24. Fuster V, Ryden L, Asinger RW, et al: ACC/AHA/ESC guidelines for the management of patients with atrial fibrillation: Executive summary. J Am Coll Cardiol 38:1231, 2001.
25. Gohlke-Barwolf C, Acar J, Oakley C, et al: Guidelines for the prevention of thromboembolic events in valvular heart disease. Eur Heart J 16:1230, 1995.
26. Manning WJ, Silverman DI, Keighley CS, et al: Transesophageal echocardiographically facilitated early cardioversion from atrial fibrillation using short-term anticoagulation: Final results of a prospective 4.5 year study. J Am Coll Cardiol 25:1354, 1995.
27. Kawaguchi AT, Kosakai Y, Sasako Y, et al : Risks and benefits of combined maze procedure for atrial fibrillation with organic heart disease. J Am Coll Cardiol 28:985, 1996.
28. Yuda S, Nakatini S, Isobe F, et al: Comparative efficacy of the maze procedure for restoration of atrial contraction in patients with and without giant left atrium associated with mitral valve disease. J Am Coll Cardiol 31,1097, 1998.
29. Nakajima H, Kobayashi J, Bando K, et al: The effect of cryo-maze procedure on early and intermediate-term outcome in mitral valve disease: Case-matched study. Circulation 106:I-46, 2002.
30. Sagie A, Freitas N, Padial LR, et al: Doppler echocardiographic assessment of long-term progression of mitral stenosis in 103 patients: Valve area and right heart disease. J Am Coll Cardiol 28:472, 1996.
31. Olesen KH: The natural history of 271 patients with mitral stenosis under medical treatment. Br Heart J 24:349, 1962.
32. Horstkotte D, Niehues R, Strauer BE: Pathomorphological aspects, aetiology, and natural history of acquired mitral valve stenosis. Eur Heart J 12(Suppl):55, 1991.
33. Orrange E, Kawanishi DT, Lopez BM, et al: Actuarial outcome after catheter balloon commissurotomy in patients with mitral stenosis. Circulation 95:382, 1997.
34. Hernandez R, Banuelos C, Alfonso F, et al: Long-term clinical and echocardiographic follow-up after percutaneous mitral valvuloplasty with the Inoue balloon. Circulation 99:1580, 1999.
35. Iung B, Garbarz E, Michaud P, et al: Late results of percutaneous mitral commissurotomy in a series of 1024 patients—Analysis of late clinical deterioration: Frequency, anatomic findings, and predictive factors. Circulation 99:3273, 1999.
36. Kang DH, Park SW, Song JK, et al: Long-term clinical and echocardiographic outcome of percutaneous mitral valvuloplasy: Randomized comparison of Inoue and double-balloon techniques. J Am Coll Cardiol 35:169, 2000.
37. Farhat MB, Ayari M, Maatzouk F, et al: Percutaneous balloon versus surgical closed and open mitral commissurotomy: Seven-year follow-up results of a randomized trial. Circulation 97:245, 1998.
38. Cannan CR, Nishimura RA, Reeder GS, et al: Echocardiographic assessment of commissural calcium: A simple predictor of outcome after percutaneous mitral balloon valvotomy. J Am Coll Cardiol 29:175, 1997.
39. Gomez-Hospital JA, Cequier A, Romero PV, et al: Partial improvement in pulmonary function after successful percutaneous balloon mitral valvotomy. Chest 117:643, 2000.
40. Padial LR, Abascal VM, Moreno PR, et al: Echocardiography can predict the development of severe mitral regurgitation after percutaneous mitral valvuloplasty by the Inoue technique. Am J Cardiol 83:1210, 1999.
41. Palacios IF, Sanchez PL, Harrell, et al: Which patients benefit from percutaneous mitral balloon valvuloplasty? Prevalvuloplasy and postvalvuloplasty variables that predict long-term outcome. Circulation 105:1465, 2002.
42. Zhang HP, Yen GS, Allen JW, et al: Comparison of late results of balloon valvotomy in mitral stenosis with versus without mitral regurgitation. Am J Cardiol 81:51, 1998.
43. Mazur W, Parilak LD, Kaluza G, et al: Balloon valvuloplasty for mitral stenosis. Curr Opin Cardiol 14:95, 1999.
44. Applebaum R, Kasliwal R, Kanojia A, et al: Utility of three-dimensional echocardiography during balloon mitral valvuloplasty. J Am Coll Cardiol 32:1405, 1998.
45. Joseph PK, Bhat A, Francis B, et al: Percutaneous transvenous mitral commissurotomy using an Inoue balloon in children with rheumatic mitral stenosis. Int J Cardiol 62:19, 1997.
46. Kothari SS, Kamath P, Juneja R, et al: Percutaneous transvenous mitral commissurtomy using Inoue balloon in children less than 12 years. Cathet Cardiovasc Diagn 43:408, 1998.
47. Zaki A, Salama M, El Masry M, Elhendy A: Five-year follow-up after percutaneous balloon mitral valvuloplasty. Am J Cardiol 83:735, 1999.
48. Iung B, Garbarz E, Michaud P, et al: Percutaneous mitral commissurotomy for restenosis after surgical commissurotomy: Late efficacy and implications for patient selection. J Am Coll Cardiol 35:1295, 2000.
49. Ben Farat M, Gamra H, Betbout F, et al: Percutaneous balloon mitral commissurotomy during pregnancy. Heart 77:564, 1997.
50. de Souza JAM, Martinez EE, Ambrose JA, et al: Percutaneous balloon mitral valvuloplasty in comparison with open mitral valve commissurotomy for mitral stenosis during pregnancy. J Am Coll Cardiol 37:900, 2001.
51. Leon MN, Harrell LC, Simosa HF, et al: Mitral balloon valvotomy for patients with mitral stenosis and atrial fibrillation: Immediate and long-term results. J Am Coll Cardiol 34:1145, 1999.
52. Cribier A, Elchaninoff H, Koning R, et al: Percutaneous mechanical mitral commissurotomy with a newly designed metallic valvulotome: Immediate results of the initial experience in 153 patients. Circulation 99:793, 1999.
53. English T: Closed mitral valvotomy. *In* Wells FC, Shapiro LM (eds): Mitral Valve Disease. 2nd ed. London, Butterworths, 1996, pp 107-113.
54. Otto CM: Surgical and percutaneous intervention for mitral stenosis. *In* Otto CM (ed): Valvular Heart Disease. 2nd ed. Philadelphia, WB Saunders, 2004, pp 272-276.
55. Edwards FH, Peterson ED, Coombs LP, et al: Prediction of operative mortality after valve replacement surgery. J Am Coll Cardiol 37:885, 2001.

Mitral Regurgitation

56. Otto CM: Evaluation and management of chronic mitral regurgitation. N Engl J Med 345:740, 2001.
57. Carabello BA: Progress in mitral and aortic regurgitation. Curr Probl Cardiol 28:553, 2003.
58. Mann JM, Davies MJ: The pathology of the mitral valve. *In* Wells FC, Shapiro LM (eds): Mitral Valve Disease. 2nd ed. London, Butterworths, 1996, pp 16-27.
59. Fox CS, Vasan RS, Parise H, et al: Mitral annular calcification predicts cardiovascular morbidity and mortality: The Framingham Heart Study. Circulation 107:1492, 2003.
60. Jeon DS, Atar S, Brasch AV, et al: Association of mitral annulus calcification, aortic valve sclerosis, and aortic root calcification with abnormal myocardial perfusion single-photon emission tomography in subjects <65 years old. J Am Coll Cardiol 38:1988, 2001.
61. Adler Y, Fink N, Tame D, et al: Association between mitral annulus calcification and carotid atherosclerotic disease. Stroke 29:1833, 1998.
62. Barber JE, Ratliff NB, Cosgrove DM, et al: Myxomatous mitral valve chordae: I. Mechanical properties. J Heart Valve Dis 10:320, 2001.
63. Lamas GA, Mitchell GF, Flaker GC, et al: Clinical significance of mitral regurgitation after acute myocardial infarction. Survival and Ventricular Enlargement Investigators. Circulation 96:827, 1997.
64. Otsuji Y, Handschumacher MD, Schwammenthal E, et al: Insights from three-dimensional echocardiography into the mechanism of functional mitral regurgitation: Direct in vivo demonstration of altered leaflet tethering geometry. Circulation 96:1999, 1997.
65. Thourani VH, Weintraub WS, Guyton RA, et al: Outcomes and long-term survival for patients undergoing mitral valve repair versus replacement: Effect of age and concomitant coronary artery bypass grafting. Circulation 108:298, 2003.
66. Dahlberg PS, Orszulak TA, Mullany CJ, et al: Late outcome of mitral valve surgery for patients with coronary artery disease. Ann Thorac Surg 76:1539, 2003.
67. 126. Rosario LB, Stevenson LW, Solomon SD, et al: The mechanism of decrease in dynamic mitral regurgitation during heart failure treatment: Importance of reduction in the regurgitant orifice size. J Am Coll Cardiol 32:1819, 1998.
68. Kizilbash AM, Willett DL, Brickner ME, et al: Effects of afterload reduction on vena contracta width in mitral regurgitation. J Am Coll Cardiol 32:427, 1998.
69. Carabello BA: Concentric versus eccentric remodeling. J Card Fail 8(Suppl):S258, 2002.
70. Sutton TM, Stewart RAH, Gerber IL, et al: Plasma natriuretic peptide levels increase with symptoms and severity of mitral regurgitation. J Am Coll Cardiol 41:2280, 2003.

71. Tallaj J, Hankes GH, Holland M, et al: Beta$_1$-adrenergic receptor blockade attenuates angiotensin II-mediated catecholamine release into the cardiac interstitium in mitral regurgitation. Circulation 108:225, 2003.
71a. Mehta RH, Supiamo MA, Oral H, et al: Compared with control subjects, the systemic sympathetic nervous system is activated in patients with mitral regurgitation. Am Heart J 145:1078, 2003.
72. Oral H, Sivasubramanian N, Dyke DB, et al: Myocardial proinflammatory cytokine expression and left ventricular remodeling in patients with chronic mitral regurgitation. Circulation 107:831, 2003.
73. Conway MA, Bottomley PA, Ouwerkerk R, et al: Mitral regurgitation: Impaired systolic function, eccentric hypertrophy, and increased severity are linked to lower phosphocreatine/ATP ratios in humans. Circulation 97:1716, 1998.
74. Akasaka T, Yoshida K, Hozumi T, et al: Restricted coronary flow reserve in patients with mitral regurgitation improves after mitral reconstructive surgery. J Am Coll Cardiol 32:1923, 1998.
75. Timmis SB, Kirsh MM, Montgomery DG, Starling MR: Evaluation of left ventricular ejection fraction as a measure of pump performance in patients with chronic mitral regurgitation. Cathet Cardiovasc Intervent 49:290, 2000.
76. Enriquez-Sarano M, Schaff HV, Tajik AJ, et al: Chronic mitral regurgitation. *In* Alpert JS, Dalen JE, Rahimtoola SH (eds): Valvular Heart Disease. 3rd ed. Philadelphia, Lippincott Williams & Wilkins, 2000, pp 113-142.
77. Matsumura T, Ohtaki E, Tanaka K, et al: Echocardiographic prediction of left ventricular dysfunction after mitral valve repair for mitral regurgitation as an indicator to decide the optimal timing of repair. J Am Coll Cardiol 42:458, 2003.
78. Flemming MA, Oral H, Rothman ED, et al: Echocardiographic markers for mitral valve surgery to preserve left ventricular performance in mitral regurgitation. Am Heart J 140:476, 2000.
79. Wisenbaugh T, Skudicky D, Sareli P: Prediction of outcome after valve replacement for rheumatic mitral regurgitation in the era of chordal preservation. Circulation 89:191, 1994.
80. Leung DY, Griffin BP, Snader CE, et al: Determinant of functional capacity in chronic mitral regurgitation unassociated with coronary artery disease or left ventricular dysfunction. Am J Cardiol 79:914, 1997.
81. Enriquez-Sarano M, Basmadjian AJ, Rossi A, et al: Progression of mitral regurgitation: A prospective Doppler echocardiographic study. J Am Coll Cardiol 34:1137, 1999.
82. Ling LH, Enriquez-Sarano M. Long-term outcomes of patients with flail mitral valve leaflets. Coron Artery Dis 11:3, 2000.
83. Rosen SF, Borer JS, Hochreiter C, et al: Natural history of the asymptomatic patient with severe mitral regurgitation secondary to mitral valve prolapse and normal right and left ventricular performance. Am J Cardiol 74:374, 1994.
84. Heinle SK, Grayburn PA: Doppler echocardiographic assessment of mitral regurgitation. Coron Artery Dis 11:11, 2000.
85. Dujardin KS, Enriquez-Sarano M, Bailey KR, et al: Grading of mitral regurgitation by quantitative Doppler echocardiography: Calibration by left ventricular angiography in routine clinical practice. Circulation 96:3409, 1996.
85a. Zoghbi WA, Enriquez-Sarano M, Foster E, et al: Recommendations for evaluation of the severity of native valvular regurgitation with two-dimensional and Doppler echocardiography. J Am Soc Echocardiogr 16:777, 2003.
86. Zhou X, Jones M, Shiota T, et al: Vena contracta imaged by Doppler color-flow mapping predicts the severity of eccentric mitral regurgitation better than color jet area: A chronic animal study. J Am Coll Cardiol 30:1393, 1997.
87. Hall SA, Brickner ME, Willett DL, et al: Assessment of mitral regurgitation severity by Doppler color-flow mapping of the vena contracta. Circulation 95:636, 1997.
88. Enriquez-Sarano M, Dujardin KS, Tribouilloy CM, et al: Determinants of pulmonary venous flow reversal in mitral regurgitation and its usefulness in determining the severity of regurgitation. Am J Cardiol 83:535, 1999.
89. Thomas L, Foster E, Schiller NB: Peak mitral inflow velocity predicts mitral regurgitation severity. J Am Coll Cardiol 31:174, 1998.
90. Thomas L, Foster E, Hoffman JIE, et al: The mitral regurgitation index: An echocardiographic guide to severity. J Am Coll Cardiol 33:2016, 1999.
91. Enriquez-Sarano M, Freeman WK, Tribouilloy CM, et al : Functional anatomy of mitral regurgitation: Accuracy and outcome implications of transesophageal echocardiography. J Am Coll Cardiol 34:1129, 1999.
92. Pu M, Thomas JD, Vandervoort PM, et al : Comparison of quantitative and semiquantitative methods for assessing regurgitation by transesophageal echocardiography. Am J Cardiol 87:66, 2001.
92a. Omram AS, Woo A, David TE, et al: Intraoperative transesophageal echocardiography accurately predicts mitral valve anatomy and suitability for repair. J Am Soc Echocardiogr 15:950, 2002.
93. De Simone R, Glombitza G, Vahl CF, et al: Three-dimensional color Doppler: A clinical study in patients with mitral regurgitation. J Am Coll Cardiol 33:1646, 1999.
94. Armstrong GP, Griffin BP: Exercise echocardiographic assessment in severe mitral regurgitation. Coron Artery Dis 11:23, 2000.
95. Kizilbash AM, Hundley WG, Willett DL, et al: Comparison of quantitative Doppler with magnetic resonance imaging for assessment of the severity of mitral regurgitation. Am J Cardiol 81:792, 1998.
96. Høst U, Kelbaek H, Hildebrant P, et al: Effect of ramipril on mitral regurgitation secondary to mitral valve prolapse. Am J Cardiol 80:655, 1997.
97. Tischler MD, Rowan M, LeWinter MM: Effect of enalapril therapy on left ventricular mass and volumes in asymptomatic chronic, severe, mitral regurgitation secondary to mitral valve prolapse. Am J Cardiol 82:242, 1998.
98. Nemoto S, Hamawaki M, De Freitas G, et al : Differential effects of the angiotensin-converting enzyme inhibitor lisinopril versus the beta-adrenergic receptor blocker atenolol on hemodynamics and left ventricular contractile function in experimental mitral regurgitation. J Am Coll Cardiol 40:149, 2002.
99. Perry GJ, Wei CC, Hankes GH, et al: Angiotensin II receptor blockade does not improve left ventricular function and remodeling in subacute mitral regurgitation in the dog. J Am Coll Cardiol 39:1374, 2002.
100. Gillinov AM, Cosgrove DM, Blackstone EH, et al: Durability of mitral valve repair for degenerative disease. J Thorac Cardiovasc Surg 116:734, 1998.
101. Braunberger E, Deloche A, Berregi A, et al: Very long-term results (>20 years) of valve repair with Carpentier's techniques in nonrheumatic mitral valve insufficiency. Circulation 104:I-8, 2001.
102. Mohty D, Orszulak TA, Schaff HV, et al: Very long-term survival and durability of mitral valve repair for mitral valve prolapse. Circulation 104:I-1, 2001.
103. Chauvand S, Fuzellier JF, Berrebi A, et al : Long-term (29 years) results of reconstructive surgery in rheumatic mitral valve insufficiency. Circulation 104:I-12, 2001.
103a. Yacoub MH, Cohn LH: Novel approaches to cardiac valve repair: From structare to function (two parts). Circulation 109:942 and 1064, 2004.
104. Phillips MR, Daly RC, Schaff HV, et al: Repair of anterior leaflet mitral valve prolapse: Chordal replacement versus chordal shortening. Ann Thorac Surg 69:25, 2000.
105. von Oppell UO, Stemmet F, Braink J, et al: Ischemic mitral valve repair surgery. J Heart Valve Dis 9:64, 2000.
106. Gillinov AM, Wierup PN, Blackstone EH, et al: Is repair preferable to replacement for ischemic mitral regurgitation? J Thorac Cardioavasc Surg 122:1125, 2001.
107. Bolling SF, Pagani FD, Deeb GM, Bach DS: Intermediate-term outcome of mitral reconstruction in cardiomyopathy. J Thorac Cardiovasc Surg 115:381, 1998.
108. Chen FY, Adams DH, Aranki SF, et al: Mitral valve repair in cardiomyopathy. Circulation 98:III-124, 1998.
109. Bishay ES, McCarthy PM, Cosgrove DM, et al: Mitral valve surgery in patients with severe left ventricular dysfunction. Eur J Cardiothorac Surg 17:213, 2000.
110. Remadi JP, Baron O, Roussel C, et al: Isolated mitral valve replacement with St. Jude medical prosthesis—Long-term results: A follow-up of 19 years. Circulation 103:1542, 2001.
111. Reardon MJ, David TE: Mitral valve replacement with preservation of the subvalvular apparatus. Curr Opin Cardiol 14:104, 1998.
112. Yun KL, Sintek CF, Miller DC, et al: Randomized trial of partial versus complete chordal preservation methods of mitral valve replacement: A preliminary report. Circulation 100:II-90, 1999.
113. Society of Thoracic Surgeons National Cardiac Surgery Database. Accessed December 10, 2003. (http://www.ctsnet.org/file/STSNationalDatabaseSpring2003Executive Summary.pdf)
114. Click RL, Schaff HV: Intraoperative transesophageal echocardiography: 5-year prospective review of impact on surgical management. Mayo Clin Proc 75:241, 2000.
114a. Savage EB, Ferguson TB Jr, DiSesa VJ: Use of mitral valve repair: Analysis of contemporary United States experience reported to the Society of Thoracic Surgeons National Cardiac Database. Ann Thorac Surg 75:820, 2003.
115. Grossi EA, Galloway AC, Miller JS, et al: Valve repair versus replacement for mitral insufficiency: When is a mechanical valve still indicated? J Thorac Cardiovasc Surg 115:389, 1998.
116. Flameng W, Herijgers P, Bogaerts K: Recurrence of mitral valve regurgitation after mitral valve repair in degenerative valve disease. Circulation 107:1609, 2003.
117. Loulmet DF, Carpentier A, Cho PW, et al: Less invasive techniques for mitral valve surgery. J Thorac Cardiovasc Surg 115:772, 1998.
118. Gillinov AM, Cosgrove DM: Minimally invasive mitral valve surgery: Mini-sternotomy with extended transseptal approach. Semin Thorac Cardiovasc Surg 11:206, 1999.
119. Greelish JP, Cohn LH, Leacche M, et al: Minimally invasive mitral valve repair suggests earlier operations for mitral valve disease. J Thorac Cardiovasc Surg 126:365, 2003.
120. Letsou GV, Reardon MJ: Minimally invasive valve surgery. Curr Opin Cardiol 13:105, 1998.
121. Goldfine H, Aurigemma GP, Zile MR, et al: Left ventricular length–force-shortening relations before and after surgical correction of chronic mitral regurgitation. J Am Coll Cardiol 31:180, 1998.
122. Krishman US, Gersony WW, Berman-Rosenzweig E, Apfel HD: Late left ventricular function after surgery for children with chronic symptomatic mitral regurgitation. Circulation 96:4280, 1997.
123. Tribouilloy CM, Enriquez-Sarano M, Schaff HV, et al: Impact of preoperative symptoms on survival after surgical correction of organic mitral regurgitation: Rationale for optimizing surgical indications. Circulation 99:400, 1999.
124. Lim E, Barlow CW, Hosseinpour AR, et al: Influence of atrial fibrillation on outcome following mitral valve repair. Circulation 104:I-59, 2001.
125. Gillinov AM, Faber C, Houghtaling PL, et al: Repair versus replacement for degenerative mitral valve disease with coexisting ischemic heart disease. J Thorac Cardioavasc Surg 125:1197, 2003.

Mitral Valve Prolapse Syndrome

126. Devereux RB: Recent developments in the diagnosis and management of mitral valve prolapse. Curr Opin Cardiol 10:107, 1995.
127. David TE, Omran A, Armstrong S, et al: Long-term results of mitral valve repair for myxomatous disease with and without chordal replacement with expanded polytetrafluoroethylene sutures. J Thorac Cardiovasc Surg 115:1279, 1998.
128. Cohn LH, Couper GS, Aranki SF, et al: Long-term results of mitral valve reconstruction for the regurgitating myxomatous mitral valve. J Thorac Cardiovasc Surg 107:143, 1994.
129. O'Rourke RA: Syndrome of mitral valve prolapse. *In* Alpert JS, Dalen JE, Rahimtoola SH (eds): Valvular Heart Disease. 3rd ed. Philadelphia, Lippincott Williams & Wilkins, 2000, pp 157-182.
130. Nishimura RA, McGoon MD: Perspectives on mitral valve prolapse. N Engl J Med 341:48, 1999.
131. Freed LA, Benjamin EJ, Levy D, et al: Mitral valve prolapse in the general population: The benign nature of the echocardiographic features in the Framingham Heart Study. J Am Coll Cardiol 40:1298, 2002.

132. Otto CM: Mitral valve prolapse. *In* Otto CM (ed): Valvular Heart Disease. 2nd ed. Philadelphia, WB Saunders, 2004, pp 368-387.
133. Becker AE, Davies MJ: Pathomorphology of mitral valve prolapse. *In* Boudoulas H, Wooley CF (eds): Mitral Valve: Floppy Mitral Valve, Mitral Valve Prolapse, Mitral Valvular Regurgitation. 2nd ed. Armonk, NY, Futura, 2000, pp 91-114.
134. Grande-Allen KJ, Griffin BP, Calabro A, et al: Myxomatous mitral valve chordae: II. Selective elevation of glycosaminoglycan content. J Heart Valve Dis 10:325, 2001.
135. Mylonakis E, Calderwood SB: Infective endocarditis in adults. N Engl J Med 345:1318, 2001.
136. Fontana MF: Mitral valve prolapse and floppy mitral valve: Physical examination. *In* Boudoulas H, Wooley CF (eds): Mitral Valve: Floppy Mitral Valve, Mitral Valve Prolapse, Mitral Valvular Regurgitation. 2nd ed. Armonk, NY, Futura, 2000, pp 283-304.
137. Schaal SF: Mitral valve prolapse: Cardiac arrhythmias and electrophysiological correlates. *In* Boudoulas H, Wooley CF (eds): Mitral Valve: Floppy Mitral Valve, Mitral Valve Prolapse, Mitral Valvular Regurgitation. 2nd ed. Armonk, NY, Futura, 2000, pp 409-430.
138. Malkowski MJ, Pearson AC: The echocardiographic assessment of the floppy mitral valve: An integrated approach. *In* Boudoulas H, Wooley CF (eds): Mitral Valve: Floppy Mitral Valve, Mitral Valve Prolapse, Mitral Valvular Regurgitation. 2nd ed. Armonk, NY, Futura, 2000, pp 231-252.
139. Langholz D, Mackin WJ, Wallis DE, et al: Transesophageal echocardiographic assessment of systolic mitral leaflet displacement among patients with mitral valve prolapse. Am Heart J 135:197, 1998.
140. Fukuda N, Oki T, Iuchi A, et al: Predisposing factors for severe mitral regurgitation in idiopathic mitral valve prolapse. Am J Cardiol 76:503, 1995.
141. Zuppiroli A, Rinaldi M, Kramer-Fox R, et al: Natural history of mitral valve prolapse. Am J Cardiol 75:1028, 1995.
142. Boudoulas H, Kolibash AJ, Wooley CF: Floppy mitral valve, mitral valve prolapse, mitral valvular regurgitation: Natural history. *In* Boudoulas H, Wooley CF (eds): Mitral Valve: Floppy Mitral Valve, Mitral Valve Prolapse, Mitral Valvular Regurgitation. 2nd ed. Armonk, NY, Futura, 2000, pp 503-540.
143. Avierinos JF, Gersh BJ, Melton LJ, et al: Natural history of asymptomatic mitral valve prolapse in the community. Circulation 106:1355, 2002.
144. Gilon D, Buonanno FS, Joffe MM, et al: Lack of evidence of an association between mitral valve prolapse and stroke in young patients. N Engl J Med 341:8, 1999.
145. Boudoulas H, Wooley CF: Floppy mitral valve/Mitral valve prolapse: Sudden death. *In* Boudoulas H, Wooley CF (eds): Mitral Valve: Floppy Mitral Valve, Mitral Valve Prolapse, Mitral Valvular Regurgitation. 2nd ed. Armonk, NY, Futura, 2000, pp 431–448.
146. Corrado D, Basso C, Rizzoli G, et al: Does sports activity enhance the risk of sudden death in adolescents and young adults? J Am Coll Cardiol 42:1959, 2003.
147. Gillinov AM, Cosgrove DM, Lytle BW, et al: Reoperation for failure of mitral valve repair. J Thorac Cardiovasc Surg 113:467, 1997.

Aortic Stenosis

148. Levinson GE, Alpert JS. Aortic stenosis. *In* Alpert JS, Dalen JE, Rahimtoola SH (eds): Valvular Heart Disease. 3rd ed. Philadelphia, Lippincott Williams & Wilkins, 2000, pp 183-211.
149. Carabello BA: Aortic stenosis. N Engl J Med 346:677, 2002.
150. Huntington K, Hunter AGW, Chan KL: A prospective study to assess the frequency of familial clustering of congenital bicuspid aortic valve. J Am Coll Cardiol 30:1809, 1997.
151. Fedak PWM, Verma S, David TE: Clinical and pathophysiological implications of a bicuspid aortic valve. Circulation 106:900, 2002.
152. Keane MG, Wiegers SE, Plappert T, et al. Bicuspid aortic valves are associated with aortic dilatation out of proportion to coexistent valvular lesions. Circulation 102:III-35, 2000.
153. Nataatmadja M, West M, West J, et al: Abnormal extracellular matrix protein transport associated with increased apoptosis of vascular smooth muscle cells in Marfan syndrome and bicuspid aortic valve thoracic aortic aneurysm. Circulation 108:II-329, 2003.
154. Rajamannan NM, Gersh B, Bonow RO: Calcific aortic stenosis: From bench to bedside—Emerging clinical and cellular concepts. Heart 89:1, 2003.
155. Otto CM, Lind BK, Kitzman DW, et al: Association of aortic valve sclerosis with cardiovascular mortality and morbidity in the elderly. N Engl J Med 341:142, 1999.
156. Olsson M, Thyberg J, Nilsson J: Presence of oxidized low-density lipoproteins in nonrheumatic stenotic aortic valves. Arterioscler Thromb Vasc Biol 19:1218, 1999.
157. Ghaisas NK, Foley JB, O'Briain DS, et al: Adhesion molecules in nonrheumatic aortic valve disease: Endothelial expression, serum levels, and effects of valve replacement. J Am Coll Cardiol 36:2257, 2000.
158. Galante A, Pietroiusti A, Vellini M, et al: C-reactive protein is increased in patients with degenerative aortic valvular stenosis. J Am Coll Cardiol 38:1078, 2001.
159. O'Brien KD, Shavelle DM, Caulfield MT, et al: Association of angiotensin-converting enzyme with low-density lipoprotein in aortic valvular lesions and in human plasma. Circulation 106:2224, 2002.
160. Mohler ER, Gannon F, Reynolds C, et al: Bone formation and inflammation in cardiac valves. Circulation 103:1522, 2001.
161. Rajamannan NM, Subramaniam M, Rickard D, et al : Human aortic valve calcification is associated with an osteoblast phenotype. Circulation 107:2181, 2003.
162. Stewart BF, Siscovick D, Lind BK, et al: Clinical factors associated with calcific aortic valve disease. J Am Coll Cardiol 29:630, 1997.
163. Palta S, Pai AM, Gill K, et al: New insights into the progression of aortic stenosis: Implications for secondary prevention. Circulation 101:2497, 2000.
164. Peltier M, Trojette F, Enriquez-Sarano M, et al: Relation between cardiovascular risk factors and nonrheumatic severe calcific aortic stenosis among patients with a three-cuspid aortic valve. Am J Cardiol 91:97, 2003.
165. Novaro GM, Iong IY, Pearce GL, et al: Effect of hydoxymethylglutaryl coenzyme A reductase inhibitors on the progression of calcific aortic stenosis. Circulation 104:2205, 2001.
166. Shavelle DM, Takasu J, Budoff MJ, et al: HMG CoA reductase inhibitor (statin) and aortic valve calcium. Lancet 359:1125, 2002.
167. Bellamy MF, Pellikka PA, Klarich KW, et al: Association of cholesterol levels, hydoxymethylglutaryl coenzyme-A reductase inhibitor treatment, and progression of aortic stenosis in the community. J Am Coll Cardiol 40:1723, 2002.
168. Rajamannan NM, Subramanian M, Sebo T, et al: Atorvastatin inhibits hypercholesterolemia-induced cellular proliferation and bone matrix production in the rabbit aortic valve. Circulation 105:2660, 2002.
169. Alpert JS: Aortic stenosis: A new face for an old disease. Arch Intern Med 163:1769, 2003.
170. Chan C: Is aortic stenosis a preventable disease? J Am Coll Cardiol 42:593, 2003.
171. Kawaguchi A, Miyatake K, Yutani C, et al: Characteristic cardiovascular manifestations in homozygous and heterozygous familial hypercholesterolemia. Am Heart J 137:410, 1999.
172. Hultgren HN: Osteitis deformans (Paget's disease) and calcific disease of the heart valves. Am J Cardiol 81:1461, 1998.
173. Hangaishi M, Taguchi J, Ikari Y, et al: Aortic valve stenosis in alkaptonuria. Circulation 98:1148, 1998.
174. Malouf JF, Enriquez-Sarano M, Pellikka PA, et al: Severe pulmonary hypertension in patients with severe aortic stenosis: Clinical profile and prognostic implications. J Am Coll Cardiol 40:789, 2002.
175. Legget ME, Kuusisto J, Healy NL, et al: Gender differences in left ventricular function at rest and with exercise in asymptomatic aortic stenosis. Am Heart J 131:94, 1996.
176. Fielitz J, Hein S, Mitrovic V, et al: Activation of the cardiac renin-angiotensin system and increased myocardial collagen expression in human aortic valve disease. J Am Coll Cardiol 37:1443, 2001.
177. Walther T, Schubert A, Falk V, et al: Left ventricular reverse remodeling after surgical therapy for aortic stenosis: Correlation to renin-angiotensin system gene expression. Circulation 106:I-23, 2002.
178. Rajappan K, Rimoldi OE, Dutka DP, et al: Mechanisms of coronary microcirculatory dysfunction in patients with aortic stenosis and angiographically normal coronary arteries. Circulation 105:470, 2002.
179. Gould KL, Carabello BA: Why angina in aortic stenosis with normal coronary arteriograms? Circulation 107:3121, 2003.
180. Julius BK, Spillmann M, Vassalli G, et al: Angina pectoris in patients with aortic stenosis and normal coronary arteries. Circulation 95:892, 1997.
181. Carabello BA: Evaluation and management of patients with aortic stenosis. Circulation 105:1746, 2002.
182. Pareti FI, Lattuada A, Bressi C, et al: Proteolysis of von Willebrand factor and shear stress-induced platelet aggregation in patients with aortic stenosis. Circulation 102:1290, 2000.
183. Vincentelli A, Susen S, Le Tourneau T, et al: Acquired von Willebrand syndrome in aortic stenosis. N Engl J Med 343:349, 2003.
184. Munt B, Legget ME, Kraft CD, et al: Physical examination in valvular aortic stenosis: Correlation with stenosis severity and prediction of clinical outcome. Am Heart J 137:298, 1999.
185. Okura H, Yoshida K, Hozumi T, et al: Planimetry and transthoracic two-dimensional echocardiography in noninvasive assessment of aortic valve area in patients with valvular aortic stenosis. J Am Coll Cardiol 30:753, 1997.
186. Kim KS, Maxted W, Nanda NC, et al: Comparison of multiplane and biplane transesophageal echocardiography in the assessment of aortic stenosis. Am J Cardiol 79:436, 1997.
187. Gilon D, Capre EG, Handschumacher MD, et al: Effect of three-dimensional valve shape on the hemodynamics of aortic stenosis: Three-dimensional echocardiographic stereolthography and patient studies. J Am Coll Cardiol 40:1479, 2002.
188. Leborgne L, Tribouilloy C, Otmani A, et al: Comparative value of Doppler echocardiography and cardiac catheterization in the decision to operate on patients with aortic stenosis. Int J Cardiol 65:163, 1998.
189. Baumgartner H, Stefenelli T, Niederberger J, et al: "Overestimation" of catheter gradients by Doppler ultrasound in patients with aortic stenosis: A predictable manifestation of pressure recovery. J Am Coll Cardiol 33:1655, 1999.
190. Garcia D, Pibarot P, Dumesnil JG, et al: Assessment of aortic valve stenosis severity: A new index based on the energy loss concept. Circulation 101:765, 2000.
191. Garcia D, Dumesnil JG, Durand LG, et al: Discrepancies between catheter and Doppler estimates of valve effective orifice area can be predicted from the pressure recovery phenomenon: Practical implications with regard to quantification of aortic stenosis severity. J Am Coll Cardiol 41:435, 2003.
192. Levine RA, Schwammenthal E: Stenosis is in the eye of the observer: Impact of pressure recovery on assessing aortic valve area. J Am Coll Cardiol 41:443, 2003.
193. John AS, Dill T, Brandt RR, et al: Magnetic resonance to assess the aortic valve area in aortic stenosis. J Am Coll Cardiol 42:519, 2003.
194. Caruthers SD, Lin SJ, Brown P, et al: Practical value of cardiac magnetic resonance imaging for clinical quantification of aortic valve stenosis: Comparison with echocardiography. Circulation 208:2236, 2003.
195. Otto CM, Burwarsh IG, Legget ME, et al: A prospective study of asymptomatic valvular aortic stenosis: Clinical, echocardiographic, and exercise predictors of outcome. Circulation 95:2262, 1997.
196. Iivanainian AM, Lindroos M, Tilvis R, et al: Natural history of aortic valve stenosis of varying severity in the elderly. Am J Cardiol 78:97, 1996.
197. Rosenhek R, Porenta G, Lang I, et al: Predictors of outcome in severe, asymptomatic aortic stenosis. N Engl J Med 343:611, 2000.
198. Amato MCM, Moffa PJ, Ramires JAF: Treatment decision in asymptomatic aortic valve stenosis: Role of exercise testing. Heart 86:381, 2001.
199. Weinschelbaum E, Stutzbach P, Oliva M, et al: Manual débridement of the aortic valve in elderly patients with degenerative aortic stenosis. J Thorac Cardiovasc Surg 87:1157, 1999.

200. Braunwald E: Aortic valve replacement: An update at the turn of the millennium. Eur Heart J 21:1032-1033, 2000.
201. Connolly HM, Oh JK, Orszulak TA, et al: Aortic valve replacement for aortic stenosis with severe left ventricular dysfunction: Prognostic indicators. Circulation 95:2395, 1997.
202. Connolly HM, Oh JK, Schaff HV, et al: Severe aortic stenosis with low transvalvular gradient and severe left ventricular dysfunction: Result of aortic valve replacement in 52 patients. Circulation 101:1940, 2000.
203. Rahimtoola SH: Severe aortic stenosis with low systolic gradient: The good and bad news. Circulation 101:1892, 2000.
204. Pereira JJ, Lauer MS, Bashir M, et al: Survival after aortic valve replacement for severe aortic stenosis with low transvalvular gradients and severe left ventricular dysfunction. J Am Coll Cardiol 39:1356, 2002.
205. Monin JL, Monchi M, Gest V, et al: Aortic stenosis with severe left ventricular dysfunction and low transvalvular pressure gradients: Risk stratification by low-dose dobutamine echocardiography. J Am Coll Cardiol 37:2102, 2001.
206. Monin JL, Quere JP, Monchi M, et al: Low-gradient aortic stenosis: Operative risk stratification and predictors for long-term outcome—A multicenter study using dobutamine stress hemodynamics. Circulation 108:319, 2003.
207. Powell DE, Tunick PA, Rosenzweig BP, et al: Aortic valve replacement in patients with aortic stenosis and severe left ventricular dysfunction. Arch Intern Med 160:1337, 2000.
208. Jolobe O: Surgery for aortic stenosis in severely symptomatic patients older than 80 years: Experience in a single UK centre. Heart 83:583, 2000.
209. Khot UN, Novaro GM, Popovic ZB, et al: Nitroprusside in critically ill patients with left ventricular dysfunction and aortic stenosis. N Engl J Med 348:1756, 2003.
209a. Rahimtoola SH: The year in valvular heart disease. J Am Coll Cardiol 43:491, 2004.
210. Zile MR, Gaasch WH: Heart failure in aortic stenosis: Improving diagnosis and treatment. N Engl J Med 348:1735, 2003.
211. Nishimura RA, Grantham A, Connolly HM, et al: Low-output, low-gradient aortic stenosis in patients with depressed left ventricular systolic function: The clinical utility of the dobutamine challenge in the catheterization laboratory. Circulation 106:809, 2002.
212. Kivdal P, Bergström R, Hörte LG, et al: Observed and relative survival after aortic valve replacement. J Am Coll Cardiol 35:747, 2000.
213. Asimakopoulous G, Edwards MB, Taylor KM: Aortic valve replacement in patients 80 years of age and older: Survival and cause of death on 1100 cases. Collective results from the UK Heart Valve Registry. Circulation 96:3403, 1997.
214. Sundt TM, Bailey MS, Moon MR, et al: Quality of life after aortic valve replacement at the age of > 80 years. Circulation 102:III-70, 2000.
215. De Paulis R, Sommariva L, Colagrande L, et al: Regression of left ventricular hypertrophy after aortic valve replacement for aortic stenosis with different valve substitutes. J Thorac Cardiovasc Surg 116:590, 1998.
216. Lamb HJ, Beyerbacht HP, de Roos A, et al : Left ventricular remodeling early after aortic valve replacement: Differential effects on diastolic function in aortic valve stenosis and aortic regurgitation. J Am Coll Cardiol 40:2182, 2002.
217. Khan SS, Siegel RJ, DeRobertis MA, et al: Regression of hypertrophy after Carpentier-Edwards pericardial aortic valve replacement. Ann Thorac Surg 69:531, 2000.
218. Hildek-Smtih DJR, Shapiro LM: Coronary flow reserve improves after aortic valve replacement for aortic stenosis: An adenosine transthoracic echocardiography study. J Am Coll Cardiol 36:1889, 2000.
219. Rajappan K, Rimoldi OE, Camici PG, et al: Functional changes in coronary microcirculation after valve replacement in patients with aortic stenosis. Circulation 107:3170, 2003.
220. Gall S Jr, Lowe JE, Wolfe WG, et al: Efficacy of the internal mammary artery in combined aortic valve replacement coronary artery bypass grafting. J Thorac Surg 69:524, 2000.
221. Cohn LH: Minimally invasive aortic valve surgery: Technical considerations and results with the parasternal approach. J Card Surg 13:302, 1998.
222. Bouchard D, Perrault LP, Carrier M, et al: Ministernotomy for aortic valve replacement: A study of the preliminary experience. Can J Surg 43:39-42, 2000.
223. Galal O, Rao PS, Al-Fadley F, Wilson AD: Follow-up result of balloon aortic valvuloplasty in children with special reference to causes of late aortic insufficiency. Am Heart J 133:418, 1997.
224. Boudjemline Y, Bonhoeffer P: Steps toward percutaneous aortic valve replacement. Circulation 105:775, 2002.
225. Cribier A, Eltchanioff H, Bash A, et al: Percutaneous transcatheter implantation of an aortic valve prosthesis for calcific aortic stenosis: First human case description. Circulation 106:3006, 2002.

Aortic Regurgitation

226. Rahimtoola SH: Aortic regurgitation. *In* Rahimtoola SH (ed): Valvular Heart Disease. Atlas of Heart Diseases. Vol. 11. Braunwald E (series ed). Philadelphia, Current Medicine, 1997, p 7.9.
227. Casselman FP, Gillinov AR, Kasirajan V, et al: Intermediate-term durability of bicuspid aortic valve repair for prolapsing leaflet. Eur J Cardiothorac Surg 15:302, 1999.
228. Olsson A, Darpo B, Bergfeldt L, Rosenqvist M: Frequency and long-term follow-up of valvar insufficiency caused by retrograde aortic radiofrequency catheter ablation procedures. Heart 81:292, 1999.
229. Bonow RO: Chronic aortic regurgitation: Role of medical therapy and optimal timing for surgery. Cardiol Clin 16:449, 1998.
230. Bonow RO: Chronic aortic regurgitation. *In* Alpert JS, Dalen JE, Rahimtoola SH (eds): Valvular Heart Disease. 3rd ed. Philadelphia, Lippincott Williams & Wilkins, 2000, pp 245-268.
231. Borer JS, Truter S, Herrold EM, et al: Myocardial fibrosis in chronic aortic regurgitation: Molecular and cellular responses to volume overload. Circulation 105:1837, 2002.
232. Otto CM: Aortic regurgitation. *In* Otto CM (ed): Valvular Heart Disease. 2nd ed. Philadelphia, WB Saunders, 2004, pp 302-335.
233. Borer JS, Bonow RO: Contemporary approach to aortic and mitral regurgitation. Circulation 108:2432, 2003.
234. Choudhry NK, Etchells EE: Does this patient have aortic regurgitation? JAMA 281:2231, 1999.
235. Chen J, Okin PM, Roman MJ, et al: Combined rest and exercise electrocardiographic repolarization findings in relation to structural and functional abnormalities in asymptomatic aortic regurgitation. Am Heart J 132:343, 1996.
236. Tribouilloy CM, Enriquez-Sarano M, Fett SL, et al: Application of the proximal flow convergence method to calculate the effective regurgitant orifice area in aortic regurgitation. J Am Coll Cardiol 32:1032, 1998.
237. Shiota T, Jones M, Agler DA, McDonald RW: New echo cardiographic windows for quantitative determination of aortic regurgitation volume using color Doppler flow convergence and vena contracta. Am J Cardiol 83:1064, 1999.
238. Tribouilloy CM, Enriquez-Sarano M, Bailey KR, et al: Assessment of severity of aortic regurgitation using the width of the vena contracta: A clinical color Doppler imaging study. Circulation 102:558, 2000.
239. Willett DL, Hall SA, Jessen ME, et al: Assessment of aortic regurgitation by transesophageal color Doppler imaging of the vena contracta: Validation against an intraoperative aortic flow probe. J Am Coll Cardiol 37:1450, 2001.
240. Zoghbi WA, Enriquez-Sarano M, Foster E, et al: Recommendations for evaluation of the severity of native valvular regurgitation with two-dimensional and Doppler echocardiography. J Am Soc Echocardiogr 16:777, 2003.
241. Borer JS, Hochreiter C, Herrold EM, et al: Prediction of indications for valve replacement among asymptomatic or minimally symptomatic patients with chronic aortic regurgitation and normal left ventricular performance. Circulation 97:525, 1998.
242. Tarasoutchi F, Grinberg M, Spina GS, et al: Ten-year clinical laboratory follow-up after application of a symptom-based therapeutic strategy to patients with severe chronic aortic regurgitation of predominant rheumatic etiology. J Am Coll Cardiol 41:1316, 2003.
243. Pohost GM, Hung L, Doyle M: Clinical use of cardiovascular magnetic resonance. Circulation 12:647, 2003.
244. Dujardin KS, Enriquez-Sarano M, Schaff HV et al: Mortality and morbidity of aortic regurgitation in clinical practice: A long-term follow-up study. Circulation 99:1851, 1999.
245. Klodas E, Enriquez-Sarano M, Tajik AJ, et al: Aortic regurgitation complicated by extreme left ventricular dilatation: Long-term outcome after surgical correction. J Am Coll Cardiol 27:670, 1996.
246. Sondergaard L, Aldershvile J, Hildebrandt P, et al: Vasodilatation with felodipine in chronic asymptomatic aortic regurgitation. Am Heart J 139:667, 2000.
247. Alehan D, Ozkutlu S: Beneficial effects of 1-year captopril therapy in children with chronic aortic regurgitation who have no symptoms. Am Heart J 135:598, 1998.
248. Scognamiglio R, Rahimtoola SH, Fasoli G, et al: Nifedipine in asymptomatic patients with severe aortic regurgitation and normal left ventricular function. N Engl J Med 331:689, 1994.
249. Klodas E, Enriquez-Sarano M, Tajik AJ, et al: Optimizing timing of surgical correction in patients with severe aortic regurgitation: Role of symptoms. J Am Coll Cardiol 30:746, 1997.
250. Borer JS: Aortic valve replacement for the asymptomatic patient with aortic regurgitation: A new piece of the strategic puzzle. Circulation 106:2637, 2002.
251. Tornos MO, Olona M, Permanyer-Miralda G, et al: Heart failure after aortic valve replacement for aortic regurgitation: Prospective 20-year study. Am Heart J 136:681, 1998.
252. Turina J, Stark T, Seifert B, et al: Predictors of the long-term outcome after combined aortic and mitral valve surgery. Circulation 100:II-48, 1999.
253. Chaliki HP, Mohty D, Avierinos JF, et al: Outcomes after aortic valve replacement in patients with severe aortic regurgitation and markedly reduced left ventricular function. Circulation 106:2687, 2002.
254. Devlin WH, Petrusha J, Briesmiester K, et al: Impact of vascular adaptation to chronic aortic regurgitation on left ventricular performance. Circulation 99:1027, 1999.
255. Odell JA, Orszulak TA: Surgical repair and reconstruction of valvular lesions. Curr Opin Cardiol 10:135, 1995.
256. Burkhart HM, Zehr KJ, Schaff HV, et al: Valve-preserving aortic root reconstruction: A comparison of techniques. J Heart Valve Dis 12:62, 2003.
257. David TE: Aortic valve repair in patients with Marfan syndrome and ascending aorta aneurysms due to degenerative disease. J Cardiovasc Surg 9(Suppl):182, 1994.
258. Leyh RG, Schmidtke C, Sievers HH, et al: Opening and closing characteristics of the aortic valve after different types of valve-preserving surgery. Circulation 100:2153, 1999.
259. Alpert JS: Acute aortic insufficiency. *In* Alpert JS, Dalen JE, Rahimtoola SH (eds): Valvular Heart Disease. 3rd ed. Philadelphia, Lippincott Williams & Wilkins, 2000, pp 269-289.
260. Eusebio J, Louie EK, Edwards DC, et al: Alterations in transmitral flow dynamics in patients with early mitral valve closure and aortic regurgitation. Am. Heart J 128:941, 1994.

Tricuspid, Pulmonic, and Multivalvular Disease

261. Ewy GA: Tricuspid valve disease. *In* Alpert JS, Dalen JE, Rahimtoola SH (eds): Valvular Heart Disease. 3rd ed. Philadelphia, Lippincott Williams & Wilkins, 2000, pp 377-392.
262. Ananthasubramaniam K, Farha A: Primary right atrial angiosarcoma mimicking acute pericarditis, pulmonary embolism, and tricuspid stenosis. Heart 81:556, 1999.
263. Møller JE, Connolly HM, Rubin J, et al: Factors associated with progression of carcinoid heart disease. N Engl J Med 348:1005, 2003.
264. Hagers Y, Koole M, Schoors D, Van Camp G: Tricuspid stenosis: A rare complication of pacemaker-related endocarditis. J Am Soc Echocardiogr 13:66, 2000.
265. Heaven DJ, Henein MY, Sutton R: Pacemaker lead related to tricuspid stenosis: A report of two cases. Heart 83:351, 2000.
266. Otto CM: Right-sided valve disease. *In* Otto CM (ed): Valvular Heart Disease. 2nd ed. Philadelphia, WB Saunders, 2004, pp 415-436.

267. Ha JW, Chung N, Jang Y, Rim SJ: Tricuspid stenosis and regurgitation: Doppler and color-flow echocardiography and cardiac catheterization findings. Clin Cardiol 23:51, 2000.
268. Del Campo C, Sherman JR: Tricuspid valve replacement: Results comparing mechanical and biological prostheses. Ann Thorac Surg 69:1295, 2000.
269. Bahl VK, Chandra S, Mishra S: Concurrent balloon dilatation of mitral and tricuspid stenosis during pregnancy using an Inoue balloon. Int J Cardiol 59:199, 1997.
270. Prieto LR, Hordof AJ, Secic M, et al: Progressive tricuspid valve disease in patients with congenitally corrected transposition of the great arteries. Circulation 98:997, 1998.
271. Kulke MH, Mayer RJ: Carcinoid tumors. N Engl J Med 858, 1999.
272. Simula DV, Edwards WD, Tazelaar HD, et al: Surgical pathology of carcinoid heart disease: A study of 139 valves from 75 patients spanning 20 years. Mayo Clin Proc 77:139, 2002.
273. Paniagua D, Aldrich HR, Lieberman EH, et al: Increased prevalence of significant tricuspid regurgitation in patients with transvenous pacemaker leads. Am J Cardiol 82:1130, 1998.
274. Reynertson MD, Kundur R, Mullen GM, et al: Asymmetry of right ventricular enlargement in response to tricuspid regurgitation. Circulation 100:465, 1999.
275. Jick H, Vasilakis C, Weinrauch LA, et al: A population-based study of appetite suppressant drugs and the risk of cardiac valve regurgitation. N Engl J Med 339:719, 1998.
276. Naschitz JE, Goldstein L, Zuckerman E, et al: Benign course of congestive cirrhosis associated with tricuspid regurgitation: Does pulsatility protect against complications of venous hypertension? J Clin Gastroenterol 30:213, 2000.
277. Kemp WE Jr, Kerins DM, Shyr Y, Byrd BF III: Optimal Albunex dosing for enhancement of Doppler tricuspid regurgitation spectra. Am J Cardiol 79:232, 1997.
278. Grossmann G, Giesler M, Stein M, et al: Quantification of mitral and tricuspid regurgitation by the proximal flow convergence method using two-dimensional colour Doppler and colour Doppler M-mode: Influence of the mechanism of regurgitation. Int J Cardiol 66:299, 1998.
279. Tribouilloy CM, Enriquez-Sarano M, Bailey KR, et al: Quantification of tricuspid regurgitation by measuring the width of the vena contracta with Doppler color-flow imaging: A clinical study. J Am Coll Cardiol 36:472, 2000.
280. Pitts WR, Lange RA, Cigarroa JE, Hillis LD: Predictive value of prominent right atrial v waves in assessing the presence and severity of tricuspid regurgitation. Am J Cardiol 83:617, 1999.
281. Sugimoto T, Okada M, Ozaki N, et al: Long-term evaluation of treatment for functional tricuspid regurgitation with regurgitant volume: Characteristic differences based on primary cardiac lesion. J Thorac Cardiovasc Surg 117:463, 1999.
282. Bajzer CT, Stewart WJ, Cosgrove DM, et al: Tricuspid valve surgery and intraoperative echocardiography: Factors affecting survival, clinical outcome, and echocardiographic success. J Am Coll Cardiol 32:1023, 1998.
283. Jamieson WRE, Edwards FH, Schwartz M, et al: Risk stratification for cardiac valve replacement. National Cardiac Surgery Database. Ann Thorac Surg 67:943, 1999.
284. Discigil B, Dearani JA, Puga FJ, et al: Late pulmonary valve replacement after repair of tetralogy of Fallot. J Thorac Cardiovasc Surg 121:344, 2001.
285. Helbing WA, de Roos A: Optimal imaging in assessment of right ventricular function in tetralogy of Fallot with pulmonary regurgitation. Am J Cardiol 82:1561, 1998.
286. Balaguer JM, Byrne JG, Cohn LH: Orthotopic pulmonic valve replacement with a pulmonary homograft as an interposition graft. J Card Surg 11:417, 1996.
287. Conte S, Jashari R, Eyskens B, et al: Homograft valve insertion for pulmonary regurgitation late after valveless repair of right ventricular outflow tract obstruction. Eur J Cardiothorac Surg 15:143, 1999.
288. Connolly HM, Schaff HV, Mullany CJ, et al: Carcinoid heart disease: Impact of pulmonary valve replacement in right ventricular function and remodeling. Circulation 106:I-51, 2002.
289. Paraskos JA: Combined valve disease. *In* Alpert JS, Dalen JE, Rahimtoola SH (eds): Valvular Heart Disease. 3rd ed. Philadelphia, Lippincott Williams & Wilkins, 2000, pp 291-337.
290. Gillinov AM, Blackstone EH, Cosgrove DM, et al: Mitral valve repair with aortic valve replacement in superior to double valve replacement. J Thorac Cardiovasc Surg 125:1372, 2003.
291. John S, Ravikumar E, John CN, Bashi VV: 25-year experience with 456 combined mitral and aortic valve replacement for rheumatic heart disease. Ann Thorac Surg 69:1167, 2000.
292. Turina J, Stark T, Seifert B, et al: Predictors of the long-term outcome after combined aortic and mitral valve surgery. Circulation 100:II-48, 1999.

Prosthetic Cardiac Valves

293. Braunwald NS, Cooper TS, Morrow AG: Complete replacement of the mitral valve. J Thorac Cardiovasc Surg 40:1, 1960.
294. Harken DE, Soroff MS, Taylor MC: Partial and complete prostheses in aortic insufficiency. J Thorac Cardiovasc Surg 40:744, 1960.
295. Starr A, Edwards ML: Mitral replacement: Clinical experience with a ball-valve prosthesis. Ann Surg 154:726, 1961.
296. Grunkemeier GL, Rahimtoola SH, Starr A: Prosthetic heart valves. *In* Rahimtoola SH (ed): Valvular Heart Disease. Atlas of Heart Diseases. Vol. 11. Braunwald E (series ed). Philadelphia, Mosby, 1997, pp 13.1-13.27.
297. Grunkemeier GL, Li HH, Naftel DC, et al: Long-term performance of heart valve prostheses. Curr Probl Cardiol 25:73, 2000.
298. Rahimtoola SH: Choice of prosthetic heart valve for adult patients. J Am Coll Cardiol 41:893, 2003.
299. Murday AJ, Hochstitzky A, Mansfield J, et al: A prospective controlled trial of St. Jude versus Starr Edwards aortic and mitral valve prostheses. Ann Thorac Surg 76:66, 2003.
300. Emery RW, Erickson CA, Arom KV, et al: Replacement of the aortic valve in patients under 50 years of age: Long-term follow up of the St. Jude medical prosthesis. Ann Thorac Surg 75:1815, 2003.
301. Jamieson WR, Fradet GJ, Miyagishima RT, et al: CarboMedics mechanical prosthesis: Performance at eight years. J Heart Valve Dis 9:678, 2000.
302. Hammermeister KE, Sethi GK, Henderson WG, et al: Outcomes 15 years after valve replacement with a mechanical versus a bioprosthetic valve: Final report of the Veterans Affairs randomized trial. J Am Coll Cardiol 36:1152, 2000.
303. Cannegieter SC, Rosendaal FR, Wintzen AR, et al: Optimal oral anticoagulant therapy in patients with mechanical heart valves. N Engl J Med 333:11, 1995.
304. Acar J, Iung B, Boissel JP, et al: AREVA, multicenter randomized comparison of low-dose versus standard-dose anticoagulation in patients with mechanical prosthetic heart valves. Circulation 94:2107, 1996.
305. Meschengieser SS, Fondevila CG, Frontroth J, et al: Low-intensity oral anticoagulation plus low-dose aspirin versus high-intensity oral anticoagulation alone: A randomized trial in patients with mechanical prosthetic heart valves. J Thorac Cardiovasc Surg 113:910, 1997.
306. Laffort P, Roudaut R, Roques X, et al: Early and long-term (one-year) effects of the association of aspirin and oral anticoagulant on thrombi and morbidity after replacement of the mitral valve with the St. Jude medical prosthesis: A clinical and transesophageal echocardiographic study. J Am Coll Cardiol 35:739, 2000.
307. Massel D, Little SH: Risks and benefits of adding anti-platelet therapy to warfarin among patients with prosthetic heart valves: A meta-analysis. J Am Coll Cardiol 37:569, 2001.
308. Lengyel M, Fuster V, Keltai M, et al: Guidelines for management of left-sided prosthetic valve thrombosis: A role for thrombolytic therapy. Consensus Conference on Prosthetic Valve Thrombosis. J Am Coll Cardiol 30:1521, 1997.
309. Schoen FJ, Levy RJ: Tissue heart valves: Current challenges and future research perspectives. J Biomed Mater Res 47:439, 1999.
310. Cohn LH, Collins JJ Jr, Rizzo RJ, et al: Twenty-year follow-up of the Hancock modified orifice porcine aortic valve. Ann Thorac Surg 66:S30, 1998.
311. Jamieson WR, Burr LH, Miyagishima RT, et al: Actuarial versus actual freedom from structural valve deterioration with the Carpentier-Edwards porcine bioprosthesis. Can J Cardiol 15:973, 1999.
312. Jamieson WRE, Lemieux MD, Sullivan JA, et al: Medtronic intact porcine bioprosthesis experience to twelve years. Ann Thorac Surg 71:S278, 2001.
313. Jamieson WR, David TE, Feindel CM, et al: Performance of the Carpentier-Edwards SAV and Hancock-II porcine bioprostheses in aortic valve replacement. J Heart Valve Dis 11:424, 2002.
314. Nollert G, Miksch J, Kreuzer E, et al: Risk factors for atherosclerosis and the degeneration of pericardial valves after aortic valve replacement. J Thorac Cardiovasc Surg 126:965, 2003.
315. Farivar RS, Cohn LS: Hypercholesterolemia is a risk factor for bioprosthetic valve calcification and explantation. J Thorac Cardiovasc Surg 126:969, 2003.
316. Westaby S, Jin XY, Katsumata T, Arifi A: Valve replacement with a stentless bioprosthesis: Versatility of the porcine aortic root. J Thorac Cardiovasc Surg 116:477, 1998.
317. Hvass U, Palatianos GM, Frassani R, et al: Multicenter study of stentless valve replacement in the small aortic root. J Thorac Cardiovasc Surg 117:267, 1999.
318. Yun KL, Sintek CF, Fletcher AD, et al: Aortic valve replacement with the Freestyle stentless prosthesis: Five year experience. Circulation 100:II-17,1999.
319. Dellgren G, Feindel CM, Bos J, et al: Aortic valve replacement with the Toronto SPV: Long-term clinical and hemodynamic results. Eur J Cardiothorac Surg 21:698, 2002.
320. Dossche K, Vanerman H, Daernen W, et al: Edwards stentless aortic valve xenograft: Early results of a multicenter clinical trial. Thorac Cardiovasc Surgeon 44:11, 1996.
321. Walther T, Falk V, Langebartels G, et al: Prospective randomized evaluation of stentless versus conventional biological aortic valves: Impact on early regression of left ventricular hypertrophy. Circulation 100:II-6, 1999.
322: Collinson J, Henein M, Flather M, et al: Valve replacement for aortic stenosis in patients with poor left ventricular function: Comparison of early changes with stented and stentless valves. Circulation 100:II-1, 1999.
323. Pibarot P, Dumesnil JG, Jobin J et al: Hemodynamic and physical performance during maximal exercise in patients with an aortic bioprosthetic valve: Comparison of stentless versus unstented bioprostheses. J Am Coll Cardiol 34:1609, 1999.
324. Le Tourneau T, Savoye C, McFadden EP, et al : Mid-term comparative follow-up after aortic valve replacement with Carpentier-Edwards and Pericarbon pericardial prostheses. Circulation 100:II-11, 1999.
325. Banbury MK, Cosgrove DM, Thomas JD, et al: Hemodynamic stability during 17 years of the Carpentier-Edwards aortic pericardial bioprosthesis. Ann Thorac Surg 73:1460, 2002.
326. Banbury MK, Cosgrove DM, White JA, et al: Age and valve size effect on the long-term durability of the Carpentier-Edwards aortic pericardial bioprosthesis. Ann Thorac Surg 72:753, 2001.
327. Aupart MR, Neville PH, Hammami S, et al: Carpentier-Edwards pericardial valves in the mitral position: Ten-year follow-up. J Thorac Cardiovasc Surg 113:492, 1997.
328. Eriksson MA, Kallner G, Rosfors S, et al: Hemodynamic performance of cryopreserved aortic homograft valves during midterm follow-up. J Am Coll Cardiol 32:1002, 1998.
329. Lund O, Chandrasekaran V, Grocott-Mason R, et al: Primary aortic valve replacement with allografts over twenty-five years: Valve-related and procedure-related determinants of outcome. J Thorac Cardiovasc Surg 117:77, 1999.
330. Willems TP, Takkenberg JJM, Sterberg WE, et al: Human tissue valves in the aortic position: Determinants of reoperation and valve regurgitation. Circulation 103:1515, 2001.
331. Palka P, Harrocks S, Lange A, et al: Primary aortic valve replacement with cryopreserved aortic allograft: An echocardiographic follow-up study of 570 patients. Circulation 105:61, 2002.
332. Frater RWM, Furlong P, Cosgrove CM, et al: Long-term durability and patient functional status of the Carpentier-Edwards Perimount Pericardial Bioprosthesis in the aortic position. J Heart Valve Dis 7:48, 1998.
333. Chambers JC, Somerville J, Stone S, Ross DN: Pulmonary autograft procedure for aortic valve disease: Long-term results of the pioneer series. Circulation 96:2206, 1997.
334. Santini F, Dyke C, Edwards S, et al: Pulmonary autograft versus homograft replacement of the aortic valve: A prospective randomized trial. J Thorac Cardiovasc Surg 113:894, 1997.

335. Elkins RC, Knott-Craig CJ, Ward KE, Lane MM: The Ross operation in children: 10-year experience. Ann Thorac Surg 65:496, 1998.
336. Carr-White GS, Kilner PJ, Hon JK, et al: Incidence, location, pathology, and significance of pulmonary homograft stenosis after the Ross operation. Circulation 104:I-16, 2001.
337. Laforest I, Dumesnil JG, Briand M, et al: Hemodynamic performance at rest and during exercise after aortic replacement: Comparison of pulmonary autografts versus aortic homografts. Circulation 106:I-57, 2002.
338. Carr-White GS, Afoke A, Birks EJ, et al: Aortic root characteristics of human pulmonary autografts. Circulation 102:III-15, 2000.
339. Luciani GB, Casali G, Favaro A, et al: Fate of the aortic root late after Ross operation. Circulation 108:II-61, 2003.
340. Schmidtke C, Bechtel JF, Noetzold A, et al: Up to seven years of experience with the Ross procedure in patients >60 years of age. J Am Coll Cardiol 36:117, 2000.
341. Rahimtoola SH: Valve prosthesis-patient mismatch: An update. J Heart Valve Dis 7:207, 1998.
342. Yun KL, Jamieson WR, Vurr LH, et al. Prosthesis-patient mismatch: Hemodynamic comparison of stented and stentless valves. Semin Thorac Cardiovasc Surg 11:98, 1999.
343. Rao V, Jamieson WR, Ivanov J, et al: Prosthesis-patient mismatch affects survival after aortic valve replacement. Circulation 102(Suppl III):III-5, 2000.
344. Blackstone EH, Cosgrove DM, Jamieson WR, et al: Prosthesis size and long-term survival after aortic valve replacement. J Thorac Cardiovasc Surg 126:783, 2003.
344a. Blais C, Dumensil JG, Baillot R, et al: Impact of valve prosthesis-patient mismatch on short-term mortality after aortic value replacement. Circulation 108:983, 2003.
344b. Pibarot P, Dumensil JG: Hemodynamic and clinical impact of prosthesis-patient mismatch in the aortic position and its prevention. J Am Coll Cardiol 36:1131, 2000.
345. Oxenham H, Bloomfield P, Wheatley DJ, et al: Twenty-year comparison of a Björk-Shiley mechanical heart valve with porcine bioprostheses. Heart 89:715, 2003.
346. Peterseim DS, Cen YY, Cheruvu S, et al: Long-term outcome after biologic versus mechanical aortic valve replacement in 841 patients. J Thorac Cardiovasc Surg 117:890, 1999.
347. Cohen G, David TE, Ivanov J, et al: The impact of age, coronary artery disease, and cardiac comorbidity on late survival after bioprosthetic aortic valve replacement. J Thorac Cardiovasc Surg 117:273, 1999.
348. Hung L, Rahimtoola SH: Prosthetic heart valves and pregnancy. Circulation 107:1240, 2003.
349. Vitale N, De Feo M, De Santo LS, et al: Dose-dependent fetal complications of warfarin in pregnant women with mechanical heart valves. J Am Coll Cardiol 33:1637, 1999.
350. Elkayam U: Pregnancy through a prosthetic heart valve. J Am Coll Cardiol 33:1642, 1999.
351. Hirsh J, Fuster V, Ansell J, et al: American Heart Association/American College of Cardiology Foundation guide to warfarin therapy. Circulation 107:1692, 2003.
352. Lucke JC, Samy RN, Atkins BZ, et al: Results of valve replacement with mechanical valves and biological prostheses in chronic renal dialysis patients. Ann Thorac Surg 64:129, 1997.
353. Herzog CA, Ma JZ, Collins AJ: Long-term survival of dialysis patients in the United States with prosthetic heart valves: Should ACC/AHA practice guidelines on valve selection be modified? Circulation105:1336, 2002.

GUIDELINES *Thomas H. Lee*

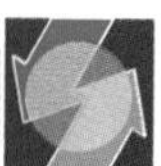

Management of Valvular Heart Disease

The American College of Cardiology and the American Heart Association (ACC/AHA) published guidelines for management of patients with valvular heart disease in 1998.[1] Other recommendations for these conditions were included in ACC/AHA guidelines for use of echocardiography,[2] ACC guidelines for assessment of athletes with cardiovascular abnormalities,[3] and AHA guidelines on cardiovascular assessment of master athletes.[4] As is the case for other ACC/AHA guidelines, the indications for various tests and procedures are divided into the following classes.

Class I: conditions for which there is evidence and/or general agreement that a given procedure or treatment is useful and effective

Class II: conditions for which there is conflicting evidence and/or a divergence of opinion about the usefulness/efficacy of a procedure or treatment

Class IIa: weight of evidence/opinion is in favor of usefulness/efficacy

Class IIb: usefulness/efficacy is less well established by evidence/opinion

Class III: conditions for which there is evidence and/or general agreement that the procedure/treatment is not useful/effective, and in some cases may be harmful

Some material from these guidelines is presented elsewhere in this book. Guidelines for prevention and treatment of infective endocarditis are summarized in the appendix to Chapter 58. Guidelines for management of anticoagulation in pregnancy are included in the appendix to Chapter 74.

The guidelines emphasize that the clinical assessment should be based on the patient's symptomatic status and findings from the physical examination. The chest radiograph and electrocardiogram (ECG), if normal, can often provide reassurance that a murmur is clinically insignificant. Echocardiography should be considered after assessment of these more routine data, and the guidelines consider echocardiography to be inappropriate (Class III) for evaluation of murmurs that experienced observers consider innocent or functional. In contrast, echocardiography was considered appropriate even in asymptomatic patients with murmurs suggesting significant valvular disease or with other signs or symptoms of cardiovascular disease (Table 57G–1).

TABLE 57G–1 ACC/AHA Guidelines for Echocardiography of Valvular Heart Disease in Adults

Indication	Class I	Class IIa	Class IIb	Class III
Echocardiography in asymptomatic patients with cardiac murmurs	1. Diastolic or continuous murmurs 2. Holosystolic or late systolic murmurs 3. Grade 3 or greater midsystolic murmurs	1. Murmurs associated with abnormal physical findings on cardiac palpation or auscultation 2. Murmurs associated with an abnormal ECG or chest radiograph		1. Grade 2 or softer midsystolic murmur identified as innocent or functional by an experienced observer 2. To detect "silent" aortic regurgitation or mitral regurgitation in patients without cardiac murmurs, then recommend endocarditis prophylaxis
Echocardiography in symptomatic patients with cardiac murmurs	1. Symptoms or signs of congestive heart failure, myocardial ischemia, or syncope 2. Symptoms or signs consistent with infective endocarditis or thromboembolism	Symptoms or signs likely due to noncardiac disease with cardiac disease not excluded by standard cardiovascular evaluation		Symptoms or signs of noncardiac disease with an isolated midsystolic "innocent" murmur

ACC = American College of Cardiology; AHA = American Heart Association; ECG = electrocardiogram.

Transthoracic echocardiography is endorsed in the ACC/AHA guidelines as the first-line test for diagnosis and follow-up of patients with mitral stenosis; transesophageal echocardiography was considered to have a potential role (Class IIa) for detection of left atrial thrombus in patients being considered for percutaneous mitral balloon valvotomy or cardioversion (Table 57G–2).

Anticoagulation was recommended for patients with mitral stenosis if they had a history of atrial fibrillation or a prior embolic event, but the guidelines were not strongly supportive of anticoagulation on the basis of left atrial dimension greater than 55 mm alone. Surgical therapy with valvotomy, valve repair, or valve replacement is indicated for patients with moderate or severe mitral stenosis (valve area < 1.5 cm^2) and New York Heart Association (NYHA) functional Class III or IV, with the choice of the procedure dictated by the anatomy. Balloon valvotomy was also endorsed for patients who were NYHA Class II. For patients with mild or no symptoms of mitral stenosis, balloon valvotomy was considered reasonably appropriate (Class IIa) in the presence of pulmonary hypertension in the absence of left atrial thrombus or moderate to severe mitral regurgitation.

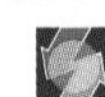

TABLE 57G–2 ACC/AHA Guidelines for Management of Patients with Mitral Stenosis

Indication	Class I	Class IIa	Class IIb	Class III
Echocardiography in mitral stenosis	1. Diagnosis of MS, assessment of hemodynamic severity (mean gradient, mitral valve area, pulmonary artery pressure), and assessment of right ventricular size and function 2. Assessment of valve morphology to determine suitability for percutaneous mitral balloon valvotomy 3. Diagnosis and assessment of concomitant valvular lesions 4. Reevaluation of patients with known MS with changing symptoms or signs	1. Assessment of hemodynamic response of mean gradient and pulmonary artery pressures by exercise Doppler echocardiography in patients when there is a discrepancy between resting hemodynamics and clinical findings	1. Reevaluation of asymptomatic patients with moderate to severe MS to assess pulmonary artery pressure	1. Routine reevaluation of the asymptomatic patient with mild MS and stable clinical findings
Transesophageal echocardiography in mitral stenosis		1. Assess for presence or absence of left atrial thrombus in patients being considered for percutaneous mitral balloon valvotomy or cardioversion 2. Evaluate mitral valve morphology and hemodynamics when transthoracic echocardiography provides suboptimal data		1. Routine evaluation of mitral valve morphology and hemodynamics when complete transthoracic echocardiographic data are satisfactory
Anticoagulation in mitral stenosis	1. Patients with atrial fibrillation, paroxysmal or chronic 2. Patients with a prior embolic event		1. Patients with severe MS and left atrial dimension ≥ 55 mm by echocardiography	All other patients with MS
Cardiac catheterization in mitral stenosis	Perform percutaneous mitral balloon valvotomy in properly selected patients	1. Assess severity of MR in patients being considered for percutaneous mitral balloon valvotomy when clinical and echocardiographic data are discordant 2. Assess pulmonary artery, left atrial, and left ventricular diastolic pressure when symptoms and/or estimated pulmonary artery pressure are discordant with the severity of MS by 2D and Doppler echocardiography 3. Assess hemodynamic response of pulmonary artery and left atrial pressures to stress when		1. Assess mitral valve hemodynamics when 2D and Doppler echocardiographic data are concordant with clinical findings

TABLE 57G–2 ACC/AHA Guidelines for Management of Patients with Mitral Stenosis—cont'd				
Indication	**Class I**	**Class IIa**	**Class IIb**	**Class III**
		clinical symptoms and resting hemodynamics are discordant		
Percutaneous mitral balloon valvotomy	1. Symptomatic patients (NYHA Classes II-IV), moderate or severe MS (mitral valve area ≤ 1.5 cm^2) and valve morphology favorable for percutaneous balloon valvotomy in the absence of left atrial thrombus or moderate to severe MR	1. Asymptomatic patients with moderate or severe MS (mitral valve area < 21.5 cm^2) and valve morphology favorable for percutaneous balloon valvotomy who have pulmonary hypertension (pulmonary artery systolic pressure > 50 mm Hg at rest or 60 mm Hg with exercise) in the absence of left atrial thrombus or moderate to severe MR 2. Patients with NYHA Class III or IV symptoms, moderate or severe MS (mitral valve area < 1.5 cm^2), and a nonpliable calcified valve who are at high risk for surgery in the absence of left atrial thrombus or moderate to severe MR	1. Asymptomatic patients, moderate or severe MS (mitral valve area < 21.5 cm^2) and valve morphology favorable for percutaneous balloon valvotomy who have new onset of atrial fibrillation in the absence of left atrial thrombus or moderate to severe MR 2. Patients in NYHA Class III or IV, moderate or severe MS (mitral valve area ≤ 1.5 cm^2), and a nonpliable calcified valve who are low-risk candidates for surgery	Patients with mild MS
Mitral valve repair for MS	1. Patients with NYHA Class III or IV symptoms, moderate or severe MS (mitral valve area ≤ 1.5 cm^2), and valve morphology favorable for repair if percutaneous mitral balloon valvotomy is not available 2. Patients with NYHA Class III or IV symptoms, moderate or severe MS (mitral valve area ≤ 1.5 cm^2), and valve morphology favorable for repair if a left atrial thrombus is present despite anticoagulation 3. Patients with NYHA Class III or IV symptoms, moderate or severe MS (mitral valve area ≤ 1.5 cm^2), and a nonpliable or calcified valve with the decision to proceed with either repair or replacement made at the time of the operation		1. Patients in NYHA Class I, moderate or severe MS (mitral valve area ≤ 1.5 cm^2), and valve morphology favorable for repair who have had recurrent episodes of embolic events on adequate anticoagulation	1. Patients with NYHA Classes I–IV symptoms and mild MS
Mitral valve replacement for mitral stenosis	1. Patients with moderate or severe MS (mitral valve area ≤ 1.5 cm^2) and NYHA Class III or IV symptoms who are not considered candidates for percutaneous balloon valvotomy or mitral valve repair	1. Patients with severe MS (mitral valve area ≤ 1 cm^2) and severe pulmonary hypertension (pulmonary artery systolic pressure > 60–80 mm Hg) with NYHA Class I or II symptoms who are not considered candidates for percutaneous balloon valvotomy or mitral valve repair		

ACC = American College of Cardiology; AHA = American Heart Association; MS = mitral stenosis; 2D = two-dimensional; NYHA = New York Association; MR = mitral regurgitation.

The ACC/AHA guidelines consider echocardiography appropriate for diagnosis of acute or chronic mitral regurgitation, as well as annual or semiannual surveillance of left ventricular function in patients with severe mitral regurgitation even if asymptomatic (Table 57G–3). Serial use of chest radiographs and ECGs are considered to be of less value. In asymptomatic patients with mild mitral regurgitation and no evidence of left ventricular dysfunction, the guidelines recommend yearly evaluations to detect worsening symptomatic status but do not support annual echocardiography. Transesophageal echocardiography is considered most appropriate for intraoperative guidance and when transthoracic studies are inadequate.

Cardiac catheterization is usually performed as a prelude to surgery in patients with mitral regurgitation. Coronary angiography is not considered routinely necessary in the ACC/AHA guidelines in patients younger than 35 years of age if there is no clinical suspicion of coronary artery disease. Left ventriculography and hemodynamic assessment are appropriate only when noninvasive studies do not provide adequate information to guide management.

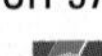

TABLE 57G–3 ACC/AHA Guidelines for Management of Patients with Mitral Regurgitation

Indication	Class I	Class IIa	Class IIb	Class III
Transthoracic echocardiography in mitral regurgitation	1. For baseline evaluation to quantify severity of MR and LV function in any patient suspected of having MR 2. For delineation of mechanism of MR 3. For annual or semiannual surveillance of LV function (estimated by ejection fraction and end-systolic dimension) in asymptomatic severe MR 4. To establish cardiac status after a change in symptoms 5. For evaluation after MVR or mitral valve repair to establish baseline status			1. Routine follow-up evaluation of mild MR with normal LV size and systolic function
Transesophageal echocardiography in mitral regurgitation	1. Intraoperative transesophageal echocardiography to establish anatomical basis for MR and to guide repair 2. For evaluation of MR patients in whom transthoracic echocardiography provides nondiagnostic images regarding severity of MR, mechanism of MR, and/or status of LV function			1. In routine follow-up or surveillance of patients with native valve MR
Coronary angiography in mitral regurgitation	1. When mitral valve surgery is contemplated in patients with angina or previous myocardial infarction 2. When mitral valve surgery is contemplated in patients with ≥1 risk factor for CAD 3. When ischemia is suspected as an etiological factor in MR		1. To confirm noninvasive tests in patients not suspected of having CAD	1. When mitral valve surgery is contemplated in patients aged <35 years and there is no clinical suspicion of CAD
Left ventriculography and hemodynamic measurements in mitral regurgitation	1. When noninvasive tests are inconclusive regarding severity of MR, LV function, or the need for surgery 2. When there is a discrepancy between clinical and noninvasive findings regarding severity of MR			1. In patients in whom valve surgery is not contemplated

TABLE 57G–3 ACC/AHA Guidelines for Management of Patients with Mitral Regurgitation—cont'd

Indication	Class I	Class IIa	Class IIb	Class III
Mitral valve surgery in nonischemic severe mitral regurgitation	1. Acute symptomatic MR in which repair is likely 2. Patients with NYHA Class II, III, or IV symptoms with normal LV function defined as ejection fraction > 0.60 and end-systolic dimension < 45 mm 3. Symptomatic or asymptomatic patients with mild LV dysfunction, ejection fraction 0.50–0.60, and end-systolic dimension 45–50 mm 4. Symptomatic or asymptomatic patients with moderate LV dysfunction, ejection fraction 0.30–0.50, and/or end-systolic dimension 50–55 mm	1. Asymptomatic patients with preserved LV function and atrial fibrillation 2. Asymptomatic patients with preserved LV function and pulmonary hypertension (pulmonary artery systolic pressure > 50 mm Hg at rest or > 60 mm Hg with exercise) 3. Asymptomatic patients with ejection fraction 0.50–0.60 and end-systolic dimension < 45 mm and asymptomatic patients with ejection fraction > 0.60 and end-systolic dimension 45–55 mm 4. Patients with severe LV dysfunction (ejection fraction < 0.30 and/or end-systolic dimension > 55 mm) in whom chordal preservation is highly likely	1. Asymptomatic patients with chronic MR with preserved LV function in whom mitral valve repair is highly likely 2. Patients with mitral valve prolapse and preserved LV function who have recurrent ventricular arrhythmias despite medical therapy	1. Asymptomatic patients with preserved LV function in whom significant doubt about the feasibility of repair exists

ACC = American College of Cardiology; AHA = American Heart Association; MR = mitral regurgitation; LV = left ventricular; MVR = mitral valve replacement; CAD = coronary artery disease; NYHA = New York Heart Association.

Surgery is considered appropriate for acute symptomatic mitral regurgitation and for patients with chronic severe mitral regurgitation and symptoms of congestive heart failure, even if they have normal left ventricular function. Even if patients are asymptomatic, surgery is appropriate when patients have mild or worse left ventricular dysfunction (ejection fraction 0.50 to 0.60 and/or end-systolic dimension 50 to 55 mm).

Mitral Valve Prolapse

Recommendations on use of echocardiography for patients with mitral valve prolapse were presented in ACC/AHA guidelines on echocardiography (Table 57G–4).[2] These guidelines emphasize that the diagnosis of mitral valve prolapse should be made by physical examination; echocardiography should be used primarily for evaluation of mitral regurgitation and ventricular compensation. Echocardiography is also considered appropriate for *excluding* the diagnosis of mitral valve prolapse in patients who have been given the diagnosis inappropriately. Serial use of echocardiography in stable patients with mild or no regurgitation is discouraged.

In general, asymptomatic athletes with mitral valve prolapse need not have any restrictions, but 2001 AHA guidelines recommended restriction of patients to low-intensity competitive sports (such as golf and bowling) if any of the following are present: (1) history of syncope, judged probably arrhythmogenic in origin; (2) family history of sudden death due to mitral valve prolapse; (3) repetitive supraventricular or complex ventricular tachyarrhythmias, particularly if exacerbated by exercise; (4) moderate to severe mitral regurgitation; and (5) prior embolic event.[4]

Antibiotic prophylaxis is considered appropriate for patients with the characteristic click-murmur complex or with echocardiographic evidence of mitral prolapse with regurgitation. Daily aspirin therapy is recommended for patients who have had cerebral transient ischemic attacks and for patients younger than 65 years of age who have atrial fibrillation without other complicating factors. Warfarin therapy is recommended for poststroke patients and older patients with atrial fibrillation accompanied by hypertension, mitral regurgitation, or a history of heart failure.

Aortic Stenosis

Doppler echocardiography is a highly appropriate test for diagnosis and assessment of aortic stenosis and for evaluation of left ventricular function in patients with this condition. The guidelines commented that yearly echocardiograms may be helpful for management of asymptomatic patients with severe aortic stenosis, but recommended intervals of 2 and 5 years for asymptomatic patients with moderate and mild aortic stenosis, respectively.

The ACC/AHA guidelines indicated that exercise testing of asymptomatic patients could be performed safely and provide useful information but emphasized the need for supervision by an experienced physician with close monitoring of blood pressure and the ECG. The Task Force on Acquired Valvular Heart Disease of the 26th Bethesda Conference recommended that competitive athletes with severe aortic stenosis be advised to limit activity to relatively low levels.[3]

The guidelines discourage catheterization solely for the purposes of confirming information available from noninvasive tests (Table 57G–5). Coronary angiography is considered appropriate in the ACC/AHA guidelines for patients with possible coronary artery disease and may be needed to assess the severity of stenosis in symptomatic patients when other data are not conclusive.

TABLE 57G–4 ACC/AHA Guidelines for Management of Patients with Mitral Valve Prolapse

Indication	Class I	Class IIa	Class IIb	Class III
Echocardiography in MVP	1. Diagnosis, assessment of hemodynamic severity of MR, leaflet morphology, and ventricular compensation in patients with physical signs of MVP 2. To exclude MVP in patients who have been given the diagnosis when there is no clinical evidence to support the diagnosis	1. To exclude MVP in patients with first-degree relatives with known myxomatous valve disease 2. Risk stratification in patients with physical signs of MVP or known MVP		1. To exclude MVP in patients in the absence of physical findings suggestive of MVP or a positive family history 2. Routine repetition of echocardiography in patients with MVP with mild or no regurgitation and no changes in clinical signs or symptoms
Antibiotic endocarditis prophylaxis for patients with MVP undergoing procedures associated with bacteremia	1. Patients with characteristic systolic click-murmur complex 2. Patients with isolated systolic click and echocardiographic evidence of MVP and MR	1. Patients with isolated systolic click, echocardiographic evidence of high-risk MVP		1. Patients with isolated systolic click and equivocal or no evidence of MVP
Aspirin and oral anticoagulants in MVP	1. Aspirin therapy for cerebral transient ischemic attacks 2. Warfarin therapy for patients aged ≥ 65 years, in atrial fibrillation with hypertension, MR murmur, or history of heart failure 3. Aspirin therapy for patients aged < 65 years in atrial fibrillation with no history of MR, hypertension, or heart failure 4. Warfarin therapy for poststroke patients	1. Warfarin therapy for transient ischemic attacks despite aspirin therapy 2. Aspirin therapy for poststroke patients with contraindications to anticoagulants	1. Aspirin therapy for patients in sinus rhythm with echocardiographic evidence of high-risk MVP	

ACC = American College of Cardiology; AHA = American Heart Association; MVP = mitral valve prolapse; MR = mitral regurgitation.

Aortic valve replacement is considered indicated in virtually all symptomatic patients with severe aortic stenosis, and the ACC/AHA guidelines were generally supportive (Class IIa) of this procedure for patients who were asymptomatic despite severe aortic stenosis but had evidence of left ventricular systolic dysfunction or exertional hypotension. However, valve replacement for asymptomatic patients was otherwise discouraged. Aortic balloon valvotomy was given qualified support only as a "bridge" to surgery in hemodynamically unstable patients who could not undergo immediate aortic valve replacement.

Aortic Regurgitation

Doppler echocardiography is a highly appropriate test for diagnosis and serial assessment of patients with aortic regurgitation (Table 57G–6). For new patients in whom the chronic nature of the lesion is uncertain, the guidelines support repeating the physical examination and echocardiogram 2 to 3 months after the initial evaluation to ensure that rapid progression is not underway. Asymptomatic patients with mild aortic regurgitation, normal left ventricular function, and little or no left ventricular dilation can be seen on an annual basis, and echocardiography can be performed every 2 to 3 years in the absence of changes in symptoms. However, the guidelines support echocardiography every 6 to 12 months for patients with severe aortic regurgitation and significant left ventricular dilation, such as end-diastolic dimension greater than 60 mm. For patients with even more advanced left ventricular dilation, echocardiography as often as every 4 to 6 months is endorsed.

Exercise testing is considered appropriate for assessment of functional capacity in patients in whom the history is not definitive, but the impact of this test on management was not otherwise strongly supported by the ACC/AHA guidelines. Radionuclide angiography was endorsed as an alternative to echocardiography for assessment of left ventricular volume and function. However, the ACC/AHA guidelines emphasized that there is no need for serial testing with both technologies. The guidelines also note that exercise ejection fraction has not been shown to have incremental value in the management of patients.

The ACC/AHA guidelines considered vasodilator therapy appropriate in patients with hypertension or left ventricular dysfunction, even if the patients were asymptomatic. However, the guidelines do not endorse vasodilator therapy in normotensive patients with normal left ventricular function and mild aortic regurgitation. The guidelines emphasize that vasodilator therapy is not an alternative to surgery for patients who are appropriate candidates for valve replacement.

TABLE 57G–5 ACC/AHA Guidelines for Management of Patients with Aortic Valve Stenosis

Indication	Class I	Class IIa	Class IIb	Class III
Echocardiography in aortic stenosis	1. Diagnosis and assessment of severity of aortic stenosis 2. Assessment of LV size, function, and/or hemodynamics 3. Reevaluation of patients with known aortic stenosis with changing symptoms or signs 4. Assessment of changes in hemodynamic severity and ventricular compensation in patients with known aortic stenosis during pregnancy 5. Reevaluation of asymptomatic patients with severe aortic stenosis	1. Reevaluation of asymptomatic patients with mild to moderate aortic stenosis and evidence of LV dysfunction or hypertrophy		1. Routine reevaluation of asymptomatic adult patients with mild aortic stenosis having stable physical signs and normal LV size and function
Cardiac catheterization in aortic stenosis	1. Coronary angiography before aortic valve replacement in patients at risk for coronary artery disease 2. Assessment of severity of aortic stenosis in symptomatic patients when aortic valve replacement is planned or when noninvasive tests are inconclusive or there is a discrepancy with clinical findings regarding severity of aortic stenosis or need for surgery		1. Assessment of severity of aortic stenosis before aortic valve replacement when noninvasive tests are adequate and concordant with clinical findings and coronary angiography is not needed	1. Assessment of LV function and severity of aortic stenosis in asymptomatic patients when noninvasive tests are adequate
Aortic valve replacement in aortic stenosis	1. Symptomatic patients with severe aortic stenosis 2. Patients with severe aortic stenosis undergoing coronary artery bypass surgery 3. Patients with severe aortic stenosis undergoing surgery on the aorta or other heart valves	1. Patients with moderate aortic stenosis undergoing coronary artery bypass surgery or surgery on the aorta or other heart valves 2. Asymptomatic patients with severe aortic stenosis and • Left ventricular systolic dysfunction, or • Abnormal response to exercise (e.g., hypotension)	1. Asymptomatic patients with severe aortic stenosis and • Ventricular tachycardia, or • Marked or excessive LV hypertrophy, or • Valve area < 0.6 cm^2	1. Prevention of sudden death in asymptomatic patients with none of the findings listed in NYHA Class II
Aortic balloon valvotomy in adults with aortic stenosis		1. A "bridge" to surgery in hemodynamically unstable patients who are at high risk for aortic valve replacement	1. Palliation in patients with serious comorbid conditions 2. Patients who require urgent noncardiac surgery	1. An alternative to aortic valve replacement

ACC = American College of Cardiology; AHA = American Heart Association; MVP = mitral valve prolapse; LV = left ventricular; NYHA = New York Heart Association.

Cardiac catheterization is not routinely needed to confirm the diagnosis or assess the severity of aortic regurgitation when echocardiographic studies are adequate. The most common appropriate indication for cardiac catheterization is the performance of coronary angiography as a prelude to surgery. Aortic valve replacement is considered clearly appropriate in patients with severe (NYHA Class III or IV) symptoms, progressive left ventricular dilation, mild-to-moderate left ventricular dysfunction, or declining exercise tolerance. The guidelines were not supportive of surgery solely because of a decline in ejection fraction during exercise.

TABLE 57G–6 ACC/AHA Guidelines for Management of Patients with Aortic Regurgitation

Indication	Class I	Class IIa	Class IIb	Class III
Echocardiography in aortic regurgitation	1. Confirm presence and severity of acute aortic regurgitation 2. Diagnosis of chronic aortic regurgitation in patients with equivocal physical findings 3. Assessment of etiology of regurgitation (including valve morphology and aortic root size and morphology) 4. Assessment of LV hypertrophy, dimension (or volume), and systolic function 5. Semiquantitative estimate of severity of aortic regurgitation 6. Reevaluation of patients with mild, moderate or severe regurgitation with new or changing symptoms 7. Reevaluation of LV size and function in asymptomatic patients with severe regurgitation 8. Reevaluation of asymptomatic patients with mild, moderate, or severe regurgitation and enlarged aortic root			1. Yearly reevaluation of asymptomatic patients with mild to moderate regurgitation with stable physical signs and normal or near-normal LV chamber size
Exercise testing in chronic aortic regurgitation	1. Assessment of functional capacity and symptomatic responses in patients with a history of equivocal symptoms	1. Evaluation of symptoms and functional capacity before participation in athletic activities 2. Prognostic assessment before aortic valve replacement in patients with LV dysfunction	1. Exercise hemodynamic measurements to determine the effect of aortic regurgitation on LV function 2. Exercise radionuclide angiography for assessing LV function in asymptomatic or symptomatic patients	1. Exercise echocardiography or dobutamine stress echocardiography for assessing LV function in asymptomatic or symptomatic patients
Radionuclide angiography in aortic regurgitation	1. Initial and serial assessment of LV volume and function at rest in patients with suboptimal echocardiograms or equivocal echocardiographic data 2. Serial assessment of LV volume and function at rest when serial echocardiograms are not used 3. Assessment of LV volume and function in asymptomatic patients with moderate to severe regurgitation when echocardiographic evidence of declining LV function is suggestive but not definitive 4. Confirmation of subnormal LV ejection fraction before recommending surgery in an asymptomatic patient with borderline echocardiographic evidence of LV dysfunction 5. Assessment of LV volume and function in patients with moderate to severe regurgitation when clinical assessment and echocardiographic data are discordant		1. Routine assessment of exercise ejection fraction 2. Quantification of AR in patients with unsatisfactory echocardiograms	1. Quantification of AR in patients with satisfactory echocardiograms 2. Initial and serial assessment of LV volume and function at rest in addition to echocardiography
Vasodilator therapy for chronic aortic regurgitation	1. Chronic therapy in patients with severe regurgitation who have symptoms and/or LV dysfunction when surgery is not recommended because of additional cardiac or noncardiac factors			1. Long-term therapy in asymptomatic patients with mild to moderate AR and normal LV systolic function 2. Long-term therapy in

TABLE 57G–6 ACC/AHA Guidelines for Management of Patients with Aortic Regurgitation—cont'd

Indication	Class I	Class IIa	Class IIb	Class III
	2. Long-term therapy in asymptomatic patients with severe regurgitation who have LV dilation but normal systolic function 3. Long-term therapy in asymptomatic patients with hypertension and any degree of regurgitation 4. Long-term ACE inhibitor therapy in patients with persistent LV systolic dysfunction after AVR 5. Short-term therapy to improve the hemodynamic profile of patients with severe heart failure symptoms and severe LV dysfunction before proceeding with AVR			asymptomatic patients with LV systolic dysfunction who are otherwise candidates for valve replacement 3. Long-term therapy in symptomatic patients with either normal LV function or mild to moderate LV systolic dysfunction who are otherwise candidates for valve replacement
Cardiac catheterization in chronic aortic regurgitation	1. Coronary angiography before AVR in patients at risk for CAD 2. Assessing severity of regurgitation when noninvasive tests are inconclusive or discordant with clinical findings regarding severity of regurgitation or need for surgery 3. Assessing LV function when noninvasive tests are inconclusive or discordant with clinical findings regarding LV dysfunction and need for surgery in patients with severe AR		1. Assessment of LV function and severity of regurgitation before AVR when noninvasive tests are adequate and concordant with clinical findings and coronary angiography is not needed	1. Assessment of LV function and severity of regurgitation in asymptomatic patients when noninvasive tests are adequate
Aortic valve replacement in chronic severe aortic regurgitation	1. Patients with NYHA Class III or IV symptoms and preserved LV systolic function, defined as normal ejection fraction at rest (ejection fraction ≥ 0.50) 2. Patients with NYHA Class II symptoms and preserved LV systolic function (ejection fraction ≥ 0.50 at rest) but with progressive LV dilation or declining ejection fraction at rest on serial studies or declining effort tolerance on exercise testing 3. Patients with Canadian Heart Association Class II or greater angina with or without CAD 4. Asymptomatic or symptomatic patients with mild to moderate LV dysfunction at rest (ejection fraction 0.25–0.49) 5. Patients undergoing coronary artery bypass surgery or surgery on the aorta or other heart valves	1. Patients with NYHA Class II symptoms and LV systolic function (ejection fraction ≥ 0.50 at rest) with stable LV size and systolic function on serial studies and stable exercise tolerance 2. Asymptomatic patients with normal LV systolic function (ejection fraction > 0.50) but with severe LV dilation (diastolic dimension > 75 mm or end-systolic dimension > 55 mm; consider lower threshold values for patients of small stature)	1. Patients with severe LV dysfunction (ejection fraction < 0.25) 2. Asymptomatic patients with normal systolic function at rest (ejection fraction > 0.50) and progressive LV dilation when the degree of dilation is moderately severe (end-diastolic dimension 70–75 mm, end-systolic dimension 50–55 mm) 3. Asymptomatic patients with normal systolic function at rest (ejection fraction > 0.50) but with decline in ejection fraction during exercise radionuclide angiography	1. Asymptomatic patients with normal systolic function at rest (ejection fraction > 0.50) but with decline in ejection fraction during stress echocardiography 2. Asymptomatic patients with normal systolic function at rest (ejection fraction > 0.50) and LV dilation when degree of dilation is not severe (end-diastolic dimension < 70 mm, end-systolic dimension < 50 mm)

ACC = American College of Cardiology; AHA = American Heart Association; LV = left ventricular; AR = aortic regurgitation; ACE = angiotensin-converting enzyme; AVR = aortic value replacement; CAD = coronary artery disease; NYHA = New York Heart Association.

Other Valvular Disease

Tricuspid valve annuloplasty is an appropriate procedure for patients with severe tricuspid regurgitation and pulmonary hypertension in patients who are undergoing surgery for mitral valve disease but not considered appropriate in patients without pulmonary artery systolic pressure of 60 mm Hg or more (Table 57G–7). The ACC/AHA guidelines otherwise offer no recommendations regarding treatment of multiple valve disease.

Anorectic Drugs

The ACC/AHA task force did not consider it possible to offer definitive diagnostic and treatment guidelines for patients who have

TABLE 57G–7 ACC/AHA Guidelines for Management of Patients with Other Valvular Heart Disease

Indication	Class I	Class IIa	Class IIb	Class III
Recommendations for surgery for tricuspid regurgitation	1. Annuloplasty for severe TR and pulmonary hypertension in patients with mitral valve disease requiring mitral valve surgery	1. Valve replacement for severe TR secondary to diseased/ abnormal tricuspid valve leaflets not amenable to annuloplasty or repair 2. Valve replacement or annuloplasty for severe TR with mean pulmonary artery pressure < 60 mm Hg when symptomatic	1. Annuloplasty for mild TR in patients with pulmonary hypertension secondary to mitral valve disease requiring mitral valve surgery	1. Valve replacement or annuloplasty for TR with pulmonary artery systolic pressure < 60 mm Hg in the presence of a normal mitral valve, in asymptomatic patients, or in symptomatic patients who have not received a trial of diuretic therapy
Patients who have used anorectic drugs (fenfluramine or dexfenfluramine or the combination of fenfluramine-phentermine or dexfenfluramine-phentermine)	1. Discontinuation of the anorectic drug(s) 2. Cardiac physical examination 3. Echocardiography in patients with symptoms, heart murmurs, or associated physical findings 4. Doppler echocardiography in patients for whom cardiac auscultation cannot be performed adequately because of body habitus	1. Repeat physical examination in 6–8 mo for those without murmurs	1. Echocardiography in all patients before dental procedures in the absence of symptoms, heart murmurs, or associated physical findings	1. Echocardiography in all patients without heart murmurs
Follow-up strategy of patients with prosthetic heart valves	1. History, physical examination ECG, chest radiograph echocardiogram, complete blood count, serum chemistries, and INR (if indicated) at first postoperative outpatient evaluation. (this evaluation should be performed 3–4 wk after hospital discharge) 2. Radionuclide angiography or magnetic resonance imaging to LV function if result of echocardiography is unsatisfactory 3. Routine follow-up visits at yearly intervals with earlier reevaluations for change in clinical status		1. Routine serial echocardiograms at time of annual follow-up visit in absence of change in clinical status	1. Routine serial fluoroscopy
Valve replacement with a mechanical prosthesis	1. Patients with expected long life spans 2. Patients with a mechanical prosthetic valve already in place in a different position than the valve to be replaced	1. Patients in renal failure, on hemodialysis, or with hypercalcemia (Class II rather than IIa) 2. Patients requiring warfarin therapy because of risk factors for thromboembolism 3. Patients ≤65 years for AVR and ≤70 years for MVR	1. Valve re-replacement for thrombosed biological valve	1. Patients who cannot or will not take warfarin therapy
Valve replacement with a bioprosthesis	1. Patients who cannot or will not take warfarin therapy 2. Patients ≥65 years needing AVR who do not have risk factors for thromboembolism	1. Patients considered to have possible compliance problems with warfarin therapy 2. Patients >70 years needing MVR who do not have risk factors for thromboembolism	1. Valve re-replacement for thrombosed mechanical valve 2. Patients <65 years	1. Patients in renal failure, on hemodialysis, or with hypercalcemia 2. Adolescent patients who are still growing

ACC = American College of Cardiology; AHA = American Heart Association; TR = tricuspid regurgitation; ECG = electrocardiogram; LV = left ventricular; AVR = aortic valve replacement; MVR = mitral valve replacement.

received anorectic drugs beyond recommending discontinuation of these agents and careful periodic examinations. The guidelines recommended echocardiography only in patients with cardiovascular symptoms, heart murmurs, or a body habitus that hindered an effective examination.

Valvular Disease in Young Adults

For adolescents and young adults with aortic stenosis, ACC/AHA guidelines recommend a lower threshold for exercise testing and cardiac catheterization to assess the risk of participation in athletics (Table 57G–8). In this population, balloon valvotomy is an effective and appropriate option. Since this procedure has little morbidity and mortality, the indications for intervention are more liberal in younger patients than in adults. The indications for management of chronic aortic regurgitation and mitral valve disease are similar to those for older adult patients. Pulmonic valvotomy is considered an appropriate intervention for patients who are symptomatic due to pulmonic stenosis and for asymptomatic patients with a peak valve gradient greater than 50 mm.

Patients with Prosthetic Heart Valves

The ACC/AHA guidelines recommend that the international normalized ratio (INR) be maintained between 2.0 and 3.0 for patients with bileaflet mechanical valves and Medtronic-Hall valves and between 2.5 and 3.5 for other disc valves and Starr-Edward valves (Table 57G–9). Aspirin therapy was considered appropriate for patients with aortic or mitral valve bioprostheses and no risk factors for thromboembolism.

The ACC/AHA guidelines indicate that admission to the hospital to give heparin before noncardiac surgery or dental care is usually unnecessary. They recommend that heparin be reserved for patients who have had a recent thrombosis or embolus, those with demonstrated thrombotic problems when previously off therapy, those with the Björk-Shiley valve, and those with three or more risk factors for thromboembolism.

After prosthetic valve implantation, asymptomatic patients need be seen only at 1-year intervals (see Table 57G–7). Routine serial echocardiograms were not strongly endorsed (Class IIb).

The ACC/AHA guidelines offer general recommendations to guide the selection of bioprosthetic versus mechanic valves. Bioprostheses are considered inappropriate in patients in renal failure, on hemodialysis, or with hypercalcemia or in adolescent patients who are still growing.

TABLE 57G–8 ACC/AHA Guidelines for Management of Valvular Heart Disease in Adolescents and Young Adults

Indication	Class I	Class IIa	Class IIb	Class III
Diagnostic evaluation of the adolescent or young adult with aortic stenosis*	1. ECG* 2. Echo-Doppler study	1. Graded exercise test† 2. Cardiac catheterization† for evaluation of gradient	1. Chest radiograph*	1. Coronary arteriography in the absence of history suggestive of concomitant CAD
Aortic balloon valvotomy in the adolescent or young adult (≤21 yr) with normal cardiac output	1. Symptoms of angina, syncope, and dyspnea on exertion, with catheterization peak gradient ≥ 50 mm Hg‡ 2. Catheterization peak gradient > 60 mm Hg 3. New-onset ischemic or repolarization changes on ECG at rest or with exercise (ST depression, T wave inversion over left precordium) with a gradient > 50 mm Hg)‡	1. Catheterization peak gradient > 50 mm Hg if patient wants to play competitive sports or desires to become pregnant		1. Catheterization gradient < 50 mm Hg without symptoms or ECG changes
Aortic valve surgery (replacement with mechanical valve, homograft, or pulmonary autograft) in the adolescent or young adult with chronic aortic regurgitation	1. Onset of symptoms 2. Asymptomatic patients with LV systolic dysfunction (ejection fraction < 0.50) on serial studies 1–3 months apart 3. Asymptomatic patients with progressive LV enlargement (end-diastolic dimension > 4 SD above normal)		1. Moderate AS (gradient >40 mm Hg) (peak-to-peak gradient at cardiac catheterization) 2. Onset of ischemic or repolarization abnormalities (ST depression, T wave inversion) over left precordium at rest	
Mitral valve surgery in the adolescent or young adult with congenital mitral regurgitation with severe MR	1. NYHA Class III or IV symptoms 2. Asymptomatic patients with LV systolic dysfunction (ejection fraction ≤ 0.60)	1. NYHA Class II symptoms with preserved LV systolic function if valve repair rather than replacement is likely	1. Asymptomatic patients with preserved LV systolic function in whom valve replacement is highly likely	

TABLE 57G–8 ACC/AHA Guidelines for Management of Valvular Heart Disease in Adolescents and Young Adults—cont'd

Indication	Class I	Class IIa	Class IIb	Class III
Mitral valve surgery in the adolescent or young adult with congenital mitral stenosis	1. Symptomatic patients (NYHA Class III or IV) and mean mitral valve gradient > 10 mm Hg on Doppler echocardiography	1. Mildly symptomatic patients (NYHA Class II) and mean mitral valve gradient > 10 mm Hg on Doppler echocardiographic study 2. Systolic pulmonary artery pressure 50 to 60 mm Hg with a mean mitral valve gradient ≥ 10 mm Hg	1. New-onset atrial fibrillation or multiple systemic emboli while receiving adequate anticoagulation	
Intervention in the adolescent or young adult with pulmonic stenosis (balloon valvotomy or surgery)	1. Patients with exertional dyspnea, angina, syncope, or presyncope 2. Asymptomatic patients with normal cardiac output (estimated clinically or determined by catheterization) and right ventricular to pulmonary artery peak gradient > 50 mm Hg	1. Asymptomatic patients with normal cardiac output (estimated clinically or determined by catheterization) and right ventricular to pulmonary artery peak gradient 40–49 mm Hg	1. Asymptomatic patients with normal cardiac output (estimated clinically or determined by catheterization) and right ventricular to pulmonary artery peak gradient 30–39 mm Hg	1. Asymptomatic patients with normal cardiac output (estimated clinically or determined by catheterization) and right ventricular to pulmonary artery peak gradient < 30 mm Hg

ACC = American College of Cardiology; AHA = American Heart Association; ECG = electrocardiogram; LV = left ventricular; CAD = coronary artery disease; AS = aortic stenosis; MR = mitral regurgitation; NYHA = New York Heart Association.

*Yearly if echo-Doppler gradient > 36 mm Hg (velocity ≥ 3 m/sec); every 2 years if echo-Doppler gradient < 36 mm Hg (peak velocity < 3 m/sec).

†If echo-Doppler gradient > 36 mm Hg (velocity > 3 m/sec) and patient interested in athletic participation or if clinical findings and echo-Doppler are disparate.

‡If gradient < 50 mm Hg, other causes of symptoms should be explored.

From Bonow RO, Carabello B, de Leon AC Jr, et al: ACC/AHA guidelines for the management of patients with valvular heart disease: Executive summary. A report of the American College of Cardiology/American Heart Association Task Force on Practice Guidelines (Committee on Management of Patients with Valvular Heart Disease). Circulation 98:1949-1984, 1998.

TABLE 57G–9 ACC/AHA Recommendations for Appropriate (Class I) Antithrombotic Therapy in Patients with Prosthetic Heart Valves

Indication	Medication	Target	Class
First 3 months after valve replacement	Warfarin	INR 2.5-3.5	I
≥3 months after valve replacement			
Mechanical valve			
AVR and no risk factor*			
Bileaflet valve or Medtronic Hall valve	Warfarin	INR 2-3	I
Other disk valves or Starr-Edwards valve	Warfarin	INR 2.5-3.5	I
AVR plus risk factor*	Warfarin	INR 2.5-3.5	I
MVR	Warfarin	INR 2.5-3.5	I
Bioprosthesis			
AVR and no risk factor*	Aspirin	80-100 mg/day	I
AVR and risk factor*	Warfarin	INR 2-3	I
MVR and no risk factor*	Aspirin	80-100 mg/day	I
MVR and risk factor*	Warfarin	INR 2.5-3.5	I

ACC = American College of Cardiology; AHA = American Heart Association; AVR = atrial valve replacement; MVR = mitral valve replacement; INR = international normalized ratio.

*Risk factors: atrial fibrillation, LV dysfunction, previous thromboembolism, and hypercoagulable condition.

References

1. Bonow RO, Carabello B, de Leon AC Jr, et al: ACC/AHA guidelines for the management of patients with valvular heart disease: Executive summary: A report of the American College of Cardiology/American Heart Association Task Force on Practice Guidelines (Committee on Management of Patients With Valvular Heart Disease). Circulation 98:1949-1984, 1998.
2. Cheitlin MD, Alpert JS, Armstrong WF, et al: ACC/AHA guidelines for the clinical application of echocardiography: A report of the American College of Cardiology/American Heart Association Task Force on Practice Guidelines (Committee on Clinical Application of Echocardiography). Circulation 95:1686-1744, 1997.
3. Cheitlin MD, Douglas PS, Parmley WW: 26th Bethesda Conference: Recommendations for Determining Eligibility for Competition in Athletes with Cardiovascular Abnormalities. Task Force 2: Acquired Valvular Heart Disease. J Am Coll Cardiol 24:874-880, 1994.
4. Maron BJ, Araujo GS, Thompson PD, et al: Recommendations for preparticipation screening and the assessment of cardiovascular disease in masters athletes. An advisory for healthcare professionals from the Working Groups of the World Heart Federation, the International Federation of Sports Medicine, and the American Heart Association Committee on Exercise, Cardiac Rehabilitation, and Prevention. Circulation 103:327-334, 2001.

CHAPTER 58

Infective Endocarditis

Adolf W. Karchmer

Infective endocarditis (IE) is a microbial infection of the endothelial surface of the heart. The characteristic lesion, the vegetation, is a variably sized amorphous mass of platelets and fibrin in which abundant microorganisms and moderate inflammatory cells are enmeshed. Heart valves are most commonly involved; however, infection may occur at the site of a septal defect or on chordae tendineae or mural endocardium. Infection of arteriovenous shunts, arterioarterial shunts (patent ductus arteriosus), or coarctation of the aorta, although actually an endarteritis, is clinically and pathologically similar to IE. Many species of bacteria and fungi, mycobacteria, rickettsiae, chlamydiae, and mycoplasmas cause IE; nevertheless, streptococci, staphylococci, enterococci, and fastidious gram-negative coccobacilli cause the majority of cases of IE.

The terms *acute* and *subacute* are often used to describe IE. Acute IE arises with marked toxicity and progresses over days to several weeks to valvular destruction and metastatic infection. In contrast, subacute IE evolves over weeks to months with only modest toxicity and rarely causes metastatic infection. Acute IE is caused typically, although not exclusively, by *Staphylococcus aureus,* whereas the subacute syndrome is more likely to be caused by viridans streptococci, enterococci, coagulase-negative staphylococci, or gram-negative coccobacilli.

EPIDEMIOLOGY

The incidence of IE remained relatively stable from 1950 through 1987 at about 4.2 per 100,000 patient-years. During the early 1980s, the yearly incidence of IE per 100,000 population was 2.0 in the United Kingdom and Wales and 1.9 in the Netherlands.[1] A higher incidence was noted from 1984 through 1999; 5.9 and 11.6 episodes per 100,000 population were reported from Sweden and metropolitan Philadelphia, respectively.[2,3] Injection drug abuse accounted for approximately half of the cases in Philadelphia. Endocarditis usually occurred more frequently in men; gender-derived ratios range from 1.6 to 2.5.The age-specific incidence of endocarditis increased progressively after 30 years of age and exceeded 14.5 to 30 cases per 100,000 person-years in the sixth through eighth decades of life.[3] From 36 to 75 percent of patients with native valve endocarditis (NVE) have predisposing conditions: rheumatic heart disease, congenital heart disease, mitral valve prolapse, degenerative heart disease, asymmetrical septal hypertrophy, or intravenous (IV) drug abuse.[2] From 7 to 25 percent of cases involve prosthetic valves.[2,3] Predisposing conditions cannot be identified in 25 to 47 percent of patients. The nature of predisposing conditions and, in part, the microbiology of IE correlate with the age of patients (Table 58-1).

CHANGE IN PATIENTS WITH INFECTIVE ENDOCARDITIS. The median age of patients has gradually increased from 30 to 40 years of age in the preantibiotic and early antibiotic eras to 47 to 69 years in recent decades.[2] Rheumatic fever with subsequent rheumatic heart disease in children and young adults has been markedly reduced in developed countries. Acquired valvular disease emerges as a risk for IE as patients enjoy greater longevity. In addition, during their later years, many of these patients require valve replacement, which places them at greater risk for endocarditis.The increasing life span of the general population results in the emergence of degenerative heart disease as a major substrate for IE. Finally, nosocomial endocarditis arises with increased frequency among elderly people, who experience high rates of hospitalization for underlying illnesses.[4]

Groups of Patients

CHILDREN. The incidence of IE among hospitalized children ranges from 1 in 4500 to 1 in 1280.[1] In the Netherlands, IE was noted in 1.7 and 1.2 per 100,000 male and female children younger than 10 years, respectively.[1] IE has been noted in neonates with increasing frequency. Among neonates, IE typically involves the tricuspid valve of structurally normal hearts and is associated with very high mortality rates. It is likely that many of these episodes arise as a consequence of infected IV and right-heart catheters as well as cardiac surgery.[5]

The vast majority of children with IE occurring after the neonatal period have identifiable structural cardiac abnormalities (see Table 58-1). In some series, rheumatic heart disease was an infrequent predisposition for IE (≤4 percent).[5] Congenital heart abnormalities, particularly those involving the aortic valve; ventricular septal defects; tetralogy of Fallot; and other complex structural anomalies associated with cyanosis are found in 75 to 90 percent of cases. Of children with IE on congenital defects, 50 percent develop infection after cardiac surgery; in these children, infection frequently involves prosthetic valves, valved conduits, or synthetic patches.[5] Secundum atrial septal defects are not associated with an increased risk for IE, nor is patent ductus arteriosus or pulmonic stenosis after repair.[6] Since 1990, mitral valve prolapse has been recognized to predispose to IE in children; it, generally in association with a regurgitant murmur, was the predisposing cardiac abnormality in 15 percent and 5 percent of cases in two series.

The clinical features and echocardiographic findings of IE in children are similar to those noted among adults with NVE or prosthetic valve endocarditis (PVE), respectively.

ADULTS. *Mitral valve prolapse* (MVP) has emerged as a prominent predisposing structural cardiac abnormality and in adults accounts for 7 to 30 percent of native valve endocarditis (NVE) in cases not related to drug abuse or nosocomial infection.[1] The frequency of MVP in IE is not entirely a direct reflection of risk but rather arises because of the frequency of the lesion in the general population, 2.4 percent of community-based samples.

The relative risk of endocarditis among patients with MVP ranges from 3.5 to 8.2. This increased risk of endocarditis is largely confined to patients with prolapse, thickened valve leaflets (>5 mm), and mitral

TABLE 58–1 Predisposing Conditions and Microbiology of Native Valve Endocarditis

Conditions and Microbiology	Children (%)		Adults (%)	
	Neonates	2 mo-15 yr	15-60 yr	>60 yr
Predisposing conditions				
RHD		2-10	25-30	8
CHD	28	75-90*	10-20	2
MVP		5-15	10-30	10
DHD			Rare	30
Parenteral drug abuse			15-35	10
Other			10-15	10
None	72†	2-5	25-45	25-40
Microbiology				
Streptococci	15-20	40-50	45-65	30-45
Enterococci		4	5-8	15
S. aureus	40-50	25	30-40	25-30
Coagulase-negative staphylococci	10	5	3-5	5-8
GNB	10	5	4-8	5
Fungi	10	1	1	Rare
Polymicrobial	4		1	Rare
Other			1	2
Culture negative	4	0-15	3-10	5

CHD = congenital heart disease; DHD = degenerative heart disease; GNB = gram-negative bacteria, frequently *Hemophilus* species, *Actinobacillus actinomycetemcomitans, Cardiobacterium hominis*; MVP = mitral valve prolapse; RHD = rheumatic heart disease.

*50% of cases follow surgery and may involve implanted devices and foreign material.

†Often tricuspid valve IE.

regurgitation murmur. Risk is also increased among men and patients older than 45 years (see Chap. 57). Among patients with MVP and a systolic murmur, the incidence of IE is 52 per 100,000 person-years, compared with a rate of 4.6 per 100,000 person-years among those with prolapse and no murmur or among the general population. The microbiology of IE engrafted on MVP is similar to that of NVE that is not associated with drug abuse. Similarly, the mortality rate of 14 percent approximates that of NVE in general.

Rheumatic heart disease was the predisposing cardiac lesion for IE in 20 to 25 percent of cases in the 1970s and 1980s. In reports from hospitals in North America and Europe in the 1980s, rheumatic heart disease predisposed to IE in only 7 and 18 percent of cases.[2] In patients with rheumatic heart disease, endocarditis occurs most frequently on the mitral valve, a site at which women are more commonly infected. The aortic valve is the next most common site for IE; infection in this setting occurs more commonly in men.

Congenital heart disease is the substrate for IE in 10 to 20 percent of younger adults and 8 percent of older adults. Among adults, the common predisposing lesions are patent ductus arteriosus, ventricular septal defect, and bicuspid aortic valve, the latter particularly found among older men (>60 years).[2]

Infection with *human immunodeficiency virus* (HIV), unless associated with endocarditis-prone behavior, i.e., IV drug abuse, is not a significant risk factor for IE. Among HIV-infected persons who are not IV drug abusers, IE is caused not only by organisms typical of NVE but also by organisms that are uniquely associated with bacteremia in this population, i.e., *Salmonella* spp. and *Streptococcus pneumoniae*. Notably, 40 percent of cases were nosocomial.[7]

In settings where NVE among adults is not skewed dramatically by infection occurring among IV drug abusers and nosocomial disease, the microbiology is notably similar to that shown in Table 58–1.[2] *Coxiella burnetii*, an uncommon cause of IE in the United States, caused 3 percent of all cases in the United Kingdom from 1976 to 1985 and is a prominent cause of IE in France.[8] *Bartonella* species have emerged as a significant cause of IE, accounting for 3 percent of cases in one report.[9]

INTRAVENOUS DRUG ABUSERS. The risk for IE among IV drug abusers, 2 to 5 percent per patient-year, is estimated to be several fold greater than that of patients with rheumatic heart disease or prosthetic valves.[10] In one study, IE was diagnosed in 74 (6.4 percent) of 1150 IV drug abusers who were hospitalized during 12 months. In metropolitan Philadelphia, 5.3 of a total of 11.6 cases of IE per 100,000 population were attributed to injection drug abuse. From 65 to 80 percent of cases of IE in this population occur in men, who typically range in age from 27 to 37 years.[11-13]

Endocarditis occurring in IV drug abusers has a unique propensity to infect right heart valves.[10-13] In clinical series, distribution of valve involvement is tricuspid in 46 to 78 percent, mitral in 24 to 32 percent, and aortic in 8 to 19 percent (as many as 16 percent of patients have infection at multiple sites).[11] In IV drug abusers, the valves were normal before infection in 75 to 93 percent of patients.[10,11] The remaining patients have preexisting aortic or mitral valve abnormalities, resulting primarily from rheumatic heart disease, congenital heart disease, or prior episodes of IE. IV drug abuse is a risk factor for recurrent NVE.

MICROBIOLOGY. The microbiology of IE occurring in IV drug abusers is unique in several respects (Table 58–2). In contrast to the etiology of NVE among adults in general, *S. aureus* causes more than 50 percent of these infections overall and 60 to 70 percent of those involving the tricuspid valve. The well-established predilection for *S. aureus* to infect normal as well as abnormal left heart valves is noted in addicts. Although the phenomenon of *S. aureus* infection of normal tricuspid valves is not unique to addicts, the high frequency is characteristic.[10] Streptococcal and enterococcal infection of previously abnormal mitral or aortic valves in addicts is comparable to that noted generally in NVE. In contrast, infection of right and left heart valves by *Pseudomonas aeruginosa* and other gram-negative bacilli and left heart valves by fungi occurs with increased frequency among drug abusers. In addition, unusual organisms, some of which are probably related to injection of contaminated materials, cause endocarditis in these patients, e.g., *Corynebacterium* species, *Lactobacillus, Bacillus cereus,* and nonpathogenic *Neisseria* species. Polymicrobial endocarditis accounts for 3 to 5 percent of cases of IE.

The clinical manifestations of IE in IV drug abusers depend on the valve or valves involved and, to a lesser degree, on the infecting organism. Tricuspid valve endocarditis, particularly when caused by *S. aureus,* arises with pleuritic chest pain, shortness of breath, cough, and hemoptysis. In 65 to 75 percent of patients, chest roentgenograms reveal abnormalities related to septic pulmonary emboli. Murmurs of tricuspid regurgitation are noted in less than half of these patients. Infection of the aortic or mitral valve in addicts clinically resembles IE seen in other patients. That caused by *S. aureus* generally arises as acute endocarditis with marked systemic toxicity. Symptoms and signs of left-sided heart failure, neurological injury, systemic emboli, metastatic infections, and the classical peripheral stigmata of IE are strongly associated with left-sided endocarditis.[10,11]

Infection with HIV has been noted in 27 to 73 percent of IV drug abusers with IE (see Chap. 61).[11-13] Among drug

TABLE 58–2 Microbiology of Endocarditis Associated with Intravenous Drug Abuse

Organisms	Number of Cases (%) of Endocarditis in Drug Addicts*			
	Right-Sided[†] *N = 346*	*Left-Sided*[†] *N = 204*	*Total*[‡] *N = 675*	*Spain (1977-1993)*[§] *N = 1529*
Streptococci[‖]	17 (5)	31 (15)	80 (12)	131 (8.5)
Enterococci	7 (2)	49 (24)	59 (9)	21 (1)
Staphylococcus aureus	267 (77)	47 (23)	396 (57)	1138 (74)
Coagulase-negative staphylococci	—	—		44 (3)
Gram-negative bacilli[¶]	17 (5)	26 (13)	45 (7)	23 (1.5)
Fungi (predominantly *Candida* species)	—	25 (12)	26 (4)	18 (1)
Polymicrobia/miscellaneous	28 (8)	20 (10)	49 (7)	48 (3)
Culture negative	10 (3)	6 (3)	20 (3)	106 (7)

*Ten patients with right- and left-sided IE are counted twice.

[†]Data from references 10 and Levine DP, Crane LR, Zervos MJ: Bacteremia in narcotic addicts at the Detroit Medical Center. Infectious endocarditis: A prospective comparative study. Rev Infect Dis 8:374, 1986. Hecht SR, Berger M: Right-sided endocarditis in intravenous drug users: Prognostic features in 102 episodes. Ann Intern Med 17:560, 1992.

[‡]Data from references 10, 11, and Sandre RM, Shafran SD: Infective endocarditis: Review of 135 cases over 9 years. Clin Infect Dis 22:276-286, 1996.

[§]Data from reference 7.

[‖]Includes viridans streptococci, *Streptococcus bovis*, other non-group A groupable streptococci, *Abiotrophia* species (nutritionally variant streptococci).

[¶]*P. aeruginosa, S. marcescens*, and Enterobacteriaceae.

abusers with IE, HIV serostatus does not significantly modify the clinical presentation, microbiology, complications, and overall survival. However, among HIV-infected drug abusers with IE, the risk of death is increased among those with a CD4 count less than 200/mm^3.[12,13]

PROSTHETIC VALVE ENDOCARDITIS. Epidemiological studies suggest that PVE constitutes 10 to 30 percent of all cases of IE in developed countries.[3,12] In metropolitan Philadelphia, 0.94 cases of IE per 100,000 population involved prosthetic valves. In six studies that observed patients undergoing valve surgery between 1965 and 1995, the cumulative incidence of PVE estimated actuarially ranged from 1.4 to 3.1 percent at 12 months and 3.0 to 5.7 percent at 5 years.[14-17] The risk of PVE over time, however, is not uniform. The risk is greatest during the initial 6 months after valve surgery (particularly during the initial 5 to 6 weeks) and thereafter declines to a lower but stable risk (0.2 to 0.35 percent per year).[14-17]

PVE has been called "early" when symptoms begin within 60 days of valve surgery and "late" with onset thereafter. These terms were established to distinguish PVE that arose early as a complication of valve surgery from infection that became symptomatic later and was more likely to be community acquired. In fact, many cases with onset between 60 days and 1 year after surgery are likely to be nosocomial and, despite their delayed presentation, derive from events during the surgical admission. Studies to identify risk factors for PVE have not resulted in a coherent picture. Data suggest that, during the initial months after valve implantation, mechanical prostheses are at greater risk of infection than bioprosthetic valves but that after 12 months the risk of infection of bioprostheses exceeds that of mechanical valves.[14-16] By 5 years after valve surgery, the rates of PVE for the two valve types are comparable.[17] Patients with antecedent NVE, particularly if the disease is active, are at increased risk for PVE.[14-16]

Microbiology. The microbiology of PVE is relatively predictable and reflects in part the presumed nosocomial or community acquisition of infection (Table 58–3). Coagulase-negative staphylococci, which when speciated are primarily *Staphylococcus epidermidis,* are the predominant causes of PVE diagnosed within 60 days after surgery. *S. aureus,* gram-negative bacilli, diphtheroids (particularly *Corynebacterium jeikeium*), and fungi (particularly *Candida* species) are also common causes of PVE during this period. Occasional cases of nosocomial PVE caused by *Legionella* species, atypical mycobacteria, mycoplasma, and fungi other than *Candida* have been reported.

TABLE 58–3 Microbiology of Prosthetic Valve Endocarditis 1975-1994

Organisms	Number of Cases (%)* with Time of Onset After Valve Surgery		
	<2 mo N = 144	*2-12 mo N = 31*	*>12 mo N = 194*
Streptococci[†]	2 (1)	3 (9)	61 (31)
Pneumococci	—	—	—
Enterococci	12 (8)	4 (12)	22 (11)
Staphylococcus aureus	32 (22)	4 (12)	34 (18)
Coagulase-negative staphylococci	47 (33)	11 (32)	22 (11)
Fastidious gram-negative coccobacilli (HACEK group)[‡]	—	—	11 (6)
Gram-negative bacilli	19 (13)	1 (3)	11 (6)
Fungi, *Candida* species	12 (8)	4 (12)	3 (1)
Polymicrobial/miscellaneous	4 (3)	2 (6)	9 (5)
Diphtheroids	9 (6)	—	5 (3)
Culture negative	7 (5)	2 (6)	16 (8)

Adapted from Karchmer AW: Infections of prosthetic valves and intravascular devices. *In* Mandell GL, Bennett JE, Dolin R (eds): Principles and Practice of Infectious Disease. 5th ed. New York, Churchill Livingstone, 2000, pp 907-917.

*Data from reference 90.

[†]Includes viridans streptococci, *Streptococcus bovis*, other non-group A groupable streptococci, *Abiotrophia* species (nutritionally variant streptococci).

[‡]Includes *Hemophilus* species, *Actinobacillus actinomycetemcomitans, Cardiobacterium hominis, Eikenella* species, and *Kingella kingae.*

Pathology. The intracardiac pathology of PVE differs notably from the largely leaflet-confined pathology of NVE. Infection on mechanical prostheses commonly extends beyond the valve ring into the annulus and periannular tissue as well as the mitral-aortic intravalvular fibrosa, resulting in ring abscesses, septal abscesses, fistulous tracts, and dehiscence of the prosthesis with hemodynamically significant paravalvular regurgitation and conduction disturbances. In autopsy experience with 74 patients, which is clearly biased toward the most severe pathology, annular invasion was noted in 85 percent, myocardial abscess in 32 percent, and valve obstruction by vegetation overgrowth, a phenomenon of PVE at the mitral site, in 19 percent.[18] Erosion through the aortic annulus to cause pericarditis occurred in 5 percent (Fig. 58–1).[18]

In clinical series encompassing 85 patients, the rate of annulus invasion was 42 percent, myocardial abscess 14 percent, valve obstruction 4 percent, and pericarditis 2 percent.[18] Bioprosthetic valve IE may result in invasive disease, comparable to that noted when PVE involves mechanical valves, as well as leaflet destruction. Among 85 patients with bioprosthetic PVE, 29 (59 percent) of 49 with infection within a year after surgery had invasive disease, in contrast to only 9 (25 percent) of 36 patients with infection occurring more than 1 year postoperatively. In surgically treated bioprosthetic IE, invasion was confirmed in 15 of 19 cases (79 percent) with onset in the initial 12 months after surgery but in only 22 of 71 bioprostheses (31 percent) when infection began more than 12 months after surgery.[19] Aortic site and clinical onset within a year of valve surgery were significantly correlated with an increased risk of invasive infection.

Signs and symptoms in patients developing PVE within 60 days of cardiac surgery may be obscured by surgery or other postoperative complications. Peripheral signs of endocarditis (5 to 14 percent) and central nervous system emboli (10 percent) occur less frequently in these patients than in those with PVE occurring later after surgery. Among patients with later onset PVE, congestive heart failure (CHF) occurs in 40 percent, cerebrovascular complications in 26 to 28 percent, and peripheral signs in 15 to 28 percent.[18,20]

HEALTH CARE–ASSOCIATED ENDOCARDITIS. Health care–associated endocarditis includes true nosocomial IE as well as IE arising in the community setting as a direct consequence of long-term indwelling devices, e.g., central venous lines, tunneled lines, and hemodialysis catheters. Hospital-acquired endocarditis unrelated to concurrent cardiac surgery makes up 5 to 29 percent of all cases of IE in various series.[4] Health care–associated IE has a predilection for abnormal native cardiac valves, normal valves including the tricuspid, transvenous pacemakers and defibrillators, and prosthetic valves.[1,17] Hemodialysis-associated *S. aureus* bacteremia is commonly associated with metastatic seeding of deep tissue sites including cardiac valves; in fact, hemodialysis is independently associated with *S. aureus* IE.[21] Infected intravascular devices and catheters give rise to 45 to 65 percent of the bacteremia that results in nosocomial IE.[4] Right-sided endocarditis was found in 5 and 7 percent of patients with central venous catheters extending into or near the right atrium and those with flow-directed pulmonary artery catheters, respectively.

The onset of health care–associated IE is usually acute, and although a changing murmur may be heard, other classical signs of endocarditis are infrequent. Mortality rates among these patients, many of whom are elderly and have serious underlying diseases, are high (40 to 56 percent).[4]

MICROBIOLOGY. Gram-positive cocci are the predominant cause of nosocomial IE. Among 82 episodes from two series, *S. aureus* caused 55 percent, coagulase-negative staphylococci 10 percent, enterococci 16 percent, streptococci 7 percent, *Candida* species 4 percent, and gram-negative bacilli 5 percent; 3 percent were culture negative.

Catheter-associated *S. aureus* bacteremia occurs with sufficient frequency to be the predominant predisposing factor for health care–associated IE.[4,21,22] In a meta-analysis of catheter-related *S. aureus* bacteremia, the mean rate of subsequent endocarditis or other deep-seated infection after short-course treatment was 6.1 percent.[21] However, when 69 patients with catheter-related *S. aureus* bacteremia were studied with transesophageal echocardiography (TEE), 16 (23 percent) were found to have IE. Only seven of the IE episodes would have been diagnosed without information from the TEE.[22] Patients with *S. aureus* catheter-related bacteremia who have abnormal heart valves, prosthetic valves, or persisting fever or bacteremia for 3 days after catheter removal and initiation of therapy are at high risk for IE.

Given the relatively high risk of IE in patients with *S. aureus* catheter-related bacteremia and its morbidity, these patients should be evaluated by echocardiography. Two decision analysis studies concluded that the most cost-effective management would proceed directly to TEE to establish the presence or absence of IE.[23,24] If, however, transthoracic echocardiography (TTE) is performed initially and is nondiagnostic, the evaluation should proceed to TEE.

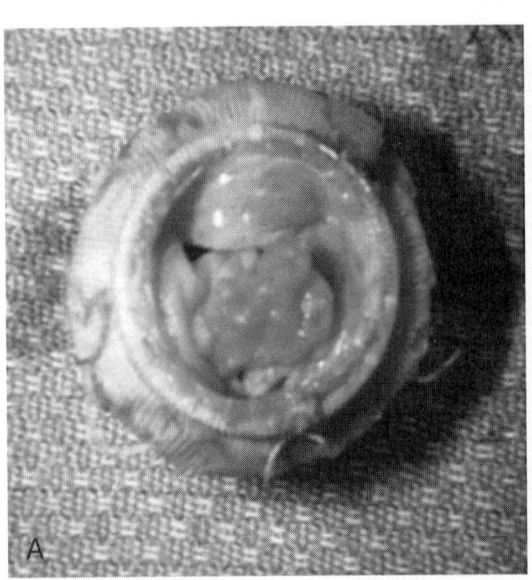

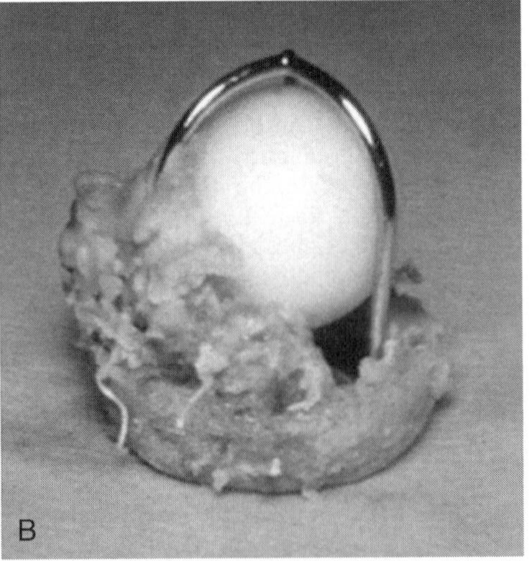

FIGURE 58–1 **A,** A large vegetation caused by *Candida albicans* partially occludes the orifice of a bioprosthetic valve removed from the mitral position. **B,** A Starr-Edwards prosthesis removed from the aortic position, where this large vegetation related to *Aspergillus* infection partially obstructed the outflow tract but also allowed regurgitation by preventing valve closure. (**A,** From Karchmer AW: Infections of prosthetic heart valves. *In* Korzeniowski OM [ed]: Cardiovascular Infection, vol x, Atlas of Infectious Diseases. Philadelphia, Churchill Livingstone, 1998, p 5.7.)

Etiological Microorganisms

VIRIDANS STREPTOCOCCI. These streptococci, which cause 30 to 65 percent of NVE cases unrelated to drug abuse, are normal inhabitants of the oropharynx, characteristically produce alpha hemolysis when grown on sheep blood agar, and are usually nontypable using the Lancefield system. Using earlier taxonomy, the species causing streptococcal NVE were distributed as follows: *Streptococcus mitior* (31 percent of cases), *Streptococcus sanguis* (24 percent), *Streptococcus bovis* (27 percent), *Streptococcus mutans* (7 percent), *Streptococcus milleri* (4 percent), *Streptococcus faecalis* (now *Enterococcus faecalis*) (7 percent), and *Streptococcus salivarius* and other species (2 percent). Another study, adjusted for the new taxonomy, has reported a similar distribution of streptococci causing IE. Nutritional variant organisms that require media supplemented with either pyridoxal hydrochloride or L-cysteine for growth and were previously speciated as *Streptococcus adjacens* or *Streptococcus defectivus* cause 5 percent of cases of streptococcal NVE. These organisms have been reclassified into a new genus, *Abiotrophia*.[25]

The viridans streptococci, other than the nutritionally variant organisms, had been in general highly susceptible to penicillin (minimum inhibitory concentration [MIC] ≤ 0.1 μg/ml for 83 percent) and are killed in an enhanced manner (synergistically) by penicillin plus gentamicin.[25]

***STREPTOCOCCUS BOVIS* AND OTHER STREPTOCOCCI.** *S. bovis* and other group D streptococci, part of the gastrointestinal tract normal flora, cause 25 to 40 percent of the episodes of streptococcal NVE.[3] Although superficially resembling the enterococci, these organisms can be easily distinguished by their biochemical characteristics. The distinction is important because group D streptococci are highly penicillin susceptible, in contrast to the relative penicillin resistance of enterococci. *S. bovis* type I NVE is frequently associated with coexistent colonic polyps or malignancy.

Group A streptococci, which can infect normal valves, cause rare episodes of endocarditis. Among IV drug abusers, group A streptococci have caused tricuspid valve IE similar to that noted with *S. aureus*. Group B organisms, *Streptococcus agalactiae*, are part of the normal flora of the mouth, genital tract, and gastrointestinal tract. Group B streptococci infect normal and abnormal valves and cause a morbid NVE syndrome with a high incidence of systemic emboli and septic musculoskeletal complications (arthritis, discitis, osteomyelitis).[26] Group G streptococci also produce a destructive, highly morbid left-sided NVE. The *S. milleri* group, now divided into three species—*Streptococcus intermedius, Streptococcus constellatus,* and *Streptococcus anginosus*—are highly pyogenic organisms that cause destructive infections and IE, similar to those caused by *S. aureus*. Although both beta-hemolytic streptococci (group A, B, C, and G) and the *S. milleri* group are invasive tissue-destroying organisms, they cause different IE syndromes.[27] IE caused by beta-hemolytic streptococci often occurs in the absence of valvular disease, has a rapid onset, and frequently results in extracardiac complications. That caused by *S. milleri* more likely occurs in the setting of valvular disease and arises less aggressively with fewer extracardiac complications. Both, however, are associated with frequent intracardiac complications, and 65 percent of patients require surgical intervention often early during therapy. Mortality rates are higher for IE caused by beta-hemolytic streptococci versus *S. milleri*, 27 and 14 percent, respectively.

***STREPTOCOCCUS PNEUMONIAE*.** Although pneumococcal bacteremia occurs frequently, *S. pneumoniae* accounts for only 1 to 3 percent of NVE cases.[28] When causing IE, *S. pneumoniae* frequently involves a previously normal aortic valve and progresses rapidly with valve destruction, myocardial abscess formation, and acute CHF.[29] The diagnosis of IE is often delayed until intracardiac complications or systemic emboli are evident. The clinical presentation, complications, and outcome of endocarditis caused by penicillin-susceptible and penicillin-resistant *S. pneumoniae* are similar. Almost half of the patients require cardiac surgery because of valve dysfunction, heart failure, or persisting fever. Mortality (35 percent) is related to left-sided heart failure and not to the penicillin susceptibility of the infecting strain.[27]

ENTEROCOCCI. *E. faecalis* and *Enterococcus faecium* cause 85 and 10 percent of cases of enterococcal IE, respectively. Enterococci, which are part of the normal gastrointestinal flora and cause genitourinary tract infection, account for 5 to 15 percent of cases of NVE and a similar percentage of PVE cases (see Tables 58-2 and 58-3).[18] Cases occur in young women as a consequence of genitourinary tract manipulation or infection and in older, predominantly male patients, who have the urinary tract as a likely portal of entry. Enterococci infect either normal or previously abnormal valves and arise as either acute or subacute IE.

Enterococci are overtly resistant to cephalosporins, semisynthetic penicillinase-resistant penicillins (oxacillin and nafcillin), and therapeutic concentrations of aminoglycosides. Most enterococci have been inhibited by modest concentrations of the cell wall–active antibiotics—penicillin, ampicillin, vancomycin, and teicoplanin (not licensed in the United States). Bactericidal antienterococcal activity can be achieved by combining an inhibitory cell wall–active agent and streptomycin or gentamicin. This bactericidal activity, called *synergy,* is essential for optimal treatment of enterococcal IE. Strains of enterococci that are highly resistant to penicillin and ampicillin, resistant to vancomycin, or highly resistant to all aminoglycosides have been identified as causes of IE. These resistant strains of enterococci may be unresponsive to standard antienterococcal agents and defy development of a synergistic bactericidal regimen. The antibiotic susceptibility of any enterococcus causing IE must be thoroughly evaluated if optimal therapy is to be assured.

STAPHYLOCOCCI. The coagulase-positive staphylococci are a single species, *S. aureus.* Of the 13 species of coagulase-negative staphylococci that colonize humans, 1, *S. epidermidis,* has emerged as an important pathogen in the setting of implanted devices and hospitalized patients. Coagulase-negative staphylococci on the surface of foreign devices have altered phenotypes, including increased resistance to the bactericidal effects of many antibiotics.

Antibiotic Resistance. In excess of 90 percent of *S. aureus* cases, whether acquired in the hospital or community, produce beta-lactamase and thus are resistant to penicillin, ampicillin, and the ureidopenicillins. These organisms are, however, susceptible to the penicillinase-resistant beta-lactam antibiotics (oxacillin, nafcillin, cefazolin, and other first-generation cephalosporins). Methicillin-resistant strains of *S. aureus* are prevalent in nosocomial settings and among some nonhospitalized populations (IV drug abusers, nursing home residents, persons hospitalized or incarcerated within the prior 6 to 12 months) and must be considered when selecting initial empirical therapy for IE.[21] Coagulase-negative staphylococci frequently produce beta-lactamase; furthermore, strains causing community-acquired infections are frequently methicillin susceptible, whereas those causing nosocomial infections, including IE, are commonly methicillin resistant.[30] Coagulase-negative staphylococci may not always phenotypically express methicillin resistance (a property called *heteroresistance*). Consequently, special testing may be required to detect this resistance.[30] Although most staphylococci, including most strains that are resistant to methicillin, remain susceptible to the glycopeptide antibiotics, vancomycin and teicoplanin, strains of *S. aureus* and coagulase-negative staphylococci with reduced susceptibility (and occasionally overt resistance) to glycopeptides have emerged as pathogens.[21]

Clinical Features. *S. aureus* is a major cause of IE in all population groups (see Tables 58-1 and 58-2). *S. aureus* IE is characterized by a highly toxic febrile illness, frequent focal metastatic infection, and a 30 to 50 percent rate of CHF and central nervous system complications.[21] A cerebrospinal fluid polymorphonuclear pleocytosis, with or without *S. aureus* cultured from the cerebrospinal fluid, is common. Heart murmurs are heard in 30 to 45 percent of patients on initial evaluation and are ultimately heard in 75 to 85 percent as a consequence of intracardiac damage. The mortality rate in nonaddicts with left-sided *S. aureus* endocarditis ranges from 16 to 65 percent overall and increases in those older than 50 years, in those with significant underlying diseases, and when IE is complicated by a major neurological event, valve dysfunction, or CHF.[21,31,32] Among addicts, left-sided *S. aureus* IE resembles that in nonaddicts. In contrast, in patients with IE limited to the tricuspid valve, complications are rare and mortality rates are only 2 to 4 percent.[11] Tricuspid staphylococcal IE occasionally results in overwhelming septic pulmonary emboli, pyopneumothorax, and severe respiratory insufficiency.

Coagulase-Negative Staphylococci. These are a major cause of PVE, particularly during the initial year after valve surgery, an important cause of nosocomial IE, and the cause of 3 to 8 percent of NVE cases, usually in the setting of prior valve abnormalities (see Tables 58-1 and 58-2).[30] The vast majority of coagulase-negative staphylococci causing PVE, when speciated, are *S. epidermidis.* In contrast, when infection involves native valves, only 50 percent of isolates are *S. epidermidis.*[30] *Staphylococcus lugdunensis,* a coagulase-negative species, has caused highly destructive, often fatal NVE and PVE. *S. lugdunensis* IE is usually community acquired, and the organism is often susceptible to many antistaphylococcal antibiotics, including penicillin.

GRAM-NEGATIVE BACTERIA. Organisms of the so-called HACEK group (*Hemophilus parainfluenzae*, *Hemophilus aphrophilus*, *Actinobacillus actinomycetemcomitans*, *Cardiobacterium hominis*, *Eikenella corrodens*, and *Kingella kingae*), which are part of the upper respiratory tract and oropharyngeal flora, infect abnormal cardiac valves, causing subacute NVE, and cause PVE that occurs a year or more after valve surgery.[33,34] In NVE, the HACEK organisms have been associated with large vegetations and a high incidence of systemic emboli.[33,34] Among the HACEK group, in descending order, *Actinobacillus actinomycetemcomitans*, *Cardiobacterium hominis*, *Hemophilus aphrophilus*, and *Hemophilus parainfluenzae* are the most common causes of IE. Although fastidious and slow growing, HACEK organisms are usually detected in blood cultures after 5 days of incubation; occasionally more prolonged incubation is required.[34]

P. aeruginosa is the gram-negative bacillus that most commonly causes endocarditis. The Enterobacteriaceae, despite causing frequent episodes of bacteremia, are implicated in only sporadic cases of IE.

Neisseria gonorrhoeae, a common cause of IE during the preantibiotic era, rarely causes endocarditis today.[35] Gonococci, similar to pneumococci, infect the aortic valve of young patients, resulting in valve destruction, abscess formation, and a probable need for valve replacement.[33-35] Although they are generally susceptible to ceftriaxone, antibiotic resistance is widespread among *N. gonorrhoeae*; accordingly, treatment must be based upon the susceptibility of the implicated isolate. Other *Neisseria* species (nongonococcal, nonmeningococcal) cause rare episodes of IE, usually in the setting of preexisting valvulopathy.[34]

OTHER ORGANISMS. *Corynebacterium* species, often called diphtheroids, although often contaminants in blood cultures, cannot be ignored when isolated from multiple blood cultures. Prolonged incubation of blood cultures is often required to isolate these slow-growing, fastidious organisms from patients with IE. They are an important cause of PVE occurring during the initial year after valve surgery and a surprisingly common cause of endocarditis involving abnormal valves.[18,35,36] *Listeria monocytogenes,* a small gram-positive rod, causes occasional cases of IE involving abnormal left heart valves and prosthetic devices,[35] most commonly in immune-compromised patients. *Tropheryma whippelii,* the cause of Whipple disease, has caused a cryptic afebrile form of IE with associated arthralgias but without diarrhea as well as valvular disease as part of typical Whipple disease.[37] The diagnosis has been established by identification of the organism in macrophages in resected valves using periodic acid–Schiff stain or by polymerase chain reaction (PCR).[34,38] Valve involvement may complicate Whipple disease more frequently than recognized. IE caused by *T. whippelii* often does not fulfill the Duke criteria for diagnosis (Table 58–4); thus, detection requires a high index of suspicion.[34,37]

The rickettsia *C. burnetii* infects humans after inhalation of desiccated materials from infected livestock or pets or contact with infected parturient animals. At variable intervals after acute infection by *C. burnetii* (Q fever), persons with abnormal mitral or aortic valves, particularly those with prosthetic valves, who have not been able to eradicate the organism develop very insidious subacute IE.[8,39] Endocarditis-prone patients with acute Q fever should receive prolonged antibiotic treatment with doxycycline plus hydroxychloroquine to prevent IE.[39] IE commonly arises with low-grade fever, fatigue, weight loss, and CHF. Hepatosplenomegaly, digital clubbing, and an immune complex vasculitis–induced purpuric rash are not uncommon. Vegetations are small, have smooth surfaces, and are not uniformly visible. On pathological examination, the vegetations of Q fever IE are nodular with a smooth surface (compared with other causes of IE) and the organisms are detected by immunohistological or Gimenez stains nearly exclusively within macrophages or by PCR.[34] The diagnosis is typically based on high antiphase I immunoglobulin G antibody titers to phase I *C. burnetii* antigens plus immunoglobulin A antibody or on demonstration of the organism in excised cardiac valves by immunohistological or Gimenez staining.[8]

Bartonella quintana and *Bartonella henselae*, which together may cause 3 percent of NVE, can be isolated from blood cultures by prolonged incubation and special techniques. In the absence of special culturing efforts, PCR detection of genetic material in excised vegetations, or serological testing, many cases would have been "culture negative."[9,34] *B. henselae*, which causes cat-scratch disease and in the HIV-infected population bacillary angiomatosis and hepatic peliosis, causes IE in patients with prior valve injury and cat exposure. In contrast, *B. quintana*, the agent of trench fever, causes IE largely in homeless people who are exposed to body lice and commonly occurs in the absence of prior valvular disease.[34] *Bartonella* IE arises insidiously; diagnosis is often delayed, and CHF and systemic emboli frequently complicate infection.[9,34] *Bartonella* infection destroys valve tissue and therapy commonly requires valve surgery.[34,40] On the basis of serological testing, *Chlamydia* species have been suggested as the cause of frequent episodes of IE. Because of the extensive serological cross-reaction between *Chlamydia* and *Bartonella*, many of these episodes have actually been *Bartonella* IE.[9,34]

FUNGI. *Candida albicans,* nonalbicans *Candida* species, *Histoplasma*, and *Aspergillus* species are the most common of the many fungal organisms identified as causing IE.[38] Unusual so-called emerging

TABLE 58–4 Diagnosis of Infective Endocarditis (Modified Duke Criteria)

Definitive Infective Endocarditis
Pathological criteria
- Microorganisms: demonstrated by culture or histology in a vegetation, *or* in a vegetation that has embolized, *or* in an intracardiac abscess, *or*
- Pathological lesions: vegetation or intracardiac abscess present, confirmed by histology showing active endocarditis

Clinical criteria, using specific definitions listed below
- Two major criteria, *or*
- One major and three minor criteria, *or*
- Five minor criteria

Possible Infective Endocarditis
One major criterion and one minor criterion or three minor criteria

Rejected
Firm alternative diagnosis for manifestations of endocarditis, *or*
Sustained resolution of manifestations of endocarditis, with antibiotic therapy for 4 days or less, *or*
No pathological evidence of infective endocarditis at surgery or autopsy, after antibiotic therapy for 4 days or less

Criteria for Diagnosis of Infective Endocarditis
Major criteria
Positive blood culture
- Typical microorganism for infective endocarditis from two separate blood cultures
  - Viridans streptococci, *Streptococcus bovis*, HACEK group *or Staphylococcus aureus* or community-acquired enterococci in the absence of a primary focus, *or*
- Persistently positive blood culture, defined as recovery of a microorganism consistent with infective endocarditis from:
  - Blood cultures (≥2) drawn more than 12 hr apart, *or*
  - All of three or a majority of four or more separate blood cultures, with first and last drawn at least 1 hr apart
- Single positive blood culture for *coxiella burnetii* or antiphase I IgG antibody titer >1:800

Evidence of endocardial involvement
- Positive echocardiogram
  - (TEE advised for PVE or complicated IE)
  - Oscillating intracardiac mass, on valve or supporting structures, *or* in the path of regurgitant jets, *or* on implanted material, in the absence of an alternative anatomical explanation, *or*
  - Abscess, *or*
  - New partial dehiscence of prosthetic valve, *or*
- New valvular regurgitation (increase or change in preexisting murmur not sufficient)

Minor criteria
Predisposition: predisposing heart condition *or* intravenous drug use
Fever ≥38.0°C (100.4°F)
Vascular phenomena: major arterial emboli, septic pulmonary infarcts, mycotic aneurysm, intracranial hemorrhage, conjunctival hemorrhages, Janeway lesions
Immunological phenomena: glomerulonephritis, Osler nodes, Roth spots, rheumatoid factor
Microbiological evidence: positive blood culture but not meeting major criterion as noted previously* *or* serologic evidence of active infection with organism consistent with infective endocarditis

IE = infective endocarditis; IgG = immunoglobulin G; PVE = prosthetic valve endocarditis; TEE = transesophageal echocardiography.

Adapted from Durack DT, Lukes AS, Bright DK: New criteria for diagnosis of infective endocarditis: Utilization of specific echocardiographic findings. Am J Med 96:200, 1994; modified per Li JS, Sexton DJ, Mick N, et al: Proposed modifications to the Duke criteria for the diagnosis of infective endocarditis. Clin Infect Dis 30:633, 2000.

*Excluding single positive cultures for coagulase-negative staphylococci and organisms that do not cause endocarditis commonly.

fungi and molds account for 25 percent of cases. Among 269 cases of fungal IE described between 1965 and 1995, 25 percent were nosocomial.[41] Risk factors include previous valve surgery, antibiotic use, injection drug abuse, intravascular catheters, surgery other than cardiac, and immunocompromised state. The last three have increased, and virtually all patients have two or more risk factors. Fever, new or changing murmurs, systemic embolization including major limb artery occlusion, neurological abnormalities, and heart failure are common symptoms. Blood cultures are positive commonly when IE is caused by *Candida* species but rarely when caused by mycelial organisms. Culture and histological examination of vegetations yield a microbiological diagnosis in 75 and 95 percent of cases, respectively, and 65 percent of embolic vegetations from peripheral arteries are diagnostic.

Pathogenesis

The interactions between the human host and selected microorganisms that culminate in IE involve the vascular endothelium, hemostatic mechanisms, the host immune system, gross anatomical abnormalities in the heart, surface properties of microorganisms, enzyme and toxin production by microorganisms, and peripheral events that initiate bacteremia. Each component of these interactions is in itself complex, influenced by many factors and not fully elucidated. These complex interactions result in a pathogenetic sequence wherein microorganisms adhere to valve surfaces, become persistent at the site of adherence, proliferate to cause local damage and vegetation growth, and ultimately disseminate hematogenously. Detailed in vitro and in vivo studies, aided by genetic manipulations, have begun to elucidate the pathogenesis of IE caused by viridans streptococci and *S. aureus*.[42] The rarity of endocarditis in spite of frequent transient asymptomatic and symptomatic bacteremia indicates that the intact endothelium is relatively resistant to infection. Endothelial damage results in platelet-fibrin deposition, which in turn is more receptive to colonization by bacteria than is the intact endothelium. It is hypothesized that platelet-fibrin deposition occurs spontaneously in persons with valvular disease and that these deposits, called nonbacterial thrombotic endocarditis (NBTE), are the sites at which microorganisms adhere during bacteremia to initiate IE.[43]

DEVELOPMENT OF NONBACTERIAL THROMBOTIC ENDOCARDITIS. Two major mechanisms appear pivotal in the formation of NBTE: endothelial injury and a hypercoagulable state. NBTE has been found in 1.3 percent of patients at autopsy and is more common with increasing age and in patients with malignancy, disseminated intravascular coagulation, uremia, burns, systemic lupus erythematosus, valvular heart disease, and intracardiac catheters.[44] NBTE deposits are found at the valve closure contact line on the atrial surfaces of the mitral and tricuspid valves and on the ventricular surfaces of the aortic and pulmonic valves, the sites of infected vegetations in patients with IE.

Three hemodynamic circumstances may injure the endothelium, initiating NBTE: (1) a high-velocity jet striking endothelium, (2) flow from a high- to a low-pressure chamber, and (3) flow across a narrow orifice at high velocity. Flow through a narrowed orifice, as a consequence of the Venturi effect, deposits bacteria maximally at the low-pressure sink immediately beyond an orifice or at the site where a jet stream strikes a surface. These are the same sites where NBTE forms as a result of hemodynamic circumstances. The superimposition of NBTE formation and preferential deposition of bacteria helps to explain the distribution of infected vegetations.[45]

CONVERSION OF NONBACTERIAL THROMBOTIC ENDOCARDITIS TO INFECTIVE ENDOCARDITIS. Bacteremia is the initiating event that ultimately converts NBTE to IE. The frequency and magnitude of bacteremia associated with daily activities and health care procedures appear related to specific mucosal surfaces and skin, the density of colonizing bacteria, the disease state of the surface, and the extent of the local trauma. Bacteremia rates are highest for events that traumatize the oral mucosa, particularly the gingiva, and progressively decrease with procedures involving the genitourinary tract and the gastrointestinal tract. A diseased mucosal surface—particularly one that is infected—is associated with an increased risk of bacteremia.

For viable circulating microorganisms to reach NBTE, they must be resistant to the complement-mediated bactericidal activity of serum.

The adherence of microorganisms to the NBTE or to apparently intact valve endothelium is a pivotal early event in the development of IE. Redundant interacting bacterial surface molecules mediate adherence to host extracellular matrix molecules on valve endothelium or NBTE. Collectively, these bacterial molecules are known as microbial surface components recognizing adhesive matrix molecules (MSCRAMMs). Streptococci that produce surface polysaccharides called glucans or dextran cause endocarditis more frequently than strains that do not produce dextran. Dextran on the surface of streptococci can be shown to mediate adherence to platelet fibrin lattices and injured valves and to facilitate development of endocarditis in experimental models.[42,44] Dextran production, however, is not universal among the major microbial causes of IE; thus, other mechanisms of adherence are likely. For example, Fim A protein of *Streptococcus parasanguis*, which belongs to a family of oral mucosal adhesins in viridans streptococci, facilitates adherence to fibrin and development of experimental endocarditis.[42]

Fibronectin, an important factor in the pathogenesis of IE, has been identified in lesions on heart valves and is produced by endothelial cells, platelets, and fibroblasts in response to vascular injury; a soluble form binds to exposed subendothelial collagen. Receptors for fibronectin, MSCRAMMs, are present on the surface of *S. aureus*; viridans streptococci; group A, C, and G streptococci; enterococci; *S. pneumoniae*; and *C. albicans*. Fibronectin has numerous binding domains and thus can bind simultaneously to fibrin, collagen, cells, and microorganisms and facilitate adherence of bacteria to the valve at the site of injury or NBTE. Fibronectin binding proteins A and B in *S. aureus* are critical in the induction of experimental endocarditis. Clumping factor (or fibrinogen-binding surface protein) of *S. aureus* also mediates the binding of these organisms to platelet fibrin thrombi and to aortic valves in models of endocarditis.[42] The glycocalyx or slime on the surface of *S. epidermidis* does not appear to function as an adhesin but may render organisms more virulent by enhancing their ability to avoid eradication by host defenses.

The mechanism by which virulent organisms colonize and infect intact valvular endothelium is less clearly understood. In elderly people, degenerative valve sclerosis may be associated with local inflammation, which in turn may promote endothelial cell binding of fibronectin and other extracellular matrix molecules. Particulate material injected during IV drug abuse might stimulate similar endothelial events. These endothelial changes could promote *S. aureus* adherence through MSCRAMMs to apparently normal valves.[42] Binding of *S. aureus* fibronectin-binding protein is required for the invasion of intact endothelial cells.[42] Multiplication of the organism intracellularly results in cell death, which in turn disrupts the endothelial surface and initiates formation of platelet-fibrin deposits and additional sites for bacterial adherence.

After adherence to NBTE or the endothelium, bacteria must persist and multiply if IE is to develop. Resistance of viridans streptococci and *S. aureus* to platelet antimicrobial proteins is associated with increased ability to cause experimental endocarditis.[42] Persistence and multiplication result in a complex dynamic process during which the infected vegetation increases in size by platelet-fibrin aggregation, microorganisms multiply and are shed into the blood, and vegetation fragments embolize. Staphylococcal and streptococcal surface proteins bind to platelets and promote aggregation and growth of the vegetation. Organisms that bind and aggregate platelets are more virulent in experimental models.[42] In addition, both streptococci and staphylococci increase local procoagulant activity by inducing fibrin-adherent monocytes to elaborate tissue factor (a tissue thromboplastin that binds to activated factor VII to initiate clotting).[42] Also, *S. aureus* can induce tissue factor production by endothelial cells, which would facilitate endocarditis development on normal valves.[42] Multiple replications of this cycle from adherence to multiplication and platelet-fibrin deposition result in clinical IE.

Pathophysiology

Aside from the constitutional symptoms of infection, which are probably mediated by cytokines, the clinical manifestations of IE result from (1) the local destructive effects of intracardiac infection; (2) the embolization of bland or septic fragments of vegetations to distant sites, resulting in infarction or infection; (3) the hematogenous seeding of remote sites during continuous bacteremia; and (4) an antibody response to the infecting organism with subsequent tissue injury caused by deposition of preformed immune complexes or antibody-complement interaction with antigens deposited in tissues.

The intracardiac consequences of IE range from trivial, characterized by an infected vegetation with no attendant tissue damage, to catastrophic, when infection is locally destructive or extends beyond the valve leaflet. Distortion or perforation of valve leaflets, rupture of chordae tendineae, and perforations or fistulas between major vessels and cardiac chambers or between chambers themselves as a consequence of burrowing infection may result in CHF that is progressive (Fig. 58–2).[46-48] Infection, particularly that involving the aortic valve or prosthetic valves, may extend into paravalvular tissue and result in abscesses and persistent fever related to antibiotic-unresponsive infection, disruption of the conduction system with electrocardiographic conduction abnormalities and clinically relevant arrhythmias, or purulent pericarditis.[48] Large vegetations, particularly at the mitral valve, can result in functional valvular stenosis and hemodynamic deterioration.[18,49] In general, intracardiac complications involving the aortic valve evolve more rapidly than those associated with the mitral valve; nevertheless, the progression is highly variable and unpredictable in individual patients.

Embolization of fragments from vegetations producing symptoms by infection or infarction is clinically evident in 11 to 43 percent of patients.[45,50-52] However, pathological evidence of emboli at autopsy is found more frequently (45 to 65 percent). Pulmonary emboli, which are often septic, occur in 66 to 75 percent of IV drug abusers with tricuspid valve IE.[10,11] The persistent bacteremia of IE, with or without septic emboli, may result in metastatic infection in any organ or tissue. These infections, which may vary in size from small miliary to large abscesses, may be manifest as local signs and symptoms or as persistent fever during therapy. IE caused by virulent organisms, particularly *S. aureus* or beta-hemolytic streptococci, is complicated more frequently by metastatic infection than that due to avirulent bacteria, e.g., viridans streptococci.[21,27] Metastatic abscesses are often small and miliary. Metastatic infection assumes particular importance when the required therapy is more than the antibiotics indicated for IE or when these infections constitute a focus that engenders relapse.

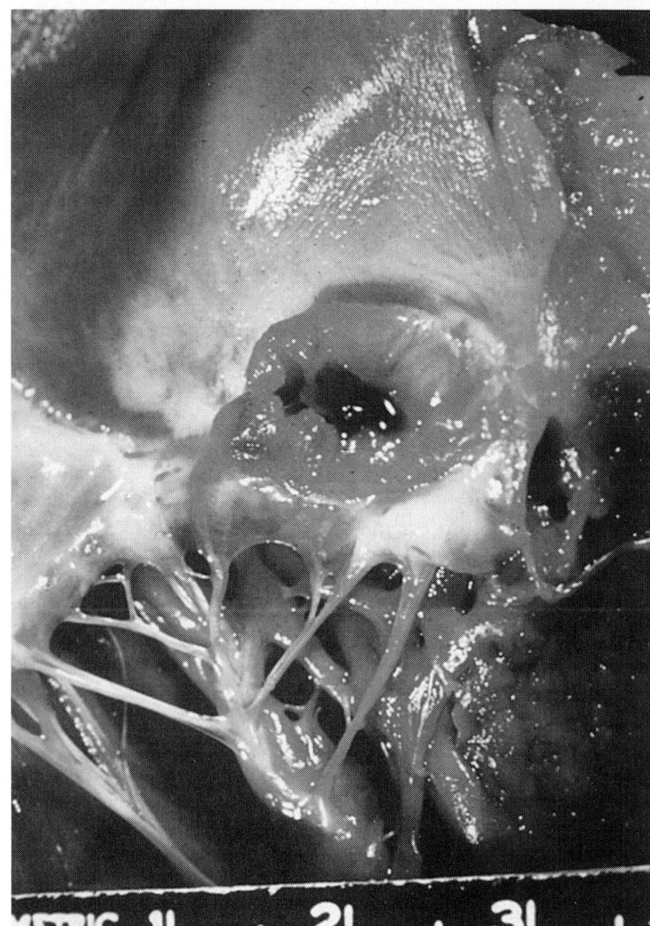

FIGURE 58–2 A normal valve with a large, bulky vegetation caused by *Staphylococcus aureus* infection. Clot is present centrally in the vegetation, obscuring a valve fenestration.

Clinical Features

The interval between the presumed initiating bacteremia and the onset of symptoms of IE is estimated to be less than 2 weeks in more than 80 percent of patients with NVE. Interestingly, in some patients with intraoperative or perioperative infection of prosthetic valves, the incubation period may be prolonged (2 to 5 or more months).[18]

Fever is the most common symptom and sign in patients with IE (Table 58–5). Fever may be absent or minimal in elderly persons or in those with CHF, severe debility, or chronic renal failure and occasionally in patients with NVE caused by coagulase-negative staphylococci.[30,53] *Heart murmurs* are noted in 80 to 85 percent of patients with NVE and are emblematic of the lesion predisposing to IE. Murmurs are commonly not audible in patients with tricuspid valve IE. Similarly, in acute NVE caused by *S. aureus,* murmurs are heard in only 30 to 45 percent of patients on initial evaluation but are ultimately noted in 75 to 85 percent. The new or changing murmurs (alterations unrelated to heart rate or cardiac output but rather regurgitant murmurs indicative of valve dysfunction) are relatively infrequent in subacute NVE and are more prevalent in acute IE and PVE.[18] They are frequently important harbingers of CHF. *Enlargement of the spleen* is noted in 15 to 50 percent of patients and is more common in subacute IE of long duration.

TABLE 58–5 Clinical Features of Infective Endocarditis

Symptoms	Percent	Signs	Percent
Fever	80-85	Fever	80-90
Chills	42-75	Murmur	80-85
Sweats	25	Changing/new murmur	10-40
Anorexia	25-55	Neurological abnormalities†	30-40
Weight loss	25-35	Embolic event	20-40
Malaise	25-40	Splenomegaly	15-50
Dyspnea	20-40	Clubbing	10-20
Cough	25	Peripheral manifestation	
Stroke	13-20	Osler nodes	7-10
Headache	15-40	Splinter hemorrhage	5-15
Nausea/vomiting	15-20	Petechiae	10-40
Myalgia/arthralgia	15-30	Janeway lesion	6-10
Chest pain*	8-35	Retinal lesion/Roth spots	4-10
Abdominal pain	5-15		
Back pain	7-10		
Confusion	10-20		

*More common in intravenous drug abusers.
†Central nervous system.

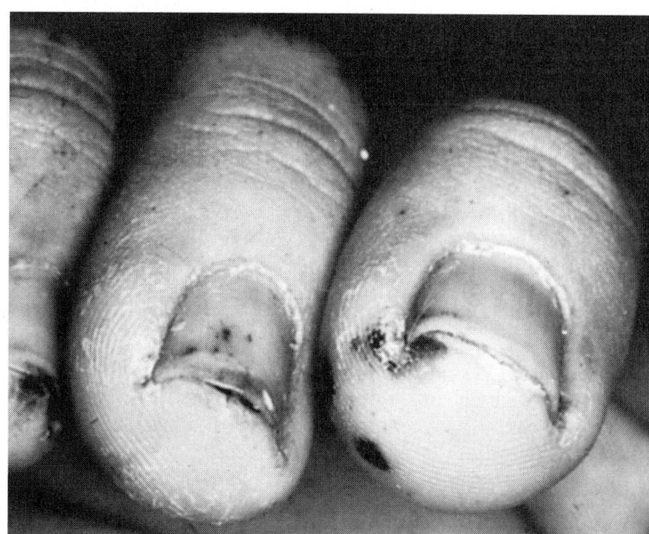

FIGURE 58–4 Subungual hemorrhages (splinter hemorrhages) and digital petechiae in a patient with infective endocarditis. (From Korzeniowski OM, Kaye D: Infective endocarditis. *In* Braunwald E [ed]: Heart Disease. 4th ed. Philadelphia, WB Saunders, 1992, p 1087.)

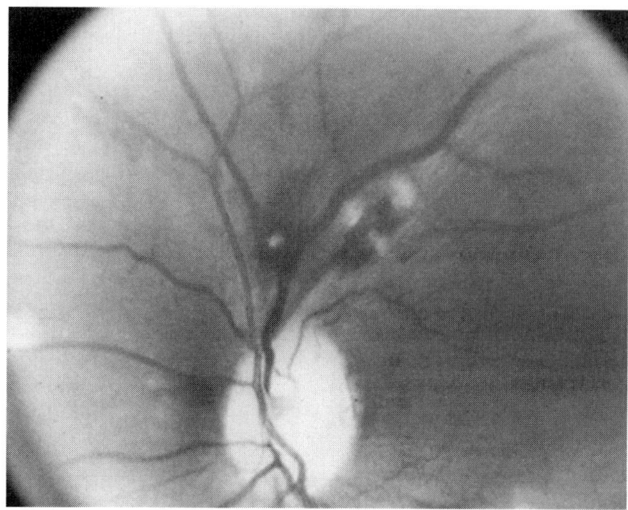

FIGURE 58–5 Roth spot (retinal hemorrhage with a clear center) in a patient with infective endocarditis. (From Korzeniowski OM, Kaye D: Infective endocarditis. *In* Braunwald E [ed]: Heart Disease. 4th ed. Philadelphia, WB Saunders, 1992, p 1087.)

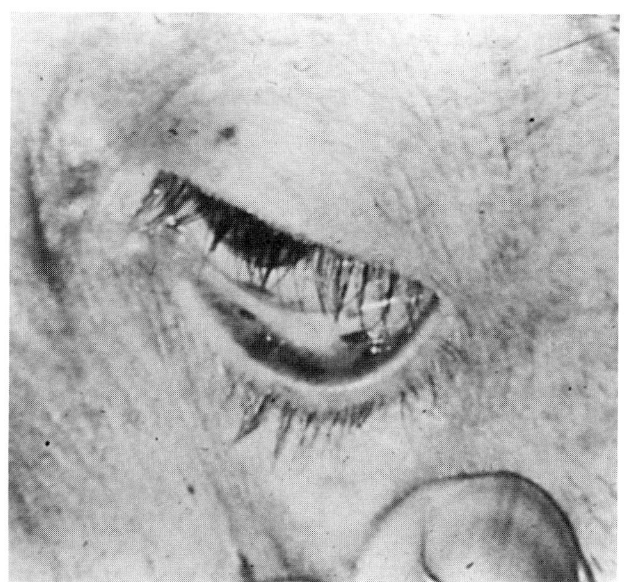

FIGURE 58–3 Conjunctival petechiae in a patient with infective endocarditis. (From Kaye D: Infective Endocarditis. Baltimore, University Park Press, 1976.)

The classical peripheral manifestations of IE are encountered less frequently today and are absent in IE restricted to the tricuspid valve.[10,54] *Petechiae* (Fig. 58–3), the most common of these manifestations, are found on the palpebral conjunctiva, the buccal and palatal mucosa, and the extremities. They are not specific for endocarditis even on the conjunctiva. *Splinter* or *subungual hemorrhages* (Fig. 58–4) are dark red, linear, or occasionally flame-shaped streaks in the nail bed of the fingers or toes. Distal lesions are probably due to trauma, whereas the more proximal ones are more likely to be related to IE. *Osler nodes* are small, tender subcutaneous nodules that develop in the pulp of the digits or occasionally more proximally in the fingers and persist for hours to several days. These, too, are not pathognomonic for IE. Janeway lesions are small erythematous or hemorrhagic macular nontender lesions on the palms and soles and are the consequence of septic embolic events. Roth spots (Fig. 58–5), oval retinal hemorrhages with pale centers, are infrequent findings in patients with IE. They have been noted in patients with collagen-vascular disease and hematological disorders, including severe anemia.

Musculoskeletal symptoms, unrelated to focal infection, are relatively common in patients with IE. These include arthralgias and myalgias, occasional true arthritis with nondiagnostic but inflammatory synovial fluid findings, and prominent back pain without evidence of vertebral body, disc space, or sacroiliac joint infection. In patients with arthritis or back pain, focal infection must be excluded because additional therapy may be required.

Systemic emboli are among the most common clinical sequelae of IE, occurring in up to 40 percent of patients, and are frequent subclinical events found only at autopsy.[45,50-52,54] Emboli often antedate diagnosis. Although embolic events may occur during or after antimicrobial therapy, the incidence decreases promptly during administration of effective antibiotic therapy.[53,55] Embolic splenic infarction may cause left upper quadrant abdominal pain and left shoulder pain. Renal emboli may occur asymptomatically or with flank pain and may cause gross or microscopic hematuria. Embolic stroke syndromes, predominantly involving the middle cerebral artery territory, occur in 15 to 20 percent of patients with NVE and PVE.[18] Coronary artery emboli are common findings at autopsy but rarely result in transmural infarction. Emboli to the extremities may produce pain and overt ischemia, and those to mesenteric arteries may cause abdominal pain, ileus, and guaiac-positive stools.

Neurological symptoms and signs occur in 30 to 40 percent of patients with IE, are more frequent when IE is caused by *S. aureus*, and are associated with increased mortality rates.[50,56,57] Embolic stroke is the most common and clinically important of the neurological manifestations. Intracranial hemorrhage occurs in 5 percent of patients with IE. Bleeding results from rupture of a mycotic aneurysm, rupture of an artery related to septic arteritis at the site of embolic occlusion, or hemorrhage into an infarct.[58] Mycotic aneurysms, with or without rupture, occur in 2 to 10 percent of patients with IE; approximately half of these involve intracranial arteries (Fig. 58–6). Cerebritis with microabscesses complicates IE caused by invasive pathogens such as *S. aureus*, but large brain abscesses are rare. Purulent meningitis complicates some episodes of IE caused by *S. aureus* or *S. pneumoniae*, but more typically the cerebrospinal fluid has an aseptic profile.[29,56] Other neurological manifestations include severe headache (a potential clue to a mycotic aneurysm), seizure, and encephalopathy.

Heart murmurs complicating IE are primarily the result of valve destruction or distortion or rupture of chordae tendineae. Intracardiac fistulas, myocarditis, or coronary artery embolization may occasionally contribute to the genesis of CHF, as obviously can underlying cardiac disease. In the absence of surgery to correct valvular dysfunction, CHF, particularly that related to aortic insufficiency, is associated with very high mortality rates.[46]

Renal insufficiency as a result of immune complex–mediated glomerulonephritis occurs in less than 15 percent of patients with IE. Azotemia as a result of this process may develop or progress during initial therapy; it usually improves with continued administration of effective antibiotic therapy. Focal glomerulonephritis and embolic renal infarcts cause hematuria but rarely result in azotemia. Renal dysfunction in patients with IE is most commonly a manifestation of impaired hemodynamics or toxicities associated with antimicrobial therapy (interstitial nephritis or aminoglycoside-induced injury).

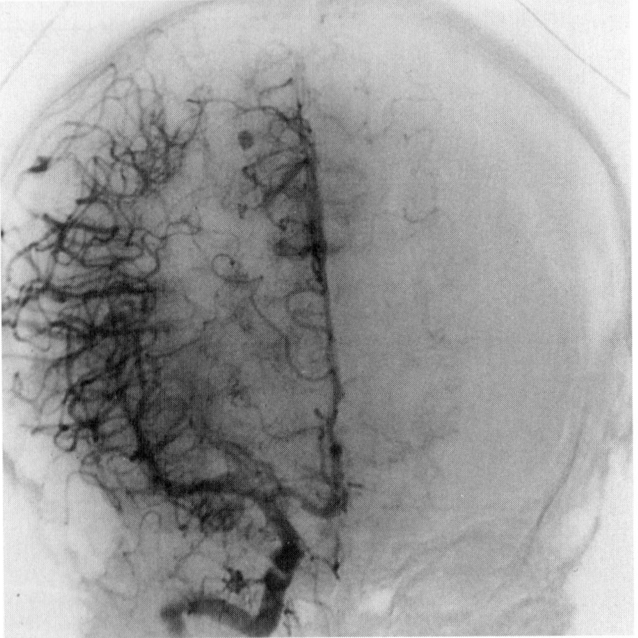

FIGURE 58–6 An irregular mycotic aneurysm of the middle cerebral artery lies laterally on the cerebral cortex. A second aneurysm is projected just lateral to the anterior cerebral artery.

Diagnosis

The symptoms and signs of endocarditis are often constitutional and, when localized, often result from a complication of IE rather than reflect the intracardiac infection itself (see Table 58–5). Consequently, if physicians are to avoid overlooking the diagnosis of IE, a high index of suspicion must be maintained. The diagnosis must be investigated when patients with fever present with one or more of the cardinal elements of IE: a predisposing cardiac lesion or behavior pattern, bacteremia, embolic phenomenon, and evidence of an active endocardial process. Because patients with prosthetic heart valves are always at risk for PVE, the presence of fever or new prosthesis dysfunction at any time warrants considering this diagnosis. In patients at risk for endocarditis, concurrent illnesses or iatrogenic events may create clusters of symptoms and signs that superficially mimic IE and require careful consideration to arrive at a correct diagnosis. Even when the illness seems typical of endocarditis, the definitive diagnosis requires positive blood cultures or positive cultures (or histology or PCR recovery of a microorganism's DNA) from the vegetation or embolus. There are many culture-negative mimics of IE: atrial myxoma, acute rheumatic fever, systemic lupus erythematosus or other collagen-vascular disease, marantic endocarditis, the antiphospholipid syndrome, carcinoid syndrome, renal cell carcinoma with increased cardiac output, and thrombotic thrombocytopenic purpura.

The modified Duke criteria provide a schema that facilitates evaluating patients for endocarditis (see Table 58–4).[59,60] Clinical and laboratory data, including echocardiography, should be collected in a manner that allows one to assess the presence or absence of the listed major and minor criteria. Finding evidence of two major or one major plus three minor or five minor criteria establishes a clinical diagnosis of "definite endocarditis," whereas finding one major plus one minor or three minor criteria indicates "possible endocarditis." When used judiciously over the entire evaluation, i.e., not limited to initial findings, these criteria are sensitive and specific for the diagnosis of IE (see Table 58–4).[59-61] Erroneous rejection of the diagnosis of endocarditis is unlikely. When these diagnostic criteria are used to guide therapy, patients who are categorized with possible endocarditis should be treated as if they have IE. Requiring at least one major criterion or three minor criteria to designate possible endocarditis reduces the potential for overdiagnosis (failure to reject the diagnosis) and the likelihood of treating uninfected patients.[60]

To use bacteremia caused by coagulase-negative staphylococci or diphtheroids (organisms that may cause IE but more often contaminate blood cultures) to support the diagnosis of endocarditis, blood cultures must be persistently positive or the organisms recovered in several sporadically positive cultures must be proved to represent a single clone.[59,60] These considerations are embodied in the diagnostic criteria (see Table 58–4).[57-59]

ECHOCARDIOGRAPHY. Inclusion of echocardiographic evidence of endocardial infection in these criteria recognizes the high sensitivity of two-dimensional echocardiography with color Doppler, especially if multiplanar TEE and TTE are combined, and the relative infrequency of false-positive studies when experienced operators use specific definitions for vegetations.[61,62] Although the sensitivity of TEE to detect vegetations in patients with suspected IE ranges from 85 to 95 percent (or higher if a follow-up study is performed), a negative study result does not preclude the diagnosis or the need for therapy if the clinical suspicion is high.[62] The likelihood of a false-negative result can be reduced to 5 to 10 percent if TEE is repeated, especially if the study is biplanar or multiplanar.[61,62] Thus, these studies help to preclude the diagnosis when the clinical suspicion is low.[61,62] Nevertheless, when the clinical suspicion is high, even these highly sensitive tests cannot preclude the diagnosis. In addition, because the echocardiogram cannot distinguish healed vegetations and valvular masses from actively infected vegetations, these guidelines are vulnerable to misidentifying as culture-negative IE the vegetations that complicate marasmus, malignancy, cryptic collagen-vascular disease, or the antiphospholipid antibody syndrome.

ESTABLISHING THE MICROBIAL CAUSE. A microbial cause of IE is established by recovering the infecting agent from the blood or by identifying it in surgically removed vegetations or embolic material. In detecting the bacteremia of IE, there is no advantage to obtaining blood cultures in relationship to fever or from arterial blood (as opposed to venous blood). In patients who have not received prior antibiotics and who will ultimately have blood culture-positive IE, it is likely that 95 to 100 percent of all cultures obtained will be positive and that one of the first two cultures will be positive in at least 95 percent of patients. Prior antibiotic therapy is a major cause of blood culture–negative IE, particularly when the causative microorganism is highly antibiotic susceptible. At least 35 percent of cases of culture-negative IE can be attributed to prior antimicrobial therapy.[63] After subtherapeutic antibiotic exposure, the time required for reversion to positive cultures is directly related to the duration of antimicrobial therapy and the susceptibility of the causative agent; days to a week or more may be required.

OBTAINING BLOOD CULTURES. Three separate sets of blood cultures, each from a separate venipuncture, obtained over 24 hours, are recommended to evaluate patients with suspected endocarditis.[61] Each set should include two flasks, one containing an aerobic medium and the other containing thioglycollate broth (anaerobic medium), into each of which at least 10 ml of blood should be placed.[64]

For optimal processing, the laboratory should be advised that endocarditis is a possible diagnosis and which, if any, unusual bacteria are suspected (*Legionella* species, *Bartonella* species, HACEK organisms). If a clinically stable patient has received an antimicrobial agent during the past several weeks, it is prudent to delay therapy so that repeated cultures can be obtained on successive days.[64] If fungal endocarditis is suspected, blood cultures should be obtained using the lysis-centrifugation method. The laboratory should be asked to save the organism causing endocarditis until successful therapy has been completed. Serological tests are occasionally used to make the presumptive etiological diagnosis of endocarditis caused by *Brucella* species, *Legionella* species, *Bartonella* species, *C. burnetii*, or *Chlamydia* species. By special techniques, including PCR, these agents and others that are difficult to recover in blood culture can be identified in blood or vegetations.[8,38,61,65]

Sustained bacteremia is typical of IE. In evaluating positive blood cultures, sustained bacteremia (persisting over 1 hour) should be distinguished from transient bacteremia. When several blood cultures obtained over 24 hours or more are positive, the diagnosis of IE must be considered. The identity of the organism is also helpful in determining the intensity with which the diagnosis is entertained. Organisms can be divided into those that commonly cause IE, those that rarely cause IE, and the intermediate-behaving organisms, e.g., enterococci and *S. aureus*, which, when in the blood, may or may not indicate IE. Finally, the presence or absence of alternative sources for the bacteremia aids in the assessment of bacteremia.

Laboratory Tests

Many other tests are inevitably performed in the evaluation of patients with suspected IE. Hematological parameters are commonly abnormal. Anemia, with normochromic normocytic red blood cell indices, a low serum iron level, and low serum iron-binding capacity, is found in 70 to 90 percent of patients. Anemia worsens with increased duration of illness and thus in acute IE may be absent. In subacute IE, the white blood cell count is usually normal; in contrast, a leukocytosis with increased segmented granulocytes is common in acute IE. Thrombocytopenia occurs only rarely.

The *erythrocyte sedimentation rate* (ESR) is elevated (average approximately 55 mm/hr) in almost all patients with IE; the exceptions are those with CHF, renal failure, or disseminated intravascular coagulation. Other tests often indicate immune stimulation or inflammation (see Pathophysiology): circulating immune complexes, rheumatoid factor, quantitative immune globulin determinations, cryoglobulins, and C-reactive protein. Although the results of these tests parallel disease activity, the tests are costly and not efficient ways to diagnose IE or monitor response to therapy. Measurement of circulating immune complexes and complement may be useful in evaluating for azotemia related to diffuse immune complex glomerulonephritis.

The *urinalysis* result is often abnormal, even when renal function remains normal. Proteinuria and microscopic hematuria are noted in 50 percent of patients.

Echocardiography (see also Chap. 11)

Evaluation of patients with clinically suspected IE by this technique frequently allows morphological confirmation of infection and increasingly aids in decisions about management.[62,66] Echocardiography should not be used as a screening test for IE in unselected patients with positive blood cultures or in patients with fevers of unknown origin when the clinical probability is low.[61,67] Nevertheless, echocardiographic evaluation should be performed in most patients with clinically suspected IE, especially those with negative blood cultures.[61] Although many patients with NVE involving the aortic or mitral valve can be imaged adequately by TTE, TEE using biplane or multiplane technology with incorporated color flow and continuous as well as pulsed Doppler is the state of the art.[67-69] TEE allows visualization of smaller vegetations and provides improved resolution compared with TTE. Not only is TEE the preferred approach in patients with clinically suspected IE in whom TTE is suboptimal, it is also the procedure of choice for imaging the pulmonic valve, patients with PVE (especially at the mitral site), and patients who are at high risk for intracardiac complications or those with signs of persistent or invasive infection despite adequate antimicrobial therapy.[61,68-70]

A decision analysis evaluation of echocardiography for diagnosis of NVE in patients with bacteremia suggests that, assuming the diagnostic enhancement of TEE over TTE is 15 percent, the most cost-effective strategy (yielding optional quality-adjusted life-years) is as follows: (1) if prior probability of IE is less than 2 percent, treat for bacteremia without echocardiography; (2) if prior probability is 2 to 4 percent, use TTE; and (3) if prior probability is 5 to 45 percent, use TEE initially in lieu of TTE. If the prior probability of IE is greater than 45 percent, therapy without echocardiography is cost effective, although studies may still be desirable to evaluate for complications and other risks.[24] The high frequency of IE patients with a high prior probability of endocarditis results in studies that demonstrate that data from TEE rarely alter clinical management plans built on data from TTE.[67,68]

TEE becomes pivotal when TTE is a technically inadequate study, when PVE is sought, and when the clinical prior probability is medium.

Another cost-effectiveness analysis suggests that in patients with clinically uncomplicated catheter-associated *S. aureus* bacteremia, evaluation with TEE to determine duration of antibiotic therapy (4 versus 2 weeks, i.e., treatment of endocarditis or not) is more cost effective than empirical selection of either duration of therapy.[23] The strategy of diagnosing IE by TTE to be followed by TEE if negative was not evaluated, but given the anticipated prior probability of IE (≥6 percent) it would probably be more costly.

The sensitivity of TTE for the detection of vegetations in NVE is approximately 65 percent. In contrast, in NVE, the sensitivity of TEE for vegetation detection ranges from 85 to 95 percent.[62] In patients with PVE, TTE is limited by the shadowing effect of the prostheses, especially in the mitral position, and its diagnostic sensitivity is reduced to 15 to 35 percent. In contrast, the sensitivity of TEE for detecting vegetations in PVE involving mechanical or bioprosthetic devices in the aortic or mitral position ranged from 82 to 96 percent.[70,71]

Despite the sensitivity of TEE in detecting vegetations in patients with proven IE, echocardiography does not itself provide a definite diagnosis. Vegetations and valve dysfunction may be demonstrated, but determination of causality requires clinical or direct anatomical and microbiological confirmation. Infectious vegetations cannot be distinguished on the echocardiogram from marantic lesions, nor can vegetations be distinguished from thrombus or pannus on prostheses. Furthermore, it is usually not possible to distinguish active from healed vegetations in NVE.[72] Thickened valves, ruptured chordae or valves, valve calcification, and nodules may be mistaken for vegetations, indicating the specificity limitations of isolated echocardiography.

Valve dysfunction caused by tissue disruption, leaflet perforation, or large obstructing vegetations can be visualized and quantitated by echocardiogram with Doppler. Some degree of regurgitation by Doppler is almost universal early in the course of NVE and PVE and does not necessarily predict progressive hemodynamic deterioration. Extension of infection beyond the valve leaflet into surrounding tissue results in abscesses in various areas of the annulus or adjacent structures, mycotic aneurysms of the sinus of Valsalva or mitral valve, intracardiac fistulas, and purulent pericarditis. Myocardial abscesses are more readily detected by TEE than TTE in patients with NVE or PVE.[70,71] The sensitivity and specificity for abscess detection were 28 percent and 98 percent for TTE, compared with 87 percent and 95 percent for TEE. TEE is also more sensitive and accurate than TTE for recognizing subaortic invasive disease and valve perforations.[73]

MAGNETIC RESONANCE AND COMPUTED TOMOGRAPHIC IMAGING. These techniques have identified paravalvular extension of infection, aortic root aneurysms, and fistulas; however, their utility relative to echocardiography has not been established.

SCINTIGRAPHY. Efforts to identify vegetations and intracardiac abscess in patients with IE and in animal models have used scintigraphy with gallium-67 citrate, indium-111-labeled granulocytes, and indium-111-labeled platelets. These efforts have not been sufficiently sensitive or anatomically localizing to be useful clinically.[74]

Treatment

Two major objectives must be achieved to treat IE effectively. The infecting microorganism in the vegetation must be eradicated. Failure to accomplish this results in relapse of infection. Also, invasive, destructive intracardiac and focal extracardiac complications of infection must be resolved if morbidity and mortality are to be minimized. The second objective often exceeds the capacity of effective antimicrobial therapy and requires cardiac or other surgical intervention.

Bacteria in vegetations multiply to population densities approaching 10^9 to 10^{10} organisms per gram of tissue, become metabolically dormant, and are difficult to eradicate. Clinical experience and animal model experiments suggest that optimal therapy should use bactericidal antibiotics or antibiotic combinations rather than bacteriostatic agents. In addition, antibiotics reach the central areas of avascular vegetations by passive diffusion. To reach effective antibiotic concentrations in vegetations, high serum concentrations must be achieved, and penetration by some agents is limited even then. Parenteral antimicrobial therapy is used whenever feasible in order to achieve suitable serum antibiotic concentrations and to avoid the potentially erratic absorption of orally administered therapy. Treatment is continued for prolonged periods to ensure eradication of dormant microorganisms.

In selecting antimicrobial therapy for patients with IE, one must consider the ability of potential agents to kill the causative organism as well as the MIC and minimum bactericidal concentration (MBC) of these antibiotics for the organism. The MIC is the lowest concentration that inhibits growth, and the MBC is the lowest concentration that decreases a standard inoculum of organisms 99.9 percent during 24 hours. For the vast majority of streptococci and staphylococci, the MIC and MBC of penicillins, cephalosporins, or vancomycin are the same or differ by only a factor of 2 to 4. Organisms for which the MBC for these antibiotics is 10-fold or greater than the MIC are occasionally encountered. This phenomenon has been termed *tolerance.*[66] Most of the tolerant strains are simply killed more slowly than nontolerant strains, and with prolonged incubation (48 hours) their MICs and MBCs are similar. Enterococci exhibit what superficially appears to be tolerance when tested against penicillins and vancomycin; however, these organisms are, in fact, not killed by these agents but are merely inhibited, even after longer incubation times. Enterococci can be killed by the combined activity of selected penicillins or vancomycin and an aminoglycoside. This enhanced antibiotic activity of the combination against enterococci, if of sufficient magnitude, is called *synergy* or a *synergistic bactericidal* effect.[66] A similar effect can be seen with these combinations against streptococci and staphylococci.

A synergistic bactericidal effect is required for optimal therapy of enterococcal endocarditis and has been used to achieve more effective therapy or effective short-course therapy of IE caused by other organisms. Tolerance in streptococci or staphylococci, although demonstrable in vivo, in animal model experiments has not been correlated with decreased cure rates or delayed responses to treatment with penicillins, cephalosporins, or vancomycin. Accordingly, the presence of tolerance in streptococci or staphylococci has not required combination therapy, and, in fact, regimens are designed using the MICs of these organisms.[75]

The regimens recommended for the treatment of IE caused by specific organisms are designed to provide high concentrations of antibiotics in serum and deep in vegetations that exceed the organism's MIC throughout most of the interval between doses. Although antibiotic concentrations in vegetations of patients with IE have been measured infrequently, the success of the recommended regimens suggests that this goal has been achieved. Accordingly, for optimal therapy, it is important that the recommended regimens be followed carefully.

Antimicrobial Therapy for Specific Organisms

The antimicrobial therapy for endocarditis should not only eradicate the causative agent but also do so while causing little or no toxicity. Therapy for a given patient requires modification to accommodate end-organ dysfunction, existing allergies, and other anticipated toxicities. With the exception of staphylococcal endocarditis, the antimicrobial regimens recommended for the treatment of NVE and PVE are similar,

TABLE 58–6 Treatment for Native Valve Endocarditis Caused by Penicillin-Susceptible Viridans Streptococci and *Streptococcus bovis* (Minimum Inhibitory Concentration ≤0.1 μg/ml)*

Antibiotic	Dosage and Route†	Duration (wk)
Aqueous penicillin G	12-18 million units/24 hr IV either continuously or every 4 hr in six equally divided doses	4
Ceftriaxone	2 gm once daily IV or IM	4
Aqueous penicillin G	12-18 million units/24 hr IV either continuously or every 4 hr in six equally divided doses	2
plus Gentamicin	1 mg/kg IM or IV every 8 hr	2
Vancomycin	30 mg/kg/24 hr IV in two equally divided doses, not to exceed 2 gm/24 hr unless serum levels are monitored	4

Modified from Wilson WR, Karchmer AW, Dajani AS, et al: Antibiotic treatment of adults with infective endocarditis due to streptococci, enterococci, staphylococci, and HACEK microorganisms. JAMA 274:1706, 1995. Copyright 1995 American Medical Association.

*For nutritionally variant streptococci (*Streptococcus adjacens, Streptococcus defectivus*), see Table 58–8.

†Dosages given are for patients with normal renal function. Vancomycin and gentamicin doses must be reduced for treatment of patients with renal dysfunction. Vancomycin and gentamicin doses are calculated using ideal body weight (men = 50 kg + 2.3 kg per inch over 5 feet; women = 45.5 kg + 2.3 kg per inch over 5 feet).

although more prolonged treatment is often advised for PVE.[18,74]

PENICILLIN-SUSCEPTIBLE VIRIDANS STREPTOCOCCI OR *STREPTOCOCCUS BOVIS.* Four regimens provide highly effective, comparable therapy for patients with endocarditis caused by penicillin-susceptible streptococci and *S. bovis* (Table 58–6). The 4-week regimens yield bacteriological cure rates of 98 percent among patients who complete therapy. Treatment with the synergistic combination of penicillin plus gentamicin for 2 weeks is as effective in selected cases as treatment with the 4-week regimens. The combination regimen is recommended for patients who have uncomplicated NVE and who are not at increased risk for aminoglycoside toxicity. Patients with endocarditis caused by nutritionally variant streptococci (*Abiotrophia* species), endocarditis involving a prosthetic valve, or endocarditis complicated by a mycotic aneurysm, myocardial abscess, perivalvular infection, or an extracardiac focus of infection should not be treated with this short-course regimen.

From 2 to 8 percent of viridans streptococci and *S. bovis* causing endocarditis are highly resistant to streptomycin (MIC >2000 µg/ml) and are not killed synergistically by penicillin plus streptomycin. These highly streptomycin-resistant strains are, however, killed synergistically by penicillin plus gentamicin. Consequently, unless a causative streptococcus can be evaluated to preclude high-level resistance to streptomycin, gentamicin is recommended for use in the short-course combination regimen.[76] Ceftriaxone 2 gm once daily plus either gentamicin (3 mg/kg) or netilmicin (4 mg/kg) given as a single daily dose for 14 days has effectively treated endocarditis caused by penicillin-susceptible streptococci.[77] Nevertheless, experience with single daily doses of aminoglycosides in the treatment of IE is limited, and these regimens are not currently recommended. The *Abiotrophia* species are generally more resistant to penicillin than other viridans streptococci.[25] Patients with endocarditis caused by these organisms are treated with regimens recommended for enterococcal endocarditis (see Table 58-8); however, outcome remains unsatisfactory.

For the treatment of streptococcal endocarditis in patients with a history of immediate allergic reactions (urticarial or anaphylactic reactions) to a penicillin or cephalosporin antibiotic, vancomycin is recommended (see Table 58-6). Patients with other forms of penicillin allergy (delayed maculopapular skin rash) may be treated cautiously with the ceftriaxone regimen (see Table 58-6) or with cefazolin, 2 gm IV every 8 hours for 4 weeks.

For patients with PVE caused by penicillin-susceptible streptococci, treatment with 6 weeks of penicillin is recommended, with gentamicin given during the initial 2 weeks.[18]

RELATIVELY PENICILLIN-RESISTANT STREPTOCOCCI. Four weeks of high-dose parenteral penicillin plus an aminoglycoside (primarily gentamicin for the reasons noted previously) during the initial 2 weeks are recommended for treatment of patients with endocarditis caused by streptococci with MICs for penicillin between 0.2 and 0.5 µg/ml (Table 58–7). Patients who cannot tolerate penicillin because of immediate hypersensitivity reactions can be treated with vancomycin alone. For those with nonimmediate penicillin hypersensitivity, effective treatment can be accomplished either with vancomycin alone or by adding gentamicin to the initial 2 weeks of the ceftriaxone regimen (see Table 58–6). Patients with endocarditis caused by streptococci that are highly resistant to penicillin (MIC > 0.5 µg/ml) should be treated with one of the regimens recommended for enterococcal endocarditis (Table 58–8).

***STREPTOCOCCUS PYOGENES*, *STREPTOCOCCUS PNEUMONIAE*, AND GROUP B, C, AND G STREPTOCOCCI.** Endocarditis caused by these streptococci has been either refractory to antibiotic therapy or associated with extensive valvular damage. Penicillin G in a dose of 3 million units IV every 4 hours for 4 weeks is recommended for the treatment of group A streptococcal endocarditis.

IE caused by group G, C, or B streptococci is more difficult to treat than that caused by penicillin-susceptible viridans streptococci. Consequently, the addition of gentamicin to the first 2 weeks of a 4-week regimen using high doses of penicillin is often advocated (see Table 58-7).[26,27] Early cardiac surgery to correct intracardiac complications is needed in almost half of these cases and may improve outcome.[26,27]

In selecting treatment for pneumococcal IE, both antibiotic resistance in the infecting strain and coexisting meningitis are important considerations.[28] The treatment of IE caused by penicillin-susceptible pneumococci (MIC = 0.6 µg/ml) with or without concomitant meningitis is penicillin G 4 million units IV every 4 hours, ceftriaxone 2 gm IV every 12 hours, or cefotaxime 4 gm IV every 6 hours. In the absence of meningitis, these regimens are effective for IE caused by pneumococci that are relatively penicillin resistant (MIC 0.1 to 1.0 µg/ml). If IE, including that

TABLE 58–7 Treatment for Native Valve Endocarditis Caused by Strains of Viridans Streptococci and *Streptococcus bovis* Relatively Resistant to Penicillin G (Minimum Inhibitory Concentration >0.1 μg/ml and <0.5 μg/ml)

Antibiotic	Dosage and Route*	Duration (wk)
Aqueous penicillin G	18 million units/24 hr IV either continuously or every 4 hr in six equally divided doses	4
plus Gentamicin	1 mg/kg IM or IV every 8 hr	2
Vancomycin	30 mg/kg/24 hr IV in two equally divided doses, not to exceed 2 gm/24 hr unless serum levels are monitored	4

*Dosages are for patients with normal renal function; see Table 58–6 footnote.

Modified from Wilson WR, Karchmer AW, Dajani AS, et al: Antibiotic treatment of adults with infective endocarditis due to streptococci, enterococci, staphylococci, and HACEK microorganisms. JAMA 274:1706, 1995. Copyright 1995 American Medical Association.

TABLE 58–8 Standard Therapy for Endocarditis Caused by Enterococci*

Antibiotic	Dosage and Route[†]	Duration (wk)
Aqueous penicillin G	18-30 million units/24 hr IV given continuously or every 4 hr in six equally divided doses	4-6
plus Gentamicin	1 mg/kg IM or IV every 8 hr	4-6
Ampicillin	12 gm/24 hr IV given continuously or every 4 hr in six equally divided doses	4-6
plus Gentamicin	1 mg/kg IM or IV every 8 hr	4-6
Vancomycin[‡]	30 mg/kg/24 hr IV in two equally divided doses not to exceed 2 gm/24 hr unless serum levels are monitored	4-6
plus Gentamicin	1 mg/kg IM or IV every 8 hr	4-6

Modified from Wilson WR, Karchmer AW, Dajani AS, et al: Antibiotic treatment of adults with infective endocarditis due to streptococci, enterococci, staphylococci, and HACEK microorganisms. JAMA 274:1706, 1995. Copyright 1995 American Medical Association.

*All enterococci causing endocarditis must be tested for antimicrobial susceptibility in order to select optimal therapy. These regimens are for treatment of endocarditis caused by enterococci that are susceptible to vancomycin or ampicillin and not highly resistant to gentamicin. These may also be used for treatment of endocarditis caused by penicillin-resistant (minimum inhibitory concentration >0.5) viridans streptococci and nutritionally variant streptococci (*S. defectivus, S. adjacens*), or enterococcal prosthetic valve endocarditis.

[†]Dosages are for patients with normal renal function. See Table 58–6, footnote.

[‡]Cephalosporins are not alternatives to penicillin/ampicillin in penicillin-allergic patients.

complicated by meningitis, is caused by a penicillin-resistant (MIC = 2.0 μg/ml) or cefotaxime-resistant (MIC = 2.0 μg/ml) pneumococcus, therapy with ceftriaxone 2 gm IV every 12 hours (or cefotaxime 4 gm IV every 4 hours) plus vancomycin 15 mg/kg IV every 12 hours is preferred. Heart failure rather than penicillin resistance is associated with mortality.

ENTEROCOCCI. Optimal therapy for enterococcal endocarditis requires synergistic bactericidal interaction of an antimicrobial targeted against the bacterial cell wall (penicillin, ampicillin, or vancomycin) and an aminoglycoside that is able to exert a lethal effect (primarily streptomycin or gentamicin). High-level resistance, defined as the inability of high concentrations of streptomycin (2000 μg/ml) or gentamicin (500 to 2000 μg/ml) to inhibit the growth of an enterococcus, is predictive of the agent's inability to exert this lethal effect and participate in the bactericidal synergistic interaction in vitro and in vivo. The standard regimens recommended for the treatment of enterococcal endocarditis (see Table 58–8) are designed to achieve bactericidal synergy. Synergistic combination therapy has resulted in cure rates of approximately 85 percent, compared with 40 percent with single-agent, nonbactericidal treatment.

Some authorities prefer gentamicin doses of 1.5 mg/kg every 8 hours; however, because this dose may be associated with an increased frequency of nephrotoxicity, others advocate doses of 1 mg/kg every 8 hours. Peak serum gentamicin concentrations of approximately 5 and 3.5 μg/ml are sought with these doses, respectively. In the absence of high-level resistance to streptomycin in a causative strain, streptomycin, 7.5 mg/kg intramuscularly (IM) or IV every 12 hours to achieve a peak serum concentration of approximately 20 μg/ml, can be substituted for gentamicin in the standard regimens. For patients allergic to penicillin, the vancomycin-aminoglycoside regimen (see Table 58–8) is recommended; alternatively, patients can be desensitized to penicillin. Desensitization may be desirable when preexisting renal dysfunction favors avoiding the potentially more nephrotoxic vancomycin-aminoglycoside combination. Cephalosporins are not effective in the treatment of enterococcal endocarditis. Therapy is administered for 4 to 6 weeks, with the longer course used to treat patients with IE that was symptomatic for more than 3 months, with complicated disease, and with enterococcal PVE. During treatment, careful clinical follow-up of patients and aminoglycoside levels is required to prevent nephrotoxicity and ototoxicity.

In the largest series to date, of 93 patients treated for enterococcal IE (66 with NVE, 27 with PVE), 75 (81 percent) were cured, 15 (16 percent) died, and 3 (3 percent) relapsed.[78] Cure was achieved with a median duration of cell wall–active antimicrobial therapy and aminoglycoside therapy of 42 and 15 days, respectively. In 39 patients who were cured, aminoglycosides were administered for 21 days or less. These favorable outcomes with regimens using foreshortened courses of aminoglycosides suggest that the aminoglycoside component of combination therapy can be reduced if toxicity becomes significant.

All enterococci causing endocarditis must be evaluated carefully in order to select effective therapy (Table 58–9). The strain causing endocarditis must be tested for high-level resistance to both streptomycin and gentamicin as well as to determine its susceptibility to penicillin, ampicillin, and vancomycin. If the strain is either resistant to achievable serum

TABLE 58–9 Strategy for Selecting Therapy for Enterococcal Endocarditis Caused by Strains Resistant to Components of the Standard Regimen 1

I. Ideal therapy includes a cell wall–active agent plus an effective aminoglycoside to achieve bactericidal synergy

II. Cell wall–active antimicrobial
   A. Determine MIC for ampicillin and vancomycin; test for beta-lactamase production (nitrocefin test)
   B. If ampicillin and vancomycin susceptible, use ampicillin
   C. If ampicillin resistant (MIC ≥ 16 μg/ml) and vancomycin susceptible, use vancomycin
   D. If beta-lactamase produced, use vancomycin or consider ampicillin-sulbactam
   E. If ampicillin resistant and vancomycin resistant (MIC ≥ 16 μg/ml), consider teicoplanin*
   F. If ampicillin resistant and highly resistant to vancomycin and teicoplanin (MIC ≥ 256 μg/ml), see IV C, D

III. Aminoglycoside to be used with cell wall–active antimicrobial
   A. If no high-level resistance to streptomycin (MIC < 2000 μg/ml) or gentamicin (MIC < 500-2000 μg/ml), use gentamicin or streptomycin
   B. If high-level resistance to gentamicin (MIC > 500-2000 μg/ml), test streptomycin. If no high-level resistance to streptomycin, use streptomycin
   C. If high-level resistance to gentamicin and streptomycin, omit aminoglycoside therapy; use prolonged therapy (8-12 wk) with cell wall–active antimicrobial if the organism is susceptible (see II A-E) or alternative therapy (see IV C, D)

IV. Alternative regimens and approaches
   A. Single-drug therapy (see III C) and surgical intervention
   B. Consider ampicillin, vancomycin (or teicoplanin), and gentamicin (or streptomycin) based on absence of high-level resistance
   C. Consider quinupristin/dalfopristin therapy for infective endocarditis caused by susceptible *Enterococcus faecium* and surgical intervention
   D. Consider linezolid therapy with or without surgical intervention
   E. Treatment with fluoroquinolones, rifampin, or trimethoprim-sulfamethoxazole of questionable efficacy
   F. Daptomycin active in vitro against vancomycin resistant enterococci but no clinical data for this entity

MIC = minimum inhibitory concentration.

*Not approved by the Food and Drug Administration for use in the United States; may be available by compassionate-use protocol.

concentrations of the cell wall–active agent or highly resistant to the aminoglycosides, synergy and optimal therapy cannot be obtained with a standard regimen that includes the inactive antimicrobial. Furthermore, high-level resistance to gentamicin predicts resistance to all other aminoglycosides except streptomycin. These susceptibility data allow selection of a bactericidal synergistic regimen, if one is possible, or alternative treatment (see Table 58–9).[46]

STAPHYLOCOCCI. More than 90 percent of coagulase-positive and coagulase-negative staphylococci are penicillin resistant. Methicillin resistance is common among coagulase-negative staphylococci and is increasingly frequent among *S. aureus*. Methicillin-resistant strains are resistant to all beta-lactam antibiotics but usually remain susceptible to vancomycin. Rare staphylococci have reduced susceptibility or resistance to vancomycin. Among staphylococci killed by cell wall–active antibiotics, the bactericidal effects of these agents can be enhanced by aminoglycosides. Combinations of semisynthetic penicillinase-resistant penicillins or vancomycin with rifampin do not result in predictable bactericidal synergism; nevertheless, rifampin has unique activity against staphylococcal infections that involve foreign material.[18] Staphylococcal infections involving prosthetic heart valves are treated differently from NVE caused by the same species (Table 58–10).[18,30,75]

STAPHYLOCOCCAL NATIVE VALVE ENDOCARDITIS. The semisynthetic penicillinase-resistant penicillins are the cornerstones of the treatment of endocarditis caused by methicillin-susceptible staphylococci. When patients have a penicillin allergy that does not induce urticaria or anaphylaxis, a first-generation cephalosporin can be used. The synergistic interaction of beta-lactam antibiotics with an aminoglycoside has not increased the cure rates for staphylococcal endocarditis; however, treatment with these combinations has modestly accelerated the eradication of staphylococci in vegetations and from the blood. To achieve this potential benefit, gentamicin may be added to beta-lactam antibiotic therapy for *S. aureus* during the initial 3 to 5 days of treatment.[75] More prolonged administration of gentamicin has been associated with nephrotoxicity and should be avoided. The role for combination therapy is less well defined in NVE caused by coagulase-negative staphylococci; pooled data suggest improved cure rates with combination therapy.[30]

In IV drug addicts, methicillin-susceptible *S. aureus* endocarditis that is uncomplicated and limited to the right heart valves has been effectively treated with 2 weeks of semisynthetic penicillinase-resistant penicillin (but not vancomycin) plus an aminoglycoside (doses as noted in Table 58–10). However, some patients with right-sided *S. aureus* during the initial week of treatment develop signs suggesting left-sided infection; these patients are not candidates for abbreviated therapy.

Endocarditis caused by methicillin-resistant staphylococci requires treatment with vancomycin (see Table 58–10). Trimethoprim-sulfamethoxazole treatment of right-sided endocarditis caused by *S. aureus* susceptible to this antimicrobial has been only moderately successful. Truly suitable alternatives to vancomycin are not available. Methicillin-resistant staphylococci are usually susceptible to linezolid and daptomycin; however, experience using either agent for treatment of endocarditis is limited. Teicoplanin, a glycopeptide antibiotic similar to vancomycin but not available in the United States, has been considered a possible alternative; however, some strains of *S. aureus* have become resistant to teicoplanin.[79]

Teicoplanin is initiated at a dose of 6 mg/kg twice daily for 3 to 4 days until a trough serum concentration of 20 to 30 μg/ml is achieved; thereafter, for optimal results this trough concentration should be maintained using a daily 10 mg/kg dose. If the methicillin-resistant strain is susceptible to gentamicin, the aminoglycoside can be used in combination with vancomycin to enhance activity against these organisms. However, the frequency of renal toxicity may also be increased by this combination. The addition of rifampin to vancomycin for treatment of methicillin-resistant *S. aureus* NVE has not been beneficial. Right-sided endocarditis caused by methicillin-resistant *S. aureus* is not treated with a 2-week regimen.

STAPHYLOCOCCAL PROSTHETIC VALVE ENDOCARDITIS. Staphylococcal infections of prosthetic heart valves should be treated with three antibiotics in combination. Rifampin provides unique antistaphylococcal activity when infection involves foreign bodies. However, rifampin-resistant staphylococci rapidly emerge when rifampin is used alone or in combination with vancomycin or beta-lactam antibiotics to treat staphylococcal PVE.[18] Consequently, staphylococcal PVE is treated with two antimicrobials plus rifampin.[18] I prefer to delay rifampin therapy briefly until treatment with two effective antistaphylococcal agents has been administered for 48 hours.

For PVE caused by methicillin-resistant staphylococci, treatment is initiated with vancomycin plus gentamicin, with rifampin added if the organism is susceptible to gentamicin. If the organism is resistant to gentamicin, an alternative aminoglycoside to which the organism is susceptible should be sought. Alternatively, if the organism is resistant to all aminoglycosides, a quinolone to which it is susceptible may be used in lieu of an aminoglycoside.[18] For treatment of PVE caused by methicillin-susceptible staphylococci, a semisyn-

TABLE 58–10 Treatment for Staphylococcal Endocarditis in the Absence of Prosthetic Material

Antibiotic	Dosage and Route*	Duration
Methicillin-susceptible staphylococci[†]		
Nafcillin or oxacillin	2 gm IV every 4 hr	4-6 wk
With optional addition of gentamicin	1 mg/kg IM or IV every 8 hr	3-5 d
Cefazolin (or other first-generation cephalosporins in equivalent dosages)[‡]	2 gm IV every 8 hr	4-6 wk
With optional addition of gentamicin	1 mg/kg IM or IV every 8 hr	3-5 d
Vancomycin[‡]	30 mg/kg/24 hr IV in two equally divided doses, not to exceed 2 gm/24 hr unless serum levels are monitored	4-6 wk
Methicillin-resistant staphylococci		
Vancomycin	30 mg/kg/24 hr IV in two equally divided doses, not to exceed 2 gm/24 hr unless serum levels are monitored	4-6 wk

Modified from Wilson WR, Karchmer AW, Dajani AS, et al: Antibiotic treatment of adults with infective endocarditis due to streptococci, enterococci, staphylococci, and HACEK microorganisms. JAMA 274:1706, 1995. Copyright 1995 American Medical Association.

*Dosages are for patients with normal renal function. See Table 58–6, footnote.

[†]For treatment of endocarditis caused by penicillin-susceptible staphylococci (minimum inhibitory concentration ≤ 0.1 μg/ml), aqueous penicillin G (18-24 million units/24 hr) can be used for 4-6 wk instead of nafcillin or oxacillin.

[‡]Cefazolin, other first-generation cephalosporins, or vancomycin may be used in selected penicillin-allergic patients.

TABLE 58–11 Treatment of Staphylococcal Endocarditis in the Presence of a Prosthetic Valve or Other Prosthetic Material

Antibiotic	Dosage and Route*	Duration (wk)
Regimen for Methicillin-Resistant Staphylococci		
Vancomycin	30 mg/kg/24 hr IV in two equally divided doses, not to exceed 2 gm/24 hr unless serum levels are monitored	≥6
plus		
Rifampin *and*	300 mg PO every 8 hr	≥6
gentamicin†	1.0 mg/kg IM or IV every 8 hr	2
Regimen for Methicillin-Susceptible Staphylococci		
Nafcillin or oxacillin	2 gm IV every 4 hr	≥6
plus		
Rifampin *and*	300 mg PO every 8 hr	≥6
gentamicin†	1.0 mg/kg IM or IV every 8 hr	2

Modified from Wilson WR, Karchmer AW, Dajani AS, et al: Antibiotic treatment of adults with infective endocarditis due to streptococci, enterococci, staphylococci, and HACEK microorganisms. JAMA 274:1706, 1995. Copyright 1995 American Medical Association.

*Dosages are for patients with normal renal function. See Table 58–6, footnote.

†Use during initial 2 wk of treatment. If strain is gentamicin resistant, see text for alternatives.

thetic penicillinase-resistant penicillin should be substituted for vancomycin in the combination regimen (Table 58–11).

Patients with a nonimmediate penicillin allergy can be treated with a first-generation cephalosporin in lieu of the semisynthetic penicillin. PVE caused by coagulase-negative staphylococci that occurs within the initial year after valve placement is often complicated by perivalvular extension of infection, and valve replacement surgery is often required to eradicate infection and maintain suitable valve function.[18] Patients with *S. aureus* PVE have frequent intracardiac complications and exceptionally high mortality rates. Cure of *S. aureus* PVE is significantly more likely if early surgical intervention is combined with appropriate combination antimicrobial therapy.[80,81]

***HEMOPHILUS PARAINFLUENZAE*, *HEMOPHILUS APHROPHILUS*, *ACTINOBACILLUS ACTINOMYCETEMCOMITANS*, *CARDIOBACTERIUM HOMINIS*, *EIKENELLA CORRODENS*, AND *KINGELLA KINGAE* (HACEK ORGANISMS).** Endocarditis caused by the HACEK group has in the past been treated with ampicillin administered alone or in combination with gentamicin. Occasional HACEK organisms that are ampicillin resistant by virtue of beta-lactamase production have been isolated. Given the marked susceptibility of both beta-lactamase–producing and non-beta-lactamase–producing HACEK strains to third-generation cephalosporins, ceftriaxone or a comparable third-generation cephalosporin is recommended for treatment of NVE or PVE caused by these organisms (Table 58–12).[75] For endocarditis caused by strains that do not produce beta-lactamase, ampicillin combined with gentamicin can be used in lieu of ceftriaxone (see Table 58–12).

OTHER PATHOGENS. Antimicrobial therapy for patients with IE caused by unusual organisms is based on limited clinical experience and data from animal models and in vitro studies. Amphotericin at full doses, often combined with 5-fluorocytosine, is recommended for treatment of *Candida* endocarditis. Several patients with *Candida* NVE and PVE without intracardiac complications are reported to have been cured by prolonged treatment with fluconazole.[82] Nevertheless, surgical intervention shortly after beginning amphotericin treatment remains the standard treatment for *Candida* endocarditis.[41,83] Prolonged or indefinite fluconazole administration has been advocated for patients treated either medically or surgically.[82,83] Although they have been used infrequently to treat IE, liposomal formulations of amphotericin may be useful because they are less toxic than amphotericin desoxycholate. New echinocandin

TABLE 58–12 Treatment for Endocarditis Caused by HACEK Microorganisms*

Antibiotic	Dosage and Route†	Duration (wk)
Ceftriaxone‡	2 gm once daily IV or IM	4
Ampicillin	12 gm/24 hr IV given continuously or every 4 hr in six equally divided doses	4
plus		
Gentamicin	1 mg/kg IM or IV every 8 hr	4

Modified from Wilson WR, Karchmer AW, Dajani AS, et al: Antibiotic treatment of adults with infective endocarditis due to streptococci, enterococci, staphylococci, and HACEK microorganisms. JAMA 274:1706, 1995. Copyright 1995 American Medical Association.

*HACEK microorganisms are *Hemophilus parainfluenzae, Hemophilus aphrophilus, Actinobacillus actinomycetemcomitans, Cardiobacterium hominis, Eikenella corrodens*, and *Kingella* species.

†Dosages are for those with normal renal function. See Table 58–6, footnote.

‡Cefotaxime or ceftizoxime in comparable doses may be substituted for ceftriaxone.

and azole agents may also offer alternatives for acute and suppressive therapy.

The antimicrobial susceptibility of corynebacteria causing endocarditis must be carefully evaluated. Many remain susceptible to penicillin, vancomycin, and aminoglycosides. Strains susceptible to aminoglycosides are killed synergistically by penicillin in combination with an aminoglycoside. *C. jeikeium,* although often resistant to penicillin and aminoglycosides, is killed by vancomycin. NVE or PVE caused by *Corynebacterium* species can be treated with the combination of penicillin plus an aminoglycoside or vancomycin, contingent on the susceptibilities of the causative strain.

The Enterobacteriaceae (*Escherichia coli* and *Klebsiella, Enterobacter, Serratia,* and *Proteus* species) are highly susceptible to third-generation cephalosporins, imipenem, and aztreonam. One of these antimicrobial agents in high doses is combined with an aminoglycoside to treat IE caused by Enterobacteriaceae.

C. burnetii IE is difficult to eradicate. Prolonged therapy (at least 4 years) using doxycycline (100 mg twice daily) or another tetracycline combined with a quinolone has been advocated. Treatment with doxycycline combined with hydroxychloroquine for 18 to 48 months (mean 31 months, median 26 months) may be more effective than longer courses of doxycycline plus a quinolone.[34,84] Surgery is important in effective treatment.

CULTURE-NEGATIVE ENDOCARDITIS. Special studies to diagnose IE caused by fastidious bacteria and other organisms must be performed (see Diagnosis). Thereafter, unless clinical or epidemiological clues suggest an etiological diagnosis, the recommended treatment for culture-negative NVE is ampicillin plus gentamicin (see standard regimen for enterococcal endocarditis, Table 58–8); because in the absence of confounding antibiotic therapy enterococci and staphylococci are unlikely causes of culture-negative NVE, ceftriaxone could be used in this regimen instead of ampicillin. For patients with culture-negative PVE, vancomycin is added to this regimen.[18] Mortality rates are lower for patients who have culture-negative endocarditis and who had received antibiotics before blood cultures were obtained and those who become afebrile during the initial week of antimicrobial treatment.[85] Marantic endocarditis should be carefully considered when treating patients for culture-negative IE. Surgical intervention should be considered for those who do not fully respond to empirical antimicrobial therapy. If surgical intervention is undertaken, a detailed microbiological and pathological examination of excised material must be performed to establish an etiologic diagnosis.

TIMING THE INITIATION OF ANTIMICROBIAL THERAPY. Current cost-containment pressures frequently result in initiation of antimicrobial therapy for suspected endocarditis immediately after blood cultures have been obtained. This practice is appropriate in the treatment of patients with acute IE that is highly destructive and rapidly progressive and of patients presenting with hemodynamic decompensation requiring urgent or emergent surgical intervention. Immediate therapy may have a favorable impact on outcome in these patients. In contrast, precipitous initiation of therapy in hemodynamically stable patients with suspected subacute endocarditis does not prevent early complications and may, by compromising subsequent blood cultures, obscure the etiological diagnosis of endocarditis. In the latter patients, it is prudent to delay antibiotic therapy briefly pending the results of the initial blood cultures. If these cultures are not positive promptly, this delay provides an important opportunity to obtain additional blood cultures without the confounding effect of empirical treatment. This opportunity is particularly important when patients have received antibiotics recently.

MONITORING THERAPY FOR ENDOCARDITIS. Patients must be carefully monitored during therapy and for several months thereafter. Failure of antimicrobial therapy, myocardial or metastatic abscess, emboli, hypersensitivity to antimicrobial agents, and other complications of therapy (catheter-related infection, thrombophlebitis) or intercurrent illness may be manifested by persistent or recurrent fever. Adverse reactions occur in 33 percent of patients treated for IE with beta-lactam antimicrobials, especially penicillin and ampicillin. The reactions include fever, rash, and neutropenia; they are increasingly frequent after 15 days of therapy.[86] Clinical events may indicate a need for potentially life-saving revision of antimicrobial therapy or adjunctive surgical therapy.

The serum concentration of vancomycin or aminoglycosides should be measured periodically. Periodic measurement allows dose adjustment to ensure optimal therapy and avoid adverse events. In addition, renal function should be monitored in patients receiving these two antimicrobials, and the complete blood count should be checked at least weekly in patients receiving high-dose beta-lactam antibiotics or vancomycin.

Repeated blood cultures should be obtained during the initial days of therapy or if fever persists to determine whether the bacteremia has been controlled. In patients with recrudescent fever after treatment, prompt cultures are essential to assess possible relapse of endocarditis.

OUTPATIENT ANTIMICROBIAL THERAPY. Technical advances allowing safe administration of complex antimicrobial regimens, combined with well-developed home care systems that provide supplies and monitor outpatient treatment, make it feasible to treat patients with endocarditis on an outpatient basis. Doing so can significantly reduce the cost of therapy. However, only patients who have responded to initial therapy and are free of fever, who are not experiencing threatening complications, who will be compliant with therapy, and who have a home situation that is physically suitable should be considered for outpatient treatment. Because most threatening complications of IE occur during the initial 2 weeks of therapy, some have suggested that treatment during this period be administered in the inpatient setting or an outpatient setting that provides daily physician oversight.[87] Furthermore, patients being treated at home must be apprised of the potential complications of endocarditis, instructed to seek advice promptly when encountering unexpected or untoward clinical events, and have assiduous clinical and laboratory monitoring. Finally, outpatient therapy must not result in compromises of antimicrobial therapy leading to suboptimal treatment.

Surgical Treatment of Intracardiac Complications

Cardiac surgical intervention has an increasingly important role in the treatment of intracardiac complications of endocarditis. Retrospective data suggest that mortality is unacceptably high when these complications are treated with antibiotics alone, whereas mortality is reduced when treatment combines antibiotics and surgical intervention.[46,88,89,89a] Accordingly, these complications have become indications for cardiac surgery (Table 58–13).

VALVULAR DYSFUNCTION. Medical therapy of NVE that is complicated by moderate to severe (New York Heart Association [NYHA] Class III and IV) CHF related to new or worsening valvular dysfunction results in mortality rates of 50 to 90 percent. Survival rates for a similar group of patients treated with antibiotics and cardiac surgery are 60 to 80 percent.[46,88] Although survival rates among surgically treated patients with PVE complicated by valvular dysfunction and CHF are 45 to 85 percent, few PVE patients with these complications are alive at 6 months when treated with antibiotics alone.[17-19] Worsening aortic valve incompetence is associated with more severe and more rapidly progressive CHF than is mitral valve incompetence. Hence, patients with aortic valve endocarditis not only account for the majority of surgically treated patients but also require surgery on a more urgent basis when heart failure supervenes. Severe mitral valve insufficiency, nevertheless, results in inexorable heart failure and ultimately requires surgical intervention. Doppler echocardiography and color flow mapping indicating significant valvular regurgitation during the initial week of endocarditis treatment do not reliably predict the patients who require valve replacement during active endocarditis. Alternatively, despite the absence of significant valvular regurgitation on early echocardiography, marked CHF may still develop. Thus, decisions about surgical intervention should be made by integrating clinical data and echocardiographic findings obtained during careful serial monitoring. On occasion, very large vegetations on the mitral valve, particularly a mitral valve prosthesis, result in significant obstruction and require surgery.[18]

TABLE 58–13 Cardiac Surgery in Patients with Infective Endocarditis

Indications
Moderate to severe congestive heart failure caused by valve dysfunction
Unstable prosthesis, prosthesis orifice obstructed
Uncontrolled infection despite optimal antimicrobial therapy
Unavailable effective antimicrobial therapy: endocarditis caused by fungi, *Brucellae, Pseudomonas aeruginosa* (aortic or mitral valves)
Staphylococcus aureus PVE with an intracardiac complication
Relapse of PVE after optimal therapy
Fistula to pericardial sac
Relative Indications*
Perivalvular extension of infection, intracardiac fistula, myocardial abscess with persistent fever
Poorly responsive *S. aureus* NVE (aortic or mitral valves)
Relapse of NVE after optimal antimicrobial therapy
Culture-negative NVE or PVE with persistent fever (≥10 d)
Large (>10 mm diameter) hypermobile vegetation (with or without prior arterial embolus)
Endocarditis caused by highly antibiotic-resistant enterococci

NVE = native valve endocarditis; PVE = prosthetic valve endocarditis.
*Surgery commonly required for optimal outcome.

UNSTABLE PROSTHESES. Dehiscence of an infected prosthetic valve is a manifestation of perivalvular infection and often results in hemodynamically significant valvular dysfunction. Surgical intervention is recommended for PVE patients with these complications.[18] The risk of invasive infection is increased among patients with onset of PVE within the year after valve implantation and those with infection of an aortic valve prosthesis. Endocarditis in these patients is often caused by invasive antimicrobial-resistant organisms; consequently, the benefit of combined medical-surgical therapy is enhanced further. Patients who appear clinically stable but who have overtly unstable and hypermobile prostheses, a finding indicative of dehiscence in excess of 40 percent of the circumference, are likely to experience progressive valve instability and warrant surgical treatment. Occasional patients with PVE caused by noninvasive, highly antibiotic-susceptible organisms, e.g., streptococci, despite a favorable clinical course during antibiotic therapy, late in treatment experience minor valve dehiscence without prosthesis instability or hemodynamic deterioration. Surgical treatment of these patients can be deferred unless clear indications arise.

UNCONTROLLED INFECTION OR UNAVAILABLE EFFECTIVE ANTIMICROBIAL THERAPY. Surgical intervention has improved the outcome of several forms of endocarditis when maximal antibiotic therapy fails to eradicate infection or, in some instances, even to suppress bacteremia. Amphotericin B is inadequate therapy for fungal endocarditis, including that caused by *Candida* species, and surgical intervention is recommended shortly after initiation of full doses of antifungal therapy. Endocarditis caused by some gram-negative bacilli, e.g., *P. aeruginosa*, *Achromobacter xylosoxidans*, may not be eradicated by maximum tolerable antibiotic therapy and may require surgical excision of the infected tissue to achieve cure. Similarly, standard therapy of endocarditis caused by *Brucella* species includes surgery because medical therapy is rarely successful.[61] Surgical intervention is recommended when patients with enterococcal endocarditis caused by a strain resistant to synergistic bactericidal therapy do not respond to initial therapy or relapse. Perivalvular invasive infection is in some instances a form of ineradicable infection. Relapse of PVE after optimal antimicrobial therapy reflects invasive disease or the difficulty in eradicating infection involving foreign devices. Patients with relapse of PVE are treated surgically.[28] In contrast, patients with NVE that relapses, unless it is associated with a highly resistant microorganism or demonstrable perivalvular infection, are often treated again with an intensified, prolonged course of antimicrobial therapy.

***S. AUREUS* PROSTHETIC VALVE ENDOCARDITIS.** Among 129 patients who had *S. aureus* PVE and who were culled from large retrospective general series of PVE, the crude mortality rate for those treated with antibiotics alone and with antibiotics plus surgery was 73 and 25 percent, respectively.[31,81,90,91] Although management strategy is undoubtedly distorted by selection bias—the most ill patients often being denied surgery—the outcomes are alarming. The overall mortality rate in 33 cases of *S. aureus* PVE treated at a single institution was 42 percent.[81] In the latter cases, when a multivariate model was used for analysis to adjust for confounding variables, the presence of intracardiac complications was associated with a 13.7-fold increased risk of death, and surgical intervention during active disease was accompanied by a 20-fold reduction in mortality. These findings do not change when the data are restricted to patients surviving a week of treatment (to correct for rejection from surgery because of imminent death) and reanalyzed. These data suggest that surgical treatment can improve outcome. Although the occurrence of central nervous system emboli is often considered to limit the opportunity for surgical intervention, in fact, appropriately timed surgery remains the preferred treatment. Thus, surgical intervention is recommended for *S. aureus* PVE with intracardiac complication and may benefit even patients with uncomplicated *S. aureus* PVE.[18,81,90]

PERIVALVULAR INVASIVE INFECTION. NVE at the aortic site and PVE are most commonly associated with perivalvular invasion with abscess or intracardiac fistula formation.[18] Invasive infection occurs in 10 to 14 percent of patients with NVE and 45 to 60 percent of those with PVE.[18] Persistent, otherwise unexplained fever despite appropriate antimicrobial therapy or pericarditis in patients with aortic valve endocarditis suggests infection extending beyond the valve leaflet. New-onset and persistent electrocardiographic conduction abnormalities, although not a sensitive indicator of perivalvular infection (28 to 53 percent), are relatively specific (85 to 90 percent).[92,93] TEE is superior to TTE for detecting invasive infection in patients with NVE and PVE. Doppler and color flow Doppler or contrast two-dimensional echocardiography optimally defines fistulas. Abscesses suspected but not detected by initial and repeated TEE may be detected by magnetic resonance imaging, including magnetic resonance angiography. Cardiac catheterization adds little to these imaging studies and is not recommended unless coronary angiography is needed.

In patients with endocarditis complicated by perivalvular extension of infection, cardiac surgery should be considered to débride invasive infection, ablate abscesses, and reconstruct anatomical damage. Surgery is warranted in patients with invasive disease that significantly disrupts cardiac structures, that is associated with CHF, that results in instability of a prosthetic valve, or that renders infection uncontrolled (persistent fever). However, it is likely that increasingly sensitive imaging techniques will elucidate invasive infections that do not require immediate surgery. Sporadic case reports of medically treated invasive infection suggest that these infections will be small, structurally nonsignificant abscesses in which the cavity is open to the circulatory stream.

LEFT-SIDED *S. AUREUS* ENDOCARDITIS. Because this infection is difficult to control, highly destructive, and associated with high mortality (25 to 47 percent), some investigators have suggested that these patients should be considered for surgical treatment when the response to antimicrobial therapy is not prompt and complete.[89] Also, patients with *S. aureus* NVE (aortic or mitral valve) and vegetations that are visible by TTE are at increased risk for arterial emboli and death and should be considered for surgery.[32] In contrast, IV drug abusers with *S. aureus* endocarditis limited to the tricuspid or pulmonary valves often experience prolonged fever during antimicrobial therapy; nevertheless, the vast majority of these patients respond to antimicrobial therapy and do not require surgery.

UNRESPONSIVE CULTURE-NEGATIVE ENDOCARDITIS. Patients who have culture-negative endocarditis and who experience unexplained persistent fever during empirical antimicrobial therapy, particularly those with PVE, should be considered for surgical intervention. If endocarditis is not marantic, persistent fever in these patients is likely to represent either unrecognized perivalvular infection or ineffective antimicrobial therapy. Causative organisms can be seen or cultured from valve-vegetation specimens in 40 to 70 percent of these patients.[91] Molecular techniques can identify additional pathogens.[65]

LARGE VEGETATIONS (>10 MM) AND THE PREVENTION OF SYSTEMIC EMBOLI. Although it was not demonstrated in all studies, in pooled data and meta-analysis, systemic embolization was increased in patients with vegetations greater than 10 mm versus those with smaller or no detectable vegetations, 33 to 37 percent versus 19 percent.[94] Larger mitral valve vegetations (>10 mm), particularly those on the anterior mitral valve leaflet, and vegetation mobility are uniquely associated with systemic emboli.[52,94-96] Although a relationship may exist between vegetation characteristics—including size, mobility, and extent (number of leaflets involved)—and embolic complications, the implications for surgical intervention are not clear. Yet to be performed are analyses examining embolic complications or outcome and vegetation characteristics but adjusted for valve dysfunction, perivalvular invasion by infection, organism, and infection site. Nevertheless, some researchers have concluded that vegetation characteristics alone might warrant surgery to prevent arterial emboli. This recommendation can be questioned, as can the recommendation for valve surgery after two major arterial emboli.[61]

In deciding to intervene with cardiac surgery to prevent arterial emboli, many factors must be considered carefully. The rate of systemic or cerebral emboli in patients with NVE and PVE decreases during the course of effective antibiotic therapy.[55,97] Also, it is not clear that surgical intervention reduces the frequency of systemic emboli.[46] Finally, the risks of morbidity and mortality caused by cerebral and coronary emboli, the major events to be prevented, must be compared with the immediate and long-term risks of valve replacement surgery or, if feasible, vegetectomy and valve repair. These risks include perioperative mortality, recrudescent endocarditis on the prosthesis, thromboembolic complications, early and late valve dysfunction requiring repeated valve replacement, the hazards of warfarin anticoagulation (including its contraindication during pregnancy), and the risk and morbidity of late-onset PVE.[85] Vegetation size alone is rarely an indication for surgery. The clinical findings and echocardiographic evidence for other intracardiac complications must be weighed against the immediate and remote hazards of cardiac surgery, including the possibility of valve preservation by vegetectomy and valve repair, when recommending therapy.[61] Thus, the risk for systemic embolization as related to vegetation size or prior systemic embolus is not an independent indication for surgical intervention but is only one of many factors to be considered when planning treatment.[55,61,97]

Repair of Intracardiac Defects

TECHNIQUES. New surgical techniques to address severe tissue destruction in NVE and PVE have been developed. Although these are beyond the scope of this discussion, examples include valve composite graft replacement of the aortic root, use of sewing skirts attached to the prostheses, and homograft replacement of the aortic valve and root with coronary artery reimplantation. Furthermore, repair of the mitral valve in patients with acute or healed endocarditis avoids the need for insertion of prosthetic materials and the associated hazards. Although tricuspid valvulectomy without valve replacement has been advocated for treatment of uncontrolled tricuspid valve infection in IV drug abusers at high risk for recidivism and recurrent endocarditis, the likelihood of refractory right-sided heart failure with time after valvulectomy makes tricuspid valve repair preferable. Cardiac transplantation has been used to salvage an occasional patient with refractory endocarditis.

TIMING OF SURGICAL INTERVENTION. When endocarditis is complicated by valvular regurgitation and significant impairment of cardiac function, surgical intervention before the development of severe intractable hemodynamic dysfunction is recommended, regardless of the duration of antimicrobial therapy.[98] Postoperative mortality correlates with the severity of preoperative hemodynamic dysfunction; consequently, this approach is justified.[94] In patients who have valvular dysfunction and in whom infection is controlled and cardiac function is compensated, surgery may be delayed until antimicrobial therapy has been completed. If infection is not controlled, surgery should be performed promptly. Similarly, if a patient who requires valve replacement in the near future has a large vegetation, indicating a high risk for systemic embolization, early cardiac surgery is appropriate (see Large Vegetations and the Prevention of Systemic Emboli).

More specific recommendations for timing of surgery have been presented.[88] Strong clinical evidence suggested emergent (same day) surgery for acute aortic regurgitation with mitral valve preclosure, sinus of Valsalva rupture into the right heart, and fistula to the pericardial sac; urgent (1 to 2 days) surgery for valve obstruction, unstable prosthesis, acute aortic or mitral regurgitation with heart failure (NYHA Class III to IV), septal perforation, perivalvular extension of infection, and no effective antimicrobial therapy; and early elective surgery for progressive paravalvular regurgitation, valve dysfunction and persistent fever, and fungal (mold or complicated yeast) IE.

To avoid worsening of neurological status or death in patients who have sustained recent neurological injury, the timing of surgical intervention may require modification. Among patients who have had a nonhemorrhagic embolic stroke, exacerbation of cerebral dysfunction occurs during cardiac surgery in 44 percent of cases when the interval between the stroke and surgery is 7 days or less, in 17 percent when the interval is 8 to 14 days, and in 10 percent or less when more than 2 weeks has elapsed. After hemorrhagic intracerebral events, the risk for neurological worsening or death with cardiac surgery persists at 20 percent even after 1 month.[99] Thus, when the response of IE to antimicrobial therapy and hemodynamic status permit, delaying cardiac surgery for 2 to 3 weeks after a significant embolic infarct and at least a month after intracerebral hemorrhage (with prior repair of a mycotic aneurysm) has been recommended.[99,100]

DURATION OF ANTIMICROBIAL THERAPY AFTER SURGICAL INTERVENTION. Inflammatory changes and bacteria visible with Gram stain have been found in vegetations removed from patients who received most or all of the standard antibiotic therapy recommended for endocarditis caused by a specific microorganism. In fact, in patients who had successfully completed standard recommended antibiotic therapy for IE—29 of 53 (55 percent) still taking antibiotics, 7 of 15 (47 percent) without antibiotics for less than a month, and 4 of 18 (22 percent) without antibiotics for 1 to 6 months—the valve or vegetation removed surgically contained visible bacteria on Gram stain or histological examination. Cultures of these valves or vegetations yielded bacteria in 5, 0, and 1 instance, respectively.[91] If valve cultures are negative, visible bacteria do not indicate that antimicrobial therapy has failed or that a full course of antibiotic therapy is needed postoperatively. The duration of antimicrobial therapy after surgery depends on the length of preoperative therapy, the antibiotic susceptibility of the causative organism, the presence of paravalvular invasive infection, and the culture status of the vegetation. In general, for endocarditis caused by relatively antibiotic-responsive organisms with negative cultures of operative specimens, preoperative plus postoperative therapy should at least equal a full course of recommended therapy; for patients with prostheses sewn into a débrided abscess cavity or with positive intraoperative cultures, a full course of therapy should be given postoperatively. Patients with PVE should receive a full course of antimicrobial therapy postoperatively when organisms are seen in resected material.[18]

Treatment of Extracardiac Complications

SPLENIC ABSCESS. Three to 5 percent of patients with IE develop a splenic abscess.[50] Although splenic defects can be identified by ultrasonography and computed tomography, these tests usually cannot reliably discriminate between abscess and infarct. Persistent fever and progressive enlargement of the lesion during antimicrobial therapy suggest that it is an abscess, which can be confirmed by percutaneous needle aspiration. Successful therapy of splenic abscesses generally requires drainage, which can sometimes be accomplished by percutaneous placement of a catheter. In patients with numerous splenic abscesses or in whom percutaneous drainage is unsuccessful, splenectomy is required.[61] Splenic abscesses should be treated effectively before valve replacement surgery. If they are not treated effectively before cardiac surgery, splenectomy should be performed as soon thereafter as surgical risks permit.[61]

MYCOTIC ANEURYSMS AND SEPTIC ARTERITIS. From 2 to 10 percent of patients with endocarditis have mycotic aneurysms; in 1 to 5 percent, the aneurysms involve cerebral vessels. Cerebral mycotic aneurysms occur at the branch points in cerebral vessels, are generally located distally over the cerebral cortex, and are found most commonly in branches of the middle cerebral artery. The aneurysms arise either from occlusion of vessels by septic emboli with secondary arteritis and vessel wall destruction or from bacteremic seeding of the vessel wall through the vasa vasorum. *S. aureus* is commonly implicated in the former and viridans streptococci in the latter.[58] Many patients with mycotic aneurysms or septic arteritis present with devastating intracranial hemorrhage. Focal deficits from embolic events, persistent focal headache, unexplained neurological deterioration or focal neurological abnormalities, or sterile meningeal irritation (cerebrospinal fluid pleocytosis) may be premonitory symptoms. Cerebral angiography is required to evaluate patients with subarachnoid hemorrhage, and this or magnetic resonance or spiral computed tomographic angiography has been recommended for patients experiencing premonitory symptoms, especially if cardiac surgery or anticoagulant therapy is planned.[61] Although rupture may occur at any point before or during antibiotic therapy, aneurysms that leak or rupture do so most commonly before or during early treatment.

Mycotic aneurysms may resolve during antimicrobial therapy[61]; however, when anatomically feasible, aneurysms that have ruptured should be repaired surgically.[101] Aneurysms that have not leaked should be monitored angiographically during antimicrobial therapy. Surgery should be considered for a single lesion that enlarges during or after antimicrobial therapy. Anticoagulant therapy should be avoided in patients with a persisting mycotic aneurysm. On rare occasions, persistent stable aneurysms may rupture after completion of standard antimicrobial therapy; however, there is no accurate estimation of risk for late rupture, and recommendations for surgical intervention are arbitrary. Nevertheless, prevailing opinion favors, whenever possible without serious neurological injury, the resection of single aneurysms that persist after therapy.[101] The potential existence of occult aneurysms in patients without neurological symptoms or in those who have had a nondiagnostic angiographic evaluation is not considered a contraindication to anticoagulant therapy after completion of antimicrobial therapy.

Extracranial mycotic aneurysms should be managed as outlined for cerebral aneurysms. Those that leak, are expanding during therapy, or persist after therapy should be repaired. Particular attention should be given to aneurysms that involve intraabdominal arteries, rupture of which could result in life-threatening hemorrhage.[61]

ANTICOAGULANT THERAPY. Patients with PVE involving devices that would usually warrant maintenance anticoagulation are continued on anticoagulant therapy.[18] Anticoagulation is not initiated as prophylaxis against IE-related thromboembolism in either patients with PVE involving devices that do not usually require this therapy or patients with NVE. Neither aspirin nor anticoagulant therapy has been shown to prevent embolization, and either might contribute to intracranial hemorrhage, particularly in the presence of a recent cerebral infarct or a mycotic aneurysm. Anticoagulant therapy in patients with NVE is limited to patients for whom there is a clear indication for this therapy and for whom there is not a known increased risk for intracranial hemorrhage. If central nervous system complications occur in patients who have IE and who are receiving anticoagulant therapy, anticoagulation should be reversed immediately.[18]

Response to Therapy

Within a week after initiation of effective antimicrobial therapy, almost 75 percent of patients with IE, including those with PVE, are afebrile and 90 percent have defervesced by the end of the second week of treatment.[18,46,97,102] The duration of fever during therapy is longer in patients with IE related to *S. aureus* or *P. aeruginosa* and culture-negative IE as well as IE characterized by microvascular phenomena and major embolic complications.[46,102] Persistence or recurrence of fever more than 7 to 10 days after initiation of antibiotic therapy identified patients with increased mortality rates and with complications of infection or therapy.[18,102] Patients with prolonged or recurrent fever should be evaluated for intracardiac complications, focal extracardiac septic complications, intercurrent nosocomial infections, recurrent pulmonary emboli (patients with right-sided IE), drug-associated fever, additional underlying illnesses, and, if appropriate, in-hospital substance abuse.

Blood cultures should be repeated in search of persistent bacteremia or the presence of additional pathogens, e.g., previously unrecognized polymicrobial IE. The antimicrobial susceptibility of the causative organism should be reevaluated, as should the adequacy of antibiotic therapy. Drug reactions have accounted for fever in 17 to 28 percent of these patients. Drug fever attributed to the antimicrobial therapy itself may warrant revision of treatment if a suitable alternative is available. In the absence of effective alternative therapy, treatment can be continued despite drug fever if the antimicrobial is not causing significant end-organ toxicity. In 33 to 45 percent of patients, persistent fever was associated with significant intracardiac complications, many of which required surgical intervention.[102]

Many clinical and laboratory features of IE are slow to resolve despite effective antimicrobial therapy. Systemic emboli occur during the early weeks of treatment, although with decreasing frequency.[55] The increased ESR and anemia may not be corrected until after therapy has been completed.

Mortality rates for large series of patients with NVE treated between 1975 and 1993 ranged from 16 to 27 percent.[1,91] Death from IE has been associated with increased age (>65 to 70 years old), underlying diseases, infection involving the aortic valve, development of CHF, renal failure, and central nervous system complications.[1,102a] The treatment of heart failure related to valve dysfunction by early surgical intervention has decreased the mortality associated with CHF, but subsequent neurological events and septic complications, e.g., uncontrolled infection and myocardial abscess, have accounted for a larger proportion of deaths and have been associated with high mortality rates.[50]

Mortality rates among patients with IE caused by viridans streptococci and *S. bovis* have ranged from 4 to 16 percent.[1] Higher mortality rates are reported with left-sided NVE caused by other organisms: enterococci, 15 to 25 percent[1]; *S. aureus*, 25 to 47 percent[1,30]; nonviridans streptococci (groups B, C, and G), 13 to 50 percent[26,27]; *C. burnetii*, 5 to 37 percent[20,76,82]; *P. aeruginosa*, Enterobacteriaceae, and fungi, greater than 50 percent.[33]

In a retrospective study of patients with NVE with NYHA Class III or IV heart failure or invasive uncontrolled infection, only 9 percent of patients treated surgically died, compared with 51 percent of those treated with antibiotics alone.[46] Mortality rates among patients with active NVE who were treated surgically have ranged from 5 to 26 percent.[103-107] Severity of heart failure, abscess, *S. aureus* infection, and decreased renal function (possibly related to heart failure) have been associated with increased postoperative mortality.[105] Nevertheless, survival rates of 85 percent can be achieved when patients with paravalvular abscesses undergo meticulous débridement and reconstructive cardiac surgery.[108]

In a large retrospective study of patients with complicated left-sided NVE, the mortality rate was 25 percent, and in a multivariate analysis the following variables were independent predictors of mortality and could be assigned a weighted mortality risk score (discrete score): abnormal mental status (4), Charlson comorbidity score = 2 (3), moderate to severe CHF (3), bacterial etiology other than viridans streptococci (*S. aureus* = 6, other = 8), and medical therapy without valve surgery (5). The model was verified in an independent cohort and the 6-month mortality rate could be predicted by total point score: less than or equal to 6 points, 6 percent; 7 to 11 points, 17 percent; 12 to 15 points, 31 percent; more than 15 points, 63 percent.[102a,109]

Outcome for patients with PVE, as contrasted with NVE, has been less desirable. Before 1980, mortality rates among patients with onset less than 60 days after surgery and later onset PVE averaged 70 and 45 percent, respectively. With the recognition that PVE was frequently complicated by invasive infection and that patients would benefit from surgical intervention, mortality rates have decreased to 33 to 45 percent, with lower rates in later onset cases.[18,108] Long-term survival was adversely affected by the presence of moderate or severe heart failure at discharge. Survival rates after aggressive surgery for PVE ranged from 75 to 85 percent and were not related to time of onset after cardiac surgery.[19,106,107]

Among patients with NVE (nonaddicts) discharged after medical or medical-surgical therapy, long-term survival was 88 percent at 5 years and 81 percent at 10 years.[91] Among patients treated surgically for NVE, survival at 5 years ranged from 70 to 80 percent.[104,107] Among patients with PVE treated surgically, survival rates at 4 to 6 years ranged from 50 to 82 percent.[19,107]

RELAPSE AND RECURRENCE. Relapse of IE usually occurs within 2 months of discontinuing antibiotic treatment. Of patients who have NVE caused by penicillin-susceptible viridans streptococci and who receive a recommended course of therapy, less than 2 percent suffer relapse. From 8 to 20 percent of patients with enterococcal IE experience relapse after standard therapy. Patients with IE caused by *S. aureus*, Enterobacteriaceae, or fungi are more likely to experience overt failure of therapy rather than relapse; nevertheless, 4 percent of patients with *S. aureus* IE suffer relapse. Relapse of fungal endocarditis at long intervals after treatment has been reported. Relapse occurs in 10 percent of patients with PVE overall and in 6 to 15 percent of those treated surgically.

Among nonaddicts with an initial episode of NVE or PVE, 4.5 to 7 percent experience one or more additional episodes.[91] Among these patients, recurrent IE shares the clinical and microbiological features and response to therapy noted in primary episodes of IE. IV drug abuse is now the most common predisposing factor for recurrent IE (43 percent of patients).

Prevention

Viridans streptococci, a common cause of NVE and late-onset PVE, are the primary target for prophylaxis used in conjunction with procedures involving the oral cavity, respiratory tract, or esophagus. Procedures involving the genitourinary and gastrointestinal tracts commonly precede the development of enterococcal endocarditis. Accordingly, the prophylaxis for endocarditis used in conjunction with procedures involving these mucosal surfaces is targeted against enterococci. When incision and drainage of infected skin or soft tissue infections are undertaken, prophylaxis is focused on *S. aureus.*

Procedures for which IE prophylaxis is recommended or not recommended have been identified by the American Heart Association and others (see Table 58G–1).[109,110] Although prophylaxis is advised for all at-risk patients who undergo dental procedures that cause gingival bleeding, extractions are the most strongly associated with subsequent IE. Because endocarditis has been reported only rarely in association with other gastrointestinal endoscopic procedures with or without biopsy, prophylaxis is not routinely recommended in this situation. Prophylaxis is not recommended with routine cardiac catheterization or TEE.[109,110]

On the basis of their frequency among patients with endocarditis compared with the general population, lesions have been assigned to high, intermediate, low, and negligible risk categories (Table 58–14).[110-113] Rheumatic heart disease is currently a less common predisposition for IE in most of the developed countries; however, the attack rate of IE among persons with rheumatic valvular disease approaches that with prosthetic valves and suggests that these lesions also entail a high risk.

The risk of IE for patients with MVP and the resulting role of prophylaxis among these patients have been controversial. MVP has been identified frequently among patients with IE. However, the risk of endocarditis among patients with MVP and a murmur of mitral regurgitation is still relatively low. It is 5- to 10-fold higher than that in the general population but 100-fold less than that among patients with rheumatic valvular heart disease. As a result, MVP with a murmur of mitral regurgitation or mitral valve thickening and prolapse defines a patient with an intermediate risk for IE and one for whom prophylaxis against endocarditis is recommended.

GENERAL METHODS. The incidence of IE can be significantly reduced by total surgical correction of some congenital lesions that otherwise predispose patients to IE, e.g., patent ductus arteriosus, ventricular septal defect, and pulmonary stenosis.[6,112] The incidence of IE remains high among patients who have undergone surgical correction of other major congenital defects, especially those involving a stenotic aortic valve.[6] Patients with persisting as well as many corrected congenital lesions and those with acquired valvular heart disease who remain at risk for IE should be given written material about their predisposing lesion, their risk for endocarditis, and the recommended antibiotic prophylaxis.

Maintaining good oral hygiene, which decreases the frequency of bacteremia that accompanies daily activities (chewing, brushing teeth), may be a more important preventive than procedure-focused chemoprophylaxis.[111] Oral hygiene and dental health should be addressed before prosthetic valves are placed electively.

Among patients at risk for IE, some activities or procedures likely to induce bacteremia should be avoided. Oral irrigating devices, which may produce bacteremia even in patients with normal gingiva, are not recommended. Similarly, the use of central intravascular catheters and urinary catheters should be minimized. Infections associated with bacteremia must be treated promptly and if possible eradicated before the involved tissues are incised or manipulated.

CHEMOPROPHYLAXIS. The widely promulgated recommendations of antimicrobial prophylaxis for endocarditis are based on circumstantial evidence supplemented by studies of prophylaxis in animal models. Studies suggest that prophylactic antibiotics prevent endocarditis by inhibiting growth of the bacteria adherent to NBTE sufficiently to allow their subsequent complete elimination by host defenses.[110,114] Experimental studies that mimic single-dose amoxicillin prophylaxis in humans suggest that adequate margins of efficacy are present after a single prophylactic dose. Nevertheless, because a more sustained inhibitory effect can be achieved through a postprocedure dose of antibiotics, this is recommended for patients in the high-risk group.[109,115]

Clinical studies supporting the efficacy of antibiotic prophylaxis for endocarditis are limited. A retrospective study of patients who had prosthetic valves and who underwent dental and surgical procedures suggested that antibiotic prophylaxis prevented PVE. However, a large case-control study failed to identify dental procedures as a risk for IE among persons with valvular abnormalities and questioned the

TABLE 58–14 Relative Risk of Infective Endocarditis Associated with Preexisting Cardiac Disorders

Relatively High Risk	Intermediate Risk	Very Low or Negligible Risk*
Prosthetic heart valves†	Mitral valve prolapse with regurgitation (murmur) or thickened valve leaflets	Mitral valve prolapse without regurgitation (murmur) or thickened valve leaflets
Previous infective endocarditis†	Pure mitral stenosis	Trivial valvular regurgitation on echocardiography without structural abnormality
Cyanotic congenital heart disease†	Tricuspid valve disease	Isolated atrial septal defect (secundum)
Patent ductus arteriosus	Pulmonary stenosis	Arteriosclerotic plaques
Aortic regurgitation	Asymmetrical septal hypertrophy	Coronary artery disease
Aortic stenosis	Bicuspid aortic valve or calcific aortic sclerosis with minimal hemodynamic abnormality	Cardiac pacemaker, implanted defibrillators
Mitral regurgitation	Degenerative valvular disease in elderly patients	Surgically repaired intracardiac lesions, with minimal or no hemodynamic abnormality, more than 6 mo after operation (atrial septal defect, ventricular septal defect, patent ductus arteriosus, pulmonary stenosis)
Mitral stenosis and regurgitation	Surgically repaired intracardiac lesions with minimal or no hemodynamic abnormality, less than 6 mo after operation	Prior coronary bypass graft surgery
Ventricular septal defect		Prior Kawasaki disease or rheumatic fever without valvular dysfunction
Coarctation of the aorta		
Surgically repaired intracardiac lesion with residual hemodynamic abnormality or prosthetic device		
Surgically constructed systemic-pulmonary shunts†		

Adapted from Durack DT: Prevention of infective endocarditis. N Engl J Med 332:38, 1995; and Dajani AS, Taubert KA, Wilson W, et al: Prevention of bacterial endocarditis: Recommendations of the American Heart Association from the Committee on Rheumatic Fever, Endocarditis, and Kawasaki Disease, Council on Cardiovascular Disease in the Young. JAMA 277:1794, 1997. Copyright 1997 American Medical Association.

*Prophylaxis against endocarditis not recommended.

†Lesions considered at highest risk for endocarditis.

TABLE 58–15 Regimens for Prophylaxis Against Endocarditis: Use with Dental, Oral, and Upper Respiratory Tract Procedures

Setting	Regimen*
Standard regimen†	Amoxicillin 3.0 gm PO 1 hr before procedure, then 1.5 gm 6 hr after initial dose
Amoxicillin/penicillin-allergic patients	Erythromycin ethylsuccinate 800 mg, or erythromycin stearate 1.0 gm, PO 2 hr before procedure, then half the dose 6 hr after initial dose *OR* Clindamycin 300 mg PO 1 hr before procedure and 150 mg 6 hr after initial dose
Patients unable to take oral medications	Ampicillin 2.0 gm IM or IV 30 min before procedure, then either ampicillin 1.0 g IM or IV, or amoxicillin 1.5 gm PO, 6 hr after initial dose
Ampicillin/amoxicillin/penicillin-allergic patients unable to take oral medications	Clindamycin 300 mg IV 30 min before procedure, then 150 mg 6 hr after initial dose
Patients considered at highest risk and not candidates for standard regimen	Use standard regimen for genitourinary and gastrointestinal procedures
Ampicillin/amoxicillin/penicillin-allergic patients considered at highest risk	Use regimen for allergic patients undergoing genitourinary and gastrointestinal procedures

*Dosages for adults. Initial pediatric dosages are as follows: Ampicillin or amoxicillin, 50 mg/kg; clindamycin, 10 mg/kg; erythromycin ethylsuccinate or erythromycin stearate, 20 mg/kg; gentamicin, 2.0 mg/kg; and vancomycin, 20 mg/kg. Follow-up doses should be one-half the initial dose. **Total pediatric dose should not exceed total adult dose.**

†Generally recommended for patients at highest risk including those with prosthetic heart valves; physician may elect more vigorous regimens.

Adapted from Dajani AS, Bisno AL, Chung KJ, et al: Prevention of bacterial endocarditis: Recommendations of the American Heart Association. JAMA 264:2919, 1990. Copyright 1990 American Medical Association.

TABLE 58–16 Regimens for Prophylaxis Against Endocarditis: Use with Genitourinary and Gastrointestinal (Except Esophageal) Procedures

Setting	Antibiotic	Regimen*
High-risk patients	Ampicillin plus gentamicin	Ampicillin 2.0 gm IV/IM plus gentamicin 1.5 mg/kg within 30 min of procedure, repeat ampicillin 1.0 gm IV/IM or give amoxicillin 1.0 gm PO 6 hr later
High-risk, penicillin-allergic patients	Vancomycin plus gentamicin	Vancomycin 1.0 gm IV over 1-2 hr plus gentamicin 1.5 mg/kg IM/IV infused or injected 30 min before procedure. No second dose recommended
Moderate-risk patients	Amoxicillin or ampicillin	Amoxicillin 2.0 gm PO 1 hr before procedure or ampicillin 2.0 gm IM/IV 30 min before procedure
Moderate-risk, penicillin-allergic patients	Vancomycin	Vancomycin 1.0 gm IV infused over 1-2 hr and completed within 30 min of procedure

*Dosing for children: ampicillin 50 mg/kg IV/IM, vancomycin 20 mg/kg IV, gentamicin 1.5 mg/kg IV/IM (children's doses should not exceed adult doses).

Adapted from Dajani AS, Taubert KA, Wilson W, et al: Prevention of bacterial endocarditis: Recommendations by the American Heart Association from the Committee on Rheumatic Fever, Endocarditis, and Kawasaki Disease, Council on Cardiovascular Disease in the Young. JAMA 277:1794-1801, 1997.

benefit of antibiotic prophylaxis for these procedures.[116] Failures of antibiotic prophylaxis unrelated to resistant bacteria have also been noted.[110]

Risk-benefit and cost-benefit analyses have raised significant questions about antibiotic prophylaxis for patients with MVP. Unless both the cost and risks of prophylaxis are very low, the cost per case of IE prevented is high and mortality or morbidity may not be reduced. From a population perspective, prophylaxis in low- to intermediate-risk settings may not be cost or risk beneficial, and prophylaxis might be reserved for patients who have high-risk cardiac lesions and who are undergoing high-risk procedures.[116] Expert committees are currently reassessing guidelines for endocarditis prophylaxis.

Even if antibiotic prophylaxis is effective as well as safe and inexpensive, only a small percentage of the cases are preventable. For example, only 55 to 75 percent of patients with NVE have preexisting endocarditis-prone valvular disease, and many are not aware of the lesion before the onset of NVE.[110,111] In addition, among patients with IE, only a small fraction (5 percent) had both a known valve lesion and a procedure within 30 days of onset of IE that would have warranted prophylaxis.[111] Nevertheless, the morbidity and mortality associated with IE are used to justify prophylaxis (Table 58–15 shows for regimens used for dental and upper respiratory tract procedures; Table 58–16 shows regimens for genitourinary and gastrointestinal procedures) in patients who have high- and intermediate-risk cardiac lesions (see Table 58–14) and who are to undergo bacteremia-inducing procedures. Penicillin-resistant flora may emerge among patients who are receiving continuous penicillin for prevention of rheumatic fever or repetitive courses of antibiotics for serial dental procedures. Consequently, a nonpenicillin prophylaxis regimen is preferred for these patients. Initiation of prophylaxis several days before a procedure encourages the emergence of antibiotic-resistant organisms at the mucosal site and is not recommended.

REFERENCES

Epidemiology

1. van der Meer JTM, Thompson J, Valkenburg HA, Michel MF: Epidemiology of bacterial endocarditis in the Netherlands. I. Patient characteristics. Arch Intern Med 152:1863, 1992.

2. Hogevik H, Olaison L, Andersson R, et al: Epidemiologic aspects of infective endocarditis in an urban population: A 5-year prospective study. Medicine (Baltimore) 74:324-339, 1995.
3. Hoen B, Alla F, Selton-Suty C, et al: Changing profile of infective endocarditis: Results of a 1-year survey in France. JAMA 288:75, 2002.
4. Fernandez-Guerrero ML, Verdejo C, Azofra J, de Gorgolas M: Hospital-acquired infectious endocarditis not associated with cardiac surgery: An emerging problem. Clin Infect Dis 20:16, 1995.
5. Baltimore RS: Infective endocarditis in children. Pediatr Infect Dis J 11:907, 1992.
6. Morris CD, Reller MD, Menashe VD: Thirty-year incidence of infective endocarditis after surgery for congenital heart defect. JAMA 279:599, 1998.
7. Miro JM, del Rio A, Mestres CA: Infective endocarditis in intravenous drug abusers and HIV-1 infected patients. Infect Dis Clin North Am 16:273, 2002.
8. Stein A, Raoult D: Q fever endocarditis. Eur Heart J 16(Suppl B):19, 1995.
9. Raoult D, Fournier PE, Drancourt M, et al: Diagnosis of 22 new cases of *Bartonella* endocarditis. Ann Intern Med 125:646, 1996.
10. Sande MA, Lee BL, Mills J, et al: Endocarditis in intravenous drug users. *In* Kaye D (ed): Infective Endocarditis. 2nd ed. New York, Raven Press, 1992, p 345.
11. Mathew J, Addai T, Anand A, et al: Clinical features, site of involvement, bacteriologic findings, and outcome of infective endocarditis in intravenous drug users. Arch Intern Med 155:1641, 1995.
12. Pulvirenti JJ, Kerns E, Benson C, et al: Infective endocarditis in injection drug users: Importance of human immunodeficiency virus serostatus and degree of immunosuppression. Clin Infect Dis 22:40, 1996.
13. Ribera E, Miro JM, Cortes E, et al: Influence of human immunodeficiency virus 1 infection and degree of immunosuppression in the clinical characteristics and outcome of infective endocarditis in intravenous drug users. Arch Intern Med 158:2043, 1998.
14. Arvay A, Lengyel M: Incidence and risk factors of prosthetic valve endocarditis. Eur J Cardiothorac Surg 2:340, 1988.
15. Calderwood SB, Swinski LA, Waternaux CM, et al: Risk factors for the development of prosthetic valve endocarditis. Circulation 72:31, 1985.
16. Agnihotri AK, McGiffin DC, Galbraith AJ, O'Brien MF: Surgery for acquired heart disease. J Thorac Cardiovasc Surg 110:1708, 1995.
17. Karchmer AW, Longworth DL: Infections of intracardiac devices. Infect Dis Clin North Am 16:477, 2002.
18. Karchmer AW: Infections of prosthetic heart valves. *In* Waldvogel F, Bisno AL (eds): Infections Associated with Indwelling Medical Devices. Washington, DC, American Society for Microbiology, 2000, pp 145-172.
19. Lytle BW, Priest BP, Taylor PC, et al: Surgery for acquired heart disease: Surgical treatment of prosthetic valve endocarditis. J Thorac Cardiovasc Surg 111:198, 1996.
20. Chastre J, Trouillet JL: Early infective endocarditis on prosthetic valves. Eur Heart J 16(Suppl B):32, 1995.
21. Petti CA, Fowler VG Jr: *Staphylococcus aureus* bacteremia and endocarditis. Infect Dis Clin North Am 16:413, 2002.
22. Fowler VG Jr, Li J, Corey GR, et al: Role of echocardiography in evaluation of patients with *Staphylococcus aureus* bacteremia: Experience in 103 patients. J Am Coll Cardiol 30:1072, 1997.
23. Rosen AB, Fowler VG Jr, Corey GR, et al: Cost-effectiveness of transesophageal echocardiography to determine the duration of therapy for intravascular catheter-associated *Staphylococcus aureus* bacteremia. Ann Intern Med 130:810, 1999.
24. Heidenreich PA, Masoudi FA, Maini B, et al: Echocardiography in patients with suspected endocarditis: A cost-effectiveness analysis. Am J Med 107:198, 1999.
25. Bouvet A: Human endocarditis due to nutritionally variant streptococci: *Streptococcus adjacens* and *Streptococcus defectivus*. Eur Heart J 16(Suppl B):24, 1995.
26. Baddour LM, Infectious Diseases Society of America Emerging Infections Network: Infective endocarditis caused by β-hemolytic streptococci. Clin Infect Dis 26:66, 1998.
27. Lefort A, Lortholary O, Casassus P, et al: Comparison between adult endocarditis due to beta-hemolytic streptococci (serogroups A, B, C, and G) and *Streptococcus milleri*: A multi-center study in France. Arch Intern Med 162:2450, 2002.
28. Martinez E, Miro JM, Almirante B, et al: Effect of penicillin resistance of *Streptococcus pneumoniae* on the presentation, prognosis, and treatment of pneumococcal endocarditis in adults. Clin Infect Dis 35:130, 2002.
29. Aronin SI, Mukherjee SK, West JC, Cooney EL: Review of pneumococcal endocarditis in adults in the penicillin era. Clin Infect Dis 26:165, 1998.
30. Whitener C, Caputo GM, Weitekamp MR, Karchmer AW: Endocarditis due to coagulase-negative staphylococci: Microbiologic, epidemiologic, and clinical considerations. Infect Dis Clin North Am 7:81, 1993.
31. Roder BL, Wandall DA, Frimodt-Moller N, et al: Clinical features of *Staphylococcus aureus* endocarditis: A 10-year experience in Denmark. Arch Intern Med 159:462, 1999.
32. Fowler VG Jr, Sanders LL, Kong LK, et al: Infective endocarditis due to *Staphylococcus aureus*: 59 prospectively identified cases with follow-up. Clin Infect Dis 28:106, 1999.
33. Hessen MT, Abrutyn E: Gram-negative bacterial endocarditis. *In* Kaye D (ed): Infective Endocarditis. 2nd ed. New York, Raven Press, 1992, p 251.
34. Brouqui P, Raoult D: Endocarditis due to rare and fastidious bacteria. Clin Microbiol Rev 14:177, 2001.
35. Berbari EF, Cockerill FR III, Steckelberg J: Infective endocarditis due to unusual or fastidious microorganisms. Mayo Clin Proc 72:532, 1997.
36. Petit AIC, Bok JW, Thompson J, et al: Native-valve endocarditis due to CDC coryneform group ANF-3: Report of a case and review of corynebacterial endocarditis. Clin Infect Dis 19:897, 1994.
37. Fenollar F, Lepidi H, Raoult D: Whipple's endocarditis: Review of the literature and comparisons with Q fever, *Bartonella* infection, and blood culture–positive endocarditis. Clin Infect Dis 33:1309, 2001.
38. Gubler JGH, Kuster M, Dutly F, et al: Whipple endocarditis without overt gastrointestinal disease: Report of four cases. Ann Intern Med 131:112, 1999.
39. Fenollar F, Fournier PE, Carrieri MP, et al: Risk factors and prevention of Q fever endocarditis. Clin Infect Dis 33:312, 2001.
40. Raoult D, Fournier PE, Vandenesch F, et al: Outcome and treatment of *Bartonella* endocarditis. Arch Intern Med 163:226, 2003.
41. Ellis ME, Al-Abdely H, Sandridge A, et al: Fungal endocarditis: Evidence in the world literature, 1965-1995. Clin Infect Dis 32:50, 2001.

Pathogenesis and Pathophysiology

42. Moreillon P, Que YA, Bayer AS: Pathogenesis of streptococcal and staphylococcal endocarditis. Infect Dis Clin North Am 16:297, 2002.
43. Weinstein L, Schlesinger JJ: Pathoanatomic, pathophysiologic and clinical correlations in endocarditis (first of two parts). N Engl J Med 291:832, 1974.
44. Livornese LL Jr, Korzeniowski OM: Pathogenesis of infective endocarditis. *In* Kaye D (ed): Infective Endocarditis. 2nd ed. New York, Raven Press, 1992, p 19.
45. Weinstein L, Schlesinger JJ: Pathoanatomic, pathophysiologic and clinical correlations in endocarditis (second of two parts). N Engl J Med 291:1122, 1974.
46. Croft CH, Woodward W, Elliott A, et al: Analysis of surgical versus medical therapy in active complicated native valve infective endocarditis. Am J Cardiol 51:1650, 1983.
47. Watanabe G, Haverich A, Speier R, et al: Surgical treatment of active infective endocarditis with paravalvular involvement. J Thorac Cardiovasc Surg 107:171, 1994.
48. Baumgartner FJ, Omari BO, Robertson JM, et al: Annular abscesses in surgical endocarditis: Anatomic, clinical and operative features. Ann Thorac Surg 70:442, 2000.
49. Douglas JL, Dismukes WE: Surgical therapy of infective endocarditis on natural valves. *In* Kaye D (ed): Infective Endocarditis. 2nd ed. New York, Raven Press, 1992, p 397.
50. Mansur AJ, Grinberg M, Lamos da Luz P, Bellotti G: The complications of infective endocarditis: A reappraisal in the 1980's. Arch Intern Med 152:2428, 1992.
51. Steckelberg JM, Murphy JG, Wilson WR: Management of complications of infective endocarditis. *In* Kaye D (ed): Infective Endocarditis. 2nd ed. New York, Raven Press, 1992, p 435.
52. DiSalvo G, Habib G, Pergola V, et al: Echocardiography predicts embolic events in infective endocarditis. J Am Coll Cardiol 37:1077, 2001.

Clinical Features and Diagnosis

53. Werner GS, Schulz R, Fuchs JB, et al: Infective endocarditis in the elderly in the era of transesophageal echocardiography: Clinical features and prognosis compared with younger patients. Am J Med 100:90, 1996.
54. Crawford MH, Durack DT: Clinical presentation of infective endocarditis. Cardiol Clin 21:159, 2003.
55. Steckelberg JM, Murphy JG, Ballard D, et al: Emboli in infective endocarditis: The prognostic value of echocardiography. Ann Intern Med 114:635, 1991.
56. Roder BL, Wandall DA, Espersen F, et al: Neurologic manifestations in *Staphylococcus aureus* endocarditis: A review of 260 bacteremic cases in nondrug addicts. Am J Med 102:379, 1997.
57. Gagliardi JP, Nettles RE, McCarty DE, et al: Native valve infective endocarditis in elderly and younger adult patients: Comparison of clinical features and outcomes with use of the Duke criteria and the Duke endocarditis data base. Clin Infect Dis 26:1165, 1998.
58. Masuda J, Yutani C, Waki R, et al: Histopathological analysis of the mechanisms of intracranial hemorrhage complicating infective endocarditis. Stroke 23:843, 1992.
59. Durack DT, Lukes AS, Bright DK: New criteria for diagnosis of infective endocarditis: Utilization of specific echocardiographic findings. Am J Med 96:200, 1994.
60. Li JS, Sexton DJ, Mick N, et al: Proposed modifications to the Duke criteria for the diagnosis of infective endocarditis. Clin Infect Dis 30:633, 2000.
61. Bayer AS, Bolger AF, Taubert KA, et al: Diagnosis and management of infective endocarditis and its complications. Circulation 98:2936, 1998.
62. Sochowski RA, Chan KL: Implication of negative results on a monoplane transesophageal echocardiographic study in patients with suspected infective endocarditis. J Am Coll Cardiol 21:216, 1993.
63. Hoen B, Selton-Suty C, Lacassin F, et al: Infective endocarditis in patients with negative blood cultures: Analysis of 88 cases from a one-year nationwide survey in France. Clin Infect Dis 20:501, 1995.
64. Towns ML, Reller LB: Diagnostic methods current best practices and guidelines for isolation of bacteria and fungi in infective endocarditis. Infect Dis Clin North Am 16:363, 2002.
65. Lisby G, Gutschik E, Durack DT: Molecular methods for diagnosis of infective endocarditis. Infect Dis Clin North Am 16:393, 2002.
66. Bayer AS, Scheld WM: Endocarditis and intravascular infections. *In* Mandell GL, Bennett JE, Dolin R (eds): Principles and Practice of Infectious Diseases. Philadelphia, Churchill Livingstone, 2000, pp 857-902.
67. Lindner JR, Case RA, Dent JM, et al: Diagnostic value of echocardiography in suspected endocarditis: An evaluation based on the pretest probability of disease. Circulation 93:730, 1996.
68. Roe MT, Abramson MA, Li J, et al: Clinical information determines the impact of transesophageal echocardiography on the diagnosis of infective endocarditis by the Duke criteria. Am Heart J 139:945, 2000.
69. Daniel WG, Mugge A: Transesophageal echocardiography. N Engl J Med 332:1268, 1995.
70. Morguet AJ, Werner GS, Andreas S, Kreuzer H: Diagnostic value of transesophageal compared with transthoracic echocardiography in suspected prosthetic valve endocarditis. Herz 20:390, 1995.
71. Daniel WG, Mugge A, Grote J, et al: Comparison of transthoracic and transesophageal echocardiography for detection of abnormalities of prosthetic and bioprosthetic valves in the mitral and aortic positions. Am J Cardiol 71:210, 1993.
72. Vuille C, Nidorf M, Weyman AE, Picard MH: Natural history of vegetations during successful medical treatment of endocarditis. Am Heart J 128:1200, 1994.

73. DeCastro S, Cartoni D, d'Amati G, et al: Diagnostic accuracy of transthoracic and multiplane transesophageal echocardiography for valvular perforation in acute infective endocarditis: Correlation with anatomic findings. Clin Infect Dis 30:826, 2000.
74. Sachdev M, Peterson GE, Jollis JG: Imaging techniques for diagnosis of infective endocarditis. Infect Dis Clin North Am 16:319, 2002.

Treatment

75. Wilson WR, Karchmer AW, Dajani AS, et al: Antibiotic treatment of adults with infective endocarditis due to streptococci, enterococci, staphylococci, and HACEK microorganisms. JAMA 274:1706, 1995.
76. Roberts SA, Lang SDR, Ellis-Pegler RB: Short-course treatment of penicillin-susceptible viridans streptococcal infective endocarditis with penicillin and gentamicin. Infect Dis Clin Pract 2:191, 1993.
77. Sexton DJ, Tenenbaum MJ, Wilson WR, et al: Ceftriaxone once daily for four weeks compared with ceftriaxone plus gentamicin once daily for two weeks for treatment of endocarditis due to penicillin-susceptible streptococci. Clin Infect Dis 27:1470, 1998.
78. Olaison L, Schadewitz K, The Swedish Society for Infectious Diseases Quality Assurance Study Group for Endocarditis: Enterococcal endocarditis in Sweden, 1995-1999: Can shorter therapy with aminoglycosides be used? Clin Infect Dis 34:159, 2002.
79. Mainardi JL, Shlaes DM, Goering RV, et al: Decreased teicoplanin susceptibility of methicillin-resistant strains of *Staphylococcus aureus*. J Infect Dis 171:1646, 1995.
80. Sett SS, Hudon MPJ, Jamieson WRE, Chow AW: Prosthetic valve endocarditis: Experience with porcine bioprostheses. J Thorac Cardiovasc Surg 105:428, 1993.
81. John MVD, Hibberd PL, Karchmer AW, et al: *Staphylococcus aureus* prosthetic valve endocarditis: Optimal management and risk factors for death. Clin Infect Dis 26:1302, 1998.
82. Nguyen MH, Nguyen ML, Yu VL, et al: *Candida* prosthetic valve endocarditis: Prospective study of six cases and review of the literature. Clin Infect Dis 22:262, 1996.
83. Nasser RM, Melgar GR, Longworth DL, Gordon SM: Incidence and risk of developing fungal prosthetic valve endocarditis after nosocomial candidemia. Am J Med 103:25, 1997.
84. Raoult D, Houpikian P, Tissot Dupont H, et al: Treatment of Q fever endocarditis: Comparison of 2 regimens containing doxycycline and ofloxacin or hydroxychloroquine. Arch Intern Med 159:167, 1999.
85. Tunkel AR, Kaye D: Endocarditis with negative blood cultures. N Engl J Med 326:1215, 1992.
86. Olaison L, Berlin L, Hogevik H, Alestig K: Incidence of β-lactam-induced delayed hypersensitivity and neutropenia during treatment of infective endocarditis. Arch Intern Med 159:607, 1999.
87. Andrews MM, von Reyn CF: Patient selection criteria and management guidelines for outpatient parenteral antibiotic therapy for native valve infective endocarditis. Clin Infect Dis 33:203, 2001.
88. Olaison L, Pettersson G: Current best practices and guidelines indications for surgical intervention in infective endocarditis. Cardiol Clin 21:235, 2003.
89. Bishara J, Leibovici L, Gartman-Israel D, et al: Long-term outcome of infective endocarditis: The impact of early surgical intervention. Clin Infect Dis 33:1636, 2001.
89a. Vikram HR, Buenconsejo J, Hasbun R, Quagliarello VJ: Impact of valve surgery on 6-month mortality in adults with complicated, left-sided native valve endocarditis: A propensity analysis. JAMA 290:3207, 2003.
90. Karchmer AW: Infections of prosthetic valves and intravascular devices. *In* Mandell GL, Bennett JE, Dolin R (eds): Principles and Practice of Infectious Diseases. New York, Churchill Livingstone, 2000, pp 907-913.
91. Morris AJ, Drinkovic D, Pottumarthy S, et al: Gram stain, culture, and histopathological examination findings for heart valves removed because of infective endocarditis. Clin Infect Dis 36:697, 2003.
92. Blumberg EA, Karalis DA, Chandrasekaran K, et al: Endocarditis-associated paravalvular abscess. Do clinical parameters predict the presence of abscess? Chest 107:898, 1995.
93. Meine TJ, Nettles RE, Anderson DJ, et al: Cardiac conduction abnormalities in endocarditis defined by the Duke criteria. Am Heart J 142:280, 2001.
94. Tischler MD, Vaitkus PT: The ability of vegetation size on echocardiography to predict clinical complications: A meta-analysis. J Am Soc Echocardiogr 10:562, 1997.
95. Cabell CH, Pond KK, Peterson GE, et al: The risk of stroke and death in patients with aortic and mitral valve endocarditis. Am Heart J 142:75, 2001.
96. Mangoni ED, Adinolfi LE, Tripodi MF, et al: Risk factors for "major" embolic events in hospitalized patients with infective endocarditis. Am Heart J 146:311, 2003.
97. Davenport J, Hart RG: Prosthetic valve endocarditis 1976-1987: Antibiotics, anticoagulation, and stroke. Stroke 21:993, 1990.
98. Reinhartz O, Herrmann M, Redling F, Zerkowski HR: Timing of surgery in patients with acute infective endocarditis. J Cardiovasc Surg 37:397, 1996.
99. Eishi K, Kawazoe K, Kuriyama Y, et al: Surgical management of infective endocarditis associated with cerebral complications: Multicenter retrospective study in Japan. J Thorac Cardiovasc Surg 110:1745, 1995.
100. Gillinov AM, Shah RV, Curtis WE, et al: Valve replacement in patients with endocarditis and acute neurologic deficit. Ann Thorac Surg 61:1125, 1996.
101. Phuong LK, Link M, Wijdicks E: Management of intracranial infections aneurysms: A series of 16 cases. Neurosurgery 51:1145, 2002.
102. Lederman MM, Sprague L, Wallis RS, Ellner JJ: Duration of fever during treatment of infective endocarditis. Medicine (Baltimore) 71:52, 1992.
102a. Hasbun R, Vikram HR, Barakat LA, et al: Complicated left-side native valve endocarditis in adults: Risk classification for mortality. JAMA 289:1933, 2003.
103. Acar J, Michel PL, Varenne O, et al: Surgical treatment of infective endocarditis. Eur Heart J 16(Suppl B):94, 1995.
104. Amrani M, Schoevaerdts JC, Eucher P, et al: Extension of native aortic valve endocarditis: Surgical considerations. Eur Heart J 16(Suppl B):103, 1995.
105. Mullany CJ, Chua YL, Schaff HV, et al: Early and late survival after surgical treatment of culture-positive active endocarditis. Mayo Clin Proc 70:517, 1995.
106. d'Udekem Y, David TE, Feindel CM, et al: Long-term results of surgery for active infective endocarditis. Eur J Cardiothorac Surg 11:46, 1997.
107. Alexiou C, Langley SM, Stafford H, et al: Surgery for active culture-positive endocarditis: Determinants of early and late outcome. Ann Thorac Surg 69:1448, 2000.
108. d'Udekem Y, David TE, Feindel CM, et al: Long-term results of operation for paravalvular abscess. Ann Thorac Surg 62:48, 1996.
109. Dajani AS, Taubert KA, Wilson W, et al: Prevention of bacterial endocarditis: Recommendations by the American Heart Association, from the Committee on Rheumatic Fever, Endocarditis, and Kawasaki Disease, Council on Cardiovascular Diseases in the Young. JAMA 277:1794, 1997.

Prevention

110. Durack DT: Prevention of infective endocarditis. N Engl J Med 332:38, 1995.
111. van der Meer JTM, Thompson J, Valkenburg HA, Michel MF: Epidemiology of bacterial endocarditis in the Netherlands. II. Antecedent procedures and use of prophylaxis. Arch Intern Med 152:1869, 1992.
112. DeGevigney G, Pop C, Delahaye JP: The risk of infective endocarditis after cardiac surgical and interventional procedures. Eur Heart J 16(Suppl B):7, 1995.
113. Spirito P, Rapezzi C, Bellone P, et al: Infective endocarditis hypertrophic cardiomyopathy. Circulation 99:2132, 1999.
114. Blatter M, Francioli P: Endocarditis prophylaxis: From experimental models to human recommendation. Eur Heart J 16(Suppl B):107, 1995.
115. Fluckiger U, Moreillon P, Blaser J, et al: Simulation of amoxicillin pharmacokinetics in humans for the prevention of streptococcal endocarditis in rats. Antimicrob Agents Chemother 38:2846, 1994.
116. Strom BL, Abrutyn E, Berlin JA, et al: Dental and cardiac risk factors for infective endocarditis: A population-based, case-control study. Ann Intern Med 129:761, 1998.

GUIDELINES *Thomas H. Lee*

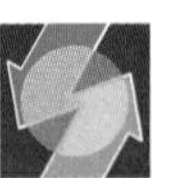

Infective Endocarditis

The American Heart Association issued guidelines for antibiotic prophylaxis to prevent infective endocarditis in 1997[1] and a scientific statement with recommendations for diagnosis and management of this condition in 1998.[2] Other guidelines with recommendations relevant to this condition include American College of Cardiology/American Heart Association (ACC/AHA) guidelines for management of valvular heart disease published in 1998[3] and guidelines for use of echocardiography published in 1997.[4]

Prevention

The 1997 AHA guidelines for antibiotic prophylaxis to prevent endocarditis represented a major departure from prior recommendations by emphasizing that most cases are not attributable to an invasive procedure. According to these guidelines, patients with preexisting cardiac disease should be divided into high-, moderate-, and negligible-risk categories on the basis of their potential outcomes if endocarditis develops (see Table 58–14). For dental work, for example, antibiotic prophylaxis is recommended just for patients with high- and moderate-risk cardiac conditions who are undergoing higher risk procedures (Table 58G–1). For nondental procedures, endocarditis prophylaxis is recommended just for high-risk patients undergoing high-risk procedures (see Table 58–14); this strategy is considered optional for medium-risk patients. Antibiotic regimens are described in Table 58–16.

The 1998 ACC/AHA guidelines for patients with valvular heart disease[3] are consistent with these recommendations, with a few caveats. The ACC/AHA guidelines recommend antibiotic prophylaxis for patients with hypertrophic cardiomyopathy only when there is latent or resting obstruction. In addition, the ACC/AHA committee expressed concern that an increased risk for endocarditis may exist

TABLE 58G–1 Dental Procedures and Endocarditis Prophylaxis

Endocarditis Prophylaxis Recommended for Patients with High- and Moderate-Risk Cardiac Conditions (see Tables 58–14 and 58–15)
Dental extractions
Periodontal procedures including surgery, scaling and root planning, probing, and recall maintenance
Dental implant placement and reimplantation of avulsed teeth
Endodontic (root canal) instrumentation or surgery only beyond the apex
Subgingival placement of antibiotic fibers or strips
Initial placement of orthodontic bands but not brackets
Intraligamentary local anesthetic injections
Prophylactic cleaning of teeth or implants where bleeding is anticipated
Endocarditis Prophylaxis not Recommended
Restorative dentistry* (operative and prosthodontic) with or without retraction cord†
Local anesthetic injections (nonintraligamentary)
Intracanal endodontic treatment; after placement and build-up
Placement of rubber dams
Postoperative suture removal
Placement of removable prosthodontic or orthodontic appliances
Taking of oral impressions
Fluoride treatments
Taking of oral radiographs
Orthodontic appliance adjustment
Shedding of primary teeth

From Dajani AS, Taubert KA, Wilson W, et al: Prevention of bacterial endocarditis: Recommendations by the American Heart Association. Circulation 96:358, 1997.

*This includes restoration of decayed teeth (filling cavities) and replacement of missing teeth.

†Clinical judgment may indicate antibiotic use in selected circumstances that may create significant bleeding.

for some patients with mitral valve prolapse without regurgitation; hence, this group was not willing to state that antibiotic prophylaxis was inappropriate for such patients. Finally, the ACC/AHA guidelines specified that antibiotic prophylaxis was not necessary in patients with physiological mitral regurgitation in the absence of a murmur.

Indications for Echocardiography

Echocardiography is strongly supported in virtually all patients with suspected or known infective endocarditis, but the 1997 ACC/AHA guidelines on echocardiography[4] do not recommend transesophageal echocardiography (TEE) as the initial test of choice in the diagnosis of native valve endocarditis (Table 58G–2). The guidelines urge use of TEE when specific questions are not adequately addressed by an initial transthoracic echocardiography (TTE) evaluation, such as if the TTE is of poor quality, if the TTE is negative despite a high clinical suspicion of endocarditis, if a prosthetic valve is involved, and if there is a high suspicion such as in a patient with staphylococcal bacteremia or in an elderly patient with valvular abnormalities that make diagnosis by TTE difficult.

Diagnosis of prosthetic valve endocarditis with TTE is more difficult than diagnosis of endocarditis of native valves. Thus, the ACC/AHA guidelines suggest a lower threshold for performance of TEE in patients with prosthetic valves and suspected endocarditis (see Table 58G–2).

Surgery for Active Endocarditis

The ACC/AHA guidelines for valvular heart disease support performance of surgery for patients with life-threatening congestive heart failure or cardiogenic shock related to active endocarditis. Indications for surgery for patients with stable endocarditis are considered less clear (see Table 58G–2).

TABLE 58G–2 ACC/AHA Guidelines for Prevention, Evaluation, and Treatment of Endocarditis

Indication	Class I	Class IIa	Class IIb	Class III
Antibiotic endocarditis prophylaxis for patients with mitral valve prolapse undergoing procedures associated with bacteremia	1. Patients with characteristic systolic click-murmur complex 2. Patients with isolated systolic click and echocardiographic evidence of MVP and MR	1. Patients with isolated systolic click, echocardiographic evidence of high-risk MVP		1. Patients with isolated systolic click and equivocal or no evidence of MVP
Echocardiography in infective endocarditis: native valves	1. Detection and characterization of valvular lesions, their hemodynamic severity, and/or ventricular compensation* 2. Detection of vegetations and characterization of lesions in patients with congenital heart disease in whom infective endocarditis is suspected 3. Detection of associated abnormalities (e.g., abscesses, shunts)* 4. Re-evaluation studies in complex endocarditis (e.g., virulent organism, severe hemodynamic lesion, aortic valve involvement, persistent fever or bacteremia, clinical change, or symptomatic deterioration) 5. Evaluation of patients with high clinical suspicion of culture-negative endocarditis*	1. Evaluation of bacteremia without a known source* 2. Risk stratification in established endocarditis*	1. Routine re-evaluation in uncomplicated endocarditis during antibiotic therapy	1. Evaluation of fever and nonpathological murmur without evidence of bacteremia

TABLE 58G–2 ACC/AHA Guidelines for Prevention, Evaluation, and Treatment of Endocarditis—cont'd

Indication	Class I	Class IIa	Class IIb	Class III
Echocardiography in infective endocarditis: prosthetic valves	1. Detection and characterization of valvular lesions, their hemodynamic severity, and/or ventricular compensation* 2. Detection of associated abnormalities (e.g., abscesses, shunts)* 3. Re-evaluation in complex endocarditis (e.g., virulent organism, severe hemodynamic lesion, aortic valve involvement, persistent fever or bacteremia, clinical change, or symptomatic deterioration) 4. Evaluation of suspected endocarditis and negative cultures* 5. Evaluation of bacteremia without a known source*	1. Evaluation of persistent fever without evidence of bacteremia or new murmur*	1. Routine re-evaluation in uncomplicated endocarditis during antibiotic therapy*	1. Evaluation of transient fever without evidence of bacteremia or new murmur
Surgery for native valve endocarditis (criteria also apply to repaired mitral and aortic allograft or autograft valves)	1. Acute AR or MR with heart failure 2. Acute AR with tachycardia and early closure of the mitral valve 3. Fungal endocarditis 4. Evidence of annular or aortic abscess, sinus or aortic true or false aneurysm 5. Evidence of valve dysfunction and persistent infection after a prolonged period (7 to 10 d) of appropriate antibiotic therapy, as indicated by presence of fever, leukocytosis, and bacteremia, provided there are no noncardiac causes for infection	1. Recurrent emboli after appropriate antibiotic therapy 2. Infection with gram-negative organisms or organisms with a poor response to antibiotics in patients with evidence of valve dysfunction	1. Mobile vegetations >10 mm	1. Early infections of the mitral valve that can probably be repaired 2. Persistent pyrexia and leukocytosis with negative blood cultures
Surgery for prosthetic valve endocarditis (criteria exclude repaired mitral and aortic allograft or autograft valves)	1. Early prosthetic valve endocarditis (first 2 mo or less after surgery) 2. Heart failure with prosthetic valve dysfunction 3. Fungal endocarditis 4. Staphylococcal endocarditis not responding to antibiotic therapy 5. Evidence of paravalvular leak, annular or aortic abscess, sinus or aortic true or false aneurysm, fistula formation, or new-onset conduction disturbances 6. Infection with gram-negative organisms or organisms with a poor response to antibiotics	1. Persistent bacteremia after a prolonged course (7 to 10 d) of appropriate antibiotic therapy without noncardiac causes for bacteremia 2. Recurrent peripheral embolus despite therapy	1. Vegetation of any size on or near the prosthesis	

ACC/AHA = American College of Cardiology/American Heart Association; AR = aortic regurgitation; MR = mitral regurgitation; MVP = mitral valve prolapse.

From Bonow RO, Carabello B, de Leon AC Jr, et al: ACC/AHA guidelines for the management of patients with valvular heart disease: Executive summary. A report of the American College of Cardiology/American Heart Association Task Force on Practice Guidelines (Committee on Management of Patients With Valvular Heart Disease). Circulation 98:1949, 1998; and Cheitlin MD, Alpert JS, Armstrong WF, et al: ACC/AHA guidelines for the clinical application of echocardiography: A report of the American College of Cardiology/American Heart Association Task Force on Practice Guidelines (Committee on Clinical Application of Echocardiography). Circulation 95:1686, 1997.

*Transesophageal echocardiography may provide incremental value in addition to information obtained by transthoracic imaging.

References

1. Dajani AS, Taubert KA, Wilson W, et al: Prevention of bacterial endocarditis: Recommendations by the American Heart Association. Circulation 96:358, 1997.
2. Bayer AS, Bolger AF, Taubert KA, et al: Diagnosis and management of infective endocarditis and its complications. Circulation 98:2936, 1998.
3. Bonow RO, Carabello B, de Leon AC Jr, et al: ACC/AHA guidelines for the management of patients with valvular heart disease: Executive summary: A report of the American College of Cardiology/American Heart Association Task Force on Practice Guidelines (Committee on Management of Patients With Valvular Heart Disease). Circulation 98:1949, 1998.
4. Cheitlin MD, Alpert JS, Armstrong WF, et al: ACC/AHA guidelines for the clinical application of echocardiography: A report of the American College of Cardiology/American Heart Association Task Force on Practice Guidelines (Committee on Clinical Application of Echocardiography). Circulation 95:1686, 1997.

CHAPTER 59

The Cardiomyopathies

Joshua Wynne • Eugene Braunwald

The cardiomyopathies constitute a group of disorders in which the dominant feature is direct involvement of the heart muscle itself. They are distinctive because they are *not* the result of pericardial, hypertensive, congenital, or valvular diseases. Although the diagnosis of cardiomyopathy requires the exclusion of these etiological factors, the features of cardiomyopathy are often sufficiently distinctive—both clinically and hemodynamically—to allow a definitive diagnosis to be made. With increasing awareness of this condition, along with improvements in diagnostic techniques, cardiomyopathy is being recognized as a significant cause of morbidity and mortality. Whether the result of improved recognition or of other factors, the incidence and prevalence of heart failure related to cardiomyopathy appear to be increasing.[1] Although coronary artery disease is the most common cause of congestive heart failure (accounting for more than two-thirds of all cases), we avoid using the term *ischemic cardiomyopathy* in this setting because the primary problem is in the coronary arteries and not the heart muscle itself. Nevertheless, some use this imprecise term to describe the condition in which coronary artery disease causes multiple infarctions, diffuse fibrosis, or severe ischemia that leads to left ventricular dilation with congestive heart failure; it may or may not be associated with angina pectoris (see Chap. 50).

A variety of schemes have been proposed for classifying the cardiomyopathies. The most widely recognized classification is that promulgated jointly by the World Health Organization (WHO) and the International Society and Federation of Cardiology (ISFC) (Table 59–1).[2] In the WHO/ISFC classification, the cardiomyopathies are classified on the basis of their predominant pathophysiological features; other diseases that affect the myocardium but that are associated with a particular cardiac disorder or are part of a generalized systemic disorder are termed *specific cardiomyopathies* (in the previous WHO/ISFC classification, they were termed *specific heart muscle diseases*).[2]

Three basic types of functional impairment have been described (Table 59–2 and Fig. 59–1): (1) *dilated* cardiomyopathy (DCM), the most common form, accounting for the majority of cardiomyopathies and characterized by ventricular dilation, contractile dysfunction, and often symptoms of congestive heart failure; (2) *hypertrophic* cardiomyopathy (HCM), recognized by inappropriate left ventricular hypertrophy, often with asymmetrical involvement of the interventricular septum, with preserved or enhanced contractile function until late in the course of the disease; and (3) *restrictive* cardiomyopathy (RCM), the least common form in Western countries, marked by impaired diastolic filling and in some cases with endocardial scarring of the ventricle.[3] The distinction between the three major functional categories is not absolute, and often there is overlap; in particular, patients with HCM also have increased wall stiffness (as a consequence of the myocardial hypertrophy) and thus manifest some of the features of an RCM.[2] Two less common forms of cardiomyopathy are recognized: *arrhythmogenic right ventricular cardiomyopathy* (ARVC) and *unclassified*; the latter includes fibroelastosis, systolic dysfunction with minimal dilation, and isolated ventricular noncompaction, an unusual disease marked by prominent endocardial thickening with prominent trabeculations and deep recesses.[4] Furthermore, ventricular dilation and systolic heart failure may occur late in the course of HCM and bear a resemblance to DCM.

Examples of what have been termed *specific cardiomyopathies* include valvular cardiomyopathy, hypertensive cardiomyopathy, and inflammatory cardiomyopathy (myocarditis with cardiac dysfunction) (see Table 59–1 and Chap. 60).[2]

Endomyocardial Biopsy

Evaluation of some patients suspected of suffering from a cardiomyopathy has been facilitated by the use of endomyocardial biopsy.[5] Using a flexible bioptome, the clinician may obtain tissue samples from the right ventricle (and left ventricle when required) through a transvenous (or transarterial) approach with ease and safety (see Chap. 17). The availability of disposable transfemoral bioptomes has further facilitated endomyocardial biopsy. Two-dimensional echocardiography may help guide the placement of the bioptome and reduce or eliminate radiation exposure. Endomyocardial biopsy results in a small tissue sample (average size 1 to 2 mm), and multiple samples (usually four or more) are required because pronounced topographical variations may be found within the myocardium. Which patients should be subjected to biopsy remains controversial, but there is general agreement that biopsy may be of benefit in certain specific situations.[6] There is little debate about its clinical utility in detecting infiltrative disorders of the myocardium and in monitoring for anthracycline cardiotoxicity and cardiac transplant rejection.[5,7]

Although on occasion endomyocardial biopsy may identify a specific etiological agent in an individual patient with cardiac disease of uncertain cause, the clinical utility of routine biopsy in cardiomyopathy is limited (particularly because no definitive pattern has been found in DCM) (Fig. 59-2).[8] It has been estimated that a specific etiological diagnosis is obtained by biopsy in fewer than 10 percent of patients with cardiomyopathy[8] and a treatable disease is found even less often.

DALLAS CRITERIA. Interpretation of biopsy specimens had been plagued by a high degree of interobserver variability; the adoption of a generally accepted set of histological definitions, the *Dallas criteria*, has improved agreement.[8] Nevertheless, there continues to be a lack of agreement about the diagnostic usefulness of any scheme that utilizes conventional histological findings—including the Dallas criteria—to evaluate a process as complex as

TABLE 59–1 Classification of the Cardiomyopathies

Disorder	Description
Dilated cardiomyopathy	Dilation and impaired contraction of the left or both ventricles. Caused by familial-genetic, viral, and/or immune, alcoholic-toxic, or unknown factors or is associated with recognized cardiovascular disease.
Hypertrophic cardiomyopathy	Left and/or right ventricular hypertrophy, often asymmetrical, which usually involves the interventricular septum. Mutations in sarcoplasmic proteins cause the disease in many patients.
Restrictive cardiomyopathy	Restricted filling and reduced diastolic size of either or both ventricles with normal or near-normal systolic function. Is idiopathic or associated with other disease (e.g., amyloidosis, endomyocardial disease).
Arrhythmogenic right ventricular cardiomyopathy	Progressive fibrofatty replacement of the right, and to some degree left, ventricular myocardium. Familial disease is common.
Unclassified cardiomyopathy	Diseases that do not fit readily into any category. Examples include systolic dysfunction with minimal dilation, mitochondrial disease, and fibroelastosis.
Specific Cardiomyopathies	
Ischemic cardiomyopathy	Arises as dilated cardiomyopathy with depressed ventricular function not explained by the extent of coronary artery obstructions or ischemic damage.
Valvular cardiomyopathy	Arises as ventricular dysfunction that is out of proportion to the abnormal loading conditions produced by the valvular stenosis and/or regurgitation.
Hypertensive cardiomyopathy	Arises with left ventricular hypertrophy with features of cardiac failure related to systolic or diastolic dysfunction.
Inflammatory cardiomyopathy	Cardiac dysfunction as a consequence of myocarditis.
Metabolic cardiomyopathy	Includes a wide variety of causes, including endocrine abnormalities, glycogen storage disease, deficiencies (such as hypokalemia), and nutritional disorders.
General systemic disease	Includes connective tissue disorders and infiltrative diseases such as sarcoidosis and leukemia.
Muscular dystrophies	Includes Duchenne, Becker-type, and myotonic dystrophies.
Neuromuscular disorders	Includes Friedreich ataxia, Noonan syndrome, and lentiginosis.
Sensitivity and toxic reactions	Includes reactions to alcohol, catecholamines, anthracyclines, irradiation, and others.
Peripartal cardiomyopathy	First becomes manifest in the peripartum period, but it is probably a heterogeneous group.

Derived from Richardson, P McKenna W, Bristow M, et al: Report of the 1995 World Health Organization/International Society and Federation of Cardiology Task Force on the Definition and Classification of Cardiomyopathies. Circulation 93:841, 1996. Copyright 1996, American Heart Association.

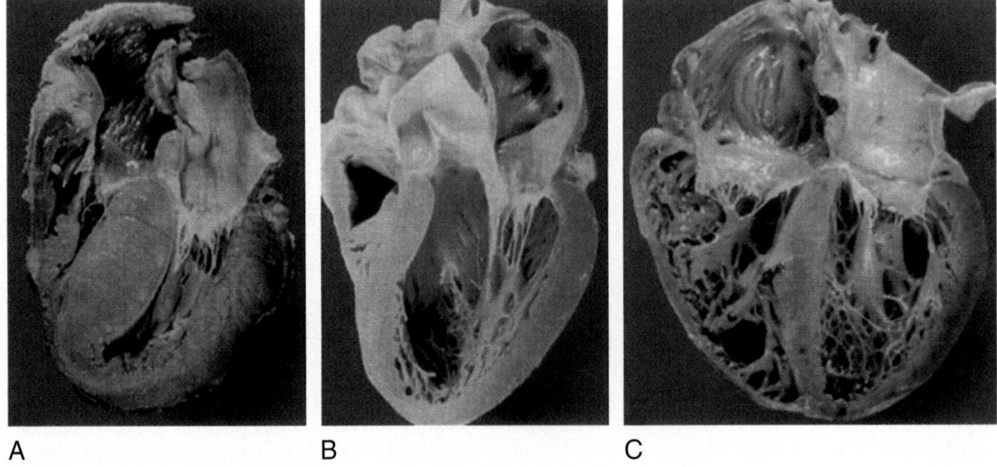

FIGURE 59–1 Gross pathological specimens of the cardiomyopathies. **A,** Hypertrophic cardiomyopathy, showing a marked increase in myocardial mass and preferential hypertrophy of the interventricular septum. **B,** Normal heart, with normal left ventricular dimensions and thickness. **C,** Dilated cardiomyopathy, showing marked increase in chamber size. Atrial enlargement is also evident in both cardiomyopathies (A and C). (From Seidman JG, Seidman C: The genetic basis for cardiomyopathy: From mutation identification to mechanistic paradigms. Cell 104:557, 2001.)

TABLE 59–2 Functional Classification of the Cardiomyopathies

Dilated	Restrictive	Hypertrophic
Symptoms		
Congestive heart failure, particularly left sided Fatigue and weakness Systemic or pulmonary emboli	Dyspnea, fatigue Right-sided congestive heart failure Signs and symptoms of systemic disease, e.g., amyloidosis, iron storage disease	Dyspnea, angina pectoris Fatigue, syncope, palpitations
Physical Examination		
Moderate to severe cardiomegaly; S_3, S_4 Atrioventricular valve regurgitation, especially mitral	Mild to moderate cardiomegaly; S_3 or S_4 Atrioventricular valve regurgitation; inspiratory increase in venous pressure (Kussmaul sign)	Mild cardiomegaly Apical systolic thrill and heave; brisk carotid upstroke S_4 common Systolic murmur that increases with Valsalva maneuver
Chest Roentgenogram		
Moderate to marked cardiac enlargement, especially left ventricular Pulmonary venous hypertension	Mild cardiac enlargement Pulmonary venous hypertension	Mild to moderate cardiac enlargement Left atrial enlargement
Electrocardiogram		
Sinus tachycardia Atrial and ventricular arrhythmias ST segment and T wave abnormalities Intraventricular conduction defects	Low voltage Intraventricular conduction defects Atrioventricular conduction defects	Left ventricular hypertrophy ST segment and T wave abnormalities Abnormal Q waves Atrial and ventricular arrhythmias
Echocardiogram		
Left ventricular dilation and dysfunction Abnormal diastolic mitral valve motion secondary to abnormal compliance and filling pressures	Increased left ventricular wall thickness and mass Small or normal-sized left ventricular cavity Normal systolic function Pericardial effusion	Asymmetrical septal hypertrophy (ASH) Narrow left ventricular outflow tract Systolic anterior motion (SAM) of the mitral valve Small or normal-sized left ventricle
Radionuclide Studies		
Left ventricular dilation and dysfunction (RVG)	Infiltration of myocardium (^{201}Tl) Small or normal-sized left ventricle (RVG) Normal systolic function (RVG)	Small or normal-sized left ventricle (RVG) Vigorous systolic function (RVG) Asymmetrical septal hypertrophy (RVG or ^{201}Tl)
Cardiac Catheterization		
Left ventricular enlargement and dysfunction Mitral and/or tricuspid regurgitation Elevated left- and often right-sided filling pressures Diminished cardiac output	Diminished left ventricular compliance "Square root sign" in ventricular pressure recordings Preserved systolic function Elevated left- and right-sided filling pressures	Diminished left ventricular compliance Mitral regurgitation Vigorous systolic function Dynamic left ventricular outflow gradient

RVG = radionuclide ventriculogram; ^{201}Tl = thallium-201.

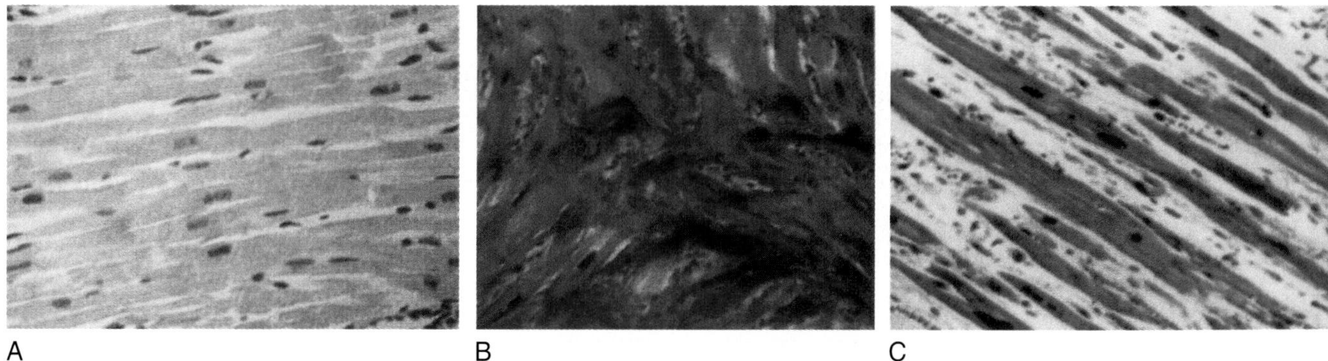

FIGURE 59–2 Histopathology of hypertrophic and dilated cardiomyopathy. **A,** The normal architecture of healthy myocardium shows orderly alignment of myocytes with minimal interstitial fibrosis. **B,** Hypertrophic cardiomyopathy, demonstrating marked enlargement and disarray of myocytes (red) with increased interstitial fibrosis (blue). **C,** Dilated cardiomyopathy, showing hypertrophy and degeneration of myocytes (dark red) without disarray. There is an increase in interstitial fibrosis (pale pink). Stains: A and C, hematoxylin and eosin; B, Masson trichrome. (From Seidman JG, Seidman C: The genetic basis for cardiomyopathy: From mutation identification to mechanistic paradigms. Cell 104:557, 2001.)

inflammatory cardiomyopathy.[9] It is hoped that newer immunohistochemical and molecular biological techniques (such as the polymerase chain reaction or in situ hybridization techniques to detect viral infection of the heart) may expand further the diagnostic utility of endomyocardial biopsy.[10]

Dilated Cardiomyopathy

Idiopathic Dilated Cardiomyopathy

DCM is a syndrome characterized by cardiac enlargement and impaired systolic function of one or both ventricles (see Figs. 59–1 and 59–2). Although it was formerly called congestive cardiomyopathy, the term *dilated cardiomyopathy* is now preferred because the earliest abnormality is usually ventricular enlargement and systolic contractile dysfunction, with the signs and symptoms of congestive heart failure often (but not invariably) developing later. In an occasional patient, the predominant finding is that of contractile dysfunction with only a minimally dilated left ventricle. In the WHO/ISFC classification scheme, this variant of DCM is placed in the *unclassified* cardiomyopathy group. Conversely, apparently normal elite athletes may demonstrate considerable ventricular enlargement with *normal* systolic performance. It is presumed that this is a physiological adaptation to intense athletic training and does not appear to represent a disease state, although the long-term consequences are not fully known.

The incidence of DCM is reported to be 5 to 8 cases per 100,000 population per year and appears to be increasing, although the true figure is probably higher as a consequence of underreporting of mild or asymptomatic cases.[11] It occurs almost three times more frequently in blacks and males as in whites and females, and this difference does not appear to be related solely to different degrees of hypertension, cigarette smoking, or alcohol use. Survival in blacks and males appears to be worse than in whites and females.[12]

Although the cause is not definable in many cases, more than 75 specific diseases of heart muscle can produce the clinical manifestations of DCM. It is likely that this condition represents a final common pathway that is the end result of myocardial damage produced by a variety of cytotoxic, metabolic, immunological, familial, and infectious mechanisms. Alcohol, for example, may lead to severe cardiac dysfunction and may produce clinical, hemodynamic, and pathological findings identical to those present in idiopathic DCM.

NATURAL HISTORY. The natural history of DCM is not well established. Many patients have minimal or no symptoms, and the progression of the disease in these patients is unclear, although there is some evidence that the long-term prognosis is not good. Nevertheless, in symptomatic patients the course is usually one of progressive deterioration, with 10 to 50 percent of patients with heart failure succumbing within a year, depending on the cohort of patients under study.[13] It has been estimated that the annual mortality rate for a typical patient with heart failure is about 11 to 13 percent.[14] A minority of patients with recent-onset DCM—perhaps about a quarter—improve spontaneously, even some sick enough initially to be considered for cardiac transplantation.

PROGNOSIS. A variety of clinical predictors of patients at enhanced risk for dying of DCM have been identified, including the presence of a protodiastolic (S_3) gallop, ventricular arrhythmias, advanced age, and the failure of the myopathic ventricle to respond to inotropic stimulation (Table 59–3).[15] However, the predictive reliability of any single feature is not high, and it may be difficult to predict with any accuracy the clinical course and outcome in an individual patient. Nevertheless, greater ventricular enlargement and worse dysfunction tend to correlate with poorer prognosis, particularly if the right ventricle is dilated and dysfunctional as well.[16]

Cardiopulmonary exercise testing can also provide useful prognostic information (see Chap. 10). Marked limitation of exercise capacity manifested by reduced maximal systemic oxygen uptake (especially when below 10 to 12 ml/kg/min) is a reliable predictor of mortality and is used widely as an indicator for consideration of cardiac transplantation (see Chap. 26).

Pathology

MACROSCOPIC EXAMINATION. This usually reveals enlargement and dilation of all four cardiac chambers; the ventricles are more dilated than the atria (see Fig. 59-1). Although the thickness of the ventricular wall is increased in some cases, the degree of hypertrophy is often less than might be expected given the severe dilation present. The development of left ventricular hypertrophy appears to have a protective or beneficial role in DCM, presumably because it reduces systolic wall stress and thus protects against further cavity dilation. The cardiac valves are intrinsically normal, and intracavitary thrombi, particularly in the ventricular apex, are not uncommon. The coronary arteries are usually normal. The right ventricle is preferentially involved in some cases of DCM, sometimes on a familial basis.

HISTOLOGICAL EXAMINATION. Microscopic study reveals extensive areas of interstitial and perivascular fibrosis, particularly involving the left ventricular subendocardium (see Fig. 59-2). Small areas of necrosis and cellular infiltrate are seen on occasion, but these are typically not prominent features. There is marked variation in myocyte size; some myocardial cells are hypertrophied, and others are atrophied. No viruses or other etiological agents have been identified with any regularity in tissue from patients with DCM. Particularly disappointing has been the failure to identify any immunological, histochemical, morphological, ultrastructural, or microbiological marker that might be used to establish the diagnosis of idiopathic DCM or to clarify its cause.

TABLE 59–3 Factors Associated with an Adverse Outcome in Dilated Cardiomyopathy

Clinical	Noninvasive	Invasive
NYHA Class III/IV	Low LV ejection fraction	High LV filling pressures
Increasing age	Marked LV dilation	
Low exercise peak oxygen consumption	Low LV mass	
Marked intraventricular conduction delay	≥Moderate mitral regurgitation	
Complex ventricular arrhythmias	Abnormal diastolic function	
Abnormal signal-averaged ECG	Abnormal contractile reserve	
Evidence of excessive sympathetic stimulation	Right ventricular dilation or dysfunction	
Protodiastolic gallop (S_3)		

ECG = electrocardiogram; LV = left ventricular; NYHA = New York Heart Association.

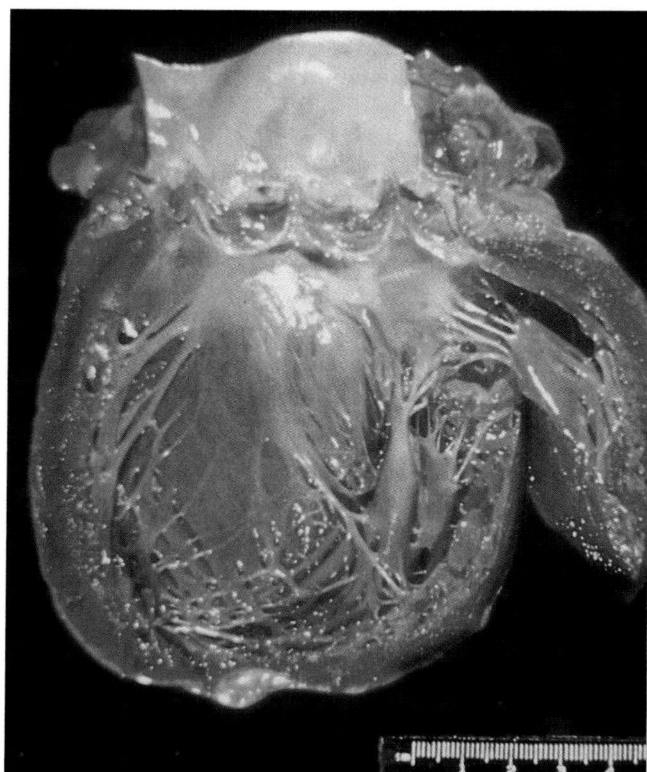

FIGURE 59–3 Gross pathology of dilated cardiomyopathy. Prominent ventricular dilatation is apparent in this heart, which has been opened so that the interior of the left ventricle can be seen. Wall thickness is normal, but the shape of the heart has become more globular. (From Kasper EK, Hruban RH, Baughman KL: Idiopathic dilated cardiomyopathy. *In* Abelmann WH, Braunwald E [eds.]. Atlas of Heart Diseases. Vol 2. Cardiomyopathies, Myocarditis, and Pericardial Disease. Philadelphia, Current Medicine, 1995, pp 3.1-3.18.)

TABLE 59–4 Molecular Defects Linked to the Various Cardiomyopathies

Genomic Defect	Cardiomyopathy: *Hypertrophic*	*Dilated*	*Restrictive*
Sarcomere			
Myosin heavy chain	M	M	
Myosin essential light chain	M		
Myosin regulatory light chain	M		
Cardiac actin	M	M	
Troponin T	M/D	D	
Troponin I	M		M
Alpha-tropomyosin	M	M	
Myosin-binding protein C	M/D		
Titin/titin-related Protein			
Titin	M	M/D	
Telethonin (T-cap)		M	
Z-disk-associated Proteins			
Muscle LIM domain protein		M	
Sarcolemma Cytoskeleton			
Dystrophin		D	
Beta-sarcoglycan		D/Dup	
Delta-sarcoglycan		M	
Alpha-dystrobrevin		M	
Metavinculin		D	
Intermediate Filaments			
Desmin		M	
Lamin A/C		M	

D = deletion; Dup = duplication; M = missense.

Adapted from Chien KR: Genotype, phenotype: Upstairs, downstairs in the family of cardiomyopathies. J Clin Invest 111:175, 2003.

Etiology

About a fourth of the cases of congestive heart failure in the United States are due to DCM; most of the remainder are caused by the sequelae of coronary artery disease or, less frequently, hypertensive heart disease.[11] More than half of all patients with the clinical picture of DCM have no identifiable etiology apparent despite rigorous evaluation and are therefore considered to have *idiopathic* DCM.[17] It is likely that this condition represents a common expression of myocardial damage that has been produced by a variety of as yet unestablished myocardial insults. Although the cause or causes remain unclear, interest has centered on three possible basic mechanisms of damage: (1) familial and genetic factors, (2) viral myocarditis and other cytotoxic insults, and (3) immunological abnormalities (Fig. 59–3).

GENETICS. Familial linkage of DCM occurs more commonly than is often appreciated. It is thought that about 25 to 30 percent of patients with DCM have an inherited form of the disease that is the result of a genetic mutation.[18] Some asymptomatic relatives of patients with DCM have subclinical left ventricular enlargement or dysfunction, or both, that may progress to overt symptomatic DMC.[19] Most familial cases demonstrate autosomal dominant transmission. More than a dozen chromosomal loci have been identified, and more are likely to be found (Table 59–4).[20] Familial DCM results from mutations in genes that encode cytoskeletal, nuclear membrane, or contractile proteins, including desmin, titin, and troponin T.[20–23] One unique form is due to mutations in the lamin A/C gene and is associated with conduction defects, variable skeletal muscle involvement, and reduced survival to adulthood.[24] Another variant affects phospholamban and leads to myocellular calcium dysregulation.[25]

However, familial DCM is genetically quite heterogeneous, and autosomal recessive and X-linked inheritance have been found as well.[26] One form of familial X-linked DCM is due to a deletion in the promoter region and the first exon of the gene that codes for the protein dystrophin, a component of the cytoskeleton of myocytes.[27] This has fueled speculation that a resulting deficiency of cardiac dystrophin is the cause of the associated DCM (see also Chap. 85).[28] Mutations involving mitochondrial DNA have been reported as well.[29]

Whether any of the patients without apparent familial linkage has a genetic predisposition to DCM remains unknown. There is great interest in using molecular genetic techniques to identify markers of disease susceptibility in asymptomatic carriers at risk for the eventual development of overt clinical DCM. An example of such a marker may be the angiotensin-converting enzyme DD genotype that is associated with an adverse clinical course in patients with DCM.[30] Even where there is no evidence of familial linkage, the failing heart demonstrates a variety of alterations in the gene and protein expression of various contractile proteins.[11]

SEQUELA OF VIRAL MYOCARDITIS (see also Chap. 60). Wide speculation exists that an episode of subclinical viral myocarditis initiates an autoimmune reaction that culminates in the development of full-blown DCM.[31] Although this hypothesis is inviting, it remains controversial.[32] In some patients who exhibit the clinical features of DCM, endomyocardial biopsy reveals evidence of an inflammatory myocarditis. The reported frequency of evidence of an inflammatory infiltrate in DCM varies widely and undoubtedly depends largely on selection of patients and the criteria used for diagnosis; using rigorous criteria, only about 15 percent (or less) of patients with DCM have biopsy evidence of myocarditis.[32] Other evidence favoring the concept that DCM is a postviral disorder includes the presence of high antibody viral titers, viral-specific RNA sequences, and apparent viral particles in patients with "idiopathic" DCM.[33] Similarly, the polymerase chain reaction generally has confirmed the presence of viral remnants in the myocardium of some patients with cardiomyopathy.[34]

AUTOIMMUNITY. Abnormalities of both humoral and cellular immunity have been found in patients with DCM,[9,35] although the findings have not been completely reproducible. It has been postulated that viral components may be incorporated into the cardiac sarcolemma, only to serve as an antigenic source that directs the immune response to attack the myocardium. On the other hand, there is speculation that antibodies might be the *result* of myocardial damage rather than the cause.[36] There appears to be an association with specific human leukocyte antigen (HLA) class II antigens (particularly DR4), suggesting that abnormalities of immunoregulation may play a role in DCM.[37] Circulating antimyocardial antibodies to a variety of antigens (including the myosin heavy chain, the beta adrenoceptor, the muscarinic receptor, sarcolemmal sodium-potassium adenosine triphosphatase, laminin, and mitochondrial proteins) have been identified.[38,39] Additional evidence for the significance of circulating antimyocardial antibodies comes from the demonstration of short- and intermediate-term clinical improvement in the manifestations of heart failure in some but not all patients treated with immunoadsorption and elimination of anti-beta$_1$-adrenergic receptor antibodies.[40–42] Conversely, a randomized trial of immune globulin in recent-onset DCM showed no benefit.[9] Thus, the precise role of either humoral or cellular immunomodulation in the pathogenesis of DCM remains unestablished.[43]

PROINFLAMMATORY CYTOKINES. A variety of proinflammatory cytokines such as tumor necrosis factor-alpha (TNF-alpha) (and the related TNF-alpha converting enzyme) are expressed in DCM and may play a role in producing contractile dysfunction; whether viral infection, autoimmune abnormalities, or other factors induce their expression is unknown.[44–46] Additional support for an etiological role of TNF-alpha in the contractile dysfunction of DCM is that the inhibition of its production by pentoxifylline results in symptomatic and functional improvement.[47] Similarly, the vasoconstrictor peptide endothelin is increased in decompensated DCM and has been implicated as a cause of the heightened vascular tone that accompanies congestive heart failure.[48,49]

OTHER POTENTIAL CAUSES. A variety of other possible causes have been proposed, although none is accepted as *the* cause of DCM. Thus, endocrine abnormalities as well as the effects of chemicals or toxins have been suggested as possible etiological factors. It has been suggested that microvascular hyperreactivity (spasm) and decreased coronary flow reserve may lead to myocellular necrosis and scarring, with resultant heart failure.[50] Apoptosis, or programmed cell death, has been demonstrated in the hearts of patients with DCM and ARVC, although there is some controversy regarding these findings in DCM.[49,51,52]

From a clinical standpoint, the more important causes of nonidiopathic DCM include alcohol and cocaine abuse (see Chap. 62),[53] human immunodeficiency virus (HIV) infection (see Chap. 61), metabolic abnormalities, and the cardiotoxicity of anticancer drugs (especially doxorubicin) (see Chap. 83).

Clinical Manifestations

HISTORY. Although patients of any age may be affected, DCM is most common in middle age and is more frequent in men than in women. Symptoms usually develop gradually in patients with DCM. Some patients are asymptomatic and yet have left ventricular dilation for months or even years. This dilation may be recognized clinically only later when symptoms develop or when routine chest roentgenography demonstrates cardiomegaly. A relatively small number of patients develop symptoms of heart failure for the first time after recovery from what appears to be a systemic viral infection. In still others, severe heart failure develops acutely during an episode of myocarditis; although some recovery occurs, chronic manifestations of diminished cardiac reserve persist and heart failure reappears months or years later. It is important to question the patient and family carefully about alcohol consumption because excessive alcohol consumption is a major cause of DCM, and its cessation may result in substantial clinical improvement.[54]

The most striking symptoms of DCM are those of left ventricular failure (see Chap. 22). Fatigue and weakness related to diminished cardiac output are common. Right-sided heart failure is a late and ominous sign and is associated with a particularly poor prognosis. Chest pain occurs in a minority of patients and may suggest concomitant ischemic heart disease. The demonstrated reduction in the vasodilator reserve of the coronary microvasculature in DCM suggests that subendocardial ischemia may play a role in the genesis of chest pain that occurs despite angiographically normal coronary arteries.[55] Chest pain secondary to pulmonary embolism and abdominal pain secondary to congestive hepatomegaly are frequent in the late stages of illness.

PHYSICAL EXAMINATION (see also Chaps. 8 and 22). Examination usually reveals variable degrees of cardiac enlargement and findings of congestive heart failure. The systolic blood pressure is usually normal or low, and the pulse pressure is narrow, reflecting a diminished stroke volume. *Pulsus alternans* is common when severe left ventricular failure is present. Cheyne-Stokes breathing may be present and is associated with a poor prognosis. The jugular veins are distended when right-sided heart failure appears, but on initial presentation most patients do not have evidence of this. Prominent a and v waves may be visible. Grossly pulsatile jugular veins with prominent regurgitant waves indicate the presence of tricuspid valvular regurgitation; this is usually a late and often ominous finding. The liver may be engorged and pulsatile. Peripheral edema and ascites are present when right-sided heart failure is advanced.

The precordium usually reveals left and, occasionally, right ventricular impulses, but the heaves are not sustained as they are in patients with ventricular hypertrophy. The apical impulse is usually displaced laterally, reflecting left ventricular dilation. A presystolic a wave may be palpable on occasion and is generated in a manner similar to that of a presystolic (S_4) gallop heard on auscultation. The second heart sound (S_2) is usually normally split, although paradoxical splitting may be detected in the presence of left bundle branch block, an electrocardiographic (ECG) finding that is not unusual in DCM. If pulmonary hypertension is present, the pulmonary component of S_2 may be accentuated and the splitting may be narrow. Presystolic gallop sounds (S_4) are common and often precede the development of overt congestive heart failure. Ventricular gallops (S_3) are the rule when cardiac decompensation occurs, and a summation gallop is heard when there is concomitant tachycardia.[56]

Systolic murmurs are common and are usually due to mitral or, less commonly, tricuspid valvular regurgitation. Mitral regurgitation results from enlargement and abnormal motion of the mitral annulus and distortion of the geometry of the subvalvular apparatus; ventricular dilation by itself plays a lesser role.[57] Gallop sounds and regurgitant murmurs can often be elicited or intensified by isometric handgrip exercise with its attendant enhancement of systemic vascular resistance and impedance to left ventricular outflow. Systemic emboli resulting from dislodgement of intracardiac thrombi from the left atrium and ventricle and pulmonary emboli that originate in the venous system of the legs are common late complications.

NONINVASIVE LABORATORY EXAMINATIONS. To identify potentially reversible causes of DCM, several basic screening biochemical tests are indicated, including determination of levels of serum phosphorus (hypophosphatemia), serum calcium (hypocalcemia), and serum creatinine and urea nitrogen (uremia); thyroid function studies (hypothyroidism and hyperthyroidism); and iron studies (hemochromatosis). It is prudent to test for HIV as well because this infection is an important and often unrecognized cause of congestive heart failure (see Chap. 61). Although not particularly useful for the diagnosis of DCM, elevated troponin T levels are predictive of a worse clinical course than normal levels.[58] The *chest roentgenogram* usually reveals generalized cardiomegaly and pulmonary vascular redistribution; interstitial and alveolar edema are less common on initial presentation. Pleural effusions may be present, and the azygos vein and superior vena cava may be dilated when right-sided heart failure supervenes.

Electrocardiography. The electrocardiogram often shows sinus tachycardia when heart failure is present. The entire spectrum of atrial and ventricular tachyarrhythmias may be seen. Poor R wave progression and intraventricular conduction abnormalities, especially left bundle branch block, are common.[59] Anterior Q waves may be present when there is extensive left ventricular fibrosis, even without a discrete myocardial scar or evidence of coronary artery disease. ST segment and T wave abnormalities are common, as are P wave changes, especially left atrial abnormality. Ambulatory monitoring demonstrates the ubiquity of ventricular arrhythmias, with the majority of monitored patients with DCM exhibiting nonsustained ventricular tachycardia.[60] There is no consensus that complex or frequent ventricular arrhythmias predict sudden (presumably arrhythmic) death, although they do appear to predict *total* mortality.[60] Perhaps ventricular arrhythmias as detected on ambulatory monitoring are a marker for the extent of myocardial damage in DCM and therefore are associated with sudden death without necessarily being its cause. In occasional cases, particularly in children, recurrent or incessant supraventricular or ventricular tachyarrhythmias may actually be the cause (rather than the result) of ventricular dysfunction.[61] In those cases, restoration of sinus rhythm or slowing of the heart rate may reverse the cardiomyopathy.[62]

Echocardiography. Two-dimensional and Doppler forms of echocardiography are useful in assessing the degree of impairment of left ventricular function and for excluding concomitant valvular or pericardial disease (see Chap. 11). In addition to examining all four cardiac valves for evidence of structural or functional abnormalities, echocardiography allows evaluation of the size of the ventricular cavity and thickness of the ventricular walls. A pericardial effusion is occasionally present. Doppler studies are useful in delineating the severity of mitral (and tricuspid) regurgitation. Patients with a pattern of left ventricular filling that simulates that seen with restrictive cardiomyopathies appear to have more advanced disease. Combining echocardiography with dobutamine infusion may identify patients with left ventricular dysfunction related to coronary artery disease by demonstrating provocable differences in regional wall motion and thus distinguish them from patients with idiopathic DCM. Furthermore, patients who demonstrate substantial contractile reserve with dobutamine infusion experience a better prognosis than those who do not.[63]

RADIONUCLIDE IMAGING. Current techniques using newer radionuclides and imaging protocols for *myocardial perfusion stress imaging* are quite reliable in making the differentiation of an ischemic from a nonischemic etiology of heart failure.[64] Like echocardiography, *radionuclide ventriculography* reveals increased end-diastolic and end-systolic left ventricular volumes, reduced ejection fraction in one or both ventricles, and wall motion abnormalities (see Chap. 13); it is used most commonly when echocardiography is technically suboptimal.

In most patients it is not necessary to carry out serial studies or batteries of noninvasive tests to observe patients with DCM and evaluate their response to treatment; adjustments in pharmacological therapies are usually based on routine bedside clinical features and symptomatic response.

CARDIAC CATHETERIZATION AND ANGIOCARDIOGRAPHY. Only certain patients with DCM require cardiac catheterization (particularly those with chest pain and a suspicion of ischemic disease or patients thought to have a treatable systemic disease such as sarcoidosis or hemochromatosis, in which myocardial biopsy is an important part of the catheterization procedure).[65] When cardiac catheterization is carried out, the left ventricular end-diastolic and pulmonary artery wedge pressures are usually elevated. Modest degrees of pulmonary arterial hypertension are common. Advanced cases may demonstrate right ventricular dilation and failure as well, with resultant elevation of the right ventricular end-diastolic, right atrial, and central venous pressures.

Left ventriculography demonstrates enlargement of this chamber, typically with a diffuse reduction in wall motion. Segmental wall motion abnormalities are not uncommon and may simulate the angiographic findings in ischemic heart disease. However, prominent localized wall motion disturbances are more characteristic of ischemic heart disease, whereas diffuse global dysfunction is more typical of DCM. The ejection fraction is reduced and the end-systolic volume is increased as a result of the impairment of left ventricular contractility. Sometimes left ventricular thrombi may be visualized within the left ventricle as intracavitary filling defects. Mild mitral regurgitation is often present. On occasion, it may be difficult to distinguish left ventricular dilation secondary to severe mitral regurgitation related to intrinsic mitral valve disease from DCM with secondary mitral regurgitation.

Coronary arteriography usually reveals normal vessels, although coronary vasodilator capacity may be impaired. This examination may be of particular value in excluding coronary artery disease in patients with abnormal Q waves on the electrocardiogram or regional left ventricular wall motion abnormalities on noninvasive evaluation. Coronary arteriography, when necessary, thus helps to distinguish between myocardial infarction as a result of obstructive coronary artery disease and extensive localized myocardial fibrosis secondary to severe DCM in the absence of coronary artery obstruction.

Management

Because the cause of idiopathic DCM, by definition, is unknown, specific therapy is not possible. Treatment, therefore, is for heart failure, as discussed in Chapters 23 and 24. Most patients should be treated with standard therapy, consisting of diuretics as needed for symptoms, angiotensin-converting enzyme inhibition, and beta-adrenergic blockade. Digoxin is considered a second-line agent, and the optimal dose is one that achieves a serum level of 0.5 to 0.8 ng/ml, as higher levels are associated with a small increase in mortality.[66]

Many of the therapeutic approaches are directed at modifying the results of the long-term activation of two interrelated systems, the adrenergic and renin-angiotensin systems. Physical, dietary, and pharmacological interventions may help to control symptoms; regular physical exercise (as tolerated) increases exercise capacity by improving endothelial dysfunction and augmenting blood flow in skeletal muscles.[67] Patients with left ventricular dysfunction not infrequently have sleep apnea, and treatment of those with obstructive sleep apnea with continuous positive airway pressure leads to an improvement in ventricular function, at least in part by reducing the increased afterload that results from the associated hypertension. Only cardiac transplantation (see Chap. 26) and specific pharmacological therapy (the vasodilators hydralazine plus nitrates, the angiotensin-converting enzyme inhibitor enalapril, the beta adrenoceptor blockers carvedilol and metoprolol, and the aldosterone receptor blocker spironolactone) have been shown to prolong life, but substantial progress has been made, with a nearly 50 percent reduction in heart failure mortality in the past decade![68]

CALCIUM ANTAGONISTS. Because of the possible link between DCM, microvascular circulatory abnormalities, and abnormal myocardial calcium handling, there has been interest in the use of calcium antagonists. These agents have generally been well tolerated when used in patients with DCM, although myocardial depression is an important potential side effect of the calcium antagonists as a group. Unfortunately, combining a calcium antagonist with traditional standard therapy does not appear to have substantial clinical benefit, nor does it reduce further the mortality in DCM. At present, the routine use of calcium antagonists in DCM is considered nonstandard and not first-line therapy.[69]

IMMUNOSUPPRESSIVES. In patients with chronic heart failure secondary to DCM and lymphocytic infiltrate on myocardial biopsy, treatment with corticosteroids and immunosuppressive agents had been advocated in the past. Unfortunately, such therapy does *not* appear to have a clinically important impact on mortality or progression to cardiac transplantation or on symptoms, exercise performance, or ejection fraction (except in the short term and perhaps in specific subgroups of DCM patients, such as those with HLA upregulation found on myocardial biopsy specimens).[70] In addition, it may be associated with significant complications.[71] Routine clinical use of immunosuppressive therapy thus cannot be recommended at present, at least until the subsets of DCM patients most likely to respond to such therapy can be identified.

BIVENTRICULAR PACING ("RESYNCHRONIZATION") (see Chaps. 24 and 31)

SURGICAL TREATMENT Surgical repair of a structurally normal but functionally incompetent mitral valve has been attempted in an increasing number of patients with DCM and prominent atrioventricular valvular regurgitation.[72] Although surgery was previously thought to be contraindicated because of the degree of preexisting cardiac dysfunction and damage (especially when valve replacement rather than repair was undertaken), some patients have shown symptomatic improvement, at least over the intermediate term.[73] The utility of left ventricular assist devices for end-stage DCM has been demonstrated (Chap. 25).[74] In appropriately selected patients, cardiac transplantation should be considered (see Chap. 26).

Alcoholic Cardiomyopathy

Chronic excessive consumption of alcohol may be associated with congestive heart failure, hypertension, cerebrovascular accidents, arrhythmias, and sudden death; it is the major cause of secondary, nonischemic DCM in the Western world and accounts for upward of one-third of all cases of DCM.[75] It is estimated that two-thirds of the adult population use alcohol to some extent, and more than 10 percent are heavy users.[76] Therefore, it is not surprising that alcoholic cardiomyopathy is a major problem. Ceasing alcohol consumption early in the course of alcoholic cardiomyopathy may halt the progression of or even reverse left ventricular contractile dysfunction. This is unlike the situation in nonalcoholic cardiomyopathy, which is often marked by progressive clinical deterioration.[77,78]

The consumption of alcohol may result in myocardial damage by three mechanisms: (1) a presumed direct toxic effect of alcohol or its metabolites; (2) nutritional effects, most commonly in association with thiamine deficiency that leads to beriberi heart disease (see Chap. 22); and (3) rarely, toxic effects related to additives in the alcoholic beverage (cobalt). There had been speculation that alcohol caused myocardial damage only through dietary deficiencies, but it is now clear that alcoholic cardiomyopathy occurs in the absence of nutritional deficiencies.

Typical Oriental beriberi may coexist with alcoholic cardiomyopathy, although it is no longer noted with any frequency. The distinguishing features of each include peripheral vasodilation and high-output heart failure, often right sided, in the former and reduced contractility with typically left-sided low-output failure in the latter.

The precise mechanisms of cardiac depression produced by alcohol are undetermined, but a direct toxic effect on striated muscle is likely (particularly because alcoholics often demonstrate concomitant skeletal myopathy and cardiomyopathy).[79] In acute studies, alcohol and its metabolite acetaldehyde have been shown to interfere with a number of membrane and cellular functions that involve the transport and binding of calcium, mitochondrial respiration, myocardial lipid metabolism, myocardial protein synthesis, and signal transduction.[80] The role that other associated electrolyte imbalances (hypokalemia, hypophosphatemia, hypomagnesemia) may play in alcohol-mediated damage has not been settled.

Because not all alcoholics develop cardiomyopathy, the relationship between the development of cardiac dysfunction and dose of alcohol is complex and probably multifactorial. There appears to be a genetic predisposition to the development of cardiomyopathy because alcoholics with the DD genotype of the angiotensin-converting enzyme are 16 times more likely to develop cardiac dysfunction than those without.[81] The cumulative dose of alcohol appears to be important in the eventual development of cardiomyopathy, and some data suggest that more moderate alcohol consumption may actually have a protective effect against the development of cardiac dysfunction and death.[82,83]

PATHOLOGY. The gross and microscopic pathological findings are nonspecific and similar to those observed in idiopathic DCM, with interstitial fibrosis, myocytolysis, evidence of small-vessel coronary artery disease, and myocyte hypertrophy.[75] Electron microscopy shows enlarged and disorganized mitochondria, with large glycogen-containing vacuoles.

Clinical Manifestations

Alcoholic cardiomyopathy most commonly occurs in men 30 to 55 years of age who have been heavy consumers of whisky, wine, or beer, usually for more than 10 years.[75] Female alcoholics who develop cardiomyopathy appear to have a lower cumulative lifetime dose of alcohol than men.[77] Although alcoholic cardiomyopathy may be observed in the homeless, malnourished, "skid row" alcoholic man, many patients are well-nourished individuals of middle and even upper socioeconomic status without liver disease or peripheral neuropathy. Accordingly, unless a high index of suspicion is maintained, it may be easy to miss a history of alcohol abuse. Persistent questioning of the patient and particularly the relatives of patients with unexplained cardiomegaly or cardiomyopathy is often required to elicit a history of alcoholism.

It is frequently possible to demonstrate mild depression of cardiac function in chronic alcoholics even before cardiac dysfunction becomes clinically manifest. Abnormalities of both systolic function (reduced ejection fraction) and diastolic function (increased myocardial wall stiffness) have been demonstrated in alcoholic patients without cardiac symptoms by a variety of invasive and noninvasive techniques.[84] Although overt alcoholic liver disease and cardiac involvement usually do not occur together, even cirrhotic patients without signs or symptoms of heart disease often have demonstrable evidence of asymptomatic myocardial disease.

The development of symptoms may be insidious, although some patients have acute and florid left-sided congestive heart failure. A paroxysm of atrial fibrillation is a relatively frequent initial presenting finding. More advanced cases demonstrate biventricular failure, with left ventricular dysfunction usually dominating. Dyspnea, orthopnea, and paroxysmal nocturnal dyspnea are frequently observed. Palpitations may be present and are usually due to supraventricular tachyarrhythmias. Syncope may occur as well and may be the result of supraventricular, or more likely ventricular, tachyarrhythmias. Angina pectoris does not occur unless there is concomitant coronary artery disease or aortic stenosis, although atypical chest pain may be seen.

PHYSICAL EXAMINATION. The cardiac findings resemble those seen in idiopathic DCM. Examination usually reveals a narrow pulse pressure, often with an elevated diastolic pressure secondary to excessive peripheral vasoconstriction. There is cardiomegaly, and protodiastolic (S3) and presystolic (S4) gallop sounds are common. An apical systolic murmur of mitral regurgitation is often found. The severity of right-sided heart failure varies, but jugular venous distention and peripheral edema are common. A concomitant skeletal muscle myopathy involving the shoulder and pelvic girdle is a frequent finding, and the degree of muscle weakness and histological abnormality in the skeletal muscles parallels that in the heart.[79]

LABORATORY EXAMINATION. The chest roentgenogram in advanced cases demonstrates considerable cardiac enlargement, pulmonary congestion, and pulmonary venous hypertension (see Chap. 12). Pleural effusions are often seen. ECG abnormalities are common and frequently are the only indication of alcoholic heart disease during the preclinical phase. Alcoholic patients without other evidence of heart disease are often seen after developing palpitations, chest discomfort, or syncope, typically after a binge of alcohol consumption on a weekend (particularly during the year-end holiday season). This has been dubbed the "holiday heart syndrome." The most common arrhythmia observed is atrial fibrillation, followed by atrial flutter and frequent ventricular premature contractions. Alcohol consumption may predispose to atrial flutter or fibrillation even in nonalcoholics. Hypokalemia may play a role in the genesis of some of these arrhythmias. Supraventricular arrhythmias are also frequently observed in patients with overt alcoholic cardiomyopathy. Sudden unexpected death is not uncommon in young adult alcoholics, and it is likely that ventricular fibrillation is responsible.

Atrioventricular conduction disturbances (most commonly first-degree heart block), bundle branch block, left ventricular hypertrophy, poor R wave progression across the precordium, and repolarization abnormalities are common ECG findings. Prolongation of the QT interval is noted frequently. ST segment and T wave changes are often restored to normal within several days after cessation of alcohol consumption.

The hemodynamic findings observed at cardiac catheterization and the assessment of left ventricular function by noninvasive methods (echocardiography and isotope angiography) resemble those in idiopathic DCM.

MANAGEMENT. The key to the long-term treatment of alcoholic cardiomyopathy is a reduction of alcohol consumption (and preferably abstinence) as early in the course of the disease as possible.[83] This may be quite effective in improving the signs and symptoms of congestive heart failure.[85] The prognosis in patients who continue to drink heavily is poor,[54] particularly if they have been symptomatic for a long time.

The management of acute episodes of congestive heart failure is similar to that of idiopathic DCM. For patients with severe congestive heart failure, it is prudent to administer thiamine on the chance that beriberi may be contributing to the heart failure. Whether to use chronic anticoagulation (as is often considered in idiopathic DCM) is a difficult question; we usually do not prescribe warfarin unless there are unequivocal and pressing indications because of the increased risk of bleeding related to noncompliance, trauma, and over-anticoagulation because of hepatic dysfunction.

COBALT CARDIOMYOPATHY

A previously unrecognized syndrome of severe congestive heart failure appeared in the mid-1960s, first in Canada and subsequently in the United States and Europe.[86] The disease was found in people who drank a particular brand of beer to which cobalt sulfate had been added as a foam stabilizer. Since cobalt was removed from the process, no more cases of the disease have been reported.

Arrhythmogenic Right Ventricular Cardiomyopathy (see also Chap. 32)

This unique cardiomyopathy (which is also called arrhythmogenic right ventricular dysplasia) is marked by myocardial cell loss with partial or total replacement of right ventricular muscle by adipose and fibrous tissue; apoptosis appears to be a principal cause of the cell death (Fig. 59–4).[87-89] ARVC is associated with reentrant ventricular tachyarrhythmias of right ventricular origin (producing a left bundle branch block configuration in the QRS complex)[90] that are often precipitated by an exercise-induced discharge of catecholamines and are a harbinger of sudden death.[88] In about one-third of the cases there is autosomal dominant inheritance of the disease,[91] and several distinct genetic mutations have been reported, including a mutation in the gene coding for the cardiac ryanodine receptor (hRYR2).[92] Another variant, found on the Greek island of Naxos, is inherited as a recessive trait but with a high degree of penetrance.[93]

ARVC is distinct from the *Uhl anomaly,* which is marked by extreme thinning of the ventricular wall.[94] The diagnosis of AVRC is based on a constellation of clinical, ECG, histological, and echocardiographic findings.[95,96] Typical features include the appearance of clinical manifestations in adolescence or early adulthood, male predominance, normal physical examination, inverted T waves in the right precordial ECG leads, symptoms of palpitations and syncope, and a risk of sudden death.[96,97] In some patients with ventricular arrhythmias of no evident cause, clinically subtle right ventricular dysplasia may be responsible.

Noninvasive and invasive evaluations demonstrate a dilated, poorly contractile right ventricle, usually with a normal left ventricle, although variable degrees of left ventricular involvement have been seen.[95,98] When left-sided involvement is present, the risk of sudden death is increased.[99] Magnetic resonance imaging (MRI) is of particular value in identifying patients with this condition[100] who in other regards may appear to be completely normal (Fig. 59–5).

MANAGEMENT. Antiarrhythmic therapy, especially with beta adrenoceptor blockers, sotalol, or amiodarone, is often effective in controlling the arrhythmias.[88] The arrhythmias may be related to abnormalities of regional right ventricular sympathetic innervation and a reduced density of beta-adrenergic receptors or impaired presynaptic catecholamine reuptake, as has been demonstrated by noninvasive scintigraphy.[101] Cryo- or catheter-based radiofrequency ablation of the presumed arrhythmogenic focus has been successful in resolving the ventricular arrhythmia in some patients unresponsive to or intolerant of antiarrhythmic drug therapy.[102] Insertion of an implantable cardioverter-defibrillator (ICD) or cardiac transplantation is reserved for patients with indications for these procedures (see Chaps. 26 and 31).[88,97]

Hypertrophic Cardiomyopathy

Although HCM was first described more than a century ago, the unique features of HCM were not studied systematically until the late 1950s.[103,104] The characteristic finding is inappropriate myocardial hypertrophy that occurs in the absence of an obvious cause for the hypertrophy (e.g., aortic stenosis or systemic hypertension), often predominantly involving the interventricular septum of a nondilated left ventricle that shows hyperdynamic systolic function (Fig. 59–6).[105,106] A distinctive clinical feature was soon recognized in some patients with HCM—a dynamic pressure gradient in the subaortic area that divided the left ventricle into a high-pressure apical region and a lower pressure subaortic region (Fig. 59–7A).[103] Although subsequent studies have shown that only a minority of patients (perhaps a fourth)[105–108] demonstrate this outflow gradient, its unique features attracted much attention and led to a myriad of terms (more than 75) used to describe the disease (among the more popular terms were *idiopathic hypertrophic subaortic* stenosis[103] and *muscular subaortic stenosis*).[109] The term *hypertrophic cardiomyopathy* is now preferred because most patients do not have an outflow gradient or "stenosis" of the left ventricular outflow tract.[106] Because hypertrophy typically occurs in the absence of a pressure gradient, the characteristic distinguishing feature of HCM is myocardial hypertrophy that is out of proportion to the hemodynamic load.

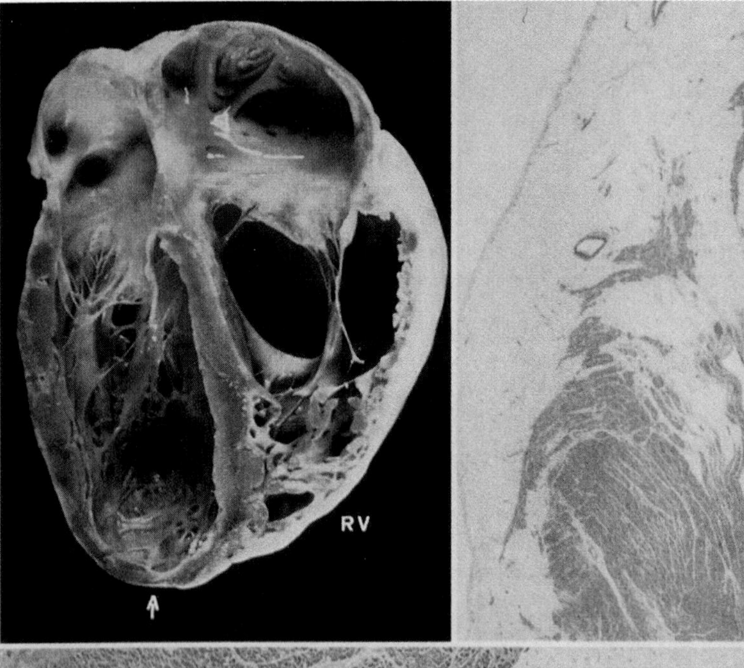

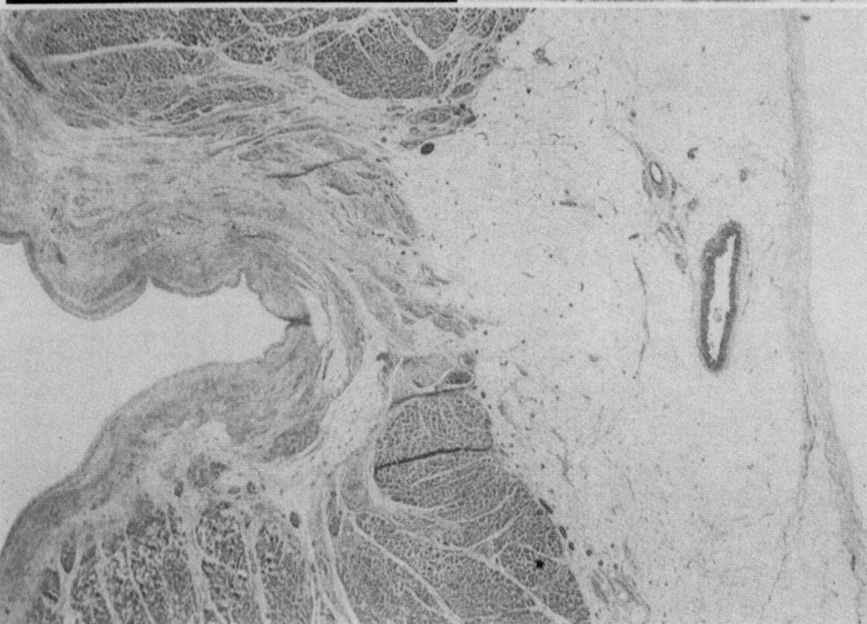

FIGURE 59–4 **Top left,** Postmortem pathological section of heart (four-chamber) in a patient with arrhythmogenic right ventricular cardiomyopathy and biventricular involvement. Severe widespread fatty infiltration of right ventricular (RV) wall is present; an apical aneurysm is present at the left ventricular level (arrow). **Top right,** Histological section at level of RV inflow (hematoxylin and eosin, ×2.5). Severe transmural fibrofatty infiltration of RV wall is present, compatible with RV dysplasia. **Bottom,** Histological section at the level of the left ventricle (outflow) (hematoxylin and eosin, ×2.5) shows focal severe fibrofatty infiltration with myocellular atrophy, compatible with left ventricular involvement. (From Pinamonti B, Pagnan L, Bussani R, et al: Right ventricular dysplasia with biventricular involvement. Circulation 98:1943-1945, 1998. Copyright 1998, American Heart Association.)

Morphological evidence of the disease is found in about one-fourth of the first-degree relatives of a patient with HCM; in many of the relatives the disease is milder than in the propositus, the degree of hypertrophy is less and is more localized, and outflow gradients are usually lacking. Symptoms are often absent or minimal, and the disease is detected only by echocardiography.

The physiological characteristics of HCM differ substantially from those of DCM. The most characteristic pathophysiological abnormality in HCM is *diastolic* rather than systolic dysfunction (see Chaps. 20 and 22).[104] Thus, HCM is characterized by abnormal stiffness of the left ventricle with resultant impaired ventricular filling. This abnormality in relaxation produces increased left ventricular end-diastolic pressure with resulting pulmonary congestion and dyspnea, the most common symptoms in HCM, despite typically hyperdynamic left ventricular systolic function. The overall prevalence of HCM is low: about 0.2 percent (1 in 500) of the general population and 0.5 percent of unselected patients referred for an echocardiographic examination.[105] It may be the most common genetically transmitted cardiac disorder.[106]

Pathology

MACROSCOPIC EXAMINATION. This typically discloses a marked increase in myocardial mass, and the ventricular cavities are small (see Figs. 59–1 and 59–6).[104] The left ventricle is usually more involved in the hypertrophic process than the right, but variable degrees of right-sided involvement may be seen.[110] The atria are dilated and often hypertrophied, reflecting the high resistance to filling of the ventricles caused by diastolic dysfunction and the effects of atrioventricular valve regurgitation. The pattern and extent of left ventricular hypertrophy in HCM vary greatly from patient to patient, and a characteristic feature is heterogeneity in the amount of hypertrophy evident in different regions of the left ventricle. A feature found in most patients with HCM is disproportionate involvement of the interventricular septum and anterolateral wall compared with the posterior segment of the free wall of the left ventricle.[106] When hypertrophy is largely localized to the anterior septum, the process has been called asymmetrical septal hypertrophy (ASH). A wide variety of other patterns of hypertrophy may be seen, and about 30 percent of patients show only localized and relatively mild hypertrophy in a single region of the ventricle.[104,106]

Differentiation of the "physiological" hypertrophy that occurs in some highly trained athletes from that seen in HCM may be difficult. Elite athletes may demonstrate left ventricular wall thicknesses up to 16 mm in the absence of HCM (normal <12 mm) along with marked ECG abnormalities.[104,111] Features that may permit differentiation of the two are the abnormal response of Doppler ultrasound–derived indices of diastolic function in response to isometric handgrip, the identification of HCM in a relative, or the simple demonstration of exceptional exercise capacity on cardiopulmonary exercise testing in normal elite athletes.[106,112]

Some patients with HCM have substantial hypertrophy in unusual locations, such as the posterior portion of the septum, the posterobasal free wall, and the midventricular level.[104] The degree of hypertrophy is dynamic in most patients and changes over time; prominent hypertrophy is rarely found in infants, and the typical patient develops hypertrophy during adolescence.[108] Development of the morphological features of HCM is unusual after the age of about 18 years,[106] although when it does occur later it is seen especially with a mutation of cardiac myosin-binding protein C.[113] There is usually an inverse relationship between the extent of hypertrophy in HCM and age. Whether this is due to premature death of younger patients with greater hypertrophy or progressive reduction in the extent of hypertrophy is unknown.[106] About 5 to 10 percent of patients eventually develop a "burned-out" phase of HCM that resembles DCM and is marked by myocardial wall thinning, ventricular dilation, systolic dysfunction, and progressive congestive heart failure.[104] Clinically silent remodeling of the ventricle may produce subtle regression of hypertrophy in some patients.[104]

Other morphological abnormalities include enlargement and elongation of the mitral valve leaflets and, in rare cases, anomalous papillary muscle insertion directly into the anterior mitral valve leaflet.[106,114,115]

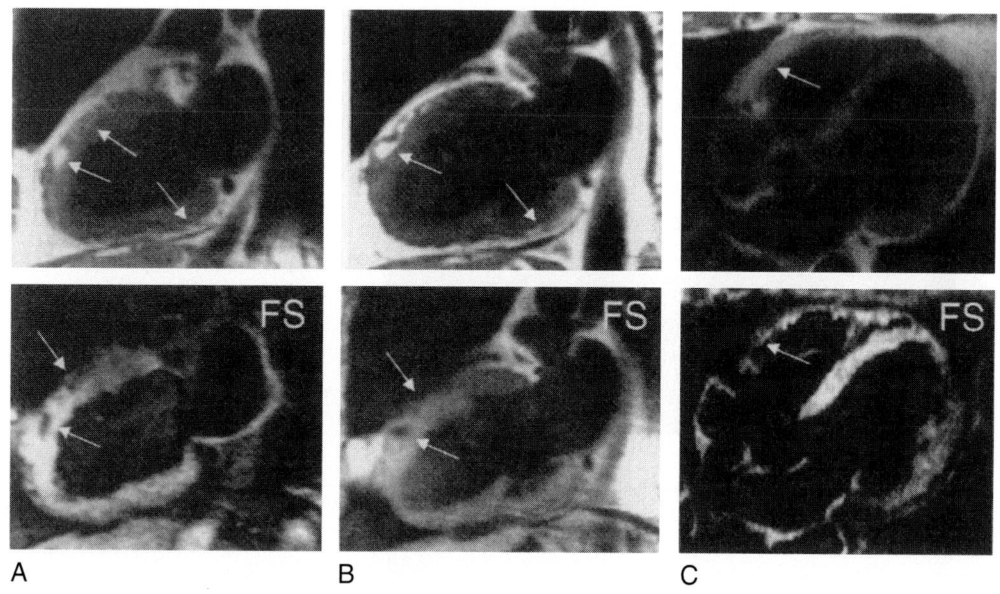

FIGURE 59–5 Magnetic resonance images before (upper panels) and after (lower panels) the application of a special imaging algorithm (fat saturation, FS) to highlight areas of fat deposition in a patient with biventricular involvement by arrhythmogenic right ventricular cardiomyopathy. The arrows (upper panels) point to areas of fatty infiltration of the anterior and inferior left **(A** and **B)** and right **(C)** ventricular myocardium. Fatty infiltration is confirmed (lower panels) by the special FS algorithm as black areas that are highlighted by arrows. (From McCrohon JA, John AS, Lorenz CH, et al: Images in cardiovascular medicine. Left ventricular involvement in arrhythmogenic right ventricular cardiomyopathy. Circulation 105:1394, 2002. Copyright 2002, American Heart Association.)

APICAL HYPERTROPHIC CARDIOMYOPATHY. A variant with predominant involvement of the apex is common in Japan and is estimated to represent a fourth of Japanese patients with HCM.[116] In other parts of the world, apical HCM is less common (<10 percent in one large Western center).[115] Typical features include a characteristic spade-like configuration of the left ventricle during angiographic study, giant negative T waves in the precordial ECG leads, absence of an intraventricular pressure gradient, mild symptoms, and a generally benign course with low mortality.[117] Nevertheless, complications may be seen, with atrial fibrillation the most common.[118]

HYPERTROPHIC CARDIOMYOPATHY IN ELDERLY PEOPLE. HCM may on occasion arise in elderly people and often demonstrates unique features, including an especially small left ventricular cavity but with relatively mild hypertrophy. Other findings include marked anterior displacement of the mitral valve, extensive submitral (annular) calcification in some patients, a left ventricular outflow gradient, and late appearance of symptoms.[119]

Gross cardiac morphological features similar to those in HCM may be seen in infants of diabetic mothers and in patients with a variety of other conditions,[104] including hyperparathyroidism, neurofibromatosis, generalized lipodystrophy, lentiginosis, pheochromocytoma, Friedreich ataxia, and Noonan syndrome. Rarely, the findings may be simulated by amyloid, glycogen storage disease, or tumor involvement of the septum.

HISTOLOGY. Microscopic findings in HCM are distinctive, with myocardial hypertrophy and gross disorganization of the muscle bundles, resulting in a characteristic whorled pattern (see Fig. 59-2); abnormalities are found in the cell-to-cell arrangement (disarray) (see Fig. 59-6) and disorganization of the myofibrillar architecture within a given cell.[120] Fibrosis is usually prominent and may be extensive enough to produce grossly visible scars. Foci of disorganized cells are often interspersed between areas of hypertrophied but otherwise normal-appearing muscle cells. Interstitial (matrix) connective tissue elements are increased. Although abnormally arranged cardiac muscle cells were initially considered specific for HCM, it is now recognized that they may be found in a variety of congenital and acquired heart conditions. What is unique about the disarray in HCM is its ubiquity and frequency. Almost all HCM patients have some degree of disarray, and most have involvement of 5 percent or more of the myocardium; in general, a third or more of the myocardium demonstrates disarray.[104,106,120] In contrast, disarray in non-HCM patients (when it occurs) usually involves less than 5 percent of the myocardium.[108] In an experimental model of HCM, myocardial regions with prominent disarray demonstrate regional contractile dysfunction related in part to the structural abnormalities themselves (as a result of the attendant abnormal geometry and length of the myocardial fibers).[121]

Abnormal intramural coronary arteries, with a reduction in the size of the lumen and thickening of the vessel wall, are common in HCM.[120] The prominence of abnormal intramural coronary arteries in areas of extensive myocardial fibrosis is consistent with the hypothesis that these abnormalities may be responsible for the development of myocardial ischemia that appears to be central to many of the clinical manifestations of HCM, including angina pectoris, arrhythmias, and sudden death.[104,106]

Etiology

Genetics of Hypertrophic Cardiomyopathy

(see also Chap. 70)

Familial HCM occurs as an autosomal dominant mendelian-inherited disease at least 50 percent of the time.[122] It is thought that some if not all of the sporadic forms of the disease are due to spontaneous mutations.[123] At least 10 different genes are associated with HCM (Fig. 59–8; see Table 59–4).[124] All of the genes encode cardiac sarcomere proteins, including components of the thick or thin filaments that have contractile, regulatory, or structural functions.[11,20,113,124] More than 150 different mutations have been discovered thus far, and most are of the missense type.[104,113.,125] It is clear that more genetic defects are yet to be identified. The precise mechanism by which the various genetic mutations culminate in the morphological and clinical features of HCM is speculative at present, but all of the mutations probably cause abnormal force generation with an attendant hypertrophic response.[11,108,126,127] The ultimate manifestations of the resulting cardiomyopathy are probably the end result of a variety of interacting factors.[20,124,128] Thus, various sarcomeric mutations (such as of troponin T, tropomyosin, or the beta-myosin heavy chain [MHC] gene) can culminate in *either* HCM or DCM (see Table 59–4),[20,22] although in some cases the apparent DCM may simply reflect the burned-out phase of HCM.[129] An occasional family with familial HCM is affected by more than one mutation.[123]

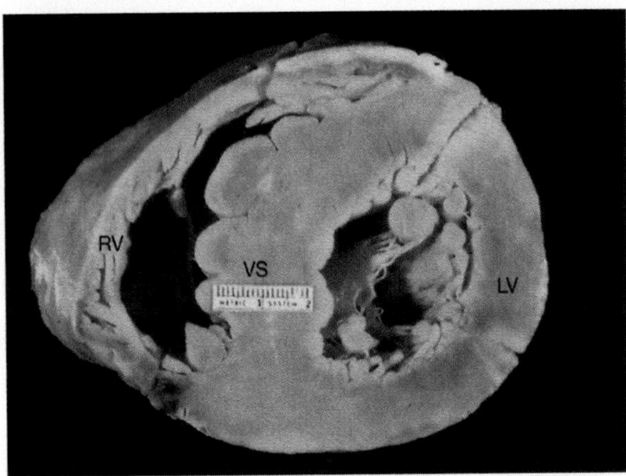

A

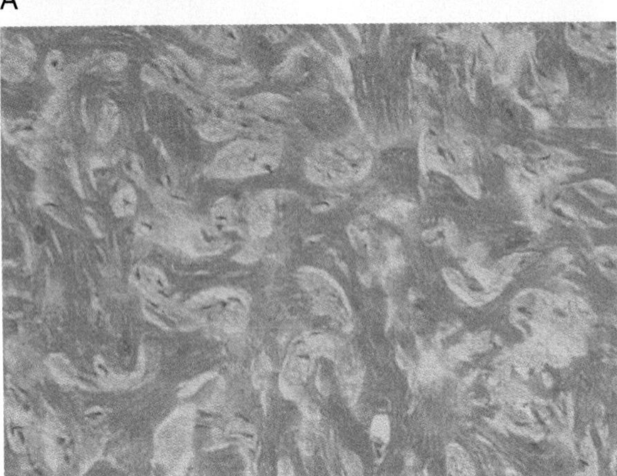

B

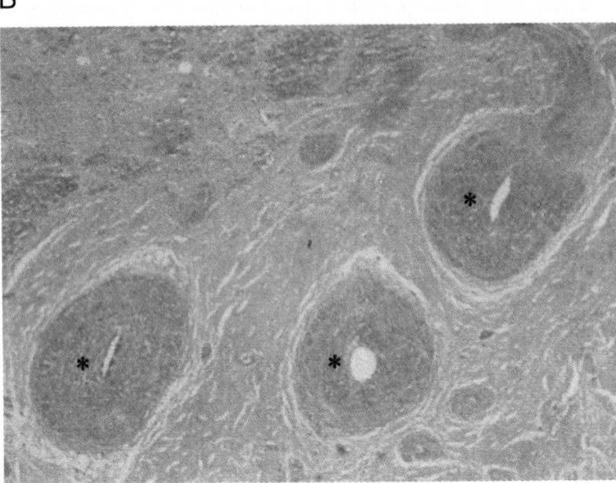

C

FIGURE 59–6 Morphological features of hypertrophic cardiomyopathy. **A,** Gross heart specimen of a 13-year-old male athlete with disproportionate thickening of the interventricular septum (VS) compared with the left ventricular (LV) free wall. **B,** Histological specimen showing marked cellular disarray with hypertrophied cells arranged in a chaotic pattern. **C,** Histological specimen showing several abnormal intramural coronary arteries, with markedly thickened walls and narrowed lumina. RV = right ventricle; hematoxylin and eosin stain in B and C; original magnifications ×50. (Adapted from Maron BJ: Hypertrophic cardiomyopathy. Curr Probl Cardiol 18:637, 1993, with permission of Mosby, Inc.)

The genetic basis of HCM was first reported by Seidman and Seidman, who reported the existence of a disease gene located on chromosome 14q11-12.[18] Subsequently they found this to be the gene encoding beta cardiac MHC. Sequencing of this gene in one family with HCM revealed that the abnormality was caused by a gene duplication in which the alpha and beta MHC genes were fused and present in an extra copy. In the second family, there was a point mutation in the beta MHC sequence that altered the myosin's arginine to glutamine. Both of these mutations affect the polypeptides crucial to the structure of myofibrils and might be responsible for the myocyte and myofibrillar disarray characteristic of familial HCM. Other disease loci that have been identified include chromosome 1q32 (encoding troponin T), chromosome 19p13 (encoding troponin I), chromosome 15q22 (encoding alpha-tropomyosin), chromosome 11p11 (encoding myosin-binding protein C), chromosomes 3p21 and 12q23-p21 (encoding essential and regulatory myosin light chains), and chromosome 15q14 (encoding actin).[18,122,130] A missense mutation of the gene that encodes a subunit of the adenosine monophosphate–activated protein kinase (*PRKAG2*) is associated with the Wolff-Parkinson-White syndrome, conduction abnormalities, and apparent left ventricular hypertrophy,[131] but this condition is due to glycogen accumulation within myocytes and thus should be regarded as a metabolic storage disease rather than a form of HCM.[104]

Most cases of familial HCM are caused by one of three mutant genes.[104] It is estimated that about 35 to 50 percent are due to mutations of the cardiac MHC gene, 15 to 25 percent due to mutations of myosin-binding protein C, 15 to 20 percent due to mutations of the cardiac troponin T gene, less than 5 percent due to mutations of the tropomyosin gene, and the remainder due to mutations of other genes.[132] There is wide variation in the phenotypic expression of a specific mutation of a given gene, with variability in clinical symptoms and the degree as well as time course of appearance of hypertrophy.[104] Of particular interest are mutations of the troponin T gene that typically result in only modest (or no) hypertrophy but indicate a poor prognosis and a high risk of sudden death (although at least one mutation has a favorable prognosis).[133,134] Several other "malignant" mutations have been described that involve the beta-MHC and tropomyosin.[135,136] Conversely, certain genes and mutations are felt to be associated with a more favorable prognosis, although the concept of a mutation-specific clinical outcome has been challenged.[137] In some patients with an abnormal gene and no echocardiographic evidence of HCM, the electrocardiogram is abnormal. Thus, otherwise unexplained abnormalities of the electrocardiogram in first-degree relatives of patients with HCM may be indicative of a carrier or preclinical state.[138]

Despite the substantial insights that molecular genetic studies have provided into the fundamental mechanisms responsible for HCM, DNA analysis for mutant genes is not yet routinely available for clinical use, although it is anticipated that it will become available in the future.[104,111] In addition, many clinicians do not adequately discuss the genetic implications of HCM with their patients, at least in part because the typical cardiologist manages only a small number of patients with HCM.[139]

Pathophysiology

SYSTOLE. Since the initial descriptions of HCM, the feature that has attracted the greatest attention is the dynamic pressure gradient across the left ventricular outflow tract (see Fig. 59–7).[103,107,139,140] Although this pressure gradient was initially attributed to a muscular sphincter action in the subaortic region or was believed by some to be an artifact,[109] it is now considered to be related to further narrowing of an already small outflow tract (narrowed by prominent septal hypertrophy and possibly abnormal location of the mitral valve) by systolic anterior motion of often elongated mitral valve leaflets against the hypertrophied septum.

There continues to be considerable controversy about the cause and significance of the outflow gradient.[109] Central to the disagreement is whether there is true obstruction to left ventricular ejection or whether the pressure gradient is simply the consequence of vigorous ventricular emptying.[141] It is now agreed that true mechanical impediment to left ventricular ejection occurs when outflow gradients are present and is the result of distal portions of the mitral valve apparatus moving anteriorly across the outflow tract and making contact with the ventricular septum in midsystole.[106,139,141] There continues to be controversy about the fundamental cause of the distinctive mitral valve systolic movement. Central to the controversy is whether the valve apparatus is displaced anteriorly because of Venturi effects and as a result of the increased ejection velocities produced by the abnormal left ventricular outflow tract orientation and geometry or whether it is *pushed* into the outflow tract as a consequence of ejection.

The pressure overload that results from the outflow gradient appears to play some role in the development of ventricular hypertrophy in HCM, perhaps involving TNF-alpha, because both myocyte hypertrophy and TNF-alpha levels are reduced after successful reduction of the gradient by septal ablation.[142,143]

DIASTOLE. Most patients with HCM demonstrate abnormalities of diastolic function (see Chaps. 20 and 21) at rest or with stress, whether or not a pressure gradient is present and whether or not they are symptomatic.[144] These abnormalities of global diastolic filling are largely independent of the extent and distribution of myocardial hypertrophy; patients with mild and apparently localized hypertrophy may demonstrate prominent diastolic dysfunction, suggesting that the myopathic process occurs in ventricular regions that are not macroscopically hypertrophied.[116] Diastolic dysfunction in turn leads to increased ventricular filling pressure despite a normal or small left ventricular cavity and appears to result from abnormalities of left ventricular relaxation and distensibility, at least in part as a direct result of the altered protein expression that occurs in many HCM patients as a consequence of genetic mutations.[145] Early diastolic filling is impaired when relaxation is prolonged, perhaps related to abnormal calcium kinetics, subendocardial ischemia, or the abnormal loading conditions found in HCM.[146] Late diastolic filling is altered when left ventricular distensibility is impaired; as a consequence, filling pressures rise. HCM may cause abnormal distensibility of the ventricle because of fibrosis or cellular disorganization.

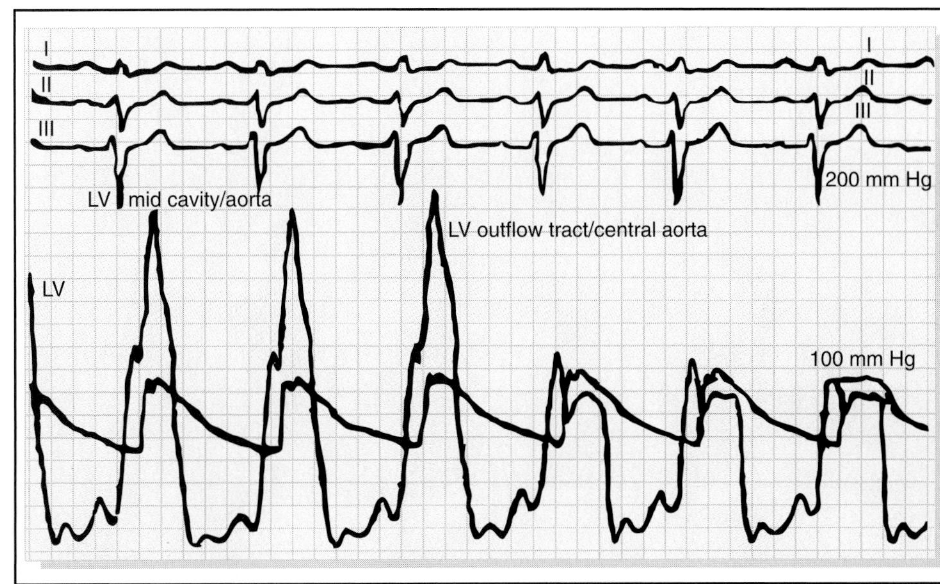

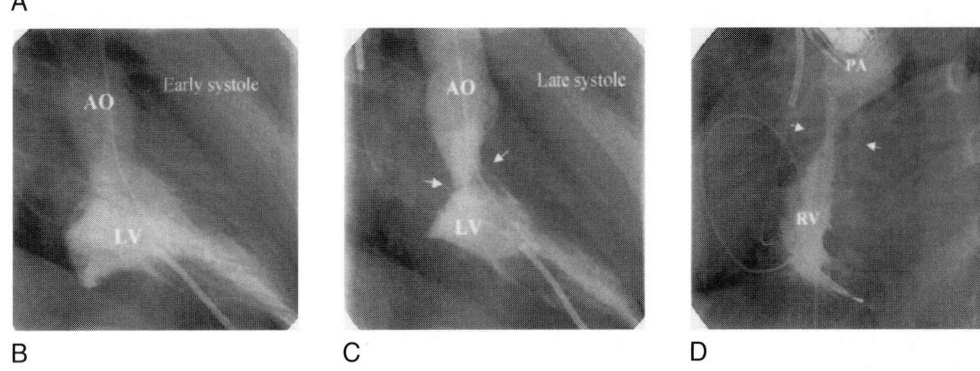

FIGURE 59–7 Hemodynamic and angiographic findings in hypertrophic cardiomyopathy with biventricular involvement. **A,** Simultaneous pressure recordings from the mid left ventricular (LV) cavity and aorta show a 100 mm Hg gradient. The aortic tracing shows a "spike-and-dome" pattern related to systolic anterior movement of the anterior leaflet of the mitral valve. The subaortic location of the gradient is confirmed as the LV catheter is pulled back from the midcavity (left) to the subaortic outflow tract (right). **B** and **C,** Left ventriculogram in the right anterior oblique projection. Arrows show systolic anterior mitral valve movement in late systole with attendant obstruction of the outflow tract. **D,** Right ventriculogram in the left lateral projection showing massive hypertrophy of the right ventricular (RV) outflow area (arrows) with an "hourglass" configuration. AO = aorta; PA = pulmonary artery. (From Doshi SN, Kim MC, Sharma SK, et al: Images in cardiovascular medicine. Right and left ventricular outflow tract obstruction in hypertrophic cardiomyopathy. Circulation 106:e3, 2002. Copyright 2002, American Heart Association.)

MYOCARDIAL ISCHEMIA. Myocardial ischemia is common and multifactorial in HCM (Table 59–5).[147] Major causes include impaired vasodilator reserve (perhaps related to the thickened and narrowed small intramural coronary arteries found in HCM)[148]; increased oxygen demand, especially in patients with outflow gradients; and elevated filling pressures with resultant subendocardial ischemia.[147,149,150] In children, compression of intramyocardial segments of the left anterior descending coronary artery (so-called myocardial bridge) has been reported to predispose to myocardial ischemia and sudden death, but this has been contested.[151]

TABLE 59–5 Possible Mechanisms for Ischemia in Hypertrophic Cardiomyopathy

Increased Myocardial Oxygen Demand	Reduced Myocardial Perfusion
Myocardial hypertrophy	Small vessel disease
Diastolic dysfunction	Abnormal vascular responses
Myocyte disarray	Myocardial bridges
Left ventricular outflow obstruction	Increased coronary vascular resistance
Arrhythmias	

From McKenna WJ, Behr ER: Hypertrophic cardiomyopathy: Management, risk stratification, and prevention of sudden death. Heart 87:169, 2002.

Clinical Manifestations

HISTORY. The majority of patients with HCM are asymptomatic or only mildly symptomatic[105,140,152] and often are identified during screening of relatives of a patient with HCM. Unfortunately, the first clinical manifestation of the disease in such individuals may be sudden death. The disease is identified most often in adults in their fourth and fifth decades; it occurs more often than is commonly suspected in elderly patients. The condition has been observed at necropsy in stillborns and both clinically and

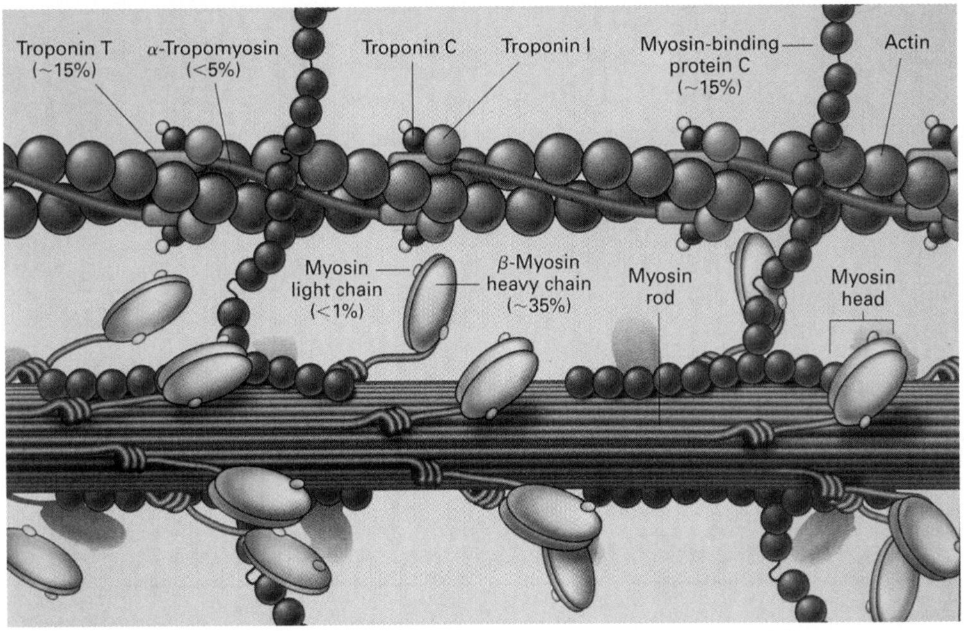

FIGURE 59–8 Drawing showing components of the sarcomere and mutations in hypertrophic cardiomyopathy. Cardiac contraction occurs when calcium binds the troponin complex (subunits C, I, and T) and alpha-tropomyosin. Actin stimulates ATPase activity in the globular myosin head and results in the production of force along actin filaments. Cardiac myosin-binding protein C binds myosin and modulates contraction. In hypertrophic cardiomyopthy, mutations may impair these and other protein interactions, result in ineffectual contraction, and produce hypertrophy. Percentages represent the estimated frequency with which a mutation causes hypertrophic cardiomyopathy. (From Spirito P, Seidman C, McKenna WJ, et al: The management of hypertophic cardiomyopathy. N Engl J Med 336:775, 1997. Copyright 1997, Massachusetts Medical Society.)

pathologically in octogenarians and is distinguished among cardiovascular diseases by its potential for clinical presentation during any phase of life.[104,140,152,153] The importance of recognizing this disorder in children at the earliest possible time is highlighted by the higher mortality rate in younger patients; death is often sudden and unexpected.[107,140] When HCM is first diagnosed in older patients, several features are distinctive and are in contrast to findings in younger patients: generally mild degrees of left ventricular hypertrophy, frequent demonstration of outflow gradients, and appearance of marked symptoms late in life (typically after age 55).[104,152] A particularly high index of suspicion of this condition must be maintained to make the clinical diagnosis in elderly people because their symptoms may easily be confused with those of coronary artery or aortic valve disease. Because syncope and sudden death have been associated with competitive sports and severe exertion in patients with HCM, it is important to diagnose this condition so that these activities may be proscribed. It appears that HCM may be more commonly unrecognized and undiagnosed in the black population than in the white population.[154]

The clinical picture varies considerably, ranging from the asymptomatic relative of a patient with recognized HCM who has a slightly abnormal echocardiogram but no other overt manifestation of the disease to the patient with incapacitating symptoms.[140] A general relationship exists between the extent of hypertrophy and the severity of symptoms, but the relationship is not absolute, and some patients have severe symptoms with only mild and apparently localized hypertrophy and vice versa. A complex interaction occurs between left ventricular hypertrophy, the left ventricular pressure gradient, diastolic dysfunction, and myocardial ischemia, which accounts for the great variability in symptoms from patient to patient.

The most common symptom is *dyspnea,* occurring in up to 90 percent of symptomatic patients. It is largely a consequence of the elevated left ventricular diastolic (and therefore left atrial and pulmonary venous) pressure, which results principally from impaired ventricular filling owing to diastolic dysfunction.[107,133,139,140] Angina pectoris (found in about three-fourths of symptomatic patients), fatigue, presyncope, and syncope are also common. Palpitations, paroxysmal nocturnal dyspnea, overt congestive heart failure, and dizziness are found less frequently, although severe congestive heart failure culminating in death may be seen. Exertion tends to exacerbate many of the symptoms. A variety of mechanisms may contribute to the production of angina pectoris (see Table 59–5). It is at least in part the result of an imbalance between oxygen supply and demand as a consequence of the greatly increased myocardial mass.[107] Abnormalities of the small coronary arteries may contribute to myocardial ischemia, particularly during exertion, and perhaps 20 percent of older patients with HCM may have concomitant atheromatous obstructive coronary artery disease. Transmural infarction may occur in the absence of narrowing of the extramural coronary arteries. Impaired diastolic relaxation may produce subendocardial ischemia as a result of prolonged maintenance of wall tension with a concomitant slower than normal decrease in the impedance to coronary blood flow. Syncope may result from inadequate cardiac output with exertion or from cardiac arrhythmias. Near-syncopal ("graying out") spells that occur in the erect posture and that can be relieved by immediately lying down are common.[140] However, in contrast to valvular aortic stenosis, syncope or near-syncope may not be an ominous finding in adult patients with HCM; some patients have a history of such episodes dating back many years without clinical deterioration.[105] In children and adolescents, however, presyncope and syncope identify patients at increased risk for sudden death (see Natural History).

PHYSICAL EXAMINATION. This may be normal (except for an S_4; see later), especially in asymptomatic patients without pressure gradients, those with mild hypertrophy, and those with the apical variant of HCM, but findings are usually prominent in patients with a left ventricular outflow tract pressure gradient.[103,104] The apical precordial impulse is often displaced laterally and is usually abnormally forceful and diffuse. Because of decreased left ventricular compliance, a prominent presystolic apical impulse that results from forceful atrial systole is often present.[140] This may result in a double apical impulse as a result of the prominent a wave. A more characteristic but less frequently recognized abnormality is a triple apical beat, the third impulse consisting of a late systolic bulge that occurs when the heart is almost empty and is performing near-isometric contraction.[140] The jugular venous pulse may demonstrate a prominent a wave, reflecting diminished right ventricular compliance secondary to massive hypertrophy of the ventricular septum. The carotid pulse typically rises briskly and then declines in midsystole as the gradient develops, followed by a secondary rise.[140] This may be appreciated on physical examination but can be demonstrated more clearly by means of indirect carotid pulse tracings. It is identical to the "spike-and-dome" configuration seen on direct arterial pressure recordings obtained during cardiac catheterization (see Fig. 59–7).

AUSCULTATION. The S_1 is normal and is often preceded by an S_4 that corresponds to the apical presystolic impulse. The S_2 is usually normally split. In some patients, however, it is narrowly split and in others, particularly those with severe outflow gradients, paradoxical splitting may be noted.[140] An S_3 may be present but does not have the same ominous significance as in patients with valvular aortic stenosis. Systolic ejection sounds related to rapid acceleration of blood flow may be found on occasion. The auscultatory hallmark of HCM associated with an outflow gradient is a systolic murmur that typically is harsh and crescendo-decrescendo in configuration; it usually commences well after S_1 and is best heard between the apex and the left sternal border.[140] It often radiates well to the lower sternal border, the axillae, and the base of the heart but not into the neck vessels. In patients with large gradients, the murmur usually reflects both left ventricular outflow tract turbulence and concomitant mitral regurgitation.[133,155] Accordingly, the murmur is often more holosystolic and blowing at the apex and in the axillae (because of mitral regurgitation) and midsystolic and harsher along the lower sternal border (because of turbulent flow across the narrowed outflow tract).[115]

The systolic murmur is labile in intensity and duration, and a variety of maneuvers may be used to augment or suppress it (Table 59–6).[133,140] A diastolic rumbling murmur, reflecting increased transmitral flow, may occur in patients with marked mitral regurgitation. The murmur of aortic regurgitation is observed in a minority of patients. It may develop after operation to correct the outflow gradient or following infective endocarditis.[156]

DIFFERENTIATION FROM VALVULAR AORTIC STENOSIS. It is important to emphasize the features of the physical examination that permit differentiation of HCM from fixed orifice obstruction, most commonly related to valvular aortic stenosis (see Chap. 57). The character of the carotid pulse and features of the murmur are most useful in this regard. Because there is obstruction to left ventricular emptying from the beginning of systole with fixed valvular stenosis, the carotid upstroke is slowed and of low amplitude (pulsus parvus et tardus). With HCM, initial ejection of blood from the left ventricle is actually enhanced, and therefore the arterial upstroke is brisk. The murmur of HCM, as opposed to that of aortic stenosis, can be reliably identified by its increase with the Valsalva maneuver and during standing from a squatting position and its decrease during squatting from a standing position, passive leg elevation, and handgrip (see Table 59–6).[115] Other features that may be helpful but are of less importance are the location of the murmur (it radiates along the carotid arteries in valvular aortic stenosis but not in HCM) and the presence and location of a systolic thrill when present (not uncommon and most prominent when present in the second right intercostal space in valvular aortic stenosis versus uncommon and in the fourth interspace along the left sternal border in HCM).

TABLE 59–6 Effects of Interventions on Outflow Gradient and Systolic Murmur in Hypertrophic Cardiomyopathy

Intervention	Contractility	Preload	Afterload
Increase in Gradient and Murmur			
Valsalva maneuver (during strain)	—	↓	↓
Standing	—	↓	—
Postextrasystole	↑	↑	—
Isoproterenol	↑	↓	↓
Digitalis	↑	↓	—
Amyl nitrite	— then ↑	↓ then ↑	↓
Nitroglycerin	—	↓	↓
Exercise	↑	↑	↑
Tachycardia	↑	↓	—
Hypovolemia	↑	↓	↓
Decrease in Gradient and Murmur			
Müller maneuver	—	↑	↑
Valsalva overshoot	—	↑	↑
Squatting	—	↑	↑
Alpha-adrenoceptor stimulation (phenylephrine)	—	—	↑
Beta-adrenoceptor blockade	↓	↑	—
General anesthesia	↓	—	—
Isometric handgrip	—	—	↑

↑ = increase; ↓ = decrease; — = no major change.

ELECTROCARDIOGRAM. This is usually abnormal in HCM and invariably so in symptomatic patients with left ventricular outflow tract gradients, showing a wide variety of patterns.[157] Entirely normal electrocardiograms are seen in only 15 to 25 percent of patients and are usually found in the presence of only localized left ventricular hypertrophy.[104] The most common abnormalities are ST segment and T wave abnormalities, followed by evidence of left ventricular hypertrophy, with QRS complexes that are tallest in the midprecordial leads.[132,158] Unfortunately, these findings are nonspecific and may be seen as well in completely healthy individuals, especially highly trained athletes in whom the abnormalities may reflect athletic conditioning itself. Only a modest relationship exists between the magnitude of left ventricular hypertrophy on electrocardiography and the degree of hypertrophy found on echocardiography.[104] Giant negative T waves in the midprecordial leads of Japanese patients are characteristic of HCM involving the apex,[115,117] but such a pattern in whites may be found with HCM involving segments other than the apex. Prominent Q waves are relatively common, occurring in 20 to 50 percent of patients.[158] The Q wave abnormalities often involve the inferior (II, III, aV_F) or precordial (V_2 to V_6) leads, or both.[132] A variety of other ECG abnormalities may occur, including abnormal electrical axis (usually left axis deviation) and P wave abnormalities (usually left atrial abnormality). Accessory atrioventricular pathways have been found in HCM, although they are uncommon. Clinically significant abnormalities of atrioventricular conduction are uncommon but may cause syncope.

ARRHYTHMIAS (see Chap. 32). Although hemodynamic or ischemic mechanisms may play a role in the death of some patients with HCM (particularly the young), many deaths, particularly those that are known to have been sudden, are probably due to ventricular tachycardia or fibrillation.[159]

Supraventricular tachyarrhythmias are common in HCM and may be found in one-fourth to one-half of patients.[160] Because of the systolic and diastolic abnormalities in this disorder, rhythm disturbances are less well tolerated. Atrial fibrillation is the most common sustained arrhythmia and eventually occurs in almost a quarter of patients; it increases in incidence with age and is associated with left atrial enlargement.[152,161] It is reasonably well tolerated by about one-third of patients but may be associated with embolic stroke, progressive congestive heart failure, and death.[162]

Ventricular arrhythmias are common in patients with HCM, occurring in more than three-fourths of patients undergoing continuous ambulatory ECG monitoring. Runs of nonsustained ventricular tachycardia are found in about one-fourth of patients with HCM, although sustained monomorphic tachycardia is uncommon.[160] In some it is a harbinger of subsequent sudden death; however, its overall predictive value in identifying patients at high risk for sudden death is limited. Treadmill testing may expose arrhythmias that are not present at rest, although continuous ambulatory monitoring is superior in detecting repetitive ventricular tachyarrhythmias. The signal-averaged electrocardiogram has not proved to be helpful in identifying patients at increased risk for sustained or lethal ventricular arrhythmia, nor has the degree of QT dispersion.[160,163] Reduced heart rate variability on ambulatory monitor recordings, a predictor of increased sudden death risk after myocardial infarction, appears to be less useful in risk stratification in patients with HCM and is not widely used.

ELECTROPHYSIOLOGICAL TESTING. The role of electrophysiological studies in identifying patients with HCM at increased risk for sudden death is controversial; despite earlier enthusiasm, it is now generally believed that it is of limited predictive value.[105,159,160] These studies may identify a variety of abnormalities in HCM patients; they induce polymorphic ventricular tachycardia in many patients with HCM, but such a response is generally believed to be nonspecific and does not identify high-risk patients.[105] Unfortunately, unlike its utility in ischemic heart disease, the predictive value of the more typical inducible sustained ventricular arrhythmias during electrophysiological testing is low in HCM. Aggressive stimulation protocols are required to induce a sustained arrhythmia in high-risk HCM patients,[159] often resulting in arrhythmias in low-risk patients as well. Tilt-table testing has shown an abnormal response consisting of an early decrease in cardiac output in some patients with HCM and a history of syncope, perhaps related to an abnormality in baroreceptor function.[164]

CHEST ROENTGENOGRAM. The findings on radiographic examination are variable; the cardiac silhouette may range from normal to markedly increased, and in most cases of apparent "cardiomegaly" the enlarged cardiac silhouette is the result of left ventricular hypertrophy or left atrial enlargement, or both.[115] Left atrial enlargement is observed frequently, especially when significant mitral regurgitation is present. Aortic root enlargement and valvular calcification are not seen unless associated diseases are present, although calcification of the mitral annulus is common in HCM.

ECHOCARDIOGRAPHY. Because echocardiography combines the attributes of high resolution and no known risk, it has been widely used in the evaluation of HCM.[115] It is useful in the study of patients with suspected HCM and also in the screening of relatives of HCM patients. The echocardiogram is of value in identifying and quantifying morphological features (i.e., distribution of septal hypertrophy), functional aspects (e.g., hypercontractile left ventricle), and (when combined with Doppler recordings) hemodynamic findings (e.g., magnitude of outflow gradient) (see Chap. 11).

Left Ventricular Hypertorphy. The cardinal echocardiographic feature of HCM is left ventricular hypertrophy (Fig. 59–9).[104] Although the characteristic feature is hypertrophy of the septum and anterolateral free wall, the echocardiogram is useful in identifying involvement of other left ventricular locations, including portions of the free wall and the apex.[106,165,166] Considerable variability exists in the degree and pattern of hypertrophy; in most patients, there is variation in the extent of hypertrophy from one left ventricular region to another.[104] Maximal hypertrophy of the septum often occurs midway between the base and apex of the left ventricle. The finding of a thickened septum that is at least 1.3 to 1.5 times the thickness of the posterior wall when measured in diastole just before atrial systole has been the time-honored criterion for the diagnosis of ASH.[133] The septum not only is relatively thicker than the posterior wall but also is typically at least 15 mm in thickness (normal < 12 mm). Although the average wall thickness detected on echocardiography is about 20 mm (i.e., almost twice normal), there is great variation, ranging from very mild hypertrophy (13 to 15 mm) to massive hypertrophy (60 mm).[104]

Outflow Tract Obstruction. A second echocardiographic feature often found in HCM is narrowing of the left ventricular outflow tract,[155] which is formed by the interventricular septum anteriorly and the anterior leaflet of the mitral valve posteriorly. The mitral valve leaflets may be abnormally large and elongated and are associated with abnormal left ventricular outflow tract geometry that culminates in the production of a pressure gradient.[115] This abnormal geometry is causally related to the mitral regurgitation that accompanies an outflow gradient; the degree of mitral regurgitation correlates with the extent of anterior and posterior leaflet malcoaptation.[167] When HCM is associated with a pressure gradient, there is abnormal systolic anterior motion of the anterior leaflet and occasionally the posterior leaflet of the mitral valve. A close relationship exists between the degree of systolic anterior motion and attendant mitral regurgitation with the magnitude of the outflow gradient.[155] Prolonged interventricular septal contact of the mitral apparatus is limited to HCM with resting pressure gradients, and a close temporal relationship exists between the onset of the pressure gradient and the onset of septal apposition of the mitral apparatus.

Three explanations have been offered for *systolic anterior motion*: (1) the mitral valve is *pulled* against the septum by contraction of abnormally oriented papillary muscles and elongated leaflets, (2) the mitral valve is *pushed* against the septum (perhaps by the left ventricular posterior wall) because of its abnormal position in the outflow tract, and (3) the mitral valve is drawn toward the septum because of the lower pressure that occurs as blood is ejected at a high velocity through a narrowed outflow tract (Venturi effect).[168] In a minority of cases (less than 15 percent), one or both papillary muscles insert anomalously directly into the anterior mitral leaflet, causing a long area of midventricular narrowing that results in an intraventricular pressure gradient.[114] Systolic anterior motion of the mitral valve and dynamic left ventricular gradients are not pathognomonic of HCM but may be found in a variety of other conditions,[104] including hypercontractile states, left ventricular hypertrophy, transposition of the great arteries, and infiltration of the septum.

OTHER ECHOCARDIOGRAPHIC FINDINGS. The following may be present: (1) a small left ventricular cavity; (2) reduced septal motion and thickening during systole, particularly of the upper septum (presumably because of the disarray of the myofibrillar architecture and abnormal contractile function); (3) normal or increased motion of the posterior wall; (4) a reduced rate of closure of the mitral valve in middiastole secondary to a decrease in left ventricular compliance or abnormal transmittal diastolic flow; (5) mitral valve prolapse; and (6) partial systolic closure or, more commonly, coarse systolic fluttering of the aortic valve related to turbulent blood flow in the outflow tract. The echocardiographic findings that accompany a left ventricular outflow tract gradient (systolic anterior motion of the mitral valve and partial closure of the aortic valve) may be quite labile, and provocative measures such as the Valsalva maneuver, pharmacologically induced vasodilation with amyl nitrite, stimulation of contractility with isoproterenol, or an induced premature ventricular contraction may be required to precipitate the findings.[115]

Abnormalities of diastolic function (see Chaps. 20 and 21) may be demonstrated by echocardiography and Doppler recordings in about 80 percent of patients with HCM, independent of the presence or absence of a systolic pressure gradient. Because the septum is typically hypokinetic, the rate of left ventricular filling is determined primarily by the rate of free wall thinning. Little relationship exists between the extent of hypertrophy and the severity of abnormalities of diastolic function.

RADIONUCLIDE SCANNING (see Chap. 13). Thallium-201 myocardial imaging, particularly when tomographic imaging (single-photon emission computed tomography [SPECT]) is performed (see Chap. 13), permits direct determination of the relative thicknesses of the septum and free wall and may be of particular value when technical constraints limit the reliability of echocardiographic evaluation in a given patient with presumed HCM. Reversible thallium defects, presumably indicative of ischemia, may be seen in HCM in the absence of obstructive coronary artery disease.[160] They may be found in adult patients with HCM and in young patients with a history of sudden death or syncope, suggesting that myocardial ischemia is playing some etiological role.[160] Fixed defects, probably indicative of myocardial scarring, occur primarily in patients with impaired systolic function (similar patchy defects can be demonstrated in hypertrophied myocardial segments by MRI in the majority of HCM patients).[169] Gated radionuclide ventriculography with blood pool labeling permits the evaluation of not only the size but also the motion of the septum and left ventricle. As with the echocardiogram, abnormal diastolic filling of the ventricle has been observed in patients with HCM (both with and without gradients) by computer analysis of the blood pool scan.[170] Because of the ease and availability of transthoracic and transesophageal echocardiography, this technique is not widely used in the evaluation of HCM.

MAGNETIC RESONANCE IMAGING (see Chap. 14). This technique may be useful for identifying HCM in cases in which the standard echocardiogram is technically inadequate and can distinguish between different causes of increased wall thickness (i.e., hypertrophy versus infiltration).[171] MRI supplemented by the contrast agent gadolinium leads to a pattern of hyperenhancement of the myocardial images in the majority of patients with HCM, presumably reflecting myocardial fibrosis or cellular disarray, or both[172] There is more hyperenhancement in patients at the highest risk for premature death, and it is hoped that the technique may aid in risk stratification of patients with HCM.[173]

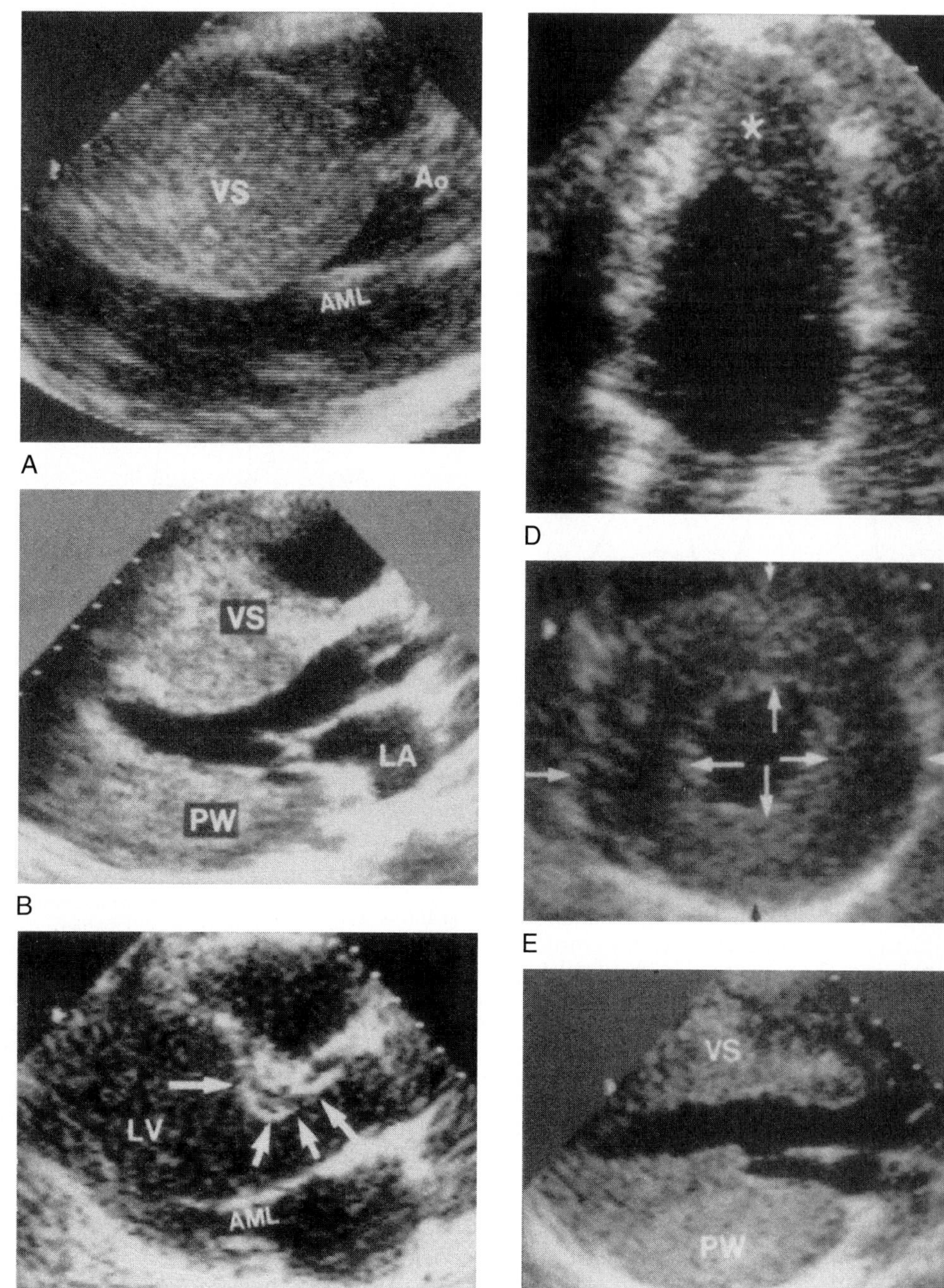

FIGURE 59–9 Heterogeneity in the pattern and extent of left ventricular wall thickening in hypertrophic cardiomyopathy (HCM) as shown by echocardiography. **A,** Massive hypertrophy of the ventricular septum (VS) with wall thickness greater than 50 mm. **B,** Distal VS thickening greater than proximal VS. **C,** Localized VS hypertrophy, confined to the immediate subaortic region. **D,** Apical HCM, with hypertrophy confined to the apex (asterisk). **E,** Concentric hypertrophy, with relatively similar thickening of VS and free wall (paired arrows). **F,** Inverted pattern of hypertrophy, with disproportionate posterior wall (PW) hypertrophy compared with the VS. A, B, C, and F = long-axis views; D = apical view; E = short-axis view. Calibration marks are 1 cm apart. Ao = aorta; AML = anterior mitral leaflet; LA = left atrium; LV = left ventricle. (From Klues HG, Schiffers A, Maron BJ: Phenotypic spectrum and patterns of left ventricular hypertrophy in hypertrophic cardiomyopathy: Morphologic observations and significance as assessed by two-dimensional echocardiography in 600 patients. J Am Coll Cardiol 26:1699, 1995.)

Hemodynamics and Angiography

CARDIAC CATHETERIZATION. Cardiac catheterization is not required for the diagnosis of HCM because noninvasive evaluation almost always suffices; it is reserved for situations where concomitant coronary artery disease is a consideration or when invasive modalities of therapy (e.g., pacemaker, percutaneous septal ablation, surgery) are being considered.[115] It discloses diminished diastolic left ventricular compliance and in some patients a systolic pressure gradient within the body of the left ventricle, which is separated from a subaortic chamber by the thickened septum and the anterior leaflet of the mitral valve that abuts the septum (see Fig. 59–7). The pressure gradient may be quite labile and may vary between 0 and 175 mm Hg in the same patient under different conditions (see later).[140] The arterial pressure tracing may demonstrate a spike-and-dome configuration similar to the carotid pulse recording (Fig. 59–10). As a consequence of diminished left ventricular compliance, the mean and particularly the a wave in the left atrial pressure pulse and the left ventricular end-diastolic pressures are usually elevated. Artifactual outflow gradients may occur if the left ventricular catheter becomes entrapped in the trabeculae of a markedly hypertrophied left ventricle.[109] Proper technique and choice of catheters with side holes should clarify the mechanism of such gradients. Cardiac output may be depressed in patients with longstanding severe gradients, but in the majority of patients it is normal; occasionally it is elevated.

Hemodynamic abnormalities in HCM are not limited to the left side of the heart. Approximately one-fourth of patients demonstrate pulmonary hypertension, which is usually mild but in some cases may be moderate to severe.[140] This is due (at least in part) to elevated mean left atrial pressures as a consequence of diminished left ventricular compliance. A pressure gradient in the right ventricular outflow tract occurs in approximately 15 percent of patients who have obstruction to left ventricular outflow[174] and appears to result from markedly hypertrophied right ventricular tissue (see Fig. 59–7).[110]

LABILITY OF GRADIENT. A feature characteristic of HCM is the variability and lability of the left ventricular outflow gradient (see Table 59–6 and Fig. 59–10).[103,107,140,175] A given patient may demonstrate a large outflow tract pressure

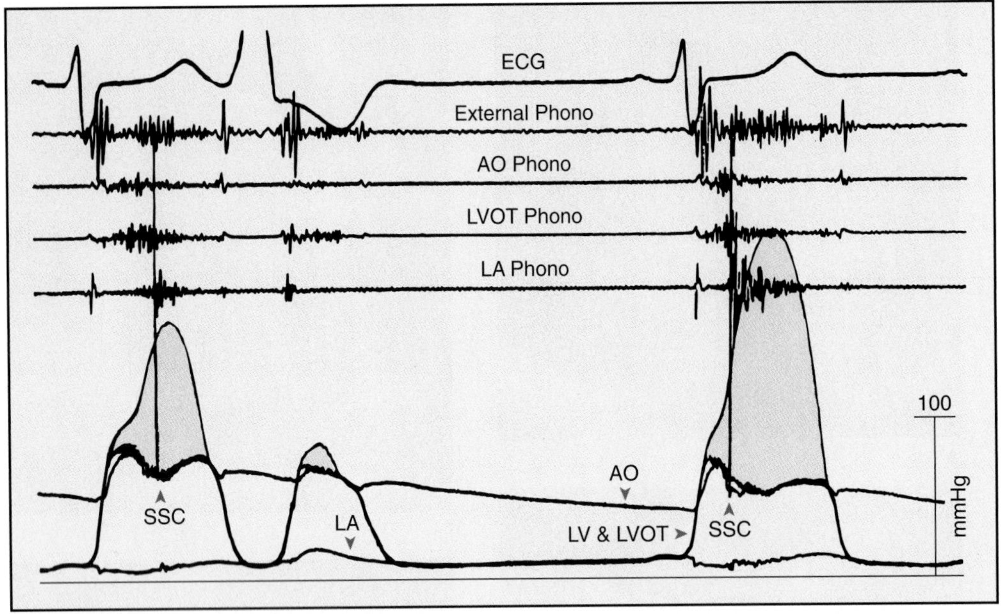

FIGURE 59–10 Hypertrophic cardiomyopathy with intracardiac pressure and phonocardiographic (phono) recordings from aorta (AO), left ventricle (LV), left ventricular outflow tract (LVOT), and left atrium (LA). Note the marked accentuation of the murmur and gradient (shaded) (in the third cycle) after a premature ventricular contraction with failure of the aortic pulse pressure to rise in the post-premature ventricular contraction beat (Brockenbrough-Braunwald sign). ECG = electrocardiogram; SSC = systolic anterior motion of the mitral valve septal contact. (From Murgo JP: Systolic ejection murmurs in the era of modern cardiology: What do we really know? J Am Coll Cardiol 32:1596, 1998.)

gradient on one occasion but have none at another time. In some patients without a resting gradient, it may be temporarily provoked. Three basic mechanisms are involved in the production of dynamic gradients, all of which act by reducing ventricular volume and presumably accentuate the apposition of the anterior mitral leaflet against the septum: (1) increased contractility, (2) decreased preload, and (3) decreased afterload.[107] In a minority of patients with HCM—perhaps about 5 percent of patients—the gradient is midventricular and may be intensified by increased contractility, which exerts a direct muscular sphincter action.[115] The stimuli that provoke or intensify left ventricular outflow tract gradients in HCM generally improve myocardial performance in normal subjects and in patients with most other forms of heart disease. Conversely, reductions in contractility or increases in preload or afterload, which increase left ventricular dimensions, reduce or abolish the left ventricular outflow gradient.

Alterations in the magnitude of the gradient are reflected by changes in the findings on physical examination, noninvasive tests, and left-sided heart catheterization. *This dynamic characteristic of HCM distinguishes it from the discrete forms of obstruction to ventricular outflow.*[140] An increase in the gradient is usually associated with a louder murmur, a longer ejection period with a more characteristic spike-and-dome configuration in the carotid pulse, and more flagrant echocardiographic evidence of systolic anterior motion of the anterior mitral leaflet. In some patients, the intensity of the murmur may *not* track with the gradient, perhaps because in many cases the murmur reflects mitral regurgitation (at least in part).[103]

A number of bedside procedures may be useful in the evaluation of suspected HCM.[140] Perhaps the most helpful is sudden standing from a squatting position.[115] Squatting results in an increase in venous return and an increase in aortic pressure, which increases ventricular volume, diminishing the gradient and decreasing the intensity of the murmur. Sudden standing has the opposite effects and results in accentuation of the gradient and the murmur.

VALSALVA MANEUVER. This is another useful bedside technique for eliciting or exacerbating the gradient.[115] After a transient increase in arterial pressure that usually lasts for four or five cardiac cycles after the onset of the strain and coincident with an increase in heart rate, the arterial systolic and pulse pressures and ventricular volume decline and the gradient (and murmur) increases. After release of the strain, a compensatory overshoot of arterial pressure and venous return with cardiac slowing occur, all of which increase ventricular volume and reduce the magnitude of the gradient and the murmur. Occasional patients may show paradoxical attenuation of the systolic murmur despite an increase in the pressure gradient, presumably related to a critical reduction in stroke volume. Inhalation of amyl nitrite also intensifies the murmur and the abnormality of the arterial pulse. Passive leg elevation, handgrip, and sudden squatting from a standing position attenuate the murmur of HCM.

POST-EXTRASYSTOLIC CHANGES. One of the most potent stimuli for enhancing the gradient is *post-extrasystolic potentiation* (see Chap. 19), which may occur after a spontaneous premature contraction or be induced by mechanical stimulation with a catheter. The resultant increase in contractility in the beat after the extrasystole is so marked that it outweighs the otherwise salutary effect of increased ventricular filling caused by the compensatory pause and produces an increase in the gradient and often of the murmur as well. A characteristic change often occurs in the directly recorded arterial pressure tracing, which, in addition to displaying a more marked spike-and-dome configuration, exhibits a pulse pressure that fails to increase as expected or actually decreases (the so-called Brockenbrough-Braunwald phenomenon) (see Fig. 59-10). This is one of the more reliable signs of dynamic obstruction of the left ventricular outflow tract. In some patients, the post-extrasystolic murmur is attenuated despite an increase in the outflow gradient, apparently because in this setting the murmur (a hybrid of outflow tract turbulence and mitral regurgitation) is mirroring to a greater degree changes in the severity of mitral regurgitation rather than changes in the outflow tract gradient.

POSITIVE INOTROPIC AGENTS. Digitalis glycosides and the beta adrenoceptor agonist isoproterenol augment the gradient because they increase myocardial contractility, whereas nitroglycerin and amyl nitrite exaggerate the gradient by decreasing arterial pressure and ventricular volume.[140] The ingestion of alcoholic beverages may exacerbate the outflow pressure gradient by producing systemic vasodilation. Hypovolemia (as a result of hemorrhage or overly aggressive diuresis) may also provoke overt obstruction to left ventricular outflow. The intensity of the murmur and the left ventricular outflow gradient may be decreased by beta adrenoceptor blockade, although the effect of the latter is often not dramatic and is of greatest hemodynamic benefit in protecting against the *increase* in the gradient that may be provoked by exercise. In most patients the severity of mitral regurgitation and the intensity of the apical blowing regurgitant murmur vary with the degree of obstruction of left ventricular outflow.[155]

ANGIOGRAPHY. Left ventriculography shows a hypertrophied ventricle; when an outflow gradient is present, the anterior leaflet of the mitral valve moves anteriorly during systole and encroaches on the outflow tract. Associated with this motion of the leaflet is mitral regurgitation, which is a constant finding in patients with gradients. The left ventricular cavity is often small, and systolic ejection is typically vigorous, resulting in virtual obliteration of the cavity at end systole (see Fig. 59-7), although the apparent hypercontractile state may relate more to reduced afterload (low end-systolic wall stress) than to enhanced inotropy. The papillary muscles are often prominent and may fill the left ventricular cavity in late systole. In patients with apical involvement, the extensive hypertrophy may convey a spade-like configuration to the left ventricular angiogram.[115]

It may be helpful to supplement angiographic evaluation of the left ventricle with simultaneous right ventriculography in a cranially angulated left anterior oblique projection to obtain optimal visualization of the size, shape, and configuration of the interventricular septum. The left septal surface either is flat or bulges into the left ventricular cavity at its middle or lower portion, in contrast to the normal findings of the septum curving toward the right ventricle.

In patients older than 45 years, obstructive coronary artery disease may be present, although the symptoms of ischemic pain are indistinguishable from those of patients with normal coronary angiograms and HCM. The left anterior descending and septal perforator coronary arteries may demonstrate phasic narrowing and associated abnormalities of coronary blood flow.[148,176]

Natural History

The clinical course in HCM is varied; in many patients symptoms are absent or mild, remain stable, and in some instances improve over a period of 5 to 10 years. The annual mortality is around 3 percent in adults seen in large referral centers but probably closer to 1 percent when all patients with HCM are included (Fig. 59–11).[104,177] The risk of sudden death is higher in children, perhaps as high as 6 percent per year.[104,152,159,160] Clinical deterioration (aside from sudden death) is usually slow. Although symptoms do not bear a predictable relationship to the severity or even the presence of a gradient, patients with gradients are more likely to develop eventual clinical deterioration than those without gradients.[177,178] The percentage of severely symptomatic patients increases with age. The onset of atrial fibrillation may lead to an increase in symptoms, although it is well tolerated in about a third of patients.[105,162] Conversion to sinus rhythm by pharmacological or electrical cardioversion should be attempted, although maintenance of sinus rhythm may be difficult.[105] Patients who develop atrial fibrillation ordinarily should be started on long-term therapy with oral anticoagulants.[104,162]

Progression of HCM to left ventricular dilation and dysfunction without a gradient (i.e., DCM) occurs in 5 to 10 percent of patients.[104,160] It appears to result, at least in part, from wall thinning and scar formation as a consequence of myocardial ischemia caused by small-vessel coronary artery disease and abnormal coronary vasodilator reserve (Fig. 59–12), although in some patients it appears to be genetically determined.[115,129] It is more likely to occur in patients with marked septal hypertrophy and generally is associated with a poor prognosis. The extent of left ventricular hypertrophy in adults usually remains stable over time, although a majority of children demonstrate increasing degrees of hypertrophy (often considerable) and adult patients (mainly women) appear to experience a very gradual degree of regression of hypertrophy over time (Fig. 59–13).[179] Whether this is the result of ventricular remodeling or an artifact related to the premature death of patients with more severe hypertrophy is unknown at present. In some children, the findings of HCM may develop despite a previous normal echocardiogram; this is not common in adults, but it may be seen in particular with

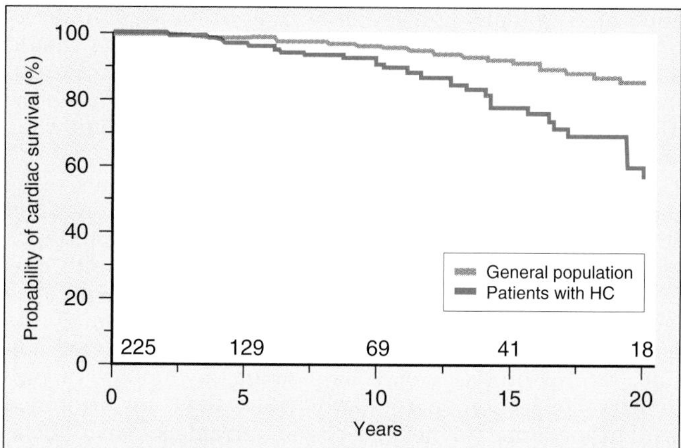

FIGURE 59–11 Kaplan-Meier survival curve of 225 community-based patients with hypertrophic cardiomyopathy (HC) and age-matched control subjects. The numbers above the horizontal axis refer to the number of patients at each follow-up period. The annual total mortality rate of the patients with HC was 1.3 percent. (From Kofflard MJ, Ten Cate FJ, van der Lee C, et al: Hypertrophic cardiomyopathy in a large community-based population: Clinical outcome and identification of risk factors for sudden cardiac death and clinical deterioration. J Am Coll Cardiol 41:987, 2003.)

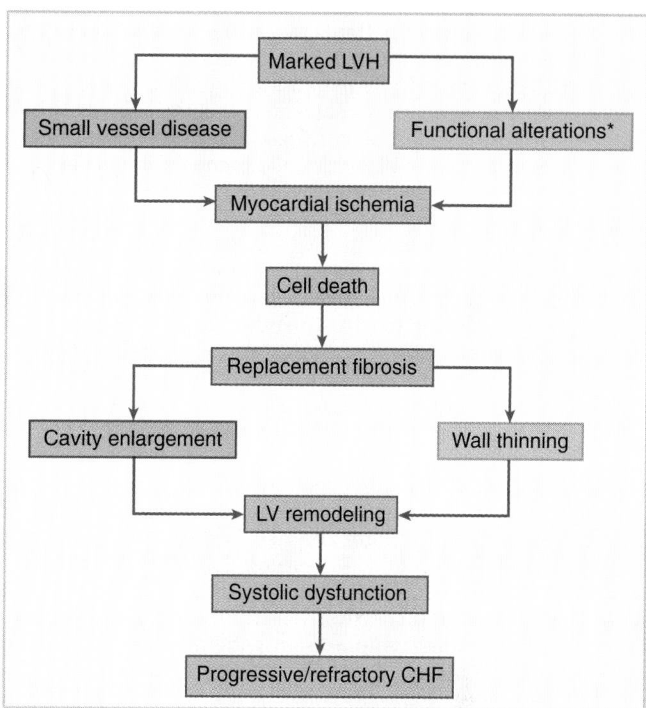

FIGURE 59–12 Hypothetical model for the pathogenesis of the end-stage phase of hypertrophic cardiomyopathy. Asterisk designates the following possibilities: (1) enhanced myocardial oxygen requirements and reduced myocardial capillary density relative to marked left ventricular (LV) hypertrophy (LVH) and (2) increased diastolic wall tension and coronary vascular resistance resulting from abnormal LV relaxation and impaired filling. CHF = congestive heart failure. (Modified from Maron BJ, Spirito P: Implications of left ventricular remodeling in hypertrophic cardiomyopathy. Am J Cardiol 81:1339-1344, 1998.)

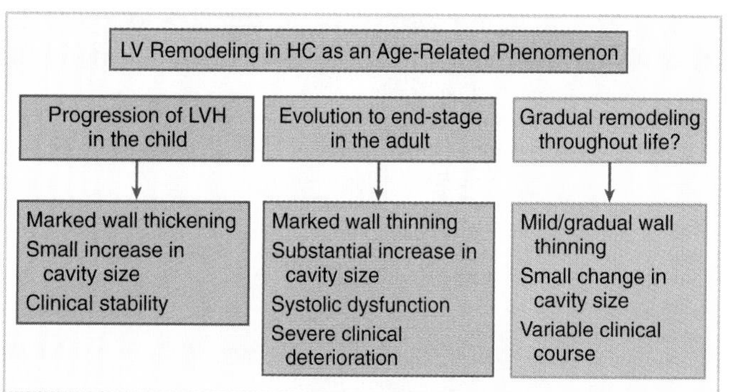

FIGURE 59–13 Patterns of left ventricular (LV) remodeling in the natural history of hypertrophic cardiomyopathy (HC). LVH = left ventricular hypertrophy. (From Maron BJ, Spirito P: Implications of left ventricular remodeling in hypertrophic cardiomyopathy. Am J Cardiol 81:1339-1344, 1998.)

the cardiac myosin-binding protein C mutation.[113] Its occurrence emphasizes that a single normal echocardiogram does *not* exclude HCM in a child or adolescent; cellular disarray and the attendant risk of sudden death may be present even in the absence of left ventricular hypertrophy. It furthermore suggests that apparently normal but at-risk postadolescent relatives of patients with HCM continue to be screened with periodic echocardiograms, perhaps at 5-year intervals.[104,160]

Many patients with HCM survive to old age, and about a quarter of all patients with diagnosed HCM are older than 75 years.[152] In such elderly HCM patients, outflow gradients are common (occurring in about 40 percent), but findings of advanced heart failure are relatively uncommon.[104]

SUDDEN DEATH. Death is most often sudden in HCM and may occur in previously asymptomatic patients, in individuals who were unaware they had the disease, and in patients with an otherwise stable course.[153,159] There is difficulty in identifying the patients at particular risk for sudden death.[180] Nevertheless, the features that most reliably identify the 10 to 20 percent of HCM patients at high risk include prior cardiac arrest or sustained ventricular tachycardia; multiple and repetitive episodes of nonsustained ventricular tachycardia[181]; young age (<30 years) at diagnosis (especially in those with extreme left ventricular hypertrophy and wall thicknesses greater than or equal to 30 mm on echocardiography); a family history of HCM with sudden death (so-called malignant family history); an abnormal blood pressure response to exercise especially in patients younger than 50 years (presumably related to subendocardial ischemia with attendant transient left ventricular systolic dysfunction)[182]; and genetic abnormalities associated with increased prevalence of sudden death (Table 59–7).[105,166,183] Prognosis correlates with the degree of hypertrophy, and patients with extreme hypertrophy (>30 mm) have almost a 40 percent risk of sudden death over a 20-year period.[165]

The presence (and severity) of an outflow tract gradient has modest predictive power for the risk of death (although not necessarily sudden), and a resting gradient on Doppler echocardiography of greater than 30 mm Hg is associated with about 1.6-fold increase in risk.[178] The degree of functional limitation and symptoms in general do not correlate with the risk of death, although syncope (especially in the young) does appear to be associated with an increased risk of sudden death.[177] It is presumed that sudden death in most patients is due to a ventricular arrhythmia, although atrial arrhythmias may play a role in sensitizing the heart so that ventricular arrhythmias appear subsequently. Bradyarrhythmias and disease of the atrioventricular conduction system may also play some role in sudden death.

TABLE 59–7 Factors Associated with an Adverse Outcome in Hypertrophic Cardiomyopathy

History of sudden cardiac death
Family history of premature death
"Malignant" causal mutations
"Malignant" modifier genes
History of syncope
Magnitude of LV hypertrophy
Extent of myocyte disarray
Extent of interstitial fibrosis
Early onset of disease
Myocardial ischemia on perfusion tomography
Abnormal blood pressure response to exercise
Nonsustained VT on Holter monitor
LV outflow tract obstruction

LV = left ventricular; VT = ventricular tachycardia.

Adapted from Marian AJ: On predictors of sudden cardiac death in hypertrophic cardiomyopathy. J Am Coll Cardiol 41:994, 2003.

Despite the difficulty in identifying patients at high risk for sudden death, the *absence* of a variety of characteristics (including the absence of severe symptoms, malignant family history, nonsustained ventricular tachycardia, marked hypertrophy, marked left atrial dilation, and abnormal blood pressure response to exercise) identifies a low-risk group that comprises more than half of all patients with HCM and requires little in the way of routine therapy.[105,166] Patients with mild hypertrophy, for example, with wall thicknesses less than 19 mm, experienced almost no sudden death mortality in one large study that spanned 20 years![165] Although avoidance of intense physical exertion is probably appropriate in this group, participation in recreational sports activities is not believed to be contraindicated.[105]

Children. The mechanism of death may be different in children with HCM because spontaneous ventricular arrhythmias and inducibility on electrophysiological testing are much less common than in adults.[154] Hemodynamic mechanisms may be involved, because younger patients are more likely to demonstrate abnormal changes in peripheral vascular resistance in response to exercise.[160,184]

Competitive Sports. Guidelines for participation in competitive sports have been developed; strenuous exertion should probably be proscribed in all patients with HCM whether or not symptoms are prominent, especially if high-risk clinical characteristics are present. Unsuspected HCM is the most common abnormality found at autopsy in young competitive athletes who die suddenly.[154] Cardiovascular screening before participation in competitive sports may identify asymptomatic patients with dormant HCM and appears to reduce the frequency of unexpected sudden death, although whether large-scale screening of athletes is administratively feasible or cost effective is not clear.[185]

Why some athletes with HCM die suddenly and others are able to continue to compete without limitation or death is not known. It has been speculated that the extent and severity of myocardial disarray may play an important role in determining prognosis, although this is not a finding that is ordinarily or easily obtainable in a living patient. Patients with marked hypertrophy are at increased risk.[159]

Pregnancy is usually well tolerated, although there is some increase in the relative risk of maternal mortality, especially in women known to be at increased risk.[186]

Management

Management of patients with HCM is directed toward alleviation of symptoms, prevention of complications, and reduction in the risk of death (Fig. 59–14). Most patients should undergo a risk assessment stratification that includes a full history and physical examination, two-dimensional echocardiography, 24- to 48-hour ambulatory (Holter) monitoring, and treadmill or bicycle exercise testing.[104]

Whether asymptomatic patients should receive drug therapy is not established because no adequate controlled studies are available.[105,109,187] Digitalis glycosides should generally be avoided unless atrial fibrillation or systolic dysfunction develops.[140] Diuretics were previously thought to be contraindicated to avoid precipitating or worsening the outflow gradient. More recent experience indicates that cautious use of diuretics may help reduce symptoms of pulmonary congestion, particularly when they are combined with beta-adrenergic blockers or calcium antagonists.[160] Beta-adrenergic agonists may improve diastolic filling but should not be used because they may produce ischemia and usually worsen the outflow gradient.[140] The majority of patients with HCM require only medical management, and at least half of all significantly symptomatic patients are improved with drug therapy.[107] Invasive interventions are needed in only 5 to 10 percent of patients and then only in patients with

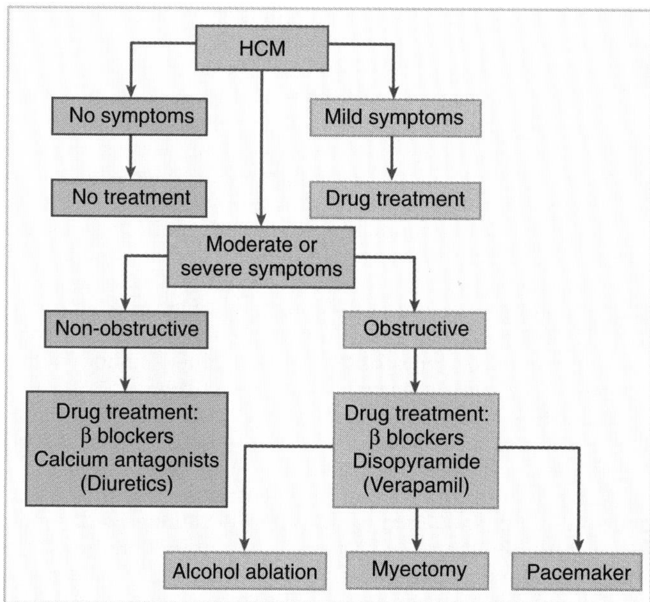

FIGURE 59–14 Clinical management algorithm for patients with hypertrophic cardiomyopathy (HCM). (From McKenna WJ, Behr ER: Hypertrophic cardiomyopathy: Management, risk stratification, and prevention of sudden death. Heart 87:169, 2002.)

outflow gradients who remain severely symptomatic despite optimal medical therapy.[105]

BETA ADRENOCEPTOR BLOCKERS. These drugs are the mainstay of medical therapy of HCM.[107,160] With their use, angina, dyspnea, and presyncope may all be improved. In patients with resting or provocable gradients, beta adrenoceptor blockade may prevent the increase in outflow obstruction that accompanies exertion, although resting gradients are largely unchanged.[105] The drugs reduce the determinants of myocardial oxygen consumption and thus angina pectoris and perhaps exert an antiarrhythmic action as well. Angina pectoris generally responds more favorably to treatment with a beta adrenoceptor blocker than does dyspnea. It has been suggested that beta adrenoceptor blockade may prevent sudden death and reduce mortality in HCM, and accordingly some use prophylactic beta adrenoceptor blockade therapy even in asymptomatic patients.[186] However, its efficacy for this purpose has not been established.[159] Beta adrenoceptor blockade also blunts the heart's chronotropic response, thus limiting the demand for increased myocardial oxygen delivery.[107] Beta adrenoceptor blockade was previously thought to have a beneficial effect on diastolic ventricular filling, but it now appears that any benefit is simply the consequence of a slower heart rate.[107] The overall clinical response to beta adrenoceptor blockade is variable, and only about one-third to two-thirds of patients experience symptomatic improvement. If beta adrenoceptor blockers are discontinued, they should probably be withdrawn slowly to avoid rebound adrenergic hypersensitivity.

CALCIUM ANTAGONISTS. These are an alternative to beta adrenoceptor blockade in the management of HCM; most of the experience has been with verapamil, with more limited use of nifedipine, diltiazem, and amlodipine.[104] No clear consensus exists as to whether therapy should be initiated first with a beta adrenoceptor blocker or a calcium antagonist, although verapamil is often effective in improving symptoms in patients who have not responded to beta adrenoceptor blockade. Exercise performance in particular may be improved when patients are changed from a beta adrenoceptor blocker to verapamil. Both the hypercontractile systolic function and the abnormalities of diastolic filling may be related to abnormal calcium kinetics,[145] and drugs that block the inward transport of calcium across the myocardial cell membrane may be able to rectify both abnormalities. Indeed, in an animal model of familial HCM, diltiazem prevented the development of the morphological features of HCM.[188]

Verapamil has been the most widely used calcium antagonist in this condition. Its use was suggested, at least in part, by the observation that it produces a protective and beneficial effect in the hereditary cardiomyopathy of the Syrian hamster, a condition marked by intracellular calcium overload in which propranolol is ineffective.[189] Although the vasodilator effects of verapamil should not be helpful in HCM, it appears that by depressing myocardial contractility, verapamil can decrease the left ventricular outflow gradient when given intravenously or orally. Perhaps more important from a symptomatic point of view, verapamil improves diastolic filling in HCM, at least in part by reducing asynchronous regional diastolic performance.[190] It also improves regional myocardial blood flow in some patients, which may contribute to the improvement in diastolic behavior.[191]

Although variable clinical responses have been reported with verapamil, about two-thirds or more of patients show increased exercise capacity and an improved symptomatic status. Sustained symptomatic improvement has been noted with the long-term administration of verapamil in ambulatory patients, although important adverse effects, including sudden death, have been observed in a small fraction of patients so treated.[105] Complications with verapamil include suppression of sinus node automaticity and inhibition of atrioventricular conduction, vasodilation, and negative inotropic effects.[160] These side effects may culminate in hypotension, pulmonary edema, and death; antiarrhythmic agents, especially quinidine, may exacerbate the deleterious hemodynamic effects of verapamil. Because of these adverse effects, it has been suggested that verapamil should not be used, or should be used only with extreme caution, in patients with high left ventricular filling pressure or symptoms of paroxysmal nocturnal dyspnea or orthopnea.[105] Unfortunately, these are usually the patients in greatest need of therapy.

The experience with other calcium channel blockers is limited. *Nifedipine* has been used in HCM, and it may have theoretical advantages over verapamil because it causes less depression of atrioventricular conduction. This may be counteracted by its more potent vasodilator action. Nifedipine may alleviate the chest pain in HCM patients. However, it should be recognized that the potent vasodilator effects of nifedipine may lead to systemic hypotension and an increase in the outflow gradient,[105] and in high doses it may depress left ventricular function. *Diltiazem* has also shown beneficial effects in HCM, producing improved diastolic function and reducing ischemia, although, like verapamil and nifedipine, it may cause an increase in the outflow gradient and a worrisome elevation of pulmonary capillary pressure.[192]

The combination of a beta adrenoceptor blocker and a calcium antagonist may be effective in patients who respond inadequately to monotherapy, although there are only anecdotal reports of the superiority of combination therapy.[105,107]

OTHER DRUGS. Disopyramide, an antiarrhythmic drug that alters calcium kinetics, has produced symptomatic improvement and a reduction or abolition of the pressure gradient in patients with HCM as a consequence of depression of left ventricular systolic performance and a reduction in ejection acceleration.[193] Particularly when combined with a beta-adrenergic blocker, it appears to be particularly efficacious in reducing outflow gradients.[140] However, long-term experience with disopyramide is limited, particularly in asymptomatic patients and those without outflow gradients, and the initial benefits appear to decrease with time.[105] Beta adrenoceptor blockers, calcium antagonists, and the conventional antiarrhythmic agents do not appear to suppress serious ventricular arrhythmias or reduce the frequency of supraventricular arrhythmias. However, amiodarone is effective in the treatment of both supraventricular[105] and ventricular tachyarrhythmias in HCM. Although there is some belief that amiodarone improves prognosis in HCM, only limited and inconclusive data are available.[105,106,159,194] Experience with sotalol is limited. We do *not* favor empirical use of amiodarone (or other antiarrhythmic agents for that matter) in unselected patients with HCM, and we worry about possible proarrhythmic effects and potential toxicity, including sudden death.

Atrial fibrillation should usually be pharmacologically or electrically converted because of the hemodynamic consequences of the loss of the atrial contribution to ventricular filling in this disorder. Amiodarone is thought to reduce the recurrence rate after successful cardioversion (based on limited data).[104] Anticoagulants should be given to patients with atrial fibrillation when no contraindication exists.[161] Infective endocarditis may occur in about 5 percent of patients but appears to be limited to those with an outflow gradient; accordingly, appropriate antibiotic prophylaxis is indicated in this group.[195] The infection usually occurs on the aortic valve or mitral apparatus, on the endocardium, or at the site of the contact lesion on the septum; thus, chronic endocardial trauma may provide a nidus for subsequent infection.

EXERCISE. Strenuous exercise should be avoided because of the risk of sudden death; almost half of deaths in HCM occur during or just after physical activity.[166] Even though many individuals with subclinical HCM exercise vigorously, the threat of sudden death is sufficiently real that competitive sports are proscribed in patients with marked hypertrophy or other factors believed to be associated with increased risk (see Table 59-7).

DDD PACING. Insertion of a dual-chamber DDD pacemaker may be useful in some patients with an outflow gradient and severe symptoms, especially elderly patients,[196,197] but it is likely that no more than 10 percent of HCM patients are candidates. Symptoms are generally improved, and the gradient appears to be reduced by an average of about 25 percent, although better symptomatic and hemodynamic results appear to follow surgery. Benefits have been described even after termination of pacing, suggesting a modification of myocardial properties. The long-term utility of pacing, however, is not known at present, and a substantial placebo effect has been demonstrated.[196,198–200] The benefit of pacing in patients without a resting outflow gradient is even more equivocal, and its use in this setting is generally not recommended at present.

ICD IMPLANTATION (see Chap. 31). In high-risk patients (especially the minority of HCM patients with sustained monomorphic ventricular tachycardia) or those with aborted sudden death, an ICD should be inserted,[201] although it may be less beneficial in HCM than in other conditions (such as coronary artery disease) with aborted sudden death.[202] Nevertheless, appropriate ICD discharges occurred in almost a quarter of the high-risk HCM patients in one large study and more than 40 percent of the subset of patients who had a device inserted for secondary prevention (i.e., after a prior cardiac arrest or spontaneous, sustained ventricular tachycardia), suggesting its efficacy in preventing sudden death.[159] However, there continues to be uncertainty about the characterization of what precisely constitutes high-risk status in consideration for ICD insertion; certainly, patients with a prior cardiac arrest or spontaneous sustained hemodynamically unstable ventricular tachycardia qualify.[201,202]

ALCOHOL SEPTAL ABLATION. A number of patients with resting or provocable outflow gradients have derived benefit (at least over the medium term) from intentional infarction of a portion of the interventricular septum by the infusion of alcohol into a selectively catheterized septal artery, with attendant reduction of the outflow gradient and mitral regurgitation, improvement in ventricular relaxation, regression of hypertrophy, and reduction in symptoms (Figs. 59–15 and 59–16).[107,203–207] Reported results of percutaneous septal reduction therapy vary from a somewhat inferior degree of gradient reduction when compared with surgical myotomy-myectomy to equivalent results, although exercise parameters may be better with surgery.[156,208,209] Both procedures improve diastolic ventricular filling.[210] It may take weeks to months for the full benefits of the procedure to become manifest.[211] Complications of the percutaneous technique include the frequent development of right bundle branch block, the precipitation of procedure-related complete heart block in half the patients, and the need for permanent pacing in about a quarter (although rates as low as 5 percent have been reported by one high-volume center).[211,212] The use of myocardial contrast echocardiography appears to improve the success rate of the procedure and reduce the need for permanent pacing after the procedure.[213] The mortality rate from the procedure in experienced centers is low (0 to 4 percent).[211,214,215]

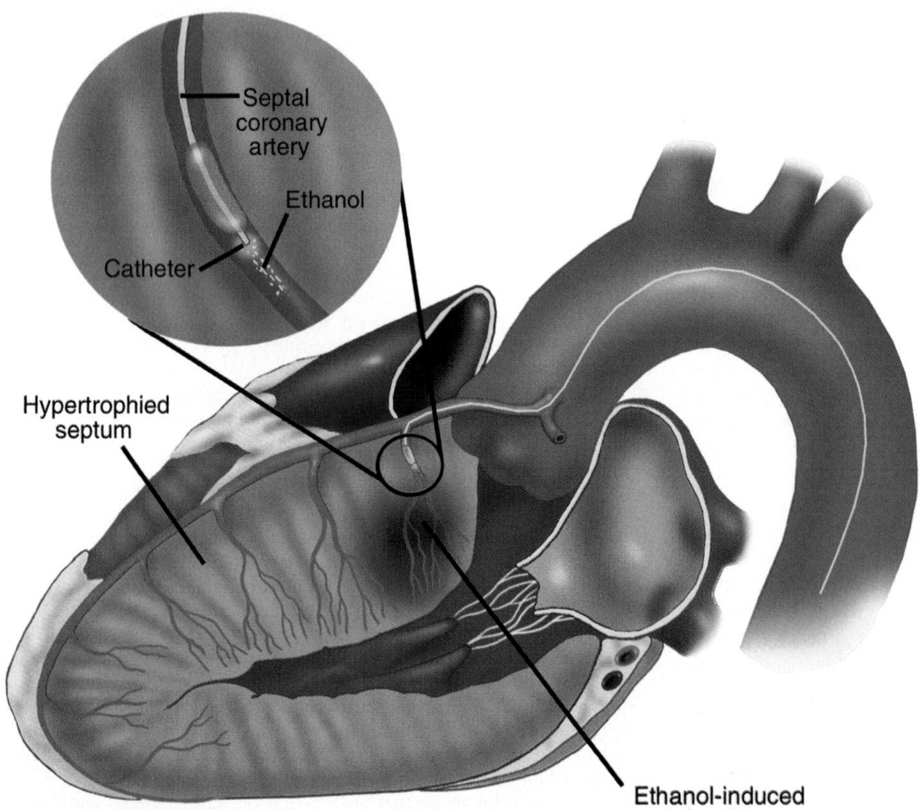

FIGURE 59–15 Drawing demonstrating technique of ethanol infusion into a septal artery in hypertrophic cardiomyopathy. The insert shows a balloon occluding the septal artery and the alcohol-induced septal infarction. (From Braunwald E: Hypertrophic cardiomyopathy—The benefits of a multidisciplinary approach. N Engl J Med 347:1306, 2002.)

SURGICAL TREATMENT. A number of surgical procedures aimed at reducing the outflow gradient have been developed. They are used most commonly in markedly symptomatic patients with gradients at rest greater than 50 mm Hg who have not responded well to medical management; such patients constitute less than 5 percent of all HCM patients.[104-106]

Myotomy-Myectomy. The most widely used operation for HCM consists of incising and resecting about 5 gm of the hypertrophied septum using a transaortic approach (the operation has been called the Morrow procedure, named after the cardiac surgeon who developed the technique).[106,216] Left transventricular as well as combined transaortic and left ventricular approaches have also been used successfully.

Operative management is facilitated by intraoperative echocardiography, and operative mortality at large centers is in the range of 2 to 3 percent or even less.[104,141,174,216] Surgery often relieves the obstruction (Fig. 59–17) as well as the mitral regurgitation.[155,211,216] Patients older than 65 as well as younger than 10 years have undergone successful operations; the operative risk is higher in older patients.[141]

Surgery results in long-term improvement in symptoms and exercise capacity in most (70 to 90 percent) patients.[104,107,211,216] Significant aortic regurgitation is an uncommon complication of the transaortic valve approach, although mild aortic regurgitation is not uncommon.[156] Myotomy-myectomy may be combined with other necessary operative procedures (particularly coronary artery bypass grafting), although the surgical risk is increased.[141] There has been enthusiasm for combining septal myotomy-myectomy with plication of the anterior leaflet of the mitral valve and reconstruction of the submitral valvular apparatus.[114,141]

Mitral Valve Replacement. Although performed less commonly than myotomy-myectomy, mitral valve replacement or repair (sometimes performed simultaneously with septal resection) has been used by some surgeons to treat HCM.[104] The rationale for this operation is that it abolishes obstruction by preventing systolic anterior motion of the mitral valve or corrects for intrinsic anatomical abnormalities of the mitral valve. It appears to be of particular value in patients with less than severe (<18 mm) hypertrophy of the upper septum or other atypical septal morphology, in those with previous myotomy-myectomy with persistent severe symptoms and obstruction, and in patients with intrinsic mitral valve disease (particularly the rare patients with HCM in whom the papillary muscles insert directly into the mitral valve leaflets).[114,141,155] In appropriate candidates not responding to maximal standard medical and surgical therapy, cardiac transplantation may be considered; this is usually required only for patients who have entered the dilated phase of HCM and have intractable symptoms of congestive heart failure.[217]

CHOICE OF THERAPY

Pharmacological therapy is the first line of treatment for symptomatic patients with HCM.[160,186] Beta adrenoceptor blockers, verapamil, and diltiazem are often used for patients without an outflow gradient (the so-called nonobstructive form), and beta adrenoceptor blockers and disopyramide are often preferred for those with a gradient.[140] A major challenge is the choice of subsequent therapy for patients who remain severely symptomatic despite maximal and optimal medical treatment, at least in part because of the paucity of studies comparing different treatment strategies.[191,195] For patients without an outflow gradient, the only established treatment option is medical because none of the interventional approaches (DDD pacing, septal ablation, or myotomy-myectomy) has an established role at this time.[195]

For severely symptomatic patients with an outflow gradient, there is no clear consensus about which intervention to choose when medical therapy has failed. Nevertheless, there are some general considerations that may be helpful in making this determination.

DDD PACING. Although the true benefit of pacing for symptom relief in HCM[196,197] is uncertain (see discussion earlier), it may be an appropriate addition to medical therapy in specific persistently symptomatic patients, including those with (1) an independent need for permanent pacing, such as those with symptomatic sinus node dysfunction or conducting system disease; (2) symptomatic or worrisome bradycardia that would otherwise preclude more aggressive treatment with pharmacological agents such as beta adrenoceptor blockers; (3) contraindications to surgery or septal ablation, including advanced age, comorbidities, or disinclination; or (4) lack of easy accessibility to a medical center skilled in septal ablation or surgery.

SEPTAL ABLATION[206]. Concern about two complications—one observed and the other theoretical—has tempered to some degree the enthusiasm for percutaneous septal ablation. A minority of patients develop heart block after the procedure and require permanent pacing. The theoretical concern is that the "therapeutic" myocardial infarction that results from the infusion of alcohol and is the mechanism of septal ablation creates myocardial scar tissue that may lead to subsequent malignant ventricular arrhythmias and sudden death. In view of these issues, septal ablation may be a preferred option for severely symptomatic patients with "obstructive" HCM if they (1) already have a pacemaker (or,

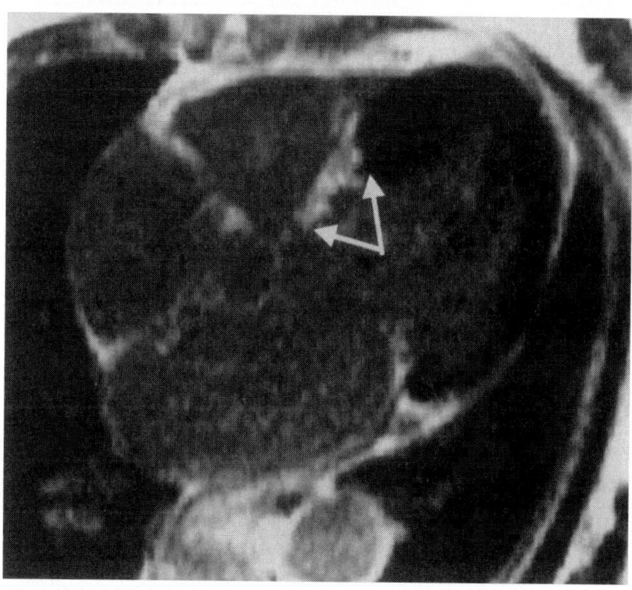

FIGURE 59–16 Magnetic resonance image after gadolinium-diethylenetriamine-pentaacetic acid contrast that demonstrates hyperenhancement (arrows) of the area of the interventricular septum that had undergone previous ablation by transcatheter alcohol infusion. (From Sievers B, Moon JC, Pennell DJ: Images in cardiovascular medicine. Magnetic resonance contrast enhancement of iatrogenic septal myocardial infarction in hypertrophic cardiomyopathy. Circulation 105:1018, 2002. Copyright 2002, American Heart Association.)

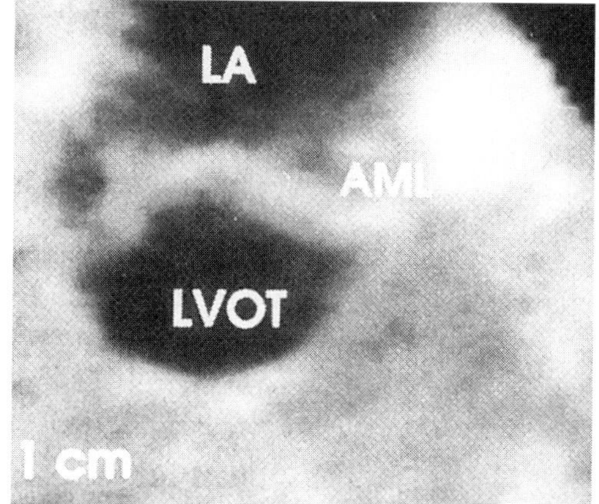

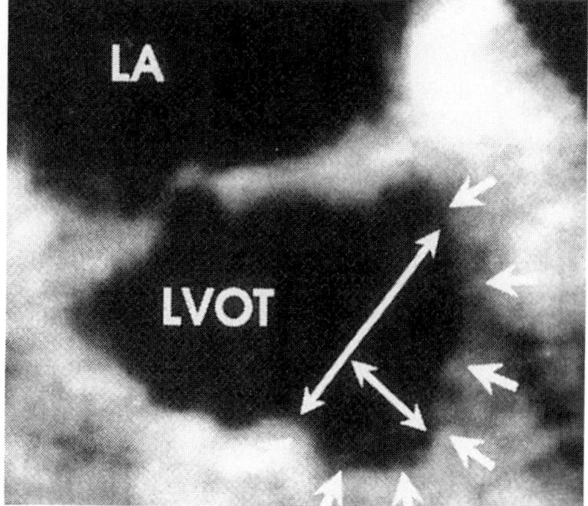

FIGURE 59–17 Three-dimensional transesophageal echocardiographic images before **(left)** and after **(right)** surgical myectomy of the left ventricular outflow tract (LVOT) in a patient with hypertrophic cardiomyopathy. The maximal width and depth of the myectomy trough are marked by large arrows. Small arrows indicate limits of myectomy trough. LA = left atrium. (From Franke A, Schondube FA, Kuhl HP, et al: Quantitative assessment of the operative results after extended myectomy and surgical reconstruction of the subvalvular mitral apparatus in hypertrophic obstructive cardiomyopathy using dynamic three-dimensional transesophageal echocardiography. J Am Coll Cardiol 31:1641, 1998.)

even better, an ICD) in place or (2) have concomitant medical conditions, advanced age, prior sternotomy, or other relative contraindications to surgery. As more favorable experience is gained with this procedure, it is being used increasingly in place of surgery in centers with skilled operators.

SURGERY. Although only a minority of patients require surgery for drug-refractory HCM,[191] it is the time-honored approach, with a 40-year experience that has demonstrated its efficacy and relative safety. It remains the "gold standard" for treating persistently symptomatic patients.[104] For these reasons, it should probably be the preferred option in younger patients, where the relatively short period of follow-up of septal ablation (3 to 5 years[331]) raises some concerns regarding long-term results. It should also be employed in failures of septal ablation.

Restrictive and Infiltrative Cardiomyopathies

Of the three major functional categories of the cardiomyopathies (dilated, hypertrophic, and restrictive), RCM is the least common form in Western countries, although nonidiopathic forms of RCM such as endomyocardial disease (Table 59–8) are common in specific geographical regions of the world.[3,218] The hallmark of the RCMs is abnormal diastolic function; the ventricular walls are excessively rigid and impede ventricular filling. Systolic function, on the other hand, is often unimpaired, even in many cases with extensive infiltration of the myocardium.[218,219] Thus, RCM bears some functional resemblance to constrictive pericarditis, which is also characterized by normal or nearly normal systolic function but abnormal ventricular filling (see Chap. 64).[218] Differentiation of the two conditions is mandatory because of the potential for successful surgical treatment of constriction.[3]

A variety of specific pathological processes may result in RCM, although the cause often remains unknown. Myocardial fibrosis (Fig. 59–18), infiltration, or endomyocardial scarring is usually responsible for the abnormal diastolic behavior; in the idiopathic variety there is often histological evidence of myocyte hypertrophy.[218,220] Myocardial involvement with amyloid (often in the setting of multiple myeloma) is a common cause of RCM, although it can be caused by a variety of other conditions (see Table 59–8). An occasional patient with a plasma cell dyscrasia may present with RCM related not to the deposition of amyloid fibrils into the myocardium but rather that of light chains.[221] Some patients may manifest the clinical features of an RCM and yet exhibit the pathological findings of left ventricular hypertrophy and fibrosis[3]; certainly, ventricular hypertrophy, especially HCM, can cause diminished ventricular compliance, but not RCM per se. RCM on occasion is inherited and has been found in association with mutations of the gene encoding troponin I (see Table 59–4); in some cases there may be an associated skeletal muscle disease.[218,222]

TABLE 59–8 Classification of Types of Restrictive Cardiomyopathy According to Cause

Myocardial
Noninfiltrative
Idiopathic cardiomyopathy*
Familial cardiomyopathy
Hypertrophic cardiomyopathy
Scleroderma
Pseudoxanthoma elasticum
Diabetic cardiomyopathy
Infiltrative
Amyloidosis*
Sarcoidosis*
Gaucher disease
Hurler disease
Fatty infiltration
Storage Disease
Hemochromatosis
Fabry disease
Glycogen storage disease
Endomyocardial
Endomyocardial fibrosis*
Hypereosinophilic syndrome
Carcinoid heart disease
Metastatic cancers
Radiation*
Toxic effects of anthracycline*
Drugs causing fibrous endocarditis (serotonin, methysergide, ergotamine, mercurial agents, busulfan)

From Kushwaha S, Fallon JT, Fuster V: Restrictive cardiomyopathy. N Engl J Med 336:267, 1997. Copyright 1997, Massachusetts Medical Society.

*These conditions are more likely than the others to be encountered in clinical practice.

HEMODYNAMICS. The clinical and hemodynamic features of restrictive heart disease simulate those of chronic constrictive pericarditis; endomyocardial biopsy, CT, and radionuclide angiography may be particularly useful in differentiating the two diseases by demonstrating myocardial scarring or infiltration (on biopsy) or thickening of the pericardium (on CT and MRI).[3] With the use of these modalities, exploratory thoracotomy should rarely be required; nevertheless, if the differentiation between constriction and RCM cannot be established with certainty, surgical exploration is in order.[218,223] The characteristic hemodynamic feature in both conditions is a deep and rapid early decline in ventricular pressure at the onset of diastole, with a rapid rise to a plateau in early diastole (although this finding is absent in some patients with RCM).[218] This dip and plateau has been termed the *square root sign* and is manifested in the atrial pressure tracing as a prominent *y* descent followed by a rapid rise and plateau. The *x* descent may also be rapid, and the combination results in the characteristic M or W waveform in the atrial pressure tracing.[218] The a wave is prominent and often of the same amplitude as the v wave. Both systemic and pulmonary venous pressures are elevated, although patients with restrictive heart disease typically have left ventricular filling pressures that exceed right ventricular filling pressure by more than 5 mm Hg; this difference is accentuated by exercise, fluid challenge, and Valsalva maneuver (although not all patients demonstrate this finding).[218]

In this respect, they differ from patients with constrictive pericarditis, in whom diastolic pressures are similar in both ventricles, usually differing by no more than 5 mm Hg. The pulmonary artery systolic pressure is often greater than 50 mm Hg in patients with RCM but is lower in constrictive pericarditis.[218] Furthermore, the plateau of the right ventricular diastolic pressure is usually at least one-third of the peak right ventricular systolic pressure in patients with constrictive pericarditis, whereas it is frequently lower in RCM.[218]

CLINICAL MANIFESTATIONS. Exercise intolerance is frequent because of the inability of patients with RCM to increase their cardiac output by tachycardia without further compromising ventricular filling. Weakness and dyspnea are often prominent. Exertional chest pain may be prominent in some patients but is usually absent. Particularly in advanced cases, the central venous pressure is elevated, with attendant peripheral edema, enlarged liver, ascites, and anasarca. *Physical examination* may reveal jugular venous distention and an S_3, S_4, or both. An inspiratory increase in venous pressure may be seen (Kussmaul sign). However, in contrast to

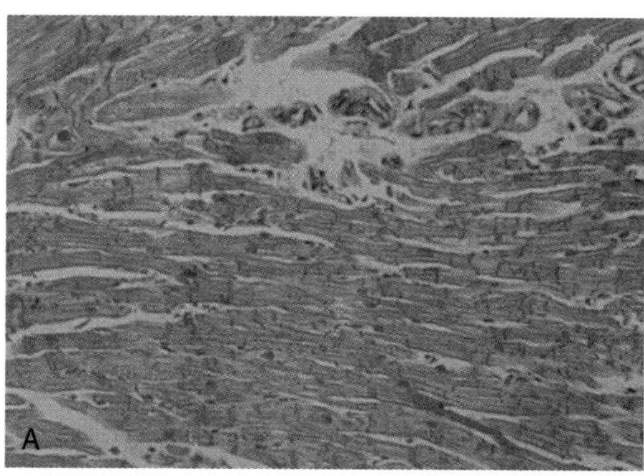

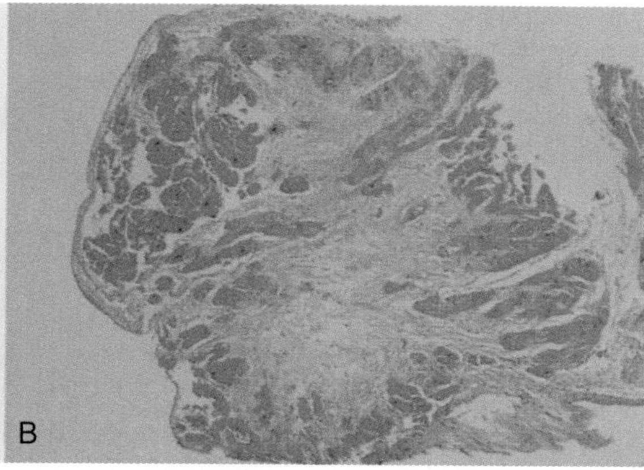

FIGURE 59–18 Endomyocardial biopsy specimens from patients with idiopathic restrictive cardiomyopathy. **A,** This histological specimen (hematoxylin and eosin, ×250) shows myocytes with slight hypertrophy but is otherwise normal. **B,** Another specimen (hematoxylin and eosin, ×40), from another patient, shows marked interstitial fibrosis, which may also occur in idiopathic restrictive cardiomyopathy. (From Kushwaha SS, Fallon JT, Fuster V: Restrictive cardiomyopathy. N Engl J Med 336:267, 1997. Copyright 1997, Massachusetts Medical Society.)

constrictive pericarditis, the apex impulse is usually palpable in RCM.[218]

LABORATORY STUDIES. The *electrocardiogram* often shows atrial fibrillation.[219] Various ancillary laboratory findings in addition to endomyocardial biopsy, CT, and MRI (see Chaps. 14 and 15) may be useful in distinguishing between constrictive and restrictive disease. Although pericardial calcification that is visible on the chest radiograph is neither absolutely sensitive nor specific for constrictive pericarditis (see Chap. 64), its presence in a patient in whom the differential diagnosis rests between RCM and constrictive pericarditis lends strong support to the latter diagnosis. The *echocardiogram* may demonstrate thickening of the left ventricular wall and an increase of left ventricular mass in patients with infiltrative disease causing RCM. The atria are almost always dilated.[219] The pattern of filling of the left ventricle differs in the two conditions, as can be demonstrated by transthoracic and transesophageal Doppler ultrasonography supplemented by tissue Doppler measurements.[218,223,224] Patients with RCM have an increased early left ventricular filling velocity, decreased atrial filling velocity, and decreased isovolumetric relaxation time.[218]

The prognosis in RCM is variable; usually it is one of relentless symptomatic progression and high mortality.[219,225] No specific therapy (other than symptomatic) is available for the idiopathic form of RCM, but several of the secondary forms may benefit from targeted treatment regimens (e.g., the cardiomyopathy related to iron overload, which is improved by removal of the iron, and Fabry disease, in which enzyme replacement therapy has demonstrated efficacy).[226,227]

Amyloidosis

ETIOLOGY AND TYPES. Amyloidosis is a disease complex that results from deposition of unique twisted beta-pleated sheet fibrils formed from various proteins by several different pathogenic mechanisms. Amyloid may be found in almost any organ, but clinically evident disease does not appear unless infiltration is extensive. Several classification systems have been used to characterize the different clinical presentations of amyloidosis. The condition with the traditional designation of *primary amyloidosis* is now known to be caused by the production of an amyloid protein composed of portions of immunoglobulin light chain (designated *AL*) by a monoclonal population of plasma cells, often as a consequence of multiple myeloma.[228] Secondary amyloidosis (also known as reactive systemic) is due to the production of a nonimmunoglobulin protein termed *AA*.

Familial Amyloidosis. This condition, inherited as an autosomal dominant trait, results from the production of a variant prealbumin serum carrier protein termed *transthyretin*; more than 80 different point mutations have been described so far.[228] It generally occurs in one of three clinical presentations: progressive neuropathy, cardiomyopathy, or nephropathy.[229] The cardiomyopathic variant typically has involvement limited to the heart and is four times more common in blacks than in whites because of a genetic variant that is found in 4 percent of the black population.[230]

Senile Systemic Amyloidosis. This form of amyloid is due to the production of either an atrial natriuretic-like protein or transthyretin and is becoming increasingly common as the average age of the population increases. Scattered deposits of amyloid localized to the aorta or atria are virtually ubiquitous in individuals older than 80 and may predispose to the development of atrial fibrillation.[231] Small deposits of amyloid may often be found in the pulmonary vessels or the vessels of other organs as well.

Cardiac Amyloidosis

Involvement of the heart is a common finding and is the most frequent cause of death in amyloidosis associated with an immunocyte dyscrasia.[232] Clinically apparent heart disease is present in one-third of patients,[233] although the heart is virtually always involved when studied pathologically.[234] In secondary amyloidosis, on the other hand, clinically significant cardiac involvement is uncommon; the myocardial deposits are typically small and perivascular and usually do not result in significant myocardial dysfunction.[235] Familial amyloidosis is associated with overt cardiac involvement in about one-fourth of the afflicted patients, usually late in the course of the disease, and often dominated by conducting system disease.[236] The clinical course is usually dominated by neurological or renal dysfunction, although death is due to heart failure or arrhythmia about half the time. Cardiac involvement in senile amyloidosis varies from small atrial deposits that do not result in functional impairment to extensive ventricular involvement with resultant cardiac failure.[231]

Cardiac amyloidosis occurs more commonly in men than in women, and it is rare before the age of 40 years. Even in the familial form, the onset of clinical cardiac disease usually does not occur before the age of 35 years and generally occurs much later in life.

PATHOLOGY. The pathological findings often include mild atrial enlargement, usually without significant ventricular dilation. The walls of both ventricles are typically firm, rubbery, noncompliant, and thickened. Amyloid is present between the myocardial fibers, often with extensive deposition in the papillary muscles. Endocardial involvement of the atria and ventricles is frequent, and disease limited to the atria may be seen.[231] Amyloidosis often results in focal thickening of or deposits on the cardiac valves, but these abnormalities do not appear to interfere with valvular function other than to produce murmurs. The intramural coronary arteries and veins frequently contain amyloid deposits in the media and adventitia, occasionally compromising the lumina of the vessels and reducing coronary flow reserve.[231,237]

CLINICAL MANIFESTATIONS. Involvement of the cardiovascular system by amyloidosis occurs in four general forms that may overlap:

1. The most common presentation of cardiac amyloidosis is that of RCM.[217] The restrictive physiology results not only from the physical presence of amyloid infiltrates in the myocardium but also from direct depression of diastolic function by circulating immunoglobulin light chains.[238] Right-sided findings dominate the clinical presentation; peripheral edema is a prominent finding, whereas paroxysmal nocturnal dyspnea and orthopnea are absent. Myopathic involvement produces the characteristic diastolic dip and plateau (square root sign) in the ventricular pressure pulse that may simulate constrictive pericarditis. In contrast to the accelerated early left ventricular diastolic filling found in constrictive pericarditis, cardiac amyloidosis is marked by an impaired rate of early diastolic filling.
2. A second common presentation is congestive heart failure related to systolic dysfunction, which is usually a late finding in cardiac amyloidosis.[239] Hemodynamic evidence of restriction of ventricular filling may not be prominent in these patients. In some patients amyloid deposition in the atria may be responsible for loss of atrial transport function despite the maintenance of electrical "sinus" rhythm, with the production of congestive heart failure. The course of this form of the disease is often one of relentless progression, usually poorly responsive to treatment. Angina pectoris occurs on occasion despite angiographically normal coronary arteries.
3. Orthostatic hypotension occurs in about 10 percent of cases. Although it is most likely due to amyloid infiltration of the autonomic nervous system or blood vessels, or both, amyloid deposition in the heart and adrenals may contribute to the pathogenesis of this variant.[240] Hypovolemia as a result of the nephrotic syndrome secondary to renal amyloidosis may worsen the postural hypotension. Frank syncope is common in amyloidosis, is often multifactorial in etiology, and is associated with emotional or physical stress.[241] When exertional, it is a dire prognostic sign, and most patients die within 3 months.[239]
4. An abnormality of cardiac impulse formation and conduction is the fourth and least common mode of presentation and may result in arrhythmias and conduction disturbances.[242] Sudden death, presumably arrhythmic in origin, is relatively common and may be preceded by episodes of syncope.[241,243]

PHYSICAL EXAMINATION. This often reveals congestive heart failure, especially right sided; a systolic murmur caused by atrioventricular valvular regurgitation may be present. Jugular venous distention, a protodiastolic gallop, hepatomegaly, peripheral edema, and a narrow pulse pressure are found in patients presenting with RCM. An S_4 is uncommon, presumably because of amyloid infiltration of the atrium with attendant reduced systolic function of the atrial myocardium.[244] Patients are typically normotensive or hypotensive; even previously hypertensive individuals usually have a fall in blood pressure as the disease progresses.

NONINVASIVE TESTING. The *chest roentgenogram* usually shows cardiomegaly in patients with systolic dysfunction, although heart size may be normal in patients with the restrictive form.[239] Pulmonary congestion may be prominent in patients with congestive heart failure. The *electrocardiogram* is often abnormal; the most characteristic feature is diffusely diminished voltage. Bundle branch block and abnormal axis deviation are common, although some patients have significant conducting system disease despite a normal QRS on ECG study.[237,242] Myocardial infarction is often simulated because of small or absent R waves in right precordial leads or, less frequently, by Q waves in the inferior leads.[239] Arrhythmias, particularly atrial fibrillation, are common and may be related to amyloid infiltration of the atrium.[231] Complex ventricular arrhythmias are found frequently in patients with cardiac amyloidosis and may be a harbinger of sudden death. The *signal-averaged electrocardiogram* can help to identify patients at increased risk for sudden death.[243] Various forms of atrioventricular conduction defects are often seen and may be associated with increased mortality, although significant infrahisian block may be apparent only on *electrophysiological testing*.[242] Abnormalities of atrioventricular conduction appear to be particularly common in familial amyloidosis with polyneuropathy. Sinus node involvement is common, and the clinical and ECG features of the sick sinus syndrome may be present (see Chap. 29).

Echocardiography (see Chap. 11). In advanced cases this most commonly reveals increased thickness of the walls of the ventricles, small ventricular chambers, dilated atria, and thickening of the interatrial septum (Fig. 59–19). Left ventricular dysfunction may be seen, especially in advanced cases, but systolic function is often surprisingly normal.[237,244] Early, unsuspected cardiac involvement may be detectable only by echocardiography or Doppler ultrasonography, although in some cases echocardiography may be falsely normal. Although the cardiac valves may be thickened, they usually move normally.[234] A pericardial effusion is common but rarely results in tamponade.[244] The appearance of the thickened cardiac walls is often distinctive on two-dimensional echocardiography, demonstrating a granular sparkling texture, presumably related to the amyloid deposit.[234,244] In some cases the pattern of increased wall thickness is nonuniform and may resemble HCM. Echocardiographic demonstration of thick left ventricular walls with concomitant low voltage on the electrocardiogram appears to distinguish cardiac amyloidosis from pericardial disease or left ventricular hypertrophy, and this distinctive voltage/mass ratio is characteristic of myocardial infiltration by amyloid (especially AL amyloid).[236] Doppler ultrasonography and radionuclide ventriculography routinely demonstrate abnormalities of diastolic function and, by estimating the degree of cardiac involvement by amyloid, provide prognostic information.[234,244]

Imaging. *Scintigraphy* with technetium-99m pyrophosphate and other agents that bind to calcium is often strongly positive with prominent amyloid involvement (Fig. 59–20), although in some patients it is falsely negative.[245] Positive scans tend to correlate with extensive cardiac involvement. Scanning with indium-labeled antimyosin antibody may also detect cardiac amyloid involvement, as may MRI.[171,246] Scanning with specialized agents has shown sympathetic denervation in patients with cardiac amyloidosis.[245]

DIAGNOSIS. Whereas two or three decades ago the clinical diagnosis of systemic amyloidosis was made correctly ante mortem in only about one-fourth of cases, with more recent clinical awareness of the disease and the utilization of *biopsy techniques* the diagnosis is now made before death in the majority of patients. An abdominal fat aspirate has been the single most useful diagnostic procedure, combining the attributes of ease of performance, sensitivity, and safety.[232,247]

Biopsy of rectum, gingiva, bone marrow, liver, kidney, and various other tissues has also been used. Endomyocardial biopsy of the right or left ventricles may be helpful in establishing the diagnosis of cardiac amyloidosis (Fig. 59–21) if the abdominal fat aspirate is negative.[232] Immunohistochemical staining of tissue samples is important to distinguish systemic senile, familial, and primary forms of amyloidosis in otherwise equivocal presentations because prognosis and management differ in the various forms[232]; unsuspected hereditary amyloidosis is found in almost 10 percent of patients thought to have the primary (AL) form.[228]

MANAGEMENT. The treatment of cardiac amyloidosis is generally unsatisfactory, although there has been some improvement in survival and functional state with the use of alkylating agents in primary (AL) amyloidosis.[248] However, the median survival is less than a year, and it is the rare patient (<5 percent) who survives for more than 5 years.[249,250] Digitalis glycosides should be used with caution because patients with cardiac amyloidosis appear to be sensitive to digitalis preparations.[251] Nevertheless, the glycosides have been used with success to control the ventricular rate in atrial fibrillation.[239] The calcium antagonists are also said to be problematic in cardiac amyloidosis and may lead to exacerbation of congestive heart failure symptoms because of an enhanced negative inotropic effect. Insertion of a permanent pacemaker may be beneficial in the short term in patients with symptomatic conducting system disease.[252] Careful use of low doses of diuretics and vasodilators may afford some symptomatic benefit, but there is a risk of hypotension and hypoperfusion with use of these agents.[218,233,239] In patients with atrial standstill related to amyloid infiltration, anticoagulation may be appropriate even in the absence of atrial arrhythmias because there is some risk of thrombus formation, presumably as a consequence of stasis in the atrium. The rare patient with a plasma cell dyscrasia and RCM caused by light-chain deposition may improve with chemotherapy.[221]

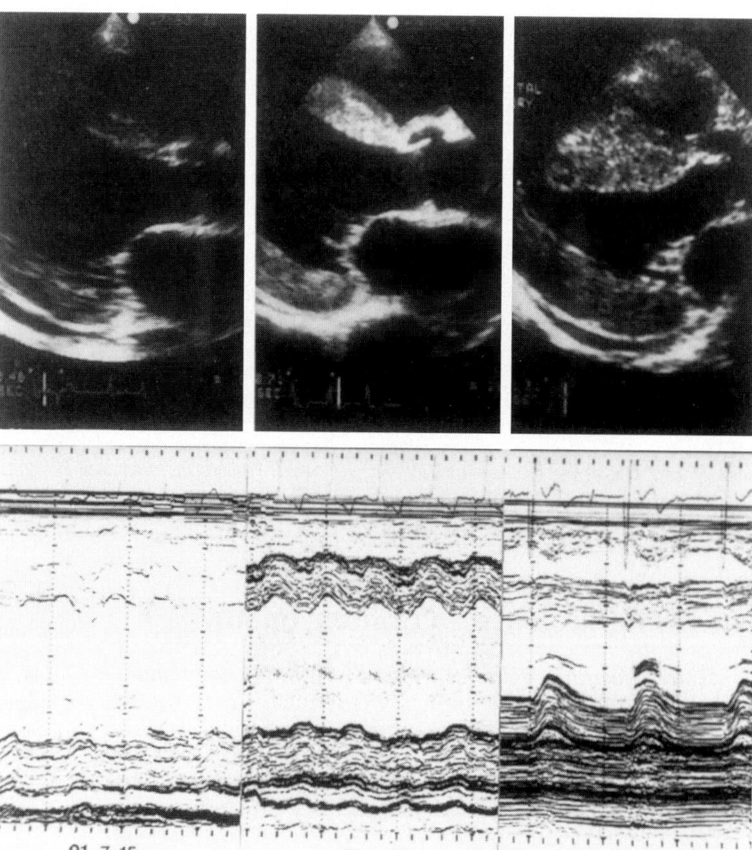

FIGURE 59–19 Serial echocardiographic findings in a patient developing cardiac amyloidosis. **Top,** Serial two-dimensional echocardiographic findings. Note the thickening of all myocardial walls and valves. **Bottom,** Serial M-mode echocardiography shows gradual increase of interventricular septal, left ventricular posterior wall, and right ventricular wall thickness. The date of the study is shown at the bottom (year.month.day). (From Youn H, Chae JS, Lee KY, et al: Images in cardiovascular medicine: Amyloidosis with cardiac involvement. Circulation 97:2093, 1998. Copyright 1998, American Heart Association.)

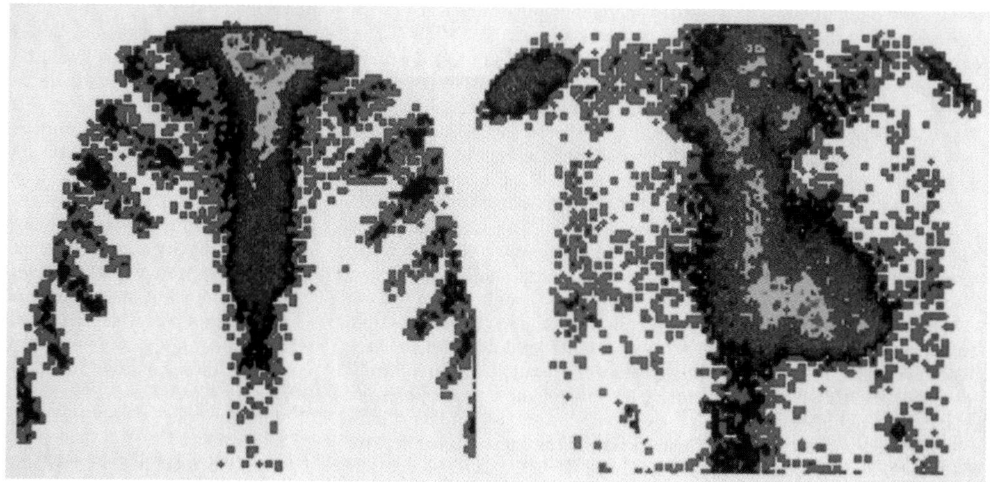

FIGURE 59–20 Nuclear scan using ^{99}Tc-methylene diphosphonate that binds to the calcium-binding site of amyloid. **Left,** Control patient, with normal uptake in bones. **Right,** Patient with familial amyloidosis, showing striking uptake by cardiac involvement. (From Singer R, Schnabel A, Strasser RH: Restrictive cardiomyopathy in familial amyloidosis TTR-Arg-50. Circulation 107:643, 2003. Copyright 2003, American Heart Association.)

Autologous bone marrow stem cell transplantation is being used with increasing frequency in primary (AL) amyloidosis, but patients with advanced cardiac amyloidosis or multiorgan involvement do not appear to reap much benefit.[253] However, selected patients (especially those with early and mild cardiac involvement) may derive some benefit from stem cell transplantation. A small number of patients have undergone cardiac transplantation, with poor long-term results (39 percent survival at 4 years in one study and 30 percent at 5 years in another) because of progressive amyloidosis in other organs or recurrence in the transplanted heart, although a few carefully selected patients have shown long-term survival and functional improvement.[218,254] No therapy is effective for the senile form, but survival is about 10 times longer than in the primary form (60 versus 6 months for patients with congestive heart failure).[244,249]

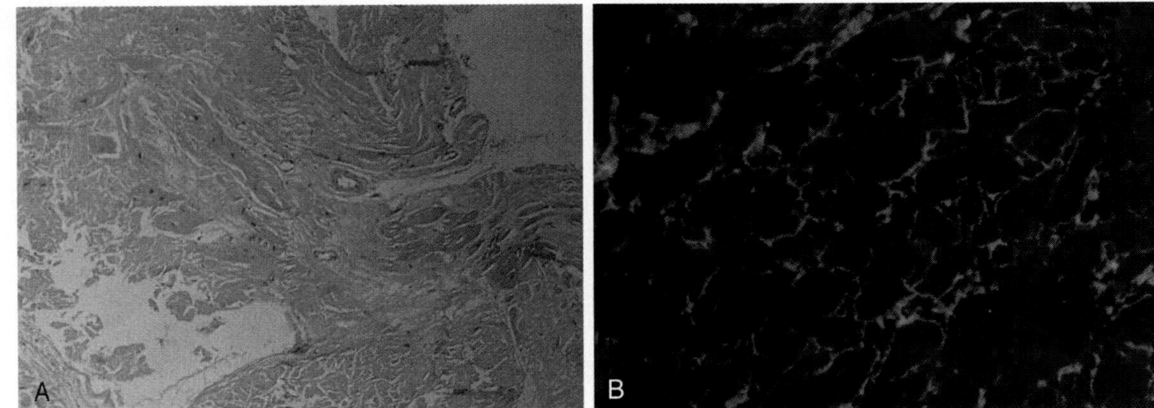

FIGURE 59–21 Endomyocardial biopsy specimens from patients with cardiac amyloidosis. **A,** This histological section (hematoxylin and eosin, ×250) shows interstitial deposition of amyloid fibrils in a specimen from the right ventricle. **B,** Immunofluorescent stain (×400) shows lambda light chains. (From Kushwaha SS, Fallon JT, Fuster V: Restrictive cardiomyopathy. N Engl J Med 336:267, 1997. Copyright 1997, Massachusetts Medical Society.)

Inherited Infiltrative Disorders Causing Restrictive Cardiomyopathy

The intramyocardial accumulation or infiltration of an abnormal metabolic product typically produces a restrictive picture with impaired diastolic ventricular filling. Systolic impairment may be seen as well but is not invariably found. A variety of infiltrative diseases, often inherited, may result in this hemodynamic picture, including the glycogenoses, the mucopolysaccharidoses, Fabry disease, and Gaucher disease.

FABRY DISEASE

This condition, also known as angiokeratoma corporis diffusum universale, is an X-linked recessive disorder of glycosphingolipid metabolism resulting from a deficiency of the lysosomal enzyme alpha-galactosidase A that is caused by one of more than 160 mutations.[227,255,256] Some mutations result in no detectable alpha-galactosidase A activity and widespread manifestations throughout the body, whereas others produce some degree of enzyme activity with attendant atypical variants of Fabry disease with involvement limited solely to the myocardium.[227,255,257] The disease is characterized by an intracellular accumulation of glycosphingolipids (especially globotriaosylceramide) with prominent involvement of the skin and kidneys as well as the myocardium in the classical form. *Histological examination* often reveals widespread involvement of the myocardium, vascular endothelium, conducting tissues, and valves, particularly the mitral valve (Fig. 59–22). The major clinical manifestations result from the accumulation of the glycolipid substrate in endothelial cells, with eventual occlusion of small arterioles.[227] The accumulation of the glycolipid occurs in the lysosomes of the cardiac tissues and is responsible for the multiple cardiovascular manifestations of Fabry disease.

CARDIAC FINDINGS. These typically include angina pectoris and myocardial infarction caused by accumulation of lipid moieties in coronary endothelial cells, but coronary arteries are usually angiographically normal. There is increased left ventricular wall thickness producing diastolic dysfunction that is usually mild, generally preserved left ventricular systolic function, and clinically unimportant mitral regurgitation.[258] Preclinical cardiac involvement (i.e., before the development of increased wall thickness) may be suggested by abnormal myocardial tissue Doppler measurements of myocardial contraction and relaxation.[259] Symptomatic cardiovascular involvement occurs eventually in most affected males, whereas female carriers are usually asymptomatic or only minimally symptomatic.[255] Systemic hypertension, mitral valve prolapse, and congestive heart failure are common clinical manifestations. ECG abnormalities may include a short PR interval, atrioventricular block, ST segment and T wave abnormalities, left ventricular hypertrophy, and QRS prolongation.[255,260] The echocardiogram usually reveals increased left ventricular wall thickness as a result of glycolipid deposition, which may simulate HCM.[256] Differentiation from other hypertrophic or restrictive processes (such as cardiac amyloidosis) may not be possible on echocardiographic grounds but may be possible with MRI (Fig. 59–23). Endomyocardial biopsy may be of considerable value in making a definitive diagnosis, as is low plasma alpha-galactosidase A activity.[260] Differentiation from HCM is important because enzyme replacement therapy for Fabry disease is safe and effective.[261] It reduces the accumulated stores of globotriaosylceramide from the heart and other tissues and produces symptomatic, clinical, and echocardiographic improvement (Fig. 59–24).[227]

GAUCHER DISEASE

Gaucher disease is an uncommon inherited disorder of glycosyl ceramide metabolism. It is secondary to a deficiency of the enzyme beta-glucosidase and results in accumulation of cerebrosides in the spleen, liver, bone marrow, lymph nodes, brain, and myocardium. Diffuse interstitial infiltration of the left ventricle by cells laden with cerebroside produces reduced left ventricular compliance and cardiac output. Clinical evidence of cardiac involvement is uncommon but when present it is characterized by left ventricular dysfunction, hemorrhagic pericardial effusion, increased left ventricular wall mass, and thickening and calcification of the left-sided valves.[262,263] Enzyme replacement therapy and liver transplantation may produce a reduction in tissue infiltration by cerebrosides with attendant clinical improvement.[262,264]

HEMOCHROMATOSIS

Hemochromatosis is characterized by excessive deposition of iron in a variety of parenchymal tissues (heart, liver, gonads, and pancreas). It may occur (1) as a familial (autosomal recessive) or idiopathic disorder, (2) in association with a defect in hemoglobin synthesis resulting in ineffective erythropoiesis, (3) in chronic liver disease, and (4) with excessive oral or parenteral intake of iron (or blood transfusions) over many years.[226] Although patients who have iron deposits in the myocardium almost always have deposits in other organs (e.g., liver, spleen, pancreas, bone marrow), the severity of myocardial involvement varies widely and only roughly parallels that in other organs. Cardiac involvement leads to a mixed DCM-RCM pattern with both systolic and diastolic dysfunction, often with associated arrhythmias.[265,266] Myocardial damage is thought to be due to direct tissue toxicity of the free iron moiety rather than simply to tissue infiltration.[267] Although cirrhosis and hepatocellular carcinoma are the most common causes of death, cardiac mortality is an important additional concern (especially in the group of patients—usually men—who present at a young age) and accounts for a third of the mortality.[267,268]

PATHOLOGICAL FINDINGS. These consist of a dilated heart with thickened ventricular walls. Myocardial iron deposits are found within the sarcoplasmic reticulum and are most common in the subepicardial region, followed by the subendocardial region, and are least common in the midmyocardial wall. They are more extensive in ventricular than in atrial myocardium. Involvement of the cardiac conducting system is common. Myocardial degeneration and fibrosis may also occur.

The severity of myocardial dysfunction is proportional to the quantity of iron present in the myocardium.[269] Extensive deposits of cardiac iron (particularly those grossly visible at postmortem examination) are invariably associated with cardiac dysfunction.

CLINICAL MANIFESTATIONS. These vary widely, depending on the extent of myocardial involvement. Some patients remain asymptomatic despite echocardiographic evidence of myocardial involvement, which is expressed initially as increased left ventricular wall thickness and later as chamber enlargement and contractile dysfunction.[269] In such cases, a variety of noninvasive techniques (CT and especially MRI) may demonstrate early subclinical myocardial involvement in which treatment is most effective.[226] Symptomatic cardiac involvement is usually associated with ECG abnormalities, including ST segment and T wave abnormalities, as well as supraventricular arrhythmias[265]; these ECG changes correlate with the degree of iron deposit in the heart.

Cardiac involvement is usually evident from the clinical and echocardiographic features; endomyocardial biopsy may be useful to confirm (but not exclude) the diagnosis. The diagnosis is aided by finding an elevated plasma iron level, a normal or low total iron-binding capacity, and markedly elevated values for serum ferritin, urinary iron, liver iron, and especially saturation of transferrin.[269] Repeated phlebotomies or the use of the chelating agent desferrioxamine may be clinically beneficial.[226,267,270]

GLYCOGEN STORAGE DISEASES

Patients may demonstrate cardiac involvement in type II, III, IV, and V glycogen storage disease, but survival to adulthood is unusual except in type III (glycogen debranching enzyme deficiency).[271] Cardiac involvement is marked most commonly by often clinically silent apparent left ventricular hypertrophy on the electrocardiogram and echocardiogram, but some patients develop overt cardiac dysfunction, arrhythmias, and a pattern of DCM.[226,267,270,272,273]

SARCOIDOSIS

Sarcoidosis is a granulomatous disorder of unknown cause, characterized by multisystem involvement. Infiltration of the lungs, reticuloendothelial system, and skin usually dominates the clinical picture, but virtually any tissue may be affected. The most important manifestation results from

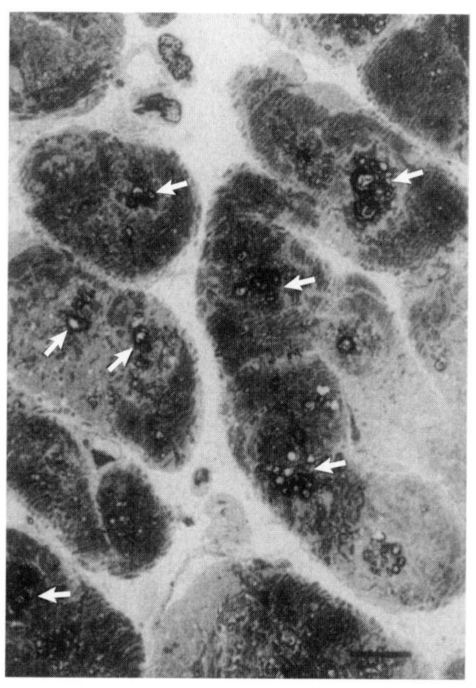

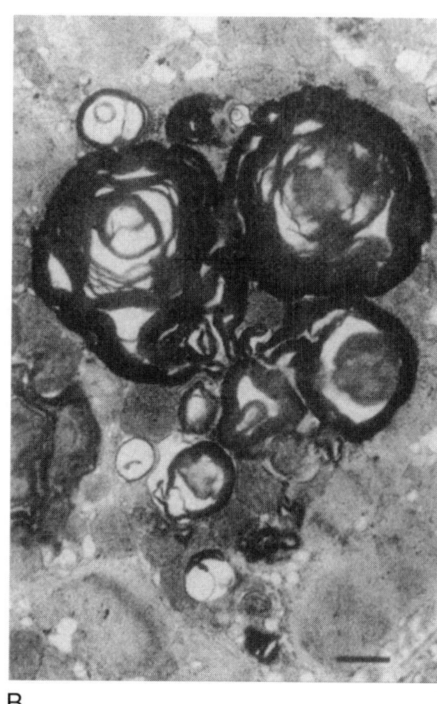

FIGURE 59–22 Transmission electron micrographs of left ventricular endomyocardial biopsy specimen of a patient with Fabry disease, showing at low **(A)** and high **(B)** magnification the perinuclear vacuoles (arrows) that consist of single membrane-bound vesicles containing concentric, lamellar, electron-dense figures, typical of glycolipid storage disease. A, ×1250 (scale bar represents 10 mm); B, ×11,000 (scale bar represents 1 μm). (From Pieroni M, Chimenti C, Ricci R, et al: Early detection of Fabry cardiomyopathy by tissue Doppler imaging. Circulation 107:1978, 2003. Copyright 2003, American Heart Association.)

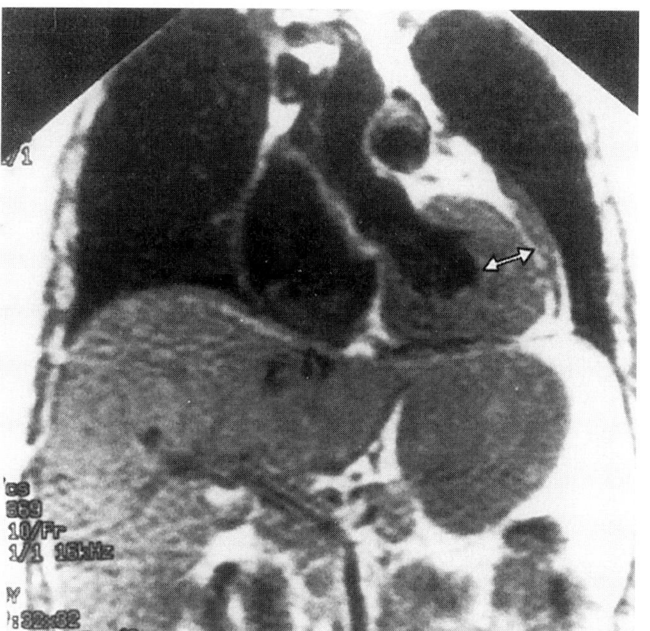

FIGURE 59–23 Cardiac magnetic resonance imaging (T1-weighted spin echo) in Fabry disease, showing marked ventricular thickening (arrow). Coronal view. (From Cantor WJ, Butany J, Iwanochko M, Liu P: Restrictive cardiomyopathy secondary to Fabry's disease. Circulation 98:1457, 1998. Copyright 1998, American Heart Association.)

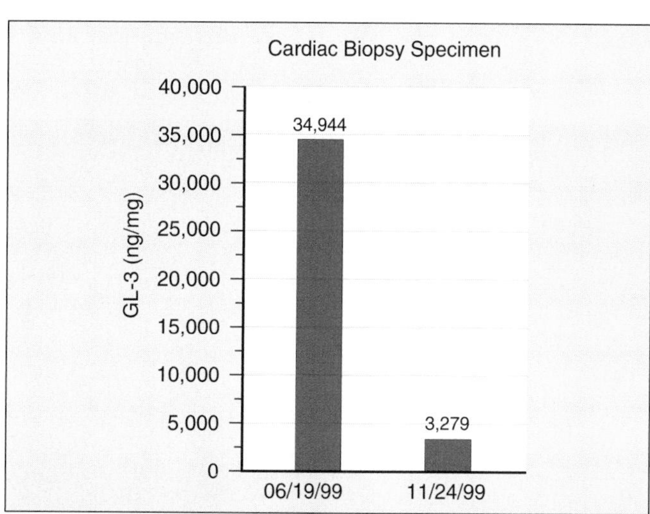

FIGURE 59–24 Marked decline in myocardial tissue levels of globotriaosylceramide (GL-3) in a patient with Fabry disease who was treated with enzyme replacement therapy. (From Waldek S: PR interval and the response to enzyme-replacement therapy for Fabry's disease. N Engl J Med 348:1186, 2003. Copyright 2003, Massachusetts Medical Society.)

pulmonary involvement. This often leads to diffuse fibrosis that may result in fatal right-sided heart failure. Primary cardiac involvement is not often recognized clinically, although it may be demonstrated at autopsy in 20 to 30 percent of cases, most of which demonstrate generalized sarcoidosis.[274,275]

Clinical manifestations of sarcoid heart disease are present in less than 5 percent of patients, although myocardial involvement may result in heart block, congestive heart failure, ventricular arrhythmias, and sudden death.[276,277] Myocardial sarcoidosis may have restrictive as well as congestive features because cardiac infiltration by sarcoid granulomas results not only in increased stiffness of the ventricular wall but also in diminished systolic contractile function.[278]

PATHOLOGY. The typical pathological feature is the presence of noncaseating granulomas, which occur in many organs (Fig. 59–25). They infiltrate the myocardium and may eventually form fibrotic scars. The granulomas may involve any region of the heart, although the left ventricular free wall and the interventricular septum are the most common sites, and extensive granulomas and scar tissue in the cephalad portion of the interventricular septum are constant findings in patients with abnormalities of the conduction system.[279] Cardiac infiltration may range from a few scattered lesions to extensive involvement. Because of the variable cardiac involvement, myocardial biopsy may be positive in as few as 20 percent of patients, and therefore a negative biopsy by no means excludes the diagnosis.[65] Transmural involvement may be seen, and large portions of the ventricular wall may be replaced by scar tissue, which may lead to aneurysm formation.[275] Although involvement of small coronary artery branches may be found in sarcoidosis, the larger conductance vessels are uninvolved.

CLINICAL MANIFESTATIONS. Sudden death is the most feared and unfortunately one of the more common manifestations of cardiac sarcoidosis. Conduction disturbances and congestive heart failure are common manifestations of symptomatic involvement in nonfatal cases, but many patients are asymptomatic despite extensive cardiac involvement.[276] Syncope is common and may reflect paroxysmal arrhythmias or conduction disturbances.[278] Atrial and ventricular arrhythmias, especially ventricular tachycardia, are observed frequently.[280] Although cor pulmonale as a consequence of pulmonary sarcoidosis accounts for some of the symptoms of heart failure, many symptoms are caused by direct myocardial involvement by granulomas and scar tissue, and patients show the clinical features of RCM or DCM, or both.[280] Cardiac dysfunction is often severe and progressive. Occasionally, patients with extensive involvement develop overt left ventricular aneurysms. Symptoms of myocardial sarcoid may be present for variable lengths of time; however, the disease may progress rapidly to death, and in some patients the interval from the onset of cardiac symptoms to death is measured in months.[276] In others, survival may be considerably longer.[278,281]

The *physical examination* may reveal findings of extracardiac sarcoid or may be totally normal. A systolic murmur reflecting mitral regurgitation is common. This appears to be more the result of left ventricular dilation than of direct sarcoid involvement of the papillary muscles.

The *electrocardiogram* is frequently abnormal and most commonly demonstrates T wave abnormalities.[275] Sarcoidosis appears to have an affinity for involvement of the atrioventricular junction and bundle of His, and thus varying degrees of intraventricular or atrioventricular block are common.[274] With extensive myocardial involvement, pathological Q waves may appear and simulate myocardial infarction (Fig. 59–26). Characteristic echocardiographic features include left ventricular dilation and dysfunction, often with regional wall motion abnormalities suggestive of ischemic heart disease; wall thinning and increased echogenicity are sometimes observed.[275,276] A small to moderate-sized pericardial effusion may be found.[280]

DIAGNOSIS. In many cases the diagnosis may be suspected in patients with bilateral hilar lymphadenopathy on chest roentgenogram in whom there is clinical or ECG evidence of myocardial disease. Endomyocardial biopsy may be useful in establishing the diagnosis, although the nonuniform involvement of the heart by sarcoidosis means that a negative biopsy does not exclude the diagnosis.[65,274] The *echocardiogram* demonstrates diffuse and often regional left ventricular wall motion abnormalities in patients with clinical cardiac involvement.[276] *Myocardial imaging* with thallium-201 or technetium-99m sestamibi may be helpful in demonstrating segmental perfusion defects that result from sarcoid infiltration of the myocardium.[274,276] Imaging may also indicate the presence of right ventricular hypertrophy in patients with right ventricular overload related to pulmonary

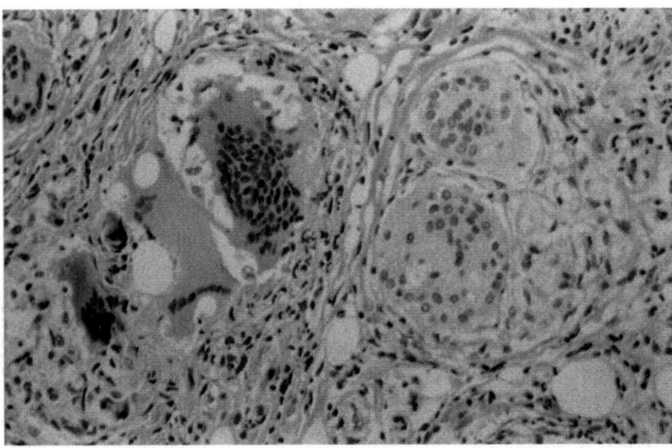

FIGURE 59–25 Typical histological findings in sarcoidosis, demonstrating many noncaseating granulomas with giant cells in skin biopsy specimen. (From Shindo T, Kurihara H, Ohishi N, et al: Images in cardiovascular medicine. Cardiac sarcoidosis. Circulation 97:1306, 1998. Copyright 1998, American Heart Association.)

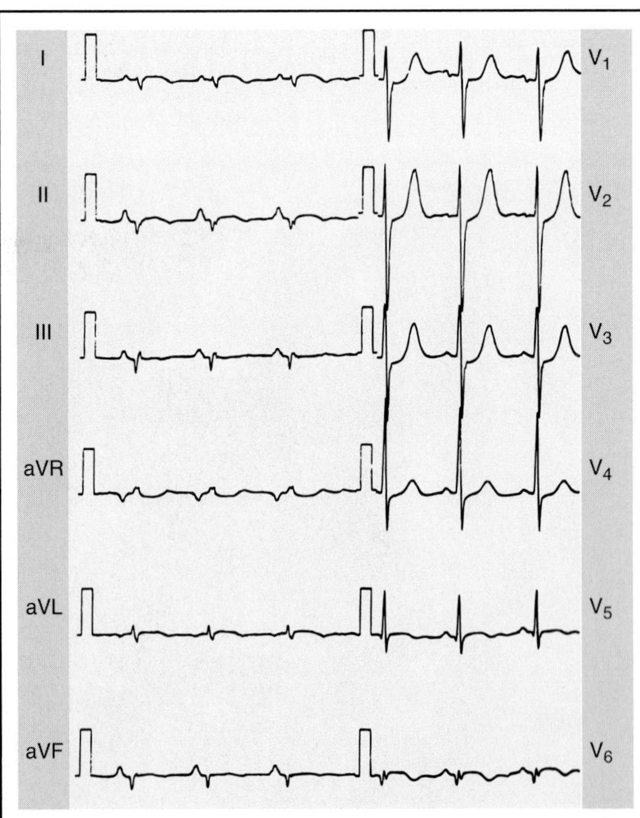

FIGURE 59–26 Electrocardiogram of a patient with cardiac sarcoidosis shows abnormal Q wave in leads II and III and aVF and ST segment elevation in V_5 and V_6. (From Shindo T, Kurihara H, Ohishi N, et al: Images in cardiovascular medicine: Cardiac sarcoidosis. Circulation 97:1306, 1998. Copyright 1998, American Heart Association.)

fibrosis and pulmonary hypertension. Uptake of technetium pyrophosphate, gallium, and labeled antimyosin antibody may aid in the diagnosis, as may MRI.[275,276,282,283]

MANAGEMENT. The treatment of myocardial sarcoidosis is difficult. Arrhythmias are often refractory to antiarrhythmic drugs. Permanent pacing may be helpful in patients with involvement of the atrioventricular conduction system. Although the matter is not settled, corticosteroids may be of some benefit in treating the conduction disturbances, arrhythmias, and myocardial dysfunction of sarcoidosis, with a suggestion of improved survival.[275,280,281] It has been suggested that further benefit may be derived from the addition of hydroxychloroquine, methotrexate, or cyclophosphamide. Because the risk of sudden death appears to be greatest in patients with extensive myocardial involvement, it may be reasonable to attempt to halt the progression of the disease with corticosteroids before irreversible fibrosis occurs.[281] Insertion of an ICD may be considered in appropriate patients at high risk for sudden death.[280] Heart or heart-lung transplantation has been used in selected patients with intractable heart failure, although recurrent sarcoid involvement of the transplanted heart can occur.[218,280]

Endomyocardial Disease

DEFINITION AND PATHOGENESIS. Endomyocardial disease (EMD) is a common form of RCM that is typically found in a geographical distribution near the equator. It is most frequent in equatorial Africa and is encountered with less frequency in South America, Asia, and nontropical countries, including the United States.[284] It is marked by intense endocardial fibrotic thickening of the apex and subvalvular regions of one or both ventricles that results in obstruction to inflow of blood into the respective ventricle, thus producing restrictive physiology.[285] For many years it had been thought that there are two variants of the disease, one occurring principally in tropical countries (termed *endomyocardial fibrosis* [EMF] or Davies disease) and the other in temperate countries (called Löffler endocarditis parietalis fibroplastica or the hypereosinophilic syndrome). However, despite the pathological similarities, there are important contrasts in clinical presentation that challenge the concept of a single disease process.[286] In addition to the geographical differences, the temperate form of the disease is a more aggressive and rapidly progressive disorder, affecting principally males, and is associated with hypereosinophilia, thromboembolic phenomena, and generalized arteritis. EMF, conversely, occurs in younger patients and has an inconstant association with an intense eosinophilia.[285,287]

DIFFERENCES BETWEEN LÖFFLER ENDOCARDITIS AND ENDOMYOCARDIAL FIBROSIS. Part of the thesis that Löffler endocarditis and EMF are different phases of a single disease is based on a theory of pathogenesis involving the toxic effect of eosinophils on the heart.[284] Under this formulation, an initial hypereosinophilia of whatever cause results in damage to the myocardium that produces the first phase of EMD: a necrotic phase, marked by an intense myocarditis, rich in eosinophils, and with an associated arteritis (i.e., Löffler endocarditis). This initial phase occurs within the first few months of illness. It may be followed by a thrombotic stage, occurring about a year after initial presentation, during which the myocarditis has receded, nonspecific thickening of the myocardium is beginning, and there is a variable degree of superimposed thrombus formation.[286] The putative last stage is one of fibrosis, presenting all of the features of EMF. The three stages—necrotic, thrombotic, and fibrotic—have been defined on the basis of postmortem material, and it is not suggested by proponents of the unified pathogenesis hypothesis that each patient with advanced disease (manifested by EMF) has necessarily passed through the earlier phases.

ROLE OF EOSINOPHILS. The possible role of eosinophils in the production of the cardiac abnormalities has intrigued investigators for years.[284] Eosinophils may damage tissues by direct invasion or by the release of toxic substances. The presence of degranulated eosinophils in the peripheral blood of patients with Löffler endocarditis suggests that the protein constituents of the eosinophil's granule may be cardiotoxic, first producing the necrotic phase of EMD, followed by the thrombotic and fibrotic phases after the disappearance of the initial eosinophilia.[284,288]

There is now, however, increasing speculation that this continuum occurs only in the temperate countries, and the endemic EMF found in tropical countries is a distinct and separate disease because a constant link with eosinophilia has been difficult to document, despite the frequency of parasitic diseases.[284,285,289] Other etiological factors have been implicated; the fibrosis of tropical EMF has been linked to the higher levels of cerium and lower concentrations of magnesium that apparently are found in endemic areas.[284,286,290,291]

Because the clinical manifestations of EMD demonstrate geographical and clinical differences, Löffler endocarditis and EMF are discussed separately, even though they are likely to be part of the same disease continuum.

Löffler Endocarditis: The Hypereosinophilic Syndrome

Marked eosinophilia of any cause may be associated with EMD. The typical patient who presents with Löffler endocarditis is a man in his fourth decade who lives in a temperate climate and has the hypereosinophilic syndrome (i.e., persistent eosinophilia with 1500 eosinophils/mm^3 for at least 6 months or until death, with evidence of organ involvement).[287,292] Cardiac involvement in the hypereosinophilic syndrome is the rule, occurring in the majority of patients.[292,293] Hypereosinophilia and cardiac involvement are also seen in the Churg-Strauss syndrome, which is differentiated by asthma or allergic rhinitis and a necrotizing vasculitis.[294] The cause of the eosinophilia in most patients with Löffler endocarditis is unknown, although in some it may be the result of leukemia, or it may be reactive (i.e., secondary to various parasitic, allergic, granulomatous, hypersensitivity, or neoplastic disorders).[292]

PATHOLOGY. In the hypereosinophilic syndrome, a variety of organs are usually involved besides the heart, including the lungs, bone marrow, and brain.[287] Cardiac involvement is often biventricular, with mural endocardial thickening of the inflow portions and apex of the ventricles.[288,293] Histological findings include variable degrees of (1) an acute inflammatory eosinophilic myocarditis involving the myocardium and endocardium; (2) thrombosis, fibrinoid change, and inflammatory reaction involving small intramural coronary vessels; (3) mural thrombosis, often containing eosinophils; and (4) fibrotic thickening of up to several millimeters.[293]

CLINICAL MANIFESTATIONS. The principal clinical features include weight loss, fever, cough, rash, and congestive heart failure. Although early cardiac involvement may be asymptomatic, overt cardiac dysfunction occurs in more than half of the patients and may be right or left sided, or both.[287] Cardiomegaly, often without overt symptoms of congestive heart failure, may be present, and the murmur of mitral regurgitation is common. Systemic embolism is frequent and may lead to neurological and renal dysfunction. Death is usually due to congestive heart failure, often with associated renal, hepatic, or respiratory dysfunction.[292]

LABORATORY EXAMINATION. The *chest roentgenogram* may reveal cardiomegaly and pulmonary congestion or, less commonly, pulmonary infiltrates. The *electrocardiogram* most commonly shows nonspecific ST segment and T wave abnormalities.[292] Arrhythmias, especially atrial fibrillation, and conduction defects, particularly right bundle branch block, may also be present.

The *echocardiogram* commonly demonstrates localized thickening of the posterobasal left ventricular wall, with absent or markedly limited motion of the posterior leaflet of the mitral valve.[287] There may be obliteration of the apex by thrombus.[293] Enlargement of the atria may be seen,[292] along with Doppler ultrasound evidence of atrioventricular regurgitation. Systolic function often is well preserved, in keeping with the restrictive picture seen in this condition.

The hemodynamic consequences of the dense endocardial scarring seen in Löffler endocarditis are those of an RCM, with abnormal diastolic filling resulting from increased stiffness of the ventricles and a reduction in the size of the ventricular cavity by organized thrombus.[287,293] Atrioventricular valvular regurgitation may occur because of involvement of the supporting apparatus of the mitral or tricuspid valves. *Cardiac catheterization* reveals markedly elevated ventricular filling pressures, and there may be evidence of tricuspid or mitral regurgitation. A characteristic feature on angiocardiography is largely preserved systolic function with obliteration of the apex of the ventricles. The diagnosis is often confirmed by percutaneous endomyocardial biopsy, but the biopsy is not invariably positive.[287]

MANAGEMENT. Medical therapy during the course of early Löffler endocarditis and surgical therapy during the later phases of fibrosis may have a positive effect on symptoms and survival.[292] Corticosteroids appear to have a beneficial effect on acute myocarditis and together with cytotoxic drugs (hydroxyurea in particular) may improve survival substantially.[218] A limited number of patients not responding to standard therapy have responded to treatment with interferon.[288,292] Routine cardiac therapy with digitalis, diuretics, afterload reduction, and anticoagulation as indicated are adjuncts in the management of these patients.[287,292] Surgical therapy appears to offer significant palliation of symptoms when the fibrotic stage has been reached.[295]

Endomyocardial Fibrosis

EMF occurs most commonly in tropical and subtropical Africa, particularly Uganda and Nigeria.[296] It is characterized by fibrous endocardial lesions of the inflow of the right or left ventricle or both and often involves the atrioventricular valves, resulting in regurgitation.[297] It is a relatively frequent cause of heart failure and death in equatorial Africa, accounting for about a quarter of all of the cases of congestive heart failure.[298]

Although most prominent in Africa, it is also found in tropical and subtropical regions in the rest of the world, typically within 15 degrees of the equator, including India, Brazil, Colombia, and Sri Lanka.[284,290] EMF is most common in specific ethnic groups, notably the Rwanda tribe in Uganda, and in people of low socioeconomic status.[296,299] The disease is equally frequent in both sexes, and, although most common in children and young adults, its reported age range is 4 to 70 years. It is most common in blacks, but cases have been reported occasionally in whites in temperate climates, rarely in the absence of prior residence in tropical areas.

PATHOLOGY. A pericardial effusion, which may be quite large, may be present. The heart is normal in size or slightly enlarged, but massive four-chamber cardiomegaly does not occur. The right atrium is often dilated, and in patients with severe right ventricular involvement there may be substantial enlargement of this chamber.[285] Indentation of the right border of the heart above the apex as a result of apical scarring may occur.

Combined right and left ventricular disease occurs in about half the cases, with pure left ventricular involvement occurring in 40 percent and pure right ventricular involvement in the remaining 10 percent. When affected, the right ventricle exhibits extensive dense fibrous thickening of the inflow tract and apex, with involvement of the papillary muscles and chordae tendineae. Involvement of the right ventricle may lead to obliteration of the apex, with a mass of thrombus and fibrous tissue filling the cavity.[297] The tricuspid valve is often distorted by the fibrous process involving the supporting structures. Right atrial thrombi occur commonly. Left ventricular involvement is similar, with fibrosis extending from the apex up the inflow portion of the left ventricle to the posterior mitral valve leaflet. The anterior leaflet of the mitral valve and the outflow portion of the left ventricle are usually spared. Thrombi often overlie the endocardial lesions, and widely distributed endocardial calcific deposits may occur.[300] The epicardial coronary arteries are free of obstructive lesions.

Histological Findings. Microscopically, the involved endocardium demonstrates a thick layer of collagen tissue on top of a layer of loosely arranged connective tissue.[301] Septa composed of fibrous and granulation tissue extend for variable distances into the myocardium. Interstitial edema is often present, but there is no prominent cellular infiltration. Small patches of fibroelastosis may occur in both ventricular outflow tracts beneath the semilunar valves but are thought to be a secondary phenomenon related to local trauma rather than a result of the basic pathological process. The intramural coronary arteries may show medial degeneration, fibrosis, and fibrin deposits.

CLINICAL MANIFESTATIONS. Because EMF may involve both ventricles or either ventricle selectively, symptoms vary. Left-sided involvement results in symptoms of pulmonary congestion, whereas predominant right-sided disease may present features of an RCM and therefore simulate constrictive pericarditis. There is often regurgitation of one or both atrioventricular valves. The onset of the disease is usually insidious, but it is sometimes ushered in by an acute febrile illness. Rarely, the disease appears to stabilize; although survival for up to 12 years has been observed, EMF is usually relentlessly progressive. Death is due to progressive myocardial failure, often associated with pulmonary congestion, infection, infarction, or sudden, unexpected cardiovascular collapse, presumably arrhythmic in origin. Survival appears to be unrelated to the site of predominant involvement (right or left ventricle), although patients presenting in advanced right-sided failure have a worse prognosis than other patients.[302]

RIGHT VENTRICULAR ENDOMYOCARDIAL FIBROSIS

Pure or predominant right ventricular involvement is characterized by fibrous obliteration of the right ventricular apex that diminishes the capacity of this chamber.[297] The fibrosis often extends to the supporting apparatus of the tricuspid valve, resulting in tricuspid regurgitation. Clinical manifestations in patients with right-sided involvement include an elevated jugular venous pressure, a prominent v wave, and a rapid *y* descent. A protodiastolic gallop sound may be heard along the lower sternal border, reflecting right ventricular dysfunction.[284] The liver is usually large and pulsatile, and ascites, splenomegaly, and peripheral edema are common. Pulmonary congestion is not present in the absence of left-sided involvement, and the pulmonary artery and pulmonary capillary wedge pressures are normal.[284] A pericardial effusion, which is sometimes quite large, may be present. The right atrium is often enlarged, sometimes massively so.

LABORATORY FINDINGS. The *electrocardiogram* is usually abnormal, with diminished QRS voltage (probably resulting from the presence of a pericardial effusion), ST segment and T wave abnormalities, and findings suggestive of right-sided enlargement, especially a qR pattern in lead V_1. Supraventricular arrhythmias are common.[284] The *chest roentgenogram* demonstrates cardiac enlargement, usually with gross prominence of the right atrium and a pericardial effusion. Calcification in the walls of the right or, less commonly, the left ventricle may be seen.[284] *Echocardiography* may demonstrate right ventricular thickening, obliteration of the apex, dilated atrium, strong echoes emanating from the endocardial surface, and abnormal septal motion in patients with tricuspid regurgitation.[284,297] At *angiography* the right ventricular apex is characteristically not visualized because of obliteration by the fibrous endocardium, but tricuspid regurgitation, right atrial enlargement, and filling defects in the right atrium caused by intraatrial thrombi are sometimes seen. Early angiographic changes that may be present before advanced disease develops include a change in the endocardial appearance, small apical filling defects, and mild tricuspid regurgitation.

LEFT VENTRICULAR ENDOMYOCARDIAL FIBROSIS

With predominant *left-sided* involvement, the EMF invades the apex of the ventricle and usually the chordae tendineae or the posterior mitral valve leaflet as well, leading to mitral regurgitation.[297] The associated murmur may be confined to late systole, as is characteristic of the papillary muscle dysfunction type of murmur, or it may be pansystolic. Findings of pulmonary hypertension may be prominent. A protodiastolic gallop is commonly heard.

LABORATORY FINDINGS The *electrocardiogram* usually shows ST segment and T wave abnormalities.[297] QRS voltage may be diminished in the presence of a pericardial effusion, although left ventricular hypertrophy may be present. There may be findings of left atrial abnormality. As with right-sided involvement, atrial fibrillation is often present and is a marker of increased mortality.[303] *Echocardiographic features* include increased echoreflectivity of the endocardium, preserved systolic wall motion in the presence of apical obliteration, dilated atrium, variable degrees of pericardial effusion, and Doppler ultrasound evidence of mitral regurgitation.[297] *Cardiac catheterization* often reveals pulmonary hypertension, with elevated left ventricular filling pressures and a reduced cardiac index. The left ventriculogram usually shows mitral regurgitation, and a filling defect related to an intracavitary thrombus within the ventricle may be present (Fig. 59–27). Coronary arteriography does not reveal obstructive disease.

BIVENTRICULAR ENDOMYOCARDIAL FIBROSIS

This form of EMF occurs more frequently than either isolated right- or left-sided disease.[295,297] If there is more than minimal right ventricular involvement, severe pulmonary hypertension does not occur and the right-sided findings dominate the clinical presentation. Typical patients with biventricular involvement may have the features of right ventricular EMF, with only a mitral regurgitant murmur to suggest left ventricular involvement. Systemic embolization may occur in up to 15 percent of patients; infective endocarditis is even less frequent and is found in less than 2 percent.

DIAGNOSIS This is based on the presence in an individual of the typical clinical and laboratory features, particularly angiography, from the appropriate geographical area. Eosinophilia may be present and may or may not reflect associated parasitic infestation.[286,296,299] Endomyocardial biopsy may occasionally be helpful in establishing the diagnosis. However, this risks dislodging a mural thrombus, with resultant embolization, and left-sided biopsy is *not* recommended. In addition, because the disease is often focal, the biopsy may miss the pathological process, particularly if a right ventricular biopsy is performed in a patient with isolated left-sided disease.

MANAGEMENT The medical treatment of EMF is often difficult and not particularly effective. In patients with advanced disease, the outlook is poor, with 35 to 50 percent 2-year mortality. Substantially better survival may be seen in less symptomatic patients who have milder forms of the disease. Digitalis glycosides may be helpful in controlling the ventricular rate in patients with atrial fibrillation,[284] but the response of congestive symptoms to treatment is disappointing, and the development of atrial fibrillation is a sign of poor prognosis.[303] Although diuretics may be useful in the early stages of the disease, they are not particularly helpful in the treatment of massive ascites in the setting of advanced right-sided heart failure and tricuspid regurgitation.[284] When EMD has reached the fibrotic stage, surgery offers the possibility of symptomatic improvement and is the treatment of choice.[295,304] Operative excision of the fibrotic endocardium and replacement of the mitral or tricuspid valves, or both, have led to substantial symptomatic improvement, especially with predominant left-sided involvement.[218,297,304] Postoperative catheterization has provided objective evidence of hemodynamic improvement with a reduction in ventricular filling pressures, an increase in cardiac output, and normalization of the angiographic appearance.[304] Operative mortality has been high, between 15 and 25 percent in the larger series,[218,295] although it appears to be lower if valve replacement can be avoided. Long-term results suggest that surgery is at best palliative, with recurrent fibrosis, continued functional limitation, and cumulative mortality limiting the overall success of an operative approach.[295]

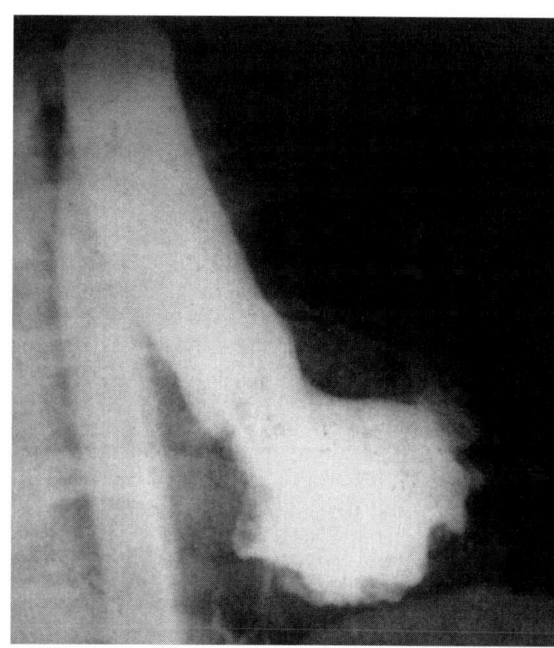

FIGURE 59–27 Left ventricular angiogram of a patient with left ventricular involvement by endomyocardial fibrosis. There is lobulated obliteration of the apex of the ventricle. (From Krishnamoorthy KM: Images in cardiology: Angiographic features of endomyocardial fibrosis. Heart 85:12, 2001.)

Carcinoid Heart Disease (see also Chap. 57)

ETIOLOGY. The carcinoid syndrome is caused by a metastasizing carcinoid tumor and is characterized by cutaneous flushing, diarrhea, bronchoconstriction, and endocardial plaques composed of a unique type of fibrous tissue. The vasomotor, bronchoconstrictor, and cardiac manifestations are related to the tumor's release of serotonin and other circulating humoral substances secreted by the tumor.[305] Virtually all patients develop diarrhea and flushing, and cardiac abnormalities are found on echocardiography in more than half; clinically apparent and severe usually right-sided disease is seen in a fourth of patients.[306,307]

Sixty to 90 percent of tumors arise in the small bowel and appendix, and the rest originate in other areas of the gastrointestinal tract and bronchus.[307] Carcinoid tumors of the ileum are the most likely to metastasize, with involvement of the regional lymph nodes and liver. Usually only carcinoid tumors that invade the liver result in carcinoid heart disease.[305] The cardiac lesions appear to be related to large circulating quantities of serotonin and its degradation product (5-hydroxyindolacetic acid), and patients with progressive cardiac disease tend to have higher levels than those without.[305] Hepatic metastases apparently allow large quantities of tumor products to reach the heart. The preferential right-sided involvement is presumably related to inactivation of the offending humoral substance or substances by the lungs.[308] In 5 to 10 percent of cases, significant left-sided valvular disease develops,[306] related in some to passage of blood directly from the right to the left side of the heart through a patent foramen ovale or less commonly to tumor involvement of the lungs.[309]

PATHOLOGY. The characteristic pathological findings are fibrous plaques that involve the "downstream" aspect of the tricuspid and pulmonic valves, the endocardium of the cardiac chambers, and the intima of the venae cavae, pulmonary artery, and coronary sinus. The fibrous tissue in the plaques results in structural and functional distortion of the valves, leading to both stenosis and regurgitation.[306,310] Histologically, the plaques consist of deposits of fibrous tissue located superficially on the endocardium, often with extension into the underlying layers. Identical morphological features have been found in some patients treated with the anorectic drugs fenfluramine and dexfenfluramine.[306] Ultrastructural and immunohistochemical studies have demonstrated that the plaques are composed of smooth muscle cells embedded in a stroma rich in acid mucopolysaccharides and collagen. Metastatic involvement of the myocardium itself is uncommon, but when it occurs, it may involve either ventricle.[311]

CLINICAL MANIFESTATIONS. Physical examination reveals a systolic murmur of tricuspid regurgitation along the left sternal border, which is a virtually ubiquitous finding; in some cases, there may be a concomitant murmur of pulmonic stenosis or regurgitation, or both.[306]

The *chest roentgenogram* is normal in half of the patients, but it may reveal enlargement of the heart and pleural effusions or nodules; the pulmonary artery trunk is typically of normal size, without evidence of poststenotic dilation as occurs in congenital pulmonic stenosis. No specific *ECG* pattern is diagnostic of carcinoid heart disease. Right atrial enlargement may be seen on occasion, but ECG evidence of right ventricular hypertrophy is usually lacking. Nonspecific ST segment and T wave abnormalities and sinus tachycardia are the most common findings, although severely symptomatic patients usually have low QRS voltage. *Echocardiography* may reveal tricuspid or pulmonary valve thickening, along with right atrial and right ventricular dilation; small pericardial effusions are present in a minority.[312]

MANAGEMENT. In patients with mild congestive heart failure, therapy includes digitalis and diuretics. Symptomatic improvement and perhaps improved survival have been noted with the use of somatostatin analogs and chemotherapy, but neither appears to slow or prevent the development of progressive cardiac disease in patients with carcinoid.[305] *Balloon valvuloplasty* of the right-sided valves has produced symptomatic improvement in some patients with stenotic tricuspid or pulmonary valves, although others have developed recurrent symptoms despite initially "successful" valvuloplasty.[307] *Surgical replacement* of the tricuspid or pulmonary valves, or both, and pulmonic valvotomy or valvectomy result in symptomatic improvement and a reduction in right ventricular dilation in severely symptomatic patients with serious valvular dysfunction, although the operative mortality is high.[306,308,309] The long-term mortality remains high regardless of treatment modality, with half the patients dead within 1 to 2 years.[308]

ENDOCARDIAL FIBROELASTOSIS

This condition is found principally in fetuses and infants and is characterized by collagen and elastin deposition, ventricular hypertrophy, and diffuse endocardial thickening.[313] The cause is unclear but endocardial fibroelastosis (EFE) is seen in association with viral infections (especially mumps), metabolic disorders, autoimmune disease, and congenital left-sided obstructive lesions.[313-315] It shares many of the clinical features of DCM and usually progresses to severe congestive heart failure and subsequent death.[316,317] EFE may be suggested on echocardiography by strong reflections from the endocardial surface of the ventricular myocardium, but such an appearance may also be seen in association with survivable left-sided lesions that do not imply the dire prognosis ordinarily associated with a diagnosis of EFE.[314]

Obesity and Heart Disease (see Chap. 79)

Diabetic Cardiomyopathy (see Chap. 51)

REFERENCES

1. Parmley WW: Surviving heart failure: Robert L. Frye lecture. Mayo Clin Proc 75:111, 2000.
2. Richardson P, McKenna W, Bristow M, et al: Report of the 1995 World Health Organization/International Society and Federation of Cardiology Task Force on the Definition and Classification of Cardiomyopathies. Circulation 93:841, 1996.
3. Artz G, Wynne J: Restrictive cardiomyopathy. Curr Treat Options Cardiovasc Med 2:431, 2000.
4. Oechslin EN, Attenhofer Jost CH, Rojas JR, et al: Long-term follow-up of 34 adults with isolated left ventricular noncompaction: A distinct cardiomyopathy with poor prognosis. J Am Coll Cardiol 36:493, 2000.
5. Veinot JP: Diagnostic endomyocardial biopsy pathology: Secondary myocardial diseases and other clinical indications—A review. Can J Cardiol 18:287, 2002.
6. Frustaci A, Pieroni M, Chimenti C: The role of endomyocardial biopsy in the diagnosis of cardiomyopathies. Ital Heart J 3:348, 2002.
7. Veinot JP: Diagnostic endomyocardial biopsy pathology—General biopsy considerations, and its use for myocarditis and cardiomyopathy: A review. Can J Cardiol 18:55, 2002.
8. Arbustini E, Gavazzi A, Dal Bello B, et al: Ten-year experience with endomyocardial biopsy in myocarditis presenting with congestive heart failure: Frequency, pathologic characteristics, treatment and follow-up. G Ital Cardiol 27:209, 1997.
9. McNamara DM, Holubkov R, Starling RC, et al: Controlled trial of intravenous immune globulin in recent-onset dilated cardiomyopathy. Circulation 103:2254, 2001.
10. Kuhl U, Lauer B, Souvatzoglu M, et al: Antimyosin scintigraphy and immunohistologic analysis of endomyocardial biopsy in patients with clinically suspected myocarditis—Evidence of myocardial cell damage and inflammation in the absence of histologic signs of myocarditis. J Am Coll Cardiol 32:1371, 1998.

Dilated Cardiomyopathy

11. Braunwald E, Bristow MR: Congestive heart failure: Fifty years of progress. Circulation 102:IV14, 2000.
12. Dries DL, Exner DV, Gersh BJ, et al: Racial differences in the outcome of left ventricular dysfunction. N Engl J Med 340:609, 1999.
13. Deedwania PC: The key to unraveling the mystery of mortality in heart failure: An integrated approach. Circulation 107:1719, 2003.
14. Konstam MA: Progress in heart failure management? Lessons from the real world. Circulation 102:1076, 2000.
15. Drozdz J, Krzeminska-Pakula M, Plewka M, et al: Prognostic value of low-dose dobutamine echocardiography in patients with idiopathic dilated cardiomyopathy. Chest 121:1216, 2002.
16. Sun JP, James KB, Yang XS, et al: Comparison of mortality rates and progression of left ventricular dysfunction in patients with idiopathic dilated cardiomyopathy and dilated versus nondilated right ventricular cavities. Am J Cardiol 80:1583, 1997.
17. Felker GM, Hu W, Hare JM, et al: The spectrum of dilated cardiomyopathy. The Johns Hopkins experience with 1,278 patients. Medicine (Baltimore) 78:270, 1999.
18. Seidman JG, Seidman C: The genetic basis for cardiomyopathy: From mutation identification to mechanistic paradigms. Cell 104:557, 2001.
19. Crispell KA, Hanson EL, Coates K, et al: Periodic rescreening is indicated for family members at risk of developing familial dilated cardiomyopathy. J Am Coll Cardiol 39:1503, 2002.
20. Chien KR: Genotype, phenotype: Upstairs, downstairs in the family of cardiomyopathies. J Clin Invest 111:175, 2003.
21. Itoh-Satoh M, Hayashi T, Nishi H, et al: Titin mutations as the molecular basis for dilated cardiomyopathy. Biochem Biophys Res Commun 291:385, 2002.
22. Li D, Czernuszewicz GZ, Gonzalez O, et al: Novel cardiac troponin T mutation as a cause of familial dilated cardiomyopathy. Circulation 104:2188, 2001.
23. Wang X, Osinska H, Dorn GW 2nd, et al: Mouse model of desmin-related cardiomyopathy. Circulation 103:2402, 2001.
24. Taylor MR, Fain PR, Sinagra G, et al: Natural history of dilated cardiomyopathy due to lamin A/C gene mutations. J Am Coll Cardiol 41:771, 2003.
25. Haghighi K, Kolokathis F, Pater L, et al: Human phospholamban null results in lethal dilated cardiomyopathy revealing a critical difference between mouse and human. J Clin Invest 111:869, 2003.
26. Sinagra G, Di Lenarda A, Brodsky GL, et al: New insights into the molecular basis of familial dilated cardiomyopathy. Ital Heart J 2:280, 2001.
27. Feng J, Yan JY, Buzin CH, et al: Comprehensive mutation scanning of the dystrophin gene in patients with nonsyndromic X-linked dilated cardiomyopathy. J Am Coll Cardiol 40:1120, 2002.
28. Vatta M, Stetson SJ, Perez-Verdia A, et al: Molecular remodelling of dystrophin in patients with end-stage cardiomyopathies and reversal in patients on assistance-device therapy. Lancet 359:936, 2002.
29. Arbustini E, Diegoli M, Fasani R, et al: Mitochondrial DNA mutations and mitochondrial abnormalities in dilated cardiomyopathy. Am J Pathol 153:1501, 1998.
30. Abraham MR, Olson LJ, Joyner MJ, et al: Angiotensin-converting enzyme genotype modulates pulmonary function and exercise capacity in treated patients with congestive stable heart failure. Circulation 106:1794, 2002.
31. Luppi P, Rudert WA, Zanone MM, et al: Idiopathic dilated cardiomyopathy: A superantigen-driven autoimmune disease. Circulation 98:777, 1998.
32. Frustaci A, Chimenti C, Calabrese F, et al: Immunosuppressive therapy for active lymphocytic myocarditis: Virological and immunologic profile of responders versus nonresponders. Circulation 107:857, 2003.
33. Fujioka S, Kitaura Y, Ukimura A, et al: Evaluation of viral infection in the myocardium of patients with idiopathic dilated cardiomyopathy. J Am Coll Cardiol 36:1920, 2000.
34. Bowles NE, Ni J, Marcus F, et al: The detection of cardiotropic viruses in the myocardium of patients with arrhythmogenic right ventricular dysplasia/cardiomyopathy. J Am Coll Cardiol 39:892, 2002.
35. Limas CJ: Cardiac autoantibodies in dilated cardiomyopathy: A pathogenetic role? Circulation 95:1979, 1997.
36. Pohlner K, Portig I, Pankuweit S, et al: Identification of mitochondrial antigens recognized by antibodies in sera of patients with idiopathic dilated cardiomyopathy by two-dimensional gel electrophoresis and protein sequencing. Am J Cardiol 80:1040, 1997.
37. McKenna CJ, Codd MB, McCann HA, et al: Idiopathic dilated cardiomyopathy: Familial prevalence and HLA distribution. Heart 77:549, 1997.
38. Liu HR, Zhao RR, Jiao XY, et al: Relationship of myocardial remodeling to the genesis of serum autoantibodies to cardiac beta(1)-adrenoceptors and muscarinic type 2 acetylcholine receptors in rats. J Am Coll Cardiol 39:1866, 2002.
39. Baba A, Yoshikawa T, Ogawa S: Autoantibodies produced against sarcolemmal Na-K-ATPase: Possible upstream targets of arrhythmias and sudden death in patients with dilated cardiomyopathy. J Am Coll Cardiol 40:1153, 2002.
40. Muller J, Wallukat G, Dandel M, et al: Immunoglobulin adsorption in patients with idiopathic dilated cardiomyopathy. Circulation 101:385, 2000.
41. Staudt A, Bohm M, Knebel F, et al: Potential role of autoantibodies belonging to the immunoglobulin G-3 subclass in cardiac dysfunction among patients with dilated cardiomyopathy. Circulation 106:2448, 2002.
42. Wallukat G, Muller J, Hetzer R: Specific removal of beta1-adrenergic autoantibodies from patients with idiopathic dilated cardiomyopathy. N Engl J Med 347:1806, 2002.
43. Pankuweit S, Portig I, Maisch B: Pathophysiology of cardiac inflammation: Molecular mechanisms. Herz 27:669, 2002.
44. Tsutamoto T, Wada A, Matsumoto T, et al: Relationship between tumor necrosis factor-alpha production and oxidative stress in the failing hearts of patients with dilated cardiomyopathy. J Am Coll Cardiol 37:2086, 2001.
45. Zwaka TP, Manolov D, Ozdemir C, et al: Complement and dilated cardiomyopathy: A role of sublytic terminal complement complex-induced tumor necrosis factor-alpha synthesis in cardiac myocytes. Am J Pathol 161:449, 2002.
46. Parthenakis FI, Patrianakos A, Prassopoulos V, et al: Relation of cardiac sympathetic innervation to proinflammatory cytokine levels in patients with heart failure secondary to idiopathic dilated cardiomyopathy. Am J Cardiol 91:1190, 2003.
47. Skudicky D, Bergemann A, Sliwa K, et al: Beneficial effects of pentoxifylline in patients with idiopathic dilated cardiomyopathy treated with angiotensin-converting enzyme inhibitors and carvedilol: Results of a randomized study. Circulation 103:1083, 2001.

48. Bristow MR: Why does the myocardium fail? Insights from basic science. Lancet 352(Suppl 1):SI8, 1998.
49. Kanoh M, Takemura G, Misao J, et al: Significance of myocytes with positive DNA in situ nick end-labeling (TUNEL) in hearts with dilated cardiomyopathy: Not apoptosis but DNA repair. Circulation 99:2757, 1999.
50. van den Heuvel AF, van Veldhuisen DJ, van der Wall EE, et al: Regional myocardial blood flow reserve impairment and metabolic changes suggesting myocardial ischemia in patients with idiopathic dilated cardiomyopathy. J Am Coll Cardiol 35:19, 2000.
51. Steenbergen C, Afshari CA, Petranka JG, et al: Alterations in apoptotic signaling in human idiopathic cardiomyopathic hearts in failure. Am J Physiol 284:H268, 2003.
52. Wencker D, Chandra M, Nguyen K, et al: A mechanistic role for cardiac myocyte apoptosis in heart failure. J Clin Invest 111:1497, 2003.
53. Lange RA, Hillis LD: Cardiovascular complications of cocaine use. N Engl J Med 345:351, 2001.
54. Nicolas JM, Fernandez-Sola J, Estruch R, et al: The effect of controlled drinking in alcoholic cardiomyopathy. Ann Intern Med 136:192, 2002.
55. Nikolaidis LA, Doverspike A, Huerbin R, et al: Angiotensin-converting enzyme inhibitors improve coronary flow reserve in dilated cardiomyopathy by a bradykinin-mediated, nitric oxide–dependent mechanism. Circulation 105:2785, 2002.
56. Wynne J: The clinical meaning of the third heart sound. Am J Med 111:157, 2001.
57. Yiu SF, Enriquez-Sarano M, Tribouilloy C, et al: Determinants of the degree of functional mitral regurgitation in patients with systolic left ventricular dysfunction: A quantitative clinical study. Circulation 102:1400, 2000.
58. Sato Y, Yamada T, Taniguchi R, et al: Persistently increased serum concentrations of cardiac troponin T in patients with idiopathic dilated cardiomyopathy are predictive of adverse outcomes. Circulation 103:369, 2001.
59. Grunig E, Benz A, Mereles D, et al: Prognostic value of serial cardiac assessment and familial screening in patients with dilated cardiomyopathy. Eur J Heart Fail 5:55, 2003.
60. Saxon LA, De Marco T: Arrhythmias associated with dilated cardiomyopathy. Card Electrophysiol Rev 6:18, 2002.
61. Umana E, Solares CA, Alpert MA: Tachycardia-induced cardiomyopathy. Am J Med 114:51, 2003.
62. Luchsinger JA, Steinberg JS: Resolution of cardiomyopathy after ablation of atrial flutter. J Am Coll Cardiol 32:205, 1998.
63. Pratali L, Picano E, Otasevic P, et al: Prognostic significance of the dobutamine echocardiography test in idiopathic dilated cardiomyopathy. Am J Cardiol 88:1374, 2001.
64. Danias PG, Ahlberg AW, Clark BA 3rd, et al: Combined assessment of myocardial perfusion and left ventricular function with exercise technetium-99m sestamibi gated single-photon emission computed tomography can differentiate between ischemic and nonischemic dilated cardiomyopathy. Am J Cardiol 82:1253, 1998.
65. Uemura A, Morimoto S, Hiramitsu S, et al: Histologic diagnostic rate of cardiac sarcoidosis: Evaluation of endomyocardial biopsies. Am Heart J 138:299, 1999.
66. Rathore SS, Curtis JP, Wang Y, et al: Association of serum digoxin concentration and outcomes in patients with heart failure. JAMA 289:871, 2003.
67. Hambrecht R, Fiehn E, Weigl C, et al: Regular physical exercise corrects endothelial dysfunction and improves exercise capacity in patients with chronic heart failure. Circulation 98:2709, 1998.
68. Bristow MR: Beta-adrenergic receptor blockade in chronic heart failure. Circulation 101:558, 2000.
69. Abraham WT, Wagoner LE: Medical management of mild-to-moderate heart failure before the advent of beta blockers. Am J Med 110(Suppl 7A):47S, 2001.
70. Wojnicz R, Nowalany-Kozielska E, Wojciechowska C, et al: Randomized, placebo-controlled study for immunosuppressive treatment of inflammatory dilated cardiomyopathy: Two-year follow-up results. Circulation 104:39, 2001.
71. Garg A, Shiau J, Guyatt G: The ineffectiveness of immunosuppressive therapy in lymphocytic myocarditis: An overview. Ann Intern Med 129:317, 1998.
72. Rothenburger M, Rukosujew A, Hammel D, et al: Mitral valve surgery in patients with poor left ventricular function. Thorac Cardiovasc Surg 50:351, 2002.
73. Bolling SF, Pagani FD, Deeb GM, et al: Intermediate-term outcome of mitral reconstruction in cardiomyopathy. J Thorac Cardiovasc Surg 115:381, 1998.
74. Rose EA, Gelijns AC, Moskowitz AJ, et al: Long term use of a left ventricular assist device for end-stage heart failure. N Engl J Med 345:1435, 2001.

Alcoholic Cardiomyopathy

75. Piano MR: Alcoholic cardiomyopathy: Incidence, clinical characteristics, and pathophysiology. Chest 121:1638, 2002.
76. Reid MC, Fiellin DA, O'Connor PG: Hazardous and harmful alcohol consumption in primary care. Arch Intern Med 159:1681, 1999.
77. Fernandez-Sola J, Estruch R, Nicolas JM, et al: Comparison of alcoholic cardiomyopathy in women versus men. Am J Cardiol 80:481, 1997.
78. Gavazzi A, De Maria R, Parolini M, et al: Alcohol abuse and dilated cardiomyopathy in men. Am J Cardiol 85:1114, 2000.
79. Preedy VR, Patel VB, Reilly ME, et al: Oxidants, antioxidants and alcohol: Implications for skeletal and cardiac muscle. Front Biosci 4:e58, 1999.
80. Duan J, McFadden GE, Borgerding AJ, et al: Overexpression of alcohol dehydrogenase exacerbates ethanol-induced contractile defect in cardiac myocytes. Am J Physiol 282:H1216, 2002.
81. Fernandez-Sola J, Nicolas JM, Oriola J, et al: Angiotensin-converting enzyme gene polymorphism is associated with vulnerability to alcoholic cardiomyopathy. Ann Intern Med 137:321, 2002.
82. Walsh CR, Larson MG, Evans JC, et al: Alcohol consumption and risk for congestive heart failure in the Framingham Heart Study. Ann Intern Med 136:181, 2002.
83. Wynne J: Stirred, not shaken. Ann Intern Med 136:247, 2002.
84. Lazarevic AM, Nakatani S, Neskovic AN, et al: Early changes in left ventricular function in chronic asymptomatic alcoholics: Relation to the duration of heavy drinking. J Am Coll Cardiol 35:1599, 2000.
85. Guillo P, Mansourati J, Maheu B, et al: Long-term prognosis in patients with alcoholic cardiomyopathy and severe heart failure after total abstinence. Am J Cardiol 79:1276, 1997.
86. Barceloux DG: Cobalt. J Toxicol Clin Toxicol 37:201, 1999.

Arrhythmogenic Right Ventricular Cardiomyopathy

87. Burke AP, Farb A, Tashko G, et al: Arrhythmogenic right ventricular cardiomyopathy and fatty replacement of the right ventricular myocardium: Are they different diseases? Circulation 97:1571, 1998.
88. Gemayel C, Pelliccia A, Thompson PD: Arrhythmogenic right ventricular cardiomyopathy. J Am Coll Cardiol 38:1773, 2001.
89. Thiene G, Basso C, Calabrese F, et al: Pathology and pathogenesis of arrhythmogenic right ventricular cardiomyopathy. Herz 25:210, 2000.
90. Pinski SL: The right ventricular tachycardias. J Electrocardiol 33(Suppl):103, 2000.
91. Hamid MS, Norman M, Quraishi A, et al: Prospective evaluation of relatives for familial arrhythmogenic right ventricular cardiomyopathy/dysplasia reveals a need to broaden diagnostic criteria. J Am Coll Cardiol 40:1445, 2002.
92. Danieli GA, Rampazzo A: Genetics of arrhythmogenic right ventricular cardiomyopathy. Curr Opin Cardiol 17:218, 2002.
93. Protonotarios N, Tsatsopoulou A, Anastasakis A, et al: Genotype-phenotype assessment in autosomal recessive arrhythmogenic right ventricular cardiomyopathy (Naxos disease) caused by a deletion in plakoglobin. J Am Coll Cardiol 38:1477, 2001.
94. Kilinc M, Akdemir I, Sivasli E: A case with Uhl's anomaly presenting with severe right heart failure. Acta Cardiol 55:367, 2000.
95. Naccarella F, Naccarelli G, Fattori R, et al: Arrhythmogenic right ventricular dysplasia: Cardiomyopathy current opinions on diagnostic and therapeutic aspects. Curr Opin Cardiol 16:8, 2001.
96. Nava A, Bauce B, Basso C, et al: Clinical profile and long-term follow-up of 37 families with arrhythmogenic right ventricular cardiomyopathy. J Am Coll Cardiol 36:2226, 2000.
97. Corrado D, Buja G, Basso C, et al: Clinical diagnosis and management strategies in arrhythmogenic right ventricular cardiomyopathy. J Electrocardiol 33(Suppl):49, 2000.
98. Patel VV, Ferrari VA, Narula N, et al: Right ventricular dysplasia in an asymptomatic young man: An uncommon case with biventricular involvement and no known family history. J Am Soc Echocardiogr 14:317, 2001.
99. Le Guludec D, Gauthier H, Porcher R, et al: Prognostic value of radionuclide angiography in patients with right ventricular arrhythmias. Circulation 103:1972, 2001.
100. Di Cesare E: MRI of the cardiomyopathies. Eur J Radiol 38:179, 2001.
101. Wichter T, Schafers M, Rhodes CG, et al: Abnormalities of cardiac sympathetic innervation in arrhythmogenic right ventricular cardiomyopathy: Quantitative assessment of presynaptic norepinephrine reuptake and postsynaptic beta-adrenergic receptor density with positron emission tomography. Circulation 101:1552, 2000.
102. Borger van der Burg AE, de Groot NM, van Erven L, et al: Long-term follow-up after radiofrequency catheter ablation of ventricular tachycardia: A successful approach? J Cardiovasc Electrophysiol 13:417, 2002.

Hypertrophic Cardiomyopathy

103. Braunwald E, Morrow AG, Cornell WP, et al: Idiopathic hypertrophic subaortic stenosis: Clinical, hemodynamic and angiographic manifestations. Am J Med 29:924, 1960.
104. Maron BJ: Hypertrophic cardiomyopathy: A systematic review. JAMA 287:1308, 2002.
105. Spirito P, Seidman CE, McKenna WJ, et al: The management of hypertrophic cardiomyopathy. N Engl J Med 336:775, 1997.
106. Maron BJ: Hypertrophic cardiomyopathy. Lancet 350:127, 1997.
107. Braunwald E, Seidman CE, Sigwart U: Contemporary evaluation and management of hypertrophic cardiomyopathy. Circulation 106:1312, 2002.
108. Marian AJ, Roberts R: The molecular genetic basis for hypertrophic cardiomyopathy. J Mol Cell Cardiol 33:655, 2001.
109. Criley JM: Unobstructed thinking (and terminology) is called for in the understanding and management of hypertrophic cardiomyopathy. J Am Coll Cardiol 29:741, 1997.
110. Mozaffarian D, Caldwell JH: Right ventricular involvement in hypertrophic cardiomyopathy: A case report and literature review. Clin Cardiol 24:2, 2001.
111. Sharma S, Maron BJ, Whyte G, et al: Physiologic limits of left ventricular hypertrophy in elite junior athletes: Relevance to differential diagnosis of athlete's heart and hypertrophic cardiomyopathy. J Am Coll Cardiol 40:1431, 2002.
112. Sharma S, Elliott PM, Whyte G, et al: Utility of metabolic exercise testing in distinguishing hypertrophic cardiomyopathy from physiologic left ventricular hypertrophy in athletes. J Am Coll Cardiol 36:864, 2000.
113. Niimura H, Bachinski LL, Sangwatanaroj S, et al: Mutations in the gene for cardiac myosin-binding protein C and late-onset familial hypertrophic cardiomyopathy. N Engl J Med 338:1248, 1998.
114. Maron BJ, Nishimura RA, Danielson GK: Pitfalls in clinical recognition and a novel operative approach for hypertrophic cardiomyopathy with severe outflow obstruction due to anomalous papillary muscle. Circulation 98:2505, 1998.
115. Wigle ED: Cardiomyopathy: The diagnosis of hypertrophic cardiomyopathy. Heart 86:709, 2001.
116. Reddy V, Korcarz C, Weinert L, et al: Apical hypertrophic cardiomyopathy. Circulation 98:2354, 1998.
117. Sakamoto T: Apical hypertrophic cardiomyopathy (apical hypertrophy): An overview. J Cardiol 37(Suppl 1):161, 2001.
118. Eriksson MJ, Sonnenberg B, Woo A, et al: Long-term outcome in patients with apical hypertrophic cardiomyopathy. J Am Coll Cardiol 39:638, 2002.
119. Niimura H, Patton KK, McKenna WJ, et al: Sarcomere protein gene mutations in hypertrophic cardiomyopathy of the elderly. Circulation 105:446, 2002.
120. Varnava AM, Elliott PM, Sharma S, et al: Hypertrophic cardiomyopathy: The interrelation of disarray, fibrosis, and small vessel disease. Heart 84:476, 2000.

121. Usyk TP, Omens JH, McCulloch AD: Regional septal dysfunction in a three-dimensional computational model of focal myofiber disarray. Am J Physiol 281:H506, 2001.
122. Mogensen J, Klausen IC, Pedersen AK, et al: Alpha-cardiac actin is a novel disease gene in familial hypertrophic cardiomyopathy. J Clin Invest 103:R39, 1999.
123. Richard P, Charron P, Carrier L, et al: Hypertrophic cardiomyopathy. Distribution of disease genes, spectrum of mutations, and implications for a molecular diagnosis strategy. Circulation 107:2227, 2003.
124. Chung MW, Tsoutsman T, Semsarian C: Hypertrophic cardiomyopathy: From gene defect to clinical disease. Cell Res 13:9, 2003.
125. Maron BJ, Moller JH, Seidman CE, et al: Impact of laboratory molecular diagnosis on contemporary diagnostic criteria for genetically transmitted cardiovascular diseases: Hypertrophic cardiomyopathy, long-QT syndrome, and Marfan syndrome: A statement for healthcare professionals from the Councils on Clinical Cardiology, Cardiovascular Disease in the Young, and Basic Science, American Heart Association. Circulation 98:1460, 1998.
126. Marian AJ: Pathogenesis of diverse clinical and pathological phenotypes in hypertrophic cardiomyopathy. Lancet 355:58, 2000.
127. McNally EM: Beta-myosin heavy chain gene mutations in familial hypertrophic cardiomyopathy: The usual suspect? Circ Res 90:246, 2002.
128. Fatkin D, McConnell BK, Mudd JO, et al: An abnormal Ca(2+) response in mutant sarcomere protein–mediated familial hypertrophic cardiomyopathy. J Clin Invest 106:1351, 2000.
129. Konno T, Shimizu M, Ino H, et al: A novel missense mutation in the myosin binding protein-C gene is responsible for hypertrophic cardiomyopathy with left ventricular dysfunction and dilation in elderly patients. J Am Coll Cardiol 41:781, 2003.
130. Moolman JA, Reith S, Uhl K, et al: A newly created splice donor site in exon 25 of the MyBP-C gene is responsible for inherited hypertrophic cardiomyopathy with incomplete disease penetrance. Circulation 101:1396, 2000.
131. Arad M, Benson DW, Perez-Atayde AR, et al: Constitutively active AMP kinase mutations cause glycogen storage disease mimicking hypertrophic cardiomyopathy. J Clin Invest 109:357, 2002.
132. Roberts R, Sigwart U: New concepts in hypertrophic cardiomyopathies, Part I. Circulation 104:2113, 2001.
133. Ho CY, Lever HM, DeSanctis R, et al: Homozygous mutation in cardiac troponin T: Implications for hypertrophic cardiomyopathy. Circulation 102:1950, 2000.
134. Anan R, Shono H, Kisanuki A, et al: Patients with familial hypertrophic cardiomyopathy caused by a Phe110Ile missense mutation in the cardiac troponin T gene have variable cardiac morphologies and a favorable prognosis. Circulation 98:391, 1998.
135. Ackerman MJ, VanDriest SL, Ommen SR, et al: Prevalence and age-dependence of malignant mutations in the beta-myosin heavy chain and troponin T genes in hypertrophic cardiomyopathy: A comprehensive outpatient perspective. J Am Coll Cardiol 39:2042, 2002.
136. Jongbloed RJ, Marcelis CL, Doevendans PA, et al: Variable clinical manifestation of a novel missense mutation in the alpha-tropomyosin (TPM1) gene in familial hypertrophic cardiomyopathy. J Am Coll Cardiol 41:981, 2003.
137. Van Driest SL, Ackerman MJ, Ommen SR, et al: Prevalence and severity of "benign" mutations in the beta-myosin heavy chain, cardiac troponin T, and alpha-tropomyosin genes in hypertrophic cardiomyopathy. Circulation 106:3085, 2002.
138. Charron P, Dubourg O, Desnos M, et al: Diagnostic value of electrocardiography and echocardiography for familial hypertrophic cardiomyopathy in a genotyped adult population. Circulation 96:214, 1997.
139. van Langen IM, Birnie E, Leschot NJ, et al: Genetic knowledge and counselling skills of Dutch cardiologists: Sufficient for the genomics era? Eur Heart J 24:560, 2003.
140. Braunwald E. Lambrew CT, Rickoff SD, et al. Idiopathic hypertrophic subaortic stenosis. I. A description of the disease based upon an analysis of 64 patients. Circulation 30(Suppl 4):3, 1964
141. Sherrid MV, Chaudhry FA, Swistel DG: Obstructive hypertrophic cardiomyopathy: Echocardiography, pathophysiology, and the continuing evolution of surgery for obstruction. Ann Thorac Surg 75:620, 2003.
142. Nagueh SF, Stetson SJ, Lakkis NM, et al: Decreased expression of tumor necrosis factor-alpha and regression of hypertrophy after nonsurgical septal reduction therapy for patients with hypertrophic obstructive cardiomyopathy. Circulation 103:1844, 2001.
143. Mazur W, Nagueh SF, Lakkis NM, et al: Regression of left ventricular hypertrophy after nonsurgical septal reduction therapy for hypertrophic obstructive cardiomyopathy. Circulation 103:1492, 2001.
144. Nagueh SF, Bachinski LL, Meyer D, et al: Tissue Doppler imaging consistently detects myocardial abnormalities in patients with hypertrophic cardiomyopathy and provides a novel means for an early diagnosis before and independently of hypertrophy. Circulation 104:128, 2001.
145. Michele DE, Gomez CA, Hong KE, et al: Cardiac dysfunction in hypertrophic cardiomyopathy mutant tropomyosin mice is transgene-dependent, hypertrophy-independent, and improved by beta-blockade. Circ Res 91:255, 2002.
146. Knollmann BC, Kirchhof P, Sirenko SG, et al: Familial hypertrophic cardiomyopathy–linked mutant troponin T causes stress-induced ventricular tachycardia and Ca^{2+}-dependent action potential remodeling. Circ Res 92:428, 2003.
147. Lazzeroni E, Picano E, Morozzi L, et al: Dipyridamole-induced ischemia as a prognostic marker of future adverse cardiac events in adult patients with hypertrophic cardiomyopathy. Echo Persantine Italian Cooperative (EPIC) Study Group, Subproject Hypertrophic Cardiomyopathy. Circulation 96:4268, 1997.
148. Krams R, Kofflard MJ, Duncker DJ, et al: Decreased coronary flow reserve in hypertrophic cardiomyopathy is related to remodeling of the coronary microcirculation. Circulation 97:230, 1998.
149. Takemura G, Takatsu Y, Fujiwara H: Luminal narrowing of coronary capillaries in human hypertrophic hearts: An ultrastructural morphometrical study using endomyocardial biopsy specimens. Heart 79:78, 1998.
150. Kyriakidis M, Triposkiadis F, Dernellis J, et al: Effects of cardiac versus circulatory angiotensin-converting enzyme inhibition on left ventricular diastolic function and coronary blood flow in hypertrophic obstructive cardiomyopathy. Circulation 97:1342, 1998.
151. Mohiddin SA, Begley D, Shih J, et al: Myocardial bridging does not predict sudden death in children with hypertrophic cardiomyopathy but is associated with more severe cardiac disease. J Am Coll Cardiol 36:2270, 2000.

Clinical Manifestations

152. Maron BJ, Casey SA, Poliac LC, et al: Clinical course of hypertrophic cardiomyopathy in a regional United States cohort. JAMA 281:650, 1999.
153. Maron BJ, Olivotto I, Spirito P, et al: Epidemiology of hypertrophic cardiomyopathy–related death: Revisited in a large non-referral-based patient population. Circulation 102:858, 2000.
154. Maron BJ, Carney KP, Lever HM, et al: Relationship of race to sudden cardiac death in competitive athletes with hypertrophic cardiomyopathy. J Am Coll Cardiol 41:974, 2003.
155. Yu EH, Omran AS, Wigle ED, et al: Mitral regurgitation in hypertrophic obstructive cardiomyopathy: Relationship to obstruction and relief with myectomy. J Am Coll Cardiol 36:2219, 2000.
156. Nagueh SF, Ommen SR, Lakkis NM, et al: Comparison of ethanol septal reduction therapy with surgical myectomy for the treatment of hypertrophic obstructive cardiomyopathy. J Am Coll Cardiol 38:1701, 2001.
157. Maron BJ: The electrocardiogram as a diagnostic tool for hypertrophic cardiomyopathy: Revisited. Ann Noninvasive Electrocardiol 6:277, 2001.
158. Runquist LH, Nielsen CD, Killip D, et al: Electrocardiographic findings after alcohol septal ablation therapy for obstructive hypertrophic cardiomyopathy. Am J Cardiol 90:1020, 2002.
159. Maron BJ, Shen WK, Link MS, et al: Efficacy of implantable cardioverter-defibrillators for the prevention of sudden death in patients with hypertrophic cardiomyopathy. N Engl J Med 342:365, 2000.
160. McKenna WJ, Behr ER: Hypertrophic cardiomyopathy: Management, risk stratification, and prevention of sudden death. Heart 87:169, 2002.
161 Maron BJ, Olivotto I, Bellone P, et al: Clinical profile of stroke in 900 patients with hypertrophic cardiomyopathy. J Am Coll Cardiol 39:301, 2002.
162. Olivotto I, Cecchi F, Casey SA, et al: Impact of atrial fibrillation on the clinical course of hypertrophic cardiomyopathy. Circulation 104:2517, 2001.
163. Maron BJ, Leyhe MJ, 3rd, Casey SA, et al: Assessment of QT dispersion as a prognostic marker for sudden death in a regional nonreferred hypertrophic cardiomyopathy cohort. Am J Cardiol 87:114, 2001.
164. Manganelli F, Betocchi S, Ciampi Q, et al: Comparison of hemodynamic adaptation to orthostatic stress in patients with hypertrophic cardiomyopathy with or without syncope and in vasovagal syncope. Am J Cardiol 89:1405, 2002.
165. Spirito P, Bellone P, Harris KM, et al: Magnitude of left ventricular hypertrophy and risk of sudden death in hypertrophic cardiomyopathy. N Engl J Med 342:1778, 2000.
166. Elliott PM, Poloniecki J, Dickie S, et al: Sudden death in hypertrophic cardiomyopathy: Identification of high risk patients. J Am Coll Cardiol 36:2212, 2000.
167. Schwammenthal E, Nakatani S, He S, et al: Mechanism of mitral regurgitation in hypertrophic cardiomyopathy: Mismatch of posterior to anterior leaflet length and mobility. Circulation 98:856, 1998.
168. Sherrid MV, Gunsburg DZ, Moldenhauer S, et al: Systolic anterior motion begins at low left ventricular outflow tract velocity in obstructive hypertrophic cardiomyopathy. J Am Coll Cardiol 36:1344, 2000.
169. Choudhury L, Mahrholdt H, Wagner A, et al: Myocardial scarring in asymptomatic or mildly symptomatic patients with hypertrophic cardiomyopathy. J Am Coll Cardiol 40:2156, 2002.
170. Losi MA, Betocchi S, Manganelli F, et al: Pattern of left ventricular filling in hypertrophic cardiomyopathy. Assessment by Doppler echocardiography and radionuclide angiography. Eur Heart J 19:1261, 1998.
171. Fattori R, Rocchi G, Celletti F, et al: Contribution of magnetic resonance imaging in the differential diagnosis of cardiac amyloidosis and symmetric hypertrophic cardiomyopathy. Am Heart J 136:824, 1998.
172. Moon JC, McKenna WJ, McCrohon JA, et al: Toward clinical risk assessment in hypertrophic cardiomyopathy with gadolinium cardiovascular magnetic resonance. J Am Coll Cardiol 41:1561, 2003.
173. Kim RJ, Judd RM: Gadolinium-enhanced magnetic resonance imaging in hypertrophic cardiomyopathy. In vivo imaging of the pathologic substrate for premature cardiac death? J Am Coll Cardiol 41:1568, 2003.
174. Fananapazir L, McAreavey D: Therapeutic options in patients with obstructive hypertrophic cardiomyopathy and severe drug-refractory symptoms. J Am Coll Cardiol 31:259, 1998.
175. Kizilbash AM, Heinle SK, Grayburn PA: Spontaneous variability of left ventricular outflow tract gradient in hypertrophic obstructive cardiomyopathy. Circulation 97:461, 1998.
176. de Gregorio C, Recupero A, Grimaldi P, et al: Noninvasive assessment of intramyocardial coronary flow in hypertrophic cardiomyopathy by high-resolution Doppler echocardiography. Ital Heart J 3:615, 2002.
177. Kofflard MJ, Ten Cate FJ, van der Lee C, et al: Hypertrophic cardiomyopathy in a large community-based population: Clinical outcome and identification of risk factors for sudden cardiac death and clinical deterioration. J Am Coll Cardiol 41:987, 2003.
178. Maron MS, Olivotto I, Betocchi S, et al: Effect of left ventricular outflow tract obstruction on clinical outcome in hypertrophic cardiomyopathy. N Engl J Med 348:295, 2003.
179. Maron BJ, Casey SA, Hurrell DG, et al: Relation of left ventricular thickness to age and gender in hypertrophic cardiomyopathy. Am J Cardiol 91:1195, 2003.
180. Doevendans PA: Hypertrophic cardiomyopathy: Do we have the algorithm for life and death? Circulation 101:1224, 2000.
181. Marian AJ: On predictors of sudden cardiac death in hypertrophic cardiomyopathy. J Am Coll Cardiol 41:994, 2003.

182. Ciampi Q, Betocchi S, Lombardi R, et al: Hemodynamic determinants of exercise-induced abnormal blood pressure response in hypertrophic cardiomyopathy. J Am Coll Cardiol 40:278, 2002.
183. Atiga WL, Fananapazir L, McAreavey D, et al: Temporal repolarization lability in hypertrophic cardiomyopathy caused by beta-myosin heavy-chain gene mutations. Circulation 101:1237, 2000.
184. Yasui K, Shibata T, Nishizawa T, et al: Response of the stroke volume and blood pressure of young patients with nonobstructive hypertrophic cardiomyopathy to exercise. Jpn Circ J 65:300, 2001.
185. Pelliccia A, Di Paolo FM, Maron BJ: The athlete's heart: Remodeling, electrocardiogram and preparticipation screening. Cardiol Rev 10:85, 2002.
186. Ostman-Smith I, Wettrell G, Riesenfeld T: A cohort study of childhood hypertrophic cardiomyopathy: Improved survival following high-dose beta-adrenoceptor antagonist treatment. J Am Coll Cardiol 34:1813, 1999.

Management

187. Autore C, Conte MR, Piccininno M, et al: Risk associated with pregnancy in hypertrophic cardiomyopathy. J Am Coll Cardiol 40:1864, 2002.
188. Semsarian C, Ahmad I, Giewat M, et al: The L-type calcium channel inhibitor diltiazem prevents cardiomyopathy in a mouse model. J Clin Invest 109:1013, 2002.
189. Paquette F, Jasmin G, Dumont L: Cardioprotective efficacy of verapamil and mibefradil in young UM-X7.1 cardiomyopathic hamsters. Cardiovasc Drugs Ther 13:525, 1999.
190. Pacileo G, De Cristofaro M, Russo MG, et al: Hypertrophic cardiomyopathy in pediatric patients: Effect of verapamil on regional and global left ventricular diastolic function. Can J Cardiol 16:146, 2000.
191. Petkow Dimitrow P, Krzanowski M, Nizankowski R, et al: Effect of verapamil on systolic and diastolic coronary blood flow velocity in asymptomatic and mildly symptomatic patients with hypertrophic cardiomyopathy. Heart 83:262, 2000.
192. Sugihara H, Taniguchi Y, Ito K, et al: Effects of diltiazem on myocardial perfusion abnormalities during exercise in patients with hypertrophic cardiomyopathy. Ann Nucl Med 12:349, 1998.
193. Sherrid MV, Pearle G, Gunsburg DZ: Mechanism of benefit of negative inotropes in obstructive hypertrophic cardiomyopathy. Circulation 97:41, 1998.
194. Cecchi F, Olivotto I, Montereggi A, et al: Prognostic value of non-sustained ventricular tachycardia and the potential role of amiodarone treatment in hypertrophic cardiomyopathy: Assessment in an unselected non-referral based patient population. Heart 79:331, 1998.
195. Spirito P, Rapezzi C, Bellone P, et al: Infective endocarditis in hypertrophic cardiomyopathy: Prevalence, incidence, and indications for antibiotic prophylaxis. Circulation 99:2132, 1999.
196. Maron BJ, Nishimura RA, McKenna WJ, et al: Assessment of permanent dual-chamber pacing as a treatment for drug-refractory symptomatic patients with obstructive hypertrophic cardiomyopathy. A randomized, double-blind, crossover study (M-PATHY). Circulation 99:2927, 1999.
197. Nagueh SF, Lakkis NM, Middleton KJ, et al: Changes in left ventricular diastolic function 6 months after nonsurgical septal reduction therapy for hypertrophic obstructive cardiomyopathy. Circulation 99:344, 1999.
198. Nishimura RA, Trusty JM, Hayes DL, et al: Dual-chamber pacing for hypertrophic cardiomyopathy: A randomized, double-blind, crossover trial. J Am Coll Cardiol 29:435, 1997.
199. Linde C, Gadler F, Kappenberger L, et al: Placebo effect of pacemaker implantation in obstructive hypertrophic cardiomyopathy. Am J Cardiol 83:903, 1999.
200. Erwin JP 3rd, Nishimura RA, Lloyd MA, et al: Dual chamber pacing for patients with hypertrophic obstructive cardiomyopathy: A clinical perspective in 2000. Mayo Clin Proc 75:173, 2000.
201. Elliott PM, Sharma S, Varnava A, et al: Survival after cardiac arrest or sustained ventricular tachycardia in patients with hypertrophic cardiomyopathy. J Am Coll Cardiol 33:1596, 1999.
202. Primo J, Geelen P, Brugada J, et al: Hypertrophic cardiomyopathy: Role of the implantable cardioverter-defibrillator. J Am Coll Cardiol 31:1081, 1998.
203. Seggewiss H, Gleichmann U, Faber L, et al: Percutaneous transluminal septal myocardial ablation in hypertrophic obstructive cardiomyopathy: Acute results and 3-month follow-up in 25 patients. J Am Coll Cardiol 31:252, 1998.
204. Kim JJ, Lee CW, Park SW, et al: Improvement in exercise capacity and exercise blood pressure response after transcoronary alcohol ablation therapy of septal hypertrophy in hypertrophic cardiomyopathy. Am J Cardiol 83:1220, 1999.
205. Park TH, Lakkis NM, Middleton KJ, et al: Acute effect of nonsurgical septal reduction therapy on regional left ventricular asynchrony in patients with hypertrophic obstructive cardiomyopathy. Circulation 106:412, 2002.
206. Gietzen FH, Leuner CJ, Obergassel L, et al: Role of transcoronary ablation of septal hypertrophy in patients with hypertrophic cardiomyopathy, New York Heart Association functional class III or IV, and outflow obstruction only under provocable conditions. Circulation 106:454, 2002.
207. Braunwald E. Hypertrophic cardiomyopathy: The benefits of a multidisciplinary approach. N Engl J Med 347:1306, 2002
208. Firoozi S, Elliott PM, Sharma S, et al: Septal myotomy-myectomy and transcoronary septal alcohol ablation in hypertrophic obstructive cardiomyopathy. A comparison of clinical, haemodynamic and exercise outcomes. Eur Heart J 23:1617, 2002.
209. Qin JX, Shiota T, Lever HM, et al: Outcome of patients with hypertrophic obstructive cardiomyopathy after percutaneous transluminal septal myocardial ablation and septal myectomy surgery. J Am Coll Cardiol 38:1994, 2001.
210. Sitges M, Shiota T, Lever HM, et al: Comparison of left ventricular diastolic function in obstructive hypertrophic cardiomyopathy in patients undergoing percutaneous septal alcohol ablation versus surgical myotomy/myectomy. Am J Cardiol 91:817, 2003.
211. Maron BJ: Role of alcohol septal ablation in treatment of obstructive hypertrophic cardiomyopathy. Lancet 355:425, 2000.
212. Seggewiss H: Percutaneous transluminal septal myocardial ablation: A new treatment for hypertrophic obstructive cardiomyopathy. Eur Heart J 21:704, 2000.
213. Faber L, Ziemssen P, Seggewiss H: Targeting percutaneous transluminal septal ablation for hypertrophic obstructive cardiomyopathy by intraprocedural echocardiographic monitoring. J Am Soc Echocardiogr 13:1074, 2000.
214. Seggewiss H: Current status of alcohol septal ablation for patients with hypertrophic cardiomyopathy. Curr Cardiol Rep 3:160, 2001.
215. Lakkis NM, Nagueh SF, Dunn JK, et al: Nonsurgical septal reduction therapy for hypertrophic obstructive cardiomyopathy: One-year follow-up. J Am Coll Cardiol 36:852, 2000.
216. Brunner-La Schonbeck MH, Rocca HP, Vogt PR, et al: Long-term follow-up in hypertrophic obstructive cardiomyopathy after septal myectomy. Ann Thorac Surg 65:1207, 1998.
217. Obeid AI, Maron BJ: Apical hypertrophic cardiomyopathy developing at a relatively advanced age. Circulation 103:1605, 2001.

Restrictive and Infiltrative Cardiomyopathies

218. Kushwaha SS, Fallon JT, Fuster V: Restrictive cardiomyopathy. N Engl J Med 336:267, 1997.
219. Ammash NM, Seward JB, Bailey KR, et al: Clinical profile and outcome of idiopathic restrictive cardiomyopathy. Circulation 101:2490, 2000.
220. Angelini A, Calzolari V, Thiene G, et al: Morphologic spectrum of primary restrictive cardiomyopathy. Am J Cardiol 80:1046, 1997.
221. Nakamura M, Satoh M, Kowada S, et al: Reversible restrictive cardiomyopathy due to light-chain deposition disease. Mayo Clin Proc 77:193, 2002.
222. Mogensen J, Kubo T, Duque M, et al: Idiopathic restrictive cardiomyopathy is part of the clinical expression of cardiac troponin I mutations. J Clin Invest 111:209, 2003.
223. Palka P, Lange A, Donnelly JE, et al: Differentiation between restrictive cardiomyopathy and constrictive pericarditis by early diastolic Doppler myocardial velocity gradient at the posterior wall. Circulation 102:655, 2000.
224. Rajagopalan N, Garcia MJ, Rodriguez L, et al: Comparison of new Doppler echocardiographic methods to differentiate constrictive pericardial heart disease and restrictive cardiomyopathy. Am J Cardiol 87:86, 2001.
225. Felker GM, Thompson RE, Hare JM, et al: Underlying causes and long-term survival in patients with initially unexplained cardiomyopathy. N Engl J Med 342:1077, 2000.
226. Hoffbrand AV: Diagnosing myocardial iron overload. Eur Heart J 22:2140, 2001.
227. Frustaci A, Chimenti C, Ricci R, et al: Improvement in cardiac function in the cardiac variant of Fabry's disease with galactose-infusion therapy. N Engl J Med 345:25, 2001.
228. Lachmann HJ, Booth DR, Booth SE, et al: Misdiagnosis of hereditary amyloidosis as AL (primary) amyloidosis. N Engl J Med 346:1786, 2002.
229. Puille M, Altland K, Linke RP, et al: ^{99m}Tc-DPD scintigraphy in transthyretin-related familial amyloidotic polyneuropathy. Eur J Nucl Med Mol Imaging 29:376, 2002.
230. Jacobson DR, Pastore RD, Yaghoubian R, et al: Variant-sequence transthyretin (isoleucine 122) in late-onset cardiac amyloidosis in black Americans. N Engl J Med 336:466, 1997.
231. Rocken C, Peters B, Juenemann G, et al: Atrial amyloidosis: An arrhythmogenic substrate for persistent atrial fibrillation. Circulation 106:2091, 2002.
232. Gertz MA, Rajkumar SV: Primary systemic amyloidosis. Curr Treat Options Oncol 3:261, 2002.
233. Wald DS, Gray HH: Restrictive cardiomyopathy in systemic amyloidosis. Q J Med 96:380, 2003.
234. Trikas A, Rallidis L, Hawkins P, et al: Comparison of usefulness between exercise capacity and echocardiographic indexes of left ventricular function in cardiac amyloidosis. Am J Cardiol 84:1049, 1999.
235. Sinha MK, Lachmann HJ, Kuriakose B, et al: An unusual cause of progressive heart failure. Lancet 357:1498, 2001.
236. Dubrey SW, Cha K, Skinner M, et al: Familial and primary (AL) cardiac amyloidosis: Echocardiographically similar diseases with distinctly different clinical outcomes. Heart 78:74, 1997.
237. Mueller PS, Edwards WD, Gertz MA: Symptomatic ischemic heart disease resulting from obstructive intramural coronary amyloidosis. Am J Med 109:181, 2000.
238. Liao R, Jain M, Teller P, et al: Infusion of light chains from patients with cardiac amyloidosis causes diastolic dysfunction in isolated mouse hearts. Circulation 104:1594, 2001.
239. Gertz MA, Lacy MQ, Dispenzieri A: Amyloidosis. Hematol Oncol Clin North Am 13:1211, 1999.
240. Pelo E, Da Prato L, Ciaccheri M, et al: Familial amyloid polyneuropathy with genetic anticipation associated to a gly47glu transthyretin variant in an Italian kindred. Amyloid 9:35, 2002.
241. Chamarthi B, Dubrey SW, Cha K, et al: Features and prognosis of exertional syncope in light-chain associated AL cardiac amyloidosis. Am J Cardiol 80:1242, 1997.
242. Reisinger J, Dubrey SW, Lavalley M, et al: Electrophysiologic abnormalities in AL (primary) amyloidosis with cardiac involvement. J Am Coll Cardiol 30:1046, 1997.
243. Dubrey SW, Bilazarian S, LaValley M, et al: Signal-averaged electrocardiography in patients with AL (primary) amyloidosis. Am Heart J 134:994, 1997.
244. Cacoub P, Axler O, De Zuttere D, et al: Amyloidosis and cardiac involvement. Ann Med Interne (Paris) 151:611, 2000.
245. Tanaka M, Hongo M, Kinoshita O, et al: Iodine-123 metaiodobenzylguanidine scintigraphic assessment of myocardial sympathetic innervation in patients with familial amyloid polyneuropathy. J Am Coll Cardiol 29:168, 1997.
246. Lekakis J, Dimopoulos M, Nanas J, et al: Antimyosin scintigraphy for detection of cardiac amyloidosis. Am J Cardiol 80:963, 1997.
247. Arbustini E, Verga L, Concardi M, et al: Electron and immuno-electron microscopy of abdominal fat identifies and characterizes amyloid fibrils in suspected cardiac amyloidosis. Amyloid 9:108, 2002.
248. Kyle RA, Gertz MA, Greipp PR, et al: A trial of three regimens for primary amyloidosis: Colchicine alone, melphalan and prednisone, and melphalan, prednisone, and colchicine. N Engl J Med 336:1202, 1997.

249. Grogan M, Gertz MA, Kyle RA, et al: Five or more years of survival in patients with primary systemic amyloidosis and biopsy-proven cardiac involvement. Am J Cardiol 85:664, 2000.
250. Sanchorawala V, Wright DG, Seldin DC, et al: Low-dose continuous oral melphalan for the treatment of primary systemic (AL) amyloidosis. Br J Haematol 117:886, 2002.
251. Jacobson DR, Ittmann M, Buxbaum JN, et al: Transthyretin Ile 122 and cardiac amyloidosis in African-Americans. 2 case reports. Tex Heart Inst J 24:45, 1997.
252. Mathew V, Olson LJ, Gertz MA, et al: Symptomatic conduction system disease in cardiac amyloidosis. Am J Cardiol 80:1491, 1997.
253. Comenzo RL, Gertz MA: Autologous stem cell transplantation for primary systemic amyloidosis. Blood 99:4276, 2002.
254. Dubrey SW, Burke MM, Khaghani A, et al: Long term results of heart transplantation in patients with amyloid heart disease. Heart 85:202, 2001.
255. Linhart A, Magage S, Palecek T, et al: Cardiac involvement in Fabry disease. Acta Paediatr Suppl 91:15, 2002.
256. Yoshitama T, Nakao S, Takenaka T, et al: Molecular genetic, biochemical, and clinical studies in three families with cardiac Fabry's disease. Am J Cardiol 87:71, 2001.
257. Perrot A, Osterziel KJ, Beck M, et al: Fabry disease: Focus on cardiac manifestations and molecular mechanisms. Herz 27:699, 2002.
258. Linhart A, Palecek T, Bultas J, et al: New insights in cardiac structural changes in patients with Fabry's disease. Am Heart J 139:1101, 2000.
259. Pieroni M, Chimenti C, Ricci R, et al: Early detection of Fabry cardiomyopathy by tissue Doppler imaging. Circulation 107:1978, 2003.
260. Sachdev B, Takenaka T, Teraguchi H, et al: Prevalence of Anderson-Fabry disease in male patients with late onset hypertrophic cardiomyopathy. Circulation 105:1407, 2002.
261. Eng CM, Guffon N, Wilcox WR, et al: Safety and efficacy of recombinant human alpha-galactosidase A—Replacement therapy in Fabry's disease. N Engl J Med 345:9, 2001.
262. Torloni MR, Franco K, Sass N: Gaucher's disease with myocardial involvement in pregnancy. Sao Paulo Med J 120:90, 2002.
263. George R, McMahon J, Lytle B, et al: Severe valvular and aortic arch calcification in a patient with Gaucher's disease homozygous for the D409H mutation. Clin Genet 59:360, 2001.
264. Schiffmann R, Brady RO: New prospects for the treatment of lysosomal storage diseases. Drugs 62:733, 2002.
265. Strobel JS, Fuisz AR, Epstein AE, et al: Syncope and inducible ventricular fibrillation in a woman with hemochromatosis. J Interv Card Electrophysiol 3:225, 1999.
266. Yalcinkaya S, Kumbasar SD, Semiz E, et al: Sustained ventricular tachycardia in cardiac hemochromatosis treated with amiodarone. J Electrocardiol 30:147, 1997.
267. Britton RS, Leicester KL, Bacon BR: Iron toxicity and chelation therapy. Int J Hematol 76:219, 2002.
268. Yang Q, McDonnell SM, Khoury MJ, et al: Hemochromatosis-associated mortality in the United States from 1979 to 1992: An analysis of multiple-cause mortality data. Ann Intern Med 129:946, 1998.
269. Anderson LJ, Holden S, Davis B, et al: Cardiovascular T2-star (T2*) magnetic resonance for the early diagnosis of myocardial iron overload. Eur Heart J 22:2171, 2001.
270. Barton JC, McDonnell SM, Adams PC, et al: Management of hemochromatosis. Hemochromatosis Management Working Group. Ann Intern Med 129:932, 1998.
271. Toda G, Yoshimuta T, Kawano H, et al: Glycogen storage disease associated with left ventricular aneurysm in an elderly patient. Jpn Circ J 65:462, 2001.
272. Lee PJ, Deanfield JE, Burch M, et al: Comparison of the functional significance of left ventricular hypertrophy in hypertrophic cardiomyopathy and glycogenosis type III. Am J Cardiol 79:834, 1997.
273. Cuspidi C, Sampieri L, Pelizzoli S, et al: Obstructive hypertrophic cardiomyopathy in type III glycogen-storage disease. Acta Cardiol 52:117, 1997.
274. Sharma OP: Diagnosis of cardiac sarcoidosis: An imperfect science, a hesitant art. Chest 123:18, 2003.
275. Shimada T, Shimada K, Sakane T, et al: Diagnosis of cardiac sarcoidosis and evaluation of the effects of steroid therapy by gadolinium-DTPA-enhanced magnetic resonance imaging. Am J Med 110:520, 2001.
276. Yazaki Y, Isobe M, Hiramitsu S, et al: Comparison of clinical features and prognosis of cardiac sarcoidosis and idiopathic dilated cardiomyopathy. Am J Cardiol 82:537, 1998.
277. Pisani B, Taylor DO, Mason JW: Inflammatory myocardial diseases and cardiomyopathies. Am J Med 102:459, 1997.
278. Okura Y, Dec GW, Hare JM, et al: A clinical and histopathologic comparison of cardiac sarcoidosis and idiopathic giant cell myocarditis. J Am Coll Cardiol 41:322, 2003.
279. Veinot JP, Johnston B: Cardiac sarcoidosis—An occult cause of sudden death: A case report and literature review. J Forensic Sci 43:715, 1998.
280. Shabetai R: Sarcoidosis and the heart. Curr Treat Options Cardiovasc Med 2:385, 2000.
281. Yazaki Y, Isobe M, Hiroe M, et al: Prognostic determinants of long-term survival in Japanese patients with cardiac sarcoidosis treated with prednisone. Am J Cardiol 88:1006, 2001.
282. Mana J: Magnetic resonance imaging and nuclear imaging in sarcoidosis. Curr Opin Pulm Med 8:457, 2002.
283. Vignaux O, Dhote R, Duboc D, et al: Detection of myocardial involvement in patients with sarcoidosis applying T2-weighted, contrast-enhanced, and cine magnetic resonance imaging: Initial results of a prospective study. J Comput Assist Tomogr 26:762, 2002.
284. Andy JJ, Ogunowo PO, Akpan NA, et al: Helminth associated hypereosinophilia and tropical endomyocardial fibrosis (EMF) in Nigeria. Acta Trop 69:127, 1998.
285. Berenguer A, Plancha E, Munoz Gil J: Right ventricular endomyocardial fibrosis and microfilarial infection. Int J Cardiol 87:287, 2003.
286. Andy JJ: Aetiology of endomyocardial fibrosis (EMF). West Afr J Med 20:199, 2001.
287. Karnak D, Kayacan O, Beder S, et al: Hypereosinophilic syndrome with pulmonary and cardiac involvement in a patient with asthma. CMAJ 168:172, 2003.
288. Baratta L, Afeltra A, Delfino M, et al: Favorable response to high-dose interferon-alpha in idiopathic hypereosinophilic syndrome with restrictive cardiomyopathy—Case report and literature review. Angiology 53:465, 2002.
289. Barbosa MM, Lamounier JA, Oliveira EC, et al: Short report: Endomyocardial fibrosis and cardiomyopathy in an area endemic for schistosomiasis. Am J Trop Med Hyg 58:26, 1998.
290. Kumari KT, Ravikumar A, Kurup PA: Accumulation of glycosaminoglycans associated with hypomagnesaemia in endomyocardial fibrosis in Kerala: Possible involvement of dietary factors. Indian Heart J 49:49, 1997.
291. Eapen JT, Kartha CC, Valiathan MS: Cerium levels are elevated in the serum of patients with endomyocardial fibrosis (EMF). Biol Trace Elem Res 59:41, 1997.
292. Corssmit EP, Trip MD, Durrer JD: Löffler's endomyocarditis in the idiopathic hypereosinophilic syndrome. Cardiology 91:272, 1999.
293. Puvaneswary M, Joshua F, Ratnarajah S: Idiopathic hypereosinophilic syndrome: Magnetic resonance imaging findings in endomyocardial fibrosis. Australas Radiol 45:524, 2001.
294. McGavin CR, Marshall AJ, Lewis CT: Churg-Strauss syndrome with critical endomyocardial fibrosis: 10 year survival after combined surgical and medical management. Heart 87:E5, 2002.
295. Moraes F, Lapa C, Hazin S, et al: Surgery for endomyocardial fibrosis revisited. Eur J Cardiothorac Surg 15:309, 1999.
296. Freers J, Masembe V, Schmauz R, et al: Endomyocardial fibrosis syndrome in Uganda. Lancet 355:1994, 2000.
297. Berensztein CS, Pineiro D, Marcotegui M, et al: Usefulness of echocardiography and Doppler echocardiography in endomyocardial fibrosis. J Am Soc Echocardiogr 13:385, 2000.
298. Amoah AG, Kallen C: Aetiology of heart failure as seen from a national cardiac referral centre in Africa. Cardiology 93:11, 2000.
299. Rutakingirwa M, Ziegler JL, Newton R, et al: Poverty and eosinophilia are risk factors for endomyocardial fibrosis (EMF) in Uganda. Trop Med Int Health 4:229, 1999.
300. Canesin MF, Gama RF, Smith DL, et al: Endomyocardial fibrosis associated with massive calcification of the left ventricle. Arq Bras Cardiol 73:499, 1999.
301. Radhakumary C, Kumari TV, Kartha CC: Endomyocardial fibrosis is associated with selective deposition of type I collagen. Indian Heart J 53:486, 2001.
302. Barretto AC, Mady C, Oliveira SA, et al: Clinical meaning of ascites in patients with endomyocardial fibrosis. Arq Bras Cardiol 78:196, 2002.
303. Barretto AC, Mady C, Nussbacher A, et al: Atrial fibrillation in endomyocardial fibrosis is a marker of worse prognosis. Int J Cardiol 67:19, 1998.
304. Schneider U, Jenni R, Turina J, et al: Long-term follow up of patients with endomyocardial fibrosis: Effects of surgery. Heart 79:362, 1998.
305. Moller JE, Connolly HM, Rubin J, et al: Factors associated with progression of carcinoid heart disease. N Engl J Med 348:1005, 2003.
306. Kulke MH, Mayer RJ: Carcinoid tumors. N Engl J Med 340:858, 1999.
307. Di Luzio S, Rigolin VH: Carcinoid heart disease. Curr Treat Options Cardiovasc Med 2:399, 2000.
308. Connolly HM, Schaff HV, Mullany CJ, et al: Carcinoid heart disease: Impact of pulmonary valve replacement in right ventricular function and remodeling. Circulation 106:I51, 2002.
309. Connolly HM, Schaff HV, Mullany CJ, et al: Surgical management of left-sided carcinoid heart disease. Circulation 104:I36, 2001.
310. Simula DV, Edwards WD, Tazelaar HD, et al: Surgical pathology of carcinoid heart disease: A study of 139 valves from 75 patients spanning 20 years. Mayo Clin Proc 77:139, 2002.
311. Pandya UH, Pellikka PA, Enriquez-Sarano M, et al: Metastatic carcinoid tumor to the heart: Echocardiographic-pathologic study of 11 patients. J Am Coll Cardiol 40:1328, 2002.
312. Denney WD, Kemp WE, Jr., Anthony LB, et al: Echocardiographic and biochemical evaluation of the development and progression of carcinoid heart disease. J Am Coll Cardiol 32:1017, 1998.
313. Nield LE, Silverman ED, Taylor GP, et al: Maternal anti-Ro and anti-La antibody-associated endocardial fibroelastosis. Circulation 105:843, 2002.
314. Mahle WT, Weinberg PM, Rychik J: Can echocardiography predict the presence or absence of endocardial fibroelastosis in infants <1 year of age with left ventricular outflow obstruction? Am J Cardiol 82:122, 1998.
315. Ni J, Bowles NE, Kim YH, et al: Viral infection of the myocardium in endocardial fibroelastosis. Molecular evidence for the role of mumps virus as an etiologic agent. Circulation 95:133, 1997.
316. Jaeggi ET, Hamilton RM, Silverman ED, et al: Outcome of children with fetal, neonatal or childhood diagnosis of isolated congenital atrioventricular block. A single institution's experience of 30 years. J Am Coll Cardiol 39:130, 2002.
317. Nield LE, Silverman ED, Smallhorn JF, et al: Endocardial fibroelastosis associated with maternal anti-Ro and anti-La antibodies in the absence of atrioventricular block. J Am Coll Cardiol 40:796, 2002.

CHAPTER 60

Myocarditis

Kenneth Lee Baughman • Joshua Wynne

Myocarditis is one of the most challenging diagnoses in cardiology. The entity is rarely recognized, the pathophysiology is poorly understood, there is no commonly accepted diagnostic gold standard, and all current treatment is controversial. Primary myocarditis is presumed to be due to either an acute viral infection or a postviral autoimmune response. Secondary myocarditis is myocardial inflammation caused by a specific pathogen. These pathogens include bacteria, spirochetes, rickettsia, fungi, protozoa, drugs, chemicals, physical agents, and other inflammatory diseases such as systemic lupus erythematosus. We will first review primary myocarditis and then consider secondary causes.

Primary Myocarditis

Many viruses can cause myocarditis (Table 60–1), including those with RNA and DNA cores. As the ability to diagnose viral myocarditis has expanded with molecular techniques, an increasingly large number of viruses have been associated with cardiac inflammation and dilated cardiomyopathy. Historically, the RNA core virus Coxsackie has been identified most frequently as responsible for myocardial or pericardial inflammation. Coxsackie virus is a member of the picornavirus family, which also includes echovirus and polioviruses. Other responsible RNA core viruses include influenza (orthomyxovirus). Responsible DNA core viruses include adenovirus, herpesvirus (varicella zoster, cytomegalovirus, and Epstein-Barr virus), and poxvirus (variola and vaccinia).[1,2]

Pathophysiology

A viral infection of the heart follows a standard progression (Fig. 60–1). Most viral pathogens enter the body through the upper respiratory or gastrointestinal tract. Susceptibility to viral infection in humans is increased by malnutrition, exercise, age (young and old), stress, and hormones.[3,4] There are undoubtedly genetic susceptibilities that alter the autoimmune response to viral infections.

The typical viral infection produces a systemic viremia and associated vascular response on days 0 to 3. During this interval, the pathogenic virus can invade the myocardium and replicate in the myocyte, causing myocytolysis. In days 5 to 10 there is a generalized macrophage and IgM antibody response associated with a histological inflammatory infiltrate.[5] An antigen-specific IgG antibody response peaks by day 14 and is associated with histological evidence of myofiber dropout and interstitial fibrosis. Each of these sequential pathophysiological stages are reviewed in further detail.

DAYS 0 THROUGH 3. The offending virus enters the upper respiratory or gastrointestinal tract and replicates, causing typical symptoms. The virus then escapes the initial portal of entry immunological response and is transported in the bloodstream to other target organs. The infection in the lungs or gut initiates a cytokine response, which may activate the cardiac immune process. The invading viral pathogen must have a mechanism by which it can enter the cardiac cell. Coxsackie virus and adenovirus share a common receptor (Coxsackie adenoviral receptor, or CAR), which serves as the docking site for the pathogenic virus.[6] Coreceptors must be present for the virus to invade the myocardium. Once the coreceptor has facilitated the binding of the virus to the CAR, the virus is transported into the myocardial cell. Once in the cell, the virus can influence cell function and present myosin-like antigens (epitopes) on the cell surface.[7]

Nuclear Factor (NF) [κ] B. NF [κ] B is an intracellular transcription factor that, when activated by cytokines, viruses, oxidants, and protein kinase, induces the production of cytokines, intracellular adhesion molecules (ICAM), and inducible nitric oxide, which are involved in the inflammatory response to viral myocarditis.[8]

DAYS 3 THROUGH 14. Dendritic cells and macrophages are present in normal myocardium and are responsible for the initial antigen-independent response to viral invasion. These immune-response cells release cytokines, interleukins, perforin, reactive oxygen species, proteases, tumor necrosis factor (TNF), and regulatory growth factors, such as transforming growth factor-beta. Dendritic cells and macrophages ingest viral agents for subsequent processing.

The viral peptide fragments, or exposed myocardial membrane antigens, are processed in the Golgi apparatus and transported to the cell surface.[3,4] These epitopes are presented to T cells in collaboration with the major histocompatibility complex (MHC) antigen, ICAM-1, as well as costimulatory signals provided by various molecules, including CD40 (a member of the TNF superfamily).

TABLE 60–1 Infectious Causes of Myocarditis

Viral	Fungal
Adenovirus	*Actinomyces*
Arbovirus (dengue fever, yellow fever)	*Aspergillus*
Arenavirus (Lassa fever)	*Blastomyces*
Coxsackie virus	*Candida*
Cytomegalovirus	*Coccidioides*
Echovirus	*Cryptococcus*
Encephalomyocarditis virus	*Histoplasma*
Epstein-Barr virus	*Nocardia*
Hepatitis B	*Sporothrix*
Herpesvirus	**Rickettsial**
Human immunodeficiency virus-1	Rocky Mountain spotted fever
Influenza virus	Q fever
Mumps virus	Scrub typhus
Poliomyelitis virus	Typhus
Rabies	**Spirochetal**
Respiratory syncytial virus	*Borrelia* (Lyme disease and relapsing fever)
Rubella virus	*Leptospira*
Rubeola virus	Syphilis
Vaccinia virus	**Helminthic**
Varicella virus	*Cysticercus*
Variola virus	*Echinococcus*
Bacterial	*Schistosoma*
Brucellosis	*Toxocara* (visceral larva migrans)
Clostridia	*Trichinella*
Diphtheria	**Protozoal**
Francisella (tularemia)	*Entamoeba*
Gonococcus	*Leishmania*
Haemophilus	*Trypanosoma* (Chagas disease)
Legionella	Toxoplasmosis
Meningococcus	
Mycobacterium (tuberculosis, avium-intracellulare, leprae)	
Mycoplasma	
Pneumococcus	
Psittacosis	
Salmonella	
Staphylococcus	
Streptococcus	
Tropheryma whippleii (Whipple disease)	

From Pisani B, Taylor D, Mason J: Inflammatory myocardial disease and cardiomyopathies. Am J Med 102:459, 1997.

The first wave of response to myocarditis is brief and is determined by the cardiotropic features of the virus as well as by the nonspecific immune response from natural killer cells, cytokines, interferon, Fas/Fas ligand, TNF, matrix metalloproteinase, elastase, endothelium, interleukins, and proteins such as perforin and apolipoprotein J/clusterin.[9-14]

The second wave of response is immunological in nature. There is initially a nonspecific IgM and macrophage response driven by activation of local macrophages and dendritic cells. Upon activation, the CD4 T cells proliferate and differentiate into effector lymphocytes and macrophages.[5] Associated with this activation is the release of cytokines, including interferon-gamma, TNF, interleukin (IL)-2, IL-3, IL-4, IL-5, IL-6, and IL-10.[9,10] Cytokines have several functions, including further proliferation and differentiation of B-lymphocytes to produce antibodies, and proliferation and differentiation of T lymphocytes (both CD4 and CD8 cells) to attract additional macrophages, lymphocytes, and other cells to the antigen-producing area. CD8 lymphocytes attach to myocytes with appropriate antigens and lyse the cell, destroying cytoplasm and nucleus. Antibodies against the myocyte enhance lysis on the activated T cell. Ultimately, the immunological response is determined by the development of TH 1 (CD4) and TH 2 (CD8) cells specific for the antigen presented and production of IgG antibodies.[15] Neutralizing antiviral antibodies and infiltrating macrophages begin to clear the virus from the myocardium within 5 to 10 days after infection. As the antibody-producing B-lymphocytes increase, their T lymphocytic counterparts decrease over the course of several weeks.

The epitope responsible for the long-term autoimmune attack on patients with virally induced cardiomyopathy is unknown. It is considered that the Coxsackie B3 virus may have a similar antigen construct to myosin. Alternatively, damage to the myocyte membrane may expose myosin, which may then contribute to the autoimmune process. Most patients with viral myocarditis clear the virus and the infected cells with minimal fibrosis and no functional deterioration in their myocardium. Other patients display a variety of responses, varying from a transient depression of myocardial function to slow evolution of a dilated cardiomyopathy.[16]

NITRIC OXIDE

The nitric oxide (NO) system may have beneficial or adverse effects in cases of myocarditis.

Furchgott demonstrated that the vascular endothelium produces a relaxing factor, subsequently named NO.[17] Three forms of NO exist in humans; endothelial cell NO (type III), macrophage NO (type II), and neuronal NO (type I). NO is an intercellular messenger that can influence vessel relaxation, platelet adhesion, and endothelial cell as well as smooth muscle cell proliferation. Inducible NO synthase (NOS) and endothelial NOS have been studied in normal and failing hearts. In normal hearts, both forms of NOS are low. In heart failure, endothelial NOS is increased and localized in the subendocardial myocytes.[18] In failing hearts with myocarditis, inducible NOS is increased in macrophages.

Nitric oxide may enhance or suppress myocardial function. Coxsackie virus B3 produces a protease IIA that cleaves dystrophin on the cardiac membrane. Dystrophin is an integral membrane glycoprotein that, when disrupted, can interfere with mechanical force generation and result in altered membrane permeability, both of which may contribute to decreased myocardial function. Viral infections result in stimulation of interferon-alpha and interferon-gamma. These cytokines induce the production of NOS by macrophages, and increased NO indeed both depresses viral replication and inhibits protease IIA, preventing myocardial dysfunction.[19,20] Excess inducible NOS, however, results in peroxynitrite, a free radical that can cause cell death. NO also stimulates cGMP, which inhibits sarcolemmal L type calcium channels, which decreases the filament response to calcium. Therefore, excess NO can depress myocardial function.[21]

DAY 14 AND BEYOND. For many years, the etiology of the progression of myocarditis to dilated cardiomyopathy has been investigated but poorly understood. There are now data to suggest that this progression may be due to viral persistence, apoptosis, autoimmune, and/or structural effects.

Viral Persistence. Molecular cardiology techniques, including detection of viral RNA by slot-blot probe hybridization, in situ probe hybridization, or polymerase chain reaction (PCR) has allowed the demonstration of persistent virus particles in patients with dilated cardiomyopathy and acute myocarditis.[22,23] Viral persistence, even without the ability to multiply, can induce dilated cardiomyopathy when matched with an activated immune system.[22] In addition to the myocardium, there is a suggestion that the skeletal muscle system may serve as a reservoir for viral infection. The patient with a skeletal infection may be asymptomatic or have symptoms of peripheral muscle infection overwhelmed by symptoms from the heart.

Apoptosis. Apoptosis may be induced by viral-mediated proteases or differentially expressed genes (Nip 21) involved in cell death by activation of a caspase pathway.[24] In addition, cytokines have been demonstrated to remain elevated for greater than 80 days, even though they first appear by 3 days and peak by 7 days after infection.[25] Cytokine expression can depress cardiac function or induce apoptosis.

Immune Responses. Myosin and Coxsackie virus capsid protein share approximately 40% identity in their amino acid sequences. This may account for the molecular mimicry that directs immunological cells against myocytes. In some patients, it is likely that the autoimmune antibody mechanism induced does not autoregulate after the clearance of the virus. This continued immune activation and myosin destruction may cause myocardial dysfunction and vasospasm.

A final mechanism of acute and chronic myocardial damage is coronary microvascular spasm, resulting in myocyte necrosis, fibrosis, calcification, and ultimately, cardiac dilation.[26] Viruses associated with viral myocarditis also can infect endothelial cells. Endothelial cell antibodies have been identified in viral myocarditis and can contribute to microvascular spasm due to interruption of endothelial cell function or nitric oxide production.[26]

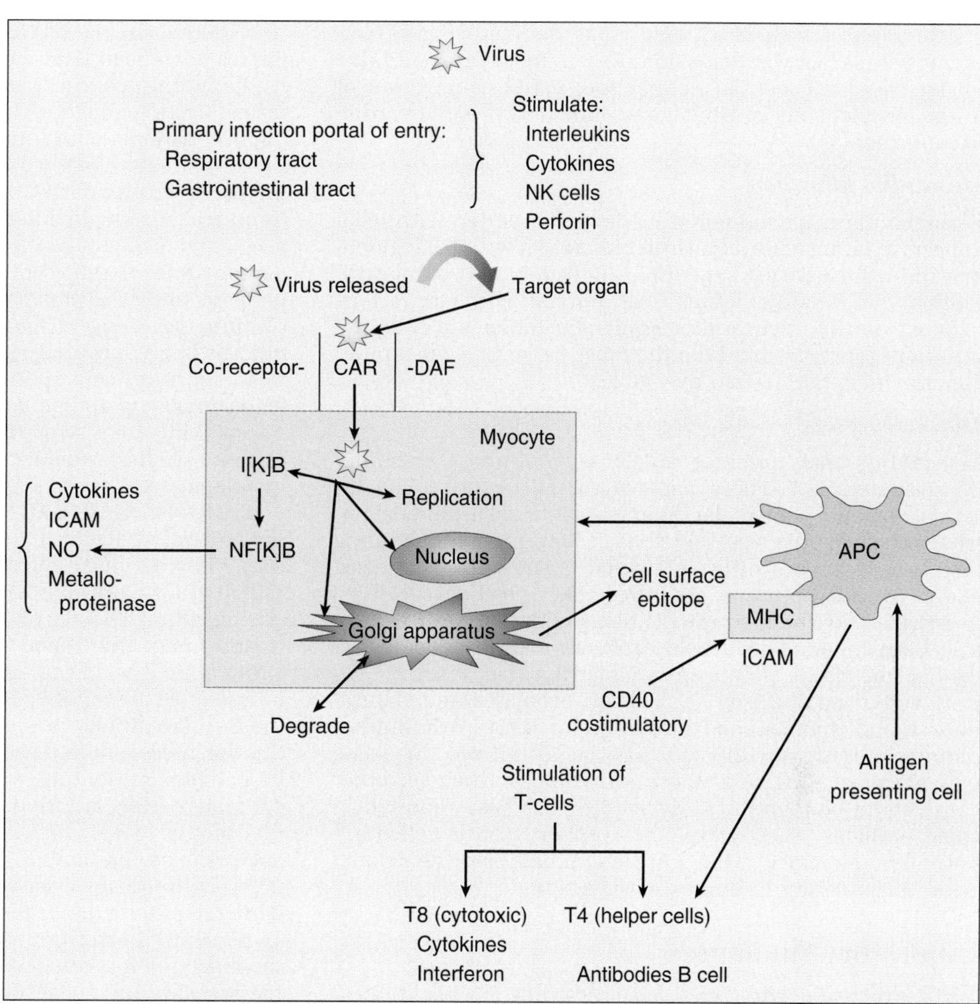

FIGURE 60–1 Pathophysiology of viral myocarditis. The virus enters the body through the respiratory or gastrointestinal tract stimulating a systemic immune response. The virus enters the myocytes through the CAR (Coxsackie adenoviral receptor) with coreceptors including DAF (decay accelerating factor). Once in the myocyte, the virus replicates and is transmitted to the nucleus, where it redirects cell activity and is released to the cell surface, where the virus can escape to infect additional cells. Dendritic cells and macrophages ingest foreign elements, including viruses, causing further enhancement of the immune response. Antigen-presenting cells expressing MHC (major histocompatibility complex) and associated with coreceptors ICAM and CD40 couple with infected myocytes displaying antigen (epitope) on their surface. The APC (antigen presenting cell) then stimulates cytotoxic cells capable of ingesting the myocyte surface or antibody-producing cells, which affect cell function or enhance membrane damage by cytotoxic cells. NK = natural killer; NO = nitric oxide.

Clinical Manifestations

Patients with myocarditis can develop a more spherical left ventricle, which is less efficient in myocardial contraction and mitral valve leaflet malcoaptation, causing additional myocardial functional deterioration.

Signs

In patients with viral myocarditis, the illness begins with the initial viral infection. The symptoms of the viral illness are due to the virus and its portal of entry (upper respiratory or gastrointestinal tract). After the viral illness, which may be unappreciated by the patient, there is a delay of days to weeks before cardiac symptoms appear, including congestive heart failure, arrhythmia (sometimes leading to sudden cardiac death), or embolic events. The latter are not infrequent in patients with acute inflammatory states because of the procoagulant effects of cytokines combined with decreased cardiac function and blood stasis.

Symptoms and signs of myocarditis and subsequent cardiac dysfunction may be protean. Symptoms include fatigue, dyspnea, chest pain (which may be pleuritic due to concomitant pericarditis), and palpitations. Signs can include sinus tachycardia, a diminished first heart sound due to decreased myocardial contraction, gallops, murmurs of mitral or tricuspid insufficiency, and, rarely, a pericardial friction rub.

Myocardial Infarction

Several authors have reported patients presenting with what appears to be an acute myocardial infarction with ST-segment elevation, positive CK and CK MB bands, and focal wall motion abnormalities (but with normal coronary arteriograms) due to myocarditis as demonstrated on endomyocardial biopsy.[27,28] Importantly, most patients' wall motion abnormalities normalized over time.[27]

Microaneurysms

Myocarditis may produce single or multiple ventricular microaneurysms.[29] These patients are characterized by (1) normal overall ventricular function, (2) nonsustained ventricular tachycardia, and (3) left heart biopsies demonstrating histological myocarditis in which standard right heart endomyocardial biopsies are infrequently positive.

Ventricular Tachycardia. Patients with myocarditis have also been reported to develop refractory ventricular tachycardia, torsade de pointes, or sudden cardiac death.[30,31] No prospective randomized trials have evaluated the natural history and spontaneous resolution of these arrhythmias. Immunosuppressive therapy has been utilized in some patients presenting with these arrhythmias when no other cause could be identified. Myocarditis has been reported in some athletes succumbing to sudden cardiac death.[32] Recently, refractory atrial fibrillation has been associated with inflammatory infiltrates in the atrium.[33]

Laboratory Findings

Electrocardiogram. The electrocardiogram is almost always abnormal in patients with myocarditis and may display changes of acute injury. More typical, however, are the presence of nonspecific ST-T wave changes. Any form of atrial or ventricular arrhythmia can be demonstrated, including atrial or ventricular premature beats, atrial or ventricular tachycardia, and atrioventricular fibrillation. In addition, patients with myocarditis may display atrial, ventricular, or intraventricular conduction delays.

Chest X-Ray. The cardiothoracic ratio is usually normal, particularly early in the illness before the development of a cardiomyopathy. Progressive compromise of left ventricular function may result in cardiomegaly. Elevation of filling pressures, regardless of the heart size, may result in findings of congestive heart failure including cephalization of blood flow or overt pulmonary edema.

Blood Studies. There are no characteristic findings on routine laboratory studies to confirm the diagnosis of myocarditis, although the white blood cell count is usually elevated.

Biomarkers of Myonecrosis. Myocardial enzymes are usually not elevated unless the patient presents acutely and displays a rapid deterioration. Cardiac specific troponin I elevation may be found in up to a third of patients, compared with less than 10% displaying CK elevations.[34] Patients with elevated enzyme levels tended to have symptoms of less than 1 month's duration.

Autoantibodies. Other immune markers have been evaluated as a means to confirm the diagnosis of myocarditis. Antibodies have been demonstrated to sarcolemma, myolemma, alpha-myosin, mitochondrial, and endothelial antigens. A number of cytokines have been demonstrated to be elevated in patients with progressive heart failure, including TNF, IL-6, and IgG3.[35,36]

NONINVASIVE STUDIES. Noninvasive imaging techniques have been used in an attempt to diagnose myocarditis, including echocardiography, nuclear scans, and magnetic resonance imaging (MRI). Echocardiography may help to identify patients with fulminant myocarditis at presentation. These patients usually have normal diastolic volumes and increased ventricular wall thickness (likely due to inflammation associated with interstitial edema).[37] Antimyosin scanning (when compared with endomyocardial biopsy) demonstrates a sensitivity of 83 percent, specificity of 53 percent, and a negative predictive value of 92 percent.[38] Gallium scanning demonstrates a sensitivity of only 36 percent but a specificity of 98 percent.[39] MRI has been used more recently; sensitivities of 100 percent and specificity between 90 and 100 percent have been claimed (Fig. 60–2).[40] These MRI data will require confirmation, particularly as most studies were accompanied by a limited number of histological analyses.

ENDOMYOCARDIAL BIOPSY. Because of the inadequacy of noninvasive means to establish the diagnosis of myocarditis, a histological diagnosis has been considered necessary to establish a secure diagnosis (which is especially important during clinical trials of therapeutic agents). The National Heart, Lung and Blood Institute Workshop reported that "idiopathic dilated cardiomyopathy is believed frequently to be a sequela of viral myocarditis, and the distinction between the two conditions is often obscured in clinical studies."[41] Studies have reported the frequency of finding myocarditis in patients presenting with cardiomyopathy or new-onset congestive heart failure who were submitted to endomyocardial biopsy to vary between 0 and 63 percent.[42,43] This variance reflects the lack of established histological criteria for myocarditis in most early studies. Later series, using standardized criteria, have displayed a prevalence between 9 and 15 percent.[44] In addition, some patients have improvement in their ejection fraction despite having negative biopsy findings for myocarditis, suggesting that they may have had myocarditis that was not histologically documented. Those with myocarditis more often have had a preceding flu-like illness,

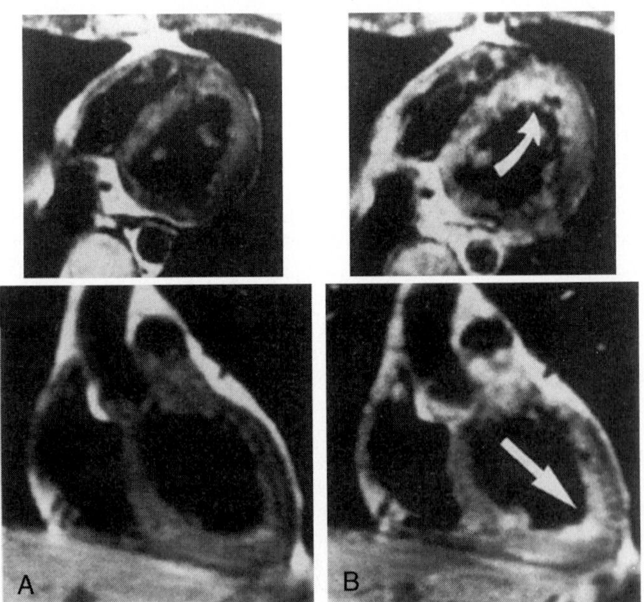

FIGURE 60–2 **A,** Precontrast T1-weighted transaxial **(upper)** and coronal **(lower)** magnetic resonance images through the left ventricle in a patient with myocarditis. **B,** Postcontrast magnetic resonance images at the same levels after contrast injection. Note enhancement of the myocardial signal in the septum and apical region (arrows). (From Matsouka H, Hamada M, Honda T, et al: Evaluation of acute myocarditis and pericarditis by Gd-DTPA enhanced magnetic resonance imaging. Eur Heart J 15:283, 1994.)

are younger, and are less frequently male, as compared with patients with idiopathic or ischemic cardiomyopathy.[44]

HISTOLOGICAL CRITERIA FOR MYOCARDITIS

In 1986, eight expert cardiac pathologists met in Dallas, Texas to establish a histopathological definition and classification for myocarditis. This classification scheme has subsequently been termed the "Dallas criteria" and has been utilized as the standard for the histological diagnosis in all subsequent studies of myocarditis (Fig. 60–3).[45] The authors defined myocarditis as "a process characterized by an inflammatory infiltrate of the myocardium with necrosis and/or degeneration of adjacent myocytes not typical of ischemic damage associated with coronary artery disease." Criteria were established to diagnose myocarditis, borderline myocarditis, or no myocarditis in the initial biopsy specimens.

Myocarditis requires an inflammatory infiltrate and damage to adjacent myocytes confirmed by light microscopy. The myocardial inflammation, both by amount and distribution, can be characterized as mild, moderate, or severe and focal, confluent, or diffuse, respectively. Similarly, the type of inflammatory infiltrate is subclassified as lymphocytic, neutrophilic, eosinophilic, giant cell, granulomatous, or mixed. Borderline myocarditis "implies the inflammatory infiltrate is too sparse, or damage to the myocyte is not demonstrable by light microscopy or both."[45] *Borderline myocarditis* does not allow an unequivocal diagnosis of myocarditis to be established, and the panel suggested re-biopsy in these cases.

Despite these seemingly straightforward criteria, subsequent publications have documented substantial interobserver and intraobserver variability. Although the endomyocardial biopsy has been considered to be the gold standard, studies have demonstrated the difficulty in making the diagnosis of myocarditis because of its focal nature.[46] Endomyocardial biopsies were performed in postmortem hearts from patients who had died from myocarditis, and the ability to establish the diagnosis was assessed. With only one biopsy of the endomyocardium in these patients with known myocarditis, histological confirmation was possible in only 17 to 28 percent of patients. With more than five biopsies, approximately two-thirds of patients had a histological diagnosis of myocarditis established. Inclusion of borderline myocarditis increased the yield by an additional 10 to 15 percent. Therefore, with approximately five biopsies, the potential to make the diagnosis of myocarditis or borderline myocarditis (when it is present) is approximately 75 to 80 percent.

Additional studies can be performed on each histological biopsy specimen to enhance the potential to establish the diagnosis of myocarditis. Common leukocyte antigen staining ensures that the mononuclear cells present in the specimen are of white cell origin. Mononuclear cells can

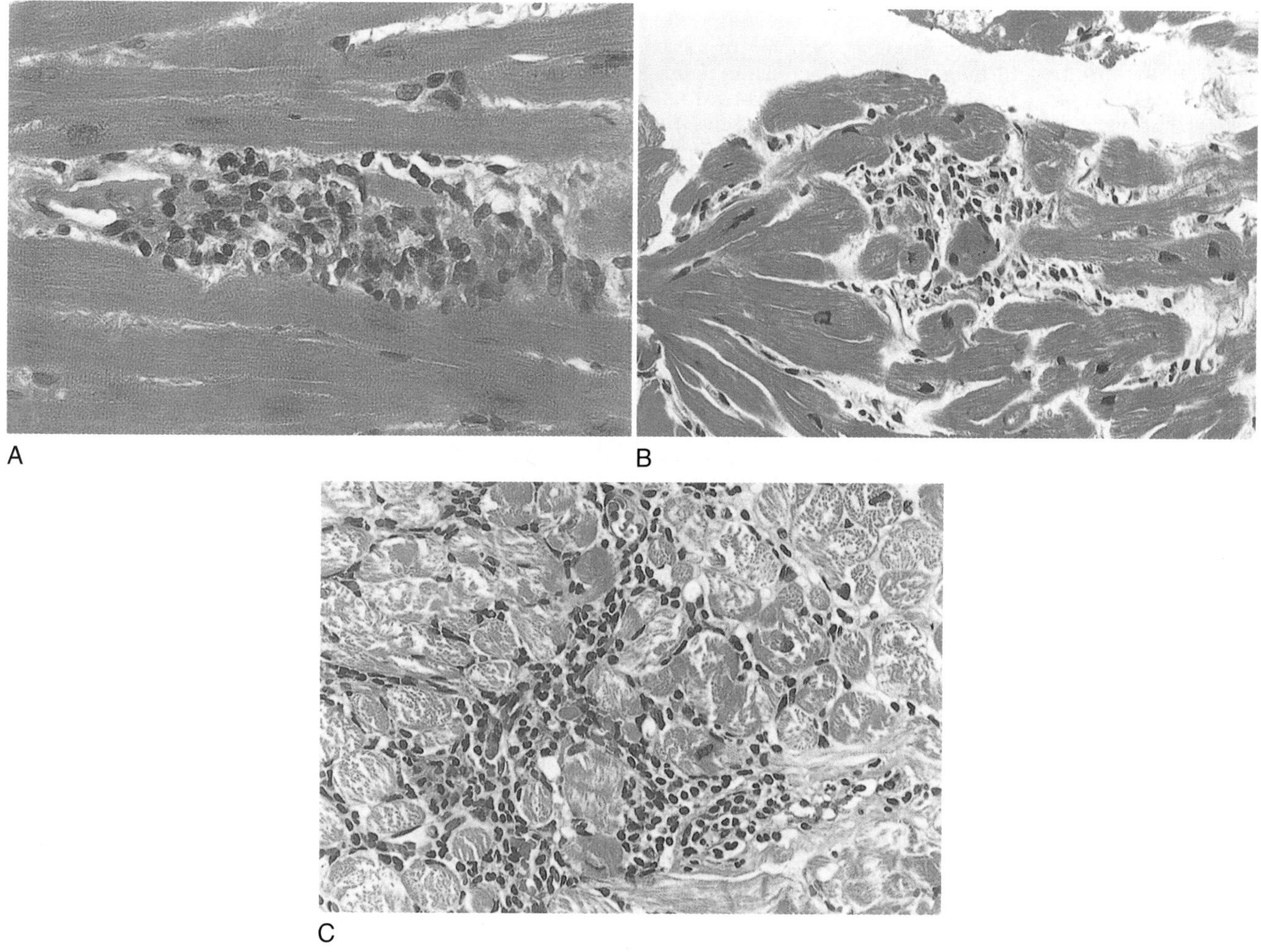

FIGURE 60–3 The diagnosis of myocarditis requires histological examination of myocardial tissue. This tissue can be obtained through endomyocardial biopsy of the interventricular septum. **A,** In this sample, longitudinally oriented myocytes are engulfed centrally by lymphocytes causing destruction of myocardial tissue. Often, sites examined immediately adjacent to the involved myofibrils appear normal. On initial biopsy, active myocarditis is defined as an inflammatory infiltrate of the myocardium with necrosis or degeneration of myocytes not typical of the ischemic changes associated with coronary artery disease. **B,** Borderline myocarditis (Dallas criteria). Borderline myocarditis is diagnosed when the inflammatory infiltrate is sparse or when myocyte damage is not demonstrated under light microscopy. This specimen demonstrates a limited mononuclear cell infiltrate not resulting in myocyte necrosis. Heart tissue from patients with idiopathic dilated cardiomyopathy reveals increased interstitial cellularity associated with myocyte hypertrophy and interstitial fibrosis (common features of myocardial response to stress). **C,** Some features of subtle myocyte degenerative changes that reflect irreversible myocyte damage. In addition to frank myocyte necrosis (see part **A**), this figure demonstrates a focus of interstitial inflammatory cells surrounding individual myocytes and small myocyte clusters. Myocytes with inflammatory cells immediately adjacent to their plasma membrane contain membrane vacuoles and irregular surface outlines. These morphological changes are similar to those noted in experimental postviral murine myocarditis during the early phases of myocyte injury. (From Herskowitz A, Ansari AA: Myocarditis. *In* Abelmann WH [ed]: Cardiomyopathies, myocarditis and pericardial disease. *In* Braunwald E [series ed]. Atlas of Heart Diseases. Vol. 2. Philadelphia, Current Medicine, 1995.)

represent myocyte nuclei, endothelial cells, or fibrous tissue. Major histocompatibility complex (MHC) antigens should be expressed in patients when there is immune upregulation. MHC class I molecules are present to some extent in virtually all nucleated cells, whereas MHC class II molecules are confined to immune system cells. In cases of myocarditis, both MHC class I and II antigens are markedly upregulated and have been used by some investigators as surrogates for the Dallas criteria for myocarditis, because MHC upregulation is more diffuse than histological inflammatory infiltrates.[47] Other histological markers of immune upregulation are being investigated, including CD40 antigen expression, NK cell and perforin upregulation, and apoptosis.[48-50]

The spontaneous improvement of some patients with Dallas criteria-negative myocarditis, the difficulties noted in establishing the histological diagnosis of myocarditis in patients with known myocarditis, and the subsequent demonstration of causative viruses by PCR in patients with histologically negative myocarditis have confirmed how rudimentary the reliance on inflammatory infiltrates or myocyte destruction has been to establish a diagnosis of myocarditis.

Antibodies are produced against important portions of the myocyte membrane (myosin, laminin, beta receptor) and mitochondria (adenine nucleotide translocator and branched chain ketoacid dehydrogenase), which may well contribute to cardiac dysfunction in this population.[51,52]

Clinical Pathological Classification of Myocarditis

In 1991, we proposed a classification system for primary (postviral) myocarditis that included fulminant, acute, (subacute) chronic active, and chronic persistent myocarditis, much as had been previously accepted for acute hepatitis (Table 60–2).[53] Patients with secondary myocarditis were excluded from this histopathological classification, including those with peripartum cardiomyopathy, human immunodeficiency virus (HIV)-related myocarditis, sarcoidosis, systemic lupus erythematosus, and ischemia with inflammation. Patients with primary myocarditis were differentiated based on their onset of illness, left ventricular function at the time of presentation, endomyocardial biopsy findings at presentation, and clinical and histological outcomes.

FULMINANT MYOCARDITIS. Patients with fulminant myocarditis have a distinct onset of the condition, usually within days of the well-identified viral illness. They present with severe left ventricular dysfunction, often cardiogenic shock requiring pressors or artificial mechanical support.[54] The left ventricles are usually not dilated, but rather thick-walled, likely a manifestation of interstitial edema. Endomyocardial biopsies in the fulminant category are unequivocally positive with severe inflammatory infiltrates and myocyte necrosis. Despite their severe decompensation at presentation, these patients typically either recover completely or die within a period of 2 weeks. Survivors show histological resolution of their myocarditis, and their hearts return to normal size and function in follow-up.

SUBACUTE MYOCARDITIS. Patients with subacute myocarditis have an indistinct onset of the disease with no clearly defined initial viral illness. They present with moderately severe ventricular dysfunction but usually mild dilation. Their biopsies reveal active or borderline myocarditis, and evidence of inflammation is often difficult to find. These patients have incomplete recovery or go on to develop progressive dilated cardiomyopathy despite complete resolution by biopsy of any inflammation. This group may have viral persistence based on the work of other investigators.

CHRONIC ACTIVE MYOCARDITIS. Patients with this form of myocarditis typically have distinctive features. Their onset is indistinct and similar to that of subacute myocarditis and they present with similar degrees of moderate left ventricular dysfunction and mild left ventricular dilation. Their biopsies at presentation and in follow-up reveal a combination of active myocarditis and active healing. Over the course of these patients' illnesses (usually 2 to 3 years), this pattern of inflammation and scarring persists and the patients ultimately develop a nondilated restrictive cardiomyopathy (see Chap. 59) with evidence of giant cell formation.

CHRONIC PERSISTENT MYOCARDITIS. Patients with chronic persistent myocarditis are usually submitted to biopsy because of non-heart failure–related symptoms of atypical chest pain or palpitations. They have no distinct onset to their illness and usually have a history of many months or years of cardiac complaints. They have no left ventricular dysfunction despite having active or borderline myocarditis on biopsy. Their clinical history is one of continued symptomatology and persistently normal left ventricular function despite ongoing inflammation.

PROGNOSIS. A follow-up study of patients with fulminant myocarditis reveals that once past the initial presentation, these patients do well and have virtually no cardiac-related morbidity or mortality (Fig. 60–4).[54] Patients with subacute myocarditis, whether meeting Dallas criteria or displaying borderline myocarditis have the same relatively poor prognosis as those with dilated cardiomyopathy. Interestingly, the rate of presentation of patients with fulminant myocarditis remained relatively constant over time, whereas the number of patients presenting with acute myocarditis declined over the period of case collection.[54] The latter finding is a mirror image of the frequency of nonpolio enteroviral infections documented by the Centers for Disease Control and Prevention over the same time interval. This suggests that there is a correlation between enteroviral infections and subacute myocarditis, which appears not to be present in patients with fulminant myocarditis. In view of their excellent long-term recovery, patients with fulminant myocarditis must be supported with whatever means necessary to provide them an opportunity to recover. This may include pressors, intraaortic balloon counterpulsation, or left ventricular assist device.[55]

TABLE 60–2 Histopathological Myocarditis Classification*

	Fulminant	Subacute	Chronic Active	Chronic Persistent
Onset	Distinct	Indistinct	Indistinct	Indistinct
Left ventricular function	Severe dysfunction	Moderate dysfunction	Moderate dysfunction	No dysfunction
Biopsy	Multiple foci	Active or borderline	Active or borderline	Active or borderline
Clinical history	Recovery or death	Incomplete dilated cardiomyopathy	Restrictive cardiomyopathy	Normal left ventricular function
Histological outcome	Complete resolution	Complete resolution	Giant cells-fibrosis	Ongoing

*Primary myocarditis is classified by clinical presentation, initial left ventricular (LV) size and function, results of endomyocardial biopsy, clinical outcome, and histological outcome into the following categories: fulminant, subacute, chronic active, and chronic persistent myocarditis. Other forms of myocarditis include giant cell myocarditis and eosinophilic myocarditis.

From Lieberman EB, Hutchins GM, Herskowitz A, et al: Clinicopathologic description of myocarditis. J Am Coll Cardiol 18:1617, 1991.

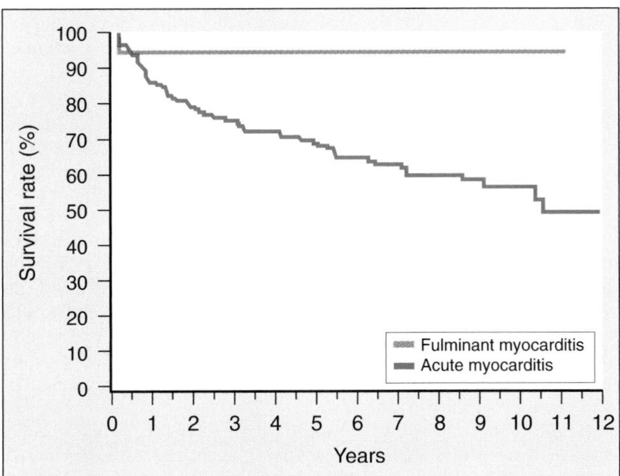

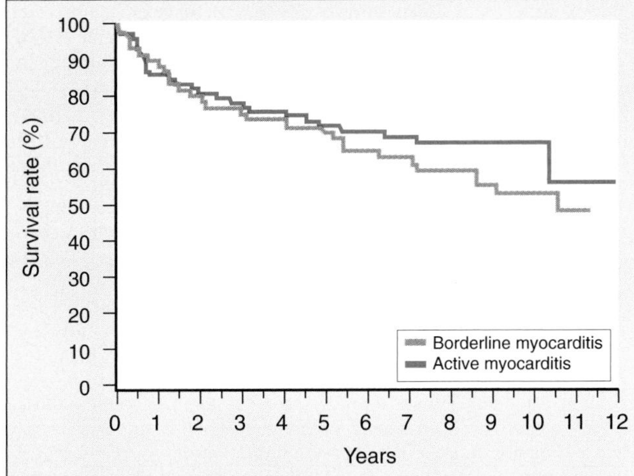

FIGURE 60–4 **A,** Unadjusted transplantation-free survival according to clinicopathological classification. Patients with fulminant myocarditis were significantly less likely to die or require heart transplantation during follow-up than were patients with acute myocarditis ($p = 0.05$ by the log-rank test). **B,** Unadjusted transplantation-free survival according to the Dallas histopathological criteria. Long-term survival did not differ significantly according to the degree of inflammation on biopsy ($p = 0.38$ by the log-rank test). (Modified from McCarthy RE 3rd, Boehmer JP, Hruban RH, et al: Long-term outcome of fulminant myocarditis as compared with acute (nonfulminant) myocarditis. N Engl J Med 342:690, 2000.)

RISKS OF ENDOMYOCARDIAL BIOPSY

In our experience, approximately 6% of those with new-onset congestive heart failure or dilated cardiomyopathy have a complication with myocardial biopsy.[56] Approximately one-half of these complications are related to venous access and the remainder to the biopsy procedure itself. Access complications include inadvertent arterial puncture, pneumothorax, vasovagal reaction, or bleeding after sheath removal.

Complications associated with the procedure include arrhythmias, cardiac conduction abnormalities, and heart perforation. Heart perforation can cause pericardial tamponade and, rarely, death. Patients with perforation report pain, which otherwise should not be experienced during the procedure. These patients may deteriorate rapidly, in part due to their degree of myocardial decompensation at the initiation of the procedure, and the rapid accumulation of blood in the pericardial space. Additionally, the rapid accumulation of blood in the pericardial space can form a clot acutely, which may interfere with pericardial evacuation attempted percutaneously. Patients who cannot be immediately resuscitated by percutaneous pericardiocentesis should have open chest evacuation of the hematoma. This requires coordination with cardiovascular surgery and preparation in the laboratory for the occurrence of these rare, but expected, complications.

The use of ultrasonographically guided techniques to identify the internal jugular vein and/or guide in vein cannulation improves the success rate and decreases the complication rate and access time.[57] The complication rate with biopsies via the femoral vein is at least equivalent to that experienced with a jugular venous procedure. Performance of left ventricular biopsies shares similar perforation complication rates, despite the greater wall thickness of the left ventricle.

Treatment

The treatment of myocarditis is controversial, and no specific therapeutic regimen has been established. All patients with myocarditis should limit their physical activity, receive standard heart failure therapy, have their arrhythmia suppressed (if indicated), and avoid vascular spasm. There have been no studies of exercise compared with rest in the management of patients with myocarditis. In animal models, acute exercise in the face of an active viral infection increases viral replication and shortens survival.[2] Patients therefore are advised to moderately limit their activities. Although activities of daily living are allowed, patients should not "work up a sweat" in sustained physical exertion. Patient should be treated for heart failure with appropriate medications, as outlined in other chapters. This includes diuretics to lower symptomatic preload excess, afterload reduction therapy (particularly with angiotensin-converting enzyme inhibitors), and beta blockers for both arrhythmia management and in hopes of improving myocardial function. Because vascular spasm is a component of myocarditis, agents that precipitate or exacerbate vascular spasm should be avoided. This may include the use of digoxin.

It has been hypothesized from animal models that calcium channel blockers are beneficial, by preventing microvascular spasm or inhibiting nitric oxide production, decreasing viral replication, decreasing T-cell activation, and diminishing interleukin production; however, there are no adequate studies upon which to base recommendations.[58] Beta blockers can stabilize myocardial membranes and prevent arrhythmia, provide antioxidants, or stimulate interleukins.[59] Angiotensin-converting enzyme inhibitors can decrease oxygen demand, protein synthesis, cardiac mass, fibrosis, inflammation, and free radical injury and, through bradykinin, dilate coronary arteries.[60]

Immunosuppressive Therapy

Immunosuppressive therapy has been proposed to treat myocarditis and new-onset cardiomyopathy in both children and adults. As hypothesized in animal models, immunoglobulin may provide an antibody to the specific virus responsible for the illness or cause a nonspecific immune response with downregulation of cytokines. Although early studies in children and adults were encouraging, the data were not from prospective, randomized trials and not all patients were submitted to endomyocardial biopsy; furthermore, the immunoglobulin treatment was not controlled.[61]

Ultimately, a multicenter prospective randomized trial in patients with new-onset cardiomyopathy (less than 6 months) and symptomatic congestive heart failure was performed.[62] All 62 patients were biopsied and only 16 percent had histological Dallas criteria myocarditis. The improvement in the ejection fraction for both treated and control groups was substantial, with a baseline ejection fraction of 25 percent rising to 41 percent in the short term and 42 percent at 1-year follow-up. The responses in both the immunoglobulin-treated and standard populations were statistically identical, and the 1-year survival rates were 92 and 88 percent, respectively. Thus, intravenous immunoglobulin therapy does *not* appear to be beneficial for adult patients with new-onset cardiomyopathy and presumed myocarditis.

Immunosuppressive therapy has been studied more extensively than any other form of treatment for myocarditis. In 1984, a compilation of 82 patients with biopsy-proven myocarditis culled from nine series was published.[63] Forty-nine of the 82 patients were reported to improve on immunosuppressive therapy (60 percent), whereas 33 percent reported no significant change and 5 percent deteriorated. Of note, however, only 1 of 21 patients (5 percent) with an acute presentation appeared to respond, whereas 20 of 22 patients with chronic disease states (91 percent) responded with an improvement in symptoms. This observation is in keeping with later reports of the inadvisability of treatment of patients with fulminant myocarditis with immunosuppressive therapy compared with the potential benefit in those with an immune complex–driven depression of heart function.

Based on these observations, two important prospective randomized trials were conducted. Parillo at the National Institutes of Health reported in 1989 the response of 102 patients with established dilated cardiomyopathy to prednisone treatment.[64] Although there was an initial improvement in the prednisone group, particularly in patients with "reactive" heart biopsies, by 9 months the increase in ejection fraction had reversed. Therefore, there seems little benefit to treating patients with an established cardiomyopathy with immunosuppressive therapy.

THE MYOCARDITIS TREATMENT TRIAL

The results of an international trial termed the Myocarditis Treatment Trial (Fig. 60–5) were reported in 1995.[65] The investigators evaluated 2233 candidates with a clinical syndrome compatible with myocarditis. Two hundred and fourteen had compatible biopsies with Dallas criteria myocarditis determined by local pathologists' interpretation. Of the 214 potential candidates for the trial, 30 were excluded with ejection fractions greater than 45 percent, 44 patients met other exclusion criteria, and 29 declined enrollment. The trial was, therefore, based on evaluation of 111 patients, with only 64 percent confirmed as having myocarditis on review by the expert panel of pathologists. Treatment was randomized to placebo versus prednisone and cyclosporin. (An initial treatment arm using prednisone and azathioprine was terminated because of low enrollment.) At 1 and 5 years of follow-up, there was no difference in survival (80 and 44 percent, respectively, for both groups combined). There was also no difference in heart function in the treated or placebo group at 28 weeks. The treated group showed an increase in ejection fraction from 24 to 34 percent, and the control group went from 26 to 32 percent.

Despite the negative results of this trial, the authors indicated that patients who responded appeared to have higher initial ejection fractions and a shorter duration of illness. The Myocarditis Treatment Trial had a sobering effect on the subsequent evaluation of myocarditis in the United States and markedly diminished the enthusiasm for endomyocardial biopsy.

OTHER TRIALS OF IMMUNOSUPPRESSIVE THERAPY

Additional data may help identify a population of patients with myocarditis who may benefit from immunosuppressive therapy. In 1984, it was suggested in a pre-Dallas criteria retrospective review that patients with more chronic forms of inflammation appear to respond more favorably to immunosuppressive therapy.[63] We evaluated 20 patients with biopsy-proven myocarditis or borderline myocarditis.[66] Both groups were treated with prednisone and azathioprine for 6 to 8 weeks and underwent repeat endomyocardial biopsy, right heart catheterization, and echocardiogram. Patients with borderline myocarditis had a greater increase in their ejection fractions in follow-up and more dramatic improvement in heart rate–corrected velocity of circumferential fiber shortening by echocardiography.

Another author recently reported the results of 84 patients with presumed myocarditis of 202 patients with cardiomyopathy evaluated by endomyocardial biopsy.[67] Patients with myocarditis were defined by demonstration of upregulation of the HLA antigen by endomyocardial biopsy rather than Dallas criteria. These patients were randomized to receive immunosuppression or a placebo. The primary endpoint of the trial (i.e., death, transplant, or hospitalization) was no different in the treated patients compared with the placebo group. The ejection fraction in the immunosuppressive group increased from 24 to 36 percent, however, while it remained virtually constant (25-27 percent) in the control group. Additionally, at the 3-month follow-up clinical improvement was noted in 72 percent of immunosuppressed patients but only 31 percent of control subjects. In another important recent trial, Italian investigators found myocarditis in 112 of 652 patients with new-onset cardiomyopathy submitted to biopsy.[68] Forty-one of these 112 patients had progressive congestive heart failure despite standard medical treatment for heart failure. These 41 patients were treated with prednisone and azathioprine. The authors noted that 20 patients responded and 21 had no response. The responders increased their ejection fraction from 26 to 47 percent and showed healed myocarditis on repeat biopsy. The 20 nonresponders showed a progressive histological evolution to dilated cardiomyopathy; 12 remained unchanged, while 3 underwent cardiac transplantation and 5 died. Cardiac autoantibodies were present in 90 percent of patients who responded and 0 percent of the nonresponders. On the other hand, viral genome was present in 85 percent of the nonresponders (enterovirus, Epstein-Barr virus, influenza A virus, and parvovirus-B19). The three responders with viral genome were all positive for hepatitis C.

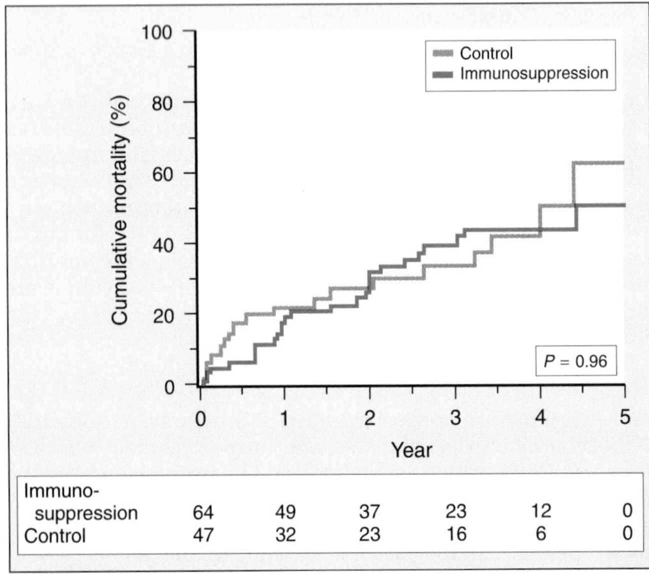

FIGURE 60–5 Actuarial mortality (defined as deaths and cardiac transplantations) in the immunosuppression and control groups. The numbers of patients at risk are shown at the bottom. There was no significant difference in mortality between the two groups. (Modified from Mason JW, O'Connell JB, Herskowitz A, et al: A clinical trial of immunosuppressive therapy for myocarditis. The Myocarditis Treatment Trial Investigators. N Engl J Med 333:269, 1995.)

The findings summarized indicate that patients with fulminant myocarditis should not be treated with immunosuppressive therapy, as their clinical course usually is one of spontaneous recovery. Patients with fulminant myocarditis, in particular, may require short-term support with intraaortic balloon counterpulsation or left ventricular assist devices. A number of case reports have documented the efficacy of this therapeutic option.[69,70] Recently, use of percutaneous cardiopulmonary support has been reported, and current trials are ongoing that compare intraaortic balloon counterpulsation with this form of cardiopulmonary support. Patients with well-established dilated cardiomyopathies do not respond to immunosuppressive therapy. There is undoubtedly a group with chronic myocardial inflammation who do respond to immunosuppressive therapy. Current data suggest that these patients have an active immune process and do not have viral persistence. Undoubtedly, our ability to identify this group of patients will improve with future investigation of endomyocardial biopsies and autoantibodies. Currently, immunosuppression therapy cannot be recommended for patients without histological confirmation of myocarditis, and then only in those who have failed to improve on standardized heart failure treatment.

Immunoabsorption of circulating antibodies in patients with myocarditis and/or dilated cardiomyopathy has been evaluated.[71] Short-term and intermediate-term studies have demonstrated the efficacy of this form of treatment, and larger prospective randomized trials are pending.

Finally, some investigators have suggested that antiviral vaccines to combat heart disease may be technologically possible, concentrating on frequently encountered viruses, including Coxsackie, adenovirus, and enteroviruses.[72]

In summary, myocarditis remains an important entity and may be a precursor to dilated cardiomyopathy in an unknown number of patients. Endomyocardial biopsy remains the key to establishing the diagnosis. Only now is our understanding of the pathophysiology adequate to allow evaluation of appropriate methods of treatment.

Giant Cell Myocarditis

CLINICAL FEATURES. Giant cell myocarditis is a relatively rare form of myocarditis first described in 1905. By 1997, only 80 cases had been reported, usually at autopsy.[73] Affected patients have an average age of 43 years, but infants as young as 6 weeks and adults as old as 88 years have been affected with the disorder. Approximately 90 percent are white. Men and women are equally affected. Patients present with rapidly progressive congestive heart failure or arrhythmias. The arrhythmias may be difficult-to-control ventricular arrhythmias or, less frequently, complete heart block. Rarely, patients present as if they are in the throes of an acute myocardial infarction.

Nearly 20 percent of patients have some other autoimmune disease, including Hashimoto thyroiditis, rheumatoid arthritis, myasthenia gravis, Takayasu arteritis, alopecia, vitiligo, pernicious anemia, Crohn disease, ulcerative colitis, idiopathic thrombocytopenic purpura, orbital myositis, and celiac disease.[74-76] The histological entity can also be associated with drug reactions and eosinophils,[77] but it is unclear whether the survival characteristics are similar for this category.[73]

Diagnosis. Patients are diagnosed by endomyocardial biopsy. The pathological assessment reveals widespread serpiginous necrosis and multifocal inflammation consisting of lymphocytes, histiocytes, and eosinophils (Fig. 60–6). Multinucleated giant cells without granuloma (particularly at the margins in the areas of myocyte necrosis) are found and characterize the condition histologically. There are conflicting reports as to whether the T cells are primarily CD4 (helper) or CD8 (cytotoxic) cells.[73] Endomyocardial biopsy has a sensitivity of approximately 80 percent in establishing the diagnosis of giant cell myocarditis in patients who are affected.[78]

Patients with giant cell myocarditis must be evaluated for bacterial, fungal, protozoal, and cytomegaloviral infection. These patients must be differentiated from those with cardiac sarcoidosis. The clinical presentation is usually dramatically different.[79,80] Patients with giant cell myocarditis have rapidly progressive symptomatology, whereas those with sarcoidosis (absent sudden cardiac death and heart block) usually present in a less abrupt fashion. Patients with giant cell myocarditis are usually white and sarcoidosis patients are usually black. Sarcoidosis patients usually present more frequently with syncope and less profound congestive heart failure. Their prognosis is much better than that of patients with giant cell myocarditis. Histologically, patients with sarcoidosis and giant cell myocarditis both have giant cells; however, only in the former case are noncaseating granulomas seen. Patients with giant cell myocarditis have myocyte destruction and, by most studies, cytotoxic CD8 cells. Sarcoidosis patients tend to have an interstitial disease without myocyte necrosis.[80]

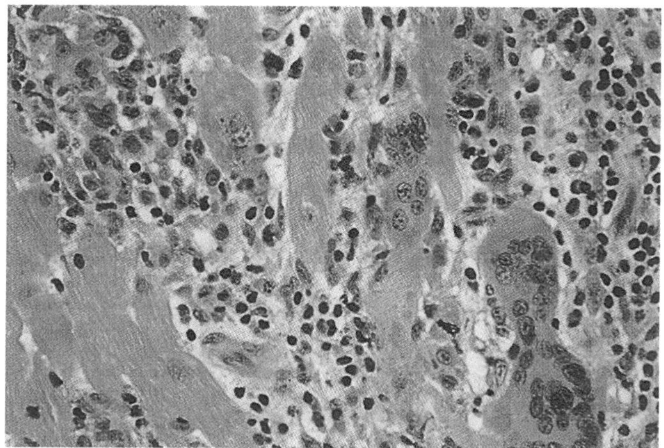

FIGURE 60–6 Giant cell myocarditis. A mixed inflammatory infiltrate, multinucleated giant cells, and extensive myocyte damage. (From Winters GL, McManus BM: Myocarditis. *In* Silver MD, et al [eds]: Cardiovascular Pathology. 3rd ed. New York, Churchill Livingstone, 2001, p 269.

PROGNOSIS. The survival of patients with giant cell myocarditis is markedly limited. In a multicenter natural history study reported by Cooper, the average survival was only 5.5 months from the onset of symptoms.[73] Cooper and others have reported an improvement in prognosis with immunosuppressive therapy. In Cooper's original study, the survival with no immunosuppressive agents was only 3 months. With use of corticosteroids alone, the survival was only 3.8 months. Additional immunosuppressive therapy (combining cyclosporin, azathioprine, or OKT_3) improved the survival to 12.3 months.[81] A subsequent report found the transplant-free survival to be 33 months in patients with combined therapy compared with patients receiving no immunosuppression. Case reports have suggested that high-dose multidrug immunosuppressive treatment may be beneficial, even to the point of including OKT_3, cyclosporin, azathioprine, and corticosteroids.[82,83] These observations are preliminary, and patients with giant cell myocarditis should be entered into the ongoing treatment trial to determine the most effective management strategy. Unfortunately, the small number of patients affected makes such a trial difficult to conduct.

Some patients are so severely affected that they will need support with a left ventricular assist device or intraaortic balloon counterpulsation as a "bridge" to transplant.[84] Thirty-eight patients with giant cell myocarditis have been reported to undergo cardiac transplantation.[85] Nine of the 38 patients had recurrence of giant cells in their endomyocardial biopsies, usually associated with rejection. This recurrence may appear up to 9 years after the transplant, but on average occurs approximately 3 years afterward. The recurrence of giant cells is usually responsive to immunosuppressive therapy in the transplanted population.

Arrhythmogenic Right Ventricular Dysplasia

Arrhythmogenic right ventricular dysplasia is discussed in Chapter 32.

Specific Agents Causing Myocarditis

Secondary Viral Myocarditis

A large number of viral pathogens cause human myocarditis. As the ability to diagnose viral causes by molecular analysis of endomyocardial biopsies has expanded, our appreciation of the frequency of myocarditis causing acute and chronic left ventricular dysfunction is increasing. The pathophysiology of secondary myocarditis is not well established but, as with primary myocarditis, is assumed to be a combination of direct viral toxicity and autoimmune damage. The pathological condition varies, depending on the cardiotrophic nature of the viral agent as well as the inflammatory and immune response, but includes lymphocytic infiltrates with myocyte damage and varying degrees of hypertrophy and fibrosis. Electrocardiographic abnormalities are common and include arrhythmias, heart block, and interventricular conduction delays. Noninvasive studies of patients with viral myocarditis document the severity of the associated left ventricular compromise and presence or absence of pericarditis. Treatment is symptomatic in most cases and is outlined in the previous section. Fortunately, most patients with secondary myocarditis resolve their illness spontaneously; however, most if not all viral agents may cause cardiomyopathy and fatalities.

HUMAN IMMUNODEFICIENCY VIRUS. See Chapter 61.

COXSACKIE VIRUS (see Primary Myocarditis). Both Coxsackie viruses A and B can produce myocarditis, although infection with coxsackie virus B is more common. Coxsackie virus B is the most frequent cause of viral myocarditis, causing more than half the cases.[86,87]

Although most infections are benign, self-limited, and subclinical, Coxsackie viral myocarditis appears to be particularly virulent in the neonate, child, and young adult. In most infections in adults, the other clinical manifestations of viral involvement predominate, such as pleurodynia, myalgia, upper respiratory tract symptoms, and arthralgias. Severe cases in the adult are characterized by myopericardial involvement with pleuritic or pericarditic chest pain, palpitations, and fever. Patients with overt myocardial involvement develop congestive heart failure with cardiomegaly and pulmonary edema.

Most patients recover completely within weeks, although the electrocardiogram (ECG) and ventricular function may require months to return to normal. Rarely, Coxsackie viral myocarditis is fatal in adults. Some patients become symptomatic after resolution of the infection, and they may present years later with dilated cardiomyopathy.[88]

Treatment. Patients with myocarditis are predisposed to ventricular and atrial thrombi due to procoagulant effects of cytokines and vascular stasis. Anticoagulation is recommended unless patients have associated pericarditis, which increases the risk for hemorrhagic pericardial tamponade.

CYTOMEGALOVIRUS. Unrecognized infection with cytomegalovirus is extremely common in childhood, and the majority of the adult population have antibodies to cytomegalovirus.[89] Primary infection after the age of 35 years is uncommon, and generalized infection usually occurs only in immunosuppressed patients with neoplastic disease, after transplantation, or with HIV infection.[90] The diagnosis of cytomegaloviral myocarditis can be suggested by the presence of viral inclusions in myocardial biopsy specimens and confirmed by the detection of viral DNA in the myocardium.[90]

VIRAL HEPATITIS. Clinical cardiac involvement in patients with hepatitis is rare; an occasional patient may develop fulminant myocarditis with congestive heart failure, hypotension, and death.[91] There are contested data implicating hepatitis C viral infection as an etiological factor in at least some cases of dilated cardiomyopathy.[92-94] The ventricles may be dilated with petechial hemorrhages. Hemorrhage into the myocardium may be a conspicuous finding.[91]

Symptomatic myocarditis is generally observed in the first to third week of illness. Patients may have dyspnea, palpitations, and anginal chest pain; fatalities have been reported.[91]

INFLUENZA. Although clinically apparent myocarditis is rare in patients with influenza, the presence of preexisting cardiovascular disease greatly increases the risk of morbidity and mortality.[95] During epidemics, 5 to 10 percent of infected patients may experience cardiac symptoms.[96]

Cardiac involvement typically occurs within 4 days to 2 weeks of the onset of the illness and may be severe, sometimes contributing to mortality.[97,98] Death may be associated with massive hemorrhagic pulmonary edema due to viral or bacterial involvement of the lungs.

MUMPS. Myocardial involvement during the course of mumps is rarely recognized.[99] The hearts of only a few patients with mumps have undergone postmortem examination, and they have been found to be both dilated and hypertrophied. Histologically, there is diffuse interstitial fibrosis, with infiltration of mononuclear cells and areas of focal necrosis.[99,100] There is speculation that prior mumps myocarditis may be involved in the development of endocardial fibroelastosis.[100] Cardiac involvement is usually unrecognized clinically, and the diagnosis of myocarditis is based on nonspecific ECG changes.[99]

RUBELLA AND RUBEOLA. Congenital cardiovascular lesions may develop in the offspring when the mother contracts rubella during the first trimester of pregnancy, with persistent ductus arteriosus and pulmonary artery maldevelopment as prominent anomalies. Rare cases of postgestational myocarditis occur, with attendant conduction defects and heart failure.[101]

Overt myocarditis is rare in patients with rubeola, although transient ECG abnormalities have been reported.[102] Congestive heart failure occurs on rare occasions, and its appearance is a poor prognostic sign, often indicating a fatal outcome.

VARICELLA. Clinical myocarditis is a rare finding in patients with varicella, although unsuspected myocarditis is common in cases of fatal varicella. Occasionally, a patient may develop overt clinical evidence of myocarditis with congestive heart failure.[103] Histological findings include rare but characteristic intranuclear inclusion bodies within the myocardial cells, along with interstitial edema, cellular infiltrates, and myonecrosis.[104]

VARIOLA AND VACCINIA. Cardiac involvement after smallpox is rare, although several cases of myocarditis associated with acute cardiac failure and death have been reported. Myocarditis with pericardial effusion and congestive heart failure has also been observed as a complication of smallpox vaccination; an immunological mechanism has been suggested, and dramatic responses to corticosteroids have been reported.[105]

OTHER VIRUSES

Other viruses causing myocarditis include the following:

Dengue[106,107]
Infectious mononucleosis[108]
Lassa fever[109]
Poliomyelitis[110]
Respiratory syncytial virus[111-113]
Enterovirus-71[114]
Parvovirus B19[115]

RICKETTSIAL MYOCARDITIS. The rickettsial diseases are frequently associated with evidence of myocardial involvement but usually it is subclinical. Transient ST segment and T wave alterations are commonly observed. The circulatory collapse that may accompany these diseases is largely a manifestation of abnormalities of the peripheral vascular bed, but a myocardial component may also be present. The basic histopathological process is a vasculitis with a periarterial interstitial infiltrate.

Other rickettsial pathogens causing myocarditis include Q fever,[116,117] Rocky Mountain spotted fever,[118] and scrub typhus.[119,120]

Bacterial Myocarditis

Virtually any bacterial agent can cause myocardial dysfunction. This occurs because of direct bacterial invasion, microabscess formation, or toxins elaborated by the pathogen. Other clinical manifestations of the infection mask or delay the appreciation of myocardial involvement, which may include atrial or ventricular arrhythmias, heart block, left or biventricular heart failure, pericarditis, or circulatory collapse. The clinician must always be alert for cardiac involvement during systemic bacterial infections.

CLOSTRIDIAL INFECTION. Cardiac involvement is common in patients with clostridial infections with multiple organ involvement. The myocardial damage results from the toxin elaborated by the bacteria but the precise actions of the toxin remain to be elucidated.[121] The pathological findings are distinctive, with gas bubbles present in the myocardium. Areas of degenerated muscle fibers are apparent, but an inflammatory infiltrate is usually absent.[121] *Clostridium perfringens* may cause myocardial abscess formation with myocardial perforation and resultant purulent pericarditis.

DIPHTHERIA. Myocardial involvement is one of the more serious complications of diphtheria and occurs in up to one half of cases.[122,123] Indeed, myocardial involvement is the most common cause of death in this infection and half of the fatal cases demonstrate cardiac involvement.[124] Cardiac damage is due to the liberation by the diphtheria bacillus of a toxin that inhibits protein synthesis by interfering with the transfer of amino acids from soluble RNA to polypeptide chains under construction. The toxin appears to have a particular affinity for the cardiac conducting system.

Because of the serious effects of the toxin on the myocardium, antitoxin should be administered as rapidly as possible.[124] Antibiotic therapy is of less urgency. The development of complete atrioventricular block is an ominous complication and mortality is high despite insertion of a transvenous pacemaker.[125]

STREPTOCOCCAL INFECTION. The most commonly detected cardiac finding after beta-hemolytic streptococcal infection is acute rheumatic fever, which is discussed in detail in Chapter 81.

Involvement of the heart by the streptococcus may produce a myocarditis that is distinct from acute rheumatic carditis. It is characterized by an interstitial infiltrate composed of mononuclear cells with occasional polymorphonuclear leukocytes; the infiltrate may be focal or diffuse and may be localized to the subendocardial or perivascular region. There may be small areas of myocardial necrosis. ECG abnormalities, including prolongation of the PR and QT intervals, occur frequently. Although these abnormalities are rarely associated with other clinical manifestations of myocardial involvement, sudden death, conduction disturbances, and arrhythmias may occur.

TUBERCULOSIS. Involvement of the myocardium by *Mycobacterium tuberculosis* (not as a complication of tuberculous pericarditis) is rare, particularly since the introduction of drugs effective against tuberculosis.[126,127] Most cases of myocardial tuberculosis are clinically silent and are diagnosed only at autopsy. Tuberculous involvement of the myocardium occurs by means of hematogenous or lymphatic spread or directly from contiguous structures and may cause nodular, miliary, or diffuse infiltrative disease. It may lead to arrhythmias, including atrial fibrillation and ventricular tachycardia, complete atrioventricular block, congestive heart failure, left ventricular aneurysms, and sudden death.[126,128,129]

WHIPPLE DISEASE. Although overt involvement is rare, intestinal lipodystrophy, or Whipple disease, is not uncommonly associated with cardiac involvement and periodic acid-Schiff-positive macrophages can be found in the myocardium, pericardium, and heart valves of patients with this disorder.[130,131] Coronary artery lesions, with smooth muscle necrosis, panarteritis, and medial scarring, can be seen. Electron microscopy has demonstrated rod-shaped structures in the myocardium similar to those found in the small intestine, and these represent the causative agent of the disease, *Tropheryma whippleii,* an agent related to the actinomycetes.[130] There may be an associated inflammatory infiltrate and foci of fibrosis. The valvular fibrosis may be severe enough to result in aortic regurgitation and mitral stenosis. Although usually asymptomatic, nonspecific ECG changes are most common; systolic murmurs, pericarditis, complete heart block, and even overt congestive heart failure may occur.[10] The cardiac manifestations of Whipple disease can be overshadowed by the prominent gastrointestinal symptoms that often are present, or it can be unappreciated.[132] Antibiotic therapy appears to be effective in treating the basic disease, but relapses can occur, often more than 2 years after initial diagnosis.

Other Bacteria

Other bacterial causes of myocarditis include the following:

Brucellosis[133]
Chlamydia[134,135]
Legionnaires disease[136]
Meningococcal infection[137,138]
Mycoplasma pneumoniae infection[139,140]
Psittacosis[141]
Salmonellosis[142,143]

Spirochetal Infections

LYME CARDITIS. Lyme disease is caused by a tickborne spirochete (*Borrelia burgdorferi*).[144] It usually begins during the summer months with a characteristic rash (erythema chronicum migrans), followed in weeks to months by neurological, joint, or cardiac involvement. Although some clinical manifestations may persist for years,[144,145] the majority of patients (90 percent) have no long-term sequelae.[145a]

About 10 percent of patients with Lyme disease develop evidence of transient cardiac involvement, the most common manifestation being variable degrees of atrioventricular block[146-149] at the level of the atrioventricular node. Syncope due to complete heart block is frequent with cardiac involvement because often there is an associated depression of ventricular escape rhythms. Ventricular tachycardia occurs uncommonly.[146] Diffuse ST segment and T wave abnormalities are transient; usually asymptomatic, left ventricular dysfunction may be found in some patients, although cardiomegaly or symptoms of congestive heart failure are rare.[147,150] A positive gallium scan can point to suspected cardiac involvement in this disease. The demonstration of spirochetes in myocardial biopsies of some patients with Lyme carditis suggests that the cardiac manifestations are due to a direct effect, although there is speculation that immune-mediated mechanisms may be involved as well.[151]

Treatment. The value of specific therapy in cases of Lyme carditis remains uncertain, and even without therapy the disease is usually self-limited, with complete recovery the rule.[152] Nevertheless, it is thought that treating the early manifestations of the disease will prevent development of late complications.[144] Patients with second-degree or complete heart block should be hospitalized and undergo continuous ECG monitoring. Temporary transvenous pacing may be required for a week or longer in patients with high-grade block. Although the efficacy of antibiotics is not established, they are used routinely in patients with Lyme carditis. Intravenous antibiotics (ceftriaxone, 2 gm, or penicillin G, 20 million units daily for 14 days) are suggested, although oral antibiotics (doxycycline, 100 mg twice daily, or amoxicillin, 500 mg three times daily for 14 to 21 days) can be used when there is only mild cardiac involvement (first-degree atrioventricular block of less than 40 msec duration).[152] Whether antiinflammatory agents (salicylates, corticosteroids) can ameliorate heart block is not clear.

OTHER SPIROCHETAL INFECTIONS CAUSING MYOCARDITIS. Other spirochetal infections include leptospirosis (Weil disease[153-155]), relapsing fever,[156] and syphilis.[157]

Fungal Infections of the Heart

Cardiac fungal infections occur most frequently in patients with malignant disease and/or those receiving chemotherapy, corticosteroids, radiation, or immunosuppressive therapy. Cardiac surgery, intravenous drug abuse, and infection with HIV are also predisposing factors for fungal cardiac involvement. Cardiac involvement may be associated with myocardial seeding by hematogenous dissemination but may also be due to direct myocardial extension from pulmonary or mediastinal infection. Rarely, coronary obstruction can occur due to fungal mycelia.

ASPERGILLOSIS. Myocardial involvement is not uncommon in patients with generalized aspergillosis, and when it occurs it is usually fatal.[158] Rarely, myocardial involvement may appear to be primary, typically after cardiac surgery. However, it is being encountered increasingly in the immunocompromised patient.[159] On pathological examination, myocardial necrosis and infarction caused by thrombosis of vessels that contain fungal mycelia are commonly seen, along with myocardial abscesses and pericardial involvement. The ECG may be normal in the face of significant myocardial damage, but T wave changes may be present. The diagnosis of *Aspergillus* infection is often difficult.[160] Identification of *Aspergillus* through open-lung biopsy, aspiration lung biopsy, transtracheal aspiration, or bronchial brush technique may be successful. Treatment is difficult and usually unsuccessful.

OTHER FUNGAL INFECTIONS. Other fungal infections causing myocarditis include the following:

Actinomycosis[160]
Blastomycosis[161]
Candidiasis[162,163]
Coccidioidomycosis[164]
Cryptococcosis[165]
Histoplasmosis[166]
Mucormycosis[167,168]

Protozoal Myocarditis

Trypanosomiasis (Chagas Disease)

Chagas disease is caused by the protozoan *Trypanosoma cruzi.* The major cardiovascular manifestation is an extensive myocarditis that typically becomes evident years after the initial infection. The disease is prevalent in Central and South America, particularly in Brazil, Argentina, and Chile, where it constitutes a major public health problem (Fig. 60–7). Upward of 20 million people are thought to be infected with the parasite and an estimated 100 million are at risk of infection.[169,170] In rare cases, the disease can be found in nonendemic areas as a consequence of transfusion with contaminated blood products; somewhat more common is emigration of patients with the disease to nonendemic areas.[171]

NATURAL HISTORY. The natural history of Chagas disease is characterized by three phases: acute, latent, and chronic. During the acute phase, the disease is transmitted to humans (usually younger than 20 years of age) through the bite of a reduviid bug (subfamily Triatominae), which harbors the parasite in its gastrointestinal tract.[169-172] This insect acquires the disease from feeding on infected animals, including the armadillo, raccoon, opossum, and skunk as well as domestic dogs and cats. The reduviid bug, popularly known in Argentina as *vinchuca,* meaning "to let oneself drop," lives in the walls and roofs of houses and, during nocturnal feedings, drops from the ceiling onto the sleeping person below. The bug then often bites the person around the eyes, and infection of the human host occurs when the trypanosomes in the animal's feces gain entry through abraded skin or through the conjunctivae.[169] Occasionally, this results in unilateral periorbital edema and swelling of the eyelid, termed the *Romaña sign,* whereas entry through the skin may result in a lesion called a *chagoma.*[169,172] Transmission can occur through blood transfusions; unfortunately, adequate screening to preclude transfusion-related disease is not possible in many areas due to financial and logistical constraints.[169]

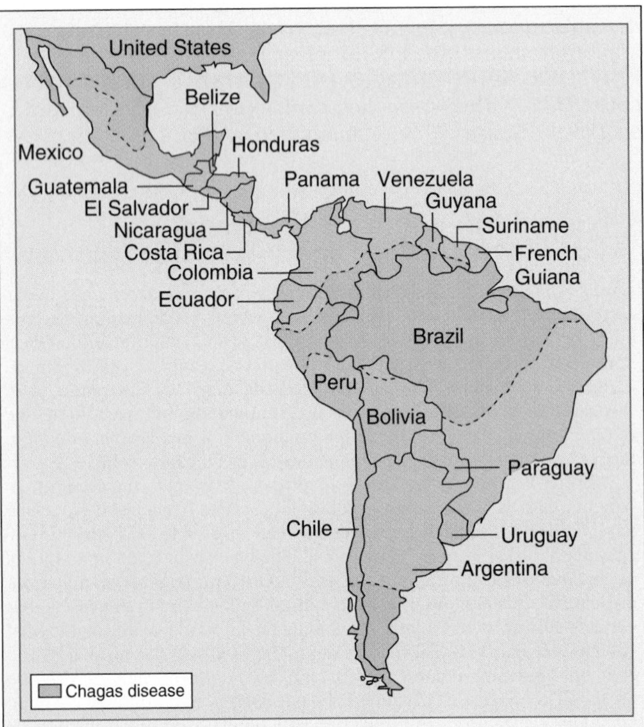

FIGURE 60–7 Distribution of Chagas disease in the Americas. (Modified from Acquatella H: Chagas' disease. *In* Abelmann WH, Braunwald E [eds]: Atlas of Heart Diseases. Vol. 2. Cardiomyopathies, Myocarditis, and Pericardial Disease. Philadelphia, Current Medicine, 1995, pp 8.1-8.18.)

ACUTE TRYPANOSOMIASIS. After inoculation, the protozoa multiply and then migrate widely throughout the body. In less than 10 percent of cases an acute illness occurs; this acute illness is fatal in about 10 percent of patients.[171,172] Pathological examination during the acute phase often reveals parasites in the cardiac fibers with a marked cellular infiltrate, particularly around cardiac cells that have ruptured and released the parasites.[172] Involvement may extend into the endocardium, resulting in thrombus formation, and into the epicardium, resulting in pericardial effusion. The pathogenesis of the myocardial lesions of acute Chagas disease appears to relate in large part to immune lysis by antibody and cell-mediated immunity directed against antigens released from *T. cruzi*–infected cells, which become adsorbed onto the surface of infected and noninfected host cells.[169] *T. cruzi* parasite growth can be regulated by inducible NOS activation and cytokine production.[173]

Clinical Manifestations. Clinical manifestations include fever, muscle pains, sweating, hepatosplenomegaly, myocarditis with congestive heart failure, pericardial effusion, and, occasionally, meningoencephalitis.[169,172] Most patients recover, and their symptoms resolve over several months. Young children most commonly develop clinical acute disease and generally are more seriously ill than adults.

LATENT AND CHRONIC TRYPANOSOMIASIS. The disease then enters a latent phase without clinical symptoms; however, there is evidence of early and progressive subclinical cardiomyopathy. ECG changes often appear at this stage and are a marker for the eventual clinical heart disease and increased mortality to become evident later. At an average of 20 years after the initial (and usually unrecognized) infestation, approximately 30 percent of infected individuals develop findings of chronic Chagas disease, the manifestations of which cover a wide spectrum from asymptomatic but seropositive patients through those with ECG abnormalities to those with advanced disease characterized by cardiomegaly, congestive heart failure, arrhythmias, thromboembolic phenomena, atypical chest pain, right bundle branch block, and sudden death.[171] In the advanced stage, cardiac dilation typically involves all the cardiac chambers, although right-sided enlargement may predominate.[171]

PATHOGENESIS. The central paradox in the pathogenesis of this disorder is the poor correlation between the level of parasitemia and the severity of disease.[174] It is not unusual to be unable to detect parasites in patients dying of Chagas disease,[175] although evidence of prior infection may be detected more frequently by the much more sensitive PCR technique.[176] *T. cruzi* antigen is frequently found in biopsy specimens of the heart from patients with chronic Chagas heart disease.[176] An autoimmune etiological mechanism has been proposed, and this may explain the lack of correlation of parasitemia with disease severity.[174,176,177] Based on animal models, it appears that self-reactive cytotoxic T lymphocytes develop after the initial infection and produce various cytokines.[174] A more vigorous Th 1 immune response and production of interferon-gamma against *T. cruzi* antigens can differentiate patients with cardiac involvement.[178,179] This response results in the lysis of normal host cells, perhaps related to cross-reacting antigens of *T. cruzi* and striated muscle.[171,180] A variety of antibodies against myocyte sarcoplasmic reticulum, laminin, and other constituents (most recently the cardiac beta receptor) have also been implicated in the pathogenesis of Chagas myocarditis.[181] It is thought that the acute phase results in the release from parasite-modified host cells of self-components that are immunogenic.[171] Another hypothesis suggests that cardiac parasympathetic denervation leads to eventual chronic Chagas disease.[171]

PATHOLOGY. Nerves and autonomic ganglia are frequently abnormal, and megaesophagus and megacolon may occur; less commonly, there is dilation of the stomach, duodenum, ureter, and bronchi. Different strains of *T. cruzi* may account for the geographical differences in the expression of Chagas disease; megaesophagus and megacolon are common in Brazil but quite uncommon in Central America and Mexico, and megaesophagus is unusual in Venezuela.[169] Lesions of the cardiac nerves are routinely found in patients with chronic Chagas disease, with evidence of cardiac parasympathetic denervation.[169] Pathological cardiac findings include cardiac enlargement with dilation and hypertrophy of all cardiac chambers. In more than half the patients, the left (and occasionally right) ventricular apex is thin and bulging, resembling an aneurysm.[182] Thrombus formation is frequent and may fill much of the apex; the right atrium also frequently contains thrombus. It has been suggested that these characteristic apical aneurysms (Fig. 60–8) may be the result of intravascular platelet aggregation leading to focal myocardial necrosis.[176]

The microscopic findings are principally those of extensive fibrosis, particularly of the left ventricle.[171,183] A chronic cellular infiltrate composed of lymphocytes, plasma cells, and macrophages often is present.[169] Increases in arteriole and capillary diameters have been reported.[183] Preferential involvement of the right bundle branch and the anterior fascicle of the left bundle branch by inflammatory and fibrotic changes explains the frequent occurrence of right bundle branch and left anterior fascicular block.[169] The basement membranes of capillaries, vascular smooth muscle cells, and myocytes are thickened.[176] It is unusual to be able to find parasites in the myofibers of autopsied patients.[182]

Clinical Manifestations. Clinical manifestations include anginal chest pain, symptomatic conducting system disease, and sudden death; chronic progressive heart failure, often predominantly right-sided, is the rule in advanced cases.[171] Thus, although pulmonary congestion is occasionally noted, the usual findings include fatigue due to diminished cardiac output, peripheral edema, ascites, and hepatic congestion. Tricuspid regurgitation is often present, particularly in patients with severe right-sided heart failure, although mitral regurgitation is frequently present as well. The S_2 is widely split, often with an accentuated pulmonic component, reflecting the combined effects of right bundle branch block and pulmonary hypertension. Autonomic dysfunction is common, with marked abnormalities in the expected reflex changes in heart rate produced by various maneuvers. Deaths result most commonly from pump failure or occur suddenly. Apical aneurysms and left ventricular dilation place patients at high risk for sudden death.[184]

Laboratory Findings. The chest radiograph often demonstrates severe cardiomegaly, with or without pulmonary venous hypertension. The serum aldolase level is usually elevated.[185] ECG abnormalities are the rule late in the course of the disease, particularly in patients who are seroreactive to *T. cruzi* antigen. Right bundle branch block, left anterior hemiblock, atrial fibrillation, and ventricular premature depolarizations are the most common findings in patients with chronic Chagas disease.[164,186] ST segment and T wave abnormalities also are common, as are Q waves; P wave abnormalities and atrioventricular block are seen less frequently.[169] Early in the disease, the ECG may be normal or nearly so. Administration of the antiarrhythmic agent ajmaline may precipitate the appearance of ECG abnormalities and thus identify patients with as yet clinically silent cardiac involvement.[169] Furthermore, electrophysiological testing of asymptomatic patients, even those with normal ECGs, may demonstrate abnormalities of the conducting system in many.

VENTRICULAR ARRHYTHMIAS. These are a prominent feature of chronic Chagas disease.[169,176,177] Frequent ventricular premature depolarizations, often with multiple morphologies, are seen frequently, and bouts of ventricular tachycardia can occur.[187] Ventricular arrhythmias are particularly common during and after exercise,[169] occurring in the majority of patients subjected to stress ECG testing (including some without any other clinical evidence of cardiac involvement). Ventricular tachycardia induced by electrophysiological testing is most common in patients with evidence of conduction abnormalities on the ECG, low ejection fraction, and apical left ventricular aneurysm, and may predict sudden death.[188] Syncope and sudden death due to ventricular fibrillation are constant threats and may develop

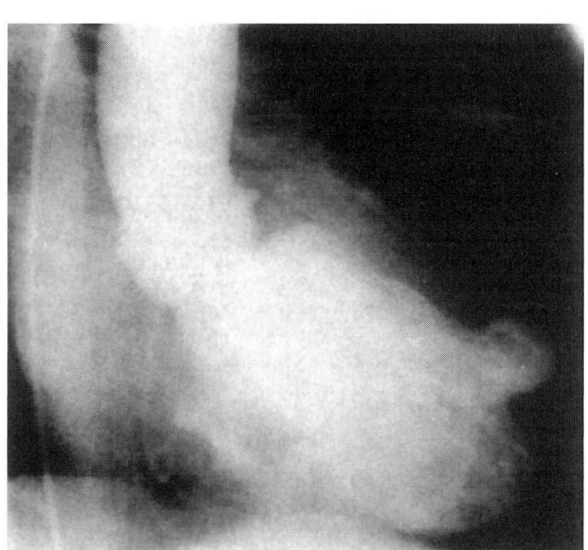

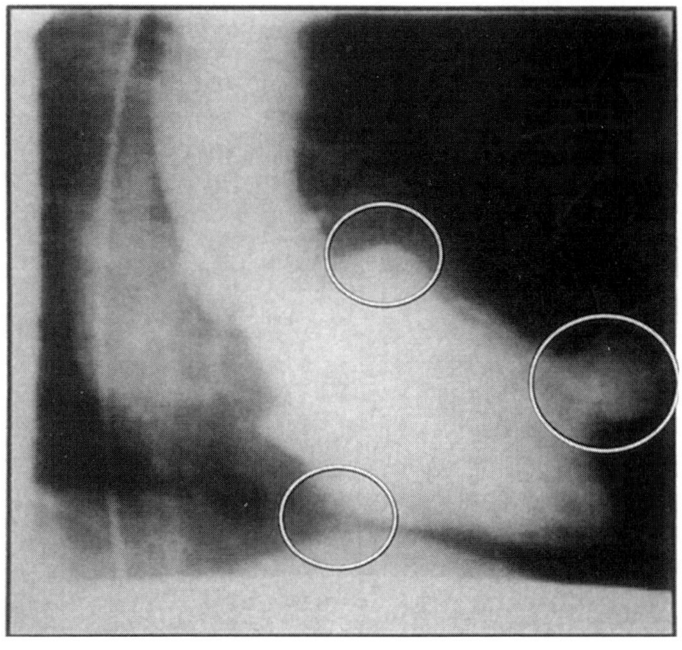

FIGURE 60–8 Left ventriculogram in the right anterior oblique view of a 55-year-old woman with chronic Chagas disease. Multiple left ventricular aneurysms are noted in anterobasal, anterior, and inferior aspects of left ventricle **(right, circled)**. (From Venegoni P, Bhatia HS: Chagas disease and ventricular arrhythmias. Circulation 96:1363, 1997. Copyright 1997, American Heart Association.)

even before cardiomegaly or heart failure.[169,189] Sinus bradycardia can also be seen, even in patients with severe heart failure when a tachycardia would be expected, presumably related to cardiac autonomic dysfunction.[169] Atrial arrhythmias, including atrial fibrillation (often with a slow ventricular response), also can occur.[169] Thromboembolic phenomena are a frequent complication, occurring in more than 50 percent of the patients.[190]

Noninvasive Imaging. The echocardiographic findings in advanced cases are those of a dilated cardiomyopathy with increased end-diastolic and end-systolic volumes and reduced ejection fraction, often with enlargement of the left atrium and right ventricle.[169] Diastolic filling of the left ventricle is frequently abnormal, even in patients without other clinical or echocardiographic evidence of cardiac involvement. In the majority of advanced cases, the echocardiographic appearance is distinctive, with left ventricular posterior wall hypokinesis and relatively preserved interventricular septal motion; an apical aneurysm is often seen on two-dimensional echocardiography. Ten to 15 percent of asymptomatic patients demonstrate apical dyskinesis. Dobutamine echocardiography may unmask chronotropic incompetence and limited myocardial contractural reserve in patients without overt heart disease.[191]

Radionuclide ventriculography may, like echocardiography, demonstrate right or left ventricular wall motion abnormalities in the absence of an overall depression of global ventricular function. Perfusion scanning with thallium-201 may show fixed defects (corresponding to areas of fibrosis) as well as evidence of reversible ischemia.[192] MRI can identify morphological and functional aspects of cardiac involvement; with the use of gadolinium as a contrast medium, it can identify patients with more active myocardial disease.[193]

Left ventricular cineangiography in advanced cases shows a dilated, hypokinetic left ventricle with one large or several apical aneurysms (Fig. 60–8) containing intracavitary thrombus, often with evidence of mitral regurgitation.[169] Coronary angiography is usually normal, although abnormalities of the coronary microcirculation have been suggested as a cause of the clinical manifestations of Chagas disease.

Serodiagnosis. The complement-fixation test (Machado-Guerreiro test) is useful in diagnosis; it has high sensitivity and specificity for the identification of chronic Chagas disease.[169] Also used in diagnosis are the indirect immunofluorescent antibody test, the enzyme-linked immunosorbent assay, and the hemagglutination test.[169] Perhaps the most widely used test in endemic areas is the detection of parasites in the blood of patients with chronic Chagas disease (which occurs in upward of 50 percent of cases) by means of xenodiagnosis.[194] The patient is bitten by reduviid bugs bred in the laboratory; the subsequent identification of parasites in the intestine of the insect is proof of infection in the human host.

MANAGEMENT. The treatment of Chagas disease remains difficult; although slowly progressive at first, once cardiac decompensation develops, there is usually a rapid and inexorable progression to death, which is usually due to arrhythmia, although congestive failure and systemic thromboembolism account for additional mortality.[195] Patients at greatest risk of mortality are those with left ventricular enlargement and especially those with impaired left ventricular function.[186,189] Patients with Chagas disease may respond to beta blockade, and there is some evidence that captopril, early in the course of disease, may alleviate disease in animal models.[196] Major efforts are aimed at interrupting transmission of the parasite to humans; such vector control methods have been generally successful.[169] They may prevent not only the initial infection but also reinfection that may play a role in determining the severity of the resulting cardiomyopathy.

Amiodarone appears to be effective in controlling the ventricular arrhythmias frequently seen in patients with Chagas disease, although whether this translates into improved survival remains to be established.[195] Implantable cardioverter defibrillators are useful, and the indications are similar to those in patients with life-threatening arrhythmias associated with other causes (see Chap. 31),[197] but this is not a practical option for the vast majority of patients (owing to financial constraints). Anticoagulation may be of some benefit in preventing recurrent thromboembolic episodes.[190] Although antiparasitic agents such as nifurtimox, benzimidazole, and itraconazole are effective in reducing parasitemia and are useful in acute disease, no evidence indicates that they are efficacious in curing the late phases of the disease.[169,198] A promising avenue of approach appears to be immunoprophylaxis, although a clinically useful vaccine is not yet available. Heart transplantations have been performed in a few patients, but the results so far appear to be inferior to those found in patients with other conditions, and neoplasms as well as episodes of parasitemia and recurrent Chagas disease may be a problem.[199-201]

Other protozoal causes of myocarditis include African trypanosomiasis,[202] toxoplasmosis,[203,204] and malaria.[205,206]

Metazoal Myocardial Diseases

ECHINOCOCCUS (HYDATID CYST). *Echinococcus* is endemic in many sheep-raising areas of the world, particularly Argentina, Uruguay, New Zealand, Greece, North Africa, and Iceland, but cardiac involvement in patients with hydatid disease is uncommon, occurring in less than 2 percent of cases.[207] The usual host of *Echinococcus granulosus* is the dog, but humans may serve as intermediate hosts (rather than the sheep, the usual intermediate host) if they accidentally ingest ova from contaminated dog feces.

When cardiac involvement is present, the cysts usually are intramyocardial in the interventricular septum or left ventricular free wall (Fig. 60–9); involvement of the right ventricle or atrium may occur.[207] Involvement of the tricuspid valve can be seen on occasion; in most cases, a single cardiac cyst is present.

A myocardial cyst can degenerate and calcify, develop daughter cysts, or rupture. Rupture of the cyst is the most dreaded complication; rupture into the pericardium can result in acute pericarditis, which may progress to chronic constrictive pericarditis.[207] Rupture into the cardiac chambers can result in systemic or pulmonary emboli.[208] Rapidly progressive pulmonary hypertension can occur with rupture of right-sided cysts, with subsequent embolization of hundreds of scolices into the pulmonary circulation. The liberation of hydatid fluid into the circulation can produce profound, fatal circulatory collapse due to an anaphylactic reaction to the protein constituents of the fluid.[207]

Symptoms depend on the location, size, and integrity of the cyst; patients may be asymptomatic or in profound circulatory collapse. It is estimated that only about 10 percent of patients with cardiac hydatid cysts have clinical manifestations.[207] The ECG may reflect the location of the cyst: T-wave changes and loss of QRS voltage can occur with left ventricular involvement, whereas atrioventricular conduction defects or right bundle branch block can be seen with involvement of the interventricular septum. Chest pain is usually due to rupture of the cyst into the pericardial space with resultant pericarditis. Large cystic masses sometimes produce right-sided obstruction.[207]

Diagnosis. Recognition of an echinococcal cyst of the heart is a relatively simple matter if there is evidence of cysts in other organs, particularly the liver and lung. However, a cardiac cyst can be an isolated, solitary finding. The chest radiograph frequently shows an abnormal cardiac silhouette or a calcified lobular mass adjacent to the left ventricle.[201] Although computed tomography (CT) and MRI may aid in the detection and localization of heart cysts, two-dimensional echocardiography is thought to be the best choice (see Fig. 60–9).[207] Eosinophilia, present in some patients, is a useful adjunctive finding. The Casoni skin test is not very helpful because both false-positive and false-negative results occur. Serological tests, including hemagglutination and complement fixation, may be more useful, but their predictive accuracy is limited.[207]

Management. Until recently, treatment for hydatid disease was limited to surgical excision.[209] Experience suggests that the benzimidazole derivatives mebendazole and albendazole are somewhat useful in the medical management of this disease.[207,210] Despite the availability of drug therapy, adjunctive surgical excision is generally recommended, even for asymptomatic patients, because of the significant risk of rupture of the cyst and its attendant serious and sometimes fatal consequences.[207] The surgical results generally have been favorable.[211]

TRICHINOSIS. Infestation with *Trichinella spiralis* is a common human finding. Mild myocarditis has been said to be a frequent finding, but recent data suggest that clinically detectable cardiac involvement occurs in only a minority of patients.[212] Symptomatic involvement is uncommon and may be responsible for the majority of fatalities.[213] Less frequently, death is due to pulmonary embolism secondary to venous thrombosis or neurological complications.

Although the parasite can invade the heart, it does not usually encyst there, and it is rare to find larvae or larval fragments in the myocardium. Nonetheless, pathological findings at autopsy can be impressive. The heart may be dilated and flabby, and a pericardial effusion may be present.[212] A prominent focal infiltrate composed of lymphocytes and eosinophils is commonly found, with occasional microthrombi in the intramural arterioles. Areas of muscle degeneration and necrosis are present.

Clinical Manifestations. Myocarditis is usually mild and goes unnoticed, but in occasional cases it is manifested by congestive heart failure and chest pain, usually appearing around the third week of the disease, when the general constitutional symptoms are abating. Physical examination findings may be normal, or there may be gross cardiomegaly with severe congestive heart failure. Sudden death can occur, usually in the fourth to eighth week of the illness.

Electrocardiographic abnormalities are detected in about 10 percent of patients with trichinosis and parallel the time course of clinical cardiac involvement, initially appearing in the second or third week and usually resolving by the seventh week of the illness. The most common ECG abnormalities are repolarization abnormalities and ventricular premature complexes.[212] The ECG changes usually resolve completely.

The diagnosis is usually based on the demonstration of a positive indirect immunofluorescent antibody test in a patient with the clinical features of trichinosis. Eosinophilia, when present, is a supportive finding. The skin test is usually but not invariably positive. Treatment is with anthelmintics and corticosteroids; dramatic improvement in cardiac function has been reported after their use.

Other metazoal causes of myocarditis include visceral larva migrans[214,215] and schistosomiasis.[216]

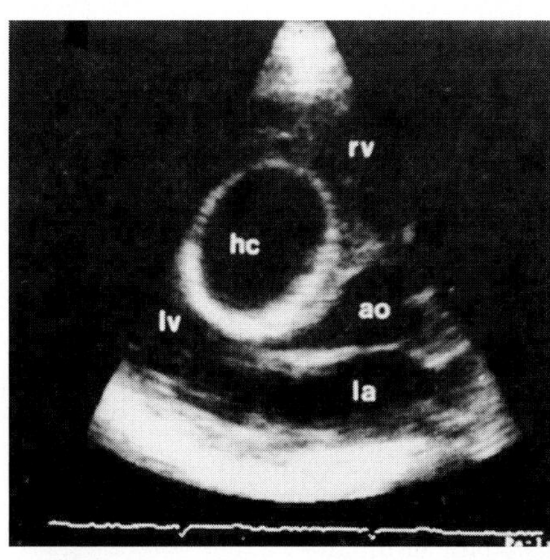

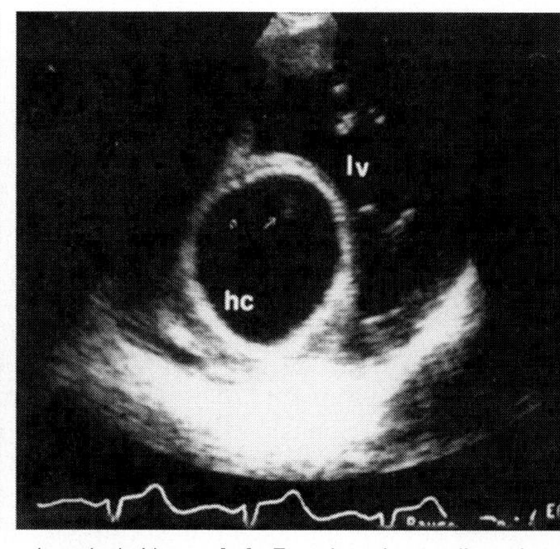

FIGURE 60–9 Involvement of interventricular septum by a hydatid cyst. **Left,** Transthoracic two-dimensional echocardiogram of parasternal long-axis view showing a 3-cm diameter hydatid cyst (hc) in the upper ventricular septum. **Right,** Transesophageal echocardiography showing a hydatid cyst (hc) having a rounded and well-contrasted capsule. ao = aorta; la = left atrium; lv = left ventricle; rv = right ventricle. (From Aupetit J, Ritz B, Ferrini M, et al: Images in cardiovascular medicine: Hydatid cyst of the interventricular septum. Circulation 95:2325, 1997. Copyright 1997, American Heart Association.)

Toxic, Chemical, Immune, and Physical Damage to the Heart

A wide variety of substances other than infectious agents can act on the heart and damage the myocardium. In some cases, the damage is acute, transient, and associated with evidence of an inflammatory myocardial infiltrate with myocyte necrosis (e.g., with the arsenicals and lithium); in other cases, a hypersensitivity reaction occurs, without prominent evidence of necrosis (e.g., with sulfonamides). Other agents that damage the myocardium can lead to chronic changes with resulting histological evidence of fibrosis and a clinical picture of a dilated cardiomyopathy. Furthermore, many offending stimuli are associated with both acute and chronic phases (e.g., alcohol, doxorubicin). The extent of myocardial damage often is related to the dose and rate of exposure to the toxin.

Numerous chemicals and drugs (both industrial and therapeutic) can lead to cardiac damage and dysfunction. Several physical agents (e.g., radiation and excessive heat) can also contribute to myocardial damage.

Toxic Agents

The cardiac effects of ethanol, cocaine, amphetamines, catecholamines, ergot, appetite suppressants, and Taxol are discussed in Chapter 62. The effects of the antineoplastic agents daunorubicin, cyclophosphamide, and 5-fluorouracil are discussed in Chapter 83. The cardiac effects of tricyclic antidepressants and phenothiazines are discussed further in Chapter 84.

TRICYCLIC ANTIDEPRESSANTS. Although sinus tachycardia, postural hypotension, disturbances in rhythm, abnormalities of atrioventricular conduction, and even sudden death can be seen in patients taking tricyclic antidepressants, particularly when they are taken as an overdose, important depression of left ventricular function usually does not occur, even in patients with preexisting heart disease.[217] There has been concern when using tricyclic antidepressants in patients with prior myocardial infarction and/or preexisting ventricular arrhythmias because these agents have a class I antiarrhythmic effect, prolong the QT interval, and might be proarrhythmic in these settings. The selective serotonin reuptake inhibitors are remarkably free of cardiovascular toxicity and do not appear to depress ventricular function.[217] They may produce side effects by interacting with the metabolism of drugs mediated through the cytochrome-P450 enzyme system.

PHENOTHIAZINES. The phenothiazines are associated with a variety of cardiac disturbances, including ECG changes, atrial and ventricular arrhythmias, and sudden death.[218,219] Postural hypotension can also be seen. The cardiac effects are largely dose dependent. ECG abnormalities can be observed with as little as 200 mg of thioridazine per day and consist of lengthening of the QT interval and T wave changes. Prolongation of the QT interval can set the stage for the emergence of ventricular arrhythmias, particularly torsades de pointes.[218,219] Higher doses may lead to frank T wave inversion and increased amplitude of the U wave. Changes in the P wave, QRS complex, and ST segment are usually absent. The ECG abnormalities and arrhythmias resolve with discontinuation of the drug, usually within 48 hours. An occasional patient requires temporary ventricular pacing.

Pathological changes in the hearts of patients who have received phenothiazines and who have died suddenly include the deposition of acid mucopolysaccharide between muscle bundles in periarteriolar regions as well as the conduction system, with myofibrillar degeneration and endothelial proliferation in the smaller blood vessels, although a direct causal relationship between drug administration and cardiomyopathic changes is only inferential. A variety of explanations have been invoked for the apparent cardiac damage, including direct toxic effects of the phenothiazines on the myocardium, stimulation of higher autonomic centers, and changes in circulating or myocardial levels of catecholamines.

CARBON MONOXIDE. Both acute and chronic carbon monoxide toxicity can occur. Although central nervous system findings usually dominate the clinical presentation, significant and occasionally fatal cardiac abnormalities have been reported, although some investigators have found no precipitation of arrhythmias following exposure.[220,221] Because carbon monoxide has a higher affinity for hemoglobin than does oxygen, reduced amounts of oxygen are delivered to the tissues. Thus, the cardiac toxicity may be partially caused by myocardial hypoxia, but a direct toxic effect of the gas on myocardial mitochondria may play an even more important role.[222] The histological features include focal areas of necrosis, most marked in the subendocardium. Focal perivascular infiltrates and punctate hemorrhages are also seen.[222]

Cardiac involvement can appear promptly after exposure or it can be delayed for up to several days. Palpitations, sinus tachycardia, and various arrhythmias, including ventricular extrasystoles and atrial fibrillation, are common.[223] Bradycardia and atrioventricular block can occur in more severe cases.[223] In patients with ischemic heart disease, angina pectoris and myocardial infarction can be precipitated. ECG ST segment and T wave abnormalities are quite common. Transient right and/or left ventricular wall motion abnormalities can be present.[222] Administration of 100 percent oxygen, bed rest, and surveillance for serious rhythm or conduction abnormalities usually permit rapid recovery.

Other Agents

Other toxic, chemical, immune, and physical agents that can be damaging to the heart include the following:

Interferon-alpha[224]
Interleukin-2[225]
Clozapine[226]
Emetine[227]
Methysergide[228]
Chloroquine[229]
Antimony compounds[230,231]
Lithium[232,233]
Hydrocarbons[234,235]
Lead[236]
Hypocalcemia[237,238]
Hypophosphatemia[239,240]
Hypomagnesemia[241,242]
Wasp stings[243]
Snake bite[244,245]
Arsenic[246]
Carnitine[247,248]
Selenium[249,250]
Scorpion sting[251,252]
Ephedra[253,254]

Hypersensitivity

Allergic reactions to a variety of agents can involve the myocardium. A number of drugs (most commonly the sulfonamides, hydrochlorothiazide, the penicillins, and methyldopa) or other sensitizers may lead to an allergic myocarditis (Table 60–3), characterized by peripheral eosinophilia and a perivascular infiltration of the myocardium by eosinophils, lymphocytes, and histiocytes; necrosis is seen on occasion.[255] Hypersensitivity myocarditis is rarely recognized clinically and is often first discovered at postmortem examination, although it is occasionally diagnosed on endomyocardial biopsy.[256] Most patients who have hypersensitivity myocarditis are not critically ill, but nevertheless may die suddenly, presumably as a consequence of an arrhythmia. Patients with hypersensitivity may develop an arteritis, and acute myocardial infarction rarely occurs.[257] An occasional patient has intense eosinophilic infiltration of the myocardium of no obvious cause, with prominent necrosis evident and findings of hemodynamic collapse; some of these patients have undiagnosed hypersensitivity myocarditis.[255] Because of the potential for significant deleterious effects, a high index of suspicion for this condition should be maintained. Therapy includes discontinuation of the offending agent and corticosteroids and/or immunosuppression therapy in severe cases.

TABLE 60–3 Principal Drugs Capable of Causing Hypersensitivity Myocarditis

Antibiotics	**Antiinflammatory**
Amphotericin B	Indomethacin
Ampicillin	Oxyphenbutazone
Chloramphenicol	Phenylbutazone
Penicillin	
Tetracycline	**Diuretics**
Streptomycin	Acetazolamide
	Chlorthalidone
Sulfonamides	Hydrochlorothiazide
Sulfadiazine	Spironolactone
Sulfisoxazole	
	Others
Anticonvulsants	Amitriptyline
Phenindione	Methyldopa
Phenytoin	Sulfonylureas
Carbamazepine	Tetanus toxoid
Antituberculous	
Isoniazid	
Paraaminosalicylic acid	

From Kounis NG, Zavras GM, Soufras GD, Kitrou MP: Hypersensitivity myocarditis. Ann Allergy 62:71, 1989.

METHYLDOPA. Although hepatitis is the most frequently encountered serious adverse reaction to methyldopa, sudden and unexpected death has been reported in a number of patients found at necropsy to have had an unsuspected myocarditis.[258] The histological findings have the characteristics of an allergic myocarditis, showing an interstitial inflammatory infiltrate with abundant eosinophils, vasculitis, and focal myocardial necrosis. ECG changes include sinus bradycardia, sinus pauses, and first- and second-degree atrioventricular block.

PENICILLIN. Allergic reactions to penicillin are fairly common, but myocardial involvement is rare.[259] Histological findings consist of a perivascular and interstitial infiltrate composed of eosinophils and mononuclear cells. Both myocardial infarction and pericarditis may occur and account for some of the ECG changes.[259] Transient ECG changes may be the only manifestation of cardiac involvement, with sinus tachycardia, ST segment elevation, and T wave inversion.

SULFONAMIDES. Use of sulfonamides can result in myocardial damage owing to a hypersensitivity vasculitis as well as a myocarditis.[255] In fatal cases, eosinophilic myocarditis, sometimes with granulomas, can be demonstrated.[258] Although usually clinically silent, myocardial involvement can produce severe and even fatal congestive heart failure. ECG changes are usually absent, but nonspecific ST segment and T wave abnormalities are sometimes seen.

TETRACYCLINE. Allergic reactions to antibiotics of the tetracycline class include fever, tachycardia, and first-degree atrioventricular block. Postmortem findings include cardiac dilation, fibrinoid muscle cell degeneration, and a diffuse interstitial and perivascular infiltrate.[255]

Physical Agents

RADIATION (see Chap. 83). The use of radiation therapy can result in a variety of cardiac complications, which are usually chronic and include pericarditis with effusion, tamponade, or constriction; coronary artery fibrosis and myocardial infarction; valvular abnormalities; myocardial fibrosis; and conduction disturbances.[260] Although the heart has been regarded as one of the organs more resistant to the effects of radiation, the clinical significance of radiation-induced heart disease is greater than often appreciated.[258] Although radiation probably results in some degree of tissue damage in all patients, clinically significant cardiac involvement occurs in the minority of patients, usually long after the radiation treatment has ended.[260] Radiation-induced cardiac damage is related to the dose of radiation, the mass of heart irradiated, and the dose schedule of the radiation.

The late cardiac damage that may follow irradiation appears to result from a long-lasting injury of the capillary endothelial cells, which leads to cell death, capillary rupture, and microthrombi.[260,261] Because of this damage to the microvasculature, ischemia results and is followed by myocardial fibrosis. In addition to microvascular damage, the major epicardial coronary arteries can become narrowed, especially at the ostia.[261,262]

Only an occasional patient manifests acute clinical cardiac abnormality with radiation therapy; typically, this consists of acute pericarditis. A mild, transient, asymptomatic depression of left ventricular function is sometimes seen early after radiation therapy. The more common clinical expressions of radiation heart disease occur months or years after the exposure. The pericardium is the most common site of clinical involvement, with findings of chronic pericardial effusion or pericardial constriction (see Chap. 64).[260] Myocardial damage occurs less frequently and is characterized by myocardial fibrosis with or without endocardial fibrosis or fibroelastosis. Left and/or right ventricular dysfunction at rest or with exercise appears to be a common, albeit usually asymptomatic, finding 5 to 20 years after radiation therapy, especially in patients in whom the now-outmoded technique of a single anteroposterior port was used.[260] Occasional patients develop usually asymptomatic left-sided (and rarely right-sided) valvular regurgitation (or on occasion stenosis) that sometimes requires valve replacement, particularly when associated with calcification of the mitral or aortic valves.[261,263,264] Often there is a latent period of a decade or more between the radiation exposure and the development of valvular deformity.[261] ECG abnormalities, heart block, accelerated atherosclerosis, and a variety of arrhythmias may be seen months or years after therapeutic radiation, although usually they are of limited clinical significance.[260,262,265]

Heat Stroke

Heat stroke results from failure of the thermoregulatory center following exposure to high ambient temperature. It is manifested principally by hyperpyrexia, renal insufficiency, disseminated intravascular coagulation, and central nervous system dysfunction.[266] However, cardiovascular abnormalities (usually ECG) appear to be common; pulmonary edema and transient right and/or left ventricular dysfunction may occur, along with hypotension and circulatory collapse. Pathological changes include dilation of the right side of the heart, particularly the right atrium. Hemorrhages of the subendocardium and the subepicardium are frequently seen at necropsy and often involve the interventricular septum and posterior wall of the left ventricle. Histological findings include degeneration and necrosis of muscle fibers as well as interstitial edema. Factors that have been implicated as possible causes of myocardial damage include direct thermal injury, myocardial hypoxia resulting from circulatory collapse, decreased coronary blood flow, and metabolic abnormalities resulting from widespread injury to other organs.

Sinus tachycardia is invariably present,[266] whereas atrial and ventricular arrhythmias usually are absent. Transient prolongation of the QT interval may be seen along with ST segment and T wave abnormalities. It can take up to several months for these repolarization abnormalities to resolve. Serum enzyme levels can be elevated and may reflect myocardial damage, at least in part, although concomitant rhabdomyolysis often is present.

Hypothermia

Low temperature can also result in myocardial damage.[267] Cardiac dilation can occur, with epicardial petechiae and subendocardial hemorrhages. Microinfarcts are found in the ventricular myocardium, presumably related to abnormalities in the microcirculation. The lesions are not caused by the low temperature per se but appear to be the result of the circulatory collapse, hemoconcentration, capillary slugging, and depressed cellular metabolism that accompany hypothermia. Clinical manifestations of hypothermia include sinus bradycardia, conduction disturbances, atrial (and occasionally ventricular) fibrillation, hypotension, a fall in cardiac output, reversible myocardial depression, and a characteristic deflection of the terminal portion of the QRS pattern (Osborn wave).[263] Treatment includes core warming (often utilizing extracorporeal blood warming), cardiopulmonary resuscitation, and management of pulmonary, hematological, and renal complications.[268,269] Notwithstanding its potential cardiac risks, mild therapeutic hypothermia appears to improve neurological outcome after cardiac arrest and is a currently accepted practice.

REFERENCES

Primary Myocarditis

1. Abelmann WH: Virus and the heart. Circulation 44:950, 1971.
2. Woodruff JF: Viral myocarditis: A review. Am J Pathol 101:425, 1980.
3. Kawai C: From myocarditis to cardiomyopathy: Mechanisms of inflammation and cell death: Learning from the past for the future. Circulation 99:1091, 1999.
4. Liu PP, Mason JW: Advances in the understanding of myocarditis. Circulation 104:1076, 2001.
5. Lange LG, Schreiner GF: Immune mechanisms of cardiac disease. N Engl J Med 330:112, 1994.
6. Liu PP, Opavsky MA: Viral myocarditis: Receptors that bridge the cardiovascular with the immune system? Circ Res 86:253, 2000.
7. Knowlton KU, Badorff C: The immune system in viral myocarditis: Maintaining the balance. Circ Res 85:559, 1999.
8. Liu PP, Le J, Nian M: Nuclear factor-kappaB decoy: Infiltrating the heart of the matter in inflammatory heart disease. Circ Res 89:850, 2001.
9. Eriksson U, Kurrer MO, Schmitz N, et al: Interleukin-6-deficient mice resist development of autoimmune myocarditis associated with impaired upregulation of complement C3. Circulation 107:320, 2003.
10. Watanabe K, Nakazawa M, Fuse K, et al: Protection against autoimmune myocarditis by gene transfer of interleukin-10 by electroporation. Circulation 104:1098, 2001.
11. Seko Y, Kayagaki N, Seino K, et al: Role of Fas/FasL pathway in the activation of infiltrating cells in murine acute myocarditis caused by Coxsackievirus B3. J Am Coll Cardiol 39:1399, 2002.
12. Bryant D, Becker L, Richardson J, et al: Cardiac failure in transgenic mice with myocardial expression of tumor necrosis factor-alpha. Circulation 97:1375, 1998.
13. Li J, Schwimmbeck PL, Tschope C, et al: Collagen degradation in a murine myocarditis model: Relevance of matrix metalloproteinase in association with inflammatory induction. Cardiovasc Res 56:235, 2002.
14. McLaughlin L, Zhu G, Mistry M, et al: Apolipoprotein J/clusterin limits the severity of murine autoimmune myocarditis. J Clin Invest 106:1105, 2000.
15. Opavsky MA, Penninger J, Aitken K, et al: Susceptibility to myocarditis is dependent on the response of alphabeta T lymphocytes to coxsackieviral infection. Circ Res 85:551, 1999.
16. Mendes LA, Picard MH, Dec GW, et al: Ventricular remodeling in active myocarditis. Myocarditis Treatment Trial. Am Heart J 138:303, 1999.
17. Finkel MS: Nitric oxide and viral cardiomyopathy. Circulation 102:2162, 2000.
18. Fukuchi M, Hussain SN, Giaid A: Heterogeneous expression and activity of endothelial and inducible nitric oxide synthases in end-stage human heart failure: Their relation to lesion site and beta-adrenergic receptor therapy. Circulation 98:132, 1998.
19. Badorff C, Fichtlscherer B, Rhoads RE, et al: Nitric oxide inhibits dystrophin proteolysis by coxsackieviral protease 2A through S-nitrosylation: A protective mechanism against enteroviral cardiomyopathy. Circulation 102:2276, 2000.
20. Lowenstein CJ, Hill SL, Lafond-Walker A, et al: Nitric oxide inhibits viral replication in murine myocarditis. J Clin Invest 97:1837, 1996.
21. Zaragoza C, Ocampo C, Saura M, et al: The role of inducible nitric oxide synthase in the host response to Coxsackievirus myocarditis. Proc Natl Acad Sci U S A 95:2469, 1998.
22. Wessely R, Henke A, Zell R, et al: Low-level expression of a mutant coxsackieviral cDNA induces a myocytopathic effect in culture: An approach to the study of enteroviral persistence in cardiac myocytes. Circulation 98:450, 1998.
23. Li Y, Bourlet T, Andreoletti L, et al: Enteroviral capsid protein VP1 is present in myocardial tissues from some patients with myocarditis or dilated cardiomyopathy. Circulation 101:231, 2000.

24. Zhang HM, Yanagawa B, Cheung P, et al: Nip21 gene expression reduces coxsackievirus B3 replication by promoting apoptotic cell death via a mitochondria-dependent pathway. Circ Res 90:1251, 2002.
25. Shioi T, Matsumori A, Sasayama S: Persistent expression of cytokine in the chronic stage of viral myocarditis in mice. Circulation 94:2930, 1996.
26. Sole MJ, Liu P: Viral myocarditis: A paradigm for understanding the pathogenesis and treatment of dilated cardiomyopathy. J Am Coll Cardiol 22:99A, 1993.

Clinical Manifestations

27. Angelini A, Calzolari V, Calabrese F, et al: Myocarditis mimicking acute myocardial infarction: Role of endomyocardial biopsy in the differential diagnosis. Heart 84:245, 2000.
28. Sarda L, Colin P, Boccara F, et al: Myocarditis in patients with clinical presentation of myocardial infarction and normal coronary angiograms. J Am Coll Cardiol 37:786, 2001.
29. Chimenti C, Calabrese F, Thiene G, et al: Inflammatory left ventricular microaneurysms as a cause of apparently idiopathic ventricular tachyarrhythmias. Circulation 104:168, 2001.
30. Badorff C, Zeiher AM, Hohnloser SH: Torsade de pointes tachycardia as a rare manifestation of acute enteroviral myocarditis. Heart 86:489, 2001.
31. Theleman KP, Kuiper JJ, Roberts WC: Acute myocarditis (predominately lymphocytic) causing sudden death without heart failure. Am J Cardiol 88:1078, 2001.
32. Maron BJ, Shirani J, Poliac LC, et al: Sudden death in young competitive athletes: Clinical, demographic, and pathological profiles. JAMA 276:199, 1996.
33. Frustaci A, Chimenti C, Bellocci F, et al: Histological substrate of atrial biopsies in patients with lone atrial fibrillation. Circulation 96:1180, 1997.
34. Smith SC, Ladenson JH, Mason JW, et al: Elevations of cardiac troponin I associated with myocarditis: Experimental and clinical correlates. Circulation 95:163, 1997.
35. Torre-Amione G, Kapadia S, Benedict C, et al: Proinflammatory cytokine levels in patients with depressed left ventricular ejection fraction: A report from the Studies of Left Ventricular Dysfunction (SOLVD). J Am Coll Cardiol 27:1201, 1996.
36. Toyozaki T, Hiroe M, Saito T, et al: Levels of soluble Fas in patients with myocarditis, heart failure of unknown origin, and in healthy volunteers. Am J Cardiol 81:798, 1998.
37. Felker GM, Boehmer JP, Hruban RH, et al: Echocardiographic findings in fulminant and acute myocarditis. J Am Coll Cardiol 36:227, 2000.
38. Dec GW, Palacios I, Yasuda T, et al: Antimyosin antibody cardiac imaging: Its role in the diagnosis of myocarditis. J Am Coll Cardiol 16:97, 1990.
39. O'Connell JB, Henkin RE, Robinson JA, et al: Gallium-67 imaging in patients with dilated cardiomyopathy and biopsy-proven myocarditis. Circulation 70:58, 1984.
40. Laissy JP, Messin B, Varenne O, et al: MRI of acute myocarditis: A comprehensive approach based on various imaging sequences. Chest 122:1638, 2002.
41. Manolio TA, Baughman KL, Rodeheffer R, et al: Prevalence and etiology of idiopathic dilated cardiomyopathy (summary of a National Heart, Lung, and Blood Institute workshop). Am J Cardiol 69:1458, 1992.
42. Dec GW Jr, Palacios IF, Fallon JT, et al: Active myocarditis in the spectrum of acute dilated cardiomyopathies: Clinical features, histologic correlates, and clinical outcome. N Engl J Med 312:885, 1985.
43. Felker GM, Hu W, Hare JM, et al: The spectrum of dilated cardiomyopathy. The Johns Hopkins experience with 1,278 patients. Medicine (Baltimore) 78:270, 1999.
44. Felker GM, Thompson RE, Hare JM, et al: Underlying causes and long-term survival in patients with initially unexplained cardiomyopathy. N Engl J Med 342:1077, 2000.
45. Aretz HT, Billingham ME, Edwards WD, et al: Myocarditis: A histopathologic definition and classification. Am J Cardiovasc Pathol 1:3, 1987.
46. Chow LH, Radio SJ, Sears TD, et al: Insensitivity of right ventricular endomyocardial biopsy in the diagnosis of myocarditis. J Am Coll Cardiol 14:915, 1989.
47. Herskowitz A, Ahmed-Ansari A, Neumann DA, et al: Induction of major histocompatibility complex antigens within the myocardium of patients with active myocarditis: A nonhistologic marker of myocarditis. J Am Coll Cardiol 15:624, 1990.
48. Seko Y, Takahashi N, Ishiyama S, et al: Expression of costimulatory molecules B7-1, B7-2, and CD40 in the heart of patients with acute myocarditis and dilated cardiomyopathy. Circulation 97:637, 1998.
49. Satoh M, Nakamura M, Satoh H, et al: Expression of tumor necrosis factor-alpha–converting enzyme and tumor necrosis factor-alpha in human myocarditis. J Am Coll Cardiol 36:1288, 2000.
50. Alter P, Jobmann M, Meyer E, et al: Apoptosis in myocarditis and dilated cardiomyopathy: Does enterovirus genome persistence protect from apoptosis? An endomyocardial biopsy study. Cardiovasc Pathol 10:229, 2001.
51. Neumann DA, Rose NR, Ansari AA, et al: Induction of multiple heart autoantibodies in mice with coxsackievirus B3- and cardiac myosin-induced autoimmune myocarditis. J Immunol 152:343, 1994.
52. Limas CJ, Goldenberg IF, Limas C: Autoantibodies against beta-adrenoceptors in human idiopathic dilated cardiomyopathy. Circ Res 64:97, 1989.
53. Lieberman EB, Hutchins GM, Herskowitz A, et al: Clinicopathologic description of myocarditis. J Am Coll Cardiol 18:1617, 1991.
54. McCarthy RE 3rd, Boehmer JP, Hruban RH, et al: Long-term outcome of fulminant myocarditis as compared with acute (nonfulminant) myocarditis. N Engl J Med 342:690, 2000.
55. Aoyama N, Izumi T, Hiramori K, et al: National survey of fulminant myocarditis in Japan: Therapeutic guidelines and long-term prognosis of using percutaneous cardiopulmonary support for fulminant myocarditis (special report from a scientific committee). Circ J 66:133, 2002.
56. Deckers JW, Hare JM, Baughman KL: Complications of transvenous right ventricular endomyocardial biopsy in adult patients with cardiomyopathy: A seven-year survey of 546 consecutive diagnostic procedures in a tertiary referral center. J Am Coll Cardiol 19:43, 1992.
57. Denys BG, Uretsky BF, Reddy PS: Ultrasound-assisted cannulation of the internal jugular vein: A prospective comparison to the external landmark-guided technique. Circulation 87:1557, 1993.

Treatment of Primary Myocarditis

58. Wang WZ, Matsumori A, Yamada T, et al: Beneficial effects of amlodipine in a murine model of congestive heart failure induced by viral myocarditis: A possible mechanism through inhibition of nitric oxide production. Circulation 95:245, 1997.
59. Nishio R, Shioi T, Sasayama S, et al: Carvedilol increases the production of interleukin-12 and interferon-gamma and improves the survival of mice infected with the encephalomyocarditis virus. J Am Coll Cardiol 41:340, 2003.
60. Rezkalla SH, Raikar S, Kloner RA: Treatment of viral myocarditis with focus on captopril. Am J Cardiol 77:634, 1996.
61. Bozkurt B, Villaneuva FS, Holubkov R, et al: Intravenous immune globulin in the therapy of peripartum cardiomyopathy. J Am Coll Cardiol 34:177, 1999.
62. McNamara DM, Holubkov R, Starling RC, et al: Controlled trial of intravenous immune globulin in recent-onset dilated cardiomyopathy. Circulation 103:2254, 2001.
63. Kereiakes DJ, Parmley WW: Myocarditis and cardiomyopathy. Am Heart J 108:1318, 1984.
64. Parrillo JE, Cunnion RE, Epstein SE, et al: A prospective, randomized, controlled trial of prednisone for dilated cardiomyopathy. N Engl J Med 321:1061, 1989.
65. Mason JW, O'Connell JB, Herskowitz A, et al: A clinical trial of immunosuppressive therapy for myocarditis. The Myocarditis Treatment Trial Investigators. N Engl J Med 333:269, 1995.
66. Jones SR, Herskowitz A, Hutchins GM, et al: Effects of immunosuppressive therapy in biopsy-proved myocarditis and borderline myocarditis on left ventricular function. Am J Cardiol 68:370, 1991.
67. Wojnicz R, Nowalany-Kozielska E, Wojciechowska C, et al: Randomized, placebo-controlled study for immunosuppressive treatment of inflammatory dilated cardiomyopathy: Two-year follow-up results. Circulation 104:39, 2001.
68. Frustaci A, Chimenti C, Calabrese F, et al: Immunosuppressive therapy for active lymphocytic myocarditis: Virological and immunologic profile of responders versus nonresponders. Circulation 107:857, 2003.
69. Kato S, Morimoto S, Hiramitsu S, et al: Use of percutaneous cardiopulmonary support of patients with fulminant myocarditis and cardiogenic shock for improving prognosis. Am J Cardiol 83:623, 1999.
70. Rockman HA, Adamson RM, Dembitsky WP, et al: Acute fulminant myocarditis: Long-term follow-up after circulatory support with left ventricular assist device. Am Heart J 121:922, 1991.
71. Felix SB, Staudt A, Landsberger M, et al: Removal of cardiodepressant antibodies in dilated cardiomyopathy by immunoadsorption. J Am Coll Cardiol 39:646, 2002.
72. Hofling K, Kim KS, Leser JS, et al: Progress toward vaccines against viruses that cause heart disease. Herz 25:286, 2000.
73. Cooper LT Jr, Berry GJ, Shabetai R: Idiopathic giant-cell myocarditis: Natural history and treatment. Multicenter Giant Cell Myocarditis Study Group Investigators. N Engl J Med 336:1860, 1997.
74. Nash CL, Panaccione R, Sutherland LR, et al: Giant cell myocarditis, in a patient with Crohn's disease, treated with etanercept—a tumour necrosis factor-alpha antagonist. Can J Gastroenterol 15:607, 2001.
75. Hyogo M, Kamitani T, Oguni A, et al: Acute necrotizing eosinophilic myocarditis with giant cell infiltration after remission of idiopathic thrombocytopenic purpura. Intern Med 36:894, 1997.
76. Frustaci A, Cuoco L, Chimenti C, et al: Celiac disease associated with autoimmune myocarditis. Circulation 105:2611, 2002.
77. Daniels PR, Berry GJ, Tazelaar HD, et al: Giant cell myocarditis as a manifestation of drug hypersensitivity. Cardiovasc Pathol 9:287, 2000.
78. Shields RC, Tazelaar HD, Berry GJ, et al: The role of right ventricular endomyocardial biopsy for idiopathic giant cell myocarditis. J Card Fail 8:74, 2002.
79. Okura Y, Dec GW, Hare JM, et al: A clinical and histopathologic comparison of cardiac sarcoidosis and idiopathic giant cell myocarditis. J Am Coll Cardiol 41:322, 2003.
80. Litovsky SH, Burke AP, Virmani R: Giant cell myocarditis: An entity distinct from sarcoidosis characterized by multiphasic myocyte destruction by cytotoxic T cells and histiocytic giant cells. Mod Pathol 9:1126, 1996.
81. Menghini VV, Savcenko V, Olson LJ, et al: Combined immunosuppression for the treatment of idiopathic giant cell myocarditis. Mayo Clin Proc 74:1221, 1999.
82. Frustaci A, Chimenti C, Pieroni M, et al: Giant cell myocarditis responding to immunosuppressive therapy. Chest 117:905, 2000.
83. Pinderski LJ, Fonarow GC, Hamilton M, et al: Giant cell myocarditis in a young man responsive to T-lymphocyte cytolytic therapy. J Heart Lung Transplant 221:818, 2002.
84. Davies RA, Veinot JP, Smith S, et al: Giant cell myocarditis: Clinical presentation, bridge to transplantation with mechanical circulatory support, and long-term outcome. J Heart Lung Transplant 21:674, 2002.
85. Scott RL, Ratliff NB, Starling RC, et al: Recurrence of giant cell myocarditis in cardiac allograft. J Heart Lung Transplant 20:375, 2001.

Secondary Myocarditis

86. Pisani B, Taylor DO, Mason JW: Inflammatory myocardial diseases and cardiomyopathies. Am J Med 102:459, 1997.
87. Hyypia T: Etiological diagnosis of viral heart disease. Scand J Infect Dis 88:25, 1993.
88. Remes J, Helin M, Vaino P, et al: Clinical outcome and left ventricular function 23 years after acute coxsackievirus myopericarditis. Eur Heart J 11:182, 1990.
89. Lowry RW, Adam E, Hu C, et al: What are the implications of cardiac infection with cytomegalovirus before heart transplantation? J Heart Lung Transplant 13:122, 1994.
90. Partanen J, Nieminen MS, Krogerus L, et al: Cytomegalovirus myocarditis in transplanted heart verified by endomyocardial biopsy. Clin Cardiol 14:847, 1991.
91. Ursell PC, Habib A, Sharma P, et al: Hepatitis B virus and myocarditis. Hum Pathol 15:481, 1984.
92. Prati D, Poli F, Farma E, et al: Multicenter study on hepatitis C virus infection in patients with dilated cardiomyopathy. J Med Virol 58:116, 1999.

93. Dalekos GN, Achenbach K, Christodoulou D, et al: Idiopathic dilated cardiomyopathy: Lack of association with hepatitis C virus infection. Heart 80:270, 1998.
94. Frustaci A, Calabrese F, Chimenti C, et al: Lone hepatitis C virus myocarditis responsive to immunosuppressive therapy. Chest 122:2611, 2002.
95. Craver RD, Sorrells K, Gohd R: Myocarditis with influenza B infection. Pediatr Infect Dis J 16:629, 1997.
96. Kaji M, Kuno H, Turu T, et al: Elevated serum myosin light chain I in influenza patients. Intern Med 40:594, 2001.
97. McGregor D, Henderson S: Myocarditis, rhabdomyolysis and myoglobinuric renal failure complicating influenza in a young adult. N Z Med J 110:237, 1997.
98. Agnino A, Schena S, Ferlan G, et al: Left ventricular pseudoaneurysm after acute influenza A myocardiopericarditis. J Cardiovasc Surg 43:203, 2002.
99. Ozkutlu S, Soylemezoglu O, Calikoglu AS, et al: Fatal mumps myocarditis. Jpn Heart J 30:109, 1989.
100. Kabakus N, Aydinoglu H, Yekeler H, Arslan IN: Fatal mumps nephritis and myocarditis. J Trop Pediatr 45:358, 1999.
101. Frustaci A, Abdulla AK, Caldarulo M, et al: Fatal measles myocarditis. Cardiologia 35: 347, 1990.
102. Degen JA: Visceral pathology in measles. Am J Med Sci 194:104, 1937.
103. Alter P, Grimm W, Maisch B: Varicella myocarditis in an adult. Heart 85:E2, 2001.
104. Tsintsof A, Delprado WJ, Keogh AM: Varicella zoster myocarditis progressing to cardiomyopathy and cardiac transplantation. Br Heart J 70:93, 1993.
105. Matthews AW, Griffiths ID: Post-vaccinial pericarditis and myocarditis. Br Heart J 36:1043, 1974.
106. Kabra SK, Juneja R, Madhulika, et al: Myocardial dysfunction in children with dengue haemorrhagic fever. Natl Med J India 11:59, 1998.
107. Wali JP, Biswas A, Chandra S, et al: Cardiac involvement in dengue haemorrhagic fever. Int J Cardiol 64:31, 1998.
108. Hebert MM, Yu C, Towbin JA, et al: Fatal Epstein-Barr virus myocarditis in a child with repetitive myocarditis. Pediatr Pathol Lab Med 15:805, 1995.
109. Cummins D, Bennett D, Fisher-Hoch SP, et al: Electrocardiographic abnormalities in patients with Lassa fever. J Trop Med Hyg 92:350, 1989.
110. Hildes JA, Schaberg A, Alcock AUW: Cardiovascular collapse in acute poliomyelitis. Circulation 12:986, 1955.
111. Thomas JA, Raroque S, Scott WA, et al: Successful treatment of severe dysrhythmias in infants with respiratory syncytial virus infections: Two cases and a literature review. Crit Care Med 25:880, 1997.
112. Olesch CA, Bullock AM: Bradyarrhythmia and supraventricular tachycardia in a neonate with RSV. J Paediatr Child Health 34:199, 1998.
113. Huang M, Bigos D, Levine M: Ventricular arrhythmia associated with respiratory syncytial viral infection. Pediatr Cardiol 19:498, 1998.
114. Ho M, Chen E, Hsu K, et al: An epidemic of enterovirus 71 infection in Taiwan. N Engl J Med 341:13, 1999.
115. Schowengerdt K, Ni J, Denfield S, et al: Association of parvovirus B19 genome in children with myocarditis and cardiac allograft rejection. Circulation 96:3549, 1997.
116. Fournier PE, Etienne J, Harle JR, et al: Myocarditis, a rare but severe manifestation of Q fever: Report of 8 cases and review of the literature. Clin Infect Dis 32:1440, 2001.
117. Raoult D, Tissot-Dupont H, Foucault C, et al: Q fever 1985-1998: Clinical and epidemiologic features of 1,383 infections. Medicine (Baltimore) 79:109, 2000.
118. Marin-Garcia J, Barrett FF: Myocardial function in Rocky Mountain spotted fever: Echocardiographic assessment. Am J Cardiol 51:341, 1983.
119. Yotsukura M, Aoki N, Fukuzumi N, et al: Review of a case of Tsutsugamushi disease showing myocarditis and confirmation of rickettsia by endomyocardial biopsy. Jpn Circ J 55:149, 1991.
120. Tsay RW, Chang FY: Serious complications in scrub typhus. J Microbiol Immunol Infect 31:240, 1998.
121. Stevens DL, Troyer BE, Merrick DT, et al: Lethal effects and cardiovascular effects of purified alpha- and theta-toxins from *Clostridium perfringens*. J Infect Dis 157:272, 1988.
122. Kadirova R, Kartoglu HU, Strebel PM: Clinical characteristics and management of 676 hospitalized diphtheria cases, Kyrgyz Republic, 1995. J Infect Dis 181(Suppl 1):S110, 2000.
123. Loukoushkina EF, Bobko PV, Kolbasova EV, et al: The clinical picture and diagnosis of diphtheritic carditis in children. Eur J Pediatr 157:528, 1998.
124. Havaldar PV, Patil VD, Siddibhavi BM, et al: Fulminant diptheretic myocarditis. Indian Heart J 41:265, 1989.
125. Dung NM, Kneen R, Kiem N: Treatment of severe diphtheritic myocarditis by temporary insertion of a cardiac pacemaker. Clin Infect Dis 35:1425, 2002.
126. O'Neill PG, Rokey R, Greenberg S, et al: Resolution of ventricular tachycardia and endocardial tuberculoma following antituberculosis therapy. Chest 100:1467,1991.
127. Afzal A, Keohane M, Keeley E, et al: Myocarditis and pericarditis with tamponade associated with disseminated tuberculosis. Can J Cardiol 16:4, 2000.
128. Chan AC, Dickens P: Tuberculous myocarditis presenting as sudden cardiac death. Forensic Sci Int 57:45, 1992.
129. Alkhuja S, Miller A: Tuberculosis and sudden death: A case report and review. Heart & Lung 30:388, 2001.
130. Silvestry FE, Kim B, Pollack BJ, et al: Cardiac Whipple disease: Identification of Whipple bacillus by electron microscopy of a patient before death. Ann Intern Med 126:214, 1997.
131. Elkins C, Shuman TA, Pirolo JS: Cardiac Whipple's disease without digestive symptoms. Ann Thorac Surg 67:250, 1999.
132. Mooney EE, Kenan DJ, Sweeney EC, et al: Myocarditis in Whipple's disease: An unsuspected cause of symptoms and sudden death. Mod Pathol 10:524, 1997.
133. Jubber AS, Gunawardana DR, Lulu AR: Acute pulmonary edema in *Brucella* myocarditis and interstitial pneumonitis. Chest 97:1008, 1990.
134. Schinkel A, Bax J, van der Wall E, et al: Echocardiographic follow-up of *Chlamydia psittaci* myocarditis. Chest 117:1203, 2000.
135. Bachmaier K, Neu N, de la Maza L, et al: Chlamydia infections and heart disease linked through antigenic mimicry. Science 283:5406, 1999.
136. Armengol S, Domingo C, Mesalles E: Myocarditis: A rare complication during Legionella infection. Int J Cardiol 37:418, 1992.
137. Garcia NS, Castelo JS, Ramos V, et al: Frequency of myocarditis in cases of fatal meningococcal infection in children: Observations on 31 cases studied at autopsy. Rev Soc Bras Med Trop 32:517, 1999.
138. Sandler MA, Pincus PS, Weltman MD, et al: Meningococcaemia complicated by myocarditis: A report of 2 cases. S Afr Med J 75:391, 1989.
139. Agarwala BN, Ruschhaupt DG: Complete heart block from *Mycoplasma pneumoniae* infection. Pediatr Cardiol 12:233, 1991.
140. Hofner G, Hofbeck M, Koch A, et al: Intrapericardial hemorrhage as a manifestation of mycoplasma pneumoniae infection. Kardiol 86:423, 1997.
141. Odeh M, Oliven A: Chlamydial infections of the heart. Eur J Clin Microbiol Infect Dis 11:885, 1992.
142. Neuwirth C, François C, Laurent N, et al: Myocarditis due to *Salmonella virchow* and sudden infant death. Lancet 354:1004, 1999.
143. Lu M, Ji B, Ouyang K: Clinical and laboratory studies with typhoid fever in 178 patients. Hunan Yi Ke Da Xue Xue Bao 22:15, 1997.

Spirochetal, Fungal, and Protozoal Myocarditis

144. Sangha O, Phillips CB, Fleischmann KE, et al: Lack of cardiac manifestations among patients with previously treated Lyme disease. Ann Intern Med 128:346, 1998.
145. Hajjar R, Kradin R: Weekly clinicopathological exercises. Case 17-2002: A 55-year-old man with second degree atrioventricular block and chest pain. N Engl J Med 346:1732, 2002.
145a. Nowakowski JN, Nadelman RB, Sell R, et al: Long-term follow-up of patients with culture-confirmed Lyme disease. Am J Med 115:91, 2003.
146. Haywood GA, O'Connell S, Gray HH: Lyme carditis: A United Kingdom perspective. Br Heart J 70:15, 1993.
147. Asch ES, Bujak DI, Weiss M, et al: Lyme disease: An infectious and postinfectious syndrome. J Rheumatol 21:454, 1994.
148. Ledford DK: Immunologic aspects of vasculitis and cardiovascular disease. JAMA 278:1962, 1997.
149. Nagi KS, Joshi R, Thakur RK: Cardiac manifestations of Lyme disease: A review. Can J Cardiol 12:503, 1996.
150. Rees DH, Keeling PJ, McKenna WJ, et al: No evidence to implicate *Borrelia burgdorferi* in the pathogenesis of dilated cardiomyopathy in the United Kingdom. Br Heart J 71:459, 1994.
151. Stanek G, Klein J, Bittner R, et al: Isolation of *Borrelia burgdorferi* from the myocardium of a patient with long-standing cardiomyopathy. N Engl J Med 322:249, 1990.
152. Rahn DW, Malawista SE: Lyme disease: Recommendations for diagnosis and treatment. Ann Intern Med 14:472, 1991.
153. Rajajee S, Shankar J, Dhattatri L: Pediatric presentations of leptospirosis. Indian J Pediatr 69:10, 2002.
154. Singh SS, Vijayachari P, Sinha A, et al: Clinico-epidemiological study of hospitalized cases of severe leptospirosis. Indian J Med Res 109:94, 1999.
155. Rajiv C, Manjuran RJ, Sudhayakumar N, et al: Cardiovascular involvement in leptospirosis. Indian Heart J 48:691, 1996.
156. Mekasha A: Louse-borne relapsing fever in children. J Trop Med Hyg 95:206, 1992.
157. Chino M, Minami T, Nishikawa K: Ruptured ventricular aneurysm in secondary syphilis. Lancet 342:935, 1993.
158. Berarducci L, Ford K, Olenick S, et al: Invasive intracardiac aspergillosis with widespread embolization. J Am Soc Echocardiogr 6:539, 1993.
159. Rueter F, Hirsch HH, Kunz F: Late *Aspergillus fumigatus* endomyocarditis with brain abscess as a lethal complication after heart transplantation. J Heart Lung Transplant 21:1242, 2002.
160. Bashour TT, Gord C, Baladi N, et al: Intracardiac actinomycosis. Am Heart J 133:467, 1997.
161. Serody JS, Mill MR, Detterbeck FC, et al: Blastomycosis in transplant recipients: Report of a case and review. Clin Infect Dis 16:54, 1993.
162. Parker JC: The potentially lethal problem of cardiac candidosis. Am J Clin Pathol 73:356, 1980.
163. Franklin WG, Simon AB, Sodeman TM: Candida myocarditis without valvulitis. Am J Cardiol 38:924, 1976.
164. Faul JL, Hoang K, Schmoker J, et al: Constrictive pericarditis due to coccidioidomycosis. Ann Thorac Surg 68:1407, 1999.
165. Lafont A, Wolff M, Marche C, et al: Overwhelming myocarditis due to *Cryptococcus neoformans* in an AIDS patient. Lancet 2:1145, 1987.
166. Kirchner SG, Hernanz-Schulman M, Stein SM, et al: Imaging of pediatric mediastinal histoplasmosis. Radiographics 11:365, 1991.
167. Jackman JD Jr, Simonsen RL: The clinical manifestations of cardiac mucormycosis. Chest 101:1733, 1992.
168. Virmani R, Connor DH, McAllister HA: Cardiac mucormycosis: A report of five patients and review of 14 previously reported cases. Am J Clin Pathol 78:42, 1982.
169. Hagar JM, Rahimtoola SH: Chagas' heart disease. Curr Probl Cardiol 20:825, 1995.
170. Rassi A Jr, Rassi A, Little WC: Chagas' heart disease. Clin Cardiol 23:883, 2000.
171. Rossi MA, Bestetti RB: The challenge of chagasic cardiomyopathy: The pathologic roles of autonomic abnormalities, autoimmune mechanisms and microvascular changes, and therapeutic implications. Cardiology 86:1, 1995.
172. Parada H, Carrasco HA, Anez N, et al: Cardiac involvement is a constant finding in acute Chagas' disease: A clinical, parasitological and histopathological study. Int J Cardiol 60:49, 1997.
173. Machado F, Martins G, Aliberti J, et al: *Trypanosoma cruzi*-infected cardiomyocytes produce chemokines and cytokines that trigger potent nitric oxide-dependent trypanocidal activity. Circulation 102:3003, 2000.

174. Reis MM, Higuchi M, de la Benvenuti LA, et al: An in situ quantitative immunohistochemical study of cytokines and IL-2R+ in chronic human chagasic myocarditis: Correlation with the presence of myocardial *Trypanosoma cruzi* antigens. Clin Immunol Immunopathol 83:165, 1997.
175. Anez N, Carrasco H, Parada H, et al: Myocardial parasite persistence in chronic chagasic patients. Am J Trop Med Hyg 60:726, 1999.
176. Bellotti G, Bocchi EA, de Moraes AV, et al: In vivo detection of *Trypanosoma cruzi* antigens in hearts of patients with chronic Chagas' heart disease. Am Heart J 131:301, 1996.
177. Bestetti RB, Muccillo G: Clinical course of Chagas' heart disease: A comparison with dilated cardiomyopathy. Int J Cardiol 60:187, 1997.
178. Cunha-Neto E, Kalil J: Heart-infiltrating and peripheral T cells in the pathogenesis of human Chagas' disease cardiomyopathy. Autoimmunity 34:187, 2001.
179. Gomes JA, Bahia-Oliveira LM, Rocha MO, et al: Evidence that development of severe cardiomyopathy in human Chagas' disease is due to a Th 1-specific immune response. Infect Immun 71:1185, 2003.
180. Higuchi MD, Ries MM, Aiello VD, et al: Association of an increase in CD8+ T cells with the presence of *Trypanosoma cruzi* antigens in chronic, human, chagasic myocarditis. Am J Trop Med Hyg 56:485, 1997.
181. Sterin-Borda L, Gorelik G, Postan M, et al: Alterations in cardiac beta-adrenergic receptors in chagasic mice and their association with circulating beta-adrenoceptor-related autoantibodies. Cardiovasc Res 41:116, 1999.
182. Rossi MA: Comparison of Chagas' heart disease to arrhythmogenic right ventricular cardiomyopathy. Am Heart J 129:626, 1995.
183. Higuchi ML, Fukasawa S, De Brito T, et al: Different microcirculatory and interstitial matrix patterns in idiopathic dilated cardiomyopathy and Chagas' disease: A three dimensional confocal microscopy study. Heart 82:279, 1999.
184. Bestetti RB, Dalbo CM, Arruda CA, et al: Predictors of sudden cardiac death for patients with Chagas' disease: A hospital-derived cohort study. Cardiology 87:481, 1996.
185. Carrasco HA, Alarçon M, Olmos L, et al: Biochemical characterization of myocardial damage in chronic Chagas' disease. Clin Cardiol 20:865, 1997.
186. Bestetti RB, Dalbo CM, Freitas QC, et al: Noninvasive predictors of mortality for patients with Chagas' heart disease: A multivariate stepwise logistic regression study. Cardiology 84:261, 1994.
187. Martinelli F, De Siqueira S, Moreira H: Probability of occurrence of life-threatening ventricular arrhythmias in Chagas' disease versus non-Chagas' disease. Pacing Clin Electrophysiol 23:1944, 2000.
188. de Paola AA, Gomes JA, Terzian AB, et al: Ventricular tachycardia during exercise testing as a predictor of sudden death in patients with chronic chagasic cardiomyopathy and ventricular arrhythmias. Br Heart J 74:293, 1995.
189. Carrasco HA, Parada H, Guerrero L, et al: Prognostic implications of clinical, electrocardiographic and hemodynamic findings in chronic Chagas' disease. Int J Cardiol 43:27, 1994.
190. Braga JC, Labrunie A, Villaca F, et al: Thromboembolism in chronic Chagas' heart disease. Rev Paul Med 113:862, 1995.
191. Acquatella H, Perez JE, Condado JA, et al: Limited myocardial contractile reserve and chronotropic incompetence in patients with chronic Chagas' disease: Assessment by dobutamine stress echocardiography. J Am Coll Cardiol 3:22, 1999.
192. Marin-Neto JA, Marzullo P, Marcassa C, et al: Myocardial perfusion abnormalities in chronic Chagas' disease as detected by thallium-201 scintigraphy. Am J Cardiol 69:780, 1992.
193. Kalil Filho R, de Albuquerque CP: Magnetic resonance imaging in Chagas' heart disease. Rev Paul Med 113:880, 1995.
194. Ferreira AW, de Avila SD: Laboratory diagnosis of Chagas' heart disease. Rev Paul Med 113:767, 1995.
195. de Paola AA, Gondin AA, Hara V, et al: Medical treatment of cardiac arrhythmias in Chagas' heart disease. Rev Paul Med 113:858, 1995.
196. Leon J, Wang K, Engman D: Captopril ameliorates myocarditis in acute experimental Chagas disease. Circulation 107:2264, 2003.
197. Muratore C, Rabinovich R, Iglesias R, et al: Implantable cardioverter defibrillators in patients with Chagas' disease: Are they different from patients with coronary disease? Pacing Clin Electrophysiol 20:194, 1997.
198. Apt W, Aguilera X, Arribada A, et al: Treatment of chronic Chagas' disease with itraconazole and allopurinol. Am J Trop Med Hyg 59:133, 1998.
199. Bocchi EA, Bellotti G, Mocelin AO, et al: Heart transplantation for chronic Chagas' heart disease. Ann Thorac Surg 61:1727, 1996.
200. Bocchi EA, Fiorelli A: The paradox of survival results after heart transplantation for cardiomyopathy caused by *Trypanosoma cruzi*. Ann Thorac Surg 71:6, 2001.
201. Bocchi EA, Higuchi ML, Vieira ML, et al: Higher incidence of malignant neoplasms after heart transplantation for treatment of chronic Chagas' heart disease. J Heart Lung Transplant 17:399, 1998.
202. Tsala Mbala P, Blackett K, Mbonifor CL, et al: Functional and immunologic involvement in human African trypanosomiasis caused by *Trypanosoma gambiense*. Bull Soc Pathol Exot Filiales 81:490, 1988.
203. Duffield JS, Jacob AJ, Miller HC: Recurrent, life-threatening atrioventricular dissociation associated with *Toxoplasma* myocarditis. Heart 76:453, 1996.
204. Montoya JG, Jordan R, Lingamneni S, et al: Toxoplasmic myocarditis and polymyositis in patients with acute acquired toxoplasmosis diagnosed during life. Clin Infect Dis 24:676, 1997.
205. Vuong PN, Richard F, Snounou G, et al: Development of irreversible lesions in the brain, heart, and kidneys following acute and chronic murine malaria infection. Parasitology 119:543, 1999.
206. Bethell DB, Phuong PT, Phuong CX, et al: Electrocardiographic monitoring in severe falciparum malaria. Trans R Soc Trop Med Hyg 90:266, 1996.
207. Salih OK, Celik SK, Topcuoglu MS, et al: Surgical treatment of hydatid cysts of the heart: A report of 3 cases and a review of the literature. Can J Surg 41:321, 1998.
208. Benomar A, Yahyaoui M, Birouk N, et al: Middle cerebral artery occlusion due to hydatid cysts of myocardial and intraventricular cavity cardiac origin: Two cases. Stroke 25:886, 1994.
209. Miralles A, Bracamonte L, Pavie A, et al: Cardiac echinococcosis: Surgical treatment and results. J Thorac Cardiovasc Surg 107:184, 1994.
210. Franchi C, Di Vico B, Teggi A: Long-term evaluation of patients with hydatidosis treated with benzimidazole carbamates. Clin Infect Dis 29:304, 1999.
211. Ozer N, Aytemir K, Kuru G, et al: Hydatid cyst of the heart as a rare cause of embolization: Report of 5 cases and review of published reports. J Am Soc Echocardiogr 14:299, 2001.
212. Lazarevic AM, Neskovic AN, Goronja M, et al: Low incidence of cardiac abnormalities in treated trichinosis: A prospective study of 62 patients from a single-source outbreak. Am J Med 107:18, 1999.
213. Compton SJ, Celum CL, Lee C, et al: Trichinosis with ventilatory failure and persistent myocarditis. Clin Infect Dis 16:500, 1993.
214. Dao AH, Virmani R: Visceral larva migrans involving the myocardium: Report of two cases and review of literature. Pediatr Pathol 6:449, 1986.
215. Abe K, Shimokawa H, Kubota T, et al: Myocarditis associated with visceral larva migrans due to *Toxocara canis*. Intern Med 41:706, 2002.
216. Morris W, Knauer CM: Cardiopulmonary manifestations of schistosomiasis. Semin Respir Infect 12:159, 1997.

Toxic, Chemical, and Physical Damage

217. Feenstra J, Grobbee DE, Remme WJ, et al: Drug-induced heart failure. J Am Coll Cardiol 33:1152, 1999.
218. Le Blaye I, Donatini B, Hall M, et al: Acute overdosage with thioridazine: A review of the available clinical exposure. Vet Hum Toxicol 35:147, 1993.
219. Schmidt W, Lang K: Life-threatening dysrhythmias in severe thioridazine poisoning treated with physostigmine and transient atrial pacing. Crit Care Med 25:1925, 1997.
220. Vanoli E, De Ferrari GM, Stramba-Badiale M, et al: Carbon monoxide and lethal arrhythmias in conscious dogs with healed myocardial infarction. Am Heart J 117:348, 1989.
221. Dahms TE, Younis LT, Wiens RD, et al: Effects of carbon monoxide exposure in patients with documented cardiac arrhythmias. J Am Coll Cardiol 21:442, 1993.
222. McMeekin JD, Finegan BA: Reversible myocardial dysfunction following carbon monoxide poisoning. Can J Cardiol 3:118, 1987.
223. Marius-Nunez AL: Myocardial infarction with normal coronary arteries after acute exposure to carbon monoxide. Chest 97:491, 1990.
224. Angulo MP, Navajas A, Galdeano JM, et al: Reversible cardiomyopathy secondary to alpha-interferon in an infant. Pediatr Cardiol 20:293, 1999.
225. Goel M, Flaherty L, Lavine S, et al: Reversible cardiomyopathy after high-dose interleukin-2 therapy. J Immunother 11:225, 1992.
226. La Grenade L, Graham D, Trontell A: Myocarditis and cardiomyopathy associated with clozapine use in the United States. N Engl J Med 345:224, 2001.
227. Ho PC, Dweik R, Cohen MC: Rapidly reversible cardiomyopathy associated with chronic ipecac ingestion. Clin Cardiol 21:780, 1998.
228. Silberstein SD: Methysergide. Cephalalgia 18:421, 1998.
229. Iglesias Cubero G, Rodriguez Reguero JJ, Rojo Ortega JM: Restrictive cardiomyopathy caused by chloroquine. Br Heart J 69:451, 1993.
230. Sundar S, Sinha PR, Agrawal NK, et al: A cluster of cases of severe cardiotoxicity among kala-azar patients treated with a high-osmolarity lot of sodium antimony gluconate. Am J Trop Med Hyg 59:139, 1998.
231. Ortega-Carnicer J, Alcazar R, De la Torre M, et al: Pentavalent antimonial-induced torsades de pointes. J Electrocardiol 30:143, 1997.
232. Groleau G: Lithium toxicity. Emerg Med Clin North Am 12:511, 1994.
233. Terao T, Abe H, Abe K: Irreversible sinus node dysfunction induced by resumption of lithium therapy. Acta Psychiatr Scand 93:407, 1996.
234. Gerhardt RT: Acute halon (bromochlorodifluoromethane) toxicity by accidental and recreational inhalation. Am J Emerg Med 14:675, 1996.
235. Brady WJ Jr, Stremski E, Eljaiek L, et al: Freon inhalational abuse presenting with ventricular fibrillation. Am J Emerg Med 12:533, 1994.
236. Kopp SJ, Barron JT, Tow JP: Cardiovascular actions of lead and relationship to hypertension: A review. Environ Health Perspect 78:91, 1988.
237. Kudoh C, Tanaka S, Marusaki S, et al: Hypocalcemic cardiomyopathy in a patient with idiopathic hypoparathyroidism. Intern Med 31:561, 1992.
238. Feldman AM, Fivush B, Zahka KG, et al: Congestive cardiomyopathy in patients on continuous ambulatory peritoneal dialysis. Am Kidney Dis 11:76, 1988.
239. Claudius I, Sachs C, Shamji T: Hypophosphatemia-induced heart failure. Am J Emerg Med 20:369, 2002.
240. Davis SV, Olichwier KK, Chakko SC: Reversible depression of myocardial performance in hypophosphatemia. Am J Med Sci 295:183, 1988.
241. Kurnik BR, Marshall J, Katz SM: Hypomagnesemia-induced cardiomyopathy. Magnesium 7:49, 1988.
242. Riggs JE, Klingberg WG, Flink EB, et al: Cardioskeletal mitochondrial myopathy associated with chronic magnesium deficiency. Neurology 42:128, 1992.
243. Wagdi P, Mehan VK, Burgi H, et al: Acute myocardial infarction after wasp stings in a patient with normal coronary arteries. Am Heart J 128:820, 1994.
244. Lalloo DG, Trevett AJ, Nwokolo N, et al: Electrocardiographic abnormalities in patients bitten by taipans (*Oxyuranus scutellatus canni*) and other elapid snakes in Papua New Guinea. Trans R Soc Trop Med Hyg 91:53, 1997.
245. Kurnik D, Haviv Y, Kochva E: A snake bite by the burrowing asp, *Atractaspis engaddensis*. Toxicon 37:223, 1999.
246. Hall JC, Harruff R: Fatal cardiac arrhythmia in a patient with interstitial myocarditis related to chronic arsenic poisoning. South Med J 82:1557, 1989.
247. Paulson DJ: Carnitine deficiency-induced cardiomyopathy. Mol Cell Biochem 180:33, 1998.
248. Ergur AT, Tanzer F, Cetinkaya O: Serum-free carnitine levels in children with heart failure. J Trop Pediatr 45:168, 1999.

249. Huttunen JK: Selenium and cardiovascular diseases: An update. Biomed Environ Sci 10:220, 1997.
250. Levy JB, Jones HW, Gordon AC: Selenium deficiency, reversible cardiomyopathy and short-term intravenous feeding. Postgrad Med J 70:235, 1994.
251. Kumar EB, Soomro RS, al Hamdani A, et al: Scorpion venom cardiomyopathy. Am Heart J 123:725, 1992.
252. Gueron M, Ilia R, Sofer S: Scorpion venom cardiomyopathy. Am Heart J 125:1816, 1993.
253. Haller CA, Jacob P 3rd, Benowitz NL: Pharmacology of ephedra alkaloids and caffeine after single-dose dietary supplement use. Clin Pharmacol Ther 71:421, 2002.
254. Samen KD, Link MS, Homoud MK, et al: Adverse cardiovascular events temporally associated with ma huang, an herbal source of ephedrine. Mayo Clin Proc 77:12, 2002.
255. Burke AP, Saenger J, Mullick F, et al: Hypersensitivity myocarditis. Arch Pathol Lab Med 115:764, 1991.
256. Getz MA, Subramanian R, Logemann T, et al: Acute necrotizing eosinophilic myocarditis as a manifestation of severe hypersensitivity myocarditis: Antemortem diagnosis and successful treatment. Ann Intern Med 115:201, 1991.
257. Galiuto L, Enriquez S, Reeder G, et al: Eosinophilic myocarditis manifesting as myocardial infarction: Early diagnosis and successful treatment. Mayo Clin Proc 72:603, 1997.
258. Webster J, Koch HF: Aspects of tolerability of centrally acting antihypertensive drugs. J Cardiovasc Pharmacol 27 (Suppl 3):S49, 1996.
259. Garty BZ, Offer I, Livni E, et al: Erythema multiforme and hypersensitivity myocarditis caused by ampicillin. Ann Pharmacother 28:730, 1994.
260. Loyer EM, Delpassand ES: Radiation-induced heart disease: Imaging features. Semin Roentgenol 28:321, 1993.
261. Gyenes G, Fornander T, Carlens P, et al: Detection of radiation-induced myocardial damage by technetium-99m sestamibi scintigraphy. Eur J Nucl Med 24:286, 1997.
262. Orzan F, Brusca A, Gaita F, et al: Associated cardiac lesions in patients with radiation-induced complete heart block. Int J Cardiol 39:151, 1993.
263. Veeragandham RS, Goldin MD: Surgical management of radiation-induced heart disease. Ann Thorac Surg 65:1014, 1998.
264. Hering D, Faber L, Horstkotte D: Echocardiographic features of radiation-associated valvular disease. Am J Cardiol 92:226, 2003.
265. Khan MH, Ettinger SM: Post mediastinal radiation coronary artery disease and its effect on arterial conduits. Catheter Cardiovasc Inter 52:242, 2001.
266. Dematte JE, O'Mara K, Buescher J, et al: Near-fatal heat stroke during the 1995 heat wave in Chicago. Ann Intern Med 129:173, 1998.
267. Danzl DF, Pozos RS: Accidental hypothermia. N Engl J Med 331:1756, 1994.
268. Walpoth BH, Walpoth-Aslan BN, Mattle HP, et al: Outcome of survivors of accidental deep hypothermia and circulatory arrest treated with extracorporeal blood warming. N Engl J Med 337:1500, 1997.
269. Lazar HL: The treatment of hypothermia. N Engl J Med 337:1545, 1997.

CHAPTER 61

Cardiovascular Abnormalities in HIV-Infected Individuals

Stacy D. Fisher • Steven E. Lipshultz

BACKGROUND

Infection with the human immunodeficiency virus (HIV) is one of the leading causes of acquired heart disease and specifically of symptomatic heart failure (Table 61-1). Cardiac complications of HIV infection tend to occur late in the disease and are therefore becoming more prevalent in our society as therapy and longevity improve.[1-5] Complicated drug therapies for HIV infection have sustained life but may lead to accelerated cardiovascular risk and atherosclerotic disease.[1,6]

Some 42 million adults and children are living with HIV or the acquired immunodeficiency syndrome (AIDS); 5 million more became infected in 2002.[7] The 2- to 5-year incidence of symptomatic heart failure ranges from 4 to 28 percent,[3,4] suggesting a prevalence of symptomatic HIV-related heart failure between 4 million and 5 million cases worldwide. Among HIV-infected children up to 10 years of age, 25 percent die with chronic cardiac disease,[8] and 28 percent experience serious cardiac events after an AIDS-defining illness.[9] The incidence of new HIV infection in the United States has decreased substantially over the last 5 years. Deaths related to HIV infection decreased 42 percent in 1996 to 1997 and 20 percent in 1997 to 1998 because of improved antiretroviral therapies and better identification and treatment of opportunistic infections. An estimated 3.1 million HIV-related deaths occurred worldwide in 2002, 15,000 in North America and 2.4 million in sub-Saharan Africa. Early in the epidemic, HIV infections were chiefly found in homosexual males; however, now most new cases occur in injection drug users and heterosexual partners of infected persons. Minority groups are overrepresented.[7]

A range of cardiac abnormalities (see Table 61–1) associated with HIV infection has been suggested by autopsy study; the conditions, in order of frequency, were pericardial effusion, lymphocytic interstitial myocarditis, dilated cardiomyopathy (frequently with myocarditis), infective endocarditis, and malignancy (myocardial Kaposi sarcoma and B-cell immunoblastic lymphoma).[10]

Left Ventricular Systolic Dysfunction (see Chap. 21)

CLINICAL PRESENTATION. In HIV-infected patients, concurrent pulmonary infections, pulmonary hypertension, anemia, portal hypertension, malnutrition, or malignancy can alter or confuse the characteristic signs that define heart failure in other populations. Thus, patients with left ventricular systolic dysfunction can be asymptomatic or can present with New York Heart Association Class III or IV heart failure.

Echocardiography is a useful test to assess left ventricular systolic function in this population and, in addition to uncovering left ventricular dysfunction, often reveals either low to normal wall thickness or left ventricular hypertrophy and a dilated left ventricular chamber.[2] Echocardiography should be performed in any patient at elevated cardiovascular risk, with any clinical manifestations of cardiovascular disease, or with unexplained or persistent pulmonary symptoms or viral coinfections at baseline and every 1 to 2 years or as clinically indicated.[6,11]

Electrocardiography (ECG) can reveal nonspecific conduction defects or repolarization changes. In one multicenter trial, 57 percent of asymptomatic HIV-infected individuals had baseline abnormalities on ECG, including supraventricular and ventricular ectopic beats.[12] The chest radiograph has low sensitivity and specificity for congestive heart failure in patients with HIV infection. Brain natriuretic peptide levels in small studies of HIV-infected patients and large populations of patients without HIV infection have been shown to correlate inversely with left ventricular ejection fraction and can be useful in the differential diagnosis of congestive cardiomyopathy in this population.[13]

Patients with encephalopathy are more likely to die of congestive heart failure than those without encephalopathy (hazard ratio 3.4).[14] HIV persists in reservoir cells in the myocardium and the cerebral cortex, even after antiretroviral therapy. These cells seem to play an important role in the development and progression of cardiomyopathy and encephalopathy. Reservoir cells may hold HIV on their surfaces for extended periods of time and cause progressive tissue damage by chronic release of cytotoxic cytokines.[15]

INCIDENCE. A 4-year observational study of 296 patients with a spectrum of HIV-related disease found 44 (15 percent) with dilated cardiomyopathy (fractional shortening <28 percent, with global left ventricular hypokinesis), 13 (4 percent) with isolated right ventricular dysfunction (right ventricle larger than left ventricle on standard two-dimensional views), and 12 (4 percent) with borderline left ventricular dysfunction (left ventricular end-systolic diameter >58 mm but fractional shortening >28 percent, or global dysfunction reported by one or two but not all three observers) (Fig. 61–1). Dilated cardiomyopathy was strongly associated with a CD4 count of less than 100 cells/ml.[4]

Left ventricular dysfunction is a common consequence of HIV infection in children. In a study of 205 children infected with HIV

TABLE 61–1 HIV-Associated Cardiovascular Disease

Type	Possible Etiologies	Incidence/Prevalence	Diagnosis	Treatment
Dilated cardiomyopathy	*Drug related:* cocaine, AZT, IL-2, doxorubicin, interferon *Infectious:* HIV, toxoplasma, coxsackievirus group B, EBV, CMV, adenovirus *Metabolic or endocrine:* selenium or carnitine deficiency, anemia, hypocalcemia, hypophosphatemia, hyponatremia, hypokalemia, hypoalbuminemia, hypothyroidism, growth hormone deficiency, adrenal insufficiency, hyperinsulinemia, hemochromatosis, pheochromocytoma, sarcoidosis, amyloidosis *Cytokines:* TNF-alpha, nitric oxide, TGF-beta, endothelin-I, interleukins *Immunodeficiency:* CD4 < 100 *Autoimmune*	Up to 8% of asymptomatic patients Up to 25% of autopsy cases Systolic > diastolic	Chest radiograph findings: nonspecific conduction abnormalities, PVCs, PACs Echocardiogram findings: low-normal LV wall thickness, increased LV mass, dilated LV, systolic LV dysfunction Possible laboratory studies: Troponin T, brain natiuretic peptide level, CD4 count, viral load, viral PCR, toxoplasma serology, thyroid-stimulating hormone, growth hormone, cortisol, carnitine, selenium, serum ACE, vanillylmandelic acid, amyloid, urine analysis, stress testing, myocardial biopsy, cardiac catheterization	Diuretics, digoxin, ACE inhibitors, beta blockers ***Adjunctive treatment in HIV+ patients*** Treatment of infection Nutritional replacement IVIg Intensify antiretroviral therapy ***Follow-up*** Serial echocardiograms
Pericardial effusion	*Bacteria: Staphylococcus, Streptococcus, Proteus, Nocardia, Klebsiella, Enterococcus, Listeria, Mycobacterium* *Viral pathogens:* HIV, HSV,CMV, adenovirus, echovirus *Other pathogens: Cryptococcus, Toxoplasma, Histoplasma* *Malignancy:* Kaposi sarcoma, lymphoma, capillary leak/wasting/malnutrition *Hypothyroidism* *Immunodeficiency* *Uremia*	11%/yr Spontaneous resolution in 42% of affected patients Approximately 30% increase in 6-mo mortality	Pericardial rub on examination Echocardiogram Fluid analysis for Gram stain and culture, malignant cells Associated pleural and peritoneal fluid analysis Pericardial biopsy	Treatment of underlying cause Pericardiocentesis Pericardial window ***Follow-up*** Serial echocardiograms Intensify antiretroviral therapy
Infective endocarditis	*Autoimmune* *Bacteria: Staphlococcus aureus* or *Staphylococcus epidermidis, Salmonella, Streptococcus, Hemophilus parainfluenzae, Pseudallescheria boydii,* HASEK *Fungal: Aspergillus fumigatus, Candida, Cryptococcus neoformans*	6% Increased incidence in IVDA regardless of HIV status	Blood cultures Echocardiogram	IV antibiotics Valve replacement
Nonbacterial thrombotic endocarditis	Valvular damage, vitamin C deficiency, malnutrition, wasting, DIC, hypercoagulable state, prolonged acquired immunodeficiency	Rare, but clinically relevant emboli in 42% of cases	Echocardiogram	Anticoagulation, treat vasculitis or underlying illness
Malignancy	Kaposi sarcoma, non-Hodgkin lymphoma, leiomyosarcoma Low CD4 count, prolonged immunodeficiency HHV-8, EBV	Approximately 1% incidence Usually metastatic in HIV+ patients	Echocardiogram, biopsy	Chemotherapy possible

TABLE 61–1 HIV-Associated Cardiovascular Disease—cont'd

Type	Possible Etiologies	Incidence/Prevalence	Diagnosis	Treatment
Right ventricle and pulmonary disease	Recurrent pulmonary infections, pulmonary arteritis, microvascular pulmonary emboli		ECG, echocardiogram Right heart catheterization	Diuretics Treat underlying lung infection or disease ± anticoagulation
Primary pulmonary HTN	Plexogenic pulmonary arteriopathy	0.5%	ECG, echocardiogram Right heart catheterization	Anticoagulation Vasodilators Prostacycline analogs
Vasculitis	Drug therapy with antibiotics and antiretrovirals	Increasing incidence	Clinical diagnosis	Systemic corticosteroids Withdrawal of causative drug
Accelerated atherosclerosis	Protease inhibitors, atherogenesis with virus-infected macrophages, chronic inflammation	Up to 8% prevalence	Stress testing Echocardiogram Lipid profile	Minimize risk factors
Autonomic dysfunction	CNS disease Drug therapy, prolonged immunodeficiency, malnutrition	Increased in patients with CNS disease	Tilt-table test Holter monitor	Procedural precautions
Arrhythmias	Drug therapy, pentamidine, autonomic dysfunction		ECG—long QT Holter monitor	Discontinue drug Procedural precautions
Lipodystrophy	Drug therapy: Protease inhibitors		Echocardiogram Lipid profile Cardiac catheterization Coronary calcium score	Lipid therapy: beware of drug interactions Aerobic exercise Altered antiretroviral therapy

ACE = angiotensin-converting enzyme; AZT = azidothymidine; CMV = cytomegalovirus; CNS = central nervous system; DIC = disseminated intravascular coagulation; EBV = Epstein-Barr virus; ECG = electrocardiogram; HHV = human herpesvirus; HIV = human immunodeficiency virus; HSV = herpes simplex virus; HTN = hypertension; IL-2 = interleukin-2; IVDA = intravenous drug abuse; IVIg = intravenous immunoglobulin; LV = left ventricular; PAC = premature atrial complex; PCR = polymerase chain reaction; PVC = premature ventricular complex; TGF = transforming growth factor; TNF = tumor necrosis factor.

by maternal-fetal transmission (enrolled at a median age of 22 months and observed with echocardiography every 4 to 6 months and ECG, Holter monitoring, and chest radiography every year), the prevalence of decreased left ventricular function (fractional shortening ≤ 28 percent) was 5.7 percent. The 2-year cumulative incidence was 15.3 percent.[3] The cumulative incidence of symptomatic congestive heart failure or the use of cardiac medications, or both, was 10 percent over 2 years.[3]

Global estimates of HIV-infected people ranged from 33.4 million to 120 million worldwide between the years 1998 and 2000. If there was a 10 percent incidence of symptomatic congestive heart failure over the 2 years, 3.34 million to 12 million cases of congestive heart failure would have presented during a 2-year interval.

PATHOGENESIS. A wide variety of possible etiologic agents have been postulated in HIV-related cardiomyopathy (see Table 61–1), including myocardial infection with HIV itself, opportunistic infections, viral infections, autoimmune response to viral infection, cardiotoxicity from therapeutic or illicit drugs, nutritional deficiencies, cytokine overexpression, and many others.

MYOCARDITIS (see Chap. 60). Myocarditis is perhaps the best studied of the possible causes. Dilated cardiomyopathy can be related to a direct action of HIV on the myocardial tissue or to proteolytic enzymes or cytokine mediators induced by HIV alone or in conjunction with coinfecting viruses.[16,17] *Toxoplasma gondii*, coxsackievirus group B, Epstein-Barr virus, cytomegalovirus, adenovirus, and HIV in myocytes have been found in biopsy specimens.

Autopsy and biopsy results have revealed only scant and patchy inflammatory cell infiltrates in the myocardium.[10,18] HIV can clearly infect myocardial interstitial cells but not the cardiac myocyte. Increased numbers of infected interstitial cells have been found in patients with confirmed myocarditis in which proteolytic enzymes or increased levels of tumor necrosis factor-alpha (TNF-α) or interleukin may injure the myocytes. Increased levels of TNF-α, inducible nitric oxide synthase, and interleukin-6 in affected patients and experimental models have been reported.[18]

Notably, HIV-related cardiomyopathy is often not associated with any specific opportunistic infection, and approximately 40 percent of patients have not experienced any opportunistic infection before the onset of cardiac symptoms.[10]

CYTOKINE ALTERATIONS. HIV infection increases the production of TNF-α, which alters intracellular calcium homeostasis and increases nitric oxide production, transforming growth factor-beta, and endothelin-1 upregulation.[14] Nitric oxide induced in high levels has been shown experimentally to have a negative inotropic effect and to be cytotoxic to myocytes.

In one study, HIV-infected individuals with dilated cardiomyopathy were much more likely to have myocarditis and had a broader spectrum of viral infections than HIV-negative patients with idiopathic dilated cardiomyopathy. Also, levels of TNF-α and induced nitric oxide synthase were higher in myocytes from the HIV-infected patients with dilated cardiomyopathy (particularly those with viral coinfections) and levels varied inversely with the CD4 count. Immunodeficiency may favor the selection of viral variants of increased pathogenicity or enhance the cardiovirulence of viral strains.[14,18]

NUTRITIONAL DEFICIENCIES. Nutritional deficiencies are common in HIV infection, particularly in late-stage disease. Poor absorption and diarrhea both lead to electrolyte imbalances and deficiencies in elemental nutrients. Deficiencies of trace elements have been associated with cardio-

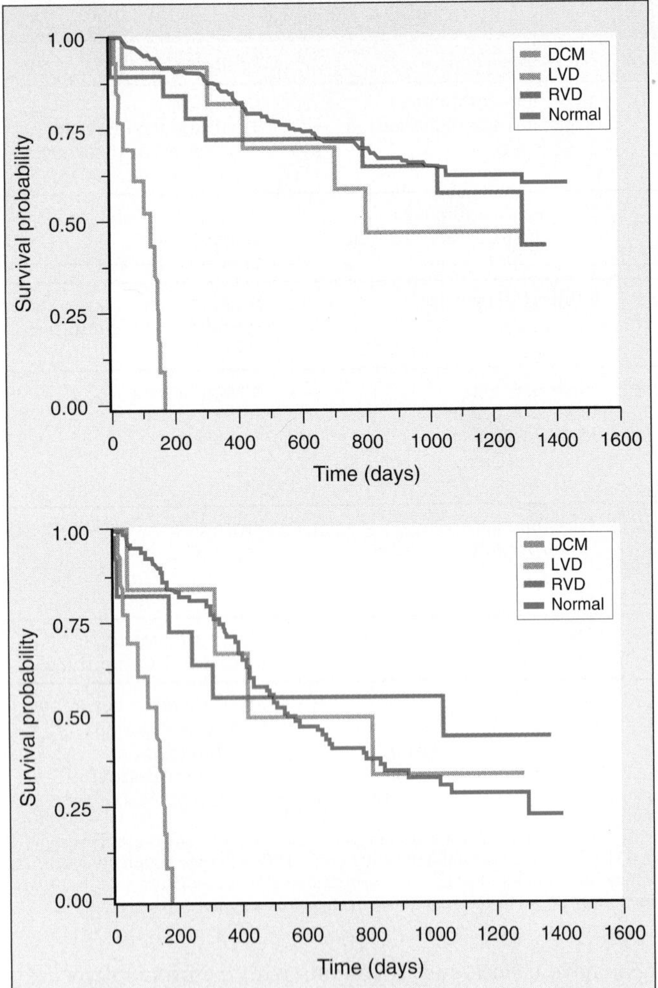

FIGURE 61–1 **Top,** Survival curves for 296 HIV-infected patients with structurally normal hearts, dilated cardiomyopathy (DCM), left ventricular dysfunction (LVD), or right ventricular dysfunction (RVD). **Bottom,** Time to death related to AIDS in 81 patients with CD4+ cell counts less than 20×10^6 cells/liter. (From Currie PF, Jacob AJ, Foreman AR, et al: Heart muscle disease related to HIV infection: Prognostic implications. Br Med J 309:1605, 1994.)

myopathy. For example, selenium deficiency increases the virulence of coxsackievirus to cardiac tissue.[10] Selenium replacement reverses cardiomyopathy and restores left ventricular function in nutritionally depleted patients. Levels of vitamin B_{12}, carnitine, and growth and thyroid hormone can also be altered in HIV disease; all have been associated with left ventricular dysfunction.

PATHOGENESIS IN CHILDREN. In children with vertically transmitted HIV infection, two mechanisms of pathogenesis have been described. One is dilation of the left ventricle with a reduction in the ratio of thickness to end-systolic dimension of the ventricle. The other is concentric hypertrophy of the muscle; with dilation, the ratio of thickness to end-systolic dimension remains normal or is increased.[2]

COURSE OF DISEASE. Patients with asymptomatic left ventricular dysfunction (fractional shortening <28 percent, with global left ventricular hypokinesis) may have transient disease by echocardiographic criteria. In one serial echocardiographic study, three of six patients with abnormal fractional shortening had normal readings after a mean of 9 months. The three with persistently depressed left ventricular function died within 1 year of baseline.[10]

PROGNOSIS. Mortality in HIV-infected patients with cardiomyopathy is increased, independent of CD4 count, age, sex, and risk group. The median survival to AIDS-related death was 101 days in patients with left ventricular dysfunction and 472 days in patients with a normal heart at a similar stage of infection (see Fig. 61–1).[4] Isolated right ventricular dysfunction or borderline left ventricular dysfunction did not place patients at risk.

In the Pediatric Pulmonary and Cardiovascular Complications of Vertically Transmitted HIV Infection (P^2C^2 HIV) study of children with vertically transmitted HIV infection (median age 2.1 years), 5-year cumulative survival was 64 percent.[9] Mortality was higher in children with baseline depressed left ventricular fractional shortening or increased left ventricular dimension, thickness, mass, wall stress, heart rate, or blood pressure. Decreased left ventricular fractional shortening and increased wall thickness were also predictive of survival after adjustment for age, height, CD4 count, HIV RNA copy number, clinical center, and encephalopathy.[2,9] Fractional shortening was abnormal for up to 3 years before death, whereas wall thickness identified a population at risk only 18 to 24 months before death. Thus, in children, fractional shortening may be a useful long-term predictor and wall thickness a useful short-term predictor of mortality.[19] Postmortem cardiomegaly was associated with echocardiographic evidence of increased left ventricular mass and documented chronically increased heart rate prior to death but not with anemia, encephalopathy, or HIV viral load.[20]

Rapid-onset congestive heart failure has a grim prognosis in HIV-infected adults and children, with over half of patients dying from primary cardiac failure within 6 to 12 months of presentation.[2,10] Chronic-onset heart failure may respond better to medical therapy in this population of patients.

THERAPY. Therapy for dilated cardiomyopathy associated with HIV infection is generally similar to therapy for nonischemic cardiomyopathy and includes diuretics, digoxin, beta blockers, aldosterone antagonists, and angiotensin-converting enzyme inhibitors as tolerated. No studies have investigated the efficacy of specific cardiac therapeutic regimens other than intravenous immunoglobulin.[19]

Opportunistic or other infections should be sought aggressively and treated with the potential to improve or resolve the cardiomyopathy. Right ventricular biopsy may be useful in identifying infectious causes of failure in order to institute targeted therapy.[6,11] However, right ventricular biopsy is probably underused.

After medical therapy is begun, serial echocardiographic studies should be performed at 4-month intervals (Fig. 61–2).[11] Monitoring recommendations for testing and timing of follow-up are based on studies relating impairment of fractional shortening to a worse prognosis. If function continues to worsen or the clinical course deteriorates, a biopsy should be considered. Patients with congestive heart failure who have not responded to 2 weeks of medical therapy may benefit from cardiac catheterization and endomyocardial biopsy, which may reveal lymphocytic infiltrates suggesting myocarditis or treatable opportunistic infections (by special stains), permitting aggressive therapy of an underlying pathogen. Tissue should be evaluated for the presence of abnormal mitochondria that could suggest benefit from an antiretroviral "drug holiday." Angiography should be selectively performed if there are risk factors for atherosclerotic disease or suggestive clinical symptoms.[11]

Intravenous immunoglobulins have had some success in acute congestive cardiomyopathy and nonspecific myocarditis in patients who are not infected with HIV.[21] Immunoglobulin therapy is beneficial in Kawasaki disease, an immunologically mediated illness with cardiac dysfunction resembling that seen with HIV disease. Monthly immunoglobulin infusions in HIV-infected pediatric patients have been associated with minimized left ventricular dysfunction, an increase in left ventricular wall thickness, and a

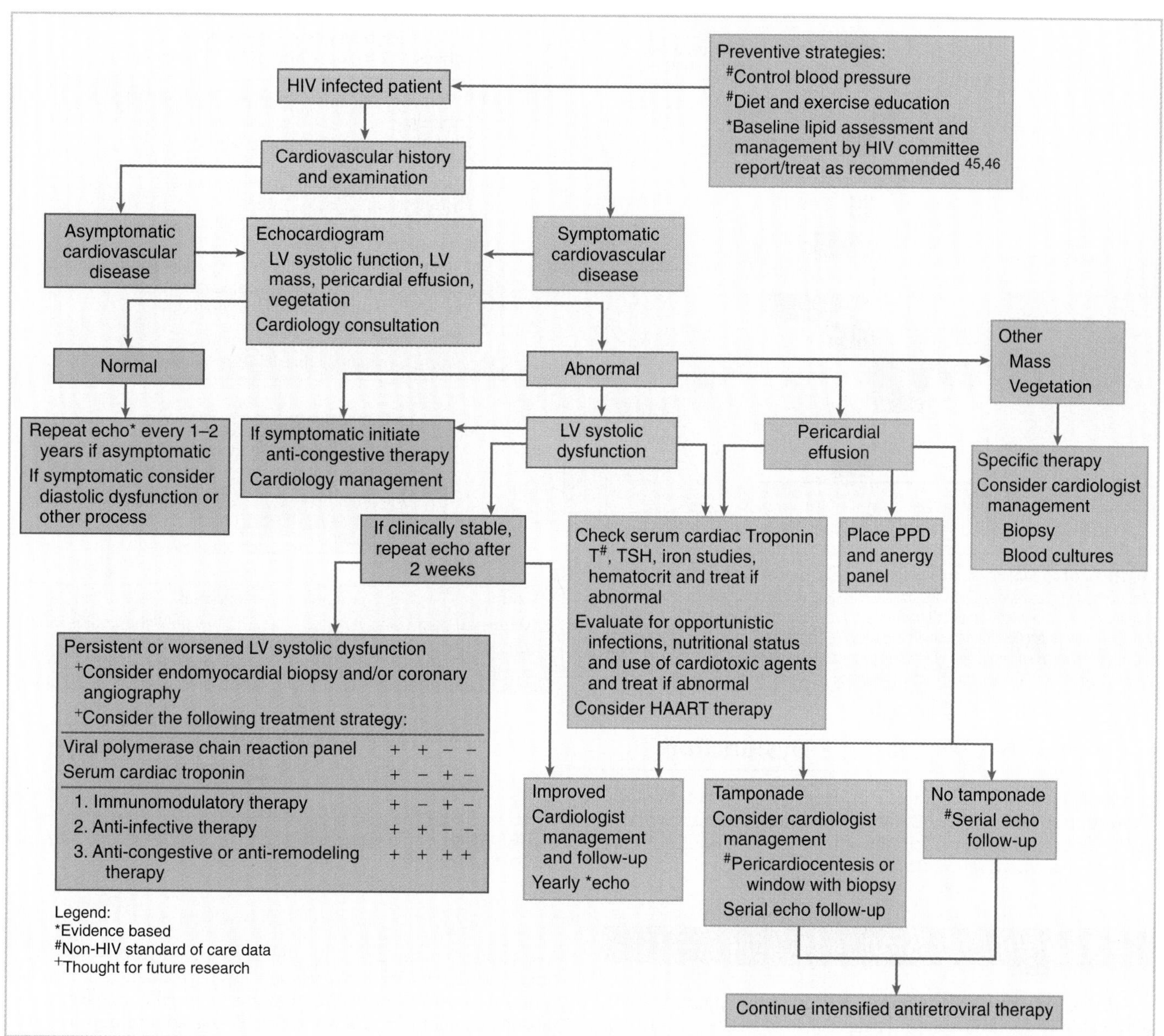

FIGURE 61–2 Cardiac dysfunction in HIV-infected patients. HAART = highly active antiretroviral therapy; LV = left ventricular; PPD = purified protein derivative; TSH = thyroid-stimulating hormone. (From Dolin R, Masur H, Saag MS [eds]: AIDS Therapy. 2nd ed. New York, Churchill Livingstone, 2003, p 817.)

reduction in peak left ventricular wall stress (Fig. 61–3), suggesting that both impaired myocardial growth and left ventricular dysfunction can be immunologically mediated.[19]

The apparent efficacy of immunoglobulin therapy may be the result of immunoglobulins removing cardiac autoantibodies or dampening the secretion or effects of cytokines and cellular growth factors. Immunomodulatory therapy may be helpful in special circumstances or in children with declining left ventricular function.

Patients should be evaluated for nutritional status and any with deficiencies should receive supplements. Supplementation with selenium, carnitine, multivitamins, or all three can be helpful, especially in anorexic patients or those with wasting or diarrhea syndromes.

Solid organ orthotopic heart transplantation has been reported in one HIV-infected man believed to have anthracycline-related cardiomyopathy, with 24 months of follow-up. His course has been complicated by more frequent and higher grade episodes of rejection than average but otherwise relatively uneventful and productive.[22] Liver and kidney transplantation in this population has also now been reported with greater frequency and generally acceptable outcomes. Transplantation therapy is not currently widely available but is an area of active consideration and discussion.

ANIMAL MODELS. Chronic pathogenic simian immunodeficiency virus (SIV) infection in rhesus macaques resulted in significant depression of left ventricular ejection fraction and extensive coronary arteriopathy suggestive of a cell-mediated immune response.[23] Notably, two-thirds of chronically infected macaques that died of SIV had myocardial pathology with lymphocytic myocarditis in 9 of 15 and coronary arteriopathy in 9 of 15 (6 alone and 3 in combination with myocarditis). Coronary arteriopathy was associated with evidence of vessel occlusion and recanalization, with associated areas of myocardial necrosis in four macaques. Two animals had marantic endocarditis and one had a left ventricular mural thrombus on pathological examination. Macaques with cardiac pathology were emaciated to a greater extent than macaques with SIV and similar periods of infection who did not experience cardiac pathology.

Transgenic mouse models with cardiac pathological changes have been created and may help to evaluate the impact of environmental factors, therapeutic or illicit drugs, or drug combinations in both the etiology and therapy of HIV-associated myocarditis.[24]

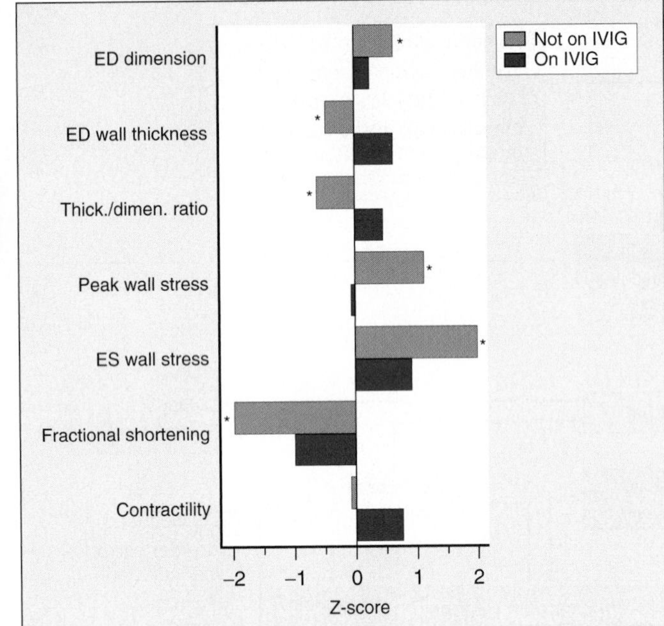

FIGURE 61–3 Mean echocardiographically measured cardiac dimensions in patients taking intravenous immunoglobulin (IVIG) and patients not taking it. All measurements are presented as age- or body surface area–adjusted Z scores. ED = end diastolic; ES = end systolic. (From Lipshultz SE, Orav EJ, Sanders SP, et al: Immunoglobulins and left ventricular structure and function in pediatric HIV infection. Circulation 92:2220, 1995. Copyright 1995, American Heart Association.)

Left Ventricular Diastolic Dysfunction

Clinical and echocardiographic findings suggest that diastolic dysfunction is relatively common in long-term survivors of HIV infection. Left ventricular diastolic dysfunction may precede systolic dysfunction.[11]

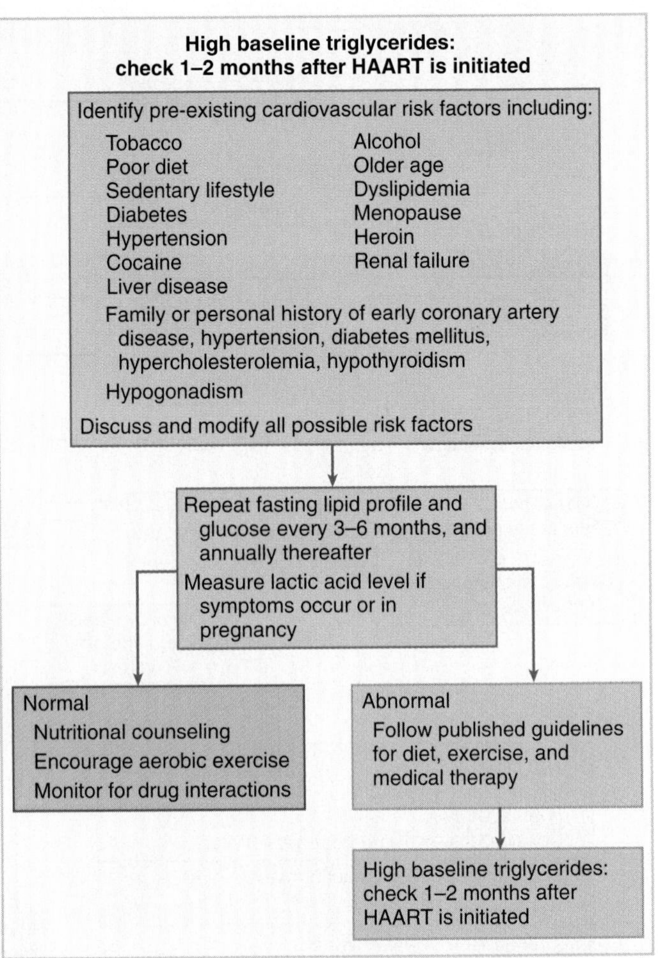

FIGURE 61–4 Cardiovascular considerations when initiating highly active antiretroviral therapy (HAART).

Pericardial Effusion (see Chap. 64)

CLINICAL PRESENTATION. HIV-infected patients with pericardial effusions generally have a lower CD4 count than those without effusions, marking more advanced disease.[10,16] Effusions are generally small and asymptomatic.

INCIDENCE. Asymptomatic pericardial effusions are common in HIV-infected patients. The 5-year Prospective Evaluation of Cardiac Involvement in AIDS (PRECIA) study found that 16 of 231 patients (59 subjects with asymptomatic HIV, 62 with AIDS-related complex, and 74 with AIDS) developed pericardial effusions.[16] Three subjects had an effusion on enrollment and 13 developed effusions during follow-up (12 of them had AIDS). Pericardial effusions were small (maximum pericardial space <10 mm at end diastole) in 80 percent and asymptomatic in 87 percent of patients with effusion. The incidence of pericardial effusion among those with AIDS was 11 percent per year.[16] The prevalence of effusion in AIDS patients rises over time, reaching a mean in asymptomatic patients of about 22 percent after 25 months of follow-up.[16]

HIV infection should be suspected whenever young patients have pericardial effusion or tamponade. In a retrospective series of cardiac tamponade cases in a city hospital, 13 of 37 patients (35 percent) had HIV infection.[10]

PATHOGENESIS. Pericardial effusion may be related to an opportunistic infection, metabolic abnormality, or malignancy (see Table 61–1), but most often a clear etiology is not found. The effusion is often part of a generalized serous effusive process also involving pleural and peritoneal surfaces. This "capillary leak" syndrome may be related to enhanced cytokine production in the later stages of HIV disease. Other causes can include uremia from HIV-associated nephropathy or drug nephrotoxicity. Fibrinous pericarditis with or without effusion is also well described, constituting 9 percent of cardiac lesions found in AIDS patients in one autopsy series.[16]

COURSE OF DISEASE AND PROGNOSIS. Effusion markedly increases mortality. For example, in the PRECIA study, it nearly tripled the risk of death among AIDS patients (Fig. 61–4).[16] Also, 2 of 16 patients with effusions developed pericardial tamponade. Pericardial effusion may, however, resolve spontaneously in up to 42 percent of patients.[10,16] Mortality was still markedly increased in patients who had an effusion.

MONITORING AND THERAPY. Screening echocardiography is recommended in HIV-infected individuals regardless of the stage of disease.[11] All HIV-infected patients with evidence of heart failure, Kaposi sarcoma, tuberculosis, or other pulmonary infections should have baseline echocardiography and ECG testing.[11] Patients should undergo pericardiocentesis if they have pericardial effusion and clinical signs of tamponade such as elevated jugular venous pressure, dyspnea, hypotension, persistent tachycardia, and pulsus paradoxus or echocardiographic signs of tamponade such as valvular inflow respiratory variation by continuous-wave Doppler study, septal bounce, right ventricular diastolic collapse, and a large effusion.

Patients with pericardial effusion without tamponade should be evaluated for treatable opportunistic infections such as tuberculosis and for malignancy. Highly active antiretroviral therapy (HAART) should be considered if therapy has not already been instituted. Repeated echocardiography is recommended after 1 month, or sooner if clinical symptoms direct (see Fig. 61–2).

Infective Endocarditis (see Chap. 58)

Injection drug users are at greater risk than the general population for infective endocarditis, chiefly of right-sided heart valves. Surprisingly, HIV-infected patients may not have a higher incidence of endocarditis than people with similar risk behaviors.

As the autoimmune response to bacterial endocarditis is often largely responsible for valvular destruction associated with endocarditis, variations in the course of the disease in HIV-infected patients may occur. For example, HIV-infected patients have a higher risk of developing salmonella endocarditis than immunocompetent patients because they are more likely to develop salmonella bacteremia during salmonella infection. However, they respond better to antibiotic therapy and may be less likely to sustain valvular damage because of their impaired immune response.[10,25]

Common organisms associated with endocarditis in HIV-infected patients include *Staphylococcus aureus* and *Salmonella* species. Fungal endocarditis with organisms such as *Aspergillus fumigatus*, *Candida* species, and *Cryptococcus neoformans* are more common in intravenous drug users with HIV than in those without it and again may be responsive to therapy (see Table 61–1).[10]

Fulminant courses of infective endocarditis with high mortality can occur in late-stage AIDS patients with poor nutritional status and severely compromised ability to fight infection, but several cases have been successfully treated with antibiotic therapy. Operative indications in HIV-infected patients with endocarditis include hemodynamic instability, failure to sterilize cultures after appropriate intravenous antibiotics, and severe valvular destruction in patients with a reasonable life expectancy after recovery from surgery.

Nonbacterial Thrombotic Endocarditis

Nonbacterial thrombotic endocarditis (or marantic endocarditis) involves large friable sterile vegetations that form on the cardiac valves. These lesions have been associated with disseminated intravascular coagulation and systemic embolization. Lesions are rarely diagnosed ante mortem; among patients who do receive the diagnosis, clinically relevant emboli occur in an estimated 42 percent of cases.[26] In the early HIV epidemic, several case series suggested a high incidence of this uncommon disorder; however, few cases have since been reported, and almost none have been found in prospective series. Marantic endocarditis should be suspected in any patient with systemic embolization, yet it should be considered rare in AIDS patients.

Treatment of nonbacterial thrombotic endocarditis should focus on reducing the underlying disease state causing coagulation abnormalities or valvular endothelial damage, or both. An anticoagulation risk-benefit assessment must be made on an individual basis.

Cardiovascular Malignancy

(see Chap. 63)

Malignancy affects many AIDS patients, generally in the later stages of disease. Cardiac malignancy is usually metastatic disease.

Kaposi sarcoma (angiosarcoma) is associated with human herpesvirus 8 and affects up to 35 percent of AIDS patients, particularly homosexuals, with an incidence inversely related to the CD4 count. Autopsy studies found that 28 percent of HIV-infected patients with widespread Kaposi sarcoma had cardiac involvement and rarely described it as a primary cardiac tumor.[27] Kaposi sarcoma has not been found invading the coronary arteries but is often an endothelial cell neoplasm with a predilection in the heart for subpericardial fat around the coronaries.[27]

Kaposi sarcoma involving the heart is generally an incidental finding at autopsy, rarely causing cardiac symptoms. Specific symptoms can be related to pericardial effusion associated with the epicardial location of the tumor. Pericardial fluid in patients with cardiac Kaposi sarcoma is typically serosanguineous without malignant cells or infection.[27] Kaposi sarcoma is difficult to treat. Most affected patients die from opportunistic infections related to the advanced stage of immunodeficiency rather than from the malignancy. Protease inhibitor use has significantly decreased the incidence of Kaposi sarcoma from the reported incidence in the pre-HAART era.[28]

Primary cardiac malignancy associated with HIV infection is generally due to cardiac lymphoma. Non-Hodgkin lymphomas are 25 to 60 times more common in HIV-infected individuals. They are the first manifestation of AIDS in up to 4 percent of new cases.[29] Patients with primary cardiac lymphoma can present with dyspnea, right-sided heart failure, biventricular failure, chest pain, or arrhythmias.[29] Cardiac lymphoma is associated with rapid progression to cardiac tamponade, symptoms of congestive heart failure, myocardial infarction, tachyarrhythmias, conduction abnormalities, or superior vena cava syndrome. Pericardial fluid typically reveals malignant cells but can be histologically normal. Systemic multiagent chemotherapy with and without concomitant radiation or surgery has been beneficial in some patients, but, overall, the prognosis is poor.[29] HAART has not substantially affected the incidence of HIV-related non-Hodgkin lymphomas.[28]

Leiomyosarcoma, associated with Epstein-Barr virus, is a rare, malignant tumor of smooth muscle origin with an increased incidence in children with AIDS. Leiomyosarcomas are largely noncardiac and often involve the arterial wall.[27] An intracardiac mass in late-stage HIV infection is associated with a uniformly poor prognosis.

Isolated Right Ventricular Disease

Isolated right ventricular hypertrophy with or without right ventricular dilation is relatively uncommon in HIV-infected individuals and is generally related to pulmonary disease that increases pulmonary vascular resistance (see Chap. 67). Possible causes include multiple bronchopulmonary infections, pulmonary arteritis from the immunological effects of HIV disease, or microvascular pulmonary emboli caused by thrombus or contaminants in injected drugs.

Pulmonary Hypertension

Primary pulmonary hypertension has been described in a disproportionate number of HIV-infected individuals, primarily in case reports. Primary pulmonary hypertension is estimated to occur in about 0.5 percent of hospitalized AIDS patients.[30,31] In one series of pulmonary hypertension associated with right ventricular hypertrophy and failure, clinical findings included dyspnea on exertion, hypoxemia, restrictive lung disease with decreased diffusing lung capacity for carbon monoxide, and right ventricular hypertrophy on ECG.[32]

Plexogenic pulmonary arteriopathy characterized by remodeling of the pulmonary vasculature with intimal fibrosis and replacement of normal endothelial structure was frequently demonstrated on lung histology. All of these patients had clear lung fields on examination and chest radiography and normal perfusion scans.

Pulmonary hypertension is often explained by lung infections, venous thromboembolism, or left ventricular dysfunction. Pulmonary hypertension found on screening echocardiography or right heart catheterization warrants further examination for treatable pulmonary infections.

Primary pulmonary hypertension has been reported in HIV-infected patients without a history of thromboembolic disease, intravenous drug use, or pulmonary infections associated with HIV.[30-33] One autopsy and one biopsy specimen revealed precapillary muscular pulmonary artery and arteriole medial hypertrophy, fibroelastosis, and eccentric intimal fibrosis without direct viral infection of pulmonary artery cells. This finding suggests mediator release from infected cells elsewhere. Primary pulmonary hypertension has also been found in hemophiliacs receiving lyophilized factor VIII, intravenous drug users, and patients with left ventricular dysfunction, obscuring any relationship with HIV.[31] It may be that HIV causes endothelial damage and mediator-related vasoconstriction of the pulmonary arteries.

In a study of 82 patients with HIV and pulmonary arterial hypertension, the CD4 count was independently associated with survival and pulmonary hypertension was the direct cause of death in 72 percent. Survival rates at 1, 2, and 3 years were 73, 60, and 47 percent, respectively. Survival rates in New York Heart Association functional Class III-IV patients at the time of diagnosis were 60, 45, and 28 percent.[32]

Therapy includes anticoagulation (on the basis of individual risk-benefit analysis) and vasodilator agents as tolerated. Safe and effective therapy has been reported using treprostinil (subcutaneous prostacyclin analog)[33] and epoprostenol in combination with antiretroviral agents.

Vasculitis

Vasculitis is being reported more often in HIV-infected patients (see Chap. 82).[34] It should be suspected in patients with fever of unknown origin, unexplained multisystem disease, unexplained arthritis or myositis, glomerulonephritis, peripheral neuropathy (especially mononeuritis multiplex), or unexplained gastrointestinal, cardiac, or central nervous system ischemia. Many types of vasculitis have been described in HIV-infected patients (see Table 61–1). Successful immunomodulatory therapy, chiefly with systemic corticosteroid therapy, has been described.

Accelerated Atherosclerosis

Accelerated atherosclerosis has been observed in young HIV-infected individuals without traditional coronary risk factors (see Chaps. 35 and 36).[35-37] Significant coronary lesions were discovered at autopsy in HIV-positive subjects 23 to 32 years of age who died unexpectedly. Cytomegalovirus was present in two of eight patients, and hepatitis B virus was found in two of eight patients. None had evidence of cocaine use.

Premature cerebrovascular disease is common in AIDS patients. An 8 percent stroke prevalence in AIDS patients was estimated in an autopsy study in the 1980s. Of the patients with stroke, 4 of 13 had evidence of cerebral emboli and 3 of those 4 had a clear cardiac source of embolus.

Protease inhibitor therapy significantly alters lipid metabolism and can be associated with premature atherosclerotic disease. Angiographically proven advanced symptomatic coronary artery disease has been reported in three men younger than 40 treated with protease inhibitors.[35] Chronic inflammatory states have also been associated with premature atherosclerotic vascular disease.

The benefits of protease inhibitor therapy and specifically HAART overall, however, have clearly been shown for morbidity and mortality endpoints with no short-term evidence of increased cardiovascular mortality.[1] Lipodystrophy including fat redistribution with increased truncal obesity, increased triglycerides and elevated small dense low-density lipoprotein, and glucose intolerance should still be recognized and treated because of an elevated 10-year cardiovascular risk.[6,11,36] Risk stratification based on traditional risk factors plus diet, alcohol intake, physical exercise, hypertriglyceridemia, cocaine use, heroin use, thyroid disease, renal disease, and hypogonadism should be considered for long-term cardiac preventive care (see Fig. 61–4).

Autonomic Dysfunction

Early clinical signs of autonomic dysfunction in HIV-infected patients include syncope and presyncope, diminished sweating, diarrhea, bladder dysfunction, and impotence (see Chap. 87). In one study, heart rate variability, Valsalva ratio, cold pressor testing, and hemodynamic responses to isometric exercise, tilt-table testing, and standing showed that autonomic dysfunction occurred in patients with AIDS-related complex and was pronounced in AIDS patients. Patients with HIV-associated nervous system disease had the greatest abnormalities in autonomic function (Fig. 61–5).[38,39]

Complications of Therapy for HIV

Potent antiretroviral medications and HAART, which generally combines three or more agents and usually includes a protease inhibitor, have clearly increased the life span and quality of life of HIV-infected patients.[1] However, protease inhibitors, particularly when used in combination therapy or in HAART, are associated with lipodystrophy, fat wasting and redistribution, metabolic abnormalities, hyperlipidemia, insulin resistance, and increased atherosclerotic risk (see Fig. 61–4). HIV-infected patients treated with protease inhibitors have reported substantial decreases in total body fat with peripheral lipodystrophy (fat wasting of the face, limbs, and buttocks) and relative conservation or enhancement of central adiposity (truncal obesity, breast enlargement, and "buffalo hump") compared with patients who have not received protease inhibitors. Lipid alterations associated with protease inhibitors include higher triglyceride, total cholesterol, insulin, lipoprotein (a), and C-peptide levels and lower high-density lipoprotein levels (all promoting an atherogenic profile).

Lipid abnormalities vary with different protease inhibitors.[40] Ritonavir had the largest adverse effects on lipids with a mean increase in total cholesterol of 2.0 mmol/liter and a mean increase in triglyceride level of 1.83 mmol/liter. More modest increases of total cholesterol without significant triglyceride increases were found in patients taking indinavir and nelfinavir. Combination with saquinavir did not further elevate the total cholesterol. Protease inhibitor therapy increased lipoprotein (a) by 48 percent in patients with elevated pretreatment values (>20 mg/dl).[40] In some cases, switching protease inhibitors may reverse both elevations in triglyceride levels and abnormal fat deposition. Low-level aerobic exercise has also been shown to help reverse lipid abnormalities.[41]

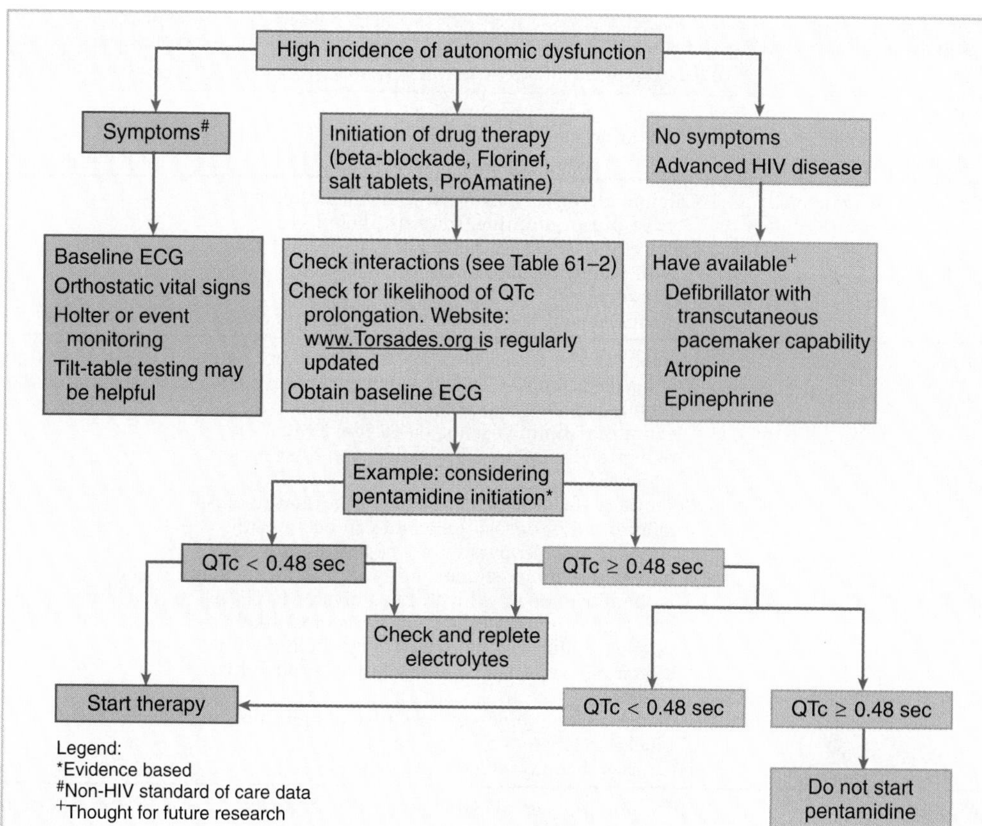

FIGURE 61–5 Evaluation and management of dysautonomia. ECG = electrocardiography. (From Dolin R, Masur H, Saag MG [eds]: AIDS Therapy. 2nd ed. New York, Churchill Livingstone, 2003, p 817.)

Zidovudine (azidothymidine [AZT], ZDV) has been implicated in skeletal muscle myopathies. In culture, AZT causes a dose-dependent destruction of human myotubes. Human cultured cardiac muscle cells treated with AZT developed mitochondrial abnormalities, and non-nucleoside reverse transcriptase inhibitors in general have been associated with altered mitochondrial DNA replication.[42] However, cardiac myopathies have not been evident in clinical data. Rarely, patients with left ventricular dysfunction have improved with cessation of AZT therapy.

A transgenic versus wild-type mouse model demonstrated cardiomyopathy with HIV infection alone, which was enhanced by AZT therapy. AZT-treated mice had mitochondrial ultrastructural damage in cardiac myocytes.[24]

Intravenous pentamidine, used to treat *Pneumocystis carinii* pneumonia in patients intolerant of trimethoprim-sulfamethoxazole, has been associated with cases of torsades de pointes and refractory ventricular tachycardia.[10,11] Recommendations for the use of intravenous pentamidine are outlined in Figure 61–5.

Multiple medication reactions and interactions have occurred during the treatment of HIV infection and are a significant cause of cardiac emergencies in HIV-infected patients. Common cardiac drug interactions are outlined in Table 61–2. Future therapies may inhibit HIV-1 cell entry and may have less toxic effects.[43]

Perinatal Transmission and Vertically Transmitted HIV Infection

Most pediatric patients with HIV are infected in the perinatal period, but HIV transmission can be minimized if mothers are given courses of AZT in the second and third trimesters or short courses before parturition.[44]

Rates of congenital cardiovascular malformations in cohorts of HIV-uninfected and HIV-infected children born to HIV-infected mothers ranged from 5.6 to 8.9 percent. These rates were 5 to 10 times higher than reported in population-based epidemiological studies but not higher than in normal populations similarly screened.[45]

In the same cohorts, serial echocardiograms performed at 4- to 6-month intervals showed subclinical cardiac abnormalities to be common, persistent, and often progressive.[2] Some had dilated cardiomyopathy (left ventricular contractility 2 SD or more below the normal mean and left ventricular end-diastolic dimension 2 SD above the mean or more) and inappropriate left ventricular hypertrophy (elevated left ventricular mass in the setting of decreased height and weight). Depressed left ventricular function correlated with immune dysfunction at baseline but not longitudinally, suggesting that the CD4 cell count may not be a useful surrogate marker of HIV-associated left ventricular dysfunction. The development of encephalopathy was highly correlated with a decline in fractional shortening.

In children with vertically transmitted HIV-1 infection, disease can progress rapidly or slowly.[46] Rapid progressors have higher heart rates, higher respiratory rates, and lower fractional shortening on serial examinations than nonrapid progressors and HIV-uninfected children who are similarly screened. Rapid progressors have higher 5-year cumulative mortality, higher HIV-1 viral loads, and lower CD8+ (cytotoxic) T-cell counts than nonrapid progressors.[46] Knowing the patterns of disease allows more aggressive therapy to be initiated earlier in rapid progressors.

TABLE 61–2 Cardiovascular Actions and Interactions of Drugs Commonly Used in HIV Therapy*

Class	Cardiac Drug Interactions	Cardiac Side Effects
Antiretroviral Nucleoside reverse transcriptase inhibitors	Zidovudine and dipyridamole	Rare—lactic acidosis, hypotension Accelerated risk with cardiopulmonary bypass Zidovudine: skeletal muscle myopathy, ?myocarditis
Nonnucleoside reverse transcriptase inhibitors	Calcium channel blockers, warfarin, beta blockers, nifedipine, quinidine, steroids, theophylline Delavirdine can cause serious toxic effects if given with antiarrhythmic drugs and calcium channel blockers Delavirdine and vasocontrictors can cause ischemia	
Protease inhibitors	Metabolized by cytochrome P450 and interact with other drugs metabolized through this pathway such as selected antimicrobials, antidepressant and antihistimine agents, cisapride, HMG CoA reductase inhibitors (lovastatin, simvastatin), and sildenafil Potentially dangerous interactions that require close monitoring or dose adjustment can occur with amiodarone, disopyramide, flecainide, lidocaine, mexiletine, propafenone, and quinidine. Ritonavir is the most potent cytochrome activator (CYP3A) and P-glycoprotein inhibitor and is most likely to interact. Indinavir, amprenavir, and nelfinavir are moderate. Saquinavir has the lowest probability to interact Calcium channel blockers, prednisone, quinine, beta blockers (1.5- to 3-fold increase). Decreases theophylline concentrations	Implicated in premature atherosclerosis, dyslipidemia, insulin resistance, diabetes mellitus, fat wasting and redistribution
Antiinfective Antibiotics	Rifampin: reduces digoxin therapeutic effect by induction of intestinal P-glycoprotein Reduces protease inhibitor concentration and effect Erythromycin: Cytochrome P450 metabolism and drug interactions Trimethoprim-sulfamethoxazole (Bactrim) increases warfarin effects	Erythromycin: orthostatic hypotension, ventricular tachycardia, bradycardia, torsades (with drug interactions) Clarithromycin: QT prolongation and torsades de pointes Trimethoprim-sulfamethoxazole: orthostatic hypotension, anaphylaxis, QT prolongation, torsades de pointes, hypokalemia Sparfloxacin (fluoroquinolones): QT prolongation
Antifungal agents	Amphotericin B: digoxin toxicity Ketoconazole or itraconazole: cytochrome P450 metabolism and drug interactions—increases levels of sildenafil, warfarin, HMG CoA reductase inhibitors, nifedipine, digoxin	Amphotericin B: hypertension, arrhythmia, renal failure, hypokalemia, thrombophlebitis, bradycardia, angioedema, dilated cardiomyopathy. Liposomal formulations still have the potential for electrolyte imbalance and QT prolongation Ketoconazole, fluconazole, itraconazole: QT prolongation and torsades de pointes
Antiviral agents	Ganciclovir: zidovudine	Foscarnet: reversible cardiac failure, electrolyte abnormalities Ganciclovir: ventricular tachycardia, hypotension
Antiparasitic		Pentamidine: hypotension, QT prolongation, arrhythmias (torsades de pointes), ventricular tachycardia, hyperglycemia, hypoglycemia, sudden death. These effects are enhanced by hypomagnesemia and hypokalemia
Chemotherapy agents	Vincristine, doxorubicin: decrease digoxin level	Vincristine: arrhythmia, myocardial infarction, cardiomyopathy, autonomic neuropathy Recombinant human interferon-alpha: hypertension, hypotension, tachycardia, acute coronary events, dilated cardiomyopathy, arrhythmias, sudden death, atrioventricular block, periperal vasodilation Contraindicated in patients with unstable angina or recent myocardial infarction Interleukin-2: hypotension, arrhythmia, sudden death, myocardial infarction, dilated cardiomyopathy, capillary leak, thyroid alterations Anthracyclines (doxorubicin, daunorubicin, mitoxantrone): myocarditis, cardiomyopathy Liposomal anthracyclines: as above for doxorubicin and also vasculitis

TABLE 61–2 Cardiovascular Actions and Interactions of Drugs Commonly Used in HIV Therapy*—cont'd

Class	Cardiac Drug Interactions	Cardiac Side Effects
Other		
Systemic corticosteroids	Corticosteroids: decrease salicylate levels and increase gastric ulceration in combination with salicylates	Corticosteroids: ventricular hypertrophy, cardiomyopathy, hyperglycemia
Pentoxifylline		Pentoxifylline: decreased triglyceride levels, arrhythmias, chest pain Megace: edema, thrombophlebitis, hyperglycemia
Megestrol acetate (Megace)		Epoetin alfa (erythropoetin): hypertension, ventricular dysfunction

*See Piscitelli and Gallicano,[47] Table 2, for cytochrome P450 isoforms and selected drugs used in the care of HIV-infected patients.
HMG CoA = 3-hydroxy-3-methylglutaryl coenzyme A.

Monitoring Recommendations

Routine, systematic cardiac evaluation including a comprehensive history and thorough cardiac examination is essential for the care of HIV-infected adults and children. The history should include traditional risk factors, environmental exposures, and therapeutic and illicit drug history. Routine blood pressure monitoring is important as HIV-infected individuals have been reported to develop hypertension at a younger age and more frequently than in the general population.[6]

Routine ECG and Holter monitoring is not warranted unless patients have symptoms such as palpitations, syncope, stroke, or dysautonomia. These tests can also be useful for baseline and monitoring before, during, and after therapies such as pentamidine that may prolong the QT interval.[6,11]

Asymptomatic cardiac disease related to HIV can be fatal, and cardiac symptoms are often disguised by secondary effects of HIV infection, so that systematic echocardiographic monitoring is warranted. We recommend a baseline echocardiogram at the time of HIV diagnosis and follow-up every 1 to 2 years (see Fig. 61–2). Symptomatic patients with HIV infection without cardiovascular abnormalities should have annual echocardiographic follow-up. Echocardiography should also be considered in patients with unexplained or persistent pulmonary symptoms and in those with viral coinfection at risk for myocarditis.[11] An international consensus panel recommended slightly less aggressive echocardiographic monitoring with a baseline for any patient at high risk or with any clinical manifestation of cardiovascular disease and serial studies repeated every 1 to 2 years or as clinically indicated.[6] Patients with cardiac symptoms should have a formal cardiac assessment including baseline echocardiography, ECG, and Holter monitoring and should begin directed therapy.[11]

In patients with left ventricular dysfunction, serum troponin assays are indicated. Serum troponin elevations warrant consideration of cardiac catheterization and endomyocardial biopsy. Myocarditis proved by biopsy warrants considering therapy with intravenous immunoglobulin.[19] Cytomegalovirus inclusions on the biopsy specimen warrant antiviral therapy, and abnormal mitochondria should encourage consideration of a drug holiday from zidovudine. Echocardiography should be repeated after 2 weeks of therapy to allow a more aggressive approach if left ventricular dysfunction persists or worsens and to encourage continued therapy if improvement has occurred.[11]

REFERENCES

Background

1. Bozzette S, Ake CF, Tam HK, et al: Cardiovascular and cerebrovascular events in patients treated for human immunodeficiency virus infection. N Engl J Med 348:702, 2003.
2. Lipshultz SE, Easley KA, Orav J, et al: Left ventricular structure and function in children infected with human immunodeficiency virus. The Prospective P²C² HIV Multicenter Study. Circulation 97:1246, 1998.
3. Starc TJ, Lipshultz SE, Easley KA, et al: Incidence of cardiac abnormalities in children with human immunodeficiency virus infection: The prospective P²C² HIV study. J Pediatr 141:327, 2002.
4. Currie PF, Jacob AJ, Foreman AR, et al: Heart muscle disease related to HIV infection: Prognostic implications. BMJ 309:1605, 1994.
5. Brannagan TH 3rd: Retroviral-associated vasculitis of the nervous system. Neurol Clin 15:927, 1997.
6. Volberding PA, Murphy RL, Barbaro G, et al: The Pavia consensus statement. AIDS 17:S170, 2003.
7. UNAIDS: AIDS epidemic update—December 2002. (http://www.unaids.org/worldaidsday/2002/press/Epiupdate.html)
8. Langston C, Cooper ER, Goldfarb J, et al: Human immunodeficiency virus–related mortality in infants and children: Data from the pediatric pulmonary and cardiovascular complications of vertically transmitted HIV (P²C²) Study. Pediatrics 107:328, 2001.
9. Al-Attar I, Orav EJ, Exil V, et al: Predictors of cardiac morbidity and related mortality in children with acquired immunodeficiency syndrome. J Am Coll Cardiol 41:1598, 2003.
10. Fisher SD, Lipshultz SE: Cardiac disease. *In* Dolin R, Masur H, Saag MS (eds): AIDS Therapy. 2nd ed. New York, Churchill Livingston, 2003, pp 814-826.

Left Ventricular Systolic Dysfunction

11. Lipshultz SE, Fisher SD, Lai WW, Miller TL: Cardiovascular risk factors, monitoring, and therapy for HIV-infected patients. AIDS 17:S96, 2003.
12. Barbaro G, Di Lorenzo G, Grisorio B, et al: Cardiac involvement in the acquired immunodeficiency syndrome: A multicenter clinical-pathological study. AIDS Res 14:1071, 1998.
13. Carrillo-Jimenez R, Treadwell TL, Goldfine H, et al: Brain natriuretic peptide and HIV-related cardiomyopathy. AIDS Read 12:501, 2002.
14. Fisher SD, Bowles NE, Towbin JA, Lipshultz SE: Mediators in HIV-associated cardiovascular disease: A focus on cytokines and genes. AIDS 17:S29, 2003.
15. Cooper ER, Hanson C, Diaz C, et al: Encephalopathy and progression of human immunodeficiency virus disease in a cohort of children with perinatally acquired human immunodeficiency virus infection. Women and Infants Transmission Study Group. J Pediatr 132:808, 1998.
16. Harmon WG, Dadlani GH, Fisher SD, Lipshultz SE: Myocardial and pericardial disease in HIV. Curr Treat Options Cardiovasc Med 4:497, 2002.
17. Shannon RP, Simon MA, Mathier MA, et al: Dilated cardiomyopathy associated with simian AIDS in nonhuman primates. Circulation 101:185, 2000.
18. Currie PF, Boon NA: Immunopathogenesis of HIV-related heart muscle disease: Current perspectives. AIDS 17:S21, 2003.
19. Lipshultz SE, Orav EJ, Sanders SP, Colan SD: Immunoglobulins and left ventricular structure and function in pediatric HIV infection. Circulation 92:2220, 1995.
20. Kearney DL, Perez-Atayde AR, Easley KA, et al: Postmortem cardiomegaly and echocardiographic measurements of left ventricular size and function in children infected with the human immunodeficiency virus. The Prospective P(2)C(2) HIV Multicenter Study. Cardiovasc Pathol 12:140, 2003.
21. McNamara DM, Rosenblum WD, Janosko KM, et al: Intravenous immune globulin in the therapy of myocarditis and acute cardiomyopathy. Circulation 95:2476, 1997.
22. Calabrese LH, Albrecht M, Young J, et al: Successful cardiac transplantation in an HIV-1-infected patient with advanced disease. N Engl J Med 348:2323, 2003.

23. Shannon RP, Simon MA, Mathier MA, et al: Dilated cardiomyopathy associated with simian AIDS in nonhuman primates. Circulation 101:185, 2000.
24. Lewis W: Use of the transgenic mouse in models of AIDS cardiomyo-pathy. AIDS 17:S36, 2003.

Infective Endocarditis

25. Nahass RG, Weinstein MP, Bartels J, Gocke DJ: Infective endocarditis in intravenous drug users: A comparison of human immunodeficiency virus type 1-negative and -positive patients. J Infect Dis 162:967, 1990.

Nonbacterial Thrombotic Endocarditis

26. Lopez JA, Ross RS, Fishbein MC, Siegel RJ: Non-bacterial thrombotic endocarditis: A review. Am Heart J 113:773, 1987.

Cardiovascular Malignancy

27. Jenson HB, Pollock BH: Cardiac cancers in HIV-infected patients. *In* Lipshultz SE (ed): Cardiology in AIDS. New York, Chapman & Hall, 1998, pp 255-263.
28. Bruno R, Sacchi P, Filice G: Overview on the incidence and the characteristics of HIV-related opportunistic infections and neoplasms of the heart: Impact of highly active antiretroviral therapy. AIDS 17:S83, 2003.
29. Duong M, Dubois C, Buisson M, et al: Non-Hodgkin's lymphoma of the heart in patients infected with human immunodeficiency virus. Clin Cardiol 20:497, 1997.

Pulmonary Hypertension

30. Seoane L, Shellito J, Welsh D, et al: Pulmonary hypertension associated with HIV infection. South Med J 94:635, 2001.
31. Saidi A, Bricker JT: Pulmonary hypertension in patients infected with HIV. *In* Lipshultz SE (ed): Cardiology in AIDS. New York, Chapman & Hall, 1998, p 187.
32. Nunes H, Humbert M, Sitbon O, et al: Prognostic factors for survival in human immunodeficiency virus–associated pulmonary arterial hypertension. Am J Respir Crit Care Med 167:1433, 2003.
33. Cea-Calvo L, Escribano Subias P, Tello De Menesses R, et al: [Treatment of HIV-associated pulmonary hypertension with treprostinil.] Rev Esp Cardiol 56:421, 2003.

Vasculitis

34. Johnson RM, Barbarini G, Barbaro G: Kawasaki-like syndromes and other vasculitic syndromes in HIV-infected patients. AIDS 17:S77, 2003.

Accelerated Atherosclerosis

35. Henry K, Melroe H, Huebsch J, et al: Severe premature coronary artery disease with protease inhibitors. Lancet 351:1328, 1998.
36. Hadigan C, Meigs JB, Wilson PW, et al: Prediction of coronary heart disease risk in HIV-infected patients with fat redistribution. Clin Infect Dis 36:909, 2003.
37. Mooser V: Atherosclerosis and HIV in the highly active antiretroviral therapy era: Towards an epidemic of cardiovascular disease? AIDS 17:S65, 2003.

Autonomic Dysfunction

38. Saidi A, Moodie D, Garson A, et al: Electrocardiography and 24-hour electrocardiographic ambulatory recording (Holter monitor) studies in children of mothers infected with human immunodeficiency virus type 1. Pediatr Cardiol 21:189, 2000.
39. Gluck T, Degenhardt E, Scholmerich J, et al: Autonomic neuropathy in patients with HIV: Course, impact of disease stage, and medication. Clin Auton Res 10:17, 2000.

Complications of Therapy for HIV

40. Periard D, Telenti A, Sudre P, et al: Atherogenic dyslipidemia in HIV-infected individuals treated with protease inhibitors. Circulation 100:700, 1999.
41. Thoni GJ, Fedou C, Brun JF, et al: Reduction of fat accumulation and lipid disorders by individualized light aerobic training in human immunodeficiency virus infected patients with lipodystrophy and/or dyslipidemia. Diabetes Metab 28:397, 2002.
42. Lewis W: Mitochondrial DNA replication, nucleoside reverse-transcriptase inhibitors, and AIDS cardiomyopathy. Prog Cardiovasc Dis 45:305, 2003.
43. Kilby JM, Eron JJ: Novel therapies based on mechanisms of HIV-1 cell entry. N Engl J Med 348:2228, 2003.

Perinatal Transmission and Vertically Transmitted HIV Infection

44. Wade NA, Birkhead GS, Warren BL, et al: Abbreviated regimens of zidovudine prophylaxis and perinatal transmission of the human immunodeficiency virus. N Engl J Med 339:1409, 1998.
45. Lai WW, Lipshultz SE, Easley KA, et al: Prevalence of congenital cardiovascular malformations in children of human immunodeficiency virus infected women: The prospective P^2C^2 HIV Multicenter Study. J Am Coll Cardiol 32:1749, 1998.
46. Shearer WT, Lipshultz SE, Easley KA, et al: Alterations in cardiac and pulmonary function in pediatric rapid human immunodeficiency virus type 1 disease progressors. Pediatrics 105:e9, 2000.
47. Piscitelli SC, Gallicano KD: Interactions among drugs for HIV and opportunistic infections. N Engl J Med 344:984, 2001.

CHAPTER 62

Toxins and the Heart

Richard A. Lange • L. David Hillis

A number of toxins can affect the cardiovascular system. This chapter considers the toxins most commonly encountered in the practice of adult cardiology, with the exception of chemotherapeutic agents, a topic discussed in Chapter 83. The toxins discussed here include agents where exposure is primarily volitional (e.g., alcohol and cocaine) as well as toxins encountered in the environment (e.g., heavy metals).

Ethanol

Some two-thirds of Americans occasionally consume ethanol, and approximately 10 percent are considered heavy consumers. Although the ingestion of a moderate amount of ethanol (usually defined as 3 to 9 drinks per week) appears to be associated with a reduced risk of cardiovascular disease, the consumption of excessive amounts has the opposite effect. When ingested in substantial amounts, ethanol may cause ventricular systolic and/or diastolic dysfunction, systemic arterial hypertension, angina pectoris, arrhythmias, and even sudden cardiac death.

Effects of Ethanol on Myocellular Structure and Function

Ethanol may cause myocardial damage via several mechanisms (Table 62–1).[1,2] First, ethanol and its metabolites, acetaldehyde and acetate, may exert a direct toxic effect on the myocardium. Second, deficiencies of certain vitamins (e.g., thiamine), minerals (e.g., selenium), or electrolytes (e.g., magnesium, phosphorus, or potassium) that sometimes occur in heavy ethanol consumers may adversely affect myocardial function. Third, certain substances that are sometimes added to alcoholic beverages, such as lead (often found in "moonshine" alcohol) or cobalt, may be toxic to the myocardium.

Ethanol impairs excitation-contraction, mitochondrial oxidative phosphorylation, and cardiac contractility by adversely affecting the function of the sarcolemmal membrane, sarcoplasmic reticulum, mitochondria, and contractile proteins. Electron microscopic studies of the hearts of experimental animals in close temporal proximity to heavy ethanol ingestion demonstrate dilated sarcoplasmic reticula and swollen mitochondria, with fragmented cristae and glycogen-filled vacuoles. With sustained exposure to ethanol, myofibrillar degeneration and replacement fibrosis appear. In addition to the effects of ethanol on the myocardial contractile apparatus, acute or chronic consumption may adversely influence myofibrillar protein synthesis. Microscopically, the hearts of chronic heavy consumers of ethanol manifest an increased accumulation of collagen in the extracellular matrix as well as increased intermolecular cross-links.

Effects of Ethanol on Organ Function

Chronic heavy ethanol ingestion may induce left ventricular diastolic and/or systolic dysfunction. Diastolic dysfunction, which is caused at least in part by interstitial fibrosis of the myocardium,[3] is often demonstrable in heavy consumers of ethanol even in the absence of symptoms or obvious signs. About half of asymptomatic chronic alcoholics have echocardiographic evidence of left ventricular hypertrophy with preserved systolic performance. By Doppler echocardiography, the left ventricular relaxation time often is prolonged, the peak early diastolic velocity decreases, and the acceleration of early diastolic flow slows—all manifestations of left ventricular diastolic dysfunction. Abnormal increases in left ventricular filling pressure during volume or pressure loading may be observed.

Ethanol may induce asymptomatic left ventricular systolic dysfunction even when it is ingested by healthy individuals in relatively small quantities, as occurs in subjects who are considered only "social" drinkers.[4] As many as 30 percent of asymptomatic chronic alcoholics have echocardiographic evidence of left ventricular systolic dysfunction.[5] With continued heavy ethanol ingestion, these subjects often develop symptoms and signs of congestive heart failure, which is due to a dilated cardiomyopathy. In fact, ethanol abuse is the leading cause of nonischemic dilated cardiomyopathy in industrialized countries, accounting for approximately half of those diagnosed with this entity. The likelihood of developing an ethanol-induced dilated cardiomyopathy correlates with the amount of ethanol consumed in a lifetime. Most men who develop an ethanol-induced dilated cardiomyopathy have consumed more than 80 gm of ethanol (i.e., 1 liter of wine, 8 standard-sized beers, or one-half pint of hard liquor) per day for at least 5 years.[6] Women appear even more susceptible to

TABLE 62–1 Mechanisms of Ethanol-Induced Myocardial Injury

• **Direct toxic effects** *Uncoupling of the excitation/contraction system* *Reduced calcium sequestration in sarcoplasmic reticulum* *Inhibition of sarcolemmal ATP-dependent Na^+/K^+ pump* *Reduction in mitochondrial respiratory ratio* *Altered substrate utilization* *Increased interstitial/extracellular protein synthesis*
• **Toxic effect of metabolites** *Acetaldehyde* *Ethyl esters*
• **Nutritional or trace metal deficiencies** *Thiamine* *Selenium*
• **Electrolyte disturbances** *Hypomagnesemia* *Hypokalemia* *Hypophosphatemia*
• **Toxic additives** *Cobalt* *Lead*

ATP = adenosine triphosphate.

ethanol's cardiotoxic effects, in that they may develop a dilated cardiomyopathy following the consumption of a smaller amount of ethanol per day and per lifetime when compared to their male counterparts.[7]

With abstinence from ethanol, left ventricular systolic and diastolic function often improve[8,9]; the earlier in the course of ethanol consumption that abstinence is initiated, the more pronounced the benefit. Even subjects with markedly symptomatic ethanol-induced dilated cardiomyopathy may manifest a substantial improvement in left ventricular systolic function and symptoms of heart failure with complete abstinence or a dramatic reduction in ethanol consumption. Although most of this improvement occurs in the first 6 months of abstinence, it often continues for as long as 2 years of observation.

Although many heavy ethanol consumers develop a dilated cardiomyopathy, others do not, thereby suggesting individual variability in susceptibility to ethanol's cardiotoxic effects. In this regard, some studies have suggested that genetic polymorphisms in the angiotensin-converting enzyme (ACE) gene may play a role in the development of ethanol-induced dilated cardiomyopathy. Subjects who are homozygous for the deletion polymorphism of the ACE gene (so-called DD) have increased plasma and cardiac levels of ACE. In the absence of ethanol consumption, these homozygous individuals reportedly have increased risk of developing left ventricular hypertrophy and idiopathic dilated cardiomyopathy. Similarly, alcoholics who are homozygous for this deletion polymorphism appear more likely to develop a dilated cardiomyopathy than alcoholic subjects without it.[10]

Ethanol and Systemic Arterial Hypertension

It is estimated that ethanol is of etiologic importance in as many as 11 percent of men with hypertension. Individuals who consume more than two drinks per day are 1.5 to 2 times more likely to have hypertension when compared to age- and gender-matched nondrinkers.[11,12] This effect is dose related and is most prominent when the daily ethanol intake exceeds five drinks (i.e., 30 gm of ethanol).[13,14] "Social" ethanol consumption is associated with a modest rise in systolic arterial pressure, whereas heavy consumption may lead to a substantial increase. Although the mechanism by which ethanol induces a rise in systemic arterial pressure is poorly understood, previous studies have demonstrated that ethanol consumption increases plasma levels of catecholamines, renin, and aldosterone, each of which may cause systemic arterial vasoconstriction. In individuals with ethanol-induced hypertension, a normalization of systemic arterial pressure often follows abstinence.

Ethanol and Lipid Metabolism

Ethanol consumption inhibits the oxidation of free fatty acids by the liver, which stimulates hepatic triglyceride synthesis and the secretion of very low-density lipoprotein cholesterol. Most commonly, therefore, ethanol consumption causes hypertriglyceridemia. In addition, it may cause an increase in the serum concentrations of total cholesterol and its low-density lipoprotein (LDL) component. Regular ethanol consumption increases the serum concentration of HDL cholesterol. Subjects with hyperlipidemia should be encouraged to limit their ethanol intake.[15]

Coronary Artery Disease

Heavy ethanol use is associated with an increased incidence of atherosclerotic coronary artery disease and resultant cardiovascular morbidity and mortality. This increase may result, at least in part, from classic coronary risk factors common in heavy ethanol consumers, such as systemic arterial hypertension, an increased left ventricular muscle mass (with concomitant diastolic and/or systolic dysfunction), and hypertriglyceridemia. In addition, heavy ethanol drinkers often smoke cigarettes. In contradistinction, mild to moderate ethanol intake (two to seven drinks per week) appears to be associated with a decreased risk of cardiovascular morbidity and mortality in both men and women. This reduced risk of cardiovascular morbidity and mortality among consumers of moderate amounts of ethanol—when compared with nondrinkers or heavy consumers—is supported by numerous retrospectively and prospectively conducted studies. The French were noted to have a reduced incidence of coronary artery disease when compared to inhabitants of other countries with similar dietary habits (the so-called French paradox).[16] Although this diminished incidence initially was attributed to the antioxidant and antithrombotic properties of red wine, similar findings subsequently were reported in mild to moderate consumers of other alcoholic beverages and in other study populations.[17] Several prospectively performed cohort studies have demonstrated that drinkers of moderate amounts of ethanol are 40 to 70 percent less likely to manifest coronary artery disease or ischemic stroke when compared to nondrinkers or heavy consumers.[17-22] Some studies have suggested that the consumption of all alcoholic beverages exerts such an effect,[17] whereas others have reported that this so-called cardioprotection is strongest with the consumption of wine.[23] The mechanism(s) by which the consumption of moderate amounts of ethanol reduces cardiovascular risk appear to be multifactorial, in that moderate consumption exerts several beneficial effects, including (1) an increase in the serum concentrations of HDL cholesterol and apolipoprotein AI; (2) inhibition of platelet aggregation; (3) a decreased serum fibrinogen concentration; (4) increased antioxidant activity (from the phenolic compounds and flavonoids contained in red wine); and (5) improved fibrinolysis (resulting from increased concentrations of endogenous tissue plasminogen activator and a concomitant decrease in endogenous plasminogen activator inhibitor activity) (Fig. 62–1).[15,24,25]

Some studies have suggested that the cardioprotective effects of moderate ethanol intake are manifest only in those who are at increased risk for coronary artery disease (i.e.,

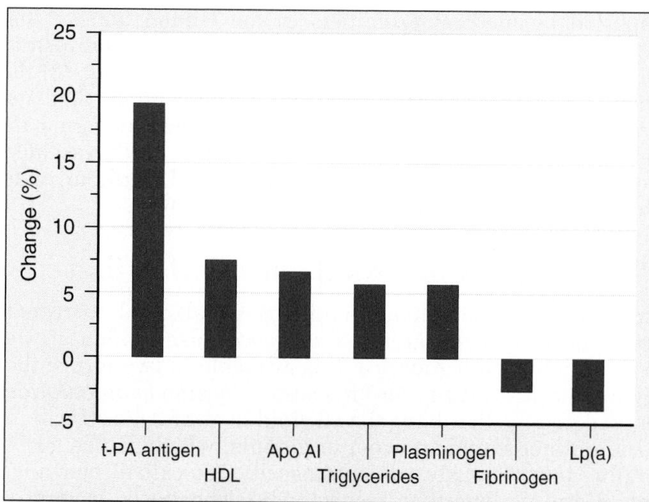

FIGURE 62–1 Percentage change in various blood variables caused by the ingestion of 30 gm of ethanol daily.[15] The ingestion of ethanol, 30 gm daily, for 1 to 9 weeks was associated with increased serum concentrations of tissue type plasminogen activator (t-PA) antigen, high-density lipoprotein (HDL) cholesterol, apolipoprotein AI (Apo AI), serum triglycerides, and serum plasminogen, as well as decreased concentrations of serum fibrinogen and lipoprotein (a) [Lp(a)]. The reduced risk of cardiovascular events seen in subjects who consume moderate amounts of ethanol may be due, at least in part, to these beneficial changes in blood variables.

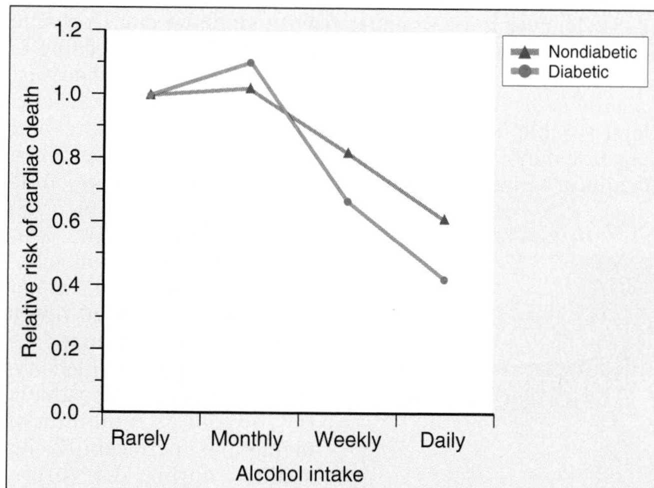

FIGURE 62–2 Ethanol consumption and relative risk of cardiac death according to diabetic status, with data from The Physicians Health Study.[28] Light to moderate alcohol consumption is associated with similar risk reductions in cardiac death among diabetic and nondiabetic men.

those > 50 to 60 years of age,[20] men with an LDL cholesterol concentration > 200 mg/dl,[26] and women with multiple risk factors for atherosclerosis).[20] Other studies have demonstrated that light to moderate ethanol consumption is associated with similar risk reductions in coronary artery disease among diabetic and nondiabetic men and women (Fig. 62–2).[27,28]

In subjects without known cardiac disease, the decrease in cardiovascular mortality associated with moderate ethanol intake results largely from a reduction in the incidence of sudden death (Fig. 62–3). Of the more than 21,000 men in the Physicians Health Study, those who consumed two to four or five or six drinks per week had a significantly reduced risk of sudden death (relative risks, 0.40 and 0.21, respectively) when compared to those who rarely or never drank.[29] In contrast, heavy ethanol consumption (i.e., six or more drinks per

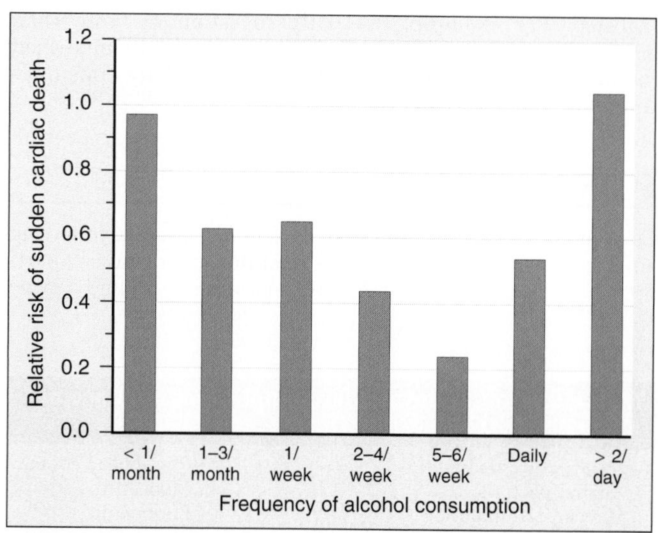

FIGURE 62–3 Ethanol consumption and the risk of sudden cardiac death among U.S. male physicians.[29] In comparison to those who had less than 1 drink per month (far left bar), those who consumed small or moderate amounts of ethanol (middle bars) had a reduced risk of sudden cardiac death. In contrast, those who consumed at least two drinks per day (far right bar) had an increased risk.

day) or binge drinking was associated with an increased risk of sudden death.

In survivors of myocardial infarction (MI), moderate ethanol consumption appears to reduce subsequent mortality.[19,30] In the setting of an acute MI, the recent ingestion of ethanol does not appear to reduce infarct size or the propensity for the subsequent appearance of an arrhythmia or heart failure.[31]

Arrhythmias

Ethanol consumption is associated with a variety of atrial and ventricular arrhythmias,[32,33] most commonly (1) atrial or ventricular premature beats, (2) supraventricular tachycardia, (3) atrial flutter, (4) atrial fibrillation, (5) ventricular tachycardia, or (6) ventricular fibrillation. The most common ethanol-induced arrhythmia is atrial fibrillation.[33] Ethanol is etiologically important in about one-third of subjects with new-onset atrial fibrillation; in those younger than 65 years of age, it may be responsible for as many as two-thirds of subjects. Most episodes occur after binge drinking, usually on weekends or holidays; hence, the term *holiday heart*. Electrophysiological testing in humans without cardiac disease has shown that ethanol enhances the vulnerability to the induction of atrial flutter and atrial fibrillation. The treatment of these ethanol-induced arrhythmias is abstinence.

Ethanol may be arrhythmogenic via several mechanisms. In many ethanol consumers, concomitant factors may predispose to arrhythmias, including cigarette smoking, electrolyte disturbances, metabolic abnormalities, or sleep apnea. Acute ethanol ingestion induces a diuresis, which is accompanied by the concomitant urinary loss of sodium, potassium, and magnesium. The presence of myocardial interstitial fibrosis, ventricular hypertrophy, cardiomyopathy, and autonomic dysfunction also may enhance the likelihood of dysrhythmias.

Sudden Death

Heavy ethanol consumption associates with an increased incidence of sudden death, irrespective of the presence of coronary artery disease. The incidence of ethanol-induced sudden death increases with age and the amount of ethanol ingested. For example, the daily ingestion of more than 80 gm of ethanol is associated with a threefold increased incidence of mortality when compared to a daily consumption of a lesser amount.

Cocaine

Cocaine is currently the most commonly used illicit drug among subjects seeking care in hospital emergency departments, and it is the most frequent cause of drug-related deaths reported by medical examiners in the United States.[34] Its widespread use is attributable to (1) its ease of administration, (2) the ready availability of relatively pure drug, (3) its relatively low cost, and (4) the misperception that its recreational use is safe. As cocaine abuse has increased in prevalence, the number of cocaine-related cardiovascular complications, including angina pectoris, MI, cardiomyopathy, and sudden death, has increased (Table 62–2).

TABLE 62–2 Cardiovascular Complications of Cocaine Use

Myocardial ischemia	Pulmonary edema
Angina pectoris	Myocarditis
Myocardial infarction	Endocarditis
Sudden death	Aortic dissection
Arrhythmias	

TABLE 62–3 Pharmacokinetics of Cocaine According to the Route of Administration

Route of Administration	Onset of Action	Peak Effect	Duration of Action
Inhalation (smoking)	3-5 sec	1-3 min	5-15 min
Intravenous	10-60 sec	3-5 min	20-60 min
Intranasal or other mucosal	1-5 min	15-20 min	60-90 min

Pharmacology and Mechanisms of Action

Cocaine (benzoylmethylecgonine) is an alkaloid extracted from the leaf of the *Erythroxylon coca* bush, which grows primarily in South America. It is available in two forms: the hydrochloride salt and the "freebase." Cocaine *hydrochloride* is prepared by dissolving the alkaloid in hydrochloric acid to form a water-soluble powder or granule, which can be taken orally, intravenously, or intranasally (so-called chewing, mainlining, or snorting, respectively). The *freebase* form is manufactured by processing the cocaine with ammonia or sodium bicarbonate (baking soda). Unlike the hydrochloride form, freebase cocaine is heat stable, so that it can be smoked. It is known as "crack" because of the popping sound it makes when heated.

Cocaine hydrochloride is well absorbed through all mucous membranes; therefore, users may achieve a high blood concentration with intranasal, sublingual, intravaginal, or rectal administration. The route of administration determines the rapidity of onset and duration of action (Table 62–3). The euphoria associated with smoking crack cocaine occurs within seconds and is short lived. Crack cocaine is considered the most potent and addictive form of the drug. Cocaine is metabolized by serum and liver cholinesterases to water-soluble metabolites (primarily benzoylecgonine and ecgonine methyl ester), which are excreted in the urine. Since cocaine's serum half-life is only 45 to 90 minutes, it is detectable in blood or urine only for several hours after its use. However, its metabolites are detectable in blood or urine for 24 to 36 hours after its administration.

When applied locally, cocaine acts as an anesthetic by virtue of its inhibition of membrane permeability to sodium during depolarization, thereby blocking the initiation and transmission of electrical signals. When given systemically, it blocks the presynaptic reuptake of norepinephrine and dopamine, thereby producing an excess of these neurotransmitters at the site of the postsynaptic receptor (Fig. 62–4). In short, cocaine acts as a powerful sympathomimetic agent.

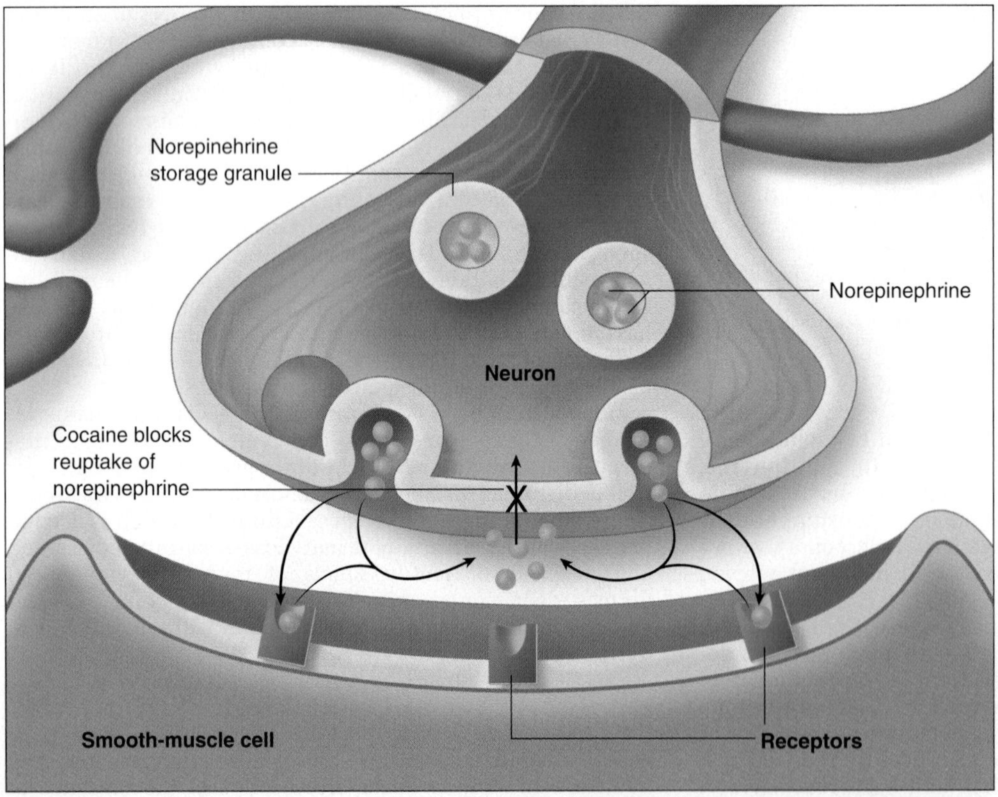

FIGURE 62–4 The mechanism by which cocaine alters sympathetic tone. Cocaine blocks the reuptake of norepinephrine by the preganglionic neuron (X), resulting in excess amounts of this neurotransmitter at receptor sites at the postganglionic site.

Cocaine-Related Myocardial Ischemia and Infarction

In 1982, Coleman and associates reported an association between cocaine use and myocardial ischemia and infarction. Subsequently, numerous reports have described cocaine-related myocardial ischemic events. In one survey of 10,085 adults, aged 18 to 45 years, 25 percent of nonfatal MI were attributed to cocaine use.[35] Cocaine-related myocardial ischemia or infarction may result from (1) increased myocardial oxygen demand in the setting of a limited or fixed oxygen supply; (2) marked coronary arterial vasoconstriction; and (3) enhanced platelet aggregation and thrombus formation (Fig. 62–5).

By virtue of its sympathomimetic effects, cocaine increases the three major determinants of myocardial oxygen demand: heart rate, left ventricular wall tension, and left ventricular contractility. At the same time, the ingestion of even small amounts of the drug causes vasoconstriction of the epicardial coronary arteries (so-called inappropriate vasoconstriction) in that the myocardial oxygen supply decreases as demand increases.[36] Cocaine induces vasoconstriction in normal and diseased coronary arterial segments, but its vasoconstrictive effect is particularly marked in the latter.[37] As a result, cocaine users with atherosclerotic coronary artery disease are probably at an especially high risk for an ischemic event after cocaine use. Cocaine-induced coronary arterial vasoconstriction primarily results from the stimulation of coronary arterial alpha-adrenergic receptors, since it is reversed by phentolamine (an alpha-adrenergic antagonist)[36] and exacerbated by propranolol (a beta-adrenergic antagonist).[38] In addition, cocaine causes increased endothelial production of endothelin (a potent vasoconstrictor) and decreased production of nitric oxide (a potent vasodilator), which also may promote vasoconstriction.

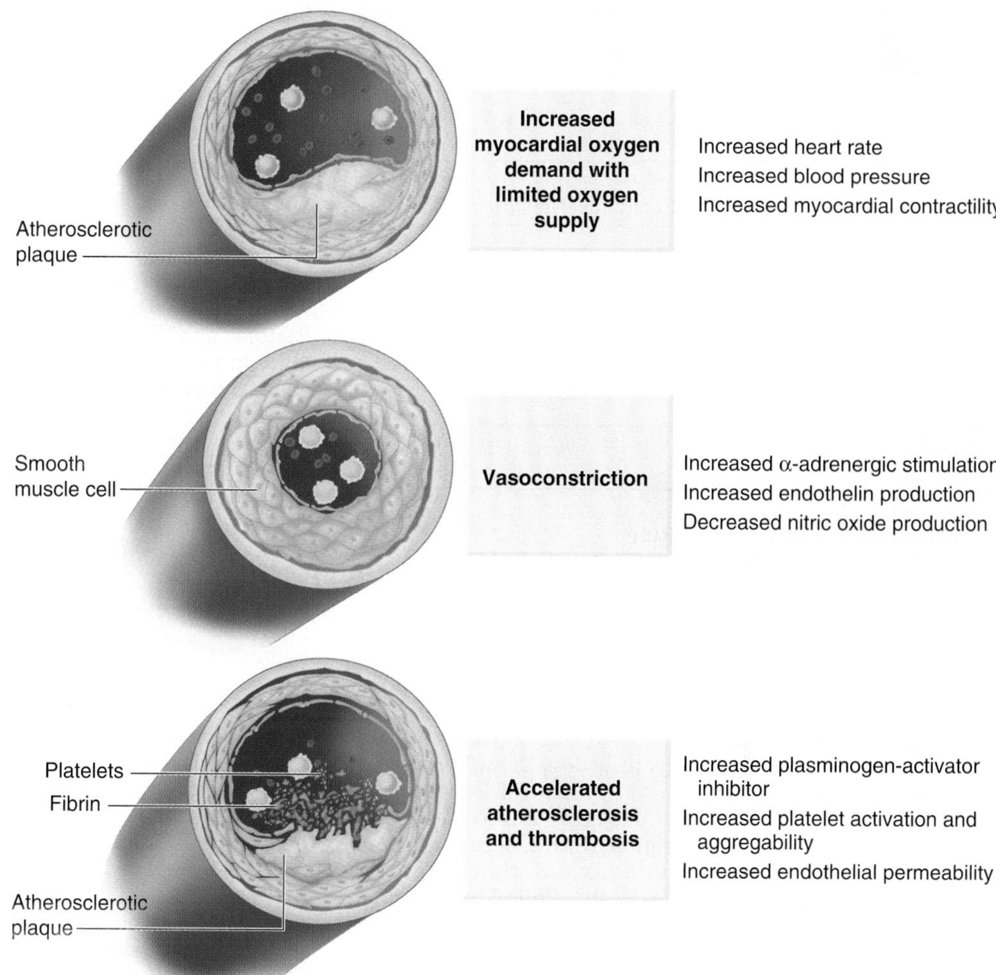

FIGURE 62–5 Mechanisms by which cocaine may induce myocardial ischemia or infarction. Cocaine may induce myocardial ischemia or infarction by increasing the determinants of myocardial oxygen demand in the setting of limited oxygen supply **(top)**, causing intense coronary arterial vasoconstriction **(middle)**, or inducing accelerated atherosclerosis and thrombosis **(bottom)**.

Cocaine use is associated with enhanced platelet activation and aggregability[39] as well as an increased concentration of plasminogen activator inhibitor,[40] which may promote thrombus formation. The presence of premature atherosclerotic coronary artery disease, which has been observed in postmortem studies of long-term cocaine users, may provide a nidus for thrombus formation. In vitro studies have shown that cocaine causes structural abnormalities in the endothelial cell barrier, increasing its permeability to LDL and enhancing the expression of endothelial adhesion molecules and leukocyte migration, all of which are associated with atherogenesis.

Chest pain is the most common cardiovascular complaint of patients seeking medical assistance following cocaine use. Approximately 6 percent of those who come to the emergency department with cocaine-associated chest pain have enzymatic evidence of myocardial necrosis.[41] Most subjects with cocaine-related MI are young, nonwhite, male cigarette smokers without other risk factors for atherosclerosis who have a history of repeated cocaine use (Table 62–4). Similar to cocaine, cigarette smoking induces coronary arterial vasoconstriction through an alpha-adrenergic mechanism. The deleterious effects of cocaine on myocardial oxygen supply and demand are exacerbated substantially by concomitant cigarette smoking: following concomitant cocaine use and smoking, heart rate and systemic arterial pressure increase markedly, and coronary arterial vasoconstriction is more intense than with either alone.[42]

The risk of MI is increased 24-fold during the 60 minutes after cocaine use by subjects considered at low risk for infarction.[43] The occurrence of MI after cocaine use appears unrelated to the amount ingested, its route of administration, and the frequency of its use: cocaine-related infarction has been reported with doses ranging from 200 to 2000 mg, after ingestion by all routes, and in habitual as well as first-time users. About half the patients with cocaine-related MI have no angiographic evidence of atherosclerotic coronary artery disease.[43] Therefore, when subjects with no or few risk factors for atherosclerosis, particularly those who are young or have a history of substance abuse, present with acute MI, urine and blood samples should be analyzed for cocaine and its metabolites.

TABLE 62–4 Characteristics of Patients with Cocaine-Induced Myocardial Infarction

• **Dose of cocaine** 5 or 6 lines (150 mg) to as much as 2 gm Serum concentration, 0.01 to 1.02 mg/liter
• **Frequency of use** Reported in chronic, recreational, and first-time users
• **Route of administration** Occurs with all routes of administration 75% of reported myocardial infarctions occurred after intranasal use
• **Age** Mean, 34 (range, 17-71) yr 20% are < 25 yr
• **Gender** 80%-90% male
• **Timing** Often within minutes of cocaine use Reported as late as 5-15 hr after use

Cardiovascular complications resulting from cocaine-related MI are relatively uncommon, with ventricular arrhythmias occurring in 4 to 17 percent, congestive heart failure in 5 to 7 percent, and death in less than 2 percent.[34] This low incidence of complications is due, at least in part, to the young age and absence of extensive multivessel coronary artery disease of most patients with cocaine-related infarction. If complications develop, most occur within 12 hours of presentation to the hospital.[44] Following hospital discharge, continued cocaine use and recurrent chest pain are common, and occasionally a patient has recurrent nonfatal or fatal MI.

Most subjects with cocaine-related myocardial ischemia or infarction have chest pain within an hour of cocaine use, at a time when the blood cocaine concentration is highest. However, an occasional individual notes the onset of symptoms several hours after the administration of the drug, when the blood cocaine concentration is low or even undetectable. With cocaine ingestion, the diameter of the coronary arteries decreases as the drug concentration increases. Then, as the drug concentration declines, the vasoconstriction resolves. Thereafter, as the concentrations of cocaine's major metabolites (benzoylecgonine and ecgonine methyl ester) rise, "delayed" (i.e., recurrent) coronary arterial vasoconstriction occurs,[45] thereby providing an explanation of why myocardial ischemia or infarction has been reported to occur several hours after drug use.

Cocaethylene

In individuals who use cocaine in temporal proximity to the ingestion of ethanol, hepatic transesterification leads to the production of a unique metabolite, cocaethylene. Cocaethylene is often detected postmortem in subjects who are presumed to have died of cocaine and ethanol toxicity. Similar to cocaine, cocaethylene blocks the reuptake of dopamine at the synaptic cleft, thereby possibly potentiating the systemic toxic effects of cocaine. In experimental animals, in fact, cocaethylene is more lethal than cocaine.[46] In humans, the combination of cocaine and ethanol has been shown to cause a substantial increase in myocardial oxygen demand. The concomitant use of cocaine and ethanol is associated with a higher incidence of disability and death than either agent alone.[47] Individuals presumably dying of a combined cocaine-ethanol overdose have been found to have much lower blood cocaine concentrations than those presumably dying of a cocaine overdose alone, thereby suggesting an additive or synergistic effect of ethanol on the catastrophic cardiovascular events induced by cocaine.

Cocaine-Induced Myocardial Dysfunction

Long-term cocaine abuse has been associated with left ventricular hypertrophy and systolic dysfunction. Several reports have described dilated cardiomyopathy in long-term cocaine abusers, and others have described profound but reversible myocardial depression after binge cocaine use. Bertolet and colleagues found that 7 percent of long-term chronic users without cardiac symptoms had radionuclide ventriculographic evidence of left ventricular systolic dysfunction.[48]

Cocaine may adversely affect left ventricular systolic function by several mechanisms.[34] First, as noted previously, cocaine may induce myocardial ischemia or infarction. Second, the profound repetitive sympathetic stimulation induced by cocaine is similar to that observed in patients with pheochromocytoma—either may induce a cardiomyopathy and characteristic microscopic changes of subendocardial contraction band necrosis. Third, the concomitant administration of adulterants or infectious agents may cause myocarditis, which has been seen on occasion in intravenous cocaine users studied at postmortem. Fourth, studies in experimental animals have shown that cocaine alters cytokine production in the endothelium and in circulating leukocytes, induces the transcription of genes responsible for changes in the composition of myocardial collagen and myosin, and induces myocyte apoptosis.

Aside from the effects of long-term cocaine use on myocardial performance, it may cause an acute deterioration of left ventricular systolic and/or diastolic function. In some subjects, this deterioration may be caused by metabolic and/or acid-base disturbances that accompany cocaine intoxication, whereas in others it may be caused by a direct toxic effect of the drug. Pitts and coworkers demonstrated that an intracoronary infusion of cocaine (in an amount sufficient to produce a concentration in coronary sinus blood similar in magnitude to the peripheral blood concentration found in abusers presumably dying of cocaine intoxication) had a deleterious effect on left ventricular systolic and diastolic function.[49] It seems feasible that cocaine or its metabolites alter the manner in which myocytes handle calcium.

Arrhythmias

Cardiac dysrhythmias may occur with cocaine use (Table 62–5), but the precise arrhythmogenic potential of the drug is poorly defined. In many instances, the dysrhythmias ascribed to cocaine occur in the setting of profound hemodynamic or metabolic derangements, such as hypotension, hypoxemia, seizures, or MI. Nonetheless, because of cocaine's sodium-channel–blocking properties and its ability to enhance sympathetic activation, it is considered a likely

TABLE 62–5 Cardiac Dysrhythmias and Conduction Disturbances Reported with Cocaine Use

Sinus tachycardia	Ventricular tachycardia
Sinus bradycardia	Ventricular fibrillation
Supraventricular tachycardia	Asystole
Bundle branch block	Torsade de pointes
Complete heart block	Brugada pattern (right bundle branch block with ST segment elevation in leads V_1 to V_3)
Accelerated idioventricular rhythm	

cause of cardiac arrhythmias.[50] The development of lethal arrhythmias with cocaine use may require an underlying substrate of abnormal myocardium: studies in experimental animals have shown that cocaine precipitates ventricular arrhythmias only in the presence of myocardial ischemia or infarction. In humans, life-threatening arrhythmias and sudden death in association with cocaine use occur most often in those with myocardial ischemia or infarction or in those with nonischemic myocellular damage. Long-term cocaine use is associated with increased left ventricular mass and wall thickness,[51] a known risk factor for ventricular dysrhythmias. In some cocaine users, such an increased mass may provide the substrate for arrhythmias.

Cocaine may affect the generation and conduction of cardiac impulses by several mechanisms. First, its sympathomimetic properties may increase ventricular irritability and lower the threshold for fibrillation. Second, it inhibits action potential generation and conduction (i.e., it prolongs the QRS and QT intervals) as a result of its sodium-channel–blocking effects. In so doing, it acts in a manner similar to that of a class I antiarrhythmic agent. Third, cocaine increases the intracellular calcium concentration, which may result in afterdepolarizations and triggered ventricular arrhythmias. Fourth, it reduces vagal activity, thereby potentiating its sympathomimetic effects.

Endocarditis

Although the intravenous administration of any illicit drug is associated with an increased risk of bacterial endocarditis, the intravenous use of cocaine appears to be accompanied by a greater risk of endocarditis than the intravenous administration of other drugs.[52] The reason for this enhanced risk of endocarditis in intravenous cocaine users is unknown, but several hypotheses have been proposed. The increase in heart rate and systemic arterial pressure that accompanies cocaine use may induce valvular injury that predisposes to bacterial invasion. Cocaine's immunosuppressive effects may increase the risk of infection. The manner in which cocaine is manufactured as well as the adulterants that are often present in it may increase the risk of endocarditis. In contradistinction to the endocarditis associated with other drugs, the endocarditis of cocaine users more often involves the left-sided cardiac valves.

Aortic Dissection

Aortic dissection or rupture has been temporally related to cocaine use; therefore, it should be considered as a possible cause of chest pain in cocaine users (see Chap. 53). In one study of 38 patients with acute aortic dissection, 14 (37 percent) were related to cocaine use, with an average interval from cocaine use to the onset of symptoms of 12 (range, 0 to 24) hours.[53] Dissection probably results from a cocaine-induced increase in systemic arterial pressure. In addition to aortic rupture, the cocaine-related rupture of mycotic and intracerebral aneurysms has been reported.

Amphetamines

Amphetamines were prescribed previously for the treatment of obesity, attention deficit disorder, and narcolepsy; at present, their use is strictly limited. The most frequently abused amphetamines are dextroamphetamine, methcathinone, methamphetamine, methylphenidate, ephedrine, propylhexedrine, phenmetrazine, and 3,4-methylenedioxymethamphetamine (MDMA, also known as *ecstasy*). *Ice* is a freebase form of methamphetamine that can be inhaled, smoked, or injected. Since amphetamines are sympathomimetic agents, their use has been associated with systemic arterial hypertension, MI, and lethal arrhythmias.[54] Similar to cocaine, amphetamines may induce intense coronary arterial vasoconstriction with or without thrombus formation.[55] Finally, subjects with dilated cardiomyopathy following repetitive amphetamine use have been described.

Catecholamines

Catecholamines, administered exogenously or secreted by a neuroendocrine tumor (e.g., pheochromocytoma or neuroblastoma), may produce acute myocarditis (with focal myocardial necrosis and inflammation), cardiomyopathy, tachycardia, and arrhythmias. Similar abnormalities have been described with the excessive use of beta-adrenoceptor agonist inhalants and methylxanthines in patients with severe pulmonary disease.[56] The secretion of large amounts of endogenous catecholamines, as may occur in subjects with subarachnoid hemorrhage, has been associated with the appearance of transient left ventricular apical dyskinesis and electrocardiographic (ECG) T wave inversions anteriorly. This entity, known as *takotsubo cardiomyopathy*, spontaneously resolves when catecholamine secretion abates.[57]

Several mechanisms may be responsible for the acute and chronic myocardial damage associated with catecholamines. They may exert a direct toxic effect on the myocardium through changes in autonomic tone, enhanced lipid mobility, calcium overload, free radical production, or increased sarcolemmal permeability. Alternatively, myocardial damage may be secondary to a sustained increase in myocardial oxygen demand and/or decrease in myocardial oxygen supply (the latter due to catecholamine-induced coronary arterial vasoconstriction or platelet aggregation).

Inhalants

The inhalants may be classified as organic solvents, organic nitrites (such as amyl nitrite or amyl butyl), and nitrous oxide. The organic solvents include toluene (airplane glue), Freon, kerosene, gasoline, carbon tetrachloride, acrylic paint sprays, shoe polish, degreasers, nail polish remover, typewriter correction fluid, adhesives, and lighter fluid. These solvents are most often inhaled by children or young adolescents. Acute or chronic inhalant use occasionally has been reported to induce cardiac abnormalities, most commonly dysrhythmias; rarely, inhalant use has been associated with myocarditis, MI,[58] and sudden death.[59] The inhalation of freon, for example, has been shown to sensitize the myocardium to catecholamines; in these individuals, fatal arrhythmias have been reported to occur when the user is startled during inhalation.[60]

Antiretroviral Agents (Protease Inhibitors)

Subjects treated with protease inhibitors have been observed to have severe hypertriglyceridemia (serum triglycerides > 1000 mg/dl) and marked elevations in lipoprotein(a) (see Chaps. 39 and 61).[61] Not surprisingly, therefore, patients who are maintained on these agents have an increased risk of atherosclerosis.[62] Dilated cardiomyopathy in association with zidovudine use has been reported.[63,64] In mice, zidovudine produces a cardiomyopathy, with pathologic changes demonstrable in the mitochondria,[65] and similar ultrastructural mitochondrial changes have been observed in myocardial biopsy specimens from HIV-infected patients treated with this agent. In one individual, zidovudine's discontinuation resulted in a reversal of cardiac dysfunction.

Ergotamine and Serotonin Agonists

Two medications used to treat subjects with migraine headaches, ergotamine and sumatriptan, have been associated with acute MI. Ergotamine causes vasoconstriction of intracerebral and extracranial arteries; rarely, its use has been associated with coronary arterial vasospasm and acute MI.[66] Its vasoconstrictor effects are exaggerated by concomitant caffeine ingestion or beta-adrenergic blocker use. Sumaptriptan, a selective 5-hydroxytryptamine agonist, also exerts its therapeutic effects by inducing cerebral arterial vasoconstriction. Several patients have been reported in whom coronary vasospasm and acute MI occurred following the administration of therapeutic doses of sumatriptan,[67] some of which were complicated by ventricular tachycardia or ventricular fibrillation and sudden cardiac death.[68]

Appetite Suppressants

Exposure to the appetite suppressants, fenfluramine or dexfenfluramine, alone or in combination with phentermine, has been implicated in the pathogenesis of certain valvular abnormalities. Fenfluramine (Pondimin), a sympathomimetic amine, promotes the release of serotonin and blocks its neuronal uptake; dexfenfluramine (Redux) is the dextroisomer of fenfluramine. Phentermine (Adipex, Fastin, Ionamin) is a noradrenergic central nervous system stimulant.

The association of appetite suppressant use and valvular abnormalities was first described in 1997, when subjects receiving the combination of fenfluramine and phentermine were noted to have unusual valvular morphology and resultant regurgitation of both left- and right-sided heart valves. All had aortic and/or mitral regurgitation, and half had tricuspid regurgitation.[69] Echocardiographic and histopathological findings resembled those described in patients with carcinoid or ergotamine-induced valvular heart disease. Grossly, the aortic and mitral valve leaflets and chordae tendineae were thickened and had a glistening white appearance. Histologically, leaflet architecture was intact; a plaque-like encasement of the leaflets and chordal structures was noted; and proliferative myofibroblasts surrounded by an abundant extracellular matrix were observed. As a result of these observations, the manufacturer withdrew fenfluramine and dexfenfluramine from the market. Since no valvular abnormalities have been associated with the use of phentermine alone, it is still available.

The risk of valvular heart disease associated with exposure to fenfluramine or dexfenfluramine, alone or in combination with phentermine, has been addressed in several studies, with the prevalence of valvular regurgitation varying from less than 1 percent to as much as 26 percent.[70-73] This apparent wide-ranging risk is attributable to differences in study type, patient populations, varying definitions of regurgitation, and differing durations of treatment with these agents. The prevalence of "significant" valvular regurgitation appears to be related directly to the duration of exposure to the anorectic agents.[72] In most subjects, the valvular abnormalities stabilize or improve after the agents are discontinued.[74]

Currently, it is recommended that all persons exposed to fenfluramine or dexfenfluramine for any period of time, alone or in combination with other agents, should undergo a thorough cardiovascular assessment to determine the presence or absence of cardiopulmonary symptoms or signs. Those with symptoms or signs suggestive of valvular disease (e.g., dyspnea or a new murmur) should undergo echocardiographic evaluation.

Pergolide (Permax)

Pergolide is a dopamine receptor agonist that is used in the treatment of subjects with Parkinson disease. During pergolide treatment, a small number of individuals have developed cardiac valvulopathy. In some of them, the symptoms or signs of valvulopathy improved with discontinuation of the drug, whereas others necessitated valve replacement surgery. Pathologically, the excised valves appeared similar morphologically and microscopically to the valvulopathy associated with the carcinoid syndrome or the use of ergot alkaloids.

Paclitaxel (Taxol) and Other Chemotherapeutic Drugs

A number of agents used in cancer chemotherapy can cause cardiac toxicity, a subject considered in detail in Chapter 83. For example, up to 29 percent of patients who receive paclitaxel as a chemotherapeutic agent develop transient asymptomatic bradycardia.[75] More substantial cardiac disturbances, including atrioventricular block, left bundle branch block, ventricular tachycardia, or myocardial ischemia, occur in up to 5 percent of subjects. When paclitaxel is given in combination with doxorubicin, the risk of cardiotoxicity may be higher: some reports have suggested that heart failure developed in as many as 20 percent of patients treated with this combination. Other chemotherapeutic agents that may cause cardiac dysfunction include doxorubicin, cyclophosphamide, trastuzumab (Herceptin),[76] and 5-fluorouracil.[77] The latter also may cause myocardial ischemia or infarction, which is thought to be caused by coronary arterial vasospasm.[78]

Environmental Exposures

Cobalt

In the mid-1960s, an acute and fulminant form of dilated cardiomyopathy was described in heavy beer drinkers. It was suggested that the cobalt chloride, which was added to the beer as a foam stabilizer, was the causative agent[79]; therefore, its addition was discontinued. Subsequently, this acute and severe form of cardiomyopathy disappeared. More recently, several reports of dilated cardiomyopathy after occupational exposure to cobalt have appeared; in these individuals, high concentrations of cobalt were demonstrated in endomyocardial biopsy specimens.[80]

Lead

Patients with lead poisoning typically have complaints that are referable to the gastrointestinal and central nervous systems. On occasion, subjects with lead poisoning have ECG abnormalities, atrioventricular conduction defects, and overt congestive heart failure; rarely, myocardial involvement may contribute to or be the principal cause of death.[81]

Mercury

Occupational exposure to metallic mercuric vapors may cause systemic arterial hypertension and myocardial failure.[82] Although some studies have suggested that a high mercury content of fish may counteract the beneficial effects of its n-3 fatty acids, thereby increasing the risk of atherosclerotic cardiovascular disease,[83,84] more recent assessments have not supported an association between total mercury exposure and the risk of coronary artery disease.[85]

Antimony

Various antimony compounds previously have been used in the treatment of patients with schistosomiasis. Their use is often associated with ECG abnormalities, including prolongation of the QT interval and T wave flattening or inversion.[86] Rarely, chest pain, bradycardia, hypotension, ventricular arrhythmias, and sudden death have been reported.

Arsenic

Arsenic exposure typically occurs from pesticide poisoning. Its cardiac manifestations include pericardial effusion, myocarditis, and various ECG abnormalities, including QT interval prolongation with T wave inversion.[87]

Carbon Monoxide

Carbon monoxide has a higher affinity for hemoglobin than does oxygen; as a result, elevated blood concentrations of carbon monoxide lead to reduced tissue oxygen delivery. Although central nervous system symptoms are the predominant manifestations of carbon monoxide poisoning, cardiac toxicity may occur because of myocardial hypoxia or a direct toxic effect of the gas on myocardial mitochondria. Such cardiac involvement may appear promptly after carbon monoxide exposure, or it may be delayed for several days. Sinus tachycardia and various arrhythmias, including ventricular extrasystoles and atrial fibrillation, are common; bradycardia and atrioventricular block may occur in more severe cases. Angina pectoris[88,89] or MI[90] may be precipitated by carbon monoxide exposure in patients with or without[91,92] underlying coronary artery disease. ECG ST segment and T wave abnormalities occur commonly, and transient ventricular dysfunction may occur. The administration of 100 percent oxygen or treatment in a hyperbaric oxygen chamber usually results in rapid recovery.

REFERENCES

Ethanol

1. Patel VB, Why HJ, Richardson PJ, et al: The effects of alcohol on the heart. Adverse Drug React Toxicol Rev 16:15, 1997.
2. Preedy VR, Patel VB, Why HJ, et al: Alcohol and the heart: Biochemical alterations. Cardiovasc Res 31:139, 1996.
3. Lazarevic AM, Nakatani S, Neskovic AN, et al: Early changes in left ventricular function in chronic asymptomatic alcoholics: Relation to the duration of heavy drinking. J Am Coll Cardiol 35:1599, 2000.
4. Kelbaek H, Gjorup T, Brynjolf I, et al: Acute effects of alcohol on left ventricular function in healthy subjects at rest and during upright exercise. Am J Cardiol 55:164, 1985.
5. Urbano-Marquez A, Estruch R, Fernandez-Sola J, et al: The greater risk of alcoholic cardiomyopathy and myopathy in women compared with men. JAMA 274:149, 1995.
6. Wilke A, Kaiser A, Ferency I, et al: [Alcohol and myocarditis]. Herz 21:248, 1996.
7. Fernandez-Sola J, Estruch R, Nicolas JM, et al: Comparison of alcoholic cardiomyopathy in women versus men. Am J Cardiol 80:481, 1997.
8. Masani F, Kato H, Sasagawa Y, et al: [An echocardiographic study of alcoholic cardiomyopathy after total abstinence]. J Cardiol 20:627, 1990.
9. Nicolas JM, Fernandez-Sola J, Estruch R, et al: The effect of controlled drinking in alcoholic cardiomyopathy. Ann Intern Med 136:192, 2002.
10. Fernandez-Sola J, Nicolas JM, Oriola J, et al: Angiotensin-converting enzyme gene polymorphism is associated with vulnerability to alcoholic cardiomyopathy. Ann Intern Med 137:321, 2002.
11. Klatsky AL: Alcohol and cardiovascular disease—more than one paradox to consider. Alcohol and hypertension: Does it matter? Yes. J Cardiovasc Risk 10:21, 2003.
12. Klatsky AL, Friedman GD, Siegelaub AB, et al: Alcohol consumption and blood pressure: Kaiser-Permanente Multiphasic Health Examination data. N Engl J Med 296:1194, 1977.
13. Thadhani R, Camargo CA Jr, Stampfer MJ, et al: Prospective study of moderate alcohol consumption and risk of hypertension in young women. Arch Intern Med 162:569, 2002.
14. Fuchs FD, Chambless LE, Whelton PK, et al: Alcohol consumption and the incidence of hypertension: The Atherosclerosis Risk in Communities Study. Hypertension 37:1242, 2001.
15. Rimm EB, Williams P, Fosher K, et al: Moderate alcohol intake and lower risk of coronary heart disease: Meta-analysis of effects on lipids and haemostatic factors. BMJ 319:1523, 1999.
16. Renaud S, de Lorgeril M: Wine, alcohol, platelets, and the French paradox for coronary heart disease. Lancet 339:1523, 1992.
17. Mukamal KJ, Conigrave KM, Mittleman MA, et al: Roles of drinking pattern and type of alcohol consumed in coronary heart disease in men. N Engl J Med 348:109, 2003.
18. Thun MJ, Peto R, Lopez AD, et al: Alcohol consumption and mortality among middle-aged and elderly U.S. adults. N Engl J Med 337:1705, 1997.
19. Muntwyler J, Hennekens CH, Buring JE, et al: Mortality and light to moderate alcohol consumption after myocardial infarction. Lancet 352:1882, 1998.
20. Fuchs CS, Stampfer MJ, Colditz GA, et al: Alcohol consumption and mortality among women. N Engl J Med 332:1245, 1995.
21. Gaziano JM, Gaziano TA, Glynn RJ, et al: Light-to-moderate alcohol consumption and mortality in the Physicians' Health Study enrollment cohort. J Am Coll Cardiol 35:96, 2000.
22. Camargo CA Jr, Stampfer MJ, Glynn RJ, et al: Moderate alcohol consumption and risk for angina pectoris or myocardial infarction in U.S. male physicians. Ann Intern Med 126:372, 1997.
23. Gronbaek M, Becker U, Johansen D, et al: Type of alcohol consumed and mortality from all causes, coronary heart disease, and cancer. Ann Intern Med 133:411, 2000.
24. Booyse FM, Parks DA: Moderate wine and alcohol consumption: Beneficial effects on cardiovascular disease. Thromb Haemost 86:517, 2001.
25. Mukamal KJ, Jadhav PP, D'Agostino RB, et al: Alcohol consumption and hemostatic factors: Analysis of the Framingham offspring cohort. Circulation 104:1367, 2001.
26. Hein HO, Suadicani P, Gyntelberg F: Alcohol consumption, serum low-density lipoprotein cholesterol concentration, and risk of ischaemic heart disease: Six-year follow-up in the Copenhagen male study. BMJ 312:736, 1996.
27. Solomon CG, Hu FB, Stampfer MJ, et al: Moderate alcohol consumption and risk of coronary heart disease among women with type 2 diabetes mellitus. Circulation 102:494, 2000.
28. Ajani UA, Gaziano JM, Lotufo PA, et al: Alcohol consumption and risk of coronary heart disease by diabetes status. Circulation 102:500, 2000.
29. Albert CM, Manson JE, Cook NR, et al: Moderate alcohol consumption and the risk of sudden cardiac death among U.S. male physicians. Circulation 100:944, 1999.
30. Mukamal KJ, Maclure M, Muller JE, et al: Prior alcohol consumption and mortality following acute myocardial infarction. JAMA 285:1965, 2001.
31. Mukamal KJ, Muller JE, Maclure M, et al: Lack of effect of recent alcohol consumption on the course of acute myocardial infarction. Am Heart J 138:926, 1999.
32. Greenspon AJ, Schaal SF: The "holiday heart": Electrophysiologic studies of alcohol effects in alcoholics. Ann Intern Med 98:135, 1983.
33. Menz V, Grimm W, Hoffmann J, et al: Alcohol and rhythm disturbance: The holiday heart syndrome. Herz 21:227, 1996.

Cocaine

34. Lange RA, Hillis LD: Cardiovascular complications of cocaine use. N Engl J Med 345:351, 2001.
35. Qureshi AI, Suri MF, Guterman LR, et al: Cocaine use and the likelihood of nonfatal myocardial infarction and stroke: Data from the Third National Health and Nutrition Examination Survey. Circulation 103:502, 2001.
36. Lange RA, Cigarroa RG, Yancy CW Jr, et al: Cocaine-induced coronary artery vasoconstriction. N Engl J Med 321:1557, 1989.
37. Flores ED, Lange RA, Cigarroa RG, et al: Effect of cocaine on coronary artery dimensions in atherosclerotic coronary artery disease: Enhanced vasoconstriction at sites of significant stenoses. J Am Coll Cardiol 16:74, 1990.
38. Lange RA, Cigarroa RG, Flores ED, et al: Potentiation of cocaine-induced coronary vasoconstriction by beta-adrenergic blockade. Ann Intern Med 112:897, 1990.
39. Kugelmass AD, Oda A, Monahan K, et al: Activation of human platelets by cocaine. Circulation 88:876, 1993.
40. Moliterno DJ, Lange RA, Gerard RD, et al: Influence of intranasal cocaine on plasma constituents associated with endogenous thrombosis and thrombolysis. Am J Med 96:492, 1994.
41. Hollander JE, Hoffman RS, Burstein JL, et al: Cocaine-associated myocardial infarction: Mortality and complications. Cocaine-Associated Myocardial Infarction Study Group. Arch Intern Med 155:1081, 1995.
42. Moliterno DJ, Willard JE, Lange RA, et al: Coronary artery vasoconstriction induced by cocaine, cigarette smoking, or both. N Engl J Med 330:454, 1994.
43. Mittleman MA, Mintzer D, Maclure M, et al: Triggering of myocardial infarction by cocaine. Circulation 99:2737, 1999.
44. Weber JE, Shofer FS, Larkin GL, et al: Validation of a brief observation period for patients with cocaine-associated chest pain. N Engl J Med 348:510, 2003.
45. Brogan WC III, Lange RA, Glamann DB, et al: Recurrent coronary vasoconstriction caused by intranasal cocaine: Possible role for metabolites. Ann Intern Med 116:556, 1992.
46. Hearn WL, Rose S, Wagner J, et al: Cocaethylene is more potent than cocaine in mediating lethality. Pharmacol Biochem Behav 39:531, 1991.
47. Randall T: Cocaine, alcohol mix in body to form even longer lasting, more lethal drug. JAMA 267:1043, 1992.
48. Bertolet BD, Freund G, Martin CA, et al: Unrecognized left ventricular dysfunction in an apparently healthy cocaine abuse population. Clin Cardiol 13:323, 1990.

49. Pitts WR, Vongpatanasin W, Cigarroa JE, et al: Effects of the intracoronary infusion of cocaine on left ventricular systolic and diastolic function in humans. Circulation 97:1270, 1998.
50. Bauman JL, DiDomenico RJ: Cocaine-induced channelopathies: Emerging evidence on the multiple mechanisms of sudden death. J Cardiovasc Pharmacol Ther 7:195, 2002.
51. Brickner ME, Willard JE, Eichhorn EJ, et al: Left ventricular hypertrophy associated with chronic cocaine abuse. Circulation 84:1130, 1991.
52. Chambers HF, Morris DL, Tauber MG, et al: Cocaine use and the risk for endocarditis in intravenous drug users. Ann Intern Med 106:833, 1987.
53. Hsue PY, Salinas CL, Bolger AF, et al: Acute aortic dissection related to crack cocaine. Circulation 105:1592, 2002.

Amphetamines

54. Waksman J, Taylor RN Jr, Bodor GS, et al: Acute myocardial infarction associated with amphetamine use. Mayo Clin Proc 76:323, 2001.
55. Costa GM, Pizzi C, Bresciani B, et al: Acute myocardial infarction caused by amphetamines: A case report and review of the literature. Ital Heart J 2:478, 2001.
56. Raper R, Fisher M, Bihari D: Profound, reversible, myocardial depression in acute asthma treated with high-dose catecholamines. Crit Care Med 20:710, 1992.
57. Akashi YJ, Nakazawa K, Sakakibara M, et al: Reversible left ventricular dysfunction "takotsubo" cardiomyopathy related to catecholamine cardiotoxicity. J Electrocardiol 35:351, 2002.

Inhalants

58. Carder JR, Fuerst RS: Myocardial infarction after toluene inhalation. Pediatr Emerg Care 13:117, 1997.
59. Shepherd RT: Mechanism of sudden death associated with volatile substance abuse. Hum Toxicol 8:287, 1989.
60. Brady WJ Jr, Stremski E, Eljaiek L, et al: Freon inhalational abuse presenting with ventricular fibrillation. Am J Emerg Med 12:533, 1994.

Antiretroviral Agents

61. Koppel K, Bratt G, Eriksson M, et al: Serum lipid levels associated with increased risk for cardiovascular disease is associated with highly active antiretroviral therapy (HAART) in HIV-1 infection. Int J STD AIDS 11:451, 2000.
62. Tabib A, Leroux C, Mornex JF, et al: Accelerated coronary atherosclerosis and arteriosclerosis in young human immunodeficiency virus–positive patients. Coron Artery Dis 11:41, 2000.
63. Domanski MJ, Sloas MM, Follmann DA, et al: Effect of zidovudine and didanosine treatment on heart function in children infected with human immunodeficiency virus. J Pediatr 127:137, 1995.
64. Herskowitz A, Willoughby SB, Baughman KL, et al: Cardiomyopathy associated with antiretroviral therapy in patients with HIV infection: A report of six cases. Ann Intern Med 116:311, 1992.
65. Lewis W, Grupp IL, Grupp G, et al: Cardiac dysfunction occurs in the HIV-1 transgenic mouse treated with zidovudine. Lab Invest 80:187, 2000.

Ergotamine and Serotonin Agonists

66. Klein LS, Simpson RJ Jr, Stern R, et al: Myocardial infarction following administration of sublingual ergotamine. Chest 82:375, 1982.
67. Mueller L, Gallagher RM, Ciervo CA: Vasospasm-induced myocardial infarction with sumatriptan. Headache 36:329, 1996.
68. Main ML, Ramaswamy K, Andrews TC: Cardiac arrest and myocardial infarction immediately after sumatriptan injection. Ann Intern Med 128:874., 1998.

Appetite Suppressants

69. Connolly HM, Crary JL, McGoon MD, et al: Valvular heart disease associated with fenfluramine-phentermine. N Engl J Med 337:581, 1997.
70. Mast ST, Gersing KR, Anstrom KJ, et al: Association between selective serotonin reuptake inhibitor therapy and heart valve regurgitation. Am J Cardiol 87:989, 2001.
71. Khan MA, Herzog CA, St Peter JV, et al: The prevalence of cardiac valvular insufficiency assessed by transthoracic echocardiography in obese patients treated with appetite-suppressant drugs. N Engl J Med 339:713, 1998.
72. Jick H, Vasilakis C, Weinrauch LA, et al: A population-based study of appetite-suppressant drugs and the risk of cardiac-valve regurgitation. N Engl J Med 339:719, 1998.
73. Weissman NJ, Tighe JF Jr, Gottdiener JS, et al: An assessment of heart-valve abnormalities in obese patients taking dexfenfluramine, sustained-release dexfenfluramine, or placebo. Sustained-Release Dexfenfluramine Study Group. N Engl J Med 339:725, 1998.
74. Weissman NJ, Panza JA, Tighe JF, et al: Natural history of valvular regurgitation 1 year after discontinuation of dexfenfluramine therapy: A randomized, double-blind, placebo-controlled trial. Ann Intern Med 134:267, 2001.

Paclitaxel and Other Chemotherapeutic Drugs

75. Arbuck SG, Strauss H, Rowinsky E, et al: A reassessment of cardiac toxicity associated with Taxol. J Natl Cancer Inst Monogr 117, 1993.
76. Keefe DL: Trastuzumab-associated cardiotoxicity. Cancer 95:1592, 2002.
77. Kuropkat C, Griem K, Clark J, et al: Severe cardiotoxicity during 5-fluorouracil chemotherapy: A case and literature report. Am J Clin Oncol 22:466, 1999.
78. Kleiman NS, Lehane DE, Geyer CE Jr, et al: Prinzmetal's angina during 5-fluorouracil chemotherapy. Am J Med 82:566, 1987.

Environmental Exposures

79. Alexander CS: Cobalt-beer cardiomyopathy: A clinical and pathologic study of twenty-eight cases. Am J Med 53:395, 1972.
80. Jarvis JQ, Hammond E, Meier R, et al: Cobalt cardiomyopathy: A report of two cases from mineral assay laboratories and a review of the literature. J Occup Med 34:620, 1992.
81. Kopp SJ, Barron JT, Tow JP: Cardiovascular actions of lead and relationship to hypertension: A review. Environ Health Perspect 78:91, 1988.
82. Marek K, Zajac-Nedza M, Rola E, et al: [Examination of health effects after exposure to metallic mercury vapors in workers engaged in production of chlorine and acetic aldehyde: I. Evaluation of general health status]. Med Pr 46:101, 1995.
83. Guallar E, Sanz-Gallardo MI, van't Veer P, et al: Mercury, fish oils, and the risk of myocardial infarction. N Engl J Med 347:1747, 2002.
84. Salonen JT, Seppanen K, Nyyssonen K, et al: Intake of mercury from fish, lipid peroxidation, and the risk of myocardial infarction and coronary, cardiovascular, and any death in eastern Finnish men. Circulation 91:645, 1995.
85. Yoshizawa K, Rimm EB, Morris JS, et al: Mercury and the risk of coronary heart disease in men. N Engl J Med 347:1755, 2002.
86. Chulay JD, Spencer HC, Mugambi M: Electrocardiographic changes during treatment of leishmaniasis with pentavalent antimony (sodium stibogluconate). Am J Trop Med Hyg 34:702, 1985.
87. Hall JC, Harruff R: Fatal cardiac arrhythmia in a patient with interstitial myocarditis related to chronic arsenic poisoning. South Med J 82:1557, 1989.
88. Allred EN, Bleecker ER, Chaitman BR, et al: Acute effects of carbon monoxide exposure on individuals with coronary artery disease. Res Rep Health Eff Inst 1, 1989.
89. Allred EN, Bleecker ER, Chaitman BR, et al: Effects of carbon monoxide on myocardial ischemia. Environ Health Perspect 91:89, 1991.
90. Fiorista F, Casazza F, Comolatti G: [Silent myocardial infarction caused by acute carbon monoxide poisoning]. G Ital Cardiol 23:583, 1993.
91. Marius-Nunez AL: Myocardial infarction with normal coronary arteries after acute exposure to carbon monoxide. Chest 97:491, 1990.
92. Ebisuno S, Yasuno M, Yamada Y, et al: Myocardial infarction after acute carbon monoxide poisoning: Case report. Angiology 37:621, 1986.

CHAPTER 63

Primary Tumors of the Heart

Marc S. Sabatine • Wilson S. Colucci • Frederick J. Schoen

With an incidence of approximately 0.02 percent in autopsy series,[1,2] primary tumors of the heart* are far less common than metastatic tumors to the heart. Nonetheless they may cause a wide variety of clinical signs and symptoms that often masquerade as many other more common cardiovascular and systemic diseases. Cardiac tumors have been misdiagnosed as other cardiac conditions (including rheumatic valvular disease, endocarditis, myocarditis, pericarditis, cardiomyopathies, and congenital heart disease), pulmonary conditions (including pulmonary emboli, pulmonary hypertension, and interstitial lung disease), cerebrovascular disease, and vasculitis. Advances in noninvasive cardiovascular imaging techniques—especially echocardiography, computed tomography (CT), and magnetic resonance imaging (MRI)—have greatly facilitated the diagnostic evaluation and permit the rapid identification of intracardiac masses (Table 63–1). Nevertheless, a high index of suspicion remains the most important element in diagnosing a cardiac tumor because the time from onset of symptoms to diagnosis can be months or even years.

Clinical Presentation

Cardiac tumors usually present with some combination of heart failure, arrhythmias, or embolic phenomena. Intracavitary tumors are more likely to cause heart failure or embolic phenomena, whereas intramural tumors are more likely to cause arrhythmias. However, all intracavitary tumors have some point of attachment and thus may be arrhythmogenic, and, if large enough, intramural tumors may bulge and partially obliterate a cardiac chamber or interfere with a ventricle's mechanical performance and thus cause heart failure. Therefore, the specific signs and symptoms produced by tumors are more closely related to their precise anatomical location, size, and effect on the surrounding structures than to their histological types.[3]

Heart Failure

Cardiac tumors may cause signs and symptoms of either backward, congestive heart failure or forward, low-output heart failure, or both. Mechanistically, these manifestations may arise from intracavitary obstruction of either filling or outflow or from intramural interference with function. Obstruction of filling or outflow can be due to cavitary obliteration as well as valvular dysfunction. Myocardial dysfunction can include both systolic dysfunction due to impaired contractility and diastolic dysfunction due to restrictive physiology.

LEFT ATRIAL TUMORS. In adults, 80 to 90 percent of primary cardiac tumors seen in the left atrium are benign myxomas. Typically intracavitary, mobile, and pedunculated, myxomas may prolapse to various degrees into the mitral valve orifice, resulting in obstruction of blood flow from the left atrium to the left ventricle as well as mitral regurgitation. The resultant signs and symptoms often mimic those of mitral valve disease, especially mitral stenosis, and include dyspnea, orthopnea, and paroxysmal nocturnal dyspnea. However, weight loss, syncope, and sudden death—manifestations that are uncommon with mitral valve disease—also occur. Furthermore, atrial fibrillation, common in advanced, symptomatic mitral stenosis, is rare in patients with atrial myxomas, presumably because atrial enlargement is uncommon. It is not unusual for the symptoms to be sudden in onset, intermittent, and related to body position.[3] Thus, although most of the symptoms produced by left atrial tumors are nonspecific, the occurrence of paroxysmal symptoms that arise characteristically in a particular body position and are out of proportion to the clinical findings should raise suspicion for a left atrial tumor.

Physical Examination. This may disclose signs of pulmonary congestion; a loud S_1, which is often widely split; an S_4, a sound rarely audible in mitral stenosis; a holosystolic murmur that is loudest at the apex and resembles mitral regurgitation; and a diastolic murmur resulting from obstruction to flow through the mitral orifice due to the tumor. The loud S_1 that occurs in patients with left atrial myxoma may be caused by the late onset of mitral valve closure resulting from either increased left atrial pressure or prolapse of the tumor through the mitral valve orifice. In some cases, an early diastolic sound (~100 msec after S_2), termed a *tumor plop,* can be identified. It is thought to be produced as the tumor strikes the endocardial wall or as its excursion is abruptly halted and its stalk tenses. Although in most cases the tumor plop occurs later than the opening snap of the mitral valve and earlier than an S_3, it is not surprising that this sound is frequently confused with either of those findings.

RIGHT ATRIAL TUMORS. Right atrial tumors frequently produce symptoms of right heart failure, including peripheral edema, ascites, and hepatomegaly.[3] As approximately half of right atrial tumors will turn out to be sarcomas, the development of right-sided heart failure may be rapidly progressive. Coincident with the development of heart failure, new systolic

*Tumors arising elsewhere in the body and metastasizing to the pericardium and heart are discussed in Chapters 64 and 83, respectively.

TABLE 63–1 Imaging Features of Cardiac Tumors

Cardiac Tumor	Echocardiography	CT	MRI
Myxoma	Mobile tumor Narrow stalk connected to fossa ovalis Heterogeneous with hypoechoic and hyperechoic foci	Narrow base of attachment Heterogeneous, low attenuation Occasionally with calcification	Heterogeneous Primarily isointense on T1, with areas of hypointensity and hyperintensity Hyperintense on T2 Heterogeneous enhancement
Papillary fibroelastoma	Mobile mass Short pedicle "Shimmering" edges	Difficult to see	Difficult to see
Lipomas	Intramural hyperechoic mass	Homogeneous Low (fat) attenuation	Hyperintense on T1 ↓ Signal with fat suppression No enhancement
Rhabdomyomas	Multiple small, lobulated hyperechoic intramural masses		Homogeneous Isointense on T1 Hyperintense on T2
Fibromas	Intramural large, solid mass Central hyperechoic foci	Homogeneous, low attenuation Calcification	Isointense on T1 Hypointense on T2 Minimal enhancement
Teratomas	Very heterogeneous Pericardial effusion	Very heterogeneous	Very heterogeneous
Hemangiomas	Hyperechoic	Heterogeneous Calcification Marked enhancement	Isointense on T1 Hyperintense on T2 Marked enhancement
Angiosarcoma	Mass protruding into right atrium Pericardial effusion	Low attenuation	Infiltrative Heterogeneous Nodular areas of hyperintensity on T1 Linear areas of enhancement
Other sarcomas	Left atrial mass Broad base of attachment to posterior atrial wall	Low attenuation ± Calcification	Infiltrative and heterogeneous Variable intensity on T1
Lymphoma	Hypoechoic masses Pericardial effusion	Low attenuation	Infiltrative Isointense to hypointense on T1 Heterogenous enhancement

Adapted from information in (1) Grebenc ML, Rosado de Christenson ML, Burke AP, et al: Primary cardiac and pericardial neoplasms: Radiologic-pathologic correlation. Radiographics 20:1073-1103, 2000; (2) Araoz PA, Mulvagh SL, Tazelaar HD, et al: CT and MR imaging of benign primary cardiac neoplasms with echocardiographic correlation. Radiographics 20:1303-1319, 2000; (3) Araoz PA, Eklund HE, Welch TJ, Breen JF: CT and MR imaging of primary cardiac malignancies. Radiographics 19:1421-1434, 1999; and (4) Frank H: Cardiac and paracardiac masses. *In* Manning WJ, Pennell DJ (eds): Cardiovascular Magnetic Resonance. New York, Churchill Livingstone, 2002, pp 342-354.

or diastolic murmurs or both may be appreciated. It is not surprising that right atrial tumors have been misdiagnosed as Ebstein's anomaly of the tricuspid valve, constrictive pericarditis, tricuspid stenosis, carcinoid syndrome, superior vena caval syndrome, and cardiomyopathy.

Physical Examination. This can reveal an elevated jugular venous pressure with prominent *a* waves and steep *y* descents, peripheral edema, evidence of superior vena cava obstruction, hepatomegaly, and ascites. An early diastolic rumbling murmur, due to obstruction to tricuspid flow, or a holosystolic murmur, secondary to tricuspid regurgitation, may demonstrate respiratory or positional variation. Because of the rarity of *isolated* rheumatic tricuspid valvular disease, the lack of other valvular findings should raise the question of a right atrial tumor. A protodiastolic tumor plop has been described and is thought to be similar in etiology to that produced by left atrial tumors.

VENTRICULAR TUMORS. Depending on which chamber is involved, intracavitary ventricular tumors may present with left- or right-sided heart failure as a result of obstruction to ventricular filling or outflow. The clinical manifestations are those typical for left- and right-sided heart failure and include dyspnea, pulmonary edema, and syncope and peripheral edema, hepatomegaly, and ascites, respectively. Systolic or diastolic murmurs and atrial or ventricular gallops may be heard and thus the cardiac findings often lead to an initial diagnosis of valvular heart disease or hypertrophic cardiomyopathy. However, whereas valvular disease is often slowly progressive, the symptoms due to cardiac tumors are often rapidly progressive. Ventricular tumors that are predominantly intramural may be asymptomatic; they can affect diastolic function mimicking a restrictive cardiomyopathy; or they can affect systolic function mimicking a dilated cardiomyopathy.

Arrhythmias

Cardiac tumors, especially those with significant intramural involvement, may cause disturbances of conduction or rhythm,[4] the precise nature of which is determined by the location of the tumor. Tumors with atrial involvement or attachment such as myxomas, sarcomas, and lipomatous hypertrophy of the septum may produce a wide variety of supraventricular tachyarrhythmias, including atrial fibrillation, atrial flutter, and ectopic atrial tachycardia. Tumors in the area of the atrioventricular (AV) node, typically angiomas and mesotheliomas, may produce AV conduction disturbances, including complete heart block, and asystole. Tumors located within the ventricular myocardium such as rhabdomyomas and fibromas can cause premature ventricular beats, ventricular tachycardia, ventricular fibrillation, and sudden cardiac death.

Embolic Phenomena

Embolization of tumor fragments or of thrombi from the surface of a tumor is a frequent and often dramatic clinical occurrence. Although myxomas are the source of most tumor emboli because of the combination of their friable consistency and intracavitary location, other types of cardiac tumors occasionally may embolize. The distribution of tumor emboli depends on the location of the tumor and the presence or absence of intracardiac shunts.

LEFT-SIDED EMBOLI. Left-sided tumors embolize to the systemic circulation, resulting in stroke, visceral infarction, peripheral limb ischemia, and peripheral vascular aneurysms. The neurological event may occasionally be the first or only clinical manifestation of a cardiac tumor. An embolic stroke in a young person without evidence of cerebrovascular disease, particularly in the presence of sinus rhythm, should raise the suspicion of intracardiac myxoma, as well as infective endocarditis. Multiple systemic emboli may mimic systemic vasculitis or infective endocarditis, especially when associated with other manifestations of a systemic illness such as fever, weight loss, arthralgias, and an elevated erythrocyte sedimentation rate (ESR). The finding at angiography of numerous vascular aneurysms secondary to tumor emboli in the cerebral, renal, femoral, and coronary arteries is not infrequent and may lead to the mistaken diagnosis of polyarteritis nodosa. Because the diagnosis of an intracardiac tumor may be made after histological examination of systemic embolic material, it is of critical importance to make every effort to recover and examine the entirety of the embolic material because what appears to be a thrombus may actually be a cardiac tumor embolism covered by thrombus.

RIGHT-SIDED EMBOLI. Right-sided cardiac tumors and left-sided cardiac tumors proximal to left-to-right intracardiac shunts may result in pulmonary emboli. Indeed, serious pulmonary hypertension and cor pulmonale due to chronic recurrent pulmonary emboli from right atrial tumors can occur.

Diagnostic Techniques

CHEST ROENTGENOGRAM. Cardiac tumors may display several findings on plain chest roentgenograms that may offer the first clue as to their presence. The cardiac contour may display generalized or specific chamber enlargement that mimics virtually any type of valvular heart disease, or may demonstrate a bizarre appearance. An enlarged cardiac contour may also be due to a pericardial effusion, which generally indicates invasion of the pericardial space by a malignant tumor. Calcification visible by roentgenographic methods may occur with several types of cardiac tumor, including rhabdomyomas, fibromas, teratomas, myxomas, hemangiomas, and osteosarcomas. However, many cardiac tumors may be entirely intracavitary, uncalcified, and not associated with any change in cardiac contour. Thus, when a cardiac tumor is suspected, a dedicated cardiac imaging study is required.

ANGIOGRAPHY. Cardiac catheterization and selective angiocardiography enabled the first antemortem diagnosis of a cardiac tumor but now are rarely necessary because echocardiography, CT, and MRI provide adequate preoperative information (see later). In several circumstances, however, the risk of cardiac catheterization is outweighed by the supplemental information it may provide. These include cases in which noninvasive evaluation has not been adequate in fully defining tumor location or attachment or when other cardiac conditions such as coronary artery disease, valvular heart disease, or pulmonary hypertension may coexist and possibly dictate a different surgical approach.

Intracavitary tumors are identified by injecting contrast material upstream to the tumor location and demonstrating a filling defect in the chamber of interest. For suspected left atrial tumors, contrast material may be injected into the pulmonary artery and then waiting for the levophase. Large intramural ventricular tumors may be identified by observing abnormalities in the typical chamber contours. Finally, highly vascular tumors may be detected on coronary angiography by seeing the characteristic tumor blush.

The major risk of angiography is peripheral embolization due to dislodgment of a fragment of tumor or of an associated thrombus. Therefore, thorough evaluation by noninvasive methods before catheterization is recommended for patients suspected of having cardiac tumors so that contrast material can be injected into the chamber proximal to the location of the tumor. Moreover, because cardiac tumors may be numerous and present in more than one chamber, all four chambers should be visualized noninvasively before cardiac catheterization whenever possible.

ECHOCARDIOGRAPHY. Echocardiography (see Chap. 11) has become the screening test of choice for cardiac tumors. In particular, two-dimensional echocardiography offers real-time, high spatial and temporal resolution imaging and thus can provide information about tumor size, attachment, and mobility (Fig. 63–1A). Continuous-mode Doppler ultrasonography may be useful for evaluating the hemodynamic consequences of valvular obstruction or incompetence caused by cardiac tumors. *Tissue harmonic imaging*, which relies on the gradual generation of harmonics as ultrasound waves propagate through tissue, results in reduced near-field and side-lobe artifacts and thus offers improved image

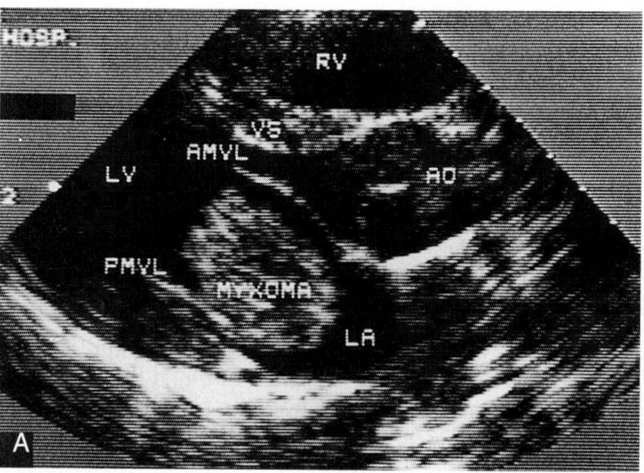

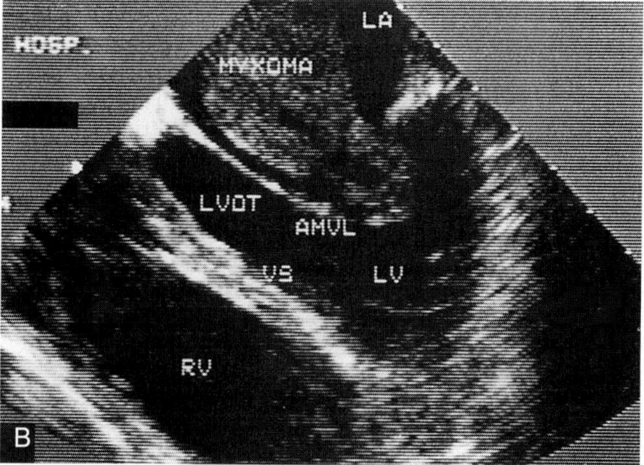

FIGURE 63–1 Transthoracic two-dimensional echocardiogram **(A)** and transesophageal two-dimensional echocardiogram **(B)** showing a left atrial (LA) mass prolapsing into and obstructing the mitral valve orifice. Note the superior resolution of the transesophageal echocardiogram. Although not visible here, the myxoma was attached to the mid-portion of the atrial septum. AO = aorta; AMVL = anterior mitral valve leaflet; PMVL = posterior mitral valve leaflet; LV = left ventricle; LVOT = left ventricular outflow tract; VS = ventricular septum. (From Allard MF, Taylor GP, Wilson JE, McManus BM: Primary cardiac tumors. *In* Goldhaber SZ, Braunwald E [eds]: Cardiopulmonary Diseases and Cardiac Tumors. Atlas of Heart Diseases. Vol 3. Philadelphia, Current Medicine, 1995, pp 15.1-15.22.)

quality. *Contrast echocardiography* uses microbubbles that are capable of transversing the pulmonary vascular bed and opacifying the left heart. This technique can be used to enhance endocardial border definition and thereby more clearly demonstrate filling defects caused by intracavitary tumors. *Myocardial contrast echocardiography,* in which the microbubbles are imaged within the myocardial capillary vascular bed, has already been used to demonstrate intracardiac mass perfusion,[5] thereby helping distinguish tumor from thrombus, and may someday be used to define the extent of intramural tumors.

Transesophageal Echocardiography. This appears to be superior to transthoracic echocardiography in many patients (see Fig. 63–1B). The potential advantages of transesophageal echocardiography include improved resolution of the tumor and its attachment, the ability to detect some masses not visualized by transthoracic echocardiography, and improved visualization of right atrial tumors.[6] Although transesophageal echocardiography does not appear warranted on a routine basis, it should be considered when the transthoracic study is suboptimal, and it is frequently used for intraoperative monitoring. *Three-dimensional transesophageal echocardiography* is a relatively new technique in which multiple cross-section images at slightly different angles are acquired by rotating a multiplane probe and using cardiac and respiratory gating.[7] The resulting volumetric data set is processed offline, and image reconstruction software is used to create a three-dimensional image that simulates intraoperative visualization.

COMPUTED TOMOGRAPHY. Recent advances in CT (see Chap. 15), including spiral, multislice spiral, and electron-beam CT (EBCT), have greatly improved its applicability to cardiac imaging.[8] A breath-hold technique is used to minimize respiratory motion artifact, and image resolution is further improved by gating the CT acquisition to the cardiac cycle. Electrocardiographic gating also allows cine-mode data to be obtained, thereby allowing assessment of mobility. Of note, data acquisition is sufficiently rapid (50 to 100 msec) for EBCT that cardiac gating is not absolutely necessary, permitting adequate imaging in patients with irregular rhythms. New rendering software has the ability to construct images in any plane and even create three-dimensional images.

CT provides a high degree of soft tissue discrimination, which is helpful in defining the degree of myocardial infiltration. CT can also be used to assess for calcification, which may be useful in the diagnosis of rhabdomyomas, fibromas, teratomas, myxomas, hemangiomas, and osteosarcomas. The administration of a contrast agent may clarify further the degree of intramural invasion (Fig. 63–2) and help differentiate a vascular tumor from an avascular thrombus. CT also allows for evaluation of the extracardiac structures. Thus, CT currently appears to be most useful in the evaluation of suspected tumors of the heart either to provide additional information when the echocardiographic data are equivocal or to determine the degree of myocardial invasion and the involvement of pericardial and extracardiac structures in lesions consistent with a malignant process.[9-11]

MAGNETIC RESONANCE IMAGING. MRI offers unsurpassed soft tissue characterization and the use of multiple, different pulse sequences presents clinicians with complementary information (see Chap. 14).[12] T1-weighted and T2-weighted dual-inversion recovery fast spin-echo sequences offer detailed morphological information, with T1-weighted images providing excellent soft tissue characterization and T2-weighted images providing superior tissue contrast and demonstration of fluid components. For complex, heterogeneous tumors such as myxomas and teratomas, studies have demonstrated excellent correlation between the MRI and pathological findings.[13] A short inversion recovery sequence permits suppression of fat signals and therefore is useful in detecting lipid-containing masses such as lipomas. Contrast enhancement with gadolinium provides information on the vascularity of the mass, often allows for better delineation of the degree of tumor infiltration within the myocardium, and assists in the differentiation of thrombus from tumor. Additionally, MRI allows for simultaneous assessment of all cardiac chambers, the pericardium, and surrounding structures. Multislice imaging can be performed in the standard cardiac axes as well as any modified axis as needed, thereby providing precise three-dimensional information (Fig. 63–3).

For evaluation of cardiac function and tumor mobility, gradient-echo sequences are used. These sequences have faster acquisition times, allowing for cine MRI. Recently developed steady-state free precession (SSFP) sequences offer even better contrast between blood and soft tissue and therefore can delineate the contour of tumors even in areas of slow

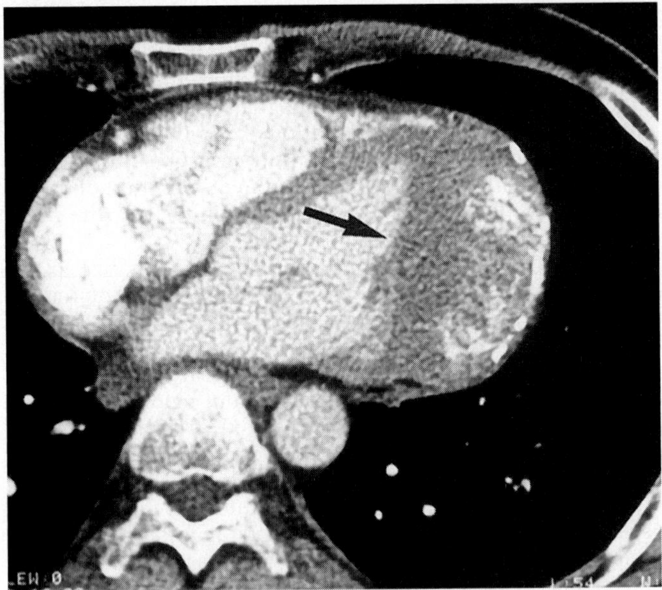

FIGURE 63–2 Contrast-enhanced electron-beam CT scan of a left ventricular fibroma. Note the coarse calcifications in the lateral wall (arrow). (From Araoz PA, Mulvagh SL, Tazelaar HD, et al: CT and MR imaging of benign primary cardiac neoplasms with echocardiographic correlation. Radiographics 20:1303-1319, 2000.)

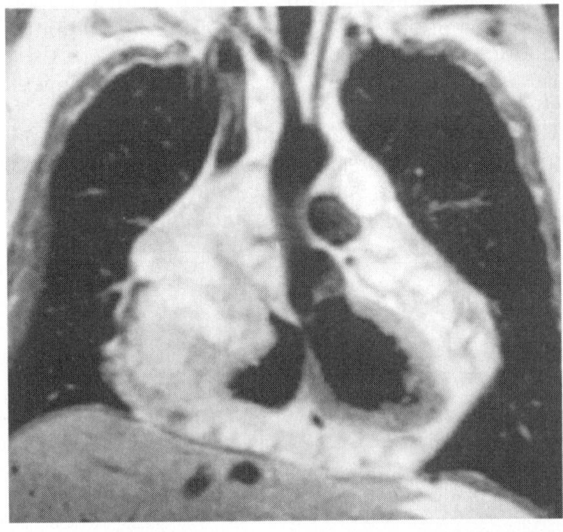

FIGURE 63–3 Coronal T2-weighted MRI of angiosarcoma demonstrating extensive circumferential cardiac involvement by the nodular, heterogeneous, hyperintense tumor, which invades the right atrium and encases the heart. (From Grebenc ML, Rosado de Christenson ML, Burke AP, et al: Primary cardiac and pericardial neoplasms: Radiologic-pathologic correlation. Radiographics 20:1073-1103, 2000.)

blood flow. With up to 50 frames per second, SSFP cine acquisitions provide excellent three-dimensional visualization of cardiac function; valve motion; and the structure, size, attachment to adjacent structures, and mobility of cardiac masses. Thus, although the current limited availability and complex interpretation of cardiac MRI may prevent it from being adopted as a universal screening tool, MRI is emerging as the imaging modality of choice for complex cardiac masses.[9-11,14]

NUCLEAR IMAGING. Because tumors are typically in a relatively hypermetabolic state, positron-emission tomography imaging using a metabolic tracer such as 2-[fluorine 18]fluoro-2-deoxy-D-glucose (FDG) has proven useful in detecting malignant tumors. A few case reports have documented its usefulness in detecting primary cardiac tumors and in differentiating tumor from thrombus.[15] Malignant tumors also typically have a high apoptotic index. In one case report, imaging with ^{99m}Tc-p-annexin-V, a marker of apoptosis, demonstrated enhancement in an area containing a known cardiac mass. Subsequent resection revealed a sarcoma that, on immunohistochemistry, stained positive for annexin V.[16]

BIOPSY. Preoperative, catheter-based biopsy is rarely done. With a few exceptions, the treatment of choice for cardiac tumors is surgical excision. Therefore, once a tumor is identified, a definitive open surgical procedure is usually planned. Thrombus, the other major diagnostic possibility when faced with an intracardiac mass, can usually be differentiated from tumor by a combination of the clinical history and imaging data. Moreover, for left-sided intracavitary lesions, the risk of an embolic complication usually precludes consideration of biopsy, and for intramural masses endomyocardial biopsy may not yield an adequate sample.

However, there are several situations in which transvenous, catheter-based biopsy is indicated.[17] In children, certain types of tumors, such as rhabdomyomas, may spontaneously regress. Therefore, biopsy of (ideally) a right-sided mass may permit a histological diagnosis to be made that would then allow surgery to be deferred. In adults, biopsy of a lesion suspicious for malignancy may be necessary to define the specific histology, particularly if the anatomical extent of the lesion is such that there would be no role for attempted surgical resection. In these cases, the biopsy data can be used to optimize chemotherapy. Transesophageal echocardiography can be used to direct the biotome.[18] Intracardiac tumors have also been sampled by fine-needle aspiration.

Treatment Options and Prognosis

Benign Tumors

In 1952, the first antemortem diagnosis of a cardiac myxoma was made,[19] raising the possibility of surgical treatment for cardiac tumors. Two years later, on July 16, 1954, Clarence Crafoord performed the first successful surgical removal of a myxoma.[20] In adults, operative excision under direct vision using cardiopulmonary bypass has now become the treatment of choice for most benign cardiac tumors and in many cases results in a complete cure. Even benign cardiac tumors are potentially lethal as a result of intracavitary or valvular obstruction, peripheral embolization, and disturbances of rhythm or conduction, and, unfortunately, it is not unusual for patients to die or experience a major complication while awaiting operation. Therefore, it is mandatory to carry out the operation promptly after the diagnosis has been established.

In rare cases, the size of a tumor and the complexity of its sites of attachment or degree of infiltration have necessitated orthotopic heart transplantation. For benign tumors, this approach carries a good prognosis with a very low recurrence rate but the usual risks of transplantation.[21] In rare cases, rather than an allogeneic transplant, autotransplantation is performed, with complete removal of the heart, ex vivo repair, and then reimplantation of the patient's excised heart.[22]

The guidelines for myxoma removal outlined by Schaff and Mullany[23] can be generalized to cover the surgical approach to most benign cardiac tumors. These include the following:

1. Minimize manipulation of the heart before cardiopulmonary bypass.
2. Examine the other cardiac chambers for additional tumors not appreciated on preoperative imaging studies. Previously this meant direct visualization, but now intraoperative transesophageal echocardiography may suffice.
3. When technically feasible, attempt to excise the entire tumor to prevent residual tumor leading to a recurrence. However, for tumors with a substantial intramural component, this may not be possible without sacrificing ventricular contractile ability, proper AV valve function, and the preservation of the conduction system. In these situations, the type of tumor and its natural history must be weighed against the risks of total excision.
4. Carefully search for any dislodged tumor fragments that could lead to the generation of peripheral emboli and dispersion of micrometastases. To reduce this risk, the tumor should be removed en bloc when possible and the chamber then irrigated well with saline.
5. Carefully inspect any cardiac valves that may have had contact with any intracavitary component of the tumor to assess for traumatic damage and the need for repair.

Malignant Tumors

Operation is not an effective treatment for most primary malignant tumors of the heart because of the large mass of cardiac tissue involved or the presence of metastases. The major role for surgery in such cases is to establish a definitive diagnosis to preclude the possibility of a curable benign tumor. Left untreated, patients with primary malignant tumors of the heart generally have a life expectancy measured in months. In some cases, palliation of hemodynamics and/or constitutional symptoms and extension of life can be achieved by aggressive therapy. To that end, disease-free survival for more than 2 years has been reported after partial resection, chemotherapy, radiation therapy, orthotopic cardiac transplantation, or various combinations of these modalities.[24] Unfortunately, most case series indicate a failure to fundamentally alter the course of primary malignant tumors of the heart, and despite maximal therapy, median survival is no better than 1 year.

Specific Cardiac Tumors

Approximately 75 percent of all cardiac tumors are benign histologically and the remainder are malignant.[25] Most benign cardiac tumors are myxomas, followed in frequency by a wide variety of other tumors (Table 63–2 and Fig. 63–4). Almost all malignant cardiac tumors are sarcomas, and of these the angiosarcoma is the most common form (Table 63–3). Some tumors are associated with systemic syndromes (Table 63–4).[26]

Myxomas

Cardiac myxomas comprise approximately 50 percent of the total in most adult clinical case series and up to 90 percent in surgical case series. The histogenesis of cardiac myxomas is uncertain, but the weight of evidence favors benign neoplasia, with the tumor probably originating from subendocardial nests of primitive mesenchymal cells that may differentiate into several cell types, including endothelial and lipidic cells. Cytogenetic analyses demonstrating clonal chromosomal abnormalities provide the best support for this concept.[27]

The mean age at the time of presentation in patients with sporadic myxoma is 50 years.[28] However, there is a wide range—the youngest reported patient was a stillborn infant

TABLE 63–2 Relative Incidence of Benign Tumors of the Heart*

	Percentage of Group		
Benign Tumors	*Adults*	*Children*	*Infants*
Myxoma	52	17	0
Papillary fibroelastoma	16	0	0
Lipoma	16	0	0
Rhabdomyoma	1	42	62
Fibroma	3	18	17
Teratoma	1	12	12
Hemangioma	6	5	4
Other tumors†	5	4	4

Sources for the data include (1) McAllister HA, Fenoglio JJ: Tumors of the cardiovascular system. *In* Hartmann WH, Cowan WR (eds): Atlas of Tumor Pathology. Second Series, Fascicle 15. Washington, DC, Armed Forces Institute of Pathology, 1978, pp 1-3; (2) Nadas AS, Ellison RC: Cardiac tumors in infancy. Am J Cardiol 21:363-366, 1968; (3) Fine G: Neoplasms of the pericardium and heart. *In* Gould SE (ed): Pathology of the Heart and Blood Vessels. 3rd ed. Springfield, Charles C Thomas, 1968, pp 851-883; (4) Lam KY, Dickens P, Chan AC: Tumors of the heart: A 20-year experience with a review of 12,485 consecutive autopsies. Arch Pathol Lab Med 117:1027-1031, 1993; and (5) Virmani R, Burke A, Farb A, Atkinson JB: Cardiovascular Pathology. Major Problems in Pathology. Vol 40. 2nd ed. Philadelphia, WB Saunders, 2001.

*Data represent collective experience of multiple investigators with a total of 447, 92, and 82 benign tumors found in adults (age > 16 years), children (age 1-16 years), and infants (age < 1 year). Lipoma includes true lipomas and lipomatous hypertrophy of the septum.

†Other tumors include cystic tumors of the atrioventricular node, endocrine tumors, and histiocytoid tumors.

TABLE 63–3 Relative Incidence of Primary Malignant Tumors of the Heart*

	Percentage of Group		
Malignant Tumors	*Adults*	*Children*	*Infants*
Angiosarcoma	28	6	0
Rhabdomyosarcoma	11	41	50
Fibrosarcoma	8	18	17
Malignant fibrous histiocytoma	6	6	0
Osteosarcoma	7	0	0
Leiomyosarcoma	5	0	17
Myxosarcoma	3	6	0
Other sarcomas†	14	12	0
Undifferentiated sarcoma	12	12	17
Lymphoma	6	0	0

See Table 63–2 footnote for sources of the data.

*Data representing collective experience of multiple investigators with a total of 250, 17, and 6 malignant tumors found in adults (age > 16 years), children (age 1-16 years), and infants (age < 1 year).

†Other sarcomas included liposarcomas, synovial, and neurogenic sarcomas.

and the oldest was a 95-year-old woman. Two-thirds of patients are female. Approximately 75 percent of myxomas occur in the left atrium, where the site of attachment is almost always in the region of the limbus of the fossa ovalis. Although myxomas may occasionally be found on the posterior left atrial wall, tumors presenting in this location should raise the suspicion of malignancy. Myxomas also may occur in the right atrium (15 to 20 percent) and, less often, in the right or left ventricle. Myxomas of the AV valves have been

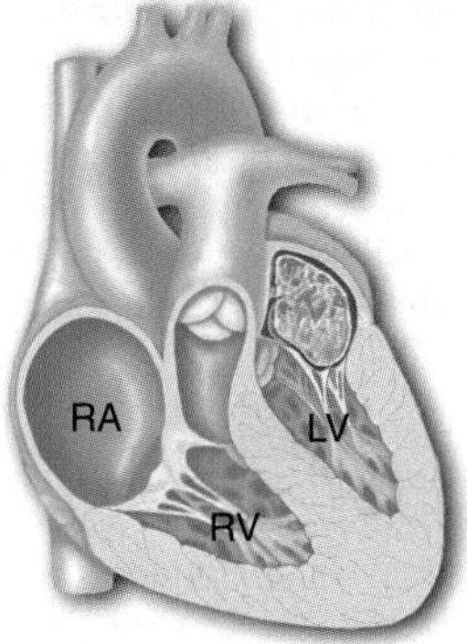

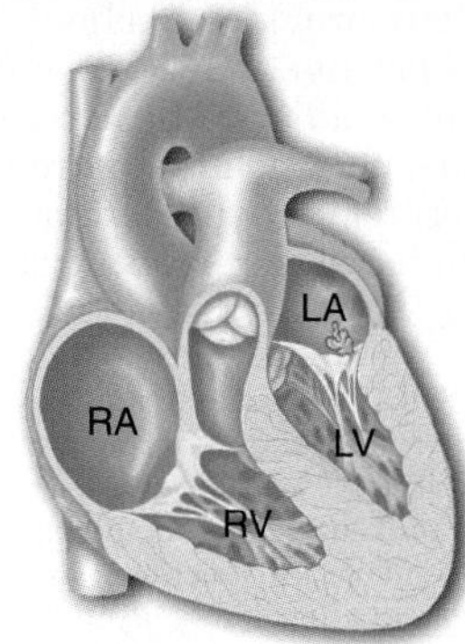

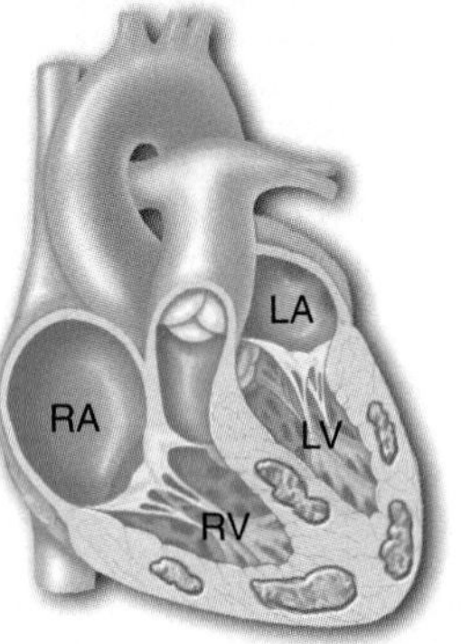

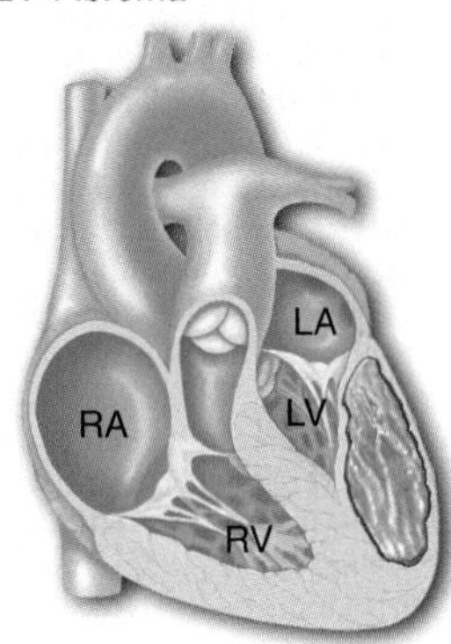

FIGURE 63–4 Characteristic appearance of the four most common benign primary cardiac tumors. **A,** Myxomas are typically a 5- to 6-cm globular mass, attached to the fossa ovalis in the left atrium, and can prolapse through the mitral valve. **B,** Papillary fibroelastomas are smaller than 1-cm, frond-like masses attached to the mitral or aortic valve. **C,** Rhabdomyomas usually present as multiple, rounded, smaller than 2-cm masses throughout the left and right ventricular myocardium. **D,** Fibromas are large, singular, 3- to 10-cm dense masses, typically found in the anterior free wall of the left ventricle.

reported. More than 90 percent of myxomas are solitary, but several myxomas within one atrium, as well as biatrial (usually extending through the foramen ovale), combined atrial and ventricular, and biventricular myxomas all have been reported. However, multiple tumors or atypical locations are more commonly seen in patients with familial myxomas (see later). The tumors average 5 to 6 cm in diameter but range from less than 1 to 15 cm or greater.[29]

CLINICAL MANIFESTATIONS. Myxomas present with one or more of the triad of intracardiac obstruction, systemic embolization, and constitutional symptoms (Table 63–5). Nearly 70 percent of patients with left atrial myxomas have cardiac symptoms, predominantly heart failure and syncope.[29] The pedunculated nature of myxomas and their predilection for the left atrium allow them to prolapse to various degrees into the mitral valve orifice, resulting in obstruction to left ventricular inflow as well as mitral regurgitation. Moreover, the recurrent collision between a left atrial myxoma and the mitral valve may cause permanent valvular damage, the so-called wrecking ball effect. In contrast to fixed mitral valve disease, the mobility of myxomas typically leads to paroxysmal symptoms of shortness of breath or syncope that may depend on body position. Large myxomas (>5 cm) are more likely to cause cardiac symptoms than their smaller counterparts.

Embolic events occur in 30 percent of patients. Of these patients, two-thirds have cerebral emboli causing transient ischemic attacks, strokes, or seizures, and half have peripheral limb emboli.[29] Cases of cardiac myxoma embolizing to coronary arteries, kidney, liver, spleen, eye, and skin have

TABLE 63–4 Syndromes Associated with Cardiac Tumors

Tumor	Syndrome	Gene	Prevalence (%): Of Syndrome Among Patients with Tumor	Prevalence (%): Of Cardiac Tumor Among Patients with Syndrome	Additional Features
Myxoma	Carney complex	*PRKAR1α*	<10	50-67	Spotty skin pigmentation, endocrine overactivity
Rhabdomyoma	Tuberous sclerosis	*TSC-1* *TSC-2*	80	50	Hamartomas, epilepsy, mental deficiency, adenoma sebaceum
Fibroma	Gorlin syndrome	*PTC*	5	<14	Nevoid basal cell carcinoma, medulloblastomas, odontogenic keratocysts, bifid ribs

TABLE 63–5 Symptoms and Signs of Cardiac Myxoma*

Variable	
Symptoms	**Incidence (%)**
Dyspnea	~70
Paroxysmal dyspnea	~25
Syncope	~20
Palpitations	~20
Chest pain	~10
Embolic event	~30
Fever	~20
Weight loss	~15
Signs	
Mitral systolic murmur	~50
Mitral diastolic murmur	~40
Loud S_1	~40
Tumor plop	~15
Laboratory Data	
Elevated ESR	~30
Anemia	~30
LA enlargement on CXR	~10

ESR = erythrocyte sedimentation rate; LA = left atrium; CXR = chest radiograph.

Sources for the data include (1) St John Sutton MG, Mercier LA, Giuliani ER, Lie JT: Atrial myxomas: A review of clinical experience in 40 patients. Mayo Clin Proc 55:371-376, 1980; (2) Burke AP, Virmani R: Cardiac myxoma: A clinicopathologic study. Am J Clin Pathol 100:671-680, 1993; (3) Bjessmo S, Ivert T: Cardiac myxoma: 40 years' experience in 63 patients. Ann Thorac Surg 63:697-700, 1997; (4) Pucci A, Gagliardotto P, Zanini C, et al: Histopathologic and clinical characterization of cardiac myxoma: Review of 53 cases from a single institution. Am Heart J 140:134-138, 2000; and (5) Pinede L, Duhaut P, Loire R: Clinical presentation of left atrial cardiac myxoma: A series of 112 consecutive cases. Medicine (Baltimore) 80:159-172, 2001.

*Summary of data representing collective experience of multiple investigators with a total of 284 cardiac myxomas.

been recorded.[30] One-fourth of patients with emboli have evidence of multiple embolic events. Compared to round and smooth tumors, polypoid, friable, and villous tumors are more than twice as likely to embolize.[29]

The third arm of the myxoma triad, constitutional symptoms, is unique among cardiac tumors. Although stated to occur in only 30 to 40 percent of patients, some investigators suggest that if searched for, they are found in up to 90 percent of patients. Symptoms include myalgias, muscle weakness, arthralgias, rash, fever, weight loss, and fatigue. Raynaud phenomenon and clubbing can be seen on physical examination. Laboratory evaluation may reveal an elevated ESR, anemia, leukocytosis, thrombocytopenia or thrombocytosis, and hypergammaglobulinemia. One can easily appreciate how a myxoma with prominent constitutional symptoms such as fever, arthralgias, Raynaud phenomenon, and an elevated ESR might initially be mistaken for collagen-vascular disease or how the combination of embolic events and fever might lead to the diagnosis of endocarditis. Rarely, myxomas are actually infected.[31]

Role of Interleukin 6. The association of constitutional symptoms with cardiac myxoma is likely due to the tumor's constitutive synthesis and secretion of interleukin (IL)-6, a cytokine that induces the acute-phase response. Increased levels of IL-6 and IL-6 messenger RNA have been found in myxoma tissue, and cultured myxoma cells have been shown to produce IL-6.[32] Patients with constitutional symptoms are more likely to have elevated levels of circulating IL-6, and in virtually all cases, serum IL-6 levels become undetectable and the autoimmune-like constitutional symptoms resolve on removal of the tumor.[33] Several cases of multiple myeloma developing in patients with cardiac myxoma have been reported, which is not unexpected given the important role IL-6 plays in promoting myeloma cell growth.

FAMILIAL MYXOMAS. These constitute 10 percent or less of all myxomas. Patients tend to present earlier (median age 20 years), are more likely to have myxomas in atypical locations, sometimes have multiple tumors, are more likely to develop recurrent tumors, and have associated dermatological and endocrine abnormalities. These observations were codified in 1985 by J. Aidan Carney, who described the "Carney complex" of myxomas, spotty skin pigmentation, and endocrine overactivity.[34] Patients with cardiac myxomas and pigmentary abnormalities had been previously described as having the NAME syndrome (*n*evi, *a*trial myxoma, *m*yxoid neurofibroma, *e*phelides)[35] or the LAMB syndrome (*l*entigines, *a*trial *m*yxoma, and *b*lue nevi).[36] However, it is now thought that these patients likely had unrecognized, subclinical endocrine abnormalities and thus had the Carney complex, which may be thought of as a form of multiple endocrine neoplasia.

Carney Complex. The diagnostic criteria for the Carney complex include having 2 of 12 recognized clinical manifestations (Table 63–6) or 1 clinical manifestation plus evidence of genetic transmission (affected first-degree relative or mutation in one of the genes linked to the Carney complex).[37] The possible clinical manifestations may be grouped into three categories: myxomas, pigmented skin lesions, and endocrine neoplasia. Cardiac myxomas are seen in half to two-thirds of patients at presentation. Although the left atrium is still the most common location for cardiac myxomas in Carney complex (~50 percent), atypical locations (right atrium ~40 percent, ventricles ~10 percent), multicentric foci (~50 percent), and recurrent tumors (10-22 percent) are far more common than in patients with nonsyndromic, isolated myxoma. In addition, one-third of patients have *mucocutaneous* myxomas at presentation, with classic sites being the eyelid, external ear canal, breast, and oropharynx. Pigmented skin lesions are the most common clinical manifestation,

TABLE 63–6 Diagnostic Criteria for Carney Complex*

Clinical Criteria

1. Spotty skin pigmentation with typical distribution (lips, conjunctiva and inner or outer canthi, vaginal and penile mucosa)
2. Myxoma (cutaneous and mucosal)
3. Cardiac myxoma
4. Breast myxomatosis or fat-suppressed MRI findings suggestive of this diagnosis
5. Primary pigmented nodular adrenocortical disease or paradoxical positive response of urinary glucocorticosteroids to dexamethasone administration during Liddle's test
6. Acromegaly due to growth hormone–producing adenoma
7. Large cell calcifying Sertoli cell tumors or characteristic calcification on testicular ultrasonography
8. Thyroid carcinoma or multiple, hyperechoic nodules on thyroid ultrasonography, in a young patient
9. Psammomatous melanotic schwannoma
10. Bule nevus, epithelioid blue nevus (multiple)
11. Breast ductal adenoma (multiple)
12. Osteochondromyxoma

Supplemental Genetic Criteria

1. Affected first-degree relative
2. Inactivating mutation of the *PRKAR1α* gene

From Stratakis CA, Kirschner LS, Carney JA: Clinical and molecular features of the Carney complex: Diagnostic criteria and recommendations for patient evaluation. J Clin Endocrinol Metab 86:4041-4046, 2001.

*A diagnosis of Carney complex requires that a patient have either 2 of the 12 clinical criteria (with histological confirmation of any suspected tumors or characteristic imaging or laboratory data) *or* 1 of the clinical criteria and 1 of the supplemental genetic criteria.

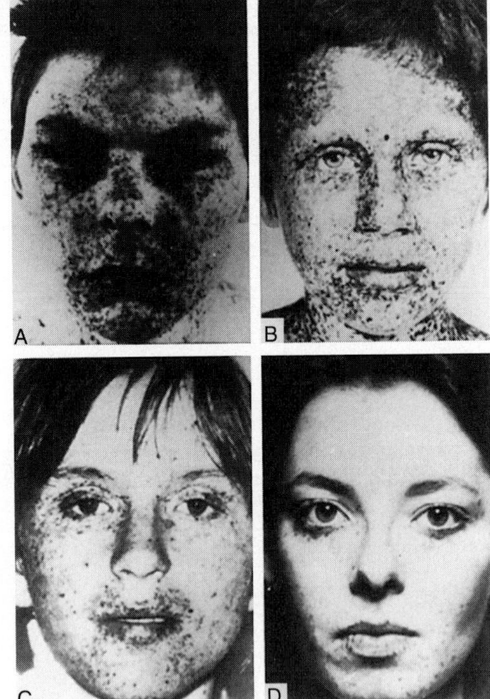

FIGURE 63–5 **A** to **D,** Four patients with extensive facial freckling, a finding associated with syndrome myxoma. Patients with this syndrome tend to be younger than patients with sporadic myxoma and have a substantially higher incidence of ventricular, multiple, biatrial, recurrent, and familial myxomas of the heart. In addition, these patients, in contrast with patients with sporadic myxoma, may have noncardiac myxomas and endocrine neoplasms. (From Vidaillet HJ Jr, Seward JB, Fyke FE, et al: "Syndrome myxoma": A subset of patients with cardiac myxoma associated with pigmented skin lesions and peripheral and endocrine neoplasms. Br Heart J 57:247, 1987.)

occurring in more than three-fourths of patients (Fig. 63–5). Blue nevi, café au lait spots, and depigmented lesions may be present at birth, but more commonly they develop in early childhood and may fade over time. Lentigines (macular melanoses) usually develop during the peripubertal period and typically involve the lips, conjunctiva, inner and outer canthi, and vaginal and penile mucosa. Endocrine abnormalities include primary pigmented nodular adrenocortical disease, growth hormone- and prolactin-producing pituitary adenomas, large cell calcifying Sertoli cell tumors, and thyroid adenoma or carcinoma. These neoplasms are identified in less than one-third of patients but are likely significantly underreported due to subclinical disease.

The Carney complex usually demonstrates autosomal dominant transmission, although such transmission may not be obvious due to incomplete penetrance and phenotypic variability even within the same family. Linkage studies have revealed two genetic loci: 2p16 and 17q22-24.[38,39] Among the families mapping to 17q, mutations in the gene encoding the protein kinase A regulatory subunit 1-α (*PRKAR1α*) have recently been identified,[40] but the cellular mechanism by which this genetic abnormality causes myxomas remains uncertain. Sporadic cardiac myxomas do not have these genetic alterations.[41]

In patients with established Carney complex, rigorous screening for the other aspects of the syndrome should be undertaken (e.g., measurement of urinary free cortisol, testicular ultrasound). Preoperatively, before resection of their cardiac myxoma, a careful search should be made in these patients for cardiac myxomas in other locations. Postoperatively, these patients should be observed closely for recurrence of myxomas. This occurs in 12 to 22 percent of such patients, and cardiac complications account for more than half the deaths in patients with Carney complex.[37] Routine echocardiographic screening of first-degree relatives of patients with familial myxomas is appropriate and should also be considered in patients with apparent sporadic myxomas but who are young or have multiple tumors.

DIAGNOSIS. On chest radiography, approximately half of patients with left atrial myxomas have evidence of left atrial enlargement or pulmonary venous hypertension, and half of patients with right atrial myxomas have evidence of calcification; however, one-third of patients have a completely normal radiograph.[42] Two-dimensional echocardiography is the imaging modality of choice, classically revealing a mobile, distensible tumor connected to the interatrial septum by a narrow stalk. Both hypoechoic and hyperechoic foci may be seen, reflecting areas of hemorrhage and calcification, respectively. Transthoracic echocardiography is usually sufficient to make the diagnosis, but if the results are suboptimal, transesophageal echocardiography should be employed. CT typically reveals a lobular, heterogeneous, low-attenuation mass with a narrow base of attachment (the stalk is usually too narrow to be visualized), and, in 14 percent of cases, punctate calcification. MRI often reveals a spherical, heterogeneous mass that is primarily isointense on T1-weighted images, with areas of hypointensity and hyperintensity, is hyperintense on T2-weighted images, and shows heterogeneous enhancement with administration of gadolinium.[42] Gradient echo-cine MRI can be used to demonstrate tumor mobility.

PATHOLOGY. On gross inspection, myxomas are gelatinous (often termed *myxoid*), smooth, and round, with a glistening surface, or they may be variably friable and either irregular or polypoid (Fig. 63–6). Areas of hemorrhage, calcification, and necrosis may be seen. The diagnosis of myxoma is now made by the observation of cords, rings, or florets of cells (often called *lipidic cells*) embedded in a myxoid stroma rich in glycosaminoglycans (Fig. 63–7).[43] Myxoma cells have a round, elongated, or polyhedral shape; scant pink cytoplasm; and an ovoid nucleus with an open chromatin pattern.

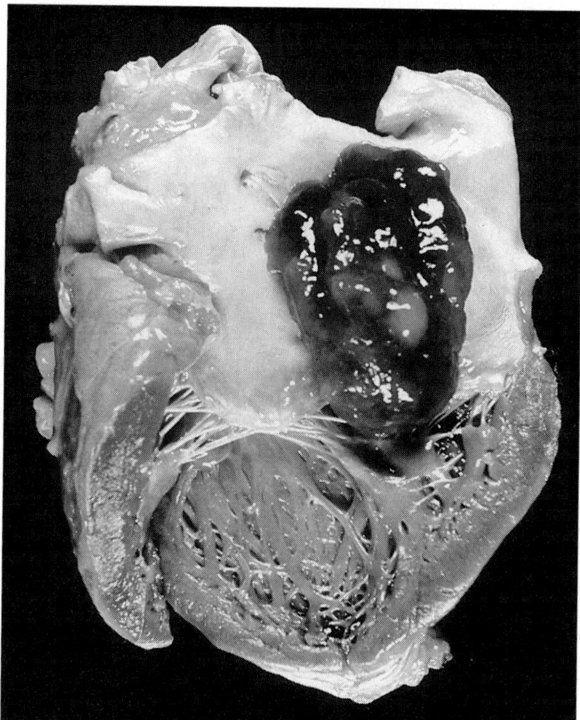

FIGURE 63–6 Photograph of the most frequent gross appearance of cardiac myxomas: a polypoid, smooth, round, hemorrhagic left atrial mass. The tumor mass nearly fills the left atrium and extends into the mitral valve orifice. (From Cotran RS, Kumar V, Robbins SL: Robbins Pathologic Basis of Disease. 5th ed. Philadelphia, WB Saunders, 1994.)

They are occasionally multinuclear. Myxoma cells have abundant fine cytoplasmic filaments similar to those of smooth muscle cells. The pathological characteristics of myxomas are well described and are independent of location or whether they are syndromic or nonsyndromic.

The cells most resemble embryonic mesenchymal cells with multipotential capabilities for cellular differentiation, including vasoformative activity and expression of vascular endothelial growth factor,[44] which can be found in the serum of patients with myxoma and resolves after excision of the tumor.[45] Myxoma cells are especially similar to embryonic endocardial cushion tissue, supporting the notion that myxomas arise from embryonic rests remaining from when the heart underwent septations. Immunohistochemical studies demonstrate positivity for vimentin, indicative of the mesenchymal derivation of the cells, as well as several neuroendocrine markers, including S-100 (89 percent of cases), protein gene product 9.5 (94 percent of cases), and calretinin (100 percent of cases).[46,47] Recent studies also demonstrate the presence of cardiomyocyte-specific transcription factors, supporting the idea that myxomas derive from mesenchymal cardiomyogenic precursor cells.[48]

Many of the morphological features of organizing mural thrombi resemble those of myxoma, including abundant loose amorphous extracellular matrix, connective tissue cells, and small vascular channels. It is difficult to distinguish between some myxomas and mural thrombi in various stages of organization; indeed, cellular intracardiac thrombi and peripheral thromboemboli occasionally receive an erroneous diagnosis of myxoma. The recent demonstration of calretinin expression in cardiac myxomas but not mural thrombi may lead to a useful tool for distinguishing myxomas from thrombi.[47] Cardiac myxomas also may be mistaken for cardiac sarcomas because a myxoid background rich in proteoglycans may be seen in both tumors. However, myxomas consist of polygonal myxoma cells that form syncytia and express S-100

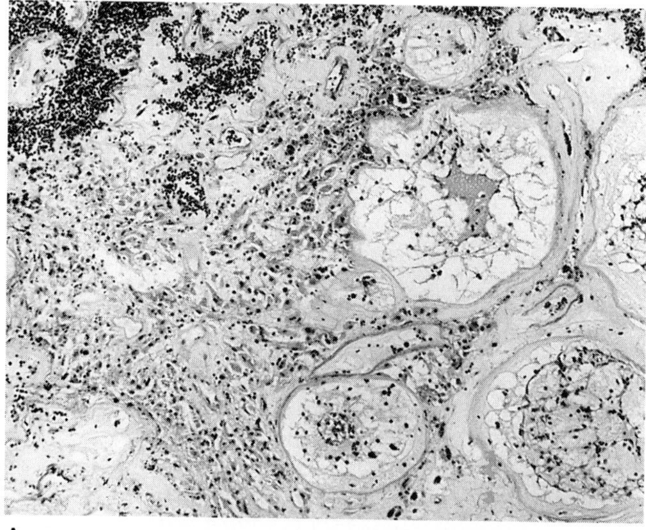

A

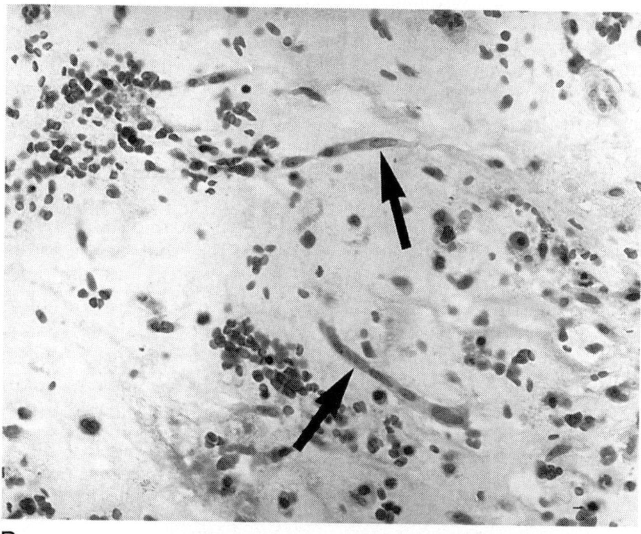

B

FIGURE 63–7 Characteristic histological features of myxoma. **A,** Low-power view demonstrating individual tumor cells, clusters, and islands scattered throughout the characteristic pale-staining granular extracellular matrix. Hemorrhage is present at upper left. Scattered inflammatory cells are also present. **B,** High-magnification view, showing individual variably rounded to elongated myxoma cells, some arranged in cords (arrows). **A,** ×50; **B,** ×400; all stained with hematoxylin and eosin.

protein, whereas sarcomas consist of spindle-shaped cells that show signs of nuclear atypia and mitoses and do not express S-100.

TREATMENT. The usual surgical approach to a typical left-sided myxoma is through the right atrium and across the interatrial septum at the fossa ovalis with en bloc resection including a rim of septum around the base. In recent case series using such techniques, operative mortality approaches 1 percent.[23] In about 1 to 5 percent of cases, a recurrence or second cardiac myxoma has been reported after resection of the initial myxoma. Possible causes of the second tumor include incomplete excision of the original tumor with regrowth; growth from a second "pretumorous" focus (i.e., a metasynchronous tumor); or intracardiac implantation from the original tumor.[49] Because of the first two possibilities, some surgeons have advocated excision of the entire region of the fossa ovalis and repair of the resultant atrial septal defect to remove presumably high concentrations of pretumorous cells thought to be located in that region. Other surgeons have reported equally successful long-term recurrence-free periods with simple excision of the tumor and a small rim at the base. More recently, minimally invasive approaches via a minithoracotomy, with and without video-assisted endoscopy, have been reported.[50] Although short-term results appear excellent, long-term data on recurrence rates are lacking.

In patients with the Carney complex, the risk of a second tumor occurring in the future is in the range of 12 to 22 percent,[37] as compared with approximately 1 percent for patients with sporadic atrial myxoma.[23,29] It is believed that tumor recurrence in these cases is from a second pretumorous focus of cells. In these high-risk patients, a careful search for additional tumors preoperatively and more extensive resection of the underlying endocardium, atrial septum, or both is recommended. Careful echocardiographic follow-up for detection of metasynchronous tumors is recommended for all patients after resection of a myxoma.

Papillary Fibroelastomas

The most common tumors of the cardiac valves, papillary fibroelastomas are benign papillomas of the endocardium. Because they are easily overlooked at autopsy, the widespread use of echocardiography has led to increased preoperative and premortem recognition, and recent series suggest they are the second most common benign tumor of the adult heart.[25] The average age at detection is 60 years, although papillary fibroelastomas have been detected in neonates as well as in patients as old as 92 years.[51,52] The incidence in men and women appears to be similar. Most patients have concomitant valvular disease, suggesting that endocardial damage from infection, inflammation, radiation, or even prior invasive cardiac procedures may predispose to papilloma formation. More than 90 percent of the time papillary fibroelastomas are single. The median diameter is 8 mm; the largest reported tumor is 40 mm. Papillary fibroelastomas can occur on any valve or, far less commonly, on papillary muscle, chordae tendineae, or in the atria. The aortic and mitral valves are most commonly involved in adults. Most often, the arterial side of semilunar valves and the atrial surface of AV valves are affected. A short pedicle is seen approximately half of the time, typically in tumors arising from the endocardium of a cardiac chamber. Whether papillary fibroelastomas are truly neoplastic, as well as their relationship to cardiac mural thrombi and endocardial injury, remains uncertain.

CLINICAL MANIFESTATIONS. Although many are clinically insignificant, papillary fibroelastomas have the potential to embolize to vital structures.[51] These tumors may mimic infective endocarditis with the combination of embolic events and an abnormal appearing valve. Despite their valvular attachment, valvular dysfunction is distinctly uncommon.[51,52] However, tumors on the aortic valve can partially obstruct a coronary arterial orifice and lead to myocardial ischemia or infarction.[53] Transthoracic echocardiography has a sensitivity of 62 percent and transesophageal echocardiography a sensitivity of 77 percent.[52] The rates approach 90 percent when tumors smaller than 2 mm are excluded. A characteristic shimmer or vibration at the tumor-blood interface, ascribed to the finger-like projections of the tumor, has been described and is best appreciated on transesophageal echocardiography.[51] Typically these tumors are too small to be seen well on CT or MRI.

PATHOLOGY. On gross inspection, papillary fibroelastomas have a characteristic frond-like appearance resembling a sea anemone (Fig. 63–8). Histologically, the tumor is covered by endothelium that surrounds an avascular core of loose connective tissue rich in glycosaminoglycans, collagen, and elastic fibers and containing smooth muscle cells (often as a fine meshwork surrounding a central collagen or dense elastic fiber core).[54] Papillary fibroelastomas may be distinguished from Lambl's excrescences, which are acellular deposits of variably organized thrombus and connective tissue covered by a single layer of endothelium that are found on heart valves at the site of endothelial damage in many adults, particularly along the closure margins of the aortic valve cusps. In contrast, papillary fibroelastomas are not usually found at valvular contact areas. However, others have argued that neither gross nor microscopic criteria can reliably distinguish the two entities and suggest that the term *papillary fibroelastoma* be used when the papilloma is large, symptomatic, or atypically situated.

TREATMENT. Most investigators recommend complete resection of papillary fibroelastomas, especially for left-sided lesions.[55] Although these tumors are small, their frond-like structure results in a relatively large and irregular surface area. The risk of embolic events may be as high as 25 percent over 3 years, and even 6 percent in asymptomatic patients in whom papillary fibroelastoma was an incidental finding.[51] Anticoagulation does not appear to protect against embolic events.[56]

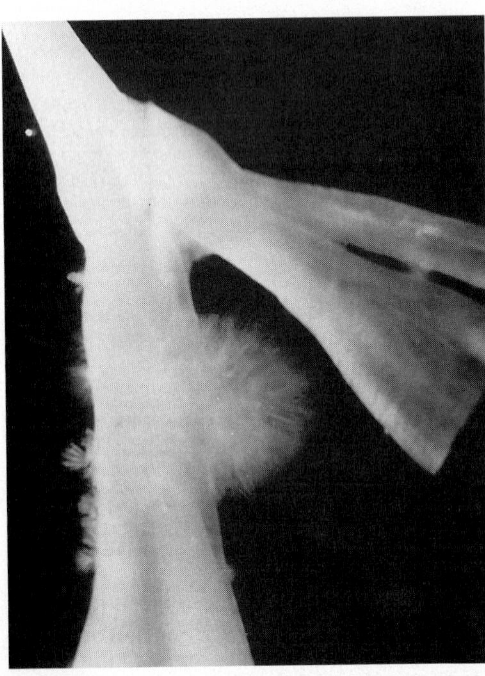

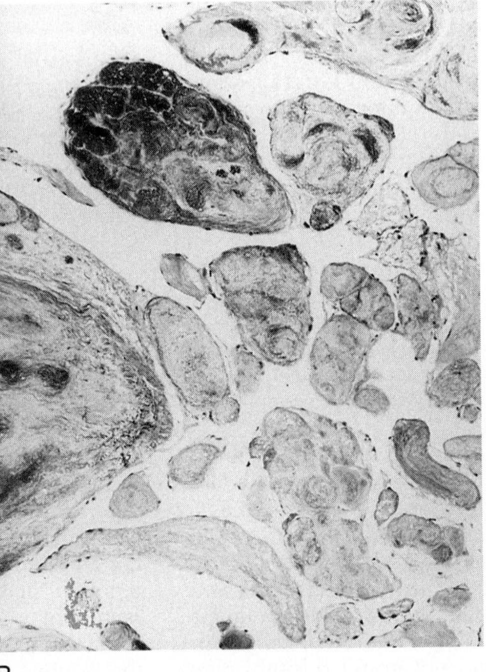

FIGURE 63–8 Papillary fibroelastoma. **A,** Gross photograph demonstrating resemblance of this lesion to a sea anemone, with myriad papillary fronds, arising from the chordae tendineae near the mitral leaflet. In this case, many lesions were present, all associated with the mitral valve apparatus. **B,** Histological appearance of papillary fibroelastoma, demonstrating the numerous papillary fronds consisting of a collagen core surrounded by elastic fibers and loose connective tissue, all covered by endocardial endothelium. ×100; stained with elastica van Gieson stain (elastin black).

More than 90 percent of tumors can be resected using a conservative, valve-sparing approach with stalk excision or quadrangular resection and valve repair using a pericardial patch.[51] Recurrences have not been reported.

LIPOMAS AND LIPOMATOUS HYPERTROPHY

True lipomas are rare and can occur at any age and with equal frequency in both sexes. They range in diameter from 1 to 15 cm, although some very large lipomas weighing up to 4.8 kg have been reported. Most tumors are sessile or polypoid and occur in the subendocardium or subpericardium, although about one-fourth are completely intramuscular.

CLINICAL MANIFESTATIONS. The most common chambers affected are the left ventricle, right atrium, and interatrial septum. Many tumors are clinically silent, however, and are found only at autopsy. Echocardiography typically reveals a homogeneous, hyperechoic mass, but these findings are not diagnostic. On CT, lipomas appear as homogeneous masses with the same attenuation as fat. The best imaging modality is MRI, on which lipoma's signal intensity strikingly decreases during fat-saturated sequences.

PATHOLOGY. Microscopically, the lesions are usually well encapsulated and composed of typical mature fat cells; they occasionally contain fibrous connective tissue (fibrolipoma), muscular tissue (myolipoma), or vacuolated brown (fetal) fat, resembling a hibernoma.

LIPOMATOUS HYPERTROPHY OF THE INTERATRIAL SEPTUM. Whereas lipomas are true neoplasms, a more common cardiac lipomatous condition termed *lipomatous hypertrophy of the interatrial septum* represents a hamartoma consisting of fatty deposition in the interatrial septum. These lesions most commonly occur in obese, elderly, female patients.[57] Lipomatous hypertrophy classically involves the anterior or superior portion of the interatrial septum, spares the fossa ovalis, and protrudes into the right atrium. On average, the septum is thickened up to 2.5 cm (the septum is usually < 1 cm thick and the upper limit of normal is generally considered to be 2 cm); however, tumors up to 10 cm in diameter have been described.[25] The thickness of the septum correlates with body weight and the thickness of adipose tissue surrounding the heart.[57]

Clinically, lipomatous hypertrophy is associated with a high incidence of atrial arrhythmias that is correlated with the degree of hypertrophy. Massive lipomatous hypertrophy can cause obstruction of the superior vena cava. Pathologically, in contrast to true lipomas, lipomatous hypertrophy consists of a *nonencapsulated* accumulation of mature and fetal adipose tissue and atypical cardiac myocytes within the interatrial septum.[58] The term *hypertrophy* is therefore a misnomer because the lesion is due to an increased number rather than increased size of adipocytes and thus represents *hyperplasia*. Lipomatous hypertrophy is easily seen on transthoracic and transesophageal echocardiography as a highly echogenic, bilobed septal mass that spares the fossa ovalis and displays the tissue signal characteristics similar to subcutaneous fat on CT and MRI.[59]

TREATMENT. Because of their progressive growth, true lipomas usually require surgical intervention with complete excision. In contrast, surgical resection of lipomatous hypertrophy of the septum is usually performed only in the setting of superior vena cava obstruction or clinically significant arrhythmias.[60] The nonneoplastic nature of these lesions permits incomplete resections that restore normal hemodynamics to be performed.[61]

RHABDOMYOMAS

These are the most common cardiac tumors of infants and children; approximately three-fourths occur in patients younger than 1 year.[62] Evidence suggests that rhabdomyomas are actually myocardial hamartomas or malformations that are composed of myocytes that resemble fetal cardiac myocytes rather than true neoplasms. They occur with equal frequency in the left and right ventricular and septal myocardium; nearly all are multiple. Approximately one-third also involve either one or both atria. They are usually small and lobulated, with diameters in the range of 2 mm to 2 cm.[63]

CLINICAL MANIFESTATIONS. The type and severity of symptoms depend on the location and size of the tumors. Tumors close to the conduction system may result in arrhythmias. Heart block is the most common manifestation, but paroxysmal supraventricular tachycardia, ventricular tachycardia, and sudden cardiac death have also been reported and may be due to reentrant circuits created by the tumor. Intracavitary tumors may lead to signs and symptoms of congestive heart failure due to obstruction of blood flow, including death in utero and a hydropic infant. Echocardiography is usually adequate for diagnosis and typically reveals multiple small, lobulated, homogeneous, hyperechoic intramural tumors.[64] On MRI, rhabdomyomas are usually isointense on T1-weighted images and hyperintense on T2-weighted images.[65]

ASSOCIATION WITH TUBEROUS SCLEROSIS. Rhabdomyomas are strongly associated with tuberous sclerosis, which is an autosomal dominant hamartoma syndrome whose causative genes (*TSC-1* and *TSC-2*) are tumor suppressor genes that encode a protein complex that regulates cell size.[66] The syndrome is characterized by hamartomas in several organs, epilepsy, mental deficiency, and adenoma sebaceum. Several studies show that at least 80 percent of patients with cardiac rhabdomyomas have tuberous sclerosis,[63] and approximately 50 percent of patients younger than 18 years of age with tuberous sclerosis have cardiac rhabdomyomas.[67]

PATHOLOGY. Rhabdomyomas are yellowish gray and range from 1 mm to several centimeters in diameter (Fig 63–9). They are circumscribed but not encapsulated; microscopically, they are easily distinguished from the surrounding myocardium as clusters of abnormal cells. The microscopic hallmark, termed the *spider cell,* is a large (≤80-μm diameter) cell containing a central cytoplasmic mass that is suspended by fine myofibrillar processes radiating to the periphery, thus giving the appearance of a spider hanging in a net.

TREATMENT. Fifty percent or more of rhabdomyomas regress spontaneously after infancy.[63,67,68] Thus, in the absence of symptoms, surgery is not indicated.[69] This is fortunate because multiple nodular rhabdomyomas, the type associated with tuberous sclerosis, are difficult to resect. In contrast, intracavitary rhabdomyomas, which may cause heart failure, tend to be sporadic tumors not associated with tuberous sclerosis and are more amenable to surgical resection.[68] If the diagnosis is in question in an asymptomatic patient, a small, isolated tumor may be resected as part of the biopsy. For larger or multiple tumors, biopsy alone should be sufficient to yield the diagnosis and, if rhabdomyoma is confirmed, allow for observation with periodic echocardiograms rather than more involved surgery.

FIBROMAS

Fibromas are benign connective tissue tumors derived from fibroblasts that occur predominantly in children and constitute the second most common type of primary cardiac tumor occurring in the pediatric age

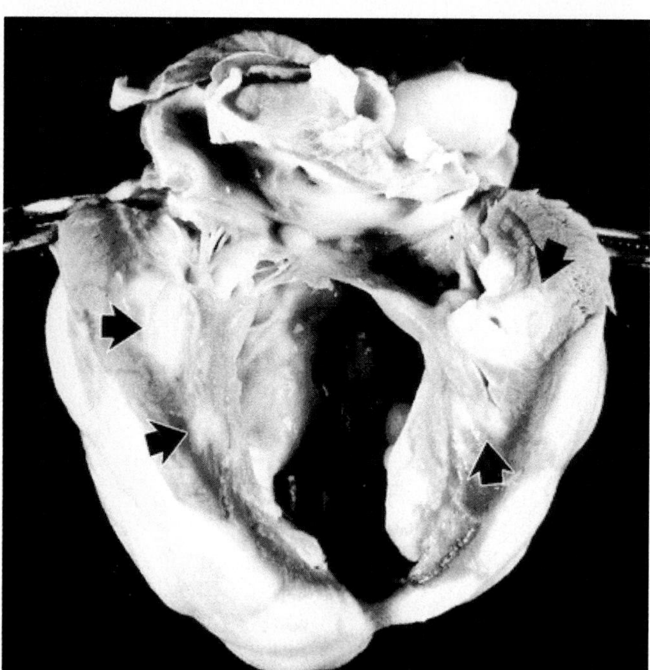

FIGURE 63–9 Photograph of a cut autopsy specimen from a 3-month-old boy with rhabdomyoma. Multiple, firm, white nodules can be seen distributed throughout the left ventricular myocardium (arrows). (From Grebenc ML, Rosado de Christenson ML, Burke AP, et al: Primary cardiac and pericardial neoplasms: Radiologic-pathologic correlation. Radiographics 20:1073-1103, 2000.)

group.[63] Most are detected in children younger than 10 years, and about one-third are diagnosed in infants younger than 1 year. Males and females appear to be equally affected. Cardiac fibromas typically are large tumors, ranging from 3 to 10 cm in diameter. They usually occur within the ventricular myocardium and much more frequently within the anterior free wall of the left ventricle or the interventricular septum than in the posterior left ventricular wall or right ventricle.[70]

CLINICAL MANIFESTATIONS. Approximately 70 percent of fibromas are symptomatic, causing mechanical interference with intracardiac flow (usually with bulky intracavitary left ventricular or right ventricular tumors), ventricular systolic function (usually with large intramyocardial left ventricular tumors), or conduction disturbances (usually with tumors arising in the interventricular septum). The most common clinical manifestations are congestive heart failure (21 percent), ventricular tachyarrhythmias (13 percent), and atypical chest pain (3.5 percent).[71] Sudden cardiac death occurs in 14 percent of patients with fibromas, typically in infants. Most symptomatic patients have cardiomegaly on their chest radiograph, with tumor calcification seen in 25 percent of cases.

Imaging. Echocardiography typically reveals an intramural, homogenous, echogenic mass. CT scanning often shows a homogeneous mass with calcification. On MRI, fibromas are usually homogeneous and isointense to hyperintense on T1-weighted images, and, owing to their dense fibrous nature, are hypointense on T2-weighted images and manifest minimal enhancement with gadolinium, although the latter finding is variable.[70]

GORLIN SYNDROME. The nevoid basal cell carcinoma, or Gorlin syndrome, is an autosomal dominant disorder characterized by multiple nevoid basal cell carcinomas, medulloblastomas, cardiac fibromas and fibrous histiocytomas and other tumors, as well as nonneoplastic features including odontogenic keratocysts, dyskeratotic pitting of the hands and feet, and a variety of skeletal abnormalities including bifid ribs.[72] In a small series of fibromas, Gorlin syndrome was identified in approximately 5 percent of patients, but many of these patients were infants in whom the other features of Gorlin syndrome might not have been apparent yet.[70] Fewer than 14 percent of patients with Gorlin syndrome have fibromas. The gene for this syndrome (*PTC*) was mapped to chromosome 9q22-31 and found to be a homolog of the *Drosophila* segment polarity gene *patched*.[73]

PATHOLOGY. Fibromas are gray, firm, circumscribed but not encapsulated, and exhibit a whorled appearance on cut sections (Fig. 63–10). Microscopically, cardiac fibromas consist of elongated fibroblasts admixed with fibrous tissue consisting mostly of collagen. Their cellularity is variable and appears to decrease with age; mitotic figures are rarely, if ever, seen.[70] Fibrous tissue is intermingled with adjacent myocardial fibers at the margins of the lesion. In older patients, fibromas may histologically resemble a scar from a healed infarct, but, unlike healed infarcts, fibromas appear as thickened or bulging masses on gross inspection. Calcification and islands of bone formation may be seen microscopically and occasionally radiographically.

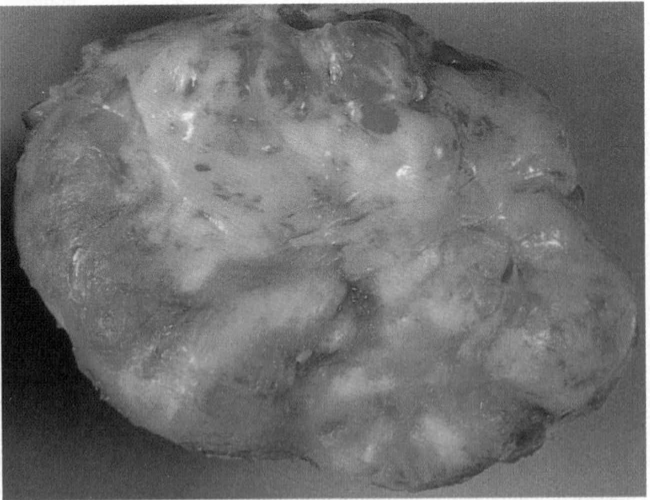

FIGURE 63–10 Photograph of an excised fibroma showing gross appearance. (From Allard MF, Taylor GP, Wilson JE, McManus BM: Primary cardiac tumors. *In* Goldhaber SZ, Braunwald E [eds]: Cardiopulmonary Diseases and Cardiac Tumors. Atlas of Heart Diseases. Vol 3. Philadelphia, Current Medicine, 1995, pp 15.1-15.22.)

TREATMENT. Surgical excision of cardiac fibromas is challenging but possible. Although these tumors lack capsules and may have extensions or satellites, it is usually possible to differentiate them from surrounding normal myocardium. Moreover, as fibromas displace rather than infiltrate the normal myocardium, reapproximation of the remaining myocardium post excision is often feasible.[71] Sometimes, though, the intramyocardial location of these tumors may preclude complete resection. Given the risk of fatal arrhythmias, resection is usually recommended even in asymptomatic cases. However, fibromas typically do not demonstrate continued growth after 1 or 2 years of age and cases of spontaneous regression have rarely been reported. Thus, patients who are able to undergo only partial resection may still do well postoperatively, and complete resection may be deferred if it will endanger the patient.

TERATOMAS

These tumors, which contain elements of all three germ cell layers, occur within the heart less frequently than they do in the anterior mediastinum.[74] Teratomas are generally observed in children and occur in the pericardium, attached to the root of the aorta or the pulmonary trunk. When located within the heart, they occur predominantly within the right atrium, right ventricle, or the interatrial or interventricular septum. Imaging studies typically reveal a heterogeneous mass with solid and cystic components.[75] They range from 0.5 to 9 cm in greatest diameter and tend to be lobulated with multiple cystic cavities containing clear, yellow, or brownish fluid.[74] On CT and MRI teratomas are very heterogeneous with areas of fat, cysts, soft tissue, calcification, and so forth.

HEMANGIOMAS

Composed of benign proliferations of endothelial cells, hemangiomas and lymphangiomas are extremely rare, with only 75 or so cases documented in the literature. Anatomically, they may occur in any part of the heart but more commonly are found in the lateral wall of the left ventricle (21 percent), the anterior wall of the right ventricle (21 percent), or the interventricular septum (17 percent).[76] Usually they are intramural, and, if in the interventricular septum or AV node, may cause complete heart block and sudden death. They may also protrude intraluminally and cause obstruction of the right ventricular outflow tract.

Hemangiomas are red, hemorrhagic, generally sessile or polypoid subendocardial nodules, ranging from 2 to 4 cm in diameter. Histologically, the tumors consist of endothelium-lined spaces that may contain blood, lymph, thrombi, or calcification; they are classified according to the predominant type of proliferating vascular channel. The natural history of these tumors is quite variable: some tumors involute, others stop growing after a certain time, and some continue to proliferate. Because there is no way to predict which course the tumor will take, resection is usually the treatment of choice. Radiation therapy has been used in instances when resection is not possible or complete,[77] and corticosteroids and interferon-alpha therapy may be considered.[78]

MISCELLANEOUS TUMORS

CYSTIC TUMOR ("MESOTHELIOMA") OF THE ATRIOVENTRICULAR NODE. Of controversial histogenesis, these small tumors (usually <15 mm in largest dimension) frequently cause death by complete heart block or ventricular fibrillation.[79] More common in women than in men, they occur at virtually any age and as poorly circumscribed, often multicystic nodules in the atrial septum, immediately cephalad to the commissure of the septal and anterior leaflets of the tricuspid valve, in the region of the AV node. These lesions are characterized by tubules and cysts lined by flat or cuboidal cells that are devoid of mitotic activity but may have secretory function.

ENDOCRINE TUMORS OF THE HEART. Approximately 2 percent of *paragangliomas* are intrathoracic, and of these, most are located in the posterior mediastinum. However, these tumors can also occur in close association with the left atrial or left ventricular epicardium, where they are thought to have arisen from sympathetic fibers to the heart or from ectopic chromaffin cells. More rarely still, paragangliomas may arise within the interatrial septum. Tumors in any of these locations may secrete catecholamines and therefore can be associated with signs and symptoms characteristic of pheochromocytoma.[80]

HISTIOCYTOID TUMORS. *Histiocytoid cardiomyopathy* (or *Purkinje cell hamartoma*) refers to a congenital collection of modified myocytes with few contractile elements. These tumors typically present as incessant ventricular tachycardia or sudden death in female infants and children.[81] *Benign fibrous histiocytomas* resemble fibromas, but with a greater number of histiocytic cells. In contrast to their malignant counterparts, mitotic figures are not seen and long-term prognosis is good.

Malignant Cardiac Tumors

About one-fourth of all cardiac tumors exhibit malignant histological characteristics and invasive or metastatic behavior. Nearly all (95 percent) of these are sarcomas, thus making these tumors second only to myxomas in overall frequency. Lymphomas account for the remaining 5 percent of primary malignant cardiac tumors.

Sarcomas

Sarcomas derive from mesenchyme and therefore may display a wide variety of morphological types, including angiosarcoma, rhabdomyosarcoma, fibrosarcoma and malignant fibrous histiocytomas, myxoid sarcomas, osteosarcoma, and others.[82] In a small case series, mutations in K-*ras* were seen in most primary cardiac sarcomas.[83] Sarcomas may occur at any age but are most common between the third and fifth decades. Except for rhabdomyosarcomas and fibrosarcomas, sarcomas are distinctly unusual in infants and children.

CLINICAL MANIFESTATIONS. The cardiac findings are determined primarily by the location of the tumor and by the extent of intracavitary obstruction.[82] Most patients present with progressive, unexplained dyspnea with evidence of heart failure, particularly of the right side. Precordial pain, uncommon in benign cardiac tumors, occurs in one-fourth of patients with sarcomas. Because of the rapid growth potential of sarcomas, they commonly extend into the pericardial space, and pericardial effusions, typically hemorrhagic and with or without tamponade physiology, are seen in one-fourth of patients. Obstruction of the superior vena cava (resulting in swelling of the face and upper extremities) and obstruction of the inferior vena cava (resulting in visceral congestion) have also been observed. In primarily intramural tumors, arrhythmias, conduction disturbances, and sudden death can occur. In older series, 75 percent of patients with cardiac sarcomas had evidence of distant metastases at the time of death; in more modern series, with superior noninvasive imaging facilitating earlier diagnosis, only 25 to 50 percent of patients have metastatic disease at the time of diagnosis. The most frequent sites are the lungs, thoracic lymph nodes, mediastinum, and vertebral column; the liver, kidneys, adrenals, pancreas, bone, spleen, and bowel are less often involved.

DIAGNOSIS. Although transthoracic echocardiography is a reasonable initial screening tool, transesophageal echocardiography may offer important clues as to the malignant nature of the lesion by showing intramyocardial and, for right atrial masses, vena caval invasion.[84] The superior soft tissue characterization possible with CT and especially MRI also allows them to determine the degree of tumor infiltration. However, there are no pathognomonic imaging signs, with most sarcomas showing heterogeneous signal intensity due to focal areas of hemorrhage and necrosis. Although pericardial involvement is common, even in those cases, pericardiocentesis may not yield malignant cells and endomyocardial or open biopsy may be needed.[85]

TREATMENT. Sarcomas proliferate rapidly and characteristically display a swift downhill course. Death is due to widespread infiltration of the myocardium, obstruction of flow within the heart, or distant metastases and most often occurs from a few weeks to 2 years after the onset of symptoms, with the median survival being 6 to 12 months. Undifferentiated tumors and those with a high mitotic rate and areas of necrosis have an especially poor prognosis.[82] Surgical excision should be considered to achieve local control and relieve symptoms. Patients who are able to undergo complete excision have a better prognosis (median survival 12 to 24 months) than those who only undergo incomplete resection (3 to 10 months).[82] Unfortunately, complete excision is possible in fewer than half of patients. Autotransplantation (i.e., cardiac explantation, ex vivo tumor resection, cardiac reconstruction and reimplantation) has been used in unusual cases to facilitate resection.[86] The benefits of chemotherapy are unclear, but based on data supporting anthracycline-based regimens in soft tissue sarcomas, adjuvant chemotherapy and/or radiation therapy is usually recommended.[87] Although orthotopic heart transplantation is a theoretical option for patients with locally unresectable disease but without evidence of metastasis, case series demonstrate that two-thirds of patients so treated will still die within 1 year, either of locally recurrent or metastatic disease.[21]

ANGIOSARCOMAS. Angiosarcomas, including Kaposi sarcomas, account for close to 30 percent of primary cardiac sarcomas.[25,82] In distinction to most other cardiac sarcomas, in which the sex distribution is equal, there appears to be a 3 : 1 male-to-female ratio among patients with angiosarcomas. These tumors have a striking predilection for the right atrium and may be either intracavitary and polypoid or diffuse and infiltrative, with sheet-like involvement of the pericardium occurring in the latter forms. Patients usually present with right-sided heart failure or tamponade as well as systemic signs such as fever and weight loss. Because these tumors are well vascularized and frequently have areas of hemorrhage and necrosis, MRI may reveal heterogeneous, nodular areas of hyperintensity, described as a "cauliflower" appearance, as well as linear areas of enhancement with gadolinium, described as a "sunray" appearance. Microscopically, angiosarcomas are characterized by ill-defined but variable anastomotic vascular channels lined with atypical, often heaped-up, endothelial cells. Approximately 25 percent of angiosarcomas contain spindled cells and the appearance of intracytoplasmic lumina containing red blood cells is a helpful diagnostic clue.[25] By electron microscopy, immature endothelial cells, primitive pericytes, and undifferentiated mesenchymal cells may be identified. Because these tumors are right sided, they tend to be discovered late and therefore have grown quite large and/or metastasized at the time of discovery. Thus they are often not amenable to complete resection and hence have a very poor prognosis even among the sarcomas.[87]

Kaposi sarcoma is a type of angiosarcoma seen in immunocompromised patients and whose pathogenesis is related to infection with human herpes virus 8. It is seen in less than 5 percent of patients with acquired immunodeficiency syndrome (AIDS) and in solid organ transplant recipients. Among those with visceral Kaposi sarcoma, rare cases of cardiac involvement have been reported, typically epicardial or pericardial, but occasionally myocardial.[88]

RHABDOMYOSARCOMAS. Embryonal rhabdomyosarcomas are the most common cardiac malignancy in infants and children and account for 10 percent of all primary cardiac sarcomas. These tumors of striated muscle often diffusely infiltrate the ventricular myocardium but may also occasionally form a polypoid extension into the cardiac chambers and therefore have been clinically mistaken for myxoma. There are usually multiple foci with occasional nodular involvement of the pericardium.[89] Rhabdomyoblasts are the histological hallmark of this tumor.

FIBROSARCOMAS. Fibrosarcomas of the heart account for 5 to 10 percent of cardiac sarcomas and have a whitish, soft "fish flesh" consistency. Fibroblastic in differentiation, they are composed of spindle-shaped cells with elongated, blunt-ended nuclei and frequent mitoses. They may contain areas of hemorrhage and necrosis and extensively infiltrate the heart, often involving more than one cardiac chamber and spreading to the pericardium.[90]

OSTEOSARCOMAS. Primary cardiac osteosarcomas comprise 5 to 10 percent of cardiac sarcomas. They almost always occur in adults and in the left atrium. Unlike myxomas, they have a broad base of attachment, typically to the posterior atrial wall. On CT, the tumors often but not invariably present as a low-attenuation mass with areas of dense calcification. Grossly, osteosarcomas are stone hard and heavily calcified.[91] Histologically, they resemble osteosarcomas of bone and may contain areas of chondrosarcoma or fibrosarcoma.

MALIGNANT FIBROUS HISTIOCYTOMAS. Previously classified as fibrosarcomas or undifferentiated sarcomas, malignant fibrous histiocytomas have a "storiform" appearance with a mix of malignant fibroblasts and histiocytes and may contain myxoid areas.[92] In modern series malignant fibrous histiocytomas account for 5 to 10 percent of sarcomas.[25] They typically involve the left atrium and can be confused with myxomas.

LEIOMYOSARCOMAS. Derived from smooth muscle cells, leiomyosarcomas account for 10 percent of cardiac sarcomas and most are located in the left atrium. Some of these tumors may actually originate in the smooth muscle lining the pulmonary veins. Patients typically present in their 30s, a decade younger than with other types of sarcoma. On CT, these tumors appear as low-attenuation masses in the left atrium. Although sessile and gelatinous, unlike myxomas these tumors usually originate from the posterior wall and may involve the pulmonary veins and mitral valve. Histologically, these tumors demonstrate fascicular growth of spindle cells that contain intracytoplasmic glycogen.

MYXOID SARCOMAS (MYXOSARCOMAS). These tumors comprise less than 5 percent of cardiac sarcomas and are usually found in the left atrium and contain extensive myxoid areas; thus, they can be confused with myxomas or thought to represent malignant transformation of a myxoma. However, the data that myxomas can undergo malignant transformation are lacking. Histologically, myxoid sarcomas are composed of spindled mesenchymal cells and lack the calcification, thrombus, and hemosiderin seen in benign myxomas.

UNDIFFERENTIATED SARCOMAS. Undifferentiated sarcomas lack specific histological features. Using strict morphological criteria and using modern immunohistochemistry, up to 25 percent of sarcomas remain unclassified.[93] These tumors are most commonly found in the left atrium.[25]

PRIMARY CARDIAC LYMPHOMAS

Primary lymphoma involving only the heart or pericardium is rare, although recently the incidence has increased due to an increased incidence of immunosuppression from AIDS and solid organ transplant. In immunocompetent patients,[94] the median age of presentation is 64 years and the male-to-female ratio is 3:1. Patients present with intractable, typically right-sided, heart failure (52 percent), precordial chest pain (17 percent), constitutional symptoms (17 percent), arrhythmias (12 percent), or tamponade (12 percent). The lymphoma usually arises from the right side of the heart (most commonly the right atrium) and half of patients have pericardial effusions, typically large.

Establishing the diagnosis of primary cardiac lymphoma is challenging.[94] Transthoracic echocardiography has only moderate sensitivity and therefore transesophageal echocardiography should be used if cardiac lymphoma is suspected. CT and MRI findings are not specific, but MRI appears to be the most sensitive diagnostic modality. A gallium-67 scan that shows marked uptake in the heart is suggestive but nonspecific.[95] Cytological analysis of pericardial fluid has reported sensitivities ranging from 14 to 67 percent.[94,96] Transvenous endomyocardial biopsy has a sensitivity of only 50 percent; open biopsy is the gold standard. On pathology, cardiac lymphoma appears as a firm, white, infiltrative process, occasionally with nodular foci that range from 3 to 12 cm in diameter. These tumors are almost universally aggressive diffuse, large B-cell lymphomas.[94]

Without treatment, the median survival of patients with cardiac lymphomas is less than 1 month. Patients treated with chemotherapy and/or radiation have median survivals on the order of 1 year.[94] Immediately after initiation of therapy patients may deteriorate due to rapid intramural tumor lysis causing heart failure,[97] arrhythmias,[98] and even cardiac rupture.[99] The long-term prognosis is almost universally dismal, although isolated cases of complete remissions after autologous stem cell transplant have been reported.[100]

REFERENCES

Clinical Presentation

1. McAllister HA, Fenoglio JJ: Tumors of the cardiovascular system. *In* Hartmann WH, Cowan WR (eds): Atlas of Tumor Pathology. Vol. Second Series, Fascicle 15. Washington, DC, Armed Forces Institute of Pathology, 1978, pp 1-3.
2. Reynen K: Frequency of primary tumors of the heart. Am J Cardiol 77:107, 1996.
3. Harvey WP: Clinical aspects of cardiac tumors. Am J Cardiol 21:328-343, 1968.
4. Kusano KF, Ohe T: Cardiac tumors that cause arrhythmias. Card Electrophysiol Rev 6:174-177, 2002.

Diagnostic Techniques

5. Tousek P, Orban M, Schomig A, Firschke C: Images in cardiovascular medicine: Real-time perfusion echocardiography of an intracardiac mass. Circulation 107:2390, 2003.
6. Shyu KG, Chen JJ, Cheng JJ, et al: Comparison of transthoracic and transesophageal echocardiography in the diagnosis of intracardiac tumors in adults. J Clin Ultrasound 22:381-389, 1994.
7. Espinola-Zavaleta N, Morales GH, Vargas-Barron J, et al: Three-dimensional transesophageal echocardiography in tumors of the heart. J Am Soc Echocardiogr 15:972-979, 2002.
8. Gerber TC, Kuzo RS, Karstaedt N, et al: Current results and new developments of coronary angiography with use of contrast-enhanced computed tomography of the heart. Mayo Clin Proc 77:55-71, 2002.
9. Grebenc ML, Rosado de Christenson ML, Burke AP, et al: Primary cardiac and pericardial neoplasms: Radiologic-pathologic correlation. Radiographics 20:1073-1103, 2000.
10. Araoz PA, Mulvagh SL, Tazelaar HD, et al: CT and MR imaging of benign primary cardiac neoplasms with echocardiographic correlation. Radiographics 20:1303-1319, 2000.
11. Araoz PA, Eklund HE, Welch TJ, Breen JF: CT and MR imaging of primary cardiac malignancies. Radiographics 19:1421-1434, 1999.
12. Hoffmann U, Globits S, Frank H: Cardiac and paracardiac masses: Current opinion on diagnostic evaluation by magnetic resonance imaging. Eur Heart J 19:553-563, 1998.
13. Masui T, Takahashi M, Miura K, et al: Cardiac myxoma: Identification of intratumoral hemorrhage and calcification on MR images. AJR Am J Roentgenol 164:850-852, 1995.
14. Frank H: Cardiac and paracardiac masses. In Manning WJ, Pennell DJ (eds): Cardiovascular Magnetic Resonance. New York, Churchill Livingstone, 2002, pp 342-354.
15. Plutchok JJ, Boxt LM, Weinberger J, et al: Differentiation of cardiac tumor from thrombus by combined MRI and F-18 FDG PET imaging. Clin Nucl Med 23:324-325, 1998.
16. Hofstra L, Dumont EA, Thimister PW, et al: In vivo detection of apoptosis in an intracardiac tumor. JAMA 285:1841-1842, 2001.
17. Veinot JP: Diagnostic endomyocardial biopsy pathology: Secondary myocardial diseases and other clinical indications—a review. Can J Cardiol 18:287-296, 2002.
18. Kang SM, Rim SJ, Chang HJ, et al: Primary cardiac lymphoma diagnosed by transvenous biopsy under transesophageal echocardiographic guidance and treated with systemic chemotherapy. Echocardiography 20:101-103, 2003.

Treatment Options and Prognosis

19. Goldberg HP, Glenn F, Dotter CT, Steinberg I: Myxoma of the left atrium: Diagnosis made during life with operative and post-mortem findings. Circulation 6:762-767, 1952.
20. Crafoord C: Discussion of Glover RP: Late results of mitral commissurotomy. *In* Lam CR (ed): Henry Ford Hospital International Symposium on Cardiovascular Surgery. Philadelphia, WB Saunders, 1955, pp 202-211.
21. Gowdamarajan A, Michler RE: Therapy for primary cardiac tumors: Is there a role for heart transplantation? Curr Opin Cardiol 15:121-125, 2000.
22. Scheld HH, Nestle HW, Kling D, et al: Resection of a heart tumor using autotransplantation. Thorac Cardiovasc Surg 36:40-43, 1988.
23. Schaff HV, Mullany CJ: Surgery for cardiac myxomas. Semin Thorac Cardiovasc Surg 12:77-88, 2000.
24. Mery GM, Reardon MJ, Haas J, et al: A combined modality approach to recurrent cardiac sarcoma resulting in a prolonged remission: A case report. Chest 123:1766-1768, 2003.

Specific Cardiac Tumors

25. Virmani R, Burke A, Farb A, Atkinson JB: Cardiovascular Pathology. Major Problems in Pathology. Vol. 40. Philadelphia, WB Saunders, 2001.
26. Vaughan CJ, Veugelers M, Basson CT: Tumors and the heart: Molecular genetic advances. Curr Opin Cardiol 16:195-200, 2001.
27. Dijkhuizen T, van den Berg E, Molenaar WM, et al: Rearrangements involving 12p12 in two cases of cardiac myxoma. Cancer Genet Cytogenet 82:161-162, 1995.
28. Yoon DH, Roberts W: Sex distribution in cardiac myxomas. Am J Cardiol 90:563-565, 2002.
29. Pinede L, Duhaut P, Loire R: Clinical presentation of left atrial cardiac myxoma: A series of 112 consecutive cases. Medicine (Baltimore) 80:159-172, 2001.
30. Reynen K: Cardiac myxomas. N Engl J Med 333:1610-1617, 1995.
31. Revankar SG, Clark RA: Infected cardiac myxoma: Case report and literature review. Medicine (Baltimore) 77:337-344, 1998.
32. Suzuki J, Takayama K, Mitsui F, et al: In situ interleukin-6 transcription in embryonic nonmuscle myosin heavy chain expressing immature mesenchyme cells of cardiac myxoma. Cardiovasc Pathol 9:33-37, 2000.
33. Parissis JT, Mentzikof D, Georgopoulou M, et al: Correlation of interleukin-6 gene expression to immunologic features in patients with cardiac myxomas. J Interferon Cytokine Res 16:589-593, 1996.
34. Carney JA, Gordon H, Carpenter PC, et al: The complex of myxomas, spotty pigmentation, and endocrine overactivity. Medicine (Baltimore) 64:270-283, 1985.

35. Atherton DJ, Pitcher DW, Wells RS, MacDonald DM: A syndrome of various cutaneous pigmented lesions, myxoid neurofibromata, and atrial myxoma: The NAME syndrome. Br J Dermatol 103:421-429, 1980.
36. Rhodes AR, Silverman RA, Harrist TJ, Perez-Atayde AR: Mucocutaneous lentigines, cardiomucocutaneous myxomas, and multiple blue nevi: The "LAMB" syndrome. J Am Acad Dermatol 10:72-82, 1984.
37. Stratakis CA, Kirschner LS, Carney JA: Clinical and molecular features of the Carney complex: Diagnostic criteria and recommendations for patient evaluation. J Clin Endocrinol Metab 86:4041-4046, 2001.
38. Stratakis CA, Carney JA, Lin JP, et al: Carney complex, a familial multiple neoplasia and lentiginosis syndrome: Analysis of 11 kindreds and linkage to the short arm of chromosome 2. J Clin Invest 97:699-705, 1996.
39. Casey M, Mah C, Merliss AD, et al: Identification of a novel genetic locus for familial cardiac myxomas and Carney complex. Circulation 98:2560-2566, 1998.
40. Kirschner LS, Carney JA, Pack SD, et al: Mutations of the gene encoding the protein kinase A type I-alpha regulatory subunit in patients with the Carney complex. Nat Genet 26:89-92, 2000.
41. Fogt F, Zimmerman RL, Hartmann CJ, et al: Genetic alterations of Carney complex are not present in sporadic cardiac myxomas. Int J Mol Med 9:59-60, 2002.
42. Grebenc ML, Rosado-de-Christenson ML, Green CE, et al: Cardiac myxoma: Imaging features in 83 patients. Radiographics 22:673-689, 2002.
43. Burke AP, Virmani R: Cardiac myxoma: A clinicopathologic study. Am J Clin Pathol 100:671-680, 1993.
44. Kono T, Koide N, Hama Y, et al: Expression of vascular endothelial growth factor and angiogenesis in cardiac myxoma: A study of fifteen patients. J Thorac Cardiovasc Surg 119:101-107, 2000.
45. Bennett KR, Gu JW, Adair TH, Heath BJ: Elevated plasma concentration of vascular endothelial growth factor in cardiac myxoma. J Thorac Cardiovasc Surg 122:193-194, 2001.
46. Pucci A, Gagliardotto P, Zanini C, et al: Histopathologic and clinical characterization of cardiac myxoma: Review of 53 cases from a single institution. Am Heart J 140:134-138, 2000.
47. Terracciano LM, Mhawech P, Suess K, et al: Calretinin as a marker for cardiac myxoma: Diagnostic and histogenetic considerations. Am J Clin Pathol 114:754-759, 2000.
48. Kodama H, Hirotani T, Suzuki Y, et al: Cardiomyogenic differentiation in cardiac myxoma expressing lineage-specific transcription factors. Am J Pathol 161:381-389, 2002.
49. Shinfeld A, Katsumata T, Westaby S: Recurrent cardiac myxoma: Seeding or multifocal disease? Ann Thorac Surg 66:285-288, 1998.
50. Ravikumar E, Pawar N, Gnanamuthu R, et al: Minimal access approach for surgical management of cardiac tumors. Ann Thorac Surg 70:1077-1079, 2000.
51. Klarich KW, Enriquez-Sarano M, Gura GM, et al: Papillary fibroelastoma: Echocardiographic characteristics for diagnosis and pathologic correlation. J Am Coll Cardiol 30:784-790, 1997.
52. Sun JP, Asher CR, Yang XS, et al: Clinical and echocardiographic characteristics of papillary fibroelastomas: A retrospective and prospective study in 162 patients. Circulation 103:2687-2693, 2001.
53. Israel DH, Sherman W, Ambrose JA, et al: Dynamic coronary ostial obstruction due to papillary fibroelastoma leading to myocardial ischemia and infarction. Am J Cardiol 67:104-105, 1991.
54. Fishbein MC, Ferrans VJ, Roberts WC: Endocardial papillary elastofibromas: Histologic, histochemical, and electron microscopical findings. Arch Pathol 99:335-341, 1975.
55. Shahian DM: Papillary fibroelastomas. Semin Thorac Cardiovasc Surg 12:101-110, 2000.
56. Nighoghossian N, Derex L, Loire R, et al: Giant lambl excrescences: An unusual source of cerebral embolism. Arch Neurol 54:41-44, 1997.
57. Shirani J, Roberts WC: Clinical, electrocardiographic and morphologic features of massive fatty deposits ("lipomatous hypertrophy") in the atrial septum. J Am Coll Cardiol 22:226-238, 1993.
58. Prior JT: Lipomatous hypertrophy of the cardiac interatrial septum: A lesion resembling hibernoma, lipo-blastomatosis and infiltrating lipoma. Arch Pathol 78:11-15, 1964.
59. Pochis WT, Saeian K, Sagar KB: Usefulness of transesophageal echocardiography in diagnosing lipomatous hypertrophy of the atrial septum with comparison to transthoracic echocardiography. Am J Cardiol 70:396-398, 1992.
60. Zeebregts CJ, Hensens AG, Timmermans J, et al: Lipomatous hypertrophy of the interatrial septum: Indication for surgery? Eur J Cardiothorac Surg 11:785-787, 1997.
61. Breuer M, Wippermann J, Franke U, Wahlers T: Lipomatous hypertrophy of the interatrial septum and upper right atrial inflow obstruction. Eur J Cardiothorac Surg 22:1023-1025, 2002.
62. Burke AP, Virmani R: Cardiac rhabdomyoma: A clinicopathologic study. Mod Pathol 4:70-74, 1991.
63. Beghetti M, Gow RM, Haney I, et al: Pediatric primary benign cardiac tumors: A 15-year review. Am Heart J 134:1107-1114, 1997.
64. Holley DG, Martin GR, Brenner JI, et al: Diagnosis and management of fetal cardiac tumors: A multicenter experience and review of published reports. J Am Coll Cardiol 26:516-520, 1995.
65. Berkenblit R, Spindola-Franco H, Frater RW, et al: MRI in the evaluation and management of a newborn infant with cardiac rhabdomyoma. Ann Thorac Surg 63:1475-1477, 1997.
66. Kwiatkowski DJ: Tuberous sclerosis: From tubers to mTOR. Ann Hum Genet 67:87-96, 2003.
67. Nir A, Tajik AJ, Freeman WK, et al: Tuberous sclerosis and cardiac rhabdomyoma. Am J Cardiol 76:419-421, 1995.
68. Bosi G, Lintermans JP, Pellegrino PA, et al: The natural history of cardiac rhabdomyoma with and without tuberous sclerosis. Acta Paediatr 85:928-931, 1996.
69. Stiller B, Hetzer R, Meyer R, et al: Primary cardiac tumours: When is surgery necessary? Eur J Cardiothorac Surg 20:1002-1006, 2001.
70. Burke AP, Rosado-de-Christenson M, Templeton PA, Virmani R: Cardiac fibroma: Clinicopathologic correlates and surgical treatment. J Thorac Cardiovasc Surg 108:862-870, 1994.
71. Parmley LF, Salley RK, Williams JP, Head GB III: The clinical spectrum of cardiac fibroma with diagnostic and surgical considerations: Noninvasive imaging enhances management. Ann Thorac Surg 45:455-465, 1988.
72. Gorlin RJ: Nevoid basal cell carcinoma syndrome. Medicine (Baltimore) 66:98-113, 1987.
73. Hahn H, Wicking C, Zaphiropoulous PG, et al: Mutations of the human homolog of *Drosophila* patched in the nevoid basal cell carcinoma syndrome. Cell 85:841-851, 1996.
74. Cox JN, Friedli B, Mechmeche R, et al: Teratoma of the heart: A case report and review of the literature. Virchows Arch A Pathol Anat Histopathol 402:163-174, 1983.
75. de Bustamante TD, Azpeitia J, Miralles M, et al: Prenatal sonographic detection of pericardial teratoma. J Clin Ultrasound 28:194-198, 2000.
76. Brizard C, Latremouille C, Jebara VA, et al: Cardiac hemangiomas. Ann Thorac Surg 56:390-394, 1993.
77. Tabry IF, Nassar VH, Rizk G, et al: Cavernous hemangioma of the heart: Case report and review of the literature. J Thorac Cardiovasc Surg 69:415-420, 1975.
78. Drolet BA, Esterly NB, Frieden IJ: Hemangiomas in children. N Engl J Med 341:173-181, 1999.
79. Cina SJ, Smialek JE, Burke AP, et al: Primary cardiac tumors causing sudden death: A review of the literature. Am J Forensic Med Pathol 17:271-281, 1996.
80. David TE, Lenkei SC, Marquez-Julio A, et al: Pheochromocytoma of the heart. Ann Thorac Surg 41:98-100, 1986.
81. Malhotra V, Ferrans VJ, Virmani R: Infantile histiocytoid cardiomyopathy: Three cases and literature review. Am Heart J 128:1009-1021, 1994.
82. Burke AP, Cowan D, Virmani R: Primary sarcomas of the heart. Cancer 69:387-395, 1992.
83. Garcia JM, Gonzalez R, Silva JM, et al: Mutational status of *K-ras* and *TP53* genes in primary sarcomas of the heart. Br J Cancer 82:1183-1185, 2000.
84. Hsieh PL, Lee D, Chiou KR, et al: Echocardiographic features of primary cardiac sarcoma. Echocardiography 19:215-220, 2002.
85. Hammoudeh AJ, Chaaban F, Watson RM, Millman A: Transesophageal echocardiography-guided transvenous endomyocardial biopsy used to diagnose primary cardiac angiosarcoma. Cathet Cardiovasc Diagn 37:347-349, 1996.
86. Conklin LD, Reardon MJ: Autotransplantation of the heart for primary cardiac malignancy: Development and surgical technique. Tex Heart Inst J 29:105-108, 2002.
87. Llombart-Cussac A, Pivot X, Contesso G, et al: Adjuvant chemotherapy for primary cardiac sarcomas: The IGR experience. Br J Cancer 78:1624-1628, 1998.
88. Burgert SJ, Strickman NE, Carrol CL, Falcone M: Cardiac Kaposi's sarcoma following heart transplantation. Catheter Cardiovasc Interv 49:208-212, 2000.
89. Raaf HN, Raaf JH: Sarcomas related to the heart and vasculature. Semin Surg Oncol 10:374-382, 1994.
90. Knobel B, Rosman P, Kishon Y, Husar M: Intracardiac primary fibrosarcoma: Case report and literature review. Thorac Cardiovasc Surg 40:227-230, 1992.
91. Reynard JS Jr, Gregoratos G, Gordon MJ, Bloor CM: Primary osteosarcoma of the heart. Am Heart J 109:598-600, 1985.
92. Laya MB, Mailliard JA, Bewtra C, Levin HS: Malignant fibrous histiocytoma of the heart: A case report and review of the literature. Cancer 59:1026-1031, 1987.
93. Donsbeck AV, Ranchere D, Coindre JM, et al: Primary cardiac sarcomas: An immunohistochemical and grading study with long-term follow-up of 24 cases. Histopathology 34:295-304, 1999.
94. Ceresoli GL, Ferreri AJ, Bucci E, et al: Primary cardiac lymphoma in immunocompetent patients: Diagnostic and therapeutic management. Cancer 80:1497-1506, 1997.
95. Hamada S, Nishimura T, Hayashida K, Uehara T: Intracardiac malignant lymphoma detected by gallium-67 citrate and thallium-201 chloride. J Nucl Med 29:1868-1870, 1988.
96. Chalabreysse L, Berger F, Loire R, et al: Primary cardiac lymphoma in immunocompetent patients: A report of three cases and review of the literature. Virchows Arch 441:456-461, 2002.
97. Chim CS, Chan AC, Kwong YL, Liang R: Primary cardiac lymphoma. Am J Hematol 54:79-83, 1997.
98. Rolla G, Bertero MT, Pastena G, et al: Primary lymphoma of the heart: A case report and review of the literature. Leuk Res 26:117-120, 2002.
99. Beckwith C, Butera J, Sadaniantz A, et al: Diagnosis in oncology. Case 1: Primary transmural cardiac lymphoma. J Clin Oncol 18:1996-1997, 2000.
100. Porcar Ramells C, Clemente Gonzalez C, Garcia Pares D, et al: [Primary cardiac lymphoma: Cytological diagnosis and treatment with response to polychemotherapy and hematopoietic precursor autotransplant. Presentation of a case a review of the literature]. An Med Interna 19:305-309, 2002.

CHAPTER 64

Pericardial Diseases

Martin M. LeWinter • Samer Kabbani

Anatomy and Physiology of the Pericardium

VISCERAL AND PARIETAL PERICARDIUM. The pericardium is composed of two layers.[1] The *visceral* pericardium is a serous membrane composed of a single layer of mesothelial cells adherent to the epicardial surface of the heart. The *parietal* pericardium is fibrous, is about 2 mm thick when measured post mortem in humans without pericardial disease, and surrounds most of the heart. The parietal pericardium is largely acellular and contains both collagen and elastin fibers. Collagen is probably the major structural component and appears as wavy bundles when the pericardium is at low levels of stretch. When it is stretched further, the bundles straighten, resulting in increased stiffness of the tissue. The visceral pericardium reflects back near the origins of the great vessels, becoming continuous with and forming the inner layer of the parietal pericardium. The pericardial space lies between these two layers. It normally contains up to about 50 ml of serous fluid. (The term pericardial *sac* refers to the parietal pericardium with its inner visceral layer.) The reflection of the visceral pericardium is a few centimeters proximal to the junctions of each of the caval vessels with the right atrium. Thus, portions of these vessels lie within the pericardial sac (Fig. 64–1). Posterior to the left atrium, the reflection occurs at the oblique sinus of the pericardium. As a result, the left atrium is largely extrapericardial.

The parietal pericardium has ligamentous attachments to the diaphragm, sternum, and other structures in the anterior mediastinum. These ensure that the heart occupies a relatively fixed position within the thoracic cavity regardless of phase of respiration and body position. The only noncardiovascular macrostructures associated with the pericardium are the phrenic nerves, which are enveloped by the parietal pericardium.

Although pericardiectomy does not result in any obvious negative consequences, the normal pericardium does have functions. As noted, it maintains the position of the heart relatively constant within the thoracic cavity. It may also function as a barrier to infection and provides lubrication between the visceral and parietal layers. The pericardium is remarkably well innervated, including mechano- and chemoreceptors and phrenic afferents.[2] The normal functions of these receptors are incompletely understood, but they probably participate in reflexes thought to result from irritation of pericardium or epicardium, or both (e.g., the Bezold-Jarisch reflex) as well as transmission of pericardial pain. The pericardium also secretes prostaglandins and related substances that may modulate epicardial-pericardial neural traffic and coronary tone by effects on coronary receptors.[3]

The best-characterized mechanical function of the normal pericardium is its *restraining* effect on cardiac volume.[4,5] This function reflects the mechanical properties of the pericardial tissue.[6] The parietal pericardium has a tensile strength similar to that of rubber. At low applied stresses approximating those at physiological or subphysiological cardiac volumes, the tissue is quite elastic (Fig. 64–2, top); i.e., small forces result in large amounts of stretch. As stretch increases, the pericardial tissue fairly abruptly becomes quite stiff and resistant to further stretch. The point on the pericardial stress-strain relationship (see Fig. 64–2, top) where this transition occurs probably corresponds to stresses present at the upper range and slightly above physiological cardiac volumes and is probably caused by straightening of the collagen bundles.

Pressure-Volume Relationship. The *pressure-volume relationship* of the pericardial sac parallels the properties of the isolated tissue[7] (see Fig. 64–2, bottom, left curve), i.e., a relatively flat, compliant segment changing relatively abruptly to a noncompliant segment, with the transition occurring in the range of the upper limit of normal total cardiac volume (in this case, for the dog). Thus, the pericardial sac has a relatively small reserve volume. As the reserve volume is exceeded, the pressure within the sac operating on the surface of the heart increases rapidly and is transmitted to the inside of the cardiac chambers. The shape of the pericardial pressure-volume relationship accounts for the fact that when a critical level of effusion is reached, relatively small amounts of additional fluid cause large increases in intrapericardial pressure and have marked effects on cardiac function; conversely, removal of small amounts of fluid in patients with tamponade can result in striking improvement.

The shape of the pericardial pressure-volume relationship suggests that the normal pericardium can restrain cardiac volume; i.e., the force exerted on the surface of the heart by the pericardium can significantly limit filling, with a component of intracavitary filling pressure representing transmission of the pericardial pressure. This relationship has been examined by directly measuring the pressure in the pericardial sac as cardiac volume is varied using devices specifically designed to measure a contact pressure between two surfaces.[8,9] These studies demonstrate a substantial contact pressure, especially when the upper limit of normal cardiac volume is exceeded. The contact pressure is proportionally more important for the right side of the heart, whose filling pressures are normally lower than those on the left. In some of these studies[9] pericardial pressure was actually found to be virtually identical to right-heart filling pressure, whereas

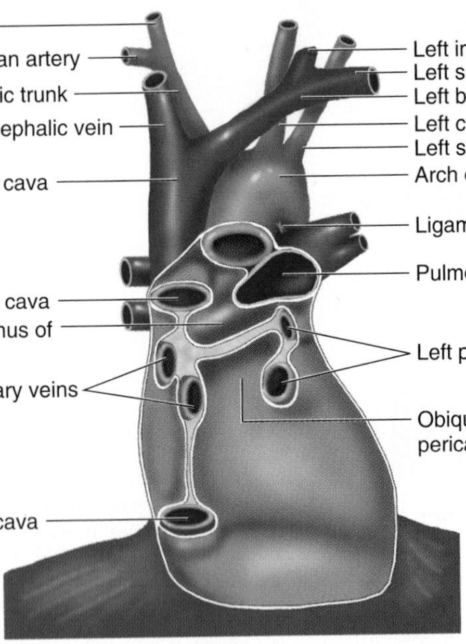

FIGURE 64–1 The pericardial reflections near the origins of the great vessels shown after removal of the heart. Note that portions of the caval vessels are within the pericardial space. (From Gabella G [sect ed]: The pericardium. *In* Gray H, Williams PL, Bannister LH [eds]: Gray's Anatomy: The Anatomical Basis of Medicine and Surgery. New York, Churchill-Livingstone, 1995, p 1471.)

in others[8] it was not as high but once again quite significant in relation to the right-heart pressure.

The pericardial contact pressure has also been estimated by quantifying the change in the right and left ventricular or right- and left-heart diastolic pressure-volume relationship before and after pericardiectomy.[4,5] Any decrease in pressure at a specified volume is the effective pericardial pressure at that volume. This method has the advantage of avoiding potential artifacts in direct pressure measurement. Studies in canine hearts using this approach[4] indicated negligible pericardial restraint at low normal filling volumes, with contact pressures in the range of 2 to 4 mm Hg at the upper end of the normal range. Contact pressure rapidly increases as filling is further augmented. With left-sided filling pressure about 25 mm Hg, estimated contact pressure is about 10 mm Hg, which accounts for a majority of the right-heart pressure at this level of filling.

Thus, it is clear that the normal pericardium can acutely restrain cardiac volume and influences measured intracavitary filling pressure. Moreover, patients undergoing pericardiotomy in conjunction with heart surgery with normal preoperative cardiac volumes were shown to have mild postoperative increases in cardiac mass and volume (as occurs with volume overload), consistent with relief of underlying, normally occurring restraint to filling by the pericardium.[10]

The normal pericardium also contributes to diastolic interaction[11] or the transmission of intracavitary filling pressure to adjoining chambers. For example, a portion of right ventricular diastolic pressure is transmitted to the left ventricle across the interventricular septum and contributes to left ventricular diastolic pressure. Because its presence increases right ventricular intracavitary pressure, the normal pericardium amplifies diastolic interaction. Thus, as cardiac volume increases above the physiological range the pericardium contributes increasingly to intracavitary filling pressures, directly because of the external contact pressure and indirectly because of increased diastolic interaction.

Passive Role of the Normal Pericardium in Heart Disease

When the cardiac chambers dilate rapidly, the restraining effect of the pericardium as well as its contribution to diastolic interaction can become markedly augmented, resulting in a hemodynamic picture with similarities to both cardiac tamponade and constrictive pericarditis. The most common example is acute right ventricular myocardial infarction (MI),[12] usually in conjunction with inferior left ventricular MI. In this situation, the right side of the heart dilates rapidly such that total heart volume exceeds the reserve volume of the pericardium. As a result of increased pericardial constraint and augmented interaction, left- and right-sided filling pressures equilibrate at elevated levels and a paradoxical pulse and inspiratory increase in systemic venous pressure (Kussmaul sign) can be observed. Other conditions in which similar hemodynamic effects are seen include acute pulmonary embolus and subacute mitral regurgitation. It is of note that these sorts of hemodynamic changes are not seen with purely left ventricular MI because of the largely extrapericardial location of the left atrium and the fact that the thicker walled left ventricle does not dilate acutely as much as the right ventricle.

Chronic cardiac dilation, as in dilated cardiomyopathy or regurgitant valvular disease, can result in cardiac volumes well in excess of the reserve volume of the normal pericardium. Despite this, exaggerated restraining effects are not ordinarily encountered. This observation implies that the pericardium undergoes chronic adaptation to accommodate marked increases in cardiac volume. In experimental chronic volume overload, the pericardial pressure-volume relationship shifts to the right and its slope decreases (see Fig. 64–2, bottom, right curve), i.e., it becomes more compliant, in association with increased pericardial area and mass and a decreased effect on the left ventricular diastolic pressure-volume relationship.[7,13] Thus, apparent growth of pericardial tissue occurs in response to chronic stretch. Presumably, a similar effect occurs with large, slowly accumulating pericardial effusions, which typically do not cause tamponade.

Acute Pericarditis

Etiology, Epidemiology, and Pathophysiology

Table 64–1 lists categories of diseases and specific conditions that can involve the pericardium. Acute pericarditis, defined as symptoms or signs resulting from pericardial inflammation of no more than 1 to 2 weeks duration, can occur in a wide variety of diseases (denoted by asterisks in Table 64–1). However, the majority of cases are idiopathic.[14,15] The term idiopathic is used to denote pericarditis for which no specific etiology can be found with routine diagnostic testing as outlined subsequently. Most such cases are presumed to be viral in etiology, but assessment of viral titers is not part of routine evaluation of sporadic cases because of cost and the fact that this knowledge does not usually alter management.

The overall incidence of acute pericarditis is impossible to define because there are undoubtedly a large number of undiagnosed cases. It is a relatively common diagnosis in the emergency department, but there are no large, modern series delineating its frequency in that setting. In one study,[16] it accounted for 1 percent of emergency department cases presenting with electrocardiographic (ECG) ST elevation, but this single criterion misses many cases. The fraction of all acute cases accounted for by idiopathic pericarditis is also uncertain and is influenced by population demographics and regional and seasonal variation in the prevalence of viral infections. However, 80 to 90 percent seems to be a reason-

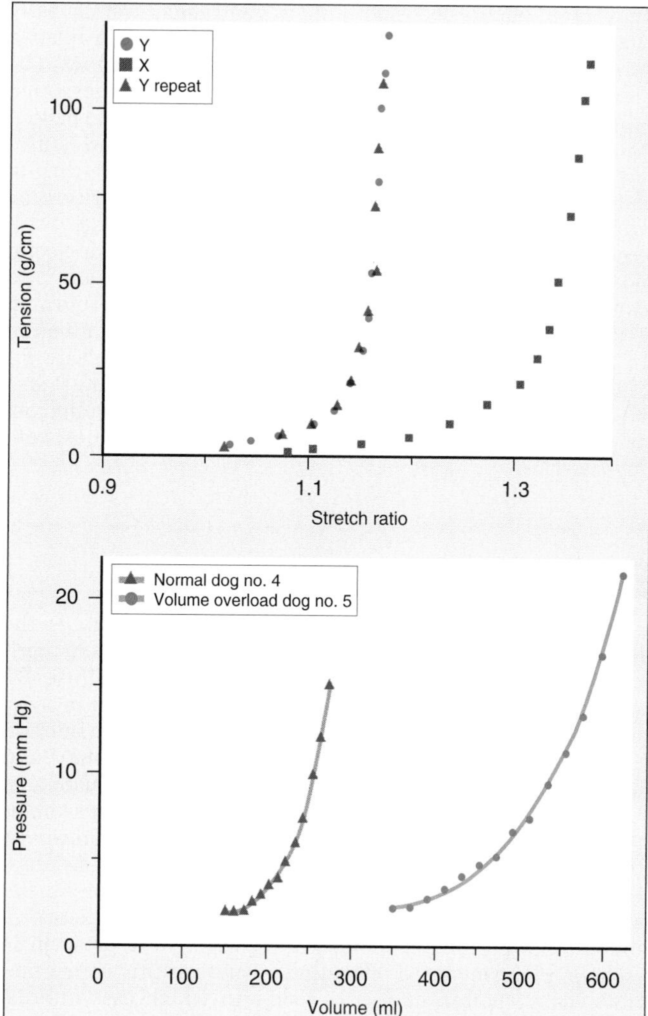

FIGURE 64–2 **Top,** Relationship between stretch and tension in vitro in normal human pericardial tissue. The tissue has been stretched in two, mutually orthogonal directions (X, Y). Note the relatively abrupt transition from a relatively flat to a steep, inelastic relationship. In addition, the tissue is anisotropic; i.e., the relation between tension and stretch depends on the direction of stretch. **Bottom,** Pressure-volume relationship of the normal canine pericardium (left) and after 4 weeks of cardiac dilation caused by volume overload (right). Note the relatively abrupt transition to a steep relationship in normal pericardium and marked shift to the right and flattening after chronic volume overload. (**Top,** From Lee M-C, Fung YC, Shabetai R, LeWinter MM: Biaxial mechanical properties of the human pericardium and canine comparisons. Am J Physiol 22:H75, 1987; **Bottom,** From Freeman G, LeWinter M: Pericardial adaptations during chronic cardiac dilation in dogs. Circ Res 54:294, 1984.)

TABLE 64–1 Categories of Pericardial Disease and Selected Specific Etiologies

Idiopathic*
Infectious Viral* (echovirus, coxsackievirus, adenovirus, cytomegalovirus, hepatitis B, infectious mononucleosis, HIV/AIDs) Bacterial* (*Pneumococcus, Staphylococcus, Streptococcus, Mycoplasma,* Lyme disease, *Hemophilus influenzae, Neisseria meningitidis*) Mycobacteria*(*Mycobacterium tuberculosis, Mycobacterium avium-intracellulare*) Fungal (histoplasmosis, coccidioidomyocosis) Protozoal
Immune-inflammatory Connective tissue disease* (systemic lupus erythematosus, rheumatoid arthritis, scleroderma, mixed) Arteritis (polyarteritis nodosa, temporal arteritis) Early post-myocardial infarction Late post-myocardial infarction (Dressler syndrome),* late post-cardiotomy/thoracotomy*, late post-trauma* Drug induced* (e.g., procainamide, hydralazine, isoniazid, cyclosporine)
Neoplastic disease Primary: mesothelioma, fibrosarcoma, lipoma, and so on Secondary*: breast and lung carcinoma, lymphomas, leukemias
Radiation induced*
Early post-cardiac surgery
Device and procedure related Coronary angioplasty, implantable defibrillators, pacemakers
Trauma Blunt and penetrating,* post-cardiopulmonary resuscitation*
Congenital Cysts, congenital absence
Miscellaneous Chronic renal failure, dialysis related Hypothyroidism Amyloidosis Aortic dissection

AIDs = acquired immunodeficiency syndrome; HIV = human immunodeficiency virus.

*Etiologies that are manifest as acute pericarditis.

able estimate.[14,15] The percentage is lower in patients with pericarditis who require hospitalization and higher in young, previously healthy patients. Tuberculous pericarditis is included in Table 64–1 as a cause of acute pericarditis but usually arises with more chronic symptoms. Bacterial pericarditis is also included because it can present with signs and symptoms of acute pericardial inflammation, but these patients are usually very sick and other components of their illness, including pericardial effusions, sepsis, and pneumonias, typically dominate the picture.

Pericarditis occurring 24 to 72 hours after transmural MI caused by local inflammation at the epicardial MI border and the delayed pericarditis of Dressler syndrome used to be common (see Chap. 46). The incidence has declined since the advent of thrombolytics and myocardial revascularization. With these exceptions, the distribution of etiologic diagnoses for acute pericarditis has changed little over time. In contrast, the epidemiology of pericardial effusion and constriction has changed considerably.

The pathophysiology of uncomplicated acute pericarditis is straightforward; all of the symptoms and signs result from inflammation of pericardial tissue. A minority of cases are complicated, as discussed later. In addition, some cases are associated with myocarditis.[17,18] Coexistent myocarditis is usually manifest only by release of biomarkers (creatine kinase, troponin I) (see Chap. 60). Occasionally, however, significant myocardial dysfunction occurs in conjunction with clinically manifest pericarditis.

History and Differential Diagnosis

Acute pericarditis almost always arises with chest pain as the chief complaint. A few cases without chest pain are diagnosed during evaluation of associated symptoms such as dyspnea or fever or incidentally in conjunction with noncardiac manifestations of systemic diseases such as rheumatoid arthritis or systemic lupus erythematosus (SLE).

The pain of pericarditis can be quite severe. It is variable in quality but often sharp and almost always pleuritic. It usually does not have the characteristic vise-like, constricting or oppressive features of ischemic discomfort. Pericardial pain typically has a relatively rapid onset and sometimes begins remarkably abruptly. It is most commonly substernal in location but can also be centered in the left anterior chest or the epigastrium. Radiation to the left arm is not unusual and can lead to confusion with myocardial ischemia. The most characteristic radiation is to the trapezius ridge, which is highly specific for pericarditis. Pericardial pain is almost always relieved by sitting forward and worsened by lying down. Associated symptoms can include dyspnea (often difficult to sort out with coexistent pleuritic pain), cough, and occasionally hiccoughs.

An antecedent history of fever or symptoms suggesting a viral syndrome are common. It is important to review the past medical history carefully for clues to specific etiologic diagnoses. Thus, a history of cancer or an autoimmune disorder, high fevers with shaking chills, skin rash, or weight loss should alert the physician to specific diseases that can cause pericarditis.

DIFFERENTIAL DIAGNOSIS. The differential diagnosis of chest pain is extensive (see Chap. 7). Diagnoses most easily confused with pericarditis include pneumonia or pneumonitis with pleurisy (which may coexist with pericarditis), pulmonary embolus or infarction, costochondritis, and gastroesophageal reflux disease. Myocardial ischemia and infarction are a major diagnostic concern. Acute pericarditis is usually relatively easily distinguished from ischemia on clinical and other grounds, but there are cases in which coronary angiography is required to resolve this issue. Other considerations include aortic dissection, intraabdominal processes, pneumothorax, and herpes zoster pain before skin lesions appear. Finally, acute pericarditis is occasionally the presenting manifestation of a preceding, clinically silent MI.

Physical Examination

Patients with uncomplicated acute pericarditis often appear quite uncomfortable and anxious and may have low-grade fever and sinus tachycardia. Other than this, the only abnormal physical finding is the pericardial friction rub, caused by contact between visceral and parietal pericardium. The classic rub is a distinctive and easily recognized auscultatory finding that is pathognomonic of pericarditis. It consists of three components corresponding to ventricular systole, early diastolic filling, and atrial contraction and has been likened to the sound made when walking on crunchy snow. The rub is usually loudest at the lower left sternal border, often extends to the cardiac apex, and is best heard with the patient leaning forward. It is often dynamic, disappearing and returning over short periods of time. Thus, it is often rewarding to listen frequently to a patient who has suspected pericarditis without an initially audible rub. Sometimes what is considered a pericardial rub in fact has only two or even one component. Labeling such findings rubs should be done with caution because the sound may actually represent a murmur.

It is important to perform a complete physical examination in a patient with acute pericarditis and look carefully for clues to specific etiologic diagnoses. The examiner must also be alert to findings indicating significant pericardial effusion, as discussed subsequently, and the presence of coexistent myocarditis.

Laboratory Testing

ELECTROCARDIOGRAM. The electrocardiogram is the most important laboratory test in the diagnosis of acute pericarditis (see Chap. 9). The classic finding is diffuse ST segment elevation (Fig. 64–3). The ST segment vector in acute pericarditis typically points leftward, anterior, and inferior. The result is ST segment elevation in all leads except aV_r and often V_1. Thus, the term "diffuse" is a slight misnomer. Usually, the ST segment is coved upward and resembles the current of injury of acute, transmural ischemia. However, the distinction between acute pericarditis and transmural ischemia is usually not difficult because of the more extensive lead involvement in pericarditis and the presence of much more prominent reciprocal ST segment depression in ischemia. However, ST elevation in pericarditis sometimes involves a smaller number of leads, in which case the distinction is more difficult. In other cases, the ST segment more closely resembles early repolarization. Here again, pericarditis usually involves more leads than typical early repolarization. As with the rub, ECG changes of acute pericarditis can be dynamic. Frequent recordings often yield a diagnosis in patients with suspected pericarditis who present initially with neither rub nor ST elevation.

PR segment depression is another common finding in acute pericarditis (see Fig. 64–3). In some cases, PR depression occurs in the absence of ST elevation and can be the initial ECG manifestation of acute pericarditis.[19] Thus, the finding is diagnostically useful in patients with neither rub nor ST elevation. In one study,[20] PR segment depression was a marker for clinically silent pericardial effusion in a series of patients referred for echocardiography, but this does not necessarily apply to those presenting with acute pericarditis.

ECG abnormalities other than ST elevation and PR depression are unusual in patients presenting soon after the onset of symptoms

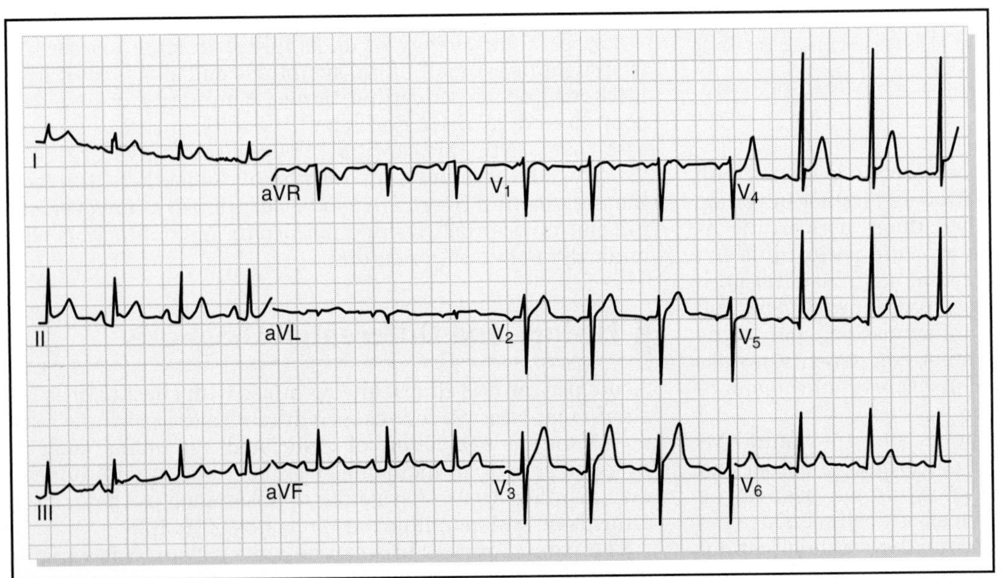

FIGURE 64–3 The electrocardiogram in acute pericarditis. Note both diffuse ST segment elevation and PR segment depression.

of acute pericarditis. Subsequent ECG changes are quite variable.[15] In some, the electrocardiogram simply reverts to normal over days or weeks. In others, the elevated ST segment passes through the isoelectric point and progresses to ST segment depression and T wave inversions in leads with upright QRS complexes. The latter changes can persist for weeks and months. They have no known significance in patients who have otherwise recovered. In patients presenting late after the onset of symptoms, these ECG changes can be difficult to distinguish from those of myocardial ischemia.

When present, ECG abnormalities other than the preceding ones should be considered carefully because they suggest diagnoses other than idiopathic pericarditis or complications. As examples, atrioventricular block may indicate Lyme disease, pathological Q waves can signify a previously silent MI with pericardial pain as its first manifestation, and low voltage or electrical alternans points toward significant effusion.

HEMOGRAM. Modest elevations of the white blood cell count, typically in the range 11,000 to 13,000/ml^3 with a mild lymphocytosis, are common in acute idiopathic pericarditis. Significantly higher counts are an alert for the presence of other etiologies. The red blood cell count should be normal. Anemia is also an alert for other etiologies. The erythrocyte sedimentation rate (ESR) should be no more than modestly elevated in acute idiopathic pericarditis. The ESR is a reasonable screening test in acute pericarditis because unusually high values may be a clue to etiologies such as autoimmune diseases or tuberculosis.

CARDIAC ENZYMES AND TROPONIN MEASUREMENTS. Several reports indicate that surprisingly large numbers of patients with a diagnosis of acute pericarditis without other evidence of myocarditis (see Chap. 60) or MI (see Chap. 46) have elevated cardiac enzymes (total creatine kinase or muscle-brain [MB] fraction) and troponin I.[17,18] These reports suggest a high incidence of concomitant, otherwise silent myocarditis. Patients with pericarditis with elevated biomarkers of myocardial injury appear to almost always have ST segment elevation. In our experience, evidence of myocardial injury in association with acute pericarditis, although it is certainly encountered, may not be as common as the relatively small studies in the literature[17,18] would suggest. Another concern in patients with elevated biomarkers is silent MI arising with subsequent pericarditis. Post-MI pericarditis usually (but not always) occurs after infarcts with pathological Q waves.

CHEST RADIOGRAPH (see Chap. 12). The chest radiograph, including the cardiac silhouette, is usually normal in uncomplicated cases of acute idiopathic pericarditis. Occasionally, small pulmonary infiltrates or pleural effusions are present, presumably related to viral or possibly mycoplasma infections. Other than this, pulmonary parenchymal or other abnormalities suggest diagnoses other than idiopathic pericarditis. Thus, bacterial pericarditis often occurs in conjunction with severe pneumonia. Tuberculous pericarditis can occur with or without associated pulmonary infiltrates. Mass lesions and enlarged lymph nodes suggestive of neoplastic disease also have great significance. Pulmonary vascular congestion may signal the presence of coexistent, severe myocarditis. Small to even moderate effusions may not cause an abnormal cardiac silhouette; thus, even modest enlargement is a cause for concern that a significant effusion is present.

ECHOCARDIOGRAPHY. The echocardiogram is normal in most patients presenting with acute idiopathic pericarditis (see Chap. 11). The main reason for performing echocardiography is to exclude an otherwise silent effusion. There are no modern data delineating the incidence of effusions in such patients. In our experience, most do not have effusions, but small ones are fairly common and not a cause for concern. Moderate or larger effusions are unusual and may signal a diagnosis other than idiopathic pericarditis. In addition to detecting effusions, echocardiography is useful in delineating whether associated myocarditis is severe enough to alter ventricular function as well as in detection of MI.

Natural History and Management

Because there have been no large, modern therapeutic trials, there are no established guidelines for management of acute pericarditis. Initial management should be focused on screening for specific etiologies that would alter management, detection of effusion and other echocardiographic abnormalities, symptomatic treatment, and appropriate treatment if a specific etiology is discovered. As initial evaluation, we recommend obtaining the laboratory data discussed previously, i.e., ECG, hemogram with ESR, chest radiograph, cardiac enzymes and troponin I, and echocardiography. In young women, it is not unreasonable to test for SLE as part of the initial evaluation.

Acute idiopathic pericarditis is a self-limited disease without significant complications or recurrence in about 70 to 90 percent of patients.[14,15] Accordingly, if the laboratory data support the diagnosis, symptomatic treatment with nonsteroidal antiinflammatory drugs (NSAIDs) should be initiated. Although indomethacin has frequently been used, ibuprofen is preferred because of its better side effect profile. The drug is administered in doses of 600 to 800 mg three times daily for 2 weeks and discontinued if pain is no longer present. Many patients have gratifying responses to the first dose or two of an NSAID. The majority respond fully to this regimen and need no additional treatment. Reliable patients with no more than small effusions who respond well to NSAIDs need not be admitted to hospital. Patients who do not respond well initially, have larger effusions, or have indications of an etiology other than idiopathic pericarditis should be hospitalized for additional observation, diagnostic testing and treatment as necessary.

Patients who respond slowly or inadequately to NSAIDs may require supplementary narcotic analgesics to allow time for a full response or a brief course of a corticosteroid, or both. For the latter, prednisone 60 mg by mouth is administered daily for 2 days with tapering to zero over a week. It is unusual not to achieve a satisfactory response to NSAIDs with narcotic analgesics or prednisone backup as necessary. Oral colchicine (1 mg daily with or without a 2- to 3-mg loading dose) can be an effective alternative to corticosteroids in patients who do not respond satisfactorily to NSAIDs. Colchicine has also been suggested as an alternative to NSAIDs for initial treatment.[21]

Complications of acute pericarditis include effusion and tamponade and constrictive pericarditis. It is not known how many patients presenting with acute pericarditis have moderate or larger effusions, but it is almost certainly less than 5 percent. As discussed earlier, a significant effusion increases the chance that a specific etiology is present. Management of effusion is discussed subsequently. The chance of developing constrictive pericarditis after a bout of acute pericarditis is also unknown but is undoubtedly extremely low. Strictly speaking, myocarditis is not a complication of pericarditis but an associated condition.

Relapsing and Recurrent Pericarditis

Perhaps 15 to 30 percent of patients with acute, apparently idiopathic pericarditis who respond satisfactorily to treatment as outlined previously suffer a relapse after completion of initial therapy.[14,15] A minority of these develop recurrent bouts of pericardial pain, which can sometimes be chronic and debilitating.[15] Recurrent pain is not necessarily associated with objective signs of pericardial inflammation. Some patients with what is initially thought to be idiopathic pericarditis manifest evidence of a specific etiology as they experience recurrences. Accordingly, a repeated evaluation for specific causes, especially autoimmune disorders, is appropriate. A pericardial biopsy to look for specific etiologic diagnoses in patients with recurrent pain without effusion is rarely if ever indicated because it is unlikely that a diagnosis would actually result or the information so obtained would alter management.

Treatment of recurrent pain is empirical. For an initial relapse, a second 2-week course of an NSAID is often effective. A course of colchicine may be at least as effective, although the optimal duration of treatment is uncertain. For bouts of recurrent pericardial pain beyond an initial relapse, we favor colchicine prophylaxis. There is now a fairly substantial favorable experience with chronic colchicine therapy as prophylaxis for recurrent pericardial pain, including that related to idiopathic pericarditis and other etiologies (e.g., postthoracotomy, SLE).[21] This experience strongly suggests that colchicine is at least as effective as chronic corticosteroid therapy, and it has a much more favorable side effect profile. The usual dose is 1 mg by mouth daily. Some recommend a 2- to 3-mg loading dose.[21] Initiation of prophylactic therapy does not preclude simultaneous use of NSAIDs or corticosteroids, although as discussed previously colchicine alone is often effective for acute episodes. The most common difficulty in using colchicine is nausea or diarrhea, or both, which in one study[21] required dose reduction or termination in 14 percent of patients.

Patients with recurrent pericardial pain despite NSAIDs and colchicine (or who cannot tolerate colchicine) are a challenging management problem. One option is a short course of prednisone as outlined earlier whenever symptoms first appear. Maintenance corticosteroid therapy should be avoided if at all possible. Nonsteroidal immunosuppressive therapy with drugs such as azathioprine and cyclophosphamide is an alternative to corticosteroids,[22] but published experience is extremely limited. In very difficult cases, low-dose maintenance therapy with these drugs may reduce the need for intermittent or maintenance corticosteroids and do so with less side effects. Pericardiectomy has occasionally been employed for recurrent pericarditis but appears to be effective in a small minority of patients at best.[23]

Pericardial Effusion and Tamponade

Etiology

Idiopathic pericarditis and any infection, neoplasm, or autoimmune or inflammatory process (including postradiation and drug induced) that can cause pericarditis can cause pericardial effusion (see Table 64–1). Effusions are common early after cardiac surgery,[24] but it is unusual for them to cause tamponade and they almost always resolve within several weeks. In addition, noninflammatory diseases, including hypothyroidism and amyloidosis, can cause effusion. Occasionally, patients with severe circulatory congestion have small to moderate transudative effusions. Bleeding into the pericardial sac occurs after blunt and penetrating trauma and as a consequence of post-MI rupture of the free wall of the left ventricle. Retrograde bleeding is an important cause of death related to dissecting aortic aneurysm (see Chap. 53). Last, occasional patients are encountered with large, silent pericardial effusions and no evidence of pericarditis.[25] Effusions in these patients are generally stable, but there is a significant incidence of tamponade over time.

Of the conditions that can cause effusion, those with a high incidence of progression to tamponade are bacterial (including mycobacteria), fungal, and human immunodeficiency virus (HIV)-associated infections (see Chap. 61), neoplastic involvement, and, of course, any form of bleeding into the pericardial space. Although large effusions related to acute idiopathic pericarditis are unusual, because of its high frequency this form of pericarditis accounts for a significant percentage of tamponade cases. Additional details of pericardial effusion pertinent to specific disease entities are discussed later in this chapter.

Pathophysiology and Hemodynamics

Formation of an effusion is simply a component of the response to inflammation when there is an inflammatory or infectious process affecting the pericardium. The latter is also probably the case with pericardial tumor implants (see Chap. 63). However, lymphomas occasionally cause effusion in association with enlarged mediastinal lymph nodes by obstructing pericardial lymph drainage. The pathophysiology of effusions in situations in which there is no obvious inflammation, for example, uremia and hypothyroidism, is poorly understood.

Cardiac tamponade is characterized by a continuum of hemodynamic events, from an effusion causing minimally detectable effects to the full-blown picture of circulatory collapse.[26a] Clinically, the most critical point occurs when an effusion reduces the volume of the cardiac chambers such that the cardiac output begins to decline. The key determinants of the hemodynamic consequences of a pericardial effusion are the level of pressure in the pericardial sac and the ability of the heart to compensate for the elevated pressure. The pressure, in turn, depends on the amount of fluid and the pericardial pressure-volume relationship. As discussed earlier, the pericardium normally has little reserve volume. As a result, relatively modest amounts of rapidly accumulating fluid can have major effects on cardiac function. Large, slowly accumulating effusions are often well tolerated, however, presumably because of chronic changes in the pericardial pressure-volume relationship as described earlier.

Compensatory Response. The compensatory response to a significant pericardial effusion includes increased adrenergic stimulation and parasympathetic withdrawal, which cause tachycardia and increased contractility.[26] Patients who cannot mount a normal adrenergic response, for example, those receiving beta-adrenergic blocking drugs, are more susceptible to the effects of a pericardial effusion. In the very late stages of tamponade, a depressor reflex with paradoxical bradycardia may supervene.[27]

Hemodynamic Consequences. The hemodynamic consequences of pericardial effusion have fascinated physiologists and physicians for many years.[26a,28,29] Non-steady-state responses to an abrupt increase in pericardial pressure provide insights into the mechanisms of the hemodynamic derangements of cardiac tamponade. Figure 64–4 shows an experiment performed in an open-chest dog in which aortic and pulmonary arterial flows (stroke volume) were measured on a beat-to-beat basis before and after a large amount of fluid was rapidly introduced into the pericardial sac over one to two cardiac cycles, indicated by the arrow. There was an immediate decrease in pulmonary arterial stroke volume but no change in aortic stroke volume. Two beats later, aortic stroke volume decreased and eventually a new steady state was achieved with equivalent decreases in aortic and pulmonary arterial stroke volume. During the time required to achieve a new steady state, pulmonary arterial stroke volume was less than aortic stroke volume. The transient inequality in left- and right-heart output resulted in net transfer of blood out of the pulmonary and into the systemic circulation and may explain the decrease in pulmonary vascularity on chest radiography in tamponade. In studies parallel to those in Figure 64–4, right-heart volume was

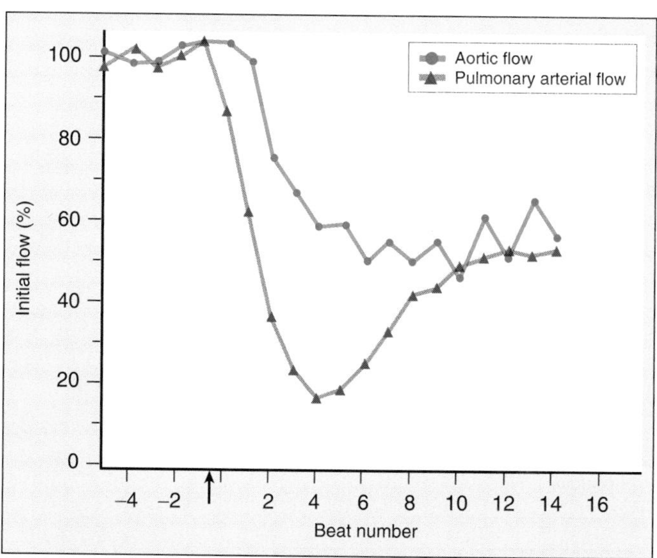

FIGURE 64–4 Beat-to-beat changes in pulmonary arterial and aortic stroke volume (as percentage of control) following abrupt production of cardiac tamponade (at arrow). Note that pulmonary arterial stroke volume decreases immediately, but there is a brief lag before aortic stroke volume decreases. Pulmonary arterial stroke volume is lower than aortic stroke volume until a new steady state is reached. (From Ditchey R, Engler R, LeWinter M, et al: The role of the right heart in acute cardiac tamponade in dogs. Circ Res 48:701, 1981.)

TABLE 64–2 Hemodynamics in Cardiac Tamponade and Constrictive Pericarditis

Finding	Tamponade	Constriction
Paradoxical pulse	Usually present	Present in ~1/3
Equal left-right filling pressures	Present	Present
Systemic venous wave morphology	Absent *y* descent	Prominent *y* descent (M or W shape)
Inspiratory change in systemic venous pressure	Decrease (normal)	Increase or no change (Kussmaul sign)
"Square root" sign in ventricular pressure	Absent	Present

shown to decrease more than left-heart volume in response to a given increase in pericardial pressure. These results show that high pericardial pressure exerts its main effect by impeding filling of the right side of the heart, with much of the effect on the left side being secondary and due to underfilling. In studies employing regional tamponade[30] the greater importance of right-heart compression was confirmed and it was also shown that compressions of the right atrium and segments of the caval vessels within the pericardial sac are independent components of the response to a pericardial effusion. These observations also provide a mechanism for the observations that atrial and ventricular diastolic collapse detected in tamponade are usually confined to the right side of the heart.[15,31]

As fluid accumulates in the pericardial sac, left- and right-sided atrial and ventricular diastolic pressures gradually rise and in severe tamponade eventually equalize at a pressure similar to that in the pericardial sac, typically 15 to 20 mm Hg (Fig. 64–5). Equalization is closest during inspiration. Thus, the pressure in the pericardial sac dictates the intracavitary filling pressure and the *transmural* filling pressures of the cardiac chambers are very low. Correspondingly, cardiac volumes progressively decline until they are very small. The small end-diastolic ventricular volume (decreased preload) accounts for the small stroke volume. Because of compensatory increases in contractility, end-systolic volume also decreases, but not enough to normalize stroke volume (hence, the importance of tachycardia in maintaining cardiac output). Under normal conditions, transmural right-heart filling pressure is lower then left-heart filling pressure (upper limit of right atrial pressure ~7 mm Hg, left atrial pressure ~12 mm Hg). It follows that as fluid accumulates, filling pressure increases more rapidly in the right than the left side of the heart until equalization is achieved.

***x* AND *y* DESCENTS.** In addition to elevated and equal intracavitary filling pressures, markedly reduced transmural filling pressures, and small cardiac volumes, two other hemodynamic abnormalities are characteristic of tamponade. One is loss of the *y* descent of the right atrial or jugular venous pressure (see Fig. 64–5). The *x* and *y* descents of the venous pressure waveform correspond to periods when venous return is increasing (in veins, pressure is the mirror image of flow). Loss of the *y* descent has been explained on the basis of the concept that total heart volume is fixed in severe tamponade.[15,32] In consequence, blood can enter the heart only when blood is simultaneously leaving. The right atrial *y* descent begins when the tricuspid valve opens, i.e., when blood is not leaving the heart. Thus, no blood can enter the heart and the *y* descent is lost. In contrast, the *x* descent occurs during ventricular ejection. Because blood is leaving the heart at this time, venous inflow can increase normally and the *x* descent is retained. Although loss of the *y* descent can be difficult to discern at the bedside, especially in sick patients with tachycardia, it can easily be appreciated in recordings of systemic venous or right atrial pressure and provides a useful clue to the presence of significant tamponade.

PARADOXICAL PULSE. The second characteristic hemodynamic finding is the paradoxical pulse (Fig. 64–6), an abnormally large decline in systemic arterial pressure during inspiration (usually defined as a >10 mm Hg drop in systolic pressure). Other causes of *pulsus paradoxus* include constrictive pericarditis, pulmonary embolus, and pulmonary disease (asthma, emphysema) with large variation in intrathoracic pressure. In severe cardiac tamponade, the arterial pulse is impalpable during inspiration. The mechanism of the paradoxical pulse is multifactorial, but respiratory changes in systemic venous return are certainly important.[15,32,33] In tamponade, in contrast to constrictive pericarditis, the normal inspiratory *increase* in systemic venous return is retained. Therefore, the normal *decline* in systemic venous pressure on inspiration is present (Kussmaul sign is absent). The increase in right-heart filling occurs, once again, under conditions in which total heart volume is fixed and left-heart volume markedly reduced to start. The interventricular septum shifts to the left in exaggerated fashion on inspiration, encroaching on the left ventricle such that its stroke volume and pressure generation are abnormally reduced (see Fig. 64–6). Although the inspiratory increase in right-heart volume (preload) causes an increase in right ventricular stroke volume, it requires several cardiac cycles to increase left ventricular filling and stroke volume and counteract the septal shift effect. Other factors that may contribute to the paradoxical pulse include increased afterload caused by transmission of negative intrathoracic pressure to the aorta and traction on the pericardium caused by the descent of the diaphragm, which increases the pericardial pressure. Associated with these complex mechanisms are the striking findings that left- and right-heart pressures and stroke volume variations are exaggerated and 180 degrees out of phase (see Fig. 64–6). Table 64–2 lists the major hemodynamic findings in cardiac tamponade and compares them with those in constrictive pericarditis.

When there are preexisting elevations in diastolic pressures or volume, or both, tamponade can occur without a paradoxical pulse. Examples are patients with left ventricular dysfunction, aortic regurgitation, and atrial septal defect.[34,35] Retrograde bleeding into the pericardial sac is a common cause of death in type I dissecting aortic aneurysms. Tamponade may occur without a paradoxical pulse because of simultaneous aortic regurgitation related to valvular disruption.

Low-Pressure Tamponade. Although left- and right-sided filling pressures are characteristically 15 to 20 mm Hg in severe tamponade, tamponade can occur at lower levels of intracavitary filling pressure, a phenomenon termed *low-pressure tamponade.*[15] Low-pressure tamponade occurs when there is a decrease in blood volume in the setting of a preexisting effusion that did not previously have significant consequences. In these conditions, a relatively modestly elevated pericardial pressure can lower transmural filling pressure to levels at which stroke volume is compromised. Because the venous pressure is only modestly elevated or even normal, the diagnosis may not be suspected. Low-pressure tamponade is typically observed during hemodialysis, where it is signaled by hypotension during a dialysis run, and in patients with blood loss and dehydration. It may also be seen when diuretics are administered to patients with effusions.

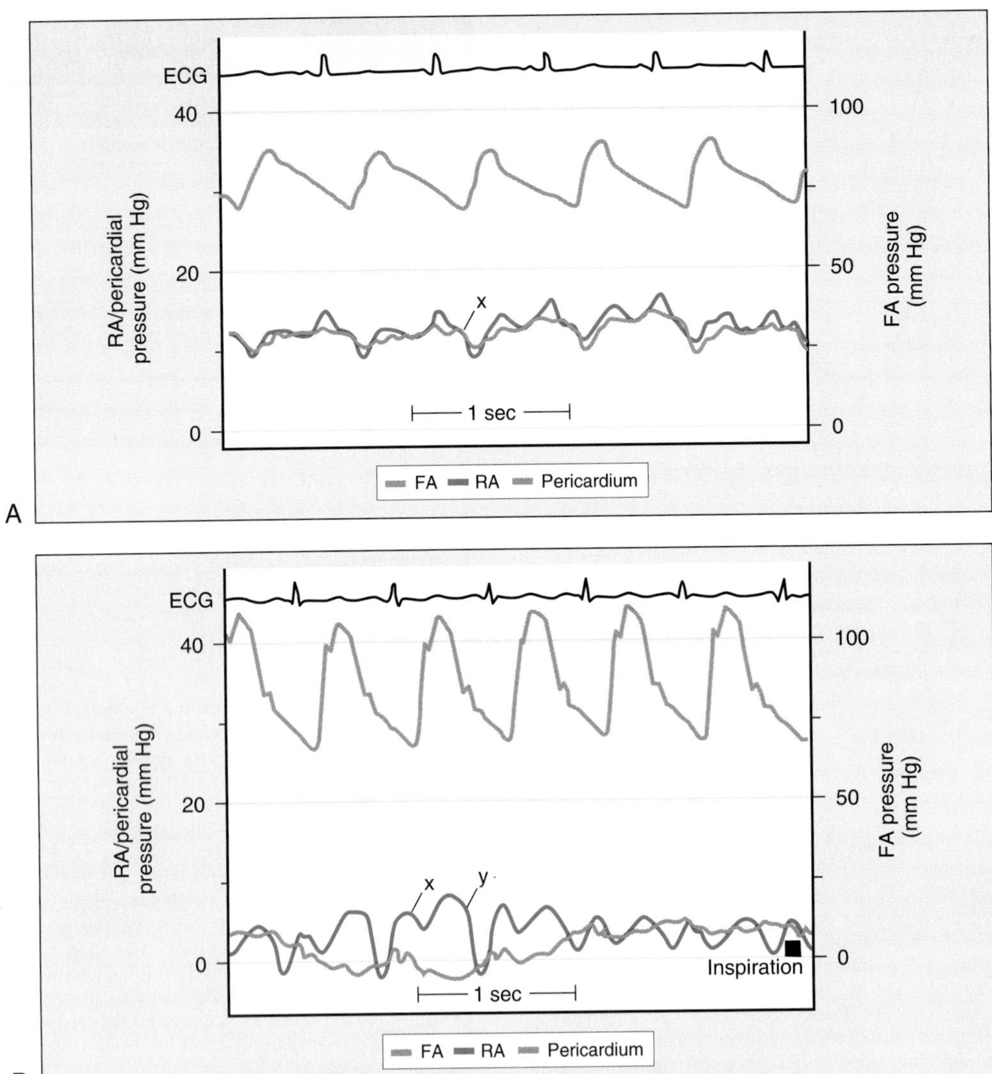

FIGURE 64–5 Femoral arterial (FA), right atrial (RA), and pericardial pressure before **(A)** and after **(B)** pericardiocentesis in a patient with cardiac tamponade. Both RA and pericardial pressure are about 15 mm Hg before pericardiocentesis. In this case there was a negligible paradoxical pulse. Note presence of *x* descent but absence of *y* descent before pericardiocentesis. Pericardiocentesis results in a marked increase in FA pressure and marked decrease in RA pressure. During inspiration, pericardial pressure becomes negative, there is clear separation between RA and pericardial pressure, and *y* descent is now evident and prominent, suggesting the possibility of an effusive-constrictive picture. (Adapted from Lorell BH, Grossman W: Profiles in constrictive pericarditis, restrictive cardiomyopathy and cardiac tamponade. *In* Baim DS, Grossman W [eds]: Grossman's Cardiac Catheterization, Angiography, and Intervention. Philadelphia, Lippincott Williams & Wilkins, 2000, p 840.)

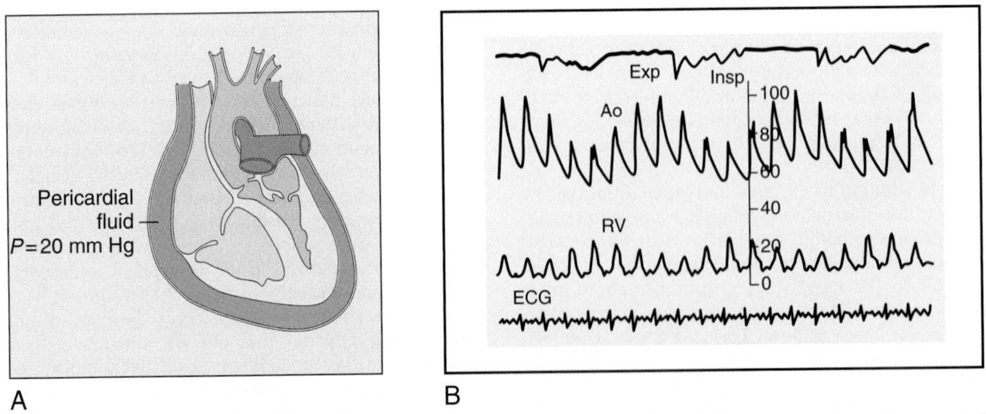

FIGURE 64–6 **A,** Schematic illustration of leftward septal shift with encroachment of left ventricular volume during inspiration in cardiac tamponade. **B,** Respiration marker and aortic and right ventricular pressure tracings in cardiac tamponade. Note paradoxical pulse and marked, 180 degrees out of phase respiratory variation in right- and left-sided pressures. Ao = aortic pressure; ECG = electrocardiogram; Exp = expiration; Insp = inspiration; RV = right ventricular pressure. (From Shabetai R: The Pericardium. New York, Grune & Stratton, 1981, p 266.)

Pericardial effusions can be loculated or localized, resulting in regional tamponade, as commonly encountered after cardiac surgery.[24,36] Regional tamponade can cause atypical hemodynamic abnormalities that can simulate heart failure, i.e., reduced cardiac output with unilateral filling pressure elevation. However, reports of the hemodynamics of regional tamponade are scarce and it is therefore difficult to generalize about this entity. Regional tamponade should be suspected whenever there are hemodynamic abnormalities in a setting in which a regional or loculated effusion is present.

Clinical Presentation

In any patient with effusion, a history pertinent to specific etiologies may be present and should be carefully sought. Occasionally, very large, asymptomatic chronic effusions are discovered when a chest radiograph is obtained for some unrelated reason.[25] As discussed earlier, specific etiologies are usually not found in these cases. Many patients with effusions also have pericardial pain. However, effusions do not by themselves cause symptoms unless tamponade is present. Patients with tamponade may complain of true dyspnea, whose mechanism is poorly understood because there is no pulmonary congestion. However, this is difficult to distinguish from tachypnea reflecting shock and respiratory alkalosis. Other symptoms reflect the extent to which the cardiac output is reduced. Usually, pericardial pain or a nonspecific sense of discomfort or both dominate the clinical picture. In our experience, patients with tamponade are almost always more comfortable sitting forward, even if they do not have pericardial pain.

A careful general physical examination in patients with pericardial effusion is critical because it may provide clues to a specific etiology. In pericardial effusion without tamponade, the cardiovascular examination is normal except that, if the effusion is very large, the cardiac impulse may be difficult or impossible to palpate and the heart sounds muffled. In addition, tubular breath sounds may be heard in the left axilla or left base because of bronchial compression.

If tamponade is present, patients usually appear uncomfortable, with signs reflecting varying degrees of reduced cardiac output and shock, including tachypnea, diaphoresis, cool extremities, peripheral cyanosis, and depressed sensorium. Hypotension is usually present, although in early stages compensatory mechanisms allow maintenance of normal blood pressure. A paradoxical pulse is the rule, but it is important to be alert to situations in which it may not be present. The paradoxical pulse is quantified using cuff sphygmomanometry by noting the difference between the pressure at which Korotkoff sounds first appear and that at which they are present with each heartbeat. In severe tamponade, the inspiratory decrease in arterial pressure is palpable and most obvious in pulses that are distant from the heart. Tachycardia is the rule unless heart rate–lowering drugs have been administered, conduction system disease coexists, or a preterminal bradycardic reflex has supervened.

The jugular venous pressure is markedly elevated, except in low-pressure tamponade, and the *y* descent is absent (see Fig. 64–5), although once again the latter can be difficult to appreciate at the bedside. The normal decrease in venous pressure on inspiration is retained. As with any large effusion, examination of the heart usually but not invariably reveals a reduced or absent cardiac impulse and, of course, a friction rub can also be present.

The clinical presentation of cardiac tamponade can be confused with the presentation of anything that can cause hypotension, shock, and elevated jugular venous pressure, including severe myocardial failure, right-sided heart failure related to pulmonary embolism or other causes of pulmonary hypertension, and right ventricular MI.

Laboratory Testing

ELECTROCARDIOGRAM. The only ECG abnormalities characteristic of pericardial effusion and tamponade are reduced voltage and electrical alternans of the QRS complex (Fig. 64–7).[15] Reduced voltage is a nonspecific finding that can be caused by several other conditions, including emphysema, infiltrative myocardial disease, and pneumothorax. Electrical alternans is virtually specific but relatively insensitive for large pericardial effusion with tamponade. It is caused by anterior-posterior swinging of the heart with each heartbeat. Its mechanism is poorly understood. When pericarditis coexists, the usual ECG findings may be present.

CHEST RADIOGRAPH (see Chap. 12). The cardiac silhouette remains normal until pericardial effusions are at least moderate in size. With moderate and larger effusions, the anteroposterior cardiac silhouette assumes a rounded, flask-like appearance (Fig. 64–8). Lateral views may reveal the pericardial fat pad sign, a linear lucency between the chest wall and the anterior surface of the heart, representing separation of parietal pericardial fat from epicardium. The lungs characteristically appear oligemic.

ECHOCARDIOGRAPHY (see Chap. 11). Because of its convenience and ease of application in critically ill patients, M-mode and two-dimensional Doppler echocardiography is currently the standard noninvasive diagnostic method for detection of pericardial effusion and noninvasive assessment of tamponade. A pericardial effusion appears as a lucent separation between parietal and visceral pericardium (Fig. 64–9). Separations should be present for the entire cardiac cycle to be classified as effusions. Small effusions are first evident over the posterobasal left ventricle. As the fluid increases it spreads anteriorly, laterally, and behind the left atrium, where its limit is demarcated by the visceral pericardial reflection. Ultimately, the separation becomes circumferential. Ordinarily, tamponade does not occur without a circumferential effusion and the diagnosis should be viewed with skepticism if this is not the case. However, in some types of pericardial disease and after cardiac surgery, effusions can be regional or loculated, or both, and, as discussed earlier, cause localized tamponade. Computed tomography (CT) and magnetic resonance (MR) are more precise than echocardiography for imaging the pericardium itself. However, frond-like or shaggy-appearing structures in the pericardial space

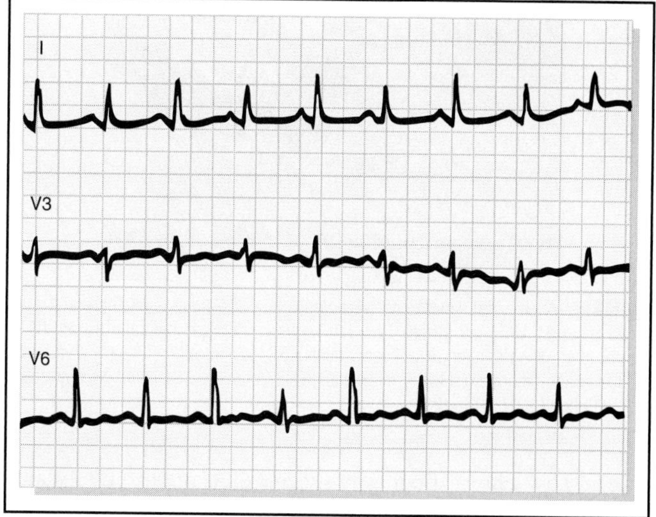

FIGURE 64–7 Electrocardiogram in cardiac tamponade showing alternans of the QRS complex. (From Shabetai R: The Pericardium. New York, Grune & Stratton, 1981, p 260.)

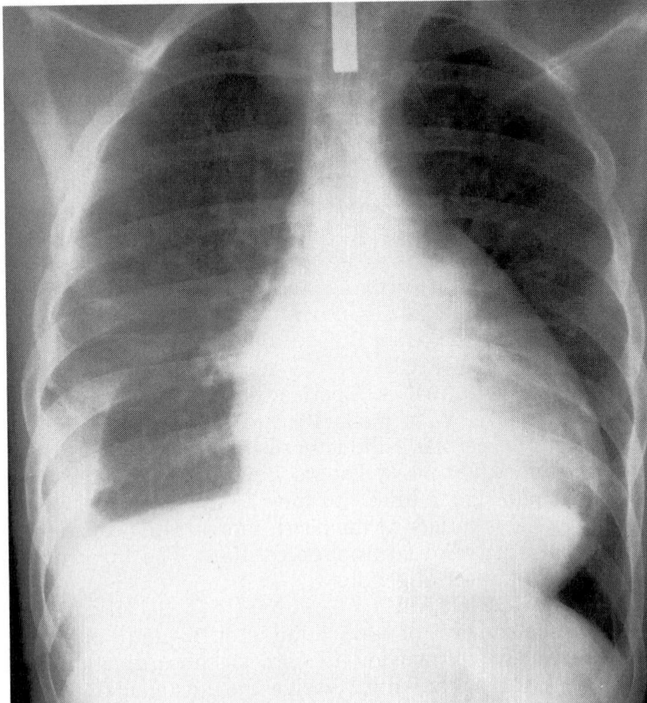

FIGURE 64–8 Anteroposterior chest radiograph of a patient with a large pericardial effusion (see text). (From Kabbani SS, LeWinter M: Cardiac constriction and restriction. *In* Crawford MH, DiMarco JP [eds]: Cardiology. St. Louis, Mosby, 2001, Sec. 5, Chap. 5, p 15.5.)

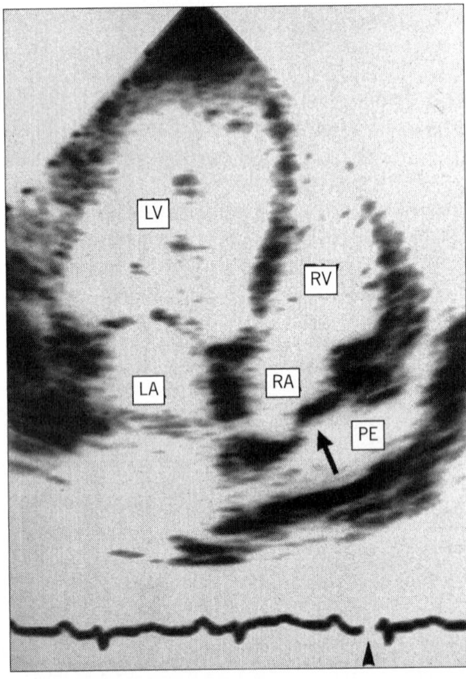

FIGURE 64–9 Two-dimensional echocardiogram of a large, circumferential pericardial effusion. LA = left atrium; LV = left ventricle; PE = pericardial effusion; RA = right atrium; RV = right ventricle. (From Kabbani SS, LeWinter M: Cardiac constriction and restriction. *In* Crawford MH, DiMarco JP [eds]: Cardiology. St. Louis, Mosby, 2001, Sec. 5, Chap. 5, p 15.5.)

detected by echocardiography suggest clots or chronic inflammatory or neoplastic pericardial processes.

As discussed previously, tamponade is best considered as a spectrum of severity of cardiac compression. Several findings indicate that tamponade is severe enough to cause some degree of hemodynamic compromise. Early diastolic collapse of the right ventricle (Fig. 64–10) and right atrium (which occurs during *ventricular* diastole) (Fig. 64–11) are sensitive and specific signs that appear relatively early during the course of tamponade.[15,30] Both occur because the pericardial pressure transiently exceeds the intracavitary pressure. A large *pleural* effusion can also elevate the pericardial pressure sufficiently to cause right ventricular collapse.[37] Left ventricular collapse[38] and left atrial collapse[39] have been reported with regional effusions after cardiac surgery but are distinctly unusual. The cardiac chambers are small and, as discussed earlier, in extreme cases the heart swings anteroposteriorly within the pericardial effusion. Distention of the caval vessels during their course outside the pericardial sac is useful as a sign of increased systemic venous pressure.

Reflecting the hemodynamic abnormalities discussed earlier, Doppler velocity recordings demonstrate exaggerated respiratory variation in right- and left-sided venous and valvular flow, with marked inspiratory increases on the right side and decreases on the left (Fig. 64–12).[28,31,35] As a result of reduced systemic venous inflow during early diastole with loss of the *y* descent, most caval and pulmonary venous inflow occurs during ventricular systole.[28,29] These changes in venous flow patterns are quite sensitive for tamponade.

In the vast majority of cases of pericardial effusion, transthoracic echocardiography provides sufficient diagnostic information to make informed management decisions. Transesophageal studies, although providing better quality images, are often impractical in sick patients. However, in intubated patients the transesophageal approach can easily be employed.

OTHER IMAGING MODALITIES. Pericardial effusion causes damping or abolition of cardiac pulsation. Accordingly, fluoroscopy is useful in the cardiac catheterization laboratory for detection of an acute effusion caused by perforations.

CT and MR imaging are useful adjuncts to echocardiography in the characterization of effusion and tamponade[15] (see Chaps. 14 and 15). Neither is ordinarily required or advisable in sick patients who require prompt management and treatment decisions. They can have an important ancillary role in situations in which hemodynamics are atypical and the presence and severity of tamponade less certain, and they are invaluable when echocardiography is technically inadequate for decision-making. Both CT and MR imaging provide more detailed quantitation and regional-spatial localization of pericardial effusion than echocardiography, and they are especially useful for loculated and regional effusions. Pericardial thickness can be measured with both, allowing indirect assessment of the severity and chronicity of inflammation. Electron beam CT is especially useful in this regard. Clues to the nature of the pericardial fluid (bloody, exudative, chylous) can also be gained, for example, from attenuation coefficients of CT images. Last, real-time CT or MR cine displays can provide information similar to that provided by echocardiography for assessment of tamponade, e.g., septal shifting, atrial and ventricular collapse.

Management of Pericardial Effusion and Tamponade

Management of pericardial effusion is dictated, first and foremost, by whether tamponade is present or has a high chance of developing in the near term. Situations in which tamponade should be considered a near-term threat include suspected bacterial or tuberculous pericarditis or bleeding into the pericardial space and any situation where there is a moderate to large effusion that is not thought to be chronic or is increasing in size, or both. When tamponade is present or threatened, clinical decision-making should be undertaken with great urgency and the threshold for pericardiocentesis should be low.

EFFUSIONS WITHOUT ACTUAL OR THREATENED TAMPONADE. In the absence of actual or threatened tamponade, management can be more leisurely. This cohort of patients includes several categories. Some have acute pericarditis with a small to moderate effusion detected as part of routine evaluation. Others undergo echocardiography because of diseases known to involve the pericardium. The remainder are asymptomatic and have effusions detected when diagnostic tests are performed for reasons other than suspected pericardial disease, for example, to evaluate an unexpectedly enlarged cardiac silhouette on chest radiography, when echocardiography is performed to assess possible cardiac disease, or when CT or MR is used to investigate thoracic pathology.

In many cases of effusion in which tamponade is neither present nor threatened, an etiology is evident or strongly suggested on the basis of the history (e.g., known neoplastic or autoimmune disease, radiation therapy) or previously obtained diagnostic tests. When a diagnosis is not clear, an assessment of specific etiologies of pericardial disease should be undertaken. This assessment should in general include the diagnostic tests recommended for acute pericarditis, a careful medication review, and anything else dictated by the clinical picture. Thus, skin testing for tuberculosis and screening for neoplastic and autoimmune diseases and infections (e.g., Lyme disease) and hypothyroidism should be considered. At the same time, careful judgment should be exercised in the selection of tests for these patients. A patient with severe heart failure and circulatory congestion with a small, asymptomatic effusion does not need extensive testing. In contrast, patients with evidence of a systemic disease deserve careful attention. Serial titers of antibodies to viruses are usually not helpful or indicated in these cases because the results may be nonspecific or negative despite a viral etiology. However, situations occasionally arise in which evidence of a viral etiology, if present, is helpful in clarifying diagnostic dilemmas,

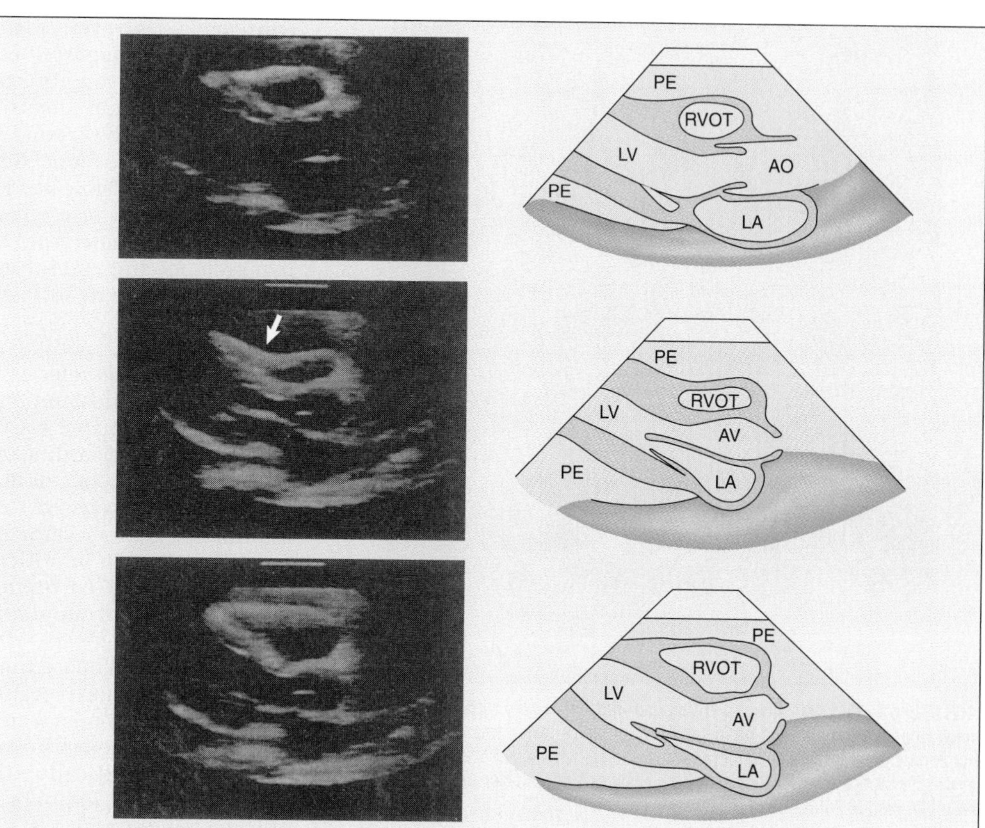

FIGURE 64–10 Two-dimensional echocardiogram illustrating diastolic collapse or indentation of the right ventricle in cardiac tamponade. **Top,** Systole; **middle,** early diastole with indentation indicated by arrow; **bottom,** late diastole with return of normal configuration. AV = aortic valve; LA = left atrium; LV = left ventricle; PE = pericardial effusion; RVOT = right ventricular outflow tract. (From Weyman AE: Principles and Practice of Echocardiography. Philadelphia, Lea & Febiger, 1994, p 1119.)

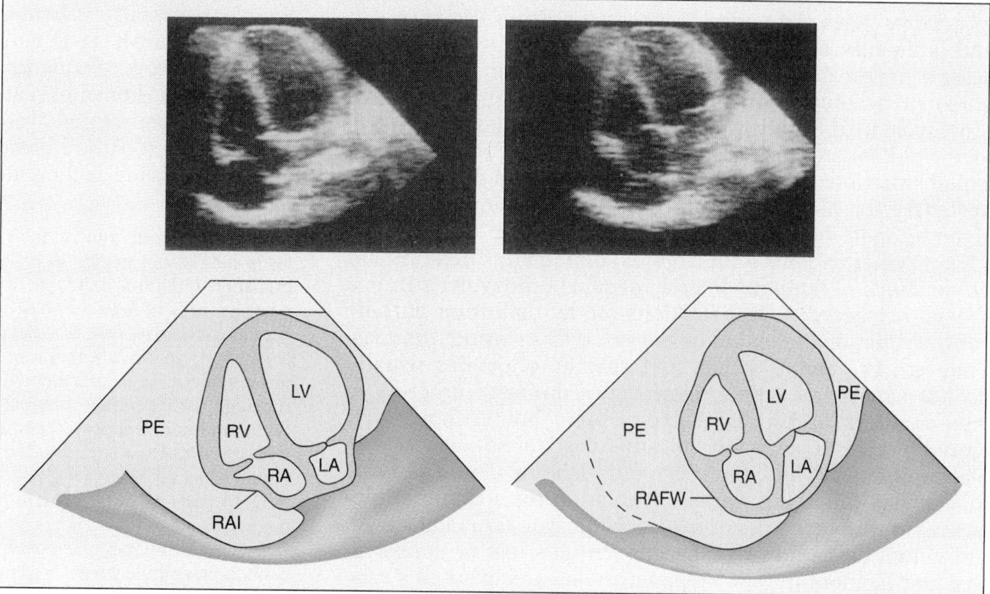

FIGURE 64–11 Two-dimensional echocardiogram illustrating right atrial collapse or indentation in cardiac tamponade. LA = left atrium; LV = left ventricle; PE = pericardial effusion; RA = right atrium; RAFW = right atrial free wall; RAI = right atrial indentation; RV = right ventricle. (From Gilliam LD: Hemodynamic compression of the right atrium: A new echocardiographic sign of cardiac tamponade. Circulation 68:294, 1983.)

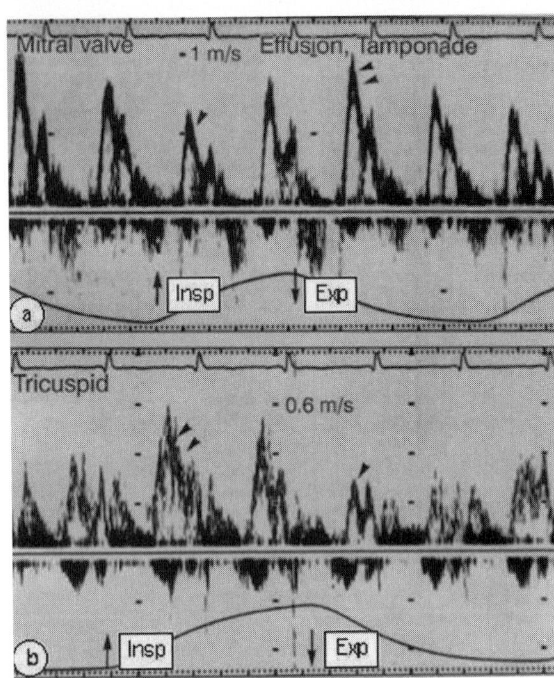

FIGURE 64–12 Transmitral and tricuspid Doppler velocity recordings in cardiac tamponade showing marked, 180 degrees out of phase respiratory variations. Exp = expiration; Insp = inspiration. (From Oh JK, Hatle LK, Mulvagh SL, Tajik AJ: Transient constrictive pericarditis: Diagnosis by two-dimensional Doppler echocardiography. Mayo Clin Proc 68:1158, 1993.)

providing reassurance, and avoiding unnecessary diagnostic testing or treatments. In these situations it is useful to save serum obtained at presentation should there be subsequent reasons for measurement of viral titers.

In this class of patients, pericardiocentesis (closed or open with biopsy) need be undertaken only for diagnostic purposes and is usually not indicated. As discussed earlier, in many cases a diagnosis either is obvious when the effusion is first noted or becomes evident as part of initial investigations. Moreover, in this setting analysis of pericardial fluid has a low yield for providing a specific diagnosis.[14,15,40] In occasional situations in which pericardiocentesis is thought to be necessary for diagnostic purposes, consideration should be given to open drainage with biopsy.

Occasional patients with large, asymptomatic effusions and no evidence of tamponade or a specific etiology constitute a special category.[25,40] The effusions are by definition chronic because tamponade would be present if this was not the case. They are in general stable, and specific etiologies usually do not emerge over time. However, a minority progress to tamponade in an unpredictable fashion. Interestingly, after closed pericardiocentesis the effusions do not necessarily reaccumulate.[25] Thus, there is a rationale for closed pericardiocentesis following routine evaluation for specific etiologies as outlined earlier. This decision can be made on an individual basis, however, because little is lost by conservative management in reliable patients who are aware of symptoms of tamponade. Before undertaking pericardiocentesis, however, a course of an NSAID, colchicine, or corticosteroids should be considered[21] as it will shrink some of these effusions.

EFFUSIONS WITH ACTUAL OR THREATENED TAMPONADE. These patients should be considered as having a true or potential medical emergency. With the exception of those who do not wish prolongation of life (mainly those with metastatic cancer), hospital admission and careful hemodynamic and echocardiographic monitoring are mandatory. Most patients require pericardiocentesis to treat or prevent tamponade. However, treatment should be carefully individualized and thoughtful clinical judgment is critical. For example, patients with acute, apparently idiopathic pericarditis or autoimmune diseases who have no more than mild tamponade can be treated with a course of prednisone and monitored in the hope that their effusions shrink rapidly. Patients with possible bacterial infections or bleeding into the pericardial sac *whose effusions are no more than moderate in size* may in some cases be suitable for initial conservative management and careful monitoring, especially because the risk of closed pericardiocentesis is increased with smaller effusions.

Hemodynamic monitoring with a balloon flotation pulmonary artery catheter is useful, especially in those with threatened or mild tamponade in whom a decision is made to defer pericardiocentesis. Hemodynamic monitoring is also helpful *after* pericardiocentesis to assess both reaccumulation and the presence of underlying constrictive disease (see Fig. 64–5), as discussed subsequently. However, insertion of a pulmonary artery catheter should not be allowed to delay definitive therapy in critically ill patients.

Intravenous Hydration. For most patients in this category, management should be directed toward urgent or emergent pericardiocentesis, with timing dependent on individual circumstances. When actual or threatened tamponade is diagnosed, intravenous hydration should be instituted, especially as some patients mistakenly receive diuretics because of an incorrect diagnosis of heart failure. In patients with tamponade who are critically ill, intravenous positive inotropes (dobutamine, dopamine) can be employed but are of limited efficacy. Hydration and positive inotropes are temporizing measures and should not be allowed to substitute for or delay pericardiocentesis.

Pericardiocentesis. In the vast majority of circumstances, closed pericardiocentesis is the initial treatment of choice. However, before proceeding it is important to be confident that there is indeed an effusion large enough to cause tamponade, especially if hemodynamics are atypical. Loculated effusions as well as effusions containing clots or fibrinous material are also of concern because the risk and difficulty of closed pericardiocentesis are increased. In these situations, if removal of pericardial fluid is thought to be necessary, an open approach should be considered for safety and to obtain pericardial tissue and create a pericardial window.

The most commonly employed approach to closed pericardiocentesis is subxiphoid needle insertion performed under echocardiographic guidance to minimize the risk of puncture of the myocardium and assess completeness of fluid removal.[41] When the needle has entered the pericardial space, a modest amount of fluid should be removed (perhaps 50 to 150 ml) in an effort to produce some degree of hemodynamic improvement. Then, a guidewire should be inserted and the needle replaced with a pigtail catheter. The catheter can then be manipulated with continuing echocardiographic guidance to maximize the amount of fluid removed. In a large, modern series from the Mayo Clinic,[41] the procedural success rate was 97 percent and the complication rate was 4.7 percent (major, 1.2 percent; minor, 3.5 percent). The procedure should be performed in the cardiac catheterization laboratory with experienced personnel in attendance unless the patient is too ill to be moved. If echocardiographic guidance is unavailable, the needle should be directed toward the right shoulder and then replaced with a catheter for subsequent fluid removal. CT fluoroscopy-guided drainage of effusions is an alternative when echocardiography cannot be used.[42]

If a pulmonary artery catheter has been inserted, right-heart, pulmonary capillary wedge, and systemic arterial pressures should be monitored before, during, and after and cardiac output measured before and after the procedure. Ideally, pressure should also be measured in the pericardial fluid. As discussed earlier, removal of relatively small amounts of fluid can result in substantial hemodynamic improvement. Hemodynamic monitoring before, during, and after pericardiocentesis is useful for several reasons. Initial measurements confirm and document the severity of tamponade. Assessment after completion establishes a baseline to assess reaccumulation, which is especially important if it is not possible to remove all fluid. As discussed in more detail subsequently, some patients presenting with tamponade have a coexisting component of constriction (i.e., effusive-constrictive pericarditis),[15] which is virtually impossible to detect when an effusion dominates the picture. Filling pressures that remain elevated after pericardiocentesis as well as the appearance of venous waveforms typical of constriction (rapid x and y descents) indicate coexistent constriction.

Following pericardiocentesis, continued hemodynamic monitoring and repeated echocardiography are recommended to check for reaccumulation. The length of continued monitoring is a matter of judgment but, typically, pulmonary artery catheter pressures are measured for about 24 hours and a follow-up echocardiogram is performed immediately before its removal. If hemodynamic changes indicating reaccumulation appear, echocardiography should be performed sooner. In most cases the intrapericardial catheter is left in place with heparinized saline in its lumen for 12 to 24 hours to facilitate repeated fluid removal. It also allows delivery of intrapericardial drugs to treat specific etiologies.

Open Pericardiocentesis. Open pericardiocentesis is occasionally preferred for the initial removal of pericardial fluid. Loculated effusions or effusions that are borderline in size are drained more safely in the operating room. Recurring effusions, especially those causing tamponade, are often initially drained using a closed approach because of logistical considerations. However, open pericardiocentesis, with biopsy and establishment of a pericardial window, is preferred for most recurrences when they are severe enough to cause tamponade. Creation of a window reliably eliminates future episodes of cardiac tamponade and provides pericardial tissue to assist in diagnosis. The surgeon should inspect the pericardium carefully and obtain multiple biopsies. Also, percutaneous balloon approaches have become available for drainage of effusions[43,44] as well as pericardioscopy and biopsy.[45] These methods appear to be quite safe and effective for producing pericardial windows, but at present they are available in only a few centers.

ANALYSIS OF PERICARDIAL FLUID (Table 64–3). Although analysis of pericardial fluid has a disappointing overall yield in identifying the etiology of pericardial disease, careful analysis can nonetheless be rewarding. *Assuming a diagnosis is not known before fluid removal*, routine pericardial fluid measurements should include specific gravity, white blood cell count and differential, hematocrit, and protein content.[14,15] Although most effusions are exudates, detection of a transudate reduces the diagnostic possibilities considerably. Blood in pericardial fluid is a nonspecific finding. Because pericardial blood usually undergoes rapid fibrinolysis, a low hematocrit does not exclude bleeding. Chylous effusions can occur after traumatic or surgical injury to the thoracic duct or obstruction by a neoplastic process. Occasionally they are idiopathic. Cholesterol-rich effusions occur in severe hypothyroidism. In certain circumstances, determination of bilirubin or cholesterol levels in pericardial fluid may be diagnostically useful.

Pericardial fluid should be routinely stained and cultured for detection of bacteria, including tuberculosis, and fungi. As much fluid as possible should be submitted for detection of malignant cells as there is a reasonably high yield for diagnosis of malignancy in patients with pericardial involvement. Elevated adenosine deaminase levels have high sensitivity and specificity for tuberculous pericardial disease.[46-48] Unless some other etiology is evident, adenosine deaminase should be a routine test because of the general difficulty of diagnosing tuberculous pericarditis and the delays involved in making a diagnosis by culture. Increased interferon-gamma in fluid also appears promising in the diagnosis of tuberculous pericarditis.[48] There may be a role for routine measurement of carcinoembryonic antigen as a general screen for malignant effusion and an adjunct to direct detection of malignant cells.[46,47]

TABLE 64–3 Routine Analysis of Pericardial Fluid
Specific gravity, white blood cell count and differential, hematocrit, protein content
Stain and culture for bacteria, including tuberculosis
Analysis for malignant cells
Adenosine deaminase
Consider: carcinoembryonic antigen, bilirubin, cholesterol

Constrictive Pericarditis

Etiology

Constrictive pericarditis represents the end stage of an inflammatory process involving the pericardium. Although virtually any of the inflammatory processes listed in Table 64–1 can cause constriction, in the industrialized world the etiology is most commonly infectious, postsurgical, or radiation injury (Table 64–4).[49] Tuberculosis was the most common cause of constrictive pericarditis in the developed world before the development of effective drug therapy. It is now much less prevalent. Although the constrictive process can follow an initial insult by as little as several months, constriction usually takes years to develop. The end result is dense fibrosis, often calcification, and adhesions of the parietal and visceral pericardium. Usually the scarring process is more or less symmetrical and impedes filling of all the heart chambers. The clinical presentation is dominated by signs and symptoms of right-sided heart failure.

Pathophysiology

The pathophysiological consequence of pericardial scarring is markedly restricted filling of all of the cardiac chambers This symmetrical effect results in elevation and equilibration of filling pressures in all chambers as well as the systemic and pulmonary veins. In early diastole the ventricles fill abnormally rapidly because of markedly elevated atrial pressures and accentuated early diastolic ventricular suction, the latter related to small end-systolic volumes. During early to mid-diastole, ventricular filling is abruptly halted when the intracardiac volume reaches the limit set by the noncompliant pericardium. As a result, almost all ventricular filling occurs very early in diastole. Systemic venous congestion results in hepatic congestion, peripheral edema, ascites, and sometimes anasarca and cardiac cirrhosis. Reduced cardiac index is also a consequence of impaired filling and results in fatigue, muscle wasting, and weight loss. In "pure" constriction, myocardial contractile function is preserved, although ejection fraction can be reduced as a consequence

TABLE 64–4 Causes of Constrictive Pericarditis
Idiopathic
Irradiation
Postsurgical
Infectious
Neoplastic
Autoimmune (connective tissue) disorders
Uremia
Posttraumatic
Sarcoid
Methysergide therapy
Implantable defibrillator patches

of reduced preload. However, the myocardium is occasionally involved in the chronic inflammation and fibrosis, leading to true contractile dysfunction that can at times be quite severe. The latter is also a predictor of a poor response to pericardiectomy.

An important contributor to the pathophysiology of constrictive pericarditis is failure of transmission of intrathoracic pressure changes during respiration to the cardiac chambers (Fig. 64–13). These changes continue to be transmitted to the pulmonary circulation. Thus, on inspiration the drop in intrathoracic pressure (and therefore pulmonary venous pressure) is not transmitted to the left side of the heart, including the left atrium. Consequently, on inspiration the small pulmonary vein to left atrial pressure gradient that normally drives left-heart filling is reduced, resulting in decreased left atrial inflow and transmitral filling. The inspiratory decrease in left ventricular filling allows an increase in right ventricular filling along with an interventricular septal shift to the left. The opposite sequence occurs with expiration.[15,50]

High systemic venous pressure and reduced cardiac output result in compensatory retention of sodium and water by the kidneys. Inhibition of atrial natriuretic peptide also contributes to renal sodium retention and further exacerbates increases in systemic venous and left-sided filling pressures.[51]

Clinical Presentation

The usual presentation consists of signs and symptoms of predominantly right-sided heart failure with normal or near-normal ventricular systolic function as assessed by echocardiography. At a relatively early stage these signs and symptoms include lower extremity edema, vague abdominal complaints, and some degree of passive hepatic congestion. As the disease becomes more severe, hepatic congestion worsens and can progress to frank jaundice, ascites or anasarca or both, and cardiac cirrhosis. Signs and symptoms ascribable to elevated pulmonary venous pressures such as exertional dyspnea, cough, and orthopnea may also appear with progressive disease. Atrial fibrillation and tricuspid regurgitation, which further exacerbates venous pressure elevation, may also appear at this stage. In the end stage of constrictive pericarditis, the effects of a chronically low cardiac output are prominent, including severe fatigue, muscle wasting, and weight loss. Rarely, initial symptoms include recurrent pleural effusions, transient ischemic attack and syncope. Clinically, severe end-stage constrictive pericarditis can be mistaken for any cause of severe right-sided heart failure as well as end-stage primary liver disease. Of course, the venous pressure is not elevated with primary liver disease.

Physical Examination

VENOUS PATTERN. Physical findings include marked elevation of jugular venous pressure with a prominent, rapidly collapsing *y* descent. This, combined with a normally prominent *x* descent, results in an M- or W-shaped venous pressure contour. At the bedside, this is best appreciated as two prominent descents with each cardiac cycle. In patients in atrial fibrillation the *x* descent is lost, leaving only the prominent *y* descent. The latter is difficult to distinguish from tricuspid regurgitation, which, as noted earlier, may itself occur as a consequence of constrictive pericarditis. The *Kussmaul sign*, an inspiratory increase in systemic venous pressure, is usually present.[15] Occasionally, the venous pressure simply fails to decrease on inspiration rather than actually increase. The Kussmaul sign reflects loss of the normal increase in right-heart venous return on inspiration even though tricuspid flow increases. These characteristic abnormalities of the venous waveform are in marked contrast to those observed in cardiac tamponade. A paradoxical pulse occurs in perhaps one-third of patients with constrictive pericarditis and is especially common when there is an effusive-constrictive picture. It is best explained by the aforementioned lack of transmission of decreased intrathoracic pressure to the left heart chambers.

PERICARDIAL KNOCK. In cases with extensive calcification and adhesion of the heart to adjacent structures, cardiac examination may reveal that the point of maximal impulse does not vary with changes in position. However, the most notable cardiac finding is the pericardial knock, which is an early diastolic sound best heard at the left sternal border or the cardiac apex, or both. It occurs slightly earlier and has a higher acoustic frequency than a third heart sound. The knock corresponds to the early, abrupt cessation of ventricular filling. Widening of second heart sound splitting may also be present. As noted previously, a significant number of patients with constrictive pericarditis have secondary tricuspid regurgitation with its characteristic systolic murmur.

Abdominal examination reveals hepatomegaly, often with palpable venous pulsations, with or without ascites. Other signs of chronic hepatic congestion may include jaundice,

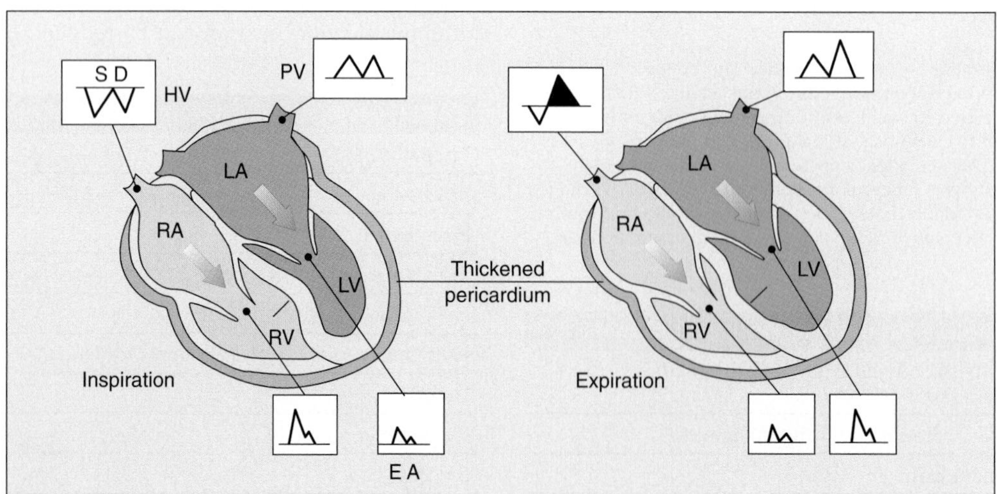

FIGURE 64–13 Schematic representation of transvalvular and central venous flow velocities in constrictive pericarditis. During inspiration the decrease in left ventricular filling results in a leftward septal shift allowing augmented flow into the right ventricle. The opposite occurs during expiration. D = diastolic venous flow; EA = mitral inflow; HV = hepatic vein; LA = left atrium; LV = left ventricle; PV = pulmonary venous flow; RA = right atrium; RV = right ventricle; S = systolic venous flow.

spider angiomata, and palmar erythema. Lower extremity edema is usually present and anasarca occurs in some cases. Patients with end-stage constrictive pericarditis may develop muscle wasting and cachexia with massive ascites and edema of the scrotum and lower extremities. The resemblance to end-stage, primary liver disease has already been noted.

Laboratory Testing

ELECTROCARDIOGRAM. There are no specific ECG findings. Nonspecific T wave abnormalities are often observed, as well as reduced voltage. Left atrial abnormality may also be present. Atrial fibrillation is present in a significant number of patients.

CHEST RADIOGRAPH (see Chap. 12). The chest radiograph frequently shows right atrial enlargement. The cardiac silhouette can be enlarged secondary to a coexisting pericardial effusion. Pericardial calcification is seen in a small number of patients and should raise suspicion of tuberculous pericarditis (Fig. 64–14). At the same time, calcification per se is by no means diagnostic of constrictive physiology. The lateral chest film is useful to detect pericardial calcification along the right heart border and in the atrioventricular groove. Isolated calcification of the left ventricular apex or posterior wall is typical of ventricular aneurysm rather than pericardial calcification. Pleural effusions are occasionally present and can be a presenting sign of constrictive pericarditis. When left-heart filling pressures are markedly elevated, pulmonary vascular congestion and redistribution can also be present.

ECHOCARDIOGRAM (see Chap. 11). M-mode and two-dimensional echocardiography findings include pericardial thickening and immobility, abrupt displacement of the interventricular septum during early diastole (septal "bounce"),[15] and signs of systemic venous congestion such as dilation of hepatic veins and distention of the inferior vena cava with blunted respiratory fluctuation. Premature pulmonic valve opening as a result of elevated right ventricular early diastolic pressure may also be observed. Exaggerated septal shifting during respiration is often present.

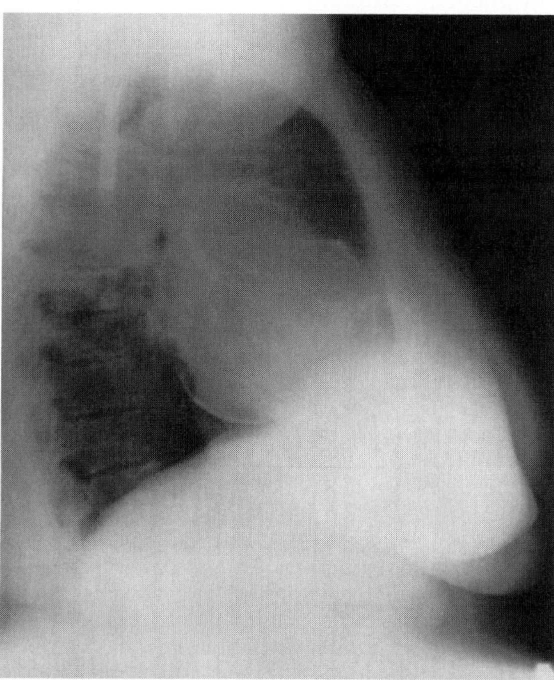

FIGURE 64–14 Chest radiograph showing marked pericardial calcifications in a patient with constrictive pericarditis.

Doppler Measurements. The role of lack of transmission of intrathoracic pressure to the cardiac chambers and resulting mitral and tricuspid inflow patterns in constrictive pericarditis has already been discussed. In accordance with these patterns, Doppler flow velocity measurements reveal exaggerated respiratory variation in both mitral inflow velocity and tricuspid-mitral inflow differences, with the latter being 180 degrees out of phase (see Fig. 64-13). Although there is some overlap with cardiac tamponade, these inflow patterns have good sensitivity and specificity for constrictive pericarditis and also help to distinguish between restrictive cardiomyopathy and constrictive pericarditis.[15,50,52] Typically, patients with pericardial constriction demonstrate an increase in mitral E velocity greater than or equal to 25 percent during expiration compared with inspiration and increased diastolic flow reversal with expiration in the hepatic veins. Mitral E wave deceleration time is usually but not always less than 160 msec. These Doppler echocardiographic findings have 88 percent sensitivity for the diagnosis of constrictive pericarditis. A subset of patients (up to 20 percent) with constriction do not exhibit typical respiratory changes, most likely because of markedly increased left atrial pressure or possibly a mixed constrictive-restrictive pattern related to myocardial involvement by the constrictive process. In patients without typical respiratory mitral-tricuspid flow velocity findings, examination after maneuvers that decrease preload (head-up tilt or sitting) can unmask the characteristic respiratory variation in mitral E velocity.[53]

A similar pattern of respiratory variation in mitral inflow velocity can be observed in chronic obstructive lung disease, right ventricular infarction, pulmonary embolism, and pleural effusion. Most of these conditions have other clinical and echocardiographic features that differentiate them from constrictive pericarditis. Superior vena caval flow velocities are particularly helpful in distinguishing between constrictive pericarditis and chronic obstructive pulmonary disease. Patients with pulmonary disease display a marked increase in inspiratory superior vena caval systolic forward flow velocity, which is not seen in constrictive pericarditis.

Transesophageal Echocardiography. Transesophageal echocardiography can be used as a valuable adjunct in assessing constrictive pericarditis. It is superior to transthoracic echocardiography for measuring pericardial thickness and has an excellent correlation with CT for this purpose.[54] Moreover, when mitral inflow velocities by transthoracic echocardiography are technically inadequate or equivocal, measurement of pulmonary venous Doppler velocities using the transesophageal approach demonstrates pronounced respiratory variation, even larger than that observed across the mitral valve.[55]

CARDIAC CATHETERIZATION AND ANGIOGRAPHY (see Chaps. 17 and 18). Right- and left-heart catheterization and coronary angiography in patients suspected of having constrictive pericarditis provide documentation of the hemodynamics of constrictive physiology and assist in the discrimination between constrictive pericarditis and restrictive cardiomyopathy.[56] Although there is limited need for contrast ventriculography in these patients, coronary angiography is used to detect occult coronary artery disease in those being considered for pericardiectomy. In addition, on rare occasions external pinching or compression of the coronary arteries or outflow tract regions by the constricting pericardium is detected.

Right- and left-heart pressures should be recorded simultaneously at equisensitive gains, with meticulous attention to calibration. Right atrial, right ventricular diastolic, pulmonary capillary wedge, and pre-a wave left ventricular diastolic pressure are elevated and equal, or nearly so, at around 20 mm Hg. Differences of more than 3 to 5 mm Hg between left- and right-heart filling pressures are rarely encountered. The right atrial pressure tracing shows a preserved x descent, a prominent y descent, and roughly equal a and v wave height, with the resultant M or W shape configuration. Both right and left ventricular pressures reveal an early, marked diastolic dip followed by a plateau ("dip and plateau" or "square root" sign) (Fig. 64-15). Pulmonary artery and right ventricular systolic pressures are usually modestly elevated, in the range 35 to 45 mm Hg. Pulmonary hypertension is not a feature of constrictive pericarditis and is indicative of coexisting cardiac or pulmonary disease. Hypovolemia, such as may occur secondary to diuretic therapy, can mask the typical hemodynamic findings. Rapid volume challenge with 1000 ml of normal saline over 6 to 8 minutes may unmask the hemodynamic features of constrictive pericarditis.[57]

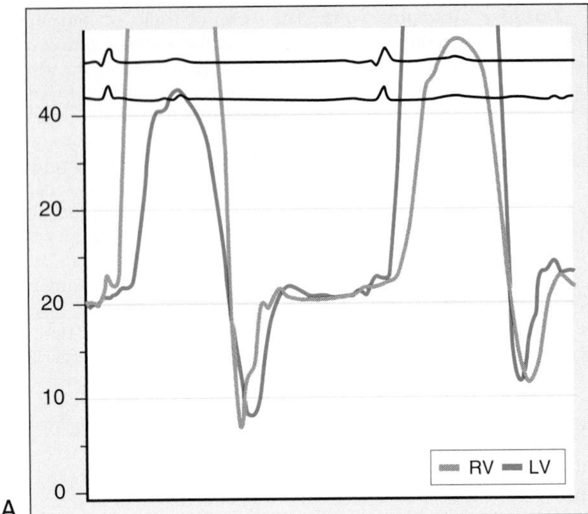

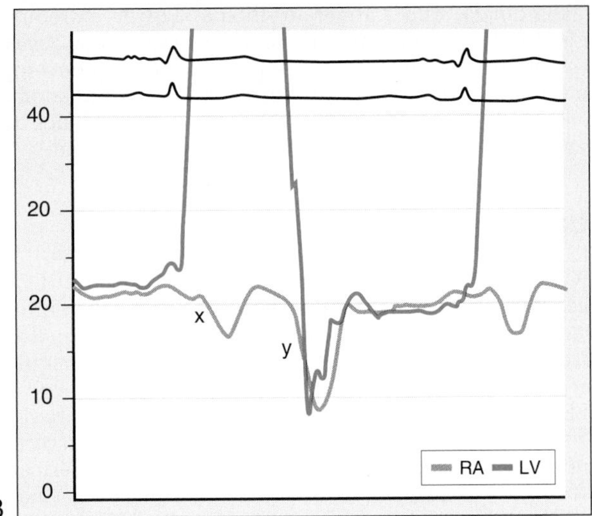

FIGURE 64–15 Pressure recordings in a patient with constrictive pericarditis. **A,** Simultaneous right ventricular (RV) and left ventricular (LV) pressure tracings with equalization of diastolic pressure as well as "dip and plateau" morphology. **B,** Simultaneous right atrial (RA) and LV pressure with equalization of RA and LV diastolic pressure. Note the prominent *y* descent. (From Vaitkus PT, Cooper KA, Shuman WP, Hardin NJ: Images in cardiovascular medicine: Constrictive pericarditis. Circulation 93:834, 1996.)

Stroke volume is almost always reduced but resting cardiac output can be preserved because of tachycardia. Depression of stroke volume is primarily related to reduced diastolic filling. In the absence of extensive coexisting myocardial involvement, left ventricular ejection fraction is normal or slightly reduced.

COMPUTED TOMOGRAPHY AND MAGNETIC RESONANCE IMAGING. CT provides detailed images of the pericardium and is especially helpful in detecting even minute amounts of pericardial calcification (Fig. 64–16). The major disadvantage of CT is the frequent need for administration of iodinated intravenous contrast material for best display of findings of pericardial pathology. The thickness of the normal pericardium measured by CT is less than 2 mm. MR imaging provides a detailed and comprehensive examination of the pericardium and heart without the need for iodinated contrast material or ionizing radiation. It is significantly less sensitive for detecting calcification than is CT. The "normal" pericardium visualized by MR imaging has been reported to be up to 4 mm in thickness. This measurement most likely reflects the entire pericardial "complex," with physiological fluid representing a significant component of the measured thickness.[58]

FIGURE 64–16 Computed tomographic scan showing increased pericardial thickness and mild calcification in a patient with constrictive pericarditis.

Demonstration of a thickened pericardium with or without calcification indicates acute or chronic pericarditis. If there is clinical evidence of impaired diastolic filling, pericardial thickening, especially if calcification is present, is virtually diagnostic of constriction. The absence of pericardial thickening argues against the diagnosis of constriction but does not completely rule it out. The pericardium can be globally thickened, but thickening is often focal. Localized compression of the heart caused by focal thickening is reported and occurs much more commonly on the right than the left side. In patients being considered for pericardiectomy, detailed descriptions of the location and severity of thickening and calcification aid the surgeon with respect to both risk stratification and planning of the operation. Additional CT and MR findings include distorted ventricular contours, hepatic venous congestion, ascites, pleural effusions, and occasionally pericardial effusion. Often there is dilation of the atria, coronary sinus, inferior vena cava, and hepatic veins. Cine acquisition (MR or electron beam CT) shows abnormal motion of the interventricular septum in early diastole.

Differentiating Constrictive Pericarditis from Restrictive Cardiomyopathy

Because their treatment is radically different, distinguishing constrictive pericarditis from restrictive cardiomyopathy is extremely important (Table 64–5). Their presentation and course overlap in many respects. An unequivocal pericardial knock points to constriction, but prominent third heart sounds in restrictive disease can confuse their bedside differentiation. ECG and chest radiographic findings are mostly nonspecific. However, a calcified pericardium indicates constrictive pericarditis and a low-voltage QRS suggests amyloidosis. There are some useful, albeit not invariably reliable, echocardiographic distinctions. Patients with restrictive cardiomyopathy usually have thick-walled ventricles because of infiltrative processes such as amyloidosis. Biatrial enlargement is also common in restriction. In constrictive pericarditis, the most distinctive finding is the ventricular septal bounce. As discussed earlier, the pericardium is usually thickened in constriction, but this may be difficult to assess

TABLE 64–5 Hemodynamic and Echocardiographic Features of Constrictive Pericarditis Compared with Restrictive Cardiomyopathy

Feature	Constriction	Restriction
Prominent *y* descent in venous pressure	Present	Variable
Paradoxical pulse	~1/3 of cases	Absent
Pericardial knock	Present	Absent
Equal right side–left side filling pressures	Present	Left at least 3–5 mm Hg > right
Filling pressures > 25 mm Hg	Rare	Common
Pulmonary artery systolic pressure > 60 mm Hg	No	Common
"Square root" sign	Present	Variable
Respiratory variation in left-right pressures or flows	Exaggerated	Normal
Ventricular wall thickness	Normal	Usually increased
Atrial size	Possible left atrial enlargement	Biatrial enlargement
Septal "bounce"	Present	Absent
Pericardial thickness	Increased	Normal

on transthoracic echocardiography. As noted, data indicate that transesophageal echocardiographic measurements of pericardial thickness correlate well with electron beam CT measurements.[54]

DOPPLER MEASUREMENTS. Doppler flow measurements are often useful in differentiating constrictive from restrictive physiology. Enhanced respiratory variation in mitral inflow velocity (>25 percent) is seen in constriction, whereas in restriction mitral inflow velocity varies by less than 10 percent (see Fig. 64–13). In restriction, pulmonary venous systolic flow is markedly blunted and diastolic flow is increased. This pattern is not observed in constriction. Hepatic veins demonstrate enhanced expiratory flow reversal with constriction, in contrast to increased inspiratory flow reversal in restriction.[15,59] Tissue Doppler echocardiography and color M-mode flow propagation have been shown to be complementary to mitral Doppler respiratory variation in distinguishing between constrictive pericarditis and restrictive cardiomyopathy.

HEMODYNAMICS. Hemodynamic differentiation between constrictive pericarditis and restrictive cardiomyopathy in the cardiac catheterization laboratory can be difficult. However, careful attention to the hemodynamic profile usually helps in making the distinction. In both conditions, right and left ventricular diastolic pressures are markedly elevated. In restrictive cardiomyopathy, however, diastolic pressure in the left ventricle is higher than in the right ventricle at rest or during exercise, usually by at least 3 to 5 mm Hg. As discussed earlier, in constrictive pericarditis left- and right-sided diastolic pressures are very close and demonstrate minimal change during exercise. Pulmonary hypertension is common with restrictive cardiomyopathy but rare in constrictive pericarditis. Marked elevation of right ventricular systolic pressure (>60 mm Hg) is usually indicative of restrictive cardiomyopathy. The absolute level of atrial or ventricular diastolic pressure elevation is also sometimes useful in distinguishing the two conditions, with extremely high pressures (>25 mm Hg) much more common in restrictive cardiomyopathy.[56]

COMPUTED TOMOGRAPHY AND MAGNETIC RESONANCE. CT (especially electron beam) and MR, because of their superior ability to provide detailed assessment of pericardial thickness and calcification, are very useful in differentiating constriction from restriction.[58] However, patients in whom constriction is present can rarely have normal pericardial thickness indicated by these imaging modalities.

Endomyocardial biopsy (or abdominal fat pad biopsy in amyloidosis) is often helpful in documenting the etiology of restrictive cardiomyopathy when an infiltrative process is involved. However, normal biopsy findings do not exclude restrictive cardiomyopathy.

The availability of the multiple diagnostic techniques that have been discussed has made it rare to have to resort to exploratory thoracotomy to distinguish between constriction and restriction. In difficult cases, however, it is often important to obtain as much diagnostic information as possible.

Management

Constrictive pericarditis is a progressive disease. Surgical pericardiectomy is the only definitive treatment. With the exception of patients with major comorbidities or severe debilitation who are considered to be at too high risk to withstand the surgery, the operation should not be delayed when the diagnosis is made. Medical management with diuretics and salt restriction is useful for symptomatic relief of fluid overload and peripheral edema, but patients ultimately become refractory. Sinus tachycardia is a compensatory mechanism. Thus, beta-adrenergic blockers and calcium antagonists that slow the heart rate should be avoided or used with great care. In patients with atrial fibrillation and a rapid ventricular response, digoxin is recommended as initial treatment to slow the ventricular rate before resorting to beta-adrenergic blockers or calcium antagonists. In general, the ventricular rate should not be allowed to drop below 80 to 90 beats/min.

PERICARDIECTOMY. Pericardiectomy is performed through a median sternotomy and involves radical excision of as much of the parietal pericardium as possible. After removal of the parietal pericardium, the visceral pericardium is inspected. Resection of the visceral pericardium should be considered if it is involved in the disease process. Most surgeons initially attempt to perform the operation without cardiopulmonary bypass. The latter should be available as back-up and is frequently required to facilitate access to the lateral and diaphragmatic surfaces of the left ventricle and allow safe removal of a maximal amount of pericardial tissue. Ultrasonic débridement is useful as an adjunct to conventional surgical débridement techniques.[60]

Hemodynamic and symptomatic improvement is achieved in some patients immediately after operation. However, in others symptomatic improvement may be delayed for weeks to months. Seventy to 80 percent of patients remain free from adverse cardiovascular outcomes at 5 years and 40 to 50 percent at 10 years after pericardiectomy.[49] Long-term results are worst in patients with radiation-induced disease. In an echocardiographic analysis, left ventricular diastolic function returned to normal in 40 percent of patients early and 57 percent late after pericardiectomy.[61] Persistence of abnormal diastolic filling was correlated with postoperative symptomatic status. Delayed or inadequate responses to pericardiectomy have been attributed to longstanding disease with myocardial atrophy or fibrosis, incomplete pericardial resection, and the development of recurrent cardiac compression by mediastinal inflammation and fibrosis. Lack of improvement after pericardiectomy may also be due to inadequate resection of visceral pericardium. Worsening of underlying tricuspid regurgitation can also cause hemodynamic deterioration after pericardiectomy.

Pericardiectomy is associated with 5 to 15 percent perioperative mortality in patients with constrictive pericarditis. Survival at 5 and 10 years is about 80 and 60 percent, respectively. Early mortality results primarily from low cardiac output, often in debilitated patients with prolonged cardiopulmonary bypass caused by difficult pericardial dissections. Sepsis, uncontrolled hemorrhage, and renal and respiratory insufficiency also contribute to early postoperative mortality.[15,61] The highest mortality occurs in patients with class III and IV preoperative symptoms. This observation supports the recommendation that pericardiectomy be performed early in the disease process, before marked clinical deterioration and myocardial damage occur.

Effusive-Constrictive Pericarditis

A significant number of patients with pericardial disease present with a syndrome that combines elements of effusion-tamponade and constriction, with a subacute or chronic course. It is common for an inflammatory effusion to dominate the picture initially, with constrictive findings prominent later. As noted earlier, these patients are sometimes identified when hemodynamics fail to normalize after pericardiocentesis. Etiologies are diverse, but the most common are probably malignancy, radiation, and tuberculosis. Physical, hemodynamic, and echocardiographic abnormalities are often mixtures of those associated with effusion and constriction and may vary considerably with time as the syndrome progresses. Diagnosis may require acquisition of pericardial fluid and biopsies if the etiology is not obvious. It is important to be cautious in performing closed pericardiocentesis in these patients when they do not have large effusions. Management is tailored to the specific etiology, if known. In our experience, it is usual for these patients to ultimately require pericardiectomy.

Specific Causes of Pericardial Disease

Bacterial Pericarditis

ETIOLOGY AND PATHOPHYSIOLOGY. Bacterial pericarditis is usually characterized by a purulent pericardial effusion. A wide variety of organisms can be causative.[15,62] Direct extension from pneumonia or empyema accounts for the majority of cases, with the most common agents being staphylococci, pneumococci, and streptococci. Hematogenous spread during bacteremia and contiguous spread after thoracic surgery or trauma are also important mechanisms of bacterial pericarditis. Hospital-acquired, penicillin-resistant staphylococcal pericarditis after thoracic surgery has increased during the past decade. There is increasing incidence of anaerobic organisms grown from pericardial fluid, the most common being *Prevotella* and *Peptostreptococcus* species and *Propionibacterium acnes*. Concomitant infection in the mediastinum or head and neck is most commonly associated with anaerobic isolates.[63,64]

Bacterial pericarditis can also result from rupture of perivalvular abscesses into the pericardial space in patients with endocarditis (see Chap. 58). Rarely, pericardial invasion spreads along fascial planes from the oral cavity, particularly periodontal and peritonsillar abscesses. The pericardium can become infected during meningococcal sepsis, producing primary meningococcal pericarditis. This can occur in the presence or absence of meningitis. In contrast to the usual purulent fluid, the *Neisseria* group can evoke a sterile effusion accompanied by systemic reactions such as arthritis, pleuritis, and ophthalmitis. This syndrome appears to have an immunological basis. It does not require antibiotic therapy and responds to antiinflammatory drugs.

CLINICAL FEATURES. The clinical presentation of bacterial pericarditis is usually high-grade fever with shaking chills and tachycardia, but one or more of these may be absent in debilitated patients. Patients may complain of dyspnea and chest pain. A pericardial friction rub is present in the majority of cases. Bacterial pericarditis can take a fulminant course with rapid development of cardiac tamponade. The disease may be unsuspected because underlying or associated illnesses such as severe pneumonia or mediastinitis after thoracic surgery dominate the clinical picture. Laboratory findings include leukocytosis with marked left shift. The pericardial fluid shows polymorphonuclear leukocytosis, low glucose, high protein, and elevated lactate dehydrogenase levels. Frank pus can occasionally be drained. The chest radiograph shows widening of the cardiac silhouette if the effusion is sufficiently large. With gas-producing organisms a lucent air-fluid interface may be observed. The electrocardiogram shows typical ST segment and T wave changes of acute pericarditis, along with low voltage if there is a large effusion. Two-dimensional echocardiography almost always demonstrates a significant pericardial effusion with or without adhesions. Cardiac tamponade is common and causes hemodynamic deterioration that can be confused with septic shock.

MANAGEMENT. Suspected or proven bacterial pericarditis should be considered a medical emergency and prompt closed pericardiocentesis or surgical drainage performed, with long-term catheter drainage if purulent fluid is obtained. Fluid should be submitted for Gram stain and cultured for aerobic and anaerobic bacteria with appropriate antibiotic sensitivity testing. Fungal and tuberculosis staining and cultures should also be performed on pericardial fluid. If not previously done, cultures of blood, sputum, urine, and recent surgical wounds should be obtained. Broad-spectrum antibiotics should be promptly started and then selected according to Gram stain and culture results. Anaerobic coverage is critical when pericardial infection secondary to head and neck infections is suspected.

Purulent pericardial effusions are likely to recur. Thus, surgical drainage with construction of a window is often needed. In patients with thick, purulent effusions and dense adhesions, extensive pericardiectomy may be required to achieve adequate drainage and prevent the development of constrictive pericarditis. *Early* surgical drainage may also help prevent late constriction. The prognosis for bacterial pericarditis is generally poor,[63,65,66] with survival in the range of 30 percent even in modern series. This poor prognosis probably reflects delays in diagnosis, disease severity, and comorbidities.[65,66]

Pericardial Disease and Human Immunodeficiency Virus (see Chap. 61)

ETIOLOGY AND PATHOPHYSIOLOGY A wide variety of pericardial disease etiologies have been reported in patients infected with HIV. It is estimated that 20 percent of patients infected with HIV have pericardial involvement. Pericardial disease is the most common cardiac manifestation of HIV disease, and the most common abnormality is a pericardial effusion.[67-69] The majority of effusions are small and asymptomatic. The effusion may be part of a generalized seroeffusive process also involving pleural and peritoneal surfaces. This "capillary leak" syndrome is probably related to enhanced cytokine expression in the later stages of HIV disease. Moderate to large effusions are more frequent in patients with more advanced stages of HIV infection. Congestive heart failure, Kaposi sarcoma, tuberculosis, and pulmonary infections are independently associated with moderate to large pericardial effusions in patients with HIV. Other forms of pericardial disease are less frequent and include involvement by various other neoplasms and classic pericarditis and myopericarditis. Constrictive pericarditis is rare in HIV patients. When present, it is usually secondary to *Mycobacterium tuberculosis*.[69]

CLINICAL FEATURES. Symptomatic patients with pericardial disease usually present with dyspnea or chest pain secondary to pericardial inflammation or a large effusion, or both. Large, symptomatic effusions are often caused by infection or a neoplasm. The most common infectious agents identified in symptomatic pericardial effusions are *M. tuberculosis* and *Mycobacterium avium-intracellulare*. However, a wide variety of organisms, often unusual, have been implicated, including *Cryptococcus neoformans*, cytomegalovirus, and *Mycobacterium kansasii*. Lymphomas and Kaposi sarcoma are the most common neoplasms associated with effusion.

MANAGEMENT. Asymptomatic patients with small to moderate pericardial effusions do not require pericardiocentesis. Most cases are idiopathic and usually remain asymptomatic or resolve spontaneously. Symptomatic, large effusions should be drained and an identifiable cause sought. One study demonstrated that pericardial effusion in HIV disease usually occurs in the context of full-blown acquired immunodeficiency syndrome and is strongly associated with a shortened survival independent of the CD4 count.[70] Mortality at 6 months for patients with pericardial effusion was ninefold greater than for patients without an effusion (Fig. 64–17).[70] The effects of highly active antiretroviral therapy on HIV-related pericardial disease have not yet been elucidated.

Tuberculous Pericarditis

ETIOLOGY AND PATHOPHYSIOLOGY. The incidence of pericardial tuberculosis has decreased markedly in the industrialized world in parallel with the deceased incidence of pulmonary tuberculosis. From 1 to 8 percent of patients with pulmonary tuberculosis develop pericardial involvement. Reflecting current epidemiology, in a modern series of cases of primary acute to subacute pericardial disease, tuberculosis was diagnosed in only 4 percent overall and in 7 percent of patients who developed cardiac tamponade. Similarly, tuberculous pericarditis was diagnosed in only 1 of 135 patients with constrictive pericarditis at the Mayo Clinic. However, pericardial tuberculosis remains a major problem in the immunocompromised host and the underdeveloped world, especially in southwest Africa. Moreover, the combination of HIV and pericardial tuberculosis is especially common in African populations. In a study of Tanzanian patients with large pericardial effusions, 14 of 14 HIV-positive patients had tuberculous pericarditis. Evidence of pericardial involvement in HIV-positive patients in African countries where both tuberculosis and HIV are endemic is usually sufficient to prompt antituberculous therapy.[71]

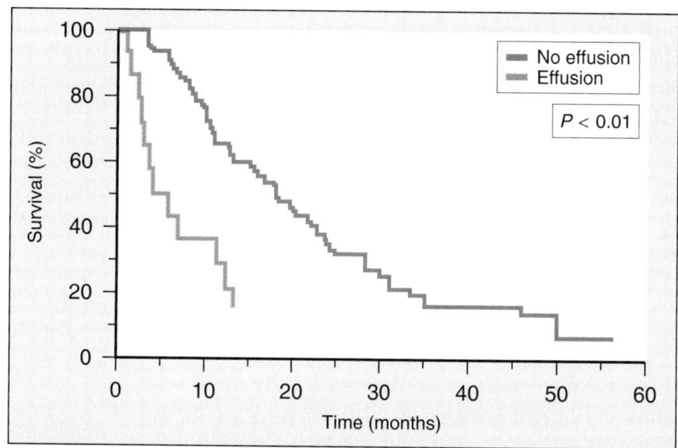

FIGURE 64–17 Kaplan-Meier survival curves in human immunodeficiency virus–positive patients with and without pericardial effusion. (From Heidenreich PA, Eisenberg MJ, Kee LL, et al: Pericardial effusion in AIDS. Incidence and survival. Circulation 92:3229, 1995.)

Pericardial involvement by tuberculosis is usually secondary to retrograde spread from peribronchial, peritracheal, or mediastinal lymph nodes or hematogenous spread from the primary focus. Less commonly, the pericardium is involved by the breakdown and contiguous spread of a necrotic lesion in the lung.

CLINICAL FEATURES. The clinical presentation of tuberculous pericarditis is usually subacute to chronic, with systemic symptoms of fever, malaise, and dyspnea in association with a pericardial effusion. Cough, night sweats, orthopnea, weight loss, and ankle edema are also common. The most common findings are radiographic cardiomegaly, pericardial rub, fever, and tachycardia. Findings related to large effusions such as paradoxical pulse, hepatomegaly, distended neck veins, pleural effusion, and distant heart sounds are common, as is severe hemodynamic compromise. Many patients are properly classified as having a subacute, effusive-constrictive syndrome, and a number develop late constrictive pericarditis despite antituberculous treatment.[72] Clinical evidence of pulmonary tuberculosis may be absent or subtle, which is one of the chief reasons the diagnosis is sometimes unsuspected.

Diagnosing tuberculous pericardial disease is notoriously difficult.[15,71,72] A definitive diagnosis is made by isolating the organism from pericardial fluid or a biopsy specimen. However, the yield for isolating the organism from pericardial fluid is relatively low. In a series of 41 patients with subacute tuberculous pericarditis, *M. tuberculosis* grew in only 4 of 13 cultures of pericardial fluid.[72] The probability of making a diagnosis is increased if both pericardial fluid and biopsy specimens are examined early in the effusive stage of the disease. Thus, there is a definite role for pericardial biopsy. Pericardial tissue reveals either granulomas or organisms in 80 to 90 percent of cases. The optimal diagnostic work-up (as well as management) of suspected tuberculous pericarditis includes a pericardial window with fluid and tissue sent for both culture and histopathological examination. The finding of granulomas without bacilli in biopsy tissue is helpful but not diagnostic of tuberculous pericarditis because granulomas can be found in rheumatoid and sarcoid pericardial disease.

A positive tuberculin skin test increases suspicion, but a negative skin test does not exclude the diagnosis and is often not useful in immunocompromised hosts. A positive skin test is also less helpful in populations with a high endemic incidence of tuberculosis. Measurement of adenosine deaminase, an enzyme produced by white blood cells in pericardial fluid, markedly improves diagnostic capabilities. Thus, in a prospective study of patients with pericardial effusion, an adenosine deaminase level greater than 40 units/liter had a sensitivity of 93 percent and a specificity of 97 percent for tuberculous pericarditis.[46] Adenosine deaminase should be routinely measured whenever tuberculous pericardial involvement is suspected. Measurement of interferon-gamma in pericardial fluid has been proposed as an additional marker for tuberculous involvement. Last, tuberculous pericarditis has also been presumptively diagnosed by polymerase chain reaction in pericardial biopsy specimens. This method offers the possibility of obtaining organism-specific results much more rapidly than do cultures.[73]

MANAGEMENT. The goals of therapy are to treat acute symptoms as well as tamponade, if present, and to prevent the progression to a constrictive stage. Antimycobacterial treatment has greatly decreased mortality. Effective multidrug therapy is mandatory. Two issues have arisen in the treatment of tuberculous pericarditis: the role of corticosteroids and the need for open surgical drainage versus closed pericardiocentesis. The most thorough study of closed pericardiocentesis versus open surgical drainage was performed in 240 South African patients with effusive tuberculous pericarditis.[74] After initial diagnostic evaluation, patients were randomly allocated to open pericardial biopsy and complete surgical drainage of fluid or percutaneous pericardiocentesis as needed. Patients were further randomly assigned to receive or not receive prednisolone. All patients were treated with isoniazid, streptomycin, rifampin, and pyrazinamide. The outcomes suggested that patients who undergo open drainage are less likely to require repeated pericardiocentesis, and there was a trend in the open drainage group toward reduced development of constriction. The role of corticosteroids was not fully elucidated. Their use did not influence the risk of death or progression to constriction but did speed the resolution of symptoms and decrease reaccumulation of fluid. There is no rationale for the use of corticosteroids when established constriction is present. No studies have addressed the use of corticosteroids in HIV-positive patients with tuberculous pericarditis. The optimal management of constrictive pericarditis related to tuberculosis is pericardiectomy.

FUNGAL PERICARDITIS

ETIOLOGY AND PATHOPHYSIOLOGY. Fungal infections are rare causes of pericarditis. They are mainly due to locally endemic organisms such as *Histoplasma* or *Coccidioides* or opportunistic fungi such as *Candida* and *Aspergillus*. Other fungi reported to cause pericardial disease include *Blastomyces*, *Cryptococcus*, and *Pneumocystis carinii*.

Histoplasmosis is the most common cause of fungal pericarditis. The organism is endemic in Ohio, the Mississippi River valley, and the western Appalachians; is acquired by inhalation; and can infect otherwise healthy patients living in the endemic areas.[75] Coccidioidomycosis is endemic in the American Southwest. The organism is acquired by inhalation of chlamydospores in an endemic area.[76] Immunocompromised patients, drug addicts, and those taking corticosteroids or potent broad-spectrum antibiotics are at increased risk for developing opportunistic fungal pericarditis.

CLINICAL FEATURES AND MANAGEMENT

Histoplasmosis. Pericardial histoplasmosis usually occurs in a previously healthy young patient. It is thought to be a noninfectious inflammatory process in response to infection confined to adjacent mediastinal lymph nodes. Accordingly, isolation of organisms from pericardial fluid is unusual. The fluid is serous, xanthochromic, or hemorrhagic. The clinical course usually begins with respiratory symptoms followed by pericardial pain. Effusion leading to cardiac tamponade occurs in almost half the cases. The diagnosis must be considered in endemic zones and is aided by rising complement fixation titers. Provided effusions are drained as needed, pericardial involvement eventually resolves with or without anti-inflammatory drugs. Antifungal agents are indicated only for disseminated histoplasmosis.

Coccidioidomycosis. Coccidioidomycosis pericarditis occurs as a complication of a progressive, disseminated form of infection. Patients are chronically ill and debilitated. Pericardial involvement does not occur in the self-limited influenza-like form of the infection. Physical findings suggestive of cardiac compression may be the first clues to the diagnosis of pericardial involvement. Treatment is directed at the disseminated fungal infection with intravenous amphotericin B. Pericardiocentesis is, of course, indicated when tamponade occurs.

Other Fungi. Pericarditis caused by opportunistic fungi such as *Candida* and *Aspergillus* usually occurs in patients who are immunosuppressed or receiving broad-spectrum antibiotics as well as patients recovering from complicated open-heart surgery. Pericardial involvement usually occurs in the setting of disseminated fungal infection. The prognosis is poor, and the diagnosis is often made at autopsy.

Uremic Pericarditis and Dialysis-Associated Pericardial Disease

(see Chap. 86)

ETIOLOGY AND PATHOPHYSIOLOGY. The incidence of classic uremic pericarditis has decreased markedly since the introduction of widespread dialysis. The pathophysiology of uremic pericarditis has never been fully elucidated, but it is clearly correlated with the levels of blood urea nitrogen (BUN) and creatinine in the blood. Toxic metabolites, hypercalcemia, hyperuricemia, and hemorrhagic, viral, and autoimmune mechanisms have been implicated.[15,77] However, there is no correlation between the development of uremic pericarditis and the level of catabolic metabolites. The acute or subacute phase is characterized by the appearance of shaggy, hemorrhagic, fibrinous exudates on both parietal and visceral surfaces with little in the way of inflammatory cellular reaction. Subacute or chronic constriction may develop with organization of the effusion and formation of thick adhesions within the pericardial space.

Dialysis-associated pericardial disease is now much more common than classic uremic pericarditis. It is characterized by de novo appearance of pericardial disease in patients undergoing chronic dialysis despite the fact that BUN and creatinine are normal or only mildly elevated. Its mechanism and relation to classic uremic pericarditis are unknown.

CLINICAL FEATURES. In modern populations of patients receiving chronic dialysis, the clinical presentation is sometimes that of acute pericarditis with chest pain, fever, leukocytosis, and pericardial friction rub. Alternatively, patients can present with an asymptomatic pericardial effusion that can cause hypotension during or after ultrafiltration (low-pressure tamponade). Although conventional cardiac tamponade with acute or subacute hemodynamic compromise can also occur, the extremely large, asymptomatic effusions typical of classic uremic pericarditis are rarely encountered today.

The electrocardiogram most often is not markedly affected and reflects a high incidence of associated abnormalities such as left ventricular hypertrophy, previous MI, or electrolyte abnormalities. The chest radiograph may demonstrate cardiac enlargement related to myocardial dysfunction and volume overload or pericardial effusion, or both. Asymptomatic effusions of small to moderate size are common in patients receiving chronic dialysis. Accordingly, the presence of typical pericardial pain or a friction rub, or both, is necessary for the diagnosis of pericarditis.

MANAGEMENT. The management of classic uremic pericarditis is intensive hemodialysis as well as drainage in patients with effusions that cause hemodynamic compromise. Patients with symptomatic pericarditis almost always respond to the initiation of intensification of dialysis. Heparin should be used cautiously during hemodialysis because of the possibility of causing hemorrhagic pericarditis with tamponade. Pericardial effusion without hemodynamic compromise resolves after several weeks of intensive hemodialysis in the majority of patients.[15]

Treatment of pericardial disease appearing de novo in patients receiving chronic dialysis is empirical. Cardiac tamponade, of course, requires drainage. In our experience, intensifying dialysis is marginally beneficial at best, presumably because these patients are already receiving most of the benefits of dialysis. Use of NSAIDs for pericardial pain is reasonable, but corticosteroids should be avoided if possible. There is no published experience with colchicine. A pericardial window may be required and is often the most effective approach in patients with recurring, hemodynamically significant effusions.

Early Post-Myocardial Infarction Pericarditis and Dressler Syndrome

(see Chap. 47)

ETIOLOGY AND PATHOPHYSIOLOGY. Early post-MI pericarditis occurs during the first 1 to 3 days and no more than a week after an MI and is due to transmural necrosis with inflammation affecting the adjacent visceral and parietal pericardium. Pericardial involvement is strongly associated with indices of infarct size. It is estimated from autopsy studies that about 40 percent of patients with large, Q wave MIs have pericardial inflammation.[78] Use of thrombolytic and mechanical revascularization therapy appears to have reduced the incidence of this form of pericarditis by at least 50 percent. On the basis of clinical criteria, the incidence in patients receiving thrombolytic therapy in the Gruppo Italiano per lo Studio della Sopravvivenza nell'Infarto Miocardico (GISSI) study was only 5 to 6 percent. Furthermore, the earlier the thrombolytic treatment is initiated, the lower the incidence of pericarditis.

Late pericarditis is characterized by pleuropericardial involvement with pericardial or pleural effusions, or both. This syndrome was initially described by Dressler and had an estimated incidence of 3 to 4 percent of MI patients in the past. However, there is a general impression that the incidence of Dressler syndrome has become markedly reduced during the reperfusion therapy era. Dressler syndrome is believed to have an autoimmune etiology because of sensitization to myocardial cells at the time of necrosis. Antimyocardial antibodies have been demonstrated in patients with the clinical syndrome,[15] although these antibodies are nonspecific. As noted previously, Dressler syndrome is a polyserositis involving the pleura and the pericardium. In contrast to that in early post-MI pericarditis, the inflammation in this syndrome is diffuse and not localized to the myocardial injury site.

CLINICAL FEATURES. Most commonly, early post-MI pericarditis is asymptomatic and identified by auscultation of a rub, usually within 1 to 3 days after presentation. Friction rubs in this setting are notoriously evanescent. Many are monophasic (usually systolic) and can be confused with a murmur of mitral regurgitation or ventricular septal defect. Acute post-MI pericarditis virtually never causes tamponade by itself. However, it can occur in association with left ventricular free wall rupture. Symptomatic patients develop pleuritic chest pain within the preceding time frame. It is important to distinguish pericardial pain from recurrent ischemic discomfort. Ordinarily, the distinction is not difficult on clinical grounds. However, the typical ECG changes of acute pericarditis are uncommon after MI. Pericardial inflammation is localized to the infarcted area; hence, the ECG changes usually involve subtle reelevation of the ST segment in the originally involved leads. An atypical T wave evolution has also been described that appears to be highly sensitive for acute post-MI pericarditis. It consists of persistent upright T waves or early normalization of inverted T waves following the MI. The presence of a pericardial effusion correlates with the presence of extensive MI but not with clinically evident pericarditis.

Dressler syndrome occurs as early as 1 week to a few months after an acute MI. Symptoms include fever and pleuritic chest pain. The physical examination may reveal pleural or pericardial friction rubs, or both. The chest radiograph may show a pleural effusion or enlargement of the cardiac silhouette, and the electrocardiogram often demonstrates ST elevation and T wave changes typical of acute pericarditis. Although pericardial effusions are common, tamponade is unusual.

MANAGEMENT. Although it is associated with relatively large, transmural MIs, early post-MI pericarditis per se is almost invariably a benign process that does not appear to affect in-hospital mortality independently. Treatment is entirely symptomatic. Augmentation of the usual low-dose aspirin administered to these patients (to 650 mg three or four times per day for 2 to 5 days) or acetaminophen can provide symptomatic relief. A brief course of prednisone may be useful in patients with unusually severe pain persisting more than 48 hours despite aspirin or acetaminophen. However, there is evidence that NSAIDs and corticosteroids interfere with the conversion of an MI into a scar, resulting in greater wall thinning and a higher incidence of post-MI rupture. Thus, these drugs should be avoided unless they are absolutely necessary. Because significant hemopericardium is extremely rare with early post-MI pericarditis and there is no evidence that heparin increases the risk, heparin administration should not be modified because of the presence of early post-MI pericarditis. However, coadministration of heparin and glycoprotein IIb/IIIa inhibitors should be done cautiously. There have been no reports of hemopericardium in patients with early post-MI pericarditis receiving dual oral antiplatelet therapy with aspirin and clopidogrel.

Although Dressler syndrome is ultimately a self-limited disorder, admission to the hospital for observation and monitoring should be considered if there is a substantial pericardial effusion or, as is often the case, other conditions, e.g., pulmonary infarction, are also being considered. Aspirin or NSAIDs are effective for symptomatic relief. A short course of prednisone, 40 to 60 mg/d with a 7- to 10-day taper, can be used in patients who do not respond to the preceding treatment or for recurrent symptoms.

POSTPERICARDIOTOMY AND POST-CARDIAC INJURY SYNDROME PERICARDITIS

Blunt or penetrating injury of the chest and heart with myocardial contusion can cause associated acute pericarditis (see Chap. 65). The pericarditis per se is rarely of clinical significance compared with other effects of the trauma. However, pericarditis can develop days to months after cardiac surgery, thoracotomy, or chest trauma. The pathogenesis of this syndrome is thought to involve production of antiheart antibodies in response to myocardial injury with resultant complement activation. A systemic inflammatory response occurs and is characterized by low-grade fever, elevated ESR, mild leukocytosis, and pleuropericardial inflammation with associated chest discomfort. The chest radiograph typically shows bilateral pleural effusions. A few patients demonstrate pulmonary infiltrates. The electrocardiogram reveals changes consistent with acute pericarditis in about 50 percent of patients. The echocardiogram usually shows a small to moderate-size pericardial effusion. Tamponade is rare. NSAIDs are first-line treatment, with an excellent response usually occurring within 48 hours of initiation. Treatment should be maintained for 2 to 3 weeks. Corticosteroid therapy is reserved for patients with unresponsive, severe, or recurrent symptoms.

RADIATION-INDUCED PERICARDITIS

Mediastinal and thoracic radiation is currently standard treatment for a variety of thoracic neoplasms. Hodgkin disease, non-Hodgkin lymphoma, and breast carcinoma are the most common neoplasms associated with radiation pericarditis (see Chaps. 63 and 83). Factors that influence the degree of injury to the pericardium include the total dose delivered, the amount of cardiac silhouette exposed, the nature of the radiation source, and the duration and fractionation of therapy. There is about a 2 percent incidence of clinically evident pericarditis in conjunction with modern techniques of radiation delivery.[79] However, the incidence can be as high as 20 percent when the entire pericardium is exposed.[15,79]

Radiation pericarditis takes one of two forms, an acute illness with chest pain and fever and a delayed form of pericardial injury that can occur years after treatment. Self-limited, asymptomatic effusions are common soon after radiation injury, but tamponade is unusual. Late manifestations of radiation injury occur from about a year to up to 20 years after exposure.[15,79] Patients can present with symptomatic pericarditis and effusion with or without cardiac compression or circulatory congestion related to constrictive pericarditis. Effusions can evolve into constriction, i.e., an effusive-constrictive syndrome.

Radiation-induced pericarditis and effusion can be confused with malignant effusions. Malignant effusions are usually associated with other evidence of disease recurrence and metastases. Hypothyroidism induced by mediastinal radiation can also contribute to pericardial effusion. Pericardiocentesis with fluid analysis for malignant cells and thyroid function tests help differentiate radiation-induced effusion from other etiologies. Large, symptomatic pericardial effusions may be drained either percutaneously or surgically. Recurrent pericardial effusions are usually best treated surgically with either a window or pericardiectomy. Pericardiectomy is, of course, the treatment of choice for patients with constrictive physiology. However, the perioperative mortality in this group of patients is higher than with idiopathic constrictive pericarditis.

METASTATIC PERICARDIAL DISEASE

Pericardial tumor implants are the usual cause of effusion in patients with known malignancies, although, as noted earlier, obstruction of lymphatic drainage by enlarged mediastinal lymph nodes is occasionally observed. The leading cause of cardiac tamponade in developed countries is malignancy. Lung (40 percent) and breast (22 percent) carcinoma and lymphomas (15 percent) are the most common causes of malignant effusion.[15] Gastrointestinal carcinoma, melanoma, and sarcomas are less common. With the advent of HIV infection, the incidence of Kaposi sarcoma and lymphomatous involvement of the pericardium have increased markedly.[69]

Pericardial tumor implants can cause pericardial pain. However, the dominant feature is usually an effusion. Effusions with elements of constriction are not unusual. An asymptomatic, incidentally discovered pericardial effusion can be the presenting sign of pericardial involvement in patients with malignant cancer. However, most patients present with symptomatic effusions or tamponade, or both. The electrocardiogram is variable but usually shows nonspecific T wave abnormalities with low-voltage QRS. ST segment elevation is somewhat unusual but can occur. In addition to echocardiography, CT and MR imaging are useful in evaluating the extent of metastatic disease to the pericardium and adjacent structures.

In most cancer patients with effusions or tamponade, it is important that metastatic involvement of the pericardium be confirmed by identification of malignant cells in pericardial fluid. Confirmation is important because of occasional cases of obstructed lymphatic drainage causing pericardial effusion, the possibility of confusion with radiation-induced disease, and the fact that other forms of pericardial disease can occur in patients who have or have had cancer. On the other hand, there are many exceptions in which clinical judgment dictates that this need not be done, especially when effusions are not large and specific treatment, e.g., instillation of drugs in the pericardial space, is not being contemplated.

It is important to evaluate the life expectancy of patients before performing pericardiocentesis and choosing treatment modalities. In terminally ill patients, drainage of effusions should be performed only to aid in relief of symptoms. However, patients with better prognoses deserve a more aggressive approach, which can be gratifying in a perhaps surprisingly large number. In a significant number of cases a single drainage provides prolonged relief as well as providing fluid for analysis. For this reason, drainage should be the initial step in the treatment of most patients, with careful attention to detection of reaccumulation. For recurrences, intrapericardial instillation of tetracycline or chemotherapeutic agents has been advocated to encourage pericardial sclerosis and has a reasonable record of success. External beam radiation therapy is an option in patients with radiation-sensitive tumors. A pericardial window or even complete surgical pericardiectomy should be considered in patients with recurrent effusions not responding to the preceding measures who continue to have a good prognosis otherwise.[80]

PRIMARY PERICARDIAL NEOPLASMS

A number of primary pericardial neoplasms have been reported. All are exceedingly rare. They include malignant mesotheliomas, fibrosarcomas, lymphangiomas, hemangiomas, teratomas, neurofibromas, and lipomas.[80,81] Because of their rarity, it is difficult to be precise about the clinical presentation and course of these neoplasms. In general, they are either locally invasive or compress cardiac structures or are detected from an abnormal cardiac silhouette on chest radiograph. Mesotheliomas and fibrosarcomas are quite lethal. Others such as lipomas are benign. CT and MR imaging are helpful in delineating the pathological anatomy of these tumors, but surgery is required for diagnosis and treatment.

AUTOIMMUNE AND DRUG-INDUCED PERICARDIAL DISEASE

Pericardial involvement can occur in almost any variety of autoimmune disease, but the great bulk of clinically recognized cases occur in rheumatoid arthritis, SLE, and progressive systemic sclerosis (scleroderma). In addition, a variety of drugs have been reported to cause pericarditis that is usually part of an autoimmune process.

RHEUMATOID ARTHRITIS. Pericardial involvement is common in rheumatoid arthritis (see Chap. 82). Older autopsy studies revealed pericardial inflammation in about 50 percent of patients. However, there are no systematic studies addressing the incidence of pericardial involvement in more contemporary patients. Clinically evident pericardial involvement is detected in up to 25 percent of patients with rheumatoid arthritis. Patients can present with chest pain, fever, and dyspnea related to acute pericarditis, which usually occurs in conjunction with exacerbation of the underlying disease. Asymptomatic large pericardial effusion or cardiac tamponade can also be the presenting manifestation of pericardial involvement in rheumatoid arthritis. The pericardial fluid is characterized by low glucose, neutrophilic leukocytosis, elevated titers of rheumatoid factor, and low complement levels. Constrictive pericarditis can also occur as the result of longstanding pericardial inflammation. In patients with joint disease exacerbation, the management of associated acute pericarditis or asymptomatic effusion is first and foremost the same as that employed to treat the exacerbation. Pericardial manifestations seem to respond well to high-dose aspirin or NSAIDs. Pericardial effusions causing cardiac tamponade should be drained, both to treat tamponade and to establish with confidence that there is no other etiology, e.g., infection, in patients who may be receiving immunosuppressive drugs. In general, the response to treatment of underlying disease exacerbations is too slow and uncertain to advocate a period of watchful waiting in the hope that effusions will shrink before drainage. Recurrent tamponade or large effusions are good indications for a pericardial window. Suppressive therapy with colchicine has also been shown to be effective for recurrent symptoms.[82]

SYSTEMIC LUPUS ERYTHEMATOSUS. Pericarditis is the most common cardiovascular manifestation of SLE,[15] and acute pericarditis can be the first manifestation of the disease. About 40 percent of patients with SLE develop pericarditis at some time, usually in conjunction with an overall flare and involvement of other serosal surfaces. Typical patients present with pleuritic chest pain, low-grade fever, and symptoms related to serosal inflammation elsewhere. The electrocardiogram often shows typical findings of acute pericarditis. The chest radiograph may show enlargement of the cardiac silhouette if pericardial effusion is present, along with pleural effusions and often parenchymal infiltrates. Pericardial effusions have high protein and low glucose contents and a white cell count below 10,000/ml. As with patients with rheumatoid arthritis, it is important to exclude purulent, fungal, or tuberculous pericarditis because the majority of these patients are being treated with immunosuppressive medications. Most patients respond to corticosteroids or immunosuppressive therapy used to treat the overall disease flare-up. Hemodynamic compromise secondary to cardiac tamponade is estimated to occur in 10 percent of patients with SLE. Accordingly, we recommend hospitalizing these patients to monitor for hemodynamic complications until clinical stability is achieved.

PROGRESSIVE SYSTEMIC SCLEROSIS (SCLERODERMA) (see Chap. 82). There is about a 10 percent incidence of acute pericarditis with chest pain and pericardial friction rub in progressive systemic sclerosis. However, pericardial involvement is found at autopsy in about 50 percent of patients. Pericardial effusion is detected by echocardiography in up to 40 percent of patients. Most effusions are small and asymptomatic, but there are occasional instances of large pericardial effusion. Late constrictive pericarditis has been described and carries a poor prognosis.[83] Treatment of acute pericarditis in patients with scleroderma is often unrewarding, with an unpredictable response to aspirin and NSAIDs. Although there is no published experience, colchicine should therefore be considered in these patients. It is important to perform right-heart catheterization in patients presenting with dyspnea or right-sided heart failure to evaluate pulmonary vascular disease, which is relatively common and can be confused with pericardial involvement.

DRUG-INDUCED PERICARDITIS

The great majority of cases of drug-induced pericardial disease occur as a component of drug-induced SLE syndromes. There have been no recent, systematic studies of the epidemiology or etiology of drug-induced SLE or drug-induced pericarditis. Therefore, it is difficult to generalize about current trends. Isoniazid and hydralazine are probably the most common current offenders. Procainamide used to be a major cause, but its use has decreased markedly in the last decade. Large effusions, tamponade, and even constriction have been reported but are rare in drug-induced SLE pericarditis. In addition to drug cessation, management is dictated by the specific elements of the SLE syndrome present as well as usual efforts aimed at detection and treatment of effusions. In rare cases, drug-induced pericarditis caused by agents such as penicillin and cromolyn has involved apparent hypersensitivity reactions with eosinophilia without an SLE picture.

PERICARDIAL DISEASE AND PERCUTANEOUS REVASCULARIZATION (see Chap. 48)

Cardiac tamponade is a rare but important complication of percutaneous revascularization. The incidence of cardiac tamponade ranges between 0.1 and 0.5 percent. The incidence has increased in the last 10 years, which is probably related to aggressive treatment of complex lesions and use of atherectomy devices and stiff or hydrophilic guidewires.

Cardiac tamponade during percutaneous revascularization is almost always a result of coronary artery perforation. Perforation can occur as a consequence of guidewire or balloon advancement. The clinical presentation is abrupt or rapidly progressive cardiac decompensation and severe hypotension. The diagnosis of perforation is made by the angiographic appearance of extravasation of dye from the coronary circulation into the pericardial space. Loss of cardiac pulsation on fluoroscopy indicates that a significant pericardial effusion is present. Management of pericardial tamponade requires sealing the coronary perforation, pericardiocentesis, and reversal of anticoagulation.[84] If the perforation cannot be managed percutaneously, emergency surgery is indicated.

HYPOTHYROID-ASSOCIATED PERICARDIAL DISEASE (see Chap. 79)

Patients with severe hypothyroidism develop pericardial effusions in perhaps 25 to 35 percent of cases.[15] These can become quite large but rarely, if ever, cause tamponade. Classically, they have high concentrations of cholesterol. The effusions gradually resolve with treatment of the thyroid condition.

CONGENITAL ANOMALIES OF THE PERICARDIUM

PERICARDIAL CYSTS. Pericardial cysts are rare, benign congenital malformations. They are usually fluid filled, located at the right costophrenic angle, and identified as an incidental finding on a chest radiograph. The diagnosis is usually confirmed by echocardiography. Patients should be managed conservatively.

CONGENITAL ABSENCE OF THE PERICARDIUM. Congenital absence of the pericardium is rare. Usually part or all of the left side of the parietal pericardium is absent, but partial absence of the right side has also been reported.[15] Partial absence of the left pericardium is often associated with other cardiac anomalies, including atrial septal defect, bicuspid aortic valve, or pulmonary malformations. It is often symptomatic and may even allow herniation of portions of the heart through the defect or torsion of the great vessels, with potentially life-threatening hemodynamic consequences. Recurrent pulmonary infections are occasionally seen. Patients can present with chest pain, syncope, or even sudden death. The electrocardiogram typically reveals an incomplete right bundle branch block. Absence of all or most of the left pericardium results in a characteristic chest radiograph, including a leftward shift of the cardiac silhouette, an elongated left heart border, and radiolucent bands between the aortic knob and the main pulmonary artery and between the left diaphragm and the base of the heart. Echocardiography reveals paradoxical septal motion and right ventricular enlargement. CT or MR imaging should be employed to establish a definitive diagnosis and elaborate the details of the defect. Appropriate surgical correction, i.e., pericardiectomy, should ordinarily be undertaken to ameliorate symptoms and eliminate the possibility of herniation.

REFERENCES

Anatomy and Physiology of the Pericardium

1. Gabella G (sect ed): The pericardium. *In* Gray H, Williams PL, Bannister LH (eds): Gray's Anatomy: The Anatomical Basis of Medicine and Surgery. New York, Churchill-Livingstone, 1995, pp 1471-1472.
2. Kostreva DR, Pontus SP: Pericardial mechanoreceptors with phrenic afferents. Am J Physiol 264:H1836, 1993.
3. Miyazaki T, Pride HP, Zipes DP: Prostaglandins in the pericardial fluid modulate neural regulation of cardiac electrophysiological properties. Circ Res 66:163, 1990.
4. Slinker BK, Bell S, Ditchey R, LeWinter MM: Pericardial pressure does not equal right heart pressure in the dog. Circulation 76:357, 1987.
5. Hamilton DR, Dani RS, Semlacher RA, et al: Right atrial and right ventricular transmural pressures in dogs and humans. Effects of the pericardium. Circulation 90:2492, 1994.
6. Lee MC, Fung YC, Shabetai R, LeWinter MM: Biaxial mechanical properties of the human pericardium and canine comparisons. Am J Physiol 22:H75, 1987.
7. Freeman G, LeWinter M: Pericardial adaptations during chronic cardiac dilation in dogs. Circ Res 54:294, 1984.
8. Freeman G, LeWinter M: Determinants of the intra-pericardial pressure in dogs. J Appl Physiol 60:758, 1986.
9. deVries G, Hamilton DR, Ter Keurs HE, et al: A novel technique for measurement of pericardial pressure. Am J Physiol 280:H2815, 2001.
10. Tischler M, Cooper K, LeWinter MM: Increased left ventricular volume and mass following coronary bypass surgery. A role for relief of pericardial constraint? Circulation 87:1921, 1993.
11. Baker AE, Dani R, Smith ER, et al: Quantitative assessment of independent contributions of pericardium and septum to direct ventricular interaction. Am J Physiol 275:H476, 1998.

Passive Role of the Normal Pericardium in Heart Disease

12. O'Rourke RA, Dell'Italia LJ: Right ventricular myocardial infarction. *In* Fuster V, Rorr R, Topol EJ (eds): Atherosclerosis and Coronary Artery Disease. Philadelphia, Lippincott-Raven, 1996, pp 1079-1096.
13. LeWinter M, Pavelec R: Influence of the pericardium on left ventricular end-diastolic pressure-segment length relations during early and late phases of experimental chronic volume overload in dogs. Circ Res 50:501, 1982.

Acute Pericarditis

14. Zayas R, Anguita M, Torres F, et al: Incidence of specific etiology and role of methods for specific etiologic diagnosis of primary acute pericarditis. Am J Cardiol 75:378, 1995.
15. Spodick DW: Pericardial diseases. *In* Braunwald E, Zipes D, Libby P (eds): Heart Disease. 6th ed. Philadelphia, WB Saunders, 2001, pp 1823-1876.
16. Brady WJ, Perron AD, Martin ML, et al: Cause of ST-segment abnormality in ED chest pain patients. Am J Emerg Med 19:25, 2001.
17. Bonnefoy E, Godon P, Kirkorian G, et al: Serum cardiac troponin I and ST-segment elevation in patients with acute pericarditis. Eur Heart J 21:798, 2000.
18. Brandt RR, Filzmaier K, Hanrath P: Circulating cardiac troponin I in acute pericarditis. Am J Cardiol 87:1326, 2001.
19. Baljepally R, Spodick DH: PR-segment depression as the initial electrocardiographic response in acute pericarditis. Am J Cardiol 81:1505, 1998.
20. Kudo Y, Yamasaki F, Doi Y, Sugiura T: Clinical correlates of PR-segment depression in asymptomatic patients with pericardial effusion. J Am Coll Cardiol 39:2000, 2002.
21. Adler Y, Finkelstein Y, Guindo J, et al: Colchicine treatment for recurrent pericarditis: A decade of experience. Circulation 97:2183, 1998.
22. Marcolongo R, Russo R, Laveder F, et al: Immunosuppressive therapy prevents recurrent pericarditis. J Am Coll Cardiol 26:1276, 1995.
23. Fowler NO, Harbin AD III: Recurrent acute pericarditis: Follow-up study of 31 patients. J Am Coll Cardiol 7:300, 1986.

Pericardial Effusion and Tamponade

24. Tsang TS, Barnes ME, Hayes SN, et al: Clinical and echocardiographic characteristics of significant pericardial effusions following cardiothoracic surgery and outcomes of echo-guided pericardiocentesis for management: Mayo Clinic experience, 1979-1998. Chest 116:322, 1999.
25. Goland S, Caspi A, Malnick S, et al: Idiopathic chronic pericardial effusion. N Engl J Med 342:1449, 2000.
26. Friedman HS, Lajam F, Zaman Q, et al: Effect of autonomic blockade on the hemodynamic findings in acute cardiac tamponade. Am J Physiol 232:H5, 1977.

26a. Spodick DH: Acute cardiac tamponade. N Engl J Med 349:684, 2003.

27. Friedman HS, Lajam F, Gomes JA, et al: Demonstration of a depressor reflex in acute cardiac tamponade. J Thorac Cardiovasc Surg 73:278, 1977.
28. Merce J, Sagrista-Sauleda J, Permanyer-Miralda G, et al: Correlation between clinical and Doppler echocardiographic findings in patients with moderate and large pericardial effusion: Implications for the diagnosis of cardiac tamponade. Am Heart J 138:759, 1999.
29. Hoit BD, Ramrakhyani K: Pulmonary venous flow in cardiac tamponade: Influence of left ventricular dysfunction and the relation to pulsus paradoxicus. J Am Soc Echocardiogr 4:559, 1991.
30. Fowler NO, Gabel M, Buncher CR: Cardiac tamponade: A comparison of right versus left heart compression. J Am Coll Cardiol 12:187, 1988.
31. Singh S, Wann LS, Schuchard GH, et al: Right ventricular and right atrial collapse in patients with cardiac tamponade—A combined echocardiographic and hemodynamic study. Circulation 70:966, 1984.
32. Shabetai R, Fowler NO, Guntheroth WG: The hemodynamics of cardiac tamponade and constrictive pericarditis. Am J Cardiol 26:480, 1970.
33. Shabetai R, Mangiardi L, Bhargava V, et al: The pericardium and cardiac function. Prog Cardiovasc Dis 22:107, 1979.
34. Winer HE, Kronzon I: Absence of paradoxical pulse in patients with cardiac tamponade and atrial septal defects. Am J Cardiol 44:378, 1979.
35. Hoit BD, Shaw D: The paradoxical pulse in tamponade: Mechanisms and echocardiographic correlates. Echocardiography 11:477, 1994.
36. Kuvin JT, Harati NA, Pandian NG, et al: Postoperative cardiac tamponade in the modern surgical era. Ann Thorac Surg 74:1148, 2002.
37. Vaska K, Wann LS, Sagar K, Klopfenstein HS: Pleural effusion as a cause of right ventricular diastolic collapse. Circulation 86:609, 1992.
38. Chuttani K, Pandian NG, Mohanty PK: Left ventricular diastolic collapse: An echocardiographic sign of regional cardiac tamponade. Circulation 83:1999, 1991.

39. Russo AM, O'Connor WH, Waxman HL: Atypical presentations and echocardiographic findings in patients with cardiac tamponade occurring early and late after cardiac surgery. Chest 104:71, 1993.
40. Merce J, Sagrista-Sauleda J, Permanyer-Miralda G, et al: Should pericardial drainage be performed routinely in patients who have a large pericardial effusion without tamponade? Am J Med 105:106, 1998.
41. Tsang TS, Enriquez-Sarano M, Freeman WK, et al: Consecutive 1127 therapeutic echocardiographically guided pericardiocenteses: Clinical profile, practice patterns, and outcomes spanning 21 years. Mayo Clin Proc 77:429, 2002.
42. Bruning R, Muehlstaedt M, Becker C, et al: Computed tomography–fluoroscopy guided drainage of pericardial effusions: Experience in 11 cases. Invest Radiol 37:328, 2002.
43. Wang HJ, Hsu KL, Chiang FT, et al: Technical and prognostic outcomes of double-balloon pericardiotomy for large malignancy-related pericardial effusions. Chest 122:893, 2002.
44. Del Barrio LG, Morales JH, Delgado C, et al: Percutaneous balloon window for patients with symptomatic pericardial effusion. Cardiovasc Intervent Radiol 25:360, 2002.
45. Maisch B, Ristic AD, Rupp H, Spodick DH: Pericardial access using the PerDUCER and flexible percutaneous pericardioscopy. Am J Cardiol 88:1323, 2001.
46. Koh KK, Kim EJ, Cho CH, et al: Adenosine deaminase and carcinoembryonic antigen in pericardial effusion diagnosis, especially in suspected tuberculous pericarditis. Circulation 89:2728, 1994.
47. Koh KK, In HH, Lee KH, et al: New scoring system using tumor markers in diagnosing patients with moderate pericardial effusions. Int J Cardiol 61:5, 1997.
48. Burgess LJ, Reuter H, Carstens ME, et al: The use of adenosine deaminase and interferon-gamma as diagnostic tools for tuberculous pericarditis. Chest 122:900, 2002.

Constrictive Pericarditis

49. Ling LH, Oh JK Schaff HV, et al: Constrictive pericarditis in the modern era: Evolving clinical spectrum and impact on outcome after pericardiectomy. Circulation 100:1380, 1999.
50. Oh JK, Hatle LK, Seward JB, et al: Diagnostic role of Doppler echocardiography in constrictive pericarditis. J Am Coll Cardiol 23:154, 1994.
51. Wolozin MW, Ortola FV, Spodick DH, Seifter JL: Release of atrial natriuretic factor after pericardiectomy for chronic constrictive pericarditis. Am J Cardiol 62:1323, 1988.
52. Klein AL, Cohen GI: Doppler echocardiographic assessment of constrictive pericarditis, cardiac amyloidosis, and cardiac tamponade. Cleve Clin J Med 59:278, 1992.
53. Oh JK, Tajik AJ, Appleton CP, et al: Preload reduction to unmask the characteristic Doppler features of constrictive pericarditis. A new observation. Circulation 96:3799, 1997.
54. Izumi C, Iga K, Sekiguchi K, et al: Usefulness of the transgastric view by transesophageal echocardiography in evaluating thickened pericardium in patients with constrictive pericarditis. J Am Soc Echocardiogr 15:1004, 2002.
55. Tabata T, Kabbani S, Murray RD, et al: Differences in the respiratory variation between pulmonary venous and mitral inflow Doppler velocities in patients with constrictive pericarditis with and without atrial fibrillation. J Am Coll Cardiol 37:1936, 2001.
56. Lorell BH, Grossman W: Profiles in constrictive pericarditis, restrictive cardiomyopathy, and cardiac tamponade. *In* Baim DS, Grossman W (eds): Cardiac Catheterization, Angiography and Intervention. Baltimore, Williams & Wilkins, 1996, pp 801-857.
57. Abdalla IA, Murray RD, Lee JC, et al: Does rapid volume loading during transesophageal echocardiography differentiate constrictive pericarditis from restrictive cardiomyopathy? Echocardiography 19:125, 2002.
58. Breen J: Imaging of the pericardium. J Thorac Imag 16:47, 2001.
59. Klein AL, Chen GI, Pietrolungo JF, et al: Differentiation of constrictive pericarditis from restrictive cardiomyopathy by Doppler transesophageal echocardiographic measurements of respiratory variation in pulmonary venous flow. J Am Coll Cardiol 22:1935, 1993.
60. Uchida T, Bando K, Minatoya K, et al: Pericardiectomy for constrictive pericarditis using the harmonic scalpel. Ann Thorac Surg 72:924, 2001.
61. Trotter MC, Chung KC, Ochsner JL, McFadden PM: Pericardiectomy for pericardial constriction. Am Surg 62:304, 1996.

Specific Causes of Pericardial Disease

62. Sagrista-Sauleda J, Barrabes JA, Permanyer-Miralda G, Soler-Soler J: Purulent pericarditis; review of a 20 year experience in a general hospital. J Am Coll Cardiol 22:1661, 1993.
63. Brook I, Frazier EH: Microbiology of acute purulent pericarditis. A 12-year experience in a military hospital. Arch Intern Med 156:1857, 1996.
64. Brook I: Pericarditis due to anaerobic bacteria. Cardiology 97:55, 2002.
65. Goodman LJ: Purulent pericarditis. Curr Treat Options Cardiovasc Med 2:343, 2000.
66. Keersmaekers T, Elshot SR, Sergeant PT: Primary bacterial pericarditis. Acta Cardiol 57:387, 2002.
67. Hakim JG, Matenga JA, Siziya S: Myocardial dysfunction in human immunodeficiency virus: An echocardiographic study of 157 patients in hospital in Zimbabwe. Heart 76:161, 1996.
68. Estok L, Wallach F: Cardiac tamponade in a patient with AIDS: A review of pericardial disease in patients with HIV infection. Mt Sinai J Med 65:33, 1998.
69. Silva-Cardoso J, Moura B, Martins L, et al: Pericardial involvement in human immunodeficiency virus infection. Chest 115:418, 1999.
70. Heidenreich P, Eisenberg M, Keel L, et al: Pericardial effusion in AIDS: Incidence and survival. Circulation 92:3229, 1995.
71. Sagrista-Sauleda J, Permanyer-Miralda G, Soler-Soler J: Tuberculous pericarditis: Ten year experience with a prospective protocol for diagnosis and treatment. J Am Coll Cardiol 11:724, 1988.
72. Barbara W, Trautner O, Rabih O: Tuberculous pericarditis: Optimal diagnosis and management. Clin Infect Dis 33:954, 2001.
73. Cegielski JP, Devlin BH, Morris AJ, et al: Comparison of PCR, culture, and histopathology for diagnosis of tuberculous pericarditis. J Clin Microbiol 35:3254, 1997.
74. Strang JI, Kakaza HHS, Gibson DG, et al: Controlled clinical trial of complete open surgical drainage and of prednisolone in treatment of tuberculous pericardial effusion in Transkei. Lancet 2:759, 1988.
75. Wheat L, Stein L, Corya BC, et al: Pericarditis as a manifestation of histoplasmosis during two large urban outbreaks. Medicine (Baltimore) 62:110, 1983.
76. Amundson DE: Perplexing pericarditis caused by coccidioidomycosis. South Med J 86:694, 1993.
77. Rostand SG, Rutsky EA: Pericarditis in end-stage renal disease. Cardiol Clin 8:701, 1998.
78. Oliva PB, Hammill SC, Talano JV: Effect of definition on incidence of postinfarction pericarditis. Is it time to redefine postinfarction pericarditis? Circulation 90:1537, 1994.
79. Tarbell N, Thompson L, Mauch P: Thoracic irradiation in Hodgkin's disease: Disease control and long-term complications. Int J Radiat Oncol Biol Phys 18:275, 1990.
80. Frankel KM: Treating malignancy-related effusions. Chest 123:1775, 2003.
81. Eren NT, Akar AR: Primary pericardial mesothelioma. Curr Treat Options Oncol 5:369, 2002.
82. Fernandez-Muixi J, Vidal F, Bardaji A: Recurrent pericarditis and cardiac tamponade in rheumatoid arthritis: Effectiveness of colchicine. Br J Rheumatol 33:596, 1994.
83. Armstrong GP, Whalley GA, Doughty RN, et al: Left ventricular function in scleroderma. Br J Rheumatol 35:983, 1996.
84. Ajuni SC, Glazier S, Blankenship L, et al: Perforation after percutaneous coronary interventions: Clinical, angiographic, and therapeutic observations. Cathet Cardiovasc Diagn 32:206, 1994.

CHAPTER 65

Traumatic Heart Disease

Kenneth L. Mattox • Anthony L. Estrera • Matthew J. Wall, Jr.

Incidence

In the United States, trauma currently is the fourth leading cause of death, and it is the leading cause of death in persons younger than 40 years of age. Thoracic trauma is responsible for 25 percent of the annual 50,000 deaths from vehicular accidents. As high a proportion as one-fourth of these deaths are due to traumatic cardiac injury. The actual incidence of cardiac injury from all of the diverse causes and classifications (including the confusing "cardiac contusion") is unknown. Cardiac injury may account for 10 percent of deaths from gunshot wounds.[1] Penetrating cardiac trauma is a highly lethal injury, with relatively few victims surviving long enough to reach the hospital. In a series of 1198 patients with penetrating cardiac injuries in South Africa, only 6 percent patients reached the hospital with any signs of life.[2] With improvements in organized emergency medical transport systems, up to 45 percent of those who sustain significant traumatic heart injury may reach the emergency department.

Blunt cardiac injuries have been reported less frequently than penetrating injuries. However, 10 to 70 percent of motor vehicle fatalities may have been the result of blunt cardiac rupture.

Etiology and Patterns of Cardiac Trauma

Categorization of traumatic heart disease is based on the mechanism of injury (i.e., penetrating, nonpenetrating [blunt], iatrogenic, metabolic, and other) (Table 65–1).

Penetrating Cardiac Trauma

Penetrating trauma is the most common cause of significant cardiac injury seen in the hospital setting, with the predominant injury being from guns and knives.[3-5] Other mechanisms, such as shotguns, ice picks, and fence impalement have also been reported.

The location of injury to the heart often correlates with the location of injury on the chest wall. Because of anterior location, the anatomical chambers at greatest risk for injury are the right and left ventricles. In a review of 711 patients with penetrating cardiac trauma, 54 percent sustained stab wounds and 42 percent had gunshot wounds. The right ventricle was injured in 40 percent of the cases, the left ventricle in 40 percent, the right atrium in 24 percent, and the left atrium in 3 percent. One-third of cardiac injuries involved multiple cardiac structures.[4] Significant intracardiac injuries involved the coronary arteries (n = 39), valvular apparatus (mitral) (n = 2), intracardiac fistulas (i.e., ventricular septal defects [VSD]) (n = 14), and unusual injuries (n = 10). Only 2 percent of patients surviving the initial injury and undergoing an operation required reoperation for a residual defect.[4]

Blunt Cardiac Trauma

Nonpenetrating or *blunt cardiac trauma* has replaced the term "cardiac contusion" and describes injury ranging from minor bruises of the myocardium to cardiac rupture. It can be caused by direct energy transferal to the heart or compression of the heart between the sternum and the vertebral column at the time of the accident, and even including cardiac contusion and cardiac rupture during external cardiac massage as a part of cardiopulmonary resuscitation (CPR). Within this spectrum, blunt cardiac injuries can manifest as free septal rupture, free wall rupture, coronary artery thrombosis, cardiac failure, complex arrhythmia, simple arrhythmia, and/or rupture of chordae tendineae or papillary muscles.[6] The incidence can be as high as three-fourths of the patients with severe bodily trauma. Causes include motor vehicle accidents, vehicular-pedestrian accidents, falls, crush injuries, blasts, assaults, CPR, and recreational events. Such injury is often associated with sternal or rib fractures. In one report, a fatal cardiac dysrhythmia occurred when the sternum was struck by a baseball,[7] which may be a form of commotio cordis (see Chap. 75).[8]

Cardiac rupture carries a significant risk of mortality. The biomechanics of cardiac rupture include[9] direct transmission of increased intrathoracic pressure to the chambers of the heart; hydraulic effect from a large force applied to the abdominal or extremity veins, causing force to be transmitted to the right atrium, resulting in rupture; decelerating force between fixed and mobile areas, which explains atriocaval tears; myocardial contusion, necrosis, and delayed rupture; and penetration from a broken rib or fractured sternum.

Blunt rupture of the cardiac septum occurs most frequently in late diastole or early systole near the apex of the heart. Multiple ruptures and disruption of the conduction system have been reported.[10] From autopsy data, blunt cardiac trauma with

TABLE 65–1 Etiology of Traumatic Heart Diseases

I. Penetrating
A. Stab wounds—knives, swords, ice picks, fence posts, wire, sporting
B. Gunshot wounds—low-high caliber, handgun, rifles, nail guns, lawnmower projectiles
C. Shotgun wounds—close range, distant
II. Nonpenetrating (Blunt)
A. Motor vehicle accident
1. Seat belt
2. Air bag
B. Vehicular-pedestrian accident
C. Falls from height
D. Crushing—industrial accident
E. Blasts—explosives, grenades
F. Assault (aggravated)
G. Sternal or rib fractures
H. Recreational—sporting events (bull goring), baseball
III. Iatrogenic
A. Catheter induced
B. Pericardiocentesis induced
IV. Metabolic
A. Traumatic response to injury
B. "Stunning"
C. Systemic inflammatory response syndrome (SIRS)
V. Others
A. Burn
B. Electrical
C. Factitious—needles, foreign bodies
D. Embolic—missiles

ventricular rupture most often involves the left ventricle, followed by the right ventricle, and, least often, the left atrium. VSD can occur, with the most common tear involving both the membranous and the muscular portions of the septum. Injury to only the membranous portion of the septum is the least common blunt VSD. Traumatic rupture of the thoracic aorta is associated with lethal cardiac rupture in almost 25 percent of cases.

Blunt pericardial rupture results from pericardial tears secondary to increased intraabdominal pressure or lateral decelerative forces. Tears occur on the left side, most often parallel to the phrenic nerve, next most often to the diaphragmatic surface of the pericardium, then to the right of the pleuropericardium, and finally to the mediastinum. Cardiac herniation with cardiac dysfunction can occur in conjunction with these tears. The heart can be displaced into either pleural cavity or even into the peritoneum. In the instance of right pericardial rupture, the heart can become torsed, leading to the surprising discovery of an "empty" pericardial cavity at resuscitative left anterolateral thoracotomy. With a left-sided cardiac herniation through a pericardial tear, a distending heart prevents the heart from returning to the pericardium, and the term *incarcerated heart* has been applied. Venous filling is impaired, and unless the cardiac herniation is reduced, hypotension and cardiac arrest can occur.

Iatrogenic Cardiac Injury

Iatrogenic cardiac injury can occur with central venous line insertion, cardiac catheterization procedures, and pericardiocentesis. Cardiac injuries caused by central venous lines usually occur with placement from either the left subclavian or the left internal jugular vein.[11] Perforation causing tamponade has also been reported with a right internal jugular introducer sheath for transjugular intrahepatic portocaval shunts. Vigorous insertion of left-sided central lines, especially during dilation of the line tract, can lead to cardiac perforations. Even appropriate technique carries a discrete rate of iatrogenic injury secondary to central venous catheterization. Common sites of cardiac injury include the superior caval-atrial junction and the superior vena cava–innominate junction. These small perforations often lead to a compensated cardiac tamponade. Drainage by pericardiocentesis is often unsuccessful, and evacuation via subxiphoid pericardial window or full median sternotomy is required. Once access to the pericardial space is gained, the site of injury has often sealed and may be difficult to find.

Complications from coronary catheterization, including perforation of the coronary arteries, cardiac perforation, and aortic dissection can be catastrophic and require emergency surgical intervention. The incidence of coronary perforation with balloon angioplasty is estimated to be 0.1 to 0.2 percent, but with advanced interventional techniques (e.g., rotablation, directional atherectomy, coronary artery stenting, and laser ablation), the incidence may be as high as 3 percent.[12]

Other potential iatrogenic causes of cardiac injury include external and internal cardiac massage, right ventricular injury during pericardiocentesis, and intracardiac injections.[13]

Metabolic Cardiac Injury

Metabolic cardiac injury refers to cardiac dysfunction in response to traumatic injury and may be associated with injuries caused by burns, electrical injury, sepsis, the systemic inflammatory response syndrome, and multisystem trauma.[14-16] The exact mechanism responsible for this dysfunction is unclear, but responses to trauma induce a mediator storm, which is a release of cytokines that may have a direct affect on the myocardium. Endotoxin, tumor necrosis factor-alpha, tumor necrosis factor-beta, interleukin-1, interleukin-6, interleukin-10, catecholamines (epinephrine, norepinephrine), cell-adhesion molecules, and nitric oxide are all possible responsible mediators.[16-18]

Metabolic cardiac injury can manifest clinically as conduction disturbances or decreased contractility leading to decreased output. Myocardial depression can occur in response to the mediator storm and can alter calcium utilization and depression of the myocyte responsiveness to beta-adrenergic stimulation.[19,20] Myocytes have altered calcium utilization in patients with injuries from burns. The activation of constitutive nitric oxide synthase can modulate cardiac responsiveness to cholinergic and adrenergic stimulation, and production of inducible nitric oxide synthase can depress myocyte contractile responsiveness to beta-adrenergic agonists. The myocardial depressive effects appear to be reversible.[16]

Treatment of metabolic cardiac injury has been supportive, with correction of the initiating insults, but some practitioners have attempted to address the involved mediators using intravenous milrinone, corticosteroids, arginine, granulocyte-macrophage colony-stimulating factor, and glutamate.[20-22] Use of an intraaortic counterpulsation balloon pump can be considered to treat such myocardial depression, but controlled series do not exist to test this hypothesis.

Burns

Cardiac complications in the early postburn period are a major cause of death. The initial cardiovascular effect of burn injury is attributable to the profound reduction in cardiac output that can occur within minutes of the injury. The overall cardiac response has been described as an ebb and flow pattern, with the initial ebb phase lasting between 1 and 3 days and marked by hypovolemia and myocardial depression, and the flow phase characterized by a prolonged period of increased metabolic demand with increased cardiac output and peripheral blood flow. The reduction in cardiac output observed in the initial period of burn injury is the result of a dramatic and rapid decrease in intravascular volume due to a "capillary leak" and of a direct myocardial depression. Hypovolemia results from the capillary leak caused by endothelial injury and may be mediated by platelet-activating factor, complement, cytokines, arachidonic acid, or oxygen free radicals. Myocardial depression manifested by a decrease in myocardial contractility and abnormalities in ventricular compliance becomes apparent with a total body surface area burn of 20 to 25 percent. Myocardial-depressant factor, tumor necrosis factor, vasopressin, oxygen free radicals, and interleukins may be responsible for the depression.

Electrical Injury

Cardiac complications are most often the cause of death after electrical injury. An estimated 1100 to 1300 deaths occur annually in the United States from electrical injury (including lighting strikes). The cardiac complications after electrical injury include immediate cardiac arrest, acute myocardial necrosis with or without ventricular failure, pseudoinfarction, myocardial ischemia, dysrhythmias, conduction abnormalities, acute hypertension with peripheral vasospasm, and asymptomatic, nonspecific abnormalities evident on an electrocardiogram (ECG). Damage from electrical injury is due to direct effects on the excitable tissues, heat generated from the current, and accompanying associated injuries (e.g., falls, explosions, or fires).

Others

Intrapericardial and intracardiac foreign bodies can cause complications of acute suppurative pericarditis, chronic constrictive pericarditis, foreign body reaction, and hemopericardium.[23] Intrapericardial foreign bodies that have been reported to result in complications include bullets, hand grenades, shrapnel, knitting needles, and hypodermic needles. Needles and similar foreign bodies have been noted after deliberate insertion by patients, usually those with psychiatric diagnoses. A report by LeMaire and colleagues[23] advocated removal of those intrapericardial foreign bodies that are greater than 1 cm in size, that are contaminated, or that produce symptoms.

Intracardiac Missiles

Intracardiac missiles are foreign bodies that are embedded in the myocardium, retained in the trabeculations of the endocardial surface, or free in a cardiac chamber or in the pericardium. These are the result of direct penetrating thoracic injury or injury to a peripheral vascular structure with embolization to the heart. Location and other conditions determine the type of complications that can occur and the treatment required. Observation might be considered when the missile is (1) right sided, (2) embedded completely in the wall, (3) contained within a fibrous covering, (4) not contaminated, and (5) producing no symptoms. Right-sided missiles can embolize to the lung, at which point they can be removed, or, in rare cases, they embolize "paradoxically" through a patent foramen ovale or atrial septal defect.[24] Left-sided missiles can manifest as systemic embolization shortly after the initial injury. Diagnosis is determined with radiographs in two projections, fluoroscopy, echocardiography, or angiography. Treatment of retained missiles is individualized. Removal is recommended for missiles that are left-sided, larger than 1 to 2 cm, rough in shape, or produce symptoms.[24] Although direct approach, either with or without cardiopulmonary bypass, has been advocated in the past, a large percentage of right-sided foreign bodies can now be removed by interventional radiologists.

Clinical Presentation and Pathophysiology

Penetrating Cardiac Trauma

Wounds involving the precordial box, the anatomical area that includes the epigastrium and precordium within 3 cm of the sternum, carry a high incidence of cardiac injury. Stab wounds present a more predictable path of injury than gunshot wounds. Patients with cardiac injury can present with a clinical spectrum from full cardiac arrest with no vital signs, to asymptomatic with normal vital signs. Up to 80 percent of stab wounds eventually manifest tamponade (see Chap. 64). The weapon injures the pericardium and heart, but as the weapon is removed, the pericardium seals and may not allow blood to escape. Rapid bleeding into the pericardium favors clotting rather than defibrination.[25] As pericardial fluid accumulates, a decrease in ventricular filling occurs, leading to a decrease in stroke volume. A compensatory rise in catecholamines leads to tachycardia and increased right-sided heart filling pressures. The limits of distensibility are reached, and the septum shifts toward the left side, further compromising left ventricular function. If this cycle persists, ventricular function can continue to deteriorate, leading to irreversible shock. As little as 60 to 100 ml of blood in the pericardial sac can produce the clinical picture of tamponade.[25]

The rate of accumulation depends on the location of the wound. Because it has a thicker wall, wounds to the right ventricle seal themselves more readily than wounds to the right atrium. Patients with injuries to the coronary arteries present with rapid onset of tamponade combined with cardiac ischemia. With injuries to the left ventricle, the decompensated state can worsen, leading to cardiac arrest. The right side of the heart can compensate for injuries, and rapid deterioration may not occur; and patients with this sort of injury can benefit from early diagnosis and immediate intervention.

The classic finding of the Beck triad (muffled heart sounds, hypotension, and distended neck veins) is seen in only 10 percent of patients. Pulsus paradoxus (a substantial fall in systolic blood pressure during inspiration) and Kussmaul sign (increase in jugular venous distention on inspiration) may be present but are not reliable signs (see Chaps. 8 and 64).[26] A very valuable and reproducible sign of pericardial tamponade is a narrowing of the pulse pressure. An elevation of the central venous pressure often accompanies rapid and cyclic hyperresuscitation with crystalloid solutions, but in such instances, there is a widening of the pulse pressure. Elevation of the central venous pressure and narrowing of the pulse pressure represents a pericardial tamponade syndrome until proven otherwise.

In contrast to stab wounds, gunshot wounds to the heart are more frequently associated with hemorrhage than with tamponade. Twenty percent of gunshot wounds to the heart manifest as tamponade. With firearms, the kinetic energy is greater and the wounds to the heart and pericardium are frequently larger. Thus, these patients present in arrest more often due to hemorrhage.[26]

Nonpenetrating Cardiac Trauma

As in penetrating cardiac trauma, clinically severe blunt cardiac trauma (e.g., cardiac rupture) manifests as either tamponade or as hemorrhage, depending on the status of the pericardium. If the pericardium is intact, tamponade develops; if it is not intact, extrapericardial bleeding occurs and hypovolemic shock ensues. Tamponade is sometimes combined with hypovolemia, thus complicating the clinical presentation.

Blunt cardiac injury can be divided into clinically significant and clinically insignificant injuries. Clinically significant injuries include cardiac rupture (ventricular or atrial), septal rupture, valvular dysfunction, and coronary thrombosis. These injuries manifest as tamponade, hemorrhage, or severe cardiac dysfunction. Septal rupture and valvular dysfunction (leaflet tear, papillary muscle, or chordal rupture) can initially appear without symptoms but later demonstrate the delayed sequela of heart failure.[25]

Blunt cardiac injury can also appear as an arrythmia, most commonly premature ventricular contractions, the precise mechanism of which is unknown. Ventricular tachycardia can occur and degenerate into ventricular fibrillation. Supraventricular tachyarrhythmias can also occur. These symptoms commonly occur within the first 24 to 48 hours after injury (see Chap. 32).

Small isolated tears in the pericardium can lead to cardiac herniation. This is a rare complication of pericardial rupture and depends on the size of the pericardial tear. If large enough, cardiac herniation can occur, leading to acute cardiac dysfunction.[25]

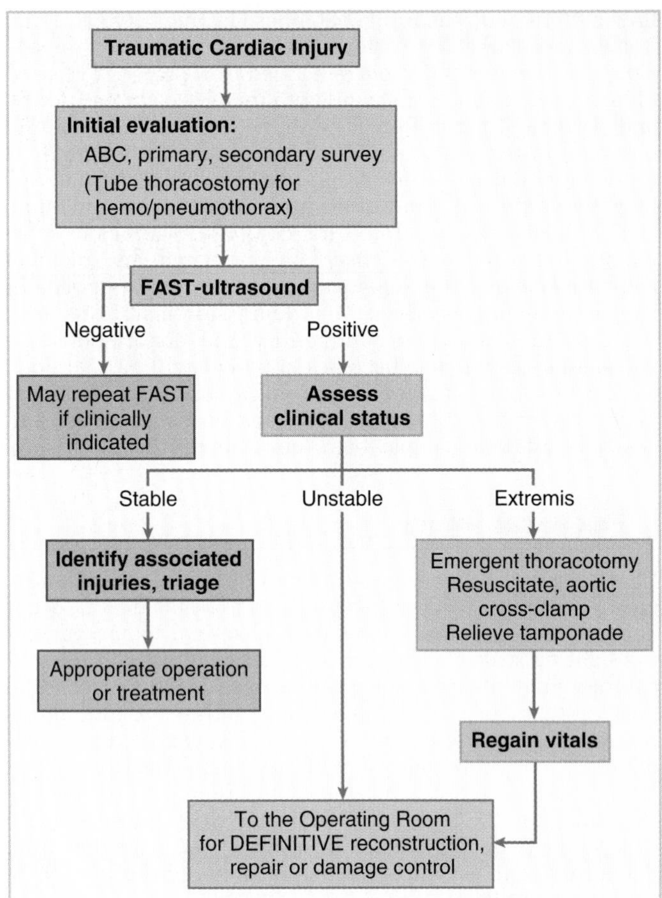

FIGURE 65–1 Algorithm for the initial assessment of traumatic cardiac injury. ABC = airway, breathing, and circulation; FAST = focused abdominal sonogram for trauma.

Evaluation

Evaluation of suspected traumatic heart injury differs, depending on the whether the presenting patient is clinically stable or in extremis.

Initial Assessment

The diagnosis of traumatic heart injury requires a high index of suspicion (Fig. 65–1). On initial presentation to the emergency center, airway, breathing, and circulation (ABCs) under Advanced Trauma Life Support (ATLS) protocol are evaluated and established.[27] Two large-bore intravenous catheters are inserted, and blood is typed and cross-matched. The patient undergoes focused abdominal sonogram for trauma (FAST) and is examined for the Beck triad of muffled heart sounds, hypotension, and distended neck veins, as well as for pulsus paradoxus and Kussmaul sign. These findings suggest cardiac injury but are present in only 10 percent of patients with cardiac tamponade. If the FAST demonstrates pericardial fluid in the unstable patient (systemic blood pressure <90 mm Hg), immediate transfer to the operating room for definitive repair or damage control is required.

Patients in extremis require immediate surgical intervention and often require emergency thoracotomy for resuscitation. The clear indications for emergency department thoracotomy by surgical personnel include the following[28,29]:

1. Salvageable postinjury cardiac arrest (e.g., patients who have witnessed cardiac arrest with high likelihood of intrathoracic injury, especially penetrating cardiac wounds)
2. Severe postinjury hypotension (i.e., systolic blood pressure <60 mm Hg) due to cardiac tamponade, air embolism, or thoracic hemorrhage

If, after resuscitative thoracotomy, vital signs are regained, the patient is transferred to the operating room for definitive repair. The patient with confirmed pericardial fluid by FAST, with normal vital signs (systemic blood pressure >90 mm Hg) may undergo a thorough evaluation to identify associated injuries. If other injuries are excluded, then open exploration may be required to exclude cardiac injury. In the absence of known causes of pericardial fluid (e.g., malignant pericardial effusion), a missed cardiac injury can lead to delayed bleeding, deterioration, or death.

Chest radiography is nonspecific, but it can identify hemothorax or pneumothorax and demonstrate an enlarged cardiac silhouette suggesting pericardial fluid. Other possibly indicated examinations include ultrasonography, central venous pressure measurements, subxiphoid pericardial window, thoracoscopy, laparoscopy, and pericardiocentesis.

ULTRASONOGRAPHY. Surgeons are increasingly performing ultrasonography for thoracic trauma, paralleling the use of ultrasonography for blunt abdominal trauma (see Chap. 11). The FAST evaluates four anatomical windows for the presence of intraabdominal or pericardial fluid (Fig. 65–2).[30] Ultrasonography in this setting is not intended to reach the precision of studies performed in the radiology suite but is merely intended to determine the presence of abnormal fluid collections, which aids in surgical decision making.[31] Ultrasonography is safe, portable, and expeditious and can be repeated as indicated.[31] If performed by a trained surgeon, the FAST examination has a sensitivity of nearly 100 percent and a specificity of 97.3 percent.[32]

To evaluate more subtle findings of blunt cardiac injury in the stable patient, transthoracic echocardiography (TTE) or

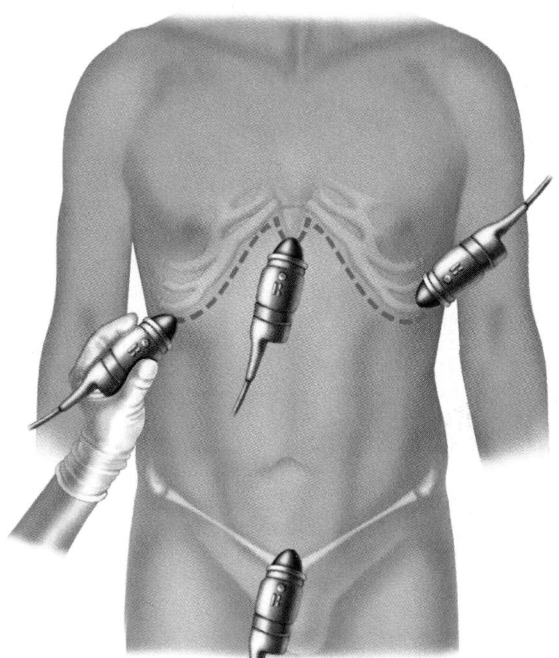

FIGURE 65–2 Focused Assessment for the Sonographic examination of the Trauma victim (FAST). (From Rozycki GS, Feliciano DV, Schmidt JA, et al: The role of surgeon performed ultrasound in patients with possible cardiac wounds. Ann Surg 223:737, 1996.)

transesophageal echocardiography (TEE) can be used. TEE is useful in identifying and characterizing valvular abnormalities and septal defects.

SUBXIPHOID PERICARDIAL WINDOW. Subxiphoid pericardial window has been performed both in the emergency department and in the operating room with the patient under either general or local anesthesia. Via a subxiphoid vertical incision, a small hole is made in the pericardium to determine the presence of blood. In a prospective study, Meyer and coworkers[33] compared the subxiphoid pericardial window with echocardiography in cases of penetrating heart injury and reported that the sensitivity and specificity of subxiphoid pericardial window were 100 percent and 92 percent, respectively, compared with 56 percent and 93 percent with echocardiography. They suggested the difference in sensitivity may have been due to the presence of hemothorax, which can confuse the pericardial and pleural space, or due to the fact that the blood had drained into the pleura.[33]

The disadvantage of a subxiphoid pericardial window is that it is an invasive procedure, and if a major injury is found, a second thoracic incision is required for definitive repair. Although there has been significant controversy in the past with regard to the indication for subxiphoid pericardial window, recent enthusiasm for ultrasonographic evaluation has almost eliminated the role of subxiphoid pericardial window in the evaluation of cardiac trauma.

PERICARDIOCENTESIS (see Chap. 64). Pericardiocentesis has had significant historical support, especially when the majority of penetrating cardiac wounds were produced by ice picks and the (surviving) patients arrived several hours and/or days after injury. In such instances, there was a natural triage of the more severe cardiac injuries and the intrapericardial blood had become defibrinated and was easy to remove. Currently, many trauma surgeons discourage pericardiocentesis for acute trauma. In general, pericardiocentesis has historically been used as a diagnostic or therapeutic maneuver to drain nonclotted pericardial fluid. In the setting of trauma, cardiac tamponade is acute and caused by hemorrhage. Clot forms quickly and is not amenable to needle drainage. Recurrence of tamponade and subsequent increase in mortality, as well as a significant incidence of false-negative results and potential for iatrogenic injury, makes pericardiocentesis a far less than optimal diagnostic tool.[13]

Indications for its use may apply in the case of iatrogenic injury caused by cardiac catheterization, at which time immediate decompression of the tamponade may be life saving, or in the trauma setting when a surgeon is not available.

Evaluation of Blunt Cardiac Injury

ELECTROCARDIOGRAPHY. In cases of blunt cardiac injury, conduction disturbances are common, and, thus, a screening 12-lead ECG could be helpful for evaluation (see Chap. 9). Sinus tachycardia is the most common rhythm disturbance seen. Other possible disturbances include T wave and ST segment changes (as seen with myocardial bruising), sinus bradycardia, first-degree atrioventricular block, right bundle branch block, right bundle branch block with hemiblock, third-degree block, atrial fibrillation, premature ventricular contractions, ventricular tachycardia, and ventricular fibrillation.

CARDIAC ENZYMES. Much has previously been written about the use of cardiac enzyme determinations in evaluating blunt cardiac injury. However, no correlation between serum assays (e.g., creatine phosphokinase myocardial band, cardiac troponin T, or cardiac troponin I) and identification and prognosis of injury has been demonstrated with blunt cardiac injury.[35-37] Therefore, cardiac enzyme assays should not be performed unless one is evaluating concomitant coronary artery disease.[32]

Treatment

Prehospital and Emergency Department

Only a small subset of patients with significant cardiac injury ever reaches the emergency department, and expeditious transport to a designated trauma facility is essential to survival. Transport times of less than 5 minutes and successful endotracheal intubation are positive factors for survival.

Definitive Treatment

Definitive treatment involves surgical exposure through a thoracotomy (Fig. 65–3A) or median sternotomy (Fig. 65–3B). The mainstays of treatment are relief of tamponade and correction of aberrant physiology, which involves correction of the acidosis and hypothermia and reestablishment of effective coronary perfusion (i.e., resuscitation of the heart).

Cardiorrhaphy should be performed by experienced surgeons (Fig. 65–4). Poor technique can result in enlargement of the lacerations or injury to the coronary arteries. If the initial treating physician is uncomfortable with the suturing technique, digital pressure can be applied until a more experienced surgeon arrives. Other techniques that have been described include the use of a Foley balloon catheter and a skin stapler (Fig. 65–5).[5]

Exposure to the heart is accomplished by a left anterolateral thoracotomy, which allows access to the pericardium and heart and exposure for aortic cross-clamping if necessary. This incision can be extended across the sternum to gain access to the right side of the chest and for better exposure of the right atrium or right ventricle. This usually requires ligation of both internal thoracic arteries. Manual access to the right hemithorax from the left side of the chest is achieved through the anterior mediastinum by blunt dissection. This maneuver allows rapid evaluation of the right side of the chest for major injuries without transecting the sternum. Once the left pleural space is entered, the lung is retracted to expose the descending thoracic aorta for cross-clamping of the pericardium for exposure. The amount of blood present in the left side of the chest indicates whether one is dealing with hemorrhage or tamponade. The pericardial sac anterior to the phrenopericardial vessels and phrenic nerve is opened, injuries are rapidly identified, and repair is performed.

In selected cases, particularly stab wounds to the precordium, median sternotomy can be used. This incision allows excellent exposure to the anterior structures of the heart, but difficulty with access to the posterior mediastinal structures and descending thoracic aorta for cross-clamping may be encountered.

Mechanical support is not often used in the acute setting.[5]

BLUNT CARDIAC INJURY. Much debate and discussion has occurred about the clinical relevance of "cardiac contusion." Most trauma surgeons conclude that this diagnosis should be eliminated because it does not affect how one treats these injuries. Thus, a normotensive patient with a normal initial ECG and suspected blunt cardiac injury is managed in emergency department or chest pain observation units, with no expected clinical significance. Patients with an abnormal ECG are admitted for monitoring and treated accordingly. Patients who present in cardiogenic shock are evaluated for a structural injury, which is then repaired.

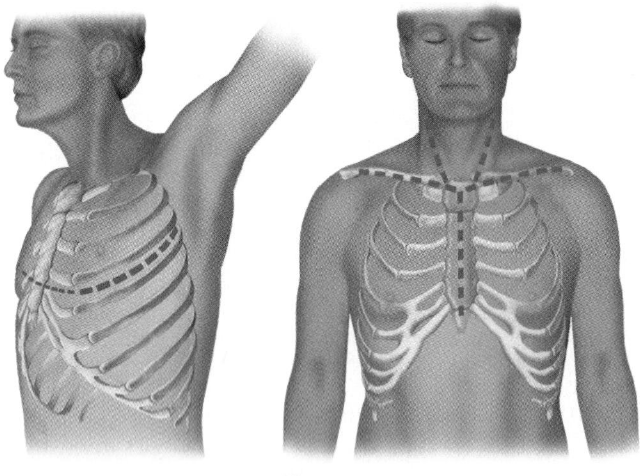

FIGURE 65–3 Incisions for cardiac injury. **A,** Left anterior thoracotomy (extension across the sternum if required). **B,** Median sternotomy (extension to the neck can be performed for exposure of the great vessels).

Results

Factors determining survival in patients with traumatic cardiac injury are mechanism of injury, location of injury, associated injuries, coronary artery involvement, presence of tamponade, length of prehospital transport, requirement for resuscitative thoracotomy, and experience of the trauma team. The overall hospital survival rate for patients with penetrating heart injuries ranges from 30 to 90 percent.

The survival rate for patients with stab wounds is 70 to 80 percent, whereas survival after gunshot wounds is between 30 and 40 percent.[26] Cardiac rupture has a worse prognosis than penetrating injuries to the heart, with a survival rate of approximately 20 percent.

COMPLICATIONS. Primary injury-related cardiac complications include coronary artery injury, valvular apparatus injury (annulus, papillary muscles, and chordae tendineae), intracardiac fistulas, arrhythmias, and delayed tamponade. These delayed sequelae have been reported to have a broad range (4 to 56 percent), depending on the definition of complication.

Coronary artery injury is a rare complication, occurring in 5 to 9 percent of patients with cardiac injures, with a 69 percent rate of mortality.[4] A coronary artery injury is most often controlled by simple ligation, but bypass grafting using saphenous vein may be required for proximal left

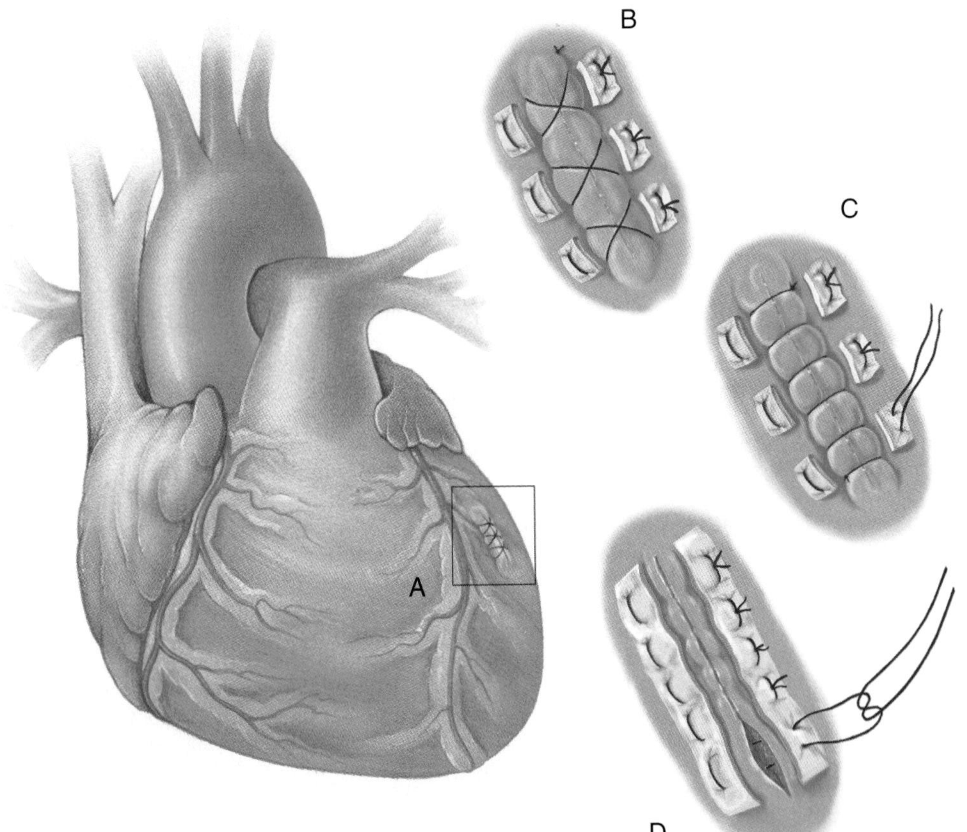

FIGURE 65–4 Technique of suture repair. **A,** Cardiorrhaphy. Should reinforcement be required, interrupted pledgeted sutures **(B)**, pledgeted sutures around previously placed staples **(C)**, or felt strips **(D)** can be used. (From Wall MJ Jr, Mattox KL, Chen CD, Baldwin JC: Acute management of complex cardiac injuries. J Trauma 42:905, 1997.)

anterior descending injuries (with total cardiopulmonary bypass).[4] With a resurrection of the old concept of coronary artery bypass grafting without cardiopulmonary bypass (off-pump bypass), this technique can theoretically be used for cases of these injuries in the highly unlikely event that the patient is hemodynamically stable.

Valvular apparatus dysfunction is rare (0.2 to 9 percent) and can occur with both blunt and penetrating trauma.[6] The aortic valve is most frequently injured, followed by the mitral and tricuspid valves. Often these injuries are identified after the initial cardiorrhaphy and resuscitation have been performed. Timing of repair depends on the patient's condition. If severe cardiac dysfunction exists at the time of the initial operation, immediate valve repair or replacement may be required; otherwise, delayed repair is advised.

Intracardiac fistulas include VSDs, atrial septal defects, and atrioventricular fistulas, with an incidence of 1.9 percent among cardiac injuries.[4] Management depends on symptoms and degree of cardiac dysfunction, with only a minority of these patients requiring repair.[12] These injuries are often identified after primary repair is accomplished, and they can be repaired after the patient has recovered from the original and associated injuries. Cardiac catheterization should be accomplished before repair so that specific anatomical sites of injury and incision planning can be accomplished.

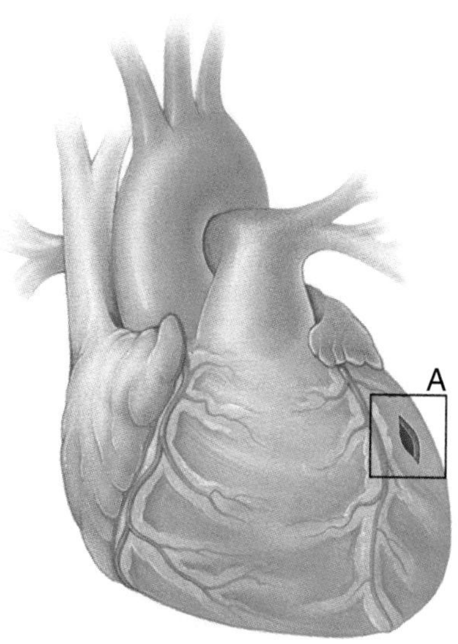

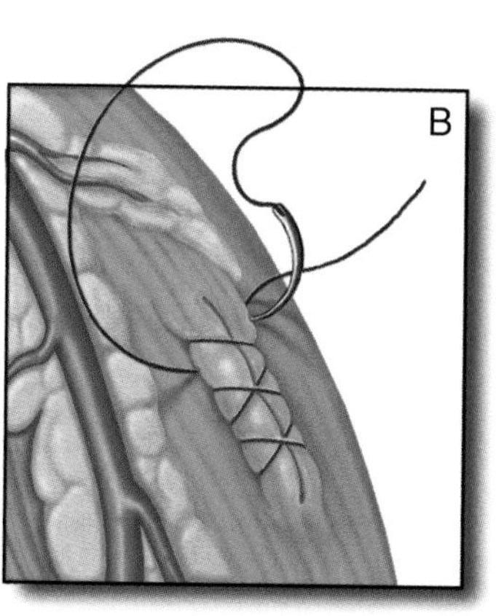

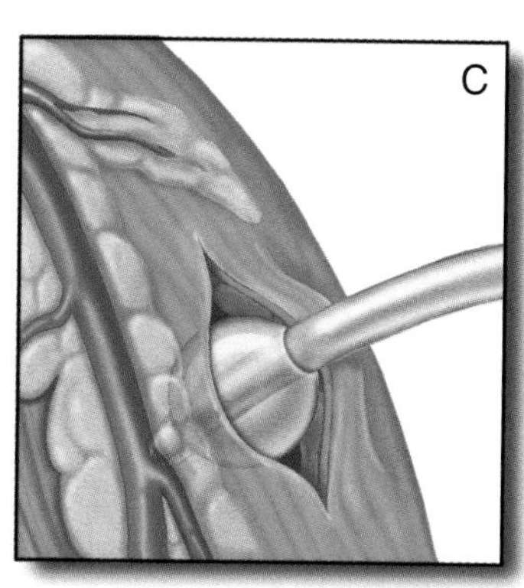

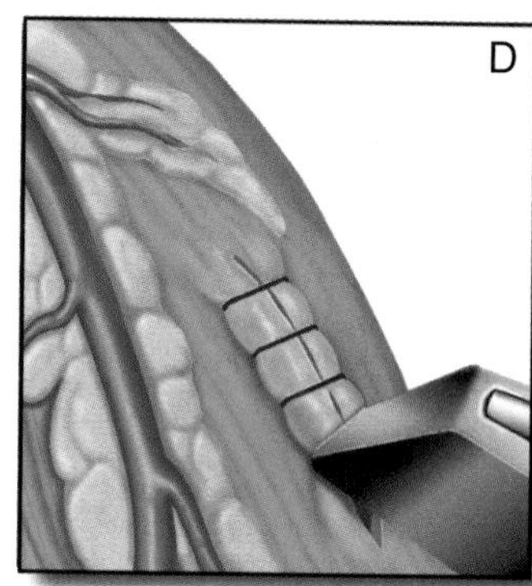

FIGURE 65–5 Temporary techniques to control bleeding. **A,** Stab wound to left ventricle. **B,** Initial management with interrupted or continuous 4-0 polypropylene sutures tied beneath the surgeon's finger. Additional techniques for complex injuries for temporary control include use of Foley balloon catheter **(C)** and skin stapler **(D)**. (From Wall MJ Jr, Mattox KL, Chen CD, Baldwin JC: Acute management of complex cardiac injuries. J Trauma 42:905, 1997.)

Arrhythmias can occur as a result of blunt injury, ischemia, or electrolyte abnormalities and are addressed according to the injury (Table 65–2) (see Chap. 32).

Delayed pericardial tamponade is very rare. It has been reported to occur as early as 1 hour after initial operation and as long as 76 days from the injury.[12]

Follow-Up

Secondary sequelae in survivors of cardiac trauma include valvular abnormalities and intracardiac fistulas.[33] These abnormalities can be identified intraoperatively by gross palpation of a thrill[15] or with the use of TEE. TEE may not be feasible, however, in the acutely injured patient. Early postoperative clinical examination and ECG findings are unreliable.[15] Thus, echocardiography is recommended during the initial hospitalization to identify occult injury and establish a baseline study. Because the incidence of late sequelae can be as high as 56 percent, follow-up echocardiography 3 to 4 weeks after injury has been recommended.[37]

In summary, the approach to the patient follows a well-defined plan. Patients with penetrating trauma arriving alive at a trauma center can have hemopericardium diagnosed by echocardiography. Urgent operation performed in the trauma resuscitation area or the operating room can result in

TABLE 65–2 Arrhythmias Associated with Cardiac Injury
Penetrating Injury
Sinus tachycardia
ST segment changes associated with ischemia
Supraventricular tachycardia
Ventricular tachycardia/fibrillation
Blunt Cardiac Injury
Sinus tachycardia
ST segment, T wave abnormalities
Atrioventricular blocks, bradycardia
Ventricular tachycardia/fibrillation
Electrical Injury
Sinus tachycardia
ST segment, T wave abnormalities
Bundle branch blocks
Axis deviation
Prolonged QT
Paroxysmal supraventricular tachycardia
Atrial fibrillation
Ventricular tachycardia, fibrillation (alternating current)
Asystole (lightnging strike)

survival. Blunt cardiac trauma can produce either minor ECG changes or frank rupture of the septum, free wall, or cardiac valves. Associated injuries are not uncommon. Stable patients can undergo evaluation in a cardiac evaluation unit, but unstable patients require rapid imaging and urgent operation. Late sequelae of fistula, coronary occlusion, and heart failure are rare and are most often detected by echocardiography within the first year after injury.

REFERENCES

1. Ivatury RR: Injury to the heart. *In* Feliciano DV, Moore EE, Mattox KL (eds): Trauma. 3rd ed. Stamford, CT, Appleton & Lange, 1996.
2. Campbell NC, Thomsen SR, Murkart DJ, et al: Review of 1198 cases of penetrating cardiac trauma. Br J Surg 84:1737, 1997.

Etiology and Patterns of Cardiac Trauma

3. Asensio JA, Berne JD, Demetriades D, et al: One hundred five penetrating cardiac injuries: A 2-year prospective evaluation. J Trauma 44:1073, 1998.
4. Wall MJ Jr, Mattox KL, Chen CD, Baldwin JC: Acute management of complex cardiac injuries. J Trauma 42:905, 1997.
5. Assencio JA, Soto SN, Forno W, et al: Penetrating cardiac injuries: A complex challenge. Injury 32:533, 2001.
6. Lin JC, Ott RA: Acute traumatic mitral valve insufficiency. J Trauma 47:165, 1999.
7. Amerongen RV, Rosen M, Winnik G, Horwitz J: Ventricular fibrillation following blunt chest trauma from a baseball. Pediatr Emerg Care 13:107, 1997.
8. Maron BJ, Link MS, Wang PJ, et al: Clinical profile of commotio cordis: An underappreciated cause of sudden death in young during sports and other activities. J Cardiovasc Electrophysiol 10:114, 1999.
9. Ivatury RR: Injury to the heart. *In* Mattox KL, Feliciano DV, Moore EE (eds): Trauma. 4th ed. New York, McGraw-Hill, 1999, pp 545-558.
10. Schaffer RB, Berdat PA, Seiler C, Carrel TP: Isolated rupture of the ventricular septum after blunt chest trauma. Ann Thorac Surg 67:853, 1999.
11. Baumgartner FJ, Rayhanabad J, Bongard FS, et al: Central venous injuries of the subclavian-jugular and innominate-caval confluences. Tex Heart Inst J 26:177, 1999.
12. Medizinische Klinik IV: Perforation und Ruptur Koronaryarterien. Herz 23:311, 1998.
13. Ivatury RR, Simon RJ, Rohman M: Cardiac complications. *In* Mattox KL (ed): Complications of Trauma. New York, Churchill Livingstone, 1994, pp 409-428.
14. Huang YS, Yang ZC, Tan BG, et al: Pathogenesis of early cardiac myocyte damage after sear burns. J Trauma 46:428, 1999.
15. Kirkpatrick AW, Chun R, Brown R, Simons RK: Hypothermia and the trauma patient. Can J Surg 42:333, 1999.
16. Sharkey SW, Shear W, Hodges M, Herzog CA: Reversible myocardial contraction abnormalities in patients with an acute non-cardiac illness. Chest 114:98, 1998.
17. Kumar A, Thota V, Dee L, et al: TNF-alpha and IL-1 are regulators for depression of in vitro myocardial cell contractility induced by serum from humans with septic shock. J Exp Med 183:949, 1996.
18. Meldrum DR, Shenkar R, Sheridan BC, et al: Hemorrhage activates myocardial NF-kappa and increases TNF-alpha in the heart. J Mol Cell Cardiol 29:2849, 1997.
19. Horton JW, Lin C, Maass D: Burn trauma and tumor necrosis factor alpha alter calcium handling by cardiomyocytes. Shock 10:270, 1998.
20. Horton JW, White J, Maass D, Sanders B: Arginine in burn injury improves cardiac performance and prevents bacterial translocation. J Appl Physiol 84:695, 1998.
21. Heinz G, Geppert A, Delle Karth G, et al: IV milrinone for cardiac output increase and maintenance: Comparison in nonhyperdynamic SIRS/sepsis and congestive heart failure. Intensive Care Med 25:620, 1999.
22. Flohe S, Borgermann J, Dominquez FE, et al: Influence of granulocyte-macrophage colony-stimulating factor (GM-CSF) on whole blood endotoxin responsiveness following trauma, cardiopulmonary bypass, and severe sepsis. Shock 12:17, 1999.
23. LeMaire SA, Wall MJ Jr, Mattox KL: Needle embolus causing cardiac puncture and chronic constrictive pericarditis. Ann Thorac Surg 65:1786, 1998.
24. Symbas PN, Symbas PJ: Missiles in the cardiovascular system. Surg Clin North Am 7:343, 1997.

Clinical Presentation and Pathophysiology

25. Ivatury RR: The injured heart. *In* Mattox KL, Moore EE, Feliciano DV (eds): Trauma. 4th ed. Stamford, CT, Appleton & Lange, 1999.
26. Brown J, Grover FL: Trauma to the heart. Chest Surg Clin North Am 7:325, 1997.

Evaluation

27. American College of Surgeons, Committee on Trauma: Advanced Trauma Life Support. Chicago, American College of Surgeons, 1997.
28. Read RA, Moore EE, Moore JB: Emergency department thoracotomy. *In* Feliciano DV, Moore EE, Mattox KL (eds): Trauma. 3rd ed. Stamford, CT, Appleton & Lange, 1996.
29. Working Group, Ad Hoc Subcommittee on Outcomes, American College of Surgeons-Committee on Trauma Practice Management Guidelines for Emergency Department Thoracotomy. J Am Coll Surg 193:303, 2001.
30. Rozycki GS, Feliciano DV, Schmidt JA, et al: The role of surgeon performed ultrasound in patients with possible cardiac wounds. Ann Surg 223:737, 1996.
31. Mattox KL, Wall MJ Jr: Newer diagnostic measures and emergency management. Chest Surg Clin North Am 7:214, 1997.
32. Rozycki GS, Schmidt JA, Oschner MG, et al: The role of surgeon-performed ultrasound in patients with possible penetrating wounds: A prospective multicenter study. J Trauma 45:190, 1998.
33. Meyer DM, Jessen ME, Grayburn PA: Use of echocardiography to detect occult cardiac injury after penetrating thoracic trauma: A prospective study. J Trauma 39:902, 1995.

Evaluation of Blunt Cardiac Injury

34. Feliciano DV, Rozycki GS: Advances in the diagnosis and treatment of thoracic trauma. Surg Clin North Am 79:1417, 1999.
35. Adams JE III, Davila-Roman VG, Bessey PQ, et al: Improved detection of cardiac contusion with cardiac troponin I. Am Heart J 131:308, 1996.
36. Ferjani M, Droc G, Dreux S, et al: Circulating cardiac troponin T in myocardial contusion. Chest 111:427, 1997.

Treatment

37. Bertinchant, JP, Polge A, Mohty D, et al: Evaluation of incidence, clinical significance and prognostic value of circulating cardiac troponin I and T elevation in hemodynamically stable patients with suspected myocardial contusion after blunt chest trauma. J Trauma 48:924, 2000.

CHAPTER 66

Pulmonary Embolism

Samuel Z. Goldhaber

Pulmonary embolism (PE) and deep venous thrombosis (DVT) account for hundreds of thousands of hospitalizations annually in the United States and afflict millions of individuals worldwide. The death rate among unselected patients is high, approximately 15 percent (Fig. 66–1).[1] Although D-dimer testing for exclusion of PE and chest computed tomography (CT) for imaging PE have revolutionized the diagnostic approach, PE and DVT nevertheless remain difficult to detect. More than 1,000,000 new cases of venous thromboembolism occur yearly in the United States, and most go unrecognized. Our understanding of the precipitants of PE has improved, especially the role of inherited hypercoagulable states and potentially modifiable risk factors such as long-haul air travel and obesity.

The most important therapeutic advance is among patients with idiopathic PE or DVT. They can now be treated safely over the long-term and at low cost to prevent most recurrent events with indefinite-duration warfarin anticoagulation. Cardiologists must provide expertise in the treatment of hemodynamically compromised patients with PE as well as those with right ventricular failure who maintain a stable blood pressure and heart rate. This requires accurate and rapid risk stratification, often with echocardiography or elevation of troponin or brain natriuretic peptide (BNP) levels, so that those patients with an adverse prognosis will be identified and treated with thrombolysis or embolectomy.

The selection of anticoagulant drugs has expanded beyond unfractionated heparin and warfarin. Low-molecular-weight heparins have improved therapeutic efficacy and can halve the rate of venous thromboembolism (VTE) in hospitalized medical patients, including those with congestive heart failure. A novel pentasaccharide drug, fondaparinux, has proved extremely effective in preventing VTE after orthopedic surgery. Oral direct thrombin inhibitors such as ximelagatran do not require serial blood testing and dose adjustment and may prove to be safer and more effective than warfarin.

Pathophysiology

Hypercoagulable States

In 1856, Rudolf Virchow postulated that a triad of factors leads to intravascular coagulation: (1) local trauma to the vessel wall, (2) hypercoagulability, and (3) stasis. Classically, the pathogenesis of PE was dichotomized as due to either unusual "inherited" (primary) or commonly "acquired" (secondary) risk factors. Now, however, it appears likely that many patients who develop PE are genetically predisposed with inherited procoagulant[2] and anticoagulant factors,[3] which often interact with a precipitating environmental stress to elicit overt thrombosis (Table 66–1).[4-13] There is also an association between atherosclerosis and the development of PE and DVT.[14]

PRIMARY HYPERCOAGULABLE STATES (see Chap. 80). Normally, a specified amount of activated protein C (aPC) can be added to plasma to prolong the activated partial thromboplastin time (PTT). Patients with "aPC resistance" have a blunted PTT prolongation and a predisposition to developing PE and DVT. The phenotype of aPC resistance is associated with a single point mutation, designated factor V Leiden, in the factor V gene.[5,6,8] Factor V Leiden triples the risk of developing VTE.[15] This genetic mutation is also a risk factor for recurrent pregnancy loss,[16] possibly due to placental vein thrombosis. Use of oral contraceptives by patients with factor V Leiden increases the risk of VTE by at least 10-fold.[17]

A single-point mutation in the 3′ untranslated region of the prothrombin gene (G-to-A transition at nucleotide position 20210) is associated with increased levels of prothrombin.[7] In the Physicians' Health Study, the prevalence of the prothrombin gene mutation was 3.9 percent, and this mutation doubled the risk of venous thrombosis.[18]

A careful family history remains the most rapid and cost-effective method of identifying a predisposition to venous thrombosis. Investigation with blood tests[19] can be misleading. For example, consumption coagulopathy due to venous thrombosis may be misdiagnosed as deficiency of antithrombin III, protein C, or protein S. Heparin administration can depress antithrombin III levels. Use of warfarin ordinarily causes a mild deficiency of protein C or S. Both oral contraceptives and pregnancy depress protein S levels.

ACQUIRED CONDITIONS THAT MAY PRECIPITATE VENOUS THROMBOSIS. Conditions that increase venous stasis or cause endothelial damage (Table 66–2) predispose to venous thrombosis, especially among patients who already have subclinical hypercoagulable states. Long-haul air travel[20] has captured the public's attention as a risk factor for PE (Fig. 66–2).

The stasis and immobilization associated with postoperative venous thrombosis may paradoxically increase after hospital discharge, because of the contemporary emphasis on minimizing the length of stay after surgery. Hospitalized patients with medical illnesses such as pneumonia or congestive heart failure are at high risk of developing VTE. There is a high prevalence of asymptomatic DVT at the time of admission of these patients.[21]

TABLE 66–1 Principal Hypercoagulable States Associated with Venous Thrombosis

Hypercoagulable State	Citation	Comments
Mutation in factor V gene (factor V Leiden)	Bertina et al[5]	Replaces arginine 506 with glutamine, rendering factor V resistant to inactivation by activated protein C
Resistance to activated protein C	Zöller et al[6]	Molecular background for resistance to activated protein C was found to be heterogeneous
Prothrombin gene mutation	Poort et al[7]	G20210A point mutation increases prothrombin levels
Mutation in protein C gene	Allaart et al[8]	Associated with protein C deficiency
Protein S deficiency	Gladson et al[9]	Protein S a cofactor for protein C
Antithrombin III deficiency	Bucciarelli et al[10]	Autosomal dominant inheritance; may cause resistance to heparin
Hyperhomocysteinemia	Langman et al[11] Ridker et al[12]	Triples risk[11]; potentiates risk from underlying factor V Leiden[12]
Antiphospholipid antibodies	Levine et al[13]	Encompasses anticardiolipin antibodies and lupus anticoagulant; associated with venous and arterial thrombosis

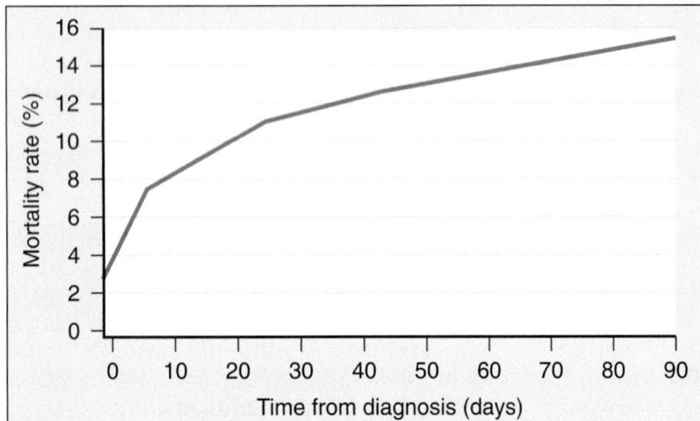

FIGURE 66–1 Overall cumulative mortality due to pulmonary embolism in the International Cooperative Pulmonary Embolism Registry (ICOPER) of 2454 patients was 11.4 percent at 2 weeks and 17.4 percent at 3 months. After exclusion of patients in whom pulmonary embolism was first discovered at autopsy, the mortality rate was 15.3 percent. (From Goldhaber SZ, Visani L, De Rosa M, for ICOPER: Acute pulmonary embolism: Clinical outcomes in the International Cooperative Pulmonary Embolism Registry [ICOPER]. Lancet 353:1386, 1999.)

TABLE 66–2 Acquired Conditions that May Precipitate Venous Thrombosis

Long-haul air travel
Surgery/immobilization/trauma
Hospitalization with medical illness such as pneumonia or congestive heart failure; stay in a medical or surgical intensive care unit
Obesity
Increasing age
Cigarette smoking
Systemic arterial hypertension
Diabetes mellitus
Use of oral contraceptives/pregnancy/postpartum state
Cancer (sometimes occult adenocarcinoma) and cancer chemotherapy
Stroke/spinal cord injury
Indwelling central venous catheter, pacemakers, and internal cardiac defibrillators

Independent risk factors for PE and DVT include surgery, trauma, hospital or nursing home confinement, cancer, and cancer chemotherapy,[22] in addition to increasing age and diabetes mellitus. In the DVT FREE prospective registry of 5451 patients with ultrasonographically confirmed DVT, the five most common comorbidities were hypertension (50 percent), surgery within 3 months (38 percent), immobility within 30 days (34 percent), cancer (32 percent), and obesity (27 percent).[23]

With respect to oral contraceptives, the risk of fatal PE in a New Zealand case-control study was estimated to be 1 per 100,000 woman-years.[24] Hormone replacement therapy with estrogen plus progestin doubles the rate of PE and DVT. This finding was proven in the Women's Health Initiative, with 16,608 women randomized to hormone replacement therapy or placebo.[25] The risk of VTE also increases with raloxifene, a selective estrogen receptor modulator.[26]

The risk of newly diagnosed cancer after a first episode of PE or DVT is two- to threefold higher than expected for at least the following 2 years.[27] When cancer is detected, it is usually at an advanced stage with a poor prognosis.

Upper extremity DT is an increasingly important clinical entity because of more frequent placement of pacemakers and internal cardiac defibrillators, as well as more frequent use of chronic indwelling catheters for chemotherapy and nutrition. Patients with upper extremity DVT are at risk for PE, superior vena caval syndrome, and loss of vascular access.[28]

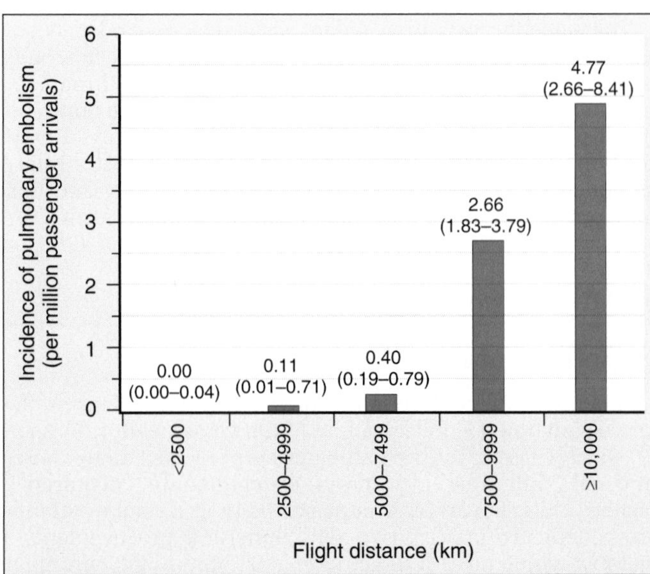

FIGURE 66–2 Incidence of pulmonary embolism increases as the distance traveled by air increases. Values shown above the bars are the number of cases per million passenger arrivals, with 95 percent confidence intervals. (From Lapostolle F, Surget V, Borron SW, et al: Severe pulmonary embolism associated with air travel. N Engl J Med 345:779, 2001.)

Relationship Between Deep Venous Thrombosis and Pulmonary Embolism

When venous thrombi detach from their sites of formation, they flow through the venous system toward the pulmonary arterial circulation. If an embolus is extremely large, it may lodge at the bifurcation of the pulmonary artery, forming a saddle embolus (Fig. 66–3, top). More commonly, a major pulmonary vessel is occluded (Fig. 66–3, bottom). Many patients with large PE do not have ultrasonographic evidence of DVT, probably because the clot has already embolized to the lungs.

RIGHT VENTRICULAR DYSFUNCTION. The extent of pulmonary vascular obstruction and the presence of underlying cardiopulmonary disease are probably the most important factors determining whether right ventricular dysfunction ensues. As obstruction increases, pulmonary artery pressure rises. The release of vasoconstricting compounds such as serotonin, reflex pulmonary artery vasoconstriction, and hypoxemia may further increase pulmonary vascular resistance and result in pulmonary hypertension.[29] The injured right ventricle releases biomarkers, including pro-brain natriuretic peptide,[30] brain natriuretic peptide,[31] and troponin,[32] all of which predict an increased likelihood of an adverse clinical outcome.

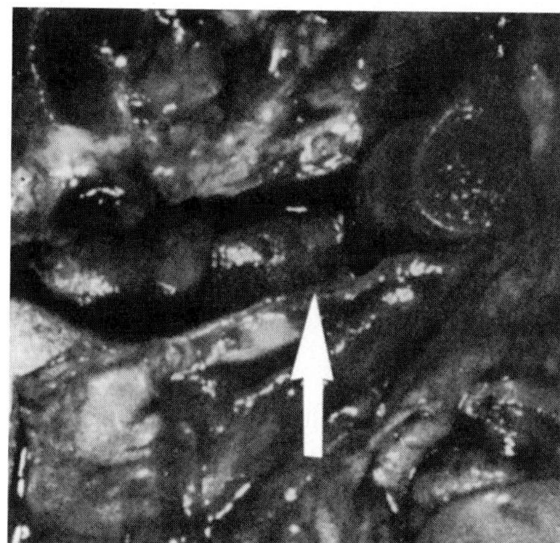

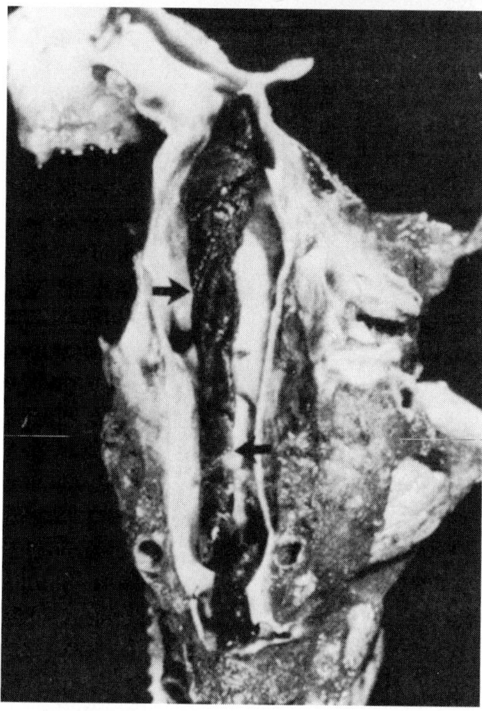

FIGURE 66–3 **Top,** Saddle embolus (arrow) at the bifurcation of the pulmonary artery. **Bottom,** Pulmonary embolus in left lower lobe pulmonary artery, with minimal attachment to the wall of the vessel. The embolus was dark red, typical of venous thrombi, and had indentations believed to represent impressions of the venous valves (arrows). (From Godleski JJ: Pathology of deep venous thrombosis and pulmonary embolism. *In* Goldhaber SZ [ed]: Pulmonary Embolism and Deep Venous Thrombosis. Philadelphia, WB Saunders, 1985, p 17.)

VENTRICULAR INTERDEPENDENCY. The sudden rise in pulmonary artery pressure reflects an abrupt increase in right ventricular afterload, with consequent elevation of right ventricular wall tension followed by right ventricular dilation and dysfunction (Fig. 66–4).[33] As the right ventricle dilates, the interventricular septum shifts toward the left, with resultant underfilling and decreased diastolic distensibility of this chamber. With underfilling of the left ventricle, systemic cardiac output and pressure both decline, potentially compromising coronary perfusion and producing myocardial ischemia.[34] Elevated right ventricular wall tension following massive PE reduces right coronary flow and increases right ventricular myocardial oxygen demand, which may result in ischemia and possibly cardiogenic shock. Perpetuation of this cycle can lead to right ventricular infarction, circulatory collapse, and death.

Summary of Pathophysiology

Pulmonary embolism can have the following pathophysiological effects: (1) increased pulmonary vascular resistance due to vascular obstruction, neurohumoral agents, or pulmonary artery baroreceptors; (2) impaired gas exchange due to increased alveolar dead space from vascular obstruction and hypoxemia from alveolar hypoventilation, low ventilation-perfusion units, and right-to-left shunting, as well as impaired carbon monoxide transfer due to loss of gas-exchange surface; (3) alveolar hyperventilation due to reflex stimulation of irritant receptors; (4) increased airway resistance due to bronchoconstriction; and (5) decreased pulmonary compliance due to lung edema, lung hemorrhage, and loss of surfactant.[35]

Diagnosis

Diagnosis of PE is more difficult than treatment or prevention. Fortunately, noninvasive diagnostic approaches have become increasingly reliable, particularly the plasma D-dimer enzyme-linked immunosorbent assay (ELISA), chest CT, and venous ultrasonography. The contemporary diagnostic strategy integrates clinical findings with various diagnostic techniques. Nevertheless, despite advances in diagnosis, major PE is missed antemortem in more than half the patients who have this condition at autopsy.[36]

CLINICAL PRESENTATION. Clinical suspicion of PE is of paramount importance in guiding diagnostic testing. Dyspnea is the most frequent symptom, and tachypnea is the most frequent sign of PE (Table 66–3). In general, severe dyspnea, syncope, or cyanosis portends a major life-threatening PE. However, pleuritic pain often signifies that the embolism is small and located in the distal pulmonary arterial system, near the pleural lining.

Pulmonary embolism should be suspected in hypotensive patients when (1) there is evidence of venous thrombosis or predisposing factors for it and (2) there is clinical evidence of acute cor pulmonale (acute right ventricular failure) such as distended neck veins, an S_3 gallop, a right ventricular heave, tachycardia, or tachypnea, especially if (3) there are echocardiographic findings of right ventricular dilation and hypokinesis or electrocardiographic (ECG) evidence of acute cor pulmonale manifested by a new S1Q3T3 pattern, new

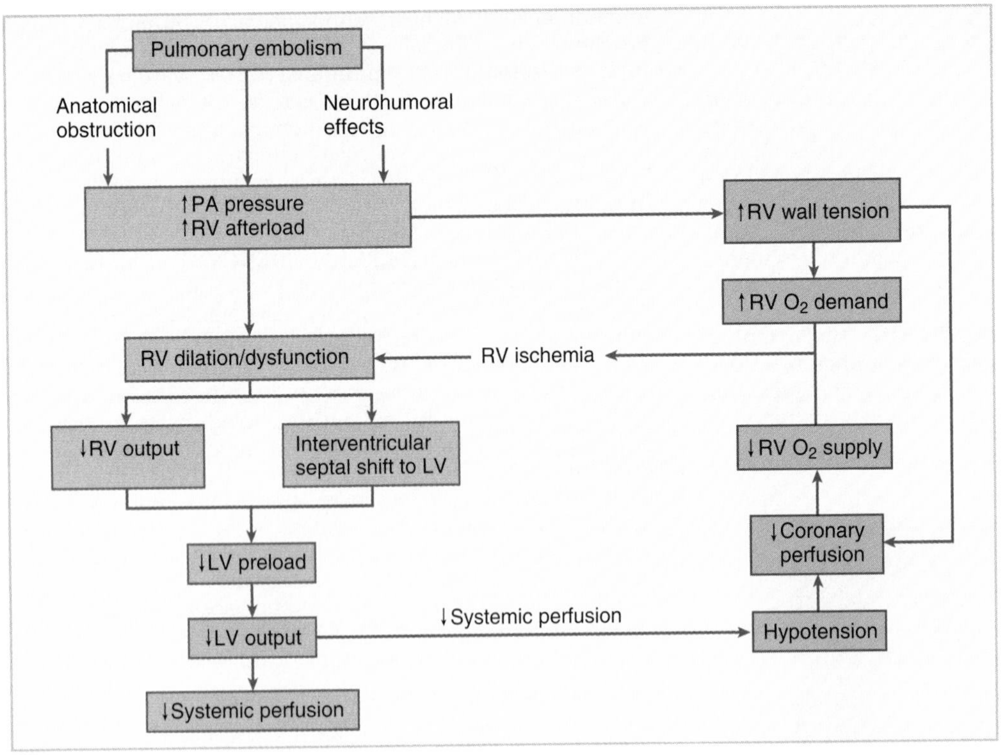

FIGURE 66–4 Pathophysiology of right ventricular dysfunction. LV = left ventricular; PA = pulmonary artery; RV = right ventricular.

incomplete right bundle branch block, or right ventricular ischemia (Fig. 66–5).

Wells and colleagues have developed a rapid seven-question bedside assessment (Table 66–4)[37] that is useful because with it almost half of their study patients could be categorized as "PE unlikely." They designated a score of 4.0 or lower as "PE unlikely." In this low-risk group, only about 5 percent of patients were subsequently diagnosed with PE.

DIFFERENTIAL DIAGNOSIS. The differential diagnosis of PE is broad and covers a spectrum from life-threatening disease such as acute myocardial infarction to innocuous anxiety states (Table 66–5). Some patients have concomitant PE and other illnesses. For example, if pneumonia or heart failure does not respond to appropriate therapy, the possibility of coexisting PE should be considered. Distinguishing between PE and primary pulmonary hypertension (see Chap. 67) warrants special vigilance. Some patients have a hybrid condition that is similar to primary pulmonary hypertension but that includes thrombi.[38] Among these patients, large central pulmonary artery thrombi can develop. It may be impossible to determine whether these thrombi formed in situ or whether they embolized to the pulmonary arteries from a separate site.

Clinical Syndromes of Pulmonary Embolism

Classification of PE into various syndromes (Table 66–6) is useful for prognostication and for deciding on subsequent clinical management.[39]

MASSIVE PULMONARY EMBOLISM. Patients with massive PE are at risk for cardiogenic shock. They have thrombosis often affecting at least half of the pulmonary arterial vasculature. Clot is almost always present bilaterally. Dyspnea is usually the most noticeable symptom, transient cyanosis is common, and systemic arterial hypotension requiring pressor support is the predominant sign. Often, these patients present without chest pain.

TABLE 66–3 Most Common Symptoms and Signs Among the 2454 Patients in the International Cooperative Pulmonary Embolism Registry (ICOPER)

Symptom or Sign	Percent
Dyspnea	82
Respiratory rate >20/min	60
Heart rate >100 beats/min	40
Chest pain	49
Cough	20
Syncope	14
Hemoptysis	7

Adapted from Goldhaber SZ, Visani L, De Rosa M, for ICOPER: Acute pulmonary embolism: Clinical outcomes in the International Cooperative Pulmonary Embolism Registry (ICOPER). Lancet 353:1386, 1999.

TABLE 66–4 Wells Clinical Bedside Scoring System for Suspected Pulmonary Embolism

Parameter	Points
Clinical signs and symptoms of DVT (minimum of leg swelling and pain with palpation of the deep veins)	3.0
An alternative diagnosis is less likely than PE	3.0
Heart rate greater than 100	1.5
Immobilization or surgery in the previous 4 weeks	1.5
Previous DVT/PE	1.5
Hemoptysis	1.0
Malignancy (on treatment, treated in the last 6 months, or palliative)	1.0

DVT = deep venous thrombosis; PE = pulmonary embolism.

Adapted from Wells PS, Anderson DR, Rodger M, et al: Derivation of a simple clinical model to categorize patients probability of pulmonary embolism: Increasing the models utility with the SimpliRED D-dimer. Thromb Haemost 83:416, 2000.

TABLE 66–5 Differential Diagnosis of Pulmonary Embolism

Myocardial infarction	Pericarditis
Pneumonia	Intrathoracic cancer
Congestive heart failure ("left-sided")	Rib fracture
Cardiomyopathy (global)	Pneumothorax
Primary pulmonary hypertension	Costochondritis
Asthma	"Musculoskeletal pain"
	Anxiety

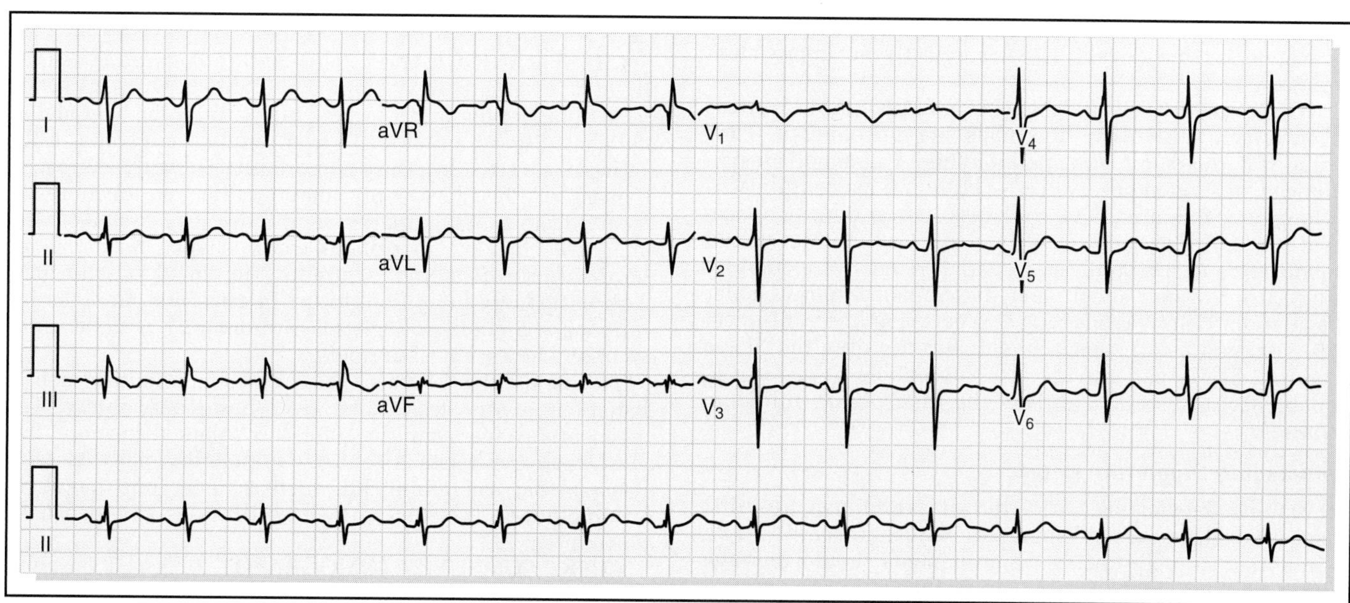

FIGURE 66–5 Electrocardiogram from a 33-year-old man who presented with a left main pulmonary artery embolism on chest computed tomographic scan. He was hemodynamically stable and had normal right ventricular function on echocardiogram. His troponin and brain natriuretic peptide levels were normal. He was managed with anticoagulation alone. On the initial electrocardiogram, he has a heart rate of 90 per minute, S1Q3T3, and incomplete right bundle branch block, with inverted or flattened T waves in Leads V1 through V4.

TABLE 66–6 Six Syndromes of Acute Pulmonary Embolism

Syndrome	Presentation	Right Ventricular Dysfunction	Therapy
Massive	Breathlessness, syncope, and cyanosis with persistent systemic arterial hypotension; typically >50 percent obstruction of pulmonary vasculature	Present	Heparin plus thrombolytic therapy or mechanical intervention
Moderate to large ("submassive")	Normal systemic arterial blood pressure; typically >30 percent perfusion defect on lung scan	Present	Heparin plus or minus thrombolytic therapy or mechanical intervention*
Small to moderate	Normal arterial blood pressure	Absent	Heparin
Pulmonary infarction	Pleuritic chest pain, hemoptysis, pleural rub, or evidence of lung consolidation; typically small peripheral emboli	Rare	Heparin and nonsteroidal antiinflammatory drugs
Paradoxical embolism	Sudden systemic embolic event such as stroke	Rare	Anticoagulation ± closure of right-to-left cardiac shunt
Nonthrombotic embolism	Most commonly air, fat, tumor fragments, or amniotic fluid	Rare	Supportive

*Therapy depends on degree of impairment of right ventricular function and presence or absence of contraindications to thrombolysis or heparin.
Adapted from Goldhaber SZ: Treatment of acute pulmonary embolism. *In* Goldhaber SZ (ed): Cardiopulmonary Diseases and Cardiac Tumors. *In* Braunwald E (series ed): Atlas of Heart Diseases. Vol 3. Philadelphia, Current Medicine, 1995, pp 7.1-7.12.

MODERATE TO LARGE ("SUBMASSIVE") PULMONARY EMBOLISM. Patients with this condition frequently have right ventricular hypokinesis, troponin or pro-BNP or BNP elevations, but normal systemic arterial pressure. Usually, one-third or more of the pulmonary artery vasculature is obstructed. These patients have various degrees of right ventricular hemodynamic instability masked by normal systemic arterial pressure. They are at risk for recurrent (and possibly fatal) PE, even with adequate anticoagulation. Most survive, but they may require escalation of therapy with pressor support or mechanical ventilation. Therefore, especially if right ventricular dysfunction persists, one should consider using thrombolytics or embolectomy.

SMALL TO MODERATE PULMONARY EMBOLISM. This syndrome is characterized by normal systemic arterial pressure, no troponin or pro-BNP release, and normal right ventricular function. Adequate anticoagulation results in an excellent clinical outcome.

PULMONARY INFARCTION. This syndrome is characterized by pleuritic chest pain that may be unremitting or may wax and wane. The pleurisy is occasionally accompanied by hemoptysis. The embolus usually lodges in the peripheral pulmonary arterial tree, near the pleura.[40] Tissue infarction usually occurs 3 to 7 days after embolism. The syndrome often includes fever, leukocytosis, an elevated erythrocyte sedimentation rate, and radiological evidence of infarction.

PARADOXICAL EMBOLISM. This syndrome often manifests with a sudden, devastating stroke and concomitant PE.[41] Although DVT is usually not detected in patients who suffer a paradoxical embolism in the presence of a patent foramen ovale, the DVT may embolize entirely to the pulmonary and systemic arteries, without residual leg or pelvic vein thrombosis. Contemporary management consists of closing the patent foramen ovale, either surgically but more often percutaneously.[42]

NONTHROMBOTIC PULMONARY EMBOLISM. Sources of embolism other than thrombus are uncommon. They include fat, tumor, air, and amniotic fluid. Fat embolism syndrome is most often observed after blunt trauma complicated by long-bone fractures.[43] Air embolus can occur during placement or removal of a central venous catheter.[44] Amniotic fluid embolism is catastrophic and characterized by respiratory failure, cardiogenic shock, and disseminated intravascular coagulation.[45] Intravenous drug abusers sometimes self-inject hair, talc, and cotton that contaminates the drug they have acquired. These patients are also susceptible to septic PE, which can cause endocarditis of the tricuspid or pulmonic valves.

Nonimaging Diagnostic Methods

To establish the diagnosis of PE, the astute clinician must first suspect this illness. Establishing the clinical probability of PE is important to help decide which patients should undergo further work-up. Many patients in whom PE is a theoretical possibility are exceedingly unlikely to have PE.

PLASMA D-DIMER ELISA. This blood-screening test relies on the principle that most patients with PE have ongoing endogenous fibrinolysis that is not effective enough to prevent PE but that does break down some of the fibrin clot to D-dimers. Although elevated plasma concentrations of D-dimers are sensitive for the presence of PE, they are not specific. Levels are elevated in patients for at least 1 week postoperatively and are also increased in patients with myocardial infarction, sepsis, cancer, or almost any other systemic illness. Therefore, the plasma D-dimer ELISA is ideally suited for outpatients or Emergency Department patients who have suspected PE but no coexisting acute systemic illness. This test is not useful for hospitalized inpatients.

At Brigham and Women's Hospital, we obtained D-dimer tests on consecutive Emergency Department patients suspected of acute PE.[46] After 1 year, 1106 assays were obtained: 559 patients had abnormally elevated D-dimer levels and 547 were within normal limits. Only 2 of the 547 patients had PE despite a normal D-dimer. Thus, the sensitivity of the D-dimer ELISA for acute PE was 96.4 percent and the negative predictive value was 99.6 percent. Similar findings have been observed in seven other urban Emergency Departments.[47] By ruling out PE with a normal D-dimer ELISA, fewer chest CT and lung scans will be required. A similar strategy works for excluding DVT, by combining a clinical risk assessment with a normal D-dimer ELISA.[48]

ARTERIAL BLOOD GASES. Among patients suspected of having PE in the Prospective Investigation of Pulmonary Embolism Diagnosis (PIOPED), there was no difference between the average PaO_2 (70 mm Hg) among those with and those without PE (72 mm Hg) at pulmonary angiography. In the subset with angiographically proven PE but no prior cardiopulmonary disease, 26 percent had a PaO_2 that was 80 mm Hg or greater.[49] Normal values of the alveolar-arterial oxygen gradient did not preclude the diagnosis of acute PE.[50] Therefore, arterial blood gas determinations should not be part of the diagnostic strategy when investigating suspected PE.

ELECTROCARDIOGRAM (see Chap. 9). The ECG helps exclude acute myocardial infarction and may raise suspicion or help confirm the diagnosis of PE among patients with ECG manifestations of right-heart strain. The converse is not true, however. Patients with massive PE may have sinus tachycardia, minor ST and T wave abnormalities, or even entirely normal ECGs. One of the most useful findings is negative T waves in precordial leads V1 through V4.[51] Other abnormalities include incomplete or complete right bundle branch block or an S1Q3T3 complex (see Fig. 66–5).[52]

Imaging Methods

CHEST RADIOGRAPHY. The chest radiograph is usually the first imaging study obtained in patients with suspected PE. Although one-fourth of patients with PE have an abnormal chest film examination, a near-normal radiograph in the setting of severe respiratory compromise is highly suggestive of massive PE. Chest x-ray abnormalities are uncommon. Focal oligemia (Westermark's sign) indicates massive central embolic occlusion. A peripheral wedge-shaped density above the diaphragm (Hampton's hump) (Fig. 66–6) usually indicates pulmonary infarction. In the International Cooperative Pulmonary Embolism Registry, cardiomegaly was the most common chest x-ray abnormality.[53]

One should always search for subtle abnormalities such as distention of the descending right pulmonary artery. The vessel often tapers rapidly after the enlarged portion. The chest radiograph can also help to identify patients with diseases that can mimic PE, such as lobar pneumonia or pneumothorax. Patients with these illnesses can also have concomitant PE.

CHEST COMPUTED TOMOGRAPHY. Chest CT has supplanted pulmonary radionuclide perfusion scintigraphy as the initial imaging test in most patients with suspected PE (Fig. 66–7).[53a] For patients with intrinsic lung disease and abnormal chest radiograph results, the chest CT scan can suggest an alternative or concomitant pulmonary disease to explain the clinical presentation. For the evaluation of suspected PE, the CT examination can include scanning of the venous system from the popliteal veins to the subsegmental pulmonary arteries. The CT examination can also provide valuable information about the size and function of the right ventricle relative to the left and can alert the clinician to the presence of right ventricular dysfunction. The latest generation of multidetector-row CT scanners permits image acquisition of the entire chest with 1 mm or submillimeter resolution with a breath-hold of less than 10 seconds.[54] With a properly performed CT scan on a multidetector row machine, it is likely that CT scanning supplants pulmonary angiography as the gold standard for PE imaging.

First-generation machines have poor resolution in the subsegmental pulmonary arteries. With first-generation machines, the sensitivity compared with pulmonary angiography is only 70 percent.[55] However, normal first-generation CT scans appear to predict a benign clinical course over the ensuing 3 months.[56]

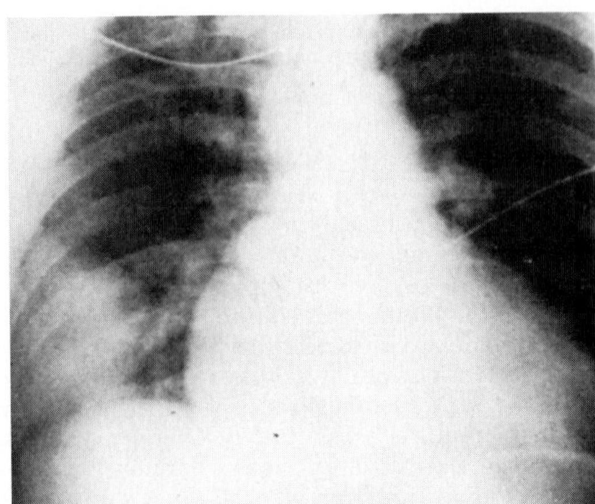

FIGURE 66–6 Posteroanterior chest film of a patient with pulmonary embolism shows a "Hampton's hump" in the right lower lung field, a homogeneous, wedge-shaped density in the peripheral field, convex to the hilum. (Courtesy of Dr. Jack L. Westcott, The New York Hospital and Cornell University Medical College.)

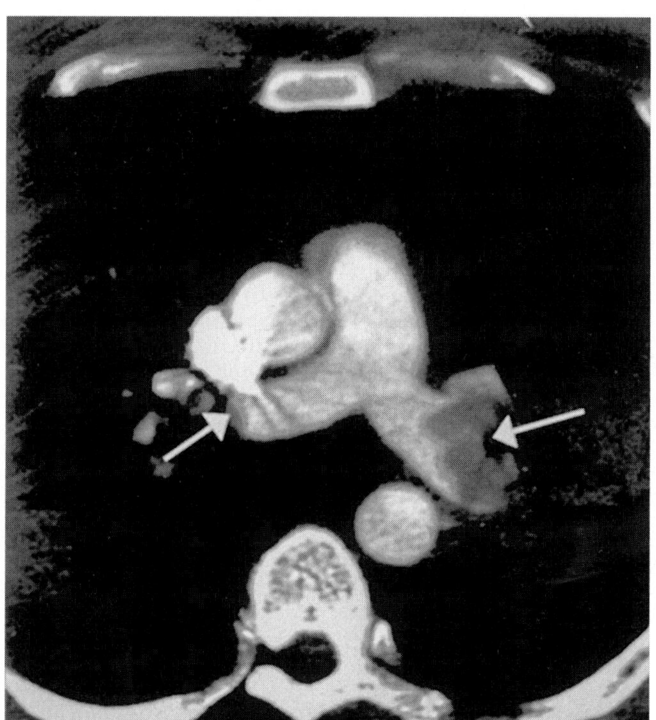

FIGURE 66–7 A 62-year-old physician suffered a massive pulmonary embolism 2 weeks after prostatectomy. Spiral chest computed tomography with contrast provided a definitive diagnosis, with a large thrombus burden apparent in the right and left main pulmonary arteries (arrows).

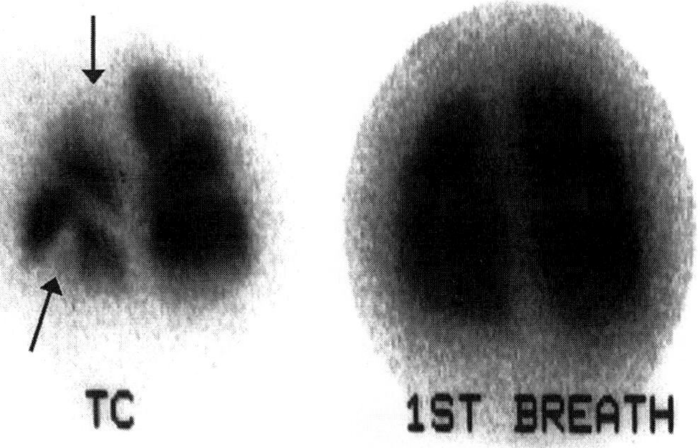

FIGURE 66–8 A 41-year-old woman presented with sudden onset of shortness of breath and retrosternal chest discomfort. Her heart rate was 168 beats/min, respiratory rate 32/min, oxygen saturation 86 percent, and blood pressure 112/70 mm Hg. She underwent a ventilation-perfusion (ventilation on the **left** and perfusion on the **right**) lung scan with xenon-133 gas (26 mCi) and technetium-99m macroaggregated albumin (3.2 mCi) in the left posterior oblique position. Numerous scattered segmental (arrows) and subsegmental perfusion defects with near normal ventilation were found. This ventilation-perfusion mismatch was interpreted as high probability for pulmonary embolism.

When ordering a CT scan, it is of paramount importance to know what generation of scanners are available. For patients suspected of massive PE, a first-generation scanner will suffice. For patients suspected of a small peripheral PE, the images should be acquired, if possible, on a newer machine with multirow detector capability. When CT scanning is preceded by D-dimer testing and venous ultrasonography of the legs, it is cost-effective in the work-up of suspected acute PE.[57]

LUNG SCANNING. Pulmonary radionuclide perfusion scintigraphy (lung scanning) is no longer the principal diagnostic imaging test when PE is suspected. Chest CT scanning with intravenous contrast has supplanted lung scanning because it provides direct and definitive results. Lung scanning is now a second-choice imaging test, usually reserved for patients with renal insufficiency, contrast allergy, or pregnancy (because of lower fetal radiation exposure than chest CT).

Perfusion scintigraphy uses radiolabeled aggregates of albumin or microspheres that are trapped in the pulmonary capillary bed. Six or eight standard views are obtained with a gamma camera. Patients with large PE may have many defects on the perfusion scan. If ventilation scanning is performed on a patient with PE but no intrinsic lung disease, a normal ventilation study result is expected, yielding a ventilation-perfusion mismatch (Fig. 66–8) and a lung scan interpreted as "high probability for PE." PE is very unlikely among patients with normal and near-normal scans. High-probability scans usually indicate acute PE, but no more than 25 percent of patients with suspected PE will have a high-probability scan.[58] Scans that fall between these extremes of the spectrum should be called "intermediate probability." Many patients with low-probability scans but high clinical suspicion for PE do, in fact, have PE at angiography.[59] Therefore, the term *low-probability* scan is a potentially lethal misnomer.[60]

TABLE 66–7	Echocardiographic Signs of Pulmonary Embolism
Direct visualization of thrombus (rare)	
Right ventricular dilation	
Right ventricular hypokinesis (with sparing of the apex)	
Abnormal interventricular septal motion	
Tricuspid valve regurgitation	
Pulmonary artery dilatation	
Lack of decreased inspiratory collapse of inferior vena cava	

MAGNETIC RESONANCE IMAGING. Gadolinium-enhanced magnetic resonance angiography (MRA) is a promising imaging test for suspected PE. When performed under ideal conditions with optimal imaging equipment, it appears to be sensitive and specific for segmental or larger PE.[61] Unlike chest CT or catheter-based pulmonary angiography, MRA does not require ionizing radiation or injection of iodinated contrast agent. Therefore, MRA can be performed safely in patients with poor renal function, at virtually no risk to the patient. Finally, magnetic resonance pulmonary angiography can include assessment of ventricular size and function, valuable in detecting patients at increased risk of an adverse clinical outcome. MRA also appears to be a promising tool for imaging leg vein thrombosis, including isolated calf vein thrombosis.[62]

ECHOCARDIOGRAPHY (see Chap. 11). Echocardiography is normal in about half of unselected patients with acute PE.[63] Therefore, echocardiography is not recommended as a routine diagnostic test for PE. However, it is a rapid, practical, and sensitive technique for detection of right ventricular overload among patients with established and large PE (Fig. 66-9). Moderate or severe right ventricular hypokinesis, persistent pulmonary hypertension, a patent foramen ovale, and free-floating thrombus in the right atrium or right ventricle help identify patients at high risk of death or recurrent thromboembolism. The frequency of echocardiographic signs of PE (Table 66-7) depends on the population being studied. For those patients in whom transthoracic imaging is unsatisfactory, transesophageal echocardiography can be carried out.[64]

Echocardiographic detection of right ventricular dysfunction at the time of presentation with PE is useful for risk stratification and prognostication.[65] Among patients with major PE, echocardiographic evidence of a patent foramen ovale signifies a high risk of death and paradoxical arterial thromboembolism.[66] Doppler echocardiography performed 6 weeks after the acute PE can identify patients with persistent pulmonary hypertension and right ventricular dysfunction. They are at high risk of developing chronic thromboembolic pulmonary hypertension.

PULMONARY ANGIOGRAPHY. Standard contrast pulmonary angiography was, for many years, considered the gold

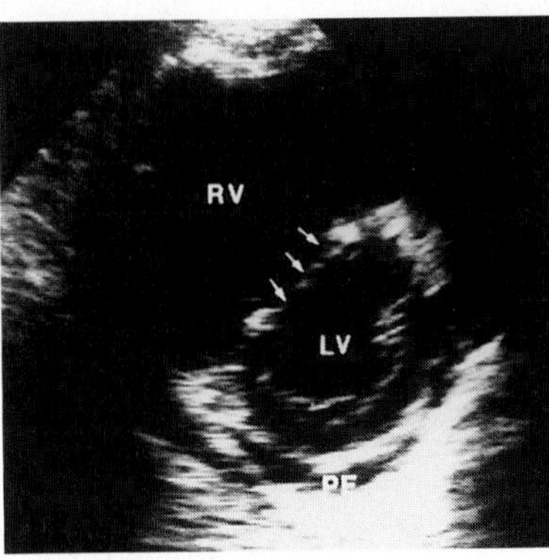

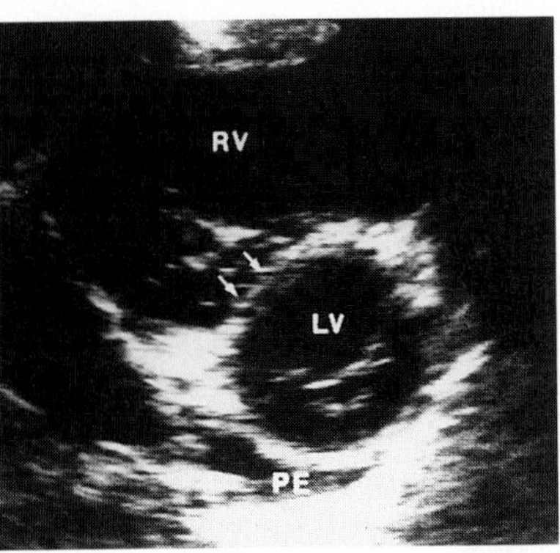

FIGURE 66–9 Parasternal short-axis views of the right ventricle (RV) and left ventricle (LV) in diastole **(left)** and systole **(right)**. Diastolic and systolic bowing of the interventricular septum (arrows) into the LV is compatible with RV volume and pressure overload, respectively. The RV is appreciably dilated and markedly hypokinetic, with little change in apparent RV area from diastole to systole. PE = small pericardial effusion. (From Come PC: Echocardiographic evaluation of pulmonary embolism and its response to therapeutic interventions. Chest 101:151S, 1992.)

standard for diagnosis but is now rarely performed because multiplanar chest CT scanning can solve most diagnostic dilemmas. However, pulmonary angiography is required when interventions are planned, such as suction catheter embolectomy, mechanical clot fragmentation, or catheter-directed thrombolysis.

The images from pulmonary angiographic evaluation can be displayed on conventional x-ray film or on a digital screen, with equivalent diagnostic accuracy.

In cases of chronic PE, CT scanning or pulmonary angiography will show arteries that appear pouched. The thrombus usually organizes with a concave edge (Fig. 66–10). Band-like defects called *webs* may be present, in addition to intimal irregularities and abrupt narrowing or occlusion of lobar vessels.

VENOUS ULTRASONOGRAPHY. The primary diagnostic criterion to establish the presence of DVT by ultrasonography is the loss of vein compressibility. Normally, the vein collapses completely when gentle pressure is applied to the skin overlying it. Upper extremity DVT can be more difficult to diagnose because the clavicle can hinder attempts to compress the subclavian vein. Venous ultrasonography is useful if it demonstrates DVT in patients with suspected PE. However, the majority of patients with PE have no imaging evidence of DVT.[67] *Therefore, if clinical suspicion of PE is high, patients without evidence of DVT should still be investigated for PE.*

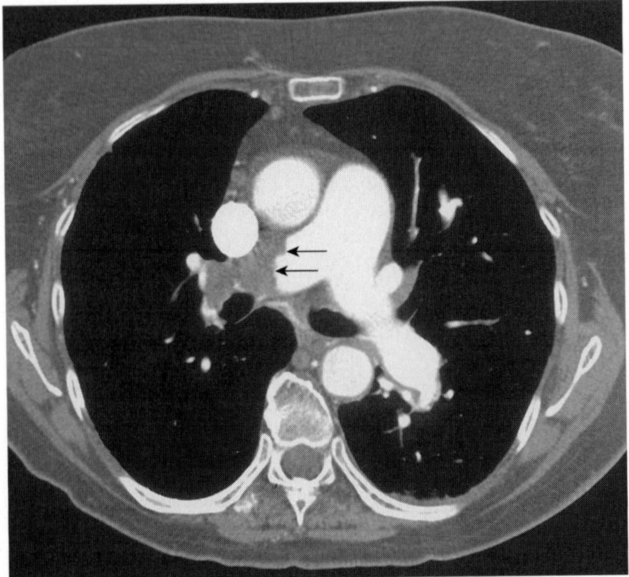

FIGURE 66–10 Chest computed tomography (CT) scan of a 59-year-old woman with chronic thromboembolic pulmonary hypertension. She has underlying antiphospholipid antibody syndrome. The chest CT scan demonstrates a large right pulmonary artery with an abrupt cut-off (arrows) in a jagged, irregular pattern due to chronic thromboembolism.

CONTRAST PHLEBOGRAPHY. Although contrast phlebography was, for many years, the gold standard for DVT diagnosis, venograms are now rarely obtained. Venography is costly and invasive and occasionally results in contrast-induced renal failure, anaphylaxis, or phlebitis. Furthermore, there is considerable disagreement in the interpretation of contrast venograms among experienced readers. DVT is usually diagnosed with ultrasonography, which is widely available, convenient, and usually accurate. Alternative modes of diagnosis are contrast-enhanced CT and magnetic resonance imaging. Consequently, we reserve contrast phlebography for situations in which we anticipate an interventional procedure such as catheter-directed thrombolysis, suction embolectomy, angioplasty, stenting, or placement of an inferior vena caval filter.

Overall Strategy: An Integrated Diagnostic Approach

A wide array of diagnostic tests is available for the investigation of suspected PE. Familiarity with each test's strengths and weaknesses (Table 66–8) as well as knowledge of the availability and reliability of specific tests at one's hospital will facilitate a concise and streamlined work-up.

At Brigham and Women's Hospital (Fig. 66–11), the initial assessment includes the history, physical examination, and ECG, with special attention to the patient's clinical milieu and risk factors for venous thromboembolism. The Wells bedside assessment score is used to semiquantitate the clinical likelihood of PE. As part of the differential diagnostic work-up, we obtain an electrocardiogram and chest radiograph. To screen for PE in the Emergency Department, we obtain a rapid turn-around plasma D-dimer ELISA. If normal, then PE is exceedingly unlikely, and the diagnosis is ordinarily considered to have been excluded at that point. If elevated, we ordinarily pursue the diagnosis of PE with chest CT scanning. For the occasional equivocal result, we next

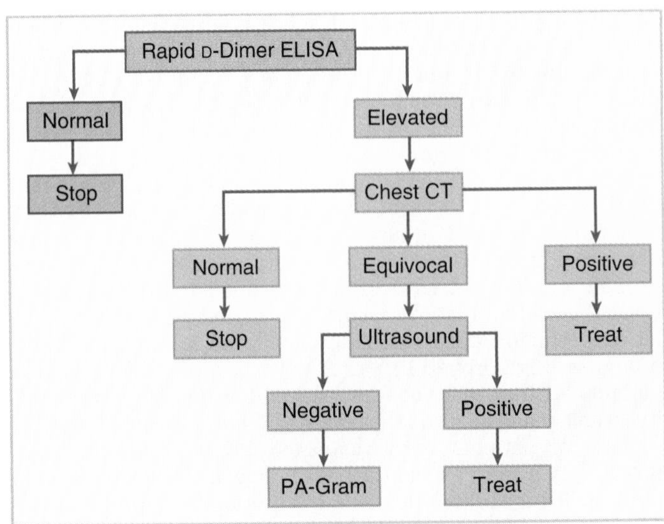

FIGURE 66–11 Emergency Department and outpatient pulmonary embolism diagnosis strategy: integrated diagnostic approach. CT = computed tomography; ELISA = enzyme-linked immunosorbent assay; PA-Gram = pulmonary arteriogram.

TABLE 66–8 Advantages and Disadvantages of Diagnostic Tests for Suspected Pulmonary Embolism

Diagnostic Test	Advantages	Disadvantages
Plasma D-dimer ELISA	A normal result in this rapid turnaround blood test makes PE exceedingly unlikely.	Level is elevated in patients with many systemic illnesses that mimic PE, such as pneumonia and myocardial infarction. Level is elevated in patients with sepsis, cancer, postoperative state, and pregnancy.
Electrocardiogram	Universally available; may indicate ominous acute cor pulmonale or benign pericarditis.	Acute cor pulmonale on electrocardiogram is not specific for PE; not a sensitive test.
Chest radiograph	Usually has minor abnormalities but occasionally pathognomonic; may indicate alternative diagnoses such as pneumothorax.	Not specific.
Chest computed tomography	New-generation scanners constitute the new gold standard for diagnosis.	Older generation scanners are insensitive for important but distal PE.
Lung scanning	High-probability scans are reliable for detecting PE; normal/near-normal scans are reliable for excluding PE.	Most scans are neither high probability nor normal/near-normal; lung scans are falling out of favor; most test results are equivocal.
Magnetic resonance imaging	Excellent for anatomy and cardiac function; the contrast agent does not cause renal failure.	In preliminary use; not widely available; experience very limited.
Echocardiography	Excellent for identifying right ventricular dilation and dysfunction that is not obvious clinically, thus providing an early warning of potentially adverse outcome.	Not specific; many patients with PE have normal echocardiograms; the test cannot reliably differentiate causes of right ventricular dysfunction.
Pulmonary angiography	Necessary for catheter-based interventions.	Invasive, costly, uncomfortable.
Venous ultrasonography	Excellent for detecting symptomatic proximal DVT; surrogate for PE.	Cannot image iliac vein thrombosis; imaging of calf is operator dependent; DVT may have embolized completely, resulting in a normal finding.
Contrast venography	Used to be gold standard; excellent for calf veins; necessary for catheter-based interventions.	Can cause chemical phlebitis; uncomfortable; costly; may fail to diagnose massive DVT because veins are filled with thrombus and cannot be opacified.

DVT = deep venous thrombosis; ELISA = enzyme-linked immunosorbent assay; PE = pulmonary embolism.

proceed to venous ultrasonography of the legs. If the ultrasonographic examination is normal and high clinical suspicion persists, a diagnostic pulmonary angiogram is obtained. An integrated diagnostic strategy that includes clinical probability assessment, chest CT, and venous ultrasonography will usually provide a noninvasive diagnosis or exclusion of PE. This approach is safe, is validated, and requires pulmonary angiography in at most 10 percent of patients.[68]

Management

Risk Stratification

Patients with PE present with a wide spectrum of illness that ranges from mild to severe. Therefore, rapid and accurate risk stratification is of paramount importance.[68a] Appropriate care can range from prevention of recurrent PE with anticoagulation alone in low-risk patients to clot dissolution or removal with thrombolysis or embolectomy in high-risk patients. High-risk patients may require intensive support with mechanical ventilation or pressors while the fundamental problem of PE is addressed with aggressive medical, interventional angiographic, or surgical therapy.

The three key components for risk stratification are (1) clinical evaluation, which can be undertaken systematically with the Geneva Prognostic Index,[69] (2) biomarkers such as troponin,[32] pro-BNP,[30] and BNP,[31] and (3) assessment of right ventricular function, usually accomplished with echocardiography.[34]

Clinical evaluation is straightforward if the patient feels perfectly well or, at the other end of the spectrum, is in cardiogenic shock. Most patients with PE, however, are moderately ill. The traditional clinical assessment and prognostication has been done by *gestalt*. However, the Geneva Prognostic Index has quantified and validated a predictive model of clinical outcome, based on a bedside history and physical examination (Tables 66–9 and 66–10). This index was used to identify low-risk patients with PE who were managed successfully as outpatients, without hospitalization.[70]

TABLE 66–9 The Geneva Point Score to Assess Pulmonary Embolism Prognosis

Variable	Point Score
Cancer	+2
Heart failure	+1
Prior DVT	+1
Hypotension	+2
Hypoxemia	+1
DVT on ultrasonogram	+1

DVT = deep venous thrombosis.

Clinical evaluation should be supplemented by cardiac biomarkers that detect microinfarction or distention of the right ventricle.[70a] These tests should be readily available with rapid turn-around in Emergency Departments, thus providing the assessment with a quantitative estimate of risk.

Right ventricular dysfunction can be detected on physical examination, by noting distended jugular veins, a systolic murmur of tricuspid regurgitation, or an accentuated P2 (see Chap. 8). In practice, obese necks often make jugular vein

TABLE 66–10 The Geneva Adverse Outcome Score

Number of Points	Number of Patients	Cumulative Percentage	Percentage of Patients with Adverse Outcome (n)
0	52	19.4	0 (0)
1	79	48.9	2.5 (2)
2	49	67.2	4.1 (2)
3	56	88.1	17.8 (10)
4	22	96.3	27.3 (6)
5	7	98.9	57.1 (4)
6	3	100	100 (3)

From Wicki J, Perrier A, Perneger TV, et al: Predicting adverse outcome in patients with acute pulmonary embolism: A risk score. Thromb Haemost 84:548, 2000.

assessment difficult, and noisy Emergency Departments can obscure the subtle auscultatory findings of right ventricular dysfunction. The electrocardiogram may show a new right bundle branch block, but often, no comparison tracing is available. Therefore, the most commonly used tool for assessing right ventricular dysfunction is echocardiography (see Chap. 11).[34]

Adjunctive measures include provision of supplemental oxygen and adequate pain relief, usually most effective with nonsteroidal antiinflammatory medications. Patients who appear toxic and hypoxic should be considered for prompt temporary mechanical ventilation. Those with impending hypotension and/or poor organ perfusion require rapid institution of an inotropic agent such as dopamine (see Chap. 23). All patients find PE to be emotionally difficult to deal with. They and their families require constant reassurance that most patients have good outcomes once the diagnosis has been established.

Prevention of Recurrent Pulmonary Embolism or Deep Venous Thromboembolism

Heparin

UNFRACTIONATED HEPARIN (see Chap. 80). Standard unfractionated heparin (UFH) is a highly sulfated glycosaminoglycan that is partially purified from porcine intestinal mucosa. Its molecular weight ranges from 3000 to 30,000 and averages 15,000. Heparin acts primarily by binding to antithrombin III (AT III), an enzyme that inhibits the coagulation factors thrombin (factor IIa), Xa, IXa, XIa, and XIIa. Heparin subsequently promotes a conformational change in AT III that accelerates its activity approximately 100- to 1000-fold. This prevents additional thrombus formation and permits endogenous fibrinolytic mechanisms to lyse clot that has already formed. However, heparin does *not* directly dissolve thrombus that already exists. The efficacy of heparin is limited because clot-bound thrombin is protected from heparin-antithrombin III inhibition. Furthermore, heparin resistance can occur because UFH binds to plasma proteins.[71] The dose response to intravenous UFH is highly variable. Even when a therapeutic activated partial thromboplastin time between 55 to 85 seconds is achieved, and the dose maintained, subsequent measurements are usually not within the desired therapeutic range.[72]

An activated PTT that is at least one and one-half times greater than the control value should provide a minimum therapeutic level of unfractionated heparin. Commonly, the therapeutic range is 60 to 80 seconds. However, there are many different PTT reagent kits and virtually no standardization of PTT levels.

Initiation of heparin therapy is discussed later (see Initiating Heparin Therapy).

LOW-MOLECULAR-WEIGHT HEPARIN. Low-molecular-weight heparins (LMWHs) are fragments of UFH that exhibit less binding to plasma proteins and endothelial cells than UFH. Therefore, LMWHs have greater bioavailability, more predictable dose response, and longer half-life than UFH.[73] The introduction of LMWHs for treatment of venous thromboembolism is revolutionizing the management of DVT and PE, especially for the majority of patients who are hemodynamically stable (Table 66–11). Large randomized trials of patients with acute DVT have compared subcutaneously administered LMWH with continuous intravenous unfractionated heparin as a bridge to full and therapeutic anticoagulation.[74] LMWH was at least as effective and safe as continuous intravenous of unfractionated heparin.

A meta-analysis of randomized trials comparing 3674 patients with acute DVT receiving LMWH versus UFH demonstrated that LMWH reduced the mortality rate over 3 to 6 months of follow-up by 29 percent (Fig. 66-12).[75] The major bleeding complication rate was reduced by 43 percent. These data were used in a cost-effectiveness analysis that showed that LMWH is highly cost-effective compared with UFH for DVT management.[76] The excellent bioavailability and subcutaneous administration of LMWH permit a strategy of weight-based LMWH dosing (without laboratory tests for dose adjustment in most instances) coupled with the possibility of outpatient therapy or an abbreviated hospitalization. It appears that the majority of ambulatory patients who present with DVT can be treated as outpatients, as long as an infrastructure, such as an Anticoagulation Clinic, has been established to ensure meticulous follow-up.

TABLE 66–11 Low-Molecular-Weight Heparins

Name	Status	Molecular Weight (Daltons)	Anti-Xa/anti-Iia ratio	Treatment Dose
Enoxaparin	FDA approved for DVT treatment	4800	3.9	1.0 mg/kg twice daily, or 1.5 mg/kg once daily
Dalteparin	FDA approved, but not for DVT treatment	5000	2.2	100 U/kg twice daily, or 200 U/kg once daily
Nadroparin	Not available in the United States	4500	3.5	4100 U twice daily for patients weighing <50 kg, 6150 U twice daily for 50-70 kg, and 9200 U twice daily for >70 kg
Reviparin	Not available in the United States	3900	3.3	3500 U twice daily for patients weighing 35-45 kg, 4200 U twice daily for 46-60 kg and 6300 U twice daily for >60 kg
Tinzaparin	FDA approved for DVT treatment	4500	1.5	175 U/Kg once daily

DVT = deep venous thrombosis; FDA = Food and Drug Administration.

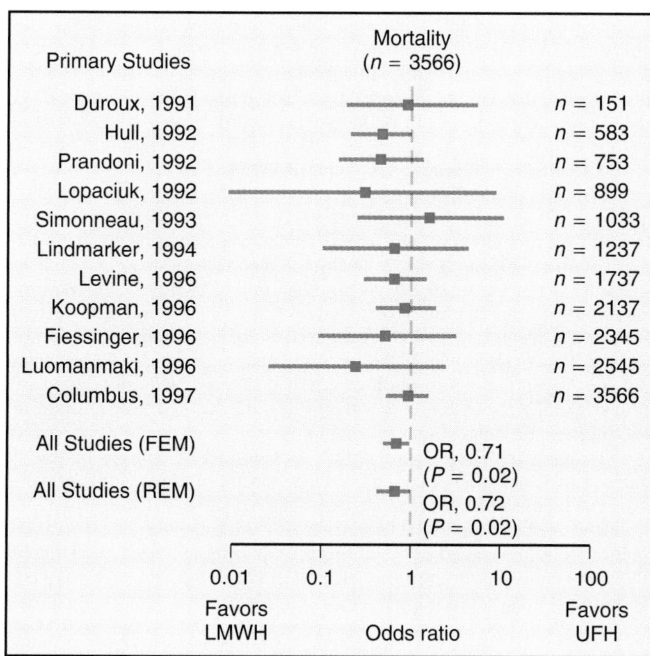

FIGURE 66–12 Meta-analysis for mortality rates comparing low-molecular-weight-heparin (LMWH) and unfractionated heparin (UFH). FEM = fixed-effects model; OR = odds ratio; REM = random-effects model. (Modified from Gould MK, Dembitzer AD, Doyle RL, et al: Low molecular weight heparins compared with unfractionated heparin for treatment of acute deep venous thrombosis: A meta-analysis of randomized, controlled trials. Ann Intern Med 130:800, 1999.)

In a randomized trial of 1137 DVT patients, the LMWH reviparin was more effective than UFH in causing thrombus regression, based on baseline and follow-up venography.[77] Reviparin reduced the recurrence rate by more than 50 percent compared with UFH. This reduction in recurrence rate correlated with successful thrombus regression on serial venography.

LMWH AS A "BRIDGE" TO WARFARIN. In patients with VTE and cancer, LMWH as monotherapy without oral anticoagulation may have advantages over traditional UFH as a "bridge" to warfarin. In one trial of 71 patients randomized to enoxaparin 1.5 mg/kg once daily versus UFH, the enoxaparin group experienced less bleeding.[78] In a larger trial of 672 patients with VTE and cancer, those randomized to dalteparin 200 U/kg once daily for 6 months had a much lower recurrence rate than patients receiving UFH: 8.8 percent versus 17.4 percent, respectively.[79]

In patients with symptomatic PE, LMWH appears at least as effective as intravenous UFH as a bridge to warfarin. Extended 3-month treatment with enoxaparin as monotherapy for symptomatic acute PE appears feasible and shortens the duration of hospitalization compared with patients receiving standard treatment.[80]

The Food and Drug Administration has approved outpatient treatment of DVT *without PE* using enoxaparin 1 mg/kg every 12 hours for a minimum of 5 days. Warfarin is usually begun on the first evening of therapy, and enoxaparin is continued until a stable and therapeutic INR of 2.0 to 3.0 is achieved. The dose of enoxaparin must be decreased in patients with renal insufficiency because LMWH is primarily renally excreted. The Food and Drug Administration approved the same enoxaparin dosing regimen for inpatient treatment of DVT *with or without PE*, as well as an alternative dosing regimen of 1.5 mg/kg once daily.

ANTI-Xa LEVELS. LMWH is usually dosed according to weight. However, if a quantitative assay is required to determine the anticoagulant effect, an anti-Xa level can be obtained. A therapeutic level for full anticoagulation is in the range of approximately 0.5 to 1.0 units/ml. Prophylactic doses of LMWH usually result in anti-Xa levels of 0.1 to 0.3 units/ml. The peak level is reached 3 to 6 hours after subcutaneous injection.

At Brigham and Women's Hospital, we assay the anti-Xa level with a HEPRN pack (Dupont) in the automated clinical analyzer used for other chemistry tests. This is a chromogenic assay based on the inhibition of factor Xa by heparin-activated antithrombin III. The plasma anti-Xa level is particularly useful in monitoring in five situations: (1) UFH anticoagulation with baseline elevated PTTs due to a lupus anticoagulant or anti-cardiolipin antibodies, (2) LMWH dosing in obese patients, (3) LMWH dosing in patients with renal dysfunction, (4) pregnancy,[81] and (5) determining the origin of an unexpected bleeding or clotting problem in patients who were receiving what appeared to be appropriate anticoagulant dosing.

INITIATING HEPARIN THERAPY. Heparin is the cornerstone of treatment for acute PE. Before heparin therapy is begun, risk factors for bleeding should be considered, such as a prior history of bleeding with anticoagulation, thrombocytopenia, vitamin K deficiency, increasing age, underlying diseases, and concomitant drug therapy. The most frequently overlooked portion of the physical examination is a rectal examination for occult blood.

Conventional anticoagulation for acute PE begins with a bolus of 5000 to 10,000 units of intravenous UFH, followed by a continuous intravenous infusion based on weight. Most patients require at least 30,000 units/24 hr. There are many nomograms, such as Raschke's,[82] to assist in adjusting the dose of continuous intravenous UFH, with guidelines provided by the patient's weight and PTT (Table 66–12). Unless a severe bleeding problem such as active gastrointestinal bleeding is detected, UFH can be started as soon as the diagnosis is suspected.

In patients with active bleeding, heparin therapy should be withheld, and nonpharmacological treatment (secondary prevention) with insertion of an inferior vena caval filter should be considered after confirmation of the diagnosis of PE. Although there is a trend toward the use of LMWH for patients who present with acute symptomatic PE, I prefer to initiate therapy with UFH if there is a possibility that the patient will require thrombolysis, catheter-based suction embolectomy, or open surgical embolectomy.

COMPLICATIONS. The most important adverse effect of heparin (UFH or LMWH) is hemorrhage. Major bleeding during anticoagulation may unmask a previously silent lesion, such as bladder or colon cancer. For most cases of moderate bleeding, cessation of heparin will suffice, and the PTT usually returns to normal within 6 hours. Resumption of heparin at a lower dose or implementing alternative therapy depends on the severity of the bleeding, the risk of recurrent thromboembolism, and the extent to which bleeding may have resulted from excessive anticoagulation.

In the event of life-threatening or intracranial hemorrhage, protamine sulfate can be administered at the time heparin is discontinued. Protamine, a strongly basic protein,

TABLE 66–12 Intravenous Unfractionated Heparin "Raschke Nomogram"

Variable	Action
Initial heparin bolus	80 U/kg bolus, then 18 U/kg/h
PTT <35 seconds (<1.2 × control)	80 U/kg bolus, then increase by 4 U/kg/h
PTT 35 to 45 seconds (1.2 to 1.5 × control)	40 U/kg bolus, then increase by 2 U/kg/h
PTT 46 to 70 seconds (1.5 to 2.3 × control)	No change
PTT 71 to 90 seconds (2.3 to 3 × control)	Decrease infusion rate by 2 U/kg/h
PTT >90 seconds (>3 × control)	Hold infusion 1 h, then decrease infusion rate by 3 U/kg/h

PTT = activated partial thromboplastin time.

From Raschke RA, Reilly BR, Guidry JR, et al: The weight-based heparin dosing nomogram compared with a "standard care" nomogram: A randomized controlled trial. Ann Intern Med 119:874, 1993.

immediately reverses anticoagulant activity by forming a stable complex with the acidic heparin. However, protamine only partially inhibits the anticoagulant activity of LMWH. For life-threatening hemorrhage, the usual dose is approximately 1 mg/100 units of heparin, administered slowly (e.g., 50 mg over 10 to 30 minutes). Protamine sulfate may cause allergic reactions, particularly in diabetic patients who have had prior exposure to protamine after using neutral protamine Hagedorn (NPH) insulin.

Heparin-induced thrombocytopenia and other complications of heparin therapy are discussed in Chapter 80.

Warfarin Sodium (see Chap. 80)

Warfarin is a vitamin K antagonist that prevents gamma carboxylation activation of coagulation factors II, VII, IX, and X. The full anticoagulant effect of warfarin may not be apparent for 5 days, even if the prothrombin time, used to monitor warfarin's effect, becomes elevated more rapidly. Elevation in the prothrombin time may initially reflect depletion of coagulation factor VII, which has a half-life of about 6 hours, whereas factor II has a half-life of about 5 days. Warfarin is a difficult drug to dose and monitor. Centralized anticoagulation clinics, staffed by nurses or pharmacists, have eased the administrative burden of prescribing warfarin and have assisted in safer and more effective anticoagulation.[83]

OVERLAP WITH HEPARIN. When warfarin therapy is initiated during an active thrombotic state, the levels of protein C and S decline, thus creating a thrombogenic potential. By overlapping heparin and warfarin for 5 days, the procoagulant effect of unopposed warfarin can be counteracted. In a Dutch study, patients with DVT were randomized to oral anticoagulation alone versus UFH plus oral anticoagulation. The recurrent DVT rate was three times higher in the group that received oral anticoagulation alone.[84]

MONITORING WARFARIN. The prothrombin time, used to adjust the dose of warfarin, should be reported according to the International Normalized Ratio (INR), not the prothrombin time ratio or the prothrombin time expressed in seconds. Not well appreciated is that warfarin can markedly increase the PTT. In a prospective cohort study, the PTT increased 16 seconds for each increase of 1.0 in the INR.[85] Unfortunately, INRs may not be a very reliable method for assessing anticoagulant effects. In a study of patients with similar INRs, there was substantial variability in tissue factor coagulation responses. This suggests that control of anticoagulation according to an INR target range may be less reliable than commonly thought.[86]

Nevertheless, from a practical viewpoint, we rely on the INR to dose warfarin. Under most circumstances, the initial dose should be 5 mg daily.[87] The dose should be reduced, however, for debilitated or elderly patients.[88] Some patients will have an extremely low warfarin requirement of 1.5 mg or less in the absence of liver dysfunction, drug interaction, or concomitant disease. They usually have CYP2CP variant alleles associated with impaired hydroxylation of S-warfarin. If not recognized when warfarin is initiated, these individuals are at a potentially high risk of bleeding complications.[89]

Warfarin is plagued by multiple drug-drug and drug-food interactions. Most antibiotics increase the INR. Even benign-sounding drugs such as acetaminophen increase the INR in a dose-dependent manner.[90] Green leafy vegetables have vitamin K and lower the INR.

COMPLICATIONS. Warfarin has a narrow therapeutic index, and the major toxic effect of warfarin is bleeding. At times, the dose response is unpredictable. The risk of bleeding increases as the INR increases. Risk factors for hemorrhage include severe hepatic or renal disease, alcoholism, drug interactions, trauma, malignant disease, and known previous bleeding sites in the gastrointestinal tract. The risk of major bleeding persists after hospital discharge and is greatest in the first 30 days following hospitalization.

Major life-threatening bleeding due to warfarin has traditionally required immediate treatment with enough cryoprecipitate or fresh frozen plasma to normalize the INR and achieve immediate hemostasis. An improved approach is to use recombinant human factor VIIa concentrate, which provides safe and rapid reversal of warfarin-induced excessive anticoagulation.[92]

Prior to "reversing" an elevated INR, it is useful to ensure that the abnormal laboratory value is "real" and not artifactual. An INR specimen that is not assayed promptly after blood collection can be spuriously high. In addition, "point of care" machines generally have higher INRs than central laboratories for patients who are intensively anticoagulated with warfarin.

To treat minor bleeding or a verified INR that exceeds 9.0 without any bleeding, vitamin K has traditionally been administered parenterally; a dose of 10 mg subcutaneously usually reverses the effects of warfarin in 6 to 12 hours. However, this approach makes patients relatively refractory to warfarin for up to 2 weeks, so that reinstitution of warfarin becomes problematic. Merely withholding one or two doses of warfarin and administering 2.5 mg of oral vitamin K is a reliable and safe method for rapidly correcting an INR that exceeds 5.0 in patients who do not have serious concomitant bleeding. Some patients with an INR less than 9.0 simply require interruption of warfarin therapy, without administration of fresh frozen plasma or vitamin K, until the INR has returned to the therapeutic range.

"Point-of-care" devices provide the INR result in 2 minutes by use of a drop of whole blood obtained from a fingertip puncture. Appropriately selected patients can self-manage their warfarin dosing at home. In a randomized trial comparing self-management with conventional management, the self-managed patients more frequently achieved their target INRs and reported an improved quality of life compared with the conventionally managed group.[93]

Optimal Duration and Intensity of Anticoagulation

There has been considerable debate about the optimal duration and intensity of anticoagulation for patients with idiopathic PE or DVT. During the past decade, a series of randomized trials[94-96a] has established that these patients benefit from either extended-duration or indefinite-duration anticoagulation.

The PREVENT Trial showed that anticoagulation can be administered safely and effectively for an indefinite period with a low-intensity target INR of 1.5 to 2.0. With this regimen, the incidence of PE and DVT was more than halved, and patients required INR testing only once every 8 weeks.[96] The benefit of low-intensity warfarin was not affected by whether the patient had factor V Leiden or the prothrombin gene mutation. Thus, the strategy of long-term, low-intensity warfarin was highly effective in preventing recurrence in all subgroups. In the ELATE study of 739 patients with idiopathic PE or DVT, indefinite-duration, full-intensity warfarin (target INR of 2.0-3.0) was more effective and as safe as indefinite-duration, low-intensity warfarin therapy (target INR of 1.5-2.0).[96a] At this time, there is no foolproof way to tell which patients with idiopathic PE or DVT are *unlikely* to require long-term anticoagulation. Therefore, we recommend 6 months of full-intensity anticoagulation (INR 2.0-3.0), followed by indefinite-duration anticoagulation for all suitable patients with idiopathic VTE (Fig. 66–13).

Inferior Vena Caval Interruption

The two major indications for placement of an IVC filter are (1) major hemorrhage that precludes anticoagulation, and (2) recurrent PE despite well-documented anticoagulation. An IVC filter prevents PE, not DVT.[97] Patients with filters after an initial PE are more than twice as likely as non-filter patients to require rehospitalization for DVT.[98] Therefore, when a filter is inserted, anticoagulation should also be used, whenever possible, to prevent further thrombosis. Some patients have an immediate contraindication to anticoagulation, but the duration of this contraindication is uncertain. Under these circumstances, placement of a nonpermanent filter may be appropriate. Temporary filters are attached to a guidewire or catheter. They can only be used for a few days because of concern for infection at the insertion site. Retrievable filters can be left in place for 10 to 14 days, or can remain perma-

- Idiopathic PE or DVT
- 6 months of warfarin, target INR = 2.0–3.0
- Age ≥ 30 years
  No surgery, trauma within 90 days
  No metastatic cancer, major GI bleeding, hemorrhagic stroke, antiphospholipid antibody syndrome
- Indefinite duration, warfarin

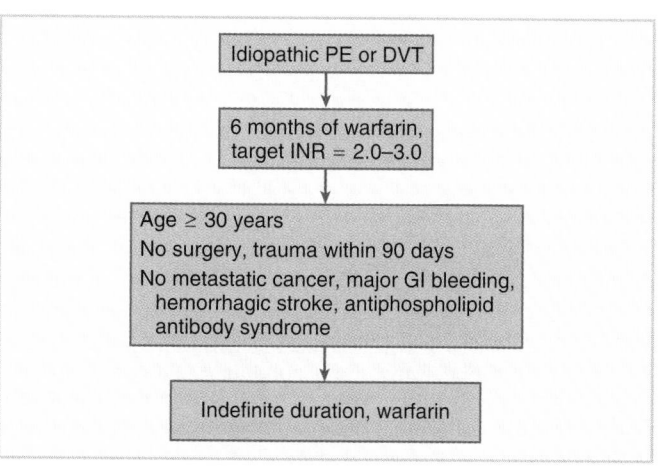

FIGURE 66–13 Optimal duration of anticoagulation for patients with idiopathic pulmonary embolism (PE) or deep venous thrombosis (DVT).

nently if necessary because of a trapped large clot or a persistent contraindication to anticoagulation.[99]

Thrombolysis

Thrombolysis is lifesaving in patients with cardiogenic shock due to massive PE (Fig. 66–14).[100] For patients with contraindications to thrombolysis, embolectomy in the Catheterization Laboratory or Operating Room can be substituted.

Thrombolysis may (1) prevent the downhill spiral of right-sided heart failure by physical dissolution of anatomically obstructing pulmonary arterial thrombus; (2) prevent the continued release of serotonin and other neurohumoral factors that might otherwise lead to worsening pulmonary hypertension; and (3) dissolve much of the source of the thrombus in the pelvic or deep leg veins, thereby decreasing the likelihood of recurrent large PE.

MAPPET-3, the largest randomized trial of thrombolytic therapy versus heparin alone, was carried out in patients with normal blood pressure but with right ventricular dysfunction or pulmonary hypertension. Tissue plasminogen activator minimized escalation of therapy—defined as the need for pressors, mechanical ventilation, cardiopulmonary resuscitation, or open-label thrombolysis—without an increase in major bleeding.[101]

The potential benefits of immediately reversing right heart failure and preventing recurrent PE must be balanced by the risk of hemorrhage. Contraindications to thrombolysis, such as intracranial disease, recent surgery, or trauma, preclude its use in some patients who can safely receive heparin alone. There is a 1 to 2 percent risk of intracranial hemorrhage.[102] Carefully screening patients for contraindications to thrombolysis is the best way to minimize bleeding risk (see Chap. 47).

At Brigham and Women's Hospital, we have coordinated five trials of PE thrombolysis. In a 101-patient trial of tissue plasminogen activator (t-PA; 100 mg as a continuous infusion over 2 hours) plus heparin versus heparin alone,[103] the initial systemic arterial systolic pressure was at least 90 mm Hg in every patient. Most importantly, no clinical episodes of PE recurred among patients receiving t-PA, but there were five (two fatal and three nonfatal) clinically suspected recurrent PEs within 14 days in patients randomized to heparin alone ($p < 0.06$). All five initially showed right ventricular hypokinesis on echocardiogram. This observation suggests that echocardiography may help identify a subgroup of patients with PE at high risk of adverse clinical outcomes if treated with heparin alone. Such patients in particular would appear to be excellent candidates for thrombolytic therapy in the absence of contraindications.

Qualitative assessment of right ventricular wall motion demonstrated that 39 percent of the t-PA recipients improved and 2.4 percent worsened, compared with 17 percent improvement and 17 percent worsening among those who received heparin alone ($p < 0.005$). Quantitative assessment showed that t-PA recipients had a significant decrease in right ventricular end-diastolic area during the 24 hours after randomization compared with none among those allocated to heparin alone ($p < 0.01$). Recipients of t-PA also had an absolute improvement in pulmonary perfusion of 14.6 percent at 24 hours, compared with 1.5 percent improvement among heparin-alone recipients ($p < 0.0001$).

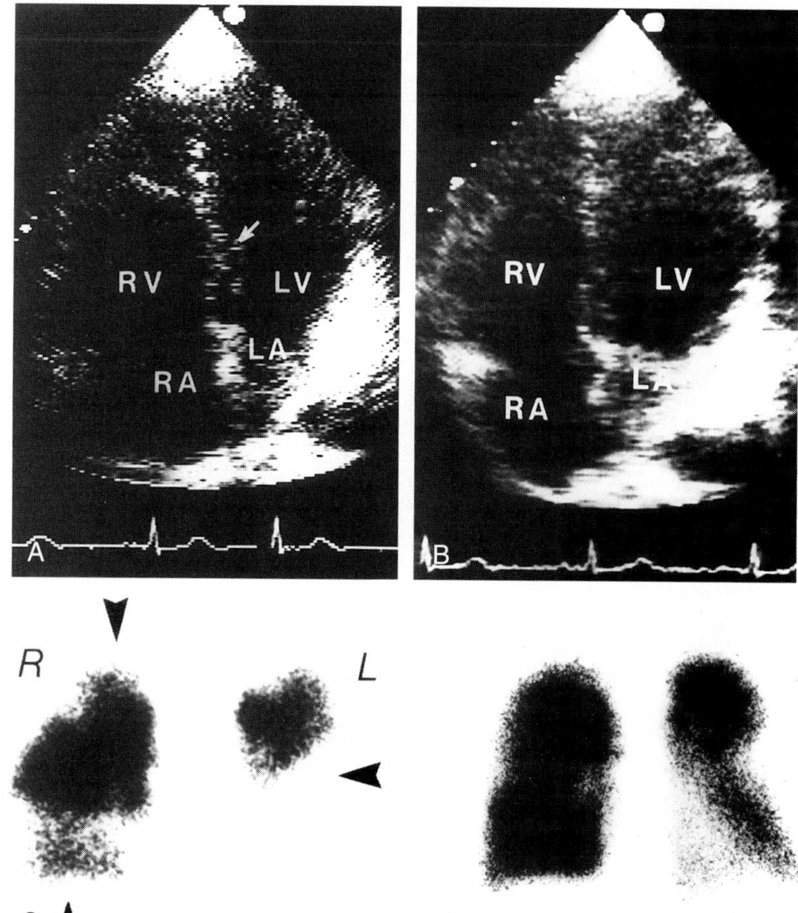

FIGURE 66–14 Echocardiograms (four-chamber view) and perfusion lung scans (anterior view) in a previously healthy 53-year-old man treated with tissue plasminogen activator (t-PA) for PE. **A,** Right ventricular (RV) enlargement before treatment. The RV end-diastolic area was 42.9 cm^2, and the interventricular septum (arrow) was displaced toward the left ventricle (LV). There was moderately severe RV hypokinesis. **B,** Three hours after initiation of t-PA therapy, the size of the RV normalized (with a planimetered area of 25.7 cm^2) and the interventricular septum resumed its normal configuration. RV wall motion normalized. **C,** The pretherapy lung scan shows absence of perfusion in the right middle lobe (lower arrowhead) and in most of the right upper lobe, particularly the apical segment of the right upper lobe (upper arrowhead). The left lung shows absence of perfusion in the lingula and anterior segment of the left upper lobe (horizontal arrowhead) and irregular perfusion in the apical-posterior segment of the left upper lobe. **D,** The posttherapy scan shows marked improvement in perfusion. LA = left atrium; RA = right atrium. (From Goldhaber SZ: Treatment of acute pulmonary embolism. *In* Goldhaber SZ [ed]: Cardiopulmonary Diseases and Cardiac Tumors. *In* Braunwald E [series ed]: Atlas of Heart Diseases. Vol 3. Philadelphia, Current Medicine, 1995, pp 3.1-3.25.)

Unlike patients receiving myocardial infarction thrombolysis, patients with PE have a wide "window" for effective use of thrombolysis. Specifically, patients who receive thrombolysis up to 14 days after new symptoms or signs maintain an effective response,[104] probably because of the bronchial collateral circulation. Therefore, patients suspected of having PE should be considered as potentially eligible for thrombolysis if they have had any new symptoms or signs within the 2 weeks before presentation.

DEEP VENOUS THROMBOSIS INTERVENTIONS

Indications for DVT thrombolysis include extensive iliofemoral or upper extremity venous thrombosis. Totally occlusive venous thrombosis usually does not lyse if the agent is administered through a peripheral vein. However, we often achieve a successful outcome with catheter-directed thrombolysis, catheter-directed suction embolectomy, venous angioplasty, venous stenting, or a combination of these interventional procedures.

VENOUS INSUFFICIENCY. Many patients with PE are plagued with chronic lower leg swelling and calf discomfort that can become problematic years after an episode of venous thromboembolism. This is known as *venous insufficiency* or *postthrombotic syndrome.*[105] In most situations, the pathophysiology is damage of venous valves from antecedent DVT. Under extreme circumstances, venous ulceration can occur, particularly in the medial malleolus. The condition is usually manageable with below-knee vascular compression stockings. However, the frequency of venous insufficiency can be halved by preventive use of sized-to-fit compression stockings of 20 to 40 mm Hg.[106]

Pulmonary Embolectomy

Emergency surgical embolectomy with cardiopulmonary bypass is reemerging as an effective and often successful strategy for managing patients with massive PE, or patients who have contraindications to thrombolysis with moderate size PE (Fig. 66–15), as well as those who require surgical excision of a right atrial thrombus or closure of a patent foramen ovale. The results of embolectomy can be optimized if patients are referred for this procedure before the onset of cardiogenic shock. At Brigham and Women's Hospital, 29 patients underwent surgical embolectomy in a 2-year period, with an 89 percent survival rate.[107] The procedure was performed without aortic cross-clamping, cardioplegic, or fibrillatory arrest on a warm, beating heart. It was imperative to avoid blind instrumentation of the fragile pulmonary arteries. Extraction was limited to directly visible clot, which was always possible throughout the segmental pulmonary arteries.

Catheter embolectomy occasionally results in extraction of massive pulmonary arterial thrombus (Fig. 66–16A). More often, multiple tiny clot fragments are suctioned through the catheter (Fig. 66–16B), with modest angiographic improvement, resulting nevertheless in rapid restoration of normal blood pressure with a decrease in hypoxemia. Interventional catheterization techniques include mechanical fragmentation of thrombus with a standard pulmonary artery catheter, clot pulverization with a rotating basket catheter, percutaneous rheolytic thrombectomy, and pigtail rotational catheter embolectomy.[108] Another approach is simultaneous mechanical clot fragmentation and pharmacological thrombolysis (Fig. 66–17).[109]

Management Approach for Acute Pulmonary Embolism

Therapy for PE should be tailored according to the patient's clinical status, the anatomical extent of the embolus, the presence of underlying cardiopulmonary disease, the presence of elevated cardiac biomarkers such as troponin, and the detection of right-sided-heart dysfunction by physical examination, electrocardiogram, and echocardiogram. High-risk patients warrant thrombolysis or embolectomy as primary therapy to dissolve or remove the thrombus, in addition to heparin anticoagulation to prevent recurrent venous thromboembolism. In low-risk patients, anticoagulation alone should suffice (Fig. 66–18).

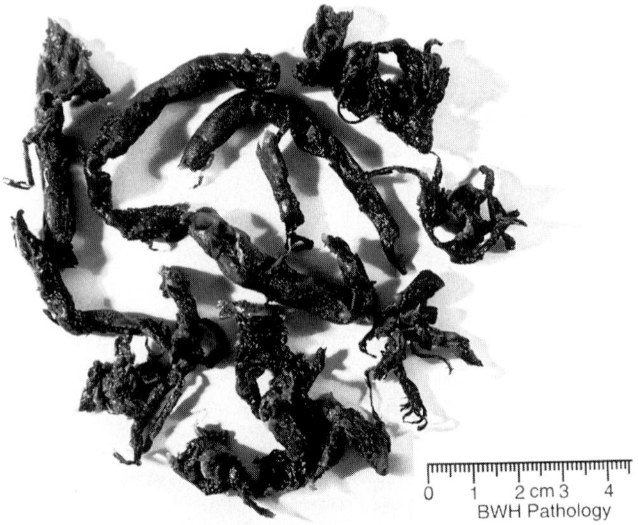

0 1 2 cm 3 4
BWH Pathology

FIGURE 66–15 A 52-year-old woman was on the medical service to treat multiple sclerosis when she became short of breath and collapsed. Her echocardiogram showed a dilated right ventricle and collapsed left ventricle. Shortly thereafter, she suffered cardiac arrest and was immediately taken to the operating room with the presumptive diagnosis of pulmonary embolism. She was placed on cardiopulmonary bypass, and massive amounts of thrombus were removed from her pulmonary arteries. She subsequently recovered uneventfully.

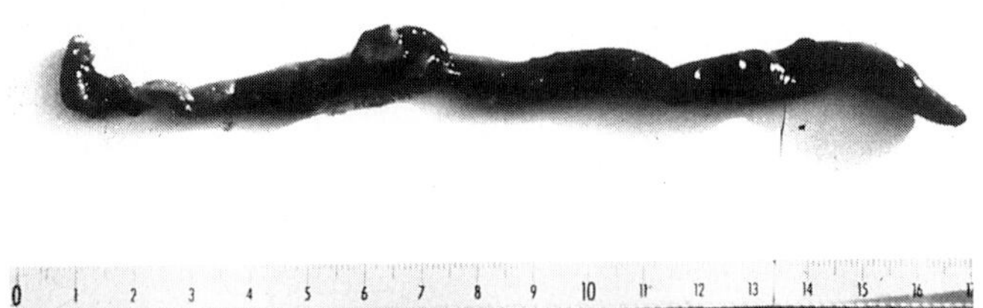

0 1 2 3 4 5 6 7 8 9 10 11 12 13 14 15

A

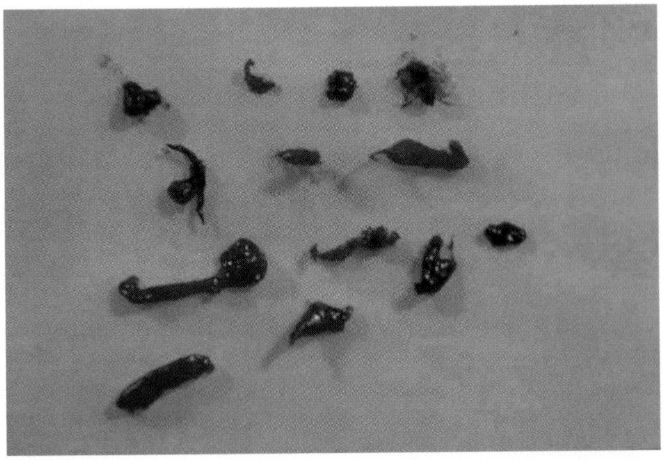

B

FIGURE 66–16 Philippe Reynaud, MD, at the Laennec Hospital in Paris, used a Greenfield embolectomy catheter to remove this 17-cm thrombus from a severely compromised patient with pulmonary embolism **(A)**. Rapid hemodynamic improvement ensued. (From Meyer G, Tamiser D, Reynaud P, Sors H: Acute pulmonary embolectomy. *In* Goldhaber SZ [ed]: Cardiopulmonary Diseases and Cardiac Tumors. *In* Braunwald E [series ed]: Atlas of Heart Diseases. Vol 3. Philadelphia, Current Medicine, 1995, pp 7.1-7.12.) Most of the time, however, suction catheter embolectomy removes multiple small clot fragments **(B)**. Despite modest angiographic improvement, marked clinical improvement often ensues.

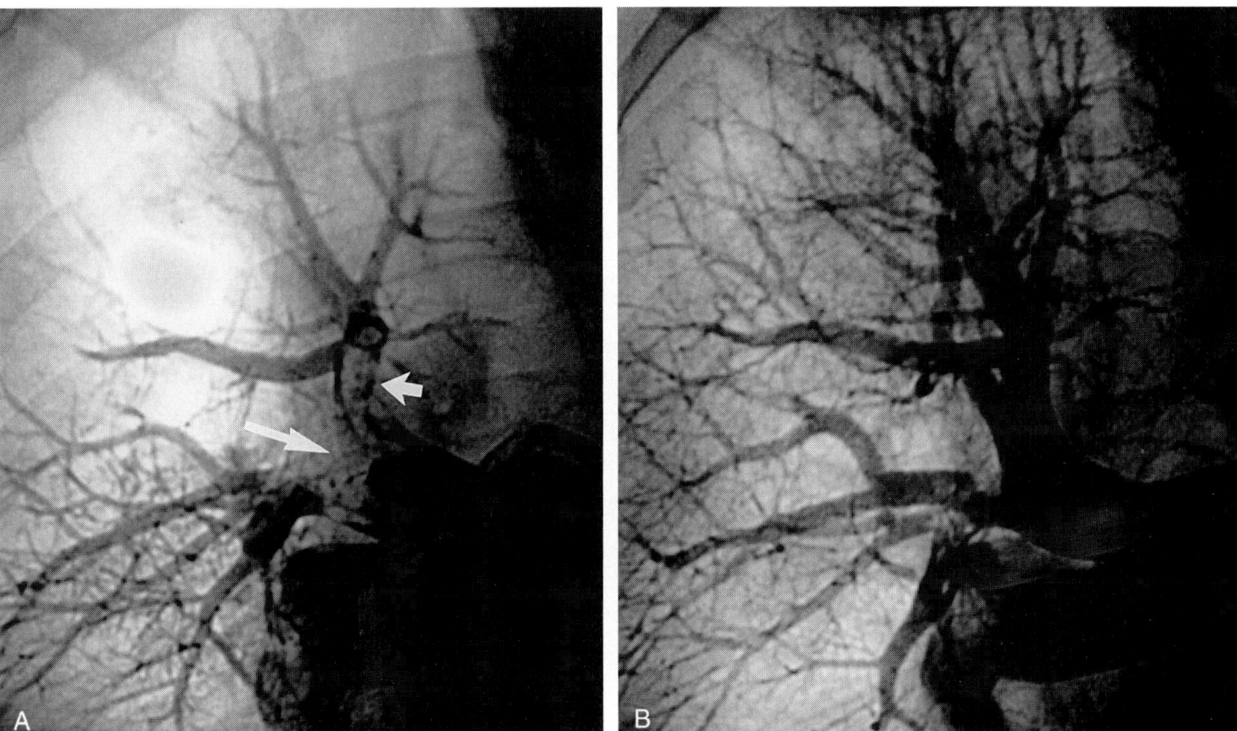

FIGURE 66–17 A 77-year-old woman had right-sided heart failure despite 3 days of full-dose heparin. Therefore, she underwent right heart catheterization and pulmonary angiography. Her pulmonary arterial pressure was 55/30 mm Hg. Seen on her baseline angiogram **(A)** were large right middle and right upper lobe pulmonary emboli (arrows). Because of relative contraindications to full-dose thrombolysis (systemic arterial hypertension and mild dementia), the patient underwent combined suction catheter embolectomy and catheter-directed thrombolysis with a bolus pulse spray of 8 mg of tissue plasminogen activator followed by an overnight infusion of 1 mg/hr. Her follow-up angiogram **(B)** shows marked improvement and reperfusion.

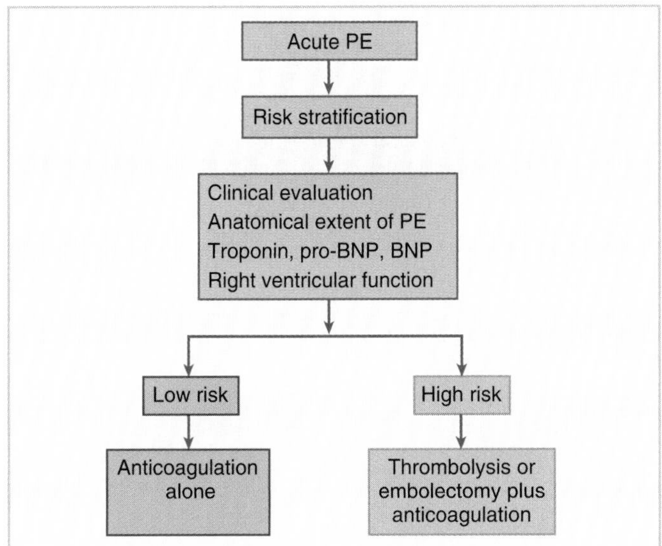

FIGURE 66–18 Management strategy for acute pulmonary embolism (PE), based on risk stratification. BNP = brain natriuretic peptide.

EMOTIONAL SUPPORT. Although PE can be as emotionally devastating as myocardial infarction, the psychological burden for patients with PE may be greater. The lay public is not familiar with PE, particularly in terms of the possibility of genetic predisposition, long-term disability, and recurrence of disease. There is a widespread lack of understanding of PE's pathophysiology[110] and treatment. By discussing the implications of PE with patients and their families, we can allay the emotional burden. For the past decade, one of my nurses and I have organized a Pulmonary Embolism Support Group for our patients. We meet at the hospital once every 3 weeks in the evening. Although these sessions have an educational component, the major emphasis is on discussing the anxieties and living difficulties that occur in the aftermath of PE.

Chronic Thromboembolic Pulmonary Hypertension (see Chap. 67; Figs 67–4 and 67–15)

Patients with chronic pulmonary hypertension due to previous PE[111] may be virtually bedridden with breathlessness due to high pulmonary arterial pressures. They should be considered for pulmonary thromboendarterectomy, which, if successful, can reduce and at times even cure pulmonary hypertension. The operation involves a median sternotomy, institution of cardiopulmonary bypass, and deep hypothermia with circulatory arrest periods. Incisions are made in both pulmonary arteries into the lower-lobe branches. Pulmonary thromboendarterectomy removes organized thrombus by establishing an endarterectomy plane in all involved vessels (Fig. 66–19).

At the University of California at San Diego, almost 2000 patients debilitated by chronic pulmonary hypertension due to PE have undergone pulmonary thromboendarterectomy with good results and at an acceptable risk. When surgery is not feasible, balloon pulmonary angioplasty can be considered. This procedure is associated with functional improvement and improved exercise tolerance.[112]

PREVENTION

Pulmonary embolism is difficult to diagnose, expensive to treat, and occasionally lethal despite therapy. Therefore, preventive measures are paramount. The concept of prophylaxis is gaining widespread acceptance, partly because of the medicolegal liability of physicians who omit prophylaxis among hospitalized patients with risk factors for venous thrombosis. Fortunately, numerous prophylaxis options are available for preventing PE and DVT in most patients (Table 66-13). The specific prophylaxis modality that is chosen is not nearly as important as upholding

TABLE 66–13 Specific Prevention Strategies for Pulmonary Embolism and Deep Venous Thrombosis

Indication	Prevention Strategy
Hospitalization with medical illness	Enoxaparin 40 mg daily or dalteparin 5000 U daily. GCS/IPC for patients with contraindications to anticoagulation. Combined LMWH or UHF *plus* GCS/IPC for patients at very high risk. Consider surveillance venous ultrasonography for medical intensive care unit patients.
General surgery	UFH 5000 U q8h, first dose 2 hr preoperatively, continued for 7 days or LMWH once daily.
Cancer surgery	Enoxaparin 40 mg daily, first dose 10-14 hr preoperatively, for 28 days.
Total hip replacement	Enoxaparin 40 mg daily, beginning preoperative evening, continuing out-of-hospital for 21-28 days. Enoxaparin 30 mg bid, first dose 12-24 hr postoperatively, until hospital discharge. Dalteparin 2500 U ≥4 hr postoperatively, then 5000 U daily until hospital discharge or for 35 days. Fondaparinux 2.5 mg 4-8 hr postoperatively, then ≥12 hr after first dose, then daily for 5-9 days. Warfarin daily, first dose 5 mg preoperative evening, adjusted to target INR of 2.0-3.0 and continued 4-6 weeks.
Total knee replacement	Enoxaparin 30 mg bid, beginning 12-24 hr postoperatively, continued for an average of 9 days. Fondaparinux 2.5 mg, first dose 4-8 hr postoperatively, second dose ≥12 hr after first dose, then daily for 5-9 days.
Hip fracture surgery	Fondaparinux 2.5 mg, first dose 4-8 hr postoperatively, second dose ≥12 hr after first dose, then daily for 5-9 days. However, if surgery is delayed >24-48 hr after admission, give first dose 10-14 hr preoperatively. Aspirin 160 mg daily for 35 days as adjunctive prophylaxis.

GCS = graduated compression stockings; IPC = intermittent pneumatic compression devices; LMWH = low-molecular-weight heparin; UFH = unfractionated heparin.

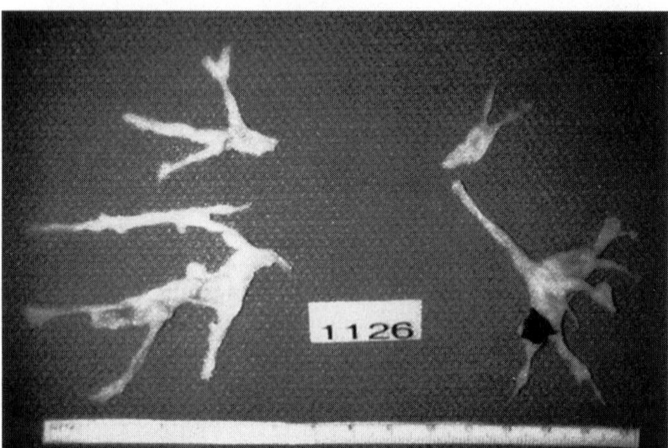

FIGURE 66–19 A 30-year-old man with chronic pulmonary embolism complained of exercise intolerance. His echocardiogram showed mild to moderate right ventricular dysfunction and enlargement. Lung scan, chest computed tomographic scan, and pulmonary angiogram showed numerous thrombi. The patient underwent pulmonary thromboendarterectomy after insertion of a prophylactic inferior vena caval filter. At surgery, a moderate amount of thromboembolic material was removed from both lungs. His pulmonary artery pressure decreased from a baseline of 35/10 mm Hg to 18/9 mm Hg before the pulmonary artery catheter was removed. He has enjoyed an excellent and uncomplicated recovery. (Courtesy of Dr. Kim M. Kerr.)

a standard that virtually all hospitalized patients receive some preventive measure appropriate to their level of risk.

American[113] and European[114] consensus conferences have provided detailed guidelines for prevention of venous thromboembolism with various mechanical measures and pharmacological agents. Computer-generated prompts increase the utilization of prophylactic measures.[115] However, even when implemented, prophylaxis may be inadequate.[116] Therefore, high-risk patients may warrant surveillance venous ultrasonography to detect "breakthrough" venous thrombi in high-risk settings.[117]

MECHANICAL MEASURES. Mechanical measures consist of graduated compression stockings and intermittent pneumatic compression devices, which enhance endogenous fibrinolysis[118] as well as increase venous blood flow. Mechanical measures are especially worthwhile among patients who have an absolute contraindication to anticoagulation.

PHARMACOLOGICAL AGENTS. Pharmacological prophylaxis options include unfractionated heparin[119] LMWH, fondaparinux,[120,121] and warfarin. Aspirin confers a slight benefit[122] but not enough to be considered a standard agent to prevent PE and DVT. For prophylaxis in the setting of total hip or knee replacement, the oral direct thrombin inhibitor ximelagatran appears promising when compared with warfarin[123] or with enoxaparin.[124] Postoperative PE often occurs several weeks after major surgery. Enoxaparin for 4 weeks postoperatively is superior to enoxaparin for 1 week postoperatively following surgery for cancer.[125] Extended-duration anticoagulation with LMWH is also worthwhile for patients undergoing total hip or knee replacement.[126]

PROPHYLAXIS STRATEGIES IN MEDICAL PATIENTS. Hospitalized medical patients are at risk for DVT and PE. The risk is greatest in intensive care units but it persists among less critically ill patients with diagnoses that include congestive heart failure, respiratory failure, pneumonia, or other serious infection. These venous thromboses can often be prevented with low, fixed, prophylactic doses of LMWH, such as enoxaparin 40 mg once daily[127] or dalteparin 5000 units once daily.[128] Nevertheless, in the DVT FREE Registry of 5451 DVT patients, 2295 of the 3894 patients (59 percent) who did not receive prophylaxis were medical patients.[23]

REFERENCES

1. Goldhaber SZ, Visani L, De Rosa M, for ICOPER: Acute pulmonary embolism: Clinical outcomes in the International Cooperative Pulmonary Embolism Registry (ICOPER). Lancet 353:1386, 1999.

Hypercoagulability

2. Ariens RA, de Lange M, Snieder H, et al: Activation markers of coagulation and fibrinolysis in twins: Heritability of the prethrombotic state. Lancet 359:667, 2002.
3. Rosendaal FR, Bovill EG: Heritability of clotting factors and the revival of the prothrombotic state. Lancet 359:638, 2002.
4. Seligsohn U, Lubetsky A: Genetic susceptibility to venous thrombosis. N Engl J Med 344:1222, 2001.
5. Bertina RM, Koeleman BPC, Koster T, et al: Mutation in blood coagulation factor V associated with resistance to activated protein C. Nature 369:64, 1994.
6. Zöller B, Dahlbäck B: Linkage between inherited resistance to activated protein C and factor V gene mutation in venous thrombosis. Lancet 343:1536, 1994.
7. Poort SR, Rosendaal FR, Reitsma PH, et al: A common genetic variation in the 3′-untranslated region of the prothrombin gene is associated with elevated plasma prothrombin levels and an increase in venous thrombosis. Blood 88:3698, 1996.
8. Allaart CF, Poort SR, Rosendaal FR, et al: Increased risk of venous thrombosis in carriers of hereditary protein C deficiency defect. Lancet 341:134, 1993.
9. Gladson CL, Scharrer I, Hach V, et al: The frequency of type heterozygous protein S and protein C deficiency in 141 unrelated young patients with venous thrombosis. Thromb Haemost 59:18, 1988.
10. Bucciarelli P, Rosendaal FR, Tripodi A, et al: Risk of venous thromboembolism and clinical manifestations in carriers of antithrombin, protein C, protein S deficiency, or activated protein C resistance: A multicenter collaborative family study. Arterioscler Thromb Vasc Biol 19:1026, 1999.
11. Langman LJ, Ray JG, Evrovski J, et al: Hyperhomocyst(e)inemia and the increased risk of venous thromboembolism: More evidence from a case-control study. Arch Intern Med 160:961, 2000.

12. Ridker PM, Hennekens CH, Selhub J, et al: Interrelation of hyperhomocyst(e)inemia, Factor V Leiden, and risk of future venous thromboembolism. Circulation 95:1777, 1997.
13. Levine JS, Branch DW, Rauch J: The antiphospholipid syndrome. N Engl J Med 346:752, 2002.
14. Prandoni P, Bilora F, Marchiori A, et al: An association between atherosclerosis and venous thromboembolism. N Engl J Med 348:1435, 2003.
15. Ridker PM, Hennekens CH, Lindpaintner K, et al: Mutation in the gene coding for coagulation factor V and risks of future myocardial infarction, stroke, and venous thrombosis in apparently healthy men. N Engl J Med 332:912, 1995.
16. Ridker PM, Miletich JP, Buring JE, et al: Factor V Leiden as a risk factor for recurrent pregnancy loss. Ann Intern Med 128:1000, 1998.
17. Vandenbroucke JP, Rosing J, Bloemenkamp KW, et al: Oral contraceptives and the risk of venous thrombosis. N Engl J Med 344:1527, 2001.
18. Ridker PM, Hennekens CH, Miletich JP: G20210A mutation in prothrombin gene and risk of myocardial infarction, stroke, and venous thrombosis in a large cohort of US men. Circulation 99:999, 1999.
19. Joffe HV, Goldhaber SZ. Laboratory thrombophilias and venous thromboembolism. Vasc Med 7:93, 2002.
20. Lapostolle F, Surget V, Borron SW, et al: Severe pulmonary embolism associated with air travel. N Engl J Med 345:779, 2001.
21. Oger E, Bressollette L, Nonent M, et al: High prevalence of asymptomatic deep vein thrombosis on admission in a medical unit among elderly patients. Thromb Haemost 88:592, 2002.
22. Heit JA, Silverstein MD, Mohr DN, et al: Risk factors for deep vein thrombosis and pulmonary embolism: A population-based case-control study. Arch Intern Med 160:809, 2000.
23. Goldhaber SZ, Tapson VF, for the DVT FREE Steering Committee: DVT FREE: A prospective registry of 5451 patients with ultrasound-confirmed deep vein thrombosis. Am J Cardiol 93:259, 2004.
24. Parkin L, Skegg DC, Wilson M, et al: Oral contraceptives and fatal pulmonary embolism. Lancet 355:2133, 2000.
25. Rossouw JE, Anderson GL, Prentice RL, et al: Risks and benefits of estrogen plus progestin in healthy postmenopausal women: Principal results From the Women's Health Initiative randomized controlled trial. JAMA 288:321, 2002.
26. Cummings SR, Eckert S, Krueger KA, et al: The effect of raloxifene on risk of breast cancer in postmenopausal women. Results from the MORE randomized trial. JAMA 281:2189, 1999.
27. Schulman S, Lindmarker P: Incidence of cancer after prophylaxis with warfarin against recurrent venous thromboembolism. Duration of Anticoagulation Trial. N Engl J Med 342:1953, 2000.

Pathophysiology

28. Joffe HV, Goldhaber SZ: Upper-extremity deep vein thrombosis. Circulation 106:1874, 2002.
29. Wood KE: Major pulmonary embolism: Review of a pathophysiologic approach to the golden hour of hemodynamically significant pulmonary embolism. Chest 121:877, 2002.
30. Kucher N, Printzen G, Doernhoefer T, et al: Low pro-brain natriuretic peptide levels predict benign clinical outcome in acute pulmonary embolism. Circulation 107:1576, 2003.
31. Kucher N, Printzen G, Goldhaber SZ: Prognostic role of BNP in acute pulmonary embolism. Circulation 107:2545, 2003.
32. Konstantinides S, Geibel A, Olschewski M, et al: Importance of cardiac troponins I and T in risk stratification of patients with acute pulmonary embolism. Circulation 106:1263, 2002.
33. Lualdi JC, Goldhaber SZ: Right ventricular dysfunction after acute pulmonary embolism: Pathophysiologic factors, detection, and therapeutic implications. Am Heart J 130:1276, 1995.
34. Goldhaber SZ: Echocardiography in the management of pulmonary embolism. Ann Intern Med 136:691, 2002.
35. Goldhaber SZ, Elliott, CE: Acute pulmonary embolism: Part I. Epidemiology, pathophysiology, and diagnosis. Circulation 108:2726, 2003.

Diagnosis

36. Pineda LA, Hathwar VS, Grant BJ: Clinical suspicion of fatal pulmonary embolism. Chest 120:791, 2001.
37. Wells PS, Anderson DR, Rodger M, et al: Derivation of a simple clinical model to categorize patients' probability of pulmonary embolism: Increasing the model's utility with the SimpliRED D-dimer. Thromb Haemost 83:416, 2000.
38. Moser KM, Fedullo PF, Finkbeiner WE, Golden J: Do patients with primary pulmonary hypertension develop extensive central thrombi? Circulation 91:741, 1995.
39. Goldhaber SZ: Treatment of acute pulmonary embolism. *In* Goldhaber SZ (ed): Cardiopulmonary diseases and cardiac tumors. *In* Braunwald E (series ed): Atlas of Heart Diseases. Vol 3. Philadelphia, Current Medicine 1995, p 3.1.
40. Dalen JE, Haffajee CI, Alpert JS, III, et al: Pulmonary embolism, pulmonary hemorrhage and pulmonary infarction. N Engl J Med 296:1431, 1977.
41. Goldhaber SZ, Polak JF: Deep vein thrombosis, pulmonary embolism, and primary pulmonary hypertension. *In* Creager MA (ed), Braunwald E (senior ed): Atlas of Vascular Disease. 2nd ed. Philadelphia, Current Medicine, 2003, pp 205-227.
42. Meier B, Lock JE: Contemporary management of patent foramen ovale. Circulation 107:5, 2003.
43. Fabian TC: Unraveling the fat embolism syndrome. N Engl J Med 329:961, 1993.
44. Muth CM, Shank ES: Gas embolism. N Engl J Med 342:476, 2000.
45. Baldisseri MR: Amniotic fluid embolism. UpToDate 2003.
46. Dunn KL, Wolf JP, Dorfman DM, et al: Normal D-dimer levels in emergency department patients suspected of acute pulmonary embolism. J Am Coll Cardiol 40:1475, 2002.
47. Kline JA, Nelson RD, Jackson RE, et al: Criteria for the safe use of D-dimer testing in emergency department patients with suspected pulmonary embolism: A multicenter US study. Ann Emerg Med 39:144, 2002.
48. Schutgens RE, Ackermark P, Haas FJ, et al: Combination of a normal D-dimer concentration and a non-high pretest clinical probability score is a safe strategy to exclude deep venous thrombosis. Circulation 107:593, 2003.
49. Stein PD, Terrin MI, Hales CA, et al: Clinical, laboratory, roentgenographic, and electrocardiographic findings in patients with acute pulmonary embolism and no preexisting cardiac or pulmonary disease. Chest 100:598, 1991.
50. Stein PD, Goldhaber SZ, Henry JW: Alveolar-arterial oxygen gradient in the assessment of acute pulmonary embolism. Chest 107:139, 1995.
51. Ferrari E, Imbert A, Chevalier T, et al: The ECG in pulmonary embolism. Predictive value of negative T waves in precordial leads—80 case reports. Chest 111:537, 1997.
52. Daniel KR, Courtney DM, Kline JA: Assessment of cardiac stress from massive pulmonary embolism with 12- lead ECG. Chest 120:474, 2001.
53. Elliott CG, Goldhaber SZ, Visani L, DeRosa M: Chest radiographs in acute pulmonary embolism. Results from the International Cooperative Pulmonary Embolism Registry. Chest 118:33, 2000.
53a. Schoepf UJ, Goldhaber SZ, Costello P: Spiral CT for acute pulmonary embolism. Circulation 109:2160, 2004.
54. Schoepf UJ, Holzknecht N, Helmberger TK, et al: Subsegmental pulmonary emboli: Improved detection with thin-collimation multi-detector row spiral CT. Radiology 222:483, 2002.
55. Perrier A, Howarth N, Didier D, et al: Performance of helical computed tomography in unselected outpatients with suspected pulmonary embolism. Ann Intern Med 135:88, 2001.
56. van Strijen MJ, de Monye W, Schiereck J, et al: Single-detector helical computed tomography as the primary diagnostic test in suspected pulmonary embolism: A multicenter clinical management study of 510 patients. Ann Intern Med 138:307, 2003.
57. Perrier A, Nendaz MR, Sarasin FP, et al: Cost-effectiveness analysis of diagnostic strategies for suspected pulmonary embolism including helical computed tomography. Am J Respir Crit Care Med 167:39, 2003.
58. Anonymous: Guidelines on diagnosis and management of acute pulmonary embolism. Task Force on Pulmonary Embolism, European Society of Cardiology. Eur Heart J 21:1301, 2000.
59. The PIOPED Investigators: Value of the ventilation/perfusion scan in acute pulmonary embolism: Results of the Prospective Investigation of Pulmonary Embolism Diagnosis (PIOPED). JAMA 263:2753, 1990.
60. Bone RC: The low-probability lung scan: A potentially lethal reading. Arch Intern Med 153:2621, 1993.
61. Oudkerk M, van Beek EJ, Wielopolski P, et al: Comparison of contrast-enhanced magnetic resonance angiography and conventional pulmonary angiography for the diagnosis of pulmonary embolism: A prospective study. Lancet 359:1643, 2002.
62. Fraser DG, Moody AR, Morgan PS, et al: Diagnosis of lower-limb deep venous thrombosis: A prospective blinded study of magnetic resonance direct thrombus imaging. Ann Intern Med 136:89, 2002.
63. Miniati M, Monti S, Pratali L, et al: Value of transthoracic echocardiography in the diagnosis of pulmonary embolism: Results of a prospective study in unselected patients. Am J Med 110:528, 2001.
64. Pruszczyk P, Torbicki A, Kuch-Wocial A, et al: Diagnostic value of transoesophageal echocardiography in suspected haemodynamically significant pulmonary embolism. Heart 85:628, 2001.
65. Grifoni S, Olivotto I, Cecchini P, et al: Short-term clinical outcome of patients with acute pulmonary embolism, normal blood pressure, and echocardiographic right ventricular dysfunction. Circulation 101:2817, 2000.
66. Konstantinides S, Geibel A, Kasper W, et al: Patent foramen ovale is an important predictor of adverse outcome in patients with major pulmonary embolism. Circulation 97:1946, 1998.
67. MacGillavry MR, Sanson BJ, Buller HR, Brandjes DP: Compression ultrasonography of the leg veins in patients with clinically suspected pulmonary embolism: Is a more extensive assessment of compressibility useful? Thromb Haemost 84:973, 2000.
68. Musset D, Parent F, Meyer G, et al: Diagnostic strategy for patients with suspected pulmonary embolism: A prospective multicentre outcome study. Lancet 360:1914, 2002.
68a. Goldhaber SZ, Elliott CG: Acute pulmonary embolism: Part II. Risk stratification, treatment, and prevention. Circulation 108:2834, 2003.

Management

69. Wicki J, Perrier A, Perneger TV, et al: Predicting adverse outcome in patients with acute pulmonary embolism: A risk score. Thromb Haemost 84:548, 2000.
70. Beer JH, Burger M, Gretener S, et al: Outpatient treatment of pulmonary embolism is feasible and safe in a substantial proportion of patients. J Thromb Haemost 1:186, 2003.
70a. Kucher N, Goldhaber SZ: Cardiac biomarkers for risk stratification of patients with acute pulmonary embolism. Circulation 108:2191, 2003.
71. Hirsh J, Anand SS, Halperin JL, Fuster V: Guide to anticoagulant therapy: Heparin: a statement for healthcare professionals from the American Heart Association. Circulation 103:2994, 2001.
72. Hylek EM, Regan S, Henault LE, et al: Challenges to the effective use of unfractionated heparin in the hospitalized management of acute thrombosis. Arch Intern Med 163:621, 2003.
73. Weitz JI: Low-molecular-weight heparins. N Engl J Med 337:688, 1997.
74. Merli G, Spiro TE, Olsson CG, et al: Subcutaneous enoxaparin once or twice daily compared with intravenous unfractionated heparin for treatment of venous thromboembolic disease. Ann Intern Med 134:191, 2001.
75. Gould MK, Dembitzer AD, Doyle RL, et al: Low-molecular-weight heparins compared with unfractionated heparin for treatment of acute deep venous thrombosis. A meta-analysis of randomized, controlled trials. Ann Intern Med 130:800, 1999.

76. Gould MK, Dembitzer AD, Sanders GD, Garber AM: Low-molecular-weight heparins compared with unfractionated heparin for treatment of acute deep venous thrombosis: A cost-effectiveness analysis. Ann Intern Med 130:789, 1999.
77. Breddin HK, Hach-Wunderle V, Nakov R, Kakkar VV: Effects of a low-molecular-weight heparin on thrombus regression and recurrent thromboembolism in patients with deep-vein thrombosis. N Engl J Med 344:626, 2001.
78. Meyer G, Marjanovic Z, Valcke J, et al: Comparison of low-molecular-weight heparin and warfarin for the secondary prevention of venous thromboembolism in patients with cancer: A randomized controlled study. Arch Intern Med 162:1729, 2002.
79. Lee AYY, Levine MN, Baker RI, et al: Low-molecular-weight heparin versus a coumarin for the prevention of recurrent venous thromboembolism in patients with cancer. N Engl J Med 349:146, 2003.
80. Beckman JA, Dunn K, Sasahara AA, Goldhaber SZ: Enoxaparin monotherapy without oral anticoagulation to treat acute symptomatic pulmonary embolism. Thromb Haemost 89:953, 2003.
81. Anticoagulation in Prosthetic Valves and Pregnancy Consensus Report Panel and Scientific Roundtable: Anticoagulation and enoxaparin use in patients with prosthetic heart valves and/or pregnancy. Clin Cardiol Consensus Rep 3: October 1, 2002.
82. Raschke RA, Reilly BR, Guidry JR, et al: The weight-based heparin dosing nomogram compared with a "standard care" nomogram: A randomized controlled trial. Ann Intern Med 119:874, 1993.
83. Grasso-Correnti N, Goldszer RC, Goldhaber SZ: The critical pathways of an anticoagulation service. Crit Pathways Cardiol 2:41, 2003.
84. Brandies DPM, Heijboer H, Buller HR, et al: Acenocoumarol and heparin compared with acenocoumarol alone in the initial treatment of proximal-vein thrombosis. N Engl J Med 327:1485, 1992.
85. Kearon C, Johnston M, Moffat K, et al: Effect of warfarin on activated partial thromboplastin time in patients receiving heparin. Arch Intern Med 158:1140, 1998.
86. Brummel KE, Paradis SG, Branda RF, Mann KG: Oral anticoagulation thresholds. Circulation 104:2311, 2001.
87. Harrison L, Johnston M, Massicotte MP, et al: Comparison of 5-mg and 10-mg loading doses in initiation of warfarin therapy. Ann Intern Med 126:133, 1997.
88. Joffe HV, Goldhaber SZ: Effectiveness and safety of long-term anticoagulation of patients ≥ 90 years of age with atrial fibrillation. Am J Cardiol 90:1397, 2002.
89. Higashi MK, Veenstra DL, Kondo LM, et al: Association between CYP2C9 genetic variants and anticoagulation-related outcomes during warfarin therapy. JAMA 287:1690, 2002.
90. Hylek EM, Heiman H, Skates SJ, et al: Acetaminophen and other risk factors for excessive warfarin anticoagulation. JAMA 279:657, 1998.
91. White RH, Beyth RJ, Zhou H, Romano PS: Major bleeding after hospitalization for deep-venous thrombosis. Am J Med 107:414, 1999.
92. Deveras RA, Kessler CM: Reversal of warfarin-induced excessive anticoagulation with recombinant human factor VIIa concentrate. Ann Intern Med 137:884, 2002.
93. Sawicki PT: A structured teaching and self-management program for patients receiving oral anticoagulation. JAMA 281:145, 1999.
94. Kearon C, Gent M, Hirsh J, et al: A comparison of three months of anticoagulation with extended anticoagulation for a first episode of idiopathic venous thromboembolism. N Engl J Med 340:901, 1999.
95. Agnelli G, Prandoni P, Santamaria MG, et al: Three months versus one year of oral anticoagulant therapy for idiopathic deep venous thrombosis. Warfarin Optimal Duration Italian Trial Investigators. N Engl J Med 345:165, 2001.
96. Ridker PM, Goldhaber SZ, Danielson E, et al: Long-term, low-intensity warfarin therapy for the prevention of recurrent venous thromboembolism. N Engl J Med 348:1425, 2003.
96a. Kearon C, Ginsberg JS, Kovacs MJ, et al: Comparison of low-intensity warfarin therapy with conventional-intensity warfarin therapy for long-term prevention of recurrent venous thromboembolism, N Engl J Med 349:631, 2003.
97. Decousus H, Leizorovicz A, Parent F, et al: A clinical trial of vena caval filters in the prevention of pulmonary embolism in patients with proximal deep-vein thrombosis. N Engl J Med 338:409, 1998.
98. White RH, Zhou H, Kim J, Romano PS: A population-based study of the effectiveness of inferior vena cava filter use among patients with venous thromboembolism. Arch Intern Med 160:2033, 2000.
99. Millward SF, Oliva VL, Bell SD, et al: Gunther Tulip Retrievable Vena Cava Filter: Results from the Registry of the Canadian Interventional Radiology Association. J Vasc Interv Radiol 12:1053, 2001.
100. Arcasoy SM, Kreit JW: Thrombolytic therapy of pulmonary embolism: A comprehensive review of current evidence. Chest 115:1695, 1999.
101. Konstantinides S, Geibel A, Heusel G, et al: Heparin plus alteplase compared with heparin alone in patients with submassive pulmonary embolism. N Engl J Med 347:1143, 2002.
102. Kanter DS, Mikkola KM, Patel SR, et al: Thrombolytic therapy for pulmonary embolism: Frequency of intracranial hemorrhage and associated risk factors. Chest 111:1241, 1997.
103. Goldhaber SZ, Haire WD, Feldstein ML, et al: Alteplase versus heparin in acute pulmonary embolism: Randomised trial assessing right-ventricular function and pulmonary perfusion. Lancet 341:507, 1993.
104. Daniels LB, Parker JA, Patel SR, et al: Relation of duration of symptoms with response to thrombolytic therapy in pulmonary embolism. Am J Cardiol 80:184, 1997.
105. Nicolaides AN: Investigation of chronic venous insufficiency: A consensus statement (France, March 5-9, 1997). Circulation 102:E126, 2000.
106. Brandjes DPM, Büller HR, Heijboer H, et al: Randomised trial of effect of compression stockings in patients with symptomatic proximal-vein thrombosis. Lancet 349:759, 1997.
107. Aklog L, Williams CS, Byrne JG, Goldhaber SZ: Acute pulmonary embolectomy: A contemporary approach. Circulation 105:1416, 2002.
108. Goldhaber SZ: Integration of catheter thrombectomy into our armamentarium to treat acute pulmonary embolism. Chest 114:1237, 1998.
109. Fava M, Loyola S, Flores P, Huete I: Mechanical fragmentation and pharmacologic thrombolysis in massive pulmonary embolism. J Vasc Interv Radiol 8:261, 1997.
110. Goldhaber SZ, Morrison RB: Pulmonary embolism and deep vein thrombosis. Circulation 106:1436, 2002.
111. Fedullo PF, Auger WR, Kerr KM, Rubin LJ: Chronic thromboembolic pulmonary hypertension. N Engl J Med 345:1465, 2001.
112. Feinstein JA, Goldhaber SZ, Lock JE, et al: Balloon pulmonary angioplasty for treatment of chronic thromboembolic pulmonary hypertension. Circulation 103:10, 2001.

Prevention

113. Geerts WH, Heit JA, Clagett GP, et al: Prevention of venous thromboembolism. Chest 119(1 Suppl):132S, 2001.
114. Prevention of venous thromboembolism: International Consensus Statement Guidelines compiled in accordance with the scientific evidence. International Angiology 20:1, 2001.
115. Durieux P, Nizard R, Ravaud P, et al: A clinical decision support system for prevention of venous thromboembolism: Effect on physician behavior. JAMA 283:2816, 2000.
116. Goldhaber SZ, Dunn K, MacDougall RC: New onset of venous thromboembolism among hospitalized patients at Brigham and Women's Hospital is caused more often by prophylaxis failure than by withholding treatment. Chest 118:1680, 2000.
117. Goldhaber SZ, Dunn K, Gerhard-Herman M, et al: Low rate of venous thromboembolism after craniotomy for brain tumor using multimodality prophylaxis. Chest 122:1933, 2002.
118. Comerota AJ, Chouhan V, Harada RN, et al: The fibrinolytic effects of intermittent pneumatic compression: Mechanism of enhanced fibrinolysis. Ann Surg 226:306, 1997.
119. Collins R, Scrimgeour A, Yusuf S, Peto R: Reduction in fatal pulmonary embolism and venous thrombosis by perioperative administration of subcutaneous heparin: Overview of results of randomized trials in general, orthopedic, and urologic surgery. N Engl J Med 318:1162, 1988.
120. Lassen MR, Bauer KA, Eriksson BI, Turpie AG: Postoperative fondaparinux versus preoperative enoxaparin for prevention of venous thromboembolism in elective hip-replacement surgery: A randomised double-blind comparison. Lancet 359:1715, 2002.
121. Bounameaux H, Perneger T: Fondaparinux: A new synthetic pentasaccharide for thrombosis prevention. Lancet 359:1710, 2002.
122. Antithrombotic Trialists' Collaboration: Collaborative meta-analysis of randomised trials of antiplatelet therapy for prevention of death, myocardial infarction, and stroke in high risk patients. BMJ 324:71, 2002.
123. Francis CW, Davidson BL, Berkowitz SD, et al: Ximelagatran versus warfarin for the prevention of venous thromboembolism after total knee arthroplasty: A randomized, double- blind trial. Ann Intern Med 137:648, 2002.
124. Eriksson BI, Agnelli G, Cohen AT, et al: Direct thrombin inhibitor melagatran followed by oral ximelagatran in comparison with enoxaparin for prevention of venous thromboembolism after total hip or knee replacement. Thromb Haemost 89:288, 2003.
125. Bergqvist D, Agnelli G, Cohen AT, et al: Duration of prophylaxis against venous thromboembolism with enoxaparin after surgery for cancer. N Engl J Med 346:975, 2002.
126. Eikelboom JW, Quinlan DJ, Douketis JD: Extended-duration prophylaxis against venous thromboembolism after total hip or knee replacement: A meta-analysis of the randomised trials. Lancet 358:9, 2001.
127. Samama MM, Cohen AT, Darmon J-Y, et al: A comparison of enoxaparin with placebo for the prevention of venous thromboembolism in acutely ill medical patients. N Engl J Med 341:793, 1999.
128. Leizorovicz A, Cohen AT, Turpie AG, et al: A randomized placebo controlled trial of dalteparin for the prevention of venous thromboembolism in acutely ill medical patients. Circulation 2004, submitted.

CHAPTER 67

Pulmonary Hypertension

Stuart Rich • Vallerie V. McLaughlin

Normal Pulmonary Circulation

Anatomy

The lung has a unique double arterial blood supply from the pulmonary and bronchial arteries, as well as double venous drainage into the pulmonary and azygos veins.[1] Inside the lung, each pulmonary artery accompanies the appropriate-generation bronchus and divides with it down to the level of the respiratory bronchiole. Additional supernumerary branches originate without relation to bronchial divisions and directly penetrate into the lung parenchyma. The diameter of the arteries decreases more rapidly than the diameter of the airways they accompany, so in the lung periphery, the diameters of the arteries are smaller than the diameters of the adjacent airways. Within the respiratory units, the pulmonary arteries and arterioles are centrally located and give rise to precapillary arterioles from which a network of capillaries radiate into the alveolar walls. The alveolar capillaries collect at the periphery of the acini and then drain into venules located within the interlobular and interlobar septa. During the passage of red blood cells through the lungs, hemoglobin is normally oxygenated to nearly full capacity and the blood is cleansed of much particulate matter and bacteria. The lungs, in addition to functioning as a blood oxygenator and filter, play a dominant role in achieving acid-base balance by excreting carbon dioxide, thereby helping to maintain optimal blood pH.

PULMONARY ARTERIES. The pulmonary arteries are classified as elastic or muscular based on the structure of the tunica media. The elastic arteries are conducting vessels, highly distensible at low transmural pressure. As the arteries decrease in size, the number of elastic laminae decreases and smooth muscle increases. Eventually, in vessels between 100 and 500 μm, elastic tissue is lost from the media and the arteries become muscular. The intima of the pulmonary arteries consists of a single layer of endothelial cells and their basement membrane. The adventitia is composed of dense connective tissue in direct continuity with the peribronchial connective tissue sheath. The muscular arteries are 500 μm in diameter or less and are characterized by a muscular media bounded by internal and external elastic laminae. In normal adults, the lumen is wide and the media is thin and represents less than 10 percent of the arterial cross-sectional area. Arterioles are precapillary arteries smaller than 100 μm in outer diameter and composed solely of a thin intima and single elastic lamina. The alveolar capillaries are lined with a continuous layer of endothelium resting on a continuous basement membrane and focally connected to scattered pericytes located beneath the basement membrane. The pulmonary circulation is characterized by high flow (the entire right ventricular output) and by low pressure and low resistance. Its wide and thin-walled vessels reflect these hemodynamic features. Thus, pulmonary vessels differ substantially from corresponding vessels in the systemic circulation (Table 67–1).

BRONCHIAL ARTERIES. These vessels ramify into a capillary network drained by bronchial veins; some empty into the pulmonary veins, and the remainder empty into the systemic venous bed. The bronchial circulation therefore constitutes a physiological "right-to-left" shunt. The function of the bronchial circulation is to provide nutrition to the airways. Normally, blood flow through this system is quite low and amounts to approximately 1 percent of the cardiac output; the resulting desaturation of left atrial blood is usually trivial. In some forms of pulmonary disease (e.g., severe bronchiectasis), however, and in the presence of many congenital cardiovascular malformations that cause cyanosis, blood flow through the bronchial circulation can increase to as much as 30 percent of left ventricular output and produce a significant right-to-left shunt.

Physiology

The normal pulmonary vascular bed offers less than one-tenth the resistance to flow offered by the systemic bed. Vascular resistance is generally quantified, by analogy to Ohm's law, as the ratio of pressure drop (ΔP in millimeters Hg) to mean flow (Q in liters

TABLE 67–1 Physiological Comparison of the Pulmonary and Systemic Circulations

Feature	Pulmonary Circulation Range	Pulmonary Circulation Mean	Systemic Circulation Range	Systemic Circulation Mean
Arterial pressure, mm Hg	25/10	15	120/80	90
Capillary pressure, mm Hg	6-9	7	10-30	17
Venous pressure, mm Hg	1-4	2	0-10	6
Arterial M/D ratio, %*	3-7	5	15-25	20
Venous M/D ratio, %*	2-5	3	3-6	5
Vascular resistance U^{m2}	1-4	3	10-25	15
Blood flow, liters/min	4-6	5	4-6	5

*M/D ratio = ratio of the medial thickness to the external diameter of the vessel.

per minute). The ratio is commonly multiplied by 79.9 (or 80 for simplification) to express the results in dynes-sec/cm^{-5}. This conversion to metric units can be avoided; that is, resistance can be expressed in millimeters Hg per liter per minute, which is sometimes referred to as hybrid units, PRU (peripheral resistance units), or Wood units (after the English cardiologist Paul Wood). The calculated pulmonary vascular resistance in normal adults is 67 ± 23 (SD) dyne-sec/cm^{-5} or 1 Wood unit.

Vascular resistance reflects a composite of variables that includes, but is not limited to, the cross-sectional area of small muscular arteries and arterioles. Other determinants are blood viscosity, the total mass of lung tissue (i.e., resistance is higher in infants and children than in adults), proximal vascular obstruction (e.g., pulmonary coarctation, pulmonary embolism, peripheral pulmonic stenosis), and extramural compression of vessels (perivascular edema).

Regulation of Vascular Tone

ADRENERGIC CONTROL. The pulmonary vasculature expresses both alpha and beta adrenoreceptors, which help regulate pulmonary vascular tone by producing vasoconstriction or vasodilation, respectively.[2] Alpha$_1$-adrenoreceptors in the pulmonary arteries have increased affinity and responsiveness to their agonists when compared with other vessels.[3] The downstream signaling events in alpha$_1$-adrenergic stimulation are an increase in ionic calcium levels and activation of protein kinase, which mediate vascular contractile and proliferative responses. The increased sensitivity of alpha$_1$-adrenoreceptors to norepinephrine in the pulmonary arteries may greatly facilitate local regulation of vascular tone in response to acute changes in oxygen concentrations, thereby adjusting regional perfusion. Stimulation of alpha$_1$-adrenoreceptors increases intracellular free calcium levels by at least two mechanisms: (1) coupling to specific G proteins on the cell membrane and (2) blockade of potassium ion channels.[4] Excessive stimulation of alpha$_1$-adrenergic receptors produces smooth muscle contraction, proliferation, and growth. Factors that produce an increase in alpha$_1$-adrenoreceptor gene synthesis, density, and activity greatly enhance pulmonary artery smooth muscle contractile and proliferative responses. Such factors include norepinephrine, appetite suppressants, and cocaine (Fig. 67–1).[5,6]

The alpha$_1$-adrenergic blocking agents phentolamine and tolazoline lower pulmonary vascular resistance, as does beta-adrenergic stimulation with isoproterenol. In contrast, beta-adrenergic blockade does not produce any change in pulmonary vascular resistance, which suggests that tonic activation of beta receptors is not necessary for maintenance of the normal low pulmonary vascular resistance. Acetylcholine is a potent relaxant of pulmonary arteries and arterioles and transiently lowers pulmonary vascular resistance in patients with elevated pulmonary vascular resistance with a major reversible component.

HYPOXIA. The hypoxic pulmonary vasoconstrictor response is an important adaptive mechanism in human physiology. Alveolar hypoxia results in local vasoconstriction so that blood flow is shunted away from hypoxic regions toward better ventilated areas of the lung, improving the ventilation-perfusion matching within the lung. Although the acute effects of this response are undoubtedly beneficial,

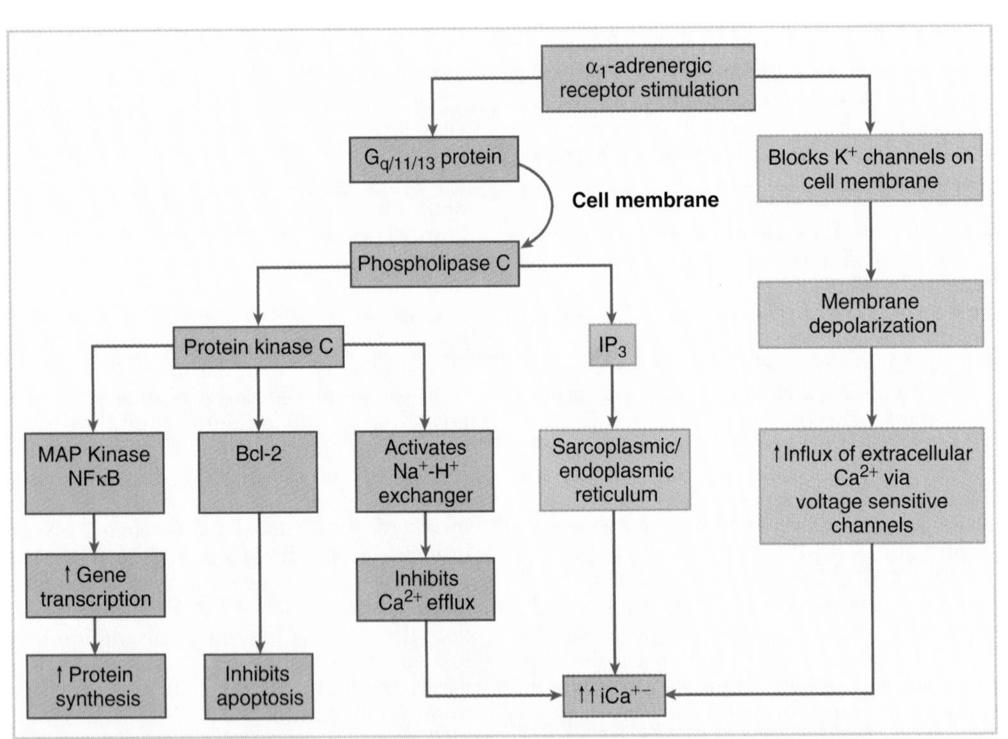

FIGURE 67–1 Signaling pathways of alpha$_1$-adrenergic receptors in smooth muscle cells that lead to pulmonary hypertension. Alpha$_1$-adrenergic receptors activate phospholipase C to produce inositol 1,4,5-triphosphate (IP$_3$), which mobilizes calcium from intracellular stores. Activation of protein kinase C also activates transcription factors such as mitogen-activated protein kinase (MAP kinase) and nuclear factor kappa-B (NFκB), which induce DNA synthesis and cell proliferation. By increasing levels of oncoprotein (Bcl-2) to inhibit apoptosis, the survival of vascular smooth muscle cells is promoted. Alpha$_1$-adrenergic receptors also couple to K$^+$ channels, which leads to entry of calcium from extracellular sources through voltage-sensitive channels. An increase in intracellular calcium is the major signal transduction mechanism responsible for producing smooth muscle contraction via the calcium calmodulin pathway, and protein kinase C activation is the major signal transduction pathway involved in the proliferation of pulmonary vascular smooth muscle cells. (From Salvi SS: α-1 Adrenergic hypothesis for pulmonary hypertension. Chest 115:1708, 1999.)

chronic hypoxemia can result in sustained elevation of pulmonary artery pressure, vascular remodeling, and the development of pulmonary hypertension.

Hypoxic pulmonary vasoconstriction can be observed in isolated pulmonary vascular smooth muscle cells.[7] The mechanism of hypoxic pulmonary vasoconstriction involves the inhibition of potassium currents and pulmonary vascular smooth muscle membrane depolarization as a result of changes in the membrane sulfhydryl redox status. Potassium, calcium, and chloride channels all play important roles in determining pulmonary vascular tone and are altered by changes in local oxygen tension in the pulmonary circulation.[8]

Increased calcium (Ca^{2+}) entry into the vascular smooth muscle cells appears to mediate hypoxic pulmonary vasoconstriction. The concentration of Ca^{2+} in the vicinity of the contractile machinery represents a balance between inflow and outflow across the cell membrane and intracellular release and uptake. Within the cell, Ca^{2+} can be mobilized from the sarcoplasmic reticulum and mitochondrial membrane, or the inner aspect of the cell membrane. Although most of the evidence favors an influx of Ca^{2+} from extracellular fluid, the relative contribution of differential mobilization from intracellular stores is unsettled. The mechanism responsible for intracellular mobilization of Ca^{2+} is also unclear.

THE ENDOTHELIUM. The vascular endothelium plays a central role as a mediator of hypoxia-induced pulmonary vasoconstriction. Balanced release of nitric oxide (NO) and endothelin by endothelial cells is a key factor in the regulation of tone in the pulmonary circulation. A reduction in NO production has been demonstrated in the chronically hypoxic piglet and rat, whereas prolonged inhalation of NO attenuates hypoxic pulmonary vasoconstriction and pulmonary vascular remodeling in rats.[9] Conversely, plasma levels of endothelin-1 are increased in association with hypoxemia in humans.[10] Endothelin receptor antagonists have been demonstrated to reduce hypoxic pulmonary vasoconstriction in animals.[11-14]

Pulmonary vascular remodeling in response to hypoxia is also meditated by a number of growth factors. Platelet-derived growth factor-A and platelet-derived growth factor-B levels are elevated in hypoxic rats, and vascular endothelial growth factor, which is an endothelial cell-specific mitogen, is upregulated during exposure to chronic hypoxia.[15,16] Vascular endothelial growth factor is likely involved in pulmonary vascular injury and endothelial cell proliferation in the setting of chronic hypoxic pulmonary vascular remodeling because of its permeability, angiogenesis, proinflammatory properties, and specificity for endothelial cells.

Hypoxia inducible factor 1[17] represents a vital link between oxygen sensing, gene transcription, and the physiological adaptation to chronic hypoxia in vivo. Hypoxia inducible factor 1 has been identified as a nuclear factor that is induced by hypoxia and bound to a site in the erythropoietin response element. Expression of hypoxia inducible factor 1 is tightly regulated by cellular oxygen tension. One of the classic adaptations to chronic hypoxia is an increased rate of erythropoiesis that is mediated by the glycoprotein growth hormone erythropoietin.

CHANGES IN ALVEOLAR OXYGENATION. These affect the oxygenation of small pulmonary arteries and arterioles by direct gaseous diffusion from the alveoli, respiratory bronchioles, and alveolar ducts in the pulmonary arterioles, even though the latter are "upstream" in relation to the alveoli. This fact, taken together with evidence for a reduction in pulmonary arterial blood volume during hypoxia, supports the view that the small pulmonary arteries and arterioles are the main sites of vasoconstriction and increased resistance in the pulmonary circulation during hypoxia. Although alveolar oxygen tension is a major physiological determinant of pulmonary arteriolar tone, a reduction in the oxygen tension in the mixed venous blood flowing through the small pulmonary arteries and arterioles may also contribute to pulmonary arterial vasoconstriction.

Acidosis significantly increases pulmonary vascular resistance and acts synergistically with hypoxia. In contrast, an increase in arterial P_{CO_2} seems to exert no direct effect but rather operates by way of the induced increase in hydrogen-ion concentration. Hypoxia and acidemia frequently coexist, and their interaction, which is clinically important, follows a predictable pattern.

Altitude. Life at high altitudes is associated with pulmonary hypertension of variable severity, reflecting the range of reactivities of different persons due to the pulmonary vasoconstrictive effect of chronic hypoxia. Altitude decreases the inspired partial pressure of oxygen (P_{O_2}) because of a decrease in barometric pressure. At sea level, P_{O_2} is on average 150 mm Hg. At high altitudes (3000 to 5500 m), P_{O_2} decreases to 80 to 100 mm Hg, and at extreme altitudes (5500 to 8840 m), P_{O_2} decreases to 40 to 80 mm Hg. Corresponding alveolar P_{O_2} (P_{AO_2}) and arterial P_{O_2} (P_{aO_2}) depend on the hypoxic ventilatory response and associated respiratory alkalosis.[18] Mild pulmonary hypertension in adult natives at high altitude occurs at rest and may increase substantially with exercise. It is not immediately reversed by breathing of oxygen, does not seem to limit exercise capacity, and is rarely the cause of right ventricular failure.

Severe pulmonary hypertension may occur with high-altitude pulmonary edema, with infantile or adult forms of subacute mountain sickness, and with chronic mountain sickness. Subjects susceptible to high-altitude pulmonary edema often present with a slight increase in pulmonary vascular resistance at rest and exercise at sea level and with an enhanced pulmonary vascular reactivity to hypoxia. Transient right ventricular dysfunction has also been described with strenuous exercise at high altitude. In one study, 5 of 14 runners who completed an ultramarathon at high altitude developed marked right ventricular dilation and hypokinesis, paradoxical septal motion, and pulmonary hypertension. These echocardiographic abnormalities had all normalized at 1-day follow-up.[19]

FETAL AND NEONATAL CIRCULATION (see Chap. 56). In the fetus, oxygenated blood enters the heart from the inferior vena cava and streams across the foramen ovale to the left atrium, left ventricle, ascending aorta, and cranial vessels. Desaturated blood returns from the superior vena cava and passes through the tricuspid valve into the right ventricle and pulmonary artery. Because the resistance of the pulmonary vascular bed in the collapsed fetal lung is extremely high, only 10 to 30 percent of the total right ventricular output passes through the lungs, the remainder being shunted across the ductus arteriosus to the descending aorta and then back to the placenta.

An abrupt change in the pulmonary circulation occurs at birth. With the first breath, expansion of the lungs and the abrupt rise in P_{O_2} of blood lead to a reversal of pulmonary arteriolar vasoconstriction and stretching and dilation of muscular pulmonary arteries and arterioles, with a marked drop in vascular resistance. This decreased resistance facilitates a large increase in pulmonary blood flow and raises left atrial volume and pressure. The latter closes the flap valve of the foramen ovale, and interatrial right-to-left shunting ordinarily ceases within the first hour of life. Normally, the ductus arteriosus closes over the next 10 hours as a result of contraction of the thick smooth muscle bundles within its wall in response to rising arterial oxygen tension and a change in the prostaglandin milieu. Following the initial dramatic fall in pulmonary vascular resistance at birth, a continuous decline occurs over the first few months of life that is associated with thinning of the media of muscular pulmonary arteries and arterioles until the normal adult pattern is achieved.

AGING. In the elderly, the main pulmonary artery becomes mildly dilated, and a few shallow atheromas commonly develop in the elastic pulmonary arteries. Mild medial thickening and eccentric intimal fibrosis are commonly identified in muscular pulmonary arteries, capillaries become slightly thicker, and veins are frequently involved by intimal hyalinization with mild luminal narrowing. Pulmonary artery pressure and pulmonary vascular resistance increase with advanced age, similar to increases that occur in systemic vascular resistance. Reduced compliance of the pulmonary vascular bed secondary to intimal fibrosis and increased wall thickness in the muscular pulmonary arteries are factors. Changes in the pulmonary arteries are also affected by reduced compliance of left ventricular filling with age that is passively reflected back on the pulmonary vascular bed.

EXERCISE. With moderate exercise, a large increase in pulmonary blood flow is normally accompanied by only a small increase in pulmonary artery pressure. Exercise results in an increase in left atrial pressure that is progressive with exercise intensity and accounts for the majority of the increase in pulmonary arterial pressure that is observed. This marked effect of downstream pressure on upstream pressure is unique to the lung circulation inasmuch as systemic arterial pressure during exercise is largely independent of right atrial pressure. Because of the high vascular compliance in the normal lung microcirculation, an increase in left atrial pressure that results from the increased flow will act to distend the small vessels, thereby accounting for the fall in pulmonary vascular resistance during exercise.[20] Microcirculatory distention increases the surface area for diffusion and slows passage of red blood cells through the lung, which facilitates oxygen transfer.

Vascular Mediators

PROSTAGLANDINS. Lung tissue is particularly active in the synthesis, metabolism, and release of a number of prostaglandins, which may play a role in the regulation of pulmonary vascular resistance.[21] Prostaglandins I_2 (PGI_2) and E_1 (PGE_1) are active pulmonary vasodilators, whereas $PGF_{2\alpha}$ and PGA_2 are pulmonary vasoconstrictors. Counterregulatory actions have been ascribed to prostacyclin (PGI_2) and thromboxane within the pulmonary circulation.

Pulmonary endothelial cells have an abundance of prostacyclin synthase, whereas platelets are replete with thromboxane synthase. Both convert the cyclic endoperoxide precursors PGG_2 and PGH_2 into specific bioactive eicosanoids. Prostacyclin is a powerful vasodilator and inhibitor of platelet aggregation through activation of adenylate cyclase. Its metabolic half-life in the bloodstream is less than one circulation time, with its metabolite 6-keto-prostaglandin $F_{1\alpha}$ having little biological activity.

Physiologically, prostacyclin is a local hormone rather than a circulating one. Release of prostacyclin by endothelial cells causes relaxation of the underlying vascular smooth muscle and prevents platelet aggregation within the bloodstream. A variety of drugs with diverse mechanisms of action are reported to stimulate prostacyclin production and include calcium channel blockers, angiotensin-converting enzyme (ACE) inhibitors, diuretics, and nitrates.[17] Thromboxane is synthesized in platelets and macrophages. It also has a short half-life. Thromboxane is a potent agonist for platelet aggregation and vasoconstriction, and it may function as a growth factor for smooth muscles by acting via protein kinase C-linked pathways.[22]

NITRIC OXIDE. The biological action of NO is similar to that of prostacyclin in the way it relaxes vascular smooth muscle. It differs, however, in that its effects are mediated by rising levels of cyclic guanosine monophosphate.[23] Endothelial NO synthase is found in the vascular endothelium of the normal pulmonary vasculature, where it is responsible for generating NO to govern vascular tone. Release of NO occurs in response to a multitude of physiological stimuli, which include thrombin, bradykinin, and shear stress.[24] Besides its direct hemodynamic effects, NO inhibits platelet activation and confers an important antithrombotic property on the endothelial surface. NO also inhibits the growth of vascular smooth muscle cells and is probably involved in vascular remodeling in response to injury.[23] NO is also important in the signal transduction of angiogenesis inasmuch as vascular endothelial growth factor receptor activation results in increased NO production (Fig. 67–2).[25]

ENDOTHELIN. Endothelin is a potent mitogenic and vasoconstrictor peptide that plays an important role in the regulation of pulmonary vascular tone. ET-1 is the predominant isoform of endothelin in the cardiovascular system, generated through the cleavage of pre-pro ET-1 to big ET-1 and then to ET-1.[26] ET-1 is found in endothelial cells and released toward the vascular smooth muscle cell, consistent with a paracrine rule, but it is also produced by smooth muscle cells and cardiomyocytes. ET-1 has vasoconstrictive and mitogenic effects, simulates the production of growth factors such as vascular endothelial growth factor and basic fibroblast growth factor, and potentiates the effects of transforming growth factor (TGF)-β and platelet-derived growth factor.[27] In the lung, ET-1 is abundantly expressed in the pulmonary vasculature and appears to play an important role in the regulation of pulmonary vascular tone. ET-1 biosynthesis is regulated by physiochemical factors such as blood flow, pulsatile stretch, hypoxia, and thrombin. Endogenous inhibitors of ET-1 synthesis include nitric oxide and prostacyclin (Fig. 67–3).

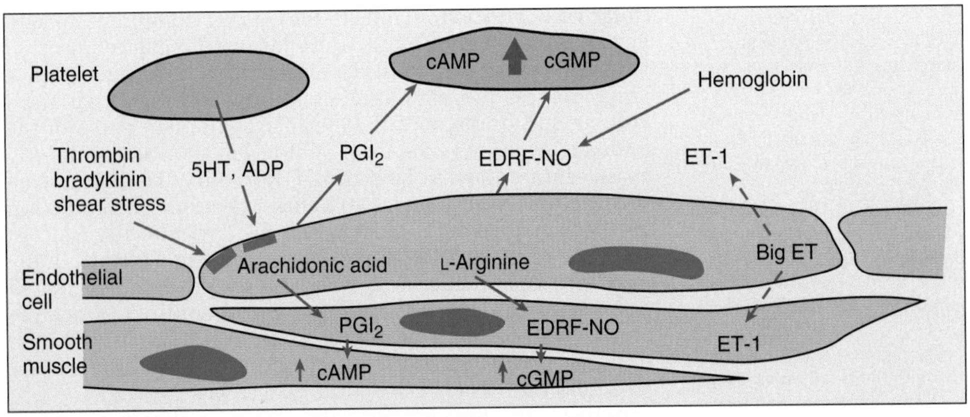

ENDOTHELIN RECEPTORS. ET-1 exerts its major vascular effects through activation of two distinct G-protein-coupled ET_A and ET_B receptors. ET_A receptors are found in the medial smooth muscle layers of the blood vessels and atrial and ventricular myocardium. When stimulated, the ET_A receptors induce vasoconstriction and cellular proliferation by increasing intracellular calcium.[28] ET_B receptors are localized on endothelial cells and to some extent on smooth muscle cells and macrophages. The activation of ET_B receptors stimulates the release of nitric oxide and prostacyclin and prevents apoptosis.[29] Normally there is a balance between production and clearance, which is mediated by the ET_B receptor such that circulating endothelin is at a low level.

In pathological states, there is upregulation of the ET_B receptors located on the smooth muscle cells that function similar to ET_A receptors, which amplify the vaso-

FIGURE 67–2 Generation of prostacyclin (PGI_2), endothelial-derived relaxing factor-nitric oxide (EDRF-NO), and endothelin-1 (ET-1) in endothelial cells. Stimulation of receptors on the cells by serotonin (5HT [5-hydroxytryptamine]) or adenosine diphosphate (ADP) released from platelets or by thrombin, bradykinin, or shear stress leads to the release of vasoactive mediators. PGI_2 relaxes vascular smooth muscle and inhibits platelet aggregation and adhesion by increasing levels of cyclic guanosine monophosphate (cGMP). The simultaneous increase in cyclic adenosine monophosphate (cAMP) and cGMP inhibits platelet aggregation. (From Vane JR, Anggard EE, Bolting RM: Regulatory functions of the vascular endothelium. N Engl J Med 323:27, 1990. Copyright 1990 Massachusetts Medical Society.)

constrictive and mitogenic effects of ET-1. There is increasing evidence that pulmonary vascular smooth cells as well as endothelial cells synthesize and release ET-1 when stimulated by cytokines. A significant correlation between serum levels of ET-1 and pulmonary vascular resistance, right atrial pressure, and oxygen saturation in patients with pulmonary hypertension has been reported.[30] An increase in expression of ET-1 mRNA in pulmonary vascular endothelial cells of patients with pulmonary hypertension has also been described.[31]

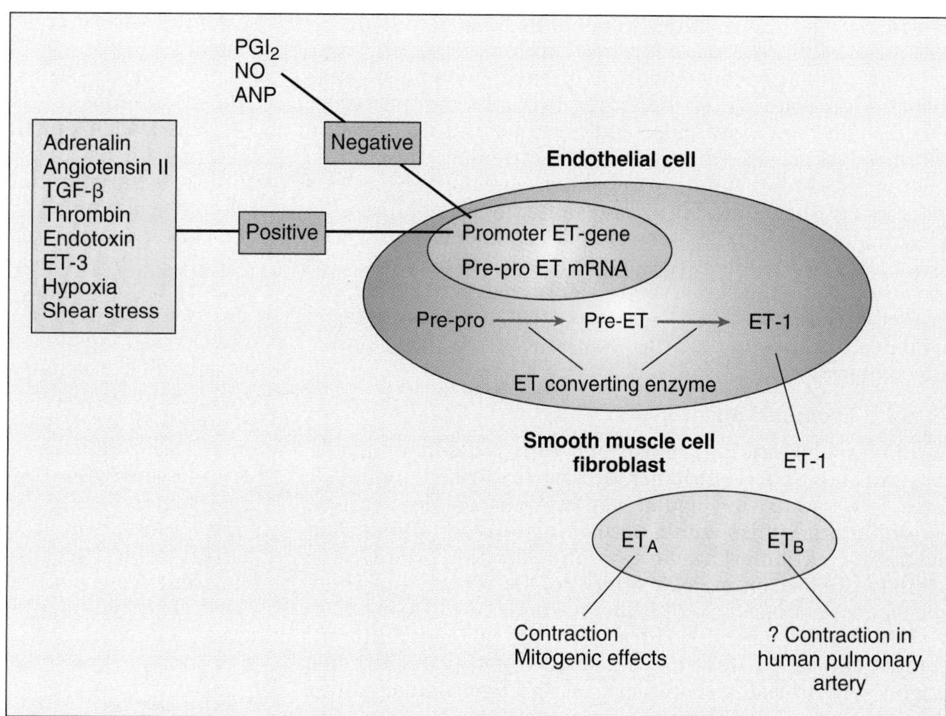

FIGURE 67–3 Regulation of the effects of endothelin (ET). ET may be active in the final stage of transduction of a number of pulmonary smooth muscle contractile and mitogenic factors. Nitric oxide (NO) and prostacyclin (PGI_2), together with atrial natriuretic peptide (ANP), inhibit expression of ET-1. ET_A receptors are involved in contraction and in mitogenic effects on smooth muscle cells and fibroblasts. The small resistance arteries in humans appear to have contraction-inducing ET_B receptors as well. TGF-β = transforming growth factor-beta. (From Higgenbottam TW, Laude EA: Endothelial dysfunction providing the basis for the treatment of pulmonary hypertension. Chest 114[Suppl]:72, 1998.)

SEROTONIN. Serotonin is an important constituent of platelet-dense granules and is released upon activation. Serotonin is a vasoconstrictor that promotes smooth muscle cell hypertrophy and hyperplasia. Normal endothelial cells respond to serotonin by enhancing the release of NO, thereby leading to vascular smooth muscle relaxation and vasodilation. In the setting of endothelial dysfunction, serotonin is unable to stimulate NO release and increases vascular smooth muscle tone, thereby leading to vasoconstriction.[32] In addition, serotonin can act as a growth factor and contribute to medial hypertrophy and promote vascular remodeling. Recently, hypoxia-dependent increased expression of the serotonin 5-hydroxytryptamine 2B receptor (5-HT 2BR) has been shown to be necessary for pulmonary hypertensive responses in mice.[33] It appears that active 5-HT 2BRs are necessary for pulmonary vascular proliferation and elastase and TGF-β dependent remodeling. Increased 5-HT receptor expression also occurs in cases of pulmonary hypertension in humans.[34]

ANGIOTENSIN II. This peptide is generated in the lung by means of enzymatic conversion of angiotensin I, a potent pulmonary vasoconstrictor. Angiotensin II stimulates cell proliferation, extracellular matrix proteins synthesis, and smooth muscle cell migration. The roles of ACE and angiotensin II in the pulmonary circulation are becoming more established. Local increases in right ventricular ACE activity and expression likely play an important role in the pathogenesis of right ventricular hypertrophy secondary to hypoxic pulmonary hypertension.[35] In chronically hypoxic rats, the development of pulmonary hypertension and right ventricular hypertrophy is associated with a significant increase in membrane-bound right ventricular ACE activity. ACE inhibitors attenuate the development of pulmonary hypertension in rats exposed to chronic hypoxia,[36] and acute hypoxic pulmonary vasoconstriction is attenuated by type 1 angiotensin II receptor blockade. Treatment of chronically hypoxic rats with ACE inhibitors also reduces right ventricular hypertrophy and fibrosis.[37]

Clinical Assessment of the Patient with Suspected Pulmonary Hypertension

History

A careful and detailed history of the patient with suspected pulmonary hypertension is often revealing. Since the earliest abnormalities in patients with pulmonary hypertension are manifest with exercise, it is characteristic that presenting symptoms are effort related. Because pulmonary hypertension can have an insidious onset, patients commonly experience dyspnea with effort that they attribute either to aging or to weight gain. With the onset of right ventricular failure, lower extremity edema from venous congestion is characteristic. Angina is also a common symptom, generally representing more advanced disease. It likely represents reduced coronary blood flow to a markedly hypertrophied right ventricle and has the typical qualities of angina from coronary artery disease. As the cardiac output becomes fixed and eventually falls, patients may have episodes of syncope or near syncope. Patients with pulmonary hypertension related to left ventricular diastolic dysfunction will characteristically have orthopnea and paroxysmal nocturnal dyspnea. Patients with underlying lung disease may also report frequent episodes of cough or wheezing. Hemoptysis is relatively uncommon in patients with pulmonary hypertension and may be associated with underlying thromboembolism and pulmonary infarction. Some patients with advanced mitral stenosis also present with hemoptysis.

Syncope is a characteristic symptom of pulmonary hypertension and is assumed to be due to a fixed cardiac output. A study on the systolic function and interactions of the left and right ventricles in patients with primary pulmonary hypertension (PPH) revealed an increased right ventricular end-diastolic volume and reduced right ventricular ejection fraction.[38] The mechanism for maintaining cardiac output with exercise was primarily through an increased heart rate inasmuch as stroke volume actually decreased. The right ventricular ejection fraction decreased with exercise, thus suggesting exercise-induced right ventricular failure. This result is expected because pulmonary artery pressure increases with exercise in patients with PPH. The left ventricular ejection fraction is maintained, but left ventricular end-diastolic volume decreases and left ventricular end-systolic volume becomes extremely small, which suggests that the left ventricle is shortening to its maximum extent. The fact that left ventricular end-diastolic and end-systolic volumes decreased whereas right ventricular end-systolic and end-diastolic volumes remained unchanged supports the concept that underfilling and not external compression accounts for the small left ventricular chamber size observed in patients with pulmonary hypertension. Syncope occurs because of exercise-induced right ventricular failure, whereby the heart rate becomes the only mechanism available to increase cardiac output, which has limited effectiveness.

Physical Examination

Cardiovascular findings consistent with pulmonary hypertension and right ventricular pressure overload include a large *a* wave in the jugular venous pulse; a low-volume carotid arterial pulse with a normal upstroke; a left parasternal (right ventricular) heave; a systolic pulsation produced by a dilated, tense pulmonary artery in the second left interspace; an ejection click and flow murmur in the same area; a closely split second heart sound with a loud pulmonic component; and a fourth heart sound of right ventricular origin. Late in the course, signs of right ventricular failure (hepatomegaly, peripheral edema, and ascites) may be present. Patients with severe pulmonary hypertension may also have prominent *v* waves in the jugular venous pulse as a result of tricuspid regurgitation, a third heart sound of right ventricular origin, a high-pitched early diastolic murmur of pulmonic regurgitation, and a holosystolic murmur of tricuspid regurgitation. Cyanosis is a late finding and usually attributable to a markedly reduced cardiac output with systemic vasoconstriction and ventilation-perfusion mismatch in the lung. Uncommonly, the left laryngeal nerve becomes paralyzed as a consequence of compression by a dilated pulmonary artery (Ortner syndrome).

CONCOMITANT ILLNESS. Patients whose pulmonary hypertension is associated with another illness often have clinical features of that disease. For example, patients with scleroderma typically report Raynaud phenomenon, dysphagia, sclerodactyly, and nonspecific arthritic symptoms. Patients with portal hypertension usually give a history of underlying chronic liver disease and may present with features that represent a blend of the high cardiac output state of cirrhosis and the low cardiac output state of pulmonary vascular disease. Many patients with congenital heart disease have a known history, but atrial septal defects in adults are frequently missed and patients may have symptoms manifest only later in life. These patients often have marked cyanosis that worsens with exercise. Patients with pulmonary venous hypertension, or pulmonary hypertension associated with lung disease, can also have extreme levels of hypoxemia. In patients with chronic obstructive pulmonary disease (COPD), the clinical signs are often obscured by hyperinflation of the chest. The jugular venous pressure may also be difficult to assess in patients with COPD because of large swings in intrathoracic pressure.

Diagnostic Tests

LABORATORY TESTS (Table 67–2). The results of these studies are usually normal in patients with pulmonary hypertension. If chronic arterial oxygen desaturation exists, polycythemia should be present. A number of investigators have reported hypercoagulable states, abnormal platelet function, defects in fibrinolysis, and other abnormalities of coagulation in patients with PPH.[39] Abnormal liver function test results

TABLE 67–2 Diagnostic Studies Useful for Elucidating Causes of Pulmonary Hypertension

Potential Cause	Diagnostic Studies
Pulmonary thromboembolic disease	Ventilation/perfusion scans, computed tomography of chest, pulmonary angiography
Pulmonary venous thrombosis or obstruction	Chest x-ray, angiography, computed tomography, magnetic resonance imaging
Congenital intracardiac shunts	Transesophageal echocardiography with contrast
Increased left atrial pressure secondary to mitral or aortic valve disease, left ventricular dysfunction, or systemic hypertension	Pulmonary artery wedge pressure, left atrial pressure (via patent foramen ovale), or LVEDP > 15 mm Hg
Pulmonary airway disease (e.g., chronic bronchitis and emphysema)	Respiratory function tests (FVC/FEV_1, chest x-ray)
Hypoxic pulmonary hypertension associated with (1) impaired ventilation, either central (CNS) or peripheral (chest wall problems or upper airway obstruction) and (2) residence at high altitude	Sleep apnea studies and respiratory function tests
Interstitial lung disease, pneumoconiosis, and fibrosis (e.g., silicosis, rheumatoid disease, and sarcoidosis)	Chest x-ray, spirometry and carbon monoxide diffusion, high-resolution chest computed tomography
Connective tissue disease (e.g., SLE, polyarteritis nodosa, scleroderma)	Serological and immunogenetic studies; skin, muscle, or other tissue biopsy: esophageal motility studies
Parasitic disease (schistosomiasis or filariasis)	Rectal biopsy, complement fixation, skin tests, blood smears
Cirrhosis with portal hypertension	Liver function tests, ultrasonography, computed tomography
Peripheral pulmonary artery stenosis (including Takayasu disease and fibrosing mediastinitis)	Selective pulmonary angiography or pressure gradient at catheterization
Sickle cell disease	Erythrocyte morphology, hemoglobin electrophoresis

CNS = central nervous system; FEV_1 = forced expiratory volume in 1 second; FVC = forced vital capacity; LVEDP = left ventricular end-diastolic pressure; SLE = systemic lupus erythematosus.

Modified from Weir EK: Diagnosis and management of primary pulmonary hypertension. *In* Weir EK, Reeves JT: Pulmonary Hypertension. Mt Kisco, NY, Futura, 1984, p 14.

can indicate right ventricular failure with resultant systemic venous hypertension.

B-type natriuretic peptide levels are elevated in patients with pulmonary hypertension and correlate positively with the pulmonary artery pressure.[40] B-type natriuretic peptide is secreted predominantly from cardiac ventricles through a constitutive pathway and is affected by the degree of myocardial stretch, damage, and ischemia in the ventricle.[41]

Uric acid levels are elevated in patients with pulmonary hypertension and correlate with hemodynamics.[42] Although the mechanism is uncertain, it may relate both to overproduction and to impaired uric acid excretion due to the low cardiac output and tissue hypoxia.

CHEST RADIOGRAPHY (see Chap. 12). Radiographic examination of the chest in patients with pulmonary hypertension shows enlargement of the main pulmonary artery and its major branches, with marked tapering of peripheral arteries. The right ventricle and atrium may also be enlarged. Fluoroscopic examination can disclose exaggerated pulsations of secondary pulmonary arterial branches reflecting an elevation in pulmonary arterial pulse pressure. However, in contrast to the plethoric peripheral lung fields in patients with left-to-right shunts, oligemia is noted in these lung regions in patients with pulmonary hypertension. The presence of pulmonary arterial hypertension in patients with COPD has been shown to be related to the width of the right descending pulmonary artery. A right descending pulmonary artery ranging from greater than 16 mm in its widest dimension to greater than 20 mm has been reported to identify patients with pulmonary arterial hypertension. In addition, a high value for the cardiothoracic ratio was 95 percent sensitive and 100 percent specific for the presence of pulmonary hypertension in patients with COPD. Dilation of the right ventricle gives the heart a globular appearance, but right ventricular hypertrophy or dilation is not easily discernible on a plain chest radiograph. Encroachment of the retrosternal air space on the lateral film may be a helpful sign to confirm that the enlarged silhouette is a result of right ventricular dilation.

ELECTROCARDIOGRAPHY (see Chap. 9). The detection of right ventricular hypertrophy by the electrocardiogram is highly specific but has a low sensitivity. The electrocardiogram in patients with PPH usually exhibits right atrial and right ventricular enlargement. A direct correlation between the amplitude of the R wave in V_1, the R/S ratio in V_2, and the level of pulmonary arterial pressure has been reported. These electrocardiographic abnormalities are usually less pronounced in patients with COPD than in patients with other forms of pulmonary hypertension because of the relatively modest degree of pulmonary hypertension that occurs and because of the effects of hyperinflation. Butler and coworkers suggested three criteria for right ventricular hypertrophy: (1) P wave amplitude less than 0.25 mV in II, III, aVF, and V_1 or V_2; (2) R wave amplitude equal to 0.2 mV in I; and (3) $A + R - PL = 0.7$ mV ($A = R$ or R' in V_1 or V_2; $R = S$ in I or V_6; $PL = S$ in V_2). A is the maximal amplitude of a positive waveform (R or R′) in leads V_1 or V_2, R is the maximal S amplitude in leads I or V_6, and PL is the S amplitude in V_1. These three criteria achieve 66 percent sensitivity in a group with right ventricular hypertrophy caused by mitral stenosis and 95 percent specificity in normal control subjects. When these criteria were evaluated in a population with pulmonary hypertension, their sensitivity was found to be even higher at 89 percent.[43]

ECHOCARDIOGRAPHY (see Chap. 11). Echocardiography usually demonstrates enlargement of the right atrium and ventricle, normal or small left ventricular dimensions, and a thickened interventricular septum.[44] Abnormal septal motion as a result of the right ventricular pressure overload is characteristic. Detection of right ventricular hypertrophy by echocardiography is limited by the ability to differentiate the right ventricular wall from its surrounding structures. Moreover, correlations between the thickness of the right ventricular wall and the right ventricular mass are poor, even when measured at autopsy. Right ventricular dysfunction is difficult to quantitate echocardiographically, but the position and curvature of the intraventricular septum gives an indication of right ventricular afterload. Echocardiographic findings that portend a poor prognosis include pericardial effusion, right atrial enlargement, and septal displacement.[45]

Doppler echocardiographic quantitation of right ventricular systolic hypertension can be obtained by measuring the velocity of the tricuspid regurgitant jet and using the Bernoulli formula (see Chap. 11). Doppler often overestimates the pulmonary artery pressure and may even suggest pulmonary hypertension in people who are normal.[46]

It is possible to estimate the pulmonary end-diastolic pressure noninvasively by summing the mean right atrial pressure and the end-diastolic gradient between the pulmonary artery and the right ventricular outflow track using the pulmonary regurgitation jet. When poor images make obtaining the estimates of peak tricuspid regurgitation velocities difficult, contrast enhancement with a saline medium should be used to improve the accuracy of the measurements. Doppler has also demonstrated left ventricular diastolic dysfunction with marked dependence on atrial contraction for ventricular filling.

RADIONUCLIDE VENTRICULOGRAPHY (see Chap. 13). Radionuclide ventriculography can provide useful information regarding right ventricular function, provided that adequate separation of the cardiac chambers can be accomplished.[47] Because radioactive counts are proportional to volume, variations in the geometric configuration of the ventricles are less important. Although pulmonary artery pressure cannot be estimated with this technique, there is an inverse relationship between pulmonary artery pressure and right ventricular ejection fraction.

LUNG SCINTIGRAPHY. A perfusion lung scan is an important test in making the correct diagnosis of pulmonary hypertension. Patients with PPH may reveal a relatively normal perfusion pattern or diffuse, patchy perfusion abnormalities. A perfusion lung scan will reliably distinguish patients with PPH from those who have pulmonary hypertension secondary to chronic pulmonary thromboembolism (Fig. 67–4).

PULMONARY FUNCTION TESTS. Although pulmonary function in patients with PPH is often completely normal, the vital capacity may be reduced to approximately 80 percent of predicted. A significant obstructive pattern is a rare finding, but hyperreactivity of the bronchial tree is common, which can lead to a misdiagnosis of asthma and could be a cause for delay in the diagnosis. In patients with PPH, the diffusing capacity for carbon monoxide (DLCO) is reduced to approximately 60 to 80 percent of predicted; there is no clear correlation between severity of the disease and the DLCO. The presence of arterial hypoxemia is due to ventilation-perfusion mismatch and/or reduced mixed venous oxygen saturations resulting from low cardiac output. The degree of arterial hypoxemia is often slight to moderate. A severe reduction of PaO_2 and SaO_2 can be due to right-to-left intra- or extracardiac shunts and/or intrapulmonary shunts. Consequently, PaO_2 and SaO_2 may vary markedly between patients with different constellations of associated abnormalities.

Approximately 20 percent of patients with systemic sclerosis have an isolated reduction in DLCO,[48] which, when severe (<55 percent of predicted) can be associated with the development of pulmonary arterial hypertension (PAH). In patients with limited systemic sclerosis, a fall in DLCO in the presence of normal lung volumes sometimes precedes PAH. A severe reduction in DLCO without changes in the pulmonary interstitium or the presence of a connective tissue

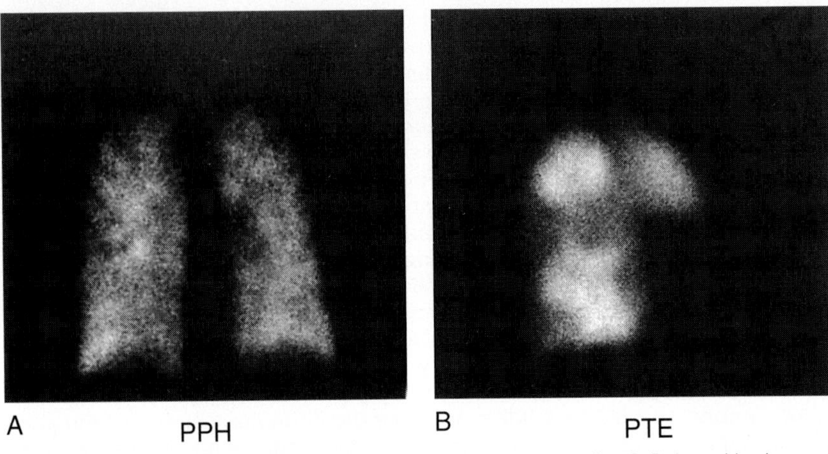

FIGURE 67–4 Perfusion lung scans in patients with pulmonary hypertension. **A,** Patient with primary pulmonary hypertension (PPH). **B,** Patient with pulmonary thromboembolism causing pulmonary hypertension (PTE). Both perfusion scans are abnormal. The scan from the patient with PPH shows a mottled distribution in a nonsegmental, nonanatomical manner. The scan from the patient with PTE reveals lobar, segmental, and subsegmental defects highly suggestive of an anatomical obstruction to pulmonary blood flow.

disease should alert the clinician to other diagnoses affecting the pulmonary vascular bed, such as pulmonary venoocclusive disease.

COMPUTED TOMOGRAPHY (see Chap. 15). Chest computed tomography (CT) scans have been used to determine the presence and severity of pulmonary hypertension based on the diameter of the main pulmonary arteries. Spiral chest CT scans have been used successfully in diagnosing chronic thromboembolic pulmonary hypertension (see Fig. 67–15). In addition to visualization of thrombi in the pulmonary vasculature with contrast enhancement, a mosaic pattern of variable attenuation compatible with irregular pulmonary perfusion can be determined in the unenhanced CT scan. Marked variation in the size of segmental vessels is also a specific feature of chronic thromboembolic disease. In some institutions, spiral CT scanning has replaced lung scintigraphy as a test to make this diagnosis.

A high-resolution CT scan of the chest is also the most accurate noninvasive means of detecting emphysema. The principal manifestation of emphysema is a hyperlucent region of lung tissue with no or only a very thin visible wall. Because CT has 10 times the density resolution of conventional radiography, it more readily distinguishes the emphysematous spaces from surrounding lung tissue. Other findings on high-resolution CT include ground-glass opacity, bullae, bronchial wall thickening, mucous plugging of bronchi and bronchioles, overinflation, air trapping (manifest as a lack of expected increase in lung opacity on exhalation scans), central arterial dilation reflecting pulmonary arterial hypertension, and modest mediastinal lymphadenopathy. CT can demonstrate emphysema in patients with little or no abnormality detected by pulmonary function tests. Because the aggregate cross-sectional area is so large, the respiratory bronchioles contribute only a small portion of the total resistance to air flow, which results in poor sensitivity of pulmonary function tests.

PULMONARY ANGIOGRAPHY. Pulmonary angiography establishes the correct diagnosis in patients with pulmonary hypertension in whom a perfusion lung scan suggests segmental or lobar defects. Typically, pulmonary angiography demonstrates large central pulmonary arteries with marked peripheral tapering. Postmortem arteriograms demonstrate the absence of "background haze" secondary to the loss of small, nonmuscular pulmonary arterioles. Although pulmonary angiography carries an increased risk in patients with pulmonary hypertension, it can be performed safely if adequate precautions are taken. Maintenance of adequate oxygenation by the administration of supplemental oxygen and the avoidance of vasovagal reactions (and rapid treatment of those that occur with intravenous atropine) should reduce the associated risk in this patient group. Placement of an arterial line for continuous arterial pressure monitoring is advised, and nonionic contrast agents appear to be better tolerated. Pulmonary wedge angiography with hand injection of small amounts of angiographic contrast material through the terminal lumen of a balloon flotation catheter is not a substitute for pulmonary angiography and may result in misleading findings.

EXERCISE TESTING (see Chap. 10). The use of a symptom-limited exercise test can be very helpful in the evaluation of patients with pulmonary hypertension.[49] Besides allowing objective assessment of the severity of symptoms, exercise testing has also been shown to be predictive of survival. The 6-minute walk test is commonly used in clinical trials as an endpoint for efficacy of therapy in patients with pulmonary hypertension. It has been correlated with workload, heart rate, oxygen saturation, and dyspnea response. In randomized clinical trials, a 6-minute walk has been shown to be an independent predictor of mortality.[50] Its drawbacks include the fact that the effort is often tester dependent and that anthropometric factors such as gait speed, age, weight, muscle mass, and length of stride can affect the test. Treadmill testing has also been used and compares with the 6-minute walk test in reflecting drug efficacy. The Naughton protocol uses a treadmill with increases in work of 1 metabolic equivalent (MET) increments at 2-minute stages to allow patients with very limited exercise tolerance to perform.[49]

Cardiopulmonary exercise testing using an upright bicycle and measurements of gas exchange has the potential to noninvasively grade the severity of exercise limitation in patients with pulmonary hypertension.[51] The breathlessness of patients with pulmonary hypertension during exercise can be related to the relative hypoperfusion of their lungs, which causes an increase in dead space ventilation manifest by a hyperbolic increase in minute ventilation. This can be exacerbated by lactic acidosis and hypoxemia as a result of their inability to increase cardiac output with exercise. Thus, dyspnea with pulmonary hypertension is attributable to worsening ventilation-perfusion mismatching, lactic acidosis, and arterial hypoxemia.[52]

CARDIAC CATHETERIZATION (see Chap. 17). Besides confirming the diagnosis and allowing the exclusion of other causes, cardiac catheterization also establishes the severity of disease and allows an assessment of prognosis. By definition, patients with PAH should have a low or normal pulmonary capillary wedge pressure. When a wedge pressure cannot be obtained, direct measurement of left ventricular end-diastolic pressure is advised. If the wedge pressure is increased, it should be correlated with left ventricular end-diastolic pressure and not attributed to a "falsely elevated" reading. It has been shown that left ventricular diastolic compliance becomes significantly impaired in patients with PAH and parallels the severity of the disease; thus, pulmonary capillary wedge pressure tends to rise slightly in the late stages of PAH, although it rarely exceed 16 mm Hg. Measurements of all right-sided pressures are properly made at end-expiration to avoid incorporating negative intrathoracic pressures.

It can be extremely difficult to pass a catheter into the pulmonary artery in patients with pulmonary hypertension because of the tricuspid regurgitation, dilated right atrium and ventricle, and low cardiac output. A specific flow-directed thermodilution balloon catheter has been developed for patients with pulmonary hypertension (American Edwards Laboratories, Irvine, CA); it has an extra port for the placement of a 0.32-inch guidewire to provide better stiffness to the catheter. The risk associated with cardiac catheterization in patients with pulmonary hypertension is extremely low in experienced hands, but deaths have been reported.

Acute Testing with Vasodilators (Table 67–3). Several vasodilators are of value in the assessment of pulmonary vasoreactivity in patients with PAH. Adenosine is an intermediate product in the metabolism of adenosine triphosphate that has potent vasodilator properties through its action on specific vascular receptors. It is believed to stimulate the endothelial cell and vascular smooth muscle receptors of the A_2 type, which induce vascular smooth muscle relaxation by increasing cyclic adenosine monophosphate. In patients with PAH, adenosine has been shown to be a potent vasodilator and predictive of the chronic effects of intravenous prostacyclin and oral calcium channel blockers.[53] Adenosine has an extremely short half-life (<5 sec), which provides a safety net by its rapid dissolution should any adverse side effects occur. It is administered intravenously as an infusion in doses of 50 μg/kg/min and titrated upward every 2 minutes until uncomfortable symptoms develop (such as chest tightness or dyspnea).

Epoprostenol has been used as an acute test of vasoreactivity in patients with PAH.[54] Like adenosine, its short half-life allows use of the drug to be discontinued if any acute adverse effects result. Also similar to adenosine, it is administered incrementally, at 2 ng/kg/min and increased every 15 to 30 minutes until systemic effects such as headache, flushing, or nausea occur, which limits the acute dose titration. Favorable acute effects from epoprostenol are predictive of a favorable response to oral calcium channel blockers.

Adenosine and epoprostenol possess potent inotropic properties, in addition to their ability to vasodilate the pulmonary vascular bed. When using these drugs for the acute testing of patients, one needs to pay particular attention to changes in cardiac output that occur in association with the changes in pulmonary arterial pressure. An increase in cardiac output with no change in pulmonary arterial pressure will result in a reduction in calculated pulmonary vascular resistance and may be erroneously interpreted as a vasodilator response.

Nitric oxide is also a useful drug to test pulmonary vasoreactivity.[55] Because it binds very rapidly to hemoglobin with high affinity and is thereby inactivated, inhalation of NO gas results in selective pulmonary vascular effects without influencing the systemic circulation.[56] Inhalation of NO by patients with PAH has been shown to produce a reduction in pulmonary vascular resistance acutely, similar to that achieved with intravenous adenosine, and to also predict the effectiveness of calcium channel blockers. NO differs importantly from adenosine and epoprostenol in that it has little effect on cardiac output. It is usually given via facemask at 20 to 40 ppm.

It must be emphasized that hemodynamic assessment of the entire circulatory system is essential when determining the influence of drugs in these patients. Small changes in pulmonary artery pressure are usually due to variability and are not related to direct drug influence. Changes in pulmonary vascular resistance cannot be directly measured but are computed by the change in pulmonary pressure and cardiac output simultaneously. Because thermodilution cardiac output—the method that is most commonly used in these patients—can be associated with large errors in reproducibility, particular care should be taken in the methodology of thermodilution used in these patients. In addition, when an underlying right-to-left shunt exists, the Fick determination of cardiac output is required.

Changes in pulmonary capillary wedge pressure can have important influences on the determination of pulmonary vascular resistance. A rising capillary wedge pressure secondary to increased cardiac output may be the first sign of impending left ventricular failure and an adverse effect of a drug, whereas the calculated pulmonary vascular resistance may become lower and suggest a beneficial effect. Right atrial pressure also reflects the filling characteristics of the right ventricle. A right atrial pressure increase in the face of rising cardiac output suggests right ventricular diastolic dysfunction. The resting heart rate is a physiological parameter of marked importance in patients with congestive heart failure, and treatments that cause an increased heart rate are likely to yield deleterious long-term results. Finally, the systemic arterial oxygen

TABLE 67–3 Hemodynamic Assessment of Vasodilators in Pulmonary Hypertension

Parameter Measured	Desired Acute Changes	Comments
Mean pulmonary artery pressure	>25% fall; ideally mean PAP below 30 mm Hg	Must not be any associated significant fall in systemic blood pressure
Pulmonary vascular resistance	>33% fall; ideally, PVR below 6 units	Should be associated with a fall in PAP *and* an increase in cardiac output. An increase in cardiac output alone may lead to future RV failure
Right atrial pressure	No change or fall	An increase in RA pressure signals impending RV failure
Pulmonary capillary wedge pressure	No change	An increase in wedge pressure suggests pulmonary venoocclusive disease or coexisting LV dysfunction
Systemic blood pressure	Minimal fall; mean arterial pressure should remain above 90 mm Hg	A significant hypotensive response makes chronic vasodilator therapy contraindicated
Cardiac output	Increase	The increase should be related to increased stroke volume and not solely due to increased heart rate
Heart rate	No significant change	A chronic increased heart rate will result in RV failure. Watch for bradycardia if high doses of diltiazem are used
Systemic arterial oxygen saturation	Increase if reduced on room air, little change if normal	A fall in systemic arterial oxygen saturation suggests lung disease or right-to-left shunting and prohibits chronic use
Pulmonary artery (mixed venous) oxygen saturation	Increase	Should reflect the increase in cardiac output and improved tissue oxygenation

LV = left ventricular; PAP = pulmonary artery pressure; PVR = pulmonary vascular resistance; RA = right atrial; RV = right ventricular.
From Rubin LJ, Rich S: Medical management. *In* Rubin LJ, Rich S (eds): Primary Pulmonary Hypertension. New York. Marcel Dekker, 1997, pp 271-286 by courtesy of Marcel Dekker, Inc.

content should be evaluated in patients with pulmonary hypertension. Effective vasodilator drugs can result in vasodilation of blood vessels supplying poorly ventilated areas of the lung and can worsen hypoxemia. This effect is particularly noticeable in patients with underlying chronic lung disease.

Classification of Pulmonary Hypertension

Pulmonary hypertension, in its simplest sense, refers to any elevation in the pulmonary arterial pressure above normal. The presence of pulmonary hypertension may reflect a serious underlying pulmonary vascular disease, which can be progressive and fatal, or simply an obligatory passive elevation in the pulmonary artery pressure in response to elevated pressures in the left heart. Consequently, an accurate diagnosis of the cause of pulmonary hypertension in a patient is essential to establish an effective treatment plan. In addition, therapies that may be beneficial in patients with some types of pulmonary hypertension may be harmful in patients with other types.

The diagnosis of pulmonary hypertension relies on establishing an elevation in pulmonary artery pressure above normal. Published norms have come from cardiac catheterizations performed in young subjects at rest without any evidence of cardiopulmonary disease. The upper limit of normal for pulmonary artery mean pressure is 19 mm Hg. However, this assumes that there are no abnormalities in downstream pressures of the left atrium or left ventricle, or an increased cardiac output. That is why a patient can have pulmonary hypertension from the standpoint of an elevated pulmonary artery pressure, but normal pulmonary vascular resistance. Recently, parameters for normal pulmonary arterial systolic pressure derived by echo-Doppler studies have been published that suggest that the upper limit of normal of pulmonary arterial systolic pressure in the general population may be higher than previously appreciated.[46]

There are patients whose resting hemodynamics are normal but in whom marked elevations in pulmonary pressure occur with exercise. It has been presumed that this represents an early stage of pulmonary vascular disease. However, because patients may have a hypertensive response to exercise with respect to the systemic vasculature, a similar type of response can occur in the pulmonary vascular disease, or reduced compliance of an otherwise normal pulmonary circulation can be difficult to ascertain.

In 1998, a new classification for pulmonary hypertension was developed at the World Symposium on Pulmonary Hypertension cosponsored by the World Health Organization. This classification catalogued clinical conditions based on common pathobiological features to serve as a guide in the clinical assessment and treatment of these patients. Recently, modifications to this classification have been proposed (Table 67–4). In addition, a functional classification patterned after the New York Heart Association functional classification for heart disease was developed to allow comparisons of patients with respect to the clinical severity of the disease process (Table 67–5).

Pulmonary arterial hypertension refers to pulmonary vascular disease affecting the arterioles, resulting in an elevation in pressure and vascular resistance. Although PPH is relatively rare, with an estimated incidence of 1 to 2 per million in the population, severe PAH associated with other conditions is more common (Table 67–6).[57] The most common etiology is associated with connective tissue disease states, primarily scleroderma, including the CREST syndrome (calcinosis cutis, Raynaud phenomenon, esophageal dysfunction, sclerodactyly, and telangiectasia), and mixed connective tissue disease. PAH is also relatively common in patients with congenital heart defects, especially those with ventricular septal defects or a patent ductus arteriosus.[58]

TABLE 67–4 Clinical Classification of Pulmonary Arterial Hypertension*

1. Pulmonary arterial hypertension
   - 1.1 Primary pulmonary hypertension
     - (a) Familial
   - 1.2 Associated with:
     - (a) Connective tissue disease
     - (b) Congenital heart disease
     - (c) Portal hypertension
     - (d) Human immunodeficiency virus infection
     - (e) Drugs/toxins
       - (1) Anorexigens
       - (2) Other
   - 1.3 Persistent pulmonary hypertension of the newborn
   - 1.4 Pulmonary veno-occlusive disease
   - 1.5 Pulmonary capillary hemangiomatosis
2. Pulmonary venous hypertension
   - 2.1 Left-sided atrial or ventricular heart disease
   - 2.2 Left-sided valvular heart disease
   - 2.3 Extrinsic compression of central pulmonary veins
     - (a) Fibrosing mediastinitis
     - (b) Adenopathy/tumors
   - 2.4 Other
3. Pulmonary hypertension associated with disorders of the respiratory system and/or hypoxemia
   - 3.1 Chronic obstructive pulmonary disease
   - 3.2 Interstitial lung disease
   - 3.3 Sleep-disordered breathing
   - 3.4 Alveolar hypoventilation disorders
   - 3.5 Chronic exposure to high altitude
   - 3.6 Neonatal lung disease
   - 3.7 Alveolar-capillary dysplasia
   - 3.8 Other
4. Pulmonary hypertension due to chronic thrombotic and/or embolic disease
   - 4.1 Thromboembolic obstruction of proximal pulmonary arteries
   - 4.2 Thromboembolic obstruction of the distal pulmonary arteries
   - 4.3 Pulmonary embolism (tumor, ova parasites, foreign material)
5. Pulmonary hypertension due to disorders directly affecting the pulmonary vasculature
   - 5.1 Inflammatory
     - (a) Schistosomiasis
     - (b) Sarcoidosis
     - (c) Histiocytosis X
     - (d) Other

*Modified from Rich S (ed): Primary Pulmonary Hypertension: Executive Summary from the World Symposium—Primary Pulmonary Hypertension 1998. Available from the World Health Organization at http://www.who.int/ncd/cvd/pph.html.

Other comorbid conditions include cirrhosis with portal hypertension and human immunodeficiency virus (HIV) infection.

COR PULMONALE. This is defined as right ventricular hypertrophy and dilation secondary to pulmonary hypertension caused by diseases of the lung parenchyma and/or pulmonary vasculature, unrelated to the left side of the heart. Chronic cor pulmonale traditionally implies pulmonary hypertension related to either obstructive or restrictive lung disease, whereas acute cor pulmonale usually refers to the development of acute pulmonary hypertension from massive pulmonary embolism.

Primary Pulmonary Hypertension

Primary pulmonary hypertension is the diagnosis given to patients with pulmonary hypertension of unexplained etiol-

TABLE 67–5 World Health Organization Functional Classification of Pulmonary Hypertension*

A. Class I—Patients with pulmonary hypertension but without resulting limitation of physical activity. Ordinary physical activity does not cause undue dyspnea or fatigue, chest pain, or syncope.

B. Class II—Patients with pulmonary hypertension resulting in slight limitation of physical activity. They are comfortable at rest. Ordinary physical activity causes undue dyspnea or fatigue, chest pain, or near syncope.

C. Class III—Patients with pulmonary hypertension resulting in marked limitation of physical activity. They are comfortable at rest. Less than ordinary activity causes undue dyspnea or fatigue, chest pain, or near syncope.

D. Class IV—Patients with pulmonary hypertension with inability to carry out any physical activity without symptoms. Patients manifest signs of right heart failure. Dyspnea and/or fatigue may even be present at rest. Discomfort is increased by any physical activity.

*Modified from Rich S (ed): Primary Pulmonary Hypertension: Executive Summary from the World Symposium—Primary Pulmonary Hypertension 1998. Available from the World Health Organization at http://www.who.int/ncd/cvd/pph.html.

ogy. Although the name of the disease stems from its distinction from pulmonary hypertension secondary to known cardiac or pulmonary causes, PPH should not be considered as only pulmonary hypertension for which no cause is found. The clinical features, usual age of onset, progression of the disease, and autopsy findings make PPH a distinct clinical entity and distinguish it from other forms of pulmonary hypertension even though its diagnosis requires careful exclusion of secondary causes. The actual incidence of PPH appears to be approximately 2 cases per million population, thus qualifying it as an orphan disease.[59]

Etiology

By definition, the precise cause of PPH is unknown, but it probably represents the clinical expression of PAH as the final common pathway from multiple biological abnormalities within the pulmonary circulation. As understanding of vascular biology improves, many studies point to abnormalities in pulmonary endothelial cell function as causing or contributing to the development of pulmonary hypertension in humans.[60] It is now understood that the endothelial cell regulates pulmonary smooth muscle cell tone. Dysfunction of the counterregulatory systems within the pulmonary vascular bed seems to be common in cases of pulmonary hypertension. The normal pulmonary vascular endothelial cell maintains the vascular smooth muscle in a state of relaxation.[61] The finding of increased pulmonary vascular reactivity and vasoconstriction in patients with PPH suggests that a marked vasoconstrictive tendency underlies the development of PPH in predisposed individuals, possibly as a result of inappropriate smooth muscle hypertrophy.

Reduced expression of NO synthase in the endothelium of patients with pulmonary hypertension has been demonstrated and correlates inversely with the extent and severity of morphological lesions.[62] Although it is unsettled whether reduced NO synthase production is a cause or a result of the disease, it is consistent with endothelial dysfunction underlying PPH as part of the disease process. Endothelin may also play an important role in the elevated pulmonary vascular tone.[63] Because it has a long half-life, subtle disturbances in production or release could lead to sustained vasoconstriction. Elevations in endothelin levels within the pulmonary vasculature of patients with various forms of pulmonary hypertension have been documented.[64] This finding suggests that regardless of whether abnormal endothelial function is the underlying cause of PPH, progression of the disease is invariably accompanied by worsening of endothelial function, which itself can promote disease progression.

A striking feature of the pulmonary vasculature in patients with PPH is intimal proliferation, and in some vessels it causes virtually complete vascular occlusion (Fig. 67–5). Several growth factors have been implicated in the development of this type of vascular pathology, including basic fibroblast growth factor from the endothelium[65] and platelet-derived growth factor and TGF-β[66] from platelets. Enhanced growth factor release, activation, and intracellular signaling may lead to smooth muscle cell proliferation and migration, as well as extracellular matrix synthesis. Even advanced lesions show evidence of in situ activity of ongoing synthesis of connective tissue proteins such as elastin, collagen, and fibronectin.[60]

An equally important etiological feature of PPH is the widespread development of in situ thrombosis of the small pulmonary arteries with intraluminal thrombin deposition. Abnormalities in platelet activation and function and biochemical features of a procoagulant environment within the pulmonary vasculature support a role of thrombosis in disease initiation in some patients.[67,68] Interactions between growth factors, platelets, and the vessel wall suggest that thrombin may play a fundamental role in many of the pathobiological processes described in patients with PPH and in disease progression.[69] A prothrombotic state can arise as a consequence of fibrinolysis, enhanced coagulation, or increased platelet activation. Platelet activation not only promotes thrombosis but also leads to the release of granules that contain mitogenic agents and vasoconstrictive substances.[70]

LOCAL HEMODYNAMICS. Several studies suggest that local hemodynamics can influence pulmonary vascular remodeling.[71] A classic example is the pulmonary hypertension that occurs in congenital systemic-to-pulmonary shunts. It is believed that endothelial cells can release mediators that induce vascular smooth muscle cell growth in response to changes in pulmonary blood flow or pressure. Experimental data suggest that medial hypertrophy can be converted to a neointimal

TABLE 67–6 Advanced Pulmonary Hypertension by Disease Category

Disease	Prevalence	Percentage of Patients with PH	Estimated Number in North America and Europe
Systemic sclerosis	190/million	33	37,620
Congenital heart defects (ASD/VSD/PDA)	300/million	15-20	31,500
Cirrhosis	1600/million	0.6	5,760
HIV related	2500/million	0.5	7,500
Primary PH	7/million	100	4,200

ASD = atrial septal defect; HIV = human immunodeficiency virus; PDA = patent ductus arteriosus; PH = pulmonary hypertension; VSD = ventricular septal defect.

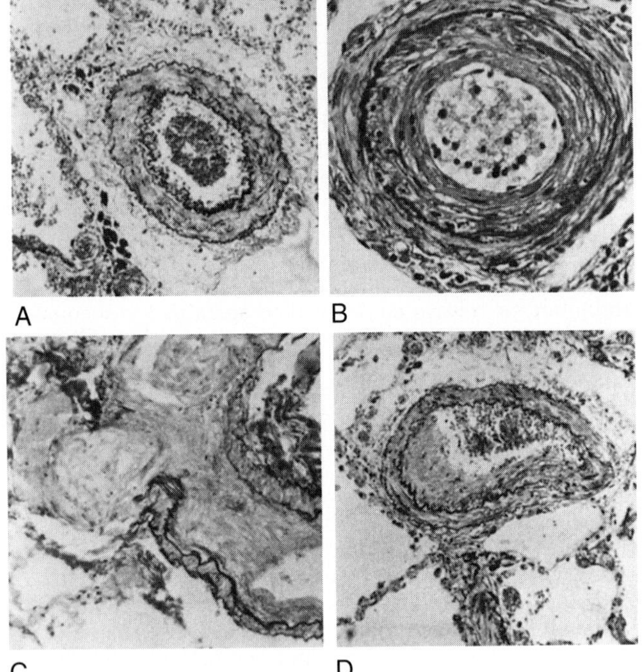

FIGURE 67–5 Photomicrographs of pulmonary arterial histological lesions seen in cases of clinically unexplained pulmonary hypertension. All slides were stained with Verhoeff-van Gieson stain. **A,** Medical hypertrophy (original magnification ×100). **B,** Concentric laminal intimal fibrosis, seen most often in association with plexiform lesions (original magnification ×200). **C,** Plexiform lesion demonstrating obstruction in the arterial lumen, aneurysmal dilation, and proliferation of anastomosing vascular channels (original magnification ×200). **D,** Eccentric intimal fibrosis, often seen in association with organized microthrombi but also present in many patients with plexiform lesions (original magnification ×100). (From Palevsky HI, Schloo BL, Pietra CC, et al: Primary pulmonary hypertension: Vascular structure, morphometry and responsiveness to vasodilator agents. Circulation 80:1207, 1989.)

pattern when pulmonary vascular injury is coupled with increased pulmonary blood flow. These neointimal lesions are composed of smooth muscle cells that are immunoreactive to anti-α smooth muscle actin antibody. It is now accepted that hemodynamic shear stress acts through the endothelium to regulate vessel tone and in the chronic restructuring of blood vessels.[71]

Endothelial denudation also results in platelet adherence to exposed tissue collagen, with release of platelet-derived smooth muscle mitogens that also have vasoconstrictor properties. This process in turn leads to an inflammatory response and thrombosis, thereby narrowing the lumen of pulmonary vessels. In a person who is susceptible—whether on a genetic or an acquired basis—intense vasoconstriction may lead to fibrinoid necrosis of the arteriolar wall and the development of plexiform lesions. Ultimately, the vessels are reduced in number, and the residua of these destroyed vessels can be seen histologically as "ghost vessels." Destruction of large numbers of pulmonary arterioles reduces the cross-sectional area of the pulmonary vascular bed, thereby producing a permanent increase in pulmonary vascular resistance and fixed pulmonary hypertension. The latter in turn damages other blood vessels and initiates a vicious circle, with progressively rising pulmonary arterial pressure.

ANGIOTENSIN-CONVERTING ENZYME. An essential role of ACE in the pathogenesis of pulmonary hypertension is strongly suggested by the presence of increased ACE immunoreactivity at sites of increased matrix gene expression in human hypertensive pulmonary arteries.[35] Further supporting a role for ACE in pulmonary vascular remodeling are observations that ACE protein and mRNA expression are focally increased in rat pulmonary arteries with medial hypertrophy from chronic hypoxia.[37]

INCREASED ACTIVITY OF ELASTOLYTIC ENZYMES. This appears to be important in the pathophysiology of pulmonary vascular disease.[72] High elastin turnover and neosynthesis of elastin have been attributed to degradation of elastin from the increased activity of serine elastase. A cause-and-effect relationship between elastase and pulmonary vascular disease was demonstrated when elastase inhibitors were shown to be effective in attenuating the development and retarding the progression of pulmonary hypertension in monocrotaline-injected hypoxic rats.[73] Progression of pulmonary hypertension may involve a series of switches in smooth muscle cell phenotype and proliferation to account for the medial hypertrophy and smooth muscle cell migration resulting in neointimal formation. Structural and functional alterations in the endothelial cell could result in loss of barrier function and allow leakage into the subendothelium of a serum factor normally excluded from this region. Enzymes released from precursor or mature smooth muscle cells could activate growth factors normally stored in the extracellular matrix, such as basic fibroblast growth factor and TGF-β, which are known to induce smooth muscle cell hypertrophy and proliferation and increase connective tissue protein synthesis. In muscular arteries, release of growth factors would result in hypertrophy of the vessel wall.

ION CHANNELS. Potassium channels are found throughout the pulmonary vascular bed.[74] They consist of voltage-dependent potassium channels and calcium-dependent potassium channels (see Chap. 27). The role of these channels has been studied primarily in the presence of acute hypoxia in animals. It is believed that potassium channels modulate adult pulmonary vascular tone. It is probable that calcium channels also serve a regulatory role in modulating vascular tone, particularly the L-type calcium channel. Inhibition of the voltage-regulated potassium channel by hypoxia or drugs can produce vasoconstriction and has been described in pulmonary artery smooth muscle cells harvested from patients with PPH. It has been suggested that defects in the potassium channel of pulmonary resistance smooth muscle cells are involved in the initiation or progression of pulmonary hypertension. A genetic defect related to potassium channels in the lungs of patients with PPH that leads to vasoconstriction may be one mechanism for the development of PPH in some patients (see Fig. 67–6).[74]

DYSFUNCTIONAL ENDOTHELIUM. The dysfunctional pulmonary hypertensive endothelial cell phenotype is characterized by uncontrolled proliferation, increased production of vasoconstrictor mediators such as endothelin, expression of 5-lipoxygenase, and decreased synthesis of prostacyclin. In patients with PPH, expression of prostacyclin synthase is reduced in pulmonary arteries ranging from 1 mm to less than 100 μm in diameter, which suggests that the reduction in prostacyclin synthesis in otherwise morphologically normal to minimally remodeled vessels may play a role in the early stages of pathogenesis. Alternatively, endothelial cells of pulmonary small arteries may become dysfunctional as the disease progresses and pulmonary artery pressure progressively rises. Loss of expression of prostacyclin synthase is one of the phenotypic alterations present in pulmonary endothelial cells in cases of severe pulmonary hypertension.[75]

SEROTONIN. This substance has also been implicated as being involved in PPH. Elevations in serotonin levels have been correlated with the pulmonary vascular pressure gradient in patients with acute respiratory distress syndrome. Children with congenital heart disease and pulmonary hypertension have increased turnover of serotonin.[76] PPH has been reported in a patient with familial platelet storage pool disease, which represents a defect in serotonin handling and release. One series reported increased serotonin in patients with pulmonary hypertension associated with the use of fenfluramine and with connective tissue disease.[77] Of interest is that after six of these patients underwent heart/lung transplantation, they had persistently elevated concentrations of plasma serotonin and decreased platelet serotonin concentrations, thus suggesting that the abnormality in platelet serotonin handling was a primary process in the evolution of their pulmonary hypertension.

Genetics

An important emerging concept in the development of PAH is that the disease develops in patients with an underlying genetic predisposition following exposure to specific stimuli, which serve as triggers. Predisposition to the development of pulmonary hypertension has been noted by the marked heterogeneity in responses of the pulmonary vasculature in a variety of disease states. Examples include the considerable variability among individuals to vasoconstrictive stimuli such as hypoxia or acidosis, which can produce marked pulmonary hypertension in one person and be essentially without effect in another. The pulmonary arterial pressure response to hypoxia is particularly great in individuals with blood group A. This variability in responsiveness of the pulmonary vascular bed undoubtedly accounts for the fact that pulmonary edema develops in only a minority of individuals on exposure to high altitude. Also, the severity of pulmonary hypertension and the level of pulmonary vascular resistance vary considerably among individuals with congenital heart disease and comparably sized ventricular septal defects. Presumably, a genetic basis underlies these differences in pulmonary vascular reactivity, just as there appears to be a genetic basis for the increased reactivity of the systemic vascular bed in essential systemic hypertension.

FAMILIAL PPH. PPH has been diagnosed in families worldwide. The prevalence of familial PPH is uncertain, but it occurs in at least 6 percent of cases, and the incidence is probably higher. Many unique features are associated with the transmission and development of PPH in families.[78] The age of onset is variable and penetrance is incomplete. Many individuals in families with PPH inherit the gene and have progeny in whom PPH never develops. The observation that fewer males are born in PPH families than in the population at large suggests that the PPH gene might influence fertilization or cause male fetal wastage. Patients with familial PPH have a similar female-to-male ratio, age of onset, and natural history of the disease as those with sporadic PPH.

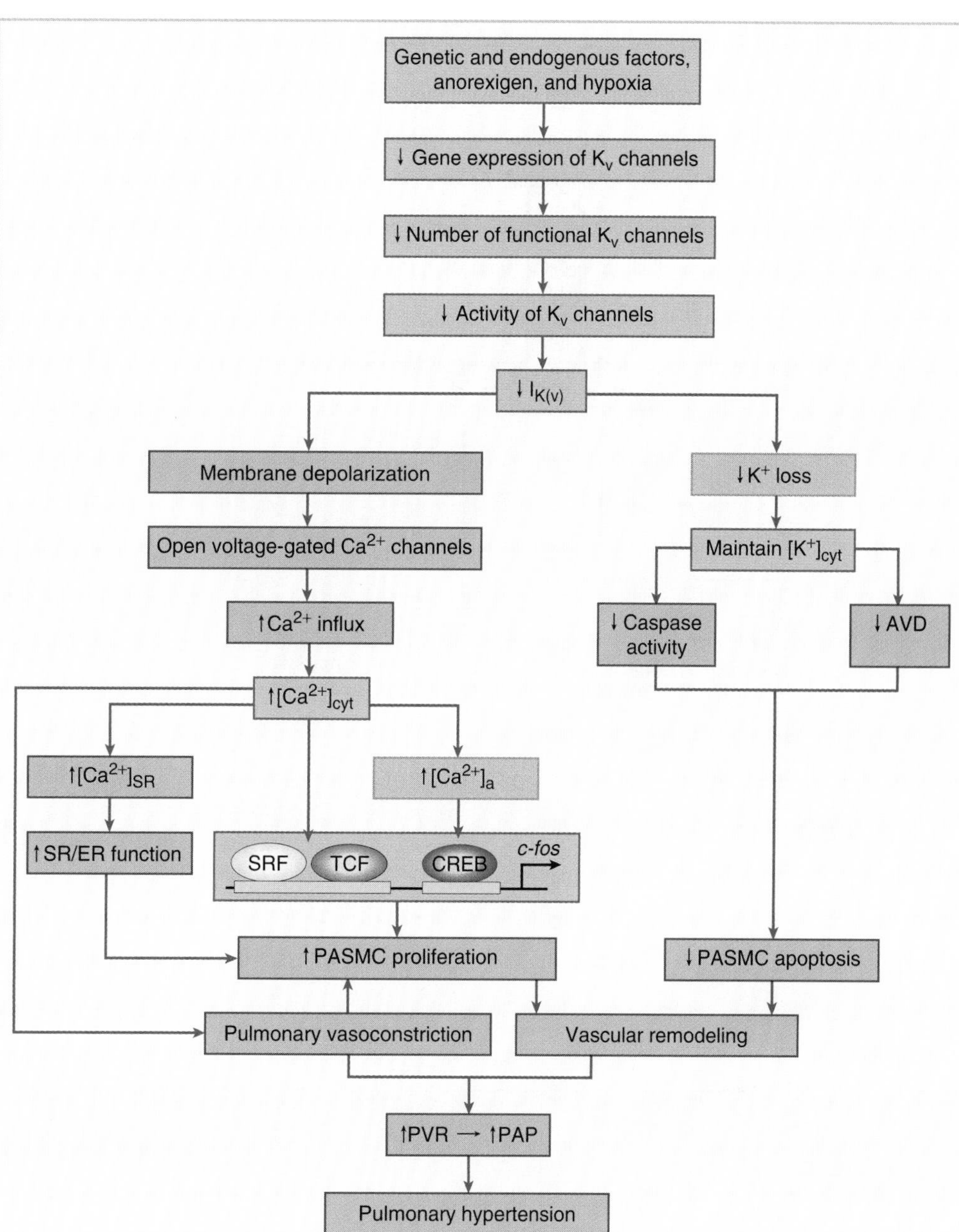

FIGURE 67–6 Schematic diagram depicting possible cellular mechanisms responsible for the development of pulmonary hypertension. The process is initiated by a series of endogenous and exogenous factors, which lead to abnormal gene transcription or expression of functional K_v channels and reduction in K_v channel activity. This leads to membrane depolarization and opening of voltage-gated Ca^{2+} channels, increasing $[Ca^{2+}]_{cyt}$. Because of the high ratio of Ca^{2+} in the SR ($[Ca^{2+}]_{SR}$) to $[Ca^{2+}]_{cyt}$ and the minimal resistance of the nuclear membrane to Ca^{2+}, a rise in $[Ca^{2+}]_{cyt}$ subsequently increases $[Ca^{2}]_{SR}$ and nuclear Ca^{2+} ($[Ca^{2+}]_n$). c-*fos* is a Ca^{2+}-responsive gene that has two Ca^{2+} elements in its promoter: the SRE (which binds with SRF), and the cyclic adenosine monophosphate response element (which binds to CREB). Activation of the early-responsive gene expression by increased $[Ca^{2+}]_{cyt}$, and $[Ca^{2+}]_n$, and the increased $[Ca^{2+}]_{SR}$ and SR/ER function stimulates pulmonary arterial smooth muscle cell (PASMC) proliferation. Increased $[Ca^{2+}]_{cyt}$ also causes increased vascular tone and vasoconstriction. Decreased IK_v, on the other hand, causes a decreased K^+ loss from the cell, maintaining sufficient K^+ in the cytosol ($[K^+]_{cyt}$). This in turn counteracts the apoptotic volume decrease (AVD) and decreases the activity of apoptotic mediators such as caspase and nucleases, leading to a reduced apoptosis of the SMCs. An increased cellular proliferation and decreased apoptosis cause vascular remodeling, ultimately leading to increased pulmonary vascular resistance (PVR), pulmonary artery pressure (PAP), and the development of pulmonary hypertension. CREB = cyclic AMP response element binding protein; SRF = serum response factor; TCF = ternary complex factor. (From Mandegar M, Yuan JX-J: Role of K^+ channels in pulmonary hypertension. Vasc Pharmacol 38:25, 2002.)

Documentation of familial PPH can be difficult, since remote common ancestry occurs in patients with apparently sporadic PPH and skip generations caused either by incomplete penetrance or by variable expression can mimic sporadic disease. Vertical transmission has been demonstrated in as many as five generations in one family and is probably indicative of a single dominant gene that is believed to be autosomal for PPH.[79] Genetic anticipation has been described in familial PPH since the early reports (Fig. 67–7). Because the clinical and pathological features of familial and sporadic PPH are virtually identical, it seems likely that the same genes are involved in both forms of the disease.

Familial PPH segregates as an autosomal dominant trait with markedly reduced penetrance. Using linkage analysis, the locus designated PPH-1 on chromosome 2q31-33 led to the discovery of the *PPH-1* gene.[80] *PPH-1* is the Human Genome Organization-approved designation DGB:1381541.[81] The low penetrance of this gene confers only about a 20 percent likelihood of development of the disease.

Bone Morphogenetic Protein Receptor Type 2 Gene. The gene (*BMPR-2*) coding for a receptor member of the TGF-β

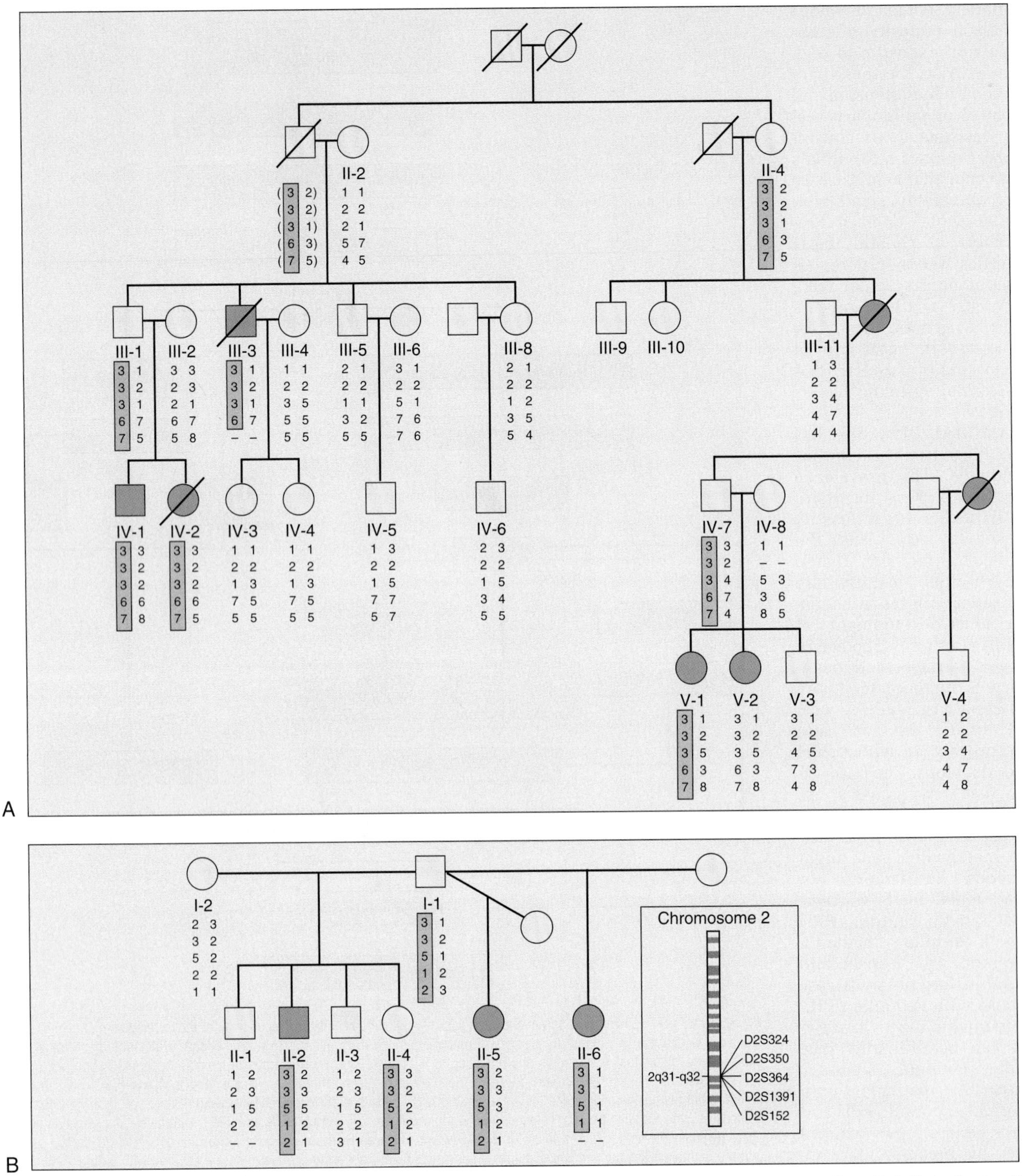

A

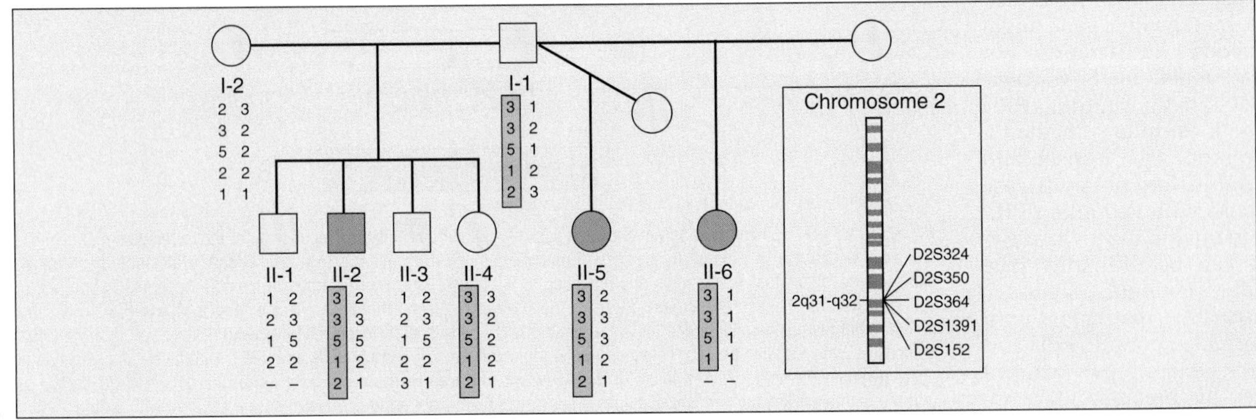

B

FIGURE 67–7 The pedigrees of two families (**A** and **B**) with familial primary pulmonary hypertension (PPH). Shaded symbols represent affected individuals. Genotyped individuals are indicated by the respective pedigree designations. The PPH-1 region on chromosome 2 (2q31-q32) contains a number of candidate genes. (From Morse JH, Jones AC, Barst RJ, et al: Mapping of familial primary pulmonary hypertension locus (*PPH-1*) to chromosome 2q31-32. Circulation 95:2603, 1997.)

family has been identified as causative of familial PPH.[82] The mutations ascribed to the locus interrupt the BMP-mediated signaling pathway, resulting in a predisposition to proliferation rather than apoptosis of cells within small pulmonary arteries. These molecular studies suggest that the target cells within the pulmonary arterial wall are sensitive to *BMPR-2* gene dosage and the TGF-β pathway mediated through *BMPR-2* is critical for the maintenance and/or normal response to injury of the pulmonary vasculature (Fig. 67–8).[83] It is clear, however, that additional factors, either environmental or genetic, are required in the pathogenesis of the disease. How defects in *BMPR-2* contribute to endothelial cell proliferation, smooth muscle cell hypertrophy, and fibroblast deposition in patients with PPH remains unknown. It is interesting to note that many patients with "sporadic" PPH actually have a kindred affected by familial PPH that can span many generations.[82] About one in four cases of sporadic PPH actually have germline mutations in the gene encoding the

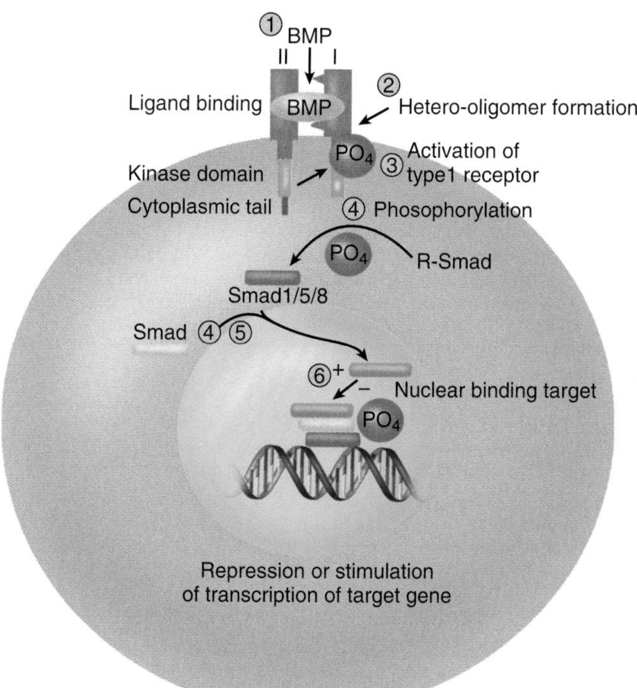

FIGURE 67–8 Bone morphogenetic protein (BMP) signaling pathway. **1** and **2,** BMPR1 and BMPR2 are present on most cell surfaces as homo-dimers or hetero-oligomers. With ligand binding, a complex of ligand, two type I receptors, and two type II receptors is formed. **3,** After ligand stimulation, the type II receptor phosphorylates the type I receptor in its juxtamembrane domain. **4,** The activated type I receptor then phosphorylates a receptor-regulated Smad (R-Smad); thus, the type I receptors determine the specificity of the signal. Smads 1, 5, and 8 are specific for BMP signaling pathway. **5,** Once activated by phosphorylation, the R-Smads interact with the common mediator Smad 4 to form hetero-oligomers that are translocated to the nucleus. **6,** In the nucleus, the Smad complex interacts with transcription factors and binds to DNA to induce or suppress transcription of target genes. Smads 6 and 7, inhibitory Smads (not shown), bind to activated type I receptors to prevent the phosphorylation of R-Smads. (From Runo JR, Loyd JE: Primary pulmonary hypertension. Lancet 361:1533, 2003.)

BMPR-2 receptor. Recent work suggesting that there are other causative genes supports the idea that there may be genetic determinants that modify the clinical expression of the disease. Endothelial cells and myofibroblast cells compose intimal lesions at the sites of pulmonary vascular expression of the *BMPR-2* receptor.[84]

Other Genetic Factors. Other factors suggested include ET-1, changes in potassium channels, sensitivity to prostacyclin, and serotonin. Adnot and colleagues demonstrated that there is overexpression of serotonin transporter (5-HTT) in pulmonary arteries and platelets from all the patients with PPH they studied and that increased activity of the 5-HTT is responsible for the associated smooth muscle hyperplasia.[85] In addition, they recently demonstrated that 5-HTT expression is elevated in cultured pulmonary artery smooth muscle cells from patients with PAH and that proliferation was also increased and related to 5-HTT expression and 5-HTT activity.[86] 5-HTT is encoded by a single gene on chromosome 17q11.2, and a variant in the upstream promotor region of the *5-HTT* gene has been described.[87] This polymorphism with long (L) and short (S) forms affects *5-HTT* expression and function, with the L-allele inducing a greater rate of *5-HTT* gene transcription than the S-allele. This L-allelic variant was found to be present in homozygous form in 65 percent of PPH patients but only in 27 percent of control subjects.[85] *5-HTT* gene polymorphism could also contribute to interindividual differences in hypoxia-induced *5-HTT* expression and potentially affects susceptibility to hypoxic PAH (Fig. 67–9).

Pathological Features

Morphological abnormalities in each cell line have been described in cases of PPH. The endothelium in particular displays marked heterogeneity in the pulmonary vascular bed. Although endothelial dysfunction has been clearly described in cases of PPH, discordance between phenotype and function is commonly noted.[88] It is not known at what stage during the evolution of PPH endothelial cell proliferation occurs. It has been proposed, however, that a somatic mutation rather than nonselective cell proliferation in response to injury accounts for the growth advantage of endothelial cells in patients with PPH.[89] Heterogeneity in the smooth muscle and fibroblast populations also contributes to discordance between phenotype and function. Interconversion between cell types (fibroblast to smooth muscle cell or endothelium to smooth muscle cell) in addition to neovascularization may occur.

Smooth muscle cell hypertrophy and increased connective tissue and extracellular matrix are found in the large muscular and elastic arteries.[72,73] In the subendothelial layer, increased thickness may be the result of recruitment and/or proliferation of smooth muscle-like cells. It is possible that precursor smooth muscle cells are in a continuous layer in the subendothelial layer along the entire pulmonary artery. These cells are similar to the pericytes that are responsible for the appearance of muscle in normally nonmuscular arteries and that contribute to intimal thickening in larger arteries. Alterations in the extracellular matrix secondary to proteolytic enzymes also play a role in the pathology of PPH. Matrix-degrading enzymes can release mitogenically active growth factors that stimulate smooth muscle cell proliferation. In addition, elastase and matrix metalloproteinases contribute to upregulation of proliferation. Degradation of elastin has also been shown to stimulate upregulation of the glycoprotein fibronectin, which in turn stimulates smooth muscle cell migration.[84]

HYPERTENSIVE PULMONARY ARTERIOPATHY. The most common vascular changes in PPH can best be characterized as a hypertensive pulmonary arteriopathy, which is present in 85 percent of cases (Table 67–7). These changes involve medial hypertrophy of the arteries and arterioles, often in conjunction with other vascular changes. Isolated medial hypertrophy is uncommon, and when present it has been assumed to represent an early stage of the disease. The intimal proliferation may be concentric laminar intimal fibrosis, eccentric intimal fibrosis, or concentric nonlaminar intimal fibrosis. The frequency of these findings differs from case to case and within regions of the same lung in the same patient. In addition, plexiform and dilation lesions, as well as a necrotizing arteritis, may be seen throughout the lungs. The fundamental nature of the plexiform lesion remains a mystery.[90] Morphologically, they represent a mass of disorganized vessels with proliferating endothelial cells, smooth muscle cells, myofibroblasts, and macrophages. Several studies have demonstrated the involvement of growth factors that have been implicated in angiogenesis.[91] Whether the plexiform lesion represents impaired proliferation or angiogenesis remains unclear.

THROMBOTIC PULMONARY ARTERIOPATHY. The other major pattern of vascular changes in PPH is that of a thrombotic pulmonary arteriopathy.[92] Typical features include medial hypertrophy of the arteries and arterioles with both eccentric and concentric nonlaminar intimal fibrosis. The presence of colander lesions, which represent recannalized thrombi, is also typical. These lesions are believed to arise as a result of primary in situ thrombosis of the small vascular arteries and not from recurrent pulmonary embolism.

On rare occasion, a diffuse pulmonary arteritis with secondary thrombosis has been reported in patients with PPH,

TABLE 67–7 Histopathological Classification of Hypertensive Pulmonary Vascular Disease

Classification	Characteristic Histopathological Features
Arteriopathy	
Isolated medial hypertrophy*	Medial hypertrophy: increase of medial muscle in muscular arteries, muscularization of nonmuscularized arterioles; no appreciable intimal or luminal obstructive lesions. No plexiform lesions.
Plexogenic pulmonary arteriopathy	Plexiform and dilation lesions. Medial hypertrophy; eccentric or concentric-laminar and nonlaminar intimal thickening; fibrinoid necrosis, arteritis, and thrombotic lesions.
Thrombotic pulmonary arteriopathy	Thrombi (fresh, organizing, or organized and colander lesions). Eccentric and concentric nonlaminar intimal thickening, varying degrees of medial hypertrophy. No plexiform lesions.
Isolated pulmonary arteritis	Active or healed arteritis. Limited to pulmonary arteries; varying degrees of medial hypertrophy, intimal fibrosis, and thrombotic lesions. No plexiform lesions. No systemic arteritis.
Venopathy	
Pulmonary venoocclusive disease	Eccentric intimal fibrosis and recanalized thrombi within pulmonary veins and venules; arterialized veins, capillary congestion, alveolar edema and siderophages, dilated lymphatics, pleural and septal edema, and arterial medial hypertrophy; intimal thickening and thrombotic lesions.
Microangiopathy	
Pulmonary capillary hemangiomatosis	Infiltrating thin-walled blood vessels throughout pulmonary parenchyma, pleura, bronchi, and walls of pulmonary veins and arteries. Medial hypertrophy and intimal thickening of muscular pulmonary arteries and arterioles.

From Pietra GG: Pathology of primary pulmonary hypertension. *In* Rubin LJ, Rich S (eds): Primary Pulmonary Hypertension. New York, Marcel Dekker, 1997, pp 19-61, by courtesy of Marcel Dekker, Inc.

*Medial hypertrophy includes muscularization of arterioles.

predominantly in children. Although the association has not been reported in patients with underlying connective tissue disease, it may reflect the vascular response to a specific but not clearly identified risk factor.

Clinical Features

NATURAL HISTORY AND SYMPTOMS. The most extensive study on the natural history of PPH was reported from the National Institutes of Health (NIH) Registry on Primary Pulmonary Hypertension from 1981 to 1987. The study included the long-term follow-up of 194 patients in whom PPH was diagnosed by established clinical and hemodynamic criteria. Sixty-three percent of the patients were female, and the mean age was 36 ± 15 years (range, 1 to 81 years) at the time of diagnosis. The mean interval from the onset of symptoms to diagnosis was 2 years, and the most common initial symptoms were dyspnea (80 percent), fatigue (19 percent), syncope or near syncope (13 percent), and Raynaud phenomenon (10 percent). No ethnic differentiation was observed, with 12.3 percent of patients being black and 2.3 percent being Hispanic.

HEMODYNAMIC CHANGES. Univariate analysis from the NIH Registry pointed to the mean right atrial pressure, mean pulmonary artery pressure, and cardiac index, as well as the diffusing capacity from carbon monoxide, as significantly related to mortality. The New York Heart Association (NYHA) classification was also strongly related to survival.

Right ventricular failure from pulmonary hypertension is a result of chronic pressure overload and associated volume overload with the development of tricuspid regurgitation. However, animal studies suggest that right ventricular ischemia may also be a common feature. The mechanism of right ventricular failure in patients with pulmonary hypertension is complex. The chronic pressure overload that induces right ventricular hypertrophy and reduced contractility has been shown to cause a reduction in coronary blood flow to the right ventricular myocardium, which can produce right ventricular ischemia, both acutely and chronically. Such right ventricular dysfunction appears to be a result of a reduction in right ventricular coronary artery driving pressure. In an interesting animal study by Vlahakes and colleagues, acute right ventricular failure secondary to right ventricular hypertension was overcome by increasing central aortic pressure, which resulted in an increase in right ventricular coronary driving pressure. Murray and Vatner reported that a moderate increase in aortic pressure was accompanied by a large increase in right ventricular myocardial perfusion only when the auto-

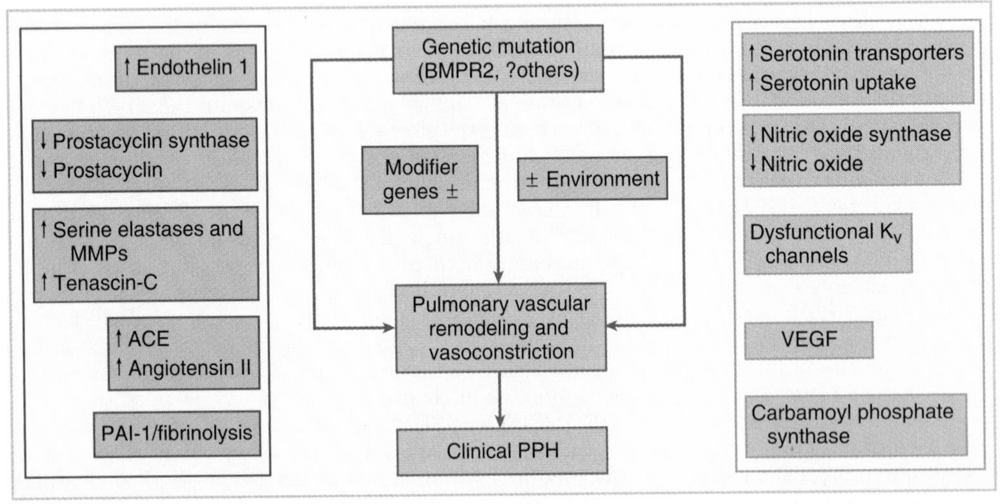

FIGURE 67–9 Proposed pathogenesis for the development of primary pulmonary hypertension (PPH). Genes implicated in the pathogenesis of PPH are bone morphogenetic protein receptor type 2 (BMPR2), prostacyclin synthase, serotonin transporters, nitric oxide synthase, serine elastases, and matrix metalloproteinases (MMPs), voltage-gated potassium (K) channels, angiotensin-converting enzyme (ACE), vascular endothelial growth factor (VEGF), carbamoyl phosphate synthase, and plasminogen activator inhibitor type 1 (PAI-1). Endothelin-1 production adds to the vasoconstriction in patients with PPH, but whether this is secondary to changes in the genes, a result of endothelial dysfunction, or a primary pathogenetic event is not clear. Pulmonary vascular remodeling results from the effects of genetics, modifying genes, and environment. (From Runo JR, Loyd JE: Primary pulmonary hypertension. Lancet 361:1533, 2003.)

nomic nervous system was blocked with an alpha blocker. Because the symptom of angina associated with PPH is characteristic of myocardial ischemia, it probably represents ongoing ischemia caused by this phenomenon.

LEFT VENTRICULAR FUNCTION. On occasion, patients with pulmonary hypertension have a reduced left ventricular ejection fraction and even regional wall motion abnormalities of the left ventricle.[93] In the past, these findings had been attributed to mechanisms related to interventricular dependence, which suggests that in some way a dysfunctional right ventricle can lead to a dysfunctional left ventricle. Clearly, the shared interventricular septum can affect the function of both ventricles. More recently, extrinsic compression of the left main coronary artery by the pulmonary artery in patients with chronic pulmonary hypertension has been described and may be associated with classic angina-like symptoms.[94,95] It is advisable to look for extrinsic compression of the left main coronary artery with coronary angiography in patients with long-standing pulmonary hypertension who have abnormal left ventricular function.

CAUSES OF DEATH. The most common cause of death in patients with PPH in the NIH Registry was progressive right-sided heart failure (47 percent). Sudden cardiac death was limited to patients who were NYHA class IV, suggesting that it is a manifestation of end-stage disease rather than a phenomenon that occurs early or unpredictably in the clinical course of the disease. The remainder of the patients died of some other medical complication, such as pneumonia or bleeding, which suggests that patients with PPH do not tolerate coexistent medical conditions well.

CLINICAL COURSE. The clinical course of patients with PPH can be highly variable. However, with the onset of overt right ventricular failure manifested by worsening symptoms and systemic venous congestion, patient survival is generally limited to approximately 6 months. Understanding the clinical course of patients with PPH is important, especially when considering major interventional therapy such as organ transplantation.

Management

LIFESTYLE CHANGES. The diagnosis of PPH does not necessarily imply total disability for the patient. However, physical activity can be associated with elevated pulmonary artery pressure inasmuch as marked hemodynamic changes have been documented to occur early in the onset of increased physical activity. For that reason, graded exercise activities, such as bike riding or swimming, in which patients can gradually increase their workload and easily limit the extent of their work, are thought to be safer than isometric activities. Isometric activities such as lifting weights or stair climbing can be associated with syncopal events and should be limited or avoided.

Pregnancy. The subject of pregnancy should also be discussed with women of childbearing age. The physiological changes that occur in pregnancy can potentially activate the disease and result in death of the mother and/or the child. Besides the increased circulating blood volume and oxygen consumption that will increase right ventricular work, circulating procoagulant factors and the risk of pulmonary embolism from deep vein thrombosis and amniotic fluid are serious concerns. Syncope and cardiac arrest have also been reported to occur during active labor and delivery, and a syndrome of postpartum circulatory collapse has been described.[96] For these reasons, surgical sterilization should be given strong consideration by women with PPH or their husbands.

DIGOXIN. Animal studies in right ventricular systolic overload show that prior administration of digoxin helps prevent the reduction in contractility of the right ventricle. Clinically, it has been shown that digoxin can exert a favorable hemodynamic effect when given acutely to patients with right ventricular failure from pulmonary hypertension.[97] An increase in resting cardiac output of approximately 10 percent was noted, which is similar to observations made in patients with left ventricular systolic failure. In addition, it was also observed that digoxin causes a significant reduction in circulating norepinephrine, which was markedly increased. Digitalis toxicity in patients with pulmonary hypertension and normal renal function is uncommon.

DIURETICS. These drugs appear to be of marked benefit in symptom relief of patients with PPH. Their traditional role has been limited to patients manifesting right ventricular failure and systemic venous congestion. However, patients with advanced PPH can have increased left ventricular filling pressures that contribute to the symptoms of dyspnea and orthopnea, which can be relieved with diuretics. Diuretics may also serve to reduce right ventricular wall stress in patients with concomitant tricuspid regurgitation and volume overload. The fear that diuretics will induce systemic hypotension is unfounded because the main factor limiting cardiac output is pulmonary vascular resistance and not pulmonary blood volume. Patients with severe venous congestion may require high doses of loop diuretics or the use of combined diuretics. In these instances, electrolytes need to be carefully watched to avoid hyponatremia and hypokalemia.

In humans, elevated plasma aldosterone concentrations are associated with endothelial dysfunction, left ventricular hypertrophy, and cardiac death. Spironolactone has been demonstrated to enhance the beneficial effect of ACE inhibition on mortality in patients with congestive heart failure.[98] Given the similarities between left and right heart failure on activation of the renin-angiotensin-aldosterone system, it seems reasonable to use aldosterone antagonists in patients with pulmonary hypertension.

SUPPLEMENTAL OXYGEN. Hypoxic pulmonary vasoconstriction can contribute to pulmonary vascular disease in patients with alveolar hypoxia from parenchymal lung disease. Supplemental low-flow oxygen alleviates arterial hypoxemia and attenuates the pulmonary hypertension in patients with these disorders. Although most patients with PPH do not exhibit resting hypoxemia, those who experience arterial oxygen desaturation with activity may benefit from ambulatory supplemental oxygen because increased oxygen extraction develops in the face of fixed oxygen delivery. Patients with severe right-sided heart failure and resting hypoxemia resulting from markedly increased oxygen extraction at rest should be treated with continuous oxygen therapy to maintain their arterial oxygen saturation above 90 percent. Patients with hypoxemia caused by a right-to-left shunt via a patent foramen ovale do not improve their level of oxygenation to an appreciable degree with supplemental oxygen.

ANTICOAGULANTS. Oral anticoagulant therapy is widely recommended for patients with PPH, although its clinical efficacy as a therapy is difficult to prove. A retrospective review of patients with PPH monitored over a 15-year period at the Mayo Clinic suggested that patients who received warfarin had improved survival over those who did not. The influence of warfarin therapy has been investigated in patients with PPH who failed to respond to high doses of calcium channel blockers.[99] Significant improvement in survival was observed in patients who received anticoagulation, with a 1-year survival rate of 91 percent and a 3-year survival rate of 47 percent as compared with 1- and 3-year rates of 62 and 31 percent, respectively, in patients who did not receive anticoagulants. The current recommendation is to use warfarin in relatively low doses, as has been recommended for prophylaxis of venous thromboembolism, with the international normalized ratio (INR) maintained at 2.0 to 3.0 times control. Given its inhibitory effects on smooth muscle proliferation, heparin might be a better anticoagulant in patients with PPH, although its use is more difficult. With the recent advent of low-molecular-weight heparins requiring once-a-day administration without the need for adjusting the dose to its antithrombotic effect, treatment with these agents is becoming a more viable alternative.

Vasodilator Therapy

Because of early reports showing a reduction in pulmonary artery pressure following the acute administration of vasodilators, it has been presumed that vasodilators are the mainstay of treatment in patients with PPH. This presumption is not supported by the published literature, however. Vasodilators are effective in a subset of patients with PPH, but many complexities regarding vasodilator administration make their use in these patients very difficult.

The final common cellular pathway by which vasodilators work is through a reduction of intracellular calcium in the vascular smooth muscle cell. The same mechanism is also attributable to cellular growth inhibition. Indeed, most vasodilators have been shown to possess growth inhibitory properties of smooth muscle cells in culture. It is likely that the chronic effects of these agents in patients with pulmonary hypertension represent both mechanisms (Fig. 67–10).

CALCIUM CHANNEL BLOCKERS. Of the vasodilators prescribed for patients with PPH, calcium channel blockers appear to have the widest use (Fig. 67–11). Early studies using conventional doses failed to demonstrate a chronic sustained benefit. Moreover, calcium channel blockers have properties that could worsen the underlying pulmonary hypertension, including negative inotropic effects on right ventricular function and reflex sympathetic stimulation, which may increase the resting heart rate. It has been reported that 10 to 20 percent of patients with PPH who are challenged with very high doses of calcium channel blockers may manifest a dramatic reduction in pulmonary artery pressure and pulmonary vascular resistance, which upon serial catheterization has been maintained for more than 5 years.[99] Importantly, the patient's quality of life is restored with improved functional class, and survival (94 percent rate at 5 years) is improved when compared with nonresponders and historical control subjects (36 percent rate). This experience suggests that a select subset of patients with PPH have the ability to have their pulmonary hyper-

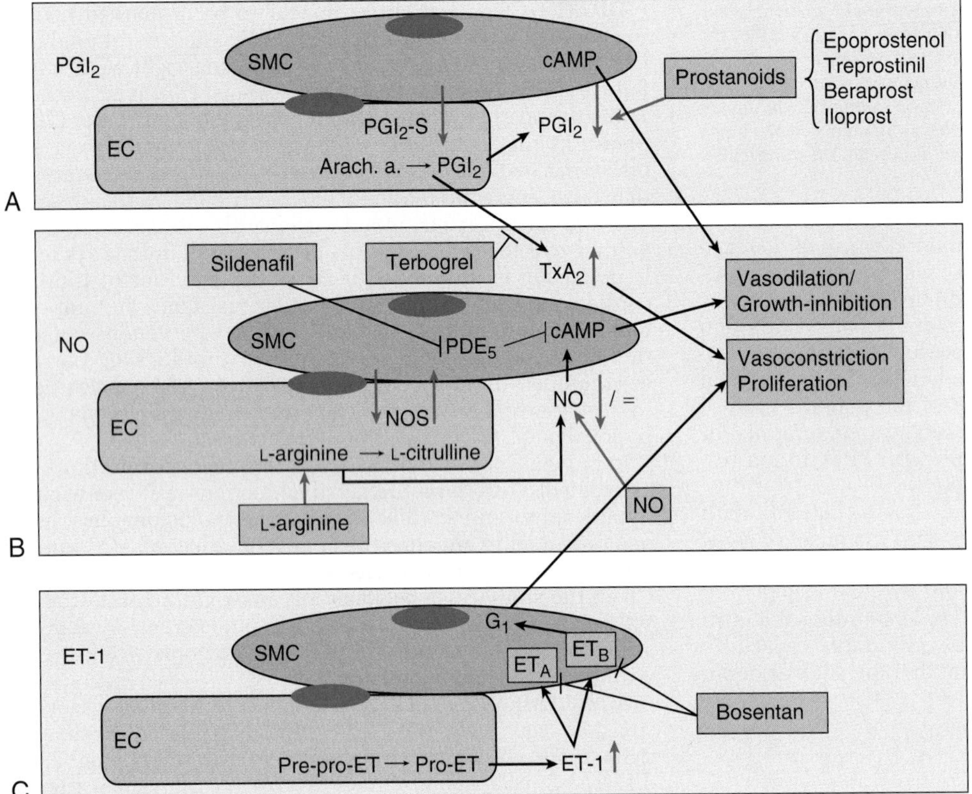

FIGURE 67–10 Endothelial dysfunction and its pharmacological correction in cases of pulmonary arterial hypertension. Arach. a. = arachidonic acid; cAMP = cyclic adenosine monophosphate; EC = endothelial cell; ET = endothelin; NO = nitric oxide; PDE = phosphodiesterase; PGI_2 = prostacyclin; S = synthase; SMC = smooth muscle cell; TxA_2 = thromboxane A_2. ↓ and ↑ denote pathobiological changes typical of pulmonary arterial hypertension. Boxes and arrows denote substances, sites, and modality of therapeutic interventions. (From Galie N, Manes A, Branzi A: Emerging medical therapies for pulmonary arterial hypertension. Prog Cardiovasc Dis 45:213, 2002.)

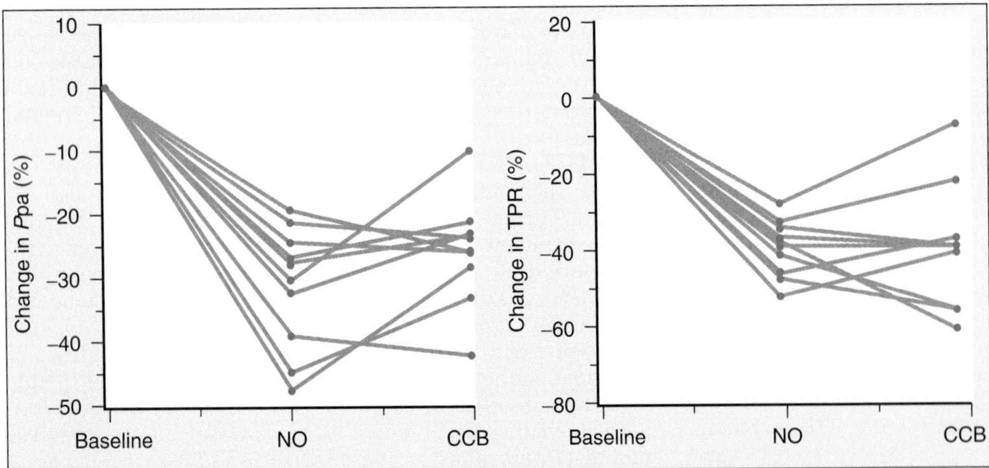

FIGURE 67–11 Comparison of individual pulmonary vasodilator response to inhaled nitric oxide (NO) and oral calcium-channel blockers (CCB) in patients with primary pulmonary hypertension (PPH). Inhalation of NO can predict acute and chronic response to oral calcium-channel blockers in PPH. P_{pa} = mean pulmonary artery pressure; TPR = total pulmonary resistance (P_{pa} divided by cardiac index). (From Sitbon O, Humbert M, Simonneau G: Primary pulmonary hypertension: Current therapy. Prog Cardiovasc Dis 45:115, 2002.)

tension reversed and their quality of life and length of survival enhanced.

It is unknown whether the response to calcium channel blockers identifies two subsets of patients with PPH, different stages of PPH, or a combination of both. However, it is essential to point out that patients who do not exhibit a dramatic hemodynamic response to calcium channel blockers do not appear to benefit from their long-term administration. Unfortunately, it is becoming common practice for physicians to prescribe calcium channel blockers at conventional doses to all patients with pulmonary hypertension, often without hemodynamic guidance. This unfortunate practice may result in quicker deterioration in these patients and should be strongly discouraged.

PROSTACYCLINS. Continuous-infusion epoprostenol has been shown in randomized clinical trials to improve quality of life and symptoms related to PPH, exercise tolerance, hemodynamics, and survival.[100-103] The initial enthusiasm for epoprostenol was based on the demonstration of pulmonary vasodilator effects when administered to experimental animals with acute pulmonary vasoconstriction. The long-term effects of epoprostenol in PPH include its vasodilator and antithrombotic effects, but its effects may also be importantly related to its ability to normalize cardiac output. Patients may have a reduction in pulmonary vascular resistance of greater than 50 percent even if no acute hemodynamic effects are noted.

Epoprostenol is administered through a central venous catheter that is surgically implanted and delivered by an ambulatory infusion system. The delivery system is complex and requires patients to learn the techniques of sterile drug preparation, operation of the pump, and care of the intravenous catheter. Most of the serious complications that have occurred with epoprostenol therapy have been attributable to the delivery system and include catheter-related infections and thrombosis and temporary interruption of the infusion because of pump malfunction. Anecdotal reports of rebound pulmonary hypertension occurring in patients in whom the infusion was interrupted suggest that great care must be taken to ensure that the infusion is never stopped.

Side effects related to epoprostenol include flushing, headache, nausea, diarrhea, and a unique type of jaw discomfort that occurs with eating. In most patients, these symptoms are minimal and well tolerated. Chronic foot pain and a poorly defined gastropathy with prolonged use develop in some patients. To date, epoprostenol has been given to patients with PPH for more than 10 years with continued favorable effectiveness. In some patients (NYHA class IV) who are critically ill, it serves as a bridge to lung transplantation by stabilizing the patient to a more favorable preoperative state. Patients who are less critically ill may do so well with epoprostenol therapy that they may delay the need to consider transplantation, perhaps indefinitely.

A high cardiac output state has been reported in a series of patients with PPH receiving chronic epoprostenol therapy and is consistent with the drug having positive inotropic effects.[104] Whether the effect is a direct one on the myocardium or indirect via neurohormonal activation has not been determined. Although most patients with PPH have reduced cardiac output on initial examination, the development of a chronic high-output state could have long-term detrimental effects on underlying cardiac function. The follow-up assessment of patients receiving intravenous epoprostenol is quite variable from medical center to medical center, but it does appear important to determine the cardiac output response to therapy periodically to optimize dosing.[105]

Long-Term Effects. The experience with epoprostenol in patients with PPH for more than 10 years has been reported by two large centers (Fig. 67–12). Survival rates over 5 years were markedly improved compared with survival in

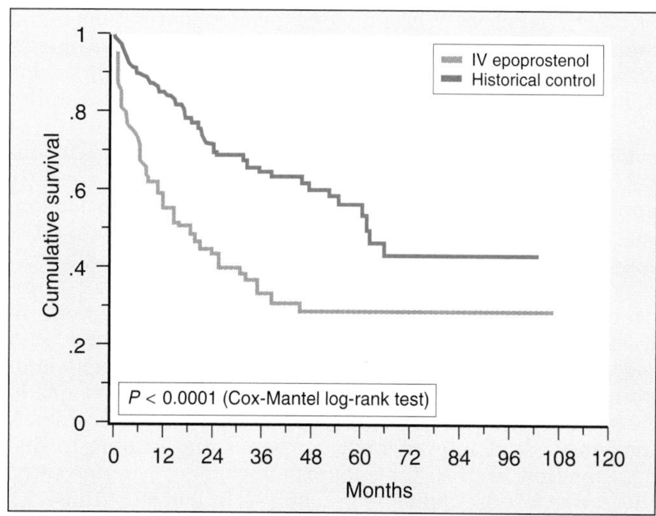

FIGURE 67–12 Kaplan-Meier survival estimates in 178 patients with primary pulmonary hypertension (PPH) from the initiation of epoprostenol therapy. For comparison, survival data are also shown for a historical group of 135 patients with PPH matched for New York Heart Association functional class and who never received epoprostenol therapy. In the population of patients treated with epoprostenol (blue line), overall survival rates at 1, 2, 3, and 5 years are 85, 75, 43, 33, and 28 percent in the historical control group (magenta line). (From Sitbon O, Humbert M, Simonneau G: Primary pulmonary hypertension: Current therapy. Prog Cardiovasc Dis 45:115, 2002.)

historical control subjects and the natural history predicted by the NIH Registry. Predictors of survival included NYHA functional class, exercise tolerance, and acute vasodilator responsiveness. Both studies provided important data for identifying patients who would do well over the long term, versus those in whom transplantation should be considered.[106,107]

Treprostinil. This is a stable prostacyclin analog, recently approved by the Food and Drug Administration, that has pharmacological actions similar to epoprostenol but differs in that it is chemically stable at room temperature and neutral pH and has a longer half-life (3-4 hours). In a large randomized clinical trial in patients with pulmonary arterial hypertension, treprostinil was effective in increasing distance walked in 6 minutes, symptoms of dyspnea associated with exercise, and hemodynamics.[108,109] Its pharmacological properties allow it to be administered through continuous subcutaneous infusion, thus eliminating the need for a central venous catheter and refrigeration during administrations. Infusion site pain was common.

Iloprost. This analog of prostacyclin has been utilized via inhalation. In randomized clinical trials, inhaled iloprost was shown to have an acute effect on hemodynamics similar to inhaled nitric oxide.[110,111] When iloprost was given chronically, patients reported an improvement in exercise, manifested by a 6-minute walk test, and in hemodynamics. Inhaled iloprost has advantages over intravenous epoprostenol in that it does not require a central venous catheter or infusion pump system or cause the attendant complications. Due to the short half-life of iloprost, however, it requires frequent (up to 12 per day) inhalations, which is very restrictive to patients on this therapy. Developments in the technology of nebulizers and the use of prostacyclin analogs with longer half-lives might allow for more widespread use of this treatment modality.

Beraprost. This is an orally active prostacyclin analog that has been evaluated in randomized double-blind placebo-controlled multicenter trials in patients with PPH. In one large European trial (the ALPHABET study), beraprost improved exercise capacity and symptoms over a 12-week period but had no significant effect on cardiopulmonary hemodynamics or functional class.[112] A similar trial conducted in the United States, however, failed to show long-term efficacy beyond 12 weeks.[113] Beraprost was associated with frequent side effects of headache, flushing, and diarrhea, which limited the ability to administer higher doses.

ENDOTHELIN RECEPTOR BLOCKERS. Bosentan is a nonselective endothelin receptor blocker that was recently approved as a treatment of pulmonary arterial hypertension. In a 12-week placebo-controlled trial of 32 patients with PAH, bosentan was superior to placebo in increasing 6-minute walk distance and hemodynamics.[114] In a large randomized clinical trial, bosentan showed a significant improvement in 6-minute walk distance after 16 weeks as compared with placebo.[115] It also was shown to lengthen the composite endpoint of time to clinical worsening, which included death, lung transplantation, hospitalization for pulmonary hypertension, lack of improvement, or worsening leading to discontinuation in need for epoprostenol therapy. Importantly, there was a dose-dependent increase in hepatic transaminases noted from the medication, with significant elevations in 14 percent of the patients randomized to the higher dose (250 mg twice a day). The Food and Drug Administration approved bosentan at the target dose of 125 mg twice a day for patients with pulmonary arterial hypertension who have World Health Organization (WHO) class III or IV disease. The investigational ET_A selective endothelin receptor antagonist, sitaxsentan, also improves exercise capacity in pulmonary arterial hypertension.[116] Further studies with this agent are ongoing (Fig. 67–13).

PHOSPHODIESTERASE-5 INHIBITORS. Sildenafil is a phosphodiesterase-5 (PDE5) inhibitor approved to treat erectile dysfunction. PDE5 inhibitors produce pulmonary vasodilation by promoting an enhanced and sustained level of cyclic guanosine monophosphate, an identical effect to inhaled NO. When tested as a single oral agent, sildenafil has been shown to be a potent and selective pulmonary vasodilator with equal efficacy to that of inhaled NO in lowering pulmonary artery pressure and pulmonary vascular resistance.[117] Sildenafil has a preferential effect on the pulmonary circulation because of the high expression of this isoform in the lung. Many anecdotal reports appear in the published medical literature on the success of sildenafil as an oral therapy for patients with primary pulmonary hypertension.[118-122] The safety and long-term effectiveness of sildenafil as a treatment of pulmonary arterial hypertension is currently under investigation and appears promising.

Invasive Techniques

ATRIAL SEPTOSTOMY. The rationale for the creation of an atrial septostomy in patients with PPH is based on experimental and clinical observations suggesting that an intraatrial defect allowing right-to-left shunting in the setting of severe pulmonary hypertension might be of benefit. Although countless patients have undergone this procedure worldwide, it should still be considered investigational.[123] Indications for the procedure include recurrent syncope and/or right ventricular failure despite maximum medical therapy, as a bridge to transplantation if deterioration occurs in the face of maximum medical therapy, or when no other option exists. Because the disease process in PPH appears to be unaffected by the procedure, the long-term effects of atrial septostomy must be considered palliative.

The rate of procedure-related mortality with atrial septostomy in patients with PPH is high, and thus the procedure should be attempted only in institutions with an established track record in the treatment of advanced pulmonary hypertension and experience in performing atrial septostomy with a low rate of morbidity. It should not be performed in a patient with impending death and severe right ventricular failure or a patient receiving maximum cardiorespiratory support. Predictors of procedure-related failure or death have been identified and include a mean right atrial pressure of greater than 20 mm Hg, a pulmonary vascular resistance index of greater than 55 units/m², or a predicted 1-year survival rate of less than 40 percent.

The mechanisms responsible for the beneficial effects of atrial septostomy remain unclear. Possibilities include increased oxygen delivery at rest and/or with exercise,

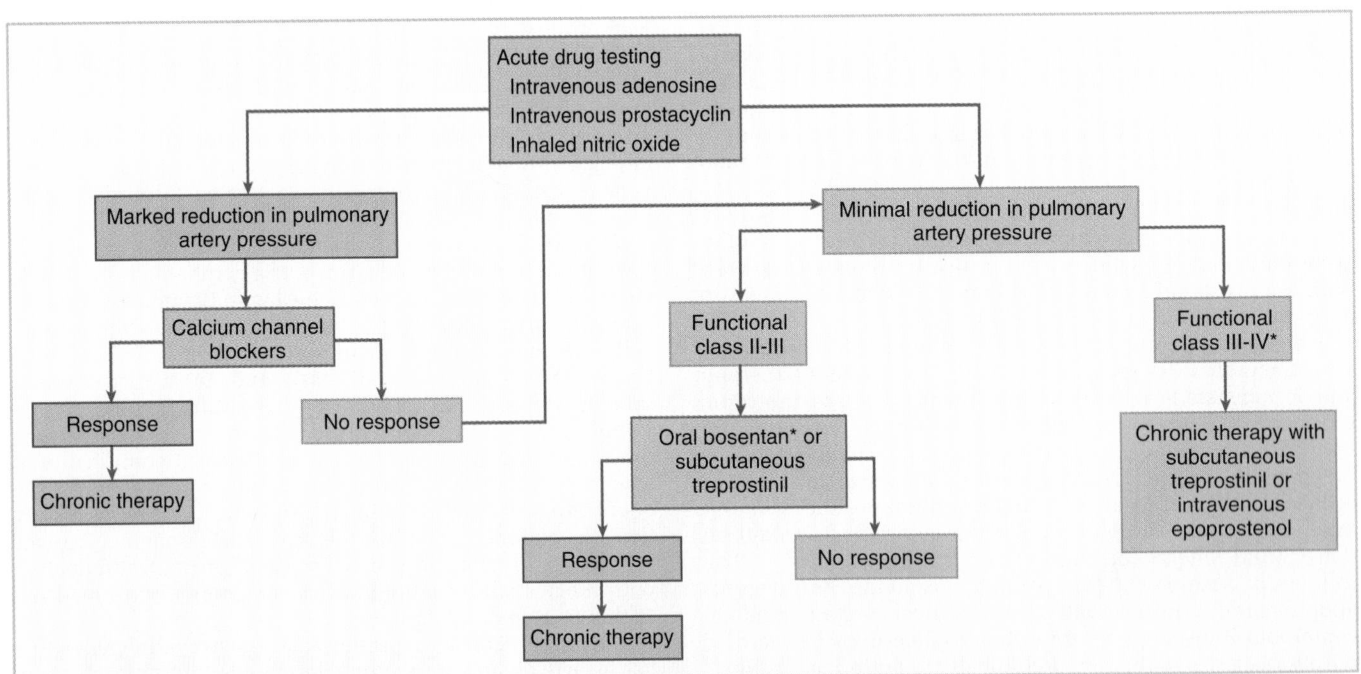

FIGURE 67–13 A treatment algorithm for pulmonary arterial hypertension (PAH) based on established clinical studies is presented. Although there is no consensus for the definition of a response to acute vasodilator testing, it appears that a reduction in mean pulmonary artery pressure below 40 mm Hg is necessary. A chronic response requires a documented improvement in resting hemodynamics, exercise tolerance, or preferably both. Patients who fail to respond chronically to epoprostenol should be considered for lung transplantation. *Bosentan is indicated for WHO functional class III and IV patients.

reduced right ventricular end-diastolic pressure or wall stress, improvement in right ventricular function by the Frank-Starling mechanism, or relief of ischemia.

HEART-LUNG AND LUNG TRANSPLANTATION (see Chap. 26). Heart-lung transplantation has been performed successfully in patients with PPH since 1981.[124] Because these patients have pulmonary vascular disease and severe right ventricular dysfunction, it was originally believed that heart-lung transplantation was the only transplantation option. Widespread application of heart-lung transplantation, however, has been limited by the number of centers with expertise to perform the procedure, the scarcity of suitable donor organs, and the very long waiting times required for patients with end-stage right-sided heart failure. Consequently, bilateral or double-lung transplantation and single-lung transplantation have been performed successfully in patients with PPH.[125] Hemodynamic studies have shown an immediate reduction in pulmonary artery pressure and pulmonary vascular resistance associated with improvement in right ventricular function.

The ages of recipients of heart-lung and lung transplantation for pulmonary hypertension have ranged from 2 months to 61 years.[126] The operative mortality rate ranges between 16 and 29 percent and is somewhat higher for recipients of a single-lung transplant. The 1-year survival rate is between 70 and 75 percent, the 2-year survival rate is between 55 and percent, and the 5-year survival rate is between 40 and 45 percent. Transplantation should be reserved for patients with pulmonary hypertension who have progressed in spite of optimal medical management (Table 67–8).[126]

Timing. In considering referral for evaluation for transplantation, the course of the disease and the waiting time must be taken into account, as well as other factors such as the anticipated waiting time before transplantation in the region and the expected survival after transplantation.[127] It is generally accepted that patients should be considered for transplantation when they have WHO functional class III or IV disease in spite of medical therapy or when treatment with prostacyclin is initiated. The major long-term complications in patients who survive the operation are the high incidence of bronchiolitis obliterans in the transplanted lungs, acute organ rejection, and opportunistic infection.[128] Although several studies have documented significant improvement in quality of life after heart-lung and lung transplantation for pulmonary hypertension, cost-effectiveness has not yet been addressed.

TABLE 67–8 General Guidelines for Selection of Lung Transplant Recipients

Indications
- Advanced obstructive, fibrotic, or pulmonary vascular disease with a high risk of death within 2 to 3 yr
- Lack of success or availability of alternative therapies
- Severe functional limitation but preserved ability to walk
- Age 55 yr or less for candidates for heart-lung transplantation, age 60 yr or less for candidates for bilateral lung transplantation, and age 65 yr or less for candidates for single-lung transplantation

Absolute Contraindications
- Severe extrapulmonary organ dysfunction, including renal insufficiency with a creatinine clearance below 50 ml/min, hepatic dysfunction with coagulopathy or portal hypertension, and left ventricular dysfunction or severe coronary artery disease (consider heart-lung transplantation)
- Acute, critical illness
- Active cancer or recent history of cancer with substantial likelihood of recurrence (except for basal cell and squamous cell carcinoma of the skin)
- Active extrapulmonary infection (including infection with human immunodeficiency virus, hepatitis B, hepatitis C)
- Severe psychiatric illness, noncompliance with therapy, and drug or alcohol dependence
- Active or recent (preceding 3 to 6 mo) cigarette smoking
- Severe malnutrition (<70% of ideal body weight) or marked obesity (>130% of ideal body weight)
- Inability to walk, with poor rehabilitation potential

Relative Contraindications
- Chronic medical conditions that are poorly controlled or associated with target organ damage
- Daily requirement for more than 20 mg of prednisone (or equivalent)
- Mechanical ventilation (excluding noninvasive ventilation)
- Extensive pleural thickening from prior thoracic surgery or infection
- Active connective tissue disease
- Preoperative colonization of the airways with pan-resistant bacteria (in patients with cystic fibrosis)

From Arcasoy SM, Kotlo RB: Lung transplantation. N Engl J Med 340:1081, 1999.

Pulmonary Arterial Hypertension Associated with Congenital Heart Disease (see Chap. 56)

It has long been known that pulmonary hypertension can develop in adults with atrial septal defect. It is presumed that chronically increased pulmonary blood flow may have effects on pulmonary endothelium through mechanical means that cause perturbations in the integrity of the vascular wall and lead to the development of pulmonary vascular disease. Increased pulmonary blood flow from hyperthyroidism and beriberi have been reported to be associated with the development of unexplained pulmonary hypertension, which suggests that high pulmonary blood flow,[129] rather than mere coincidence, is the basis for the development of pulmonary hypertension in patients with pretricuspid shunts such as atrial septal defect or anomalous pulmonary venous drainage.

If a congenital cardiovascular defect causes pulmonary hypertension from the time of birth, the small, muscular arteries of the fetal lung may undergo delayed or only partial involution, with subsequent persistently high levels of pulmonary vascular resistance. This is especially true in lesions in which a left-to-right shunt enters the right ventricle or pulmonary artery directly (i.e., a post-tricuspid valve shunt, such as ventricular septal defect or patent ductus arteriosus): These patients experience a higher incidence of severe and irreversible pulmonary vascular damage than do those in whom the shunt is proximal to the tricuspid valve (pretricuspid shunts, as in atrial septal defect and partial anomalous pulmonary venous drainage). In the latter category, pulmonary hypertension may result from a large pretricuspid left-to-right shunt, which enhances the risk of pulmonary vascular damage.

Pathology

The extent of reversibility of pulmonary vascular obstructive disease in the presence of congenital heart disease varies. From an anatomical point of view, reversible conditions are those in which the decreased pulmonary arteriolar cross-sectional area is the result of medial hypertrophy and vasoconstriction; irreversibility is associated with the presence of necrotizing arteritis and plexiform lesions in these small vessels.

The classification by Heath and Edwards of six grades of structural change is widely used to assess the potential reversibility of pulmonary vascular disease and is summarized as follows: Grade I is characterized by hypertrophy of the media of small muscular pulmonary arteries and arterioles. In grade II, intimal cellular proliferation is added to the medial hypertrophy. Grade III is characterized by advanced medial thickening with hypertrophy and hyperplasia, together with progressive intimal proliferation and concentric fibrosis that result in obliteration of many arterioles and small arteries. In grade IV, dilation and so-called plexiform lesions of the muscular pulmonary arteries and arterioles are observed. The latter consist of a plexiform network of capillary-like channels within a dilated segment of a muscular pulmonary artery. The channels are separated by proliferating endothelial cells that often contain thrombi; indeed, the network of capillary channels may constitute recanalization of a thrombus. Grade V changes include complex plexiform, angiomatous, and cavernous lesions and hyalinization of intimal fibrosis. Finally, grade VI is characterized by the presence of necrotizing arteritis.

Clinical Considerations

EISENMENGER SYNDROME. This refers to any anomalous circulatory communication that leads to obliterative pulmonary vascular disease, including pretricuspid and posttricuspid shunts. Health-Edwards grade IV to VI changes are usual in these patients; occasionally, lesser anatomical changes predominate and may be reversible after successful corrective surgery. The long-term prognosis of patients with the Eisenmenger syndrome is substantially better than that of patients with other conditions associated with pulmonary hypertension.[130] Patients with the Eisenmenger syndrome have an 80 percent survival rate at 10 years, a 77 percent survival rate at 15 years, and a 42 percent survival rate at 25 years.[131,132] Survival is typically related to mean right atrial pressure and pulmonary vascular resistance.

When pulmonary vascular resistance has increased so that it equals or exceeds systemic resistance and the anatomical changes of the pulmonary vessels are predominantly those of grades IV to VI, surgical closure of the anomalous circulatory communication will be associated with a prohibitive immediate risk and, if the patient survives, will usually fail to relieve pulmonary hypertension. Surgery may in fact hasten death in most survivors who had either balanced shunts or predominant right-to-left shunts, because closure of the right-to-left communication merely increases the load on an already overburdened right ventricle. Structural changes in the pulmonary vascular bed are evident in pulmonary arteriograms, which reveal dilated central pulmonary arteries and narrowing of the peripheral branches. These changes can be evaluated by means of quantitative analysis of the pulmonary wedge angiogram.

TREATMENT. Intravenous epoprostenol therapy has been shown to improve exercise tolerance, quality of life, and hemodynamics in patients with congenital heart disease, irrespective of the severity or duration of the condition.[133,134] It is effective in patients who have had previous surgical repair of their defect and in those who have not. No increased incidence of systemic side effects has been noted in patients who have a persistent right-to-left shunt. In patients who have bidirectional shunts, the use of epoprostenol may be a therapeutic strategy to enable a patient who is considered inoperable to become eligible for surgery at a later date. Treprostinil has also been used effectively in patients with congenital heart disease.

Pulmonary Arterial Hypertension Associated with Connective Tissue Diseases (see Chap. 82)

Scleroderma, including the CREST syndrome, is the most common cause of pulmonary hypertension in connective tissue disease states.[57] Scleroderma is associated with pulmonary hypertension in as many as one-third of patients and CREST syndrome in as many as 50 percent. The high incidence suggests that periodic screening with echocardiography in these patients may be a reasonable practice. Although pulmonary hypertension may occur as a result of entrapment and obstruction of the pulmonary microvasculature by interstitial inflammation or fibrosis, patients initially seen with severe pulmonary hypertension usually do not have evidence of interstitial lung disease and have a pulmonary vasculature with histological features that resemble those of PPH.[135] Patients with systemic lupus erythematosus also have pulmonary hypertension, although less commonly than patients with scleroderma. Mixed connective tissue disease is a less common form of connective tissue disease, but pulmonary hypertension may occur in as many as two-thirds of these patients. Pulmonary hypertension has also been described in patients with polymyositis, dermatomyositis, and rheumatoid arthritis.

Because connective tissue diseases may have an insidious onset and slowly progressive course, early recognition of the symptoms of pulmonary hypertension may be difficult. Although easy fatigability may be a feature of the connective tissue disease, it may also be an initial symptom of pulmonary hypertension. Dyspnea is still the most common initial symptom and should not be attributed to advancing age. Syncope, presyncope, or peripheral edema represents advanced pulmonary hypertension and right-sided heart failure. Physical findings of an elevated jugular venous pressure and an increased pulmonic component of the second heart sound along with a right ventricular fourth heart sound are typical features of pulmonary hypertension and warrant an evaluation for pulmonary hypertension. A murmur of tricuspid regurgitation generally reflects more advanced disease. Arterial hypoxemia is characteristic and should also prompt an evaluation of possible pulmonary hypertension in these patients.

The prognosis of patients with connective tissue disease in whom pulmonary hypertension develops is very poor.[133] Conventional therapy with digitalis, diuretics, and supplemental oxygen is used, and anticoagulation has been recommended to provide a survival benefit similar to the practice in PPH. Although the use of oral vasodilators has been disappointing, intravenous epoprostenol has demonstrated therapeutic efficacy manifested by improved exercise tolerance, hemodynamics, and sense of well-being.[136] In patients with associated Raynaud phenomenon, it may provide relief of digital ischemia. Subcutaneous treprostinil and oral bosentan are also approved treatments of pulmonary hypertension associated with connective tissue diseases.

Pulmonary Arterial Hypertension Associated with Portal Hypertension

Pulmonary abnormalities have been commonly associated with the development of hepatic cirrhosis and portal hypertension[137] and include hypoxemia and intrapulmonary shunting, portal-pulmonary shunting, impaired hypoxic pulmonary vasoconstriction, and pulmonary hypertension. Although the relative risk associated with the development of pulmonary hypertension in patients with portal hypertension is unknown, a large postmortem study from the Johns Hopkins Hospital showed that the prevalence of unexplained or pulmonary hypertension in patients with cirrhosis was 5.6 times higher than that of PPH alone. A modest increase in pulmonary artery systolic pressure is not unusual in patients with cirrhosis and portal hypertension. The increase in pulmonary artery pressure is usually passive and relates to the increase in cardiac output and/or blood volume and is associated with near-normal pulmonary vascular resistance. Published studies indicate a strong association between portal hypertension and pulmonary hypertension regardless of whether liver disease is present.[138,139] Although the mechanisms are uncertain, several possibilities are consistent. Portal hypertension itself induces numerous modifications in the vascular media that may trigger a cascade of intracellular signals and/or cause activation or repression of various genes in endothelial and smooth muscle cells. Increased levels of several vasoactive mediators, cytokines, and growth factors have been demonstrated in patients with portal hypertension, including serotonin and interleukin-1.[139] Other angiogenic factors such as hepatocyte growth factor or vascular endothelial growth factor may be involved in pulmonary artery remodeling.

Patients in whom PPH develops in association with cirrhosis appear to be similar to patients without cirrhosis, with the sole exception that they tend to have higher cardiac output and consequently lower calculated systemic and pulmonary vascular resistance, which is characteristic of the cirrhotic state. Treatment of portal pulmonary hypertension generally follows the guidelines developed for treating patients with PPH. Although severe pulmonary hypertension is considered a contraindication to liver transplantation because of the risk of irreversible right-sided heart failure, successful liver transplantation has been reported in patients with very mild pulmonary hypertension treated successfully with intravenous epoprostenol.[140,141]

PULMONARY ARTERIAL HYPERTENSION ASSOCIATED WITH HUMAN IMMUNODEFICIENCY VIRUS INFECTION

Although well documented, it remains unclear how HIV infection results in an increased incidence of PPH in HIV-infected patients.[142,143] A direct pathogenic role of HIV seems unlikely inasmuch as no viral constituents have been detected in the vascular endothelium of these patients. On the other hand, reports of pulmonary arteriopathy with intimal proliferation in monkeys experimentally infected with the simian immunodeficiency virus and in a murine model of acquired immunodeficiency syndrome suggest a pathogenetic link between infection with an immunodeficiency virus and the development of PPH, possibly mediated by release of inflammatory mediators or by autoimmune mechanisms.[142] A large case-control study of HIV-associated PPH was recently conducted in the Swiss HIV Cohort Study.[143] The cumulative incidence was 0.6 percent within the entire HIV-infected population. PPH was diagnosed in patients in all stages of HIV infection and without an obvious relationship to immune deficiency. The clinical and hemodynamic features of these patients were similar to those of patients with PPH.

PULMONARY ARTERIAL HYPERTENSION RELATED TO ANOREXIGENS

Several anorexigenics have been demonstrated to cause pulmonary hypertension in humans. The first observation was made in 1967, when an epidemic of PPH was associated with the use of aminorex in Europe coincident with its introduction in the general population. The mechanism by which aminorex causes pulmonary hypertension remains uncertain, but it has similarities to both adrenaline and ephedrine in its chemical structure. The clinical features of pulmonary hypertension were identical to those attributed to PPH.

The association between the use of fenfluramine appetite suppressants and the development of PPH was established in the International Primary Pulmonary Hypertension Study (IPPHS), a case-control study conducted in Europe in 1992 to 1994.[59] The study resulted in severe restriction of the use of appetite suppressants in Europe, only to see their use popularized in the United States. Ultimately, the marked increase in the number of cases of PPH and cardiac valvulopathy ascribed to the use of fenfluramine drugs in the United States led to their withdrawal in 1997. Unfortunately, in the majority of patients, the development of pulmonary hypertension has been progressive despite withdrawal of the appetite suppressants.[144,145] Although the drugs mainly identified in the IPPHS were the fenfluramines, anorexigenics such as amphetamine were also implicated.

The mechanism by which the fenfluramines and aminorex produce pulmonary hypertension has been investigated. Experimental studies have demonstrated that these drugs can cause pulmonary vasoconstriction by inhibiting voltage-gated potassium channels in the smooth muscle cells of resistance-level pulmonary arteries.[146] Although the degree of pulmonary vasoconstriction noted was small, it increased dramatically when NO synthase was inhibited. One recent study compared NO production in patients with PPH and patients with pulmonary hypertension associated with the use of anorexigens.[147] It appears that the latter group had a deficiency in basal NO production when compared with patients with PPH, which suggests that NO may be a compensatory product of the pulmonary arterial endothelium that increases in pulmonary hypertension to counteract the effects of chronic vasoconstriction.

Because of the consistent association with anorexigenics and unexplained pulmonary hypertension, clinicians should be exceedingly careful in the use of these drugs in the future, especially in patients who may have increased susceptibility to the development of pulmonary hypertension. Although treatment is similar to that of PPH, prognosis may be worse.[148]

PERSISTENT PULMONARY HYPERTENSION OF THE NEWBORN

Three forms of persistent pulmonary hypertension of the newborn have been described. In the hypertrophic type, the muscular tissue of the pulmonary arteries is hypertrophied and extends peripherally to the acini. Medial hypertrophy causes narrowing of the arteries and an increase in pulmonary pressure and reduction in pulmonary blood flow. It is believed to be the result of sustained fetal hypertension from chronic vasoconstriction due to chronic fetal distress. In the hypoplastic type, the lungs including the pulmonary arteries are underdeveloped, usually as the result of a congenital diaphragmatic hernia or prolonged leakage of amniotic fluid.[149,150] The cross-sectional area of the pulmonary vascular bed is inadequate for normal neonatal pulmonary blood flow. In the reactive type, lung histology is presumably normal but vasoconstriction causes pulmonary hypertension. High levels of vasoconstrictive mediators such as thromboxane, norepinephrine, and leukotrienes may be responsible and may result in a streptococcal infection or acute asphyxia at birth.

Although persistent pulmonary hypertension of the newborn can vary in severity, severe cases are usually life threatening. It is usually associated with severe hypoxemia and the need for mechanical ventilation. Echocardiographic findings of severe pulmonary hypertension and right-to-left shunting at the level of the ductus arteriosus or foramen ovale are common. Inhaled nitric oxide has provided encouraging results through improvement in oxygenation in these patients (see Fig. 67–9). Intravenous epoprostenol has also been used and may even have additive effects to that of inhaled NO.[151] Alveolar capillary dysplasia is a very rare cause of persistent pulmonary hypertension of the newborn and is characterized by a developmental abnormality in the pulmonary vasculature. The antemortem diagnosis can be made only with open-lung biopsy. Despite aggressive treatment with NO, epoprostenol, and even extracorporeal membrane oxygenation, survival in the setting of alveolar capillary dysplasia is rare.[152]

PULMONARY VENOOCCLUSIVE DISEASE

Pulmonary venoocclusive disease is a rare form of PPH. The histopathological diagnosis is based on the presence of obstructive eccentric fibrous intimal pads within the pulmonary veins and venules. Arterialization of the pulmonary veins is often present and associated with alveolar capillary congestion. Other changes of chronic pulmonary hypertension such as medial hypertrophy and muscularization of the arterioles with eccentric intimal fibrosis may also be seen. The pulmonary venous obstruction explains the increased pulmonary capillary wedge pressure described in patients in the late stages of the disease and the increase in basilar bronchovascular markings described on the chest radiograph. These clinical findings, along with a perfusion lung scan showing diffuse, patchy nonsegmental abnormalities, is suggestive of the diagnosis on a clinical basis.[153] The chest CT scan may be very helpful, revealing smooth interlobular septal thickening, ground-glass opacities, and a mosaic attention pattern. The treatment of pulmonary venoocclusive disease is unsatisfactory. Anecdotal reports of success with calcium blockers or epoprostenol have been tempered by reports of these treatments producing fulminant pulmonary edema. Any therapy needs particularly close supervision, and early referral of the patient for lung transplantation should be considered.

PULMONARY CAPILLARY HEMANGIOMATOSIS

Pulmonary capillary hemangiomatosis was first described in 1978 as a very rare cause of pulmonary hypertension.[154] Because of the few reports in the medical literature, it is hard to characterize this abnormality. The typical chest radiographic appearance is a diffuse bilateral reticular nodular pattern associated with enlarged central pulmonary arteries.[155] Ventilation-perfusion scans are often abnormal and may show matched or unmatched defects. The most characteristic finding on high-resolution CT scan is diffuse bilateral thickening of the interlobular septa and small centrilobular, poorly circumscribed, nobular opacities.[156] Diffuse ground-glass opacities have also been described. Histological findings often include irregular small nodular foci of thin-walled capillary-sized vessels that diffusely invade the lung parenchyma, the bronchiolar walls, and the adventitia of large vessels. These nodular lesions are often associated with alveolar hemorrhage. Changes of hypertensive arteriopathy manifest by intimal fibrosis and medial hypertrophy are also common. Most patients appear to be young adults and present with dyspnea and/or hemoptysis. It is very difficult to distinguish pulmonary capillary hemangiomatosis from PPH clinically. A hereditary form with probable autosomal recessive transmission has been reported.

The clinical course of patients with this condition is usually one of progressive deterioration leading to severe pulmonary hypertension, right-sided heart failure, and death. Intravenous epoprostenol has been used, but it has been reported with the associated development of severe pulmonary edema.[157] The only definitive treatment for these patients is bilateral lung transplantation.

Pulmonary Venous Hypertension

PATHOPHYSIOLOGY. Increased resistance to pulmonary venous drainage is a mechanism common to several conditions of diverse causes in which pulmonary hypertension occurs. Altered resistance to pulmonary venous drainage may be the result of diseases affecting the left ventricle or pericardium, mitral or aortic valves, or rare entities such as cor triatriatum and left atrial myxoma.

The severity of pulmonary hypertension depends, in part, on the performance of the right ventricle. In response to an acute stress such as pulmonary embolism, the normal right ventricle of an adult living at sea level can achieve systolic pulmonary pressures of 45 to 50 mm Hg, above which right ventricular failure supervenes. Systolic pressures exceeding these levels can be generated only by a hypertrophied right ventricle. If right ventricular infarction or ischemia has occurred or if the right and left ventricles are both affected by a myopathic process, right ventricular failure occurs at lower pulmonary artery pressure and severe elevations in pulmonary artery pressure may not develop despite an increase in pulmonary vascular resistance.

In the presence of a normal right ventricle, an increase in left atrial pressure initially results in a fall in both pulmonary vascular resistance and the pressure gradient across the lungs. These reductions may reflect distention of a population of compliant small vessels, recruitment of additional vascular channels, or both. With further increases in left atrial pressure, pulmonary arterial pressure rises along with pulmonary venous pressure, so that at a constant pulmonary blood flow, the pressure gradient between the pulmonary artery and veins and pulmonary vascular resistance remains constant. When pulmonary venous pressure approaches or exceeds 25 mm Hg on a chronic basis, a disproportionate elevation in pulmonary artery pressure occurs, so that the pressure gradient between the pulmonary artery and veins rises while pulmonary blood flow remains constant or falls, which is indicative of an elevation in pulmonary vascular resistance that is due, in part, to pulmonary vasoconstriction. Such patients may have some of the pathological features of PPH (see later) and it may be this subgroup that benefits from therapy directed at pulmonary hypertension.

Pulmonary Arterial Vasoconstriction. Considerable variability in pulmonary arterial vasoconstriction occurs in response to pulmonary venous hypertension. Marked reactive pulmonary hypertension with pulmonary artery systolic pressures in excess of 80 mm Hg occurs in somewhat less than one-third of patients whose pulmonary venous pressures are elevated in excess of 25 mm Hg. The fact that severe reactive pulmonary hypertension develops in less than one-third of patients with severe mitral stenosis suggests a broad spectrum of pulmonary vascular reactivity to chronic increases in pulmonary venous pressure.

The mechanisms involved in elevating pulmonary vascular resistance are unclear. In addition to hypertrophy of the media of the vasculature, a neural component may be present. An elevation in pulmonary venous pressure may also narrow or close airways, which may diminish ventilation and lead to hypoxia and vasoconstriction, and interstitial pulmonary edema secondary to pulmonary venous hypertension may encroach on the vascular lumen.

PATHOLOGY. Structural changes in the pulmonary vascular bed develop in association with chronic pulmonary venous hypertension, irrespective of its origin. At the ultrastructural level, these changes include swelling of pulmonary capillary endothelial cells, thickening of their basal lamina, and wide separation of groups of connective tissue fibrils, indicative of interstitial edema. With persistence of the edema, reticular and elastic fibrils proliferate and the alveolar capillaries become embedded in dense connective tissue. The permeability of interendothelial junctions depends on pulmonary capillary pressure, with leakage of large molecules (40,000 to 60,000 daltons) occurring at capillary pressures in excess of approximately 30 mm Hg.

Light microscopic examination of the lungs of patients with pulmonary venous hypertension shows distention of pulmonary capillaries, thickening and rupture of the basement membranes of endothelial cells, and transudation of erythrocytes through these ruptured membranes into the alveolar spaces, which contain fragments of disintegrating erythrocytes. Pulmonary hemosiderosis is commonly observed and may progress to extensive fibrosis. In the late stages of pulmonary venous hypertension, areas of hemorrhage may be scattered throughout the lungs, edema fluid and coagulum may collect in the alveolar spaces, and widespread organization and fibrosis of pulmonary alveoli may be present. Occasionally, particularly in patients with chronic pulmonary venous hypertension caused by mitral valve disease, the alveolar spaces become ossified. Pulmonary lymphatics may become markedly distended and give the appearance of lymphangiectasis, particularly when pulmonary venous pressure chronically exceeds 30 mm Hg. Structural alterations in the small pulmonary arteries, arterioles, and venules include medial hypertrophy, intimal fibrosis, and rarely, necrotizing arteritis. However, plexiform lesions are not seen.

CAUSES. Pulmonary hypertension secondary to elevation of the pulmonary venous pressure occurs in left ventricular dysfunction (see Chaps. 21 and 22), mitral and aortic valve disease (see Chap. 57), cardiomyopathy (see Chap. 59), cor triatriatum (see Chap. 56), and pericardial disease (see Chap. 64).

Pulmonary Hypertension Associated with Disorders of the Respiratory System

Diseases of the lung parenchyma are a common cause of pulmonary hypertension. The pathogenic mechanisms that can lead to pulmonary hypertension in this setting are shown in Table 67–9.

Chronic Obstructive Pulmonary Disease

Chronic obstructive pulmonary disease is the fourth leading cause of death in the United States, affecting more than 16 million people. The incidence, morbidity rate, and mortality rate of COPD vary widely among countries and are rising. The variation is possibly related to differences in exposure to risk factors as well as to differences in individual susceptibility.

TABLE 67–9 Potential Pathogenetic Mechanisms Leading to Pulmonary Arterial Hypertension and Cor Pulmonale

Mechanisms	Example
Primary	
Anatomical decrease in cross-sectional area (vessel destruction; encroachment on lumen by hypertrophy) of the pulmonary resistance vessels	Interstitial fibrosis and granuloma
Vasoconstriction of pulmonary resistance vessels	Hypoxia and acidosis
Contributory	
Large increments in pulmonary blood flow	Exercise
Increased pressures on the left side of the heart and pulmonary veins	Left ventricular failure or pulmonary venoocclusive disease
Increased viscosity of the blood	Secondary polycythemia or chronic hypoxia
Unproved	
Compression of pulmonary resistance vessels by raised alveolar pressures in their vicinity	Asthmatic bronchitis
Bronchial arterial-pulmonary arterial anastomoses	Expanded bronchial circulation

From Fishman AP: Pulmonary hypertension and cor pulmonale. *In* Fishman AP: Pulmonary Diseases and Disorders. 2nd ed. New York, McGraw-Hill, 1988, p 1001.

Chronic obstructive pulmonary disease is a heterogeneous group of diseases that share a common feature: the airways are narrowed, which causes the inability to exhale completely. Although there are numerous disorders that fall under the heading of COPD, the two largest components are emphysema and chronic bronchitis. While clear-cut distinctions between these components can often be made, there is considerable overlap as to the dominant abnormality in the individual patient in whom features of both may be manifest. Chronic bronchitis is a condition associated with excessive tracheal bronchial mucus production sufficient to cause cough with expectoration for at least 3 months of the year for more than 2 consecutive years. Emphysema is defined as the permanent, abnormal distention of the air spaces distal to the terminal bronchi, with destruction of the alveolar septa. In lungs from patients with COPD studied at postmortem, the major site of air flow obstruction has been shown to be in the small airways.

Definitions of COPD have been prepared by expert panels of the American Thoracic Society,[158] the European Respiratory Society,[159] the British Thoracic Society,[160] and the Global Initiative for Chronic Obstructive Lung Disease (GOLD).[161] Despite some subtle differences, all four expert panels make essentially the same key points:

1. Irreversible air flow obstruction is a cardinal feature of COPD.
2. Although limited reversibility of airflow obstruction in response to bronchodilator drugs is common, absence of such reversibility does not preclude bronchodilator treatment.
3. Neither asthma with complete reversibility nor chronic airflow obstruction due to other diagnosable conditions such as cystic fibrosis, obliterative bronchiolitis, or panbronchiolitis are included in the definition of COPD.
4. Tobacco smoking is the major, but not the only, risk factor for COPD.
5. The cause of irreversible airflow obstruction in patients with COPD is the presence in the lungs of bronchiolitis or small airway disease and emphysema, which are present to a variable mix among patients.

Of all of these definitions, the GOLD definition has gained widespread acceptance because of its simplicity and emphasis on spirometry as the standard for the diagnosis of airflow obstruction.

RISK FACTORS. Cigarette smoking is the most commonly identified correlate with COPD and accounts for 80 to 90 percent of the risk of developing COPD.[162] It has been estimated that 15 percent of one-pack-per-day smokers and 25 percent of two-pack-per-day smokers develop COPD during their lifetime. Other potential environmental causes include air pollution, occupational exposures, and infection. It is likely that there are important interactions between environmental factors and a genetic predisposition to COPD. Individuals who are homozygous for alpha$_1$-antitrypsin deficiency develop severe emphysema in the third and fourth decades of life. Dusty occupational environments are well-established risks but probably not major factors in North America.

PATHOGENESIS. A chronic inflammatory process is involved in COPD that differs from that seen in asthma, with different inflammatory cells, mediators, inflammatory effects, and responses to treatment.[163] Most inflammation in cases of COPD occurs in the peripheral airways (bronchioles) and lung parenchyma. There is increased destruction of lung parenchyma and an increased number of macrophages and T-lymphocytes, which are predominantly CD8+ (cytotoxic) T cells.[164] Importantly, eosinophils are not prominent as they are in asthma, except during an exacerbation.[165] Other inflammatory mediators that are elevated in patients with COPD include leukotriene B_4, which is chemotactic for neutrophils, tumor necrosis factor (TNF)-alpha, and interleukin-8.[166] Macrophages also appear to play an important role, since the cells are five to 10 times more numerous, are activated, are localized to the sites of damage, and also have the capacity to produce the pathological changes of COPD.[167] Macrophages also appear to be activated by cigarette smoke and other irritants to release neutrophil-chemotactic factors such as leukotriene B_4 and interleukin-8. Neutrophils and macrophages also release multiple proteinases that break down connective tissue in the lung parenchyma, resulting in emphysema, and stimulate mucus secretion (Fig. 67–14).[168]

Protease-Antiprotease Imbalance. This likely contributes to the pathophysiology of COPD.[167] In this condition, the balance appears to be tipped in favor of increased proteolysis because of either an increase in proteases, including neutrophil elastase, cathepsins, and matrix metalloproteinases, or a deficiency of the antiproteases, which may include alpha$_1$-antitrypsin in the lung parenchyma and airways, epithelium-derived secreting leukoprotease inhibitor in the airways, or at least three tissue inhibitors of matrix metalloproteinases (called TIMP-1, TIMP-2, and TIMP-3).[168] There is accumulating evidence that oxidative stress may have an important role in COPD,[169] possibly exacerbating the condition through several mechanisms, including the activation of transcription factor nuclear factor-κB and oxidative damage of the antiproteases, thus enhancing inflammation and proteolytic injury.

Systemic Effects of COPD. These include increased circulating concentrations of interleukin-6 and of acute phase proteins such as C-reactive protein.[170,171] Weight loss in patients with COPD has been associated with increased circulating levels of TNF-α and soluble TNF receptors and with increased release of TNF-α from circulating cells. The subsequent elevation of circulating levels of leptin may lead to weight loss and skeletal muscle wasting in COPD patients.[172] The low-grade systemic inflammation that is present in patients with moderate to severe airflow obstruction is thought to play a role in the increased cardiovascular risk for COPD patients.[173]

PATHOPHYSIOLOGY OF PULMONARY HYPERTENSION. Most commonly, pulmonary hypertension in COPD patients is due to multiple factors, including pulmonary vasoconstriction caused by alveolar hypoxia, acidemia, and hypercarbia; the compression of pulmonary vessels by the high lung volume; the loss of small vessels in the vascular bed in regions of the emphysema and lung destruction; and

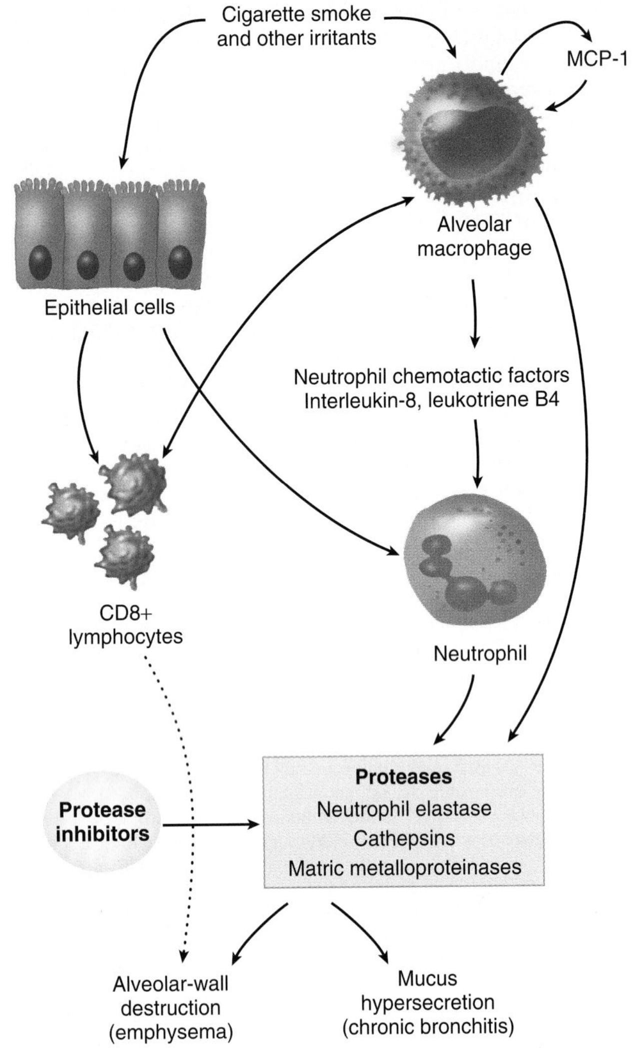

Cigarette smoke and other irritants
MCP-1
Epithelial cells
Alveolar macrophage
Neutrophil chemotactic factors Interleukin-8, leukotriene B4
CD8+ lymphocytes
Neutrophil
Protease inhibitors
Proteases
Neutrophil elastase
Cathepsins
Matric metalloproteinases
Alveolar-wall destruction (emphysema)
Mucus hypersecretion (chronic bronchitis)

FIGURE 67–14 Inflammatory mechanisms in chronic obstructive pulmonary disease. Cigarette smoke and other irritants activate macrophages and airway epithelial cells in the respiratory tract, which release neutrophil chemotactic factors, including interleukin-8 and leukotriene B_4. Neutrophils and macrophages then release proteases that break down connective tissue in the lung parenchyma, resulting in emphysema, and also stimulate mucus hypersecretion. Proteases are normally counteracted by protease inhibitors, including alpha$_1$-antitrypsin, secretory leukoprotease inhibitor, and tissue inhibitors of matrix metalloproteinases. Cytotoxic T cells (CD8+ lymphocytes) may also be involved in the inflammatory cascade. MCP-1 denotes monocyte chemotactic protein 1, which is released by and affects macrophages. (From Barnes PJ: Chronic obstructive pulmonary disease. N Engl J Med 343:269, 2000.)

increased cardiac output and blood viscosity from polycythemia secondary to hypoxia. Of these, hypoxia is the most important factor and is associated with pathological changes that occur characteristically in the peripheral pulmonary arterial bed. The intima of small pulmonary arteries develop accumulations of vascular smooth muscle cells that are laid down longitudinally along the length of the vessels. Intimal thickening appears to be an early event that occurs in association with progressive air flow limitation. Medial hypertrophy in the muscular pulmonary arteries, and less commonly fibrinoid necrosis in these vessels, has also been reported in patients with COPD with chronic pulmonary arterial hypertension. Thus, structural change, rather than hypoxic vasoconstriction, is required for the development of sustained pulmonary hypertension in patients with COPD.

Changes in airway resistance may augment pulmonary vascular resistance in patients with COPD by increases in the alveolar pressure. The normal linear relationship between pressure and flow in the pulmonary circulation changes when alveolar pressure is elevated. The effect of airway resistance on pulmonary artery pressure may be particularly important when ventilation increases (such as in cases of acute exacerbation of COPD). In patients with COPD, even the small increases in flow that occur during mild exercise may increase pulmonary artery pressure significantly.

Alveolar hypoxia is a potent arterial constrictor in the pulmonary circulation that reduces perfusion with respect to ventilation in an attempt to restore PaO_2. In patients with COPD, there is a positive correlation between the $PaCO_2$ and the pulmonary artery pressure. Polycythemia, which may develop in response to chronic hypoxemia, increases the blood viscosity, which may also contribute to the severity of pulmonary arterial hypertension. Pulmonary arterial thrombosis may also occur in patients with COPD and may be a result of peripheral airway inflammation.

Evaluation of the Patient with Chronic Obstructive Pulmonary Disease

The diagnosis of COPD should be considered in patients with chronic cough, sputum production, dyspnea, or history of exposure to risk factors for the disease. Key indicators for considering a diagnosis of COPD are listed in Table 67–10. Although an important part of patient care, physical examination is relatively insensitive for diagnosing pulmonary hypertension and COPD. Clinical signs are often obscured by hyperinflation of the chest. Spirometry is the gold standard by which to diagnose and categorize COPD. Spirometry should measure the maximal volume of air forcibly exhaled from the point of maximal inhalation (FVC) and the volume of air exhaled during the first second of this maneuver (FEV_1). The

TABLE 67–10 Key Indicators for Considering a Diagnosis of Chronic Obstructive Pulmonary Disease (COPD)*

Stage	Characteristics
Chronic cough	Present intermittently or every day Often present throughout the day; seldom only nocturnal
Chronic sputum production	Any pattern of chronic sputum production may indicate COPD
Dyspnea that is:	Progressive (worsens over time) Persistent (present every day) Described by the patients as: "increased effort to breath," "heaviness," "air hunger," or "gasping" Worse on exercise Worse during respiratory infections
History of exposure to risk factors, especially:	Tobacco smoke Occupational dusts and chemicals Smoke from home cooking and heating fuels

Adapted from Pauwels RA, Buist AS, Calverley PM, et al: Global strategy for the diagnosis, management, and prevention of chronic obstructive pulmonary disease. Am J Respir Crit Care Med 163:1256, 2001.

*Consider COPD and performs spirometry if any of these indicators are present. These indicators are not diagnostic by themselves, but the presence of multiple key indicators increases the probability of a diagnosis of COPD. Spirometry is needed to establish a diagnosis of COPD.

ratio of these two components (FEV_1:FVC) should then be calculated. Patients with COPD typically show a decrease in both FEV_1 and FVC. An FEV_1:FVC ratio of less than 70 percent and a post-bronchodilator FEV_1 of less than 80 percent of predicted confirms the presence of airflow limitation that is not fully reversible. However, even patients who do not demonstrate reversibility with a short-acting bronchodilator can benefit symptomatically from long-term bronchodilator treatment.

ECHOCARDIOGRAPHY. Although echocardiography is an invaluable tool in the evaluation of most forms of pulmonary hypertension, its utility is more limited in cases of COPD because hyperinflation of the lungs and marked respiratory variations in intrathoracic pressures often result in suboptimal images. In a recent study, Doppler echocardiography was used to estimate systolic pulmonary artery pressure in a cohort of 374 lung transplantation candidates.[174] Of these patients, 68 percent had obstructive lung disease, 28 percent had interstitial lung disease, and 4 percent had pulmonary vascular disease. The prevalence of pulmonary hypertension was 18 percent among the COPD population, 59 percent among those with interstitial lung disease, and 100 percent among those with pulmonary vascular disease. Estimation of the systolic pulmonary artery pressure was possible in only 44 percent of the patients. Although the correlation between systolic pulmonary artery pressure estimated by echocardiography and that measured at the time of cardiac catheterization was good, 52 percent of the pressure measurements were found to be inaccurate, defined as a more than 10 mm Hg difference compared with the measured pressure at the time of cardiac catheterization. Furthermore, 48 percent of patients were misclassified as having pulmonary hypertension by echocardiography. Sensitivity, specificity, and positive and negative predictive values of systolic pulmonary artery pressure estimation by echocardiography for the diagnosis of pulmonary hypertension were 85, 55, 52, and 87 percent, respectively. Although the right ventricle was adequately visualized in nearly all of the patients, detection of right ventricular abnormalities did not enhance the poor positive predictive value of the Doppler echocardiogram. Given the inaccuracy of the echocardiogram in patients with pulmonary disease, an elevated estimated systolic pulmonary artery pressure obtained by echocardiogram must be interpreted with caution, because approximately half of the time it will represent a false-positive finding.

The largest hemodynamic characterization of patients with severe emphysema included 120 patients evaluated for participation in the National Emphysema Treatment Trial at 3 of the 17 participating centers.[175] These patients had severe airflow limitation with an FEV_1 of 27 percent of predicted, residual volume of 225 percent of predicted, and diffusing capacity of 27 percent of predicted. In 77.5 percent of the patients, pulmonary artery systolic pressure was between 30 and 45 mm Hg, whereas only 13.3 percent had a pulmonary artery systolic pressure of greater than 45 mm Hg. The mean pulmonary artery pressure was greater than 35 mm Hg in only 5 percent of patients.

In patients with mild COPD, right ventricular end-diastolic pressure and right ventricular stroke work, which were normal at rest, increased during exercise because of an increase in work against a higher pulmonary artery pressure.

Severe pulmonary arterial hypertension is uncommon in the presence of COPD. In a review of 500 patients with pulmonary hypertension, only 6 were found to have severe elevation in mean pulmonary artery pressure (>50 mm Hg), which was not related to the severity of their underlying lung disease.[176] This observation suggests that a different biological mechanism results in changes in the pulmonary vascular bed in susceptible patients and that severe pulmonary hypertension occurs in the presence of lung disease rather than as a result of the lung disease. Therefore, patients who present with severe pulmonary hypertension should be evaluated for another disease process that is responsible for the high pulmonary arterial pressures before it is attributed to the COPD.

Prognosis and Predictors of Survival

Chronic obstructive pulmonary disease is usually a progressive disease, and a patient's lung function can be expected to deteriorate over time, even with the best available care. Although pulmonary hypertension progresses slowly in patients with COPD, its presence confers a poor prognosis. For example, Weitzenblum and coworkers showed a 72 percent 4-year survival rate in patients with normal pulmonary artery pressure compared with a 49 percent survival rate in those with an elevated pulmonary artery pressure (mean >20 mm Hg).[177]

A study with a 10-year follow-up conducted on a cohort of 870 patients with severe COPD concluded that: (1) patients with COPD have a high mortality rate from acute respiratory failure, cor pulmonale, and lung cancer; (2) patients' age at the time of diagnosis influences the death risk; (3) patients who need long-term oxygen treatment have a higher death risk than those who do not; (4) the higher the FEV_1 or PaO_2 at the time of diagnosis, the lower the death risk; (5) patients who need and use long-term oxygen treatment have a lower death risk those who need it but do not use it properly; and (6) patients with a partial reversible airway obstruction who regularly attend the clinic for planned checkups have a lower death risk than those who have the same characteristics but do not show adherence to the care program.[178] In another study of 166 patients treated with long-term oxygen therapy, the overall survival rates were 78.3 and 67.1 percent at 2 and 3 years, respectively. A multivariate analysis showed an independent predictive power for right ventricular systolic pressure, age, and FEV_1.[179] Once endotracheal intubation is necessary, the prognosis is usually poor and the survival after 1 year is usually lower than 40 percent.[180] Pulmonary embolism is a common cause of death, with the frequency estimated to be approximately 11 percent.[181] Among patients with COPD in the intensive care unit, pulmonary embolism was the most frequent cause of death, at 40.6 percent.

Management

The overall approach to the management of stable COPD should revolve around a stepwise increase in treatment, depending on the severity of the disease. Disease severity is determined by the severity of symptoms and air flow limitation as well as other factors, including the frequency and severity of exacerbations, complications, respiratory failure, and comorbid factors, including cardiovascular disease and sleep-related disorders, in addition to the general health status of the patient. Patient education is paramount to effective treatment of COPD.

SMOKING CESSATION. The importance of smoking cessation cannot be overemphasized. The annual rate of decline of FEV_1 in smokers is approximately 80 ml per year, in contrast to 25 to 30 ml per year in nonsmokers. The Lung Health Study reported that patients who stopped smoking had a small improvement in FEV_1 (57 ml) after 1 year.[182] Thereafter, the rate of decline in lung function is similar to that of age-matched nonsmokers. The short-term success rates with smoking cessation are variable (18-77 percent), but success is more likely if the patient abstains from smoking within the first 2 weeks of entry into a program.

Numerous effective pharmacotherapies for smoking cessation now exist. They are generally recommended when counseling alone is not sufficient to help the patient to quit smoking. Numerous studies indicate that nicotine replacement therapy in any form (gum, inhaler, nasal spray, transdermal patch, sublingual tablets, or lozenges) reliably increases long-term smoking abstinence rates.[183] The antidepressants bupropion or nortriptyline have also been shown to increase long-term smoking cessation rates, although fewer data are available.[184]

PULMONARY REHABILITATION. The goals of pulmonary rehabilitation in COPD patients are to reduce symptoms, improve quality of life, and increase physical and emotional participation in everyday activities. Although a large study of 200 patients with disabling COPD demonstrated no difference in hospital admission among the patients randomized to receive rehabilitation versus the control patients, the rehabilitation group showed greater improvements in walking ability and general and disease-specific health status.[185]

PHARMACOLOGICAL TREATMENT. Pharmacological therapy is used to prevent and control symptoms, reduce the frequency and severity of exacerbations, improve health status, and improve exercise tolerance (Table 67–11). Although none of these medications has been demonstrated to modify the long-term decline in lung function, this should not preclude the use of these therapies to control symptoms.

Bronchodilators and Corticosteroids. Bronchodilators are central to the management of COPD and can be used either on an as-needed basis for relief of persistent or worsening symptoms or on a regular basis to help prevent and reduce symptoms. The choice of a beta-2 agonist, anticholinergic agent, theophylline, or combination therapy depends on the availability and individual response in terms of symptom relief and side effects. A combination of a short-acting beta-2 antagonist and an anticholinergic agent in stable COPD patients produces greater and more sustained improvements in FEV_1 than either agent alone and does not produce evidence of tachyphylaxis over 90 days of treatment.[186,187] Such combinations are commercially available. Prolonged treatment with corticosteroids does not modify the long-term decline in lung function in patients with COPD and should primarily be used in those who have a documented spirometric response to inhaled corticosteroids.[188]

Other Pharmacological Treatments. The use of vasodilators has been disappointing in the treatment of COPD patients, even those with pulmonary hypertension. No agent other than oxygen has been shown convincingly to vasodilate the pulmonary circulation in patients with COPD. Because of potential for worsening ventilation-perfusion mismatch, vasodilators may worsen hypoxemia. Data regarding the use of digoxin in COPD patients is insufficient to make recommendations, although short-term intravenous digoxin improved cardiac output and reduced circulating norepinephrine levels in patients with right ventricular dysfunction due to PPH.[97] Influenza and pneumococcal vaccines are recommended for prophylaxis..

OXYGEN. Hypoxemia is a common finding in patients with advanced COPD and is easily corrected with low-flow supplemental O_2. In key clinical trials, long-term O_2 therapy clearly improved the survival of hypoxemic patients with COPD.[189,190] The British study[191] compared the effect of treatment with oxygen for approximately 15 hours per day with the effects of no O_2 therapy, whereas the NIH study compared nocturnal O_2 therapy (about 12 hours per day) to "continuous" O_2 therapy (at least 19 hours per day).[189] In each study, the mean baseline PaO_2 when the patients were breathing ambient air was 51 mm Hg; the mean FEV_1 was 0.7 to 0.8 liters.

Oxygen therapy was beneficial in both studies. In the British study, 19 of 42 (45 percent) O_2-treated patients died within 5 years, whereas 30 of 45 (67 percent) untreated patients died. In the NIH study, the mortality rate after 1 year was 20.6 percent in the group receiving nocturnal O_2 and 11.9 percent in the group receiving continuous oxygen therapy; and after 2 years, mortality rates were 40.8 and 22.4 percent, respectively.[189] The relative risk of death for nocturnal O_2 therapy compared with continuous O_2 was 1.94. O_2 therapy is therefore effective, and continuous therapy is more effective than nocturnal therapy only.

HEMODYNAMIC EFFECTS OF OXYGEN. How oxygen therapy improves survival is unknown. Two major hypotheses have been proposed: (1) O_2 relieves pulmonary vasoconstriction, decreasing pulmonary vascular resistance and thus enabling the right ventricle to increase stroke volume; and (2) oxygen therapy improves arterial oxygen content, providing enhanced oxygen delivery to the heart, brain, and other vital organs. These two hypotheses are not mutually exclusive, and each one has supporting evidence. Oxygen therapy clearly alleviates the progressive pulmonary hypertension of untreated COPD. Patients who exhibit a significant decrease in pulmonary artery pressure (>5 mm Hg) after acute oxygen therapy (28 percent O_2 for 1 day) have better survival than patients who do not respond acutely when both groups of patients are subsequently treated with long-term continuous oxygen therapy.[190] Enhanced right ventricular performance during short-term oxygen therapy may also be the direct result of improved tissue (e.g., myocardial) oxygenation rather than decreased pulmonary vascular resistance.[191]

RECOMMENDATIONS FOR OXYGEN THERAPY. Criteria for chronic home oxygen therapy are shown in Table 67–12. Long-term oxygen therapy is warranted if the resting PaO_2 remains less than 55 mm Hg after a 3-week stabilization period on maximal medical therapy (e.g., bronchodilators, antimicrobial agents, diuretics). Patients with a PaO_2

TABLE 67–11 Therapy at Each Stage of Chronic Obstructive Pulmonary Disease (COPD)

Stage	Characteristics	Recommended Treatment
All		Avoidance of risk factors Influenza vaccination
0: At risk	Chronic symptoms (cough, sputum) Exposure to risk factors	
I: Mild COPD	$FEV_1/FVC < 70\%$ $FEV_1 \geq 80\%$ predicted With or without symptoms	Short-acting bronchodilator when needed
II: Moderate COPD	IIA $FEV_1/FVC < 70\%$ 50% < FEB1 < 80% predicted With or without symptoms	Regular treatment with one or more bronchodilators Inhaled glucocorticosteroids if significant symptoms and lung function response or if repeated exacerbations Rehabilitation
	IIB $FEV_1/FVC < 70\%$ $30\% \leq FEV_1 > 50\%$ predicted With or without symptoms	Regular treatment with one or more bronchodilators Inhaled glucocorticosteroids if significant symptoms and lung function response or if repeated exacerbations Rehabilitation
III: Severe COPD	$FEV_1/FVC < 70\%$ $FEV_1 < 30\%$ predicted or presence of respiratory failure or right heart failure	Regular treatment with one or more bronchodilators Inhaled glucocorticosteroids if significant symptoms and lung function response or if repeated exacerbations Treatment of complications Rehabilitation Long-term oxygen therapy if respiratory failure Consider surgical treatments

Adapted from Pauwels RA, Buist AS, Calverley PM, et al: Global strategy for the diagnosis, management, and prevention of chronic obstructive pulmonary disease. Am J Respir Crit Care Med 163:1256, 2001.

TABLE 67–12 Indications for Home Oxygen

Absolute
PaO_2 ≤55 mm Hg or SaO_2 ≤88%
PaO_2 55-59 mm Hg or SaO_2 = 89% in the presence of any of the following
Dependent edema suggesting congestive heart failure
P pulmonale on the ECG (P wave <3 mm in standard leads II, III, or aVF)
Erythrocytosis (hematocrit >56%)
Specific Situations
During exercise
PaO_2 <55 mm Hg or O_2 saturation <88% with low level of exertion
During sleep
PaO_2 <55 mm Hg or O_2 saturation <88% with associated complications, such as pulmonary hypertension, excessive daytime sleepiness, and cardiac arrhythmias

Adapted from ATS Statement: Comprehensive outpatient management of COPD. Am J Respir Crit Care Med 152(Suppl):S84, 1995.

above 55 mm Hg should be considered for oxygen therapy if they are polycythemic or have clinical evidence (e.g., electrocardiogram, physical examination) of pulmonary hypertension. Hypoxemia should be documented after the stabilization period to avoid the cost of long-term oxygen therapy in patients who do not require it. O_2 has been shown to delay the onset of fatigue in exercising muscles, thus improving ventilatory endurance and exercise capacity.[191] In addition, it decreases dyspnea and minute ventilation for a given workload.[192] Nocturnal oxygen therapy may be important in patients with sleep desaturation. Daily activities, such as walking, washing, and eating, are associated with transient oxygen desaturation in patients with moderate to severe COPD, even in the absence of resting hypoxemia[193]; this desaturation can be relieved with O_2.

NONINVASIVE VENTILATION. Noninvasive positive-pressure ventilation has been reported to improve gas exchange, sleep efficiency, quality of life, and functional status in patients with restrictive lung disease and chronic respiratory failure; however, its usefulness in patients with COPD is not as well established. Uncontrolled studies have demonstrated that noninvasive positive pressure ventilation used at home may improve oxygenation and reduce hospital admissions in patients with severe COPD and hypercapnia and improve long-term survival, although large controlled clinical trials are now needed.[194] The combination of noninvasive positive pressure ventilation and long-term O_2 therapy may be more effective,[195] but again large trials are needed before this approach can be recommended.

LUNG VOLUME REDUCTION SURGERY. Volume reduction surgery, which was originally described by Brantigan, has been advocated in selected patients with advanced emphysema. The surgical technique involves removing 20 to 30 percent of the volume of each lung by means of sternotomy, sequential thoracotomy, or thoracoscopy to reduce the severe hyperinflation commonly seen in patients with severe COPD.

A randomized trial comparing the results of lung volume reduction surgery with medical therapy for severe emphysema has been completed.[196] A total of 1218 patients with severe emphysema who underwent pulmonary rehabilitation were randomly assigned to undergo lung volume reduction surgery or to receive continued medical therapy. An interim analysis determined that patients with a FEV_1 of less than 20 percent of predicted and either homogeneous distribution of emphysema on CT scan or carbon monoxide diffusing capacity that was 20 percent or less of the predicted value were at high risk for death after lung volume reduction surgery with a low probability of functional benefit.[197] Such patients were subsequently excluded from entry into the trial. Overall, there was a death rate of 0.11 per person-year in both treatment groups, although it was determined that certain subgroups might benefit. Among patients with predominantly upper lobe emphysema and low exercise capacity, the mortality rate was lower in the surgery group than in the medical therapy group. Among patients with non-upper lobe emphysema and high exercise capacity, the mortality rate was higher in the surgery group than in the medical therapy group.

Exercise Capacity. Despite the lack of survival advantage, exercise capacity improved by more than 10 watts in 28, 22, and 15 percent of patients in the surgery group after 6, 12, and 24 months, respectively, as compared with 4, 5, and 3 percent of patients in the medical therapy group. Patients in the surgery group were also significantly more likely to have improvements in 6-minute walk distance, percentage of predicted value for FEV_1, general and health-related quality of life, and degree of dyspnea. Thus, patients with predominantly upper lobe emphysema and a low maximal workload have a lower mortality rate and a greater probability of improvement in exercise capacity with lung volume reduction surgery and should be considered for the procedure. In contrast, patients with predominantly non-upper lobe emphysema and high maximal workload had a higher mortality rate and little functional improvement, regardless of treatment received. These symptomatic improvements after lung volume reduction surgery appear to wane with time, and long-term data from the large National Emphysema Treatment Trial may be enlightening. Lung volume reduction is a palliative procedure that does not halt, but only slows, the rate of functional decline for COPD. The disease will still progress, and symptoms will likely worsen.

LUNG TRANSPLANTATION (see Chap. 26)**.** COPD is the most common indication for lung transplantation worldwide. In 1995, approximately 60 percent of single lung and 30 percent of bilateral lung transplants were performed on patients with COPD.[198] Lung transplantation is a viable treatment option in patients with advanced pulmonary parenchymal or pulmonary vascular disease who have exhausted medical management. Both the number of patients waiting for lung transplantation and the waiting period have increased. Because of the scarcity of organ donors, the waiting time is now approximately 18 to 24 months in the United States. Patient selection and timing of referral for lung transplantation should take into account this waiting period. Selection criteria are outlined in Table 67–8. Both single-lung transplantation and bilateral lung transplantation result in significant improvement in postoperative lung function, exercise capacity, and quality of life.[199] The choice of the procedure needs to be individualized. In general, single-lung transplantation is used for emphysema because of the scarcity of organ donors, lower perioperative morbidity and mortality rates, and comparable improvement in exercise capacity compared with bilateral lung transplantation.[200] However, postoperative spirometry, single breath diffusing capacity, and arterial oxygen tension are all significantly higher in bilateral lung transplantation compared with single-lung transplantation, which may benefit young patients with emphysema because the higher pulmonary reserve will offset any decline in lung function due to infection or rejection. In most centers, bilateral lung transplantation is reserved for patients with suppurative lung disease or pulmonary vascular disease. The 1-year and 5-year survival rates for single and bilateral lung transplantation for emphysema are approximately 80 percent and 40 percent, respectively.

Interstitial Lung Diseases

Interstitial lung diseases represent a variety of conditions that involve the alveolar walls, perialveolar tissue, and other contiguous supporting structures.[201-203] Pulmonary hypertension occurs in patients with a variety of interstitial lung diseases and is often associated with obliteration of the pulmonary vascular bed by lung destruction and fibrosis. The mechanism for pulmonary hypertension may be related to hypoxemia, a loss of effective pulmonary vasculature from lung destruction, and/or by indirectly triggering a pulmonary vasculopathy. Interstitial lung disease may be due to environmental inhalant exposures, such as to asbestos, drugs, and chemotherapeutic agents, to radiation, and to recurring aspiration pneumonias. A large number of patients have interstitial lung disease of unknown origin, the most common being idiopathic pulmonary fibrosis and interstitial lung disease associated with connective tissue diseases.

Adult Cystic Fibrosis

Cystic fibrosis is the most common lethal genetic disease in white persons and occurs in approximately 1 of every 2000 live births. As the disease progresses, patients develop disabling lung disease and eventually respiratory failure, pulmonary hypertension, and cor pulmonale. The pathophysiology of pulmonary hypertension in cystic fibrosis is believed to be related to progressive destruction of the lung parenchyma and the pulmonary vasculature and to pulmonary vasoconstriction secondary to hypoxemia.[204] The development of pulmonary hypertension in patients with cystic fibrosis carries a grave prognosis. The mean survival time from the onset has been reported to be as short as 8 months. Typically, patients have severe hypoxemia, which may be a result of and a causative factor in the disease.

One study evaluated patients with cystic fibrosis and pulmonary hypertension in depth.[205] Right ventricular hypertrophy appears to be a precursor of right ventricular failure and an indicator of the onset of pulmonary hypertension. The severity of the pulmonary hypertension appeared to correlate significantly with declining pulmonary function, as well as with the degree of oxygen desaturation with exercise. In this study, patients who developed pulmonary hypertension had a much worse prognosis (average survival, 15 months) compared with those without pulmonary hypertension (average survival, 33 months). Once lung function is severely limited (FEV_1 <40 percent of predicted), the prevalence of pulmonary hypertension may be as a high as 40 percent. Because hypoxemia is universally found, supplemental oxygen is considered to be the mainstay of treatment in this group.

Sleep-Disordered Breathing (see Chap. 68)

PULMONARY HYPERTENSION. Observational studies have demonstrated a wide variation in the incidence of pulmonary hypertension as a complication of sleep apnea with a wide range of severity. The percentage has ranged from 17 to 73 percent, although these studies had variable entry criteria and some included patients with coexistent COPD.[206] The diagnosis of pulmonary hypertension in obstructive sleep apnea patients is also clouded by the coexistence of systemic hypertension, obesity, and diastolic dysfunction. Successful treatment with continuous positive airway pressure improves pulmonary hemodynamics in patients with obstructive sleep apnea,[207] supporting the relationship between these two disease entities. Acute pulmonary hemodynamic changes during obstructive apneas have been well defined; however, the extent to which these translate into persistent daytime pulmonary hypertension remains less certain.

ALVEOLAR HYPOVENTILATION DISORDERS

Alveolar hypoventilation disorders are characterized by hypoxemia and mechanical disorders of the ventilatory system which, in concert, may cause pulmonary hypertension.

CHEST WALL DISORDERS. Thoracovertebral deformities that can result in restrictive pulmonary syndromes, chronic alveolar hypoventilation, and pulmonary hypertension include idiopathic kyphoscoliosis, spinal tuberculosis, congenital spinal developmental abnormalities, spinal cord injury and other childhood myelopathies, ankylosing spondylitis, or other congenital and acquired muscular skeletal conditions, such as pectus excavatum. Kyphoscoliosis is a relatively common disorder of the spine and its articulations. When severe, it can have a profound impact on pulmonary function, characterized by a severe restrictive pattern on pulmonary function testing. In addition, there can be associated inspiratory muscle weakness that appears related to the increased elastic load from reduced lung and chest wall compliance. Scoliosis that appears before the age of 5 years has the worst respiratory prognosis. An angulation of greater than 100 degrees is considered very severe and is strongly associated with chronic alveolar hypoventilation.[208] Pulmonary compliance is often reduced by 50 percent or more as a result of lung underdevelopment and chronic lung hypoinflation. Patients can also have both central and obstructive apneas and hypopneas.

Pulmonary hypertension frequently occurs in patients with thoracovertibular deformities. Pulmonary hypertension is related to the reduction of the vascular bed because of hypoventilation and hypoxia. Symptoms are commonly slowly progressive. Hypoxemia can be seen from ventilation-perfusion mismatch or underlying atelectasis. In patients with advanced disease, intermittent positive-pressure breathing and noninvasive ventilation have been used successfully, as well as supplemental oxygen in patients who are hypoxemic.[209]

NEUROMUSCULAR DISEASE. The development of right-sided heart failure is an unusual manifestation of respiratory failure solely due to respiratory muscle weakness. It usually develops in response to the hypoxic and hypercapnic stimuli in patients with chronic forms of these disorders. Weakness of the respiratory muscles can be caused by either generalized muscle diseases, such as myopathic infiltrating diseases or muscular dystrophy (see Chap. 85), or more commonly by such neurological disorders as a cord lesion at or below the third cervical vertebra, amyotrophic lateral sclerosis, myasthenia gravis, poliomyelitis, and Guillain-Barré syndrome. The diagnosis of respiratory muscle weakness is confirmed by the finding of a restrictive ventilatory defect and a marked impairment of maximal respiratory pressures. Nocturnal ventilatory support, with either positive or negative pressure, has become established as effective therapy in appropriate cases, and its beneficial effects are well recognized.[210]

DIAPHRAGMATIC PARALYSIS. Bilateral diaphragmatic paralysis is an uncommon and rarely recognized cause of pulmonary hypertension. Diaphragmatic paralysis is a result of phrenic nerve injury, which can be traumatic or secondary to an underlying motor neuron disease. It may occur after cardiac surgery, as a manifestation of Lyme disease,[211] after radiation therapy,[212] or as a manifestation of other neurological disorders. When an affected patient is upright, ventilation may be normal or almost so, but when the patient is supine, gas exchange deteriorates. The diagnosis may be suspected in a patient with supine breathlessness, a disturbed sleep pattern, paradoxical motion of the abdomen on inspiration, and a low vital capacity in the upright position.

Patients with nontraumatic bilateral diaphragmatic paralysis may go unrecognized until they present either with respiratory failure or pulmonary hypertension. The diagnosis can be suspected when the vital capacity is reduced by more than 40 percent of predicted and paradoxic motion of the hemidiaphragms is noted on fluoroscopy.[213] Patients can also have unilateral paralysis of the diaphragm, which is more common but is associated with fewer symptoms and physiological abnormalities. The treatment should always be directed toward correcting the underlying chronic neuromuscular disease, if present, and addressing nocturnal hypoventilation with noninvasive ventilatory techniques. Intermittent positive airway pressure is an effective therapy.[214]

Pulmonary Hypertension due to Chronic Thrombotic or Embolic Obstruction of the Pulmonary Arteries (see Chap. 66)

Pulmonary thromboembolism, as a single event or as repeated events, rarely leads to the development of chronic pulmonary hypertension. In a subset of patients (believed to be less than 0.1 percent of all patients suffering from pulmonary embolism), however, the outcome is unusual. Rather than having inherent fibrinolytic resolution of the thromboembolism with restoration of vascular patency, the thromboemboli in these patients fail to resolve adequately. They undergo organization and incomplete recanalization and become incorporated into the vascular wall. Commonly, they are in the subsegmental, segmental, and lobar vessels, although it is believed that chronic thromboembolism tends to propagate retrograde, leading to slowly progressive vascular obstruction.

An identifiable hypercoagulable state is found in only a minority of patients. The lupus anticoagulant is present in 10 to 20 percent of patients with chronic thromboembolic pulmonary hypertension, whereas inherited deficiencies of protein C, protein S, and antithrombin III as a group can be identified in up to 5 percent of this population.[215] The development of a pulmonary hypertensive arteriopathy, similar to that seen in patients with other forms of pulmonary hypertension, has been documented in unobstructive lung regions as well as in vessels distal to partially or completely occluded proximal pulmonary arteries. These small vessel changes therefore appear to be a significant contributor to the hemodynamic progression seen in many patients. It appears that the vast majority of these patients have suffered one major thromboembolic event rather than multiple recurrences.

Chronic thromboembolic pulmonary hypertension involving the proximal pulmonary arteries is a well-characterized entity. The slowly progressive nature of the course of chronic thromboembolic pulmonary hypertension allows right ventricular hypertrophy to ensue and compensate for the increased pulmonary vascular resistance. However, owing to either progressive thrombosis or vascular changes in the "uninvolved" vascular bed,[216] the pulmonary hypertension becomes progressive and the patient manifests the clinical symptoms of dyspnea, fatigue, hypoxemia, and right-sided heart failure.

Patient Evaluation

The findings on clinical examination of patients with chronic thromboembolic pulmonary hypertension are similar to those of other patients with pulmonary hypertension, with the exception of the following features: These patients tend to have lower cardiac outputs than patients with PPH, which is often reflected in the reduced carotid arterial pulse volume. In addition, on occasion, bruits can be heard over areas of the lung that represent vessels with partial occlusions, but they must be carefully listened for.[217] It is important to make the diagnostic distinction between patients with chronic thromboembolic pulmonary hypertension and those with other forms of pulmonary hypertension, because the treatments are so different. For the former group, a potentially curative therapy through thromboendarterectomy is available, whereas for the latter group effective pharmacological regimens are now evolving. The symptoms and physical findings of chronic thromboembolic pulmonary hypertension are nonspecific and similar to those of patients with PPH.

PERFUSION LUNG SCAN. The perfusion lung scan is usually adequate to identify patients with this entity and is an important reason why lung scans are recommended for all patients who present with pulmonary hypertension (see Fig. 67–4). However, the lung scan typically underestimates the severity of the central pulmonary arterial obstruction.[218] Therefore, patients who present with one or more mismatched segmental or larger defects should undergo pulmonary angiography. This continues to be the gold standard for defining the pulmonary vascular anatomy and is performed to determine whether chronic thromboembolic obstruction is present, to determine its location and surgical accessibility, and to rule out other diagnostic possibilities. Maturation and organization of clot results in vessel retraction and partial recanalization, resulting in several angiographic patterns suggestive of chronic thromboembolic disease: pouch defect; pulmonary webs or bands; intimal irregularities; abrupt narrowing of major pulmonary vessels; and obstruction of main, lobar, or segmental pulmonary arteries, frequently at their point of origin.[219] Since chronic thromboembolic pulmonary hypertension is usually bilateral, the presence of unilateral central pulmonary artery obstruction should prompt consideration of other diagnoses, such as pulmonary vascular tumors or extravascular compression from a lung carcinoma, hilar or mediastinal adenopathy, or mediastinal fibrosis. Pulmonary angiography can be performed safely in these patients if careful attention is given to the hemodynamic state. Nonionic contrast medium has been demonstrated to cause no major hemodynamic effects, even in patients with severe chronic thromboembolic pulmonary hypertension,[220] and is preferred. Hypotension and/or bradycardia should be immediately treated with atropine.

COMPUTED TOMOGRAPHY. CT scanning can be a great aid in diagnosing chronic thromboembolic pulmonary hypertension (Fig. 67–15). Using high-resolution nonenhanced CT, areas of increased attenuation that do not obscure the vessels and that have a ground-glass appearance have been characterized as a mosaic pattern corresponding to hypoperfusion of the lung. Although this pattern is consistent with chronic thromboembolic pulmonary hypertension, it may also be seen in patients with cystic fibrosis, those with bronchiectasis, and lung transplant recipients, but it is virtually never seen in patients with PPH.[221] The contrast-enhanced CT features suggestive of chronic thromboembolic pulmonary hypertension include evidence of organized thrombus lining the pulmonary vessels in an eccentric or concentric fashion; enlargement of the right ventricle and central pulmonary arteries; variation in size of segmental arteries (relatively smaller in the affected segments compared to uninvolved segments); bronchial artery collaterals; and parenchymal changes to pulmonary infarcts. Marked variation in the size of the segmental vessels is more specific for chronic thromboembolic pulmonary hypertension and is believed to represent involvement of the segmental vessels due to thromboemboli. It has been reported that these findings might also be mimicked in patients with fibrosing mediastinitis.

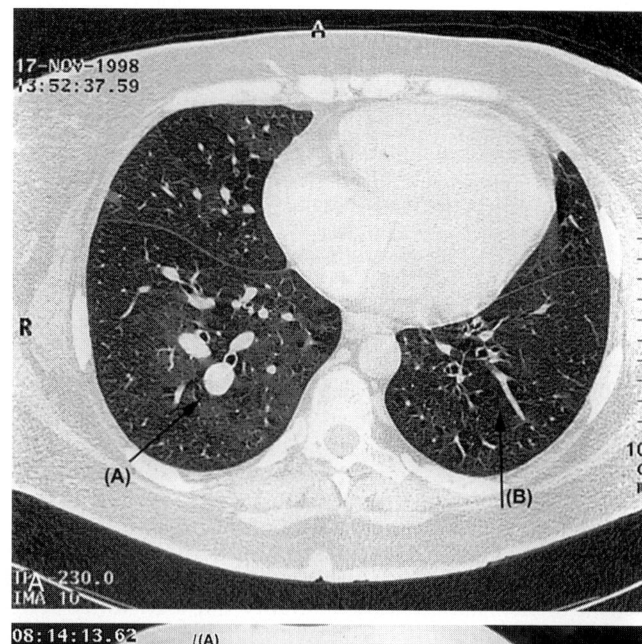

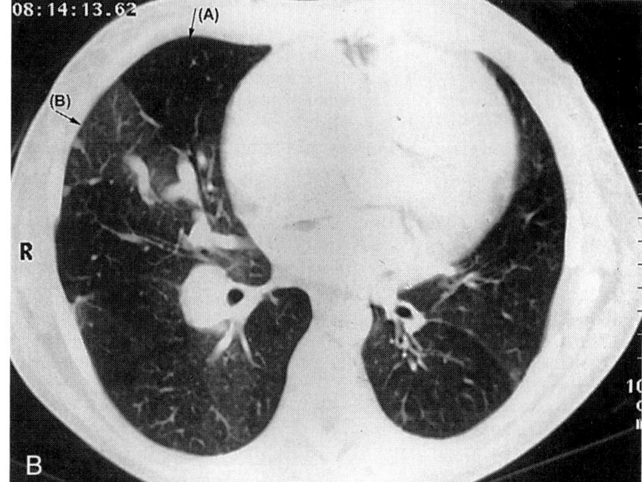

FIGURE 67–15 Chest computed tomographic scans in a patient with chronic thromboembolic pulmonary hypertension. **A,** Helical scan with contrast medium enhancement of the pulmonary vasculature shows a marked disparity in vessel size between the involved vessels (A), which are enlarged from thrombus, and the uninvolved vessels (B). **B,** Non-contrast-enhanced high-resolution scan illustrates a marked mosaic pattern manifest by differences in density of regions of the lung parenchyma reflecting the perfused areas (B) and the nonperfused areas (A), also consistent with underlying thromboembolic disease.

CARDIAC CATHETERIZATION. Patients with chronic thromboembolic pulmonary hypertension tend to have higher right atrial pressures and lower cardiac outputs than comparable patients with PPH for the same level of pulmonary artery pressure. Because this is a disease that generally is progressive, the hemodynamic indications for surgical intervention are an elevation of pulmonary artery pressure and pulmonary vascular resistance for a period of more than 3 months despite adequate anticoagulation.

Treatment

Pulmonary thromboendarterectomy is considered in patients who are symptomatic and have evidence of hemodynamic or ventilatory impairment at rest or with exercise.[222] Operability is determined by the location and extent of proximal thromboemboli (see Fig. 66–19). Thrombi must involve the main, lobar, or proximal segmental arteries. It is important to evaluate whether the amount of surgically accessible thrombus is compatible with a degree of hemodynamic impairment. Failure to significantly reduce the pulmonary vascular resistance with endarterectomy, usually a result of the small vessel arteriopathy that may accompany this disease, is associated with a higher perioperative mortality rate and worse long-term outcome.[223]

Patients undergoing surgery usually have a preoperative pulmonary vascular resistance of greater than 4 Wood units and typically in the range of 10 to 12 Wood units. It is also important to assess the comorbid conditions preoperatively. Although severe left ventricular dysfunction is the only absolute contraindication to pulmonary thromboendarterectomy, advanced age, severe right ventricular dysfunction, and other significant comorbid illnesses increase the perioperative morbidity and mortality risks.[224] Right ventricular dysfunction is not considered a contraindication to surgery, because right ventricular function has been noted to improve once the obstruction of the pulmonary blood flow is removed. It is a true endarterectomy requiring establishment of a dissection plane at the level of the media. The procedure is performed on cardiopulmonary bypass and usually requires periods of complete circulatory arrest to allow for a bloodless field and define an adequate endarterectomy plane.

An operative classification of thromboembolic disease has recently been established and may be useful in terms of prognostication.[225] Among 202 patients who underwent pulmonary thromboendarterectomy, intraoperative classification of thromboembolism was defined as follows: type 1 (37.6 percent), thrombus in the main lobar pulmonary arteries; type 2 (40 percent), intimal thickening and fibrosis proximal to the segmental arteries; type 3 (18.8 percent), disease within distal segmental arteries only; and type 4 (3.4 percent), distal arteriolar vasculopathy without visible thromboembolic disease. Although all four patient groups were similar with respect to age, preoperative pulmonary artery pressures, and pulmonary vascular resistance, patients with proximal thromboembolic disease (groups 1 and 2) had a significantly greater improvement in pulmonary artery systolic pressure and pulmonary vascular resistance. There was also a greater increase in postoperative cardiac index and decrease in right ventricular systolic pressure in these patients as compared with those who had disease within the segmental or distal branches (groups 3 and 4). Although in previous series the operative mortality rate has been reported to be fairly high, the 1-month survival rate in patients who fell into groups 1 and 2 was 98.7 and 97.5 percent, respectively, whereas the 1-month survival rate in patients classified in groups 3 and 4 was 86.8 and 85.7 percent, respectively.

POSTOPERATIVE MANAGEMENT. Postoperative management can be extremely challenging. Patients in whom a large volume of central thrombus is removed, associated with back-bleeding from the distal vascular segments and an immediate fall in the pulmonary artery pressure, usually have an extremely good postoperative course and long-term follow-up. Patients in whom small amounts of thrombus can be removed, in whom the thrombus becomes fragmented at the time of thromboendarterectomy, or in whom there is no distal back-bleeding from the segment where the thrombus was removed usually have a difficult postoperative course. In addition, a lack of significant fall in pulmonary artery pressure and an increase in cardiac output portends a difficult postoperative recovery.

These patients may need mechanical ventilation and inotropic support for days to weeks during periods of slow recovery. Much of their mortality risk appears to be related to severe right ventricular dysfunction, which actually becomes initially worsened during the surgical procedure. Reperfusion injury, which is manifest by profound hypoxemia and pulmonary infiltrates corresponding to the segments where thrombus was removed, occurs in approximately 15 to 20 percent of patients and can be extensive. The only effective management of this complication is sustained assisted ventilation and oxygen supplementation. Attempts to reverse this with corticosteroids or other agents have not been successful. Other complications include atrial fibrillation, pneumonia, delirium, pneumothorax, pancreatitis, clostridium difficile, colitis, and gastrointestinal bleeding.

Those survivors who have a good result, with a significant reduction in postoperative pulmonary vascular resistance at 48 hours, can expect to realize an improvement in functional class and exercise tolerance.[226] Life-long anticoagulation with a goal INR ratio of 2.5 to 3.5 is indicated postoperatively.

PPH VERSUS CHRONIC THROMBOEMBOLIC PULMONARY HYPERTENSION. There are patients whose clinical presentation and evaluation findings are virtually identical to those of patients with PPH but who on autopsy have widespread thrombotic lesions throughout their pulmonary vasculature. It is unclear whether they represent PPH with an excessive tendency toward thrombosis or chronic thromboembolic pulmonary hypertension with persistent thromboemboli only at the arteriolar level. Often their lung scan will show a perfusion pattern characterized by a diffuse mottled abnormality. Because of the poor outcomes after surgery of patients with very distal thromboembolic disease, medical management has been attempted. Both the oral prostacyclin analog beraprost sodium and the phosphodiesterase inhibitor sildenafil have been reported in small case series to improve hemodynamics and exercise tolerance in patients with nonoperable chronic thromboembolic pulmonary hypertension.[227,228]

SICKLE CELL DISEASE

Cardiovascular abnormalities are prominent as part of the clinical spectrum of sickle cell disease. Evidence of right ventricular dysfunction, presumably resulting from pulmonary hypertension, is a poorly characterized complication. In one series of 60 consecutive patients undergoing echocardiography, the incidence of pulmonary hypertension in the setting of sickle cell disease was 20 percent. The mortality rate was also significantly greater in patients with pulmonary hypertension than in those without (42 vs. 8 percent; $p = 0.03$). One must always consider left ventricular dysfunction as a cause of pulmonary hypertension in patients with sickle cell disease because the elevation of pulmonary artery pressure is most often associated with elevation of the pulmonary capillary wedge pressure.[229] Patients with sickle cell disease can also have an increased risk of thromboembolism, and pulmonary thromboendarterectomy may be indicated in certain situations.[230] Sickle cell disease can rarely affect the lungs by causing embolization of bone marrow elements. Generally, the smaller pulmonary arteries, arterioles, and capillaries are affected. It can be associated with pulmonary infarction or local perivascular fibrosis.

Pulmonary Hypertension due to Disorders Directly Affecting the Pulmonary Vasculature

SCHISTOSOMIASIS

Although schistosomiasis is extremely rare in North America, hundreds of millions of people are affected worldwide, particularly in developing countries. The development of pulmonary hypertension almost always occurs in the setting of hepatosplenic disease and portal hypertension.[231] Clinical features appear when ova embolize to the lungs, where they induce formation of delayed hypersensitivity granulomas. In addition, deposition of fibrous tissue causes narrowing, thickening, and occlusion of the pulmonary arterioles. Histologically, focal changes related directly to the presence of schistosome ova may be located either within the alveolar tissue or within the pulmonary arteries, and plexiform or angiomatoid lesions may be found. Fibrosis surrounds most focal lesions. The clinical symptoms and radiographic findings in these patients who develop pulmonary hypertension are not distinctive. In developing countries, this condition can be confused with primary pulmonary hypertension.

The diagnosis of schistosomiasis-induced pulmonary hypertension is confirmed by finding the parasite ova in the urine or stools of persons with symptoms. However, the insidious onset of pulmonary vascular disease years after infection makes finding these parasite ova difficult. Active infections are treated with praziquantel, which kills the adult worms and stops further destruction of tissue by ova deposition.[232] Reversal of pathological lesions in the lungs after therapy has not been documented.

SARCOIDOSIS

Sarcoidosis is a multisystemic granulomatous disease of unknown origin characterized by an enhanced cellular immune response at the sites of involvement. Although any organ can be involved, sarcoidosis most commonly affects the lungs and intrathoracic lymph nodes.[233] The clinical manifestation and natural history of sarcoidosis vary greatly, but the lung is involved in more than 90 percent of patients. The most common presenting symptoms are cough and shortness of breath, which is of a progressive nature.[234] As the disease progresses in the lung parenchyma, extensive interstitial fibrosis is the result. In addition, obstructive airway disease, fibrocystic disease, bronchiectasis, endobronchial granulomas, and lobar atelectasis are common consequences of lung involvement.

Cardiac involvement from sarcoidosis appears to be more common than previously thought and may be present in up to one-third of the cases. Consequently, patients presenting with dyspnea should undergo a thorough cardiac evaluation for the possibility of cardiac involvement. Noncaseating granulomas may infiltrate the myocardium and leave fibrotic scars; and if enough of the myocardium is involved, the patients will develop clinical features of a restrictive cardiomyopathy. Patients with cardiac involvement from sarcoidosis also present with varying degrees of heart block, arrhythmias, and/or clinical features of biventricular diastolic heart failure. Sudden death can be a common manifestation of cardiac sarcoid, and it is one of the most feared sequelae. The prognosis of patients with cardiac involvement from sarcoidosis is variable but can be quite poor. Usually a trial of corticosteroids is given in the hope that it will alter the natural history of the disease.

The echocardiogram often demonstrates either diffuse or regional wall motion abnormalities in patients with cardiac involvement. It is not uncommon, however, to find the features of pulmonary hypertension. Pulmonary hypertension detected by echo-Doppler techniques may be the result of restrictive cardiomyopathy from sarcoid and needs to be clearly distinguished from pulmonary hypertension from direct pulmonary vascular involvement, because the clinical management of these two conditions differs dramatically.

Pulmonary hypertension is most commonly the result of chronic severe fibrocystic sarcoidosis.[235] Patients have chronic progressive dyspnea with effort, a chest radiograph demonstrating severe diffuse interstitial fibrotic lung disease, and pulmonary function tests that reflect severe restrictive physiology and hypoxemia. In these cases, the resulting pulmonary hypertension is usually mild to moderate and typical of patients presenting with restrictive lung disease of any cause.

MANAGEMENT. Management is generally focused on reversing any acute exacerbations of the lung disease and giving supplemental oxygen when indicated. Some patients with sarcoidosis, however, have mild to moderate restrictive lung disease with severe pulmonary hypertension, presumed from granulomatous vasculitis of the pulmonary vessels. It is critically important in the cardiopulmonary evaluation of the patient presenting with underlying sarcoidosis and dyspnea to distinguish whether the symptoms are from chronic interstitial lung disease, restrictive cardiomyopathy, or pulmonary vascular disease.[236] Although the traditional treatment of these patients has been unsatisfactory, it was recently demonstrated that some patients have a very favorable response to intravenous epoprostenol therapy.[133] Although interstitial lung involvement from sarcoidosis can result in mild pulmonary hypertension, a subset of patients present with severe pulmonary hypertension believed to be due to direct pulmonary vascular involvement. It appears that, as with other, secondary causes, these patients are predisposed to the development of pulmonary vascular disease that is triggered in some way by the sarcoid disease process. Although the use of intravenous epoprostenol chronically may reverse the right-sided heart failure and dramatically improve these patients' pulmonary hemodynamics, it will have no impact on any underlying fibrotic lung disease and/or hypoxemia, which still may render the patients symptomatic and dyspneic.

REFERENCES

Normal Pulmonary Circulation

1. Pietra G: The pathology of primary pulmonary hypertension. *In* Rubin LJ, Rich S (eds): Primary Pulmonary Hypertension. New York, Marcel Dekker, 1997, pp 19-61.
2. Salvi SS: Alpha1-adrenergic hypothesis for pulmonary hypertension. Chest 115:1708, 1999.
3. Bevan R: Influence of adrenergic innervation on vascular growth and mature characteristics. Am Rev Respir Dis 140:147, 1989.
4. Takizawa T, Hara Y, Saito T, et al: Alpha-1-adrenoceptor stimulation partially inhibits ATP-sensitive K^+ current in guinea pig ventricular cells: Attenuation of the action potential shortening induced by hypoxia and K^+ channel openers. J Cardiovasc Pharmacol 28:799, 1996.
5. Weir EK, Reeve HL, Huang JM, et al: Anorexic agents aminorex, fenfluramine, and dexfenfluramine inhibit potassium current in rat pulmonary vascular smooth muscle and cause pulmonary vasoconstriction. Circulation 94:2216, 1996.
6. Bento AC, de Moraes S: Effects of estrogen pretreatment of the spare α_1-adrenoceptors and the slow and fast components of the contractile response of the isolated female rat aorta. Gen Pharmacol 23:565, 1992.
7. Kourembanas S, Morita T, Christou H, et al: Hypoxic responses of vascular cells. Chest 114:25S, 1998.
8. Weir E, Reeve H, Peterson D, et al: Pulmonary vasoconstriction, oxygen sensing, and the role of ion channels. Chest 114:17, 1998.
9. Horstman D, Frank D, Rich G: Prolonged inhaled NO attenuates hypoxic, but not monocrotaline-induced, pulmonary vascular remodeling in rats. Anesth Analg 86:74, 1998.
10. Cargill R, Kiely D, Clark R, Lipworth B: Hypoxaemia and release of endothelin-1. Thorax 50:1308, 1995.
11. Peng W, Michael J, Hoidal J, et al: ET-1 modulates KCa-channel activity and arterial tension in normoxic and hypoxic human pulmonary vasculature. Am J Physiol 275:L729, 1998.
12. Bialecki R, Stinson-Fisher C, Murdoch W, et al: A novel orally active endothelin-A receptor antagonist, ZD1611, prevents chronic hypoxia-induced pulmonary hypertension in the rat. Chest 114:91S, 1998.
13. Haleen S, Schroeder R, Walker D, et al: Efficacy of CI-1020, an endothelin A receptor antagonist, in hypoxic pulmonary hypertension. J Cardiovas Pharmacol 31:S331, 1998.
14. Holm P, Liska J, Franco-Cereceda A: The ETA receptor antagonist, BMS-182874, reduces acute hypoxic pulmonary hypertension in pigs in vivo. Cardiovasc Res 37:765, 1998.
15. Christou H, Yoshida A, Arthur V, et al: Increased vascular endothelial growth factor production in the lungs of rats with hypoxia-induced pulmonary hypertension. Am J Respir Cell Mol Biol 18:768, 1998.
16. Partovian C, Adnot S, Eddahibi S, et al: Heart and lung VEGF mRNA expression in rats with monocrotaline- or hypoxia-induced pulmonary hypertension. Am J Physiol 275:H1948, 1998.
17. Semenza GL, Agani F, Iyer N, et al: Hypoxia-inducible factor 1: From molecular biology to cardiopulmonary physiology. Chest 114:40S, 1998.
18. Naeije R: Pulmonary circulation at high altitude. Respiration 64:429, 1997.
19. Davila-Roman VG, Guest TM, Tuteur PG, et al: Transient right but not left ventricular dysfunction after strenuous exercise at high altitude. J Am Coll Cardiol 30:468, 1997.
20. Cacciapuoti F, D'Avino M, Lama D, et al: Hemodynamic changes in pulmonary circulation induced by effort in the elderly. Am J Cardiol 71:1481, 1993.
21. Vane JR, Anggard EE, Botting RM: Regulatory functions of the vascular endothelium. N Engl J Med 323:27, 1990.
22. Murtha YM, Allen BM, Orr JA: The role of protein kinase C in thromboxane A2-induced pulmonary artery vasoconstriction. J Biomed Sci 6:293, 1999.
23. Cooper CJ, Landzberg MJ, Anderson TJ, et al: Role of nitric oxide in the local regulation of pulmonary vascular resistance in humans. Circulation 93:266, 1996.
24. Cooper CJ, Jevnikar FW, Walsh T, et al: The influence of basal nitric oxide activity on pulmonary vascular resistance in patients with congestive heart failure. Am J Cardiol 82:609, 1998.
25. Bouloumie A, Schini-Kerth VB, Busse R: Vascular endothelial growth factor upregulates nitric oxide synthase expression in endothelial cells. Cardiovasc Res 41:773, 1999.
26. Cacoub P, Dorent R, Nataf P, et al: Endothelin-1 in the lungs of patients with pulmonary hypertension. Cardiovasc Res 33:196, 1997.
27. Gray MO, Long CS, Kalinyak JE, et al: Angiotensin II stimulates cardiac myocyte hypertrophy via paracrine release of TGF-beta 1 and endothelin-1 from fibroblasts. Cardiovasc Res 40:352, 1998.
28. Wort S, Woods M, Warner T, et al: Endogenously released endothelin-1 from human pulmonary artery smooth muscle promotes cellular proliferation. Am J Respir Cell Mol Biol 25:104, 2001.
29. Dupuis J, Jasmin J, Prie S, Cernacek P: Importance of local production of endothelin-1 and of the ET_B receptor in the regulation of pulmonary vascular tone. Pulm Pharmacol Therap 13:135, 2000.
30. Rubens C, Ewert R, Halank M, et al: Big endothelin-1 and endothelin-1 plasma levels are correlated with the severity of primary pulmonary hypertension. Chest 120:1562, 2001.
31. Peifley K, Winkles J: Angiotensin II and endothelin-1 increase fibroblast growth factor-2 mRNA expression in vascular smooth muscle cells. Biochem Biophys Res Commun 242:202, 1998.
32. Fanburg B, Lee S:A new role for an old molecule: Serotonin as a mitogen. Am J Physiol 272:L795, 1997.
33. Eddahibi S, Hanoun N, Lanfumey L, et al: Attenuated hypoxic pulmonary hypertension in mice lacking the 5-hydroxytryptamine transporter gene. J Clin Invest 105:1555, 2000.
34. MacLean MR, Herve P, Eddahibi S, Adnot S: 5-hydroxytryptamine and the pulmonary circulation: Receptors, transporters and relevance to pulmonary arterial hypertension. Br J Pharmacol 131:161, 2000.
35. Schuster DP, Crouch EC, Parks WC, et al: Angiotensin converting enzyme expression in primary pulmonary hypertension. Am J Respir Crit Care Med 154:1087, 1996.
36. Okada K, Bernstein ML, Zhang W, et al: Angiotensin-converting enzyme inhibition delays pulmonary vascular neointimal formation. Am J Respir Crit Care Med 158:939, 1998.

37. Morrell NW, Atochina EN, Morris KG, et al: Angiotensin converting enzyme expression is increased in small pulmonary arteries of rats with hypoxia-induced pulmonary hypertension. J Clin Invest 96:1823, 1995.

Clinical Assessment of the Patient with Suspected Pulmonary Hypertension

38. Noutens M, Wolfkiel CJ, Chemka EV, et al: Understanding right and left ventricular systolic function and interactions at rest and with exercise in primary pulmonary hypertension. Am J Cardiol 73:379, 1995.
39. Wolf M, Boyer-Neumann C, Parent F, et al: Thrombotic risk factors in pulmonary hypertension. Eur Respir J 15:395, 2000.
40. Nagaya N, Nishikimi T, Okano Y, et al: Plasma brain natriuretic peptide levels increase in proportion to the extent of right ventricular dysfunction in pulmonary hypertension. J Am Coll Cardiol 31:202, 1998.
41. Wada A, Tsutamato T, Maeda Y, et al: Endogenous atrial natriuretic peptide inhibits endothelin-1 secretion in dogs with severe congestive heart failure. Am J Physiol 270:H1819, 1996.
42. Nagaya N, Uematsu M, Satoh T, et al: Serum uric acid levels correlate with the severity and the mortality of primary pulmonary hypertension. Am J Respir Crit Care Med 160:487, 1999.
43. Behar JV, Howe CM, Wagner NB, et al: Performance of new criteria for right ventricular hypertrophy and myocardial infarction in patients with pulmonary hypertension due to cor pulmonale and mitral stenosis. J Electrocardiol 24:231, 1991.
44. Zompatori M, Battaglia M, Rimondi M, et al: Hemodynamic estimation of chronic cor pulmonale by Doppler echocardiography. Clinical value and comparison with other noninvasive imaging techniques. Rays 22:73, 1997.
45. Raymond RJ, Hinderliter AL, Willis PW, et al: Echocardiographic predictors of adverse outcomes in primary pulmonary hypertension. J Am Coll Cardiol 39:1214, 2002.
46. McQuillan B, Picard M, Leavitt M, Weyman A: Clinical correlates and reference intervals for pulmonary artery systolic pressure among echocardiographically normal subjects. Circulation 104:2797, 2001.
47. Jain D, Zaret B: Assessment of right ventricular function: Role of nuclear imaging techniques. Cardiol Clin 10:23, 1992.
48. Steen VD, Graham G, Conte C, et al: Isolated diffusing capacity reduction in systemic sclerosis. Arthritis Rheum 35:765, 1992.
49. Butler J, Chomsky D, Wilson J: Pulmonary hypertension and exercise intolerance in patients with heart failure. J Am Coll Cardiol 34:1802, 1999.
50. Wax D, Garofano R, Barst R: Effects of long-term infusion of prostacyclin on exercise performance in patients with primary pulmonary hypertension. Chest 116:914, 1999.
51. Sun X-G, Hansen J, Oudiz R, Wasserman K: Exercise pathophysiology in patients with primary pulmonary hypertension. Circulation 104:429, 2001.
52. Myers J, Gullestad L, Vagelos R, et al: Clinical, hemodynamic, and cardiopulmonary exercise test determinants of survival in patients referred for evaluation of heart failure. Ann Intern Med 129:286, 1998.
53. Nootens M, Schrader B, Kaufmann E, et al: Comparative acute effects of adenosine and prostacyclin in primary pulmonary hypertension. Chest 107:54, 1995.
54. Raffy O, Azarian R, Brenot F, et al: Clinical significance of the pulmonary vasodilator response during short-term infusion of prostacyclin in primary pulmonary hypertension. Circulation 93:484, 1996.
55. Ricciardi MJ, Knight BP, Martinez FJ, Rubenfire M: Inhaled nitric oxide in primary pulmonary hypertension: A safe and effective agent for predicting response to nifedipine. J Am Coll Cardiol 32:1068, 1998.
56. Krasuski R, Warner J, Wang A, et al: Inhaled nitric oxide selectively dilates pulmonary vasculature in adult patients with pulmonary hypertension, irrespective of etiology. J Am Coll Cardiol 36:2204, 2000.
57. Mitchell H, Bolster MB, LeRoy EC: Scleroderma and related conditions. Med Clin North Am 81:129, 1997.

Primary Pulmonary Hypertension

58. Brickner M, Hillis L, Lange R: Congenital heart disease in adults: First of two parts. N Engl J Med 342:256, 2000.
59. Abenhaim L, Moride Y, Brenot F, et al: Appetite-suppressant drugs and the risk of primary pulmonary hypertension. N Engl J Med 335:609, 1996.
60. Botney MD, Liptay MJ, Kaiser LR, et al: Active collagen synthesis by pulmonary arteries in human primary pulmonary hypertension. Am J Pathol 143:121, 1993.
61. Higenbottam TW, Laude EA: Endothelial dysfunction providing the basis for the treatment of pulmonary hypertension. Chest 114(Suppl):72, 1998.
62. Giaid A, Saleh D: Reduced expression of endothelial nitric oxide synthase in the lungs of patients with pulmonary hypertension. N Engl J Med 333:214, 1995.
63. Giaid A: Nitric oxide and endothelin-1 in pulmonary hypertension. Chest 114(Suppl):208, 1998.
64. Stewart DJ, Levy RD, Cernacek P, Langleben D: Increased plasma endothelin-1 in pulmonary hypertension: Marker or mediator of disease? Ann Intern Med 114:464, 1991.
65. Lindner V, Lappi DA, Baird A, et al: Role of basic fibroblast growth factor in vascular lesion formation. Circ Res 68:106, 1991.
66. Botney MD, Bahadori L, Gold LI: Vascular remodeling in primary pulmonary hypertension. Potential role for transforming growth factor-beta. Am J Pathol 144:286, 1994.
67. Welsh CH, Hassell KL, Badesch DB, et al: Coagulation and fibrinolytic profiles in patients with severe pulmonary hypertension. Chest 110:710, 1996.
68. Morse JH, Barst RJ, Fotino M, et al: Primary pulmonary hypertension, tissue plasminogen activator antibodies, and HLA-DQ7. Am J Respir Crit Care Med 155:274, 1997.
69. Ware JA, Helstad DD: Platelet-endothelium interactions. N Engl J Med 328:628, 1993.
70. Nakonechnicov S, Gabbasov Z, Chazova I, et al: Platelet aggregation in patients with primary pulmonary hypertension. Blood Coagul Fibrinolysis 7:225, 1996.
71. Botney MD: Role of hemodynamics in pulmonary vascular remodeling: Implications for primary pulmonary hypertension. Am J Respir Crit Care Med 159:361, 1999.
72. Rabinovitch M: Insights into the pathogenesis if primary pulmonary hypertension from animal models. *In* Rubin LJ, Rich S (ed): Primary Pulmonary Hypertension. New York, Marcel Dekker, 1997, pp 63-82.
73. Rabinovitch M: Elastase and the pathobiology of unexplained pulmonary hypertension. Chest 114:213, 1998.
74. Yuan JX, Aldinger AM, Juhaszova M, et al: Dysfunctional voltage-gated K^+ channels in pulmonary artery smooth muscle cells of patients with primary pulmonary hypertension. Circulation 98:1400, 1998.
75. Tuder R, Cool C, Geraci M, et al: Prostacyclin synthase expression is decreased in lungs from patients with severe pulmonary hypertension. Am J Respir Crit Care Med 159:1925, 1999.
76. Breuer J, Georgaraki A, Sieverding L, et al: Increased turnover of serotonin in children with pulmonary hypertension secondary to congenital heart disease. Pediatr Cardiol 17:214, 1996.
77. Herve P, Launay JM, Scrobohaci ML, et al: Increased plasma serotonin in primary pulmonary hypertension. Am J Med 99:249, 1995.
78. Loyd JE, Newman JH: Familial primary pulmonary hypertension. *In* Rubin LJ, Rich S (ed). Primary Pulmonary Hypertension. New York, Marcel Dekker, 1997, pp 151-162.
79. Barst R, Loyd JE: Genetics and immunogenetic aspects of primary pulmonary hypertension. Chest 114(Suppl):231, 1998.
80. Deng Z, Haghighi F, Helleby L, et al: Fine mapping of *PPH1*, a gene for familial primary pulmonary hypertension, to a 3-cM region on chromosome 2q33. Am J Respir Crit Care Med 161:1055, 2000.
81. Morse JH, Jones AC, Barst RJ, et al: Mapping of familial primary pulmonary hypertension locus (*PPH1*) to chromosome 2q31-q32. Circulation 95:2603, 1997.
82. Newman J, Wheeler L, Lane K, et al: Mutation in the gene for bone morphogenetic protein receptor II as a cause of primary pulmonary hypertension in a large kindred. N Engl J Med 345:319, 2001.
83. Rudarakanchana N, Flanagan J, Chen H, et al: Functional analysis of bone morphogenetic protein type II receptor mutations underlying primary pulmonary hypertension. Hum Mol Genet 11:1517, 2002.
84. Atkinson C, Stewart S, Upton PD, et al: Primary pulmonary hypertension is associated with reduced pulmonary vascular expression of type II bone morphogenetic protein receptor. Circulation 105:1672, 2002.
85. Eddahibi S, Humbert M, Fadel E, et al: Serotonin transporter overexpression is responsible for pulmonary artery smooth muscle hyperplasia in primary pulmonary hypertension. J Clin Invest 108:1141, 2001.
86. Eddahibi S, Humbert M, Fadel E, et al: Hyperplasia of pulmonary artery smooth muscle in primary and secondary pulmonary hypertension is causally related to serotonin transporter overexpression. Am J Respir Crit Care Med 165:A97, 2002.
87. Lesch K-P, Engel D, Heils A, et al: Association of anxiety-related traits with a polymorphism in the serotonin transporter gene regulatory region. Science 274:1527, 1996.
88. Voelkel NF, Tuder RM, Weir EK: Pathophysiology of primary pulmonary hypertension: From physiology to molecular mechanisms. *In* Rubin LJ, Rich S (ed): Primary Pulmonary Hypertension. New York, Marcel Dekker, 1997, pp 83-129.
89. Lee SD, Shroyer KR, Markham NE, et al: Monoclonal endothelial cell proliferation is present in primary but not secondary pulmonary hypertension. J Clin Invest 101:927, 1998.
90. Tuder R: Plexiform lesions in primary pulmonary hypertension may represent an abnormal form of angiogenesis. Semin Respir Crit Care Med 15:207, 1994.
91. Tuder RM, Groves B, Badesch DB, Voelkel NF: Exuberant endothelial cell growth and elements of inflammation are present in plexiform lesions of pulmonary hypertension. Am J Pathol 144:275, 1994.
92. Wagenvoort CA, Mulder PG: Thrombotic lesions in primary plexogenic arteriopathy: Similar pathogenesis or complication? Chest 103:844, 1993.
93. Nagaya N, Satoh T, Ishida Y, et al: Impaired left ventricular myocardial metabolism in patients with pulmonary hypertension detected by radionuclide imaging. Nucl Med Commun 18:1171, 1997.
94. Patrat JF, Jondeau G, Dubourg O, et al: Left main coronary artery compression during primary pulmonary hypertension. Chest 112:842, 1997.
95. Kawut SM, Silvestry FE, Ferrari VA, et al: Extrinsic compression of the left main coronary artery by the pulmonary artery in patients with long-standing pulmonary hypertension. Am J Cardiol 83:984, A10, 1999.
96. Weiss BM, Zemp L, Seifert B, Hess OM: Outcome of pulmonary vascular disease in pregnancy: A systematic overview from 1978 through 1996. J Am Coll Cardiol 31:1650, 1998.
97. Rich S, Seidlitz M, Dodin E, et al: The short-term effects of digoxin in patients with right ventricular dysfunction from pulmonary hypertension. Chest 114:787, 1998.
98. Weber K: Aldosterone in congestive heart failure. N Engl J Med 345:1689, 2001.
99. Rich S, Kaufmann E, Levy PS: The effect of high doses of calcium-channel blockers on survival in primary pulmonary hypertension. N Engl J Med 327:76, 1992.
100. Barst RJ, Rubin LJ, Long WA, et al: A comparison of continuous intravenous epoprostenol (prostacyclin) with conventional therapy for primary pulmonary hypertension. The Primary Pulmonary Hypertension Study Group. N Engl J Med 334:296, 1996.
101. Barst RJ, Maislin G, Fishman AP: Vasodilator therapy for primary pulmonary hypertension in children. Circulation 99:1197, 1999.
102. Shapiro SM, Oudiz RJ, Cao T, et al: Primary pulmonary hypertension: Improved long-term effects and survival with continuous intravenous epoprostenol infusion. J Am Coll Cardiol 30:343, 1997.
103. McLaughlin VV, Genthner DE, Panella MM, Rich S: Reduction in pulmonary vascular resistance with long-term epoprostenol (prostacyclin) therapy in primary pulmonary hypertension. N Engl J Med 338:273, 1998.
104. Rich S, McLaughlin V: The effects of chronic prostacyclin therapy on cardiac output and symptoms in primary pulmonary hypertension. J Am Coll Cardiol 34:1184, 1999.

105. Robbins IM, Christman BW, Newman JH, et al: A survey of diagnostic practices and the use of epoprostenol in patients with primary pulmonary hypertension. Chest 114:1269, 1998.
106. Sitbon O, Humbert M, Nunes H, et al: Long-term intravenous epoprostenol infusion in primary pulmonary hypertension. J Am Coll Cardiol 40:780, 2002.
107. McLaughlin V, Shillington A, Rich S: Survival in primary pulmonary hypertension. The impact of epoprostenol therapy. Circulation 106:1477, 2002.
108. McLaughlin V, Gaine S, Barst R, et al: Efficacy and safety of treprostinil: An epoprostenol analog for primary pulmonary hypertension. J Cardiovasc Pharmacol 41:293, 2003.
109. Simonneau G, Barst RJ, Galie N, et al: Continuous subcutaneous infusion of treprostinil, a prostacyclin analogue, in patients with pulmonary arterial hypertension: A double-blind, randomized, placebo-controlled trial. Am J Respir Crit Care Med 165:800, 2002.
110. Hoeper M, Schwarze M, Ehlerding S, et al: Long-term treatment of primary pulmonary hypertension with aerosolized iloprost, a prostacyclin analogue. N Engl J Med 342:1866, 2000.
111. Olschewski H, Simonneau G, Galie N, et al: Inhaled iloprost for severe pulmonary hypertension. N Engl J Med 347:322, 2002.
112. Galie N, Humber M, Vachiery J-L, et al: Effects of beraprost sodium, an oral prostacyclin analogue, in patients with pulmonary arterial hypertension: A randomized, double-blind, placebo-controlled trial. J Am Coll Cardiol 39:1496, 2002.
113. Barst RJ, McGoon M, McLaughlin VV, et al: Beraprost therapy for pulmonary arterial hypertension. J Am Cell Cardiol 41:2119, 2003.
114. Channick R, Simonneau G, Sitbon O, et al: Effects of the dual endothelin-receptor antagonist bosentan in patients with pulmonary hypertension: A randomised placebo-controlled study. Lancet 358:1119, 2001.
115. Rubin L, Badesch D, Barst R, et al: Bosentan therapy for pulmonary arterial hypertension. N Engl J Med 346:896, 2002.
116. Barst RJ, Langleben D, Frost A, et al: Sitaxsentan therapy for pulmonary arterial hypertension. Am J Respir Crit Care Med 169:441, 2004.
117. Michelakis E, Tymchak W, Lien D, et al: Oral sildenafil is an effective and specific pulmonary vasodilator in patients with pulmonary arterial hypertension. Circulation 105:2398, 2002.
118. Ghofrani H, Wiedemann R, Rose F, et al: Sildenafil for treatment of lung fibrosis and pulmonary hypertension: A randomised controlled trial. Lancet 360:895, 2002.
119. Sitbon O, Humbert M, Simonneau G: Primary pulmonary hypertension: Current therapy. Prog Cardiovasc Dis 45:115, 2002.
120. Wilkens H, Guth A, Konig J, et al: Effect of inhaled iloprost plus oral sildenafil in patients with primary pulmonary hypertension. Circulation 104:1218, 2001.
121. Wensel R, Opitz C, Anker S, et al: Assessment of survival in patients with primary pulmonary hypertension. Circulation 106:319, 2002.
122. Ghofrani HA, Rose F, Schermuly RT, et al: Oral sildenafil as long-term adjunct therapy to inhaled iloprost in severe pulmonary arterial hypertension. J Am Coll Cardiol 42:158, 2003.
123. Rich S, Dodin E, McLaughlin VV: Usefulness of atrial septostomy as a treatment for primary pulmonary hypertension and guidelines for its application. Am J Cardiol 80:369, 1997.
124. Arcasoy SM, Kotloff RM: Lung transplantation. N Engl J Med 340:1081, 1999.
125. Trulock EP: Lung transplantation. Am J Respir Crit Care Med 155:789, 1997.
126. Maurer JR, Frost AE, Estenne M, et al: International guidelines for the selection of lung transplant candidates. Transplantation 66:951, 1998.
127. Rich S, McLaughlin VV: Lung transplantation for pulmonary hypertension: Patient selection and maintenance therapy while awaiting transplantation. Semin Thorac Cardiovasc Surg 10:135, 1998.

Pulmonary Arterial Hypertension with Associated Conditions

128. Sundaresan S: The impact of bronchiolitis obliterans on late morbidity and mortality after single and bilateral lung transplantation for pulmonary hypertension. Semin Thorac Cardiovasc Surg 10:152, 1998.
129. Okura H, Takatsu Y: High-output heart failure as a cause of pulmonary hypertension. Intern Med 33:363, 1994.
130. Clabby ML, Canter CE, Moller JH, Bridges ND: Hemodynamic data and survival in children with pulmonary hypertension. J Am Coll Cardiol 30:554, 1997.
131. Hopkins WE, Ochoa LL, Richardson GW, Trulock EP: Comparison of the hemodynamics and survival of adults with severe primary pulmonary hypertension or Eisenmenger syndrome. J Heart Lung Transplant 15:100, 1996.
132. Vongpatanasin W, Brickner ME, Hillis LD, Lange RA: The Eisenmenger syndrome in adults. Ann Intern Med 128:745, 1998.
133. McLaughlin VV, Genthner DE, Panella MM, et al: Compassionate use of continuous prostacyclin in the management of secondary pulmonary hypertension: A case series. Ann Intern Med 130:740, 1999.
134. Rosenzweig EB, Kerstein D, Barst RJ: Long-term prostacyclin for pulmonary hypertension with associated congenital heart defects. Circulation 99:1858, 1999.
135. Palevsky HI, Gurughagavatula I: Pulmonary hypertension in collagen vascular disease. Compr Ther 25:133, 1999.
136. Badesch DB, Tapson VF, McGoon MD, et al: Continuous intravenous epoprostenol for pulmonary hypertension due to the scleroderma spectrum of disease: A randomized controlled trial. Ann Intern Med 132:425, 2000.
137. Lange PA, Stoller JK: The hepatopulmonary syndrome. Ann Intern Med 122:521, 1995.
138. Kuo PC, Plotkin JS, Johnson LB, et al: Distinctive clinical features of portopulmonary hypertension. Chest 112:980, 1997.
139. Herve P, Lebrec D, Brenot F, et al: Pulmonary vascular disorders in portal hypertension. Eur Respir J 11:1153, 1998.
140. Kuo P: Pulmonary hypertension: Considerations in the liver transplant candidate. Transpl Int 9:141, 1996.
141. Schott R, Chaouat A, Launoy A, et al: Improvement of pulmonary hypertension after liver transplantation. Chest 115:1748, 1999.
142. Humbert M, Monti G, Fartoukh M, et al: Platelet-derived growth factor expression in primary pulmonary hypertension: Comparison of HIV seropositive and HIV seronegative patients. Eur Respir J 11:554, 1998.
143. Opravil M, Pechere M, Speich R, et al: HIV-associated primary pulmonary hypertension. A case control study. Swiss HIV Cohort Study. Am J Respir Crit Care Med 155:990, 1997.
144. Simonneau G, Fartoukh M, Sitbon O, et al: Primary pulmonary hypertension associated with the use of fenfluramine derivatives. Chest 114(Suppl):195, 1998 .
145. Rich S, Rubin L, Walker AM, et al: Anorexigens and pulmonary hypertension in the United States: Results from the surveillance of North American pulmonary hypertension. Chest 117:870, 2000.
146. Weir EK, Reeve HL, Huang JM, et al: Anorexic agents aminorex, fenfluramine, and dexfenfluramine inhibit potassium current in rat pulmonary vascular smooth muscle and cause pulmonary vasoconstriction. Circulation 94:2216, 1996.
147. Archer SL, Djaballah K, Humbert M, et al: Nitric oxide deficiency in fenfluramine- and dexfenfluramine-induced pulmonary hypertension. Am J Respir Crit Care Med 158:1061, 1998.
148. Rich S, Shillington A, McLaughlin V: Comparison of survival in patients with pulmonary hypertension associated with fenfluramine to patients with primary pulmonary hypertension. Am J Cardiol 92:1366, 2003.
149. Hulsmann AR, van den Anker JN: Evolution and natural history of chronic lung disease of prematurity. Monaldi Arch Chest Dis 52:272, 1997.
150. Langer JC: Congenital diaphragmatic hernia. Chest Surg Clin North Am 8:295, 1998.
151. Roberts JD Jr, Fineman JR, Morin FC III, et al: Inhaled nitric oxide and persistent pulmonary hypertension of the newborn. N Engl J Med 336:605, 1997.
152. Steinhorn RH, Cox PN, Fineman JR, et al: Inhaled nitric oxide enhances oxygenation but not survival in infants with alveolar capillary dysplasia. J Pediatr 130:417, 1997.
153. Valdes L, Gonzalez-Juanatey JR, Alvarez D, et al: Diagnosis of pulmonary veno-occlusive disease: New criteria for biopsy. Respir Med 92:979, 1998.
154. Masur Y, Remberger K, Hoefer M: Pulmonary capillary hemangiomatosis as a rare cause of pulmonary hypertension. Pathol Res Pract 192:290, discussion 296, 1996.
155. Lippert JL, White CS, Cameron EW, et al: Pulmonary capillary hemangiomatosis: Radiographic appearance. J Thorac Imaging 13:49, 1998.
156. Dufour B, Maitre S, Humbert M, et al: High-resolution CT of the chest in four patients with pulmonary capillary hemangiomatosis or pulmonary venoocclusive disease. AJR Am J Roentgenol 171:1321, 1998.
157. Humbert M, Maitre S, Capron F, et al: Pulmonary edema complicating continuous intravenous prostacyclin in pulmonary capillary hemangiomatosis. Am J Respir Crit Care Med 157:1681, 1998.

Pulmonary Hypertension Associated with Disorders of the Respiratory System

158. American Thoracic Society: Standards for the diagnosis and care of patients with chronic obstructive disease [official statement]. Am J Respir Crit Care Med 152:S77, 1995.
159. Siafakas NM, Vermeire P, Pride NB, et al: Optimal assessment and management of chronic obstructive pulmonary disease (COPD). European Respiratory Society Task Force. Eur Respir J 8:1398, 1995.
160. British Thoracic Society Group of the Standards of Care Committee: BTS guidelines for the management of chronic obstructive pulmonary disease. COPD Guidelines Group of the Standards of Care Committee of the BTS. Thorax 52:S1, 1997.
161. Pauwels RA, Buist AS, Calverley PM, et al: Global strategy for the diagnosis, management, and prevention of chronic obstructive pulmonary disease. NHLBI/WHO Global Initiative for Chronic Obstructive Lung Disease (GOLD) Workshop summary. Am J Respir Crit Care 163:1256, 2001.
162. Sherrill DL, Lebowitz MD, Burrows B: Epidemiology of chronic obstructive pulmonary disease. Clin Chest Med 11:375, 1990.
163. Barnes PJ: Mechanisms in COPD: Differences from asthma. Chest 117:10S, 2000.
164. Saetta M, Di Stefano A, Turato G, et al: CD8+ T-lymphocytes in peripheral airways of smokers with chronic obstructive pulmonary disease. Am J Respir Crit Care Med 157:822, 1998.
165. Saetta M, Di Stefano A, Maestrelli P, et al: Airway eosinophilia in chronic bronchitis during exacerbations. Am J Respir Crit Care Med 150:1646, 1994.
166. Keatings VM, Collins PD, Scott DM, et al: Differences in interleukin-8 and tumor necrosis factor-alpha in induced sputum from patients with chronic obstructive pulmonary disease or asthma. Am J Respir Crit Care Med 153:530, 1996.
167. Stockley RA: Neutrophils and protease/antiprotease imbalance. Am J Respir Crit Care Med 160:S49, 1999.
168. Shapiro SD, Senior RM: Matrix metalloproteinases: Matrix degradation and more. Am J Respir Cell Mol Biol 20:1100, 1999.
169. Repine JE, Bast A, Lankhorst I: Oxidative stress in chronic obstructive pulmonary disease. Oxidative Stress Study Group. Am J Respir Crit Care Med 156:341, 1997.
170. Di Francia M, Barbier D, Mege JL, et al: Tumor necrosis factor-alpha levels and weight loss in chronic obstructive pulmonary disease. Am J Respir Crit Care Med 150:1453, 1994.
171. Schols AM, Buurman WA, Staal van den Brekel AJ, et al: Evidence for a relation between metabolic derangements and increased levels of inflammatory mediators in a subgroup of patients with chronic obstructive pulmonary disease. Thorax 51:819, 1996.
172. Schols AM, Creutzberg EC, Buurman WA, et al: Plasma leptin is related to proinflammatory status and dietary intake in patients with chronic obstructive pulmonary disease. Am J Respir Crit Care Med 160:1220, 1999.
173. Sin DD, Man SF: Why are patients with chronic obstructive pulmonary disease at increased risk of cardiovascular diseases? The potential role of systemic inflammation in chronic obstructive pulmonary disease. Circulation 107:1514, 2003.

174. Arcasoy SM, Christie JD, Ferrari VA, et al: Echocardiographic assessment of pulmonary hypertension in patients with advanced lung disease. Am J Respir Crit Care Med 167:735, 2003.
175. Scharf SM, Iqbal M, Keller C, et al: Hemodynamic characterization of patients with severe emphysema. Am J Respir Crit Care Med 166:314, 2002.
176. Stevens D, Sharma K, Rich S, et al: Severe pulmonary hypertension associated with COPD. [abstract]. Am J Respir Crit Care Med 159:A155, 1999.
177. Weitzenblum E, Hirth C, Ducolone A, et al: Prognostic value of pulmonary artery pressure in chronic obstructive pulmonary disease. Thorax 36:752, 1981.
178. Piccioni P, Caria E, Bignamini E, et al: Predictors of survival in a group of patients with chronic airflow obstruction. J Clin Epidemiol 51:547, 1998.
179. Dallari R, Barozzi G, Pinelli GP, et al: Predictors of survival in subjects with chronic obstructive pulmonary disease treated with long-term oxygen therapy. Respiration 61:8, 1994.
180. Braghiroli A, Zaccaria S, Ioli F, et al: Pulmonary failure as a cause of death in COPD. Monaldi Arch Chest Dis 52:170, 1997.
181. Filipecki S, Kober J, Kaminski D, Tomowsi W: Pulmonary thromboembolism. Monaldi Arch Chest Dis 52:492, 1997.
182. Anthonisen N, Connett J, Kiley J, et al: Effects of smoking intervention and the use of an inhaled anticholinergic bronchodilator on the rate of decline of FEV_1: The Lung Health Study. JAMA 272:1497, 1994.
183. Lancaster T, Stead L, Silagy C, Sowden A: Effectiveness of interventions to help people stop smoking: Findings from the Cochrane Library. BMJ 321:355, 2000.
184. Jorenby DE, Leischow SJ, Nides MA, et al: A controlled trial of sustained-release bupropion, a nicotine patch, or both for smoking cessation. N Engl J Med 340:685, 1999.
185. Griffiths TL, Burr ML, Campbell IA, et al: Results at 1 year of outpatient multidisciplinary pulmonary rehabilitation: A randomised controlled trial. Lancet 355:362, 2000.
186. The COMBIVENT Inhalation Solution Study Group: Routine nebulized ipratropium and albuterol together are better than either alone in COPD. Chest 112:1514, 1997.
187. Gross N, Tashkin D, Miller R, et al: Inhalation by nebulization of albuterol-ipratropium combination (Dey combination) is superior to either agent alone in the treatment of chronic obstructive pulmonary disease. Dey Combination Solution Study Group. Respiration 65:354, 1998.
188. The Lung Health Study Research Group: Effect of inhaled triamcinolone on the decline in pulmonary function in chronic obstructive pulmonary disease. N Engl J Med 343:1902, 2000.
189. Nocturnal Oxygen Therapy Trial Group: Continuous or nocturnals oxygen therapy in hypoxemic chronic obstructive lung disease. Ann Intern Med 93:931, 1980.
190. Ashutosh K, Mead G, Dunsky M: Early effects of oxygen administration and prognosis in chronic obstructive pulmonary disease and cor pulmonale. Am Rev Respir Dis 127:399, 1983.
191. Dewan NA, Bell CW: Effect of low flow and high flow oxygen delivery on exercise tolerance and sensation of dyspnea: A study comparing the transtracheal catheter and nasal prongs. Chest 105:1061, 1994.
192. Meduri GU, Abou-Shala N, Fox RC, et al: Noninvasive face mask mechanical ventilation in patients with acute hypercapnic respiratory failure. Chest 100:445, 1991.
193. Soguel Schenkel N, Burdet L, de Muralt B, et al: Oxygen saturation during daily activities in chronic obstructive pulmonary disease. Eur Respir J 9:2584, 1996.
194. Antonelli M, Conti G, Rocco M, et al: A comparison of noninvasive positive-pressure ventilation and conventional mechanical ventilation in patients with acute respiratory failure. N Engl J Med 339:429, 1998.
195. Meecham Jones DJ, Paul EA, Jones PW, et al: Nasal pressure support ventilation plus oxygen compared with oxygen therapy alone in hypercapnic COPD. Am J Respir Crit Care Med 152:538, 1995.
196. National Emphysema Treatment Trial Research Group: A randomized trial comparing lung-volume-reduction surgery with medical therapy for severe emphysema. N Engl J Med 348:2059, 2003.
197. National Emphysema Treatment Trial Research Group: Patients at high risk of death after lung-volume-reduction surgery. N Engl J Med 345:1075, 2001.
198. Trulock EP, Edwards LB, Taylor DO, et al: The registry of the International Society for Heart and Lung Transplantation: Twentieth official adult lung and heart-lung transplant report-2003. J Heart Lung Transplant 22:625, 2003.
199. Lynch JP, Trulock EP: Lung transplantation in chronic airflow limitation. Med Clin North Am 80:657, 1996.
200. Low DE, Trulock EP, Kaiser LR, et al: Morbidity, mortality, and early results of single versus bilateral lung transplantation for emphysema. J Thorac Cardiovasc Surg 103:1119, 1992.
201. Katzenstein AL, Myers JL: Idiopathic pulmonary fibrosis: Clinical relevance of pathologic classification. Am J Respir Crit Care Med 157:1301, 1998.
202. Ryu JH, Colby TV, Hartman TE: Idiopathic pulmonary fibrosis: Current concepts. Mayo Clin Proc 73:1085, 1998.
203. Idiopathic pulmonary fibrosis: Diagnosis and treatment: International consensus statement. Am J Respir Crit Care Med 161:646, 2000.
204. Coffey MJ, FitzGerald MX, McNicholas WT: Comparison of oxygen desaturation during sleep and exercise in patients with cystic fibrosis. Chest 100:659, 1991.
205. Fraser KL, Tullis DE, Sasson Z, et al: Pulmonary hypertension and cardiac function in adult cystic fibrosis: Role of hypoxemia. Chest 115:1321, 1999.
206. Marrone O, Bonsignore MR: Pulmonary hemodynamics in obstructive sleep apnea. Sleep Med Rev 6:175, 2002.
207. Sajkov D, Wang T, Saunders NA, et al: Continuous positive airway pressure treatment improves pulmonary hemodynamics in patients with obstructive sleep apnea. Am J Resp Crit Care Med 165:152, 2002.
208. Leger P: Long-term noninvasive ventilation for patients with thoracic cage abnormalities. Respir Care Clin North Am 2:241, 1996.
209. Simonda A: Nasal intermittent positive pressure ventilation in neuromuscular and chest wall disease. Monaldi Arch Chest Dis 48:156, 1993.
210. Robert D, Gerard M, Leger P, et al: Domiciliary ventilation by tracheostomy for chronic respiratory failure. Rev Fr Mal Respir 11:923, 1983.
211. Faul JL, Ruoss S, Doyle RL, Kao PN: Diaphragmatic paralysis due to Lyme disease. Eur Respir J 13:700, 1999.
212. De Vito EL, Quadrelli SA, Montiel GC, Roncoroni AJ: Bilateral diaphragmatic paralysis after mediastinal radiotherapy. Respiration 63:187, 1996.
213. Gierada D, Slone R, Fleishman M: Imaging evaluation of the diaphragm. Chest Surg Clin North Am 8:237, 1998.
214. Lin MC, Liaw MY, Huang CC, et al: Bilateral diaphragmatic paralysis: A rare cause of acute respiratory failure managed with nasal mask bilevel positive airway pressure (BiPAP) ventilation. Eur Respir J 10:1922, 1997.

Pulmonary Hypertension due to Chronic Thrombotic or Embolic Obstruction of the Pulmonary Arteries

215. Wolf M, Boyer-Neumann C, Parent F, et al: Thrombotic risk factors in pulmonary hypertension. Eur Respir J 15:395, 2000.
216. Moser KM, Auger WR, Fedullo PF, Jamieson SW: Chronic thromboembolic pulmonary hypertension: Clinical picture and surgical treatment. Eur Respir J 5:334, 1992.
217. Auger WR, Moser KM: Pulmonary flow murmurs: A distinctive physical sign found in chronic pulmonary thromboembolic disease. Clin Res 37:145A, 1989.
218. Ryan KL, Fedullo PF, Davis GB, et al: Perfusion scan findings understate the severity of angiographic and hemodynamic compromise in chronic thromboembolic pulmonary hypertension. Chest 93:1180, 1988.
219. Auger WR, Fedullo PF, Moser KM, et al: Chronic major-vessel thromboembolic pulmonary artery obstruction: Appearance at angiography. Radiology 182:393, 1992.
220. Pitton MB, Duber C, Mayer E, Thelen M: Hemodynamic effects of nonionic contrast bolus injection and oxygen inhalation during pulmonary angiography in patients with chronic major-vessel thromboembolic pulmonary hypertension. Circulation 94:2485, 1996.
221. King M, Ysrael M, Bergin C: Chronic thromboembolic pulmonary hypertension: CT findings. AJR Am J Roentgenol 170:955, 1998.
222. Daily PO, Dembitsky WP, Iversen S, et al: Risk factors for pulmonary thromboendarterectomy. J Thorac Cardiovasc Surg 99:670, 1990.
223. Jamieson SW, Kapelanski DP: Pulmonary endarterectomy. Curr Probl Surg 37:165, 2000.
224. Thistlethwaite PA, Mo M, Madani MM, et al: Operative classification of thromboembolic disease determines outcome after pulmonary endarterectomy. J Thorac Cardiovasc Surg 124:1203, 2002.
225. Thistlethwaite PA, Mo M, Madani MM, et al: Operative classification of thromboembolic disease determines outcome after pulmonary endarterectomy. J Thorac Cardiovasc Surg 124:1203, 2002.
226. Mayer E, Dahm M, Hake U, et al: Mid-term results of pulmonary thromboendarterectomy for chronic thromboembolic pulmonary hypertension. Ann Thorac Surg 61:1788, 1996.
227. Ono F, Nagaya N, Okumura H, et al: Effect of orally active prostacyclin analogue on survival in patients with chronic thromboembolic pulmonary hypertension without major vessel obstruction. Chest 123:1583, 2003.
228. Ghofrani HA, Schermuly RT, Rose F, et al: Sildenafil for long-term treatment of nonoperable chronic thromboembolic pulmonary hypertension. Am J Respir Crit Care Med 167:1139, 2003.
229. Norris SL, Johnson C, Haywood LJ: Left ventricular filling pressure in sickle cell anemia. J Assoc Acad Minor Phys 3:20, 1992.

Pulmonary Hypertension due to Disorders Directly Affecting the Pulmonary Vasculature

230. Yung GL, Channick RN, Fedullo PF, et al: Successful pulmonary thromboendarterectomy in two patients with sickle cell disease. Am J Respir Crit Care Med 157:1690, 1998.
231. Morris W, Knauer CM: Cardiopulmonary manifestations of schistosomiasis. Semin Respir Infect 12:159, 1997.
232. Barbosa MM, Lamounier JA, Oliveira EC, et al: Pulmonary hypertension in schistosomiasis mansoni. Trans R Soc Trop Med Hyg 90:663, 1996.
233. Sheffield EA: Pathology of sarcoidosis. Clin Chest Med 18:741, 1997.
234. Nagai S, Shigematsu M, Hamada K, Izumi T: Clinical courses and prognoses of pulmonary sarcoidosis. Curr Opin Pulm Med 5:293, 1999.
235. Lynch JP 3rd, Kazerooni EA, Gay SE: Pulmonary sarcoidosis. Clin Chest Med 18:755, 1997.
236. Mana J, Badrinas F: Prognosis of sarcoidosis: An unresolved issue. Sarcoidosis 9:15, 1992.

CHAPTER 68

Sleep Disorders and Cardiovascular Disease

Meir H. Kryger

There is a complex interaction between the cardiovascular system and sleep. Sleep disorders, such as sleep apnea, can cause abnormal cardiovascular function and disease; cardiovascular disease, for example, congestive heart failure (see Chap. 21), can cause a sleep disorder. In addition, some cardiovascular disorders seem to be linked to a specific sleep state or time of day, such as coronary vasoconstriction (see Chap. 17) occurring during rapid eye movement sleep, and sudden death (see Chap. 33) occurring in the early morning hours during awakening. In this chapter, the most common sleep problems likely to be encountered by a cardiologist in clinical practice are reviewed, including obstructive sleep apnea syndrome and Cheyne-Stokes respiration. Cardiac physiology and pathophysiology during sleep and less common cardiovascular problems that are impacted by sleep and its disorders are reviewed elsewhere.[1]

Sleep Physiology

Using neurophysiological monitoring, sleep is divided into two types: (1) rapid eye movement (REM) sleep, which makes up about one-fourth of the night in young adults and (2) non-rapid eye movement (NREM) sleep, which makes up the remaining three-fourths.[2] During REM sleep, which is the time of the most intense dreaming, monitoring reveals that people are not moving and there are at times marked increases in activity in certain parts of the brain and brain stem. When the increased activity is in the region of the oculomotor nuclei, then the REMs occur. Because there are more abnormal cardiovascular events in REM than NREM sleep, it is possible that when the increased activity passes through the parts of the nervous system that control the cardiovascular system, instability in cardiovascular function might occur. NREM sleep is subdivided, again based on neurophysiological criteria, into stage 1 sleep, a transition between wakefulness and deeper sleep, which makes up in normal subjects roughly 5 percent of the night; stage 2 sleep, determined by the presence of characteristic waves (spindles and K complexes), which makes up half of the night; and stages 3 and 4, that together are often called *slow-wave sleep*, or *delta sleep*, which make up roughly a quarter of the night. During NREM sleep, most physiological functions appear to be normally controlled except for a dip in blood pressure that can occur with a transition from wakefulness to sleep. Thereafter, blood pressure and heart rate and rhythm do not vary a great deal unless an arousal (a brief awakening) occurs.

In contrast to the tight regulation in NREM sleep, during REM sleep, control of many physiological control systems, for example cardiovascular regulation and thermoregulation, may be more erratic (e.g., variability in heart rate and blood pressure), or virtually absent (e.g., thermoregulation). Superimposed on the change in physiology directly related to the sleep state are time-related changes in physiological systems, whether the person is awake or asleep. These are the circadian influences. For example, there appear to be circadian influences on myocardial ischemic threshold that are present even during the awake state (see Chap. 44). This circadian effect may explain the increased propensity to develop adverse cardiovascular events at certain times of the day. For example, even though one would expect the reduction in demands on the cardiovascular system during sleep to markedly reduce cardiovascular events, 20 percent of myocardial infarctions (see Chap. 46), 15 percent of sudden deaths (see Chap. 33), and 29 percent of episodes of atrial fibrillation (see Chap. 32) occur between midnight and 6:00 AM. Over the 24-hour period new onset of myocardial infarction, sudden cardiac death, and thrombotic stroke are most likely to occur between early and mid-morning.[3] Thus, abnormal cardiovascular physiology can be impacted by sleep state, circadian rhythm, and sleep pathology.

Types of Sleep Apnea

Sleep apnea refers to the cessation of breathing during sleep. In one type of apnea, *obstructive apnea*, the cessation is caused by obstruction in the upper airway. In *central apnea*, the cessation of breathing is caused by a reduction of impulses from the central nervous system to the muscles of respiration. Some patients have features of both. Cardiologists are likely to encounter many patients with sleep apnea in their practice. Obstructive sleep apnea is a common condition that causes cardiovascular morbidity. Cheyne-Stokes respiration, a form of central sleep apnea, is found in about 40 percent of cases of heart failure.

Obstructive Sleep Apnea Syndrome

Obstructive sleep apnea syndrome is characterized by repetitive upper airway obstruction during sleep, resulting in profound effects on cardiovascular function, gas exchange, and continuity of sleep. These in turn result in important clinical consequences that affect several organ systems (especially the cardiovascular system) and create a poor quality of life.

Epidemiology and Risk Factors

Obstructive sleep apnea occurs in all age groups and both genders.[4,5] Although it was previously believed that sleep apnea was rare in women, it is now thought to be much more common in that group. It has been estimated that 4 percent of adult men and 2 percent of adult women have obstructive sleep apnea syndrome. It has been estimated that 1 to 3 percent of children have sleep apnea, with the most common etiology being adenotonsillar hypertrophy. The mean age of presentation in adults in most series is between 48 and 51 years. Any disorder that can compromise the upper airway, including obesity, retrognathia (mandible too far posterior), micrognathia (small mandible), mass lesions in the airway, or nasal obstruction, can lead to obstructive sleep apnea syndrome. About 70 to 80 percent of adults with obstructive sleep apnea syndrome have obesity as the main cause of their problem.

Physiological Changes during Sleep in Obstructive Sleep Apnea

When patients with obstructive sleep apnea stop breathing during sleep, a reduction in arterial oxygen saturation (SaO_2) occurs, along with activation of the sympathetic and parasympathetic nervous systems. The episodes of sleep apnea by definition exceed 10 seconds in duration and, in our laboratory, average about 25 seconds in NREM sleep and about 35 seconds in REM sleep. On the average, patients spend 20 percent of sleep time with an SaO_2 of less than 90 percent.

CARDIAC RHYTHM. The changes in autonomic nervous system activity result in a slowing of the heart rate during the episodes of apnea and a speeding up of the heart rate once breathing resumes. Cardiac arrhythmias (see Chap. 32) are much more common in those patients who have more severe sleep apnea as measured by the apnea/hypopnea index, which is the number of abnormal breathing events per hour of sleep. The most common arrhythmias seen are bradyarrhythmias and ventricular extrasystoles.[6,7] In one series, almost 80 percent of cases had some rhythm abnormality, and 18 percent had a clinically significant abnormal rhythm including recurrent sinus pauses, asystolic periods lasting 6 seconds or longer, or ventricular extrasystoles.[7] The ventricular arrhythmias are not usually related to bradycardia and may be most frequent during the most severe hypoxemia. The bradyarrhythmias are likely related to increased vagal tone since they have been reported to be reversed by atropine and are more common during REM sleep.[6] Patients with the rhythms just mentioned, in whom the diagnosis of sleep apnea–induced bradyarrhythmia is not apparent, may end up having unnecessary cardiac pacemakers inserted and are best treated with continuous positive airway pressure (CPAP).[8] In cardiac disease patients who are at high risk for arrhythmias and have a low left ventricular ejection fraction (LVEF) (see later), coexistent sleep apnea increases the risk of ventricular arrhythmias.[9]

BLOOD PRESSURE. Systemic blood pressure increases during the apneic episodes, although in elderly patients the blood pressure may fall.[10] Pulmonary artery pressure can also increase in the presence of severe hypoxemia and some patients can develop cor pulmonale (see Chap. 67).[11-13]

VENTILATION. In the most severe cases, the abnormalities in ventilation during sleep can partially persist into the wakefulness period and patients can develop awake-hypoventilation documented by an elevated PCO_2. The combination of awake-respiratory failure, cor pulmonale, and obesity is the hallmark of the obesity-hypoventilation syndrome previously called *Pickwickian syndrome* (see Chap. 67).[13] Obesity does not have to be present for hypoventilation to occur in people with upper airway obstruction; hypoventilation causing right-sided cardiac failure has been described, for example, in children with enlarged tonsils. Some patients with obesity-hypoventilation syndrome do not actually develop apnea during sleep but instead have continuous hypoventilation with severe hypoxemia during wakefulness and sleep.[13]

AROUSALS. To resume unobstructed breathing, patients have a neurological arousal (a brief awakening), which results in an increase in the tone of the upper airway dilating muscles; this has the effect of opening the obstructed or occluded airway. These arousals result in markedly abnormal sleep structure; in particular, most patients have a decrease or absence of slow wave sleep and a reduction in REM sleep, which lead to the most common symptom—excessive daytime sleepiness.

Daytime Clinical Consequences of Sleep Apnea

Sleep apnea has its major clinical effects on the neurological and cardiovascular systems. The abnormal sleep causes severe daytime sleepiness and, in some patients, impaired daytime cognitive function. The latter may be responsible for an increased automobile accident rate.[14-16] Sleep apnea is associated with systemic hypertension (see Chap. 37), pulmonary hypertension (see Chap. 67), ischemic heart disease (see Chap. 46), and heart failure and stroke.[17-20] There is now no doubt that sleep apnea is a risk factor for systemic hypertension independent of age, gender, and body mass index.[20,21] Patients with sleep apnea are two or three times more likely than control groups to have arterial hypertension and are two or three times more likely to be treated with antihypertensive medications.[19,22] Patients with "idiopathic" hypertension are highly likely to include a substantial proportion of patients with obstructive sleep apnea, and this is particularly true in patients whose hypertension is resistant to therapy or difficult to control.[23] *Therefore, the clinical cardiologist should consider sleep apnea in the evaluation of hypertensive patients.*

Clinical Features

The most common presenting symptoms found in patients with obstructive sleep apnea include excessive daytime sleepiness, snoring, and the observation by others that the patient stops breathing during sleep. In most patients the snoring and observed apneas are present most nights. Other common symptoms in these patients include awakening with headache, sensation of choking, poor memory and concentration, and poor performance at work. There is frequently an associated history of arterial hypertension, and a previous history of depression and hypothyroidism are common, especially in women.[24]

Diagnosis

Patients with suspected obstructive sleep apnea syndrome should receive an overnight sleep study that has sufficient channels to be able to confirm the presence and type (central versus obstructive) of apnea, oxygenation, and sleep structure (Fig. 68–1). The latter measurement is particularly important because some patients, particularly women, can have a mild variant of obstructive sleep apnea called *upper airway resistance syndrome* in which the obstructions to inspiration are not sufficiently severe or long to be classed as an apnea (by definition 10 seconds), but would be sufficiently severe to disrupt sleep quality and result in many of the earlier mentioned pathophysiology and symptoms.

As part of the sleep evaluation, if a sleep breathing disorder is confirmed, the patient will also be studied using a ventilatory assist device, either CPAP or bilevel positive airway pressure (BiPAP) to determine the optimal settings for the equipment. These devices can stent the airway open and thus prevent the episodes of obstruction.

Indications for Treatment

It is recommended that all patients with polysomnographically proven obstructive sleep apnea with an apnea/hypopnea index exceeding 20 be treated, since that level of apnea has been associated with an increased death rate without treatment. Because hypertension has been associated with an apnea/hypopnea index higher than 15, some have recommended that patients be treated if the apnea/hypopnea index exceeds this level. Many authorities also recommend treating patients who have a proven apnea/hypopnea index higher than 5, if in addition they have known complications attributable to sleep apnea, including excessive daytime sleepiness and cardiovascular disease (Table 68–1). U.S. government guidelines for reimbursement for CPAP by Medicare and Medicaid Services in the United States have recently changed to reflect this latter indication.[25]

THERAPY. The principles of treatment of obstructive sleep apnea are first to reduce the risk factors, and then if a specific anatomic cause of the apnea is found, to treat that abnormality if possible and, if no abnormality is found, to use a ventilatory assistance device to reverse the obstruction (Fig. 68–2).

General Measures. Since 70 to 80 percent of obstructive sleep apnea patients are obese, weight loss is a critical component of any treatment plan for the obese patient. Because many of the patients also have hypertension and diabetes (see Chap. 40), this approach should help those conditions as well. Patients do not have to achieve their ideal weight for the apnea to resolve most of the time. It seems as though for many patients there is a threshold, and once the threshold is reached, the apnea improves dramatically even though they may continue to still snore and to be overweight.

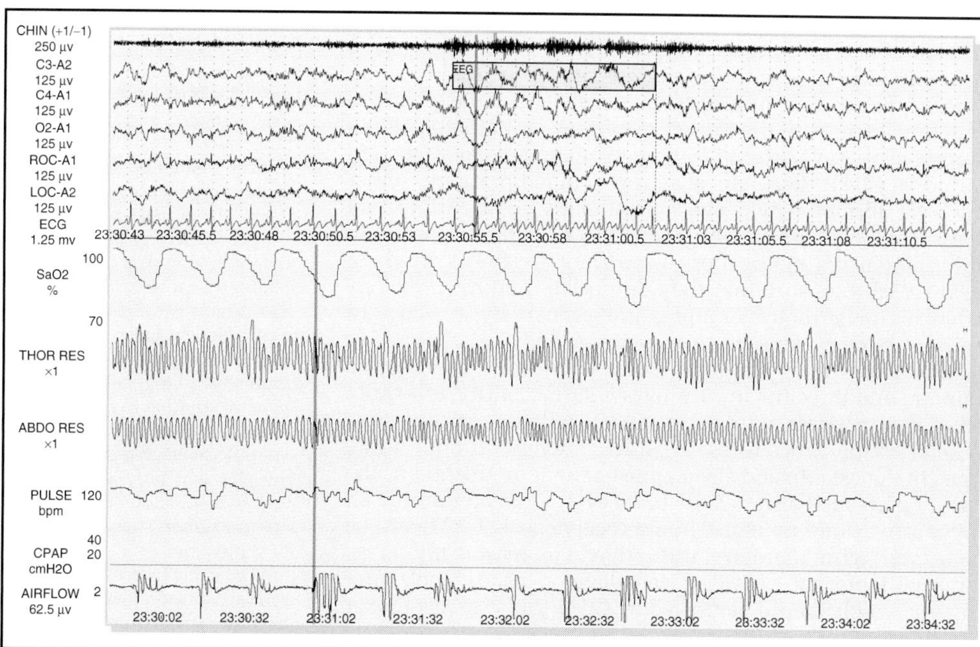

FIGURE 68–1 This is a fragment of an overnight sleep study from a patient with severe obstructive sleep apnea syndrome. The top seven channels represent about 30 seconds of data and show the information used to stage sleep and the electrocardiogram (ECG). The top channel is the chin electromyogram; the next three are used for the electroencephalogram (EEG), the next two for eye movements, followed by the ECG. The bottom six channels represent about 5 minutes of data and show the information used to document apnea type. The channels from top to bottom are oxyhemoglobin saturation (SaO_2), thoracic movement (THOR RES), abdominal movement (ABDO RES), pulse rate (bpm), continuous positive airway pressure (CPAP), and nasal airflow. There are 14 apneic episodes in this segment. The episodes are associated with efforts to breathe seen in the chest wall and abdomen, but notice the intermittent cessation of airflow in the bottom channel. The vertical blue line in each segment corresponds to an identical moment in time. Notice that resumption of breathing occurs right after an arousal on EEG (the yellow box). Also note the marked variability in pulse rate.

Avoidance of Alcohol and Sedatives. Because alcohol can make a patient much more sleepy and dramatically worsen the episodes of apnea, patients should be encouraged to avoid drinking alcohol. The same advice can be given about the use of hypnotic or sedative drugs.

Specific Anatomical Treatment. If nasal obstruction or anatomical obstruction of the pharyngeal airway caused by lesions such as enlarged tonsils are present, the patient should be referred to a specialist to assess them to see whether they are candidates for surgical treatment. If the patient has significant retrognathia or micrognathia, the patient may benefit from the use of an oral appliance worn at night, which brings the lower jaw upward and forward. Sometimes the patient can benefit from reconstructive surgery of the mandible.

TABLE 68–1 Indications for CPAP Treatment

Treatment is indicated if either of the following criteria* is met:

AHI ≥ 15 events per hr

or

AHI ≥ 5 and ≤14 events per hr with documented symptoms of excessive daytime sleepiness, impaired cognition, mood disorders or insomnia, or documented hypertension, ischemic heart disease, or history of stroke

AHI = apnea/hypopnea index; CPAP = continuous positive airway pressure.

*If these criteria are met, CPAP therapy will be covered under Medicare in adult patients with obstructive sleep apnea. See http://cms.hhs.gov/mcd/index_list.asp?list_type=ncd for complete description at medicare coverage in the List of National Coverage Determinations.

Ventilatory Assist Devices. CPAP and BiPAP are the most widely used treatments and the treatment of first choice in patients with obstructive sleep apnea syndrome. The principle of these devices is that the positive pressure splints the pharyngeal airway open, counteracting its tendency to collapse during inspiration. The treatment is usually highly effective, although compliance appears to be between 50 and 70 percent, which is probably comparable to that of many other medical treatments. Treatment with nasal CPAP has been shown to improve quality of life, cognitive function, and arterial hypertension.[26-29]

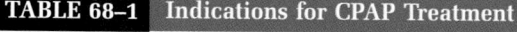

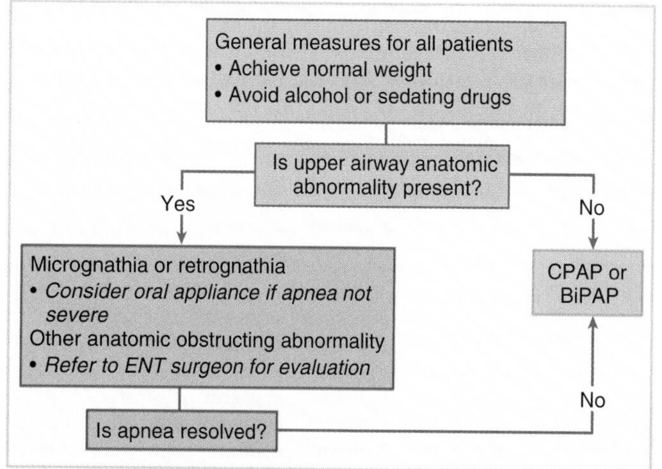

FIGURE 68–2 Approach to treatment of typical obstructive sleep apnea syndrome. ENT = ear, nose, throat; CPAP = continuous positive airway pressure; BiPAP = bilevel positive airway pressure.

Additional Issues of Particular Interest to Cardiologists. Arrhythmias and arterial hypertension were mentioned earlier. Difficult-to-control hypertension can be due to sleep apnea.[30] Thus it is appropriate to ask about sleep apnea symptoms in newly diagnosed hypertensive patients. When patients who have arterial hypertension and sleep apnea are started on CPAP, there can be a drop in blood pressure, sometimes to normotensive levels. Clinicians should routinely measure blood pressure in hypertensive patients receiving antihypertensive medication when they are first started on nasal CPAP to ensure that they do not become hypotensive. If they do lower their blood pressure excessively, a change in their antihypertensive drugs may be needed.

Anesthesia and Surgery. Because sleep apnea is so common and it results in cardiovascular morbidity, it is quite likely that patients with sleep apnea will undergo cardiac catheterization procedures or cardiac surgery. In both situations, in the established sleep apnea patient on treatment, the use of opiate analgesia results in an even more compromised upper airway and patients should receive nasal CPAP and be monitored with oximetry until they are reasonably alert. Some patients not on CPAP can develop heart block after surgery, which should be treated by CPAP and not pacemaker insertion.[31]

Patients who have had coronary artery bypass grafting (see Chap. 50) or other surgical procedures involving the chest can have a great deal of pain at the incision site when continued on nasal CPAP in the postoperative period. Such patients may benefit from switching (at least temporarily) from a CPAP to a BiPAP system. With the latter modality of airway support, in which the pressure during inspiration is higher than during expiration, patients find the application of pressure less painful, in our experience.

Sleep Abnormalities in Patients with Left Ventricular Cardiac Failure (Central Sleep Apnea)

In 1818, Cheyne first described repetitive cycles of apneas followed by hyperpneas in what is now called *Cheyne-Stokes respiration*.[32] Although this form of central apnea, characterized by a waxing and waning of ventilation, occurs in other conditions, such as after some cerebrovascular accidents, renal disease, and exposure to high altitude, it is generally most often linked to left ventricular cardiac failure (see Chap. 21). Cheyne-Stokes respiration in heart failure can cause sleep-onset insomnia and paroxysmal nocturnal dyspnea and treatment of the heart failure can ameliorate the breathing pattern.[33] More recent studies have shown that although Cheyne-Stokes respiration is by far the most common abnormal breathing pattern in heart failure, a significant number of patients have obstructive sleep apnea as their primary sleep breathing problem. In this section we focus primarily on Cheyne-Stokes respiration.

EPIDEMIOLOGY. About 40 percent of all the heart failure patients with an LVEF less than 0.45 have been reported to have Cheyne-Stokes respiration, whereas 10 percent have obstructive sleep apnea.[34] Those with obstructive sleep apnea were more obese and were more likely to have a snoring history. The consequences (apnea/hypopnea index, number of arousals per hour of sleep, and degree of hypoxemia) were similar in those with central or obstructive sleep apnea. Risk factors for Cheyne-Stokes respiration in heart failure include male gender, age older than 60 years, the presence of atrial fibrillation, and hypocapnia.[35] The presence of Cheyne-Stokes respiration is an indicator of poor prognosis.[36]

PATHOPHYSIOLOGY. Many theories and models have been proposed to explain the mechanisms that start and maintain the Cheyne-Stokes respiration pattern in left ventricular failure.[37] These mechanisms include heightened ventilatory response to carbon dioxide, alkalemia, prolonged circulation time, and effect of sleep state, all of which alone or in combination can be used to explain a periodic breathing pattern. Cheyne-Stokes respiration decreases during REM sleep, the time when chemical control of breathing is the most blunted, suggesting that chemical drives are necessary to perpetuate the abnormal breathing pattern. Sleep is not a necessary condition for Cheyne-Stokes respiration since it can occur during wakefulness.

The breathing pattern in Cheyne-Stokes respiration can be almost monotonously repetitive over long periods of time. Cheyne-Stokes respiration is present in the average patient with left-sided heart failure about half the night and might even be present while the patient is awake. Some trigger starts and another stops this breathing pattern. What seems to trigger Cheyne-Stokes respiration is an event that initially destabilizes breathing, perhaps a sigh, a deep breath, or an arousal. One can hypothesize that in response to the event, a temporary hyperventilation results in hypocapnia, which is sensed by the chemical ventilatory control system, which results in a reduction in output to the respiratory muscles, which then results in hypoventilation or apnea. Once Cheyne-Stokes respiration starts, it is perpetuated by the chemical ventilatory control systems that lead to repetitive overshooting and undershooting of ventilation.

The cycle time of the Cheyne-Stokes breathing pattern seems related to the circulation time. It has been predicted in models and shown in experiments that cycle time (the time between peaks of hyperpnea) is roughly four times the circulation time and therefore people with severe heart failure and a long circulation time will have a long cycle time. Thus, it is as though the breathing pattern goes on "autopilot." The breathing pattern normalizes when the main perpetuating factor, the ventilatory control of breathing, becomes blunted, as occurs during REM sleep.

One would expect that all patients with very low LVEF would have Cheyne-Stokes respiration, but this is not the case. Some patients with very low LVEFs do not have Cheyne-Stokes respiration, whereas some with LVEFs higher than 0.40 might have Cheyne-Stokes respiration. Thus, it is not the ejection fraction *per se* that determines whether Cheyne-Stokes respiration will be present but rather an interaction of the pathogenic mechanisms mentioned earlier.

PHYSIOLOGICAL CONSEQUENCES OF CHEYNE-STOKES RESPIRATION

Arousals. When Cheyne-Stokes respiration occurs at sleep onset, the episodes of decreased ventilation or apnea can cause an arousal. Thus, patients with Cheyne-Stokes respiration frequently complain of insomnia and have difficulty falling asleep.

Arousals from sleep are common with Cheyne-Stokes respiration. The arousals typically occur not at the end of apnea, which is the situation in patients with obstructive sleep apnea, but instead during the peak of hyperpnea. Not all episodes of Cheyne-Stokes breathing are associated with an arousal, however. The arousals are believed to be related to the increased work of breathing during the peak of hyperpnea.

Hypoxemia. Hypoxemia commonly occurs with Cheyne-Stokes respiration, and the lowest oxygen saturation occurring in a cycle usually coincides with the peak of hyperpnea. This is quite different from the situation in obstructive sleep apnea during which the lowest oxygen saturations are found immediately before breathing resumes. The reason why oxygen saturation is lowest when the patient is breathing the most, rather than at the end of the apneic episodes, is because patients with heart failure usually have a prolonged circulation time, and once breathing resumes, it takes longer for oxygenated blood to go from the lungs to peripheral tissues.

Additional Physiological Changes. There can be a substantial oscillation in systemic blood pressure[38] in association with Cheyne-Stokes respiration. The hypoxemia, and the increased systemic blood pressure, likely place an important burden on an already compromised cardiovascular system, whereas the changes in the central nervous system can lead to cognitive impairment.

CLINICAL FEATURES. The most common symptom of patients with Cheyne-Stokes respiration, besides the symptoms of the underlying cardiovascular disease, is severe insomnia, which can be of the sleep-onset type (i.e., an inability to fall asleep) as well as the sleep maintenance type (i.e., difficulty staying asleep). The insomnia can be particularly stressing for the patient because they can, in addition, have severe sleepiness. Thus, they can have the combination of being quite sleepy yet being unable to fall or stay asleep.

When patients with Cheyne-Stokes respiration awaken during the night, sometimes at the end of a long apneic episode, they can have severe shortness of breath consistent with paroxysmal nocturnal dyspnea (see Chap. 22). Severe cough and unpleasant dreams can precede these episodes of nocturnal dyspnea.[39] Some patients are short of breath when lying flat, and the shortness of breath can be relieved somewhat on sitting up or using several pillows (orthopnea). Some patients complain of symptoms consistent with angina pectoris that might awaken them.

Some patients also have a movement disorder that can lead to the symptoms of restless legs syndrome and periodic contractions of some muscle groups during sleep. This can also contribute to the sleeplessness of some of the patients. During the daytime the patients may complain of severe daytime sleepiness and may have markedly impaired cognitive function.

CLINICAL ASSESSMENT. All patients with heart disease should be asked about symptoms of sleep disorders. These questions should include how long it takes the patients to fall asleep, how often they wake up during sleep, have they been observed to snore, have they been observed to stop breathing during sleep, and do they have symptoms of paroxysmal nocturnal dyspnea, orthopnea, or angina. We have found, in our own practice, that some patients who do not normally have nocturia can have significant nocturia on nights in which they develop an arrhythmia (e.g., sustained atrial fibrillation). Some patients have palpitations that awaken them.

MANAGEMENT OF HEART FAILURE. With improvement in heart failure, Cheyne-Stokes respiration can resolve.[33] The cornerstone of management is the treatment of the heart failure (see Chap. 23); nocturnal symptoms can be a marker that the heart failure may not be under optimal control.

If, with what is considered to be optimal heart failure control, the patient still has symptoms of disturbed sleep (sleep-onset or sleep-maintenance insomnia), the patient should have a comprehensive overnight sleep study—polysomnography.

DIAGNOSIS. Polysomnography can be extremely helpful in deciding on treatment (Fig. 68–3). The sleep study should confirm that an abnormal breathing pattern is present and should be able to distinguish the reduced respiratory efforts in Cheyne-Stokes respiration from the findings seen in obstructive apnea. About 80 percent of heart failure patients with a sleep breathing problem have the findings of Cheyne-Stokes respiration, whereas 20 percent have the obstructive type. Many such patients also have periodic movements in sleep, which may also be a factor in disrupting sleep. The sleep study should also be able to yield information about the severity of hypoxemia, whether cardiac arrhythmias are present, and the extent of sleep disruption.

Our practice is to perform a split-night study in which patients have a baseline assessment for 3 to 4 hours so the diagnosis can be documented, followed by application of treatment for the remainder of the night. If Cheyne-Stokes respiration is confirmed, we first start the patient on oxygen at roughly 2 to 3 liters/min to assess its impact on the breathing pattern. If the patient has an element of obstructive sleep apnea, we would instead assess the patient using nasal CPAP or BiPAP.

Studying a patient who is still recovering from a bout of heart failure may not help in determining optimal treatment. The sleep evaluation should occur when the patient is on optimal treatment and stable. We do not recommend screening studies in this situation. Oximetry alone or many screening systems cannot differentiate apnea type (central or obstructive) and cannot determine whether a patient is actually sleeping, and they do not store the electrocardiogram.

TREATMENT OF ABNORMAL SLEEP BREATHING PATTERN. Treatment of sleep breathing abnormalities in heart failure (Fig. 68–4) is an area of great current research interest. If the patient is found to have obstructive sleep apnea (which is present in about 10 percent of heart failure patients), then CPAP treatment as outlined earlier should be instituted.

Administration of nocturnal oxygen,[40,41] nasal CPAP or BiPAP,[42-45] or more complex ventilatory assist modes[46] have

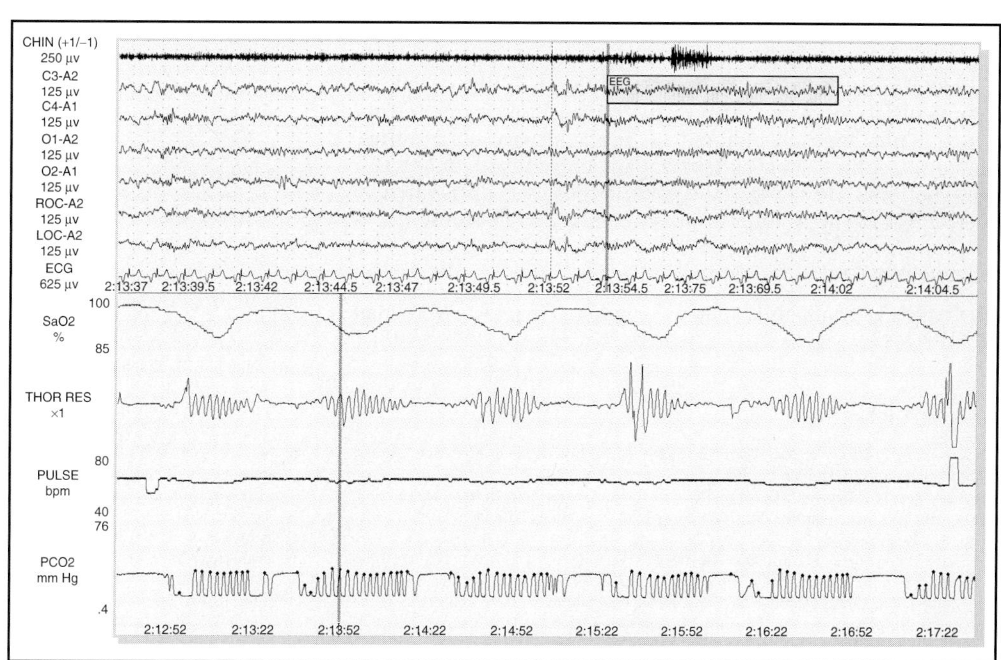

FIGURE 68–3 This is a fragment of an overnight sleep study from a patient with severe left ventricular failure who eventually had a heart transplant. The top eight channels represent about 30 seconds of data and show the information used to stage sleep and the electrocardiogram. The top channel is the chin electromyogram; the next four are used for the electroencephalogram (EEG), the next two for eye movements, followed by the electrocardiogram. The bottom four channels represent about 5 minutes of data and show the information used to document apnea type. The channels from top to bottom are oxyhemoglobin saturation, thoracic movement, pulse rate, and oronasal P_{CO_2} (see the Fig. 68–1 legend for abbreviations). There are six apneic episodes in this segment of Cheyne-Stokes respiration. Note the hyperpneas following each apnea. The apneic episodes are associated with decreased or absent efforts to breathe seen in the chest wall, and notice the intermittent cessation of airflow in the bottom channel. The vertical blue line in each segment corresponds to an identical moment in time. Notice that resumption of breathing occurs before an arousal on EEG (the yellow box), and that the nadir of Sa_{O_2} occurs during the peak of hyperpnea. Also note the lack of variability in pulse rate.

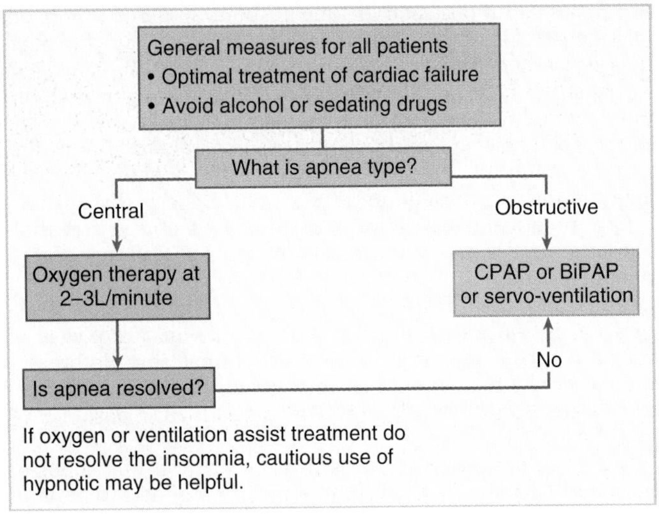

General measures for all patients
• Optimal treatment of cardiac failure
• Avoid alcohol or sedating drugs

What is apnea type?

Central → Oxygen therapy at 2–3L/minute

Obstructive → CPAP or BiPAP or servo-ventilation

Is apnea resolved? No →

If oxygen or ventilation assist treatment do not resolve the insomnia, cautious use of hypnotic may be helpful.

FIGURE 68–4 Approach to treatment of sleep disorders in left ventricular failure. CPAP = continuous positive airway pressure; BiPAP = bilevel positive airway pressure.

been suggested, and positive short-term results have been reported with them. In those patients who have obstructive sleep apnea, CPAP reduces daytime systolic blood pressure, heart rate, and the left ventricular end-systolic dimension and improves the LVEF.[42] In patients with heart failure and central apnea, CPAP and BiPAP may improve cardiac function by reducing afterload, and ongoing clinical trials will help determine the role of these treatments in the treatment of heart failure. Until long-term outcome trials are developed, the clinician must weigh the following factors in determining treatment choices: patient comfort and acceptance of treatment, response to treatment, and what is available in the local medical community.

If drug therapy with hypnotic agents is contemplated, published studies to date suggest that there is little risk of hypoventilation in patients with Cheyne-Stokes respiration who do not have an element of upper airway obstruction. Benzodiazepines such as temazepam may improve sleep in these patients. However, if the patient does have upper airway obstruction, using hypnotics may worsen the obstruction.

Acknowledgment

Dr. Kryger's work on this chapter was supported in part by NIH Grant R01 HL63342-01A1.

REFERENCES

1. Kryger M, Roth T, Dement WC: Principles and Practice of Sleep Medicine. 4th ed. Philadelphia, WB Saunders, 2004.
2. Carskadon MA, Dement WC: Normal human sleep: An overview. *In* Kryger M, Roth T, Dement WC: Principles and Practice of Sleep Medicine. 4th ed. Philadelphia, WB Saunders, 2004 (in press).
3. Verrier R: Sleep-related cardiovascular risk. *In* Kryger M, Roth T, Dement WC: Principles and Practice of Sleep Medicine. 4th ed. Philadelphia, WB Saunders, 2004 (in press).
4. Young T, Peppard PE, Gottlieb DJ: Epidemiology of obstructive sleep apnea: A population health perspective. Am J Respir Crit Care Med 165:1217-1239, 2002.
5. Kapsimalis F, Kryger MH: Gender and obstructive sleep apnea syndrome: I. Clinical features. Sleep 25:412-419, 2002.
6. Koehler U, Becker HF, Grimm W, et al: Relations among hypoxemia, sleep stage, and bradyarrhythmia during obstructive sleep apnea. Am Heart J 139:142-148, 2000.
7. Harbison J, O'Reilly P, McNicholas WT: Cardiac rhythm disturbances in the obstructive sleep apnea syndrome. Chest 118:591-595, 2000.
8. Stegman SS, Burroughs JM, Henthorn RW: Asymptomatic bradyarrhythmias as a marker of sleep apnea: Appropriate recognition and treatment may reduce the need for pacemaker therapy. Pacing Clin Electrophysiol 19:899-904, 1996.
9. Fichter J, Bauer D, Arampatzis S, et al: Sleep-related breathing disorders are associated with ventricular arrhythmias in patients with an implantable cardioverter-defibrillator. Chest 122:558-561, 2002.
10. Weiss JW, Launois SH, Anand A, Garpestad E: Cardiovascular morbidity in obstructive sleep apnea. Prog Cardiovasc Dis 41:367-376, 1999.
11. Sajkov D, Wang T, Saunders NA, et al: Continuous positive airway pressure treatment improves pulmonary hemodynamics in patients with obstructive sleep apnea. Am J Respir Crit Care Med 165:152-158, 2002.
12. Kessler R, Chaouat A, Weitzenblum E, et al: Pulmonary hypertension in the obstructive sleep apnea syndrome: Prevalence, causes, and therapeutic consequences. Eur Respir J 9:787-794, 1996.
13. Kessler R, Chaouat A, Schinkewitch P, et al: The obesity-hypoventilation syndrome revisited: A prospective study of 34 consecutive cases. Chest 120:369-376, 2001.
14. Roth T, Roehrs TA: Etiologies and sequelae of excessive daytime sleepiness. Clin Ther 18:562-576, 1996.
15. Naegele B, Pepin J-L, Levy P, et al: Cognitive executive dysfunction in patients with obstructive sleep apnea syndrome (OSAS) after CPAP treatment. Sleep 21:392-397, 1998.
16. George CF, Smiley A: Sleep apnea and automobile crashes. Sleep 22:790-795, 1999.
17. Smith R, Ronald J, Delaive K, et al: What are obstructive sleep apnea patients being treated for prior to this diagnosis? Chest 121:164-172, 2002.
18. Shamsuzzaman AB, Somers VK: Fibrinogen, stroke and obstructive sleep apnea: An evolving paradigm of cardiovascular risk. Am J Respir Crit Care Med 162:2018-2020, 2000.
19. D'Alessandro R, Magelli C, Gamberini G, et al: Snoring every night as a risk factor for myocardial infarction: A case control study. BMJ 300:1557-1558, 1990.
20. Nieto FJ, Young TB, Lind BK, et al: Association of sleep disordered breathing, sleep apnea, and hypertension in a large community-based study: Sleep Heart Health Study. JAMA 283:1829-1836, 2000.
21. Peppard PE, Young T, Palta M, Skatrud J: Prospective study of the association between sleep-disordered breathing and hypertension. N Engl J Med 342:1378-1384, 2000.
22. Otake K, Delaive K, Walld R, et al: Cardiovascular medication use in patients with undiagnosed obstructive sleep apnoea. Thorax 57:417-422, 2002.
23. Logan AG, Perlikowski SM, Mente A, et al: High prevalence of unrecognized sleep apnoea in drug-resistant hypertension. J Hypertens 19:2271-2277, 2001.
24. Shepertycki M, Kryger M: Effect of gender on clinical features of OSAS. Sleep 26:A221, 2004.
25. Web site for the List of National Coverage Determinations [NCDs] in the Indexes for the Medicare Coverage Databases. On the site, scroll down to "continuous positive airway pressure" (http://cms.hhs.gov/mcd/index_list.asp?list_type=ncd).
26. Engleman HM, Kingshott RN, Wraith PK, et al: Randomized placebo-controlled crossover trial of continuous positive airway pressure for mild sleep apnea/hypopnea syndrome. Am J Respir Crit Care Med 159:461-467, 1999.
27. Redline S, Adams N, Strauss ME, et al: Improvement of mild sleep-disordered breathing with CPAP compared with conservative therapy. Am J Respir Crit Care Med 157:858-865, 1998.
28. Faccenda JF, Mackay TW, Boon NA, Douglas NJ: Randomized placebo-controlled trial of continuous positive airway pressure on blood pressure in the sleep apnea-hypopnea syndrome. Am J Respir Crit Care Med 163:344-348, 2001.
29. White J, Cates C, Wright J: Continuous positive airways pressure for obstructive sleep apnoea. Cochrane Database Syst Rev CD001106, 2002.
30. Grote L, Hedner J, Peter JH: Sleep-related breathing disorder is an independent risk factor for uncontrolled hypertension. J Hypertens 18:679-685, 2000.
31. Block M, Jacobson LB, Rabkin RA: Heart block in patients after bariatric surgery accompanying sleep apnea. Obes Surg 11:627-630, 2001.
32. Cheyne J: A case of apoplexy in which the fleshy part of the heart was converted into fat. Dublin Hosp Rep 2:216-223, 1818.
33. Harrison TR, King CE, Calhoun JA, Harrison WG Jr: Congestive heart failure: XX. Cheyne-Stokes respiration as the cause of paroxysmal dyspnea at the onset of sleep. Arch Intern Med 53:891-910, 1934.
34. Javaheri S, Parker TJ, Liming JD, et al: Sleep apnea in 81 ambulatory male patients with stable heart failure: Types and their prevalences, consequences, and presentations. Circulation 97:2154-2159, 1998.
35. Sin DD, Fitzgerald F, Parker JD, et al: Risk factors for central and obstructive sleep apnea in 450 men and women with congestive heart failure. Am J Respir Crit Care Med 160:1101-1106, 1999.
36. Lanfranchi PA, Braghiroli A, Bosimini E, et al: Prognostic value of nocturnal Cheyne-Stokes respiration in chronic heart failure. Circulation 99:1435-1440, 1999.
37. Javaheri S: A mechanism of central sleep apnea in patients with heart failure. N Engl J Med 341:949-954, 1999.
38. Trinder J, Merson R, Rosenberg JI, et al: Pathophysiological interactions of ventilation, arousals, and blood pressure oscillations during Cheyne-Stokes respiration in patients with heart failure. Am J Respir Crit Care Med 162:808-813, 2000.
39. Harrison TR, King CE, Calhoun JA, Harrison WG Jr: Congestive heart failure: XVIII. Clinical types of nocturnal dyspnea. Arch Intern Med 53:561-573, 1934.
40. Javaheri S, Ahmed M, Parker TJ, Brown CR: Effects of nasal O_2 on sleep-related disordered breathing in ambulatory patients with stable heart failure. Sleep 22:1101-1106, 1999.
41. Franklin KA, Eriksson P, Sahlin C, Lundgren R: Reversal of central sleep apnea with oxygen. Chest 111:163-169, 1997.
42. Kaneko Y, Floras JS, Usui K, et al: Cardiovascular effects of continuous positive airway pressure in patients with heart failure and obstructive sleep apnea. N Engl J Med 348:1233-1241, 2003.
43. Kohnlein T, Welte T, Tan LB, Elliott MW: Assisted ventilation for heart failure patients with Cheyne-Stokes respiration. Eur Respir J 20:934-941, 2002.
44. Krachman SL, D'Alonzo GE, Berger TJ, Eisen HJ: Comparison of oxygen therapy with nasal continuous positive airway pressure on Cheyne-Stokes respiration during sleep in congestive heart failure. Chest 116:1550-1557, 1999.
45. Mansfield DR, Gollogly NC, Kaye DM, et al: Controlled trial of continuous airway pressure in obstructive sleep apnea and heart failure. Am J Respir Crit Care Med 169:329-331, 2004.
46. Pepperell JC, Maskell NA, Jones DR, et al: A randomized controlled trial of adaptive ventilation for Cheyne-Stokes breathing in heart failure. Am J Respir Crit Care Med 168:1109-1114, 2003.

PART VIII

Molecular Biology and Genetics

CHAPTER 69

Principles of Cardiovascular Molecular Biology and Genetics

Elizabeth G. Nabel

Molecular biology and genetics now form the solid foundation of cardiovascular science and medicine. In the past two decades, the concepts of molecular biology and genetics have permeated all aspects of medicine. The principles of these disciplines are a cornerstone of medical school curricula. Molecular genetic approaches are routinely used in physician-scientists' laboratories to test hypotheses about cardiovascular disease. Physicians have access to an array of molecular and genetic tools to guide the diagnosis and treatment of patients. Many therapeutic agents are now produced using recombinant DNA technology.

The breakthroughs in our understanding of the genetic basis of cardiovascular disease have been equally impressive. Our appreciation of the mechanism by which single genes cause disease, even when the diseases are uncommon, has led to an understanding of the pathogenesis of more common cardiovascular diseases. With completion of sequencing of the Human Genome Project, genomic discoveries in cardiovascular diseases now occur at a rapid pace. How these discoveries will be translated to the care of patients with cardiovascular disease is currently difficult to predict.

This chapter highlights the basic principles of molecular biology and genetics. It is designed as a brief review and reference source, intended to prepare the reader for discussions of specific cardiovascular applications in other chapters throughout the text. References are provided for a general coverage on a topic as well as an in-depth coverage of each subject.

Principles of Cell Biology and the Cell Cycle

All living organisms are composed of cells, and all cells arise from preexisting cells.[1,2] Cells are organized into compartments. Prokaryotes, such as bacteria, contain a single cell compartment bounded by a membrane or membranes. Eukaryotes, such as mammals, are defined by the division of each cell into a nucleus that contains the genetic material, surrounded by a cytoplasm, which in turn is bounded by the plasma membrane that marks the periphery of the cell. The cytoplasm also contains other discrete compartments, also bounded by membranes. To define the execution of genetic instructions in a cell, we must consider the nature of the various compartments and how they function to create regions with different properties.

The mammalian cell is a highly compartmentalized structure (Fig. 69–1). The outer membrane, called the *plasma membrane*, is a lipid bilayer intended to exclude an aqueous environment, such as extracellular fluid.[3] The plasma membrane is studded with a class of transmembrane proteins called *receptors*. A receptor has a binding site that recognizes some ligand on the exterior side of the membrane. Binding of the ligand usually triggers a change in the protein, which is transmitted to the

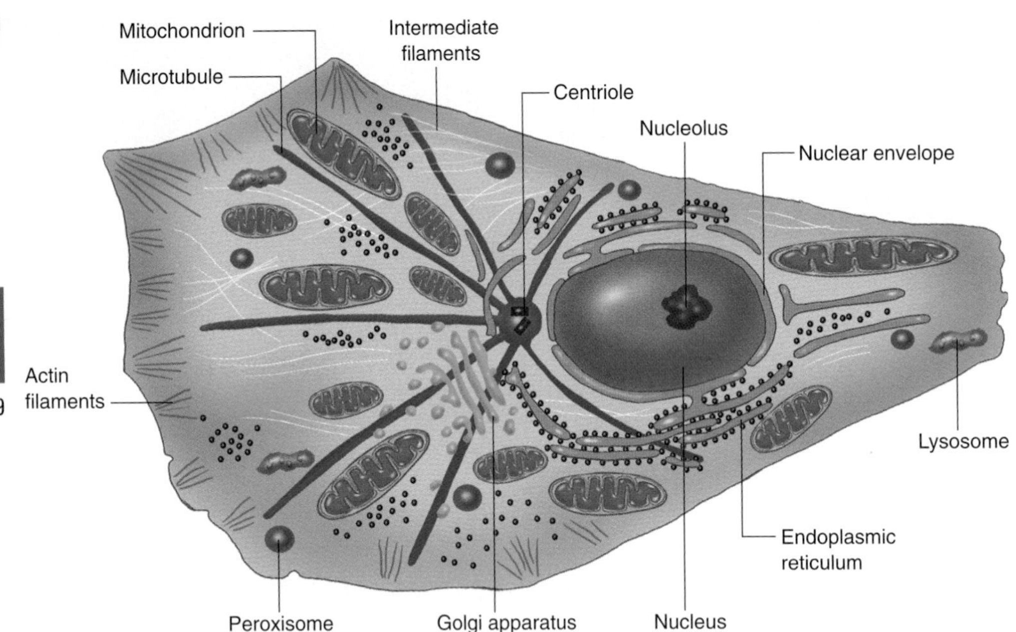

FIGURE 69–1 Structure of a mammalian cell. Schematic illustration of a cell, demonstrating structures common to most cells.

cytoplasmic face by a conformational change in the receptor protein, or as movement of the whole protein into the interior. This change, in turn, triggers other changes within the cell, and thus provides a means for responding to the environment. This type of relationship is called *signal transduction*.[4]

The cytoplasm contains networks of membranes. Membrane sheets make up the endoplasmic reticulum (ER) and the Golgi apparatus.[5] ER consists of a continuous sheet of highly folded membranes extending from the outer nuclear membrane. ER can be divided into two types, which are part of the same membrane sheet. Rough ER has ribosomes, the small particles concerned with the synthesis of proteins, on its surface, whereas smooth ER does not. The Golgi apparatus consists of stacks of separate cisternae. Proteins that have been modified in ER enter the Golgi apparatus, undergo further modifications, and then exit. A major function of the ER and Golgi apparatus is to sort proteins according to destination, using signals inherent in the protein sequence. This process of directing proteins to their final destination is called *protein sorting* or *trafficking*.[6] Mitochondria are specialized organelles in the cytoplasm that generate energy stored in the form of adenosine triphosphate from the oxidation of carbon-containing compounds such as sugars or fats. Lysosomes are membrane-enclosed bodies that contain hydrolytic enzymes, which further process proteins within the cell. Cell shape is determined by the cytoskeleton, which contains networks of protein fibers extending across and around the cell. The three classes of fibers are actin filaments, microtubules, and intermediate filaments.

The most important feature of the nucleus is the genetic material. It has a granular appearance, due to chromatin, that is easily recognized with certain stains. Between cell divisions, chromatin forms a single dense mass. When a cell divides, its chromatin can be seen to consist of a discrete number of thread-like particles, called chromosomes.[7] A common feature of cells, except those that have reached a final, specialized state of development (*terminal differentiation*), is their ability to divide. Many structural changes occur within a cell during division. There is extensive reorganization of membranes and the cytoskeleton. The cell is organized by a new structure, called the *spindle*, the function of which is to allow the distribution of chromosomes to daughter cells. The result of these changes is that many of the former activities of the cell—gene expression, protein synthesis and secretion, cell motility—come to a halt.[8]

The cell cycle, the period between the release of a newly formed cell as a progeny of a division and its own subsequent division into two daughter cells, consists of two parts.[9] Interphase, a relatively long period, represents the time during which the cell engages in its synthetic activities and reproduces its subcellular components. During interphase, the cell has a discrete nuclear compartment, containing a compact mass of chromatin. Mitosis is a short period of time during which the actual division into two daughter cells is accomplished. During mitosis, the internal organization of the cell is replaced by the spindle, and individual chromosomes are apparent. The products of the series of mitotic divisions that generate the organism are called the *somatic cells*. During embryonic development, many or most of the somatic cells proceed through the cell cycle. In the adult organism, many cells are terminally differentiated and no longer divide. They remain in a stationary phase in which there is no DNA synthesis, equivalent to a perpetual interphase.

Mitosis recapitulates the chromosome constitution of the cell. Each daughter cell starts its life with two copies of each chromosome. These copies are called *homologues*. The total number of chromosomes is called the *diploid set* and has 2n members (see Chap. 70). During interphase, a growing cell duplicates its chromosomal material. At the beginning of mitosis, each chromosome appears to split longitudinally to generate two copies, called *sister chromatids*. The cell now contains 4n chromosomes, organized as 2n pairs of sister chromatids. The process of mitosis consists of four phases: prophase, metaphase, anaphase, and telophase, ending in cytokinesis, in which the cell divides and each daughter has the same complete set of chromosomes, one member of each pair derived from each parent (Fig. 69–2). Each phase consists of distinct movements of the centromere, the central, constriction region of the chromosome. These movements are essential to separation of the pairs of chromosomes into each daughter cell and completion of cell division.

Just before mitosis, double-stranded chromosomal breaks or other DNA damage is repaired by a series of cell cycle checkpoints.[10] Under normal conditions, cellular DNA is repaired, and the cell completes mitosis. Cells in which DNA is not repaired undergo apoptosis, or programmed cell death.[11] This mechanism allows the perpetuation of cell division in which chromosomal DNA is intact. Carcinogenesis results when cell division escapes checkpoint control, and cells with double-stranded DNA break or other forms of damaged DNA divide uncontrollably and metastasize to other sites in the organism.

The essential proteins in cell cycle checkpoint control are the cyclins and the cyclin-dependent kinases (CDKs) (Fig. 69–3). The CDKs are holoenzyme complexes that contain cyclin regulatory subunits and CDK catalytic subunits.[12] Four distinct phases of the cell cycle are regulated by cyclin-CDK complexes: Gap 1 or G1 phase, DNA replication or S phase, Gap 2 or G2 phase, and mitosis or M phase. Restriction point control in G1 phase is mediated by two CDKs, the cyclin D- and cyclin E-dependent kinases. The D-type cyclins (D1, D2, and D3) interact combinatorially with two catalytic partners, CDK4 and CDK6, early in G_1 to yield at least six holoenzymes expressed in tissue-specific patterns.[13] Cyclin E enters into a complex with its catalytic partner CDK2 and collaborates with the cyclin D-dependent kinases to complete phosphorylation of the retinoblastoma tumor-suppressor protein (Rb) late in G1, which results in transit through the G1-S checkpoint into S phase.[14]

Endogenous inhibitors of the cyclins-CDKs, termed the *cyclin-dependent kinase inhibitors* or CKIs, are expressed throughout G1 to inhibit phosphorylation and activation of cyclin-CDK complexes, resulting in G1 arrest.[15] The CKIs function to prevent transition through the G1 checkpoint and inhibit mitosis, leading to growth arrest of cells. CKIs are classified into two families on the basis of their structures and CDK targets. The CIP/KIP proteins are broadly acting inhibitors that alter the activities of cyclin-D, cyclin E- and cyclin A-dependent kinases. This family includes p21(Cip1), p27(Kip1), and p57(Kip2). All three contain characteristic motifs in their amino-terminal regions that bind cyclin and CDK substrates. p21(Cip1) functions as a downstream effector of the transcription factor and tumor suppressor gene, p53, to cause DNA damage repair and/or promote apoptosis. p27(Kip1) is a potent inhibitor of cell proliferation in normal and diseased tissues and is a critical mediator in tissue injury, inflammation, and wound repair.[16] The INK4 (*in*hibitor of CD*K4*) family of proteins consists of INK4A (p16), INK4B (p15), INK4C (p18), and INK4D (p19).[17] These CKIs contain multiple ankyrin repeats, bind only to CDK4 and CDK6 and not to other CDKs, and specifically inhibit the catalytic subunits of CDK4 and CDK6. The INK proteins are important regulators of tumor growth and in developmental biology, but they play a lesser role in cardiovascular diseases.

Injury to the heart or blood vessels leads to a remodeling process that is adaptive under normal conditions or maladaptive in conditions of disease pathophysiology (see Chaps. 35 and 71). In response to physiological stimuli, vascular smooth muscle cells (VSMCs) within the media proliferate and migrate into the intima to form a multilayered vascular wound or *neointima.* Normally, this is a self-limited process that results in a well-healed vascular wound and preservation of luminal blood flow. In certain vascular diseases, however, VSMC proliferation becomes excessive, leading to a pathological lesion in the blood vessel, which in turn produces clinical symptoms. These diseases are often characterized by systemic or local inflammation, which exacerbates the VSMC proliferative response. The CIP/KIP CKIs are important regulators of tissue remodeling in the vasculature.[18] p27(Kip1) is constitutively expressed in VSMCs and endothelial cells of arteries and is downregulated after vascular injury or exposure of VSMCs and endothelial cells to mitogens. After a proliferative burst, VSMCs synthesize and secrete extracellular matrix molecules, which signal to VSMCs and endothelial cells, leading to induction of p27(Kip1) and p21(Cip1), and suppression of cyclin E-CDK2. Expression of the CIP/KIP CKIs leads to cell cycle arrest and inhibition of cell division.[19] p27(Kip1) is also an important regulator of tissue inflammation through its effects on T-lymphocyte proliferation. In the vasculature, p27(Kip1) mediates vascular repair through its regulation of proliferation, inflammation, and bone marrow progenitor cells. Genetic deletion of p27(Kip1) in mice results in a benign hyperplasia of epithelial and mesodermal cells in multiple organs, including the heart and vasculature.

p21(Cip1) is required for growth and differentiation in the heart, bone, skin, and kidney, and it confers susceptibility to apoptosis.[20] This CKI functions in a p53-dependent and p53-

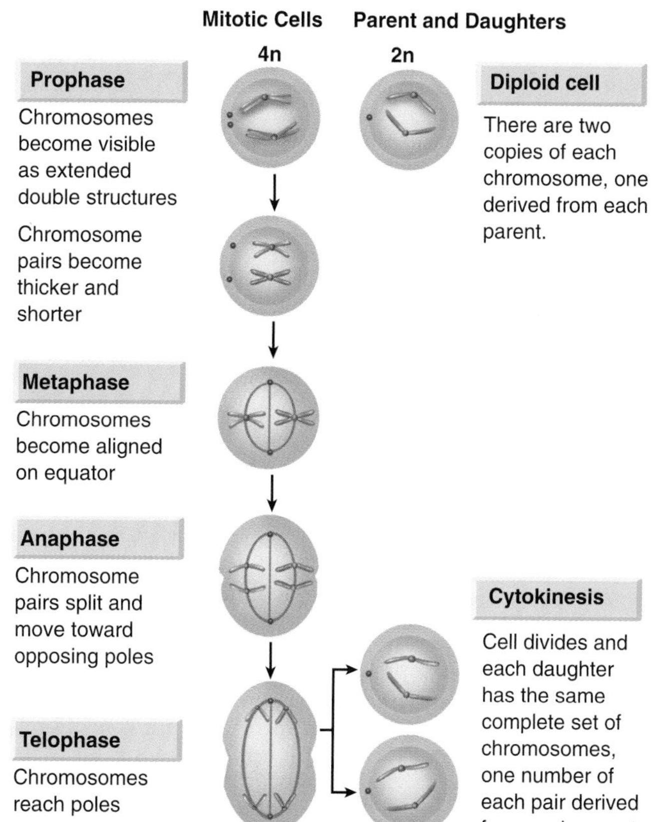

FIGURE 69–2 Process of mitosis in a mammalian cell in which the genetic material is duplicated and distributed during cell division (see text).

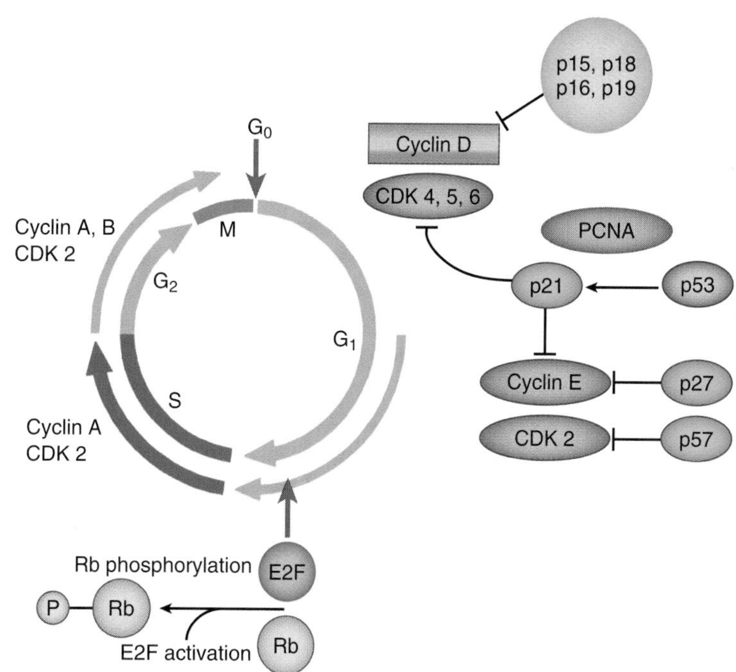

FIGURE 69–3 The mammalian cell cycle. The cyclins, cyclin-dependent kinases, and cyclin-dependent kinase inhibitors active in each phase are shown (see text for explanation and abbreviations).

independent manner. In the heart, p21(Cip1) is expressed independent of p53 in cardiac myocytes; overexpression of p21(Cip1) within myocytes leads to hypertrophy.

Most human cancer cells sustain mutations that alter the functions of p53 or Rb by direct mutation of gene sequences or by targeting genes that act epistatically to prevent their normal function. Rb limits cell proliferation by preventing entry into S phase. The mechanism is blockage of E2F transcription factors from activating genes required for DNA replication and nucleotide metabolism. p53 is mutated in more than 50 percent of human cancers. The protein accumulates in response to cellular stress from DNA damage, hypoxia, and oncogene activation. p53 initiates a transcriptional program that triggers cell cycle arrest or apoptosis.[21] When activated by p53, p21(Cip1) induces apoptosis in tumor and other cells.

The cell cycle functions as the major regulator of cell division. DNA replication and cytokinesis depend on normal functioning of the cell cycle. The cyclins, CDKS, and CKIs are, secondarily, important mediators of carcinogenesis, tissue inflammation, and wound repair.

The Genetic Code: DNA, RNA, and Protein

DNA

Deoxyribonucleic acid (DNA) is the building block of human life (Fig. 69–4). Its double helical structure is deceptively simple, yet the rules encoded within this structure specify the form and function of all cells within an organism. DNA consists of two long strands of polynucleotides that twist around each other clockwise to form an unbroken double helix. Alternating deoxyribose-phosphate groups form the backbone of the helix, with the phosphate group making a 5′-3′ phosphodiester bond between the fifth carbon of one pentose ring and the third carbon of the next pentose ring (Fig. 69–5). Nucleic acid bases attached to the sugar groups of each strand face each other within the helix, perpendicular to the strand axis. The order of the nucleic acids specifies the eventual sequence of the protein product of the gene. There are only four bases: the purines adenine and guanine (A and G) and the pyrimidines cytosine and thymine (C and T). During assembly of the double helix, a purine can pair only with a pyrimidine, and a pyrimidine with a purine. Each base pair (bp) forms one of the rungs in the twisted ladder of the DNA molecule, which can be millions of bases long. The two strands of DNA, which are held together by hydrogen bonds between complementary base pairs, have opposite chemical polarities. One strand is oriented in a 5′ to 3′ direction, while the other is in a 3′ to 5′ direction. Enzymes that recognize specific DNA sequences also recognize the polarity of the strand. An enzyme "reads" the nucleotide sequences on the two strands in opposite directions. Because the structure of the helical backbone is invariant, enzymes responsible for DNA copying, cleavage, and repairing strand breaks can act anywhere along the length of the DNA strand.

An important consequence of the A-T and G-C pairing is that the sequence of nucleotides on one strand of the double helix determines the sequence on the complementary strand. This base pairing rule is critical for the storage, retrieval, and

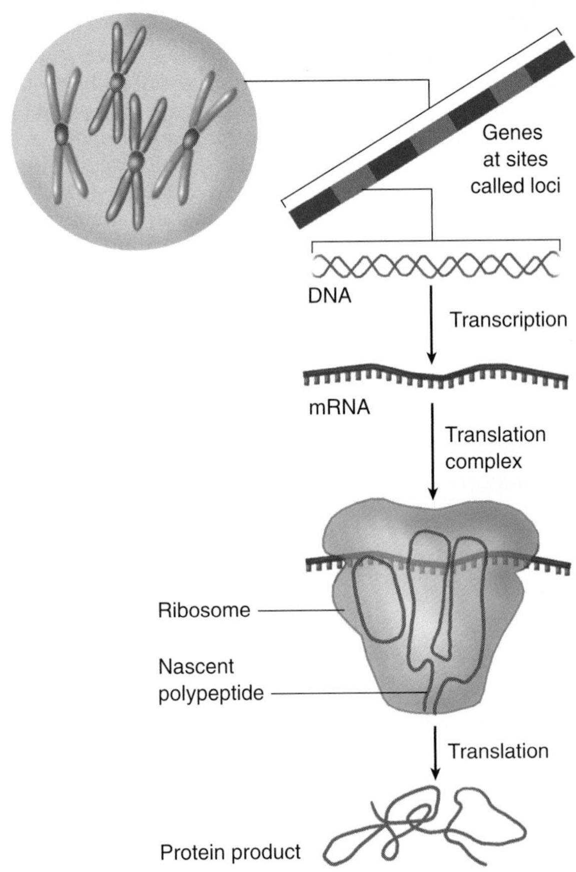

FIGURE 69–4 Depiction of the storage of genetic information in homologous chromosomes, which contain genes made up of DNA and genetic expression involving transcription of DNA into RNA, which is translated on a ribosome into protein.

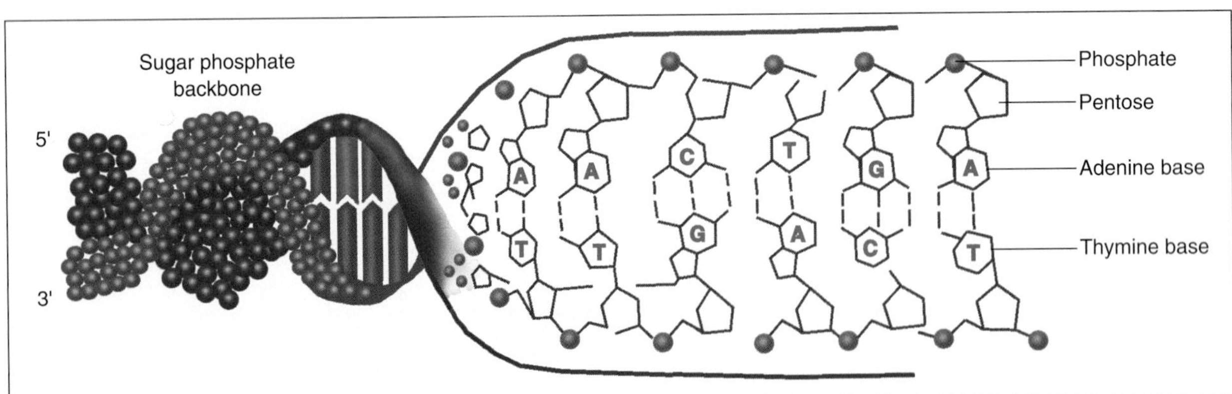

FIGURE 69–5 Schematic representation of the DNA double helix. The specificity of genetic information is carried in the four bases—guanine, adenine, thymine, and cytosine—that extend inward from a sugar-phosphate background and form pairs with complementary bases on the opposing strand.

transfer of genetic material, whether it be for duplication of DNA into a daughter cell, repair of a damaged DNA strand, or reading as a template for RNA transcription.

Chromosomes are long double helical strands of DNA tightly coiled into compacted, discrete lengths by nuclear proteins. Each chromosome varies in length and base pair composition. In human cells, the nucleus contains 23 different pairs of chromosomes, each with a specific length and base pair sequence. The combined DNA sequences (approximately 3×10^9) on all the chromosomes within a cell comprise the genome.[22,23] The information carried within the genome is identical in all cells of an organism and varies little between members of a species. Indeed, the genome of humans, *Homo sapiens*, is approximately 99 percent identical.[24]

During cell division, enzymes called *polymerases* unwind the DNA helix in each chromosome and copy each of the two strands separately along their entire length. Each daughter cell, then, inherits a double-stranded DNA molecule containing one old and one new strand. Each of these strands can in turn generate a new strand that faithfully reproduces the original template. This fidelity of DNA replication is essential for accurate transfer of genetic information. Errors in this process are a common source of gene mutations, which are inherited in successive rounds of cell division.

A gene is a section of base sequences used as a template for the copying process of transcription and, therefore, is the fundamental unit of inherited DNA information. Genes comprise only a small fraction of all the DNA carried on a chromosome. Only 1 to 2 percent of its bases encode proteins, and the full complement of protein-coding sequences still remains to be established. The human genome contains an estimated 30,000 distinct genes.[22,23] The protein coding information contained within a single gene is not continuous but instead is encoded in multiple discontinuous packets called *exons*. Between these exons are variably sized stretches of DNA called *introns*. The function of these introns is not known. They probably contain the bulk of the regulatory information controlling the expression of the approximately 30,000 protein-coding genes, and myriad other functional elements, such as non-protein-coding genes and the sequence determinants of chromosome dynamics. Even less is known about the function of the roughly half of the genome that consists of highly repetitive sequences or of the remaining noncoding, nonrepetitive DNA.

RNA

The first step in the expression of genetic information is transcription, which serves to carry the genetic information out of the nucleus into the cytoplasm where the synthesis of proteins occurs. In this process, transcription of DNA to RNA requires the expression of a gene template called messenger RNA (mRNA) in the nucleus (Fig. 69–6). A specialized enzyme, RNA polymerase, copies one of the two DNA strands (the antisense strand), creating a complementary stretch of sequence that is an exact copy of the sense strand. RNA structure differs slightly from DNA. One of the RNA bases, uracil, replaces the DNA base thymine, and the RNA sugar phosphate component ribose replaces DNA deoxyribose. Ribose renders the RNA molecule much more susceptible to degradation than the more stable deoxyribose. This allows RNAs to respond more rapidly to shifts in cellular signaling and move quickly to the cytoplasm for protein production.

From Genes to Proteins

The process of converting a gene to a protein involves two major steps: transcription of the DNA by RNA in the nucleus and translation of the RNA into protein in the cytoplasm.

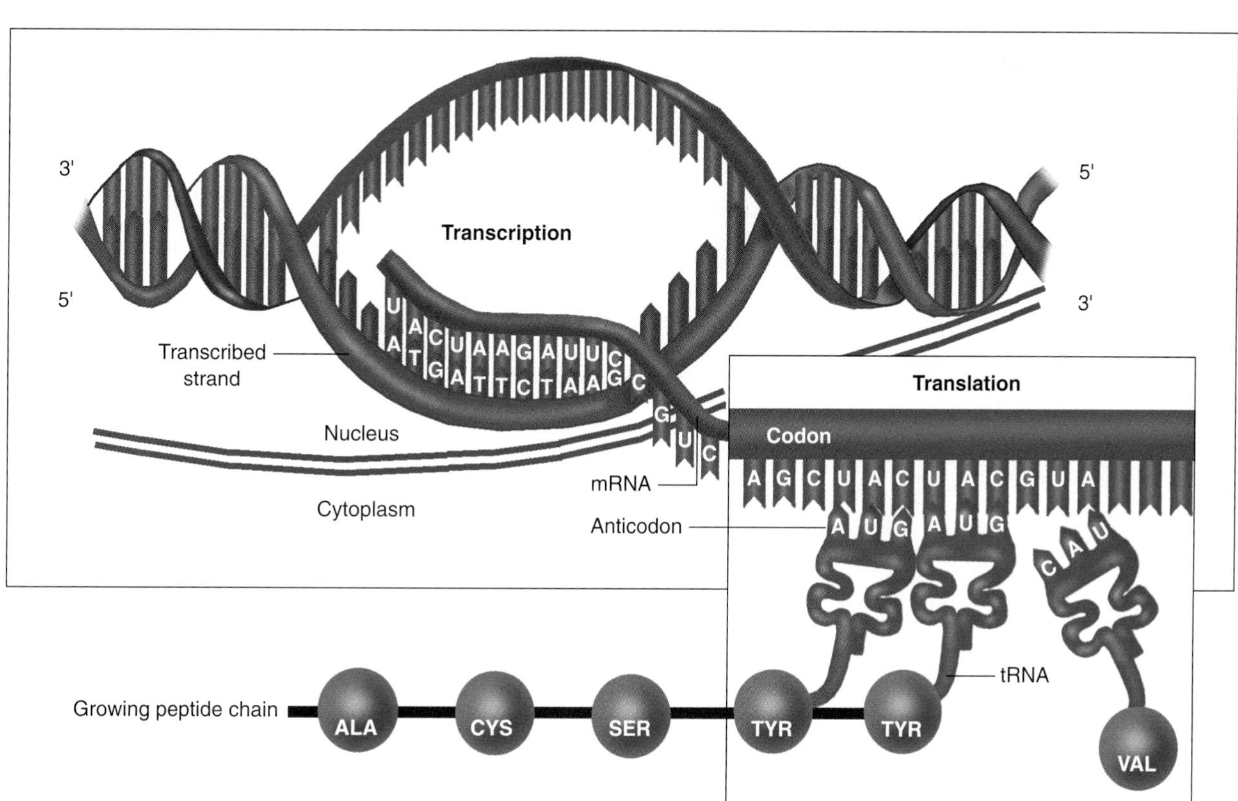

FIGURE 69–6 The flow of genetic information. Transcription in the nucleus creates a complementary ribonucleic acid copy from one of the DNA strands in the double helix. mRNA is transported into the cytoplasm, where it is translated into protein.

This is a complex and highly regulated process. Transcription begins in the nucleus by copying of the DNA sequence of the gene into mRNA (see Fig. 69–6). The single-stranded RNA is modified at both ends. At the 5′ end, a nucleotide structure called a *cap* is added to increase translation efficiency by allowing ribosomes to bind to RNA. At the 3′ end, a nucleotide recognizes an A/T rich sequence in a noncoding region and trims the transcript downstream by about 20 bp. An enzyme that adds a stretch of adenosine to form a polyA tail, which stabilizes the transcript, modifies the newly cleaved 3′ end. The transcript then undergoes splicing to remove intronic sequences. This is a highly regulated process, since unspliced transcripts are highly unstable and are cleared rapidly from the cell. Splicing is an important control point in gene expression. It must be absolutely precise, since the deletion or addition of a single nucleotide at the splice junction would throw out of frame the subsequent three-base codon translation of the RNA. The full significance of RNA splicing is not completely understood, but it must represent a critical point in the regulation of gene expression due to the large expanses of intron sequences and the inability of transcripts to leave the nucleus until their introns are removed.

Once in the cytoplasm, mRNA provides a template for translation or protein synthesis. Translation occurs on a macromolecular complex, like an assembly line, called *ribosomes.* The ribosomes read and translate the nucleotide sequence in mRNA into an amino acid sequence; that is, the four base mRNA code is translated into the 20 amino acid alphabet of proteins. This genetic code is remarkably simple and has been conserved in most organisms. Every three RNA nucleotides encodes for a single amino acid; therefore, the codon is a triplet of bases (Fig. 69–7). Permutations of the four RNA nucleotides results in 64 different triplets (4 × 4 × 4), so that any one of the 20 amino acids can be specified by more than one codon. One of the triplets, AUG, specifies methionine, which is the amino acid that starts each protein. Three other triplets, UAA, UGA, and UAG, program the ribosome to end translation and are therefore called *stop codons.*

The conversion of a codon into an amino acid requires an adapter molecule, called *transfer RNA* (tRNA), to decode mRNA. Each tRNA uses a unique three-base sequence or anticodon to line up with the complementary codon in mRNA (see Fig. 69–6). Ribosomal enzymes link adjoining amino acids, which frees them from the tRNA adapters and adds them to the growing amino acid chain. The order of the amino acids is specified by the order of the codons on the corresponding mRNA template. Translation then completes the transfer of information from DNA in the nucleus to a unique protein structure.

Since the genetic code is preserved across species, human genetic sequences can be transferred into bacteria, yeast, or insect cells, where the sequences will be faithfully replicated and decoded into RNA and protein. This principle constitutes the basis of recombinant DNA technology, which is used to produce recombinant proteins for research and therapeutic purposes (tissue plasminogen activator is an example).

The process of gene expression requires controlled and precise regulation at multiple steps. Only a small number of genes are expressed within a cell at a given time. One set of genes is constitutively expressed in most cells and are referred to colloquially as "housekeeping genes." These genes are necessary for cell replication, energy generation, and survival functions. A second set of genes are expressed in a lineage-specific manner, i.e., within certain cells. These genes are required for cell-specific functions, such as contractility. The precise regulation of lineage-specific genes determines the unique identity and function of a particular cell. Another set of genes is expressed in response to environmental stimuli. These sets of controls are required to produce the complex and dynamic patterns of gene expression, which allow an organism to respond to internal and external signals.

First Base	Second Base: U	C	A	G
U	UUU, UUC: Phe UUA, UUG: Leu	UCU, UCC, UCA, UCG: Ser	UAU, UAC: Tyr UAA, UAG: TERM	UGU, UGC: Cys UGA: TERM UGG: Trp
C	CUU, CUC, CUA, CUG: Leu	CCU, CCC, CCA, CCG: Pro	CAU, CAC: His CAA, CAG: Gin	CGU, CGC, CGA, CGG: Arg
A	AUU, AUC, AUA: Ile AUG: Met	ACU, ACC, ACA, ACG: Thr	AAU, AAC: Asn AAA, AAG: Lys	AGU, AGC: Ser AGA, AGG: Arg
G	GUU, GUC, GUA, GUG: Val	GCU, GCC, GCA, GCG: Ala	GAU, GAC: Asp GAA, GAG: Glu	GGU, GGC, GGA, GGG: Gly

FIGURE 69–7 The genetic code. The amino acids corresponding to each nucleotide triplet in the mRNA are shown. There is a single start codon (AUG) and three stop codons (UAG, UAA, UGA).

Principles and Techniques of Molecular Biology

Recombinant DNA technologies developed in the 1970s as a response to the need for sufficient quantities of DNA for biochemical analysis. The method refers to the clipping of a segment out of surrounding DNA using sequence-specific endonucleases known as *restriction enzymes.* The segment then can be inserted at will into a vector that permits copying it millions of times (see later). The success of recombinant DNA techniques fueled most of the advances in molecular biology over the past 30 years. Many of these techniques are now commonplace in research laboratories. These approaches are routinely used for analysis of gene structure, expression, and organization; regulatory pathways by which cells control gene expression; and discovery of novel genes and therapeutics. These advances have changed the face of medical research. Genetic engineering in which an organism is modified to include new genes designed with desired characteristics is in routine practice in many research laboratories. Recombinant DNA technologies are used to mass-produce therapeutic proteins, such as recombinant tissue plasminogen activator. The ability to manipulate the human genome has opened up new possibilities for the development of diagnostic tests and new therapies. Yet, the techniques of molecular biology, like the structure of DNA itself, are surprisingly simple. The basic approaches are described here; the reader is guided to in-depth reviews for a primer on how to perform the techniques.[25]

Cloning DNA

Molecular cloning provides a means to produce millions of copies of a DNA sequence or gene within bacterial cells. A DNA fragment is first inserted into a cloning vector. The most commonly used vectors are small circular DNA molecules called *plasmids* or bacterial viruses called *phage*. The vectors also contain genetic information that allows the bacterial cell to replicate the DNA sequence. After insertion of a DNA sequence, the plasmid or phage vector is introduced into a bacterial cell. The growing bacterial culture replicates the vector containing the DNA sequence in hundreds of copies per cell, yielding multiple identical clones of the original DNA sequence. The vectors are then harvested from the bacterial culture using the same restriction enzymes used to insert the DNA sequence into the vector.

The molecular biologist uses restriction endonucleases derived from bacteria as molecular scissors that cut DNA motifs at predictable sequences. Each restriction enzyme recognizes a specific nucleotide sequence. These recognition sites occur randomly along the DNA of any organism and consist of a short symmetric sequence motif called a *palindrome*, which is repeated in opposing orientation on both strands of the double helix DNA. For example, the enzyme EcoRI from the bacteria *Escherichia coli* recognizes and cuts the sequence GAATTC in double-strand DNA at GA and AG junctions. Most restriction enzymes cleave their palindromic sequence asymmetrically, leaving a single-stranded overhang on each end of the cut. These "sticky" ends have unique and complementary sequences that can be used to connect a fragment of human DNA with complementary ends of DNA from another source. An enzymatic reaction connects the continuous double-stranded DNA to form a smooth splice. These principles are used to construct various DNA rearrangements for multiple purposes, such as gene cloning, generating knock-out mice, or constructing recombinant DNA therapies.

Blotting Techniques

Blotting is a tool that permits identification of DNA, RNA, or protein by its molecular size. Analysis of DNA is referred to as a Southern blot; RNA identification is a Northern blot; and protein isolation is a Western blot. The principles of blotting techniques are straightforward.[25] A mixture of molecules to be analyzed is subjected to gel electrophoresis, which separates different species according to size and/or electrical charge (Fig. 69–8). An agarose gel is used in which the molecules are loaded into wells at one end. The gel is submerged into buffer and subjected to an electrical current. The molecules migrate across the electrical field. Since DNA and RNA are acids that carry a negative charge, they migrate toward the positive pole of the gel. The agarose matrix hinders the migration of larger molecules, so that the molecules also separate by size. When the electrophoresis is completed, the gel is removed from the buffer, and a nylon filter and dry absorbent material are placed on top. The buffer from the gel is blotted into the absorbent material carrying with it the separated molecules, which remain on the nylon filter. The filter is treated to permanently fix the molecules on its surface, creating a mirror image of the original gel. The filter is then bathed with a tagged molecule that recognizes (hybridizes to) the molecule of interest (the probe) and washed to remove the unbound probe. For Southern (DNA) and Northern (RNA) blots, the probe is a small fragment of nucleic acid that carries a complementary sequence to the molecule being investigated. The nucleic acid is tagged with a radioactive element detectable by exposure to x-ray film or other techniques.

The position of the hybridized probe, which appears as a band, provides an estimate of the size of DNA or RNA segment. By running parallel lanes of molecular markers of known size, the precise size of the DNA or RNA element is determined. For protein identification (Western blot), the probe consists of a tagged antibody that recognizes the target protein. Size markers are also run in the gel to identify the size of the protein.

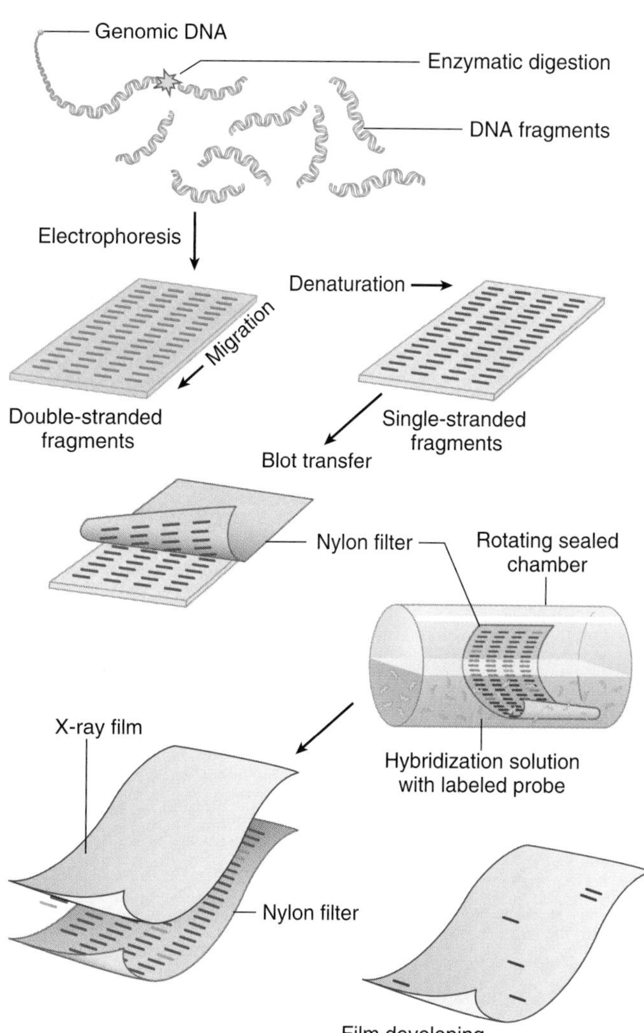

FIGURE 69–8 Blotting DNA. The process of Southern blotting to identify genomic DNA is shown.

Blotting techniques are also used for other purposes, including to map the position of restriction sites in a specific gene following restriction enzyme digestion, and in cytogenetic analysis to compare restriction sites in genomic DNA from a test and reference sample.

Polymerase Chain Reaction

Polymerase chain reaction (PCR) is an amplification procedure that takes place within a test tube (Fig. 69–9). The segment of DNA or RNA to be amplified is combined in a test tube with two short oligonucleotide primers (chemically synthesized single-stranded DNA fragments). The primers initiate the amplification, which then proceeds in a series of cycles in which the original DNA, called the *template*, is separated into single strands. The separation of the strands allows the primers to bind or anneal to the respective complementary sequences at each end of the single strands. A heat-stable DNA polymerase enzyme adds nucleotide bases at the ends of each primer, reading across the single DNA strand, generating a complementary copy of the single strand. By the time the polymerase has reached the end of the single

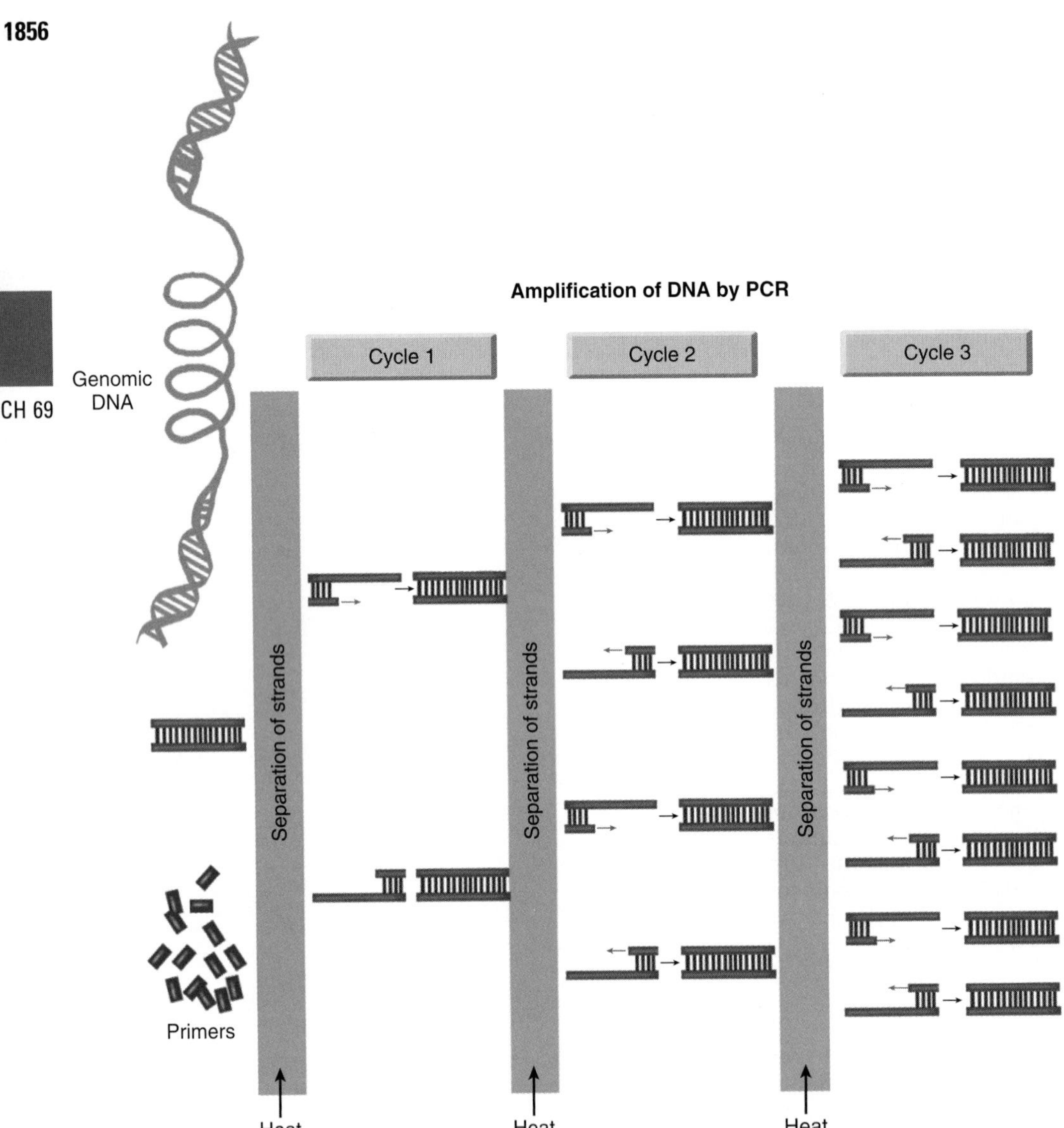

FIGURE 69–9 DNA amplification with the polymerase chain reaction (PCR). Synthetic primers corresponding to the 5′ and 3′ ends of the DNA sequence are chemically synthesized. The double-stranded DNA is melted by heating to 92°C, followed by cooling to 72°C to anneal the primers. A heat-stable DNA polymerase amplifies each strand of the target sequence, producing two copies of the DNA sequence. The process is repeated multiple times to achieve amplification of the target sequence.

strand, a new double-stranded sequence has been generated. The cycle begins again, heating and separating the double strand, followed by the generation of a new strand by the primer and polymerase. Each round of PCR amplification doubles the number of DNA templates. It is possible to create millions of copies of a DNA segment in several hours by PCR, even when the starting material is a single copy of DNA. The entire amplification is carried out in a sealed test tube or well in a specially designed machine that can be programmed to automatically heat and cool the sample. PCR has now become a commonplace tool to generate a sufficient quantity of identical genetic material for analysis.

Principles of Molecular Genetics

Genotype and the Identification of Disease-Causing Genes

The discovery of the structure and function of DNA in 1953 laid the foundation for molecular genetics.[26] The completion of sequencing of the human genome has added considerably to this foundation.[22,23] Clinicians now have at hand the tools of molecular genetics with which they can pursue diagnoses and treatments. In this regard, three concepts prove particularly useful in cardiovascular genetics: genotype, genomics, and proteomics. Genotype is the composite of DNA sequences within an individual's set of genes, or the complete sequence of an individual's DNA on all 23 pairs of chromosomes. Genomics is the expression of gene sequences as RNA. The focus of genomics is "Which genes are expressed?" Proteomics is the study of proteins expressed within a cell or organism and seeks to understand the networks of protein-protein interactions.

Historically, the field of genetics focused on monogenic disorders, i.e., diseases caused by a single gene deletion or mutation (see Chap. 70). With the newer tools of genomics and proteomics, attention has turned to the evaluation of the genetic susceptibility to complex disease traits, such as coronary artery disease and hyperlipidemias. Understanding the genetic basis of complex diseases requires knowledge of gene sequences, the proteins encoded by the genes, and the functions of the proteins. However, it is becoming increasingly clear that complex cardiovascular problems will not be resolved by deriving the nucleotide sequence of the human genome or from unraveling the approximately 30,000 loci that encode the corresponding proteins or regulate other genes. Considerable work is required to define precisely the molecular mechanisms by which changes in an individual gene or set of genes specify or confer risk for a specific disease phenotype.

Monogenic Disorders

Medical genetics has classically focused on single gene or monogenic diseases, where the cause of the disease is traced to a missing or mutated gene. Approximately 1000 disease-causing genes have been identified.[27] Monogenic disorders are rare and typically are inherited in a mendelian or autosomal manner. Interestingly, our understanding of the mechanism by which single genes cause disease, even though these mechanisms are uncommon, has led to an understanding of the pathogenesis of more common cardiovascular diseases.

Our current understanding of genetic factors in cardiovascular disease is reviewed in more detail elsewhere (see Chap. 70).[28] Briefly, each gene exists in two copies, known as *alleles*. An individual is homozygous at a given locus if the two alleles are identical, or heterozygous if the alleles are different. The specific alleles present at a given loci represent the genotype for those genes. Viewed more broadly, a genotype is a composite of the genetic factors responsible for creating a phenotype. A phenotype, in turn, is the visible or measurable properties resulting from a genotype, such as coronary artery disease or obesity. Phenotype can also be defined as the effect of gene action, whether due to a single gene or the entire genotype.

Differences in nucleotide sequences, either between two individuals or among all individuals within a population, constitutes genetic *variation*. Differences that arise in nucleotide sequences and lead to a structural change in the proteins they encode are called *mutations*. A mutation is defined as occurring in less than 1 percent of a given population.[29] Approximately 16,000 mutations in single-gene disorders have been identified.[27] Examples of mutations include missense, nonsense, frame shift, deletion, and insertion (Fig. 69–10). Missense mutations result from substitutions of one or more nucleotides in such a way as to change the primary sequence of the encoded protein. These missense mutations alter the function of the protein by changing its primary structure. A nonsense mutation introduces a premature stop codon into a gene, resulting in a truncated gene product that can display alterations in function and can be unstable. Insertions or deletions of nucleotides add or subtract amino acids from the resulting proteins, if the nucleotide changes lead to an addition or deletion of a triplet. Frame-shift mutations occur when codons of a gene are read in the wrong reading frame. These mutations typically cause abnormal protein structure due to the introduction of out-of-frame termination codons, which lead to premature termination of proteins. Mutations in introns and exons cause splicing errors that also lead to alterations in protein structure or premature termination. Finally, mutations in the promoters or enhancers of genes can lead to alterations in the levels of expression of a protein, or the temporal or spatial patterns of gene expression of a protein.

Wild-type Sequence							
...	AUG	GCC	TAC	GTT	CGA	CCC	...
...	Met	Ala	Tyr	Val	Arg	Pro	...
Missense							
	AUG	ACC	TAC	GTT	CGA	CCC	
	Met	Thr	Tyr	Val	Arg	Pro	
Nonsense							
	AUG	GCC	TAG	GTT	CGA	CCC	
	Met	Ala	Stop				
Frameshift							
	AUG	GCC	TAC	•TTC	CGA	CCC	
	Met	Ala	Tyr	Phe	Asp	...	
Deletion							
	AUG	GCC	TAC	GTT	...	CCC	
	Met	Ala	Tyr	Val	–	Pro	
OR							
	AUG	GCC	TA•	G	TT	CCC	
	Met	Ala	Stop	⟶			
Insertion							
	AUG	GCC	AAA	TAC	GTT	CGA	CCC
	Met	Ala	Lys	Tyr	Val	Arg	Pro
OR							
	AUG	GCC	ATA	CGT	TCG	ACC	...
	Met	Ala	Ile	Arg	Ser	Thr	...

FIGURE 69–10 Different types of mutations that alter the structure and expression of human genes.

A variety of mutations have been found in monogenic cardiovascular diseases (see Chap. 70). For example, while the primary defect in familial hypercholesterolemia is a deficit of low-density lipoprotein receptors (LDLRs), more than 600 mutations in the LDLR gene have been identified in patients with this disorder.[30] Likewise, hypertrophic cardiomyopathy, an autosomal dominant disease, is caused by mutations in the genes encoding proteins of the myocardial-contractile apparatus. Multiple causative mutations in at least 10 different sarcomeric proteins have been identified, including cardiac beta-myosin heavy chain, cardiac myosin-binding protein, cardiac troponin T, cardiac troponin I, alpha-tropomyosin, essential and regulatory light chains, and cardiac actin.[31] Other monogenic cardiovascular disorders include familial long Q-T syndrome,[32] venous thrombosis due to factor V Leiden,[33] and inherited forms of hypertension.[34]

Complex Trait Analysis

Polymorphisms are common variations, defined as being present in more than 1 percent of the population. Single nucleotide polymorphisms (SNPs) are nucleotide substitutions that do not alter a protein structure (Fig. 69–11). SNPs are very useful markers to map genes to chromosomal loci.[35] An SNP may be a marker of disease susceptibility, i.e., it can associate with a disease due to either a direct effect of the SNP on the disease or linkage with a nearby susceptibility locus.[36] There are an estimated 1.4 million SNPs in the human genome.[37] Putative and confirmed SNPs are accessible through several public databases, such as dbSNP, a database maintained by the National Center for Biotechnology Information.[38]

A haplotype is a set of SNPs grouped by genetic regions and inherited en bloc within a given population. Haplotypes may have a true association with a disease or may only appear to be associated due to confounding factors.[39] If a SNP is associated with a disease, it is likely that the SNP is

Wild-type Sequence							
...	AUG	GCC	TAC	GTT	CGA	CCC	...
...	Met	Ala	Tyr	Val	Arg	Pro	...
Polymorphism							
...	AUG	GCA	TAC	GTT	CGA	CCC	...
...	Met	Ala	Tyr	Val	Arg	Pro	...

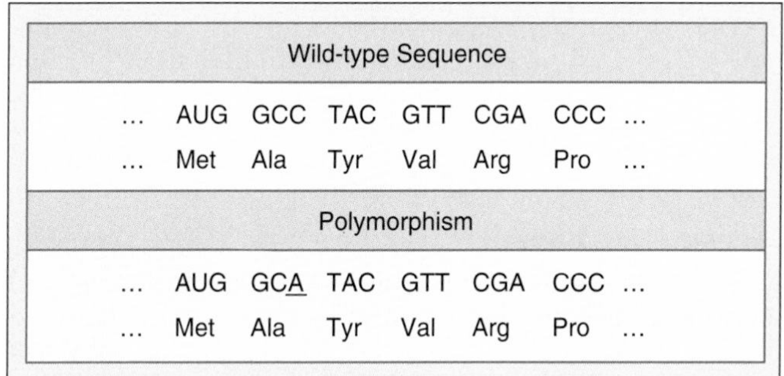

FIGURE 69–11 A polymorphism is a nucleotide substitution that does not alter the primary amino acid structure of the resulting protein.

inherited as part of a haplotype in which other SNPs are also statistically associated with the disease. This nonrandom association of alleles is called *linkage disequilibrium*. Linkage disequilibrium exists when alleles at two distinct locations in the genome are inherited together more frequently than expected. Since a SNP may simply be a marker of disease predisposition rather than a causal agent, demonstration of altered gene function must be shown in order to prove causality.

An international effort is underway to identify all SNPs on all 22 somatic chromosomes in 300 individuals from diverse backgrounds in Asia, Africa, Europe, and the Americas. This project, called the Haplotype Map or HapMap, was initiated in October 2002 to construct a genome-wide map of SNP clusters based on DNA samples from different human populations.[40] The HapMap will provide a SNP roadmap for performing linkage analysis, association studies, and evaluation of SNP partners for contribution to a disease. SNPs, then, provide insight into the genetic basis for disease for several reasons: direct causal agents of altered gene function; markers of disease, regardless of causality; and genome-wide markers for genetic studies due their presence at high density throughout the genome.[41,42]

Linkage Analysis and Association Studies

Two types of genetic studies examine inheritance: linkage analysis and association studies. Linkage studies are performed in families to study coinheritance of two traits passed down from parent to child.[43] Sets of polymorphic markers or SNPs are used to identify the location of the two alleles on a chromosomal locus. The genes encoding the two traits typically reside in close proximity to each other, and hence, the traits, or alleles, are linked. Linkage is determined by a LOD score, or the *l*ogarithm of the *od*ds that markers are linked at a particular distance, divided by the odds that they are linked at 50 percent coinheritance (not linked at all). Linkage analysis is commonly used to identify and study mendelian traits.[44] Allele-sharing methods are also used to compare similarity of alleles in closely affected individuals, such as affected sibling pairs.

Population-based association studies are useful for investigations of common disorders without clear mendelian inheritance.[45] Association studies often employ a case control approach in which an experimental and reference group are compared. Careful consideration of the most appropriate control population is necessary to draw valid conclusions and infer gene function from these studies. Case control studies should be sufficiently powered with a large enough sample size to achieve statistical significance. In this approach, known SNPs in candidate genes are investigated, using the alleles of a given SNP as variables, which are then associated with the presence or absence of disease or a particular outcome. If SNPs in a candidate gene are not known, then the gene is directly sequenced in a subset of the study and in control populations to determine which SNPs are differentially represented in the two populations. Confirmation of SNPs is then performed in the remainder of the population using PCR-based techniques. A limitation of this approach is the bias inherent in selection of candidate genes. Only those genes known or of interest are often chosen for investigation. In contrast, identification of genes by positional cloning has frequently led to unanticipated discoveries.

Genome-Wide Scans

Genome-wide scans of SNPs are newer techniques performed on high-throughput platforms and assay for several thousand SNPs simultaneously.[46-48] By taking advantage of the physical distribution of SNPs through the genome, chromosomal regions between SNPs are associated with a disease. With this technique, SNPs can be identified as biomarkers of disease. This approach will be an active area of research in the coming years.

Genomics

Genomics is the study of gene function through the parallel measurements of genomes, most commonly using the techniques of microarrays and serial analysis of gene expression (SAGE). Microarray usage in drug discovery is expanding, and its applications include basic research and target discovery, biomarker determination, pharmacology, toxicogenomics, target selectivity, development of prognostic tests, and disease-subclass determination.

The basic technique involves extraction of RNA from biological samples in either normal or test states (Fig. 69–12).[49] The RNA is copied, while incorporating either fluorescent nucleotides or a tag that is later stained with fluorescence. The labeled RNA is then hybridized to a microarray for a period of time, after which the excess is washed off and the microarray is scanned under laser light. The end result is 4000 to 5000 measurements of gene expression per biological sample. Because a complete experiment might involve any number up to hundreds of microarrays, the resultant RNA-expression data sets can vary greatly in size.

cDNA Microarrays

cDNA microarrays are created from probe cDNA libraries (500-5000 bases) by spotting a cDNA corresponding to an individual gene or probe at a precise location on a microscope slide. Each microarray measures two samples and provides a relative measurement level for each RNA molecule. Target RNAs labeled with a fluorescent dye are hybridized to the cDNA microarray surface, along with a control sample. The two RNA samples compete for binding to each probe. RNA that matches the cDNA sequence hybridizes to the cDNA spot on the microscope slide. The fluorescent labels are laser activated, and the signal intensities from fluorescent probes binding cDNA spots are compared. The comparison reflects the ratios of RNA abundance for each expressed gene. Normalization strategies that allow for standardization of interarray comparisons are applied, followed by analytical methods, as described previously.

Oligonucleotide Arrays

Oligonucleotide arrays are created by attachment of synthetic nucleotide probes (12-80-mer oligonucleotides) representa-

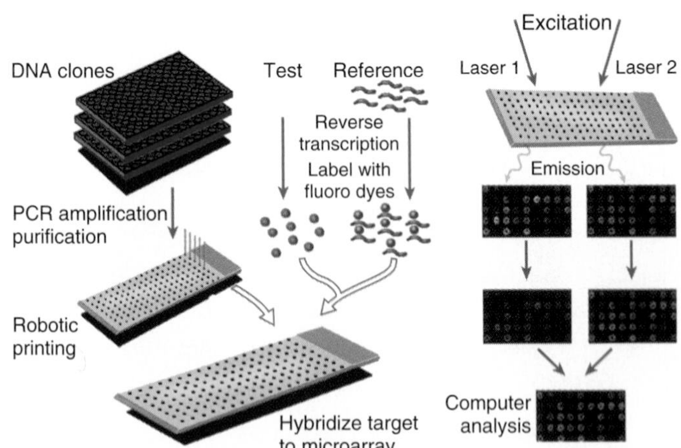

FIGURE 69–12 Detection of differential expression of mRNA from cells or tissues using gene expression profiling. After mRNA is isolated from cells or tissues, it is analyzed by hybridization to fluorescent-labeled cDNA clones imprinted onto a microscope slide. The fluorescent labels are laser activated, and the signal intensities from fluorescent probes binding cDNA spots are compared.

tive of unique portions of genes to an array surface. cDNA is synthesized from the experimental mRNA sample, followed by an in vitro transcription step to create biotin-labeled cRNA, which hybridizes to the microarray target. The microarray is treated with a fluorescent dye tagged to avidin (a protein that binds tightly to biotin) and subjected to laser activation. With oligonucleotide arrays, each microarray measures a single sample and provides an absolute measurement level of each RNA molecule. Signal intensities are measured as a reflection of expression level for each gene.

SAGE

SAGE is a technique for characterization of gene expression based on direct sequencing of transcripts. Its major strength is determination and analysis of transcripts when the sequence is unknown. SAGE requires approximately 10-fold larger quantities of mRNA for analysis and hence is much more labor intensive than some array platforms, even with automated sequencers, since the simplest two-sample comparison requires sequencing of approximately 1.5×10^6 bases. This factor alone poses difficulties when RNA abundance is low, whereas a major advantage is its higher sensitivity for changes in expression level.[50,51]

After acquisition of data by image processing, data are analyzed in three steps: normalization, filtering, and computation. Normalization accounts for technical factors, such as array manufacturing, differences in dye incorporation, and irregularities in probe distribution during hybridization, and is performed to allow meaningful comparisons between individual arrays. Filtering of data refers to the selection of those data likely to represent significant findings. Typical criteria for filtering include assessment of signal quality and fold-change in gene expression level. Differential gene expression in microarray analysis is often defined by a 1.5- to 2-fold difference in relative gene expression level.

Determination of similarity and dissimilarity is a critical component of the data analysis. Two general approaches are used: supervised and unsupervised. Supervised methods are employed for finding genes with expression levels that are significantly different between groups of samples, and finding genes that accurately predict a characteristic of the sample. Two commonly used supervised techniques include "nearest neighbors" and "support vector machines." Users of unsupervised methods try to find internal structure or relationships in a data set instead of trying to determine how best to predict a correct answer. Four commonly used unsupervised techniques include hierarchical clustering, self-organizing maps, relevance networks, and principal-component analysis. These analytical methods are described in detail elsewhere.[52] These computational approaches are then followed by a statistical analysis. Before any microarray data are taken at face value, significant findings should be validated with independent testing of RNA expression levels using quantitative reverse transcription PCR or conventional Northern blotting techniques.

Proteomics

Proteomics is the study of proteins expressed by the genome. Genomics and proteomics should be viewed as complementary components of the genetic spectrum, beginning with DNA and ending with modified proteins (Fig. 69–13). Proteins are the final product of the human genome and ultimately define human biology. Proteins are responsible for biological form and function. It is estimated that there are six to seven times as many proteins as genes (approximately 200,000) in humans, due to splicing, exchange of structural cassettes among genes during transcription, and posttranslational modifications. The field of proteomics seeks to understand the complex interactions of all proteins expressed

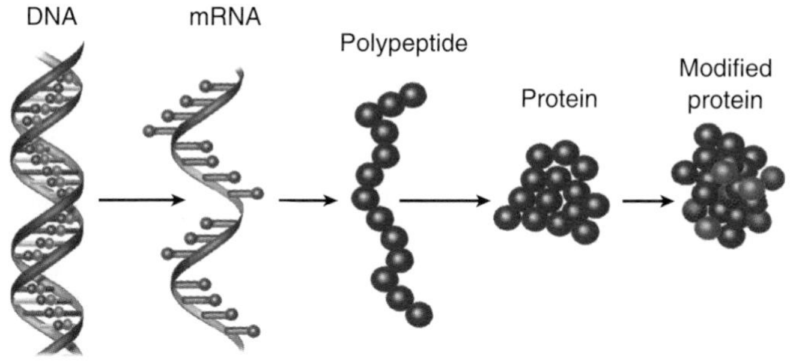

FIGURE 69–13 Relationship of the genome to the proteome. Examples of common posttranslational modifications include the addition to amino acids (blue balls) of sugars (glycosylation), phosphorylation, and prenylation depicted by the red and green balls.

within a tissue or organism under normal or perturbed conditions. Indeed, human proteomics is in its infancy.[53]

The methods for proteome analysis are still under development and validation. However, there are five basic elements to any proteomic analysis: sample acquisition, protein extraction, protein separation, protein sequence determination, and sequence comparison to reference databases for protein identification.[54] Sample acquisition is straightforward, involving obtaining a tissue biopsy or a plasma sample from an individual (under informed consent). Protein extraction is generally performed by chemical methods, generally with methanol, to remove all DNA, RNA, carbohydrates, and lipids. Extracted proteins must be separated for identification, and this step has traditionally been performed by two-dimensional gel electrophoresis. In the first dimension, proteins are separated by mass, and in the second dimension, they are separated by isoelectric point or net charge. Because most spots on a two-dimensional gel contain multiple protein constituents, alternate methods for separating and identifying proteins have evolved, including liquid chromatography. Liquid chromatography utilizes solid- and liquid-phase media to separate proteins according to biochemical properties, including molecular mass, isoelectric point, or hydrophobicity. These liquid chromatography separations can be performed in series to improve resolution. Other types of chromatographic columns can be used to improve sensitivity and specificity, such as affinity chromatography in which a column contains antibodies specific to certain functions to achieve the desired separation. Following separation, the protein is identified, generally using some form of mass spectrometry (Fig. 69–14). Mass spectrometry converts proteins or peptides to charged species that can be separated on the basis of their mass-to-charge ratio. Several types of mass spectrometry ionization methods are in use, including electrospray ionization and matrix-assisted laser desorption ionization (MALDI). Peptide sequences identified with these methods must next be analyzed by comparison with known database sequences to determine the unequivocal identity of the protein. Once proteins in a given proteome have been identified, their relative abundance levels are determined to compare relative abundance of proteins in a normal or diseased state. Finally, a thorough analysis of a proteome should include some measure of function, whether it is in cultured cells or in animal models. This approach is similar to functional genomic analysis, in which it is critical to gauge the importance of a gene or mutation through determination of gene function.

Proteomic analysis is currently limited by sensitivity, specificity, and throughput. However, this field and its methodologies are developing rapidly. The application of proteomics to cardiovascular disease holds great promise for understanding the function of the cardiovascular system in all its complexity.

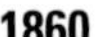

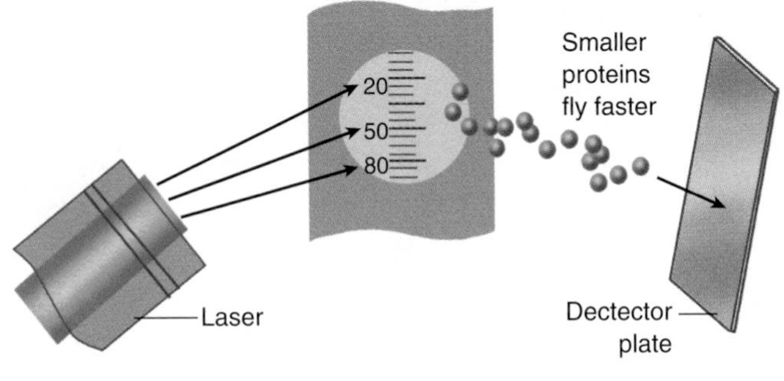

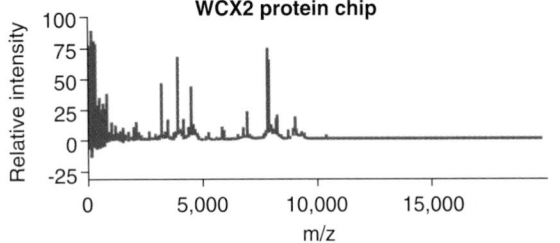

FIGURE 69–14 Mass spectrometry to identify separated proteins. A sample of serum or plasma is applied to the surface of a protein-binding chip, and the chip is irradiated with a laser where bound proteins are launched as ions. A time of flight to detection by an electrode is a measure of the mass-to-charge ratio (m/z) of the ion, which is displayed graphically.

Genetic Modification of Mice to Study Human Cardiovascular Disease

The techniques for generating genetically modified mice has had a tremendous impact on cardiovascular research. The mouse is a small animal with a short gestation period (21 days). Yet, there is remarkable conservation of the molecular pathways that control cardiovascular development and function between mice and humans. Similar genes and signaling pathways regulate the development of the heart and vasculature in both species.[55] With completion of sequencing of the mouse and human genome, comparative genetics is now possible.[56] For these reasons, genetically modified mice have become an essential animal model to study cardiovascular genetics, developmental biology, and physiology. Limitations of mouse models to study human cardiovascular disease are evident, but due to the simplicity of genetic manipulation in the mouse, it has become a standard starting place for hypothesis testing prior to evaluation in a larger animal. This section briefly describes the principles of four approaches to genetic modification in the mouse: transgenics, gene deletion or "knockout," conditional knockout, and studying mouse physiology. The reader is referred to other sources for in-depth reviews.[57]

Transgenic Mice

Creation of a transgenic mouse involves four steps: cloning of the gene of interest; fusion of the gene to transcriptional regulatory sequences that program its expression in all tissues of the mouse or in specific tissues; injection of the purified transgene into the male pronucleus of a fertilized one-cell mouse embryo; and reimplantation of the injected embryo into a foster mother. The injected transgene randomly integrates into a chromosome of the fertilized embryo, resulting in a founder mouse that expresses the injected transgene and that passes the transgene to 50 percent of its progeny. Comparative studies can then be performed between the transgenic mouse and nontransgenic littermate mouse as a control. Production of a founder transgenic mouse is now routinely performed in many laboratories and is accomplished generally in less than a month. Similar techniques have been used to create transgenic rabbits, rats, and pigs.

Refinements of these techniques have facilitated more sophisticated transgenic models. Cell-specific promoters program transgene expression exclusively in cardiomyocytes, endothelial cells, and vascular smooth muscle cells, creating a transgenic mouse with restricted expression in the cardiovascular system. While overexpression of a transgene results in a gain-of-function, it is also possible to eliminate the function of a single gene by overexpressing a dominant-negative mutant of that gene whose encoded protein interferes with the function of the wild-type protein. Expression of a transgene can also be turned on or off by administration of a simple drug like tetracycline using a tet operon system.[58] These mice allow precisely timed transgene expression as well as a comparison in the same animal of the phenotypes of transgene on and off states.

Gene Inactivation or Knockout Approaches

Gene deletion is a complementary approach to transgenesis for studying the role of a specific gene in mouse development and physiology (Fig. 69–15). In gene deletion studies, the expression of one or more genes is "knocked out" to produce a loss-of-function mutant mouse. The knockout approach involves the following steps: construction of a targeting vector containing the gene of interest with a deletion or nonsense mutation; transfection of a pluripotent mouse embryonic stem cell with the targeting vector; homologous recombination between the targeting construct and one copy of the endogenous gene, producing an embryonic stem cell with a homozygous deletion of the gene of interest; injection of the mutant embryonic stem cell into a fertilized mouse blastocyst; and implantation of the blastocyst into a foster mother. The resulting mouse pup is a chimera in which all tissues, including the gonads, are derived in part from the mutant embryonic stem cells and in part from the wild-type cells of the injected blastocysts. This chimeric animal is bred to a wild-type animal, and fertilization of a wild-type egg with a mutant sperm from the chimera produces a heterozygous knockout mouse in which one copy of the gene of interest in all cells is mutant and the other copy is wild-type. Heterozygous animals are then bred with each other to produce homozygous knockouts that have deletions of the gene of interest in all cells. The absence of the gene in the knockout animal produces a specific phenotype that reveals the direct function of the gene in development and normal and perturbed physiology. Creation of a knockout mouse is technically more challenging that transgenesis and often takes 9 to 12 months to complete.

Conditional Knockout Mice

Inactivation of important genes commonly results in early embryonic lethal phenotypes that are difficult to analyze and understand. As a result, methods have been developed to delete genes in a tissue-specific fashion and/or to inactivate genes at different times in development. In addition, it is often of interest to produce specific mutations of genes rather than to eliminate their expression completely. Homologous recombination is also used to introduce specific mutations into wild-type genes; the difference in technique is that these "knock-ins" utilize a targeting construct containing a mutant gene rather than a gene deletion. Other homologous recombination approaches permit introduction of a distinct or unrelated gene into a foreign genetic locus to regulate the new gene under the control of the promoter of the targeted locus.

Another approach to tissue-specific gene deletion is use of a bacterial phage recombination system called Cre-lox.[59] A P1

Electroporation of ES cells targeting vector

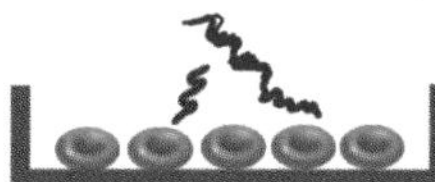

Picking drug-resistant ES cell clones

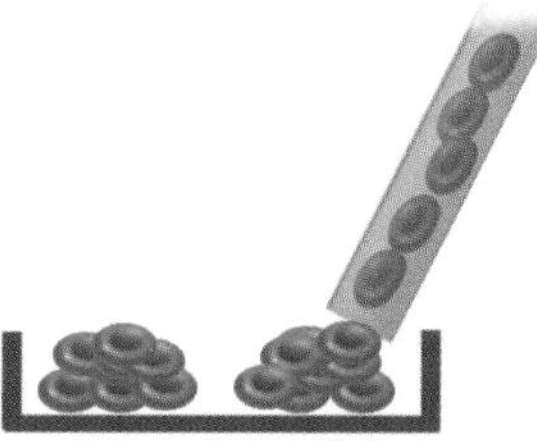

Southern blot identification of a targeting event

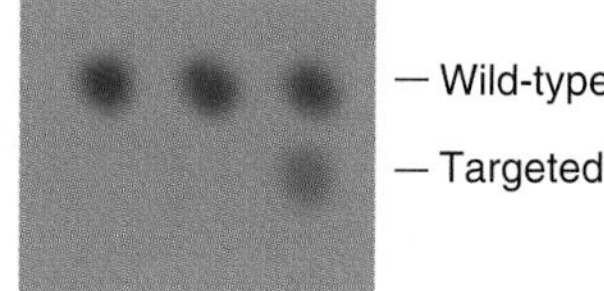

Generation of chimeric mice

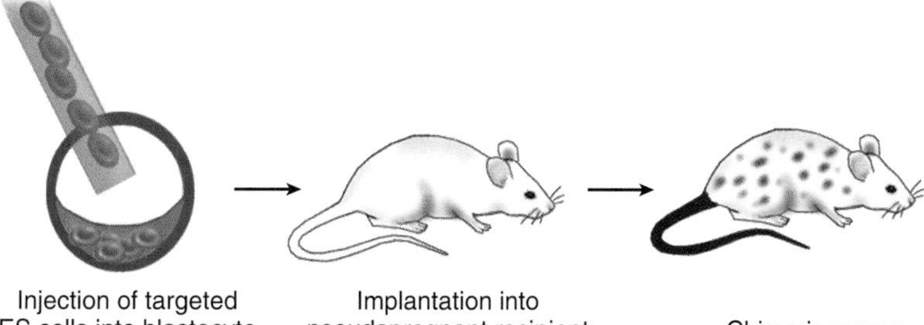

Breeding chimera to obtain knockout heterozygotes

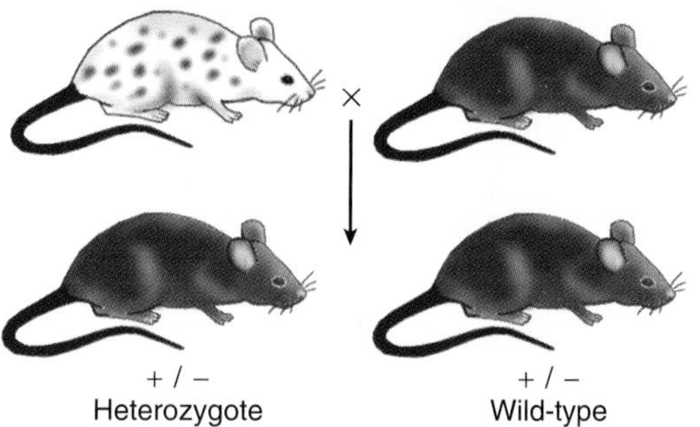

Breeding heterozygotes to obtain knockout heterozygotes

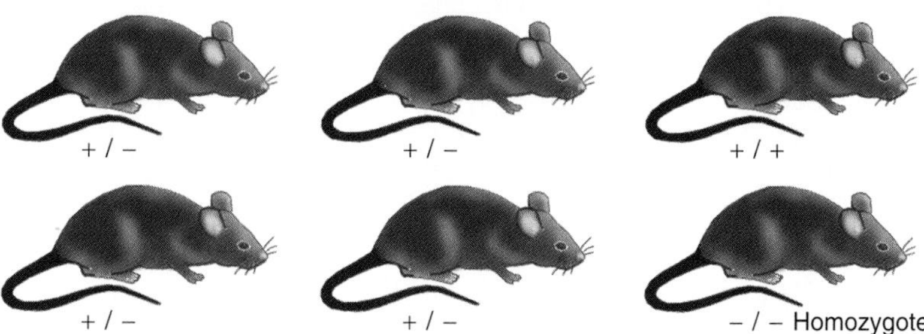

FIGURE 69–15 Scheme for generating heterozygous and homozygous gene knockout mice by homologous recombination in mouse embryonic stem (ES) cells.

bacteriophage encodes an enzyme called Cre that catalyzes recombination of DNA between two specific sequences (called loxP sites) that signal recombination. This system has been adapted in mice by producing a targeting construct in which the gene of interest is *flanked* by *lox*P sites (a "floxed allele"). Mice homozygous for the floxed allele are bred with transgenic mice that express the Cre recombinase in a tissue-specific manner (e.g., endothelial cells, vascular smooth muscle cells, cardiomyocytes). The resulting mice have a deletion of the gene of interest only in the tissue expressing the Cre recombinase. By placing the Cre transgene under the control of a tetracycline responsive promoter, gene deletion is programmed only following tetracycline feeding.

Studies of Mouse Physiology

Realizing the advantage of the potential of mouse genetics requires technologies that can characterize the phenotype of mutant mice. The mouse is technically challenging because the heart and blood vessels are very small in size and the resting mouse heart beat is greater than 500 beats/min. Miniaturized instrumentation and microsurgical techniques have helped solve these problems.[60,61] It is now possible to obtain a wide variety of physiological measurements in anesthetized and intubated mice, including aortic blood pressures, left ventricular pressure tracings, and cardiac hemodynamics before and after infusions of pharmacological agents, such as dobutamine or isoproterenol. Noninvasive imaging of the heart and vasculature has improved substantially, and two-dimensional echocardiograms are now routine in fetal and adult mice. Magnetic resonance imaging renders clear images of cardiac structure and function. These noninvasive techniques are used to measure end-systolic and end-diastolic left ventricular dimensions, left ventricular wall thickness and mass, and shortening fraction. Myocardial infarctions produced by coronary artery ligation, wire injuries to vessels that simulate angioplasty, and aortic banding to induce left ventricular hypertrophy are commonly performed in gene modified mice. Exercise testing, 24-hour electrocardiogram recordings on conscious mice using implanted transducers, and electrophysiological studies to detect inducible cardiac arrhythmias are also standard techniques. With the availability of techniques to study cardiovascular physiology, genetically modified mice now provide an accurate and convenient way to evaluate the function of specific genes in cardiovascular disease.

Gene- and Cell-Based Therapies

Gene transfer is the introduction and expression of recombinant genes in mammalian cells. Gene transfer aims to introduce recombinant genes into target cells to study the mechanisms and consequences of gene expression. Genes are transfected into cells using vectors. The recombinant gene undergoes transcription into RNA and translation into protein by host enzymes, culminating in the expression of the recombinant protein. The recombinant protein remains intracellular or is secreted into the extracellular space or circulation. Gene expression is transient or stable, depending on whether integration into chromosomes occurs. The efficiency of DNA uptake and gene expression, often referred to as *transfection efficiency*, depends on many factors, including delivery of DNA to the cell, uptake of DNA into the cytoplasm, degradation of DNA in endosomes, release of DNA from endosomes into the cytoplasm, transport to the nucleus, and persistence in the nucleus.

In vivo gene transfer is performed by cell-mediated or direct gene transfer methods. Cell-mediated or ex vivo gene transfer involves removing autologous cells from the host and transfecting the cells with the vector in vitro.[62] Genetically modified cells are reintroduced into the host by infusion or injection. Ex vivo gene transfer permits the introduction of recombinant genetic material into a specific cell—for example, endothelial or smooth muscle cells—and analysis of recombinant gene expression within that cell type.

In vivo gene transfer employs the direct introduction of recombinant genes into target cells and tissues.[63] Targeted gene transfer in the vasculature has been performed with cell-specific promoters to achieve gene expression within endothelial cells or smooth muscle cells.[64] Both ex vivo and in vivo gene transfer approaches have been employed in the development of animal models of vascular disease and in clinical trials of gene transfer to the cardiovascular system.

Vectors

Transfection of appropriate target cells represents the critical first step in gene transfer. As a result, development of gene transfer methods has represented a significant area of research in the field. Both viral and nonviral vectors have been employed in vascular gene transfer studies. A common feature of these methods is the efficient delivery of genes into cells. Vectors differ, however, in the processing of foreign DNA and the frequency of integration into chromosomal DNA. In the case of retroviral and lentiviral vectors, the transferred sequences are stably integrated into the chromosomal DNA of the target cell. These vectors have been considered most often for ex vivo gene therapy. Other methods of gene transfer result primarily in the introduction of foreign DNA into target cell nuclei in an unintegrated form. These methods result in high, but transient, gene expression. These vectors, including adenovirus, adeno-associated virus, and cationic liposomes, have been employed predominantly for in vivo gene transfer studies.

Retroviruses

Retroviruses were the first vectors employed in gene transfer studies, dating back to the 1980s. Initial interest in retroviruses as vectors arose from the observation that these vectors stably transduce nearly 100 percent of proliferating target cells in culture. Retroviral vectors were used initially in vascular gene transfer studies, primarily in ex vivo studies, but their use has been limited by low transfection efficiencies. Retroviral vectors have been used recently in clinical gene therapy studies for treatment of severe combined immune deficiency (SCID). Unfortunately, in one trial, two children experienced the complication of retroviral insertion into an oncogenic site of chromosome X, leading to leukemia.[65]

Adenovirus

Adenovirus type 2 and type 5 are the two serotypes used for vectors in cardiovascular gene transfer. The adenovirus genome is linear, double-stranded DNA, approximately 36 kb in length, which is divided into 100 map units, each of which is 360 base pairs in length. The DNA contains short inverted terminal repeats (ITRs) at the end of the genome that are required for viral DNA replication. The gene products are organized into early (E1-E4) and late (L1-L5) regions, based on expression before or after initiation of DNA replication. Adenoviruses have a lytic life cycle characterized by attachment to an adenoviral glycoprotein receptor on mammalian cells and entry into cells by receptor-mediated endocytosis. Adenoviral capsid proteins protect adenoviruses from lysosomal degradation, and viral DNA translocates to the nucleus. Expression of viral genes depends on cellular transcription factors and expression of the adenoviral E1 region, which encodes a transactivator of viral gene expression. During lytic infection, the viral genome replicates to several thousand copies per cell. The viral genome associates with core proteins and is packaged into capsids by self-assembling of major capsid proteins.

The adenovirus genome is rendered replication-deficient to generate a vector. Vectors are constructed by homologous recombination in a cell line known as 293 cells by cotransfection of (1) a bacterial plasmid containing the cDNA of interest and a small region of adenoviral genome deleted from E1A and E1B regions (these regions regulate adenoviral transcription and are required for viral replication), and (2) an incomplete adenoviral genome. Homologous recombination between the two DNAs generates a recombinant genome in which the foreign gene replaces the E1 region. Viral stock is further propagated in 293 cells to high titer, generally 10^9 to 10^{10} plaque-forming units (pfu) per milliliter.

Adenoviral vectors have several additional advantages, including efficient infection of mammalian cells and expression in nondividing cells in vitro and in vivo. These vectors are relatively stable and can be grown and concentrated to a high titer. Extrachromosomal replication of the vector greatly reduces the chance of mutation by random integration and dysregulation of host cellular genes. However, a number of shortcomings limit their use as gene transfer vectors. Gene expression in vascular and myocardial cells following adenoviral infection is short-lived, persisting for only several weeks.[66-68] Host immune response to adenoviral proteins is a major limitation to their in vivo use. Although low levels of neutralizing antibodies do not appear to have adverse clinical effects, it remains to be determined whether host immune responses to the adenovirus will preclude repeated administrations of the same serotype of adenovirus. First-generation recombinant adenoviral vectors (deletion of E1A and E1B genes and partial deletion of E3 genes) have been used clinically in gene therapy studies, even though in animal models these vectors are often associated with tissue inflammation, particularly in the liver and lung.[69] Direct exposure of diseased liver to high-titer adenoviral vectors is highly toxic, and in one case, unfortunately lethal.[70] Inactivation of the E2A gene has been associated with longer gene expression and less inflammation in lung and liver. In arterial gene transfer studies employing adenoviral vectors, mononuclear inflammatory cell infiltrates have been observed in the adventitia of peripheral[71] and pulmonary[68] arteries, but no necrosis or vasculitis was observed. Infection of pulmonary arteries with adenovirus was associated with mild degrees of perivascular inflammation; however, pulmonary arteries instilled with saline or liposomes also exhibited mild accumulation of perivascular mononuclear cells.[68] Despite the limitations of immune responses to adenoviral capsid proteins, adenoviral vectors are attractive vehicles for in vivo gene transfer in animal models because of the efficiency of transfection. Whether adenoviral vectors will be used clinically remains to be seen.

Adeno-Associated Virus

Adeno-associated virus (AAV) is a defective human parvovirus that has attractive features as a gene transfer vector. This viral vector is prepared at high titers, is not normally pathogenic in humans, and infects many cell types in vitro.[72] The AAV genome is a single-stranded, linear, 5 kb DNA molecule. The wild-type AAV integrates in a site-specific fashion into a single 7 kb region on human chromosome 19. The AAV genome is flanked by 145 base pair–inverted terminal repeats containing the sequences required for packaging, DNA replication, and integration. The coding region contains two open reading frames, which are deleted and replaced with one or more cDNAs plus transcriptional regulatory units during vector construction.[73] AAV vectors accept transgene cassettes of only 4 to 5 kb; this limits the types of transgenes that can be used. Propagation of AAV vectors requires complex packaging, including AAV Rep and Cap proteins and five adenoviral proteins (E1A, E1B, E2A, E4, and VA). These complex packaging requirements have precluded construction of a helper cell line for AAV. Currently, vectors are constructed by cotransfection of cells with the AAV vector and a nonpackageable plasmid containing the AAV Rep and Cap proteins. This is followed by infection of the transfected cells with wild-type or mutant helper adenovirus. AAV is separated from contaminating adenovirus by heat treatment and equilibrium density gradation centrifugation. Protocols for constructing AAV vectors are described elsewhere.[72]

The AAV vectors infect multiple cell types in vitro, but their utility in vivo has not been established. Transduction of vascular endothelial and smooth muscle cells remains unknown.[74] Further limitations include a lack of packaging cell lines and a requirement for coinfection with adenovirus, making it difficult to prepare large quantities of pure AAV vectors. Deletion of viral genes during vector construction limits the ability of these vectors to integrate in a site-specific manner but does raise the possibility of insertional mutagenesis. AAV vectors are theoretically attractive, but considerable work is required before they can be implemented clinically.

Cationic Liposomes

Cationic lipids are preparations of positively charged lipids that spontaneously complex with negatively charged DNA to form DNA-lipid conjugates. The lipid component facilitates delivery of DNA to cells by fusion with plasmid membrane or with endosomal membranes after endocytosis. Following release from endosomes, plasmid DNA is maintained in an extrachromosomal form. Cationic liposomes have been employed in arterial gene transfer studies in many animal models, including rats, rabbits, dogs, and pigs. Advantages of cationic liposomes include a favorable safety profile, a lack of viral coding sequences, and no cDNA size constraints. Minimal biochemical, hemodynamic, or cardiac toxicity has been associated with their use in animals or humans.[75] These vectors are straightforward to prepare for experimental and clinical use. The limitations include a low transfection efficiency and short-term gene expression.

Polymers

Nucleic acids and drugs have been applied to polymer gels coated onto stents or balloons and directly applied to arteries. Hydrogel catheters were developed to transmit plasmid DNA to rabbit arteries in vivo and to humans in clinical gene therapy trials.[76] Over time, other polymers were developed associated with stenting of arteries, but many early polymers were associated with intense inflammatory reactions. Newer formulations have been successfully used in the development of drug-eluting stents.[77,78]

Animal Models

Gene transfer is a useful approach to introduce nucleic acids to somatic cells of an animal to define gene function, dissect disease pathophysiology, or achieve a therapeutic effect. Over the past decade, gene transfer has been employed in many animal models of cardiovascular disease.[79] Gene- and cell-based approaches have been used, including a recent interest in combining gene transfer with stem cell based therapies.[80,81] Gene transfer as a tool to induce vascular growth is an illustrative example.

Vascular growth proceeds through the stages of angiogenesis, arteriogenesis, and lymphangiogenesis. Angiogenesis is the sprouting of new blood vessels from preexisting vessels. Arteriogenesis is the enlargement of muscular collateral blood vessels from preexisting arteriolar anastomoses and is often referred to as "collateralization." Lymphangiogenesis is the generation of new lymphatic vessels from preexisting ones. It has been widely used in preclinical and clinical studies. Two splice variants of vascular endothelial growth factor (VEGF A), $VEGF_{165}$ and $VEGF_{121}$, have angiogenic properties in animal models[82] and have been evaluated in clinical trials.[83] Placental growth factor (PlGF) also has angiogenic activity in animals. PlGF binds to VEGFR-1 and has been implicated in angiogenesis under pathological conditions.[84] Interestingly, PlGF also promotes angiogenesis and arteriogenesis through mobilization of hematopoietic stem cells and endothelial progenitor cells from the bone marrow. The clinical relevance of VEGF, PlGF, and endothelial progenitor cells in the clinical treatment of ischemia remains undetermined, although there have been recent efforts at transducing stem cells with VEGF to enhance angiogenesis.[85,86] Other growth factors have been evaluated for their angiogenic properties in gene transfer models. Hypoxia-inducible transcription factor-1-alpha activates several angiogenic growth factors, including VEGF-A, VEGFR-2, insulin-like growth factor-2, and erythropoietin.[87] A leucine zipper transcription factor that activated VEGF transcription has also been recently described.[88]

The hypothesis that overexpression of growth factors will result in therapeutic vascular growth has been tested in several animal models of peripheral and myocardial ischemia, including ex vivo transduction of stem cells and endothelial progenitor cells.[82,86,89] Adenoviral-mediated VEGF and fibroblast growth factor delivery and vascular growth has been demonstrated in the myocardium and skeletal muscle by the proliferation and enlargement of capillaries, although cessation of therapy (or extinction of the transgene) leads to regression of most of the vessels. Expression of VEGF for more than 4 weeks leads to sufficient vascular remodeling that new vessel growth persists for several months after VEGF treatment is withdrawn.[90] In animal models, hemodynamic factors and persistence of blood flow are important for stabilization of the newly formed vessels. Furthermore, the predictive value of a preclinical animal model is inversely related to the animal size. Many applications and vectors work well in smaller animals, such as mice and rats, but scaling up to larger animals, such as pigs, dogs, and sheep, has proved difficult. Demonstration of efficacy in young, normal animals may not predict responses in older human patients with chronic diseases. Indeed, vascular growth is impaired in elderly and diabetic animals.[91] Many of the beneficial biological effects reported in animals may not be achievable in humans, given the limitations of current vectors.

Clinical Trials

Cardiovascular gene therapy trials have had a checkered course. Many phase I trials have been completed, but few have proceeded to phase II studies. Concerns have been raised about the use of adenoviral vectors, even for cardiac or vascular applications, as well as low transfection efficiencies in vivo. The majority of studies have focused on stimulation of angiogenesis and arteriogenesis to improve perfusion of myocardial or skeletal muscle. Three phases of therapeutic angiogenesis trials have been conducted to date. Initial phase I trials employed plasmid DNA[76,92,93] and adenoviruses[94,95] to induce angiogenesis for peripheral or myocardial ischemia. These trials evaluated the safety of vectors and catheter or direct injection delivery in small numbers of patients. Consistent findings were evident: no serious adverse events were encountered attributable to the gene vector or delivery device. With this demonstration of safety, phase I/II trials evaluated larger numbers of patients with soft efficacy endpoints.[96-104] No major adverse events were reported, and while positive efficacy findings were reported, many of these trials were not controlled. Collectively, however, the following clinical insights accrued. Placebo effects are common in treated patients, perhaps due to altered hemodynamics or improved clinical care. Meaningful clinical endpoints were not always predefined and hence cast doubt on efficacy data. The absence of controlled, randomized studies also did not help the field move forward. Recently, a third phase of clinical trials has been initiated with placebo-controlled studies, including larger numbers of patients and well-defined clinical endpoints.[105-114] Data from these phase III studies and long-term follow-up are essential in determining whether a gene therapy product will be approved by the Food and Drug Administration and clinically used to treat myocardial and/or peripheral ischemia. Improved understanding of the pharmacokinetics is essential.[115] Investigators must proceed with carefully conducted and evaluated trials.

Future Directions

Molecular and cellular biology are now part of mainstream cardiovascular research. These approaches have advanced our understanding of the pathogenesis of cardiovascular diseases, have led to the development of extremely useful animal models, and have provided the basic principles for molecular therapies. Cardiovascular research is now turning to molecular genetics as the next scientific arena in which major advances will occur. To date, we have begun to understand the mechanisms by which single genes cause cardiovascular disease. These mechanisms have provided great insight into the pathophysiology of complex common cardiovascular disorders. The next major challenge in the field of molecular genetics is to understand with greater clarity genetic susceptibility to common cardiovascular diseases. Genotyping, genomics, and proteomics are approaches with promise but are incompletely developed at this time. The information gleaned from these techniques will only be as good as the characterization of clinical phenotypes by thoughtful, observant physicians who detect unusual patterns of disease in their patients. While many investigators remain hopeful, we do not know the role that genetic or cell-based therapies will play in the practice of clinical cardiology. The efforts of many physician-scientists and clinical investigators are required to conduct careful, well-considered studies. Only then can the promise of molecular genetics be realized and applied to the care of cardiovascular patients.

REFERENCES

1. Alberts B, Johnson A, Lewis J, et al: Molecular Biology of the Cell. New York, Garland Science, 2002.
2. Lewin B. Genes VII. Oxford, Oxford University Press, 2000.
3. Edidin M: Lipids on the frontier: A century of cell-membrane bilayers. Nat Rev Mol Cell Biol 4:414, 2003.
4. Shi Y, Massague J: Mechanisms of TGF-beta signaling from cell membrane to the nucleus. Cell 113:685, 2003.
5. Weis K: Regulating access to the genome: Nucleocytoplasmic transport throughout the cell cycle. Cell 112:441, 2003.
6. Bonifacino JS, Lippincott-Schwartz J: Coat proteins: Shaping membrane transport. Nat Rev Mol Cell Biol 4:409, 2003.
7. Williams RR, Fisher AG: Chromosomes, positions please! Nat Cell Biol 5:388, 2003.
8. Eichler EE, Sankoff D: Structural dynamics of eukaryotic chromosome evolution. Science 301:793, 2003.
9. Page SL, Hawley RS: Chromosome choreography: The meiotic ballet. Science 301:785, 2003.
10. Cline SD, Hanawalt PC: Who's on first in the cellular response to DNA damage? Nat Rev Mol Cell Biol 4:361, 2003.
11. Lawen A: Apoptosis: An introduction. Bioessays 25:888, 2003.
12. Roberts JM: Evolving ideas about cyclins. Cell 98:129, 1999.
13. Sherr CJ: The Pezcoller lecture: Cancer cell cycles revisited. Cancer Res 60:3689, 2000.
14. Roberts JM, Sherr CJ: Bared essentials of CDK2 and cyclin E. Nat Genet 35:9, 2003.
15. Sherr CJ, Roberts JM: CDK inhibitors: Positive and negative regulators of G1-phase progression. Genes Dev 13:1501, 1999.

16. Conqueret O: New roles for p21 and p27 cell-cycle inhibitors: A function for each cell compartment? Trends Cell Biol 13:65, 2003.
17. Lowe SW, Sherr CJ: Tumor suppression by Ink4a-Arf: Progress and puzzles. Curr Opin Genet Dev 13:77, 2003.
18. Nabel EG: CDKs and CKIs: Molecular targets for tissue remodeling. Nat Rev Drug Discov 1:587, 2002.
19. Nabel EG, Boehm M, Akyurek LM, et at: Cell cycle signaling and cardiovascular disease. Cold Spring Harb Symp Quant Biol 67:163, 2002.
20. Gartel AL, Tyner AL: The role of the cyclin-dependent kinase inhibitor p21 in apoptosis. Mol Cancer Ther 1:639, 2002.
21. Vogelstein B, Lane D, Levine AJ: Surfing the p53 network. Nature Nov 408:307, 2000.
22. Lander ES, Linton LM, Birren B, et al: Initial sequencing and analysis of the human genome. Nature 409: 860, 2001.
23. Venter JC, Adams MD, Myers EW, et al: The sequence of the human genome. Science 291:1304, 2001.
24. Collins FS, Green ED, Guttmacher AE, et al: A vision for the future of genomics research. Nature 422:835, 2003.
25. Sambrook J, Russell DW: Molecular cloning: A laboratory manual. Cold Spring Harbor, Cold Spring Harbor Laboratory, 2001.
26. Watson JD, Crick FHC: Molecular structure of nucleic acids: A structure for deoxyribose nucleic acid. Nature 171:737, 1953.
27. NCBI: Online Mendelian Inheritance in Man. Available at: http://www.ncbi.nlm.nih.gov/omim
28. Nabel EG: Cardiovascular disease. N Engl J Med 349:60, 2003.
29. Wang DG, Fan JB, Siao CJ, et al: Large-scale identification, mapping, and genotyping of single-nucleotide polymorphisms in the human genome. Science 280:1077, 1998.
30. Goldstein JL, Hobbs HH, Brown MS: Familial hypercholesterolemia. *In* Scriver CR, Beaudet AL, Sly WS, et al (eds): The Metabolic & Molecular Bases of Inherited Disease. New York, McGraw-Hill, 2001.
31. Seidman JG, Seidman C: The genetic basis for cardiomyopathy: From mutation identification to mechanistic paradigms. Cell 104:557, 2001.
32. Keating MT, Sanguinetti MC: Molecular and cellular mechanisms of cardiac arrhythmias. Cell 104:569, 2001.
33. Ridker PM, Stampfer MJ: Assessment of genetic markers for coronary thrombosis: Promise and precaution. Lancet 353:687, 1999.
34. Lifton RP, Gharavi AG, Geller DS: Molecular mechanisms of human hypertension. Cell 104:545, 2001.
35. Riva A, Kohane IS: SNPper: Retrieval and analysis of human SNPs. Bioinformatics 18:1681-1685, 2002.
36. Cargill M, Altshuler D, Ireland J, et al: Characterization of single-nucleotide polymorphisms in coding regions of human genes. Nat Genetics 22:231, 1999.
37. Sachidanandam R, Weissman D, Schmidt SC, et al: A map of human genome sequence variation containing 1.42 million single nucleotide polymorphisms. Nature 409:928, 2002.
38. NCBI: Single Nucleotide Polymorphism. Available at: http://www.ncbi.nlm.nih.gov/SNP/
39. Sabeti PC, Reich DE, Higgins JM, et al: Detecting recent positive selection in the human genome from haplotype structure. Nature 419:832, 2002.
40. Couzin J: Human Genome. HapMap launched with pledges of $100 million. Science 298:941, 2002.
41. Syvänen A: Accessing genetic variation: Genotyping single nucleotide polymorphisms. Nat Rev Genet 2:930, 2001.
42. Wang DG, Fan J, Siao C, et al: Large-scale identification, mapping, and genotyping of single-nucleotide polymorphisms in the human genome. Science 280:1077, 1998.
43. Zwick ME, Cutler DJ, Chakravarti A: Patterns of genetic variation in Mendelian and complex traits. Annu Rev Genomics Hum Genet 1:387, 2000.
44. Glazier AM, Nadeu JH, Altman TJ: Finding genes that underlie complex traits. Science 298:2345, 2002.
45. Lohmueller KE, Pearce CL, Pike M, et al: Meta-analysis of genetic association studies supports a contribution of common variants to susceptibility to common disease. Nat Genet 33:177, 2003.
46. Mohike KL, Erdos MR, Scott LJ, et al: High-throughput screening for evidence of association by using mass spectrometry genotyping on DNA pools. PNAS 99:16928, 2002.
47. Storey JD, Tibshirani R: Statistical significance for genomewide studies. PNAS 100:9440, 2003.
48. Kennedy GC, Matsuzaki H, Dong S, et al: Large-scale genotyping of complex DNA. Nat Biotechnol 21:1233, 2003.
49. Butte A: The use and analysis of microarray DNA. Nat Rev Drug Disc 1:951, 2002.
50. Velculescu VE, Vogelstein B, Kinzler KW: Analysing uncharted transcriptomes with SAGE. Trends Genet 16:423, 2000.
51. Patino WD, Mian OY, Hwang PM: Serial analysis of gene expression: Technical considerations and applications to cardiovascular biology. Circ Res 91:565, 2002.
52. Lockhart DJ, Winzeler EA: Genomics, gene expression and DNA arrays. Nature 405:827, 2000.
53. Loscalzo J: Proteomics in cardiovascular biology and medicine. Circulation 108:380, 2003.
54. Arrell DK, Neverova I, Van Eyk JE: Cardiovascular proteomics: Evolution and potential. Circ Res 88:763, 2001.
55. Fishman MC, Olson EN, Chien KR: Molecular advances in cardiovascular development. *In* Chien KR, Braunwald E (eds): Molecular Basis of Cardiovascular Disease: A Companion to Braunwald's Heart Disease. Philadelphia, WB Saunders, 1999, pp 115-134.
56. Mouse Genome Sequencing Consortium: Initial sequencing and comparative analysis of the mouse genome. Nature 420:520, 2002.
57. Young SG, Lusis AJ, Hammer RE: Genetically modified animal models in cardiovascular research. *In* Chien KR, Braunwald E (eds): Molecular Basis of Cardiovascular Disease: A Companion to Braunwald's Heart Disease. Philadelphia, WB Saunders, 1999, pp 37-85.
58. Gossen M, Bujard H: Tight control of gene expression in mammalian cells by tetracycline-responsive promoters. Proc Natl Acad Sci U S A 89:5547, 1992.
59. Gu H, Marth JD, Orban PC, et al: Deletion of a DNA polymerase β gene segment in T cells using cell type-specific gene targeting. Science 265:103, 1994.
60. Chien KR: Cardiac muscle diseases in genetically engineered mice: Evolution of molecular physiology. Am J Physiol 269:h755, 1995.
61. Duckers HJ, Boehm M, True AL, et al: Heme oxygenase-1 protects against vascular constriction and proliferation. Nat Med 7:693, 2001.
62. Nabel EG, Plautz G, Boyce FM, et al: Recombinant gene expression in vivo within endothelial cells of the arterial wall. Science 244:1342, 1989.
63. Nabel EG, Plautz G, Nabel GJ: Site-specific gene expression in vivo by direct gene transfer into the arterial wall. Science 249:1285, 1990.
64. Akyürek LM, Yang Z-Y, Aoki K, et al: SM22 a promoter targets gene expression to vascular smooth muscle cells in vitro and in vivo. Mol Med 11:983, 2000.
65. Marshall E: Second child in French trial is found to have leukemia. Science 299:320, 2003.
66. Lemarchand P, Jones M, Yamada I, Crystal RG: In vivo gene transfer and expression in normal uninjured blood vessels using replication-deficient recombinant adenovirus vectors. Circ Res 72:1132, 1993.
67. Guzman RJ, Lemarchand P, Crystal RG, et al: Efficient gene transfer into myocardium by direct injection of adenovirus vectors. Circ Res 73:1202, 1993.
68. Muller DW, Gordon D, San H, et al: Catheter-mediated pulmonary vascular gene transfer and expression. Circ Res 75:1039, 1994.
69. Yang Y, Nunes FA, Berencsi K, et al: Cellular immunity to viral antigens limits E1-deleted adenoviruses for gene therapy. Proc Natl Acad Sci U S A 91:4407, 1994.
70. Somia N, Verma IM: Gene therapy: Trials and tribulations. Nat Rev Genet 1:91, 2002.
71. Ohno T, Gordon D, San H, et al: Gene therapy for vascular smooth muscle cell proliferation after arterial injury. Science 265:781, 1994.
72. Tal J: Adeno-associated virus-based vectors in gene therapy. J Biomed Sci 7:279, 2000.
73. Rolling F, Samulski RJ: AAV as a viral vector for human gene therapy. Generation of recombinant virus. Mol Biotechnol 3:9, 1995.
74. Lynch CM, Hara PS, Leonard JC, et al: Adeno-associated virus vectors for vascular gene delivery. Circ Res 80:497, 1997.
75. San H, Yang ZY, Pompili VJ, et al: Safety and short-term toxicity of a novel cationic lipid formulation for human gene therapy. Hum Gene Ther 4:781, 1993.
76. Isner JM, Pieczek A, Schainfeld R, et al: Clinical evidence of angiogenesis after arterial gene transfer of phVEGF165 in patient with ischaemic limb. Lancet 348:370, 1996.
77. Sousa JE, Serruys PW, Costa MA: New frontiers in cardiology: Drug-eluting stents: Part I. Circulation 107:2274, 2003.
78. Sousa JE, Serruys PW, Costa MA: New frontiers in cardiology: Drug-eluting stents: Part II. Circulation 107:2383, 2003.
79. Baskir R, Vale PR, Isner JM, Losordo DW: Angiogenic gene therapy: Pre-clinical studies and phase I clinical data. Kidney Int 61:110, 2002.
80. Mangi AA, Noiseux N, Kong D, et al: Mesenchymal stem cells modified with Akt prevent remodeling and restore performance of infarcted hearts. Nat Med 9:1195, 2003.
81. Hill JM, Dick AJ, Raman VK, et al: Serial cardiac magnetic resonance imaging of injected mesenchymal stem cells. Circulation 108:1009, 2003.
82. Isner JM: Myocardial gene therapy. Nature 415:234, 2002.
83. Yla-Herttuala S, Martin JF: Cardiovascular gene therapy. Lancet 355:213, 2000.
84. Lutun A, Tjwa M, Moons L, et al: Revascularization of ischemic tissues by PlGF treatment, and inhibition of tumor angiogenesis, arthritis and atherosclerosis by anti-Flt1. Nat Med 8:831, 2002.
85. Iwaguro H, Yamaguchi J, Kalka C, et al: Endothelial progenitor cell vascular endothelial growth factor gene transfer for vascular regeneration. Circulation 105:672, 2002.
86. Nabel EG: Stem cells combined with gene transfer for therapeutic vasculogenesis. Circulation 105:672, 2002.
87. Vincent KA, Shyu KG, Luo Y, et al: Angiogenesis is induced in a rabbit model of hindlimb ischemia by naked DNA encoding an HIF-1alpha/VP16 hybrid transcription factor. Circulation 102:2255, 2000.
88. Rebar EJ, Huang Y, Hickey R, et al: Induction of angiogenesis in a mouse model using engineered transcription factors. Nat Med 8:1427, 2002.
89. Yla-Herttuala S, Alitalo K: Gene transfer as a tool to induce therapeutic vascular growth. Nat Med 9:694, 2003.
90. Dor Y, Djonov V, Abramovitch R, et al: Conditional switching of VEGF provides new insights into adult neovascularization and pro-angiogenic therapy. EMBO J 21:1939, 2002.
91. Schratzberger P, Walter DH, Rittig K, et al: Reversal of experimental diabetic neuropathy by VEGF gene transfer. J Clin Invest 107:1083, 2001.
92. Baumgartner I, Pieczek A, Manor O, et al: Constitutive expression of phVEGF165 after intramuscular gene transfer promotes collateral vessel development in patients with critical limb ischemia. Circulation 97:1114, 1998.
93. Isner JM, Baumgartner I, Rauh G, et al: Treatment of thromboangiitis obliterans (Buerger's disease) by intramuscular gene transfer of vascular endothelial growth factor: Preliminary clinical results. J Vasc Surg 28:964, 1998.
94. Laitinen M, Makinen K, Manninen H, et al: Adenovirus-mediated gene transfer to lower limb artery of patients with chronic critical leg ischemia. Hum Gene Ther 9:1481, 1998.
95. Losordo DW, Vale PR, Symes JF, et al: Gene therapy for myocardial angiogenesis: Initial clinical results with direct myocardial injection of phVEGF165 as sole therapy for myocardial ischemia. Circulation 98:2800, 1998.
96. Symes JF, Losordo DW, Vale PR, et al: Gene therapy with vascular endothelial growth factor for inoperable coronary artery disease. Ann Thorac Surg 68:830, 1999.

97. Vale PR, Losordo DW, Milliken CE, et al: Left ventricular electromechanical mapping to assess efficacy of phVEGF(165) gene transfer for therapeutic angiogenesis in chronic myocardial ischemia. Circulation 102:965, 2000.
98. Laitinen M, Hartikainen J, Kiltunen MO, et al: Catheter-mediated vascular endothelial growth factor gene transfer to human coronary arteries after angioplasty. Hum Gene Ther 11:263, 2000.
99. Vale PR, Losordo DW, Milliken CE, et al: Randomized, single-blind, placebo-controlled pilot study of catheter-based myocardial gene transfer for therapeutic angiogenesis using left ventricular electromechanical mapping in patients with chronic myocardial ischemia. Circulation 103:2138, 2001.
100. Rajagopalan S, Shah M, Luciano A, et al: Adenovirus-mediated gene transfer of VEGF(121) improves lower-extremity endothelial function and flow reserve. Circulation 104:753, 2001.
101. Sarkar N, Ruck A, Kallner G, et al: Effects of intramyocardial injection of phVEGF-A165 as sole therapy in patients with refractory coronary artery disease—12-month follow-up: Angiogenic gene therapy. J Intern Med 250:373, 2001.
102. Comerota AJ, Throm RC, Miller KA, et al: Naked plasmid DNA encoding fibroblast growth factor type 1 for the treatment of end-stage unreconstructible lower extremity ischemia: Preliminary results of a phase I trial. J Vasc Surg 35:930, 2002.
103. Losordo DW, Vale PR, Hendel RC, et al: Phase 1/2 placebo-controlled, double-blind, dose-escalating trial of myocardial vascular endothelial growth factor 2 gene transfer by catheter delivery in patients with chronic myocardial ischemia. Circulation 105:2012, 2002.
104. Shyu KG, Chang H, Wang BW, Kuan P: Intramuscular vascular endothelial growth factor gene therapy in patients with chronic critical leg ischemia. Am J Med 114:85, 2003.
105. Henry TD, Annex BH, McKendall GR, et al: The VIVA trial: Vascular endothelial growth factor in ischemia for vascular angiogenesis. Circulation 107:1359, 2003.
106. Simons M, Annex BH, Laham RJ, et al: Pharmacological treatment of coronary artery fibroblast growth factor-2: Double-blind, randomized, controlled clinical trial. Circulation 105:788, 2002.
107. Lederman RJ, Mendelsohn FO, Anderson RD, et al: TRAFFIC Investigators. Therapeutic angiogenesis with recombinant fibroblast growth factor-2 for intermittent claudication (the TRAFFIC study): A randomized trial. Lancet 359:2058, 2002.
108. Seiler C, Pohl T, Wustmann K, et al: Promotion of collateral growth by granulocyte-macrophage colony-stimulating factor in patients with coronary artery disease: A randomized, double-blind, placebo-controlled study. Circulation 104:2012, 2001.
109. Grines CL, Watkins MW, Helmer G, et al: Angiogenic Gene Therapy (AGENT) trial in patients with stable angina pectoris. Circulation 105:1291, 2002.
110. Makinen K, Manninen H, Hedman M, et al: Increased vascularity detected by digital subtraction angiography after VEGF gene transfer to human lower limb artery: A randomized, placebo-controlled, double-blinded phase II study. Mol Ther 6:127, 2002.
111. Hedman M, Hartikainen J, Syvanne M, et al: Safety and feasibility of catheter-based local intracoronary vascular endothelial growth factor gene transfer in the prevention of postangioplasty and in-stent restenosis and in the treatment of chronic myocardial ischemia: Phase II results of the Kuopio Angiogenesis Trial (KAT). Circulation 107:2677, 2003.
112. Stewart DJ, et al: A phase 2, randomized, multicenter, 26-week study to assess the efficacy and safety of BIOBYPASS (AdGVVEGF121) delivered through minimally invasive surgery versus maximum medical treatment in patients with severe angina, advanced coronary artery disease, and no options for revascularizations. Circulation 106:23, 2002.
113. Rajagopalan S, Mohler E 3rd, Lederman RJ, et al: Regional Angiogenesis with Vascular Endothelial Growth Factor Trial. Regional angiogenesis with vascular endothelial growth factor (VEGF) in peripheral arterial disease: Design of the RAVE trial. Am Heart J 145:1114, 2003.
114. Kastrup J: Euroinject One trial. Late breaking clinical trials sessions, American College of Cardiology 2003, Chicago. J Am Coll Cardiol 41:1603, 2003.
115. Pislaru S, Janssens SP, Gersh BJ, Simari RD: Defining gene transfer before expecting gene therapy: Putting the horse before the cart. Circulation 106:631, 2002.

CHAPTER 70

Genetics and Cardiovascular Disease

Reed E. Pyeritz

Genetic Factors in Disease

Genes contribute to both the cause and the pathogenesis of virtually any abnormality of human physiology and behavior, including, of course, disorders of the heart and the vascular system. This statement carries two messages in addition to the obvious one. First, disease associated with even the most "environmental" of causes, such as trauma, malnutrition, and drug abuse, depends on the human body's response to the insult. How the stress of the initial insult is expressed (the *phenotype*) and how the patient suffers and perhaps recovers depend, to various and yet often poorly defined degrees, on the patient's *genotype*. This idea seems self-evident and verges on the trite, but it is frequently neglected. Some environmental insults, such as massive trauma or poisoning, are lethal to all, regardless of genotype. Nonetheless, as developments in fields such as pharmacogenetics and ecogenetics are defining genetic susceptibilities to human disease better and more simply, physicians must become increasingly attuned to the importance of the genotype.[1]

Second, the introductory statement emphasizes that genetic factors have roles in *both* cause and process; etiology and pathogenesis, although related, are conceptually distinct.[2] For example, the cause of sickle cell anemia is clearly a single mutant gene, but whether a patient homozygous for this mutation expresses all, some, or none of the manifestations of the disease depends on many other genetic and nongenetic factors. Conversely, the cause of pneumococcal pneumonia is equally evident, but the severity and resolution of the disease depend on the patient's immune competence (which in turn depends on genetic and nongenetic factors) as much as on treatment with an antibiotic.

The genotype, therefore, can be detrimental in at least two distinct ways. First, mutant genes can so upset embryology or physiology that a clinical abnormality occurs. Whereas the phenotype of any particular mutation depends on a host of factors, including which homeostatic systems are available to modulate the action of the defect, the genotype has the principal role in causing the disease. This class of mutations is usually referred to as *genetic diseases*. Second, a mutation can facilitate the action of an extrinsic cause in producing disease. Inherited susceptibilities are part of the pathogenesis of disease and are one reason for taking a patient's family history. Until recently, clinicians could do little to pursue tantalizing facts, such as several relatives' suffering myocardial infarction before age 50. The long-touted prospect of detecting a patient's inherited susceptibilities and intervening before irreversible clinical sequelae occur is becoming reality.

Two caveats are important. First, a considerable gap exists between identifying an apparently inherited susceptibility and prescribing an intervention of proven benefit. For example, several years ago a parental history of sudden death was found to identify middle-aged men at increased risk of sudden death, independent of myocardial infarction.[3] However, effective clinical use of this association will require understanding the pathological factors and conducting outcome studies of potential interventions. Second, the risk of "genetic determinism" remains ever-present. A recent study examined public perceptions of "a gene for heart disease"[4]; the concept was interpreted correctly by the majority of the sample, but an important minority thought in terms of an absolute risk that denoted inevitability.

Disorders Due to Microscopic Alterations in Chromosomes

The estimate of the total number of human genes has been revised downward, from 100,000 to about 35,000, as a result of the Human Genome Project. Two copies (termed *alleles*) of each gene are arrayed along 23 pairs of *chromosomes*. Twenty-two of the chromosomes are called *autosomes* (numbered 1 through 22), and the 23rd pair is the *sex chromosomes*, X and Y. Females have two X chromosomes and males have an X and a Y chromosome. Both autosomal alleles are potentially active in specifying RNA copies of their DNA sequences; whether a gene is active depends on the cell type, the developmental stage of the organism, and the regulatory molecules that interact with promoter and enhancer nucleotide sequences that control transcription of the gene. In cells with two X chromosomes (i.e., in all females, in persons with Klinefelter syndrome in which two Xs and one Y

TABLE 70–1 Genomic Disorders (Contiguous Gene Syndromes)

	Symbol	Genetic Defect	Cardiovascular Abnormalities
Syndromes with Cardiovascular Involvement			
Arteriohepatic dysplasia	AHD	del 20p11.23-p12.2	Peripheral pulmonic stenosis/hypoplasia
Cat-eye syndrome	CES	dup 22q11	Total anomalous pulmonary venous return
DiGeorge sequence	DGS	del 22q11	Truncus arteriosus, right aortic arch, TOF, PDA
Miller-Dieker syndrome	MDS	del 17p13	PDA ± complex anomalies
Prader-Willi syndrome	PWS/AS	del 15q12	Cor pulmonale (secondary to obesity and central apnea)
WAGR syndrome		del 11p13	Hypertension (secondary to Wilms tumor)
Syndromes without Frequent Cardiovascular Involvement			
Angelman syndrome	AS	del 15q12*	
Smith-Magenis syndrome	SMS	del 17p11.2	

*The deletion is often indistinguishable at the cytogenetic level from that of the Prader-Willi syndrome; genetic imprinting of locus *UBE3A* is thought to account in part for the phenotypic differences. In Prader-Willi syndrome, the deleted chromosome is always the chromosome 15 inherited from the father, whereas in Angelman syndrome, the deletion affects the maternal chromosome 15.

PDA = patent ductus arteriosus; TOF = tetralogy of Fallot; WAGR = Wilms tumor, aniridia, genitourinary, and retardation.

occur, and in persons with some other rare conditions), only one X is entirely active after early embryogenesis.

Human chromosomes can be examined by culturing cells capable of mitosis; T lymphocytes obtained from venous blood are the usual source, but fibroblasts, cells from chorionic villi, amniocytes, and leukocyte precursors present in bone marrow are also used clinically. Chromosomes are distinguished from one another by their size, shape (determined by the position of a constriction called the *centromere,* which functions as the attachment of the mitotic apparatus), and characteristic banding pattern as revealed by any of several staining techniques. The chromosomes are photographed, cut out, and arranged in pairs, from 1 through 22 and the sex chromosomes, in a display called the *karyotype.* This display and its interpretation are the end results of a clinical study of a patient's chromosomes. The chromosome constitution of a cell is designated by first specifying the number of chromosomes present (46 being normal in diploid cells), then specifying the sex chromosomes, and finally describing any abnormalities. For example, a normal male is designated 46,XY, and a female with an extra chromosome 21 is designated 46,XX,+21.

ANEUPLOIDY. Chromosome aberrations, especially too many or too few chromosomes (*aneuploidy*), are extremely common in human embryos; more than one-half of all conceptuses are spontaneously aborted in early pregnancy, and at least one-half of them are aneuploid. Among live-born infants, about 0.5 percent have a chromosome aberration.

Gain or loss of chromosomes generally happens by nondisjunction, or the failure of a homologous pair of chromosomes to separate. Absence of one chromosome is termed *monosomy;* all autosomal monosomies are embryonic lethals, as is presence of only a Y sex chromosome. The presence of three chromosomes is *trisomy,* and the presence of an entire extra set of chromosomes (for a total of 69) is *triploidy.* The most common autosomal aneuploidy, trisomy 21 associated with Down syndrome, and aneuploidy for sex chromosomes all are compatible with survival into adulthood.

CHROMOSOME REARRANGEMENTS. A chromosome can break and rejoin within itself, potentially giving rise to an *inversion* of genetic material. Often no apparent phenotypic effect occurs in people with an inversion, but because inversions can disrupt chromosome pairing during meiosis, their offspring may have more profound aberrations.

DELETIONS AND DUPLICATIONS. Just as their names imply, these aberrations are losses or gains of chromosomal material. Many clinical syndromes have been associated with aberrations of specific chromosome regions.[5] The smallest deletion detectable by light microscopy is associated with loss of considerable DNA, on the order of 1 million base pairs, so more than one gene is potentially disrupted or lost.

A number of conditions, each initially thought to be due to a mutation in a single locus, are associated with small interstitial chromosome aberrations affecting a cluster of genes (Table 70–1). So rather than pleiotropic manifestations of one mutation, these conditions are likely due to the effects of absences of several, and perhaps many, loci on one chromosome, and therefore are best thought of as *genomic disorders.* In the past, they were referred to as *contiguous gene syndromes.*[6] In the regions of the genome where these deletions occur, repetitive nucleotide sequences appear to predispose to aberrant recombination, and this accounts for their surprising incidence.[7] In addition, such defects are potentially heritable, and the occurrence of the disorder in a family behaves as a Mendelian dominant. Several interstitial deletions are both relatively common and important causes of congenital heart disease.

Disorders Due to Changes in Single Nuclear Genes (see Chap. 69)

Mutations of genes located on the 22 pairs of autosomes and the two sex chromosomes produce phenotypes inherited according to the two principal tenets of Mendel: alleles segregate and nonalleles assort. The first statement refers to gametes receiving only one of the two alleles at a given locus as a result of meiosis. The second statement describes the results of recombination, the meiotic process of rearranging DNA between the two chromosomes of the pair (*homologous chromosomes*); if two loci are widely spaced along a chromosome, their chances of being separated by recombination are 50-50, and they are said to be *unlinked.*

The Human Genome Project, begun in 1990, had goals to map all expressed genes, to create a physical map of overlapping pieces of DNA composing the entire genome, and finally, to sequence all 3.2 billion nucleotides in the haploid complement of human DNA. The project was completed well ahead of schedule, and more than 95 percent of the entire sequence now exists in public databases.[8] More than 12,000 individual loci have been identified, either on the basis of the phenotype that mutations in single genes produce, or through understanding the normal product or function of the gene.[9] The presumption of single-gene defects is based in most instances on the pattern of inheritance in families; segregation of the phenotype according to Mendelian principles is the central piece of evidence. For an increasing number of loci, however, molecular genetic techniques have mapped the phenotype to a narrow chromosome region or to a single gene, or even revealed the actual alteration in nucleotide sequence (see Chap. 69) (Table 70–2).[10] The range of known Mendelian variation in humans and information about gene mapping and molecular defects are routinely catalogued and available on-line.[11]

Of the more than 10,000 loci that have been clearly identified on the basis of either an abnormal phenotype or a normal product, 17.4 percent involve the heart.[11] Many others involve other parts of the cardiovascular system. Thousands

Text continued on p. 1873

TABLE 70–2 Mendelian Conditions that Involve the Cardiovascular System with Known Genetic Defects or Gene Mapping of the Phenotype

Phenotype	Gene Symbol	OMIM No.*	Gene Map Locus
Cardiomyopathies			
Adhalinopathy, primary	*SGCA*	600119	17q12-q21.33
Arrhythmogenic RV dysplasia-1	*ARVD1*	107970	14q23-q24
Arrhythmogenic RV dysplasia-2	*ARVD2*	600996	1q42-q43
Arrhythmogenic RV dysplasia-3	*ARVD3*	602086	14q12-q22
Arrhythmogenic RV dysplasia-4	*ARVD4*	602087	2q32.1-q32.3
Arrhythmogenic RV dysplasia-5	*ARVD5*	604400	3p23
Arrhythmogenic RV dysplasia-6	*ARVD6*	604401	10p12-p14
Becker and Duchenne muscular dystrophies	*DMD*	310200	Xp21.2
Emery-Dreifuss muscular dystrophy	*EMD*	310300	Xp28
Emery-Dreifuss muscular dystrophy	*LMNA*	150330	1q21.2-q21.3
Endocardial fibroelastosis-2	*TAZ*	302060	Xq28
FDC	*ACTC*	102540	15q14
FDC-1A	*CMD1A*	115200	1p11-q11
FDC-1B	*CMD1B*	600884	9q13
FDC-1C	*CMD1C*	601493	10q21-q23
FDC-1E	*CMD1E*	601154	3p25-p22
FDC-1F	*CMD1F*	602067	6q23
FDC-1G	*CMD1G*	604145	2q31
FDC-1H	*CMD1H*	604288	2q14-q22
FDC-2	*CMD1D*	601494	1q32
FDC, X-linked	*DMD*	310220	Xp21.2
FDC-3A	*TAZ*	302060	Xq28
FHC-1	*MYH7*	160760	14q12
FHC-2	*TNNT2*	191045	1q32
FHC-3	*TPM1*	191010	15q22.1
FHC-4	*MYBPC3*	600958	11p11.2
FHC	*TNNI3*	191044	19q13.4
FHC with WPW	*CMH6*	600858	7q3
FHC, mid-LV type	*MYL2*	160781	12q23-q24.3
FHC, mid-LV type	*MYL3*	160790	3p
Friedreich ataxia	*FRDA*	229300	9q13
Muscular dystrophy, Duchenne-like	*SGCA*	600119	17q12-q21.33
Myotonic dystrophy	*DMPK*	160900	19q13.2-q13.3
Myotonic dystrophy 2	*DM2*	602668	3q
Noncompaction of LV	*TAZ*	302060	Xq28
Developmental Disorders			
Alagille syndrome	*JAG1*	601920	20p12
Atrial septal defect, secundum	*ASDI*	108800	6p21.3
Atrial septal defect with AV conduction defects	*CSX*	600584	5q34
AV canal defect-1	*AVSD*	600309	1p31-p21
Bannayan-Zonana syndrome	*PTEN*	601728	10q23.3
Cardiac valve dysplasia-1	*CVD1*	314400	Xq28
Cat-eye syndrome	*CECR*	115470	22q11

Continued

TABLE 70–2 Mendelian Conditions that Involve the Cardiovascular System with Known Genetic Defects or Gene Mapping of the Phenotype—cont'd

Phenotype	Gene Symbol	OMIM No.*	Gene Map Locus
Conotruncal cardiac defects	*CTHM*	217095	22q11
DiGeorge sequence and velocardiofacial syndrome	*DGCR*	188400	del22q11
Down syndrome	*DCR*	190685	21q22.3
Ellis–van Creveld syndrome	*EVC*	225500	4p16
Goldenhar syndrome	*GHS*	141400	7p
Heterotaxy, X-lined visceral	*ZIC3*	306955	Xq26.2
Holt-Oram syndrome	*TBX5*	601620	12q24.1
Keutel syndrome	*MGP*	154870	12p13.1-p12.3
Left-right axis malformation	*TGFB4*	601877	1q42.1
Noonan syndrome	*NSI*	163950	12q24
Progeria	*LMNA*	176670	1q21.1
Total anomalous pulmonary venous return	*TAPVR1*	106700	4p13-q12
Turner syndrome	*RPS4X*	312760	Xq13.1
Werner syndrome	*WRN*	277700	8p12-p11.2
Williams syndrome	*ELN*	194050	del7q11
Wolf-Hirschhorn syndrome	*WHCR*	194190	4p16.3
Disorders of Blood Pressure			
Bartter syndrome	*SLC12A1*	600839	15q15-q21.1
Bartter syndrome with deafness	*BSND*	602522	1p31
Bartter syndrome, type 2	*KCNJ1*	600359	11q24
Bartter syndrome, type 3	*CLCNKB*	602023	1p36
Dysautonomia, familial	*DYS*	223900	9q31-q33
Hypertension, essential	*SAH*	145505	16p13.11
Hypertension, essential	*PNMT*	171190	17q21-q22
Hypertension, essential	*AGTR1*	106165	3q21-q25
Hypertension, essential	*GNB3*	139130	12p13
Hypertension, essential	*AGT*	106150	1q42-q43
Hypertension, low renin	*HSD11B2*	218030	16q22
Hypertension, salt resistant	*NPR3*	108962	5p14-p12
Hypertension, with brachydactyly	*HTNB*	112410	12p12.2-p11.2
Liddle syndrome	*SCNN1B*	600760	16p13-p12
Liddle syndrome	*SCNN1G*	600761	16p13-p12
Mineralocorticoid excess	*HSD11B2*	218030	16p22
Orthostatic hypotensive disorder	*OHDS*	143850	18q
Pheochromocytoma	*SDHB* *VHL* *RET* *SDHD*	185470 193300 164761 602690	1p36.1-p35 3p26-p25 10q11.2 11q23
Polycystic kidney disease, adult 1	*PKD1*	601313	16p13.3-p13.12
Polycystic kidney disease, adult 2	*PKD2*	173910	4q21-q23
Preeclampsia, susceptibility to	*NOS3*	163729	7q36
Preeclampsia, susceptibility to	*AGT*	106150	1q42-q43
Preeclampsia/eclampsia	*PEE*	189800	4q25-q34
Pulmonary hypertension, familial	*PPH1*	178600	2q31-q32

TABLE 70–2 Mendelian Conditions that Involve the Cardiovascular System with Known Genetic Defects or Gene Mapping of the Phenotype—cont'd

Phenotype	Gene Symbol	OMIM No.*	Gene Map Locus
Disorders of Coagulation and Thrombosis			
Antithrombin III deficiency	*AT3*	107300	1q23-q25
Antithrombin Pittsburgh defect	*PI*	107400	14q32.1
Coumarin resistance	*CYP2A6*	122720	19q13.2
Defective thromboxane A2 receptor	*TBXA2R*	188070	19p13.3
Dysfibrinogenemia, α type	*FGA*	134820	4q28
Dysfibrinogenemia, β type	*FGB*	134830	4q28
Dysfibrinogenemia, γ type	*FGG*	134850	4q28
Dysprothrombinemia	*F2*	176930	11p11-q12
Factor H deficiency	*HF1*	134370	1q32
Factor V deficiency	*F5*	227400	1q23
Factor VII deficiency	*F7*	227500	13q34
Factor X deficiency	*F10*	227600	13q34
Factor XI deficiency	*F11*	264900	4q35
Factor XII deficiency	*F12*	234000	5q33-qter
Factor XIIIA deficiency	*F13A1*	134570	6p25-p24
Factor XIIIB deficiency	*F13B*	134580	1q31-q32.1
Glanzmann thrombasthenia, type A	*ITGA2B*	273800	17q21.32
Glanzmann thrombasthenia, type B	*ITGB3*	173470	17q21.32
GNAQ deficiency	*GNAQ*	600998	9q21
Hemophilia A	*F8C*	306700	Xq28
Hemophilia B	*F9*	306900	Xq27.1-q27.2
PAI1 deficiency	*PAI1*	173360	7q21.3-q22
Plasmin inhibitor deficiency	*PLI*	262850	17pter-p12
Plasminogen activator deficiency	*PLAT*	173370	8p12
Plasminogen deficiency	*PLG*	173350	6q26
Platelet α/δ storage pool deficiency	*SELP*	173610	1q23-q25
Platelet disorder, familial with myeloid malignancy	*FPDMM*	601399	21q22.1-q22.2
Platelet glycoprotein IV deficiency	*CD36*	173510	7q11.2
Platelet-activating factor acetylhydrolase deficiency	*PAFAH*	601690	6p21.2-p12
Protein C inhibitor deficiency	*PCI*	601841	14q32.1
Protein S deficiency	*PROS1*	176880	3p11.1-q11.2
Thrombocythemia, essential	*THPO*	600044	3q26.3-q27
Thrombocytopenia, neonatal	*ITGA2B*	273800	17q21.32
Thrombocytopenia, Paris-Trousseau	*TCPT*	188025	11q23
Thrombocytopenia, X-linked	*WAS*	301000	Xp11.23-p11.22
Thrombophilia	*HRG*	142640	3q27
Thrombophilia	*PAI1*	173360	7q21.3-q22
Thrombophilia	*HCF2*	142360	22q11
Thrombophilia	*THBD*	188040	20p11.2
Thrombophilia	*PLG*	173350	6q26
Thromboxane synthase deficiency	*TBXAS1*	274180	7q34
Vitamin K–dependent coagulation defect	*GGCX*	137167	2p12
von Willebrand disease	*VWF*	193400	12p13.3
Warfarin sensitivity	*CYP2C9*	601130	10q24

Continued

TABLE 70–2 Mendelian Conditions that Involve the Cardiovascular System with Known Genetic Defects or Gene Mapping of the Phenotype—cont'd

Phenotype	Gene Symbol	OMIM No.*	Gene Map Locus
Disorders of Lipid Metabolism			
Abetalipoproteinemia	*MTP*	157147	4q22-q24
Abetalipoproteinemia	*APOB*	107730	2p24
Apo A-I and Apo C-III deficiency	*APOA1*	107680	11q23
Apo A-II deficiency	*APOA2*	107670	1q21-q23
Apo B-100 ligand defect	*APOB*	107730	2p24
Cerebrotendinous xanthomatosis	*CYP27A1*	213700	2q33-qter
Combined familial hyperlipidemia	*LPL*	238600	8p22
HMG-CoA synthetase-2 deficiency	*HMGCS2*	600234	1p13-p12
Hypercholesterolemia, familial	*LDLR*	143890	19p13.2-p13.1
Hypercholesterolemia, familial 3	*FH3*	603776	1p34.1-p32
Hypertriglyceridemia	*APOC3*	107720	11q23
Hypertriglyceridemia	*APOA1*	107680	11q23
Hypoalphalipoproteinemia	*APOA1*	107680	11q23
Hypobetalipoproteinemia	*APOB*	107730	2p24
Sitosterolemia	*STSL*	210250	2p21
Tangier disease	*HDLDT1*	205400	9q31
Wolman disease	*LIPA*	278000	10q24-q25
Metabolic Disorders with Primary Effects in the Cardiovascular System			
Carnitine acetyltransferase deficiency	*CRAT*	600184	9q34.1
Carnitine deficiency, systemic	*SLC22A5*	603377	5q33.1
Metabolic Disorders with Secondary Effects in the Cardiovascular System			
Amyloidosis	*APOA1*	107680	11q23
Amyloidosis, cerebroarterial	*APP*	104760	21q21.3-q22.05
Cerebral amyloid angiopathy	*CST3*	105150	20p11.2
Cerebrovascular disease, occlusive	*AACT*	107280	14q32.1
Coronary spasm, susceptibility to	*NOS3*	163729	7q36
Fabry disease	*GLA*	301500	Xq22
Gaucher disease with calcification	*GBA*	230800	1q21
Glycogen storage disease II (Pompe)	*GAA*	232300	17q25.2-q25.3
Hemochromatosis	*HFE*	235200	6p21.3
Homocystinuria	*CBS*	236200	21q22.3
Homocystinuria, MTHFR deficiency	*MTHFR*	236250	1p36.3
Menkes syndrome	*ATP7A*	300011	Xq12-q13
Mucopolysaccharidosis I	*IDUA*	252800	4p16.3
Mucopolysaccharidosis II	*IDS*	309900	Xq28
Mucopolysaccharidosis IVA	*GALNS*	253000	16q24.3
Mucopolysaccharidosis IVB	*GLB1*	230500	3p21.33
Mucopolysaccharidosis VI	*ARSB*	253200	5q11-q13
Mulibrey nanism	*MUL*	253250	17q22-q23
Pseudoxanthoma elasticum	*PXE*	264800	16p13.1
Neoplastic Disorders			
Carney (NAME) complex	*CNC*	160980	2p16
Paraganglioma, familial nonchromaffin 1	*PGL1*	168000	12q23

TABLE 70–2 Mendelian Conditions that Involve the Cardiovascular System with Known Genetic Defects or Gene Mapping of the Phenotype—cont'd

Phenotype	Gene Symbol	OMIM No.*	Gene Map Locus
Paraganglioma, familial nonchromaffin 2	*PGL2*	601650	11q13.1
von Hippel–Lindau syndrome	*VHL*	193300	3p26-p25
Primary Disorders of Rhythm and Conduction			
Heart block, progressive familial-1	*HB1*	113900	19q13.2-q13.3
Jervell and Lange-Nielsen syndrome	*KCNQ1*	192500	11p15.5
Jervell and Lange-Nielsen syndrome	*KCNE1*	176261	21q22.1-q22.2
Long-QT syndrome-1	*KCNQ1*	192500	11p15.5
Long-QT syndrome-2	*KCNH2*	152427	7q35-q36
Long-QT syndrome-3 and ventricular fibrillation, idiopathic	*SCN5A*	600163	3p24-p21
Long-QT syndrome-4	*LQT4*	600919	4q25-q27
Long-QT syndrome-5	*KCNE2*	603796	21q22.1
Ventricular tachycardia, idiopathic	*GNAI2*	139360	3p21
Primary Disorders of Vasculature			
Aneurysm, familial and Ehlers-Danlos, vascular type	*COL3A1*	120180	2q31
Arterial calcification of infancy	*ENPP1*	208000	6q22-q23
Cerebral arteriopathy with subcortical infarcts and leukoencephalopathy	*NOTCH3*	600276	19p13.2-p13.1
Cerebral cavernous malformations-1	*CCM1*	116860	7q11.2-q21
Cerebral cavernous malformations-2	*CCM2*	603284	7p15-p13
Cerebral cavernous malformations-3	*CCM3*	603285	3q25.2-q27
Fibromuscular dysplasia of arteries	*COL3A1*	120180	2q31
Hemangioma, capillary infantile	*HC1*	602089	5q31-q33
Hemiplegic migraine, familial	*CACNA1A*	601011	19p13
Hemiplegic migraine, familial 2	*MHP2*	602481	1q21-q23
Hemiplegic migraine, familial, susceptibility to	*MFTS*	300125	Xq
Hereditary hemorrhagic telangiectasia-1	*ENG*	131195	9q34.1
Hereditary hemorrhagic telangiectasia-2	*ALK1*	601284	12q11-q14
Lymphedema, hereditary	*FLT4*	136352	5q35.3
Marfan syndrome	*FBN1*	134797	15q21.1
Moyamoya disease	*MYMY*	252350	3p26-p24.2
Supravalvular aortic stenosis	*ELN*	130160	7q11.2
Venous malformations, multiple	*TEK*	600221	9p21

*Refers to the entry for the locus in http://www.ncbi.nlm.nih.gov/Omim/.

AV = atrioventricular; FDC = familial dilated cardiomyopathy; FHC = familial hypertrophic cardiomyopathy; LV = left ventricle; RV = right ventricle.

Disorders may have been mapped by the phenotype, by the gene, or both. The annotations p and q refer to band patterns in chromosomes detected cytochemically that mark specific regions.

of loci have been mapped to a specific region of the genome. Many of these loci, when mutated, cause Mendelian disorders, and the genetic map of these loci represents the "morbid anatomy of the human genome." Some of the cardiovascular and hemostatic disorders that were mapped by mid-2003 are shown in Figure 70–1. Knowledge of the molecular etiology of the monogenic disorders, most of which are relatively rare, will undoubtedly lead to improved understanding of the cause, pathogenesis, and treatment of more common conditions.[10,12]

Another product of the Human Genome Project is the identification and cataloging of tens of thousands of single nucleotide polymorphisms (SNPs), nonpathological alterations in 1 nucleotide that occur in all humans at a prevalence of about 1 per 1100 nucleotides. Two types of genetic analyses can be performed using SNPs: linkage and association. Association analyses have been especially common in studies of common cardiovascular disease; however, most investigations of individual phenotypes, such as myocardial infarction, have produced conflicting results.[13] Improved precision will require both larger numbers of subjects and careful attention to control populations, since the frequency and distribution of SNPs depend highly on ethnicity. Increasingly, studies of common conditions are melding large

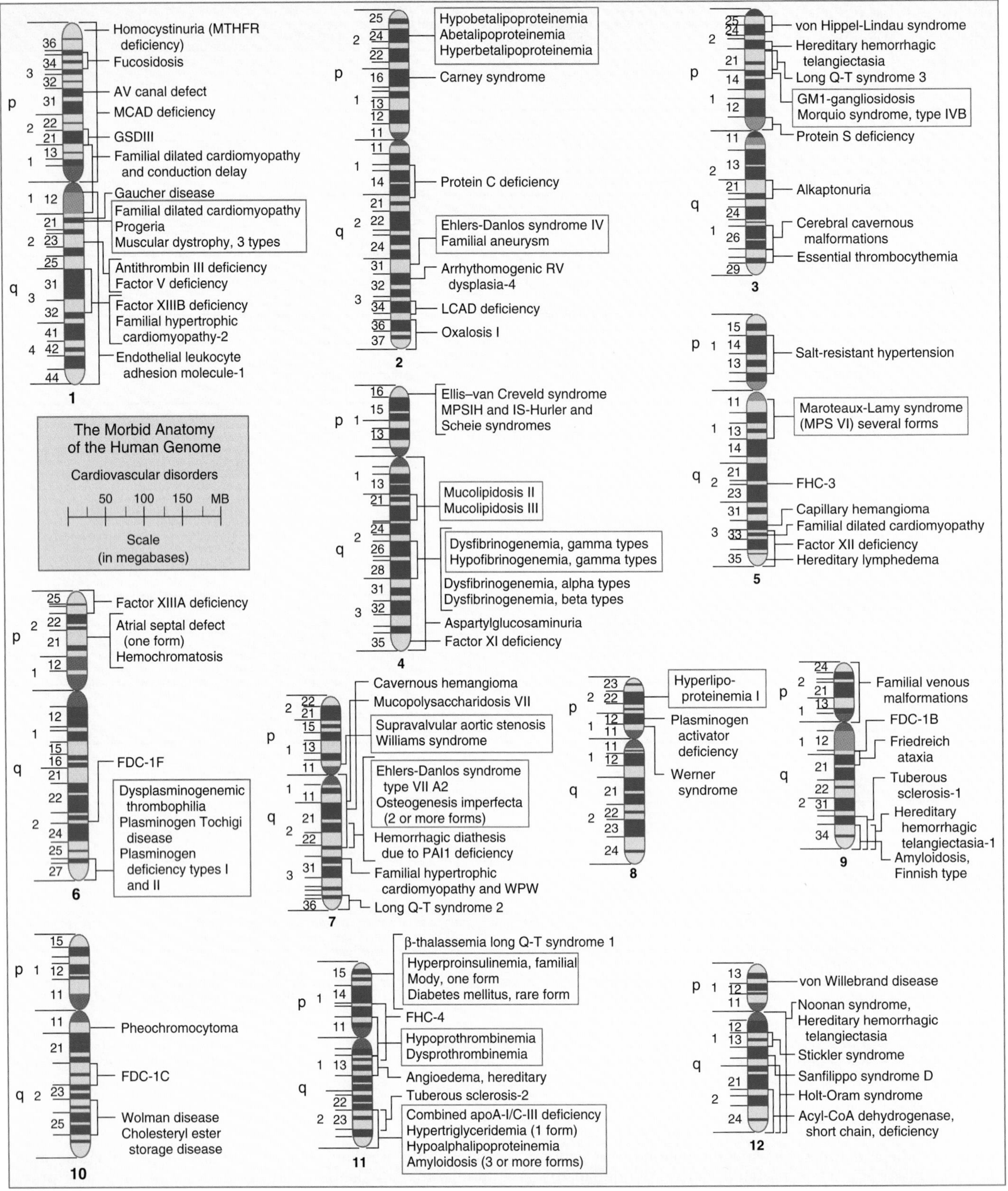

FIGURE 70–1 Chromosomal location of human genes associated with some disorders of the cardiovascular system. These genes affect the structure, function, and metabolism of the heart and blood vessels and hemostasis and have been identified by the deleterious effects of mutations. Numerous additional genes that encode structural proteins important to the cardiovascular system have been identified but not yet associated with disease. In the figure, brackets next to the chromosome show the regional localization of the gene causing a particular disorder. Brackets next to two or more disorders indicate that all of the genes causing the disorders map to the same region. Disorders surrounded by boxes are caused by different mutations at the same gene.

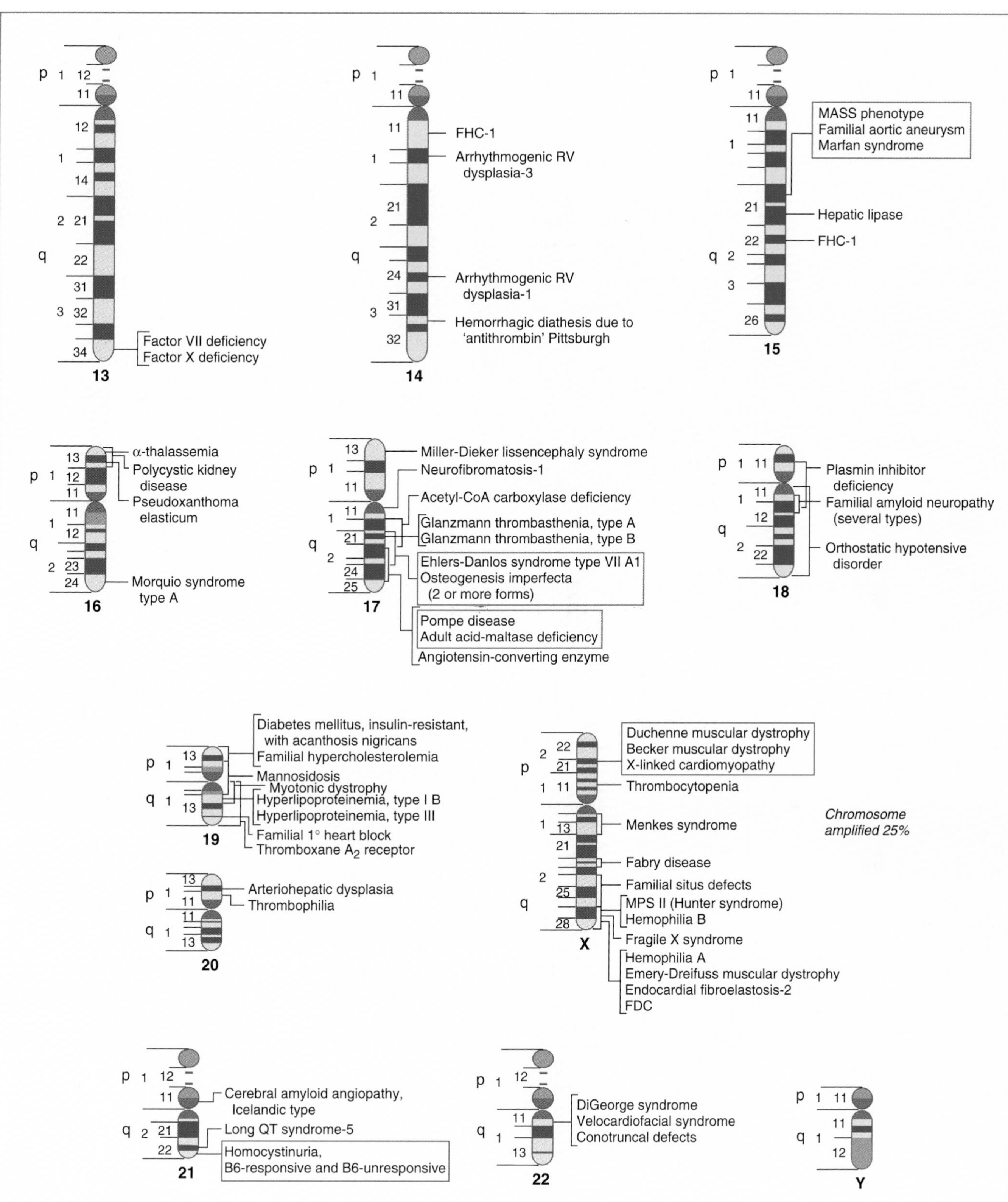

FIGURE 70–1, cont'd

databases of medical history, genealogy, and genotypes based on SNPs.[9,14]

Dominance and Recessiveness

The related concepts of dominance and recessiveness are characteristics of the phenotype, *not of the gene.* A phenotype is dominant when the patient is *heterozygous* for a mutation, i.e., when one copy of the mutant allele and one copy of the normal allele are present. This holds for genes on both autosomes and the X chromosome. A phenotype is recessive when the patient has two mutant alleles at the locus causing the condition. If the mutant alleles are identical, the patient is *homozygous* at that locus, a situation usually present either when the allele is identical by descent through both parents (i.e., the parents had a common ancestor and are *consanguineous*) or when the mutant allele is common in the population (e.g., the most prevalent mutation for cystic fibrosis and the mutation for sickle cell anemia). Biochemical and molecular genetic assessment of mutant alleles has shown that the majority of recessive phenotypes are due to two distinct mutant alleles, a situation termed a *genetic compound,* indicative of the widespread heterogeneity in mutations at each locus. Males have but one X chromosome, and each locus is therefore *hemizygous;* a mutant locus is always expressed in the phenotype of a male. Dominance and recessiveness for X-linked traits refer to expression in heterozygous and homozygous women, respectively.

Whether a disorder is called dominant or recessive depends on how carefully the phenotype is assessed and how it is defined. For example, familial hypercholesterolemia is a relatively common hereditary disorder caused by defects in the receptor for low-density lipoprotein (LDL; see Chap. 39). The vast majority of patients are heterozygous for a mutant allele at the *LDLR* locus on chromosome 19, and the disease is inherited as a Mendelian dominant trait. However, if a man and a woman, each heterozygous for an *LDLR* mutation, produce a child, that child has a 25 percent risk of inheriting both of the mutant alleles and thereby is either homozygous or a genetic compound for *LDLR.* Such a child has a much more severe form of familial hypercholesterolemia that is inherited as a Mendelian recessive trait. Similarly, homozygosity for the sickle hemoglobin mutation at the β-globin locus on chromosome 11 produces the familiar autosomal recessive disease sickle cell anemia. However, heterozygosity for the same mutation rarely produces disease but rather sickling of erythrocytes if they are examined under conditions of low oxygen tension; this phenotype is transmitted as a dominant trait.

AUTOSOMAL RECESSIVE INHERITANCE. Nearly all deficiencies of enzymatic activity—the classic inborn errors of metabolism first defined by Archibald Garrod in 1903—cause recessive phenotypes. Most homeostatic systems, which include all metabolic pathways, have sufficient flexibility to function well if one of the enzymatic steps functions at half-normal efficiency, as would occur in the case of heterozygosity for a mutant allele at a structural gene for an enzyme. However, homeostasis cannot cope if two mutant alleles cause a reduction in enzymatic activity to a few percent or less of normal activity. The characteristics of autosomal recessive inheritance, features common to such phenotypes, and a typical pedigree are shown in Figure 70–2.

AUTOSOMAL DOMINANT INHERITANCE. Only a few enzyme deficiencies but many disorders of development and structure are inherited as dominant traits. The reasons for this are several. One possibility is that developmental homeostasis has a limited repertoire of responses to stress, and when a structural or regulatory macromolecule is reduced to only one-half normal amount, the system cannot cope. Another possibility, illustrated by mutations in procollagen molecules, pertains to gene products that must interact before becoming functional; an aberrant protein combined with a normal one would be a defective multimer, and the effect of being heterozygous for a mutation would be magnified—a *dominant-negative effect.*[2,15] The characteristics of autosomal dominant inheritance, features common to many such phenotypes, and a typical pedigree are shown in Figure 70–3.

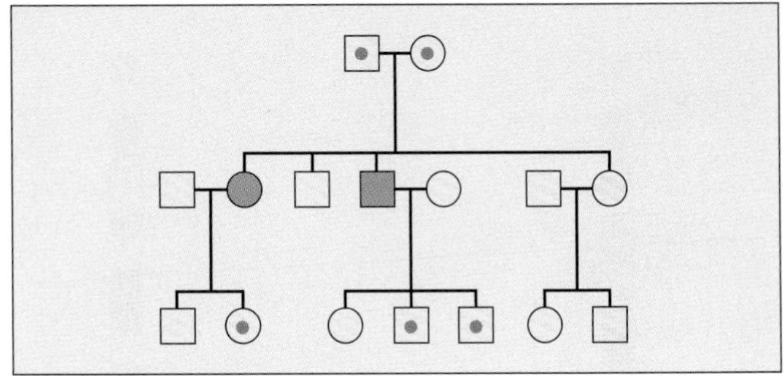

FIGURE 70–2 *Characteristics of autosomal recessive inheritance:*
A single generation is affected.
Both sexes are affected equally frequently.
Each parent is heterozygous (a carrier).
Each offspring of two carriers has a 25 percent chance of being affected, a 50 percent chance of being a carrier, and a 25 percent chance of inheriting neither mutant allele.
Two-thirds of clinically normal offspring are carriers.
The rarer the phenotype, the greater is the likelihood of consanguinity.
Characteristics of autosomal recessive phenotypes:
Often due to enzyme deficiencies.
Often more severe than dominant disorders.
Often early age of onset.

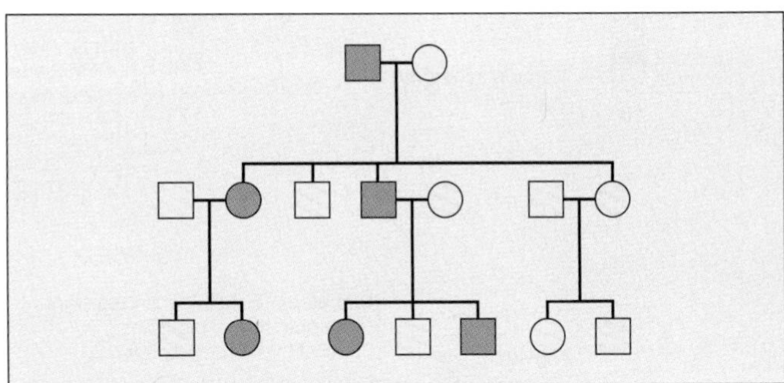

FIGURE 70–3 *Characteristics of autosomal dominant inheritance:*
Several generations are affected.
Both sexes are affected equally frequently.
In familial cases, only one parent need be affected.
Male-to-male transmission occurs.
Offspring of an affected parent has a 50 percent chance of being affected.
The frequency of sporadic cases is higher, the more severe the condition.
Paternal age has an effect in sporadic cases.
Characteristics of autosomal dominant phenotypes:
Often associated with malformations.
Often pleiotropic.
Usually variable.
Often age dependent.

Most human dominant traits are *incomplete,* because the heterozygote is less severely affected than the homozygote. Defects of *LDLR* are illustrative: the heterozygote has classic type IIa hyperlipidemia whereas the homozygote has a quantitatively worse form of the same disease. It may well be that homozygosity for most alleles that cause dominant disorders is incompatible with life.

X-LINKED INHERITANCE. The characteristics of X-linked inheritance, features common to such phenotypes, and a typical pedigree are shown in Figure 70–4. Whereas virtually

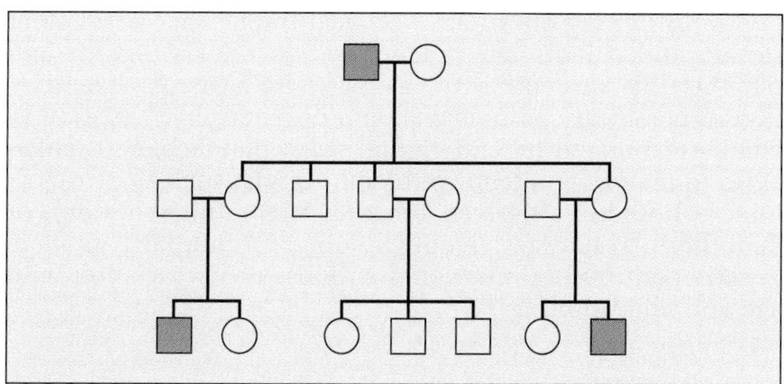

FIGURE 70–4 *Characteristics of X-linked inheritance:*
No male-to-male transmission.
All daughters of affected males are carriers.
Sons of a carrier mother have a 50 percent chance of being affected; daughters have a 50 percent chance of being carriers.
Some mothers of an affected male are not heterozygotes in all cells of their body, but they may have more affected sons if germinal mosaicism is present.
Characteristics of X-linked phenotypes:
More severe in males.
Heterozygous females may be unaffected.
Variable, especially in females.

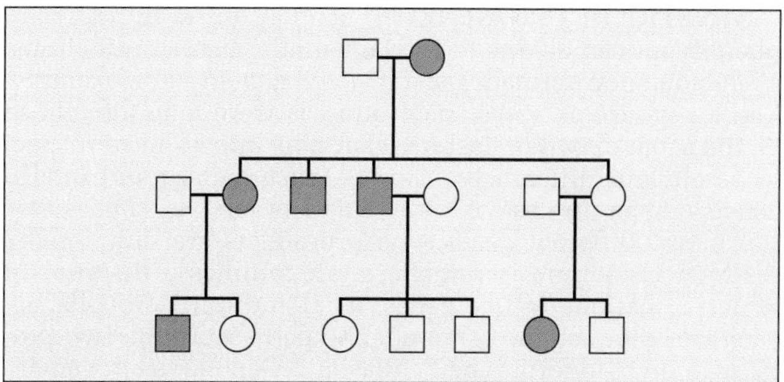

FIGURE 70–5 *Characteristics of disorders due to a mutation of the mitochondrial chromosome:*
Both sexes are equally frequently and severely affected.
Transmission is only through women; offspring of affected men are unaffected.
All offspring of an affected woman may be affected.
Variability of expression can be extreme in a family, including apparent nonpenetrance.
Phenotypes may be age dependent.

TABLE 70–3 Causes of Variability of Gene Expression

Genetic background	Physiological rearrangements
Age dependence	Variation in X inactivation*
Sex influence	Endogenous complementation*
Sex limitation	Maternal factors
Modifying loci:	Effects of mitochondrial genome
Hypostasis and epistasis	Intrauterine environment
Gene alteration	Imprinting
Somatic mutation	Exogenous and ecological factors
Somatic amplification	Ecology—temperature, diet
Transpositions and rearrangements	Teratogens
	Medical intervention
Mutations	Chance

*Pertains to female heterozygotes for X-linked disorders.

all diseases due to mutations on the X chromosome are more severe in hemizygous males, women heterozygous for the same mutations often show some manifestations, albeit less severe and of later age of onset. For example, most women carriers of alpha-galactosidase A deficiency (Fabry disease) eventually develop cerebrovascular disease or renal failure because of the accumulation of glycosphingolipid.

MITOCHONDRIAL INHERITANCE. Energy generation through oxidative phosphorylation occurs in mitochondria in the cytoplasm of most cell types. Numerous mitochondria, each containing a single chromosome, exist in each cell. Some of the enzymes of oxidative phosphorylation are encoded by genes on the nuclear chromosomes and the proteins transported into the mitochondrion; the rest of the proteins are encoded by genes on the mitochondrial chromosome. Thus, genetic defects of oxidative phosphorylation can be due to mutations of genes on the autosomes or the X chromosome, and the resulting diseases behave as Mendelian recessive traits, or they can be due to mutations of genes on the mitochondrial chromosome, in which case the resulting diseases do not behave as Mendelian traits.[16] The differences are explicable by the events of conception. The spermatocyte contributes few if any mitochondria to the zygote, and the effective complement of mitochondria that will ever be present in the fetus is derived from the mitochondria already present in the cytoplasm of the oocyte. Thus, phenotypes due to mutations of the mitochondrial chromosome show *maternal inheritance,* the characteristics of which are shown in Figure 70–5.

Principles of Clinical Genetics

PLEIOTROPY. Most mutant alleles have effects on more than one organ system, and a Mendelian phenotype frequently displays numerous, often diverse manifestations. For example, Marfan syndrome is defined by abnormalities in the eye, skeleton, skin, heart, and aorta, and until the recognition of a defect in extracellular microfibrils, the findings could not be linked either etiologically or pathogenetically.

VARIABILITY. The effects of the same mutant allele on phenotype can be different among people heterozygous (for dominant traits), homozygous (for autosomal recessive traits), or hemizygous (for X-linked traits) for the allele. Variability can be described in terms of the frequency of a particular pleiotropic manifestation among patients with the mutation; the severity of the phenotype; and the age of onset of manifestations. If a person has the mutant allele or alleles but shows no phenotypic effect, the trait is called *nonpenetrant.* To an important degree, whether a clinical phenotype is called nonpenetrant depends on the sensitivity of the techniques used for detection. For example, two decades ago, based on bedside examination, cardiovascular abnormalities were thought to affect about half of people with Marfan syndrome; echocardiography now reveals aortic dilation in more than 90 percent. The term *incomplete penetrance* should not be used with reference to individuals but rather to indicate that prevalence of the phenotype is less than 100 percent of people known to carry the mutation. The Holt-Oram syndrome (see Chap. 56) is an instructive example. In this autosomal dominant syndrome of reduction anomalies of the upper limb and congenital heart defect, patients in the same family can have only arm anomalies, only a heart defect, or both. Moreover, the severity of the reduction defect varies widely, from a proximally placed thumb to near total absence of the arm. The cardiac feature is incompletely penetrant because only about 50 percent of patients have it, but in any individual with the Holt-Oram allele, the heart is either structurally normal or not.

Numerous genetic and environmental factors can affect expression of a gene (Table 70–3), and it is often impossible to determine which of these factors are most important in a specific patient or particular disease. However, the pervasiveness of variable expression emphasizes that phenotypes determined by single genes are to some extent really "multifactorial."

GENETIC HETEROGENEITY. Similar or even identical phenotypes can be due to fundamentally distinct mutations, a phenomenon termed *genetic heterogeneity.* For example, Marfan syndrome and homocystinuria were long thought to be the same disorder, despite what now appear in retrospect to be obvious differences in inheritance pattern and intelligence.[17] As in the case of these two disorders, the causes may lie in two different genes whose products are functionally distinct. Osteogenesis imperfecta exemplifies a disorder in which mutations in two genes, α1(I) and α2(I) procollagen, each can produce the same phenotype because the two proteins interact to form type I collagen.[18] Genetic heterogeneity is pervasive at the intragenic level of analysis; except for sickle cell anemia, hemochromatosis, and achondroplasia, virtually all single-gene disorders are due to a wide variety of mutations at a given locus.

Nonpathological Variation in the Cardiovascular System

CARDIAC STRUCTURE AND PHYSIOLOGY. All aspects of the ontogeny of the cardiovascular system are dictated by the genome. If, as seems most credible, few genes have a large effect and many have small contributions, any specific aspect of "normal" cardiovascular phenotype—size, shape, function—exhibits multifactorial inheritance. In other words, to the extent that any given phenotype can be quantified, it shows a normal distribution within the population, and near-relatives are more similar to each other than they are to distant relatives and the rest of the population. The twin method should demonstrate a higher concordance of the trait in monozygotic than dizygotic twins. However, surprisingly few phenotypes have been examined.

Preliminary data on left ventricular dimensions measured echocardiographically showed higher correlations between parent and child than between matched control subjects, suggesting a genetic contribution; however, as in many such studies, the effect of shared environment was not estimated. In an attempt to minimize environmental contributions, left ventricular sizes of twins who were not exercise-trained were compared; the mean intrapair differences in echocardiographic dimensions were less in the monozygotic than in the dizygotic twins and nontwin siblings. The caliber and branch geometry of coronary arteries show familial resemblance, and both parameters are much more similar in monozygotic twins than in other relatives. Further support for the importance of genetic factors in normal development derives from studies that demonstrate ethnic differences in structure. For example, the thickness of the intima and the media of coronary arteries of children who died of noncardiovascular causes varied significantly with the ethnicity of the child.

Measures of cardiac electrophysiology show familial resemblance. Studies of both nuclear families[19] and twins suggest a genetic contribution to resting heart rate, conduction times, and repolarization time. Polymorphic variation in the beta-1 adrenergic receptor is associated with resting heart rate.[20] Genetic control of normal cardiovascular function has been especially difficult to study because of the multitude of environmental (training, diet), stochastic (age), and clinical (subtle, unrecognized pathological condition) issues that confound comparisons of relatives and control subjects. Thus far, no strong genetic contribution to an individual's response to physical conditioning has emerged.

VASCULAR SYSTEM. All members of certain inbred animal strains show little variation in arterial anatomy, especially branch angles, and considerable variation with other strains of the same species. Except for the studies of coronary arterial anatomy already noted, similar studies of humans have not been reported.

One intriguing question of clinical importance is whether certain individuals are predisposed to arterial spasm and whether this susceptibility has a genetic basis. An examination of hereditary pathological and polymorphic variation in factors elaborated by endothelial cells, platelets, and leukocytes to maintain patency of blood vessels, such as prostacyclin, endothelium-derived relaxing factor (nitric oxide), or endothelin-1, may prove enlightening.[21,22] Similarly, is there genetic contribution to arterial stiffness or its variation with age and conditioning?[23]

Cardiovascular Disorders Associated with Chromosome Aberrations

Chromosome aberrations occur in 0.5 percent of the population at birth and are common findings in tumors. Visible alterations of the amount of chromosomal material cause primarily structural defects of the cardiovascular system that are evident in the newborn. The frequency of chromosome aberrations among live-born children with congenital heart defects has been found to range from 5 to 13 percent. Upward of 40 percent of all fetuses with heart defects detected by ultrasonography at 18 to 20 weeks' gestation have chromosome aberrations; most are spontaneously aborted. Most forms of aneuploidy and most duplications and deletions of more than a chromosome band are associated with defects of the cardiovascular system (see Tables 70–1 and 70–4).[24] Exceptions are 47,XXX, 47,XYY, and 47,XXY (Klinefelter syndrome), in which the incidence of congenital heart disease is probably not elevated over the population baseline.

ANEUPLOIDY. How the abnormal phenotypes caused by autosomal aneuploidy develop remains controversial. One view holds that disturbance of the dosage of the genes present on the specific aneuploid chromosome segments is the central issue. The other view is that any aneuploid state disturbs developmental homeostasis in a nonspecific manner. The former theory predicts some distinctiveness of phenotype among the trisomy syndromes that occur in live-born children, whereas the latter predicts shared manifestations. At a coarse level, the clinical pictures are similar, with grave problems of the craniofacies, central nervous system, genitalia, distal limbs, and heart usually present. However when a more refined examination of the phenotypes is obtained, considerable distinctiveness emerges.

The three most common autosomal trisomies—13, 18, and 21—can be distinguished readily at the bedside. In all three, membranous ventricular and atrial septal defects are common. However, the detailed accounting of cardiovascular lesions among large numbers of patients with these trisomies reveals important differences that suggest aneuploidy exerts more than a global effect on development. In this and most other analyses of congenital heart defects, the system of classification based on the presumed pathogenetic mechanisms proves most instructive and is a useful approach to comparing different causative factors (Table 70–4).

About one-quarter of the defects in trisomies 13 and 18 are due to cell migration abnormalities, and two-thirds are flow lesions; when combined, these two mechanisms account for considerably more of these classes of defects than in the general population with congenital heart disease. By contrast, in trisomy 21, left-sided flow lesions are much less common, whereas abnormal closure of endocardial cushions is strikingly frequent. Indeed, in contrast to endocardial cushion defects without a chromosome 21 anomaly, left-sided flow lesions rarely occur in patients with Down syndrome and endocardial cushion defects. Furthermore, the high incidence of endocardial cushion defects and low incidence of

TABLE 70–4 Cardiovascular Manifestations Associated with Chromosome Aberrations

Chromosome Aberration	Eponym	Cardiovascular Manifestations
Triploidy		
69,XXX (or XXY or XYY)		>50% have CHD: ASD and VSD
Aneuploidy		
+13	Patau	~80% have CHD; 75% of CHD is complex: PDA, VSD, ASD, PS, AS, dextrocardia, CoA
+18	Edwards	~90% have CHD: most CHD is complex: VSD, PDA, ASD, bicuspid PV and AV, CoA
+21	Down	~40% have CHD: ECD, TOF; MVP in ~20%; AR
+8 mosaicism		~25% have CHD, most of little clinical consequence: VSD, PDA, CoA, PS
+9 mosaicism		~70% have CHD, usually complex: VSD, PDA, PLSVC
45,X	Turner	~10% have clinically important CHD: 50% of these have CoA; mild CoA is likely much more common; also AS, ARD, VSD, ASD, dextrocardia
47,XXX		CHD not increased
47,XXY	Klinefelter	CHD possibly slightly increased; ? mild conduction changes; venous thromboembolic disease
47,XYY		CHD not increased; ? mild conduction changes
Deletions		
4p–	Wolf-Hirschhorn	~50% have CHD, usually complex: VSD, ASD, PDA, PS
5p–	Cri du chat	~20% have CHD, usually single: VSD, PDA, ASD, PS
7q–		~20% have CHD, various, often complex
13q–		CHD common, often severe, but depends on region deleted
18p–		CHD uncommon
18q–		~25% have CHD, usually single, of little consequence: VSD, PDA, ASD, PS
ring 18		~20% have CHD: CoA, PA hypoplasia, HLH, PLSVC
Duplications		
4p trisomy		~10% have CHD, usually single: no defect predominates
9p trisomy		>10% have CHD: VSD, ASD, AS, PS
10p trisomy		~30% have CHD, usually single: no defect predominates
10q24-qter trisomy		~50% have CHD, usually complex: ECD, VSD, TOF
22pter-q11 trisomy or tetrasomy	Cat eye	~50% have CHD, usually complex: TAPVR, VSD, TOF
Other Aberrations		
Marker Xq27.3	Fragile X syndrome	~50% have aortic root dilatation, MVP, or both

AR = aortic regurgitation; ARD = aortic root dilation; AS = aortic stenosis; ASD = atrial septal defect; AV = aortic valve; CHD = congenital heart defect(s); CoA = coarctation of aorta; ECD = endocardial cushion defect; HLH = hypoplastic left heart; MVP = mitral valve prolapse; PA = pulmonary artery; PDA = patent ductus arteriosus; PLSVC = persistence of left superior vena cava; PS = valvular pulmonic stenosis; PV = pulmonic valve; TAPVR = total anomalous pulmonary venous return; TOF = tetralogy of Fallot; VSD = ventricular septal defect.

conotruncal and distal aortic anomalies have suggested a distinct pathogenetic mechanism in trisomy 21, potentially involving cell adhesiveness and the extracellular matrix.

TRISOMY 21–DOWN SYNDROME. This most common phenotype due to a human chromosome aberration occurs about once in every 600 births. Most patients have trisomy 21, and the risk of this aberration is exponentially related to maternal age: the risk is lowest for young women and rises steeply after age 35, reaching 4 percent for women older than 45. A small minority (3 percent) of cases of Down syndrome result from an extra copy of all or part of the long arm of chromosome 21 translocated to another chromosome. This situation is relatively more common in mothers younger than 30 years. The phenotypes of the two forms of Down syndrome do not differ. The phenotype tends to be less severe if the trisomy is mosaic (3 percent of Down syndrome) as a result of a mitotic nondisjunctional error in the embryo.

The most common causes of morbidity and mortality in patients with Down syndrome are congenital heart defects (present in 40 to 50 percent of cases),[25] hematological malignant disease, and duodenal atresia. If patients either escape or survive these problems, survival into the fifth decade and beyond is likely but is complicated by progressive dementia of the Alzheimer type. Premature aging may also affect the vasculature, although definitive studies are lacking.

The most characteristic cardiac anomaly in patients with Down syndrome is a defect of closure of the endocardial cushions (see Chap. 56). Complicating the clinical problems in such patients and those with simple septal defects is a seeming predisposition to pulmonary hypertension in the presence of elevated pulmonary blood flow. About one-third of congenital heart defects are complex, and affected individuals tend, not surprisingly, to be the most ill patients. Mitral valve prolapse (MVP) is found with a frequency exceeding that in age- and gender-matched control subjects. The aortic and pulmonary valve cusps seem predisposed to fenestrations in adulthood. In the neonate with Down syndrome, the physical examination has a sensitivity of 80 percent for detecting cardiovascular anomalies; echocardiography detects some additional infants who have normal physical examination findings but who will later require cardiac surgery.[26]

Through the study of individuals trisomic for only a portion of the long arm of chromosome 21, the region crucial to the development of heart defects has been narrowed to 5.5 megabases (mb) of DNA in band 21q22.3; a locus in this region, *DSCAM*, that encodes a cell adhesion molecule is a leading candidate gene for this aspect of the Down syndrome phenotype.[27]

Medical treatment of patients with Down syndrome has undergone evolution to more aggressive measures in recent years. Objections and hesitations on medical, societal, and ethical grounds to operative repair of heart defects in Down syndrome have been mollified substantially.[28] More follow-up data are becoming available, and early and late postoperative survival in patients with Down syndrome appears to be comparable to that in other patients with similar defects.

TRISOMY 18. Edwards syndrome is the second most common autosomal trisomy. Most cases are due to meiotic disjunction, and there is a strong relationship to maternal age. Routine prenatal diagnostic testing of women older than 34 years would detect all aneuploid fetuses in them, but this would represent only one-third of all autosomal trisomies; in the United States, less than one-half of all women of this advanced age undergo definitive testing. Prenatal detection of trisomies followed by termination of pregnancy is currently having a small but measurable impact on decreasing the incidence of Down, Edwards, and Patau syndromes.

Although the severity of the phenotype rarely enables survival beyond a few months, 5 to 10 percent of patients live to 1 year and a few survive to adulthood, perhaps because of undetected mosaicism for a chromosomally normal cell line.[29,30] However, central nervous system function is far less than in patients with Down syndrome and leads to complex medical management and supportive care for long-term survivors.[28]

Cardiovascular defects occur in at least 90 percent of cases and contribute to death. Complex lesions, usually involving septal defects, dysplastic valves that are rarely hemodynamically important, patent ductus arteriosus (PDA), and persistence of the left superior vena cava are common. Right ventricular enlargement is common and may indicate not only shunting from left to right but pulmonary hypertension due to anomalies of the pulmonary vasculature. As in Down syndrome, transposition of the great arteries is virtually unknown in patients with trisomy 18. Invasive diagnostic procedures or aggressive supportive measures should be undertaken only rarely in patients with Edwards syndrome.

TRISOMY 13. Patau syndrome occurs in about 0.01 percent of live births and in progressively higher frequencies in stillbirths and spontaneous abortions. The external phenotype is usually severe but occasionally not as characteristic as that of other trisomies; survival beyond a few weeks is rare, and the causes of death involve several organ systems, especially the heart. Cardiovascular anomalies occur a bit less frequently than in trisomy 18 and have a slightly different spectrum.[28] Septal defects are the most common isolated lesions, dextrocardia and bicuspid semilunar valves occur in association with other anomalies, and accessory papillary muscles occur in 30 percent of fetuses with trisomy 13.[31]

Median survival is about 10 days, but 5 to 10 percent survive to 1 year, and a very few live beyond one decade.[30,32] Patients who survive beyond 1 month often are mosaic for a chromosomally normal cell line; thus, prognosis is fraught with uncertainty until detailed analysis is completed. Whether invasive cardiological studies are performed or aggressive management is undertaken can be determined by the severity of involvement of other organ systems, especially the brain, pending cytogenetic investigation.

TURNER SYNDROME. About 1 in every 2500 females lacks an X chromosome and has a 45,X karyotype, which is by far the most common cause of Turner syndrome. The frequency of a nonmosaic 45,X karyotype is much higher in spontaneous abortuses than in live-borns, and probably less than 2 percent of such conceptuses come to term. The clinical phenotype is variable and often mild; typically, the diagnosis is not suspected until a child's short stature is evaluated or a woman complains of amenorrhea. Many cases are mosaic for cell lines with 46,XX or 46,XY constitutions. Various structural aberrations involving the X chromosome can cause partial or complete Turner syndrome.

Among patients with the 45,X karyotype, reported frequencies of congenital cardiovascular defects vary from 20 to 50 percent, depending on how patients were ascertained. Fifty to 70 percent of those with cardiovascular defects have clinically important aortic coarctation, usually of the postductal form. As noninvasive imaging studies of asymptomatic patients become routine, the frequency of coarctation may increase. Various other cardiac malformations may occur, either singly or combined with coarctation. However, there is strong support for left-sided flow abnormalities as a major pathogenetic mechanism. Bicuspid aortic valve, dilation of the ascending aorta (with a risk of dissection and histopathologic examination showing elastic fiber disruption), or both occur even in the absence of coarctation,[33] and hypoplastic left heart has been reported. Partial anomalous pulmonary venous drainage without an atrial septal defect is fairly common and should be suspected when echocardiography detects right ventricular overload.

Postmortem examination of midtrimester abortuses with 45,X showed a higher incidence of left-sided flow lesions than found at birth, suggesting an association between the pathogenesis of the cardiovascular anomalies and the uniform presence of lymphatic obstruction at the base of the heart. In fetuses with Turner phenotype that do not survive, the size of the heart is reduced, perhaps representing a mild but generalized form of hypoplastic left heart, the most severe form of left-sided flow defects.[34] The fetal hydrops common in cases of severe, fetal Turner syndrome could be due to inadequate cardiac function, rather than its cause. Blood pressure elevation is common, even without coarctation or after its repair; a high frequency of renal anomalies is one likely cause but not the sole explanation for the prevalence of hypertension. Elevated blood pressure is strongly associated with dilation of the ascending aorta, so aggressive treatment is warranted on several accounts.[33]

In about two-thirds of cases, the retained X chromosome derives from the oocyte (maternal X). Because entire chromosomes or regions of a chromosome may be differentially regulated (imprinted)[35] by passage through oogenesis versus spermatogenesis, could some of the variability in phenotype among patients with Turner syndrome be due to the origin of the retained X or the origin of the lost X? In a study of 63 patients, 10 had severe cardiovascular features, and 9 of them had retained the maternal X.[36] This is an idea worthy of further investigation. Women with mosaic karyotypes are less likely to have cardiovascular defects. Some studies also suggest a "critical region" of the X chromosome, which, when deleted, results in most of the features of Turner syndrome.[37]

Management of both children[38] and adults[39] with Turner syndrome requires careful and routine attention to the cardiovascular system. Chronic treatment of children with human growth hormone to increase mature height has no apparent deleterious effect on cardiac performance.[40]

Congenital Heart Disease (see Chap. 56)

In the past few decades, the reported incidence of structural heart defects in newborns has increased from 5 to 7 per 1000 in live births, probably as the result of increased diagnostic sensitivity (especially cross-sectional and Doppler echocardiography and magnetic resonance imaging), including prenatally.[40-42] Supporting this explanation is the lack of change over the same period in the incidence of critical defects diagnosed neonatally at 3.1 to 3.5 per 1000.[40,43] This enhanced resolving power of noninvasive methods should prove particularly useful in the study of familial structural defects, because apparently unaffected relatives can be evaluated for subclinical evidence of anomalies. Few investigations to date have capitalized on this approach.[44]

As is evident from the previous section, gross aberrations of chromosomes produce an extensive and varied array of structural heart disease, an observation as true for spontaneous abortuses as for live-born children. Unfortunately, cytogenetic aberrations have provided few clues about etiology and pathogenesis of congenital malformations.[45,46] Better understanding comes from investigating the other two mechanisms by which genes cause congenital heart defects: multifactorial processes and mutations of single genes. In addition to the Mendelian syndromes discussed later, evidence for the involvement of genes of large effect derives, in part, from studies of incidence of congenital heart disease in populations with a high rate of inbreeding. The increased occurrence of defects in offspring of consanguineous matings suggests that mutations in one or more genes, when homozygous, strongly predispose to abnormal cardiovascular development.

MULTIFACTORIAL PROCESSES. The empirical risks of recurrence of congenital heart defects have increased in recent years,[47] in keeping with the overall higher incidence noted earlier. However, this conclusion has been criticized because the studies focused on the offspring of women probands, in whom the recurrence risk appears higher than in men with congenital heart defects.[48] In addition to this unexplained maternal influence, other factors may be at work. For example, improved detection of subtle lesions, more faithful reporting of patients, and the assiduousness of epidemiologists may have shown a systematic variation. More patients with cardiovascular problems now survive[48] to bear children due to improved medical and surgical care; their offspring might be at increased risk because of the severity of the parents' problems, but some evidence refutes this idea.

The familial aggregation of congenital heart defects supports many of the predictions of the threshold liability model of multifactorial inheritance.[43,49] In most studies, whether focused on populations or families, defects were classified by their pathological findings; for example, all ventricular septal defects were considered as one group. There has been bias in reporting families in which one type of defect aggregates, leading to many reports of "familial atrial septal defect," "familial cardiomyopathy," and so on, although not all septal defects or cardiopathies have the same structure on careful scrutiny, let alone the same cause.[50,51]

TABLE 70–5 Classification of Congenital Heart Defects Based on Pathogenetic Mechanisms

Pathogenetic Mechanism	Examples of Defects
Embryonic blood flow defects	
Left-sided lesions	HLH; bicuspid aortic valve; IAA type A; CoA; PDA
Right-sided lesions	Secundum ASD; PS
Mesenchymal tissue migration defects	TOF; D-TGA
Extracellular matrix defects	ECD
Abnormal cellular death	Ebstein anomaly; muscular VSD
Defects of looping and situs	L-TGA
Abnormalities of targeted growth	TAPVR

ASD = atrial septal defect; CoA = coarctation of aorta; ECD = endocardial cushion defect; HLH = hypoplastic left heart; IAA = interrupted aortic arch; PDA = patent ductus arteriosus; PS = valvular pulmonic stenosis; TAPVR = total anomalous pulmonary venous return; TGA = transposition of great arteries; TOF = tetralogy of Fallot; VSD = ventricular septal defect.

A major advance has been the movement to examine familial aggregation of defects based on presumed pathogenesis.[41] The scheme developed by Clark[52] and since modified and expanded (Table 70–5), has become widely used. Under this approach, some anatomically distinct lesions are related by common pathogenesis; if the pathogenetic mechanism has substantial genetic control, then the occurrence of distinct defects in the same family would still be consistent with a genetic model. Alternatively, defects unrelated by pathogenesis would require a different interpretation. This model rationalizes examination of apparently unaffected relatives, which increases the chances of detecting subtle manifestations of defective development of cardiovascular structures. Such investigation, in addition to targeted testing for single-gene mutations or chromosomal microdeletions, is now fundamental to genetic counseling for all congenital heart disease.[53]

ERRORS IN MESENCHYMAL TISSUE MIGRATION. Included in this category is a wide range of anomalies of the outflow tract, some due to failure of fusion and others due to failure of septation. Relatives of probands with interruption of the aortic arch type B or truncus arteriosus, both uncommon conotruncal malformations, had 2.5 percent and 6.6 percent incidences, respectively, of congenital heart defects. Both recurrence rates were higher than expected. The frequency of congenital malformations was much lower in relatives of patients with other forms of interrupted aortic arch. Moreover, relatives of probands with truncus arteriosus and other defects had a recurrence rate of 13 percent, the majority in the spectrum of conotruncal lesions. Here is an instance in which refined empirical risk data should improve the accuracy of genetic counseling.

Categorizing anatomical defects by presumed pathogenesis emphasizes that all ventricular septal defects are not alike. However, even within an embryologically circumscribed category, the situation is complex. Many perimembranous ventricular septal defects and tetralogy of Fallot can be considered errors in mesenchymal tissue migration. Evidence exists for the effects of major genes (e.g., as yet unidentified ones in the 22q11 region,[54] *JAG1*,[55,56] the gene that when mutated also causes Alagille syndrome[57,58] and *NKX2.5*[59,60]), and for multifactorial effects.[61]

CONOTRUNCAL DEVELOPMENT. Considerable progress has been made during the past few years in identifying a region of chromosome 22 that has a major role in development of the conotruncus, the branchial arches, and the face. Interest was first stimulated by detection of small deletions involving 22q11 in patients with DiGeorge sequence. This condition includes developmental anomalies of the fourth branchial arch and derivatives of the third and fourth pharyngeal pouches. Hypoplasia of the thymus and parathyroids causes immune deficiency and hypocalcemia. The cardiac defects range from tetralogy of Fallot to ventricular septal defect, truncus arteriosus, interrupted aorta type B, and right aortic arch, and are often lethal. Deletion of 22q11 accounts for about 90 percent of instances of DiGeorge sequence.[53]

Subsequently, patients with velocardiofacial syndrome (VCF, also called Shprintzen-Goldberg syndrome) and what has been called in Japan the *conotruncal anomaly face syndrome* were found to have deletions in the same region, albeit generally smaller ones than in patients with DiGeorge syndrome. Because the deletion is often too small to be detected by routine cytogenetics, fluorescent in situ hybridization (FISH) with a DNA probe for the region is the assay of choice. The VCF syndrome is unlike DiGeorge syndrome and includes an abnormal but characteristic facies, cleft palate, pharyngeal insufficiency, and conotruncal cardiac defects.

This same region of chromosome 22 has been examined in patients with familial occurrence of various congenital cardiac defects and in patients with nonfamilial occurrence, nonsyndromic conotruncal defects; an important fraction of patients in both categories have submicroscopic deletions of 22q11.[54,62-64] Thus, a gene or genes in this region account for much of the recurrence risk of defects due to mesenchymal tissue migration abnormalities. Further, accurate counseling about recurrence risks for this broad range of defects necessitates FISH or molecular analysis for the presence of a deletion in the proband and, if present, in both parents. Deletion of 22q11 occurs in about 13 per 100,000 live births and is, after trisomy 21, the second most common genetic cause of congenital heart disease.[65]

Investigation of a strain of Keeshond dogs prone to conotruncal defects has shown that a single gene can be responsible for pathogenetically related defects of widely varying severity.

FLOW DEFECTS. Left-sided flow lesions comprise a spectrum that includes hypoplastic left heart, congenital aortic stenosis, bicuspid aortic valve, interrupted aortic arch type A, and aortic coarctation. Various components of this spectrum can be present in the same patient. Data from the Baltimore-Washington Infant Study,[41] a population-based case-control study of congenital cardiovascular malformations, were used to show that in first-degree relatives of probands with isolated hypoplastic left heart, the incidence of bicuspid aortic valve was 12 percent; most of the cases were asymptomatic and unrecognized before they were detected by echocardiography as part of this investigation. In an exceptional family, four instances of aortic coarctation occurred in four generations. Coarctation, even when repaired, poses an important risk factor for a woman during pregnancy.[66]

The association of coarctation of the aorta, bicuspid aortic valve, and dilation of the ascending aorta, which may occur as part of Turner syndrome (see earlier discussion), is well known in the general population. Several intriguing questions about the genetics and pathogenesis of this association need to be addressed. To what extent is the ascending aorta intrinsically abnormal and hence predisposed to dilate, and to what extent is the dilation simply a result of abnormal turbulence created by a bicuspid aortic valve? Some patients with this association also have subtle evidence of a systemic connective tissue abnormality, reminiscent of Marfan syndrome, in support of the former hypothesis. Furthermore, some people with a bicuspid aortic valve and neither stenosis nor regurgitation develop aneurysms. It will be of interest to extend the study of left-sided flow lesions to include probands with coarctation or congenital aortic stenosis and to evaluate close relatives with techniques capable of detecting the entire range of flow defects.

EXTRACELLULAR MATRIX ABNORMALITIES. Enough is known about the biochemistry and cell biology of cardiac embryology to state with some confidence that the extracellular matrix ("connective tissue") has an important role. The endocardial cushions have received the most attention as an area where defects in the extracellular matrix might produce malformations.[52] The high frequency of endocardial cushion defects and atrioventricular septal defects in patients with Down syndrome has been noted. Of interest is the finding of increased adhesiveness of fibroblasts from patients with trisomy 21, a phenomenon that could reflect interaction with the extracellular matrix. The distinctiveness of endocardial cushion defects in patients with normal chromosomes and in those with trisomy 21 has been suggested because of differences in associated cardiovascular malformations.[50] However, of six families in which the proband had an endocardial cushion defect, three had recurrence of the same type of defect in a relative, including two with trisomy 21. Atrioventricular septal defects (AVSD) are also seen in patients with a number of other conditions, including deletions of the short arm of chromosome 3 (3p–). A gene in this region, *CRELD1*, has been found to be mutated in some families with AVSD in multiple generations.[67]

SITUS AND LOOPING DEFECTS. This is an area fraught with difficulties of nomenclature, diagnosis, and heterogeneity of both etiology and pathogenesis.[68] In analysis of clinical data, the most informative approach but clearly arduous because of the large amount of data required, would be to categorize probands and their relatives by the type of situs (solitus, inversus, dextroversion, or levoversion; see Chap. 56) and each of those by the presence or absence of other cardiac and visceral defects. This has not been done on epidemiological cohorts, and relatives in family studies have rarely been subjected to evaluations sufficient to characterize their phenotypes in detail. However, when careful family studies are performed, evidence for genetic contribution to specific defects may emerge, e.g., in cases of complete transposition of the great arteries.[69]

Many variable phenotypes are grouped in a category, *heterotaxy*, that accounts for 3 to 4 percent of all congenital heart defects. Several Mendelian phenotypes point to single genes that have a major effect on determining laterality. In the autosomal recessive Kartagener syndrome, a randomization of lateralization of the heart (situs solitus and situs inversus are equally likely in homozygotes) coexists with a defect in ciliary motility, which leads to sinusitis, bronchiectasis, and sperm immotility.[70]

Heterotaxy with splenic and other cardiac defects, particularly of the position of the great vessels, can be inherited as autosomal recessive, autosomal dominant, and X-linked recessive traits.[11] Some of the families with these apparently single-gene disorders have concordance of phenotype, but many do not, suggesting that in some cases various types of situs defects, polysplenia, and asplenia are different manifestations of the same mutation.

In recent years, investigation of molecular embryology has shed increasing light on cardiovascular development and maldevelopment.[71] The determination of laterality and defects involving heterotaxy have been especially revealing in both mice and humans.[72,73] In mice, the *inv* locus has long been associated with left/right asymmetry, and the gene was recently cloned.[74] In humans, mutations of two genes thus far, one encoding the activin receptor type IIB[75] and one encoding the connexin43 gap junction protein, have been associated with defects of laterality.

Few data define the recurrence risks of defects in the *cell death* (e.g., Ebstein anomaly) and *abnormal targeted growth* (e.g., anomalous pulmonary venous return) categories. Data from the Baltimore-Washington Infant Study do not show an increased risk of any cardiovascular defect in the relatives of a proband with a defect in either of these categories.[41]

DISORDERS OF UNCLEAR CAUSE. A number of disorders include an important likelihood of malformation of the cardiovascular system but are of unclear cause (Table 70–6). Familial recurrence is low enough to be incompatible with multifactorial inheritance. Several of these disorders deserve comment.

Certain congenital cardiac defects and other malformations occur together more frequently than expected by chance; this *association* of defects suggests a common cause, pathogenesis, or both, but the following disorders and those in Table 70–7 remain enigmatic on most of these counts. Designation as a *sequence* implies that some evidence exists for a common developmental problem to account for the features.

CHARGE Association (see Table 70-6). Patients with this condition by definition have congenital heart defects. The spectrum of cardiovascular malformations suggests not so much a common pathogenetic scheme as a common time of abnormal development. During gestational days 32 to 45, cardiac septation, fusion of the endocardial cushions and membranous ventricular septum, and formation of the outflow tracts and valves occur. An environmental insult or a breakdown in developmental homeostasis during this period could result in the malformation spectrum of this disorder. The defects in other systems could also arise during this embryological window and would be consistent with either environmental or intrinsic factors.

VACTERL Association (see Table 70-6). This condition has expanded over the years to include *v*ertebral, *v*entricular septal, *a*nal, *c*ardiac, *t*racheoesophageal, *r*enal, and *l*imb defects. Omitted from the mnemonic is the single umbilical artery often present. Cardiac defects are present in about one-half of patients with more than two components of this association but usually are not life-threatening. VACTERL

TABLE 70–6 Disorders of Uncertain Cause and Inheritance that are Associated with a High Incidence of Cardiovascular Abnormalities

Disorder and Phenotype	OMIM No.*	Cardiovascular Abnormalities†
Aase syndrome (congenital anemia, triphalangeal thumbs)	205600	VSD
Bilateral left-sidedness sequence (polysplenia syndrome)	208530	ASD
Bilateral right-sidedness sequence (asplenia syndrome; Ivemark syndrome)	208530	Situs inversus, ECD, VSD
CHARGE association (*c*oloboma, *h*eart anomaly, choanal *a*tresia, *r*etardation, *g*enital, and *e*ar anomalies)	214800	TOF, PDA, ECD, VSD
Cornelia de Lange syndrome (short stature, retardation, synophrys, hypertrichosis, micromelia, genital anomalies)	122470	~20% Have CHD: VSD, PDA, ASD, PLSVC, TOF
DiGeorge sequence‡ (abnormalities of derivatives of third and fourth pharyngeal pouches and fourth branchial arch: hypoplastic thymus with cellular immune deficiency, hyoplastic parathyroids with hypocalcemia)	188400	CHD in ~100%: aortic arch anomalies (especially IAA type B and right-sided aortic arch); PDA, TOF
Goldenhar syndrome (abnormalities of derivatives of first and second branchial arches: hemifacial microsomia, microtia, vertebral anomalies)	141400, 164210, 257700	~50% have CHD: VSD, TOF, PDA, CoA, right-sided aortic arch, PLSVC
Klippel-Feil sequence (short neck, limited rotation of the head, cervical anomalies)	118100 148900, 214300	Variable estimates (5%-70%) of CHD: VSD, dextrocardia
Kabuki make-up syndrome (dwarfism, peculiar facies, scoliosis, mental retardation)	147920	30% have CHD: ASD, VSD, TOF, CoA, PDA
Pallister-Hall syndrome (hypothalamic hamartoblastoma, hypopituitarism, imperforate anus, postaxial polydactyly)	146510	ECD
Poland sequence (unilateral absence of sternocostal pectoralis major, ipsilateral synbrachydactyly)	173800	~10% have dextrocardia or dextroversion
Rubinstein-Taybi syndrome (short stature, retardation, microcephaly, characteristic facies, broad thumbs)	180849	~20% have CHD: ECD, ASD, TOF, PDA, VSD
VATER association (*v*ertebral defects, *a*nal atresia, *t*racheo *e*sophageal fistula, *r*adial dysplasia, renal anomaly)	192350	VSD

*None of these disorders is evidently due to a mutation in a single gene; however, most are listed in Online Mendelian Inheritance in Man (www.ncbi.nlm.nih.gov/omim)[8] and the OMIM no. is provided as a ready source to the literature.

†Listed in approximate order of decreasing frequency.

‡90% of cases associated with del(22q11); likely a contiguous gene deletion defect.

ASD = atrial septal defect; CHD = congenital heart defect(s); CoA = coarctation of aorta; ECD = endocardial cushion defect; IAA = interrupted aortic arch; PDA = patent ductus arteriosus; PLSVC = persistence of left superior vena cava; TOF = tetralogy of Fallot; VSD = ventricular septal defect.

TABLE 70–7 Congenital Heart Defects Occasionally Showing Familial Aggregation Consistent with Mendelian Inheritance

Defect	OMIM No.*
Aneurysm, intracranial berry	105800
Aneurysm, abdominal aortic	100070
Angioma	106050, 106070, 206570
ASD, ostium primum	209400
ASD, ostium secundum	108800, 108900, 178650
Bicuspid aortic valve	109730
Conotruncal defect	231060
Dextrocardia	244400, 304750
Ebstein anomaly	224700
Endocardial fibroelastosis	226000, 227280, 305300
Hemangioma	106070, 140800, 140900, 234800
Hemangioma, cavernous	116860, 140850
Hypoplastic left heart	140500, 241550
Hypoplastic right heart	277200
Lymphedema, congenital	153000, 153100, 153400, 214900, 247440
Mitral valve prolapse	157700
Patent ductus arteriosus	169100
Pulmonary venous return, anomalous	106700
Pulmonic stenosis	126190, 178650, 193520, 265500, 265600, 270460
Subaortic stenosis	271950, 271960
Tetralogy of Fallot	187500
Ventricle, single	234750

*Data from Online Mendelian Inheritance in Man (www.ncbi.nlm.nih.gov/omim).
ASD = atrial septal defect.

association occasionally occurs in relatives.[76] Although infants with this condition often fail to thrive initially, the long-term prognosis for health and mental function is good, so aggressive management of the multiple malformations is warranted. It is important to separate as soon as possible those patients who have the features of trisomy 18 or 13q chromosome aberrations, as prognosis in these cases is distinctly unfavorable.

Mendelian Disorders

Some congenital cardiovascular defects segregate in occasional families as predicted of a Mendelian phenotype. Strong bias favors reporting such occurrences, and equally strong is a temptation to conclude that, at least in some cases, the defect is caused by mutation in a single gene. However, rarely and by chance alone, a multifactorial trait recurs in a family in a pattern mimicking Mendelian segregation. This potential confusion and the resultant uncertainty in counseling patients and families pertains equally well to disturbances of conduction and rhythm, various cardiomyopathies, vascular anomalies, and hypertension, all discussed subsequently. The true cause of the cardiovascular diseases in such families may not become clarified until each is investigated in detail, in concert with efforts to map and sequence the entire human genome.

The subject of this section can therefore be parsed into three broad classes of conditions: congenital cardiac defects that occasionally seem to be inherited as Mendelian traits (see Table 70–7), pleiotropic Mendelian syndromes that always or frequently affect the structure of the cardiovascular system (Table 70–8), and Mendelian syndromes that occasionally affect the cardiovascular system (Table 70–9).

PATENT DUCTUS ARTERIOSUS. Most instances of PDA are sporadic occurrences, and a strong association with prematurity and all of its antecedents is noted. However, in a number of families that have been described, PDA occurs as an autosomal dominant trait. In some pedigrees, mild facial dysmorphism segregates with PDA; because the facial features differ among families, the number of syndromes remains unclear.[77] Some families with autosomal dominant PDA are predisposed to aortic dissection.[78] In other families, PDA occurs as a recessive trait, and a locus at 12q24 has been implicated.[79]

FAMILIAL ATRIAL SEPTAL DEFECT. Two Mendelian forms of atrial septal defect exist as autosomal dominant traits.[80] One has no associated problems and has been described in few pedigrees. Mutations in *GATA4* have been described recently in several families.[81]

The second, more common condition is associated with atrioventricular conduction delay.[82] The defect is of the secundum type, and relatives do not seem to be at increased risk of other cardiac malformations. The severity of heart block rarely progresses to third degree. The electrocardiographic abnormality in a patient with apparently sporadic atrial septal defect should prompt a detailed family history and evaluation of close relatives. Attention should be directed to the upper limbs, particularly the thumbs, to rule out the Holt-Oram syndrome; radiographic examination of the upper limbs of the proband is helpful on this account.

In patients with atrial septal defect due to aneuploidy (a syndrome with extracardiac features), when one of the autosomal dominant forms is excluded, the recurrence risk of secundum atrial septal defect is about 3 percent, a value that conforms closely to the multifactorial threshold model. Several pleiotropic Mendelian conditions have defects of the atrial septum as frequent manifestations.

HOLT-ORAM SYNDROME. This autosomal dominant condition, first elaborated in 1960, shows marked variability within a pedigree. The cardinal manifestations are dysplasia of the upper limbs and atrial septal defect. In heterozygotes for the mutation, arm deformity ranges from undetectable through distally placed thumbs and hypoplastic thenar eminences, triphalangeal thumbs, anomalies of the carpus, and radial aplasia, to phocomelia and hypoplasia of the clavicles and shoulders. Upper-extremity deformity is usually bilateral but may be asymmetrical in severity, with the left side more affected. Similarly, the atrial involvement ranges from none to a large secundum defect with early, severe hemodynamic compromise. Other cardiac malformations have been reported, with ventricular septal defects and PDA the most frequent. The skeletal and cardiac manifestations are not correlated in individuals, and how a parent is affected is not a reliable predictor of effects on offspring. Prenatal diagnosis by ultrasonography was reported in a fetus with severe limb abnormalities; a large septal defect could presumably be detected as well. Other manifestations include dermatoglyphic abnormalities, pectus excavatum, hypoplastic peripheral arteries, and cardiac conduction disturbance, the last usually involving the atrioventricular node and present in patients with septal defects. Although the Holt-Oram syndrome bears some resemblance to the VACTERL association, the clear Mendelian nature and lack of more extensive organ system involvement of the former indicate that the two conditions do not represent a pathogenetic spectrum.

TABLE 70–8 Mendelian Disorders with Congenital Defects of Cardiovascular Structure as Frequent Manifestations

Descriptive Name	Eponym	OMIM No.*	Cardiovascular Abnormalities
Adult polycystic kidney disease		173900	MVP, dilated aortic root, intracranial berry aneurysm
Arteriohepatic dysplasia	Alagille syndrome	118450	PPS
Cataract and cardiomyopathy		212350	HCM
Chondroectodermal dysplasia	Ellis–van Creveld syndrome	225500	ASD (ostium primum), common atrium
Deafness, mitral regurgitation, and short stature	Forney syndrome	157800	MR
Familial collagenoma syndrome		115250	DCM
Heart-hand syndrome	Holt-Oram syndrome	142900	ASD (ostium secundum), VSD, MVP, HLH
Keratosis palmoplantaris	Mal de Meleda syndrome	248300	DCM, dysrhythmia
Malignant hyperthermia and skeletal defects	King syndrome	145600	Malignant hyperthermia→cardiac arrest
Noonan syndrome		163950	PS, HCM
Pulmonic stenosis and deafness		178651	PS
Smith-Lemli-Opitz syndrome		270400	PDA, ASD, VSD, TOF, ECD, CoA
Velocardiofacial syndrome	Shprintzen syndrome	192430	TOF, tortuous retinal vasculature

*Data from Online Mendelian Inheritance in Man (www.ncbi.nlm.nih.gov/omim).

ASD = atrial septal defect; CoA = coarctation of aorta; DCM = dilated cardiomyopathy; ECD = endocardial cushion defect; HCM = hypertrophic cardiomyopathy; HLH = hypoplastic left heart; MR = mitral regurgitation; MVP = mitral valve prolapse; PDA = patent ductus arteriosus; PPS = peripheral pulmonic stenosis; PS = valvular pulmonic stenosis; TOF = tetralogy of Fallot; VSD = ventricular septal defect.

TABLE 70–9 Mendelian Disorders with Cardiovascular Abnormalities as Occasional Manifestations

Syndrome	Eponym	OMIM No.*	Cardiovascular Abnormalities
Acrocephalosyndactyly type I	Apert syndrome	101200	PS, PPS, VSD, EFE
Acrocephalopolysyndactyly type II	Carpenter syndrome	201000	PDA, VSD, PS, TGA
Hereditary angioedema		106100	Coronary arteritis
Imperforate anus with hand, foot, and ear anomalies	Townes-Brocks syndrome	107480	Sporadic cases have CHD: VSD, ASD
Mandibulofacial dysostosis	Treacher Collins syndrome	154500, 248390	10% have CHD: variable
Neuronal ceroid lipofuscinosis	Batten disease	204200	HCM
Orofacial digital syndrome type II	Mohr syndrome	252100	Variable
Short rib–polydactyly syndrome	Saldino-Noonan syndrome	263530	TGA, ECD, hypoplastic right heart
Thrombocytopenia–absent radius syndrome	TAR syndrome	274000	TOF

*Data from Online Mendelian Inheritance in Man (www.ncbi.nlm.nih.gov/omim).

ASD = atrial septal defect; CHD = congenital heart defect(s); ECD = endocardial cushion defect; EFE = endocardial fibroelastosis; HCM = hypertrophic cardiomyopathy; PDA = patent ductus arteriosus; PS = valvular pulmonic stenosis; PPS = peripheral pulmonic stenosis; TGA = transposition of great arteries; TOF = tetralogy of Fallot; VSD = ventricular septal defect.

The diagnosis of Holt-Oram syndrome is most likely to be missed in a patient with an unknown or unremarkable family history, a secundum septal defect, and minimal or no thumb anomaly. In any "sporadic" case of an atrial septal defect, the patient and the parents should be carefully examined for limb malformations and the family history studied in detail. Detection of a subtle limb defect alters the recurrence risk in offspring of the proband from the empirical risk of an isolated septal defect of 3 percent to the 50 percent of an autosomal dominant trait.

Mutations in the *TBX5* gene, a transcriptional regulator, cause one form of Holt-Oram syndrome.[83] The effect of different mutations on expression of the transcription factor does not appear to correlate with the marked differences seen in limb and cardiac development in different families.[84] Not all families with Holt-Oram syndrome are linked to this locus at 12q2, so at least one additional gene can cause this spectrum of defects.

ELLIS–VAN CREVELD SYNDROME (Fig. 70–6). This rare autosomal recessive chondrodysplasia is found among the old-order Amish because of a founder effect and consanguinity. Short stature, metaphyseal dysplasia, dysplastic nails and teeth, and postaxial polydactyly are the pleiotropic manifestations, in addition to congenital heart disease. Congenital heart disease is present in more than one-half of homozygotes, and most of the defects affect the atrial septum. The majority are defects of endocardial cushion closure, including ostium primum defects of widely varying size up to

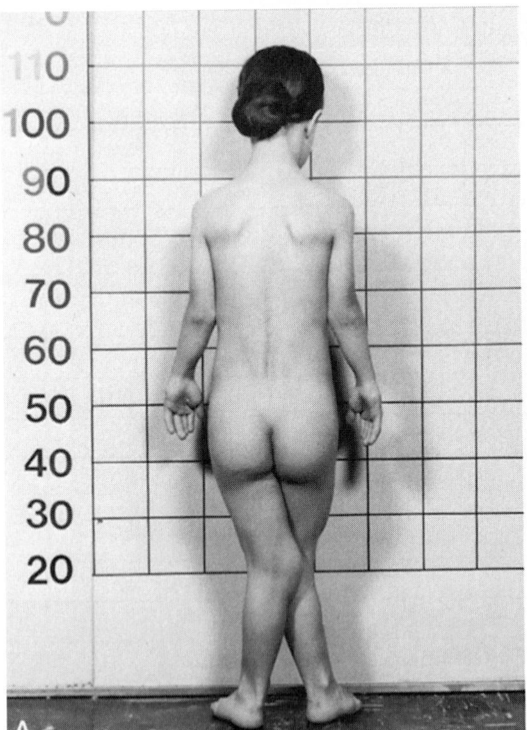

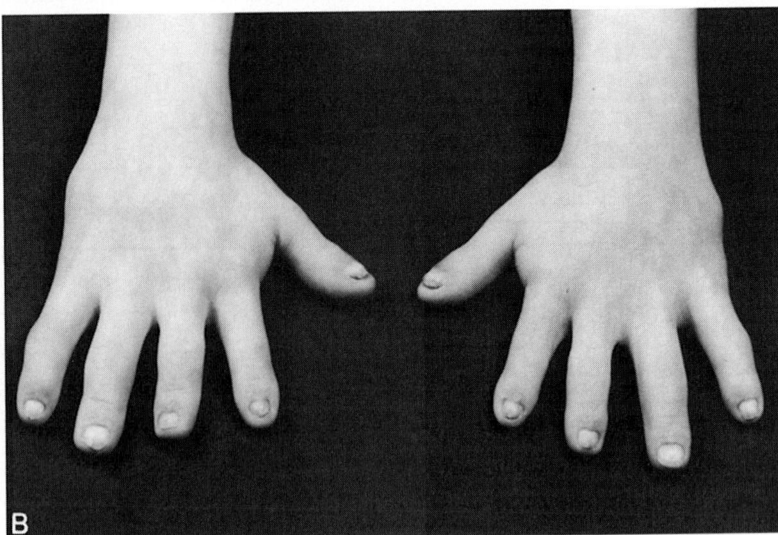

FIGURE 70–6 Ellis–van Creveld syndrome in a young woman. **A,** Note short stature, joint contractures at the elbows, and marked genu valgum. **B,** The fingers are short and the nails dysplastic. Note the protuberances along the ulnar edges of the hands where sixth digits were amputated.

a single atrium. This disorder has long been thought to be due to a yet unknown defect in the extracellular matrix, which would fit with the high frequency of endocardial cushion lesions. However, defects thought to be due to abnormal embryonic flow (coarctation, hypoplastic left heart, and patent ductus arteriosus) occur in about 20 percent of cases. The gene maps to 4p16 in patients of all ethnic derivations. A gene of unknown function within this locus, termed *EVC*, is mutated in some, but not all, patients.[85] A second gene in this chromosomal region, called *EVC2*, is mutated in patients of Ashkenazi ethnicity.[86] The finding that two closely linked genes cause the same condition is distinctly unusual. Ellis–van Creveld syndrome can be diagnosed prenatally by detection of polydactyly by ultrasonography.

FAMILIAL ATRIOVENTRICULAR CANAL DEFECTS. This spectrum of defects occasionally occurs in an autosomal dominant pattern in families and is unassociated with features in other systems. Because the cardiac defect is suggestive of that in Down syndrome, linkage to chromosome 21 markers was pursued, to no avail. In a large kindred that showed variable expression of nonsyndromic atrioventricular canal defects, analysis of shared markers among persons clearly affected identified a region on chromosome 1 (1p31-p21) that must harbor a gene that effects susceptibility to failure of closure of the endocardial cushions.[87]

VENTRICULAR SEPTAL DEFECT. This malformation does not seem to be inherited as an isolated Mendelian malformation, and no syndromes include it as a common, isolated manifestation.[80]

SUPRAVALVULAR AORTIC STENOSIS. This congenital lesion, which can be asymptomatic and detected long after birth because of an ejection murmur, occurs in at least three settings. It can be a sporadic anomaly, a component of Williams syndrome, or an autosomal dominant trait associated with peripheral pulmonic stenoses and a diffuse arteriopathy.

Williams syndrome is usually sporadic but, in more instances than previously recognized, is a highly variable autosomal dominant condition. The full spectrum includes infantile hypercalcemia, abnormal (elfin) facies (see Fig. 56–33), mental deficiency, short stature, numerous peripheral pulmonic stenoses, and supravalvular aortic stenosis. Although patients usually survive the problems of infancy and show catch-up growth, progressive problems of joint contractures, genitourinary and gastrointestinal dysfunction, hypertension, and psychosocial adjustment define the long-term prognosis.[88]

Supravalvular aortic stenosis (SVAS) is due to heterozygosity for a mutation in tropoelastin (discussed later). Because elastic fibers are intrinsic to the media of elastic and muscular arteries, a diffuse, progressive arteriopathy develops, with thickening of the wall and reduction of the lumen. The natural history of the arterial disease is just emerging as patients with Williams syndrome live longer and are monitored prospectively. A predisposition to cerebrovascular disease seems certain. Virtually all tested patients with Williams syndrome have a deletion of the long arm of chromosome 7.[89,90] Those with SVAS have a deletion involving the tropoelastin locus.[91] The crucial gene or genes involved in the rest of the Williams phenotype lie telomeric to the tropoelastin locus; considerable effort is currently directed at identifying the genes that have a role in development of the face, in calcium metabolism, and in development of personality and cognitive capability. Cultured cells from patients with either Williams syndrome or SVAS make less elastin than normal, but the cells have a higher than normal rate of proliferation, a finding that may explain the thickening of the arterial media seen in both conditions.[92]

Autosomal dominant SVAS is an entity distinct from Williams syndrome, although some patients have subtle defects in personality and intelligence. Peripheral pulmonary artery stenoses may be present but rarely cause hemodynamic problems. The aortic lesion requires surgery in less than half of patients.

MITRAL VALVE PROLAPSE (see Chap. 57). This trait is of heterogeneous cause and pathogenesis, although it has been called the most common abnormality of human heart valves. MVP is, equally clearly, not always an abnormality.[93,94] The heritable forms of MVP can be classified into three groups. The first is a familial form with minimal extracardiac involvement. The second is clinically variable, an autosomal dominant condition that merges at one end of its spectrum with Marfan syndrome; it could just as well be discussed as a heritable disorder of connective tissue. The third category is composed of the various Mendelian syndromes that include MVP as a pleiotropic manifestation. In all of these categories, prolapse of the tricuspid valve is a frequent accompaniment.

The first category, which some have called MVP syndrome or familial MVP, includes a condition centered on the mitral valve. The development of actual prolapse shows the age- and gender-dependent behavior characteristic of the idiopathic form. Formal genetic studies in most families confirm autosomal dominance with variable expression. This category has been partitioned into those patients with billowing of the mitral leaflets and those with excessive systolic mitral annular expansion; because this phenotype breeds relatively true, two distinct autosomal dominant forms may exist. The cause, or causes, of these entities is unknown. Moreover, when and how the phenotype of this condition can be distinguished from the sporadic cases of MVP and the cases with obvious evidence of a systemic disorder of connective tissue are unclear. The only consistent extracardiac manifestations are excessive arm span in women and relatively low body weight and systolic pressure. Recently, MVP has been mapped to three genetic loci; none of the genes has been identified. Two are autosomal loci, 11p15.4 and 16p11.2-p12.1.[95,96] Susceptibility to myxomatous degeneration of all cardiac valves can be inherited as an X-linked trait that maps to Xq28.[97]

Many clinical geneticists and cardiologists have referred patients with a suspicion of Marfan syndrome or Ehlers-Danlos syndrome. Some of these patients do not meet minimal diagnostic criteria for a recognized connective tissue disorder[98] but clearly have extracardiac features consistent with a defect of the extracellular matrix described later. MVP is commonly but not always present; when it is present and when evidence of a systemic abnormality of connective tissue is lacking, the patient should be considered to have *primary MVP* (see above). The clinical spectrum of the patients with syndromic MVP includes abnormal striae atrophicae, excessive arm span and leg length, joint hypermobility, pectus excavatum, scoliosis, reduction in thoracic kyphosis ("straight back"), myopia, and mild aortic root dilation.[99] Aortic dilation beyond 3 SD above the mean for body surface area, aortic dissection, ectopia lentis, or a family history of any of these three features *removes* a patient from this category. For the remainder of patients, the acronym MASS phenotype (*m*itral valve, *a*orta, *s*kin, and *s*keletal) describes what certainly is a heterogeneous grouping of patients and families. The aorta is mentioned specifically because of the appropriate concern that progressive dilation and dissection will occur; in fact, neither has been the case, although prospective evaluation has been unsystematic. Many of the associations between MVP and deformity of the thoracic cage and spontaneous pneumothorax are explained by the MASS phenotype.

Finally, MVP frequently accompanies Marfan syndrome, several of the Ehlers-Danlos syndromes, and cutis laxa and occurs more often than expected in patients with osteogenesis imperfecta, Larsen syndrome, pseudoxanthoma elasticum, and other Mendelian syndromes (see Table 70–13). In addition, occasional families with otherwise unclassified heritable disorders of connective tissue have prominent involvement of the mitral apparatus, with myxomatous deterioration, calcification, or both.[100]

NOONAN SYNDROME. Among the pleiotropic Mendelian syndromes with frequent cardiovascular involvement, Noonan syndrome is important because of its relatively high prevalence and clinical variability. This autosomal dominant condition has been called the male Turner syndrome in the past because of the short stature, cubitus valgus, neck webbing, congenital lymphedema, and congenital heart defects that coexist in the 45,X Turner syndrome. However, Noonan syndrome is distinct, but not simply because both men and women are affected. Patients with Noonan syndrome often have an unusual deformity of the sternum, mental dullness, hypertelorism, ptosis, and cryptorchidism. The cardiovascular defects, although widely varied, do not include an increased incidence of coarctation of the aorta. Due to the dysmorphism of the facies and the cardiac involvement, Noonan syndrome is often classified, along with William, LEOPARD, King, and Watson syndromes, as a cardiofacial syndrome.

The entire phenotype of Noonan syndrome is highly variable, and affected persons can escape clinical problems (or accurate diagnosis) even if they have obvious manifestations. Similarly, a wide range of cardiovascular involvement can occur. *Valvular pulmonic stenosis* was the first defect identified, and Noonan syndrome should always be considered in a patient with this lesion. The valve cusps are thickened and dysplastic, even in the absence of hemodynamic compromise. Obstruction to right-sided flow can also occur in patients with Noonan syndrome because of pulmonary artery hypoplasia or infundibular subvalvular changes. The latter finding reflects a generalized predisposition to hypertrophic cardiomyopathy, often asymmetrical, that can affect either ventricle. *Atrial septal defect* occurs in about one-third of patients, usually in association with pulmonic stenosis. *Ventricular septal defects* and *patent ductus arteriosus* each occur in about 10 percent. Congenital anomalies of coronary arteries are found occasionally and unexpectedly during evaluation of more obvious defects. The electrocardiogram often shows left anterior hemiblock and a deep precordial S wave, a pattern not common in pulmonic stenosis of other causes.

Lymphatic dysplasia, especially of the lower limbs, is common but causes clinical difficulties in less than 20 percent of cases. Although evidence of lymphedema often disappears during childhood, chylothorax and a protein-losing enteropathy represent the severe end of the spectrum.

Noonan syndrome shares features with other cardiofacial syndromes, and in sporadic cases (which account for 50 percent of Noonan syndrome), diagnosis can be difficult. All are autosomal dominant, so genetic counseling is somewhat easier. Affected males have reduced reproductive capabilities because of testicular abnormalities. Susceptibility to malignant hyperthermia can be detected by family history, elevated skeletal muscle creatine kinase levels, or muscle biopsy. Noonan syndrome occurs with a relatively high frequency, estimated to be as great as 1 per 1000. Mutations in the gene *PTPN11*, mapped to 12q24.2-q24.31, causes Noonan syndrome in about one-half of instances, so interlocus genetic heterogeneity is likely.[101] Intriguing issues that may shed light on both cause and pathogenesis are the overlap in phenotype with type I neurofibromatosis (the gene for which is on chromosome 17), and the frequent coexistence of Noonan syndrome and deficiency of coagulation factor XI.

Teratogenic Effects

A teratogen is any agent that adversely affects embryonic or fetal development, such as infectious vectors, radiation, drugs, and other chemicals (Table 70–10).[102,103] Teratogenic effects on the cardiovascular system are considered in this chapter for several reasons. First, the phenotypes are often reminiscent of those caused by chromosomal aberrations and single-gene mutations. Second, clinical geneticists and dysmorphologists are involved in diagnosing, managing, and investigating both teratogenic and genetic syndromes. Finally, an organism's response to an encounter with a potential teratogen is largely determined by its genome. The entire field of ecogenetics and part of pharmacogenetics are concerned with these issues.

TABLE 70–10 Cardiovascular Defects Associated with Prenatal Exposure to Teratogens

Teratogen	Cardiovascular Abnormalities*
Ethanol	~50% have CHD: VSD (~50% close spontaneously), TOF, ASD, ECD, absence of a pulmonary artery
Hydantoin	~10% have CHD: VSD, ASD, PS
Lithium	<3% have Ebstein anomaly
Phenylalanine	~20% have CHD: TOF
Retinoic acid	>50% have CHD: TGA, TOF, VSD, IAA
Rubella	>50% have CHD: PDA with or without ASD, VSD, PPS, IAA
Trimethadione	~50% have CHD: complex combinations most frequent (involving VSD, ASD, PDA, AS, PS), VSD, TOF
Valproic acid	>50% have CHD: left- and right-sided flow lesions: CoA, HLH, ASD, VSD, pulmonary atresia
Vitamin D	Supravalvular aortic stenosis is the cardinal manifestation; PPS
Warfarin	~10% have CHD: PDA, PS; rarely, intracranial hemorrhage.

*Among patients with the full clinical spectrum associated with each teratogen; cardiovascular defects listed in decreasing order of prevalence.

AS = aortic stenosis; ASD = atrial septal defect; CHD = congenital heart defect(s); CoA = coarctation of aorta; ECD = endocardial cushion defect; HLH = hypoplastic left heart; IAA = interrupted aortic arch; PDA = patent ductus arteriosus; PPS = peripheral pulmonic stenosis; PS = valvular pulmonic stenosis; TGA = transposition of great arteries; TOF = tetralogy of Fallot; VSD = ventricular septal defect.

The abilities to resist disruption of normal human embryogenesis and development involve systems quite distinct from physiological homeostasis and related only in part with developmental homeostasis. Genetic susceptibilities to teratogens can be illustrated by diverse mechanisms: reduced or inaccurate repair of radiation-induced DNA damage; enhanced receptiveness to viral entry or replication; immune deficiencies that prevent inactivation of infectious vectors or maintenance of immunity; slow inactivation of a compound that exerts a direct deleterious effect; or rapid conversion of an inoffensive drug to a teratogenic metabolite. These types of hereditary variation can be determined by single genes, with susceptibility inherited as a Mendelian trait, or by many genes, each of small effect. Either situation can account for the well-known fact that only a fraction of pregnancies exposed to a given agent are affected adversely. Variation in dose and timing of exposure also confound interpretation of epidemiological and family data. It is not surprising, then, that the actual appearance of the abnormal phenotype is not amenable to traditional pedigree analysis. Rather, examination of the biochemical susceptibilities have proved, and will continue to prove, more enlightening.

Some teratogens, such as warfarin, have a clear action that explains how the pleiotropic manifestations emerge. The action of other teratogens, such as alcohol, is obscure. Finally, in some teratogenic syndromes, such as that in offspring of women with diabetes mellitus, the actual offensive agent is unclear, and numerous pathogenetic mechanisms seem to pertain. Regardless of cause and pathogenetic mechanism, the phenotypes of many teratogens often share manifestations, especially prenatal growth retardation, abnormalities of the craniofacies, and mental retardation.[91] The following syndromes have prominent consequences on the cardiovascular system.

FETAL ALCOHOL SYNDROME. Ethanol is the most common teratogen to which the human embryo and fetus are exposed. The period of greatest vulnerability is the first trimester, and the risks are related clearly to the amount of alcohol consumed; the risk that fetal alcohol syndrome will occur in an offspring of a chronic alcoholic woman is 30 to 50 percent. The features are highly variable and include growth retardation, mild to moderate mental retardation, hyperactivity, short palpebral fissures, a smooth philtrum with a thin upper lip, and small distal phalanges.[104] Congenital heart defects occur in more than one-half of children with the full spectrum of the phenotype; ventricular septal defects are most common and often insignificant, but atrial septal defects, tetralogy of Fallot, and aortic coarctation can occur.

FETAL HYDANTOIN SYNDROME. Virtually all antiseizure medications can affect the fetus. Hydantoin was the first to be identified as a teratogen. The risk to the fetus depends in part on the genotype of the fetus; defects in arene oxidase predispose to the full syndrome. The features include prenatal and postnatal growth retardation, mild mental retardation, a broad face with a short nose, short distal phalanges with small nails, and hip dislocation. Cardiovascular defects, which are an inconstant part of the syndrome, include septal defects, right- and left-sided flow defects, and a single umbilical artery.

RETINOIC ACID EMBRYOPATHY. Isotretinoin was not recognized as a teratogen until after it was licensed for the treatment of acne. The vulnerable period extends from the first week through the fourth month of gestation. Isotretinoin increases the risks of miscarriage and stillbirth. The phenotype includes anomalies of the craniofacies and gross neuroanatomical disruption. Cardiovascular defects are common and emphasize various conotruncal malformations. Live-born infants often succumb to the cardiac and brain anomalies. Although the mechanism of action is not certain, vitamin A derivatives such as retinoic acid function as morphogens during embryogenesis, serving as signals for cell migration. The fact that the cardiovascular defects are primarily those of rotation and folding suggests disruption of a normal developmental homeostatic system.

WARFARIN EMBRYOPATHY. Coumarin-related vitamin K antagonists are usually prescribed for various cardiovascular problems in women of childbearing age and can cause diverse cardiovascular and other organ damage to the fetus. Coumarin interferes with embryogenesis directly when administered during gestational weeks 6 through 9. The most pronounced effects are on cartilage because of inhibition of enzymes of extracellular matrix metabolism. Congenital cardiac defects perhaps increase in frequency but fit no specific pathogenetic mechanism. The second pattern of coumarin effects involves exposure during the second and third trimesters and includes spontaneous abortion, stillbirth, and various central nervous system defects. The last are not due simply to intracranial hemorrhage as was once assumed.

What predisposes to the adverse fetal effects of coumarin remains undetermined. First, more than 75 percent of women who take coumarin derivatives throughout pregnancy have normal offspring; reassuring most women while identifying those at risk for adverse effects has obvious advantages. Second, placing all pregnant women on a regimen of heparin is not an acceptable solution, because heparin can cause stillbirth or premature fetal loss in about 20 percent of exposures, is not as effective as coumarin in some indications for anticoagulation, and is more difficult to administer and regulate.

MATERNAL PHENYLKETONURIA. The inborn error of metabolism phenylketonuria (PKU) produces severe mental retardation unless the phenylalanine content of the diet is markedly reduced soon after birth.[105] Deficiency of phenylalanine hydroxylase in the fetus produces no harm because fetal blood levels of phenylalanine are regulated by the heterozygous mother's enzyme. Because neonatal screening for this disease is now routine in all states, virtually all patients receive treatment and grow to adulthood with average intelligence. Many patients discontinue the rigorous dietary therapy during adolescence, when the elevated phenylalanine levels have far less deleterious effects. The embryopathy occurs when a woman with homozygous deficiency for phenylalanine hydroxylase becomes pregnant and her fetus is exposed to high levels of the amino acid, which overwhelm its ability to metabolize. The result is highly predictable if the mother does not restart dietary restriction of phenylalanine for the entire gestation: moderate to severe mental retardation, prenatal and postnatal growth retardation, microcephaly, and various cardiovascular defects in 15 to 20 percent of cases. This condition can largely be prevented by effective counseling of female patients with PKU.

FETAL RUBELLA EFFECTS (see Chap. 56). About 50 percent of fetuses become infected with the rubella virus when the mother is infected during the first trimester. An infected fetus not only suffers varied and severe interference with development and organogenesis but also acquires a chronic viral illness that can persist for years. The most common features of the embryopathy are mental deficiency, deafness, cataract, and cardiovascular defects. PDA is common, as are septal defects. Peripheral pulmonary stenosis and fibromuscular proliferation of medium and small arteries often improve postnatally.

Cardiomyopathies (see Chap. 59)

Each of the three clinical categories of primary cardiomyopathy—hypertrophic, dilated, and restrictive—can be caused by mutations in single genes as judged by Mendelian inheritance of a consistent phenotype in numerous families. Many other Mendelian and mitochondrial disorders also cause cardiomyopathies as a secondary consequence of their basic metabolic disturbance.

Hypertrophic Cardiomyopathy

In more than four decades since the recognition of hypertrophic cardiomyopathy as a clinical entity, many aspects of its natural history, pathology, and management have been clarified substantially.[106-111] The phenotype is most clearly defined anatomically and histologically and consists of myocardial hypertrophy without secondary cause; cellular and myofiber disarray; myocardial fibrosis; and mediointimal proliferation of small coronary arteries. None of these features is pathognomonic; for example, myofiber disorganization is present in the normal human heart during embryogenesis and in congenital heart defects that place strain on the right-sided circulation.

About half of probands with idiopathic hypertrophic cardiomyopathy of any segment of the left ventricle have affected first-degree relatives, and the phenotype in those families is inherited as an autosomal dominant, familial hypertrophic cardiomyopathy (FHC). There is wide variability of expression within a family, in part due to the age dependence of the trait.[107] Later generations of relatives in adolescence and childhood may not have developed echocardiographic evidence of hypertrophy. Hence, pedigree screening by phenotype for clinical, counseling, or investigative purposes should not be considered complete until the following criteria are satisfied: two-dimensional echocardiography is used to ensure that segmental hypertrophy is detected; a person at risk has normal echocardiographic findings and no evidence of electrocardiographic abnormality or important dysrhythmia after about age 20; and a person of any age has left ventricular hypertrophy without any other explanation, such as hypertension or aortic stenosis.

Familial hypertrophic cardiomyopathy is a disease of the sarcomere, with primary defects of thick and thin filaments now defined. Mutations of at least 10 and perhaps more loci cause FHC (see Table 70–2).[112] The first gene identified was the cardiac beta-myosin heavy chain gene (*MYH7*). Depending on the population studied, about 50 percent of all FHC mutations occur in *MYH7*, and many mutations have been described.[113,114] Patients with neither parent affected may also have *MYH7* mutations, suggesting that the genetic alteration occurred in the egg or sperm of a parent. The likelihood of germline mosaicism is suggested strongly by two siblings with FHC and the same mutation in *MHY7*, even though neither parent shows the mutation in leukocyte DNA.[115] Mutations that alter the charge of the beta-myosin heavy chain generally carry a worse prognosis in terms of age of detection, electrocardiographic abnormalities, and sudden death.[116-118] Thus, defining the specific gene involved, followed by the specific mutation, likely has clinical importance.[119] However, because of the substantial technical challenges and expense of identifying the specific mutation in any given patient with FHC, genetic testing is not yet routine.[120] A recent survey of families with FHC found that in 82 percent, a mutation in either *MYH7* or *MYBPC3* was responsible, a finding that should facilitate a systematic approach to molecular testing.[112] How the mutant protein interacts with other components of the sarcomere of both cardiac and skeletal muscle to produce the phenotype is another area of active research,[121] as is the generation and characterization of animal models of FHC. Both approaches suggest that abnormal signaling by calcium ions in the sarcomere and diminished myocardial energetics and contractile reserve represent common pathways to aberrant myocyte growth and myocardial remodeling.[122,123] The importance of presymptomatic and even prehypertrophy diagnosis through mutation analysis in families will become more important as improved methods of therapy evolve.[124] Apparent cases of sporadic noncompaction of the left ventricle may represent the first recognizable instance of FHC in a family.[125]

Although intergenic and intragenic heterogeneity account for much of the interfamilial variability in the FHC phenotype, considerable variation remains among relatives who share the same mutation. Both environmental and genetic factors have impacts. A possible example of the latter is the angiotensin I–converting enzyme (ACE) genotype, with different polymorphic variants of ACE associated with more or less hypertrophy. Prognosis also depends on the degree of involvement of the cardiac microvasculature; patients unable to increase blood flow in response to dipyridamole were more likely to have an unfavorable outcome.[126]

Dilated Cardiomyopathy

The prevalence of idiopathic dilated cardiomyopathy (DCM) is about double that of the hypertrophic form, or about 2 to 8 per 100,000. Approximately one-half of patients who are evaluated for unexplained DCM are left with the "idiopathic" designation.[127] Although numerous occurrences of familial dilated cardiomyopathy (FDC) are reported, few investigations have been conducted of an unselected series of probands for clinical and subclinical evidence of cardiac disease. Thus, it is unclear what fraction of patients with idiopathic DCM have a Mendelian disease, how many have a new mutation for a Mendelian disease, and how many have phenocopies of nongenetic causes. Estimates of a positive family history, which could suggest a Mendelian condition or a shared environmental cause, range from 7 to 30 percent.[113]

Because of the risk of severe dysrhythmia in patients with DCM, early detection of individuals with the disorder can be life saving. Echocardiography sensitively detects affected relatives with subclinical disease. Individuals who have equivocal left ventricular enlargement or dysfunction can have ambulatory electrocardiographic monitoring and, if the diagnosis is still uncertain, can have serial examinations. Certainly every patient with idiopathic DCM should have a detailed family history taken; about 20 percent reveal an affected relative.[128] If any close relative has a history consistent with cardiomyopathy, dysrhythmia, or sudden death at a relatively young age, counseling about the risk of a familial disease and the potential benefits of pedigree screening should be offered. The majority of instances of FDC fit autosomal dominant inheritance, but X-linked, autosomal recessive, and mitochondrial forms exist.[107,129-131] Clinical variability characterizes virtually all pedigrees; variation in severity, clinical phenotype, and age of onset is typical.

Considerable progress has been made in the past few years in defining the causes of many of the autosomal dominant forms of FDC. Mutations that affect either force generation or force transmission can result in the DCM phenotype. Histological examination of myocardium generally shows nonspecific hypertrophy and fibrosis. By electron microscopy, however, mitochondria are distinctly abnormal, a finding not seen in cases of congestive heart failure due to other causes. Although various mutations of the mitochondrial chromosome can cause dilated cardiomyopathy, including childhood onset, the inheritance pattern in most cases does not suggest maternal transmission.[131]

Some pedigrees show convincing evidence of X-linkage of dilated cardiomyopathy. At least three loci have been identified. In Barth syndrome, cardiac involvement is associated with skeletal myopathy, proportionate short stature, and neutropenia. The cause is mutation of the (*TAZ*) gene at Xq28. Mutations of this gene can also cause isolated FDC and noncompaction of the left ventricle.[107,132]

Many males with Duchenne and some with Becker muscular dystrophy develop myocardial dysfunction.[133] In the Becker form, right ventricular involvement may be unassociated with left ventricular dysfunction. Deletion of exon 49 of the dystrophin gene predisposes to cardiomyopathy. This pleiotropic feature in a disease that manifests as a skeletal myopathy prompted evaluation of the dystrophin locus in pedigrees with apparently isolated cardiomyopathy. Mutations in the 5′ end of the dystrophin gene have been found to account for some instances of X-linked dilated cardiomyopathy. Why some dystrophin mutations are selectively expressed in cardiac muscle (and others in brain) is unclear.

Emery-Dreifuss muscular dystrophy is distinguishable clinically from the Duchenne and Becker forms by absence of pseudohypertrophy of skeletal muscle, early involvement of the arms with elbow contractures, and early onset of cardiac conduction abnormalities and atrial dysrhythmia.[133,134] Autosomal dominant and X-linked recessive forms occur. In the latter, female heterozygotes are also commonly affected, albeit more mildly than males. The disease was mapped to the distal region of Xq28, and a previously unknown gene, called *emerin*, was found to be mutated. Hearts show replacement of myocardium, especially in the atria, with fat and fibrosis. Even though the conduction system is not primarily affected histologically, sudden death is common in both hemizygous men and heterozygous women; thus, carrier detection can be life saving.

The dominant form of Emery-Dreifuss muscular dystrophy is caused by mutations in the lamin A/C gene.[135] Both emerin and lamin A/C are expressed in the nuclear membrane of skeletal and heart muscle. Mutations in lamin A/C cause a number of diverse syndromes, including Hutchinson-Gilford progeria.[136]

Autosomal recessive forms of limb-girdle muscular dystrophy with DCM have been found to be due to mutations in the genes encoding β- and δ-sarcoglycan, and mutations in the same genes, when heterozygous, cause autosomal dominant FDC.[137,138]

The arrhythmogenic right ventricular dysplasias are distinct from idiopathic DCM but share some features with most of the FDCs in that they are generally autosomal dominant, and conduction defects, dysrhythmia, and sudden death can precede the appearance of overt heart failure.[139,140]

TABLE 70–11 Disorders Associated with Restrictive Cardiomyopathy

Phenotype	OMIM No.*
Primary endocardial fibroelastosis	
Familial endocardial fibroelastosis	226000, 305300
Faciocardiorenal syndrome	227280
Secondary endocardial fibroelastosis	
As a Relatively Common Manifestation	
Maternal lupus erythematosus	
Pseudoxanthoma elasticum	177850, 264800
Systemic carnitine deficiency	212140
Trisomy 18	
As a Relatively Infrequent Manifestation	
Cornelia de Lange syndrome	122470
Rubinstein-Taybi syndrome	268600
Secondary Infiltrative Cardiomyopathy	
Familial amyloidoses I and III	176300
Fabry disease	301500
Gaucher disease type I	230800
Glycogen storage disorder II	232300
Glycogen storage disorder III	232400
Hemochromatosis	235200
Mucopolysaccharidosis IH	252800
Mucopolysaccharidosis II	309900

*Data from Online Mendelian Inheritance in Man (www.ncbi.nlm.nih.gov/omim).

Restrictive Cardiomyopathy

Restrictive cardiomyopathy is primarily a defect of diastolic function.[141] The pathogenesis of the majority of cases of restrictive cardiomyopathy involves infiltration or replacement of the myocardium or both. The causes are varied and can be nongenetic or genetic; the latter are mostly metabolic diseases with secondary effects on the heart and are summarized in Table 70–11; some are reviewed subsequently. One form of restrictive cardiomyopathy that has primary genetic forms among many other causes is endocardial fibroelastosis. Other mutations produce restriction through pericardial constriction. Isolated pedigrees of primary myocardial fibrosis without secondary cause and leading to restrictive hemodynamics are not classifiable.

Endocardial Fibroelastosis

This abnormality is characterized by thickening of the endocardium, which leads to decreased compliance and impaired diastolic function. Primary forms, discussed here, are unassociated with other cardiac anomalies (see Table 70–9). In infants, there is often an indolent course of failure to thrive, tachypnea, and tachycardia, until a precipitant such as an upper respiratory infection leads to rapid cardiac decompensation. Treatment of children with primary endocardial fibroelastosis is ineffective; cardiac transplantation now offers some hope. Autopsy shows enlargement of the left ventricle and perhaps other chambers, no abnormality of lung vessels, and collapse of the left lower lobe. Histopathological study reveals extensive deposition of extracellular matrix, primarily collagen and elastic fibers, in the endocardium.

X-linked recessive inheritance is the most firmly established of the single-gene causes. Some pedigrees show mainly small, contracted cardiac chambers, whereas others have chamber dilation; both are compatible with the functional pathophysiology described by the term *restrictive*. Males are affected earlier and more severely by both forms, and death in infancy is not unusual. The condition must be distinguished from X-linked dilated cardiomyopathy and Barth syndrome. Morphological abnormalities of mitochondria occur on ultrastructural studies of heart and leukocytes. Insufficient longitudinal experience is recorded to know whether females heterozygous for this mutation develop a dilated or restrictive cardiomyopathy later in life.

Several pedigrees suggestive of autosomal recessive inheritance of primary endocardial fibroelastosis were reported before the routine availability of laboratory methods to diagnose metabolic derangements, especially defects in fatty acid catabolism. The occurrence of hydrocephalus, endocardial fibroelastosis, and neonatal cataracts may be due to a single gene mutation but could represent sequelae of a viral infection. Endocardial fibroelastosis can be a prominent finding at autopsy in patients with autosomal dominant dilated cardiomyopathy; whether the endocardial changes are primary, representing yet another Mendelian form of this disorder, or secondary remains unclear.

Restrictive cardiomyopathy often occurs with both hemodynamic evidence of impaired diastolic filling and wall thickening; any of the conditions causing pseudohypertrophy of the myocardium can eventually exhibit restrictive pathophysiology. Hemochromatosis and the amyloidoses, both hereditary and acquired forms, are especially likely to present in this manner. Connective tissue replaces myocytes or infiltrates the interstitium in a number of conditions. Fibrosis of the myocardium may cause pseudohypertrophy, but the clinical consequences are more those of restriction. Restrictive pathophysiology often accompanies fibrosis of the myocardium, at least in the early stages. Replacement of myocytes or infiltration of the interstitium by collagen and proteoglycan occurs in various conditions, such as muscular dystrophies and disorders that predispose to ischemia due to coronary artery occlusion, such as diabetes mellitus, hemoglobinopathies associated with sickling, Fabry disease, and the mucopolysaccharidoses. Severe fibrosis may produce considerable thickening of the myocardium, or pseudohypertrophy. Finally, a number of hereditary conditions associate with endocardial fibroelastosis (see Table 70-11).

CONSTRICTIVE PERICARDITIS (see Chap. 64). Two rare autosomal recessive disorders include fibrous thickening of the pericardium as a manifestation. In both, signs and symptoms of constrictive pericarditis develop insidiously, and treatment by pericardiotomy is life saving. One condition was first described in Finland and given the name *MULIBREY nanism,* a combination of a mnemonic for *mu*scle, *li*ver, *br*ain, and *ey*e and an archaic word for dwarfism (nanism). Growth failure from an early age is common, and growth does not improve once pericardial constriction is abated. Subsequently, more than a dozen patients, generally with consanguineous parents, have been reported from around the world.[142] The gene in which mutations occur maps to 17q22-q23 and encodes an apparent zinc-finger transcription factor of unclear function.[143]

The arthropathy-camptodactyly syndrome previously had been reported because of the skeletal and rheumatological manifestations before pericardial effusion and fibrous thickening of the pericardium were recognized as manifestations. The disease locus was mapped in consanguineous kindreds by homozygosity by descent to 1q25-q31, and mutations occur in the gene, *CACP,* that encodes a secreted proteoglycan.[144,145]

Cardiomyopathies Secondary to Other Causes

INBORN ERRORS OF METABOLISM. These can affect the left ventricle by various mechanisms (Table 70–12) and produce diverse anatomical, histological, and functional disturbances. The most common anatomical result is an apparent hypertrophic cardiomyopathy, which is actually pseudohypertrophic because the thickened walls are not due to myocardial cell hypertrophy but to cellular or interstitial infiltration by metabolites. Abnormalities of both systolic and diastolic function result, outflow obstruction may occur, and in some cases the hemodynamic characteristics resemble a restrictive cardiomyopathy. The offending metabolite may be an incompletely degraded macromolecule such as glycogen (glycogen storage disorder II [Pompe disease] and glycogen storage disorder III), proteoglycan and glycosaminoglycan (mucopolysaccharidoses I, III, IV, VI, and VII),[146] sphingolipid (Fabry disease,[147] Tay-Sachs disease, Farber disease, Refsum disease, and Gaucher disease), glycoprotein (fucosidosis and mannosidosis), and amyloid (familial amyloidoses I and III) or a small molecule such as iron in hemochromatosis. Some of these disorders are discussed later. True myocardial hypertrophy occurs as a part of Mendelian syndromes, such as Noonan syndrome, von Recklinghausen neurofibromatosis, Costello syndrome[148] and LEOPARD syndrome,[149] and monogenic errors of metabolism, notably those producing hyperthyroidism and pheochromocytoma. Any of the Mendelian disorders that cause hypertension may, over time, produce true myocardial hypertrophy.

Dilated cardiomyopathy often results from inborn errors of energy production, especially fatty acid metabolism. Various disorders associated with carnitine deficiency, mitochondrial and peroxisomal dysfunction, and muscle dysfunction can manifest with symptoms of congestive heart failure or dysrhythmia.

Primary Disorders of Rhythm and Conduction

See Chapter 28.

Disorders of Connective Tissue

The two broad classes of connective tissue disorders are those due to mutations in single genes that determine or somehow affect components of the extracellular matrix and those due to extrinsic factors affecting the extracellular matrix, such as rheumatoid arthritis and systemic lupus erythematosus. The former category includes many disorders that affect the cardiovascular system. Susceptibility to so-called acquired disorders of connective tissue is, in part, determined by genes, and this specific aspect is reviewed below.

Mendelian Disorders of the Extracellular Matrix

Close to 200 distinct phenotypes now make up this category, which was first defined less than four decades ago with fewer than 10 disorders. Several reviews and textbooks describe the phenotypes, genetics, and causes of many of the conditions (Table 70–13).[18,150,151]

Marfan Syndrome

This autosomal dominant disorder is relatively frequent (2-3 per 10,000) and occurs in all races and ethnic groups.[15,151] Even with the discovery of the genetic and biochemical bases of the condition, the diagnosis of Marfan syndrome outside families with the classic phenotype remains entirely clinical. Current criteria (Table 70–14) depend on the manifestations in the cardinal organ systems—the eye, the skeleton, the heart, and the aorta—and other systems as well as the family history (Fig. 70–7).[98,151] The presence of manifestations more specific for Marfan syndrome, such as aortic dilation, aortic dissection in a nonhypertensive young person, ectopia lentis, and dural ectasia, clearly is more important diagnostically

TABLE 70–12 Mendelian Errors of Metabolism with Manifestations in the Cardiovascular System

Disorder	Eponym or Common Name	OMIM No.*	Pathogenesis
Aminoacidopathies			
Alkaptonuria	Ochronosis	203500	Deposition of homogentisic acid in connective tissue
Cystinosis, nephropathic type		219800	Lysosomal storage
Homocystinuria		236200	Unknown
Oxalosis I	Hyperoxaluria	259900	Vascular and tissue accumulation of oxalate
Defects in Fatty Acid Metabolism			
Carnitine transport defect	Primary carnitine deficiency	212140	Lipid myopathy; defective energy generation
MCAD deficiency		201450	Lipid myopathy; defective energy generation
LCAD deficiency		201460	Lipid myopathy; defective energy generation
Glycogen Storage Disorders			
GSD II	Pompe	232300	Lysosomal storage
GSD II	Adult acid maltase deficiency	232300	Lysosomal storage
GSD III	Forbes; debrancher deficiency	232400	Intracellular glycogen accumulation; fibrosis
GSD VIII	GSD of the heart	306000	
Glycoproteinoses			
Fucosidosis, severe		230000	Lysosomal storage
Fucosidosis, mild		230000	Lysosomal storage
Mannosidosis		248500	Lysosomal storage
Aspartylglycosaminuria		208400	Lysosomal storage
Mucolipidoses			
ML II	I-cell	252500	Lysosomal storage
ML III	Pseudo-Hurler polydystrophy	252500	Lysosomal storage
Mucopolysaccharidoses			
MPS IH	Hurler	252800	Lysosomal storage
MPS IS	Scheie	252800	Lysosomal storage
MPS IH/S	Hurler-Scheie	252800	Lysosomal storage
MPS II	Hunter	209900	Lysosomal storage
MPS III A	Sanfilippo A	252900	Lysosomal storage
MPS III B	Sanfilippo B	252920	Lysosomal storage
MPS III C	Sanfilippo C	252930	Lysosomal storage
MPS III D	Sanfilippo D		Lysosomal storage
MPS IV A	Morquio A	253000	Lysosomal storage
MPS IV B	Morquio B	253010	Lysosomal storage
MPS VI	Maroteaux-Lamy	253200	Lysosomal storage
MPS VII	Sly	253220	Lysosomal storage
Sphingolipidoses			
Fabry		301500	Cellular accumulation of trihexosyl ceramide, especially in endothelium
Farber		228000	Histiocytic infiltration
Gaucher, adult form		230800	Cellular accumulation of glucocerebroside
Miscellaneous Disorders			
Acid lipase deficiency	Wolman	278000	↑ Cholesterol; foam cell infiltration
Cholesterol ester storage disease		278000	↑ Cholesterol; foam cell infiltration
Geleophysic dysplasia		231050	Lysosomal storage
Hereditary angioedema		106100	Complement and kinin activation

*Data from Online Mendelian Inheritance in Man (www.ncbi.nlm.nih.gov/omim).
†Gene symbol; for chromosomal locus see Table 70–2.
‡Naturally occurring mutants; does not include transgenic and knockout rodent models.

Cardiovascular Involvement	Biochemical Defect	Gene Locus[†]	Animal Model[‡]
AS; atherosclerosis	Homogentisate oxidase	*HGD*	
Hypertension from renal failure, vascular wall thickening	Cystinosin	*CTNS*	
Early CAD; venous thrombosis; pulmonary embolism	Cystathionine β-synthase	*CBS*	
Conduction defect; vascular occlusions; Raynaud phenomenon	Peroxisomal alanine-glyoxylate aminotransferase	*AGT*	
DCM: ECF	Solute carrier 22	*OCTN2*	Syrian hamster
DCM	Medium-chain acyl-CoA dehydrogenase	*ACADM*	
DCM	Long-chain acyl-CoA dehydrogenase	*ACADL*	
Pseudohypertrophic CM; short PR interval; ECF	α-1,4-glucosidase	*GAA*	Canine and bovine
Primarily skeletal muscle; respiratory insufficiency; cor pulmonale	α-1,4-glucosidase	*GAA*	
Pseudohypertrophic CM	Amylo-1,6-glucosidase	*AGL*	
DCM	Phosphorylase kinase	*PHKA2*	
Myocardial thickening	α-Fucosidase	*FUCA1*	
Angiokeratoma	α-Fucosidase	*FUCA1*	
Myocardial thickening; valvular thickening; conduction disturbance	α-Mannosidase	*MANB*	
Valvular thickening	Aspartylglycosylamine aminohydrolase	*AGA*	
Same as MPS IH	Acetylglucosamine-1-phosphotransferase	*GNPTA*	
Valvular thickening and dysfunction, especially AS, AR	Acetylglucosamine-1-phosphotransferase	*GNPTA*	
Early CAD; PH and OAD→CP; valvular dysfunction, especially MR, AR; pseudohypertrophic CM	α-L-Iduronidase	*IDUA*	Canine and feline
Valvular dysfunction, especially AS	α-L-Iduronidase	*IDUA*	
Same as MPS IH	α-L-Iduronidase	*IDUA*	
Same as MPS IH; less severe in mild MPS II variant	Sulfoiduronate sulfatase	*IDS*	
Valvular thickening and occasional dysfunction	Heparan sulfate sulfatase	*SGSH*	
Valvular thickening and occasional dysfunction	*N*-Acetyl-α-D-glucosaminidase	*NAGLU*	
Valvular thickening and occasional dysfunction	Acetyl-CoA; α-glucosaminidase *N*-acetyltransferase	*MPS3C*	
Valvular thickening and occasional dysfunction	*N*-Acetylglucosamine-6-sulfatase	*GNS*	
Valvular dysfunction, especially AR	Galactosamine-6-sulfatase	*GALNS*	
Milder than MPS IV A	β-Galactosidase	*GLBI*	
Same as MPS IH	Arylsulfatase B	*ARSB*	Feline
Valvular thickening	β-Glucuronidase	*GUSB*	Murine and canine
Early CAD, valvular thickening and dysfunction; pseudohypertrophic CM; short PR interval; arteriolar occlusion; angiokeratoma	α-Galactosidase A	*GLA*	
Nodular thickening of valves	Ceramidase	*ASAH*	
PH→CP; interstitial infiltration of myocytes by Gaucher cells; constrictive pericarditis	β-Glucocerebroside	*GBA*	
Atherosclerosis	Lysosomal acid lipase	*LIPA*	
Atherosclerosis; PH	Lysosomal acid lipase	*LIPA*	
Valvular dysfunction	?		
Angioedema	C1 esterase inhibitor	*CINH*	

AR = aortic regurgitation; AS = aortic stenosis; CAD = coronary artery disease; CM = cardiomyopathy; CP = cor pulmonale; DCM = dilated cardiomyopathy; ECF = endocardial fibroelastosis; GSD = glycogen storage disease; MPS = mucopolysaccharoidoses; MR = mitral regurgitation; OAD = obstructive airway disease; PH = pulmonary hypertension.

TABLE 70–13 Cardiovascular Manifestations of Heritable Disorders of Connective Tissue

Disorder	OMIM No.*	Cardiovascular Manifestations
Cutis laxa	219100 123700	PS, PPS, CP MVP
Ehlers-Danlos, classic form	130000, 130010	MVP, occasional aortic root dilatation
Ehlers-Danlos, hypermobile form	130020	MVP
Ehlers-Danlos, vascular form	130050	Arterial rupture, MVP, occasionally aortic dissection and arterial aneurysms, easy bruising
Ehlers-Danlos, ocular-scoliotic form	225400	MVP
Ehlers-Danlos, tenascin-X deficiency[151a]	606408	MVP, easy bruising
Osteogenesis imperfecta I	166200	MVP, mild aortic root dilatation
Osteogenesis imperfecta II	166210	CP, arterial calcification
Osteogenesis imperfecta III	259420	MVP
Osteogenesis imperfecta IV	166220	Aortic root dilatation
Marfan syndrome	154700	MVP, aortic root dilatation, aortic dissection
MASS phenotype	157700	MVP, mild aortic root dilatation
Pseudoxanthoma elasticum	177850	Arteriolar sclerosis, claudication, myocardial infarction, endocardial fibroelastosis

CP = cor pulmonale; MVP = mitral valve prolapse; PPS = peripheral pulmonic stenosis; PS = valvular pulmonic stenosis.
*Data from Online Mendelian Inheritance in Man (www.ncbi.nlm.nih.gov/omim).

TABLE 70–14 Diagnostic Criteria for Marfan Syndrome

Phenotypic Manifestations*	
Skeleton	Joint hypermobility, tall stature, pectus excavatum, reduced thoracic kyphosis, scoliosis, arachnodactyly, dolichostenomelia, pectus carinatum, erosion of the lumbosacral vertebrae from dural ectasia[d]
Eye	Myopia, retinal detachment, elongated globe, precocious cataracts, ectopia lentis[d]
Cardiovascular	Mitral valve prolapse, endocarditis, dysrhythmia, dilated mitral annulus, mitral regurgitation, tricuspid valve prolapse, aortic regurgitation, aortic dissection,[d] dilation of the aortic root[d]
Pulmonary	Apical blebs, spontaneous pneumothorax
Skin and integument	Inguinal hernias, incisional hernias, striae atrophicae
Central nervous system	Attention deficit disorder, hyperactivity, verbal-performance discrepancy, dural ectasia,[d] anterior pelvic meningocele[d]
Family history	*If the family history is positive* for a close relative clearly affected by Marfan syndrome, to make the diagnosis in the patient, a major criterion should be present as well as findings in one other system. *If the family history is negative or unknown,* to make the diagnosis, the patient should have one major criterion and manifestations in two other systems.

*Manifestations are listed within each organ system in increasing specificity for Marfan syndrome, although none is completely specific; those indicated by[d] are the most specific and constitute major criteria.[141]

than features common in other connective tissue disorders and in the general population, such as scoliosis, joint hypermobility, myopia, and MVP.

The most common cardiovascular features are MVP and dilation of the sinuses of Valsalva.[151] Associated clinical problems of mitral regurgitation, aortic regurgitation, and aortic dissection account, if untreated, for most of the early mortality that results in an average age of death in the fourth and fifth decades of life.[152] Children tend to be more severely affected by mitral valve disease, whereas aortic problems are progressive and more likely in adolescence and beyond.

MITRAL VALVE INVOLVEMENT. MVP (see Chap. 57) is age dependent and more common in women with Marfan syndrome. The incidence reaches 60 to 80 percent when patients are studied by two-dimensional echocardiography, and the valve leaflets generally have an elongated and redundant appearance. Progression of severity, as judged by the appearance or worsening of mitral regurgitation by clinical and echocardiographic criteria, occurs in at least one-quarter of patients, a much higher rate than in MVP found in the general population. The mitral annulus dilates and contributes to the regurgitation, as do stretching and occasional rupture of chordae. About 10 percent of patients with marked prolapse have calcification of the mitral annulus. Standard treatment for chronic mitral regurgitation is indicated, but coexistent aortic root dilation usually requires that increasing inotropy be avoided. When mitral regurgitation becomes severe enough to warrant surgical intervention, two considerations must be added to the balance: (1) repair of the mitral apparatus is often successful and durable in patients with Marfan syndrome.[153] Repair is less easily accomplished when the cusps are extremely redundant, there is marked chordal damage, or the annulus is heavily calcified; (2) the aorta may be enlarged enough to permit concomitant repair. With Marfan syndrome, as with virtually all of the heritable disorders of connective tissue, there is an increased susceptibility to dehiscence of prosthetic mitral valves, regardless of the care taken in placing them.

AORTIC ROOT INVOLVEMENT (see Chap. 53). The sinuses of Valsalva are often dilated at birth, and the rate of progression varies widely among patients in general and also among relatives (Fig. 70–8). Thus, predicting long-term risks of developing aortic regurgitation (which clearly is positively associated with aortic root diameter), suffering aortic dissection (which is less clearly associated with diameter), or requiring aortic surgery is fraught with uncertainty.[154] Transthoracic echocardiography is sufficient for detecting and monitoring changes in diameter, because in the absence of dissection, dilation is limited to the proximal ascending aorta, and the rate of change is slow, measured in millimeters per year. Rare exceptions of principal dilation of the thoracic aorta can be monitored with transesophageal echocardiography or magnetic resonance imaging. Patients with dilation less than 1.5 times the mean diameter predicted for their body size can be observed annually; as the diameter increases, more frequent evaluation is necessary. Aortic regurgitation often appears in adults at a diameter of 50 mm but may be absent at diameters of more than 60 mm. The risk of dissection increases with the size of the aorta and fortunately occurs infrequently below a diameter of 55 mm in the adult. Many physicians have adopted the criterion of a 50 to 55 mm maximal aortic root dimension for performing elective surgery in adult patients with Marfan syndrome, regardless of the severity of the aortic regurgitation,[153] although patients with a family history of aortic dissection should have surgery at the lower end of this range. The perioperative results of both elective and emergency repair of the aortic root have been excellent and a marked improvement from the precomposite graft era that ended in the mid-1970s. Long-term results of operation are limited by the problems of endocarditis and anticoagulation common to all prosthetic valves, but in the absence of chronic aortic dissection appear favorable for patients with Marfan syndrome.[153,155]

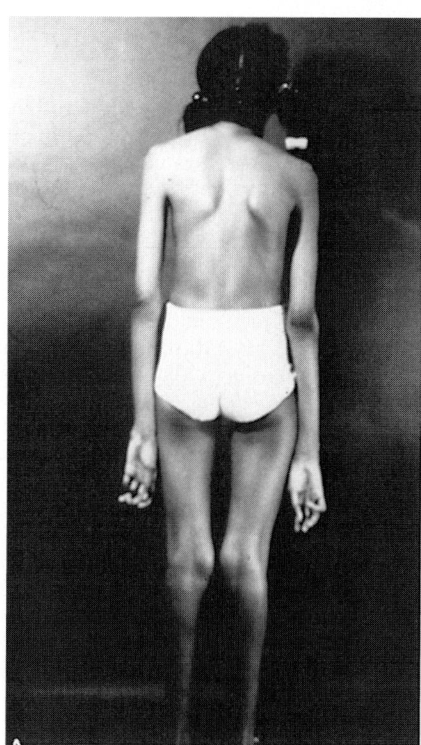

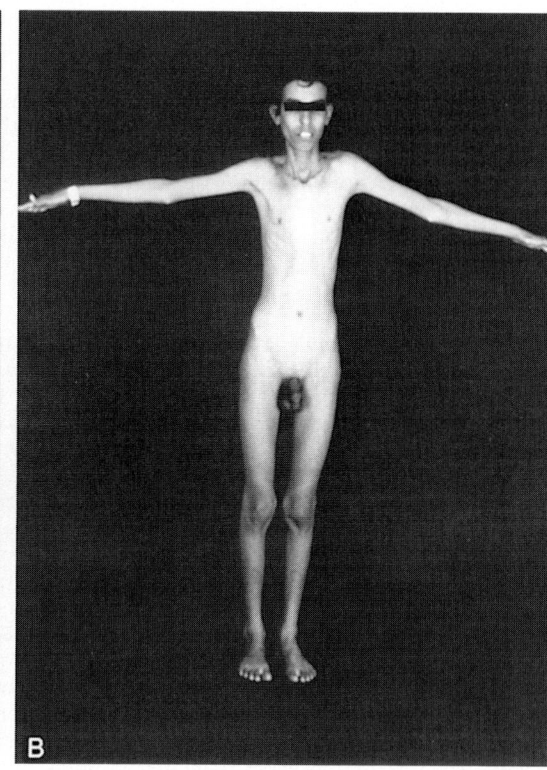

FIGURE 70–7 External phenotype of patients with Marfan syndrome, showing long extremities and digits, tall stature, and pectus carinatum.

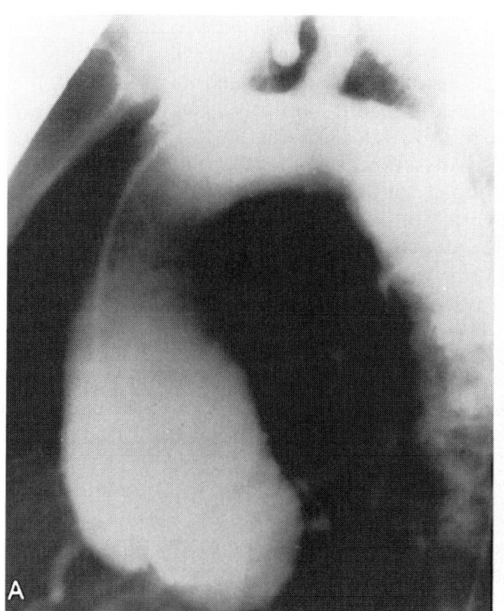

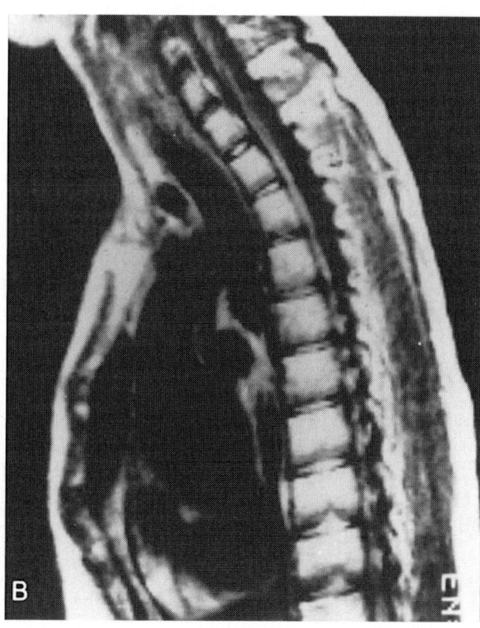

FIGURE 70–8 Dilation of the aortic root in Marfan syndrome. **A,** Lateral angiogram of the ascending aorta showing dilation of the sinuses of Valsalva and proximal ascending aorta and relatively normal caliber of the ascending aorta. **B,** Lateral magnetic resonance imaging scan of the same patient.

Several approaches to repairing the dilated or dissected aortic root while preserving the native aortic valve have been developed.[156] Findings at both short- and, now, long-term follow-up of patients with Marfan syndrome who have undergone this repair have been quite favorable.[153,157] The operation must be performed before the root is widely dilated and the valve commissures and cusps markedly stretched. This approach is increasingly being taken in all patients when the maximal root dimension reaches 50 mm, and it is an especially suitable procedure for women of childbearing age who want to consider pregnancy, as well as for all others in whom anticoagulation is contraindicated.

THORACIC ABNORMALITIES. Severe *pectus excavatum* can complicate cardiovascular surgery by hampering exposure of the heart by median sternotomy. For elective cardiovascular surgery, repair of the sternal deformity some months in advance permits sufficient healing of the costochondral junctions that a stable and functionally and cosmetically improved thoracic cage will facilitate further surgery and postoperative recovery. Simultaneous repair of cardiac and sternal defects, although possible, is a long procedure, and intraoperative bleeding from bone can be considerable due to the anticoagulation associated with cardiopulmonary bypass.

AORTIC DISSECTION (see Chap. 53). This complication usually begins just above the coronary ostia (type A in the Stanford scheme) and extends the entire length of the aorta (type I in DeBakey scheme). About 10 percent of dissections begin distal to the left subclavian artery (type B or III), but dissection rarely is limited to the abdominal aorta. Angiography, magnetic resonance imaging, and transesophageal echocardiography all have a role in the diagnosis of acute dissection in patients with Marfan syndrome; the capabilities and experience of the medical center and the stability of the patient are important determinants of the approach. Because many acute dissections of the ascending aorta in patients with Marfan syndrome have a stuttering course that culminates in death due to rupture or hemopericardium, rapid transfer to a facility prepared to perform immediate repair is essential.

Not all acute dissections in patients with Marfan syndrome involve severe, tearing chest pain that radiates to the back; indeed, some extensive dissections have been occult. This experience reinforces the need for a high index of suspicion by physicians whenever a tall, nearsighted young person with a thoracic cage deformity arrives at an emergency department with vague complaints of lightheadedness, chest or abdominal discomfort, or a murmur of aortic regurgitation. Similarly, patients known to have Marfan syndrome and their close relatives need education about the signs and symptoms of aortic dissection. In general, the management of acute and chronic dissection in patients with Marfan syndrome follows standard practice, with several departures. First, all dissections of the ascending aorta should be repaired promptly, preferably with a composite graft. Second, regular evaluation with magnetic resonance imaging is important, as the diameter of any region of dissected aorta is likely to expand over time. Third, reduction of systolic blood pressure and administration of negative-inotropic doses of beta-adrenergic blockers should be even more strictly adhered to than in dissections without a connective tissue abnormality. In most instances, any region of the aorta should be repaired when complications of further dissection, branch vessel occlusion, or dilation beyond about 50 mm occur. A staged approach to total replacement of the Marfan aorta is now both feasible and successful.

DYSRHYTHMIAS. Some patients develop serious ventricular or supraventricular dysrhythmia.[152] The latter often accompanies chronic mitral regurgitation, but the former may be of high grade and difficult to suppress when only MVP is present. Some patients have the syndrome of autonomic dysfunction, atypical chest pain, and palpitations seen in some patients with MVP unassociated with a flagrant connective tissue abnormality.

VENTRICULAR FUNCTION. Occasional patients with Marfan syndrome who have no clinically important valvular abnormalities develop moderate-to-severe left ventricular dysfunction. While this could represent the unlikely coincidence of Marfan syndrome and idiopathic dilated cardiomyopathy, we have speculated that certain fibrillin mutations could have a detrimental effect on myocardial function.[151] Evidence for and against this hypothesis has recently been produced.[158,159] Further study appears warranted.

MANAGEMENT. Routine cardiological management of Marfan syndrome is multifaceted: regular clinical and echocardiographic examinations; routine endocarditis prophylaxis for dental and other procedures; restriction of activity from heavy weightlifting, contact sports, and any exertion at maximal capacity; and long-term beta-adrenergic blocking agent therapy form the basic approach, with individual variation often appropriate. Support for the role of beta-adrenergic antagonists comes from several prospective studies that show a reduction in the rate of aortic dilation and the risk of aortic dissection in patients treated with negatively inotropic doses of propranolol or atenolol.[160] However, short-term administration of propranolol to patients with large sinus of Valsalva aneurysms, although reducing heart rate and peak systolic pressure, did not improve the impedance characteristics recorded in the ascending aorta. However, given studies that emphasize the importance of central pulse pressure to aortic dilation,[161] use of beta-adrenergic blocking agents seems warranted.

A woman with Marfan syndrome has two concerns about pregnancy (see Chap. 74). The first is the 50:50 risk that any child will inherit the condition; prenatal diagnosis can currently be attempted in selected situations. The second is the risk of dissection that the hemodynamic stresses of pregnancy place on the aorta. Several dozen case reports attest to the heightened incidence of dissection during the third trimester, parturition, and the first month postpartum. However, serious aortic dilation was present in the majority of instances. Prospective evaluation of 21 women through 45 pregnancies confirmed our earlier recommendation that the cardiovascular risks are relatively low if the aortic diameter does not exceed 40 mm and cardiac function is not compromised, a view shared by other investigators.[162]

ETIOLOGY. Marfan syndrome is caused by mutations in the gene that encodes fibrillin-1 (*FBN1*), the major constituent of microfibrils, which are components of the extracellular matrix that are widely dispersed and perform numerous functions.[151] Microfibrils and tropoelastin form elastic fibers. Fragmentation and disorganization of elastic fibers in the aortic media have long been a histological marker (inappropriately called *cystic medial necrosis*) of Marfan syndrome, although similar microscopic pathological lesions occur in familial aortic aneurysms and aging aortas of the normal population. A defect in microfibrils explains all of the pleiotropic manifestations of Marfan syndrome.

Several hundred distinct mutations in *FBN1*, the gene that encodes fibrillin-1, occur in different families, and only a few have emerged, by chance, in unrelated patients.[163,164] Because *FBN1* is such a large gene (approximately 9000 nucleotides in the mRNA, dispersed in 65 exons over 240kb of chromosome 15q21.1), finding a mutation is still not a simple matter.[165,166] Once the mutation is identified, diagnosis in that family is straightforward. In families with several alive and cooperative affected members, linkage analysis can be used for presymptomatic and prenatal diagnosis. The use of molecular testing is confounded, however, by the discovery that autosomal dominant ectopia lentis, familial tall stature, MASS phenotype, and familial aortic aneurysm all are phenotypes caused by mutations in *FBN1* and are exactly the conditions clinicians are interested in excluding in their patients of questionable diagnosis.[163]

Mutations in *FBN1* have distinct effects on microfibril formation: some affect synthesis, others secretion, and yet others incorporation of fibrillin-1 monomers into the extracellular matrix. Studies in mice deficient in fibrillin-1 suggest that microfibrils have an important role in embryological development through interaction with transforming growth factor-beta (TGF-β). Mutations in fibrillin may result in inappropriate or excessive activation of TGF-β signaling.[167]

MITRAL VALVE PROLAPSE AND THE MASS PHENOTYPE. This heterogeneous group of conditions, described earlier, likely contains large numbers of patients and families who have a defect of the extracellular matrix underlying the phenotypes. Some, but not all, have mutations in *FBN1*.[151,163]

Ehlers-Danlos Syndrome

Ehlers-Danlos syndrome is a group of heterogeneous conditions linked by variable involvement of the skin and the joints, with hyperelasticity and fragility of the former occurring with hypermobility of the latter (Fig. 70-9).[168] Mitral valve prolapse is clearly increased in frequency in most of the clinical types, but the occurrence of aortic root dilation is controversial. A recent study found that 25 to 30 percent of patients with the classic and hypermobile forms of Ehlers-Danlos syndrome had mild dilation of the aortic root,[169] a finding counter to what a previous survey had shown.[170]

The most serious cardiovascular problems occur in patients with the vascular form of Ehlers-Danlos syndrome with spontaneous rupture of large- and medium-caliber arteries.[171] Various defects of type III collagen caused the phenotype in virtually all patients studied.[172] Analysis of collagen production by cultured skin fibroblasts should be used to confirm the diagnosis.[18] True aneurysms form rarely; rather, a rupture without dissection usually occurs as a catastrophic event. Most prone are the abdominal aorta and its branches, the great vessels of the aortic arch, and the large arteries of the limbs. False aneurysms and fistulas may be one result in those patients who do not die of the initial rupture. Vascular surgery is difficult, as the normal-appearing vessels around the rent fail to hold sutures. As a consequence, elective surgery to repair vascular anomalies, such as false aneurysms, that are causing no immediate problem is contraindicated in most cases. The vascular form of Ehlers-Danlos syndrome is often sporadic but, when familial, is usually autosomal dominant.[173] Prenatal diagnosis is possible by examining collagen production in amniocytes. However, pregnancy is particularly hazardous to women with this condition because of vascular rupture, although some mutations may not be as dangerous.[172,174]

Pseudoxanthoma Elasticum

Pseudoxanthoma elasticum (PXE) is a clinically variable and genetically heterogeneous disorder caused by mutations in the gene *ABCC6*, which encodes a membrane protein of unclear function. Histopathological examination of affected tissues shows fragmentation and calcification of elastic fibers. The skin, eyes, gastrointestinal system, and cardiovascular system are the organs most severely affected.[175] The skin shows highly characteristic raised yellowish papules (pseudoxanthoma) overlying areas of flexural stress, such as the neck, cubital and popliteal fossae, and groin (Fig. 70-10). Breaks in the elastic lamella, Bruch membrane of the choroid, produce the fundoscopic finding of angioid streaks. Gastrointestinal hemorrhage is common and potentially fatal; mucosal arterioles bleed, and because the calcified elastic fibers prevent effective vessel retraction, hemostasis is difficult. Selective arterial embolization was life saving in one instance. The heart is affected in a number of ways. Endocardial fibroelastosis is common, but because primarily the atria are involved, a restrictive cardiomyopathy is uncommon. One patient with marked endocardial fibroelastosis was helped by resection of calcified elastic bands within the left ventricle. Mitral valve prolapse may be increased in frequency but is rarely a clinical problem. Coronary artery disease with myocardial ischemia and infarction is a common cause of early death.

Elastic and muscular arteries, including the coronaries, develop a type of arteriosclerosis similar to Mönckeberg; progressive luminal narrowing occurs and can produce complete occlusion. This is initially most evident at the radial and ulnar arteries, where absence of pulses and a positive Allen test result are noted early in the course. Interestingly, carotid-femoral pulse wave velocity was not increased in patients with PXE, and radial artery stiffness was reduced in female patients.[176] Because narrowing progresses slowly, collateral arteries form, and peripheral ischemia is a late complication. Because the arterial stenoses tend to be

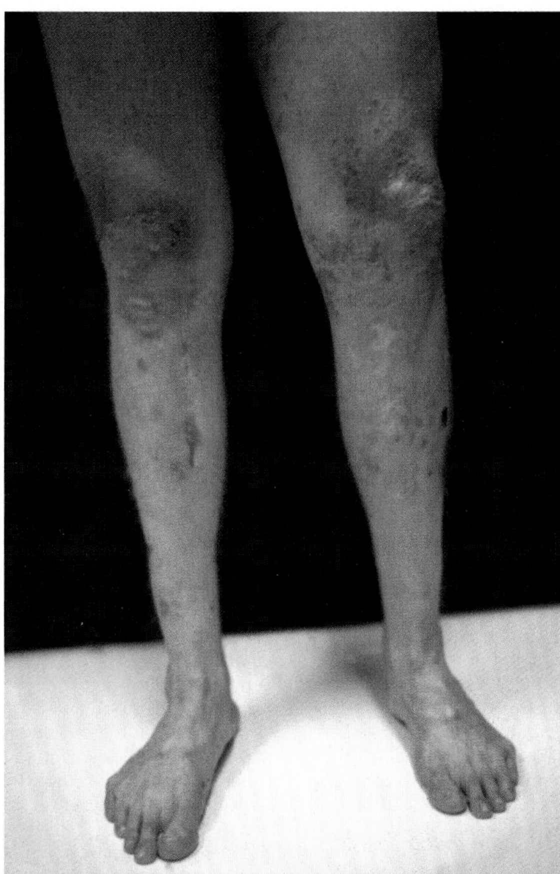

FIGURE 70–9 Legs of a patient with Ehlers-Danlos syndrome type IV who died of rupture of the subclavian artery. Note the mild joint hypermobility and the striking dermal abnormalities—elastosis perforans serpiginosa and thin, atrophic scars over areas of recurrent trauma.

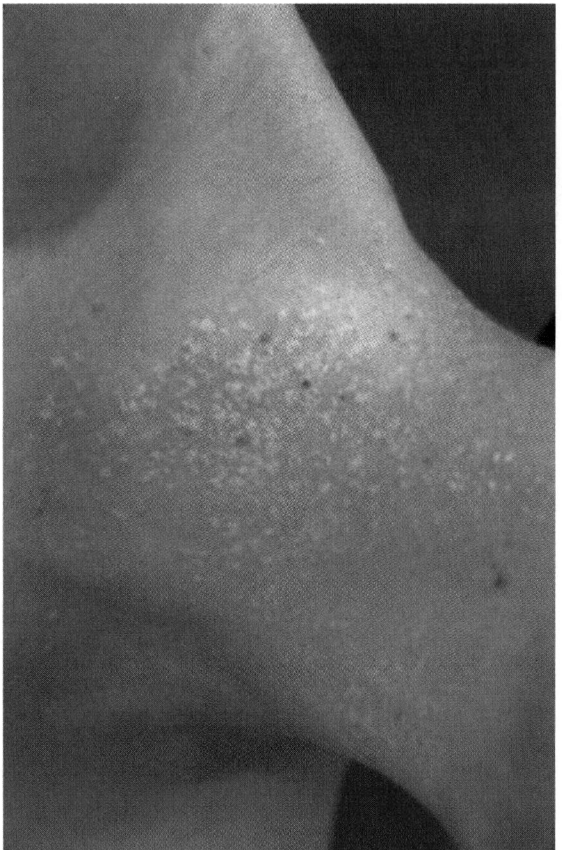

FIGURE 70–10 Skin of a young man with pseudoxanthoma elasticum. The neck is a typical location to notice the raised, yellowish papules from which the name of the condition derives.

diffuse, bypassing them often involves extensive surgery. Hypertension and all risk factors for atherosclerosis should be aggressively controlled.

Genetic Susceptibility to Acquired Disorders of Connective Tissue

Genetic factors are clearly implicated in the susceptibility to many of the rheumatic disorders and to specific complications of specific conditions. The cardiovascular manifestations of these disorders are particularly interesting in this regard. For example, study of HLA-DR antigen frequencies suggests that immune-response factors are involved in the pathogenesis of chronic rheumatic heart disease in black patients.

Inborn Errors of Metabolism that Affect the Cardiovascular System

Hundreds of biochemical defects that affect human metabolism have direct or secondary impact on the cardiovascular system (see Table 70–12).[177] Several examples are reviewed, selected for their relevance to clinical practice or their instructive lessons about pathophysiology.

Aminoacidopathies

Inborn errors of amino acid metabolism result in the accumulation of precursors and a deficit of end products, either or both of which can be detrimental.

ALKAPTONURIA. An intermediate of tyrosine catabolism polymerizes to homogentisic acid, which readily accumulates in the extracellular matrix.[178] Over many years, connective tissue of cartilage, heart valves, and arteries becomes increasingly abnormal. Aortic stenosis and arteriosclerosis are the cardiological sequelae.

HOMOCYSTINURIA. This condition is caused by a deficiency of cystathionine beta-synthase; the pathogenesis of the pleiotropic manifestations is largely unknown.[17,179,180] Perhaps the amino acid sulfhydryl groups bind to collagen, fibrillin, and other macromolecules and interfere with cross-linking. The clinical features, once confused with Marfan syndrome, include tall stature, skeletal deformity, ectopia lentis, mental retardation, psychiatric disturbances, and a predilection for venous and arterial thromboses. Those patients with mutations that render the enzyme activity able to be increased by pharmacological doses of pyridoxine are less severely affected; early treatment can prevent most aspects of the phenotype.[181] Patients unresponsive to pyridoxine can be helped by a low-protein diet to reduce intake of methionine and by oral betaine, a cofactor essential for remethylation of homocysteine.

Myocardial infarction, pulmonary embolism, and stroke are the most common causes of death. The pathogenesis of the vascular complications was once thought to involve abnormal platelet function, but platelet survival in untreated patients is normal. Growing evidence supports a susceptibility of heterozygotes, who have none of the external phenotype of the disease, to atherosclerosis.[182] Various actions of homocysteine on endothelial receptors, stimulation of smooth muscle growth, and production of extracellular matrix components are being explored for clinical relevance.[183] Current therapeutic approaches are focused on maintaining physiological levels of the cofactors involved in metabolism of sulfurated amino acids, folate and vitamins B_6 and B_{12}.

Disorders of Fatty Acid Metabolism

Although most organs can metabolize fatty acids when faced with hypoglycemia, only the heart depends on fatty acids as the primary source of energy generation. Thus, it is not surprising that virtually all genetic defects in fatty acid metabolism, including generalized defects in mitochondria and peroxisomes, are associated with myocardial dysfunction.[184] Other substrates—glucose, lactate, and oxaloacetate—also generate energy in myocardial cells by entry into mitochondria and the tricarboxylic acid (Krebs) cycle. Thus, defects in conversion of pyruvate to acetyl coenzyme A and in any point along the tricarboxylic acid cycle and the respiratory chain have a major impact on myocardial energy generation. Quite likely, some sporadic and familial instances of idiopathic cardiomyopathy represent undiagnosed or undefined metabolic disorders.

CARNITINE DEFICIENCIES. Carnitine is a required cofactor for entry of long-chain fatty acids into mitochondria and is both synthesized endogenously and available from dietary sources.[185] Deficiency of carnitine effectively blocks metabolism of long-chain fatty acids throughout the body and hepatic metabolism of ketones. Because of their relative dependence on fatty acids, muscle cells, including myocytes, suffer out of proportion to other tissue when carnitine levels are low for any reason. Cytoplasmic inclusions of lipid are characteristic findings in myocytes and hepatocytes.

Several Mendelian defects produce primary or secondary carnitine deficiency. An autosomal recessive defect in carnitine palmitoyltransferase I leads to increased plasma carnitine and a skeletal muscle myopathy with little effect on the heart.[185] So-called systemic carnitine deficiency can have various causes: primary deficiency of intake, synthesis, or function, and secondary deficiency, the majority now known to be a result of defects in fatty acid metabolism. The latter group of conditions usually does not respond to pharmacological doses of carnitine.[185]

Primary carnitine deficiency usually manifests in infancy with hypoglycemia, coma, and congestive heart failure due to dilated cardiomyopathy. In the few cases reported, problems largely resolve with carnitine treatment; they can be prevented from recurring by oral supplementation with L-carnitine. Primary systemic carnitine deficiency is due to a defect in carnitine transport, which leads to excessive urinary loss and affects muscle but not liver.[186] Thus, muscle cells still may be relatively deficient in carnitine, despite supplementation, and long-term prognosis is uncertain.

DEFECTS OF BETA-OXIDATION. At least 20 steps are involved when a molecule of free fatty acid leaves the plasma, enters beta-oxidation in the mitochondrion, and generates electrons and acetyl-CoA[185] At each turn of the oxidation spiral, two carbons are removed from the fatty acid, and the enzymes involved in this step are specific for substrates of only certain chain length: long-chain, medium-chain, and short-chain acetyl-CoA dehydrogenases, or LCAD, MCAD, and SCAD. Thus far, patients with defects in nine of the steps have been characterized.

Patients homozygous for these generally autosomal recessive disorders develop episodic hypoketotic hypoglycemia, usually associated with fasting or intercurrent illness. Deficiency of MCAD is the most common cause and occurs in about 1 of every 7000 newborns in the United States. Hypoglycemic crises can rapidly progress to coma and death, and 50 to 60 percent of affected infants die in the first 2 years of life.[186] Because infants between episodes or before a fatal crisis appear normal, MCAD deficiency accounts for a proportion of so-called sudden infant deaths.[180] Histopathological examination shows microvesicular accumulation of fat in cardiac and skeletal muscle. One mutation in MCAD (A985G) accounts for a large percentage of all alleles that predispose to this lethal disorder, and various approaches to newborn screening are being investigated.

MITOCHONDRIAL MYOPATHIES. All of the enzymes of fatty acid oxidation are encoded by genes located on nuclear chromosomes, but the components of the electron transport chain are encoded by both nuclear and mitochondrial genes. Several syndromes involving various types of myopathies have been shown to be due to mutations in the mitochondrial chromosome.[16] The *Kearns-Sayre* syndrome includes pigmentary degeneration of the retina, ophthalmoplegia, and cardiomyopathy as its most prominent manifestations; all of the affected tissues rely nearly exclusively on oxidative phosphorylation for energy generation.

The MELAS syndrome (*m*yopathy, *e*ncephalopathy, *l*actic *a*cidosis, and *s*troke-like episodes) is due to mutations in mitochondrial transfer RNA genes. In addition to the features that define the acronym, hypertrophic cardiomyopathy and diffuse coronary angiopathy are common. Various other mtDNA mutations are associated with hypertrophic or dilated cardiomyopathy.[131]

Variations in both the actual mutations and the fraction of abnormal mitochondria in the cells of the different organs (heteroplasmy) account for many of the clinical differences in phenotype, severity, and age of onset among patients with this disorder. Inheritance is maternal for patients with mitochondrial mutations; apparent autosomal recessive and dominant inheritance may indicate that mutations of nuclear genes can impair electron transport similarly to mitochondrial mutations. Some patients have been treated with moderate success over the short term with coenzyme Q and with cardiac transplantation in one case.

Glycogenoses

Several of the glycogen storage disorders affect cardiac muscle.

GLYCOGEN STORAGE DISEASE II. This autosomal recessive condition is due to deficiency of the lysosomal enzyme α-1,4-glucosidase and results in the lysosomal accumulation of glycogen in most tissues. Several allelic variants occur.[187] The condition with infantile onset is called *Pompe disease,* and cardiac involvement is profound.[185] Infants with Pompe disease appear well initially but soon fail to thrive and develop hypotonia, tachypnea, and tachycardia; the disease progresses during the first year to irreversible congestive heart failure and death due to pneumonia or cardiopulmonary failure. Auscultation typically reveals no murmurs until late in the course when obstruction develops, and hypoglycemia does not appear because the nonlysosomal pathway of glycogen catabolism is intact. The diagnosis is suggested by massive cardiomegaly on examination and chest radiography and by characteristic echocardiographic abnormalities of a short PR interval and markedly increased QRS voltage. Echocardiography shows tremendously thickened (pseudohypertrophic) ventricles, and Doppler interrogation or catheterization may reveal subaortic and subpulmonic pressure gradients characteristic of obstructive cardiomyopathy.

Reduced diastolic function of a restrictive cardiomyopathy develops eventually, and endocardial fibroelastosis is common. With these findings, the diagnosis of Pompe disease is virtually certain, but it can be confirmed by analysis of α-1,4-glucosidase activity in cultured fibroblasts. Prenatal diagnosis is possible by enzymatic assay of amniocytes. Treatment is supportive, but cardiac transplantation could correct the cardiac problem; unfortunately, involvement of other organs, including the lungs, liver, and skeletal muscle, might eventually prove just as serious as the cardiomyopathy. Bone marrow transplantation might be a solution if performed early in the course. An animal model of α-1,4-glucosidase deficiency exists in cattle and develops cardiac pathology typical of human Pompe disease.

Cardiomyopathy may develop in the juvenile-onset form of α-1,4-glucosidase deficiency, but it is not invariable because of allelic heterogeneity. In one sibship without cardiac involvement, three brothers had extensive hepatic, skeletal muscle, and arterial smooth muscle accumulation of glycogen, and each died of rupture of a basilar artery aneurysm. The adult-onset form usually presents with insidious onset of respiratory insufficiency, and clinically important cardiac disease is rare.

GLYCOGEN STORAGE DISEASE III. The striking clinical variability in phenotype associated with deficiency of α-1,4-glucosidase is due in large part to the extensive array of mutations that occur at the *GAA* locus. This autosomal recessive deficiency of amylo-1,6-glucosidase results in infantile- and juvenile-onset syndromes of muscle weakness, wasting, and hepatomegaly. Clinical cardiac disease is not common, although both cytoplasmic (nonlysosomal) and intermyofibril glycogen is routinely present in the heart and causes pseudohypertrophy and increased voltage on electrocardiography. The diagnosis has been established by enzymatic assay of an endomyocardial biopsy specimen.

GLYCOGEN STORAGE DISEASE IV. This is caused by deficiency of α-1,4-glucan: α-1,4-glucan 6-glycosyl transferase. It usually causes a fatal disorder of early childhood characterized by hepatic failure; although extensive deposition of polysaccharide occurs in the heart, death intervenes before cardiac symptoms appear. In the most severe form, the fetus has hydrops and generalized muscle degeneration.[188] As with all of the glycogen storage diseases, extensive allelic heterogeneity results in milder forms of the classic disorders. Patients with diagnosis later in adolescence tend to have more severe cardiomyopathy. Liver transplantation has been life saving in some cases and has, somewhat surprisingly, resulted in a reduction of glycogen deposits in the heart and skeletal muscles.

AMP-ACTIVATED PROTEIN KINASE DEFICIENCY. Mutations in the gene *PRKAG2*, which encodes the γ-2 regulatory subunit of the enzyme that controls the uptake of glucose by various cells, are associated with potentially severe cardiovascular manifestations.[189] Cardiac hypertrophy is an inconstant finding, but conduction defects and dysrhythmia, especially preexcitation, are common. Myocardial histopathology shows accumulation of glycogen in myocyte vacuoles and interstitial fibrosis.

CARDIAC PHOSPHORYLASE KINASE DEFICIENCY. Few cases of this enzyme deficiency have been reported: deposition of glycogen is confined to the heart, which may be massively thickened and enlarged, and leads to early death.

GLYCOPROTEINOSES. This group of disorders results in the lysosomal accumulation of various compounds that cannot be catabolized further because of the specific enzyme deficiency (see Table 70–12). Some have prominent cardiac pathological findings, generally of pseudohypertrophy and valvular thickening, which manifest with congestive failure, valvular dysfunction, conduction defects, or dysrhythmia.[190]

Hematological Disorders

HEMOCHROMATOSIS. This autosomal recessive disorder of unknown cause results in iron deposition in many tissues, including the myocardium. The manifestations include diabetes mellitus, skin hyperpigmentation, hypogonadism, hepatic failure with cirrhosis, hepatoma, and congestive heart failure; severity is less and age of onset later in women due to the autophlebotomy provided by menstruation.[191] The cause of the most common form of hereditary hemochromatosis is a gene, *HFE,* closely linked to the major histocompatibility locus on chromosome 6. One specific mutation accounts for a large proportion of the mutant alleles among white patients.[192] Fully 10 percent of the population is heterozygous for a hemochromatosis mutation. On the one hand, this allele prevalence might suggest that, at an incidence of 2 to 3 per 1000, hemochromatosis is underdiagnosed. On the other hand, a large population survey suggests that homozygosity for the mutation has markedly reduced penetrance.[193] The allele frequency has given rise to interest in population screening by molecular genetic techniques, but for now traditional clinical laboratory approaches are appropriate.[194] Diagnosis depends on finding increased serum iron, ferritin, and, especially, transferrin saturation in the absence of any obvious cause of excessive iron intake.

Cardiac involvement often appears first as dysrhythmia or congestive heart failure. Dysrhythmia, conduction abnormalities, and low QRS voltage are typical electrocardiographic findings; cardiomegaly is seen on chest radiography, and a dilated cardiomyopathy with reduced systolic function can be documented on echocardiography. Occasional patients have a restrictive pattern on cardiac catheterization. Treatment by repeated phlebotomy is most effective if begun before organ damage is irreversible. If a patient with congestive heart failure has not yet developed serious compromise in other organs, cardiac transplantation can be contemplated, as can combined heart-liver replacement.

HEMOGLOBINOPATHIES. Sickle cell disease and other hemoglobinopathies associated with sickling can produce ischemia and infarction in numerous organs by occlusion of small vessels; however, the heart is relatively resistant.[195] Nonetheless, the combination of chronic hypoxemia and anemia produces a sustained high-output state that leads to congestive heart failure in many adults. The cardiovascular system can also be compromised by systemic hypertension due to renal infarction, pulmonary embolism and infarction (the chest pain of which often causes concern about myocardial ischemia), pulmonary hypertension, stroke, and hemosiderosis from chronic transfusions.

In addition to a hyperdynamic congestive failure, iron overload is the principal risk to the myocardium in cases of decreased erythrocyte production of other causes (thalassemias) and increased erythrocyte consumption (hemolytic anemias) requiring repeated transfusions. Treatment with daily injections of deferoxamine can, if begun early, prevent the development of severe cardiac and hepatic disease. Development of an oral iron chelator would greatly improve compliance and efficacy. In patients with beta-thalassemia, heart failure can occur from an autoimmune mechanism, the risks for which depend on the patient's immunogenetic profile.[196] Various approaches to management of sickle cell disease, including hydroxyurea, show promise.[197] Combined heart-liver transplantation has been used in a case of end-stage organ failure with homozygous beta-thalassemia. Both sickle cell disease and thalassemias are associated with diffuse defects in elastic tissue, manifest in the skin and arteries, among other organs.[198,199]

Mucopolysaccharidoses and Disorders of Targeting Lysosomal Enzymes

Many of the specific disorders included in the groupings *mucopolysaccharidoses* and *disorders of targeting lysosomal enzymes* share phenotypic manifestations and are caused by various defects in the ability of lysosomes to catabolize proteoglycan and glycosaminoglycan. Short stature, progressive coarsening of facial features, a skeletal dysplasia termed *dysostosis multiplex*, corneal clouding, and protean effects on the cardiovascular system are common (Fig. 70–11).[200] Only MPS IS (Scheie syndrome), the mild form of MPS IH (mild Hunter syndrome), MPS IV (Morquio syndrome), and MPS VI (Maroteaux-Lamy syndrome) carry minimal or no mental impairment.

CARDIOVASCULAR MANIFESTATIONS. The cardiovascular complications of these disorders (see Table 70–12), which are all progressive and usually insidious, arise from engorgement of cells and tissues with macromolecular storage material. First, the ventricular walls become pseudohypertrophic, and systolic function gradually deteriorates. The electrocardiogram shows reduced QRS voltages; rarely is any conduction disturbance present. Second, coronary arteries narrow because of intimal and medial thickening. Myocardial infarction is common in MPS IH and the severe form of MPS II, although the patients are usually too impaired mentally to report classic symptoms, and the diagnosis is made postmortem. Third, valve leaflets thicken and cause progressive dysfunction oddly specific for individual disorders. For example, aortic stenosis is common in patients with MPS IS, and mitral regurgitation is frequently found in patients with MPS IH and MPS IV. Finally, narrowing of the upper and middle airways causes obstructive apnea, chronic hypoxemia and hypercarbia, pulmonary hypertension, and eventually cor pulmonale.[201]

MANAGEMENT. Treatment of children with those conditions that cause mental retardation has in the past been supportive. Increasing experience with bone marrow transplantation in many of the conditions shows that in the survivors of the transplant, somatic accumulation of mucopolysaccharide can be reduced, with clinical improvement in cardiopulmonary function.[200] However, improvement of central nervous system function has been marginal or absent. Nonetheless, bone marrow transplantation may have a role, especially in cases of MPS IV and MPS VI, in which cardiopulmonary compromise can greatly shorten otherwise productive lives. Attempts at cardiovascular surgery, indeed of any procedure requiring general anesthesia, are fraught with risks of difficult intubation, hyperextension of the neck with cervical cord damage (the odontoid process is often hypoplastic), and prolonged efforts to wean from mechanical ventilation.[201] Enzyme replacement therapy is being developed for most of the MPS disorders and received Food and Drug Administration (FDA) approval for MPS I in 1993. However, the enzyme does not cross the blood-brain barrier, and therapy is indicated only for the somatic manifestations.[202]

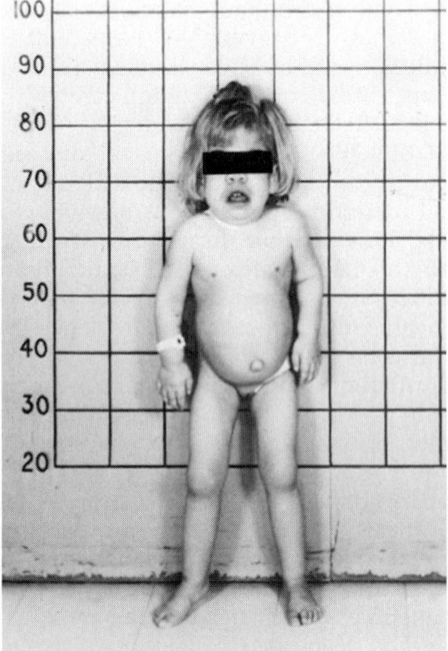

FIGURE 70–11 Hurler syndrome in a 4-year-old girl. Note the short stature and coarse facial features.

Sphingolipidoses

FABRY DISEASE. This X-linked condition deserves comment because the diagnosis is often not made until adulthood, when serious end-organ damage has occurred.[203,204] As a result of deficiency of alpha-galactosidase A, ceramide trihexoside and other glycosphingolipids accumulate in lysosomes of many cells and organs, especially endothelial cells, glomerular and tubular cells of the kidneys, and the heart. Microangiopathy causes the characteristic skin lesion, angiokeratoma, and may contribute, along with primary nerve involvement, to acroparesthesias and painful crises. Proteinuria and hypertension precede renal failure, which often has led to death in male subjects and often requires long-term dialysis or renal transplantation by the fourth decade. A successful kidney allograft does not correct the systemic metabolic defect, and the disease usually progresses in other organs. Infusion of purified human α-galactosidase A, which received FDA approval in 2003, reduces tissue storage of glycosphingolipid.[205,206]

CARDIAC MANIFESTATIONS. Structural and functional cardiac involvement is qualitatively similar to that in the mucopolysaccharidoses. Thickening of the myocardium is pseudohypertrophy due to deposition of glycosphingolipid in lysosomes; the diagnosis has been made by endocardial biopsy during the evaluation of unexplained ventricular hypertrophy or frank obstructive cardiomyopathy. Chronic hypertension can exaggerate left ventricular dysfunction, as can ischemia and infarction due to diffuse luminal narrowing of the coronary arteries. Echocardiography is useful for serial documentation of myocardial function. Although valvular thickening and MVP are common, hemodynamically important mitral regurgitation is not. The pulmonary vasculature becomes narrowed and right-sided pressures rise, but cor pulmonale is rarely a problem. The electrocardiogram often shows a shortened PR interval, increased left ventricular voltages, and dysrhythmia. Medium-sized arteries throughout the body develop luminal narrowing, with cerebrovascular disease the most common cause of death after renal failure.

Heterozygous females generally show some clinical manifestations, especially in the eyes, and at much later ages than hemizygous males develop renal, cerebrovascular, and cardiac disease.[204] Prenatal diagnosis is possible, and a detailed family history and genetic counseling are essential whenever the disease is found. Various mutations occur in the gene for alpha-galactosidase A and account for much of the clinical variability.

Familial Amyloidoses (see Chap. 59)

Various disorders, defined initially by clinical phenotype and due to progressive accumulation of amyloid in organs and tissues, are beginning to be categorized by the underlying biochemical and genetic defects.[207] The several conditions termed *familial amyloidosis with polyneuropathy* and originally classified as separate autosomal dominant disorders are now known to be due to different mutations in the same gene encoding transthyretin, a thyroxine- and retinol-binding protein also called *prealbumin*. Amyloidosis that occurs in the absence of a positive family history is often the first diagnosable case of familial amyloidosis.[208] Although polyneuropathy dominates the early course during young adulthood, renal failure and restrictive cardiomyopathy supervene later and cause death in most cases. Pulmonary hypertension can be a late complication.[209] The age of onset, severity, and predilection for kidney and cardiac involvement are determined by the type of mutation, with male subjects affected earlier and more severely. Autonomic dysfunction is common, reflected in reduced heart rate variability.[210]

Liver transplantation can prevent progression of the disease and potentially reverse some tissue accumulation but may not prevent progression of cardiomyopathy.[211] When the myocardium is severely infiltrated, combined liver-heart transplant offers the only hope.

Neuromuscular Disorders

See Chapter 85.

Cardiac Tumors (see Chap. 63)

The three most common tumors that originate in the heart are myxomas, fibromas, and rhabdomyomas. All occur as part of hereditary syndromes and as sporadic events. The new occurrence of any of these tumors, especially in a child, may represent the first manifestation of a systemic condition, so a detailed general examination and family history are always indicated.[212,213] For example, 51 to 86 percent of cardiac rhabdomyomas occur because of tuberous sclerosis.[214] Tumors due to hereditary disorders tend to be multiple and to recur after resection. An example is the NAME syndrome (for *n*evi, *a*trial myxoma, *m*yxoid neurofibromata, and *e*phelides; the acronym ignores the numerous endocrine tumors), also called *Carney complex*, in which many myxomas can occur throughout the myocardium.[215-217]

Inherited Disorders of the Circulation

Hereditary Hemorrhagic Telangiectasia

Hereditary hemorrhagic telangiectasia (HHT), an autosomal dominant condition often called *Osler-Rendu-Weber disease*, is more common than is appreciated. Because of marked intrafamilial and interfamilial variability, the condition can remain undiagnosed in affected patients for years despite mild manifestations.[218,219] Mucocutaneous telangiectases, 0.5 to 3 mm in diameter, occur on the tongue, lips, and fingertips most commonly. Small and moderate-sized arteriovenous fistulas occur in the nose, leading to recurrent epistaxis, in the gastrointestinal system, where they cause recurrent bleeding and occult anemia, and in the lungs, resulting in hypoxemia, hemoptysis, polycythemia, clubbing, paradoxical embolization through the right-to-left shunt, and a hyperdynamic circulation. Less common sites of vascular malformations are the brain,[220] liver, and kidneys. Diffuse ectasia of the coronary arteries was noted in one patient, and hemorrhagic pericarditis with tamponade in another.[221] Bleeding is facilitated, even in the presence of normal platelet function and clotting function, because of the lack of resistance channels in the telangiectatic lesions.

Patients with HHT and their close relatives should be screened for pulmonary arteriovenous malformations (PAVM) with a contrast echocardiogram.[222] Appearance of "bubbles" in the left atrium after 4 to 10 cardiac cycles is virtually pathognomonic of a shunt in the lung. A positive contrast echocardiogram should be followed by spiral computed tomography to document the number, size, and location of PAVMs. A low oxygen saturation should prompt angiography and therapeutic balloon occlusion of the feeding arteries of any sizable malformation to prevent systemic embolization, especially to the brain.[223] In a few patients, epistaxis and gastrointestinal blood loss have been reduced by antifibrinolytic therapy with danazol or aminocaproic acid.[224] Controlled trials of various approaches to chronic management, taking into account clinical and genetic variables, are sorely needed. Whether to screen all patients with HHT for cerebral vascular malformations and, if so, at what age screening should be started are both unclear.[225]

At least three genes are capable of causing HHT, and two have been mapped to 9q33-q34 and to 3p22. The former locus, *ENG*, encodes a TGF-β-binding protein called endoglin, and various mutations segregate with HHT in different families. The other locus, *ALK1*, encodes an activin receptor–like kinase, which is a member of the serine-threonine kinase receptor family, expressed in endothelial cells. This suggests that defects in this gene might affect development or repair of vessels.[226] Not all families link to these two genes, so a third locus is being sought. Thus, by mutation detection or linkage analysis, presymptomatic and prenatal diagnosis are available to a large number of patients with a potentially life-threatening disorder.

von Hippel–Lindau Syndrome

The features of this autosomal dominant condition involve malformations and abnormal growth of small blood vessels. Retinal angioma, hemangioblastoma of the cerebellum, and hemangioma of the spinal cord occur in association with renal cell carcinoma, pancreatic and epididymal cystadenomas, and pheochromocytoma. Secondary hypertension due to renal disease and pheochromocytoma, which is often bilateral, occurs and predisposes to subarachnoid hemorrhage. The cause is a tumor suppressor gene, *VHL*, at 3p26-p25. Patients inherit a germline mutation (and there is great diversity among families in the actual mutations) that is present in all cells. When a somatic mutation in the normal allele occurs in a susceptible cell, such as in the renal parenchyma or adrenal medulla, the cell becomes functionally homozygous for a lack of the gene product, and the cascade toward neoplasia is initiated.[227] How this gene product stimulates or permits angiomatous malformations is unclear.

Disorders Primarily Affecting Arteries

Mendelian disorders are associated with a diverse array of arterial pathological findings, and some were described or catalogued earlier in this chapter. This section deals with two categories of disorders caused by a single mutant gene: pleiotropic syndromes better known for affecting organ systems other than the vasculature, and primary abnormalities of arteries.

ADULT POLYCYSTIC KIDNEY DISEASE. Adult polycystic kidney disease (APKD) is a relatively common autosomal dominant disease that affects 0.5 million people and accounts for 8 to 10 percent of all long-term hemodialysis in the United States. Development of renal cysts is age-dependent, and presymptomatic detection of heterozygotes, even by ultrasonography, can be uncertain into adulthood. About one-half of patients are hypertensive, one-half have hepatic cysts, one-half eventually develop severe renal failure, and an unknown (but probably high) fraction have colonic diverticula. Elevated plasma renin levels contribute to hypertension long before renal failure occurs. The cardiovascular manifestations include MVP in one-quarter, mild dilation of the aortic root, occasional thoracic and abdominal aneurysms, and a predisposition to regurgitation of the aortic, mitral, and tricuspid valves. The association of diverticula, organ cysts, and cardiovascular lesions reminiscent of, but milder than, Marfan syndrome suggests some involvement of the extracellular matrix.

The most serious vascular problem is typical berry aneurysms of the cerebral circulation that occur in about 10 percent of heterozygotes but may remain asymptomatic throughout life. Hypertension predisposes to subarachnoid hemorrhage. How to screen for and treat intracranial aneurysms in patients without neurological symptoms remains controversial. Cerebral angiography carries higher risks in patients with APKD because of dissection and heightened vascular reactivity. Magnetic resonance imaging detects most saccular aneurysms down to 2 to 3 mm in diameter. Whether to attempt prophylactic repair when a small aneurysm is detected has not been investigated systematically. Without question, aggressive blood pressure control is indicated in any patient with APKD.

At least three genes cause APKD. The greatest portion of cases are due to mutations in a gene called *PBP* at the *PKD1* locus (16p13.3).[228] In most of the remaining families, the disease maps to the *PKD2* locus in the region 4q23-q23. Families affected by mutations in *PKD2* tend to develop renal failure later and have a milder course.[229] In both *PKD1* and *PKD2* cases, the multiorgan cysts develop when a somatic mutation occurs in the normal allele at the respective mutant locus, analogous to the two-hit model so familiar with tumorigenesis.[230] A French Canadian family with disease typical of *PKD1* is unlinked to either locus, indicating that a *PKD3* gene exists. Patients with mutations in *PKD1* and *PKD2* show marked intrafamilial variability. Discovering some of the factors that affect this variability could suggest novel approaches to modifying disease progression.[231]

ARTERIOHEPATIC DYSPLASIA. An autosomal dominant disorder of marked variability, *Alagille syndrome* causes neonatal jaundice due to aplasia of intrahepatic bile ducts and congestive heart failure in the most severely affected infants but may be asymptomatic in heterozygous relatives.[58,232] The cardiovascular findings include peripheral pulmonic and systemic arterial stenoses in the majority, occasionally associated with septal defects or PDA.[233-235] A diffuse vasculopathy is present in some patients.[56] Renal disease can produce hypertension. The locus was initially mapped by studying chromosomes and finding in some patients that part or all of band 20p12 was missing (an interstitial deletion). The *Jagged1* gene, which mapped to this exact region, was then identified as the cause.

ARTERIAL ANEURYSM, ECTASIA, OR DISSECTION (see Chap. 53). Pedigrees abound in which dilation of the aortic root, aneurysm of the abdominal aorta, aortic dissection without dilation, or a combination of these problems occurs in an autosomal dominant pattern without evidence of a recognized heritable disorder of connective tissue.[236,237] Because of the variable presentation and natural history of the aortic disease, presymptomatic detection of presumed heterozygotes is uncertain, as is reassurance of relatives at risk who are of childbearing age and would prefer not to pass this condition to offspring.

The association of dissection of the ascending aorta with bicuspid aortic valve and aortic coarctation is well known, although the cause and pathogenesis remain unclear. In such cases, the aortic wall shows abnormalities of elastic fibers. A person with a congenitally bicuspid aortic valve or aortic coarctation should be screened for dilation of the aortic root, and first-degree relatives should be screened for both lesions. This recommendation is based, in part, on the bicuspid aortic valve being a congenital heart defect of the left-sided flow category, with a relatively high recurrence risk.

In two families with autosomal dominant transmission of arterial aneurysms and mildly increased skin fragility and bruisability, different mutations in the gene encoding type III procollagen occurred. Thus, depending on the mutation, deficiency of type III collagen can cause the vascular form of Ehlers-Danlos syndrome or a form of the much subtler but just as deadly syndrome, familial arterial rupture. For these families in which the mutations have been defined, reliable presymptomatic and prenatal diagnoses are at hand. However, suggestions that mutations in type III collagen would account for the majority of aortic aneurysms, including abdominal aneurysms in the elderly, have proved unfounded.

Families with aneurysm, dissection, or both of the thoracic aorta have been studied extensively in the past few years. Linkage to three loci, 3p25-p24.2, 5q13-q14, and 11q23.2-q24, has been reported.[238-240] A predisposition to cervical arterial dissection in young people was found to be associated with diffuse lentiginosis in several families, with a suggestion of autosomal recessive inheritance. An association is also noted between cervical dissection and intracranial hemorrhage, which is increased when congenital cardiovascular defects are present, especially bicuspid aortic valve or aortic coarctation. Formal genetic analysis of 91 families ascertained through a proband with abdominal aortic aneurysm suggests that an autosomal recessive predisposition exists for late-onset aneurysms. This study and others[241] provide a rationale for offering ultrasonographic screening to siblings of patients with abdominal aortic dilation.

FAMILIAL ARTERIAL TORTUOSITY. This is a rare, possibly autosomal recessive condition of unknown cause. Paradoxically, diffuse ectasia of all systemic arteries occurs with peripheral pulmonic stenoses.[242]

FAMILIAL INTRACRANIAL HEMORRHAGE. In addition to APKD, three syndromes predispose to subarachnoid or cerebral hemorrhage. Berry aneurysms without pleiotropic manifestations in other organs are a rare but well-documented autosomal dominant trait. How aggressively near relatives should be screened for intracranial aneurysms remains controversial because of the relatively low risk of hemorrhage compared with the morbidity and mortality of current surgical techniques for repairing defects.[243-245] A defect in type III collagen was suggested by linkage analysis, but sequence analysis of the gene in 55 unrelated patients found no mutations.

The cerebral arterial type of familial amyloidosis (type VI) is an autosomal dominant condition caused by a defect in the proteinase inhibitor cystatin O. This disease is rare outside Iceland and Holland. The walls of cerebral arteries are thickened by a material resembling amyloid, and the vessels become tortuous and fragile. Recurrent cerebral hemorrhage is common in the fifth and sixth decades of life.

Familial hemangiomas have been reported infrequently to occur as an autosomal dominant condition. The brain and retina are the principal sites of vascular malformation, although cutaneous lesions occur in some pedigrees. The intracranial hemangioma can be large and the patient can present with varied neurological symptoms, including hemorrhage. A more benign familial disorder of primarily isolated cutaneous hemangiomas also exists.[246]

FAMILIAL ARTERIAL OCCLUSIVE DISEASES.[247] Fibromuscular dysplasia of the renal and other arteries occurs in cases of von Recklinghausen neurofibromatosis and, along with pheochromocytoma, can be a cause of hypertension. Severe deficiency of alpha 1-antiprotease is another cause of fibromuscular dysplasia. The arterial lesion can occur by itself in families and produce stroke, myocardial infarction, intermittent claudication, and hypertension as early as childhood. Inheritance is most consistent with autosomal dominance.

Familial hypoplasia of the carotid arteries, familial arteriopathy caused by concentric thickening of systemic and pulmonic arteries, familial moyamoya disease (which has been mapped to 3p24.2-p26),[248] and generalized arterial calcification of infancy all are rare, possibly Mendelian, syndromes of unknown cause.

Cerebral autosomal dominant arteriopathy with subcortical infarcts and leukoencephalopathy (CADASIL) is due to mutations in the *NOTCH3* gene.[249] Characteristic inclusions occur in vascular smooth muscle cells, and the deep, perforating cerebral arterioles develop occlusions that produce insidious onset of symptoms and transient ischemic attacks.

FAMILIAL HEMIPLEGIC MIGRAINE. The migraine syndrome is commonly familial and occurs in many generations. A severe form, associated with recurrent hemiplegia, is inherited as an autosomal dominant trait and is due to mutations in a sodium channel gene.[250] However, some families with hemiplegic migraine and others with simple migraine are unlinked to this locus. In the same region of 19p is a locus causing autosomal dominant cerebral arteriopathy with subcortical infarcts. Whether the two conditions are related through allelism is unclear.

FAMILIAL PULMONARY HYPERTENSION (see Chap. 67). Primary pulmonary hypertension (PPH) is occasionally familial. Inheritance is most consistent with an autosomal dominant predisposition with sex influence favoring expression in females.[251,252] Mutations in the *BMPR2* gene at 2q33 cause the disease in many of the families.[253]

Pulmonary hypertension can occur in patients with neurofibromatosis due to pulmonary fibrosis, and in patients with hereditary hemorrhagic telangiectasia caused by mutations in *ALK1*.

Disorders Primarily Affecting Veins

VARICOSE VEINS. Although a familial susceptibility to varicosities of the lower extremities clearly exists and favors women in a ratio of 2 : 1, Mendelian inheritance has not been confirmed. Marfan syndrome, various Ehlers-Danlos syndromes, and an autosomal recessive condition featuring distichiasis (a double row of eyelashes) predispose to varicose veins.

ATRETIC VEINS. Some patients with the Klippel-Trénaunay syndrome of cutaneous hemangioma and hemihypertrophy have atresia of the deep venous system. The concomitant superficial varicosities should not be stripped, lest the remaining venous drainage of the lower extremity be removed. This is a confusing syndrome that overlaps with several others; Mendelian inheritance is uncertain.[254] Renal arterial aneurysm and hemangioma occurred in one patient.

CAVERNOUS ANGIOMAS. Cavernous angiomas represent at least 15 percent of vascular malformations of the central nervous system, and familial occurrence is common. These are not arteriovenous malformations but primarily a tortuous collection of veins. Seizure is the most common presenting feature, followed by headache, stroke, and progressive neurological deficit. Magnetic resonance (T2-weighted) imaging is the procedure of choice because it is sensitive; arteriography is not likely to detect the venous malformation. In some families, hepatic angiomas are an important feature. Three genetic loci have been mapped to 7q, 7p and 3q; the locus on 7q is *KRIT1*, of unclear function.[255-257]

ARTERIOVENOUS MALFORMATIONS. The most common Mendelian causes of arteriovenous malformations (AVMs) are the various forms of hereditary hemorrhagic telangiectasia. However, AVMs, especially of the brain, are relatively common findings,[258] and other genetic susceptibilities exist, such as the Parkes Weber syndrome.[254]

Disorders Primarily Affecting Lymphatics

Several forms of hereditary lymphedema exist,[259,260] with the best studied inherited as autosomal dominant conditions. An early-onset form bears the eponym *Nonne-Milroy lymphedema* and can cause a protein-losing enteropathy and pleural effusion. A form called *Meige lymphedema* does not appear until about the time of puberty and is most severe in the legs, although one family with late-onset edema had involvement of the arms and face. Considerable intrafamilial variability in age of onset is noted, however, and whether two or more distinct conditions exist remains unclear. Mutations in one of the receptors for vascular endothelial growth factor, *VEGFR3*, have been found in some families.[261,262] Lymphedema associated with distichiasis is due to mutations in *FOXC2*, which encodes a transcription factor, and hypotrichosis-lymphedema-telangiectasia syndrome is caused by mutations in another transcription factor gene, *SOX18*.[263]

Genetic Factors Predisposing to Atherosclerosis (see Chaps. 36 and 39)

Various genetic factors, in addition to the well-studied errors of lipid metabolism, clearly predispose to atherosclerosis.[264] A few genes aside from those involved in lipid metabolism have such a prominent impact as to be identifiable from the family history. Two genes recently found to predispose to coronary artery disease are *ABCC6*, the gene that also causes pseudoxanthoma elasticum,[265] and *KLOTHO*, a gene of unclear function.[266] However, genes that predispose to hypertension and diabetes mellitus; control arterial diameter, reactivity, and branching angles; affect platelet adhesiveness, thrombosis, and fibrinolysis; and regulate endothelial and smooth muscle function all can be considered candidate genes for study in families predisposed to atherosclerosis. Screening numerous genes for common mutations and polymorphisms that convey risk information will be increasingly possible.[267-269]

Abnormal Regulation of Blood Pressure (see Chap. 37)

Blood pressure is a quantifiable trait that shows continuous variation within the population. Although many genes and environmental factors undoubtedly affect a person's blood pressure, familial transmission of some arbitrarily defined disease "hypertension" follows neither Mendelian nor multifactorial inheritance.[270,271] Various cybernetic systems operate to maintain the blood pressure within tolerable limits. When this physiological homeostasis goes awry or its limits are too lax, pathological and clinical consequences occur.[272] For example, sensitivity of the baroreflex was impaired in patients who had untreated essential hypertension and a positive family history of hypertension compared with hypertensive patients with no family history and to nonhypertensive control subjects. The complexities of such systems are considerable, and two approaches have been taken in recent years to focus the analysis.[271,272] One involves a candidate-gene approach in humans, based on loci known to be involved in physiological pathways; the second involves naturally occurring and experimentally created strains of animals.

STUDIES OF HUMANS. All the classic approaches to detecting genetic influences in diseases—twin studies, familial aggregation, adoption—confirm that genes have a role, but less than 5 percent of patients with hypertension have a defined genetic cause.[273]

Occasional families show striking Mendelian segregation of hypertension without being associated with one of the identifiable syndromes listed in Table 70–15. One example, in which early, severe hypertension is inherited as an autosomal dominant trait, is Liddle syndrome. Because of hypokalemia, aldosteronism was suspected, but both aldosterone and renin levels were low. Attention then focused on sodium resorption in the distal nephron and its regulation. Mutations discovered in the beta subunit of the epithelial sodium channel render the channel insensitive to the usual regulators.

Another example of successful application of the candidate gene approach is investigation of glucocorticoid-remediable

TABLE 70–15 Mendelian Disorders Associated with Abnormal Blood Pressure

Disorder	OMIM No.*	Pathogenesis
Primarily Elevated Blood Pressure		
Adrenal hyperplasia IV	202010	11-β-hydroxylase deficiency→ ↑ 11-deoxycorticosterone
Adrenal hyperplasia V	202110	17-α-hydroxylase deficiency→ ↑ 11-deoxycorticosterone
Aldosteronism	103900	↑ Aldosterone
Alport syndrome	104200 301050	Renal failure
Amyloidosis, familial visceral (amyloidosis VIII)	105200	Nephropathy
Arterial calcification of infancy	208000	Arteriosclerosis
Arterial fibromuscular dysplasia	135580	Renal artery stenosis→ ↑ renin
Arteriohepatic dysplasia	118450	Renal dysplasia; renal arterial stenosis
Bartter syndrome	241200	Secondary to hyperaldosteronism
Fabry disease	301500	Renal failure; renal arterial stenosis; arteriolar stenosis→ ↑ peripheral resistance
Liddle syndrome	177200	Defective epithelial sodium channel→ ↓ K^+ ↓ aldosterone, ↓ renin, ↓ angiotensin
Multiple endocrine neoplasia I	131100	Adrenocortical adenoma→ ↑ Cushing syndrome
Multiple endocrine neoplasia II	171400	Pheochromocytoma→ ↑ catecholamines
Nail-patella syndrome	161200	Nephropathy
Neurofibromatosis type I	162200	Pheochromocytoma→ ↑ catecholamines; renal arterial fibromuscular dysplasia
Paraganglioma	168000	↑ Catecholamines
Pheochromocytoma, familial	171300	↑ Catecholamines
Polycystic kidney disease, adult	173900, 173910	↑ Renin; renal failure
Porphyria, acute intermittent	176000	?, but only during acute attacks
Pseudohypoaldosteronism, type I	264350	Aldosterone receptor deficiency
Pseudohypoaldosteronism, type II	145260	Defective renal secretion of potassium
Pseudoxanthoma elasticum	177850, 264800	Arteriosclerosis
Riley-Day syndrome	223900	Dysautonomia
von Hippel–Lindau syndrome	193300	Pheochromocytoma→ ↑ catecholamines
Wilms tumor	194070, 194071, 194090	?
Primarily Low Blood Pressure†		
Dopamine β-hydroxylase deficiency	223360	↑ Synthesis of epinephrine
Fabry disease	301500	↓ Peripheral vascular tone
Hyperbradykininism	143850	↑ Bradykinin
Pelizaeus-Merzbacher, late-onset	169500	?
Peripheral motor neuropathy and dysautonomia	252320	?
Pheochromocytoma, familial	171300	↑ Catecholamines (epinephrine)
Shy-Drager syndrome	146500	Primary autonomic insufficiency

*Data from Online Mendelian Inheritance in Man (www.ncbi.nlm.nih.gov/omim).

†Does not include hypovolemia, obstruction of blood flow, and cardiogenic causes of hypotension, each of which subsumes numerous hereditary disorders as primary causes.

aldosteronism. The phenotype was mapped to chromosome 8q21, a region already known to contain two candidate genes, aldosterone synthase and 11β-hydroxylase. By honing in on these loci, mutations creating a chimeric gene by unequal recombination were found to be the cause. As a result of the fusion, aldosterone synthase comes under regulation of adrenocorticotropic hormone. The actual frequency of such mutational events is considerably higher than suspected in the population, and the molecular means are now available to assess the epidemiology of what will likely be a common cause of early hypertension.

Angiotensinogen, the gene for which is in the region 1q42-q43, is a logical candidate gene to investigate because of the central role of its product in blood pressure regulation. Several polymorphic variants involving single amino acid substitutions occur; at positions 174 and 235, either methionine (M) or threonine (T) can exist. The special effects of these polymorphisms on activity, if any, are unclear, but persons homozygous for the 235T allele have plasma angiotensinogen levels 20 percent higher than those with the 235M alleles. Some but not all studies have found an association between the 174M and 235T alleles and hypertension. The importance of these polymorphisms seems to depend on the subject's ethnic background.[274]

The ACE gene, at 17q23, contains a common insertion/deletion polymorphism termed I and D, respectively, that permits both association and linkage studies. The three possible genotypes are DD, ID, and II, and the plasma level of ACE is highest, for unclear reasons, in persons who are DD and lowest in those who are II. The DD genotype has been associated with predisposition to coronary artery disease and myocardial infarction, which may account for a relative decrease of hypertensive patients with the DD genotype at older ages.

Pregnancy is a clear risk factor for hypertension. A susceptibility locus for preeclampsia has been identified.[275,276]

The opposite of hypertension, inappropriate control of pressure on the low side, also has numerous genetic bases (see Table 70–15).[277,278] A number of Mendelian conditions, most of which are rare, cause major deviations of blood pressure from an appropriate physiological range (see Table 70–15). These disorders are likely to be underdiagnosed.

REFERENCES

1. Childs B: Genetic Medicine: A Logic of Disease. Baltimore, Johns Hopkins University Press, 1999.
2. Murphy EA, Pyeritz RE: Pathogenetics. *In* Rimoin DL, Connor JM, Pyeritz RE, Korf BR (eds): Principles and Practice of Medical Genetics. 4th ed. New York, Churchill Livingstone, 2002, pp 439-455.
3. Jouven X, Desnos M, Guerot C, et al: Predicting sudden death in the population. The Paris prospective study I. Circulation 99:1978, 1999.
4. Bates BR, Templeton A, Achter PJ, et al: What does "A gene for heart disease" mean? A focus group study of public understandings of genetic risk factors. Am J Med Genet 119A:156, 2003.
5. Pai GS, Lewandowski RC Jr, Borgaonkar D: Handbook of Chromosomal Syndromes. New York, John Wiley & Sons, 2002.
6. Shaffer LG, Ledbetter DH, Lupski JR: Molecular cytogenetics of contiguous gene syndromes: Mechanisms and consequences of gene dosage imbalance. *In* Scriver CR, Beaudet AL, Sly WA, Valle D (eds): The Metabolic and Molecular Bases of Inherited Disease. 8th ed. New York, McGraw-Hill, 2001, pp 1291-1326.
7. Bayés M, Magano LF, Rivera N, et al: Mutational mechanisms of Williams-Beuren syndrome deletions. Am J Hum Genet 73:131, 2003.
8. The International Human Genome Sequencing Consortium: Initial sequencing and analysis of the human genome. Nature 409:860, 2001.
9. Collins FS, Green ED, Guttmacher AE, et al: A vision for the future of genomics research. Nature 422:835, 2003.
10. Pyeritz RE: Genetic approaches to cardiovascular disease. *In* Chien KR, Breslow JL, Leiden JM, et al (eds): Molecular Basis of Cardiovascular Disease. Philadelphia, WB Saunders, 1999, pp 19-36.
11. Online Mendelian Inheritance in Man. Available at www.ncbi.nlm.nih.gov/omim
12. Epstein JA, Rader DJ, Parmacek MS: Perspective: Cardiovascular disease in the postgenomic era—lessons learned and challenges ahead. Endocrinology 143:2045, 2002.
13. Hirschhorn JN, Lohmueller K, Byrne E, et al: A comprehensive review of genetic association studies. Genet Med 4:45, 2002.
14. Lachmeijer AMA, Arngrímsson R, Bastiaans EJ, et al: A genome-wide scan for preeclampsia in the Netherlands. Eur J Hum Genet 9:758, 2001.
15. Pyeritz RE: Marfan syndrome and related disorders of connective tissue. Annu Rev Med 51:481, 2000.
16. Wallace DC, Lott MT: Mitochondrial genetics. *In* Rimoin DL, Connor JM, Pyeritz RE, Korf BR (eds): Principles and Practice of Medical Genetics. 4th ed. New York, Churchill Livingstone, 2002, pp 299-409.
17. Pyeritz RE: Homocystinuria. *In* Beighton P (ed): McKusick's Heritable Disorders of Connective Tissue. 5th ed. St. Louis, CV Mosby, 1993, p 137.
18. Byers PH: Disorders of collagen biosynthesis and structure. *In* Scriver CR, Beaudet AL, Sly WA, Valle D (eds): The Metabolic and Molecular Bases of Inherited Disease. 8th ed. New York, McGraw-Hill, 2001, pp 5241-5286.
19. Friedlander Y, Lapidos T, Sinnreich R, Kark JD: Genetic and environmental sources of QT interval variability in Israeli families: The kibbutz settlements family study. Clin Genet 56:200, 1999.
20. Ranade K, Jorgenson E, Sheu WH-H, et al: A polymorphism in the β1 adrenergic receptor is associated with resting heart rate. Am J Hum Genet 70:935, 2002.
21. Wang XL, Mahaney MC, Sim AS, et at: Genetic contribution of the endothelial constitutive nitric oxide synthase gene to plasma nitric oxide levels. Arterioscler Thromb Vasc Biol 17:3147, 1997.
22. Rudic RD, Sessa WC: Human Genetics '99: The cardiovascular system: Nitric oxide in endothelial dysfunction and vascular remodeling: Clinical correlates and experimental links. Am J Hum Genet 64:673, 1999.
23. Zannad F, Visvikis S, Gueguen R, et al: Genetics strongly determines the wall thickness of the left and right carotid arteries. Hum Genet 103:183, 1998.

Cardiovascular Disorders Associated with Chromosome Aberrations

24. van Karnebeek CDM, Hennekam RCM: Associations between chromosomal anomalies and congenital heart defects: A database search. Am J Med Genet 84:158, 1999.
25. Freeman SB, Taft LF, Dooley KJ, et al: Population-based study of congenital heart defects in Down syndrome. Am J Med Genet 80:213, 1998.
26. McElhinney DB, Straka M, Goldmuntz E, et al: Correlation between abnormal cardiac physical examination and echocardiographic findings in neonates with Down syndrome. Am J Med Genet 113:238, 2002.
27. Barlow GM, Chen X-N, Shi ZY, et al: Down syndrome congenital heart disease: A narrowed region and a candidate gene. Genet Med 3:91, 2001.
28. Tolmie JL: Down syndrome and other autosomal trisomies. *In* Rimoin DL, Connor JM, Pyeritz RE, Korf BR (eds): Principles and Practice of Medical Genetics. 4th ed. New York, Churchill Livingstone, 2002, pp 1129-1183.
29. Kelly M, Robinson BW, Moore JW: Trisomy 18 in a 20-year-old woman. Am J Med Genet 112:397, 2002.
30. Rasmussen SA, Wong LY, Yang Q, et al: Population-based analyses of mortality in trisomy 13 and trisomy 18. Pediatrics 111:777, 2003.
31. Wax JR, Pinette MG, Blackstone J, et al: Isolated multiple bilateral echogenic papillary muscles: A unique sonographic feature of trisomy 13. Obstet Gynecol 99:902, 2002.
32. Tunca Y, Kadandale JS, Pivnick EK: Long-term survival in Patau syndrome. Clin Dysmorphol 10:149, 2001.
33. Elsheikh M, Casadei B, Conway GS, et al: Hypertension is a major risk factor for aortic root dilatation in women with Turner's syndrome. Clin Endocrinol 54:69, 2001.
34. Lin AE: The heart of Turner syndrome: Small matters. Teratology 66:63, 2002.
35. Gravholt CH: Medical problems of adult Turner's syndrome. Horm Res 56(suppl 1):44, 2001.
36. Sapienza C, Hall JG: Genome imprinting in human disease. *In* Scriver CR, Beaudet AL, Sly WA, Valle D (eds): The Metabolic and Molecular Bases of Inherited Disease. 8th ed. New York, McGraw-Hill, 2001, pp 417-432.
37. Jacobs P, Dalton P, James R, et al: Turner syndrome: A cytogenetic and molecular study. Ann Hum Genet 61:471, 1997.
38. Zinn AR, Tonk VS, Chen Z, et al: Evidence for a Turner syndrome locus or loci at Xp11.2-p22.1. Am J Hum Genet 63:1757, 1998.
39. Frías JL, Davenport ML, et al: Health supervision for children with Turner syndrome. Pediatrics 111:692, 2003.
40. Radetti G, Crepaz R, Milanesi O, et al: Cardiac performance in Turner's syndrome patients on growth hormone therapy. Horm Res 55:240, 2001.

Congenital Heart Disease

41. Ferencz C, Loffredo CA, Correa-Villaseñor A, Wilson P: Genetic and Environmental Risk Factors of Major Cardiovascular Malformations: The Baltimore-Washington Infant Study 1981-1989. Armonk, NY, Futura, 1997.
42. Wong SF, Chan FY, Cincotta RB, et al: Factors influencing the prenatal detection of structural congenital heart diseases. Ultrasound Obstet Gynecol 21:19, 2003.
43. Lin AE, Herring AH, Scharenberg K, et al: Cardiovascular malformations: Changes in prevalence and birth status, 1972-1990. Am J Med Genet 84:102, 1999.
44. Pyeritz RE, Murphy EA: The genetics of congenital heart disease: Perspectives and prospects. J Am Coll Cardiol 13:1458, 1989.
45. Devriendt K, Matthijs G, Dael RV, et al: Delineation of the critical deletion region for congenital heart defects on chromosome 8p23.1. Am J Hum Genet 64:1119, 1999.
46. Clayton-Smith J, Donnai D: Human malformations. *In* Rimoin DL, Connor JM, Pyeritz RE, Korf BR (eds): Principles and Practice of Medical Genetics. 4th ed. New York, Churchill Livingstone, 2002, pp 488-500.
47. Siu SC, Colman JM, Sorensen S, et al: Adverse neonatal and cardiac outcomes are more common in pregnant women with cardiac disease. Circulation 105:2179, 2002.

48. Romano-Zelekha O, Hirsh R, Blieden L, et al: The risk for congenital heart defects in offspring of individuals with congenital heart defects. Clin Genet 59:325, 2001.
49. Anderson NH, Dominiczak AF: Genetic analysis of complex traits. *In* Rimoin DL, Connor JM, Pyeritz RE, Korf BR (eds): Principles and Practice of Medical Genetics. 4th ed. New York, Churchill Livingstone, 2002, pp 410-424.
50. Digilio MC, Marino B, Toscanno A, et al: Atrioventricular canal defect without Down syndrome: A heterogeneous malformation. Am J Med Genet 85:140, 1999.
51. Marino B, Digilio MC: Inlet ventricular septal defect is not a partial atrioventricular septal defect. Am J Med Genet 87:195, 1999.
52. Clark EB: Mechanisms in the pathogenesis of congenital cardiac malformations. *In* Pierpont MEM, Moller JH (eds): Genetics of Cardiovascular Disease. Boston, Martinus Nihjoff, 1986, p 3.
53. Hoess K, Goldmuntz E, Pyeritz RE: Genetic counseling for congenital heart disease: New approaches for a new decade. Curr Cardiol Rep 4:68, 2002.
54. Goldmuntz E, Clark BJ, Mitchell LE, et al: Frequency of 22q11 deletions in patients with conotruncal defects. J Am Coll Cardiol 32:492, 1998.
55. Eldadah ZA, Hamosh A, Biery NJ, et al: Familial tetralogy of Fallot caused by mutation in the jagged-1 gene. Hum Molec Genet 10:163, 2001.
56. McElhinney DB, Krantz ID, Bason L, et al: Analysis of cardiovascular phenotype and genotype-phenotype correlation in individuals with a *JAG1* mutation and/or Alagille syndrome. Circulation 106:2567, 2002.
57. Krantz ID, Smith R, Colliton RP, et al: *Jagged1* mutations in patients ascertained with isolated congenital heart defects. Am J Med Genet 84:56, 1999.
58. Krantz ID: Alagille syndrome: Chipping away at the tip of the iceberg. Am J Med Genet 112:160, 2002.
59. Benson DW, Silberbach GM, Kavanaugh-McHugh A, et al: Mutations in the cardiac transcription factor *NKX2.5* affect diverse cardiac developmental pathways. J Clin Invest 104:1567, 1999.
60. Kasahara H, Lee B, Schott J-J, et al: Loss of function and inhibitory effects of human CSX/NKX2.5 homeoprotein mutations associated with congenital heart disease. J Clin Invest 106:299, 2000.
61. Ewing CK, Loffredo CA, Beaty TH: Paternal risk factors for isolated membranous ventricular septal defects. Am J Med Genet 71:42, 1997.
62. Funke B, Puech A, Saint-Jore B, et al: Isolation and characterization of a human gene containing a nuclear localization signal from the critical region for velo-cardiofacial syndrome on 22q11. Genomics 53:146, 1998.
63. Hokanson JS, Pierpont ME, Hirsch B, et al: 22q11.2 microdeletions in adults with familial tetralogy of Fallot. Genet Med 3:61, 2001.
64. Maeda J, Yamagashi H, Matsuoka R, et al: Frequent association of 22q11.2 deletion with tetralogy of Fallot. Am J Med Genet 92:269, 2000.
65. Goodship J, Cross I, LiLing J, Wren C: A populations study of chromosome 22q11 deletions in infancy. Arch Dis Child 79:348, 1998.
66. Beauchesne LM, Connolly HM, Ammash NM, et al: Coarctation of the aorta: Outcome of pregnancy. J Am Coll Cardiology 38:1728, 2001.
67. Robinson SW, Morris CD, Goldmuntz E, et al: Missense mutations in *CRELD1* are associated with cardiac atrioventricular septal defects. Am J Hum Genet 72:1047, 2003.
68. Kathiriya IS, Srivastava D: Left-right asymmetry and cardiac looping: Implications for cardiac development and congenital heart disease. Am J Med Genet 97:271, 2000.
69. Digilio MC, Casey B, Toscano A, et al: Complete transposition of the great arteries: Patterns of congenital heart disease in familial precurrence. Circulation 104:2809, 2001.
70. Afzelius BA, Mossberg B, Bergström SE: Immotile-cilia syndrome (primary ciliary dyskinesia), including Kartagener syndrome. *In* Scriver CR, Beaudet AL, Sly WA, Valle D (eds): The Metabolic and Molecular Bases of Inherited Disease. 8th ed. New York, McGraw-Hill, 2001, pp 4817-4828.
71. Solloway MJ, Harvey RP: Molecular pathways in myocardial development: A stem cell perspective. Cardiovasc Res 58:265, 2003.
72. Casey B: Two rights make a wrong: Human left-right malformations. Hum Mol Genet 7:1565, 1998.
73. Towbin JA, Casey B, Belmont J: Human Genetics '99: The cardiovascular system: The molecular basis of vascular disorders. Am J Hum Genet 64:678, 1999.
74. Mochizuki T, Saijoh U, Tsuchiya K, et al: Cloning of *inv*, a gene that controls left/right asymmetry and kidney development. Nature Genet 395:177, 1998.
75. Kosaki R, Gebbia M, Kosaki K, et al: Left-right axis malformations associated with mutations in *ACVR2B*, the gene for human activin receptor type IIB. Am J Med Genet 82:70, 1999.
76. Nezarati MM, McLeod DR: VACTERL manifestations in two generations of a family. Am J Med Genet 82:40, 1999.
77. Slavotinek A, Clayton-Smith J, Super M: Familial patent ductus arteriosus: A further case of CHAR syndrome. Am J Med Genet 71:229, 1997.
78. Glancy DL, Wegmann M, Dhurandhar RW: Aortic dissection and patent ductus arteriosus in three generations. Am J Cardiol 87:813, 2001.
79. Mani A, Meraji S-M, Houshyar R, et al: Finding genetic contributions to sporadic disease: A recessive locus at 12q24 commonly contributes to patent ductus arteriosus. Proc Natl Acad Sci U S A 99:15054, 2002.
80. Vaughan CJ, Basson CT: Molecular determinants of atrial and ventricular septal defects and patent ductus arteriosus. Am J Med Genet 97:304, 2001.
81. Garg V, Kathiriya IS, Barnes R, et al: GATA4 mutations cause human congenital heart defects and reveal an interaction with TBX5. Nature 424:443, 2003.
82. Schott J-J, Benson DW, Basson CT, et al: Congenital heart disease caused by mutations in the transcription factor NKX2-5. Science 281:108, 1998.
83. Basson CT, Huang T, Lin RC, et al: Different TBX5 interactions in heart and limb defined by Holt-Oram syndrome mutations. Proc Natl Acad Sci U S A 96:2919, 1999.
84. Brassington A-ME, Sung SS, Toydemir RM, et al: Expressivity of Holt-Oram syndrome is not predicted by *TBX5* genotype. Am J Hum Genet 73:74, 2003.
85. Ruiz-Perez VL, Ide SE, Strom TM, et al: Mutations in a new gene in Ellis-van Creveld syndrome and Weyers acrodental dysostosis. Nature Genet 24:283, 2000.
86. Galdzicka M, Patnala S, Hirshman MG, et al: A new gene, *EVC2*, is mutated in Ellis-van Creveld syndrome. Molec Genet Metabolism 77:291, 2002.
87. Sheffield VC, Pierpont ME, Nishimura D, et al: Identification of a complex congenital heart defect susceptibility locus by using DNA pooling and shared segment analysis. Hum Molec Genet 6:117, 1997.
88. Broder K, Reinhardt E, Ahern J, et al: Elevated ambulatory blood pressure in 20 subjects with Williams syndrome. Am J Med Genet 83:356, 1999.
89. Tassabehji M, Metcalfe K, Karmiloff-Smith A, et al: Williams syndrome: Use of chromosomal microdeletions as a tool to dissect cognitive and physical phenotypes. Am J Hum Genet 64:118, 1999.
90. Francke U: Williams-Beuren syndrome: Genes and mechanisms. Hum Molec Genet 8:1947, 1999.
91. Metcalfe K, Rucka AK, Smoot L, et al: Elastin: Mutational spectrum in supravalvular aortic stenosis. Eur J Hum Genet 8:955, 2000.
92. Urbán Z, Riazi S, Seidl TL, et al: Connection between elastin haploinsfficiency and increased cell proliferation in patients with supravalvular aortic stenosis and Williams-Beuren syndrome. Am J Hum Genet 71:30, 2002.
93. Nishimura RA, McGoon MD: Perspectives on mitral-valve prolapse. N Engl J Med 341:48, 1999.
94. Freed LA, Levy D, Levine RA, et al: Prevalence and clinical outcome of mitral-valve prolapse. N Engl J Med 341:1, 1999.
95. Freed LA, Acierno JS Jr, Dai D, et al: A locus for autosomal dominant mitral valve prolapse on chromosome 11p15.4. Am J Hum Genet 72:1551, 2003.
96. Disse S, Abergel E, Berrebi A, et al: Mapping of a first locus for autosomal dominant myxomatous mitral-valve prolapse to chromosome 16p11.2-p12.1. Am J Hum Genet 65:1242, 1999.
97. Kyndt F, Schott JJ, Trochu JN, et al: Mapping of X-linked myxomatous valvular dystrophy to chromosome Xq28. Am J Hum Genet 62:627, 1998.
98. DePaepe A, Deitz HC, Devereux RB, et al: Revised diagnostic criteria for the Marfan syndrome. Am J Med Genet 62:417, 1996.
99. Glesby MJ, Pyeritz RE: Association of mitral valve prolapse and systemic abnormalities of connective tissue: A phenotypic continuum. JAMA 262:523, 1989.
100. James PA, Aftimos S, Skinner JR: Familial mitral valve prolapse associated with short stature, characteristic face, and sudden death. Am J Med Genet 119A:32, 2003.
101. Musante L, Kehl HG, Majewski F, et al: Spectrum of mutations in *PTPN11* and genotype-phenotype correlation in 96 patients with Noonan syndrome and five patients with cardio-facio-cutaneous syndrome. Eur J Hum Genet 11:201, 2003.
102. Friedman JM, Hanson JW: Clinical teratology. *In* Rimoin DL, Connor JM, Pyeritz RE, Korf BR (eds): Principles and Practice of Medical Genetics. 4th ed. New York, Churchill Livingstone, 2002, pp 1011-1045.
103. Shepard TH: Catalog of Teratogenic Agents. 10th ed. Baltimore, Johns Hopkins Press, 2001.
104. Bagheri MM, Burd L, Martsolf JT, Klug MG: Fetal alcohol syndrome. J Perinat Med 26:263, 1998.
105. Scriver CR, Kaufman S: Hyperphenylalaninemia: Phenylalanine hydroxylase deficiency. *In* Scriver CR, Beaudet AL, Sly WA, Valle D (eds): The Metabolic and Molecular Bases of Inherited Disease. 8th ed. New York, McGraw-Hill, 2001, pp 1667-1724.
106. Seidman JG, Seidman C: The genetic basis for cardiomyopathy: From mutation identification to mechanistic paradigms. Cell 104:557, 2001.
107. Vosberg H-P, McKenna WJ. Cardiomyopathies. *In* Rimoin DL, Connor JM, Pyeritz RE, Korf BR (eds): Principles and Practice of Medical Genetics. 4th ed. New York, Churchill Livingstone, 2002, pp 1342-1416.
108. Maron, BJ, Casey SA, Poliac LC, et al: Clinical course of hypertrophic cardiomyopathy in a regional United States cohort. JAMA 281:650, 1999.
109. Maron BJ: Hypertrophic cardiomyopathy. JAMA 287:1308, 2002.
110. McKenna W, Behr ER: Hypertrophic cardiomyopathy: Management, risk stratification, and prevention of sudden death. Heart 87:169, 2002.
111. Braunwald E, Seidman CE, Sigwart U: Contemporary evaluation and management of hypertrophic cardiomyopathy. Circulation 106:1312, 2002.
112. Richard P, Charron P, Carrier L, et al: Hypertrophic cardiomyopathy: Distribution of disease genes, spectrum of mutations, and implications for a molecular diagnosis strategy. Circulation 107:2227, 2003.

Cardiomyopathies

113. Semsarian C, Seidman J, Seidman CE: Molecular genetics of inherited cardiomyopathies. *In* Chien KR (ed): Molecular Basis of Cardiovascular Disease. 2nd ed. Philadelphia, Saunders, 2004, pp 293-305.
114. Fung DCY, Yu B, Littlejohn T, et al: An online locus-specific mutation database for familial hypertrophic cardiomyopathy. Hum Mutat 14:326, 1999.
115. Forissier J-F, Richard P, Briault S, et al: First description of germline mosaicism in familial hypertrophic cardiomyopathy. J Med Genet 37:132, 2000.
116. Jeschke B, Uhl K, Weist B, et al: A high risk phenotype of hypertrophic cardiomyopathy associated with a compound genotype of two mutated β-myosin heavy chain genes. Hum Genet 102:299, 1998.
117. Tesson F, Richard P, Charron P, et al: Genotype-phenotype analysis in four families with mutations in β-myosin heavy chain gene responsible for familial hypertrophic cardiomyopathy. Hum Mutat 12:385, 1998.
118. Richard P, Isnard R, Carrier L, et al: Double heterozygosity for mutations in the β-myosin heavy chain and in the cardiac myosin binding protein C genes in a family with hypertrophic cardiomyopathy. J Med Genet 36:542, 1999.

119. Yu B, French JA, Jeremy RW, et al: Counseling issues in familial hypertrophic cardiomyopathy. J Med Genet 35:183, 1998.
120. Maron BJ, Moller JH, Seidman CE, et al: Impact of laboratory molecular diagnosis on contemporary diagnostic criteria for genetically transmitted cardiovascular diseases: Hypertrophic cardiomyopathy, long-QT syndrome, and Marfan syndrome. Circulation 98:1460, 1998.
121. Lim D-S, Roberts R, Marian AJ: Expression profiling of cardiac genes in human hypertrophic cardiomyopathy: Insight into the pathogenesis of phenotypes. J Am Coll Cardiol 38:1175, 2001.
122. Fatkin D, McConnell BK, Mudd JO, et al: An abnormal Ca^{2+} response in mutant sarcomere protein-mediated familial hypertrophic cardiomyopathy. J Clin Invest 106:1351, 2000.
123. Javadpour MM, Tardiff JC, Pinz K, Ingwall JS: Decreased energetics in murine hearts bearing the R92Q mutation in cardiac troponin T. J Clin Invest 112:768, 2003.
124. Maron BJ, Shen W-K, Link MS, et al: Efficacy of implantable cardioverter-defibrillators for the prevention of sudden death in patients with hypertrophic cardiomyopathy. N Engl J Med 342:365, 2000.
125. Sasse-Klaassen S, Gerull B, Oechslin E, et al: Isolated noncompaction of the left ventricular myocardium in the adult is an autosomal dominant disorder in the majority of patients. Am J Med Genet 119A:162, 2003.
126. Cecchi F, Olivotto I, Gistri R, et al: Coronary microvascular dysfunction and prognosis in hypertrophic cardiomyopathy. N Engl J Med 349:1027, 2003.
127. Felker GM, Thompson RE, Hare JM, et al: Underlying causes and long-term survival in patients with initially unexplained cardiomyopathy. N Engl J Med 342:1077, 2000.
128. Legius E, Schollen E, Matthijs G, Fryns J-P: Fine mapping of Noonan/cardiofacio-cutaneous syndrome in a large family. Eur J Hum Genet 6:32, 1998.
129. Maeda M, Holder E, Lowes B, et al: Dilated cardiomyopathy associated with deficiency of the cytoskeletal protein metavinculin. Circulation 95:17, 1997.
130. Jung M, Poepping I, Perrot A, et al: Investigation of a family with autosomal dominant dilated cardiomyopathy defines a novel locus on chromosome 2q14-q22. Am J Hum Genet 65:1068, 1997.
131. Vilarinho L, Santorelli FM, Rosas MJ, et al: The mitochondrial A3243G mutation presenting as severe cardiomyopathy. J Med Genet 34:607, 1997.
132. Digilio MC, Marino B, Bevilacqua M, et al: Genetic heterogeneity of isolated noncompaction of the left ventricular myocardium. Am J Med Genet 85:90, 1999.
133. Emery AEH: Duchenne and other X-linked muscular dystrophies. *In* Rimoin DL, Connor JM, Pyeritz RE, Korf BR (eds): Principles and Practice of Medical Genetics. 4th ed. New York, Churchill Livingstone, 2002, pp 3266-3284.
134. Bushby KMD: Autosomally inherited muscular dystrophies. *In* Rimoin DL, Connor JM, Pyeritz RE, Korf BR (eds): Principles and Practice of Medical Genetics. 4th ed. New York, Churchill Livingstone, 2002, pp 3285-3302.
135. Morris GE, Manilal S: Heart to heart: From nuclear proteins to Emery-Dreifuss muscular dystrophy. Hum Molec Genet 8:1847, 1999.
136. De Sandre-Giovannoli A, Bernard R, Cau P, et al: Lamin A truncation in Hutchinson-Gilford Progeria. Science 300:2055, 2003.
137. Barresi R, Di Blasi C, Negri T, et al: Disruption of heart sarcoglycan complex and severe cardiomyopathy caused by β sarcoglycan mutations. J Med Genet 37:102, 2000.
138. Sylvius N, Duboscq-Bidot L, Bouchier C, et al: Mutational analysis of the β- and δ-sarcoglycan genes in a large number of patients with familial and sporadic dilated cardiomyopathy. Am J Med Genet 120A:8, 2003.
139. Tiso N, Stephan DA, Nava A, et al: Identification of mutations in the cardiac ryanodine receptor gene in families affected with arrhythmogenic right ventricular cardiomyopathy type 2 (ARVD2). Hum Molec Genet 10:189, 2001.
140. Rampazzo A, Beffagna G, Nava A, et al: Arrhythmogenic right ventricular cardiomyopathy type 1 (ARVD1): Confirmation of locus assignment and mutation screening of four candidate genes. Eur J Hum Genet 11:69, 2003.
141. Ammash NM, Seward JB, Bailey KR, et al: Clinical profile and outcome of idiopathic restrictive cardiomyopathy. Circulation 101:2490, 2000.
142. Lipsanen-Nyman M, Perheentupa J, Rapola J, et al: Mulibrey heart disease. Clinical manifestations, long-term course, and results of pericardiectomy in a series of 49 patients born before 1985. Circulation 107:2810, 2003.
143. Avela K, Lipsanen-Nyman M, Idanheimo N, et al: Gene encoding a new RING-B-box-Coiled-coil protein is mutated in mulibrey nanism. Nature Genet 25:298, 2000.
144. Bahabri SA, Suwairi WM, Laxer RM, et al: The camptodactyly-arthropathy-coxa vara-pericarditis syndrome: Clinical features and genetic mapping to human chromosome 1. Arthritis Rheum 41:730, 1998.
145. Marcelino J, Carpten JD, Suwairi WM, et al: CACP, encoding a secreted proteoglycan, is mutated in camptodactyly-arthropathy-coxa vara-pericarditis syndrome. Nature Genet 23:319, 1999.
146. Van Hove JLK, Wevers RA, Van Cleemput J, et al: Late-onset visceral presentation with cardiomyopathy and without neurological symptoms of adult Sanfilippo A syndrome. Am J Med Genet 118:282, 2003.
147. Kampmann C, Baehner F, Ries M, et al: Cardiac involvement in Anderson-Fabry disease. J Am Soc Nephrol 13:S147, 2002.
148. Lin AE, Grossfeld PD, Hamilton RM, et al: Further delineation of cardiac abnormalities in Costello syndrome. Am J Med Genet 111:115, 2002.
149. Coppin BD, Temple IK: Multiple lentigines syndrome (LEOPARD) syndrome or progressive cardiomyopathic lentiginosis. J Med Genet 24:582, 1997.

Disorders of Connective Tissue

150. Royce PM, Steinmann B (eds): Connective Tissue and Its Heritable Disorders: Molecular, Genetic and Medical Aspects. 2nd ed. New York, Wiley-Liss, 2002.
151. Pyeritz RE: Disorders of fibrillins and microfibrilogenesis: Marfan syndrome, MASS phenotype, contractural arachnodactyly and related conditions. *In* Rimoin DL, Connor JM, Pyeritz RE, Korf BR (eds): Principles and Practice of Medical Genetics. 4th ed. New York, Churchill Livingstone, 2002, pp 3977-4020.
151a. Schalkwijk J, Zweers MC, Steijlen PM, et al: A recessive form of the Ehlers-Danlos syndrome caused by tenascin-X deficiency. N Engl J Med 345:1167, 2001.
152. Yetman AT, Bornemeier RA, McCrindle BW: Long-term outcome in patients with Marfan syndrome: Is aortic dissection the only cause of sudden death? J Am Coll Cardiol 41:329, 2003.
153. Gott VL, Greene PS, Alejo DE, et al: Surgery for ascending aortic disease in Marfan patients: A multi-center study. N Engl J Med 340:1307, 1999.
154. van Karnebeek CDM, Naeff MSJ, Mulder BJM, et al: Natural history of cardiovascular manifestations in Marfan syndrome. Arch Dis Child 84:129, 2001.
155. Lepore V, Jeppsson A, Radberg G, et al: Aortic surgery in patients with Marfan syndrome: Long-term survival, morbidity and function. J Heart Valve Dis 10:25, 2001.
156. De Oliveira NC, David TE, Ivanov J, et al: Results of surgery for aortic root aneurysm in patients with Marfan syndrome. J Thorac Cardiovasc Surg 125:789, 2003.
157. Miller DC: Valve-sparing aortic root replacement in patients with the Marfan syndrome. J Thorac Cardiovasc Surg 125:773, 2003.
158. Porciani MC, Giurlani L, Chelucci A, et al: Diastolic subclinical primary alterations in Marfan syndrome and Marfan-related disorders. Clin Cardiol 25:416, 2002.
159. Chatrath R, Beauchesne LM, Connolly HM, et al: Left ventricular function in the Marfan syndrome without significant valvular regurgitation. Am J Cardiol 91:914, 2003.
160. Shores J, Borger KR, Murphy EA, et al: Chronic β-adrenergic blockade protects the aorta in the Marfan syndrome: A prospective, randomized trial of propranolol. N Engl J Med 330:1335, 1994.
161. Jondeau G, Boutouyrie P, Lacolley P, et al: Central pulse pressure is a major determinant of ascending aorta dilatation in Marfan syndrome. Circulation 99:2677, 1999.
162. Lipscomb KJ, Clayton-Smith J, Clarke B, et al: Outcome of pregnancy in women with Marfan's syndrome. Br J Obstet Gynaecol 104:210, 1997.
163. Pyeritz RE, Dietz HC: The Marfan syndrome and other fibrillinopathies. *In* Royce PM, Steinmann B (eds): Connective Tissue and Its Heritable Disorders: Molecular, Genetic and Medical Aspects. 2nd ed. New York, Wiley-Liss, 2002, pp 585-626.
164. Collod-Beroud G, Beroud C, Ades L: Marfan Database (3rd ed): New mutations and new routines for the software. Nucl Acids Res 26:229, 1998.
165. Yuan B, Thomas JP, von Kodolitsch Y, Pyeritz RE: Comparison of heteroduplex analysis, direct sequencing and enzyme mismatch cleavage for detecting mutations in a large gene, FBN1. Hum Mutat 14:440, 1999.
166. Korkko J, Kaitila I, Lonnqvist L, et al: Sensitivity of conformation sensitive gel electrophoresis in detecting mutations in Marfan syndrome and related conditions. J Med Genet 39:34, 2002.
167. Neptune ER, Frischmeyer PA, Arking DE, et al: Dysregulation of TGF-α activation contributes to pathogenesis in Marfan syndrome. Nature Genet 33:407, 2003.
168. Beighton P, De Paepe A, Steinmann B, et al: Ehlers-Danlos syndromes: Revised nosology, Villefranche, 1997. Am J Med Genet 77:31, 1998.
169. Wenstrup RJ, Meyer RA, Lyle JS, et al: Prevalence of aortic root dilation in the Ehlers-Danlos syndrome. Genet Med 4:112, 2002.
170. Dolan AL, Mishra MB, Chambers JB, et al: Clinical and echocardiographic survey of the Ehlers-Danlos syndrome. Br J Rheumatol 36:459, 1997.
171. Pyeritz RE: Ehlers-Danlos syndrome. N Engl J Med 342:730, 2000.
172. Gilchrist D, Schwarze U, Shields K, et al: Large kindred with Ehlers-Danlos syndrome type IV due to a point mutation (G571S) in the *COL3A1* gene of type III procollagen: Low risk of pregnancy complications and unexpected longevity in some affected relatives. Am J Med Genet 82:305, 1999.
173. Pepin M, Schwarze U, Superti-Furga A, Byers PH: Clinical and genetic features of Ehlers-Danlos syndrome type IV, the vascular type. N Engl J Med 342:673, 2000.
174. Lind J, Wallenburg HCS: Pregnancy and the Ehler-Danlos syndrome: A retrospective study in a Dutch population. Acta Obstet Gynecol Scand 81:293, 2002.
175. Uitto J, Pulkkinen L: Heritable disorders of elastic tissue: Cutis laxa, pseudoxanthoma elasticum and related disorders. *In* Rimoin DL, Connor JM, Pyeritz RE, Korf BR (eds): Principles and Practice of Medical Genetics. 4th ed. New York, Churchill Livingstone, 2002, pp 4044-4070.
176. Germain DP, Boutouyrie P, Laloux B, et al: Arterial remodeling and stiffness in patients with pseudoxanthoma elasticum. Arterioscler Thromb Vasc Biol 23:836, 2003.

Inborn Errors of Metabolism that Affect the Cardiovascular System

177. Wilcken DEL: Overview of inherited metabolic disorders causing cardiovascular disease. J Inherit Metab Dis 26:245, 2003.
178. La Du BN: Alkaptonuria: *In* Scriver CR, Beaudet AL, Sly WA, Valle D (eds): The Metabolic and Molecular Bases of Inherited Disease. 8th ed. New York, McGraw-Hill, 2001, pp 2109-2124.
179. Mudd SH, Levy HL, Skovby F: Disorders of transsulfuration. *In* Scriver CR, Beaudet AL, Sly WA, Valle D (eds): The Metabolic and Molecular Bases of Inherited Disease. 8th ed. New York, McGraw-Hill, 2001, pp 2007-2056.
180. Kraus JP, Janosik M, Kozich V, et al: Cystathionine β-synthase mutations in homocystinuria. Hum Mutat 13:362, 1999.
181. Wilcken DEL, Wilcken B: The natural history of vascular disease in homocystinuria and the effects of treatment. J Inher Metab Dis 20:295, 1997.
182. Eikelboom JW, Lonn E, Genest J Jr, et al: Homocyst(e)ine and cardiovascular disease: A critical review of the epidemiologic evidence. Ann Intern Med 131:363, 1999.
183. Majors A, Ehrhart LA, Pezacka EH: Homocysteine as a risk factor for vascular disease. Enhanced collagen production and accumulation by smooth muscle cells. Arterioscler Thromb Vasc Biol 17:2074, 1997.

184. Darras BT, Friedman NR: Metabolic myopathies: A clinical approach; Part II. Pediatr Neurol 22:171, 2000.
185. Roe CR, Ding J: Mitochondrial fatty acid oxidation disorders. *In* Scriver CR, Beaudet AL, Sly WA, Valle D (eds): The Metabolic and Molecular Bases of Inherited Disease. 8th ed. New York, McGraw-Hill, 2001, pp 2297-2326.
186. Goodman SI: Organic acidemias and disorders of fatty acid oxidation. *In* Rimoin DL, Connor JM, Pyeritz RE, Korf BR (eds): Principles and Practice of Medical Genetics. 4th ed. New York, Churchill Livingstone, 2002, pp 2550-2565.
187. Chen Y-T: Glycogen storage diseases. *In* Scriver CR, Beaudet AL, Sly WA, Valle D (eds): The Metabolic and Molecular Bases of Inherited Disease. 8th ed. New York, McGraw-Hill, 2001, pp 1521-1552.
188. Cox PM, Brueton LA, Murphy KW, et al: Early-onset fetal hydrops and muscle degeneration in siblings due to a novel variant of type IV glycogenosis. Am J Med Genet 86:187, 1999.
189. Arad M, Benson DW, Perez-Atayde AR, et al: Constitutively active AMP kinase mutations cause glycogen storage disease mimicking hypertrophic cardiomyopathy. J Clin Invest 109:357, 2002.
190. Leroy JG: Oligosaccharidoses and allied disorders. *In* Rimoin DL, Connor JM, Pyeritz RE, Korf BR (eds): Principles and Practice of Medical Genetics. 4th ed. New York, Churchill Livingstone, 2002, pp 2677-2711.

191. Beutler E, Bothwell TH, Charlton RW, Motulsky AG: Hereditary hemochromatosis. *In* Scriver CR, Beaudet AL, Sly WA, Valle D (eds): The Metabolic and Molecular Bases of Inherited Disease. 8th ed. New York, McGraw-Hill, 2001, pp 3127-3162.
192. Olynyk JK, Cullen DJ, Aquilia S, et al: A population-based study of the clinical expression of the hemochromatosis gene. N Engl J Med 341:718, 1999.
193. Beutler E, Felitti VJ, Koziol JA, et al: Penetrance of 845G → A(C282Y) *HFE* hereditary haemochromatosis mutation in the USA. Lancet 359:211, 2002.
194. Burke W, Thomson E, Khoury MJ, et al: Hereditary hemochromatosis: Gene discovery and its implications for population-based screening. JAMA 280:172, 1998.
195. Weatherall DJ, Clegg JB, Higgs DR, et al: The hemoglobinopathies. *In* Scriver CR, Beaudet AL, Sly WA, Valley D (eds): The Metabolic and Molecular Bases of Inherited Disease. 8th ed. New York, McGraw-Hill, 2001, pp 4571-636.
196. Kremastinos DT, Flevari P, Spyropoulou M, et al: Association of heart failure in homozygous β-thalassemia with the major histocompatibility complex. Circulation 100:2074, 1999.
197. Steinberg MH: Management of sickle cell disease. N Engl J Med 340:1021, 1999.
198. Tsomi K, Karagiorga-Lagana M, Karabatsos F, et al: Arterial elastorrhexis in β-thalassaemia intermedia, sickle cell thalassaemia and hereditary sperocytosis. Eur J Haematol 67:135, 2001.
199. Aessopos A, Farmakis D, Loukopoulos D: Elastic tissue abnormalities resembling pseudoxanthoma elasticum in β thalassemia and the sickling syndromes. Blood 99:30, 2002.
200. Spranger J: Mucopolysaccharidoses. *In* Rimoin DL, Connor JM, Pyeritz RE, Korf BR (eds): Principles and Practice of Medical Genetics. 4th ed. New York, Churchill Livingstone, 2002, pp 2666-2676.
201. Semenza GL, Pyeritz RE: Respiratory complications of the mucopolysaccharide storage disorders. Medicine 67:209, 1988.
202. Kakkis ED, Muenzer J, Tiller GE, et at: Enzyme-replacement therapy in mucopolysaccharidosis I. New Engl J Med 344:182, 2001.
203. Percy AK: Gangliosidoses and related lipid storage diseases. *In* Rimoin DL, Connor JM, Pyeritz RE, Korf BR (eds): Principles and Practice of Medical Genetics. 4th ed. New York, Churchill Livingstone, 2002, pp 2712-2751.
204. Desnick RJ, Brady R, Barranger J, et al: Fabry disease, an under-recognized multisystemic disorder: Expert recommendations for diagnosis, management, and enzyme replacement therapy. Ann Intern Med 138:338, 2003.
205. Schiffmann R, Murray GJ, Treco D, et al: Infusion of α-galactosidase A reduces tissue globotriaosylceramide storage in patients with Fabry disease. Proc Natl Acad Sci U S A 97:365, 2000.
206. Hopkin RJ, Bissler J, Grabowski, GA: Comparative evaluation of α-galactosidase A infusions for treatment of Fabry disease. Genet Med 5:144-53, 2003.
207. Boerkoel CN III, Lupski JR: Hereditary motor and sensory neuropathies. *In* Rimoin DL, Connor JM, Pyeritz RE, Korf BR (eds): Principles and Practice of Medical Genetics. 4th ed. New York, Churchill Livingstone, 2002, pp 3303-3320.
208. Lachmann HJ, Booth DR, Booth SE, et al: Misdiagnosis of hereditary amyloidosis as AL (primary) amyloidosis. N Engl J Med 346:1786, 2002.
209. Dingli D, Utz JP, Gertz MA: Pulmonary hypertension in patients with amyloidosis. Chest 120:1735, 2001.
210. Morelli S, Carmenini E, Sgreccia A, et al: Heart rate variability and familial amyloidosis. Inter J Cardiol 83:295, 2002.
211. Olofsson BO, Backman C, Karp K, et al: Progression of cardiomyopathy after liver transplantation in patients with familial amyloidotic polyneuropathy, Portuguese type. Transplantation 73:745, 2002.
212. Roach ES, DiMario FJ, Kandt RS, Northrup H: Tuberous sclerosis complex consensus conference: Recommendations for diagnostic evaluation. J Child Neurol 14:401, 1999.
213. Sperling D, Smith M: Novel 23-base-pair duplication mutation in TSC1 exon 15 in an infant presenting with cardiac rhabdomyomas. Am J Med Genet 84:346, 1999.
214. Astrinidis A, Khare L, Carsillo T, et al: Mutational analysis of the tuberous sclerosis gene *TSC2* in patients with pulmonary lymphangioleiomyomatosis. J Med Genet 37:55, 2000.
215. Harris NL, McNeely WF, Shepard JO, et al: Presentation of case 11-2002, MGH. N Engl J Med 346:1152, 2002.
216. Basson CT, MacRae CA, Korf B, Merliss A: Genetic heterogeneity of familial atrial myxoma syndromes (Carney complex). Am J Cardiol 79:994, 1997.
217. Groussin L, Kirschner LS, Vincent-Dejean C, et al: Molecular analysis of the cyclic AMP-dependent protein kinase A (PKA) regulatory subunit 1A (*PRKAR1A*) gene in patients with Carney complex and primary pigmented nodular adrenocortical disease (PPNAD) reveals novel mutations and clues for pathophysiology: Augmented PKA signaling is associated with adrenal tumorigenesis in PPNAD. Am J Hum Genet 71:1433, 2002.

Inherited Disorders of the Circulation

218. Shovlin CL, Guttmacher AE, Buscarini E, et al: Diagnostic criteria for hereditary hemorrhagic telangiectasia (Rendu-Osler-Weber syndrome). Am J Med Genet 91:66, 2000.
219. McDonald JE, Miller FJ, Hallam SE, et al: Clinical manifestations in a large hereditary hemorrhagic telangiectasia (HHT) type 2 kindred. Am J Med Genet. 93:320, 2000.
220. Fulbright RK, Chaloupka JC, Putman CM, et al: MR of hereditary hemorrhagic telangiectasia: Prevalence and spectrum of cerebrovascular malformations. Am J Neuroradiol 19:477, 1998.
221. Kopel L, Lage SG: Cardiac tamponade in hereditary hemorrhagic telangiectasia. Am J Med 105:252, 1998.
222. Lee WL, Graham AF, Pugash RA, et al: Contrast echocardiography remains positive after treatment of pulmonary arteriovenous malformations. Chest 123:351, 2003.
223. Lee DW, White RI Jr, Egglin TK, et al: Embolotherapy of large pulmonary arteriovenous malformations: Long-term results. Ann Thorac Surg 64:930, 1997.
224. Longacre AV, Gross CP, Gallitelli M, et al: Diagnosis and management of gastrointestinal bleeding in patients with hereditary hemorrhagic telangiectasia. Am J Gastroenterol 98:59, 2003.
225. Easey AJ, Wallace GM, Hughes JM, et al: Should asymptomatic patients with hereditary haemorrhagic telangiectasia (HHT) be screened for cerebral vascular malformations? J Neurol Neurosurg Psychiatry 74:743, 2003.
226. Marchuk DA, Srinivasan S, Squire TL, et al: Vascular morphogenesis: Tales of two syndromes. Hum Molec Genet 12:R97, 2003.
227. Prowse AH, Webster AR, Richards FM, et al: Somatic inactivation of the VHL gene in Von Hippel-Lindau disease tumors. Am J Hum Genet 60:765, 1997.
228. Watnick T, Phakdeekitcharoen B, Johnson A, et al: Mutation detection of *PKD1* identifies a novel mutation common to three families with aneurysms and/or very-early-onset disease. Am J Hum Genet 65:1561, 1999.
229. Hateboer N, van Dijk MA, Bogdanova N, et al: Comparison of phenotypes of polycystic kidney disease types 1 and 2. Lancet 353:103, 1999.
230. Koptides M, Hadjimichael C. Koupepidou P, et al: Germinal and somatic mutations in the PKD2 gene of renal cysts in autosomal dominant polycystic kidney disease. Hum Molec Genet 8:509, 1999.
231. Peters DJM, Breuning MH: Autosomal dominant polycystic kidney disease: Modification of disease progression. Lancet 358:1439, 2001.
232. Piccoli DA, Spinner NB: Alagille syndrome and the Jagged1 gene. Sem Liver Dis 21:525, 2001.
233. Woolfenden AR, Albers GW, Steinberg GK, et al: Moyamoya syndrome in children with Alagille syndrome: Additional evidence of a vasculopathy. Pediatrics 103:505, 1999.
234. Yuan Z-R, Kohsak T, Ikegaya T, et al: Mutational analysis of the Jagged 1 gene in Alagille syndrome families. Hum Molec Genet 7:1363, 1998.
235. Li L, Krantz ID, Deng Y, et al: Alagille syndrome is caused by mutations in human Jagged1, which encodes a ligand for Notch1. Nature Genet 16:243, 1997.
236. Biddinger A, Rocklin M, Coselli J, Milewicz DM: Familial thoracic aortic dilatations and dissections: A case control study. J Vasc Surg 25:506, 1997.
237. Milewicz DM, Chen H, Park E-S, et al: Reduced penetrance and variable expressivity of familial thoracic aortic aneurysms/dissections. Am J Cardiol 82:474, 1998.
238. Guo D, Hasham S, Kuang SQ, et al: Familial thoracic aortic aneurysms and dissections: Genetic heterogeneity with a major locus mapping to 5q13-14. Circulation 103:2461, 2001.
239. Vaughan CJ, Casey M, He J, et al: Identification of a chromosome 11q23-2-q24 locus for familial aortic aneurysm disease, a genetically heterogeneous disorder. Circulation 103:2469, 2001.
240. Hasham SN, Willing MC, Guo DC, et al: Mapping a locus for familial thoracic aortic aneurysms and dissections. Circulation 107:3184, 2003.
241. Multicentre Aneurysm Screening Study Group: Multicentre aneurysm screening study (MASS): Cost effectiveness analysis of screening for abdominal aortic aneurysms based on four year results from randomized controlled trial. BMJ 325:1135, 2002.
242. Franceschini P, Guala A, Licata D, et al: Arterial Tortuosity syndrome. Am J Med Genet 91:141, 2000.
243. Caplan LR: Should intracranial aneurysms be treated before they rupture? N Engl J Med 339:1774, 1998.
244. Magnetic Resonance Angiography Study Group: Risks and benefits of screening for intracranial aneurysms in first-degree relatives of patients with sporadic subarachnoid hemorrhage. N Engl J Med 241:1344, 1999.
245. Gaist D, Væth M, Tsiropoulos I, et al: Risk of subarachnoid haemorrhage in first degree relatives of patients with subarachnoid haemorrhage: Follow up study based on national registries in Denmark. BMJ 320:141, 2000.
246. Walter JW, Blei F, Anderson JL, et al: Genetic mapping of a novel familial form of infantile hemangioma. Am J Med Genet 82:77, 1999.
247. Iadecola C: Genetics of cerebrovascular disease. N Engl J Med 339:216, 1998.
248. Ikeda H, Sasaki T, Yoshimoto T, et al: Mapping of a familial Moyamoya disease gene to chromosome 3p24.2-p26. Am J Hum Genet 64:533, 1999.
249. De Lange RPJ, Bolt J, Reid E, et al: Screening British CADASIL families for mutations in the *NOTCH3* gene. J Med Genet 37:224, 2000.
250. Ducros A, Denier C, Joutel A, et al: Recurrence of the T666M calcium channel *CACNA1A* gene mutation in familial hemiplegic migraine with progressive cerebellar ataxia. Am J Hum Genet 64:89, 1999.
251. Trembath RC, Harrison R: Insights into the genetic and molecular basis of primary pulmonary hypertension. Pediatr Res 53:883, 2003.
252. Runo JR, Loyd JE: Primary pulmonary hypertension. Lancet 361:1533, 2003.

253. Deng Z, Morse JH, Slager SL, et al: Familial primary pulmonary hypertension (gene PPH1) is caused by mutations in the bone morphogenetic protein receptor-II gene. Am J Hum Genet 67:737, 2000.
254. Cohen MM Jr: Klippel-Trenaunay syndrome. Am J Med Genet 93:171, 2000.
255. Craig HD, Gunel M, Cepeda O, et al: Multilocus linkage identifies two new loci for a Mendelian form of stroke, cerebral cavernous malformation, at 7p15-13 and 3q25.2-27. Hum Molec Genet 7:1851, 1998.
256. Zhang J, Clatterbuck RE, Rigamonti D, et al: Mutations in KRIT1 in familial cerebral cavernous malformations. Neurosurgery 46:1272, 2000.
257. Cavé-Riant F, Denier C, Labauge P, et al: Spectrum and expression analysis of *KRIT1* mutations in 121 consecutive and unrelated patients with cerebral cavernous malformations. Eur J Hum Genet 10:733, 2002.
258. Arteriovenous Malformation Study Group: Arteriovenous malformations of the brain in adults. N Engl J Med 340:1812-1818, 1999.
259. Ferrell RE, Pyeritz RE: Hereditary disorders of the lymphatic and venous systems. *In* Rimoin DL, Conner JM, Pyeritz RE, Korf B (eds): Principles and Practice of Medical Genetics, 4th ed. Edinburgh: Churchill Livingstone, 2002, pp 1546-1560.
260. Van Balkom IDC, Alders M, Allanson J, et al: Lymphedema-lymphangiectasia-mental retardation (Hennekam) syndrome: A review. Am J Med Genet 112:412, 2002.
261. Ferrell RE, Levinson KL, Esman JH, et al: Hereditary lymphedema: Evidence for linkage and genetic heterogeneity. Hum Molec Genet 7:2073, 1998.
262. Evans AL, Brice G, Sotirova V, et al: Mapping of primary congenital lymphedema to the 5q35.3 region. Am J Hum Genet 64:547, 1999.
263. Irrthum A, Devriendt K, Chitayat D, et al: Mutations in the transcription factor gene *SOX18* underlie recessive and dominant forms of hypotrichosis-lymphedema-telangiectasia. Am J Hum Genet 72:1470, 2003.
264. Asad R, Thompson PD, Pyeritz RE: Genetic factors in occlusive arterial disease. *In* Rimoin DL, Conner JM, Pyeritz RE, Korf B (eds): Principles and Practice of Medical Genetics, 4th ed. New York, Churchill Livingstone, 2002, pp 1519-1545.
265. Trip MD, Smulders YM, Wegman JJ, et al: Frequent mutation in the ABCC6 gene (*R1141X*) is associated with a strong increase in the prevalence of coronary artery disease. Circulation 106:773, 2002.
266. Arking DE, Becker DM, Yanek LR, et al: KLOTHO allele status and the risk of early-onset occult coronary artery disease. Am J Hum Genet 72:1154, 2003.
267. von Kodolitsch Y, Pyeritz RE, Rogan PK: Splice site mutations in atherosclerosis candidate genes: Relating individual information to phenotype. Circulation 100:693, 1999.
268. Hacia JG, Collins FS: Mutational analysis using oligonucleotide microarrays. J Med Genet 36:730, 1999.
269. Elston RC: Linkage and association. Genet Epidemiol 15:565, 1998.
270. Hunt SC, Hopkins PN, Lalouel J-M: Hypertension. *In* King RA, Rotter JI, Motulsky AG (eds): The Genetic Basis of Common Diseases. 2nd ed. New York, Oxford University Press, 2002, pp 127-154.
271. Jeunemaitre X, Gimenez-Roqueplo A-P, Disse-Nicodeme S, Corvol P: Molecular basis of human hypertension. *In* Rimoin DL, Connor JM, Pyeritz RE, Korf BR (eds): Principles and Practice of Medical Genetics. 4th ed. New York, Churchill Livingstone, 2002, pp 1475-1479.
272. Halushka MK, Fan JB, Bentley K, et al: Patterns of single-nucleotide polymorphisms in candidate genes for blood-pressure homeostasis. Nature Genet 22:239, 1999.
273. Lifton RP, Gharavi AG, Geller DS: Molecular mechanisms of human hypertension. Cell 104:545, 2001.
274. Niu T, Xu X, Rogus J, et al: Angiotensinogen gene and hypertension in Chinese. J Clin Invest 101:188, 1998.
275. Arngrimsson R, Hayward C, Nadaud S, et al: Evidence for a familial pregnancy-induced hypertension locus in the eNOS-gene region. Am J Hum Genet 61:354, 1997.
276. Arngrimsson R, Siguroardottir S, Frigge ML, et al: A genome-wide scan reveals a maternal susceptibility locus for pre-eclampsia on chromosome 2p13. Hum Molec Genet 8:1799, 1999.
277. DeStefano AL, Baldwin CT, Burzstyn M, et al: Autosomal dominant orthostatic hypotensive disorder maps to chromosome 18q. Am J Hum Genet 63:1425, 1998.
278. Schwartz F, Baldwin CT, Baima J, Gavras H: Mitochondrial DNA mutations in patients with orthostatic hypotension. Am J Med Genet 86:145, 1999.

CHAPTER 71

Myocardial Regeneration

Piero Anversa • Annarosa Leri

Two distinct forms of myocardial regeneration occur in the adult heart after injury. The first is restricted to the unaffected portion of the myocardium and uses the growth reserve of the viable tissue. The process of generating new myocardial mass involves hypertrophy of terminally differentiated myocytes and replication of myocytes that have retained the ability to reenter the cell cycle and divide.[1] The second requires the repair of necrotic lost myocardium that can be accomplished only by cellular therapy. This novel procedure has been performed recently using exogenous primitive cells of various sources (Fig. 71–1). The expansion of the surviving myocardium by replication of parenchymal cells imposes a different view of the growth of the heart, whereas tissue reconstitution from nonresident cells demands that these cells be capable of developing myocytes and coronary vessels in an orderly manner to rebuild functionally competent new myocardium.[2]

Growth Reserve of the Heart

If the adult heart were a static organ, its biology would be rather simple. Shortly after birth, myocytes would cease to divide and would acquire a state of terminal differentiation.[3] The total number of parenchymal cells would become established at this time, and this cell population would remain constant throughout life. According to this paradigm, the myocardium would constitute a steady-state tissue because its most distinctive cellular compartment would persist intact until death of the individual. Although nature continuously teaches us the simplicity of natural events, the biological model of the postnatal heart as a lethargic organ is unrealistic. The evidence that has accumulated on the dynamic state of the cellular population of the heart[1,2,4] has forced us to deal with complexity.

As the basic components of a tissue, cells represent autonomous agents that are driven by built-in programs and also sense the chemical and mechanical signals dictated by the surrounding microenvironment. The integration of intrinsic and extrinsic cues regulates cell migration, growth, differentiation, and death, which constitute the basic processes of organ homeostasis. These notions, valid for any organ or tissue in the organism, have only recently been applied to the heart. Therefore, the new concept of cardiac development, maturation, aging, and disease must include these fundamental biological principles of myocardial homeostasis. These principles are critical for the identification of novel therapeutic strategies for the repair of the injured heart.

Aging, cardiac diseases, and, most apparently, ischemic injury and myocardial infarction are characterized by scattered or segmental loss of myocytes by apoptotic and necrotic death.[1,4] The lack of restoration of the myocyte compartment has been cited as unequivocal proof of the postmitotic condition of the old and damaged heart. This phenomenon is actually common to other organs, including highly proliferating tissues. A decline in the number of parenchymal cells as a function of age and pathological damage occurs in the bone marrow, immune system, testis, retinal epithelium, cochlea, liver, brain, and peripheral nervous system. Similarly, infarcts of the intestine, brain, skin, kidney, and liver evolve in a manner identical to the heart.[5] Additionally, as in the heart, other organs respond to stress by an increase in cell-replicative growth. However, this reaction is often unsuccessful and does not reestablish tissue homeostasis.[6] Cell death may exceed cell division, and cell regeneration may occur preferentially in the unaffected region of all organs, precluding effective repair.

The behavior of the heart, therefore, fits into a common model of organ growth. During development and physiological turnover of a tissue, cells divide for a defined number of rounds, ultimately reaching terminal differentiation. The process of commitment of primitive cells into more specialized units involves an increased restriction in their proliferative potential that culminates in cell cycle withdrawal. A precise coordination between cells entering a quiescent nondividing state and cells reaching terminal differentiation and functional competence is required to ensure proper performance of any organ, including the heart. Moreover, maintenance of cell cycle arrest in fully mature cells is crucial for tissue architecture and function. The preservation of the differentiated state of myocytes must be tightly regulated. In fact, the heart would fail if most of its parenchymal cells were involved not in contractile activity but in cell replication. Mitotic division is restricted to small amplifying myocytes that possess a minimal amount of myofibrils distributed at the periphery of the cell in the subsarcolemmal region (Fig. 71–2). This observation illustrates the new paradigm.

The old paradigm is strongly engrained among cardiologists and cardiovascular scientists who accept the principles that the heart can survive and exert its pump function throughout life with the same cells present at birth.[3] Because of this misconception, research in the past 50 years has focused on understanding the molecular control of myocyte hypertrophy,[7] with acrimonious objections to information supporting the replicative capacity of the adult heart.[8] The demonstration of myocyte cytokinesis during development was considered a biological curiosity rather than a relevant component of the physiological turnover of the normal heart. Concurrently, the identification of myocyte division in the overloaded ventricle was not recognized as

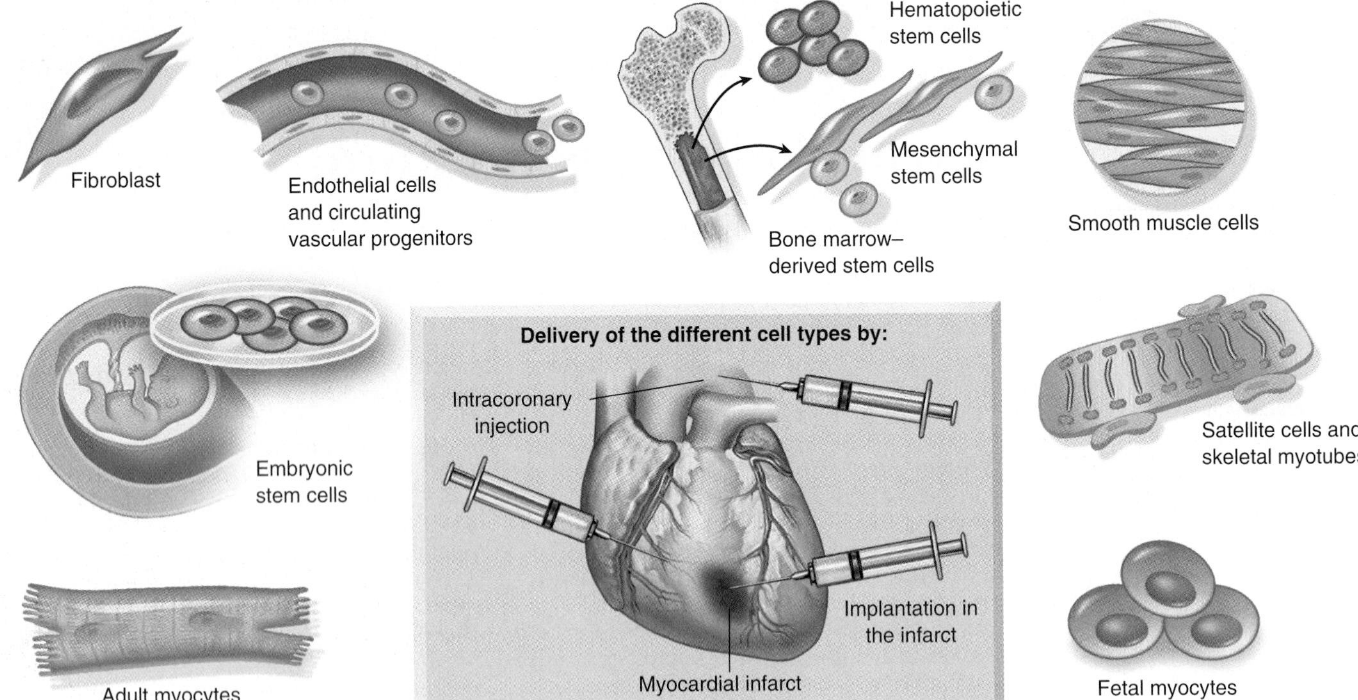

FIGURE 71–1 Myocardial repair. A variety of cell types from different origins have been employed in an attempt to repair and improve the function of the infarcted heart. The various cell populations used for this purpose are depicted here.

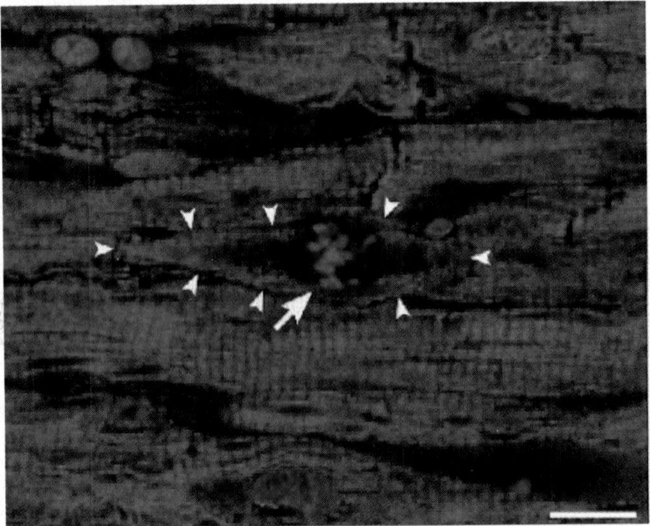

FIGURE 71–2 Dividing myocyte. In a small myocyte (alpha-sarcomeric actin = red), there is a nucleus in mitosis (propidium iodide [PI] = green; arrow) characterized by a cluster of metaphase chromosomes. The mitotic myocyte shows myofibrillar structures located at the periphery of the cell (arrowheads). This section derives from the heart of a patient affected by end-stage ischemic myopathy. Confocal microscopy, bar = 10 μm.

an important growth mechanism dramatically affecting the remodeling of the pathological heart. According to the established view, new cells cannot replace dead myocytes. This belief has delayed the understanding of the cellular response of the diseased heart. The answer to this conundrum has been provided by a series of findings that urge a reinterpretation of the biology of the heart, perennially viewed as a postmitotic organ.[3]

Identification of Myocyte Proliferation in the Damaged Heart

Cardiac regeneration by myocyte multiplication cannot be restricted to the detection of karyokinesis and cytokinesis, which are rapid events difficult to capture. The analysis of duplicating cells includes identification of cells and their nuclei in various phases of the cell cycle. Probes are available, and an accurate evaluation of the number of cycling myocytes can be obtained. This involves the identification of myocytes that express cyclins and cyclin-dependent kinases, replicate DNA, traverse the cell cycle, and divide. These approaches have provided information on the dynamic state of cell regeneration in the normal and pathological heart.[9,10] (For an extended discussion and pictorial representation of the cell cycle, see Chap. 69.)

The presence of myofibrils in cycling myocytes indicates that a subpopulation of partially differentiated parenchymal cells can divide in the adult organ. The basic cell cycle machinery of myocytes has its core in the cyclins and cyclin-dependent kinases. Key regulators of G_1 progression are the group of D cyclins that are synthesized during the G_0-G_1 transition. However, kinase activity becomes apparent only in mid-G_1. The increase in cyclin D_2 and cyclin D_2-associated kinase in myocytes demonstrates that these cells have left the quiescent state and have reentered the cell cycle.[11] The enhanced expression of cyclin A and cdk2 activity is followed by activation of cyclin B and cdc2, which promote the progression of myocytes in S phase and G_2-M before cytokinesis.[11]

Markers capable of recognizing different phases of the cell cycle or present during the entire cell cycle have been identified. DNA synthesis can be detected by modified nucleotides, including bromodeoxyuridine (BrdU). Immunofluorescence can visualize the incorporation of BrdU in the DNA; this technique has been used to assess cell proliferation (Fig.

71-3). This methodology visualizes cells undergoing DNA synthesis. Therefore, cells in S phase or in which DNA damage is repaired show BrdU labeling.[12] An obvious limitation of this procedure is that the chances that a cycling cell will incorporate the nucleotide are restricted to the period of exposure to the marker. Additionally, cells at the G_1-S boundary are not labeled and the G_1 phase may be particularly long, resulting in an underestimation of the actual number of cycling cells.

Expression of the proliferating cell nuclear antigen (PCNA) is associated with cell proliferation, being low in quiescent cells and high in cycling cells.[13] An increase in PCNA is observed in late G_1, and a further increase occurs in S phase. G_2-M cells show a markedly reduced level of PCNA immunofluorescence. PCNA acts as a sliding clamp that allows DNA polymerase δ and ε to move quickly along the DNA while remaining tightly bound.[13] Moreover, PCNA is an integral component of DNA repair,[13] limiting its utilization as a marker of cell proliferation in many pathological conditions where cell multiplication is coupled with cell death and DNA damage. In the myocardium, increased PCNA transcription has been linked to DNA synthesis, DNA repair, and myocyte proliferation. In the presence of ventricular failure following acute myocardial infarction or in conditions of global ischemia, PCNA and histone-H_3 messenger RNA levels are upregulated in myocytes, and the distribution of PCNA protein in the cells correlates closely with the regional variations in diastolic wall stress in the injured ventricle. PCNA labeling of myocytes occurs in the human heart affected by terminal failure in combination with the appearance of myocyte nuclear and cell division.[14]

Ki67 is a nuclear protein present only in proliferating cells (see Fig. 71-3). This antigen is expressed during late G_1, S, G_2, prophase, and metaphase, declining progressively in anaphase and telophase.[15] Of relevance, Ki67 is absent in quiescent cells and is not involved in DNA repair. The function of this protein is largely unknown. The localization of Ki67 in the outer dense compartment of the nucleolus suggests a participation in ribosome biogenesis, required only when a rapid production of these organelles is necessary, such as during the cell cycle. Additionally, the C-terminal domain of Ki67 has the ability to bind DNA sequences rich in adenine and thymine, and may work as a transcription factor. A certain similarity with the consensus sequences of p53, an inhibitor of the cell cycle, and the stretches of nucleotides that Ki67 binds in vitro has been reported.[16] These findings have favored intriguing speculations concerning the potential opposite role that these two proteins may play in the cell cycle. In contrast to markers of S phase, Ki67 protein expression reflects a physiological state of the cell and is closely coupled with cell proliferation. The evaluation of Ki67 labeling of nuclei offers a sensitive approach for the analysis of the degree of cell multiplication. This nuclear protein recognizes cells in all the active phases of the cell cycle. Additionally, there is not a single example of a Ki67-positive cell that cannot divide.[15]

More recently, Cdc6 and the minichromosome maintenance (MCM) family of proteins have been employed as novel markers of cell multiplication (see Fig. 71-3). Eukaryotic cells possess control mechanisms to restrict DNA replication to one in the entire cell cycle. At the level of DNA, the origin recognition complex (ORC) determines where replication can initiate, and this allows Cdc6 to recruit MCM proteins. At this stage, the DNA is licensed to replicate.[17] During M-G_1 transition, a multiprotein complex is assembled at the ORC and awaits a signal to initiate DNA synthesis. As cells progress from the G_1 to S, this complex is activated. In late S phase, the dissociation of Cdc6 and MCM from chromatin ensures that DNA is replicated only once during a single division cycle. Despite the restriction of DNA replication to S phase, changes in the proteins associated with ORC occur throughout the cell cycle. Thus, Cdc6 and MCM recognize cells throughout G_1, S, and late mitosis, including anaphase and telophase.[17] Both Cdc6 and MCM are downregulated in terminally differentiated and quiescent cells.

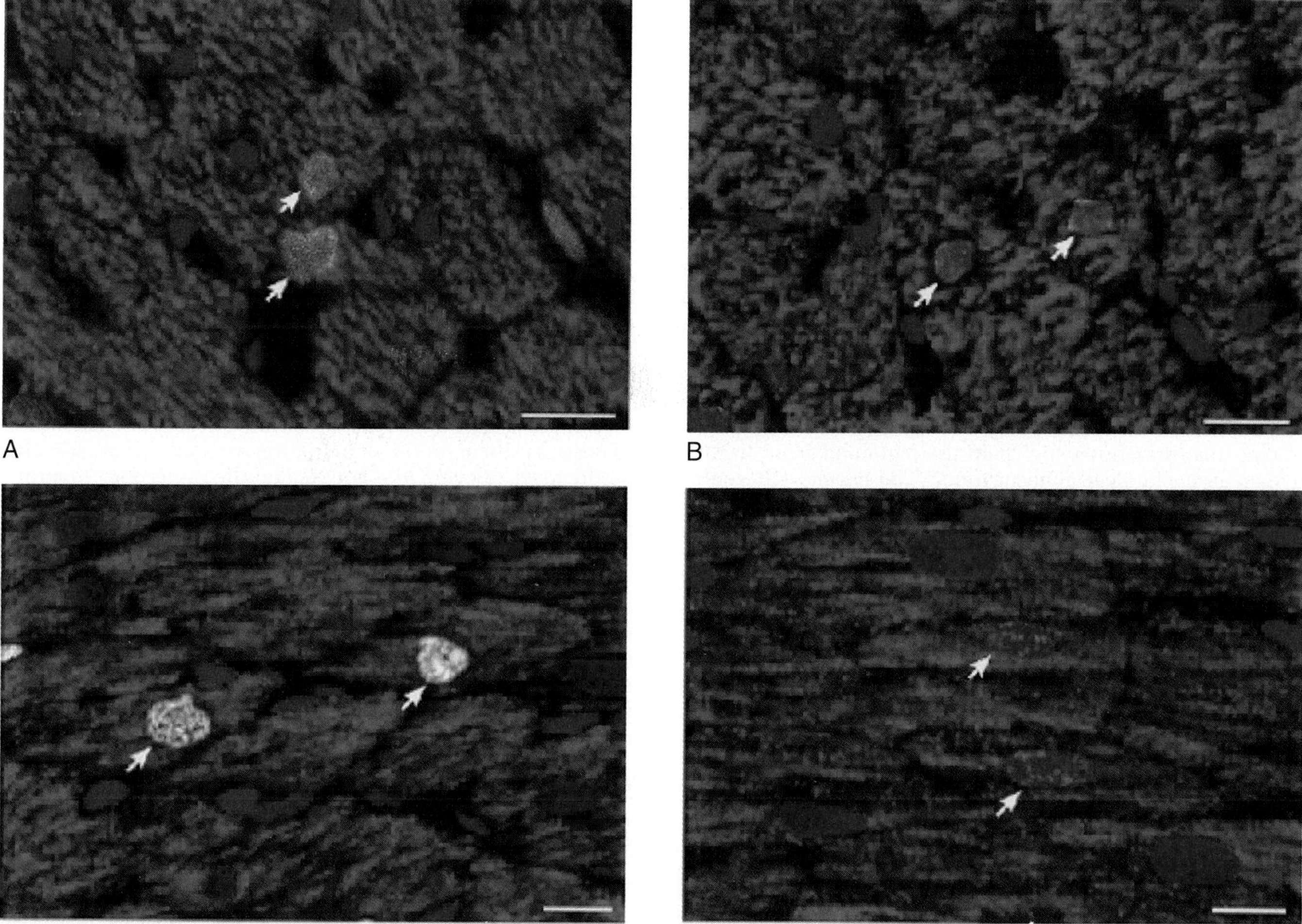

FIGURE 71–3 Markers of replicating myocytes. In each panel, two myocyte nuclei are positive for BrdU (**A,** yellow), Ki67 (**B,** green), MCM5 (**C,** white), and Cdc6 (**D,** magenta). Arrows point to cycling myocytes. Myocyte cytoplasm is recognized by alpha-sarcomeric actin (red) and nuclei by propidium iodide (blue). These sections derive from the ventricle of a Fischer rat. Confocal microscopy, bar = 10 μm.

On the basis of the earlier discussion, identification and quantification of the replicating pool in a given tissue or cell population require utilization of specific markers able to recognize molecules expressed only during the cell cycle and absent during quiescence. Colabeling with antibodies against contractile proteins recognizes dividing myocytes by high-resolution confocal microscopy.[9,10] Mitosis, the most impressive event within the cell cycle, is characterized by the formation of the mitotic spindle, with the bipolar shooting out of chromosomes, and the identification of the actomyosin contractile ring, which constricts and pinches off the membrane to form two daughter cells. These findings have shown unequivocally that adult cardiac myocytes undergo karyokinesis and cytokinesis. All stages of mitosis have been identified in myocytes and, thereby, mitotic indices have been computed by examining large areas of myocardium by confocal microscopy.

Magnitude of Myocyte Regeneration in the Damaged Heart

Evaluation of a myocyte mitotic index provides an important gauge of the rapidity and intensity of the response of the growth reserve of the heart to stressful conditions. The interpretation of the myocyte mitotic index is influenced by variables that are difficult to predict. For example, the time required for the completion of karyokinesis and cytokinesis of myocytes in vivo is unknown. Similarly, whether aging, ventricular loading, or disease states influence the duration of this nuclear or cellular event remains to be established. These determinants could attenuate or enhance myocardial growth and play a critical role in the adaptation of the heart to acute and chronic changes in wall stress. On this basis, the degree of myocyte division has been evaluated separately in acute and chronic heart failure of ischemic origin.

A myocyte mitotic index has been measured in myocyte nuclei of control and acutely infarcted human hearts by confocal microscopy. A value of $11/10^6$ myocytes was determined in control intact left ventricles, while a 47-fold higher value of $520/10^6$ myocytes was detected in the infarcted ventricles ($775/10^6$ in the border zone and $264/10^6$ in the remote myocardium). The expression of Ki67 was also measured. In comparison with $489/10^6$ myocytes in normal hearts, myocardial infarcts resulted in an 84-fold, $40{,}997/10^6$, and 28-fold, $13{,}799/10^6$, increase in the number of myocyte nuclei labeled by Ki67 in the region bordering and remote from infarction, respectively. Thus, the number of Ki67-positive myocyte nuclei was three times higher in the region adjacent to than distant from the dead myocardium.[9] The normal left ventricle contains 5.5×10^9 myocytes, and this value decreases to 3.8×10^9 myocytes after a 30 percent infarct. The fraction of mitotic myocytes implies that 60,500 myocytes are in mitosis in the normal left ventricle and 1,976,000 in the infarcted left ventricle. Since mitosis lasts approximately 30 minutes, a 30 percent infarct would be replaced in less than 3 weeks if this level of myocyte regeneration persisted with time.[9]

The degree of cell division detected acutely after infarction suggests that, in the absence of a change in the rate of cell regeneration, 17×10^9 myocytes would be formed over a period of 6 months. Essentially, all left ventricular myocytes would be replaced three times in half a year. A relationship exists between the number of myocyte nuclei expressing Ki67 and the number of myocyte nuclei in mitoses. The number of cycling myocytes measured by Ki67 labeling is 50 times as high as the number of mitotic myocytes. On the assumption that mitosis is completed in 30 minutes, the duration of the myocyte cell cycle in vivo should be approximately 25 hours. When MCM5 labeling of myocyte nuclei and the myocyte mitotic index are considered (our unpublished results), the computed length of the cell cycle is nearly 45 hours. This is because Ki67 is expressed only late in G_1 and MCM5 is expressed during the entire G_1 phase.[15,17]

A mitotic index of $150/10^6$ myocytes has been found in the left ventricle of postinfarcted hearts in end-stage cardiac failure.[18] In the presence of 3.8×10^9 left ventricular myocytes, a mitotic index of $150/10^6$ implies that 570,000 cells are in mitosis and 4.9×10^9 myocytes are formed in 6 months. Similar results have been obtained in patients with end-stage dilated cardiomyopathy.[18] Therefore, myocyte regeneration is attenuated in chronically decompensated hearts, suggesting that the duration of the disease and the persistence of a high loading state lead to a progressive utilization of the proliferative cell reserve of the myocardium, and this phenomenon may promote terminal failure.

In spite of these various approaches that provide relevant indices of myocyte multiplication, by definition, myocyte proliferation corresponds to an absolute increase in the number of parenchymal cells in the ventricle or the heart. However, myocyte loss, an event common to aging and cardiac diseases, complicates the estimation of the real number of newly formed myocytes. Myocyte loss results in an underestimation of myocyte hyperplasia, and myocyte hyperplasia leads to an underestimation of the magnitude of myocyte death in the heart. Thus, myocyte proliferation may be obscured by myocyte loss, and the measurement of cell number may not give unequivocal evidence of cell regeneration. This consideration pertains to several forms of heart failure, particularly of ischemic origin. Thus, the quantitative estimation of the actual number of newly generated myocytes presents a difficult challenge whether it concerns physiological or pathological conditions of the adult heart.[19]

Quantitative measurements of myocyte proliferation in the overloaded heart in animal models have documented increases in the number of myocytes that varied from 20 to 45 percent.[4] These values are significantly lower than those obtained in the decompensated human heart in which myocyte number is more than doubled in conditions of extreme hypertrophy with a heart weight of nearly 2 pounds.[19] In human hearts weighing more than 500 gm, myocyte proliferation has been identified as the prevailing mechanism of increased muscle mass.[19] Because of the contribution of myocyte death in heart failure, these levels of cell regeneration can be interpreted only as minimal indices of the actual magnitude of myocyte proliferation in the pathological heart. The remarkable degrees of myocyte reconstitution in the diseased heart emphasize the importance of defining the origin of the newly formed myocytes. This information is critical for the potentiation of a cellular process that could have relevant therapeutic implications for "mending the broken heart." Myocardial regeneration is the most promising form of remedy for the damaged failing heart.

The challenging results discussed earlier indicate that the old paradigm concerning the growth property of adult myocytes should be changed to the new paradigm that recognizes that myocytes can undergo cellular hypertrophy and cell division. This new view raises questions about the factors conditioning distinct growth reactions of the myocyte compartment. The critical issue is myocyte replication since myocyte hypertrophy can be interpreted as a terminally differentiated cell that has exercised the ability only to expand the myofibrillar and nonmyofibrillar components of the cytoplasm. Conversely, several feasible mechanisms of myocyte regeneration can be proposed, as follows:

1. The adult heart contains a subpopulation of partially differentiated myocytes, which can engage in a limited number of doublings before they acquire a mitotic block.
2. Resident primitive cells cluster in specific regions of the heart and, following activation, migrate to sites of cell turnover, where they replicate and differentiate, or

translocate to the proximity of areas of damage, where they undergo proliferation and differentiation.

3. Circulating progenitor cells mobilized from the bone marrow might reach the myocardium through the systemic circulation and, after homing, are conditioned by the local microenvironment to commit themselves to cardiac cell lineages, replacing myocytes and vascular structures (Fig. 71–4).
4. These three pathways could conceivably operate in combination.

Recent observations favor the possibility that primitive cells reside in the heart and possess the ability to differentiate and generate myocytes and coronary vessels.[1,2,20,21] However, this is still an issue of great controversy and intense study. The available data do not allow an indisputable answer to this important question.

Attenuation of Myocyte Replication

The mechanisms that cause the progressive decrease in myocyte proliferation in the diseased heart are unknown but point to a critical reduction in telomeric length possibly mediated by a chronic decline in telomerase activity. During the S phase of the cell cycle, the semiconservative model of DNA replication encounters an intrinsic obstacle consisting of the inability of conventional DNA polymerase to complete the synthesis of the lagging strand of the replication fork of the DNA double helix. This end-replication problem would cause progressive loss of genetic material and DNA shortening.[22] In eukaryotic cells a specialized DNA polymerase and protective caps called *telomeres* preserve the integrity of chromosomes. Telomeres are chromatin structures bound to an array of proteins localized at the ends of chromosomes. Telomerase is a ribonucleoprotein that acts as a reverse transcriptase extending the 3′ chromosomal ends by using its own RNA as a template.[22] Synthesis of telomeric repeats by telomerase prevents loss of DNA and allows complete duplication of DNA (Fig. 71–5).

Telomerase activity is a property of dividing cells. In germ cells, this protein ensures telomere length and unlimited proliferative potential. Somatic cells, with stem cell–like characteristics such as hematopoietic and basal epithelial cells, are telomerase competent.[23] Telomerase does not operate in somatic replicating cells. The telomeric DNA, which is lost in each cell cycle, exceeds that synthesized.[24] However, telomeres are essential for chromosomal stability and, thereby, cell viability.[22,24] Telomere shortening coupled with cell division in the absence of telomerase activity is one of the major causes of telomere dysfunction in human cells.[24] Telomerase activity, however, does not necessarily prevent telomere erosion, which is also influenced by the telomeric proteins TRF1 and TRF2. Loss of these proteins leads to telomere instability, which is as critical as telomeric shortening in determining the destiny of a cell.[25] Telomere erosion to a critically short length results in end-to-end fusions or chromatin anaphase bridges and triggers cell arrest and/or apoptosis. This phenomenon can occur in cardiomyocytes (see Fig. 71–5). Average telomeric length varies between 9 and 10 kilobase pairs[26] in both dogs and humans,[27] and is approximately 30 to 40 kilobase pairs in mice, and undetermined as yet in rats.[24]

The proliferative history of a cell is written on telomeres: telomere erosion tells us the number of past divisions experienced by a somatic cell and, most important, its residual proliferative potential. However, average telomeric length provides only an approximate indication of the actual length of individual telomeres. This is because loss of DNA and telomeric shortening do not affect all telomeres homogeneously. Shortening preferentially occurs in a fraction of telomeres, and the shortest telomere present in a cell is critical for cell viability and chromosome integrity.[24] The identification in myocytes of specific chromosomes with shortest telomeres may clarify issues related to myocyte growth and death; the fate of a myocyte may be determined by its shortest telomere. Telomeric shortening has been detected in a subpopulation of myocytes in the old rat heart affected by chronic cardiac failure[28] in combination with an age-dependent decrease in telomerase activity.[29] Conversely, this enzyme activity is increased in acute cardiac failure in dogs preserving telomeric length in myocytes.[27]

Thus, cardiomyocyte hypertrophy and regeneration constitute the growth reserve mechanisms of the heart during aging and cardiac diseases. Cellular growth, however, is controlled by telomeric length and telomerase activity. The relative impact of these factors on myocyte growth can be better characterized when telomerase function is repressed. Knockout mice in which the RNA component of telomerase has been deleted have a severe attenuation in myocyte regeneration.[30] Because of the complete lack of telomerase activity, these mice exhibit shortening of telomeres at a rate of 3 to 5 kilobase pairs per cell cycle. This mutation severely affects cell death and markedly enhances cardiomyocyte renewal. The expression of the tumor suppressor p53 with activation of myocyte apoptosis becomes apparent when the mean length of telomeres is reduced by 55 to 65 percent to nearly 14 kilobase pairs. These phenomena result in pathological cardiac remodeling and ventricular decompensation at 6 to 8 months after birth, underlining the importance of the absence

Mechanisms of Myocardial Regeneration

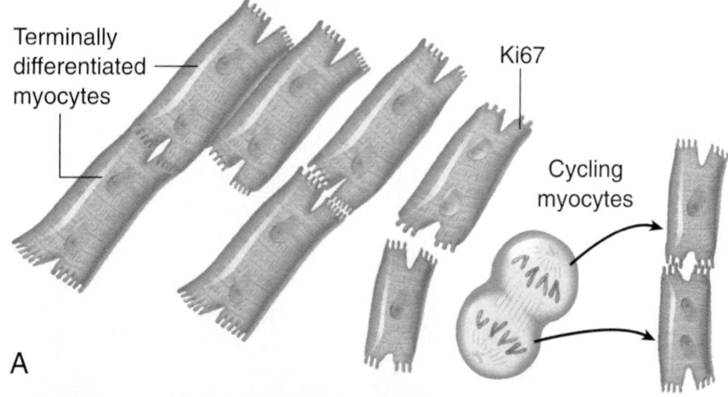

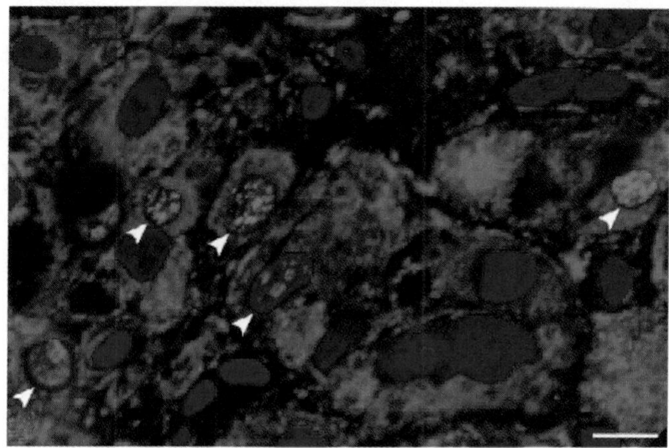

FIGURE 71–4 Mechanisms of myocardial regeneration. Several potential mechanisms of myocardial reconstitution are shown in schematic forms in **A, C,** and **E** and by confocal microscopy of tissue sections in **B, D,** and **F**. **A** schematically illustrates terminally differentiated myocytes and dividing or cycling myocytes. **B** shows a group of small developing myocytes expressing the cell cycle marker, Ki67 (green, arrowheads) in their nuclei. The myocyte cytoplasm is recognized by alpha-sarcomeric actin (red) and nuclei by propidium iodide (PI) (blue). This image corresponds to a human heart in end-stage failure. Confocal microscopy, bar = 10 μm. *Continued*

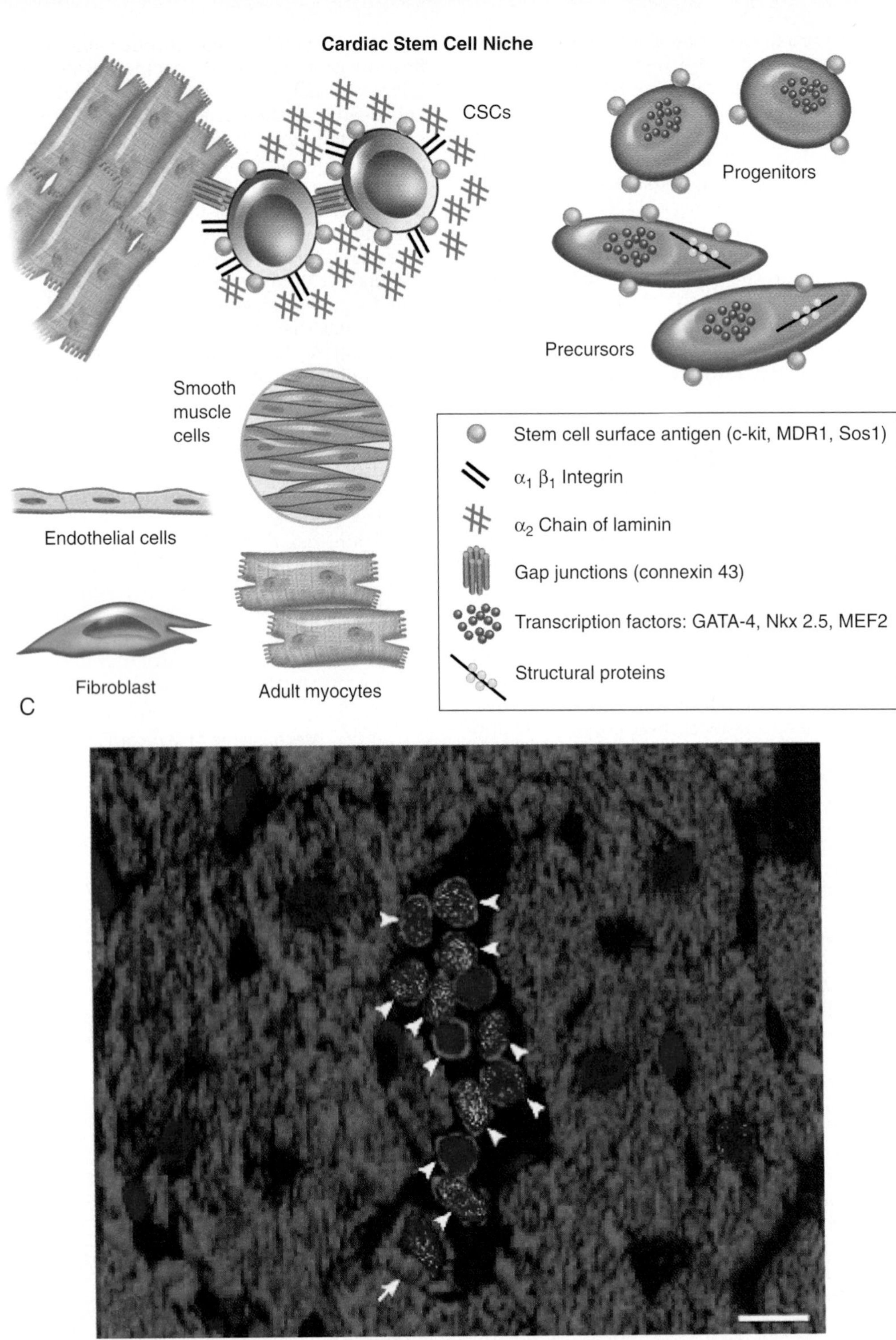

FIGURE 71–4, cont'd **C** illustrates schematically a cardiac stem cell (CSC) niche containing primitive cells, progenitors, and precursors. Primitive cells express stem cell surface antigens and integrin receptors. Progenitors are similar to primitive cells but also express cardiac or myocyte transcription factors. Precursor cells are similar to primitive and progenitor cells but contain in their cytoplasm structural proteins such as alpha-sarcomeric actin and cardiac myosin heavy chain. These cells lose the surface antigens and progressively become fully differentiated myocytes. A similar pattern of growth occurs in endothelial cells, smooth muscle cells, and fibroblasts. **D** demonstrates some of the aspects of cell differentiation illustrated in C. A cluster of primitive cells expressing the stem cell surface antigen c-kit (green) is documented within the ventricular myocardium. Nine (arrowheads) of the 12 c-kit positive cells express GATA-4 (white) in their nuclei. The nucleus of a small maturing myocyte is positive for GATA-4 (arrow). The myocyte cytoplasm is recognized by alpha-sarcomeric actin (red) and nuclei by PI (blue). This section corresponds to the ventricle of a Fischer rat. Confocal microscopy, bar = 10 μm.

of myocyte division in the development of heart failure.[30] This observation demonstrates the pivotal role of myocyte regeneration in the preservation of the performance of the heart under physiological conditions. Any imposition of an abnormal load might potentiate this impaired adaptation of the "nonmitotic heart" and favor precocious cardiac failure and death of the organism.

In summary, efforts have been made in the past 10 years to identify the mechanisms of myocyte growth in the pathological heart. Myocyte hypertrophy and proliferation in

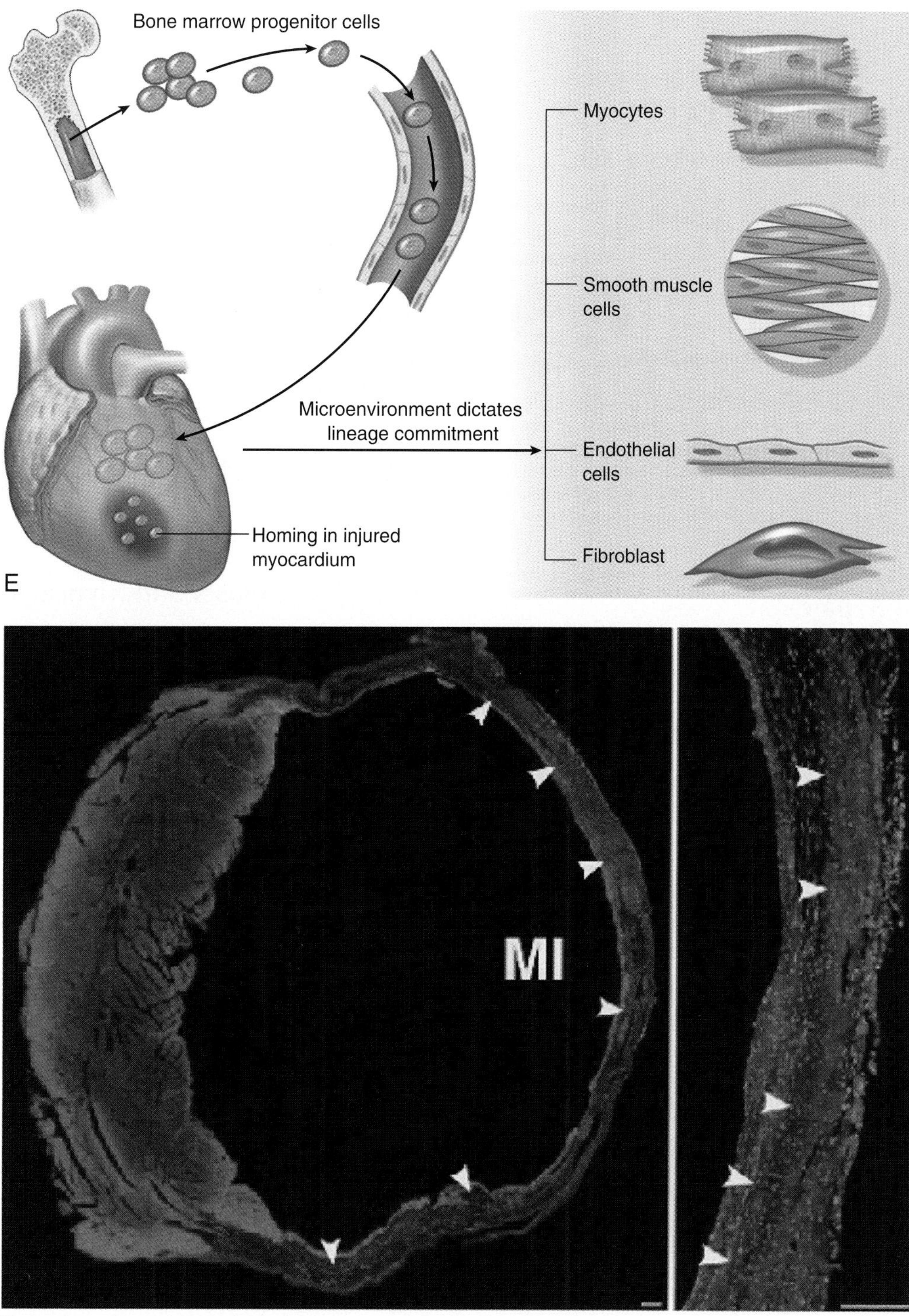

FIGURE 71–4, cont'd **E** presents in a schematic form the repair of infarcted myocardium by circulating and bone marrow–mobilized progenitor cells. **F** demonstrates the actual regeneration of infarcted myocardium 27 days after the increase in circulating progenitor cells mediated by the systemic administration of cytokines in mice. The regenerating band indicated by arrowheads in the large transverse section is shown at higher magnification in the adjacent panel. New myocytes are identified by the red fluorescence of cardiac myosin. Green-yellow fluorescence reflects PI labeling of nuclei. Confocal microscopy, bar = 200 μm. (**A** to **F**, From Orlic D, Kajstura J, Chimenti S, et al: Mobilized bone marrow cells repair the infarcted heart, improving function and survival. Proc Natl Acad Sci U S A 98:10344-10349, 2001.)

combination with myocyte death, apoptotic and necrotic in nature, constitute the fundamental elements of cardiac remodeling. Improvement in methodology enabled experiments that have disproved the dogma introduced more than 60 years ago that all myocytes are terminally differentiated. There is a group of myocytes that expresses the molecular components required for entry into the cell cycle and the regulation of their progression through S, G_2, karyokinesis, and cytokinesis. The recognition that myocyte hypertrophy and regeneration, and myocyte necrosis and apoptosis, occur in the diseased heart has significantly enhanced our understanding of the plasticity of the myocardium and the critical role played by cell death and cell division in the complex transition from cardiac hypertrophy to heart failure.

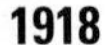

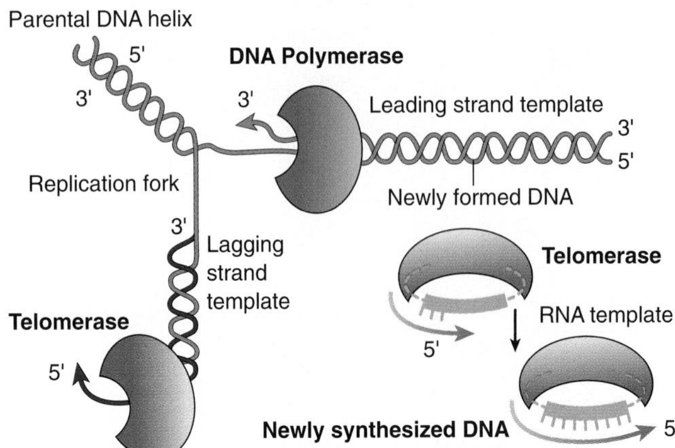

FIGURE 71–5 The end-replication problem. During cell division, conventional DNA polymerase cannot complete the synthesis of the lagging strand of the replication fork of the DNA double helix. This end-replication problem would cause progressive shortening of the DNA. However, telomerase, which is a reverse transcriptase, extends the 3′ chromosomal ends using its own RNA as a template. Synthesis of telomeric repeats by telomerase protects from loss of nucleic acid, allowing complete replication of DNA.

Myocardial Repair

Repair of damaged tissues and organs implies two distinct but interconnected processes: dead cells must be replaced by newly generated ones, and the newborn cells have to differentiate and become organized in a complex pattern that, ideally, restores the original structure of the injured tissue. However, this dual process usually occurs only during physiological cell turnover, in the absence of damage. For example, the bone marrow replenishes the blood with terminally differentiated cells, and the cells nested in the bulge of the hair follicle replace dead keratinocytes in the epidermis. Conversely, ischemic injury results in scar formation in all tissues, whether parenchymal cells are highly proliferating, slow cycling, or terminally differentiated. In the skin, which is an organ characterized by elevated levels of cell proliferation, wound healing leads to substitution of the damaged area with fibrotic tissue. The scarred portion of the skin does not possess the properties of the unaffected skin in terms of cellular composition, architecture, and biochemical and physical function. It is unknown why lesions of various etiologies cannot be repaired with complete *restitutio ad integrum*. Whether this depends on the accumulation of transforming growth factor-beta–like molecules (chalones) with massive inhibition of cell proliferation, chemorepellents of migrating cells (which could initiate the actual reconstitution of the damaged region), or inflammatory cytokines promoting leukocytes and fibroblast infiltration has not been identified. The need to overcome this biological obstacle of high clinical importance has stimulated the search for novel approaches to the replacement of dead cells with new functionally competent cells.

Several interventions have been used in the attempt to induce regeneration of damaged ventricular myocardium after infarction or cryoinjury in animal models. These therapeutic strategies have used a variety of cell types, including fetal cardiomyocytes and tissues, skeletal myoblasts, embryo-derived endothelial cells, bone marrow–derived immature myocytes, fibroblasts, smooth muscle cells, and bone marrow c-kit positive and negative primitive cells.[1,2,5,31,32] Promising results have been obtained with several of these cell types. Positive effects, including the successful survival of the implanted cells that occasionally integrated structurally and functionally with the host myocardium, have been reported. At times an improvement in cardiac performance has been found. Currently, however, there is no consensus but rather a vigorous debate on the most promising form of cellular therapy for myocardial injury.

Several problems confound the interpretation of attempts to ameliorate cardiac anatomy, function, or loading conditions with interventions involving fibroblasts, smooth muscle cells, and the other cell types indicated earlier. With the exception of bone marrow cells (BMCs) and neonatal myocytes, which generate cardiomyocytes and vascular structures,[33-35] it remains an open question how cell populations with no or minimal angiogenic properties furnish novel therapeutic tools of the decompensated heart of ischemic and nonischemic origin. Most important, the question concerning the reconstitution of scarred tissue into contracting myocardium has been addressed only peripherally. The ultimate form of cell therapy has to include an approach that can interfere and substitute acutely dead myocardium and areas of nonmechanically active scarred postischemic myocardium. Some specific therapeutic strategies are discussed in some detail because of their popularity and recent application to humans.[36-42] Questions are also raised in terms of the feasibility of these initial clinical trials in view of the data available from animal work.

Skeletal Myoblasts and Myocardial Repair

The first attempt to enwrap infarcted myocardium with a patch of skeletal muscle in humans was performed in the 1930s. Fifty years passed before large sheets of skeletal muscle tissue were positioned on the epicardial surface of the ischemic area and stimulated by a pacemaker. This surgical procedure, known as *dynamic cardiomyoplasty*, has prompted investigators to experimentally use individual myogenic cells instead of whole pieces of tissue. The new approach has been called *cellular cardiomyoplasty*. Isolated skeletal myoblasts or satellite cells have been directly injected into the ischemic zone or delivered through the coronary circulation.[43-46] Myogenic cells were obtained from the musculature of the limbs or abdomen of animals, which were subsequently exposed to ligation of the main left coronary artery or cryoinjury. The myogenic cells expanded in vitro were then injected in the infarcted or damaged portion of the ventricle to restore contractile function (Fig. 71–6). The autologous origin of the cells to be implanted constituted an obvious advantage compared with approaches of cardiac repair. The need for immunosuppressive therapy and the risk of immune rejection were circumvented. Moreover, skeletal myoblasts resist ischemia better than cardiomyocytes,[42] enhancing their survival in a region of the ventricle supplied by an occluded vessel. For these reasons, clinical trials of skeletal myoblast implantation have begun in patients with acute myocardial infarction injection of skeletal myoblasts during surgical revascularization.[42] Thus, two forms of treatment are applied simultaneously.

This intervention usually enhances cardiac function. However, it is difficult to establish whether the implanted cells constitute an active graft, which dynamically contributes to myocardial contractility, or a passive graft, which reduces negative remodeling by decreasing the stiffness of the scarred portion of the wall. Findings from different groups of investigators reflect these two possibilities. Hagège and collaborators report an improvement of systolic function in humans,[42] whereas Taylor and colleagues observe an amelioration of diastolic performance in animals.[45] Engraftment of other cell types, such as fibroblasts and embryonic cardiomyocytes, also improved diastolic function,[31,32] independent of their different origins. The elastic properties of the implanted myoblasts could, therefore, account for much of the improvement in ventricular hemodynamics. The lack of integration of skeletal myoblasts with surrounding viable

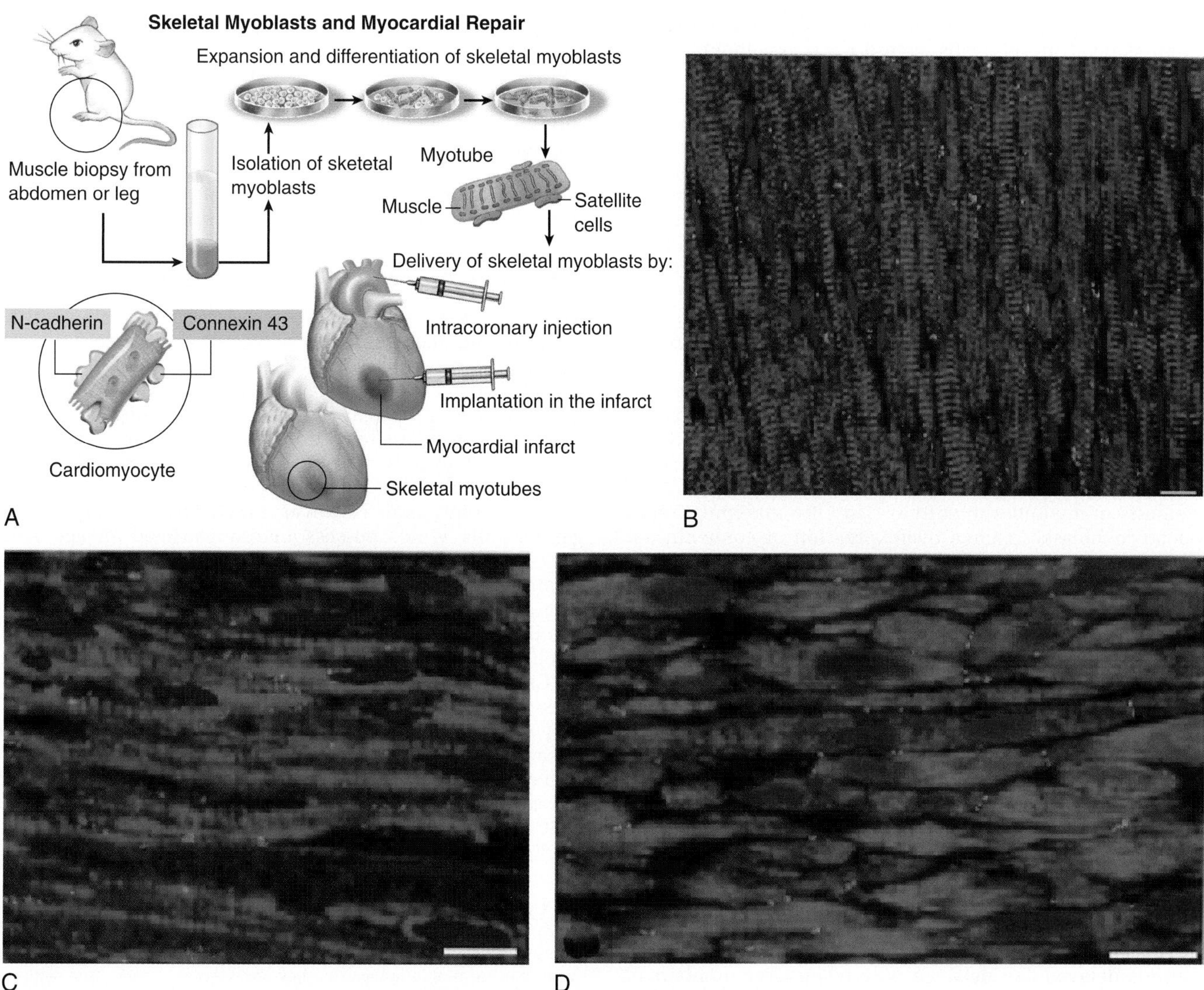

FIGURE 71–6 Skeletal myoblasts and myocardial injury. Schematic illustration of the different steps implicated in the preparation of skeletal myoblasts prior to injection **(A)**. The consequences of this form of intervention are also shown. Two critical proteins, connexin 43 and N-cadherin, are not expressed in implanted myoblasts. This deficiency does not allow electrical and mechanical coupling between injected skeletal myoblasts and between skeletal myoblasts and surrounding cardiomyocytes. **B** to **D,** Distribution of connexin 43 (green) is shown in adult mouse heart **(B)** and in regenerating tissue after infarction (**C,** green). Similarly, myocytes in the reconstituting myocardium possess N-cadherin (**D,** green). The myocyte cytoplasm is recognized by cardiac myosin antibody labeling (red) and nuclei are stained by propidium iodide (blue). Confocal microscopy, bar = 10 μm. (**C,** From Orlic D, Kajstura J, Chimenti S, et al: Mobilized bone marrow cells repair the infarcted heart, improving function and survival. Proc Natl Acad Sci U S A 98:10344-10349, 2001.)

tissue supports the likelihood of a passive graft. The absence of functional interaction between the graft and the spared myocardium represents a serious concern and limitation in the use of skeletal myoblasts for the repair of a dead region of the heart. Analysis of the graft-host organ interface has failed to provide evidence of mechanical or electrical coupling between skeletal myoblasts and resident cardiac myocytes. The microenvironment of the heart has apparently not permitted the desired effect of changing the biology of skeletal muscle cells into cardiomyocytes.

To appreciate the inherent problems with the therapeutic efficacy of skeletal myoblasts, a few comments on the role of the plasma membrane of cardiomyocytes in myocardial contractility may be helpful. Nexuses and fasciae adherentes of the intercalated discs constitute the intercellular junctions responsible, respectively, for electrical and mechanical coupling of myocytes (see Fig. 71–6). Nexuses or gap junctions are composed of clusters of intercellular channels at the interface of the cells.[47] By regulating the direct exchange of ions and small molecules between cells, these channels participate in various cellular processes, including differentiation, development, metabolic homeostasis, and electrical connection.[48] The connexins, a protein family with 15 distinct isoforms, form gap junctions. The rodent heart expresses at least three connexin proteins. Connexin 43 is the most abundant and localizes in both atrial and ventricular myocardium but not in pacemaker cells and the conduction system.[48] The fascia adherens or intermediate junction is a specialized region that provides strong cell-to-cell adhesion mediated by the cadherin/catenin complex through linkage to the actin cytoskeleton. This structure constitutes the site of attachment of myofibrils and aids the transmission of contraction across the plasma membrane of neighboring cells.[49] N-cadherin, a member of the Ca^{2+}-dependent cell-to-cell adhesion molecule family, is one of the distinctive components of the fascia adherens in the heart.[50] Cadherins act as adhesion-activated cell receptors.[50] The inhibition of N-cadherin causes myocytes to lose contact with adjacent cells, disrupting the organization of myofibrils. The integrity of the intercalated disc is, therefore, essential for the myocardium to function as a syncytium and to guarantee a synchronous contraction of its parenchymal cells.

Connexin 43 and N-cadherin are consistently absent in grafted skeletal muscle cells from 3 days to 3 months after surgery in both animal models and treated patients.[42] Thus, the grafts are unable to establish persistent electrical and mechanical interactions with the spared myocardium in vivo. A layer of dense, scarred tissue often separates the cardiomyocytes from the implanted skeletal muscle cells opposing the integration of these two cell populations in the infarcted heart. To evaluate whether the presence of this physical obstacle prevented the graft from making structural association with myocytes, skeletal myoblasts were injected in normal hearts. Although cardiac and skeletal muscle cells were nested together and there was a minimal amount of scarring, connexin 43 and N-cadherin did not develop in myoblasts and no direct communication was created with myocytes. Murry and collaborators[44] detected structures resembling adherens junctions and tight junctions exclusively in skeletal muscle cells. Unfortunately, in spite of an initial excitement, these structures correspond to low-resistance junctions, which commonly occur during fusion of myoblasts in myotubes in culture.[51] In vitro manipulation of skeletal myoblasts to force overexpression of connexin 43, has led to the appearance of gap junctions on the surface of cultured cells.[52] However, the efficacy of this approach remains to be shown in vivo. The absence of synchronous contraction may be one of the factors responsible for the episodes of arrhythmia in infarcted patients treated with skeletal myoblasts.[42]

Before skeletal myoblasts are employed for treatment, the cell population is expanded for 2 to 3 weeks in vitro. This necessity prevents the immediate clinical application of this form of therapy, and the delay may be critical in determining the number of surviving cells after implantation. The heart tissue shows extensive inflammation at this time, and the environment may be hostile for homing of skeletal myoblasts. Moreover, adult human myoblasts divide only 20 to 25 times before reaching senescence,[53] and the success of skeletal myoblast implantation is related to the number of donor cells. For this reason, the improvement in function in end-stage failure is delayed and detected only when large numbers of cells are administrated. A similar outcome has been found in patients with Duchenne myopathy. The need for a large quantity of cells has been attributed to acute and extensive cell death during the first week of engraftment.

During in vitro expansion and following introduction in the heart, myoblasts parallel the normal developmental process characterized by cell cycle withdrawal and myogenic differentiation with formation of myotubes.[44] The state of terminal differentiation rapidly acquired by skeletal myoblasts limits any possible proliferation of the implanted cells. The absence of cell turnover has a negative impact on the long-term efficacy of this kind of cellular cardiomyoplasty. Damaged cells within the graft cannot be replaced, impairing the mechanical and elastic properties of the graft and, ultimately, cardiac function. High-proliferative potential could be achieved with the implantation of immortalized myogenic cell lines. However, the risk of tumor formation precludes any clinical application.

Although this pioneer work with skeletal myoblasts has highlighted the need and importance of cellular therapy for ischemic heart disease, cardiac repair demands that the injured portion of the ventricular wall be replaced by tissue that has the same structural and functional properties of the lost myocardium. Complex manipulations of skeletal myoblasts have to be developed before these cells acquire the capability of reconstituting healthy functioning myocardium. The target of regenerative medicine must be the restoration of a tissue composed of parenchymal cells and vessels organized in an orderly manner, which resembles the native organ. In the cardiac microenvironment, the plasticity of skeletal muscle cells is quite limited. The only modification consists of a switch from fast-twitch muscle to slow-twitch muscle.[42] This phenotypic change is characterized by the expression of slow-twitch myosin isoforms,[44] suggesting that the cardiac milieu alters in part the developmental program of the implanted cells. However, transdifferentiation of skeletal myoblast in cardiac myocytes has never been observed. Conversely, the myocardial environment is permissive for a normal maturation of myogenic cells into skeletal myotubes.

Mesenchymal Stem Cells and Cardiac Repair

The bone marrow contains several cell types. In addition to differentiated cells, such as stroma, vascular cells, adipocytes, osteoblasts, and osteoclasts, a pool of primitive immature cells reside in the bone marrow. This class of cells has stem cell properties and is rather heterogeneous; it is composed of hematopoietic stem cells (HSCs) and mesenchymal stem cells[54] (MSCs). The bone marrow, followed by the peripheral and cord blood, constitutes the main source of MSCs in adulthood. However, MSCs or mesenchymal progenitor cells, which possess a more restricted lineage developmental potential, have been identified in tissues distant from the bone marrow. The oval cells of the liver, prostatic stem cells, metanephric mesenchymal cells, precursors of the Leydig cells in the testis, primitive osteoprogenitors, and satellite cells of the skeletal muscle have been classified as MSCs.[54] Not all studies agree that MSCs actually reside in these mesenchymal tissues. A "long-distance" traffic of MSCs may operate from the bone marrow through the blood stream.[54] Alternatively, embryonic primordia may be stored in a quiescent state in organs of mesodermal origin and participate in tissue repair in response to injury. We focus on MSCs of bone marrow origin, which have been used for cardiac repair.

Human and murine MSCs have been extensively characterized in vitro. MSCs are isolated from bone marrow aspirates and density gradient. These cells adhere quickly to the culture dish and grow as fibroblast-like cells, forming colonies that become visible 1 week after plating.[55] Following removal of HSCs and nonadherent cells, only a small percentage of the initial BMC population consists of MSCs, ranging from 0.001 to 0.01 percent. MSCs undergo a relatively few population doublings, from 4 to 20, maintaining the original normal karyotype and a constant level of telomerase activity.[54,55] Telomeric shortening does not occur in MSCs in culture. During the in vitro phase of amplification, MSCs usually do not differentiate spontaneously. However, by culturing them in distinct media containing different cytokines and growth factors, MSCs differentiate into multiple mesenchymal phenotypes, such as adipocytes, chondrocytes, and osteocytes.[54,55] The immunophenotype of MSCs has partially been defined. MSCs express adhesion receptors,[54,55] including CD29, CD44, CD71, CD90, CD106, CD120a, and CD124, and surface antigens[54] that are not present in HSCs, stromal hybridoma 2 (SH2), SH3, and SH4. These surface antigens have been identified in SH cell lines. They constitute early markers of undifferentiated MSCs and disappear with lineage commitment.[54] MSCs, however, are negative for markers of the hematopoietic lineage, including CD34 and the common leukocyte antigen CD45.[55]

This population of BMCs differentiates in cardiomyocytes in vitro. By dilution technique, clones of MSCs have been obtained.[56] Clonogenic cells have a fibroblast-like shape, but after stimulation with 5-aza-cytidine, which is a DNA demethylating agent that promotes the reactivation of gene expression, the morphology of nearly 30 percent of the cells changes from a spindle shape to a ball-like form and, with time, to a rod shape. Subsequently, the differentiating cells fuse together in a syncytium that resembles a myotube.[57] In spite of this characteristic that mimics the organization of skeletal muscle, MSC-derived cardiomyogenic cells exhibit markers of fetal cardiac myocytes.[57] The beta isoform of myosin heavy chain is expressed much more than the alpha isoform. Similarly, alpha skeletal actin predominates with respect to alpha cardiac actin. Myosin light chain-2v is also present. Specific transcription factors of the cardiac and myocyte lineage can be detected; they include GATA-4, Nkx2.5, and HAND1/2.[58] Alternative splicing forms of the *MEF2* gene are observed. From early to late passages, MEF2A and MEF2B are replaced by MEF2C and MEF2D.[57,58] The differentiation of this cardiomyogenic cell line seems to recapitulate the developmental program of gene expression during prenatal life, which is tightly regulated by the turning on and off of multiple genes. Finally, these cells express functionally competent alpha- and beta-adrenergic and muscarinic receptors on the membrane.[59] Cells beat spontaneously and synchronously in vitro, and the rate of contraction increases after exposure to isoproterenol, whereas the addition of a selective $beta_1$ blocker inhibits contractile activity.[59] The synchrony of contraction is most likely due to the formation of intercalated discs. The same phenomenon is observed when cardiomyogenic cells derived from MSCs are cocultured with neonatal myocytes.[60] Mechanical and electrical coupling between the two cell types has been observed in vitro. Intercalated discs have been identified in functionally competent myocytes by electron microscopy.

MSC-derived cardiomyogenic cells have been used for cardiac repair after experimental myocardial infarction. Four weeks after coronary artery occlusion in pigs, 100×10^6 autologous bone marrow stromal cells, which had been expanded and induced to differentiate in vitro, were injected in the infarcted region of the ventricular wall.[61] One month later, islands of cardiac-like tissue and new capillaries were found within the scarred tissue. Wall motion reappeared in the infarcted myocardium, suggesting that cell implantation led to partial reconstitution of dead myocardium that had positive consequences on the hemodynamics and anatomy of the damaged heart. Myocardial regeneration reduced cavitary volume, increased the thickness of the infarcted wall, and improved the contractile performance.[61] Similar results have been obtained in a model of ischemia reperfusion injury in pigs.[62] Two weeks after a 60-minute occlusion of the left anterior descending coronary artery, 6×10^7 labeled MSCs were directly injected in the infarcted area. By placing ultrasonic crystals within the ischemic region, the recovery of contractile activity could be followed during the entire period of observation. Systolic and diastolic function ameliorated and wall thinning was markedly reduced after 1 month. Cotransplantation of human MSCs and human fetal cardiomyocytes in infarcted pigs resulted in a greater improvement in cardiac function than with MSCs alone.[63]

Before discussing other results obtained with the injection of MSCs after infarction, it might be relevant to compare the efficacy of skeletal myoblasts and MSCs as distinct forms of therapy for the infarcted heart. In both cases, cells must be collected and expanded before utilization. The time factor can influence the engraftment of MSCs in the damaged area and how the changes in the microenvironment of the infarcted tissue interfere with cell growth and differentiation. However, MSCs possess the ability to generate myocytes and coronary vessels and, thereby, new myocardium.[61,63] MSCs should therefore have a greater therapeutic impact on cardiac repair than skeletal myoblasts. The latter does not differentiate into myocytes, and the creation of vascular structures by implantation of skeletal myoblasts remains to be demonstrated.

A number of other experiments have been performed in rats, utilizing MSC transplantation following cryoinjury of the myocardium.[64] BrdU-labeled cells were injected in the scar, which, 5 weeks later, contained muscle cells positive for troponin I, confirming their myocyte commitment. Additionally, large vascular structures and capillary profiles were detected in the area of damage.[64] The growing myocardium reduced the dimension of the scar in association with an improvement in peak systolic pressure and developed pressure of the treated infarcted rats. An alternative route of administration of MSCs has been attempted with the expectation that, if successful, the new procedure would have greater clinical relevance. Bone marrow stromal cells have been delivered directly through the coronary circulation.[65] However, MSCs differentiated into fibroblasts in the region of the scar and into cardiomyocytes in the surviving myocardium. This study emphasizes the importance of the microenvironment in guiding the developmental pathway of MSCs in vivo. These observations agree with in vitro reports of the medium-dependent specific lineage commitment engaged by MSCs.[54]

A lower degree of engraftment of MSCs has been found in the normal heart. In the study by Wang and collaborators,[66] MSCs implanted within the healthy rat ventricular myocardium were identified only at the site of injection. Conversely, in the paper by Toma and colleagues,[67] implanted cells were scattered throughout the myocardium, but they failed to accumulate in clusters. Only individual cells randomly distributed were detected up to 60 days after the intervention. Thus, in the absence of injury MSCs appear to remain in a viable partially quiescent state. In fact, they participate minimally in the physiological turnover of myocytes. In this regard, a relevant unexpected finding was that MSCs expressed connexin 43, forming gap junctions between engrafted cells and resident myocytes within the host myocardium.[66] A systemic infusion of MSCs was performed in lethally irradiated and nonconditioned adult baboons.[68] Transplantation was significantly more successful in animals exposed to irradiation. A broad distribution of MSCs was detected with a preferential engraftment in the gastrointestinal tract, kidney, lung, liver, thymus, and skin. Unfortunately, the heart was not harvested; therefore, no information is available regarding colonization of MSCs to the myocardium in nonhuman primates.

Recent work has identified a rare cell population within the MSC compartment of the bone marrow in mice.[55] These cells have been classified as multipotent adult progenitor cells (MAPCs). MAPCs can undergo more than 120 population doublings without modification of morphology or immunophenotype. Membrane antigens on MAPCs are not specific for a previously known progenitor cell. They share some characteristic with HSCs and some others with MSCs. MAPCs express low levels of Flk-1, Sca-1 and Thy-1, and higher levels of CD13 and stage-specific antigen I. In a manner similar to MSCs, MAPCs lack CD34, CD44, CD45, and the major histocompatibility complex classes I and II.[55] The surface antigen c-kit is typically present in HSCs and MSCs, although its level is lower in the latter group of stem cells.[54] A unique property of MAPCs is that c-kit is absent in this highly purified progenitor cell population. Whether this difference helps or hinders growth and commitment of MAPCs has not yet been determined.

In this regard, during embryogenesis in the blastocyst, MAPCs give rise to essentially all somatic tissues in the organism, including the myocardium. However, MAPCs only partly maintained this property following in vivo injection in the systemic circulation. The ability to differentiate into cardiac and skeletal muscle, kidney, skin, and brain tissues is lost, raising questions whether the therapeutic applications of these progenitor cells as a source of repair of several important vital organs. This limitation is particularly significant because similar results were obtained in intact and irradiated injured animals.

In summary, it is currently difficult to reach definitive conclusions concerning the use of MSCs and MAPCs for myocardial regeneration. The observations made so far require confirmation, and specific experimental protocols aiming at target organs have to be developed and tested. The actual potential of MSCs and progenitor cells in tissue reconstitution remains an open, important question.

Bone Marrow Cells and Myocardial Repair

In addition to MSCs, the bone marrow possesses a blood-forming stem cell. This is a rare cell population that corresponds to true HSCs, which are responsible for the permanent long-term reconstitution of hematopoiesis. These cells are few and their phenotype is well established.[69] HSCs are lineage negative, Sca-1-positive, c-kit-positive, and Thy1.1-low. The plasticity of HSCs defined by their ability to generate tissues different from the organ of origin has recently been challenged.[70] A major problem in tissue regeneration including the myocardium is the lack of purity of bone marrow donor cells. This heterogeneity raises questions regarding the type of BMC that actually promotes the repair of an injured portion of an organ. Moreover, the use of enriched cell preparations and the difficulty of obtaining an actually pure and uniform cell population have cast doubts on the actual plasticity of HSCs. Alternative explanations have been offered, varying from the possibility of in vivo cell fusion to models based on the notion of preexisting heterogeneity of primitive cells within the bone marrow. In the first case, the replacement of damaged tissue in the liver and intestinal epithelia in vivo has been shown to be the consequence of fusion of BMCs with the existing cells, which then reacquire primitive properties.[71-73] This sequence, however, does not seem to operate in the heart.[1] In the second case, the bone marrow is viewed as a reservoir that contains progenitor cells in an early stage of commitment to multiple cell lineages.[74] Physiological turnover or discrete areas of injury may transmit signals to these poorly differentiated cells, which migrate from the bone marrow to these sites where they become activated and substitute for the old cell or repair the damage.

In spite of uncertainty about the mechanisms of cardiac repair, the use of BMCs in the management of myocardial infarction has advantages over other approaches employed in animals and humans. As discussed, at least in part, in the previous sections, efforts have been made to restore function in the infarcted myocardium by transplanting cultured fetal myocytes or tissue, adult myocytes, skeletal myoblasts, and bone marrow–derived immature cardiomyocytes. When incorporation of the engrafted cells or tissue was successful, some improvement in ventricular performance occurred. However, these approaches failed to reconstitute healthy myocardium, integrated structurally and functionally with the spared portion of the wall. This limitation was particularly evident with skeletal myoblasts. Moreover, the formation of vessels in the implants remained an unresolved problem. With the exception of skeletal myoblasts obtained from the recipient, the use of cyclosporine was required to prevent rejection. These issues have tempered the enthusiasm for this pioneering work and stimulated the search for new therapeutic strategies for the regeneration of dead myocardium.

The growth potential of adult HSCs or less purified BMCs injected in the circulation or locally delivered in areas of injury[33,75,76] raises the possibility that these primitive cells sense signals from lesions, migrate to regions of damage, and ultimately result in the reconstitution of the damaged tissue.[33,75,76] On this basis, an enriched population of lineage-negative, c-kit–positive BMCs were implanted into the viable myocardium in the proximity of an acute infarct in mice.[33] In less than 2 weeks, numerous small cardiomyocytes and vascular structures developed within the infarcted zone and replaced a large fraction of the dead myocardium. Myocytes expressed connexin 43, and the newly formed arterioles and capillaries were connected with the primary coronary circulation and were uniformly distributed within the regenerated portion of the ventricular wall. BMCs developed functioning myocardium, reduced infarct size, and ameliorated cardiac performance.[33]

Cytokines and growth factors appear to participate in the mobilization of stem cells and their translocation to damaged organs. This issue is highly relevant clinically because it might permit the application of strategies that do not require local implantation of exogenous stem cells or their preventive storage from the recipient. It is well established that SCF and granulocyte colony–stimulating factor induce a marked increase in the total number of circulating HSCs.[75] Mobilization by cytokines of HSCs into the circulation results in their localization to the infarcted portion of the ventricle, promoting regeneration of parenchymal cells and vascular structures and de novo reconstitution of viable myocardium (see Fig. 71–4). Therefore, two independent approaches have been identified for the regeneration of infarcted myocardium. A partial recovery was accomplished by autologous BMC implantation in dogs with chronic infarcts[77] and following the intravenous injection of CD34-positive BMCs in rats with acute myocardial injury.[78] The number of microvessels increased in both cases, mostly in the border zone. Angiogenesis and wall thickening improve cardiac performance.

On the basis of these few initial studies of myocardial regeneration and before the long-term consequences of BMC implantation could be established in animals, this procedure was translated to humans. Patients with acute myocardial infarcts have been treated with intracoronary delivery of BMCs at the time of reperfusion of the occluded vessel.[38,40,41,79] The immunophenotype of the administered cells in infarcted heart was established only in one case, in which the cells employed were AC133 positive.[40] AC133-positive bone marrow–derived cells are CD34 negative and have a high potential for angiogenesis.[40] In all trials, echocardiography showed a marked increase in ejection fraction and coronary blood flow. In some patients, wall motion recovered in the previously akinetic region and signs of myocardial viability were detected by fluorodeoxyglucose-positron emission tomography. Patients have been followed up to 6 months or 1 year after surgery. Malignant neoplasms have not been detected. In contrast to coronary infusion, six patients with acute infarcts were treated with local myocardial implantation of BMCs. Early after the intervention, ventricular arrhythmia developed in two cases and pericardial effusion in two others. At 16 months, the six patients were alive and reported a noticeable improvement in exercise capacity.[40] Finally, eight patients with refractory stable angina received an injection of BMCs through a catheter, which was guided to the ischemic areas by nonfluoroscopic left ventricular electromechanical mapping. The cells were a mixed population of primitive and early committed cells: about 8 percent exhibited only CD34, and the remaining were CD3-positive T cells, CD11b-positive/D15-positive granulocyte precursors, and granulocyte colony–forming units. The episodes of angina were reduced and the thickness of the target wall was improved.[41] With the exception of this study, the major limitation of these small clinical trials is that the delivery of bone marrow–derived cells is done simultaneously with revascularization of the ischemic region, complicating interpretation of the results. Therefore, the success of BMC therapy as a novel treatment of the ischemic myopathy is unresolved.

REFERENCES

1. Nadal-Ginard B, Kajstura J, Leri A, et al: Myocyte death, growth and regeneration in cardiac hypertrophy and failure. Circ Res 92:139-150, 2003.
2. Anversa P, Nadal-Ginard B: Myocyte renewal and ventricular remodeling. Nature 415:240-243, 2002.
3. Chien KR, Olson EN: Converging pathways and principles in heart development and disease. Cell 110:153-162, 2002.
4. Anversa P, Kajstura J: Ventricular myocytes are not terminally differentiated in the adult mammalian heart. Circ Res 83:1-14, 1998.
5. Anversa P, Leri A, Kajstura J, et al: Myocyte growth and cardiac repair. J Mol Cell Cardiol 34:91-105, 2002.
6. Conlon I, Raff M: Size control in animal development. Cell 96:235-244, 1999.
7. Molkentin JD, Dorn GW II: Cytoplasmic signaling pathways that regulate cardiac hypertrophy. Annu Rev Physiol 63:391-426, 2001.
8. Taylor DA, Hruban R, Rodriguez ER, et al: Cardiac chimerism as a mechanism for self-repair: Does it happen and if so to what degree? Circulation 106:2-4, 2002.
9. Beltrami AP, Urbanek K, Kajstura J, et al: Evidence that human cardiac myocytes divide after myocardial infarction. N Engl J Med 344:1750-1757, 2001.
10. Quaini F, Urbanek K, Beltrami AP, et al: Chimerism of the transplanted heart. N Engl J Med 346:5-15, 2002.
11. Setoguchi M, Leri A, Wang S, et al: Activation of cyclins and cyclin-dependent kinases, DNA synthesis, and myocyte mitotic division in pacing-induced heart failure in dogs. Lab Invest 79:1545-1558, 1999.
12. Dolbeare F: Bromodeoxyuridine: A diagnostic tool in biology and medicine: III. Proliferation in normal, injured and diseased tissue, growth factors, differentiation, DNA replication sites and in situ hybridization. Histochem J 28:531-575, 1996.
13. Larsen JK, Landberg G, Roos G: Detection of proliferating cell nuclear antigen. Methods Cell Biol 63:419-431, 2001.
14. Quaini F, Cigola E, Lagrasta C, et al: End-stage cardiac failure in humans is coupled with the induction of PCNA and nuclear mitotic division in myocytes. Circ Res 75:1050-1063, 1994.
15. Scholzen T, Gerdes J: The Ki-67 protein: from the known to the unknown. J Cell Physiol 182:311-322, 2000.
16. MacCallum DE, Hall PA: The biochemical characterization of the DNA binding activity of pKi67. J Pathol 191:286-298, 2000.
17. Stoeber K, Tlsty TD, Happerfield L, et al: DNA replication licensing and human cell proliferation. J Cell Sci 114:2027-2041, 2001.
18. Kajstura J, Leri A, Finato N, et al: Myocyte proliferation in end-stage cardiac failure in humans. Proc Natl Acad Sci U S A 95:8801-8805, 1998.

19. Anversa P, Olivetti G: Cellular basis of physiological and pathological myocardial growth. *In* Page E, Fozzard HA, Solaro RJ (eds): Handbook of Physiology. Chicago, Oxford University Press, 2002, pp 75-144.
20. Anversa P, Kajstura J, Nadal-Ginard B, et al: Primitive cells and tissue regeneration. Circ Res 92:579-582, 2003.
21. Nadal-Ginard B, Kajstura J, Anversa P, et al: A matter of life and death. J Clin Invest 111:1457-1459, 2003.
22. Cong YS, Wright WE, Shay JW: Human telomerase and its regulation. Microbiol Mol Biol Rev 66:407-425, 2002.
23. Allsopp RC, Morin GB, DePinho R, et al: Telomerase is required to slow telomere shortening and extend replicative lifespan of HSC during serial transplantation. Blood 102:517-520, 2003.
24. Hande MP, Samper E, Lansdorp P, et al: Telomere length dynamics and chromosomal instability in cells derived from telomerase null mice. J Cell Biol 144:589-601, 1999.
25. Smogorzewska A, van Steensel B, Bianchi A, et al: Control of human telomere length by TRF1 and TRF2. Mol Cell Biol 20:1659-1668, 2000.
26. Nakamura K, Izumiyama-Shimomura N, Sawabe M, et al: Comparative analysis of telomere lengths and erosion with age in human epidermis and lingual epithelium. J Invest Dermatol 119:1014-1019, 2002.
27. Leri A, Barlucchi L, Limana F, et al: Telomerase expression and activity are coupled with myocyte proliferation and preservation of telomeric length in the failing heart. Proc Natl Acad Sci U S A 98:8626-8631, 2001.
28. Kajstura J, Pertoldi B, Leri A, et al: Telomere shortening is an in vivo marker of myocyte replication and aging. Am J Pathol 156:813-819, 2000.
29. Leri A, Malhotra A, Liew CC, et al: Telomerase activity in rat cardiac myocytes is age and gender dependent. J Mol Cell Cardiol 32:385-390, 2000.
30. Leri A, Franco S, Zacheo A, et al: Ablation of telomerase and telomere loss leads to cardiac dilatation and heart failure associated with p53 upregulation. EMBO J 22:131-139, 2003.
31. Gepstein L: Derivation and potential applications of human embryonic stem cells. Circ Res 91:866-876, 2002.
32. El Oakley RM, Ooi OC, Bongso A, et al: Myocyte transplantation for myocardial repair: A few good cells can mend a broken heart. Ann Thorac Surg 71:1724-1733, 2001.
33. Orlic D, Kajstura J, Chimenti S, et al: Bone marrow cells regenerate infarcted myocardium. Nature 410:701-705, 2001.
34. Hirschi KK, Goodell MA: Hematopoietic vascular and cardiac fates of bone marrow–derived stem cells. Gene Therapy 9:648-652, 2002.
35. Reffelmann T, Dow JS, Dai W, et al: Transplantation of neonatal cardiomyocytes after permanent coronary artery occlusion increases regional blood flow of infarcted myocardium. J Mol Cell Cardiol 35:607-613, 2003.
36. Hamano K, Mishida M, Hirata K, et al: Local implantation of autologous bone marrow cells for therapeutic angiogenesis in patients with ischemic heart disease: Clinical trial and preliminary results. Jpn Circ J 65:845-847, 2001.
37. Assmus B, Schachinger V, Teupe C, et al: Transplantation of progenitor cells and regeneration enhancement in acute myocardial infarction (TOPCARE-AMI). Circulation 106:3009-3017, 2002.
38. Strauer BE, Brehm M, Zeus T, et al: Repair of infarcted myocardium by autologous intracoronary mononuclear bone marrow cell transplantation in humans. Circulation 106:1913-1918, 2002.
39. Beran G: Autologous stem cells injection in a patient after acute myocardial infarction. Heart Surg Forum 6:9, 2002.
40. Stamm C, Westphal B, Kleine HD, et al: Autologous bone-marrow stem-cell transplantation for myocardial regeneration. Lancet 361:45-46, 2003.
41. Tse HF, Kwong YL, Chan JKF, et al: Angiogenesis in ischaemic myocardium by intramyocardial autologous bone marrow mononuclear cell implantation. Lancet 361:47-49, 2003.
42. Hagège AA, Carrion C, Menasché P, et al: Viability and differentiation of autologous skeletal myoblast grafts in ischaemic cardiomyopathy. Lancet 361:491-492, 2003.
43. Koh GY, Klug MG, Soonpaa MH, et al: Differentiation and long-term survival of C2C12 myoblast grafts in heart. J Clin Invest 92:1548-1554, 1993.
44. Murry CE, Wiseman RW, Schwartz SM, Hauschka SD: Skeletal myoblast transplantation for repair of myocardial necrosis. J Clin Invest 98:2512-2523, 1996.
45. Taylor DA, Atkins BZ, Hungspreugs P, et al: Regenerating functional myocardium: Improved performance after skeletal myoblast transplantation. Nat Med 4:929-933, 1998.
46. Suzuki K, Murtuza B, Suzuki N, et al: Intracoronary infusion of skeletal myoblasts improves cardiac function in doxorubicin-induced heart failure. Circulation 104:I213-I217, 2001.
47. Kumar NM, Gilula NB: The gap junction communication channel. Cell 84:381-388, 1996.
48. Spray DC, Suadicani SO, Srinivas M, et al: Gap junctions in the cardiovascular system. *In* Page E, Fozzard HA, Solaro RJ (eds): Handbook of Physiology. Chicago, Oxford University Press, 2002, pp 169-212.
49. Luo Y, Radice GL: Cadherin-mediated adhesion is essential for myofibril continuity across the plasma membrane but not for assembly of the contractile apparatus. J Cell Sci 116:1471-1479, 2003.
50. Yap AS, Kovacs EM: Direct cadherin-activated cell signaling: A view from the plasma membrane. J Cell Biol 160:11-16, 2003.
51. Bonincontro A, Cametti C, Hausman RE, et al: Changes in myoblast membrane electrical properties during cell-cell adhesion and fusion in vitro. Biochim Biophys Acta 903:89-95, 1987.
52. Suzuki K, Brand NJ, Allen S, et al: Overexpression of connexin 43 in skeletal myoblasts: Relevance to cell transplantation to the heart. J Thorac Cardiovasc Surg 122:759-766, 2001.
53. Decary S, Mouly V, Hamida CB, et al: Replicative potential and telomere length in human skeletal muscle: Implications for satellite cell–mediated gene therapy. Hum Gene Ther 8:1429-1438, 1997.
54. Minguell JJ, Erices A, Conget P: Mesenchymal stem cells. Exp Biol Med 226:507-520, 2001.
55. Jiang Y, Jahagirdar BN, Reinhardt RL, et al: Pluripotency of mesenchymal stem cells derived from adult marrow. Nature 418:41-49, 2002.
56. Colter DC, Sekiya I, Prockop DJ: Identification of a subpopulation of rapidly self-renewing and multipotential adult stem cells in colonies of human marrow stromal cells. Proc Natl Acad Sci U S A 98:7841-7845, 2001.
57. Makino S, Fukuda K, Miyoshi S, et al: Cardiomyocytes can be generated from marrow stromal cells in vitro. J Clin Invest 103:697-705, 1999.
58. Fukuda K: Development of regenerative cardiomyocytes from mesenchymal stem cells for cardiovascular tissue engineering. Artif Organs 25:187-193, 2001.
59. Hakuno D, Fukuda K, Makino S, et al: Bone marrow–derived regenerated cardiomyocytes (CMG cells) express functional adrenergic and muscarinic receptors. Circulation 105:380-386, 2002.
60. Tomita S, Nakatani T, Fukuhara S, et al: Bone marrow stromal cells contract synchronously with cardiomyocytes in a coculture system. Jpn J Thorac Cardiovasc Surg 50:321-324, 2002.
61. Tomita S, Mickle DA, Weisel RD, et al: Improved heart function with myogenesis and angiogenesis after autologous porcine bone marrow stromal cell transplantation. J Thorac Cardiovasc Surg 123:1132-1140, 2002.
62. Shake JG, Gruber PJ, Baumgartner WA, et al: Mesenchymal stem cell implantation in a swine myocardial infarct model: Engraftment and functional effects. Ann Thorac Surg 73:1919-1925, 2002.
63. Min JY, Sullivan MF, Yang Y, et al: Significant improvement of heart function by cotransplantation of human mesenchymal stem cells and fetal cardiomyocytes in postinfarcted pigs. Ann Thorac Surg 74:1568-1575, 2002.
64. Tomita S, Li RK, Weisel RD, et al: Autologous transplantation of bone marrow cells improves damaged heart function. Circulation 100:II247-II256, 1999.
65. Wang JS, Shum-Tim D, Chedrawy E, Chiu RC: The coronary delivery of marrow stromal cells for myocardial regeneration: Pathophysiologic and therapeutic implications. J Thorac Cardiovasc Surg 122:699-705, 2001.
66. Wang JS, Shum-Tim D, Galipeau J, et al: Marrow stromal cells for cellular cardiomyoplasty: Feasibility and potential clinical advantages. J Thorac Cardiovasc Surg 120:999-1005, 2000.
67. Toma C, Pittenger MF, Cahill KS, et al: Human mesenchymal stem cells differentiate to a cardiomyocyte phenotype in the adult murine heart. Circulation 105:93-98, 2002.
68. Devine SM, Cobbs C, Jennings M, et al: Mesenchymal stem cells distribute to a wide range of tissues following systematic infusion into non-human primates. Blood 101:2999-3001, 2003.
69. Kondo M, Wagers AJ, Manz MG, et al: Biology of hematopoietic stem cells and progenitors: Implications for clinical applications. Annu Rev Immunol 21:759-806, 2003.
70. Wagers AJ, Sherwood RI, Christensen JL, et al: Little evidence for developmental plasticity of adult hematopoietic stem cells. Science 297:2256-2259, 2002.
71. Spees JL, Olson SD, Ylostalo J, et al: Differentiation, cell fusion, and nuclear fusion during ex vivo repair of epithelium by human adult stem cells from bone marrow stroma. Proc Natl Acad Sci U S A 100:2397-2402, 2003.
72. Vassilopoulos G, Wang PR, Russell DW: Transplanted bone marrow regenerates liver by cell fusion. Nature 422:901-904, 2003.
73. Wang X, Willenbring H, Akkari Y, et al: Cell fusion is the principal source of bone marrow–derived hepatocytes. Nature 422:897-901, 2003.
74. Orkin SH, Zon LI: Hematopoiesis and stem cells: Plasticity versus developmental heterogeneity. Nat Immunol 3:323-328, 2002.
75. Orlic D, Kajstura J, Chimenti S, et al: Mobilized bone marrow cells repair the infarcted heart, improving function and survival. Proc Natl Acad Sci U S A 98:10344-10349, 2001.
76. Jackson KA, Majka SM, Wang H, et al: Regeneration of ischemic cardiac muscle and vascular endothelium by adult stem cells. J Clin Invest 107:1395-1402, 2001.
77. Hassink RJ, Brutel de la Riviere A, Mummery CL, et al: Transplantation of cells for cardiac repair. J Am Coll Cardiol 41:711-717, 2003.
78. Kawamoto A, Tkebuchava T, Yamaguchi J, et al: Intramyocardial transplantation of autologous endothelial progenitor cells for the therapeutic neovascularization of myocardial ischemia. Circulation 107:461-468, 2003.
79. Strauer BE, Brehm M, Zeus T, et al: Repair of infarcted myocardium by autologous intracoronary mononuclear bone marrow cell transplantation in humans. Circulation 106:1913-1918, 2002.

PART IX

Cardiovascular Disease in Special Populations

CHAPTER 72

Cardiovascular Disease in the Elderly

Janice B. Schwartz • Douglas P. Zipes

Demographics and Epidemiology[1]

The proportion of people aged 65 years and older in the United States is projected to increase from 12.4 percent (35 million) of the population in 2000 to 19.6 percent in 2030 (71 million) and to 82 million in 2050. The number of people older than 80 years is projected to double from 9.3 million in 2000 to 19.5 million in 2030 and to more than triple by 2050. Women represented 59 percent of persons older than 65 years in 2000 and are estimated to make up 56 percent of the older population in 2030 (Fig. 72-1). If current projections hold, there will be increases in the percentage of racial minorities. From 2000 to 2030, the proportion of persons older than 65 years who are members of racial minority groups (i.e., black, Native American–Alaska Native, Asian–Pacific Islander) is expected to increase from 11.3 to 16.5 percent and the proportion of Hispanic people is expected to increase from 5.6 to 10.9 percent. Almost half of people older than 65 years in the United States in 2000 had after-tax incomes at the poverty level (41 percent of 65- to 74-year-olds and 56 percent of those older than 75 years); and this trend is likely to continue.[2] Global trends are similar, with the worldwide population older than 65 years projected to increase to 973 million or 12.0 percent in 2030 and make up about 20 percent of the population in 2050. Increases will be greatest in undeveloped nations. Estimates are for twice as many women as men older than 80 years and three times as many women as men older than 90.

Cardiovascular disease is the most frequent diagnosis in elderly people and is the leading cause of death in both men and women older than 65 years. Hypertension occurs in one-half to two-thirds of people older than 65 years, and heart failure (HF) is the most frequent hospital discharge diagnosis among older Americans. The profile of these common cardiovascular diseases in older patients differs from that in younger patients. Systolic, but not diastolic, blood pressure increases with aging, and systolic hypertension becomes a stronger predictor of cardiovascular events, especially in women. HF with preserved systolic function becomes more common at older ages and is more common in women than men. Coronary artery disease (CAD) is more likely to involve multiple vessels and left main artery disease and is equally likely in women and men older than 65 years. Equal numbers of older men and women present with acute myocardial infarction (AMI) until age 80, after which more women present. More than 80 percent of all deaths attributable to cardiovascular disease occur in people older than 65 years, with approximately 60 percent of deaths in patients older than 75 years.

Furthermore, cardiovascular disease in older people is not seen in isolation. Eighty percent of older Americans have at least one chronic medical condition and half have at least two. Arthritis affects about 60 percent of persons older than 65 years, and diabetes affects about 20 percent (Fig. 72–2). Ear, nose, and throat problems, vision disorders, and orthopedic problems are also common. As U.S. adults live longer, the prevalence and incidence of dementia that impairs memory, decision-making capability, orientation to physical surroundings, and language also increase. The prevalence of Alzheimer's disease is estimated as 10 percent in community-dwelling whites older than 65 years and is higher in black and Hispanic populations. By age 80, approximately 40 percent of people may be affected.[3] One-third of Medicare

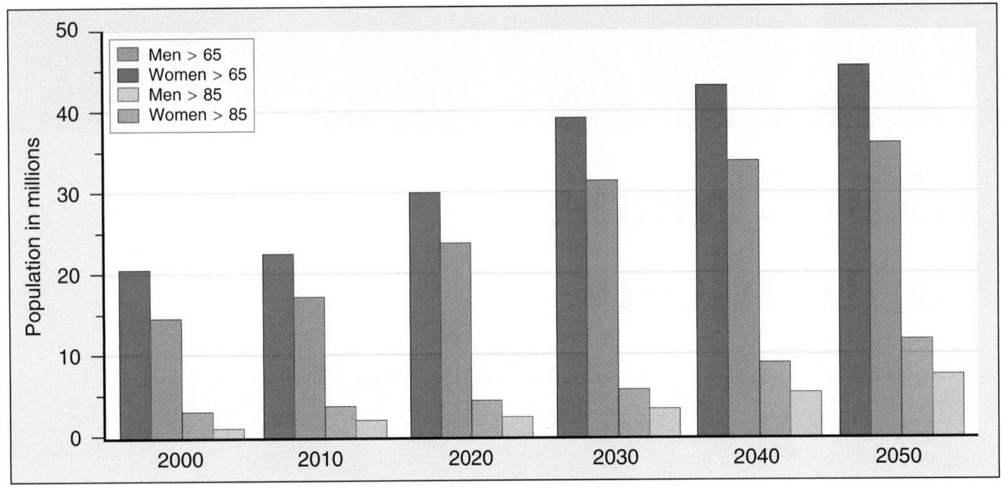

FIGURE 72–1 U.S. population estimates projected from 2000 to 2050. Dark pink bars represent numbers of women older than 65 years, dark blue bars represent numbers of men older than 65 years, light pink bars represent numbers of women older than 85 years, and light blue bars represent numbers of men older than 85 years, in millions of people. (From the U.S. Census Bureau.)

beneficiaries with Alzheimer's disease have CAD, one-quarter have had a stroke, and 22 percent have diabetes.[4]

The high morbidity and mortality from cardiovascular disease in elderly persons warrant aggressive approaches to treatment that have been shown to be effective in older patients. Compelling data demonstrate reduced morbidity and mortality rates for the treatment of hypertension, HF, atrial fibrillation, and lipid abnormalities in older patients 60 to 74 years of age, although data on minorities and women are limited.[5] Few trials of cardiovascular therapies have enrolled significant numbers of men or women older than 75 years, elderly patients with multisystem disease, or elderly patients with cognitive impairment, and none have addressed cardiovascular therapies in the nursing home population. The projected increase in numbers of older people from previously understudied and undertreated groups presents both medical and economic challenges for cardiovascular disease treatment.

PATHOPHYSIOLOGY

No universal definition of "elderly" and no accurate biomarker for aging exist. Although physiological changes associated with aging do not appear at a specific age and do not proceed at the same pace in all individuals, most definitions of elderly are based on chronological age. The World Health Organization uses 60 years of age to define "elderly," and most U.S. classifications use the age of 65 years. Gerontologists subclassify older age groups into young old (60 to 74 years), old old (75 to 85 years), and very old (over 85 years of age). Clinicians often separate older patients into two subgroups—those 65 to 80 years of age and those older than 80 years—to highlight the frailty, reduced capacity (physical and mental), and presence of multiple disorders that are more common after 80 years of age.

Hallmarks of cardiovascular aging in humans[6-8] include progressive increases in systolic blood pressure, pulse pressure (Fig. 72-3), pulse wave velocity, and left ventricular mass and increased incidence of CAD and atrial fibrillation. Reproducible age-related decreases are seen in rates of early left ventricular diastolic filling, maximal heart rates (Fig. 72-4), maximal cardiac output (see Fig. 72-4), maximal aerobic capacity or maximal oxygen consumption (VO_{2max}), exercise-induced augmentation of ejection fraction, reflex responses of heart rate, heart rate variability, and vasodilation in response to beta-adrenergic stimuli or endothelium-mediated vasodilator compounds (Fig. 72-5).

Cellular, enzymatic, and molecular alterations in the arterial vessel wall include migration of activated vascular smooth muscle cells into the intima, with increased matrix production related to altered activity of matrix metalloproteinases, angiotensin II, transforming growth factor beta, intercellular cell adhesion molecules, and production of collagen and collagen cross-linking. Loss of elastic fibers, increases in fibronectin, and calcification are also observed. These processes lead to arterial dilation and increased intimal thickness resulting in increased vascular stiffness. Increased arterial stiffness is manifested by increases in pulse wave velocity away from the heart and increased and earlier pulse wave reflections back toward the heart (often estimated as the aortic augmentation index). In both animal and human models of aging, endothelial cell production of nitric oxide (NO) decreases with age; there is decreased endothelial cell mass associated with increased cell senescence and apoptosis and increased NO consumption because of an age-dependent increase in vascular superoxide anion production. These changes contribute to reduced endothelial cell NO-mediated vasodilatory responses of the peripheral and coronary vasculature. Vascular responses to beta-adrenergic agonists and alpha-adrenergic blockade are also reduced with aging. In contrast, responses to non-endothelium-derived compounds such as nitrates or nitroprusside are preserved with aging but may vary by vascular bed or be altered by diseases such as hypertension or diabetes.

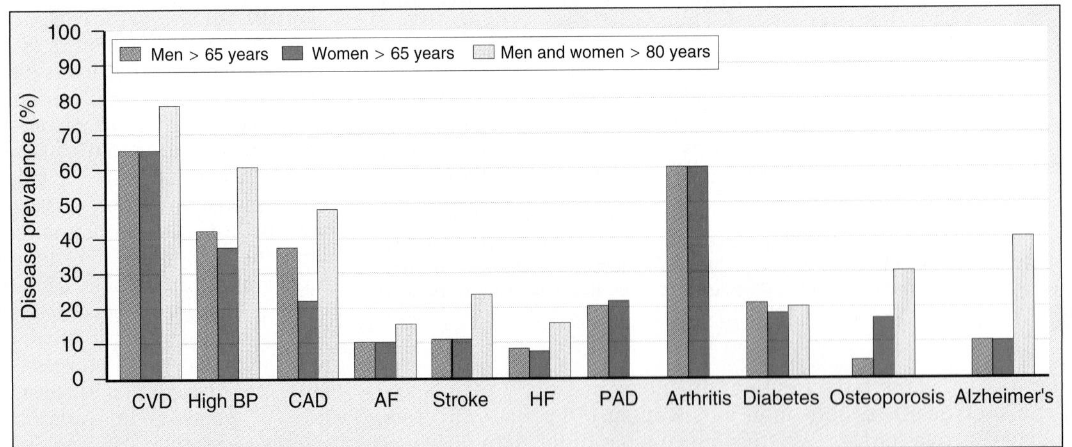

FIGURE 72–2 Prevalence of cardiovascular and other common chronic medical illnesses in older persons in the United States. Data are percentages. AF = atrial fibrillation; CAD = coronary artery disease; CVD = cardiovascular disease; HF = heart failure; High BP = hypertension (all forms); PAD = peripheral artery disease. Blue bars represent data for men older than 65 years, pink bars represent women older than 65 years, and yellow bars represent men and women older than 80 years.

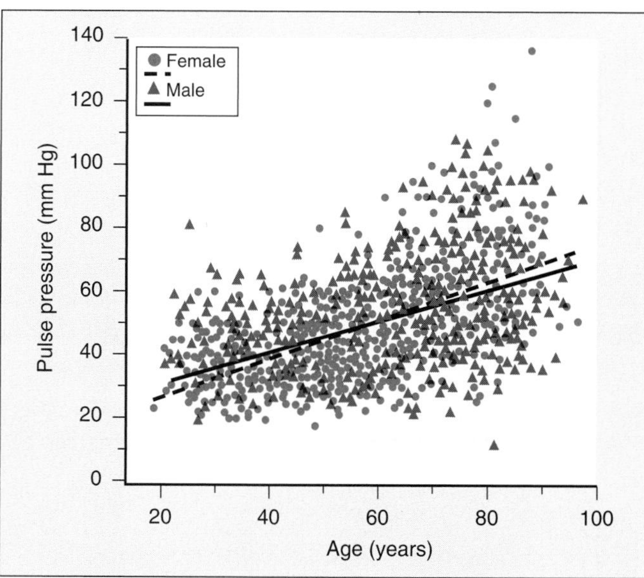

FIGURE 72–3 Pulse pressure (systolic minus diastolic pressure) with aging in apparently healthy subjects enrolled in the Baltimore Longitudinal Study of Aging. (From Pearson JD, Morrell CH, Brant LJ, et al: Age-associated changes in blood pressure in a longitudinal study of healthy men and women. J Gerontol Med Sci 53:M177, 1997.)

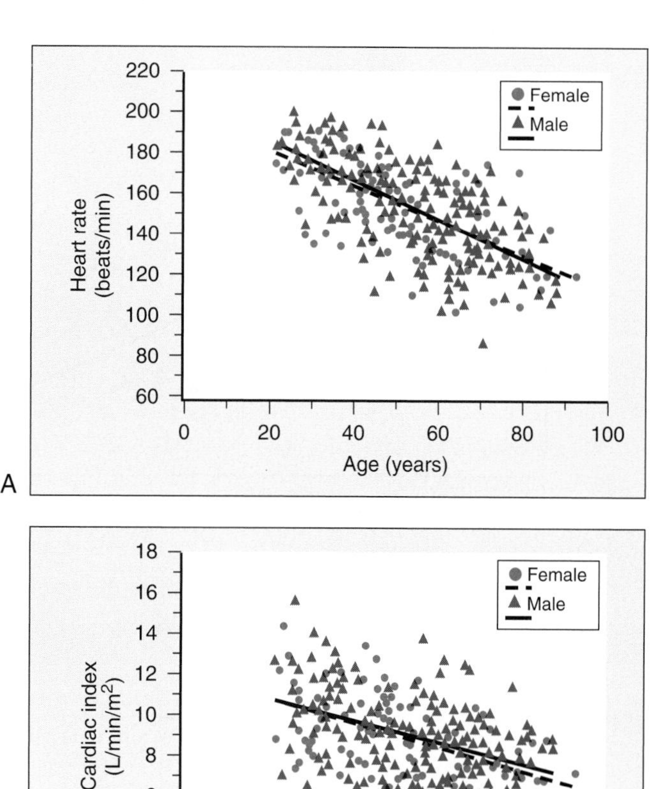

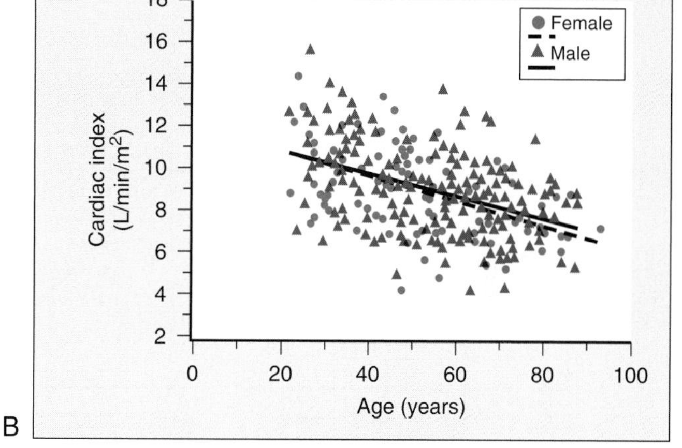

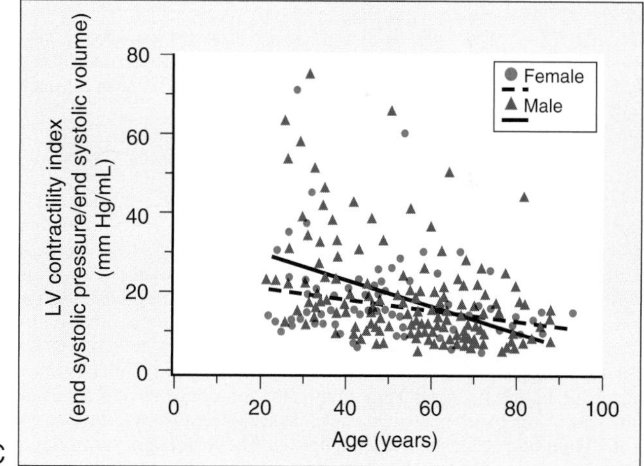

FIGURE 72–4 Maximum exercise heart rate **(A)**, cardiac index **(B)**, and left ventricular (LV) contractility index **(C)** in men and women in the Baltimore Longitudinal Study of Aging who had been prescreened to exclude clinical and occult cardiovascular disease. (From Fleg JL, O'Connor FC, Gerstenblith G, et al: Impact of age on the cardiovascular response to dynamic upright exercise in healthy men and women. J Appl Physiol 78:890, 1995.)

Changes in the extracellular matrix of the myocardium parallel those in the vasculature with increased collagen, increased fibril diameter and collagen cross-linking, an increase in the ratio of type I to type III collagen, decreased elastin content, and an increase in fibronectin. There may also be a shift in the balance between matrix metalloproteinases and tissue inhibitors of matrix metalloproteinases that favors increased production of extracellular matrix. Fibroblast proliferation is induced by growth factors, in particular angiotensin, transforming growth factors, tumor necrosis factor-alpha, and platelet-derived growth factor. These changes are accompanied by cell loss and altered cellular function.[9,10] In the atria, decreased sinus node cells and extracellular matrix changes contribute to sinus node dysfunction and atrial fibrillation. Collagen, elastic tissue, and calcification changes in or near the central fibrous body and the atrioventricular (AV) node or proximal bundle branches contribute to conduction abnormalities and annular valvular calcification. In the ventricle, collagen deposition and extracellular matrix changes contribute to loss of cells, hypertrophy of myocytes with changes in myosin subforms, and altered myocardial calcium handling.[11] Changes in myocardial calcium handling include reduced or delayed inactivation of L-type transmembrane calcium current, decreased and delayed intracellular ionized calcium uptake by cardiac myocyte sarcoplasmic reticulum (in part due to reduced sarcoendoplasmic reticulum calcium adenosine triphosphatase [SERCA2] activity), and reduced and delayed outwardly directed potassium rectifier current activation. The result is prolongation of the membrane action potential and inward calcium current with prolongation of both contraction and relaxation.[9,11,12]

Age-related changes are also seen in the intravascular environment. Increases in fibrinogen; coagulation factors V, VIII, and IX; and other coagulation proteins are seen without countering increases in anticoagulant factors. Platelet phospholipid content is altered and platelet activity is increased with increased binding of platelet-derived growth factor to the arterial wall in older individuals compared with younger individuals. Increased levels of plasminogen activator inhibitor 1 (PAI-1) are seen with aging, especially during stress, resulting in impaired fibrinolysis. Circulating prothrombotic inflammatory cytokines, especially interleukin-6, also increase with age and may play a role in the pathogenesis of acute coronary syndromes. Adipose cells associated with obesity are also sources of PAI-1 and inflammatory cytokines. All these changes also potentiate development of atherosclerosis.[9,13,14]

Consistent changes in the autonomic nervous system (see Chap. 87) accompany aging and influence cardiovascular function. For the beta-adrenergic system, age-related changes include decreased receptor numbers, altered G protein coupling, and altered G protein–mediated signal transduction. Age-related decreases in alpha-adrenergic platelet receptors and decreased alpha-adrenergic–mediated arterial vasoreactivity of forearm blood vessels occur, but alpha-adrenergic–mediated changes in human hand veins appear to be preserved. Dopaminergic receptor content and dopaminergic transporters decrease and cardiac contractile responses to dopaminergic stimulation may be blunted with aging. Decreased sensitivity and responses to parasympathetic stimulation are seen in cardiac and vascular tissues, but increased central nervous system effects are frequently seen in models of aging. The combined age-related autonomic changes lead to decreased baroreflex function and responses to physiological stressors with increased sensitivity to parasympathetic stimulation of the central nervous system.[6,7,9,15-20]

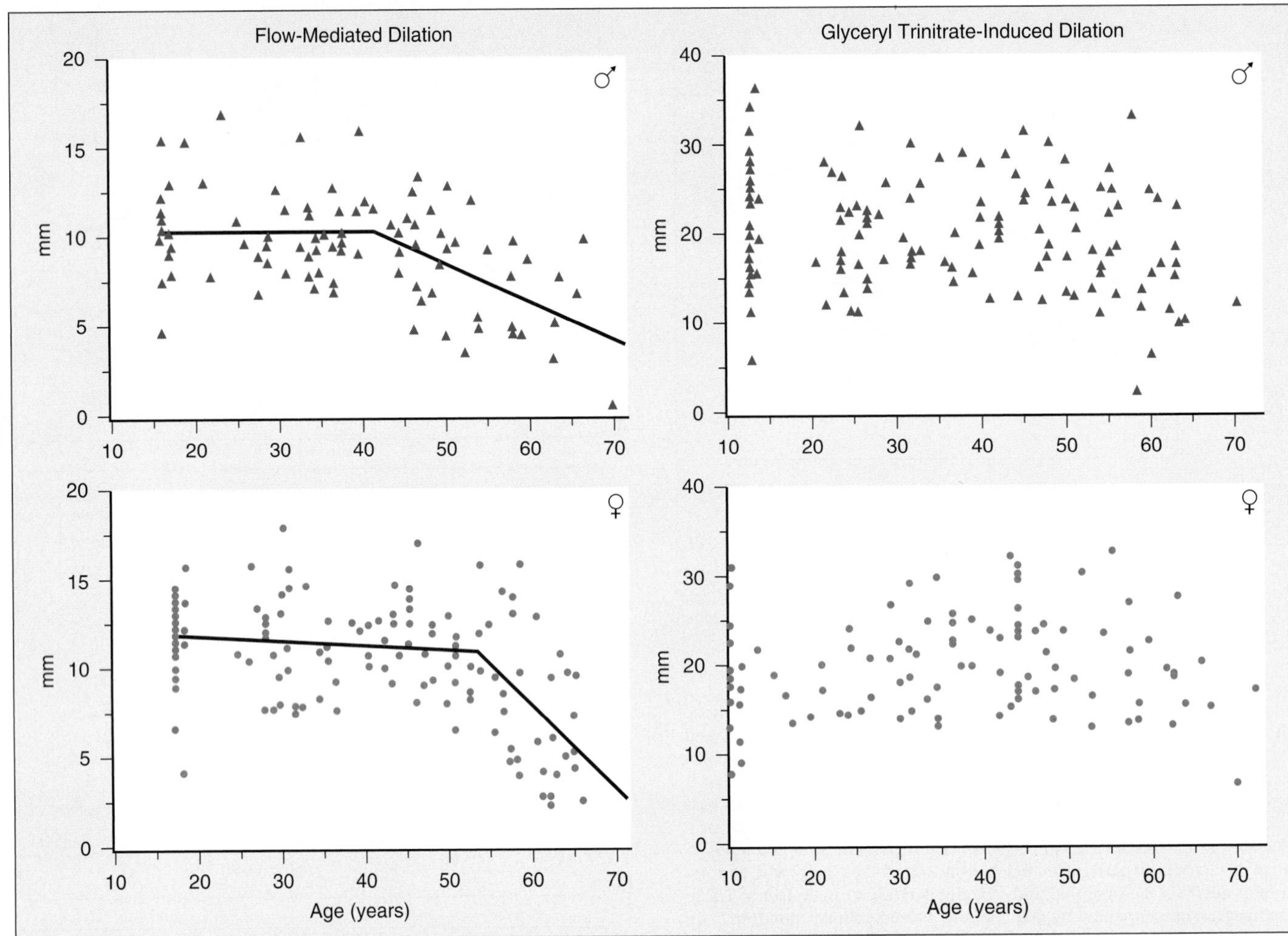

FIGURE 72–5 Endothelial (flow)-mediated and nonendothelial (glyceryl trinitrate)-induced arterial dilation in apparently healthy men and women. Age-associated declines are seen in flow-mediated dilation but not in glyceryl trinitrate–induced dilation. Age-related changes occur earlier in men than women. (From Celermajer DS, Sorensen KE, Spiegelhalter DJ, et al: Aging is associated with endothelial dysfunction in healthy men years before the age-related decline in women. J Am Coll Cardiol 24:471, 1994.)

Several unifying hypotheses for age-related changes throughout the body have been proposed and include cumulative oxidative damage, inflammatory responses to cellular stress or infection, and programmed cell death. Some of the age-related cardiovascular changes can be partially, if not totally, reversed. Exercise improves endothelial function, measures of arterial stiffness, and baroreceptor function in older people. Pharmacological approaches with antiinflammatory and antioxidant vitamin administration have not been successful, although dietary antioxidant intake has been associated with slowing of age-related changes in the vasculature, and medications such as angiotensin-converting enzyme (ACE) inhibitors, aldosterone antagonists, or beta blockers may influence the vascular and cardiac remodeling associated with hypertension, atherosclerosis, or HF.[21-29] Agents that directly target collagen cross-linking and inflammation are being evaluated.

Age-related changes create a cardiovascular system faced with increased pulsatile load and one that is less able to increase output in response to stress. Age-related changes also limit maximal capacity and decrease reserve capacity, contributing to lower thresholds for symptoms in the presence of cardiovascular diseases that become more common with increasing age. Table 72-1 summarizes age-related cardiovascular changes contrasted with cardiovascular disease.

Medication Modifications

The vast majority of therapeutic interventions for elderly people are pharmacological, making appropriate drug selection and modification of dosing regimens for the older patient important (see Chap. 5).

LOADING DOSES OF MEDICATIONS. On average, body size decreases with aging and body composition changes, resulting in decreased total body water, intravascular volume, and muscle mass. Age-related changes are continuous but most pronounced after 75 to 80 years. Women tend to weigh less and have smaller body and intravascular volumes and muscle mass than men at all ages. Higher serum concentrations of medications are found in older patients, and especially older women, if initial doses are the same as those in younger patients. Weight adjustments for loading doses of the cardiovascular drugs digoxin, lidocaine, and other type I antiarrhythmic drugs, and type III antiarrhythmic drugs; aminoglycoside antibiotics; chemotherapy regimens; and unfractionated heparin are standard. When fibrinolytic drugs have been administered without weight-based dosage adjustments, increased risk of intracranial hemorrhage (ICH) resulted with older age, smaller body weight, and female sex (in addition to hypertension and prior cerebrovascular disease).[30,31] Increased risk of bleeding in older patients is also seen after administration of "standard" doses of low-molecular-weight heparins in combination with other lytic agents. In contrast, increased risk of intracranial bleeding in older patients was not seen in trials using weight-based dosing.[32]

Routine dosage-weight adjustments should be made in loading doses of medications, especially those with low therapeutic-to-toxicity ratios, resulting in doses that are usually lower in older patients, especially older women.

TABLE 72–1 Differentiation Between Age-Associated Changes and Cardiovascular Disease in Older People

Organ	Age-Associated Changes	Cardiovascular Disease
Vasculature	Increased intimal thickness Arterial stiffening Increased pulse pressure Increased pulse wave velocity Early central wave reflections Decreased endothelium-mediated vasodilation	Systolic hypertension Coronary artery obstruction Peripheral artery obstruction Carotid artery obstruction
Atria	Increased left atrial size Atrial premature complexes	Atrial fibrillation
Sinus node	Decreased maximal heart rate Decreased heart rate variability	Sinus node dysfunction, sick sinus syndrome
Atrioventricular node	Increased conduction time	Type II block, third-degree block
Valves	Sclerosis, calcification	Stenosis, regurgitation
Ventricle	Increased left ventricular wall tension Prolonged myocardial contraction Prolonged early diastolic filling rate Decreased maximal cardiac output Right bundle branch block Ventricular premature complexes	Left ventricular hypertrophy Heart failure (with or without preserved systolic function) Ventricular tachycardia, fibrillation

CHRONIC MEDICATION ADMINISTRATION

RENAL CLEARANCE. Renal clearance by all routes (glomerular filtration, renal tubular reabsorption, and secretion) decreases with age and is lower in women than in men at all ages. There is considerable intersubject variability, but a general estimate is a 10 percent decline in glomerular filtration per decade with 15 to 25 percent lower rates in women than in men. Algorithms to estimate creatinine clearance or glomerular filtration often include age, sex, weight, serum creatinine concentrations, and, more recently, race as variables.[33] Two useful formulas to estimate glomerular filtration or creatinine clearance in people during stable conditions are:

Creatinine clearance = (140 − age [yr] × weight [kg])/(creatinine × 72)

multiplied by 0.85 for women[34]

Glomerular filtration = $186.3 \times (\text{creatinine})^{-1.154} \times (\text{age})^{-0.203} \times$ 1.212 (if black) × 0.742 (if female)[35]

Significant decreases in renal elimination can be present in older patients in the presence of normal serum creatinine measurements. The algorithms predict that most women older than 70 have stage 3 renal function or moderate renal failure (National Kidney Foundation 2001 guidelines, available at http://www.kidney.org). With elevations of serum creatinine, severe renal impairment is likely to be present. Estimates of renal clearance are recommended before prescribing renally cleared medications, in determining risks for procedures, and before administration of contrast agents or other potentially nephrotoxic agents in older patients. They are not, however, accurate if the patient is clinically unstable.

HEPATIC (AND INTESTINAL) CLEARANCE. Most studies show decreases in oxidative drug metabolism or clearance by the cytochrome P450 (CYP) system with aging, suggesting that lower amounts of drug per unit time (or day) should be given to older patients compared with younger patients. Cardiovascular drugs showing such age-related changes in hepatic clearance include alpha blockers (doxazosin, prazosin, terazosin), some beta blockers (metoprolol, propranolol, timolol), calcium channel blockers (dihydropyridines, diltiazem, verapamil), several 3-hydroxy-3-methylglutaryl coenzyme A (HMG CoA) reductase inhibitors (atorvastatin, fluvastatin), and the benzodiazepine midazolam. Variability in age-related changes is marked, however, and the effects of disease states, gender, race, and medication interactions are usually greater than those of age in populations of patients.[36,37] CYP drug clearance is usually faster in men than women, even after correction for weight, suggesting that women should receive lower dosages per unit time and weight than men. The exceptions are CYP3A substrates such as midazolam and nifedipine that are cleared more rapidly in women. Additional information on sex-specific medication adjustments has been reviewed.[38,39]

Genetic variation in drug metabolism exists, and allelic variants for most of the CYP pathways have been described that affect drug clearance as well as responses.[40,41] Encainide, metoprolol, and warfarin are metabolized by the polymorphic CYP2D6 enzyme that can produce distinct phenotypes of ultrarapid, rapid, slow, and ultraslow drug clearance. Pharmacogenetic variants can also explain some of the variability in metabolism and toxicity with the HMG CoA reductase inhibitor simvastatin.[42] It is currently difficult to estimate the clinical impact of genetic polymorphisms of drug-metabolizing enzymes (or receptors or transcription-regulating elements), and routine pharmacogenomic screening is not recommended at present.[43] Further information can be found at the National Institutes of Health–sponsored Pharmacogenetics Research Network (www.pharmgkb.org or www.imm.ki.se/CYPalleles/). Data on CYP pathways of human metabolism have been reviewed,[44] and updates are available in a searchable data base (www.gentest.com).

Drugs metabolized by the conjugative reactions of glucuronidation (morphine, diazepam), sulfation (methyldopa), or acetylation (procainamide) do not appear to be affected by aging but show disease-related effects, and clearance is consistently lower in women than in men.

ELIMINATION HALF-LIVES. In general, elimination half-lives of drugs increase with age, so that the time between dosage adjustments needs to be increased in older patients before the full effect of a given dose can be assessed. Conversely, increased time is needed for complete drug elimination from the body and dissipation of the drug effects.

Age-related changes in protein binding of drugs are not usually found. Changes in free drug concentrations related to drugs competing for binding sites can occur, although these changes are predicted to be transitory.[45] Clinically significant examples involve warfarin and changes in anticoagulation when additional drugs are added to therapy. For example, markedly increased prolongation of coagulation times can occur when amiodarone is added to warfarin therapy (see Chap. 30). Drug interactions must be considered whenever an agent is added to warfarin therapy. Table 72–2 summarizes general guidelines for drug dosing in older patients.

ADVERSE DRUG EVENTS AND DRUG INTERACTIONS. Adverse drug events are estimated to affect millions of people per year and account for up to 5 percent of hospital admissions.[46] Cardiovascular medications such digoxin, warfarin, diuretics, and calcium channel blockers are among those most frequently cited as responsible for "preventable" adverse drug events in community-dwelling elderly people and hospitalized elderly patients.[47,48] The odds ratio of severe adverse drug events with cardiovascular medications has been reported to be 2.4 times that of other medications in hospitalized patients.[49] In adult patients in ambulatory primary care settings, selective serotonin reuptake inhibitors (SSRIs), beta blockers, ACE inhibitors, and nonsteroidal anti-inflammatory drugs (NSAIDs) have been identified in adverse

TABLE 72–2	Guidelines for Drug Dosing in Older Patients

In general, loading doses should be reduced—weight (or body surface area) can be used to estimate loading dose requirements; doses in women are usually less than those in men.
Base doses of renally cleared drugs on estimates of glomerular filtration or creatinine clearance (or, if not possible, initiate with lower doses than in younger patient); reduce doses of hepatically cleared drugs.
Time between dosage adjustments and evaluation of dosing changes should be longer in older patients than in younger patients.
Routine use of strategies to avoid drug interactions is essential.
Assessment of adherence and attention to factors contributing to nonadherence should be part of the prescription process.

drug events.[50] In nursing home patients, drugs associated with adverse drug events are more frequently antibiotics, anticoagulants, antipsychotic drugs, antidepressants, antiseizure medications, or opioids.[51] Adverse drug effects may arise with "atypical" symptoms in the older patient, such as mental status changes and impaired cognition with digitalis excess.

The strongest risk factor for adverse drug-related events is the number of drugs prescribed, independent of age. Chronic administration of four drugs is associated with a risk of adverse effects of 50 to 60 percent; administration of eight or nine drugs increases the risk to almost 100 percent (Fig. 72–6). Although the goal is to prescribe as few drugs as possible for elderly patients, the presence of multiple diseases and multidrug regimens for common cardiovascular diseases often results in polypharmacy. A national survey of noninstitutionalized people older than 65 years found that over 40 percent used 5 or more different medications each week and 12 percent used 10 or more different medications per week.[52] American College of Cardiology/American Heart Association (ACC/AHA) guidelines for the pharmacological treatment of patients after uncomplicated myocardial infarction and for the management of chronic HF recommend use of four or five drugs.[53,54] Strategies that minimize the chance of drug interactions and adverse drug effects are thus essential.

PHARMACOKINETIC INTERACTIONS. Pharmacokinetic interactions that alter the concentration of concomitantly administered medications are more likely if drugs that are metabolized by or inhibit the same pathway are coadministered. Table 72–3 lists some examples of cardiovascular drugs by metabolic pathway with examples of inducers and inhibitors (see also Table 5–1, Chap. 5). The most potent inhibitors of the CYP oxidative enzymes are amiodarone (all CYP isoforms), the azole antifungal drugs itraconazole and ketoconazole (CYP3A), and protease inhibitors (CYP3A), followed by erythromycin (CYP3A) and terfenadine (CYP3A). Oral hypoglycemic agents are commonly prescribed drugs for elderly patients, and coadministration of sulfonamide antibiotics with sulfonylureas can lead to hypoglycemia, in part because of CYP2C9 inhibition. Some drugs are administered as prodrugs and metabolized to active agents (cardiovascular examples include many ACE inhibitors and clopidogrel). Inhibition of the antiplatelet effects of clopidogrel by coadministration of atorvastatin, which decreases clopidogrel activation (CYP3A), has been reported,[55] although the clinical significance is not entirely clear.[55a]

Inducibility of hepatic enzyme activity can lower concentrations of medications and lead to ineffective therapy. The antituberculous drug rifampin is the most potent inducer of CYP1A and CYP3A. With mandatory screening of nursing home residents for tuberculosis, treatment with rifampin may be initiated. Dosages of coadministered drugs cleared by CYP1A and CYP3A may need to be increased during rifampin administration and decreased upon discontinuation of rifampin. The clinical importance of this interaction was recognized with markedly decreased cyclosporine levels during rifampin coadministration. Reduced clopidogrel inhibition of platelet aggregation by atorvastatin has also been reported after rifampin administration.[55] Other significant hepatic enzyme inducers include dexamethasone and phenytoin (CYP2C); caffeine, cigarette smoke, lansoprazole, and omeprazole (CYP1A); and St. John's wort (CYP3A). Diet-drug and herb-drug interactions also occur.[56,57]

Despite the predictability of some of these interactions, many hospital admissions of elderly patients for drug toxicity involve administration of drugs known to interact.[58] Because of the multiplicity of potential interactions, release of new medications, and discovery of new interactions, use of pharmacy or computerized and on-line tools that provide comprehensive up-to-date information and guidelines for avoiding drug interactions is highly recommended. Available tools include the *Physician's Desk Reference* (PDR; traditional, pocket, or on-line versions), PDR handbook of drug interactions (traditional, computer version, or handheld computer version available free of charge at www.PDR.net), the Clinical Pharmacology modules (computer-based), the Medical Letter and the Medical Letter Drug Interactions Program (computer-based), Epocrates for the handheld computer (available free of charge at <www.epocrates.com>), and online pharmacology texts or data bases (the Food and Drug Administration: www.fda.gov/cder, drug reactions section; or www.druginteractions.org), among others. Many individual hospitals or health care systems and pharmacies provide internal reference sources. Information organized by CYP pathways is accessible in a searchable human P450 metabolism data base (www.gentest.com). Specialized clinics, use of specific algorithms, and computer-based dosage programs to monitor oral anticoagulant therapy in outpatients, especially, have been shown to reduce bleeding-related complications.[59]

Other approaches that have been shown to reduce adverse drug reactions in older patients include involvement of pharmacy-trained individuals to assess the appropriateness of doses and medication counseling using

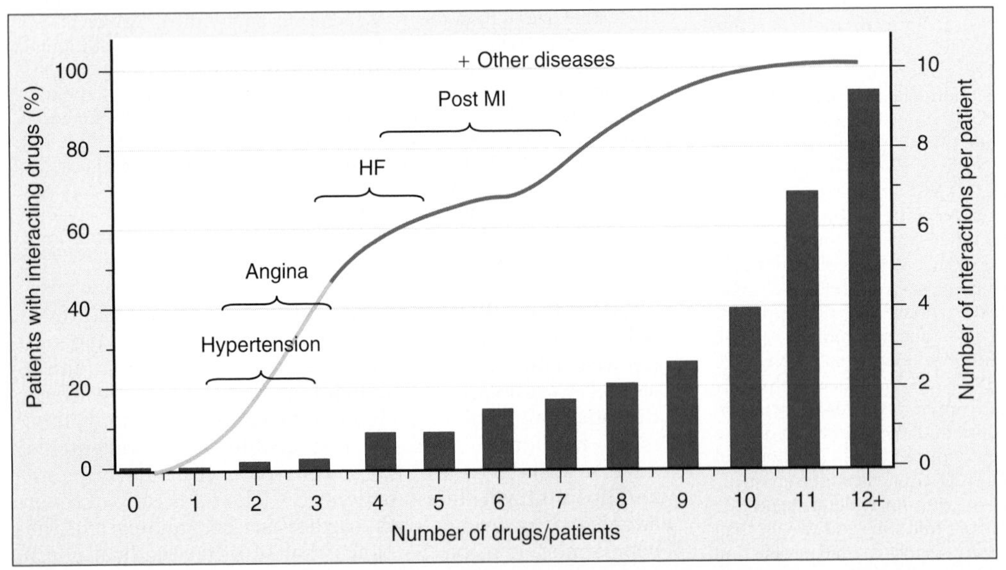

FIGURE 72–6 Relationship between the number of drugs consumed and drug interactions. Current guidelines for the pharmacological management of patients with heart failure (HF) or myocardial infarction (post MI) place them at higher risk for drug interactions (≥4 drugs). (From Schwartz JB: Clinical Pharmacology, American College of Cardiology Self-Assessment Program V, 2003 as modified from Nolan and O'Malley, Age Aging, 1989, and Denham, Br Med Bull, 1990.)

TABLE 72–3 Major Routes of Cytochrome P450 (CYP) Metabolism of Cardiovascular and Commonly Administered Drugs in Elderly People*

Enzyme Isoform	Cardiovascular	Other Substrates	Inducers[†]	Inhibitors[†]
CYP1A2	Carvedilol	Acetaminophen	Rifampin	Cimetidine
	Fluvastatin	Caffeine	Omeprazole	Grapefruit juice
	Guanabenz	Imipramine	Cigarette smoke	Irbesartan, losartan
	Mexiletine	Mirtazapine	Charbroiled, pan-fried meat	Fluoroquinolones
	Pimobendan	Nicotine		Fluvoxamine
	Propranolol	Tacrine	Lansoprazole	Mexiletine
		Testosterone		Omeprazole
		Theophylline		Ticlodipine
				Cholecalciferol
CYP2C				
2C8/9 (Polymorphic)	ARB's (irbesartan, losartan)	Acenocoumarol	Dexamethasone	Azole antifungals
	Fluvastatin	Celecoxib	Phenobarbital	Amiodarone
	Torsemide	Fluoxetine	Phenytoin	Cimetidine
	Warfarin	Glipizide	Rifampin	Fluconazole
		NSAIDs	Secobarbital	Isoniazid
		(diclofenac, flurbiprofen		Sulfaphenazole
		ibuprofen, meloxicam,		Ticlodipine
		naproxen, piroxicam)		
		Phenytoin		
		Tamoxifen		
		Tolbutamide		
2C19 (Polymorphic)		Cyclophosphamide	Rifampin	Ketoconazole
		Diazepam	Phenobarbital	Fluoxetine
		Lansoprazole		Fluvoxamine
		Omeprazole, pantoprazole		Fluconazole
		Phenytoin		Lansoprazole
		Progesterone		Omeprazole
		Selegiline		Ticlodipine
		Sulfamethoxazole		
		Tricyclic antidepressants (amitriptyline, clomipramine)		
		Venlafaxine		
CYP2D6 (Polymorphic)	Beta blockers	Amitriptyline	Haloperidol	Amiodarone
	(carvedilol, metoprolol,	Codeine		Ticlodipine
	propranolol, timolol)	Dextromethorphan		Quinidine
	Flecainide	DHEA		
	Metoprolol	Haloperidol		Chlorpheniramine
	Mexiletine	Omeprazole		Cimetidine
	Pindolol	Ondansetron		Clomipramine
	Procainamide	Paroxetine		Desipramine
	Propafenone	Risperidone		Flecainide
		SSRI antidepressants		Fluoxetine
		Tamoxifen		Haloperidol
		Tolterodine		Lansoprazole
		Tramadol		Methadone
		Tricyclic antidepressants		Paroxetine
		(desipramine, imipramine)		
		Venlafaxine		
CYP3A4	Beta blockers (bisoprolol,	Alprazolam	Rifampin	Ketoconazole
	metoprolol)	Astemizole		Itraconazole
	Cilostazol	Carbamazepine		Protease inhibitors
	Clopidogrel	Cisapride	Bosentan	Amiodarone
	Dihydropyridines (nifedipine,	Colchicine	Nitric oxide	Nefazodone
	amlodipine, felodipine,	Clozapine	St. John's wort	Mibefradil
	isradipine, nicardipine,	Cyclosporine		
	nisoldipine)	Diazepam		Fluvoxamine
	Diltiazem	Diclofenac		Cimetidine
	Eplerenone	Erythromycin		Grapefruit juice
	Fenofibrate	Estradiol, ethinylestradiol		Cyclosporine
	Flosequinan	Fentanyl		Erythromycin
	HMG CoA reductase Inhibitors	Itraconazole		Verapamil
	(atorvastatin, lovastatin,	Ketoconazole		Diltiazem
	pravastatin, simvastatin)	Medroxyprogesterone		Doxorubicin
	Gemfibrozil	Midazolam		Losartan
	Lidocaine	Mirtazapine		Quinidine
	Losartan	Nefazodone		Antibiotics
	Propafenone	Paclitaxel		(fluroquinolones, e.g.,

Continued

TABLE 72–3 Major Routes of Cytochrome P450 (CYP) Metabolism of Cardiovascular and Commonly Administered Drugs in Elderly People*—cont'd

Enzyme Isoform	Cardiovascular	Other Substrates	Inducers†	Inhibitors†
	Quinidine Verapamil Vesnarinone	Protease inhibitors Rifampin Salmeterol Sildenafil Sulfinpyrazone Tamoxifen Terfenadine Theophylline Triazolam Troglitazone Zolpidem		ciprofloxacin; macrolides, e.g., clarithromycin, troleandomycin)

ARB = angiotensin receptor blocker; DHEA = dehydroepiandrosterone; HMG CoA = 3-hydroxy-3-methylglutaryl coenzyme A; NSAID = nonsteroidal antiinflammatory drug; SSRI = selective serotonin reuptake inhibitor.

*Examples cite major pathway only for drugs that are substrates of multiple CYP pathways.

†In approximate order of potency.

multidisciplinary care team members. A major limitation to the success of all of these approaches is the frequent lack of complete and readily accessible information on medication consumption and disease state information, especially for the older patient with multiple diseases and physicians. Integrated medical record and pharmacy information and interactive data bases have been recommended by numerous panels investigating strategies to reduce adverse drug events and improve medication therapy but are not widely available.[60,61]

ADVERSE PHARMACODYNAMIC EFFECTS. Age-related changes in cardiovascular physiology and dynamics affect pharmacodynamics (see Table 72–1).[6,7,62] Greater age-related sensitivity to parasympathetic stimulation may explain the increased frequency of adverse effects such as urinary retention, constipation, and fecal impaction in older patients who receive drugs with anticholinergic properties (e.g., disopyramide). Gastrointestinal transit time is generally increased in elderly people, and constipation is a frequent complaint of hospitalized, less active, and institutionalized elderly persons. Drug-induced constipation and bowel obstruction can occur in older patients receiving bile acid sequestrants, anticholinergic medications, opiates, and verapamil.

Pharmacodynamic drug interactions are most likely to occur between drugs acting on the same system. A classical example of additive effects that can produce hypotension and postural hypotension in elderly people is the coadministration of direct vasodilators or nitrates combined with alpha blockers, beta blockers, calcium channel blockers, ACE inhibitors, diuretics, or sildenafil. Additional examples are combinations of amiodarone, beta-adrenergic blocking drugs, digoxin, diltiazem, or verapamil producing bradycardia and bleeding caused by increased inhibition of platelet and clotting factors with combinations of aspirin, NSAIDs (including cyclooxygenase 2 [COX-2] selective inhibitors), warfarin, or clopidogrel. Increased potassium concentrations caused by combined administration of ACE inhibitors and potassium-sparing diuretics in older patients are cited as causes of serious adverse drug reactions.[63] Combinations of NSAIDs, including selective COX-2 inhibitors, with ACE inhibitors can also decrease potassium excretion and cause hyperkalemia in the older patient or can cause a decrease in renal function.[64]

Examples of pharmacodynamic interactions with antagonistic effects include increased angina when a beta-agonist or theophylline is given to patients with CAD receiving beta blockers or nondihydropyridine calcium channel antagonists and loss of hypertension control when a drug such as fludrocortisone acetate is given for postural hypotension.

INAPPROPRIATE PRESCRIBING IN ELDERLY PATIENTS. Long-acting benzodiazepines, sedative and hypnotic agents, long-acting oral hypoglycemic agents, selected analgesics, antiemetics, and gastrointestinal antispasmodics are usually considered inappropriate in elderly patients on the basis of an unfavorable risk-to-benefit ratio.[65,66] Although most cardiovascular medications are not considered inappropriate for the older patient, more recent definitions of inappropriate drug use include failure to consider drug-disease interactions and failure to adjust drug dosages for age-related changes, drug duplication, drug-drug interactions, and duration of use. Using these criteria, most drug utilization review studies conclude that inappropriate drug prescribing occurs in a significant fraction of older patients. Explicit criteria for appropriate prescribing of digoxin, calcium channel blockers, and ACE inhibitors in older patients have been developed by expert consensus panels[67] and are accessible at www.ahrqpubs@ahrq.gov. It is pertinent that initial drug dose recommendations from resources such as the PDR may not be the minimally effective dose established by studies done after drug marketing approval or in guideline statements.[68]

ADHERENCE. Adherence taking medications is commonly thought to be lower in older patients than younger patients. In one report, hospitalization for decompensated congestive HF was attributed to medication noncompliance in 42 percent of elderly patients.[69] Contributing factors include the cost of medications; difficulty with understanding directions because of either small print of written directions, hearing impairment, or impaired memory; inadequate instructions; complex dosing regimens; difficulties with packaging materials; and insufficient eduction of the patient, family, or caregiver on medication use. Of these, the most limiting are thought to be the cost of medications, poor education of the patient regarding medications, and cognitive impairment in elderly patients, especially those living alone.[70] In a study of Medicare beneficiaries with CAD, use of HMG CoA reductase inhibitors was directly related to drug payment coverage.[71] It is of note that physicians routinely overestimate patients' adherence taking medications.[72] Assessment of adherence should be part of care and issues related to potential contributors to medication nonadherence should be addressed by prescribing health care professionals. Unfortunately, there are few trials of interventions to improve medication adherence with resources usually available in clinical settings.[73] Strategies to overcome these obstacles include programs for low-income seniors, visual or memory aids, medication dispensing tools, use of geriatric-friendly packaging, assessment of cognitive status and patients' understanding, and inclusion of caregivers or family members in discussion regarding medications.

Vascular Disease

HYPERTENSION (see Chaps. 37 and 38)

Prevalence and Incidence. Diastolic (>90 mm Hg) or systolic (>140 mm Hg) hypertension, or both, occurs in one-half to two-thirds of people older than 65 years. The prevalence varies by race (or genetics) and is slightly higher in black and Hispanic people than in non-Hispanic whites.[74] The profile of hypertension is altered by aging.[75] Systolic hypertension becomes more prevalent with aging, whereas diastolic blood pressure is relatively constant from 50 to 80 years of age with average diastolic pressures higher in men than women from ages 50 to 80 years. Systolic blood pressure rises with aging in both men and women but rises more steeply in women. Systolic blood pressure is lower in women than in men until about age 50 (average age of menopause) but rises to levels equal to those of men by age 65 years. "Isolated" systolic hypertension, without elevation of diastolic blood pressure, is present in about 8 percent of sexagenarians and more than 25 percent of the population older than 80 years. A large percentage of people are unaware that they have hypertension, and hypertension is not controlled in many older patients.[76]

Treatment. The cardiovascular benefits of treatment of systolic as well as diastolic hypertension in older patients have been well established in randomized clinical trials (Table 72–4). The Systolic Hypertension in the Elderly (SHEP) trial[77] also reported reduced rates of dementia in the open blind extended follow-up phase.[78] A comprehensive profile of older patients and responses to antihypertensive strategies, however, is still being elucidated. Most available data suggest that thiazide diuretics are as efficacious as any drug for first-line treatment of hypertension in elderly people[79] and offer advantages of use that include health outcomes and price as well as preservation of bone mineral density in older adults.[80,81] There may also be a role for ACE inhibitors compared with diuretics as first-line therapy in some older white men.[82] Neither the alpha blocker doxazosin nor dihydropyridine calcium channel blockers compare favorably with other first-line strategies for older patients with HF; and blacks may benefit less from ACE inhibitors (see Chaps. 37 and 38 for further discussion of hypertensive subgroups). Because most older patients require second (or third) medications to reach target blood pressures, treatment decisions for elderly patients with hypertension should focus on control of blood pressure and extend beyond first-line therapy.

Consideration of conditions that are highly prevalent in elderly people in the choice of antihypertensive therapy can optimize effects; minimize adverse effects, cost, and the number of medications; and increase adherence. In addition to recommendations based on concomitant cardiovascular diseases recognized in hypertension treatment guidelines (Table 72–5),[83,84] other conditions in elderly people warrant consideration. In older people, arthritis is second in prevalence to cardiovascular disease and NSAIDs are among the most frequently consumed drugs (prescription and over the counter). In addition to the potential for adverse renal effects or hyperkalemia when NSAIDs are given in combination with ACE inhibitors, angiotensin receptor blockers, or aldosterone antagonists, loss of blood pressure control and HF have been precipitated by nonselective NSAIDs as well as COX-2-selective NSAIDs. Age-related bone loss is accelerated in older men and women and is the major contributing cause of

TABLE 72–4 Trials of Blood Pressure Reduction in Elderly People

				Risk Reduction (%)			
Trial	***N***	**Age (yr)**	**Type**	***Stroke***	***CAD***	***HF***	***All CVD***
HDFP	2374	60-69	D	44	15	NR	16
Australian	582	60-69	D	33	18	NR	31
EWPHE	840	>60	D (+S)	36	20	22	29
Coope	884	60-79	D (+S)	42	−3	32	24
STOP-HTN	1627	70-84	D (+S)	47	13	51	40
MRC	4396	65-74	D (+S)	25	19	NR	17
SHEP	4736	≥60	S	33	27	55	32
Syst-Eur	4695	≥60	S	42	26	36	31
STONE	1632	60-79	S	57	6	68	60
Syst-China	2394	≥60	S	38	33	38	37

Age = age at study entry; CAD = coronary artery disease; all CVD = all cardiovascular disease composite endpoint; D = diastolic; EWPHE = European Working Party on High Blood Pressure in the Elderly; HDFP = Hypertension Detection and Follow-up Program; HF = heart failure; MRC = Medical Research Council; NR = not reported; S = systolic; SHEP = Systolic Hypertension in the Elderly Program; STONE = Shanghai Trial of Hypertension in the Elderly; Syst-China = Systolic Hypertension in China; Syst-Eur = Systolic Hypertension in Europe; type = type of hypertension.

References: randomized trials of pharmacological blood pressure reduction in the elderly: (1) HDFP: Five-year findings of the hypertension detection and follow up program: I. Reduction in mortality of persons with high blood pressure, including mild hypertension. JAMA 242:2562, 1979. Five-year findings of the hypertension detection and follow-up program: II. Mortality by race, sex and age. Hypertension detection and follow-up program cooperative. JAMA 242:2572, 1979. (2) Treatment of mild hypertension in the elderly: A study initiated and administered by the National Heart Foundation of Australia. Med J Austr 2:398, 1981. (3) Amery A, Birkenhäger W, Brixko P, et al: Mortality and morbidity results from the European Working Party on High Blood Pressure in the Elderly trial. Lancet 1:1349, 1985. (4) Coope J, Warrender TS: Randomised trial of treatment of hypertension in elderly patients in primary care. BMJ 293:1145, 1986. (5) Dahlöf B, Lindholm LH, Hansson L, et al: Morbidity and mortality in the Swedish Trial in Old Patients with Hypertension (STOP-hypertension). Lancet 338:1281, 1991. (6) MRC Working Party: Medical Research Council trial of treatment of hypertension in older adults: Principal results. BMJ 304:405, 1992. (7) SHEP Cooperative Research Group: Prevention of stroke by antihypertensive drug treatment in older persons with isolated systolic hypertension: Final results of the Systolic Hypertension in the Elderly Program (SHEP). JAMA 265:3255, 1991. (8) Syst-Eur: Staessen J, Fagard R, Thijs L, et al: Randomised double-blind comparison of placebo and active treatment for older patients with isolated systolic hypertension. Lancet 350:757, 1997. (9) Gong L, Zwang W, Zhu Y: Shanghai Trial of Nifedipine in the Elderly. Seventh European Meeting on Hypertension; June 9-12 1995; Milan. (10) Liu L, Wang JG, Gong L, et al for the Systolic Hypertension in China (Syst-China) Collaborative Group: Comparison of active treatment and placebo for older patients with isolated systolic hypertension. J Hypertens 16:1823, 1998.

TABLE 72–5 Considerations for Pharmacologic Therapy of Older Patients with Hypertension and Other Disorders

Hypertension Plus	Efficacy Considerations	Toxicity and Adverse Effect Considerations
Arthritis	—	ACE, ARB, aldosterone antagonist interactions with NSAIDs
Atrial fibrillation	Beta blocker,* calcium channel blocker (non-DHP),* amiodarone	Interactions with warfarin
Atrioventricular block	—	Beta blockers, non-DHP calcium channel blockers
Carotid disease or stroke	Calcium channel blocker,* ACE†	
Constipation	—	Verapamil
Coronary artery disease	Beta blocker,*,† calcium channel blocker*,†	Nitrates and postural hypotension
Dementia	Clonidine‡	
Diabetes	ACE,*,† ARB,*,† calcium channel blocker (non-DHP),† beta blocker†	
Gout		Diuretics
Heart failure	ACE,*,† ARB*,† + loop diuretic,*,† ± beta blocker,*,† ± aldosterone antagonist*,†,§	Calcium channel blockers (possible) ACE, ARB, aldosterone antagonist, and hyperkalemia
Hyponatremia	—	Diuretic (especially with SSRI)
Incontinence	—	Diuretic
Myocardial infarction	Beta blocker,*,† ± ACE,*,† ± aldosterone antagonist†	ACE, ARB, aldosterone antagonist, and hyperkalemia
Osteoporosis	Thiazides and bone density preservation	—
Peripheral artery disease	Calcium channel blocker (DHP)*	Beta blocker (if severe)
Postural hypotension	Thiazide‖	Alpha blocker, calcium channel blockers (DHP)
Prostatic hypertrophy	Alpha blocker*	
Renal failure	ACE,*,† ARB,*,† ACE + ARB; loop diuretic*	Aldosterone antagonists
Ventricular arrhythmias	Beta blocker*	Thiazide, loop diuretics, and hypokalemia

*Recommendations for first-line therapy from the European Society of Cardiology guidelines for the management of arterial hypertension.[84]

†Recommendations for second-line agents usually added to thiazide diuretics from the Seventh Report of the Joint National Committee on Prevention, Detection, Evaluation, and Treatment of High Blood Pressure.[83]

‡Only available transdermal formulation for patients unable to swallow or who refuse oral medications.

§Systolic heart failure only.

‖Nursing home patients.

ACE = angiotensin-converting enzyme inhibitor; ARB = angiotensin receptor blocking inhibitor; DHP = dihydropyridine; NSAID = nonsteroidal antiinflammatory drug; SSRI = selective serotonin reuptake inhibitor.

osteoporosis. Osteoporosis is a major risk factor for fractures in older people, and the lifetime risk of osteoporotic fracture in Americans is estimated as 40 percent for women and 13 percent for men. Thiazide administration has been associated with higher bone mineral density and a reduction in risk of hip fractures in epidemiological studies and preservation of bone mineral density compared with placebo in older adults.[81]

Effects of thiazides plus other agents have been evaluated in hypertension trials involving elderly patients. The Losartan Intervention for Endpoint reduction in hypertension study (LIFE) involving primarily whites with systolic hypertension and left ventricular hypertrophy found similar myocardial event and death rates with thiazides plus losartan compared with thiazides plus beta blockers, with more strokes and new-onset diabetes in the beta blocker arm.[85] The Study on Cognition and Prognosis in the Elderly (SCOPE) compared effects of low-dose diuretic therapy combined with either candesartan or placebo.[86] The combined incidence of cardiovascular death, nonfatal myocardial infarction, and nonfatal stroke did not differ; but candesartan plus thiazide was associated with a reduction in stroke risk compared with the thiazide plus placebo group. No difference in the rate of cognitive decline was seen between groups.

The older patients for whom thiazide diuretics may not be the best choice include patients with urinary frequency problems—stress incontinence, urinary frequency with or without incontinence related to prostatic hypertrophy, overactive bladders—and patients needing assistance with toileting. These patients may be more compliant with drugs that do not increase urinary frequency. Table 72–5 presents suggested antihypertensive regimens in older patients based on the presence of hypertension and concomitant diseases. Additional data on frequent geriatric problems and medications to use or avoid are available at www.geriatricsatyourfingertips.com.

Additional Considerations. Both the Seventh Report of the Joint National Committee on Prevention, Detection, Evaluation, and Treatment of High Blood Pressure (JNC 7)[83] and the European Guidelines for the Management of Arterial Hypertension[84] recommend lower initial drug dosages and slower medication titration in older patients and point out the need to monitor for postural hypotension.

A decrease in standing systolic blood pressure is estimated to be present in 15 percent of 70- to 74-year-old community-dwelling men or women and up to 30 percent of patients with systolic hypertension.[87] Postural hypotension of greater than 20 mm Hg or 20 percent of systolic pressure is a risk factor for falls and fractures that are associated with significant morbidity and mortality.[88] Antihypertensive medications add to the risk of postural hypotension, as do many antiparkinsonian agents, antipsychotic agents, or tricyclic antidepressant drugs. Postural blood pressure changes should be assessed (after more than 5 minutes supine, immediately after standing, and 2 minutes after standing) in older patients and volume depletion avoided.

Postprandial falls in both systolic and diastolic blood pressure occur in hospitalized, institutionalized,[89] and community-dwelling elderly persons.[90] The greatest fall occurs about 1 hour after eating, and the blood pressure returns to fasting levels 3 to 4 hours after eating. Blood pressure should be measured at least 4 hours after meals, and vasoactive medications with rapid absorption and peaks should not be administered with meals.

Smaller trials have shown weight loss and sodium restriction to be effective in patients from 65 to 75 years of age.[91] Manipulation of dietary calcium can also reverse some of the age-related change in blood pressure.[92]

The optimal blood pressure target is not known for the very old. Patients older than 80 years are a heterogeneous group. Meta-analyses of randomized trial data have concluded that there are cardiovascular morbidity benefits without mortality benefit for treatment of hypertension in patients older than 80 years[93] but have also reported a slightly higher overall risk of death in treated hypertensives older than 80 years compared with reduced deaths in patients aged 60 to 80 years.[94]

The frailest and oldest people may reside in long-term care facilities. It is estimated that 30 to 70 percent are hypertensive and 30 percent have postural hypotension. Diuretic therapy appears to be effective in controlling systolic blood pressure in these patients and may also decrease postural hypotension.[95]

Table 72–6 summarizes the approach to hypertension in older patients.

CORONARY ARTERY DISEASE (see Chaps. 47 to 50)

Prevalence and Incidence. Both the prevalence and severity of atherosclerotic CAD increase with age in men and women. Autopsy studies show that more than half of people older than 60 years have significant CAD with increasing prevalence of left main or triple-vessel CAD with older age. Using electrocardiographic (ECG) evidence of myocardial infarction, abnormal echocardiogram, carotid intimal thickness, or abnormal ankle-brachial index as measures of subclinical vascular disease in community-dwelling elderly people in the Cardiovascular Health Study, abnormalities were detected in 22 percent of women and 33 percent of men aged 65 to 70 years and 43 percent of women and 45 percent of men older than 85 years.[96-98] The lifetime risk of developing symptomatic CAD is estimated as 1 in 3 for men and 1 in 4 for women, with onset of symptoms about 10 years earlier in men than women and with hypertension, diabetes, and lipid abnormalities influencing individual risk.[99] By 80 years of age, similar frequencies of symptomatic CAD of about 20 to 30 percent are seen in men and women. Because of the increasing proportion of women at older ages, however, population studies show more absolute numbers of women with angina compared with men in the community.

TABLE 72–6 Approach to Hypertension in Older Patients

Systolic as well as diastolic hypertension should be treated • Diastolic target is <90 mm Hg • Systolic target is <140 mm Hg • Individualization is needed for patients older than 80 years
Initial therapy is often a low dose of a thiazide diuretic or is based on concomitant diseases (cardiac and noncardiac)
Drug dosing regimens should be reduced for age- and disease-related changes in drug metabolism and for drug-drug interactions
Patients should be monitored for postural hypotension • Blood pressure should be measured at least 4 hr from meals
Patients should be monitored for adverse effects and drug interactions, especially • Hypovolemia with diuretics • Hyperkalemia with angiotensin-converting enzyme, angiotensin receptor blocker, aldosterone antagonists • Renal function

Diagnosis

HISTORY. Angina symptoms are more likely to be absent or ischemia silent in older patients compared with young patients. Symptoms are also more likely to be termed “atypical” in older patients because the description differs from the classical description of substernal pressure with exertion. Symptoms may be described primarily as dyspnea, shoulder or back pain, weakness, fatigue (in women), or epigastric discomfort and may be precipitated by concurrent illnesses. Some older patients describe symptoms with effort but others may not because of limited physical exertion or altered manifestations of pain related to concomitant diabetes or possible age-related changes. Symptoms in these patients may occur at rest or during mental stress. Memory impairment may also limit the accuracy of the history. Lack of symptoms during evidence of myocardial ischemia on electrocardiography (silent ischemia) has been reported in 20 to 50 percent of patients 65 years of age or older.

TESTING FOR ISCHEMIA (see Chap. 50). The high prevalence of resting ST-T abnormalities in older people results in a modest age-associated reduction in specificity of exercise electrocardiography. Treadmill exercise testing can provide prognostic information in patients able to exercise sufficiently and can also provide information regarding functional capacity and exercise tolerance. Exercise results can be enhanced by the use of modified protocols beginning with low-intensity exercise. The ACC/AHA Guidelines on Exercise Testing estimate a slightly higher sensitivity (84 percent) and lower specificity (70 percent) in patients older than 75 years than in younger patients.[100] Echocardiography and nuclear testing can be used to overcome some of the limitations of ECG interpretation. In older patients unable to exercise, pharmacological agents such as dipyridamole or adenosine can be used with nuclear scintigraphy to assess myocardial perfusion at rest and after vasodilation; or agents such as dobutamine can be combined with echocardiography to assess ventricular function at rest and during increased myocardial demand.[101] Because of the high prevalence of coronary calcification with or without coronary flow decrease in the older population, electron beam cinetomography has little prognostic role in the older patient.

Treatment. Therapeutic goals and management goals that have been established for chronic stable angina are targeted primarily at risk reduction and symptom relief without modification for older patients[102] (see Chap. 50). No age restriction is considered for treatment of patients with CAD unless life expectancy is less than 2 years. Most data on lipid lowering for elderly people come from trials of HMG CoA reductase inhibitors (Table 72–7), with only the Heart Protection Study enrolling significant numbers of women and including patients older than 73.[103] The Heart Protection Study of low-density lipoprotein (LDL) cholesterol lowering with the HMG CoA reductase inhibitor simvastatin in patients with CAD from 40 to 80 years of age with concomitant disease demonstrated decreased total mortality in prespecified subgroups of women, patients older than 75, diabetics, and patients without elevated LDL cholesterol levels. Of the two large primary prevention trials of lipid lowering with HMG CoA reductase inhibitors, one enrolled only men up to age 64 and the other had an upper age cutoff of 73 years.[104,105] Thus, there are no published data about the use of cholesterol-lowering drugs for primary prevention in patients older than 75, especially women.

The incidence of rhabdomyolysis is low with HMG CoA reductase inhibitors, but risk factors for statin-induced myopathy include older age (>80 and women more than men), smaller body frame and frailty, multisystem disease (including chronic renal insufficiency, especially related to diabetes), the perioperative period, coadministration of certain medications (fibrates, nicotinic acid, cyclosporine,

TABLE 72–7 Secondary Prevention Trials of Lipid-Lowering Therapy with Elderly Participants

Study	Patients	*N*	% Older than 65 (*n*) (%, Women, *n*)	Drug (Dose)	Major Results
Scandinavian Simvastatin Survival Study (4S) Trial	CAD	4444	23% (1021) (19%, 827)	Simvastatin (20-40 mg/d)	Reduced all-cause and CAD mortality, CAD events, coronary revascularization, and stroke
Cholesterol and Recurrent Events (CARE) Trial	Post-MI	4159	31% (1283) (14%, 576)	Pravastatin (40 mg/d)	Reduced CAD mortality, death or events, coronary revascularization, and stroke
Long-Term Intervention with Pravastatin in Ischaemic Disease (LIPID) Study	Post-MI or unstable angina	9014	39% (3514) (17%, 1516)	Pravastatin (40 mg/d)	Reduced all-cause mortality, CAD death or events, coronary revascularization, and stroke
Veterans Affairs Cooperative Studies Program High-Density Lipoprotein Cholesterol Intervention Trial (VA-HIT)	CAD + high cholesterol and low HDL	2531	76%*(1936) (0, 0)	Gemfibrozil (1200 mg/d)	Reduced death from cardiovascular cause, no difference in coronary revascularization rates
Heart Protection Study (HPS)	CAD + other vascular disease, diabetes or hypertension	>20,000	28%† (5806) (33%, 5082)	Simvastatin (40 mg/d)	Reduced all-cause mortality, reduced cardiovascular events, reduced coronary revascularizations, and reduced stroke

*Age older than 60.
†Age older than 70.
CAD = coronary artery disease; MI = myocardial infarction.
References: Randomised trial of cholesterol lowering in 4444 patients with coronary heart disease: The Scandinavian Simvastatin Survival Study (4S). Lancet 344:1383, 1994. Miettinen T, Pyorala K, Olsson A, et al: Cholesterol-lowering therapy in women and elderly patients with myocardial infarction or angina pectoris. Findings from the Scandinavian Simvastatin Survival Study (4S). Circulation 96:4211, 1997. Sacks F, Pfeffer M, Moye L, et al: The effect of pravastatin on coronary events after myocardial infarction in patients with average cholesterol levels. Cholesterol and Recurrent Events Trial investigators. N Engl J Med 335:1001, 1996. Lewis S, Moye L, Sacks F, et al: Effect of pravastatin on cardiovascular events in older patients with myocardial infarction and cholesterol levels in the average range. Results of the Cholesterol and Recurrent Events (CARE) Trial. Ann Intern Med 129:681, 1998. The Long-Term Intervention with Pravastatin in Ischaemic Disease (LIPID) Study Group: Prevention of cardiovascular events and death with pravastatin in patients with coronary heart disease and a broad range of initial cholesterol levels. N Engl J Med 339:1349, 1998. Rubins H, Robins S, Collins D, et al for the Veterans Affairs High-density Lipoprotein Cholesterol Intervention Trial Study Group: Gemfibrozil for the secondary prevention of coronary heart disease in men with low levels of high-density lipoprotein cholesterol. N Engl J Med 341:410, 1999. Heart Protection Study Collaborative Group: MRC/BHF Heart Protection Study of cholesterol lowering with simvastatin in 20,536 high-risk individuals: A randomised placebo-controlled trial. Lancet 360:7, 2002.

azole antifungals, macrolide antibiotics, erythromycin, clarithromycin, nefazodone, verapamil, amiodarone), and alcohol abuse. Symptoms of myopathy may be difficult to differentiate from other types of pain in the older patient, and myopathy may not be recognized because of cognitive impairment or the presence of other musculoskeletal disorders. The smallest effective dose should be used and signs and symptoms monitored, and there should be a low threshold for laboratory tests. Muscle strength testing may be helpful in evaluating symptoms in older patients, including simple assessments of the ability to rise from a chair or climb stairs.

SPECIAL CONSIDERATIONS. Marked vasodilation related to rapid absorption or higher peak effects of isosorbide dinitrates can exacerbate postural hypotension, and agents with smooth concentration versus time profiles such as mononitrates or transdermal formulations may be preferred for daily administration, although cost may be prohibitive. Beta blockers have not been shown to increase the occurrence of depression in randomized trials, but beta blockers that are not lipophilic (e.g., atenolol, nadolol) may produce fewer central nervous system effects. Calcium channel blockers, especially the dihydropyridines, can produce pedal edema more frequently in the older patient. Shorter acting formulations can produce or exacerbate postural hypotension and should be avoided. Verapamil can exacerbate constipation, especially in inactive elderly persons. Beta blockers and nondihydropyridine calcium channel blockers both should be avoided in the presence of sinus node disease.

REVASCULARIZATION. There is increasing experience with both percutaneous coronary intervention (PCI) and coronary artery bypass grafting (CABG) in older patients. Half of all PCI and CABG procedures are performed in patients older than 65 years, with one-third of coronary artery revascularization procedures performed in patients older than 70 years. Randomized trials have demonstrated efficacy and successful outcomes in patients, including limited numbers of older patients (Table 72–8) (see Chap. 48). The largest enrollment of patients older than 75 years to date (109 patients) was in the Bypass Angioplasty Revascularization Investigation (BARI) trial involving patients with multivessel disease. Patients aged 65 to 80 had higher early morbidity and mortality after CABG compared with PCI but greater angina relief and fewer repeated procedures after CABG. Stroke was more common after CABG than after percutaneous transluminal coronary angioplasty (PTCA; 1.7 versus 0.2 percent), and HF and pulmonary edema were more common after PTCA (4.0 versus 1.3 percent). The 5-year survival rate was over 80 percent for both procedures (86 percent after CABG and 81.4 percent after PTCA) in these highly selected patients.[106] Women and minorities were underrepresented. Reports from the National Cardiovascular Revascularization Network also show increased early mortality rates after revascularization procedures in older patients, with a more rapid rise in the mortality risk in patients older than 75 years (Fig. 72–7).[107,108] Registry data suggest an in-hospital mortality risk of PCI of less than 1 percent in patients younger than 60 years that

TABLE 72–8 Representation of Elderly Patients with Coronary Artery Disease in Trials of Revascularization

Trial Name	Enrollment Year(s)	Treatment Comparisons	Number Enrolled	Age Inclusion	Number Enrolled ≥75 yr of Age
CASS	1970s	CABG vs. medical	780	Age ≤65 yr	0
VA	1970s	CABG vs. medical	686	None	0
European	1970s	CABG vs. medical	767	Age <65 yr	0
RITA	1980s-1990s	CABG vs. PCI	1011	None	22
EAST	1980s-1990	CABG vs. PCI	392	None	36
GABI	1986-1991	CABG vs. PCI	359	Age <75 yr	0
CABRI	1980s-1990s	CABG vs. PCI	1054	Age ≤75 yr	0
BARI	Late 1980s-1990s	CABG vs. PCI	1829	Age <80 yr	109
ERACI	1980s	CABG vs. PCI	127	Age <76	N/A (few)
ACME	Late 1980s	PCI vs. medical	328	N/A (mean = 60)	N/A
ARTS	1997-1998	PCI + stent vs. CABG	1205	Age ≤83 yr	70†
TIME	1996-2000	PCI or CABG vs. medical	282	>75 yr	282

ACME = Angioplasty Compared to Medicine Study (VA study); ARTS = Arterial Revascularization Therapy Study Trial; BARI = Bypass Angioplasty Revascularization Investigation; CABG = coronary artery bypass graft; N/A = not available; CABRI = Coronary Artery versus Bypass Revascularization Investigation; CASS = Coronary Artery Surgery Study; EAST = Emory Angioplasty versus Surgery Trial; ERACI = Argentine Randomized Trial of Percutaneous Transluminal Coronary Angioplasty versus Coronary Artery Bypass Surgery in Multivessel Disease; European = European Coronary Surgery Study; GABI = German Angioplasty versus Bypass Surgery Trial; PCI = percutaneous coronary intervention; RITA = Randomized Intervention Treatment of Angina; TIME = Trial of Invasive versus Medical Therapy in Elderly patients; VA = VA Cooperative Study of Coronary Artery Bypass for Stable Angina.

†Personal communication.

increases to about 4 percent in patients older than 75 years. Data for small numbers of patients older than 90 years suggest limited clinical benefit despite procedural success. Early CABG mortality rates increase from less than 2 percent in patients younger than 60 years to between 6 and 8 percent in patients older than 75 years; rates approaching 10 percent have been reported in patients older than 80 years. Elderly women are at highest risk, in part because of comorbid conditions.

Nonfatal complications with procedures also increase with age. PCI is associated with a slightly less than 1 percent risk of permanent stroke or coma and CABG is associated with a 3 to 6 percent incidence of permanent stroke or coma in patients older than 75 years. In the immediate postoperative period, longer durations of ventilatory support, greater need for inotropic support and intraaortic balloon placement, greater incidence of bleeding, delirium, renal failure, perioperative infarction, and infection are seen in older patients compared with younger patients. The highest rates of complications are usually seen in older women and in patients undergoing emergency procedures.

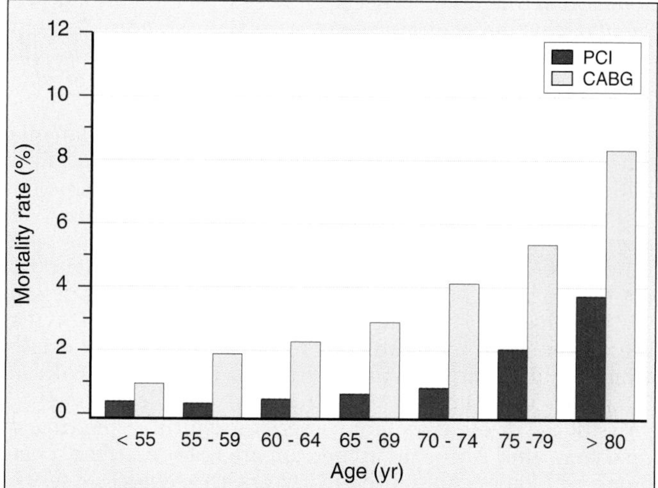

FIGURE 72–7 In-hospital mortality rates reported for revascularization procedures by age group. CABG = coronary artery bypass graft surgery; PCI = percutaneous intervention of all types. (Data from the National Cardiovascular Revascularization Network as reported by Alexander K, Anstrom K, Muhlbaier L, et al: Outcomes of cardiac surgery in patients ≥ 80 years: Results from the National Cardiovascular Network. J Am Coll Cardiol 35:731, 2000 and available at www.sgcard.org.)

In addition to the increased immediate mortality and morbidity associated with revascularization in older patients, the duration of disability and rehabilitation after procedures is usually longer for older persons. Preoperative considerations for older patients should address the potential need for in-home assistance or extended-care hospitalization. Postoperative considerations should also include evaluation for depression (see later). A current unknown is the precise risk of postoperative cognitive impairment in older patients, although neuropsychological testing detects impairment in significant numbers of patients after CABG.[109]

The Trial of Invasive versus Medical Therapy in Elderly patients (TIME) study compared invasive (PCI or CABG) versus optimized medical therapy in CAD patients older than 75 years with angina refractory to standard therapy.[110] Although the initial analysis at 6 months showed an advantage for revascularization, the advantage was no longer present at 1 year. Revascularization presented an early risk of death and complications and optimized medical therapy carried a chance of later events (hospitalization and revascularization) without a clear advantage of either strategy. This is the only revascularization study to enroll significant numbers of patients older than 75 years (see Table 72-8) and enroll significant numbers of women (40 percent). Data remain limited on comparisons involving stents, drug-eluting stents, and off-pump surgery in older groups.

Special Considerations. The ACC/AHA coronary bypass surgery and PCI guidelines conclude that age alone should not be used as the sole criterion when considering revascularization procedures (see www.acc.org or www.americanheart.org).[111] There is a clear role for individualized prognostic information based on multiple clinical factors and respect for patients' preferences in the decision-making process.[107-109,112] The possibility of disability or prolonged hospitalization after interventions must be considered. Recurrent angina or myocardial infarction may not be viewed as having the same negative impact as a stroke by many older patients. For the patient unable to make decisions, involvement of family members or agents is key to choices reflecting the prior wishes of the patient.

Acute Myocardial Infarction (see Chaps. 46 and 47). About 60 percent of hospital admissions for AMI are of people older than 65 years. With increasing age, the gender composition of patients presenting with AMI changes from predominantly men presenting in middle age, to equal number of men and women presenting between the ages of 75 to 84, to the majority of patients with AMI being women at ages older than 80 years. A review of the national Cooperative Cardiovascular Project (CCP) cohort of Medicare beneficiaries further characterized elderly patients presenting with AMI.[113] As age increases past 65 years, there are more patients with functional limitation, HF, prior coronary disease, and renal insufficiency; more women; and lower proportions of diabetics, smokers, or patients with prior revascularization. As age increased from 65 to more than 85 years, the proportion presenting with chest pain and ST elevation on electrocardiography within 6 hours of symptom onset also decreased. Mortality is at least threefold higher in patients older than 85 years than in patients younger than 65 years. Thus, the older old patient with AMI differs from both middle-aged and younger elderly patients.[114]

DIAGNOSIS. Chest pain or discomfort is the most common complaint in older as well as younger patients, but older patients may also present with sudden pulmonary edema or neurological symptoms such as syncope, stroke, or confusion. The electrocardiogram is also more likely to be nondiagnostic (because of baseline abnormalities of ventricular hypertrophy, intraventricular conduction, or pacing). The combination of atypical symptoms and nondiagnostic ECG findings increases the importance of rapid laboratory testing for circulating markers of myocardial damage such as troponin.

TREATMENT

THROMBOLYSIS. Randomized clinical trials of the effects of thrombolysis enrolled few patients older than 75 to 80 years. For patients up to the age of 75 years, most trials showed that fibrinolytic therapy is associated with a survival advantage similar to or greater than that seen in younger patients with ST elevation myocardial infarction. Population-based studies have suggested that community-dwelling elderly patients older than 75 years treated with thrombolytics, however, have an increased risk of ICH of approximately 1.4 percent[115] and some subgroups may not have an overall benefit.[116,117] Those with a high risk for ICH include patients older than 75 years, women, blacks, small patients (<65 kg in women and <80 kg for men), those with prior stroke, patients with systolic blood pressure greater than 160 mm Hg, and patients administered tissue plasminogen activator as compared with other agents. Cardiac rupture risk with thrombolysis is also increased in patients older than 70 years and in women, with an incidence of 0.5 to 2 percent.[32,118,119] The risk of cardiac rupture does not appear to be related to the intensity of anticoagulation. Complication rates of minor and major bleeding are also higher in older patients than younger patients. The ACC/AHA guidelines for management of myocardial infarction published in 1999 recommended thrombolytic administration in patients younger than 75 years with acute ischemic symptoms associated with ST elevation or left bundle branch block who present within 12 hours of symptom onset but acknowledged disagreement on recommendations for patients with this presentation who are older than 75 years[54] (accessible at www.acc.org; www.americanheart.org).

Fibrinolytic agents, especially fibrin-specific agents, are also associated with increased stroke risk related to ICH in the over 75 to 80 age group. Most agents are administered in combination with low-molecular-weight heparin, and dosage adjustments for weight may decrease risks of bleeding.

ANTIPLATELET AGENTS. Trial data show that aspirin reduces mortality in patients older than 70 years and aspirin is recommended for routine administration to older patients with AMI, although older patients have been less likely to receive aspirin than younger patients. The addition of clopidogrel to aspirin after non-ST-segment elevation myocardial infarction reduced major event rates by 20 percent, with similar absolute reductions in patients younger and older than 65 years; there are no significant data on patients older than 75 years. Newer glycoprotein (GP) IIb/IIIa inhibitors appear efficacious in patients older than 70 years, although net benefit may decline with increasing age. In clinical trials, bleeding risk was increased about twofold with GP IIb/IIIa inhibitors, with the risk being about 2 percent. Registry data estimate the increased risk of bleeding to be similar, with about a twofold greater (or 2 percent) risk in patients undergoing PCI who receive GP IIb/IIIa inhibitors compared with patients who do not.[120] A review of the Food and Drug Administration adverse event reports related to GP IIb/IIIa inhibitor administration found deaths in patients with a mean age of 69 to be associated with excessive bleeding, with intracranial bleeding the most common site.[121] It appears that older age is associated with an increased bleeding risk with GP IIb/IIIa inhibitors as well as aspirin and thrombolytics.

INVASIVE STRATEGIES. Results from several studies and data base reviews suggest that primary angioplasty in experienced centers is associated with improved outcomes compared with thrombolytic strategies in elderly patients with ST elevation AMI.[122,123] Primary angioplasty is associated with increased bleeding at the access site as well as increased transfusion requirements in the elderly. PCI procedures are also associated with an increased risk for contrast agent–mediated renal dysfunction in older patients that is an important predictor of adverse outcomes. The benefits of angioplasty compared with those of fibrinolysis have not been convincingly demonstrated in very elderly patients but are being investigated. Reperfusion strategies in elderly patients with acute coronary syndromes are under investigation by the Primary Angioplasty in Myocardial Infarction (PAMI) group.[124]

BETA BLOCKERS. Beta blocker administration is recommended for all patients with AMI regardless of age in the absence of contraindications. Age-related dosage adjustments are appropriate.

ANGIOTENSIN-CONVERTING ENZYME INHIBITORS. In the presence of left ventricular systolic dysfunction or anterior wall myocardial infarction, ACE inhibitors are recommended within the first 24 hours of onset of AMI. ACE inhibitors are recommended after 24 hours for all other patients with myocardial infarction, especially those with reduced left ventricular ejection and prior myocardial infarction. As with other agents in elderly people, smaller initial doses and slower titration are indicated, as is close monitoring of renal function.

Mortality rates are usually higher in older women than men with AMI, as are adverse outcomes with thrombolytics, fibrinolytics, and GP IIb/IIIa inhibitors.[114]

Post-Myocardial Infarction. Recommendations for administration of aspirin, beta blockers, ACE inhibitors, and lipid-lowering drugs for the post-myocardial infarction patient are based on clinical trial data showing benefit in populations that have included elderly patients. Data suggest that these agents are underutilized in older patients, especially women and minorities. Analyses of care delivery to Medicare recipients estimate that 24 percent of eligible patients 65 years of age or older are not prescribed aspirin at the time of discharge after AMI, and 50 percent are not prescribed a beta blocker.[125] Patients older than 75 years are even less likely to receive these therapies than patients 65 to 74 years of age. In contrast, calcium antagonist drugs may be more frequently prescribed in older than younger post-myocardial infarction patients. There is no role for routine administration of antiarrhythmic agents after myocardial infarction (with the exception of beta blockers).

ANTIDEPRESSANTS. Depression is considered relatively common in elderly persons, affecting 10 percent of community-dwelling older people. The prevalence of depression in patients after myocardial infarction is estimated at 20 percent for major depression to 27 percent for minor depression. Studies have shown associations between depression, low perceived social support, and increased cardiac morbidity and mortality in post-myocardial infarction patients[126] and patients undergoing CABG.[127,128] Individual trials of counseling interventions in patients with depression have not shown cardiac benefit, but meta-analyses suggest benefit.[129] Trials have addressed the efficacy and safety of SSRI antidepressant therapy in patients with depression after acute coronary syndromes or myocardial infarction. The Sertraline Antidepressant Heart Attack Randomized Trial (SADHART) involving depressed patients with unstable angina or myocardial infarction compared placebo with sertraline.[130] A small benefit was seen with sertraline that reached significance for patients with recurrent depression. A larger randomized trial, the Enhancing Recovery in Coronary Heart Disease Patients (ENRICHD) trial, compared interventions of cognitive therapy or cognitive therapy combined with an SSRI (sertraline) with "usual" care in patients diagnosed with depression early after myocardial infarction.[131] The intervention group showed increased quality of life and overall function without reduction in cardiac events or mortality after 2 years of treatment. Many patients assigned to usual care also received antidepressants (20.6 percent in the usual care group versus 28 percent in the intervention group). A post hoc analysis of all participants found SSRI use associated with reduced rates of death (hazard ratio = 0.58) and the combined endpoint of death or nonfatal myocardial infarction (hazard ratio = 0.57) without evidence of improvement of depression. General recommendations for all older patients with chronic medical diseases include screening for depression. Initial screening can take the form of a simple two-question test or the geriatric depression screen for older patients followed by additional evaluation for patients with answers suggesting the presence of depression.[132]

MODIFICATIONS IN THERAPY. Analyses showed that older post-myocardial infarction patients who were prescribed beta blockers had a greater risk of rehospitalization with HF if given high doses compared with low doses.[133] It is possible that higher use of beta blockers in the post-myocardial infarction regimen of older patients might be reached if recommendations were for lower and better tolerated doses of these drugs.

HORMONE REPLACEMENT THERAPY. Randomized trials comparing administration of hormone replacement therapy in the form of combined estrogen and progesterone or estrogen alone have shown overall lack of cardiovascular morbidity or mortality benefit and potential harm for both secondary and primary prevention in postmenopausal women.[134-135b] Estrogen with progesterone also increases both the risk of breast cancer and the invasiveness of tumors. Unopposed estrogen therapy has been associated with an increased risk of uterine cancer. The role of selective estrogen receptor modulators in prevention or treatment of vascular disease is under evaluation.

REHABILITATION PROGRAMS (see Chap. 43). The feasibility of and improvement with intensive exercise interventions have been shown for the frailest elderly people residing in the community as well as the nursing home.[136,137] The Cardiac Rehabilitation in Advanced Age (CR-AGE) trial compared hospital-based with home-based cardiac rehabilitation in cognitively intact patients from age 46 to 86 with recent myocardial infarction.[138] Similar improvement in total work capacity and health-related quality of life was seen with home-based rehabilitation compared with hospital-based rehabilitation in all age groups without improvement in the control group. The improvement, however, was somewhat smaller in those older than 75. Benefits decreased over time after hospital rehabilitation but were maintained with home cardiac rehabilitation. Complications were similar across groups; costs, however, were lower in the home rehabilitation group.

Table 72–9 summarizes the approach to the older patient with CAD.

TABLE 72–9 Approach to the Older Patient with Coronary Artery Disease

Morbidity and mortality from CAD and CAD treated medically or with revascularization increases with age and more steeply at ages older than 75 years. After age 70 to 75 years, there are few data to suggest clear advantages of one method of treatment of CAD over another.

Anticipated procedural complication rates should reflect the age and health status of the patient, not complication rates from series of younger patients.

Decisions regarding medical therapy versus revascularization or for PCI versus CABG should be based on the role of CAD in the context of the individual older patient's overall health, life style, projected life span, and preferences.

CABG = coronary artery bypass graft; CAD = coronary artery disease; PCI = percutaneous coronary intervention.

CAROTID ARTERY DISEASE AND STROKE

Prevalence and Incidence. Stroke is the third leading cause of death and leading cause of disability in the United States. The risk of stroke increases with age. Data from the Framingham Study estimate the 10-year probability of stroke as 11 percent in men at age 65 years and 7 percent in women at age 65. At age 80, the probability increases to 22 and 24 percent for men and women, respectively. One in 15 people older than 65 years reports a history of transient ischemic attacks (TIAs). Fifteen percent of patients with stroke report a prior TIA. The short-term risk of stroke after TIA appears to be higher than the risk after a completed stroke. Age older than 60, diabetes, longer duration of TIAs, and TIAs accompanied by weakness increase the risk of stroke after TIA. Carotid stenosis is responsible for about 25 percent of strokes. Risk factors for stroke and TIAs are the same as for other atherosclerotic diseases.

Diagnosis. The diagnosis of TIA is made following a spell of neurological impairment lasting less than 24 hours that is produced by ischemia in a discrete vascular territory in the brain, and the diagnosis is usually based on clinical history alone. Neurological deficits are not present unless there has been prior stroke or disease. Diagnosis of significant carotid disease is usually made in the presence of a stenosis greater than 70 to 80 percent defined by noninvasive imaging with Doppler ultrasonography or magnetic resonance angiography or less frequently with computed tomographic angiography (see Chap. 15). Carotid bruits may or may not be present and carotid disease may be asymptomatic.

Treatment. Preventive and secondary treatment is targeted at modifiable risk factors.[139] Increasing attention has been directed at antiplatelet or anticoagulant therapy in high-risk patients such as those with TIAs, prior stroke, or atrial fibrillation (see Chap. 30) and after myocardial infarction as well as carotid artery interventions for patients with severe lesions or symptomatic disease.[140-142]

STROKE PREVENTION

ANTIPLATELET DRUGS. Aspirin reduces the long-term risk of stroke, as well as cardiovascular events, after stroke or TIA and is considered standard therapy after a stroke regardless of the patient's age. The role of other agents such as the thienopyridine drugs ticlopidine and clopidogrel that inhibit platelet aggregation by blocking platelet adenosine diphosphate receptors is less clear. Ticlopidine-induced hematological side effects have limited its clinical use. Clopidogrel has substantially lower rates of hematological side effects than ticlopidine but is considerably more expensive than aspirin. Secondary prevention trials with clopidogrel that enrolled stroke patients found reductions in composite endpoints that included stroke, but the effect was not as great as the reduction in peripheral artery disease events.[143] Combined aspirin and extended-release dipyridamole has been reported to prevent more strokes than placebo or either aspirin or dipyridamole alone but was associated with greater gastrointestinal intolerance, headache, cost, and drug discontinuation.[144] A comparison of warfarin and aspirin did not find significant differences in the prevention of recurrent ischemic stroke or death or occurrence of serious adverse events.[145]

In most reports, bleeding complications with antiplatelet drugs are more frequent in older than in younger patients. No dose-response relationship was observed for the protective effects of aspirin from 50 to 1500 mg/d, but larger doses increased the risk of gastrointestinal bleeding.[146,147] Although the minimally effective dose for aspirin has not been determined, lower doses are recommended for older patients in particular.

WARFARIN. Antithrombotic prophylaxis should be determined individually on the basis of the estimated risk for stroke during aspirin therapy and the risk for bleeding during anticoagulation. For older patients at moderate and higher risk for stroke, anticoagulation with warfarin is appropriate, unless contraindicated. The target International Normalized Ratio (INR) is 2 to 3. Both initial and maintenance warfarin doses are usually lower in older adults than middle-aged patients, with initiation of warfarin at the estimated maintenance dosage (usually less than 5 mg/d in elderly persons) recommended, followed by frequent monitoring (www.americangeriatrics.org). See Table 72–10 for a summary of the approach to anticoagulation in the older patient.

ACUTE STROKE MANAGEMENT. Data support administration of aspirin in the acute stroke setting but do not support use of unfractionated or low-molecular-weight heparin, heparinoids, streptokinase, or recombinant urokinase. The overall benefit of recombinant tissue plasminogen activator may outweigh the bleeding risk in highly selected patients. Blood pressure management in the setting of acute stroke remains controversial, with aggressive reduction in pressure not generally recommended.[142]

SURGICAL AND ENDOVASCULAR APPROACHES. Several clinical trials have demonstrated that carotid endarterectomy in symptomatic patients with 70 to 99 percent internal carotid artery stenosis who have had a stroke or TIA attributable to the stenosis is safe and effective in reducing the risk of ipsilateral carotid ischemia. Surgery has performed better than medical treatment in preventing disabling ipsilateral stroke (Fig. 72–8).[148] Its benefit is less certain in patients with stenosis of 50 to 69 percent. In asymptomatic patients with carotid stenoses, carotid endarterectomy is less likely to benefit the patient. To achieve a net beneficial effect of carotid endarterectomy versus medical therapy alone, the combined mortality and morbidity rate should be less than 3 percent for asymptomatic patients and less than 6 to 7 percent for symptomatic patients. Increased risk of perioperative stroke or death is associated with surgery for completed stroke (versus TIA), female sex, age older than 75 years, systolic blood pressure higher than 180 mm Hg, and a history of peripheral vascular disease.[149] Intracranial vascular disease and bilateral carotid disease also increase the risk of stroke or death.

During the past few years, carotid angioplasty and stenting have evolved as an alternative to carotid endarterectomy, particularly in patients who are known to have a higher operative complication rate or technical contraindications to surgery such as previous neck surgeries, radiation, or restenosis after endarterectomy.[150]

Table 72–11 summarizes the general approach to the older patient with stroke.

TABLE 72–10 Approach to Anticoagulation in Older Patients

Obtain complete medication and nutraceutical intake data to anticipate warfarin requirements, interactions, contraindications, and necessary adjustment
Educate patient, family, and/or caregivers on diet, alcohol effects, and drug interactions and need for monitoring and communication
Initiate at low doses—often at 2 mg/d, not to exceed 5 mg/d
Monitor closely and titrate slowly; consider use of
- anticoagulation clinics and/or
- fingerstick self-testing programs (patient, family, or caregiver)

Consider warfarin effects of all medication, supplement, and diet changes
Use preventive measures for osteoporosis

PERIPHERAL ARTERY DISEASE

Prevalence and Incidence. Lower extremity peripheral arterial disease (PAD) is common among older men and women (see Chap. 54). The frequency of intermittent claudication increases with age from 0 to 6 percent of people aged 45 to 54 years to about 9 percent of patients aged 65 to 74 years. When an ankle brachial index of 0.9 is used to

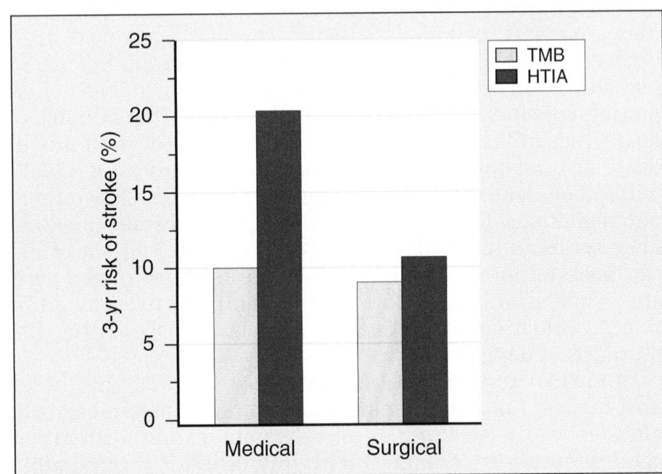

FIGURE 72–8 Three-year risk of ipsilateral stroke in patients with at least 50 percent stenosis and transient monocular blindness (TMB) or hemispheric transient ischemic attack (HTIA) in the North American Symptomatic Carotid Endarterectomy Trial (NASCET). (Data from Benevente O, Eliasziw M, Streifler J, et al: Prognosis after transient monocular blindness associated with carotid stenosis. N Engl J Med 345:1084, 2000.)

TABLE 72–11 Approach to the Older Patient with Stroke

Modifiable risk factors of hypertension, elevated lipids, smoking, physical inactivity, and obesity should be treated; older patients with atrial fibrillation should have anticoagulation (in the absence of contraindications).
Aspirin should be administered in the acute stroke setting and for secondary prevention with lower doses recommended for the older patient.
Warfarin should be considered for patients with strokes while receiving aspirin in the absence of contraindications and with moderate to high likelihood of recurrent stroke.
Anticoagulation with unfractionated or low-molecular-weight heparin, heparinoids, streptokinase, or urokinase is not recommended for acute stroke. Recombinant tissue plasminogen activator may have a role in selected patients.
Carotid endarterectomy benefits symptomatic patients with 70-99% internal carotid artery stenosis who have had a stroke or transient ischemic attack attributable to the stenosis. Definitive conclusions regarding carotid angioplasty cannot be made at this time.

identify PAD, significant PAD is diagnosed in 17 to 20 percent of men and 21 percent of women older than 55, with somewhat higher rates in blacks compared with whites. Individuals with PAD have approximately the same relative risk of death from cardiovascular causes as patients with coronary or cerebrovascular disease.[96,151]

Diagnosis. Intermittent claudication is the earliest and most frequent presenting symptom in about one-third of patients with PAD. More than half of patients with abnormal ankle brachial index measurements indicating PAD have "atypical" leg discomfort.[152] About 20 percent of patients with PAD are asymptomatic. PAD is about equally prevalent in older men and women. Screening for PAD with the ankle brachial index is recommended in all patients older than 70 years, patients 50 to 69 years of age who smoke or have diabetes, patients with leg pain with exertion, those with abnormal results on vascular examinations of the leg, and patients with coronary, carotid, or renal arterial disease.

Treatment. Therapy in PAD should be directed at reduction of cardiovascular risk factors, exercise, and weight loss in overweight patients and improvement of symptoms and walking impairment with pharmacological or surgical intervention, if necessary (see Chap. 54). There are no age restrictions to therapeutic approaches.[153-156] Surgical recovery times, however, are longer in older patients. Table 72–12 presents the general approach to the older patient with PAD.

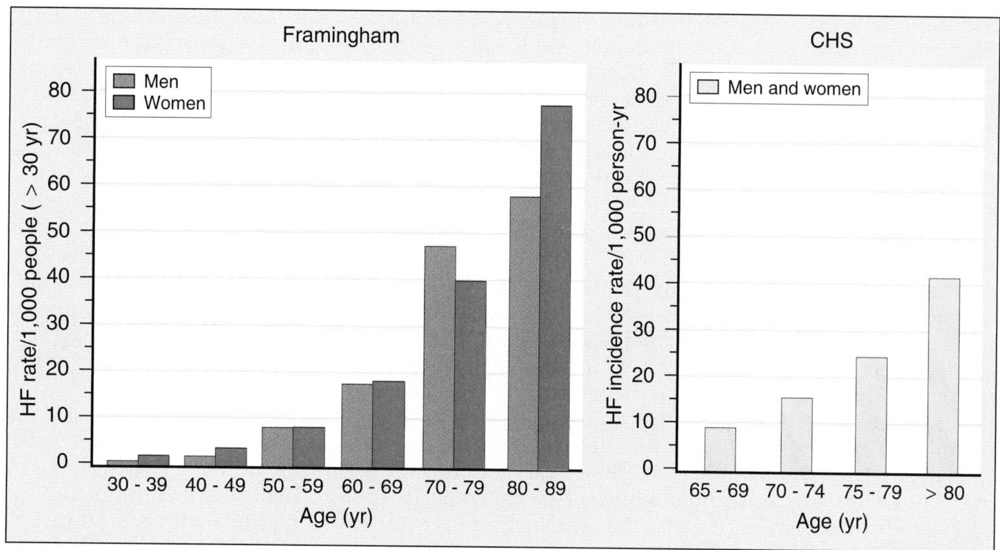

FIGURE 72–9 Prevalence and incidence rates of heart failure (HF) with aging in longitudinal studies. Prevalence rates of HF by age for men (blue) and women (pink) in the Framingham Study are shown in the **left panel** and incidence rates of congestive heart failure by age, from the Cardiovascular Health Study (CHS) are shown in the **right panel.** (Framingham data from Ho K, Pinsky J, Kannel W, Levy D: The epidemiology of heart failure: Framingham Study. J Am Coll Cardiol 22(Suppl A):6A, 1993; CHS data from Gottdiener J, Arnold A, Aurigemma G, et al: Predictors of congestive heart failure in the elderly: The Cardiovascular Health Study. J Am Coll Cardiol 35:1628, 2000.)

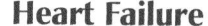

Heart Failure

Prevalence and Incidence. HF has become primarily a disorder of the elderly. HF contributes to at least 20 percent of hospital admissions of patients older than 65 years, with approximately three-quarters of hospitalizations for HF occurring in older patients. HF was reported as one of their medical conditions by 0.1 percent of people at ages 18 to 39 years, by about 4 percent aged 65 to 74 years, and by about 6 percent at ages 75 to 105 years in a national health interview survey.[157] In the Cardiovascular Health Study of independent community-dwelling subjects aged 66 to 103 years ($n = 4842$), HF defined by physician report and medical record review developed at a rate of 19.3 per 1000 patient-years. The incidence increased from 10.6 per 1000 person-years in participants 65 to 69 years of age at the initial evaluation to 42.5 per 1000 person-years in those older than 80 years[158] (Fig. 72–9). Asymptomatic left ventricular systolic dysfunction is estimated to occur in another 3 to 5 percent of the community with higher prevalences at older ages.[159]

HF of any type is associated with a reduction in life span as well as decreased quality of life and recurrent hospitalizations. Although HF treatments are improving, average 5-year mortality is approximately 50 percent for HF patients with systolic dysfunction and approximately 25 percent for HF patients with preserved systolic function.[160,161] In general, prognosis is worse in patients older than 65 years (Fig. 72–10).[162]

TABLE 72–12 Approach to the Older Patient with Peripheral Artery Disease

Treatment of cardiovascular risk factors, aspirin, and supervised walking-based exercise programs are first-line therapy.
Medications can improve symptoms (cilostazol > clopidogrel > pentoxifylline; cilostazol should not be used in patients with heart failure).
Estrogen and progesterone should be avoided in women with PAD.
Revascularization options include percutaneous interventions for iliac disease but long-term efficacy requires surgical approaches at the femoropopliteal and infrapopliteal level.
Surgical morbidity and mortality increase with age and postoperative recovery times can be prolonged. All are highest in the setting of surgery for critical ischemia or limb salvage.

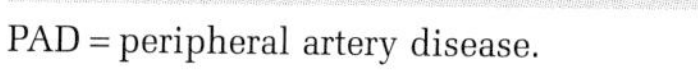
PAD = peripheral artery disease.

Age-Related Changes in Ventricular Function (see Chap. 19). In contrast to the etiology in middle-aged patients with HF, factors other than systolic function contribute to HF in the elderly population. Signs and symptoms of HF in older

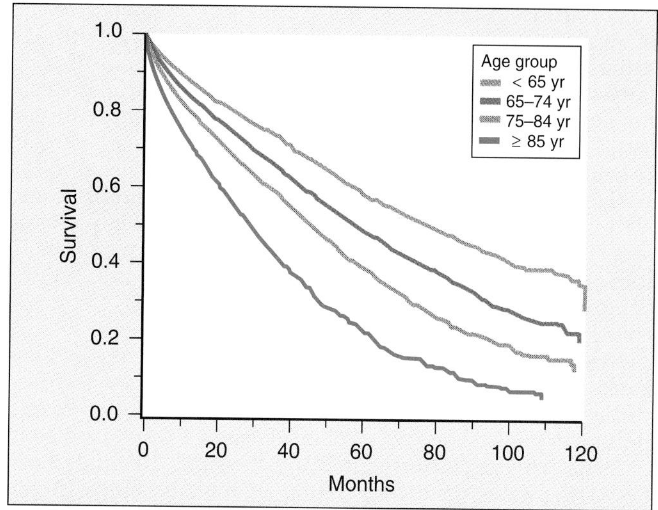

FIGURE 72–10 Age-stratified mortality (adjusted for gender and race) for patients with a diagnosis of heart failure in the Resource Utilization Among Congestive Heart Failure (REACH) study of 29,686 health care recipients during the years 1989 to 1999. (From McCullough P, Philbin E, Spertus J, et al: Confirmation of a heart failure epidemic: Findings from the Resource Utilization Among Congestive Heart Failure [REACH] study. J Am Coll Cardiol 39:60, 2002.)

patients often occur in the presence of preserved left ventricular function.[163-165] Preserved left ventricular systolic function may be seen in 40 to 80 percent of older patients with HF and is almost twice as frequent in women as men.[166,167] Although HF with preserved systolic function has a slightly better prognosis than HF with abnormal function, there is a fourfold higher mortality risk compared with that of subjects free of HF.[168]

Diagnosis. Exercise intolerance is the primary symptom in chronic HF of either systolic or diastolic etiology. Dyspnea and fatigue are prominent symptoms in patients with HF, but fatigue also accompanies many chronic illnesses such as pulmonary disease, thyroid abnormality, anemia, or depression. Complaints of shortness of breath, orthopnea or development of nocturnal cough, or paroxysmal nocturnal dyspnea suggest the presence of HF. Despite these possible symptoms and complaints associated with HF, less than half of patients with moderate or severe diastolic or systolic dysfunction as measured by Doppler echocardiography had recognized HF in a community-based study.[164] Potential explanations for unrecognized HF in older patients include the nonspecificity of complaints of fatigue, with symptoms ascribed to aging, reduction in activities to avoid symptoms, and memory impairment leading to poor historical information. Physical examination may not be as definitive as in younger individuals. Peripheral edema can be due to age-related changes in venous tone, decreased skin turgor, or prolonged sedentary states. Evaluation of volume status on the basis of neck veins may also be difficult in the older patient. Rales and a third heart sound may be present only during episodes of acute decompensation, and differentiation of HF from pneumonia may be difficult in older patients, who are less likely to present with temperature elevations. With diastolic HF, fourth heart sounds may be present but third heart sounds are seldom present. Chest radiography shows pulmonary congestion during acute exacerbations and for some time after an episode; cardiomegaly is present in systolic HF but may or may not be present in diastolic HF. Because of the difficulties with diagnosing HF in the older patient by physician examination or by conventional radiography, use of echocardiography and serum markers of HF takes on greater diagnostic importance.[169]

Treatment. Most data regarding therapy for CHF are from studies of younger middle-aged men with systolic dysfunction resulting from ischemic CAD and few major medical comorbidities. Guidelines[53] are available at www.acc.org and www.americanheart.org. The elderly population with HF differs markedly from patients who have been enrolled in large trials of systolic HF treatment, and clinical trial data are not available to guide treatment of the older patient with diastolic HF. Conceptually, strategies that have demonstrated benefit for systolic HF may benefit patients with diastolic HF. Because the direct applicability of clinical trial findings and HF treatment guidelines to the majority of older HF patients, especially women and those residing in long-term care facilities, is unknown, it is important to consider care in the context of the individual patients and their goals, comorbid conditions, and estimated life expectancy.

SYSTOLIC HEART FAILURE. Pharmacological therapy is targeted at control of systolic and diastolic hypertension (see earlier), use of diuretics to control pulmonary congestion and pulmonary edema, and control of ventricular response rate in patients with atrial fibrillation. Most systolic HF trials have tested therapies on a background of digitalis and diuretic administration. Efficacy of the addition of ACE and angiotensin receptor blockers has been demonstrated in trials that have included elderly patients, and these agents have additional efficacy in diabetes, which is present in at least 10 percent of the older population.[85,170-172] Caution and close monitoring are necessary with use of ACE inhibitors in elderly persons, especially when given at "full doses" used in studies of younger patients. Beta blockers are usually considered next and can be instituted at low doses during periods of clinical stability. Direct vasodilators are efficacious but may have less of a role in older patients with increased likelihood of orthostatic hypotension. Studies of aldosterone antagonists and selective aldosterone blockers have enrolled limited numbers of older patients, especially minorities or women. Benefit may be seen with these drugs used at lower doses in patients with severe HF,[173] but age-related decreases in renal function increase the risk for hyperkalemia.[174] Data for natriuretic peptides in older patients are also lacking. Sex differences in HF etiology and prognosis have been suggested, but there are no sex-specific therapeutic recommendations to date.[175-177]

NONPHARMACOLOGICAL STRATEGIES. Dietary sodium restriction is advised and moderate physical activity should be encouraged if feasible. Cardiac resynchronization therapy can decrease hospitalizations and reduce mortality in selected patients with symptomatic systolic HF and prolonged cardiac repolarization or QRS intervals on the electrocardiogram (see Chap. 31).[178] Revascularization therapies are considered in the setting of ischemia. The few highly selected patients older than 65 years who have received cardiac transplantation appear to have survival times similar to those of younger patients, with slightly more morbidity and mortality related to the surgical procedure but lower rates of rejection than younger patients (see Chap. 26).

DIASTOLIC HEART FAILURE. Diuretics are advised for therapy of diastolic HF in the ACC/AHA guidelines for the evaluation and management of heart failure.[53] Digoxin was associated with symptomatic improvement and decreased hospitalizations (without mortality benefit) in the Digitalis Investigation Group study in patients with diastolic as well as systolic HF,[179] although its risk/benefit ratio in women has been questioned.[177] Small studies of HF in elderly persons with preserved left ventricular function suggest that ACE inhibitors or angiotensin receptor blockers may improve functional class, exercise duration, ejection fraction, diastolic filling, and left ventricular hypertrophy. Although calcium channel antagonists are often proposed for diastolic HF, supportive data are limited. Data are also lacking on nitrates, but some clinicians find them helpful in reducing orthopnea if given at bedtime. Finally, spironolactone and other aldosterone antagonists have not been tested in patients with diastolic HF. Studies of angiotensin II antagonists are ongoing (for a comprehensive review see reference 180).

ADDITIONAL CONSIDERATIONS. Education and involvement of the patient, family members, or caregivers is key to the management of older patients with HF. Recognition of warning signs of worsening failure, understanding of medication regimens, diet adjustments, and the role of regular moderate physical activity should be emphasized. Reliance cannot be on classical symptoms of HF, and weight should be measured daily with a mechanism for rapid communication of information and timely adjustment of diuretic dosages in order to prevent exacerbations of HF. Multidisciplinary team approaches with contacts with the patient between office visits can be highly beneficial, and use of primary care preventive strategies such as influenza vaccination can reduce hospitalizations for HF in older people.[181]

For very old patients or those with progressive symptoms of severe HF, goals of improving symptoms and quality of life and preventing acute exacerbations and hospitalization rather than prolongation of life become the emphasis. Hospice programs may have special expertise in the management of symptoms such as dyspnea with opiates and in providing support for family and caregivers as well as the patient with advanced HF (see Table 72–13 for the approach to the older patient with HF).

TABLE 72–13 Approach to the Older Patient with Heart Failure

Symptoms may be relatively nonspecific in the older patient.
Diagnosis may be facilitated by use of echocardiography or serum markers of heart failure.
Recognize that heart failure may be present in the older patient with preserved systolic function, especially older women.
Treat symptoms with a goal of improving quality of life as well as morbidity.
- Control blood pressure—systolic and diastolic.
- Control atrial fibrillation rate.
- Promote physical activity.
- Adjust medications for age- and disease-related changes in kinetics and dynamics.

Educate and involve patients, family members, or caregivers in management of heart failure.
- Monitor weight.
- Consider use of multidisciplinary team approaches.

Arrhythmias

PATHOPHYSIOLOGY AND AGE-RELATED ELECTROCARDIOGRAPHIC CHANGES. Cell loss and collagen infiltration occur in the area of the sinus node and throughout the atria, the central fibrous body, and cytoskeleton of the heart with increasing age. Changes are most marked in the area of the sinus node with destruction of as many as 90 percent of cells by age 75 years. The correlation between pathology and sinus node function, however, is poor, and sinus node function is preserved in most elderly patients although sinoatrial conduction is decreased. Collagen infiltration and fibrosis are of lesser magnitude in the area of the AV node and more marked in the left and right bundle branches. Conduction times through the AV node increase with aging with the site of delay above the His bundle. Despite age-related collagen infiltration, His-Purkinje conduction times are not usually increased by aging alone.

Resting heart rate is not altered by age, but maximal heart rate (see Fig. 72-4) and beat-to-beat variability in heart rate decrease with age because of age-related decreases in sinus node responses to beta-adrenergic and parasympathetic stimulation (see Chap. 87). On the surface electrocardiogram, the PR interval increases and the R, S, and T wave amplitude decrease. The QRS axis shifts leftward. This shift may reflect increased left ventricular mass or interstitial fibrosis of the anterior fascicular radiation. Right bundle branch block is found in 3 percent of healthy people older than 85 years and up to 20 percent of centenarians; it is found in 8 to 10 percent of older patients with heart disease but is not associated with cardiac morbidity or mortality. The presence of left bundle branch block increases with age and is more likely to be associated with cardiovascular disease. Similarly, nonspecific intraventricular conduction delays become more frequent with increasing age and are usually related to underlying myocardial disease. Repolarization times throughout the myocardium increase with age, and surface ECG QT intervals increase.

Atrial ectopy has been found on ECG recordings in 10 percent of community-dwelling elderly people without known cardiac disease and up to 80 percent during 24-hour ambulatory ECG recordings. Brief episodes of atrial tachyarrhythmias were seen in up to 50 percent of 24-hour ambulatory electrocardiograms of community-dwelling elderly people. Premature ventricular complexes also increase in prevalence and frequency with age. Ventricular ectopic beats are seen on ECG recordings in 6 to 11 percent of elderly people without known cardiovascular disease and as many as 76 percent on 24-hour ambulatory ECG recordings. In the absence of cardiac disease, these age-related changes have not been associated with subsequent cardiovascular events (see Table 72-1).

SINUS NODE DYSFUNCTION. Bradycardia related to sinus node dysfunction or AV conduction disease, or both, is more common as age increases. The mean age of patients undergoing permanent pacemaker implantation is about 74 years, with 70 percent of new pacemaker recipients being older than 70 years, and in the United States 85 percent of pacemaker implantations are in patients older than 65 years. The most common indication is for sinus node dysfunction.

ATRIOVENTRICULAR CONDUCTION DISEASE. First-degree AV block is diagnosed in 6 to 10 percent of healthy elderly people. Higher degree AV block is less common. Transient type II AV block occurs on 0.4 to 0.8 percent of 24-hour ambulatory ECG recordings of community-dwelling elderly people and transient third-degree AV block in less than 0.2 percent. These arrhythmias usually represent advanced conduction system disease requiring pacemaker implantation (see Chaps. 29 and 30).

ATRIAL ARRHYTHMIAS

Atrial Fibrillation. Atrial fibrillation is seen on 24-hour ambulatory recordings in 10 percent of community-dwelling older patients. The incidence of atrial fibrillation doubles with each decade beginning at age 60, so that by ages 80 to 89 years the incidence of atrial fibrillation is currently estimated to be 8 to 10 percent. Approximately one-half of patients with atrial fibrillation in the United States are older than 75 years. Atrial fibrillation in the population is increasing, however, and a 2.5-fold increase in the prevalence of atrial fibrillation over the next 50 years has been predicted (see Chap. 32).[182]

The focus of therapy in the older patient should be on anticoagulation to prevent stroke and recurrent stroke and rate control to improve symptoms. Rarely, rhythm control is needed to provide symptom relief. Patients should receive anticoagulation with warfarin in the absence of contraindications (see Table 72–10). The target INR is 2 to 2.5 in older patients in whom close monitoring of INRs can be performed. Low fixed warfarin doses of 1 mg/d are not efficacious. Patients older than 75 may require less than half the dose of middle-aged patients for equivalent anticoagulation. Warfarin dosing guidelines for elderly patients recommend initiation of warfarin at the estimated maintenance dosage of warfarin, usually less than 5 mg/d (www.americangeriatrics.org). Drug interaction information should be consulted whenever warfarin is being initiated or a drug is added to or deleted from a patient's medication regimen.

Chronic warfarin administration may contribute to osteoporosis. Vitamin K plays a role in bone metabolism, and oral anticoagulation with warfarin antagonizes vitamin K. In analyses of women receiving chronic oral anticoagulation compared with nonanticoagulated cohorts, increased risk of osteoporosis and higher rates of vertebral and rib fractures were associated with oral anticoagulation for more than 12 months.[183] Measures to prevent osteoporosis should accompany long-term anticoagulation with warfarin (calcium and vitamin D in most; bisphosphonates, calcitonin if needed) (Table 72–14).

TABLE 72–14 Approach to the Older Patient with Atrial Fibrillation

Atrial fibrillation is frequent in elderly people and confers a risk of stroke but the patient may be unaware of its presence, suggesting that routine examinations or electrocardiographic evaluations be targeted toward detection of atrial fibrillation.
Anticoagulation is the chief weapon against stroke.
- Both greater potential benefit and risk for fatal intracranial bleeding are present at ages older than 75 years, especially in women.
- Careful attention to anticoagulation monitoring is needed.
- Aspirin does not usually provide stroke risk reduction in older patients because of higher likelihood of the presence of cardiovascular diseases but has overall bleeding complication rates similar to those with warfarin.

Rate control produces equivalent benefits with lower costs than attempts at rhythm control.
- Useful agents for elderly patients include digoxin (rest control), beta blockers, nondihydropyridine calcium channel blockers, and amiodarone with dose adjustments for age, weight, and concomitant diseases.

VENTRICULAR ARRHYTHMIAS. Treatment of premature ventricular contractions with most type 1 antiarrhythmic agents either has been of no benefit or has decreased survival. If patients have symptoms, administration of a beta blocker may be helpful. Sustained ventricular tachycardia and ventricular fibrillation require treatment in patients of any age (see Chap. 30).

Valvular Disease (see also Chap. 57)

PATHOPHYSIOLOGY AND AGE-RELATED CHANGES. Age-related changes in the fibromuscular skeleton of the heart include myxomatous degeneration and collagen infiltration termed sclerosis. Sclerosis of the aortic valve is present in as many as 30 percent of elderly persons,[184] with the prevalence of sclerosis detected on echocardiography increasing as age increased from 65 to more than 85 years in the Cardiovascular Health Study.[185] Further age-related changes include calcification of the aortic valve leaflets, aortic annulus, base of the semilunar cusps, and the mitral annulus. Aortic valve calcium detected by electron beam computed tomography increases over time[186] with progression from valvular sclerosis to stenosis with a transvalvular pressure gradient in a significant percentage of patients (Table 72–15).[187] Aortic sclerosis appears to parallel atherosclerotic progression in other vessels.[188-190] This may explain the increased risk of myocardial infarction and death from cardiovascular causes in patients with aortic sclerosis without evidence of stenosis.[184] Risk factors identified for progression include hypertension, hyperlipidemia, smoking, end-stage renal disease, congenital bicuspid valves, and, in some series, diabetes, shorter stature, and male sex. In older patients, fibrosis with valve calcification is now the most common etiology of valvular stenoses, especially at the aortic position. Ischemic or hypertensive disease has become the most common etiology of valvular regurgitation, especially at the mitral valve. Similarly, pulmonary or tricuspid regurgitation in elderly persons is usually secondary to pulmonary hypertension and dilation of the right ventricle resulting from left ventricular ischemia, HF, or pulmonary disease. Less common etiologies of mild to moderate mitral or aortic regurgitation are ruptured chordae, endocarditis, trauma, aortic dissection, and rheumatic heart disease.

Infective endocarditis is seen with about equal frequency in younger and older patients but is more likely to be associated with nosocomial infections with the use of intravascular catheters or other devices, the presence of prosthetic implants, pacemaker leads, atheromas, or mitral annular calcification in older patients. Polymicrobial infections are uncommon in elderly people, and the most frequent pathogens are group D streptococci and enterococcus, *Staphylococcus epidermidis*, and *Streptococcus viridans* (see Chap. 58).

Treatment for symptomatic valvular disease relies on surgical approaches. Surgery in patients 70 to 80 years of age is increasingly common, but experience with those older than 90 years is limited and there is a high surgical mortality rate.

AORTIC STENOSIS. The prevalence of aortic stenosis in patients older than 65 years is estimated as 2 percent for severe stenosis, 5 percent for moderate stenosis, and 9 percent for mild stenosis. Aortic stenosis in more than 90 percent of older patients involves calcification of the aortic annulus and semilunar cusps of trileaflet valves without commissural fusion. The pathophysiological consequences of aortic stenosis are independent of etiology and include left ventricular hypertrophy, elevated left ventricular diastolic pressures, and decreased stroke volume in patients of all ages. For any given degree of aortic stenosis, left ventricular hypertrophy and decreased left ventricular compliance are greater in patients older than 65 than in younger patients. Approximately 50 percent of patients with severe aortic stenosis have significant CAD, further influencing left ventricular function, symptoms, and morbidity.

Diagnosis. Symptoms can be exertional angina, syncope, or HF and may be precipitated by atrial arrhythmias such as atrial fibrillation. Symptoms may be absent in inactive older patients or may not be elicited from patients with memory impairment. Physical findings of calcific aortic valve stenosis in older patients differ from those seen with rheumatic aortic stenosis and do not accurately reflect the degree of stenosis. The age-related arterial changes of decreased compliance and increased stiffness mask carotid artery findings associated with rheumatic aortic stenosis in younger individuals (see Chap. 8). The carotid artery upstroke and peak may appear normal and carotid amplitude may be unaltered or increased even in the presence of severe calcific stenosis. The presence of decreased carotid upstroke and volume (in the absence of carotid disease) usually indicates severe stenosis. Aortic sclerosis and aortic stenosis both produce systolic ejection murmurs. The volume of the murmur depends on flow as well as the pressure gradient and does not reflect the severity of stenosis. It may be absent in low-output states reflecting severe aortic valve obstruction. The murmur may be high pitched and musical as opposed to harsh and low in frequency. The loudness of the second heart sound may be preserved. Hypertension is common in elderly people, making left ventricular hypertrophy on electrocardiography or ventricular enlargement on chest radiography similarly of

TABLE 72–15 Prevalence of Aortic Valve Abnormalities Detected by Echocardiography in the Cross-Sectional Cardiovascular Health Study of 5201 Medicare Subjects Older than 65 Years

	Aortic Valve Abnormality*			
Subjects	***None***	***Sclerosis***	***Stenosis***	***Valve Replacement***
All subjects	3736 (72%)	1329 (26%)	88 (2%)	23 (0.4%)
Women	2249 (76%)	641 (22%)	43 (1.5%)	12 (0.4%)
Men	1487 (67%)	688 (31%)	45 (2%)	11 (0.5%)
65-74 yr old	2684 (78%)	697 (20%)	43 (1.3%)	16 (0.5%)
Women	1654 (82%)	344 (17%)	20 (1.0%)	9 (0.4%)
Men	1030 (73%)	353 (25%)	23 (1.6%)	7 (0.5%)
75-84 yr old	962 (62%)	542 (35%)	37 (2.4%)	7 (0.5%)
Women	546 (66%)	259 (31%)	22 (2.7%)	3 (0.4%)
Men	416 (58%)	283 (39%)	15 (2.1%)	4 (0.6%)
85+ yr old	90 (48%)	90 (48%)	8 (4%)	0 (0%)
Women	49 (56%)	38 (43%)	1 (1%)	0
Men	41 (41%)	52 (52%)	7 (7%)	0

From Stewart BF, Siscovick D, Lind BK, et al: Clinical factors associated with calcific aortic valve disease. Cardiovascular Health Study. J Am Coll Cardiol 29:630, 1997.

*Data are expressed as number (%) of subjects.

TABLE 72–16 Approach to the Older Patient with Suspected Valvular Disease

Physical examination cannot reliably assess the severity of valvular lesions in most older patients.
Doppler echocardiography is the clinical standard for diagnosis and evaluation of the severity of valve lesions.
- Differentiates sclerosis from stenosis
- Quantitates regurgitation
- Assesses calcification of valves and supporting structures

Age is a predictor of worse outcomes for the natural history of valvular lesions as well as surgical approaches.
Surgery is definitive therapy for valvular lesions with age, coronary artery disease, additional diseases, projected life span, and desired life style as factors in evaluating surgical options.

little diagnostic help. Thus, Doppler echocardiography has become the clinical standard for diagnosis of aortic stenosis in elderly patients. In the setting of low cardiac output, maneuvers (vasodilators, inotropes) to increase output may be helpful in quantifying stenosis. Catheterization is less commonly used to make the diagnosis, but coronary angiography is usually performed to evaluate CAD in older patients before surgical interventions.

Management. Management (Table 72–16) is similar to that of younger patients, with recognition of the increased likelihood of concomitant coronary disease and diseases of other organs (see Chap. 57).[191] Antibiotic prophylaxis should be used to prevent bacterial endocarditis. Risk factors should be treated, and current concepts support aggressive lipid lowering in patients with calcific aortic sclerosis and stenosis.[186,192,193]

Surgical morbidity and mortality are related to the severity and duration of aortic stenosis, presence or absence of HF or CAD, concomitant diseases (especially renal), urgency of the procedure, and complexity of the procedure. Combined valve replacement and CABG is associated with higher perioperative morbidity and mortality than isolated valve replacement. Estimates of operative mortality are in the range of 5 to 10 percent for selected older patients who have undergone valve replacement with or without CABG. Perioperative renal failure, pulmonary insufficiency, stroke, late cognitive impairment, and late death rates are higher than in younger individuals. Postoperative hospitalization and rehabilitation times are usually longer for older patients. Appropriate selection of patients includes assessment of the burden of disease in addition to that of valve disease, anticipated life span independent of valve disease, and symptom status. The frailer the patient and the more comorbidities, the more likely that the risk of perioperative mortality will outweigh the potential of benefit. Biological tissue valves are frequently implanted in elderly patients on the basis of a number of factors including shorter anticipated life expectancy, longer bioprosthesis durability with older age, and avoidance of chronic anticoagulation.[194,195] Estimated structural failure rates of current bioprosthetic valves are about 1 percent per patient-year in patients older than 65 years, and mechanical valves should be considered for younger old patients or those with longer estimated lifespans.[195]

Aortic balloon valvuloplasty has been used in symptomatic patients who were not surgical candidates. No studies have directly compared surgery with balloon valvuloplasty, but observed mortality rates for patients after aortic valvuloplasty are similar to those for patients with severe symptomatic aortic stenosis who do not undergo surgery. Valvuloplasty may improve hemodynamics and symptoms initially but is associated with high procedural morbidity and mortality, with rapid restenosis and recurrence of symptoms within months in most series. It may serve as a bridge to valve surgery in hemodynamically unstable patients (cardiogenic shock), patients undergoing emergent noncardiac surgery, and patients with severe comorbidities who are too ill to undergo cardiac surgery.[196]

Asymptomatic patients with aortic stenosis should be educated concerning signs and symptoms related to aortic stenosis and observed regularly for development of symptoms. Risk of sudden death in asymptomatic patients with aortic stenosis is estimated as 3 to 5 percent. Operative mortality in older patients exceeds this rate; thus, asymptomatic patients with severe aortic stenosis are not usually recommended for surgical interventions.

AORTIC REGURGITATION. The prevalence of aortic regurgitation also increases with age. Mild aortic regurgitation was detected by Doppler echocardiography in 13 percent of patients older than 80 years and moderate or severe regurgitation in 16 percent in one series.[197] Causes of aortic regurgitation in older patients include primary valvular disease (myxomatous or infective) or aortic root disease and dilation secondary to hypertension or dissection. Significant aortic regurgitation in older patients is usually seen in combination with aortic stenosis. When infective aortic regurgitation occurs in elderly patients, the clinical manifestations may be insidious and nonspecific and symptoms fewer than in younger patients with endocarditis. Central nervous system symptoms are common and may predict a less favorable clinical outcome. Patients who have acute HF and pulmonary congestion as the manifestation of aortic valve endocarditis have a mortality rate of 50 to 80 percent. Age is a predictor of worse outcome for the natural history of aortic regurgitation. The estimated life span of older patients with chronic severe aortic regurgitation who do not undergo valve replacement was estimated as 2 years after the onset of HF in earlier observational studies.

Aortic regurgitation can be diagnosed by the presence of the classic diastolic murmur on physical examination. The finding of a widened pulse pressure usually associated with aortic regurgitation in younger patients is of limited diagnostic value in the older patient because age-related changes in the vasculature usually produce a widened pulse pressure in older people. Doppler echocardiography is the usual method of quantitation of the regurgitation and assessment of ventricular function.

MITRAL ANNULAR CALCIFICATION. Mitral annular calcification is an age-related chronic degenerative process that is seen more commonly in women than men and in people older than 70 years. An increased prevalence of mitral annular calcification is seen in patients with systemic hypertension, increased mitral valve stress, mitral valve prolapse, raised left ventricular systolic pressure, aortic valve stenosis, chronic renal failure, secondary hyperparathyroidism, atrial fibrillation, and aortic atherosclerosis. As with aortic calcific processes, mitral annular calcification is associated with risk factors for the development of coronary atherosclerosis and may reflect generalized atherosclerosis.[189,190] Mitral annular calcification may produce mitral stenosis, mitral regurgitation, infective endocarditis, atrial arrhythmias, or heart block. It is an independent risk factor for systemic embolism and stroke, with the risk of stroke directly related to the degree of mitral annular calcification.

MITRAL STENOSIS. Symptoms and presentation are the same as in younger patients and include exertional dyspnea, orthopnea, paroxysmal nocturnal dyspnea, and pulmonary edema or right-sided HF. Physical findings of calcific mitral stenosis differ from those of rheumatic mitral stenosis, and neither a loud first heart sound nor an opening snap is usually heard. The characteristic diastolic rumbling murmur is usually present. Quantification of stenosis is usually accomplished by Doppler echocardiography.

MITRAL REGURGITATION. Myxomatous degenerative and ischemic papillary muscle dysfunction or rupture related to CAD and myocardial infarction as etiologies of mitral regurgitation (MR) in the older patient are increasing. Rheumatic mitral disease is declining, and endocarditis etiology is unchanged. MR may also be seen in the setting of left ventricular dilation related to HF.

Patients with acute MR present with HF and pulmonary edema, but this may also be the initial presentation for medical care of the older patient with chronic MR. Chronic MR may be asymptomatic, especially in the sedentary patient. In symptomatic patients, initial complaints are usually easy fatigability and decreasing exercise tolerance because of low forward cardiac output followed by dyspnea on exertion, orthopnea, paroxysmal nocturnal dyspnea, and dyspnea at rest as left ventricular function fails. Right-sided HF may also occur. Findings on examination are not altered by age, and a holosystolic murmur is usually present. Doppler echocardiography can quantitate the MR. Increasingly, transesophageal echocardiography plays a role in defining the structure of the mitral valve apparatus and evaluation of endocarditis.

Medical treatment is age independent and includes afterload reduction, diuretics as needed for HF, management of atrial fibrillation, and antibiotic prophylaxis. When symptoms cannot be controlled, surgical options are based on left ventricular function and the extent of comorbid diseases. Age older than 65 has been reported to be a predictor of hospital mortality with isolated mitral valve surgery. The presence of CAD and need for combined valve replacement and CABG also increase surgical morbidity and mortality. Survival at 5 years may be as low as 50 percent. Mitral valve repair is preferred to mitral valve replacement when possible in the older patient. Series reporting results of mitral valve repair (alone and with CABG) estimate early death rates in patients older than 70 of 9 percent.[198]

Additional Considerations. Drug-induced valve disease is uncommon, but there are case reports of fibroproliferative lesions producing valvular insufficiency or regurgitation in older patients receiving chronic treatment with the antiparkinsonian dopamine receptor agonist pergolide.[199,200]

REFERENCES

Demographics and Epidemiology

1. Trends in aging—United States and worldwide. MMWR Morb Mortal Wkly Rep 52(6):101, 2003.
2. U.S. Census Bureau: Income 2001 (http://www.census.gov/hhes/income ed).
3. Clark C, Karlawish J: Alzheimer disease: Current concepts and emerging diagnostic and therapeutic strategies. Ann Intern Med 138:400, 2003.
4. Alzheimer's Disease and Dementia. A Growing Challenge. Washington, DC, National Academy on an Aging Society; September 2000.
5. Harris D, Douglas P: Enrollment of women in cardiovascular clinical trials funded by the National Heart, Lung, and Blood Institute. N Engl J Med 343:475, 2000.

Pathophysiology

6. Lakatta E, Levy D: Arterial and cardiac aging: Major shareholders in cardiovascular disease enterprises: Part II: The aging heart in health: Links to heart disease. Circulation 107:346, 2003.
7. Lakatta E, Levy D: Arterial and cardiac aging: Major shareholders in cardiovascular disease enterprises: Part I: Aging arteries a "set up" for vascular disease. Circulation 107:139, 2003.
8. Kass D: Age-related changes in ventricular-arterial coupling: Pathophysiologic implications. Heart Fail Rev 7:51, 2002.
9. Lakatta E: Arterial and cardiac aging: Major shareholders in cardiovascular disease enterprises: Part III: Cellular and molecular clues to heart and arterial aging. Circulation 107:490, 2003.
10. Anversa P, Nadal-Ginard B: Myocyte renewal and ventricular remodelling. Nature 415:240, 2002.
11. Lakatta E, Sollott S: Perspectives on mammalian cardiovascular aging: Humans to molecules. Comp Biochem Physiol A Mol Integr Physiol 132:699, 2002.
12. Zhou Y, Lakatta E, Xiao R: Age-associated alterations in calcium current and its modulation in cardiac myocytes. Drugs Aging 13:159, 1998.
13. Wilkerson W, Sane D: Aging and thrombosis. Semin Thromb Hemost 28:555, 2002.
14. Willerson J: Systemic and local inflammation in patients with unstable atherosclerotic plaques. Prog Cardiovasc Dis 44:469, 2002.
15. Schwartz J: Dopaminergic responses in the Fischer 344 rat heart: Preserved chronotropic and dromotropic responses with aging. J Gerontol Med Sci 52:M36, 1997.
16. Supiano M, Hogikyan R, Sidani M, et al: Sympathetic nervous system activity and α-adrenergic responsiveness in older hypertensive humans. Am J Physiol 276:E519, 1999.
17. Seals D, Esler M: Human ageing and the sympathoadrenal system. J Physiol 528:407, 2000.
18. Rehman H, Masson E: Neuroendocrinology of ageing. Age Ageing 30:279, 2001.
19. Kaasinen V, Rinne J: Functional imaging studies of dopamine system and cognition in normal aging and Parkinson's disease. Neurosci Biobehav Rev 26:785, 2002.
20. Jones P, Christou D, Jordan J, Seals D: Baroreflex buffering is reduced with age in healthy men. Circulation 107:1770, 2003.
21. The ATBC Study Group: Incidence of cancer and mortality following alpha-tocopherol and beta-carotene supplementation. JAMA 290:476, 2003.
22. Liem A, Reynierse-Buitenwerf R, Zwinderman A, et al: Secondary prevention with folic acid: Effects on clinical outcomes. J Am Coll Cardiol 41:2105, 2003.
23. Salonen J: Clinical trials testing cardiovascular benefits of antioxidant supplementation. Free Radic Res 36:1299, 2002.
24. Waters D, Alderman E, Hsia J, et al: Effects of hormone replacement therapy and antioxidant vitamin supplements on coronary atherosclerosis in postmenopausal women. A randomized controlled trial. JAMA 288:2432, 2002.
25. Gruppo Italiano per lo Studio della Sopravivenza nell'Infarto miocardico (GISSI)-Prevenzione Investigators: Dietary supplementation with n-3 polyunsaturated fatty acids and vitamin E after myocardial infarction: Results of the GISSI-Prevenzione trial. Lancet 354:447, 1999.
26. Gale C, Ashurst H, Powers H, Martyn C: Antioxidant vitamin status and carotid atherosclerosis in the elderly. Am J Clin Nutr 74:402, 2001.
27. Miquel J: Can antioxidant diet supplementation protect against age-related mitochondrial damage? Ann NY Acad Sci 959:508, 2002.
28. Remme W: Aldosterone and myocardial infarction—Are aldosterone antagonists needed to prevent remodelling or does ACE inhibition suffice? Cardiovasc Drugs Ther 15:297, 2001.
29. Hansson L: ACE inhibition and left ventricular remodelling. Eur Heart J 18:1203, 1997.

Medication Modifications

30. Gurwitz J, Gore J, Goldberg R, et al: Risk for intracranial hemorrhage after tissue plasminogen activator treatment for acute myocardial infarction. Participants in the National Registry of Myocardial Infarction 2. Ann Intern Med 129:597, 1998.
31. Van de Werf F, Barron H, Armstrong P, et al: Incidence and predictors of bleeding events after fibrinolytic therapy with fibrin-specific agents. Eur Heart J 22:2253, 2001.
32. Van de Werf F: ASSENT-3: Implications for future trial design and clinical practice. Eur Heart J 23:911, 2002.
33. Levey A, Bosch J, Lewis J, et al: A more accurate method to estimate glomerular filtration rate from serum creatinine: A new prediction equation. Ann Intern Med 130:461, 1999.
34. Cockcroft DW, Gault MH: Prediction of creatinine clearance from serum creatinine. Nephron 16:31, 1976.
35. Manjunath G, Sarnak M, Levey A: Prediction equations to estimate glomerular filtration rate: An update. Curr Opin Nephrol Hypertens 10:785, 2001.
36. Kang D, Verotta D, Krecic-Shepard M, et al: Population analyses of sustained release verapamil in patients: Age, race, and sex effects. Clin Pharmacol Ther 73:31, 2003.
37. Krecic-Shepard M, Park K, Barnas C, et al: Race and sex influence clearance of nifedipine: Results of a population study. Clin Pharmacol Ther 68:130, 2000.
38. Schwartz J: Gender-specific implications for cardiovascular medication use in the elderly: Optimizing therapy for older women. Cardiol Rev 11:275, 2003.
39. Schwartz J: The influence of sex on pharmacokinetics. Clin Pharmacokinet 42:107, 2003.
40. Evans W, Relling M: Pharmacogenomics: Translating functional genomics into rational therapeutics. Science 286:487, 1999.
41. Weinshilboum R: Inheritance and drug response. N Engl J Med 348:529, 2003.
42. Mulder A, van Lijf H, Bon M, et al: Association of polymorphism in the cytochrome CYPD6 and the efficacy and tolerability of simvastatin. Clin Pharmacol Ther 70:546, 2001.
43. Roden DM, Brown NJ:. Preprescription genotyping: Not yet ready for prime time, but getting there. Circulation 103:1608, 2001.
44. Rendic S: Summary of information on human CYP enzymes: Human P450 metabolism data. Drug Metab Rev 34:83, 2002.
45. Benet L, Hoener B: Changes in plasma protein binding have little clinical relevance. Clin Pharmacol Ther 71:115, 2002.
46. Kohn LT, Corrigan JM, Donaldson MS (eds): To Err Is Human: Building a Safer Health System. Washington, DC, National Academies Press, 2000.
47. Onder G, Padone C, Landi F, et al: Adverse drug reactions as cause of hospital admission: Results from the Italian Group of Pharmacoepidemiology in the Elderly (GIFA). J Am Geriatr Soc 50:1962, 2002.
48. Gurwitz JH, Field TS, Harrold LR, et al: Incidence and preventability of adverse drug events among older persons in the ambulatory setting. JAMA 289:1107, 2003.
49. Bates D, Miller E, Cullen D, et al for the ADE Prevention Study Group: Patient risk factors for adverse drug events in hospitalized patients. Arch Intern Med 159:2553, 1999.
50. Gandhi TK, Weingart SN, Borus J, et al: Adverse drug events in ambulatory care. N Engl J Med 348:1556, 2003.
51. Field TS, Gurwitz JH, Avom J, et al: Risk factors for adverse drug events among nursing home residents. Arch Intern Med 161:1629, 2001.
52. Kaufman D, Kelly JP, Rosenberg L, et al: Recent patterns of medication use in the ambulatory adult population of the United States. The Slone survey. JAMA 287:337, 2002.
53. Hunt SA, Baker DW, Chin MH, et al: ACC/AHA guidelines for the evaluation and management of chronic heart failure in the adult: Executive summary: A report of the

American College of Cardiology/American Heart Association Task Force on Practice Guidelines (Committee to revise the 1995 Guidelines for the Evaluation and Management of Heart Failure). J Am Coll Cardiol 38:2101, 2001.

54. Ryan TJ, Antman EM, Brooks NH, et al: 1999 update: ACC/AHA Guidelines for the Management of Patients with Acute Myocardial Infarction: Executive Summary and Recommendations. A report of the American College of Cardiology/American Heart Association Task Force on Practice Guidelines (Committee on Management of Acute Myocardial Infarction). Circulation 100:1016, 1999.
55. Lau WC, Waskell LA, Watkins PB, et al: Atorvastatin reduces the ability of clopidogrel to inhibit platelet aggregation: A new drug-drug interaction. Circulation 107:32, 2003.
55a. Saw J, Steinhubl SR, Berger PB, et al: Lack of adverse clopidogrel-atorvastatin clinical interaction from secondary analysis of a randomized, placebo-controlled clopidogrel trial. Circulation 108:921, 2003.
56. De Smet P: Herbal remedies. N Engl J Med 347:2046, 2002.
57. Ioannides C: Pharmacokinetic interactions between herbal remedies and medicinal drugs. Xenobiotica 32:451, 2002.
58. Juurlink DN, Mamdani M, Kopp A, et al: Drug-drug interactions among elderly patients hospitalized for drug toxicity. JAMA 289:1652, 2003.
59. Schulman S. Care of patients receiving long-term anticoagulant therapy. N Engl J Med 349:675, 2003.
60. Institute of Medicine: Workshop on Pharmacokinetics and Drug Interactions in the Elderly and Special Issues in Elderly African-American Populations. Washington, DC, National Academy of Sciences, 1997.
61. Re-engineering the medication-use system. Am J Health Syst Pharm 57:537, 2000.
62. Pugh K, Wei J: Clinical implications of physiological changes in the aging heart. Drugs Aging 18:263, 2001.
63. Juurlink D, Mamdani M, Kopp A, et al: Drug-drug interactions among elderly patients hospitalized for drug toxicity. JAMA 289:1652, 2003.
64. Brater D: Anti-inflammatory agents and renal function. Semin Arthritis Rheum 32(3 Suppl 1):33, 2002.
65. Beers M: Explicit criteria for determining potentially inappropriate medication by the elderly. Arch Intern Med 157:1531, 1997.
66. Hanlon JT, Schmader KE, Boult C, et al: Use of inappropriate prescription drugs by older people. J Am Geriatr Soc 50:26, 2002.
67. Zhan C, Sangl J, Bierman AS, et al: Potentially inappropriate medication use in the community-dwelling elderly: Findings from the 1996 Medical Expenditure Panel Survey. JAMA 286:2866, 2001.
68. Cohn J: Adverse drug effects, compliance, and initial doses of antihypertensive drugs recommended by the Joint National Committee vs. the Physician's Desk Reference. Arch Intern Med 161:880, 2001.
69. Michalsen A, Konig G, Thimme W: Preventable causative factors leading to hospital admission with decompensated heart failure. Heart 80:437, 1998.
70. Salas M, Int'Veld BA, van der Linden PD, et al: Impaired cognitive function and compliance with antihypertensive drugs in elderly: The Rotterdam Study. Clin Pharmacol Ther 70:561, 2001.
71. Federman AD, Adams AS, Ross-Degnan D, et al: Supplemental insurance and use of effective cardiovascular drugs among elderly medicare beneficiaries with coronary heart disease JAMA 286:1732, 2001.
72. Barat I, Andreasen F, Damsgaard EMS: Drug therapy in the elderly: What doctors believe and patients actually do. Br J Clin Pharmacol 51:615, 2001.
73. McDonald HP, Garg AX, Haynes RB: Interventions to enhance patient adherence to medication prescriptions: Scientific review. JAMA 288:2868, 2002.

Vascular Disease

74. Hajjar I, Kotchen T: Trends in prevalence, awareness, treatment, and control of hypertension in the United States, 1988-2000. JAMA 290:199, 2003.
75. Franklin S, Gustin WT, Wong N, et al: Hemodynamic patterns of age-related changes in blood pressure. The Framingham Heart Study. Circulation 96:308, 1997.
76. Hyman D, Pavlik V: Characteristics of patients with uncontrolled hypertension in the United States. N Engl J Med 345:479, 2001.
77. Staessen J, Fagard R, Thijs L, et al: Randomised double-blind comparison of placebo and active treatment for older patients with isolated systolic hypertension. The Systolic Hypertension in Europe (Syst-Eur) Trial Investigators. Lancet 350:757, 1997.
78. Forette F, Seux ML, Staessen JA, et al for the Syst-Eur Investigators: The prevention of dementia with antihypertensive treatment. Arch Intern Med 162:2046, 2002.
79. The ALLHAT Collaborative Group: Major outcomes in high-risk hypertensive patients randomized to angiotensin-converting enzyme inhibitor or calcium channel blocker vs diuretic: The Antihypertensive and Lipid-Lowering Treatment to Prevent Heart Attack Trial (ALLHAT). JAMA 288:2981, 2002.
80. Psaty B, Lumley T, Furberg C, et al: Health outcomes associated with various antihypertensive therapies used as first-line agents. A network meta-analysis. JAMA 289:2534, 2003.
81. Lacroix A, Ott S, Ichikawa L, et al: Low-dose hydrochlorothiazide and preservation of bone mineral density in older adults. A randomized double-blind, placebo-controlled trial. Ann Intern Med 133:516, 2000.
82. Wing LM, Reld CM, Ryan P, et al for the Second Australian National Blood Pressure Study Group: A comparison of outcomes with angiotensin-converting-enzyme inhibitors and diuretics for hypertension in the elderly. N Engl J Med 348:583, 2003.
83. Chobanian AV, Bakris GL, Black HR, et al and the National High Blood Pressure Education Program Coordinating Committee: The Seventh Report of the Joint National Committee on Prevention, Detection, Evaluation, and Treatment of High Blood Pressure. The JNC 7 report. JAMA 289:2560, 2003.
84. Guidelines Committee: 2003 European Society of Hypertension–European Society of Cardiology guidelines for the management of arterial hypertension. J Hypertens 21:1011, 2003 (available on line at http://www.eshonline.org/documents/2003_guidelines.pdf).
85. Dahlof B, Devereux RB, Kjeldsen SE, et al: Cardiovascular morbidity and mortality in the Losartan Intervention For Endpoint reduction in hypertension study (LIFE): A randomised trial against atenolol. Lancet 359:995, 2002.
86. Lithell H, Hansson L, Skoog I, et al for the SCOPE Study Group: The Study on Cognition and Prognosis in the Elderly (SCOPE): Principal results of a randomized double-blind intervention trial. J Hypertens 21:875, 2003.
87. Fagard R: Epidemiology of hypertension in the elderly. Am J Geriatr Cardiol 11:23, 2002.
88. Tinetti M: Preventing falls in elderly persons. N Engl J Med 348:42, 2003.
89. Kohara K, Uemura K, Takata Y, et al: Postprandial hypotension: Evaluation by ambulatory blood pressure monitoring. Am J Hypertens 11:1358, 1998.
90. Smith N, Psaty B, Rutan G, et al: The association between time since last meal and blood pressure in older adults: The Cardiovascular Health Study. J Am Geriatr Soc 51:824, 2003.
91. Whelton P, Appel L, Espeland M, et al: Sodium reduction and weight loss in the treatment of hypertension in older persons: A randomized controlled trial of nonpharmacologic interventions in the elderly (TONE). JAMA 279:878, 1998.
92. Hajjar I, Grim C, Kotchen T: Dietary calcium lowers the age-related rise in blood pressure in the United States: The NHANES III Survey. J Clin Hypertens 5:122, 2003.
93. Gueyffler F, Bulpitt C, Boissel J-P, et al: Antihypertensive drugs in very old people: A subgroup meta-analysis of randomised controlled trials. INDANA Group. Lancet 353:793, 1999.
94. Goodwin J: Embracing complexity: A consideration of hypertension in the very old. J Gerontol Med Sci 58A:653, 2003.
95. Auseon A, Ooi W, Hossain M, Lipsitz L: Blood pressure behavior in the nursing home: Implications for diagnosis and treatment of hypertension. J Am Geriatr Soc 47:2377, 1999.
96. Kuller L, Fisher L, McClelland R, et al: Differences in prevalence of and risk factors for subclinical vascular disease among black and white participants in the Cardiovascular Health Study. Arterioscler Thromb Vasc Biol 18:283, 1998.
97. Newman AB, Shemanski L, Manolio TA, et al: Ankle-arm index as a predictor of cardiovascular disease and mortality in the Cardiovascular Health Study. Arterioscler Thromb Vasc Biol 19:538, 1999.
98. Kuller L, Borhani N, Furberg C, et al: Prevalence of subclinical atherosclerosis and cardiovascular disease and association with risk factors in the Cardiovascular Health Study. Am J Epidemiol 139:1164, 1994.
99. Wilson P, D'Agostino R, Levy D, et al: Prediction of coronary heart disease using risk factor categories. Circulation 97:1837, 1998.
100. Gibbons R, Balady G, Bricker J, et al: ACC/AHA 2002 Guideline Update for Exercise Testing: A Report of the American College of Cardiology/American Heart Association Task Force on Practice Guidelines (Committee on Exercise Testing). Available on the Web sites of the American College of Cardiology (www.acc.org) and the American Heart Association(www.americanheart.org), 2002.
101. Fleg J: Stress testing in the elderly. Am J Geriatr Cardiol 10:308, 2001.
102. Gibbons R, Abrams J, Chatterjee K, et al: ACC/AHA 2002 guideline update for the management of patients with chronic stable angina—Summary article: A report of the American College of Cardiology/American Heart Association Task Force on Practice Guidelines (Committee on the Management of Patients with Chronic Stable Angina). Circulation 107:149, 2003.
103. Heart Protection Study Collaborative Group: MRC/BHF Heart Protection Study of cholesterol lowering with simvastatin in 20,536 high-risk individuals: A randomised placebo-controlled trial. Lancet:7, 2002.
104. Downs J, Clearfield M, Weis S, et al: Primary prevention of acute coronary events with lovastatin in men and women with average cholesterol levels. Results of AFCAPS/TexCAPS. JAMA 279:1615, 1998.
105. Shepherd J, Cobbe S, Ford I, et al: Prevention of coronary heart disease with pravastatin in men with hypercholesterolemia. N Engl J Med 333:1301, 1995.
106. Mullany C, Mock M, Brooks M, et al: Effect of age in the Bypass Angioplasty Revascularization Investigation (BARI) randomized trial. Ann Thorac Surg 67:396, 1999.
107. Alexander K, Galanos A, Jollis J, et al: Post-myocardial infarction risk stratification in elderly patients. Am Heart J 142:37, 2001.
108. Batchelor W, Anstrom K, Muhlbaier L, et al: Contemporary outcome trends in the elderly undergoing percutaneous coronary interventions: Results in 7,472 octogenarians. National Cardiovascular Network Collaboration. J Am Coll Cardiol 36:723, 2000.
109. Newman MF, Kirchner J, Phillips-Bute B, et al: Neurological Outcome Research Group and the Cardiothoracic Anesthesiology Research Endeavors Investigators. Longitudinal assessment of neurocognitive function after coronary-artery bypass surgery. N Engl J Med 344:395, 2001.
110. Pfisterer M, Buser P, Osswald S, et al for the Trial of Invasive versus Medical Therapy in Elderly patients (TIME) Investigators: Outcome of elderly patients with chronic symptomatic coronary artery disease with an invasive vs. optimized medical treatment strategy. One-year results of the randomized TIME trial. JAMA 289:1117, 2003.
111. Eagle K, Guyton R, Davidoff R, et al: ACC/AHA Guidelines for Coronary Artery Bypass Graft Surgery: Executive Summary and Recommendations. A Report of the American College of Cardiology/American Heart Association Task Force on Practice Guidelines (Committee to Revise the 1991 Guidelines for Coronary Artery Bypass Graft Surgery). Circulation 100:1464, 1999.
112. Vaccarino V, Lin Z, Kasl S, et al: Gender differences in recovery after coronary artery bypass surgery. J Am Coll Cardiol 41:307, 2003.
113. Mehta R, Rathore S, Radford M, et al: Acute myocardial infarction in the elderly: Differences by age. J Am Coll Cardiol 38:736, 2001.
114. Rich MW, PRICE-2 Organizing Committee, PRICE-2 Investigators: Executive summary: Second Pivotal Research in Cardiovascular Syndromes in the Elderly (PRICE-II) Symposium. Acute coronary syndromes in the elderly: Mechanisms and management. Am J Geriatr Cardiol 12:307, 2003.

115. Brass LM, Lichtman JH, Wang Y, et al: Intracranial hemorrhage associated with thrombolytic therapy for elderly patients with acute myocardial infarction: Results from the Cooperative Cardiovascular Project. Stroke 31:1802, 2000.
116. Berger A, Radford M, Wang Y, et al: Thrombolytic therapy in older patients. J Am Coll Cardiol 36:366, 2000.
117. Thiemann D, Coresh J, Schulman S, et al: Lack of benefit for intravenous thrombolysis in patients with myocardial infarction who are older than 75 years. Circulation 101:2239, 2000.
118. Becker RC, Hochman JS, Cannon CP, et al: Fatal cardiac rupture among patients treated with thrombolytic agents and adjunctive thrombin antagonists: Observations from the Thrombolysis and Thrombin Inhibition in Myocardial Infarction 9 Study. J Am Coll Cardiol 33:479, 1999.
119. Angeja B, Rundle A, Gurwitz J, et al: Death or nonfatal stroke in patients with acute myocardial infarction treated with tissue plasminogen activator. Am J Cardiol 87:627, 2001.
120. Horwitz P, Berlin J, Sauer W, et al: Registry Committee of the Society for Cardiac Angiography Interventions. Bleeding risk of platelet glycoprotein IIb/IIIa receptor antagonists in broad-based practice (results from the Society for Cardiac Angiography and Interventions Registry). Am J Cardiol 91:803, 2003.
121. Brown D: Deaths associated with platelet glycoprotein IIb/IIIa inhibitor treatment. Heart 89:535, 2003.
122. Weaver W, Simes R, Betriu A, et al: Comparison of primary coronary angioplasty and intravenous thrombolytic therapy for acute myocardial infarction: A quantitative review. JAMA 278:2093, 1997.

123. Berger A, Schulman K, Gersh B, et al: Primary coronary angioplasty vs thrombolysis for the management of acute myocardial infarction in elderly patients. JAMA 282:341, 1999.
124. Rich MW: Executive summary: Second Pivotal Research in Cardiovascular syndromes in the Elderly (PRICE-2) symposium. Acute coronary syndromes in the elderly: Mechanisms and management. Am J Geriatr Cardiol 12:305, 2003.
125. Berwen D, Galusha D, Lewis J, et al: National and state trends in quality of care for acute myocardial infarction between 1994-1995 and 1998-1999. Arch Intern Med 163:1430, 2003.
126. Bush D, Ziegelstein R, Tayback M, et al: Even minimal symptoms of depression increase mortality risk after acute myocardial infarction. Am J Cardiol 88:337, 2001.
127. Scheir M, Matthews K, Owens J, et al: Optimism and rehospitalization after coronary artery bypass graft surgery. Arch Intern Med 159:829, 1999.
128. Connerney I, Shapiro P, McLaughlin J, et al: Relation between depression after coronary artery bypass surgery and 12-month outcome: A prospective study. Lancet 358:1766, 2001.
129. Dusseldorp E, van Elderen T, Maes S, et al: A meta-analysis of psychoeducational programs for coronary heart disease patients. Health Psychol 18:506, 1999.
130. Glassman A, O'Connor C, Califf R, et al: Sertraline treatment of major depression in patients with acute MI or unstable angina. JAMA 288:701, 2002.
131. Berkman LF, Blumenthal J, Burg M, et al: Effects of treating depression and low perceived social support on clinical events after myocardial infarction. The Enhancing Recovery in Coronary Heart Disease Patients (ENRICHD) Randomized Trial. JAMA 289:3106, 2003.
132. Whooley M, Avins A, Miranda J, Browner W: Case-finding instruments for depression: Two questions are as good as many. J Gen Intern Med 12:439, 1997.
133. Rochon P, Tu J, Anderson G, et al: Rate of heart failure and 1-year survival for older people receiving low-dose beta-blocker therapy after myocardial infarction. Lancet 356:639, 2000.
134. Grady D, Herrington D, Vittner V, et al: Cardiovascular disease outcomes during 6.8 years of hormone therapy. Heart and Estrogen/Progestin Replacement Study Follow-up (HERS II). JAMA 288:49, 2002.
135. Risks and Benefits of Estrogen Plus Progestin in Healthy Postmenopausal Women: Principal results from the Women's Health Initiative Randomized Controlled Trial. JAMA 288:321, 2002.
135a. Tanne JH: Oestrogen only arm of women's health initiative trial is stopped. BMJ 328:602, 2004.
135b. National Institutes of Health: NIH News. www.nhlbi.nih.gov/new/press/04-03-02.htm.
136. Binder F, Schechtman K, Ehsani A, et al: Effects of exercise training on frailty in community-dwelling older adults: Results of a randomized, controlled trial. J Am Geriatr Soc 50:2089, 2002.
137. Baum E, Jarjoura D, Polen A, et al: Effectiveness of a group exercise program in a long-term care facility: A randomized pilot trial. J Am Med Dir Assoc 4:74, 2003.
138. Marchionni N, Fattirolli F, Fumagalli S, et al: Improved exercise tolerance and quality of life with cardiac rehabilitation of older patients after myocardial infarction. Results of a randomized, controlled trial. Circulation 107:2201, 2003.
139. Straus S, Majumdar S, McAlister F: New evidence for stroke prevention. Scientific review. JAMA 288:1388, 2002.
140. Albers G, Hart R, Lutsep H, et al: AHA Scientific Statement. Supplement to the guidelines for the management of transient ischemic attacks. A statement from the Ad Hoc Committee on Guidelines for the Management of Transient Ischemic Attacks, Stroke Council, American Heart Association. Stroke 30:2502, 1999.
141. Johnston S: Transient ischemic attack. N Engl J Med 347:1687, 2002.
142. Adams HJ, Adams R, Brott T, et al: Stroke Council of the American Stroke Association. Guidelines for the early management of patients with ischemic stroke: A scientific statement from the Stroke Council of the American Stroke Association. Stroke 34:1056, 2003.
143. Committee CS: A randomized, blinded, trial of clopidogrel vs. aspirin in patients at risk of ischemic events (CAPRIE). Lancet 348:1329, 1996.
144. Diener H, Cunha L, Forbes C, et al: European Stroke Prevention Study-2. Dipyridamole and acetylsalicylic acid in the secondary prevention of stroke. J Neurol Sci 143:1, 1996.
145. Mohr J, Thompson J, Lazar R, et al: A comparison of warfarin and aspirin for the prevention of recurrent ischemic stroke. N Engl J Med 345:1444, 2001.
146. Antiplatelet Trialists' Collaboration: Collaborative meta-analysis of randomised trials of antiplatelet therapy for prevention of death, myocardial infarction and stroke in high risk patients. BMJ 324:71, 2002.
147. Johnson E, Lanes S, Wentwork CI, et al: A metaregression analysis of the dose-response effect of ASA on stroke. Arch Intern Med 159:1284, 1999.
148. Barnett H, Meldrum H, Eliasziw M: North American Symptomatic Carotid Endarterectomy Trial (NASCET) collaborators. The appropriate use of carotid endarterectomy. CMAJ 166:1169, 2002.
149. Rothwell P, Slattery J, Warlow C: Clinical and angiographic predictors of stroke and death from carotid endarterectomy: Systematic review. BMJ 315:1571, 1997.
150. Hanel R, Xavier A, Kirmani J, et al: Management of carotid artery stenosis: Comparing endarterectomy and stenting. Curr Cardiol Rep 5:153, 2003.
151. Ouriel K: Peripheral arterial disease. Lancet 358:1257, 2001.
152. McDermott M, Greenland P, Liu K, et al: Leg symptoms in peripheral arterial disease. Associated clinical characteristics and functional impairment. JAMA 286:1599, 2001.
153. Dormandy J, Rutherford R: Management of peripheral arterial disease (PAD). J Vasc Surg 31:S1, 2000.
154. Hiatt W: Medical treatment of peripheral arterial disease and claudication. N Engl J Med 344:1608, 2001.
155. Trans Atlantic Inter-Society Consensus (TASC): Management of peripheral arterial disease (PAD). Eur J Vasc Endovasc Surg Suppl A(Sec A-D):S1, 2000.
156. Trans Atlantic Inter-Society Consensus (TASC): Management of peripheral arterial disease (PAD). Int Angiol 19(Suppl 1):1, 2000.

Heart Failure

157. Ni H: Prevalence of self-reported heart failure among US adults: Results from the 1999 National Health Interview Survey. Am Heart J 146:1, 2003.
158. Gottdiener J, Arnold A, Aurigemma G, et al: Predictors of congestive heart failure in the elderly: The Cardiovascular Health Study. J Am Coll Cardiol 35:1628, 2000.
159. Wang T, Levy D, Benjamin E, Vasan R: The epidemiology of "asymptomatic" left ventricular systolic dysfunction: Implications for screening. Ann Intern Med 138:907, 2003.
160. Gottdiener J, McClellan R, Marshall R, et al: Outcome of congestive heart failure in elderly persons: Influence of left ventricular systolic function. The Cardiovascular Health Study. Ann Intern Med 137:631, 2002.
161. MacCarthy P, Kearney M, Nolan J, et al: Prognosis in heart failure with preserved left ventricular systolic function: Prospective cohort study. Br Med J 327:78, 2003.
162. Croft J, Giles W, Pollard R, et al: Heart failure survival among older adults in the United States: A poor prognosis for an emerging epidemic in the Medicare population. Arch Intern Med 159:505, 1999.
163. Vasan R, Larson M, Benjamin E, et al: Congestive heart failure in subjects with normal versus reduced let ventricular ejection fraction: Prevalence and mortality in a population-based cohort. J Am Coll Cardiol 33:1948, 1999.
164. Redfield M, Jacobsen S, Burnett J, et al: Burden of systolic and diastolic ventricular dysfunction in the community. Appreciating the scope of the heart failure epidemic. JAMA 289:194, 2003.
165. Senni M, Tribouilloy C, Rodeheffer R, et al: Congestive heart failure in the community. Circulation 98:2282, 1998.
166. Kitzman DW, Gardin JM, Gottdiener JS, et al, Cardiovascular Health Study Research Group: Importance of heart failure with preserved systolic function in the elderly. CHS Research Group. Am J Cardiol 87:413, 2001.
167. Masoudi F, Havranek E, Smith G, et al: Gender, age, and heart failure with preserved left ventricular systolic function. J Am Coll Cardiol 41:217, 2003.
168. Philbin E, Erb T, Jenkins P: The natural history of heart failure with preserved left ventricular systolic function. J Am Coll Cardiol 29(2 Suppl A):245, 1997.
169. European Study Group on Diastolic Heart Failure: How to diagnose diastolic heart failure. Eur Heart J 19:990, 1998.
170. Garg R, Yusuf S, Trials C, GoAI: Overview of randomized trials of angiotensin converting enzyme inhibitors on mortality and morbidity in heart failure. JAMA 273:1450, 1995.
171. Flather M, Yusuf S, Kober L, et al for the ACE-Inhibitor Myocardial Infarction Collaborative Group: Long-term ACE-inhibitor therapy in patients with heart failure or left-ventricular dysfunction: A systematic overview of data from individual patients. Lancet 355:1575, 2000.
172. MacMahon S: The Blood Pressure Lowering Treatment Trialists' Collaboration: Second cycle of analyses. Program and abstracts of the 13th European Meeting on Hypertension, June 13-17, 2003, Milan, Italy.
173. Pitt B, Zannad F, Remme W, et al: The effect of spironolactone on morbidity and mortality in patients with severe heart failure. N Engl J Med 341:709, 1999.
174. Shlipak M: Pharmacotherapy for heart failure in patients with renal insufficiency. Ann Intern Med 139:917, 2003.
175. Petrie M, Dawson N, Murdoch D, et al: Failure of women's hearts. Circulation 99:2334, 1999.
176. Simon T, Mary-Krause M, Funck-Brentano C, Jaillon P: Sex differences in the prognosis of congestive heart failure. Results from the Cardiac Insufficiency Bisoprolol Study (CIBIS II). Circulation 103:375, 2001.
177. Rathore S, Wang Y, Krumholz H: Sex-based differences in the effect of digoxin for the treatment of heart failure. N Engl J Med 347:1403, 2002.
178. Bradley E, Baughman K, Berger R, et al: Cardiac resynchronization and death from progressive heart failure. A meta-analysis of randomized controlled trials. JAMA 289:730, 2003.
179. The effect of digoxin on mortality and morbidity in patients with heart failure. The Digitalis Investigation Group. N Engl J Med 336:525, 1997.
180. Kitzman D: Diastolic heart failure in the elderly. Heart Fail Rev 7:17, 2002.
181. Nichol K, Nordin J, Mullooly J, et al: Influenza vaccination and reduction in hospitalizations for cardiac disease and stroke among the elderly. N Engl J Med 348:1322, 2003.

Arrhythmias

182. Tsang T, Petty G, Barnes M, et al: The prevalence of atrial fibrillation in incident stroke cases and matched population controls in Rochester, Minnesota. Changes over three decades. J Am Coll Cardiol 42:93, 2003.
183. Caraballo P, Heit J, Atkinson E, et al: Long-term use of oral anticoagulants and the risk of fracture. Arch Intern Med 159:1750, 1999.

Valvular Disease

184. Otto C, Lind B, Kitzman D, et al: Association of aortic-valve sclerosis with cardiovascular mortality and morbidity in the elderly. N Engl J Med 341:142, 1999.
185. Stewart BF, Siscovick D, Lind BK, et al: Clinical factors associated with calcific aortic valve disease. Cardiovascular Health Study. J Am Coll Cardiol 29:630, 1997.
186. Shavelle D, Takasu J, Budoff M, et al: HMG CoA reductase inhibitor (statin) and aortic valve calcium. Lancet 359:1125, 2002.
187. Faggiano P, Antonini-Canterin F, Erlicher A, et al: Progression of aortic valve sclerosis to aortic stenosis. Am J Cardiol 91:99, 2003.
188. Pohle K, Maffert R, Ropers D, et al: Progression of aortic valve calcification. Association with coronary atherosclerosis and cardiovascular risk factors. Circulation 104:1927, 2001.
189. Atar S, Jeon D, Luo H, Siegel R: Mitral annular calcification: A marker of severe coronary artery disease in patients under 65 years old. Heart 89:161, 2003.
190. Adler Y, Herz I, Vaturi M, et al: Mitral annular calcium detected by transthoracic echocardiography is a marker for high prevalence and severity of coronary artery disease in patients undergoing coronary angiography. Am J Cardiol 81:784, 1998.
191. ACC/AHA guidelines for the management of patients with valvular heart disease. A Report of the American College of Cardiology/American Heart Association Task Force on Practice Guidelines (Committee on Management of Patients With Valvular Heart Disease). J Am Coll Cardiol 32:1486, 1998.
192. Peltier M, Trojette F, Enriquez-Sarano M, et al: Relation between cardiovascular risk factors and nonrheumatic severe calcific aortic stenosis among patients with a three-cuspid aortic valve. Am J Cardiol 91:97, 2003.
193. Bellamy M, Pellikka P, Klarich K, et al: Association of cholesterol levels, hydroxymethylglutaryl coenzyme-A reductase inhibitor treatment, and progression of aortic stenosis in the community. J Am Coll Cardiol 40:1723, 2002.
194. Cohen G, David T, Ivanov J, et al: The impact of age, coronary artery disease, and cardiac comorbidity on late survival after bioprosthetic aortic valve replacement. J Thorac Cardiovasc Surg 117:273, 1999.
195. Helft G, Tabone X, Georges J, et al: Late results with bioprosthetic valves in the elderly. J Card Surg 14:252, 1999.
196. Kauterman K, Michaels A, Ports T: Is there any indication for aortic valvuloplasty in the elderly? Am J Geriatr Cardiol 12:190, 2003.
197. Aronow W, Ahn C, Kronzon I: Comparison of echocardiographic abnormalities in African-American, Hispanic, and white men and women aged > 60 years. Am J Cardiol 87:1131, 2001.
198. Lee R, Sundt TI, Moon M, et al: Mitral valve repair in the elderly: Operative risk for patients over 70 years of age is acceptable. J Cardiovasc Surg 44:157, 2003.
199. Pritchett A, Morrison J, Edwards WD, et al: Valvular heart disease in patients taking pergolide. Mayo Clin Proc 77:1280, 2002.
200. Flowers C, Racoosin J, Lu S, Beitz J: The US Food and Drug Administration's registry of patients with pergolide-associated valvular heart disease. Mayo Clin Proc 78:730, 2003.

CHAPTER 73

Cardiovascular Disease in Women

Nancy K. Sweitzer • Pamela S. Douglas

More women die every year from cardiovascular disease than from any other cause (Fig. 73–1), yet women worry more about breast cancer than heart disease.[1,2] Women with heart disease may present differently than men, have unique underlying pathophysiologies, and have distinctive risk-benefit profiles with commonly accepted therapies. Heart disease is far more age dependent in women than in men; women with cardiovascular disease are older and have more comorbidities. This fact, in turn, makes diagnostic and treatment procedures more problematic in women. In addition, many effective pharmacological strategies are underutilized, and there is a lack of gender-specific data on numerous therapies. The fact that heart disease is on the decline in men but not women highlights our failure to treat this large segment of the population optimally (Fig. 73–2).

Gender and Mechanisms of Cardiovascular Disease

Genes and Hormones

Although men and women differ by only 1 chromosome out of 46, the impact on health and disease is large. Outside the reproductive systems, the heart and circulation are perhaps most affected. Clinicians have long known of the apparent "protection" of younger, premenopausal women from ischemic heart disease, and this protection has been attributed to estrogen.[3,4] The biological plausibility of this connection is indisputable—gonadal hormones do alter many pathophysiological processes thought to be fundamental to the development of atherosclerosis,[5] including thrombosis and inflammation.[6] Further, nuclear estrogen receptors are present in cardiac myocytes of both males and females, a potential explanation for gender differences in gene regulation.[7] However, these physiological differences have failed to translate into a useful pharmacopoeia. A series of experimental trials have failed to demonstrate any utility of estrogen therapy for either the primary or secondary prevention of vascular disease in men or women.[8-10] Many questions shade these results, and it may well be that in the future we will learn how to better harness the power of estrogens, through use of altered compounds, new delivery routes, and even pharmacogenomics, but for now, estrogens are not indicated in the treatment or prevention of atherosclerosis.

Gender, Genomics, and the Vulnerable Plaque

The differences between men and women in atherosclerosis are not limited to gonadal hormones. Research has shown some fundamental variation in the underlying mechanisms of disease. A Japanese study assayed a large population of myocardial infarction survivors for the presence of 71 single-nucleotide polymorphisms in candidate genes known to be relevant to the pathophysiology of atherosclerosis. Two were found to be significantly more prevalent in men—connexin37 and p22^{phox}—and two different genes were relevant in women—plasminogen activator inhibitor 1 (PAI-1) and stromelysin-1—suggesting that the genetic basis underlying coronary heart disease (CHD) varies by gender.[11]

Such genetic differences are manifest in the physiology of atherosclerosis, including plaque components (more cellular and fibrous tissue in women),[12] endothelial function (estrogen-induced coronary vasodilation),[13,14] and hemostasis (higher fibrinogen and factor VII levels in women).[15] Although coronary thrombosis is overwhelmingly the most likely cause of myocardial infarction in both genders (only rarely are infarctions due to spasm or syndrome X), women are twice as likely to have plaque erosion (37 percent in women versus 18 percent in men), whereas men have plaque rupture as the underlying cause of the infarction (82 percent in men versus 63 percent in women).[16]

Gender Differences in Ventricular Remodeling

Even after the onset of established clinical disease, compensation differs between men and women. In pressure overload syndromes (hypertension and aortic stenosis), female rats express different cardiac genes.[7] Women with aortic stenosis or hypertension tend to have more vigorous hypertrophy, with greater left ventricular mass, and better preserved systolic function and contractile reserve than men. In ischemic syndromes, animal studies suggest that females show less hypertrophy but also less pathological remodeling and dilation.[17] Apoptosis and

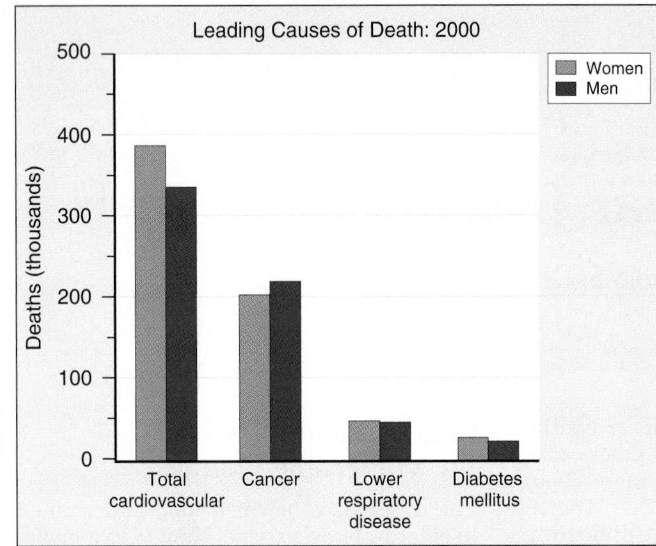

FIGURE 73–1 Number of deaths related to four leading causes of death in women and men in the United States in 2000, ranked in order for women. (Modified from the American Heart Association Heart Disease and Stroke Statistics—2003 Update; 2002. Available at http://www.americanheart.org/downloadable/heart/1059017971148 2003HDSStatsBookREV7-03.pdf. Accessed August 15, 2003.)

myocyte necrosis in response to aging, injury, or stress are more pronounced in males than in females.[18]

Gender Roles and Psychosocial Aspects of Cardiovascular Disease

It is important to recognize that, as patients, there are differences between the genders.[19] Because women are older and have a greater burden of risk factors and concomitant disease, they are more frail and less likely to recover fully from cardiovascular events. Women's greater longevity and our society's gender roles combine to make women caregivers to men with atherosclerotic disease but often leave the same women without social, emotional, or financial support at the time of their own illness.[20] Women, as well as their caregivers, may underestimate the importance of atherosclerotic disease and fail to implement preventive strategies fully or even recognize and act on symptoms appropriately. These factors have a significant, negative impact on optimal care delivery for women.[21]

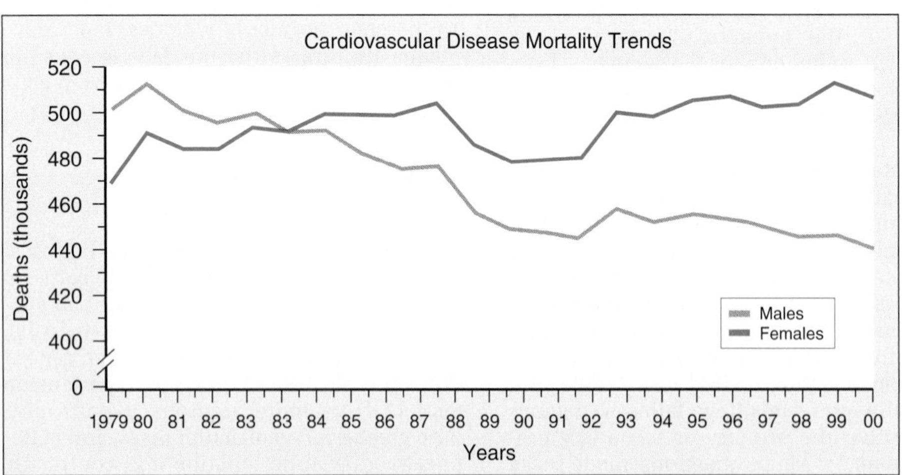

FIGURE 73–2 Trends in cardiovascular disease mortality in males and females in the United States from 1979 to 2000. (From the American Heart Association Heart Disease and Stroke Statistics—2003 Update; 2002. Available at http://www.americanheart.org/downloadable/heart/10590179711482003HDSStatsBookREV7-03.pdf. Accessed August 15, 2003.)

Atherosclerotic Vascular Disease

Risk Factors for Coronary Heart Disease in Women and Their Modification

Diabetes Mellitus and Metabolic Syndrome

Diabetes is associated with a greater incremental risk in women, completely eliminating the "female advantage."[22] The American Heart Association awards double weight to diabetes in women when calculating CHD risk,[23] similar to the weight given a systolic blood pressure of 173 mm Hg or above or a cholesterol level of 316 mg/dl or above. More than in men, diabetes dramatically increases the mortality of myocardial infarction in women (Fig. 73–3). Type 2 diabetes is associated with obesity, abdominal body fat distribution, hypertension, atherogenic dyslipidemia, and insulin resistance, all of which have been associated with higher CHD risk.[22] This complex of abnormalities, termed "metabolic syndrome," alters hepatic metabolism, lipoprotein levels, and circulating insulin levels.[24] More so than in men, obesity and body fat distribution appear to be independent coronary artery disease risk factors in women.[22] Diabetes is also linked with endothelial dysfunction and a variety of platelet abnormalities. Data from the Diabetes Control and Complications Trial suggest that intensive diabetes therapy reduces cardiovascular complications in men and women younger than 40 years.[25]

Hypertension

More than 25 million American women have high blood pressure, and cardiovascular risk related to hypertension rises steeply with age in females.[26] Further, although women have fewer cardiovascular events, the population risk attributable to hypertension is higher for women than men because of the increased incidence with age and the longevity of women.[27] Nonpharmacological interventions effectively decrease blood pressure in women, including a low-salt diet, physical activity, and weight loss. However, compliance with such changes is low (~10 percent)[28] and blood pressure increases again when physical activity decreases or weight is regained. Most trials have shown equal efficacy of blood pressure lowering to prevent cardiovascular events in men and women. The Seventh Joint National Committee on Prevention, Detection, Evaluation, and Treatment of High Blood Pressure includes a single set of guidelines for both men and women, stating that "large, long-term clinical trials of antihypertensive treatment have not demonstrated clinically significant gender differences in blood pressure response and outcomes."[29] Although it is clear that hypertension in women should be treated as aggressively as in men, it is possible that the optimal choice of antihypertensive agent may differ. The Antihypertensive and Lipid-Lowering Treatment to Prevent Heart Attack Trial (ALLHAT) demonstrated superiority of diuretic therapy in the prespecified female cohort, as in the trial as a whole.[30] The Second

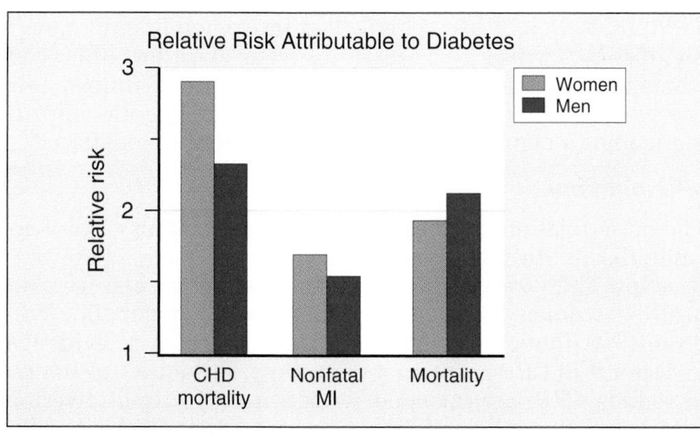

FIGURE 73–3 Relative risks of coronary heart disease (CHD) mortality, nonfatal myocardial infarction (MI), and total mortality attributable to diabetes in women compared with men. (Modified from Grady D, Chaput L, Kristof M: Diagnosis and Treatment of Coronary Heart Disease in Women: Systematic Reviews of Evidence on Selected Topics. Evidence Report/Technology Assessment No. 81. AHRQ Publication No. 03-0037. Rockville, Md, Agency for Healthcare Research and Quality, May 2003.)

Australian National Blood Pressure Study Group found that angiotensin-converting enzyme (ACE) inhibitor therapy decreased cardiovascular endpoints relative to hydrochlorothiazide in men but not in women.[31] The numbers of women included in trials are often too small to draw conclusions.

Smoking

Tobacco contributes to 17 percent of all female deaths in the United States and results in more deaths from CHD and stroke than any other cause.[32] The combination of accelerated atherosclerosis and propensity to vascular thrombosis induced by cigarette smoking is responsible for a six- to ninefold increased risk of myocardial infarction among female smokers compared with nonsmokers. There is a similar increase in stroke risk. The combination of cigarette smoking and oral contraceptive use appears to be particularly potent at increasing the risk of arterial thrombosis. Cigarettes have an antiestrogenic effect and induce an unfavorable lipid profile, leading women to lose their "natural" protection against atherosclerotic vascular disease. Currently available methods to assist with quitting may be less effective in women, perhaps because of a greater behavioral component and less nicotine addiction in women smokers.[33] Environmental exposure to tobacco smoke increases the risk of cardiovascular disease in women, and assessment of environmental exposure is an important part of risk assessment.[34]

Lipids

The average lipid profile in women is affected by hormonal status and changes throughout life. Young women have lower low-density lipoprotein (LDL) cholesterol levels and higher high-density lipoprotein (HDL) cholesterol levels than men of the same age.[35,36] As women age, LDL cholesterol increases, HDL cholesterol decreases, and the risk of CHD climbs.[37] Elevated total cholesterol and LDL levels are only weakly associated with CHD in women and only in women 65 years old or younger. Instead, HDL cholesterol is closely and inversely associated with CHD risk. Triglycerides are an independent predictor of CHD, particularly in older women. Lipoprotein(a), a composite of LDL, apolipoprotein B-100, and apolipoprotein(a), is also associated with higher cardiac risk in women.[35] Initial modification of a high-risk lipoprotein profile is generally accomplished by the same life-style changes and medications in men and women, although dietary interventions may be less effective in women.[38]

Multiple trials have demonstrated efficacy of 3-hydroxy-3-methylglutaryl coenzyme A (HMG CoA) reductase inhibitors, or statins, in both primary and secondary prevention of coronary events and death in women with both elevated and normal cholesterol, supporting the persistent theory that there are benefits of these agents independent of LDL-lowering effects (Fig. 73–4).[39] Women have generally not been included in trials of other classes of lipid-lowering agents, such as the bile acid sequestrant cholestyramine and the fibrate gemfibrozil. In addition, there are no data from large trials on the efficacy of lipid-lowering agents targeted more specifically at altering the HDL and triglyceride lipid subfractions, which appear more important in women. It seems reasonable to apply strategies shown to be successful in men, recognizing that optimal care of women with dyslipidemia may eventually be different from that of men.

Estrogen

The presence of estrogen in the premenopausal female population, the obvious protection this group enjoys against cardiovascular events, and documentation of estrogen receptors in cardiomyocytes and vascular tissues in both men and women led to tremendous enthusiasm for use of postmenopausal hormone replacement therapy as a preventive measure against atherosclerotic heart disease. This enthusiasm was bolstered by multiple observational studies suggesting improved longevity and decreased cardiac events in postmenopausal women receiving hormone replacement therapy as well as mechanistic data supporting biological plausibility.[40,41] Multiple randomized controlled trials in the past 3 years have refuted this hypothesis and provided strong evidence of an increase in cardiovascular risk (Fig. 73–5), particularly in the first year after beginning therapy, combined with increased risk of breast cancer, thromboembolic disease, and stroke, resulting in a withdrawal of prior recommendations.[8,9,42] In the Women's Health Initiative Study, use of estrogen alone, without a progestin, neither caused nor prevented cardiac events, although it did increase the risk of stroke and decrease the risk of hip fracture.[42a] Other studies documenting progression of atherosclerosis during hormone replacement therapy have confirmed the lack of benefit. Hormone replacement therapy has no place in prevention of heart disease in women at present.

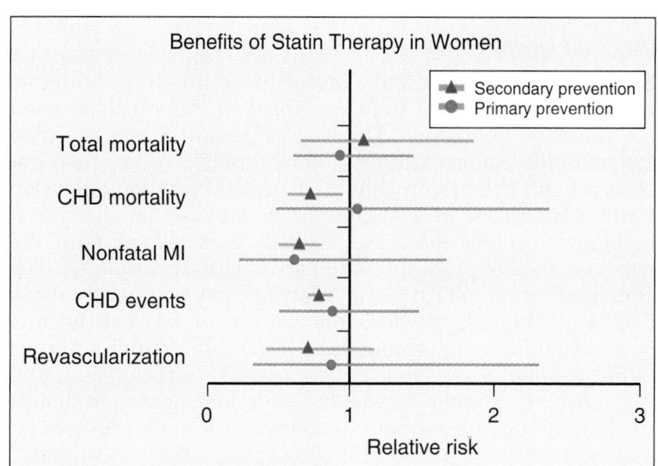

FIGURE 73–4 Risk reduction in multiple cardiovascular endpoints attributable to lipid-lowering therapy with statins in women with and without preexisting atherosclerotic disease. Summary odds ratios with 95 percent confidence intervals are presented. CHD = coronary heart disease; MI = myocardial infarction. (Modified from Grady D, Chaput L, Kristof M. Diagnosis and Treatment of Coronary Heart Disease in Women: Systematic Reviews of Evidence on Selected Topics. Evidence Report/Technology Assessment No. 81. AHRQ Publication No. 03-0037. Rockville, Md, Agency for Healthcare Research and Quality, May 2003.)

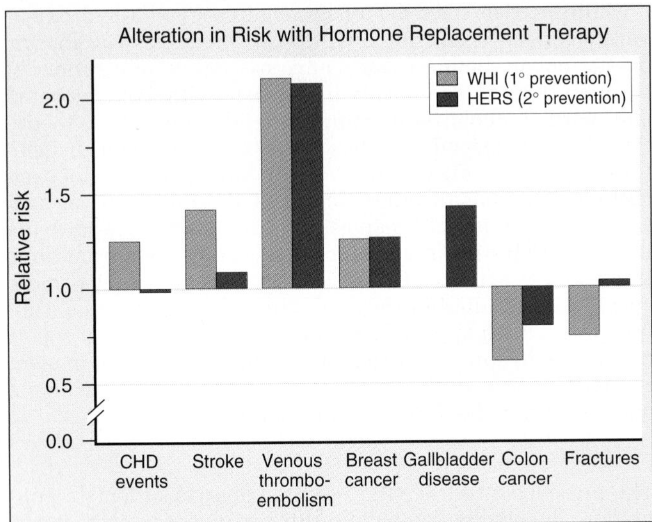

FIGURE 73–5 Relative risks of significant medical endpoints in large randomized controlled trials of postmenopausal hormone replacement therapy. CHD = coronary heart disease; WHI = Women's Health Initiative. (Modified from Grady D, Herrington D, Bittner V, et al: Cardiovascular disease outcomes during 6.8 years of hormone therapy: Heart and Estrogen/progestin Replacement Study follow-up [HERS II]. JAMA 288:49, 2002; and Rossouw JE, Anderson GL, Prentice RL, et al: Risks and benefits of estrogen plus progestin in healthy postmenopausal women: Principal results from the Women's Health Initiative randomized controlled trial. JAMA 288:321, 2002.)

Many questions about estrogen remain unanswered. Would alternative formulations of either estrogen or progesterone be of benefit? Does starting therapy immediately at menopause eliminate risk? Can genotype predict the risk-benefit profile of estrogen therapy? In addition, if the estrogen hypothesis is indeed a fallacy, what does afford the protection in the premenopausal female population? Several candidates have been suggested, although none have substantial scientific support: lower iron levels and higher oxytocin levels, for example.[3,43] Estrogen therapy is associated with impressive changes in so many risk factors, including lower LDL, higher HDL, improved glucose tolerance, and reductions in weight and waist circumference, that an understanding of the mechanism of increased risk is likely to revolutionize yet again our understanding of the atherosclerotic process.

Diet and Obesity

Excess caloric intake and obesity are a growing epidemic worldwide, and more than one-third of American women are classified as obese.[22] The Nurses' Health Study revealed a sevenfold higher cardiovascular mortality in the heaviest women, and the Framingham Offspring study demonstrated a dramatic rise in risk factors for cardiovascular disease at body mass indices above 20.[44] Obesity is associated with elevated C-reactive protein (CRP), particularly in women.[45] The combination of obesity and diabetes appears particularly deadly in women, as does the pattern of fat distribution. Abdominal fat accumulation is an important predictor of type 2 diabetes mellitus, hypertriglyceridemia, hypertension, and CHD. Among women, a waist-to-hip ratio greater than 0.88 is predictive of a substantially increased risk of cardiovascular events, as is a waist circumference of more than 38 inches.[46]

Physical Activity

Physical inactivity is more prevalent among women than men.[47] There is a strong inverse association between physical activity and coronary events in women.[48] Physical activity also has a salutary effect on other cardiovascular risk factors, including hypertension, obesity, and diabetes mellitus. The effect of regular exercise to increase HDL cholesterol and induce weight loss may be less in women than in men.[49] Significant barriers to regular exercise exist for American women, particularly older women. Caregiving duties, low energy, and lack of peers seen exercising are cited as impeding women's compliance with exercise recommendations.[50]

Inflammation

The close relationship between inflammation and cardiovascular risk is discussed in depth elsewhere (see Chap. 36). Baseline CRP levels predict future cardiovascular risk in healthy women, particularly those with metabolic syndrome.[51] Although we currently lack clinical trial evidence in support of CRP as a target of therapy, the ability of statins to reduce CRP is associated with benefit in lipid-lowering trials[52] and the ability of oral estrogen to raise CRP is associated with harm.[9,10]

Psychosocial Factors (see also Chap. 84)

The interaction of psychosocial and behavioral factors and heart disease is complex and has not been rigorously studied. Several cardiovascular risk factors are related to behavior (obesity, smoking, exercise), yet modification may be more difficult for women than for men, with caregiving roles often blamed for this failure. Perceived stress and lack of situational control have been found to increase CHD risk in both genders.[20,53] Social networks and support influence CHD outcome both independently and through the likelihood of compliance with therapeutic strategies (e.g., cardiac rehabilitation), and their impact may be greater in women, who are more likely to live alone. Although depression increases cardiac risk in both women and men, a causal relationship is unclear, as is the impact of treatment.[54]

Emerging Risk Factors

Many newer markers of increased cardiovascular risk apply equally to men and women, including abnormal endothelial reactivity, increased pulse pressure (thought to be a surrogate for increased vascular stiffness), factor V Leiden mutation, hyperhomocysteinemia, and elevated fibrinogen.[55,56] Estrogen increases fibrinogen levels, explaining the increased risk of vascular thrombosis associated with exogenous estrogen therapy. Although several members of the coagulation and fibrinolysis cascade have been proposed as possible risk factors, most recently through genetic polymorphisms,[56] current data support a role for these factors as modifiers of risk rather than causal. Whether targeting any of these emerging risk factors for intervention produces a reduction in cardiovascular events is unknown.

Strategies for Primary Prevention

Improvement in prevention of coronary artery disease in women requires earlier awareness and identification of risk. An overwhelming majority of women are unaware of their cardiovascular risk, and physicians do little to educate them.[1,21] Health care providers neglect to perform a formal assessment of cardiovascular risk with simultaneous education of the patient at risk about the real chance that she will experience cardiac disease and her role in altering modifiable risk factors. Identification of clustered risk factors, with aggressive treatment of hypertension and dyslipidemia, is imperative. Smoking cessation should be advised for every woman, regardless of overall risk profile. Early identification of glucose intolerance, abdominal adiposity, and metabolic syndrome, with aggressive behavior modification aimed at weight loss, is increasingly recognized as important. The role of aspirin is controversial in primary prevention in women, as most trials included only men. In the absence of compelling data, it is recommended that low-dose aspirin be considered as therapy only in women with a high estimated risk (>10 percent in 10 years).[23] The importance of encouraging life-style modification at each encounter with young women so that they may approach menopause with heart healthy behaviors in place is underscored by Nurses' Health Study data, which predict an 86 percent risk reduction in women who adopt healthy life styles including smoking cessation, achievement of ideal body weight, regular physical exercise, and a low-fat diet.[57]

Evaluation of Chest Pain

Clinical Syndromes and Natural History

Differences in presentation and disease manifestations between men and women exist and should be considered in the evaluation of chest pain. Women are on average 5 to 10 years older and have more comorbidities at the time of their first presentation with CHD. Angina is the most common first symptom of CHD in women, who are less likely than men to present initially with a concrete event such as myocardial infarction or sudden cardiac death (Fig. 73–6A).[2] Perhaps even more than in men, the prevalence of angiographic coronary disease varies dramatically according to the nature of the chest pain, age, and coronary risk factors. As illustrated in Figure 73–6B, typical or classic angina (defined as exertional substernal discomfort relieved rapidly by rest or nitroglycerin) is commonly due to atherosclerosis in women, particularly older women. Atypical chest pain (exertional substernal discomfort with atypical radiation or not relieved rapidly by rest or nitroglycerin) is less likely to be associated with angiographic coronary disease in women, particularly younger women, than in men.[53,58] Although equally likely to have effort angina, women with CHD are more likely than men to experience atypical symptoms, such as pain at rest, during sleep, or with mental stress. These differences make a gender-based approach essential in the recognition and assessment of acute and chronic ischemic syndromes.

The reasons for these differences are unclear. Although most women have typical angiographic findings of atherosclerosis, women have higher prevalences of vasospastic angina, microvascular angina, and abnormal coronary vasodilator reserve (syndrome X). These syndromes are associated with atypical chest pain patterns, have distinct treatments, and have a more favorable prognosis than epicardial coronary disease.[19,53] Finally, noncoronary chest pain syndromes are more common in women, further complicating clinical assessment of chest pain in females.

Women with undiagnosed chest pain have a better prognosis than men with chest pain because of a lower prevalence of atherosclerosis in women with chest pain. However, when a diagnosis of atherosclerotic disease is made conclusively (e.g., by a history of myocardial infarction), women are at equal and perhaps greater risk for adverse outcomes (Fig. 73–7). In subjects older than 65 with exertional chest pain, women and men have the same relative risks of CHD death (2.7 versus 2.4). Mortality after myocardial infarction is worse in women younger than 60 than that in men, reinforcing the fact that once an atherosclerotic etiology for the chest pain syndrome is identified, the prognosis is no different between the genders. The presence of elevated troponin in a woman with unstable angina predicts a worse outcome (Fig. 73–8), with a positive serum troponin predicting a greater increase in risk of death or myocardial infarction in women than in men.[59]

Noninvasive Diagnostic Testing

The general principles underlying noninvasive diagnostic testing do not differ in men and women.[60] Resting electrocardiography reveals a higher prevalence of repolarization (ST-T wave) abnormalities in women with suspected coronary disease than in men (32 versus 23 percent). Treadmill exercise testing is associated with a higher false-positive rate and a lower false-negative rate than in men (12 versus 40 percent), suggesting that routine testing reliably excludes the presence of CHD in women with negative tests. Variables that may alter test accuracy are resting ST-T wave abnormalities,

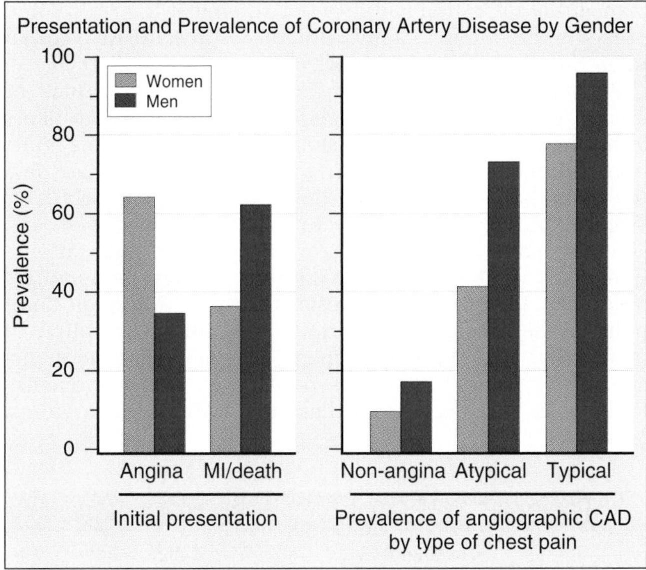

FIGURE 73–6 **A,** Differences in presenting symptom of coronary artery disease by sex. **B,** Prevalence of angiographically documented coronary artery disease (CAD) according to chest pain syndrome. Typical angina was defined as exertional substernal discomfort relieved rapidly by rest or nitroglycerin (NTG). Probable angina was similar to typical angina but varied in an important respect (atypical radiation, not relieved by NTG or rest). Nonanginal pain did not fit the preceding descriptions. MI = myocardial infarction. (Data from Kannel WB, Feinleib M: Natural history of angina pectoris in the Framingham study. Prognosis and survival. Am J Cardiol 29:154, 1972; and Chaitman BR, Bourassa MG, Davis K, et al: Angiographic prevalence of high-risk coronary artery disease in patient subsets [CASS]. Circulation 64:360, 1981.)

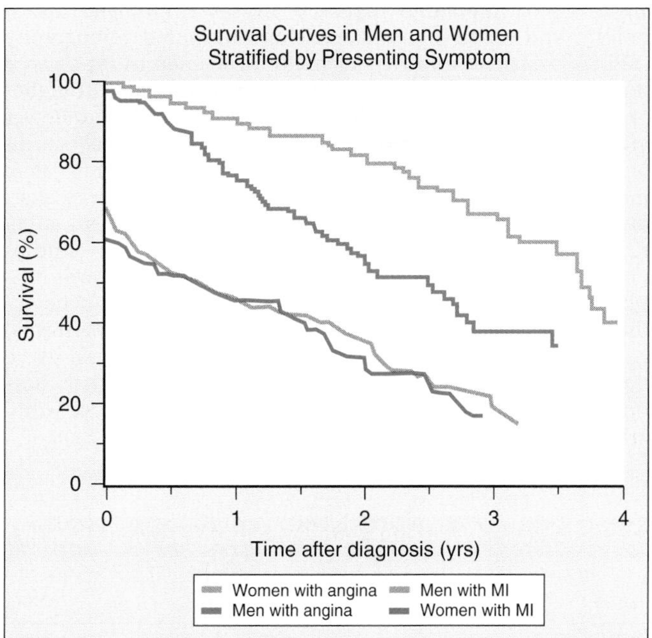

FIGURE 73–7 Survival curves of men and women 60 to 69 years of age presenting with angina, contrasted with those of men and women with documented coronary artery disease. The population of women with angina is more heterogeneous and includes more patients without an atherosclerotic etiology. MI = myocardial infarction. (From Hayes SN, Gersh BJ: *In* Douglas PS [ed]: Cardiovascular Health and Disease in Women. 2nd ed. Philadelphia, WB Saunders, 2002. Redrawn from Orencia A, Bailey K, Yawn BP, Kottke TE: Effect of gender on long-term outcome of angina pectoris and myocardial infarction/sudden unexpected death. JAMA 269:2392, 1993.)

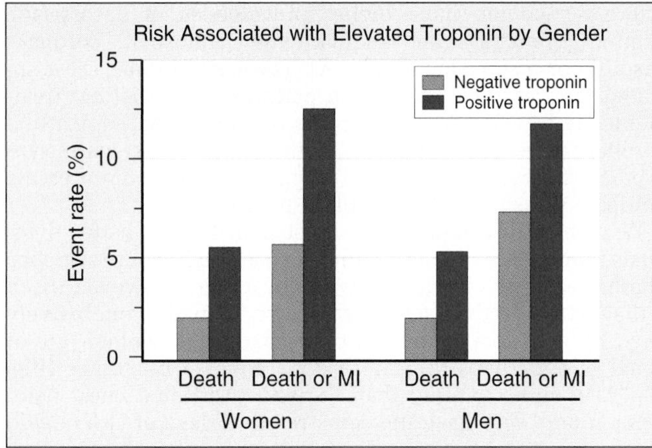

FIGURE 73–8 Impact of serum troponin level on risk of death and myocardial infarction (MI) in both men and women presenting with acute coronary syndromes. (Modified from Grady D, Chaput L, Kristof M: Diagnosis and Treatment of Coronary Heart Disease in Women: Systematic Reviews of Evidence on Selected Topics. Evidence Report/Technology Assessment No. 81. AHRQ Publication No. 03-0037. Rockville, Md, Agency for Healthcare Research and Quality. May 2003.)

peak exercise heart rate, number of diseased vessels, age, drug use (digitalis, diazepam), hyperventilation, conduction abnormalities, left ventricular hypertrophy, mitral valve prolapse, vasospasm, and hormonal influences. False-negative studies may be the result of gender-specific characteristics, including reduced exercise tolerance and the higher prevalence of single-vessel disease in women. The exercise component also provides useful prognostic information in women.[61]

The addition of imaging to electrocardiographic stress testing markedly improves its accuracy in women, as noted by meta-analyses[62,63] and reviews (see also Chaps. 10 and 13). Planar thallium scans during treadmill exercise testing suggest only moderate increases in sensitivity and specificity,[62] and single-photon emission computed tomography (SPECT) may not improve accuracy in women as much as it does in men.[64] Breast attenuation is reduced by use of higher energy isotopes such as technetium 99m sestamibi and newer algorithms for attenuation correction.[65] Exercise echocardiography improves diagnostic accuracy in women,[62] even more so than in men.[63] Meta-analyses[62,63] have shown exercise echocardiography to have similar sensitivity and superior specificity compared with nuclear perfusion studies (Table 73–1), with the accuracy of exercise electrocardiography and exercise nuclear studies, but not exercise echocardiography, showing gender dependence. Several formal cost-effectiveness models show stress echocardiography to dominate over nuclear techniques,[66,67] suggesting that diagnostic testing strategies employing exercise echocardiography as the first test might be superior (see also Chap. 15).

Coronary Angiography

Women are more likely than men to experience vascular and renal complications from diagnostic angiography, possibly because of more advanced age, higher prevalence of diabetes, and smaller body size. The incidences of myocardial infarction, stroke, and death complicating coronary angiography are similar in men and women.[68]

Gender Bias in the Diagnosis of Ischemic Heart Disease

A study in 1987 reporting that men with positive nuclear exercise tests were 6.3 times more likely to be referred to cardiac catheterization than women gave rise to concerns that female patients were receiving inadequate or inappropriate care, a conclusion that has been both substantiated and refuted by subsequent studies. Although awareness of the importance of CHD in women is growing, discrepancies still exist, and both gender and race influence management of chest pain.[69]

Less aggressive treatment strategies in women do not represent optimal care, nor can they be attributed solely to the difficulties in diagnosing coronary disease in women. In one study, subsequent CHD event rates after diagnostic testing were higher in women, whether they had a normal initial test (1.6 percent/yr death or myocardial infarction versus 0.8 percent in men) or an abnormal one (14.3 percent/yr versus 6.0 percent/yr). Revascularization was protective in both male and female patients, and untreated women had a worse prognosis. These data demonstrate not only a gender-based difference in clinical practice but also a worse outcome in women treated less aggressively.

Management of Symptomatic Coronary Heart Disease in Women

Acute Coronary Syndromes

Women have a different clinical presentation and hospital course following acute coronary syndromes and acute myocardial infarction and respond differently to medical and procedural therapies. Gender differences in acute myocardial infarction have been reviewed.[70-72]

Women suffering from an acute coronary syndrome or myocardial infarction are likely to be older; are more likely to have a history of hypertension, diabetes, unstable angina, hyperlipidemia, and congestive heart failure; and are less likely to be smokers than their male counterparts.[70,72,73] Women are also more likely to experience jaw, neck, and shoulder pain; abdominal pain; nausea; vomiting; palpitations; fatigue; and dyspnea in addition to chest pain and are less likely to report diaphoresis than men. Although chest pain is the single most common presenting symptom of myocardial infarction in women,[70] women seem more susceptible to "silent" infarction, particularly elderly women.[74] Perhaps in part because of these more atypical symptoms,

TABLE 73–1 Predictive Value of Noninvasive Testing in Women with Coronary Artery Disease*

Type of Study	Sensitivity	Specificity	Likelihood Ratio for Positive Test	Likelihood Ratio for Negative Test
Myocardial perfusion imaging	0.77 (0.69-0.81)	0.71 (0.69-0.78)	2.54 (1.95-3.32)	0.36 (0.28-0.46)
Exercise echocardiography	0.82 (0.73-0.89)	0.60 (0.48-0.71)	2.06 (1.53-2.77)	0.29 (0.18-0.47)

*Summary of data from good-quality clinical trials to determine clinical utility of noninvasive diagnostic testing in detection of coronary artery disease in women presenting with chest pain syndromes. Estimates with 95% confidence intervals are presented.

Modified from Grady D, Chaput L, Kristof M: Diagnosis and Treatment of Coronary Heart Disease in Women: Systematic Reviews of Evidence on Selected Topics. Evidence Report/Technology Assessment No. 81. AHRQ Publication No. 03-0037. Rockville, Md, Agency for Healthcare Research and Quality, May 2003.

women seek medical attention more slowly and even after hospital arrival may experience greater delays in receiving care. Physician uncertainty about the true clinical diagnosis is more common for women than men with acute myocardial infarction, and misdiagnosis is more likely.[75]

Women with infarction have higher risk initial presentations, with greater prevalences of tachycardia, rales, heart block, and a higher Killip class.[73] Women are less likely to be admitted to a coronary care unit or to be hospitalized in an institution in which catheterization is available. Most studies, but not all, find that women with acute infarction are less likely to undergo diagnostic catheterization during their hospital stay, even after controlling for age and a variety of clinical characteristics. Whether this distinction exists only for patients with equivocal indications for catheterization and whether it extends to lower rates of angioplasty and bypass surgery among catheterized patients are unclear. Women have higher rates of in-hospital complications from infarction, including bleeding, stroke, shock, myocardial rupture, and recurrent chest pain, than do men, although most of these differences appear attributable to age and comorbidities.

Mortality

Mortality in non-Q-wave myocardial infarction appears to be similar to that in men, but women with unstable angina are less likely to have angiographic CHD, reinfarction, or death.[76] In acute ST elevation myocardial infarction, early or in-hospital mortality in women is greater than in men, and adjustment for age or clinical characteristics, or both, reduces but does not eliminate this difference. In part, this gap may be due to a higher rate of prehospital sudden death in men, but this cannot explain the twofold greater mortality in women younger than 50 years compared with similarly aged men. Mortality 1 to 3 years after hospital discharge is also increased in younger women, although it is similar in postmenopausal women and men.[77]

Thrombolysis and Acute Medical Treatment

Because men and women show similar rates of intracoronary thrombosis on pretreatment angiography, it is not surprising that the efficacy of thrombolysis is equivalent with similar infarct-related artery patency and preservation of left ventricular function. However, whereas mortality is similar, complication rates, particularly hemorrhagic stroke and recurrent myocardial infarction, appear to be higher in women. In contrast to older studies, eligible women now seem to receive thrombolytic therapy at rates equal to those of men, but women more frequently have contraindications to thrombolysis.[78] Primary angioplasty is equally, if not more, effective in women, in part because of the greater reduction in hemorrhagic stroke. Despite a greater risk profile in women, percutaneous revascularization is as safe and effective in women as it is in men.[79]

Although there are physiological reasons to suspect that women may benefit from use of low-molecular-weight heparin and clopidogrel, adequate trial data assessing efficacy in women are unavailable. Use of glycoprotein IIb/IIIa inhibitors confers benefit in addition to that of aspirin in unstable coronary syndromes in women but not in men, provided there is evidence of injury (elevated troponin). Women do not appear to benefit in the absence of positive biomarkers. This finding suggests that, in women, platelets may play a more important role or may require more aggressive inhibition. Several studies, including Treat Angina with Aggrastat and determine Cost of Therapy with an Invasive or Conservative Strategy–Thrombolysis in Myocardial Infarction 18 (TACTICS-TIMI 18),[80] demonstrated equivalent benefit in men and women of an early invasive strategy over aggressive medical therapy alone even though women have a higher likelihood of no angiographic stenoses (17 versus 9 percent) and a lower likelihood of left main coronary disease. Other studies have suggested that the benefit in women is dependent upon the invasive strategy—women do not benefit when coronary artery bypass graft (CABG) surgery is used.[81]

Percutaneous Revascularization

Data show the efficacy of coronary artery stenting to be similar in men and women in both the short and long term.[82] The likelihood of angiographic success is similar in men and women in newer series, with lower success rates in women reported in older studies. However, the proportional risk of death from procedural complications remains greater in women, with higher complication and mortality rates, including groin complications, acute vessel closure, hemorrhagic complications, and death.[83] The difference in outcome has been variously attributed to women's older age, smaller body size, greater severity of angina, more fragile vessels, and greater burden of comorbidity. Care must be taken in the dosing of antiplatelet and anticoagulant therapies in women to minimize the incidence of hemorrhagic side effects.[72]

Surgical Therapies

In 2000, nearly 150,000 women had CABG in the United States, approximately 30 percent of the total number of CABG surgeries performed. Gender differences in outcome following CABG are well established and, although decreasing over time, persist in the new millennium.[84] In-hospital mortality is 1.4 to 4.4 times higher, particularly for younger women (<60 years) and low- and medium-risk patients, with no difference in highest risk patients, suggesting nonanatomical factors as the proximate cause.[85] Women are less likely to receive internal mammary grafts or undergo complete revascularization and are more likely to experience the complications of heart failure, perioperative infarction, and hemorrhage. Neurological complications of CABG, including stroke, transient ischemic attack, and coma, are more frequent in women.[86] Rehospitalization rates for women are two times those for men in the first 2 months after CABG.[84]

The causes of higher operative mortality and morbidity appear to be multiple, including technical factors such as smaller body size and coronary diameter, advanced age, comorbidities such as diabetes and hypertension, and clinical factors such as the urgency of the procedure. However, controlling for these eliminates only a small portion of the excess risk, with about 70 percent of the risk unaccounted for in well-controlled multivariate analyses.[85] Disease-related factors such as the extent and severity of angiographic stenoses and left ventricular dysfunction are consistently more favorable in women. Current data on "off-pump" CABG (OPCAB) appear to demonstrate a clear reduction in neurological events in both men and women compared with those associated with traditional coronary bypass techniques,[87] but the marked reduction in length of stay for men undergoing OPCAB may not be seen in women.[88]

After CABG, women have a lower likelihood of being free of angina than do men and experience greater physical disability and less return to work.[89,90] Rates of long-term survival, infarction, and reoperation are similar. Quality of life is worse for women, even when measures are adjusted for premorbid level of function.[84] The worse outcomes following CABG in women are related to more depression, slower recovery of normal physical function, greater physical symptoms, and a higher perceived degree of functional impairment. Much of this gap appears to be related to societal roles of women. Women undergoing CABG are more likely than men to be single and of lower socioeconomic class and thus lack adequate social support. In addition, women who have served as household managers return to this function rapidly after surgery and do not enjoy as extensive a recovery period free from obligations.

Adjunctive Medical Treatment and Secondary Prevention

Women with acute infarction are more likely than men to be treated with nitrates, digoxin, and diuretics and less likely to receive thrombolytics, antiarrhythmics, antiplatelet agents, ACE inhibitors, and beta blockers despite evidence for similar benefit in women.[73] Calcium channel blockade was not effective in either men or women. Although the Coronary Artery Surgery Study (CASS) showed that women treated medically had better 12-year survival with angiographically documented zero-, one-, or two-vessel disease than men with similar anatomy, other studies suggest that undertreatment of women is related to a worse outcome.[91]

Data from the Heart and Estrogen/progestin Replacement Study (HERS) provide the most extensive and distressing snapshot of the current state of secondary prevention in women with known CHD.[92] At the start of the study, only 33 percent of patients were receiving beta blockers, 53 percent were receiving lipid-lowering drugs, and 83 percent were receiving aspirin or other antiplatelet agents. Women at greatest risk were less likely to be taking aspirin ($p < 0.001$) or lipid-lowering drugs ($p = 0.006$). During the study period, the rate of aspirin use by participants actually fell. Current data on secondary prevention of coronary artery disease in women are summarized in Table 73–2.

Lipid lowering is efficacious in women with atherosclerotic disease, with several statin trials showing reductions in cardiac events and death.[39,93] Newer observational studies suggest benefit of aspirin in secondary prevention but still await confirmation by a randomized clinical trial. Diabetic, elderly, and symptomatic women appeared to benefit most, as did women with prior myocardial infarctions. Aspirin and other antiplatelet agents also reduced vascular events in women. Two studies suggest that men may experience more benefit than women when treated with ACE inhibitors after infarction. In contrast, administration of a beta-blocking agent clearly provides substantial improvement in postinfarction survival in women equal to, if not greater than, that in men.

After hospital discharge, women are less likely to be scheduled for exercise tests or referred for cardiac rehabilitation, and recovery from infarction appears delayed with slower return to work and full resumption of all activities and more sleep disturbance and psychiatric and psychosomatic complaints.[84]

Peripheral Arterial Disease

Peripheral arterial disease (PAD) is understudied from a gender-specific perspective. Although men have a higher reported prevalence of PAD, there is widespread failure to recognize PAD in women with documented reduction in ankle brachial index (ABI).[94,95] With noninvasive testing, the incidence of clinically significant PAD is equal in women and men at risk. Women with PAD have a higher incidence of confounding comorbidities, including osteoarthritis and spinal stenosis, and more often present with symptoms other than classical claudication or no symptoms.[94,96] They also have substantially increased mortality compared with age-matched healthy women, often because of myocardial ischemia.[95] Although all elderly women should receive a careful examination of peripheral pulses, ABI screening is recommended in women older than 60 at risk for PAD, including those with known atherosclerotic disease elsewhere, current smokers, and diabetics.

The risk factors for PAD are similar to those for CHD; however, diabetes and cigarette smoking have particularly strong associations with PAD. There are few data comparing evaluation or treatment between women and men, although women are less likely to be actively exercising or treated with aspirin or lipid-lowering agents, at least in part because of failure to recognize the disease.

Women with reduced ABI are less likely than men to have had prior revascularization. About a third of lower extremity revascularization procedures and amputations are performed in women. The rates of graft patency and long-term survival are significantly lower in women than in men.[97]

Hemostasis, Thrombosis, and Stroke

Gender and Hemostasis

The clotting and fibrinolysis systems are complex and intensively regulated (see also Chap. 80). Although genetic polymorphisms for many of the proteins involved in these

TABLE 73–2 Secondary Prevention of Coronary Artery Disease in Women*

Strategy	Level of Evidence	Reduction in Endpoints (%)	Underuse?
Lipid lowering	A	30-50	Y
Aspirin	A	20-25	Y
Beta blockers			
After MI	A	20-30	Y
With LV dysfunction	A	10-40	Y
ACE inhibitors			
After MI	A	5-10†	Y
With LV dysfunction	A	25-30†	Y
Smoking cessation	B	65	Y
Hypertension	C	?	?
Cardiac rehabilitation	C	?	Y
Hormone replacement therapy	A	Increase	N/A

*Summary of current data on secondary prevention of coronary artery disease in women, including level of evidence by American Heart Association criteria, reduction in endpoints noted in trials, and level of adoption by the medical community.

†Although the effect is probably positive, the 95% confidence interval crosses 1.0.

ACE = angiotensin-converting enzyme; LV = left ventricular; MI = myocardial infarction.

Modified from Grady D, Chaput L, Kristof M: Diagnosis and Treatment of Coronary Heart Disease in Women: Systematic Reviews of Evidence on Selected Topics. Evidence Report/Technology Assessment No. 81. AHRQ Publication No. 03-0037. Rockville, Md, Agency for Healthcare Research and Quality, May 2003.

cascades have been described, all identified to date are autosomal rather than gender linked. There are no identifiable differences in platelet function between the genders, although platelet levels in women fluctuate during the menstrual cycle.[15] Levels and function of several of the proteins involved in hemostasis do appear to be hormonally regulated. Fibrinogen and factor VII are slightly higher in women, and fibrinogen levels in women increase with age. Young women have higher plasma tissue plasminogen activator levels and lower PAI-1 levels than men, and levels of both increase with age in women. Changes in levels and activity of these and other factors are well described with alterations in the hormonal milieu seen with pregnancy, use of birth control pills and other exogenous estrogens, and hormonal cancer chemotherapy. On balance, the hemostatic profile in women appears slightly more thrombogenic, perhaps to protect against fetal hemorrhage, and is probably responsible for the increased rate of venous thromboembolism seen in women.[15]

Risk Factors and Their Modification

Hypertension and smoking are the most significant risk factors for stroke in women, although hyperlipidemia, diabetes, and obesity are also important predictors of stroke risk.[47,96] Nontraditional risk factors are increasingly being implicated in stroke risk, including homocysteine and, in young women, antiphospholipid antibody syndrome.[98] Single-gender studies in the last several years have shown that physical activity, a diet rich in omega-3 fatty acids, and intake of whole grains (but not processed grains) protect against ischemic stroke in women. Elevated serum levels of CRP in patients with an otherwise benign risk profile predict future stroke risk in both men and women. Abdominal obesity is also a predictor of stroke and is associated with elevated CRP levels. Aggressive treatment of hypertension with multiple agents has been shown to reduce the risk of first stroke, and treatment with angiotensin II receptor antagonists and diuretics reduces the risk of recurrent stroke even in patients without significant blood pressure elevation.[99] The Heart Outcomes Prevention Evaluation Study (HOPE) demonstrated a significant reduction in stroke risk with ramipril in both men and women with high risk for vascular disease, independent of blood pressure lowering effects.[100] In both trials, nearly 50 percent of treated patients were female.

In contrast to its effect in men, aspirin use does not appear to prevent first stroke in women,[101,102] but it may reduce the risk of recurrent stroke by approximately 25 percent. In patients with cardioembolic stroke, the risk reduction associated with aspirin therapy is 20 percent and that of warfarin is 60 percent for recurrent events. Elderly women in atrial fibrillation are less likely to be prescribed warfarin than men of the same age and more likely to receive aspirin therapy.[103] Multiple studies have demonstrated that physicians overestimate the risks associated with warfarin therapy, especially in elderly women.[104] Lipid-lowering therapy with HMG CoA reductase inhibitors is effective in both primary and secondary prevention of stroke.[39] Although experimental data suggest that estrogen is neuroprotective, estrogen as secondary prevention had no effect on stroke rate[8,10] and in the Women's Health Initiative trial of primary prevention there was a small increase in stroke risk among estrogen and progesterone users.

Clinical Syndromes, Natural History, and Treatment

Stroke incidence is approximately equal in both genders; however, 61 percent of all deaths associated with stroke occur in women.[47] Atherothrombotic stroke, which is strongly related to atherosclerotic disease, is the most common type of stroke in men, whereas the predominant stroke type in women is cardioembolic, typically related to atrial fibrillation. Significant carotid stenosis is found more frequently in men.[97] Hemorrhagic stroke occurs at roughly equal rates in men and women and accounts for 15 percent of all strokes. Subarachnoid hemorrhages are much more common in premenopausal women than in any other age group and are more often fatal in women than in men.[47,96]

Women are older when they have their first stroke and have more comorbidities. Stroke in women is more often complicated by congestive heart failure, typically in the presence of preserved systolic function. Treatment of acute ischemic stroke with thrombolytic therapy has apparently equal efficacy in both genders, although there is an increased risk of hemorrhage in women.[105]

Approximately one-third of carotid endarterectomies are performed in women.[97] The postoperative stroke rate is higher in women, perhaps because of smaller vessel size. Long-term outcome after carotid endarterectomy has not been extensively studied, but 5-year survival was higher in women than men in one study.[106] Women are more likely to develop recurrent carotid stenosis but have no increase in late stroke.[97] Following all types of stroke, women have more prolonged recovery, less often have adequate family support, and, as a result, account for a substantial portion of stroke victims requiring some type of long-term care.[107]

Arrhythmias

Gender and Cardiac Electrophysiology

(see also Chaps. 27 and 30)

Bazett first recognized a gender difference in the electrocardiogram between men and women in 1920, reporting higher heart rates and longer corrected QT intervals in women. Both gender and estrogen status affect the electrocardiogram in women. At birth and throughout life, the heart rate of a female is higher than that of a male. This difference has been ascribed variously to higher intrinsic parasympathetic tone in females, training effects related to higher fitness levels in men, intrinsic differences in quantities or kinetics, or both, of cardiac ion channels, and differences in cell coupling.[108] Estrogen modulates cardiac electrophysiology both in vitro and in vivo. Estrogen, but not dihydrotestosterone, prolongs action potential duration in ventricular myocytes. There is a direct effect of estrogen on both the rapidly and slowly activating inward-rectifying potassium channels (IK_r, IK_s). This gender difference in potassium channels has been tied to the higher incidence of drug-induced torsades de pointes among women. Estradiol-17β also reduces L-type calcium channel current rapidly through nongenomic mechanisms. Females with congenital long-QT syndrome have a different distribution of disease than men, with a larger number of women exhibiting the LQT2 subtype. Presentation of congenital long-QT syndrome in women commonly occurs during puberty or pregnancy. The postpartum period is a time of particular risk for women with this disorder, demonstrating the profound impact that fluctuating levels of sex steroids can have on channel biology and electrophysiology.[109]

Syncope (see also Chap. 34)

Women with syncope are older than men, less likely to have left ventricular dysfunction, and more often have a noncardiac etiology of the syncope identified.[110] Women with syncope have significantly higher cardiac event–free survival rates, with a cardiac event rate of 6 percent in more than 9 months of follow-up in one study compared to 21 percent in men.[110] Neurocardiogenic syncope is the most commonly identified type of syncope in women. Contrary to the usual teaching, this type of syncope is common among elderly patients, with a positive tilt-table test in approximately 30 percent of patients with unexplained syncope.[111] Older subjects with positive tilt-table tests are more likely to have a pure vasodepressor response without bradycardia, and midodrine has been proposed as the therapy of choice. Women have higher anxiety scores than men with neurocardiogenic syncope and also higher scores than women without positive tilt-table tests.[112] It is important to assess a woman with syncope fully before attributing the event to an underlying psychiatric disorder, as anxiety commonly coexists with electrophysiological abnormalities in women.

Atrial Arrhythmias

Palpitations are a common complaint with a large differential diagnosis. It is often difficult, particularly in women, to distinguish treatable atrial arrhythmias from other causes of palpitations. Inappropriate sinus tachycardia may arise as palpitations and an exaggerated heart rate response to mild exercise and has an almost 90 percent female prevalence.[113] Gender-specific dysregulation of the autonomic input to the sinus node is thought to be the etiology. Beta blockers are often poorly tolerated; selective sinus node ablation may be curative.

Among paroxysmal supraventricular tachycardias (PSVTs), electrocardiographic findings of Wolff-Parkinson-White syndrome are approximately 3.5 times more common in males than in females, whereas concealed bypass tracts occur with similar frequency in both genders. Two-thirds of patients with atrioventricular nodal tachycardia are female. Atrial fibrillation is 1.5 times more common in men than in women. In patients without overt heart disease, the incidence of atrial fibrillation increases with age in the male but not the female population. The incidence of paroxysms of atrial arrhythmias shows a distinct variance with phase of the menstrual cycle in women, again providing evidence for significant hormonal effects.[114]

Inappropriate and missed diagnoses among women with atrial arrhythmias are common. In 107 patients with documented PSVT, the disorder was unrecognized after initial evaluation in 59 patients (55 percent), including 68 percent of women.[115] In these patients the median time to diagnosis after presentation was 3.3 years, with symptoms attributed to panic, anxiety, or stress more often among women than men (65 versus 32 percent; $p < 0.04$). These investigators also looked at the prevalence of panic disorder according to the *Diagnostic and Statistical Manual of Mental Disorders*, fourth edition (DSM-IV), among patients with documented PSVT and found that 88 percent of patients had four or more symptoms of panic attack and 67 percent met DSM-IV criteria for panic disorder. Clearly, a history of palpitations must be thoroughly investigated before ascribing the complaint to an anxiety disorder, particularly in women. Among women with documented PSVT, multiple episodes of palpitations occurring frequently are the rule, with 75 percent of patients experiencing episodes at least monthly, making diagnosis less difficult if the proper level of suspicion is maintained. There is no evidence that the response of women to accepted therapy differs from that of men. However, few therapies have been tested in significant populations of women.

Ventricular Arrhythmias and Sudden Cardiac Death (see also Chap. 33)

Ventricular arrhythmias and sudden cardiac death are less common in women than in men. Approximately one in five sudden deaths occurs in women, and the etiology of sudden death more commonly is noncardiac among women, including a higher percentage of drug-related causes.[108] Among survivors of cardiac arrest, 80 percent of men are found to have coronary artery disease compared with 45 percent of women.

Women account for 70 percent of cases of torsades de pointes, probably because of their longer baseline QT interval. In addition, women have a higher risk of significant QT prolongation when exposed to drugs known to delay myocardial repolarization (Table 73–3) (see also Chap. 5). Despite this marker of increased risk, men die of sudden cardiac death at a much higher rate. This difference has been postulated to be the result of increased QT dispersion in men compared with women. It is possible that the combination of ischemia and increased QT dispersion is particularly lethal.[114]

When clinically significant ventricular arrhythmias have been documented, gender does not affect the subsequent clinical course. Mortality, defibrillator discharges, and arrhythmia-free survival are comparable among female and male survivors of sudden death. Nevertheless, risk stratification of women for ventricular arrhythmia is even more difficult than that of men because ventricular premature beats and nonsustained ventricular tachycardia do not carry the same negative prognostic implications, even after myocardial infarction. The optimal method of risk stratification is

TABLE 73–3 Drugs and Conditions Associated with QT Prolongation and Polymorphic Ventricular Tachycardia, Particularly in Women

Pharmaceutical Agents	
Antibiotics	Erythromycin; Clarithromycin; Azithromycin; Trimethoprim; Clindamycin; Ketoconazole*; Pentamidine; Halofantrine; Amantadine; Foscarnet; Moxifloxacin; Gatifloxacin
Psychiatric Drugs	Thioridazine; Chlorpromazine; Prochlorperazine; Quetiapine; Mesoridazine; Pimozide; Risperidone; Haloperidol; Tricyclic antidepressants; Fluoxetine; Paroxetine; Citalopram; Sertraline; Venlafaxine
Antiarrhythmic Agents	Quinidine; Procainamide; Disopyramide; *N*-Acetyl-procainamide; Sotalol; Ibutilide; Amiodarone; Dofetilide; Adenosine†
Other Agents	Astemizole; Terfenadine; Cisapride; Famotidine; Salmeterol; Indapamide; Nicardipine; Isradipine; Moexipril/hydrochlorothiazide; Bepridil; Probucol; Chloral hydrate; Sumatriptan; Dolasetron; Felbamate; Droperidol; Methadone
Toxins	Taxine (yew); Arsenic; Organophosphorus insecticides
Physiological Conditions	Intracranial hemorrhage; Liquid protein diets; Complete atrioventricular block; Pacemaker malfunction; Hypokalemia; Hypocalcemia; Hypomagnesemia; Hypothyroidism; Acute myocardial infarction; Human immunodeficiency virus infection

*Particularly in combination with terfenadine.

†In the setting of long-QT syndrome.

unclear.[114] Women survivors of sudden death have higher ejection fractions than men and are less often inducible at electrophysiological study. The Multicenter Unsustained Tachycardia Trial (MUSST), Multicenter Automatic Defibrillator Implantation Trials (MADIT I and MADIT II), and Amiodarone Versus Implantable Defibrillators (AVID) trial together enrolled less than 500 women, making gender-specific analysis impossible because of small numbers.[108]

Valvular Heart Disease

The epidemiology of several types of valvular heart disease demonstrates clear gender differences, but no data are available about variability in response to medical or surgical treatment (see also Chap. 57).

Mitral Valve Prolapse

Mitral valve prolapse is thought to be a genetic disorder with gender, body size, mean blood pressure, and thoracic geometry influencing the phenotype. Although clinically recognizable disease has a female predominance as high as 70 percent, major complications, most notably infective endocarditis and severe mitral regurgitation, have a strong male predominance.[116] The associations between mitral valve prolapse and chest pain, dyspnea at rest, anxiety, and panic attacks are related to a higher prevalence of these conditions in the female population rather than to the disease. There are, however, clear associations between mitral valve prolapse and midsystolic clicks, mitral systolic murmurs, thoracic bone abnormalities, low body weight, low systolic blood pressure, and palpitations. The majority of women with echocardiographic evidence of mitral valve prolapse have a benign natural history. The presence of a significant mitral valve murmur should prompt further diagnostic evaluation, including a prescription for antibiotic prophylaxis at the time of dental or other high-risk procedures (see also Chap. 58).

Rheumatic Valvular Disease

Development of mitral stenosis with a classic rheumatic deformity is more common in women than in men, although aortic disease is less common.[116] Women with rheumatic mitral stenosis often present during pregnancy, as the narrowed mitral orifice becomes limiting in the setting of increased cardiac output and relative tachycardia. Hemoptysis is a more common presenting feature of mitral stenosis in women than in men. There is no evidence that response to percutaneous balloon valvotomy or surgical valve replacement varies by gender, although the issue has not been closely studied.

Nonrheumatic Aortic Valve Disease

Bicuspid aortic valves have a nearly 3:1 male predominance, and aortic valve surgery among patients younger than 65 occurs predominantly in men. There is some evidence that women with bicuspid valves have less propensity to progression to stenosis or regurgitation and require surgical intervention less frequently.[116] In patients 65 or older, there is a twofold higher prevalence of calcific aortic valve disease in men than in women.[117]

Marfan Syndrome

Because Marfan syndrome is an autosomal dominant disorder, incidence, therapy, and outcome do not differ by gender. However, pregnancy increases the risk of aortic dissection, particularly in the presence of any abnormality of the aortic root.[116]

Heart Failure

Clinical Syndromes and Natural History

Given that the genetic and physiological responses to myocardial stress or injury clearly differ between men and women (see earlier), it is not surprising that the clinical spectrum and epidemiology of heart failure also differ. Women develop heart failure at a later age, are less likely to have had a prior myocardial infarction, and are more likely to have hypertension, diabetes, and obesity. In the Medicare population, 80 percent of patients with heart failure and preserved systolic function are women.[118] Alcoholic cardiomyopathy is encountered less frequently in women than in men, but this may be due to the lower prevalence of alcoholism among women because data suggest that alcohol may be more toxic to the myocardium in women, with a lower total dose required to produce cardiomyopathy.[119]

Diagnosis of heart failure may be more difficult in women than in men, in part because of higher prevalences of fluid retention and shortness of breath of noncardiac origin. Women prescribed diuretic therapy meet diagnostic criteria for heart failure less often than men. This difference seems to be related to higher rates of obesity in women and is not explained purely by the presence of diastolic abnormalities.[120] Following a diagnosis of heart failure, men more frequently undergo echocardiographic study, stress testing, and catheterization and are more likely to be referred to specialists.[120]

The prognosis in women with heart failure differs from that in men. Heart failure with preserved systolic function has been thought to have a better prognosis than that associated with systolic dysfunction, although the mortality in patients with preserved systolic function is four times that of age-matched patients without heart failure[121] and has been suggested to be equal to that of patients with systolic dysfunction in the modern era.[122] Because of this, general population studies show an improved prognosis for women with heart failure. However, women enrolled in the Studies of Left Ventricular Dysfunction (SOLVD) trial, all of whom had significant systolic dysfunction, had a distinctly worse prognosis than the men. The heterogeneity of populations and underlying disease in various studies probably explains discrepancies in the literature.

Medical Therapy

There is a disturbing uncertainty about the efficacy of many established therapies in women with heart failure. Clinical trials have focused almost exclusively on patients with systolic dysfunction and typically enrolled younger patients and patients with an ischemic etiology disproportionately, thus having a heavy predominance of male subjects and failing to address treatment of diastolic dysfunction.

Conclusive evidence for a reduction in mortality and morbidity with ACE inhibitor therapy in systolic dysfunction exists only for men because of the small numbers of women enrolled and the lack of prespecified analyses by gender. Adverse events are more common in women receiving ACE inhibitor therapy, perhaps in part because of the failure to account for body size when determining dosing regimens in the major clinical trials.[120] Meta-analyses have demonstrated improvement in outcomes in women treated with ACE inhibitors but suggested that the effect may be less than in men.[123] Beta-adrenergic blocking agent therapy appears equally effective for both genders with systolic dysfunction and symptoms of heart failure.[124]

A concerning report demonstrated an increased risk of death in women randomly assigned to digoxin therapy in the Digitalis Investigation Group (DIG) trial, with a smaller reduction in hospitalizations than was seen in men.[125] This may be due in part to higher serum digoxin levels in the physically smaller female population. However, there was an increase in the risk of both death from heart failure and death from other cardiovascular causes, which is difficult to explain solely on the basis of toxicity of the medication. Diuretic therapy has been associated with a greater risk of hypokalemia in women.[126] Combined with the longer basal QTc interval in women this raises the question of greater risk of iatrogenic arrhythmia. No studies have addressed this issue.

There are currently no gender-specific data on the use of newer therapies, such as aldosterone blockade, or therapies used in acutely decompensated patients, such as intravenous natriuretic peptides, inotropes, or inodilators, although the ongoing Acute Decompensated Heart Failure National Registry (ADHERE), collecting data on patients hospitalized with acutely decompensated heart failure, should provide some insight.

Surgical Therapies and Transplantation

Far fewer women than men have undergone cardiac transplantation, which is in part due to the older average age of women with heart failure as well as differences in patients' desires for transplantation.[127] There is no evidence of inherent bias against females in selection of candidates for transplantation, although age and body weight restrictions commonly employed reduce the numbers of eligible women. There are no gender-specific data on use or outcomes of high-risk surgical procedures or ventricular assist devices in women.

Issues of Death and Dying in Women

A growing body of literature suggests that women choose different paths from men when faced with chronic or terminal illness (see also Chap. 6).[128,129] Women are more concerned about comfort and have a greater fear of technology and associated suffering, avoiding therapies perceived as heroic or experimental. Women and men with heart failure and chronic disability both choose quality of life over longer life.[130] Although cardiology has justifiably focused on major life-saving advances, increasing attention is being paid to therapies that may improve but not necessarily lengthen life. Gender-specific aspects of palliative care and assisting the dying patient with cardiac disease remain relatively unexplored.

REFERENCES

1. Wenger NK: Coronary heart disease and women: magnitude of the problem. Cardiol Rev 10:211, 2002.
2. Kannel WB: The Framingham Study: Historical insight on the impact of cardiovascular risk factors in men versus women. J Gend Specif Med 5:27, 2002.

Gender and Mechanisms of Cardiovascular Disease

3. Sullivan JL: Are menstruating women protected from heart disease because of, or in spite of, estrogen? Relevance to the iron hypothesis. Am Heart J 145:190, 2003.
4. Mikkola TS, Clarkson TB: Estrogen replacement therapy, atherosclerosis, and vascular function. Cardiovasc Res 53:605, 2002.
5. Mendelsohn ME: Genomic and nongenomic effects of estrogen in the vasculature. Am J Cardiol 90:3F, 2002.
6. Zanger D, Yang BK, Ardans J, et al: Divergent effects of hormone therapy on serum markers of inflammation in postmenopausal women with coronary artery disease on appropriate medical management. J Am Coll Cardiol 36:1797, 2000.
7. Weinberg EO, Thienelt CD, Katz SE, et al: Gender differences in molecular remodeling in pressure overload hypertrophy. J Am Coll Cardiol 34:264, 1999.
8. Hulley S, Grady D, Bush T, et al: Randomized trial of estrogen plus progestin for secondary prevention of coronary heart disease in postmenopausal women. Heart and Estrogen/progestin Replacement Study (HERS) Research Group. JAMA 280:605, 1998.
9. Manson JE, Hsia J, Johnson KC, et al: Estrogen plus progestin and the risk of coronary heart disease. N Engl J Med 349:523, 2003.
10. Grady D, Herrington D, Bittner V, et al: Cardiovascular disease outcomes during 6.8 years of hormone therapy: Heart and Estrogen/progestin Replacement Study follow-up (HERS II). JAMA 288:49, 2002.
11. Yamada Y, Izawa H, Ichihara S, et al: Prediction of the risk of myocardial infarction from polymorphisms in candidate genes. N Engl J Med 347:1916, 2002.
12. Burke AP, Farb A, Malcom GT, et al: Effect of risk factors on the mechanism of acute thrombosis and sudden coronary death in women. Circulation 97:2110, 1998.
13. English JL, Jacobs LO, Green G, et al: Effect of the menstrual cycle on endothelium-dependent vasodilation of the brachial artery in normal young women. Am J Cardiol 82:256, 1998.
14. Sader MA, McCredie RJ, Griffiths KA, et al: Oestradiol improves arterial endothelial function in healthy men receiving testosterone. Clin Endocrinol (Oxf) 54:175, 2001.
15. Weksler B: Hemostasis and thrombosis. *In* Douglas PS (ed): Cardiovascular Health and Disease in Women. 2nd ed. Philadelphia, WB Saunders, 2002, pp 157-177.
16. Arbustini E, Dal Bello B, Morbini P, et al: Plaque erosion is a major substrate for coronary thrombosis in acute myocardial infarction. Heart 82:269, 1999.
17. Crabbe DL, Dipla K, Ambati S, et al: Gender differences in post-infarction hypertrophy in end-stage failing hearts. J Am Coll Cardiol 41:300, 2003.
18. Guerra S, Leri A, Wang X, et al: Myocyte death in the failing human heart is gender dependent. Circ Res 85:856, 1999.
19. Mosca L, Manson JE, Sutherland SE, et al: Cardiovascular disease in women: A statement for healthcare professionals from the American Heart Association. Writing Group. Circulation 96:2468, 1997.
20. Wenger NK: Social support and coronary heart disease in women: The challenge to learn more. Eur Heart J 19:1603, 1998.
21. Mosca L, Jones WK, King KB, et al: Awareness, perception, and knowledge of heart disease risk and prevention among women in the United States. American Heart Association Women's Heart Disease and Stroke Campaign Task Force. Arch Fam Med 9:506, 2000.

Atherosclerotic Vascular Disease

22. Skerrett PJ, Spelsberg A, Manson JE: Carbohydrate metabolism, obesity, and diabetes mellitus. *In* Douglas PS (ed): Cardiovascular Health and Disease in Women. 2nd ed. Philadelphia, WB Saunders, 2002, pp 39-70.
23. Pearson TA, Blair SN, Daniels SR, et al: AHA Guidelines for Primary Prevention of Cardiovascular Disease and Stroke: 2002 Update: Consensus Panel Guide to Comprehensive Risk Reduction for Adult Patients Without Coronary or Other Atherosclerotic Vascular Diseases. American Heart Association Science Advisory and Coordinating Committee. Circulation 106:388, 2002.
24. Wheatcroft SB, Williams IL, Shah AM, et al: Pathophysiological implications of insulin resistance on vascular endothelial function. Diabet Med 20:255, 2003.
25. Sowers JR: Diabetes mellitus and cardiovascular disease in women. Arch Intern Med 158:617, 1998.
26. Franklin SS: Definition and epidemiology of hypertensive cardiovascular disease in women: The size of the problem. J Hypertens 20(Suppl 2):S3, 2002.
27. Gueyffier F, Boutitie F, Boissel JP, et al: Effect of antihypertensive drug treatment on cardiovascular outcomes in women and men. A meta-analysis of individual patient data from randomized, controlled trials. The INDANA Investigators. Ann Intern Med 126:761, 1997.
28. Silaste ML, Junes R, Rantala AO, et al: Dietary and other non-pharmacological treatments in patients with drug-treated hypertension and control subjects. J Intern Med 247:318, 2000.
29. Chobanian AV, Bakris GL, Black HR, et al: The Seventh Report of the Joint National Committee on Prevention, Detection, Evaluation, and Treatment of High Blood Pressure: The JNC 7 report. JAMA 289:2560, 2003.
30. Major outcomes in high-risk hypertensive patients randomized to angiotensin-converting enzyme inhibitor or calcium channel blocker vs diuretic: The Antihypertensive and Lipid-Lowering Treatment to Prevent Heart Attack Trial (ALLHAT). JAMA 288:2981, 2002.
31. Wing LM, Reid CM, Ryan P, et al: A comparison of outcomes with angiotensin-converting-enzyme inhibitors and diuretics for hypertension in the elderly. N Engl J Med 348:583, 2003.
32. Bolego C, Poli A, Paoletti R: Smoking and gender. Cardiovasc Res 53:568, 2002.
33. Bohadana A, Nilsson F, Rasmussen T, et al: Gender differences in quit rates following smoking cessation with combination nicotine therapy: Influence of baseline smoking behavior. Nicotine Tob Res 5:111, 2003.
34. Steenland K, Thun M, Lally C, et al: Environmental tobacco smoke and coronary heart disease in the American Cancer Society CPS-II cohort. Circulation 94:622, 1996.
35. LaRosa JC: Lipids. *In* Douglas PS (ed): Cardiovascular Health and Disease in Women. 2nd ed. Philadelphia, WB Saunders 2002, pp 23-28.
36. Third Report of the National Cholesterol Education Program (NCEP) Expert Panel on Detection, Evaluation, and Treatment of High Blood Cholesterol in Adults (Adult Treatment Panel III) final report. Circulation 106:3143, 2002.
37. Bittner V: Lipoprotein abnormalities related to women's health. Am J Cardiol 90:77i, 2002.
38. Mosca LJ: Contemporary management of hyperlipidemia in women. J Womens Health Gend Based Med 11:423, 2002.
39. MRC/BHF Heart Protection Study of cholesterol lowering with simvastatin in 20,536 high-risk individuals: A randomised placebo-controlled trial. Lancet 360:7, 2002.
40. Mendelsohn ME, Karas RH: The protective effects of estrogen on the cardiovascular system. N Engl J Med 340:1801, 1999.

41. Manson JE, Martin KA: Clinical practice. Postmenopausal hormone-replacement therapy. N Engl J Med 345:34, 2001.
42. Rossouw JE, Anderson GL, Prentice RL, et al: Risks and benefits of estrogen plus progestin in healthy postmenopausal women: Principal results from the Women's Health Initiative randomized controlled trial. JAMA 288:321, 2002.
42a. Women's Health Initiative Study: Available at http://www.nhlbi.nih.gov/whi/
43. Pickering TG: Men are from Mars, women are from Venus: Stress, pets, and oxytocin. J Clin Hypertens (Greenwich) 5:86, 2003.
44. Manson JE, Willett WC, Stampfer MJ, et al: Body weight and mortality among women. N Engl J Med 333:677, 1995.
45. Visser M, Bouter LM, McQuillan GM, et al: Elevated C-reactive protein levels in overweight and obese adults. JAMA 282:2131, 1999.
46. Rexrode KM, Carey VJ, Hennekens CH, et al: Abdominal adiposity and coronary heart disease in women. JAMA 280:1843, 1998.
47. Heart Disease and Stroke Statistics—2003 Update. Dallas, American Heart Association, 2002 (http://www.americanheart.org/downloadable/heart/10590179711482003HDSStatsBookREV7-03.pdf).
48. Manson JE, Hu FB, Rich-Edwards JW, et al: A prospective study of walking as compared with vigorous exercise in the prevention of coronary heart disease in women. N Engl J Med 341:650, 1999.
49. Mensink GB, Ziese T, Kok FJ: Benefits of leisure-time physical activity on the cardiovascular risk profile at older age. Int J Epidemiol 28:659, 1999.
50. King AC, Castro C, Wilcox S, et al: Personal and environmental factors associated with physical inactivity among different racial-ethnic groups of U.S. middle-aged and older-aged women. Health Psychol 19:354, 2000.
51. Ridker PM, Buring JE, Cook NR, et al: C-reactive protein, the metabolic syndrome, and risk of incident cardiovascular events: An 8-year follow-up of 14 719 initially healthy American women. Circulation 107:391, 2003.
52. Ridker PM, Rifai N, Clearfield M, et al: Measurement of C-reactive protein for the targeting of statin therapy in the primary prevention of acute coronary events. N Engl J Med 344:1959, 2001.
53. Hayes SN, Gersh BJ: Chronic stable angina. *In* Douglas PS (ed): Cardiovascular Health and Disease in Women. 2nd ed. Philadelphia, WB Saunders, 2002, pp 291-315.
54. Bankier B, Littman AB: Psychiatric disorders and coronary heart disease in women—A still neglected topic: Review of the literature from 1971 to 2000. Psychother Psychosom 71:133, 2002.
55. Nguyen VH, McLaughlin MA: Coronary artery disease in women: A review of emerging cardiovascular risk factors. Mt Sinai J Med 69:338, 2002.
56. Donati MB, Zito F, Castelnuovo AD, et al: Genes, coagulation and cardiovascular risk. J Hum Hypertens 14:369, 2000.
57. Stampfer MJ, Hu FB, Manson JE, et al: Primary prevention of coronary heart disease in women through diet and lifestyle. N Engl J Med 343:16, 2000.
58. Kyker KA, Limacher MC: Gender differences in the presentation and symptoms of coronary artery disease. Curr Womens Health Rep 2:115, 2002.
59. Grady D, Chaput L, Kristof M: Diagnosis and Treatment of Coronary Heart Disease in Women: Systematic Reviews of Evidence on Selected Topics. Evidence Report/Technology Assessment No. 81. (Prepared by the University of California, San Francisco-Stanford Evidence-based Practice Center under Contract No 290-97-0013.) AHRQ Publication No. 03-0037. Rockville, Md, Agency for Healthcare and Research and Quality, May 2003.
60. Lualdi JC, Douglas PS: Considerations in the selection of noninvasive testing for the diagnosis of coronary artery disease. Cardiol Rev 6:278, 1998.
61. Alexander KP, Shaw LJ, Shaw LK, et al: Value of exercise treadmill testing in women. J Am Coll Cardiol 32:1657, 1998.
62. Kwok Y, Kim C, Grady D, et al: Meta-analysis of exercise testing to detect coronary artery disease in women. Am J Cardiol 83:660, 1999.
63. Fleischmann KE, Hunink MG, Kuntz KM, et al: Exercise echocardiography or exercise SPECT imaging? A meta-analysis of diagnostic test performance. JAMA 280:913, 1998.
64. Hansen CL, Kramer M, Rastogi A: Lower accuracy of TI-201 SPECT in women is not improved by size-based normal databases or Wiener filtering. J Nucl Cardiol 6:177, 1999.
65. Taillefer R, DePuey EG, Udelson JE, et al: Comparative diagnostic accuracy of Tl-201 and Tc-99m sestamibi SPECT imaging (perfusion and ECG-gated SPECT) in detecting coronary artery disease in women. J Am Coll Cardiol 29:69, 1997.
66. Kuntz KM, Fleischmann KE, Hunink MG, et al: Cost-effectiveness of diagnostic strategies for patients with chest pain. Ann Intern Med 130:709, 1999.
67. Kim C, Kwok YS, Saha S, et al: Diagnosis of suspected coronary artery disease in women: A cost-effectiveness analysis. Am Heart J 137:1019, 1999.
68. Steen MK, Jacobs AK, Freney D, et al: Gender related differences in complications during coronary angiography. Circulation 86:I-254, 1992.
69. Schulman KA, Berlin JA, Harless W, et al: The effect of race and gender on physicians' recommendations for cardiac catheterization. N Engl J Med 340:618, 1999.
70. Devon HA, Zerwic JJ: Symptoms of acute coronary syndromes: Are there gender differences? A review of the literature. Heart Lung 31:235, 2002.
71. Leopold JA, Jacobs AK: Catheter-based revascularization strategies for acute coronary syndromes in women. Rev Cardiovasc Med 2:181, 2001.
72. Hochman JS, Tamis-Holland JE: Acute coronary syndromes: Does gender matter? JAMA 288:3161, 2002.
73. Collins L, Douglas, PS: Acute coronary syndromes. *In* Douglas PS (ed): Cardiovascular Health and Disease in Women. 2nd ed. Philadelphia, WB Saunders, 2002, pp 316-342.
74. de Bruyne MC, Mosterd A, Hoes AW, et al: Prevalence, determinants, and misclassification of myocardial infarction in the elderly. Epidemiology 8:495, 1997.
75. Lundberg V, Wikstrom B, Bostrom S, et al: Exploring gender differences in case fatality in acute myocardial infarction or coronary death events in the northern Sweden MONICA Project. J Intern Med 251:235, 2002.
76. Hochman JS, Tamis JE, Thompson TD, et al: Gender, clinical presentation, and outcome in patients with acute coronary syndromes. Global Use of Strategies to Open Occluded Coronary Arteries in Acute Coronary Syndromes IIb Investigators. N Engl J Med 341:226, 1999.
77. Vaccarino V, Krumholz HM, Yarzebski J, et al: Gender differences in 2-year mortality after hospital discharge for myocardial infarction. Ann Intern Med 134:173, 2001.
78. Kaplan KL, Fitzpatrick P, Cox C, et al: Use of thrombolytic therapy for acute myocardial infarction: Effects of gender and age on treatment rates. J Thromb Thrombolysis 13:21, 2002.
79. Mehilli J, Kastrati A, Dirschinger J, et al: Gender-based analysis of outcome in patients with acute myocardial infarction treated predominantly with percutaneous coronary intervention. JAMA 287:210, 2002.
80. Cannon CP, Weintraub WS, Demopoulos LA, et al: Comparison of early invasive and conservative strategies in patients with unstable coronary syndromes treated with the glycoprotein IIb/IIIa inhibitor tirofiban. N Engl J Med 344:1879, 2001.
81. Wallentin L, Lagerqvist B, Husted S, et al: Outcome at 1 year after an invasive compared with a non-invasive strategy in unstable coronary-artery disease: The FRISC II invasive randomised trial. FRISC II Investigators. Fast Revascularisation during Instability in Coronary artery disease. Lancet 356:9, 2000.
82. Glaser R, Herrmann HC, Murphy SA, et al: Benefit of an early invasive management strategy in women with acute coronary syndromes. JAMA 288:3124, 2002.
83. Malenka DJ, O'Rourke D, Miller MA, et al: Cause of in-hospital death in 12,232 consecutive patients undergoing percutaneous transluminal coronary angioplasty. The Northern New England Cardiovascular Disease Study Group. Am Heart J 137:632, 1999.
84. Vaccarino V, Lin ZQ, Kasl SV, et al: Gender differences in recovery after coronary artery bypass surgery. J Am Coll Cardiol 41:307, 2003.
85. Vaccarino V, Abramson JL, Veledar E, et al: Gender differences in hospital mortality after coronary artery bypass surgery: Evidence for a higher mortality in younger women. Circulation 105:1176, 2002.
86. Hogue CW Jr, Barzilai B, Pieper KS, et al: Gender differences in neurological outcomes and mortality after cardiac surgery: A society of thoracic surgery national database report. Circulation 103:2133, 2001.
87. Stamou SC, Jablonski KA, Pfister AJ, et al: Stroke after conventional versus minimally invasive coronary artery bypass. Ann Thorac Surg 74:394, 2002.
88. Capdeville M, Chamogeogarkis T, Lee JH: Effect of gender on outcomes of beating heart operations. Ann Thorac Surg 72:S1022, 2001.
89. Jacobs AK: Coronary revascularization in women in 2003: Gender revisited. Circulation 107:375, 2003.
90. Ott RA, Gutfinger DE, Alimadadian H, et al: Conventional coronary artery bypass grafting: Why women take longer to recover. J Cardiovasc Surg (Torino) 42:311, 2001.
91. Schwartz LM, Fisher ES, Tosteson NA, et al: Treatment and health outcomes of women and men in a cohort with coronary artery disease. Arch Intern Med 157:1545, 1997.
92. Vittinghoff E, Shlipak MG, Varosy PD, et al: Risk factors and secondary prevention in women with heart disease: The Heart and Estrogen/progestin Replacement Study. Ann Intern Med 138:81, 2003.
93. Miettinen TA, Pyorala K, Olsson AG, et al: Cholesterol-lowering therapy in women and elderly patients with myocardial infarction or angina pectoris: Findings from the Scandinavian Simvastatin Survival Study (4S). Circulation 96:4211, 1997.
94. McDermott MM, Greenland P, Liu K, et al: Gender differences in peripheral arterial disease: Leg symptoms and physical functioning. J Am Geriatr Soc 51:222, 2003.
95. Higgins JP, Higgins JA: Epidemiology of peripheral arterial disease in women. J Epidemiol 13:1, 2003.
96. Langer RD, Criqui MH: Stroke and peripheral vascular disease in women. *In* Douglas PS (ed): Cardiovascular Health and Disease in Women. 2nd ed. Philadelphia, WB Saunders, 2002, pp 445-459.
97. Norman PE, Semmens JB, Lawrence-Brown M, et al: The influence of gender on outcome following peripheral vascular surgery: A review. Cardiovasc Surg 8:111, 2000.

Hemostasis, Thrombosis, and Stroke

98. Brey RL, Stallworth CL, McGlasson DL, et al: Antiphospholipid antibodies and stroke in young women. Stroke 33:2396, 2002.
99. Randomised trial of a perindopril-based blood-pressure-lowering regimen among 6,105 individuals with previous stroke or transient ischaemic attack. Lancet 358:1033, 2001.
100. Yusuf S, Sleight P, Pogue J, et al: Effects of an angiotensin-converting-enzyme inhibitor, ramipril, on cardiovascular events in high-risk patients. The Heart Outcomes Prevention Evaluation Study Investigators. N Engl J Med 342:145, 2000.
101. Hansson L, Zanchetti A, Carruthers SG, et al: Effects of intensive blood-pressure lowering and low-dose aspirin in patients with hypertension: Principal results of the Hypertension Optimal Treatment (HOT) randomised trial. HOT Study Group. Lancet 351:1755, 1998.
102. de Gaetano G: Low-dose aspirin and vitamin E in people at cardiovascular risk: A randomised trial in general practice. Collaborative Group of the Primary Prevention Project. Lancet 357:89, 2001.
103. Humphries KH, Kerr CR, Connolly SJ, et al: New-onset atrial fibrillation: Gender differences in presentation, treatment, and outcome. Circulation 103:2365, 2001.
104. Stafford RS, Singer DE: Recent national patterns of warfarin use in atrial fibrillation. Circulation 97:1231, 1998.
105. Kent DM, Ruthazer R, Selker HP: Are some patients likely to benefit from recombinant tissue-type plasminogen activator for acute ischemic stroke even beyond 3 hours from symptom onset? Stroke 34:464, 2003.
106. Schneider JR, Droste JS, Golan JF: Carotid endarterectomy in women versus men: Patient characteristics and outcomes. J Vasc Surg 25:890; discussion 897, 1997.
107. Holroyd-Leduc JM, Kapral MK, Austin PC, et al: Gender differences and similarities in the management and outcome of stroke patients. Stroke 31:1833, 2000.

108. Beauregard LA: Incidence and management of arrhythmias in women. J Gend Specif Med 5:38, 2002.
109. Rashba EJ, Zareba W, Moss AJ, et al: Influence of pregnancy on the risk for cardiac events in patients with hereditary long QT syndrome. LQTS Investigators. Circulation 97:451, 1998.
110. Freed LA, Eagle KA, Mahjoub ZA, et al: Gender differences in presentation, management, and cardiac event-free survival in patients with syncope. Am J Cardiol 80:1183, 1997.
111. McGavigan AD, Hood S: The influence of gender and age on response to head-up tilt-table testing in patients with recurrent syncope. Age Ageing 30:295, 2001.
112. Cohen TJ, Thayapran N, Ibrahim B, et al: An association between anxiety and neurocardiogenic syncope during head-up tilt table testing. Pacing Clin Electrophysiol 23:837, 2000.
113. Zimetbaum P, Josephson ME: Evaluation of patients with palpitations. N Engl J Med 338:1369, 1998.
114. Larsen JA, Kadish AH: Effects of gender on cardiac arrhythmias. J Cardiovasc Electrophysiol 9:655, 1998.
115. Lessmeier TJ, Gamperling D, Johnson-Liddon V, et al: Unrecognized paroxysmal supraventricular tachycardia. Potential for misdiagnosis as panic disorder. Arch Intern Med 157:537, 1997.

Valvular Heart Disease

116. Devereux RB: Valvular heart disease. *In* Douglas PS (ed): Cardiovascular Health and Disease in Women. 2nd ed. Philadelphia, WB Saunders, 2002, pp 405-425.
117. Stewart BF, Siscovick D, Lind BK, et al: Clinical factors associated with calcific aortic valve disease. Cardiovascular Health Study. J Am Coll Cardiol 29:630, 1997.

Heart Failure

118. Masoudi FA, Havranek EP, Smith G, et al: Gender, age, and heart failure with preserved left ventricular systolic function. J Am Coll Cardiol 41:217, 2003.
119. Fernandez-Sola J, Nicolas-Arfelis JM: Gender differences in alcoholic cardiomyopathy. J Gend Specif Med 5:41, 2002.
120. Petrie MC, Dawson NF, Murdoch DR, et al: Failure of women's hearts. Circulation 99:2334, 1999.
121. Vasan RS, Larson MG, Benjamin EJ, et al: Congestive heart failure in subjects with normal versus reduced left ventricular ejection fraction: Prevalence and mortality in a population-based cohort. J Am Coll Cardiol 33:1948, 1999.
122. Redfield MM, Jacobsen SJ, Burnett JC Jr, et al: Burden of systolic and diastolic ventricular dysfunction in the community: Appreciating the scope of the heart failure epidemic. JAMA 289:194, 2003.
123. Shekelle PG, Rich MW, Morton SC, et al: Efficacy of angiotensin-converting enzyme inhibitors and beta-blockers in the management of left ventricular systolic dysfunction according to race, gender, and diabetic status: A meta-analysis of major clinical trials. J Am Coll Cardiol 41:1529, 2003.
124. Ghali JK, Pina IL, Gottlieb SS, et al: Metoprolol CR/XL in female patients with heart failure: Analysis of the experience in Metoprolol Extended-Release Randomized Intervention Trial in Heart Failure (MERIT-HF). Circulation 105:1585, 2002.
125. Rathore SS, Wang Y, Krumholz HM: Gender-based differences in the effect of digoxin for the treatment of heart failure. N Engl J Med 347:1403, 2002.
126. Schwartz JB: Congestive heart failure medications: Is there a rationale for gender-specific therapy? J Gend Specif Med 3:17, 2000.
127. Aaronson KD, Schwartz JS, Goin JE, et al: Gender differences in patient acceptance of cardiac transplant candidacy. Circulation 91:2753, 1995.

Issues of Death and Dying in Women

128. Crawford BM, Meana M, Stewart D, et al: Treatment decision making in mature adults: Gender differences. Health Care Women Int 21:91, 2000.
129. Bookwala J, Coppola KM, Fagerlin A, et al: Gender differences in older adults' preferences for life-sustaining medical treatments and end-of-life values. Death Stud 25:127, 2001.
130. Lewis EF, Johnson PA, Johnson W, et al: Preferences for quality of life or survival expressed by patients with heart failure. J Heart Lung Transplant 20:1016, 2001.

CHAPTER 74

Pregnancy and Cardiovascular Disease

Uri Elkayam

Cardiovascular Physiology During Pregnancy and the Puerperium

Pregnancy and the peripartum period are associated with important cardiocirculatory changes[1] that can lead to marked clinical deterioration in the woman with heart disease. Hemodynamic changes occurring during pregnancy are summarized in Table 74–1.

BLOOD VOLUME. Blood volume increases substantially during pregnancy, starting as early as the sixth week and rising rapidly until midpregnancy, when the rise continues but at a much slower rate (Fig. 74-1).[1] The degree of maximum volume expansion varies considerably in the individual patient (20 to 100 percent) and averages 50 percent. This increase is reported to correlate with fetal weight, placental mass, weight of the products of conception, and maternal and neonatal weight.[1] A higher increment in blood volume is reported in multigravidas and in women with multiple pregnancies. Because increase in plasma volume is more rapid than increase in red blood cell mass (see Fig. 74-1), hemoglobin concentration falls during pregnancy gradually until week 30, causing the "physiological anemia of pregnancy" with hematocrit levels that can be as low as 33 to 38 percent, a condition that can be partially corrected with iron therapy. Changes in blood volume during pregnancy are attributable to estrogen-mediated stimulation of the renin-aldosterone system,[2] which results in sodium and water retention. Changes in other hormones, including deoxycorticosterone, prostaglandin, estrogen, prolactin, placental lactogen, growth hormone, and adrenocorticotropic hormone, may also be involved in water retention during pregnancy.

CARDIAC OUTPUT, STROKE VOLUME, AND HEART RATE. Cardiac output during pregnancy is estimated to increase by approximately 50 percent.[1] It begins to rise around the fifth week and increases rapidly until the 24th week, when it levels off or continues to rise slightly (Fig. 74-2; see Table 74-1).[1,3] During the third trimester, body position can substantially influence cardiac output, which increases in the lateral position and declines in the supine position owing to caval compression by the gravid uterus and decreased venous return to the heart. The increase in cardiac output early in pregnancy is predominantly due to augmentation in stroke volume, whereas in the third trimester it is largely due to an accelerated heart rate and stroke volume does not change or even declines as a result of caval compression (Fig. 74-3). Increase in cardiac output seems to be enhanced in subsequent pregnancies.[3]

Heart rate peaks during the third trimester with an average increase of 10 to 20 beats/min (see Fig. 74-2),[3,4] although on occasion it may be markedly faster. Pregnancy with multiple fetuses is associated with an even higher heart rate.

BLOOD PRESSURE AND SYSTEMIC VASCULAR RESISTANCE. Systemic arterial pressure begins to fall during the first trimester, reaches a nadir in midpregnancy, and returns toward pregestational levels before term (see Table 74-1).[3] Because diastolic blood pressure decreases substantially more than systolic pressure, the pulse pressure widens.[1] Reduction in blood pressure is caused by a decline in systemic vascular resistance related to reduced vascular tone,[5] probably mediated by (1) gestational hormonal activity, increased levels of circulating prostaglandins and atrial natriuretic peptides,[1] as well as endothelial nitric oxide; (2) increased heat production by the developing fetus; and (3) the creation of a low-resistance circulation in the pregnant uterus.

SUPINE HYPOTENSIVE SYNDROME OF PREGNANCY. The supine hypotensive or the uterocaval syndrome of pregnancy occurs with significant decreases in heart rate and blood pressure in up to 11 percent of pregnant women.[1] These hemodynamic changes are associated with weakness, lightheadedness, nausea, dizziness, and even syncope and are explained by acute occlusion of the inferior vena cava by the enlarged uterus. When the supine position is abandoned, these hemodynamic effects and symptoms are usually promptly relieved.

HEMODYNAMIC CHANGES DURING LABOR AND DELIVERY. Hemodynamics are altered substantially during labor and delivery secondary to anxiety, pain, and uterine contractions.[1] Oxygen consumption increases threefold; cardiac output rises progressively during labor because of increases in both stroke volume and heart rate, and it is higher in the lateral position. Both systolic and diastolic blood pressures increase markedly during contractions, with greater augmentation during the second stage.[1] The supine position is associated with a 20 percent reduction in stroke volume, cardiac output, and mean arterial pressure and a marked increase in systemic vascular resistance compared with the lateral position. Hemodynamic changes during labor and delivery are greatly influenced by the form of anesthesia and analgesia. Reduction of pain and apprehension by local, caudal, or epidural anesthesia may limit hemodynamic changes and the rise in oxygen consumption.

HEMODYNAMIC EFFECTS OF CESAREAN SECTION. To avoid the hemodynamic changes associated with vaginal delivery, cesarean section is frequently recommended for women with cardiovascular disease. However, this form of delivery can also be associated with considerable hemodynamic fluctuations related largely to intubation, drugs used for anesthesia and analgesia, larger extent of blood loss, the relief of caval compression, extubation, and postoperative awakening.[1]

HEMODYNAMIC CHANGES POST PARTUM. A temporary increase in venous return may occur immediately after delivery because of relief of caval compression and, in addition, blood shifting from the contracting uterus into the systemic circulation (autotransfusion). This change in effective blood volume occurs despite blood loss during delivery and can result in a substantial rise in ventricular

TABLE 74–1 Cardiocirculatory Changes During Normal Pregnancy

	Changes at Various Times (Weeks)					
Parameter	***5***	***12***	***20***	***24***	***32***	***38***
Heart rate	↑	↑↑↑	↑↑↑	↑↑↑	↑↑↑↑	↑↑↑↑
Systolic blood pressure	↔	↓	↓	↔	↑	↑↑
Diastolic blood pressure	↔	↓	↓↓	↓	↔	↑↑
Stroke volume	↑	↑↑↑↑↑	↑↑↑↑↑↑	↑↑↑↑↑↑	↑↑↑↑↑	↑↑↑↑↑
Cardiac output	↑↑	↑↑↑↑↑↑	↑↑↑↑↑↑↑	↑↑↑↑↑↑↑	↑↑↑↑↑↑↑	↑↑↑↑↑↑↑
Systemic vascular resistance	↓↓	↓↓↓↓↓	↓↓↓↓↓↓	↓↓↓↓↓↓	↓↓↓↓↓↓	↓↓↓↓↓
Left ventricular ejection fraction	↑	↑↑	↑↑	↑↑	↑	↑

↑, ≤5%; ↑↑, 6-10%; ↑↑↑, 11-15%; ↑↑↑↑, 16-20%; ↑↑↑↑↑, 21-30%; ↑↑↑↑↑↑, >30%; ↑↑↑↑↑↑↑, >40%.

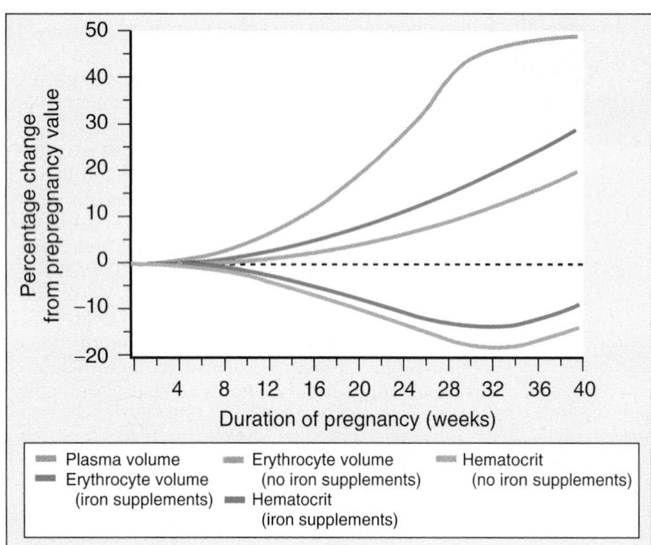

FIGURE 74–1 Changes in plasma volume, erythrocyte volume, and hematocrit during pregnancy. The increase in plasma volume is more rapid than the increase in erythrocyte volume, causing the "physiological anemia of pregnancy," which can be partially corrected with iron supplements. (From Pitkin RM: Nutritional support in obstetrics and gynecology. Clin Obstet Gynecol 19:489, 1976.)

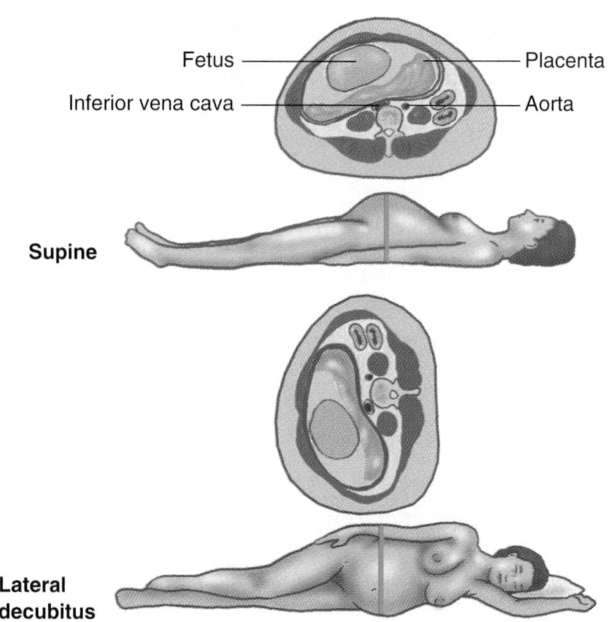

FIGURE 74–3 Venocaval compression of the inferior vena cava and abdominal aorta by the gravid uterus can lead to reduced venous return and thus to decreased cardiac output. (From Lee W, Shah PK, Amin DK, et al: Hemodynamic monitoring of cardiac patients during pregnancy. *In* Elkayam U, Gleicher N [eds]: Cardiac Problems in Pregnancy. 2nd ed. New York, Alan R. Liss, 1990, p 61.)

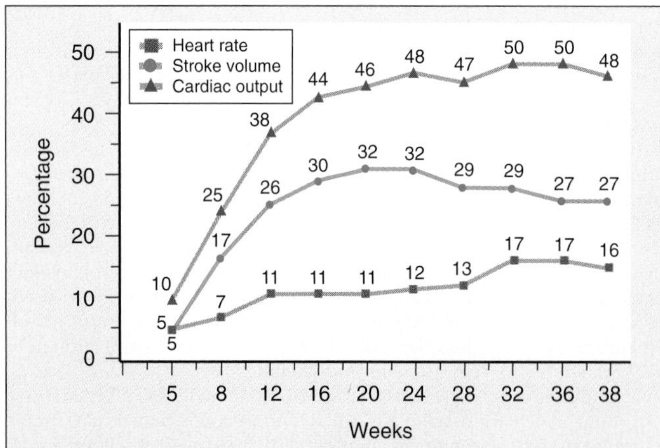

FIGURE 74–2 Percent changes of heart rate, stroke volume, and cardiac output measured in the lateral position throughout pregnancy compared with prepregnancy values. (Modified from Robson SC, Hunter S, Boys RJ, Dunlop W: Serial study of factors influencing changes in cardiac output during human pregnancy. Am J Physiol 256:H1060, 1989.)

filling pressure, stroke volume, and cardiac output and may lead to clinical deterioration.[6] Both heart rate and cardiac output return to prelabor values by 1 hour after delivery and mean blood pressure and stroke volume by 24 hours after delivery. Hemodynamic adaptation to pregnancy persists post partum and gradually returns to prepregnancy values within 12 to 24 weeks after delivery.[1]

Cardiovascular Evaluation During Pregnancy

History and Physical Examination

Normal pregnancy is often accompanied by symptoms of fatigue, decreased exercise capacity, hyperventilation, dyspnea, palpitations, lightheadedness, and even syncope (Table 74–2).[7] In addition, augmentation of jugular venous pulsation related to increased blood volume and leg edema (often observed in late pregnancy) could lead to an erroneous diagnosis of heart failure or overestimation of its severity.

TABLE 74–2 Cardiac Symptoms and Findings During Normal Pregnancy

Symptoms
Decreased exercise capacity
Tiredness
Dyspnea
Orthopnea
Palpitations
Lightheadedness
Syncope

Physical Findings
Inspection
Hyperventilation
Peripheral edema
Distended neck veins with prominent a and v waves and brisk *x* and *y* descents
Capillary pulsation
Precordial palpation
Brisk, diffuse, and displaced left ventricular impulse
Palpable right ventricular impulse
Palpable pulmonary trunk impulse
Auscultation
Pulmonary basilar rales
Increased first heart sound with exaggerated splitting
Exaggerated splitting of second heart sound
Midsystolic ejection-type murmurs at the lower left sternal edge and over the pulmonary area radiating to suprasternal notch and more to the left than right side of neck
Continuous murmurs (cervical venous hum, mammary souffle)
Diastolic murmurs (rare)

Systemic arterial pulses are full and collapsing and are similar to those palpated in patients with aortic regurgitation or hyperthyroidism. A left ventricular impulse is easily detected in most women in late pregnancy and is hyperactive and brisk. Right ventricular heave is usually present during the second and third trimesters, and the pulmonary trunk and pulmonic valve closure are often palpable. This group of findings may result in difficulty in assessing the presence or severity, or both, of pulmonary hypertension.

CARDIAC AUSCULTATION. Especially after the first trimester, auscultation often reveals an increased first heart sound (S_1) with exaggerated splitting that may be misinterpreted as a fourth heart sound (S_4) or as a systolic click.[7] The second heart sound (S_2) is often increased in late pregnancy and can exhibit persistent splitting when the patient is examined in the lateral position. These changes in S_2 may be interpreted as signs of pulmonary hypertension (loud P_2) or atrial septal defect (systolic murmur and splitting of S_2). Auscultation of the third and fourth heart sounds is uncommon in normal pregnancy.

Innocent Systolic Murmurs. These can be heard in most pregnant women and are the result of the hyperkinetic circulation of pregnancy. Murmurs are usually midsystolic and soft, are heard best at the lower left sternal edge and over the pulmonic area, and radiate to the suprasternal notch and more to the left than to the right side of the neck.[7] Not uncommonly, the benign murmur of pregnancy may be louder or longer and may sound like those associated with atrial septal defect or stenosis of one of the semilunar valves. In such cases an echocardiographic and Doppler evaluation is warranted to rule out an abnormal cardiac condition. Two benign continuous murmurs that may be heard during gestation are the cervical venous hum and mammary souffle. The venous hum is usually heard maximally over the right supraclavicular fossa but can radiate to the contralateral area and sometimes to the area below the clavicle. The mammary souffle may be either systolic or continuous, is heard over the breast late in gestation or in the lactating period, and is caused by increased flow in the mammary arteries. Characteristically, the murmur decreases or vanishes when pressure is applied to the stethoscope or when the patient moves to the upright position. Diastolic murmurs may be heard in normal pregnant women because of increased blood flow through the atrioventricular valve. Such a finding, however, is infrequent in the healthy pregnant woman and therefore requires careful diagnostic work-up to rule out organic disease.

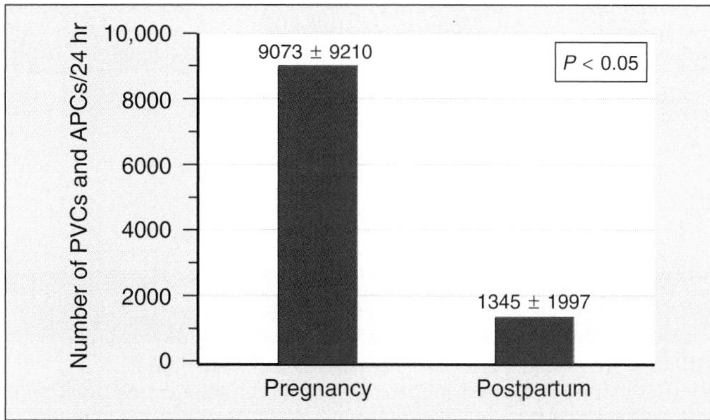

FIGURE 74–4 Total number of ventricular and atrial premature beats as recorded over 24 hours in nine healthy women with palpitations during pregnancy and in the postpartum period. APC = atrial premature complex; PVC = premature ventricular complex. (Modified from Shotan A, Ostrzega E, Mehra A, et al: Incidence of arrhythmias in normal pregnancy and relation to palpitations, dizziness, and syncope. Am J Cardiol 79:1061, 1997.)

TABLE 74–3 Electrocardiographic Findings During Normal Pregnancy

QRS axis deviation
Small Q wave and inverted P wave in lead III (abolished by inspiration)
ST segment and T wave changes (ritodrine tocolysis, cesarean section)
Frequent sinus tachycardia
Higher incidence of arrhythmias
Increased R/S ratio in leads V_2 and V_1

Laboratory Examinations

ELECTROCARDIOGRAPHY (see Chap. 9). In normal pregnancy, the QRS axis may shift to either the left or the right, but it usually stays within normal limits (Table 74–3).[7] A small Q wave and an inverted P wave in lead III that vary with respiration as well as a greater R wave amplitude in leads V_1 and V_2 and an inverted T wave in V_2 can be present. ST segment depression mimicking myocardial ischemia but not associated with wall motion abnormalities has been described between induction of anesthesia and the end of surgery in patients undergoing cesarean section. Increased susceptibility to arrhythmias during pregnancy is manifested by the frequent finding of sinus tachycardia and atrial or ventricular premature beats (Fig. 74–4),[8] and an increased incidence of paroxysmal supraventricular tachycardia during normal pregnancy and several cases of ventricular tachycardia have been reported in healthy women (see Chap. 32).

CHEST RADIOGRAPHY. Although the radiation dose associated with a routine chest radiograph is minimal, because of the potential for adverse biological effects from

TABLE 74–4 Chest Radiograph Findings During Normal Pregnancy

Straightening of the left upper cardiac border
Horizontal position of the heart
Increased lung markings
Small plural effusion in early postpartum period

TABLE 74–5 Doppler and Echocardiographic Findings During Normal Pregnancy

Slightly increased systolic and diastolic left ventricular dimensions (when patient examined in the lateral position)
Unchanged or slightly improved left ventricular systolic function
Moderate increase in size of right atrium, right ventricle, and left atrium
Progressive dilation of pulmonary, tricuspid, and mitral valve annuli
Functional pulmonary, tricuspid, and mitral regurgitation
Small pericardial effusion

any amount of radiation the pelvic area should be shielded by protective lead material.[9]

Changes seen on chest films in normal pregnancy can simulate those of cardiac disease and should be interpreted with caution (Table 74–4).[7] Straightening of the left upper cardiac border because of prominence of the pulmonary conus is often seen. The heart may seem enlarged because of its horizontal positioning secondary to the elevated diaphragm. In addition, an increase in lung markings can simulate a pattern of flow redistribution seen with increased pulmonary venous pressure. Pleural effusion can be found early post partum; it is usually small and is resorbed 1 to 2 weeks after delivery.

DOPPLER ECHOCARDIOGRAPHY (see Chap. 5) (Table 74–5). Gestational use of both maternal and fetal cardiac ultrasonography is considered safe.[10] Transesophageal echocardiography has been increasingly used in pregnancy and seems to be well tolerated by both mother and fetus. Pericardial effusion, usually small or minimal, has been noted in normal pregnant women late in pregnancy.[7] There is a progressive increase in all cardiac chamber dimensions with an approximately 20 percent increase in the size of the right atrium and the right ventricle, 12 percent increase in left atrial size, and 10 percent increase in left ventricular size. Post partum, these changes gradually return toward baseline but may remain different from prepregnancy values for several months.[3] In addition, there is early and progressive dilation of mitral, tricuspid, and pulmonary annuli, which is associated with an increase in valvular regurgitation.

STRESS TESTING. An exercise test using bicycle ergometry or a treadmill can be carried out during pregnancy to help establish the diagnosis of ischemic heart disease and to assess functional capacity and cardiac reserve.[7] Although maximal exercise has been reported to be safe by some investigators,[11] a low-level exercise protocol allowing heart rate to increase to 70 percent of the maximal predicted heart rate with fetal monitoring is preferred when stress testing is indicated.[7]

RADIATION. Exposure of the embryo to irradiation during the first 10 days after conception would most likely either have no effect or lead to resorption.[9] Irradiation during organ formation (days 10 to 50) may have a teratogenic effect, whereas after completion of organogenesis it may cause intrauterine growth retardation, central nervous system abnormalities, and possibly an increased incidence of childhood cancer or leukemia.

Routine chest radiography is associated with radiation of 20 millirads to the chest. Standard fluoroscopy can deliver 1 to 2 rads/min to the chest and high-level fluoroscopy or cine as much as 5 to 10 rads/min. The amount of radiation scattered to the uterus and absorbed by the embryo is less than 5 percent of radiation absorbed by the directly radiated tissue. Direct irradiation to the fetus should be avoided and can be prevented by covering the patient with a lead apron during radiographic procedures. The use of a lead apron, however, is of little help in reducing fetal irradiation associated with Compton-scattered photons.

Radiation to the fetus from nuclear medicine procedures is mainly due to distribution of radiopharmaceuticals to the bladder or the placenta or directly across the placental barrier. The expected radiation with thallium-201 or technetium-99m–labeled sestamibi diagnostic procedures is less than 1 rad per examination. Cardiac function studies with technetium-99m–labeled red blood cells are associated with fetal radiation of 1 to 2 rads, peripheral contrast radiographic venography with 0.5 rad or less, and pulmonary scintigraphy with technetium-macroaggregated albumin with 0.05 rad or less.

Current recommendations related to intrauterine radiation exposure are as follows[9]:

- Less than 5 rads—patient can be reassured of very low likelihood of risk.
- Five to 10 rads—patient should be counseled regarding low risk of problems.
- Ten to 15 rads during first 6 weeks—individual considerations for termination of pregnancy should be made.
- More than 15 rads—termination of pregnancy recommended.

MAGNETIC RESONANCE IMAGING. The technique has been used increasingly during pregnancy for the diagnosis of fetal anomalities.[12] Although magnetic resonance imaging poses no known risks to the fetus and its use for diagnosis of fetal disease has increased, its safety has not been fully established. Currently, the U.S. Food and Drug Administration recommends prudence in using magnetic resonance imaging during pregnancy.

PULMONARY ARTERY CATHETERIZATION. Hemodynamic monitoring with the aid of a pulmonary artery catheter can be of great help in managing patients at high risk during pregnancy, labor, delivery, and the postpartum period. The ability to insert and position the flotation catheter with pressure monitoring without the need for fluoroscopy makes it particularly attractive for use during pregnancy. Hemodynamic monitoring is recommended throughout labor and delivery for any patient with symptomatic cardiac disease during pregnancy or with the potential for deterioration because of valvular, myocardial, or ischemic heart disease. Because significant circulatory changes that may lead to hemodynamic deterioration occur in the early postpartum period,[1] hemodynamic monitoring should be continued for at least several hours after delivery to ensure stability.

CARDIAC CATHETERIZATION. Cardiac catheterization may be indicated in rare instances of cardiac decompensation when sufficient information cannot be obtained by noninvasive techniques, especially if cardiac surgery, percutaneous coronary intervention, or balloon valvuloplasty is being considered. Although this technique provides high-quality images, it is associated with a relatively high dose of radiation.[9] To minimize radiation to the pelvic and abdominal areas, the brachial rather than the femoral approach is preferred, fluoroscopy and cine time should be reduced to the minimum required, and direct irradiation to the fetus should be avoided.

Pregnancy in Women with Congenital Heart Disease

Because of increased survival of children with congenital heart disease (see Chap. 56), pregnancy has become more common in this population of patients.[13,14] Preconception evaluation should include careful history and assessment of risk for both the mother and the fetus.[15] The patient should be counseled regarding contraceptive alternatives,[16] potential maternal and fetal risks of pregnancy,[17-19] and, when appropriate, expected long-term maternal morbidity and survival as well as the risk of congenital malformations in the offspring.[20] In addition, guidance concerning anticoagulation and prophylactic antibiotics, if needed, should be provided.

MATERNAL AND FETAL OUTCOME. In general, a good maternal outcome can be expected in most cases with noncyanotic congenital heart disease. Maternal outcome is determined by the nature of the disease, surgical repair, presence and severity of cyanosis, increased pulmonary vascular resistance, maternal functional capacity, myocardial dysfunction, left ventricular obstruction, and history of arrhythmias or other prior cardiac events.[14,19] An unfavorable outcome, including development of congestive heart failure, arrhythmias, and hypertension, is commonly seen in patients with impaired functional status and those with cyanosis.[17] Other reported complications include angina, infective endocarditis, and thromboembolic phenomena.[13,19] Pregnant women with congenital heart disease have an increased risk for neonatal complications including fetal wastage, low birth weight for gestational age, prematurity, congenital heart disease, and respiratory distress syndrome.[19] The risk of fetal and neonatal complications is increased in patients with cyanotic heart disease.[13,21] Fetal wastage was reported in 45 percent of cyanotic mothers compared with 20 percent of acyanotic mothers with congenital heart disease.[21] In addition, low birth weight for gestational age and prematurity are common in cyanotic mothers and correlate with maternal hemoglobin and hematocrit values.[13,21] Risk of congenital heart disease is increased for the offspring of mothers with congenital heart disease with a reported incidence of 4 to 8 percent,[19] and there are many noncardiac congenital malformations as well as mental and physical impairments in children born to mothers with congenital heart disease.[19]

LABOR AND DELIVERY. Elective induction of labor when fetal maturity is confirmed may be used in high-risk patients for better planning, hemodynamic monitoring, and availability of expert personnel during labor and delivery.[13] Vaginal delivery is preferred for most patients, and cesarean section is indicated in the stable patients only for obstetric reasons. Oxygen should be given to hypoxemic mothers, and blood gas monitoring is recommended in most patients with impaired functional capacity, cardiac dysfunction, pulmonary hypertension, and cyanotic malformations. Hemodynamic monitoring should be considered in selected patients, and blood volume loss must be anticipated and treated promptly.

ANTIBIOTIC PROPHYLAXIS. Official recommendations by the American Heart Association suggest that antibiotic prophylaxis for an uncomplicated delivery is unnecessary except for cases with prosthetic heart valves or a surgically constructed systemic-to-pulmonary shunt.[22] Because of difficulties in predicting complicated deliveries and potential devastating consequences of endocarditis,[23] antibiotic prophylaxis for vaginal delivery in all patients with congenital heart disease (except those with an isolated secundum type of atrial septal defect and those 6 months or more after repair of septal defects or surgical ligation and division of patent ductus arteriosus) seems reasonable.

ATRIAL SEPTAL DEFECT AND PATENT FORAMEN OVALE. Atrial septal defect is usually well tolerated in pregnancy even in patients with large left-to-right shunts. A retrospective review of 163 pregnancies in 80 women with atrial septal defect reported higher incidences of miscarriage, preterm delivery, and cardiac symptoms in cases in which pregnancy occurred before surgical correction.[24] The development of pulmonary hypertension and atrial arrhythmias rarely occurs in women of childbearing age. Because endocarditis is rare, antibiotic prophylaxis is not indicated in patients with secundum-type atrial septal defect. Recommendations concerning pregnancy in patients with atrial septal defect should be made on an individual basis, considering accompanying lesions, functional status, and the level of pulmonary vascular resistance. Paradoxical embolism leading to stroke has been reported in patients with patent foramen ovale during pregnancy.[25,26] In one of the cases, percutaneous closure of the patent foramen ovale was performed during pregnancy guided by echocardiography.[26]

VENTRICULAR SEPTAL DEFECT. Women with isolated ventricular septal defect usually tolerate pregnancy well, although congestive heart failure and arrhythmias have been reported.[13,14,18] The risk posed by pregnancy after closure of an uncomplicated ventricular septal defect should not differ from that in patients without heart disease. The incidence of ventricular septal defect in offspring has been reported to be 4 to 11 percent.[17] Marked reduction in blood pressure during or after delivery as a result of blood loss or anesthesia can lead to shunt reversal in patients with pulmonary hypertension. The use of vasopressors and volume replacement to stabilize blood pressure should prevent further complications.

PATENT DUCTUS ARTERIOSUS. Maternal outcome in patients with patent ductus arteriosus with left-to-right shunt is usually favorable,[13,14,18] but clinical deterioration and congestive heart failure can occur in some patients. There were no maternal deaths among a large number of patients with patent ductus arteriosus.[17] The need for surgical intervention during pregnancy is rare. A fall in systemic vascular resistance during gestation and hypotension early post partum can lead to shunt reversal in women with pulmonary hypertension. Peripartum decreases in systemic blood pressure should be corrected by means of vasopressor agents. Postoperative pregnancy is well tolerated by the mother, and recurrence of patent ductus arteriosus in the fetus is rare (<1 percent).[27]

CONGENITAL AORTIC VALVE DISEASE. Most patients with mild aortic stenosis have a favorable outcome of pregnancy.[6,13,14] At the same time, however, moderate or severe aortic stenosis is likely to be associated with symptomatic deterioration during pregnancy, may lead to maternal morbidity and even mortality, and is associated with important effects on the fetus including intrauterine growth retardation, premature delivery, and reduced birth weight.[6]

Symptoms usually develop in the second or third trimester and most commonly arise as exertional dyspnea, but chest pain, lightheadedness, and syncope may also occur. An increased incidence of cardiac defects has been reported in liveborn infants of mothers with left ventricular outflow obstruction.[13] Because of the risk involved, patients with severe aortic stenosis (aortic valve area <1.0 cm^2) should consider undergoing valve replacement before becoming pregnant. Optional management strategies for a pregnant patient with severe aortic stenosis include (1) early abortion followed by valve replacement and repeated pregnancy and (2) continuation of pregnancy and planning for percutaneous balloon valvuloplasty or surgical intervention in patients who show clinical deterioration not controlled by medical therapy. Both replacement of the aortic valve and percutaneous balloon valvuloplasty have been performed successfully in pregnant women with aortic stenosis.[28] These procedures, however, are not free of complications. Although valvuloplasty obviates the general anesthesia and cardiopulmonary bypass required for surgery, it can be associated with prolonged radiation exposure and hemodynamic fluctuations that can lead to immediate and late fetal complications. Surgical replacement of the aortic valve during pregnancy can be associated with an increased incidence of maternal complications and fetal loss.[29] These procedures should therefore be considered only for symptomatic patients with severe disease not manageable by medical therapy and should be avoided when possible during the first trimester.

COARCTATION OF THE AORTA. Both maternal and fetal outcomes are usually favorable in cases with aortic coarctation.[30,31] At the same time, however, cases of severe hypertension, congestive heart failure, and aortic dissection have been reported.[13,30-32] Systemic hypertension is common during pregnancy in women with a significant coarctation gradient.[31] Congenital heart disease was reported in 3 to 4 percent of newborns born to women with corrected coarctation.[30,31] Because increased incidences of hypertension and infective endocarditis in the mother and of congenital heart disease in the fetus have been shown in cases with surgically uncorrected compared with corrected coarctation,[13] it seems advisable to correct aortic coarctation before pregnancy.

Measures to reduce the incidence of aortic dissection and rupture of cerebral aneurysms during pregnancy consist of limiting physical activity and controlling blood pressure. Because beta blockade may decrease the risk of these events by reduction of aortic wall tension, beta blockers should be the antihypertensive drugs of choice. Excessive blood pressure reduction, however, may compromise uteroplacental blood flow and should be avoided. Surgical correction of coarctation has been performed successfully during pregnancy[30] and may be indicated in patients with severe, uncontrollable systolic hypertension or heart failure. No information is available on pregnancy in women with aortic coarctation following percutaneous dilation.

PULMONIC STENOSIS. Isolated pulmonic stenosis is usually well tolerated during pregnancy.[6] When possible, however, severe stenosis should be corrected before conception. In the rare instance of progressive right ventricular failure or symptoms clearly related to the stenotic valve, or in a patient with an intracardiac shunt at either the atrial or ventricular level with cyanosis, percutaneous balloon valvotomy should be considered during pregnancy.

TETRALOGY OF FALLOT. Hemodynamic changes associated with pregnancy may cause clinical deterioration in women with surgically uncorrected or only partially corrected tetralogy of Fallot. Increase in blood volume and venous return to the right atrium raises right ventricular pressure, which, combined with a fall in systemic vascular resistance, can produce or exacerbate right-to-left shunt and cyanosis. Labor and delivery are particularly important because a fall in blood pressure can also increase right-to-left shunt and the degree of cyanosis. Maternal hematocrit above 60 percent, arterial oxygen saturation below 80 percent, right ventricular hypertension, and syncopal episodes are poor prognostic signs. Pregnancies in women with cyanosis are associated with high rates of spontaneous abortion, premature delivery, and fetal growth retardation.[13,14,21]

Close monitoring of systemic blood pressure and blood gases during labor and delivery is recommended for cyanotic or symptomatic patients. The incidence of cardiac defects reported in the infants ranges between 3 and 17 percent.[17]

The risk of pregnancy in patients with good surgical repair is similar to that in the general population. Patients who have undergone only palliative procedures and have residual problems, such as pulmonic regurgitation, right ventricular outflow obstruction, and right ventricular dilation and dysfunction, are still at higher risk for the development of heart failure and arrhythmias during pregnancy.[33] Patients who have undergone shunt procedures to improve cyanosis may develop pulmonary hypertension, which increases the risk of pregnancy.[34] Because maternal and fetal outcomes seem to be markedly improved after surgical repair, this procedure should be performed before conception.[13,35] Because revision of an incompletely repaired defect is recommended in patients with residual ventricular septal defect when the pulmonary/systemic flow ratio is greater than 1.5:1.0, in those with right ventricular outflow obstruction (right ventricular systolic pressure >60 mm Hg), and in those with right ventricular failure related to pulmonic regurgitation, such revision should be performed before conception in a woman who plans to conceive. To determine the risk of defects in the fetus, patients with tetralogy of Fallot should be tested with fluorescent in situ hybridization to rule out 22q11 deletion syndrome. Negative results of this test indicates a low risk of a defect in the fetus.[36]

EISENMENGER SYNDROME. This condition continues to be associated with a high risk of maternal morbidity and mortality. Two reviews involving 55 and 65 women, respectively, reported maternal mortality of approximately 40 percent.[13,37] The cause of maternal death is often unclear; it usually occurs between the first few days and the first few weeks after delivery and is preceded by desaturation and hemodynamic and clinical deterioration.[38-41] Diffuse fibrinoid necrosis of pulmonary arterioles has been found in some patients,[42] and pulmonary embolism has been reported at necropsy.[42] Eisenmenger syndrome is also associated with a poor fetal outcome, with a high incidence of fetal loss, prematurity, intrauterine growth retardation, and perinatal death.[13,34]

Because of the high risk of maternal mortality, patients with Eisenmenger syndrome should be advised against pregnancy. Sterilization may be considered prior to pregnancy, and early abortion should be recommended for patients who are already pregnant. Management of a pregnant patient who decides to proceed to term must include close follow-up for early detection of clinical deterioration. To prevent an increased incidence of peripartum thromboembolism, anticoagulant therapy seems indicated in the third trimester of gestation and for 4 weeks post partum. Because premature delivery is common, women with Eisenmenger syndrome should be hospitalized for any sign of premature uterine activity. For this reason and to ensure restriction of activity and close follow-up, early elective hospitalization is recommended. Spontaneous labor is preferred to induction and should lower the chance of prematurity or the need for cesarean section. Blood pressure, electrocardiographic, and blood gas monitoring are essential during labor and delivery to ensure early detection and correction of problems; high concentrations of oxygen may be helpful. Most patients in stable condition tolerate vaginal delivery; however, an attempt should be made to shorten the second stage of labor by the use of forceps or vacuum extraction. Because of the higher risk of fetal distress during vaginal delivery and potential need for emergency cesarean section, a planned cesarean section is often preferred. Insertion of a Swan-Ganz catheter may be difficult and associated with the development of arrhythmias, and its routine use is not recommended. Inhaled nitric oxide has been used successfully to reduce pulmonary pressure and improve oxygenation during labor and the early postpartum period in two patients with Eisenmenger syndrome.[38,39] Patients gave birth to live infants but died 2 and 21 days post partum.

EBSTEIN ANOMALY. Pregnancy in women with noncyanotic Ebstein anomaly is well tolerated. In cyanotic cases, pregnancy is associated with increased risks of maternal heart failure, prematurity, and fetal loss.[35] The approach to labor and delivery in symptomatic or cyanotic patients with Ebstein anomaly includes antibiotic prophylaxis, oxygen administration, hemodynamic and blood gas monitoring, and efforts to prevent a drop in systemic blood pressure in response to peripheral vasodilation or blood loss.

COMPLEX CYANOTIC CONGENITAL HEART DISEASE. The more widespread use of palliative and corrective surgical procedures for complex cyanotic congenital cardiac anomalies has allowed more women who are so affected to reach childbearing age.[13] Although successful pregnancies have been reported in patients with partially corrected and uncorrected cyanotic heart disease, pregnancy is associated with increased risk in these patients. A report of 96 pregnancies in 44 patients with cyanotic heart disease without pulmonary hypertension demonstrated cardiovascular complications in 32 percent of the patients.[21] These complications included heart failure, thromboembolic events, supraventricular tachycardia, and peripartum bacterial endocarditis resulting in postpartum maternal death in one patient. In addition, a high incidence of fetal wastage (57 percent), premature deliveries, small-for-gestational-age newborns, and both cardiac and noncardiac congenital malformations have been reported.

More than 100 pregnancies in women with intraatrial repair for transposition of the great arteries have been reported without maternal mortality.[43] Pregnancy seems to be well tolerated in asymptomatic patients or those with only mild symptoms (Class II) prior to pregnancy. Worsening of systemic ventricular function during pregnancy or shortly thereafter has been reported in 10 percent of cases.

A report describing the experience in 60 pregnancies in 22 women with congenitally corrected transposition of great arteries indicated a successful outcome in most cases.[44] The rate of fetal loss and maternal morbidity was, however, increased. Morbidity included congestive heart failure, worsening valve regurgitation, endocarditis, and myocardial infarction. Because of the small number of cases, the risk of congenital heart disease in the offspring of women with congenitally corrected transposition is uncertain.

A report by Canobbio and colleagues[45] on patients after the Fontan operation indicated that a good pregnancy outcome was possible with small babies. Other reports, however, described thromboembolic complications with right atrial thrombus leading to embolic obstruction of the connection and to death.[42]

Valvular Heart Disease (see Chap. 57)

MITRAL STENOSIS. This condition is the most common rheumatic valvular lesion in pregnancy.[46,47] A majority of patients with moderate to severe mitral stenosis (mitral valve area <1.5 cm^2) demonstrate worsening of one or two classes in New York Heart Association functional status during gestation (Fig. 74–5).[6,46] Although mitral stenosis is often accompanied by some degree of mitral regurgitation, hemodynamic problems are related predominantly to flow obstruction. The pressure gradient across the narrowed mitral valve may increase greatly secondary to the physiological increase in heart rate and blood volume of pregnancy. Increased left atrial pressure can result in atrial arrhythmias that may lead to an acceleration of ventricular rate and further elevation of left atrial pressure. In addition, decreased serum colloid osmotic pressure during pregnancy and excessive peripartum intravenous fluid administration can both predispose to pulmonary edema. Studies have demonstrated a high incidence of worsening of functional class and the development of heart failure which led to the need for hospitalizations and either starting or increasing the dose of cardiac medications in patients with moderate to severe mitral stenosis (Figs. 74–6 and 74–7).[6,48] In addition, there was a marked increase in the rate of prematurity, fetal growth retardation, and low neonatal birth weight in these cases. Despite a marked increase in maternal morbidity, mortality is rare and is mostly due to standard care.[6,49]

Treatment. The therapeutic approach to patients with significant mitral stenosis should aim to reduce the heart rate and decrease left atrial pressure. Both heart rate and symptoms can be controlled effectively by restricting physical activity and administering beta-adrenergic receptor blockers. In patients with atrial fibrillation, digoxin may also be useful for control of ventricular rate. Left atrial pressure can be reduced by a decrease in blood volume through restriction of salt intake and the use of oral diuretics; aggressive use of diuretic agents should, however, be avoided to prevent hypovolemia and reduction of uteroplacental perfusion.

Although careful medical therapy allows successful completion of pregnancy in the great majority of women,[46] repair or replacement of the valve during pregnancy may be indicated in some patients with severe symptoms in spite of adequate medical therapy. The use of percutaneous mitral balloon valvuloplasty during pregnancy has been reported in an increasing number of pregnant patients with mitral stenosis.[50-53] In the majority of cases, hemodynamic and symptomatic improvement has been achieved without apparent untoward maternal and fetal effects. Follow-up for several

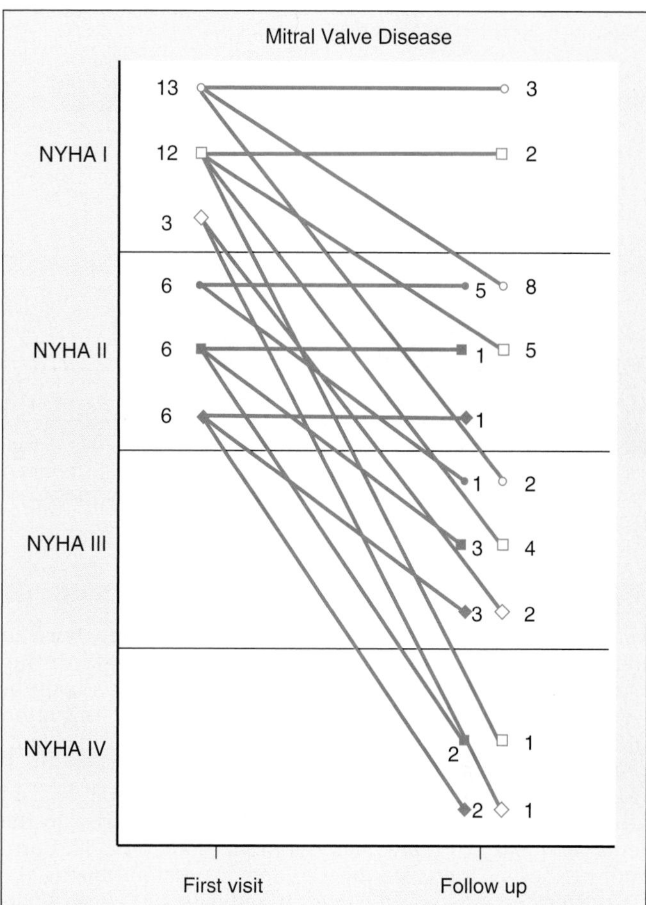

FIGURE 74–5 Change in New York Heart Association (NYHA) functional class between first visit and follow-up during pregnancy in patients with predominant mitral valve disease. Circles = mild mitral stenosis; squares = moderate mitral stenosis; diamonds = severe mitral stenosis; open symbols = NYHA functional Class I on presentation; closed symbols = NYHA functional Class II on presentation. (From Hameed A, Karaalp IS, Tummala PP, et al: The effect of valvular heart disease on maternal and fetal outcome of pregnancy. J Am Coll Cardiol 37:893, 2001.)

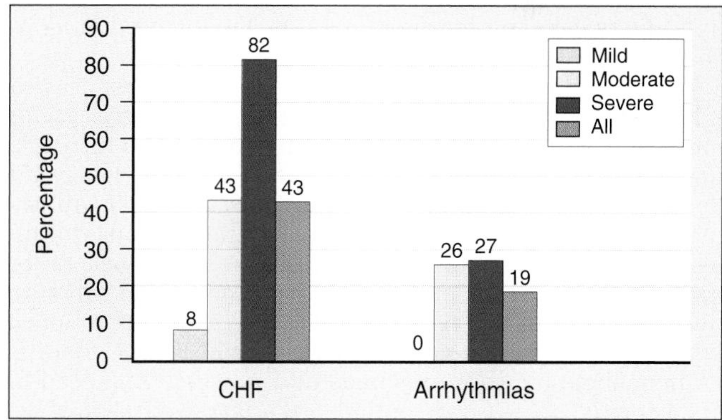

FIGURE 74–6 Percent development of symptoms of congestive heart failure (CHF) and arrhythmias during pregnancy in 46 patients with mitral stenosis. (From Hameed A, Karaalp IS, Tummala PP, et al: The effect of valvular heart disease on maternal and fetal outcome of pregnancy. J Am Coll Cardiol 37:893, 2001.)

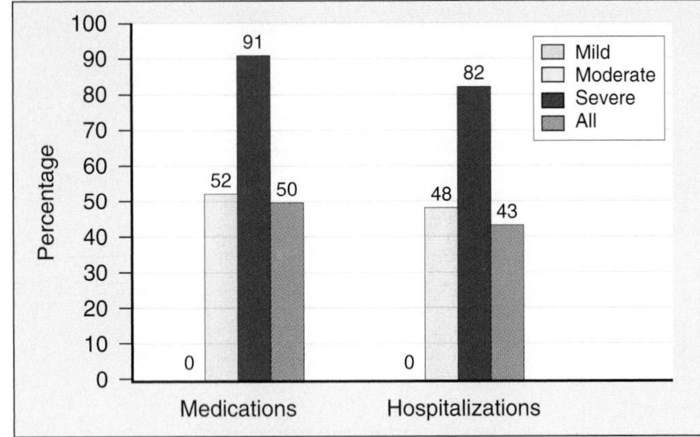

FIGURE 74–7 Percent usage of new cardiac medications or increase in their dose and hospitalizations during pregnancy in 46 patients with mitral stenosis. (From Hameed A, Karaalp IS, Tummala PP, et al: The effect of valvular heart disease on maternal and fetal outcome of pregnancy. J Am Coll Cardiol 37:893, 2001.)

years has shown normal development of children born to mothers who had mitral valve balloon valvuloplasty during pregnanacy.[52,53] At the same time, however, serious complications have occasionally been reported, including initiation of maternal arrhythmias leading to fetal distress, cardiac tamponade requiring surgical intervention, systemic embolization, uterine contraction, and even precipitous labor. In addition, this procedure is associated with some risk to the fetus secondary to unavoidable ionizing radiation. The procedure should, therefore, be avoided if possible during the first trimester and should be performed by experienced operators with adequate abdominal and pelvic shielding with minimum radiation exposure and under echocardiographic guidance, when possible.

Mitral valve repair or replacement should be considered during pregnancy only in cases with severe mitral stenosis (mitral valve area <1.0 cm^2) refractory to optimal medical therapy or when close follow-up during pregnancy, labor, and delivery is not possible. When valve replacement is indicated, selection of the type of prosthesis should be based on its hemodynamic profile and durability and the need for anticoagulation.

Vaginal delivery can be permitted in most patients with mitral stenosis.[6] In symptomatic patients and those with moderate or severe stenosis (mitral valve area <1.5 cm^2), hemodynamic monitoring is recommended during labor and delivery. Initiation of monitoring at onset of labor allows hemodynamic optimization by means of intravenous diuretics, digoxin (in case of atrial fibrillation), beta blockers, or nitroglycerin and prevention of a rise in left atrial pressure during labor and delivery. With delivery and thus relief of venocaval obstruction caused by the gravid uterus, there is an immediate increase in venous return, which may lead to a substantial increase in pulmonary artery wedge pressure and pulmonary edema.[1,6] For this reason, hemodynamic monitoring should be continued for at least several hours post partum.

Epidural anesthesia is the most appropriate form of analgesia in patients with mitral stenosis for both vaginal and abdominal delivery. This form of anesthesia is often associated with a significant fall in pulmonary arterial and left atrial pressures related to systemic vasodilation.[54] With this approach, the great majority of patients with mitral stenosis, even if it is severe, can be delivered with few complications.

MITRAL REGURGITATION. This condition is usually well tolerated in pregnancy, presumably because of left ventricular unloading secondary to the physiological fall in systemic vascular resistance.[1] In symptomatic patients, drug therapy with diuretics is indicated, and digoxin may be useful in those with impaired left ventricular systolic function. Hydralazine has been shown to be safe for use during pregnancy,[55] and it may be used for further reduction of left ventricular afterload and prevention of hemodynamic worsening associated with isometric exercise during labor. Because of risk of fetal loss, surgery should be avoided if possible during pregnancy and considered only in patients with severe heart failure and hemodynamic compromise in spite of adequate medical management.

AORTIC STENOSIS. Rheumatic aortic stenosis is rare during pregnancy and occurs in conjunction with mitral valve disease in approximately 5 percent of pregnant patients with rheumatic valvular disease.[46] Although most patients with aortic stenosis and valve area greater than 1.5 cm^2 tolerate pregnancy well, patients with more severe stenosis may demonstrate clinical deterioration with exertional dyspnea, near-syncope, or syncope and pulmonary edema.[6] Development of serious symptoms during pregnancy, especially if resistant to medical therapy, may require termination of pregnancy or repair of the valve either surgically (valve replacement) or by percutaneous balloon valvuloplasty.[56]

AORTIC REGURGITATION. Aortic regurgitation in young women may be due to a bicuspid aortic valve, rheumatic disease, previous endocarditis, or dilated aortic annulus. Like mitral regurgitation, aortic regurgitation is well tolerated during pregnancy, probably because of reduced systemic vascular resistance and increased heart rate, which results in shortening of diastole. In symptomatic patients, diuretics, digoxin, and hydralazine for left ventricular afterload reduction can be safely used.

Other Conditions Affecting the Valves, Aorta, and Myocardium

MITRAL VALVE PROLAPSE. The prevalence of mitral valve prolapse in the general population has been found to be 2.4 percent, and mitral valve prolapse was reported in approximately 1.2 percent of pregnant women.[57,58] Because of the high incidence of systolic functional murmurs and wide splitting of the first heart sound during pregnancy, mitral valve prolapse may be falsely diagnosed and needs to be confirmed by echocardiographic criteria.[57] At the same time, the incidence of prolapse-related auscultatory and echocardiographic findings may decrease during gestation as a result of an increase in left ventricular end-diastolic volume.[58]

For the few patients with mitral valve prolapse with chest pain or cardiac arrhythmias, the emphasis should be on reassurance and attempts to avoid the use of medications during pregnancy. Beta-adrenergic blocking agents are recommended when therapy is indicated for arrhythmias. Patients with mitral valve prolapse, especially those with a thickened mitral valve and mitral regurgitation, are at increased risk for infective endocarditis. Although antibiotic prophylaxis for uncomplicated vaginal delivery has not been uniformly recommended,[22] the development of bacteremia during vaginal delivery and cesarean section cannot always be predicted. For this reason, prophylaxis for labor and delivery in patients with mitral valve prolapse accompanied by valve thickening or regurgitation, or both, seems warranted.

MARFAN SYNDROME. Pregnancy in women with Marfan syndrome poses a twofold problem: (1) cardiovascular complications and (2) a high risk of having a child who inherits the condition.[59,60] Cardiovascular complications during pregnancy include dilation of the ascending aorta, which may lead to the development of aortic regurgitation and congestive heart failure, and proximal and distal dissections of the aorta with possible involvement of the iliac and coronary arteries. The risk of aortic dissection is significantly higher in patients with a dilated aorta or a history of previous dissection. Patients with Marfan syndrome who have only minor involvement of the cardiovascular system and aortic diameter less than 40 mm usually tolerate pregnancy well. The majority of complications are developed in the later phase of pregnancy. Marfan syndrome may also be responsible for obstetric complications including cervical incompetence, abnormal placental site, and postpartum hemorrhagic complications.[61]

The management of pregnancy in women with Marfan syndrome should include preconception counseling to discuss potential maternal and fetal risks.[59] Women with significant cardiac involvement—in particular, dilation of the aorta and previous history of aortic dissection—are at high risk for complications during gestation and should be advised against conception or, if they are already pregnant, advised to have an early abortion. In contrast, the risk in patients without cardiac complications and with a normal aortic diameter is significantly lower. Still, a favorable outcome is not guaranteed, and aortic dissection can occur, albeit infrequently, in patients with a normal-sized aorta.[59,60] Because of reported progressive dilation during gestation, preconception echocardiographic assessment of the aorta and periodic follow-up during pregnancy are highly recommended.[62] Because aneurysms and dissections of the aorta can occasionally involve the descending aorta, the use of transesophageal echocardiography seems preferred to transthoracic examination. During pregnancy, vigorous physical activity should be avoided. Beta blockers, which have been shown to reduce the rate of aortic dilation and the risk of complications in patients with Marfan syndrome, should be administered. In case of substantial dilation or dissection of the aorta during pregnancy, depending on the stage of pregnancy, therapeutic abortion, early delivery, or surgical intervention should be considered.[59,60,62,63] A number of patients have been reported to have successful full-term pregnancies without complications after an elective aortic root replacement.[64] In women with aortic dilation, aortic dissection, or other cardiac complications, abdominal delivery by cesarean section should be the preferred mode of delivery to minimize hemodynamic changes associated with vaginal delivery.[43,59,61]

Cardiomyopathies

HYPERTROPHIC CARDIOMYOPATHY. Reported experience in approximately 350 pregnancies in 200 women with hypertrophic cardiomyopathy (see Chap. 59) has suggested a favorable outcome in most cases but at the same time a potential for increased morbidity and even mortality.[65-67] Worsening of symptoms and increased shortness of breath and fatigue have been reported in approximately 15 to 20 percent of cases and are more common in women with symptoms prior to pregnancy[67]; chest pain, palpitations, dizzy spells, and syncope have also been reported. In addition, isolated cases of arrhythmias have been described, including poorly tolerated resistant supraventricular tachycardia with fetal distress,[65] atrial fibrillation leading to hemodynamic deterioration requiring electrical cardioversion, and ventricular fibrillation treated by electric shock. Pregnancy-related maternal mortality is low in patients with hypertrophic cardiomyopathy, but it is increased compared with that in the general population[67] and is due to ventricular arrhythmias.[65] Although fetal outcome is in general favorable, women with symptoms before pregnancy have an increased risk of fetal prematurity compared with healthy women.[67] The risk of inheriting the disease may be as high as 50 percent in familial cases and less in sporadic cases.[65]

The therapeutic approach to the pregnant patient with hypertrophic cardiomyopathy depends on the presence of symptoms and left ventricular outflow obstruction. In the symptomatic patient with obstructive hypertrophic cardiomyopathy, an attempt should be made to avoid blood loss and use of drugs that can lead to vasodilation or sympathetic stimulation during labor and delivery. Indications for drug therapy during gestation include arrhythmias and symptoms of heart failure. Symptoms associated with elevated left ventricular filling pressure should be treated with beta-adrenergic blocking agents, and diuretics and calcium antagonists may be added if beta blockers alone are not sufficient.[65] Because of the potential arrhythmogenic effect of pregnancy, implantation of an automatic defibrillator before pregnancy should be considered in patients with history of syncope, life-threatening arrhythmias, or a family history of death caused by the same condition.[65]

Vaginal delivery has been shown to be safe in women with hypertrophic cardiomyopathy.[65] In those with symptoms of outflow obstruction, the second stage of labor may be shortened by the use of forceps. The use of prostaglandins to induce uterine contractions may be risky in a patient with obstructive hypertrophic cardiomyopathy owing to their vasodilatory effect, whereas oxytocin should be well tolerated. Because tocolytic agents with beta-adrenergic receptor activity may worsen left ventricular outflow tract obstruction, other medications such as magnesium sulfate are preferred. Similarly, spinal and epidural anesthetics should be used with caution in obstructive hypertrophic cardiomyopathy because of their vasodilatory effect, and excessive blood loss should be avoided and if it occurs it should be replaced promptly with intravenous fluid or blood.[68]

Because the risk for infective endocarditis is increased in hypertrophic cardiomyopathy, especially the obstructive form, and in patients with mitral valve abnormalities, antibiotic prophylaxis should be considered for labor and delivery.

PERIPARTUM CARDIOMYOPATHY. Peripartum cardiomyopathy is a form of dilated cardiomyopathy with left ventricular systolic dysfunction that results in signs and symptoms of heart failure (see Chaps. 21 to 23).[69,70] The syndrome has been defined by the following four criteria: (1) the development of cardiac failure in the last month of pregnancy or within 5 months of delivery, (2) absence of an identifiable cause for the cardiac failure, (3) absence of recognizable heart disease prior to the last month of pregnancy, and (4) left ventricular systolic dysfunction demonstrated by classical echocardiographic criteria, such as depressed shortening fraction or ejection fraction.[70] However, there have been reports of an early presentation of peripartum cardiomyopathy during the second and third trimesters of pregnancy in a large minority of patients.[71] The incidence of the disease in the United States is not known and has been reported to range between 1 per 4000 and 1 per 15,000 deliveries; the incidence is higher in Haiti and in certain parts of Africa.[69,70,72]

Peripartum cardiomyopathy can occur at any age but is more common in women older than 30 years. In the United States, it involves women of various ethnic groups and it is related to first and second pregnancies in almost 60 percent of cases.[73] There is a strong relation between the development of peripartum cardiomyopathy, gestational hypertension, twin pregnancy, and the use of tocolytic therapy.[70,73]

Common symptoms and signs are shortness of breath, fatigue, chest pain, palpitations, weight gain, peripheral edema, peripheral or pulmonary embolization, and arrhythmias. Physical examination often reveals an enlarged heart, S_3, and murmurs of mitral and tricuspid regurgitation. The electrocardiogram may show tachycardia, ST-T wave changes, conduction abnormalities, and arrhythmias. Chest radiography usually shows cardiomegaly, pulmonary venous congestion with interstitial or alveolar edema, and occasionally pleural effusion. Doppler echocardiography commonly demonstrates enlargement of all four cardiac chambers, with marked reduction in left ventricular systolic function. Small to moderate pericardial effusion and mitral, tricuspid, and pulmonic regurgitation may be evident. The clinical presentation and hemodynamic changes are indistinguishable from those found in other forms of dilated cardiomyopathy.

The clinical course of peripartum cardiomyopathy varies, with 50 to 60 percent of patients showing complete or near-complete recovery of clinical status and cardiac function, usually within the first 6 months post partum[73]; the rest of the patients demonstrate either further clinical deterioration, leading to cardiac transplantation or premature death, or persistent left ventricular dysfunction and chronic heart failure.[69,70,74]

Management. Acute heart failure should be treated vigorously with oxygen, diuretics, digitalis, and vasodilator agents. The use of hydralazine as an afterload-reducing agent is safe during pregnancy.[55] The use of organic nitrates, dopamine, dobutamine, or milrinone has been reported in pregnancy in a limited number of cases, but the use of nesiritide during pregnancy has not been reported. Nitroprusside has been used successfully during pregnancy, but experiments in animals have shown a potential for fetal toxicity.[55] Angiotensin-converting enzyme inhibitors have a teratogenic effect, may cause fetal renal dysfunction, and should therefore not be used during pregnancy.[75] Because of the increased incidence of thromboembolic events, anticoagulant therapy is recommended.[76,77] Because the disease may be reversible, the temporary use of an intraaortic balloon pump or left ventricular assist device may help stabilize the patient's condition pending improvement. A small retrospective study of intravenous immune globulin showed a favorable effect on recovery of left ventricular dysfunction in patients with peripartum cardiomyopathy.[78] Similarly, the use of pentoxifylline in addition to standard care was reported to lead to a significant improvement in outcome in patients with peripartum cardiomyopathy.[79] Further evaluation of these therapies seems warranted. Because of continuous clinical deterioration, some patients with peripartum cardiomyopathy may need to undergo cardiac transplantation. Reports comparing results of cardiac transplantation in age-matched females with peripartum cardiomyopathy and idiopathic cardiomyopathy showed favorable and comparable long-term survival in both groups.[74] The rate of mortality in patients with peripartum cardiomyopathy was reported to be 10 and 32 percent in two reports.[80,81]

Subsequent pregnancies in women with peripartum cardiomyopathy are often associated with relapse, leading to left ventricular dysfunction, symptomatic deterioration, and even death (Fig. 74–8). Although the likelihood of such relapse is greater in patients with persistently abnormal cardiac function, it has also been reported in women in whom left ventricular function is restored after the first episode.[82] A survey on the risk of subsequent pregnancy in women with history of peripartum cardiomyopathy reported no mortality in patients with normal left ventricular ejection but 19 percent mortality in patients with a depressed left ventricular ejection fraction (25 percent in those who did not have an abortion [Fig. 74–8]). For these reasons, subsequent pregnancies should be discouraged in patients with peripartum cardiomyopathy who have persistent cardiac dysfunction; women with recovered cardiac function can also not be guaranteed an event-free pregnancy, and recurrence of the disease is possible. The risk of mortality in such cases, however, seems to be small.[82]

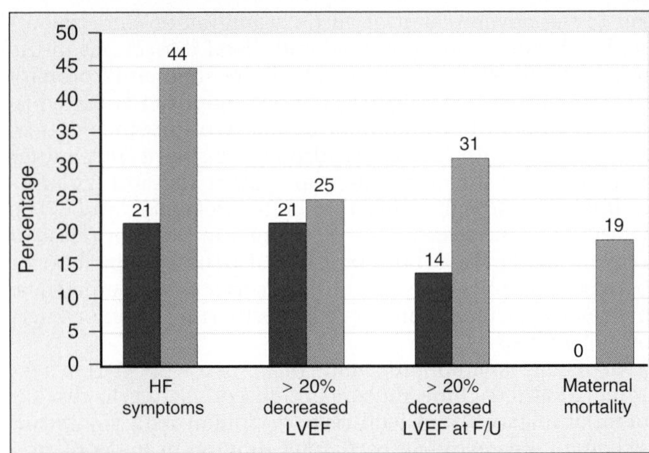

FIGURE 74–8 Maternal complications associated with subsequent pregnancy in women with a history of peripartum cardiomyopathy who did not have an abortion. F/U = follow-up; HF = heart failure; LVEF = left ventricular ejection fraction. (Modified from Elkayam U, Tummala PP, Rao K, et al: Maternal and fetal outcomes of subsequent pregnancies in women with peripartum cardiomyopathy. N Engl J Med 344:1567, 2001.)

Hypertension in Pregnancy (see Chap. 38)

Hypertensive disorders of pregnancy are a major cause of maternal and perinatal morbidity and mortality. Most adverse events are attributable to the preeclampsia syndrome, which is characterized by new-onset hypertension with proteinuria during pregnancy and is more common in women with chronic hypertension.[83,84] In general, hypertension in pregnancy is defined as blood pressure greater than 140 mm Hg systolic and 90 mm Hg diastolic on at least two occasions 6 hours apart. Hypertension complicates 8 to 10 percent of all pregnancies and is an important cause of maternal mortality and morbidity, including abruptio placentae, pulmonary edema, respiratory failure, disseminated intravascular coagulation, cerebral hemorrhage, hepatic failure, and acute renal failure. Fetal complications include prematurity, intrauterine growth retardation, stillbirth, and neonatal death.[83,84] Hypertensive disorders in pregnancy can be divided into three broad categories: chronic hypertension, gestational hypertension, and preeclampsia-eclampsia.[83-85]

CHRONIC HYPERTENSION. Chronic hypertension is defined as hypertension that precedes pregnancy. It can be assumed when elevated blood pressure is detected before the 20th gestational week, and it can also be diagnosed in retrospect when blood pressure fails to become normal 12 weeks after delivery.[86] It occurs in 1 to 5 percent of pregnancies and is associated with increased complications (15 percent), such as fetal growth retardation, premature delivery, abruptio placentae, acute renal failure, and hypertensive crisis; most of these complications occur in patients older than 30 years with a longer duration of hypertension or those who develop superimposed preeclampsia. Drug therapy is recommended for patients with high-risk characteristics of preeclampsia[87] (severe hypertension with evidence of end-organ involvement, a poor obstetric history, renal insufficiency, diabetes, or collagen-vascular disease) (Table 74–6). High-risk patients also require frequent monitoring of blood and urine chemistry and of fetal growth. In low-risk patients (blood pressure between 140 and 160 systolic and 90 and 110 diastolic, normal physical examination, normal electrocardiogram and echocardiogram, and no proteinuria), antihypertensive therapy has not been shown to prevent development of preeclampsia or affect fetal outcome.[64]

GESTATIONAL HYPERTENSION. Gestational hypertension is defined as hypertension induced by pregnancy

TABLE 74–6 Antihypertensive Drugs in Pregnancy

Class	Drug	Starting Dose	Maximum Dose
	Drugs for Long-Term Treatment of Hypertension		
Central $alpha_2$-agonist	Methyldopa Clonidine	250 mg tid 0.1-0.3 mg bid	4 g/d 1.2 mg/d
$Alpha_1$-adrenergic blocker	Prazosin	1 mg bid	20 mg/d
Calcium channel blocker	Nifedipine	10 mg qid	120 mg/d
Beta-adrenergic blocker	Atenolol	100 mg qd	100 mg/bid
Alpha/beta-adrenergic blocker	Labetalol	100 mg tid	2400 mg/d
Diuretics	Hydrochlorothiazide	25 mg qd	50 mg/d
Class	**Drug**	**Dose**	
	Drugs for Acute Treatment of Severe Hypertension		
Arterial dilator	Hydralazine Diazoxide	5-10 mg IV q 15-30 min 30-60 mg IV q 10-15 min	
Calcium channel blocker	Nifedipine	10-20 mg PO q 30 min	
Alpha/beta-adrenergic blocker	Labetalol	20-40-80 mg IV q 10-20 min (up to 300 mg)	
Arterial/venous dilator	Sodium nitroprusside	(50 mg/250 ml saline): 0.5-5.0 μg/kg/min	

beginning after 20 weeks of gestation and resolving by the sixth postpartum week.[86] Gestational hypertension is further classified as transient hypertension (hypertension without proteinuria) and preeclampsia (hypertension with proteinuria). Transient hypertension usually arises in the late third trimester with return of blood pressure to normal by the 10th postpartum day. It should be noted that the presence of proteinuria can occur late in the course of preeclampsia and the distinction between transient hypertension and preeclampsia can be difficult and can often be made only retrospectively. For this reason, in uncertain situations, preeclampsia should be considered and seizure prophylaxis should be instituted empirically in patients with blood pressure greater than 160/110 mm Hg. Pregnancy outcome is usually favorable in cases with transient hypertension, and use of antihypertensive therapy should be reserved for patients with blood pressure greater than 160/110 mm Hg.

PREECLAMPSIA-ECLAMPSIA. Preeclampsia is a pregnancy-specific syndrome that usually occurs after 20 weeks of gestation and is defined by the de novo appearance of hypertension (systolic blood pressure >140 mm Hg or diastolic blood pressure of ≥90 mm Hg) accompanied by new-onset proteinuria, defined as 300 mg or more per 24 hours. In the absence of proteinuria, the disease is highly suspect when increased blood pressure is accompanied by symptoms of headache, blurred vision, pulmonary edema, and abdominal pain or abnormal laboratory tests, specifically low platelet counts and abnormal liver enzymes. Preeclampsia is reversible and usually regresses within 24 to 48 hours post partum. In a minority of cases, postpartum eclampsia with hypertension, proteinuria, and convulsions occurs within 10 days after delivery. The maternal and fetal outcome for preeclampsia superimposed on existing hypertension is worse than that for de novo preeclampsia.

Management (see Table 74–6). The majority of women with chronic hypertension in pregnancy with a systolic blood pressure of 140 to 160 mm Hg or a diastolic blood pressure up to 110 mm Hg are at low risk for cardiovascular complications and are candidates for nondrug therapy. Most of the risk associated with chronic hypertension occurs in the setting of superimposed preeclampsia (25 percent of cases).

Indications for drug therapy include blood pressure exceeding 150 to 160 mm Hg systolic or 100 to 110 mm Hg diastolic or the presence of target organ damage, such as left ventricular hypertrophy or renal insufficiency. Methyldopa is the preferred therapy; alternatively, an effective prepregnancy regimen can be continued with the exception of converting enzyme inhibitors or angiotensin receptor antagonists.[75]

Delivery is the only definitive treatment for preeclampsia, and there is no evidence that any other therapy alters the underlying pathophysiology or improves perinatal outcome. All women with the diagnosis of preeclampsia should be considered for delivery at 40 weeks of gestation. Delivery may be indicated for women with mild disease and a favorable cervix for induction at 38 weeks of gestation and should be considered in women with severe preeclampsia beyond 32 to 34 weeks of gestation. Delivery is indicated even in women with fetal gestational age between 23 and 32 weeks if there are worsening maternal symptoms, laboratory evidence of end-organ dysfunction, or fetal deterioration.

Patients with stable, mild preeclampsia may be observed until fetal pulmonary maturity is verified or until after 37 weeks of gestation with cervical ripening.[86] There is no evidence of a need for or benefit from antihypertensive drug therapy in this subgroup of patients. Severe preeclampsia can be rapidly progressive, leading to sudden deterioration of the status of both mother and fetus. Patients with severe preeclampsia who are at or past 34 weeks of gestation should be delivered promptly. Patients with severe preeclampsia who are at 23 to 34 weeks of gestation should be treated with bed rest, intravenous magnesium sulfate for seizure prophylaxis, blood pressure control, fetal assessment, and corticosteroids for acceleration of fetal lung maturity. Indications for delivery include eclampsia; resistant, severe hypertension (refractory to maximum doses of three antihypertensive drugs); completion of 34 weeks of gestation; HELLP syndrome (hemolysis, elevated liver enzymes, and low platelet count); and abnormal fetal testing. Because of potential risks to the mother and fetus, conservative management of severe preeclampsia has been recommended only at tertiary perinatal centers under close maternal and fetal monitoring.

The primary goal of treatment is to prevent maternal cerebral complications. The recommended goal of therapy is reduction of mean blood pressure below 126 mm Hg but not less than 105 mm Hg and diastolic blood pressure between 90 and 105 mm Hg. Use of intravenous hydralazine is recommended as initial therapy; a 5-mg bolus is given intravenously over 1 to 2 minutes. After 20 minutes, subsequent doses are dictated by the initial response; when the desired effect is obtained, the drug is repeated as necessary. If this therapy is not effective or is associated with maternal side effect (tachycardia, headache, nausea), labetalol (given in divided doses [20 mg intravenonsly and, if needed, followed by 40 mg and 3 doses of 80 mg in intervals of 10 to 20 minutes] or continuous infusion of 1 to 2 mg/min as needed) or nifedipine should be given. In rare cases, intravenous nitroglycerin or nitroprusside may be needed after failure of hydralazine, labetalol, and nifedipine.

Pregnancy after Cardiac Transplantation (see Chap. 26)

A study conducted to determine the outcome of pregnancy in cardiac allograft recipients identified 47 pregnancies in 35 heart transplant recipients that resulted in 35 live births (74 percent).[88] Therapeutic abortion was performed in five cases owing to a short interval between transplantation and conception. Maternal hemodynamic changes during gestation seemed well tolerated, and rejection episodes were rare. At the same time, however, a higher incidence of maternal complications was reported, including chronic hypertension, preeclampsia, worsening kidney failure, premature rupture of membranes, and infections. Although fetal loss does not seem to be increased, an increased incidence of preterm deliveries and fetal growth retardation and cesarean sections has been reported. No maternal deaths were reported during pregnancy, but the incidence of late death was high compared with that in age-matched healthy women. None of the newborns was found to have congenital malformations, supporting a lack of teratogenic effect of immunosuppressive agents.[89] The limited available information suggests, therefore, that pregnancy in women after cardiac transplantation is not associated with increased maternal mortality; however, it results in increased maternal morbidity, preterm deliveries, and fetal growth retardation.

Coronary Artery Disease

(see Chaps. 46 to 50)

Pathogenesis

Although clinical manifestations of coronary artery diseases are expected to be encountered during pregnancy with increasing frequency because of increasing maternal age and fertility,[90,91] these are still rare among women of childbearing age, and the occurrence of peripartum acute myocardial infarction is anecdotal.[92]

Risk factors for coronary artery disease in women younger than 50 years include cigarette smoking, high levels of total plasma cholesterol, low levels of high-density lipoproteins, lipoprotein (a), diabetes mellitus, hypertension, a family history of coronary artery disease, toxemia of pregnancy, and the use of oral contraceptives.[91-93] The combination of heavy smoking or hypertension and concurrent use of oral contraceptives has been shown to be a powerful predictor of acute myocardial infarction. Women who have had very low birth weight babies or preterm delivery also seem to be at an increased risk for coronary artery disease.[94]

In the assessment of risk factors for coronary artery disease during pregnancy, it should be noted that total cholesterol, low-density lipoprotein cholesterol, and triglyceride levels are significantly increased during pregnancy.[95]

Acute Myocardial Infarction

Acute myocardial infarction has been reported at any stage of pregnancy and at ages between 16 and 45. The highest incidence, however, occurs in the third trimester and in women older than 33 years. In addition, acute myocardial infarction has been noted to occur more commonly in multigravidas and its location to be more commonly in the anterolateral wall. Most maternal deaths occurred either at the time of infarction or within 2 weeks.[92]

Although atherosclerotic disease seems to be the primary cause of acute myocardial infarction,[92] peripartum acute myocardial infarction is often associated with normal coronary angiograms and has been suggested to be due to a decrease in coronary perfusion caused by spasm or in situ thrombosis. A coronary atheroma with ruptured fibrous cap demonstrated by intravascular ultrasonography, in spite of a normal coronary vessel angiogram in a patient who experienced an acute myocardial infarction during cesarean section, may suggest plaque rupture as a cause of infarction in some of these patients.[96] Although the presence of spasm has not been documented and its cause is not clear, it has been suggested as a mechanism of myocardial infarction in some instances with pregnancy-induced hypertension and with the administration of ergot derivatives, bromocriptine, oxytocin, and prostaglandin[97] used to suppress lactation or uterine bleeding and in patients with pheochromocytoma. Coronary arterial dissection mostly in the immediate postpartum period has been commonly associated with peripartum acute myocardial infarction.[92,98] The dissection involves the left anterior descending artery in approximately 80 percent of cases and the right coronary artery in most other cases. Other potential causes of acute myocardial infarction during pregnancy have been collagen-vascular disease, Kawasaki disease (see Chap. 82), sickle cell anemia, and hemostatic abnormalities.[92]

DIAGNOSIS. The diagnostic approach to ischemic myocardial disease in pregnancy is influenced to some extent by whether a diagnostic procedure could harm the fetus and by normal changes seen during pregnancy that may mimic pathological changes. T wave inversion, Q wave in lead III, and increased R/S ratio in leads V_1 and V_2 are commonly seen in normal pregnancy. ST segment depressions, not associated with chest pain or echocardiographic wall motion abnormalities, have been described during elective cesarean section and can mimic myocardial ischemia.

Because fetal bradycardia has been reported during maximal exercise in normal women, a submaximal exercise protocol with fetal monitoring is recommended for the evaluation of ischemic myocardial disease during pregnancy.[7]

Radionuclide myocardial perfusion scans and radionuclide ventriculography expose the fetus to some radiation[9] and should be used only when the potential benefit seems to outweigh the risk. For similar reasons, cardiac catheterization involving fluoroscopy and cineangiography should be used only when relevant information cannot be obtained by other, noninvasive methods. The diagnosis of myocardial ischemia and infarction has been reported to be delayed during pregnancy because of the low level of suspicion.[92] Concentrations of myoglobin, creatine kinase, and creatine kinase with muscle and brain subunits (CK-MB) were found to be increased twofold 30 minutes after delivery, whereas the level of troponin I remained below the cutoff value for discriminating myocardial infarction. For this reason, troponin should be used to diagnose myocardial infarction after delivery.[99]

MANAGEMENT. Both maternal and fetal considerations should influence the therapeutic approach to ischemic heart disease during pregnancy. Morphine sulfate does not cause congenital defects. Because it crosses the placenta, it can cause neonatal respiratory depression when given shortly before delivery.[92] Available reports on the use of thrombolytic therapy during pregnancy do not support a teratogenic effect, and the majority of reported cases resulted in favorable maternal and fetal outcomes.[92] This therapy, however, is associated with risk of maternal hemorrhage, especially when given at the time of delivery. Because of their safety in pregnancy, beta blockers appear to be the drugs of choice. The use of organic nitrates and calcium antagonists in patients with acute myocardial ischemia or infarction has been described in a limited number of patients. These drugs should be given cautiously to prevent maternal hypotension and potential fetal distress. Use of high-dose aspirin during pregnancy is debatable because it has been reported to cause fetal growth retardation and bleeding in the neonate and in the mother.[100] Although the use of low-dose aspirin is considered safe during pregnancy,[101,102] a large-scale randomized study demonstrated that prolonged use of 100 mg of aspirin started in the second trimester of pregnancy was associated with increased bleeding complications and lower birth weight compared with placebo.[102]

Coronary reperfusion by means of percutaneous transluminal coronary angioplasty or coronary artery bypass graft surgery[92,93] has been reported to be successful during pregnancy, although experience is still limited. Such procedures should be avoided during the first trimester, if possible, owing to the potential deleterious fetal effects related to ionizing radiation as well as cardiopulmonary bypass.

Risk stratification after acute myocardial infarction during pregnancy should be determined by noninvasive methods. Total cholesterol, low-density lipoprotein cholesterol, and triglyceride levels are significantly increased during pregnancy.[95] Coronary angiography should be done only in cases in which coronary angioplasty or bypass surgery seems indicated during pregnancy.

Management of the Pregnancy. Management should focus on reducing cardiovascular stress during pregnancy and the peripartum period.[92] Termination of pregnancy may be preferred in patients with severe ischemia or heart failure in the early phase of gestation. During labor, adequate analgesia and supplemental oxygen should be given, and, if desired, cardiac output can be increased by placing the patient in the left lateral decubitus position. Labor in the supine position, however, may decrease venous return and thus reduce right and left ventricular filling pressures. Low forceps can be used to shorten the second stage of labor. Pulmonary artery catheterization with hemodynamic monitoring can help in the early detection and correction of hemodynamic abnormalities during labor and delivery. Although elective cesarean section is not indicated in every case, it should be used in patients with active ischemia or hemodynamic instability despite adequate medical therapy. Continued hemodynamic monitoring is advisable for several hours post partum to detect hemodynamic worsening associated with the postpartum hemodynamic changes described earlier.

Arrhythmias

Pregnancy is associated with an increased incidence of arrhythmias in women both with and without structural heart disease (see Chaps. 29 to 32).[8,103,104] In healthy women, multiple and even frequent atrial and ventricular premature complexes may occur, usually without effect on either the mother or the fetus (see Fig. 74–4).[8] There is also a strong suggestion of an increased frequency of paroxysmal supraventricular tachycardia during pregnancy.[104]

Atrial flutter and fibrillation are rare during normal pregnancy and are usually associated with rheumatic mitral valve disease.[6,104,105] Reports have described atrial fibrillation during gestation accompanied by treatment with terbutaline and magnesium sulfate and in the presence of preexcitation.[103,104,106,107] Ventricular tachycardia is a rare occurrence in pregnancy and the puerperium. It has been reported in women with normal hearts,[104] but it is usually associated with structural heart disease, drugs, electrolyte abnormalities, or eclampsia.[106,108-110]

Although palpitations, dizziness, and even syncope are relatively common symptoms in normal pregnancy, they are rarely associated with cardiac arrhythmias.[8] Cardiac arrhythmias, however, when they occur, can be hemodynamically significant during gestation even in patients with a normal heart. Reduction in blood pressure occasionally associated with such arrhythmias can result in fetal bradycardia and the need for immediate treatment with antiarrhythmic drugs, electric cardioversion, or urgent cesarean section. The effect of pregnancy on women with the hereditary long-QT syndrome has been reported (see Chap. 28).[111] The postpartum interval was associated with a significant increase in the risk for cardiac events, including death, aborted cardiac arrest, and syncope. Treatment with beta-adrenergic blockers was independently associated with a decrease in the risk for cardiac events.

Complete heart block has been described during pregnancy and is usually congenital. Patients with complete heart block may remain asymptomatic during pregnancy and have uncomplicated labor and delivery without treatment. Symptomatic patients with conduction abnormalities, including bifascicular block, second-degree atrioventricular block, and complete heart block, have been treated during pregnancy with either temporary or permanent pacemakers; and numerous pregnancies have been reported in patients after pacemaker implantation.[104,112]

MANAGEMENT OF ARRHYTHMIAS. A complete evaluation is indicated in patients with arrhythmias during pregnancy to rule out a treatable cause such as electrolyte imbalance, thyroid disease, and arrhythmogenic effects of drugs, alcohol, caffeine, and cigarette smoking. An identified cause should be treated and antiarrhythmic drug therapy initiated only if the arrhythmia persists and is symptomatic, hemodynamically important, or life threatening. When drug therapy seems necessary, the smallest therapeutic dose of drugs known to be safe for the fetus should be used (Table 74–7). Therapeutic blood levels and the indication for continuous drug therapy should be reevaluated periodically. Because of the unpredictable exposure to ionizing radiation, electrophysiological evaluation and catheter ablation procedures are usually postponed until the postpartum period but have been reported during pregnancy.[113] If delay of such procedures is undesirable, an attempt should be made to minimize radiation and use echocardiographic guidance whenever possible. Synchronized electrical cardioversion has been performed safely during all stages of pregnancy[114,115] and can be used in patients with tachyarrhythmias unresponsive to drug therapy that are associated with hemodynamic decompensation. Insertion of an implantable cardioverter-defibrillator has not been reported during pregnancy; however, pregnancies in women with an implantable cardioverter-defibrillator have been reported to be uneventful.[116]

Other Cardiovascular Disorders

AORTIC DISSECTION (see Chap. 53). A predisposition for aortic dissection during gestation has been suggested.[117] Over the past 50 years, more than 200 cases of aortic dissection in association with pregnancy have been reported; most cases occur in women with Marfan syndrome,[59,60,118] and cases of aortic dissection in women with systemic hypertension, coarctation of the aorta, Turner syndrome, and the use of crack cocaine have been reported.[119-121] Pregnancy-related aortic dissection may be due to increased hemodynamic stress and alterations in the structure of the vascular wall[117] and seems to occur most often in the third trimester and peripartum period.

Transesophageal echocardiography provides a powerful and safe tool for establishing the diagnosis of aortic dissection.[122] During pregnancy, this method is preferable to computed tomography, which involves radiation exposure, and to magnetic resonance imaging, whose safety during gestation has not been fully established.

The combination of intravenous nitroprusside and beta-adrenergic blocking agents is currently recommended to control hypertension in nonpregnant patients with aortic dissection[123] and has been used successfully during pregnancy. However, because nitroprusside can result in fetal toxicity, it should be used only post partum or in patients refractory

TABLE 74–7 Cardiovascular Drugs in Pregnancy

Drug	Use in Pregnancy	Potential Side Effects	Breast Feeding	Risk Factors
Adenosine	Maternal and fetal arrhythmias	No side effects reported; data on use during first trimester are limited.	Data NA	C
Amiodarone	Maternal arrhythmias	IUGR, prematurity, congenital goiter, hypothyroidism and hyperthyroidism, transient bradycardia, and prolonged QT in the newborn.	Not recommended	C
Angiotensin-converting enzyme inhibitors	Hypertension	Oligohydramnios, IUGR, prematurity, neonatal hypotension, renal failure, anemia, death, skull ossification defect, limb contractures, patent ductus arteriosus.	Compatible	C
Beta blockers	Hypertension, maternal arrhythmias, myocardial ischemia, mitral stenosis, hypertrophic cardiomyopathy, hyperthyroidism, Marfan syndrome	Fetal bradycardia, low placental weight, possible IUGR, hypoglycemia, no information on carvedilol.	Compatible, monitoring of infant's heart rate recommended	Acebutolol B Labetalol C Metoprolol C Propranolol C Atenolol D
Digoxin	Maternal and fetal arrhythmias, heart failure	No evidence for unfavorable effects on the fetus.	Compatible	C
Diltiazem	Myocardial ischemia, tocolysis	Limited data. Increased incidence of major birth defects.	Compatible	C
Disopyramide	Maternal arrhythmias	Limited data. May induce uterine contraction and premature delivery.	Compatible	C
Diuretics	Hypertension, congestive heart failure	Hypovolemia → reduced uteroplacental perfusion, fetal hypoglycemia, thrombocytopenia, hyponatremia, hypokalemia. Thiazide diuretics can inhibit labor and suppress lactation.	Compatible	C
Flecainide	Maternal and fetal arrhythmias	Limited data. Two cases of fetal death after successful treatment of fetal SVT reported, relation to flecainide uncertain.	Compatible	C
Lidocaine	Local anesthesia, maternal arrhythmias	No evidence for unfavorable fetal effects; high serum levels may cause central nervous depression at birth.	Compatible	C
Nifedipine	Hypertension, tocolysis	Fetal distress related to maternal hypotension reported.	Compatible	C
Nitrates	Myocardial infarction and ischemia, hypertension, pulmonary edema, tocolysis	Limited data. Use is generally safe, few cases of fetal heart rate deceleration and bradycardia have been reported.	Data NA	C
Procainamide	Maternal and fetal arrhythmias	Limited data. No fetal side effects reported.	Compatible	C
Propafenone	Fetal arrhythmias	Limited data. Fetal death reported after direct intrauterine administration in fetuses with fetal hydrops.	Data NA	C
Quinidine	Maternal and fetal arrhythmias	Minimal oxytoxic effect, high doses may cause premature labor or abortion. Transient neonatal thrombocytopenia and damage to eighth nerve reported.	Compatible	C
Sodium nitroprusside	Hypertension, aortic dissection	Limited data. Potential thiocyanate fetal toxicity, fetal mortality reported in animals.	Data NA	C
Sotalol	Maternal arrythmias, hypertension, fetal tachycardia	Limited data. Two cases of fetal death and two cases of significant neurological morbidity in newborns reported as well as bradycardia in newborns.	Compatible, monitoring of infant's heart rate recommended	B
Verapamil	Maternal and fetal arrhythmias, hypertension, tocolysis	Limited data. Other than a single case of fetal death of uncertain cause, no adverse fetal or newborn effects have been reported.	Compatible	C

IUGR = intrauterine growth retardation; NA = not available; SVT = supraventricular tachycardia.

to other drugs during pregnancy and can be substituted by hydralazine, nitroglycerin, or labetolol.[55] To avoid blood pressure elevation associated with labor and vaginal delivery in women with aortic dissection, cesarean section is recommended.[118]

TAKAYASU ARTERITIS (see Chap. 82)

Because Takayasu arteritis often occurs in young women, there is a high likelihood of pregnancy in patients with this condition.[123] Review of the literature revealed information on pregnancies in more than 60 women with Takayasu disease.[123,124] The majority of more recently published cases have had favorable maternal outcomes, although increase in blood pressure during pregnancy with or without superimposed preeclampsia, development of heart failure, and progression of renal insufficiency have been described.[124] Although a favorable fetal outcome has been reported in many cases, the incidence of fetal growth retardation, premature deliveries, and fetal loss is increased.[123,124] The mode of delivery in the majority of cases was vaginal, and forceps were often used to expedite the second stage of labor. Cesarean section delivery has been performed mainly for obstetrical indications or maternal hypertension and vascular disorders. In the great majority of patients, abdominal delivery has been performed under epidural anesthesia with favorable results.

PRIMARY PULMONARY HYPERTENSION (see Chap. 67)

Primary pulmonary hypertension is one of the few cardiovascular conditions that in pregnancy continues to be associated with high maternal mortality, estimated to be 30 to 40 percent.[125,126] Clinical deterioration or death during pregnancy cannot be predicted on the basis of the patient's preconceptual clinical status. Symptomatic deterioration usually occurs in the second or third trimester and may be manifested by fatigue, exertional dyspnea, syncope, chest pain, palpitations, nonproductive cough, hemoptysis, and leg edema. Worsening of symptoms during pregnancy led to early hospitalization in many reported cases.[125-129] Death often occurs a few hours to several days post partum, usually related to sudden death or progressive right ventricular failure.[130,131] Although the exact cause of death in patients with primary pulmonary hypertension is not clear, right ventricular ischemia and failure caused by an increase in pulmonary vascular resistance after delivery, cardiac arrhythmias, and pulmonary embolism are potential mechanisms. In addition to high maternal risk, primary pulmonary hypertension is associated with poor fetal outcome with high incidences of prematurity, fetal growth retardation, and fetal loss.[125]

Because of the high risk to both mothers with primary pulmonary hypertension and their fetuses, pregnancy should be discouraged in these patients and tubal ligation should be considered. In addition, early abortion should be considered in patients who become pregnant. The incidence of premature delivery is increased in patients with primary pulmonary hypertension, and should, therefore, be anticipated. Because of the beneficial effect of anticoagulation in patients with primary pulmonary hypertension[34] and the increased incidence of thromboembolism during pregnancy, such therapy is recommended throughout gestation or at least during the third trimester and early postpartum phase. Hemodynamic monitoring and blood gas measurements should be performed continuously during labor and delivery. Oxygen should be provided to prevent hypoxemia, and inhaled nitric oxide or prostaglandins administered either by inhalation or intravenously may be useful to lower pulmonary vascular resistance.[131-133]

Because of the high rate of early postpartum maternal death, close monitoring is recommended for several days post partum. Successful use of vasodilators including inhaled nitric oxide and intravenous and inhaled prostaglandins to lower pulmonary pressure during labor, delivery, and the early postpartum period has been reported.[131-133] In addition, a successful maternal and fetal outcome has been reported in one case treated with intravenous epoprostenol for 4 weeks prior to and then during cesarean section delivery; the drug was continued after the delivery.[128]

Cardiac Surgery During Pregnancy

Because heart disease that requires surgery is usually diagnosed and treated before pregnancy, cardiac surgery during gestation is uncommon.[29] The experience continues to be anecdotal and usually limited to urgent, life-threatening conditions in which surgery cannot be delayed and delivery is not desired, mostly because of fetal immaturity.[93,134,135] The effects of anesthesia and the surgical procedure, especially cardiopulmonary bypass, on the placental circulation and fetal outcome are still not well understood.[136] A review of the literature published between 1984 and 1996[137] identified 161 cases of various cardiovascular operations, 137 with and 24 without cardiopulmonary bypass. Surgery during pregnancy resulted in a high fetal-neonatal mortality of 30 percent. Week of gestation at time of surgery, surgery with cardiopulmonary bypass, longer duration, and temperature of cardiopulmonary bypass did not influence fetal-neonatal outcome. Operations performed during pregnancy resulted in a moderately high maternal mortality of 6 percent, and surgery performed immediately after delivery was associated with even higher mortality of 12 percent. Hospitalization after the 27th gestational week and emergency surgery were associated with poor maternal outcome. Nine percent maternal mortality was reported in cases that involved valvular surgery and 22 percent in cases of aortic or arterial dissection repairs and pulmonary embolectomies. Maternal risk associated with peripartum cardiovascular surgery therefore seems higher than the risk of similar surgery in nonpregnant patients.

Because of high incidence of fetal wastage and moderate increase in maternal risk, surgery should be recommended only for patients who do not respond to medical therapy and should be performed if possible after delivery.[138] To minimize the risk of teratogenicity, surgery should be avoided during the first trimester. Because heart surgery is indicated after failure of medical therapy, many of these patients are hemodynamically unstable and require hemodynamic evaluation and optimization before and monitoring during surgery. Anesthetic agents should be selected on the basis of their hemodynamic effects and fetal safety. When the patient is at or near term, abdominal delivery by cesarean section can be performed before cardiac surgery when fetal maturity has been confirmed.[138] Fetal heart monitoring should be performed continuously during surgery by experienced personnel.

Pregnancy in Patients with Prosthetic Heart Valves

VALVE SELECTION. The selection of a prosthetic heart valve for women of childbearing age remains difficult.[139-141] New-generation mechanical valves offer excellent durability, low risk of reoperation, and superior hemodynamic profile. However, the need for anticoagulation is associated with an increased risk of maternal bleeding and fetal loss.[142] Tissue valves have an inferior hemodynamic profile, especially with small valve sizes in the aortic position, and are associated with a high incidence of deterioration in young patients; deterioration may be further accelerated during pregnancy, with an expected rate of valve replacement as high as 30 to 50 percent within 10 years.[139,140] Although homograft valves and new pericardial valves appear to have better hemodynamics, information regarding pregnancy in women with these valves is limited.[141,143] In the nonpregnant population, homograft valves have been reported to have the same rate of deterioration as porcine, bioprosthetic valves.[144] An evaluation of long-term follow-up of young women with a prosthetic heart valve reported a substantially higher rate of reoperation in bioprosthetic valves compared with homografts in the aortic position (60 versus 30 percent).[145] Long-term follow-up of nonpregnant patients undergoing the Ross procedure also showed high rates of reoperation of 24 and 38 percent at 10 and 20 years, respectively, and mortality of 15 and 39 percent.[146]

Risks associated with pregnancy in women with prosthetic valves are related mainly to the increased hemodynamic burden and incidence of thromboembolic events as well as to untoward fetal effects caused by cardiovascular drugs and anticoagulation. Experience in more than 1000 pregnancies indicates that most patients who are asymptomatic or mildly symptomatic before gestation tolerate the hemodynamic burden of pregnancy, although decreased functional capacity and need to start or increase drug therapy are not uncommon.[140]

Increased thromboembolic events have been reported during pregnancy in women with mechanical prosthetic heart valves, with incidences as high as 10 to 15 percent (Fig. 74–9). Approximately two-thirds of these patients presented with valve thrombosis, which led to death in 40 percent of them.[139] Thromboembolism, however, has been reported mostly with older generation mechanical prostheses in the mitral position.[139] Heparin has been considered the anticoagulant of choice during pregnancy because of its proven safety for both the patient and the fetus.[147] Reports of an increased incidence of mechanical valve thrombosis during use of subcutaneous heparin in pregnancy[139] have raised concern regarding the effectiveness of heparin in pregnant women with mechanical heart valves.

ANTICOAGULATION. Thromboembolic prophylaxis for women at higher risk (old-generation prosthetic heart valve in the mitral position, atrial fibrillation, history of thromboembolic event despite adequate anticoagulation level) seems to be best achieved with oral anticoagulation (International Normalized Ratio of 3.0 to 4.5) for the first 35 weeks. An alternative therapy for patients electing to avoid warfarin in the first gestational trimester is unfractionated or low-molecular-weight heparin with close monitoring and appropriate dose adjustment for the first trimester, followed by warfarin between 13 and 36 weeks and then heparin until delivery. A high heparin intensity should be used in patients at high risk. Because peak levels cannot always predict trough levels, anticoagulation should aim at predose antifactor Xa levels higher than 0.55 units/ml or a midinterval activated partial thromboplastin time of 2.5 to 3.5 seconds (predose = 2.0 seconds) with unfractionated heparin and higher than 0.7 units/ml with low-molecular-weight heparin.

Oral anticoagulants cross the placenta and can be harmful to the fetus. Exposure during the first 8 to 12 weeks can be associated with a teratogenic effect leading to warfarin embryopathy (depressed nasal bridge, nasal hypoplasia, small nasal bones, hypoplastic alae nasi, telecanthus, upper airway obstruction related to choanal stenosis, and punctate epiphyseal dysplasia of the long bones and the cervical and lumbar vertebrae plates). Use of warfarin during pregnancy can also lead to fetal intracranial bleeding and is associated with a high rate of fetal loss, mostly because of spontaneous abortion.[142,147] One study suggested a relationship between fetal complications and warfarin dose with most of the fetal adverse effects occurring in women treated with warfarin at doses higher than 5 mg/d.[149] This relationship, however, has not been confirmed by other studies.[150,151]

A review of the literature showed the occurrence of warfarin embryopathy in 6.4 percent of women with prosthetic heart valves treated with warfarin throughout pregnancy.[142] The risk of embryopathy was eliminated by substitution of warfarin with heparin started at or prior to 6 weeks and continued until 12 weeks of gestation. The use of warfarin was also associated with a high frequency of spontaneous abortions (25 percent), congenital fetal anomalies (6 percent), and fetal wastage (34 percent) (Fig. 74–10).

Low-molecular-weight heparins have several potential advantages over unfractionated heparin, including a lower frequency of heparin-induced thrombocytopenia and osteoporosis, superior absorption from the subcutaneous injection site and bioavailability, and a two- to fourfold greater half-life and, therefore, a more predictable and sustained anticoagulant effect.[143]

There is substantial experience with the use of low-molecular-weight heparins in pregnancy, mostly for venous thromboembolism prophylaxis.[152,153] Limited information, however, is available regarding the use of low-molecular-weight heparin in pregnant patients with mechanical prosthetic heart valves, and several of the reports have described pregnancies complicated by valve thrombosis[154-158]; most of these cases, however, were associated with inadequate doses or subtherapeutic anti-Xa levels, or both.[159]

The latest recommendations as published by the American College of Chest Physicians for anticoagulation in pregnant patients with prosthetic heart valves[160] are as follows:

- Aggressive adjusted dose of unfractionated heparin, given every 12 hours subcutaneously throughout pregnancy; midinterval activated partial thromboplastin time maintained at two times control levels, or anti-Xa heparin level maintained at 0.35 to 0.70 IU/ml.
- Low-molecular-weight heparin throughout pregnancy, in doses adjusted according to weight, or as necessary to maintain a 4-hour postinjection anti-Xa heparin level of about 1.0 IU/ml.
- Unfractionated or low-molecular-weight heparin, as above, until the 13th week; change to warfarin until the middle of the third trimester, then restart heparin therapy until delivery.

Our recommendations are similar but further emphasize the need for frequent and careful monitoring of the predose level

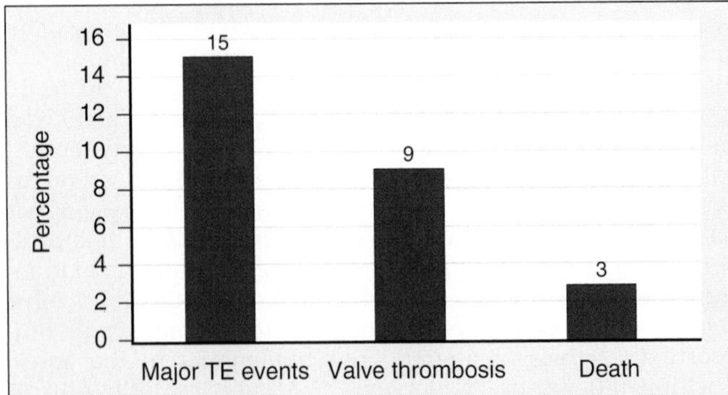

FIGURE 74–9 Incidence of major thromboembolic (TE) events during pregnancy in 326 pregnancies of women with mechanical prosthetic heart valves. (Modified from Elkayam U: Pregnancy through a prosthetic heart valve. J Am Coll Cardiol 33:1642, 1999.)

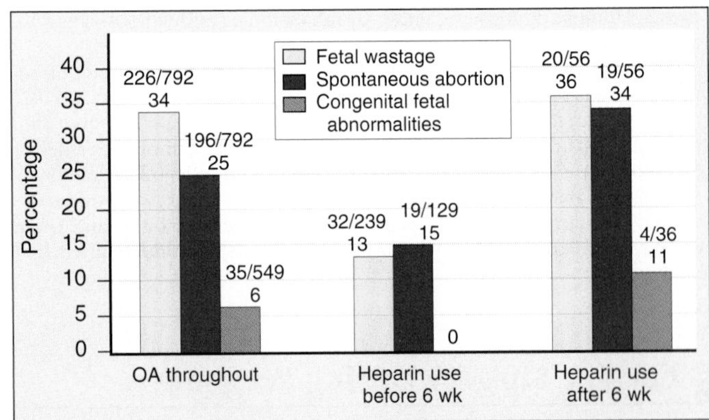

FIGURE 74–10 Frequency of fetal complications reported with various anticoagulation regimens. OA = oral anticoagulation. (Modified from Chan WS, Anand S, Ginsberg JS: Anticoagulation of pregnant women with mechanical heart valves: A systematic review of the literature. Arch Intern Med 160:191, 2000.)

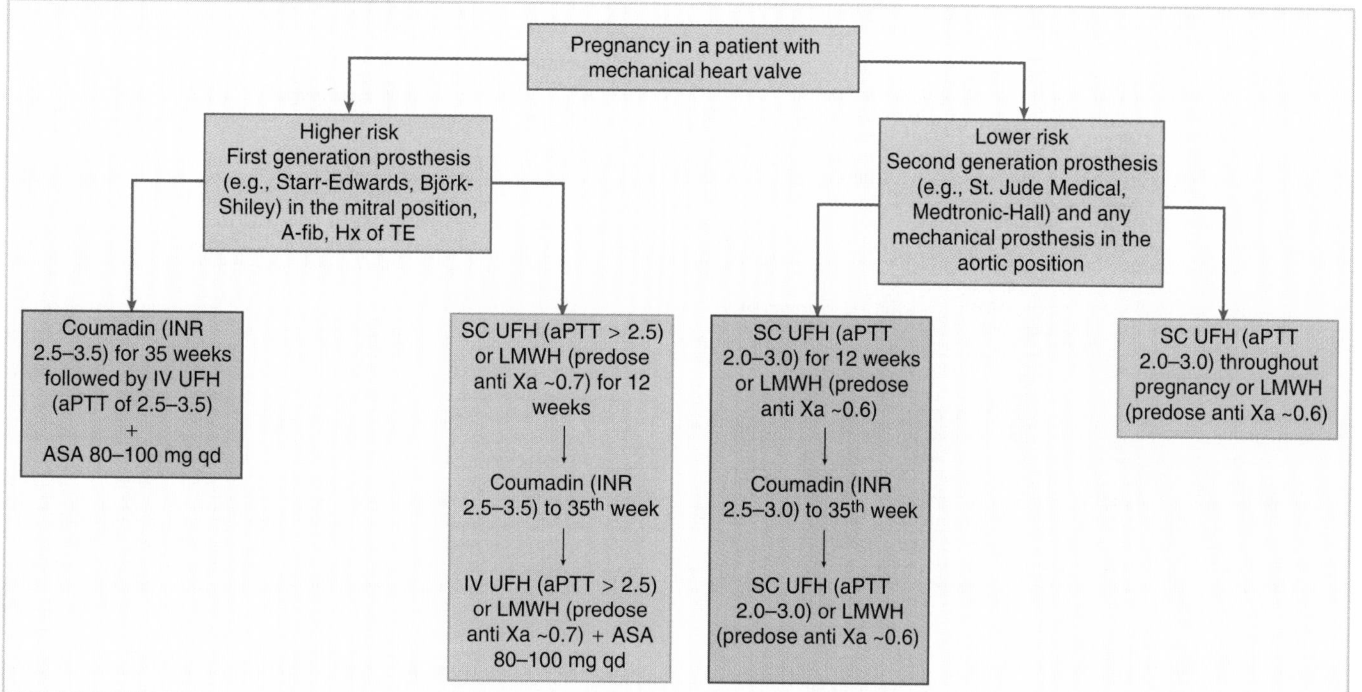

FIGURE 74–11 Recommended approach for anticoagulation prophylaxis in women with mechanical prosthetic heart valves during pregnancy. A-fib = atrial fibrillation; aPTT = activated partial thromboplastin time; ASA = acetylsalicylic acid; Hx =history; INR = International Normalized Ratio; LMWH = low-molecular-weight heparin; SC = subcutaneous; TE = thromboembolism; UFH = unfractionated heparin. (Elkayam U, Singh H, Irani A: Anticoagulation in pregnant women with prosthetic heart valves. Submitted for publication.)

of anticoagulation to ensure persistent thromboembolic prophylaxis in this high-risk group of patients (Fig. 74–11).[148,159]

Because of a high incidence of premature labor in patients with prosthetic heart valves, warfarin should be substituted for heparin at the 35th or 36th week to avoid onset of labor during warfarin therapy. The switch from warfarin to heparin should be performed in the hospital. In lower risk patients, including those with an aortic prosthetic valve and second-generation prosthesis in the mitral position, subcutaneous heparin therapy may be used throughout pregnancy (activated partial thromboplastin time of 2.0 to 3.0 seconds). A change from subcutaneous injections of heparin to an intravenous drip prior to elective delivery may be advisable because it allows discontinuation of therapy 4 hours before expected delivery. A higher level of anticoagulation seems justified in patients with mechanical prostheses in the mitral position, in patients with more than one mechanical prosthesis, in patients with atrial fibrillation, and in patients with a history of systemic embolization. The intensity of anticoagulation should be monitored frequently and immediately corrected if needed. Because a small dose of aspirin is safe during pregnancy[101] and can reduce the incidence of systemic embolization or death when added to oral anticoagulation, 80 mg of aspirin may be added to maximize the antithrombotic effect.

REFERENCES

Cardiovascular Physiology During Pregnancy and the Puerperium

1. Elkayam U, Gleicher N: Hemodynamic and cardiac function during normal pregnancy and the puerperium. *In* Elkayam U, Gleicher N (eds): Cardiac Problems in Pregnancy. 3rd ed. New York, Wiley-Liss, 1998, pp 3-20.
2. Brown MA, Gallery ED: Volume homeostasis in normal pregnancy and preeclampsia: Physiology and clinical implications. Baillieres Clin Obstet Gynecol 8:287, 1994.
3. Clapp JF III, Capeless E: Cardiovascular function before, during and after the first and subsequent pregnancies. Am J Cardiol 80:1469, 1997.
4. Mesa A, Jessurun C, Hernandez A, et al: Left ventricular diastolic function in normal human pregnancy. Circulation 99:511, 1999.
5. Poppas A, Shroff SG, Korcarz CE, et al: Serial assessment of the cardiovascular system in normal pregnancy. Circulation 95:2407, 1997.
6. Hameed AB, Karaalp IS, Tummala PP, et al: The effect of valvular heart disease on maternal and fetal outcome in pregnancy. J Am Coll Cardiol 37:893, 2001.

Cardiovascular Evaluation During Pregnancy

7. Elkayam U, Gleicher N: Cardiac evaluation during pregnancy. *In* Elkayam U, Gleicher N (eds): Cardiac Problems in Pregnancy. 3rd ed. New York, Wiley-Liss, 1998, pp 23-32.
8. Shotan A, Ostrzega E, Mehra A, et al: Incidence of arrhythmias in normal pregnancy and relation to palpitations, dizziness and syncope. Am J Cardiol 79:1061, 1997.
9. Colletti PM, Lee K: Cardiovascular imaging in the pregnant patient. *In* Elkayam U, Gleicher N (eds): Cardiac Problems in Pregnancy. 3rd ed. New York, Wiley-Liss, 1998, pp 33-36.
10. Allan L: Antenatal diagnosis of heart disease. Heart 83:367, 2000.
11. Veille JC, Kitzman D, Millsaps PD, et al: Left ventricular diastolic filling response to stationary bicycle exercise during pregnancy and the postpartum period. Am J Obstet Gynecol 185:822, 2001.
12. Colletti PM: Computer-assisted imaging of the fetus with magnetic resonance imaging. Comput Med Imaging Graph 20:491, 1996.

Pregnancy in Women with Congenital Heart Disease

13. Warnes CA, Elkayam U: Congenital heart disease and pregnancy. *In* Elkayam U, Gleicher N (eds): Cardiac Problems in Pregnancy. 3rd ed. New York, Wiley-Liss, 1998, pp 39-53.
14. Siu SC, Colman JM: Heart disease and pregnancy. Heart 85:710, 2001.
15. Swan L, Hillis WS, Cameron A: Family planning requirements of adults with congenital heart disease. Heart 78:9, 1997.
16. Kjos SL: Fertility control in the cardiac patient. *In* Elkayam U, Gleicher N (eds): Cardiac Problems in Pregnancy. 3rd ed. New York, Wiley-Liss, 1998, pp 451-456.
17. Sin SC, Sermer M, Harrison DA, et al: Risk and predictors for pregnancy-related complications in women with heart disease. Circulation 96:2789, 1997.
18. Zuber M, Gautschi N, Oechslin E, et al: Outcome of pregnancy in women with congenital shunt lesions. Heart 81:271, 1999.
19. Siu SC, Colman JM, Sorensen S, et al: Adverse neonatal and cardiac outcomes are more common in pregnant women with cardiac disease. Circulation 105:2179, 2002.
20. Ardinger RH Jr: Genetic counseling in congenital heart disease. Pediatr Ann 26:99, 1997.
21. Presbitero P, Somerville J, Stone S, et al: Pregnancy in cyanotic congenital heart disease: Outcome of mother and fetus. Circulation 89:2673, 1994.
22. Dajani AS, Taubert KA, Wilson W, et al: Prevention of bacterial endocarditis. Recommendations by the American Heart Association. JAMA 277:1794, 1997.
23. Ebrahimi R, Leung CY, Elkayam U, Reid CL: Infective endocarditis. *In* Elkayam U, Gleicher N (eds): Cardiac Problems in Pregnancy. 3rd ed. New York, Wiley-Liss, 1998, pp 191-198.
24. Actis Dato GM, Rinaudo P, Revelli A et al: Atrial septal defect and pregnancy: A retrospective analysis of obstetrical outcome before and after surgical correction. Minerva Cardioangiol 46:63, 1998.

25. Kozelj M, Novak-Antolic Z, Grad A, et al: Patent foramen ovale as a potential cause of paradoxical embolism in the post partum period. Eur J Obstet Gynecol Reprod Biol 84:55, 1999.
26. Daehnert I, Ewert P, Berger F, et al: Echocardiographically guided closure of a patent foramen ovale during pregnancy after recurrent strokes. J Interv Cardiol 14:191, 2001.
27. Actis Dato GM, Cavaglia M, Aidala E, et al: Patent ductus arteriosus. Follow up of 677 operated cases 40 years later. Minerva Cardioangiol 47:245,1999.
28. Bhargava B, Agarwal R, Yadav R, et al: Percutaneous balloon aortic valvuloplasty during pregnancy: Use of the Inoue balloon and the physiologic antegrade approach. Cathet Cardiovasc Diagn 45:422, 1998.
29. Cohen RG, Castro LJ: Cardiac surgery during pregnancy. *In* Elkayam U, Gleicher N (eds): Cardiac Problems in Pregnancy. 3rd ed. New York, Wiley-Liss, 1998, pp 277-284.
30. Saidi AS, Bezold LI, Altman CA, et al: Outcome of pregnancy following intervention for coarctation of the aorta. Am J Cardiol 82:786, 1998.
31. Beauchesne LM, Connolly HM, Ammash NM, et al: Coarctation of the aorta: Outcome of pregnancy. J Am Coll Cardiol 38:1728, 2001.
32. Plunkett MD, Bond LM, Geiss DM: Staged repair of acute type I aortic dissection and coarctation in pregnancy. Ann Thorac Surg 69:1945, 2000.
33. Therrian J, Marx GR, Gatzoulis MA: Late problems in tetralogy of Fallot—Recognition, management, and prevention. Cardiol Clin 20:395, 2002.
34. Weiss BM, Hess OM: Pulmonary vascular disease and pregnancy: Current controversies, management strategies, and perspectives. Eur Heart J 21:104, 2000.
35. Sawhney H, Suri V, Vasishta K, et al: Pregnancy and congenital heart disease—Maternal and fetal outcome. Aust NZ J Obstet Gyneol 38:266, 1998.
36. Burn J, Brennan P, Little J, et al: Recurrence risks in offspring of adults with major heart defects: Results from first cohort of British collaborative study. Lancet 351:311, 1998.
37. Branko WM, Otto H: Perioperative cardiovascular evaluation for noncardiac surgery: Congenital heart disease and heart disease in pregnancy deserve better guidelines. Circulation 95:530, 1997.
38. Goodwin TM, Gherman RB, Hameed A, Elkayam U: Favorable response of Eise menger's syndrome to inhaled nitric oxide during pregnancy. Am J Obstet Gynecol 180:64, 1999.
39. Lust KM, Boots RH, Dooris M, Wilson J: Management of labor in Eisenmenger syndrome with inhaled nitric oxide. Am J Obstet Gynecol 181:419, 1999.
40. Kansaria JJ, Salvi VS: Eisenmenger syndrome in pregnancy. J Postgrad Med 46:101, 2000.
41. Somerville J: The Denolin Lecture: The woman with congenital heart disease. Eur Heart J 19:1766, 1998.
42. Lao TT, Sermer M, Colman JM: Pregnancy after the Fontan procedure for tricuspid atresia: A case report. J Reprod Med 41:287, 1996.
43. Genomi M, Jenni R, Hoerstrup SP, et al: Pregnancy after atrial repair for transposition of the great arteries. Heart 81:276, 1999.
44. Connolly HM, Grogan M, Warnes CA: Pregnancy among women with congenitally corrected transposition of great arteries. J Am Coll Cardiol 33:1692, 1999.
45. Canobbio MM, Mair DD, van der Velde M, Koos BJ: Pregnancy outcome after the Fontan repair. J Am Coll Cardiol 28:763, 1996.

Valvular Heart Disease

46. Essop MR, Sareli P: Rheumatic valvular disease and pregnancy. *In* Elkayam U, Gleicher N (eds): Cardiac Problems in Pregnancy. 3rd ed. New York, Wiley-Liss, 1998, pp 55-60.
47. Reimold SC, Rutherford JD: Valvular heart disease in pregnancy. N Engl J Med 349:52, 2003.
48. Barbosa PJ, Lopes AA, Feitusa GS, et al: Prognostic factors of rheumatic mitral stenosis during pregnancy and puerperium. Arq Bras Cardiol 75:215, 2000.
49. Naidoo DP, Desai DK, Moodley J: Maternal death due to pre-existing cardiac disease. Cardiovasc J S Afr 13:17, 2002.
50. Birincioglu CL, Kucuker SA, Yapar EG, et al: Perinatal mitral valve interventions: A report of 10 cases. Ann Thorac Surg 67:1312, 1999.
51. de Souza JA, Martinez EE, Ambrosa JA, et al: Percutaneous balloon mitral valvuloplasty in comparison with open mitral valve commissurotomy for mitral stenosis during pregnancy. J Am Coll Cardiol 37:900, 2001.
52. Mangione JA, Lourenco RM, dos Santos ES, et al: Long-term follow-up of pregnant women after percutaneous mitral valvuloplasty. Catheter Cardiovasc Interv 50:413, 2000.
53. Kinsara AJ, Ismail O, Fawzi ME: Effect of balloon mitral valvuloplasty during pregnancy on childhood development. Cardiology 97:155, 2002.
54. Kubota N, Morimoto Y, Kemmotsu O: Anesthetic management for cesarean section in a patient with mitral stenosis and pulmonary hypertension. Masai Jpn J Anesthesiol 52:177, 2003.
55. Calvin SE: Use of vasodilators during pregnancy. *In* Elkayam U, Gleicher N (eds): Cardiac Problems in Pregnancy. 3rd ed. New York, Wiley-Liss, 1998, pp 391-398.
56. Bhargava B, Agarwal R, Yadar R, et al: Percutaneous balloon aortic valvuloplasty during pregnancy: Use of the Inoue balloon and the physiologic antegrade approach. Cathet Cardiovasc Diagn 45:422, 1998.

Other Conditions Affecting the Valves, Aorta, and Myocardium

57. Freed LA, Levy D, Levine RA, et al: Prevalence and clinical outcome of mitral-valve prolapse. N Engl J Med 341:1, 1999.
58. Rayburn WF: Mitral valve prolapse and pregnancy. *In* Elkayam U, Gleicher N (eds): Cardiac Problems in Pregnancy. 3rd ed. New York, Wiley-Liss, 1998, pp 175-182.
59. Elkayam U, Ostrzega E, Shotan A, Mehra A: Marfan syndrome and pregnancy. *In* Elkayam U, Gleicher N (eds): Cardiac Problems in Pregnancy. 3rd ed. New York, Wiley-Liss, 1998, pp 211-221.
60. Lind J, Wallenburg HC: The Marfan syndrome and pregnancy: A retrospective study in a Dutch population. Eur J Obstet Gynecol Reprod Biol 98:28, 2001.
61. Paternoster DM, Santarossa C, Vettore N, et al: Obstetric complications in Marfan's syndrome. Minerva Ginecol 50:441, 1998.
62. Uchida T, Ogino H, Ando M, et al: Aortic dissection in pregnant women with the Marfan syndrome. Jpn J Thorac Surg 55:693, 2001.
63. Gott VL, Greene PS, Alejo DE, et al: Replacement of the aortic root in patients with Marfan's syndrome. N Engl J Med 340:1307, 1999.
64. Oakley C, Child A, Jung B, et al: Expert consensus document on management of cardiovascular diseases during pregnancy. Eur Heart J 24:761, 2003.

Cardiomyopathies

65. Elkayam U, Dave R: Hypertrophic cardiomyopathy and pregnancy. *In* Elkayam U, Gleicher N (eds): Cardiac Problems in Pregnancy. 3rd ed. New York, Wiley-Liss, 1998, pp 211-221.
66. Probst V, Langlard JM, Desnos M, et al: Familial hypertrophic cardiomyopathy. French study of the duration and outcome of pregnancy. Arch Mal Coeur Vaiss 95:81, 2002.
67. Autore C, Conte MR, Piccinirino M, et al: Risk associated with pregnancy in hypertrophic cardiomyopathy. J Am Coll Cardiol 40:1864, 2002.
68. Autore C, Brauneis S, Fabrizio A, et al: Epidural anesthesia for cesarean section in patients with hypertrophic cardiomyopathy: A report of three cases. Anesthesiology 90:1205, 1999.
69. Lang RM, Lampert MB, Poppas A, et al: Peripartal cardiomyopathy. *In* Elkayam U, Gleicher N (eds): Cardiac Problems in Pregnancy. 3rd ed. New York, Wiley-Liss, 1998, pp 87-100.
70. Pearson GD, Veille JC, Rahimtoola S, et al: Peripartum cardiomyopathy: National Heart, Lung, and Blood Institute and Office of Rare Diseases (National Institutes of Health) workshop recommendations and review. JAMA 283:1183, 2000.
71. Akhter WM, Shotan A, Hameed A, et al: Pregnancy associated cardiomyopathy: Early versus late presentation. J Am Coll Cardiol 41:1039, 2003.
72. Fett JD: Peripartum cardiomyopathy. Insights from Haiti regarding a disease of unknown etiology. Minn Med 85:46, 2002.
73. Akhter WM, Shotan A, Hameed A, et al: Pregnancy associated cardiomyopathy: Clinical profile in 137 patients diagnosed in the U.S. J Am Coll Cardiol 41:1136, 2003.
74. Aziz TM, Burgess MI, Acladious NN, et al: Heart transplantation for peripartum cardiomyopathy: A report of three cases and a literature review. Cardiovasc Surg 7:565, 1999.
75. Shotan A, Widerhorn J, Hurst A, Elkayam U: Risks of angiotensin-converting enzyme inhibition during pregnancy: Experimental and clinical evidence, potential mechanisms, and recommendations for use. Am J Med 96:451, 1994.
76. Ford RF, Barton JR, O'Brien JM, et al: Demographics, management, and outcome of peripartum cardiomyopathy in a community hospital. Am J Obstet Gynecol 182:1036, 2000.
77. Carlson KM, Browning JE, Eggleston MK, et al: Peripartum cardiomyopathy presenting as lower extremity arterial thromboembolism; a case report. J Reprod Med 45:351, 2000.
78. Bozkurt B, Villaneuva FS, Halubkov R, et al: Intravenous immune globulin in the therapy of peripartum cardiomyopathy. J Am Coll Cardiol 34:177, 1999.
79. Sliwa K, Skudicky D, Candy G, et al: The addition of pentoxifylline to conventional therapy improves outcome in patients with peripartum cardiomyopathy. Eur J Heart Fail 4:305, 2002.
80. Sliwa K, Skudicky D, Bergemann A, et al: Peripartum cardiomyopathy: Analysis of clinical outcome, left ventricle function, plasma levels of cytokines and Fas/APO-O. J Am Coll Cardiol 35:701, 2000.
81. Felker GM, Thompson RE, Hare JM, et al: Underlying causes and long-term survival in patients with initially unexplained cardiomyopathy. N Engl J Med 342:1077, 2000.
82. Elkayam U, Tummala PP, Rao K, et al: Maternal and fetal outcomes of subsequent pregnancies in women with peripartum cardiomyopathy. N Engl J Med 344:1567, 2001.

Hypertension in Pregnancy

83. Roberts JM, Pearson G, Cutler J, et al: Summary of the NHLBI working group on research on hypertension during pregnancy. Hypertension 41:437, 2003.
84. Report of the national high blood pressure education program working group on high blood pressure in pregnancy. Am J Obstet Gynecol 183:S1, 2000.
85. Higgins JR, de Swiet M: Blood pressure measurement and classification in pregnancy. Lancet 357:131, 2001.
86. Chari RS, Frangieh AY, Sibai BM: Hypertension during pregnancy: Diagnosis, pathophysiology, and management. *In* Elkayam U, Gleicher N (eds): Cardiac Problems in Pregnancy. 3rd ed. New York, Wiley-Liss, 1998, pp 257-273.
87. Roberts JM, Cooper DW: Pathogenesis and genetics of pre-eclampsia. Lancet 357:53, 2001.
88. Branch KR, Wagoner LE, McGrory CH, et al: Risks of subsequent pregnancies on mother and newborn in female heart transplant recipient. J Heart Lung Transplant 17:698, 1998.
89. Alami WS, Young JB: Pregnancy after cardiac transplantation. *In* Elkayam U, Gleicher N (eds): Cardiac Problems in Pregnancy. 3rd ed. New York, Wiley-Liss, 1998, pp 327-337.

Coronary Artery Disease

90. Paulson RJ, Boostanfar R, Saadat P, et al: Pregnancy in the sixth decade of life. JAMA 288:2320, 2002.
91. Rutherford JD: Coronary artery disease in the childbearing age. *In* Elkayam U, Gleicher N (eds): Cardiac Problems in Pregnancy. 3rd ed. New York, Wiley-Liss, 1998, pp 121-130.
92. Roth A, Elkayam U: Acute myocardial infarction and pregnancy. *In* Elkayam U, Gleicher N (eds): Cardiac Problems in Pregnancy. 3rd ed. New York, Wiley-Liss, 1998, pp 131-151.
93. Hameed AB, Tummala PP, Godwin TM, et al: Unstable angina during pregnancy in two patients with premature coronary atherosclerosis and aortic stenosis in association with familial hypercholesterolemia. Am J Obstet Gynecol 182:1152, 2000.
94. Sattar N, Greer IA: Pregnancy complications and maternal cardiovascular risk: Opportunities for intervention and screening? BMJ 325:157, 2002.
95. Brizzi P, Tonalo G, Esposito F, et al: Lipoprotein metabolism during normal pregnancy. Am J Obstet Gynecol 181:430, 1999.
96. Kulka PJ, Scheu C, Tryba M, et al: Coronary artery plaque disruption as cause of acute myocardial infarction during cesarean section with spinal anesthesia. J Clin Anesth 12:335, 2000.
97. Chen FG, Koh KF, Chong YS: Cardiac arrest associated with sulprostone: Use during cesarean section. Anaesth Intensive Care 26:298, 1998.
98. Lerakis S, Manoukian S, Martin RP: Transesophageal echo detection of post partum coronary artery dissection. J Am Soc Echocardiogr 14:1132, 2001.

99. Shivvers SA, Wians FH Jr, Keffer JH, Ramin SM: Maternal cardiac troponin I levels during normal labor and delivery. Am J Obstet Gynecol 180:122, 1999.
100. Ginsberg JS, Hirsch J: Use of antithrombotic agents during pregnancy. Chest 114:524S, 1998.
101. Cartis S, Sibai B, Houth J, et al: Low-dose aspirin to prevent preeclampsia in women at high risk. National Institute of Child Health and Human Development, network of maternal-fetal medicine unit. N Engl J Med 338:701, 1998.
102. Subtil D, Goeusse P, Puech F, et al: Aspirin (100 mg) used for prevention of pre-eclampsia in nulliparous women: The Essai Regional Aspirine Mere-Enfant Study. Int J Obstet Gynecol 110:475, 2003.

Arrhythmias

103. Wolbrette D: Treatment of arrhythmias during pregnancy. Curr Womens Health Rep 3:135, 2003.
104. Leung CY, Brodsky MA: Cardiac arrhythmias and pregnancy. *In* Elkayam U, Gleicher N (eds): Cardiac Problems in Pregnancy. 3rd ed. New York, Wiley-Liss, 1998, pp 155-175.
105. Desai DK, Adanlawo M, Naidoo DP, et al: Mitral stenosis in pregnancy: A four year experience at King Edward VIII hospital, Durban, South Africa BJOG 107:953, 2000.
106. Braden GL, Von Oeyen PT, Germain MJ, et al: Ritodrine and terbutaline-induced hypokalemia in preterm labor: Mechanisms and consequences. Kidney Int 51:1867, 1997.
107. Carson MP, Fisher AJ, Scorza WE: Atrial fibrillation in pregnancy associated with oral terbutaline. Obstet Gynecol 100:1096, 2002.
108. Onagawa T, Ohkuchi A, Ohki R, et al: Woman with postpartum ventricular tachycardia and hypomagnesemia. J Obstet Gynecol Res 29:92, 2003.
109. Palma EC, Saxenberg V, Vijayaraman P, et al: Histopathological correlation of ablation lesions guided by noncontact mapping in a patient with peripartum cardiomyopathy and ventricular tachycardia. Pacing Clin Electrophysiol 24:1812, 2001.
110. Mela T, Galvin JM, McGovern BA: Magnesium deficiency during lactation as a precipitant of ventricular tachyarrhythmias. Pacing Clin Electrophysiol 25:231, 2002.
111. Rashba EJ, Zareba W, Moss AJ, et al: Influence of pregnancy on the risk for cardiac events in patients with hereditary long QT syndrome. Circulation 97:451, 1998.
112. Sharma JB, Malhotra M., Pundir P: Successful pregnancy outcome with cardiac pacemaker after complete heart block. Int J Gynaecol Obstet 68:145, 2000.
113. Dominguez A, Iterralde P, Hermosillo AG, et al: Successful radio frequency ablation of an accessory pathway during pregnancy. Pacing Clin Electrophysiol 22:131, 1999.
114. Brown O, Davidson, N, Palmer J: Cardioversion in the third trimester of pregnancy. Aust NZ J Obstet Gynecol 41:241, 2001.
115. Oktay C, Kesapli M, Altekin E: Wide-QRS complex tachycardia during pregnancy: Treatment with cardioversion and review. Am J Emerg Med 20:492, 2002.
116. Olufolabi AJ, Charlton GA, Allen SA, et al: Use of implantable cardioverter defibrillator and anti-arrhythmic agents in a parturient. Br J Anaesth 89:652, 2002.

Other Cardiovascular Disorders

117. Elkayam U, Hameed A: Vascular dissections and aneurysms during pregnancy. *In* Elkayam U, Gleicher N (eds): Cardiac Problems in Pregnancy. 3rd ed. New York, Wiley-Liss, 1998, p 201.
118. Brar HB: Anaesthetic management of a cesarean section in a patient with Marfan's syndrome and aortic dissection. Anaesth Intensive Care 29:67, 2001.
119. Plunkett MD, Bond LM, Geiss DM: Staged repair of acute type I aortic dissection and coagulation in pregnancy. Ann Thorac Surg 69:1945, 2000.
120. Garvey P, Elovitz M, Landsberger EJ: Aortic dissection and myocardial infarction in a pregnant patient with Turner syndrome. Obstet Gynecol 91:864, 1998.
121. Madu EC, Shala B, Baugh D: Crack-cocaine–associated aortic dissection in early pregnancy; a case report. Angiology 50:163, 1999.
122. Nienaberg CA, Eagle KA: Aortic dissection: New frontiers in diagnosis and management Part II: Therapeutic management and follow up. Circulation 108:772, 2003.
123. Elkayam U, Hameed A: Takayasu's arteritis and pregnancy. *In* Elkayam U, Gleicher N (eds): Cardiac Problems in Pregnancy. 3rd ed. New York, Wiley-Liss, 1998, p 237.
124. Sharma BK, Jain S, Vasishta K: Outcome of pregnancy in Takayasu arteritis. Int J Cardiol 75:S159, 2000.
125. Elkayam U, Dave R, Bokhari SWH: Primary pulmonary hypertension in pregnancy. *In* Elkayam U, Gleicher N (eds): Cardiac Problems in Pregnancy. 3rd ed. New York, Wiley-Liss, 1998, p 183.
126. Weiss BM. Zemp L. Seifert B, Hess OM: Outcome of pulmonary vascular disease in pregnancy: A systematic overview from 1978 through 1996. J Am Coll Cardiol 31:1650, 1998.
127. Satoh H, Masuda Y, Izuta S, et al: Pregnant patient with primary pulmonary hypertension: General anesthesia and extracorporeal membrane oxygenation support for termination of pregnancy. Anesthesiology 97:1638, 2002.
128. Stewart R, Tuazon D, Olson G, et al: Pregnancy and primary pulmonary hypertension; successful outcome with epoprostenol therapy. Chest 119:973, 2001.
129. Wong PS, Constantinides S, Kanellopoulos V, et al: Primary pulmonary hypertension in pregnancy. J R Soc Med 94:523, 2001.
130. Takeuchi K, Yokota H, Moriyama T, et al: Two cases of primary pulmonary hypertension diagnosed during pregnancy. J Perinat Med 26:248, 1998.
131. Monnery L, Nanson J, Charlton G: Primary pulmonary hypertension in pregnancy; a role for novel vasodilators. Br J Anaesth 87:295, 2001.
132. Decoene C, Bourzoufi K, Moreau D, et al: Use of inhaled nitric oxide for emergency cesarean section in a woman with unexpected primary pulmonary hypertension. Can J Anaesth 48:584, 2001.
133. Weiss BM, Maggiorini M, Jenni R, et al: Pregnant patient with primary pulmonary hypertension; inhaled pulmonary vasodilators and epidural anesthesia for cesarean delivery. Anesthesiology 92:1191, 2000.
134. Fabricius AM, Autschbach R, Doll N, et al: Acute aortic dissection during pregnancy. Thorac Cardiovasc Surg 49:56, 2001.
135. Ceresoli G, Passoni P, Benussi S, et al: Primary cardiac sarcoma in pregnancy: A case report and review of the literature. Am J Clin Oncol 22:460, 1999.
136. Mul TF, van Herwerden LA, Cohen-Overbeek TE, et al: Hypoxic-ischemic fetal insult resulting from maternal aortic root replacement, with normal fetal heart rate at term. Am J Obstet Gynecol 179:825, 1998.
137. Weiss BM, von Segesser LK, Alon E, et al: Outcome of cardiovascular surgery and pregnancy: A systematic review of the period 1984-1996. Am J Obstet Gynecol 179:1643, 1998.
138. Akashi H, Tayama K, Fujino T, et al: Surgical treatment for acute type A aortic dissection in pregnancy: A case of aortic root replacement just after cesarean section. Jpn Circ J 64:729, 2000.
139. Elkayam U: Pregnancy through a prosthetic heart valve. J Am Coll Cardiol 33:1642, 1999.
140. Elkayam U, Khan SS: Pregnancy in the patient with artificial heart valve. *In* Elkayam U, Gleicher N (eds): Cardiac Problems in Pregnancy. 3rd ed. New York, Wiley-Liss, 1998, pp 61-78.
141. Hung L, Rahimtoola SH: Prosthetic heart valves and pregnancy. Circulation 107:1240, 2003.
142. Chan WS, Ananad S, Ginsberg JS: Anticoagulation of pregnant women with mechanical heart valves: A systemic review of the literature. Arch Intern Med 160:191, 2000.
143. Dore A, Somerville J: Pregnancy in patients with pulmonary autograft valve replacement. Eur Heart J 18:1659, 1997.
144. Grunkemeir GL, Li HH, Naftel DC, et al: Long term performance of heart valve prosthesis. Curr Probl Cardiol 25:73, 2000.
145. North RA, Sadler L, Stewart AW, et al: Long-term survival and valve-related complications in young women with cardiac valve replacement. Circulation 99:2669, 1999.
146. Chambers JC, Somerville J, Stone S, et al: Pulmonary autograft procedure for aortic valve disease: Long-term results of the pioneer series. Circulation 96:2206, 1997.
147. McGehee W: Anticoagulation in pregnancy. *In* Elkayam U, Gleicher N (eds): Cardiac Problems in Pregnancy. 3rd ed. New York, Wiley-Liss, 1998, pp 407-417.
148. Elkayam U, Singh H, Irani A: Anticoagulation in pregnant women with prosthetic heart valves. Submitted for publication.
149. Vitale N, Defeo M, De Santo LS, et al: Dose-dependent fetal complications of warfarin in pregnant women with mechanical heart valves. J Am Coll Cardiol 33:1637, 1999.
150. Meschengieser SS, Fondevila CG, Santarelli MT, et al: Anticoagulation in pregnant women with mechanical valves prostheses. Heart 82:23, 1999.
151. Sadler L, McCowan L, White H, et al: Pregnancy outcomes and cardiac complications in women with mechanical bioprosthetic and homograft valves. Br J Obstet Gynaecol 17:245, 2000.
152. Laurent P, Dussarat GV, Bonal J, et al: Low molecular weight heparins: A guide to their optimum use in pregnancy. Drugs 62:463, 2002.
153. Ensom MH, Stephenson MD: Low molecular-weight heparins in pregnancy. Pharmacotherapy 19:1013, 1999.
154. Rowan JA, McCowan LM, Raudkivi PJ, et al: Enoxaparin treatment in women with mechanical heart valve during pregnancy. Am J Obstet Gynecol 185:633, 2001.
155. Arnaout MS, Kazma H, Khalil A, et al: Is there a safe anticoagulation protocol for pregnant women with prosthetic valves? Clin Exp Obstet Gynecol 25:101, 1998.
156. Berndt N, Khan I, Gallo R: A complication in anticoagulation using low-molecular weight heparin in a patient with a mechanical valve prosthesis. A case report. J Heart Valve Dis 9:844, 2000.
157. Saw J, Thompson E, Macdonald I: Mechanical valve thrombosis during pregnancy. Can J Cardiol 17:95, 2001.
158. Oles D, Berryessa R, Campbell K, et al: Emergency redo mitral valve replacement in a 27-year-old pregnant female with a clotted prosthetic mitral valve, preoperative fetal demise and postoperative ventricular assist device: A case report. Perfusion 16:159, 2001.
159. Sheshadi N, Goldhaber SZ, Elkayam U, et al: The clinical challenge of bridging anticoagulation in patients with mechanical prosthetic heart valves. Am Heart J (in press).
160. Ginsberg JS, Greer I, Hirsh J: Use of antithrombotic agents during pregnancy. Chest 119:122S, 2001.

GUIDELINES *Thomas H. Lee*

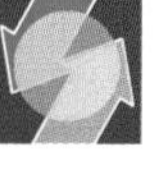

Pregnancy

Recommendations for management of heart disease in pregnancy are included in the 1998 American College of Cardiology/American Heart Association (ACC/AHA) guidelines on valvular disease[1] and in the 2003 ACC/AHA Scientific Statement on warfarin therapy.[2] These guidelines do not recommend routine antibiotic prophylaxis in patients with valvular heart disease undergoing uncomplicated vaginal delivery or cesarean section unless infection is suspected. For high-risk patients, such as those with prosthetic heart valves or prior histories of endocarditis, antibiotics are considered optional.

TABLE 74G–1 Guidelines for Anticoagulation During Pregnancy in Patients with Mechanical Prosthetic Valves

Indication	Class I	Class IIa	Class IIb	Class III
Anticoagulation during pregnancy in patients with mechanical prosthetic valves: Weeks 1 through 35	1. The decision whether to use heparin during the first trimester or to continue oral anticoagulation throughout pregnancy should be made after full discussion with the patient and her partner; if she chooses to change to heparin for the first trimester, she should be made aware that heparin is less safe for her, with a higher risk of both thrombosis and bleeding, and that any risk to the mother also jeopardizes the baby.[2] 2. High-risk women (a history of thromboembolism or an older generation mechanical prosthesis in the mitral position) who choose *not* to take warfarin during the first trimester should receive continuous unfractionated heparin intravenously in a dose to prolong the midinterval (6 hours after dosing) aPTT to two to three times the control value. Transition to warfarin can occur thereafter.	1. In patients receiving warfarin, INR should be maintained between 2.0 and 3.0 with the lowest possible dose of warfarin, and low-dose aspirin should be added.	1. Women at low risk (no history of thromboembolism, newer low-profile prosthesis) may be managed with adjusted-dose subcutaneous heparin (17,500 to 20,000 units b.i.d.) to prolong the midinterval (6 hours after dosing) aPTT to two to three times the control value.	
Anticoagulation during pregnancy in patients with mechanical prosthetic valves: After the 36th week		1. Warfarin should be stopped no later than week 36 and heparin substituted in anticipation of labor. 2. If labor begins during treatment with warfarin, a cesarian section should be performed. 3. In the absence of significant bleeding, heparin can be resumed 4 to 6 hours after delivery and warfarin begun orally.		

aPTT = activated partial thromboplastin time; INR = International Normalized Ratio.

Complex guidelines were offered in the 1998 ACC/AHA guidelines on valvular heart disease for management of anticoagulation in pregnant patients with mechanical prosthetic heart valves (Table 74G–1). These guidelines reflect high complication rates in pregnant women managed with subcutaneous heparin and support use of intravenous heparin during the first trimester. After the 36th week of pregnancy, transition from warfarin to heparin is recommended in anticipation of labor.

The 2003 Scientific Statement on anticoagulation notes a dilemma for physicians managing anticoagulation for pregnant patients. Three options are available:

1. Heparin or low-molecular-weight heparin throughout pregnancy,
2. Warfarin throughout pregnancy, changing to heparin or low-molecular-weight heparin at 38 weeks' gestation with planned labor induction at about 40 weeks, or
3. Heparin or low-molecular-weight heparin in the first trimester of pregnancy, switching to warfarin in the second trimester, continuing it until about 38 weeks' gestation, and then changing to heparin or low-molecular-weight heparin at 38 weeks with planned labor induction at about 40 weeks.

These strategies are complicated by the fact that low-molecular-weight heparin is not approved by the U.S. Food and Drug Administration (FDA) for use in any patients with mechanical prosthetic heart valves, and the FDA has issued an advisory warning against use of enoxaparin (Lovenox) in pregnant women with mechanical prosthetic heart valves. The guidelines note that some data indicate that low-molecular-weight heparin appears to be safe in nonpregnant patients with mechanical heart valves, but the expert panel could not recommend its use directly given the status of FDA-approved indications.

References

1. Bonow RO, Carabello B, de Leon AC Jr, et al: ACC/AHA guidelines for the management of patients with valvular heart disease: Executive summary: A report of the American College of Cardiology/American Heart Association Task Force on Practice Guidelines (Committee on Management of Patients With Valvular Heart Disease). Circulation 98:1949, 1998.
2. Hirsh J, Fuster V, Ansell J, Halperin JL: American Heart Association/American College of Cardiology Foundation guide to warfarin therapy. Circulation 107:1692, 2003.

CHAPTER 75

Cardiovascular Disease in Athletes

Barry J. Maron

Over the past several years interest has heightened considerably among medical practitioners and the lay public regarding the causes of sudden deaths in trained athletes, as well as the clinical significance of cardiac symptoms such as syncope and arrhythmias.[1-4] Catastrophic events in athletes are always unexpected, and although relatively uncommon, often achieve high visibility and convey a particularly devastating impact on the community.[2] Indeed, the possibility that young, highly trained high school, college, or even professional athletes may harbor potentially lethal heart disease[1-8] or are susceptible to sudden death under a variety of circumstances[1,2,9,10] may seem counterintuitive. Over the last several years, a large measure of clarification has resulted with regard to the causes of sudden death during sporting activities, as well as the most appropriate diagnostic and management strategies for this distinct subset of the population with a unique life style.

Causes of Sudden Death

Young Athletes (≤35 Years)

Although the overall athlete population is at low risk,[2] a number of largely congenital (usually unsuspected) cardiovascular diseases, each relatively uncommon in the general population, have been causally linked to exercise-related sudden death in young trained athletes or asymptomatic individuals with active sports-related life styles (Figs. 75–1 and 75–2).[1,2,6,7,11] Indeed, any cardiac disease capable of causing sudden death in young nonathletes can also be responsible for such events in athletes.

Based on autopsy surveys, about 80 percent of deaths in young athletes can be linked to structural cardiovascular disease.[1,2,6,7] In the United States, hypertrophic cardiomyopathy (HCM) has consistently been the single most common cause of such sudden deaths, accounting for about one-third of these events due to cardiovascular disease.[2] HCM is a relatively common genetic cardiac disease (1:500 in the general population) characterized by an asymmetrically hypertrophied and nondilated left ventricle with heterogeneous clinical, morphological, and genetic expression (see Chap. 59).[12,13] Indeed, HCM is the most common cause of sudden cardiac death in young individuals, frequently occurring with physical exertion. Sudden death due to ventricular tachyarrhythmias (see Chap. 32) probably emanates from an electrically unstable (and largely unpredictable) myocardial substrate,[1,2,6,7,11] evidenced by the histopathological markers of disorganized myocardial architecture and replacement scarring (a consequence of microvascular abnormalities and bursts of myocardial ischemia).[12] High-risk HCM patients are considered for primary prevention of sudden death with prophylactic implantation of cardioverter-defibrillators (see Chap. 31).[14]

In addition, not infrequently, hearts are encountered at autopsy with increased left ventricular mass (and wall thickness) and nondilated ventricular cavities, in which other objective morphological findings are suggestive of HCM, although not sufficient to permit definitive diagnosis.[1] In the absence of clinical data, it is uncertain whether such cases represent relatively mild morphological expressions of HCM or possibly unusual examples of marked physiological left ventricular hypertrophy associated with deleterious consequences.

The second most frequent causes of athletic field deaths, accounting for about 20 percent, are congenital coronary artery anomalies of wrong sinus origin (most commonly, left main coronary artery from right sinus of Valsalva) (Fig. 75–3); the mirror image malformation, anomalous right coronary from the left aortic sinus, has also been occasionally incriminated in such deaths (see Chap. 56).[1,2,15] These coronary anomalies may be more common than previously regarded, but diagnosis requires a high index of clinical suspicion, which is crucial given that surgical correction is possible.[15] Diagnosis of the coronary anomalies should be aroused in any young athlete with a history of chest pain or syncope, particularly if symptoms are triggered by exercise.[15,16] Suspicion may be raised with transthoracic echocardiography and identification possible with transesophageal echocardiography, multislice CT imaging, or magnetic resonance imaging (MRI) (see Chaps. 11, 14, and 15), ultimately with full confirmation achieved by coronary arteriography. Large, clinically identified patient cohorts with anomalous coronary artery and long-term follow-up (with or without surgery) are not presently available. Patients usually do not demonstrate abnormalities on 12-lead or exercise electrocardiogram (ECG) since myocardial ischemia is episodic,[15] thereby limiting the power for detection during preparticipation screening. Most likely mechanisms for myocardial ischemia include the acute-angled take-off and kinking at the origin of the left main coronary artery or compression, during exercise, of the anomalous artery between aorta and pulmonary trunk.

In addition, a diverse array of about 15 other congenital or acquired diseases account for only 5 percent or less of all athletic field deaths.[1,2] An unexpectedly high occurrence of premature atherosclerotic coronary artery disease has, however, been noted in some surveys of young athletes and is probably underrecognized in this population (see Chap. 46). Uncommon causes of sudden death include valvular heart disease (aortic stenosis or myxomatous mitral valve degeneration) (see Chap. 57), dilated cardiomyopathy (see Chap. 59), arrhythmogenic right ventricular cardiomyopathy (ARVC)

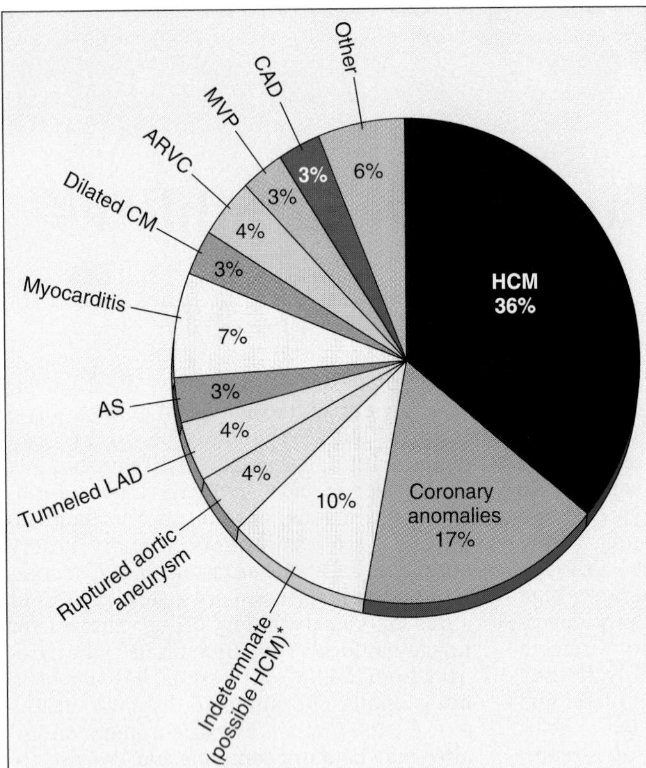

FIGURE 75–1 Causes of sudden cardiac death in young competitive athletes (median age, 17 years) based on systematic tracking in the U.S. Registry. In an additional 2 percent of the patients, no evidence of cardiovascular disease sufficient to explain death was identified at necropsy; *hearts with increased weight and some morphological features consistent with (but not diagnostic of) hypertrophic cardiomyopathy (HCM). LAD = left anterior descending coronary artery; AS = aortic stenosis; CM = cardiomyopathy; ARVC = arrhythmogenic right ventricular cardiomyopathy; MVP = mitral valve prolapse; CAD = coronary artery disease. (Adapted from Maron BJ, Thompson PD, Puffer JC, et al: Cardiovascular preparticipation screening of competitive athletes: A statement for health professionals from the Sudden Death Committee [Clinical Cardiology] and Congenital Cardiac Defects Committee [Cardiovascular Disease in the Young], American Heart Association. Circulation 94:850-856, 1996.)

(see Chap. 32), apparent coronary artery hypoplasia and other rare coronary anomalies, Marfan syndrome (see Chap. 56), and myocarditis (see Chap. 60).

Myocarditis is challenging to diagnose clinically (or at autopsy in the healed phase) and may be manifest only by ECG abnormalities, including heart block and ventricular arrhythmias, in the absence of symptoms. Although the inflammatory process of myocarditis is usually triggered by viral agents (most often enterovirus, but not uncommonly adenovirus), chronic cocaine ingestion can provoke a similar clinical and pathological profile (see Chap. 62).[2,9] Diagnosis is enhanced by testing endomyocardial biopsy specimens for viral genome by the polymerase chain reaction.

Athletes with Marfan syndrome can participate successfully in strenuous competitive sports for many years without experiencing a catastrophic event, presumably before aortic dilation becomes marked and the predisposition to dissection or rupture increases critically. Marfan syndrome may be underdiagnosed, particularly in populations of elite basketball players. ARVC is an uncommon familial cardiac disease, associated with ventricular or supraventricular tachyarrhythmias and sudden death, and characterized largely by diffuse or segmental right ventricular abnormalities with myocyte death, fibrous and adipose tissue replacement and myocarditis[7] resulting in chamber enlargement and systolic dysfunction, and T-wave inversion and epsilon waves in the right precordial ECG leads.[17] In athletes with heart disease, primary ventricular tachyarrhythmias are the predominant mechanism of sudden death, although in Marfan syndrome, demise is usually due to dissection and a ruptured aorta (associated with disruption of aortic media with decreased numbers of elastic fibers), or occasionally an arrhythmia.

Only about 2 percent of young athletes show normal cardiac structure without a definitive cause of death at autopsy.[1] Such deaths are probably due to conditions unassociated with gross or histological cardiac abnormalities, such as ion-channel disorders (long-QT and Brugada syndromes), Wolff-Parkinson-White syndrome, abnormalities of conducting system and microvasculature, catecholaminergic polymorphic ventricular tachycardia or right ventricular outflow tract tachycardia (see Chaps. 29 to 32), coronary vasospasm (see Chap. 46), and subtle morphological forms of HCM or ARVC.[2,7,18,19]

In addition, intramural tunneled coronary arteries (short segments of left anterior descending surrounded by myocardium) are occasionally the sole abnormality found at autopsy.[20] It remains unresolved as to whether these bridged coronary arteries are simply variants of normal or have pathophysiological significance in triggering myocardial ischemia and sudden death during exertion in otherwise healthy young individuals or patients with HCM. Sudden and unexpected arrhythmic death, nonfatal stroke, and acute myocardial infarction in trained athletes have also been attributed to illicit substance abuse with cocaine, anabolic steroids, or dietary and nutritional supplements (particularly ephedrine-containing compounds).[9,10]

Reports from the Veneto region of northeastern Italy provide an alternative profile for the causes of athletic field deaths, with ARVC the most common.[2,7] This unusual prevalence could possibly be due in part to genetic predisposition or, alternatively, the Italian national preparticipation athlete screening program, which probably identifies and disqualifies from competition disproportionately fewer athletes with ARVC than those with other diseases more readily identified during screening (e.g., HCM).[21]

Older Athletes (>35 Years)

Older athletes can also harbor occult cardiac disease and die suddenly and unexpectedly related to participation in athletic activities, usually road racing (including marathon), jogging, rugby, squash, and golf.[4,8] Unlike young athletes, the cause of death in most older conditioned athletes is atherosclerotic coronary artery disease (see Chaps. 47 and 50), with the remainder due to nonischemic diseases such as HCM or valvular heart disease. Many older athletes who have died of coronary heart disease had known risk factors, cardiovascular symptoms, or prior myocardial infarction (or coronary interventions) and severe atherosclerotic narrowing of two or three major extramural arteries with myocardial scarring. Although no strategies are in place for systematically screening older athletes in organized sports, it has been recommended that competitors in master's sports[8] with at least a moderate cardiovascular risk profile for coronary artery disease (≥1 independent risk factors) should undergo, in addition to history and physical examination, exercise (stress) testing before initiating training or competition.

There is overwhelming evidence that the cardiovascular benefits attributable to consistent exercise represent a primary prevention strategy for coronary artery disease in asymptomatic middle-aged and older persons. Although habitual exercise appears to mitigate the likelihood of sudden death in trained individuals (with unsuspected or known coronary artery disease), such events are triggered paradoxically with increased frequency when associated with vigorous exertion in untrained persons.[22] This supports the recommendation in sedentary persons for gradual entry into conditioning programs.[8]

COMMOTIO CORDIS

Virtually instantaneous cardiac arrest may result during sports activities from a relatively modest innocent-appearing and nonpenetrating blunt blow to the chest in the *absence* of underlying cardiovascular disease or structural injury to the chest wall or heart itself (i.e., commotio cordis).[5] Such occurrences are produced either by a projectile (most commonly a baseball, softball, or hockey puck) or by bodily contact with another athlete. The blow to the chest may be delivered with a wide range in velocities but is usually not perceived as particularly unusual for the sporting event nor of sufficient magnitude to result in death. A common scenario is that of a young baseball player struck in the chest (while batting) by a pitched ball thrown from a standard distance. However,

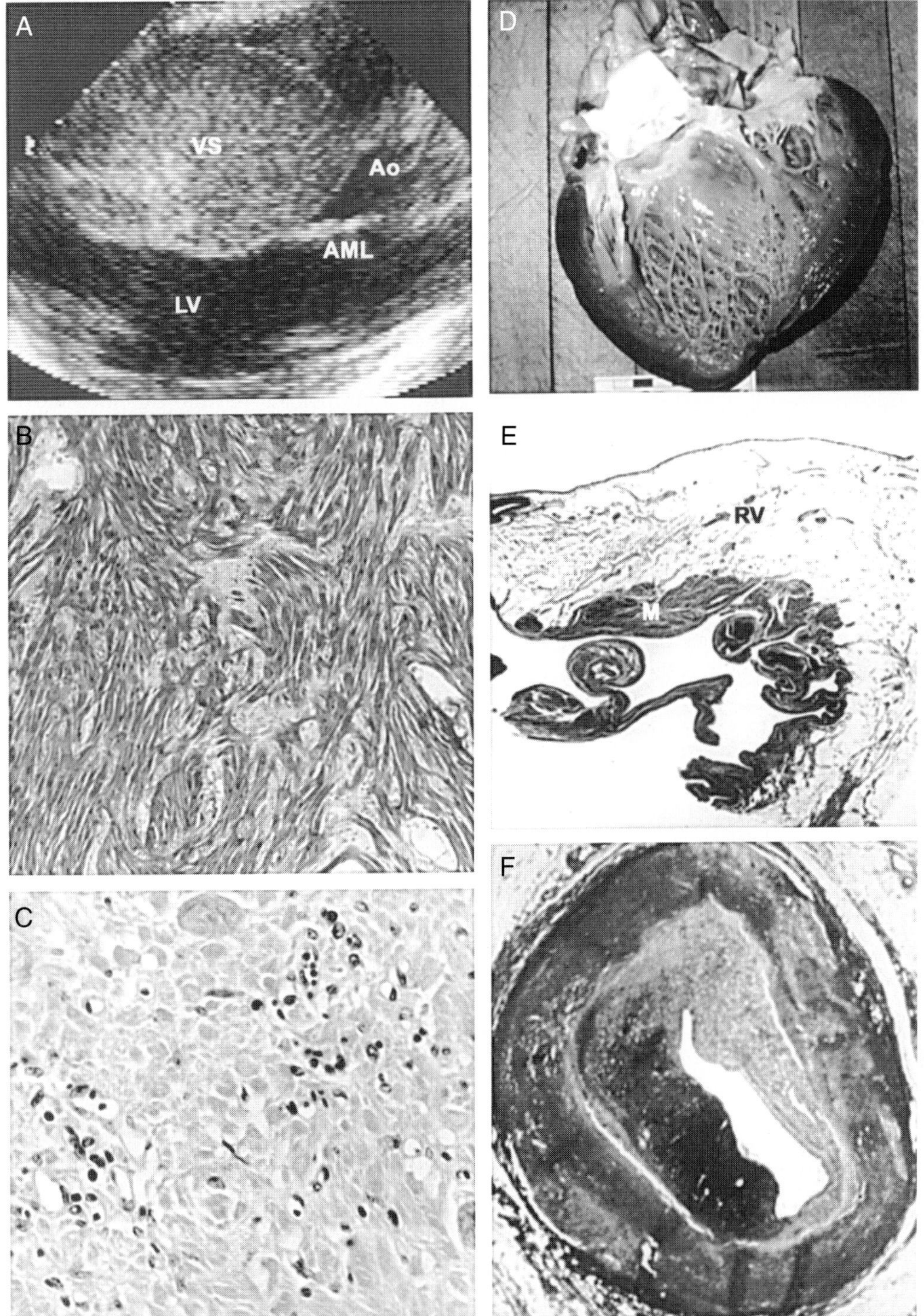

FIGURE 75–2 Causes of sudden cardiac death in young competitive athletes. **A,** Hypertrophic cardiomyopathy. Two-dimensional echocardiogram in parasternal long-axis view showing extreme asymmetrical thickening of the ventricular septum (VS) (i.e., 53 mm). LV = left ventricle; Ao = aorta; AML = anterior mitral leaflet. **B,** Hypertrophic cardiomyopathy. Histopathology showing the substrate of disorganized cardiac muscle cells and chaotic architectural pattern; hematoxylin and eosin stain. **C,** Myocarditis. Area of left ventricular myocardium with clusters of inflammatory mononuclear cells; hematoxylin and eosin stain, ×400. **D,** Idiopathic dilated cardiomyopathy, showing greatly enlarged left ventricular cavity. **E,** Arrhythmogenic right ventricular cardiomyopathy. Histological section of right ventricular (RV) wall showing extensive fatty replacement adjacent to a small area of residual myocytes (M); hematoxylin and eosin stain. **F,** Premature coronary artery disease. Portion of right coronary artery with atherosclerotic narrowing and ruptured plaque. (**A** to **F,** From Maron BJ: Sudden death in young athletes. N Engl J Med 349:1064-1075, 2003.)

many of these events occur in purely recreational situations at home or on the playground (some even unrelated to sports) with the fatal injuries often produced by family members.

Commotio cordis is most common in young children (mean age 13 years) with characteristically pliable chest walls that probably facilitate transmission of the chest impact energy to the myocardium.[5] There appear to be two other major determinants of a commotio cordis event: (1) the chest impact is located directly over the heart; and (2) the timing of the blow occurs precisely in a narrow 20-msec window during repolarization, just prior to the T wave peak, involving activation of the K^+-ATP channel.[23]

Certain measures aimed at prevention of commotio cordis during sports have been considered. Softer-than-normal ("safety") baseballs reduced the risk for ventricular fibrillation in an experimental model, suggesting that modification of athletic equipment could prevent sudden death; however, such projectiles do not provide absolute protection in

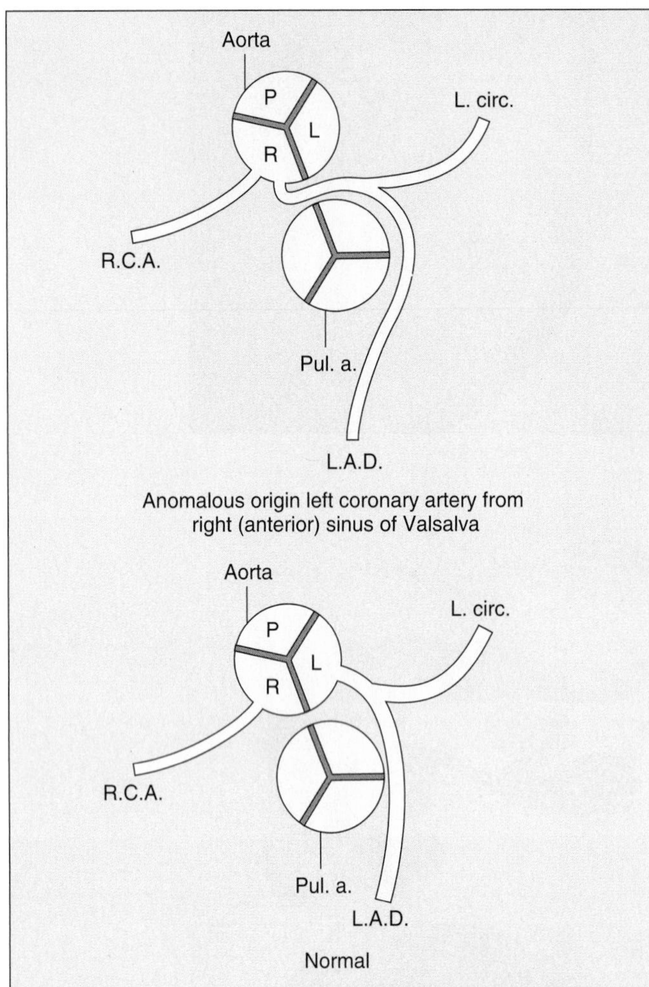

FIGURE 75–3 Congenital coronary artery anomaly of wrong aortic sinus origin, which may cause sudden death in young athletes. **Top,** Anomalous origin of the left main coronary artery arising from right (anterior) sinus of Valsalva. Note acute leftward bend of left main coronary artery at its origin and its posterior course between aorta and pulmonary artery trunk (Pul a.). **Bottom,** Normal coronary artery anatomy is shown for comparison. L.A.D. = left anterior descending; L. circ. = left circumflex; L = left sinus; R = right sinus; P = posterior sinus; R.C.A. = right coronary artery. (From Maron BJ, Epstein SE, Roberts WC: Causes of sudden death in competitive athletes. J Am Coll Cardiol 7:204-214, 1986.)

the field.[5] Greater use of chest barriers that effectively cover the precordium would theoretically protect against commotio cordis in young people competing in sports such as baseball, ice hockey, karate, and lacrosse. However, the infrequency of commotio cordis events remains an obstacle to documenting the effectiveness of any protective intervention.

Commotio cordis events are not uniformly fatal, with reported survival of 15 percent, usually associated with prompt cardiopulmonary resuscitation and defibrillation.[5] With enhanced public awareness of this syndrome and more widespread dissemination of automatic external defibrillators, effective emergency measures are likely to be implemented more rapidly on the athletic field, avoiding many future catastrophes.

Frequency and Demographics of Sudden Death in Athletes

Based largely on data assembled from U.S. populations, a profile of young competitive athletes with sudden death has emerged.[1,2,6] In young athletes, the frequency of sudden unexpected death due to cardiovascular disease during competitive sports appears to be low, occurring in about 1:200,000 individual student athletes per academic year and in about 1:70,000 over a 3-year high school career.[2] In comparison, older athletes have somewhat higher rates of exercise-related sudden death, reported to be from 1:15,000 to 1:50,000 per year.[2] Such estimates suggest that the intense and persistent public interest in these tragic events is disproportionate to their significance in numerical terms. However, such data are limited, and there is circumstantial evidence that the overall importance of this public health problem may have been underestimated. Regardless of prevalence, however, the social and emotional impact of an athlete dying suddenly (often fueled by the news media) is substantial, given the widely held perception that trained athletes epitomize the healthiest element of our society.[2]

Sudden death due to cardiovascular disease has been reported in a wide variety of sports, most commonly basketball and football in the United States[1,2] and soccer in Europe,[7,15,21] and is much more common in males (9:1), probably due to the overall lower participation rates of females and their absence from certain competitive sports (e.g., football). HCM is the most common cause of sudden cardiac death in previously undiagnosed young African American male athletes, contrasting sharply with the underrepresentation of African Americans in clinically identified HCM populations.[6] This suggests HCM is underdiagnosed in African Americans and that socioeconomic status and ethnicity may impact significantly on the access to cardiovascular diagnosis and ultimately the clinical identification of this disease.

The association of sudden death and unsuspected cardiovascular disease in young athletes does not appear coincidental.[24] Vigorous physical exertion in the context of competitive sports can act as a trigger for lethal ventricular arrhythmias and sudden death on the athletic field in certain susceptible athletes with underlying structural heart disease.[1-4,6,24] Indeed, most deaths in young athletes (i.e., 90 percent) occur on the athletic field during training or competition, predominantly in the late afternoon and early evening hours corresponding to the peak period of the day for intense physical activity, particularly with organized team sports.[1] Sudden cardiac death is not, however, limited to competitive athletes since similar tragedies can occur in young people during recreational or even sedentary activities.

Clinical Evaluation of Young Athletes

Young trained athletes present a unique challenge for cardiological assessment due to the many diverse alterations in cardiac physiology, structure, rhythm, and ECG pattern that can result from chronic conditioning and occasionally mimic pathological conditions.[2,4] Furthermore, despite the absence of cardiac symptoms, such highly conditioned individuals can in fact harbor unsuspected cardiovascular disease.[1,2,6,7]

Suspicion of cardiovascular disease in a trained athlete may arise by virtue of findings on preparticipation screening, onset of symptoms such as syncope, or fortuitously by recognition of a heart murmur on routine examination.[2,11] Thereafter, the preferred strategy should focus on systematically targeting with testing each of the heart diseases known to cause sudden death in young people until a cardiovascular abnormality is identified or each is effectively excluded (with priority afforded the most common). Since most of these causes of sudden death in young athletes are structural and functional abnormalities (e.g., HCM, coronary anomalies, valvular heart disease, ARVC, and myocarditis), tests such as echocardiography and possibly MRI become important implements in the differential diagnosis. Standard 12-lead

ECG (see Chap. 9) targets ion-channel diseases such as long-QT and Brugada syndromes,[11,18] and arrhythmia on ambulatory (Holter) ECG (see Chap. 29) may raise suspicion of diseases such as myocarditis, which otherwise may have subtle expression. The list of diseases shown in Table 75–1 serves as the basis for this differential diagnosis in athletes suspected as having cardiovascular disease.

Episodes of impaired consciousness including syncope, near-syncope, or frequent dizziness (as well as palpitations) are challenging symptoms in young athletes.[16] These symptoms, particularly when exertional, require careful investigation (initially with history, physical examination, ECG, echocardiography, and ambulatory Holter monitoring) to resolve the critical diagnostic distinction between structural heart disease and the physiological causes of impaired consciousness such as neurocardiogenic (neurally mediated) (see Chap. 34), hypotension, carotid sinus hypersensitivity, dehydration, supraventricular tachycardia, or hyperventilation.[16] Since this assessment has important clinical implications, aggressive differential diagnosis with a high index of suspicion is necessary to define the cause of syncope and initiate treatment when appropriate. Pathological causes of syncope should be excluded first, since physiological etiologies are often a matter of clinical judgment or a diagnosis of exclusion employing exercise and tilt-table testing, serial Holter ECGs, or implanted loop-monitor recordings.

TABLE 75–1 Causes of Sudden Death in 387 Young Athletes*

Cause	No. of Athletes (%)
Hypertrophic cardiomyopathy	102 (26)
Commotio cordis	77 (20)
Coronary artery anomalies	53 (14)
LVH—indeterminate etiology†	29 (7)
Myocarditis	20 (5)
Ruptured aortic aneurysm (Marfan syndrome)	12 (3)
ARVC	11 (3)
Tunneled (bridged) coronary artery‡	11 (3)
Aortic valve stenosis	10 (2.5)
Atherosclerotic CAD	10 (2.5)
Dilated cardiomyopathy	9 (2)
Myxomatous mitral valve degeneration	9 (2)
Asthma (or other pulmonary)	8 (2)
Heat stroke	6 (1.5)
Drug abuse	4 (1)
Other cardiovascular	4 (1)
Long-QT syndrome¶	3 (1)
Cardiac sarcoidosis	3 (1)
Trauma§	3 (1)
Ruptured cerebral artery	3 (1)

*From the registry of the Minneapolis Heart Institute Foundation.[1,5,6]
†Findings at autopsy suggestive of hypertrophic cardiomyopathy, but insufficient to be diagnostic.
‡In the absence of any other cardiac abnormality.
§Involving structural bodily injury.
¶Documented on clinical evaluation.
ARVC = arrhythmogenic right ventricular cardiomyopathy; CAD = coronary artery disease; LVH = left ventricular hypertrophy.

Asymptomatic trained athletes without structural heart disease are subject to certain arrhythmias or conduction alterations, largely due to the heightened vagal tone that accompanies physical conditioning, and which usually do not require invasive investigation or specific treatment. These arrhythmias include sinus arrhythmia or tachycardia or bradyarrhythmia, premature atrial or ventricular couplets, supraventricular tachycardia, junctional rhythm, and first degree or Wenckebach (Mobitz type I) atrioventricular block (see Chaps. 31 and 32).[4] Also, complex ectopy on ambulatory Holter ECG monitoring including frequent ventricular or supraventricular premature complexes, couplets, and even nonsustained ventricular tachycardia does not confer ominous prognosis nor usually require drug treatment in athletes without structural heart disease, but it may be challenging to distinguish such benign arrhythmias from those caused by inflammatory myocardial disease.[25]

Athlete's Heart

"Athlete's heart" due to endurance (dynamic; aerobic) or isometric (static; power) sports involves a complex and heterogeneous profile of physiological, morphological, and ECG alterations secondary to systematic and often intense physical training.[2] Physiological adaptations include increased stroke volume and cardiac output, arteriovenous oxygen difference, and maximum oxygen consumption as well as reduced basal heart rate. Conditioning often triggers structural remodeling, usually with modest alterations in dimensions: increased left ventricular mass, left and right ventricular and atrial chamber enlargement, and occasionally increased left ventricular wall thickness, all in the presence of preserved systolic and diastolic function.[26-31] This physiological form of hypertrophy (i.e., athlete's heart) is generally regarded as a benign adaptation to systematic training unassociated with adverse cardiovascular consequences. Physiological increases in cardiac mass vary in magnitude according to sporting discipline, with the most extreme left ventricular cavity dimensions and/or wall thicknesses reported with rowing, cross-country skiing, cycling, and swimming,[26,29,30] although paradoxically less pronounced with ultraendurance sports.[27,29] Isometric training (e.g., weight lifting or wrestling) is associated with left ventricular wall thickness that is normal in absolute terms (≤12 mm) but disproportionately large in relation to cavity size. Abnormal cardiac dimensions associated with athletic training are related to body surface area or lean body mass and consequently are less pronounced in female athletes.[26,29] Other physiological adaptations include a variety of abnormal 12-lead ECG patterns in about 40 percent of athletes, sometimes reminiscent of cardiac disease with greatly increased precordial voltages, Q waves, and repolarization abnormalities (see Chap. 9).[31] ACE/DD genotype has been associated with the magnitude of exercise-induced left ventricular hypertrophy in endurance athletes.[2]

Athlete's Heart and Cardiovascular Disease

Clinical distinctions between physiological athlete's heart and pathological conditions have critical implications for trained athletes, since cardiovascular disease may be the basis for disqualification from intense competitive sports to reduce the risk for sudden death or disease progression.[32,33] Alternatively, overdiagnosis can lead to unnecessary restriction, depriving athletes of the psychological or monetary benefits of sports.[2]

Indeed, adaptations of athlete's heart can mimic cardiovascular disease when cardiac dimensions fall outside

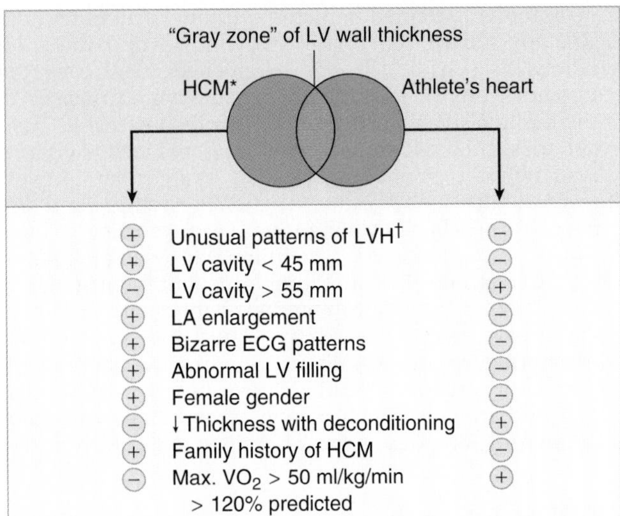

FIGURE 75–4 Chart depicting the criteria used to distinguish hypertrophic cardiomyopathy (HCM) from athlete's heart when the left ventricular (LV) wall thickness is within the shaded "gray zone" of overlap (13 to 15 mm), consistent with both diagnoses. *Assumed to be the nonobstructive form of HCM in this discussion, since the presence of substantial mitral valve systolic anterior motion would confirm, per se, the diagnosis of HCM in an athlete. †May involve a variety of abnormalities, including heterogeneous distribution of left ventricular hypertrophy (LVH) in which asymmetry is prominent, and adjacent regions may be of greatly different thicknesses, with sharp transitions evident between segments; also, patterns in which the anterior ventricular septum is spared from the hypertrophic process and the region of predominant thickening may be in the posterior portion of septum or anterolateral or posterior free wall. ↓ = decreased; LA = left atrial; ECG = electrocardiograph. (From Maron BJ, Pelliccia A, Spirito P: Cardiac disease in young trained athletes: Insights into methods for distinguishing athlete's heart from structural heart disease with particular emphasis on hypertrophic cardiomyopathy. Circulation 91:1596-1601, 1995.)

clinically accepted partition values, most frequently raising a differential diagnosis with hypertrophic and dilated cardiomyopathies or ARVC.[7,12,26] For example, about 2 percent of highly trained adult male athletes show mildly increased left ventricular wall thicknesses of 13 to 15 mm, which define a "gray zone" where extreme expressions of athlete's heart and mild morphological forms of HCM overlap (Fig. 75–4).[2,32] Such diagnostic ambiguity can often be resolved with noninvasive testing, such as the response of cardiac mass to short periods of deconditioning, or assessment of diastolic filling with Doppler echocardiography.[32] DNA-based laboratory testing strategies are not presently available on a routine clinical basis to provide definitive diagnostic resolution between genetic heart disease and athlete's heart.

Extreme cardiac dimensions evident in some highly trained athletes unavoidably raise the consideration of whether such adaptations are truly physiological and innocent. For example, about 15 percent of highly trained athletes show striking left ventricular cavity enlargement (end-diastolic dimension ≥ 60 mm) similar to that found in dilated cardiomyopathy[26]; after deconditioning, incomplete reversal with substantial residual chamber dilation is not uncommonly evident, suggesting the possibility that extreme physiologically induced ventricular remodeling could have adverse clinical consequences over long periods of time.[30]

Preparticipation Screening for Cardiovascular Abnormalities

Detection of cardiovascular disease with the potential for significant morbidity or sudden death is an objective of large population preparticipation screening in high school- and college-age athletes.[11] Although the degree to which screening reduces risk for sudden death is unknown, it is nevertheless a widely held practice with the potential for identifying athletes with heart disease.[11]

Athletic screening for both U.S. high school- and college-aged student athletes customarily includes a personal and family history and physical examination.[11] However, the effectiveness of these routine evaluations has been questioned.[34,35] For high school athletes, approved history and physical questionnaires (that serve to guide the examiners) are suboptimal or nonexistent in about 40 percent of the states. Indeed, in one retrospective study, potentially lethal cardiovascular abnormalities were suspected by preparticipation history and physical examination in only 3 percent of high school and college athletes who ultimately died suddenly of these diseases. An American Heart Association consensus panel[11] proposed more comprehensive and targeted preparticipation screening to enhance the likelihood that important cardiovascular abnormalities would be suspected and subsequently identified by cardiovascular testing. Improved design of history and physical examination screening would undoubtedly result in the detection of greater numbers of athletes unknowingly harboring clinically relevant cardiovascular abnormalities, and represents the most practical future strategy for preparticipation screening. History and physical screening alone can be expected to result in the identification of many athletes, such as those with aortic stenosis or other valvular heart disease, HCM with outflow obstruction, Marfan syndrome, and premature coronary artery disease.[11]

By virtue of being abnormal in up to 95 percent of HCM patients,[12] the 12-lead ECG empowers preparticipation screening programs to identify many previously undiagnosed athletes with HCM (and other) diseases.[21] Indeed, although the addition of noninvasive testing (e.g., echocardiography or ECG) to the screening process would undoubtedly enhance detection of several diseases capable of causing sudden death, this is probably an unrealistic aspiration on a national scale in the United States due to prohibitive cost-efficacy considerations and other practical obstacles. Routine preparticipation screening of single athletes (or small groups) in office practice involves a noninvasive cardiovascular evaluation initially, including ECG and echocardiography.

APPROACH TO THE PATIENT

Athletes presenting with impaired consciousness (syncope, near-syncope, or frequent dizziness) or palpitations, and asymptomatic athletes with suspicious findings on preparticipation screening (e.g., heart murmur or family history of sudden death), should be systematically assessed by initially excluding those cardiovascular diseases known to cause sudden death in young athletes: most commonly HCM, congenital coronary anomalies of wrong sinus origin (which requires a high index of suspicion), and premature atherosclerotic coronary artery disease. In addition to the history and physical examination, noninvasive clinical assessment can include echocardiography, ECG and MRI, and ambulatory (Holter) monitoring when appropriate. If structural heart disease is excluded, physiological causes of syncope such as neurocardiogenic (neurally mediated) conditions should be investigated by stress exercise, tilt-table testing, and implanted loop-monitor recording. Older athletes, for whom the primary consideration is atherosclerotic coronary artery disease, should undergo exercise stress testing before initiating training or competition, particularly when risk factors are evident or following long periods of sedentary life style.

Eligibility Considerations for Athletes with Cardiovascular Disease

When a cardiovascular abnormality is identified in a trained athlete, several considerations arise, including (1) the level of risk for sudden death incurred by continued participation in competitive sports; (2) the likelihood that this risk will be reduced by withdrawing the athlete from training and competition; and (3) the appropriate criteria to be used for formulating eligibility or disqualification decisions.

The 26th Bethesda Conference[33] affords prospective, expert consensus panel recommendations for athletic eligibility and disqualification, taking into account the severity of relevant cardiovascular abnormalities, as well as the intensity of sports training and competition.

The risks associated with sports and the extent to which disqualification reduces sudden death risk cannot be determined with precision for individual participants. However, the temporary or permanent withdrawal of selected athletes with cardiovascular disease from competitive athletics is widely regarded as a prudent strategy.[33] Fundamental to these recommendations are the premises that intense physical activity places athletes with heart disease at increased risk for sudden death and that the unique pressures of organized sports do not permit athletes to exert strict control over their level of exertion and reliably discern when cardiac symptoms arise and it is prudent to terminate competition.[33]

For example, under the Bethesda guidelines,[33] young athletes with unequivocal HCM are discouraged from participation in most competitive sports with the exception of those of low intensity (e.g., golf and bowling). However, the medical disqualification process can become polarized when the personal freedoms and aspirations of the athlete conflict with the physician mandate to protect patients from circumstances that provoke an unacceptable risk for morbidity and mortality.[2,3] Advocating the return of athletes with ventricular arrhythmias to competition based on the implantation of a cardioverter-defibrillator is not advised.

REFERENCES

1. Maron BJ, Shirani J, Poliac LC, et al: Sudden death in young competitive athletes: Clinical, demographic, and pathological profiles. JAMA 276:199-204, 1996.
2. Maron BJ: Sudden death in young athletes. N Engl J Med 349:1064-1075, 2003.
3. Maron BJ, Mitten MJ, Quandt EK, et al: Competitive athletes with cardiovascular disease—the case of Nicholas Knapp. N Engl J Med 339:1632-1635, 1998.
4. Estes NAM, Link MS, Cannom D, et al: Report of the NASPE Policy Conference on Arrhythmias and the Athlete. J Cardiovasc Electrophysiol 12:1208-1219, 2001.
5. Maron BJ, Gohman TE, Kyle SB, et al: Clinical profile and spectrum of commotio cordis. JAMA 287:1142-1146, 2002.
6. Maron BJ, Carney KP, Lever HM, et al: Relationship of race to sudden cardiac death in competitive athletes with hypertrophic cardiomyopathy. J Am Coll Cardiol 41:974-980, 2003.
7. Corrado D, Basso C, Thiene G, et al: Spectrum of clinicopathologic manifestations of arrhythmogenic right ventricular cardiomyopathy/dysplasia: A multicenter study. J Am Coll Cardiol 30:1512-1520, 1997.
8. Maron BJ, Araújo CGS, Thompson PD, et al: Recommendations for preparticipation screening and the assessment of cardiovascular diseases in masters athletes. An Advisory for Healthcare Professionals from the Working Groups of the World Heart Federation, the International Federation of Sports Medicine, and the American Heart Association Committee on Exercise, Cardiac Rehabilitation, and Prevention. Circulation 103:327-334, 2001.
9. Lange RA, Hillis LD: Cardiovascular complications of cocaine use. N Engl J Med 345:351-358, 2001.
10. Samenuk D, Link MS, Homoud MK, et al: Adverse cardiovascular events temporally associated with ma huang, an herbal source of ephedrine. Mayo Clin Proc 77:12-16, 2002.

Causes of Sudden Death

11. Maron BJ, Thompson PD, Puffer JC, et al: Cardiovascular preparticipation screening of competitive athletes: A statement for health professionals from the Sudden Death Committee (Clinical Cardiology) and Congenital Cardiac Defects Committee (Cardiovascular Disease in the Young), American Heart Association. Circulation 94:850-856, 1996.
12. Maron BJ: Hypertrophic cardiomyopathy: A systematic review. JAMA 287:1308-1320, 2002.
13. Seidman JG, Seidman CE: The genetic basis for cardiomyopathy: From mutation identification to mechanistic paradigms. Cell 104:557-567, 2001.
14. Maron BJ, Shen W-K, Link MS, et al: Efficacy of implantable cardioverter-defibrillators for the prevention of sudden death in patients with hypertrophic cardiomyopathy. N Engl J Med 342:365-373, 2000.
15. Basso C, Maron BJ, Corrado D, Thiene G: Clinical profile of congenital coronary artery anomalies with origin from the wrong aortic sinus leading to sudden death in young competitive athletes. J Am Coll Cardiol 35:1493-1501, 2000.
16. Goldschlager N, Epstein AE, Grub BP, et al: Etiologic considerations in the patient with syncope and an apparently normal heart. Arch Intern Med 163:151-162, 2003.
17. McKenna WJ, Thiene G, Nava A, et al: Diagnosis of arrhythmogenic right ventricular dysplasia/cardiomyopathy. Br Heart J 71:215-218, 1994.
18. Brugada J, Brugada R, Antzelevitch C, et al: Long-term follow-up of individuals with the electrocardiographic pattern of right bundle branch block and ST segment elevation in precordial leads V_1 to V_3. Circulation 105:73-78, 2002.
19. Priori SG, Napolitano C, Memmi M, et al: Clinical and molecular characterization of patients with catecholaminergic polymorphic ventricular tachycardia. Circulation 106:69-74, 2002.
20. Yetman AJ, McCrindle BW, MacDonald C, et al: Myocardial bridging in children with hypertrophic cardiomyopathy—a risk factor for sudden death. N Engl J Med 339:1201-1209, 1998.
21. Corrado D, Basso C, Schiavon M, et al: Screening for hypertrophic cardiomyopathy in young athletes. N Engl J Med 339:364-369, 1998.
22. Albert CM, Mittleman MA, Chae CU, et al: Triggering of sudden death by vigorous exertion. N Engl J Med 343:1355-1361, 2000.

Commotio Cordis

23. Link MS, Wang PJ, Pandian NG, et al: An experimental model of sudden death due to low-energy chest-wall impact (commotio cordis). N Engl J Med 338:1805-1811, 1998.

Frequency and Demographics of Sudden Death in Athletes

24. Corrado D, Basso C, Rizzoli G, et al: Does sports activity enhance the risk of sudden death in adolescents and young adults? J Am Coll Cardiol 42:1959-1963, 2003.

Clinical Evaluation of Young Athletes

25. Biffi A, Pelliccia A, Verdile L, et al: Long-term clinical significance of frequent and complex ventricular tachyarrhythmias in trained athletes. J Am Coll Cardiol 40:446-452, 2002.

Athlete's Heart

26. Pelliccia A, Culasso F, Di Paolo F, et al: Physiologic left ventricular cavity dilatation in elite athletes. Ann Intern Med 130:23-31, 1999.
27. Douglas PS, O'Toole ML, Katz SE, et al: Left ventricular hypertrophy in athletes. Am J Cardiol 80:1384-1388, 1997.
28. Abernethy WB, Choo JK, Hutter AM Jr: Echocardiographic characteristics of professional football players. J Am Coll Cardiol 41:280-284, 2003.
29. Pluim BM, Zwinderman AH, van der Laarse A, van der Wall EE: The athlete's heart: A meta-analysis of cardiac structure and function. Circulation 100:336-344, 1999.
30. Pelliccia A, Maron BJ, de Luca R, et al: Remodeling of left ventricular hypertrophy in elite athletes after long-term deconditioning. Circulation 105:944-949, 2002.
31. Pelliccia A, Maron BJ, Culasso F, et al: Clinical significance of abnormal electrocardiographic patterns in trained athletes. Circulation 102:278-284, 2000.
32. Maron BJ, Pelliccia A, Spirito P: Cardiac disease in young trained athletes: Insights into methods for distinguishing athlete's heart from structural heart disease with particular emphasis on hypertrophic cardiomyopathy. Circulation 91:1596-1601, 1995.
33. Maron BJ, Mitchell JH: 26th Bethesda Conference: Recommendations for determining eligibility for competition in athletes with cardiovascular abnormalities. J Am Coll Cardiol 24:845-899, 1994.

Preparticipation Screening for Cardiovascular Abnormalities

34. Glover DW, Maron BJ: Profile of preparticipation cardiovascular screening for high school athletes. JAMA 279:1817-1819, 1998.
35. Pfister GC, Puffer JC, Maron BJ: Preparticipation cardiovascular screening for U.S. collegiate student-athletes. JAMA 283:1597-1599, 2000.

CHAPTER 76

Medical Management of the Patient Undergoing Cardiac Surgery

David H. Adams • Farzan Filsoufi • Elliott M. Antman

Continued advances in cardiac surgery make operative repair of a variety of cardiac lesions a viable therapeutic alternative for numerous patients with cardiovascular disease. These advances include improvements in tools for assessment of perioperative risk, surgical and anesthesia techniques for myocardial revascularization, valve repair and replacement, and repair of complex congenital cardiac defects, as well as new approaches to management of patients with left ventricular dysfunction and cardiac arrhythmias.[1-3a,3b] Advances relating to minimally invasive cardiac surgical procedures have added additional options in the comprehensive care of patients with surgical cardiovascular disease.[4-10] Perioperative medical and surgical supportive measures have progressed, including the proliferation of intraoperative transesophageal echocardiography,[11] ventricular assist devices, pharmacological supportive strategies, glucose management algorithms, and comprehensive blood conservation programs. Evidence suggests that translation of these improvements into routine surgical practice and institution of regular quality-control surveillance measures have led to a reduction in risk-adjusted operative mortality for coronary artery bypass grafting (CABG) to less than 2 percent for the general population and 2 to 4 percent for the Medicare population.[12-15] However, the profile of patients referred for surgery has also changed and includes more patients with advanced age, depressed left ventricular function, multiple comorbidities, prior revascularization operations or multiple percutaneous interventions, and failed acute interventional procedures, which has led to higher mortality rates in tertiary care referral centers that are called on to operate on such patients with greater frequency.[16-27]

This chapter summarizes the information required by the cardiologist, whose important responsibilities include collaboration with the surgical team for both preoperative and postoperative care, especially care of the medical complications that may develop.

Preoperative Evaluation

GENERAL MEDICAL CONDITION. Except for life-threatening conditions (e.g., proximal aortic dissection, cardiogenic shock caused by ruptured papillary muscle in acute myocardial infarction, penetrating wound of the heart), it behooves the consulting cardiologist to assess the overall medical condition of the patient and advise the surgical team if postponement of the operation seems warranted (Table 76–1). Particular attention should be paid to the patient's potential for development of one or more of the following complications: (1) bleeding during cardiopulmonary bypass while heparinized or while anticoagulated after insertion of a mechanical heart valve prosthesis or in the setting of postoperative atrial fibrillation; (2) deterioration in renal function; (3) arrhythmias due to electrolyte imbalance; (4) sepsis from incompletely treated pulmonary, urinary tract, or dental infection or dermatological infection over the sternum or saphenous vein harvest site; (5) need for prolonged ventilatory support postoperatively because of underlying pulmonary disease or preoperative malnutrition; and (6) exacerbation of a neurological deficit because of carotid artery disease or prior stroke.[28-37] When perioperative intraaortic balloon pump support may be needed, the iliofemoral circulation should be assessed bilaterally. Of note, the use of sheathless, small-caliber balloon pump catheters reduces the risk of limb ischemia.[38] Despite the increased risk of perioperative morbidity and mortality, recent data indicate that patients with combined coronary artery disease and peripheral vascular disease have a greater likelihood of long-term survival and freedom from myocardial infarction with CABG versus medical therapy, particularly in the presence of two- and three-vessel coronary artery disease.[39]

The *protein-calorie malnutrition* associated with cardiac cachexia has been shown to compromise cardiac function and is associated with a greater risk of respiratory failure, sepsis, and prolonged hospitalization. If the clinical situation allows, patients with cardiac cachexia should receive a few weeks of preoperative nutritional support before undergoing elective cardiac surgery.

RISK FACTORS FOR CARDIAC MORBIDITY AND MORTALITY. Risk factors for morbidity and mortality after coronary revascularization surgery have been analyzed extensively.[40-46] A relatively new but widely used, simple clinical severity scoring system (EuroSCORE) is shown in Tables 76–2 to 76–4. This simple additive scoring system has been validated in different patient cohorts in both Europe and the United States. Recently a full logistic version of EuroSCORE has been developed and is capable of even more accurate risk prediction for a particular patient undergoing cardiac surgery (Table 76–5).[47-51] Patients with low-risk scores may be candidates for "fast-track" cost-saving measures such as admission on the day of surgery or early extubation postoperatively; however, those with higher-risk scores will likely experience increased morbidity, require longer intensive care unit (ICU) stays and more consultations by specialists, and consume a greater proportion of medical resources overall. Furthermore, clinical

TABLE 76–1 Preoperative Laboratory Evaluation of Patients Undergoing Cardiac Surgery

Preoperative Laboratory Test	Abnormal Finding	Comment
Complete blood count	1. Anemia, especially Hct <35% 2. WBC >10,000	1. Anticipate that hemodilution will occur on cardiopulmonary bypass and blood loss will occur intraoperatively. In stable patients, preoperative iron supplementation (weeks) or erythropoietin therapy (days) should be considered. Patients with unstable angina, congestive heart failure, aortic stenosis, and left main coronary artery disease should be advised against autologous donation of blood in the preoperative period. 2. Search for possible infection.
Coagulation screen	1. Prolonged bleeding time 2. Elevated PT and/or PTT 3. Thrombocytopenia	Any of these laboratory abnormities suggest that the patient is at risk for bleeding postoperatively and may have excessive chest tube drainage. Corrective measures (e.g., vitamin K, fresh frozen plasma, platelet transfusions) should be considered preoperatively, and surgery may need to be postponed. Hematological consultation may be required if there is reason to suspect an inherited defect in coagulation (e.g., von Willebrand factor deficiency) or heparin-induced thrombocytopenia.
Chemistry profile	1. Elevated BUN/creatine 2. Potassium <4.0 mEq/liter and/or magnesium <2.0 mEq/liter 3. Abnormal liver function tests	1. Abnormal renal function that may worsen in the perioperative period (caused by nonpulsatile flow on cardiopulmonary bypass and potential low flow postoperatively); may necessitate temporary or even permanent hemodialysis. 2. Electrolyte deficits may place the patient at risk of arrhythmias perioperatively and should be corrected before induction of anesthesia. 3. Patient may clear anesthetic agents as well as other cardioactive drugs more slowly. Low albumin level may indicate a state of relative malnutrition that may need to be corrected with nutritional support perioperatively.
Stool Hematest	Positive for occult blood	Because heparinization will take place while on the cardiopulmonary bypass apparatus, the patient may be at risk for GI bleeding perioperatively. The source of GI heme loss should be investigated perioperatively if clinical circumstances permit. The potential for bleeding in the future may influence the choice of prosthetic valve inserted.
Pulmonary function	Reduced VC or prolonged FEV_1	Anticipate longer than usual process of waning from ventilator postoperatively if FEV_1 <65% of VC or FEV_1 <1.5-2.0 liters. Obtain baseline arterial blood gas analysis on room air to help guide respiratory management postoperatively.
Thyroid function	These tests are not ordered routinely but should be performed in cases of suspected hypothyroidism or hyperthyroidism, known thyroid dysfunction during replacement therapy, and atrial fibrillation in patients who have not undergone evaluation of thyroid function.	Hypothyroid patients require prolonged period of ventilatory support postoperatively because of slower clearance of anesthetic agents. Hyperthyroid patients have a hypermetabolic state that places them at increased risk of myocardial ischemia, vasomotor instability, and poorly controlled ventricular rate in atrial fibrillation.
Echocardiography	1. Decreased LV ejection fraction 2. Decreased RV function 3. Aortic stenosis 4. Aortic insufficiency 5. Mitral insufficiency 6. LV aneurysm 7. Ventricular septal defect	1. Patients with decreased LV function are at higher perioperative risk for surgery. Selected patients should undergo viability assessment. 2. RV function increases perioperative risk and identification may lead to preoperative assessment of reversibility of pulmonary hypertension. 3. Mild to moderate aortic stenosis (gradient <25 mm Hg) may be treated by prophylactic valve replacement in selected low-risk patients. 4. Ventricular dimension helps guide decisions to perform valve replacement in addition to revascularization in patients with combined aortic regurgitation and coronary disease. 5. Moderate or severe mitral regurgitation may warrant valve exploration in patients undergoing coronary revascularization. 6. This may alert surgeons to the need of aneurysmectomy in selected patients. 7. Identification suggests the need for early surgical intervention.
Cardiac catheterization	1. Elevated LV end-diastolic pressure and pulmonary capillary wedge pressure 2. Elevated right atrial pressure	1. May remain elevated in the early postoperative period and indicate a need for careful attention to maintenance of adequate preload postoperatively. 2. May reflect tricuspid regurgitation or RV dysfunction from prior infarction. Such patients require vigorous volume expansion postoperatively to maintain adequate cardiac output.

TABLE 76–1 Preoperative Laboratory Evaluation of Patients Undergoing Cardiac Surgery—cont'd

Preoperative Laboratory Test	Abnormal Finding	Comment
	3. Elevated pulmonary artery pressure (and pulmonary vascular resistance)	3. Fixed pulmonary vascular resistance should be suspected when the pulmonary artery diastolic pressure exceeds the mean pulmonary capillary wedge pressure. Vigorous oxygenation and pharmacological support with a pulmonary vasodilator (isoproterenol, prostaglandin E) are important in such cases. Patients with a pulmonary artery diastolic pressure equal to the pulmonary capillary wedge pressure usually have more rapid resolution of pulmonary hypertension postoperatively.
	4. LV mural thrombus	4. Increased risk of stroke perioperatively.
	5. Status of internal mammary arteries	5. Highly desirable arterial conduits for planned revascularization surgery.[40,41] Particular care is required during reoperation if patent internal mammary artery bypass is in place from previous surgery.
	6. Status of saphenous vein grafts	6. "Pseudoextravasation" of dye outside the lumen in a patent graft with slow flow probably represents thrombus-filled atherosclerotic aneurysm of the graft.
Vascular Doppler	1. Carotid stenosis	1. Suggests and increased risk of perioperative stroke. If symptomatic or if stenosis >80%, consideration for combined or staged carotid surgery.
	2. Aortic iliac disease	2. May contraindicate insertion of an intraaortic balloon pump and suggests increased risk of peripheral vascular complications.
	3. Absent or varicosed veins	3. In patients with severe varicosities or who have undergone venous stripping, alternative conduits such as bilateral internal mammary arteries or radial grafts must be considered.

BUN = blood urea nitrogen; FEV_1 = volume of air expired in 1 second; GI = gastrointestinal; Hct = hematocrit; LV = left ventricular; PT = prothrombin time; PTT = partial prothrombin time; RV = right ventricular; VC = vital capacity; WBC = white blood cell count.

TABLE 76–2 Risk Factors, Definitions, and Weights (Score)

Risk Factor	Definition	Score
Patient-Related Factors		
Age	Per 5 years or part thereof >60 yr)	1
Sex	Female	1
Chronic pulmonary disease	Long-term use of bronchodilators or steroids for lung disease	1
Extracardiac arteriopathy	Any one or more of the following: claudication, carotid occlusion or >50% stenosis, previous or planned intervention on the abdominal aorta, limb arteries, or carotid arteries	2
Neurological dysfunction	Disease severely affecting ambulation or day-to-day functioning	2
Previous cardiac surgery	Requiring opening of the pericardium	3
Serum creatinine	>200 μmol/liter preoperatively	2
Active endocarditis	Patient still receiving antibiotic treatment for endocarditis at the time of surgery	3
Critical preoperative state	Any one or more of the following: ventricular tachycardia or fibrillation or aborted sudden death, preoperative cardiac massage, preoperative ventilation before arrival in the operating room, preoperative inotropic support, intraaortic balloon counterpulsation, or preoperative acute renal failure (anuria or oliguria <10 ml/hr)	3
Cardiac-Related Factors		
Unstable angina	Rest angina requiring IV nitrates until arrival in the operating room	2
LV dysfunction	Moderate or LVEF 0.30-0.50 Poor or LVEF <0.30	1 3
Recent myocardial infarct	<90 days	2
Pulmonary hypertension	Systolic PA pressure >60 mm Hg	2
Operation-Related Factors		
Emergency	Carried out on referral before the beginning of the next working day	2
Other than isolated CABG	Major cardiac procedure other than or in addition to CABG	2
Surgery on thoracic aorta	For disorder of ascending, arch, or descending aorta	3
Postinfarct septal rupture		4

CABG = coronary artery bypass grafting; IV = intravenous; LV = left ventricular; LVEF = LV ejection fraction; PA = pulmonary artery.

severity scoring helps to identify patients at high risk for operative mortality (score > 6). By assembling and reviewing the data necessary for accurate assessment of a patient's operative risk, cardiologists can help with the appropriate clinical triage of patients, contain hospital costs, and facilitate consultations with other medical specialists (e.g., dialysis team) as needed. Patients at increased risk of mediastinal infection include the elderly and those with morbid obesity, diabetes mellitus, malnutrition, severe pulmonary disease that is likely to lead to prolonged postoperative ventilatory support, or macromastia in women.[52-54]

VENTRICULAR DYSFUNCTION. An especially important aspect of the preoperative evaluation of a cardiac surgical patient involves estimating the extent of underlying ventricular dysfunction. Un-revascularized viable myocardium after myocardial infarction likely serves as a substrate for recurrent ischemic events.[55-61] Also, patients with severe multivessel disease and akinetic myocardial zones who have chronic congestive heart failure as a result of hibernating myocardium (see Chap. 50) experience improved ventricular function after CABG.[55] Contemporary techniques that should be used for assessing myocardial viability in dysfunctional regions include imaging procedures that correlate perfusion with cell membrane integrity (thallium reperfusion), metabolic activity (positron-emission tomography), regional myocardial strain (magnetic resonance imaging), or contractile reserve (stress echocardiography) (see Chap. 16).[55-57,61] Clinicians should rely on imaging modalities with which they are most familiar and that are available at their institution. In addition to viability, the same imaging modalities can localize akinetic or dyskinetic segments. Patients with severe ventricular dysfunction as well as regional wall akinesia or dyskinesia may benefit from surgical ventricular restoration (Dor procedure) designed to restore mechanically the left ventricle to a more normal size and shape.[58]

The possibility of *right ventricular dysfunction* deserves careful consideration (see Table 76–1), particularly in patients with preoperatively elevated pulmonary artery systolic pressure (>60 mm Hg), a history of inferoposterior left ventricular infarction (which may be associated with right ventricular infarction), or longstanding tricuspid regurgitation. Patients with right ventricular dysfunction should receive an inotropic agent with vasodilating actions such as milrinone (0.5 μg/kg/min) or dobutamine (5 μg/kg/min) in addition to supplemental oxygen perioperatively in an attempt to lower pulmonary vascular resistance and improve right ventricular systolic performance. Intravenous nitrate infusions in the perioperative period have also been shown to reduce pulmonary hypertension and ameliorate right ventricular failure. Inhaled agents, including aerosolized prostacyclin and nitric oxide, can lower pulmonary vascular resistance and improve perioperative right ventricular performance.[62] Recombinant human B-type natriuretic peptide (BNP) is a promising new agent with pharmacological properties favorable for the treatment of right sided heart failure. Its ability to reduce markedly pulmonary vascular resistance and central venous pressure with mild systemic vasodilation may aid the management of selected patients.[63,64]

Patients with mitral regurgitation and severe heart failure should undergo preoperative afterload reduction with such agents as oral angiotensin-converting enzyme (ACE) inhibitors and intravenous sodium nitroprusside to a systolic pressure of about 90 to 100 mm Hg. Potential contraindications to such preoperative afterload reduction include concomitant severe aortic stenosis and hemodynamically significant cerebral or renal vascular disease. In these patients, early intervention with intraaortic balloon counterpulsation may be useful. This population may also benefit from preoperative tailored therapy with BNP in an ICU setting with pulmonary artery catheter monitoring to document lowering of pulmonary artery pressures and improved cardiac output. Intraaortic balloon support is also commonly used in the setting of severe decompensation from acute mitral regurgitation secondary to conditions such as papillary muscle rupture. Infarct-related ventricular septal defect may also require pharmacological and intraaortic balloon support in the perioperative period.

TABLE 76–3 Logistic Regression Model of EuroSCORE in the 1995 Pilot Study

Variables	Beta Coefficient
Age (continuous)	0.0666354
Female	0.3304052
Serum creatinine >200 μmol/liter	0.6521653
Extracardiac arteriopathy	0.6558917
Pulmonary disease	0.4931341
Neurological dysfunction	0.841626
Previous cardiac surgery	1.002625
Recent myocardial infarction	0.5460218
LVEF 0.30-0.50	0.4191643
LVEF <0.30	1.094443
Systolic pulmonary pressure >60 mm Hg	0.7676924
Active endocarditis	1.101265
Unstable angina	0.5677075
Emergency operation	0.7127953
Critical preoperative state	0.9058132
Ventricular septal rupture	1.462009
Other than isolated coronary surgery	0.5420364
Thoracic aortic surgery	1.159787
Constant (β_0)	−4.789594

LVEF = left ventricular ejection fraction. Full definitions of these variables are published and can be seen on-line (http://www.euroscore.org).

TABLE 76–4 Application of Scoring System

			95% Confidence Limits for Mortality	
EuroSCORE	**Patients**	**Died**	***Observed***	***Expected***
0-2 (low risk)	4,529	36 (0.8%)	(0.56-1.10)	(1.27-1.29)
3-5 (medium risk)	5,977	182 (3.0%)	(2.62-3.51)	(2.90-2.94)
6 plus (high risk)	4,293	480 (11.2%)	(10.25-12.16)	(10.93-11.54)
Total	14,799	698 (4.7%)	(4.37-5.06)	(4.72-4.95)

TABLE 76–5 EuroSCORE Risk Profile: 66-year-old Female with COPD, Recent Myocardial Infarction for Isolated CABG

		Additive EuroSCORE	Logistic EuroSCORE $\beta i\ Xi$
Patient Factors			
Age	**66 yr**	2	**0.546775405**
Sex	☐ Female		
Chronic pulmonary disease	☑ Yes	1	**0.4931341**
Extracardiac arteriopathy	☐ Yes		
Neurological dysfunction	☐ Yes		
Previous cardiac surgery	☐ Yes		
Serum creatinine >200 μmol/liter	☐ Yes		
Active endocarditis	☐ Yes		
Critical preoperative state	☐ Yes		
Cardiac Factors			
Unstable angina	☐ Yes		
LV dysfunction moderate or LVEF 30-50%	☐ Moderate		
LV dysfunction poor or LVEF <30	☐ Poor		
Recent myocardial infarct	☑ Yes	2	**0.5460218**
Pulmonary hypertension	☐ Yes		
Operation Factors			
Emergency	☐ Yes		
Other than isolated CABG	☐ Yes		
Surgery on thoracic aorta	☐ Yes		
Postinfarct septal rupture	☐ Yes		
EuroSCORE		5	**3.90%**

Downloaded from http://euroscore.org.
CABG = coronary artery bypass grafting; COPD = chronic obstructive pulmonary disease; LV = left ventricular; LVEF = LV ejection fraction.

RISK OF MYOCARDIAL ISCHEMIA. Acute thrombolytic and interventional catheterization treatment regimens for acute myocardial infarction may not successfully restore coronary perfusion because of inadequate thrombolysis, reocclusion of the infarct-related artery following initially successful thrombolysis, or dissection/acute thrombosis of the target vessel during angioplasty.[65,66] Identification of patients for referral for emergency bypass surgery and decisions regarding the timing of such surgery remain a challenging clinical problem, particularly in view of the high perioperative mortality rate for patients who require surgery within 24 to 48 hours of thrombolysis.[66,67]

Potential indications for emergency bypass surgery following failed attempts at reperfusion in acute myocardial infarction include significant left main stenosis and inability to maintain patency of the infarct-related artery, severe multivessel coronary artery disease with anatomy unsuitable for angioplasty and ischemic dysfunction of the noninfarct zones, and inability to maintain patency of an infarct-related artery that places a large amount of myocardium in jeopardy (proximal left anterior descending) in patients with an infarct of less than 6 hours' duration. Although some clinical reports suggest that patients in cardiogenic shock who undergo urgent revascularization have improved survival in comparison to those who are not revascularized, these series suffer from potential selection bias, and definitive recommendations regarding the management of patients with cardiogenic shock and acute myocardial infarction must await the results of ongoing randomized trials.[65]

Patients who are referred for emergency revascularization surgery should be supported by an intraaortic balloon pump and, if technically feasible, an intracoronary perfusion catheter. Other methods for mechanical assistance of the failing circulation are described in Chapter 25. Because patients who undergo emergency bypass surgery within 6 to 12 hours of administration of a thrombolytic agent are at greater risk for intraoperative and postoperative hemorrhage, they should receive a hemostatic agent such as aprotinin (2 million kallikrein-inhibiting units [KIU] over a 20-minute period, followed by a continuous infusion of 500,000 KIU/hr).[68]

Patients with other manifestations of an acute coronary syndrome such as active, unstable angina may also be in tenuous hemodynamic balance as they proceed to the operating room, particularly if significant left main coronary artery stenosis or severe three-vessel coronary artery disease coexists with left ventricular dysfunction and/or mitral regurgitation. Delays while awaiting surgery and the time between the induction of anesthesia and the institution of cardiopulmonary bypass are high-risk periods during which a vicious spiral of myocardial ischemia and low-output syndrome can rapidly develop. Such patients should be protected by an intraaortic balloon pump inserted preoperatively and an infusion of nitroglycerin.

The risk of recurrent myocardial ischemia must be carefully weighed against the risk of early surgical intervention in patients sustaining a transmural myocardial infarction. Recent data suggest that the risk of coronary bypass surgery is high during the first several days following transmural injury, and a waiting period of 4 to 7 days should be sought unless patients are experiencing active, ongoing refractory myocardial ischemia or hemodynamic instability.[69,70] Preoperative intra-aortic balloon support may be extremely useful in stabilizing patients in the clinical setting of transmural injury.[71]

ANESTHESIA FOR CARDIAC SURGERY. The details of the practice of cardiac anesthesia are beyond the scope of this chapter and are available in other sources (see Chap. 77).[72,73] High-dose synthetic narcotics that do not cause vasodilation, such as fentanyl and sufentanil, have replaced morphine in many centers. Most cardiac units currently employ early extubation protocols for patients with low or moderate risk. Advantages of early extubation include a decrease in respiratory complications, ventilatory support, and length of stay in the ICU. To achieve early extubation within 6 hours of surgery, anesthetic techniques have included combinations of inhalational anesthetics, such as enflurane and isoflurane, together with low to moderate amounts of intravenous opioids, such as fentanyl and sufentanil, along with the intravenous anesthetic propofol. The newer, inhaled anesthetics that have replaced nitrous oxide still have the potential to cause vasodilation. Patients with critical aortic stenosis, critical mitral stenosis, and large right-to-left shunts may experience a dramatic reduction in cardiac output because ventricular stroke volume falls with a reduction in preload. Preoperative volume expansion and even administration of vasopressor agents may be necessary to avoid this problem.

Special attention in the perioperative setting should be focused on controlling heart rate and preventing intraoperative anemia or hypothermia to decrease the risk of myocardial injury and in-hospital mortality in patients undergoing CABG (Fig. 76–1).[74-76]

RHYTHM DEVICES AND CARDIAC SURGERY. Patients with high-grade (third-degree or type II second-degree) atrioventricular block and hemodynamic compromise (systolic pressure < 90 mm Hg) are at high risk during general anesthesia unless a temporary transvenous pacemaker wire or a flow-directed pacing system is inserted perioperatively. In a patient with a permanent pacemaker, its specifications (model, mode, and settings) and, if possible, a statement regarding the pacemaker dependency of the patient should be noted in the medical record (see Chap. 31). The possibility of postoperative malfunction in the permanent pacing system because of the effects of anesthesia, electrocautery, and surgical manipulation of the leads (e.g., during atrial cannulation) should be anticipated. Clinicians should have the appropriate pacemaker programming equipment available postoperatively because many problems (secondary to electromagnetic interference from the electrocautery apparatus) can be quickly resolved by interrogation of the generator and reprogramming in the recovery area. Patients with previously implanted cardioverter-defibrillator devices should have their unit disabled prior to surgery to minimize the risk of inappropriate shocks from sensing of electrocautery signals intraoperatively. Until the device is reactivated in the postoperative period, equipment for rapid external defibrillation should be available.

PERIOPERATIVE DRUG THERAPY. With the exception of oral anticoagulation with warfarin, most medications can and should be continued up to the time of surgery. Clinical trials of patients receiving saphenous vein bypass grafts demonstrated the importance of initiating antiplatelet therapy in the perioperative period. Because of the increased risk of postoperative bleeding, in the past some surgical groups discontinued aspirin use for several days preoperatively in elective cases. Because of the risk of "breakthrough" episodes of ischemia if aspirin therapy is discontinued preoperatively, most cardiologists currently prefer to continue it up to the time of surgery and rely on preoperative donations of autologous red blood cells, cell-saver techniques, autotransfusion of shed blood intraoperatively, and antitibrinolytic drugs such as aprotinin to minimize the need for and potential hazards of homologous blood transfusion. If aspirin is withheld preoperatively, it should be restarted within 24 to 48 hours after surgery to reduce the risk of vein graft occlusion. Warfarin therapy should be stopped 2 to 3 days preoperatively and, if necessary, treatment with heparin or low-molecular-weight heparin initiated.

Although definitive data are not available, we usually continue both aspirin and clopidogrel up to the time of surgery in patients who have undergone implantation of a stent in the coronary circulation within the preceding 2 weeks to minimize the risk of stent thrombosis preoperatively. For patients who have had a stent implanted more than 2 weeks prior to surgery, we discontinue clopidogrel administration but continue aspirin up to the time of surgery. For patients receiving long-term clopidogrel as secondary prevention for vascular disease, we discontinue use of the drug 5 to 7 days preoperatively when feasible.

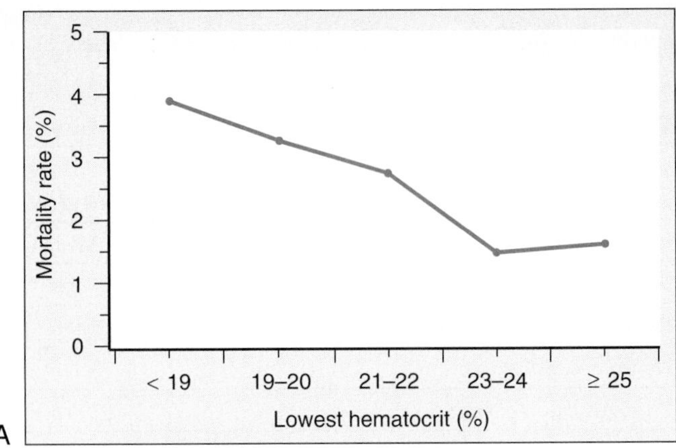

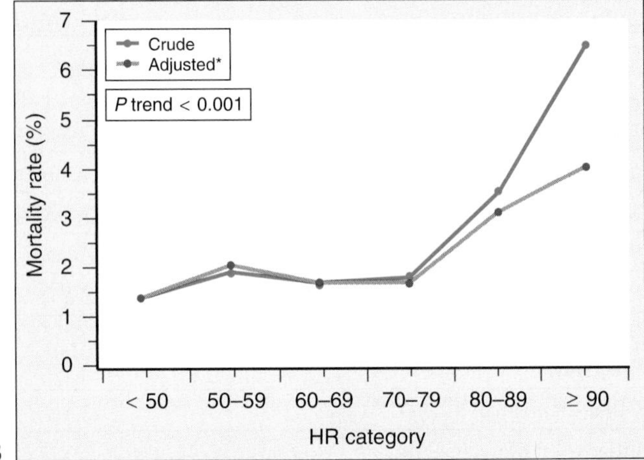

FIGURE 76–1 Intraoperative variables factors influencing mortality in coronary artery bypass patients. **A,** Adjusted mortality rates by lowest hematocrit on cardiopulmonary bypass. **B,** Preinduction heart rate (HR) and in-hospital mortality crude and adjusted rates. In both **A** and **B,** rates are adjusted for the following variables: age, sex, body surface area, comorbidity score, prior coronary artery bypass graft, ejection fraction, left ventricular end-diastolic pressure, and priority at surgery. (**A,** From DeFoe GR, Ross CS, Olmstead EM, et al: Lowest hematocrit on bypass and adverse outcomes associated with coronary artery bypass grafting. Ann Thorac Surg 71:769-776, 2001; and **B,** From Fillinger MP, Surgenor SD, Hartman GS, et al: The association between heart rate and in-hospital mortality after coronary artery bypass graft surgery. Anesth Analg 85:1483-1488, 2002.)

To minimize the risk of intraoperative bleeding, if patients are undergoing percutaneous intervention and have normal renal function and if cardiac surgery is likely to take place within the ensuing 24 to 48 hours, we prefer to use a short-acting intravenous glycoprotein IIb/IIIa inhibitor such as eptifibatide or tirofiban rather than a long-acting agent such as abciximab. Treatment with the short-acting agent is usually discontinued 6 to 12 hours preoperatively to permit platelet function to return toward normal. We prefer to use abciximab in patients with renal dysfunction since the small, short-acting inhibitors are cleared predominantly through renal elimination. When abciximab is used, we discontinue the infusion at least 12 hours prior to surgery.

For patients who have received an intravenous glycoprotein IIb/IIIa inhibitor and must proceed urgently to cardiac surgery, the antiplatelet effects of abciximab may be reversed by platelet transfusions.[77] In contrast, the high excess of free drug versus bound drug in the case of eptifibatide or tirofiban limits the ability of platelet transfusions to restore normal platelet function. In cases in which urgent removal of eptifibatide or tirofiban from the circulation is desired, hemodialysis may be necessary.

Calcium channel antagonists previously prescribed for control of ischemic heart disease should be continued up to the time of surgery to reduce the chance of myocardial ischemia from withdrawal of the drug. In the case of diltiazem and verapamil, the dose may need to be reduced because these agents may provoke bradycardia and a low-output syndrome postoperatively, especially if a beta-blocking agent or amiodarone is given concurrently or if the patient is elderly. Profound atropine- and isoproterenol-resistant bradyarrhythmias may occur postoperatively in patients treated with these calcium channel antagonists, particularly when the patient has not yet recovered from the hypothermia that is imposed intraoperatively; temporary dual-chamber pacing support should be available to manage such patients. Postoperative systemic hypotension is also common in patients receiving preoperative ACE inhibitors, and pharmacological strategies to increase systemic vascular resistance including vasopressin or norepinephrine maybe useful in selected patients.[78]

CONTINUATION OF ANTIARRHYTHMICS. With the exception of amiodarone, antiarrhythmic drugs that have been prescribed for hemodynamically compromising or life-threatening ventricular tachyarrhythmias should be continued up to the time of surgery because of the risk of breakthrough of a potentially lethal ventricular arrhythmia in the preoperative period.

Patients with a documented history of resuscitation from sudden cardiac death who are receiving amiodarone should continue to receive this drug up to the time of surgery. However, in cases in which amiodarone was prescribed for a less overtly life-threatening arrhythmia (e.g., atrial fibrillation), the maintenance dosage has been more than 200 mg/d, and the patient has a history of lung disease, we would consider omission of the drug for at least 3 months before subjecting the patient to elective cardiopulmonary bypass.

IMPLANTABLE CARDIOVERTER-DEFIBRILLATORS. Prophylactic implantation of cardioverter-defibrillators at the time of CABG in patients at high risk for ventricular arrhythmias (ejection fraction ≤ 0.35, abnormal signal-averaged electrocardiogram [ECG]) does not improve survival according to the results of the CABG-PATCH trial.[78a]

Intraoperative Management

Despite increased risks, particularly related to age and advanced disease, cardiac surgery patients today enjoy markedly improved outcomes when compared with patients operated on 10 years ago. Important intraoperative surgical advances that have contributed to this improved outcome include epiaortic echocardiographic scanning in patients with ascending aortic atherosclerosis (Fig. 76–2), transesophageal echocardiography, retrograde blood cardioplegia, carbon dioxide insufflation to prevent air embolization, vacuum-assisted venous drainage, and performance of all vascular anastomoses with a single aortic cross-clamp under cardioplegic arrest.[15] Emphasis on modern strategies to ensure blood conservation and minimize hemostatic complications has significantly decreased or eliminated homologous blood exposure for most patients undergoing cardiac surgery (Fig. 76–3).

Until the past decade, nearly all cardiac surgical procedures were performed via a standard median sternotomy with the use of cardiopulmonary bypass and cardiac arrest to provide a bloodless, motionless surgical field. Cardiac surgeons have now adopted less invasive approaches to coronary and valvu-

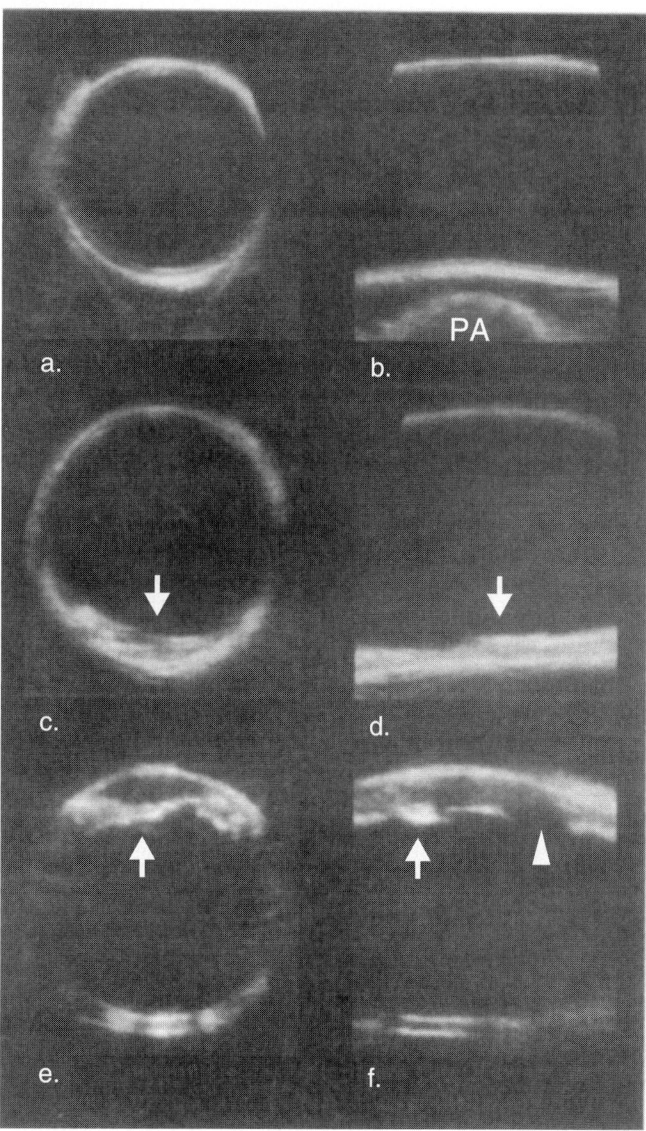

FIGURE 76–2 Ultrasonographic images of the ascending aorta, demonstrating transverse (a, c, and e) and longitudinal scans (b, d, and f). Panels a and b illustrate a normal patient. Panels c and d reveal a moderate arteriosclerosis (arrow). Panels e and f demonstrate typical severe arteriosclerosis (arrow) and ulcerated plaque (arrowhead) of the ascending aorta. PA = pulmonary artery. (From Goto T, Baba T, Matsuyama K, et al: Aortic atherosclerosis and postoperative neurological dysfunction in elderly coronary surgical patients. Ann Thorac Surg 75:1912-1918, 2003.)

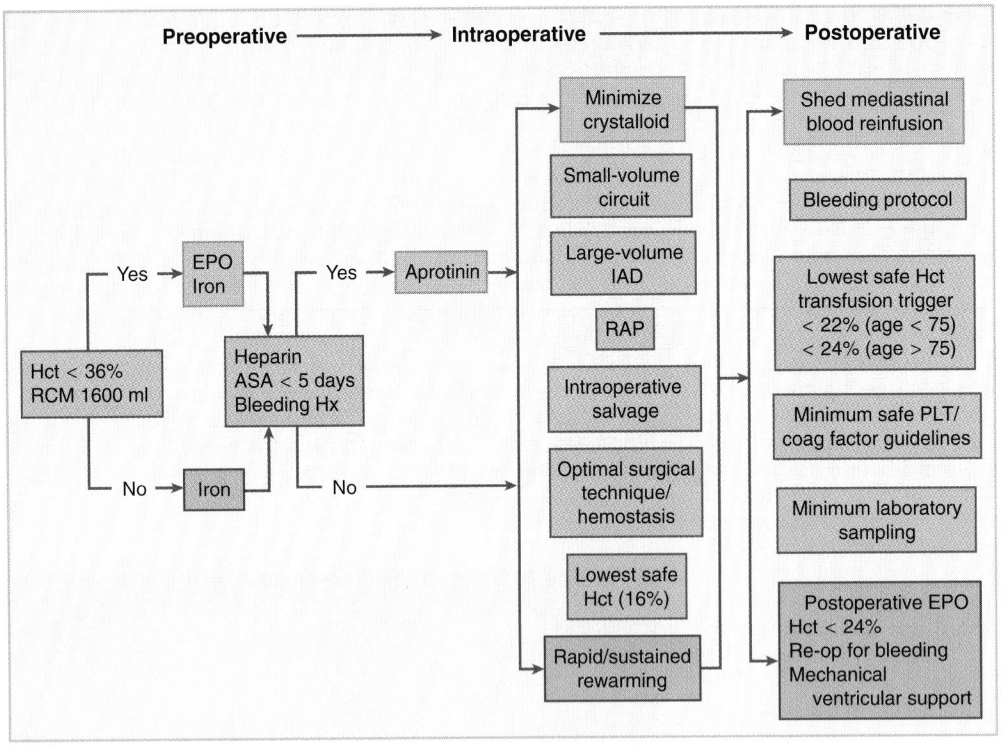

FIGURE 76–3 Multimodality algorithm designed to optimize blood conservation in cardiac surgical patients. Preoperative, intraoperative, and postoperative strategies all are important to eliminate the requirement for homologous blood transfusion. ASA = aspirin; coag = coagulation; EPO = erythropoietin; Hct = hematocrit; Hx = history; IAD = intraoperative autologous donation; PLT = platelet; RAP = retrograde autologous priming; RCM = red blood cell mass. (From Rosengart TK: Open heart surgery without transfusion in high-risk patients. Am J Cardiol 83:31B-37B, 1999.)

lar heart disease. The impetus for this change has been to decrease overall surgical trauma associated with full sternotomy and cardiopulmonary bypass without compromising the efficacy and safety of procedures. In valvular heart disease, cardiopulmonary bypass is essential, and therefore the focus has been on reducing trauma through a variety of less invasive incisions (Fig. 76–4). In coronary surgery, smaller incisions have also been used with or without cardiopulmonary bypass, particularly to perform single-vessel bypass to the left anterior descending artery. Recent technical advances in myocardial stabilization (Fig. 76–5) have now focused attention on off-pump multivessel coronary bypass through a full sternotomy.[79] This approach is particularly appealing in selected high-risk patients, including those with ascending aortic atherosclerosis, renal dysfunction, and severe pulmonary disease. Continued adoption of less invasive cardiac surgical techniques can be anticipated if ongoing clinical trials demonstrate medium- and long-term results comparable to those obtained with standard techniques.[79-86b]

Postoperative Management

Fluid, Electrolyte, and Acid-Base Balance

Extracorporeal circulation is associated with an increase in extracellular fluid and total exchangeable sodium, along with a decrease in exchangeable potassium. The cumulative experience in many centers has led to the following basic principles of management:

1. For the first 48 hours after surgery, free water is limited to about 1000 ml/d and intravenous fluids are administered in the form of dextrose (5%) in water. Sodium replacement varies with volume needs but is usually limited to 4 gm/liter.
2. Serum potassium levels can fluctuate dramatically; therefore, frequent measurement of serum potassium is indicated, especially in diabetic patients. We attempt to maintain serum potassium in the range of 4.5 ± 0.5 mEq/liter and magnesium at 2.0 mEq/liter or greater to minimize cardiac arrhythmias.
3. Serum glucose levels are frequently elevated (250 to 400 mg/dl), as a result of glucose-containing intravenous solutions and surgically induced increases in cortisol and catecholamine levels. Contemporary series have shown the importance of tight control of postoperative blood glucose levels to decrease morbidity following coronary bypass surgery. Protocols to maintain aggressively serum glucose levels to less than 150 mg/dl by continuous insulin infusion should be utilized in postoperative patients.[87-89]
4. Mild metabolic acidosis or metabolic alkalosis may be present for the first 24 hours postoperatively, particularly during rewarming. These acid-base abnormalities usually do not require correction in the absence of preoperative renal dysfunction or development of acute renal failure postoperatively. Significant metabolic acidosis (pH < 7.35) should be avoided during the rewarming phase, particularly if patients are dependent on an inotropic agent. Hyperventilation (pco_2 < 35 mm Hg) and treatment with sodium bicarbonate should be instituted.
5. Serum total calcium, phosphorus, and magnesium levels are frequently depressed for about 24 to 48 hours in normally convalescing patients, partly because of the effects of hemodilution. Hypocalcemia and hypomagnesemia may predispose to the development of cardiac arrhythmias, and replacement therapy is generally warranted.

Respiratory Management

EFFECTS OF ANESTHESIA, STERNOTOMY, AND CARDIOPULMONARY BYPASS ON PULMONARY FUNCTION. To optimize respiratory management, four broad areas should be considered (Table 76–6). Most all patients experience alveolar dysfunction after open-heart surgery because of right-to-left intrapulmonary shunting of blood from various intrinsic alveolar abnormalities (e.g., atelectasis, edema, infection) and pulmonary vascular events (e.g., extravasation of fluid, inhibition of hypoxia-induced vasoconstriction).[90] Central respiratory drive and respiratory muscle function are depressed postoperatively because of a combination of pharmacological effects and mechanical derangements of thoracic function. Patients with preexisting pulmonary disease may experience more profound depression of respiratory function, necessitating vigorous pulmonary toilette.

EARLY EXTUBATION. Historically, most postoperative cardiac surgery patients received between 6 and 18 hours of ventilatory support. Early extubation protocols have now been widely adopted in cardiac ICUs, and stable patients are extubated within 4 hours (Table 76–7). Advantages of early extubation include improved patient mobility with early transition to step-down units.

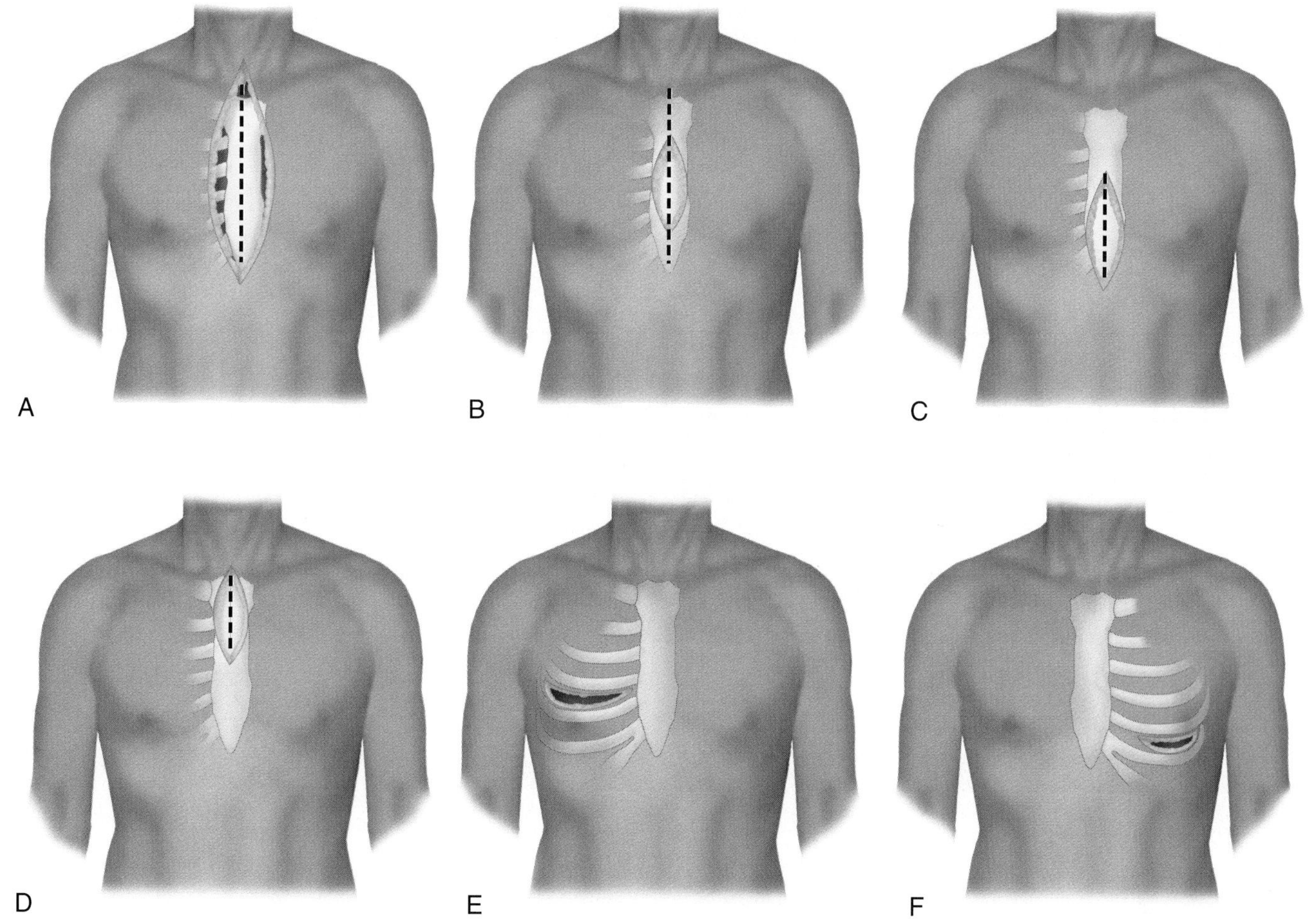

A B C

D E F

FIGURE 76–4 Schematic representation of traditional incision and sternotomy **(A)** compared with a variety of less invasive incisions (dotted lines represent chest wall incisions). Limited skin incision/full sternotomy **(B)** is gaining in popularity because of improved cosmetics and reduced trauma from the limited chest wall retraction. Partial lower or upper sternotomy **(C** and **D)** has been used predominantly in valve procedures. Limited right anterior thoracotomy **(E)** is a useful approach, particularly in mitral valve reoperations. Left anterior small thoracotomy **(F)** is currently used in robotic-assisted coronary bypass surgery.

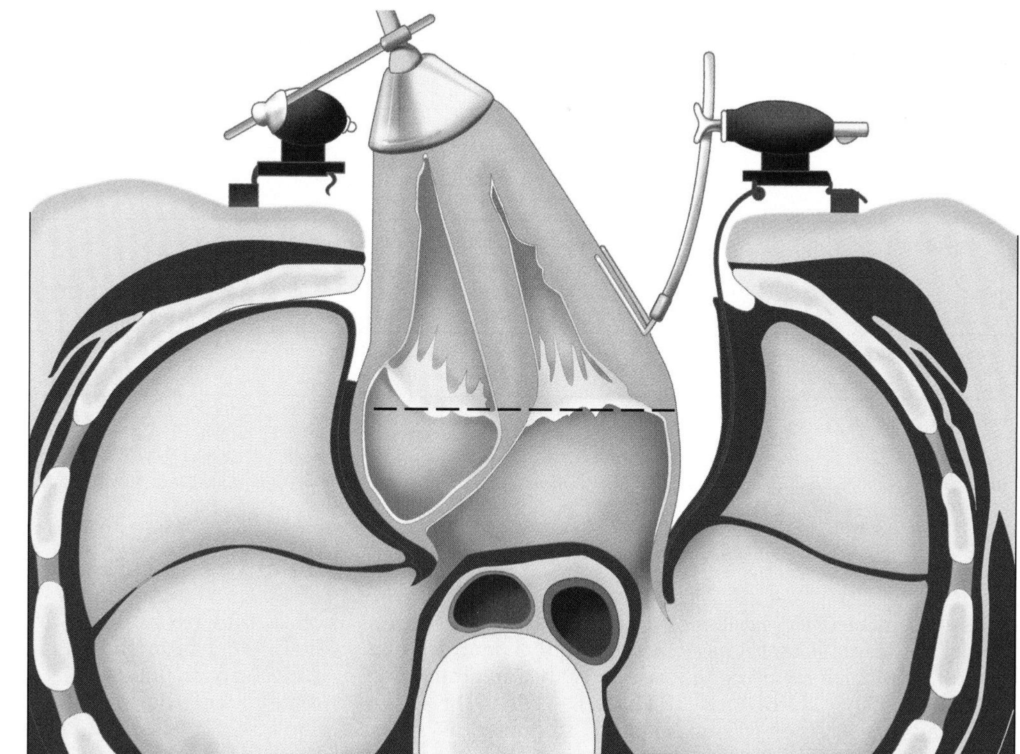

FIGURE 76–5 Off-pump coronary bypass surgery on the beating heart has been greatly facilitated by the development of positioning devices and platform stabilization systems. Positioning devices using apical suction cups **(left, top)** now allow optimal exposure of the posterolateral circulation while minimizing hemodynamic compromise. Platform stabilization systems **(right, top)** provide isolated immobilization during the performance of distal anastomoses.

TABLE 76–6 Abnormalities of Respiratory Function After Cardiac Surgery

Effects of Anesthesia, Thoracic Surgery, and Cardiopulmonary Bypass on Pulmonary Function	Potential Causes
Alveolar dysfunction (e.g., widened alveolar-arterial oxygen gradient because of right-to-left intrapulmonary shunting)	Scattered regions of atelectasis with preserved perfusion Pulmonary edema (e.g., cardiogenic, noncardiogenic "postpump" alveolar capillary leak) Pleural effusion Pneumothorax Infection Inhibition of hypoxic pulmonary vasoconstriction by anesthetic agents Exacerbation of ventilation/perfusion mismatch by vasodilating agents used postoperatively (e.g., nitroprusside)
Decreased central respiratory drive	General anesthetics Narcotic analgesics Cerebral insult in perioperative period
Decreased respiratory muscle function	Thoracic pain (incision, chest tubes) Persistent effects of muscle relaxants Age Obesity Depressed cardiac function Primary diaphragmatic dysfunction (e.g., phrenic nerve injury)
Exacerbation of underlying chronic pulmonary disease	Increase in airway resistance Increased secretions and worsening bronchitis Pneumonia Ventilatory management

TABLE 76–7 Cardiac Surgery Early Extubation Protocol

Definition	Extubation Within 4 hr after Surgery
Patient selection	
Inclusion criteria	All patients ≤80 yr old, LV ejection fraction >0.50
Excusion criteria	High inotropic requirement, postoperative bleeding or ischemia, severe pulmonary hypertension
Anesthetic management	
Intraoperative	Low-dose synthetic narcotics and inhalation agents
Postoperative	Muscle relaxant reversal Propofol 0.1 ml/kg/hr Minimize narcotic use
Ventilatory management	
Postoperative	SIMV mode Check ABGs and decrease ventilatory support every 20 min Always keep between pH 7.35 and 7.45 Always keep $pO_2 > 75$ mm Hg
Exubation guidelines	
Oxygenation	$pO_2 > 75$ mm Hg at an $FIO_2 \leq 0.50$
Respiratory drive	$pCO_2 < 45$ mm Hg and pH > 7.35 Spontaneously breathing
Mechanics	Respiratory rate < 25 breaths/min Negative inspiratory pressure > 20 cm H_2O Tidal volume > 8 ml/kg Vital capacity > 10 ml/kg
Airway protection	Alert with gag reflex Absence of heavy secretions
Cardiovascular	Cardiac index > 2.0 liter/min·m^{-2} MAP > 80 and < 120 mm Hg

ABG = arterial blood gas; LV = left ventricular; MAP = mean arterial pressure; SIMV = synchronized intermittent mandatory ventilation.

Special Problems

Failure to meet early extubation criteria may result from a variety of factors. Careful assessment usually identifies one or more etiologies resulting in respiratory dysfunction.

INCREASED ALVEOLAR-ARTERIAL GRADIENT. An increased alveolar-arterial gradient postoperatively is a serious problem that demands thorough evaluation. The ventilator settings should be checked and a chest radiograph obtained to ascertain the position of the tip of the endotracheal tube (to exclude, for example, intubation of the right main stem bronchus) and to rule out pneumothorax, lobar atelectasis or pneumonia, or a large pleural effusion. Hemodynamic monitoring by means of a pulmonary artery catheter can rarely cause pulmonary hemorrhage from overinflation of the balloon, and bronchoscopy may need to be performed to diagnose and manage the problem (e.g., occlusion of the bronchus draining the bleeding segment of the lung).

PULMONARY EDEMA. The most common cause of pulmonary edema postoperatively is elevated pulmonary venous pressure arising from left ventricular dysfunction. Patients with increased risk of pulmonary edema require aggressive diuresis, as well as vasodilator/inotropic and possibly intraaortic balloon support. Mechanical ventilation with positive end-expiratory pressure (PEEP) is used until the patient's ventricular function improves. A less common cause of postoperative respiratory failure is residual mitral regurgitation in a patient not undergoing concomitant mitral valve surgery at the time of other cardiac surgery. Repeat surgery may be needed if pulmonary edema persists despite attempts to control mitral regurgitation medically.[91,92]

In a few patients, pulmonary edema after cardiac surgery is due to adult respiratory distress syndrome. In its most extreme form, this disorder is associated with a generalized condition characterized by increased capillary permeability, interstitial edema, fever, leukocytosis, renal dysfunction, and occasionally hemodynamic collapse.

UNDERLYING CHRONIC LUNG DISEASE. General surgical preparation of patients with obstructive lung disease, including antibiotics, bronchodilators, and cessation of cigarette smoking, may help minimize the risk of respiratory failure from postoperative atelectasis and pneumonia. Inhaled bronchodilators should be continued postoperatively. Refractory patients may require a short course of corticosteroids (e.g., methylprednisolone 0.5 mg/kg every 6 hours for 3 days) to be weaned from the ventilator. Previous enthusiasm for intravenous methylxanthines has waned because of evidence of limited efficacy and the risk of agitation, arrhythmias, and grand mal seizures. Intravenous theophylline should therefore be reserved for extremely refractory cases and administered in a dose of 0.4 mg/kg/hr, with careful monitoring of plasma levels to maintain them in the range of 10 to 15 μg/ml.[93]

We have successfully operated on patients with severe respiratory compromise, including those with a forced expiratory volume in 1 second (FEV_1) of less than 0.8 liters who require home oxygen therapy. All patients with severe pulmonary dysfunction are considered for early extubation. It is important to maintain the arterial carbon dioxide tension close to the patient's baseline level to ensure an adequate respiratory drive.

DIAPHRAGMATIC FAILURE. Diaphragmatic dysfunction after cardiac surgical procedures usually occurs as a result of injury to the phrenic nerve. An elevated hemidiaphragm may be seen on postoperative radiographs in 25 percent of patients who undergo myocardial preservation, including topical ice slush and harvesting of an internal mammary artery.[94] A simple bedside test of diaphragmatic function is to ask the patient to protrude the umbilicus, a movement that requires diaphragmatic functional integrity. Of note, an elevated hemidiaphragm is not usually associated with increased postoperative morbidity or mortality.

Recovery of the hemidiaphragm to normal position occurs in 80 percent of patients at 1 year and nearly all patients by 2 years postoperatively. Clinically important diaphragmatic dysfunction caused by unilateral or bilateral phrenic nerve injury develops in less than 1 percent of patients after cardiac surgery.

Evidence of diaphragmatic failure includes an inability to wean the patient from the ventilator, vital capacity less than 500 ml, and paradoxical movement of the diaphragm on fluoroscopy (abnormal "sniff" test) or ultrasonography.

PROLONGED VENTILATORY INSUFFICIENCY. Patients who fail to be weaned from the ventilator within 48 hours require special attention. Because of the risk of stress-induced gastritis, H_2 receptor blockers (e.g., ranitidine 50 mg intravenously every 8 to 12 hours) or a mucosal cytoprotective agent (sucralfate 1 gm orally two to four times per day) is administered. Nutritional support is critical to provide metabolic needs and prevent the catabolism of respiratory muscles. Pressure support ventilation strategies are particularly useful for patients in need of prolonged ventilation. Barotrauma is minimized and patient comfort is improved while permitting incremental weaning in small steps.

High-compliance, low-pressure cuff (<20 mm Hg) endotracheal tubes have reduced the risk of mechanical complications (e.g., tracheal stenosis) and permit patients to remain intubated for several weeks. Nonetheless, we believe that patients requiring prolonged ventilatory support beyond 10 to 14 days benefit from a decision to proceed with early tracheostomy.[95] Tracheostomy provides improved patient comfort and greater pulmonary toilet and enhances weaning by minimizing pulmonary dead space. Percutaneous tracheostomy offers the advantage of bedside insertion with minimal surgical trauma and is particularly useful in patients with reasonable ventilatory mechanics but heavy secretions. Recent data suggest that early tracheostomy does not increase the risk of mediastinitis.

Hypertension

Postoperative hypertension has been defined variably in the literature,[96] but we consider it to be present if systolic pressure exceeds 140 mm Hg. The incidence of postoperative hypertension ranges from 40 to 60 percent. It occurs more commonly in patients with a preoperative history of hypertension, prior maintenance therapy with a beta-adrenergic antagonist, and well-preserved left ventricular function.[97] Postoperative hypertension is especially frequent after CABG and surgical relief of left ventricular outflow tract obstruction (e.g., aortic valve replacement, correction of coarctation of the aorta).

The mechanism of postoperative hypertension probably varies from patient to patient but usually includes (1) a "rebound" effect from withdrawal of beta-adrenergic antagonist administered preoperatively; (2) excessive sympathetic nervous system activity with elevated levels of circulating catecholamines (especially norepinephrine); (3) pressor reflexes originating in the heart, great vessels, or coronary arteries; and (4) a drop in aortic pressure proximal to the site of the corrected coarctation with resultant stimulation of aortic and carotid baroreceptors by apparent "hypotension." The renin-angiotensin system is stimulated and peripheral resistance is increased. Sudden exposure of vascular beds downstream from the coarctation to "undamped" aortic pressure can also cause mesenteric arteritis. Other frequent causes of transient hypertension in postoperative cardiac surgery patients include anxiety, pain, hypoxia, and pharyngeal manipulation. The adverse consequences of elevated systemic pressure include an increased risk of postoperative bleeding, suture line disruption, and aortic dissection; elevated left ventricular afterload and a consequent reduction in left ventricular output; and injury to aortocoronary bypass grafts, or postoperative stroke.

Management

Although a variety of agents may be used for treating acute postoperative hypertension, we prefer those that are rapidly acting and titratable and have a short half-life. Nitroglycerin is our first-choice agent, beginning at a dose of 25 μg/min and titrating up to a dose of 300 μg/min. Sodium nitroprusside (0.5 to 2 μg/kg/min) may be required in hypertension refractory to nitroglycerin therapy. Because of its prominent vasodilatory effects, sodium nitroprusside should be administered with caution for the first 3 to 4 hours after surgery since volume shifts may occur during the rewarming phase. Reflex tachycardia is a common side effect of sodium nitroprusside. The ultra-short-acting beta blocker esmolol (50 to 250 μg/kg/min) may be useful in patients with a hyperdynamic circulation. It is initially preferred over longer-acting beta blockers when evaluating patient tolerance to beta blockade (e.g., moderately severe left ventricular dysfunction). The need for transition to oral antihypertensive therapy is assessed on an individual basis; patients with a

TABLE 76–8 Diagnosis of Myocardial Infarction After Cardiac Surgery

Diagnostic Finding	Comment
Symptoms	
Early (<24 hr postop)	Not reliable because of residual effects of anesthesia and postoperative analgesics
Late (>24 hr postop)	Potentially reliable but may be confused with incisional pain and pleuritic pain from chest tubes, pericarditis
Electrocardiogram	
New, persistent Q waves	Most reliable diagnostic finding, but only if the Q waves persist on serial EGGs over several days
Evolutionary ST-T changes	Supportive data favoring the diagnosis or MI only if a typical evolutionary pattern is observed. Because of the effects of cardiopulmonary bypass, hypothermia, postoperative pericarditis, mediastinal chest tubes, and medications (e.g., digitalis), a variety of nonspecific ST-T wave abnormalities may be seen and should not be relied on for diagnosing perioperative MI
Myocardial-specific enzymes	
Total CK	Elevated total CK levels postoperatively may arise from multiple sources, including skeletal muscle in the thorax and calf, as well as myocardium
CK-MB	Myocardial-specific CK may be released from ischemia occurring during cardiopulmonary bypass, as well as myocardial and aortic incisions made intraoperatively (e.g., right atrium for cannulation of the cavae). Because of the nearly universal release of CK-MB, a diagnosis of MI should not be made unless CK-MB is significantly elevated (e.g., >30 units/liter)
Echocardiogram	A regional wall motion abnormality is a helpful finding, particularly if it can be shown to be a new finding by comparison with a peroperative study. Paradoxical motion of the high anterior portion of the interventricular septum is a common finding postoperatively in the absence of MI and should not be taken as the sole evidence of new perioperative myocardial necrosis

CK = creatine kinase; MI = myocardial infarction; ECG = electrocardiogram; postop = postoperative.

preoperative history of hypertension usually require chronic treatment.

Perioperative Myocardial Infarction (see Chap. 46)

Despite modern intraoperative myocardial protection and improvements in surgical technique, some degree of ischemia occurs nearly uniformly during CABG. Only a minority of patients (5 to 15 percent of patients undergoing CABG), however, actually experience a *perioperative myocardial infarction,* even in tertiary care centers currently operating on higher-risk patients, including those with failed percutaneous procedures.[98-100] Potential causes of myocardial ischemia and infarction in the perioperative period include incomplete revascularization; diffuse atherosclerotic disease of the distal coronary arteries; spasm, embolism, or thrombosis of the native coronary vessels or bypass grafts[101-103]; technical problems with graft anastomoses; inadequate myocardial preservation intraoperatively; increased myocardial oxygen needs, as in left ventricular hypertrophy; and hemodynamic derangements in the postoperative period (e.g., hypotension, hypertension, tachycardia). Although initially one might suspect that perioperative myocardial infarction results from occlusion of bypass grafts placed to circumvent diseased coronary arteries, autopsy studies have shown that bypass grafts are usually patent in patients dying of a perioperative myocardial infarction. This observation lends support to the concept that poor myocardial protection or a mismatch between myocardial oxygen supply and demand postoperatively accounts for much of the infarction noted.

DIAGNOSIS. The diagnosis of a myocardial infarction after cardiac surgery is more difficult than at other times because of the nonspecific ST-T wave abnormalities on ECG and nearly universal elevation of creatine kinase (CK) levels postoperatively. A number of diagnostic findings (Table 76–8) must be carefully interpreted and then integrated as shown in the algorithm displayed in Table 76–9. A 12-lead ECG should be obtained immediately on the patient's arrival in the ICU after surgery and no less frequently than once every 24 hours for the first few postoperative days. Measurements of total CK and CK-MB should be made every 8 hours for the first 24 to 36 hours if perioperative myocardial infarction is suspected.

Troponin. Experience with more sensitive serum markers of cardiac injury suggest that cardiac-specific troponin I and troponin T are elevated postoperatively in virtually all patients who undergo CABG.[104,105] Patients who experience a perioperative myocardial infarction release greater quantities of troponin such that serum measurements may remain 10- to 20-fold higher than the upper limit of the reference interval for at least 4 to 5 days postoperatively. Even in patients not experiencing perioperative myocardial infarctions by conventional diagnostic criteria, the relative increase in proteins such as cardiac troponin I over preoperative baseline values is greater than that of CK-MB, which suggests that troponin measurements can detect small amounts of myocardial tissue damage that are not detected by CK-MB.

Electrocardiography. The ECG is the most reliable tool for diagnosing a perioperative myocardial infarction. New and persistent Q waves accompanied by new, persistent, and evolutionary ST-T wave abnormalities are the most helpful criteria. Pathological Q waves resulting from perioperative myocardial infarction may appear with an earlier time course (i.e., immediately on arrival from the operating room) than in a nonrevascularized patient.

Echocardiography. Bedside echocardiograms (transthoracic and if necessary transesophageal) play an important role in establishing the diagnosis of a perioperative myocardial infarction by detecting new regional wall motion abnormalities in cases in which the ECG or serum marker measurements are unclear. It is especially helpful to compare new echocardiograms with the preoperative studies that are almost always available.

RISKS AND CONSEQUENCES OF PERIOPERATIVE INFARCTION. Variables that have been found to correlate with the development of perioperative myocardial infarction in patients undergoing CABG include emergency surgery, aortic cross-clamp time greater than 100 minutes, a recent myocardial infarction (within the prior week), intraoperative tachycardia, intraoperative anemia on cardiopulmonary bypass, left ventricular hypertrophy, and a history of previ-

TABLE 76–9 Algorithm for Diagnosis of Perioperative Myocardial Infarction After Cardiac Surgery

New Qs on ECG	CK-MB >30 IU/Liter	New RWMA On Echo*	Diagnosis	Comment
Yes	Yes	Yes	Definite MI	
Yes	Yes	No	Probable MI	New zone of necrosis not evident on Echo. The persistence of new Q waves and abnormally elevated CK-MB suggests that Q waves are not a "benign" postoperative finding
Yes	No	Yes	Definite MI	CK-MB peak probably missed because of infrequent sampling
Yes	No	No	Possible MI	New Q waves may be false-positive finding
No	Yes	Yes	Probable MI	Non-Q-wave MI
No	Yes	No	MI unlikely	Small non-Q-wave MI cannot be entirely excluded
No	No	Yes	MI unlikely	Removal of "restraining" effect of pericardium may result in new RWMAs, especially in high anterior septal area
No	No	No	No MI	Although small patchy areas of necrosis may be seen histologically, these abnormalities are probably not of clinical significance

Echo = echocardiography; MI = myocardial infarction; RWMA = regional wall motion abnormality; ECG = electrocardiogram.
*Perioperative echocardiography is not *required* for the diagnosis of a perioperative MI but can provide useful supportive data or aid in the diagnosis in unclear cases, especially if obtained acutely.

ous revascularization (either percutaneous transluminal coronary angioplasty or CABG).[100]

Patients with a perioperative myocardial infarction have increased hospital mortality (~10 to 15 percent) when compared with patients undergoing CABG who have not sustained a perioperative myocardial infarction (~1 percent).[100] Characteristics of patients who are especially at risk of increased short-term mortality after a perioperative myocardial infarction include age older than 65 years, unstable angina preoperatively, a myocardial infarction within 1 week before surgery, left ventricular aneurysm, intraventricular conduction disturbance (e.g., left bundle branch block), and the need for reoperation for bleeding. About two-thirds of the postoperative mortality is due to pump failure and one-third is due to malignant ventricular tachyarrhythmias. Perioperative myocardial infarction also adversely affects the long-term prognosis, particularly if associated with inadequate revascularization and depressed left ventricular function.[106]

MANAGEMENT OF MYOCARDIAL ISCHEMIA AFTER CABG. Patients with evidence of myocardial ischemia after coronary bypass surgery require an integrated assessment of clinical findings and laboratory tests on an individualized basis to define the appropriate management strategy. At the center of the decision pathway are the 12-lead ECG and hemodynamic observations (Fig. 76–6). Patients with ST elevations and a low cardiac index require intraaortic balloon pump support. Echocardiography may disclose new wall motion abnormalities that may necessitate coronary angiography and a percutaneous revascularization procedure or surgical reexploration in selected patients.

Low-Output Syndrome and Shock States

RECOGNITION. Sometimes, diagnosis of low-output syndrome and a shock state after cardiac surgery is difficult. Because cold extremities and mottled skin may result from hypothermia postoperatively, these observations lack sufficient specificity. Although reduced systolic pressure is the most striking manifestation of this disorder, low-output syndrome may be present even if the arterial systolic pressure exceeds 100 mm Hg because increased systemic vascular resistance (>1500 dyne-sec$\cdot$cm^{-2}) may be supporting the peripheral perfusion pressure. It is important to recognize this syndrome because of the strong relationship between cardiac index in the early postoperative period and the probability of cardiac death after surgery. Common clinical features of the low-output syndrome and shock states after cardiac surgery include cold extremities, mottled skin, reduced systolic pressure (<90 mm Hg), decreased urine output (<30 ml/hr), low cardiac index (<2.0 liter/min$\cdot$m^{-2}), low mixed venous oxygen saturation (<50 percent), and acidosis.

One should assess hemodynamic findings and integrate them with bedside echocardiographic recordings to confirm the diagnosis of low-output syndrome and attempt to segregate the findings into one of the patterns (*reduced preload, cardiogenic shock,* or *sepsis*) in Table 76–10. Although the hemodynamic findings among these patterns overlap and the coexistence of multiple disorders (e.g., bradycardia and hypovolemia) may blur the distinction between patterns, they offer a clinically useful approach to the evaluation of a patient with low-output syndrome. In addition to the specific treatment measures discussed later, a number of general measures are applicable to all patients who are in a shock-like condition after cardiac surgery, including prompt correction of any electrolyte and acid-base disturbances, transfusion to a hematocrit over 30 percent for improved oxygen-carrying capacity of the blood, and a "low threshold" for mechanical ventilatory support to minimize the work of breathing and thereby reduce total-body oxygen needs.

REDUCED PRELOAD

Hypovolemia. Low ventricular filling pressure, normal systemic vascular resistance, and a reduced cardiac index, coupled with echocardiographic demonstration of small ventricular volume with preserved systolic function, are indicative of *hypovolemia*. Possible causes include bleeding, excessive diuresis, the "leaky capillary state" associated with the postpump syndrome, and less frequently, inadequate vascular volume because of insufficient return of fluids at the conclusion of cardiopulmonary bypass. Rarely, adrenocortical insufficiency as a result of perioperative hemorrhage into the adrenal glands has been reported as a cause of hypovolemic hypotension after cardiac surgery.

Therapeutic maneuvers include the administration of intravenous fluids (normal saline solution, lactated Ringer solution), transfusion with packed red blood cells if the hemoglobin is less than 8 gm/dl, and administration of colloid-type volume expanders. It is also important to discontinue any vasodilators or antihypertensives that may have been prescribed during a period when the patient was hypertensive. While waiting for these measures to take effect, the patient may require transient infusion of a vasoconstrictor (usually phenylephrine) or an inotropic pressor (usually dopamine or epinephrine).

VASODILATION. Inhibition of sympathetic tone by the effects of anesthetic agents may cause peripheral vasodilation. In combination with the increased venous capacitance that may occur during rewarming, a low-output syndrome may develop as a result of markedly reduced systemic vascular resistance (<1000 dyne·sec·cm^{-5}). This situation is best treated by intravenous infusion of a vasoconstrictor such as norepinephrine in a dose of 1 to 10 μg/min until the systemic vascular resistance returns to a normal level. In patients not responsive to norepinephrine, commonly associated with preoperative ACE inhibition, the addition of intravenous vasopressin in a dose of 0.05 to 6 units per minute can restore normal systemic vascular resistance.

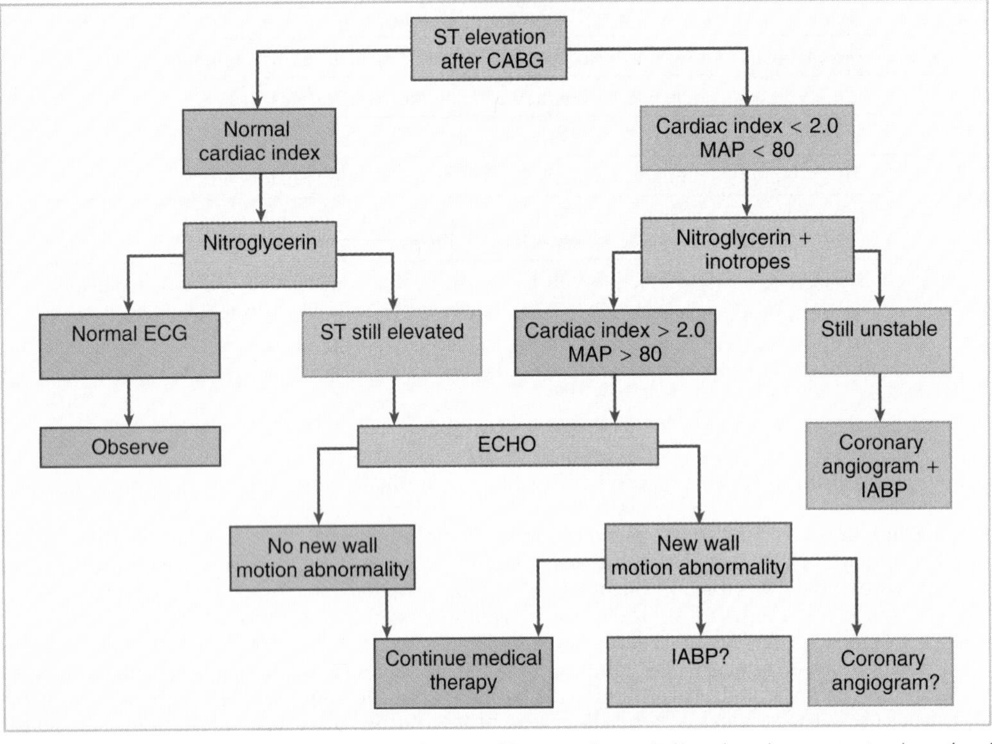

FIGURE 76–6 Myocardial ischemia after coronary bypass grafting occurs frequently. Hemodynamic assessment and ensuring of adequate coronary and systemic perfusion dictate early management strategies. Echocardiographic evaluation helps further tailor postoperative care. CABG = coronary artery bypass grafting; ECG = electrocardiogram; ECHO = echocardiography; IABP = intraaortic balloon pumping; MAP = mean arterial pressure.

CARDIOGENIC SHOCK. When right ventricular and left ventricular filling pressures are in the normal range and systemic vascular resistance is not reduced, a frequent cause of a cardiac index less than 2 liter/min·m^{-2} is *bradycardia.* Because the cardiac index is the product of stroke volume and heart rate, this abnormality is easily corrected by atrial or atrioventricular pacing at 85 to 100 beats/min.

LEFT VENTRICULAR FAILURE. The pattern of predominant *left ventricular failure* in the early postoperative state is characterized by a disproportionately elevated pulmonary capillary wedge pressure in comparison to right atrial pressure, a low cardiac index, and normal or elevated systemic

TABLE 76–10 Hemodynamic Disturbances Following Cardiac Surgery

	Reduced Preload		Bradycardia (Inappropriately Slow HR Postoperatively)
	Hypovolemia	*Vasodilation*	
Hemodynamics			
RA	<8	<8	≤10
PCW	<15	<15	>15
CI	<2.0	<2.0	<2.0
SVR	<1200	<1000	>1200
Other			HR <60
Echocardiogram	Small ventricular chambers with vigorous systolic contraction unless LV dysfunction was present preoperatively	Small ventricular chambers with normal systolic contraction unless LV dysfunction was present preoperatively	Normal-sized ventricular chambers with vigorous systolic contraction, albeit at a slow rate
Management	IV fluids Transfusion if Hgb ≤ 10 Inotropes	Vasopressors	Cardiac pacing

CI = cardiac index; Hgb = hemoglobin; HR = heart rate; IV = intravenous; LV = left ventricular; PAD = pulmonary artery diastolic; PCW = pulmonary capillary wedge; RA = right arterial; RV = right ventricular; SVR = systemic vascular resistance; TR = tricuspid regurgitation.

vascular resistance. Echocardiography usually reveals a dilated, poorly contractile left ventricle, often exhibiting multiple regional wall motion abnormalities.

Diagnosis. The differential diagnosis of left ventricular failure after cardiac surgery includes the following conditions (which may coexist in the same patient): preoperative left ventricular dysfunction, inadequate surgical correction of the cardiac lesion (e.g., residual left ventricular outflow tract obstruction after repair of idiopathic hypertrophic subaortic stenosis, residual ventricular septal defect), complication of a surgical procedure (e.g., prosthetic valve leak or thrombosis, depression of stroke volume after correction of mitral regurgitation caused by elevation of afterload), dysrhythmia, depressant effect of a pharmacological agent (e.g., antiarrhythmic drug), acid-base or electrolyte disturbance, or myocardial ischemia and/or infarction. Bedside echocardiography can usually help identify mechanical disorders such as prosthetic valve dysfunction and dysrhythmias,[107] and metabolic abnormalities and toxic drug levels can be readily recognized by ECG and laboratory measurements.

Management. The objectives of hemodynamic management of patients with *left ventricular failure* postoperatively are to correct hypotension if present, increase forward left ventricular output, and return left and right ventricular filling pressures to the normal range. These variables are intimately related, and treatment may require careful titration of several intravenous agents for pharmacological support of the failing circulation. Boluses of calcium chloride (0.5 to 1 gm) increase myocardial contractility, but the effect is modest and short-lived. A continuous infusion of dopamine (5 to 10 μg/kg/min) or epinephrine (1 to 10 μg/min) is preferable if the primary goal is to increase systemic arterial pressure and cardiac output. Dobutamine (2 to 5 μg/kg/min), amrinone (bolus of 0.75 mg/kg and infusion of 5 to 10 μg/kg/min), or milrinone (bolus of 50 μg/kg/min and infusion of 0.375 to 0.75 μg/kg/min) also augment cardiac output and should be selected if a reduction in ventricular filling pressure is desired; systemic arterial pressure is usually unchanged or may even drop slightly because of the peripheral vasodilatory effects of these drugs. A commonly used combination is dopamine (2 μg/kg/min) to achieve greater renal perfusion in conjunction with dobutamine (2 to 5 μg/kg/min) for augmentation of cardiac output. If the mean arterial pressure is 90 mm Hg or higher, vasodilator therapy with nitroglycerin increases forward cardiac output and lowers pulmonary capillary wedge pressure further. When hypotension is profound (e.g., systolic pressure < 70 mm Hg), norepinephrine or epinephrine 1 to 10 μg/min or vasopressin 1 to 6 units per minute may be necessary to prevent coronary hypoperfusion.

We prefer to use an intraaortic balloon pump (see Chap. 25) for mechanical support of the circulation along with pharmacotherapy early in the course of management of postoperative left ventricular failure that does not respond to the initial pharmacological maneuvers already discussed. This protocol has the advantages of avoiding a continuous upward titration of the dose of sympathomimetic inotropic agents and vasoconstrictors associated with downregulation of beta-adrenergic antagonist receptors and diminished perfusion of the renal, mesenteric, and coronary vascular beds. Also, intraaortic balloon counterpulsation does not increase myocardial oxygen demand. The intraaortic balloon pump is contraindicated in the presence of severe aortic regurgitation and if an abdominal aortic aneurysm is present. In patients with severe peripheral vascular disease, balloon placement via the ascending aorta should be considered. Delayed sternal closure is another important adjunct in the management of cardiogenic shock following surgery (Fig. 76–7).[108,109] If the patient fails to improve despite a combination of intraaortic balloon pumping, open-chest management, and pharmacotherapy, a ventricular assist device may be inserted for temporary support or as a "bridge" to recovery or cardiac transplantation.[110-112] Serial evaluations of left ventricular function over time and under different loading conditions and supportive measures are best obtained with transesophageal echocardiograms.

Cardiogenic Shock			
LV Failure	*RV Failure*	*Cardiac Tamponade*	*Sepsis*
≥10	>10	>15	<10
>20	≤15	>15	<15
<2.0	<2.0	<2.0	≥2.0
>1000	>1000	>1000	<1000
	PCW > 15 if LV failure is present	RA = PCW = PAD (within 5 mm Hg) unless "asymmetrical" tamponade occurs because of pericardial clots	Narrow A – VO_2 difference
Dilated LV with reduced systolic performance; regional wall motion abnormalities may reflect old or new myocardial ischemia and/or infarction	Dilated RA and RV with reduced RV systolic contraction TR often present on Doppler study IV contractile performance is variable	Small cardiac chambers with diastolic collapse of RA and RV Systolic contraction of RV and LV usually normal unless dysfunction was present preoperatively or coexistent LV or RV failure has occurred postoperatively	Small ventricular chambers with normal or slightly depressed contractile function (myocardial depressant factor)
Search for correctible lesion, offending agent, or laboratory abnormality Inotropes Vasopressors and vasodilators Mechanical assistance	Supplemental O_2 Pulmonary vasodilators Nitrous oxide Inotropes Mechanical assistance	Reexploration Supportive measures: IV fluids, inotropes	IV fluids Antibiotics Vasopressors Inotropes

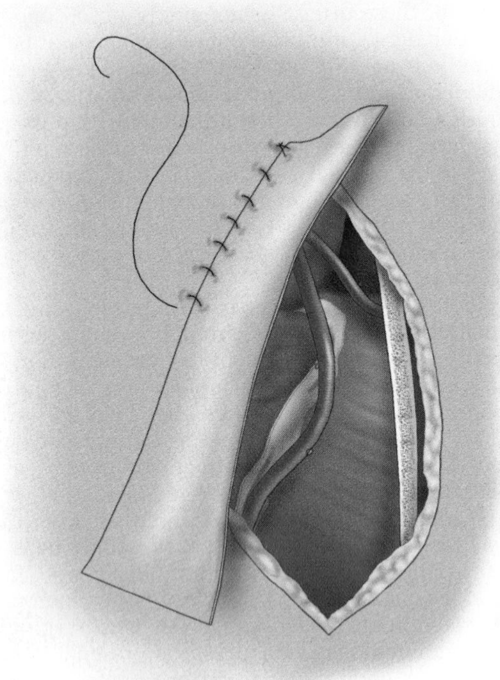

FIGURE 76–7 A patient in a low-output state may not tolerate immediate sternal closure, particularly in the setting of significant mediastinal and myocardial edema associated with prolonged cardiopulmonary bypass. Profuse coagulapathy represents an additional indication for open-chest management. After resolution of edema and recovery of myocardial function, the patient is returned to the operating room for a standard sternal closure.

RIGHT VENTRICULAR FAILURE. The pattern of predominant *right ventricular failure* is characterized by a disproportionate elevation in right atrial pressure in comparison to pulmonary capillary wedge pressure. In severe cases of postoperative right ventricular failure, right atrial pressure may exceed 20 mm Hg while pulmonary capillary wedge pressure remains equal to or less than 15 mm Hg. When left ventricular failure is present simultaneously, the difference between right atrial and pulmonary capillary wedge pressure lessens and differentiation from cardiac tamponade becomes difficult. Bedside echocardiography can aid the proper diagnosis (see Table 76–10).

Postoperatively, predominant right ventricular failure may be seen as a result of one or more of the following conditions: elevated pulmonary vascular resistance (persistently elevated from preoperative elevations in pulmonary artery pressure; postoperative hypoxia, pulmonary embolus, or pneumothorax), primary right ventricular ischemia/infarction,[113] or a mechanical lesion (tricuspid regurgitation, residual shunt flow, right ventriculotomy).

Massive pulmonary embolism occurs rarely after cardiac surgery (see Chap. 66). The diagnosis should be suspected when sudden deterioration in oxygenation occurs in association with confusion, systemic hypotension, tachycardia, ECG abnormalities (unexplained right axis deviation, right bundle branch block, a right ventricular strain pattern), and elevation of right atrial pressure. Angiographic confirmation of the diagnosis is not usually necessary. Expeditious noninvasive investigation by echocardiography is advisable in patients in whom the diagnosis remains uncertain.

Management. Hemodynamic management of predominant right ventricular failure should focus on improvement in right ventricular output to allow adequate filling of the left ventricle. Supplemental oxygen and hyperventilation to decrease P_{CO_2} levels help lower pulmonary artery pressure. Bradycardia (>60 beats/min) is corrected by atrial or atrioventricular pacing, isoproterenol (1 to 2 μg/min in an average adult) increases right ventricular contractility and also causes pulmonary vasodilation. Pulmonary hypertension may also be reduced by prostaglandin E_1 or intravenous nitroglycerin. In postoperative patients with massive pulmonary embolism and severe right ventricular dysfunction, emergency pulmonary embolectomy and placement of an inferior vena caval filter can be life-saving.

CARDIAC TAMPONADE (see Chap. 64). Postoperative echocardiography has shown that virtually all patients have pericardial effusion after cardiac surgery and that many such effusions are asymmetrical and loculated.[114] Even with mediastinal drains in place, cardiac tamponade can develop postoperatively; recognition of this condition requires a high index of suspicion and assessment of hemodynamics at the bedside.

Recognition. Important clinical features of tamponade, such as diminished heart sounds and pulsus paradoxus, may be obscured by mechanical ventilation. Asymmetrical, loculated accumulation of blood and clots in the mediastinum and pericardial space may cause isolated tamponade of one or two cardiac chambers and produce unusual elevations in diastolic pressure (e.g., right atrial tamponade with elevation of central venous pressure without an increase in right ventricular end-diastolic pressure or pulmonary capillary wedge pressure). Bedside transthoracic and transesophageal echocardiography is usually helpful for diagnosing pericardial effusions and assessing the hemodynamic significance of fluid collections.[115] Diastolic collapse of the right atrium and right ventricle is an indication of a hemodynamically significant external compressive force and should prompt urgent treatment.

Treatment. Although pericardiocentesis may be helpful in non-perioperative tamponade, it is unlikely to be successful in evacuating the organized pericardial and mediastinal material that develops after cardiac surgery; subxiphoid drainage and/or emergency resternotomy is preferred. Supportive measures that can be attempted in the interim include volume expansion with intravenous fluids (Plasmanate, whole blood) and inotropic agents (epinephrine).

SEPTIC SHOCK. Low ventricular filling pressure, markedly reduced systemic vascular resistance, and a normal or unexpectedly high cardiac index in the setting of hypotension and a shocklike state should raise suspicion of the early stages of *sepsis.* With progression of septic shock, a capillary leak syndrome develops (hypovolemia) and myocardial depression may occur and result in a somewhat reduced contractile pattern of the ventricles on echocardiography. Combined therapy with intravenous fluids, antibiotics, and inotropic agents is required to interrupt the vicious cycle of hypotension, acidosis, and diminished coronary perfusion. Most patients in a septic state during the first several days after cardiac surgery are infected with a skin organism (e.g., indwelling catheters) or from seeding the bloodstream from a pulmonary or urinary source. Broad antibiotic coverage (e.g., vancomycin plus ceftazidime) should be instituted. Because the offending organism is likely to be resistant to the prophylactic antibiotic given preoperatively, it is wise to not include it as one of the empirical antibiotics selected to treat sepsis.

Perioperative Arrhythmias (see Chaps. 30 and 32)

EVALUATION AND TREATMENT. There appear to be two peaks in the incidence of arrhythmias perioperatively: the first occurs in the operating room (most commonly during induction of anesthesia, weaning from cardiopulmonary bypass, or rewarming), and the second occurs in the ICU between the second and fifth postoperative days. The electrophysiological mechanisms underlying perioperative arrhythmias are incompletely understood, but they can probably be ascribed to a combination of the effects of circulating catecholamines, alterations in autonomic nervous system tone, transient electrolyte imbalance, myocardial ischemia or infarction, and mechanical irritation of the heart.

APPROACH TO THE PATIENT. Several factors may predispose to the development of arrhythmias, including ventilatory dysfunction, fever, electrolyte imbalance (hypokalemia, hypomagnesemia, hypocalcemia), anemia, myocardial ischemia or infarction, low cardiac output and reflex increase in sympathetic tone, hypertension, pericardial inflammation, and toxic effects of cardioactive medications (e.g., digitalis toxicity, bradycardia induced by diltiazem). *Every effort should be made to seek and eliminate any of the factors that may be provoking the arrhythmia.*

Although antiarrhythmic drug therapy and direct-current cardioversion are traditional methods for treating postoperative arrhythmias, cardiac pacing techniques have a number of advantages, including more rapid onset and offset of action, avoidance of potential drug toxicity (especially proarrhythmia), elimination of the need for anesthesia (required for cardioversion), reduced anxiety for the patient, greater safety in patients receiving digitalis, and perhaps most important, the ability to repeat the pacing protocol if the arrhythmia should recur, a not infrequent event. In addition to terminating arrhythmias, cardiac pacing can be used to suppress arrhythmias in many patients by atrial, atrioventricular sequential, or ventricular stimulation at a critical rate (e.g., 85 to 100 beats/min).

Surface Electrocardiogram. The value of a 12-lead ECG and simultaneously recorded multiple standard ECG lead rhythm strips cannot be overemphasized if one is attempting to analyze a wide-complex tachycardia. Unfortunately, a number of the criteria for differentiating supraventricular tachycardia with aberrant conduction from ventricular tachycardia (see Chap. 32) may not apply to postoperative patients because of previous or newly acquired infarction patterns, transient conduction defects (seen in 5 to 15 percent of patients in the early recovery period), and nonspecific repolarization patterns.

Epicardial Electrodes. It is desirable to place two wires on the free wall of the right atrium and a bipolar wire on the right ventricle intraoperatively to allow for bipolar atrial recording and pacing or dual-chamber pacing. The advantages of bipolar pacing include a smaller stimulus artifact, the ability to record a bipolar atrial electrogram during ventricular pacing, and a reduced likelihood of precipitating undesired atrial arrhythmias if an atrial wire is used as the indifferent electrode during unipolar ventricular pacing. Schematic diagrams showing the typical intrathoracic positioning of the atrial and ventricular wires are shown in Figure 76–8. In patients with severe heart failure, placement of biventricular pacing wires should be considered for postoperative support.[116,117]

Supraventricular Arrhythmias

ATRIAL PREMATURE DEPOLARIZATIONS. The hemodynamic consequences of atrial premature depolarizations are almost always minor, and one should resist the urge to suppress them with antiarrhythmic drugs. Instead, they should be considered a signal that the patient is possibly hypoxic or that an electrolyte or acid-base imbalance is present and a warning that the patient is at risk for more serious arrhythmia such as atrial fibrillation or atrial flutter. In the absence of such correctable abnormalities, one may want to administer a beta-adrenergic antagonist to inhibit the effects of circulating catecholamines and also to slow the ventricular rate if atrial fibrillation should develop.

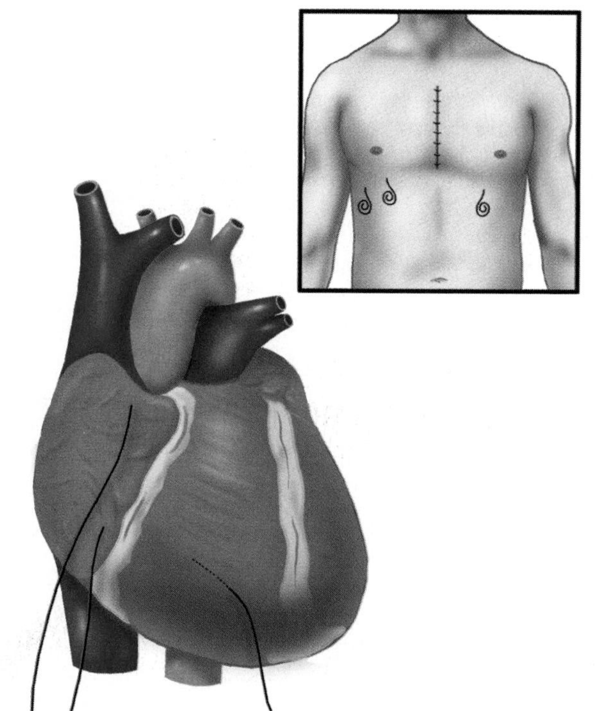

FIGURE 76–8 Epicardial electrodes in patients undergoing cardiac surgery. The precise number and location of pacing wires may vary among institutions and also according to the complexity of the operation (e.g., no atrial wires for routine coronary artery bypass surgery but both atrial and ventricular wires for valve surgery). In the example shown, the two atrial wires exit to the patient's right while the bipolar ventricular wire exits to the left.

ATRIAL FLUTTER. Control of the ventricular rate in atrial flutter is more difficult than in atrial fibrillation because of the limited number of ventricular responses to atrial activation (usually 2:1, 4:1, but rarely an odd-numbered multiple). Atrial flutter may be difficult to terminate with antiarrhythmic agents. Ibutilide 0.01 mg/kg up to 1 mg given intravenously over 10 minutes is useful as a first-line treatment of atrial flutter. Torsade de pointes can occur in up to 8 percent of cases, so patients post-ibultilide must be closely monitored during treatment with this drug. If ibultilide is unsuccessful, cardioversion with energy of 25 to 50 watt-seconds delivered as a single discharge can be expected to terminate atrial flutter in more than 90 percent of patients. Atrial flutter can also be terminated by rapid atrial pacing with the temporary epicardial atrial wires placed at the time of surgery (Fig. 76–9). The likelihood of success increases if one uses sufficiently rapid rates of pacing (up to 140 percent of the spontaneous atrial rate), a sufficient duration of pacing (10 to 30 seconds) with adequate strength (5 to 20 mA), and pretreatment of the patient with procainamide. To achieve the high drive rates required, a special stimulator is used.

ATRIAL FIBRILLATION. Although atrial fibrillation is an extremely common arrhythmia following cardiac surgery, etiology, predictors, and optimal management strategy remain elusive.[118-126] Even after prophylactic therapy with beta-adrenergic blockers, transient symptomatic atrial fibrillation occurs in at least 25 to 30 percent of patients after CABG and in 50 percent of patients following valvular surgery; atrial fibrillation appears with greatest incidence on the second or third postoperative day. Because of the hazards of postoperative atrial fibrillation, considerable effort has been devoted to identifying preoperative factors associated with an increased risk of postoperative arrhythmia.[118,121,123] Such factors include advanced age, male gender, hyperten-

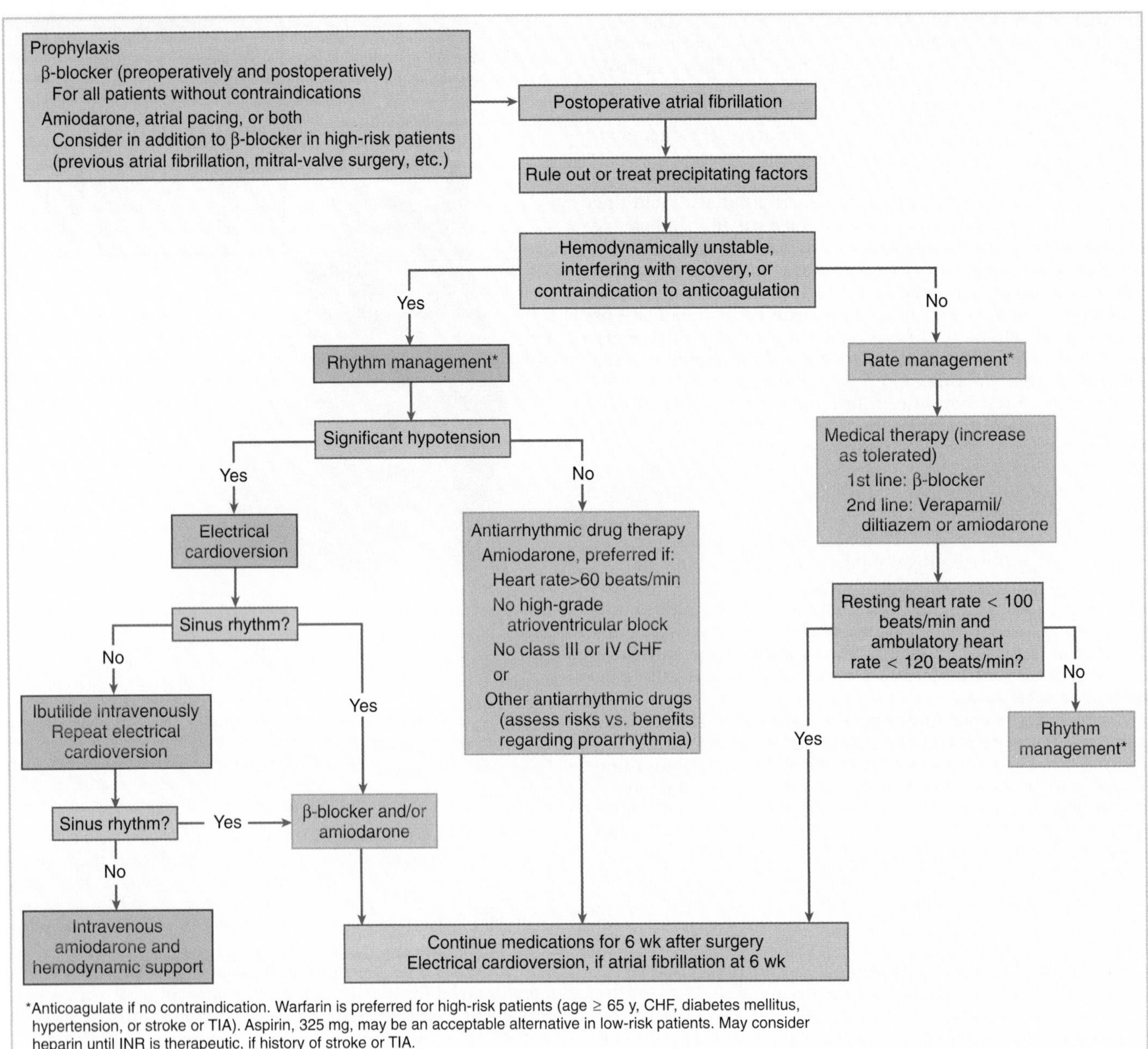

FIGURE 76–9 Algorithm for the prevention and management of atrial fibrillation after cardiac surgery. CHF = congestive heart failure; TIA = transient ischemic attack. (From Maisel WH, Rawn JD, Stevenson WG: Atrial fibrillation after cardiac surgery. Ann Intern Med 135:1061-1073, 2001.)

sion, intraaortic balloon pump, postoperative pneumonia, and mechanical ventilation for longer than 24 hours. A prolonged P wave duration recorded on a signal-averaged ECG and greater than 70 percent narrowing of the lumen of the right coronary artery may predict an increased risk of postoperative atrial fibrillation. However, for a substantial number of patients with postoperative atrial fibrillation, no apparent preoperative risk factor can be identified. Perhaps patients undergoing cardiac operations are vulnerable to postoperative atrial fibrillation because of mild nonuniformity in the distribution of their trial refractory periods. Intraoperative atrial ischemia associated with rapid rewarming of the atria during prolonged periods of cold cardioplegic arrest may increase the dispersion of refractoriness in the atria of such patients and thereby increase the risk of postoperative atrial fibrillation.

An algorithm for the prevention and management of atrial fibrillation after cardiac surgery is shown in Figure 76–9. Because of difficulties in reliably identifying patients at risk for atrial fibrillation preoperatively, it is common clinical practice to provide prophylactic therapy to most patients undergoing CABG. Beta-adrenergic blocking agents are most suitable for prophylaxis against atrial fibrillation. In the *absence* of an ejection fraction less than 30 percent, severe bronchospastic lung disease, or bradyarrhythmias, we advocate the use of prophylactic beta blockers in patients undergoing CABG. Conclusive data regarding the use of prophylactic antiarrhythmic therapy to prevent postoperative atrial fibrillation are lacking, although prophylactic amiodarone in selected patients has appeared promising in several clinical trials.[119,120,124] Unless hemodynamic collapse is present, in which case direct-current cardioversion should be performed, the initial treatment of choice in a postoperative patient is to slow the ventricular rate. Provided that the patient's ventricular function is adequate, acute intravenous administration of beta-adrenergic blocking agents (e.g., metoprolol 5 mg every 5 minutes for up to three doses), verapamil (5-mg bolus every 5 to 10 minutes for three or four doses), diltiazem (0.25- to 0.35-mg/kg bolus over a period of 2 minutes), or amiodarone (loading dose of 150-mg bolus, then 1 mg/min infusion for 6 hours, then 0.5 mg/min) is a more desirable option. Esmolol, an ultrashort-acting cardioselective beta blocker, when administered intravenously in a dose of 50 to 250 mg/kg/min, provides the option of rapid onset; in the event of hemodynamic deterioration, the effects of the drug are usually dissipated within 15 to 30 minutes after discontinuation of the infusion. In addition, the probability of conversion to sinus rhythm with esmolol appears to be better than with other agents such as verapamil.[127]

ANTICOAGULANTS. Epidemiological observations suggest that the development of postoperative atrial fibrillation is associated with a marked increase in the risk of stroke (odds ratio 3.0) and prolonged hospitalization. No consensus has been reached regarding anticoagulation recommendations in patients with postoperative atrial fibrillation. The risk of hemorrhage in the early postoperative period must be weighed against the risk of systemic thromboembolism. When atrial fibrillation develops beyond the second postoperative day, we generally advocate adherence to the guidelines established for nonsurgical patients and initiate anticoagulation (intravenous heparin followed by oral warfarin) in patients who have been in the arrhythmia for more than 48 hours, especially if the patient has a history of systemic embolism or if mitral valve disease or cardiomyopathy is present.

Beyond control of the ventricular rate acutely, the two treatment strategies for management of postoperative atrial fibrillation are similar to those for nonsurgical patients: chronic anticoagulation while administering rate-controlling agents versus restoration of sinus rhythm and attempts at suppression of recurrence of atrial fibrillation. Because large-scale clinical trial data are not available to guide decision making in this area, therapeutic approaches must be individualized. Ibutilide can acutely convert post-CABG atrial fibrillation when administered intravenously, albeit with a small risk (<2 percent) of torsades de pointes.[128] Procainamide is frequently used for the treatment of atrial fibrillation after open-heart surgery, although present evidence indicates that it has limited effectiveness in suppressing recurrence of atrial fibrillation.[129] Furthermore, any treatment decision formulated during hospitalization should be readdressed at the first postoperative visit (typically 4 to 6 weeks) to determine whether it is still a desirable course of action once the inflammation and metabolic alterations of the postoperative state have dissipated. Patients with depressed left ventricular function or striking ventricular hypertrophy who experience troublesome dyspnea and/or hypotension when in atrial fibrillation postoperatively are suitable candidates for a trial of restoration of sinus rhythm.

Patients with rheumatic heart disease and a preoperative history of atrial fibrillation often require permanent suppressive antiarrhythmic therapy despite successful aortic or mitral valve surgery even if sinus rhythm is present during the early postoperative period.

PAROXYSMAL SUPRAVENTRICULAR TACHYCARDIA. The reentrant forms of paroxysmal supraventricular tachycardia (PSVT)—atrioventricular nodal reentry tachycardia and atrioventricular reentry tachycardia—occur less frequently in postoperative patients than does atrial fibrillation or atrial flutter and, fortunately, retain their responsiveness to vagal maneuvers and pharmacotherapy designed to inhibit atrioventricular nodal conduction. The antiarrhythmic agent adenosine, an endogenous nucleoside, has a number of features that make it the drug of choice for treating PSVT in postoperative patients (see Chaps. 30 and 32). A rapid (2-second) intravenous bolus of 6 mg terminates about 60 percent of episodes of PSVT within 20 seconds; a subsequent bolus of 12 mg administered 1 to 2 minutes later terminates PSVT in virtually all patients who failed to respond to the lower dose. Because adenosine is rapidly transported into the cell or degraded enzymatically to inosine, the physiological effects of adenosine are dissipated in less than 5 minutes. Untoward reactions such as flushing, chest pain, or dyspnea, although common, are mild and short lived. PSVT may also be diagnosed by atrial recordings and terminated by burst atrial pacing or randomly delivered ventricular or atrial premature depolarizations that invade the reentrant circuit and interrupt the arrhythmia.

CARDIOVERSION. Direct-current cardioversion should be used in postsurgical patients with the following additional considerations. The recent cardiotomy with resultant pericardial and mediastinal inflammation, the presence of chest tubes and/or pleural effusions, and elevated catecholamine levels after surgery all may contribute to higher energy requirements for reversion of arrhythmias such as atrial fibrillation than are commonly required in patients who have not recently undergone cardiac surgery. To achieve the maximum transcardiac spread of current after median sternotomy, the anterior paddle should be placed to the *right* of the sternum between the third and sixth intercostal space, and the other paddle should be positioned in the fourth to sixth intercostal space as far in the left axilla as possible or in a posterior location under the tip of the left scapula. Firm pressure is applied to the paddles to maintain contact with the chest wall as the discharge buttons are depressed.

Ventricular Arrhythmias

VENTRICULAR PREMATURE DEPOLARIZATIONS. Isolated ventricular premature depolarizations (VPDs) commonly occur after cardiac surgery. An increase in the frequency of VPDs may be seen in patients with a preoperative history of VPDs, or they may appear de novo in patients with no history of ventricular arrhythmias. Although a fall in arterial pressure may be associated with isolated VPDs, this decreased pressure is usually extremely brief and of no significant hemodynamic consequence to the patient unless prolonged periods of bigeminy occur.

Management. We advocate a conservative approach focusing on prompt detection and correction of provocative factors (e.g. ischemia, hypoxia, metabolic derangement, or catheter initiation), liberal use of beta-adrenergic antagonists in patients with an ejection fraction greater than 0.30, and overdrive atrial or atrioventricular sequential pacing between 85 and 100 beats/min. We restrict suppressive antiarrhythmic therapy to patients with a preoperative history of serious ventricular tachyarrhythmias. If the decision is made to suppress VPDs in a patient without a history of symptomatic ventricular arrhythmias, the treatment period should be brief (6 to 24 hours) and the patient should not be automatically converted to treatment with an oral antiarrhythmic drug regimen without careful reconsideration of the indications for treatment.

VENTRICULAR TACHYCARDIA. Many of the same arguments cited earlier for isolated VPDs apply to paroxysms of nonsustained ventricular tachycardia. No definitive guidelines are available, but we believe that symptomatic episodes of nonsustained ventricular tachycardia in the absence of correctable factors and attempts at overdrive atrial or atrioventricular sequential pacing are indications for antiarrhythmic therapy, especially if the episodes are associated with hemodynamic compromise. *Sustained ventricular tachycardia* is a serious emergency that should be handled in an orderly approach. If the clinical situation permits, a 12-lead ECG should be obtained for future reference and confirmation of the diagnosis; simultaneous recording of surface ECG leads with electrograms from the epicardial wires may be helpful in establishing the mechanism of a wide-complex tachycardia.

Attempts at acute conversion of the tachycardia include the following maneuvers in the sequence listed: thumpversion, burst ventricular pacing, and boluses of antiarrhythmic agents (lidocaine 100 mg, procainamide up to 500 to 1000 mg over a period of 20 minutes, or amiodarone 75 to 150 mg infused over a 10-minute period). In urgent circumstances, synchronized direct-current cardioversion with a low-energy shock (25 to 50 watt-seconds) may be used. Unsynchronized shocks of 100 to 200 watt-seconds should be administered if the tachycardia rate is greater than 160 beats/min and/or has a sinusoidal waveform on ECG. After conversion, a search for correctable disorders should be undertaken, and if none is found, a continuous infusion of lidocaine (2 mg/min), procainamide (2 mg/min), or amiodarone (1 mg/min for 6 hours followed by a maintenance infusion of 0.5 mg/min).

VENTRICULAR FIBRILLATION. As in nonsurgical patients, ventricular fibrillation must be promptly treated with an unsynchronized direct-current shock. Ventricular fibrillation can often be reverted with shocks of 200 watt-seconds, provided that the intervention is performed promptly. It should be possible to defibrillate postoperative patients in the ICU expeditiously; therefore, the higher energies (360 to 400 watt-seconds) used in the "field" are probably unnecessary, at least initially. Because of the small number of patients experiencing unexpected sustained, hemodynamically compromising ventricular tachycardia or ventricular fibrillation, epidemiological data on provocative factors and the prognosis of these arrhythmias are difficult to evaluate. Unexplained ventricular tachycardia or ventricular fibrillation occurring within 24 hours after CABG is associated with very high in-hospital mortality, probably resulting from perioperative ischemia, infarction, and/or pump failure. Episodes of ventricular tachycardia or ventricular fibrillation occurring more than 24 hours after bypass surgery have a slightly less ominous prognosis and may be due to reperfusion of previously ischemic zones, early postoperative occlusion of coronary bypass grafts, or transmembrane shift of electrolytes during the process of recovery.[130]

Risk stratification of patients experiencing ventricular tachycardia or ventricular fibrillation postoperatively should include assessment of left ventricular function, coronary arteriography if ischemia/infarction is suspected, and consideration of an electrophysiological study to establish the most appropriate course of therapy. Because of the numerous metabolic fluxes taking place in the early postoperative period, electrophysiological study should, if possible, be postponed until at least 5 to 7 days following surgery. Serious consideration should be given to use of an implantable cardioverter-defibrillator in patients without an identifiable reversible cause of their arrhythmia, particularly those with a depressed ejection fraction (see Chap. 31).

ATRIOVENTRICULAR JUNCTIONAL RHYTHMS. Nonparoxysmal atrioventricular junctional rhythms (rate > 45 beats/min) can be seen after mitral or aortic valve surgery. Trauma and tissue swelling from surgical débridement and suture placement are believed to be the provocative mechanisms. Such rhythms are typically transient (≤48 hours) and easily treated with atrial or atrioventricular sequential pacing at a rate above that of the intrinsic junctional mechanism.

Bradyarrhythmias

Sinus bradycardia or sinus arrest with emergence of a slow atrioventricular junction escape rhythm can occur postoperatively when one or more of the following factors are present: advanced age, hypothermia, drug effects (diltiazem, beta blocker, digitalis, procainamide), preoperative sinus node dysfunction, intraoperative trauma to the sinus node, and postoperative elevation in vagal tone.[131] In addition to modifying the dose or discontinuing the use of offending drugs (such as those noted earlier), atrial pacing at 85 to 100 beats/min should be initiated to maintain adequate cardiac output and urine flow.

Although a new conduction defect may develop in up to 45 percent of patients following cardiac surgery, most are transient and related to myocardial hypothermia, perioperative electrolyte shifts, or surgical trauma during valve repair/replacement or closure of septal defects.[132] The risk of permanent, complete heart block postoperatively is increased in patients with preoperative conduction disturbances or multiple valve replacements and in those who have had previous valve surgery. However, implantation of a permanent epicardial pacing lead is rarely needed at the time of surgery because of the ease of implantation of a transvenous endocardial system postoperatively. An exception would be patients who are undergoing tricuspid valve replacement with a mechanical prosthesis, especially if they are simultaneously undergoing an aortic or mitral valve operation. Because of the contraindication to passing a transvenous lead through the mechanical tricuspid prosthesis, the surgical team should be alerted to the need for placement of permanent epicardial leads intraoperatively.

MANAGEMENT. The decision to insert a permanent pacemaker (see Chap. 31) after cardiac surgery should be based on the hemodynamic consequences of bradycardia in the individual patient rather than on a specific heart rate. Most new conduction defects resolve in the early postoperative period, but some persist for as long as 2 weeks. Few data are available to guide the decision about timing of implantation of a permanent pacemaker. We are willing to monitor a younger patient (<65 years) following CABG with a temporary pacing system postoperatively to see whether a conduction defect resolves. However, we have a low threshold for implanting a permanent pacemaker following aortic or mitral valve surgery or if antiarrhythmic therapy or beta-adrenergic blocker treatment is contemplated because these pharmacological measures might "stress" a diseased conduction system. We advocate early insertion of a permanent pacemaker in elderly patients with symptomatic bradycardia because the recuperative process is facilitated, the period of relative immobilization and ECG monitoring is minimized, and hospital stay is shortened. Finally, we are more aggressive about implantation of permanent pacemakers in patients with persistent advanced atrioventricular block than in those with isolated sinus bradycardia.

Hemostatic Disturbances (see Chap. 80)

EXCESSIVE BLEEDING. Multifactorial derangement of the hemostatic system develops in all patients who undergo cardiopulmonary bypass. These abnormalities are caused by exposure of the blood to artificial surfaces, hemodilution, and the effects of heparin (Table 76–11).[133] Platelet dysfunction is the most significant hemostatic abnormality that occurs after cardiopulmonary bypass, although diminution of coagulation factor levels may assume greater significance in patients with preoperative deficiencies in hemostasis. These abnormalities are increased in the setting of prolonged cardiopulmonary bypass times and the use of deep hypothermic circulatory arrest. Administration of the following drugs before surgery may predispose the patient to excessive bleeding: aspirin and other antiplatelet agents, nonsteroidal antiinflammatory agents, thrombolytic agents, certain antibiotics (carbenicillin, ticarcillin, moxalactam, cefamandole, third-generation cephalosporins), dextran, amrinone, quinidine, cytotoxic agents, gold, phenylbutazone, and fish oils. Other clinical conditions associated with increased postoperative hemorrhage include chronic renal failure, active endocarditis, and chronic hepatic congestion. The most obvious evidence of

TABLE 76–11 Hemostatic Disturbances Following Cardiopulmonary Bypass

Abnormality	Cause
Exposure of blood to artificial surfaces	
1. Platelet dysfunction A. Prolonged bleeding time B. Decreased adhesiveness	1. Depletion of platelet alpha granules, reduced response to wounds, and increased plasma levels of platelet factor 4 and beta-thromboglobulin
2. Inflammatory response	2. Activation of the complement, coagulation, fibrinolytic, and kallikrein cascades; activation of neutrophils with degranulation and protease enzyme release; oxygen free radical production; and synthesis of cytokines (tumor necrosis factor, IL-1, IL-6, IL-8)
Hemodilution	
1. Thrombocytopenia	1. Priming of extracorporeal bypass circuit with crystalloid solutions. Heparin-mediated immune thrombocylopenia may occur in about 5% of patients*
2. Coagulation factor depletion	2. Most coagulation factor levels are reduced by hemodilution by about 50%; factor V is reduced to 20-30% of normal and factor VIII is relatively unaffected. Factor levels usually return to normal within 12 hr after completion of cardiopulmonary bypass. Although plasminogen and fibrinogen levels are decreased by about 50%, fibrin degradation products usually do not appear in the plasma during bypass
Heparinization	Thrombus formation is inhibited and excessive bleeding is avoided intraoperatively by maintaining the activated clotting time between 400 and 480 sec

IL = interleukin.

*Reversal of heparin effects is accomplished with protamine sulfate. Vascular collapse has been reported in some patients during protamine treatment. To avoid the problem of heparin-induced thrombocytopenia and because heparin may not effectively inhibit all the thrombin generated during cardiopulmonary bypass ("heparin rebound"), novel antithrombins are being evaluated as alternatives to heparin during surgery.

bleeding in a postoperative cardiac surgical patient is by means of chest tube drainage. "Acceptable" rates of bleeding are usually less than 100 ml/hr. We advocate return to the operating room because of excessive bleeding include more than 500 ml/hr for 1 hour, more than 300 ml/hr for 3 hours, and 200 to 300 ml/hr for 4 hours. These criteria may be tempered by correctable extenuating circumstances, such as uncontrolled hypertension postoperatively, failure to achieve normothermia, or an abnormal coagulation status that is being corrected. In contrast, select patients undergoing minimally invasive surgery may be returned for exploration earlier if no explanation for excessive blood loss is obvious. Emergency medical maneuvers that can be attempted after sending coagulation studies to the laboratory include the use of PEEP up to 10 cm H_2O for mediastinal tamponade, empirical "correction" of putative platelet dysfunction with desmopressin acetate (DDAVP, a synthetic analog of arginine vasopressin that increases plasma levels of von Willebrand factor) 0.3 μg/kg infused over a period of 15 to 30 minutes, and empirical administration of a small dose of protamine sulfate 25 to 50 mg because heparin may be liberated from the patient's fat stores as rewarming occurs.

Once the coagulation profile returns, additional therapy in the form of platelet transfusions for a platelet count less than 100,000/mm^3 and fresh frozen plasma to correct an elevated prothrombin time can be prescribed. Aprotinin therapy (2×10^5 KIU loading bolus followed by infusion of 0.5×10^5 KIU/hr for 4 hours) is helpful in cases of excessive postoperative bleeding by virtue of its ability to inhibit fibrinolysis and preserve platelet glycoprotein Ib and von Willebrand factor activity.[134] When monitoring bleeding from a chest tube, it is important to be alert to sudden cessation of hemorrhage, which may indicate that the chest tubes have clotted and the fluid is now draining into the mediastinum or the pleural spaces. Serial chest radiographs may be helpful while observing a patient during a bleeding episode. With correct medical management, less than 2 percent of patients need to return to the operating room for control of bleeding, preferably within 3 to 4 hours of the original surgery, before hemodynamic destabilization occurs and large volumes of blood products are administered.

HYPERCOAGULABLE DISORDERS. Management of patients with hypercoagulable syndromes requiring cardiac surgery poses special challenges.[135-140] Common (factor V Leiden) and uncommon (antithrombin deficiency, proteins C and S deficiency) syndromes have different risk associations for venous thrombosis ranging between 2.5% (factor V Leiden) and 25% (antithrombin deficiency) (see Chap. 80). Surgery is a known trigger for thrombosis, and therefore aggressive prophylaxis with subcutaneous unfractionated heparin or low-molecular-weight heparin is warranted in the postoperative setting. If patients are on long-term anticoagulation, warfarin therapy should be switched to heparin therapy 3 to 5 days prior to surgery. As soon as adequate postoperative hemostasis is ensured, restarting heparin therapy within 2 days of surgery is recommended with simultaneous resumption of warfarin therapy. Patients with antiphospholipid antibody syndrome (lupus, anticoagulant/anticardiolipin antibodies, history of arterial or venous thrombosis, and/or recurrent fetal loss) can have associated valvular heart disease requiring surgery. Anticoagulation monitoring during cardiopulmonary bypass may be challenging, and preoperative in vitro testing to identify the most reliable assay for heparin monitoring may be warranted. In the postoperative setting aggressive anticoagulation is again recommended to prevent thromboembolic complications. In patients undergoing deep hypothermic circulatory arrest, particularly during aortic reconstructive surgery, cases of catastrophic circulatory thrombosis have been reported in patients with hypercoagulable states also receiving antifibrinolytics. We recommend factor V Leiden screening if circulatory arrest is planned, with avoidance of antifibrinolytics in patients who screen positive.[141]

HEPARIN-INDUCED THROMBOCYTOPENIA (see Chap. 80). Heparin-induced thrombocytopenia (HIT) is an immune-mediated, potentially life-threatening thrombotic complication that occurs in 3 percent of patients receiving heparin for 5 or more days.[142] HIT is a clinicopathological diagnosis that should be suspected in any patient who experiences a 50% or greater decrease in platelet count from baseline or a 30% or greater decrease in platelet count and associated thrombotic complication while on heparin for at least 5 days. Antibodies to heparin-platelet factor 4 cause platelet activation, aggregation and thrombin formation resulting often in deep venous thrombosis, pulmonary embolism, or cerebral sinus thrombosis. In general, thrombo-

TABLE 76–12 Anticoagulation Guidelines for Antithrombotic Therapy in Cardiac Surgery Patients

Surgery	Anticoagulant	INR*
Mitral mechanical valve	Warfarin	2.5-3.5
Aortic mechanical valve	Warfarin	2.0-3.0
Tricuspid mechanical valve	Warfarin	2.5-3.0
Atrial fibrillation	Warfarin	2.0-2.5
Mitral tissue valve	Warfarin	2.0-3.0 for 6 wk
Mitral valve repair	Warfarin	2.0-3.0 for 6 wk
Tricuspid tissue valve	Warfarin	2.0-3.0 for 6 wk
Tricuspid repair	Warfarin	2.0-3.0 for 6 wk
LV thrombus	Warfarin	2.0-3.0 for 6 mo
LV aneurysm repair	Warfarin	2.0-3.0 for 6 wk
Aortic tissue valve	ASA (80 mg/d)	
Coronary artery bypass	ASA 325 mg/d, 81 mg/d if taking warfarin	

ASA = acetylsalicylic acid (aspirin); LV = left ventricular.
*The target international normalized ratio (INR) is the midpoint of the range.

cytopenia resolves within 1 week of heparin discontinuation, but the prothrombotic state can persist for up to 1 month. Diagnostic tests for HIT are discussed in Chapter 80. In patients with suspicion of HIT, heparin should be stopped and, if a strong indication for anticoagulation persists, another antithrombotic agent (lepirudin, argatroban) should be initiated.[143-146] In patients with HIT, warfarin initiation should be done in the presence of lepirudin or argatroban due to warfarin's association with limb gangrene when used as the sole agent. HIT antibodies are usually undetectable 100 days after the cessation of heparin therapy, and if these antibodies are negative and the patient requires reoperative cardiac surgery, unfractioned heparin can be reused for cardiopulmonary bypass.

ANTITHROMBOTIC THERAPY IN CARDIAC SURGICAL PATIENTS. A wide spectrum of patients recovering from cardiac surgery may require either short- or long-term antithrombotic therapy (Table 76–12). Furthermore, the intensity of therapy is dictated by the estimated risk of thromboembolism. Variables that may have an impact on the risk of thromboembolism include insertion of a prosthetic valve (mechanical more than bioprosthetic), valve location (mitral more than aortic), the presence of atrial fibrillation, size of the left atrium, history of thromboembolism, left atrial thrombi visualized at surgery, and ventricular wall motion abnormalities associated with mural thrombi.

Neurological Complications

Neurological complications after cardiac surgery are quite common, particularly in the elderly, if one is attentive to the subtle cognitive (short-term memory loss, lack of concentration) and psychological (depression, increased sense of dependency) changes seen early after surgery.[29,147-149] A positive and supportive attitude on the part of the staff and enlistment of the aid of family members help minimize these problems. Although many patients return to their preoperative state by 4 to 6 weeks after surgery, about 10 percent continue to show deterioration in neuropsychological functioning over the next 6 months, especially if they are older than 65 years of age.[29,149] More serious neurological complications such as stroke occur in 1 to 5 percent of patients but may be seen in as many as 10 percent of patients older than 65.[29]

Symptomatic visual defects may be seen after cardiac surgery and result from retinal emboli, occipital lobe infarction, or anterior ischemic optic neuropathy. Risk factors for cerebrovascular accident or transient ischemic attack after cardiac surgery include preoperative carotid bruit, previous cerebrovascular accident or transient ischemic attack, postoperative atrial fibrillation, prolonged cardiopulmonary bypass (>2 hours), and preoperative left ventricular mural thrombus.[29]

Measures that decrease the risk of stroke in patients undergoing cardiac surgery include preoperative carotid scanning in high-risk patients, use of a soft-flow aortic cannula that minimizes disruption of aortic plaques, precise management of cardiopulmonary bypass with increased mean arterial pressure in elderly patients, and a strict strategy of minimal aortic manipulation if epiaortic ultrasound scanning reveals significant aortic atherothrombotic disease (see Fig. 76–3).[15]

Neuropathies in the upper extremities can occur after cardiac operations. A pattern of injury involving predominantly the ulnar nerve and medial antebrachial cutaneous nerve suggests that the lesion involves brachial plexus compression or a traction injury. The average duration of symptoms after such an injury is 2 months, but some patients show a slower time course of improvement extending over 6 to 12 months.

Infection

FEVER. Despite its nonspecific nature, fever is the most common initial clinical sign of a postoperative infection. It should be emphasized, however, that patients who experience a normal course of convalescence continue to show an elevated temperature for up to 6 days postoperatively. In the absence of infection, such early fevers probably result from alterations in blood components after cardiopulmonary bypass such as activation of polynuclear neutrophils and complement system. In addition to infectious causes, fevers that occur beyond 6 days may be due to drug reactions, phlebitis at the site of intravenous lines, atelectasis, pulmonary emboli, or the postpericardiotomy syndrome.

WOUND AND INCISION

Infections of the leg wound are typically manifested by fever, induration, pain, erythema, local warmth, and drainage from the suture line. The usual infectious agents include *Staphylococcus, Streptococcus,* and aerobic Gram-negative bacilli. Wound aspiration and Gram stain should be used to guide antibiotic treatment. More advanced cases require wound débridement and open drainage. Techniques of minimally invasive saphenous vein harvesting now make it possible to avoid a long leg incision, which decreases the risk of postoperative leg infection (Fig. 76–10).[150]

Recurrent bacterial cellulitis in the leg used for saphenous vein harvest may be a recalcitrant problem that appears months to years after surgery. Antibiotic courses directed against staphylococcal and streptococcal species for each individual occurrence may be insufficient, and a long-term course of antibiotic therapy may be needed. It is important to search for evidence of superficial fungal infections in the affected leg because persistent tinea pedis infection can cause recurrent lower extremity cellulitis. If a fungal infection is identified, treatment with topical miconazole or clotrimazole should be given in addition to antibacterial therapy.

Mediastinitis

Mediastinitis and sternal osteomyelitis are among the most serious complications of median sternotomy.[52,151,152] If one excludes operations that occur after thoracic trauma, it is estimated that mediastinitis occurs in about 2 percent of patients who undergo median sternotomy.

Most cases of mediastinitis occur within 2 weeks after sternotomy. Important diagnostic features of patients in whom mediastinitis develops early after cardiac surgery include persistent fever in excess of 101°F beyond the fourth postoperative day, a systemic toxic condition, leukocytosis, bacteremia, and a purulent discharge from the sternal wound. Recognition of mediastinitis requires a high index of suspicion

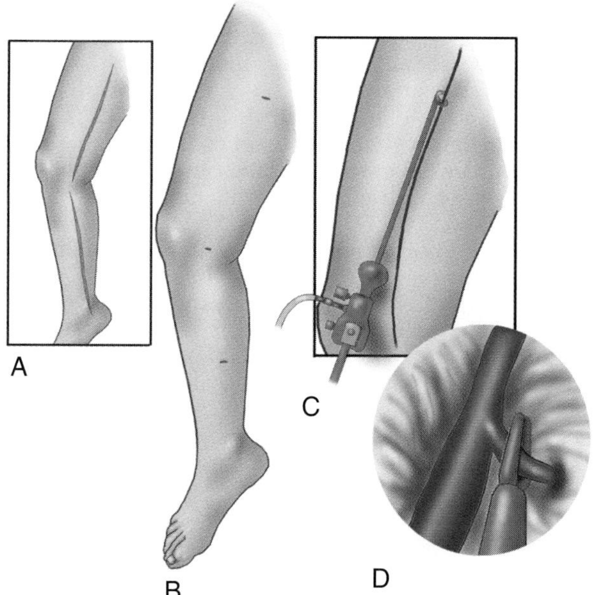

FIGURE 76–10 Minimally invasive approaches to saphenous vein harvesting have significantly reduced incisional morbidity. Traditional harvesting requires long leg incisions **(A)**, as compared with the less invasive videoscopic harvesting **(B)**. A dissection cannula is introduced through a small incision **(C)**, and branches are later divided **(D)** under videoscopic guidance.

and a vigorous, repetitive search for evidence of sternal wound drainage in patients who are persistently febrile late into the first week after surgery and who have no other obvious focus of infection, such as pneumonia or urinary tract infection. The diagnosis can be confirmed by needle aspiration from the subxiphoid approach followed by Gram stain and culture.

Risk Factors

Risk factors for the development of mediastinitis include prolonged cardiopulmonary bypass time, excessive postoperative bleeding with reexploration for control of hemorrhage, and diminished cardiac output in the postoperative period. The incidence of mediastinitis maybe increased when both internal mammary arteries are mobilized bilaterally for use as bypass conduits.[153] Therefore, many surgeons prefer to use only the left internal mammary artery, particularly in elderly diabetic patients, who may already be predisposed to delayed sternal wound healing. If both internal mammary arteries are utilized in this subgroup, they should be harvested without a large pedicle (skeletonized grafts) to preserve sternal vascularization.[35]

The spectrum of microorganisms that cause mediastinitis includes *Staphylococcus aureus* and *Staphylococcus epidermidis* in about 50 percent of patients and a variety of Gram-negative bacilli in about 40 percent of cases.[153,154] Mixed infections and fungal infections are rare. The organism isolated frequently is resistant to the prophylactic antibiotic used preoperatively, especially if the isolate includes a gram-negative bacillus or a beta-lactamase–producing *S. aureus*.

Diagnosis of Sternal Wound Infection

Definitive diagnosis requires exploration of the wound and culture of suspicious areas. In the past, closed (débridement, reclosure, and antibiotic irrigation) and open (débridement, packing, closure by secondary intent) approaches were commonly used. To facilitate functional recovery, we now favor early plastic surgical flap techniques to allow for immediate primary closure with vascularized tissue.[155] Regardless of the sternal closure strategy used, bacterial-specific intravenous antibiotics are typically administered for 6 weeks.

ANTIBIOTIC PROPHYLAXIS. Perioperative antibiotic prophylaxis benefits patients undergoing cardiac surgery.[156] Although the antibiotic regimen varies, in part related to local differences in microbiological flora and personal preference, it is directed against gram-positive cocci (the most frequent causative pathogens in infections after cardiac surgery) and usually contains a cephalosporin. A commonly used regimen consists of 1 gm of cefazolin intravenously 30 minutes before the skin incision and then repeated at 8-hour intervals for 48 hours after surgery.

PROSTHETIC VALVE ENDOCARDITIS (see Chaps. 57 and 58). Prosthetic valve endocarditis is a rare but extremely serious complication of cardiac surgery, frequently arising from nosocomial bacteremias.[33] It is estimated to occur in only 2 to 4 percent of patients; about half of the cases are classified as "early" (<60 days from the date of surgery) and half as "late" (>60 days from the date of surgery). Pooled data from several series indicate that the organism responsible for early prosthetic valve endocarditis includes a *Staphylococcus* species in about 50 percent of cases. The remainder of early cases of prosthetic valve endocarditis are caused by Gram-negative bacilli, dipthteroids, and fungi.[33,157]

Management. Features of prosthetic valve endocarditis that have been associated with increased mortality include invasive infection (i.e., extension into the myocardium); congestive heart failure resulting from dysfunction of the prosthesis; and the presence of antibiotic-resistant, virulent microorganisms or a fungal organism.[33,157] Appropriate antibiotic therapy for prosthetic valve endocarditis is discussed in Chapter 58, but practically all patients will require removal of the infected prosthesis.

VIRAL. Viral infections that occur after cardiac surgery are almost exclusively the result of infectious complications of transfusion therapy and, with the exception of human immunodeficiency virus, primarily result in hepatitis. The incidence of viral infections after cardiac operations is decreasing as a result of a reduction in the number of transfusions of blood bank products (e.g., cell-saver techniques and preoperative autologous blood donations) and improved screening techniques in contemporary blood bank practice. Cytomegalovirus infection is a febrile syndrome that typically occurs 1 month postoperatively. It is characterized by high-spiking fevers, abnormalities in liver function tests, and arthralgias. A self-limited illness, it is best treated with antipyretics and supportive fluid therapy.

FUNGAL. Fungal infections that involve the heart are rare. They are typically seen in cases of fungemia and are usually fatal. Although the problem of fungemia is well described in immunocompromised hosts (e.g., heart transplant recipient), in an autopsy study of 60 patients with fungal infections of the heart, 25 percent of cases occurred in association with conventional valvular surgery. About half of fungal infections of the heart are confined to the endocardium, and half involve both the endocardium and the myocardium. Extracardiac involvement is common, with spread of infection to the lungs, cerebrospinal fluid, urine, and skin. The most commonly encountered organisms, in descending order of frequency, are *Candida, Aspergillus,* and *Cryptococcus* species. Patients who appear to be at particular risk of fungal involvement of the heart are those who have received corticosteroids and long courses of antibiotic treatment postoperatively.

Peripheral Vascular Complications

Most adults who undergo cardiac surgery—especially coronary revascularization—have atherosclerosis of the peripheral arteries (e.g., iliofemoral system) and may experience lower extremity ischemia after surgery because of low flow in the perioperative period with in situ thrombosis, embolism from the heart or aorta, or vascular compromise from an intraaortic balloon pump catheter (see also Chaps. 54 and 55). Management consists of anticoagulation and removal of indwelling catheters, if clinically feasible. Thrombectomy and even revascularization surgery of the lower extremities (e.g., femorofemoral, femoropopliteal, or axillofemoral by pass) may be required to salvage threatened limbs.

Asymptomatic deep venous thrombosis of the calf can develop before hospital discharge in about one-third to one-half of patients who receive saphenous vein bypass grafts. Occasionally, these thrombi propagate to the proximal leg veins; only rarely do they cause massive pulmonary embolism. The best preventive strategy is rigorous perioperative prophylaxis against venous thromboembolism in all patients, including unfractionated or low-molecular-weight heparin.

Other Complications

PERICARDITIS (see Chap. 64). Pericardial friction rubs are commonly audible in the early postoperative period and probably result from local inflammation and mechanical irritation from the mediastinal chest tubes. The friction rubs usually subside by the second or third postoperative day and are asymptomatic because of the narcotic analgesics prescribed at that stage of recovery. Although pericardial rubs develop in some patients toward the end of the first postoperative week, they are usually benign, do not indicate a need for prolongation of hospitalization, and do not require treatment. A separate clinical syndrome that appears late in the first postoperative month is *postpericardiotomy syndrome.* The relationship between postpericardotomy syndrome and chronic constrictive pericarditis is not firmly established, but a number of patients with *postoperative constrictive pericarditis* have a history of postpericardiotomy syndrome.

RENAL FAILURE (see Chap. 86). All patients who undergo cardiac surgery experience a reduction in renal blood flow and the glomerular filtration rate as a consequence of both anesthesia and cardiopulmonary bypass. Risk factors for the development of persistent renal failure after cardiac surgery include a preoperative history of renal dysfunction or left ventricular dysfunction, prolonged bypass time (>180 minutes), prolonged aortic cross-clamping (>60 minutes), perioperative hypotension, advanced age (>70 years), and the development of medical complications postoperatively.[158,159]

Most cases of acute renal failure after cardiac surgery result from renal ischemia that lowers the glomerular filtration rate directly (prerenal disease) or, if severe or prolonged, can induce acute tubular necrosis. Possible additional contributory factors include sepsis, nephrotoxic drugs, radiocontrast material injection, embolization of cholesterol or other atheromatous debris in the renal circulation, increased urine free hemoglobin levels from hemolysis while undergoing cardiopulmonary bypass, and the effects of ACE inhibitors on glomerular capillary pressure. The detrimental effects of ACE inhibitors are most likely to occur when renal perfusion pressure is low because of renal artery stenosis or systemic hypotension caused by cardiac failure.

Urine output is variable in patients with postoperative acute renal failure. Anuria is uncommon and, if present, should raise the suspicion of urinary tract obstruction (e.g., occluded Foley catheter). More commonly, patients are either oliguric (<400 mg/d) or nonoliguric. Oliguric acute renal failure occurs less frequently than nonoliguric renal failure, usually reflects more severe renal injury, and is associated with a greater probability of requiring dialysis during the acute phase.

Differentiation Between Prerenal Azotemia and Acute Tubular Necrosis. Important diagnostic studies in all patients with acute renal failure include urinalysis and estimation of pulmonary capillary wedge pressure and cardiac output by means of pulmonary artery catheterization. Prerenal azotemia should be suspected if the urine sodium level is less than 20 mEq/liter, the fractional excretion of sodium is less than 1 percent, and urine osmolality is greater than 500 mOsm/liter. Acute tubular necrosis should be suspected if the urine sodium level is greater than 40 mEq/liter, fractional excretion of sodium is greater than 2 percent, and urine osmolality is less than 350 mOsm/liter.

Treatment. Essential elements of therapy for both prerenal azotemia and acute tubular necrosis include optimization of intravascular fluid volume and cardiac output. The latter is best accomplished with vasodilators and inotropic agents rather than vasoconstrictors to avoid further reductions in renal blood flow.

It is prudent to undertake a trial of furosemide and mannitol (only if the patient can tolerate the volume load of the latter) within the first 12 to 24 hours after the development of oliguria. The aim of such therapy is to increase urine output. Because of the renal-vasodilating effects of dopamine (2 to 3 μg/kg/min), patients with both oliguric and nonoliguric renal failure may experience an increase in urine output.

If oliguria persists beyond 12 hours, a number of supportive measures must be initiated, including careful attention to electrolyte balance, specifically avoiding hyperkalemia; avoidance of excessive free water administration, which might lead to hyponatremia; correction of acidosis (adding bicarbonate to daily fluids); and adjustment of medication dosages for delayed excretion if the drug is cleared by renal mechanisms. The care team should remain alert for pericarditis, refractory hyperkalemia, uremic encephalopathy, or colitis. Continuous arteriovenous hemofiltration can be used to remove excess fluid.

Cardiac Surgery in Patients with Chronic Renal Failure. Patients with chronic renal failure who undergo surgery have an increased risk of exacerbation of renal dysfunction perioperatively. Deterioration in renal function may require temporary or even permanent hemodialysis, and these eventualities should be addressed with the patient and the cardiac surgical team preoperatively. Surgery can be safely performed in patients who are already maintained by hemodialysis, but careful coordination of the surgical and dialysis schedules is essential to minimize postoperative problems with fluid and electrolyte management.[158]

GASTROINTESTINAL COMPLICATIONS. Serious gastrointestinal complications after cardiac surgery are rare (occurring in about 1 percent of patients) and can usually be handled by a conservative approach. Only about 0.5 percent of patients who undergo cardiac surgery require a general surgical operation for a gastrointestinal complication. Complications that may require intervention include upper or lower gastrointestinal bleeding, cholecystitis, and mesenteric ischemia. Patients with circulatory compromise on high-dose pressors and those who require intraaortic balloon pump support are more likely to have gastrointestinal complications. Despite their relative rarity, gastrointestinal complications are associated with significant mortality (approaching 40 percent in some series), thus highlighting the need for careful monitoring and repeated physical examination in high-risk patients. Most complications occur within 7 days of surgery.

Rehabilitation and Preparation for Discharge (see Chap. 43)

A coordinated, multidisciplinary cardiac exercise program is essential to overcome the physical deconditioning and psychosocial upheaval associated with cardiac surgery. Emphasis should be placed on early mobilization and progressively more patient self-care, including initiation of these measures in the ICU during the first 24 hours postoperatively. After transfer out of the ICU, the patient should be encouraged to engage in low-density (2 to 3 metabolic equivalent threshold) isotonic activities such as walking and range-of-motion exercises.[160] The nursing staff should monitor the patient's progress while being alert to any undue acceleration in heart rate (>120 beats/min) or hemodynamically compromising arrhythmias.

Patients should also participate in an education program focusing on instructions regarding postoperative medications and initiation of secondary measures targeted at preventing graft occlusion and progression of atherosclerosis.[161] Because of the overwhelming evidence indicating that platelet inhibition can prevent graft occlusion, all patients undergoing bypass surgery should receive long-term therapy with aspirin unless contraindicated. Clopidogrel may be useful in aspirin-intolerant patients, but there is no evidence of significant benefit from the routine use of either dipyridamole or sulfinpyrazone. Fast-track discharge protocols are now standard, and uncomplicated patients are typically discharged on the fifth postoperative day.[162,163]

REFERENCES

1. Braunwald E, Antman EM, Beasley JW, et al: ACC/AHA 2002 guideline update for the management of patients with unstable angina and non-ST-segment elevation myocardial infarction—summary article: A report of the American College of Cardiology/American Heart Association Task Force on Practice Guidelines (Committee on the Management of Patients With Unstable Angina). J Am Coll Cardiol 40:1366-1374, 2002.
2. Bech-Hanssen O, Caidahl K, Wall B, et al: Influence of aortic valve replacement, prosthesis type, and size on functional outcome and ventricular mass in patients with aortic stenosis. J Thorac Cardiovasc Surg 118:57-65, 1999.
3. Di Carli MF, Maddahi J, Rokhsar S, et al: Long-term survival of patients with coronary artery disease and left ventricular dysfunction: Implications for the role of myocardial viability assessment in management decisions. J Thorac Cardiovasc Surg 116:997-1004, 1998.

3a. Rahimatoola SH: The year in valvular heart disease. J Am Coll Cardiol 43:491, 2004.

3b. Schinkel AFL, Plodermans D, Vanoverschelde J-LL, et al: Incidence of recovery of contractile function following revascularization in patients with ischemic left ventricular dysfunction. Am J Cardiol 93:14, 2004.

4. Trachiotis GD, Weintraub WS, Johnston TS, et al: Coronary artery bypass grafting in patients with advanced left ventricular dysfunction. Ann Thorac Surg 66:1632-1639, 1998.
5. Bigger JT Jr: Prophylactic use of implanted cardiac defibrillators in patients at high risk for ventricular arrhythmias after coronary artery bypass graft surgery. Coronary Artery Bypass Graft (CABG) Patch Trial Investigators. N Engl J Med 337:1569-1575, 1997.
6. Aklog L, Adams DH, Couper GS, et al: Techniques and results of direct-access minimally invasive mitral valve surgery: A paradigm for the future. J Thorac Cardiovasc Surg 116:705-715, 1998.
7. Machler HE, Bergmann P, Anelli-Monti M, et al: Minimally invasive versus conventional aortic valve operations: A prospective study in 120 patients. Ann Thorac Surg 67:1001-1005, 1999.
8. Magovern JA, Benckart DH, Landreneau RJ, et al: Morbidity, cost, and six-month outcome of minimally invasive direct coronary artery bypass grafting. Ann Thorac Surg 66:1224-1229, 1998.
9. Allen KB, Griffith GL, Heimansohn DA, et al: Endoscopic versus traditional saphenous vein harvesting: A prospective, randomized trial. Ann Thorac Surg 66:26-32, 1998.
10. Filsoufi F, Aklog L, Adams DH: Minimally invasive CABG. Curr Opin Cardiol 16:306-309, 2001.
11. Byrne JG, Aklog L, Adams DH: Assessment and management of functional or ischaemic mitral regurgitation. Lancet 335:1743-1744, 2000.
12. Katz NM, Gersh BJ, Cox JL: Changing practice of coronary bypass surgery and its impact on early risk and long-term survival. Curr Opin Cardiol 13:465-475, 1998.
13. Aldea GS, Gaudiani JM, Shapira OM, et al: Effect of gender on postoperative outcomes and hospital stays after coronary artery bypass grafting. Ann Thorac Surg 67:1097-1103, 1999.
14. Mullany CJ, Mock MB, Brooks MM, et al: Effect of age in the Bypass Angioplasty Revascularization Investigation (BARI) randomized trial. Ann Thorac Surg 67:396-403, 1999.
15. Filsoufi F, Adams DH: Surgical approaches to coronary artery disease. Curr Treat Options Cardiovasc Med 4:55-63, 2002.
16. Blanche C, Khan SS, Chaux A, et al: Cardiac reoperations in octogenarians: Analysis of outcomes. Ann Thorac Surg 67:93-98, 1999.
17. Adams DH, Chen RH, Kadner A, et al: Impact of small prosthetic valve size on operative mortality in the elderly after aortic valve replacement for aortic stenosis: Does gender matter? J Thorac Cardiovasc Surg 118:815-822, 1999.
18. Jamieson WR, Edwards FH, Schwartz M, et al: Risk stratification for cardiac valve replacement. National Cardiac Surgery Database. Database Committee of The Society of Thoracic Surgeons. Ann Thorac Surg 67:943-951, 1999.
19. Lazar HL, Jacobs AK, Aldea GS, et al: Factors influencing mortality after emergency coronary artery bypass grafting for failed percutaneous transluminal coronary angioplasty. Ann Thorac Surg 64:1747-1752, 1997.
20. Gott JP, Thourani VH, Wright CE, et al: Risk neutralization in cardiac operations: Detection and treatment of associated carotid disease. Ann Thorac Surg 68:850-857, 1999.
21. Duarte IG, Murphy CO, Kosinski AS, et al: Late survival after valve operation in patients with left ventricular dysfunction. Ann Thorac Surg 64:1089-1095, 1997.
22. Couper GS, Dekkers RJ, Adams DH: The logistics and cost-effectiveness of circulatory support: Advantages of the ABIOMED BVS 5000. Ann Thorac Surg 68:646-649, 1999.
23. Erickson LC, Torchiana DF, Schneider EC, et al: The relationship between managed care insurance and use of lower-mortality hospitals for CABG surgery. JAMA 283:1976-1982, 2000.
24. Alexander KP, Anstrom KJ, Muhlbaier LH, et al: Outcomes of cardiac surgery in patients age ≥ 80 years: Results from the National Cardiovascular Network. J Am Coll Cardiol 35:731-738, 2000.
25. Byrne JG, Karavas AN, Filsoufi F, et al: Aortic valve surgery after previous CABG with functioning IMA grafts. Ann Thorac Surg 73:779-784, 2002.
26. Byrne JG, Karavas AN, Adams DH, et al: The preferred approach for mitral valve surgery after CABG: Right thoracotomy, hypothermia and avoidance of LIMA-LAD graft. J Heart Valve Dis 10:584-590, 2001.
27. Adams DH, Filsoufi F, Byrne JG, et al: Mitral valve repair in redo cardiac surgery. J Card Surg 17:40-45, 2002.

Preoperative Evaluation

28. Akins CW: Combined carotid endarterectomy and coronary revascularization operation. Ann Thorac Surg 66:1483-1484, 1998.
29. Scarborough JE, White W, Derilus FE, et al: Neurologic outcomes after coronary artery bypass grafting with and without cardiopulmonary bypass. Semin Thorac Cardiovasc Surg 15:52-62, 2003.
30. Levinson MM, Rodriguez DI: Endarterectomy for preventing stroke in symptomatic and asymptomatic carotid stenosis: Review of clinical trials and recommendations for surgical therapy. Heart Surg Forum 2:147-168, 1999.
31. Allie DE, Lirtzman M, Malik AP, et al: Rapid-staged strategy for concomitant critical carotid and left main coronary disease with left ventricular dysfunction: IABP use. Ann Thorac Surg 66:1230-1235, 1998.
32. Aranki SF, Adams DH, Rizzo RJ, et al: Determinants of early mortality and late survival in mitral valve endocarditis. Circulation 92(Suppl 2):143-149, 1995.
33. Filsoufi F, Adams DH: Surgical treatment of mitral valve endocarditis. *In* Cohn LH, Edmunds LH (eds): Cardiac Surgery in the Adult. 2nd ed. New York, McGraw-Hill, 2003, pp 987-997.
34. Leavitt BJ, O'Connor GT, Olmstead EM, et al: Use of the internal mammary artery graft and in-hospital mortality and other adverse outcomes associated with coronary artery bypass surgery. Circulation 103:507-512, 2001.
35. Uva MS, Braunberger E, Fisher M, et al: Does bilateral internal thoracic artery grafting increase surgical risk in diabetic patients? Ann Thorac Surg 66:2051-2055, 1998.
36. Engoren M, Buderer NF, Zacharias A, Habib RH: Variables predicting reintubation after cardiac surgical procedures. Ann Thorac Surg 67:661-665, 1999.
37. Milas BL, Jobes DR, Gorman RC: Management of bleeding and coagulopathy after heart surgery. Semin Thorac Cardiovasc Surg 12:326-336, 2000.
38. Meharwal ZS, Trehan N: Vascular complications of intra-aortic balloon insertion in patients undergoing coronary revascularization: Analysis of 911 cases. Eur J Cardiothorac Surg 21:741-747, 2002.
39. Rihal C, Eagle K, Mickel M, et al: Surgical therapy for coronary artery disease among patients with combined coronary artery and peripheral vascular disease. Circulation 91:46, 1995.
40. Higgins T, Estafanous F, Lloyd F, et al: Stratification of morbidity and mortality outcome by preoperative risk factors in coronary artery bypass patients: A clinical severity score. JAMA 207:2344, 1992.
41. Edwards FH, Carey JS, Grover FL, et al: Impact of gender on coronary bypass operative mortality. Ann Thorac Surg 66:125-131, 1998.
42. Athanasiou T, Al-Ruzzeh S, Del Stanbridge R, et al: Is the female gender an independent predictor of adverse outcome after off-pump coronary artery bypass grafting? Ann Thorac Surg 75:1153-1160, 2003.
43. Ferraris VA, Ferraris SP: Risk factors for postoperative morbidity. J Thorac Cardiovasc Surg 111:731-741, 1996.
44. Tu JV, Jaglal SB, Naylor CD, Steering Committee of the Provincial Adult Cardiac Care Network of Ontario: Multicenter validation of a risk index for mortality, intensive care unit stay, and overall hospital length of stay after cardiac surgery. Circulation 91:677, 1995.
45. Brooks MM, Jones RH, Bach RG, et al: Predictors of mortality and mortality from cardiac causes in the Bypass Angioplasty Revascularization Investigation (BARI) randomized trial and registry. Circulation 101:2682-2689, 2000.
46. Vogt A, Grube E, Glunz HG, et al: Determinants of mortality after cardiac surgery: Results of the Registry of the Arbeitsgemeinschaft Leitender Kardiologischer Krankenhausarzte (ALKK) on 10,525 patients. Eur Heart J 21:28-32, 2000.
47. Roques F, Nashef SA, Michel P, et al: Risk factors and outcome in European cardiac surgery: Analysis of the EuroSCORE multinational database of 19,030 patients. Eur J Cardiothorac Surg 15:816-822, 1999.
48. Nashef SA, Roques F, Michel P, et al: European system for cardiac operative risk evaluation (EuroSCORE). Eur J Cardiothorac Surg 16:9-13, 1999.
49. Geissler HJ, Hölzl P, Marohl S, et al: Risk stratification in heart surgery: Comparison of six score systems. Eur J Cardiothoracic Surg 17:400-406, 2000.
50. Nashef SA, Roques F, Hammill BG, et al: Validation of European system for cardiac operative risk evaluation (EuroSCORE) in North American cardiac surgery. Eur J Cardiothoracic Surg 22:101-105, 2002.
51. Roques F, Michel P, Goldstone AR, et al: The logistic EuroSCORE. Eur Heart J 24:881-882, 2003.
52. Borger MA, Rao V, Weisel RD, et al: Deep sternal wound infection: Risk factors and outcomes. Ann Thorac Surg 65:1050-1056, 1998.
53. Pevni D, Mohr R, Lev-Run O, et al: Influence of bilateral skeletonized harvesting on occurrence of deep sternal wound infection in 1,000 consecutive patients undergoing bilateral internal thoracic artery grafting. Ann Surg 237:277-280, 2003.

54. Braxton JH, Marrin CA, McGrath PD, et al: Mediastinitis and long-term survival after coronary artery bypass graft surgery. Ann Thorac Surg 70:2004-2007, 2000.
55. Pasquet A, Lauer MS, Williams MJ, et al: Prediction of global left ventricular function after bypass surgery in patients with severe left ventricular dysfunction: Impact of preoperative myocardial function, perfusion, and metabolism. Eur Heart J 21:125-136, 2000.
56. Reichek N: MRI myocardial tagging. J Magn Reson Imaging 10:609-616, 1999.
57. Bogaert J, Bosmans H, Maes A, et al: Remote myocardial dysfunction after acute anterior myocardial infarction—impact of left ventricular shape on regional function: A magnetic resonance myocardial tagging study. J Am Coll Cardiol 35:1525-1534, 2000.
58. Athanasuleas CL, Stanley AW, Buckberg GD, et al: Surgical anterior ventricular endocardial restoration (SAVER) for dilated ischemic cardiomyopathy. Semin Thorac Cardiovasc Surg 13:448-458, 2001.
59. Salati M, Lemma M, Di Mattia DG, et al: Myocardial revascularization in patients with ischemic cardiomyopathy: Functional observations. Ann Thorac Surg 64:1728-1734, 1997.
60. Bax JJ, Schinkel AFL, Boersma E, et al. Early versus delayed revascularization in patients with ischemic cardiomyopathy and substantial viability: Impact on outcome. Circulation 108:II39-II42, 2003.
61. Qin JX, Shiota T, McCarthy PM, et al. Importance of mitral valve repair associated with left ventricular reconstruction for patients with ischemic cardiomyopathy: A real-time three-dimensional echocardiography study. Circulation 108:II241-II246, 2003.
62. Fullerton DA, Jones SD, Jaggers J, et al: Effective control of pulmonary vascular resistance with inhaled nitric oxide after cardiac operation. J Thorac Cardiovasc Surg 111:753-762, 1996.
63. Moazami N, Damiano RJ, Bailey MS, et al: Nesiritide (BNP) in the management of postoperative cardiac patients. Ann Thorac Surg 75:1974-1976, 2003.
64. Young JB, Abraham WT, Stevenson LW, et al: Intravenous nesiritide vs nitroglycerin for treatment of decompensated congestive heart failure. JAMA 287:1531-1540, 2002.
65. Alvarez JM: Emergency coronary bypass grafting for failed percutaneous coronary artery stenting: Increased costs and platelet transfusion requirements after the use of abciximab. J Thorac Cardiovasc Surg 115:472-473, 1998.
66. Tardiff BE, Califf RM, Morris D, et al: Coronary revascularization surgery after myocardial infarction: Impact of bypass surgery on survival after thrombolysis. GUSTO Investigators. Global Utilization of Streptokinase and Tissue Plasminogen Activator for Occluded Coronary Arteries. J Am Coll Cardiol 29:240-249, 1997.
67. Braxton JH, Hammond GL, Letsou GV, et al: Optimal timing of coronary artery bypass graft surgery after acute myocardial infarction. Circulation 92:66, 1995.
68. Misfeld M, Dubbert S, Eleftheriadis S, et al: Fibrinolysis-adjusted perioperative low-dose aprotin reduces blood loss in bypass operations. Ann Thorac Surg 66:792-799, 1998.
69. Lee DC, Oz MC, Weinberg AD, et al: Optimal timing of revascularization: Transmural versus nontransmural acute myocardial infarction. Ann Thorac Surg 71:1197-1202, 2001.
70. Lee DC, Oz MC, Weinberg AD, et al: Appropriate timing of surgical intervention after transmural acute myocardial infarction. J Thorac Cardiovasc Surg 125:115-119, 2003.
71. Stone GW, Ohman EM, Miller MF, et al: Contemporary utilization and outcomes of intra-aortic balloon counterpulsation in acute myocardial infarction. J Am Coll Cardiol 41:1940-1945, 2003.
72. Kouchoukos NT, Blackstone EH, Doty DB, et al: Anesthesia for cardiovascular surgery. *In* Kirklin J, Barratt-Boyes B (eds): Cardiac Surgery. New York, Churchill Livingstone, 2003, p 163.
73. Savino JS, Floyd TE, Cheung AT: Cardiac anesthesia. *In* Cohn LH, Edmunds LH (eds): Cardiac Surgery in the Adult. New York, McGraw-Hill, 2003, p 249.
74. DeFoe GR, Ross CS, Olmstead EM, et al: Lowest hematocrit on bypass and adverse outcomes associated with coronary artery bypass grafting. Northern New England Cardiovascular Disease Study Group. Ann Thorac Surg 71:769-776, 2001.
75. Fillinger MP, Surgenor SD, Hartman GS, et al: The association between heart rate and in-hospital mortality after coronary artery bypass surgery. Anesth Analg 95:1483-1488, 2002.
76. DeFoe GR, Krumholz CF, DioDato CP, et al: Lowest core body temperature and adverse outcomes associated with coronary artery bypass surgery. Perfusion 18:127-133, 2003.
77. Lemmer JH Jr, Metzdorff MT, Krause AH Jr, et al: Emergency coronary artery bypass graft surgery in abciximab-treated patients. Ann Thorac Surg 66:90-95, 2000.
78. Morales DL, Garrido MJ, Madigan JD, et al: A double-blind randomized trial: prophylactic vasopressin reduces hypotension after cardiopulmonary bypass. Ann Thorac Surg 75:926-930, 2003.
78a. Bigger JT Jr, Whang W, Rottman JN, et al: Mechanisms of death in the CABG PATCH trial: A randomized trial of implantable cardiac defibrillator prophylaxis in patients with high risk of death after coronary bypass graft surgery. Circulation 99:1416, 1999.
79. Cartier R, Brann S, Dagenais F, et al: Systematic off-pump coronary artery revascularization in multivessel disease: Experience of three hundred cases. J Thorac Cardiovasc Surg 119:221-229, 2000.
80. Berger PB, Alderman EL, Nadel A, Schaff HV: Frequency of early occlusion and stenosis in a left internal mammary artery to left anterior descending artery bypass graft after surgery through a median sternotomy on conventional bypass: Benchmark for minimally invasive direct coronary artery bypass. Circulation 100:2353-2358, 1999.
81. Al-Ruzzeh S, Ambler G, Asimakopoulos, et al: Off-pump coronary artery bypass (OPCAB) surgery reduces risk-stratified morbidity and mortality: A United Kingdom multi-center comparative analysis of early outcome. Circulation 108:II1-II8, 2003.
82. Magee MJ, Coombs LP, Peterson ED, et al: Patient selection and current practice strategy for off-pump coronary artery bypass surgery. Circulation 108:II9-II14, 2003.
83. Sharony R, Bizekis CS, Kanchuger M, et al: Off-pump coronary artery bypass grafting reduces mortality and stroke in patients with atheromatous aortas: A case control study. Circulation 108:II15-II20, 2003.
84. Sharony R, Grossi EA, Saunders PC, et al: Minimally invasive aortic valve surgery in the elderly: A case-control study. Circulation 108:II43-II47, 2003.
85. Casselman FP, Slycke SV, Wellens F, et al: Mitral valve surgery can now routinely be performed endoscopically. Circulation 108:II48-II54, 2003.
86. Argenziano M, Oz MC, Kohmoto T, et al: Totally endoscopic atrial septal defect repair with robotic assistance. Circulation 108:II191-II194, 2003.
86a. Athanasion T, Al-Ruzzeh S, Kumar P, et al: Off-pump myocardial revascularization is associated with less incidence of stroke in elderly patients. Ann Thorac Surg 77:745, 2004.
86b. Khan NE, De Souza A, Mister R, et al: A randomized comparison of off-pump and on-pump multivessel coronary-artery bypass surgery. N Engl J Med 350:1, 2004.

Postoperative Management

87. Thourani VH, Weintraub WS, Stein B, et al: Influence of diabetes mellitus on early and late outcome after coronary artery bypass grafting. Ann Thorac Surg 67:1045-1052, 1999.
88. Fish LH, Weaver TW, Moore AL, et al: Value of postoperative blood glucose in predicting complications and length of stay after coronary artery bypass grafting. Am J Cardiol 92:74-76, 2003.
89. Furnary AP, Gao G, Grunkemeier GL, et al: Continuous insulin infusion reduces mortality in patients with diabetes undergoing coronary artery bypass grafting. J Thorac Cardiovasc Surg 125:1007-1021, 2003.
90. Canver CC, Chanda J: Intraoperative and postoperative risk factors for respiratory failure after coronary bypass. Ann Thorac Surg 75:853-857, 2003.
91. Adams DH, Filsoufi F, Aklog L: Surgical treatment of the ischemic mitral valve. J Heart Valve Dis Suppl 1:S21-S25, 2002.
92. Aklog L, Filsoufi F, Flores KQ, et al: Does coronary artery bypass grafting alone correct moderate ischemic mitral regurgitation? Circulation 104(Suppl 1):I68-I75, 2001.
93. ZuWallack RL, Mahler DA, Reilly D, et al: Salmeterol plus theophylline combination therapy in the treatment of COPD. Chest 119:1661-1670, 2001.
94. Katz MG, Katz R, Schachner A, Cohen AJ: Phrenic nerve injury after coronary artery bypass grafting: Will it go away? Ann Thorac Surg 65:32-35, 1998.
95. Stamenkovic SA, Morgan IS, Pontefract DR, Campanella C: Is early tracheostomy safe in cardiac patients with median sternotomy incisions? Ann Thorac Surg 69:1152-1154, 2000.
96. Vuylsteke A, Feneck RO, Jolin-Mellgard A, et al: Perioperative blood pressure control: A prospective survey of patient management in cardiac surgery. J Cardiothorac Vasc Anesth 14:269-273, 2000.
97. Cooper TJ, Clutton BTH, Jones SN, et al: Factors relating to the development of hypertension after cardiopulmonary bypass. Br Heart J 54:91, 1985.
98. Hamm CW, Reimers J, Ischinger T, et al: A randomized study of coronary angioplasty compared with bypass surgery in patients with symptomatic multivessel coronary disease. German Angioplasty Bypass Surgery Investigation (GABI). N Engl J Med 331:1037, 1994.
99. King SE, Lembo NJ, Weintraub WS, et al: A randomized trial comparing coronary angioplasty with coronary bypass surgery. Emory Angioplasty Versus Surgery Trial (EAST). N Engl J Med 331:1044, 1994.
100. Greaves S, Rutherford J, Aranki S, et al: Current incidence and determinants of perioperative myocardial infarction in coronary artery surgery. Am Heart J 132:572-573, 1996.
101. Myers MG, Fremes SE: Prevention of radial artery graft spasm: A survey of Canadian surgical centres. Can J Cardiol 19:677-681, 2003.
102. Muneretto C, Negri A, Manfredi J, et al: Safety and usefulness of composite grafts for total arterial myocardial revascularization: A prospective randomized evaluation. J Thorac Cardiovasc Surg 125:826-835, 2003.
103. Obarski TP, Loop FD, Cosgrove DM, et al: Frequency of acute myocardial infarction in valve repairs versus valve replacement for pure mitral regurgitation. Am J Cardiol 65:887, 1990.
104. Fransen EJ, Diris JH, Maessen JG, et al: Evaluation of "new" cardiac markers for ruling out myocardial infarction after coronary artery bypass grafting. Chest 122:1316-1321, 2002.
105. Kim LJ, Martinez EA, Faraday N, et al: Cardiac troponin I predicts short-term mortality in vascular surgery patients. Circulation 106:2366-2371, 2002.
106. Nalysnyk L, Fahrbach K, Reynolds MW, et al: Adverse events in coronary artery bypass graft (CABG) trials: A systematic review and analysis. Heart 89:767-772, 2003.
107. Joffe II, Jacobs LE, Lampert C, et al: Role of echocardiography in perioperative management of patients undergoing open heart surgery. Am Heart J 131:162, 1995.
108. Anderson CA, Filsoufi F, Aklog L, et al: Liberal use of delayed sternal closure for postcardiotomy hemodynamic instability. Ann Thorac Surg 73:1484-1488, 2002.
109. Shalabi RI, Amin M, Ayed AK, et al: Delayed sternal closure is a life-saving decision. Ann Thorac Cardiovasc Surg 4:220-223, 2002.
110. Frazier OH, Myers TJ, Westaby S, et al: Use of the Jarvik 2000 left ventricular assist system as a bridge to heart transplantation or as destination therapy for patients with chronic heart failure. Ann Surg 237:631-637, 2003.
111. Richenbacher WE, Naka Y, Raines EP, et al: Surgical management of patients in the REMATCH trial. Ann Thorac Surg 75:S86-S92, 2003.
112. Radovancevic B, Vrtovec B, Frazier OH: Left ventricular assist devices: An alternative to medical therapy for end-stage heart failure. Curr Opin Cardiol 18:210-214, 2003.
113. Costachescu T, Denault A, Guimond JG, et al: The hemodynamically unstable patient in the intensive care unit: Hemodynamic vs. transesophageal echocardiographic monitoring. Crit Care Med 30:1214-1223, 2002.
114. Kuvin JT, Harati NA, Pandian NG, et al: Postoperative cardiac tamponade in the modern surgical era. Ann Thorac Surg 74:1148-1153, 2002.
115. Schmidlin D, Schuepbach R, Bernard E, et al: Indications and impact of postoperative transesophageal echocardiography in cardiac surgical patients. Crit Care Med 29:2143-2148, 2001.
116. Mizuno T, Tanaka H, Makita S, et al: Biventricular pacing with coronary bypass and Dor's ventriculoplasty. Ann Thorac Surg 75:998-999, 2003.

117. DeRose JJ, Ashton RC, Belsley S, et al: Robotically assisted left ventricular epicardial lead implantation for biventricular pacing. J Am Coll Cardiol 41:1414-1419, 2003.
118. Aranki S, Shaw D, Adams D, et al: Predictors of atrial fibrillation following coronary artery surgery: Current trends and impact on hospital resources. Circulation 94:390-397, 1996.
119. Redle JD, Khurana S, Marzan R, et al: Prophylactic oral amiodarone compared with placebo for prevention of atrial fibrillation after coronary artery bypass surgery. Am Heart J 138:144-150, 1999.
120. Daoud EG, Strickberger SA, Man KC, et al: Preoperative amiodarone as prophylaxis against atrial fibrillation after heart surgery. N Engl J Med 337:1785-1791, 1997.
121. Ascione R, Caputo M, Calori G, et al: Predictors of atrial fibrillation after conventional and beating heart surgery: A prospective, randomized study. Circulation 102:1530-1535, 2000.
122. Creswell LL, Damiano RJ: Postoperative atrial fibrillation: An old problem crying for new solutions. J Thorac Cardiovasc Surg 121:638-641, 2003.
123. Maisel WH, Rawn JD, Stevenson WG: Atrial fibrillation after cardiac surgery. Ann Intern Med 135:1061-1073, 2001.
124. Crystal E, Kahn S, Roberts R, et al: Long-term amiodarone therapy and the risk of complications after cardiac surgery: Results from the Canadian Amiodarone Myocardial Infarction Arrhythmia Trial (CAMIAT). J Thorac Cardiovasc Surg 125:633-637, 2003.
125. Klein AL, Grimm RA, Murray RD, et al: Use of transesophageal echocardiography to guide cardioversion in patients with atrial fibrillation. N Engl J Med 344:1411-1420, 2001.
126. Gaita F, Riccardi R, Gallotti R: Surgical approaches to atrial fibrillation. Card Electrophysiol Rev 6:401-405, 2002.
127. Mooss AN, Wurdeman RL, Mohiuddin SM: Esmolol versus diltiazem in the treatment of postoperative atrial fibrillation/atrial flutter after open heart surgery. Am Heart J 140:176-180, 2000.
128. VanderLugt JT, Mattioni T, Denker S, et al: Efficacy and safety of ibutilide fumarate for the conversion of atrial arrhythmias after cardiac surgery. Circulation 100:369-375, 1999.
129. Raitt MH, Dolack GL, Kino K, et al: Procainamide has limited effectiveness for the treatment of atrial fibrillation after open heart surgery. Circulation 90(Supp 1):376, 1994.
130. Willems S, Weiss C, Meinertz T: Tachyarrhythmias following coronary artery bypass graft surgery: Epidemiology, mechanisms, and current therapeutic strategies. Thorac Cardiovasc Surg 45:232-237, 1997.
131. Koplan BA, Stevenson WG, Epstein LM, et al: Development and validation of a simple risk score to predict the need for permanent pacing after cardiac valve surgery. J Am Coll Cardiol 41:795-801, 2003.
132. Emlein G, Huang S, Pires L, et al: Prolonged bradyarrhythmias after isolated coronary artery bypass graft surgery. Am Heart J 126:1084, 1993.
133. Morse DS, Adams DH, Magnani B: Platelet and neutrophil activation during cardiac surgical procedures: Impact of cardiopulmonary bypass. Ann Thorac Surg 65:691-695, 1998.
134. Levi M, Cromheecke ME, de Jonge E, et al: Pharmacological strategies to decrease excessive blood loss in cardiac surgery: A meta-analysis of clinically relevant endpoints. Lancet 354:1940-1947, 2000.
135. Kearon C, Crowther M, Hirsh J: Management of patients with hereditary hypercoagulable disorders. Annu Rev Med 51:169-185, 2000.
136. Clagett GP, Anderson FA Jr, Geerts W, et al: Prevention of venous thromboembolism. Chest 114(5 Suppl):531S-560S, 1998.
137. Garcia-Torres R, Amigo MC, de la Rosa A, et al: Valvular heart disease in primary antiphospholipid syndrome (PAPS): Clinical and morphological findings. Lupus 5:56-61, 1996.
138. Brenner B, Blumenfeld Z, Markiewicz W, et al: Cardiac involvement in patients with primary antiphospholipid syndrome. J Am Coll Cardiol 18:931-936, 1991.
139. Levine JS, Branch DW, Rauch J: The antiphospholipid syndrome. N Engl J Med 346:752-763, 2002.
140. Hogan WJ, McBane RD, Santrach PJ, et al: Antiphospholipid syndrome and perioperative hemostatic management of cardiac valvular surgery. Mayo Clin Proc 75:971-976, 2000.
141. Fanashawe MP, Shore-Lesserson L, Reich DL: Two cases of fatal thrombosis after aminocaproic acid therapy and deep hypothermic circulatory arrest. Anesthesiology 95:1525-1527, 2001.
142. Ginsberg JA, Crowther MA, White RH, et al: Anticoagulation therapy. Hematology (Am Soc Hematol Educ Program) 339-357, 2001.
143. Greinacher A, Völpel H, Janssens U, et al: Recombinant hirudin (lepirudin) provides safe and effective anticoagulation in patients with heparin-induced thrombocytopenia: A prospective study. Circulation 99:73-80, 1999.
144. Sun Y, Greilich PE, Wilson SI, et al: The use of lepirudin for anticoagulation in patients with heparin-induced thrombocytopenia during major vascular surgery. Anesth Analg 92:344-346, 2001.
145. Verme-Gibboney CN, Hursting MJ: Argatroban dosing in patients with heparin-induced thrombocytopenia. Annu Pharmacother 37:970-975, 2003.
146. Koster A, Kuppe H, Hetzer R, et al: Emergent cardiopulmonary bypass in five patients with heparin-induced thrombocytopenia type II employing recombinant hirudin. Anesthesiology 89:777-780, 1998.
147. Taggart DP, Browne SM, Halligan PW, Wade DT: Is cardiopulmonary bypass still the cause of cognitive dysfunction after cardiac operations? J Thorac Cardiovasc Surg 118:414-420, 1999.
148. Puskas JD, Winston AD, Wright CE, et al: Stroke after coronary artery operation: Incidence, correlates, outcome, and cost. Ann Thorac Surg 69:1053-1056, 2000.
149. Newman MF, Kirchner JL, Phillips-Bute B, et al: Longitudinal assessment of neurocognitive function after coronary artery bypass surgery. N Engl J Med 344:395-402, 2001.
150. Carpino PA, Khabbaz KR, Bojar RM, et al: Clinical benefits of endoscopic vein harvesting in patients with risk factors for saphenectomy wound infections undergoing coronary artery bypass grafting. J Thorac Cardiovasc Surg 119:69-76, 2000.
151. The Parisian Mediastinitis Study Group: Risk factors for deep sternal wound infection after sternotomy: A prospective, multicenter study. J Thorac Cardiovasc Surg 111:1200-1207, 1996.
152. Braxton JH, Marrin CA, McGrath PD, et al: Mediastinitis and long-term survival after coronary artery bypass graft surgery. Ann Thorac Surg 70:2004-7, 2000.
153. He GW, Ryan WH, Acuff TE, et al: Risk factors for operative mortality and sternal wound infection in bilateral internal mammary artery grafting. J Thorac Cardiovasc Surg 107:196-202, 1994.
154. Milano CA, Georgiade G, Muhlbaier LH, et al: Comparison of omental and pectoralis flaps for poststernotomy mediastinitis. Ann Thorac Surg 67:377-381, 1999.
155. Rand RP, Cochran RP, Aziz S, et al: Prospective trial of catheter irrigation and muscle flaps for sternal wound infection. Ann Thorac Surg 65:1046-1049, 1998.
156. Hall J, Christiansen K, Carter M, et al: Antibiotic prophylaxis in cardiac operations. Ann Thorac Surg 56:916, 1993.
157. Niwaya K, Knott-Craig CJ, Santangelo K, et al: Advantage of autograft and homograft valve replacement for complex aortic valve endocarditis. Ann Thorac Surg 67:1603-1608, 1999.
158. Liu JY, Birkmeyer NJ, Sanders JH, et al: Risks of morbidity and mortality in dialysis patients undergoing coronary artery bypass surgery. Circulation 102:2973-2977, 2000.
159. Boldt J, Brenner T, Lehmann A, et al: Is kidney function altered by the duration of cardiopulmonary bypass? Ann Thorac Surg 75:906-912, 2003.

Rehabilitation and Preparation for Discharge

160. Fletcher G, Balady G, Froelicher V, et al: Exercise standards: A statement for healthcare professionals from the American Heart Association. Circulation 91:580, 1995.
161. Daida H, Yokoi H, Miyano H, et al: Relation of saphenous vein graft obstruction to serum cholesterol levels. J Am Coll Cardiol 25:193, 1995.
162. Walji S, Peterson RJ, Neis P, et al: Ultra-fast track hospital discharge using conventional cardiac surgical techniques. Ann Thorac Surg 67:363-370, 1999.
163. Ovrum E, Tangen G, Schiott C, et al: Rapid recovery protocol applied to 5,658 consecutive "on-pump" coronary bypass patients. Ann Thorac Surg 70:2008-2012, 2000.

CHAPTER 77

Anesthesia and Noncardiac Surgery in Patients with Heart Disease

Lee A. Fleisher • Kim A. Eagle

Cardiovascular morbidity and mortality represent a significant risk in the patient with known, or risk factors for, cardiovascular disease undergoing noncardiac surgery. Perioperative cardiovascular complications not only have implications in the immediate postoperative period but also may influence outcome over the subsequent 1 to 2 years. Over the past three decades there has been a steady progression of knowledge, from the identification of those at greatest risk, to randomized trials to identify strategies to reduce perioperative cardiovascular complications. However, much of the practice of management of the high-risk patient remains dependent on information from the nonsurgical arena. To disseminate best practices, guidelines have been developed to provide information for management of high-risk patients. This chapter attempts to distill this information, incorporating the available guidelines.

Assessment of Preoperative Risk for Noncardiac Surgery in Patients with Cardiovascular Disease

Ischemic Heart Disease

There are numerous care systems by which a patient may be evaluated prior to noncardiac surgery. The patient may be seen by his or her primary caregiver or a cardiologist. However, there are many patients who are evaluated only by the surgeon or anesthesiologist immediately before surgery. The stress of noncardiac surgery may raise heart rate and has been associated with a high incidence of symptomatic and asymptomatic myocardial ischemia. Therefore, the clinical evaluation of the patient may identify stable or unstable coronary artery disease (CAD). Patients with acute coronary syndromes, such as unstable angina or decompensated heart failure of ischemic origin, are at high risk for the development of further decompensation, myocardial necrosis, and death during the perioperative period. Such patients clearly warrant further evaluation and medical stabilization. If the noncardiac surgery is truly emergent, there are several case series utilizing intraaortic balloon bump counterpulsation as a means of providing short-term myocardial protection in addition to maximal medical therapy.

If the patient does not demonstrate unstable symptoms, the identification of known or symptomatic stable CAD or risk factors for CAD can guide the need for further diagnostic evaluation or changes in perioperative management. In determining the extent of the preoperative evaluation, it must be remembered that testing should not be performed unless the results would affect perioperative management. These management changes include cancellation of surgery because of prohibitive risk compared with benefit, delay of surgery for further medical management, coronary interventions before noncardiac surgery, utilization of an intensive care unit (ICU), and changes in monitoring.

Patients with stable angina represent a continuum from mild angina with extreme exertion to dyspnea with angina after walking up a few stairs. The patient who manifests angina only after strenuous exercise often does not demonstrate signs of left ventricular dysfunction and generally can be stabilized with adequate medical therapy, particularly treatment with beta-blocking agents. In contrast, a patient with dyspnea on mild exertion would be at high risk for perioperative ventricular dysfunction, myocardial ischemia, and possible myocardial infarction (MI). Such patients have a high probability of having extensive CAD, and additional monitoring or cardiovascular testing should be contemplated, depending upon the surgical procedure and institutional factors.

Traditionally, coronary risk assessment for noncardiac surgery in patients with a prior MI was based upon the time interval between the MI and surgery. Multiple studies demonstrated an increased incidence of reinfarction after noncardiac surgery if the prior MI was within 6 months of the operation. With improvements in perioperative care, this time interval has been shortened.[1] However, the intervening time interval is less relevant in the current era of thrombolytics, angioplasty, and routine coronary risk stratification after an acute MI. Although some patients with a recent MI may continue to have myocardium at risk for subsequent ischemia and infarction, most patients in the United

States have had their critical coronary stenosis evaluated and opened or bypassed or are receiving maximal medical therapy. The American Heart Association/American College of Cardiology Task Force on Perioperative Evaluation of the Cardiac Patient Undergoing Noncardiac Surgery has suggested that the highest risk cohort consists of patients within 6 weeks of their MI, a time period during which plaque and myocardial stabilization occur. After that period, risk stratification is based upon the presentation of disease (i.e., those with active ischemia are at highest risk).[2,3]

Hypertension

In the 1970s, a series of case studies changed the prevailing thought that antihypertensive agents should be discontinued before surgery, and suggested that poorly controlled hypertension was associated with untoward hemodynamic responses and that antihypertensive agents should be continued perioperatively. However, several large prospective studies did not establish mild to moderate hypertension as an independent predictor of postoperative cardiac complications such as cardiac death, postoperative MI, heart failure, or arrhythmias. Therefore, much of the approach to the patient with hypertension relies on management strategies from the nonsurgical literature.

More severe hypertension of a chronic nature, e.g., diastolic blood pressure higher than 110 mm Hg, should be controlled before any elective noncardiac surgery.[2] In contrast, a patient who is normally well controlled at home may demonstrate a markedly elevated blood pressure preoperatively because of anxiety. Although these patients are at increased risk for intraoperative hemodynamic lability, particularly with induction, most anesthesiologists proceed with surgery in the absence of other signs or symptoms of end-organ dysfunction.

A hypertensive crisis in the postoperative period, defined as a diastolic blood pressure higher than 120 mm Hg and clinical evidence of impending or actual end-organ damage, poses a definite risk of MI or cerebrovascular accident. Diagnostic criteria include papilledema or other evidence of increased intracranial pressure, myocardial ischemia, or acute renal failure. Several precipitants of hypertensive crises have been identified, including preeclampsia or eclampsia, pheochromocytomas, abrupt clonidine withdrawal prior to surgery, the use of chronic monoamine oxidase inhibitors with or without sympathomimetic drugs in combination, and inadvertent discontinuation of antihypertensive therapy.

Chronic hypertension may indirectly predispose patients to perioperative myocardial ischemia because CAD is more prevalent in these patients. Even in the absence of CAD, patients with chronic hypertension may have episodes of myocardial ischemia, perhaps related to impaired coronary vasodilator reserve and autoregulation such that higher arterial pressures are required to maintain adequate perfusion of vital organs. Because of vascular stiffness, hypertensive patients are also predisposed to hypotension and hence lower filling pressures. Thus, hypertensive patients with known peripheral and coronary vascular disease must have preoperative blood pressure levels monitored and maintained.

The Study of Perioperative Ischemia Research Group trial, in which patients had continuous perioperative electrocardiographic monitoring, showed that a history of hypertension was one of five independent predictors of postoperative ischemia and one of three independent predictors of increased postoperative mortality. Patients with a history of hypertension had almost twice the risk of postoperative myocardial ischemia and almost four times the risk of postoperative death compared with patients without hypertension in the first 48 hours postoperatively.

Thus, whether patients with mild to moderate hypertension should be considered at greater than average risk of perioperative myocardial ischemia remains uncertain due to often conflicting reports from the last 20 years. Surgery generally need not be postponed or canceled in the otherwise uncomplicated patient with mild to moderate hypertension.[2] Antihypertensive medications should be continued perioperatively,[2] and blood pressure should be maintained near preoperative levels to reduce the risk of myocardial ischemia. In patients with more severe hypertension, such as diastolic blood pressure higher than 110 mm Hg, the potential benefits of delaying surgery in order to optimize antihypertensive medications should be weighed against the risk of delaying the surgical procedure. With rapid-acting intravenous agents, blood pressure can usually be controlled within a matter of several hours. Weksler and colleagues studied 989 chronically treated hypertensive patients who presented for noncardiac surgery with diastolic blood pressure between 110 and 130 mm Hg and who had no previous MI, unstable or severe angina pectoris, renal failure, pregnancy-induced hypertension, left ventricular hypertrophy, previous coronary revascularization, aortic stenosis, preoperative dysrhythmias, conduction defects, or stroke.[4] The control group had their surgery postponed and remained in hospital for blood pressure control, and the study patients received 10 mg of nifedipine intranasally delivered. They observed no statistically significant differences in postoperative complications, suggesting that this subset of patients without significant cardiovascular comorbidities can proceed with surgery despite elevated blood pressure on the day of surgery.

Isolated systolic hypertension (systolic blood pressure greater than 160 mm Hg and diastolic blood pressure less than 90 mm Hg) has been identified as a risk factor for cardiovascular complications in the general population, and successful treatment reduces the future risk of stroke. However, only one study has directly assessed the relationship between cardiovascular disease and preoperative isolated systolic hypertension. In a multicenter study of patients undergoing coronary artery bypass grafting (CABG), isolated systolic hypertension was associated with a 30 percent increased incidence of cardiovascular complications compared with those in normotensive individuals.[5] Because it is unknown whether these findings can be generalized to noncardiac surgery and whether treatment will affect outcome, definition of the best approach requires further study. Treatment of systolic hypertension in elderly people is particularly challenging because the diastolic pressures are often low and unusually sensitive to hypovolemia.

Heart Failure

Heart failure has been associated in several studies with perioperative cardiac morbidity after noncardiac surgery.[6] Cohn and Goldman identified a third heart sound or other signs of heart failure as portending the most significant perioperative risks. For patients who present for noncardiac surgery with signs or symptoms of heart failure, its underpinnings need to be characterized before major noncardiac surgery. The goal of the preoperative evaluation should be identification of the underlying myocardial disease and assessment of the severity of systolic and diastolic dysfunction. Treatment of decompensated hypertrophic cardiomyopathy is very different from that of dilated cardiomyopathy, and the preoperative evaluation can influence perioperative management. In particular, this assessment may influence perioperative fluid and vasopressor management. Ischemic cardiomyopathy is of greatest concern because the patient has a substantial risk for developing further ischemia, leading to myocardial necrosis and potentially a downward spiral. In such patients, a pulmonary artery catheter or intraoperative transesophageal echocardiography could be indicated.

Obstructive hypertrophic cardiomyopathy was formerly regarded as a high-risk condition associated with high perioperative morbidity. A retrospective review of perioperative care in 35 patients concluded that the risk of general anesthesia and major noncardiac surgery is low in such patients. However, this study did suggest that spinal anesthesia may be relatively contraindicated in view of the sensitivity of cardiac output to hypovolemia in this condition. Haering and colleagues studied 77 patients with asymmetrical septal hypertrophy who were retrospectively identified from a large data base.[7] Forty percent of patients had one or more adverse perioperative cardiac events, including one patient who had an MI and ventricular tachycardia that required emergent cardioversion; the majority of the events were perioperative congestive heart failure. There were no perioperative deaths. Important independent risk factors for adverse outcome in all patients include major surgery and increasing duration of surgery. Unlike the findings in the original cohort of patients, the type of anesthesia was not an independent risk factor.

Valvular Heart Disease

The presence of critical aortic stenosis associates with a very high risk of cardiac decompensation in patients undergoing elective noncardiac surgery. The presence of any of the classical triad of angina, syncope, and heart failure in a patient with aortic stenosis should alert the clinician to the need for further evaluation and potential interventions, usually valve replacement. However, many patients with severe or critical aortic stenosis may be asymptomatic, and preoperative patients with aortic systolic murmurs warrant a careful history and physical examination and often further evaluation. There are several case series of patients with critical aortic stenosis demonstrating that, when necessary, noncardiac surgery can be performed with acceptable risk.[8] For the most part, these cases have included patients with few or no symptoms but a valve area less than 0.5 cm^2. Alternatively, aortic valvuloplasty represents an option for occasional patients. Although the long-term outcome of patients who undergo aortic balloon valvuloplasty is generally poor,[9] primarily because of restenosis, this procedure may be used for temporary benefit in noncardiac surgery in patients who cannot undergo valve replacement in the short term. The considerable procedure-related morbidity and mortality risk must be carefully considered before recommending this strategy as a means of trying to lower the risk of noncardiac surgery.

Mitral valve disease tends to cause less risk of perioperative complications than aortic stenosis. However, occult mitral stenosis from rheumatic heart disease is still encountered on occasion and can lead to severe left-sided heart failure in the presence of tachycardia or volume loading, or both. In contrast to aortic valvuloplasty, mitral valve balloon valvuloplasty often yields reasonable short- and long-term benefit, especially in younger patients with predominant mitral stenosis but without severe mitral valve leaflet thickening or significant subvalvular fibrosis and calcification.[10] In the perioperative patient with a functioning prosthetic heart valve, the major issues are antibiotic prophylaxis and anticoagulation. All patients with prosthetic valves who are undergoing procedures that can cause transient bacteremia should receive prophylaxis.[11,12]

In patients with prosthetic valves, the risk of increased bleeding during a procedure in a patient receiving antithrombotic therapy must be weighed against the increased risk of a thromboembolism caused by stopping the therapy. The common practice for patients with a mechanical prosthetic valve in place undergoing noncardiac surgery is the cessation of anticoagulants 3 days prior to surgery. This allows the International Normalized Ratio (INR) to fall to less than 1.5 times normal. The oral anticoagulants can then be resumed on postoperative day 1. Using a similar protocol, Katholi and colleagues observed no perioperative episodes of thromboembolism or hemorrhage in 25 patients. An alternative approach in patients at high risk for thromboembolism is conversion to heparin during the perioperative period. The heparin can be discontinued 4 to 6 hours prior to surgery and resumed shortly thereafter. Current prosthetic valves may involve a lower incidence, and the risk of heparin may outweigh the benefit in the perioperative setting. According to the American Heart Association/American College of Cardiology guidelines, heparin usually can be reserved for those who have had a recent thrombosis or embolus (arbitrarily within 1 year), those with demonstrated thrombotic problems when previously not receiving therapy, those with the Björk-Shiley valve, and those with more than three risk factors (atrial fibrillation, previous thromboembolism, hypercoagulable condition, and mechanical prosthesis).[13] A lower threshold for recommending heparin should be considered for patients with mechanical valves in the mitral position, in whom a single risk factor would be sufficient evidence of high risk. Subcutaneous low-molecular-weight heparin offers an alternative outpatient approach.[14] It is critical to have a discussion between the surgeon and cardiologist regarding the optimal perioperative management.

Congenital Heart Disease in Adults

(see also Chap. 56)

Congenital heart disease afflicts some 500,000 to 1 million adults in the United States alone. The nature of the underlying anatomy and any anatomical correction affect the perioperative plan and incidence of complications, including infection, bleeding, hypoxemia, hypotension, and paradoxical embolization. A major concern in the patient with congenital heart disease is the development of pulmonary hypertension and Eisenmenger syndrome. It has been thought traditionally that regional anesthesia should be avoided in these patients because of the potential for sympathetic blockade and worsening of the shunt. However, a review of the published literature incorporating 103 cases found that overall perioperative mortality was 14 percent; patients receiving regional anesthesia had a mortality of 5 percent, whereas those receiving general anesthesia had a mortality of 18 percent.[15] The authors concluded that most deaths probably occurred as a result of the surgical procedure and disease and not anesthesia. Although perioperative and peripartum mortalities were high, many anesthetic agents and techniques had been used with success. Patients with congenital heart disease are at risk for infective endocarditis and should receive antibiotic prophylaxis. A review discusses the anesthetic management of these patients in detail.[16]

Arrhythmias

Cardiac arrhythmias are common in the perioperative period, particularly in elderly patients or patients under-going thoracic surgery. Predisposing factors include pain (e.g., from hip fractures), severe anxiety, and other situations that heighten adrenergic tone. A prospective study of 4181 patients 50 years of age or older demonstrated supraventricular arrhythmia in 2 percent of patients during and 6.1 percent after surgery. Perioperative atrial fibrillation raises several concerns, including stroke.[17] Therefore, early treatment to restore sinus rhythm or control the ventricular response and anticoagulation is indicated. Amar and colleagues evaluated the prophylactic value of intravenous

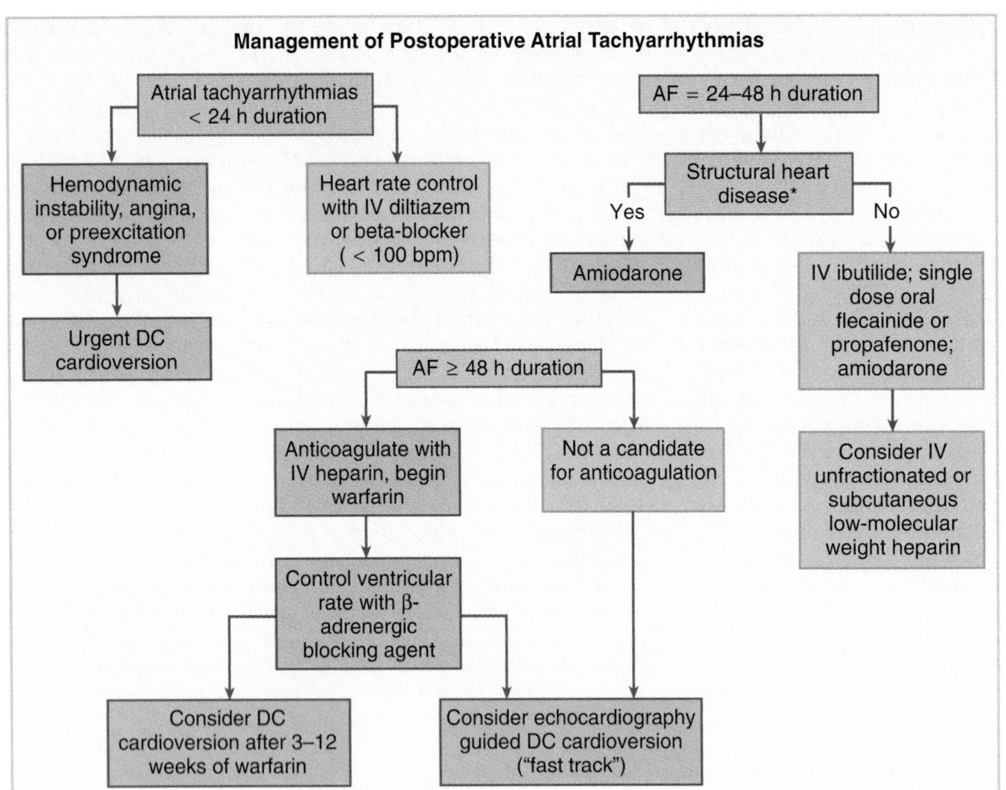

FIGURE 77–1 Proposed algorithm for the treatment of postoperative atrial tachyarrhythmias. AF = atrial fibrillation or flutter; bpm = beats/min; DC = direct current. *Structural heart disease is defined as the presence of one of the following: left ventricular hypertrophy with wall thickness greater than 1.4 cm, mitral valve disease, coronary artery disease, or heart failure. (From Amar D: Perioperative atrial tachyarrhythmias. Anesthesiology 97:1618, 2002.)

diltiazem in a randomized, placebo-controlled trial involving high-risk thoracic surgery and reported that prophylactic diltiazem reduced the incidence of clinically significant atrial arrhythmias.[18] Balser and colleagues studied 64 cases of postoperative supraventricular tachyarrhythmia.[19] After adenosine administration, patients who remained in supraventricular tachyarrhythmia were prospectively randomly assigned to receive either intravenous diltiazem or intravenous esmolol for ventricular rate control. The authors reported that intravenous esmolol produced a more rapid (2-hour) conversion to sinus rhythm than intravenous diltiazem. The literature has been reviewed and an algorithm for treatment produced (Fig. 77–1).[17]

Although ventricular arrhythmias were originally identified as a risk factor for perioperative morbidity, subsequent studies have not confirmed this finding. O'Kelly studied a consecutive sample of 230 male patients with known CAD or at high risk for CAD undergoing major noncardiac surgical procedures. Preoperative arrhythmias were associated with the occurrence of intraoperative and postoperative arrhythmias. However, nonfatal MI and cardiac death did not occur significantly more frequently in those with prior perioperative arrhythmias. Amar and colleagues studied 412 patients undergoing major thoracic surgery and determined that the incidence of nonsustained ventricular tachycardia is 15 percent but is not associated with poor outcome.[20] Despite this finding, the presence of an arrhythmia in the preoperative setting should provoke a search for underlying cardiopulmonary disease, ongoing myocardial ischemia or infarction, drug toxicity, or metabolic derangements.

Conduction abnormalities can increase perioperative risk and may require the placement of a temporary or permanent pacemaker. On the other hand, patients with intraventricular conduction delays, even in the presence of a left or right bundle branch block, and no history of advanced heart block or symptoms rarely progress to complete heart block perioperatively. Since transthoracic pacing units have become available, the need for temporary transvenous pacemakers has decreased.

Decision to Undergo Diagnostic Testing

The American College of Cardiology/American Heart Association Guidelines on Perioperative Cardiovascular Evaluation for Noncardiac Surgery proposed an algorithm based upon expert opinion, which has been reaffirmed in an update published in 2002.[2,3] A stepwise bayesian strategy that relies on assessment of clinical markers, prior coronary evaluation and treatment, functional capacity, and surgery-specific risk is outlined below. Successful use of the algorithm requires an appreciation for different levels of risk attributable to certain clinical circumstances, levels of functional capacity, and types of surgery.

Multiple studies have attempted to identify clinical risk markers for perioperative cardiovascular morbidity and mortality. As described earlier, patients with unstable coronary syndromes and severe valvular disease are at the highest risk. Patients with known, stable CAD are at intermediate risk. Through the use of large cohort studies and multivariate analyses, both diabetes and chronic renal insufficiency (creatinine >2.0 mg/dl) also have been associated with increased perioperative cardiovascular complications that place the patients at intermediate risk. Several clinical risk markers for cardiovascular disease, each associated with variable levels of perioperative risk, have been classified as "low risk factors." The classification of perioperative clinical risk markers for the purpose of assessing the need for further testing is shown in Table 77–1.

As described with regard to angina pattern, exercise tolerance is one of the strongest determinants of perioperative risk and the need for invasive monitoring.[21] In one study of outpatients referred for evaluation before major noncardiac procedures, patients were asked to estimate the number of blocks they could walk and flights of stairs they could climb without experiencing cardiac symptoms.[21] Patients who could not walk four blocks and climb two flights of stairs were considered to have poor exercise tolerance and were found to have twice as many perioperative cardiovascular complications as those with better functional status. The likelihood of a serious complication occurring was related inversely to the number of blocks that could be walked or flights of stairs that could be climbed. Several scales based upon activities of daily living have been proposed as a means of assessing exercise tolerance. One such scale (the Duke Activity Scale Index [DASI]) is advocated in the guidelines (Table 77–2).[2]

The type of surgical procedure itself has a significant impact on perioperative risks and the amount of preoperative preparation required for safe performance of anesthesia. For surgical procedures that are not associated with significant stress or a high incidence of perioperative myocardial ischemia or morbidity, the costs of the evaluation are often greater than any perceived benefits from the information gained by preoperative assessment. For example, outpatient procedures cause little morbidity and mortality. In such patients, perioperative management is rarely changed by the cardiovascular status unless the patient demonstrates unstable angina or overt congestive heart failure. In contrast, surgery for vascular disease is associated with a high risk of morbidity and ischemic potential. Intraabdominal, thoracic, and orthopedic procedures are considered to involve intermediate risk (Table 77–3).

In addition to the risk of the surgical procedure itself, risk is correlated with the surgical volume in a given center. Several studies have demonstrated differential mortality rates in both cancer and vascular surgery, with higher mortality seen in low-volume centers. Therefore, surgical mortality rates may be very institution specific, which may influence the decision to perform further perioperative evaluations and interventions.

The stepwise approach advocated in the American College of Cardiology/American Heart Association Task Force Guidelines on Perioperative Evaluation of the Cardiac Patient Undergoing Noncardiac Surgery is shown in Figure 77–2.[2,3]

TABLE 77–1 Clinical Predictors of Increased Perioperative Cardiovascular Risk (Myocardial Infarction, Congestive Heart Failure, Death)

Major
Unstable coronary syndromes
- Recent myocardial infarction* with evidence of important ischemic risk by clinical symptoms or noninvasive study
- Unstable or severe† angina (Canadian class III or IV)‡

Decompensated congestive heart failure
Significant arrhythmias
- High-grade atrioventricular block
- Symptomatic ventricular arrhythmias in the presence of underlying heart disease
- Supraventricular arrhythmias with uncontrolled ventricular rate

Severe valvular disease

Intermediate
Mild angina pectoris (Canadian class I or II)
Prior myocardial infarction by history or pathological Q waves
Compensated or prior congestive heart failure
Diabetes mellitus
Chronic renal insufficiency

Minor
Advanced age
Abnormal electrocardiogram (left ventricular hypertrophy, left bundle branch block, ST-T abnormalities)
Rhythm other than sinus (e.g., atrial fibrillation)
Low functional capacity (e.g., inability to climb one flight of stairs with a bag of groceries)
History of stroke
Uncontrolled systemic hypertension

*The American College of Cardiology National Database Library defines recent myocardial infarction as greater than 7 days but less than or equal to 1 month (30 days).
†May include "stable" angina in patients who are unusually sedentary.
‡Campeau L: Grading of angina pectoris. Circulation 54:522, 1976.
From Eagle KA, Berger PB, Calkins H, et al: ACC/AHA guideline update for perioperative cardiovascular evaluation for noncardiac surgery: Executive summary: A report of the American College of Cardiology/American Heart Association Task Force on Practice Guidelines (Committee to Update the 1996 Guidelines on Perioperative Cardiovascular Evaluation for Noncardiac Surgery). J Am Coll Cardiol 39:542, 2002.

TABLE 77–3 Cardiac Risk* Stratification for Noncardiac Surgical Procedures

High (Reported Cardiac Risk Often >5%)
Emergent major operations, particularly in elderly people
Aortic and other major vascular
Peripheral vascular
Anticipated prolonged surgical procedures associated with large fluid shifts and/or blood loss

Intermediate (Reported Cardiac Risk Generally <5%)
Carotid endarterectomy
Head and neck
Intraperitoneal and intrathoracic
Orthopedic
Prostate

Low† (Reported Cardiac Risk Generally <1%)
Endoscopic procedures
Superficial procedure
Cataract
Breast

*Combined incidence of cardiac death and nonfatal myocardial infarction.
†Do not generally require further preoperative cardiac testing.
From Eagle KA, Berger PB, Calkins H, et al: ACC/AHA guideline update for perioperative cardiovascular evaluation for noncardiac surgery: Executive summary: A report of the American College of Cardiology/American Heart Association Task Force on Practice Guidelines (Committee to Update the 1996 Guidelines on Perioperative Cardiovascular Evaluation for Noncardiac Surgery). J Am Coll Cardiol 39:542, 2002.

TABLE 77–2 Estimated Energy Requirement for Various Activities*

METs	Activities	METs	Activities
1 MET ↓	Can you take care of yourself? Eat, dress, or use the toilet? Walk indoors around the house? Walk a block or two on level ground at 2-3 mph or 3.2-4.8 km/hr? Do light work around the house like dusting or washing dishes?	4 METs ↓	Climb a flight of stairs or walk up a hill? Walk on level ground at 4 mph or 6.4 km/hr? Run a short distance? Do heavy work around the house like scrubbing floors or lifting or moving heavy furniture? Participate in moderate recreational activities like golf, bowling, dancing, doubles tennis, or throwing a baseball or football?
4 METs		>10 METs	Participate in strenuous sports like swimming, singles tennis, football, basketball, or skiing?

*Adapted from the Duke Activity Status Index and AHA Exercise Standards.
MET = metabolic equivalent.
From Eagle KA, Berger PB, Calkins H, et al: ACC/AHA guideline update for perioperative cardiovascular evaluation for noncardiac surgery: Executive summary: A report of the American College of Cardiology/American Heart Association Task Force on Practice Guidelines (Committee to Update the 1996 Guidelines on Perioperative Cardiovascular Evaluation for Noncardiac Surgery). J Am Coll Cardiol 39:542, 2002.

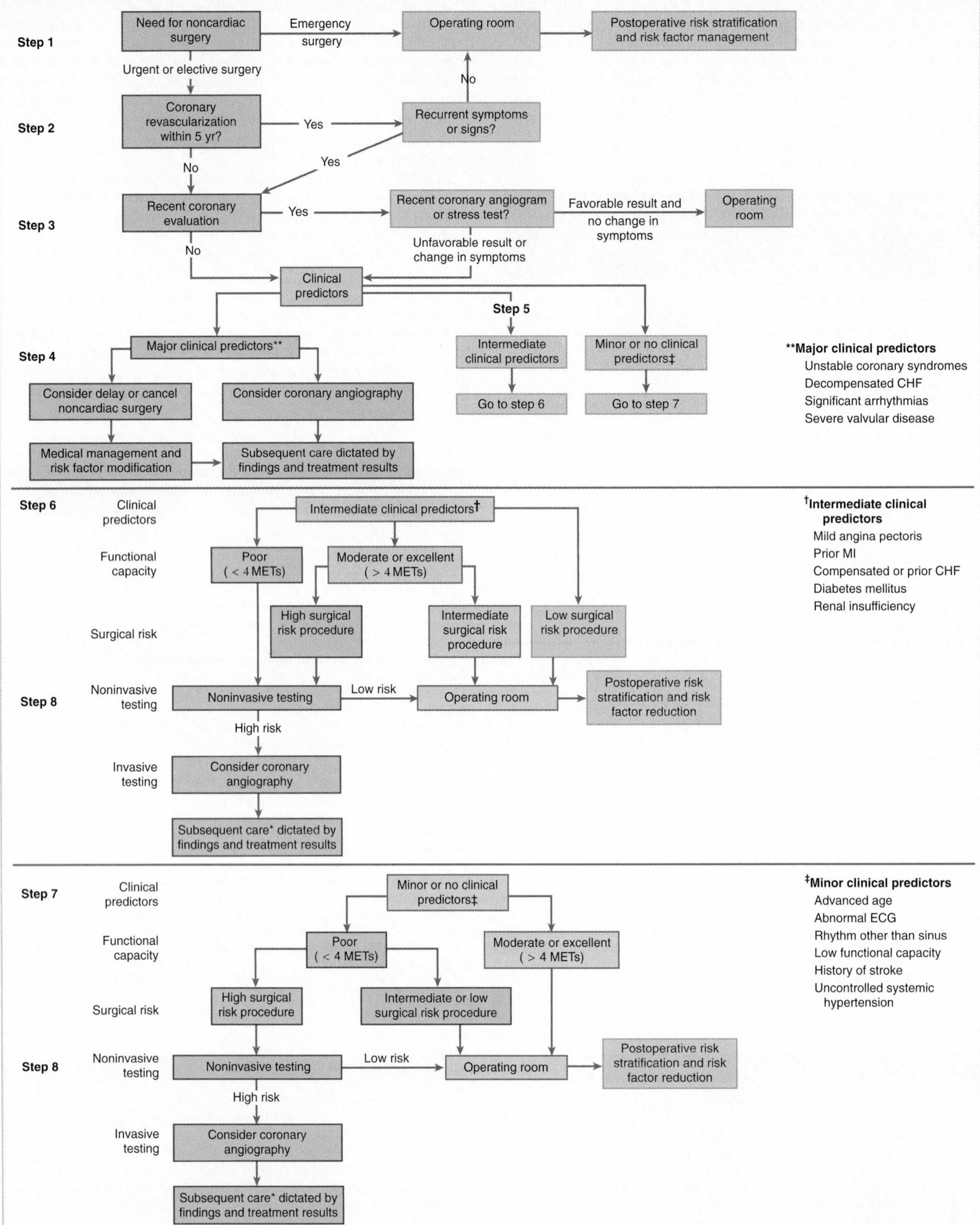

FIGURE 77–2 The American Heart Association/American College of Cardiology Task Force on Perioperative Evaluation of Cardiac Patients Undergoing Noncardiac Surgery has proposed an algorithm for decisions regarding the need for further evaluation. This represents one of multiple algorithms proposed in the literature. It is based upon expert opinion and incorporates eight steps. First, the clinician must evaluate the urgency of the surgery and the appropriateness of a formal preoperative assessment. Next, he or she must determine whether the patient has had a previous revascularization procedure or coronary evaluation. Patients with unstable coronary syndromes should be identified, and appropriate treatment should be instituted. The decision to have further testing depends on the interaction of the clinical risk factors, surgery-specific risk, and functional capacity. CHF = congestive heart failure; ECG = electrocardiogram; MET= metabolic equivalent; MI = myocardial infarction. (From Eagle KA, Berger PB, Calkins H, et al: ACC/AHA guideline update for perioperative cardiovascular evaluation for noncardiac surgery—Executive summary: A report of the American College of Cardiology/American Heart Association Task Force on Practice Guidelines [Committee to Update the 1996 Guidelines on Perioperative Cardiovascular Evaluation for Noncardiac Surgery]. J Am Coll Cardiol 39:542, 2002.)

First, the clinician must evaluate the urgency of the surgery and the appropriateness of a formal preoperative assessment. Next, the clinician must determine whether the patient has undergone a previous coronary revascularization procedure or coronary evaluation. Patients with unstable coronary syndromes should be identified and appropriate treatment instituted. Finally, the decision to undergo further testing depends upon the interaction of the clinical risk factors, surgery-specific risk, and functional capacity. High clinical risk markers include acute coronary syndromes and severe valvular disease. *Intermediate predictors* of increased risk are the factors that have been associated with higher perioperative risk in multiple studies. The guidelines currently consider mild angina pectoris, prior MI, compensated or prior congestive heart failure, chronic renal insufficiency, and diabetes mellitus as intermediate risk factors. *Minor predictors* of risk are those associated with CAD but whose relationship with perioperative cardiac complications is less well established. These include advanced age, an abnormal electrocardiogram, rhythm other than sinus, low functional capacity, history of stroke, and uncontrolled systemic hypertension; of these, low functional status is the most important. For patients at intermediate clinical risk, both exercise tolerance and the extent of the surgery are taken into account with regard to the need for further testing. No preoperative cardiovascular testing should be performed if the results would not change perioperative management.

Since the publication of the algorithm in 1996, several studies have suggested that this stepwise approach to the assessment of CAD is both effective and cost-effective.[22-24] Licker and colleagues compared data from two consecutive 4-year periods (1993 to 1996 [control period] versus 1997 to 2000 [intervention period]). Implementation of the American College of Cardiology/American Heart Association guidelines was associated with increased use of preoperative stress myocardial imaging (44.3 versus 20.6 percent; $p < 0.05$) and coronary revascularization (7.7 versus 0.8 percent; $p < 0.05$).[24] During the intervention period, there was a significant decrease in the incidence of cardiac complications (from 11.3 to 4.5 percent) and an increase in event-free survival at 1 year after surgery (from 91.3 to 98.2 percent). Froehlich and colleagues compared 102 historical control patients with 94 patients after guideline implementation and 104 patients later after guideline implementation.[23] Both resource utilization and costs were reduced after guideline implementation, and the effect was sustained for 2 years. We performed a small randomized trial involving 99 patients undergoing elective vascular surgery.[25] Patients at low or intermediate clinical risk were randomly assigned to testing or no testing, with no difference in perioperative or long-term outcome. The vast majority of these patients were highly functional and given perioperative beta blocker therapy, suggesting that exercise capacity can help determine the need for further diagnostic testing preoperatively.

Tests to Improve Identification and Definition of Cardiovascular Disease

Several noninvasive diagnostic methods have been proposed to evaluate the extent of coronary artery disease before noncardiac surgery. The exercise electrocardiogram has traditionally served to evaluate individuals for the presence of coronary artery disease. However, as outlined earlier, patients with excellent exercise tolerance in daily life rarely benefit from further testing. Patients with poor exercise capacity may not achieve heart rate and blood pressure adequate for diagnostic purposes on electrocardiographic stress tests. Such patients often require concomitant imaging.

A substantial number of high-risk patients either are unable to exercise or have contraindications to exercise. In surgical patients, this phenomenon is most evident in patients undergoing vascular surgery with claudication or an abdominal aortic aneurysm; both conditions associate with a high rate of perioperative cardiac morbidity. Therefore, pharmacological stress testing has become popular, particularly as a preoperative test in patients undergoing vascular surgery. Several authors have shown that the presence of a redistribution defect on dipyridamole or adenosine thallium or sestamibi imaging in patients undergoing peripheral vascular surgery predicts postoperative cardiac events. Pharmacological stress imaging is best employed in patients at moderate clinical risk. Several strategies may increase the predictive value of such tests. The redistribution defect can be quantitated, with larger areas of defect associated with increased risk. In addition, both increased lung uptake and left ventricular cavity dilation indicate ventricular dysfunction with ischemia. Several investigative groups have demonstrated that the delineation of "low-" and "high-" risk scintography (larger area of defect, increased lung uptake, and left ventricular cavity dilation) markedly improved the test's predictive value.[26] They demonstrated that patients with high-risk thallium scans had particularly increased risk for perioperative morbidity and long-term mortality.

Stress echocardiography has also been widely employed as a preoperative test.[27] One advantage of this test is that it assesses dynamically myocardial ischemia in response to increased inotropy and heart rate, such as may occur during the perioperative period. The presence of new wall motion abnormalities that occur at a low heart rate is the best predictor of increased perioperative risk, with large areas of defect being of secondary importance.[27]

Boersma and colleagues investigated the value of dobutamine stress echocardiography with respect to the extent of wall motion abnormalities and the ability of preoperative beta blocker treatment to attenuate risk in patients undergoing major aortic surgery. They assigned one point for each of the following characteristics: age older than 70 years, current angina, myocardial infarction, congestive heart failure, prior cerebrovascular disease, diabetes mellitus, and renal failure.[28] As the total of number of clinical risk factors increases, perioperative cardiac event rates also increase.

Which diagnostic test should be used (see also Chap. 16)? Several groups have published meta-analyses examining the various preoperative diagnostic tests. Mantha and colleagues demonstrated good predictive values of ambulatory electrocardiographic monitoring, radionuclide angiography, dipyridamole thallium imaging, and dobutamine stress echocardiography. Shaw and coworkers also demonstrated excellent predictive values for both dipyridamole thallium imaging and dobutamine stress echocardiography.[29] Although studies suggested the superior predictive value of dobutamine stress echocardiography, there was significant overlap of the confidence intervals with other tests. However, an important determinant with respect to the choice of preoperative testing is the expertise at the local institution. Another factor is whether assessment of valve function or myocardial thickness is of interest, in which case echocardiography may be preferred. Stress nuclear imaging may have slightly higher sensitivity, but stress echocardiography may be less likely to be falsely positive. The role in preoperative risk assessment of newer stress imaging modalities for preoperative assessment utilizing magnetic resonance imaging, 16-slice computed tomographic imaging, and position-emission tomography is rapidly evolving.

Overview of Anesthesia Used in Cardiac Patients Undergoing Noncardiac Surgery

There are three classes of anesthetics: general, regional, and local or sedation or monitored anesthetic care (MAC). General anesthesia can be defined best as a state including unconsciousness, amnesia, analgesia, immobility, and attenuation of autonomic responses to noxious stimulation. General anesthesia can be achieved with inhalational agents, intravenous agents, or a combination (frequently termed a balanced technique). In addition, general anesthesia can be achieved with or without an endotracheal tube. Laryngoscopy and intubation were traditionally thought to associate with the greatest stress and risk for myocardial ischemia, but extubation may involve greater risk. Alternative methods for delivering general anesthesia are through a mask or a laryngeal mask airway, a newer device that fits above the epiglottis and does not require laryngoscopy or intubation.

There are five currently approved inhalational anesthetic agents in the United States in addition to nitrous oxide, although enflurane and halothane are rarely utilized today. All inhalational agents have reversible myocardial depressant effects and lead to decreases in myocardial oxygen demand. The degree to which they depress cardiac output is a function of their concentration, effects on systemic vascular resistance, and effects on baroreceptor responsiveness. Therefore, they differ in their specific effects on heart rate and blood pressure.

Isoflurane causes negative inotropic effects, potent vascular smooth muscle relaxation, and minimal effects on baroreceptor function. Desflurane has the fastest onset and is used commonly in the outpatient setting. Sevoflurane's onset and offset of action are intermediate between those of isoflurane and desflurane. Its major advantage is that it is extremely pleasant smelling and therefore is used frequently as the agent of choice in children.

There have been several issues regarding the safety of the inhalational agents in patients with CAD. Isoflurane, because of its vasodilating properties, can cause a coronary artery steal leading to myocardial ischemia in an animal model. Several clinical cases have reported an association between myocardial ischemia and isoflurane, leading to an editorial suggesting that isoflurane should not be used in patients with CAD. However, several large-scale randomized and nonrandomized studies of the use of inhalational agents in patients undergoing CABG have not demonstrated any increased incidence of myocardial ischemia or infarction in patients receiving isoflurane compared with other inhalation agents or narcotic-based techniques. In a subsequent analysis of one of the randomized trials, the patients who were found to have steal-prone anatomy on coronary angiography did not have a higher incidence of myocardial ischemia. On the basis of the accumulated data from human studies, most anesthesiologists do not believe that isoflurane use presents a major threat of coronary steal, and it has become the most widely used anesthetic for patients, including those with CAD.

There are theoretical concerns regarding the safety of desflurane. Desflurane has been shown to be associated with airway irritability and led to tachycardia in volunteer studies. In a large-scale study comparing a narcotic-based anesthetic and a desflurane-based anesthetic, the desflurane group had a significantly higher incidence of myocardial infarction, although there was no difference in the incidence of MI. Including a narcotic with desflurane can prevent this tachycardia. Ongoing studies aim to determine the safety profile of desflurane in patients undergoing major vascular surgery. Sevoflurane has been studied in comparison with isoflurane in one randomized trial involving patients at high risk for cardiovascular disease. No difference in the incidence of myocardial ischemia was observed; however, the incidence of MI was too low to detect any difference. Overall, at this time no single inhalation anesthetic seems best for the patient with CAD.

There are theoretical advantages of the use of inhalational anesthetics in patients with CAD. Several investigative groups have demonstrated in vitro and in animal models that these agents have protective effects on the myocardium similar to those of ischemic preconditioning.[30,31] This favorable effect on myocardial oxygen demand would serve to offset the theoretical effects of coronary steal in patients with chronic coronary occlusion.

High-dose narcotic techniques offer the advantage of hemodynamic stability and lack of myocardial depression. In 1969, Lowenstein and colleagues proposed a high-dose narcotic technique for patients undergoing CABG. Narcotic-based anesthetics were frequently considered the "cardiac anesthesia" and advocated for use in all high-risk patients including those undergoing noncardiac surgery. The disadvantage of these traditional high-dose narcotic techniques is the requirement for postoperative ventilation. An ultra-short-acting narcotic (remifentanil) has been introduced into clinical practice, obviating the need for prolonged ventilation. It has been used in patients undergoing cardiac surgery and shown to facilitate early extubation.

Despite the theoretical advantages of a high-dose narcotic technique, several large-scale trials in patients undergoing CABG showed no difference in survival or major morbidity compared with the inhalation-based technique. This observation has led in part to the abandonment of high-dose narcotics in much of cardiac surgery and an emphasis on early extubation. Most anesthesiologists use a "balanced" technique that involves the administration of lower doses of narcotics with an inhalational agent. This approach allows the anesthesiologist to derive the benefits of each of these agents while minimizing the side effects.

An alternative mode of delivering general anesthesia is the intravenous agent propofol. Propofol is an alkyl phenol that can be used for both induction and maintenance of general anesthesia. It can result in profound hypotension because of reduced arterial tone with no change in heart rate. The major advantage of propofol is its rapid clearance with few residual effects on awakening; however, because it is quite expensive, its current use tends to be limited to operations of brief duration. Despite its hemodynamic effects, it has been used extensively to facilitate early extubation after coronary artery bypass surgery.

Current evidence indicates that there is no one best general anesthetic technique for patients with CAD undergoing noncardiac surgery and has led to the abandonment of the concept of a "cardiac anesthetic."

Spinal and Epidural Anesthesia

Regional anesthesia includes the techniques of spinal and epidural anesthesia as well as peripheral nerve blocks. Each technique has advantages and risks. Peripheral techniques, such as brachial plexus or Bier blocks, offer the advantage of having minimal or no hemodynamic effects. In contrast, spinal or epidural techniques can produce sympathetic blockade, which can reduce blood pressure and slow heart rate. Spinal anesthesia and lumbar or low thoracic epidural anesthesia can also evoke reflex sympathetic activation above the blockade, which might lead to myocardial ischemia.

The primary clinical difference between epidural and spinal anesthesia is the ability to provide continuous anesthesia or analgesia through placement of an epidural catheter as opposed to a single dose in spinal anesthesia, although some clinicians place a catheter in the intrathecal space. Although the speed of onset depends upon the local anesthetic agent used, spinal anesthesia and its associated autonomic effects occur sooner than the same agent administered epidurally. Because a catheter is usually left in place for epidural anesthesia, it can be more easily titrated. Epidural catheters can also be used postoperatively to provide analgesia.

A great deal of research has compared regional versus general anesthesia for patients with CAD, particularly patients undergoing infrainguinal bypass surgery. Overall mortality was reduced by about a third in patients allocated to neuraxial blockade, although the findings were controversial because most of the benefit was observed in older studies.[32] There were also reductions in MI and renal failure. Currently available evidence does not provide definitive data regarding one best anesthetic technique for patients undergoing high-risk noncardiac surgery.

Monitored Anesthesia Care

Monitored anesthesia care (MAC) encompasses local anesthesia administered by the surgeon with or without sedation. In a large-scale cohort study, MAC was associated with increased 30-day mortality in a univariate analysis compared with general anesthesia, although it did not remain significant in multivariate analysis when patients' comorbidity was taken into account.[33] The major issue with MAC is the ability to block the stress response adequately because inadequate analgesia associated with tachycardia may be worse than the potential hemodynamic effects of general or regional anesthesia. Since the introduction of the newer short-acting intravenous agents, general anesthesia essentially can now be administered without an endotracheal tube. This can allow the anesthesiologist to provide intense anesthesia for short or peripheral procedures without the potential effects of endotracheal intubation and extubation, blurring the distinction between general anesthesia and MAC.

Intraoperative Hemodynamics and Myocardial Ischemia

Over the past two decades, numerous studies have explored the relationship between hemodynamics, perioperative ischemia, and MI. Tachycardia is the strongest predictor of perioperative ischemia. Although traditionally heart rate higher than 100 beats/min has been defined as the lower limit for tachycardia, slower heart rates may result in myocardial ischemia. As described below, control of heart rate using beta blockers does decrease the incidence of myocardial ischemia and infarction.[34-37]

Although there has been concern about intraoperative hypotension in patients with CAD, there is no evidence to support such a contention. In CABG, the vast majority of episodes of intraoperative ischemia do not correlate with hemodynamic changes.[38] In the absence of tachycardia, hypotension has not been shown to be associated with myocardial ischemia.

Postoperative Management of Patients with Cardiac Disease after Noncardiac Surgery

Overview of the Postoperative Response to Surgery

To determine the best approach to preoperative testing, it is important to understand the pathophysiology of perioperative cardiac events. A full discussion of the pathophysiology of perioperative myocardial infarction has been published.[39]

All surgical procedures cause a stress response, although the extent of the response depends on the extent of the surgery and the use of anesthetics and analgesics to reduce the response. The stress response can lead to increases in heart rate and blood pressure, which can precipitate episodes of myocardial ischemia in areas distal to coronary artery stenoses. Prolonged myocardial ischemia (either prolonged individual episodes or cumulative duration of shorter episodes) has been associated with myocardial necrosis and perioperative MI and death.[39] Identification of patients with a high risk of coronary artery stenoses, through either history or cardiovascular testing, can lead to implementation of strategies to reduce morbidity from supply-demand mismatches.[40] As described previously, beta-blocking agents can reduce the increased demand and coronary revascularization may be of utility in improving supply-related issues in patients with critical stenoses.

A major mechanism of MI in the nonoperative setting is plaque rupture of a noncritical coronary stenosis with subsequent coronary thrombosis (see Chap. 35). Because the perioperative period is marked by tachycardia and a hypercoagulable state, plaque disruption and thrombosis may occur quite commonly. As the nidus for the thrombosis is a noncritical stenosis, preoperative cardiac evaluation may fail to identify such a patient before surgery, although control of heart rate may decrease the propensity of the plaque to rupture. The areas distal to the noncritical stenosis would not be expected to have collateral coronary flow, and therefore any acute thrombosis may have a greater detrimental effect than it would in a previously severely narrowed vessel. Preoperative cardiovascular testing clearly does not identify these patients. However, if the postoperative MI is due to a prolonged increase in myocardial oxygen demand in patients with one or more critical fixed stenoses, one would expect preoperative testing to identify such patients.

Some evidence supports both mechanisms. There have been several autopsy and postinfarction angiography studies after surgery. Ellis and colleagues demonstrated that one-third of all patients sustained events in areas distal to noncritical stenoses.[41] Dawood and colleagues demonstrated that fatal perioperative myocardial infarction occurs predominantly in patients with multivessel coronary disease, especially left main and three-vessel disease; however, the severity of preexisting underlying stenosis did not predict the resulting infarct territory.[42] This analysis suggests that fatal events occur primarily in patients with advanced fixed stenoses but that the infarct may be triggered by plaque rupture in a coexisting mild or only moderate stenosis of the area of diseased vessel.

Postoperative Intensive Care

Increasing evidence suggests that patients cared for in ICUs staffed by dedicated intensivists have improved outcomes. Pronovost and colleagues performed a systematic review of the literature on physician staffing patterns and clinical outcomes in critically ill patients.[43] They divided ICU physician staffing into low-intensity (no intensivist or elective intensivist consultation) and high-intensity (mandatory intensivist consultation or closed ICU [all care directed by intensivist]) groups. High-intensity staffing was associated with lower hospital mortality in 16 of 17 studies (94 percent) and with a pooled estimate of the relative risk for hospital mortality of 0.71 (95 percent confidence interval [CI], 0.62 to 0.82). High-intensity staffing was associated with lower ICU mortality in 14 of 15 studies (93 percent) and with a pooled estimate of the relative risk for ICU mortality of 0.61 (95 percent CI, 0.50 to 0.75). High-intensity staffing reduced hospital length of stay (LOS) in 10 of 13 studies and reduced ICU LOS in 14 of 18 studies without case-mix adjustment. High-intensity staffing was associated with reduced hospital LOS in two of four studies and ICU LOS in both studies that adjusted for case mix. No study found increased LOS with high-intensity staffing after case-mix adjustment. High-intensity versus low-intensity ICU physician staffing is associated with reduced hospital and ICU mortality and hospital and ICU LOS.

Postoperative Pain Management

There is interest in the value of postoperative analgesia regimens in reducing perioperative cardiac morbidity. The value of postoperative analgesia has been reviewed elsewhere.[44] Because postoperative tachycardia and catecholamine surges probably promote myocardial ischemia or coronary plaque rupture, or both, and postoperative pain is associated with tachycardia and increased catecholamines, effective postoperative analgesia may reduce cardiac complications. In addition, there is growing interest in the role of postoperative analgesia in reducing the hypercoagulable state. Epidural anesthesia may reduce platelet aggregability compared with general anesthesia. It is unclear whether this is related to intraoperative or postoperative management.

Future research will focus on how best to deliver postoperative analgesia to maximize the potential benefits in reducing complications.

Surveillance and Implications of Perioperative Cardiac Complications

The optimal and most cost-effective strategy for monitoring high-risk patients for major morbidity after noncardiac surgery is unknown. Myocardial ischemia and infarctions that occur postoperatively are usually silent, most likely because of the confounding effects of analgesics and postoperative surgical pain. Creatine kinase with muscle and brain subunits (CK-MB) is also less specific for myocardial necrosis postoperatively because this marker can rise during aortic surgery and after mesenteric ischemia. Further confounding the issue, most perioperative MIs are non-Q-wave in nature, and nonspecific ST-T wave changes are common after surgery with or without MI. Therefore, the diagnosis of a perioperative MI is particularly difficult using these traditional tests.

The approach to detection of perioperative MI has evolved with the use of troponins T and I. Adams and colleagues studied 108 patients undergoing high-risk surgery and obtained measures of CK-MB, total CK, and cardiac troponin I; daily electrocardiograms; and pre- and postoperative echocardiograms. Eight patients undergoing vascular surgery sustained a perioperative MI, as confirmed by the presence of new segmental-wall motion abnormalities. All eight patients had elevations of cardiac troponin I, and six patients had elevated CK-MB. Troponin I had a specificity of 99 percent and CK-MB a specificity of 81 percent. Lee and coworkers measured CK-MB and troponin T levels in 1175 patients undergoing noncardiac surgery and created receiver operating characteristic curves.[45] They found that troponin T had similar performance for diagnosing perioperative MI, but a significantly better correlation for major cardiac complications developing after an acute MI. Metzler and associates examined the sensitivity of troponin assay at variable cutoff levels—a value greater than 0.6 ng/ml demonstrated a positive predictive value of 87.5 percent and a negative predictive value of 98 percent.[46]

Traditionally, perioperative MI were associated with 30 to 50 percent short-term mortality. However, more recent series have reported a fatality rate associated with perioperative MIs as less than 20 percent.[39] This improvement may be due to more reliable detection of small nonfatal MIs. There also appears to be a shift in the timing of a perioperative MI. Studies from the 1980s suggested a peak incidence on the second and third postoperative days. Badner and colleagues, using troponin I as a marker for MI, suggested that the immediate and first postoperative days were the time of highest incidence.[47] This has been confirmed in other studies. Again, it is likely that this change is related to more robust surveillance methods, not a fundamental shift in how or when myocardial ischemia or infarction occurs.

Increasing evidence suggests that a perioperative MI or biomarker elevation predicts a worse long-term outcome. Lope-Jimenez and coworkers found that abnormal troponin T levels were associated with an increased incidence of cardiovascular complications within 6 months of surgery.[48] Kim and associates studied perioperative troponin I levels in 229 patients having aortic or infrainguinal vascular surgery or lower extremity amputation.[49] Twenty-eight patients (12 percent) had postoperative troponin I greater than 1.5 ng/mL, which was associated with a 6-fold increased risk of 6-month mortality and a 27-fold increased risk of MI. Furthermore, they observed a dose-response relation between troponin I concentration and mortality.

Strategies to Reduce Perioperative Cardiac Risk of Noncardiac Surgery

Coronary Artery Bypass Grafting

Coronary revascularization provides one means of reducing the perioperative risk of noncardiac surgery. There are currently no randomized trials of coronary revascularization, although there is an ongoing trial in the Veterans Affairs (VA) hospitals.[50] Some evidence exists that prior successful preoperative revascularization may decrease postoperative cardiac risk two- to fourfold in patients undergoing elective vascular surgery. The strongest evidence comes from the Coronary Artery Surgery Study (CASS) Registry, which enrolled patients from 1978 to 1981. The operative mortality for patients with CABG prior to noncardiac surgery was 0.9 percent but was significantly higher at 2.4 percent in patients without prior CABG. However, there was a 1.4 percent mortality rate associated with the CABG procedure itself.

Eagle and colleagues reported on a long-term analysis of patients entered into CASS.[51] They studied patients assigned for more than 10 years to medical or surgical therapy for CAD who underwent 3368 noncardiac operations in the years following assignment of coronary treatment. The reported rate of perioperative MI and death was stratified by type of surgical procedure. Specifically, low-risk surgeries such as skin, breast, urological, and minor orthopedic procedures were associated with a total morbidity and mortality less than 1 percent regardless of coronary treatment type, and prior revascularization did not affect outcome. Intermediate-risk surgery such as abdominal or thoracic surgery or carotid endarterectomy was associated with a combined morbidity and mortality of 1 to 5 percent with a small but significant improvement in outcome in patients who had undergone prior revascularization. The most significant improvement in outcome was in patients undergoing major vascular surgery such as abdominal or lower extremity revascularization. In this cohort, mortality after noncardiac surgery was reduced by two-thirds in patients who had had bypasses. However, this observational study did not randomly allocate patients and was undertaken in the 1970s and 1980s, before significant advances in medical, surgical, and percutaneous coronary strategies.[51]

The length of time between the coronary revascularization and noncardiac surgery most likely affects its protective effect. Back and colleagues studied 425 consecutive patients undergoing 481 elective major vascular operations at an academic VA Medical Center.[52] Coronary revascularization was classified as recent (CABG, <1 year; percutaneous transluminal coronary angioplasty [PTCA], <6 months) in 35 cases (7 percent), prior (1 year ≤ CABG < 5 year, 6 months ≤ PTCA < 2 year) in 45 cases (9 percent), and remote (CABG, ≥ 5 year; PTCA, ≥ 2 year) in 48 cases (10 percent). Outcomes in patients with previous PTCA were similar to those after CABG ($p = 0.7$). Significant differences in adverse cardiac events and mortality were found between patients with CABG within 5 years or PTCA within 2 years (6.3 and 1.3 percent, respectively), individuals with remote revascularization (10.4 and 6.3 percent), and nonrevascularized patients stratified as high risk (13.3 and 3.3 percent) or intermediate and low risk (2.8 and 0.9 percent). The authors concluded that previous coronary revascularization (CABG, <5 years; PTCA, <2 years) may provide only modest protection against adverse cardiac events and mortality following major arterial reconstruction.

An alternative approach to examining the optimal strategy for medical care in the absence of clinical trials is the construction of a decision analysis.[53] Such models assume that patients with significant CAD would undergo CABG prior to noncardiac surgery. The models found that the optimal decision was sensitive to local morbidity and mortality rates within the clinically observed range. These models suggest that preoperative testing for the purpose of coronary revascularization is not the optimal strategy if perioperative morbidity and mortality are low. If long-term survival is included in the models, coronary revascularization may lead to improved overall outcome and be a cost-effective intervention,[53] particularly in patients with significant left main or three-vessel coronary stenoses, or both.

Percutaneous Coronary Interventions

Several cohort studies have examined the benefit of percutaneous coronary intervention (PCI) before noncardiac surgery. Posner and colleagues utilized an administrative data set of patients who underwent PCI and noncardiac surgery in Washington State.[54] They matched patients with coronary disease undergoing noncardiac surgery with and without prior PCI and looked at cardiac complications. In this nonrandomized design, they noted a significantly lower rate of 30-day cardiac complications in patients who underwent PCI at least 90 days before the noncardiac surgery. PCI within 90 days of noncardiac surgery did not improve outcome. Although the explanation for these results is unknown, they may support the notion that PCI performed "to get the patient through surgery" may not improve perioperative outcome because cardiac complications may not occur in patients with stable or asymptomatic coronary stenosis and PCI may actually destabilize coronary plaques that become manifest in the days or weeks after noncardiac surgery. Hassan and colleagues evaluated the effect of multivessel angioplasty on subsequent noncardiac surgery in the Bypass Angioplasty Revascularization Investigation (BARI).[55] A total of 501 patients had noncardiac surgery a median of 29 months after the most recent revascularization procedure. Mortality and nonfatal MI occurred in 4 of the 250 surgery-assigned patients and 4 of the 251 angioplasty-assigned patients. Therefore, there does not appear to be an optimal choice of revascularization procedure for multivessel disease among patients who appear to be acceptable candidates for either strategy, although a larger scale study is necessary to confirm these findings.

PCI using coronary stenting poses several special issues. Kaluza and colleagues reported on the outcome in 40 patients who underwent prophylactic coronary stent placement less than 6 weeks before major noncardiac surgery requiring general anesthesia.[56] There were 7 MIs, 11 major bleeding episodes, and 8 deaths. All deaths and MIs, as well as 8 of 11 bleeding episodes, occurred in patients subjected to surgery fewer than 14 days after stenting. Four patients expired after undergoing surgery 1 day after stenting. The time between stenting and surgery appeared to be the main determinant of outcome, and the authors recommend that a minimum of 2 weeks, and preferably 4 weeks, elapse before elective surgery. Wilson and colleagues reported on 207 patients who underwent noncardiac surgery within 2 months of stent placement.[57] A total of 8 patients died or suffered an MI, all of whom were among the 168 patients undergoing surgery 6 weeks after stent placement. No events occurred in the 39 patients undergoing surgery 7 to 9 weeks after stent placement. These authors suggested that, whenever possible, noncardiac surgery should be delayed 6 weeks after stent placement has been performed, by which time stents are generally endothelialized, and a course of antiplatelet therapy to prevent stent thrombosis has been completed. For patients who must proceed to noncardiac surgery within the first 6 weeks of a PCI, balloon angioplasty without stent implantation may be the preferred strategy.

Pharmacological Interventions

Beta-Blocking Agents

Beta blockers are the best-studied medical treatment. They reduced perioperative cardiac morbidity, as shown in two well-designed randomized trials, and reduced surrogate endpoints of biomarker release and myocardial ischemia in other trials. Mangano and colleagues administered atenolol or placebo beginning the morning of surgery and continuing for 7 days postoperatively in a cohort of 200 patients with known coronary disease or risk factors for CAD undergoing high-risk noncardiac surgery.[34] They demonstrated a marked reduction in the incidence of perioperative myocardial ischemia but no differences in the rates of perioperative MI. There was a marked improvement in survival at 6 months in the atenolol group, which continued for at least 2 years.

The authors speculated that the lower incidence of myocardial ischemia was the result of less plaque destabilization with a resultant reduction in subsequent MI or death in the 6 months after noncardiac surgery. There were issues of randomization and uneven distribution of risk factors and treatment at baseline and upon discharge with beta blockers that may, at least in part, account for the findings. However, Poldermans and colleagues studied the perioperative use of bisoprolol versus routine care in elective major vascular surgery in the Dutch Echocardiographic Cardiac Risk Evaluation Applying Stress Echocardiography (DECREASE) trial.[37] This medication was started at least 7 days preoperatively, titrated to achieve a resting heart rate less than 60 beats/min, and continued postoperatively for 30 days. Of note, the study was confined to patients with at least one clinical marker of cardiac risk (prior MI, diabetes, angina pectoris, heart failure, age older than 70 years, or poor functional status) and evidence of inducible myocardial ischemia on a preoperative dobutamine stress echocardiogram. Patients with extensive regional wall abnormalities (large zones of myocardial ischemia) were excluded. Bisoprolol reduced perioperative MI or cardiac death by some 80 percent in this high-risk population. Because of the selection criteria, the efficacy of bisoprolol in the highest risk group, those who would be considered for coronary revascularization or modification or cancellation of the surgical procedure, cannot be determined from this trial. However, the event rate in the placebo group (nearly 40 percent) suggests that all but the highest risk patients were enrolled in the trial.

Boersma and colleagues reevaluated the use of dobutamine stress echocardiography with respect to the extent of wall motion abnormalities and use of beta blockers during surgery for the entire cohort of patients screened for the DECREASE trial.[28] They assigned one point for each of the following characteristics: age older than 70 years, current angina, MI, congestive heart failure, prior cerebrovascular disease, diabetes mellitus, and renal failure. As the total number of clinical risk factors increased, perioperative cardiac event rates also increased (Fig. 77-3). When the risk of death or MI was stratified by perioperative beta blocker usage, there was no significant improvement in those without any of the prior risk factors. In those with a risk factor score between 1 and 3, which represented more than half of all patients, the rate of cardiac events fell from 3 to 0.9 percent with effective beta blockade. Most important, in those with less than three risk factors, constituting 70 percent of the population, beta blocker therapy was very effective in reducing cardiac events in those with new wall motion abnormalities in one to four segments (33 versus 2.8 percent), having a smaller effect in those without new wall motion abnormalities (5.8 versus 2 percent). Beta blockers were not protective in patients with new wall motion abnormalities in more than five segments. The group with risk factors and extensive wall motion abnormalities on preoperative stress echocardiography may be the group to consider for prophylactic coronary revascularization.

On the basis of the accumulated evidence for the benefit of beta blockers in the perioperative period and that for the nonoperative benefit of beta blockers for CAD and heart failure, several groups have advocated prophylactic beta blockade in high-risk patients undergoing high-risk surgery. The American Heart Association/American College of Cardiology guidelines recommend treatment with a beta-blocking agent for patients previously receiving these agents and patients with positive stress tests undergoing major vascular surgery. They

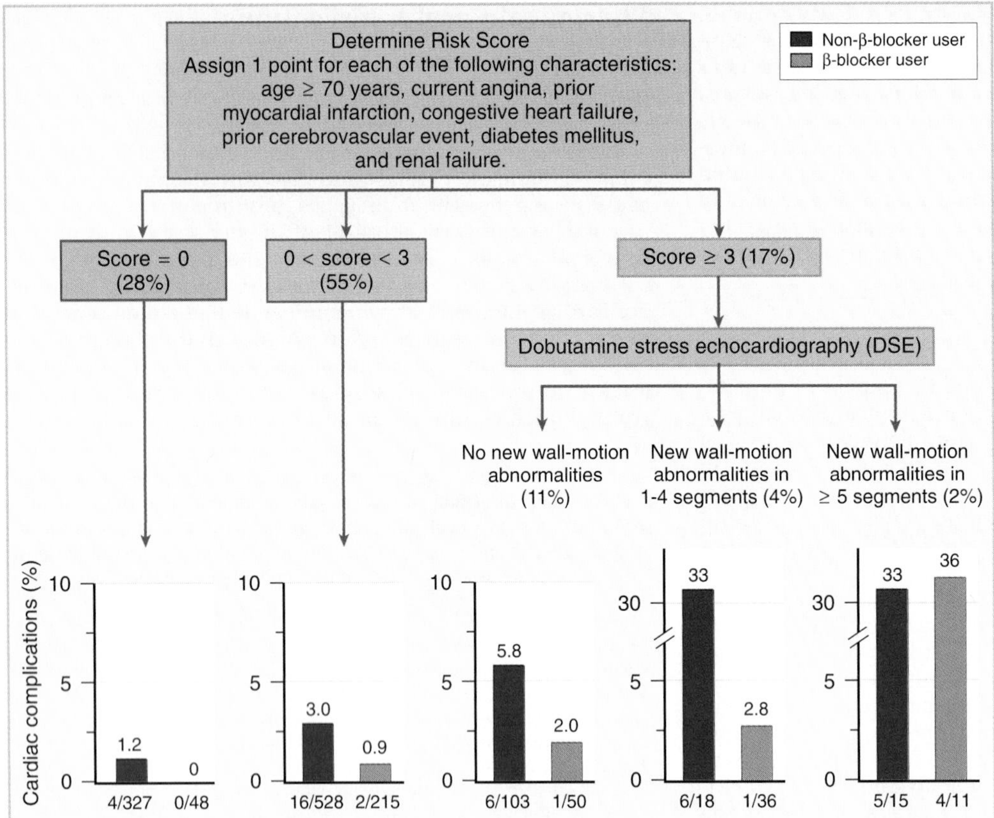

FIGURE 77–3 Perioperative cardiac risk and death in different populations of patients enrolled in the Dutch Echocardiographic Cardiac Risk Evaluation Applying Stress Echocardiography (DECREASE) trial. Risk is defined according to clinical risk and use of beta blockers in the randomized and nonrandomized cohorts of individuals. Patients with risk factors and a positive stress test demonstrating one to four areas of regional wall motion abnormality on dobutamine stress echocardiography were randomly assigned to perioperative bisoprolol titrated preoperatively to a heart rate less than 60 beats/min or to standard care. For all other patients who were not randomly assigned but were receiving preoperative beta blockers, the medication was switched to bisoprolol targeted to a heart rate less than 60 beats/min. (From Poldermans D, Boersma E, Bax JJ, et al: The effect of bisoprolol on perioperative mortality and myocardial infarction in high-risk patients undergoing vascular surgery. Dutch Echocardiographic Cardiac Risk Evaluation Applying Stress Echocardiography Study Group. N Engl J Med 341:1789, 1999.)

also recommend (level IIa evidence) prophylactic beta blocker administration in patients with known or major risk factors for CAD, although the strength of evidence is weaker and therefore the recommendation is based upon the general knowledge of beta blockers and cardiac disease. A report from the Agency for Healthcare Research and Quality has also suggested that prophylactic beta blocker treatment in patients with known risk factors for CAD is supported by the strongest forms of evidence.[58] Auerbach and Goldman have published recommendations regarding the use of beta-blocking drugs in the perioperative setting. These recommendations have led many institutions to develop protocols for implementation of perioperative beta-blocking agents.[59]

We have proposed an algorithm concerning beta blocker use (Fig. 77–4).[60] Several authors have demonstrated that the majority of patients presenting for noncardiac surgery and even for vascular surgery have not been started on beta blockers. One concern of the anesthesiologists is related to the acute administration of a beta-blocking agent on the morning of surgery. The combined effect of acute heart rate decrease coupled with the induction of anesthesia in a patient who had previously been beta blocker–naive has been associated anecdotally with marked bradycardia and hypotension. Treatment of these events could lead to wide swings in heart rate and blood pressure and less heart rate control than desired. The approach to the use of beta blockers depends on the preoperative status, the type of surgery, the cardiac risk factors, and any results of cardiac stress testing. If patients are receiving beta blockers preoperatively, it is important to continue perioperative beta blockers including intravenous administration in those unable to take the medication by mouth. If patients are undergoing vascular surgery and preoperative diagnostic imaging demonstrates areas at risk for myocardial ischemia, it would be important to initiate beta blocker therapy several days or more in advance and titrate to a heart rate of 60 to 70 beats/min.

Ideally, the beta blocker therapy should be initiated more than 7 days in advance, similar to the schedule in the Poldermans protocol, because there is a basal level of drug leading to modification of beta-adrenergic receptors. For a patient with a negative stress test and high clinical risk undergoing nonvascular surgery or vascular surgery, initiation of beta blockers several days in advance by the internist, cardiologist, or other primary care provider would be appropriate to ensure a stable beta blocker level on the day of surgery. If several days of beta blocker therapy cannot be achieved, the potential risks of new-onset beta blocker therapy during induction of general, epidural, or spinal anesthesia may outweigh the benefits of beginning drug therapy on the morning of surgery. Because the study by Mangano did not demonstrate any difference in outcome and the approach of Raby and colleagues[35] demonstrated similar efficacy with respect to perioperative ischemia, we suggest inducing general anesthesia or providing regional anesthesia prior to starting beta blocker therapy. If the induction is associated with tachycardia, administration of esmolol would be appropriate. After adequate anesthesia and analgesia are achieved, the heart rate should be controlled and maintained below 80 beats/min, as in the study by Poldermans, using short- and long-acting beta blocker therapy. If the patient is initially unstable, esmolol should be first-line therapy with eventual conversion to long-acting agents.

Alpha$_2$-Agonists

Several randomized trials have evaluated prophylactic alpha$_2$-agonists as a means of reducing perioperative cardiac morbidity. Wallace and colleagues published an abstract evaluating alpha$_2$-agonists compared with placebo in high-risk patients undergoing noncardiac surgery.[36] They reported results similar to those of Mangano and colleagues and demonstrated marked improvement in 2-year survival in the alpha$_2$-agonist group. Licker and colleagues reported on a cardioprotection protocol involving preoperative alpha$_2$-agonist administration and intra- and postoperative beta blocker administration compared with historical control studies that did not use preoperative testing or this pharmacological protocol. They reported markedly improved perioperative and long-term survival and reduced perioperative troponin levels in the more contemporary group employing the cardioprotection protocol. A meta-analysis of published studies demonstrated that perioperative clonidine reduced cardiac ischemic episodes in patients with known or at risk for coronary arterial disease without increasing the incidence of bradycardia, although the studies were underpowered to evaluate the efficacy for reduction of perioperative cardiac morbidity.[61]

Nitroglycerin

Only two randomized trials have evaluated the potential protective effect of prophylactic nitroglycerin in reducing perioperative cardiac complications after noncardiac surgery. In a small study by Coriat and colleagues involving patients undergoing carotid endarterectomy, high-dose (1 μg/kg/min) nitroglycerin was more effective than lower dose (0.5 μg/kg/min) nitroglycerin in reducing the incidence of myocardial ischemia, but MI did not occur in either group. The anesthetic used in this study was an oxygen-pancuronium-fentanyl anesthetic, and therefore inhalational agents, which may be cardioprotective and cause coronary vasodilation, were not administered. Dodds studied nitroglycerin versus placebo using a balanced anesthetic technique and reported no difference in the rates of myocardial ischemia or infarction. Taken together, the evidence suggests that prophylactic nitroglycerin does not reduce the incidence of perioperative cardiac morbidity, although neither trial was powered to detect a modest benefit of nitroglycerin. As these agents have considerable hemodynamic effects, it would seem prudent to avoid the prophylactic use of nitroglycerin, although there are clear indications for use as treatment when myocardial ischemia develops.

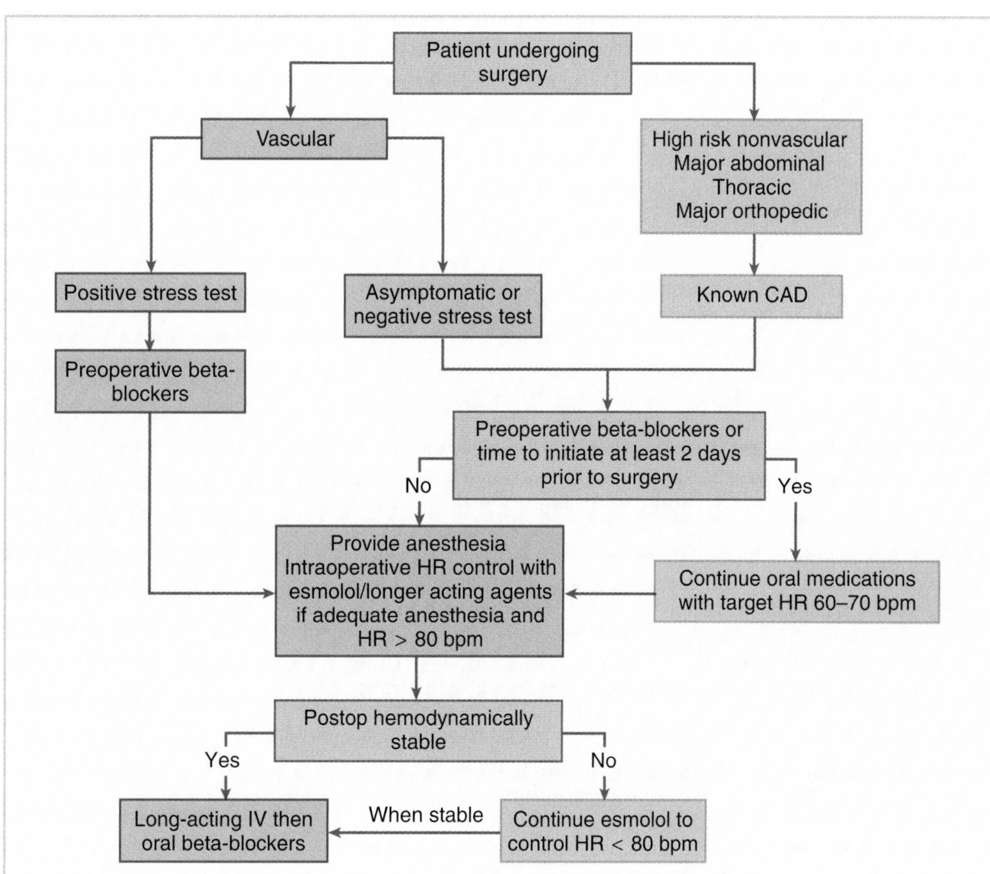

FIGURE 77–4 One proposed algorithm for the administration of beta blockers. CAD = coronary artery disease; HR = heart rate. (From Fleisher LA: Optimizing perioperative outcomes. International Anesthesia Research Society Refresher Course, Cleveland, Ohio, 2003.)

NONPHARMACOLOGICAL INTERVENTIONS

TEMPERATURE. Frank and colleagues completed a randomized trial of regional versus general anesthesia for lower extremity vascular bypass procedures and noted an association between hypothermia (temperature less than 35° C) and myocardial ischemia. They subsequently performed a randomized trial involving 300 high-risk patients undergoing a diverse group of intermediate- and high-risk procedures and randomly assigned patients to maintenance of normothermia or routine care. They observed a significantly reduced incidence of perioperative cardiac morbidity and mortality within 24 hours of surgery in the group that was kept normothermic.

Monitoring

Multiple studies have demonstrated the correlation between perioperative ST segment changes and major cardiac events, as described previously. Furthermore, the duration, either cumulative or continuous, of perioperative ST changes strongly predicts poor outcomes. Therefore, ST segment monitoring has become standard during the intraoperative and ICU periods for high-risk patients. However, patients at low to moderate risk may also develop ST segment changes. These changes may not reflect true myocardial ischemia, as suggested in one series.[62]

The period of greatest risk may be the time when the patient is in the ward and unmonitored. Many of the monitoring companies have developed ST segment telemetry monitors, but they have not been tested to any large degree in the perioperative period. This issue of whether early treatment of prolonged ST segment changes leads to improved outcome is not yet clarified. Until such studies are completed, the efficacy of such monitors remains debatable.

The value of pulmonary artery catheterization for noncardiac surgery has engendered controversy. Several small randomized trials did not demonstrate significant reductions in major cardiac morbidity and mortality in patients undergoing aortic surgery. A large-scale cohort study performed by Polanczyk and colleagues in which patients who had pulmonary catheters placed were matched with those who did not, using a propensity score, was also unable to demonstrate any significant benefit.[63] In fact, they observed an increased incidence of congestive heart failure and untoward noncardiac outcomes in the pulmonary artery catheter group. In a subsequent study, a total of 1994 patients were randomly assigned to goal-directed therapy guided by a pulmonary catheter or standard care without the use of a pulmonary catheter for patients undergoing urgent or elective major surgery.[64] There was no difference in survival, but there was a higher rate of pulmonary embolism in the catheter group compared with the standard care group. Therefore, current evidence does not support the routine use of pulmonary artery catheterization for high-risk patients undergoing major noncardiac surgery. Further work is required to understand whether these results can be generalized to the high-risk vascular surgical population and to determine the benefits of pulmonary artery catheters in specific clinical situations.

Transesophageal echocardiography (TEE) is another means of assessing intraoperative cardiac function. It is an extremely sensitive noninvasive tool for monitoring intraoperative wall motion abnormalities and fluid status. In patients undergoing aortic cross-clamping, TEE proved to have significantly better sensitivity for detecting intraoperative ischemia than electrocardiography. For noncardiac surgery, a study of TEE, 2-lead electrocardiography, and 12-lead electrocardiography demonstrated minimal additive value of TEE over 2-lead electrocardiography. Although TEE for routine monitoring of intraoperative ischemia in noncardiac surgery may have minimal additive value over ST segment recording for predicting which patients will sustain perioperative morbidity, TEE monitoring may be valuable to guide treatment in patients with unstable hemodynamics where filling status or myocardial function or both are uncertain.

Transfusion Threshold

There is a great deal of controversy regarding the optimal hemoglobin level at which to transfuse high-risk noncardiac surgical patients. No randomized trials have evaluated the optimal transfusion threshold, although there is a great deal of anecdotal evidence. Several small cohort studies have shown that hematocrits in the range 27 to 29 percent represent the point below which there is an increased incidence of myocardial ischemia and potentially MI. Data from a large-scale trial of transfusion triggers in the ICU were unable to document increased morbidity and mortality with a transfusion threshold of hemoglobin less than 7 gm/dl, but there were trends for increased morbidity in the subset of patients with ischemic heart disease. In the setting of acute MI, Wu demonstrated that lower hemoglobin levels, particularly below 10 gm/dl, are associated with increased mortality within 30 days. Therefore, there is accumulating evidence to suggest that patients with known ischemic heart disease who have not had revascularization should be maintained perioperatively with a hemoglobin greater than 9 gm/dl.

REFERENCES

Assessment of Preoperative Risk for Noncardiac Surgery in Patients with Cardiovascular Disease

1. Rivers SP, Scher LA, Gupta SK, et al: Safety of peripheral vascular surgery after recent acute myocardial infarction. J Vasc Surg 11:70, 1990.
2. Eagle KA, Brundage BH, Chaitman BR, et al: Guidelines for perioperative cardiovascular evaluation for noncardiac surgery. Report of the American College of Cardiology/American Heart Association Task Force on Practice Guidelines (Committee on Perioperative Cardiovascular Evaluation for Noncardiac Surgery). J Am Coll Cardiol 27:910, 1996.
3. Eagle KA, Berger PB, Calkins H, et al: ACC/AHA guideline update for perioperative cardiovascular evaluation for noncardiac surgery—Executive summary: A report of the American College of Cardiology/American Heart Association Task Force on Practice Guidelines (Committee to Update the 1996 Guidelines on Perioperative Cardiovascular Evaluation for Noncardiac Surgery). J Am Coll Cardiol 39:542, 2002.
4. Weksler N, Klein M, Szendro G, et al: The dilemma of immediate preoperative hypertension: To treat and operate, or to postpone surgery? J Clin Anesth 15:179, 2003.
5. Aronson S, Boisvert D, Lapp W: Isolated systolic hypertension is associated with adverse outcomes from coronary artery bypass grafting surgery. Anesth Analg 94:1079, 2002.
6. Cohn SL, Goldman L: Preoperative risk evaluation and perioperative management of patients with coronary artery disease. Med Clin North Am 87:111, 2003.
7. Haering JM, Comunale ME, Parker RA, et al: Cardiac risk of noncardiac surgery in patients with asymmetric septal hypertrophy. Anesthesiology 85:254, 1996.
8. Torsher LC, Shub C, Rettke SR, et al: Risk of patients with severe aortic stenosis undergoing noncardiac surgery. Am J Cardiol 81:448, 1998.
9. Otto C, Mickel M, Kennedy J, et al: Three-year outcome after balloon aortic valvuloplasty: Insights into prognosis of valvular aortic stenosis. Circulation 89:642, 1994.
10. Palacios I, Tuzcu M, Weyman A, et al: Clinical follow-up of patients undergoing percutaneous mitral balloon valvotomy. Circulation 91:671, 1995.
11. Dajani A, Taubert K, Wilson W, et al: Prevention of bacterial endocarditis. Recommendations by the American Heart Association. JAMA 277:1794, 1997.
12. Leport C, Horstkotte D, Burckhardt D: Antibiotic prophylaxis for infective endocarditis from an international group of experts towards a European consensus. Group of Experts of the International Society for Chemotherapy. Eur Heart J 16(Suppl B):126, 1995.
13. Bonow RO, Carabello B, de Leon AC Jr, et al: Guidelines for the management of patients with valvular heart disease: Executive summary. A report of the American College of Cardiology/American Heart Association Task Force on Practice Guidelines (Committee on Management of Patients with Valvular Heart Disease). Circulation 98:1949, 1998.
14. Ezekowitz MD: Anticoagulation management of valve replacement patients. J Heart Valve Dis 11(Suppl 1):S56, 2002.
15. Martin JT, Tautz TJ, Antognini JF: Safety of regional anesthesia in Eisenmenger's syndrome. Reg Anesth Pain Med 27:509, 2002.
16. Galli KK, Myers LB, Nicolson SC: Anesthesia for adult patients with congenital heart disease undergoing noncardiac surgery. Int Anesthesiol Clin 39:43, 2001.
17. Amar D: Perioperative atrial tachyarrhythmias. Anesthesiology 97:1618, 2002.
18. Amar D, Roistacher N, Rusch VW, et al: Effects of diltiazem prophylaxis on the incidence and clinical outcome of atrial arrhythmias after thoracic surgery. J Thorac Cardiovasc Surg 120:790, 2000.
19. Balser JR, Martinez EA, Winters BD, et al: Beta-adrenergic blockade accelerates conversion of postoperative supraventricular tachyarrhythmias. Anesthesiology 89:1052, 1998.
20. Amar D, Zhang H, Roistacher N: The incidence and outcome of ventricular arrhythmias after noncardiac thoracic surgery. Anesth Analg 95:537, 2002.
21. Reilly DF, McNeely MJ, Doerner D, et al: Self-reported exercise tolerance and the risk of serious perioperative complications. Arch Intern Med 159:2185, 1999.
22. Bartels C, Bechtel J, Hossmann V, et al: Cardiac risk stratification for high-risk vascular surgery. Circulation 95:2473, 1997.
23. Froehlich JB, Karavite D, Russman PL, et al: American College of Cardiology/American Heart Association preoperative assessment guidelines reduce resource utilization before aortic surgery. J Vasc Surg 36:758, 2002.
24. Licker M, Khatchatourian G, Schweizer A, et al: The impact of a cardioprotective protocol on the incidence of cardiac complications after aortic abdominal surgery. Anesth Analg 95:1525, 2002.
25. Falcone RA, Nass CM, Jermyn RM, et al: The value of preoperative pharmacological stress testing before vascular surgery using ACC/AHA guidelines: A prospective, randomized pilot trial. J Cardiothoracic Vasc Anesth 17: 694, 2003.
26. Fleisher LA, Rosenbaum SH, Nelson AH, et al: Preoperative dipyridamole thallium imaging and Holter monitoring as a predictor of perioperative cardiac events and long-term outcome. Anesthesiology 83:906, 1995.
27. Poldermans D, Arnese M, Fioretti PM, et al: Improved cardiac risk stratification in major vascular surgery with dobutamine-atropine stress echocardiography. J Am Coll Cardiol 26:648, 1995.
28. Boersma E, Poldermans D, Bax JJ, et al: Predictors of cardiac events after major vascular surgery: Role of clinical characteristics, dobutamine echocardiography, and beta-blocker therapy. JAMA 285:1865, 2001.
29. Shaw LJ, Eagle KA, Gersh BJ, et al: Meta-analysis of intravenous dipyridamole-thallium-201 imaging (1985 to 1994) and dobutamine echocardiography (1991 to 1994) for risk stratification before vascular surgery. J Am Coll Cardiol 27:787, 1996.

Overview of Anesthesia Used in Cardiac Patients Undergoing Noncardiac Surgery

30. Toller WG, Kersten JR, Pagel PS, et al: Sevoflurane reduces myocardial infarct size and decreases the time threshold for ischemic preconditioning in dogs. Anesthesiology 91:1437, 1999.
31. Chen Q, Camara AK, An J, et al: Sevoflurane preconditioning before moderate hypothermic ischemia protects against cytosolic [Ca^{2+}] loading and myocardial damage in part via mitochondrial K(ATP) channels. Anesthesiology 97:912, 2002.
32. Rodgers A, Walker N, Schug S, et al: Reduction of postoperative mortality and morbidity with epidural or spinal anaesthesia: Results from overview of randomised trials. BMJ 321:1493, 2000.
33. Cohen M, Duncan PG, Tate RB: Does anesthesia contribute to operative mortality? JAMA 260:2859, 1988.
34. Mangano DT, Layug EL, Wallace A, et al: Effect of atenolol on mortality and cardiovascular morbidity after noncardiac surgery. Multicenter Study of Perioperative Ischemia Research Group. N Engl J Med 335:1713, 1996.
35. Raby KE, Brull SJ, Timimi F, et al: The effect of heart rate control on myocardial ischemia among high-risk patients after vascular surgery. Anesth Analg 88:477, 1999.
36. Wallace A, Layug B, Tateo I, et al: Prophylactic atenolol reduces postoperative myocardial ischemia. McSPI Research Group. Anesthesiology 88:7, 1998.
37. Poldermans D, Boersma E, Bax JJ, et al: The effect of bisoprolol on perioperative mortality and myocardial infarction in high-risk patients undergoing vascular surgery. Dutch Echocardiographic Cardiac Risk Evaluation Applying Stress Echocardiography Study Group. N Engl J Med 341:1789, 1999.
38. Leung JM, O'Kelly BF, Mangano DT, et al: Relationship of regional wall motion abnormalities to hemodynamic indices of myocardial oxygen supply and demand in patients undergoing CABG surgery. Anesthesiology 73:802, 1990.

Postoperative Management of Patients with Cardiac Disease after Noncardiac Surgery

39. Landesberg G: The pathophysiology of perioperative myocardial infarction: Facts and perspectives. J Cardiothorac Vasc Anesth 17:90, 2003.
40. Fleisher LA, Eagle KA: Clinical practice. Lowering cardiac risk in noncardiac surgery. N Engl J Med 345:1677, 2001.
41. Ellis SG, Hertzer NR, Young JR, et al: Angiographic correlates of cardiac death and myocardial infarction complicating major nonthoracic vascular surgery. Am J Cardiol 77:1126, 1996.
42. Dawood MM, Gutpa DK, Southern J, et al: Pathology of fatal perioperative myocardial infarction: Implications regarding pathophysiology and prevention. Int J Cardiol 57:37, 1996.
43. Pronovost PJ, Angus DC, Dorman T, et al: Physician staffing patterns and clinical outcomes in critically ill patients: A systematic review. JAMA 288:2151, 2002.
44. Kehlet H, Holte K: Effect of postoperative analgesia on surgical outcome. Br J Anaesth 87:62, 2001.
45. Lee TH, Thomas EJ, Ludwig LE, et al: Troponin T as a marker for myocardial ischemia in patients undergoing major noncardiac surgery. Am J Cardiol 77:1031, 1996.
46. Metzler H, Gries M, Rehak P, et al: Perioperative myocardial cell injury: The role of troponins. Br J Anaesth 78:386, 1997.

47. Badner NH, Knill RL, Brown JE, et al: Myocardial infarction after noncardiac surgery. Anesthesiology 88:572, 1998.
48. Lopez-Jimenez F, Goldman L, Sacks DB, et al: Prognostic value of cardiac troponin T after noncardiac surgery: 6-month follow-up data. J Am Coll Cardiol 29:1241, 1997.
49. Kim LJ, Martinez EA, Faraday N, et al: Cardiac troponin I predicts short-term mortality in vascular surgery patients. Circulation 106:2366, 2002.

Strategies to Reduce Perioperative Cardiac Risk of Noncardiac Surgery

50. McFalls EO, Ward HB, Krupski WC, et al: Prophylactic coronary artery revascularization for elective vascular surgery: Study design. Veterans Affairs Cooperative Study Group on Coronary Artery Revascularization Prophylaxis for Elective Vascular Surgery. Control Clin Trials 20:297, 1999.
51. Eagle KA, Rihal CS, Mickel MC, et al: Cardiac risk of noncardiac surgery: Influence of coronary disease and type of surgery in 3368 operations. CASS Investigators and University of Michigan Heart Care Program. Coronary Artery Surgery Study. Circulation 96:1882, 1997.
52. Back MR, Stordahl N, Cuthbertson D, et al: Limitations in the cardiac risk reduction provided by coronary revascularization prior to elective vascular surgery. J Vasc Surg 36:526, 2002.
53. Glance LG: Selective preoperative cardiac screening improves five-year survival in patients undergoing major vascular surgery: A cost-effectiveness analysis. J Cardiothorac Vasc Anesth 13:265, 1999.
54. Posner KL, Van Norman GA, Chan V: Adverse cardiac outcomes after noncardiac surgery in patients with prior percutaneous transluminal coronary angioplasty. Anesth Analg 89:553, 1999.
55. Hassan SA, Hlatky MA, Boothroyd DB, et al: Outcomes of noncardiac surgery after coronary bypass surgery or coronary angioplasty in the Bypass Angioplasty Revascularization Investigation (BARI). Am J Med 110:260, 2001.
56. Kaluza GL, Joseph J, Lee JR, et al: Catastrophic outcomes of noncardiac surgery soon after coronary stenting. J Am Coll Cardiol 35:1288, 2000.
57. Wilson SH, Fasseas P, Orford JL, et al: Clinical outcome of patients undergoing noncardiac surgery in the two months following coronary stenting. J Am Coll Cardiol 42:234, 2003.

Perioperative Management in High-Risk Patients

58. Shojania KG, Duncan BW, McDonald KM, et al: Safe but sound: Patient safety meets evidence-based medicine. JAMA 288:508, 2002.
59. Auerbach AD, Goldman L: Beta-blockers and reduction of cardiac events in noncardiac surgery: Scientific review. JAMA 287:1435, 2002.
60. Fleisher LA: Optimizing perioperative outcomes. International Anesthesia Research Society Refresher Course, Cleveland, Ohio, 2003.
61. Nishina K, Mikawa K, Uesugi T, et al: Efficacy of clonidine for prevention of perioperative myocardial ischemia: A critical appraisal and meta-analysis of the literature. Anesthesiology 96:323, 2002.
62. Fleisher LA, Zielski MM, Schulman SP: Perioperative ST-segment depression is rare and may not indicate myocardial ischemia in moderate-risk patients undergoing noncardiac surgery. J Cardiothorac Vasc Anesth 11:155, 1997.
63. Polanczyk CA, Rohde LE, Goldman L, et al: Right heart catheterization and cardiac complications in patients undergoing noncardiac surgery: An observational study. JAMA 286:309, 2001.
64. Sandham JD, Hull RD, Brant RF, et al: A randomized, controlled trial of the use of pulmonary-artery catheters in high-risk surgical patients. N Engl J Med 348:5, 2003.

GUIDELINES *Thomas H. Lee*

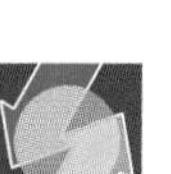

Reducing Cardiac Risk with Noncardiac Surgery

Guidelines on the assessment and management of perioperative cardiovascular risk for patients undergoing noncardiac surgery were published by an American College of Cardiology/American Heart Association (ACC/AHA) task force in 1996 and updated in 2002.[1] Guidelines were also published by the American College of Physicians (ACP) in 1997,[2] but these guidelines preceded more recent research that has shifted the focus of management from noninvasive risk stratification to risk reduction through strategies such as use of perioperative beta blockade.[3]

Both ACC/AHA and ACP guidelines emphasize the importance of a directed history and physical examination, including assessment of patient functional capacity. Clinicians are urged to give attention to noncardiac comorbid conditions as well as cardiac issues. The ACC/AHA guidelines noted but did not endorse any single risk prediction decision aid; instead, these guidelines recommended a stepwise algorithm to identify patients most appropriate for noninvasive testing for further risk stratification (see Fig. 77–2).

The ACC/AHA guidelines also offer a simple alternative approach for clinicians to decide whether noninvasive cardiac testing is needed (Fig. 77G–1). The guidelines recommend noninvasive testing if any two of these three factors are present:

Intermediate clinical predictors are present (Canadian class 1 or 2 angina, prior myocardial infarction based on history or pathological Q waves, compensated or prior heart failure, or diabetes)

Poor functional capacity (less than 4 metabolic equivalents)

High surgical risk procedure (emergency major operations; aortic repair or peripheral vascular surgery; prolonged surgical procedures with large fluid shifts or blood loss)

Ancillary Testing

ACC/AHA recommendations for utilization of tests in patients undergoing noncardiac surgery are summarized in Table 77G–1. The routine 12-lead electrocardiogram (ECG) is supported for use in patients with high or intermediate clinical risk factors, including diabetes, or recent chest pain. The guidelines recommend restraint in the use of ECGs in asymptomatic patients undergoing low-risk procedures. Routine use of echocardiography to assess left ventricular function is discouraged unless patients have heart failure or dyspnea of unknown etiology. Similarly, routine use of exercise or pharmacological stress testing in asymptomatic patients without evidence of coronary artery disease is considered a class III indication (not supported by evidence).

The recommendations for use of coronary angiography (see Table 77G–1) reflect the goal of improving the patient's long-term cardiovascular prognosis and of minimizing the chances of the patient having an acute complication during the planned procedure. In general, the same indications that are used to determine whether a nonsurgical patient warrants coronary angiography should be used in the preoperative setting, but the threshold for performing angiography should decrease if the patient is to undergo a higher risk surgical procedure.

Risk Reduction Interventions

The guidelines emphasize that "It is almost never appropriate to recommend coronary bypass surgery or other invasive interventions such as coronary angioplasty in an effort to reduce the risk of noncardiac surgery when they would not otherwise be indicated." Thus, most of the attention of the guidelines is given to medical therapies and monitoring interventions for higher risk patients. Beta blockers receive strong support for patients with high cardiac risk who are undergoing vascular surgery. Evidence for use of alpha$_2$-agonists was considered less convincing.

Intraoperative nitroglycerin was supported for patients with acute ischemic syndromes who must undergo noncardiac procedures on a presumably urgent basis. The guidelines warn that prophylactic use of nitroglycerin must take into account the anesthetic plan and patient's hemodynamics and must recognize that vasodilation and hypovolemia can readily occur during anesthesia and surgery. The ACC/AHA task force did not find sufficient evidence to weight risks versus benefits of intraaortic balloon counterpulsation for patients with myocardial ischemic syndromes or routine use of transesophageal echocardiography.

The guidelines acknowledge data (primarily from observational studies) questioning the value of pulmonary artery catheterization for patients undergoing noncardiac surgery but note expert opinion that this procedure might provide valuable information in patients at highest risk for and from hemodynamic shifts with major procedures (Table 77G–2). These recommendations preceded a large randomized controlled trial that did not find benefit from pulmonary artery catheterization in elderly high-risk surgical patients.[4] There was some

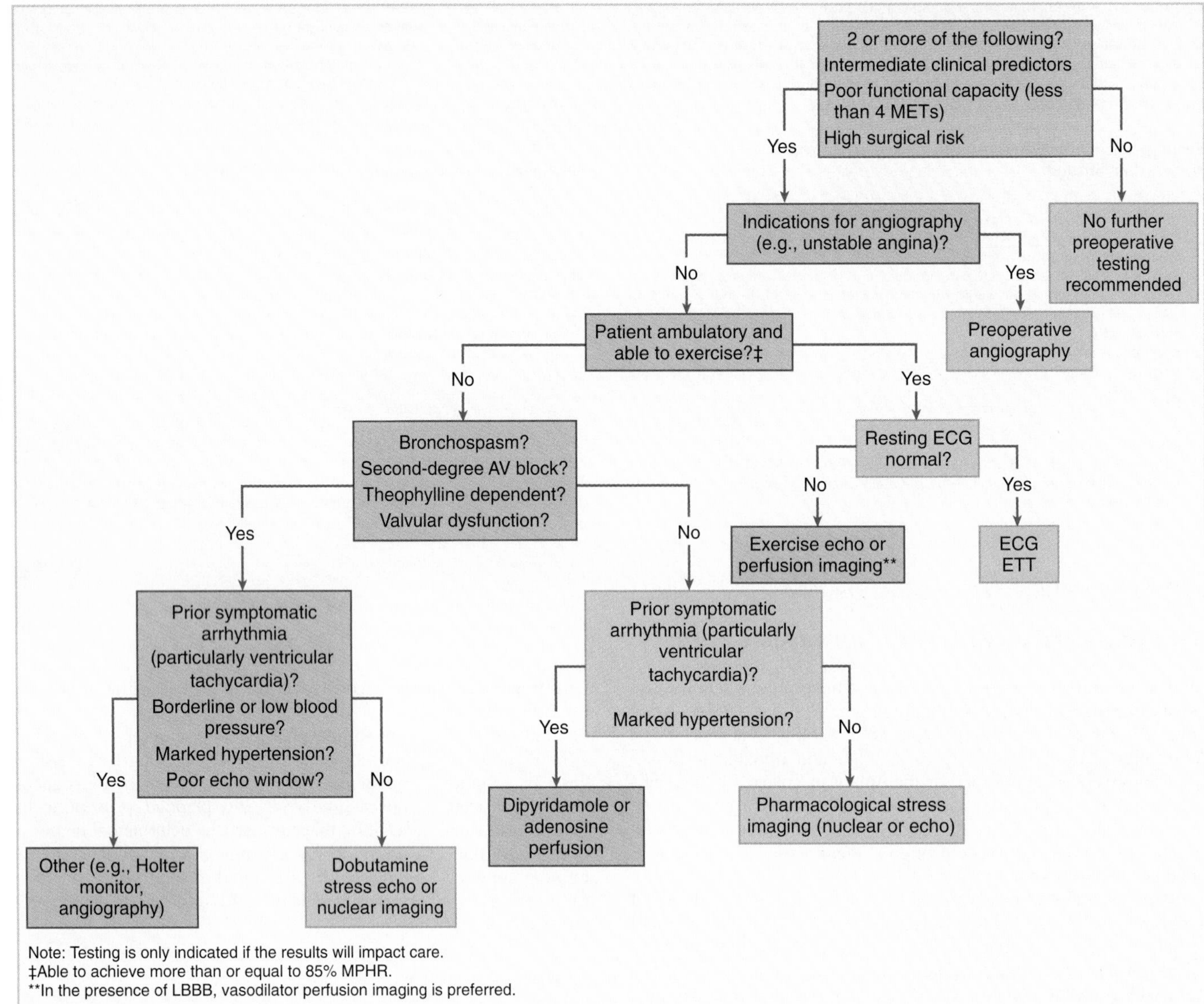

FIGURE 77G–1 Supplemental preoperative evaluation. AV = atrioventricular; ECG = electrocardiogram; ETT = exercise tolerance test; MET = metabolic equivalent. (From Eagle KA, Berger PB, Calkins H, et al: ACC/AHA guideline update for perioperative cardiovascular evaluation for noncardiac surgery: A report of the American College of Cardiology/American Heart Association Task Force on Practice Guidelines [Committee to Update the 1996 Guidelines on Perioperative Cardiovascular Evaluation for Noncardiac Surgery]. 2002. American College of Cardiology Web site. Available at: http://www.acc.org/clinical/guidelines/perio/dirIndex.htm.)

TABLE 77G–1 American College of Cardiology/American Heart Association Recommendations for Use of Ancillary Tests in Patients Undergoing Noncardiac Surgery

Indication	Class I (Indicated)	Class IIa (Good Supportive Evidence)	Class IIb (Weak Supportive Evidence)	Class III (Not Indicated)
Preoperative 12-lead rest ECG	1. Recent episode of chest pain or ischemic equivalent in clinically intermediate- or high-risk patients scheduled for an intermediate- or high-risk operative procedure.	1. Asymptomatic persons with diabetes mellitus.	1. Patients with prior coronary revascularization. 2. Asymptomatic male older than 45 yr or female older than 55 yr with two or more atherosclerotic risk factors. 3. Prior hospital admission for cardiac causes.	1. As a routine test in asymptomatic subjects undergoing low-risk operative procedures.
Preoperative noninvasive evaluation of left ventricular function	1. Patients with current or poorly controlled heart failure.	1. Patients with prior heart failure and patients with dyspnea of unknown origin.		1. As a routine test of left ventricular function in patients without prior heart failure.
Exercise or pharmacological stress testing	1. Diagnosis of adult patients with intermediate pretest probability of CAD. 2. Prognostic assessment of patients undergoing initial evaluation for suspected or proven CAD; evaluation of subjects with significant change in clinical status. 3. Demonstration of proof of myocardial ischemia before coronary revascularization. 4. Evaluation of adequacy of medical therapy; prognostic assessment after an acute coronary syndrome (if recent evaluation unavailable).	1. Evaluation of exercise capacity when subjective assessment is unreliable.	1. Diagnosis of CAD patients with high or low pretest probability; those with resting ST depression less than 1 mm, those undergoing digitalis therapy, and those with ECG criteria for left ventricular hypertrophy. 2. Detection of restenosis in high-risk asymptomatic subjects within the initial months after PCI.	1. For *exercise* stress testing, diagnosis of patients with resting ECG abnormalities that preclude adequate assessment, e.g., preexcitation syndrome, electronically paced ventricular rhythm, rest ST depression greater than 1 mm, or left bundle branch block. 2. Severe comorbidity likely to limit life expectancy or candidacy for revascularization. 3. Routine screening of asymptomatic men or women without evidence of CAD. 4. Investigation of isolated ectopic beats in young patients.
Coronary angiography in perioperative evaluation before (or after) noncardiac surgery	Patients with suspected or known CAD: 1. Evidence for high risk of adverse outcome based on noninvasive test results. 2. Angina unresponsive to adequate medical therapy. 3. Unstable angina, particularly when facing intermediate-risk* or high-risk* noncardiac surgery. 4. Equivocal noninvasive test results in patients at high clinical risk† undergoing high-risk* surgery.	1. Multiple markers of intermediate clinical risk† and planned vascular surgery (noninvasive testing should be considered first). 2. Moderate to large region of ischemia on noninvasive testing but without high-risk features and without lower LVEF. 3. Nondiagnostic noninvasive test results in patients of intermediate clinical risk† undergoing high-risk* noncardiac surgery. 4. Urgent noncardiac surgery while convalescing from acute MI.	1. Perioperative MI. 2. Medically stabilized class III or IV angina and planned low-risk or minor* surgery.	1. Low-risk* noncardiac surgery with known CAD and no high-risk results on noninvasive testing. 2. Asymptomatic after coronary revascularization with excellent exercise capacity (greater than or equal to 7 METs). 3. Mild stable angina with good left ventricular function and no high-risk noninvasive test results. 4. Noncandidate for coronary revascularization owing to concomitant medical illness, severe left ventricular dysfunction (e.g., LVEF less than 0.20), or refusal to consider revascularization. 5. Candidate for liver, lung, or renal transplantation older than 40 yr as part of evaluation for transplantation, unless noninvasive testing reveals high risk for adverse outcome.

CAD = coronary artery disease; ECG = electrocardiogram; HF = heart failure; LVEF = left ventricular ejection fraction; MET = metabolic equivalent; MI = myocardial infarction; PCI = percutaneous coronary intervention.

From Eagle KA, Berger PB, Calkins H, et al: ACC/AHA guideline update for perioperative cardiovascular evaluation for noncardiac surgery: A report of the American College of Cardiology/American Heart Association Task Force on Practice Guidelines (Committee to Update the 1996 Guidelines on Perioperative Cardiovascular Evaluation for Noncardiac Surgery). 2002. American College of Cardiology Web site. Available at: http://www.acc.org/clinical/guidelines/perio/dirIndex.htm.

*Cardiac risk according to type of noncardiac surgery. High risk: emergent major operations, aortic and major vascular surgery, peripheral vascular surgery, or anticipated prolonged surgical procedure associated with large fluid shifts and blood loss; intermediate risk: carotid endarterectomy, major head and neck surgery, intraperitoneal and intrathoracic surgery, orthopedic surgery, or prostate surgery; and low risk: endoscopic procedures, superficial procedures, cataract surgery, or breast surgery.

†Cardiac risk according to clinical predictors of perioperative death, MI, or HF. High clinical risk: unstable angina, acute or recent MI with evidence of important residual ischemic risk, decompensated HF, high degree of atrioventricular block, symptomatic ventricular arrhythmias with known structural heart disease, severe symptomatic valvular heart disease, or patient with multiple intermediate-risk markers such as prior MI, HF, and diabetes; intermediate clinical risk: Canadian Cardiovascular Society class I or II angina, prior MI by history or ECG, compensated or prior HF, diabetes mellitus, or renal insufficiency.

TABLE 77G–2 American College of Cardiology/American Heart Association Recommendations for Use of Interventions in Patients Undergoing Noncardiac Surgery

Indication	Class I (Indicated)	Class IIa (Good Supportive Evidence)	Class IIb (Weak Supportive Evidence)	Class III (Not Indicated)
Perioperative medical therapy	Beta blockers required in the recent past to control symptoms of angina or patients with symptomatic arrhythmias or hypertension. Beta blockers: patients at high cardiac risk owing to the finding of ischemia on preoperative testing who are undergoing vascular surgery.	Beta blockers: preoperative assessment identifies untreated hypertension, known coronary disease, or major risk factors for coronary disease.	$Alpha_2$-agonists: perioperative control of hypertension, or known CAD or major risk factors for CAD.	Beta blockers: contraindication to beta blockade. $Alpha_2$-agonists: contraindication to $alpha_2$-agonists.
Intraoperative nitroglycerin	High-risk patients previously taking nitroglycerin who have active signs of myocardial ischemia without hypotension.	As a prophylactic agent for high-risk patients to prevent myocardial ischemia and cardiac morbidity, particularly in those who have required nitrate therapy to control angina.		Patients with signs of hypovolemia or hypotension.
Intraoperative use of pulmonary artery catheters		Patients at risk for major hemodynamic disturbances that are most easily detected by a pulmonary artery catheter who are undergoing a procedure that is likely to cause these hemodynamic changes (e.g., suprarenal aortic aneurysm repair in a patient with angina) in a setting with experience in interpreting the results.	Either the patient's condition or the surgical procedure (but not both) places the patient at risk for hemodynamic disturbances (e.g., supraceliac aortic aneurysm repair in a patient with a negative stress test).	No risk of hemodynamic disturbances.
Perioperative ST segment monitoring		When available, proper use of computerized ST segment analysis in patients with known CAD or undergoing vascular surgery may provide increased sensitivity to detect myocardial ischemia during the perioperative period and may identify patients who would benefit from further postoperative and long-term interventions.	Patients with single or multiple risk factors for CAD.	Patients at low risk for CAD.

CAD = coronary artery disease.

From Eagle KA, Berger PB, Calkins H, et al: ACC/AHA guideline update for perioperative cardiovascular evaluation for noncardiac surgery: A report of the American College of Cardiology/American Heart Association Task Force on Practice Guidelines (Committee to Update the 1996 Guidelines on Perioperative Cardiovascular Evaluation for Noncardiac Surgery). 2002. American College of Cardiology Web site. Available at: http://www.acc.org/clinical/guidelines/perio/dirIndex.htm.

support for use of ST segment monitoring to detect perioperative ischemia, but the guidelines acknowledge that no studies have shown that this intervention improves outcome when therapy is based upon the resulting data.

Perioperative surveillance for acute coronary syndromes using routine ECGs and cardiac serum biomarkers was considered unnecessary in clinically low-risk patients undergoing low-risk operative procedures. In patients with high or intermediate clinical risk who have known or suspected coronary artery disease and who are undergoing high- or intermediate-risk surgical procedures, the guidelines recommend performance of ECGs at baseline, immediately after the surgical procedure, and daily on the first 2 days after surgery. For detection of myocardial injury, cardiac troponin measurements 24 hours postoperatively and on day 4 or hospital discharge (whichever comes first) were recommended.

References

1. Eagle KA, Berger PB, Calkins H, et al: ACC/AHA guideline update for perioperative cardiovascular evaluation for noncardiac surgery: A report of the American College of Cardiology/American Heart Association Task Force on Practice Guidelines (Committee to Update the 1996 Guidelines on Perioperative Cardiovascular Evaluation for Noncardiac Surgery). 2002. American College of Cardiology Web site (http://www.acc.org/clinical/guidelines/perio/dirIndex.htm).
2. American College of Physicians: Guidelines for assessing and managing the perioperative risk from coronary artery disease associated with major noncardiac surgery. Ann Intern Med 127:309, 1997.
3. Grayburn PA, Hillis LD: Cardiac events in patients undergoing noncardiac surgery: Shifting the paradigm from noninvasive risk stratification to therapy. Ann Intern Med 138:506, 2003.
4. Sandham JD, Hull RD, Brant RF, et al: A randomized, controlled trial of the use of pulmonary-artery catheters in high-risk surgical patients. N Engl J Med 348:5, 2003.

CHAPTER 78

Heart Disease in Varied Populations

Clyde W. Yancy

The Changing Demographics of the US Population

Cardiovascular disease remains the leading cause of death and disability in the United States, and its burden permeates the entirety of the US population. In the past, we have been comfortable extracting data from large epidemiological surveys, such as The Framingham Study, and from major clinical trials and applying those data to all persons at risk for heart disease. These databases have typically been overrepresented by predominantly white male study cohorts. Clinically naive assumptions have been made that the data discovered would be applicable to all persons, irrespective of gender, race, or ethnicity. However, current literature now strongly suggests that certain dissimilarities between cardiovascular disease in white populations and the other racial/ethnic populations in the United States do exist and that these differences are clinically relevant.

The need to focus on these dissimilarities has less to do with inclusiveness and more to do with the changing demographics of the United States. The United States is in the midst of a remarkable shift in population demographics. Currently, African Americans account for 14 percent of the US population and Hispanic Americans account for 13 percent. Asian Americans and Native Americans make up a smaller cohort of the US population, but together these four racial/ethnic or "varied" populations account for approximately 30 percent of the US population. The diversity of the American population is expected to increase over the next two to three decades. By 2050, the white non-Hispanic population may reach a nadir of 52.5 percent, compared to 75.7 percent in 1990, while Hispanic Americans may account for 22.5 percent and African Americans for 15.7 percent of the population. Asians and Pacific Islanders will account for 10.3 percent and American Indians and Alaska Natives will add 1.1 percent.[1] Thus, the epidemiology, pathophysiology, and treatment of heart disease in varied populations will have a major effect on the cardiovascular milieu in the United States.

DISTRIBUTION OF KNOWN RISK FACTORS FOR HEART DISEASE IN VARIED POPULATIONS

Hypertension. Within the varied populations, the incidence of known risk factors for cardiovascular disease is alarmingly high. The Third National Health and Nutrition Examination Survey (NHANES III) provides data on the distribution of hypertension among non-Hispanic white, non-Hispanic black, and Hispanic American groups. At least 33 million whites are hypertensive; nearly 6 million African Americans and 1.3 million Hispanic Americans are also affected with hypertension (see Chap. 37). Crude prevalence rates of hypertension for African Americans are 29.9 percent for men and 27.3 percent for women. For non-Hispanic whites, hypertension affects 25.6 percent of men and 23.8 percent of women, and for Hispanic Americans, it affects 14.6 percent of men and 14 percent of women. The higher prevalence of hypertension in African Americans is also accompanied by a worse disease severity. The prevalence of stage 3 hypertension (>180/110 mm Hg) is 8.5 percent for African Americans and 1 percent for whites. The mean systolic blood pressure and diastolic blood pressure for all African Americans is 125/75 mm Hg, which compares to a mean of 122/74 mm Hg for all whites. For hypertensive African Americans, the difference in blood pressure versus normotensive African Americans is 30/20 mm Hg, whereas for hypertensive whites, the difference is 23/15 mm Hg.[2]

Diabetes Mellitus. Diabetes is a deadly risk factor for cardiovascular disease and currently affects 17 million Americans (see Chap. 40). The incidence of the disease has increased 49 percent in the past decade; this is likely attributable to the alarming incidence of obesity. Among patients 40 to 74 years of age, the prevalence of diabetes is 11.2 percent for whites, 18.2 percent for African Americans, and 20.3 percent for Hispanic Americans. Despite the higher incidence of diabetes in Hispanic Americans, mortality rates due to diabetes are highest in African Americans, at 28.4 per 100,000 for men and 39.1 per 100,000 for women. This compares to 23.4 and 25.7 for white men and women, respectively.[3] Hypertension is concomitantly present in 75.4 percent of African American diabetic persons, 70.7 percent of Hispanic Americans with diabetes, and 64.5 percent of whites affected with diabetes.[4]

Metabolic Syndrome. Insulin resistance along with obesity, hypertension, and dyslipidemia constitutes the metabolic syndrome, which is associated with excessive cardiovascular disease (see Chap. 40). Using the NCEP ATP III criteria applied to the NHANES III database, the incidence of the metabolic syndrome is 22 percent overall for the US population over the age of 20 years but increases to more than 40 percent in elderly populations[5] and is highest in the varied populations. Hispanic Americans have the highest incidence of the metabolic syndrome, at 31.9 percent overall and 35 percent among Hispanic American women (Fig. 78–1). Of note, despite the high incidence of insulin resistance and the metabolic syndrome, Hispanic Americans have a lower prevalence of hypertension than African Americans. When the influence of obesity, body fat distribution, and insulin concentrations is followed prospectively in whites and Hispanic Americans, each factor is independently associated with the development of hypertension, with the greatest risk in subjects with the highest body mass index (BMI) (>30) and the highest insulin concentration (>95 pmol/liter). There does not appear to be an additional cardiovascular disease risk for Hispanic ethnicity versus white ethnicity, however.[6]

Obesity. The incidence of obesity (BMI > 25 is defined as overweight and BMI > 30 is defined as obese) in the US population is alarming, and the varied populations are disproportionately affected by this crisis (see Chap. 41). At the current rate of growth, the prevalence of obesity will be 40 percent by 2015.[7] The prevalence of both overweight and obesity is higher in African Americans and Hispanic Americans than in whites. The mean BMIs for African Americans, Hispanic Americans, and whites are 29.2, 28.6, and 26.3, respectively. African American women are on average 17 pounds heavier than white women of comparable age and socioeconomic status. Six of the 15 states with the highest prevalence of hypertension are in the

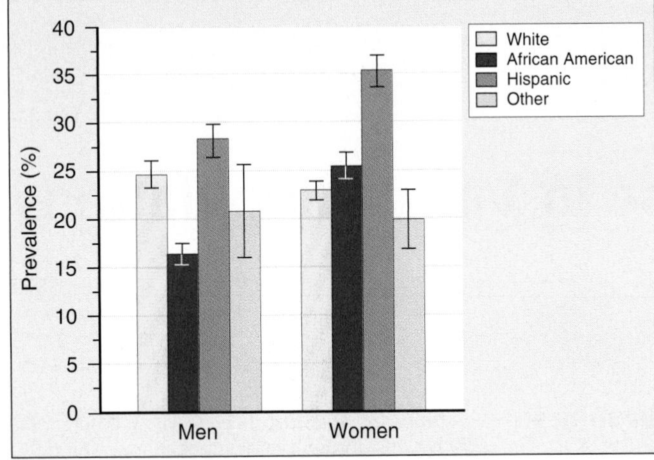

FIGURE 78–1 Age-adjusted prevalence of the metabolic syndrome among 8814 US adults aged at least 20 years, by sex and race or ethnicity, according to the National Health and Nutrition Examination Survey III, 1988-1994. Data are presented as percentage (shaded bars) and standard error (bracket). (From Ford ES, Giles WH, Dietz WH: Prevalence of the metabolic syndrome among US adults. JAMA 287:356, 2002.)

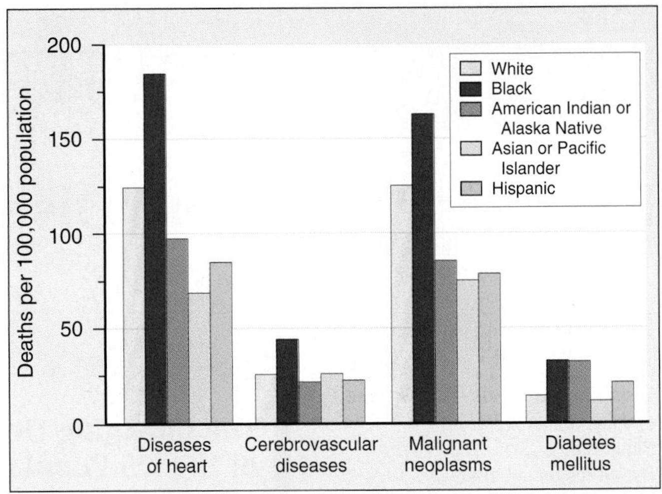

FIGURE 78–2 Age-adjusted death rates for selected causes of death by ethnicity, United States, 1950-1998. (From Smedley BD, Stith AY, Nelson AR [eds]: Unequal treatment: Confronting racial and ethnic disparities in health care. The Institute of Medicine. Washington, DC, National Academies Press, 2002, p 83.)

southeastern region of the United States (corresponding with the "stroke belt"). The highest prevalence of obesity is in African American women, at 44 percent, and in the Southeast, 71 percent of African American women are obese.[7,8]

The International Collaborative Study on Hypertension in Blacks (ICSHIB) demonstrated an important interaction of body mass index and hypertension across the course of the African Diaspora. Seven populations of West African origin were identified. A striking linear relationship was noted between BMI and the percentage of the respective population with hypertension, varying from less than 15 percent incidence of hypertension in Africans in Nigeria with a mean BMI of less than 24, to a hypertension incidence of nearly 35 percent in the Chicago area, where the mean BMI was 29.[9] Overall, 22 percent of the US population is physically inactive, but 40 percent of African American women are physically inactive. Data taken from the CARDIA study demonstrate that African American women have a higher BMI (by at least 2.7), higher energy intake, lower levels of physical activity, and lower overall physical fitness than white women.[10] Thus, the influence of obesity and physical inactivity on the development of hypertension and subsequent heart disease in African Americans is great.

Dyslipidemia is an important modifiable risk factor for heart disease in the United States, and correction of lipid disorders results in a decrease in the incidence of heart disease (see Chap. 39). Several reports have suggested that African Americans have lower low-density lipoprotein (LDL) cholesterol concentrations and less hypercholesterolemia. The Coronary Artery Risk Development in Young Adults study (CARDIA) identified the prevalence of LDL levels in young adults. An LDL cholesterol greater than 160 mg/dl was seen in 10 percent of young African American men and 5 percent of young African American women, which compared to 9 percent of young white men and 4 percent of young white women. High-density lipoprotein (HDL) levels were higher in African American men than in white men.[10]

Dietary Variations. In addition to greater energy intake, individuals in varied populations have several important dietary variations that are potentially associated with an increased incidence of cardiovascular disease. These dietary alterations include greater sodium consumption, less potassium consumption, and less calcium intake. The Treatment of Mild Hypertension Study (TOMHS) demonstrated dissimilar urinary Na^+ and $Na^+:K^+$ ratios for African Americans versus whites, especially at lower socioeconomic levels. This difference is related to dietary electrolyte intake, and the higher intake of dietary sodium is linked to the incidence of hypertension.[11] The recommended daily intake of sodium is quite low at 20 to 40 mmol. Currently, sodium consumption in the United States averages 140 to 150 mmol/day (8-10 gm/day) and is highest in African Americans and Hispanic Americans. Whereas there is a direct relationship between sodium intake and hypertension, there is an inverse relationship between potassium intake and hypertension.[12] African Americans consume a diet low in potassium. Low potassium consumption is typically associated with concurrent high sodium intake, caloric intake, and alcohol consumption; such diets are common in industrialized countries. African Americans also consume a diet low in calcium and perhaps lower in magnesium as well. The intake of calcium and magnesium is associated with lower blood pressures. The Dietary Approaches to Stop Hypertension Trial (DASH) tested the potential benefit of a diet rich in fruits, vegetables, and low-fat dairy products and low in saturated and total fats in control subjects and in patients with known hypertension. The diet led to an increase in potassium intake from 1700 mg/day to 4100 mg/day and a corresponding drop in sodium intake. The impact of the DASH diet was greatest in those subjects with the highest sodium intake, achieving a 12 mm Hg reduction in blood pressure in African Americans, which is equivalent to the results expected from pharmacological intervention with a single drug to control blood pressure.[13]

Left Ventricular Hypertrophy. In the setting of hypertension, the rates of left ventricular hypertrophy are highest in African Americans, at 31 percent versus 10 percent in whites, and the pattern of hypertrophy is more of the concentric type—a type known to be associated with increased cardiovascular events.[14] Left ventricular mass is correlated with systolic blood pressure and is a predictor of heart disease (see Chap. 37). The CARDIA study demonstrated a higher incidence of increased left ventricular mass in young adult African Americans and a close relationship between obesity, systolic blood pressure elevation, and left ventricular mass. Smoking rates are generally higher in African Americans and Hispanic Americans and may be increasing in teens and young adults.

Other risk factors for heart disease, such as hypertriglyceridemia, hyperuricemia, microalbuminuria, and elevated tissue plasminogen activator inhibitor-1 levels, may demonstrate subtle differences in these varied populations, but adequate data points are not available to make definitive comment.

Cardiovascular Mortality in Varied Populations

Heart disease is the leading cause of death for all cohorts of the US population, including the varied population. Of these groups, African Americans experience the highest rates of mortality from heart disease (Fig. 78–2). The mortality rate for African Americans is 1.6 times that of whites, a ratio that is identical to the black/white mortality ratio in 1950.[15] Hispanic Americans are twice as likely as all others to die from diabetes and Native Americans die disproportionately from diabetes as well. The average annual death rate due to heart disease expressed as deaths per 100,000 in the 45- to 64-year age range is 404 for African Americans, 219 for whites, 188 for Native Americans, 143 for Hispanic Americans, and 90 for Asian/Pacific Islanders. For the 65- to 74-year age range, the corresponding numbers are 1278 for African Americans,

871 for whites, 650 for Native Americans, 614 for Hispanic Americans, and 443 for Asian/Pacific Islanders. In women, cardiovascular disease is the leading cause of death, affecting 41 percent of white women, 41 percent of African American women, 33 percent of Hispanic American women, and 37 percent of Asian American women.[16,17]

The prevalence of coronary heart disease is higher in African Americans, with a prevalence of 7.1 percent and 9.0 percent, respectively, for men and women, as compared with 6.9 percent and 5.4 percent for white men and women. Death rates per 100,000 due to coronary heart disease are 272 and 193 for African American men and women, compared with 249 and 153 for white men and women.[16,17] In fact, death rates due to coronary heart disease in African Americans are the highest in the world.[18] Death rates from stroke are also higher in African Americans. Compared with whites, young African Americans have a threefold increased risk of ischemic stroke and a fourfold higher risk of stroke death. The death rate due to stroke is highest in the southeastern United States.[16] In addition, the five states with the highest rate of deaths due to congestive heart failure are also in the southeastern United States, and of the 15 states with the highest rates of end-stage renal disease (ESRD), 10 are in the Southeast.[8]

The prevalence of coronary heart disease in Mexican Americans is 7.2 percent for men and 6.8 percent for women, and the prevalence of myocardial infarction is 4.1 percent for men and 1.9 percent for women. This compares to 5.2 percent and 2.0 percent for white men and women and 4.3 percent and 3.3 percent for African American men and women. Death rates are similar for Hispanic Americans and whites (Table 78–1).[16]

Disparities in Cardiovascular Care and Outcomes in Varied Populations

The foregoing information clearly establishes important population differences regarding risk and outcomes for cardiovascular disease. The complete explanation for these differential outcomes is lacking but is likely to be a complex interplay of social, political, physiological, and genetic variances in these populations. These differences are best captured by an evaluation of the disparities in health care for the different racial and ethnic groups. *Disparities* in health care refers to differences in the quality of health care that are not due to access-related factors or clinical needs, preferences (patient choices), or appropriateness of the intervention (Fig. 78–3).[19] This is to be distinguished from *discrimination,* which implicates biases, prejudices, and stereotyping. Disparities may emanate from decisions made by the patient, provider, or health care system.

Members of ethnic minority groups have been found to refuse coronary artery bypass surgery (CABG) at a higher rate than others, but not sufficiently so to account for major differences in outcomes.[20] Greater issues are pertinent at the level of the health care delivery system. Language barriers are important obstacles for many patients. Nearly 14 million Americans are not proficient in English, and one in five Spanish-speaking persons report not seeking health care because of language issues. Nearly 8 million Hispanic Americans do not speak English well. One in 20 Native Americans does not speak English well, and among Asian Americans, the language barrier varies from 1 percent in persons of Hawaiian origin, to 15 percent for persons of Japanese origin and 55 percent for persons of Cambodian origin.[21] In addition to language barriers, lack of health insurance and geographic isolation both contribute further to disparities.

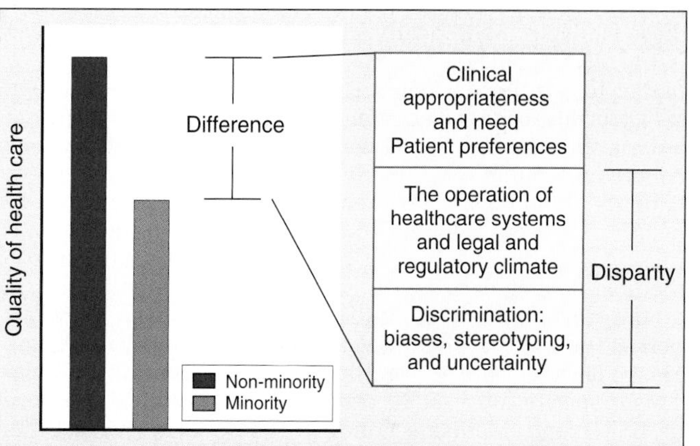

FIGURE 78–3 Differences, disparities, and discrimination: populations with equal access to health care. (From Gomes C, McGuire TG: Identifying the sources of racial and ethnic disparities in health care use. The Institute of Medicine Report. Washington, DC, National Academies Press, 2001.)

TABLE 78–1 Coronary Heart Disease and Angina Pectoris

Population Group	Prevalence CHD	Prevalence MI	Incidence CHD	Incidence MI	Mortality CHD	Mortality MI
Total population	12,900,000	7,600,000	1,100,000	540,000	515,204	192,898
Total males	6,300,000	4,700,000	660,000	330,000	260,574	100,306
Total females	6,600,000	2,900,000	440,000	210,000	254,630	92,585
White males	6.9%	5.2%	—	—	230,951	89,383
White females	5.4%	2.0%	—	—	224,449	81,201
Black males	7.1%	4.3%	68,200	—	24,625	9,045
Black females	9.0%	3.3%	47,700	—	26,640	10,067
Mexican-American males	7.2%	4.1%	—	—	—	—
Mexican-American females	6.8%	1.9%	—	—	—	—

CHD = coronary heart disease: includes heart attack angina pectoris (chest pain) or both; MI = myocardial infarction (heart attack).

Prevalence: NHANES III (1988-1994). CDC/NCHS: data for white and black males and females are for non-Hispanics. Total population data are for Americans age 20 and older: percentages for racial/ethnic groups are age-adjusted for age 20 and older. Incidence: ARIC (1987-1994). NHLBI. Mortality: CDC/NCHS: data for white and black males and females include Hispanics.

From American Heart Association: Heart Disease and Stroke Statistics—2003 Update. Dallas, American Heart Association, 2002.

Providers can contribute to disparities in health care as well through subconscious stereotyping, clinical uncertainty due to cultural ignorance, and delay in referral for indicated procedures. It has been demonstrated that physicians have lower rates of referrals for cardiac catheterization in African American women than in white men, white women, and African American men despite similar articulation of symptoms and reasonable indications for further evaluation.[22]

Because of the interdigitation of patient, system, and provider issues, Americans belonging to ethnic minority groups undergo cardiovascular procedures at a lower rate. In a survey of 4 million patients with acute myocardial infarction as indexed in the National Hospital Discharge Survey (NHDS), African American men and women have been demonstrated to undergo coronary angiography and CABG at much lower rates.[23] A separate Medicare survey suggested that there is a fourfold difference in the rate of CABG between whites and African Americans, even after adjusting for age and gender. These differences were most striking in the southeastern United States.[23] An analysis of Hispanic Americans and whites with a diagnosis of myocardial infarction revealed that Hispanic Americans were discharged on 38 percent fewer medications. Similarly, they were less likely to receive percutaneous coronary interventions.[24] Studies done at Veterans Administration hospitals are quite intriguing, as these facilities theoretically have removed any access to care issues. Nonetheless, referral for cardiac procedures was higher for whites. Of note, African Americans refused invasive procedures twice as often. Differences in rates of thrombolytic therapy and CABG were also observed, with African Americans much less likely to receive either strategy.[25] Patients with ESRD have access to Medicare funding for health care needs, which should theoretically reduce disparities. A longitudinal survey of health care disparities from Medicare beneficiaries with ESRD is quite compelling. Prior to the development of ESRD, white Americans were 300 percent more likely to undergo cardiac catheterization, angioplasty, or CABG after controlling for socioeconomic variables. This disparity fell to a 40 percent difference after the onset of ESRD and Medicare funding. These data suggest that similar health care funding could significantly diminish certain health care disparities in cardiovascular care.

The disproportionate risk for cardiovascular disease and apparent disparities in care are most evident in African American women. The Heart and Estrogen/Progestin Replacement Study (HERS) evaluated 2699 women, of whom 218 were African American. HERS evaluated women in a longitudinal study over 4 years to determine the health risks and benefits of hormone replacement therapy. Despite a definite twofold increase in cardiovascular event rates, African American women had less optimal control of hypertension and LDL cholesterol and lesser use of aspirin and statins.[26]

Hypertension in Varied Populations

No segment of the US population is devoid of excessive cardiovascular risk due to the consequences of hypertension (see Chap. 37). This risk is especially evident in the varied populations, however.

Hispanic Americans

A paradox exists in Hispanic Americans. Despite a higher incidence of diabetes and obesity, the prevalence of hypertension in Hispanic Americans is lower than in the general population. Hypertension among Hispanic Americans varies by gender and by the country of origin. Puerto Rican origin is associated with the highest incidence of hypertension, followed by Cuban origin and Mexican origin. When Hispanic Americans of Mexican origin are affected by hypertension, control of blood pressure can be more difficult.[27] The lower incidence of hypertension in Hispanic Americans of Mexican origin versus other Hispanic Americans is postulated to be due to a modernization phenomenon, implicating acclimatization to a Western lifestyle as a factor in the development of hypertension. In Puerto Rico, urban men with a high school education have a blood pressure 8 mm Hg higher than less educated men. This is not the same experience seen in other North American ethnic groups, in which education is associated with lower blood pressure measurements. For persons younger than 45 years, the prevalence of hypertension is twice the rate seen in the mainland United States. Death rates due to heart disease have increased by 72 percent over the last three decades while otherwise falling in the remainder of the United States. The incidence of ESRD is higher in Puerto Rico than in any other region of Latin America.[28]

Americans of South Asian Descent

Americans with ancestry from the Indian subcontinent have a major health problem with hypertension. Hypertension is a significant concern in the Indian subcontinent and is an important cardiovascular risk for South Asians worldwide. The World Health Organization has reported that Indian men in the age range of 40 to 55 years have the highest blood pressure among populations from 20 other developing countries. The prevalence of hypertension in Indian countries has increased from less than 2 percent in 1950 to nearly 20 percent currently. This increased risk is further exacerbated with emigration to North America and varies directly with the degree of urbanization. The Study of Health Assessment and Risk in Ethnic Groups (SHARE) done in Canada reported that South Asians had the highest self-reported incidence of hypertension.[29] Coincident with the hypertension risk is a growing risk of diabetes, dyslipidemia (perhaps related to a genetic predisposition to a low HDL level), and obesity. Tobacco consumption is likewise increasing in South Asians, and per capita fat consumption has increased. Taken together, the confluence of these risk factors contributes not only to the alarming rate of hypertension but also to the increasing rate of symptomatic coronary artery disease (CAD).[30]

African Americans

Hypertension in African Americans represents the most prolific variance in heart disease and cardiovascular disease risk factors in the varied populations. African Americans experience the highest prevalence of hypertension, perhaps in the world, with nearly 35 percent of all African Americans affected by hypertension.[31] It is estimated that 5.6 million African Americans have hypertension, a number that eclipses the total number of persons affected with congestive heart failure. The Hypertension and Detection Follow-up Program found that severe hypertension (diastolic blood pressure > 115 mm Hg) was five to seven times more likely to be present in African Americans than in white Americans.[31] The differential experience of hypertension is evident in childhood, with higher recorded blood pressures noted prior to the age of 10 years in black children as compared with white children.[32] The consequences of hypertension in African Americans are quite pathological, with a 50 percent higher frequency of heart failure,[33] a sixfold higher incidence of developing ESRD due to hypertension,[31] a 38 percent higher risk of stroke, and a higher risk of death due to stroke.[17] Overall, mortality due to hypertension and its consequences is four to five times more likely in African Americans than in whites.[31]

Hypertensive heart disease is manifest as left ventricular hypertrophy, which separately is a risk factor for sudden death and coronary events. The CARDIA study demonstrated that left ventricular mass is higher and independently correlated with systolic blood pressure in young African American males.[31,34] The Veterans Administration Cooperative Monotherapy Hypertension Trial determined that left ventricular hypertrophy diagnosed by electrocardiographic criteria is noted in 31 percent of African American hypertensive patients, as compared with 10 percent of white hypertensive patients.[35] The presence of increased left ventricular mass is associated with an increased rate of death and is thus a contributor to the excess rate of morbidity and mortality due to cardiovascular disease seen in African Americans. It is noted that CAD is the leading putative cause of heart failure in whites, but pooled data from published clinical trials suggest that hypertension may be the leading imputed cause of heart failure in blacks.[33]

Variances in the pathophysiology of stroke may also be extant. African Americans typically have more occlusive disease in the large and medium-sized intracranial arteries, whereas whites typically have more occlusive disease in the extracranial arteries. The incidence of hemorrhagic stroke is also higher. Similar observations have been made in the setting of ESRD. Hypertensive nephrosclerosis is the leading cause of ESRD for African Americans, and they disproportionately populate the hemodialysis cohort. For African Americans aged 20 to 44 years, hypertension-related ESRD is 20-fold higher than in whites. African Americans have been noted to lack the nocturnal dip in blood pressure and to have an earlier onset of proteinuria. Both of these findings are associated with a higher incidence of hypertension-induced nephrosclerosis.[36]

Several purported mechanisms may explain in part the excess burden of hypertension in African Americans. Peripheral vascular resistance may be higher in some African Americans with hypertension. Small studies have also demonstrated that vasodilatory responses are blunted in African Americans in a manner suggesting subtle differences in nitric oxide homeostasis.[37] Plasma renin activity is lower in African Americans than in age-matched white hypertensive patients,[38] urinary kallikrein excretion is lower, and insulin levels are higher.[33]

Much has been written about salt sensitivity in African Americans, including a theoretical assertion that Darwinian influences during the African Diaspora (active slave trading from West Africa to North America) led to selective pressure favoring genes that promote salt retention that now predispose to hypertension. This is an unproven but nevertheless prevalent theory.[39,40] Rates of hypertension in rural West Africa are the lowest in the world, but populations of West African origin in the Caribbean and in North America demonstrate dramatic rises in blood pressure that are linearly related to increases in body mass index (Fig. 78–4).[40] It is evident, however, that some African Americans do appear to be more salt sensitive than others. Salt restriction leads to a greater reduction in systolic blood pressure in African Americans (approximately 12 mm Hg) than in whites.[41] A genetic basis for sodium sensitivity may exist. The epithelial sodium channel is responsible for the final reabsorption of filtered sodium from the distal nephron and has now been found to have at least eight single nucleotide polymorphisms. One of these polymorphisms (T594M), is found only in people of West African descent and is four times more likely in hypertensive African Americans than in normotensive African Americans.[42] Unfortunately, variations in a single gene are not likely to be responsible for more than 2 to 4 percent of the difference in hypertension seen between ethnic groups.[40] Yet another very attractive candidate polymorphism related to the excess risk of hypertension-related cardiovascular disease in African Americans is noted within the inflammatory cytokines. Transforming growth factor beta-1 (TGF-β_1) is a proinflammatory cytokine associated with stimulation of fibrosis, extracellular matrix turnover, glomerular hyperplasia, and left ventricular hypertrophy. TGF-β_1 is overexpressed in African Americans, with higher circulating levels noted. A described polymorphism at codon 25 of the TGF-β_1 gene that involves the substitution of arginine for proline is associated with higher TGF-β_1 levels and is seen more frequently in African Americans.[43] Angiotensin-converting enzyme (ACE) inhibitors and angiotensin receptor blockers both reduce angiotensin-II-mediated stimulation of TGF-β_1, and this may be of clinical importance in the treatment of hypertension in African Americans. Beta blockers are reportedly less effective as monotherapy for hypertension in African Americans,[44] but data exist that suggest a strong correlation between visceral obesity in African American women and sympathetic nervous system activity.[45]

THERAPY FOR HYPERTENSION IN AFRICAN AMERICANS. The therapy for hypertension for all persons should be focused clearly on goal blood pressure reduction and the prevention of cardiovascular disease related to hypertension (see Chap. 38). The treatment of hypertension is similar for

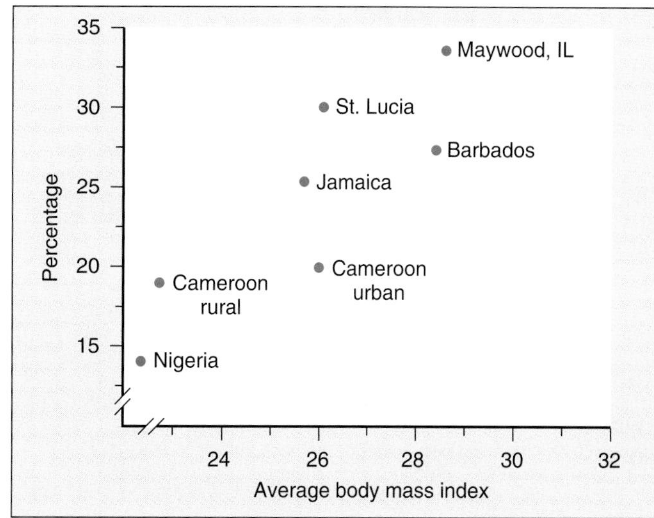

FIGURE 78–4 Hypertension prevalence across the African Diaspora. (From Cooper R, Rotimi C, Ataman S: The prevalence of hypertension in seven populations of West African origin. Am J Public Health 87:160, 1997.)

all demographic groups.[44] Within the African American group, the responsiveness to monotherapy with ACE inhibitors, angiotensin receptor blockers, and beta blockers may be less than the responsiveness to diuretics and calcium channel blockers, but these differences are corrected when diuretics are added to the neurohormonal antagonists. The African American Study of Kidney Disease and Hypertension (AASK) prospectively addressed the impact of three antihypertensive drug classes on decline of glomerular filtration rate in cases of hypertension. Diabetic patients were excluded. In patients with established hypertension-induced nephrosclerosis and reduced glomerular filtration rate (20-60 ml/min per 1.73 m^2), a clinical composite that included 50 percent reduction in glomerular filtration rate, ESRD, or death was most favorably affected by an ACE inhibitor as compared with either a beta blocker or a calcium channel blocker (Table 78–2). It was noted in this study that African American patients with hypertension uniformly required a multidrug regimen to achieve adequate blood pressure control.[46] An algorithm to guide ideal management of high blood pressure in African Americans is depicted in Figure 78–5[47] and its features are highlighted in Table 78–3. The reader is advised to note the lower goal blood pressure reduction.

Ischemic Heart Disease in Varied Populations

All of the varied populations are experiencing increasing rates of ischemic heart disease related to the concurrent and often disproportionate presence of risk factors for CAD (see Chap. 36). Rates for CAD are increasing in Asian Americans, Hispanic Americans, Native Americans, and Americans of South Asian origin. It is important to note that the rates of CAD in these groups are approaching the rates seen in whites but do not exceed those rates. This is not the case, however, for African Americans.

African Americans have the highest rate of overall mortality due to CAD of any ethnic group in the United States. The risk for sudden cardiac death is higher and the onset of disease occurs approximately 5 years earlier. The usual presentation is more likely to be unstable angina or a non-ST segment elevation myocardial infarction rather than a typical ST segment elevation event.[48] Despite this increased incidence of disease, the presence of obstructive epicardial CAD on angiograms is less. Not infrequently, angiographic studies show normal epicardial vessels but autopsy studies demon-

TABLE 78–2 Analyses of Clinical Event Composite Outcomes

	Lower vs Usual Blood Pressure Goal Intervention		Drug Intervention					
			Ramipril vs Metoprolol		Metoprolol vs Amlodipine		Ramipril vs Amlodipine*	
Outcomes‡	*% Risk Reduction (95% Confidence Interval)*†	*p Value*	*% Risk Reduction (95% Confidence Interval)*†	*p Value*	*% Risk Reduction (95% Confidence Interval)*†	*p Value*	*% Risk Reduction (95% Confidence Interval)*†	*p Value*
GFR event, ESRD, or death	2 (−22 to 21)	0.85	22 (1 to 38)	0.04	20 (−10 to 41)	0.17	38 (14 to 56)	0.004
GFR event or ESRD	−2 (−31 to 20)	0.87	22 (−2 to 41)	0.07	24 (−9 to 47)	0.13	40 (14 to 59)	0.006
ESRD or death	12 (−13 to 32)	0.31	21 (−5 to 40)	0.11	42 (17 to 60)	0.003	49 (26 to 65)	<0.001
ESRD alone	6 (−29 to 31)	0.72	22 (−10 to 45)	0.16	59 (36 to 74)	<0.001	59 (36 to 74)	<0.001

ESRD = end-stage renal disease; GFR = glomerular filtration rate.

*Secondary comparison described in previous publication.

†All risk reductions adjusted for prespecified covariates: baseline proteinuria, mean arterial pressure, sex, history of heart disease, and age. Risk difference for ESRD or death composite and ESRD alone also adjusted for baseline GFR.

‡GFR event, ESRD, or death: main secondary composite clinical outcome with 340 events, including 179 declining GFR events, 84 additional participants with ESRD events, and 77 deaths; GFR event or ESRD: composite endpoint with 263 events, including 179 declining GFR events and 84 additional participants with ESRD events; ESRD, or death composite endpoint with 251 events, including 171 ESRD events and 80 deaths; and ESRD alone: endpoint with 171 events and deaths censored in this analysis.

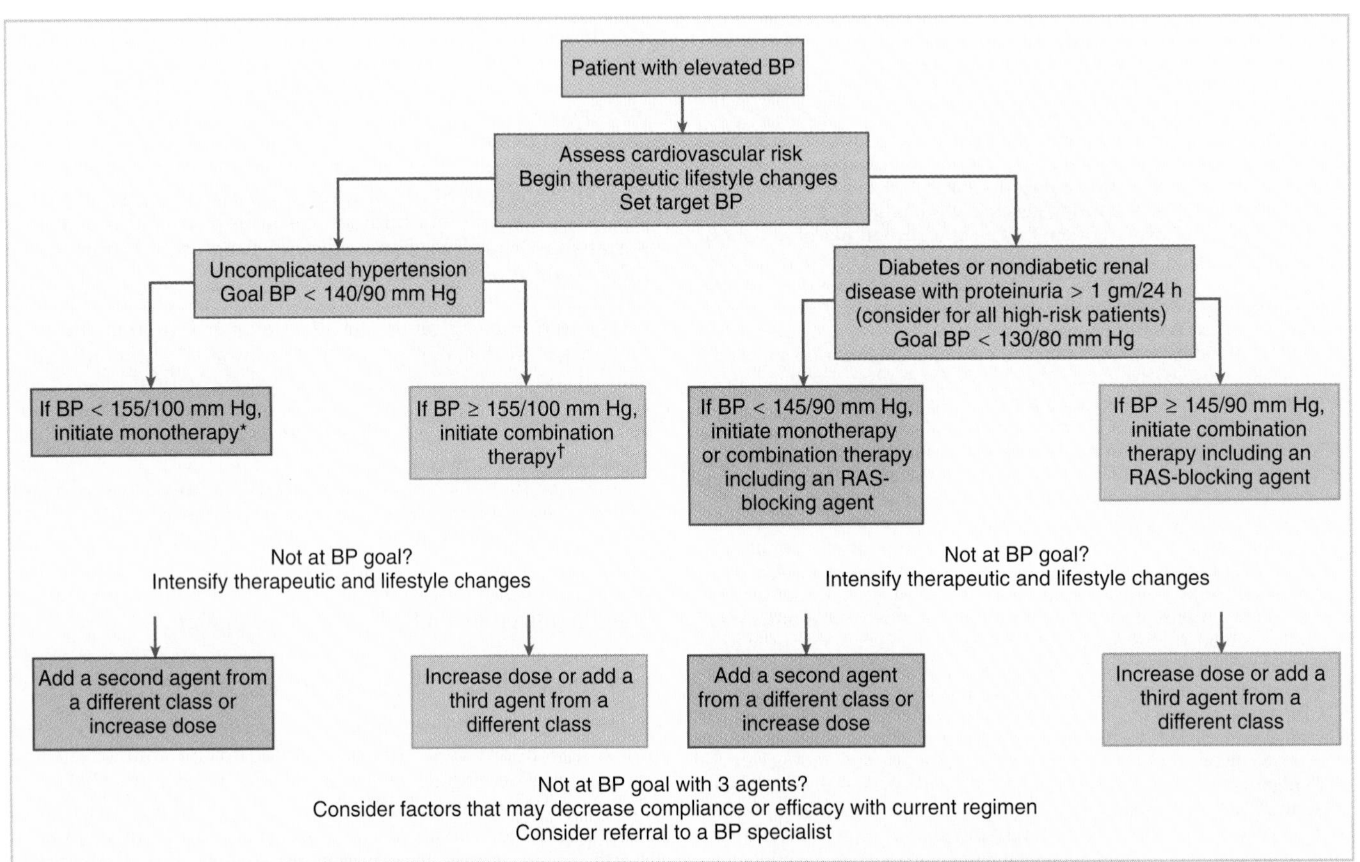

FIGURE 78–5 Clinical algorithm for achieving target blood pressure (BP) in African American patients with high BP. *Initiate monotherapy at the recommended starting dose with an agent from any of the following classes: diuretics, beta blockers, calcium channel blockers, angiotensin-converting enzyme inhibitors, or angiotensin II receptor blockers. †Initiate low-dose combination therapy with any of the following combinations: beta blocker/diuretic, angiotensin-converting enzyme inhibitor/diuretic, angiotensin-converting enzyme inhibitor/calcium channel blocker, or angiotensin II receptor blocker/diuretic. RAS = renin-angiotensin system.

strate a greater extent of atherosclerosis in African Americans despite a lesser degree of obstructive CAD.[49] As described earlier, interventions with thrombolytic therapy, percutaneous coronary interventions, and CABG are all less frequently administered.

The reason for the excess prevalence of CAD in African Americans is less likely related to pathophysiological variances, as suggested in the discussion on hypertension, and more likely due to the overabundance of cardiovascular risk factors. Obesity, left ventricular hypertrophy, type 2 diabetes, and physical inactivity are all more common in African Americans. Total cholesterol levels may be less in African Americans and HDL levels higher. Lipoprotein (a) levels are higher, by two- to threefold, in African Americans, but the

TABLE 78–3 Ideal Management of Hypertension in African Americans

Increase dietary potassium intake
Limit dietary sodium intake to <2.4 gm/day
Increase physical activity
Weight loss
All antihypertensive medications and combinations are effective
Multiple drug combinations may be required to achieve control
ACE inhibitors and beta blockers as monotherapy may be less effective but should be used when indicated (e.g., renal disease, heart failure, post-myocardial infarction)
Thiazide diuretics and calcium channel blockers may have greater blood pressure lowering efficacy
There is a higher incidence of angioedema when using ACE inhibitors

ACE = angiotensin-converting enzyme.

From Douglas JG, Bakris GL, Epstien M, et al: Management of high blood pressure in African Americans; consensus statement of the Hypertension in African Americans Working Group of the International Society of Hypertension in Blacks. Arch Intern Med 163:525, 2003.

TABLE 78–4 Polymorphisms Associated with Heart Failure

Genetic Polymorphism	Clinical Implications
Beta-1 adrenergic receptor; Gly-389	Subsensitive beta-1 receptor; decreased affinity for agonist and less cAMP generation
Beta-1 adrenergic receptor; ARG-389/alpha 2C Del322-325 receptor	Presence of both polymorphisms is associated with increased risk for heart failure in blacks; RR 10.11 when both are present
Enos	Subsensitive nitric oxide system
Aldosterone synthase	? Excessive fibrosis
Transforming growth factor beta-1	40% higher transforming growth factor beta-1 levels; higher endothelin levels?; more fibrosis
G Protein 825-T Allele	Marker of low renin hypertension, left ventricular hypertrophy, and stroke

From Yancy CW: Does race matter in heart failure? Am Heart J 146:203, 2003. See references 57-61.

relationship of lipoprotein (a) to coronary events remains unclear and may vary according to ethnicity. The relationship between total cholesterol, plaque formation, and coronary events may be weaker.[50]

The excess prevalence of left ventricular hypertrophy likely confounds the ischemic burden in the setting of CAD and may relate to excess mortality and sudden death. Mechanisms to support this theory are not yet clear. The increase in left ventricular mass with a disproportionately less robust vascular supply may lead to a lower threshold for arrhythmias and more damage due to ischemic events.[48] Endothelin-1 is a potent vasoconstrictor that has been demonstrated to be present in higher levels in African Americans.[51] Endothelin is stimulated by TGF-β_1, which, as described, is higher in hypertensive African Americans. The confluence of left ventricular hypertrophy and endothelial dysfunction may contribute to a greater risk of ischemia-related injury.

Importantly, there are no described differences in the presentation of acute coronary syndromes for any ethnic group, nor any described variations in treatment regimens or responses to standard medical and revascularization strategies. As such, no differences should be contemplated in the management of varied populations presenting with symptomatic CAD.

Heart Failure in Varied Populations

Heart failure has become one of the most pervasive cardiovascular illnesses in the United States (see Chap. 21). The prevalence of heart failure is increasing, as is the burden of excess mortality and morbidity—a burden that is once again borne in a disproportionate way by the demographics of varied populations. Although data for most ethnic groups are lacking in the realm of heart failure, data regarding African Americans are quite compelling and controversial.

Heart failure occurs in African Americans at a greater frequency, perhaps 50 percent higher overall and more than 100 percent higher in African American women than in whites. There are several striking differences in the natural history of heart disease in African Americans. The disease occurs at an earlier age; there is usually more profound left ventricular systolic dysfunction at the time of onset; and the clinical class is usually of more advanced severity.[33] The overall incidence of heart failure within the US population is 2 percent, but it occurs in 3 percent of the African American population. The issues regarding excess mortality and morbidity in African Americans with heart failure remain unresolved. The original data from the Studies of Left Ventricular Dysfunction (SOLVD) suggested a higher mortality rate,[52] but a reanalysis of African American and white cohorts matched for disease severity and left ventricular dysfunction demonstrated only an excess rate of hospitalization.[53] Data from the SOLVD prevention trial clearly demonstrated a higher incidence of heart failure, which is consistent with epidemiological surveys, but a similar responsiveness to ACE inhibitors.[54]

Based on the foregoing discussion, it is not surprising to discover that the leading putative cause of left ventricular dysfunction in African Americans with heart failure is hypertension. A survey of published clinical trials and registries suggests that the incidence of hypertension as the likely cause of heart failure in this population varies from approximately 30 percent to nearly 60 percent (Fig. 78-6).[33] True cause and effect is lacking, because few if any mechanistic data support the conversion from hypertensive heart disease to systolic dysfunction. Data from spontaneously hypertensive salt-sensitive animals suggest that the conversion from left ventricular hypertrophy to overt heart failure is associated with an increase in the progenitors of endothelin.[55] Although data do exist from the Systolic Hypertension in the Elderly Trial to justify therapy for hypertension as an effective means of preventing heart failure, these data are most pertinent for systolic hypertension of the elderly (which included 14 percent African Americans).[56] Similar inferences for the treatment of diastolic hypertension in African Americans are conjectural and not yet supported by definitive data.

A genomic basis to explain the differential epidemiology and natural history of heart failure in African Americans is under active investigation. Several candidate polymorphisms have emerged as plausible culprit genetic variations, but the relationship of these genes to the environment and the complex interplay of multiple physiological systems makes these discussions largely theoretical until additional data from large cohorts of the population are evaluated (Table 78-4).[57-61]

Data regarding the response to medical therapy for heart failure affecting African Americans emanate from post-hoc analyses of the African American subgroups in major clinical trials in heart failure. These analyses are all compromised by their retrospective nature, inconsistent sample sizes, and differences in disease expression between the African American and white cohorts. As such, the analyses yield provocative inferences and generate new hypotheses but do not alter current treatment recommendations (Table 78-5).[52-54,62-65]

Taken in aggregate, the data from Table 78–5 demonstrate that all approved therapeutic strategies for heart failure are effective and yield improved outcomes (see Chap. 23). There should be no reluctance to treat African Americans with

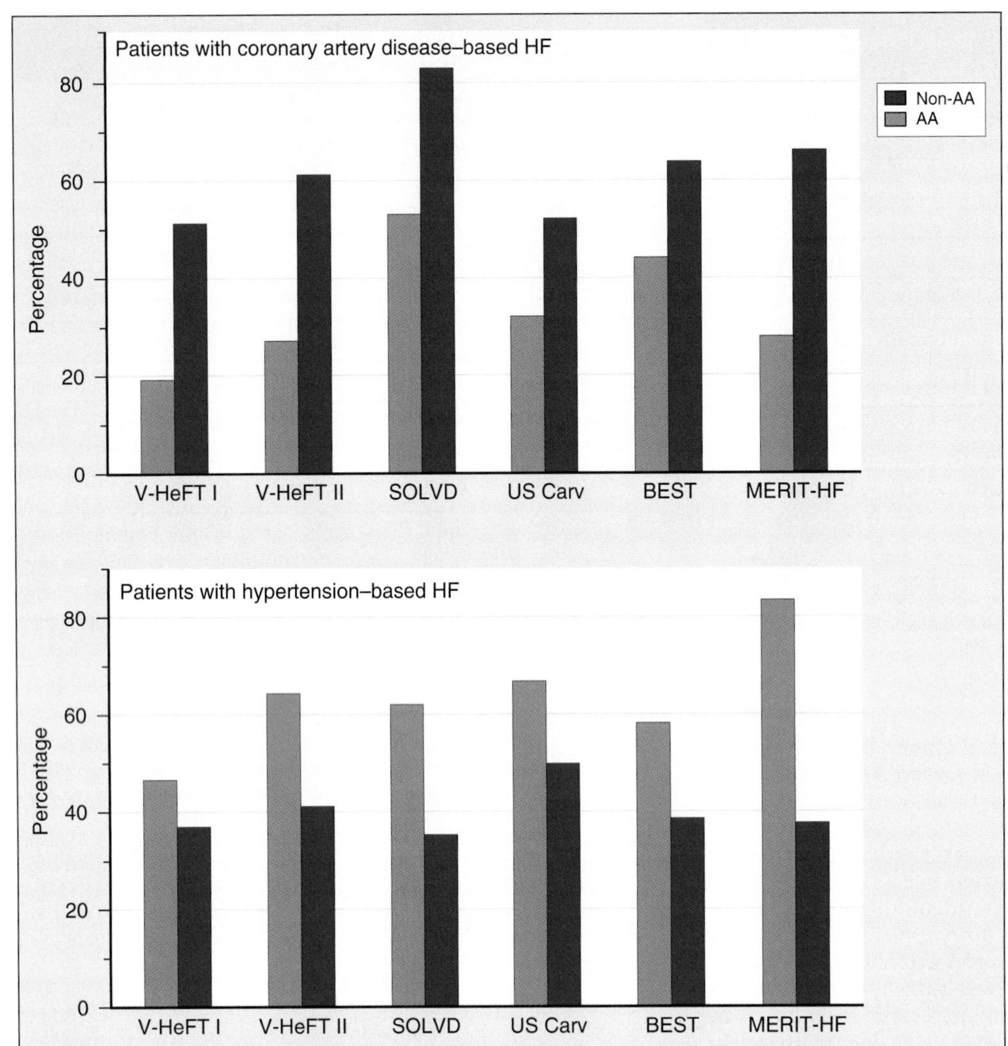

FIGURE 78–6 Etiology of heart failure (HF) in African Americans (AA). (Data from The BEST Investigators: N Engl J Med 344:1659, 2001 [BEST]; MERIT-HF Study Group: Lancet 353:2001, 1999 [MERIT]; The SOLVD Investigators: N Engl J Med 325:293, 1991 [SOLVD]; Packer M, et al: N Engl J Med 334:1349, 1996 [US Carv]; Cohn JN, et al: N Engl J Med 314:1547, 1986 [V-HeFT I]; Cohn JN, et al: N Engl J Med 325:303, 1991 [V-HeFT II].)

heart failure using any of the current treatment modalities. The data regarding beta blocker efficacy are least consistent. The analysis from the Beta Blocker Evaluation of Survival Trial was interpreted to mean that African American patients responded less well to beta blocker therapy and may have failed to benefit.[63] Given the presence of intrinsic sympathomimetic activity in this compound, it is more likely that these results are drug specific and not class specific. The number of African Americans exposed to extended release metoprolol in clinical trials has been insignificant, and subgroup analysis has been unrewarding.[64] However, the experience with carvedilol given in combination with ACE inhibitors to African Americans with all classes of heart failure are quite encouraging and are consistent with salutary outcomes. These data represent the strongest basis for recommended use of ACE inhibitors and beta blockers as primary therapy for heart failure in African Americans as in all other patients (Fig. 78–7).[65]

The African American Heart Failure Trial, A-HeFT, will prospectively identify the clinical benefit of therapy with a proprietary combination of isosorbide dinitrate and hydralazine as adjunctive therapy for heart failure in African Americans already receiving ACE inhibitors and beta blockers. A-HeFT will test the hypothesis that subtle differences in nitric oxide homeostasis are contributory to the excess cardiovascular risk seen in African Americans and that exogenous administration of a nitric oxide donor/antioxidant will overcome this perturbation. This first prospective trial in heart failure affecting African Americans will similarly address a number of additional questions regarding the natural history, epidemiology, and genetic profile of this disease.[66]

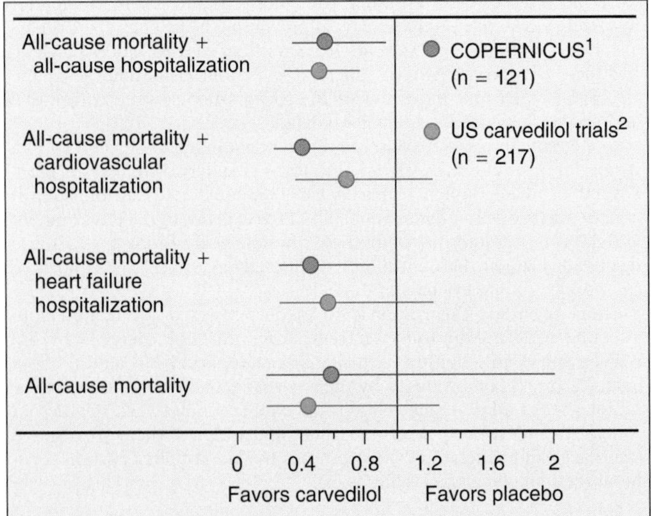

FIGURE 78–7 Effect of carvedilol in African American patients with heart failure. [1] Mean duration, 10.5 months. [2] Mean duration, 6.5 months. (Data from Packer M: Presentation at American Heart Association Scientific Sessions 2000 [COPERNICUS]; and Yancy CW: N Engl J Med 344:1358, 2001 [US Carvedilol Trials].)

The Construct of Race in Medicine

The inclusion of race or ethnicity in any discussion of medicine is problematic. Race is neither scientific nor physiological. The heterogeneity within race is similar to the heterogeneity between races,[67] and the very real requirements for the perpetuation of race, that is, intermarriage and similar environmental surroundings, are rapidly disappearing in the United States. Even the genomic debates are overshadowed by the observation that all persons share more than 99 percent of the same genetic code and that the variance between races is in approximately 0.1 percent of the code. Whether this one

TABLE 78–5 Clinical Trials of Heart Failure Therapy

Study	% of African American Subjects	Design	Intervention	Results
V-HeFT I	29	Double-blind RCT; primary endpoint: mortality	Placebo vs. hydralazine/isosorbide nitrate Background: diuretics and digoxin	Annual mortality rate decreased from 17.9 to 9.7%; $p = 0.04$
V-HeFT II	27	Double-blind RCT; primary endpoint: mortality	Hydralazine/isosorbide dinitrate vs. enalapril Background: diuretics and digoxin	Annual mortality rate decreased from 12.9 to 12.8%; $p =$ NS
SOLVD—treatment	12	Double-blind RCT; primary endpoint: mortality	Placebo vs. enalapril in NYHA Class II/III heart failure	No mortality difference in blacks vs. nonblacks in a matched population regarding LVEF and clinical trial participation; RR 0.92 vs. 0.95; higher hospitalization rate for blacks; RR 0.95 vs. 0.54; $p = 0.005$
SOLVD—prevention	9.8	Double-blind RCT; primary endpoint: mortality	Placebo vs. enalapril in NYHA Class I/II HF	No difference in the prevention of heart failure using enalapril; statistically significant difference in the incidence of heart failure; RR 1.81; $p < 0.001$
BEST	23	Double-blind RCT; primary endpoint: all-cause mortality	Placebo vs. bucindolol in NYHA Class III and IV; randomization stratified for women and blacks Background: diuretics, ACE inhibitors; digoxin at investigator's discretion	Nonsignificant 17% increase in risk of death on bucindolol; $p = 0.27$
MERIT-HF	<5	Double-blind RCT; primary endpoint: mortality	Placebo vs. metoprolol succinate in NYHA Class II/IV; mostly II/III	Insufficient numbers to ascertain efficacy
US Carvedilol Trials Program	20	Four concurrent trials; double-blind RCT design; mortality was not a predetermined endpoint	Placebo vs. carvedilol in NYHA Class II-IV; mostly II/III with protocol participation determined by 6-minute walk time; background: diuretics, ACE inhibitors, and digoxin at investigator's discretion	Similar efficacy between black and nonblack groups; reduction in death for any cause or hospitalization for any cause—48%; reduction in worsening of heart failure—54%
COPERNICUS	5	Double-blind RCT design; primary endpoint: all-cause mortality	Placebo vs. carvedilol in NHYA Class III/IV; LVEF < 0.25 (mean 0.19)	Similar efficacy between black and nonblack groups despite small number of blacks

From Yancy CW: Does race matter in heart failure? Am Heart J 146:203, 2003.
See references 52-54 and 62-65.
ACE = angiotensin-converting enzyme; LVEF = left ventricular ejection fraction; NYHA = New York Heart Association; RCT = randomized controlled trial; RR = relative risk.

tenth of a percent matters is the crux of all of the genomic investigations.

The inclusion of race in medicine need always respect the limitations and variability of race-specific data. Race is usually a self-designation, and not all individuals can be easily classified. Some may actually acknowledge more than one racial designation. Race is less likely to be a "risk factor" and much more likely to be a "risk marker." Race provides a clustering of events that occur because of similar environmental factors and unique physiological variables (e.g., obesity and hypertension) affecting a given population. Discussions of race must rigorously avoid polarization and perpetuation of disparate health care.[68]

Clinical Messages

1. The demographics of the US population is changing. Varied populations—that is, African Americans, Asian Americans, Hispanic Americans, and Native Americans—now make up 30 percent of the population but will soon constitute 50 percent of the US population.
2. Cardiovascular disease affects the varied populations in a striking way. African Americans have the highest rate of mortality due to cardiovascular disease.
3. Risk factors are especially prevalent in the varied populations; African Americans are at risk due to hypertension, obesity, and physical inactivity; Hispanic Americans are at risk due to obesity and diabetes; and emigrant Asian Americans, especially those of South Asian origin, are at risk due to hypertension and urbanization. Native Americans are at risk due to diabetes.

4. Disparate outcomes in cardiovascular disease occur in varied populations because of issues related to access to care, insurance deficits, and persistent bias in health care decision-making.
5. The treatment of hypertension is effective in all individuals; decisions regarding therapy should be based on the absence or presence of compelling indications for aggressive therapy, such as diabetes, renal insufficiency, post-myocardial infarction, and heart failure, and less so on race.
6. African Americans with hypertension are at high risk for complications due to hypertension, especially renal disease and heart failure, and should be treated aggressively, including with lower goal blood pressure reductions and earlier use of either combination agents or multiple drug classes. Although the response to ACE inhibitors, angiotensin receptor blockers, and beta blockers may be less, these differences are overcome with the concomitant use of diuretics, and these agents should be utilized preferentially in African Americans to reduce cardiovascular disease, stroke, and renal disease.
7. Ischemic heart disease occurs at a lower frequency in Hispanic Americans and at a similar frequency for Asian Americans as whites. Ischemic heart disease occurs at a *higher* frequency in African Americans, even though epicardial obstructive CAD is noted less frequently. Hypertension and left ventricular hypertrophy are the leading risk factors. Acute coronary syndromes in African Americans are more likely to include unstable angina and non-ST segment elevation myocardial infarction presentations. Multivessel CAD is the usual angiographic discovery when epicardial disease is present. Thrombolytic therapy, percutaneous coronary interventions, and CABG are applied less frequently in African Americans, especially women, thus contributing to disparate outcomes.
8. Heart failure is notably different in African Americans. The disease occurs at an earlier age, with more advanced left ventricular dysfunction and worse clinical class severity. The incidence of heart failure is higher in African Americans and morbidity is much worse, yet the mortality risk may be similar. The response to neurohormonal antagonists for heart failure is likely to be similar for all patients, and data regarding the use of beta blockers and ACE inhibitors are consistent with good outcomes in African Americans. The A-HeFT trial will further address the benefit of nitrates and hydralazine as adjunctive therapy for heart failure in African Americans.
9. A genomic basis for the differential expression of cardiovascular disease in varied populations may exist, and candidate single nucleotide polymorphisms have been discovered. The exact contribution of these genomic variations to the clinical expression of cardiovascular disease is not yet clear and much more investigation is required.
10. Any use of race/ethnicity in medicine should be done so with caution. The heterogeneity within races is similar to the heterogeneity between races and clinical decision-making should continue to be made on an individual basis.

REFERENCES

1. Barnett E, Casper ML, Halverson JA, et al: Men and Heart Disease: An Atlas of Racial and Ethnic Disparities in Mortality, 1st ed. Morgantown, WV, Office for Social Environment and Health Research, West Virginia University, 2001.

Risk Factors for Cardiovascular Disease

2. Winkleby MA, Kraemer HC, Ahn DK, Varady AN: Ethnic and socioeconomic differences in cardiovascular disease risk factors. JAMA 280:356, 1998.
3. National Center for Health Statistics (NCHS): Fast stats. 2002. (http://www.cdc.gov/nchc/fastats/)
4. Geiss LS, Rolka DB, Engelgau MN: Elevated blood pressure among US adults with diabetes, 1988-94. Am J Prev Med 22:42, 2002.
5. Ford ES, Giles WH, Dietz WH: Prevalence of the metabolic syndrome among US adults. JAMA 287:356, 2002.
6. Ferrannini E, Natali A, Capaldo B, et al: Insulin resistance, hyperinsulinemia and blood pressure. Hypertension 30:1144, 1997.
7. Must A, Spadano J, Coakley EH: The disease burden associated with overweight and obesity. JAMA 282:1523, 1999.
8. Hall WD, Ferrario CM, Moore MA: Hypertension related morbidity and mortality in the southeastern United States. Am J Med Sci 313:195, 1997.
9. Cooper R, Rotimi C, Ataman S: The prevalence of hypertension in seven populations of West African origin. Am J Public Health 87:160, 1997.
10. Flack JM, Ferdinand KC, Nasser SA: Epidemiology of hypertension and cardiovascular disease in African Americans. J Clin Hypertens 5(1 Suppl 1):5, 2003.
11. Ganguli MC, Grimm RH, Svendsen KH: Higher education and income are related to a better Na:K ratio in blacks. Baseline results of the Treatment of Mild Hypertension Study (TOMHS) data. Am J Hypertens 10:979, 1997.
12. Stamler J, Sacks FM, Svetkey LP, Vollmer WM, for the DASH-Sodium Collaborative Research Group: Effects on blood pressure of reduced dietary sodium and the Dietary Approaches to Stop Hypertension (DASH) diet. N Engl J Med 344:3, 2001.
13. INTERSALT Study: Background, methods, findings and implications. Am J Clin Nutrit 65:626S, 1997.
14. Levy D: Left ventricular hypertrophy risk. *In* Hypertension Primer. Dallas, American Heart Association, 2003, pp 243-246.

Cardiovascular Disease Mortality

15. Williams DR, Rucker TD: Understanding and addressing racial disparities in health care. Health Care Financing Rev 21:75, 2000.
16. American Heart Association: 2002 Heart and Stroke Statistics—Update. Dallas, American Heart Association, 2001.
17. American Heart Association: 2003 Heart Disease and Stroke Statistics—Update. Dallas. American Heart Association, 2002.
18. Gillum RF: The epidemiology of cardiovascular disease in black Americans. N Engl J Med 335:1597, 1996.

Cardiovascular Disease Disparities

19. Gomes C, McGuire TG: Identifying the sources of racial and ethnic disparities in health care use. The Institute of Medicine Report, Washington DC, National Academies Press, 2001.
20. Hannan EL, van Ryn M, Burke J, et al: Access to coronary artery bypass surgery by race/ethnicity and gender among patients who are appropriate for surgery. Med Care 37:68, 1999.
21. Robert Wood Johnson Foundation: New survey shows language barriers causing many Spanish-speaking Latinos to skip care. *In* Smedley BD, Stith AY, Nelson AR (eds): Unequal Treatment: Confronting Racial and Ethnic Disparities in Healthcare. Institute of Medicine, National Academy of Sciences, 2003, pp 88-90.
22. Schulman KA, Berlin JA, Harless W: The effect of race and sex on physicians' recommendations for cardiac catheterization. N Engl J Med 340:618, 1999.
23. Smedley BD, Stith AY, Nelson AR (eds): Unequal Treatment: Confronting Racial and Ethnic Disparities in Healthcare. Institute of Medicine, National Academy of Sciences, 2003, pp 43-44.
24. Ramsey DJ, Goff DC, Wear ML, et al: Sex and ethnic differences in use of myocardial revascularization procedures in Mexican Americans and Non-Hispanic Whites; The Corpus Christi Heart Project. J Clin Epidemiol 50:603, 1997.
25. Petersen LA, Wright SM, Petersen ED, Daley J: Impact of race and cardiac care and outcomes in veterans with acute myocardial infarction. Med Care 40(Suppl I):I-86, 2002.
26. Jha AK, Varosy PD, Kanaya AM, et al: Differences in medical care and disease outcomes among black and white women with heart disease. Circulation 108:1098, 2003.

Hypertension

27. Haffner SM: Hypertension in the San Antonio Heart Study and the Mexico City Diabetes Study: Clinical and metabolic correlates. Public Health Rep 111:11, 1996.
28. Crespo CJ, Smit E, Garcia Palmieri MR: Hypertension in Hispanic Americans. *In* Izzo JL, Black HR (eds): Hypertension Primer, 3rd ed. Philadelphia, Lippincott Williams & Wilkins, 2003.
29. Anand SS, Yusuf S, Vuksan V: Differences in risk factors, atherosclerosis and cardiovascular disease between ethnic groups in Canada: The Study of Health Assessment and Risk in Ethnic Groups (SHARE). Lancet 356:279, 2000.
30. Deewania PC, Gupta R: Hypertension in South Asians. *In* Izzo JL, Black HR (eds): Hypertension Primer, 3rd ed. Philadelphia, Lippincott Williams & Wilkins, 2003.
31. Rahman M, Douglas JG, Wright JT: Pathophysiology and treatment implications of hypertension in the African American population. Endocrinol Metab Clin North Am 26:125, 1997.
32. Berenson GS, Voors AW, Webber LS, et al: Racial differences of parameters associated with blood pressure levels in children: The Bogalusa Heart Study. Metabolism 28:1218, 1979.
33. Yancy CW: Heart failure in African Americans: A cardiovascular enigma. J Card Fail 6:183, 2000.
34. Gardin JM, Wagenknecht LE, Anton-Culver H, et al: Relationship of cardiovascular risk factors to echocardiographic left ventricular mass in healthy young black and white adult men and women: The CARDIA study. Circulation 92:380, 1995.
35. Gottdiener JS, Reda DJ, Materson BJ, et al: Importance of obesity, race and age to the cardiac structural and functional effects of hypertension. The Department of Veterans Affairs Cooperative Study Group on Antihypertensive Agents. J Am Coll Cardiol 24:1492, 1994.
36. Kotchen TA, Piering AW, Cowley AW, et al: Glomerular hyperfiltration in hypertensive African-Americans. Hypertension 35:822, 2000.
37. Stein CM, Lang CC, Nelson R, et al: Vasodilation in black Americans: Attenuated nitric oxide-mediated responses. Clin Pharmacol Ther 62:436, 1997.
38. Kaplan NM: Kaplan's Clinical Hypertension, 8th ed. Philadelphia, Lippincott Williams & Wilkins, 2002.
39. Grim CE, Robinson M: Salt, slavery and survival—Hypertension in the African Diaspora. Epidemiology 14:120, 2003.
40. Cooper RS, Rotimi CN, Ward R: The puzzle of hypertension in African Americans. Sci Am 280:56, 1999.
41. Sacks FM, Svetkey LP, Vollmer WM, et al: Effects on blood pressure of reduced dietary sodium and the Dietary Approaches to Stop Hypertension (DASH) diet. DASH-Sodium Collaborative Research Group. N Engl J Med 344:3, 2001.
42. Baker EH: Association of hypertension with T594M mutation in beta subunit of epithelial sodium channels in black people resident in London. Lancet 351:1388, 1998.
43. August P, Leventhal B, Suthanthiran M: Hypertension-induced organ damage in African Americans: Transforming growth factor-beta 1 excess as a mechanism for increased prevalence. Curr Hypertens Rep 2:184, 2000.

44. Chobanian AV, Bakris GL, Black HR, et al: The Seventh Report of the Joint National Committee on Prevention, Detection, Evaluation and Treatment of High Blood Pressure. The JNC 7 report. JAMA 289:2560, 2003.
45. Nesbitt S, Victor RG: Pathogenesis of hypertension in African Americans. Congest Heart Fail 10:24, 2004.
46. Wright JT, Bakris G, Green T, et al: Effect of blood pressure lowering and antihypertensive drug class on progression of hypertensive kidney disease. Results from the AASK Trial. JAMA 19:2421, 2002.
47. Douglas JG, Bakris GL, Epstein M, et al: Management of high blood pressure in African Americans. Arch Intern Med 163:525, 2003.

Ischemic Heart Disease

48. Clark LT, Ferdinand KC, Flack JM, et al: Coronary heart disease in African Americans. Heart Dis 3:97, 2001.
49. Strong JP, Malcom GT, Oalmann MC, Wissler RW: The PDAY study: Natural history, risk factors, and pathobiology. Pathobiological Determinants of Atherosclerosis in Youth. Ann N Y Acad Sci 811:226, 1997.
50. Sorlie PD, Sharrett AR, Patsch W, et al: The relationship between lipids/lipoproteins and atherosclerosis in African Americans and whites: The Atherosclerosis Risk in Communities study. Ann Epidemiol 9:149, 1999.
51. Ergul S, Parish DC, Puett D, et al: Racial differences in plasma endothelin-1 concentrations in individuals with essential hypertension. Hypertension 28:652, 1996.

Heart Failure

52. Dries DL, Exner DV, Gersh BJ, et al: Racial differences in the outcome of left ventricular dysfunction. N Engl J Med 341:298, 1999.
53. Exner DV, Dries DL, Domanski MJ, et al: Lesser response to angiotensin-converting-enzyme inhibitor therapy in black as compared with white patients with left ventricular dysfunction. N Engl J Med 344:1351, 2001.
54. Dries DL, Strong MH, Cooper RS, Drazner M: Efficacy of angiotensin-converting enzyme inhibition in reducing progression from asymptomatic left ventricular dysfunction to symptomatic heart failure in black and white patients. J Am Coll Cardiol 40:311, 2002.
55. Iwanaga Y, Kihara Y, Hasegawa K, et al: Cardiac endothelin-1 plays a critical role in the functional deterioration of left ventricles during the transition from compensatory hypertrophy to congestive heart failure in salt-sensitive hypertensive rats. Circulation 98:2065, 1998.
56. Kostis JB, Davis BR, Cutler J, et al, for the SHEP Cooperative Research Group: Prevention of heart failure by antihypertensive drug treatment in older persons with isolated systolic hypertension. JAMA 278:212, 1997.
57. August P: TGF Beta-1 overexpressed in African American hypertensives. Proc Natl Acad Sci U S A 97:3479, 2000.
58. McNamara DM, Holubkov R, Janosko K, et al: Genetic Risk Assessment of Cardiac Events, GRACE, Circulation 103:1644, 2001.
59. Mason DA, Moore JD, Green SA, Liggett SB: A gain of function polymorphism in a G-protein coupling domain of the human beta-1 adrenergic receptor. J Biol Chem 274:12670, 1999.
60. Small KM, Wagoner LE, Levin AM, et al: Synergistic polymorphisms of beta 1 and alpha 2C adrenergic receptors and the risk of congestive heart failure. N Engl J Med 347:1135, 2002.
61. Turner ST, Schwartz GL, Chapman AB, Boperwinkle E: C825T polymorphism of the G protein beta-3 subunit and antihypertensive response to a thiazide diuretic. Hypertension 37:739, 2001.
62. Carson P, Ziesche S, Johnson G, et al: Racial differences in response to therapy for heart failure: Analysis of the vasodilator-heart failure trials. Vasodilator-Heart Failure Trial Study Group. J Card Fail 5:178, 1999.
63. The Beta-Blocker Evaluation of Survival Trial Investigators: A trial of the beta-blocker bucindolol in patients with advanced chronic heart failure. N Engl J Med 344:1659, 2001.
64. MERIT-HF Study Group: Effect of metoprolol CR/XL in chronic heart failure: Metoprolol CR/XL Randomised Intervention Trial in Congestive Heart Failure (MERIT-HF). Lancet 353:2001, 1999.
65. Yancy CW, Fowler MB, Colucci WS, et al: Race and the response to adrenergic blockade with carvedilol in patients with heart failure. N Engl J Med 344:1358, 2001.
66. Franciosa JA, Taylor AL, Cohn JN, et al, for the A-HeFT Investigators: African American Heart Failure Trial (A-HeFT): Rationale, design, and methodology. J Card Fail 8:128, 2002.

Race in Medicine

67. American Anthropological Association: American Anthropological Association statement on race, 1998. (http:/www.aaanet.org/stmts/racepp.htm)
68. Kaplan JB, Bennett T: Use of race and ethnicity in biomedical publication. JAMA 289:2709, 2003.

PART X

Cardiovascular Disease and Disorders of Other Organ Systems

CHAPTER 79

Endocrine Disorders and Cardiovascular Disease

Irwin Klein

Throughout medical science, there are very few areas where basic science investigation links as closely to clinical observations and therapy as in the field of cardiovascular endocrinology. As our knowledge of the cellular and molecular effects of various hormones evolves, we can better understand the clinical manifestations that arise from both excess hormone secretion and glandular failure leading to hormone deficiency states. More than 200 years ago, Caleb Hillier Parry described a woman with goiter and palpitations whose "each systole shook the whole thorax." He was the first to suggest that there was a connection between diseases of the heart and enlargement of the thyroid gland. The cardiovascular abnormalities associated with pathological changes of endocrine glands were recognized prior to the understanding of the specific hormones produced by these glands. This chapter reviews the broad spectrum of cardiac disease states that arise from changes in specific endocrine function. This approach allows us to explore the cellular mechanisms by which various hormones can produce changes in the cardiovascular system through actions on the cardiac myocyte, vascular smooth muscle cells, and other target cells and tissues.

Pituitary Gland

The pituitary gland is made up of two distinct anatomical portions. The anterior portion, or adenohypophysis, contains six different cell types, five of which produce polypeptide or glycoprotein hormones; the sixth classically has been referred to as nonsecretory chromophobic cells. Of these cell types, the somatotrophic cells, which secrete human growth hormone (hGH), and the corticotrophic cells, which produce adrenocorticotropic hormone (ACTH), have been linked to cardiac disease. The posterior pituitary, or neurohypophysis, is the anatomical location of the nerve terminals that secrete vasopressin (antidiuretic hormone) or oxytocin.

Growth Hormone

In adults, excessive growth hormone secretion before the fusion of the bone epiphysis leads to gigantism, whereas increased secretion of hGH after maturation of the long bones leads to acromegaly. The growth-promoting factor obtained from extracts of the pituitary gland was first identified by Evans and Long in the early 1920s. Almost 50 years later, the protein sequence and structure of hGH were first identified and its role as one member of a family of growth-promoting (somatic) factors emerged.

Growth hormone exerts its cellular effects through two major pathways. The first involves hormone binding to specific growth hormone receptors on target cells. These receptors have been identified in heart, skeletal muscle, fat, liver, and kidney and in many additional cell types throughout fetal development.[1] The second growth-promoting effect of hGH results from stimulation of synthesis of the insulin-like growth factor type 1

(IGF-1). This protein is produced primarily in the liver, but other cell types can produce IGF-1 under the influence of hGH.

Shortly after the identification of the IGF family, it was proposed that most actions of growth hormone were mediated through this second messenger. Clinical disease activity of patients with growth hormone excess (acromegaly) correlates better with serum levels of IGF-1 than with hGH. The ability to promote glucose uptake and cellular protein synthesis gave rise to the term insulin-like. IGF-1 binds to its cognate IGF-1 receptor, which is present in virtually all cell types. Transgenic experiments have demonstrated that the presence of IGF-1 receptors on cell types associates closely with the ability of those cells to divide. Ingenious studies in which the IGF-1 receptor was overexpressed in cardiac myocytes reportedly produced an increased myocyte number, mitotic rate, and the ability of the postdifferentiated myocytes to replicate.[2] The harnessing of this action holds potential benefit for genetic manipulation and repair of the diseased myocardium.

Acute changes in cardiovascular hemodynamics result from the infusion of both hGH and IGF-1. The acute increases in cardiac contractility and cardiac output may be due, at least in part, to a decrease in systemic vascular resistance and cardiac afterload.[3] Short-term administration of both hGH and IGF-1 does not increase blood pressure, implying that the increase in cardiac output is indeed a result of changes in systemic vascular resistance.[4-6]

Cardiovascular Manifestations of Acromegaly

Acromegaly is a relatively uncommon condition, and approximately 900 new cases are diagnosed each year in the United States. Acromegaly and pituitary-dependent human gigantism associate with markedly increased morbidity and mortality primarily resulting from cardiovascular disease. Untreated acromegaly, identified by its characteristic clinical signs and symptoms and by increased hGH secretion, markedly shortens life expectancy, with less than 20 percent of patients surviving beyond 60 years. Multiple studies implicate increased neoplasia arising from the gastrointestinal tract, colon polyps, colon cancer, and pulmonary disease in this increased mortality.[7] However, the cardiovascular and cerebral vascular changes including hypertension, cardiomegaly, congestive heart failure, and cerebral vascular accidents continue to be the major events that limit survival.[8] First recognized by Pierre Marie in 1886, cardiovascular involvement in acromegaly is a chronic insidious process.

The cardiovascular and hemodynamic effects of acromegaly are highly variable and differ among patients depending upon age, severity of disease, and disease duration.[9] In patients diagnosed with less than 5 years of disease activity, changes in systolic or diastolic blood pressure were not significant, but echocardiographic determination of left ventricular mass index increased almost 35 percent and cardiac index increased 24 percent. Measures of systolic function including stroke index increased significantly, and systemic vascular resistance increased by 20 percent.[10] Left ventricular diastolic function was normal. These studies stand in marked contrast to the reports that longer duration of acromegaly produces left ventricular dysfunction and cardiomyopathy.[8,9]

Known cardiac disease risk factors including hypertension, insulin resistance, diabetes mellitus, and hyperlipidemia frequently occur in patients with acromegaly. Although initial reports suggested that impairment of cardiac function in longstanding acromegaly was due to accelerated atherosclerosis, a postmortem study revealed significant coronary artery disease in only 11 percent of patients who died from disease-related causes. Angiography demonstrates the presence of either normal or dilated coronary arteries in most cases. Thallium stress testing is positive in less than 25 percent of patients and overall allows us to conclude that atherosclerosis and ischemic heart disease are unlikely to account for the marked degrees of biventricular cardiac hypertrophy, cardiac failure, and cardiovascular mortality associated with acromegaly.[11]

Rather specific functional and histological myocyte changes appear to arise in the setting of prolonged excess serum levels of hGH and IGF-1.[9,12] As many as two-thirds of acromegalic patients have echocardiographic criteria for left ventricular hypertrophy (LVH).[7,8] The right ventricle also increases in mass in acromegaly, indicating a more generalized process beyond systemic hypertension.[10] Asymmetrical septal hypertrophy, initially thought to be common in patients with acromegaly, is an unusual finding. There appears to be an increased prevalence of both aortic and mitral valve disease, which persists despite disease cure.[13] Individual patients with dilation of the aortic root and defects of the cardiac conduction system have been reported.[8,14]

Histological evaluation of acromegalic cardiac tissue reveals that there is an increase in myocyte size (hypertrophy) without an increase in cell number.[15] Acromegaly produces interstitial fibrosis and infiltration of a variety of inflammatory cells including mononuclear cells consistent with myocarditis.[8,11] The absence of cell necrosis in the presence of an inflammatory reaction has raised the question of whether part of these histological findings can be explained by IGF-1–promoted programmed cell death (apoptosis). A study of acromegalic patients with diastolic dysfunction indicated apoptotic cell death in endomyocardial biopsies.[16]

Given the breadth of pathological involvement of the heart in acromegaly, it is not surprising that there are associated functional changes.[10-12] Whereas approximately 10 percent of newly diagnosed patients have signs and symptoms of cardiac compromise, this percentage increases markedly with disease duration.[17] Some studies report a low incidence of overt left ventricular failure, suggesting that supervening factors including hypertension, type 2 diabetes, and hyperlipidemia are needed to impair function.[11] In acromegaly, LVH and congestive heart failure can occur in longstanding disease without hypertension, indicating that high levels of growth hormone or IGF-1, or both, can produce cardiac myopathic changes per se.[12,14] Successful therapy reverses many if not all of these findings.[18,19]

Electrocardiographic (ECG) abnormalities including left axis deviation, septal Q waves, ST-T wave depression, abnormal QT dispersion, and conduction system defects occur in as many as 50 percent of acromegalic patients. A variety of dysrhythmias including atrial and ventricular ectopic beats, sick sinus syndrome, and supraventricular and ventricular tachycardias have been described.[8,15] The finding in a signal average electrocardiogram of a fourfold increase in complex ventricular arrhythmias and late potentials, thought to be predictors of ventricular irritability, was also more common in patients with active acromegaly than in treated patients.[14] In contrast, exercise stress testing with ECG monitoring did not show inducible rhythm disturbances or evidence of ischemia, suggesting that left ventricular rhythm disturbances were not related to any underlying ischemia.

Secondary hypertension associated with acromegaly has been reported in 20 to 40 percent of patients.[7,8] Given the overall high prevalence rate of hypertension in the adult population and the insidious onset of acromegaly, it is difficult to determine whether the occurrence of hypertension is secondary or merely coincidental. The improvement with therapy, however, suggests that they are related.[19] Although epidemiological studies of survival in acromegaly initially suggested that hypertension was not an independent risk factor for mortality, a survey of patients who died of the disease demonstrated that mean blood pressures were higher than in those who survived.[7] The mechanism underlying hypertension in acromegaly is not clearly understood. Newly diagnosed patients with a short duration of disease had systolic and diastolic blood pressures no different from those of age- and sex-matched control subjects, but cardiac index was significantly increased. It does appear that the arterial intimal thickness is increased in patients with longstanding acromegaly, and these changes respond to hGH lowering.[8]

Growth hormone administration promotes sodium retention and volume expansion and appears to have a potent antinatriuretic effect independent of any effect on aldosterone.[20] Studies of the renin-angiotensin-aldosterone system show a failure to inhibit renin release optimally by volume expansion. When angiotensin II inhibitors are given to patients with acromegaly, there is a paradoxical increase in blood pressure.[11] The role of hyperinsulinemia in the hypertension of acromegaly has been questioned. Increased serum insulin can contribute to urinary sodium retention, impairment of endothelium-dependent vasodilation, and increased sympathetic activity.[21] There are rare associations of acromegaly with aldosterone-secreting adrenal adenomas and with pheochromocytoma.

Diagnosis

In 99 percent of cases, acromegaly arises from benign adenomas of the anterior pituitary gland.[7,19] At the time of diagnosis, the majority of these neoplasms are classified as macroadenomas (>10 mm), and patients have had clinical evidence of disease for more than 10 years. The diagnosis can be confirmed by demonstrating a serum growth hormone level greater than 5 ng/dl and a serum IGF-1 level greater than 300 μIU/ml measured 1 hour after a 100-gm glucose load. In the majority of patients, fasting growth hormone levels are higher than 10 ng/ml. Tumor localization can be established by magnetic resonance imaging dedicated to the pituitary gland. Rarely, growth hormone–releasing hormone can be secreted, causing diffuse hyperplasia of the pituitary. The existence of such changes must lead to the consideration of a neoplastic lesion residing in other parts of the endocrine system.

Therapy

Transsphenoidal surgery with resection of the adenoma is the procedure of choice for initial management. If hGH or IGF-1 or both remain elevated, radiotherapy in older patients, or dopamine or somatostatin receptor agonists in younger patients, can be used to restore serum growth hormone and IGF-1 levels to normal. Octreotide acetate, a pharmacological analog of somatostatin, is effective in the vast majority of patients in lowering hGH to less than 5 ng/ml. It may be primary therapy in selected cases. The cardiovascular complications of acromegaly including hypertension, LVH, and left ventricular dysfunction improve with treatment, and survival is significantly better in patients who achieve clinical and biochemical disease remission. A growth hormone receptor antagonist, pegvisomant, can normalize IGF-1 levels in long-term therapy and may play a role in somatostatin-resistant patients.[18,19]

Adrenocorticotropic Hormone and Cortisol

The adrenal corticotropic cells in the anterior pituitary synthesize a large protein (pro-opiomelanocortin) that is processed within the corticotropic cell into a family of smaller proteins that include alpha-melanocyte-stimulating hormone (αMSH), beta-endorphin, and ACTH. ACTH in turn binds to specific cells within the adrenal gland. The adrenal gland is anatomically divided into two major segments: the cortex and the medulla. The cortex zona glomerulosa produces aldosterone, the zona fasciculata produces primarily cortisol and some androgenic steroids, and the zona reticularis also produces cortisol and androgens. Synthesis of cortisol in the zona fasciculata and zona reticularis is primarily regulated by ACTH.[22] The zona glomerulosa shows a much lesser degree of ACTH responsiveness and responds primarily to angiotensin II by increased aldosterone secretion.

Cushing Disease

Excess cortisol secretion and its attendant clinical disease states can arise either from excess pituitary release of ACTH (Cushing disease) or through the adenomatous or rarely malignant neoplastic process arising in the adrenal gland itself (Cushing syndrome). Well-characterized conditions of both adrenal glucocorticoid and mineralocorticoid excess appear to result from the excessively high levels of (ectopic) ACTH produced by small cell carcinoma of the lung, carcinoid tumors, pancreatic islet cell tumors, medullary thyroid cancer, and other adenocarcinomas and hematological malignancies.[22]

Cortisol, a member of the glucocorticoid family of steroid hormones, binds to monomeric receptors located within the cytoplasm of many cell types (Fig. 79-1). The unliganded glucocorticoid receptors are bound to heat shock protein complexes. After binding cortisol, the receptors dissociate from these complexes, homodimerize or occasionally heterodimerize, translocate to the nucleus, and function as transcription factors. A variety of cardiac genes contain glucocorticoid response elements in their promoter regions that confer glucocorticoid responsiveness.[23] These genes include those that encode the voltage-gated potassium channel as well as protein kinases, which phosphorylate and regulate voltage-gated sodium channels. This expression may in turn be chamber specific.[24]

The cardiac effects of glucocorticoid excess in Cushing disease arise from both the direct effects of glucocorticoids on the heart and the effects of glucocorticoids on the liver, skeletal muscle, and fat tissue.[25] Accelerated atherosclerosis can result from abnormal glucose metabolism with hyperglycemia and hyperinsulinemia, hypertension, and altered clotting and platelet function. The mechanism for cortisol-mediated hypertension is multifactorial.[26] Studies have shown that, in contrast to the findings in aldosterone-induced hypertension, the central administration of glucocorticoids lowers blood pressure. Thus, cortisol-mediated hypertension appears not to result from activation of the mineralocorticoid receptor. In addition, antagonism of glucocorticoid effects through its cytosolic receptor can block cortisol-induced elevations of glucose and insulin but not those related to blood pressure.[27,28] Interestingly, one study suggested that inhibition of sodium retention is also insufficient to block the cortisol-mediated rise in blood pressure, pointing to the changes in vascular reactivity, systemic vascular resistance, and nitric oxide–mediated vasodilation as candidates for the hypertensive effect.[24,26]

The rise in serum glucose and the development of insulin resistance may give rise to activation of proinflammatory cytokines such as tumor necrosis factor-alpha and interleukin-6, which may underlie the accelerated atherosclerosis of insulin resistance found in other endocrine disease states.[27] Thus, while acting classically as an antiinflammatory hormone, cortisol excess can promote inflammation and accelerate atherosclerosis by producing insulin resistance, changes in corticosteroid-binding protein, and regulation of a variety of proinflammatory cytokines. The centripetal obesity characteristic of glucocorticoid excess resembles that seen in the insulin resistance syndromes. Excess androgen production resulting from increased ACTH stimulation of the adrenal cortex may also accelerate atherosclerosis in both men and women.[22]

The increased cardiovascular morbidity and mortality of Cushing syndrome can be explained in large part by cerebrovascular disease, peripheral vascular disease, coronary artery disease with myocardial infarction, and chronic congestive heart failure.[25,29] These are all changes that would be expected in the setting of accelerated atherosclerosis resulting from hypertension and hyperlipidemia.[30] Studies of left ventricular structure and function have shown hypertrophy and impaired contractility in 40 percent of patients.[31] In addition, the marked muscle weakness resulting from corticosteroid-induced skeletal myopathy contributes to impaired exercise tolerance.

Patients with Cushing disease can exhibit a variety of ECG changes. There appears to be a direct correlation between

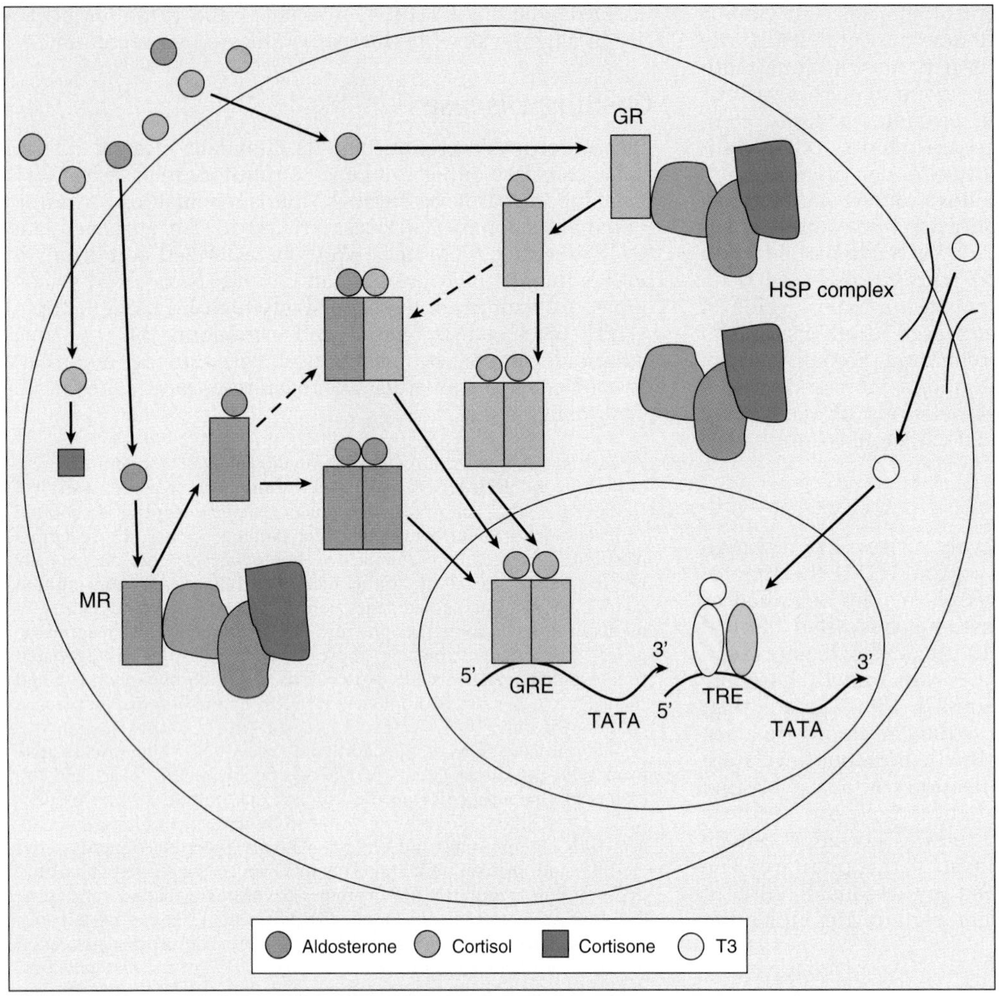

FIGURE 79–1 Scheme of a generalized nuclear hormone receptor mechanism of action. The mineralocorticoid receptor (MR) has similar affinities for aldosterone and cortisol. Circulating levels of cortisol are 100 to 1000 times greater than that of aldosterone. In MR-responsive cells, the enzyme 11beta-hydroxysteroid dehydrogenase metabolizes cortisol to cortisone, thereby allowing aldosterone to bind to MR. MR and the glucocorticoid receptor (GR) are cytoplasmic receptors that, after binding ligand, translocate to the nucleus and bind to glucocorticoid response elements (GREs) in the promoter regions of responsive genes. Triiodothyronine (T_3) enters the cell by facilitated diffusion and binds to thyroid hormone receptors (TRs), which are bound to thyroid hormone response elements (TREs) in the promoter regions of T_3-responsive genes. (Courtesy of Dr. S. Danzi.)

adrenal cortisol production rates and the duration of the PR interval. The underlying mechanism may be related to either the expression or the regulation of the voltage-gated sodium channel (SCN5A). Changes in electrocardiograms, specifically PR and QT intervals, may also arise as a result of the direct (nongenomic) effects of glucocorticoids on the voltage-gated potassium channel (Kv1.5) in a variety of excitable tissues.[24,25,32]

A particular complex of cardiac and adrenal lesions, referred to as the Carney complex, combines Cushing syndrome, cardiac myxoma, and a variety of pigmented dermal lesions (not café-au-lait).[33] This monogenic autosomal dominant trait maps to the q2 region of chromosome 17. Myxomas most commonly occur in the left atrium but can occur throughout the heart, at young ages, and be multicentric.

Diagnosis

Diagnosis of Cushing disease and syndrome requires demonstration of increased cortisol production, best accomplished by a 24-hour urinary free cortisol test.[22] ACTH measurements to determine whether the disease is pituitary, adrenal, or ectopically based and anatomical localization with magnetic resonance imaging of the suspected lesions confirm the laboratory tests.

Treatment

The treatment of excess cortisol production depends on the underlying mechanisms. In Cushing disease, transsphenoidal hypophysectomy can partially or completely reverse the increased ACTH production by the anterior pituitary. Cushing syndrome requires surgical removal of one (adrenal adenoma, adrenal carcinoma) or both (multiple nodular) adrenal glands. Immediately after surgery, it is necessary to replace both cortisol and mineralocorticoid (fludrocortisone) to prevent adrenal insufficiency. Treatment of the ectopic ACTH syndrome requires identification and treatment of the neoplastic process. Patients treated with exogenous steroids (e.g., prednisone, methylprednisolone) in doses above 10 mg/d for periods in excess of 1 month often develop clinical signs and symptoms of Cushing syndrome.[22] In nonsurgical patients, the adrenal enzyme inhibitor ketoconazole can reverse excess cortisol production. Even mild or subclinical degrees of Cushing syndrome (adrenal incidentaloma) appear to increase the risk for cardiovascular disease.[34]

Hyperaldosteronism

Aldosterone production by the zona glomerulosa is under the control of the renin-angiotensin system.[35] Renin secretion responds to changes in intravascular volume. Aldosterone synthesis and secretion are primarily regulated by angiotensin II, which binds to the angiotensin II type I receptor on the cells of the zona glomerulosa.[22,35]

The mechanism of action of aldosterone on target tissues resembles that reported for glucocorticoids (see Fig. 79–1).[36] Aldosterone is taken up into cells and binds to the mineralocorticoid receptor, which then translocates to the nucleus and promotes the expression of aldosterone-responsive genes.[28] In addition to kidney cells, where they control sodium transport, in vitro studies have demonstrated mineralocorticoid receptors in rat cardiac myocytes, which respond to stimulation with an increase in protein synthesis.[36-38] It is not clear whether these changes correspond to any relevant in vivo cardiac effects. Genetically engineered mice with an inactive mineralocorticoid receptor gene show classical features of mineralocorticoid deficiency and require sodium supplementation to survive. The aldosterone antagonists spironolactone and eplerenone compete for receptor binding in the cytosol (see Fig. 79–1).[39]

A variety of tissue-specific responses to aldosterone appear to be mediated at the level of the cell membrane and have been referred to as "nongenomic." Although these effects usually require a higher concentration of the hormone, they can change Na^+/H^+ transport and in vitro studies of cardiac myocytes have demonstrated a nongenomic effect on the Na^+/K^+ pump.[32]

Whereas the major cause of increased serum aldosterone is the physiological response to the activation of the renin-angiotensin system, there are well-recognized aldosterone-producing benign adrenal adenomas (Conn syndrome).[22,40] Primary hyperaldosteronism augments sodium retention, causes hypertension, increases renal loss of magnesium and potassium, decreases arterial compliance with a rise in systemic vascular resistance and resulting vascular damage, and alters the sympathetic and parasympathetic neural regulation. Many of the changes in the heart and cardiovascular system in hyperaldosteronism result from the associated hypertension. The degree of LVH, however, exceeds that expected from the hypertension alone, perhaps because of the increase in volume as well as pressure load resulting from increased aldosterone action.[41,42] The hyperaldosterone-mediated hypokalemia and much of the associated hypertension respond to the surgical removal of a unilateral (or occasionally bilateral) benign adrenal adenoma.

Addison Disease

Long before recognition that the glands situated just above the upper pole of each kidney (suprarenal) synthesize and secrete glucocorticoids and mineralocorticoids, Thomas Addison described the association of atrophy with loss of function of these structures with marked changes in the cardiovascular system. The hypovolemia, hypotension, and acute cardiovascular collapse resulting from renal sodium wasting, hyperkalemia, and loss of vascular tone are the hallmarks of acute Addisonian crisis, one of the most severe endocrine emergencies. Adrenal insufficiency most commonly arises from bilateral loss of adrenal function on an autoimmune basis; as a result of infection, hemorrhage, or metastatic malignancy; or in selected cases as a result of inborn errors of steroid hormone metabolism. In contrast, secondary adrenal insufficiency, which results from pituitary-dependent loss of ACTH secretion, leads to a fall in glucocorticoid production while mineralocorticoid production, including aldosterone production, remains at relatively normal levels. Studies have addressed the issue of relative hypothalamic-pituitary-adrenal insufficiency in acutely ill patients.[43] This issue has reopened the question of the need for stress dose cortisol treatment of patients with critical illness.

Addison disease can occur at any age. The noncardiac symptoms including increased pigmentation, abdominal pain with nausea and vomiting, and weight loss can be chronic, whereas the tachycardia, hypotension, and electrolyte abnormalities are harbingers of impending cardiovascular collapse and crisis.[44] Blood pressure measurements uniformly show low diastolic pressure (<60 mm Hg) with significant orthostatic changes reflecting volume loss. Laboratory findings of hyponatremia and hyperkalemia indicate loss of aldosterone production (renin levels are high). The hyperkalemia can alter the electrocardiogram producing low-amplitude P waves and peaked T waves.[45] In newly diagnosed, untreated patients with Addison disease, both left ventricular end-systolic and end-diastolic dimensions were reduced compared with control values. Cardiac atrophy is an unusual condition. It is seen in malnutrition related to anorexia, in astronauts after prolonged space flight, in populations with sodium-deficient diets, and characteristically with Addison disease (teardrop heart) (Fig. 79–2). This atrophic process is in response to decreases in cardiac workload because restoration of normal plasma volume with both mineralocorticoid and glucocorticoid replacement increases ventricular mass.[46]

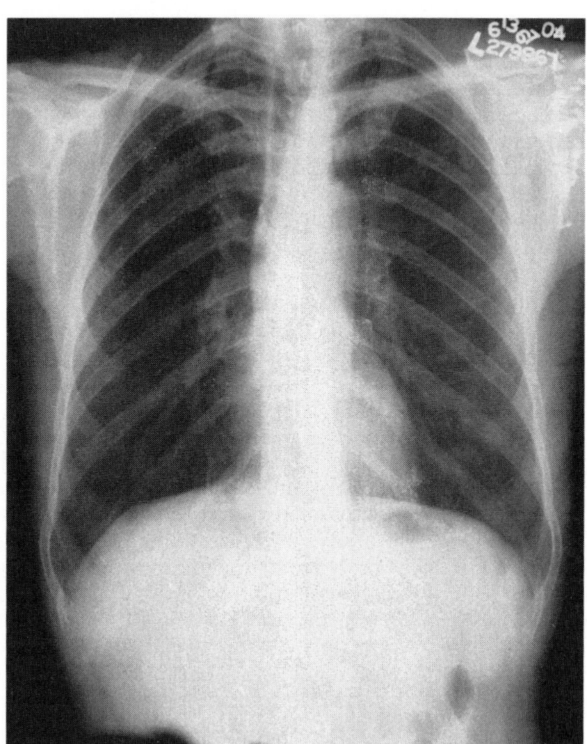

FIGURE 79–2 Routine chest radiograph of a patient with Addison disease related to tuberculosis. In addition to the small cardiac silhouette, there are calcified lymph nodes in the hilum of the right lung. (Courtesy of Dr. J. B. Naidich.)

Diagnosis

Acute adrenal insufficiency characteristically occurs in the setting of an acute stress, infection, or trauma in a patient with chronic adrenal insufficiency. It can also result from bilateral adrenal hemorrhage in patients with severe systemic infection or disseminated intravascular coagulation. Secondary adrenal insufficiency can occur in the setting of hypopituitarism, which in most situations is chronic; however, acute changes related to pituitary hemorrhage (apoplexy) or pituitary inflammation (lymphocytic hypophysitis) have been observed. Patients treated with long-term suppressive doses of corticosteroids (>10 mg of prednisone for more than 1 month) can develop acute adrenal insufficiency should such treatment be stopped precipitously.

The diagnosis is established when, in the morning or during severe stress, cortisol levels are low (<8 μg/dl) and fail to rise above 20 μg/dl 30 minutes after an intravenous injection of 0.25 mg of cosyntropin.

Treatment

Management of acute Addisonian crisis needs to address three major issues. The first is adequate hydrocortisone replacement, 100 mg given as an initial intravenous bolus and then 100 mg every 8 hours for the first 24 hours, tapering the dose for the next 72 to 96 hours. The second is restoration of the intravascular fluid deficit using large volumes of normal saline with 5 percent dextrose. Last is the need to identify and treat any underlying precipitating cause, including infection, acute cardiac or cerebral ischemia, or intraabdominal emergency. Chronic treatment is with oral corticosteroid and mineralocorticoid (fludrocortisone 0.1 mg/d) replacement.[22,46]

Parathyroid Disease

Diseases of the parathyroid glands can produce cardiovascular disease and alter cardiac function by two mechanisms. The first is through changes in the secretion of parathyroid hormone (PTH), a protein hormone that exerts effects on the heart, vascular smooth muscle cells, and endothelial cells.[47] The second is by way of changes in serum calcium. There is an exquisitely sensitive negative feedback mechanism by which serum ionized calcium regulates the synthesis and secretion of PTH.

PTH can bind to its cell surface receptor and alter the spontaneous beating rate of neonatal cardiac myocytes by an increase in intracellular cyclic adenosine monophosphate (AMP). PTH can also alter calcium influx and cardiac contractility in adult cardiac myocytes. In vascular smooth muscle cells, this alteration causes vasodilation. In addition to PTH, there is a parathyroid hormone–related peptide (PTHrP) that is structurally related to PTH and is synthesized and secreted in a variety of tissues including cardiac myocytes. PTHrP was first characterized as the humoral substance secreted by malignant tumors producing hypercalcemia. Interestingly, PTHrP can bind to the PTH receptor on cardiac cells and stimulate cyclic AMP accumulation and contractile activity and regulate L-type calcium currents. Thus, in a variety of paraneoplastic syndromes characterized by hypercalcemia, the direct effects of PTHrP on the heart and systemic vasculature can be manifested.[47]

HYPERPARATHYROIDISM

Classical primary hyperparathyroidism producing hypercalcemia most often arises as a result of the adenomatous enlargement of one of four parathyroid glands. The cardiovascular actions of hypercalcemia include an increase in cardiac contractility, a shortening of the ventricular action potential duration primarily through changes in phase 2, and blunting of the T wave and changes in the ST segment occasionally suggesting cardiac ischemia.[48] The QT interval is shortened, and occasionally accompanied by decreases in the PR interval as well. Treatment with digitalis glycosides appears to increase sensitivity of the heart to hypercalcemia.

Hypercalcemia has been linked to pathological changes in the heart including the myocardial interstitium, the conducting system, and calcific deposits in the valve cusps and annuli. Although initially observed in fairly longstanding and severe hypercalcemia, so-called metastatic calcifications can also occur in secondary parathyroid disease arising from chronic renal failure in which the serum calcium-phosphorus product constant is exceeded.[49]

Presumably as a result of the direct effect of calcium on vascular smooth muscle tone, patients with primary hyperparathyroidism have increased arterial pressure. Because PTH exerts a direct vasodilator effect and increased dietary calcium has been linked with a decrease in arterial pressure, the mechanisms that link PTH to blood pressure are complex.[47,48]

A simultaneous increase in serum immunoreactive PTH (best represented by the intact PTH assay) with an elevation of serum calcium establishes the diagnosis of primary hyperparathyroidism. Other causes include hypercalcemia of malignancy with an increased level of PTHrP or direct bone metastasis and neoplastic (lymphoma) or nonneoplastic (sarcoidosis) diseases leading to an increase in synthesis and release of 1,25-dihydroxyvitamin D_3. Treatment of hyperparathyroidism is the surgical removal of the parathyroid adenoma.

HYPOCALCEMIA

Low serum levels of total and ionized calcium directly alter myocyte function. Hypocalcemia prolongs phase 2 of the action potential duration and the QT interval. Severe hypocalcemia can potentially impair cardiac contractility and gives rise to a diffuse musculoskeletal syndrome including tetany and rhabdomyolysis. Primary hypoparathyroidism is a rare disease that can be seen after surgical removal of the parathyroid glands, in the setting of polyglandular dysfunction syndromes, as the result of glandular agenesis (DiGeorge) syndrome, and in the rare but interesting heritable disorder pseudohypoparathyroidism.

The most common cause of low serum calcium is chronic renal failure, and PTH levels are high (secondary hyperparathyroidism). In such patients it appears that the chronic effects of high levels of PTH on the heart and cardiovascular system predominate. Thus, the ability of PTH to stimulate G protein–coupled receptors may contribute to the LVH commonly observed in patients with chronic renal failure.[47] Systemic vascular resistance is often low, potentially reflecting the vasodilatory action of PTH. In patients with chronic renal failure, however, a variety of other important cardiovascular variables including anemia, accelerated atherosclerosis, hypertension, and changes in other vasoactive hormones contribute to the overall picture. Whether direct actions of the markedly elevated levels of PTH can produce alterations in myocyte physiology sufficient to cause further impairment of contractile function remains speculative.

Thyroid Gland

The thyroid gland and the heart share a close relationship arising in embryology. In ontogeny, the thyroid and heart Anlage migrate together. The close physiological relationship is affirmed by predictable changes in cardiovascular function across the entire range of thyroid disease states. In fact, cardiovascular manifestations are some of the most common and characteristic findings of hyperthyroidism.[50] To approach the diagnosis and management of thyroid hormone–mediated cardiac disease states, it is important to understand the cellular mechanisms of thyroid hormone action on the heart and vascular smooth muscle cells.[51]

CELLULAR MECHANISMS OF THYROID HORMONE ACTION ON THE HEART

Under the regulation of thyroid stimulating hormone (thyrotropin, TSH), the thyroid gland has the unique property of concentrating serum iodide and through a series of enzymatic steps synthesizes predominantly tetraiodothyronine (T_4, 85 percent) and a smaller percentage of triiodothyronine (T_3, 15 percent) (Fig. 79-3).[52] The major source of T_3 synthesis is conversion by 5′ monodeiodination primarily in the liver and to a lesser degree in the kidney.[53] A variety of studies have confirmed that T_3 is the active form of thyroid hormone and accounts for the vast majority of biological effects, including stimulation of tissue thermogenesis, alterations in the expression of various cellular proteins, and actions on the heart and vascular smooth muscle cells.[50,54] Serum free T_3 in turn is available to be taken up by a process of facilitated diffusion within cells, where it appears to pass without additional protein binding to the cell nucleus (Fig. 79-4). Most data indicate that the cardiac myocyte cannot metabolize T_4 to T_3 and therefore, all nuclear actions and changes observed in gene expression result from changes in blood levels of T_3. The cardiac myocyte expresses both the alpha and beta isoforms of the thyroid hormone receptors (TRs), which arise from two separate genes. These genes give rise to splice variants $TRalpha_1$ and $TRalpha_2$, of which only the former binds thyroid hormone, as well as $TRbeta_1$, $TRbeta_2$, and $TRbeta_3$[54] (see Fig. 79-1). It has been suggested, although direct confirmatory data are lacking, that $TRalpha_1$ is the predominant T_3 binding isoform in the heart and that isoform specificity may in turn determine myocyte-specific gene expression.[51,54] Similarly to the steroid and retinoic acid family of receptor proteins, the TRs act by binding as either homodimers or heterodimers to the thyroid hormone response elements in a promoter region of specific genes.[54] Binding to the promoter regions can either activate or repress gene expression.[55]

The cardiac proteins transcriptionally regulated by thyroid hormone are listed in Table 79-1. They include structural as well as regulatory proteins and also a variety of cardiac membrane ion channels and cell surface receptors, thus providing a molecular mechanism to explain many of the diverse effects of thyroid hormone on the heart. The first reported and the best studied to date have been the myosin heavy chain isoforms alpha and beta.[56] However, in the human ventricle, myosin isoform expression is primarily beta and there appears to be little if any alteration in isoform expression accompanying thyroid disease states.[57] There are changes in myosin heavy chain isoform expression in the human atria in a variety of disease states including congestive heart failure, and it remains to be determined whether these changes are thyroid hormone mediated.[58]

The sarcoplasmic reticulum calcium-activated adenosine triphosphatase (ATPase) is an important ion pump that determines the magnitude of myocyte calcium cycling (see also Chap. 19). The reuptake of calcium into the sarcoplasmic reticulum early in diastole in part determines the rate at which the left ventricle relaxes (isovolumetric relaxation time).[50] The activity of sarcoendoplasmic reticulum Ca^{2+}-ATPase (SERCA2), in turn, is regulated by the polymeric protein phospholamban, with its ability to inhibit SERCA activity further modified by the level of phosphorylation of the individual phospholamban monomers.[59] Inotropic agents that enhance cardiac contractility through increases in myocyte cyclic AMP do so by stimulating the phosphorylation of phospholamban. Thyroid hormone inhibits the genetic expression of phospholamban and increases phospholamban phosphorylation,[60] and genetically engineered animals deficient in phospholamban do not further increase cardiac contractility after exposure to excess thyroid hormone.[59] These data indicate that thyroid hormone exerts most of its direct effects on cardiac contractility by regulating calcium cycling through the SERCA-phospholamban system both transcriptionally and post-transcriptionally. Somewhat in conflict with these conclusions is the observation that patients with a homozygous deletion of phospholamban develop a dilated cardiomyopathy.[61] This molecular mechanism can explain why diastolic function varies inversely across the entire spectrum of thyroid disease states (Fig. 79–5).[50,62,63] In addition, beta-adrenergic blockade of the heart in hyperthyroidism does not decrease the rapid diastolic relaxation, further dissociating the thyroid hormone from the adrenergic effects of thyrotoxicosis.[50]

Changes in other myocyte genes, including Na^+, K^+-ATPase, account for the increase in basal oxygen consumption of the experimental hyperthyroid heart as well as explain the decrease in digitalis sensitivity of hyperthyroid patients. A variety of studies have shown that thyroid hormone can regulate the genetic expression of its own nuclear receptors within the cardiac myocyte (see Table 79–1).

In addition to the well-characterized nuclear effects of thyroid hormone, a growing body of cardiac responses to thyroid hormone appear to be mediated through nongenomic mechanisms,[64] as suggested by their relatively rapid onset of action (faster than can be accounted for by changes in gene expression and protein synthesis) and failure to be affected by inhibitors of gene transcription. The significance of these diverse actions remains to be established. They may alter the functional properties of membrane ion channels and pumps including the sodium channel and the inward-rectifying potassium current (I_k).

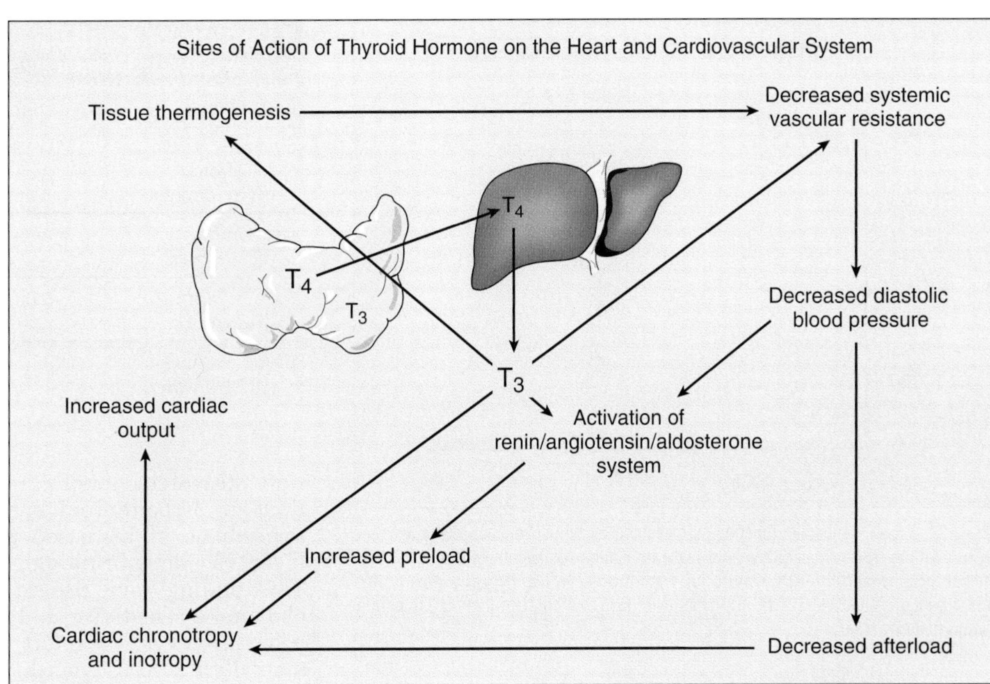

FIGURE 79–3 Schematic representation of thyroid hormone metabolism and the effects of triiodothyronine (T_3) on the heart and systemic vasculature.

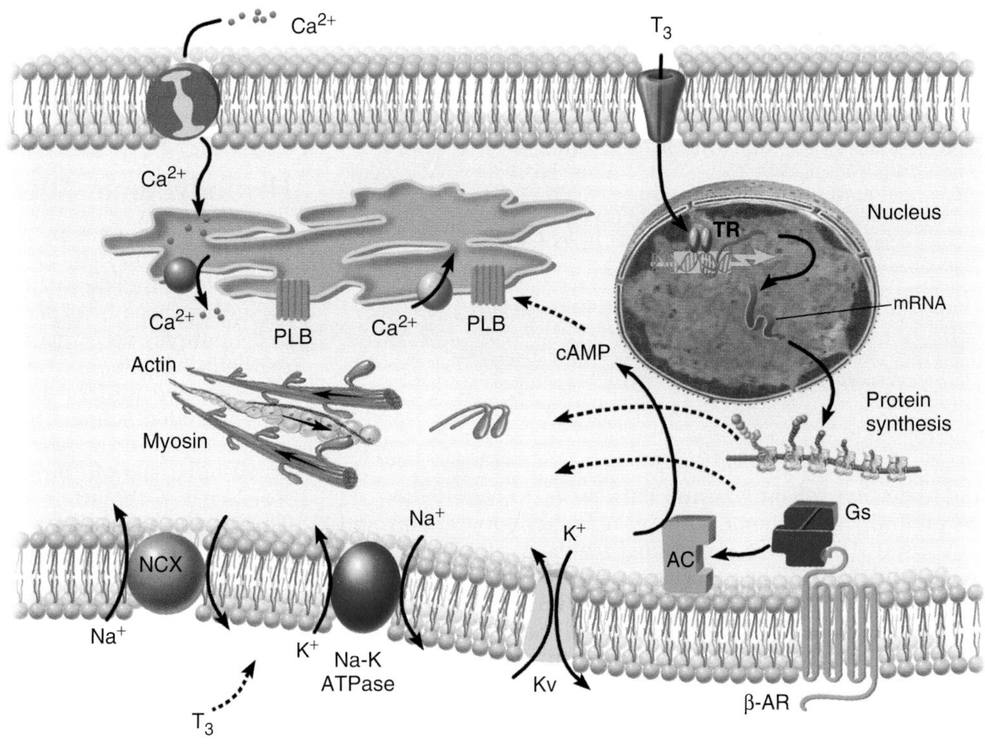

FIGURE 79–4 Triiodothyronine (T_3) enters the cell and binds to nuclear T_3 receptors. The complex then binds to thyroid hormone response elements (TREs) and regulates transcription of specific genes. Nonnuclear T_3 actions on ion channels for sodium (Na^+), potassium (K^+), and calcium (Ca^{2+}) ions are indicated. ATPase = adenosine triphosphatase; cAMP = cyclic adenosine monophosphate; mRNA = messenger RNA; TR = T_3 receptor protein; AC = adenylyl cyclase; β-AR = beta adrenergic receptor; Kv = voltage-gated potassium channel; NCX = sodium channel; PLB = phospholamban.

Thyroid Function Testing

A number of sensitive and specific laboratory tests can establish a diagnosis of thyroid disease with a high degree of precision. Serum TSH is the most widely used and most sensitive measure for the diagnosis of both hypothyroidism

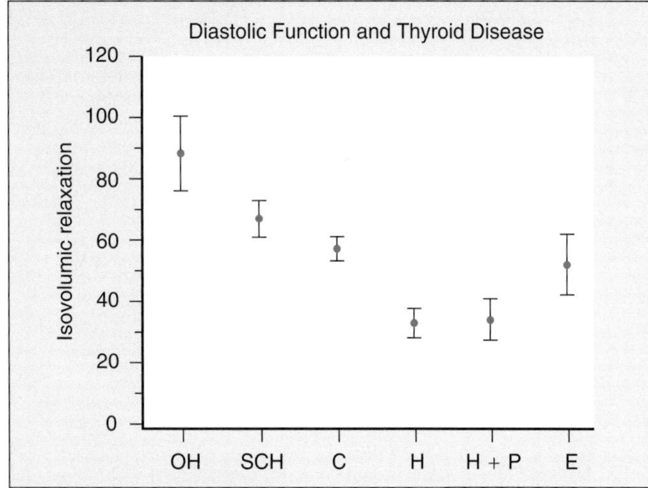

FIGURE 79–5 Diastolic function as measured by the isovolumic relaxation time varies over the entire range of thyroid disease including overt hypothyroidism (OH), subclinical hypothyroidism (SCH), control (C), hyperthyroidism (H), hyperthyroidism after beta-adrenergic blockade (H + P), and hyperthyroidism after treatment to restore normal thyroid function studies (E).

TABLE 79–1 Thyroid Hormone Regulation of Cardiac Gene Expression

Positively Regulated	Negatively Regulated
Alpha-myosin heavy chain	Beta-myosin heavy chain
Sarcoplasmic reticulum Ca^{2+}-ATPase	Phospholamban
Na^+, K^+-ATPase	Na^+/Ca^{2+} exchanger
Voltage-gated potassium channels (Kv1.5, Kv4.2, Kv4.3)	Thyroid hormone receptor alpha1
Atrial and brain natriuretic peptide	Adenylyl cyclase (AC) types V, VI
Malic enzyme	Guanine nucleotide–binding protein G_i
Beta-adrenergic receptor	
Guanine nucleotide–binding protein G_s	
Adenine nucleotide transporter 1	

ATPase = adenosine triphosphatase.

and hyperthyroidism.[65] Serum TSH levels uniformly increase (>5 μIU/mL) in patients with primary hypothyroidism and conversely, because of the normal feedback of excess levels of T_4 (and T_3) on the pituitary synthesis and secretion of TSH, the levels are low (<0.01 to 0.001 μIU/mL) in hyperthyroidism. Measures of free T_4 (and rarely free T_3) can be useful when coexistent hepatic, nutritional, or genetic disease may alter thyroxine-binding globulin content. Autoimmune thyroid diseases (Hashimoto and Graves) can be further diagnosed by the use of serological measures of antithyroid antibodies, most specifically antithyroid peroxidase or antithyroglobulin antibodies.

Thyroid Hormone–Catecholamine Interaction

Early observations of the heart in hyperthyroidism emphasize the similarity to that of hyperadrenergic states and moreover suggest enhanced sensitivity to catecholamines in this setting. This postulate forms the basis for the test described by Goetsch in 1918 in which hyperthyroidism could be diagnosed by demonstrating a marked cardioacceleration and blood pressure response to subcutaneous doses of epinephrine. Measurements of circulating catecholamine concentrations in hyperthyroid subjects revealed that despite the appearance of increased adrenergic signs and symptoms, levels of epinephrine and norepinephrine were decreased. This finding gave rise to the concept of enhanced catecholamine sensitivity, and molecular measures of increased beta$_1$-adrenergic receptors on cardiac myocytes in experimentally induced hyperthyroidism support this mechanism. A carefully controlled study of subhuman primates, however, has clearly demonstrated that there is no increase in sensitivity of the heart or cardiovascular system to catecholamines in experimental hyperthyroidism.[66] Accompanying the increased levels of beta$_1$-adrenergic receptors and guanosine triphosphate binding proteins, thyroid hormone decreases the genetic expression of cardiac-specific (V, VI) adenylyl cyclase catalytic subunit isoforms and thereby maintains cellular response to beta-adrenergic agonists within normal limits.[67]

TABLE 79–2 Cardiovascular Changes with Thyroid Disease

Parameter	Normal	Hyperthyroid	Hypothyroid
Systemic vascular resistance (dyne-cm) sec^{-5}	1500-1700	700-1200	2100-2700
Heart rate (beats/min)	72-84	88-130	60-80
Cardiac output (liter/min)	5.8	>7.0	<4.5
Blood volume (% of normal)	100	105.5	84.5

Hemodynamic Alterations in Thyroid Disease

Predictable changes in myocardial contractility and cardiovascular hemodynamics occur across the entire spectrum of thyroid disease (Table 79–2; see Fig. 79–5).[50] Multiple studies including those in experimental animals as well as invasive and noninvasive measurements in patients indicate that T_3 regulates cardiac inotropy and chronotropy through a variety of direct and indirect mechanisms.[50,68-70] Figure 79–3 shows the integrated schema by which T_3 acts on tissues throughout the body to increase tissue thermogenesis. Direct effects on vascular smooth muscle cells decrease systemic vascular resistance of the arterioles of the peripheral circulation.[68,71] There is a decrease in mean arterial pressure and activation of the renin-angiotensin-aldosterone system and an increase in renal sodium reabsorption. The increase in plasma volume coupled with an increase in erythropoietin leads to an increase in blood volume and a rise in cardiac preload.[70] Thus, a decrease in systemic vascular resistance (by as much as 50 percent), coupled with increases in venous return and preload, increases cardiac output. Cardiac output may more than double in hyperthyroidism and conversely may decrease by as much as 30 to 40 percent in hypothyroidism. Studies using positron-emission tomography (PET) measurements of acetate metabolism have demonstrated that the marked increase in cardiac output in hyperthyroidism is accomplished with no change in energy efficiency.[72]

T_3 appears to reduce systemic vascular resistance by both direct effects on vascular smooth muscle cells and changes in the vascular endothelium potentially involving the synthesis and secretion of nitric oxide.[68] The vasodilatory effect of T_3 can be observed within hours after administration of T_3 to patients undergoing coronary artery bypass grafting as well as patients with chronic congestive heart failure.[58,71] Arterial

TABLE 79–3 Cardiovascular Symptoms of Hyperthyroidism	
Palpitations	Anginal-like chest pain
Exercise intolerance	Peripheral edema
Dyspnea	Congestive heart failure

compliance also falls in hypothyroidism and may explain why mean arterial and diastolic pressures are low and peak systolic pressures increase.[69] Thus, the combination of increased cardiac output and decreased arterial compliance, which may be more pronounced in older patients with some degree of arterial vascular disease, leads to systolic hypertension in as many as 30 percent of patients.[69] In hypothyroidism, systemic vascular resistance may be increased by as much as 30 percent. Mean arterial pressure rises with as many as 20 percent of patients having significant diastolic hypertension.[69] Even mild hypothyroidism may decrease endothelium-derived relaxing factors.[73] The diastolic hypertension of hypothyroidism is frequently associated with a low renin level and a decrease in hepatic synthesis of renin substrate. This leads to a characteristically low level of salt sensitivity, again reinforcing the importance of an increase in systemic vascular resistance underlying the mechanism for diastolic hypertension.[74]

Hyperthyroidism

Cardiovascular symptoms are an integral and often the predominant clinical presentation of patients with hyperthyroidism (Table 79–3). Palpitations resulting from an increase in the rate and force of cardiac contractility are present in the majority of patients.[75] The increase in heart rate results from both an increase in sympathetic tone and a decrease in parasympathetic stimulation.[75] It is common to observe heart rates higher than 90 beats/min both at rest and during sleep; the normal diurnal variation in heart rate is blunted and the increase during exercise is exaggerated. Many hyperthyroid patients experience exercise intolerance and exertional dyspnea, in part because of weakness in skeletal and respiratory muscle.[76] In the setting of a low vascular resistance and increased preload, cardiac functional reserve is compromised and cannot rise further to accommodate the demands of submaximal or maximal exercise.[77]

A subset of thyrotoxic patients can experience angina-like chest pain. In older patients with known or suspected coronary artery disease, the increase in cardiac work associated with the increase in cardiac output and cardiac contractility of hyperthyroidism can produce myocardial ischemia, which can respond to beta-adrenergic blocking agents or the restoration of a euthyroid state. In rare patients, usually younger women, a syndrome of chest pain at rest associates with ischemic ECG changes. Cardiac catheterization has demonstrated that the majority of these patients have angiographically normal coronary arteries; however, coronary vasospasm has been reported similar to that found in variant angina. Myocardial infarction rarely develops, and these patients appear to respond to calcium channel blockers or nitroglycerin.

Atrial Fibrillation

The most common rhythm disturbance in patients with hyperthyroidism is sinus tachycardia.[75] Its clinical impact, however, is overshadowed by that of patients with atrial fibrillation resulting from thyrotoxicosis. The prevalence of atrial fibrillation and the less common forms of supraventricular tachycardia in this disease ranges between 2 and 20 percent.[78,79] When compared with a prevalence of atrial fibrillation of 2.3 percent in a control population with normal thyroid function, the prevalence of atrial fibrillation in overt hyperthyroidism was 13.8 percent.[79] It was reported that in more than 13,000 hyperthyroid patients the prevalence of atrial fibrillation was less than 2 percent, perhaps because of earlier recognition and disease treatment. When the same group of patients was analyzed for age distribution, it was seen that there was a stepwise increase in prevalence in each decade, peaking at about 15 percent in patients older than 70 years.[78] The latter study confirms essentially all reports that atrial fibrillation related to hyperthyroidism is more common with advancing age. In a study of unselected patients presenting with atrial fibrillation, less than 1 percent of cases were caused by overt hyperthyroidism.[80] Thus, the yield of abnormal thyroid function testing including a low serum TSH appears to be low in patients with new-onset atrial fibrillation. However, the ability to restore thyrotoxic patients to a euthyroid state and sinus rhythm justifies TSH testing in all patients with the recent onset of otherwise unexplained atrial fibrillation or other supraventricular arrhythmias.

Treatment of atrial fibrillation in the setting of hyperthyroidism includes beta-adrenergic blockade using one of a variety of $beta_1$-selective or nonselective agents to control the ventricular response. This symptomatic measure can be accomplished rapidly, but the treatments leading to a restoration of the euthyroid state require more time. Digitalis has been used to control the ventricular response in hyperthyroidism-associated atrial fibrillation; however, because of the increased rate of digitalis clearance as well as decreased sensitivity of the drug action resulting from high cellular levels of Na^+,K^+-ATPase and the presence of decreased parasympathetic tone, patients usually require higher doses of this medication. Anticoagulation in patients with hyperthyroidism and atrial fibrillation is controversial.[50,81] The potential for systemic or cerebral embolization must be weighed against the risk of bleeding and complications related to this therapy. Whether hyperthyroid patients are at increased risk for systemic embolization is not totally resolved. In a retrospective study of patients with hyperthyroidism, it was age rather than the presence of atrial fibrillation that was the main risk factor for embolization. Retrospective analysis of large series of patients did not demonstrate a prevalence of thromboembolic events greater than the reported risk of major bleeding from warfarin treatment.[81] Thus, in younger patients with hyperthyroidism and atrial fibrillation in the absence of other heart disease, hypertension, or other independent risk factors for embolization, the benefits of anticoagulation have not been proved and may well be outweighed by the risk. Aspirin provides an alternative for lowering risk for embolic events in young people and can be used safely.

Successful treatment of hyperthyroidism with either radioiodine or antithyroid drugs and restoration of normal serum levels of T_4 and T_3 associates with reversion to sinus rhythm in two-thirds of patients within 2 to 3 months.[78] In older patients or in the setting of atrial fibrillation of longer duration, the rate of reversion to sinus rhythm is lower and therefore electrical or pharmacological cardioversion should be attempted but only after the patient has been rendered euthyroid. The majority of patients (90 percent) can be restored to sinus rhythm by either electrical cardioversion or pharmacological measures, and many remain in sinus rhythm for periods up to 5 years or more. In a regimen in which disopyramide 300 mg/d was added for 3 months after successful cardioversion, patients were more likely to remain in sinus rhythm than those not treated.[81]

Heart Failure

The cardiovascular alterations in hyperthyroidism include increased resting cardiac output and enhanced cardiac contractility (Fig. 79–6; see Table 79–2). Despite this, a minority

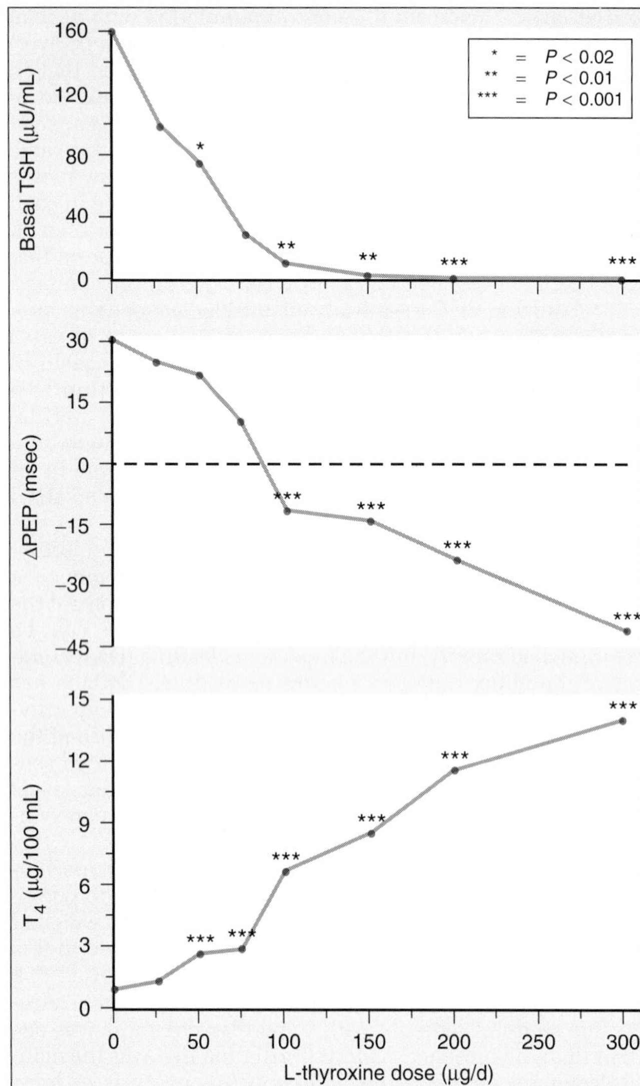

FIGURE 79–6 Response to stepwise L-thyroxine sodium treatment of hypothyroid patients as assessed by serum thyrotropin (TSH), serum tetraiodothyronine (T_4), and the improvement in left ventricular contractility as measured noninvasively by the preejection period (PEP). (From Crowley WF Jr, Ridgway EC, Bough EW, et al: Noninvasive evaluation of cardiac function in hypothyroidism. Response to gradual thyroxine replacement. N Engl J Med 296:1, 1977.)

of patients present with symptoms including dyspnea on exertion, orthopnea, and paroxysmal nocturnal dyspnea as well as signs demonstrating peripheral edema, neck vein distention, and an S_3 indicative of heart failure (see Table 79–3). This complex of findings coupled with a failure to increase the left ventricular ejection fraction with exercise has suggested the possibility of a hyperthyroid cardiomyopathy. The term often used in this setting, "high-output failure," is inappropriate; although resting cardiac output is as much as two to three times normal, the exercise intolerance appears to be a result not of cardiac failure but rather of skeletal muscle weakness.[50,76] High-output states, however, can increase renal sodium reabsorption, expand plasma volume, and cause development of peripheral edema, pleural effusions, and neck vein distention. Interestingly, although systemic vascular resistance falls with hyperthyroidism, the pulmonary vascular bed is not similarly affected and as a result of the increase in output to the pulmonary circulation, there is an increase in pulmonary artery pressures. This effect results in a rise in mean venous pressure, neck vein distention, hepatic congestion, and peripheral edema of the type associated with primary pulmonary hypertension or right-sided heart failure.[69]

Patients with longstanding hyperthyroidism and marked sinus tachycardia or atrial fibrillation can experience the development of low cardiac output, impaired cardiac contractility with a low ejection fraction, an S_3, and pulmonary congestion, all consistent with congestive heart failure.[50] Review of such cases suggests that impairment in left ventricular function is the result of a prolonged high heart rate and the development of rate-related heart failure. When the left ventricle becomes dilated, mitral regurgitation may also develop. Recognition of this entity is important because treatments aimed at slowing heart rate or controlling the ventricular response in atrial fibrillation appear to improve left ventricular function even before initiation of antithyroid therapy.[50] Because these patients are critically ill, they should be managed in an intensive care unit setting. Some patients with hyperthyroidism (similar to the overall congestive heart failure population) do not tolerate initiation of beta-adrenergic blocking drugs in full doses, and treatment can be started with lower doses of short-acting beta-blocking drugs in conjunction with classical forms of treatment of acute congestive heart failure, including diuresis.

The increase in rate pressure product and oxygen consumption that results from hyperthyroidism can impair cardiac function in older patients with known or suspected ischemic, hypertensive, or valvular heart disease. It is important to recognize promptly the cardiac manifestations of hyperthyroidism in older patients as they may have a higher risk for adverse cardiovascular and cerebral vascular outcomes.[82]

Treatment

Treatment of patients with thyrotoxic cardiac disease should include a beta-adrenergic antagonist to lower the heart rate to 10 or 15 percent above normal. This treatment causes the tachycardia-mediated component of ventricular dysfunction to improve, whereas the direct inotropic effects of thyroid hormone persist (see Fig. 79–4).[50] The rapid onset of action and the improvement in many of the signs and symptoms of hyperthyroidism indicate that most patients with overt symptoms should receive beta-blocking agents. Definitive therapy then can be accomplished safely with iodine-131 alone or in combination with an antithyroid drug.

Hypothyroidism

In contrast to the dramatic clinical signs and symptoms of hyperthyroidism, the cardiovascular findings of hypothyroidism are more subtle. Mild degrees of bradycardia, diastolic hypertension, a narrow pulse pressure and a relatively quiet precordium, and decreased intensity of the apical impulse are characteristic. Hemodynamic changes of hypothyroidism are diametrically opposite to those of hyperthyroidism (see Table 79–2) and explain many of the findings on physical examination. Despite the decrease in cardiac output and contractility of the hypothyroid myocardium, studies of myocardial metabolism using PET scan methodology have shown that the hypothyroid myocardium is energy inefficient. The oxygen cost of work increases primarily as a result of the increase in afterload.[83] Treatment of hypothyroid patients with restoration of a euthyroid state resolves these changes in parallel with a return of systemic vascular resistance to lower levels.

Hypothyroidism also produces increases in total and low-density lipoprotein (LDL) cholesterol as well as apolipoprotein B.[84] Although thyroid hormone can alter cholesterol metabolism through multiple mechanisms, including a decrease in biliary excretion, it appears that changes in LDL metabolism related to decreases in LDL receptor number are a primary mechanism. Thus, the finding of a direct relationship between the level of TSH as a measure of hypothyroidism and serum total cholesterol and LDL cholesterol is not surprising.[85]

Serum creatine kinase (CK) is elevated by 50 percent to 10-fold in as many as 30 percent of patients with hypothyroidism. Analysis of isoform specificity indicates that more than 96 percent is the muscle form (MM), consistent with a skeletal muscle origin of increased enzyme release.[86] In contrast to the half-life of CK after acute myocardial infarction (12 hours), the half-life in hypothyroidism after initiation of standard oral thyroid hormone replacement is approximately 10 to 14 days. Pericardial effusions can occur, consistent with observation that patients with hypothyroidism have an increase in volume of distribution of albumin and a decrease in lymphatic clearance function. Occasionally, the pericardial effusions are quite large, causing the appearance of cardiomegaly on routine chest radiographs. Echocardiography demonstrates small to moderate effusions in as many as 30 percent of overtly hypothyroid patients. The presence of pericardial fluid in hypothyroid patients does not compromise cardiac output, cardiac tamponade is exceedingly rare, and the effusion resolves over a period of weeks to months after initiation of thyroid hormone replacement.

As a result of changes in ion channel expression, the electrocardiogram in hypothyroidism is characterized by sinus bradycardia, low voltage, and prolongation of the action potential duration and the QT interval. The latter, in turn, predisposes patients to ventricular arrhythmias, and there are case reports of patients with acquired torsades de pointes that has improved or completely resolved with thyroid hormone replacement.[50]

As a result of increases in risk factors, including hypercholesterolemia, hypertension, and elevated levels of homocysteine, patients with hypothyroidism may have increased risk for atherosclerosis and coronary and systemic vascular disease.[87] Studies have shown increases in abdominal aortic atherosclerosis in patients with even mild hypothyroidism.[88] Small autopsy series have shown an increase in coronary artery disease, but only in patients with both hypertension and hypercholesterolemia. Whether patients with hypothyroidism have an increase in coronary artery disease is an important clinical issue. Noninvasive studies including thallium scanning have demonstrated abnormalities in perfusion suggestive of myocardial ischemia, but these defects appear to resolve with thyroid hormone treatment and may not reflect flow limitation related to fixed stenoses.

In patients younger than 50 years, it is possible to initiate full replacement doses of L-thyroxine (0.1 to 0.15 mg/d) without concern about untoward cardiac effects. In patients older than 50 with known or suspected coronary artery disease, the issue is more complicated. In patients with known coronary artery disease and a coexistent diagnosis of hypothyroidism, three major issues need to be addressed.

The first issue is whether coronary artery revascularization is required before initiating thyroid hormone replacement. If patients are not candidates for percutaneous intervention, coronary artery bypass grafting can be accomplished in patients with unstable angina, left main coronary artery disease, or three-vessel disease with impaired left ventricular function, even in the setting of overt hypothyroidism. Rarely, a patient is so profoundly hypothyroid that bleeding times and partial thromboplastin times are prolonged, requiring preoperative supplementation of clotting factors. Thyroid hormone replacement can be delayed until the postoperative period, when it can be administered in full dose either parenterally or orally.[71]

The second issue concerns patients with known stable cardiac disease in whom cardiac revascularization is not clinically indicated. Treatment of such patients should begin with low doses (12.5 μg) of L-thyroxine with doses increased stepwise (12.5 to 25 μg) every 6 to 8 weeks until serum TSH is normal. Thyroid hormone replacement in this setting and its ability to lower systemic vascular resistance and lower afterload as well as improve myocardial efficiency can actually decrease clinical signs of myocardial ischemia. Beta-adrenergic blocking agents are an ideal concomitant therapy to control heart rate.

The third issue concerns the group of patients who, although potentially at risk for coronary artery disease, exhibit no clinical signs or symptoms. In this group, thyroid hormone replacement can be started at low doses generally in the range of 25 to 50 μg/d and increased 25 μg every 6 to 8 weeks until serum TSH is normal. Should signs or symptoms of ischemic heart disease develop, the same recommendations apply as to patients with known underlying heart disease.

In all patients, thyroid hormone replacement should continue until serum TSH is normal and the patients are clinically euthyroid. The concept that these patients benefit from maintenance of "mild hypothyroidism" is not supported by the known effects of thyroid hormone on the heart and cardiovascular system. Thyroid hormone replacement should be accomplished with purified preparations of levothyroxine sodium. Preparations containing T_4 with T_3 (thyroid extract) or the existing purified preparations of T_3 do not offer benefit. The short half-life of T_3 and the inability to maintain serum levels within normal range in patients so treated can add to cardiac risk.[89]

Diagnosis

Hashimoto disease, radioiodine therapy for Graves disease, and iodine deficiency (in parts of the world where that remains a public health problem) are the leading causes of hypothyroidism and produce diagnostic elevations in serum TSH.[65] Thus, the finding of elevated TSH is sufficient to establish the diagnosis and form the basis for treatment. In routine practice, additional testing with a serum T_4 and T_3 resin uptake test is confirmatory. The prevalence of hypothyroidism is estimated as 3 to 4 percent for overt disease and 7 to 10 percent for the milder forms of disease. Thus, TSH screening can be advised for all adults and particularly patients demonstrating hypertension, hypercholesterolemia, hypertriglyceridemia, coronary or peripheral vascular disease, unexplained pericardial or pleural effusions, and a variety of musculoskeletal syndromes.[52]

Treatment

The response to treatment of hypothyroidism is predictable, especially from a cardiovascular perspective. Stepwise thyroid hormone replacement using levothyroxine sodium (Levoxyl, Synthroid) produces an incremental decrease in serum TSH, serum cholesterol, and serum CK and an improvement in left ventricular performance. Full replacement is accomplished when serum TSH is normal.[65] In the rare condition of myxedema coma, which is characterized by severe and longstanding hypothyroidism with the development of hypothermia, altered mental status, hypotension, bradycardia, and hypoventilation, the need for thyroid hormone replacement is more emergent and treatment can be accomplished with either T_4 at 100 μg/d or T_3 at 25 μg/d administered intravenously. These patients often require intensive care unit monitoring with volume repletion, gentle warming, and ventilatory support in the presence of CO_2 retention. Administration of hydrocortisone (100 mg every 8 hours) should be undertaken until results of serum cortisol testing are obtained. When patients are treated in this manner, hemodynamics including systemic vascular resistance, cardiac output, and heart rate improve within 24 to 48 hours.

SUBCLINICAL THYROID DISEASE

In contrast to overt symptomatic thyroid disease, subclinical thyroid disease implies the absence of classical hyper- or hypothyroidism-related symptoms in patients with thyroid dysfunction. The definition has been further refined to include the demonstration of an abnormal TSH level in the presence of normal serum levels of total T_4 and free T_4.[65] With the advent of widespread TSH screening, the magnitude of subclinical thyroid disease may exceed that of overt disease by three- to fourfold.[85]

Subclinical Hypothyroidism

Subclinical hypothyroidism, defined by a TSH level above the upper range of the reference population (usually >5 μIU/ml), is seen in as many as 9 percent of unselected populations and prevalence clearly increases with advancing age.[85] In contrast to younger patients, in whom there is a strong female predilection, this difference is lost in older populations. Studies of lipid metabolism, atherosclerosis, cardiac contractility, and systemic vascular resistance are altered in subclinical hypothyroidism. Cholesterol levels rise in parallel with increments in TSH elevations starting at 5 μIU/L. In a large study of women in Rotterdam, it was noted that atherosclerosis and myocardial infarction were increased with odds ratios of 1.7 and 2.3, respectively, in women with subclinical hypothyroidism. Interestingly, the presence of antithyroid antibodies indicated heightened risk.[88] Restoration of serum TSH to normal after thyroid hormone replacement improved lipid levels, lowered systemic vascular resistance, and improved cardiac contractility.[90] In patients with subclinical hypothyroidism, isovolumetric relaxation times are prolonged while systolic contractile function is unchanged (see Fig. 79-6). Replacement with L-thyroxine sodium at a mean dose of 68 μg/d (range 50 to 100 μg/d) restored isovolumetric relaxation times to normal, and compared with those in the same patients before therapy, systemic vascular resistance declined and systolic function was significantly improved.[91] A variety of studies have indicated that the changes in systemic vascular resistance may result from alterations in endothelium-dependent vasodilation.[73,87] Taking these findings together, it seems appropriate to recommend thyroid hormone replacement for all patients with subclinical hypothyroidism from a cardiovascular perspective. The lack of untoward cardiac effects observed when serum TSH levels have been restored to normal indicates that the potential benefits far outweigh the risks of treatment.[50]

Subclinical Hyperthyroidism

Subclinical hyperthyroidism is diagnosed when serum TSH is low (<0.1 μIU/ml) and both T_4 and T_3 are normal.[65] The significance of subclinical hyperthyroidism was conclusively established from a study of atrial fibrillation in patients 60 years of age or older in the Framingham cohort.[92] Prevalence of atrial fibrillation after 10 years was 28 percent in the patients with subclinical hyperthyroidism compared with 11 percent in patients with normal thyroid function with a relative risk of 3.1 (Fig. 79-7). A population-based study of more than 1000 individuals with subclinical hyperthyroidism not receiving L-thyroxine therapy or antithyroid medication demonstrated that a TSH level less than 0.5 was associated with twofold increased mortality with relative risk of 2.3 to 3.3 from all causes, which in turn was largely accounted for by increases in cardiovascular mortality.[93]

Whereas the cardiovascular changes are well established, the management of patients with subclinical hyperthyroidism is controversial. Therapy can be individualized with regard to three specific groups. The first group includes patients receiving thyroid hormone replacement for hypothyroidism in whom the low TSH is thought to be the result of excess medication and reduction of the dose is indicated. The second group includes patients with a prior diagnosis of thyroid cancer currently receiving L-thyroxine for the purpose of TSH suppression. In younger patients or those with more advanced disease (stage 3 or 4), beta-adrenergic blocking agents can reverse many if not all of the cardiovascular manifestations including heart rate control, LVH, and atrial ectopy. In older patients or patients with milder disease, the degree of TSH suppression can be relaxed by lowering the T_4 dosage.[94]

The third group includes patients in whom subclinical hyperthyroidism results from endogenous thyroid gland overactivity, including Graves disease, chronic thyroiditis, nodular goiter, or autonomously functioning adenoma. In this category, younger patients appear to have few or no untoward effects but older patients are potentially at risk from atrial fibrillation. In patients older than 60 years, antithyroid therapy (methimazole [Tapazole] 5 to 10 mg/d) can produce improvement, and in patients who do respond consideration should be given to the use of radioiodine for definitive treatment.[50]

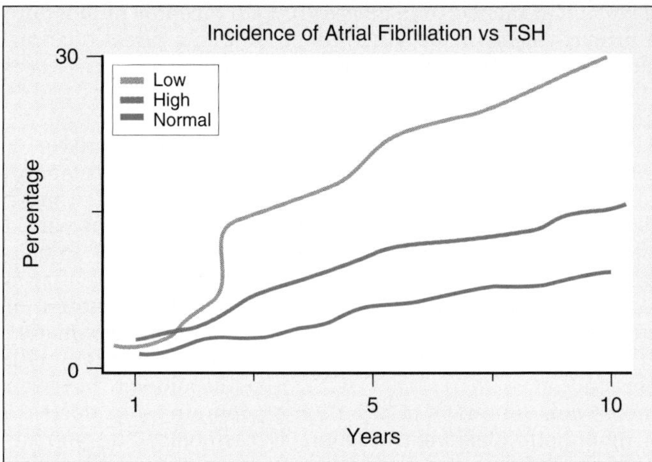

FIGURE 79–7 Atrial fibrillation in subclinical hyperthyroidism. Low thyrotropin (TSH) designates patients who have serum TSH less than 0.1 μIU/ml. (Adapted from Sawin CT: Subclinical hyperthyroidism and atrial fibrillation. Thyroid 12:501, 2002.)

Amiodarone and Thyroid Function

Amiodarone is an iodine-rich antiarrhythmic agent effective in the treatment of both ventricular and atrial tachyarrhythmias. It is currently used extensively in patients with a variety of cardiac diseases. As a result of the 30 percent by weight iodine content, this drug commonly causes abnormalities in thyroid function testing in patients treated for either short or long periods of time.[95] Similarly to other iodinated drugs, amiodarone inhibits the 5′ monodeiodination of T_4 in both the liver and the pituitary. Inhibition of T_4 metabolism in the liver decreases serum T_3 and increases serum T_4 while serum TSH levels initially remain normal. With more chronic treatment and as the total iodide content of the body rises, there is a potential for inhibition of T_4 synthesis and release from the thyroid gland, producing a rise in TSH. In patients with underlying goiter, autoimmune thyroid disease, or enzymatic defects in thyroid hormone biosynthesis and in some patients without any risk factors there is a progression to overt chemical and clinical hypothyroidism with a marked rise in serum TSH.[95] The overall prevalence of hypothyroidism in amiodarone-treated patients is reported to be between 15 and 20 percent. It is important to note that the symptoms of hypothyroidism in this setting can be quite subtle and significant hypothyroidism can occur even in their absence.

Thyroid function should be measured every 3 months in all patients receiving amiodarone. The effect on thyroid function does not depend on dose and can occur any time after initiating treatment and, because of the high lipid solubility and long half-life of the drug, for periods up to a year after discontinuation of therapy.[95]

Less common but perhaps more challenging is the development of amiodarone-induced thyrotoxicosis. Although it was initially not observed in the iodine-replete American population, the experience from Italy suggested that it occurred with a prevalence as high as 10 percent.[95] The onset was often sudden and could occur shortly after drug initiation, during chronic treatment, or up to 1 year after stopping therapy. Although the pathogenesis is multifactorial, early studies distinguished two forms of amiodarone-induced thyrotoxicosis. Type I occurs primarily in patients with preexisting thyroid disease and most commonly in iodine-deficient areas. These patients may rarely have an increase in 24-hour radioiodine uptake measures and frequently some measures of thyroid autoimmunity, including antithyroid antibodies. Color flow Doppler sonography of the thyroid gland has a "characteristic" appearance consistent with other forms of autoimmune thyroid disease. In contrast, type II disease was identified as a form of thyroiditis presumably mediated by a variety of proinflammatory cytokines including interleukin-6.[96] This disease is primarily a destructive process causing release of preformed thyroid hormone, which may continue for periods of weeks and months and is most often associated with low to absent radioiodine uptake. Further experience has shown that these two types have substantial overlap for many of the distinguishing parameters.

Because of the increased thyroidal and total body iodine content, use of iodine-131 is almost always ineffective. Similarly, treatment with antithyroid drugs has marginal effectiveness. Corticosteroids (prednisone 20 to 40 mg/d) have been recommended and proved to be of benefit, perhaps with increased utility in patients with type II disease in whom serum levels of interleukin-6 are high.[95] Alternatively, corticosteroids can be instituted in all patients; when they are effective, the response usually occurs within 1 week of initiating treatment. Treatment can then be tapered over 3 months leading to disease remission.[95] In patients unresponsive to glucocorticoids with evidence of hyperthyroidism including weight loss, tachycardia, palpitations, worsening angina, or other untoward cardiac effects, treatment with a combination of antithyroid therapy (methimazole 10 to 30 mg/d) and potassium perchlorate is variably effective.[97] Treatment can cause significant side effects including bone marrow toxicity resulting from the potassium perchlorate. A report confirms that total thyroidectomy can be performed safely and is an effective means of rapidly reversing the hyperthyroidism. Preoperative treatment with beta-adrenergic blocking drugs is indicated, and there have been no reported cases of resulting thyroid storm.[98]

An important issue is whether amiodarone-mediated thyroid dysfunction should mandate discontinuation of the drug. Because certain patients require amiodarone therapy to manage critical arrhythmias and the duration of drug retention in the body in lipid-soluble stores is in excess of 6 months, it seems prudent to continue amiodarone therapy while making separate management plans to deal with the thyroid dysfunction.

CHANGES IN THYROID HORMONE METABOLISM THAT ACCOMPANY CARDIAC DISEASE

In addition to the changes in thyroid function, which can result from classical thyroid disease, there are primary alterations in serum total and free T_3 and occasionally serum T_4 that accompany a variety of acute and chronic illnesses including sepsis, starvation, and cardiac disease.[99] In the absence of thyroid gland abnormality, changes in serum T_3 levels result from alterations in thyroid hormone metabolism. These cases have been referred to as "nonthyroidal illness." The mechanism for this decrease in serum T_3 is multifactorial and in part related to a decrease in 5′ monodeiodination in the liver.

A wide variety of acute and chronic cardiac diseases can alter thyroid hormone metabolism associated with marked declines in serum T_3. A population-based study of patients with cardiac disease has shown that a low serum T_3 level is a strong predictor of all-cause and cardiovascular mortality.[100] Following uncomplicated acute myocardial infarction, serum T_3 levels fall by about 20 percent and reach a nadir after approximately 96 hours. Experimental myocardial infarction in animal models produces a similar decrease in serum T_3, and replacement of T_3 levels to normal has been reported to increase left ventricular contractile function.[58]

Both children and adults undergoing cardiac surgery with cardiopulmonary bypass demonstrate a predictable fall in serum T_3 in the perioperative period.[101] Although treatment strategies using acute administration of intravenous T_3 to adults after coronary artery bypass grafting have resulted in an improvement in cardiac output and a fall in systemic vascular resistance, there was no alteration in overall mortality.[71] When the prevalence of atrial fibrillation was studied in this group of patients, however, it was shown to be decreased by as much as 50 percent compared with that in age-matched control subjects.[102] Pediatric cardiac patients, especially those undergoing surgery in the neonatal period, demonstrate an even greater decline in serum T_3 that can last for longer periods of time. The low postoperative T_3 level identifies patients at increased risk for morbidity and mortality.[103] A prospective randomized study has shown, especially in neonates, that the degree of therapeutic intervention and the need for postoperative inotropic agents are decreased by the administration of T_3 in doses sufficient to restore serum T_3 levels to normal.[104]

In patients with chronic congestive heart failure, the fall in serum T_3 is proportional to the severity of heart failure as assessed by the New York Heart Association classification.[58] As many as 30 percent of patients with heart failure have a low serum T_3, which occurs in both patients treated with amiodarone and those who are not.[58,100] In view of the deleterious effects of hypothyroidism on the myocardium, T_3 replacement may be of benefit. Human studies using a novel form of T_3 that is capable of restoring serum T_3 levels to normal and avoiding the peaks and valleys of drug levels associated with existing drug preparations are required to answer this question.[58]

Pheochromocytoma

Pheochromocytomas are primarily benign tumors arising from neuroectodermal chromaffin cells primarily within the adrenal medulla and abdomen, but they may arise anywhere within plexus of sympathetic adrenergic nerves. Although the prevalence is probably less than one per 2000 cases of diastolic hypertension, the importance of pheochromocytoma derives from the dramatic way in which symptoms can arise. Various autopsy studies have shown that in 75 percent of patients the diagnosis was not clinically suspected and in more than half it was thought to be a factor contributing to mortality.[105]

A variety of tumor characteristics have been established.[106] Most pheochromocytomas are 1 cm or greater in size, the vast majority arise as a unilateral adrenal lesion, and extraadrenal tumors are more common in children. Although most tumors are sporadic, approximately 10 percent are familial, and the latter are more often bilateral or occur in an extraadrenal location. When pheochromocytoma coexists with medullary thyroid carcinoma or occasionally with hyperparathyroidism, it is a designated multiple endocrine neoplasia (MEN) syndrome type II. These patients have a mutation in the RET proto-oncogene. In patients with MEN IIB, pheochromocytomas coexist with medullary thyroid cancer and mucosal neuromas are frequently seen on the lips and tongue. Pheochromocytoma may be present in up to 1 percent of patients with neurofibromatosis, and in von Hippel–Lindau disease pheochromocytoma develops in association with cerebellar or retinoangiomas.[107]

The clinical presentation of pheochromocytoma is characterized by headache, palpitations, excessive sweating, tremulousness, chest pain, weight loss, and a variety of other constitutional complaints. Hypertension may be episodic but is most commonly constant and is paradoxically associated with orthostatic hypotension upon arising in the morning. The paroxysmal attacks and classical symptoms result from episodic excess catecholamine secretion.[105]

The first onset of hypertension related to pheochromocytoma can be at the time of elective surgical intervention for an unrelated condition. As a result of norepinephrine release with an increase in systemic vascular resistance, cardiac output is increased minimally if at all despite increases in heart rate. The electrocardiogram can show LVH as well as the presence of inverted T waves, suggesting a left ventricular strain pattern. Although ventricular and atrial ectopy and episodes of supraventricular tachycardia can occur, there is little to distinguish the LVH from that of essential hypertension.[105]

There are reports of impaired left ventricular function and cardiomyopathy in patients with pheochromocytoma. The underlying mechanism is complex and includes increased left ventricular work and LVH from associated hypertension, potential adverse effects of excess catecholamines on myocyte structure and contractility, and changes in coronary arteries including thickening of the media presumably potentially impairing blood flow to the myocardium. Histological evidence of myocarditis is present post mortem in patients with previously diagnosed or undiagnosed disease.[105] The possibility of catecholamine-stimulated tachycardia in turn mediating left ventricular dysfunction should be addressed because treatments designed to slow the heart rate may rapidly improve left ventricular function.

Release of catecholamines from pheochromocytomas involves diffusion out of chromaffin cells as well as release from storage vessels, accounting for the demonstration of chromogranin A in the circulation. The primary catecholamine released is norepinephrine, but increases in epinephrine can also be measured. Demonstration of elevated serum dopamine implies the possibility of malignant transformation, which in turn suggests that the tumor may arise in an extraadrenal site. Rarely, pheochromocytoma can arise within the heart, presumably from chromaffin cells, which are part of the adrenergic autonomic paraganglia.[108]

Diagnosis

The diagnosis is established by demonstrating an increase in norepinephrine or epinephrine or its metabolites in serum or blood. Quantitative 24-hour urinary metanephrines are the most reliable for screening, and plasma catecholamines, when obtained under proper conditions, are also fairly sensitive.[108,109] A variety of provocative tests have been used to increase plasma catecholamines in patients with episodic disease. In contrast, the clonidine suppression test is safe and suppresses plasma norepinephrine by more than 50 percent in essential hypertensive patients but not in those with pheochromocytoma.[106] Imaging modalities include magnetic resonance imaging, which has a high degree of specificity, and computed tomographic scanning, which has a high degree of sensitivity because adrenal lesions are of sufficient size to be detected. Further studies with isotopic precursors of catecholamine biosynthesis, including [^{131}I]metaiodobenzylguanidine (MIBG), are useful for confirming that anatomical lesions are producing catecholamines.

Treatment

Definitive treatment of pheochromocytoma requires removal of the lesion. Accurate preoperative localization has reduced operative mortality and eliminates the need for exploratory laparotomy. Endoscopic procedures are now standard.[110] Preoperative pharmacological management includes 7 to 14 days of alpha-adrenergic blockade, usually with prazosin or phenoxybenzamine. Beta-adrenergic blocker therapy is considered contraindicated before establishing sufficient alpha blockade. If supraventricular arrhythmias or unremitting tachycardia is present, beta$_1$-selective agents such as atenolol are preferred.[109] Operative intervention requires constant blood pressure monitoring, and the use of intravenous phentolamine or sodium nitroprusside may be required to treat episodic hypertension.[105,110] Postoperative management includes the use of large volumes of crystalloid-containing fluids to maintain blood volume and prevent hypotension. Glucose may be needed to replace depleted liver glycogen stores. In patients who are not candidates for surgical treatment, metyrosine can decrease catecholamine synthesis and improve the majority of cardiovascular signs and symptoms.[105,110]

REFERENCES

Pituitary Gland

1. Lu C, Schwartzbauer G, Sperling MA, et al: Demonstration of direct effects of growth hormone on neonatal cardiomyocytes. J Biol Chem 276:22892, 2001.
2. Reiss K, Cheng W, Ferber A, et al: Overexpression of insulin-like growth factor-1 in the heart is coupled with myocyte proliferation in transgenic mice. Proc Natl Acad Sci USA 93:8630, 1996.
3. Napoli R, Guardasole V, Angelini V, et al: Acute effects of growth hormone on vascular function in human subjects. J Clin Endocrinol Metab 88:2817, 2003.
4. Colao A, Marzullo P, Di Somma C, et al: Growth hormone and the heart. Clin Endocrinol (Oxf) 54:137, 2001.
5. Brevetti G, Marzullo P, Silvestro A, et al: Early vascular alterations in acromegaly. J Clin Endocrinol Metab 87:3174, 2002.
6. Chanson P, Megnien JL, del Pino M, et al: Decreased regional blood flow in patients with acromegaly. Clin Endocrinol (Oxf) 49:725, 1998.
7. Melmed S, Ho K, Klibanski A, et al: Clinical review 75: Recent advances in pathogenesis, diagnosis, and management of acromegaly. J Clin Endocrinol Metab 80:3395, 1995.
8. Clayton RN: Cardiovascular function in acromegaly. Endocr Rev 24:272, 2003.
9. Bruch C, Herrmann B, Schmermund A, et al: Impact of disease activity on left ventricular performance in patients with acromegaly. Am Heart J 144:538, 2002.
10. Colao A, Spinelli L, Cuocolo A, et al: Cardiovascular consequences of early-onset growth hormone excess. J Clin Endocrinol Metab 87:3097, 2002.
11. Lopez-Velasco R, Escobar-Morreale HF, Vega B, et al: Cardiac involvement in acromegaly: Specific myocardiopathy or consequence of systemic hypertension? J Clin Endocrinol Metab 82:1047, 1997.
12. Minniti G, Jafrain-Rea ML, Moroni C, et al: Echocardiographic evidence for a direct effect of GH/IGF-1 hypersecretion on cardiac mass and function in young acromegalics. Clin Endocrinol (Oxf) 49:101, 1998.
13. Colao A, Spinelli L, Marzullo P, et al: High prevalence of cardiac valve disease in acromegaly: An observational, analytical, case-control study. J Clin Endocrinol Metab 88:3196, 2003.
14. Herrmann BL, Bruch C, Saller B, et al: Acromegaly: Evidence for a direct relation between disease activity and cardiac dysfunction in patients without ventricular hypertrophy. Clin Endocrinol (Oxf) 56:595, 2002.
15. Ciulla M, Arosio M, Barelli MV, et al: Blood pressure–independent cardiac hypertrophy in acromegalic patients. J Hypertens 17:1965, 1999.
16. Frustaci A, Chimenti C, Setoguchi M, et al: Cell death in acromegalic cardiomyopathy. Circulation 99:1426, 1999.
17. Damjanovics SS, Neskovic AN, Petakov MS, et al: High output heart failure in patients with newly diagnosed acromegaly. Am J Med 112:610, 2002.
18. Trainer PJ, Drake WM, Katznelson L, et al: Treatment of acromegaly with the growth hormone-receptor antagonist pegvisomant. N Engl J Med 342:1171, 2000.
19. Melmed S, Casanueva FF, Cavagnini R, et al: CONSENSUS: Guidelines for acromegaly management. J Clin Endocrinol Metab 87:4054, 2002.
20. Fazio S, Cittadini A, Biondi B, et al: Cardiovascular effects of short-term growth hormone hypersecretion. J Clin Endocrinol Metab 85:179, 2000.
21. Maison P, Demolis P, Young J, et al: Vascular reactivity in acromegalic patients: Preliminary evidence for regional endothelial dysfunction and increased sympathetic vasoconstriction. Clin Endocrinol (Oxf) 53:445, 2000.
22. Orth DN, Kovacs WJ, DeBold CR: The adrenal cortex. *In* Wilson JD, Foster DW, Kronenberg HM, Larsen PR (eds): Williams Textbook of Endocrinology. Philadelphia, WB Saunders, 1998, pp 517-664.
23. Wallerath T, Witte K, Schafer SC, et al: Down-regulation of the expression of endothelial NO synthase is likely to contribute to glucocorticoid-mediated hypertension. Proc Natl Acad Sci USA 96:13357, 1999.
24. Whitworth JA, Mangos GJ, Kelly JJ: Cushing, cortisol, and cardiovascular disease. Hypertension 36:912, 2000.
25. Colao A, Pivonello R, Spiezia S, et al: Persistence of increased cardiovascular risk in patients with Cushing's disease after five years of successful cure. J Clin Endocrinol Metab 84:2664, 1999.
26. Kelly JJ, Mangos G, Williamson PM, et al: Cortisol and hypertension. Clin Exp Pharmacol Physiol 25(Suppl):S51, 1998.
27. Fernandez-Real J, Ricard W: Insulin resistance and chronic cardiovascular inflammatory syndrome. Endocr Rev 24:278, 2003.
28. Mortensen RM, Williams GH: Aldosterone action. *In* DeGroot L, Jameson L (eds): Endocrinology. Philadelphia, WB Saunders, 2001, p 1783.
29. Suzuki T, Shibata H, Ando T, et al: Risk factors associated with persistent postoperative hypertension in Cushing's syndrome. Endocr Res 26:791, 2000.
30. Faggiano A, Pivonello R, Spiezia S, et al: Cardiovascular risk factors and common carotid artery caliber and stiffness in patients with Cushing's disease during active disease and 1 year after disease remission. J Clin Endocrinol Metab 88:2527, 2003.
31. Muiesan ML, Lupia M, Salvetti M, et al: Left ventricular structural and functional characteristics in Cushing's syndrome. J Am Coll Cardiol 41:2275, 2003.
32. Norman WN, Wehling M (eds): Proceedings of the First International Meeting on Rapid Responses to Steroid Hormones. Steroids 64:3, 1999.
33. Basson CT: Case records of the Massachusetts General Hospital, case 11-2002. N Engl J Med 346:1152, 2002.
34. Ambrosi B, Sartorio A, Pizzocaro A, et al: Evaluation of haemostatic and fibrinolytic markers in patients with Cushing's syndrome and in patients with adrenal incidentaloma. Exp Clin Endocrinol Diabetes 108:294, 2000.
35. Carey RM, Siragy HM: Newly recognized components of the renin-angiotensin system: Potential roles in cardiovascular and renal regulation. Endocr Rev 24:261, 2003.
36. Young MJ, Funder JW: Mineralocorticoid receptors and pathophysiological roles for aldosterone in the cardiovascular system. J Hypertens 20:1465, 2002.
37. White PC: Aldosterone: Direct effects on and production by the heart. J Clin Endocrinol Metab 88:2376, 2003.
38. Mihailidou AS, Buhagiar KA, Rasmussen HH: Na^+ influx and Na^+-K^+ pump activation during short-term exposure of cardiac myocytes to aldosterone. Am J Physiol 274:C175, 1998.

39. Pitt B, Zannad F, Remme WJ, et al: The effect of spironolactone on morbidity and mortality in patients with severe heart failure. N Engl J Med 341:709, 1999.
40. Rossi GP, Sacchetto A, Pavan E, et al: Remodeling of the left ventricle in primary aldosteronism due to Conn's adenoma. Circulation 95:1471, 1997.
41. Pessina AC, Sacchetto A, Rossi GP: Left ventricular anatomy and function in primary aldosteronism and renovascular hypertension. Adv Exp Med Biol 432:63, 1997.
42. Shigematsu Y, Hamada M, Okayama H, et al: Left ventricular hypertrophy precedes other target-organ damage in primary aldosteronism. Hypertension 29:723, 1997.
43. Cooper MS, Stewart PM: Corticosteroid insufficiency in acutely ill patients. N Engl J Med 348:727, 2003.
44. Espinosa G, Santos E, Cervera R, et al: Adrenal involvement in the antiphospholipid syndrome: Clinical and immunologic characteristics of 86 patients. Medicine (Baltimore) 82:106, 2003.
45. Bhattacharyya A, Jagadeesan S, Wolstenholme RJ, et al: Acute adrenocortical crisis and an abnormal electrocardiogram. Hosp Med 60:908, 1999.
46. Fallo F, Betterle C, Budano S, et al: Regression of cardiac abnormalities after replacement therapy in Addison's disease. Eur J Endocrinol 140:425, 1999.

Parathyroid Disease

47. Schluter K, Piper HM: Cardiovascular actions of parathyroid hormone and parathyroid hormone–related peptide. Cardiovasc Res 37:34, 1998.
48. Stefenelli T, Abela C, Frank H, et al: Cardiac Abnormalities in patients with primary hyperparathyroidism: Implications for follow-up. J Clin Endocrinol Metab 82:106, 1997.
49. Stefenelli T, Mayr H, Bergler-Klein J, et al: Primary hyperparathyroidism: Incidence of cardiac abnormalities and partial reversibility after successful parathyroidectomy. Am J Med 95:197, 1993.

Thyroid Gland

50. Klein I, Ojamaa K: Thyroid hormone and the cardiovascular system. N Engl J Med 344:501, 2001.
51. Dillmann WH: Cellular action of thyroid hormone on the heart. Thyroid 12:447, 2002.
52. Levey GS, Klein I: Disorders of the thyroid. *In* Stein JH (ed): Internal Medicine. 5th ed. St. Louis, Mosby, 1998, pp 1323-1349.
53. Pachucki J, Hopkins J, Peeters R, et al: Type 2 iodothyronine deiodinase transgene expression in the mouse heart causes cardiac-specific thyrotoxicosis. Endocrinology 142:13, 2001.
54. Harvey CB, Williams GR: Mechanism of thyroid hormone action. Thyroid 12:441, 2002.
55. Danzi S, Klein I: Thyroid hormone–regulated cardiac gene expression and cardiovascular disease. Thyroid 12:467, 2002.
56. Morkin E: Control of cardiac myosin heavy chain gene expression. Microsc Res Tech 50:522, 2000.
57. Reiser PJ, Portman MA, Ning X, et al: Human cardiac myosin heavy chain isoforms in fetal and failing adult atria and ventricles. Am J Physiol 280:H1814, 2001.
58. Ojamaa K, Ascheim D, Hryniewicz K, et al: Thyroid hormone therapy of cardiovascular disease. Cardiovasc Rev Rep 23:20, 2002.
59. Carr AN, Kranias EG: Thyroid hormone regulation of calcium cycling proteins. Thyroid 12:453, 2002.
60. Ojamaa K, Kenessey A, Klein I: Thyroid hormone regulation of phospholamban phosphorylation in the rat heart. Endocrinology 141:2139, 2000.
61. Haghighi K, Kolokathis F, Pater L, et al: Human phospholamban null results in lethal dilated cardiomyopathy revealing a critical difference between mouse and human. J Clin Invest 111:869, 2003.
62. Biondi B, Palmieri EA, Lombardi G, et al: Subclinical hypothyroidism and cardiac function. Thyroid 12:505, 2002.
63. Virtanen VK, Saha HH, Groundstroem KW, et al: Thyroid hormone substitution therapy rapidly enhances left-ventricular diastolic function in hypothyroid patients. Cardiology 96:59, 2001.
64. Davis PJ, Davis FB: Nongenomic actions of thyroid hormone on the heart. Thyroid 12:459, 2002.
65. Demers LM, Spencer CA: Laboratory medicine practice guidelines, laboratory support for the diagnosis and monitoring of thyroid disease. Thyroid 13:3, 2003.
66. Hoit BD, Khoury SF, Shao Y, et al: Effects of thyroid hormone on cardiac beta-adrenergic responsiveness in conscious baboons. Circulation 96:592, 1997.
67. Ojamaa K, Klein I, Sabet A, et al: Changes in adenylyl cyclase isoforms as a mechanism for thyroid hormone modulation of cardiac beta-adrenergic receptor responsiveness. Metabolism 49:275, 2000.
68. Park KW, Kai HB, Ojamaa K, et al: The direct vasomotor effect of thyroid hormones on rat skeletal muscle resistance arteries. Anesth Analg 85:734, 1997.
69. Danzi S, Klein I: Thyroid hormone and blood pressure regulation. Curr Hypertens Rep 5:513, 2003.
70. Biondi B, Palmieri EA, Lombardi G, et al: Effects of thyroid hormone on cardiac function: The relative importance of heart rate, loading conditions, and myocardial contractility in the regulation of cardiac performance in human hyperthyroidism. J Clin Endocrinol Metab 87:968, 2002.
71. Klemperer JD, Klein I, Gomez M, et al: Thyroid hormone treatment after coronary-artery bypass surgery. N Engl J Med 333:1522, 1995.
72. Bengel FM, Lehnert J, Ibrahim T, et al: Cardiac oxidative metabolism, function, and metabolic performance in mild hyperthyroidism: A noninvasive study using positron emission tomography and magnetic resonance imaging. Thyroid 13:471, 2003.
73. Taddei S, Caraccio N, Virdis A, et al: Impaired endothelium-dependent vasodilatation in subclinical hypothyroidism: Beneficial effect of levothyroxine therapy. J Clin Endocrinol Metab 88:3731, 2003.
74. Marcisz C, Jonderko G, Kucharz EJ: Influence of short-time application of a low sodium diet on blood pressure in patients with hyperthyroidism or hypothyroidism during therapy. Am J Hypertens 14:995, 2001.
75. Cacciatori V, Bellavere F, Pessarossa A, et al: Power spectral analysis of heart rate in hyperthyroidism. J Clin Endocrinol Metab 81:2828, 1996.
76. Klein I, Levey GS: The cardiovascular system in thyrotoxicosis. *In* Braverman LE, Utiger RD (eds): Werner and Ingbar's the Thyroid: A Fundamental and Clinical Text. 8th ed. Philadelphia, Lippincott Williams & Wilkins, 2000, pp 596-604.
77. Kahaly GJ, Kampmann C, Mohr-Kahaly S: Cardiovascular hemodynamics and exercise tolerance in thyroid disease. Thyroid 12:473, 2002.
78. Shimizu T, Koide S, Noh JY, et al: Hyperthyroidism and the management of atrial fibrillation. Thyroid 12:489, 2002.
79. Auer J, Scheibner P, Mische T, et al: Subclinical hyperthyroidism as a risk factor for atrial fibrillation. Am Heart J 142:838, 2001.
80. Forfar JC: Atrial fibrillation and the pituitary-thyroid axis: A re-evaluation. Heart 77:3, 1997.
81. Nakazawa H, Lythall DA, Noh J, et al: Is there a place for the late cardioversion of atrial fibrillation? A long-term follow-up study of patients with post-thyrotoxic atrial fibrillation. Eur Heart J 21:327, 2000.
82. Franklyn JA, Maisonneuve P, Sheppard MC, et al: Mortality after the treatment of hyperthyroidism with radioactive iodine. N Engl J Med 338:712, 1998.
83. Bengel FM, Nekolla SC, Ibrahim T, et al: Effect of thyroid hormones on cardiac function, geometry, and oxidative metabolism assessed noninvasively by positron emission tomography and magnetic resonance imaging. J Clin Endocrinol Metab 85:1822, 2000.
84. Bakker S, ter Maaten JC, Popp-Snijders C, et al: The relationship between thyrotropin and low density lipoprotein cholesterol is modified by insulin sensitivity in healthy euthyroid subjects. J Clin Endocrinol Metab 86:1206, 2001.
85. Canaris GJ, Manowitz NR, Mayor G, et al: The Colorado thyroid disease prevalence study. Arch Intern Med 160:526, 2000.
86. Klein I, Ojamaa K: Thyroid (neuro) myopathy. Lancet 356:614, 2000.
87. Cappola AR, Ladenson PW: Hypothyroidism and atherosclerosis. J Clin Endocrinol Metab 88:2438, 2003.
88. Hak AE, Pols HAP, Visser TJ, et al: Subclinical hypothyroidism is an independent risk factor for atherosclerosis and myocardial infarction in elderly women: The Rotterdam Study. Ann Intern Med 132:270, 2000.
89. Danzi S, Ojamaa K, Klein I: Triiodothyronine-mediated myosin heavy chain gene transcription in the heart. Am J Physiol 284:H2255, 2003.
90. Monzani F, Di Bello V, Caraccio N, et al: Effect of levothyroxine on cardiac function and structure in subclinical hypothyroidism: A double blind, placebo-controlled study. J Clin Endocrinol Metab 86:1110, 2001.
91. Biondi B, Fazio S, Palmieri EA, et al: Left ventricular diastolic dysfunction in patients with subclinical hypothyroidism. J Clin Endocrinol Metab 84:2064, 1999.
92. Sawin CT: Subclinical hyperthyroidism and atrial fibrillation. Thyroid 12:501, 2002.
93. Parle, JV, Maisonneuve P, Sheppard MC, et al: Prediction of all-cause and cardiovascular mortality in elderly people from one low serum thyrotropin result: A 10-year cohort study. Lancet 358:861, 2001.
94. Burmeister LA, Flores A: Subclinical thyrotoxicosis and the heart. Thyroid 12:495, 2002.
95. Martino E, Bartalena L, Bogazzi F, et al: The effects of amiodarone on the thyroid. Endocr Rev 22:240, 2001.
96. Wiersinga WM: Amiodarone and the thyroid. *In* Weetman AP, Grossman A (eds): Pharmacotherapeutics of the Thyroid Gland. Berlin, Springer Verlag, 1997, pp 225-287.
97. Bogazzi F, Bartalena L, Cosci C, et al: Treatment of type II amiodarone-induced thyrotoxicosis by either iopanoic acid or glucocorticoids: A prospective, randomized study. J Clin Endocrinol Metab 88:1999, 2003.
98. Williams M, Lo Gerfo P: Thyroidectomy using local anesthesia in critically ill patients with amiodarone-induced thyrotoxicosis: A review and description of the technique. Thyroid 12:523, 2002.
99. DeGroot LJ: Dangerous dogmas in medicine: The nonthyroidal illness syndrome. J Clin Endocrinol Metab 84:151, 1999.
100. Iervasi G, Pingitore A, Landi P, et al: Low-T3 syndrome: A strong prognostic predictor of death in patients with heart disease. Circulation 107:708, 2003.
101. Portman MA, Fearneyhough C, Ning W, et al: Triiodothyronine repletion in infants during cardiopulmonary bypass for congenital heart disease. J Thorac Cardiovasc Surg 120:604, 2000.
102. Klemperer JD, Klein I, Ojamaa K, et al: Triiodothyronine therapy lowers the incidence of atrial fibrillation after cardiac operations. Ann Thorac Surg 61:1323, 1996.
103. Mainwaring RD, Capparelli E, Schell K, et al: Pharmacokinetic evaluation of tri-iodothyronine supplementation in children after modified Fontan procedure. Circulation 101:1423, 2000.
104. Chowdhury D, Parnell V, Ojamaa, K, et al: Usefulness of triiodothyronine (T3) treatment after surgery for complex congenital heart disease in infants and children. Am J Cardiol 84:1107, 1999.
105. Bravo EL: Pheochromocytoma. Cardiol Rev 10:44, 2002.
106. Manger WM, Gifford RW: Pheochromocytoma. J Clin Hypertens (Greenwich) 4:62, 2002.
107. Pacak K, Linehan WM, Eisenhofer G, et al: Recent advances in genetics, diagnosis, localization, and treatment of pheochromocytoma. Ann Intern Med 134:315, 2001.
108. Lenders JW, Pacak K, Eisenhofer G: New advances in the biochemical diagnosis of pheochromocytoma: Moving beyond catecholamines. Ann NY Acad Sci 970:29, 2002.
109. Schiff RL, Welsh GA: Perioperative evaluation and management of the patient with endocrine dysfunction. Med Clin North Am 87:175, 2003.
110. Eigelberger MS, Duh QY: Pheochromocytoma. Curr Treat Options Oncol 2:321, 2001.

CHAPTER 80

Hemostasis, Thrombosis, Fibrinolysis, and Cardiovascular Disease

Barbara A. Konkle • Andrew I. Schafer

Basic Mechanisms of Hemostasis and Thrombosis

The human hemostatic system has evolved as a remarkably orchestrated scheme of linked activities designed to preserve the integrity of blood circulation. Hemostasis is regulated to promote blood fluidity under normal circumstances. It is also prepared to clot blood with speed and precision to arrest blood flow and prevent exsanguination whenever and wherever the integrity of the circulation is disrupted. Finally, hemostasis has the capability to restore blood flow and perfusion upon subsequent healing of a damaged vessel. The major components of the hemostatic system are (1) the vessel wall itself, (2) plasma proteins (the coagulation and fibrinolytic factors), and (3) platelets (and probably other formed elements of blood, such as monocytes and red blood cells). These constituents function virtually inseparably (Fig. 80–1). Although this chapter discusses them individually, it is important to recognize the interdependence of the actions of the vessel wall, plasma clotting factors, and platelets.

Vascular Endothelium

Endothelial cells arise from hemangioblasts, which collect in blood islands, the precursors of blood vessels, in the yolk sac of the developing embryo.[1] Hemangioblasts differentiate into both primitive endothelial cells (angioblasts) and hematopoietic cells.[2] The endothelial cell progenitors that arise from hemangioblasts can form new blood vessels (a process termed *vasculogenesis*) under the influence of vascular endothelial growth factors and their tyrosine kinase receptors, as well as other tyrosine kinase receptors and their ligands. Endothelial cell precursors may actually circulate in adult human blood, and their numbers may increase as they participate in neovascularization (*angiogenesis*) of target tissues in response to ischemia, injury, tumor growth, and other pathological processes. Endothelial cell progenitors enter the adult circulation from bone marrow-derived angioblasts as well by shedding from the vessel wall.[3]

A monolayer of endothelial cells lines the intimal surface of the entire circulatory tree, thereby representing the only stationary cell type that components of blood ever come in contact with under normal circumstances. The endothelial surface of the adult human is enormous; it is composed of about 1 to 6×10^{13} cells, weighs approximately 1 kg, and covers a surface area equivalent to about six tennis courts.[4] Yet as recently as the first half of the 20th century, endothelial cells were viewed simply as barriers of blood flow, acting "merely in a negative manner," "similarly to a layer of paraffin or oil."[5] Today, we recognize that endothelium is a dynamic organ with complex metabolic capabilities, including the ability to control vascular permeability, the flow of biologically active molecules and nutrients, cell-cell and cell-matrix interactions within the vessel wall, blood flow and vascular tone, interactions of blood cells, the inflammatory response, and angiogenesis.

Endothelium is also an ideal regulator of hemostasis.[6] It possesses a remarkable repertoire of activities that permit it to transform rapidly from a potent antithrombotic to a prothrombotic surface wherever the need arises. Indeed, attempts to reproduce these properties clinically—for example, in cardiovascular prostheses, extracorporeal circuits, and bypass grafts—by pharmacological or even gene transfer methods have proved suboptimal.

Normal, quiescent endothelium constitutively displays a potent antithrombotic (thromboresistant) surface to blood (Fig. 80–2). It expresses anticoagulant, profibrinolytic, and platelet inhibitory properties. Whenever endothelium is activated or perturbed, however, it rapidly transforms to a prothrombotic surface that actually promotes coagulation, inhibits fibrinolysis, and activates platelets. These are not entirely uniform phenomena, however. Throughout the circulatory tree, even within a single organ, there is marked heterogeneity in the phenotype of endothelial cells. With respect to hemostasis, for example, endothelial cells from different tissues are heterogeneous in their expression of the various antithrombotic and prothrombotic mediators. Vascular bed–specific phenotypic characteristics of endothelium may account for the distinctively focal nature of thrombosis in the face of systemic abnormalities of hemostasis.[7,8] This endothelial heterogeneity depends on both genetic and environmental factors. Exposure to different microenvironmental stimuli, including variable hemodynamic forces, extracellular matrix composition, and cellular and humoral mediators, contributes significantly to the heterogeneity of endothelial phenotypes that develops throughout the circulation.

The specific antithrombotic and prothrombotic properties of endothelial cells

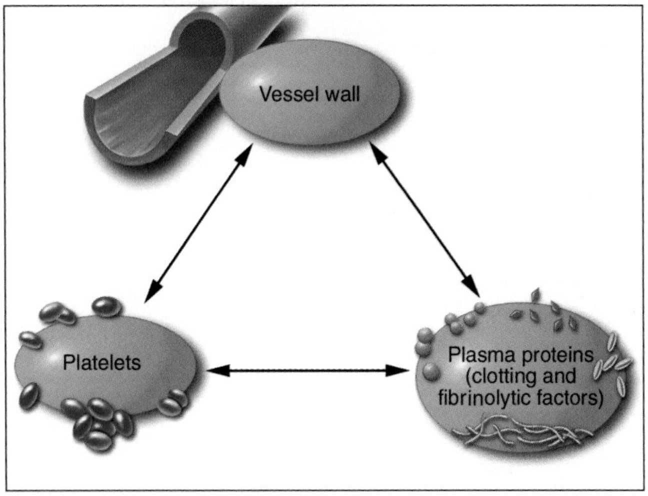

Vessel wall

Platelets

Plasma proteins (clotting and fibrinolytic factors)

FIGURE 80–1 Interactions between the major components of the hemostatic system: the vessel wall, plasma proteins (clotting and fibrinolytic factors), and platelets.

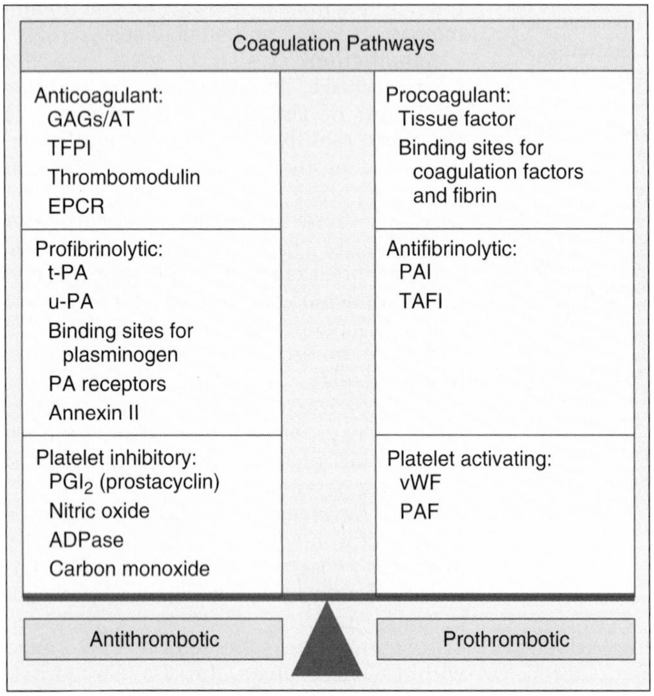

Coagulation Pathways

Antithrombotic	Prothrombotic
Anticoagulant: GAGs/AT TFPI Thrombomodulin EPCR	Procoagulant: Tissue factor Binding sites for coagulation factors and fibrin
Profibrinolytic: t-PA u-PA Binding sites for plasminogen PA receptors Annexin II	Antifibrinolytic: PAI TAFI
Platelet inhibitory: PGI_2 (prostacyclin) Nitric oxide ADPase Carbon monoxide	Platelet activating: vWF PAF

FIGURE 80–2 Balance of antithrombotic and prothrombotic properties of vascular endothelium. In general, antithrombotic properties dominate in quiescent endothelium under normal physiological conditions. In contrast, prothrombotic properties are expressed whenever endothelium is perturbed or activated. AT = antithrombin; EPCR = endothelial cell protein C receptor; GAGs = glycosaminoglycans; PAF = platelet-activating factor; PAI = plasminogen activator inhibitor; TAFI = thrombin-activatable fibrinolysis inhibitor; TFPI = tissue factor pathway inhibitor; t-PA = tissue-type plasminogen activator; u-PA = urokinase-type plasminogen activator; vWF = von Willebrand factor. (Modified from Rosendaal FR: Venous thrombosis: A multicausal disease. Lancet 353:1167, 1999.)

are described in more detail in the following sections (see Fig. 80–2). The hemostatic conversion of the vessel wall is triggered by mechanical damage or by perturbation and activation of the vascular cells by agents such as cytokines, bacterial endotoxin, hypoxia, and hemodynamic forces.

Similarly, a delicate balance exists in the capability of endothelial cells to modulate vascular tone (Fig. 80–3). An important physiological vasodilator released by endothelial cells is nitric oxide (NO), a gas synthesized from the terminal guanidino nitrogen atoms of L-arginine by the action of a group of enzymes known as nitric oxide synthases (NOSs). The major isoform of NOS present in endothelial cells, eNOS, is constitutively active and is further activated by stimuli that increase intracellular calcium, including several receptor-dependent agonists (e.g., thrombin) and hemodynamic forces (shear stress and cyclic stretch).[9] NO acts as a potent vasodilator as well as an inhibitor of platelet adhesion and platelet aggregation by stimulating soluble guanylate cyclase and thereby elevating intracellular levels of cyclic guanosine monophosphate in vascular smooth muscle cells and platelets. Prostaglandin I_2 (PGI_2, prostacyclin) is a major endothelium-derived oxygenation product of arachidonic acid, synthesized by the sequential actions of cyclooxygenase (COX) and prostacyclin synthase.[10,11] Prostacyclin, like NO, is both a vasodilator and an inhibitor of platelet aggregation (but not adhesion), exerting these actions by stimulating adenylate cyclase and thereby elevating intracellular cyclic adenosine monophosphate in target vascular smooth muscle and platelets. Endothelium-derived hyperpolarizing factor[12] and carbon monoxide, a byproduct of heme metabolism to biliverdin by heme oxygenases,[13] are also direct vasodilators elaborated by endothelial cells. Endothelial ecto-adenosine diphosphatase (ADPase), or CD39,[14] is a membrane-associated platelet inhibitor but may also indirectly promote vasodilation by generating adenosine. These vasodilator properties of endothelium are counterbalanced by endothelium-derived vasoconstrictors, including platelet-activating factor, endothelin-1, and thromboxane A_2 (TXA_2).[15,16]

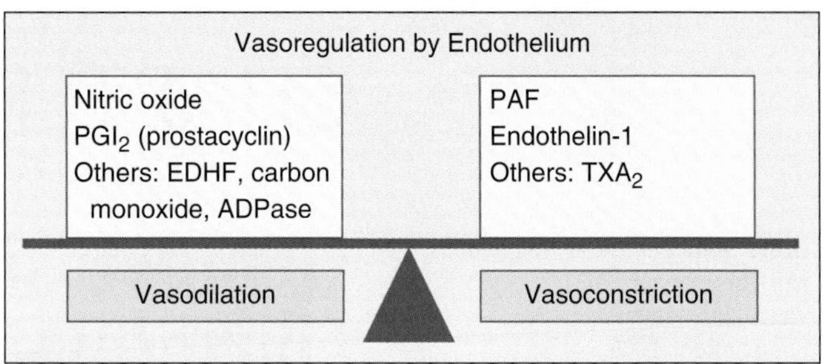

FIGURE 80–3 Regulation of vascular tone by the balance of endothelium-derived vasodilators and vasoconstrictors. ADPase = adenosine diphosphatase; EDHF = endothelium-derived hyperpolarizing factor; PAF = platelet-activating factor; TXA_2 = thromboxane A_2.

In many cases, endothelium-derived vasodilators also inhibit platelets and, conversely, endothelium-derived vasoconstrictors can also activate platelets. The net effect of vasodilation and inhibition of platelet function is to promote blood fluidity, whereas the net effect of vasoconstriction and platelet activation is to promote hemostasis. Thus, blood fluidity and hemostasis can be exquisitely regulated by the balance of antithrombotic/prothrombotic and vasodilatory/vasoconstrictor properties of endothelial cells, which are often coordinately modulated by their relative states of quiescence and activation (see Figs. 80–2 and 80–3).[6]

Coagulation

Plasma coagulation proteins ("clotting factors") normally circulate in plasma in their biologically inactive zymogen (or proenzyme) forms. When the thromboresistant nature of the vascular system is altered, by either mechanical injury or inflammatory and other systemic stimuli (e.g., coronary plaque rupture in patients who develop unstable angina), the coagulation system is activated. If the physiological antithrombotic defenses can be overwhelmed, the result will be the formation of hemostatic thrombi composed of platelets and fibrin. In cases in which focal vascular injury triggers

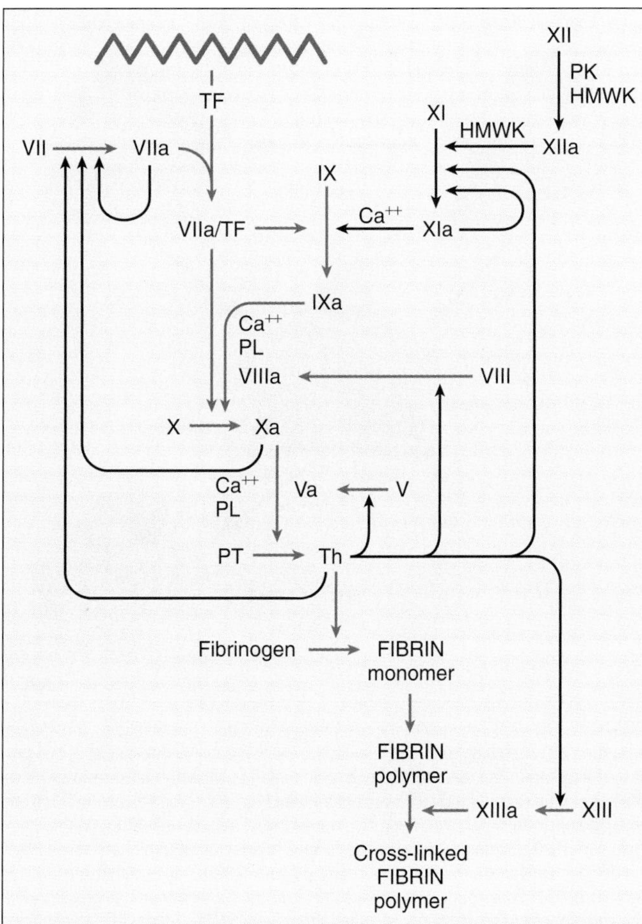

FIGURE 80–4 The coagulation cascade. This scheme emphasizes recent understanding of the importance of the tissue factor pathway in initiating clotting in vivo, the interactions between pathways, and the pivotal role of thrombin in sustaining the cascade by feedback activation of coagulation factors. HMWK = high-molecular-weight kininogen; PL = phospholipid; PT = prothrombin; TF = tissue factor; PK = prekallikrein; Th = thrombin. (Modified from Schafer AI: The primary and secondary hypercoagulable states. *In* Schafer AI [ed]: Molecular Mechanisms of Hypercoagulable States. Austin, TX, Landes Bioscience, 1997, pp 1-48.)

activation of the coagulation system, the occlusive hemostatic thrombus will be precisely localized at and limited to the site of damage.

The sequence of coagulation protein reactions that culminate in the formation of fibrin was originally described as a "waterfall" or a "cascade" (Fig. 80–4). The coagulation cascade is a highly coordinated and regulated series of linked enzymatic reactions that involves the sequential activation of plasma zymogens to serine proteases. Each protease then catalyzes the subsequent zymogen-protease transition by cleavage of peptide bonds. This creates a biochemical amplifier in which a small initiating stimulus rapidly generates high levels of the end-product fibrin. Our understanding of the coagulation cascade has been refined with the recognition that it actually involves a series of linked enzymatic multiprotein complexes, each consisting of a serine protease, one or more cofactor proteins, divalent cations, and a cellular surface (e.g., platelet membranes) on which these components can be assembled.[17,18]

Two pathways of blood coagulation have been recognized: the so-called extrinsic or tissue factor pathway and the so-called intrinsic or contact activation pathway. These two pathways of activation of the coagulation cascade converge to form a "common" pathway, which leads to the generation of the pivotal coagulation enzyme thrombin. Thrombin not only catalyzes the conversion of fibrinogen to fibrin but also serves an important role in sustaining the cascade by feedback activation of coagulation factors at several strategic sites (see Fig. 80–4).

EXTRINSIC PATHWAY. Coagulation in vivo is probably initiated through the extrinsic pathway. The immediate trigger is the injury-induced expression of tissue factor, an integral membrane glycoprotein on the surfaces of activated endothelial cells and circulating blood cells (particularly leukocytes), cells that normally do not express tissue factor activity on their surfaces.[18,19] Alternatively, vascular damage can expose blood to tissue factor expressed within the vessel wall, such as activated smooth muscle cells in atheromata, and constitutively by adventitial fibroblasts. The serine protease factor VIIa (activated factor VII) circulates in blood at trace levels but possesses very poor enzymatic activity in its free form. Exposure of blood to cell surface tissue factor activates coagulation by binding this free factor VIIa. The tissue factor/factor VIIa complex then acts as a bimolecular enzyme to accelerate the conversion of factor VII to VIIa, thereby generating more tissue factor/factor VIIa complexes and amplifying this initial hemostatic response.[20] Factor Xa and thrombin can also induce factor VII activation (see Fig. 80–4); in fact, these two enzymes may be kinetically preferred over the tissue factor/factor VIIa complex as physiological activators of factor VII. The final reaction in the extrinsic pathway is the activation of factor X to factor Xa. This can be catalyzed directly by the tissue factor/factor VIIa complex. Alternatively, this complex can activate factor X indirectly by initially converting factor IX to factor IXa (providing communication between the extrinsic and intrinsic pathways of coagulation), which then activates factor X. This indirect route of factor X activation is probably the one that is favored kinetically.

INTRINSIC PATHWAY. This pathway of coagulation is triggered by the autoactivation of factor XII to its active serine protease form (factor XIIa) on "negatively charged" surfaces, optimally in the presence of two other contact activation proteins, prekallikrein and high-molecular-weight kininogen.[21] A physiological negatively charged surface for contact activation of factor XII and the intrinsic pathway of coagulation has not been identified. However, this pathway is important in in vitro activation of coagulation, and knowledge of this pathway is necessary for interpretation of coagulation laboratory testing. In this pathway, factor XIIa converts the zymogen factor XI to its corresponding serine protease, factor XIa. Factor XIa, in turn, serves as an activator of factor IX to IXa. The final step in the intrinsic pathway is the activation of the plasma zymogen factor X to factor Xa by factor IXa, a reaction that requires the activated form of the plasma cofactor, factor VIIIa. Factor VIIIa is generated by thrombin-induced limited proteolysis of factor VIII.

The most compelling support that coagulation is not initiated by the intrinsic pathway is the clinical observation that individuals with inherited deficiencies of any of the contact activation factors (factor XII, prekallikrein, high-molecular-weight kininogen) do not have a bleeding tendency. Thus, it has been argued that this system has little to do with the initiation of hemostasis. In fact, these proteins may play important roles in other physiological systems, such as vasoregulation, and as antithrombotic and profibrinolytic agents.[22] In contrast, individuals with deficiencies of factors XI, IX, or VIII do have clinical bleeding tendencies and, therefore, these proteins in the intrinsic pathway do appear to play important roles in hemostasis. Therefore, the participation of factor XI in hemostasis probably does not depend on its activation by factor XIIa but rather on its positive feedback activation by thrombin. Thus, this positive feedback loop (see Fig. 80–4) would permit factor XIa to function in the propagation and amplification, rather than in the initiation, of the coagulation cascade.

COMMON PATHWAY. Factor Xa, which can be formed through the actions of either the tissue factor/factor VIIa complex or factor IXa (with factor VIIIa as a cofactor), initiates the common pathway of coagulation by converting the inactive plasma zymogen prothrombin to thrombin, the pivotal protease of the coagulation system. The essential cofactor for this reaction is factor Va, a plasma protein that shares about 30 percent sequence identity with the other plasma coagulation cofactor, factor VIIIa. Like the homologous factor VIIIa, factor Va is produced by thrombin-induced limited proteolysis of factor V. As noted earlier and further described later, thrombin is a multifunctional enzyme, but its major role in the common pathway is to convert soluble plasma fibrinogen to an insoluble fibrin matrix.[23] Fibrin polymerization involves an orderly process of intermolecular associations. Thrombin also activates factor XIII (fibrin-stabilizing factor) to factor XIIIa, a transglutaminase that covalently cross-links and thereby stabilizes the fibrin clot.

The coagulation cascade that culminates in fibrin formation would occur extremely inefficiently and slowly in fluid phase plasma. However, the assembly of these clotting factors on activated cell membrane surfaces greatly accelerates their reaction rates and also serves to localize blood clotting to sites of vascular injury.[18,24,25] In addition, proteases in the coagulation factor complexes assembled on cell surfaces are sequestered from inactivation by their physiological antithrombotic regulators (described later), further enhancing the efficiency of membrane-dependent reactions. The critical cell membrane components on which these coagulation reactions proceed are acidic phospholipids. These phospholipid species are not normally exposed on resting cell membrane surfaces. However, when platelets, monocytes, and endothelial cells are activated by vascular injury or inflammatory stimuli, the procoagulant head groups of the membrane anionic phospholipids translocate to the surfaces of these cells, making them available to support and promote the plasma coagulation reactions.[26]

PHOSPHOLIPID-ASSOCIATED ENZYME COMPLEXES. Major membrane phospholipid-associated enzyme complexes in the coagulation cascade include the "Xase" (or tenase) and "prothrombinase" complexes (Fig. 80–5). Each complex consists of a serine protease enzyme, its zymogen substrate, and its cofactor assembled in association with each other on the membrane surface. The extrinsic Xase complex consists of the tissue factor/factor VIIa enzyme complex and its zymogen substrates, factor IX and factor X. The intrinsic Xase complex consists of factor IXa as the enzyme, factor X as its substrate, and factor VIIIa as the cofactor. The prothrombinase complex consists of factor Xa as the enzyme, prothrombin (factor II) as its substrate, and factor Va as the cofactor. Factor IXa generated by the extrinsic Xase complex becomes the enzyme of the intrinsic Xase complex. Factor Xa generated by either the extrinsic Xase or the intrinsic Xase complex becomes the enzyme of the prothrombinase complex. These successive reaction complexes of coagulation most likely occur by diffusion of products along the same cell membrane surface.

The final enzyme product, thrombin, detaches from cell membranes and circulates in the blood to serve its multiple purposes. A major terminating reaction (see Fig. 80–5) involves membrane assembly of the protein Case complex in which free thrombin (factor IIa) binds to the integral membrane protein, thrombomodulin, which serves as the site for activation of protein C, a major antithrombotic protein discussed later in the chapter.

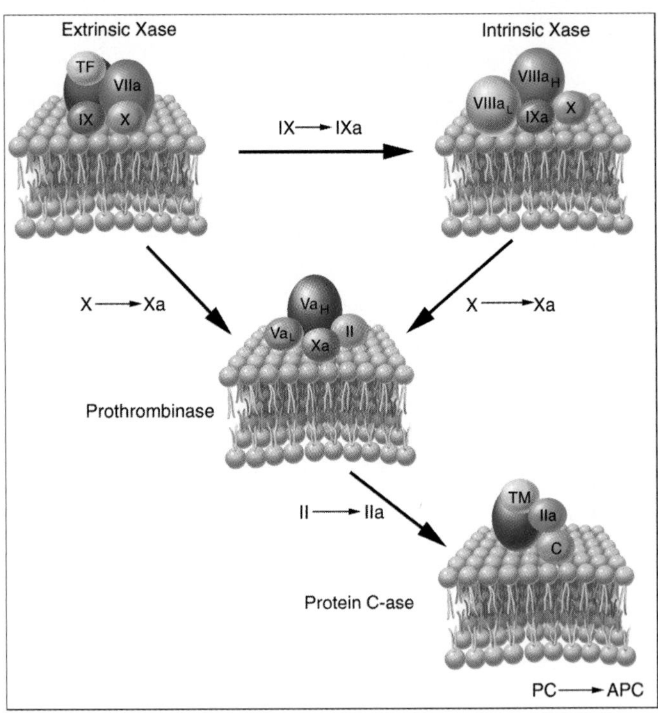

FIGURE 80–5 Schematic representation of the phospholipid membrane-associated enzyme complexes of coagulation. Each vitamin K–dependent serine protease (factors VIIa, IXa, and Xa and α-thrombin [IIa]) is shown in association with its cofactor protein (tissue factor [TF], factors VIIIa and Va, and thrombomodulin [TM]) and zymogen substrate(s) (factors IX and X, prothrombin [II] and protein C [C]) on the membrane surface. The cofactor proteins, factor VIIIa and factor Va, are characterized by a two-domain structure and consist of heavy (H) and light (L) chains that are bridged together by Ca^{2+} ions. Both domains are required for cofactor-membrane association and cofactor-protease binding. (Modified from Jenny NS, Mann KG: Coagulation cascade: An overview. *In* Loscalzo J, Schafer AI [eds]: Thrombosis and Hemorrhage. 2nd ed. Baltimore, Williams & Wilkins, 1998, pp 3-27.)

Anticoagulant (Antithrombotic) Mechanisms

Several physiological antithrombotic mechanisms act in concert to prevent clotting under normal circumstances. Optimal activity of each of the anticoagulant systems depends on the integrity of vascular endothelium. Thus, these physiological mechanisms operate to preserve blood fluidity in the intact circulation and also to limit blood clotting to specific focal sites of vascular injury.

Endothelial PGI_2, nitric oxide, ADPase, and carbon monoxide are physiological platelet-inhibitory mediators (see Fig. 80–2). Other anticoagulant systems are designed to limit fibrin accumulation. Several of these mechanisms, including antithrombin, the protein C/protein S/thrombomodulin system, and tissue factor pathway inhibitor (TFPI), act at different sites in the coagulation cascade to dampen fibrin accumulation. Fibrin that forms despite these anticoagulant defenses is then degraded by the fibrinolytic system. The sites of action of the major physiological antithrombotic pathways are shown in Figure 80–6.

ANTITHROMBIN. Antithrombin (or antithrombin III), the major plasma protease inhibitor of thrombin and the other clotting factors in the intrinsic and common pathways of coagulation, is a single-chain glycoprotein synthesized primarily in the liver and belonging to the serine protease inhibitor (*serpin*) family of proteins.[27,28] Antithrombin neutralizes thrombin and other activated coagulation factors by forming a complex between the active site of the enzyme and the reactive center (Arg393 and Ser394) of antithrombin. The rate of formation of these inactivating complexes increases by a factor of several thousand in the presence of heparin. This is the major anticoagulant mechanism of action of heparin (see later). Heparin and heparan sulfate proteoglycans are actually present as endogenous components of the vessel wall. Thus, antithrombin inactivation of thrombin and other

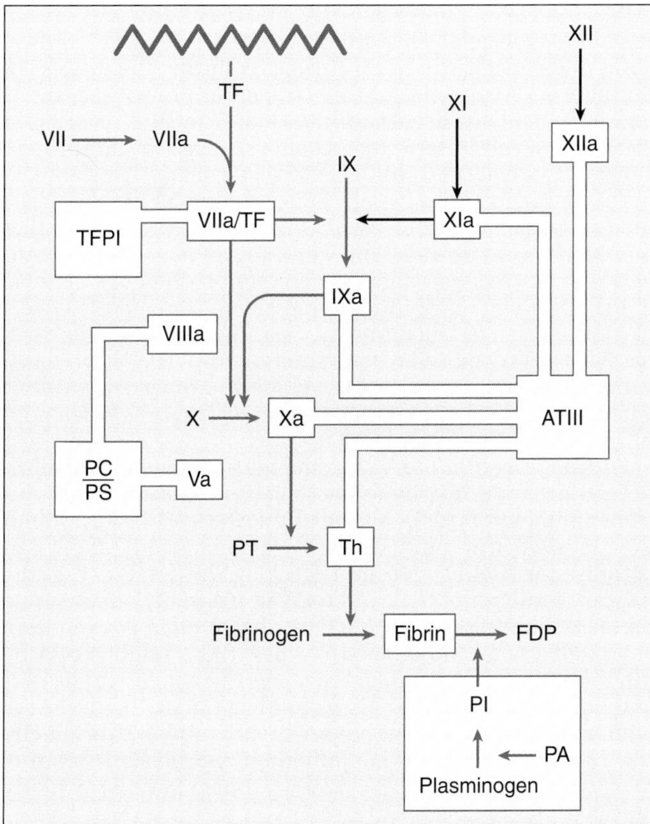

FIGURE 80–6 Sites of action of the four major physiological antithrombotic pathways: antithrombin (AT); protein C/protein S (PC/PS); tissue factor pathway inhibitor (TFPI); and the fibrinolytic system, consisting of plasminogen, plasminogen activator (PA), and plasmin (PI). (From Schafer AI: The primary and secondary hypercoagulable states. *In* Schafer AI [ed]: Molecular Mechanisms of Hypercoagulable States. Austin, TX, Landes Bioscience, 1997, pp 1-48.)

activated clotting factors probably occurs physiologically on vascular surfaces, where heparins are present to catalyze these reactions, rather than in fluid phase plasma. Inherited quantitative or qualitative deficiencies of antithrombin lead to a lifelong predisposition to venous thromboembolism.

PROTEIN Z. Protein Z–dependent protease inhibitor (ZPI) is a recently described, heparin-independent inhibitor of factor Xa.[29] Protein Z is a vitamin K–dependent protein that circulates in plasma in a complex with ZPI. Inhibition of factor Xa by ZPI, a member of the serpin superfamily of proteinase inhibitors, is enhanced 1000-fold by protein Z. The potential roles of protein Z and ZPI deficiency in thrombosis are under study.[29]

PROTEIN C/PROTEIN S/THROMBOMODULIN. Protein C is another plasma glycoprotein synthesized by the liver, which becomes an anticoagulant when it is activated by thrombin through cleavage of an Arg169-Leu170 bond in its heavy chain.[30] The thrombin-induced activation of protein C occurs physiologically on thrombomodulin, a transmembrane proteoglycan binding site for thrombin on endothelial cell surfaces.[31,32] Thrombomodulin thus serves an antithrombotic function both by binding and thereby removing thrombin from the circulation and by promoting the generation of anticoagulantly active protein C. The binding of protein C to its receptor on endothelial cells (endothelial cell protein C receptor) allows its concentration in proximity to the thrombin-thrombomodulin complex, therefore enhancing its efficiency of activation. Activated protein C acts as an anticoagulant by cleaving multiple bonds and thereby destroying the membrane-bound activated forms of coagulation factors V (Va) and VIII (VIIIa). This reaction is accelerated by a cofactor, protein S. Like protein C, protein S is a glycoprotein that undergoes vitamin K–dependent posttranslational carboxylations to form gamma-carboxyglutamic acid (Gla) residues that allow it to bind to negatively charged phospholipid surfaces. Protein S acts as a cofactor by increasing the affinity of activated protein C for phospholipids in the formation of the membrane-bound protein Case complex (see Fig. 80–5).[32] Quantitative or qualitative deficiencies of protein C or protein S, or resistance to the action of activated protein C by a specific mutation at its target cleavage site in factor Va (factor V Leiden), lead to hypercoagulable states.[28,33]

TISSUE FACTOR PATHWAY INHIBITOR. Tissue factor pathway inhibitor is a plasma protease inhibitor that regulates the tissue factor–induced extrinsic pathway of coagulation.[34] Unlike other coagulation inhibitors, which are members of the serpin family, TFPI is a multivalent Kunitz-type serine protease inhibitor. This structure permits TFPI to exert dual inhibitory actions against both tissue factor/factor VIIa (mediated by its Kunitz-1 domain binding to factor VIIa) and factor Xa (mediated by its Kunitz-2 binding to factor Xa) (see Fig. 80–6). Circulating plasma TFPI is bound to lipoproteins. TFPI can also be released by heparin from endothelial cells, where it is bound to glycosaminoglycans, and from platelets. The heparin-mediated release of TFPI may play a role in the anticoagulant effects of unfractionated and low-molecular-weight heparins.[35] Recent studies have demonstrated impairment of TFPI activity[36] and antibodies to TFPI in patients with antiphospholipid antibody syndrome.[37] Lipoprotein (a) [Lp(a)] has been shown to bind and inactivate TFPI, a novel mechanism by which Lp(a) may promote thrombosis.[38] Low levels of TFPI have also been recently reported to constitute a risk factor for venous thrombosis.[39]

THE FIBRINOLYTIC SYSTEM. Any thrombin that escapes the inhibitory effects of the physiological anticoagulant systems described earlier is available to convert fibrinogen to fibrin. In response, the endogenous fibrinolytic system is then activated to dispose of intravascular fibrin and thereby maintain or reestablish the patency of the circulation (Fig. 80–7). Just as thrombin is the key protease enzyme of the coagulation system, plasmin is the major protease enzyme of the fibrinolytic system, acting to digest fibrin to fibrin degradation products. Plasminogen, the inactive zymogen form of plasmin, is synthesized primarily in the liver and circulates in plasma in high (micromolar) concentrations. This single-chain glycoprotein has significant sequence homology with

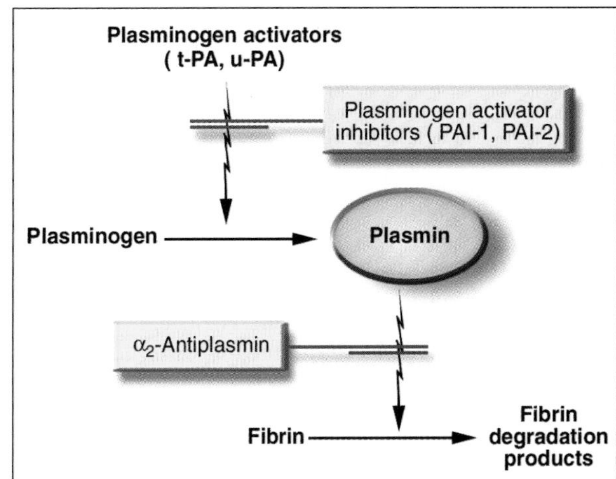

FIGURE 80–7 Scheme of the fibrinolytic system and its control. See text for explanation of abbreviations.

apolipoprotein A. Elevated plasma levels of lipoprotein A are associated with atherosclerotic cardiovascular risk (see Chap. 36).[40] Indeed, one possible atherogenic mechanism for Lp(a) might be to inhibit fibrinolysis by competing with plasminogen for plasmin generation.

Plasminogen Activators. Plasminogen activators cleave the Arg560-Val561 bond of plasminogen to generate the active enzyme plasmin, a two-chain molecule that derives its heavy chain (or A chain) from the amino-terminal region and its light chain (or B chain) from the carboxy-terminal region of plasminogen. The enzyme-active site of plasmin is localized in the B chain, whereas the A chain contains lysine-binding sites. The lysine-binding sites of plasmin (and plasminogen) permit it to bind to fibrin, so that physiological fibrinolysis is "fibrin specific."[17,41] Plasmin, a serine protease whose actions reach beyond fibrinolysis, plays important roles in tissue remodeling, wound healing, angiogenesis, and cell migration.[42]

The major physiological plasminogen activators that convert plasminogen to plasmin are tissue-type plasminogen activator (t-PA) and urokinase-type plasminogen activator (u-PA).[41] Both are serine proteases that are released by endothelial cells into plasma in trace concentrations. Plasmin can convert t-PA from its single-chain form to a two-chain molecule, in which the heavy and light chains are disulfide bonded. Both single-chain and two-chain forms of t-PA can convert plasminogen to plasmin. In contrast, single-chain u-PA (scu-PA) has little enzyme activity and must be converted to its disulfide bonded, two-chain active form by hydrolysis of a Lys158-Ile159 bond. t-PA and u-PA are released from endothelial cells by a variety of humoral factors (e.g., growth factors, hormones, and cytokines), as well as hemodynamic forces, but many of these stimuli also induce the release of plasminogen activator inhibitors.

Both plasminogen (through its lysine-binding sites) and t-PA possess specific affinity for fibrin and thereby bind selectively to clots. In the absence of fibrin, t-PA activates plasminogen to plasmin relatively slowly. Fibrin provides a surface for the sequential binding of t-PA and plasminogen. The assembly of a ternary complex, consisting of fibrin, plasminogen, and t-PA, promotes the localized interaction between plasminogen and t-PA and thereby greatly accelerates the rate of plasminogen activation to plasmin. Moreover, partial degradation of fibrin by plasmin exposes new plasminogen and t-PA binding sites in carboxy-terminus lysine residues of fibrin fragments, further enhancing these reactions. Thus, early fibrin digestion by plasmin further accelerates fibrinolysis, thereby amplifying the process. This creates a highly efficient mechanism to generate plasmin focally on the fibrin clot, which then becomes plasmin's substrate for digestion to fibrin degradation products. Thus, the fibrin surface itself is an important regulator of its own degradation by providing binding sites for fibrinolytic proteins.

In addition to its interactions with fibrin, components of the fibrinolytic system are also efficiently assembled on cell surfaces, similar to the coagulation system, to localize and kinetically optimize the generation of plasmin.[42,43] The surface of endothelial cells contain specific binding sites for plasminogen and t-PA, identified with annexin II, and other cell surfaces to catalyze plasminogen activation. u-PA receptors (u-PAR) also localize on endothelial cells and other cell types. The capacity of endothelial cells to synthesize and release plasminogen activators and then to bind these and other components of the fibrinolytic system provides a powerful paracrine mechanism to concentrate and activate fibrinolysis in proximity to intravascular thrombi contiguous to sites of endothelial damage. At the same time, receptors for the fibrinolytic proteins are also present on the surfaces of other cell types, including platelets and leukocytes that accumulate within thrombi.[42]

Plasmin cleaves fibrin at different rates at different sites of the fibrin molecule. This orderly process leads to the generation of characteristic fibrin fragments during the process of fibrinolysis. At the end of this sequential proteolysis, the D and E domains of fibrin are liberated. The sites of plasmin cleavage of fibrin are the same as those in fibrinogen. However, when plasmin acts on covalently cross-linked fibrin, D-dimers are released; hence, D-dimers can be measured in plasma as a relatively specific test of fibrin (rather than fibrinogen) degradation. Fibrin(ogen) degradation products may have potent anticoagulant and antiplatelet actions, thereby further contributing to the net antithrombotic effects of fibrinolysis. D-Dimer assays can be used as sensitive markers of blood clot formation, and some have been validated for clinical use to exclude the diagnosis of deep venous thrombosis and pulmonary embolism in selected populations (see Chap. 66).[44,45]

Fibrinolytic Inhibitors. Physiological regulation of fibrinolysis occurs primarily at two levels: (1) plasminogen activator inhibitors (PAIs), specifically PAI-1 and PAI-2, inhibit the physiological plasminogen activators, and (2) alpha$_2$-antiplasmin inhibits plasmin (see Fig. 80–7). PAI-1 is the primary inhibitor of t-PA and u-PA in plasma.[46,47] This serine protease inhibitor is a single-chain glycoprotein derived from endothelial cells and other cell types. PAI-1 inhibits t-PA by the formation of a complex between the active site of t-PA and the "bait" residues (Arg346-Met347) of PAI-1. PAI-2, which also belongs to the serpin superfamily, was originally identified in trophoblastic epithelium and hence is referred to as *placental-type PAI.*[48] Pregnant women have particularly elevated plasma levels of PAI-2.

Alpha$_2$-antiplasmin is a single-chain glycoprotein serpin that is synthesized predominantly by the liver. It is the main inhibitor of plasmin in human plasma, forming a 1:1 stoichiometric complex with plasmin that inactivates the enzyme.[41] Alpha$_2$-macroglobulin also inhibits plasmin, but at a much slower rate than alpha$_2$-antiplasmin; therefore, alpha$_2$-macroglobulin is of questionable importance in the physiological regulation of fibrinolysis.

Further regulation of fibrinolysis occurs by a unique feedback mechanism of thrombin generation via the thrombin-activatable fibrinolysis inhibitor (TAFI).[49] TAFI is activated by thrombin, a reaction that is increased more than 1000-fold in the presence of thrombomodulin. TAFI suppresses fibrinolysis through the removal of carboxy-terminal lysine residues on fibrin monomers, eliminating plasminogen and t-PA binding sites that normally serve to augment t-PA mediated conversion of plasminogen to plasmin. Elevated TAFI levels may constitute a mild risk factor for venous thrombosis.[50]

Platelets

Platelets, cytoplasmic fragments released into blood from bone marrow megakaryocytes, circulate with an average life span of 7 to 10 days.[51] These terminal cell fragments lack nuclei and therefore have limited capacity to synthesize new protein. The antithrombotic properties of intact vascular endothelium include potent platelet inhibitors (Figs. 80–2 and 80–8A). These inhibitors include PGI$_2$, NO, and carbon monoxide, which are labile molecules that are released by endothelial cells and act locally as autocoids, and ADPase, an ectonucleotidase of endothelial membranes that breaks down platelet-activating ADP.

PLATELET ADHESION. Vascular intimal injury diminishes locally the antiplatelet properties of endothelium, whereas previously cryptic, thrombogenic subendothelial substances (e.g., collagen) become exposed to flowing blood. Circulating platelets recognize sites of vascular disruption and adhere to the site of injury (Fig. 80–8B). Adhesion results

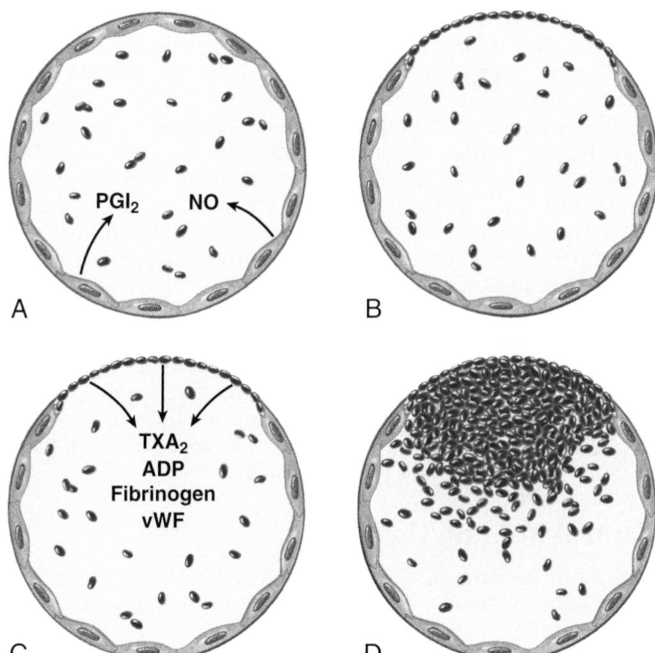

FIGURE 80–8 Sequence of events in platelet activation. **A,** Under normal conditions, a monolayer of endothelial cells lines the intimal surface of the circulatory tree, releasing platelet-inhibitory mediators such as PGI_2 (prostacyclin) and nitric oxide (NO). **B,** At a site of vascular injury (depicted from 11 o'clock to 1 o'clock), endothelium is lost and platelets undergo "adhesion" (platelet–vessel wall interactions) to subendothelial structures that are now exposed (e.g., collagen). **C,** Adherent platelets are activated and release granule constituents (e.g., ADP, fibrinogen, von Willebrand factor) and thromboxane A_2 (TXA_2). **D,** Substances released from activated platelets recruit additional platelets from the circulation to the site of injury and mediate the process of platelet "aggregation" (platelet-platelet interactions), resulting in the formation of an occlusive platelet plug.

in the formation of a monolayer of platelets that are attached to the denuded vascular intimal surface. Platelet adhesion (i.e., platelet–vessel wall interaction) is mediated primarily by von Willebrand factor (vWF), a multimeric protein consisting of a wide spectrum of polymerized subunits that create a mature protein with a molecular mass that ranges from about 550 to more than 10,000 Da, one of the largest soluble proteins in plasma.[52] vWF is synthesized by both endothelial cells and megakaryocytes, where it is stored in Weibel-Palade bodies and alpha granules, respectively, before its regulated secretion.[53] Released vWF is present in both plasma and in the extracellular matrix of the subendothelial vessel wall, to which the platelets are anchored. The large vWF multimers serve as the primary "molecular glue" to attach platelets to a damaged vessel wall with sufficient strength to withstand the high levels of shear stress that would tend to detach them with the flow of blood. The receptor for vWF on the platelet surface is localized in membrane glycoprotein (Gp) Ib, part of the platelet membrane Gp Ib/IX-V complex.[54] Higher levels of shear stress on the arterial side of the circulation promote the interaction between vWF and platelet membrane Gp Ib, probably through subtle shear-induced changes in the vWF molecule and/or its platelet receptor.[54,55] A Gp Ib–vWF dependent platelet adhesion to intact "activated" mesenteric venule endothelium under low-flow conditions has been described.[56] Platelet adhesion is also facilitated by direct binding to subendothelial collagen by means of specific platelet membrane collagen receptors, including $\alpha_2\beta_1$ integrin (also known as Gp Ia/IIa) and the immunoglobulin superfamily member Gp VI.[57,58] Under conditions of high shear stress in small arteries, Gp Ib and Gp VI may act in concert to rapidly tether platelets to the exposed extracellular matrix of the injured vessel wall through their respective ligands, vWF and collagen.[59] Subsequently, the generation of intracellular signals from Gp Ib and Gp VI leads to platelet activation (see next paragraph) and activation of integrin receptors to reinforce the initial adhesion.

PLATELET ACTIVATION. Adherent platelets then become activated (Fig. 80–8C). The platelet activation process results from the combined actions of several agonists that bind to their respective membrane receptors on adherent platelets and transmit platelet-activating intracellular signals.[60,61] These platelet stimuli include humoral mediators in plasma (e.g., epinephrine, thrombin), mediators released from activated cells (e.g., ADP, serotonin), and vessel wall extracellular matrix constituents that come in contact with adherent platelets (e.g., collagen, vWF). Several of these stimuli can activate platelets synergistically and may also act in concert with shear forces to which platelets are simultaneously exposed. Activated platelets undergo the release reaction, during which they secrete prepackaged constituents of their cytoplasmic granules: ADP, adenosine triphosphate, and serotonin from the dense granules; soluble adhesive proteins (fibrinogen, vWF, thrombospondin, fibronectin), growth factors (including platelet-derived growth factor, transforming growth factor-alpha, and transforming growth factor-beta), and procoagulants (platelet factor 4, factor V) from the alpha granules. Simultaneously, activated platelets synthesize de novo and release the potent platelet activator and vasoconstrictor TXA_2. TXA_2 is the major cyclooxygenase product of arachidonic acid metabolism in platelets. As described later in the section on antiplatelet agents, aspirin inhibits cyclooxygenase and thereby blocks TXA_2 synthesis in platelets. TXA_2 acts in concert with several of the substances released from granules to induce the activation of additional platelets in the microenvironment of the developing thrombus.[60,62]

AGGREGATION. The products of the platelet release reaction, including secreted granule constituents and TXA_2, mediate the final phase of platelet activation, the process of aggregation (Fig. 80–8D).[60,61] During platelet aggregation (platelet-platelet interaction), additional platelets are recruited from the circulation to the site of vascular injury, leading to the formation of an occlusive platelet thrombus. As discussed earlier, the platelet plug is anchored and stabilized by the fibrin mesh that develops simultaneously as the product of the coagulation cascade. At lower shear levels (e.g., in the venous circulation), the "molecular glue" that mediates aggregation is fibrinogen, which can be derived either from plasma or from the alpha-granule releasate of activated platelets. At higher shear levels (e.g., in arteries), vWF itself, which is also the ligand that mediates platelet adhesion, can substitute for fibrinogen as the ligand of aggregation. Fibrinogen or vWF binds to specific platelet membrane receptors that are located in the Gp IIb/IIIa integrin complex. Integrins are widely distributed on the surfaces of adherent eukaryotic cells. All receptors in the integrin superfamily contain an alpha and a beta subunit. Individual integrins can often bind to more than one ligand; thus, platelet Gp IIb/IIIa can recognize both fibrinogen and vWF, as well as some other adhesive proteins.

The Gp IIb/IIIa complex is the most abundant receptor on the platelet surface. Its alpha subunit (Gp IIb) is expressed specifically on platelets, but its $beta_3$ subunit (Gp IIIa) is shared by other integrins, including receptors on vascular cells. The heterodimeric, ligand-binding Gp IIb/IIIa complexes are not normally exposed in their active forms on the surfaces of quiescent circulating platelets. However, platelet activation converts Gp IIb/IIIa into competent receptors by means of specific signal transduction pathways,[63] enabling Gp IIb/IIIa to bind fibrinogen and vWF. The binding of these adhesive proteins requires that they contain the specific tripeptide sequence Arg-Gly-Asp (RGD). Recognition of

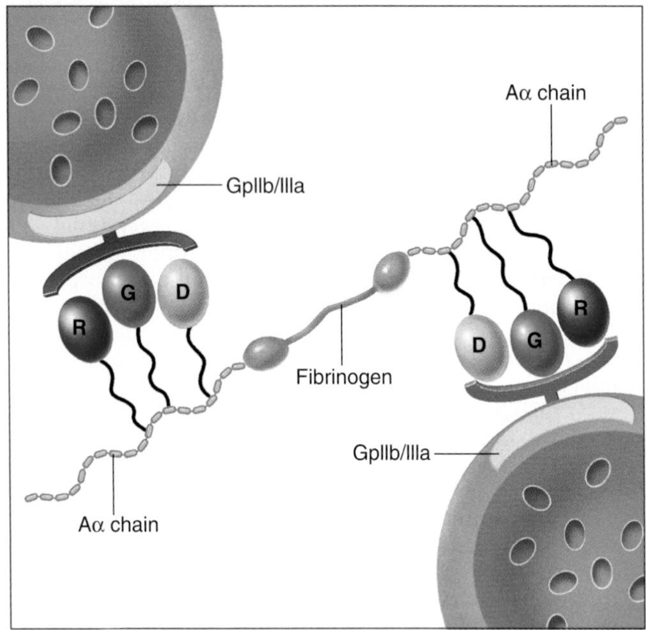

FIGURE 80–9 Linkage of two activated platelets by fibrinogen, which binds to its receptors in the platelet Gp IIb/IIIa complex by means of tripeptide RGD (arginine-glycine-aspartic acid) sequences located on the α chains of dimeric fibrinogen. The high density of Gp IIb/IIIa complexes on the surfaces of activated platelets permits the rapid formation of a network of fibrinogen bridges, leading to platelet aggregation at the site of vascular injury. (In regions of high shear stress, such as in diseased coronary arteries, von Willebrand factor may replace fibrinogen as the primary aggregating ligand. Like fibrinogen, the von Willebrand factor molecule has RGD sequences that mediate this process.) The result of platelet aggregation is the formation of an occlusive platelet thrombus. (From Schafer AI: Antiplatelet therapy with glycoprotein IIb/IIIa receptor inhibitors and other novel agents. Tex Heart Inst J 24:90, 1997.)

fibrinogen and other ligands by the active Gp IIb/IIIa complex involves the RGD tripeptide sequence (located at positions 95-97 and 572-574 of each of the two A-alpha chains of fibrinogen). When two activated platelets with functional Gp IIb/IIIa receptors each bind the same fibrinogen molecule, a fibrinogen bridge is created between the two platelets (Fig. 80–9). Because the surface of each platelet has about 50,000 Gp IIb/IIIa fibrinogen binding sites, numerous activated platelets recruited to the site of vascular injury can rapidly form an occlusive aggregate by means of a dense network of intercellular fibrinogen bridges.[64] In addition to its RGD sequences, the gamma chains of fibrinogen also contain a 12-amino acid residue (dodecapeptide HHLGGAKQAGDV) that also has the ability to bind to the platelet Gp IIb/IIIa receptor. These events of ligand binding to activated platelet membrane Gp IIb/IIIa receptors, which mediate the process of platelet aggregation, have served as targets for antiplatelet therapy with Gp IIb/IIIa antagonists.[65]

Central Role of Thrombin

Thrombin plays a pivotal role in coordinating, integrating, and regulating hemostasis. Depending on the circumstances, it can either promote or prevent blood clotting. This multifaceted effect of thrombin has been referred to as the *thrombin paradox*.[66] The balance of prothrombotic and antithrombotic activities of thrombin depends on at least three variables: (1) the concentration of free thrombin in blood, (2) the presence or absence of endothelial cells at thrombin's site of action, and, (3) the physiological state of the endothelium, if present.

When free thrombin is available in blood at high concentrations, particularly at a site of vascular injury where the antithrombotic influence of endothelium is lost, thrombin potently induces clotting (Fig. 80–10). This enzyme catalyzes several coagulation factor activation reactions that lead to fibrin formation, factor XIII activation to promote fibrin cross-linking, and activation and aggregation of platelets. In fact, under these procoagulant conditions, reciprocal, interdependent, and mutually self-amplifying interaction occurs between thrombin generation and platelet activation. Membranes of activated platelets facilitate thrombin generation by providing a surface for the assembly of coagulation factors and cofactors (Fig. 80–11; see earlier description). Conversely, thrombin is a potent activator of platelets, stimulating the availability of additional activated platelet surface for further thrombin generation. Thus, this reciprocal interaction between thrombin and platelets promotes and amplifies the formation of a tightly focused hemostatic plug composed of platelets and fibrin.

At lower concentrations of thrombin and in the presence of intact, "nonactivated," or

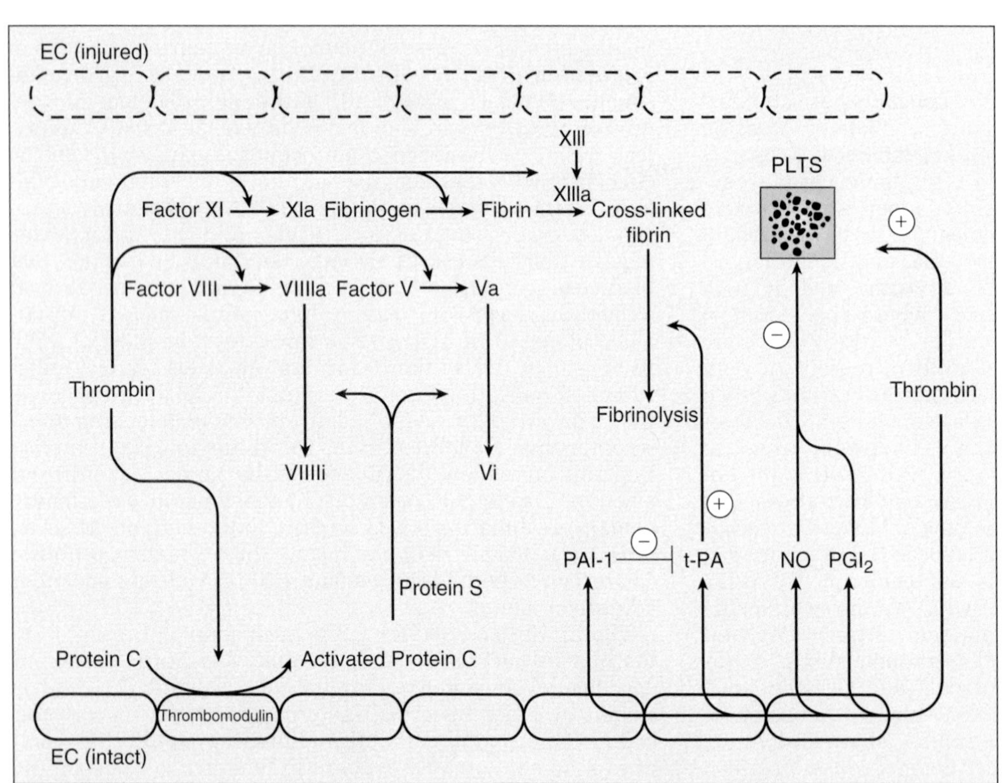

FIGURE 80–10 Central role of thrombin in modulating the state of blood coagulability, depending on the presence or absence of intact endothelial cells (EC) at its site of action. In the presence of intact EC (lower part of figure), free thrombin is removed from the circulation by EC thrombomodulin, and the antithrombotic effects of thrombin predominate: activation of protein C, release of tissue-type plasminogen activator (t-PA), and release of platelet-inhibitory nitric oxide (NO) and prostaglandin I_2 (PGI_2) by intact EC. In the absence of intact EC (upper part of figure), free thrombin is available in blood at higher concentrations and its prothrombotic effects predominate: activation of coagulation factors, fibrin formation and cross-linking, and activation of platelets (PLTS). PAI-1 = plasminogen activator inhibitor-1.

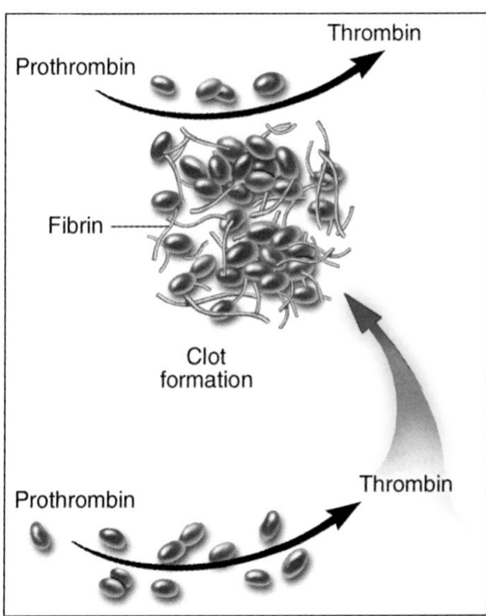

FIGURE 80–11 Reciprocal interaction between thrombin generation and platelet activation. The oval objects represent platelets. Membranes of activated platelets facilitate thrombin generation by providing a surface for assembly of coagulation factors. Conversely, thrombin is a potent activator of platelets, thus acting to promote and amplify activation of the coagulation system. This reciprocal interaction results in the accelerated and tightly focused formation of a hemostatic plug composed of platelets and fibrin. (From Schafer AI: The primary and secondary hypercoagulable states. *In* Schafer AI [ed]: Molecular Mechanisms of Hypercoagulable States. Austin, TX, Landes Bioscience, 1997, pp 1-48.)

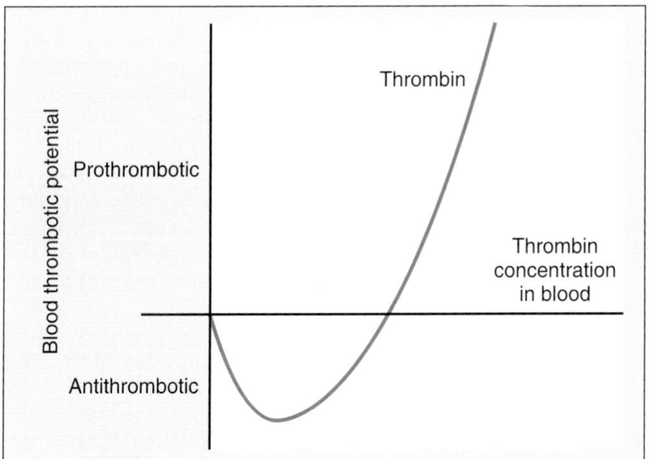

FIGURE 80–12 The thrombin paradox. At low concentrations of thrombin, protein C is activated, and elevated activated protein C exhibits antithrombotic activity. At increasingly higher levels of thrombin, the procoagulant properties of thrombin become dominant and prothrombotic potential is markedly increased. (Adapted from Griffin JH: The thrombin paradox. Nature 378:337, 1995.)

"noninflamed" endothelium, the antithrombotic effects of thrombin predominate (see Fig. 80–10). Low levels of thrombin stimulate increased levels of the endogenous circulating anticoagulant, activated protein C.[67,68] Accordingly, a J-shaped curve describes the relationship between the thrombotic potential of blood and free thrombin concentration (Fig. 80–12).[66] Furthermore, in the presence of normal endothelial cells in the intact circulation (see Fig. 80–10), endothelial thrombomodulin removes free thrombin from blood and low concentrations of thrombin stimulate t-PA release and the release of antiplatelet PGI_2 and NO from endothelial cells. Inflammation results in decreased endothelial thrombomodulin expression, diminishing its antithrombotic effect.[69] Thus, thrombin plays a central role in modulating the state

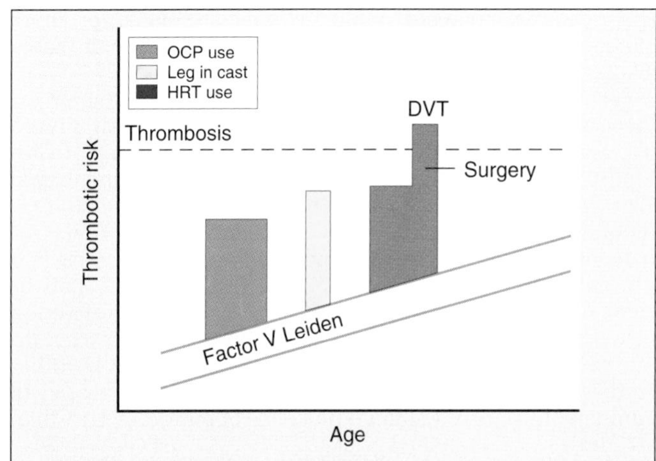

FIGURE 80–13 Thrombotic risk over time. Shown schematically is an individual's thrombotic risk over time. An underlying factor V Leiden mutation provides a "theoretically" constant increased risk. The thrombotic risk increases with age and, intermittently, oral contraceptive (OCP), hormone replacement (HRT) use, or other events increase that risk further. At some point, the cumulative risk may increase to the threshold for thrombosis and result in deep venous thrombosis (DVT). Note: The magnitude and duration of risk portrayed in the figure is meant for example only and may not precisely reflect the relative risk determined by clinical study. (Modified from Rosendaal FR: Venous thrombosis: A multicausal disease. Lancet 353:1167, 1999.)

of blood coagulability, depending on its free concentration in blood and the presence or absence of intact nonactivated endothelial cells at its site of action.

Thrombophilic Disorders

Pathological arterial or venous thromboembolism results from a complex interplay of inherited and acquired risk factors. An individual's likelihood of suffering a thrombotic event over his or her lifetime results from a combination of risk factors; an example is illustrated in Figure 80–13. Although an individual's risk at any given time cannot currently be completely defined, research is moving toward that goal. The major risk factor for arterial thrombosis in adults is atherosclerosis (see Chap. 35). This section focuses on inherited and acquired risk factors for venous or both venous and arterial thrombosis, as listed in Table 80–1.

Inherited Thrombophilia

FACTOR V LEIDEN. Factor V Leiden is the most common inherited thrombophilia, with a prevalence in whites of approximately 5 percent and as high as 20 to 40 percent in patients with venous thromboembolism (VTE), depending on selection criteria.[70,72] Factor V Leiden results from a single mutation (G1691A) in the factor V gene, which results in an arginine at amino acid 506 being replaced by a glutamine. This site is one of three activated protein C (APC) cleavage sites in factor V, by which APC, with free protein S as a cofactor, inactivates factor V and thus inhibits blood clot formation (see Fig. 80–6). Individuals heterozygous for this mutation have an approximately three- to eightfold increased risk of VTE, and those homozygous for the mutation have an approximately 50- to 80-fold increased risk of VTE. Interestingly, it appears to be a stronger risk factor for deep venous thrombosis (DVT) than for pulmonary embolism (see Chap. 66). Some investigators have speculated that a more adherent clot is formed in these individuals, which is therefore less likely to embolize. Although the mutation is most common in patients of European descent, and rare in sub-Saharan Africa and Asia, its prevalence in the United States in African Americans is approximately 1 percent, and among Asian

Americans 0.5 percent, which is as common as or more common than protein C, protein S, or AT deficiency (Table 80–2).[72-74]

Factor V Leiden does not appear to be a risk factor for myocardial infarction or ischemic stroke. This is supported by large cohort studies, including the Physician's Health Study, the Cardiovascular Health Study, and the Copenhagen City Heart Study. A meta-analysis evaluated 18 studies, including 4623 patients with myocardial infarction (7.4 percent with factor V Leiden) and 12,856 control subjects (7.4 percent with factor V Leiden).[75] One study found a statistically significant increased risk of early myocardial infarction in women who smoked cigarettes but not in women who did not smoke.[76] This finding has not been confirmed by other studies. The risk of ischemic stroke is also not increased in adults with factor V Leiden but may be in children (see Chap. 36).[72]

Women with the factor V Leiden mutation have an enhanced risk of thrombosis with hormonal therapy, including oral contraceptives and postmenopausal hormone replacement.[71,77-79] The risk of VTE with oral contraceptive use in women heterozygous for the mutation is increased 20- to 50-fold, compared to three- to fivefold in women without thrombophilia. A higher risk is seen in women using third-generation versus second-generation oral contraceptives, presumably due to the synthetic progestins used in the third-generation preparations. Since young women have a low underlying risk of DVT (approximately 1 in 10,000 per year), the number of women who will actually suffer a DVT, even when risk is increased significantly, is low in this age group. The risk of VTE in women receiving hormone replacement therapy is increased 13- to 14-fold, versus two- to fourfold in women without factor V Leiden or other identified underlying thrombophilia. Hormone-induced VTE in thrombophilic women occurs earlier after initiation of therapy than in women without an identified thrombophilia.

The factor V Leiden mutation accounts almost exclusively for the inherited form of the laboratory phenomenon of APC resistance. Rare cases of other factor V mutations affecting APC cleavage have been reported.[72] APC resistance was first described as impairment of APC-mediated prolongation of the aPTT in the plasma of selected thrombophilic patients.[80] In the absence of factor V Leiden, this abnormality has been associated with an increased risk of thrombosis, but the testing cannot be well standardized and the clinical utility of this finding is unclear. APC resistance is acquired in patients with many conditions, including hormone therapy, pregnancy, and antiphospholipid antibody syndrome, but its role in the pathogenesis of thrombosis in patients with these conditions has not been defined. Many laboratories use a factor V–specific APC resistance test that is highly sensitive and specific for the factor V Leiden mutation. Only other factor V mutations affecting APC cleavage and, rarely, lupus anticoagulants have been reported to produce false-positive results in this assay.

PROTHROMBIN GENE MUTATION. In 1996, a polymorphism in the 3′ untranslated region of the prothrombin gene (PT G20210A) was found to be associated with a two- to threefold increased risk of VTE.[28,81] This mutation is found predominantly in whites (1-6 percent), is uncommon in African Americans (0.2 percent) and is rare in other racial groups.[81,82] Although this mutation is not in the coding region of the prothrombin gene, it appears to result in increased prothrombin levels, probably by an increase in mRNA. Overall, studies do not show a greater risk of VTE recurrence in individuals heterozygous for either the factor V Leiden or the PT G20210A mutations. Thus, these states alone do not modify general recommendations for duration of anticoagulation after a single episode of VTE.

Like factor V Leiden, PT G20210A is associated with an increased risk of venous but not arterial thrombosis. Because PT G20210A is such a mild risk factor, thrombosis usually occurs in the setting of additional risk factors, either genetic or acquired. The risk of VTE is increased in patients heterozygous for both the factor V Leiden and PT G20210A mutations above that for either mutation alone. Since both are common in white populations, homozygous and compound heterozygous states are seen.

Hormonal therapy further increases the thrombotic risk in patients with PT G20210A. The VTE risk in patients heterozygous for this mutation who use OCP is increased 16-fold.[83] In addition, a markedly increased risk of cerebral

TABLE 80–1 Risk Factors for Thrombosis

Venous	Venous and Arterial
Inherited	Inherited
Factor V Leiden	Homocysteinuria
Prothrombin G20210A	Dysfibrinogenemia
Antithrombin deficiency	
Protein C deficiency	Mixed
Protein S deficiency	Hyperhomocysteinemia
Elevated factor VIII activity	
Acquired	Acquired
Age	Malignancy
Previous thrombosis	Antiphospholipid antibody syndrome
Immobilization	Hormonal therapy (oral contraceptives and hormone replacement therapy)
Major surgery	Polycythemia vera
Pregnancy and puerperium	Essential thrombocythemia
Hospitalization	Paroxysmal nocturnal hemoglobinuria
Activated protein C resistance, nongenetic	
Unknown*	
Elevated factor VII, IX, XI, von Willebrand factor	
Elevated levels of thrombin-activatable fibrinolysis inhibitor	
Low levels of tissue factor pathway inhibitor	

*Unknown whether risk factor is inherited or acquired.

TABLE 80–2 Ethnic Distribution of Inherited Thrombophilia in the United States (Prevalence %)

	Factor V Leiden	PT G20210A	↓Protein C*	↓Protein S*	↓AT*
White Americans	3-7	1-3	0.2-0.5	0.1-1	0.02-0.04
African Americans	~1	0-0.2			
Hispanic Americans	~2	†			
Asian Americans	~0.05	†			
Native Americans	~1	†			

*The prevalence of protein C, protein S, or AT deficiency is not known to vary by ethnic origin of the population tested.
†Unknown.

venous thrombosis, a rare clinical event, has been reported in women using oral contraceptives who are heterozygous for this mutation.[84]

ANTITHROMBIN DEFICIENCY. Antithrombin deficiency was the first described inherited risk factor for thrombosis.[27,28] Inherited antithrombin deficiency can be due to a quantitative (type I) or a qualitative (type II) abnormality, the latter manifest by decreased function with a normal protein level. Complete antithrombin deficiency has not been described and is likely incompatible with life. Patients with inherited type I deficiency carry the highest risk of thrombosis with a likelihood of thrombosis, based on small cohort studies, of up to 85 percent by the age of 50 years. Population studies do not support such a high risk. The discrepancy is likely due to a number of factors, including issues with testing, acquired antithrombin deficiency not carrying the same risk of thrombosis, and possible additional unrecognized genetic defects in the most affected families. In antithrombin-deficient individuals who present with thrombosis, anticoagulation is usually continued indefinitely.

While rare instances of arterial thrombosis have been reported, antithrombin deficiency is predominantly a risk for VTE. Venous thrombosis at unusual sites (including the portal and mesenteric veins) has been reported. Evaluation for antithrombin deficiency should not be done in patients with arterial thrombosis alone, except in unusual circumstances.

PROTEIN C AND S DEFICIENCIES. As described previously, free protein S serves as a cofactor for activated protein C in the inactivation of factor V and factor VIII (see Fig. 80–6). Homozygous deficiency of either protein C or S manifests in infancy as purpura fulminans. The risk of thrombosis in individuals heterozygous for these mutations is unclear, as reports vary, but is probably increased approximately 10-fold.[28,33,85] There appears to be substantial variability between affected families, which may be secondary to additional inherited factors. Factor V Leiden can be a significant cofactor in the increased thrombotic risk in families with protein C or protein S deficiency. Because factor V Leiden is so common, at least in white populations, a combination of these defects can occur and the combined effect may be enhanced by a "double-hit" of the same anticoagulant pathway. While rare cases of arterial thrombosis, particularly for protein S deficiency, have been reported, deficiencies of these proteins are predominantly, if not exclusively, risk factors for VTE. Therefore, determination of levels of protein C and protein S should not be included in an evaluation of adult patients with arterial thrombosis only.

Acquired deficiencies, not clearly associated with a thrombotic risk, and difficulties in laboratory testing, make diagnosis of these deficiencies challenging.[33,85] Ideally, an inherited deficiency is confirmed in family members. Proteins C and S are affected by vitamin K deficiency, warfarin ingestion, and liver disease, all of which tend to reduce their levels. Mildly decreased protein C levels can be an early marker of liver disease. Approaches to diagnosing protein C or protein S deficiency in patients on warfarin have been proposed by comparing values with other vitamin K–dependent factors. However, relationships between factor levels in patients on warfarin have significant interpatient variability, and this approach has not been validated.

Functional protein S assays are used as initial testing for protein S deficiency in many laboratories.[85] This test is known to have a significant false-positive rate and should not be used alone to diagnose protein S deficiency without further testing or family studies. Acquired protein S deficiency, particularly a low free protein S level, occurs in a number of settings, including pregnancy, inflammatory states, and hormone use. Although a decreased level of free protein S with a normal total protein S level is frequently an acquired

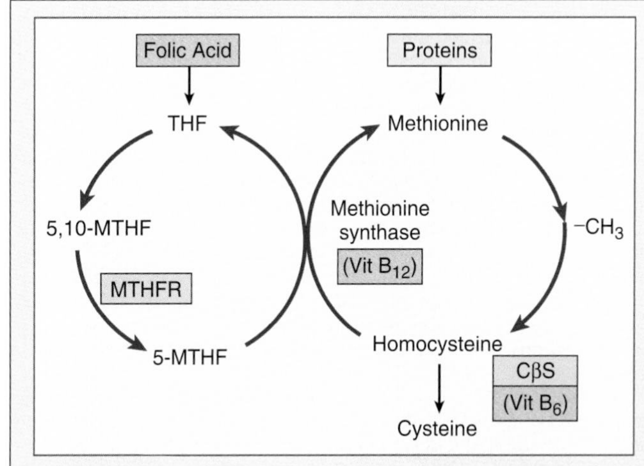

FIGURE 80–14 Homocysteine metabolism. Metabolism of homocysteine can occur through remethylation to methionine, a reaction that requires the enzyme methionine synthase and the cofactor, vitamin B12, or through transsulfuration to cysteine, via initial condensation with serine to form cystathionine, in a reaction catalyzed by cystathionine-β-synthase (CβS) followed by hydrolysis by the enzyme γ-cystathionase to cysteine and α-ketobutyrate. Both steps in the transsulfuration pathway require vitamin B6 as a cofactor. In the liver, remethylation also occurs with betaine as the methyl donor (not shown). Methyltetrahydrofolate is derived from the reduction of 5,10-methylene-tetrathydrofolate in a reaction catalyzed by methylene-tetrahydrofolate reductase (MTHFR). Enzymes in which mutations occur that may increase thrombotic risk are depicted in blue. Vitamins, supplementation with which is used for therapy, are depicted in red. MTHF = methylene-tetrahydrofolate; THF = tetrahydrofolate.

condition, individuals with inherited deficiency may have a similar picture (type III deficiency or type I in older individuals), making the distinction difficult. A diagnosis of protein S deficiency should be made with caution in individuals taking medications or in those with conditions known to affect protein S levels.

HOMOCYSTEINE. Homocysteine is a sulfhydryl amino acid formed from the demethylation of dietary methionine (Fig. 80–14).[86] Homocysteine can be remethylated to methionine by donation of a methyl group from (1) methyltetrahydrofolate (MTHF) in a reaction catalyzed by methionine synthase using vitamin B12 as an essential cofactor, or from (2) betaine. MTHF is derived from the reduction of 5-10, methylene tetrahydrofolate in a reaction catalyzed by MTHF reductase (MTHFR). Homocysteine is also condensed with serine to form cystathionine, a reaction catalyzed by cystathionine beta-synthase (CβS). Vitamin B6 is an essential cofactor in this reaction.

Patients with severe deficiencies in the enzymes methionine synthase, MTHFR, and, particularly, CβS can have marked elevations in plasma homocysteine (hyperhomocysteinemia) and suffer from premature atherosclerosis and arterial and venous thrombosis.[86] Homocysteinuria, due almost exclusively to homozygous CβS deficiency, is rare, with a frequency in the general population of 1 in 250,000, and is manifest by mental retardation, ectopic lenses, and skeletal abnormalities, as well as premature atherosclerosis and thrombosis. Approximately 25 percent of affected individuals will suffer a vascular occlusive event by 16 years of age and approximately 50 percent will do so by 29 years of age. In a review of reported cases, 51 percent were VTE, 32 percent were cerebrovascular accidents, 11 percent were peripheral vascular disease, and 4 percent were myocardial infarctions. Pathogenic effects of markedly elevated homocysteine levels are supported by in vitro studies and include induction of smooth muscle proliferation, accelerated oxidation of low-density lipoprotein cholesterol, direct endothelial toxicity, impairment of endothelial derived NO, decreased synthesis of heparan sulfate, proteoglycan synthesis, and induction of proinflammatory changes including increased tissue factor synthesis, decreased cell-surface expression of thrombomodulin, and increased expression of vascular adhesion molecule-1.[86,87]

The strong association of markedly elevated homocysteine levels with atherosclerotic and thrombotic disease prompted the evaluation of the effects of less marked elevations of homocysteine[88] (see Chap. 36). Mild (16-24 μmol/liter) or moderate (25-100 μmol/liter) hyperhomocysteinemia usually results from mutations in MTHFR and/or acquired dietary deficiencies of vitamin B12, folic acid, or vitamin B6, which are cofactors in homocysteine metabolism. The relationship of hyperhomocysteinemia to atherosclerotic vascular disease has been evaluated primarily by retrospective case-control studies but also by some prospective studies. One meta-analysis of 27 retrospective case-control studies demonstrated that for each 5 μmol/liter incremental rise in total plasma homocysteine, the odds ratios for coronary artery disease and cerebrovascular disease were 1.6 and 1.5, respectively. However, when studied prospectively, the relationship has not been found to be as strong, and a meta-analysis of prospective studies suggested at best a weak association.[86]

In assessing VTE risk, two meta-analyses found a 2.5 to 3 pooled odds ratio of VTE in individuals with an elevated fasting homoscysteine level.[86,89] While MTHFR mutations that can result in higher plasma homocysteine levels are common, it is the fasting plasma homocysteine levels, and not the presence of specific mutations, that correlate with increased thrombotic risk.[90] In a recent study evaluating genetic (five common functional polymorphisms in MTHFR) and nutritional factors contributing to hyperhomocysteinemia, the genetic contribution to the variance in homocysteine levels was estimated to be approximately 9 percent, compared with approximately 35 percent that could be attributed to low levels of folate and vitamin B12.[91] In evaluating patients for hyperhomocysteinemia, methionine loading to detect elevated plasma homocysteine not detected by fasting studies is probably not needed. Many small studies evaluating thrombophilic factors have reported that elevated homocysteine levels further increase the risk of thrombosis in individuals with other causes of thrombophilia.[92]

Elevated plasma homocysteine levels are usually responsive to vitamin supplementation, particularly folic acid supplementation. Implementation of folic acid fortification programs results in decreased rates of folic acid deficiency.[93] While vitamin supplementation can biochemically correct hyperhomocysteinemia, the clinical efficacy of such intervention in preventing thrombotic and vascular complications is currently under study. However, since oral supplementation with folic acid, vitamin B12, and vitamin B6 is an easily tolerated treatment, inclusion of fasting homocysteine levels in a thrombophilia evaluation and institution of treatment, if they are elevated, seems warranted.

OTHERS. Recent studies have provided data that increased levels of procoagulants may be associated with an increased risk of thrombosis.[94] The strongest association is with elevated factor VIII levels.[95] Persistently elevated factor VIII levels, remote from acute events, can be inherited, and in that setting have been found to increase the risk of VTE fivefold (individuals with factor VIII >150 U/dl versus those with factor VIII <100 U/dl). As a risk factor for thrombosis, factor VIII levels are independent of vWF levels. Elevated vWF levels were found to be a risk factor for VTE independent of factor VIII levels in one study,[96] but not in another.[97] Elevated factor VIII levels may increase the risk of VTE recurrence, with the highest levels imparting the greatest risk. One study found a 37 percent likelihood of recurrence at 2 years in individuals with factor VIII levels above the 90th percentile of the normal range.[98] Since factor VIII is an acute-phase reactant, it is important that if testing is performed, this be done remote from an acute event.

Elevated fibrinogen levels are associated with an increased risk of atherothrombotic disease, but not VTE. However, this likely reflects an inflammatory response, and inherited factors resulting in increased fibrinogen have not been clearly associated with an increased risk of thrombosis (see Chap. 36).[94,96] Also, lowering fibrinogen levels has not been shown to decrease risk. Increased prothrombin (factor II) levels not due to the prothrombin G20210A mutation has been associated with an increased risk of thrombosis, similar to that seen in individuals with the PT G20210A mutation.[83] Elevated factor IX, XI, or VII levels may be weakly associated with an increased risk of VTE.[94,96] Other than for factor VIII, there is no evidence that levels of these factors should alter management of VTE at this time. In the future, multiple levels may be assessed in a multifactorial approach to thrombotic risk. Until such an approach is validated in clinical study, testing these factors as part of a routine thrombophilia evaluation cannot be recommended.

Inherited heparin cofactor II deficiency is currently not considered a strong risk factor for thrombosis, although it may contribute to thrombotic risk when combined with other thrombophilias. Routine testing of patients with thromboembolic disease for heparin cofactor II deficiency is not recommended. Qualitative abnormalities of fibrinogen (dysfibrinogenemias) are usually associated with no clinical manifestations, although both mild bleeding symptoms and venous or arterial thrombosis have been reported. These are inherited in an autosomal dominant fashion. Because thrombosis-related dysfibrinogenemia is so rare, its inclusion in a thrombophilia evaluation is not routine.[99] Plasminogen deficiency, previously proposed as a thrombophilic condition, has not been substantiated in studies of deficient families.

Acquired Thrombophilia

Most instances of VTE are at least partially due to acquired conditions. Age itself is a strong risk factor for VTE, with the underlying risk in octogenarians (baseline risk of approximately 1 in 100 per year) 100-fold that of young children (baseline risk of approximately 1 in 100,000 per year).[71] Thrombotic risk in acquired situations as assessed in the Leiden Thrombophilia Study are shown in Table 80–3. Malignancy is strongly associated with thrombosis and should always be considered in adults who present with thrombosis, particularly if it is apparently "idiopathic" in individuals without a family history of thrombosis. Evaluations in these individuals beyond age-appropriate recommended cancer screening has not been shown to prolong survival.[100] Many individuals presenting with thrombosis and diagnosed with malignancy have abnormalities on physical examination or routine laboratory or radiological studies. A frequent laboratory finding in this setting is unexplained anemia. Individuals with myeloproliferative disorders, notably polycythemia vera and essential thrombocythemia, have an increased risk of venous and arterial thrombosis, and a complete blood cell count should be part of a thrombophilia evaluation. Although uncommon, essential thrombocythemia has been reported as a cause of myocardial infarction, particularly in young women.

HORMONAL THERAPY. Hormonal therapy carries an increased risk of VTE, and this risk may be increased significantly in thrombophilic women, as discussed earlier in this chapter (see also Chap. 73). Second-generation oral contraceptives and hormone replacement therapy increase the risk of thrombosis two- to fourfold.[79,101,102] Because middle-aged women have an underlying risk of VTE approximately 10-fold greater than that of young women, they are more likely to experience thrombosis when placed on hormonal therapy. Third-generation oral contraceptives, which contain less estrogen and a different progestin, are associated with a twofold increased risk of VTE compared to second-generation products. This surprising finding of increased risk, which has been confirmed in a number of large studies, is presumably due to the progestins in the third-generation preparations. Oral contraceptive use is associated with an increased risk of peripheral arterial disease[103] and a modest increase in myocardial infarction.[104] The pathogenesis of hormone-induced thrombosis is not clear. Estrogens have many differ-

TABLE 80–3 Thrombosis Risk in Acquired Situations: Data from the Leiden Thrombophilia Study

Risk Factor	Patients (n = 474), n (%)	Controls (n = 474), n (%)	Odds Ratio	95% Confidence Interval
Surgery	85 (18)	17 (3.6)	5.9	3.4-10.1
Hospitalization	59 (12)	6 (1.3)	11.1	4.7-25.9
Immobilization	17 (3.6)	2 (0.4)	8.9	2.0-38.2
Pregnancy	8 (5.0)	2 (1.3)	4.2	0.9-19.9
Puerperium	13 (8.2)	1 (0.6)	14.1	1.8-109
Oral contraceptives	109 (70)	65 (38)	3.8	2.4-6.0

From the Leiden Thrombophilia Study, a population based case-control study. Cases were unselected consecutive patients aged 18-70 years with a first objectively diagnosed deep vein thrombosis, and controls were acquaintances of cases or spouses of (other) cases. Controls were matched for age and sex and subjects with active malignancies were excluded. Time window for surgery, hospitalization (without surgery), and immobilization (not in the hospital, immobilized >13 days) was 1 year preceding the index date. For puerperium, it was delivery 30 days or less before the index date and for pregnancy and oral contraceptives it was at the index date. Data on pregnancy, puerperium, and oral contraceptive use refer to women of childbearing age only.

Adapted from Bauer KA, Rosendaal FR, Heit JA: Hypercoagulability: Too many tests, too much conflicting data. Hematology. Am Soc Hematol Edu Program Book 353, 2002.

ent effects on the coagulation system that include increases in procoagulant factors, reductions in free protein S and antithrombin, and acquired protein C resistance. Hormone-induced increases in fibrinolytic activity do not counterbalance this procoagulant effect.[101]

ANTIPHOSPHOLIPID ANTIBODY SYNDROME (APS). APS is defined by a characteristic constellation of clinical and laboratory abnormalities, including an increased risk of thrombosis.[105-107] Clinical findings can include unexplained venous or arterial thrombosis and pregnancy morbidity, including repeated miscarriages or fetal growth retardation. These are associated with persistent antibodies to certain phospholipid binding proteins. These antibodies, and particularly antibodies to the phospholipid cardiolipin (anticardiolipin antibodies, ACA), can be induced by infections or drugs, but in those settings they are not clearly associated with thrombosis. "True" APS likely results from an autoimmune reaction, either not associated with a defined autoimmune disorder, designated primary APS, or associated with an autoimmune disease, such as systemic lupus erythematosus, designated secondary APS.

In the 1990s, work from a number of laboratories clarified that the antibodies found in individuals with this syndrome were actually directed against phospholipid-binding proteins, not against the phospholipid itself. Actually, most positive ACA reactions require beta$_2$-glycoprotein 1 (β_2GP1) in the assay. β_2GP1 is an abundant protein in bovine and human plasma and thus is present in many assays without specifically being added. Antibodies against other phospholipid-binding proteins, most notably against prothrombin, but also against protein C, protein S, annexin V, and tissue factor pathway inhibitor, can also be found in patients with this syndrome. The role these autoantibodies play in the pathogenesis of APS has not been elucidated, although many studies are under way. Two mechanisms proposed whereby antiphospholipid antibodies promote thrombosis are as follows: (1) interfering with phospholipid-dependent anticoagulant pathways, including APC and TFPI functions, and (2) binding to cell surfaces and inducing cell activation.[107]

Patients with APS may have antibodies that react only in an immunoassay, as described, or that interfere with phospholipid dependent tests (termed *lupus anticoagulants*), or both. The presence of antibodies to β_2GP1 appear to be better predictors of thrombosis than antibodies to prothrombin, but testing for anti-β_2GP1 antibodies has not clearly been shown to improve the diagnosis of APS over the use of ACA determinations alone. Anti-prothrombin antibodies do not prevent conversion of prothrombin to thrombin but may result in prothrombin deficiency, which rarely is associated with bleeding, in contrast to the more characteristic thrombotic tendency of APS. A pattern of positive ACA and negative anti-β_2GP1 antibodies is seen in cases of infection, and in that setting it has not been associated with thrombosis.

A number of laboratory tests are used to diagnose lupus anticoagulants.[105,108] Many of these tests have been developed to detect lupus anticoagulants by modifications that make them more sensitive to interactions of the antibody with the phospholipid component of the assay. The aPTT can be prolonged, depending on the strength of the lupus anticoagulants and the aPTT reagent used. A widely used test, which when yielding positive results probably correlates best with an increased risk of thrombosis, is the dilute Russell viper venom test (dRVVT). Russell viper venom activates factor X directly, and results of the test are affected by underlying conditions or drugs that decrease common pathway factors. Prolongation of the dRVVT corrects with mixing with normal plasma if the prolongation is due to factor deficiency, which could be inherited, or it could be secondary to liver disease, vitamin K deficiency, or warfarin therapy. Heparin functions as an inhibitor and the finding does not correct when mixed with normal plasma, resulting in a false-positive test result. Many dRVVT assay procedures absorb out heparin, eliminating this problem; however, if positive values are found in a patient on heparin, the test should be repeated with the patient off heparin at a later date to confirm the finding. Laboratory confirmation of a lupus anticoagulant requires prolongation of a phospholipid-dependent test that does not correct with mixing but does correct with the addition of the correct phospholipid, usually a hexagonal phase phospholipid or platelet membranes (platelet neutralization procedure).

Antiphospholipid antibody syndrome can be manifest by arterial and/or venous thrombosis. Recurrence rates in patients with "true" APS have been reported to be as high as 70 percent, making this an indication for long-term anticoagulation. Patients with systemic lupus erythematosus or rheumatoid arthritis with persistently positive ACA or lupus anticoagulant have a higher rate of venous and arterial thrombosis than those without these laboratory findings. Recent studies have raised questions about the need for routine warfarin anticoagulation in these individuals above an international normalized ratio (INR) of 2 to 3, as previously proposed. However, there is a subset of patients who will develop recurrent arterial or venous thrombosis, even at higher levels of anticoagulation, who require alternative prophylactic approaches.

Diagnosis of APS based on laboratory findings, particularly ACA or anti-β_2GP1 antibody positivity alone, is problematic. The association of IgM ACA or anti-β_2GP1 antibodies or low titer IgG antibodies with thrombosis has not been documented by clinical study.[105-110] Many individuals without evidence of underlying disease have circulating ACA, including approximately 7 percent of normal blood donors. In data from the Physician's Health Study, there was no difference in the incidence of arterial or venous thrombosis in subjects testing positive versus those testing negative for ACA. In a recent meta-analysis of published studies (1988-2000), lupus anticoagulants and, less strongly, IgG ACA at medium or high titer, were associated with thrombosis.[110]

Most, but not all, patients who are positive for lupus anticoagulants also have ACA or anti-β_2GP1 antibodies. β_2GP1 has a weak affinity for binding to physiological procoagulant phospholipids. In the presence of such phospholipids, some anti-β_2GP1 antibodies can cross-link two phospholipid-bound β_2GP1 molecules, thereby attaching these with high affinity to the phospholipid surface.[107] It has been postulated that only anti-β_2GP1 antibodies with lupus anticoagulant activity can do this. If this mechanism were involved in the pathogenesis of APS, this would be consistent with the stronger association of thrombosis with lupus anticoagulant than with positive anti-β_2GP1 antibodies or ACA detected by immunoassay only.

Antithrombotic Drugs

Heparin and Related Drugs

Because its onset of action is practically immediate when administered parenterally, heparin is the anticoagulant of choice when rapid anticoagulation is required.[111] Commercial preparations of unfractionated heparin consist of a heterogeneous mixture of glycosaminoglycans, with molecular weights ranging from 3000 to 30,000.[35] However, only about one-third of the molecules in these products are anticoagulantly active. Heparin exerts its anticoagulant effect by interacting with antithrombin (Fig. 80–15). A specific pentasaccharide sequence in heparin accounts for its ability to bind with high affinity to lysine sites on antithrombin. In the absence of heparin, antithrombin binds to and neutralizes thrombin and other activated clotting factors (see earlier) slowly; however, heparin-bound antithrombin undergoes a conformational change that dramatically accelerates its ability to bind to and neutralize these factors. In these reactions, arginine reactive centers in antithrombin bind to the enzyme active center serines of thrombin and other serine protease coagulation factors, thereby inhibiting their activities. Heparin then dissociates from these complexes and can be reused to bind to other antithrombin molecules. Heparin thus acts as a true catalyst in accelerating the neutralization of thrombin and other activated clotting factors by antithrombin.[112] Fibrin-bound thrombin is relatively protected from inactivation by the heparin/ antithrombin complex.

Heparin is poorly absorbed from the gastrointestinal tract and therefore is administered parenterally. The complex pharmacokinetics of unfractionated heparin is due to its nonspecific binding to many plasma proteins (including some acute-phase reactants) and to vascular and blood cells. Provided that the doses used are adequate, the efficacy and safety of heparin are comparable when administered by continuous intravenous infusion or by subcutaneous injection.[112] Intermittent intravenous injections of heparin are associated with more bleeding complications than is continuous intravenous infusion.

UNFRACTIONATED HEPARIN MONITORING. Because of unfractionated heparin's often unpredictable pharmacokinetics and its narrow therapeutic range, therapy with this agent requires laboratory monitoring for proper dosing.[111] This is performed conventionally with the activated partial thromboplastin time (aPTT), a test sensitive to the inhibitory effects of heparin on thrombin, factor Xa, and factor IXa. For the treatment of DVT or pulmonary embolism, weight-based nomograms have been recommended because this approach results in more prompt anticoagulation without an increased risk of bleeding compared with other approaches. Treatment is initiated with an 80 U/kg bolus, followed by 18 U/kg/hr, with a target aPTT that has been standardized in the laboratory to reflect heparin levels measured by anti-Xa levels of 0.3 to 0.7 U/ml. The aPTT is sensitive over a heparin range of 0.1 to 1.0 U/ml. Because the aPTT becomes immeasurably prolonged at heparin concentrations of more than 1.0 U/ml, this test is unsuitable for monitoring heparin dosage during percutaneous coronary interventions (angioplasty and stenting) and during cardiac bypass surgery, in which patients require higher levels of anticoagulation with heparin. In these procedures, heparin can be monitored by the activated clotting time, because this test provides a graded response to heparin concentrations in the range of 1 to 5 U/ml. Low-dose subcutaneous unfractionated heparin has also been used to prevent (rather than treat) venous thromboembolism in high-risk patients. Doses of 5000 U every 8 or 12 hours generally

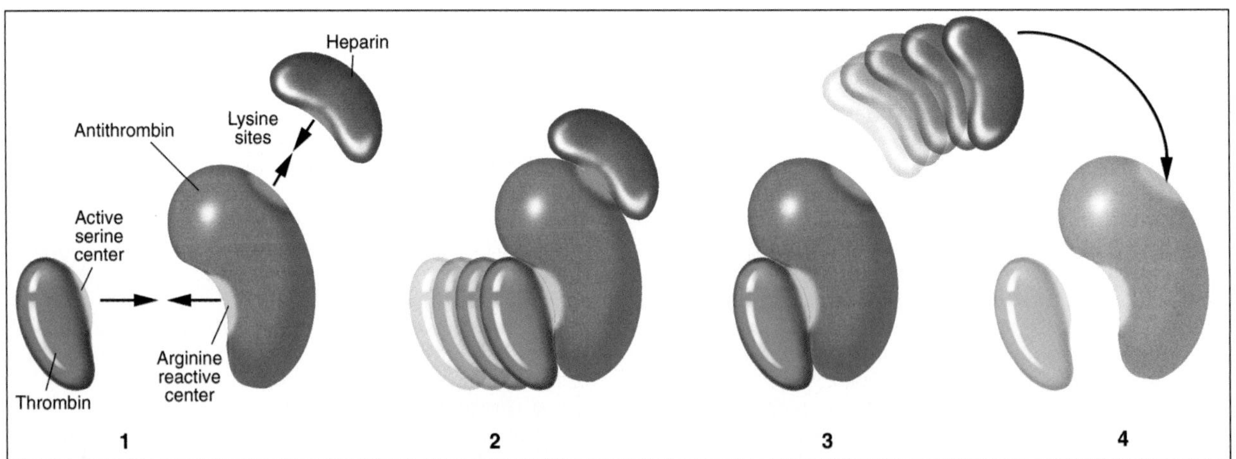

FIGURE 80–15 Mechanism of heparin action. See text for explanation. (Modified from Rosenberg RD: Hemorrhagic disorders: I. Protein interactions in the clotting mechanism. *In* Beck WS [ed]: Hematology. 5th ed. Cambridge, MIT Press, 1991, pp 507-542.)

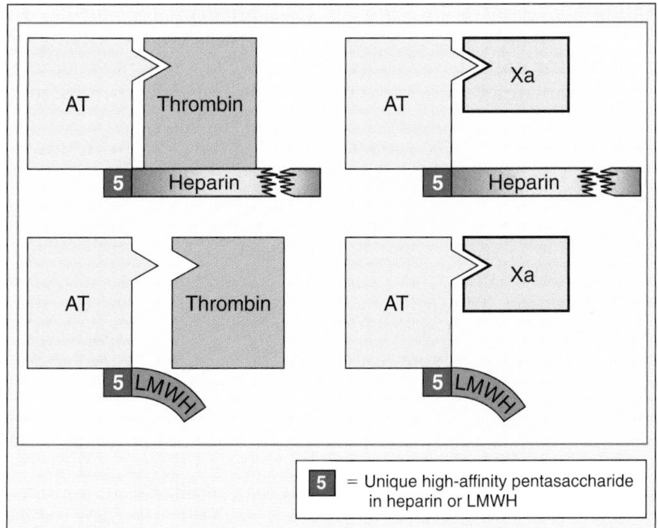

FIGURE 80–16 Mechanisms of inhibitory action of unfractionated heparin (heparin) and low-molecular-weight heparin (LMWH) on thrombin and factor Xa. Both unfractionated heparin and LMWH bind to antithrombin (AT) through a high-affinity pentasaccharide sequence (5) that both types of heparin contain. Inhibition of thrombin (left side of figure) requires formation of a ternary complex of heparin with both antithrombin and thrombin. Unfractionated heparins have sufficient length (≥18 saccharide residues, including the pentasaccharide sequence) to accomplish this, but LMWHs do not. In contrast, inhibition of factor Xa (right side of figure) requires that heparin bind only to antithrombin, which unfractionated heparin and LMWH can catalyze equally effectively through their common pentasaccharide sequences. Thus, LMWH (but not unfractionated heparin) inactivates factor Xa selectively relative to thrombin.

do not prolong the aPTT and therefore do not require monitoring in this setting.

LOW-MOLECULAR-WEIGHT HEPARINS. Low-molecular-weight heparins (LMWH) are manufactured from standard, unfractionated heparin by chemical or enzymatic depolymerization that yields fragments about one-third the size of unfractionated heparin.[35,111] Inhibition of thrombin requires that heparin bind to both antithrombin and thrombin, thereby forming a ternary complex (Fig. 80–16). Ternary complex formation requires that heparin contain at least 18 saccharide residues, including the high-affinity pentasaccharide sequence that binds to antithrombin. In contrast, inhibition of factor Xa requires that heparin bind only to antithrombin; hence, only the pentasaccharide sequence of heparin is needed for this simpler reaction. Most heparin chains in LMWH preparations have fewer than 18 saccharide units and therefore are of insufficient length to bind to both antithrombin and thrombin. However, the shorter heparin fragments in LMWH are able to catalyze the inhibition of factor Xa by antithrombin, provided that they contain the essential pentasaccharide sequence. Thus, the effects of LMWH in the coagulation cascade are restricted to relatively selective inactivation of factor Xa, whereas standard (unfractionated) heparin has equivalent inhibitory activity against factor Xa and thrombin.

Low-molecular-weight heparin has theoretical advantages over standard heparin for several additional reasons[113] First, unlike unfractionated heparin, it can inhibit platelet-bound factor Xa and therefore should be a more effective anticoagulant. Second, LMWH binds less readily to plasma proteins (including acute phase reactants) and vascular and blood cells, and LMWH is more resistant to neutralization by platelet factor 4; this produces a longer plasma half-life, more predictable bioavailability, and more favorable pharmacokinetics than standard heparin. Third, LMWH has less pronounced effects on platelet function and vascular integrity, properties that presumably contribute to its lower risk of bleeding complications than standard heparin. The longer plasma half-life and more predictable anticoagulant response of LMWH preparations allow their administration as fixed-dose, once-daily or twice-daily subcutaneous injections, without need for laboratory monitoring. The convenience of use of LMWH has been extended to outpatient management of patients with uncomplicated acute venous thromboembolism, a situation that previously required continuous intravenous heparin infusion in the hospital. Although several LMWH preparations have been approved for use in North America and Europe, they are prepared by different depolymerization methods and have somewhat different molecular compositions, pharmacological properties, and anticoagulant profiles.[114,115] Therefore, caution may need to be exercised in the interchangeability of these LMWH products.

COMPLICATIONS OF HEPARIN AND LMWH. The major complication of heparin is bleeding. Early studies suggested that treatment with LMWH caused significantly less bleeding than with unfractionated heparin; however, data from more recent and larger studies do not show as great a difference in bleeding risks between the two preparations (see Chap. 47). Factors that predispose to increased bleeding risk include advanced age, serious concurrent illness, heavy consumption of alcohol, concomitant use of aspirin, and renal failure.[35] LMWHs are cleared by renal excretion and should be used with caution in patients with renal insufficiency. In the TIMI 11A trial, a multicenter dose-ranging trial to evaluate the safety of enoxaparin in the treatment of patients with non-ST-segment elevation acute coronary syndrome, patients with a creatine clearance of less than 40 ml/min had higher trough and peak anti-Xa activity and were more likely to have major hemorrhagic events than subjects with normal renal function.[116]

Due to the relatively short half-life of unfractionated heparin, simple discontinuation is usually adequate to control bleeding complications. Protamine sulfate can be used in emergency situations with serious bleeding. Protamine, a strongly basic protein, practically instantaneously neutralizes heparin, which is highly negatively charged. Protamine is effective in neutralizing the antithrombin activity of LMWH but does not completely reverse its anti-factor X activity.

Two distinct types of thrombocytopenia are associated with heparin therapy.[117] The more common form, which may occur in up to 15 percent of patients receiving therapeutic doses of heparin, is a benign and self-limited side effect. This dose-dependent, non-immune-mediated type of thrombocytopenia rarely causes severe reductions in the platelet count or clinical complications and usually does not require discontinuation of heparin. In contrast, the immune form of heparin-induced thrombocytopenia (HIT) can, paradoxically, cause serious, limb- and life-threatening arterial as well as venous thrombosis (HITT). The mechanism in these cases is the interaction of antibody (usually IgG) with a complex of heparin and platelet factor 4 on the surfaces of platelets from which platelet factor 4 is released upon activation (Fig. 80–17A).[117,118] This complex results in the activation of platelets and monocytes through their FcγIIa receptors or on the surface of endothelial cells where released platelet factor 4 also binds (Fig. 80–17B).[119]

In HIT, patients develop absolute or relative (greater than 50 percent drop in platelet count) thrombocytopenia in a reproducible and diagnostic manner.[120] Thrombocytopenia begins at least 4 days after the initiation of heparin and rarely occurs more than 14 days after this time point. The exceptions are patients who received heparin within the recent past, usually within the past 3 months, and have circulating anti-heparin/platelet factor 4 antibodies. In those individuals, re-exposure to heparin can abruptly decrease platelet

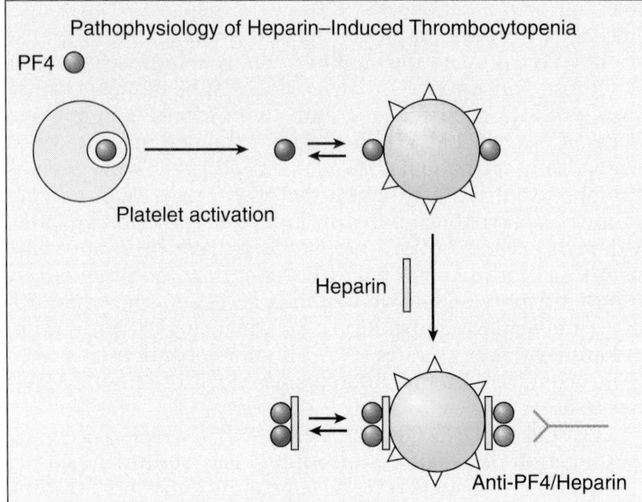

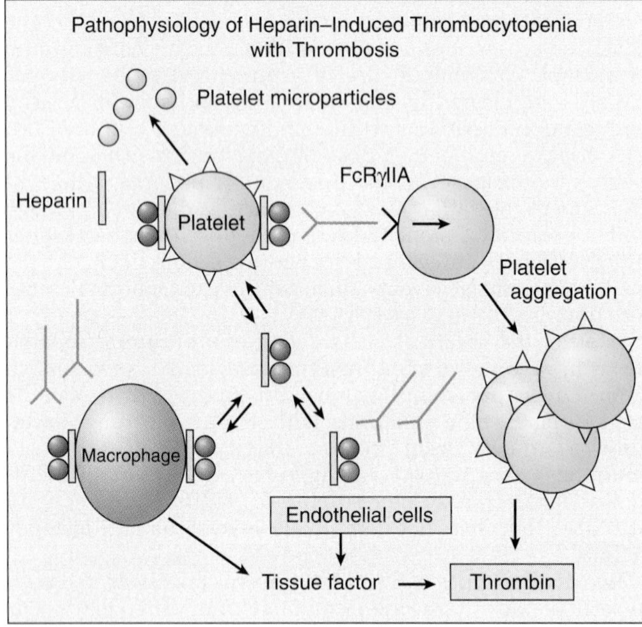

FIGURE 80–17 **A,** Pathophysiology of HIT. With platelet activation, platelet factor 4 (PF4) is released from the platelet α-granule and binds the surface of the activated platelet. PF4, a very basic protein, can complex with circulating negatively charged heparin, forming an antigenic complex. **B,** Pathophysiology of HITT. PF4/heparin antibodies can activate coagulation by a number of mechanisms, including (1) activation of platelets via the platelet FCRγlla receptor resulting in platelet microparticle formation and the provision of a phospholipid surface for coagulation and (2) activation of endothelial cells and monocytes resulting in tissue factor expression, initiation of coagulation, and ultimately thrombin formation, which results in amplification of coagulation and further platelet activation. (Courtesy of D. Cines, University of Pennsylvania, Philadelphia, PA.)

count, and systemic reactions can occur. Except in this circumstance, prior exposure to heparin does not alter the time course of HIT. The decline in platelet count in HIT is usually moderate, with a typical nadir of 50,000 to 60,000/mm^3. However, HIT can cause severe thrombocytopenia even in the absence of thrombosis; and, conversely, heparin-induced thrombosis can actually occur with a normal platelet count. Immune-mediated HIT is not heparin dose-dependent and can develop with low-dose heparin or even with heparin flushes or the use of heparin-bonded catheters. Delayed-onset HIT has been described recently, a clinical scenario in which patients present a few weeks after heparin exposure with thrombosis and strongly positive testing for HIT, with or without thrombosis.[121,122] The pathogenesis of this variant is unclear but may result from ongoing antigenic stimulation, possibly from vascular wall bound complexes.

No single definitive laboratory test can ascertain the diagnosis of HIT, and HIT remains a clinical diagnosis supported by laboratory testing.[117] Laboratory testing for HIT can involve functional assays in which the heparin-induced activation of platelets in vitro is tested by aggregation, serotonin release, or platelet activation markers. Alternatively, enzyme immunoassays of antibody-heparin-platelet factor 4 complexes can be used to test for HIT. The latter have a high sensitivity but low specificity for HIT. Up to 70 percent of patients undergoing cardiopulmonary bypass surgery will develop anti-heparin/platelet factor 4 antibodies, whereas only 2 percent of those individuals will actually develop HIT.[123] Platelet activation assays, notably the serotonin-release assay, are more specific but less sensitive. In general, a negative immunoassay result excludes HIT, although false-negative results have been reported early in the presentation while the patient is still receiving heparin, presumably due to antigen to antibody excess. Therefore, if the initial test finding is negative in patients strongly suspected of HIT, treatment modifications should still be made and laboratory testing should be repeated a few days later.

When HIT is suspected, any source or route of heparin being administered to the patient must be discontinued immediately. LMWH therapy can result in HIT, although the incidence is approximately one-tenth that seen with unfractionated heparin. HIT is associated with a marked hypercoagulable state, and as many as 30 to 50 percent of individuals with HIT will develop thrombosis in the 30 days after diagnosis.[117] For this reason, patients with HIT should be assessed for thrombosis and, even in its absence, should be considered for anticoagulant therapy. Two direct thrombin inhibitors have been studied and have efficacy as anticoagulants in this setting: recombinant hirudin (lepirudin)[124] and argatroban,[125] a small-molecule synthetic antithrombin. LMWHs should not be substituted for heparin because they have strong cross-reactivity with HIT sera.

Other side effects of heparin include cumulative dose-dependent osteoporosis, skin necrosis, alopecia, hypersensitivity reactions, and hypoaldosteronism.[126] Heparin is the anticoagulant of choice during pregnancy; unlike warfarin, it does not cross the placenta and is not teratogenic. However, warfarin may be needed in women with mechanical heart valves who are at high risk of thromboembolism, at least in the periods of low risk of teratogenicity, because of the increased effectiveness of warfarin in this setting (see Chap. 57).[127]

OTHER GLYCOSAMINOGLYCAN-DERIVED DRUGS. Heparan sulfate, dermatan sulfate, and proteoglycans are endogenous heparin-like molecules with antithrombotic activity.[128] Several of these endogenous glycosaminoglycans have been developed as clinical anticoagulants.[128,129] Danaparoid (Orgaran), a mixture of low-molecular-weight anticoagulant glycosaminoglycans, predominantly heparan sulfate (84 percent) and dermatan sulfate (12 percent), was recently removed from the US market.[130] Dermatan sulfate, a naturally occurring glycosaminoglycan, promotes the inactivation of thrombin by heparin cofactor II. Like direct thrombin inhibitors (see later), and unlike standard and low-molecular-weight heparins, dermatan sulfate can inactivate fibrin-bound thrombin.[128] Heparins that can be absorbed orally are under development and some have entered clinical trials, although their efficacy has yet to be documented.

Fondaparinux, a chemically synthesized methoxy-derivative of the naturally occurring antithrombin-binding pentasaccharide, selectively catalyzes the inactivation of factor

Xa by antithrombin without inhibiting thrombin (see Fig. 80–15). Once-daily treatment with fondaparinux (2.5 mg subcutaneously) initiated in the early postoperative period is more effective than an LMWH preparation in preventing venous thromboembolism after hip or knee surgery, without increasing the risk of bleeding.[131,132] Fondaparinux is administered by subcutaneous injection, and its elimination half-life of 17 to 21 hours allows once-daily dosing. Unlike unfractionated heparin and LMWH, it does not bind platelets or platelet factor 4, nor does it result in release of TFPI. Since it does not bind platelet factor 4, an association with HIT would not be expected, and it may become a therapeutic option in this setting. There is no known antidote for reversal of the anticoagulant effect of fondaparinux. Even with a low bleeding risk, given its long half-life, this may become an issue in the clinical management of patients receiving this drug. In the completed studies, clinical situations requiring rapid reversal of the anticoagulant effect were not reported. Additional synthetic pentasaccharides for anticoagulation are under clinical study, including the drug idraparinux, which has a longer half-life than fondaparinux.

Warfarin

Warfarin (Coumadin) is the most frequently used oral anticoagulant.[133] Oral anticoagulants, which are derivatives of coumarins, exert their anticoagulant actions as vitamin K antagonists. The reduced form of vitamin K, vitamin KH_2, is normally required as a cofactor for the gamma-carboxylation of glutamic acid residues in coagulation factors II (prothrombin), VII, IX, and X[134] (Fig. 80–18). This posttranslational modification of these clotting factors is necessary for them to function physiologically in the coagulation cascade by allowing them to bind to and form calcium-dependent complexes on cellular phospholipid surfaces. Oral anticoagulants block the reductase enzymes that are required to recycle vitamin K epoxide to vitamin KH_2 after the gamma-carboxylation reaction, thereby depleting the active vitamin K cofactor.

Warfarin is rapidly and almost completely absorbed from the gastrointestinal tract and circulates bound to albumin with a mean plasma half-life of approximately 40 hours. Metabolism is affected by inherited allelic variants of P450 CYP2C9, which catalyzes the conversion of S-warfarin to its inactive metabolite. Subjects homozygous for the least active alleles are more likely to require a low warfarin dose and to experience warfarin-related bleeding complications.[135] Numerous drugs alter the anticoagulant response to warfarin by pharmacokinetic or pharmacodynamic interactions. Drugs such as phenylbutazone, erythromycin, fluconazole, cimetidine, amiodarone, clofibrate, isoniazid, and propranolol increase warfarin levels, whereas drugs such as cholestyramine, barbiturates, rifampin, and sucralfate decrease warfarin levels. Dietary variations in vitamin K likewise alter warfarin's anticoagulant effects; high vitamin K intake in the diet (including nutritional supplements and vitamin preparations) reduces the anticoagulant response to warfarin. Conversely, liver disease, malabsorption, and hypermetabolic states enhance the anticoagulant effect of warfarin.

MONITORING. Oral anticoagulant therapy requires laboratory monitoring with the prothrombin time test. Commercially available thromboplastin reagents that are used in the prothrombin time assay vary considerably in their clotting ability. This problem previously created major variability in the prothrombin time values reported by different laboratories. To standardize prothrombin time reporting, the INR is now used. The INR corrects for differences in the thromboplastin reagents used by different laboratories. The optimal therapeutic range of warfarin for the prevention of venous thromboembolism and systemic embolism from atrial fibrillation and tissue heart valves targets an INR of 2.0 to 3.0. Higher intensity anticoagulation (INR, 2.5-3.5) is required in patients with mechanical prosthetic heart valves.

"Loading doses" of warfarin should not be employed in initiating oral anticoagulation. Although warfarin has a rapid onset of action, its optimal antithrombotic effect requires several days. The activity of all four of the vitamin K–dependent clotting factors must be inhibited to achieve clinically effective anticoagulation. The effects of warfarin require depletion of circulating clotting factors that are already gamma-carboxylated and hence biologically active when warfarin is started. The vitamin K–dependent clotting factors have different half-lives, with factor VII having the shortest. Therefore, the initial increase in the INR is predominantly due to a decrease in functional factor VII. A large "loading dose" of warfarin (i.e., 10 mg or more per day) will thus create a selective, severe factor VII deficiency state, while still failing to provide antithrombotic effect. In addition, a precipitous reduction in the plasma level of protein C, a vitamin

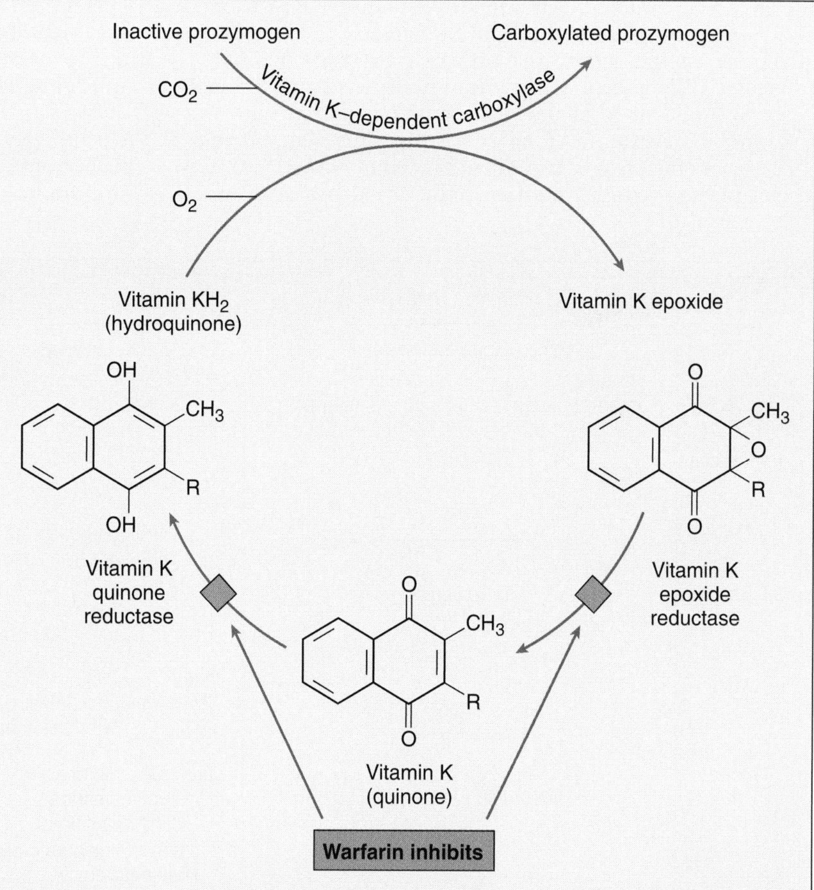

FIGURE 80–18 Vitamin K cycle and its inhibition by warfarin. Warfarin inhibits vitamin K epoxide reductase and vitamin K quinone reductase and so blocks the conversion of vitamin K epoxide to vitamin KH_2. Vitamin KH_2 is a cofactor for the carboxylation of inactive proenzymes (factors II, VII, IX, and X) to their active forms. (From Furie B, Furie BC: Molecular basis of vitamin K–dependent gamma-carboxylation. Blood 75:1753, 1990.)

K–dependent anticoagulant (rather than clotting) factor, which has the shortest half-life of all vitamin K–dependent proteins, can lead to a transient paradoxical hypercoagulable state during the first 36 hours of warfarin therapy (see later).[136,137] Therefore, the initial dose of warfarin should approximate the chronic maintenance dose that is anticipated, generally in the range of 4 to 6 mg/d in most adults.

COMPLICATIONS. Skin necrosis, a very rare complication that occurs within the first few days of starting warfarin therapy, tends to occur in patients with underlying inherited protein C or protein S deficiency. As noted earlier, it is likely related to the initial precipitous decrease in protein C levels (especially in individuals who may already have a congenitally low level of protein C). This leads to a transient prothrombotic imbalance, particularly with the use of large loading doses of warfarin. Warfarin should be avoided in pregnant patients, if possible, because of its potential to cause embryopathy and peripartum neonatal and maternal bleeding complications.

As with heparin, bleeding complications are the most frequent adverse effects of warfarin. For an individual patient, the cumulative risk of bleeding complications relates directly to the intensity and duration of anticoagulant therapy.[138] Major bleeding on warfarin occurs at a rate of 5 to 7 percent per year.[139] As noted earlier, the INR can vary despite a stable, chronic dose of warfarin as a function of changes in either medications or diet. When the INR exceeds the therapeutic range, discontinuing or reducing the dose of warfarin is usually sufficient; stopping warfarin generally normalizes the INR within about 3 days. If more rapid reversal of warfarin effect is required due to extreme elevations of the INR or clinical bleeding, vitamin K can be administered orally or parenterally. Vitamin K given orally has been shown to be superior to that given by subcutaneous injection, as the latter is ineffective in some patients.[140] However, particularly when vitamin K is given at higher doses, a transient resistance to re-anticoagulation with warfarin may be encountered subsequently. Emergency reversal of warfarin effect can be rapidly achieved by infusion of fresh frozen plasma (usually starting with 2 to 4 units). A single dose of recombinant factor VIIa reduced the prothrombin level in a small number of patients who had an elevated INR with serious bleeding (n = 4), required a procedure (n = 5), or were at high risk of bleeding and had an INR greater than 10 (n = 4).[141] Clinical efficacy was reported, although larger trials are needed to determine the efficacy and safety of this drug in this setting. Algorithms for the management of elevated INR with or without bleeding have been proposed.[136]

Thrombin Inhibitors and Other Specific Coagulation Inhibitors

Newly developed anticoagulants specifically target inactivation of thrombin, factor Xa, factor IXa, and the factor VIIa/tissue factor complex, as well as inactivation of factors VIIIa and Va by enhancement of the protein C anticoagulant pathway.[142-146] The sites of action of these anticoagulants are shown in Figure 80–19. Except for the direct thrombin inhibitors, most of these agents still await evaluation in phase 3 trials.

THROMBIN INHIBITORS. Direct thrombin inhibitors inactivate both free (fluid-phase) thrombin and fibrin-bound thrombin. In this respect, these agents differ from heparin and its low-molecular-weight derivatives, which require complex formation with antithrombin and thus are weak inhibitors of clot-bound thrombin.[142-144]

The thrombin molecule has distinct functional domains. The "active site" of thrombin is the catalytic site that possesses serine protease activity. "Exosite 1" of thrombin serves to dock substrates in the proper orientation and is the binding site for fibrin(ogen). Direct thrombin inhibitors interact with one or both of these sites. Hirudin and bivalirudin are more specific for thrombin than active-site inhibitors because they are bivalent, binding to thrombin at both the active site and exosite 1. In contrast, low-molecular-weight thrombin inhibitors such as argatroban and efegatran bind only to the active site of thrombin. Because the active site of thrombin is structurally similar to other serine proteases, these active-site inhibitors are less selective for thrombin than the bivalent inhibitors.

Hirudin, the prototype of the direct thrombin inhibitors, is a 65-amino acid polypeptide originally isolated from the saliva of *Hirudo medicinalis*, the medicinal leech. Hirudin is now produced by recombinant DNA technology (lepirudin). It binds tightly to thrombin, forming a slowly reversible, 1:1 stoichiometric complex. In this complex, the amino-terminus of hirudin binds to the active site and its carboxy-terminal binds to exosite 1 of thrombin.

Bivalirudin (formerly Hirulog) is a synthetic 20-amino acid polypeptide composed of a peptide sequence (D-Phe-Pro-Arg-Pro) that is directed at the active site of thrombin, linked to a dodecapeptide analog of the exosite 1–binding carboxy-terminal of hirudin. Thus, like hirudin, bivalirudin interacts bivalently with both the active

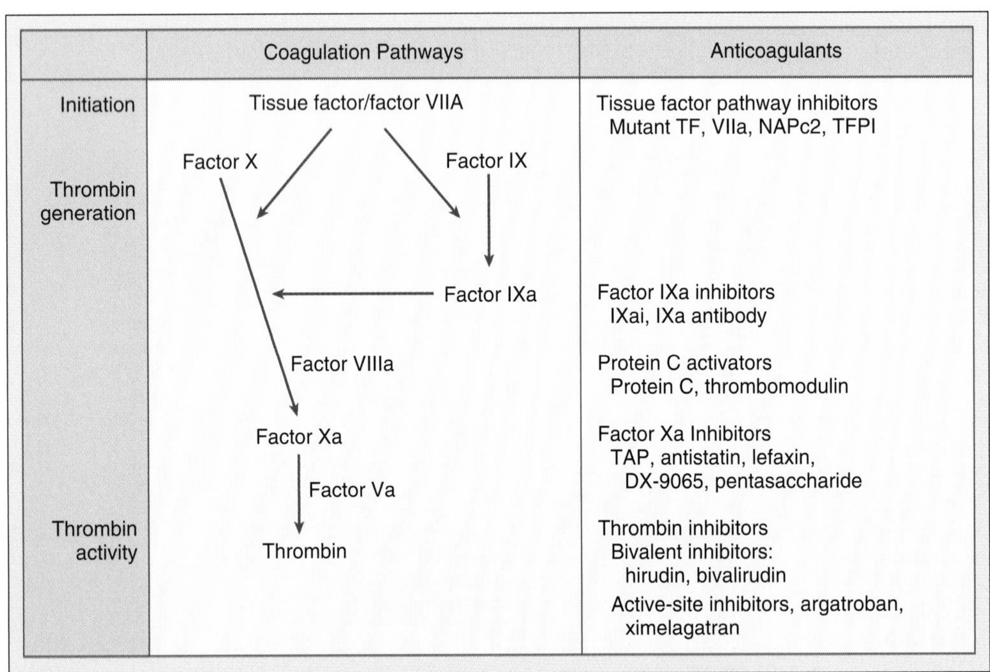

FIGURE 80–19 Activation and inhibitors of coagulation. New anticoagulants act by inhibiting the tissue factor pathway (initiation), thrombin generation, and thrombin activity. Ximelagatran is the product of the active thrombin inhibitor melagatran. (Modified from Hirsh J, Weitz JI: New antithrombotic agents. Lancet 353:1431, 1999.)

site and exosite 1 of thrombin, forming a 1:1 stoichiometric complex. However, once bound, thrombin cleaves the Arg-Pro bond and thereby removes the active site-binding part of bivalirudin, leaving only a low-affinity, weaker inhibitory interaction with thrombin. Consequently, the potent thrombin inhibitory effect of bivalirudin is short lived, conferring on it a potential safety advantage.

Several low-molecular-weight direct thrombin inhibitors have been developed. These less-specific agents target only the active site of thrombin. Argatroban is the prototype of the noncovalent class of these active site inhibitors, which also includes napsagatran, inogatran, and melagatran.

Direct thrombin inhibitors have theoretical advantages over heparin. First, as noted earlier, they can inactivate clot-bound thrombin. Second, unlike heparin, they do not bind to plasma proteins. Therefore, they have the pharmacokinetic advantage of a more predictable anticoagulant response. This may permit their administration without laboratory monitoring, which has not been true for the currently available parenterally administered agents due to their narrow therapeutic window and their use in combination with other anticoagulants, such as for coronary procedures.[144] However, laboratory monitoring may not be needed for the oral agents under development and in clinical study (see later). Clinical trial results and clinical experience suggest that the bleeding risk with the parenteral agents is greater than that seen with heparin. Because of their short half-lives, discontinuation of the drug is usually adequate to control bleeding symptoms.

Orally administered direct thrombin inhibitors have been developed and one, ximelagatran, is in phase 3 clinical trials. After oral administration, ximelagatran is rapidly absorbed and converted to its active metabolite melagatran, a small molecule direct thrombin inhibitor. In clinical trials, ximelagatran is given by twice-daily dosing and without laboratory monitoring. Efficacy in prevention of VTE after total knee arthroplasty has been reported, without increased bleeding risk as compared with warfarin.[146] Phase II trials showed promising results in the treatment of DVT,[147] and large international randomized controlled trials in thromboprophylaxis in atrial fibrillation and in the treatment of DVT were completed in 2003. Melagatran is excreted renally, and patients with significant renal impairment have not been included in clinical trials. Additional oral direct thrombin inhibitors are in clinical development.

OTHER SPECIFIC COAGULATION INHIBITORS. Inhibitors of factor Xa (see Fig. 80–19) include tick anticoagulant peptide (TAP), antistatin, and lefaxin.[145,148] The latter two are extracts of the salivary glands of two species of leeches. All are potent and specific factor Xa inhibitors that are available in recombinant forms. DX-9065 is a synthetic, low-molecular-weight, reversible factor Xa inhibitor that has oral bioavailability. Experimental agents that are inhibitors of factor IXa include a monoclonal antibody and active site-blocked-factor IXa.[149] Specific inhibitors of the tissue factor pathway under study include a soluble mutant form of tissue factor that has decreased cofactor function for factor VIIa-induced activation of factor X; active-site-blocked factor VIIa (VIIai), which competes with factor VII for tissue factor binding; NAPc2, a small, nematode-derived anticoagulant protein that binds to factor X and inhibits factor VIIa within the factor VII/tissue factor complex; and recombinant TFPI.[150] Protein C activators that have been studied as therapeutic anticoagulants include plasma and recombinant forms of protein C and recombinant soluble thrombomodulin. Recombinant human activated protein C, or drotrecogin alfa (activated), has antithrombotic, antiinflammatory, and profibrinolytic properties. A randomized, double-blind, placebo-controlled trial showed that this agent significantly reduced mortality in patients with severe sepsis, although with an increased risk of bleeding.[151]

Thrombolytic (Fibrinolytic) Drugs (see Chap. 47)

The common mechanism of action of currently available thrombolytic (fibrinolytic) agents, including streptokinase, urokinase, and alteplase (recombinant tissue-type plasminogen activator [rt-PA]), involves the conversion of the inactive plasma zymogen, plasminogen, to the active fibrinolytic enzyme, plasmin (see Fig. 80–7). Plasmin has relatively weak substrate specificity and can degrade not only fibrin but also any protein that has an arginyl-lysyl bond available for enzymatic attack, including fibrinogen. Indiscriminate plasmin lysis of both fibrin and fibrinogen can produce a systemic state of fibrin(ogen)olysis (or "systemic lytic state"), which might cause a serious systemic bleeding tendency, so attempts have been made to develop thrombolytic agents that generate plasmin preferentially at the fibrin surface in a preformed thrombus ("fibrin-specific agents"). Plasmin associated with fibrin is protected from rapid inhibition by alpha$_2$-antiplasmin (see earlier) and can thereby effectively degrade the fibrin of a clot. Thus, the biochemical strategy was to develop fibrinolytic agents that bind to fibrin and thereby produce only fibrin-bound plasmin from fibrin-bound plasminogen.

Streptokinase and urokinase induce a systemic lytic state, with extensive systemic activation of the fibrinolytic system, deplete alpha$_2$-antiplasmin, and degrade circulating fibrinogen. In contrast, the physiological plasminogen activators t-PA and scu-PA activate plasminogen preferentially at the fibrin surface. The promise of a marked reduction in the risk of hemorrhage with "second-generation" fibrin-specific agents has not been fulfilled in large clinical trials, however. This may be due to the inability of plasmin to discriminate between fibrin in pathological thrombi, which is the desired target, and fibrin in physiological hemostatic plugs, the lysis of which will induce bleeding.

STREPTOKINASE. Streptokinase is isolated from hemolytic streptococci and is produced from bacterial cultures. The mechanism of activation of plasminogen by streptokinase is unique among plasminogen activators in that streptokinase itself possesses no enzymatic activity.[152,153] Streptokinase forms a complex with plasminogen, and it is the streptokinase-plasminogen complex that actually possesses enzymatic activity toward plasminogen. The streptokinase-plasminogen complexes are thereby converted to streptokinase-plasmin complexes, and the enzyme active sites in the streptokinase-plasmin complexes are the same as those in plasmin. The streptokinase-plasmin(ogen) complexes activate circulating and fibrin-bound plasminogen relatively indiscriminately, producing a systemic lytic state.

Because of its bacterial source, streptokinase is antigenic. Most individuals have preexisting antibodies resulting from previous streptococcal infection. The administration of streptokinase stimulates the rapid formation of high titers of neutralizing antistreptokinase antibodies, which are sufficient to neutralize standard doses of streptokinase. Although antibody titers may return to near-baseline levels as early as 2 years after a single dose, once streptokinase has been used, subsequent thrombolytic treatment should be with an immunologically unrelated agent because of the uncertain efficacy of repeated treatment. Streptokinase causes transient hypotension in many patients and significant allergic reactions in some, including a serum sickness–type syndrome, fever, rash, and bronchospasm.

UROKINASE. Urokinase, or two-chain urokinase-type plasminogen activator (tcu-PA), is a trypsin-like serine protease composed of two polypeptide chains linked by a disulfide bridge.[152,153] Urokinase is produced from cultures of human fetal kidney cells. It directly activates plasminogen to plasmin, leading to relatively nonspecific degradation of fibrin, fibrinogen, and other plasma proteins, depletion of circulating alpha$_2$-antiplasmin, and a systemic lytic state. Urokinase is not antigenic and does not cause allergic reactions.

TISSUE-TYPE PLASMINOGEN ACTIVATOR. Tissue-type plasminogen activator is a naturally occurring molecule released from vascular endothelial cells. For therapeutic thrombolysis, it is produced commercially by recombinant DNA technology (rt-PA; alteplase) and, as a "second-generation" agent, it is relatively fibrin specific.[152,153]

Tissue-type plasminogen activator, a single-chain serine protease, activates plasminogen directly. Fibrin significantly enhances the efficiency of plasminogen activation by t-PA. The basis for the relative fibrin specificity of t-PA action is described previously in the section on the fibrinolytic system. Briefly, fibrin provides a surface for the sequential binding of enzyme (t-PA) and substrate (plasminogen). The assembly of this ternary complex thereby promotes the activation of plasminogen to plasmin that is efficiently localized to the fibrin clot; fibrin then becomes the substrate for lysis by the plasmin that is generated on its surface.

Tissue-type plasminogen activator is converted by plasmin to a disulfide-linked two-chain form by hydrolysis of the Arg 275-Ile276 bond; alteplase consists mainly of the single-chain form of t-PA. Both the single-chain and two-chain forms of t-PA are cleared from plasma according to a two-compartment model, with initial half-lives of 3 to 6 minutes and terminal half-lives of 40 to 50 minutes. The currently preferred dosage regimen of fibrin-selective alteplase for coronary thrombolysis consists of weight-adjusted, accelerated ("front-loaded") administration (see Chap. 47). The front-loaded administration of alteplase achieves a mean steady-state plasma concentration during the initial 30 minutes that is 45 percent higher than that achieved with standard infusion, although it does not alter the plasma half-life.

VARIANTS OF PLASMINOGEN ACTIVATORS. These thrombolytic agents have been engineered to favorably alter the pharmacokinetic and functional properties of currently used drugs. They are designed to have prolonged half-lives, improved enzymatic efficiency, enhanced local concentrations in the clot by altered binding to fibrin and stimulation by fibrin, and resistance to plasma protease inhibitors.[153]

Variants of u-PA have been developed and evaluated in clinical study.[153] Saruplase is an unglycosylated, single-chain recombinant u-PA. Clinical trials have demonstrated similar efficacy of this drug to other thrombolytics, but in some studies, increased bleeding complications occurred. M23 is a single-chain molecule composed of the kringle and protease domain of saruplase and the carboxy-terminal fragment of the direct thrombin inhibitor hirudin, providing both fibrinolytic and antithrombotic activity.

A number of t-PA mutants have been developed. These can be divided into those in which amino acid substitutions have been made (monteplase, tenecteplase) and deletion mutants (reteplase, lanoteplase, pamiteplase). In monteplase, there is a cysteine to serine substitution at position 84, resulting in an increased half-life of the drug compared to native t-PA. Tenecteplase contains amino acid substitutions at three sites: threonine at position 103 is replaced by asparagine; asparagine at position 117 is replaced by glutamine; and four amino acids, lysine, histidine, arginine, and arginine, are replaced by alanine-alanine-alanine-alanine at positions 296 through 299. Tenecteplase is characterized by a prolonged half-life, increased fibrin specificity, and increased resistance to inhibition by PAI-1.[154,155]

Reteplase (r-PA) is a single-chain nonglycosylated deletion variant of t-PA, containing only the kringle-2 and serine protease domains. This deletion mutant has a prolonged half-life and, therefore, can be administered by bolus injection. Another third-generation drug is lanoteplase (n-PA), which retains kringle-1, kringle-2, and protease domains and also has a glutamine substituted for asparagines at position 117. It has an even longer half-life (37 min) and can be administered by single-bolus, weight-adjusted injection.[155] Pamiteplase is a modified t-PA with deletion of the kringle-1 domain and a point substitution of glutamine for arginine at position 274. These modifications make the drug resistant to plasmin-mediated cleavage.

The t-PA of saliva from the vampire bat *Desmodus rotundus* (bat-PA) has potent and relatively fibrin-specific thrombolytic properties.[153,156] Different molecular forms of bat-PA have been purified, characterized, cloned, and expressed. These are being evaluated in preclinical ex vivo and animal studies.

Antibody targeting of thrombolytic agents is a potentially powerful approach to localizing the actions of these drugs to specific components of different types of thrombi (e.g., directed at platelet antigens in arterial thrombi, or thrombin in recently formed thrombi). This can be achieved by conjugating plasminogen activators with monoclonal antibodies that are specific, for example, for fibrin but do not cross-react with fibrinogen. These bifunctional molecules are engineered to contain both a highly specific antigen-binding site that concentrates the drug at the clot and an effector site that promotes thrombolysis.

Antiplatelet Agents

The sequence of events involved in the process of platelet activation is described in detail in the previous section on platelets (Figs. 80–8 and 80–20). Inhibition of platelet function can be targeted at any one of these activation steps.[157,158] Platelet blockade would be expected to be most effective if it is directed at either the initial (adhesion) (see Fig. 80–20A) or final (aggregation) (see Fig. 80–20D) points in the sequence. Antiplatelet agents targeted at any one of the intermediate events should be less potent, because platelet adhesion is followed by the binding of several specific agonists to their respective receptors and the activation of several simultaneous intracellular pathways (e.g., ADP release, TXA_2 synthesis) that act in concert to induce the final step of platelet aggregation. Therefore, pharmacological interruption of only one of these intermediate steps (e.g., with aspirin, antithrombins, clopidogrel) may permit platelet activation through alternative, uninhibited pathways. Agents that block the interaction of vWF with its platelet membrane Gp Ib receptor should inhibit adhesion (see Fig. 80–20A) as well as the subsequent downstream cascade of platelet activation events, including secretion of mitogens into the vessel wall and platelet aggregation. Therapeutic approaches to inhibit adhesion could involve anti-vWF or anti-Gp Ib monoclonal antibodies or agents that interfere with vWF-platelet Gp-Ib binding. These strategies have yet to be translated to clinical practice, however. In contrast, considerable clinical evidence has now validated powerful therapeutic strategies to block the final step of platelet aggregation that is mediated by the interaction of fibrinogen (or vWF) with its platelet Gp IIb/IIIa receptors (see Fig. 80–20D).

ASPIRIN. Aspirin (acetylsalicylic acid), known for more than 50 years to have antithrombotic efficacy, has stood the test of time as an effective, inexpensive, and relatively safe drug for the prevention of various thrombotic and vascular disorders, particularly in the arterial circulation where platelets are the predominant participants in the thrombotic process.[159] Until recently, aspirin has been essentially the only available, clinically effective antiplatelet drug. However, there are several clinical settings in which aspirin fails to provide full (or even partial) antithrombotic benefit.[160]

Aspirin is readily absorbed from the stomach and upper small intestine and is then hydrolyzed to release free acetyl groups. This moiety acetylates serine residues at position 529 of cyclooxygenase (COX; prostaglandin G/H synthase), which leads to irreversible inactivation of the enzyme (Fig. 80–21). Inactive, acetylated COX cannot function to catalyze the oxygenation of arachidonic acid to prostaglandin G_2. Aspirin thereby blocks the formation of TXA_2, a potent mediator of platelet aggregation and vasoconstrictor. Because anucleate platelets essentially are unable to synthesize new, unacetylated COX, aspirin blocks the function of platelets exposed to it for their remaining lifetime (normally 7 to 10 days) in the circulation. This accounts for the lengthy therapeutic effect of aspirin despite its plasma half-life of only 20 minutes.

The inhibitory effects of aspirin on platelet TXA_2 production and ex vivo aggregation are rapid, with maximal effects achieved within 15 to 30 minutes of oral administration of a dose as low as 81 mg. A single oral dose of 100 mg of aspirin almost completely suppresses platelet TXA_2 synthesis in both normal individuals and patients with cardiovascular disease. Daily administration of only 30 to 50 mg of aspirin exerts a cumulative effect and likewise results in almost complete inhibition of platelet TXA_2 production within 7 to 10 days. These aspirin effects on platelet TXA_2 formation generally correlate well with inhibition of ex vivo platelet aggregability and prolongation of the skin bleeding time. Although platelet function remains impaired for 4 to 7 days after a single dose of aspirin, reflecting the life span of irreversibly inhibited platelets, the prolonged bleeding time generally returns to normal within 24 to 48 hours of aspirin ingestion. This discrepancy is due to the release from bone marrow into the circulation of a sufficient cohort of uninhibited platelets after the elimination of aspirin from blood to restore normal in vivo hemostasis (bleeding time) even before complete normalization of ex vivo platelet function.

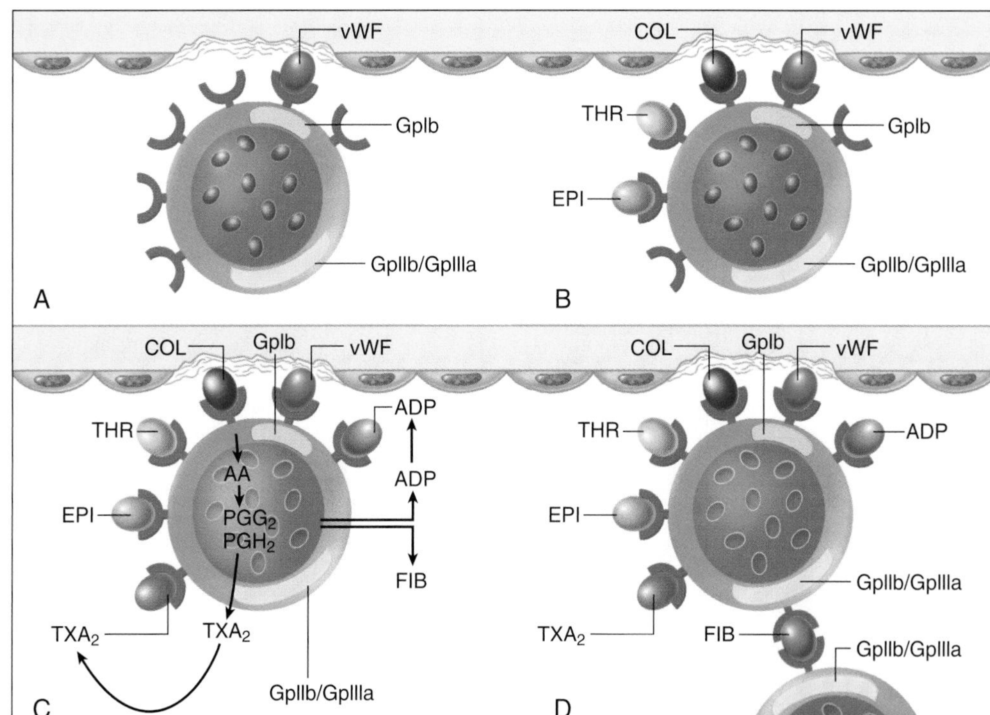

FIGURE 80–20 Sequence of events in platelet activation, with potential targets for antiplatelet therapy. **A,** Platelet adhesion to the injured vascular intimal surface is mediated by von Willebrand factor (vWF) binding to its receptor on platelet membrane Gp Ib. **B,** Adherent platelets are also anchored to the damaged vessel wall by binding of subendothelial collagen (COL) to its platelet surface COL receptors. Other platelet stimuli in blood, including thrombin (THR) and epinephrine (EPI), bind to their respective receptors. **C,** In response to these different stimuli, adherent platelets are activated and release thromboxane A_2 (TXA_2) and adenosine diphosphate (ADP), which bind to their own respective platelet receptors and amplify the activation process. **D,** Platelet aggregation is mediated by fibrinogen (FIB) binding to its receptors on adjoining platelets, forming fibrinogen bridges. The FIB receptor is formed by the complexing of Gp IIb/IIIa in the membrane of activated platelets. AA = arachidonic acid; PGG_2 and PGH_2 = labile prostaglandin endoperoxides. (Modified from Schafer AI: Antiplatelet therapy with glycoprotein IIb/IIIa receptor inhibitors and other novel agents. Tex Heart Inst J 24:90, 1997.)

Aspirin also inhibits COX in vascular endothelial cells, leading to suppression of platelet inhibitory and vasodilatory endothelium-derived PGI_2; this would be expected to offset the antiplatelet effects of aspirin. Attempts to design "platelet selective" aspirin regimens have not translated to clinical feasibility. Nevertheless, there is ample evidence that the antithrombotic effects of aspirin predominate in vivo, possibly due to mechanisms in addition to platelet TXA_2 inhibition.

Up to 50 percent of individuals exhibit a relative state of "aspirin resistance."[161] This phenomenon is defined as suboptimal inhibition of ex vivo platelet function or TXA_2 blockade in response to conventional doses of aspirin. "Aspirin resistance" has not yet been conclusively linked to aspirin "treatment failure," so its clinical relevance requires further study. Potential mechanisms may include pharmacodynamic interactions with other drugs (see next section), extraplatelet sources of TXA_2, or COX polymorphisms that lead to interindividual variability in response.[162]

NON-ASPIRIN NONSTEROIDAL ANTIINFLAMMATORY DRUGS (NSAIDS). Non-aspirin NSAIDs likewise inhibit COX. Unlike aspirin, however, these other NSAIDs inhibit the enzyme reversibly, and therefore their durations of TXA_2 and platelet inhibitory action depend on the clearance of the drugs from the circulation.[163] Thus, there is considerable variability in the extent and duration of the effects of various NSAIDs on ex vivo platelet aggregation and bleeding time prolongation. Non-aspirin NSAIDs reversibly inhibit COX by preventing its arachidonic acid substrate from gaining access to the active site of the enzyme.

COX-1, the constitutive isoform of COX, is present in platelets and produces TXA_2. Aspirin and the traditional NSAIDs are nonselective inhibitors of both COX-1 and COX-2. The newer COX-2-specific inhibitors are designed to maximize the antiinflammatory effects mediated by the COX-2 isoform, while minimizing the common side effects (e.g., bleeding) attributed to the COX-1 isoform. Therefore, the antiplatelet potency of the new COX-2 inhibitors is several orders of magnitude lower than that of aspirin and the standard NSAIDs, and generally cannot be assumed to afford antithrombotic protection. In fact, in clinical reports, COX-2 ingestion may promote, or at least not provide protection from, thromboembolism.[164] Concerns have been raised about the cardiovascular safety of long-term use of these agents because of their inhibition of COX-2-dependent PGI_2 production.[165]

Interaction of NSAIDs with COX may prevent acetylation of the enzyme by aspirin. This suggests that the concomitant administration of nonselective NSAIDs (e.g., ibuprofen), but not COX-2-selective NSAIDs, may actually antagonize the

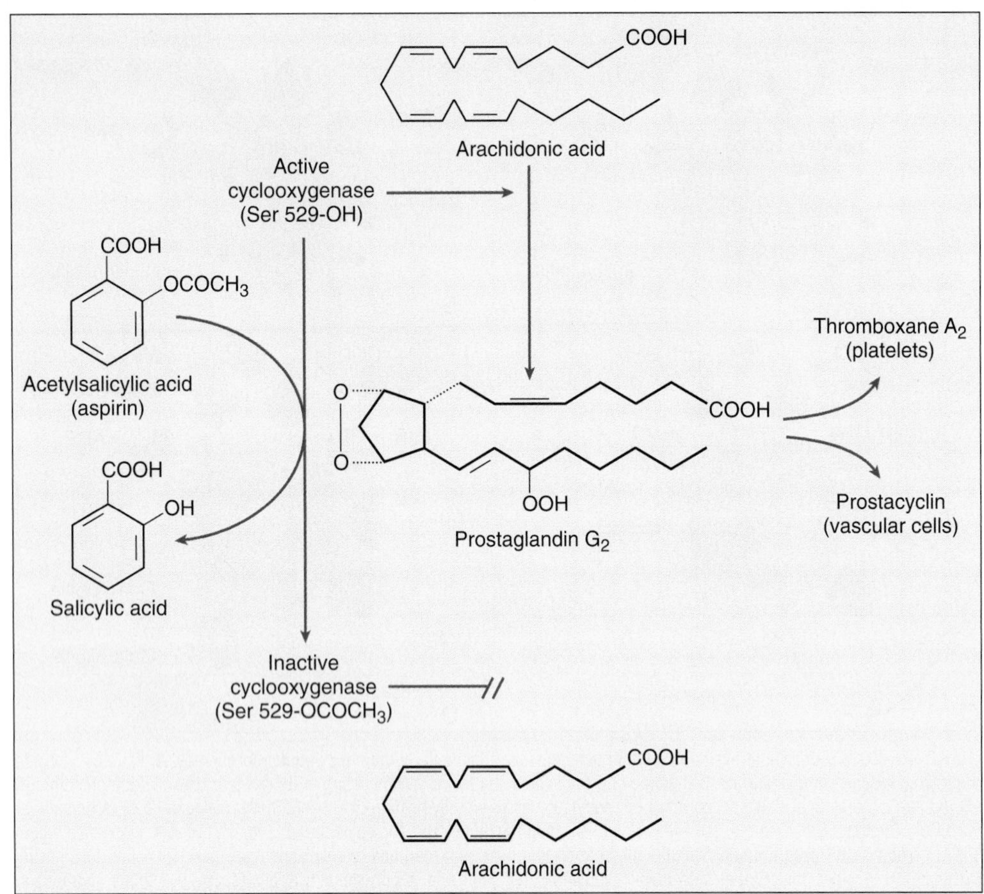

FIGURE 80–21 Aspirin (acetylsalicylic acid) inhibition of cyclooxygenase (prostaglandin-G/H synthase). Aspirin acetylates serine at position 529 of cyclooxygenase, rendering the enzyme inactive. Acetylated cyclooxygenase does not function to catalyze the oxygenation of arachidonic acid to prostaglandin G_2. Aspirin thereby blocks the formation of thromboxane A_2 (in platelets) and prostacyclin (in vascular cells). (From Loscalzo J, Schafer AI: Anticoagulants, antiplatelet agents, and fibrinolytics. *In* Loscalzo J, Creager MA, Dzau MV [eds]: Vascular Medicine: A Textbook of Vascular Biology and Diseases. Philadelphia: Lippincott Williams & Wilkins, 1996.)

effects of aspirin on COX by competitive interaction and consequently blunt aspirin's antiplatelet efficacy.[166] The mechanism of this pharmacodynamic interaction is competition between aspirin and NSAIDs for a common docking site within the COX channel, which aspirin binds to in platelets prior to irreversible acetylation of Ser529.[167]

OTHER THROMBOXANE INHIBITORS. Figure 80–20C illustrates other opportunities to interrupt platelet TXA_2 synthesis and/or action in addition to COX blockade. The reduced incidence of atherosclerotic cardiovascular disease in Greenland Eskimos has been attributed, at least in part, to their diets rich in fish oils containing omega-3 polyunsaturated fatty acids. A major omega-3 fatty acid in fish oils is eicosapentaenoic acid, which incorporates into phospholipids of cell membranes and competes with arachidonic acid as substrate for COX. The product of eicosapentaenoic acid oxygenation is TXA_3, an eicosanoid that is devoid of the potent platelet-activating and vasoconstrictor actions of arachidonic acid-derived TXA_2. Large and often unpalatable doses (>10 gm eicosapentaenoic acid daily) of medicinal fish oils are required to simulate changes in platelet membrane fatty acid content attained with Eskimo diets and thereby produce antiplatelet actions. Thromboxane synthase inhibitors (e.g., dazoxiben) and TXA_2 receptors antagonists (e.g., vapiprost), as well as dual thromboxane synthase/TXA_2 receptor inhibitors (e.g., ridogrel), have been developed but generally have not been found to be superior to aspirin in limited clinical trials.[158]

CLOPIDOGREL AND TICLOPIDINE. Clopidogrel (Plavix) and ticlopidine (Ticlid) are structurally related thienopyridine derivatives. Clopidogrel is largely replacing ticlopidine in clinical practice because of its more favorable side-effect profile and more rapid onset of action. These drugs produce their antiplatelet effects by inhibiting the ADP-dependent pathway of platelet activation.[158,168] After oral administration, both drugs require modification to active forms. They exert a permanent effect on a platelet protein, which is the ADP receptor itself or a platelet membrane component closely related to the ADP receptor. As ADP receptor blockers, these drugs inhibit ADP-induced platelet aggregation (see Fig. 80–20C).

Presumably because they must be converted to an active form in vivo, clopidogrel and ticlopidine have a relatively slow onset of antiplatelet action. On repeated daily dosing of 75 mg clopidogrel, partial inhibition of platelet aggregation occurs from the second day of treatment and reaches steady-state inhibition after 4 to 7 days. Ticlopidine has a slower onset of antiplatelet effect than clopidogrel. Using a larger loading dose of clopidogrel (300-400 mg) results in platelet inhibition within hours of adminstration.[169] The antiplatelet activity of clopidogrel and ticlopidine persists for 4 to 8 days after discontinuation of the drug, reflecting the circulating lifetime of platelets and consistent with an irreversible antiplatelet effect, as is the case with aspirin. Individual variability in platelet inhibition and the occurrence of "clopidogrel resistance" (similar to aspirin resistance) has been described, but the clinical relevance of these phenomena is as yet unclear.[162]

Ticlopidine can cause severe neutropenia, which is usually reversible with discontinuation of the drug, in up to 1 percent of patients.[158] The risk of this adverse effect is much lower (about 0.1 percent) with clopidogrel. In addition, thrombotic thrombocytopenic purpura, a serious and sometimes fatal disorder, is a rare complication of therapy with both ticlopidine and clopidogrel. Thrombotic thrombocytopenic purpura typically occurs within 2 to 8 weeks of initiation of the thienopyridine and was noted in 0.02 percent of patients receiving ticlopidine after coronary stenting.[170-172] Other side effects, including gastrointestinal symptoms, pruritus, urticaria, and bleeding, also appear to occur less often with clopidogrel than with ticlopidine.

PHOSPHODIESTERASE INHIBITORS

Dipyridamole. The mechanism of antiplatelet action of dipyridamole is unclear. Although this drug can stimulate PGI_2 synthesis, potentiate the platelet inhibitory effects of PGI_2, raise platelet cyclic adenosine monophosphate levels by inhibiting phosphodiesterase, and block uptake of adenosine into vascular and blood cells, these potential antiplatelet actions generally do not occur at therapeutically achievable drug concentrations.[158] Unlike aspirin, dipyridamole does not prolong the bleeding time or inhibit ex vivo platelet aggregation at therapeutic doses. Although numerous clinical trials have failed to demonstrate antithrombotic efficacy of dipyridamole when it is used alone in any clinical setting, it may enhance the effect of warfarin in preventing systemic embolization from mechanical heart valve prostheses and add to the beneficial effect of aspirin in preventing the progression of peripheral occlusive arterial disease or, when used in a sustained-release preparation, in the secondary prevention of ischemic stroke.[173]

Cilostazol. Cilostazol is a quinolone derivative that is a potent inhibitor of platelet phosphodiesterase-3 and has vasodilatory effects. It may be beneficial in the treatment of intermittent claudication due to peripheral vascular disease, an indication for which it has been approved by the Food and Drug Administration.[158]

GLYCOPROTEIN IIB/IIIA ANTAGONISTS. Regardless of the stimulus for their activation, the aggregation of platelets is finally regulated through their membrane binding sites for fibrinogen in the Gp IIb/IIIa receptor complex (see Fig. 80–20D). This provides the rationale for pharmacological intervention directed against the platelet Gp IIb/IIIa complex. The role of the platelet Gp IIb/IIIa complex in platelet activation is discussed in more detail earlier in the section on platelets. Because Gp IIb/IIIa antagonists do not block TXA_2 production by activated platelets, concomitant use of aspirin may enhance their antithrombotic efficacy.

Platelet Gp IIb/IIIa antagonists generally belong to one of the following classes: (1) monoclonal antibody against Gp IIb/IIIa; (2) peptide (peptidomimetic) antagonists, many of which contain the RGD sequence that can compete with fibrinogen for its Gp IIb/IIIa binding site; and (3) nonpeptide (nonpeptide-mimetic) antagonists of Gp IIb/IIIa. Three drugs currently available for coronary intervention or acute coronary syndromes represent the prototypes for these groups: abciximab (c7E3 Fab, ReoPro), a monoclonal antibody; eptifibatide (Integrilin), a peptide antagonist; and tirofiban (Aggrastat), a nonpeptide mimetic (see Chaps. 47, 48, and 52). These agents are approved for intravenous administration.[157,158,174] Although these agents have similar mechanisms of action (i.e., inhibition of ligand binding to the receptor), it should not be assumed that they react at the same site within the receptor or that the consequences of their binding to Gp IIb/IIIa are identical. Monoclonal antibody has a relatively extended duration of antiplatelet action, whereas the peptides and nonpeptide mimetics have a shorter elimination half-life.

Abciximab is the Fab fragment of a monoclonal antibody to Gp IIb/IIIa that has been humanized (mouse/human chimera) to reduce immunogenicity.[175] Abciximab is not specific to platelet Gp IIb/IIIa: it cross-reacts with the related integrin, alpha$_v$-beta$_3$, the vitronectin receptor that is present on vascular cells. This cross-reactivity was originally considered to be of potential therapeutic benefit in the prevention of coronary restenosis and inhibition of thrombin generation. Abciximab is currently administered as an intravenous bolus followed by infusion for 12 to 24 hours for coronary interventions. Because abciximab is derived from an antibody, concern has been raised about repeat administration. However, data indicate that readministration is safe and efficacious and that the same indications for first-time use can apply to subsequent readministration.[176]

Eptifibatide is a synthetic cyclic heptapeptide that contains a modified lysine-glycine-aspartic acid (KGD), rather than RGD, sequence that recognizes the binding site of platelet Gp IIb/IIIa (see Fig. 80–9). The rationale for eptifibatide is that the substitution of a single lysine (K) for arginine (R) makes this agent specific for the platelet Gp IIb/IIIa integrin. Whether this is an advantageous or a disadvantageous property (see earlier) has yet to be definitely determined. Eptifibatide is not immunogenic and is safe for repeated administration.[177]

Tirofiban (Aggrastat) is a nonpeptide mimetic. In contrast to the RGD (or KGD) peptidomimetics, which inhibit platelet aggregation by binding competitively to the RGD recognition site of Gp IIb/IIIa, the nonpeptides mimic the structural steric and charge characteristics of the RGD sequence.[158]

The clinical experience with oral Gp IIb/IIIa antagonists has been disappointing. The lack of clinical benefit for these agents as compared with the established efficacy with intravenous inhibitors may be in part due to inadequate in vivo platelet Gp IIb/IIIa blockade. Oral Gp IIb/IIIa antagonists may also cause paradoxical platelet activation. Ligand-mimetic Gp IIb/IIIa blockers can have intrinsic platelet-activating properties or can stimulate outside-inside signal transduction, leading to paradoxical platelet aggregation. These ligand-mimetic properties of Gp IIb/IIIa antagonists may also cause thrombocytopenia (see later).[178]

Complications. Bleeding complications with currently approved intravenous platelet Gp IIb/IIIa antagonists have primarily involved vascular access puncture sites in patients undergoing percutaneous intervention. Reduction and weight-adjustment in adjunctive heparin dosing in patients undergoing coronary interventions have reduced the incidence of these bleeding problems. No increase in intracerebral hemorrhage has been observed with the Gp IIb/IIIa antagonists. Therefore, the need for platelet transfusion to treat life-threatening bleeding is extremely rare, particularly with the short-acting agents such as eptifibatide and tirofiban. Severe thrombocytopenia (platelet count $<20{,}000/\mu l$) occurs in 0.1 to 0.5 percent of patients treated with the intravenous agents, and the incidence appears to be slightly higher with abciximab.[158] A precipitous decrease in platelet count may occur within 1 to 2 hours of initial exposure, or there may be a significant decline several days after initiation of therapy. Preexisting antibodies appear to play a role in some cases of thrombocytopenia induced by these agents, and in the future, pretreatment detection of these antibodies may select for patients at greater risk of thrombocytopenia.[179,180] Alterations in platelet Gp IIb/IIIa, similar to those induced by these drugs, may occur in some patients with intermittent platelet activation, such as from atherosclerosis, leading to neo-antigen and subsequent antibody formation.[181]

REFERENCES

Basic Mechanisms of Hemostasis and Thrombosis

1. Hajjar KA: The endothelium in thrombosis and hemorrhage. *In* Loscalzo J, Schafer AI (eds): Thrombosis and Hemorrhage, 3rd ed. , Lippincott Williams & Wilkins, 2003, pp 206-209.
2. Kubo H, Alitalo K: The bloody fate of endothelial stem cells. Genes Dev 17:322, 2003.
3. Carmeliet P: Angiogenesis in health and disease. Nature Med 9:653, 2003.
4. Cines DB, Pollak ES, Buck CA, et al: Endothelial cells in physiology and in the pathophysiology of vascular disorders. Blood 91:3527, 1998.
5. Schafer AI: Preface. *In* Schafer AI (ed): Molecular Mechanisms of Hypercoagulable States. Austin, Landes Bioscience, 1997.
6. Schafer AI: Vascular endothelium: In defense of blood fluidity. J Clin Invest 99:1143, 1997.
7. Rosenberg RD, Aird WC: Vascular-bed-specific hemostasis and hypercoagulable states. N Engl J Med 340:1555, 1999.
8. Edelberg JM, Christie PD, Rosenberg RD: Regulation of vascular bed–specific prothrombotic potential. Circ Res 89:117, 2001.
9. Cook JP: Flow, NO, and atherogenesis. Proc Natl Acad Sci U S A 100:1420, 2003.
10. Davidge ST: Prostaglandin H synthase and vascular function. Circ Res 89:650, 2001.
11. Smyth EM, FitzGerald GA: Human prostacyclin receptor. Vitam Horm 65:149, 2002.
12. Busse R, Edwards G, Feletou M, et al: EDHF: Bringing the concepts together. Trends Pharmacol Sci 23:374, 2002.
13. Durante W, Schafer AI: Carbon monoxide and vascular cell function. Int J Mol Med 2:255, 1998.

14. Marcus AJ, Broekman MJ, Drosopoulos JH, et al: Metabolic control of excessive extracellular nucleotide accumulation by CD39/ectonucleotidase-1: Implications for ischemic vascular diseases. J Pharmacol Exp Ther 305:9, 2003.
15. Busse R, Fleming I: Regulation of endothelium-derived vasoactive autacoid production by hemodynamic forces. Trends Pharmacol Sci 24:24, 2003.
16. Schiffrin EL: A critical review of the role of endothelial factors in the pathogenesis of hypertension. J Cardiovac Pharmacol 38(Suppl 2):S3, 2001.
17. Walsh PN, Ahmad SS: Proteases in blood clotting. Essays Biochem 38:95, 2002.
18. Mann KG, Butenas S, Brummel K: The dynamics of thrombin formation. Arteriosler Thromb Vasc Biol 23:17, 2003.
19. Morrissey JH: Tissue factor: An enzyme cofactor and a true receptor. Thromb Haemost 86:66, 2001.
20. Edgington TS, Dickinson CD, Ruf W: The structural basis of function of the TF VIIa complex in the cellular initiation of coagulation. Thromb Haemost 78:401, 1997.
21. Kitchens CS: The contact system. Arch Pathol Lab Med 126:1382, 2002.
22. Colman RW, Schmaier AH: Contact system: A vascular biology modulator with anticoagulant, profibrinolytic, antiadhesive, and proinflammatory attributes. Blood 90:3819, 1997.
23. Mosesson MW: Fibrinogen structure and fibrin clot assembly. Semin Thromb Hemost 24:169, 1998.
24. Schafer AI: The primary and secondary hypercoagulable states. *In* Schafer AI (ed); Molecular Mechanisms of Hypercoagulable States. Austin, Landes Bioscience, 1997, pp 1-48.
25. Walsh PN, London FS, Ahmad SS: The assembly of the factor X-activating complex on activated human platelets. J Thromb Haemost 1:48, 2003.
26. Zwaal RF, Comfurius P, Beevers EM: Lipid-protein interactions in blood coagulation. Biochim Biophys Acta 1376:433, 1998.
27. Kottke-Marchant K, Duncan A: Antithrombin deficiency. Arch Pathol Lab Med 126:1326, 2002.

28. Crowther, MA, Kelton JG: Congenital thrombophilic states associated with venous thrombosis: A qualitative overview and proposed classification system. Ann Intern Med 138:128, 2003.
29. Broze GJ Jr: Protein Z-dependent regulation of coagulation. Thromb Haemost 86:8, 2001.
30. Simmonds RE, Rance J, Lane DA: Regulation of coagulation. *In* Loscalzo J, Schafer AI (eds): Thrombosis and Hemorrhage, 3rd ed. Philadelphia, Lippincott Williams & Wilkins, 2003, pp 35-61.
31. Weiler H, Isermann BH: Thrombomodulin. J Thromb Haemost 1:1515, 2003.
32. Esmon CT: Regulation of blood coagulation. Biochim Biophys Acta 1477:349, 2000.
33. Kottke-Marchant K, Comp P: Laboratory issues in diagnosing abnormalities of protein C, thrombomodulin, and endothelial cell protein C receptor. Arch Pathol Lab Med 126:1337, 2002.
34. Bajaj MS, Birktoft JJ, Steer SA, Bajaj SP: Structure and biology of tissue factor pathway inhibitor. Thromb Haemost 86:959, 2001.
35. Morris TA: Heparin and low molecular weight heparin: Background and pharmacology. Clin Chest Med 24:39, 2003.
36. Adams MJ, Donohoe S, Mackie IJ, Machin SJ: Anti-tissue factor pathway inhibitor activity in patients with primary antiphospholipid syndrome. Br J Haematol 114:375, 2001.
37. Forastiero RR, Martinuzzo ME, Broze GJ Jr: High titers of autoantibodies to tissue factor pathway inhibitor are associated with the antiphospholipid syndrome. J Thromb Haemost 1:718, 2003.
38. Caplice NM, Panetta C, Peterson TE, et al: Lipoprotein(a) binds and inactivates tissue factor pathway inhibitor: A novel link between lipoproteins and thrombosis. Blood 98:2980, 2001.
39. Dahm A, van Hylekama Vlieg A, Bendz B, et al: Low levels of tissue factor pathway inhibitor (TFPI) increase the risk of venous thrombosis. Blood 101:4387, 2003.
40. Kostner KM, Kostner GM: Lipoprotein (a): Still an enigma? Curr Opin Lipidol 13:391, 2002.
41. Vaughan DE, Declerck PJ: Regulation of fibrinolysis. *In* Loscalzo J, Schafer AI (eds): Thrombosis and Hemorrhage, 3rd ed. Philadelphia, Lippincott Williams & Wilkins, 2003, pp 105-119.
42. Taubman MB: Interactions of coagulation and fibrinolytic proteins with the vessel wall. *In* Loscalzo J, Schafer AI (eds): Thrombosis and Hemorrhage. 3rd ed. Philadelphia, Lippincott Williams & Wilkins, 2003, pp 266-277.
43. Longstaff C: Plasminogen activation on the cell surface. Frontiers Biosci 7:244, 2002.
44. Oswald CT, Menon V, Stouffer GA: The use of D-dimer in emergency room patients with suspected deep vein thrombosis: A test whose time has come. J Thromb Haemost 1:635, 2003.
45. Schutgens REG, Haas FJLM, Gerritsen WBM, et al: The usefulness of five D-dimer assays in the exclusion of deep venous thrombosis. J Thromb Haemost 1:976, 2003.
46. Eitzman DT, Ginsberg D: Of mice and men: The function of plasminogen activator inhibitors (PAIs) in vivo. Adv Exp Med Biol 425:131, 1997.
47. Vaughn DE: Plasminogen activator inhibitor-1: A common denominator in cardiovascular disease. J Invest Med 46:370, 1998.
48. Astedt B, Lindoff C, Lecander I: Significance of the plasminogen activator inhibitor of placental type (PAI-2) in pregnancy. Semin Thromb Hemost 24:431, 1998.
49. Bouma BN, Meijers JCM: Thrombin activatable fibrinolysis inhibitor (TAFI, plasma procarboxypeptidase B, procarboxypeptidase R, procarboxypeptidase U). J Thromb Haemost 1:1566, 2003.
50. van Tiburg NH, Rosendaal FR, Bertina RM: Thrombin activatable fibrinolysis inhibitor and the risk for deep vein thrombosis. Blood. 95:2855, 2000.
51. Kaushansky K: Thrombopoietin. N Engl J Med 339:746, 1998.
52. Ruggeri ZM: Structure of von Willebrand factor and its function in platelet adhesion and thrombus formation. Baillieres Best Practice Clin Haematol 14:257, 2001.
53. de Wit TR, van Mourik JA: Biosynthesis, processing and secretion of von Willebrand factor: Biological implications. Baillieres Best Practice Clin Haematol 14:241, 2001.
54. Andrews RK, Shen Y, Gardiner EE, et al: The glycoprotein Ib-IX-V complex in platelet adhesion and signaling. Thromb Haemost 82:357, 1999.
55. McEver RP: Adhesive interaction of leukocytes, platelets, and the vessel wall during hemostasis and inflammation. Thromb Haemost 86:746, 2001.
56. Andre P, Denis CV, Ware J, et al: Platelets adhere to and translocate on von Willebrand factor presented by endothelium in stimulated veins. Blood 96:3322, 2000.
57. Savage B, Almus-Jacobs F, Ruggeri ZM: Specific synergy of multiple substrate receptor interactions in platelet thrombus formation under flow. Cell 94:657, 1998.
58. Nakamura T, Kambayashi J, Okuma M: Activation of the Gp IIb/IIIa complex induced by platelet adhesion to collagen is mediated by both alpha$_2$-beta$_1$ integrin and Gp VI. J Biol Chem 274:11897, 1999.
59. Nieswandt B, Watson SP: Platelet-collagen interactions: Is Gp VI the central receptor? Blood 102:449, 2003.
60. Ruggeri ZM: Platelets in atherothrombosis. Nature Med 8:1227, 2002.
61. Kroll MH, Resendiz JC: Mechanisms of platelet activation. *In* Loscalzo J, Schafer AI (eds): Thrombosis and Hemorrhage. 3rd ed. Philadelphia, Lippincott Williams & Wilkins, 2003, pp 187-205.
62. Thomas DW, Mannon RB, Mannon PJ, et al: Coagulation defects and altered hemodynamic responses in mice lacking receptors for thromboxane A_2. J Clin Invest 102:1994, 1998.
63. Jackson SP, Nesbitt WS, Kulkarni S: Signaling events underlying thrombus formation. J Thromb Haemost 1:1602, 2003.
64. Bennett JS: Platelet-fibrinogen interactions. Ann New York Acad Sci 936:340, 2001.
65. Schafer AI: Antiplatelet therapy with glycoprotein IIb/IIIa receptor inhibitors and other novel agents. Tex Heart Inst J 24:90, 1997.
66. Griffin JH: The thrombin paradox. Nature 378:337, 1995.
67. Hanson SR, Griffin JH, Harker LA, et al: Antithrombotic effects of thrombin-induced activation of endogenous protein C in primates. J Clin Invest 92:2003, 1993.
68. Mann KG, Butenas S, Brummel K: The dynamics of thrombin formation. Arterioscler Thromb Vasc Biol 23:17, 2003.
69. Esmon CT: Inflammation and thrombosis. J Thromb Haemost 1:1343, 2003.

Thrombophilic Disorders

70. Price DT, Ridker PM: Factor V Leiden mutation and the risks for thromboembolic disease: A clinical perspective. Ann Intern Med. 127:895, 1997.
71. Bauer KA, Rosendaal FR, Heit JA: Hypercoagulability: Too many tests, too much conflicting data. Hematology. Am Soc Hematol Educ Program Book 353-38168, 2002.
72. Press RD, Bauer KA, Kujovich JL, Heit JA: Clinical utility of factor V Leiden (R506Q) testing for the diagnosis and management of thromboembolic disorders. Arch Pathol Lab Med 126:1304, 2002.
73. Ridker PM, Miletich JP, Hennekens, Buring JE: Ethnic distribution of factor V Leiden in 4047 men and women. JAMA 277:1305, 1997.
74. Dowling NF, Austin H, Dilley A, et al: The epidemiology of venous thromboembolism in Caucasians and African-Americans: The GATE study. J Thromb Haemost 1:80, 2003.
75. Juul K, Tybjaerg-Hansen A, Steffensen R, et al: Factor V Leiden: The Copenhagen city heart study and 2 meta-analyses. Blood 100:3, 2002.
76. Rosendaal FR, Siscovick DS, Schwartz SM, et al: Factor V Leiden (resistance to activated protein C) increases the risk of myocardial infarction in young women. Blood 89:2817, 1997.
77. MacGillavry MR, Prins MH: Oral contraceptives and inherited thrombophilia: A gene-environment interaction with a risk of venous thrombosis. Sem Thromb Hemost 29:219, 2003.
78. Bauer KA: Hormone replacement therapy and the factor V Leiden mutation. Arterioscler Throm Vasc Biol 22:879, 2002.
79. Rosendaal FR, Van Hylckama Vlieg A, Tanis BC, Helmerhorst FM: Estrogens, progestogens and thrombosis. J Haemost Thromb 1:1371, 2003.
80. Dahlback B: The discovery of activated protein C resistance. J Thromb Haemost 1:3, 2003.
81. McGlennen RC, Key NS: Clinical and laboratory management of the prothrombin G20210A mutation. Arch Pathol Lab Med 126:1319, 2002.
82. Dilley A, Austin H, Hooper WC, et al: Prevalence of the prothrombin 20210 G-to-A variant in blacks: Infants, patients with venous thrombosis, patients with myocardial infarction, and control subjects. J Lab Clin Med 132:452, 1998.
83. Legnani C, Cosmi B, Valdre L, et al: Venous thromboembolism, oral contraceptives and high prothrombin levels. J Thromb Haemost 1:112, 2002.
84. Martinelli I, Sacchi E, Landi G, et al: High risk of cerebral-vein thrombosis in carriers of a prothrombin-gene mutation and in users of oral contraceptives. N Engl J Med 338:1793, 1998.
85. Goodwin AJ, Rosendaal FR, Kottke-Marchant K, Bovill EG: A review of the technical, diagnostic, and epidemiologic considerations for protein S assays. Arch Pathol Lab Med 126:1349, 2002.
86. Key NS, McGlennen RC: Hyperhomocyst(e)inemia and thrombophilia. Arch Pathol Lab Med 126:1367, 2002.
87. Langman LJ, Ray JG, Evrovski J, et al: Hyperhomocyst(e)inemia and the increased risk of venous thromboembolism: more evidence from a case-control study. Arch Intern Med 160:961, 2000.
88. Mangoni AA, Jackson SH: Homocysteine and cardiovascular disease: Current evidence and future prospects. Am J Med 112:556, 2002.
89. Ray JG: Meta-analysis of hyperhomocysteinemia as a risk factor for venous thromboembolic disease. Arch Intern Med 158:2101, 1998.
90. Ray JG, Shmorgun D, Chan WS: Common C677T polymorphism of the methylenetetrahydrofolate reductase gene and the risk of venous thromboembolism: Meta-analysis of 31 studies. Pathophys Haemost Thromb 32:51, 2002.

91. Kluijtmans LAJ, Young IS, Boreham CA, et al: Genetic and nutritional factors contributing to hyperhomocysteinemia in young adults. Blood 101:2483, 2003.
92. Keijzer MBAJ, den Heijer M, Blom HJ, et al: Interaction between hyperhomocysteinemia, mutated methylenetetrahydrofolate reductase (MTHFR) and inherited thrombophilic factor in recurrent venous thrombosis. Thromb Haemost 88:723, 2002.
93. Ray JG, Vermeulen MJ, Boss SC, Cole DE: Declining rate of folate insufficiency among adults following increased folic acid food fortification in Canada. Can J Public Health. Rev Can Sante Publique 93:249, 2002.
94. Chandler WL, Rodgers GM, Sprouse JT, Thompson AR: Elevated hemostatic factor levels as potential risk factor for thrombosis. Arch Pathol Lab Med 126:1405, 2002.
95. Kamphuisen PW, Eikenboom JCJ, Bertina RM: Elevated factor VIII levels and the risk of thrombosis. Arterioscler Thromb Vasc Biol 21:731, 2001.
96. Tsai AW, Cushman M, Rosamond WD, et al: Coagulation factors, inflammation markers, and venous thromboembolism: the longitudinal investigation of thromboembolism etiology (LITE). Am J Med 113:636, 2002.
97. Koster T, Blann AD, Briet E, et al: Role of clotting factor VIII in effect of von Willebrand factor on occurrence of deep-vein thrombosis. Lancet 345:152, 1995.
98. Kyrle PA, Minar E, Hirschl M, et al: High plasma levels of factor VIII and the risk of recurrent venous thromboembolism. N Engl J Med 343:457, 2000.
99. Haynes T: Dysfibrinogenemia and thrombosis. Arch Pathol Lab Med 126:1387, 2002.
100. Rickles FR, Levine MN: Hemostatic and thrombotic disorders of malignancy. *In* Kitchens CS, Alving BM, Kessler CM (eds): Consultative Hemostasis and Thrombosis. Philadelphia, WB Saunders, 2002, pp 325.
101. Stein S, Konkle BA: Thrombotic risk of oral contraceptives, postmenopausal hormone replacement, and selective estrogen receptor modulators (SERMs). *In* Kitchens CS, Alving BM, Kessler CM (eds): Consultative Hemostasis and Thrombosis. Philadelphia, WB Saunders, 2002, pp 427-436.
102. Vandenbroucke JP, Rosing J, Bloemenkamp K, et al: Oral contraceptives and the risk of venous thrombosis. N Engl J Med 344:1527, 2001.
103. van den Bosch MAAJ, Kemmeren JM, Tanis BC, et al: The RATIO study: Oral contraceptives and the risk of peripheral arterial disease in young women. J Thromb Haemost 1:439, 2002.
104. Tanis BC, van den Bosch MAAJ, Kemmeren JM, et al: Oral contraceptives and the risk of myocardial infarction. N Engl J Med 345:1787, 2001.
105. Levine JS, Branch DW, Rauch J: The antiphospholipid syndrome. N Engl J Med 346:752, 2002.
106. Galli M, Barbui T: Antiphospholipid syndrome: Definition and treatment. Semin Thromb Hemost 29:195, 2003.
107. Arnout J, Vermylen J: Current status and implications of autoimmune antiphospholipid antibodies in relation to thrombotic disease. J Thromb Haemost 1:931, 2002.
108. Triplett DA: Antiphospholipid antibodies. Arch Pathol Lab Med 126:1424, 2002.
109. Previtali S, Barbui T, Galli M: Anti-β2-glycoprotein 1 and anti-prothrombin antibodies in antiphospholipid-negative patients with thrombosis. Thromb Haemost 88:729, 2002.
110. Galli M, Luciani D, Bertolini G, Barbui T: Lupus anticoagulants are stronger risk factors for thrombosis than anticardiolipin antibodies in the antiphospholipid syndrome: A systematic review of the literature. Blood 101:1827, 2003.

Antithrombotic Drugs

111. Hirsh J, Warkentin TE, Shaughnessy S, et al: Heparin and low-molecular-weight heparin: Mechanisms of action, pharmacokinetics, dosing, monitoring, efficacy and safety. Chest 119:64S, 2001.
112. Ginsberg JS: Pharmacology of heparin-related compounds and coumarin derivatives. *In* Loscalzo J, Schafer AI (eds): Thrombosis and Hemorrhage. 3rd ed. Philadelphia, Lippincott Williams & Wilkins, 2003, pp 937-948.
113. Schafer AI: Low-molecular-weight heparin for venous thromboembolism. Hosp Pract 31:99, 1997.
114. Nenci GG: Low molecular weight heparins: Are they interchangeable? No. J Thromb Haemost 1:12, 2003.
115. Prandoni P: Low molecular weight heparins: Are they interchangable? Yes. J Thromb Haemost 1:10, 2003.
116. Becker RC, Spencer FA, Gibson M, et al: Influence of patient characteristics and renal function on factor Xa inhibition pharmacokinetics and pharmacodynamics after enoxaparin administration in non-ST-segment elevation acute coronary syndromes. Am Heart J 143:753, 2002.
117. McCrae KR, Cines DB: Drug-induced thrombocytopenias. *In* Loscalzo J, Schafer AI (eds): Thrombosis and Hemorrhage. 3rd ed. Philadelphia, Lippincott Williams & Wilkins, 2003, pp 457-475.
118. Aster RH: Heparin induced thrombocytopenia and thrombosis. N Engl J Med 332:1374, 1995.
119. Arepally GM, Poncz M, Cines DB: Immune vascular injury in heparin-induced thrombocytopenia. *In* Warkentin TE, Greinacher A (eds): Heparin-Induced Thrombocytopenia. 2nd ed. New York, Marcel Dekker, 2001, pp 215-230.
120. Warkentin TE, Kelton JG: Temporal aspects of heparin-induced thrombocytopenia. N Engl J Med 344:1286, 2001.
121. Warkentin TE, Kelton JG: Delayed-onset heparin-induced thrombocytopenia and thrombosis. Ann Intern Med 135:502, 2001.
122. Warkentin TE, Bernstein RA: Delayed-onset HIT and cerebral thrombosis after a single administration of unfractionated heparin. N Engl J Med 348:1067, 2003.
123. Warkentin TE, Sheppard JL, Horsewood P, et al: Impact of the patient population on the risk for heparin-induced thrombocytopenia. Blood 96:1703, 2000.
124. Greinacher A, Volpel H, Janssens U, et al: Recombinant hirudin (lepirudin) provides safe and effective anticoagulation in patients with heparin-induced thrombocytopenia: A prospective study. Circulation 99:73, 1999.
125. Lewis BE, Walenga JM, Wallis DE: Anticoagulation with Novastan (argatroban) in patients with heparin-induced thrombocytopenia and thrombosis syndrome. Semin Thromb Hemost 23:197, 1997.
126. Warkentin TE: Nonhemorrhagic complications of antithrombotic therapy. *In* Spandorfer J, Konkle B, Merli G (eds): Management and prevention of thrombosis in primary care. New York, Oxford University Press, 2001, pp 202-220.
127. Ginsberg J, Chan WS, Bates S, Kaatz S: Anticoagulation of pregnant women with mechanical heart valves. Arch Intern Med. 163:694, 2003.
128. Freedman JE, Loscalzo J: New antithrombotic strategies. *In* Loscalzo J, Schafer AI (eds): Thrombosis and Hemorrhage. 3rd ed. Philadelphia, Lippincott Williams & Wilkins, 2003, pp 978-995.
129. Bates SM, Weitz JI: The new heparins. Coron Artery Dis 9:65, 1998.
130. Ibbotson T, Perry CM: Danaparoid: A review of its use in thromboembolic and coagulation disorders. Drugs 62:2283, 2002.
131. Eriksson BI, Bauer KA, Lassen MR, et al: Fondaparinux compared with enoxaparin for the prevention of venous thromboembolism after hip-fracture. N Engl J Med 345:1298, 2001.
132. Bauer KA, Eriksson BI, Lassen MR, et al: Fondaparinux compared with enoxaparin for the prevention of venous thromboembolism after elective major knee surgery. N Engl J Med 345:1305, 2001.
133. Keller C, Matzdorff AC, Kemkes-Matthes B: Pharmacology of warfarin and clinical implications. Semin Thromb Hemost 25:13, 1999.
134. Furie B, Furie BC: Molecular basis of vitamin K-dependent gamma-carboxylation. Blood 75:1753, 1990.
135. Aithal GP, Day CP, Kesteven PJL, Daly AK: Association of polymorphisms in the cytochrome P450 CYP2C9 with warfarin dose requirement and risk of bleeding complications. Lancet 353:717, 1998.
136. Hirsh J, Dalen JE, Anderson D, et al: Oral anticoagulants: Mechanism of action, clinical effectiveness, and optimal therapeutic range. Chest 119(Suppl): 8S, 2001.
137. Harrison L, Johnston M, Massicotte MP, et al: Comparison of 5-mg and 10-mg loading doses in initiation of warfarin therapy. Ann Intern Med 126:133, 1997.
138. Levine MN, Raskob G, Landefeld S, et al: Hemorrhagic complications of anticoagulant treatment. Chest 119(Suppl):108S, 2001.
139. Schafer AI: Venous thrombosis as a chronic disease. N Engl J Med 340:955, 1999.
140. Crowther MA, Douketis JD, Schnurr T, et al: Oral vitamin K lowers the international normalized ratio more rapidly than subcutaneous vitamin K in the treatment of warfarin-associated coagulopathy: A randomized, controlled trial. Ann Intern Med 137:251, 2002.
141. Deveras RAE, Kessler CM: Reversal of warfarin-induced excessive anticoagulation with recombinant human factor VIIa concentrate. Ann Intern Med 137:884, 2002.
142. Heit JA: Mapping out the future in venous thromboembolism and acute coronary syndromes. Semin Thromb Hemost 28:33, 2002.
143. Hirsh J: New anticoagulants. Am Heart J 142(2 Suppl):S3, 2001.
144. Kaplan KL, Francis CW: Direct thrombin inhibitors. Semin Hematol 39:187, 2002.
145. Samama MM: Synthetic direct and indirect factor Xa inhibitors. Thromb Res106:V267, 2002.
146. Francis CW, Davidson BL, Berkowitz SD, et al: Ximalagatran versus warfarin for the prevention of venous thromboembolism after total knee arthroplasty. Ann Intern Med 137:648, 2002.
147. Eriksson H, Wahlander K, Gustafsson D, et al: A randomized, controlled, dose-guiding study of the oral direct thrombin inhibitor ximelagatran compared with standard therapy for the treatment of acute deep vein thrombosis. J Thromb Haemost 1:41, 2002.
148. Hauptmann J, Stürzebecher J: Synthetic inhibitors of thrombin and factor Xa: From bench to bedside. Thromb Res 93:203, 1999.
149. Bauer KA: Selective inhibition of coagulation factors: Advance in antithrombotic therapy. Semin Thromb Hemost 28:15, 2002.
150. Golino P: The inhibitors of the tissue factor: Factor VII pathway. Thromb Res 106:V257, 2002.
151. Bernard GR, Vincent J-L, Laterre P-F, et al: Efficacy and safety of recombinant human activated protein C for severe sepsis. N Engl J Med 344:699, 2001.
152. Collen D: Thrombolytic therapy. Thromb Haemost 78:742, 1997.
153. Leopold JA, Loscalzo J: Pharmacology of thrombolytic agents. *In* Loscalzo J, Schafer AI (eds): Thrombosis and Hemorrhage. 3rd ed. Philadelphia, Lippincott Williams & Wilkins, 2003, pp 949-977.
154. Tanswell P, Modi N, Combs D, Danays T: Pharmacokinetics and pharmacodynamics of tenecteplase in fibrinolytic therapy of acute myocardial infarction. Clin Pharmacokinet 45:1229, 2002.
155. Al-Shwafi KA, de Meester A, Pirenne B, Col JJ: Comparative fibrinolytic activity of front-loaded alteplase and the single-bolus mutants tenecteplase and lanoteplase during treatment of acute myocardial infarction. Am Heart J 145:127, 2003.
156. Toschi L, Bringmann P, Petri T, et al: Fibrin selectivity of the isolated protease domains of tissue-type and vampire bat salivary gland plasminogen activators. Eur J Biochem 252:108, 1998.
157. Bennett JS, Mousa S: Platelet function inhibitors in the year 2000. Thromb Haemost 85:395, 2001.
158. Bennett JS: Novel platelet inhibitors. Annu Rev Med 52:161, 2001.
159. Mehta P: Aspirin in the prophylaxis of coronary artery disease. Curr Opin Cardiol 17:552, 2002.
160. Folts JD, Schafer AI, Loscalzo J, et al: A perspective on the potential problems with aspirin as an antithrombotic agent: A comparison of studies in an animal model with clinical trials. J Am Coll Cardiol 33:295, 1999.
161. Patrono C: Aspirin resistance: Definition, mechanisms and clinical read-outs. J Thromb Haemost 1:1710, 2003.
162. Schafer AI: Genetic and acquired determinants of individual variability of response to antiplatelet drugs. Circulation 108:910, 2003.
163. Schafer AI: Effects of nonsteroidal anti-inflammatory therapy on platelets. Am J Med 106:25S, 1999.

164. McAdam B, Catella-Lawson F, Mardini L, et al: Systemic biosynthesis of prostacyclin by cyclooxygenase (COX)-2: The human pharmacology of a selective inhibitor of COX-2. Proc Natl Acad Sci U S A 96:272, 1999.
165. FitzGerald GA, Patrono C: The coxibs, selective inhibitors of cyclooxygenase-2. N Engl J Med 345:433, 2001.
166. Catella-Lawson F, Reilly MP, Kapoor SC, et al: Cyclooxygenase inhibitors and the antiplatelet effects of aspirin. N Engl Med 345:1809, 2001.
167. Patrono C, Coller B, Fitzgerald GA, et al: Platelet-active drugs: The relationship among dose, effectiveness, and side effects. Chest 119(1 Suppl):395, 2001.
168. Jneid H, Bhatt DL, Corti R, et al: Aspirin and clopidogrel in acute coronary syndromes. Arch Intern Med 163:1145, 2003.
169. Gurbel PA, Cummings CC, Bell CR, et al: Onset and extent of platelet inhibition by clopidogrel loading in patients undergoing elective coronary stenting: The plavix reduction of new thrombus occurrence (PRONTO) trial. Am Heart J 145:239, 2003.
170. Chen DK, Kim JS, Sutton DM: Thrombotic thrombocytopenic purpura associated with ticlopidine use: A report of 3 cases and review of the literature. Arch Intern Med 159:311, 1999.
171. Steinhubl SR, Tan WA, Foody JM, et al: Incidence and clinical course of thrombotic thrombocytopenia purpura due to ticlopidine following coronary stenting. EPISTENT Investigators. Evaluation of platelet IIb/IIIa inhibitor for stenting. JAMA 281:806, 1999.
172. Bennett CL, Connors JM, Carwile JM, et al: Thrombotic thrombocytopenic purpura associated with clopidogrel. N Engl J Med 342:1773, 2000.
173. De Schryver EL, Algra A, van Gijn J: Dipyridamole for preventing stroke and other vascular events in patients with vascular disease. Cochrane Database of Systematic Reviews CD001820, 2003.
174. Plow EF, Cierniewski CS, Xiao Z et al: Alpha IIbbeta3 and its antagonism at the new millennium. Thromb Haemost 86:34, 2001.
175. Bhatt DL, Lincoff AM: Abciximab. *In* Sasahara AA, Loscalzo J (eds): New Therapeutic Agents in Thrombosis and Thrombolysis. 2nd ed. New York, Marcel Dekker, 2003, pp 349-369.
176. Tcheng JE, Kereiakes DJ, Braden GA, et al: Readministration of abciximab: Interim report of the ReoPro Readministration Registry. Am Heart J 138:33, 1999.
177. Lorenz TJ, Macdonald F, Kitt MM: Nonimmunogenieity of eptifibatide, a cyclic heptapeptide inhibitor of platelet glycoprotein IIb-IIIa. Clin Ther 21:128, 1999.
178. Peter K, Bode C: Procoagulant activities of glycoprotein IIb/IIIa receptor blockers: *In* Sasahara AA, Loscalzo J (eds): New Therapeutic Agents in Thrombosis and Thrombolysis. 2nd ed. New York, Marcel Dekker, 2003, pp 401-411
179. Curtis BR, Swyers J, Divgi A, McFarland JG, Aster RH: Thrombocytopenia after second exposure to abciximab is caused by antibodies that recognize abciximab-coated platelets. Blood 99:2054, 2002.
180. Billheimer JT, Dicker IB, Wynn R, et al: Evidence that thrombocytopenia observed in humans treated with orally bioavailable glycoprotein IIb/IIIa antagonists is immune mediated. Blood 99:3540, 2002.
181. Abrams CS, Cines DB: Platelet glycoprotein IIb/IIIa inhibitors and thrombocytopenia: Possible link between platelet activation, autoimmunity and thrombosis. Thromb Haemost 88:888, 2002.

CHAPTER 81

Rheumatic Fever

Adnan S. Dajani

Rheumatic fever (RF) is generally classified as a connective tissue disease or collagen-vascular disease. Its anatomical hallmark is damage to collagen fibrils and to the ground substance of connective tissue. The rheumatic process is expressed as an inflammatory reaction that involves many organs, primarily the heart, the joints, and the central nervous system. The clinical manifestations of acute RF follow a group A streptococcal (group A strep) infection of the tonsillopharynx after a latent period of approximately 3 weeks. The major importance of acute RF is its ability to cause fibrosis of heart valves, leading to crippling hemodynamics of chronic heart disease.

RF is the most common cause of acquired heart disease in children and young adults worldwide. Although the incidence of RF declined sharply in many developed countries, the disease remains a major problem in many developing countries. The precise reasons for the fluctuations in the incidence of the disease remain only partly understood. Although RF has been studied extensively, the pathogenesis of the disease is not well defined.

EPIDEMIOLOGY

The incidence of RF and prevalence of rheumatic heart disease are markedly variable in different countries.[1,2] At the beginning of the 20th century, the incidence of RF in the United States exceeded 100 per 100,000 population; it ranged between 40 and 65 per 100,000 between 1935 and 1960 and is currently estimated as less than 2 per 100,000. Beginning in 1984, several outbreaks of acute RF were reported from a number of geographically distinct areas in the United States.[2] These focal outbreaks were not associated with a national increase in the incidence of RF. The decline in the incidence of RF in industrialized countries is in sharp contrast to the persistent high incidence of the disease in nonindustrialized countries.

In many developing countries, the incidence of acute RF approaches or exceeds 100 per 100,000.[1] In keeping with the falling incidence of RF in industrialized countries, the prevalence of rheumatic heart disease has declined. Table 81-1 compares the prevalence of rheumatic heart disease in school-age children in different regions of the world.

The decline in incidence of RF and prevalence of rheumatic heart disease has been attributed to several factors. Although the decline preceded the introduction of antimicrobial agents for the treatment of streptococcal pharyngitis, the use of these agents may have enhanced the rate of this decline. Improved economic standards, better housing conditions, decreased crowding in homes and schools, and access to medical care are often credited, at least in part, for the marked decline in RF.[1] Epidemiological observations show periodic shifts in the appearance and disappearance of specific M types in a particular geographical location. Such shifts may be another explanation for the decline and resurgence of RF in some parts of the world.

Because of the causal relationship between RF and group A strep pharyngitis, the epidemiologies of the two illnesses are very similar. Initial attacks of RF occur most commonly between the ages of 6 and 15 years, and RF rarely occurs before the age of 5 years. The risk of RF is increased in populations at high risk for streptococcal pharyngitis, such as military recruits, persons living in crowded conditions, and those in close contact with school-age children. The incidence of RF is equal in male and female patients. The seasonal incidence of RF also parallels that of streptococcal pharyngitis. The peak incidence of RF in Europe and the United States is in spring. Although RF used to be considered a disease of temperate climates, it is now more common in warm tropical climates, particularly in developing countries.

Pathogenesis

The evidence that group A streptococcus is the agent causing initial and recurrent attacks of RF is strong but indirect. It is based on clinical, epidemiological, and immunological observations. Factors that contribute to the pathogenesis of RF are related to both the putative causative agent and the host (Table 81–2).

THE ETIOLOGICAL AGENT. An untreated group A strep tonsillopharyngitis is the antecedent event that precipitates RF. RF does not follow streptococcal skin infection (impetigo). Proper antimicrobial treatment of streptococcal pharyngitis with eradication of the organism virtually eliminates the risk of RF. In situations conducive to epidemic streptococcal pharyngitis (such as the military population, crowding), as many as 3 percent of untreated acute streptococcal sore throats may be followed by RF. Endemic infections result in much lower attack rates. It has been well documented that about one-third of all cases of acute RF follow mild, almost asymptomatic pharyngitis. The lack of symptomatic pharyngitis was particularly striking in most of the more recent outbreaks of acute RF in which the majority of patients (58 percent) had no history of pharyngitis.[2] This is an alarming observation because primary prevention of acute RF relies on identification and proper treatment of streptococcal pharyngitis.

The major factors that are related to the risk of RF are the magnitude of the immune response to the antecedent streptococcal pharyngitis and persistence of the organism during convalescence. Variations in the rheumatogenicity of group A strep strains are a factor influencing the attack rate of RF.[3] The concept that RF is associated with infections with virulent encapsulated (mucoid) strains capable of inducing strong type-specific immune responses to M protein and other streptococcal antigens[4] has been strengthened by observations made during the outbreaks of acute RF in the mid-1980s. The streptococci isolated from patients with RF and their sibling contacts during these outbreaks were primarily strains belonging to M types 1, 3, 5, 6, and 18.[5] M proteins of rheumatogenic streptococci show distinct structural characteristics. They share a long terminal antigenic domain[6-8] and contain epitopes that are shared with human heart tissue, particularly sarcolemmal membrane proteins and cardiac myosin.

THE HOST. Although only a small proportion of individuals with untreated streptococcal pharyngitis may develop RF (3 percent), the incidence of the disease after

TABLE 81–1 Rheumatic Heart Disease in School-Age Children

Location	Prevalence Per 1000
United States	0.6
Japan	0.7
Asia (other)	0.4–21.0
Africa	0.3–15.0
South America	1.0–17.0

TABLE 81–2 Pathogenesis of Rheumatic Fever Group A Streptococcus

Tonsillopharyngeal infection, no other sites

Intensity of the infection
- Brisk antibody response
- Persistence of the organism

Rheumatogenic strains
- M types 1, 3, 5, 6, 14, 18, 19, 27, and 29
- Distinct structural characteristics of M proteins
  - Long terminal antigenic domain
  - Epitopes shared with human heart tissue
- Heavily encapsulated, forming mucoid colonies
- Resistance to phagocytosis
- Does not produce opacity factor

Susceptible Host

Genetic predisposition
- Presence of specific B-cell alloantigen

High incidence of class II HLA antigens

HLA = human leukocyte antigen.

streptococcal pharyngitis in patients who have had a previous episode of RF is substantially greater (about 50 percent). Numerous epidemiological studies also indicate familial predisposition to the disease. These observations and more recent studies strongly suggest a genetic basis for susceptibility to RF. A specific B-cell alloantigen, identified by monoclonal antibodies, has been described in almost all patients (99 percent) with RF but in only a small number (14 percent) of control subjects. Furthermore, susceptibility to RF has been linked with human leukocyte antigen (HLA) DR 1, 2, 3, and 4 haplotypes in various ethnic groups.

PATHOLOGY

The acute phase of RF is characterized by exudative and proliferative inflammatory reactions involving connective or collagen tissue. Although the disease process is diffuse, it affects primarily the heart, joints, brain, and cutaneous and subcutaneous tissues.

The basic structural change in collagen is fibrinoid degeneration. The interstitial connective tissue becomes edematous and eosinophilic, with fraying, fragmentation, and disintegration of collagen fibers. This change is associated with infiltration of mononuclear cells including large modified fibrohistiocytic cells (Aschoff cells). Some of the histiocytes are multinucleated and form Aschoff giant cells.

The Aschoff nodule in the proliferative stage is considered pathognomonic of rheumatic carditis. These nodules have been found almost invariably in the autopsies of patients who died of rheumatic carditis; however, more recent observations indicate that Aschoff nodules are observed in only 30 to 40 percent of biopsy specimens from patients with primary or recurrent episodes of RF.[9] Aschoff bodies may be seen in any area of the myocardium but not in other affected organs such as joints or brain. They are most often noted in the interventricular septum, the wall of the left ventricle, or the left atrial appendage. Aschoff nodules persist for many years after a rheumatic attack, even in patients with no evidence of recent or active inflammation.

TABLE 81–3 Guidelines for the Diagnosis of Initial Attacks of Rheumatic Fever (Jones Criteria, Updated 1992)

Major Manifestations	Minor Manifestations
Carditis	Clinical findings
Polyarthritis	Arthralgia
Chorea	Fever
Erythema marginatum	Laboratory findings
Subcutaneous nodules	Elevated acute phase reactants Erythrocyte sedimentation rate C-reactive protein Prolonged PR interval

Supporting Evidence of Antecedent A Streptococcal Infection

Positive throat culture or rapid streptococcal antigen test

Elevated or rising streptococcal antibody titer

From Dajani AS, Ayoub EM, Bierman FZ, et al: Guidelines for the diagnosis of rheumatic fever: Jones criteria, updated 1992. JAMA 268:2069, 1992. Copyright 1992 American Medical Association.

Inflammation of valvular tissue accounts for the more commonly recognized clinical manifestations of rheumatic carditis. Initial inflammation leads to valvular insufficiency. The extravasation of lymphocytes through the valvular endothelium may initiate the pathological process.[10] The histological findings in endocarditis consist of edema and cellular infiltration of the valvular tissue and the chordae tendineae. Hyaline degeneration of the affected valve leads to the formation of verrucae at its edge, preventing total approximation of the leaflets. Fibrosis and calcification of the valve occur if inflammation persists. This process may eventually lead to valvular stenosis.

Diagnosis

No specific clinical, laboratory, or other test establishes the diagnosis of RF. In 1944, T. Duckett Jones formulated his criteria for the diagnosis of RF, which are still valuable. They have been modified, revised, edited, and updated by the Committee on Rheumatic Fever, Endocarditis, and Kawasaki Disease of the Council on Cardiovascular Disease in the Young (American Heart Association)[11] and, more recently, they have been reaffirmed.[12] The most recent guidelines (Table 81–3) emphasize the diagnosis of *initial attacks* of RF. Dividing clinical and laboratory findings into major and minor manifestations is based on the diagnostic importance of a particular finding. If supported by evidence of preceding group A strep infection, the presence of two major manifestations or of one major and two minor manifestations indicates a high probability of acute RF.

Major Clinical Manifestations

CARDITIS. Rheumatic carditis is a pancarditis affecting the endocardium, myocardium, and pericardium to various degrees. Clinically, rheumatic carditis is almost always associated with a murmur of valvulitis. The severity of carditis is variable. In its most severe form, death from cardiac failure may occur. More commonly, carditis is less intense, and the predominant effect is subsequent scarring of the heart valves. Evidence of carditis may be subtle; signs of valvular involvement may be mild and transient and may be easily missed on auscultation. Baseline studies, including electrocardiograms, echocardiograms, and Doppler studies,[12,13] should be obtained in patients in whom RF is suspected. The use of echocardiographic abnormalities in the recognition of carditis in patients without a heart murmur is controversial.[12,14]

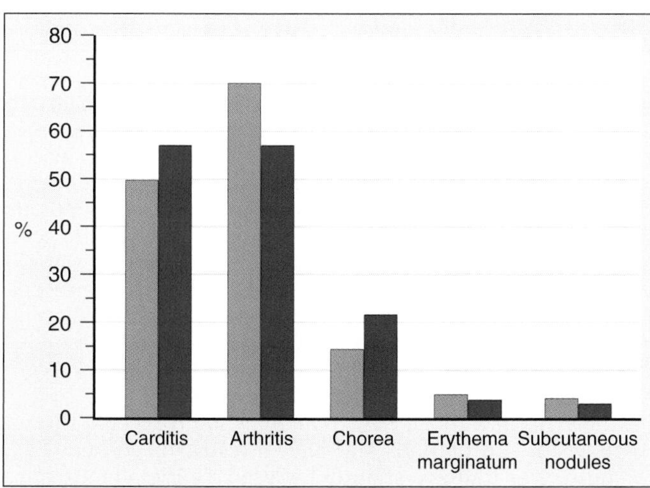

FIGURE 81–1 Relative frequency of major manifestations of rheumatic fever in earlier (blue) and more recent (purple) reports in the 1980s.

Patients who show no clear evidence of carditis on initial examination should be closely monitored for a few weeks to assess cardiac involvement.

Carditis is often regarded as the most specific manifestation of RF. It is noted in at least 50 percent of patients with acute RF (Fig. 81–1). More recent outbreaks in the United States suggested that the frequency of carditis was somewhat higher than traditionally reported, which may be due in part to more sophisticated diagnostic methods.[2] In one report, carditis was diagnosed in 72 percent of cases by auscultation and in 91 percent of cases by Doppler ultrasonography. The risk of overdiagnosing valvular incompetence by echocardiography should be emphasized, and overreliance on this tool in diagnosing rheumatic carditis should be avoided.

Valvulitis (endocarditis) involving mitral and aortic valves and the chordae of the mitral valve is the most characteristic component of rheumatic carditis. Mitral regurgitation is the hallmark of rheumatic carditis. Aortic regurgitation is less common and usually associated with mitral regurgitation. The pulmonic and tricuspid valves are rarely involved. Residual valvular damage is a major concern in patients with RF and may lead to intractable cardiac failure requiring surgical intervention. Valvular abnormalities, especially aortic and mitral regurgitation, rather than myocardial damage appear to be dominant in causing cardiac dysfunction.[12,14]

Myocarditis or pericarditis in the *absence* of valvulitis is *not* likely to be due to RF. Tachycardia is an early sign of myocarditis but may also be due to fever or cardiac failure. Transient arrhythmias may occur in patients with myocarditis. Severe myocarditis or valvular regurgitation may lead to cardiac failure. Cardiac enlargement occurs when severe hemodynamic changes result from valvular, myocardial, or pericardial disease.

ARTHRITIS. Polyarthritis is the most common major manifestation of RF (see Fig. 81–1) but the least specific. It is almost always asymmetrical and migratory and involves larger joints (knees, ankles, elbows, and wrists). Swelling, redness, heat, severe pain, limitation of motion, and tenderness to touch are characteristic. The arthritis of RF is benign and does not result in permanent joint deformity. Joint fluid shows findings characteristic of inflammation (not infection). In untreated cases, arthritis usually lasts 2 to 3 weeks. A striking feature of rheumatic arthritis is its dramatic response to salicylates.

Some patients may develop arthritis and other multisystem manifestations after acute streptococcal pharyngitis that do not fulfill the Jones criteria for the diagnosis of acute RF. This "syndrome" has been referred to as poststreptococcal reactive arthritis (PSRA). The arthritis of PSRA does not respond dramatically to antiinflammatory agents. Some patients with PSRA may have silent or delayed-onset carditis[15]; therefore, these patients should be carefully observed for several months for the subsequent development of carditis.

CHOREA. Sydenham chorea, St. Vitus dance, or chorea minor occurs in about 20 percent of patients with RF (see Fig. 81–1). The rheumatic inflammatory process in the central nervous system specifically involves the basal ganglia and caudate nuclei. Chorea is a *delayed* manifestation of RF, usually appearing 3 months or longer after the onset of the precipitating streptococcal infection. This period is in sharp contrast to the latent period of carditis or arthritis, which is usually 3 weeks. Thus, chorea is frequently the only manifestation of RF. Furthermore, evidence of a recent group A strep infection may be difficult to document, and other supporting historical, clinical, or laboratory findings to fulfill the Jones criteria may be lacking. The diagnosis of RF can be made in a patient with chorea without strictly adhering to the Jones criteria.

Sydenham chorea is characterized clinically by purposeless and involuntary movements, muscle incoordination and weakness, and emotional lability. The manifestations are more evident when a patient is awake and under stress and may disappear during sleep. All muscles, but primarily muscles of the face and extremities, may be involved. Speech may be affected, being explosive and halting. Handwriting deteriorates, and patients become uncoordinated and easily frustrated. The symptoms of Sydenham chorea must be distinguished from tics, athetosis, conversion reactions, hyperkinesis, and behavior problems. Symptoms usually resolve in 1 to 2 weeks, even without treatment. Patients with RF, and especially those with Sydenham chorea, are at higher risk for the development of neuropsychiatric disorders, including obsessive-compulsive and depressive disorders.[16]

ERYTHEMA MARGINATUM. This distinctive rash is a rare manifestation of RF, occurring in less than 5 percent of patients. It is an evanescent, erythematous, macular, nonpruritic rash with pale centers and rounded or serpiginous margins. Lesions vary greatly in size and occur mainly on the trunk and proximal extremities, not on the face. The rash may be induced by application of heat.

SUBCUTANEOUS NODULES. These are firm, painless, freely movable nodules that measure 0.5 to 2 cm. They are rarely seen in patients with RF (about 3 percent); when present, they are most often seen in patients with carditis. They are usually located over extensor surfaces of the joints (particularly elbows, knees, and wrists), in the occipital portion of the scalp, or over spinous processes. The overlying skin is freely movable, shows no discoloration, and is not inflamed.

Minor Manifestations

CLINICAL FINDINGS. Fever and arthralgia are nonspecific, common findings in patients with acute RF. Their diagnostic value is limited because they are encountered commonly in various other diseases. They are used to support the diagnosis of RF when only a single major manifestation is present. Fever is noted during the acute stages of the disease and has no characteristic pattern. Arthralgia is pain in one or more large joints without objective findings on examination and must not be considered a minor manifestation if arthritis is present. Epistaxis and abdominal pain may also occur but are not included as minor diagnostic criteria for RF.

LABORATORY FINDINGS. Elevated acute phase reactants offer objective but nonspecific indications of tissue inflammation. The erythrocyte sedimentation rate (ESR) and

C-reactive protein (CRP) level are almost always elevated during the acute stages of the disease in patients with carditis or polyarthritis but are usually normal in patients with chorea. The ESR is useful in monitoring the course of the disease; it usually returns to normal as the rheumatic activity subsides. The ESR may be elevated in patients with anemia and may be suppressed to normal levels in patients with congestive cardiac failure. Unlike the ESR, the CRP level is unaffected by anemia or cardiac failure.

A common finding in patients with acute RF is a prolonged PR interval for age and rate on electrocardiography. This finding alone is not diagnostic of carditis and does not correlate with the ultimate development of chronic rheumatic cardiac disease. Other findings on electrocardiography include tachycardia, atrioventricular block, and QRS-T changes suggestive of myocarditis; these changes are not considered minor manifestations.

Leukocytosis may be observed in the acute stages of RF, but the leukocyte count is variable and not dependable. Anemia is usually mild or moderate and normocytic normochromatic in morphology (anemia of chronic inflammation). Chest roentgenograms are useful in assessing cardiac size; however, normal findings on a chest roentgenogram do not preclude the presence of carditis. Pericarditis, pulmonary edema, and increased pulmonary vascularity are also detected by this examination. Echocardiography may be helpful in detecting endocardial, myocardial, and pericardial involvement. Antimyosin antibody imaging has been reported to be useful in the detection of rheumatic carditis.[17]

Antecedent Group A Streptococcal Infection

A number of illnesses mimic acute RF, and no laboratory test or tests establish a specific diagnosis of RF. It is therefore important to establish an antecedent streptococcal infection by demonstrating group A streptococcus in the tonsillopharynx or an elevated or rising streptococcal antibody titer. *Evidence of an antecedent streptococcal infection is required for confirmation of the initial diagnosis of acute RF.*

At the time of diagnosis of acute RF, only about 11 percent of patients have throat cultures positive for group A streptococcus.[2] The paucity of positive cultures is due, in part, to elimination of the organism by host defense mechanisms during the latent period between the onset of the infection and the subsequent development of RF. Several rapid group A strep antigen detection tests are commercially available. These tests vary in method. Most have a high degree of specificity but low sensitivity in a clinical setting. A negative test result does not preclude the presence of group A streptococcus in the pharynx. A positive throat culture result or rapid antigen test does not distinguish between a recent infection that can be associated with acute RF and chronic pharyngeal carriage of the organism.

Because the presence of group A streptococci in the pharynx may not represent active infection, elevated or rising antistreptococcal antibody titers provide more reliable evidence of a recent streptococcal infection than does a positive culture or a positive rapid antigen test result. The most commonly used antibody tests are the antistreptolysin O (ASO) and antideoxyribonuclease B (anti-DNase B) tests. The ASO test is usually performed first, and if results are not elevated, the anti-DNase B test is done. Elevated titers for both tests may persist for several weeks or months. ASO titers rise and fall more rapidly than anti-DNase B titers. A commercially available slide agglutination test measures antibodies to several streptococcal antigens. It is simple to perform, rapid, and widely available; however, the test is not well standardized and not very reproducible and is not recommended as a definitive test for evidence of a preceding group A strep infection.

Treatment

GENERAL. Whenever possible, patients should be admitted to a hospital for close observation and appropriate workup. Bed rest is generally considered important because it lessens joint pain. Ambulation may be attempted when fever abates and acute phase reactants return to normal. Patients should be allowed to return to a reasonably active life with normal physical activity. Strenuous physical exercise should be avoided, however, particularly if carditis was present. Although throat cultures are rarely positive for group A streptococcus at the time of onset of RF, patients should receive a 10-day course of penicillin therapy. Patients allergic to penicillin should be treated with erythromycin.

If heart failure intervenes, patients should receive diuretics, oxygen, and digitalis and have a restricted sodium diet. Digitalis preparations should be used cautiously because cardiac toxicity may occur with conventional dosages.

ANTIRHEUMATIC THERAPY. There is no specific treatment for the inflammatory reactions initiated by RF. Supportive therapy is aimed at reducing constitutional symptoms, controlling toxic manifestations, and improving cardiac function.

Patients with mild or no carditis usually respond well to salicylates. Salicylates are particularly effective in relieving joint pain; such pain usually abates within 24 hours of starting salicylates. Indeed, if joint pain persists after salicylate treatment, the diagnosis of RF may be questionable and patients should be re-evaluated. Because no specific diagnostic tests for RF exist, antiinflammatory therapy should be withheld until the clinical picture has become sufficiently clear to allow a diagnosis. Early administration of antiinflammatory agents may suppress clinical manifestations and prevent appropriate diagnosis. For optimal antiinflammatory effect, serum salicylate levels around 20 mg percent are required. Aspirin, at doses of 100 mg/kg/d, given four to five times daily, usually results in adequate serum levels to achieve a clinical response. Optimal salicylate therapy must be individualized, however, to ensure adequate response and avoid toxicity. Tinnitus, nausea, vomiting, and anorexia are common dose-related toxicities associated with salicylism. Side effects can subside after a few days of treatment despite continuation of the medication.

Patients with significant cardiac involvement—particularly those with pericarditis or congestive heart failure—respond more promptly to corticosteroids than to salicylates. Patients who do not respond to adequate doses of salicylates may occasionally benefit from a trial course of corticosteroids. Prednisone, 1 to 2 mg/kg/d, is the usual agent.

There is no evidence that salicylate, corticosteroids, or intravenous immunoglobulin therapy affects the course of carditis or diminishes the incidence of residual heart disease.[18-20] Therefore, the duration of therapy with antiinflammatory agents is arbitrarily based on an estimate of the severity of the episode and the promptness of the clinical response.

Mild attacks with little or no cardiac involvement can be treated with salicylates for about 1 month or until there is sufficient clinical and laboratory evidence of inflammatory inactivity. In more severe cases, therapy with corticosteroids may be continued for 2 to 3 months. The medication is then gradually reduced over the next 2 weeks. Even with prolonged therapy, some patients (approximately 5 percent) continue to demonstrate evidence of rheumatic activity for 6 months or more. A "rebound," manifested by reappearance of mild symptoms or of acute phase reactants, may occur in some patients after antiinflammatory medications have been discontinued, usually within 2 weeks. Modest symptoms usually subside without treatment; more severe symptoms may require treatment with salicylates. Some physicians recommend the use of salicylates (aspirin, 75 mg/kg/d) during the period when corticosteroids are being tapered and believe that such an approach may reduce the likelihood of a rebound.

Information about the use of salicylates other than aspirin is limited. In patients who cannot tolerate aspirin or who are allergic to it, a trial of other nonsteroidal agents may be warranted. Aspirin preparations that are coated or that contain alkali or buffers may also be tried; however, little evidence shows that such preparations are better tolerated, and some may have undesirable side effects.

Prevention

Primary Prevention

Prevention of primary attacks of RF depends on prompt recognition and proper treatment of group A strep tonsillopharyngitis. Eradication of group A streptococcus from the throat is essential. Although appropriate antimicrobial therapy started up to 9 days after the onset of acute streptococcal pharyngitis is effective in preventing primary attacks of RF, early therapy is advisable because it reduces both morbidity and the period of infectivity. In selecting a regimen for the treatment of group A strep pharyngitis, various factors should be considered, including bacteriological and clinical efficacy, ease of adherence to the recommended regimen (frequency of daily administration, duration of therapy, palatability), cost, spectrum of activity of the selected agent, and potential side effects.[21]

Penicillin is the antimicrobial agent of choice for the treatment of group A strep pharyngitis, except in patients with history of allergy to penicillin.[22] Penicillin has a narrow spectrum of activity, has longstanding proven efficacy, and is the least expensive regimen. Group A streptococcus resistant to penicillin has not been documented. Penicillin can be administered intramuscularly or orally (Table 81–4), depending on the patient's likely adherence to an oral regimen.

Intramuscular benzathine penicillin G is preferred, particularly for patients who are unlikely to complete a 10-day course of oral therapy and for patients with a personal or family history of RF or rheumatic heart disease. Benzathine penicillin G injections should be given as a single dose in a large muscle mass. This formulation is painful; injections that contain procaine penicillin in addition to benzathine penicillin G are less painful. Less discomfort is associated with intramuscular benzathine penicillin G if the medication is warmed to room temperature before administration.

The oral antibiotic of choice is penicillin V (phenoxymethyl penicillin). Patients should take oral penicillin regularly for an entire 10-day period, although they are likely to be asymptomatic after the first few days. Although the broader spectrum amoxicillin is often used for treatment of group A strep pharyngitis, it offers no microbiological advantage over penicillin.

Oral erythromycin is acceptable for patients allergic to penicillin. Treatment should also be prescribed for 10 days. Erythromycin estolate (20 to 40 mg/kg/d in two to four divided doses) or erythromycin ethyl succinate (40 mg/kg/d in two to four divided doses) is effective in treating streptococcal pharyngitis. The maximal dose of erythromycin is 1 gm/d. Although strains of group A streptococci resistant to erythromycin are prevalent in some areas of the world and have resulted in treatment failures, they are uncommon in most parts of the United States.

The macrolide azithromycin has susceptibility similar to that of erythromycin against group A streptococcus but may cause fewer gastrointestinal side effects. Azithromycin can be administered once daily and produces high tonsillar tissue concentrations. A 5-day course of azithromycin is acceptable as a second-line therapy for the treatment of patients with group A strep pharyngitis. The recommended dosage is 500 mg as a single dose on the first day followed by 250 mg once daily for 4 days.

A 10-day course of an oral cephalosporin is an acceptable alternative, particularly for penicillin-allergic patients. Narrower spectrum cephalosporins, such as cefadroxil or cephalexin, are probably preferable to the broader spectrum cephalosporins such as cefaclor, cefuroxime, cefixime, and cefpodoxime. Some penicillin-allergic persons (<15 percent) are also allergic to cephalosporins, and these agents should

TABLE 81–4 Prevention of Rheumatic Fever

Agent	Dose	Route	Duration
Primary Prevention			
Benzathine penicillin G	600,000 units for patients ≤27 kg 1,200,000 units for patients >27 kg *or*	IM	Once
Pencillin V	Children: 250 mg 2-3 times daily Adolescents and adults: 500 mg 2-3 times daily	PO	10 d
For patients allergic to penicillin:			
Erythromycin	40 mg/kg/d 2-4 times daily (maximum 1 gm/d)	PO	10 d
Secondary Prevention			
Benzathine penicillin G	1,200,00 units every 3-4 wk *or*	IM	See Table 81–5
Penicillin V	250 mg b.i.d. *or*	PO	See Table 81–5
Sulfadiazine	0.5 gm once daily for patients ≤27 kg (60 lb) 1.0 gm once daily for patients >27 kg (60 lb)	PO	See Table 81–5
For patients allergic to penicillin and sulfadiazine:			
Erythromycin	250 mg b.i.d.	PO	See Table 81–5

Modified from Dajani AS, Taubert K, Ferrieri P, et al: Treatment of streptococcal pharyngitis and prevention of rheumatic fever. Pediatrics 96:758, 1995, with permission.

not be used by patients with immediate (anaphylactic-type) hypersensitivity to penicillin.

A 10-day course with an oral cephalosporin is superior to 10 days of oral penicillin in eradicating group A streptococcus from the pharynx. Reports suggest that a 5-day course with selected oral cephalosporins is comparable to a 10-day course of oral penicillin in eradicating group A streptococcus from the pharynx.

Secondary Prevention

Patients who have suffered a previous attack of RF and who develop streptococcal pharyngitis are at high risk for a recurrent attack of RF. A group A strep infection need not be symptomatic to trigger a recurrence. Furthermore, RF can recur even when a symptomatic infection is optimally treated. For these reasons, prevention of recurrent RF requires continuous antimicrobial prophylaxis rather than recognition and treatment of acute episodes of streptococcal pharyngitis. Continuous prophylaxis is recommended for patients with a well-documented history of RF (including cases manifested solely by Sydenham chorea) and those with definite evidence of rheumatic heart disease. Such prophylaxis should be initiated as soon as acute RF or rheumatic heart disease is diagnosed. A full therapeutic course of penicillin (as outlined in Table 81–4) should first be given to patients with acute RF to eradicate residual group A streptococci even if a throat culture is negative at that time. Streptococcal infections occurring in family members of rheumatic patients should be treated promptly.

CONTINUOUS ANTIMICROBIAL PROPHYLAXIS. Continuous prophylaxis provides the most effective protection from RF recurrences. Risk of recurrence depends on several factors. Risk increases with several previous attacks, whereas the risk decreases as the interval since the most recent attack lengthens. The likelihood of acquiring a streptococcal upper respiratory tract infection is an important consideration. Patients with increased exposure to streptococcal infections include children and adolescents; parents of young children; teachers, physicians, nurses, and allied health personnel in contact with children; military recruits; and others in crowded housing. A higher risk of recurrences in economically disadvantaged populations has been demonstrated.

Physicians must consider each individual situation when determining the appropriate duration of prophylaxis. Patients who have had rheumatic carditis are at a relatively high risk for recurrences of carditis and are likely to sustain increasingly severe cardiac involvement with each recurrence. Therefore, patients who have had rheumatic carditis should receive long-term antibiotic prophylaxis, perhaps for life. Duration of prophylaxis depends on whether residual valvular disease is present or absent (Table 81–5). Prophylaxis should continue even after valve surgery, including prosthetic valve replacement. Patients who have had RF without carditis are at considerably less risk of cardiac involvement with a recurrence. Therefore, prophylaxis may be discontinued in these individuals after several years.[23] In general, prophylaxis should continue until 5 years have elapsed since the last RF attack or age 21 years, whichever is longer. The decision to discontinue prophylaxis or reinstate it should be made after discussion with the patient of potential risks and benefits and careful consideration of the epidemiological risk factors enumerated earlier.

An injection of 1,200,000 units of a long-acting penicillin preparation every 4 weeks is the recommended regimen for secondary prevention in most circumstances in the United States (see Table 81–4). In countries where the incidence of RF is particularly high, in special circumstances, or in certain high-risk individuals, such as patients with residual rheumatic carditis, the administration of benzathine penicillin G every 3 weeks is recommended.[24] Long-acting penicillin is of particular value in patients with a high risk of recurrence of RF. The advantages of benzathine penicillin G must be weighed against inconvenience to patients and pain of injection, which cause some patients to discontinue prophylaxis.

TABLE 81–5 Duration of Secondary Prophylaxis in Patients with Rheumatic Fever

Category	Duration
Rheumatic fever with carditis and residual valvular disease	At least 10 yr after last episode and at least until age 40 Sometimes lifelong prophylaxis
Rheumatic fever with carditis but no residual valvular disease	10 yr or well into adulthood, whichever is longer
Rheumatic fever without carditis	5 yr or until age 21, whichever is longer

From Dajani AS, Taubert K, Ferrieri P, et al: Treatment of streptococcal pharyngitis and prevention of rheumatic fever. Pediatrics 96:758, 1995, with permission.

Successful oral prophylaxis depends primarily on patients' adherence to prescribed regimens. Patients need careful and repeated instructions about the importance of continuing prophylaxis. Most failures of prophylaxis occur in nonadherent patients. Even with optimal adherence, risk of recurrence is higher in individuals receiving oral prophylaxis than in those receiving intramuscular benzathine penicillin G.[21] Oral agents are more appropriate for patients at lower risk for rheumatic recurrence. Accordingly, some physicians switch patients to oral prophylaxis when they have reached late adolescence or young adulthood and have remained free of rheumatic attacks for at least 5 years.

Penicillin V is the preferred oral agent (see Table 81–4). There are no published data about the use of other penicillins, macrolides, or cephalosporins for secondary prevention of RF. Although sulfonamides are not effective in eradication of group A streptococci, they do prevent infection. Sulfadiazine and sulfisoxazole appear to be equivalent; the use of sulfisoxazole is acceptable on the basis of extrapolation from data demonstrating that sulfadiazine has proven effectiveness in secondary prophylaxis. The recommended dose of sulfisoxazole is the same as that for sulfadiazine. Sulfonamide prophylaxis is contraindicated in late pregnancy because of transplacental passage of the drugs and potential competition with bilirubin for albumin binding sites. Erythromycin is recommended for patients who are allergic to penicillin and sulfisoxazole.

Infective Endocarditis Prophylaxis

(see also Chap. 58)

Patients with rheumatic valvular heart disease also require additional short-term antibiotic prophylaxis before certain surgical and dental procedures to prevent possible development of infective endocarditis. Patients with prosthetic valves or previous endocarditis are at particularly high risk. *Antibiotic regimens used to prevent recurrences of acute RF are inadequate for prevention of bacterial endocarditis.* The current recommendations of the American Heart Association concerning prevention of bacterial endocarditis should be followed.[25] Because alpha-hemolytic streptococci in the oropharynx may have developed resistance to oral penicillin being used for secondary prevention of RF, the agent selected to prevent endocarditis should not be a penicillin. Patients who have had RF but who do not have evidence of rheumatic heart disease do not need endocarditis prophylaxis.

GENERAL REFERENCES

Narula J, Virmanil R, Reddy KS, et al: Rheumatic Fever. American Registry of Pathology. Washington, DC, Armed Forces Institute of Pathology, 1999.

Jones TD: Diagnosis of rheumatic fever. JAMA 126:481, 1944.

REFERENCES

1. World Health Organization: Rheumatic fever and rheumatic heart disease. WHO Technical Report Series 764. Geneva, World Health Organization, 1998.
2. Dajani AS: Current status of nonsuppurative complications of group A streptococci. Pediatr Infect Dis J 10:S25, 1991.
3. Stollerman GH: Rheumatogenic group A streptococci and the return of rheumatic fever. Adv Intern Med 35:1, 1990.
4. Stollerman GH: Rheumatogenic streptococci and autoimmunity. Clin Immunol Immunopathol 61:131, 1991.
5. Kaplan EL, Johnson DR, Cleary PP: Group A streptococcal serotypes isolated from patients and sibling contacts during the resurgence of rheumatic fever in the United States in the mid-1980s. J Infect Dis 159:101, 1989.
6. Bessen D, Jones KF, Fischetti VA: Evidence for two distinct classes of streptococcal M protein and their relationship to rheumatic fever. J Exp Med 169:269, 1989.
7. Stollerman GH: Rheumatic fever in the 21st century. J Clin Infect Dis 33:806, 2001.
8. Smoot JC, Barbian KD, Van Gompel JJ, et al: Genome sequence and comparative microarray analysis of serotype M18 group A streptococcus strains associated with acute rheumatic fever outbreaks. Proc Natl Acad Sci USA 99:4668, 2002.
9. Narula J, Chopra P, Talwar KK, et al: Does endomyocardial biopsy aid in the diagnosis of active rheumatic carditis? Circulation 88:2198, 1993.
10. Roberts S, Kosanke S, Terrence Dunn S, et al: Pathogenic mechanisms in rheumatic carditis: Focus on valvular endothelium. J Infect Dis 183:507, 2001.
11. Dajani AS, Ayoub EM, Bierman FZ, et al: Guidelines for the diagnosis of rheumatic fever: Jones criteria, updated 1992. JAMA 268:2069, 1992.
12. Ferrieri P for the Jones Criteria Working Group: Proceedings of the Jones Criteria Workshop. Circulation 106:2521, 2002.
13. Veasy LG: Time to take soundings in acute rheumatic fever. Lancet 357:1994, 2001.
14. Gentles TL, Colan SD, Wilson NJ, et al: Left ventricular mechanics during and after acute rheumatic fever: Contractile dysfunction is closely related to valve regurgitation. J Am Coll Cardiol 37:201, 2001.
15. Schaffer FM, Agarwal R, Helm J, et al: Poststreptococcal reactive arthritis and silent carditis: A case report and review of the literature. Pediatrics 93:837, 1994.
16. Mercadente MT, Busatto GF, Lombroso PJ, et al: The psychiatric symptoms of rheumatic fever. Am J Psychiatry 157:2036, 2000.
17. Narula J: Usefulness of antimyosin antibody imaging for the detection of active rheumatic myocarditis. Am J Cardiol 84:946, 1999.
18. Cilliers AM, Manyemba J, Saloojee H: Anti-inflammatory treatment for carditis in acute rheumatic fever (Cochrane review). Cochrane Database Syst Rev 2:CD003176, 2003.
19. Voss LM, Wilson NJ, Neutze JM, et al: Intravenous immunoglobulin in acute rheumatic fever: A randomized controlled trial. Circulation 103:401, 2001.
20. Rullan E, Sigal LH: Rheumatic fever. Curr Rheumatol Rep 3:445, 2001.
21. Dajani AS: Adherence to physicians' instructions as a factor in managing streptococcal pharyngitis. Pediatrics 97:976, 1996.
22. Dajani AS, Taubert K, Ferrieri P, et al: Treatment of streptococcal pharyngitis and prevention of rheumatic fever. Pediatrics 96:758, 1995.
23. Berrios X, del Campo E, Guzman B, et al: Discontinuing rheumatic fever prophylaxis in selected adolescents and young adults. Ann Intern Med 118:401, 1993.
24. Lue HC, Wu MH, Wang JK, et al: Long-term outcome of patients with rheumatic fever receiving benzathine penicillin G prophylaxis every three weeks versus every four weeks. J Pediatr 125:812, 1994.
25. Dajani AS, Taubert KA, Wilson W, et al: Prevention of bacterial endocarditis: Recommendations by the American Heart Association. JAMA 277:1794, 1997.

CHAPTER 82

Rheumatic Diseases and the Cardiovascular System

Brian F. Mandell • Gary S. Hoffman

General Principles

Systemic rheumatological conditions often involve the cardiovascular system. They may first come to medical attention because of constitutional symptoms, muscle or joint pain, fever, regional or visceral ischemia, or organ failure. Rheumatological events that affect the heart and vessels vary from inapparent to catastrophic. Although cardiologists or cardiothoracic surgeons are usually not the initial source of care, in certain instances they may be the first to recognize that cardiovascular disease may have a primary immunological basis. Examples include patients with the vasculitides, who may present with claudication, aortic aneurysms, or ischemic heart disease (Takayasu or giant cell arteritis), and patients with systemic lupus erythematosus, who may first require medical attention for treatment of pericarditis.

Vasculitis

Discrimination between the various forms of rheumatic diseases and vasculitis begins with the concept of *primary* (i.e., the primary process is immune dysregulation without a known trigger) versus *secondary* (i.e., the cause is known and inflammation- or immune-mediated injury requires treatment or removal of the causative agent). Not knowing which group a patient fits into can lead to inappropriate use of immunosuppressive therapy that may have adverse or lethal consequences. Examples of secondary vasculitides include vasculitis secondary to sepsis, particularly endocarditis; drug toxicity and poisonings; malignancies; cardiac myxomas; and multifocal emboli from large-vessel aneurysms (Table 82–1). Each can mimic vasculitis or cause multifocal ischemia or infarction with accompanying vasculitis.

The greatest certainty in the diagnosis of primary vasculitis is in the setting of classic clinical and laboratory patterns, e.g., a 70-year-old woman with new-onset severe headache, temporal region pain, hip and shoulder girdle stiffness, visual aberration (amaurosis or blindness), and a high sedimentation rate. This picture would be so compatible with giant cell arteritis as not to require biopsy evidence of the diagnosis. Unfortunately, many patients with vasculitis do not present with such recognizable features. Instead, one may have to depend on combinations of less typical clues. A patient with ischemic digits, active urinary sediment, and peripheral neuropathy is likely to have vasculitis, especially if the previously noted secondary causes of vasculitis and its mimics have already been ruled out. The presence of a purpuric rash, particularly if it is palpable (Fig. 82–1), furthers the probability of this diagnosis, which can be confirmed by a simple skin biopsy. Such features occurring in the setting of an established autoimmune disease (e.g., rheumatoid arthritis, systemic lupus erythematosus, Sjögren syndrome, or relapsing polychondritis) enhance the likelihood of vasculitis being present. The physician must still distinguish primary from secondary causes.

Approach to Proving the Diagnosis of Vasculitis

Definitive proof of the diagnosis depends on visualizing vasculitic lesions in affected tissue. The greatest success in achieving a tissue diagnosis comes from biopsy of abnormal or symptomatic sites. In patients with proven vasculitis, the yield from biopsies of clinically normal sites is considerably less than 20 percent. Therefore, a biopsy of apparently normal tissue is not recommended. Biopsies of abnormal organs provide diagnostically useful information in more than 65 percent of cases. Biopsies of involved viscera have less than 100 percent yield because needle and organ-penetrating biopsies often do not directly visualize the affected tissue, and uniform involvement of vessels in affected viscera is uncommon.

A biopsy may not be practical in certain circumstances, such as systemic illness with symptoms of visceral ischemia, carotidynia, or findings of unequal pulses or blood pressures. Because biopsy of large vessels is usually impractical, angiography may be helpful. In this setting, vascular stenoses or aneurysms, or both, that cannot be explained on the basis of atherosclerosis may provide sufficient circumstantial evidence to proceed with treatment for primary systemic vasculitis.

Forms of Vasculitis Relevant to Cardiologists and Cardiovascular Surgeons

Takayasu Arteritis

Takayasu arteritis (TA) is an idiopathic large-vessel vasculitis of young individuals that affects the aorta and its major branches.

EPIDEMIOLOGY. Women are affected about 10 times more often than men. The median age at onset is 25 years. Although TA is best known to occur in Asia, the distribution of the disease is worldwide and it has been reported among people of all races

TABLE 82–1 Diagnosis of Vasculitis: Diseases That Can Mimic Primary Systemic Vasculitis

Sepsis, especially endocarditis
Drug toxicity or poisoning Cocaine Amphetamines Ephedra Phenylpropanolamine
Coagulopathy Anticardiolipin antibody syndrome Disseminated intravascular coagulation
Malignancy (solid organ or "liquid" tumors)
Cardiac myxoma
Multifocal emboli from large-vessel aneurysms (cholesterol, mycotic)
Ehlers-Danlos syndrome (vascular ectatic type)
Fibromuscular dysplasia

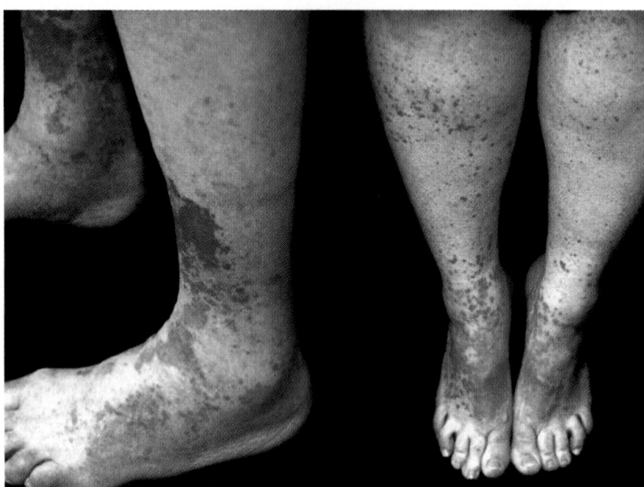

FIGURE 82–1 Palpable purpura. Vascular inflammation at the level of capillaries and venules leads to exudation of formed elements and the color and texture of lesions noted in these patients. The legs on the right are those of a young woman with Henoch-Schönlein vasculitis or purpura. The elderly man on the left has a similar lesion. However, in this case it was associated with hepatitis C virus (HCV), acquired in the course of transfusions for heart surgery. HCV infection led to cryoglobulinemia and *secondary* vasculitis. The treatment for each patient is quite different. The one with Henoch-Schönkin purpura, who does not have extracutaneous disease, requires only reassurance and monitoring for her usually self-limiting problem, whereas the patient with HCV and vasculitis requires antiviral therapy.

and ethnicities. The incidence of TA is estimated to be 2.6 per 1,000,000 persons in the United States and 1.26 per 1,000,000 in northern Europe.[1] Autopsy series from Japan point to a higher incidence, with 1 in every 3000 autopsies having features of TA.[2]

PATHOGENESIS. Although the cause of TA is unknown, studies of acute lesions reveal mononuclear cell infiltrates that appear to have reached the vessel wall through the vasa vasorum and subsequently migrate to the macroluminal intima (Fig. 82–2A, left). These cells are predominantly macrophages and T, gamma-delta, cytotoxic, and natural killer lymphocytes. There is also a small admixture of B lymphocytes. The presence of a variety of cytokines, including interleukin-6 (IL-6) and tumor necrosis factor (TNF), in these granulomatous lesions has suggested a variety of therapeutic approaches using biological agents. The finding of the mycobacterial heat shock protein, HSP-65, in the affected media and vasa vasorum of TA-affected vessels is intriguing. However, it is uncertain whether this is an epiphenomenon or a primary or intermediate step in TA pathogenesis.[3]

CLINICAL FEATURES. In TA, arterial stenoses occur three to four times more often than aneurysms. Claudication (>60 percent upper versus ~30 percent lower extremities) is the most common complaint, and bruits (~80 percent) and blood pressure and pulse asymmetries (60 to 80 percent) are the most common findings. Aneurysms are most common and clinically most significant in the aortic root, where they can lead to valvular regurgitation (~20 percent) (Fig. 82–2A, left, and B). Hypertension is most often due to renal artery stenosis but can also be associated with suprarenal aortic stenosis or a chronically damaged, rigid aorta. Cardiac, renal, and central nervous system vascular diseases are the principal causes of severe morbidity and mortality. Estimates of mortality range from a low of about 3 percent at 8 years[4] to about 35 percent at 5 years follow-up.[1,4]

Symptoms of large-vessel abnormalities or the finding of hypertension, especially in young patients, necessitates examination of extremity pulses and blood pressures for asymmetry and a search for bruits. Increasing extremity or visceral ischemia, malaise, myalgias, arthralgias, night sweats, and fever may indicate active disease. When such symptoms occur in the setting of an elevated erythrocyte sedimentation rate (ESR), active disease is assumed to be present. Yet, many patients may not have any constitutional or new vascular symptoms, and as many as 50 percent may have normal ESRs and still experience progressive disease.[1,4] The following findings indicate that active TA can occur in this setting:

1. New vascular abnormalities on sequential angiographic studies in patients who were thought to be in remission and
2. The presence of inflammatory changes in arterial biopsy specimens from patients in whom surgery was performed because of critical flow abnormalities in the setting of clinically "quiescent" disease.[1,4]

Until we are better able to judge the degree of disease activity in TA, outcomes will be compromised. Studies using refinements in magnetic resonance and positron-emission tomography imaging techniques may enable the clinician to detect qualitative abnormalities in the vessel wall that imply inflammatory change.[5] These abnormalities may then be followed sequentially to determine response to therapy.

The cardiac sequelae of TA are more often due to aortic regurgitation and inadequately treated hypertension than to arteritis affecting the coronary vessels.[1,4] When coronary artery vasculitis is detected (<5 percent), it is most frequent in the ostial regions. However, more distal involvement has also been reported and both types of lesions may occur in the same patient. These observations underscore the importance of considering vasculitis in the differential diagnosis for young patients with ischemic symptoms.

DIFFERENTIAL DIAGNOSIS. Certain congenital diseases cause abnormalities of tissue matrix and aortic regurgitation (e.g., Marfan syndrome, Ehlers-Danlos syndrome). However, these conditions are not associated with stenotic lesions in large vessels, the most common feature of TA. "Inborn" genetic errors that affect matrix structure are also not associated with systemic symptoms, abnormal acute phase reactants, anemia, or thrombocytosis, which may be present with large-vessel vasculitis. The young female predominance of TA distinguishes it from typical atherosclerosis, a disease much more likely to affect the lower extremity large vessels than the arms and the abdominal aorta than the aortic root. Infectious causes of large-vessel aneurysms (e.g., bacterial, syphilitic, mycobacterial, and fungal) must be considered in either gender and all age groups but usually are not associated with vascular stenoses affecting the arch vessels. Certain "autoimmune" diseases may be complicated by large-vessel vasculitis, but they are readily discerned by their associated characteristics (e.g., systemic lupus, Cogan syndrome, Behçet disease, spondyloarthropathies) and characteristic age preferences (e.g., Kawasaki disease and giant cell arteritis of the elderly). Sarcoidosis can closely mimic TA. Making the correct diagnosis depends on other characteristic features of sarcoidosis being present (e.g., proliferative synovitis, skin lesions, Bell palsy, hilar adenopathy).

There are no specific diagnostic tests for TA. The diagnosis is based on clinical features in conjunction with vascular imaging abnormalities. In patients who undergo vascular surgery, histopathological abnormalities may further support the diagnosis.

TREATMENT. Approximately 50 percent of patients with TA respond to corticosteroid therapy (e.g., prednisone 1 mg/kg/d), with subsequent resolution of symptoms and stabilization of abnormalities noted on arteriography. However, relapse can occur in more than 40 percent of patients with tapering of corticosteroid therapy. Corticosteroid-resistant patients or those with relapses may respond to the addition of daily therapy with cyclophosphamide (~2 mg/kg) or weekly therapy with methotrexate (~20 mg).[6] About 40 percent of patients who are treated with a cytotoxic agent and corticosteroid achieve remission, but in time about half of these patients also have relapses, leading to the need for chronic immunosuppressive therapy in at least 25 percent of all patients with TA.[1,4,6] Such unsatisfactory results have led to ongoing studies that seek to take advantage of new insights into pathogenesis. Preliminary studies have demonstrated that treatment designed to block TNF may dramatically benefit most patients (14 of 15) with TA who have had relapses during tapering of steroid therapy.[7]

A discussion of pharmacological therapy for TA addresses only one important aspect of care. Other important issues include treatment of the anatomical effects of vascular lesions. Patients with TA may have signs of clinical deterioration related to fixed critical stenoses or aneurysms. Hypertension affects about 40 to 90 percent of patients.[1,4] In Asia, India, and Mexico, TA is one of the most common causes of hypertension in adolescents and young adults. One of the most common errors in clinical management is related to the physician not knowing whether blood pressure recordings in an extremity are representative of aortic root pressure. Because more than 90 percent of patients have stenotic lesions and the most common sites of stenosis are the subclavian and innominate arteries, blood pressure in one or both arms may underestimate pressure in the aorta. Elevated aortic root pressure, when unrecognized and untreated, enhances the risks of hypertensive complications. This potential dilemma can best be appreciated when angiographic procedures include intravascular pressure recordings. These observations emphasize the importance of knowing the distribution and severity of all vascular lesions. In the setting of renal insufficiency, the potential of contrast agents to cause further renal impairment may limit exploration of the extent of all potential vascular lesions. However, if contraindications are not present, patients should have the entire aorta and its primary branches included in vascular imaging studies. Magnetic resonance angiography lacks the ability to measure intravascular pressures. If the clinical examination does not suggest that lesions affecting extremity-recorded blood pressures are present and extremity pressures are equal, a magnetic resonance study may be sufficient to delineate other vascular lesions without resorting to catheter-guided angiography.

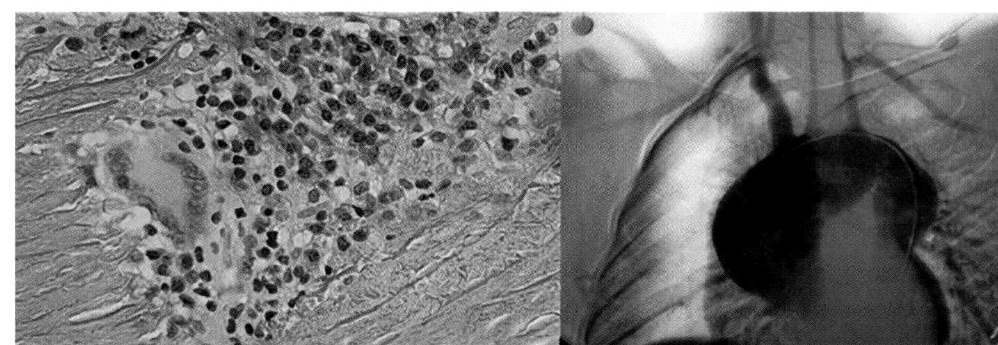

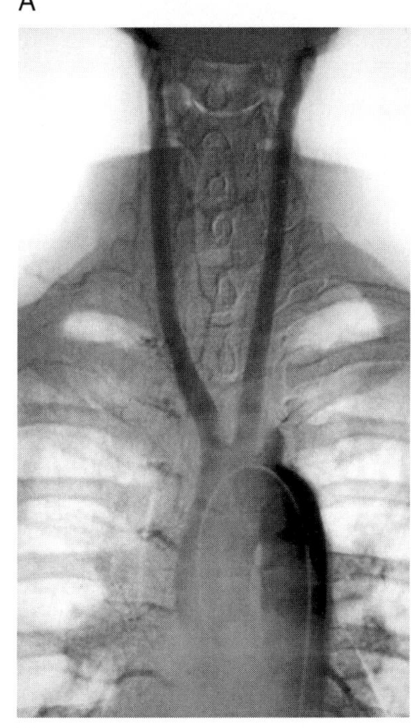

FIGURE 82–2 Takayasu arteritis. **A,** Granulomatous inflammation and medial destruction **(left)** have led to marked aortic root dilation **(right)** in a 17-year-old female high school student who developed symptoms of congestive heart failure and exertional angina. She also had diffuse narrowing of the left common carotid artery and irregular dilation of the innominate artery. **B,** Occlusion of both subclavian arteries has led to leg pressures being the only reliable measure of central aortic pressure.

Whenever feasible, anatomical correction of clinically significant lesions should be considered, especially in the setting of renal artery stenosis and hypertension. In about 20 percent of patients, aortic root involvement may lead to valvular insufficiency, angina, and congestive heart failure (Fig. 82-3).[1,4] Severe or progressive changes may require aortic surgery, with or without valve replacement. Although it is always preferable to operate on patients in remission, because judgment of TA activity may be difficult, *all* such surgeries should include obtaining vascular specimens for histopathological evaluation. Findings from surgical specimens should guide the need for postoperative immunosuppressive treatment.

The care of patients with TA requires a team approach that includes clinicians familiar with the proper use of immunosuppressive therapies, vascular imaging or intervention specialists, and, in the setting of critical stenoses or aneurysms, cardiovascular physicians and surgeons. For most patients, medical and surgical therapies provide important palliation.

Giant Cell Arteritis of the Elderly

Giant cell arteritis (GCA) and TA are the principal diseases associated with sterile granulomatous inflammation of large and medium-sized vessels.

EPIDEMIOLOGY. In the United States, GCA affects approximately 18 people per 100,000 population, and the affected people are older than 50 years (mean = 74 years). Although it is not understood, it is particularly interesting

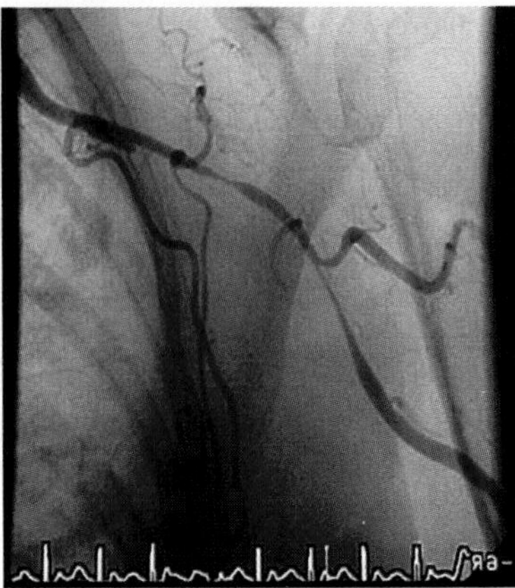

FIGURE 82–3 Giant cell arteritis. "Takayasu-like" lesions involving the subclavian and axillary arteries in a case of giant cell arteritis are shown.

that the incidence of GCA is much greater in northern latitudes. For example, in Iceland and Denmark, the incidence is 27 and 21 per 100,000, respectively, in the age group older than 50 years. Although women predominate in frequency of being affected (2 to 3:1), this predominance is not as striking as in TA (6 to 10:1). The demographic characteristics of patients with GCA are the same as those of patients with polymyalgia rheumatica, and in fact 30 to 50 percent of patients with GCA may concurrently have features of polymyalgia rheumatica.[8]

PATHOGENESIS. Although the cause of GCA remains unknown, much has been learned over the past 10 years about the inflammatory lesion. It begins in the adventitia, where the vasa vasorum are the conduit for the mononuclear cells (macrophages and Th1-type lymphocytes) that mediate vascular injury. Dendritic cells participate in the process by presenting to lymphocytes the putative antigen that is believed to "drive" GCA. This concept is supported by the finding of clonality of approximately 4 percent of T lymphocytes in the vessel wall. Clonality is not found in peripheral blood lymphocytes, enhancing the likelihood that a responsible antigen is presented in the adventitia or media. Vascular lesions are initially rich in proinflammatory cytokines such as IL-1, IL-6, TNF, and interferon-gamma. Intermediate lesions harbor mediators of matrix destruction (e.g., metalloproteinases, reactive oxygen and nitrogen species). In later stages, growth factors such as platelet-derived growth factor (PDGF) and fibroblast growth factor participate in stimulating myointimal proliferation, leading to vessel stenosis. Preliminary reports of improvement of GCA with anti-TNF treatment suggest that the cytokines play a pathogenetic role. The use of other anticytokine therapies that target the Th1 pathway merits evaluation in the future and may shed further light on the pathogenesis of GCA.[8]

CLINICAL FEATURES. The most characteristic features of GCA are new onset of atypical and often severe headaches, scalp and temporal artery tenderness, acute visual loss, polymyalgia rheumatica, and pain in the muscles of mastication (Table 82–2). Conjunction of such abnormalities with an increase in ESR supports a clinical diagnosis of GCA and treatment, even without temporal artery biopsy. The diagnosis is doubtful if dramatic improvement does not occur within 24 to 72 hours. In the instances in which typical features are not present but the diagnosis is suggested by vague systemic symptoms and atypical headache in the setting of a normal or elevated sedimentation rate, and all other reasonable diagnoses have been ruled out, the specific findings of a positive biopsy would be helpful in guiding treatment. The yield of positive temporal artery biopsies in patients clinically diagnosed with GCA has been estimated to be about 50 to 80 percent, depending in part on the size of the biopsy and whether bilateral samples have been obtained.[9]

TABLE 82–2 Giant Cell Arteritis: Clinical Profile

Abnormality	Frequency (%)
Atypical headache	60-90
Tender temporal artery	40-70
Systemic symptoms not attributable to other diseases	20-50
Fever	20-50
Polymyalgia rheumatica	30-50
Acute visual abnormalities	12-40
Transient ischemic attacks or stroke	5-10
Claudication	
"Jaw"	30-70
Extremities	5-15
Aortic aneurysm	15-20
Dramatic response to corticosteroid	~100
Positive temporal artery biopsy	~50-80

GCA may produce clinically apparent aortitis in at least 15 percent of cases and involve the primary branches of the aorta, especially the subclavian arteries, in a similar number of individuals.[10,11] Postmortem studies suggest that large-vessel involvement is far more common than clinically appreciated. Consequently, some patients with GCA may present with features that resemble those of TA. Among elderly people with inflammatory large-vessel disease, the same considerations and precautions must be applied in GCA as in TA: the need to identify an extremity that provides a reliable blood pressure that is equivalent to aortic root pressure and follow-up including careful observation for new bruits, pulse and blood pressure asymmetry, and the possible development of aortic aneurysms.

Studies have demonstrated that patients with GCA were more than 17 times more likely than age-matched control subjects to have thoracic aortic aneurysms and about 2.5 times more likely than age-matched control subjects to have abdominal aortic aneurysms[10,11] (see also Chap. 53). Fifty-five percent of patients with thoracic aortic aneurysms died as a result of those lesions. Because aneurysms were found either in the course of routine care or at postmortem examination, these may be conservative estimates. The finding of large-vessel disease, including aortic aneurysms, in elderly persons with GCA should not merely be assumed to be secondary to atheromatous disease. It is not surprising that about half of all patients with GCA have objective features of cardiac disease. However, it appears that myocardial infarction related to GCA is rare or rarely appreciated because histopathological findings in coronary arteries are infrequently sought in patients whose mean age is 74 years.

DIFFERENTIAL DIAGNOSIS. Mimics of GCA include other vasculitides that may cause musculoskeletal pain, headache, visual aberrations, fever, and malaise. These include Wegener granulomatosis (WG), Churg-Strauss vasculitis, and microscopic polyangiitis, and it is relatively simple to rule these out on the basis of more characteristic features of those illnesses (e.g., upper or lower airway disease, or both, and features of small-vessel vasculitis). Rarely, the GCA phenotype may be part of a paraneoplastic process. If polymyalgia rheumatica is the most compelling symptom of GCA, the differential also includes polymyositis and proximal-onset rheumatoid arthritis.

No precise serological test exists for GCA. Diagnosis is based on a clinically compatible presentation, concurrent highly abnormal acute phase reactants (>80 percent of cases), a positive temporal artery biopsy (50 to 80 percent of cases), or angiographic abnormalities of large vessels (see Fig. 82-3) that are compatible with GCA.

TREATMENT. Corticosteroids continue to be the most effective therapy for GCA. Prednisone (~0.7 to 1 mg/kg/d) reduces symptoms within 1 to 2 days and often eliminates symptoms within a week. About 2 to 4 weeks after clinical and laboratory parameters, particularly the ESR, have become normal, tapering of corticosteroid can begin. Unfortunately, the ESR does not always become normal even with disease control and should not be relied on as the only measure of disease activity. Occasional patients may either not achieve complete remission or not be able to have corticosteroid tapered. Cytotoxic or immunosuppressive agents have been recommended for such individuals by some authors, but the utility of these agents has not been proved in controlled comparative trials.[12]

Idiopathic Aortitis

Aortitis is a recognized feature of TA and GCA. It may also occur in diseases such as Behçet disease, Cogan syndrome, and in children as a complication of Kawasaki disease. Occasionally, it is an unanticipated finding in patients undergoing surgery for aortic valve regurgitation, aneurysm resection, or coarctation.[13] Little is known about the frequency and clinical characteristics of idiopathic aortitis. (Aortitis in the context of retroperitoneal fibrosis is a separate topic that is not discussed in this section.)

EPIDEMIOLOGY. A 20-year review of pathological specimens from consecutive aortic surgeries at the Cleveland Clinic Foundation revealed that 52 (4.3 percent) of 1204 specimens were classified as idiopathic aortitis. Sixty-seven percent of patients with idiopathic aortitis were women.[13]

PATHOGENESIS. Unless the patient with idiopathic aortitis had a past history of GCA or TA, the mechanisms of disease have remained unexplored.

CLINICAL FEATURES. In our series, 96 percent of cases with idiopathic aortitis had findings limited to the thoracic aorta. These data are similar to those from large postmortem series in which aortas have been examined in spite of the absence of overt aortic disease during life. In 96 percent of our cases, symptoms of systemic illness were not present at the time of surgery. In 69 percent of cases, idiopathic aortitis was not related to a current or past history of systemic disease. However, in 31 percent (16 of 52), aortitis was associated with a past history of GCA, TA, systemic lupus, WG, or a variety of other disorders. Thus, a past history of these illnesses and reports that they are presumably in remission become suspect in the setting of a newly recognized thoracic root aneurysm.

DIFFERENTIAL DIAGNOSIS. Patients with idiopathic aortitis vary in age from children to very elderly individuals. Consequently, differential diagnostic considerations might include Kawasaki disease, TA, GCA, systemic lupus, sarcoidosis, Cogan syndrome, Behçet disease, spondyloarthropathies, rheumatoid arthritis, rheumatic fever, and aortitis related to infectious agents (e.g., tuberculosis, syphilis, mycotic and bacterial agents). Symptoms or findings of these diseases may immediately allow prioritization of diagnostic choices. However, some processes may be clinically silent and diagnosis may be aided by ancillary laboratory studies (e.g., RPR, antinuclear antibody), skin tests (e.g., purified protein derivative), cultures, and special stains of surgical specimens. Because idiopathic aortitis is a syndrome that requires ruling out all causes of aortitis that may have specific therapies (e.g., antibiotics), it should be clear that no diagnostic tests for this entity exist apart from histopathological ones.

TREATMENT. In our experience with 36 patients, observed for a mean period of 42 months and analyzed retrospectively, new aneurysms were identified among 6 of 25 patients who were not treated with glucocorticosteroids and none of 11 patients who were treated with glucocorticosteroids. Although these results suggest that such therapy is indicated in this setting, there were marked variations of dose and duration of therapy that led to uncertainty about corticosteroid efficacy. Because only 17 percent of all patients subsequently developed new aneurysms over 3.5 years, we do not feel that all such patients require medical treatment.[13] These observations suggest that inflammatory disease may be isolated to the aortic root in most patients. To justify treatment, one would have to prove the existence of ongoing inflammatory disease. We approach this by routine history and physical examination, laboratory evaluation (complete blood count, ESR, C-reactive protein), and imaging studies (magnetic resonance angiography or imaging of the entire aorta and its primary branches). Because new lesions may occur over time, patients with idiopathic aortitis identified at the time of surgery should be periodically evaluated for recurrence. If proof of recurrent disease is present, treatment should be pursued, as recommended for TA and GCA. Although proof of the effectiveness of this approach is lacking, it can be defended on the basis of the similarities of these conditions and demonstrated efficacy in GCA and TA.

Kawasaki Disease

Kawasaki disease (KD) is an acute febrile systemic illness of childhood. It is the principal cause of acquired heart disease in children in Japan and the United States.

EPIDEMIOLOGY. KD was first described more than 35 years ago.[14] It occurs primarily in children younger than 4 to 5 years. Peak incidence is in children younger than 2 years. Boys are affected 1.5 times more often than girls. KD almost never occurs beyond age 8 years (mean age in Japan is 12 months and in the United States 2.8 years). Although all racial groups can be affected, Asian children have the highest incidence of KD (50 to 200 per 100,00 children younger than 5 years versus 6 to 15 per 100,000 in the United States). Asian Americans have a higher incidence of KD than blacks, in whom the incidence exceeds that of whites.[15] Although siblings of patients with KD are infrequently affected, KD does affect siblings more often than the general age-matched population (2.1 percent versus 0.19 percent). When siblings are affected, symptoms often occur shortly after their family member became ill. This finding raises questions about an infectious etiology in the setting of an immunological predisposition.[15-18]

PATHOGENESIS. Fever, rash, conjunctivitis, adenopathy, and geographical clustering suggest an infectious cause. However, no agent has yet been identified. The following scenarios remain possible:

1. An undiscovered pathogen is responsible for KD.
2. A known infectious agent plays a role in triggering an abnormal immune response, but the pathogen itself is cleared.
3. A pathogen triggers disease by molecular mimicry to normal host antigens.
4. A sequence of stochastic events leads to clinically apparent disease, but by the time the patient presents, the most critical early features of pathogenesis have disappeared.

The essential absence of disease in neonates invites speculation about protection related to maternal antibodies, and the rarity of KD in adults suggests that protection may occur through acquired immunity.[16,17]

The acute phase of illness is characterized by widespread evidence of immunoinflammatory activation. This evidence includes high levels of acute phase reactants, leukocytosis with a left shift, lymphocytosis with a predominance of polyclonal B cells, and thrombocytosis that frequently reaches 1,000,000/mm^3. Blood T lymphocytes, including CD4+ and CD8+ cells, increase in number and show signs of activation. In spite of these observations, children with acute KD are often anergic, indicating T-cell dysfunction. Increased blood levels of a broad range of cytokines and fragments of endothelial cell adhesion molecules indicate widespread immune activation. Cytokine-mediated endothelial cell activation and factors cytotoxic to endothelial cells may play an important early role in pathogenesis. Pathology specimens reveal vasculitis with endothelial cell edema, necrosis, desquamation, and a changing profile of leukocytes in the vessel wall (first neutrophils and later macrophages and T lymphocytes). After months, the inflammatory infiltrate diminishes, and as it fades, myointimal proliferation may produce stenoses or wall weakening may lead to aneurysm formation. In either case, the stage is set for subsequent thrombosis.[16,17]

CLINICAL FEATURES. The most prominent features are included in the case definition guidelines of the Centers for Disease Control and Prevention (Table 82–3). These guidelines lack any specific, single serological diagnostic test. The illness is usually self-limiting within 4 to 8 weeks, and mortality is 2 percent.

Cardiac abnormalities include pericardial effusions (~30 percent), myocarditis, mitral regurgitation (~30 percent), aortic regurgitation (infrequent), congestive heart failure, and atrial and ventricular arrythmias.[16,17] Electrocardiographic findings include decreased R wave voltage, ST segment depression, and T wave flattening or inversion. Slowed conduction may be seen with prolonged PR or QT prolongation. Deaths usually result from acute coronary artery thrombosis in aneurysms that form after vasculitis. Noninvasive techniques disclose coronary artery aneurysms in about 20 percent of patients, compared with 60 percent shown by angiography. Aneurysms usually appear 1 to 4 weeks after onset of fever. New aneurysms seldom form after 6 weeks. Aneurysms are more common in the proximal than distal

coronary arteries. Although larger aneurysms (>8 mm) (Fig. 82–4) are among the most susceptible to later thrombosis and occlusion, leading to infarction and even sudden death, endothelial abnormalities and intimal proliferation in smaller lesions (<4 mm) may lead to cardiac ischemia as well. Myocardial infarction is most common in the first year after illness but can occur in young adults as well.[16,17]

Data from postmortem studies have also demonstrated vasculitis of the aorta and celiac, carotid, subclavian, and pulmonary arteries. Rare case reports of gut vasculitis in KD exist.[17,18] Gastrointestinal morbidity may depend more on small-vessel than large-vessel disease.

DIFFERENTIAL DIAGNOSIS. Given the resemblance of KD to infectious diseases, competing diagnoses include bacterial, spirochetal (e.g., leptospirosis), rickettsial (e.g., Rocky Mountain spotted fever), and viral illnesses. Drug reactions, poisonings (e.g., mercury), juvenile rheumatoid arthritis, systemic lupus, other vasculitides, and malignancies, especially lymphomas and leukemias, may also share aspects of KD.[17]

TABLE 82–3 CDC Case Definition of Kawasaki Syndrome

Fever ≥5 days, without other explanation, plus at least four of the following:

1. Bilateral conjunctival injection
2. Mucous membrane changes: injected or fissured lips; injected pharynx or "strawberry" tongue
3. Extremity abnormality: erythema of palms/soles, edema of hands/feet or generalized, or peripheral desquamation (hands, feet)
4. Rash (polymorphous)
5. Cervical lymphadenopathy (usually a single node >1.5 cm)

Associated manifestations
- Irritability
- Sterile pyuria, meatitis
- Perineal erythema and desquamation
- Arthralgias, arthritis
- Abdominal pain, diarrhea
- Aseptic meningitis
- Hepatitis
- Obstrucive jaundice
- Hydrops of gallbladder
- Uveitis
- Sensorineural hearing loss
- Cardiovascular changes

Note: 80% of cases <4 years old; rare >8 years old.
CDC = Centers for Disease Control and Prevention.
Adapted from Barron KS: Kawasaki disease. *In* Hoffman GS, Weyand CM (eds): Inflammatory Disease of Blood Vessels. New York, Marcel Dekker, 2002, pp 305-319.

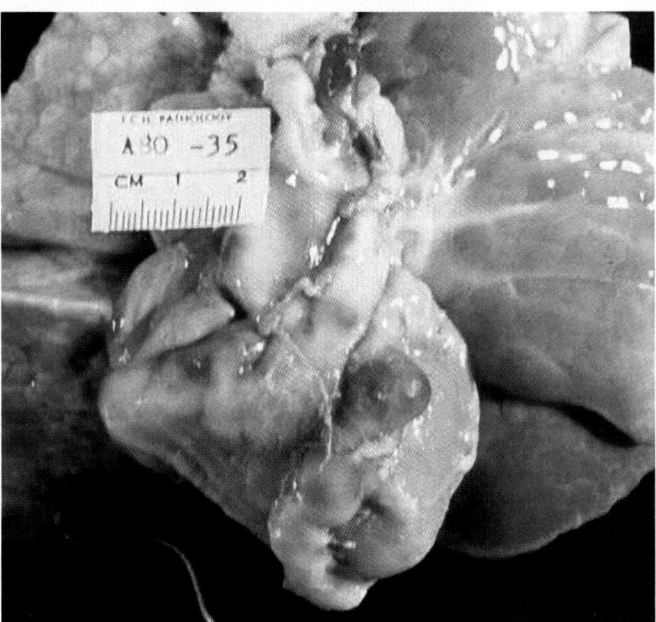

FIGURE 82–4 Giant coronary artery aneurysms related to Kawasaki disease. Note the bulbous protrusion from the left anterior descending coronary artery. (Courtesy of Dr. Karyl Barron.)

TREATMENT. Before the use of high doses of aspirin and intravenous gamma globulin, coronary artery aneurysms were relatively common. However, such treatment appears to have reduced the incidence of aneurysms to less than 10 percent.[16] The current standard of care consists of 2 gm/kg of intravenous gamma globulin as a single infusion. Treatment provided within the first 10 days of illness shows efficacy most convincingly. Aspirin (80 to 100 mg/kg/d until the patient is afebrile) has both antiinflammatory and antithrombotic effects. After fever subsides, the dose of aspirin is reduced (3 to 5 mg/kg/d) to achieve primarily antiplatelet effects. This treatment should continue until the platelet count and other inflammatory parameters return to normal (about 8 weeks). Long-term, low-dose aspirin is recommended in children with echocardiogram-demonstrated aneurysms, although the efficacy of such therapy has not been proved in controlled studies.

A small subset of patients with KD resist conventional therapy. They constitute a group that is most prone to aneurysm formation and long-term disease sequelae. The use of corticosteroids in this group and other patients remains controversial. The reported increased frequency of coronary artery aneurysms in an early report of corticosteroid-treated patients has not been seen by others.[16]

Recommendations for long-term follow-up by the American Heart Association include consideration of anticoagulation therapy in children with multiple giant aneurysms and known obstructive lesions and evaluation by stress testing during adolescence. Severe coronary artery lesions have been treated by bypass, but if disease is widespread and bypass is not possible, transplantation should be considered.[16]

Vasculitis of Small or Medium-Sized Vessels That May Affect the Cardiovascular System

Churg-Strauss Syndrome (Allergic Angiitis and Granulomatosis)

Churg-Strauss syndrome (CSS) is a rare syndrome that typically includes a history of asthma, eosinophilia, pulmonary infiltrates, upper airway inflammation, and a variable frequency of renal, neurological, cutaneous, and cardiac involvement. Histopathological observations of involved lesions reveal eosinophilic, granulomatous infiltrates and vasculitis.

EPIDEMIOLOGY. The most generous estimate of the annual incidence of CSS is 2.4 cases per 1,000,000 persons per year. Those affected may be children or adults, with the peak age being 35 to 50 years. Significant gender bias does not exist.[19]

PATHOGENESIS. The cause of CSS remains unknown. Nonetheless, authorities have recommended withdrawal of any newly introduced drugs or treatments (e.g., desensitization) and avoidance of new environmental stimuli (e.g., farms, industry, if relevant to the medical history). A role for leukotriene antagonists, as used in the treatment of asthma, in precipitating CSS is a subject of controversy. Most would agree that if such an agent were introduced just before the emergence of CSS, it should be discontinued. Whether antineutrophil cytoplasmic antibodies (ANCAs) play a role in CSS is uncertain. ANCAs occur in 30 to 60 percent of cases, suggesting that if they play a role, it is not an essential one. Most often the immunofluorescent pattern for ANCAs in CSS is perinuclear (P pattern), but in a minority of cases it can be cytoplasmic (C). The specific antigen targeted by ANCA is usually myeloperoxidase, but in some cases it is proteinase 3 and the corresponding immunofluorescent pattern is C.

The granulomatous nature of CSS lesions suggests an involvement of Th1 lymphocytes and macrophages, whereas ANCA, if relevant, and eosinophils argue for a role of Th2-biased lymphocytes. The latter are a source of IL-5, which increases eosinophil production and release from the bone marrow.

CLINICAL FEATURES. By definition, the diagnosis requires a past or present history of asthma. Nonetheless, rare cases have been recognized with only a history of allergies and allergic rhinitis. Systemic symptoms are present in 70 to 100 percent of cases from different series. Chest imaging reveals infiltrates, usually multifocal, in 30 to 75 percent. Much less often, pulmonary nodules may be seen, as in WG; however, in CSS nodules are unlikely to cavitate, a finding that is common in WG. Cardiac disease in CSS is the most common cause of death. It is reported in 15 to 55 percent and may include pericarditis, myocarditis, and coronary arteritis. Congestive heart failure occurs in 15 to 30 percent of cases. Gastrointestinal ischemia (~5 percent) contributes significantly to morbidity and mortality. It may be manifest by frank blood from the rectum, melena, or bowel perforation. Many more patients have abdominal pain (30 to 60 percent) for which the ultimate cause is suspected to be CSS. The small intestine and colon are the sites more often affected. Peripheral neurological abnormalities (sensory or motor or both) affect more than two-thirds of patients. Although these features are not life-threatening, they can be a source of profound morbidity. Musculoskeletal symptoms and rashes may be seen in about one-half of all patients, and renal disease (glomerulonephritis) is seen in at least one-third.[19]

DIFFERENTIAL DIAGNOSIS. CSS may be confused with WG. However, patients who suffer from WG do not have an unusually high frequency of allergies and asthma and striking eosinophilia (although in some patients with WG eosinophils can be approximately 10 percent of the total white blood cell count). In WG, the most common ANCA pattern is C and antibody is usually directed to proteinase 3 (70 to 80 percent of ANCA-positive cases). Pulmonary nodules may cavitate in WG, an event that would be rare in CSS.

Other considerations in the differential are parasitic infections (especially helminths, larvae and adults, e.g., hookworm, ascaris, *Trichinella*, *Strongyloides*, filaria, flukes) that may produce chronic eosinophilia by stimulating IL-5 in affected organs. Because helminths may migrate through the lungs, infiltrates and bronchospasm may result, producing a picture of eosinophilic pneumonia and asthma. Idiopathic hypereosinophilic syndrome (HES) is a diagnosis to be considered only after all other causes of eosinophilia have been ruled out. In some cases it is part of a leukoproliferative syndrome and may be associated with splenomegaly, cytogenetic abnormalities, myelofibrosis, myelodysplasia, anemia, and abnormal red blood cell forms. When such findings are not present, the absence of vasculitis and asthma distinguishes HES from CSS. HES is of particular interest to cardiologists because of the risks of cardiac fibrosis, ventricular apical necrosis, and intraventricular thrombus formation. Emboli from the ventricles may lead to pulmonary infarction or systemic circulatory events, including stroke and peripheral occlusive lesions. Myocarditis and cardiac fibrosis may lead to a restrictive cardiomyopathy.

TREATMENT. Corticosteroids (most often prednisone, 1 mg/kg/d orally) usually produce dramatic improvement. In patients with critical organ system involvement (heart, brain, kidneys, gut) it may be prudent to provide "pulse" intravenous therapy (1 gm/d of methylprednisolone) for 1 to 3 days. Although recommended, this regimen has never been the subject of controlled clinical trials. Patients who are critically ill should also receive a second agent (most often cyclophosphamide). Cyclophosphamide is utilized daily in a dose of 2 mg/kg, assuming normal renal function. In the presence of renal impairment, the dose must be proportionately reduced to avoid severe bone marrow suppression. Long-term cyclophosphamide therapy carries many risks. Although once the standard of care, cyclophosphamide is now utilized to induce remission and then after 3 to 6 months, while corticosteroids are being tapered, if remission continues, cyclophosphamide is switched to maintenance therapy with either daily azathioprine or weekly methotrexate.

Polyarteritis Nodosa

Polyarteritis nodosa (PAN) is a nongranulomatous disease of only medium-sized arteries. The old literature on PAN has been a source of confusion to modern students of vasculitis. The older series included patients with both PAN and microscopic polyangiitis (MPA), a disease that can have features of PAN but is defined by the presence of small-vessel vasculitis (capillaries, venules, and arterioles). In modern parlance, cases of nongranulomatous vasculitis with glomerulonephritis (renal capillaritis) and pulmonary infiltrates (alveolitis or capillaritis) would be considered MPA and not PAN. The Chapel Hill Consensus Conference (CHCC) on Nomenclature set forth these guidelines.[20] The guidelines also stress that PAN and MPA are not immune complex mediated and not secondary forms of vasculitis, as might be due to infections, hepatitis viruses, or systemic lupus and other rheumatological diseases.

EPIDEMIOLOGY. Because not all authors adhere strictly to the CHCC guidelines, it is difficult to know the incidence of PAN. Even liberal application of these guidelines indicates that PAN is a rare disease, with an annual incidence of less than 1 per 100,000. Some authors include vasculitis related to hepatitis, mediated by immune complexes and cryoglobulins, in this figure. Men and women are equally affected. PAN may affect people of any age, but the incidence peaks between 40 and 60 years of age.

PATHOGENESIS. When one properly excludes cases associated with hepatitis, the etiology of medium-sized vessel vasculitis compatible with PAN is unknown. The histopathology of lesions varies and often evolves in time, at first having a predominance of neutrophils and later mononuclear cells. Granulomas and increased numbers of eosinophils *are not* present. Necrotizing changes may follow, with weakening of the vessel wall and aneurysm formation, or myointimal proliferation, causing stenosis and occlusion.

CLINICAL FEATURES. Systemic symptoms are present in at least 50 percent of all patients in different series. Any organ system can be involved. However, if one adheres to CHCC guidelines, several features should not be included because they reflect microvascular (capillary-venule) disease: palpable purpura, pulmonary infiltrates or hemorrhage, and glomerulonephritis. In contrast, these may be findings in MPA.

PAN would more typically include deep skin inflammatory changes that may produce painful nodules (similar to erythema nodosum) or progress to infarction and gangrene (30 to 50 percent), neuropathy (especially mononeuritis multiplex, 20 to 50 percent), renal infarction and insufficiency (~10 to 30 percent), hypertension (~30 percent), segmental pulmonary infarctions (<40 percent), and cardiac disease (10 to 30 percent, congestive failure, angina, infarction, pericarditis). Although musculoskeletal symptoms occur in more than 50 percent of all PAN patients, they are not a helpful differential diagnostic feature. As was noted for CSS, poor prognostic markers include ischemia or infarction of critical organs (brain, gut, kidneys, and heart). Although clinically apparent heart disease may affect less than one-third of cases, postmortem examination may reveal medium-size vessel vasculitis or consequences of hypertension (left ventricular hypertrophy, congestive heart failure) in up to 75 percent.[19]

DIFFERENTIAL DIAGNOSIS. The preceding discussion of epidemiology and classification addressed this issue. However, it is important to reemphasize that certain infections may cause inflammation of medium-sized vessels. All patients with clinical findings that resemble those of PAN should be tested for hepatitis B and C. A PAN-like presentation is most often associated with hepatitis B virus and cryoglobulinemia, whereas an MPA-like presentation occurs more frequently in association with hepatitis C virus infection and cryoglobulinemia. Rarely, infection with human immunodeficiency virus (HIV) may arise in this fashion. In immunocompromised hosts, cytomegalovirus should also be sought as a possible cause of small- and medium-sized vessel disease. The PAN-MPA–like spectrum obligates a search for bacterial and fungal infections as causes of endocarditis or endovascular vegetations. Use and abuse of vasoactive drugs (e.g., cocaine, amphetamines, ephedrine) should also be considered (see also Chap. 62). Subsequent sections discuss sarcoidosis with vasculitis, another disease that can affect vessels of any size. PAN is not associated with ANCA. No serological diagnostic tests exist for PAN. The diagnosis depends on biopsy or angiographic proof of medium-sized vessel inflammation (Fig. 82–5).

TREATMENT. The guidelines for treatment are the same as those for CSS. Not all patients with PAN require the addition of a cytotoxic agent (cyclophosphamide, methotrexate, or azathioprine). However, in the setting of critical organ disease, one should not hesitate to employ these agents.

Other primary vasculitides such as hypersensitivity vasculitis, Henoch-Schönlein purpura, and WG may all have cardiac consequences. However, because vasculitis-mediated heart disease is infrequent in these disorders, they are not addressed further. The principles of treatment are similar to those noted for CSS and PAN, with the exception that WG therapy always requires the addition of a cytotoxic agent.[19]

Rheumatoid Arthritis

Rheumatoid arthritis (RA) is the most common form of chronic inflammatory polyarthritis. Rheumatoid factor is present in approximately 70 percent of patients. Its presence does not confirm the diagnosis of RA; it is frequently present in other diseases including chronic viral hepatitis and bacterial endocarditis. Systemic complications of RA include pericarditis, pleuritis, vasculitis, compressive neuropathies, interstitial lung disease, and Sjögren and Felty syndromes.

EPIDEMIOLOGY. RA affects approximately 1 to 3 percent of the population. Some cases of milder disease are probably not diagnosed. Patients with a positive circulating rheumatoid factor or human leukocyte antigen (HLA) DR4 are more likely to have severe erosive joint disease and extraarticular manifestations. The disease affects patients of all ages but is most frequently diagnosed in patients during the third to fifth decade of life.

PATHOGENESIS. As in most of the systemic rheumatic diseases, the exact etiology is unknown. There is a genetic predisposition, but this is seemingly polygenic. There may be an infectious trigger, but no agent has been proved to cause disease. An abnormal T-cell response triggers macrophage activation. TNF, IL-1, and other cytokines are required to sustain the chronic inflammatory response.

CLINICAL FEATURES. The hallmark of RA is a chronic symmetrical polyarthritis that affects small and large joints, especially the metacarpal phalangeal joints and wrists, while sparing the lumbar and thoracic spine and the distal interphalangeal joints. Characteristic radiographic damage to the joints can be documented in the majority of patients and may occur quite early in the course of the disease. RA affects the pericardium in approximately 50 percent of patients, as indicated by echocardiographic and necropsy studies. Chronic, asymptomatic effusive pericardial disease is more common than acute pericarditis.[21] Although the frequency of symptomatic pericarditis among outpatients with RA has been estimated as less than 0.5 percent, in a series of 41 selected patients with severe RA, 75 percent had symptoms compatible with acute pericarditis. Patients with rheumatoid pericardial disease are generally older and have longstanding RA. The electrocardiogram is usually normal in patients with chronic pericardial disease but may show characteristic changes in acute pericarditis. Coexistent small pleural effusions are common and may reflect rheumatoid

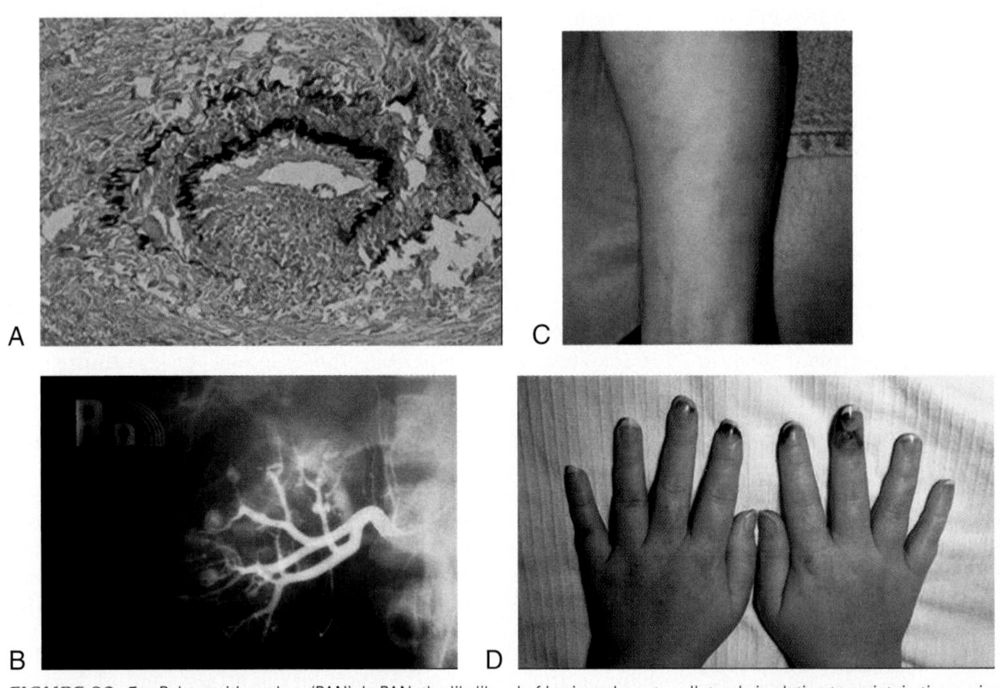

FIGURE 82–5 Polyarteritis nodosa (PAN). In PAN, the likelihood of having adequate collateral circulation to maintain tissue viability following vasoocclusion is less than that in other vasculitides. **A,** A section of a muscular artery shows destruction of the internal elastic lamina (from 5 o'clock to 8 o'clock) as well as intimal thickening and stenosis. Although aneurysms may be visually more striking on angiography, vascular occlusive lesions **(B)** may contribute to high-renin hypertension and renal failure. **C,** Palpable subcutaneous nodules are shown that were painful on the patient's forearms. **D,** Infarcts on the fingers caused by severe digital artery involvement are shown.

serositis or hemodynamic effects of the pericarditis. Pericardial calcification has been reported, mimicking tuberculous pericarditis. Limited data have been published on the nature of pericardial fluid in RA. Fluid is frequently blood tinged with leukocyte counts ranging from scant to more than 30,000/mm^3, generally with a neutrophil predominance. Glucose may be quite low compared with serum glucose values, similar to the markedly depressed glucose levels reported in rheumatoid pleural effusions. The presence of rheumatoid factor in the fluid does not confirm the diagnosis of RA pericarditis. Constrictive pericarditis can occur and must be distinguished from restrictive cardiomyopathy, which is rarely a complication of secondary amyloidosis in patients with longstanding RA. Treatment of clinical pericarditis includes the use of nonsteroidal antiinflammatory drugs (NSAIDs), intensified systemic immunosuppressive therapy, pericardial steroid injections, or pericardiocentesis if hemodynamic compromise occurs. If systemic therapy is ineffective or already at an intense level, recurrent pericardial effusions may require a pericardial window. Constriction should be surgically treated. Chest pain related to costochondritis is far more common than pericarditis. The use of aggressive medical therapy early in the course of rheumatoid disease may decrease the frequency of pericardial involvement.

Patients with RA have a decreased life expectancy. The leading cause of death is cardiovascular disease.[22] Potential risk factors for coronary artery disease (CAD) in patients with RA include the chronic systemic inflammatory state; the use of corticosteroids, which may accelerate atherosclerosis; and possibly the use of methotrexate, which can elevate levels of circulating homocysteine. The relative contributions of these factors to acceleration of CAD are not clear (see Chap. 36). Significant ischemic disease may be clinically silent because of the relative inactivity of patients with severe RA. Special consideration should be given to the patient with RA about to undergo major noncardiac surgery. Although currently unsupported by adequate data, it is reasonable to consider longstanding RA as an intermediate risk factor in preoperative risk assessment, similar to considerations of renal insufficiency or diabetes in the American Heart Association guidelines. Coronary arteritis is a rarely reported complication of RA.

RA does not usually cause clinically significant myocarditis or congestive heart failure. Secondary amyloidosis is rare in rheumatoid disease but can cause cardiomyopathy and heart block. Tachyarrhythmias can occur as a result of rheumatoid pericarditis. Focal cardiac involvement with rheumatoid nodules has been well described and has been associated with conduction block. All levels of block have been described and, once established, usually do not respond to antiinflammatory and immunosuppressive therapies.

Autopsy studies have indicated frequent involvement of the cardiac valves and aorta, but these are rarely of clinical significance. Slowly progressive granulomatous valvulitis may be difficult, if not impossible, to distinguish from disease unrelated to RA. A rapidly progressive inflammatory valvulitis of the aortic valve advancing to need for valve replacement over less than 5 years has been described.[23] Rheumatoid aortitis, with involvement of the aortic valve, has been reported, but aortitis is not frequently recognized before death. RA does not cause primary pulmonary hypertension. However, secondary pulmonary hypertension may result from rheumatoid lung disease.

DIFFERENTIAL DIAGNOSIS. RA, in the absence of characteristic radiographic erosive changes, remains a diagnosis of exclusion. Other conditions that can cause a symmetrical small- and large-joint polyarthritis include chronic hepatitis B and C, systemic lupus erythematosus, several vasculitides including PAN and WG, and crystal-induced arthropathies. Early or acute RA can also be confused with bacterial endocarditis and other infections such as parvovirus or rubella. Lyme disease (*Borrelia* infection), which can be associated with cardiac conduction disease, causes an oligoarticular large joint arthritis that does not mimic RA.

TREATMENT. Current regimens for the treatment of RA emphasize aggressive disease-modifying therapy as soon as the diagnosis is made. Combination therapy with agents including methotrexate, sulfasalazine, leflunomide, hydroxychloroquine, and low-dose prednisone is frequently employed. NSAIDs are no longer the mainstay of therapy. Antagonists of TNF are extremely effective agents, although cost and the unknown long-term effects of therapy are concerns in their use. The increased use of effective therapy may be associated with a decreased incidence of extraarticular complications of RA. Notable is the concern about increased cardiac morbidity with the use of anti-TNF therapies in patients with severe congestive heart failure.

HLA-B27–Associated Spondyloarthropathies

The rheumatoid factor–negative spondyloarthropathies include ankylosing spondylitis (AS), psoriatic arthritis, inflammatory bowel disease–associated arthritis, and postinfectious reactive arthritis (including Reiter syndrome).

EPIDEMIOLOGY. The vast majority of whites with AS and many patients with other spondyloarthropathies have the HLA-B27 gene. Although individuals may carry this gene and not have spondyloarthritis, patients with arthritis share several features that distinguish them from patients with RA. Although females do suffer from these disorders, AS and reactive arthritis are male-dominant diseases. The spondyloarthropathies are distinctly less common than RA.

PATHOGENESIS. The seronegative spondyloarthropathies have been historically grouped together because of some shared clinical characteristics and the disproportionate presence of the B27 antigen. Studies with transgenic rats expressing the human B27 antigen have shown that these animals, when raised in a non-germ-free environment, exhibit inflammation of skin, spine, and other tissues similar to that seen in patients. This finding strongly supports the role that B27 plays in the pathogenesis of the inflammation. It has been proposed that the presence of the B27 gene permits an abnormal immune response to gut or mucosal bacterial antigens that are cross-reactive with tissue antigens present in joints, skin, and other tissues. The abnormal response includes breaking of tolerance to specific self-antigens and perpetuation of localized inflammation. This theory has not been confirmed, and the antigens have not been reproducibly delineated. Because not all patients with spondyloarthropathies have the B27 antigen, either there are alternative pathogenic mechanisms or the current ability to define the B27 specificity at a molecular level is limiting our full understanding of its role in the pathogenesis.

CLINICAL FEATURES. In these conditions, unlike RA, the entire spine, not just the cervical region, may be involved. Sacroiliac joint involvement is frequent and may be the only musculoskeletal manifestation. Large peripheral joints are commonly involved but, unlike that in RA, involvement tends to be asymmetrical. There is frequently inflammation of the tendons, ligaments, or joint capsules at the point of insertion into bone (enthesis, thus the term "enthesitis"). Diffuse tendon sheath involvement may produce "sausage" digits. Ninety percent of American whites with AS and approximately 60 percent of patients with inflammatory bowel–related spondylitis have the HLA-B27 gene. The carriage rate of HLA-B27 in healthy American whites is approximately 10 percent. It is much lower in blacks and Asians. Presence of the gene predisposes to anterior uveitis, cardiac conduction disease, and proximal aortitis. Thus, some patients with psoriatic arthritis, enteropathic arthritis, and reactive arthritis including Reiter syndrome as well as AS are predisposed to these complications. Patients may express extraskeletal B27-related complications without overt rheumatic disease. Most important, the HLA-B27 gene is *not* a diagnostic test.

Pericarditis, although reported, is not characteristic of the spondyloarthropathies. CAD does not occur at an increased rate, and coronary arteritis is not expected. Diastolic dysfunction has been reported[24] in patients who have HLA-B27 but is rarely of clinical significance. Cardiac conduction disease has been well described in patients with AS as well as Reiter syndrome. It has been estimated that up to one-third of patients with AS experience conduction disease. Atrioventricular conduction block may initially be intermittent but tends to progress. Conduction disease is more common in male patients, and as many as 20 percent of males with permanent pacemakers carry the HLA-B27 gene. Conduction disease may be the only abnormality associated with the HLA-B27 gene. Electrophysiological studies indicate that the level of block is usually at the atrioventricular node, not fascicular.[25] Atrial fibrillation may occur more commonly than expected in patients with the HLA-B27 gene.

Aortic root disease, with involvement of the aortic valve, has been reported in up to 100 percent of AS patients in autopsy series and 82 percent in a transesophageal echocardiographic study of patients with AS. Characteristic findings have included thickening of the aortic root with subsequent dilation. Aortic cusp nodularity with proximal thickening constitutes the "subaortic bump." The subaortic bump was found in 74 percent of 44 patients with AS[26] using transesophageal echocardiography. In this study, aortic regurgitation developed in 50 percent of patients, and 20 percent of patients had congestive heart failure, underwent valve replacement, had a stroke, or died compared with only 3 percent of age- and sex-matched volunteers. The aortic lesions progressed in 24 percent of patients and resolved in an additional 20 percent of patients over approximately a 2-year follow-up. The severity of aortic root disease was associated with the patients' age and duration of spondylitis. Dilation and stiffening of the aortic root may contribute to the aortic regurgitation. Hence, the regurgitant murmur, as in syphilitic aortitis, may be best heard along the right sternal border. There seems to be a unique B27-associated syndrome of aortic regurgitation and atrioventricular conduction block.

DIFFERENTIAL DIAGNOSIS. The B27-associated spondyloarthropathies are characterized by inflammation of the spine, with morning stiffness of the involved areas. Unlike that in RA, the peripheral arthritis is asymmetrical and usually involves large joints. The specific spondyloarthropathies are suggested by their associated extraarticular features (e.g., psoriasis, balanitis, urethritis, oral or genital ulcers or both). Cardiac involvement seems more linked to the presence of the HLA-B27 gene than to any specific rheumatic disorder.

TREATMENT. For years the spondyloarthropathies have been treated symptomatically, with marginal success, with NSAIDs and physical therapy. Modification of the disease course had not been expected from such therapy. The disease-modifying drugs used successfully in patients with RA (methotrexate, sulfasalazine) had minimal efficacy in relieving the symptoms and findings of spinal inflammation, although they were variably successful in treating peripheral arthritis. The B27 extraarticular manifestations were treated, as needed, with corticosteroids (uveitis) or surgery (aortic regurgitation or aortitis). The anti-TNF agents (etanercept, infliximab, adalimumab) have been found to have dramatic clinical efficacy in treating the symptoms of spondylitis; whether they will have a salubrious effect in treating or preventing the cardiovascular and ocular manifestations is currently unknown.

Systemic Lupus Erythematosus

Systemic lupus erythematosus (SLE) is a systemic autoimmune disease characterized by the presence of immune complexes and antinuclear antibodies (ANAs) and a constellation of clinical features, which may include serositis, arthritis, glomerulonephritis, central nervous system dysfunction, hemolytic anemia, thrombocytopenia, and leukopenia. Antiphospholipid antibodies (APLAs) are present in more than 20 percent of patients with lupus and may predispose the individual patient to arterial and venous thrombosis, pulmonary hypertension, or miscarriage (see also Chap. 80).

EPIDEMIOLOGY. SLE is more common in women and can occur at any age. Both idiopathic and drug-induced lupus have cardiac manifestations. Drug-induced lupus is well recognized following treatment with various cardiac medications including procainamide, quinidine, and hydralazine.

PATHOGENESIS. More than 90 percent of patients with SLE have ANAs; however, the presence of even high titers of ANA is *not* diagnostic of SLE. Antibodies to double-stranded DNA are present in approximately 50 to 70 percent of patients with idiopathic SLE and is more common in those with glomerulonephritis. SLE is an immune complex disorder, with immunoglobulin and complement deposition in involved organs, including the heart. The view of SLE as only an immune complex disorder is probably an oversimplification because (1) removal of complexes by apheresis has not been shown to alter the course of the disease, (2) immune deposits can be found in tissue (skin, heart) without resultant inflammation, and (3) T-cell hyperreactivity is an acknowledged component of SLE. Some lupus animal models have been associated with retroviral infections, but there are no consistently demonstrable viral agents in humans with SLE. Twin studies have suggested important roles for genetic factors.

CLINICAL FEATURES. Pericarditis is the most common cardiac problem in SLE.[27] Imaging and autopsy series demonstrate pericardial involvement in more than 60 percent of patients, and clinically significant pericarditis occurs in less than 30 percent. Unexplained chest pain is common in patients with SLE but is more likely due to etiologies other than pericarditis. Pericarditis may occur as the initial manifestation of SLE, appear at any point during the disease course, or occur as a complication of chronic renal disease. Pericardial fluid has generally demonstrated a neutrophil predominance, elevated protein, and a low or normal glucose level. Complement levels in pericardial fluid tend to be low, but this is not a characteristic unique to SLE. The fluid is indistinguishable from that obtained from patients with bacterial pericarditis, and thus infection must be excluded. Pericardial tamponade may occur at any point in the course of SLE, including the initial presentation. When effusions occur in the setting of chronic renal failure, it is difficult to distinguish uremic from lupus pericarditis. Pericarditis, as well as tamponade, can occur with drug-induced lupus. Constrictive pericarditis, presumably as a sequela of lupus pericarditis, has been reported.

Coronary arteritis, resulting in ischemic syndromes, rarely occurs in patients with SLE. The distinction between CAD and coronary arteritis may require sequential angiographic studies, with documentation of more rapid change in luminal images than is usually seen with CAD. Despite the young age of many patients with lupus, atherosclerosis remains the most common cause of ischemic cardiac disease. The prevalence of subclinical CAD is quite high, as determined by scintigraphy, electron beam computed tomography, and autopsy studies. Angina or myocardial infarction occurs in less than 20 percent of patients. As patients live longer with their disease, the prevalence of clinical cardiovascular events will increase. The most common cause of death in patients with longstanding SLE is cardiovascular disease. There are reports of young patients with SLE suffering myocardial infarction as the initial manifestation of their CAD. Middle-aged women with lupus are more than 50 times more likely to have a myocardial infarction[28] than age- and gender-matched control subjects. Risk factors include disease duration, period of time treated with corticosteroids, postmenopausal status, and hypercholesterolemia.

Additional causes of acute coronary syndromes in SLE include thrombosis, often related to the presence of APLA, and embolism from nonbacterial vegetative endocarditis (Libman-Sacks). The presence of APLA predisposes to thrombosis in some patients and has been associated in some echocardiographic studies with valve thickening and nonbacterial endocarditis. Antiendothelial cell antibodies may accelerate atherogenesis. The presence of APLA independently predicted CAD in a subset analysis of the Helsinki heart study.[29] Treatment of ischemic disease in patients with SLE is similar to that in patients with "routine" atherosclerotic disease, but because the mechanism for the increased risk of cardiovascular events is unknown and thus untreatable, an extremely aggressive approach to reducing known risk factors is warranted. The rare patient with coronary arteritis should be treated aggressively with high-dose corticosteroids, and patients with thrombotic disease related to APLA should receive long-term high-dose anticoagulation. Aspirin is *not* sufficient as an anticoagulant. Thrombocytopenia is common in patients with APLA and may complicate therapy.

Myocardial dysfunction in lupus is usually multifactorial and may result from immunological injury, ischemia, valvular disease, or coexistent problems such as hypertension. Acute myocarditis is infrequent but can be the initial presentation of SLE. Patients with peripheral skeletal myositis are reportedly at increased risk for myocarditis. Measurement of troponin I may be of value in documenting cardiac involvement, but the muscle-brain (MB) fraction of creatine kinase (CK) may be significantly elevated in the presence of skeletal myositis even in the absence of myocarditis. Noninvasive studies have demonstrated abnormal systolic and diastolic function in patients with active SLE. These changes are usually reversed with control of disease activity. Acute or chronic congestive heart failure related to SLE, in the absence of other confounding factors, is not common. Endomyocardial biopsy of the patient with cardiomyopathy and suspected lupus may not provide a specific diagnosis of lupus. The biopsy generally reveals patches of myocardial fibrosis, sparse interstitial mononuclear cell infiltrates, and occasional myocyte necrosis with some immune complex deposition even in areas devoid of inflammatory changes. If acute left ventricular failure occurs in patients with active SLE, in the absence of CAD or valve disease, a trial of corticosteroid therapy is indicated.

Tachyarrhythmias can occur in patients with SLE secondary to pericarditis or ischemia. Sinus tachycardia may be the earliest manifestation of myocarditis. A gallium scan may be abnormal in lupus myocarditis, but this has not been studied in adequate numbers of patients to be validated. Abnormal heart rate variability may be due to autonomic dysfunction or to occult myocarditis. Abnormal myocardial single-photon emission computed tomography scans have been noted, even among some patients with a normal resting echocardiogram.[30] Unexplained sinus tachycardia, which resolves with treatment of SLE, can occur in the presence of active lupus, even when evidence of cardiac dysfunction is absent. Occult pulmonary embolism should always be considered as a cause of tachycardia in patients with SLE, especially in the presence of APLA.

Babies born to mothers with SLE and other systemic autoimmune diseases have an increased incidence of congenital complete heart block. The pathogenic mechanism is the transmission of maternal anti-Ro and anti-La antibodies in utero causing myocardial inflammation and fibrosis of the conduction system.[31] The risk for development of complete heart block in infants born to mothers carrying the antibodies is low. However, women with systemic autoimmune diseases, known to be associated with these antibodies, should be screened before pregnancy for their presence. If the antibodies are present, the women should be observed throughout pregnancy with ultrasound studies to detect fetal complete heart block or hydrops. Heart block usually appears after the first trimester of pregnancy and is almost always irreversible. If it is recognized early, dexamethasone in utero *may* be successful in reversing myocarditis. Data to support this intervention are limited. Pacemaker placement is frequently necessary in the infant and may be required shortly after delivery.

Valvular involvement in SLE is common. Recognized 50 years ago as noninfectious vegetations (Libman-Sacks endocarditis), valvular abnormalities have been shown by transesophageal studies in more than 50 percent of patients with SLE.[32] Valvular thickening is the most common echo finding, followed by vegetations and valvular insufficiency. The vegetations are generally located on the atrial side of the mitral valve and the arterial side of the aortic valve. The vegetations are usually nonmobile. Over time, the lesions may resolve or worsen; fibrosis may cause retraction of the valve, resulting in insufficiency. Less commonly, the vegetations on the valve may occlude the orifice, causing stenosis. Valvulitis (Fig. 82–6), with valve fenestrations and rapidly progressing dysfunction, has been described. There are descriptions of mitral and aortic valve replacement in patients with SLE.[33] Valve repair has also been described.[34] Recurrence of valve disease, particularly thrombosis, may affect prosthetic valves. The nonbacterial vegetations rarely embolize and cause stroke syndromes. Several studies have demonstrated an increased prevalence of cardiac valve dysfunction in the presence of APLA with or without SLE. Because vegetations may occur in APLA-negative patients with SLE, there appear to be multiple mechanisms by which heart valves are affected in patients with lupus. Because of the high prevalence of valvular abnormalities in patients with SLE, it has been suggested that all patients with SLE receive antibiotic prophylaxis for endocarditis. Adequate studies do not exist to allow objective evaluation of this proposal.

On the basis of Doppler echocardiography, pulmonary artery hypertension is common in SLE.[35] Clinically significant pulmonary hypertension is less common. Etiologies for the development of pulmonary hypertension include thromboembolic disease related to APLA, intimal proliferation of the pulmonary artery, chronic vasospastic disease associated with peripheral Raynaud disease, and rarely arteritis of the pulmonary vessels. Successful heart-lung transplantation has been reported in a patient with SLE and progressive pulmonary hypertension. Aortitis can rarely occur in SLE.[36]

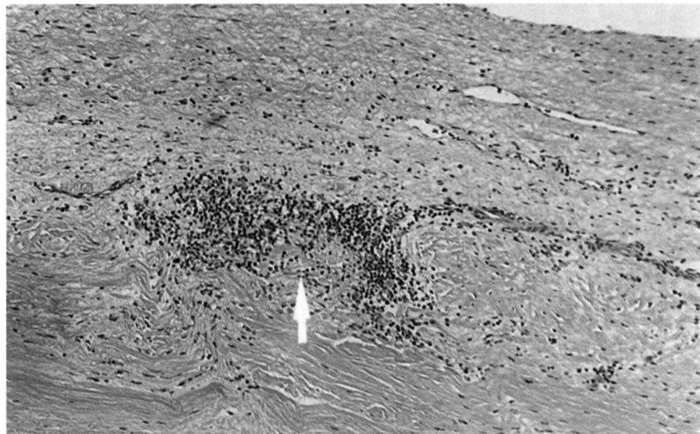

FIGURE 82–6 Valvulitis in systemic lupus erythematosus (SLE). Patients with SLE can experience valve dysfunction caused by bland vegetations (Libman-Sacks endocarditis), valve-associated thrombosis, and rarely true valvulitis. This photomicrograph illustrates aortic valve valvulitis that was discovered at the time of surgery for aortitis and aortic insufficiency (×400). The white arrow indicates a cluster of infiltrating leukocytes.

DIFFERENTIAL DIAGNOSIS. Among the most common features of SLE are ANAs (>90 percent), arthralgias and arthritis (60 to 90 percent), constitutional symptoms (50 to 75 percent), rash (50 to 80 percent), Raynaud vasospasm (30 to 60 percent), and glomerulonephritis (30 to 75 percent). More characteristic features that further enhance diagnostic likelihood include "butterfly" rash, sun-sensitive skin eruptions, discoid skin lesions, hemocytopenias (especially thrombocytopenia and leukopenia), antibodies to double-stranded DNA and Sm (anti-Smith), hypocomplementemia, and characteristic findings on biopsies of involved sites. Diseases that are occasionally confused with SLE include dermatomyositis, infections, lymphomas, thrombotic thrombocytopenic purpura (TTP), idiopathic thrombocytopenic purpura (ITP), Still disease, and sarcoidosis. The pattern of cardiac involvement in SLE is not diagnostic of this disorder.

TREATMENT. There is no single treatment for SLE per se. The specific manifestations are managed on an individual basis. Life-threatening organ involvement is controlled by high-dose corticosteroids, often with the addition of cyclophosphamide. Patients with mild pericarditis without threat of hemodynamic compromise are generally treated with NSAIDs unless there is a contraindication to such therapy, such as renal insufficiency. Corticosteroids are used for more severe disease. If prompt response to steroid therapy does not occur, large sterile pericardial effusions, particularly those accompanied by fever or hemodynamic compromise or both, are best treated with drainage and, if recurrent, consideration of a pericardial window. Arteritis and myocarditis are treated with high-dose corticosteroids with or without adjunctive cyclophosphamide or azathioprine. Corticosteroids may be used for acute valvulitis, and the indications for surgery are the same as for other causes of valvular dysfunction.

Antiphospholipid Antibody Syndrome

(see also Chap. 80)

APLA syndrome is defined as the presence of either APLA or a lupus anticoagulant *and* a history of otherwise unexplained recurrent venous or arterial thrombosis or frequent second- or third-trimester miscarriages. Mild thrombocytopenia, hemolytic anemia, and livedo reticularis are commonly present. APLAs are quite common (10 to 30 percent) in SLE, although not all of these patients exhibit the clinical syndrome. Low to moderate levels of APLA can also be found in association with a number of infectious and other autoimmune diseases, usually without clinical consequence. In the absence of an underlying systemic disease, APLA syndrome is termed primary.

EPIDEMIOLOGY. The true prevalence of the APLA syndrome is unknown. The presence of a lupus anticoagulant or APLA does not define the clinical syndrome, which requires a coincident clinical thrombotic or embolic event or events.

PATHOGENESIS. See Chapter 80.

CLINICAL FEATURES. Venous thromboembolic disease is the most common manifestation and most often occurs in the legs and lungs. Arterial thrombosis most often leads to stroke but can occur in a wide range of locations. Primary APLA syndrome is not associated with pericarditis, myocarditis, or conduction disease. Cardiac manifestations include thrombotic CAD, intracardiac thrombi, and nonbacterial endocarditis.[37] Heart valve abnormalities occur in approximately 30 percent of patients with primary APLA syndrome and include thrombotic masses extending from the valve ring or leaflets, vegetations, or thickening. The mitral valve is affected more frequently than the aortic valve, and regurgitation is far more common than stenosis (Fig. 82–7). Most valvular involvement is clinically silent. The first manifestation of valvular involvement with APLA syndrome may be a thromboembolic event such as stroke. The incidence of superimposed bacterial endocarditis is not known. Clinically significant valvular or intracardiac masses are treated by high-dose anticoagulation with warfarin,[38] with or without the addition of aspirin. Full-dose heparin therapy is probably also effective. Management of heparin dosing in the setting of a lupus anticoagulant, which prolongs the baseline partial thromboplastin time, may require consultation with the coagulation laboratory.[39] Vegetations may resolve with anticoagulation therapy over several months,[40] but spontaneous resolution has also been noted. Patients with APLA are at risk for myocardial infarction and reocclusion after angioplasty or bypass grafting. Aggressive prophylactic anticoagulation should be employed perioperatively in patients with APLA and previous thrombosis. Pulmonary hypertension can

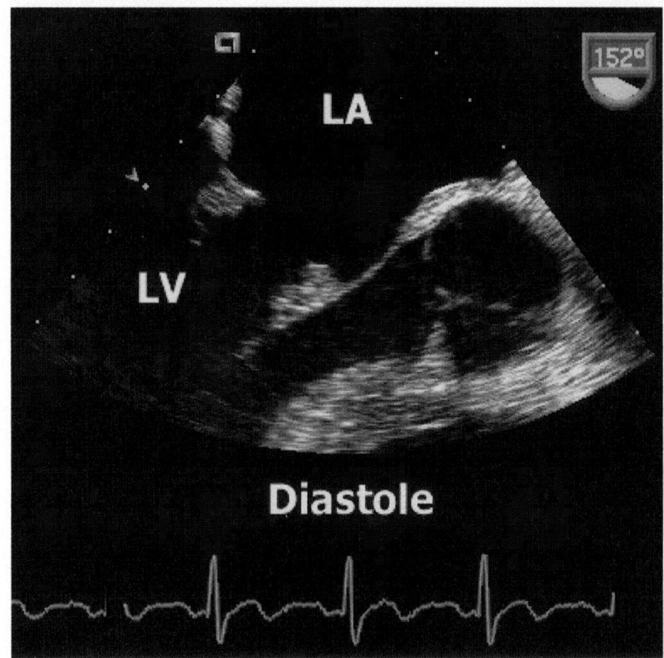

A

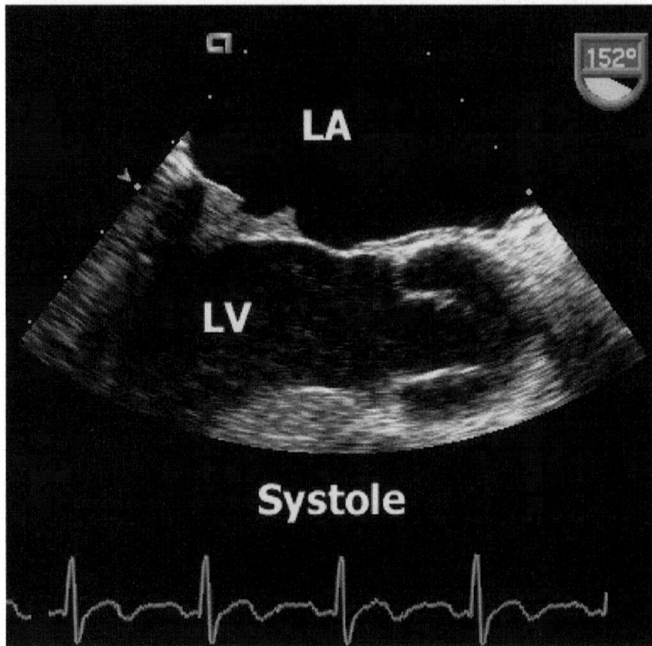

B

FIGURE 82–7 **A** and **B,** Transesophageal echocardiogram demonstrating large sterile vegetations in a 41-year-old man with a previous history of deep venous thrombosis, symptoms of dyspnea on exertion, and a holosystolic apical murmur. A transthoracic echocardiogram demonstrated severe mitral regurgitation. The presence of apposing lesions on both the anterior (right) and posterior (left) leaflets of the mitral valve, also known as "kissing" vegetations, is characteristic of the anticardiolipin antibody syndrome. LA = left atrium; LV = left ventricle. (Courtesy of Dr. Mario Carcia, Cleveland Clinic, Cleveland, OH.)

occur in patients with APLA secondary to chronic thromboembolic disease. It has also been proposed that APLA can directly stimulate pulmonary artery intimal proliferation.

DIFFERENTIAL DIAGNOSIS. The differential diagnosis of APLA syndrome includes SLE, TTP, ITP, and frequently occult neoplasia. SLE can involve the heart, as discussed earlier. TTP can cause coronary ischemia but not valvular disease, and occult neoplasia has been associated with nonbacterial thrombotic endocarditis.

TREATMENT. The primary therapy of APLA syndrome is anticoagulation, generally to a level similar to that used for patients with prosthetic valves. Monitoring of the anticoagulation level can be difficult in the presence of a prolonged partial thromboplastin time, but use of weight-based algorithms and low-molecular-weight heparin while waiting for a full warfarin effect makes it easier. There are no long-term controlled studies of the effect of chronic anticoagulation and valve disease. Valve replacement can be successfully accomplished in these patients; the indications for surgery are the same as in other patients. The consideration of the type of valve may be influenced by the need for lifelong anticoagulation in these patients, independent of the valve surgery.

Scleroderma (Progressive Systemic Sclerosis, CREST Syndrome)

Scleroderma and its variants are characterized by the presence of microvascular occlusive disease with vasospasm and intimal proliferation and various patterns of cutaneous and parenchymal fibrosis. Although early lesions are inflammatory, the most obvious clinical manifestations are due to enhanced extracellular matrix accumulation (fibrosis).

EPIDEMIOLOGY. Scleroderma, particularly progressive systemic sclerosis (PSS), is a rare disease that affects less than 1 to 19 per million persons per year. An increased prevalence occurs in certain populations such as the Choctaw Native Americans. The average age of onset is 45 to 65 years. Children are infrequently affected. Among younger individuals, there is a female bias (~7:1 versus 3:1 for entire scleroderma cohorts).

PATHOGENESIS. The cause of scleroderma is unknown. An increased frequency of autoimmune disorders and autoantibodies among relatives of patients suggests the importance of genetic factors. Nonetheless, the presence of scleroderma is extremely rare in both members of twin pairs, indicating that if inheritance plays a role, it is complex, almost certainly polygenic, and perhaps influenced by environmental factors. The influence of environmental factors is supported by the association of scleroderma-like conditions with exposures to "tainted" oils (rapeseed oil) and drugs (certain preparations of L-tryptophan).

The earliest lesions are mononuclear infiltrates, primarily T lymphocytes, surrounding terminal vessels. Endothelial injury and vascular leak probably account for the edema seen in the early stages of scleroderma in some patients. Immunocyte and endothelial cell activation is subsequently associated with release of cytokines (e.g., transforming growth factor-beta, PDGF, IL-4) that is linked to an increase in fibroblast production of extracellular matrix, especially types I and III collagen and glycosaminoglycans.

More than 90 percent of patients have ANA positivity in both PSS and the more limited CREST (*c*alcinosis, *R*aynaud phenomenon, *e*sophageal dysmotility, *s*clerodactyly, *t*elangiectasia) variant. This observation demonstrates a likely role for both T-cell and B-cell dysregulation.

CLINICAL FEATURES. Raynaud phenomenon usually precedes skin "hardening" and occurs in more than 90 percent of patients, again providing testimony to the initial and critical role of vascular dysfunction. Common features among patients with either limited (CREST) or generalized scleroderma are arthralgias (>90 percent), proximal weakness (>60 percent), esophageal dysmotility (>80 percent), telangiectasias (90 percent with CREST, ~60 percent with generalized disease), and pulmonary fibrosis (35 percent with CREST, 70 percent generalized). Renal crisis[41] is 20-fold more common in generalized disease than in CREST (20 percent versus 1 percent). Calcinosis may occur in both subtypes but is twice as common in the CREST variant (40 percent versus 20 percent). Generalized scleroderma (PSS) is distinguished by proximal cutaneous fibrosis. Thus, the term "limited" is not meant to indicate the absence of risk of visceral disease; it refers only to the distribution of skin lesions. The pattern of visceral involvement differs somewhat between CREST and PSS.

Pericardial involvement is common in PSS and includes fibrinous pericarditis in up to 70 percent of patients at autopsy.[42] Echocardiography demonstrates small pericardial effusions in less than 40 percent of patients. Acute pericarditis syndromes, including significant effusions, also occur.[43] The presence of moderate or large pericardial effusions is an independent risk factor for mortality. Pericarditis with effusions may require corticosteroid therapy, but there is concern about the risk of inducing scleroderma renal crisis with the use of corticosteroids

Necropsy and endomyocardial biopsies demonstrate the presence of patchy fibrosis, occasionally with contraction band necrosis. These findings may result from intermittent, intense ischemia produced by microvascular occlusion, perhaps related to vasospasm. The epicardial coronary arteries are generally angiographically normal. However, approximately 80 percent of PSS and 65 percent of CREST patients have fixed perfusion defects on scintigraphic imaging. Myocardial infarctions have been documented in PSS patients who have angiographically normal coronary arteries. Ventricular conduction abnormalities are common and, along with a septal pseudoinfarct pattern, correlate with reduced myocardial function with exercise. Electrical abnormalities can be found throughout the conduction system, and ventricular ectopy is present in more than 60 percent of patients. Patients with scleroderma, especially those with a history of palpitations or syncope, are susceptible to sudden death. The risk of sudden death is increased in patients with coexistent skeletal myositis. Primary valvular disease is not common. Renal crisis[41] may be associated with variable degree of hypertension, rapidly rising creatinine, microangiopathy, thrombocytopenia, and left ventricular failure. Treatment is with angiotensin-converting enzyme inhibitors, not corticosteroids.

Pulmonary hypertension occurs in both limited scleroderma and PSS and is a major clinical problem. It may be due to intrinsic pulmonary artery disease or secondary to interstitial fibrosis.[44] Patients with CREST, as well as PSS, should have periodic echocardiograms to screen for asymptomatic pulmonary hypertension.

DIFFERENTIAL DIAGNOSIS. Initially, prior to skin hardening or sclerodactyly, SLE, RA, or severe primary Raynaud disease can be confused with early scleroderma. Buerger disease does not lead to thick, tight skin and is more often seen in male smokers but can cause Raynaud phenomenon and digital necrosis (see also Chap. 54). Cryoglobulinemia and its primary causes (hepatitis, malignancy, other systemic autoimmune diseases) should be excluded in patients presenting with principally vascular symptoms and ischemic lesions. Eosinophilic fasciitis, carcinoid syndrome, and several paraneoplastic syndromes can rarely cause some diagnostic confusion. In time, the emergence of typical scleroderma features enables clarification of the diagnosis.

TREATMENT. At present, there is no proven effective treatment to limit the underlying mechanisms responsible for progression of PSS. Anecdotes and uncontrolled studies have suggested that cyclophosphamide may alter pulmonary progression and improve mortality. Controlled trials have been planned for the future.

Treatment of Raynaud vasospasm is symptomatic. Gastric reflux is often severe and can be improved by avoiding food and liquid intake before reclining, not assuming a fully horizontal position (wedged pillows for beds or raising the head of the bed), and aggressive antacid regimens with proton pump inhibitors. Renal crisis usually responds to aggressive control of blood pressure; angiotensin-converting enzyme inhibitors are the initial agents of choice. A few of the complications (myositis, alveolitis, and pericarditis) may respond to corticosteroids. Conduction disease and arrhythmias are treated as they would be in the absence of PSS. Pulmonary hypertension may respond to vasodilator therapy with endothelin antagonists or prostanoids.

Polymyositis and Dermatomyositis

Myositis with resultant weakness of proximal more than distal skeletal muscles characterizes polymyositis (PM) and dermatomyositis. CK is usually elevated. Respiratory muscles can be involved in severe cases. Both can be associated with fever and interstitial lung disease. Other visceral organ involvement is uncommon in adults. Dermatomyositis involves characteristic skin lesions, which include extensor surface erythema; Gottron papules overlying knuckles, elbows, and knees; edema of the eyelids; and a photosensitive diffuse papular eruption with scaling. Dermatomyositis, in a minority of older patients, may be a paraneoplastic syndrome.

EPIDEMIOLOGY. The incidence of inflammatory myositis is about 2 to 10 new cases per million population per year. People in all races and ethnic groups may have PM or dermatomyositis. There is an overall predilection that favors females, 2.5:1. In children there is less gender bias (1:1), and when myositis coexists with other autoimmune diseases (e.g., SLE, scleroderma—"overlap syndromes") gender bias is enhanced (10:1 females). When myositis coexists with malignancy in the adult population (mean age = 60), there is no gender bias.

Inflammatory myositis can affect patients of all ages. Juvenile dermatomyositis has no association with malignancy, but it may be associated with visceral arteritis that can cause bowel ischemia.

PATHOGENESIS. The cause of these disorders is unknown. Involved muscles are infiltrated with lymphocytes, and the lymphocyte subsets and histopathological pattern of inflammation differ between the two disorders. Autoantibodies are demonstrable, and certain antibody profiles may be associated with specific clinical patterns of presentation of PM and response to therapy; but at present these autoantibodies cannot be used reliably to dictate therapeutic decisions. The increased frequency of other autoimmune diseases in relatives, as in scleroderma and lupus, suggests at least some genetic component in the pathogenesis.

CLINICAL FEATURES. Both diseases affect skeletal muscle but can also affect the heart. Pericarditis is not common but can occur when PM is part of an overlap syndrome with other autoimmune diseases such as SLE or PSS. Coronary arteritis and ischemic CAD are rarely part of these overlap syndromes. Localized or generalized myocardial dysfunction is commonly found by echocardiographic assessment but infrequently causes clinical failure. The cardiomyopathy may be steroid responsive. Corticosteroid myopathy, a complication of treatment that can mimic PM although with a normal CK, generally affects skeletal but not respiratory or cardiac muscle. PM and dermatomyositis frequently affect the conduction system. In an electrocardiographic study of 77 patients, 23 percent had conduction block,[45] which can occur in the absence of cardiomyopathy and usually in the absence of symptoms. Pulmonary hypertension can occur but is usually secondary to interstitial lung disease.

DIFFERENTIAL DIAGNOSIS. PM is recognized by either the presence of chronically elevated CK or proximal weakness. Statin therapy can cause myopathy and occasionally elevated CK and thus can mimic PM. Myalgias are more common than in PM and weakness less common. Other drugs can also induce elevations in CK, and drug-induced myopathy should always be considered before proceeding with diagnostic tests for PM (electromyography, biopsy). Hypothyroidism can mimic PM and is easily ruled out by appropriate laboratory studies. Inclusion body myositis causes an elevated CK but is usually more indolent than PM and frequently involves the distal muscles. The distinction is important because it is less responsive to therapy. Polymyalgia rheumatica is not associated with an increase in muscle enzymes and may be associated with GCA. Dermatomyositis is recognized by one of several characteristic rashes, although SLE can closely mimic dermatomyositis in some patients.

TREATMENT. There are no controlled trials to guide treatment decisions. Nonetheless, initial therapy of inflammatory myositis when an underlying malignancy is not identified includes high doses of daily oral corticosteroids. In severe disease, i.e., in the setting of proximal dysphagia or myocarditis, a pulse regimen of several grams of methylprednisolone is often prescribed. Many clinicians frequently use a second agent (methotrexate, azathioprine, cyclosporine, tacrolimus) along with corticosteroids from the outset or if the patient demonstrates a chronic requirement for high-dose corticosteroid therapy. Long-term immunosuppressive therapy is frequently required. Refractory cases may respond to the addition of high-dose intravenous immunoglobulin therapy.

Sarcoidosis

Sarcoidosis is a granulomatous inflammatory disease of unknown etiology that primarily affects the lung parenchyma but can cause significant adenopathy, arthropathy, myositis, fever, and renal, liver, skin, eye, and cardiac disease.

EPIDEMIOLOGY. Sarcoidosis can affect men and women of all ages. The peak incidence is in the second to fourth decades. Few cases are diagnosed in childhood. The prevalence varies with the degree of vigilance applied to screening and the susceptibility of populations. In Sweden the prevalence is 64 per 100,000, and that in the United States has been variably reported as 10 to 40 per 100,000. The manifestations of the disease are seemingly different in different populations. Scandinavians seem more predisposed to acute sarcoid presentations. There appears to be a preponderance of cases with cardiac involvement reported from Japan. Blacks and Hispanic Americans are more susceptible to severe multisystem disease.

PATHOGENESIS. The etiology of sarcoidosis is unknown. A multicenter U.S study of sarcoidosis found limited evidence to support an environmental or occupational exposure etiology for sarcoidosis. In contrast, studies have linked infectious agents including mycobacterial and propionibacterial organisms with sarcoidosis. Evidence of polyclonal B-cell activation in the blood and several reports of transmission of sarcoidosis to recipients of organs donated by patients with sarcoidosis also support the presence of a transmissible agent, despite the general successful use of immunosuppressive therapy. Analysis of tissue involved with sarcoidosis reveals that T helper lymphocytes drive the granulomatous inflammatory response. There is evidence for a genetic predisposition to sarcoidosis, including familial clustering and shared HLA haplotypes in different populations.

CLINICAL PRESENTATION. Pericarditis has frequently been described, and necropsy studies have documented cardiac involvement in 27 percent of patients. Clinically significant pericarditis is uncommon. The granulomatous, infiltrative disease of the myocardium is often asymptomatic but can cause arrhythmias, conduction disease, and rarely otherwise unexplained congestive heart failure. Granulomatous infiltration may be patchy, and there is a predilection toward involvement of the left ventricle, particularly the upper septal area. This distribution influences the likelihood of obtaining a diagnostic right-sided endomyocardial biopsy. Gallium imaging may be helpful in determining the need for and duration of immunosuppressive therapy, but this has not been proved in any formal trial. Sarcoid dilated cardiomyopathy may be difficult to distinguish from idiopathic cardiomyopathy or occasionally from giant cell myocarditis. Conduction disease is more common than pump dysfunction in patients with sarcoidosis.[46] Biopsy may help to distinguish sarcoidosis from idiopathic or giant cell myocarditis, but the diagnostic yield of endomyocardial biopsy is low.[47] Sarcoidosis is, at least anecdotally, somewhat steroid responsive. Pulmonary artery hypertension and cor pulmonale can occur in sarcoidosis, generally as a result of pulmonary fibrosis. Systemic vasculitis is an uncommon complication of sarcoidosis. Its prevalence remains unknown. Sarcoid vasculitis can affect small- to large-caliber vessels, including the aorta. The latter presentation can easily be confused with Takayasu arteritis (Fig. 82–8). Black patients appear predisposed to large-vessel involvement.

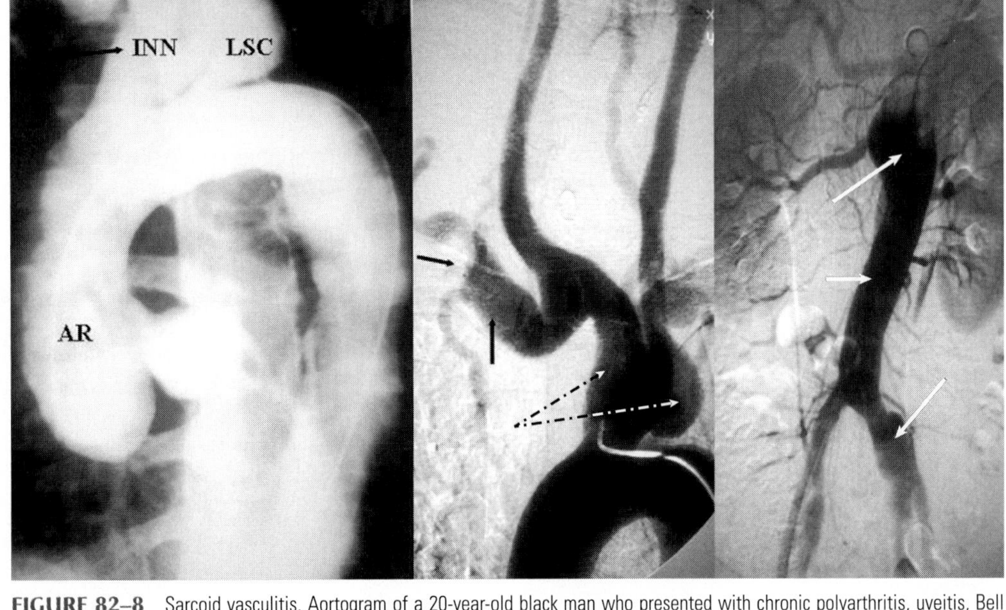

FIGURE 82–8 Sarcoid vasculitis. Aortogram of a 20-year-old black man who presented with chronic polyarthritis, uveitis, Bell palsy, and upper extremity claudication. The angiogram shows aneurysmal dilation of the innominate and proximal subclavian arteries (dotted arrows), the entire aortic root (AR, **left**), occlusion of both subclavian vessels (arrows) associated with arm claudication **(middle)**, and stenosis of the iliac vessels **(right)**. Note that sarcoid vasculitis can mimic Takayasu arteritis (TA). However, TA is associated with stenoses three to four times more often than aneurysms. Therefore, this angiographic picture should raise the differential diagnosis of TA. INN = innominate artery; LSC = left subclavian artery.

DIFFERENTIAL DIAGNOSIS. Clinically, there are many mimics of systemic sarcoidosis including chronic viral hepatitis, granulomatous hepatitis, SLE, Still disease, lymphoma, HIV infection, fungal infections, and Sjögren syndrome. When tissue specimens are available, special stains and cultures should be used to seek fungal and mycobacterial infection. Cardiac sarcoidosis is usually diagnosed by the presence of otherwise unexplained cardiomyopathy or conduction disease in the presence of documented pulmonary or hepatic sarcoidosis. Despite the inherent sampling errors, myocardial biopsy is desirable whenever reasonable.

TREATMENT. Although corticosteroid therapy may be palliative for all forms of sarcoidosis, including vasculitis, relapses of the disease are common and often preclude total withdrawal of treatment. Myocardial involvement is generally treated with long-term therapy, and frequently "steroid-sparing" therapies such as methotrexate are added. Morbidity from disease and treatment is common. There are no controlled trials of therapeutic interventions in cardiac sarcoid, and specifically there are no data to guide the duration of therapy. The serum angiotensin-converting enzyme level is an imperfect guide to therapy.

REFERENCES

Takayasu Arteritis

1. Kerr GS, Hallahan CW, Giordano J, et al: Takayasu's arteritis. Ann Intern Med 120:919, 1994.
2. Hashimoto Y, Tanaka M, Hata A, et al: Four years followup study in patients with Takayasu arteritis and severe aortic regurgitation; assessment by echocardiography. Int J Cardiol 54(S):173, 1997.
3. Seko Y, Sato O, Takagi A, et al: Restricted usage of T-cell receptor V alpha-V beta genes in infiltrating cells in aortic tissue of patients with Takayasu's arteritis. Circulation 93:1788, 1996.
4. Hoffman GS: Treatment of resistant Takayasu's arteritis. Rheum Dis Clin North Am 21:73, 1995.
5. Tso E, Flamm SD, White RD, et al: Takayasu's arteritis: Utility of magnetic resonance imaging in diagnosis and treatment. Arthritis Rheum 46:1634, 2002.
6. Hoffman GS, Leavitt RY, Kerr GS, et al: Treatment of Takayasu's with methotrexate. Arthritis Rheum 37:578, 1994.
7. Hoffman GS, Merkel PA, Tan-Ong M, et al: Anti-tumor necrosis factor therapy in patients with Takayasu's arteritis. Arthritis Rheum 2004 (in press).

Giant Cell Arteritis

8. Weyand CM, Goronzy JJ: Medium and large vessel vasculitis. N Engl J Med 349:160, 2003.
9. Rodriguez-Valverde V, Sarabia JM, Gonzalez-Gay MA, et al: Risk factors and predictive models of giant cell arteritis in polymyalgia rheumatica. Am J Med 102:331, 1997.
10. Evans J, Hunder GG: The implications of recognizing large-vessel involvement in elderly patients with giant cell arteritis. Curr Opin Rheumatol 9:37, 1997.
11. Evans JM, O'Fallon WM, Hunder GG: Increased incidence of aortic aneurysm and dissection in giant cell (temporal) arteritis. Ann Intern Med 122:502, 1995.
12. Hoffman GS, Cid MC, Hellmann DB, et al: A multicenter, randomized, double-blind, placebo-controlled trial of adjuvant methotrexate treatment for giant cell arteritis. Arthritis Rheum 46:1309, 2002.

Idiopathic Aortitis

13. Rojo-Leyva F, Ratliff N, Cosgrove DM, Hoffman GS: Study of 52 patients with idiopathic aortitis from a cohort of 1,204 surgical cases. Arthritis Rheum 43:901, 2000.

Kawasaki Disease

14. Kawasaki T: Acute febrile mucocutaneous lymph node syndrome with accompanying specific peeling of the fingers and the toes [in Japanese]. Allergy 16:178, 1967.
15. Davis RL, Waller PL, Mueller BA, et al: Kawasaki syndrome in Washington State: Race-specific incidence rates and residential proximity to water. Arch Pediatr Adolesc Med 149:66, 1995
16. Barron K: Kawasaki disease: Etiology, pathogenesis and treatment. Cleve Clin J Med 69(Suppl II):SII69, 2002.
17. Barron KS: Kawasaki disease. *In* Hoffman GS, Weyand CM (eds): Inflammatory Disease of Blood Vessels. 1st ed. New York, Marcel Dekker, 2002, pp 305-319.
18. Bell DM, Brink EW, Nitzkin JL, et al: Kawasaki's syndrome: Description of two outbreaks in the United States. N Engl J Med 304:1568, 1981.

Churg-Strauss Syndrome, Polyarteritis Nodosa

19. Guillevin L, Lhote F, Gayraud M, et al: Prognostic factors in polyarteritis nodosa and Churg-Strauss syndrome. Medicine (Baltimore) 75:17, 1996.
20. Jennette JC, Falk RJ, Andrassy K, et al: Nomenclature of systemic vasculitides: The proposal of an International Consensus Conference. Arthritis Rheum 37:187, 1994.

Rheumatoid Arthritis

21. Kitas G, Banks MJ, Bacon PB: Cardiac involvement in rheumatoid disease. Clin Med 1:18, 2001.
22. Van Doornum S, McColl G, Wicks IP: Accelerated atherosclerosis. An extraarticular feature of rheumatoid arthritis? Arthritis Rheum 46:862, 2002.
23. Levine AJ, Dimitri WR, Bonser RS: Aortic regurgitation in rheumatoid arthritis necessitating aortic valve replacement. Eur J Cardiothoracic Surg 15:213, 1999.

HLA-B27–Associated Spondyloarthropathies

24. Lautermann D, Braun J: Ankylosing spondylitis—Cardiac manifestations. Clin Exp Rheumatol 20:S11, 2002.
25. Bergfeldt L: HLA-B27-associated cardiac disease. Ann Intern Med 127:621, 1997.
26. Roldan CA, Chavez J, Wiest PW, et al: Aortic root disease associated with ankylosing spondylitis. J Am Coll Cardiol 32:1397, 1998.

Systemic Lupus Erythematosus

27. Moder KG, Miller TD, Tazelaar HD: Cardiac involvement in systemic lupus erythematosus. Mayo Clin Proc 74:275, 1999.

28. Manzi S, Meilahn EN, Rairie JE, et al: Age-specific incidence rates of myocardial infarction and angina in women with systemic lupus erythematosus: Comparison with the Framingham study. Am J Epidemiol 145:408, 1997.
29. Vaarala O, Manttari M, Manninen V, et al: Anti-cardiolipin antibodies and risk for myocardial infarction in a prospective cohort of middle-aged men. Circulation 91:23, 1995.
30. Laganà B, Schillaci O, Tubani L, et al: Lupus carditis: Evaluation with technetium-99m MIBI myocardial SPECT and heart rate variability. Angiology 50:143, 1999.
31. Finkelstein Y, Adler Y, Harel L, et al: Anti-Ro (SSA) and anti-La (SSB) antibodies and complete congenital heart block. Ann Med Interne (Paris) 148:204, 1997.
32. Roldan CA, Shively BK, Crawford MH: An echocardiographic study of valvular heart disease associated with systemic lupus erythematosus. N Engl J Med 335:1424, 1996.
33. Morin AM, Boyer A, Nataf P, Gandjbakhch I: Mitral insufficiency caused by systemic lupus erythematosus requiring valve replacement: Three case reports and a review of the literature. Thorac Cardiovasc Surg 44:313, 1996.
34. Kalangos A, Panos A, Sezerman O: Mitral valve repair in lupus valvulitis—Report of a case and review of the literature. J Heart Valve Dis 4:202, 1995.
35. Winslow TM, Ossipov MA, Fazio GP, et al: Five-year follow-up study of the prevalence and progression of pulmonary hypertension in systemic lupus erythematosus. Am Heart J 129:510, 1995.
36. Peguero A, Rabb H, Morgan M, et al: Lupus aortitis and aneurysm. Case report and review of the literature. J Clin Rheumatol 5:32, 1999.

Antiphospholipid Antibody Syndrome

37. Hojnik M, George J, Ziporen L, Shoenfeld Y: Heart valve involvement (Libman-Sacks endocarditis) in the antiphospholipid syndrome. Circulation 92:1579, 1996.
38. Khamashta MA, Buadrado MJ, Mujic F, et al: The management of thrombosis in the antiphospholipid-antibody syndrome. N Engl J Med 332:992, 1985.
39. Bartholomew J: Dosing of heparin in the presence of a lupus anticoagulant. J Clin Rheumatol 4:307, 1998.
40. Agirbasli MA, Hansen DE, Byrde BF: Resolution of vegetations with anticoagulation after myocardial infarction in primary antiphospholipid syndrome. Echocardiography 10:877, 1997.

Scleroderma

41. Steen VD: Scleroderma renal crisis. Rheum Dis Clin North Am 22:861, 1996.
42. Byers RJ, Marshall DAS, Freemont AJ: Pericardial involvement in systemic sclerosis. Ann Rheum Dis 45:393, 1997.
43. Deswal A, Follansbee WP: Cardiac involvement in scleroderma. Rheum Dis Clin North Am 22:841, 1996.
44. Koh ET, Lee P, Gladman DD, Abu-Shakra M: Pulmonary hypertension in systemic sclerosis: An analysis of 17 patients. Br J Rheumatol 35:989, 1996.

Polymyositis and Dermatomyositis

45. Stern R, Godblold J, Chess Q, Kagen L: ECG abnormalities in polymyositis. Arch Intern Med 144:2185, 1984.

Sarcoidosis

46. Yazaki Y, Isobe M, Hiramitsu S, et al: Comparison of clinical features and prognosis of cardiac sarcoidosis and idiopathic dilated cardiomyopathy. Am J Cardiol 82:537, 1998.
47. Uemura A, Morimoto SI, Hiramissu S, et al: Histologic diagnostic rate of cardiac sarcoidosis: Evaluation of endomyocardial biopsies. Am Heart J 138:299, 1999.

CHAPTER 83

The Patient with Cardiovascular Disease and Cancer

Karen Antman • Andrew R. Marks

Cardiovascular disease and cancer are both common; therefore, many patients with cardiovascular disease also have cancer. Because of overlapping risk factors such as obesity, hormone replacement therapy, and, particularly, smoking, heart disease patients are likely to have a higher risk of cancer than the general population.[1,2] Certainly cardiac transplant patients are at significant risk for squamous skin cancers[3–6] and Kaposi sarcoma.[7] Exercise, healthy body weight, and moderate wine intake may decrease the risk of both coronary heart disease and cancer.[8,9]

Cardiac complications of cancer such as pericardial tamponade or superior vena cava syndrome are frequent first manifestations of advanced neoplasia. Cancer treatments frequently compromise cardiac function. Radiation ports that include the heart for the treatment of lymphoma or lung or breast cancers can, rarely, produce late coronary artery disease or constrictive pericarditis. Oncolytic drugs, most frequently anthracyclines, paclitaxel, and trastuzumab, but also cyclophosphamide, 5-fluorouracil, and others, result in cardiotoxicity.

Although cardiac resuscitation is often attempted in patients with end-stage cancer, the chance of meaningful survival and even discharge in this setting is low. In one series, 22 percent of cancer patients with a sudden unanticipated cardiac arrest survived to be discharged from the hospital, but 0 of 171 patients with cardiac arrest from end-stage cancer survived.[10] Expert care of patients with both cancer and heart disease requires a basic knowledge of oncology.

Direct Complications of Neoplasia

Primary cardiac malignancies are rare[11-13] (see Chap. 63). Metastases to various cardiac structures are common. Tumor involvement can occur via hematogenous spread leading to multiple nodules involving all cardiac structures, possibly obstructing outflow tracts[14]; via direct invasions from primary lung or mediastinal tumors or metastases to mediastinal lymph nodes; or by direct intravascular spread up the inferior vena cava, most commonly from renal or uterine primary tumors.[15,16] Pericardial metastases occur in one third or more of dying patients, and metastases to the myocardium develop in about 10 percent, particularly in lung cancer patients with mediastinal lymph node involvement.

Cardiac Tamponade and Constrictive Pericarditis

A pericardial effusion with cardiac compression becomes a life-threatening medical emergency when it causes cardiac tamponade.[17–19] A thickened, fibrotic pericardium restricts diastolic filling and the diastolic volume of the heart in cases of constrictive pericarditis. Patients with large pericardial effusions from metastases may report dull chest pain, edema, fever, dyspnea, or cough. Distant heart sounds, pulsus paradoxus, jugular vein distention, and a narrow pulse pressure are characteristic on examination (see Chap. 64). The electrocardiogram (ECG) classically shows low voltage and perhaps electrical alternans. The chest radiograph often shows an enlarged cardiac silhouette. Echocardiography confirms the presence of a large pericardial effusion. Right atrial and ventricular collapse indicates tamponade.

The development of increased intrapericardial pressure depends on the rate of fluid accumulation and the volume of the effusate. Pericardiocentesis can be life saving, but pericardiectomy may be required to prevent rapid reaccumulation of fluid. Fluid should be sent for cytology even in the absence of a history of cancer.

ETIOLOGY. Cardiac tamponade can occur due to pericardial fluid accumulation that may be associated with pericarditis. Pericarditis can result from neoplasms, including metastases.[18,19] The differential diagnosis should include viral pericarditis, uremia, Dressler syndrome after myocardial infarction, iatrogenic cardiac perforation, bacterial infection, radiation therapy, aortic dissection, and others. The pericardium is frequently involved in metastatic lung cancer, breast cancer, leukemia, Hodgkin disease, and non-Hodgkin lymphoma, which account for the majority of cases of malignant pericarditis. Acute pericarditis can occur during radiation treatment of a mediastinal tumor adjacent to the pericardium due to inflammatory necrosis and usually does not cause chronic inflammation. Chronic constrictive pericarditis is becoming increasingly important in patients with breast cancer or lymphoma because of prolonged survival. Chemotherapeutic agents, including doxorubicin (Adriamycin), daunorubicin, cyclophosphamide, and others, may cause an acute form of pericarditis.

DIAGNOSIS. Patients with cancer can present with cardiac tamponade or constrictive pericarditis that is secondary either to a neoplastic process or to the therapy for a cancer. The diagnosis of malignant pericarditis depends on the documentation of pericardial inflammation and the clinical association with a neoplasm. Patients with pericarditis and neoplasm may have symptoms from radiation therapy. Many patients with advanced neoplastic disease are prone to infections that can cause pericarditis, and additional instrumentation with intravascular ports for chemotherapy substantially increases the risk of infections. Constrictive pericarditis should be suspected in patients with increased central venous pressure or unexplained pleural effusion, ascites, shortness of breath, and edema.

An important finding on physical examination is the Kussmaul sign, which is a paradoxical rise in the jugular venous pulse on inspiration. This finding is caused by increased pericardial fluid or a noncompliant pericardium. Normally, during inspiration, there is an increase in the "a" wave of the jugular venous pulse and a decrease in the mean jugular venous pressure as a result of the increased filling of the right-sided chambers associated with the decrease in intrathoracic pressure. The differential diagnosis for the Kussmaul sign includes cardiac tamponade, constrictive pericarditis, restrictive cardiomyopathy, severe right-sided heart failure, and right ventricular infarction.

TREATMENT. Cytological examination of pericardial fluid is diagnostic for malignant pericarditis in about 85 percent of cases.[19] Pericardial biopsy provides a histological diagnosis in up to 90 percent of cases. Removal of pericardial fluid can be therapeutic as well as diagnostic.[20] However, pericardial fluid often reaccumulates and may require insertion of a draining catheter, removal of the pericardium (pericardiectomy), or sclerosis with agents that induce scar formation, including tetracycline instilled into the pericardial space. Control often requires systemic treatment of the underlying malignancy with chemotherapy, although intrapericardial chemotherapy can be effective.[18] Radiotherapy can be helpful in patients with lymphoma or breast cancer but is limited in patients with less radiosensitive diseases by the radiation tolerance of normal cardiac structures.

Superior Vena Cava Obstruction

Superior vena cava syndrome (SVCS) occurs when obstruction of the thin-walled superior vena cava (SVC) interrupts venous return of blood from the head, upper extremities, and thorax to the right atrium. The SVC is encircled by lymph nodes that drain from the right thoracic cavity and the lower left thorax (Fig. 83–1). SVCS often manifests with slowly progressive symptoms worsening over weeks and recruitment of collateral circulation via the azygos, internal mammary, paraspinous, subcutaneous, or lateral thoracic veins and the esophageal venous complex. When symptoms occur abruptly, SVCS can constitute a medical emergency.[21]

SYMPTOMS. Obstruction of the SVC is a distressing manifestation of malignant or benign disease. Clinically, patients report the progressive development of shortness of breath (60 percent), facial swelling (50 percent), cough (24 percent), arm swelling (18 percent), chest pain (15 percent), and dysphagia (9 percent) as well as distorted vision, hoarseness, nausea, headache, and loss of consciousness. Physical findings include venous distention over the neck (66 percent) and chest wall (54 percent) (Fig. 83–2), facial edema (46 percent), plethora (19 percent), and cyanosis (19 percent) as well as dyspnea, orthopnea, stridor, and syncope. Symptoms may be exacerbated by lying in a supine position or bending forward. Patients with this syndrome can be uncomfortable or may develop life-threatening complications such as laryngeal or cerebral edema.

ETIOLOGY. Seventy-five to 85 percent of cases of SVCS result from neoplasia (Table 83–1), with lung cancer accounting for the majority of cases.[22,23] Of patients with lung cancer, 2 to 5 percent develop SVCS. However, 10 to 20 percent of patients with small cell lung cancer (SCLC), which constitutes only 20 percent of lung cancers, develop SVCS, accounting for almost 40 percent of patients with SVCS and lung cancer. Of patients with lung cancer–associated SVCS, 80 percent have right-sided primary lesions.

Lymphoma is the second most common cause of neoplasia associated with SVCS, comprising 2 to 21 percent of SVCS patients. Diffuse large cell lymphoma is the most common form (64 percent), followed by lymphoblastic lymphoma (33 percent). Similar to patients with lung

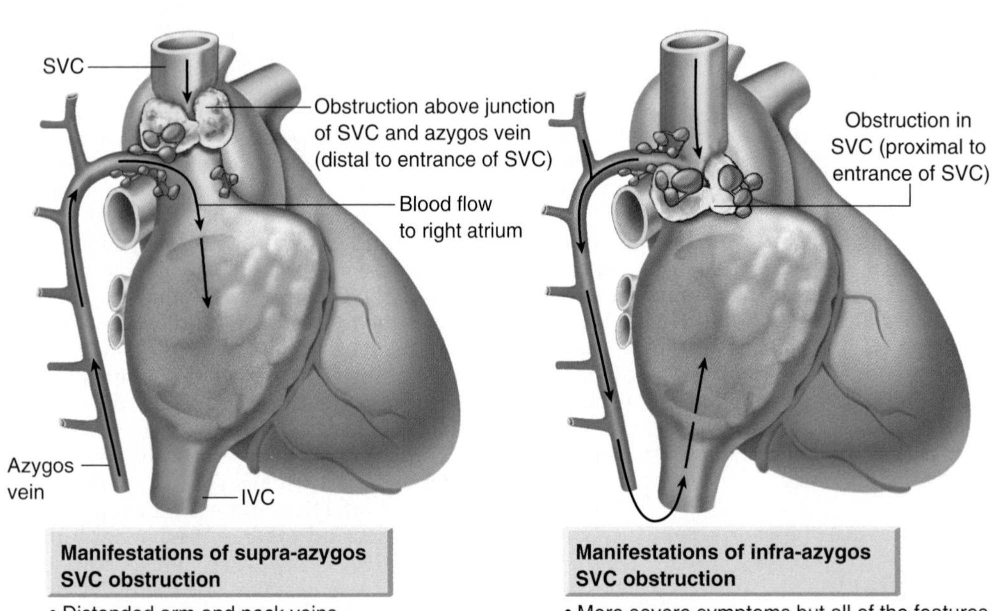

FIGURE 83–1 Anatomy of superior vena cava (SVC) syndrome. Lymph nodes may obstruct blood return above the entrance of the azygos vein **(A)**, resulting in edema of the face, neck, and arms and distended veins in the neck and arms and over the upper chest. Obstruction below the return of the azygos vein **(B)** results in retrograde flow through the azygos via collateral veins to the inferior vena cava (IVC), resulting in all the symptoms and signs in **A** plus dilation of the veins over the abdomen as well. (Modified from Skarin AT [ed]: Atlas of Diagnostic Oncology, 3rd ed. Philadelphia, Elsevier Science, 2003.)

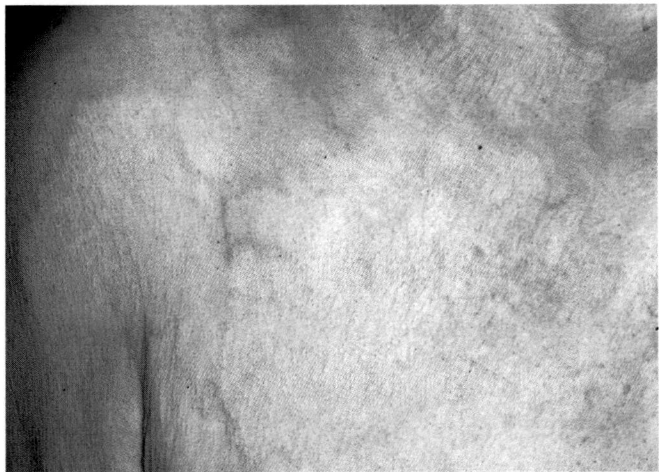

FIGURE 83–2 Distended veins in the skin over the chest wall of a patient with superior vena cava syndrome. (From Skarin AT [ed]: Atlas of Diagnostic Oncology, 3rd ed. Philadelphia, Elsevier Science, 2003.)

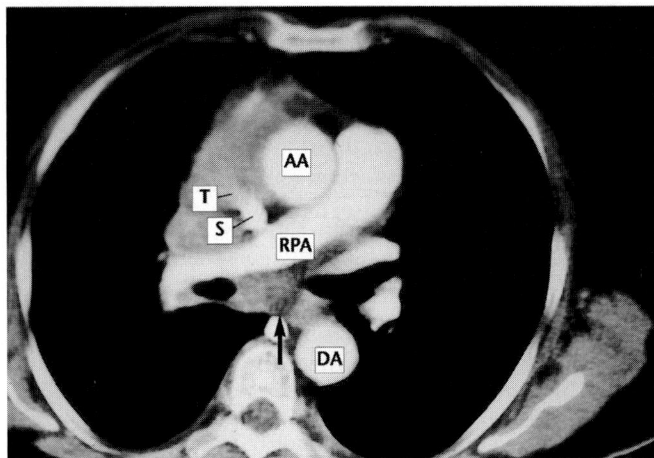

FIGURE 83–3 Superior vena cava syndrome in a case of diffuse large cell lymphoma. Computed tomography image with intravenous contrast at the level of the right pulmonary artery (RPA) showing tumor (T) infiltrating into the area of the superior vena cava (S), which is narrowed. Tumor is also present in the subcarinal space (arrow). AA = ascending aorta; DA = descending aorta. (From Skarin AT [ed]: Atlas of Diagnostic Oncology, 3rd ed. Philadelphia, Elsevier Science, 2003.)

TABLE 83–1 Malignancies Associated with Superior Vena Cava (SVC) Syndrome in Adults*

Neoplastic Diagnosis	Percentage of SVC	Percentage of Disease-Associated SVC
Lung cancer, stage 3B or 4:	48-81	
Small cell lung cancer		15-45
Squamous cell cancer		20-25
Adenocarcinoma		5-25
Large cell carcinoma		4-30
Lymphoma:	2-21	
Diffuse large cell lymphoma		64
Lymphoblastic lymphoma		33
Breast cancer	11	

*Include lung cancer, lymphomas, and metastases from other solid tumors. Seventy-five percent to 85% of patients with SVC have neoplastic disease.

cancer, only 1 to 5 percent of patients with lymphoma develop SVCS (21 percent of lymphoblastic lymphomas and 7 percent of diffuse large cell lymphomas). Of patients with primary mediastinal B-cell lymphoma with sclerosis, 57 percent developed SVCS. Although Hodgkin lymphoma often involves the mediastinum, SVCS rarely develops. Thymoma and germ cell tumors are other primary mediastinal malignancies that occasionally cause SVCS. The most common metastatic disease that causes SVCS is breast cancer, accounting for 11 percent of SVCS cases.

DIFFERENTIAL DIAGNOSIS. Benign causes of SVC obstruction not associated with neoplasia result from mediastinal fibrosis caused by radiotherapy or histoplasmosis, tuberculosis, collagen-vascular disease, arteriovenous shunts, or SVC thrombosis as a complication of central venous catheters, pacemaker leads, peritoneovenous shunts, Swan-Ganz catheters, or hyperalimentation catheters. Pacemakers and implantable cardioverter defibrillators result in up to 30 percent of local venous thrombosis, in some cases associated with infection; however, SVC obstruction is uncommon and relates to acute or previous lead infection or retention of a severed lead.[24]

In children with SVCS, up to 70 percent of cases are iatrogenic, developing after correction surgery for congenital heart disease, ventriculoatrial shunt to decompress hydrocephalus, and SVC catheterization for parenteral nutrition. Other benign causes include granulomas, congenital anomalies, and mediastinal fibrosis secondary to histoplasmosis. Neoplasia-associated SVCS in children results from lymphomas, acute lymphoblastic leukemia, rhabdomyosarcoma, neuroblastoma, and other solid tumors.[21]

DIAGNOSTIC PROCEDURES. In a patient with characteristic symptoms of SVC obstruction, physical evaluation is usually informative and raises a high level of suspicion. In patients with SVCS due to neoplasia, 60 percent lack a prior history of cancer. A mass is generally present on chest radiograph, with superior mediastinal widening and often pleural effusions. Computed tomography (CT) provides critical additional information (Fig. 83–3).

Imaging. Although the clinical picture usually makes diagnosis straightforward, patients with SVC obstruction frequently require imaging evaluation for assessment and therapy planning. Chest radiography in two planes reveals abnormal mediastinal widening suspicious of lymphoma or other mediastinal masses. Lesions in the lung fields or pleural effusions strongly suggest lung malignancy. Sonographic analysis is used to assess the extrathoracic systemic veins for thrombosis, and Doppler analysis may reveal the lack of transmitted right heart pulsations or dampened pulsations, which raises the suspicion of intrathoracic venous obstruction.

Most patients with suspected SVCS undergo contrast-enhanced CT when the modality is available. CT can document the presence of obstruction and establish the level, extent, and therapeutic options by mapping collateral and patent vasculature to aid interventional access and documenting any pulmonary emboli. Increased imaging of patients with neoplasm has identified many asymptomatic patients with "impending" SVC obstruction. The CT scan can illustrate the strategic relationship of growing tumor masses or the development of nonocclusive, early intraluminal thrombus. Magnetic resonance imaging can also perform this role effectively. If neoplasm was diagnosed previously, earlier radiation therapy may prevent SVCS. If CT is not an option, a venogram of the arms can provide additional information for therapeutic decisions.

The causes of SVCS include intraluminal, mural, and extraluminal obstruction. Intraluminal causes include bland and neoplastic thrombus as well as direct tumor extension. Bland thrombus is usually associated with intravenous lines or infected pacemaker leads, although it is an uncommon cause of complete occlusion. A paraneoplastic bland thrombus can also occur, and tumor vascularization can be used to differentiate a bland from a neoplastic thrombus. Mural causes include benign stenoses related to renal dialysis and strictures resulting from radiation therapy. Extraluminal causes are usually direct compression by bronchogenic tumors or malignant lymphadenopathy and represent the most common causes detected by imaging.

Oncological Intervention. Because the underlying cause will guide any therapeutic recommendations, obtaining tissue samples is essential to establishing the cause of SVCS. Sputum cytology can establish the diagnosis in almost half of patients. Biopsy of enlarged lymph nodes, when present, is frequently a relatively noninvasive method to obtain reliable tissue diagnosis. Thoracentesis can establish the diagnosis of malignancy in 70 percent of patients with pleural effusions. A diagnosis is made in most of the remaining cases with bronchoscopy, including brushing, washing, and biopsy samples. A marrow biopsy may be diagnostic of lymphoma or SCLC. If the diagnosis remains obscure, percutaneous transthoracic CT-guided fine-needle biopsy is a safe and effective method of diagnosis. When other methods have been unsuccessful, mediastinoscopy has a high diagnostic yield but at a somewhat higher risk of complications (5 percent).

MANAGEMENT. During medical evaluation and before institution of specific therapy, oxygen is administered to reduce the cardiac output and venous pressure, and head elevation, diuretics, and a low-salt diet are used to reduce edema. Dehydration increases the risk of further thrombosis, however. In patients with SVCS caused by malignant tumors, radiotherapy and chemotherapy are the most common first-line treatment options. Steroids can decrease inflammation or tumor-associated obstruction, but may obscure the diagnosis of lymphoma. Anticoagulation has not been proved to provide benefit in patients with neoplasia-associated SVCS and may interfere with diagnostic biopsies and interventions. Percutaneous transluminal angioplasty or stent insertion may relieve symptoms without obscuring the diagnosis.

Vascular Interventions. Endovascular stenting or angioplasty and thrombolysis can provide prompt relief of symptoms, particularly for patients with palliative treatment.[25] Balloon venoplasty and stenting, which may be augmented by catheter-applied thrombolysis, are prompt treatment options to decrease morbidity or to prevent impending SVC obstruction. Despite the historical concern that invasive diagnostic procedures in the setting of increased intrathoracic venous pressure would result in severe bleeding and complications of anesthesia, complication rates in experienced centers have proved acceptably low. Ideally, there is a remaining lumen for passage of a guidewire. Balloon angioplasty is undertaken and one or more stents are placed. The results of stent insertion are excellent, with a high percentage of technical success and rapid relief of symptoms. Adjuvant radiation therapy can be given. In the case of a preexisting paraneoplastic thrombus, the risk of stent thrombosis remains.

Surgical treatment involves the insertion of a bypass graft between the left innominate or jugular vein and the right atrial appendage, using an autologous or Dacron graft. However, this operation is very invasive and difficult. Therefore, it should be avoided if possible and, if necessary, performed only in patients with a relatively long life expectancy. In the chronic situation devoid of vascular interventions, patients may develop a network of chest wall and azygos/hemiazygos collateral vessels that effectively restore venous return to the right heart.[26]

Oncological Treatment of SVCS. The goal is to determine as rapidly as possible the histological type of the primary lesion and to institute curative therapy for lymphomas, germ cell tumors, and even SCLC and to provide palliation for advanced non-small-cell lung cancers and other metastatic solid tumors (Table 83–2). The prognosis of patients who present with SVCS depends greatly on the prognosis of the underlying neoplasm. Combination chemotherapy with or without radiation therapy relieves SVCS symptoms within 1 to 2 weeks in cases of newly diagnosed SCLC and lymphoma.

TABLE 83–2 Yields of Various Procedures for Diagnosis in Patients with Superior Vena Cava Syndrome

Procedure	% Diagnostic
Thoracotomy	98
Mediastinoscopy	90
Thoracentesis	71
Lymph node biopsy	67
Bronchoscopy	52
Sputum cytology	49

Treatment of SCLC with both chemotherapy and radiation significantly decreases the risk of SVCS recurrence over chemotherapy alone but may not improve survival. In some series of patients with SCLC, presentation with SVCS indicated a more favorable prognosis. SVCS secondary to lymphoma is rarely an emergency that requires treatment before histological diagnosis and complete staging. Chemotherapy provides both local and systemic therapy. Consolidation with radiation therapy may be appropriate for patients with large mediastinal masses (>10 cm). Dysphagia, hoarseness, and stridor are poor prognostic signs. Non-small-cell lung cancers and breast or other cancers metastatic to SVC lymph nodes are generally managed with radiation therapy or percutaneous transluminal angioplasty or stent insertion, or both.

Valvular Heart Disease in the Cancer Patient

Cardiac valves can be involved directly by primary or metastatic tumor, by bacterial or candidal infections, with nonbacterial thrombotic endocarditis, by trauma from semipermanent catheters inserted to facilitate treatment, and as a late effect of radiation therapy (see section on radiation complications).

Nonbacterial thrombotic endocarditis complicates the course of various malignancies, most commonly adenocarcinomas from the gastrointestinal tract and lung.[27] Morbidity and mortality mainly result from systemic embolism. Two hundred nonselected ambulatory patients with solid tumors evaluated for evidence of thromboembolic events and for plasma D-dimer levels were compared with a control group of 100 consecutive patients without overt heart disease referred to echocardiography for the detection of an occult arterial embolic source. Of 38 cancer patients with cardiac valvular vegetations from the group of 200, the valves affected were mitral (n = 19), aortic (n = 18), and tricuspid (n = 1). Primary lesions were lymphoma (n = 10), lung (n = 9), and pancreatic (n = 3). Thromboembolism to extremities was diagnosed in 4 patients, cerebrovascular accidents were diagnosed in 2, and 4 patients had silent segmental left ventricular wall motion abnormalities on echocardiography. Nine of 38 patients (24 percent) with vegetations developed thromboembolism, as compared with 13 of 162 patients without vegetations (8 percent; $p = 0.013$). D-Dimer levels were increased in 19 of 21 patients (90 percent) with thromboembolism and in 76 of 149 patients without thromboembolism

(51 percent; $p = 0.001$).[27] Treatment of cancer-associated nonbacterial thrombotic endocarditis remains difficult.

Ischemic Heart Disease and Malignancy

Cancer patients are at a higher risk for coronary artery disease due to prior radiation to the heart (see later), extrinsic compression by tumor of a coronary artery, or even tumor emboli within a coronary artery. Hypercoagulable states particularly associated with mucin-secreting adenocarcinomas also increase the risk of a coronary thrombosis.

Arrhythmias

Arrhythmias in cancer patients result from cardiomyopathies due to drugs or radiation (see later), electrolyte imbalance (particularly potassium wasting) from renal complications of antineoplastic and antibiotic drugs, and hypoxia from underlying chronic obstructive pulmonary disease,[28] pulmonary or pleural involvement with tumor, or infection with large pleural or pericardial effusions.[28] Rhythm disturbances, sinus tachycardia, ST segment and T wave changes, atrial fibrillation or flutter, and complete heart block can result. Cervical lymph node involvement can rarely lead to carotid sinus syncope.

Indirect Cardiovascular Complications of Cancer

Hyperviscosity

ERYTHROCYTOSIS. Elevated red blood cell mass can occur from a variety of stimuli. Polycythemia vera is a clonal chronic myeloproliferative disorder characterized by an increase in red blood cell mass with or without elevated leukocytes and platelets. Hyperviscosity is in part related to decreased red blood cell membrane fluidity and deformability.[29] An increased sensitivity of hematopoietic progenitor cells to regulatory factors such as erythropoietin; dysregulation of the *SHP1* gene, which encodes an intracellular phosphatase involved in cell signaling pathways; and mutations in the erythropoietin receptor gene are possible mechanisms for the development of polycythemia vera.

Patients with polycythemia vera have a 30 percent risk of thrombosis (extremity deep venous thrombosis, hepatic vein thrombosis [Budd-Chiari syndrome], pulmonary embolism, or coronary occlusions). Cerebrovascular occlusion and basilar artery insufficiency develop. Mitral valve thickening or nonbacterial vegetations also occur. Reduced cerebral blood flow caused by the erythrocytosis is associated with confusion and abnormal mental status, visual disturbances, dizziness, and headache.

Phlebotomy should maintain the hematocrit in the 40 to 45 percent range. Hydroxyurea is often used if phlebotomy alone is insufficient. Phlebotomy alone increases the risk of thrombosis, but hydroxyurea can, rarely, result in leukemia.

THROMBOCYTOSIS. Reactive thrombocytoses, which appropriately develop after surgery or in pregnancy, are not associated with an increased risk of thrombosis. However, essential thrombocytosis, a myeloproliferative disorder, increases the risk of both hemorrhage and thrombosis. Hydroxyurea, used to lower the platelet count, also reduces the risk of myocardial infarction.

LEUKOCYTOSIS. Although very high white blood cell counts associated with acute and chronic lymphoid leukemia generally do not cause significant hyperviscosity, leukemic white blood cell counts greater than 100,000/μl in patients with acute myeloid leukemia can cause leukostasis producing thrombosis and hemorrhages in microcapillaries of the brain (encephalopathy) and lung (pulmonary infiltrates and hypoxia). Hydroxyurea, definitive antileukemic chemotherapy, central nervous system radiation, and leukophoresis are used to limit complications. Patients with chronic myeloid leukemia often tolerate high white blood cell counts without leukostatic/thrombotic complications.

PLASMA PROTEINS. Multiple myeloma and Waldenström macroglobulinemia are clonal proliferations of plasma cells that elaborate a single immunoglobulin, the M-component. The immunoglobins produced are IgG and IgM, respectively. Congestive heart failure can result from anemia and expanded plasma volume as well as increased viscosity from circulating immunoglobulins. Hyperviscosity is more likely at any given IgM level compared to a similar IgG level. Most patients with Waldenström disease have elevated serum viscosity, but symptoms such as headache, dizziness, blurry vision, diplopia, and ataxia are uncommon (15 to 20 percent). Retinal examination can reveal distention of vessels with constrictions, especially of veins (a "sausage links" or "box car" effect) (Fig. 83–4). Symptoms can progress to confusion, stroke, or coma. Hyperviscosity syndrome, confirmed by measurements of serum viscosity, requires immediate reduc-

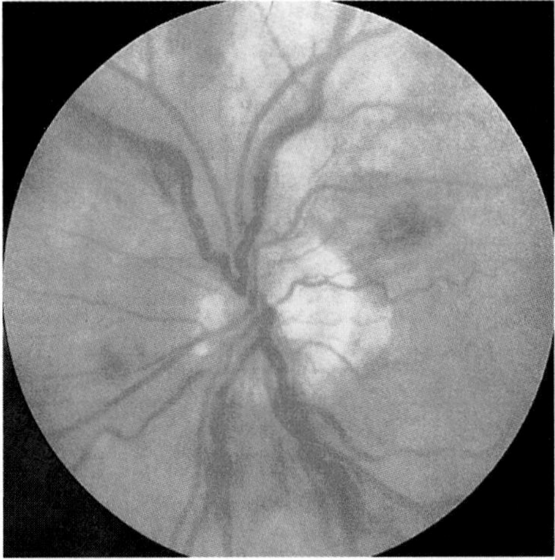

A

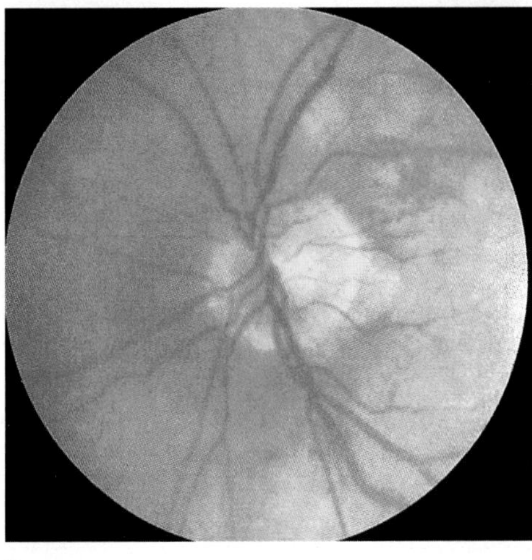

B

FIGURE 83–4 Waldenström macroglobulinemia (hyperviscosity syndrome). **A,** The retina of a patient who presented with blurred vision, headache, and dizziness exhibits gross distention of vessels, particularly the veins, which show bulging and constriction (the "linked sausage" effect), as well as areas of hemorrhage. **B,** After plasmapheresis, the vascular diameters are normal and the hemorrhagic areas have cleared. (From Skarin AT [ed]: Atlas of Diagnostic Oncology, 3rd ed. Philadelphia, Elsevier Science, 2003.)

tion in the M-component, generally with plasmapheresis and chemotherapy.

Cryoglobulins, immunoglobulins that aggregate at temperatures below 37°C, are associated with a variety of inflammatory conditions as well as with lymphoma and infections, particularly hepatitis C.[30] Severe hypertension from peripheral vasculitis can lead to renal failure, stroke, and cardiovascular events.

Cardiac Complications of Chemotherapy

Oncolytic drugs, most frequently anthracyclines, paclitaxel, and trastuzumab, but also cyclophosphamide, 5-fluorouracil, and others, result in cardiotoxicity.[31–34] Some hormone therapies are associated with increased risks of myocardial infarction and cardiomyopathies (Table 83–3).

Anthracycline Cardiotoxicity

ACUTE MANIFESTATIONS. Acute anthracycline toxicity includes arrhythmias, myocardial dysfunction, and pericardial effusions.

CHRONIC OR LATE CARDIOTOXICITY. Late cardiomyopathy was reported soon after anthracyclines were introduced—with congestive heart failure in up to 30 percent in patients who had received more than 500 mg/m^2 of doxorubicin (Adriamycin).[35] In randomized trials, congestive heart failure (CHF) developed significantly more often in the anthracycline arms of the studies, thus establishing cardiomyopathy due to anthracyclines. Endomyocardial biopsy studies documented a correlation between cumulative anthracycline dose and myocardial pathological condition.[36] Based on these studies, cumulative anthracycline doses are now generally kept lower than 450 mg/m^2, resulting in a risk of clinical symptoms of about 3 percent of cases. The risk is up to 26 percent for cumulative doses of 550 mg/m^2.[37] Measurably decreased function is found in asymptomatic patients (Fig. 83–5).

Although anthracycline-associated cardiomyopathy can develop as late as decades after the last anthracycline therapy, it classically produces congestive heart failure within a median of 3 months after the last anthracycline dose. Tachycardia and fatigue are followed by shortness of breath, pulmonary edema, and cardiac dilation. Associated arrhythmias include ventricular tachycardia or fibrillation, heart block, and occasional sudden death. Autopsy reveals fibrosis and hypertrophy of remaining myocytes. Cardiac function in patients who progress to this state but survive generally improves over a period of years.

In a retrospective study at M.D. Anderson Cancer Center, 682 consecutive women with metastatic breast cancer received doxorubicin by bolus infusion. Doxorubicin-associated CHF developed in 33 of 538 patients aged 50 to 64 years and in 13 of 144 aged 65 years and older after cumulative doses of 410 mg/m^2 (range, 150-550 mg/m^2) and 400 mg/m^2 (range, 100-570 mg/m^2), respectively, a median of 5 (range, <1-65 months) and 9 months (range, <1-28 months) after the last dose of doxorubicin. No risk factors could be identified. Thus, in this study, patients older than 65 years had no added risk of developing congestive heart failure.[38]

TABLE 83–3 Cardiotoxicity of Antineoplastic Agents

Implicated Agent	Comments
Anthracyclines	
Doxorubicin or daunorubicin	CHF at cumulative doses above 450 mg/m^2, arrhythmias
Mitoxantrone, idarubicin	CHF, decreases in left ventricular ejection fraction
Alkylating agents	
Cyclophosphamide	Produces a hemorrhagic myopericarditis 1-2 weeks after marrow transplant doses
Busulfan	Endocardial fibrosis
Cisplatin	Acute myocardial ischemia
Other cytotoxics	
Paclitaxel (Taxol)	Exacerbates anthracycline-associated CHF, bradycardia
5-Fluorouracil	Angina/myocardial infarction
Vincristine, vinblastine, vinorelbine (Navelbine)	Myocardial infarction
Biologics	
Trastuzumab (Herceptin)	Exacerbates anthracycline-associated CHF
Interferons	Exacerbates underlying cardiac disease
Interleukin-2	Acute myocardial injury, ventricular arrhythmias, hypotension
Hormones	
Megestrol (progestin)	Cardiomyopathy
Estramustine (androgen antagonist [Emcyt])	Myocardial infarction, CHF
Goserelin (gonadotropin-releasing hormone analog [Zoladex])	Myocardial infarction, CHF
Diethylstilbestrol (estrogen)	Myocardial infarction
Toremifene (antiestrogen [Fareston])	Myocardial infarction
Bicalutamide (antiandrogen [Casodex])	Angina, CHF, myocardial infarction
All-*trans*-retinoic acid	Myocardial dysfunction, heart failure, fever, shortness of breath, pleural and pericardial effusions, pulmonary infiltrates, and peripheral edema
Hematopoietic growth factors	
Granulocyte macrophage colony-stimulating factor (sargramostim [Leukine])	Capillary leak syndrome
Antiemetic	
Granisetron	Sinus bradycardia, atrioventricular block and increased PR interval or a Wenckebach block (Mobitz I).

CHF = congestive heart failure.

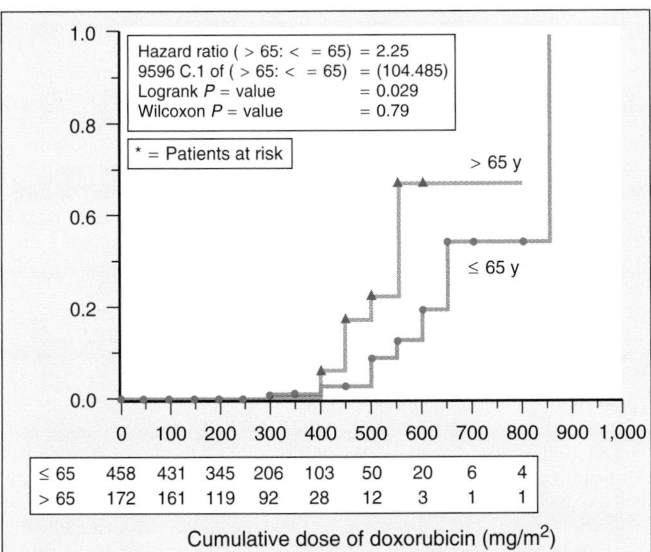

FIGURE 83–5 Risk of doxorubicin-associated congestive heart failure by patient age: Cumulative doxorubicin dose at onset of doxorubicin-associated congestive heart failure in 630 patients according to patient age older or younger than 65 years (y). (Redrawn from Swain SM, Whaley FS, Ewer MS: Congestive heart failure in patients treated with doxorubicin: A retrospective analysis of three trials. Cancer 97:2869, 2003.)

Children are at increased risk.[39,40] In a Roswell Park Cancer Institute study of 15-year survivors of childhood or adolescent cancer, cardiac mortality exceeded that expected, particularly for men after doxorubicin treatment. Risk was not ameliorated by treatment era (1960-1970 or 1971-1984).[41]

A Finnish group studied serum *N*-terminal atrial natriuretic peptide (NT-ANP) in 43 children during and in 48 children after chemotherapy for cancer. Cumulative anthracycline doses ranged between 0 and 600 mg/m^2 (median 225 mg/m^2). Cardiac evaluation included an ECG and echocardiographic assessment of systolic and diastolic left ventricular function. During chemotherapy, serum NT-ANP levels rose compared to controls but varied markedly in the same individuals. Serum NT-ANP levels were highest in patients after bone marrow transplantation or cardiac irradiation.[42]

In a Japanese study of 34 children (18 boys and 16 girls) who had received doxorubicin, plasma ANP and brain natriuretic peptide (BNP) were assayed at the first echocardiogram for cardiac function; 8 (23.5 percent) had left ventricular dysfunction. Both ANP and BNP were significantly elevated in comparison with healthy controls ($p < 0.01$) or patients with normal cardiac function ($p < 0.05$) and correlated significantly with systolic but not diastolic function. Plasma ANP and BNP levels may provide early markers for doxorubicin-induced cardiotoxicity in children.[43]

MECHANISMS. Despite many hypotheses, no mechanism underlying doxorubicin cardiotoxicity has proved definitive. Doxorubicin binds to cardiolipin in the inner mitochondrial membrane and interrupts synthesis of adenosine triphosphate (ATP). The doxorubicin-cardiolipin complex promotes transfer of electrons through doxorubicin-producing reactive oxygen species. Resulting peroxides lead to mitochondrial membrane damage. Glutathione peroxidase is depleted, which is particularly important in myocytes that lack catalase. The iron-doxorubicin complex disrupts the sarcoplasmic reticulum. Doxorubicinol also disturbs calcium transport.

PREVENTION. Limiting the cumulative dose of doxorubicin to less than 450 mg/m^2 provides the first line of defense against cardiotoxicity.[37] Anthracycline toxicity is also associated with peak dose per course. For tumors that require high doses of doxorubicin per course, the dose can be divided over several days or given by continuous infusion. Smaller weekly doses also provide an effective antitumor dose density but with lower peak doses. Liposome-encapsulated anthracycline decreases the risk of cardiac toxicity in clinical trials. Dexrazoxane (Zinecard or Cardioxane), an iron chelator, has been protective in randomized trials.[44,45] Other anthracycline analogs may have lower rates of cardiotoxicity for given level of efficacy, but this has been difficult to prove.

Patients are generally monitored for falling left ventricular ejection fractions with noninvasive techniques.[46] Troponin and natriuretic peptide levels as well as single-photon emission computed tomography scans have been monitored as well but are not established.[43,47,48]

MANAGEMENT. Management includes afterload reduction and angiotensin II converting enzyme inhibitors; selective beta-receptor blockers such as metoprolol may also be useful in patients with congestive heart failure. Malignant arrhythmias may also require treatment.

Trastuzumab (Herceptin) Cardiotoxicity

Amplification of the gene encoding the ErbB2 (Her2/neu) receptor tyrosine kinase, a coreceptor for neuroregulin signaling, promotes the progression of several forms of breast cancer.[49] Trastuzumab (Herceptin) is a humanized monoclonal antibody specific for the extracellular domain of ErbB2 and has been approved by the United States Food and Drug Administration to treat breast cancers that overexpress ErbB2. In a large-scale trial, treatment with trastuzumab led to marked improvement in survival.[50] However, 7 percent of patients receiving trastuzumab as a second-line therapy, following anthracycline treatment as a first-line therapy, develop cardiac dysfunction.[50,51] Such observations suggest an important role for ErbB2 signaling as a modifier of human heart failure. Trastuzumab-related cardiomyopathy likely results from downregulation of ErbB2 signaling, which appears to protect against the development of dilated cardiomyopathy.[52] Myocardial levels of ErbB2 receptors decrease during the transition from hypertrophy to decompensated heart failure.[53] Previous studies have shown that neuroregulins promote cardiomyocyte cell survival in vitro,[54] and ErbB2 signaling may prevent myocytic apoptosis and slow cardiac remodeling in cases of heart failure.[52]

In clinical trials, trastuzumab is effective as a single agent in the treatment of breast cancer but can also have additive or synergistic effects when used in combination with chemotherapeutic agents. Because the majority of patients with breast cancer receive anthracycline treatment, the incidence of cardiomyopathy in trastuzumab-treated patients in the absence of concurrent or prior anthracycline treatment remains uncertain. When trastuzumab is combined with anthracyclines, the incidence of cardiac dysfunction is 28 percent.[50,51,55] Trastuzumab appears to increase the sensitivity of heart muscle cells to anthracycline toxicity.[52] The essential role of ErbB2 signaling in the development of the embryonic heart and the slowing of cardiac myocyte cell death in heart failure models suggests that trastuzumab-related cardiac dysfunction is not mediated by immunological mechanisms or drug-drug interaction. Currently, the use of trastuzumab is restricted to treatment of metastatic breast cancer. Clinical trials are underway to test the effectiveness of trastuzumab in other forms of ErbB2-overexpressing cancers, such as breast cancer at earlier stages, as well as lung, prostate, and ovarian cancers.[51,56]

Cyclophosphamide at Conventional and Marrow Transplant Doses

The alkylating agents cyclophosphamide and ifosfamide can cause an acute myopericarditis, particularly in the setting of bone marrow transplantation.[47,57–60] Risk is associated with peak dose and thus can be decreased by dividing the transplant doses of cyclophosphamide over 2 to 4 days. Prior exposure to imatinib (Gleevec) may increase cardiotoxicity.[61] Cardiomyopathy develops a median of 10 days after administration of high-dose cyclophosphamide, with tachycardia, dyspnea, pulmonary edema, and impressive cardiac dilation. Atrioventricular conduction abnormalities have also been reported.[62] Patients who survive can have normal ejection fractions months later.

Taxanes

Taxanes can cause sinus bradycardia, transient atrioventricular conduction delays from first-degree to complete heart block, and ventricular tachycardia. Combinations of paclitaxel with doxorubicin for breast cancer have produced congestive heart failure at cumulative doses of doxorubicin that are generally safe when the drug is used as a single agent. Paclitaxel may delay the elimination of doxorubicin, thus prolonging exposure.

In a retrospective Cleveland Clinic study of the medical records of patients with gynecological cancer, 15 patients with major cardiac risk factors had been treated with paclitaxel either as a single agent or in combination with cisplatin or carboplatin. Cardiac function after paclitaxel remained stable in all patients.[63] Thus, paclitaxel is probably relatively safe despite significant cardiac risk, including ischemic heart disease.

Docetaxel (Taxotere) can also produce arrhythmias but to date has not caused documented cardiotoxicity.[64,65] In 24 women with breast cancer who received docetaxel 100 mg/m^2 after prior therapy with anthracyclines monitored before docetaxel treatment and after three to four courses of docetaxel, the number of cardiac extrasystoles during docetaxel infusion did not increase and the number of ventricular extrasystoles decreased from 14 to 7 during and to 5 after the first infusion (p = 0.02). Heart rate, heart rate variability (HRV), and extrasystoles were similar before and after three to four courses of docetaxel, as were circadian variations in heart rate.[64] The antitumor activity and lack of cardiotoxicity with docetaxel, its ease of outpatient administration, and its linear pharmacokinetics make it attractive for use in combination with doxorubicin or other anthracyclines.[65,66]

Doxorubicin and Paclitaxel Combinations

Because doxorubicin and paclitaxel both have substantial activity against breast cancer, combining the two agents seemed worthy of study. At the Istituto Nazionale Tumori (Milano, Italy), 35 women with metastatic breast cancer with no prior chemotherapy received a fixed dose of doxorubicin (60 mg/m^2) with paclitaxel (125-200 mg/m^2) for a maximum of eight cycles. The complete response rate was high (41 percent; confidence interval [CI], 24-59 percent), as was the overall response rate (94 percent; CI, 79-99 percent); however, six women (18 percent) developed clinically reversible CHF after a median dose of 480 mg/m^2 total doxorubicin.[67]

The same investigators used pooled data from 10 doxorubicin and paclitaxel trials to estimate the risk of CHF. Of 657 patients, 31 (4.7 percent) developed CHF at a median of 7 months (range, 0.3-25 months) from the start of therapy. The risk of CHF was similar in women receiving doxorubicin and paclitaxel or doxorubicin monotherapy. CHF developed in 5 percent or less at a total doxorubicin dose of 380 mg/m^2 or less but occurred in more than 25 percent in patients with a cumulative doxorubicin dose of more than 440 mg/m^2 in both groups. CHF was stable in 29 patients at a median of 17 months (range, 4-31 months) after diagnosis.

Left ventricular ejection fraction (LVEF) progressively decreased in patients who received doxorubicin and paclitaxel, especially at a cumulative doxorubicin dose of more than 380 mg/m^2. LVEF decreased more frequently in patients who later developed CHF, but LVEF was not altered in most CHF patients prior to symptoms. LVEF recovered after discontinuation of doxorubicin in 25 of 67 women with LVEF of less than 50 percent.[68]

In an M.D. Anderson Hospital study of 82 women with no prior anthracycline or taxane therapy and normal cardiac function, patients received bolus doxorubicin 60 mg/m^2, followed by paclitaxel 200 mg/m^2, as either 1- or 3-hour infusions for six or seven cycles. A response was achieved in 58 percent of the patients (3.8 percent had complete response). The median survival was 31 months. Multiple gated acquisition cardiac scans were performed at baseline and after administration of total doxorubicin doses of 60 to 180 mg/m^2, 200 to 300 mg/m^2, 310 to 360 mg/m^2, and 420 mg/m^2. Median ejection fractions were 62, 60, 58, 52, and 32 percent, respectively. The ejection fraction fell by 15 percent or more in 15 patients (18 percent) to an ejection fraction of 50 percent or less. Eight of the 15 patients (53 percent) developed clinical congestive heart failure: 4 of 74 (5.4 percent) with a dose 360 mg/m^2 or less versus 4 of 8 (50 percent) at a total doxorubicin dose of 420 mg/m^2 (p = 0.002).[32]

In a multicenter Belgian study, 275 women with metastatic breast carcinoma and no prior anthracycline use were randomized to either doxorubicin (60 mg/m^2) followed 30 minutes later by a 3-hour infusion of paclitaxel (175 mg/m^2) (AT), or a standard doxorubicin and cyclophosphamide regimen (AC; 60/600 mg/m^2). Treatments were repeated every 3 weeks for six cycles. Congestive heart failure developed in three patients in the AT arm and in one patient in the AC arm (p = 0.62). Decreased left ventricular ejection fraction to less than normal occurred in 33 percent of AT and 19 percent of AC patients but did not predict clinical CHF.

Bolus doxorubicin and a 3-hour paclitaxel infusion had dramatic antitumor activity, but with an unacceptable risk of cardiac toxicity. When the total doxorubicin dose was limited to less than 360 mg/m^2, cardiac toxicity did not exceed that of similar cumulative doses of single-agent doxorubicin.[69] Paclitaxel appears to decrease the clearance of doxorubicin by approximately 30 percent when the two drugs are administered in close succession. Thus, up to six courses of therapy with doxorubicin 60 mg/m^2 and paclitaxel 175 mg/m^2 by 3-hour infusion appears safe, and therapy can be continued with single-agent paclitaxel. Patients should be selected carefully and monitored for changes in ejection fraction.[31,32,59,66,68,70,71]

All-*Trans*-Retinoic Acid Syndrome

All-*trans*-retinoic acid, used for the treatment of acute promyelocytic leukemia, can produce retinoic acid syndrome (myocardial dysfunction, heart failure, fever, shortness of breath, pleural and pericardial effusions, pulmonary infiltrates, and peripheral edema).[72]

Other Agents

5-Fluorouracil can produce heart failure[73] or acute cardiac ischemia in a small percentage of patients, generally during or immediately after administration of the agent. Acute myocardial infarction is rare; arrhythmias and ventricular dysfunction have been reported as well as sudden death. ECG changes disappear if the infusion is discontinued. Symptoms have recurred with rechallenge. Angiography has documented normal coronary arteries in some patients with ischemic symptoms and acutely abnormal ECGs. At postmortem examination, some but not all patients are found to have had acute infarcts.

Cisplatin occasionally produces arrhythmia and angina. Tamoxifen does not significantly alter cardiovascular risks.[74]

The hematopoietic growth factors such as granulocyte macrophage colony-stimulating factor (GM-CSF) (sargramostin [Leukine]) can cause a capillary leak syndrome with edema and effusions, generally at doses above those usually prescribed.

About 10 percent of patients on interferon develop abnormalities of cardiac rhythm or conduction, ischemia, or infarction, particularly those with preexisting ischemic heart disease, although ischemic changes and arrhythmias have been documented during interferon treatment in patients with no prior heart disease. Cardiomyopathy has occasionally developed in patients receiving years of treatment with interferon.

Interleukin-2 can produce capillary leak syndrome similar to that of the cytokines. Patients have experienced myocardial infarction during or immediately after treatment, even those with documented normal coronary arteries. Sepsis-like states appear to be associated with elevated levels of tumor necrosis factor-alpha during interleukin-2 infusion.[75]

Granisetron, an antiemetic agent, occasionally produces sinus bradycardia, atrioventricular block, and increased PR interval or Wenckebach block (Mobitz I).

Cardiac Complications of Radiation Therapy

Radiation therapy treatment volumes that include portions of the heart are part of standard therapy for many malignancies, most commonly lymphomas, breast, esophageal, and lung cancers. Risks of serious acute and late clinical effects on the heart may follow either curative or palliative radiation therapy. Increased cardiac mortality among irradiated patients may offset any potential reduced risk of recurrence or of death from cancer. Alternatively, substandard radiation doses to avoid cardiac toxicity could increase relapse risk. Concurrent or sequential cardiotoxic chemotherapy agents may substantially increase the incidence of radiation-associated cardiotoxicity. Nevertheless, clinically significant radiation cardiotoxicity is rare even with older radiation therapy techniques.[76]

Cardiac complications after radiation to ports that include the heart can affect pericardium, myocardium, valves, coronary arteries and the conduction system as well as damage pacemakers. Clinical manifestations can be acute or delayed by decades and correlate with cardiac radiation dose volume.[77] Initially, pericarditis and pericardial effusions were the most common cardiac complications, but with newer equipment and techniques, coronary artery disease is becoming the most common long-term risk of cardiac radiation. Risk is associated with the volume of the heart irradiated, dose, and dose fractionation. Computerized blocking can be used to decrease the exposure of the heart when increasing levels of radiation are required. Cardiac toxicity due to radiation therapy is uncommon and should become increasingly rare with modern equipment.

In a study conducted in the University Hospital in Lund, Sweden, of 90 patients younger than 50 years of age at the time of adjuvant radiotherapy after mastectomy examined at least 10 years later, the cardiovascular derangements identified included 14 patients with abnormal ECG, 5 with positive exercise test results, 6 with positive myocardial scintigraphic findings, 14 with thickened valve cusps, 20 with mild valvular regurgitation, and 6 with diastolic dysfunction (abnormal relaxation in 4 patients, and 2 with restrictive filling abnormalities). All patients had normal systolic function.[76]

Prevention of Cardiac Radiation Toxicity

Left-sided radiation fields for the treatment of breast, lung, or esophageal cancer or lymphoma often include the heart within the treatment volume. Radiation therapy techniques to preserve radiation dosage to the target and reduce late morbidity and decrease irradiated cardiac volume and thus possibly reduce associated cardiovascular toxicity and mortality include sophisticated three-dimensional planning,[78] optimal patient positioning,[78] and deep inspiratory maneuvers designed to minimize cardiac volume in the radiation field.[79,80] Extended blocking of cardiac volume decreases cardiac risk[81] but may compromise treatment efficacy.

PERICARDIAL COMPLICATIONS OF CARDIAC IRRADIATION. The spectrum of pericardial complications includes pericarditis during and up to several years after radiation and late constrictive pericarditis.[48,82,83] Given its high incidence in patients treated for Hodgkin disease with mantle radiotherapy, radiation-associated hypothyroidism must be considered in the differential diagnosis of constrictive pericarditis.

Low radiation doses to even a substantial volume of pericardium in the field carry a small risk of 2 to 5 percent. Pathologically, the pericardium becomes thickened and effusion develops. Small blood vessels proliferate, and collagen replaces pericardial tissue.

Acute pericarditis during radiation, associated with pain and fever, does not correlate with late pericardial damage. Pericarditis can be delayed for several years after mediastinal radiation. Symptoms can start with pain and fever, and there can be ST segment changes and a decrease in QRS voltage on the ECG. The chest radiograph may show a pericardial effusion with an enlarged cardiac silhouette sometimes resulting in tamponade, which requires pericardiocentesis.

Steroids may be helpful in treating radiation-associated pericardial disease, but symptoms can reemerge during tapering of the steroid drug. The rate of mortality due to pericardiectomy has been reported to be high, in the range of 20 to 35 percent, because of fibrosis and underlying radiation-associated cardiomyopathy.

MYOCARDIAL RADIATION TOXICITY. During and after radiation, left ventricular dysfunction can be documented with decreased filling and a decreased LVEF. Interactions with anthracyclines can occur, but when cumulative doses of anthracyclines are kept to standard levels, the risk remains low despite later radiotherapy. Restrictive cardiomyopathy can be difficult to distinguish from constrictive pericarditis. Pathological examination reveals interstitial fibrosis proportional to the radiation dose. Valvular disease includes abnormalities and new murmurs, but associated symptoms are few. Mitral and aortic valves are most commonly affected, with fibrous thickening of the valvular endocardium developing decades after radiation.

Investigators from Southern Hospital, Stockholm, Sweden evaluated the incidence of myocardial infarction in 960 women after mastectomy randomized to preoperative radiation therapy, postoperative radiation therapy, or surgery alone. At a median follow-up of 20 years (range, 17-23 years), 58 patients had had an acute myocardial infarction, with no significant difference between the three treatment groups. However, patients with the highest cardiac radiation dose-volumes had a relative risk of myocardial infarction of 1.3 (95 percent CI, 0.7-2.6) compared with surgical controls; the relative risk for those receiving intermediate and low dose-volumes was less than 1.0. The risk of death for patients in the high dose-volume group compared with surgical controls was 2.5 for ischemic heart disease (95 percent CI, 1.1-5.7; $p = 0.03$) and 2.0 for any cardiovascular disease (95 percent CI, 1.0-3.9; $p = 0.04$). Difference emerged after 4 to 5 years and continued to increase through 10 to 12 years. Increased risk of death from ischemic heart disease but no excess risk of myocardial infarction implies a mechanism such as radiation-associated microvascular damage.[77]

In contrast, the incidence of myocardial infarction for a Canadian cohort of 2128 breast cancer patients with a median follow-up of 10 years was similar to that in an age-matched general population of Ontario women. At least one definite or possible myocardial infarction occurred in 26 patients with left-sided and 23 patients with right-sided breast cancer. Fatal myocardial infarctions occurred in 8 patients with left-sided and 6 with right-sided cancers. No other cardiac abnormalities were found in excess among patients with left-sided cancers as compared with right-sided lesions. Thus, the investigators found no excess morbidity or mortality from coronary artery disease among women treated with radiation therapy to the left breast.[82]

CONDUCTION SYSTEM AND PACEMAKERS. Electrical abnormalities include complete bundle branch block developing a decade after radiation doses due to fibrosis of the conduction system. Implanted pacemakers have been damaged by radiation as well, and pacemaker function requires careful monitoring.

CORONARY ARTERY DISEASE. Coronary artery disease has emerged as a late risk of cardiac radiation. Coronary spasm can also occur in patients with angiographically normal–appearing coronary arteries. Deaths have occurred in up to 1 percent of patients irradiated with curative intent for Hodgkin disease and after patients have been irradiated for breast cancer.

Risks of Radiation and Drug-Associated Cardiotoxicity

Cardiac function must be monitored when patients receive combinations of radiation and drugs known to cause dysfunction.[48,84] In a Duke University study of 20 patients with left-sided breast cancer who underwent cardiac perfusion imaging using single-photon emission computed tomography before doxorubicin chemotherapy (10 patients), before radiation, and 6 months after radiation, 60 percent of the patients had new perfusion defects 6 months after radiation. The defects were dose dependent, with minimal changes at 0 to 10 Gy but a 20 percent decrease in regional perfusion at 41 to 50 Gy. Two patients developed transient pericarditis, although none had myocardial infarction or clinical congestive heart failure. Follow-up was insufficient to determine whether these perfusion changes were transient, permanent, or associated with later clinical dysfunction.[48]

In a Dana-Farber Cancer Institute study, 299 women with breast cancer were randomized to 5 versus 10 cycles of adjuvant cyclophosphamide (500 mg/m^2) and doxorubicin (45 mg/m^2) intravenously every 21 days; 122 patients also received radiation. At a median follow-up of 6.0 years (range, 0.5 to 19.4 years), the rate of cardiac events per 100 patient-years was significantly higher for the patients who received 10 cycles than for those who received 5 cycles (1.7 [CI, 1.0-2.8] vs. 0.5 [CI, 0.1 to 1.2]; $p = 0.02$]. Cardiac risk in patients receiving 5 months of chemotherapy did not differ significantly from that of women in the Framingham Heart Study, irrespective of cardiac radiation dose-volume. In women receiving 10 chemotherapy cycles, however, cardiac events were significantly increased (relative risk, 3.6; $p < 0.00003$) compared with the Framingham population, particularly for women who also received moderate and high dose-volume cardiac radiation.[85]

In a retrospective analysis of 825 women entered in randomized adjuvant chemotherapy trials with or without doxorubicin (Adriamycin) at the Istituto Nazionale Tumori (Milan, Italy), 360 women (44 percent) also received breast irradiation. Congestive heart failure occurred in 4 women after doxorubicin-containing chemotherapy (2.6 percent of those who received both doxorubicin and radiation to the left breast) and was fatal in 2. Cardiac events were documented in 6.8 percent, more frequently in women who received left breast radiation and in those older than 55 years of age.[86]

Cardiac Neoplasm and Acquired Immunodeficiency Syndrome

(see also Chap. 61)

KAPOSI SARCOMA. In patients with acquired immunodeficiency syndrome (AIDS) and human immunodeficiency virus (HIV) infection, Kaposi sarcoma and malignant lymphoma have been described as malignant neoplasms that affect the heart. The incidence of Kaposi sarcoma involving the heart ranged from 12 to 28 percent in retrospective autopsy findings. During HIV infection, cardiac involvement with Kaposi sarcoma usually occurs as a part of disseminated Kaposi sarcoma. AIDS-related metastatic Kaposi sarcoma involves either the visceral layer of pericardium or the subepicardial fat, where it can involve the subepicardial adipose tissue adjacent to a major coronary artery with involvement of the adventitia of the ascending aorta or pulmonary trunk. Pericardial and myocardial involvement can also occur. Fatal cardiac tamponade and pericardial constriction can complicate cardiac Kaposi sarcoma.[87] Pericardiocentesis has no diagnostic role and is a high-risk procedure in this group of patients. In patients with AIDS in whom the clinician has a high index of suspicion of Kaposi sarcoma pericardial effusion, a transthoracoscopic pericardial window can provide decompression and establish the pathological diagnosis.[88] Kaposi sarcoma generally responds well to chemotherapy.[7]

LYMPHOMA. Intermediate- or high-grade lymphoma is among the diagnostic criteria for AIDS. Cardiac involvement with non-Hodgkin lymphoma, usually derived from B cells, is typically high grade and is often disseminated early in patients with AIDS. Involvement of the heart by disseminated lymphoma is more common than primary cardiac lymphoma.[89] Patients usually have nonspecific symptoms, but rapid progression of cardiac dysfunction can present as intractable congestive heart failure, pericardial effusion, cardiac arrhythmia, or cardiac tamponade. Masses commonly infiltrate the pericardium with or without extension into the myocardium in cases of aggressive HIV-related lymphomas. Patients with mechanical obstruction can benefit from surgical resection. The prognosis of patients with HIV-associated cardiac lymphoma is generally poor, although combination chemotherapy can produce clinical remission.[90]

Summary

Because cardiovascular disease and cancer are both common, the cardiologist will care for many patients with cancer or a history of cancer. Because of overlapping risk factors such as obesity, hormone therapy, and, in particular, smoking, patients with coronary artery disease also have an elevated risk of cancer.

Cardiac complications of cancer such as pericardial tamponade or superior vena cava syndrome are frequent first manifestations of advanced neoplasia. Cancer treatments frequently compromise cardiac function. Radiation ports that include the heart for the treatment of lymphoma or lung or breast cancers can rarely produce late coronary artery disease or constrictive pericarditis. Oncolytic drugs, most frequently anthracyclines, paclitaxel, and trastuzumab, but also cyclophosphamide, 5-fluorouracil, and others, result in cardiotoxicity. Conversely, cardiac transplant patients have significant risk for lymphoma, squamous skin cancers, and Kaposi sarcoma, likely related to immunosuppressive therapy. The dismal outcome of cardiac resuscitation in patients with end-stage cancer requires careful coordination of end-of-life planning between the patients and families and the cardiology and oncology teams. Increased monitoring and heightened awareness of the cardiovascular complications of cancer can improve quality of life and survival in many with oncologic diseases.

REFERENCES

1. Reicher-Reiss H, Jonas M, Goldbourt U, et al: Selectively increased risk of cancer in men with coronary heart disease. Am J Cardiol 87:459, A6, 2001.

2. Kuller LH, Matthews KA, Meilahn EN: Estrogens and women's health: Interrelation of coronary heart disease, breast cancer and osteoporosis. J Steroid Biochem Mol Biol 74:297, 2000.
3. Gjersvik P, Hansen S, Moller B, et al: Are heart transplant recipients more likely to develop skin cancer than kidney transplant recipients? Transpl Int 13(Suppl 1):S380, 2000.
4. Caforio AL, Fortina AB, Piaserico S, et al: Skin cancer in heart transplant recipients: Risk factor analysis and relevance of immunosuppressive therapy. Circulation 102:III222, 2000.
5. Jensen P, Moller B, Hansen S: Skin cancer in kidney and heart transplant recipients and different long-term immunosuppressive therapy regimens. J Am Acad Dermatol 42:307, 2000.
6. Fortina AB, Caforio AL, Piaserico S, et al: Skin cancer in heart transplant recipients: Frequency and risk factor analysis. J Heart Lung Transplant 19:249, 2000.
7. Antman K, Chang Y: Kaposi's sarcoma. N Engl J Med 342:1027, 2000.
8. Calle EE, Rodriguez C, Walker-Thurmond K, Thun MJ: Overweight, obesity, and mortality from cancer in a prospectively studied cohort of U.S. adults. N Engl J Med 348:1625, 2003.
9. Gronbaek M, Becker U, Johansen D, et al: Type of alcohol consumed and mortality from all causes, coronary heart disease, and cancer. Ann Intern Med 133:411, 2000.
10. Ewer MS, Kish SK, Martin CG, et al: Characteristics of cardiac arrest in cancer patients as a predictor of survival after cardiopulmonary resuscitation. Cancer 92:1905, 2001.

Direct Complications of Neoplasia

11. Veinot JP, Burns BF, Commons AS, Thomas J: Cardiac neoplasms at the Canadian Reference Centre for Cancer Pathology. Can J Cardiol 15:311, 1999.
12. Grebenc ML, Rosado de Christenson ML, Burke AP, et al: Primary cardiac and pericardial neoplasms: Radiologic-pathologic correlation. Radiographics 20:1073, quiz 1110, 2000.
13. Eren NT, Akar AR: Primary pericardial mesothelioma. Curr Treat Options Oncol 3:369, 2002.
14. Youn HJ, Jung SE, Chung WS, et al: Obstruction of right ventricular outflow tract by extended cardiac metastasis from esophageal cancer. J Am Soc Echocardiogr 15:1541, 2002.
15. Bissada NK, Yakout HH, Babanouri A, et al: Long-term experience with management of renal cell carcinoma involving the inferior vena cava. Urology 61:89, 2003.
16. Nam MS, Jeon MJ, Kim YT, et al: Pelvic leiomyomatosis with intracaval and intracardiac extension: A case report and review of the literature. Gynecol Oncol 89:175, 2003.

Cardiac Tamponade and Constrictive Pericarditis

17. Ortega-Carnicer J, Benezet J, Porras L: Lung cancer presenting as cardiac tamponade associated with transmural myocardial ischaemia. Resuscitation 51:317, 2001.
18. Bishiniotis TS, Antoniadou S, Katseas G, et al: Malignant cardiac tamponade in women with breast cancer treated by pericardiocentesis and intrapericardial administration of triethylenethiophosphoramide (thiotepa). Am J Cardiol 86:362, 2000.
19. Wang PC, Yang KY, Chao JY, et al: Prognostic role of pericardial fluid cytology in cardiac tamponade associated with non-small cell lung cancer. Chest 118:744, 2000.
20. Okamoto H, Shinkai T, Yamakido M, Saijo N: Cardiac tamponade caused by primary lung cancer and the management of pericardial effusion. Cancer 71:93, 1993.

Superior Vena Cava Obstruction

21. Case records of the Massachusetts General Hospital: Weekly clinicopathological exercises. Case 33-2000. A seven-year-old girl with the superior vena cava syndrome after treatment for a peripheral rhabdomyosarcoma. N Engl J Med 343:1249, 2000.
22. Wudel LJ Jr, Nesbitt JC: Superior vena cava syndrome. Curr Treat Options Oncol 2:77, 2001.
23. Kvale PA, Simoff M, Prakash UB: Lung cancer: Palliative care. Chest 123:284S, 2003.
24. Teo N, Sabharwal T, Rowland E, et al: Treatment of superior vena cava obstruction secondary to pacemaker wires with balloon venoplasty and insertion of metallic stents. Eur Heart J 23:1465, 2002.
25. Lanciego C, Chacon JL, Julian A, et al: Stenting as first option for endovascular treatment of malignant superior vena cava syndrome. AJR Am J Roentgenol 177:585, 2001.
26. Kovacs RG, Aguayo SM: Images in clinical medicine: Superior vena cava syndrome. N Engl J Med 329:1007, 1993.

Valvular Heart Disease in the Cancer Patient

27. Edoute Y, Haim N, Rinkevich D, et al: Cardiac valvular vegetations in cancer patients: A prospective echocardiographic study of 200 patients. Am J Med 102:252, 1997.

Arrhythmias

28. Sekine Y, Kesler KA, Behnia M, et al: COPD may increase the incidence of refractory supraventricular arrhythmias following pulmonary resection for non-small cell lung cancer. Chest 120:1783, 2001.

Indirect Cardiovascular Complications of Cancer

Hyperviscosity

29. Ambrus JL, Ambrus CM, Dembinsky W, et al: Thromboembolic disease susceptibility related to red cell membrane fluidity in patients with polycythemia vera and effect of phlebotomies. J Med 30:299, 1999.
30. Dammacco F, Sansonno D, Piccoli C, et al: The cryoglobulins: An overview. Eur J Clin Invest 31:628, 2001.

Cardiac Complications of Chemotherapy

Anthracycline Cardiotoxicity

31. Biganzoli L, Cufer T, Bruning P, et al: Doxorubicin-paclitaxel: A safe regimen in terms of cardiac toxicity in metastatic breast carcinoma patients. Results from a European Organization for Research and Treatment of Cancer multicenter trial. Cancer 97:40, 2003.
32. Giordano SH, Booser DJ, Murray JL, et al: A detailed evaluation of cardiac toxicity: A phase II study of doxorubicin and one- or three-hour-infusion paclitaxel in patients with metastatic breast cancer. Clin Cancer Res 8:3360, 2002.
33. Tham YL, Verani MS, Chang J: Reversible and irreversible cardiac dysfunction associated with trastuzumab in breast cancer. Breast Cancer Res Treat 74:131, 2002.
34. Keefe DL: Cardiovascular emergencies in the cancer patient. Semin Oncol 27:244, 2000.
35. Von Hoff DD, Layard MW, Basa P, et al: Risk factors for doxorubicin-induced congestive heart failure. Ann Intern Med 91:710, 1979.
36. Bristow MR, Mason JW, Billingham ME, Daniels JR: Doxorubicin cardiomyopathy: Evaluation by phonocardiography, endomyocardial biopsy, and cardiac catheterization. Ann Intern Med 88:168, 1978.
37. Swain SM, Whaley FS, Ewer MS: Congestive heart failure in patients treated with doxorubicin: A retrospective analysis of three trials. Cancer 97:2869, 2003.
38. Ibrahim NK, Hortobagyi GN, Ewer M, et al: Doxorubicin-induced congestive heart failure in elderly patients with metastatic breast cancer, with long-term follow-up: The M.D. Anderson experience. Cancer Chemother Pharmacol 43:471, 1999.
39. Li CK, Sung RY, Kwok KL, et al: A longitudinal study of cardiac function in children with cancer over 40 months. Pediatr Hematol Oncol 17:77, 2000.
40. Lanzarini L, Bossi G, Laudisa ML, et al: Lack of clinically significant cardiac dysfunction during intermediate dobutamine doses in long-term childhood cancer survivors exposed to anthracyclines. Am Heart J 140:315, 2000.
41. Green DM, Hyland A, Chung CS, et al: Cancer and cardiac mortality among 15-year survivors of cancer diagnosed during childhood or adolescence. J Clin Oncol 17:3207, 1999.
42. Tikanoja T, Riikonen P, Perkkio M, Helenius T: Serum N-terminal atrial natriuretic peptide (NT-ANP) in the cardiac follow-up in children with cancer. Med Pediatr Oncol 31:73, 1998.
43. Hayakawa H, Komada Y, Hirayama M, et al: Plasma levels of natriuretic peptides in relation to doxorubicin-induced cardiotoxicity and cardiac function in children with cancer. Med Pediatr Oncol 37:4, 2001.
44. Venturini M, Michelotti A, Del Mastro L, et al: Multicenter randomized controlled clinical trial to evaluate cardioprotection of dexrazoxane versus no cardioprotection in women receiving epirubicin chemotherapy for advanced breast cancer. J Clin Oncol 14:3112, 1996.
45. Lopez M, Vici P, Di Lauro K, et al: Randomized prospective clinical trial of high-dose epirubicin and dexrazoxane in patients with advanced breast cancer and soft tissue sarcomas. J Clin Oncol 16:86, 1998.
46. Mitani I, Jain D, Joska TM, et al: Doxorubicin cardiotoxicity: Prevention of congestive heart failure with serial cardiac function monitoring with equilibrium radionuclide angiocardiography in the current era. J Nucl Cardiol 10:132, 2003.
47. Morandi P, Ruffini PA, Benvenuto GM, et al: Serum cardiac troponin I levels and ECG/Echo monitoring in breast cancer patients undergoing high-dose ($7\ g/m^2$) cyclophosphamide. Bone Marrow Transplant 28:277, 2001.
48. Hardenbergh PH, Munley MT, Bentel GC, et al: Cardiac perfusion changes in patients treated for breast cancer with radiation therapy and doxorubicin: Preliminary results. Int J Radiat Oncol Biol Phys 49:1023, 2001.

Herceptin Cardiotoxicity

49. Klapper LN, Kirschbaum MH, Sela M, Yarden Y: Biochemical and clinical implications of the ErbB/HER signaling network of growth factor receptors. Adv Cancer Res 77:25, 2000.
50. Slamon DJ, Leyland-Jones B, Shak S, et al: Use of chemotherapy plus a monoclonal antibody against HER2 for metastatic breast cancer that overexpresses HER2. N Engl J Med 344:783, 2001.
51. Baselga J: Current and planned clinical trials with trastuzumab (Herceptin). Semin Oncol 27:27, 2000.
52. Crone SA, Zhao YY, Fan L, et al: ErbB2 is essential in the prevention of dilated cardiomyopathy. Nat Med 8:459, 2002.
53. Rohrbach S, Yan X, Weinberg EO, et al: Neuregulin in cardiac hypertrophy in rats with aortic stenosis: Differential expression of erbB2 and erbB4 receptors. Circulation 100:407, 1999.
54. Zhao YY, Sawyer DR, Baliga RR, et al: Neuregulins promote survival and growth of cardiac myocytes: Persistence of ErbB2 and ErbB4 expression in neonatal and adult ventricular myocytes. J Biol Chem 273:10261, 1998.
55. Sparano JA: Cardiac toxicity of trastuzumab (Herceptin): Implications for the design of adjuvant trials. Semin Oncol 28:20, 2001.
56. Agus DB, Bunn PA Jr, Franklin W, et al: HER-2/neu as a therapeutic target in non-small cell lung cancer, prostate cancer, and ovarian cancer. Semin Oncol 27:53, discussion 92, 2000.

Cyclophosphamide at Conventional and Marrow Transplant Doses

57. Gralow JR, Livingston RB: University of Washington high-dose cyclophosphamide, mitoxantrone, and etoposide experience in metastatic breast cancer: Unexpected cardiac toxicity. J Clin Oncol 19:3903, 2001.
58. Nieto Y, Cagnoni PJ, Bearman SI, et al: Cardiac toxicity following high-dose cyclophosphamide, cisplatin, and BCNU (STAMP-I) for breast cancer. Biol Blood Marrow Transplant 6:198, 2000.
59. Klein JL, Rey PM, Dansey RD, et al: Cardiac sequelae of doxorubicin and paclitaxel as induction chemotherapy prior to high-dose chemotherapy and peripheral blood progenitor cell transplantation in women with high-risk primary or metastatic breast cancer. Bone Marrow Transplant 25:1047, 2000.
60. Brockstein BE, Smiley C, Al-Sadir J, Williams SF: Cardiac and pulmonary toxicity in patients undergoing high-dose chemotherapy for lymphoma and breast cancer: Prognostic factors. Bone Marrow Transplant 25:885, 2000.

61. Sohn SK, Kim JG, Kim DH, Lee KB: Cardiac morbidity in advanced chronic myelogenous leukaemia patients treated by successive allogeneic stem cell transplantation with busulphan/cyclophosphamide conditioning after imatinib mesylate administration. Br J Haematol 121:469, 2003.
62. Ando M, Yokozawa T, Sawada J, et al: Cardiac conduction abnormalities in patients with breast cancer undergoing high-dose chemotherapy and stem cell transplantation. Bone Marrow Transplant 25:185, 2000.

Taxanes

63. Markman M, Kennedy A, Webster K, et al: Paclitaxel administration to gynecologic cancer patients with major cardiac risk factors. J Clin Oncol 16:3483, 1998.
64. Ekholm E, Rantanen V, Syvanen K, et al: Docetaxel does not impair cardiac autonomic function in breast cancer patients previously treated with anthracyclines. Anticancer Drugs 13:425, 2002.
65. Syvanen K, Ekholm E, Anttila K, Salminen E: Immediate effects of docetaxel alone or in combination with epirubicin on cardiac function in advanced breast cancer. Anticancer Res 23:1869, 2003.
66. Valero V, Perez E, Dieras V: Doxorubicin and taxane combination regimens for metastatic breast cancer: Focus on cardiac effects. Semin Oncol 28:15, 2001.

Doxorubicin and Paclitaxel Combinations

67. Gianni L, Munzone E, Capri G, et al: Paclitaxel by 3-hour infusion in combination with bolus doxorubicin in women with untreated metastatic breast cancer: High antitumor efficacy and cardiac effects in a dose-finding and sequence-finding study. J Clin Oncol 13:2688, 1995.
68. Gianni L, Dombernowsky P, Sledge G, et al: Cardiac function following combination therapy with paclitaxel and doxorubicin: An analysis of 657 women with advanced breast cancer. Ann Oncol 12:1067, 2001.

69. Hortobagyi GN, Willey J, Rahman Z, et al: Prospective assessment of cardiac toxicity during a randomized phase II trial of doxorubicin and paclitaxel in metastatic breast cancer. Semin Oncol 24:S17, 1997.
70. Perez EA: Doxorubicin and paclitaxel in the treatment of advanced breast cancer: Efficacy and cardiac considerations. Cancer Invest 19:155, 2001.
71. Doxorubicin/paclitaxel combination does not expose breast cancer patients to excessive cardiac risk. Oncology (Huntingt) 15:830, 2001.

All-Trans-Retinoic Acid Syndrome

72. Tallman MS, Andersen JW, Schiffer CA, et al: Clinical description of 44 patients with acute promyelocytic leukemia who developed the retinoic acid syndrome. Blood 95:90, 2000.

Other Agents

73. David JS, Gueugniaud PY, Hepp A, et al: Severe heart failure secondary to 5-fluorouracil and low-doses of folinic acid: Usefulness of an intra-aortic balloon pump. Crit Care Med 28:3558, 2000.
74. Reis SE, Costantino JP, Wickerham DL, et al: Cardiovascular effects of tamoxifen in women with and without heart disease: Breast cancer prevention trial. National Surgical Adjuvant Breast and Bowel Project Breast Cancer Prevention Trial Investigators. J Natl Cancer Inst 93:16, 2001.
75. Caorsi C, Quintana E, Valdes S, Munoz C: Continuous cardiac output and hemodynamic monitoring: High temporal correlation between plasma TNF-alpha and hemodynamic changes during a sepsis-like state in cancer immunotherapy. J Endotoxin Res 9:91, 2003.

Cardiac Complications of Radiation Therapy

76. Gustavsson A, Bendahl PO, Cwikiel M, et al: No serious late cardiac effects after adjuvant radiotherapy following mastectomy in premenopausal women with early breast cancer. Int J Radiat Oncol Biol Phys 43:745, 1999.
77. Gyenes G, Rutqvist LE, Liedberg A, Fornander T: Long-term cardiac morbidity and mortality in a randomized trial of pre- and postoperative radiation therapy versus surgery alone in primary breast cancer. Radiother Oncol 48:185, 1998.
78. Canney PA, Deehan C, Glegg M, Dickson J: Reducing cardiac dose in post-operative irradiation of breast cancer patients: The relative importance of patient positioning and CT scan planning. Br J Radiol 72:986, 1999.
79. Chen MH, Cash EP, Danias PG, et al: Respiratory maneuvers decrease irradiated cardiac volume in patients with left-sided breast cancer. J Cardiovasc Magn Reson 4:265, 2002.
80. Sixel KE, Aznar MC, Ung YC: Deep inspiration breath hold to reduce irradiated heart volume in breast cancer patients. Int J Radiat Oncol Biol Phys 49:199, 2001.
81. Gagliardi G, Lax I, Soderstrom S, et al: Prediction of excess risk of long-term cardiac mortality after radiotherapy of stage I breast cancer. Radiother Oncol 46:63, 1998.
82. Vallis KA, Pintilie M, Chong N, et al: Assessment of coronary heart disease morbidity and mortality after radiation therapy for early breast cancer. J Clin Oncol 20:1036, 2002.
83. Muren LP, Maurstad G, Hafslund R, et al: Cardiac and pulmonary doses and complication probabilities in standard and conformal tangential irradiation in conservative management of breast cancer. Radiother Oncol 62:173, 2002.

Risks of Radiation and Drug-Associated Cardiotoxicity

84. Zambetti M, Moliterni A, Materazzo C, et al: Long-term cardiac sequelae in operable breast cancer patients given adjuvant chemotherapy with or without doxorubicin and breast irradiation. J Clin Oncol 19:37, 2001.
85. Shapiro CL, Hardenbergh PH, Gelman R, et al: Cardiac effects of adjuvant doxorubicin and radiation therapy in breast cancer patients. J Clin Oncol 16:3493, 1998.
86. Valagussa P, Zambetti M, Biasi S, et al: Cardiac effects following adjuvant chemotherapy and breast irradiation in operable breast cancer. Ann Oncol 5:209, 1994.

Cardiac Neoplasm and AIDS

87. Chyu KY, Birnbaum Y, Naqvi T, et al: Echocardiographic detection of Kaposi's sarcoma causing cardiac tamponade in a patient with acquired immunodeficiency syndrome. Clin Cardiol 21:131, 1998.
88. Rerkpattanapipat P, Wongpraparut N, Jacobs LE, Kotler MN: Cardiac manifestations of acquired immunodeficiency syndrome. Arch Intern Med 160:602, 2000.
89. Roberts WC: Primary and secondary neoplasms of the heart. Am J Cardiol 80:671, 1997.
90. Duong M, Dubois C, Buisson M, et al: Non-Hodgkin's lymphoma of the heart in patients infected with human immunodeficiency virus. Clin Cardiol 20:497, 1997.

CHAPTER 84

Psychiatric and Behavioral Aspects of Cardiovascular Disease

Arthur J. Barsky

Daily life offers ample empirical evidence of an intimate relationship between the psyche and the heart. Intense emotions such as anxiety, anger, elation, and sexual arousal are accompanied by predictable increases in heart rate and blood pressure. Our everyday speech is filled with cardiac metaphors—the heart "races" with excitement, "pounds" in eager anticipation, "stands still" in dread, "aches" with grief. Many cultures have regarded the heart as the seat of emotion, the origin of love, the source of courage, or the abode of the soul. Generous people have "big hearts" and stingy people are "heartless." When you first met your first love, your heart "skipped a beat," and you were "broken hearted" when you parted ways soon thereafter. We attend funerals with a "heavy heart" and offer our "heartfelt" condolences. The interaction of heart and psyche is bidirectional. Emotions and stressful experiences affect the heart directly through the autonomic nervous system and indirectly via neuroendocrine pathways. Conversely, cardiac activity and function can reach conscious awareness and may be experienced as symptoms.

Psychiatric and Behavioral Aspects of Coronary Heart Disease

Type A Behavior Pattern and Anger

Clinicians have long observed that many patients with coronary heart disease (CHD) seem to be compulsive, driven overachievers who are unable to relax and are quick to feel angry and frustrated when things do not proceed as planned. These observations were reinforced in the 1960s by Friedman and Rosenman, who advanced the concept of type A behavior. Type A behavior is suffused with a sense of ambition, time urgency, and anger and hostility; type A people are excessively competitive and aggressive, with an extreme drive for achievement—impatient people leading fast-paced lives in continual and strenuous pursuit of a goal. This was contrasted with type B individuals, who are relaxed, unhurried, less aggressive, and who do not get as upset when thwarted. Large-scale, prospective studies in the 1970s and 1980s conducted on initially healthy individuals showed that those with type A behavior pattern, compared to type B individuals, had a significantly elevated rate of developing CHD and myocardial infarction at 5- to 8.5-year follow-up and had more extensive CHD at the time of angiography. Although some subsequent studies replicated these findings,[1] a number failed to support the association.

These contradictory findings led to a search for a specific component of type A behavior that might be more closely associated with CHD. This work suggested that anger and/or suppressed anger are the pathogenic components of type A personality. Anger, hostility, antagonistic interactions, cynicism, and mistrust have now been associated in long-term, prospective studies with the incidence of CHD, coronary events, and total mortality. For example, in a sample of 2890 middle-aged men followed prospectively for more than 8 years, suppressed anger was a significant predictor of a major cardiac event, and this relationship persisted after controlling for physiological, psychosocial, and behavioral risk factors.[2] In a prospective study of young adults, high levels of hostility were associated with subsequent coronary artery calcification,[3] and cross-sectional studies also report an association between the degree of hostility and the severity of CHD.[4] In large, prospective studies of initially healthy individuals, higher levels of anger were associated with a twofold to threefold increased incidence of developing CHD, after adjusting for other biological risk factors.[5]

Some studies, however, have failed to find an association between anger and CHD, and in general it appears that hostility and anger may predispose more to the initial cardiac event than adversely influencing the course of already established CHD. It is unclear to what degree hostility's effect may be mediated through its effect on other risk factors such as lack of social support, smoking, obesity, and alcohol use. The combination of both anger and low social support may be particularly hazardous.[6] Possible associations between anger and race, socioeconomic status, and gender also represent potential confounds. Although more research is necessary, it does appear that anger and hostility play some role in the development of CHD.

Depression and Anxiety

DEPRESSION. Depression is prevalent in CHD patients but is consistently underdiagnosed by their cardiologists and primary care physicians. Clinically significant depressive symptoms are found in 40 to 65 percent of patients following a myocardial infarction, and major depressive disorder is found in 15 to 25 percent of such patients.[7,8] In one study, 31.5 percent of patients with myocardial infarction experienced major depression while in the hospital or in the year following discharge.[9] The prevalence of depression is also elevated in patients with stable CHD who have not had a recent myocardial infarction and in patients who have undergone coronary artery bypass grafting (CABG).[10] Depression is often chronic: Three-fourths of the patients with major depression 2 weeks after a myocardial infarction remain depressed 3 months later. Although most subjects in these studies have been men, the risk of depression in women with CHD is twice as high as that of men.

Depression is important in itself because of the considerable suffering it imposes. In addition, depression exacerbates and amplifies cardiac symptoms. Depressed CHD patients have more severe cardiac symptoms than nondepressed CHD patients, even after controlling for the severity of cardiac disease[11]: They have more angina during exercise treadmill testing, terminate the treadmill test sooner, and have more persistent angina following myocardial infarction. Depression adversely affects compliance with medical therapy, and it is detrimental to cardiac rehabilitation. Depression also predicts a slower resumption of activities, poorer social readjustment, a lower likelihood of returning to work, and poorer quality of life following myocardial infarction.[12] In a 1-year, prospective study of patients who had undergone catheterization for documented CHD, physical functioning and interference with activities were better predicted by baseline depression and anxiety than by the number of stenosed vessels, even after controlling for medical comorbidity and treatment.[13]

Depression both worsens the prognosis of established CHD and constitutes a risk factor for the development of CHD in healthy individuals; that is, it confers an increased risk of cardiac mortality in both those with and without CHD at baseline.[14] In patients with documented CHD, depression predicts future cardiac events and is associated with significantly elevated rates of cardiac mortality (primarily as a result of sudden cardiac death [SCD]).[7] This risk is elevated for women as well as men and is not limited to major depressive disorder but also includes milder depressive symptoms. Thus, there is a continuous, linear relationship between the severity of depression and the risk of subsequent cardiac events.[15] Major depressive disorder at the time of cardiac catheterization is a significant predictor of subsequent myocardial infarction, angioplasty, CABG, and death in patients with evidence of CHD, and this effect is independent of disease severity, ejection fraction, and smoking. Depression prior to undergoing CABG surgery is an independent predictor of rehospitalization, continued surgical pain, and failure to resume previous activity.[16] Following myocardial infarction, depression increases the risk of reinfarction, cardiac arrest, and death, after adjusting for CHD severity.[7]

In an important longitudinal study of 222 patients, baseline depression was a significant predictor of cardiac mortality 6 and 18 months after myocardial infarction, and this association persisted after controlling statistically for the effects of baseline left ventricular dysfunction, Killip class, previous myocardial infarction, and frequency of premature ventricular complexes.[7] For longer follow-up periods, from 5 to 15 years, the relative risk of recurrent myocardial infarction or cardiac mortality associated with depression is between 1.5 and 6, after controlling for disease severity, smoking, diabetes, and age in multivariate analyses.[15] The degree of risk associated with depression is as great as that associated with traditional risk factors (e.g., cholesterol, smoking, hypertension) and is largely independent of them. In some studies, however, the association between depression and post-myocardial reinfarction is no longer significant when adjusted for all other predictors of cardiac mortality and for possible confounds (e.g., fatigue) that are common to both CHD and depression.[17] Much of the increased cardiac mortality associated with depression appears to be attributable to SCD due to arrhythmias. This suggests that the effect of depression may be more arrhythmogenic than atherogenic. An interaction effect may exist, in which the co-occurrence of depression with ventricular arrhythmias constitutes a particularly ominous prognostic factor. Conversely, optimism seems to have a positive influence on prognosis; optimism at the time of CABG is associated with a lower rate of rehospitalization for cardiac events over the subsequent 6 months, after controlling for sociodemographic differences and disease severity.[18]

Depression as a Risk Factor. Depression also appears to be a risk factor for the development of CHD in healthy individuals, though the evidence here is somewhat less conclusive. In prospective studies of initially healthy, community residents without a history of CHD, depression has been associated with an adjusted relative risk between 1.5 and 2 for the subsequent development of CHD, myocardial infarction, and cardiac death over periods from 6 to 40 years in men and in women, and this risk is largely independent of the more traditional risk factors.[19] A dose-response relationship seems to exist such that the more severely depressed the patient is, the greater the risk of developing CHD.

In *summary*, depression is a negative prognostic indicator for patients with established CHD and a risk factor for the development of CHD in healthy individuals. It is associated with increased morbidity, mortality, disability, and impaired quality of life. Both major depressive disorder and less severe depressive symptoms are significant in this regard. The degree of risk associated with major depression is comparable to that associated with other, established risk factors and is largely independent of them.

Several behavioral and physiological mechanisms may mediate the relationship between depression and CHD. Depression may operate through its influence on lifestyle and behavior[20]: Depressed individuals take poorer care of themselves; are less physically active; pay less attention to diet; drink more alcohol; smoke more and have worse quitting rates; have less motivation and energy to exercise regularly; and may be less likely to seek medical care. Depression is associated with poorer adherence to the medical regimen and to cardiac risk factor modification and rehabilitation, and depressed patients are more likely to drop out of exercise programs. For reasons that remain unclear, patients with a range of psychiatric disorders, including depression, undergo revascularization procedures (percutaneous transluminal coronary angioplasty and CABG) less frequently than those without psychiatric disorders, even after adjusting for disease severity.[21]

Pathophysiological Mechanisms. Several pathophysiological mechanisms may link depression and CHD.[22] First, depression results in autonomic arousal and hypothalamic-adrenocortical and sympathoadrenal hyperactivity. Depressed patients show hyperactivity of the hypothalamic-pituitary-adrenocortical axis and hypercortisolemia, and corticosteroids have atherogenic effects, including the induction of high blood pressure and increases in cholesterol and free fatty acids,[22] as well as possible effects on arterial endothelial function.[23] In addition, there is hypersecretion of norepinephrine in depression, and plasma catecholamines stimulate heart rate, blood pressure, and myocardial oxygen consumption. Catecholamines are also proarrhythmic, and an increased incidence of ventricular tachyarrhythmias has been found in depressed patients. (This observation is compatible with the finding that SCD accounts for a large share of the excess cardiac mortality found in depressed CHD patients.)[15,24] Second, depressed cardiac patients exhibit diminished heart rate variability,[25] resulting from a relative increase in sympathetic tone and/or a relative decrease in parasympathetic tone, which increases the risk of fatal arrhythmias. Third, depression may be accompanied by changes in platelet aggregability.[22,26] Serotonin plays a major role in depression, and it is also known to influence thrombogenesis and enhance platelet activation and responsiveness to other thrombogenic agents. Serotonin reuptake inhibitor antidepressants appear to normalize this platelet hyperactivity seen in depression.

ANXIETY. Chronically high levels of anxiety, panic disorder, and phobic anxiety appear to be both a risk factor for developing CHD and a negative prognostic influence on the course of established disease.[24] In the former instance, several prospective studies of initially healthy men and women reveal that those who are highly anxious at the outset are more likely to subsequently develop arteriosclerotic plaques, carotid artery intimal thickening, nonfatal myocardial infarction, and cardiac death.[27] Anxiety may also worsen the course of established CHD. Thus high levels of anxiety following myocardial infarction appear to confer a 2.5-fold to fivefold increased risk of recurrent ischemia, reinfarction, ventricular fibrillation, and SCD. In one study, for example, anxiety was an independent predictor of cardiac events following myocardial infarction, after adjusting for the influence of depression. In another study, higher levels of anxiety in patients hospitalized for myocardial infarction were independent predictors of more in-hospital ischemic and arrhythmic complications.[28] It remains unclear whether anxiety is more closely related to arrhythmias and SCD than to arteriosclerosis and infarction.

Possible mechanisms explaining these associations include sympathetic nervous system upregulation with increased catecholamine production and decreased vagal activity, microvascular angina, and idiopathic cardiomyopathy.

Psychosocial Factors

Psychosocial, cultural, and environmental factors increase the risk of CHD, either independently or in combination. These include social isolation and lack of social support, life stresses (such as job strain), and sociodemographic characteristics. These psychosocial risk factors tend to be associated with each other and often co-occur. For example, job strain and socioeconomic position may be inversely correlated, and depression is associated with social isolation. Furthermore, these psychosocial factors tend to be associated with unhealthy lifestyle behaviors. For example, life stress may be correlated with smoking, increased alcohol consumption, and body weight, and people with fewer social supports are less likely to stop smoking or adhere to the medical regimen.

SOCIAL ISOLATION, LACK OF SOCIAL SUPPORT, AND SOCIAL DISRUPTION. Population-based, cross-sectional surveys reveal that social integration (e.g., being married, having regular contact with friends, and belonging to organizations) is associated with lower levels of CHD. Conversely, social isolation and low social support (living alone, having few friends or family members, and not belonging to organizations, clubs, or churches) is associated with an increased incidence of CHD and a poorer outcome following first diagnosis of CHD.[29] In a recent prospective study of 430 CHD patients, those with fewer than four people in their social network had a 2.4 times greater risk of cardiac mortality after adjusting for differences in age, disease severity, psychological distress, smoking, and income.[30] Social support and depression seem to interact, such that high levels of social support blunt the impact of depression on cardiac mortality.[31]

Animal studies also suggest a protective role for social support against atherogenesis. When research personnel fondle laboratory rabbits placed on an atherogenic diet, the development of coronary atherosclerosis is retarded. Crowding and social disruption of animal colonies, as well as isolation of individual laboratory animals, increase the rates of atherogenesis.

Several mediating mechanisms have been proposed to explain this relationship between social integration and CHD. First, concerned and supportive others may encourage healthy behaviors and adherence to the medical regimen and provide a motivation for altering unhealthy behavioral risk factors; conversely, loneliness may foster unhealthy behaviors such as smoking and drinking. Second, social support, by providing comfort, encouragement, and consolation, may attenuate and buffer the individual's emotional and/or physiological response to environmental stress. Finally, significant others can provide practical assistance that mitigates the impact of stressful life events, for example, lending money, doing errands, and providing transportation.

LIFE STRESS AND JOB STRAIN. The relationship between life stress and CHD has long been of interest. Animal work is provocative in this regard. In studies ranging from mice to primates, stressful experimental paradigms that increase aggression and fear and that disturb stable social hierarchies and decrease social affiliation are associated with atherosclerosis. Thus, dominant male monkeys fed an atherogenic diet develop coronary atherosclerosis at a higher rate when repeatedly moved from one social group to another rather than when left in a single, stable group.

In humans, two different forms of stress have received particular attention: major life events that tax one's abilities to adapt (e.g., getting divorced, moving, encountering financial difficulties, or being involved in a lawsuit) and minor, recurrent irritants and frustrations. Some studies of individuals undergoing major, stressful life events have found an association with the incidence of myocardial infarction, the development of CHD, or cardiac mortality, but other prospective studies have not. At present, the evidence remains inconclusive.

When turning to recurrent daily stresses, job strain and work-related pressures have received considerable attention. *Job strain* is defined as the combination of high demands with little autonomy or control over one's working conditions, routine, or schedule. Job strain has been associated with an increased risk of CHD in previously healthy people,[32] but its impact on the progress of already established CHD is less clear. Cross-sectional studies in the United States and Europe disclose that both men and women workers with high job strain have a higher prevalence of CHD and higher incidence of myocardial infarction than do those with low job strain. Longitudinal studies also provide some support for this hypothesis.[33,33a] In a longitudinal study of 12,517 Swedish men over a 14-year period, low levels of control over one's work conditions were an independent risk factor for cardiovascular disease mortality.[34] After adjusting for age, smoking, exercise, and social class, workers with low levels of control over their jobs had a relative risk of 1.83 for cardiovascular mortality. Workers with both low control over their work and low levels of social support had a relative risk of 2.62 for cardiovascular mortality. Marital stress has been found to exert a negative prognostic influence on CHD in women and may be even more important than job stress for women.[35]

SOCIODEMOGRAPHIC CHARACTERISTICS. Lower socioeconomic status (whether assessed by education, occupation, or income) prospectively predisposes healthy people to an increased risk of CHD and CHD patients to a poorer prognosis. The decline in cardiovascular disease mortality over the past 30 years in the United States has been more pronounced among those of higher socioeconomic status, and the reasons for this are not clear. Because beneficial health habits (including not smoking and weight control) tend to be associated with socioeconomic status, they may play a role. Poorer nutrition and difficulty obtaining medical care may contribute, and hostility and depression may be weakly inversely correlated with social position. Stressful life events, greater job strain, lack of social support, and diminished sense of self-control may mediate the relationship between socioeconomic status and CHD. There are also complex racial and ethnic differences in cardiovascular disease that remain poorly understood. Because race and ethnicity tend to be confounded with differences in socioeconomic position, it has been difficult to isolate their effects.

Acute Mental Stress

Acute mental stress has negative cardiovascular consequences. Cardiovascular mortality rises in the month following the death of a loved one, and the incidence of cardiac events rises immediately after natural disasters and among civilians subjected to military attack. The direct cardiovascular effects of acute mental stress have been observed during daily life and with laboratory paradigms of experimental stress. Experimental stress (induced, for example, by public speaking or accomplishing difficult intellectual tasks under time pressure or in frustrating circumstances) reliably increases heart rate, blood pressure, and myocardial oxygen demands. The effect of acute mental stress on the heart already damaged by preexisting CHD has been studied with relatively sensitive measures of myocardial ischemia such as regional myocardial perfusion and wall motion abnormalities. Such stress precipitates myocardial ischemia in 30 to 60 percent of CHD patients.[36]

Mental stress-induced ischemia occurs at lower heart rates and at a lower levels of myocardial work than does exercise-induced ischemia, suggesting that decreases in myocardial perfusion may play a role in mental stress-induced ischemia. In a representative study, 59 percent of CHD patients (and 8 percent of controls) exhibited wall motion abnormalities during periods of experimentally induced stress. One third of the CHD patients had a decrease of at least 5 percent in ejection fraction. Mental stress–induced ischemia is more likely to be "silent," or asymptomatic, than is ischemia induced by exercise. In the study just referred to, 83 percent of mental stress-induced ischemic episodes were asymptomatic.

When CHD patients are monitored during daily life, mental challenges unaccompanied by strenuous physical exertion are frequently associated with transient myocardial ischemia. Such ischemia has been observed, for example, while driving and during public speaking. Although most ischemic episodes during daily life do not appear to be precipitated by psychological or mental stress, a sizable minority (perhaps as many as one fourth) are.

CHD patients who exhibit mental stress-induced ischemia appear to be at increased risk of subsequent fatal and nonfatal cardiac events.[37] This relationship persists after other risk factors (including age, left ventricular function, and prior myocardial infarction) have been taken into account.

Acute stress may promote ischemic heart disease in a number of ways. First, stress increases myocardial oxygen demands as a result of its hemodynamic effects. Second, vasospasm may reduce coronary blood flow, especially in more severely diseased vessels. Third, the stress response increases circulating cortisol and catecholamines, which activate platelets and promote platelet aggregation and which increase cholesterol and decrease high-density lipoproteins. The net result of these actions is to increase cardiac demand while at the same time decreasing coronary blood supply and to promote plaque rupture and thrombus formation.

Sudden Emotion

The work on anger, depression, and anxiety discussed earlier deals with the long-term consequences and sequelae of enduring, persistent emotions. There is also a body of work on the immediate and acute effects of sudden, intense, negative emotion. Because much of this work focuses on arrhythmias and SCD, it will be reviewed in the next section. However, mental activities leading to intense anger or frustration and, to a lesser degree, to anxiety and sadness can trigger myocardial ischemia.[38] The relative risk for myocardial infarction in the 1 to 2 hours following an episode in which the patients report feeling very angry is between 2.3 and 9.[39] Because these intense, negative emotional states involve sympathetic arousal, they may act by triggering coronary vasospasm, rupture of atherosclerotic plaques, and increased platelet aggregation. Anger and hostility in particular have been associated with increased platelet adhesion.[40] Hostility is also associated with decreased parasympathetic arousal during ambulatory monitoring. When anger is experimentally induced, patients scoring higher on hostility scales exhibit greater sympathetic nervous system–mediated cardiovascular responses than those who are less hostile.[41]

Arrhythmias and Sudden Cardiac Death

Increasing evidence links mentally stressful and emotionally powerful events with lethal arrhythmias and SCD. Intense, overwhelming emotions such as fear and anger have been associated with both benign and lethal arrhythmias, including ventricular premature complexes, ventricular tachycardia, and ventricular fibrillation. This effect is most evident in hearts that are already diseased, ischemic, or electrically unstable. There are at least three lines of investigation into the arrhythmogenic potential of stress and intense emotion: retrospective case series of psychological distress immediately preceding lethal arrhythmias or SCD; psychophysiological experiments demonstrating that arrhythmias immediately follow sudden, intense emotion or acute stress; and investigations of the neural control of cardiac rate and rhythm.

OBSERVATIONAL STUDIES. has long been suspected that acutely stressful events and sudden, intense emotion can precipitate fatal arrhythmias and SCD, and there are many anecdotal case reports of SCD following immediately after severe psychological stress and intense emotional arousal. Careful psychiatric interviews of patients hospitalized after ventricular tachycardia or ventricular fibrillation revealed that 21 percent had undergone a major emotional disturbance or psychological trigger in the preceding 24 hours. These included interpersonal conflicts, bereavement, public humiliation, marital separation, and business losses. Studies like these suffer from retrospective bias and selective recall, inadequate or absent control groups, and sampling bias. When taken together, however, they nonetheless suggest that acute stress (perhaps in conjunction with other factors such as preexisting CHD) has the power on occasion to precipitate lethal arrhythmias and contribute to SCD.

STRESS AND ARRHYTHMIAS. Other research has probed the link between emotionally provocative daily stresses and arrhythmias. Healthy subjects manifest ventricular ectopy during driving, public speaking, and stressful interviews. Among cardiac patients undergoing ambulatory monitoring, daily life stresses are associated with ectopy. Experimentally induced psychological stress has been shown to lower the ventricular vulnerable period and the threshold for ventricular fibrillation and to increase the frequency of ventricular ectopic beats in patients with preexisting ventricular arrhythmias. Thus it is clear that stressful experiences and events can produce rhythm changes in both normal subjects and CHD patients. The clinical importance of this remains to be established, but the combination of severe, acute mental distress and a myocardium made vulnerable by preexisting disease can result in lethal arrhythmias and SCD.

The link between stress and arrhythmias has been explored in experimental animal work. When dogs are subjected to aversive restraint and electric shock, there is a 49 to 66 percent decrease in the repetitive extrasystole threshold. If a coronary artery occlusion is first produced experimentally, then the same stressful paradigm induces spontaneous ventricular fibrillation. Similarly, when pigs with a coronary artery occlusion are placed in a stressful environment, there is a high incidence of spontaneous ventricular fibrillation.

Some psychiatric disorders, particularly anxiety and depressive disorders, may predispose to SCD. The empirical evidence, however, remains scanty. In one study, psychiatric distress after myocardial infarction predicted ventricular arrhythmias in the year following the infarct, although subsequent work failed to confirm these findings. Depressed patients with CHD have an increased incidence of significant ventricular arrhythmias.[24] Post-myocardial infarction depression in particular has been linked to SCD, and much of its negative influence on cardiac mortality in patients with CHD is mediated through SCD. However, a number of methodological problems make this work difficult to interpret, and on balance the evidence at this time must be considered equivocal.

Sociocultural and sociodemographic factors may also play a role in SCD. The inverse relationship between socioeconomic status and cardiac mortality in general is especially robust for SCD, although this may well be confounded by an association between social position and access to emergency medical care. Other work has disclosed that cardiac mortality is significantly higher immediately after, as compared with immediately before, an important religious holiday. There are also well-recognized, culture-specific syndromes in which sudden death follows highly ritualized events with a powerful, culture-specific significance, such as "voodoo death."

NEURAL INFLUENCES ON RATE AND RHYTHM. A number of pathways mediate the neural control of heart rate and rhythm. First, activation of the hypothalamic-adrenomedullary axis increases myocardial irritability and decreases the threshold for inducing ventricular fibrillation. Second, direct sympathetic innervation of the heart exerts a proarrhythmic effect, increasing ventricular ectopy and lowering the threshold for inducing ventricular arrhythmias, especially in the heart with preexisting ischemic damage or electrical instability. Animal work provides evidence of cortical and brain stem influence over cardiac rhythm: Pathways run from the frontal cortex and hypothalamus to the brain stem nuclei controlling cardiovascular function. Thus, stimulation of the lateral and posterior hypothalamus lowers the ventricular fibrillation threshold, and blockade of these corticofrontal pathways raise it. In humans, electrocardiographic (ECG) changes in rhythm and/or repolarization are seen in patients suffering cerebrovascular accidents involving the cortex. Finally, extreme stress and acute psychological trauma can cause myocardial necrosis. In animal models, large quantities of catecholamines, either exogenously administered or stress induced, can result in myofibrillar degeneration and myocardial necrosis. On pathological examination, widespread calcification is found, the result of peroxidation of myocardial lipid membranes and blockage of the calcium-channel pump. This same lesion has also been reported in humans who died suddenly at the peak of extreme psychic stress and trauma.

Implantable cardioverter-defibrillators are increasingly used in the treatment of potentially lethal arrhythmias (see Chap. 31). Although these devices are medically efficacious and generally meet with a high degree of patient acceptance, in a substantial minority of patients (probably between 25 and 50 percent) the implantation of the device results in significant emotional distress (anxiety, depression, anger, withdrawal).[42]

Psychiatric and Behavioral Aspects of Hypertension and Heart Failure

Hypertension (see Chap. 37)

Stress, conditioned learning, and autonomic arousal all can elevate blood pressure. Stimulation of brain sites with connections to the sympathetic nervous system have a pressor effect, and many of these sites are in turn connected with higher centers involved in the perception of the environment. However, the transient elevations of blood pressure seen in stressful and provocative situations may be unrelated to the persistent, sustained elevation that constitutes the disease of hypertension.

STRESS AND BLOOD PRESSURE. Stressful environments and challenging or aversive situations transiently increase the blood pressure both of normotensive and hypertensive individuals. This has been demonstrated in field studies using ambulatory monitoring of blood pressure during daily life and in laboratory studies assessing blood pressure reactivity to a discrete stimulus or specific experimental stressor. Some individuals exhibit greater cardiovascular reactivity than others, consistently responding to psychological stressors with greater increases in blood pressure and heart rate, more vasoconstriction and catecholamine secretion, and a more prolonged recovery phase. These individual differences in cardiovascular reactivity emerge early in life and are thought to be stable and enduring. Such hyperreactivity to stress has long been believed to predispose the individual to the eventual development of hypertension (and atherosclerosis), but the empirical evidence remains inconclusive. Several large epidemiological surveys of initially normotensive individuals have found that exaggerated blood pressure responses to psychological and physical stress predict the subsequent development of essential hypertension on long-term follow-up.[43] However, a number of questions remain about the hypothesis that an exaggerated stress response predisposes individuals to hypertension: cardiovascular reactivity may vary over time; it may vary within the same individual depending on the nature of the stress; and it is not yet clear that transient blood pressure increases in response to such stressors are the precursors of pathological, sustained hypertension.

In surveys examining the relationship between naturally occurring stress and blood pressure, stress has been associated with the onset or worsening of essential hypertension. Job strain in particular has been associated with an elevated prevalence and incidence of hypertension in men (this is less clear in women), and the blood pressures of people in more stressful occupations tend to be higher than those in less stressful jobs. However, it appears that such chronic stress requires the co-occurrence of other etiological factors (e.g., genetic endowment, dietary factors, or psychological characteristics) to cause sustained hypertension. This situation may be analogous to that emerging from animal work: Repeated exposure to stress can lead to sustained hypertension in animals that are predisposed to hypertension by genetic endowment or salt ingestion, but not in healthy animals free of such predisposing factors.

PSYCHOLOGICAL STATES. Anger and anxiety are accompanied by increases in peripheral vascular resistance and blood pressure, and anger has long been thought to contribute to the development of essential hypertension. Hostile individuals respond to provocation, conflict, and disagreement with larger increases in blood pressure than people who are less hostile,[44] and there have been reports of higher levels of anger and suppressed anger among hypertensive patients.[45] Other studies, however have failed to detect an association between anger or aggression and hypertension.[46] The relationship between anger and hypertension may be stronger in some minority groups than in non-minorities. In sum, the evidence linking anger and hypertension remains equivocal. Recent work has focused on the more-difficult-to-measure construct of repressed or *suppressed* emotion (particularly anger), and there are reports of an association between emotional inhibition and essential hypertension. Although one meta-analysis concluded that there appears to be an association between suppressed anger and resting blood pressure, overall, this literature must still be considered inconclusive.

Other work has examined the role of anxiety. There is some evidence that chronically anxious persons develop greater increases in systolic blood pressure over the ensuing years and may also be at increased risk of developing essential hypertension.[47] However, although several prospective studies confirmed this association, others have not.[16,48] Finally, the possible etiological role of depression has also been investigated. The prevalence of hypertension is reported to be higher in depressed community residents, depressed medical patients, and depressed psychiatric patients than in nondepressed comparison groups. In a recent, large, population-based study, the symptoms of depression and anxiety were significantly associated with the development of hypertension, even after adjusting for sociodemographic characteristics, smoking and alcohol use, and blood pressure at inception.[49]

Based on this work, relaxation training, meditation, and blood pressure and heart rate biofeedback have been employed to treat hypertension. Relaxation techniques and meditation apparently decrease blood pressure by lowering total vasoconstrictor tone and peripheral resistance, but it is unclear to what degree the treatment effect persists after the discontinuation of active treatment. Several expert groups and consensus panels have concluded that the benefits of such psychological treatments for hypertension have not yet been conclusively demonstrated.[50] On the other hand, several meta-analyses suggest that they are beneficial.[51] For example, a recent, small, controlled trial of individualized stress management reported statistically significant and clinically meaningful reductions of systolic and diastolic blood pressure at 6-month follow-up.[52] Some of the confusion is because the empirical findings seem to vary depending on the study design, methods, and measurements. Although these behavioral techniques may not be very effective when used alone, they may provide some incremental benefit when used to augment conventional antihypertensive therapy, perhaps enabling the physician to lower the doses of antihypertensives. This is important since nonadherence to the antihypertensive medication regimen is common and constitutes a major impediment to effective treatment. Relaxation training, meditation, and biofeedback may be most suitable for those patients who report a subjective sense of stress in their lives and for those who are attracted to the idea of psychological treatments for medical conditions.[52]

SOCIOCULTURAL FACTORS. Epidemiological and animal studies suggest a relationship between high blood pressure and sociocultural conditions. Individuals in more crowded and stressful living and working environments tend to show increased levels of catecholamines, increased cardiovascular reactivity, and higher blood pressures. Essential hypertension tends to be less prevalent in societies with stronger cultural traditions and more commonly shared value systems, and in those that are safer and more stable, than in societies with more disintegration, higher crime rates, and less stable social orders. In societies undergoing transition, conflict, or disintegration, blood pressures tend to rise over time, but many factors (e.g., changes in diet) may be contributing. Animal studies seem to corroborate these findings: Mice subjected to crowding or exposed to repeated threat from cats develop sustained high blood pressure.

Heart Failure (see Chap. 22)

The psychiatric and behavioral aspects of congestive heart failure (CHF) have only recently been subjected to study. CHF patients report high levels of psychological distress and diminished quality of life.[53] It appears that the same sorts of psychosocial factors that affect the course and outcome of CHD also influence CHF. Stress and emotional distress have been linked to the onset and exacerbation of CHF, perhaps by increasing heart rate and blood pressure and/or by provoking myocardial ischemia in patients with preexisting CHD. It has been suggested that left ventricular function is impaired during psychological stress,[54] and stress-induced heart failure has been described. In patients with idiopathic cardiomyopathy, experimental psychological stress (mental arithmetic) has been shown to induce changes in left ventricular diastolic function.

Depression has received particular attention in CHF patients because of its high prevalence in the elderly and because it appears to worsen the medical outcome. Approximately one-fourth of patients hospitalized for CHF have major depression.[55-57] Depression is an independent predictor of hospital admission and of increased medical care utilization in CHF.[56,58] It may also predict subsequent mortality.[55,56] Depression may also predispose to the development of CHF; in a prospective study of 2500 elderly community residents who were initially free of heart failure, depression at inception independently increased the risk of developing CHF in women, but not in men, over a 14-year follow-up period.[59] Research in this area is complicated by difficulty in differentiating the symptoms of CHF from those of depressive disorder. The anorexia, fatigue, weakness, and insomnia (resulting from orthopnea and paroxysmal nocturnal dyspnea) accompanying CHF can be confused with the symptoms of depression, and the cardiac cachexia of end-stage CHF may also suggest severe depression. When CHF is severe enough to cause cerebral ischemia, then cognitive dysfunction, confusion, and delirium with psychotic symptoms may result. This may at times be difficult to distinguish from anxiety disorder and panic.

Social support is an important moderator of the clinical course of CHF. Elderly women hospitalized with CHF who were without sources of emotional support had a more than threefold increase in the risk of cardiovascular events in the ensuing year than comparable patients with emotional support.[60] Elderly men without emotional support were not at increased risk. Social isolation was also found to be a significant predictor of mortality in CHF patients over a 2-year follow-up period, while controlling for depression, age, and disease severity.[60a]

Cardiac Symptoms: Chest Pain and Palpitations

Chest Pain (see Chaps. 7 and 45)

Chest pain, the classic symptom of CHD, is a nonspecific, insensitive, and unreliable indicator of ischemia. Pain does not bear a fixed, one-to-one relationship to demonstrable pathology; many patients with chest pain have no heart disease, and conversely, ischemia and infarction are often asymptomatic. Approximately one-fourth of myocardial infarctions are silent, and 70 to 80 percent of out-of-hospital, ischemic episodes in CHD patients are asymptomatic. Conversely, no cardiac cause can be found to explain most complaints of chest pain. Even in patients with documented CHD, two-thirds of chest pain episodes occur in the absence of ST segment depression indicative of ischemia, and approximately one-third of revascularized patients continue to have chest pain. Even among patients undergoing coronary angiography for chest pain, 10 to 30 percent have minimal or no angiographic evidence of CHD.

The absence of demonstrable heart disease does not mean that the patient's chest pain is either inconsequential or self-limited. Follow-up studies of chest pain patients with negative angiography and/or negative exercise stress testing reveal persistent distress and disability and a generally poor response to conventional antiischemic therapy. Although rates of myocardial infarction and of cardiac morbidity and mortality remain low, these patients continue to exhibit elevated levels of symptoms, disability, and medical care utilization. At least half continue to report recurrent chest pain, the persistent belief that they have serious heart disease, and impaired functioning (at work, socially, and in daily activities), at levels that are comparable to that of patients with CHD.

Psychological, psychiatric, and behavioral factors mediate some of this variance in symptoms among CHD patients. Thus, emotional distress is highly correlated with reports of chest pain in both those with and without CHD.[13] Mood and daily activities may account for as much of the variability in ambulatory patients' reports of chest pain as does ST depression indicative of ischemia.[61] Several psychological factors differentiate chest pain patients with and without demonstrable cardiac disease. Generalized psychological distress and body awareness is higher in patients with chest pain and normal coronary arteries than in chest pain patients with CHD. When those with normal angiography or normal stress tests are compared to those with positive tests, the former group is younger, more likely to be female, somatizes more, and has more psychological distress and a higher prevalence of diagnosable psychiatric disorder. Patients with medically unexplained chest pain, when compared to chest pain patients with abnormal angiographic findings have elevated rates of panic disorder (~35 to 50 percent vs. 5 percent) and of major depression (~35 to 40 percent vs. 5 to 8 percent). Of course, cardiac and psychiatric disorders are not mutually exclusive and therefore not infrequently co-occur. Thus, 5 to 23 percent of patients with angiographic evidence of CHD also have panic disorder. These cases of psychiatric and cardiac comorbidity pose especially difficult diagnostic dilemmas, and it is in these patients that panic disorder is most likely to be overlooked. The chest pain seen in panic disorder is more likely to be atypical in clinical character and to be accompanied by palpitations, dizziness, paresthesias, and multiple other somatic symptoms.

Palpitations (see Chap. 29)

Palpitations are among the most common symptoms encountered in medical practice, reported by 16 percent of primary care patients. Yet this subjective sensation corresponds poorly to demonstrable abnormalities of cardiac rate or rhythm. Most palpitations are not accompanied by arrhythmias, and most arrhythmias are not perceived and reported as palpitations. When patients complaining of palpitations undergo 24-hour, ambulatory ECG monitoring, 39 to 85 percent manifest a rhythm disturbance (most being benign and clinically insignificant). Approximately three-fourths of these patients with arrhythmias report at least one palpitation during 24 hours of monitoring, but in less than 15 percent of them are their symptoms coincident with the arrhythmia. Thus, accurate symptom reports occur in less than 10 percent of all patients being monitored.

A high proportion of patients with palpitations either have a psychiatric cause for their symptom or no etiology can be established. In a careful survey of 190 patients presenting with palpitations, 31 percent were judged to have a psychiatric basis for their presenting symptom and no etiology could be established in an additional 16 percent. The most common psychiatric cause of palpitations is panic disorder, found in more than one-fourth of ambulatory medical patients complaining of palpitations. In one study, 31 percent of 229 such patients had panic disorder or panic attacks, and in another study, 28 percent of patients complaining of palpitations had lifetime panic disorder and 19 percent had current panic disorder.

Palpitations that have no demonstrable cardiac basis may nonetheless be persistent and disturbing. In an observational 1-year follow-up study, 75 percent of palpitation patients reported recurrent symptoms, 19 percent reported impairment of their work performance, and 37 percent reported impairment in their role functioning at home. In another study, 84 percent of palpitation patients remained symptomatic 6 months after initially presenting and had an elevated rate of medical care utilization.

Panic attacks and arrhythmias may be difficult to distinguish clinically. Both may present as palpitations, shortness of breath, and light-headedness, and both not infrequently occur in those who are young and otherwise healthy. Frank syncope, however, is unusual in panic disorder, and if there have been multiple episodes, panic attacks are more stereotyped and more consistent from episode to episode. Recurrent panic attacks tend to lead to agoraphobia, in which the patient first becomes apprehensive about, and then avoids, being left alone, trapped in large crowds, and journeying far from home. Conversely, to make matters more difficult, the sympathetic arousal that may accompany an arrhythmia (and other acute cardiac events such as pulmonary emboli, acute valvular dysfunction, and myocardial ischemia as well) may be experienced and reported by the patient as acute anxiety or panic rather than as a cardiac event.

Delay and Denial of Cardiac Symptoms

Myocardial infarction patients commonly rationalize, ignore, or deny their symptoms, so that the average interval between the onset of symptoms and arrival in an emergency department is between 3 and 9 hours. Such delay poses a serious problem since a high proportion of myocardial infarction deaths occur soon after the event, and the newer therapies to preserve myocardial tissue require early intervention (see Chap. 47). Delay is greater in women and in the elderly[62] and (paradoxically) in those with a history of previous myocardial infarction.[63] A crucial determinant of the extent of delay is the length of time before the myocardial infarction sufferer informs another person of his or her symptoms; once the patient tells someone else, medical attention is usually obtained promptly.

Psychiatric Care of the Cardiac Patient

Acute Care of the Hospitalized Patient

ANXIETY. The onset or sudden progression of cardiac disease is terrifying. Pain and physical discomfort, the specter of sudden death or prolonged invalidism, and the knowledge that one has a chronic and potentially lethal disease all are profoundly distressing. The initial reaction is almost always one of anxiety. Fears of premature and sudden death loom, and worries about physical, sexual, social, and occupational incapacity materialize and plague patients. They may become terrified of any physical activity or strong emotion, fearing that these will trigger sudden death. As time passes, anxiety may be replaced with despondency and a heightened sense of physical vulnerability and of one's mortality. The individual may come to feel useless, damaged, or diminished. Patients may believe that their job performance and future livelihood have been irrevocably compromised, that they have become worn out and decrepit, and that they face a meager and empty future. They may feel guilty and blame themselves for falling ill, ascribing their plight to their failure to exercise enough, diet sufficiently, or maintain other "healthy" habits. All of this may presage a clinically significant, depressive episode.

Several psychiatric and behavioral problems commonly arise in patients while they are hospitalized for an acute cardiac event. The hospitalization itself (in particular, admission to the coronary care or intensive care unit) can be frightening and stressful. Patients suddenly find themselves in an unfamiliar, alien and frightening world, surrounded by fearsome machines with blinking lights and beeping alarms, subjected to painful procedures and tests about which they know little and understand less, while their lives seemingly hang in the balance from moment to moment. They are cut off from family, friends, neighbors, and all that is familiar. Sustained sleep is next to impossible, and many are afraid to fall asleep believing that the heart is in greater jeopardy during sleep. Their worst fears are substantiated if they witness the death or cardiac arrest of another patient.

Hospitalized patients should be kept well informed about what is transpiring, what is being done medically for them, and why. They should be told what to expect before procedures are carried out; the functions of equipment should be explained; and the effects and (especially) side effects of medications should be described in advance. The patient should be reassured that anxiety is a normal and entirely appropriate reaction. Early and frequent family visitation generally helps the patient to feel supported. Anxiolytics are often prescribed because anxiety is not only uncomfortable but its concomitant sympathetic arousal can be medically dangerous. Benzodiazepines are most commonly used for this purpose and should be prescribed on a regular, round-the-clock (rather than as-needed) basis. In the elderly and in those with compromised liver function, the shorter-acting benzodiazepines (e.g., oxazepam or lorazepam) are preferred, because they are cleared primarily by the kidney. The pharmacology of anxiolytics is discussed in the following section.

DELIRIUM AND COGNITIVE IMPAIRMENT. Delirium is frequent in hospitalized cardiac patients, especially following cardiac surgery. The delirious patient is confused, disoriented to time and place, has impaired memory and attention, has delusional ideas, and experiences perceptual disturbances such as illusions or hallucinations. The sleep-wake cycle is disrupted, and the level of consciousness and arousal is disturbed, so that the patient may be either stuporous and obtunded, or hyperalert and agitated. The onset of delirium may be insidious (e.g., insomnia, mild nocturnal confusion, and restlessness) and go unnoticed by the staff, or it may be dramatic and abrupt. The patient begins to misinterpret sensory information (e.g., mistaking a shadow for someone lurking in a corner of his or her room) and becomes suspicious and increasingly frightened. As confusion, fear, and excitement mount, frank paranoia sets in and the patient may become agitated, disruptive, belligerent, and out of control. This is a psychiatric emergency, because in their confusion and frenzy, delirious patients may harm themselves accidentally, fall, or pull out therapeutic life-lines, catheters, and implanted devices. The incidence of delirium after cardiac surgery is between 10 and 30 percent,[64] typically following a lucid interval of 3 to 5 days following surgery. The risk factors for postcardiotomy delirium are advanced age (>70 years of age); more extensive aortic atherosclerosis (large atheromas may be liberated by surgical manipulation of the aorta); a prior history of neurological disease, particularly preexisting cerebrovascular disease; a history of pulmonary disease, with the concomitant risks of poorer cerebral oxygenation and more hypoxia; and higher doses of narcotics and sedatives.[65]

Treatment of Delirium. This rests on rapid identification and correction of its underlying cause, medication for behavioral control if necessary, and supportive measures to provide comfort and safety. The etiological search is paramount. This means checking for cerebral hypoperfusion or hypoxia, acid-base disturbance, inadequate hydration, fluid and electrolyte imbalance, renal or hepatic failure, endocrine dysfunction, infection, and nutritional deficiency. Alcohol or drug withdrawal is a frequent cause, and the history must be searched carefully with this possibility in mind. Medications must be carefully reviewed because anticholinergics, narcotics, sedative-hypnotics, and H_2 blockers are common causes of delirium. Common offenders include cimetidine, digoxin, aminophylline, anticonvulsants, and all sedatives and hypnotics.

If the patient is agitated, disruptive, or confused enough to require behavioral control, high-potency antipsychotic drugs can be administered. Haloperidol has been widely used for this purpose and is safe and effective in critically ill patients, whether given orally or parenterally (including intravenously in emergency situations). Mild, delirious agitation is treated with 0.5 to 2 mg of haloperidol, moderate delirium with 5 to 10 mg; and the severely delirious patient can be given 10 or more mg of haloperidol. If the agitation persists unabated after 20 to 30 minutes, twice the original dose may be readministered. It has a minimal effect on heart rate, blood pressure, and respiration, and extrapyramidal effects are rare when it is administered intravenously. Parenteral droperidol is sometimes used. If excitement, hyperarousal, and motor agitation are especially prominent, the antipsychotic may be supplemented with a short-acting benzodiazepine such as lorazepam. The newer, "atypical" antipsychotics are increasingly used to treat delirium.[66] They appear to be safe and effective but have not yet been studied definitively. Antipsychotic agents are discussed in the following section.

Supportive measures should be undertaken to calm, orient, and comfort the delirious patient. He or she should be reoriented frequently by the staff, and a clock and calendar should be prominently displayed to aid in this process. It is helpful to preserve as much of a normal day-night cycle as is feasible considering the hospital routine. Family visitation should be encouraged because it is helpful in reassuring and calming the patient and in reducing paranoia. Familiar objects, such as family photographs, should be prominently displayed and plainly visible. Staff need to continually reintroduce themselves, educate the patient about what they are doing, and repeatedly explain the situation. Physical restraint should be employed whenever necessary to prevent self-harm or harm to the staff.

Longer-term cognitive changes also occur following cardiac surgery. These often involve memory, arithmetic skills, and the sequencing of complex actions. Neurocognitive testing of patients following CABG disclosed cognitive decline in 53 percent at discharge, 36 percent at 6 weeks, and in 24 percent of patients 6 months after discharge.[67] This study lacked a noncardiac surgery comparison group, however.

Convalescence and Recovery after Hospitalization

In the weeks and months after hospital discharge, depression is common. It is often self-limited, gradually diminishing as the patient resumes his or her old activities and as the specter of the acute episode and the hospitalization recede into the past. Frank discussion of the patient's concerns and specific information about common myths and fears are helpful. Lingering anxiety may lead patients to avoid activities or situations that they fear will provoke symptoms or even sudden death. Early, progressive mobilization is the best antidote. The patient may be dismayed by the degree of exhaustion resulting from even mild exertion, and although this easy fatigability is actually the result of deconditioning, it is mistakenly interpreted as evidence of permanent cardiac damage. As a result, exercise may be assiduously avoided, further exacerbating the problem.

Patients are often apprehensive about returning to work because of the stress it engenders. Many believe that strong emotions can be lethal and try to protect themselves by assiduously avoiding all situations or activities that arouse strong feelings, such as sexual activity or watching sports on television. Sexual activity in particular is diminished, and sexual dysfunction is common in both women and men with cardiac disease. Such concerns should be elicited by the physician and then discussed frankly and openly. Recommendations about proscribed and prescribed activities should be as specific as possible; simply saying "use your judgment" or "do it in moderation" is not helpful. Group meetings in which cardiac patients share common concerns, provide mutual support, obtain educational information, and guide the progressive resumption of activities are helpful.

TREATMENT. If depression lasts more than several weeks and meets diagnostic criteria for major depressive disorder, as happens in one-third or more of patients in the year after myocardial infarction,[9] pharmacotherapy is indicated. If left untreated, depression imposes a serious psychosocial burden, medical rehabilitation and recovery are impeded, and the depression itself is likely to become chronic. Because of this, and its negative effect on cardiac outcomes, increasing emphasis is being placed on the prompt detection and treatment of post-myocardial infarction depression. The Sertraline Antidepressant Heart Attack Randomized Trial (SADHART) was a double-blind, randomized, placebo-controlled trial of a selective serotonin reuptake inhibitor (SSRI) for major depressive disorder in patients hospitalized for myocardial infarction or unstable angina. At 6-month follow-up, when compared with placebo, the more severely depressed patients who received active drug were less depressed, although the less severely depressed patients did not show a treatment effect. There was a 20 percent reduction in life-threatening cardiac events (including nonfatal myocardial infarction and death) among those on active drug, but this difference in cardiac outcomes was not statistically significant due to the number of patients in the trial. In a case-controlled study of smokers hospitalized for myocardial infarction, SSRI administration was associated with a lowered risk of recurrent myocardial infarction, suggesting that treatment of depression may reduce its negative prognostic influence on cardiac outcomes.[68] Thus it remains to be definitively demonstrated that the treatment of depression following myocardial infarction significantly improves cardiac outcomes. The pharmacotherapy of depression is discussed in the following section.

Interest in psychosocial interventions for depression and/or social isolation has also been high. In one study of 435 post-myocardial infarction patients, a nursing-based psychosocial intervention reduced 1-year cardiac mortality, and the incidence of recurrent myocardial infarction was significantly lower at 7-year follow-up. However, two subsequent, large, randomized trials of multimodal interventions delivered by nurses or health visitors failed to improve depression or cardiac outcomes.[69] In the Montreal Heart Attack Readjustment Trial (M-HART), a supportive and educational home nursing intervention was provided to the most psychologically distressed post-myocardial infarction patients. This rather limited intervention was compared to usual care. At 1-year follow-up, the intervention had no effect on psychological distress and no overall effect on cardiac mortality, while it was actually associated with a *higher* mortality rate among women.[70] However, a subgroup analysis revealed that those patients whose psychological distress did improve with treatment did have more favorable long-term cardiac outcomes.[71] In the Enhancing Recovery in Coronary Heart Disease (ENRICHD), 2500 recent myocardial infarction patients with depression and/or low social support randomly received either cognitive behavior therapy (and SSRI antidepressants if indicated) or care as usual. Preliminary results suggest that there was no benefit in terms of cardiac outcomes or mortality, and outcomes appear worse for women. At the least, one can safely conclude from these studies that when the psychosocial treatment fails to improve depression (because the patient population is not sufficiently depressed or the treatment is not effective enough), then it does not improve cardiac outcomes. There is also a suggestion that women may benefit less from these psychosocial interventions in terms of cardiac outcomes than men.

Over the long term, some cardiac patients adopt a persistent coping style that is maladaptive and dysfunctional. They may ignore and deny their illness entirely, maintaining that nothing serious has happened at all. They may refuse to acknowledge any limitations or adhere to a therapeutic regimen and generally overdo things. Alternatively, they may capitulate completely to their illness and retreat into unwarranted invalidism, becoming "cardiac cripples" who are preoccupied with their health, terrified by every benign twinge or cramp, and living a life of psychological invalidism and disability. Each of these profoundly maladaptive coping patterns deserves psychotherapeutic attention.

Cardiac Rehabilitation Programs (see Chap. 43)

Cardiac rehabilitation programs seek to modify biobehavioral risk factors and retard the progression of the disease. These psychosocial, educational, and behavioral programs include various components. Almost all emphasize a formal program of graduated, progressive, aerobic exercise. Most assist patients in smoking cessation, curtailing alcohol abuse, lowering saturated fat intake, and controlling weight.

Most cardiac rehabilitation programs also include psychosocial interventions.[72] These involve the identification of psychosocial stressors and problems (depression, anxiety, anger, social isolation), individual or group counseling to deal with them, and instruction in stress reduction and stress management. The latter often entails relaxation training, which generally combines elements of progressive muscle relaxation, diaphragmatic breathing, and the use of calming mental imagery.

It is difficult to evaluate the effectiveness of these heterogeneous psychotherapeutic, psychosocial, and behavioral programs because they vary so widely in quality, content, design, and intensity. Many intervention trials are flawed by small sample size, high dropout rates, lack of randomization, insufficient long-term follow-up, and inadequate comparison or control groups. In addition, as standard cardiac care improves so substantially, it becomes more difficult to demonstrate the incremental benefit of these programs in terms of hard cardiac endpoints. Nonetheless, there are now a substantial number of intervention trials and several careful meta-analyses assessing the incremental benefit of adding a specific psychosocial component to cardiac rehabilitation programs. These studies generally indicate that, when compared to rehabilitation programs without such components, these programs further reduce psychological distress and anxiety and depressive symptoms, and improve coping skills and quality of life.[72] The empirical evidence also suggests that they lead to significantly lower rates of cardiac death and nonfatal, recurrent myocardial infarction.[73,74] When these psychological interventions have been found ineffective against cardiac endpoints, they have at the same time failed to lower psychosocial distress, depression, and anxiety.[74] The cardiac benefits of psychosocial treatment generally seem less clear for women and perhaps for older patients as well.

Psychopharmacology in the Cardiac Patient

Cardiovascular Aspects of Psychotropic Agents

ANTIDEPRESSANTS (Table 84–1)

Selective Serotonin Reuptake Inhibitors. The SSRIs have superseded the tricyclic antidepressants (TCAs) as the first-line agents for treating the cardiac patient with major depressive disorder. Their efficacy is comparable to that of the older TCAs; they are better tolerated, safer in overdose, and have less pharmacological action on the heart. The data thus far suggest that the SSRIs have minimal cardiovascular effects and a large margin of safety in treating patients with even very severe heart disease.[75] The SSRIs have little anticholinergic, antihistaminic, or noradrenergic activity and appear to inhibit platelet aggregation.

In healthy patients, the SSRIs have no adverse effects on cardiac contractility or conduction and there is no evidence of cardiotoxicity in overdose. In cardiac populations, they do not appear to cause significant ECG or blood pressure changes, although they can slow heart rate. Only rarely do they produce a clinically significant degree of sinus bradycardia. Because the SSRIs interfere with platelet aggregation, they can increase bleeding time. The SSRIs do have the potential to interact with a number of medications used in cardiac patients. They inhibit hepatic cytochrome P450 isoenzymes,[76] a series of isoenzymes involved in the oxidative metabolism of many drugs. These include lipophilic beta blockers (e.g., metoprolol and propranolol), calcium-channel blockers, type IC antiarrhythmics, angiotensin-converting enzyme (ACE) inhibitors, anticonvulsants, antihistamines, benzodiazepines, TCAs, codeine, and warfarin. The SSRIs therefore can raise the blood levels of these other agents when coadministered. Caution should be exercised when giving SSRIs to patients on these medications, and in particular the prothrombin time of patients receiving both warfarin and an SSRI should be monitored closely. Because the SSRIs are highly protein bound, they may displace other protein-bound drugs when coadministered, thereby increasing their bioavailability. This interaction can occur with warfarin and digitoxin, but it does not appear to be clinically significant in magnitude.

Tricyclic Antidepressants. TCAs were previously the mainstay of antidepressant pharmacotherapy and remain effective agents that are still widely employed. However, their multiple cardiovascular side effects and their potential lethality in overdose are disadvantages in patients with cardiac disease. TCAs act on adrenergic and serotoninergic neurons in the central nervous system and, in the periphery, have anticholinergic properties. They also have quinidine-like effects and produce alpha-adrenergic receptor blockade. They affect heart rate, rhythm, conduction, contractility, and blood pressure. Accordingly, these agents are not generally used in the presence of rhythm or conduction disturbances, severe CHF, or within 4 to 6 weeks of a myocardial infarction. Among the TCAs, the tertiary amines (e.g., imipramine and amitriptyline) are associated with more side effects, and the secondary amines (e.g., nortriptyline) have a preferable side effect profile in cardiac patients.[77]

The TCAs are type IA antiarrhythmic agents (see Chap. 30) and accordingly depress cardiac conduction, decrease ventricular irritability, and suppress ectopic activity. They slow atrial and ventricular depolarization; increase the QT, PR, and QRS intervals; and decrease T wave amplitude. In the absence of preexisting conduction abnormalities, this action is unlikely to be clinically significant at therapeutic doses. However, second-degree heart block, sick sinus syndrome, bundle branch block, a prolonged QT interval, and the concurrent administration of antiarrhythmic agents all are considered contraindications to their use. In contrast to this antiarrhythmic effect, the TCAs can on occasion be arrhythmogenic, probably by virtue of their prolongation of the QT interval and/or an increase in myocardial norepinephrine resulting from their peripheral inhibition of norepinephrine reuptake. Although the most common such arrhythmias are atrial and ventricular premature beats, these may give way to more malignant ventricular arrhythmias. These toxic, proarrhythmic effects are seen primarily in overdose, and are more likely in those with preexisting CHD, a prolonged QT interval, electrical instability, or a recent myocardial infarction. The TCAs also elevate heart rate 5 to 20 beats/min as a result of their anticholinergic blockade. Although this does not pose a problem in relatively healthy patients, it may be a consideration in those with heart disease.

TCAs produce postural hypotension in up to 20 percent of patients. In the elderly, in whom orthostatic hypotension can produce cerebral hypoperfusion and lead to falls and fractures, this side effect can be crucial. Blood pressure and pulse should be monitored for signs of orthostasis in patients treated with TCAs, especially when initiating treatment and when adjusting the dose. Elderly patients should be advised to stand up slowly after lying or sitting for prolonged periods. The magnitude of this effect is related to the magnitude of pretreatment orthostatic hypotension, and it is more likely to be clinically significant in patients with CHF, impaired left ventricular function, or volume depletion or who are taking antihypertensive medications. Caution is indicated when treating patients with poor ejection fractions because in animal studies TCAs exert a depressant effect on myocardial contractility, although in humans this effect is evident only at toxic doses and only rarely aggravates CHF.

Other Antidepressants. *Bupropion*, a non-TCA that acts on both the dopamine and norepinephrine systems, causes less hypotension than the TCAs; does not affect cardiac conduction or contractility; and is safely used in patients with cardiac disease. It does not exacerbate ventricular arrhythmias or conduction block in patients with these conditions. An additional benefit of bupropion in cardiac patients is that it is apparently effective in smoking cessation. An increased incidence of seizures is seen at higher doses, and bupropion may occasionally elevate blood pressure and heart rate, though rarely to a clinically significant degree. Because it inhibits the cytochrome P450 isoenzymes, bupropion can raise the levels of beta blockers and type 1C antiarrhythmics when administered concurrently.

Venlafaxine affects the reuptake of both serotonin and norepinephrine. It appears to have few cardiovascular actions and no effect on the ECG.[78] At higher doses venlafaxine has been associated with an elevation in blood pressure and pulse. Unlike the SSRIs, it does not inhibit cytochrome P450

TABLE 84–1 Antidepressants

Agent	Starting Dose	Maximum Dose	Side Effects		Cardiovascular Effects
Serotonin Reuptake Inhibitors					
Sertraline	12.5-25 mg/d	200 mg/d	Sexual dysfunction Nausea, diarrhea,headache, anxiety, agitation, insomnia, somnolence, sedation, tremor		Benign bradycardia
Fluoxetine	5-10 mg/d	80 mg/d			
Paroxetine	10 mg/d	50 mg/d			
Tricyclics					
Amitriptyline	10-25 mg h.s.	300 mg/d	Sedation, somnolence	Dry mouth Blurry vision Constipation Urinary retention Postural hypotension Weight gain	Increased QT, PR, QRS intervals Decreased T wave amplitude Tachycardia Arrhythmias Postural hypotension
Imipramine	10-25 mg h.s.	300 mg/d			
Nortriptyline	10 mg/d	150 mg/d	Anxiety, insomnia		
Desipramine	25 mg/d	300 mg/d			
Psychostimulants					
Methylphenidate	2.5 mg b.i.d.	20 mg b.i.d.	Anxiety, agitation Insomnia Anorexia Paranoia		Tachycardia (mild) Hypertension (mild)
Other Agents					
Bupropion	75 mg/d	150 mg t.i.d.	Anorexia, nausea Anxiety, agitation Insomnia Seizures		
Venlafaxine	25 mg b.i.d.	125 mg t.i.d.	Nausea Headache Sexual dysfunction Anxiety, insomnia Somnolence Dizziness		Hypertension (dose related) Tachycardia (dose related)
Trazodone	25 mg/d	300 mg b.i.d.	Sedation Nausea Headache Priapism (rare)		Postural hypotension
Mirtazapine	15 mg q.h.s.	45 mg q.h.s.	Sedation, somnolence Weight gain Dry mouth, anticholinergic effects Dizziness Agranulocytosis (rare)		Tachycardia (mild)

isoenzymes and is not highly protein bound; it may therefore be useful in patients on cardiac medications.

Trazodone, a triazolopyridine antidepressant, is often used in low doses as a hypnotic. Cardiovascular complications from trazodone are rare. It has few, if any, antiarrhythmic properties, although it has rarely been associated with heart block and ventricular arrhythmias. Because of its weak alpha-adrenergic blockade, it may also produce orthostatic hypotension. Nefazodone, a closely related drug, can also occasionally produce orthostatic hypotension and has significant P450 isoenzyme inhibition, and it can therefore increase the levels of concurrently administered calcium-channel blockers, quinidine, and lidocaine.

Mirtazapine is a tetracyclic antidepressant with a complex mechanism of action. It has not been studied in patients with cardiovascular disease, but in noncardiac populations it does not affect blood pressure or cardiac conduction. It has no anticholinergic activity, but it may increase heart rate slightly.[78a]

Psychostimulants such as dextroamphetamine and methylphenidate are used to treat depression in medically compromised and elderly patients. These agents tend to be used when depression is life threatening, when immediate treatment response is crucial (because they have a rapid onset of action), and in depressions with prominent anergia and apathy. Although there is considerable clinical support for their use, empirical evidence of their sustained efficacy over time is lacking. Serious cardiovascular side effects such as tachycardia, hypertension, and arrhythmias are relatively rare, but caution must be exercised when administering these medications to patients with significant hypertension, tachycardia, or ventricular ectopy, and blood pressure and heart rate should be monitored.

NEUROLEPTICS (Table 84–2). Neuroleptic or antipsychotic drugs are used in the treatment of schizophrenia, organic psychoses, and mood disorders that are refractory or have psychotic features. They are also widely used for agitation, confusion, excitement, and behavioral dyscontrol in geriatric patients. Neuroleptic drugs generally affect cardiac conduction and rhythm and produce hypotension. They have alpha-adrenergic blocking and quinidine-like properties, along with anticholinergic activity. They can produce prolongation of the PR and QT intervals, ST segment depression, T wave changes, ventricular arrhythmias, and heart block. Increasing attention has been devoted to their potential to increase the QT interval, leading in rare instances to torsades de pointes. *Thioridazine* is most frequently implicated in this

TABLE 84–2 Neuroleptic (Antipsychotic) Agents

Agent	Starting Dose	Maximum Dose	Side Effects	Cardiovascular Effects
Haloperidol	0.5 mg/d	>10 mg q.i.d.	Akathisia Dystonia Parkinsonism Tardive dyskinesia Neuroleptic malignant syndrome Rash Anticholinergic effects	Tachycardia QT interval prolongation Torsades de pointes
Clozapine	12.5 mg q.h.s. or b.i.d.	200-300 mg t.i.d.	Dizziness Somnolence Weight gain Hypersalivation Seizures Agranulocytosis Anticholinergic effects	Tachycardia Postural hypotension
Olanzapine	2.5-5 mg/d	20 mg/d	Sedation Constipation Weight gain Seizures Akathisia Extrapyramidal symptoms	Postural hypotension (mild) QT interval prolongation
Risperidone	0.25-0.5 mg/d	>6 mg/d	Somnolence Fatigue Nausea, diarrhea Weight gain Sexual dysfunction Nasal congestion Extrapyramidal symptoms	Hypotension QT interval prolongation Tachycardia

respect.[79] Although the quinidine-like effects of the neuroleptics are usually negligible, they can become significant in patients already taking type I antiarrhythmics or in those with hypokalemia or with clinically significant conduction delays. When administering a low-potency neuroleptic along with an antiarrhythmic, the ECG should be monitored for conduction delays. The lower potency neuroleptics produce more orthostatic hypotension (by means of alpha-adrenergic blockade) and tachycardia (by means of anticholinergic action), and this is of particular concern in the elderly and in the acute myocardial infarction patient.[80] Orthostasis is more likely to be a problem when these agents are combined with antihypertensives.

The higher potency neuroleptic agents, such as *haloperidol* and the piperazine phenothiazines, produce less of these effects and are therefore preferred in the presence of significant cardiac disease (especially conduction problems) and after cardiac surgery. Haloperidol in particular has been frequently used with safety and efficacy in severely ill cardiac patients. Oral haloperidol does not significantly affect the ECG, and intravenous haloperidol is used in acute emergencies such as agitated deliria. Administration can on rare occasions result in torsades de pointes and even SCD, and the QT interval should therefore be monitored during aggressive intravenous haloperidol therapy.

Experience with the newer "atypical" antipsychotics in cardiac patients is much more limited but suggests a generally similar profile. *Clozapine* can cause tachycardia and orthostatic hypotension and has significant anticholinergic activity (along with a risk of myelosuppression and agranulocytosis). There are reports of an infrequent association of clozapine with myocarditis and cardiomyopathy.[81] This risk is greatest in the first month of therapy.[82] *Olanzapine* produces mild orthostatic hypotension but has little effect on the ECG. *Risperidone* produces hypotension and has a quinidine-like effect, prolonging the QT interval, although this may not be of clinical significance. *Ziprasidone* has been associated with QT prolongation and is not recommended in patients with recent myocardial infarction, heart failure, QT prolongation, or arrhythmias. Thus it is clear that the new atypical neuroleptics, like the phenothiazines and haloperidol, can prolong QT interval.[79] However, the relationship to torsades de pointes and SCD is less clear since the tendency to prolong the QT interval is not closely associated with the tendency to cause torsades de pointes.[79] Recently, concern with atypical antipsychotics has focused on the incidence of new-onset diabetes and increased glucose levels in patients with preexisting diabetes, on hyperlipidemia, and on the weight gain seen in patients on these agents.

MOOD STABILIZERS (Table 84–3)

Lithium. Lithium exerts minimal cardiotoxicity at therapeutic doses in most patients and can be used safely in cardiac disease if initiated at a low dose, increased gradually, and monitored carefully. Clinically significant, cardiovascular side effects of lithium are rare; they may include sinus node dysfunction and increases in ventricular irritability. Benign, reversible T wave changes (including inversion and flattening) are common with lithium administration and are not clinically significant. The major toxic effects of lithium are neural (confusion, sedation), and the primary concern in cardiac patients is lithium toxicity resulting from decreased renal clearance or hypovolemia. This is of concern in patients with CHF, and it is exacerbated by their diuretics and restricted sodium intake. Sodium depletion decreases renal clearance of lithium. In the kidney, lithium is filtered out at the glomerulus and then reabsorbed in the proximal tubules. Sodium depletion, such as with diuretics, causes an increased proximal reabsorption of sodium, and lithium is reabsorbed more efficiently at the same time. A given lithium dose thus results in a higher blood level. Lithium may still be administered to the patient on diuretics, but levels must be monitored and dosage may need to be reduced. The elderly also require lower lithium doses because of a decline in the glomerular filtration rate. On rare occasion, lithium may worsen arrhythmias in patients with sinus node dysfunction.

TABLE 84–3 Mood Stabilizers

Agent	Staring Dose	Maximum Dose	Side Effects	Cardiovascular Effects
Lithium	300 mg b.i.d.	2100 mg/d (titrate against serum concentration)	Drowsiness, sedation Confusion Nausea, diarrhea Metallic taste Polyuria/polydipsia Tremor Hypothyroidism	T wave inversion or flattening Sinus node dysfunction Ventricular irritability
Carbamazepine	100 mg b.i.d.	1600 mg/d	Dizziness Drowsiness, sedation Ataxia Diplopia, blurred vision Rash Nausea Leukopenia Hyponatremia	Depressed cardiac conduction
Valproate	250 mg b.i.d.	3500 mg/d-4500 mg/d	Nausea, vomiting, anorexia Sedation Confusion Weight gain Tremor	

TABLE 84–4 Benzodiazepines

Agent	Starting Dose	Maximum Dose	Side Effects
Short-Acting Benzodiazepines			
Oxazepam	10 mg b.i.d.	120 mg/d	Sedation, drowsiness Slowed psychomotor function Exacerbation of underlying cognitive impairment Ataxia/falls in elderly Respiratory depression Tolerance/addiction Amnesia
Lorazepam	0.5 mg b.i.d.	10 mg/d	
Long-Acting Benzodiazepines			
Diazepam	2-5 mg q.d.	60 mg/d	
Chlordiazepoxide	5 mg q.d.	100 mg/d	
Clonazepam	0.25 mg/d	6 mg/d	
Alprazolam	0.25 mg b.i.d.	8 mg/d	

Anticonvulsants. These drugs are increasingly prescribed to stabilize the mood of patients with bipolar disorder (manic-depressive illness). Their use in cardiac patients has not yet been systematically studied. It is known that carbamazepine has quinidine-like effects and can aggravate heart block,[83] and it may also exacerbate CHF. *Carbamazepine* can also produce hyponatremia, and this effect is potentiated by other causes of hyponatremia, such as diuretics and CHF. *Valproate*, although not yet studied widely in cardiac populations, does not appear to have adverse cardiac effects. It can, however, lower the platelet count, decrease fibrinogen levels, and increase the prothrombin time. *Lamotrigine* is increasingly used in refractory depression and appears to have no significant cardiac effects nor impact on the cytochrome P450 system. *Topiramate* may have a role in the treatment of mania and anxiety. It is renally excreted, and care must be taken to ensure adequate hydration.

Benzodiazepines (Table 84–4). Benzodiazepines have anxiolytic, sedative, anticonvulsant, and muscle relaxant properties. Anxiety disorders, especially panic disorder and generalized anxiety disorder, are prevalent in patients with cardiac disease. Panic disorder is treated either with a benzodiazepine with antipanic efficacy (such as clonazepam, lorazepam, or alprazolam) or an antidepressant. Generalized anxiety disorder can also be treated with benzodiazepines, buspirone, or SSRIs. Hospitalized cardiac patients are acutely anxious and benzodiazepines are widely used in coronary care units. They can decrease respiratory drive in patients with chronic obstructive pulmonary disease and chronic hypercapnia but are free of cardiac side effects and are safe in seriously ill cardiac patients, even in the period immediately after myocardial infarction.

Benzodiazepines with longer half-lives and/or active metabolites (e.g., diazepam, flurazepam, clonazepam, chlordiazepoxide) accumulate in the body with repeated administration. A steady state is reached slowly, and clearance of the drug after discontinuation is prolonged. Thus the benzodiazepines with shorter half-lives and fewer active metabolites (lorazepam, oxazepam) are generally preferable, particularly in the elderly. Intramuscular absorption of these agents, other than lorazepam and midazolam, is erratic and unpredictable. The most prominent side effects are sedation, fatigue, memory complaints, and psychomotor impairment. In hospitalized patients and in the elderly, these effects can result in frank oversedation or delirium. Patients with preexisting cognitive impairment or organic brain syndromes often react to benzodiazepines with further confusion, increased memory loss, behavioral disinhibition, and belligerence. Ambulatory patients should be cautioned about driving and participating in activities requiring a high degree of alertness.

Psychiatric Side Effects of Cardiovascular Drugs

ANTIHYPERTENSIVES. Many antihypertensive agents have central nervous system side effects. Depression is not uncommon with methyldopa, clonidine, reserpine, and guanethidine. Therefore, calcium-channel blockers and ACE inhibitors may be preferable in the hypertensive patient with a history of depression. Abrupt discontinuation of antihypertensive agents can cause anxiety, agitation, and vivid dreams. *Methyldopa* is a relatively common cause of insomnia.

BETA-ADRENERGIC RECEPTOR ANTAGONISTS. There is a longstanding clinical impression that beta blockers can cause depression. Although there are reports that patients maintained on these agents have an elevated rate of concurrent antidepressant pharmacotherapy, other studies have failed to find an association between beta-blocker use and depression. Some of the confusion may stem from the fact that these agents cause sedation, lethargy, fatigue, and impotence, side effects that may be confused with depression. Depression may be more likely in those with a past history of depressive disorder, with the more lipophilic agents (e.g., propranolol, metoprolol), and when using higher doses. Beta blockers also occasionally cause vivid dreams and nightmares, hallucinations, and other psychotic symptoms, particularly in the elderly.

CALCIUM-CHANNEL BLOCKERS. In general, calcium-channel blockers do not have prominent psychiatric side effects. There are isolated case reports of depression associated with their administration, but this has not been demonstrated conclusively. Care should be taken when these agents are coadministered with the psychotropic drugs that inhibit the cytochrome P450 system, such as nefazodone and high doses of fluoxetine and paroxetine.

ANGIOTENSIN-CONVERTING ENZYME INHIBITORS. These inhibitors appear to have relatively few central nervous system side effects, although they may, on rare occasion, induce depression.

ANTIARRHYTHMICS. *Lidocaine* is a relatively common cause of anxiety, confusion, disorientation, hallucinations, and central nervous system excitement. Confusion, hallucinations, and delirium have also been reported with high doses of quinidine. Procainamide may cause depression, hallucinations, and other psychotic symptoms.

DIGITALIS. Anxiety, depression, visual illusions (e.g., yellow halos), and confusion may be the first signs of digitalis toxicity, but psychiatric symptoms may emerge at therapeutic levels as well.

DIURETICS. Diuretics can induce cognitive mental status changes by causing electrolyte imbalance (e.g., hyponatremia) or hypovolemia, and a secondary mood disorder may also occur, often characterized by anorexia, lethargy, and weakness.

Interactions of Psychotropic and Cardiac Drugs (Table 84–5)

Because many cardiac and psychotropic agents lower blood pressure, additive hypotensive effects are not uncommon, as for example between the TCAs and antihypertensives. Many psychotropic agents slow conduction and prolong the PR, QRS, and QT intervals, and synergistic effects can occur when they are used in conjunction with antiarrhythmic medications, resulting in heart block or the long-QT syndrome. Extreme caution is required if atypical neuroleptics are administered concomitantly with other drugs that increase

TABLE 84–5 Interactions of Psychotropic and Cardiac Drugs

Medication	Effect on Cardiac Agent
Interactions Involving Tricyclic Antidepressants	
Type IA antiarrhythmics	Potentiate delay in cardiac conduction; heart block
Antihypertensives: guanethidine, clonidine, reserpine	Antagonize antihypertensive effect; potentiate orthostatic hypotension
Sublingual nitrates	Oral absorption hindered by dry mouth
Alpha-adrenergic blocking agents	Potentiate antihypertensive effect
Interactions Involving Serotoninergic Antidepressants	
Lipophilic beta blockers	Increase blood levels due to decreased hepatic degradation
Calcium channel blockers	Increase blood levels due to decreased hepatic degradation
Type IC antiarrhythmics	Increase blood levels due to decreased hepatic degradation
Angiotensin-converting enzyme inhibitors	Increase blood levels due to decreased hepatic degradation
Warfarin	Increase blood levels due to decreased hepatic degradation
Digitoxin	Increase bioavailability due to displacement from protein-binding sites
Warfarin	Increase bioavailability due to displacement from protein-binding sites
Medication	**Effect on Psychotropic Agent**
Interactions Involving Lithium	
Diuretics that cause sodium loss	Increase blood lithium levels
Calcium channel blockers	Enhance lithium toxicity; bradycardia
Angiotensin-converting enzyme inhibitors	Enhance lithium toxicity
Methyldopa	Enhance lithium toxicity
Medication	**Effect on Psychotropic or Cardiac Agent**
Interactions Involving Carbamazepine	
Calcium channel blockers	Enhance carbamazepine toxicity
Antiarrhythmics	Potentiate delay in cardiac conduction

the QT interval such as *ketoconazole, quinidine,* and *cisapride*. There are several interactions between the TCAs and cardiac medications: The TCAs interfere with neuronal reuptake of clonidine and guanethidine and thus antagonize their antihypertensive action. They may potentiate the antihypertensive action of prazosin, and the dry mouth induced by TCAs may hinder the absorption of sublingual nitrates.

SSRIs are bound to plasma proteins and can displace other protein-bound drugs, thereby increasing the level of active drug and resulting in possible toxicity. This is particularly salient with *warfarin* and *digitoxin*, although the clinical significance of these interactions is not yet clear. As noted earlier, diuretics may raise *lithium* levels into the toxic range. This can generally be dealt with by reducing the lithium dose, although during acute diuresis the proper adjustment of lithium is difficult because of the massive shifts in sodium and fluid balance.

There are reports of idiosyncratic toxic reactions and of bradycardia when lithium is coadministered with the calcium-channel blockers *verapamil* and *diltiazem* and of lithium toxicity precipitated by the use of ACE inhibitors. *Methyldopa* seems to have a number of interactions with psychotropic agents, including possible toxicity when combined with lithium. The metabolic degradation of *carbamazepine* may be inhibited by calcium-channel blockers, thereby increasing the risk of carbamazepine toxicity. Carbamazepine and antiarrhythmics may have additive effects in slowing cardiac conduction.

REFERENCES

Psychiatric and Behavioral Aspects of Coronary Heart Disease

1. Kawachi I, Kubzansky LD, Spiro A, et al: Prospective study of a self-report type A scale and risk of coronary heart disease: Test of the MMPI-2 type A scale. Circulation 98:405-412, 1998.
2. Gallacher JE, Yarnell JW, Sweetnam PM, et al: Anger and incident heart disease in the Caerphilly study. Psychosom Med 61:446-454, 1999.
3. Iribarren C, Sidney S, Bild DE, et al: Association of hostility with coronary artery calcification in young adults: The Cardia Study. JAMA 283:2546-2551, 2000.
4. Siegman AW, Townsend ST, Civelek AC, et al: Antagonistic behavior, dominance, hostility, and coronary disease. Psychosom Med 62:248-257, 2000.
5. Chang PP, Ford DE, Meoni LA, et al: Anger in young men and subsequent premature cardiovascular disease: The precursors study. Arch Intern Med 162:901-906, 2002.
6. Angerer P, Siebert U, Kothny W, et al: Impact of social support, cynical hostility, and anger expression on progression of coronary atherosclerosis. J Am Coll Cardiol 36:1781-1788, 2000.
7. Frasure-Smith N, Lespérance F, Talajic M: Depression following myocardial infarction. Impact on 6-month survival. JAMA 270:1819-1825, 1993.
8. Glassman AH, O'Connor CM, Califf RM, et al: Sertaline treatment of major depression in patients with acute MI or unstable angina. JAMA 288:701-709, 2002.
9. Lespérance F, Frasure-Smith N, Talajic M: Major depression before and after myocardial infarction: Its nature and consequences. Psychosom Med 58:99-110, 1996.
10. McKhann GM, Borowicz LM, Goldsborough MA, et al: Depression and cognitive decline following coronary artery bypass grafting. Lancet 349:1282-1284, 1996.
11. Sullivan M, LaCroix A, Russo J, et al: Depression in coronary heart disease: What is the appropriate diagnostic threshold? Psychosomatics 40:285-292, 1999.
12. Carney RM, Jaffe AS: Treatment of depression following acute myocardial infarction. JAMA 288:750-751, 2002.
13. Sullivan MD, LaCroix AZ, Baum C, et al: Functional status in coronary artery disease: A one-year prospective study of the role of anxiety and depression. Am J Med 103:348-356, 1997.
14. Penninx BWJH, Beekman ATF, Honig A: Depression and cardiac mortality: Results from a community-based longitudinal study. Arch Gen Psychiatry 58:221-227, 2001.
15. Lespérance F, Frasure-Smith N, Talajic M, et al: Five-year risk of cardiac mortality in relation to initial severity and one-year changes in depression symptoms after myocardial infarction. Circulation 105:1049-1053, 2002.
16. Burg MM, Benedetto MC, Rosenberg R, et al: Presurgical depression predicts medical morbidity 6 months after coronary artery bypass graft surgery. Psychosom Med 65:111-118, 2003.
17. Ziegelstein RC: Depression in patients recovering from myocardial infarction. JAMA 286:1621-1627, 2001.
18. Scheier MF, Matthews KA, Owens JF, et al: Optimism and rehospitalization after coronary artery bypass surgery. Arch Intern Med 159:829-835, 1999.
19. Rugulies R: Depression as a predictor for coronary heart disease: A review and meta-analysis. Am J Prev Med 23:51-61, 2002.
20. Rutledge T, Reis SE, Olson M, et al: Psychosocial variables are associated with atherosclerosis risk factors among women with chest pain: The WISE Study. Psychosom Med 63:282-288, 2001.
21. Druss RG, Bradford DW, Rosenheck RA: Mental disorders and use of cardiovascular procedures after myocardial infarction. JAMA 283:506-511, 2000.
22. Musselman DL, Evans DL, Wemeroff CB: The relationship of depression to cardiovascular disease: Epidemiology, biology, and treatment. Arch Gen Psychiatry 55:580-592, 1998.
23. Broadley AJM, Korszun A, Jones CJH, et al: Arterial endothelial function is impaired in treated depression. Heart 88:521-524, 2002.
24. Januzzi JL, Stern TA, Pasternak RC, et al: The influence of anxiety and depression on outcomes of patients with coronary artery disease. Arch Intern Med 160:1913-1925, 2000.
25. Carney RM, Blumenthal JA, Stein PK, et al: Depression, heart rate variability, and acute myocardial infarction. Circulation 104:2024-2028, 2001.
26. Musselman DL, Marzec UM, Manatunga A: Platelet reactivity in depressed patients treated with paroxetine: Preliminary findings. Arch Gen Psychiatry 57:875-882, 2000.
27. Paterniti S, Zureik M, Ducimetière P, et al: Sustained anxiety and 4-year progression of carotid atherosclerosis. Arterioscler Thromb Vasc Biol 21:136-141, 2001.
28. Moser DK, Dracup K: Is anxiety early after myocardial infarction associated with subsequent ischemic and arrhythmic events? Psychosom Med 58:395-401, 1996.
29. King KB: Psychologic and social aspects of cardiovascular disease. Ann Behav Med 19:264-270, 1997.
30. Brummett BH, Barefoot JC, Siegler IC, et al: Characteristics of socially isolated patients with coronary artery disease who are at elevated risk for mortality. Psychosom Med 63:267-272, 2001.
31. Frasure-Smith N, Lespérance F, Gravel G, et al: Social support, depression, and mortality during the first year after myocardial infarction. Circulation 101:1919-1924, 2000.
32. Bosma H, Peter R, Siegrist J, et al: Two alternative job stress models and the risk of coronary heart disease. Am J Public Health 88:68-74, 1998.
33. Wamala SP, Mittleman MA, Schenck-Gustafsson K, et al: Potential explanations of the educational gradient in women: A population-based case-control study of Swedish women. Am J Public Health 89:315-321, 1999.

33a. Wamala SP, Mittleman MA, Horsten M, et al: Job stress and the occupational gradient in coronary heart disease risk in women. The Stockholm Female Coronary Risk Study. Soc Sci Med 51:481-489, 2000.

34. Johnson JV, Stewart W, Hall EM, et al: Long-term psychosocial work environment and cardiovascular mortality among Swedish males. Am J Public Health 86:324-331, 1996.
35. Orth-Gomér K, Wamala SP, Horsten M, et al: Marital stress worsens prognosis in women with coronary heart disease. JAMA 284:3008-3014, 2000.
36. Krantz DS, Kop WJ, Santiago HT, et al: Mental stress as a trigger of myocardial ischemia and infarction. Cardiol Clin 14:271-287, 1996.
37. Jiang W, Babyak M, Krantz DS, et al: Mental stress–induced myocardial ischemia and cardiac events. JAMA 21:1651-1656, 1996.
38. Gullette ECD, Blumenthal JA, Babyak M, et al: Effects of mental stress on myocardial ischemia during daily life. JAMA 277:1521-1526, 1997.
39. Möller J, Hallqvist J, Diderichsen F, et al: Do episodes of anger trigger myocardial infarction? A case-crossover analysis in the Stockholm Heart Epidemiology Program (SHEEP). Psychosom Med 61:842-849, 1999.
40. Markowitz JH: Hostility is associated with increased platelet activity in coronary heart disease. Psychosom Med 60:586-591, 1998.
41. Suarez EC, Kuhn CM, Schanberg SM, et al: Neuroendocrine, cardiovascular, and emotional responses of hostile men: The role of interpersonal challenge. Psychosom Med 60:78-88, 1998.
42. Heller SS, Ormont MA, Lidagoster L: Psychosocial outcome after ICD implantation: A current perspective. Pacing Clin Electrophysiol 21:1207-1215, 1998.

Psychiatric and Behavioral Aspects of Hypertension and Heart Failure

43. Weidner G, Kohlmann C, Horsten M, et al: Cardiovascular reactivity to mental stress in the Stockholm Female Coronary Risk Study. Psychosom Med 63:917-924, 2001.
44. Smith TW, Gallo LG: Hostility and cardiovascular reactivity during marital interaction. Psychosom Med 61:436-445, 1999.
45. Perini C, Muller FB, Rauchfliesch U, et al: Psychosomatic factors in borderline hypertensive subjects and offspring of hypertensive parents. Hypertension 16:627-634, 2002.
46. Friedman R, Schwartz JE, Schnall PL, et al: Psychological variables in hypertension: Relationship to casual or ambulatory blood pressure in men. Psychosom Med 63:19-31, 2001.
47. Jonas BS, Franks P, Ingram DD: Are symptoms of anxiety and depression risk factors for hypertension? Longitudinal evidence from the National Health and Nutrition Survey I Epidemiologic Follow-up Study. Arch Fam Med 6:43-49, 1997.
48. Shinn EH, Poston WSC, Kimball KT, et al: Blood pressure and symptoms of depression and anxiety: A prospective study. Am J Hypertens 14:660-664, 2001.
49. Jonas BS, Lando JF: Negative affect as a prospective risk factor for hypertension. Psychosom Med 62:188-196, 2000.
50. The Sixth Report of the Joint National Committee on Prevention, Detection, Evaluation, and Treatment of High Blood Pressure. Arch Intern Med 157:2413-2446, 1997 [published correction appears in Arch Intern Med 158:573, 1998.]
51. Linden W, Chambers LA: Clinical effectiveness of non-drug therapies for hypertension: A meta-analysis. Ann Behav Med 16:35-45, 1994.
52. Linden W, Lenz JW, Con AH: Individualized stress management for primary hypertension: A randomized trial. Arch Intern Med 161:1071-1080, 2001.
53. MacMahon K, Lip GYH: Psychological factors in heart failure: A review of the literature. Arch Intern Med 162:509-516, 2002.
54. Feenstra J, Grobee DE, Jonkman FAM, et al: Prevention of relapse in patients with congestive heart failure: The role of precipitating factors. Heart 80:432-436, 1998.
55. Koenig HG: Depression in hospitalized older patients with congestive heart failure. Gen Hosp Psychiatry 20:29-43, 1998.

56. Jiang W, Alexander J, Christopher E, et al: Relationship of depression to increased risk of mortality and rehospitalization in patients with congestive heart failure. Arch Intern Med 161:1849-1856, 2001.
57. Freedland KE, Rich MW, Skala JA, et al: Prevalence of depression in hospitalized patients with congestive heart failure. Psychosom Med 65:119-128, 2003.
58. Sullivan M, Simon G, Spertus J, et al: Depression-related costs in heart failure care. Arch Intern Med 162:1860-1866, 2002.
59. Williams SA, Kasl SV, Heiat A, et al: Depression and risk of heart failure among the elderly. Psychosom Med 64:6-12, 2002.
60. Krumholtz HM, Butler J, Miller J, et al: Prognostic impact of emotional support for elderly patients hospitalized with heart failure. Circulation 97:958-964, 1998.
60a. Murberg TA, Bru E: Social relationships and mortality in patients with congestive heart failure. J Psychosom Res 51:521-527, 2001.
61. Krantz DS, Hedges SM, Gabbay FH, et al: Triggers of angina and ST segment depression in ambulatory patients with coronary artery disease: Evidence for uncoupling of angina and ischemia. Am Heart J 128:703-712, 1994.
62. Leizorovicz A, Haugh MC, Mercier C, et al: Pre hospital and hospital time delays in thrombolytic treatment in patients with suspected myocardial infarction. Eur Heart J 18:248-253, 1997.
63. Meischke H, Larsen MP, Eisenberg MS: Gender differences in reported symptoms for acute myocardial infarction: Impact of prehospital delay time interval. Am J Emerg Med 16:363-366, 1998.

Psychiatric Care of the Cardiac Patient

64. Selnes OA, McKhann GM: Coronary-artery bypass surgery and the brain. N Engl J Med 344:451-452, 2001.
65. Roach GW, Kanchuger M, Mangano CM, et al: Adverse cerebral outcomes after coronary bypass surgery. N Engl J Med 335:1857-1863, 1996.
66. Schwartz TL, Masand PS: The role of atypical antipsychotics in the treatment of delirium. Psychosomatics 43:171-174, 2002.
67. Newman MF, Kirchner JL, Phillips-Bute B, et al: Longitudinal assessment of neurocognitive function after coronary-artery bypass surgery. N Engl J Med 344:395-402, 2001.
68. Sauer WH, Berlin JA, Kimmel SE: Selective serotonin reuptake inhibitors and myocardial infarction. Circulation 104:1894-1898, 2001.
69. Taylor CB, Miller NH, Smith PM, et al: The effect of a home-based, case-managed, multifactorial risk-reduction program on reducing psychological distress in patients with cardiovascular disease. J Cardiopulm Rehabil 17:157-162, 1997.
70. Frasure-Smith N, Lespérance F, Prince RH, et al: Randomized trial of home-based psychosocial nursing intervention for patients recovering from myocardial infarction. Lancet 350:473-479, 1997.
71. Cossette S, Frasure-Smith N, Lespérance F: Clinical implications of a reduction in psychological distress on cardiac prognosis in patients participating in a psychosocial intervention program. Psychosom Med 63:257-266, 2001.
72. Ades PA: Cardiac rehabilitation and secondary prevention of coronary heart disease. N Engl J Med 345:892-902, 2001.
73. Dusseldorp E, van Elderen T, Maes S, et al: A meta-analysis of psychoeducational programs for coronary heart disease patients. Health Psychol 18:506-519, 1999.
74. Linden W: Psychological treatments in cardiac rehabilitation: Review of rationales and outcomes. J Psychosom Res 48:443-454, 2000.

Psychopharmacology in the Cardiac Patient

75. Roose SP, Glassman AH, Attia E, et al: Cardiovascular effects of fluoxetine in depressed patients with heart disease. Am J Psychiatry 155:650-655, 1998.
76. Harvey AT, Preskorn SH: Cytochrome P450 enzymes: Interpretation of their interactions with selective srotonin reuptake inhibitors: I. J Clin Psychopharmacol 16:273-285, 1996.
77. Nelson JC, Kennedy JS, Pollock BG, et al: Treatment of major depression with nortriptyline and paroxetine in patients with ischemic heart disease. Am J Psychiatry 156:1024-1028, 1999.
78. Beliles K, Stoudemire A: Psychopharmacologic treatment of depression in the medically ill. Psychosomatics 39:S2-S19, 1998.
78a. Nelson JC: Safety and tolerability of the new antidepressants [review]. J Clin Psychiatry 58(Suppl 6):26-31, 1997.
79. Glassman AH, Bigger JT: Antipsychotic drugs: Prolonged QTc interval, torsade de pointes, and sudden death. Am J Psychiatry 158:1774-1782, 2001.
80. Stoudemire A, Moran MF: Psychopharmacology in the medically ill patient. *In* Schatzberg AF, Nemeroff CB (eds): Textbook of Psychopharmacology. Washington, DC, American Psychiatric Press, 1998, pp 931-959.
81. Killian JG, Kerr K, Lawrence C, et al: Myocarditis and cardiomyopathy associated with clozapine. Lancet 354:1841-1845, 1999.
82. Lieberman JA: Maximizing clozapine therapy: Managing side effects. J Clin Psychiatry 59(Suppl 3):38-43, 1998.
83. Benassi E, Bo GP, Cociot L, et al: Carbamazepine and cardiac conduction disturbances. Ann Neurol 22:280-281, 1999.

CHAPTER 85

Neurological Disorders and Cardiovascular Disease

William J. Groh • Douglas P. Zipes

Cardiovascular disease that occurs secondary to an underlying neurological disorder is related either to a direct involvement of the heart or to induced neurohormonal abnormalities that act on the heart. In several neurological disorders, the cardiovascular manifestations can be responsible for a greater risk of morbidity and mortality than the neurological manifestations. This chapter reviews those neurological disorders associated with important cardiovascular sequelae.

Muscular Dystrophies

The muscular dystrophies are a diffuse group of heritable disorders in which direct involvement of cardiac muscle and/or the cardiac conduction system is present to a variable degree. The muscular dystrophies can be classified into the following types:

1. X-linked—Duchenne and Becker muscular dystrophy
2. Myotonic muscular dystrophy
3. Emery-Dreifuss muscular dystrophy and associated disorders
4. Limb-girdle muscular dystrophy
5. Facioscapulohumeral muscular dystrophy

Duchenne and Becker Muscular Dystrophies

GENETICS. Both Duchenne and Becker muscular dystrophy are X-linked recessive disorders in which the genetic locus has been identified as an abnormality in the dystrophin gene. The dystrophin protein and dystrophin-associated glycoproteins provide a structural link between the myocyte cytoskeleton and extracellular matrix functioning to link contractile proteins to the cell membrane.[1] Dystrophin messenger RNA is expressed predominantly in skeletal, cardiac, and smooth muscle with lower levels in brain. Its absence can lead to membrane fragility resulting in myofibril necrosis and eventual loss of muscle fibers with fibrotic replacement. Abnormalities in dystrophin and in dystrophin-associated glycoproteins underlie the degeneration of cardiac and skeletal muscle in several inherited myopathies, including X-linked dilated cardiomyopathy.[2] Beyond the inherited disorders, the loss of dystrophin plays a role in myocyte failure in many cardiomyopathies including those associated with coronary artery disease.[3] In Duchenne muscular dystrophy, dystrophin is nearly absent, whereas in Becker muscular dystrophy, dystrophin is present but reduced in size or amount. This leads to the characteristic rapidly progressive skeletal muscle disease in Duchenne and the more benign course in Becker muscular dystrophy. The heart as a muscle is involved in both disorders.

CLINICAL PRESENTATION. Duchenne muscular dystrophy is the most common inherited neuromuscular disorder, with an incidence of 30 per 100,000 live male births. Patients typically become symptomatic before 5 years of age, presenting with skeletal muscle weakness that progresses such that the boy becomes wheelchair bound before 13 years of age (Fig. 85–1).[4] Death occurs commonly by age 20 to 25 years primarily from respiratory failure or cardiac arrest. Becker muscular dystrophy is less common (3 per 100,000 live male births) and has a more variable presentation of skeletal muscle weakness (Fig. 85–2) and a better prognosis, with most patients surviving to age 40 to 50 years.

In both Duchenne and Becker muscular dystrophy, elevated serum creatinine kinase activity is observed, over 10-fold and 5-fold normal values, respectively.

CARDIOVASCULAR MANIFESTATIONS. Virtually all patients with Duchenne muscular dystrophy develop a cardiomyopathy (see Chap. 59), but clinical recognition may be masked by severe skeletal muscle weakness. Preclinical cardiac involvement is present in one-fourth by 6 years of age, with the onset of clinically apparent cardiomyopathy after the age of 10 years being common. Predilection for involvement in the posterobasal and posterolateral left ventricle has been observed (Fig. 85–3). As with the skeletal muscle weakness, cardiac involvement in Becker muscular dystrophy is more variable than in Duchenne muscular dystrophy, ranging from none or subclinical to severe cardiomyopathy requiring transplant. Cardiac involvement in Becker muscular dystrophy is independent of the severity of skeletal muscle involvement, with some but not all investigators observing increased likelihood of cardiovascular disease in older individuals.[5] More than one-half of patients with subclinical or benign skeletal muscle disease were noted to have cardiac involvement if carefully evaluated.[6] In follow-up studies, progression in the severity of cardiac involvement is common. Cardiomyopathy can initially solely involve the right ventricle.

Thoracic deformities and a high diaphragm can alter the cardiovascular examination in Duchenne muscular dystrophy. A reduction in the anteroposterior chest dimension is commonly responsible for a systolic impulse displaced to the left sternal border, a grade 1–3/6 short midsystolic murmur in the second left interspace, and a loud pulmonary component of the second heart sound. In both Duchenne and Becker muscular dystrophy, mitral regurgitation is commonly observed. The presence of mitral regurgitation is related to posterior papillary muscle dysfunction in Duchenne

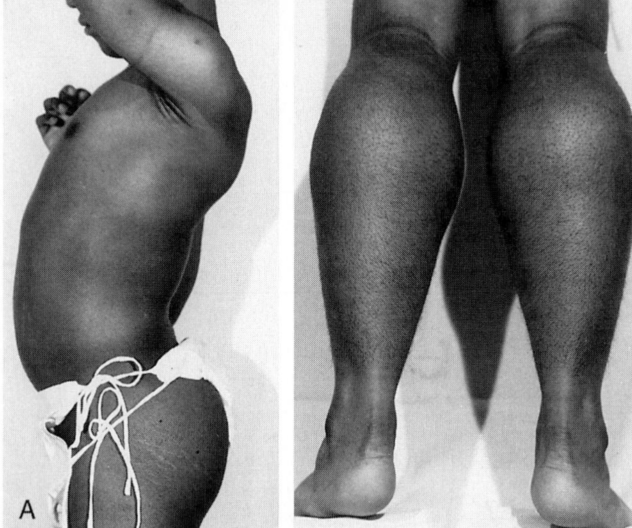

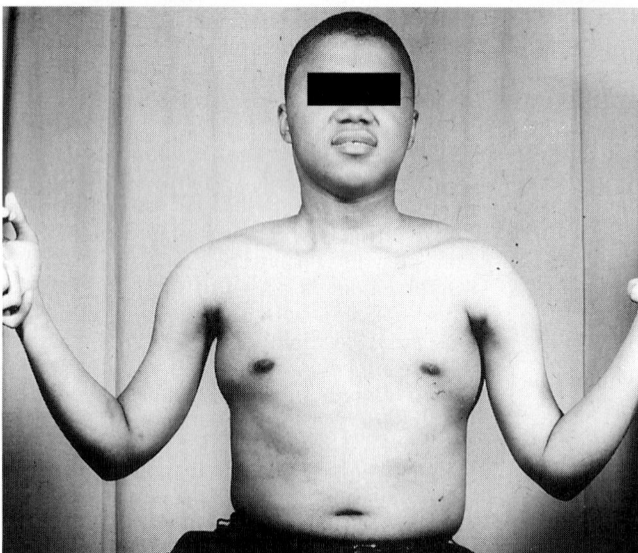

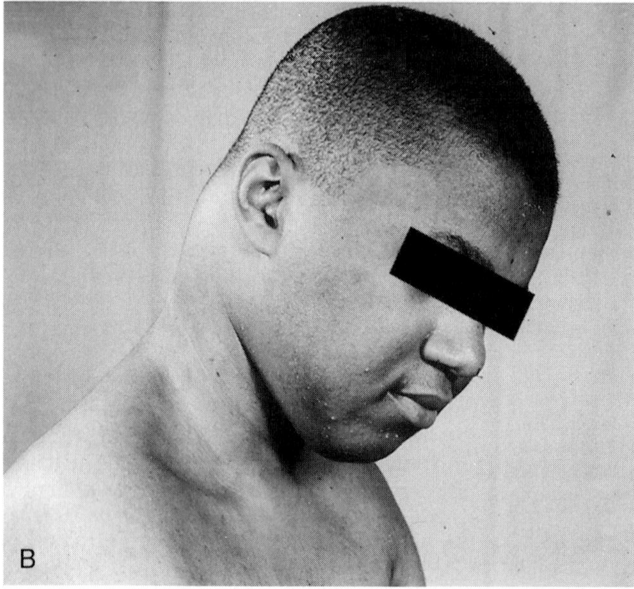

FIGURE 85–1 **A,** Classic X-linked muscular dystrophy. **Left,** Exaggerated lumbar lordosis. **Right,** Calf pseudohypertrophy and shortening of the Achilles tendons. **B,** Seventeen-year-old boy with Duchenne muscular dystrophy. There is striking enlargement (hypertrophy/pseudohypertrophy) of the deltoid and pectoralis major muscles **(upper panel)** and of the trapezius **(lower panel)**. There was also striking enlargement of both calves (not shown). (**A** and **B,** Courtesy of Joseph K. Perloff, MD.)

muscular dystrophy and to mitral annular dilation in Becker muscular dystrophy.[7]

Female carriers of Duchenne and Becker muscular dystrophy are at increased risk of dilated cardiomyopathy.[8]

ELECTROCARDIOGRAPHY. In patients with Duchenne muscular dystrophy the electrocardiogram (ECG) is abnormal in 90 percent, demonstrating a distinctive pattern of tall R waves and an increased RS amplitude in V_1 and deep narrow Q waves in the left precordial leads related to the characteristic posterolateral left ventricular involvement (Fig. 85–4). In patients with Becker muscular dystrophy, ECG abnormalities are present in up to 75 percent.[5] The ECG abnormalities observed include tall R waves and an increased RS amplitude in V_1, similar to that seen in Duchenne muscular dystrophy, but may also show frequent incomplete right bundle branch block. This may be related to early involvement of the right ventricle. In patients with congestive heart failure, left bundle branch block is common (Fig. 85–5).

ARRHYTHMIAS (see Chap. 32)**.** In Duchenne muscular dystrophy, arrhythmias secondary to disturbances in both rhythm and conduction are observed. Persistent or labile sinus tachycardia is the most recognized abnormality. The pathogenesis of this tachycardia is unknown but does not appear related to abnormal autonomic function. Atrial arrhythmias including atrial fibrillation and atrial flutter occur commonly as a preterminal rhythm. Abnormalities in atrioventricular conduction have been observed. Up to 10 percent of individuals have PR intervals less than 120 milliseconds, while an additional 10 percent have prolonged PR intervals. Ventricular arrhythmias, primarily ventricular premature complexes, occur on monitoring in 30 percent. More complex ventricular arrhythmias have been reported, more commonly in individuals with severe muscle disease. Sudden death occurs in Duchenne muscular dystrophy, primarily in patients with severe skeletal muscle weakness. Whether the sudden death is primarily arrhythmic in nature is not clear. Several follow-up studies have shown a correlation between sudden death and complex ventricular arrhythmias.

Arrhythmic manifestations in Becker muscular dystrophy tend to correspond to the degree of the associated dilated cardiomyopathy but are not well characterized. Distal conduction system disease with complete heart block and bundle branch reentry ventricular tachycardia has been observed (see Chaps. 30 through 32).[9]

TREATMENT AND PROGNOSIS. Duchenne muscular dystrophy is a progressive disorder with respiratory or cardiac death common by age 20 to 25 years. Steroids and steroid derivatives have shown promise in delaying disease progression.[4] Gene replacement therapy holds future promise. A primary cardiac etiology for death occurs in about one-fourth of patients, with an equal distribution of death from progressive heart failure and sudden death. Intravenous verapamil used for preterminal atrial arrhythmias can lead to acute respiratory failure.

In Becker muscular dystrophy or female carriers of Duchenne muscular dystrophy, it is not known whether therapy to decrease myocardial wall stress is beneficial in preventing or delaying progression to cardiac failure. Once heart failure is established, conventional therapy is indicated. Cardiac transplantation has been reported.[10]

Myotonic Muscular Dystrophy

GENETICS. Myotonic muscular dystrophy (dystrophica myotonia, Steinert disease) is an autosomal dominant inherited disorder characterized by reflex and percussion myotonia, weakness and atrophy of distal skeletal muscles as well as systemic manifestations of early balding, gonadal atrophy, cataracts, mental retardation, and cardiac involvement (Fig. 85–6).[11] The genetic abnormality responsible is an amplified and unstable trinucleotide (cytosine-thymine-guanine [CTG]) repeat found on the long arm of chromosome 19 (myotonic dystrophy type 1). In individuals without myotonic dystrophy, between 5 and 37 copies of the CTG repeat are present. In individuals with myotonic dystrophy, 50 to several thousand CTG repeats are observed. A direct correlation exists between an increasing number of CTG repeats and earlier age of onset and increasing severity of neuromuscular involvement. Cardiac involvement, including conduction disease and arrhythmias, also correlates with the length of CTG repeat expansion.[12] The mechanism by which an amplified CTG repeat leads to the characteristic involvement in myotonic dystrophy is multifactorial.[13-15]

Proximal myotonic myopathy, or myotonic dystrophy type 2, is a disorder similar to myotonic dystrophy type 1 but with typically less severe muscular involvement.[16,17] Cardiac abnormalities including conduction disease have been reported in proximal myotonic myopathy but also appear much less common than in myotonic dystrophy type 1.[18] The differences in the reported prevalence of cardiac involvement in proximal myotonic myopathy are likely related to genetic heterogeneity in the clinical syndrome. A repeat expansion at a separate genetic loci (3q21) has been identified as being responsible for proximal myotonic myopathy in many but not all families.[19,20] The remainder of the section focuses on the more common myotonic dystrophy type 1, hereafter referred to as *myotonic dystrophy*.

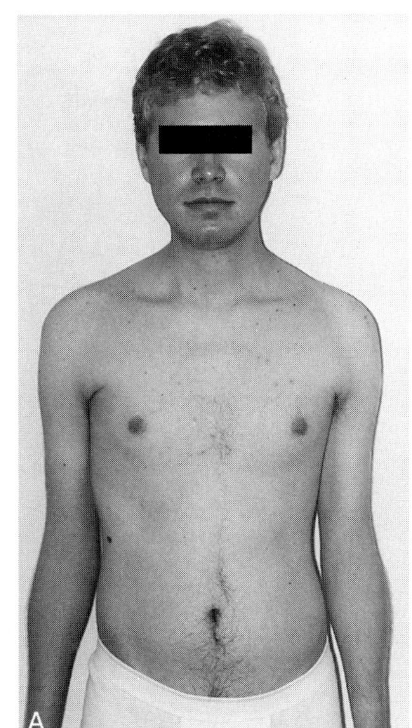

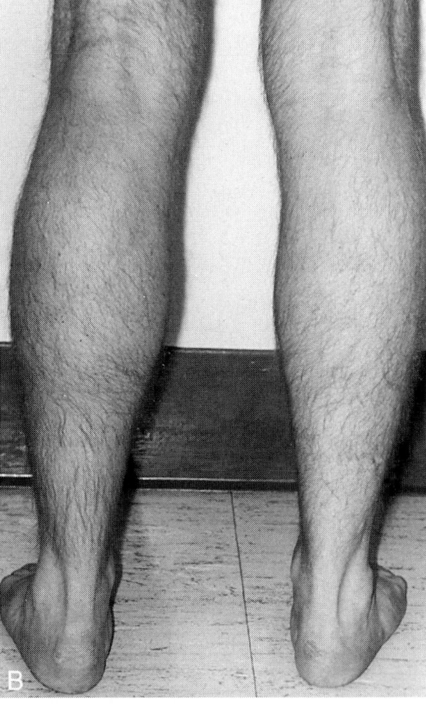

FIGURE 85–2 Late-onset, slowly progressive Becker muscular dystrophy in a 22-year-old man. **A,** There is dystrophy of the shoulder girdle, arms, and pelvic girdle (last not shown). **B,** Asymmetrical calf pseudohypertrophy, greater on the left than on the right. Dystrophy of proximal leg muscles is not shown. (**A** and **B,** Courtesy of Joseph K. Perloff, MD.)

CLINICAL PRESENTATION. Myotonic dystrophy is the most common inherited neuromuscular disorder in patients presenting as adults. The global incidence has been estimated to be 1 in 8000, although it is higher in certain populations, such as French Canadians and lower to nonexistent in other populations, such as African blacks. The age at onset of symptoms and diagnosis averages 20 to 25 years. Common early manifestations are weakness in the muscles of the face, neck, and distal extremities. On examination, myotonia (delayed muscle relaxation) can be demonstrated in the grip, thenar muscle group, and tongue (Fig. 85–7). Diagnosis when the individual is asymptomatic is possible using electromyography and genetic testing. Symptomatic myotonic dystrophy tends to present at an earlier age and with increasing severity in successive generations. This property is called *anticipation* and is related to the increasing amplification of CTG repeat length in successive generations. In general, cardiac symptoms occur after the onset of skeletal muscle weakness but can be the initial manifestation of the disease.

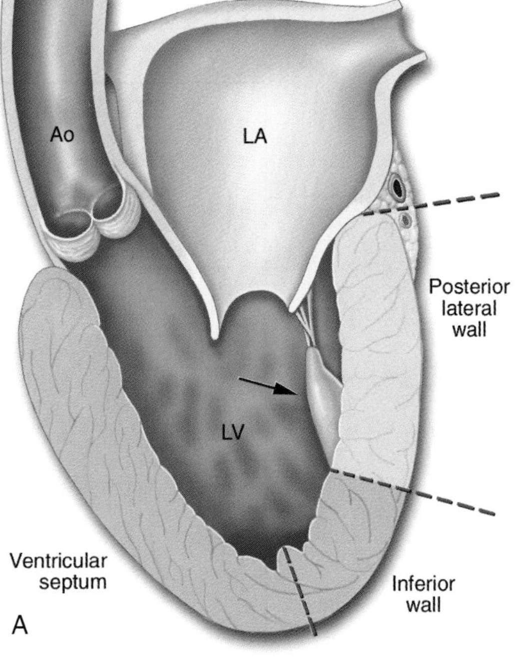

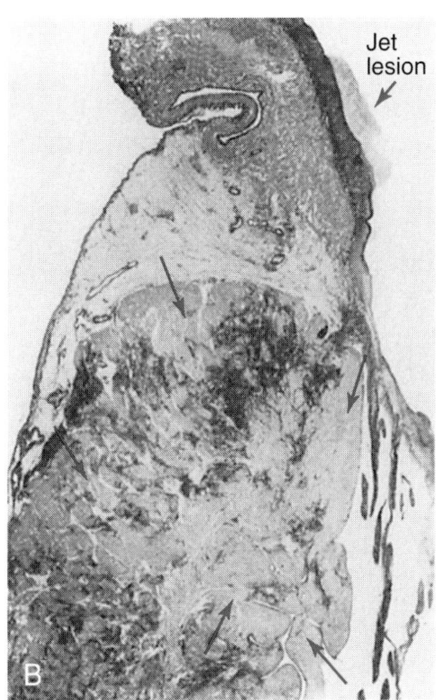

FIGURE 85–3 **A,** Schematic illustration showing the typical posterobasal myocardial involvement with lateral extension in classic Duchenne muscular dystrophy. The posterolateral papillary muscle is involved (arrow). **B,** Necropsy section showing posterobasal involvement (long arrows) of the left ventricle in a boy with classic Duchenne muscular dystrophy. The posterolateral papillary muscle was involved, resulting in mitral regurgitation and the jet lesion shown at upper right (arrow). LA = left atrium; LV = left ventricle; Ao = aorta. (**A** and **B,** Courtesy of Joseph K. Perloff, MD.)

CARDIOVASCULAR MANIFESTATIONS. Cardiac pathology is commonly seen in myotonic dystrophy primarily involving degeneration (fibrosis and fatty infiltration) of the specialized conduction tissue including the sinus node, atrioventricular node, and His-Purkinje system. Degenerative changes are observed in working atrial and ventricular tissue but only rarely progress to a symptomatic dilated cardiomyopathy (Fig. 85–8). It is not surprising, based on the preferential degeneration of conduction tissue, that the

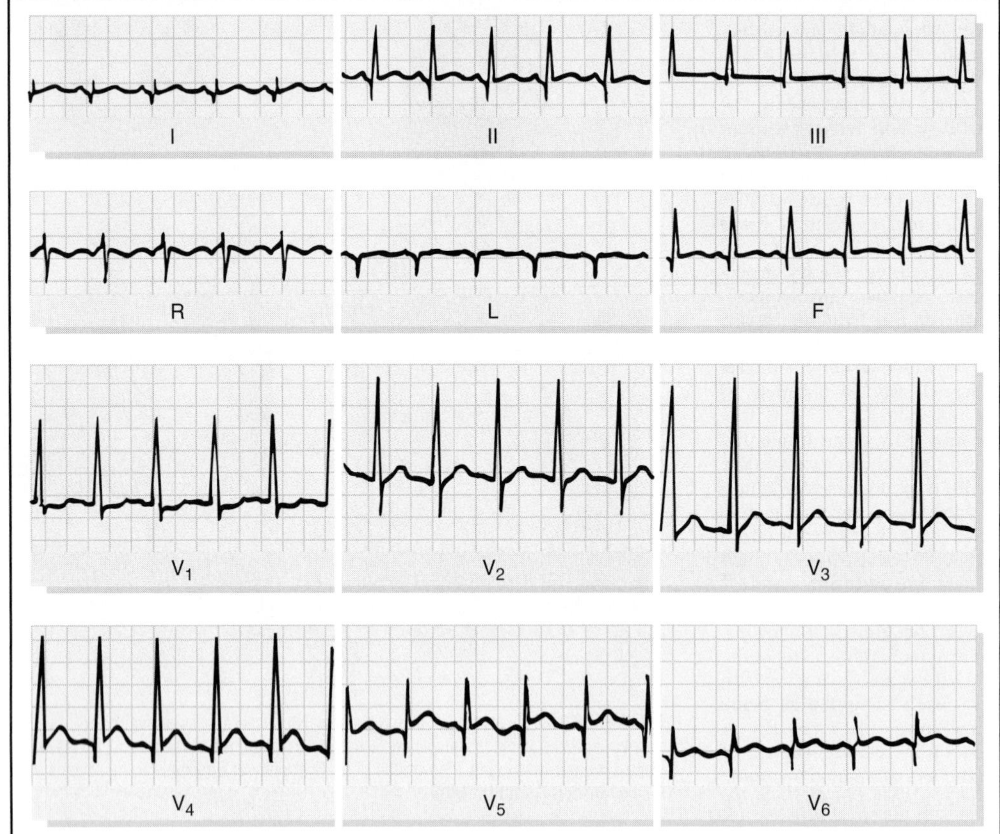

FIGURE 85–4 Electrocardiogram from a 12-year-old boy with classic Duchenne muscular dystrophy. Sinus tachycardia is observed. The QRS complex is typical of Duchenne dystrophy, showing tall R waves in lead V_1 and deep, narrow Q waves in leads I, aVL, and V_4 to V_6. (Courtesy of Charles Fisch, MD, Indiana University School of Medicine, Indianapolis, IN.)

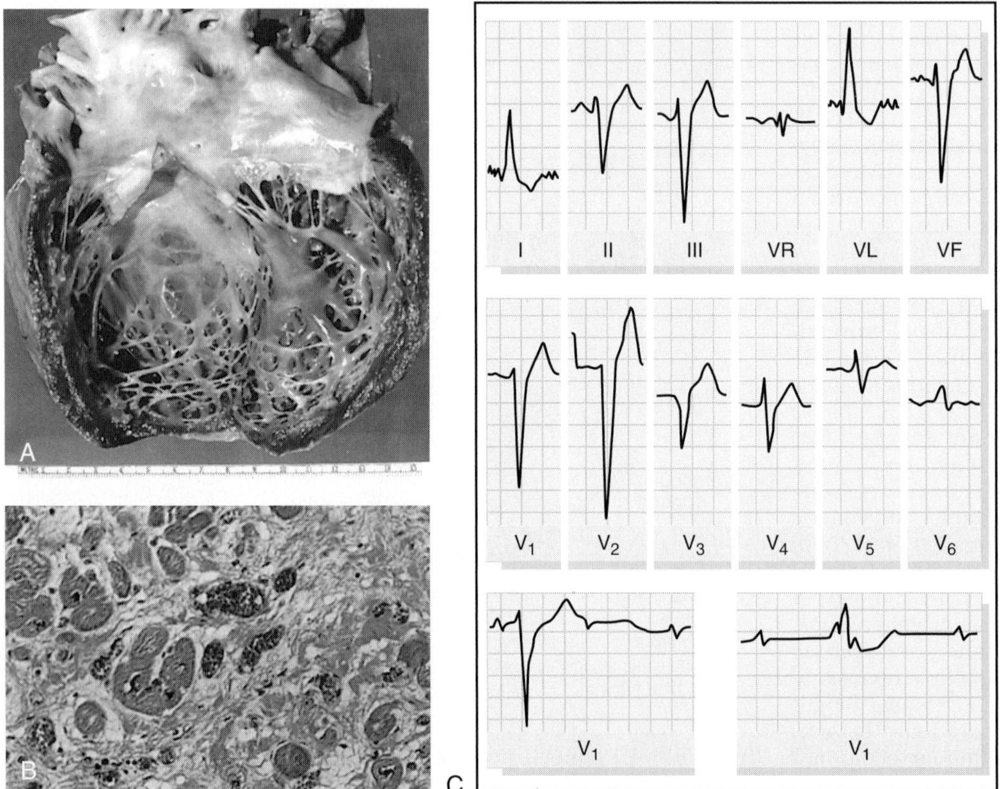

FIGURE 85–5 Gross and microscopic cardiac pathological specimens and the electrocardiogram from a 45-year-old man with late-onset, slowly progressive Becker muscular dystrophy. **A,** Dilated, flabby left ventricle with focal endocardial thickening. **B,** Microscopic section from the left ventricle shows marked confluent scarring with variations in fiber size; there was no significant coronary artery disease. **C,** Electrocardiogram recorded at age 40 years. The 12-lead tracing shows left axis deviation, a QRS of 0.14 second, small Q waves in leads I and aVL, and loss of R waves in leads V_2 and V_3. The lower tracings, taken 4 years later (a year before death), show complete heart block with a variable QRS configuration. (**A** to **C,** From Perloff JK, de Leon AC Jr, O'Doherty D: The cardiomyopathy of progressive muscular dystrophy. Circulation 33:625, 1966.)

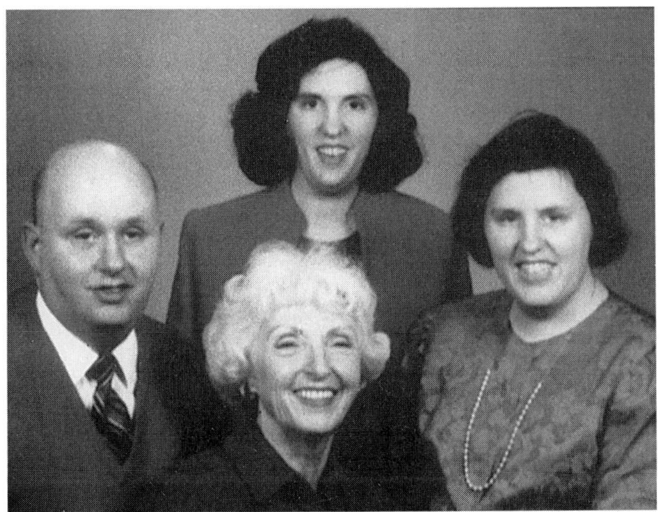

FIGURE 85–6 Myotonic muscular dystrophy in three siblings. Note the unaffected mother (front). Premature balding (left) and characteristic thin facies (rear) are demonstrated.

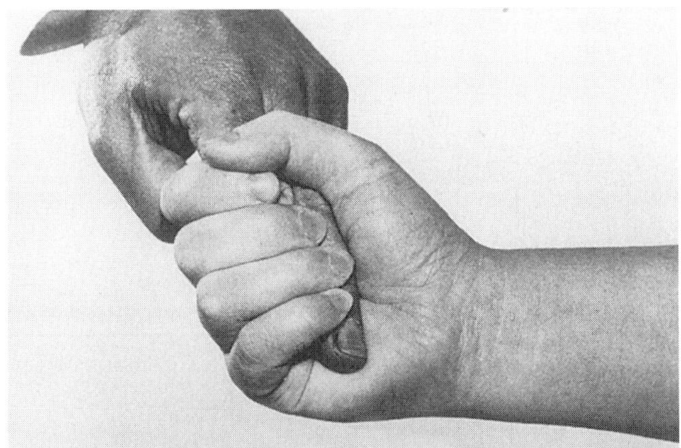

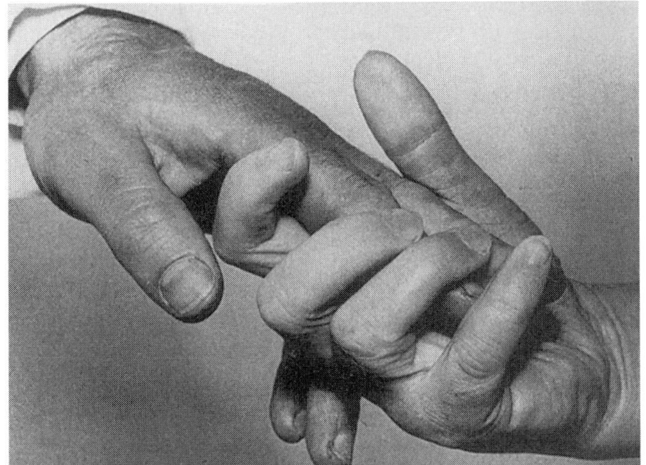

FIGURE 85–7 Grip myotonia in myotonic muscular dystrophy. Inability to release **(bottom)** after exerting grip **(top)**. (From Engel AG, Franzini-Armstrong C [eds]: Myology: Basic and Clinical. 2nd ed. Vol. II. New York, McGraw-Hill, 1994, p 1195.)

primary cardiac manifestations of myotonic dystrophy are arrhythmias.

Electrocardiography. The majority of adult patients with myotonic dystrophy have ECG abnormalities. In a large, unselected myotonic population followed in a U.S. neuromuscular clinic setting, 65 percent of patients had an abnormal ECG.[12] Abnormalities included first-degree atrioventricular

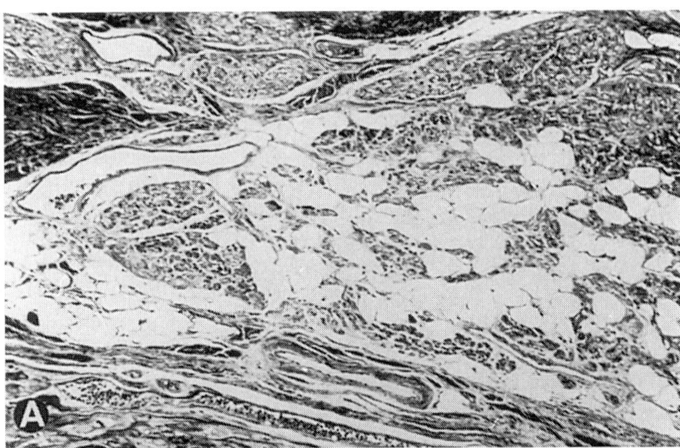

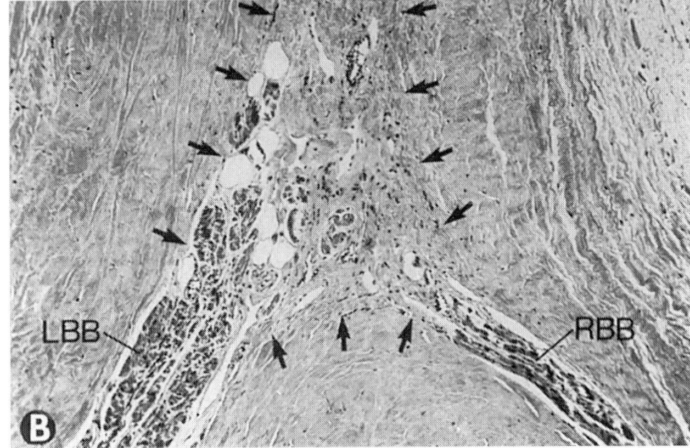

FIGURE 85–8 Histopathology of the atrioventricular bundle in myotonic dystrophy. **A,** Fatty infiltration in a 57-year-old man (Masson trichrome stain, ×90). **B,** Focal replacement fibrosis and atrophy in a 48-year-old woman. Arrows demarcate expected size and shape of the branching atrioventricular bundle (hematoxylin-eosin stain, ×90). LBB = left bundle branch; RBB = right bundle branch. (**A** and **B,** From Nguyen HH, Wolfe JT III, Holmes DR Jr, Edwards WD: Pathology of the cardiac conduction system in myotonic dystrophy: A study of 12 cases. J Am Coll Cardiol 11:662, 1988.)

block in 42 percent, right bundle branch block in 3 percent, left bundle branch block in 4 percent, and nonspecific intraventricular conduction delay in 12 percent. Q waves not associated with a known myocardial infarction are common. ECG abnormalities often progress over time (Fig. 85–9).

Echocardiography. Left ventricular systolic and diastolic dysfunction, left ventricular hypertrophy, and mitral valve prolapse have been reported in myotonic dystrophy patients at a higher prevalence than expected in an age-matched population.[21] The prevalence of symptomatic heart failure is estimated at 6 percent.

Arrhythmias. Patients with myotonic dystrophy demonstrate a wide range of arrhythmias. At cardiac electrophysiological study, the most common abnormality found is a prolonged His-ventricular interval, observed in 56 to 90 percent of selected patients.[22] Conduction system disease can progress to symptomatic atrioventricular block and necessitate pacemaker implantation. The prevalence of permanent cardiac pacing in patients with myotonic dystrophy varies widely between studies based on referral patterns and the indications used for implant. In a large, unselected myotonic population seen in a U.S. neuromuscular clinic setting, 3 percent had received a pacemaker.[12] In France, where early prophylactic pacemaker implantation in myotonic patients is practiced commonly, up to one-half of all myotonic patients receive a pacemaker.[22] Recent pacing guidelines have recognized that asymptomatic conduction abnormalities in neuromuscular diseases such as myotonic dystrophy may warrant special consideration for pacing.[23]

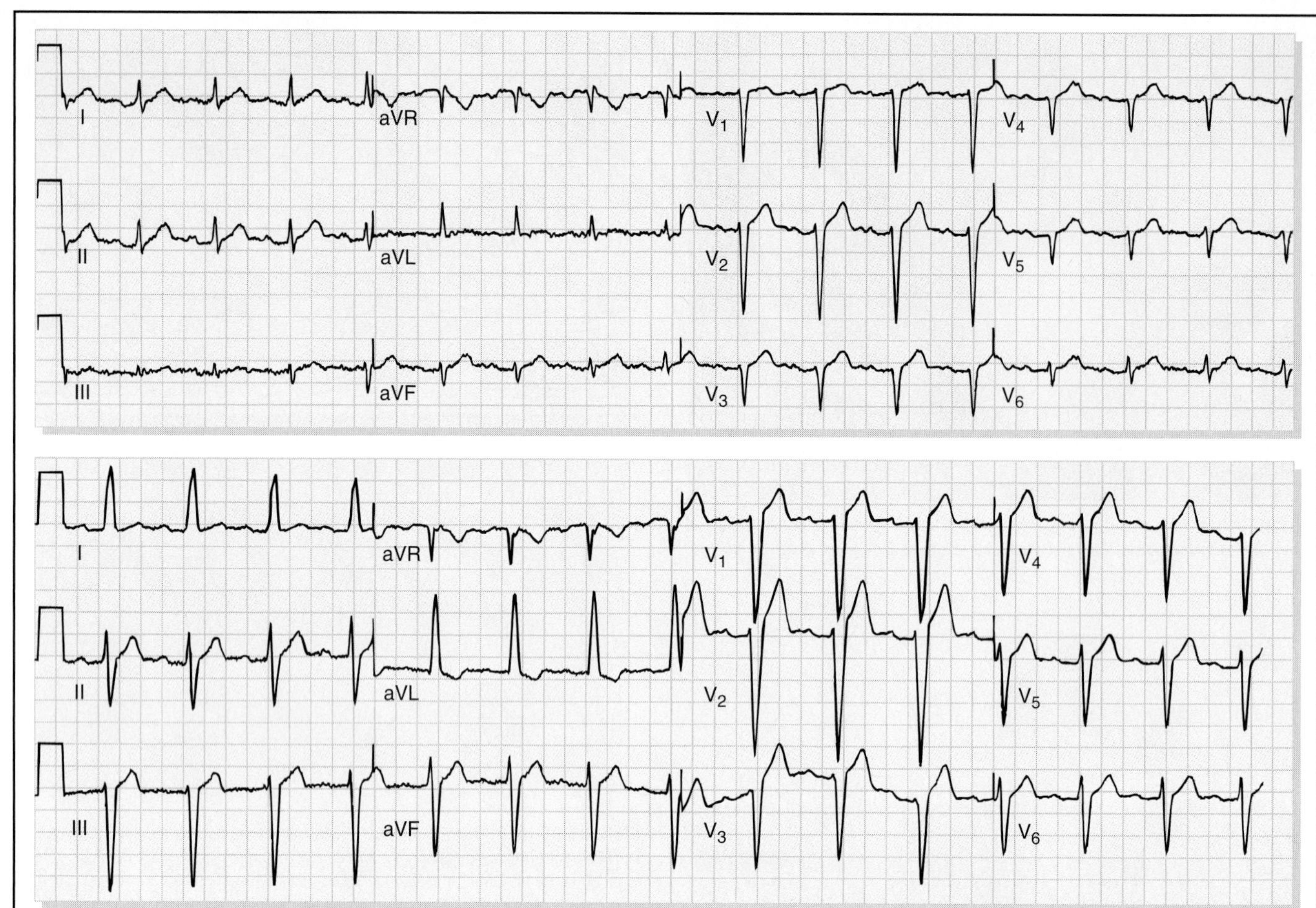

FIGURE 85–9 Electrocardiograms obtained 1 year apart in a 36-year-old man with myotonic dystrophy (the top set is older). Note the abnormal Q waves in the precordial leads. An increasing PR interval and QRS duration are observed consistent with increasing severity of conduction disease.

Atrial arrhythmias, primarily atrial fibrillation and atrial flutter, are the most common arrhythmias observed in myotonic dystrophy, being seen in approximately 4 percent of a general population.[12] Ventricular tachycardia can occur in patients with myotonic dystrophy. In at least two reports and a series of 6 patients, the ventricular tachycardia observed was related to reentry in the diseased distal conduction system, as characterized by bundle branch reentry and interfascicular reentry tachycardia (see Chaps. 27 and 32).[24] Therapy with right bundle branch and/or fascicular radiofrequency ablation resulted in absence of further inducible ventricular tachycardia.

The incidence of sudden death in patients with myotonic dystrophy is substantial and is believed to be primarily caused by arrhythmias. In a registry of 180 myotonic dystrophy patients from the Netherlands collected from 1950 to 1997, 29 percent of all deaths were classified as sudden presumably secondary to arrhythmias.[25] This was secondary only to pneumonia (31 percent) as a cause of death. In a 10-year study of mortality in a cohort of 367 patients from Quebec, 75 (20 percent) of patients died.[26] In these 75 deaths, 31 percent were characterized as secondary to cardiovascular causes, with 11 percent sudden. The mechanisms leading to sudden death in myotonic dystrophy are not clear. Distal conduction disease producing atrioventricular block can result in the lack of an appropriate escape rhythm and asystole or bradycardia-mediated ventricular fibrillation. Sudden death can occur in myotonic dystrophy despite previous permanent cardiac pacing, implicating the role of ventricular arrhythmias.

TREATMENT AND PROGNOSIS. Cardiac management in individuals with myotonic dystrophy is not well established. In the unusual patient in whom a dilated cardiomyopathy does develop, standard therapy including angiotensin-converting enzyme inhibitors and beta blockers has improved symptoms.[27] Patients presenting with symptoms indicative of arrhythmias such as syncope and palpitations should undergo an extensive evaluation, including cardiac electrophysiological study, to determine an etiology. A low threshold for permanent pacing is warranted. An appropriate level of screening for patients who do not manifest cardiac symptoms is unclear. Yearly ECGs and consideration for 24-hour ambulatory monitoring have been recommended. Whether significant or progressive ECG abnormalities require intervention such as prophylactic pacing or cardiac electrophysiological study is unclear. In one study, a combined arrhythmic endpoint was predicted by ECG markers indicative of conduction disease.[28] Trials encompassing more patients by using a multicenter approach have been recommended.[29] Certain families may be more prone to arrhythmic manifestations of myotonic dystrophy. Anesthesia in individuals with myotonic dystrophy can increase the risk of atrioventricular block and other arrhythmias. Careful monitoring during the perioperative period with a low threshold for prophylactic temporary pacing is recommended.

In patients presenting with wide complex tachycardia, cardiac electrophysiological study with particular evaluation for bundle branch reentry tachycardia should be done. The use of class I antiarrhythmic agents in suppressing ventricular tachycardia in myotonic dystrophy has had limited efficacy. Sotalol may be more effective. Implantable cardioverter-defibrillators are being used in myotonic patients.[30]

The course of neuromuscular abnormalities in myotonic dystrophy is highly variable. Death from progressive weakness and respiratory difficulty can occur in advanced skeletal muscle disease. Other individuals may be only minimally limited by weakness to ages of 60 to 70 years. Sudden death may significantly reduce survival in patients with myotonic dystrophy including those minimally symptomatic from a neuromuscular status. What evaluation and interventions are appropriate and the degree of effectiveness to decrease the risk of sudden death are unclear.

Emery-Dreifuss Muscular Dystrophy and Associated Disorders

GENETICS AND CARDIAC PATHOLOGY. Emery-Dreifuss muscular dystrophy is a rare familial disorder in which skeletal muscle symptoms are often mild but with cardiac involvement that is common and life threatening. The disease is classically inherited in an X-linked recessive fashion, but there is heterogeneity in that families have been reported that fit an autosomal dominant and recessive inheritance pattern. The gene responsible for the X-linked recessive Emery-Dreifuss muscular dystrophy, *STA*, encodes a nuclear membrane protein termed *emerin*.[31] The lack of emerin in skeletal and cardiac muscle is responsible for the disease phenotype.[32] Mutations in genes encoding two other nuclear membrane proteins, lamins A and C, have been identified as being responsible for a variety of other disorders with a phenotypic expression related to X-linked Emery-Dreifuss muscular dystrophy. The disorders include autosomal dominant and recessive Emery-Dreifuss muscular dystrophy, autosomal dominant dilated cardiomyopathy with conduction disease, autosomal dominant limb-girdle muscular dystrophy with conduction disease, and lipodystrophy with associated cardiac abnormalities.[33-37]

The mechanisms by which abnormalities in emerin and lamins A and C lead to cardiac involvement in Emery-Dreifuss muscular dystrophy and the associated disorders are not clear. The nuclear membrane proteins provide structural support for the nucleus as well as interact with the cell's cytoskeleton. One group of investigators have reported that emerin localizes to cardiac desmosomes and fasciae adherentes, possibly accounting for the predominance of conduction disease.[38] Localization of emerin in intercalated discs has not been observed by others.[39] Mutations in the tail regions of lamins A and C are responsible for most of the cases of autosomal dominant Emery-Dreifuss muscular dystrophy with a phenotype of both cardiac and skeletal muscle involvement.[33] Mutations in the rod domain of the lamins A and C gene primarily cause isolated cardiac disease including dilated cardiomyopathy, conduction system degeneration, and atrial and ventricular arrhythmias.[36] A rod domain deletion mutation has been reported as being responsible for a phenotype consistent with autosomal dominant Emery-Dreifuss muscular dystrophy.[40]

CLINICAL PRESENTATION. Emery-Dreifuss muscular dystrophy is characterized by a triad of (1) early contractures of the elbow, Achilles tendon, and posterior cervical muscles; (2) slowly progressing muscle weakness and atrophy primarily in humeroperoneal muscles; and (3) cardiac involvement. The disorder has been labeled *benign X-linked muscular dystrophy* to differentiate the slowly progressive muscular weakness from that of Duchenne muscular dystrophy. A definitive diagnosis can be made in Emery-Dreifuss muscular dystrophy and in carriers using antiemerin antibodies.[41]

In the autosomal dominant and recessive inheritance of Emery-Dreifuss muscular dystrophy, a more variable phenotypic expression and penetrance is typically observed.[34]

A mutation in the lamins A and C gene is also responsible for an autosomal dominantly–inherited familial partial lipodystrophy characterized by marked loss of subcutaneous fat, diabetes, hypertriglyceridemia, and cardiac abnormalities.[37]

CARDIOVASCULAR MANIFESTATIONS. Arrhythmias and dilated cardiomyopathy are the major manifestations of cardiac disease in Emery-Dreifuss muscular dystrophy and the associated disorders. In X-linked recessive Emery-Dreifuss muscular dystrophy, abnormalities in impulse generation and conduction are exceedingly frequent. ECGs are generally abnormal by age 20 to 30 years, commonly showing first-degree atrioventricular block. The atria appear to be involved earlier than the ventricles, with atrial fibrillation and atrial flutter, or more classically, permanent atrial standstill and junctional bradycardia, observed. Abnormalities in impulse generation or conduction are present in virtually all individuals by age 35 to 40 years, and pacing is often required. Ventricular arrhythmias, including sustained ventricular tachycardia and ventricular fibrillation, have been reported. Invasive cardiac electrophysiological study data are limited in this rare condition. Mild prolongation of the His-ventricular interval, atrial, atrioventricular nodal, and ventricular refractory periods have been observed. Sudden death (presumed cardiac) before 50 years of age is common. The incidence of sudden death may decrease with prophylactic pacing. Female carriers of X-linked recessive Emery-Dreifuss muscular dystrophy do not develop skeletal muscle disease, but late cardiac disease, including conduction abnormalities and sudden death, can occur.

Although arrhythmic disease is the most common presentation of cardiac involvement in X-linked recessive Emery-Dreifuss muscular dystrophy, a dilated cardiomyopathy can develop. The dilated cardiomyopathy is more common in patients in whom survival has been improved with pacemaker implantation. Both autopsy and endomyocardial biopsy have shown abnormal cardiac fibrosis.

Patients with disorders caused by lamins A and C mutations typically present at the ages of 20 to 40 years with cardiac conduction disease, atrial fibrillation, and dilated cardiomyopathy.[33-37] Skeletal muscle disease is typically subclinical or absent. Progression of a cardiomyopathy to an extent that heart transplant is required has been observed. Sudden death in those patients with a dilated cardiomyopathy is common. Permanent pacing is often required for symptomatic heart block.

TREATMENT AND PROGNOSIS. Affected patients should be monitored for development of ECG conduction abnormalities and other arrhythmias. Atrioventricular block can occur with anesthesia. In X-linked recessive Emery-Dreifuss muscular dystrophy, permanent pacing is recommended once conduction disease is evident, and it can be life saving. Whether similar pacing recommendations should be followed in patients with disorders caused by lamins A and C mutations is not clear. History, examination, and cardiac imaging for evaluation of left ventricular function is appropriate in all of the patients with Emery-Dreifuss muscular dystrophy and the associated disorders. Patients with left ventricular dysfunction should benefit from appropriate pharmacological therapy. These patients appear to benefit from heart transplant. Sudden death even in patients with pacemakers is common. Whether prophylactic implantable cardioverter-defibrillators should be considered in certain subgroups of patients is not clear. Female carriers of X-linked recessive Emery-Dreifuss muscular dystrophy develop conduction disease, and ECG monitoring on a routine basis is appropriate.

Limb-Girdle Muscular Dystrophy

GENETICS. Limb-girdle muscular dystrophy constitutes a group of disorders with a limb–pelvic girdle distribution of weakness but with otherwise heterogeneous inheritance and genetic etiology.[42] Inheritance is autosomal recessive (limb-girdle muscular dystrophy type 2), with many of the cases sporadic or autosomal dominant (limb-girdle muscular dystrophy type 1). At least 15 different gene abnormalities have been reported. The genes involved encode dystrophin-associated glycoproteins.[43]

CLINICAL PRESENTATION. The onset of muscle weakness is variable but usually occurs before 30 years of age. The recessive disorders tend to cause earlier weakness than the dominant disorders. Creatine kinase levels are typically moderately elevated. Patients commonly present with complaints of difficulty with walking or running secondary to pelvic girdle involvement. As the disease progresses, involvement of the shoulder muscles and then more distal muscles occurs, with sparing of facial involvement. Slow progression to severe disability and death can occur.

CARDIOVASCULAR MANIFESTATIONS. As with many of the features of limb-girdle muscular dystrophy, there is heterogeneity also observed in the presence and degree of cardiac involvement.

Limb-girdle muscular dystrophy types 2C to 2F are autosomal recessive disorders caused by mutations in a subunit of the sarcoglycan subcomplex.[42] These sarcoglyconopathy disorders are associated with a dilated cardiomyopathy.[44-48] ECGs in these patients have shown abnormalities such as an increased R wave in V_1, consistent with a pattern of dystrophin-related cardiomyopathy, similar to that observed in Duchenne muscular dystrophy. With ECG or echocardiographic evaluations, cardiac abnormalities have been detected in up to 80 percent of patients. A smaller proportion of patients are symptomatic related to the cardiac involvement. A severe cardiomyopathy, including presentation with heart failure in childhood, may occur.[44,47,48] Sudden death associated with the cardiomyopathy has been reported. The mechanisms by which sarcoglycan abnormalities lead to a dilated cardiomyopathy are not clear. Recent studies support abnormalities in vascular supply to the myocardium rather than a direct myopathic effect.[49-51]

The autosomal dominant limb-girdle muscular dystrophy type 1B is caused by mutations in the gene encoding lamins A and C, similar to that observed in Emery-Dreifuss muscular dystrophy.[35] It is not surprising that the clinical phenotype is also similar to Emery-Dreifuss muscular dystrophy, with mild skeletal muscle symptoms and more severe cardiac involvement, primarily arrhythmic in nature.[52] Affected patients develop atrioventricular block by early middle age often necessitating pacing. Sudden death, believed to be cardiac, is common, including in those in whom pacing was previously instituted. A dilated cardiomyopathy can occur.

TREATMENT AND PROGNOSIS. Because of the heterogeneous nature of limb-girdle muscular dystrophy, specific recommendations for routine cardiac evaluation and therapy are difficult to formulate. Genetic testing can determine those with sarcoglyconopathies or lamins A and C mutations who are at the highest risk for cardiac involvement. In these patients (and families), cardiac evaluation for arrhythmias and ventricular dysfunction should be done. Whether standard heart failure therapy will decrease the progression of cardiomyopathy is unclear. Prophylactic pacing in those with lamins A and C mutations after conduction disease is observed should be considered. The high risk of sudden death in spite of pacing may point toward the implantable cardioverter-defibrillator as being a more appropriate electrical therapy.

Facioscapulohumeral Muscular Dystrophy

GENETICS. Facioscapulohumeral muscular dystrophy is the third most common type of muscular dystrophy after Duchenne and myotonic, with a prevalence of 1 per 20,000 persons.[53] It is an autosomal dominant disorder in which the genetic locus has been mapped to chromosome 4q35. Genetic heterogeneity has been reported. The diagnosis can be confirmed by a 4q35 *Eco*RI allele size of 38 kilobases or less.[54] Neither the definitive gene nor the gene product responsible for facioscapulohumeral muscular dystrophy has been identified.

CLINICAL PRESENTATION. Muscle weakness tends to follow a slowly progressive but variable course, presenting with facial and/or shoulder girdle muscle weakness and progressing to involve the pelvic musculature (Fig. 85–10). Major disability affecting walking eventually occurs in 20 percent of individuals.

CARDIOVASCULAR MANIFESTATIONS. Cardiac involvement in facioscapulohumeral muscular dystrophy is reported but does not constitute as significant of a problem in prevalence or severity as in other muscular dystrophies. In some series no evidence of cardiac abnormalities were found. Other series have reported a propensity toward arrhythmias, primarily atrial in origin, with atrioventricular conduction abnormalities less common.[55]

TREATMENT AND PROGNOSIS. Because significant clinical cardiac involvement is rare in facioscapulohumeral

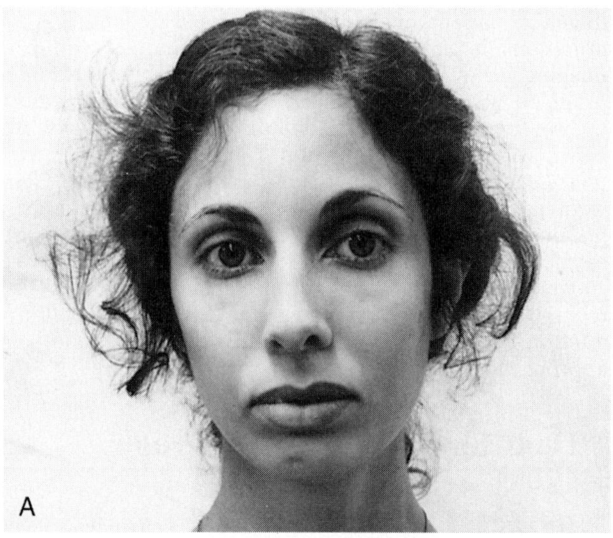

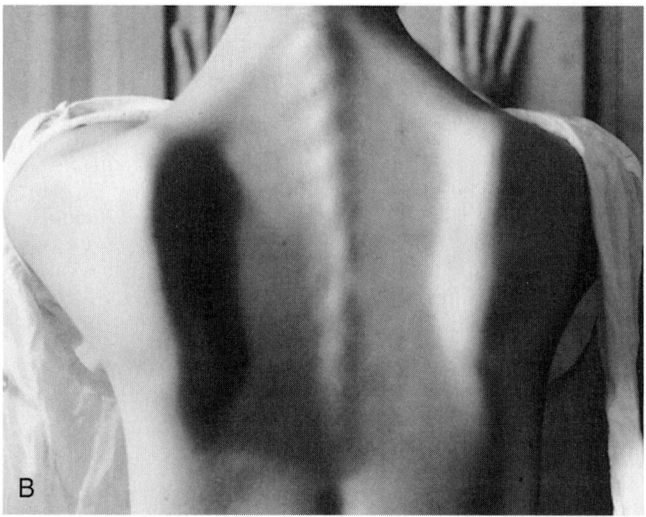

FIGURE 85–10 Facioscapulohumeral muscular dystrophy in a 32-year-old woman. **A,** The face is in repose (myopathic) with dimpling of the corners of the mouth. **B,** Typical winging of the scapulae. (**A** and **B,** Courtesy of Joseph K. Perloff, MD.)

muscular dystrophy, specific monitoring or treatment recommendations are not well defined. One group has recommended yearly ECGs.[55]

Friedreich Ataxia

GENETICS. Friedreich ataxia is an autosomal recessive spinocerebellar degenerative disease characterized clinically by ataxia of the limbs and trunk, dysarthria, loss of deep tendon reflexes, sensory abnormalities, skeletal deformities, diabetes mellitus, and cardiac involvement.[56] The disease is linked to chromosome 9, with the gene mutation affecting the encoding of a 210-amino acid protein, frataxin. Frataxin is a mitochondrial protein important in iron homeostasis and respiratory function. Messenger RNA for frataxin is highly expressed in the heart. The mutation responsible for Friedreich ataxia is an amplified trinucleotide (guanine-adenine-adenine [GAA]) repeat found in the first intron of the gene encoding frataxin. Whereas normal individuals have fewer than 33 repeats, patients with Friedreich ataxia have 66 to 1500 GAA repeats. In 95 percent of patients, both alleles of the gene have the expanded repeat. In 5 percent of patients, a point mutation occurs on one allele in association with an expanded repeat on the other. The GAA repeat disrupts transcription severely decreasing frataxin synthesis. The decrease in frataxin leads to mitochondrial dysfunction, poor cellular response to oxidative stress, and apoptosis.[57] Endomyocardial biopsies in patients with Friedreich ataxia have shown deficient function in mitochondrial respiratory complex subunits and in aconitase, an iron-sulfur protein involved in iron homeostasis.[58] Abnormal cardiac bioenergetics appear to result from the abnormalities in respiratory function and iron handling.[59] As the GAA triplet size increases an earlier age of symptom onset, increasing severity of neurological symptoms and worsening left ventricular hypertrophy by echocardiography are observed.[60]

CLINICAL PRESENTATION. The estimated prevalence of Friedreich ataxia is 1 in 50,000. Neurological symptoms usually manifest around puberty and almost always before age 25 years. Progressive loss of neuromuscular function, with the individual wheelchair bound 10 to 20 years after symptom onset, is the norm. Neurological symptoms precede cardiac symptoms in most but not all cases.

CARDIOVASCULAR MANIFESTATIONS. Friedreich ataxia is commonly associated with a concentric hypertrophic cardiomyopathy (see Chap. 59) (Fig. 85–11). Less commonly, asymmetrical septal hypertrophy is observed. The presence of a left ventricular outflow gradient associated with the septal hypertrophy has been reported. Presentation with a dilated cardiomyopathy is more rare but can occur (Fig. 85–12). The dilated cardiomyopathy appears to occur as a progressive transition from a hypertrophic cardiomyopathy. The prevalence of hypertrophy varies between studies but does increase in prevalence with a younger age at diagnosis and with increasing GAA trinucleotide repeat length.[60,61] Up to 95 percent of neurologically symptomatic patients have abnormalities on ECG and echocardiographic evaluations.

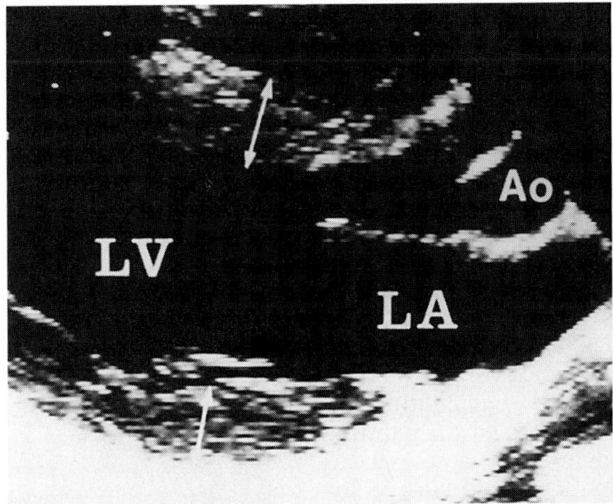

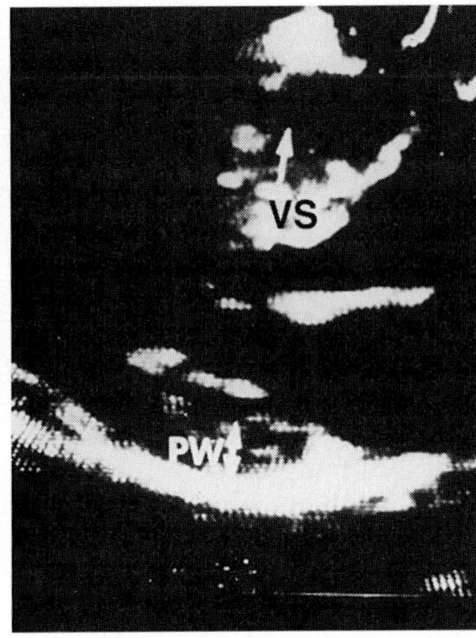

FIGURE 85–11 **A,** Two-dimensional echocardiogram (parasternal long axis diastolic frames) from a 14-year-old girl with Friedreich ataxia and concentric hypertrophy (arrows) of the LV. **B,** Two-dimensional echocardiogram (parasternal long axis) from a 17-year-old boy with Friedreich ataxia and hypertrophic cardiomyopathy characterized by disproportionate thickness (arrows) of the VS compared with the PW. LV = left ventricle; Ao = aorta; LA = left atrium; PW = posterior wall; VS = ventricular septum. (**A** and **B,** From Perloff JK: Cardiac manifestations of neuromuscular disease. *In* Abelmann WH [ed]: Cardiomyopathies, Myocarditis, and Pericardial Disease. *In* Braunwald E [series ed]: Atlas of Heart Diseases. Vol 2. Philadelphia, Current Medicine, 1995.)

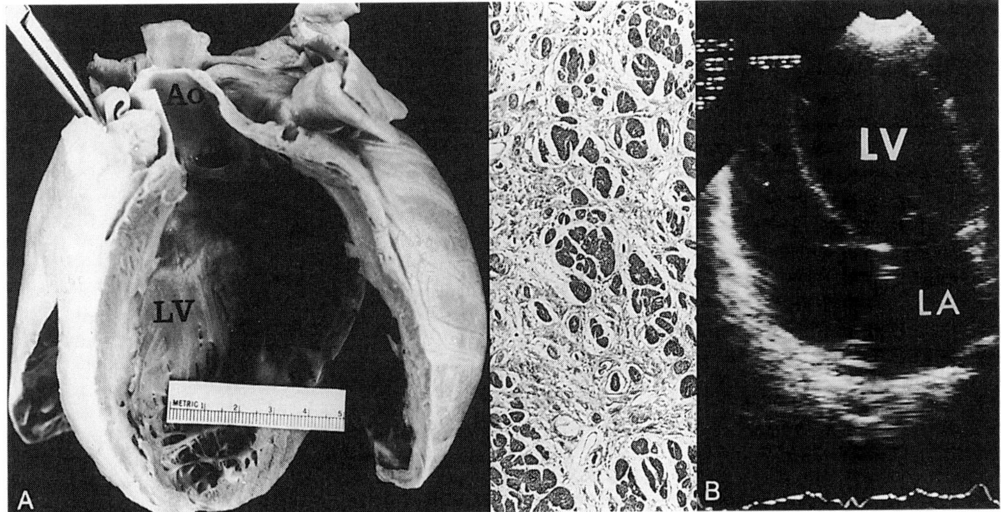

FIGURE 85–12 **A,** Gross and histological specimens from a 17-year-old boy with Friedreich ataxia whose echocardiogram progressed from normal at age 13 years to a minimally dilated, hypocontractile left ventricle 3 to 4 years later. The gross specimen shows a mildly dilated LV with normal wall thickness; the walls were flabby. The microscopic section from the LV free wall (middle panel) shows marked connective tissue replacement. Although specifically sought, small-vessel coronary artery disease was not identified. **B,** Two-dimensional echocardiogram (apical window) showing the mildly dilated, thin-walled LV. LA = left atrium; LV = left ventricle. (**A** and **B,** From Child JS, Perloff JK, Bach PM, et al: Cardiac involvement in Friedreich ataxia. J Am Coll Cardiol 7:1370, 1986.)

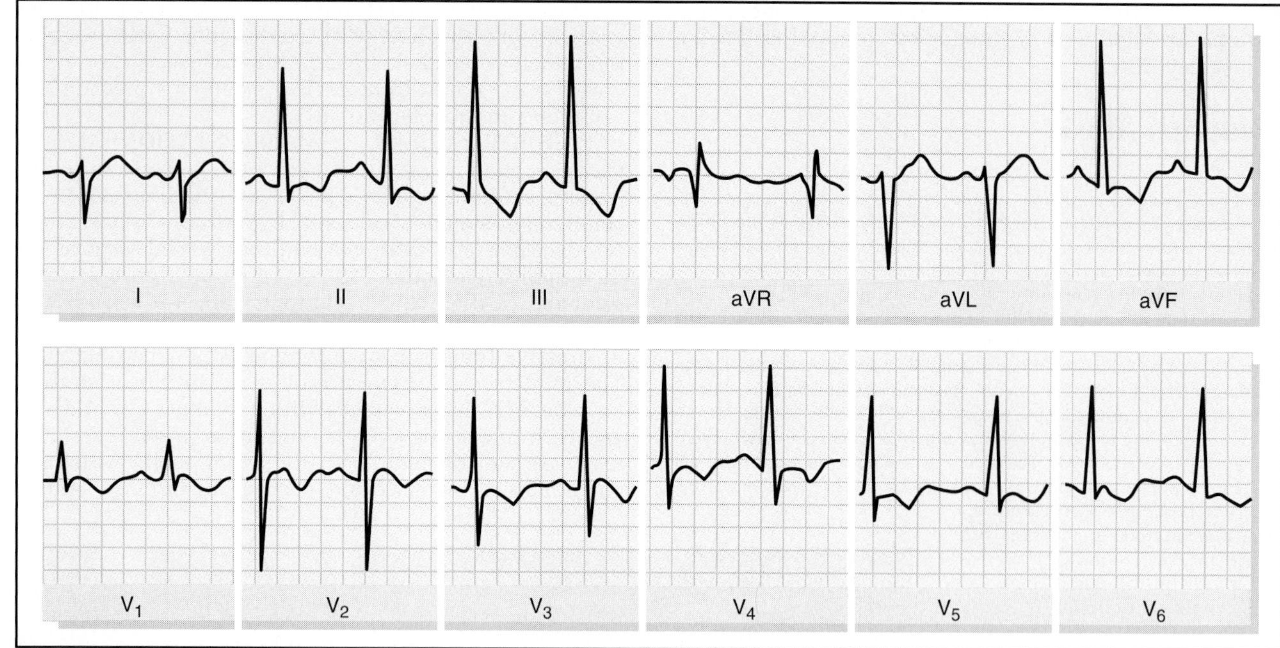

FIGURE 85–13 Electrocardiogram from a 34-year-old man with Friedreich ataxia. Widespread ST and T changes are observed. (Courtesy of Charles Fisch, MD, Indiana University School of Medicine, Indianapolis, IN.)

Findings are primarily consistent with ventricular hypertrophy. Left ventricular hypertrophy is not always present on ECGs despite echocardiographic evidence. Widespread T wave inversions are common (Fig. 85–13).

Arrhythmias occur in Friedreich ataxia but are less common than what might be expected, considering the high incidence of cardiac involvement. Atrial arrhythmias including atrial fibrillation and flutter are associated with the progression to a dilated cardiomyopathy. Ventricular tachycardia, again in the setting of a dilated cardiomyopathy, has been observed. The hypertrophic cardiomyopathy of Friedreich ataxia is not associated with serious ventricular arrhythmias as observed in the other types of heritable hypertrophic cardiomyopathies. Myocardial fiber disarray is not commonly observed in the hypertrophic cardiomyopathy of Friedreich ataxia. Sudden death has been reported, but a mechanism has not been well characterized.

Endomyocardial biopsies in Friedreich ataxia have demonstrated myocyte hypertrophy and interstitial fibrosis. Histopathological examination has revealed myocyte hypertrophy and degeneration, interstitial fibrosis, active muscle necrosis, bizarre pleomorphic nuclei, and periodic acid–Schiff-positive deposition in both large and small coronary arteries. Degeneration and fibrosis in cardiac nerves and ganglia and the conduction system have also been observed. Deposition of calcium salts and iron has been reported.

TREATMENT AND PROGNOSIS. Idebenone, a free radical scavenger, was reported to significantly decrease overall left ventricular mass in one-half of Friedreich ataxia patients treated in an unblinded, noncontrolled trial for 6 months.[62] No characteristics were found that separated responders from nonresponders. In patients with depressed left ventricular function at the initiation of idebenone therapy most showed improvement. Idebenone decreases markers of oxidative DNA damage in patients with Friedreich ataxia.[63] Whether an improvement in neurological outcome will result is unclear.

In general, progressive neurological dysfunction is the norm in Friedreich ataxia, with death from respiratory failure or infection in the fourth or fifth decades. Cardiac death occurs primarily in those developing a dilated cardiomyopathy. These patients tend do poorly, with rapid progression to end-stage congestive heart failure.

Less Common Neuromuscular Diseases Associated with Cardiac Manifestations

The Periodic Paralyses

GENETICS. The primary periodic paralyses are rare, nondystrophic, autosomal dominant disorders that result from abnormalities in ion channel genes. They can be classified into hypokalemic, hyperkalemic (potassium-sensitive), and normokalemic periodic paralyses, with several subclassifications in each.[64]

Hypokalemic periodic paralysis is characterized by episodic attacks of weakness in association with decreased serum potassium levels. Penetrance is complete in males and approximately 50 percent in females. Hypokalemic periodic paralysis has been mapped to chromosome 1q31-32 with subsequent identification of mutations in the alpha$_1$ subunit of the dihydropyridine-sensitive calcium channel. The disease may be genetically heterogeneous, as observed with the identification of a family with hypokalemic periodic paralysis and a mutation in the skeletal muscle sodium channel (SCN4A).[65]

Hyperkalemic periodic paralysis also manifests with episodic weakness but with symptoms worsening with potassium supplementation. Complete penetrance is observed. Potassium levels are usually high but may be normal during an attack. Hyperkalemic periodic paralysis is due primarily to mutations in the alpha subunit of SCN4A found on chromosome 17.[66] Multiple different mutations in this gene have been reported and result in a potassium-sensitive failure of inactivation in the sodium channel. Hyperkalemic periodic paralysis is genetically heterogeneous.

Andersen syndrome is a distinct potassium-sensitive periodic paralysis associated with dysmorphic features of low-set ears, micrognathia, and clinodactyly as well as a long-QT interval and ventricular arrhythmias (Fig. 85–14).[67] Andersen syndrome is linked to chromosome 17q23 with the mutation responsible in the *KCNJ2* gene encoding an inward rectifier potassium channel (Kir2.1).[68-70] Andersen syndrome has been given an alternate long-QT syndrome 7 nomenclature.

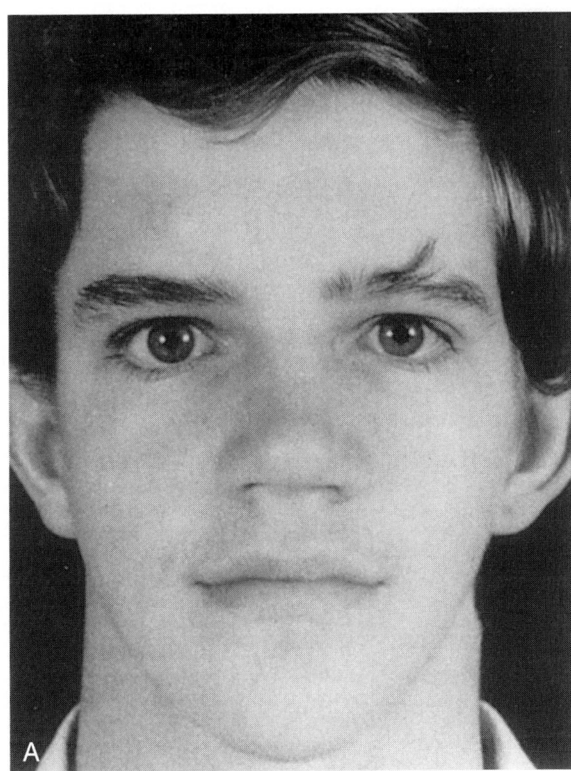

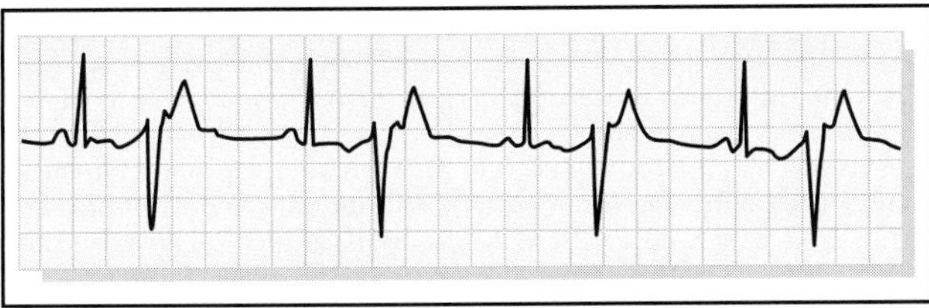

FIGURE 85–14 Andersen syndrome in a 22-year-old man. **A,** Characteristic low-set ears and hypoplastic mandible. **B,** Electrocardiographic recording revealing ventricular bigeminy. (**A** and **B,** From Tawil R, Ptacek LJ, Pavlakis SG, et al: Andersen's syndrome: Potassium-sensitive periodic paralysis, ventricular ectopy, and dysmorphic features. Ann Neurol 35:326, 1994.)

CLINICAL PRESENTATION. The primary manifestation of the periodic paralyses is episodic weakness. Attacks of weakness tend to be more severe and of longer duration with hypokalemic periodic paralysis than with hyperkalemic periodic paralysis. In both diseases, cold and rest after exercise can trigger an attack. Ingestion of carbohydrates can trigger an attack in hypokalemic periodic paralysis but may ameliorate an attack in hyperkalemic periodic paralysis.

CARDIOVASCULAR MANIFESTATIONS. The periodic paralyses are associated with ventricular arrhythmias. Arrhythmias occur primarily in hyperkalemic periodic paralysis and Andersen syndrome. Bidirectional ventricular tachycardia has been observed independent of digitalis intoxication. The episodes of bidirectional ventricular tachycardia are independent of attacks of muscle weakness, do not correlate with serum potassium levels, and can convert to sinus rhythm with exercise. Ventricular ectopy is common.

A prolonged QT interval can be observed. In some reports, this is episodic and associated with weakness, hypokalemia, or antiarrhythmic therapy. In other cases, a prolonged QT interval can be constant. Andersen syndrome is typically associated with a prolonged QT interval. Ventricular arrhythmias have been reported but are less likely in Andersen syndrome than other long-QT syndromes.

Sudden death has been reported in the periodic paralyses.

TREATMENT AND PROGNOSIS. The episodes of weakness typically respond to measures that work to normalize potassium levels. Weakness in hyperkalemic periodic paralysis can respond to mexiletine. Weakness in hypokalemic periodic paralysis can respond to acetazolamide. Treatment of electrolytes usually does not improve arrhythmias, or if it does, only transiently. Improvement in symptomatic nonsustained ventricular tachycardia associated with a prolonged QT interval has been reported with beta-blocker therapy. Class 1A antiarrhythmic agents can worsen muscle weakness and exacerbate arrhythmias associated with a prolonged QT interval. Bidirectional ventricular tachycardia, not associated with a prolonged QT interval, may not respond to beta-blocker therapy. Amiodarone has been observed to decrease episodes of sustained polymorphic ventricular tachycardia in Andersen syndrome.

MITOCHONDRIAL DISORDERS

GENETICS. The mitochondrial disorders are a heterogeneous group of diseases resulting from abnormalities in mitochondrial DNA and function.[71] The number of distinct disorders is extensive. Mitochondrial DNA is inherited maternally, and most of these disorders are thus transmitted from mother to children of both sexes. Some of the disorders occur sporadically or are inherited in an autosomal fashion. Disease severity can vary between patients and family members because both mutant and normal mitochondrial DNA can be present in tissue in a variable proportion. It is not surprising, based on the important metabolic function of mitochondria, that these disorders manifest with systemic pathology. Tissue with a high respiratory workload such as brain, skeletal muscle, and cardiac muscle are especially affected.

Mitochondrial disorders, which have cardiac manifestations, present as several clinical phenotypes, consisting of chronic progressive external ophthalmoplegia, which includes Kearns-Sayre syndrome; myoclonus epilepsy with red ragged fibers (MERRF); mitochondrial myopathy, encephalopathy, lactic acidosis, and stroke-like episodes (MELAS); and Leber hereditary optic neuropathy. Other, more rare mitochondrial point mutation disorders, present primarily with cardiac manifestations, typically a hypertrophic or dilated cardiomyopathy.[72] Chronic progressive external ophthalmoplegia is primarily a sporadic disease, whereas the others listed are maternally inherited.

CLINICAL PRESENTATION. *Kearns-Sayre syndrome* is characterized by the clinical triad of progressive external ophthalmoplegia, pigmentary retinopathy, and atrioventricular block (Fig. 85–15). Diabetes, deafness, and ataxia can also be associated. Clinical features of MERRF include myoclonus, seizures, ataxia, dementia, and skeletal muscle weakness. MELAS is the most common of the maternally inherited mitochondrial disorders and is characterized by encephalopathy, subacute stroke-like events, migraine-like headaches, recurrent emesis, extremity weakness, and short stature. *Leber hereditary optic neuropathy* manifests as a severe, subacute, painless loss of central vision, predominantly affecting young men.

CARDIOVASCULAR MANIFESTATIONS. In chronic, progressive external ophthalmoplegia, most commonly in Kearns-Sayre syndrome, cardiac involvement manifests primarily as conduction abnormalities.[73] A dilated cardiomyopathy has also been reported.[74] In Kearns-Sayre syndrome, atrioventricular block is common, usually presenting after eye involvement. The His-ventricular interval is prolonged, consistent with distal conduction disease. Pacing is often required before 20 years of age. An increased prevalence of preexcitation has also been reported.

Leber hereditary optic neuropathy can be associated with a short PR interval on the ECG and preexcitation. Supraventricular tachycardia has been reported.

In MERRF and MELAS, cardiac involvement manifesting as hypertrophic (symmetrical or asymmetrical) or dilated cardiomyopathy is observed. Other disorders caused by mitochondrial point mutations can present with a similar cardiac phenotype.[74] Patients can present with chest pain with ECG abnormalities and myocardial perfusion defects. Whether the dilated cardiomyopathy represents a progression from the hypertrophic cardiomyopathy or a separate syndrome is not clear. The dilated cardiomyopathy can result in heart failure and death.

Preexcitation has been described with MELAS.

TREATMENT AND PROGNOSIS. In Kearns-Sayre syndrome, the prophylactic implantation of a pacemaker has been advocated when distal conduction disease is evident. Pacing appears to improve survival.[73] The

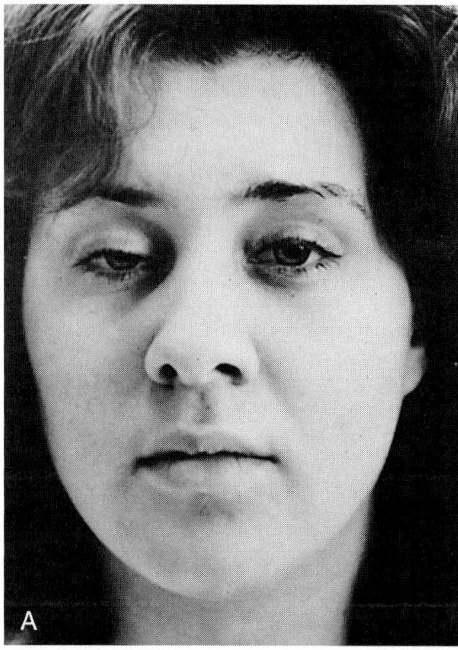

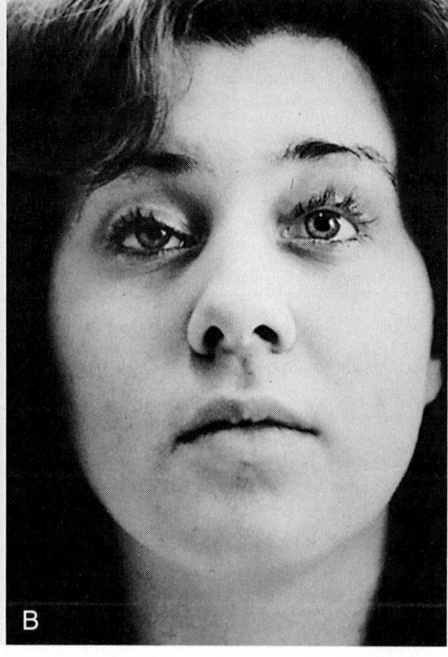

FIGURE 85–15 An 18-year-old girl with Kearns-Sayre syndrome and bilateral asymmetrical ptosis. Within 24 months, her electrocardiogram changed from normal to bifascicular block (complete right bundle branch block and left anterior fascicular block). **A,** Asymmetrical ptosis when the patient looks straight ahead. **B,** Ptosis of the right lid persists when the patient looks up. She also had typical pigmentary retinopathy. (**A** and **B,** Courtesy of Joseph K. Perloff, MD.)

degree of distal conduction disease that warrants prophylactic pacing is not clear. In Leber hereditary optic neuropathy, a baseline ECG may be prudent. In the other mitochondrial disorders, an understanding of the potential for cardiac involvement is necessary. Screening echocardiography has been recommended.[72] Whether other specific screening evaluations are warranted in these disorders is uncertain.

SPINAL MUSCULAR ATROPHY

GENETICS AND CLINICAL PRESENTATION. The spinal muscular atrophies are a group of lower motor neuron disorders presenting as progressive, symmetrical muscular weakness.[75,76] The disorders are inherited in an autosomal recessive fashion or are sporadic. The spinal muscular atrophies are classified clinically by the age of symptom onset and disease severity. *Type I (Werdnig-Hoffman disease)* and *type II* have early childhood onset with severe limitation of life span. *Type III (Kugelberg-Welander disease)* is characterized by later onset and slower progression, typically with survival to adulthood.

The spinal muscular atrophies link to chromosome 5q13. Mutations in two genes, *SMN* (survival of motor neuron) and *NAIP* (neuronal apoptosis inhibitory protein), are responsible for most cases.[77,78]

CARDIOVASCULAR MANIFESTATIONS. Cardiac involvement in spinal muscular atrophies includes coexisting complex congenital heart disease, cardiomyopathy, and arrhythmias. Congenital heart disease has been associated with types I and III spinal muscular atrophies. The most common abnormality is atrial septal defect, with other abnormalities reported. In spinal muscular atrophy type III, a dilated cardiomyopathy may occur with endomyocardial biopsies demonstrating fibrosis. Progression leading to a fatal outcome has been reported. Arrhythmic abnormalities including atrial standstill, atrial fibrillation, atrial flutter, and atrioventricular block may be the most common cardiac manifestation in these diseases. Permanent pacing for atrial standstill and atrioventricular block has been reported.

TREATMENT AND PROGNOSIS. The skeletal muscle involvement in spinal muscular atrophy types I and II limit life span to such a significant degree that treatment of associated cardiac abnormalities is often not indicated. In spinal muscular atrophy type III, awareness of the potential for associated cardiac abnormalities is necessary. Permanent pacing may be required.

GUILLAIN-BARRÉ SYNDROME

CLINICAL PRESENTATION. Guillain-Barré syndrome is an acute inflammatory demyelinating neuropathy characterized by peripheral, cranial, and autonomic nerve dysfunction.[77] It is the most common acquired demyelinating neuropathy, with an annual incidence of 1.7 per 100,000 population. In two-thirds of affected patients, an acute viral or bacterial illness, typically respiratory or gastrointestinal, precedes the onset of neurological symptoms by 5 days to 3 weeks. The disorder typically presents with symmetrical limb weakness that can progress to involve cranial and respiratory muscles. Approximately one-third of individuals require assisted ventilation.

CARDIOVASCULAR MANIFESTATIONS. Cardiac involvement in Guillain-Barré syndrome is related to accompanying autonomic nervous system dysfunction that manifests as hypertension, orthostatic hypotension, resting sinus tachycardia, loss of heart rate variability, ECG ST abnormalities, and both bradycardia and tachycardias. Significant autonomic nervous system dysfunction occurs primarily in severe cases of Guillain-Barré syndrome. Microneurographic recordings have shown increased sympathetic outflow during the acute illness that normalizes with recovery.

Life-threatening arrhythmias are common in severe cases of Guillain-Barré syndrome, primarily those requiring assisted ventilation. Arrhythmias observed include asystole, symptomatic bradycardia, rapid atrial fibrillation, and ventricular tachycardia/fibrillation. Deaths due to arrhythmias occur. Asystole was commonly associated with tracheal suctioning.

TREATMENT AND PROGNOSIS. In addition to supportive care, early plasmapheresis and intravenous immunoglobulin can improve recovery. In patients requiring ventilation, cardiac rhythm monitoring is mandatory. If serious bradycardia or asystole is observed, temporary or permanent pacing can improve survival. Atropine or isoproterenol during tracheal suctioning can be of benefit. The mortality rate in individuals hospitalized with Guillain-Barré syndrome is as high as 20 percent. In individuals who recover from Guillain-Barré syndrome, autonomic function also recovers and long-term arrhythmia risk has not been observed.

MYASTHENIA GRAVIS

CLINICAL PRESENTATION. Myasthenia gravis is a disorder of neuromuscular transmission resulting from production of antibody targeted against the nicotinic acetylcholine receptor. The primary symptom, fluctuating weakness, usually begins with the eye and facial muscles and later can involve the large muscles of the limbs. Patients can present at any age, typically at a younger age in women and an older age in men. Myasthenia gravis is usually associated with hyperplasia or a benign or malignant tumor (thymoma) of the thymus gland. The prevalence in the United States is 1 per 33,000 persons.

CARDIOVASCULAR MANIFESTATIONS. A myocarditis can be associated with myasthenia gravis, especially that occurring with thymoma. A cardiac muscle antibody is believed to be responsible. Up to 16 percent of patients with myasthenia gravis have cardiac manifestations not explained by another etiology. Presentation is typically with arrhythmic symptoms including atrial fibrillation, atrioventricular block, asystole, and unexplained sudden death. Autopsy findings were consistent with myocarditis.

TREATMENT AND PROGNOSIS. Myasthenia gravis is treated with anticholinesterase and immunosuppressive agents. Thymectomy is often indicated. Anticholinesterase agents may slow heart rate and cause hypotension. Whether immunosuppressive agents or thymectomy improve associated cardiac disease is unknown. Use of quinidine or propranolol in patients with myasthenia gravis may precipitate an acute exacerbation of weakness.

Acute Cerebrovascular Disease

CARDIOVASCULAR MANIFESTATIONS. Acute cerebrovascular diseases, including subarachnoid hemorrhage, other stroke syndromes and head injury, can be associated with severe cardiac manifestations.[78] The mechanism by which this occurs appears to be related to abnormal autonomic nervous system function, primarily a markedly increased sympathetic and parasympathetic output (see Chap. 87). Hypothalamic stimulation can reproduce the ECG changes observed in acute cerebrovascular disease. ECG changes associated with hypothalamic stimulation or blood in the subarachnoid space can be diminished with spinal cord transection, stellate ganglion blockade, vagolytics, and adrenergic blockers.

ECG abnormalities are observed in as high as 80 to 90 percent of individuals with subarachnoid hemorrhage. Abnormalities including ST elevation and depression, T wave inversion, and pathologic Q waves are observed.[79] Peaked inverted T waves and a prolonged QT interval can occur in 25 to 40 percent of patients (Fig. 85–16). Hypokalemia is observed in up to 50 percent of patients with subarachnoid hemorrhage, and this increases the likelihood of QT interval prolongation. Other stroke syndromes are often associated with abnormal ECGs but whether these are related to the stroke syndrome or to underlying intrinsic cardiac disease is often difficult to discern. A prolonged QT interval is more common in subarachnoid hemorrhage than other stroke syndromes. Closed-head trauma can cause similar ECG abnormalities as subarachnoid hemorrhage including a prolonged QT interval.

Myocardial damage with liberation of myocardial enzymes and subendocardial hemorrhage or fibrosis at autopsy can occur in the setting of acute cerebrovascular disease. Like the ECG changes, these abnormalities are believed to be related to local myocardial catecholamine excess.

Neurogenic pulmonary edema can accompany the acute neurological insult. The edema can have both a cardiogenic component, related to systemic hypertension, and a noncardiogenic (pulmonary capillary leak) component.

Life-threatening arrhythmias can occur in the setting of acute cerebrovascular disease. Ventricular tachycardia or fibrillation has been observed in patients with subarachnoid hemorrhage and head trauma. A torsades de pointes–type of ventricular tachycardia can occur (Fig. 85–17). Often this is observed in the setting of a prolonged QT interval and hypokalemia. Stroke syndromes, other than subarachnoid hemorrhage, appear to be only rarely associated with serious ventricular tachycardias. Atrial arrhythmias including atrial fibrillation and regular supraventricular tachycardia have been observed. Atrial fibrillation is most common in individuals presenting with what is believed to be an acute thromboembolic stroke. Separating an effect from the cause can be difficult. Bradycardias including sinoatrial block, sinus arrest, and atrioventricular block occur in up to 10 percent of individuals with subarachnoid hemorrhage.

TREATMENT AND PROGNOSIS. Beta-adrenergic blockers appear effective in decreasing myocardial damage and in controlling both supraventricular and ventricular arrhythmias associated with subarachnoid hemorrhage and head trauma. Beta-adrenergic blockers can increase the likelihood of bradycardia. Life-threatening arrhythmias occur primarily in the first day following the neurological event. Continuous ECG monitoring during this period is indicated. Careful monitoring of potassium levels especially in patients with subarachnoid hemorrhage is warranted. Refractory ventricular arrhythmias have been controlled effectively with stellate ganglion blockade. ECG abnormalities reflect adverse intracranial factors but do not appear to portend a poor cardiovascular outcome.

Head injury (blunt trauma or gunshot wound) and cerebrovascular accident are the leading causes of brain death in individuals being considered as heart donors. These donors can manifest ECG abnormalities, hemodynamic instability,

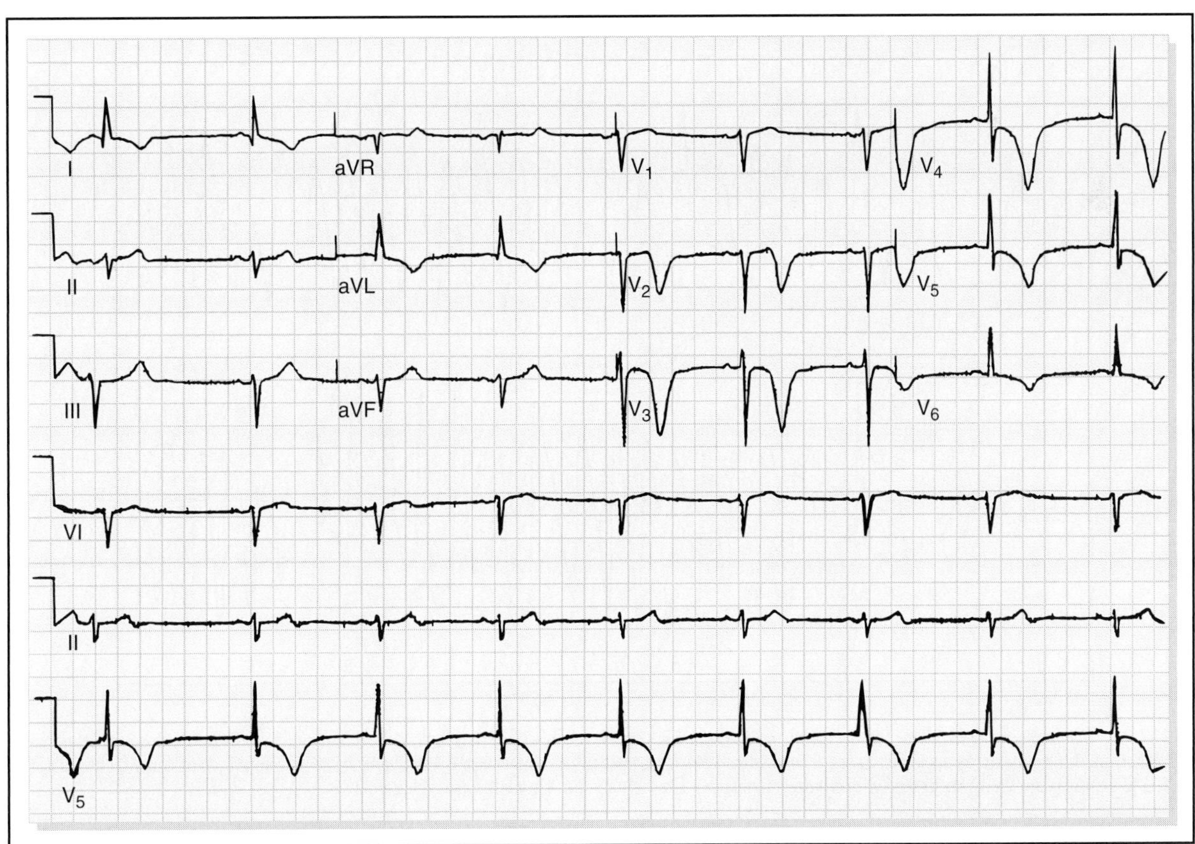

FIGURE 85–16 Electrocardiogram from a patient with cerebral hemorrhage. Deep and symmetrical T wave inversions are observed. (Courtesy of Charles Fisch, MD, Indiana University School of Medicine, Indianapolis, IN.)

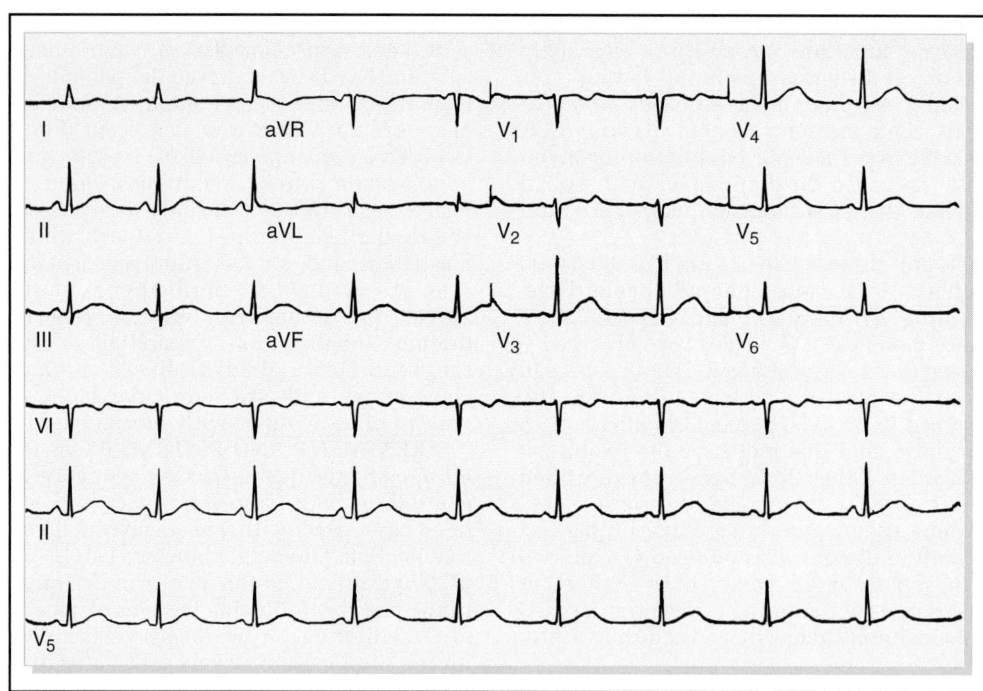

A

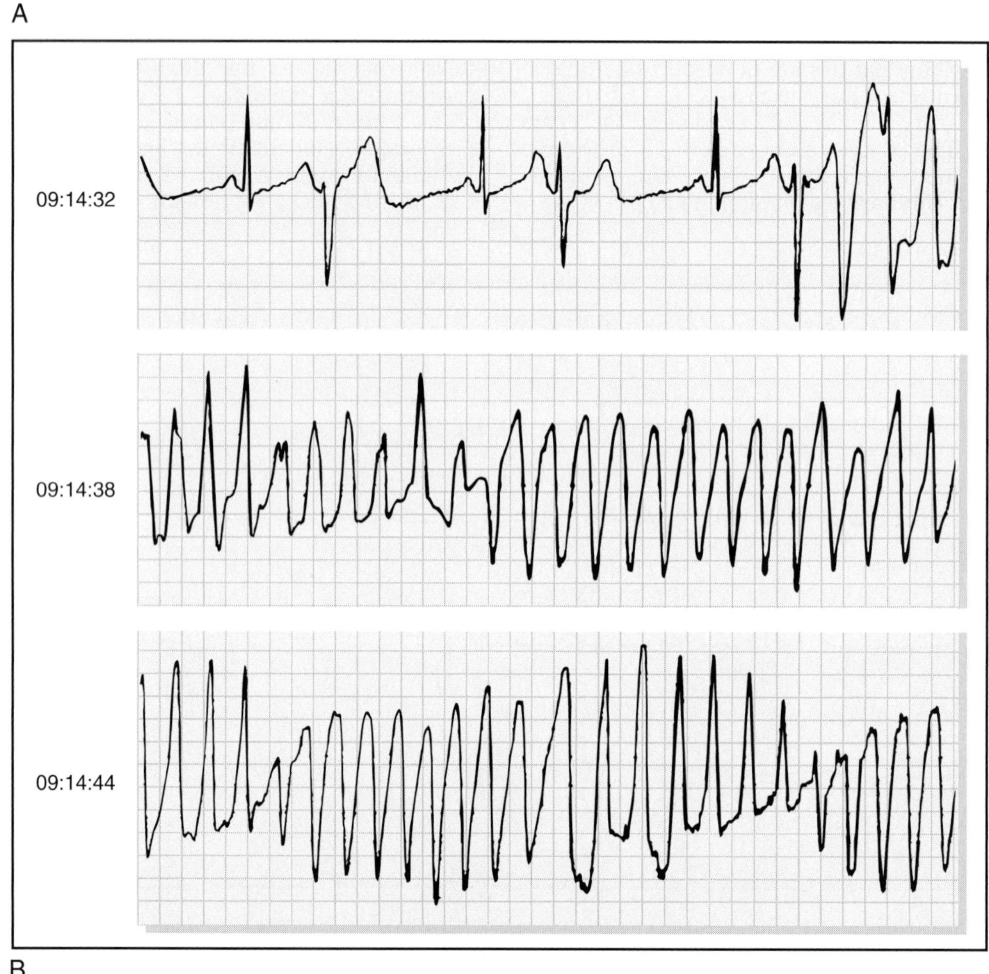

B

FIGURE 85–17 A 49-year-old patient with cerebral hemorrhage. **A,** Electrocardiogram recorded within 3 hours of admission and 4 hours after onset of symptoms. QT interval prolongation is observed. **B,** Electrocardiographic monitoring 6 hours after admission. Ventricular bigeminy precedes the onset of polymorphic ventricular tachycardia. Cardioversion was required. The patient was subsequently treated with a beta-adrenergic blocker without further ventricular tachycardia.

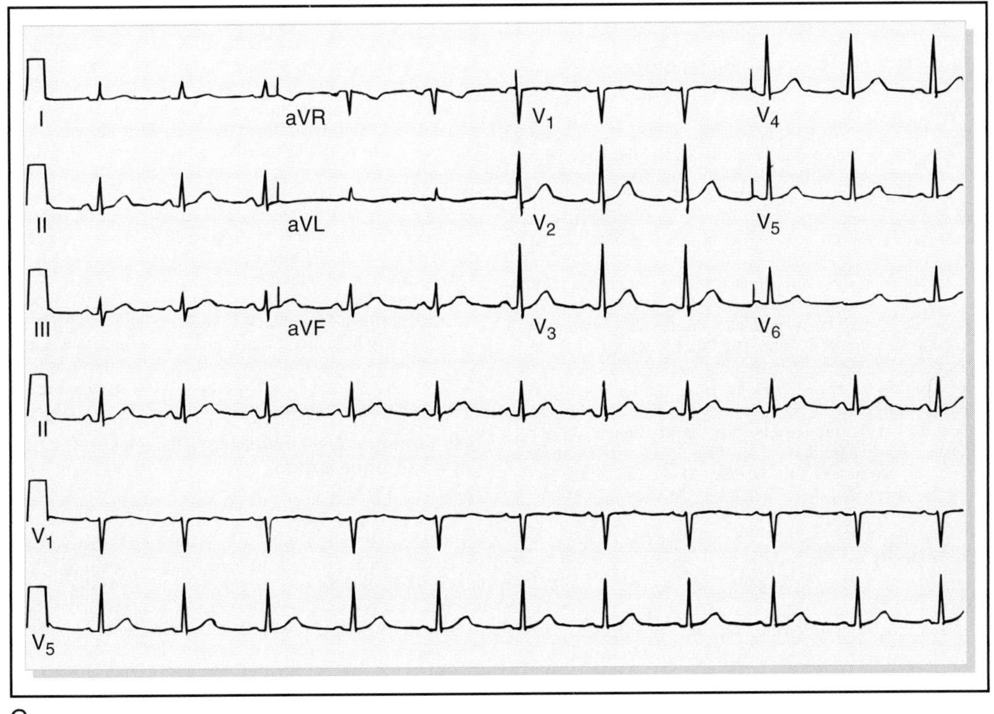

FIGURE 85–17, cont'd **C,** Electrocardiogram done 2 weeks after admission. The QT interval has normalized.

and myocardial dysfunction related primarily to adrenergic storm and not to intrinsic cardiac disease. Experimental studies on whether contractile performance recovers with transplantation are still controversial.[80] Optimization of volume status and inotropic support with careful echocardiographic evaluation and possibly left heart catheterization can allow the use of some donor hearts that would have otherwise been rejected.

REFERENCES

Duchenne and Becker Muscular Dystrophies

1. Towbin JA: The role of cytoskeletal proteins in cardiomyopathies. Curr Opin Cell Biol 10:131-9, 1998.
2. Ortiz-Lopez R, Li H, Su J, et al: Evidence for a dystrophin missense mutation as a cause of X-linked dilated cardiomyopathy. Circulation 95:2434-40, 1997.
3. Kaprielian RR, Stevenson S, Rothery SM, et al: Distinct patterns of dystrophin organization in myocyte sarcolemma and transverse tubules of normal and diseased human myocardium. Circulation 101:2586-94, 2000.
4. Biggar WD, Klamut HJ, Demacio PC, et al: Duchenne muscular dystrophy: Current knowledge, treatment, and future prospects. Clinical Orthop 88-106, 2002.
5. Hoogerwaard EM, de Voogt WG, Wilde AA, et al: Evolution of cardiac abnormalities in Becker muscular dystrophy over a 13-year period. J Neurol 244:657-63, 1997.
6. Melacini P, Fanin M, Danieli GA, et al: Myocardial involvement is very frequent among patients affected with subclinical Becker's muscular dystrophy. Circulation 94:3168-75, 1996.
7. Saito M, Kawai H, Akaike M, et al: Cardiac dysfunction with Becker muscular dystrophy. Am Heart J 132:642-7, 1996.
8. Hoogerwaard EM, Bakker E, Ippel PF, et al: Signs and symptoms of Duchenne muscular dystrophy and Becker muscular dystrophy among carriers in The Netherlands: A cohort study. Lancet 353:2116-9, 1999.
9. Negri SM, Cowan MD: Becker muscular dystrophy with bundle branch reentry ventricular tachycardia. J Cardiovasc Electrophysiol 9:652-4, 1998.
10. Case records of the Massachusetts General Hospital: Weekly clinicopathological exercises. Case 22-1998. A 22-year-old man with a cardiac transplant and creatine kinase elevation. N Engl J Med 339:182-90, 1998.

Myotonic Muscular Dystrophy

11. New nomenclature and DNA testing guidelines for myotonic dystrophy type 1 (DM1). The International Myotonic Dystrophy Consortium (IDMC). Neurology 54:1218-21, 2000.
12. Groh WJ, Lowe MR, Zipes DP: Severity of cardiac conduction involvement and arrhythmias in myotonic dystrophy type 1 correlates with age and CTG repeat length. J Cardiovasc Electrophysiol 13:444-8, 2002.
13. Tapscott SJ: Deconstructing myotonic dystrophy. Science 289:1701-2, 2000.
14. Tapscott SJ, Thornton CA: Biomedicine. Reconstructing myotonic dystrophy. Science 293:816-7, 2001.
15. Berul CI, Maguire CT, Aronovitz MJ, et al: DMPK dosage alterations result in atrioventricular conduction abnormalities in a mouse myotonic dystrophy model. J Clin Invest 103:R1-7, 1999.
16. Abbruzzese C, Krahe R, Liguori M, et al: Myotonic dystrophy phenotype without expansion of (CTG)n repeat: An entity distinct from proximal myotonic myopathy (PROMM)? J Neurol 243:715-21, 1996.
17. Meola G, Sansone V, Marinou K, et al: Proximal myotonic myopathy: A syndrome with a favourable prognosis? J Neurol Sci 193:89-96, 2002.
18. von zur Muhlen F, Klass C, Kreuzer H, et al: Cardiac involvement in proximal myotonic myopathy. Heart 79:619-21, 1998.
19. Ranum LP, Rasmussen PF, Benzow KA, et al: Genetic mapping of a second myotonic dystrophy locus. Nature Genet 19:196-8, 1998.
20. Liquori CL, Ricker K, Moseley ML, et al: Myotonic dystrophy type 2 caused by a CCTG expansion in intron 1 of ZNF9. Science 293:864-7, 2001.
21. Finsterer J, Gharehbaghi-Schnell E, Stollberger C, et al: Relation of cardiac abnormalities and CTG-repeat size in myotonic dystrophy. Clin Genet 59:350-5, 2001.
22. Lazarus A, Varin J, Ounnoughene Z, et al: Relationships among electrophysiological findings and clinical status, heart function, and extent of DNA mutation in myotonic dystrophy. Circulation 99:1041-6, 1999.
23. Gregoratos G, Abrams J, Epstein AE, et al: ACC/AHA/NASPE 2002 guideline update for implantation of cardiac pacemakers and antiarrhythmia devices. Circulation 106:2145-61, 2002.
24. Merino JL, Carmona JR, Fernandez-Lozano I, et al: Mechanisms of sustained ventricular tachycardia in myotonic dystrophy: Implications for catheter ablation. Circulation 98:541-546, 1998.
25. de Die-Smulders CE, Howeler CJ, Thijs C, et al: Age and causes of death in adult-onset myotonic dystrophy. Brain 121:1557-63, 1998.
26. Mathieu J, Allard P, Potvin L, et al: A 10-year study of mortality in a cohort of patients with myotonic dystrophy. Neurology 52:1658-62, 1999.
27. Stollberger C, Finsterer J, Keller H, et al: Progression of cardiac involvement in patients with myotonic dystrophy, Becker's muscular dystrophy and mitochondrial myopathy during a 2-year follow-up. Cardiology 90:173-9, 1998.
28. Colleran JA, Hawley RJ, Pinnow EE, et al: Value of the electrocardiogram in determining cardiac events and mortality in myotonic dystrophy. Am J Cardiol 80:1494-1497, 1997.
29. Phillips MF, Harper PS: Cardiac disease in myotonic dystrophy. Cardiovasc Res 33:13-22, 1997.
30. Hadian D, Lowe MR, Scott LR, et al: Use of an insertable loop recorder in a myotonic dystrophy patient. J Cardiovasc Electrophysiol 13:72-3, 2002.

Emery-Dreifuss Muscular Dystrophy and Associated Disorders

31. Nigro V, Bruni P, Ciccodicola A, et al: SSCP detection of novel mutations in patients with Emery-Dreifuss muscular dystrophy: Definition of a small C-terminal region required for emerin function. Hum Mol Genet 4:2003-4, 1995.
32. Nagano A, Koga R, Ogawa M, et al: Emerin deficiency at the nuclear membrane in patients with Emery-Dreifuss muscular dystrophy. Nature Genet 12:254-9, 1996.

33. Bonne G, Di Barletta MR, Varnous S, et al: Mutations in the gene encoding lamin A/C cause autosomal dominant Emery-Dreifuss muscular dystrophy. Nature Genet 21:285-8, 1999.
34. Di Barletta MR, Ricci E, Galluzzi G, et al: Different mutations in the LMNA gene cause autosomal dominant and autosomal recessive Emery-Dreifuss muscular dystrophy. Am J Hum Genet 66:1407-12, 2000.
35. Muchir A, Bonne G, van der Kooi AJ, et al: Identification of mutations in the gene encoding lamins A/C in autosomal dominant limb girdle muscular dystrophy with atrioventricular conduction disturbances (LGMD1B). Hum Mol Genet 9:1453-9, 2000.
36. Fatkin D, MacRae C, Sasaki T, et al: Missense mutations in the rod domain of the lamin A/C gene as causes of dilated cardiomyopathy and conduction-system disease. N Engl J Med 341:1715-24, 1999.
37. van der Kooi AJ, Bonne G, Eymard B, et al: Lamin A/C mutations with lipodystrophy, cardiac abnormalities, and muscular dystrophy. Neurology 59:620-3, 2002.
38. Cartegni L, di Barletta MR, Barresi R, et al: Heart-specific localization of emerin: New insights into Emery-Dreifuss muscular dystrophy. Hum Mol Genet 6:2257-64, 1997.
39. Manilal S, Sewry CA, Pereboev A, et al: Distribution of emerin and lamins in the heart and implications for Emery-Dreifuss muscular dystrophy. Hum Mol Genet 8:353-9, 1999.
40. Felice KJ, Schwartz RC, Brown CA, et al: Autosomal dominant Emery-Dreifuss dystrophy due to mutations in rod domain of the lamin A/C gene. Neurology 55:275-80, 2000.
41. Manilal S, Sewry CA, Man N, et al: Diagnosis of X-linked Emery-Dreifuss muscular dystrophy by protein analysis of leucocytes and skin with monoclonal antibodies. Neuromusc Disord 7:63-6, 1997.

Limb-Girdle Muscular Dystrophy

42. Mathews KD, Moore SA: Limb-girdle muscular dystrophy. Curr Neurol Neurosci Rep 3:78-85, 2003.
43. Beckmann JS, Brown RH, Muntoni F, et al: 66th/67th ENMC sponsored international workshop: The limb-girdle muscular dystrophies, 26-28 March 1999, Naarden, The Netherlands. Neuromusc Disord 9:436-45, 1999.
44. Fadic R, Sunada Y, Waclawik AJ, et al: Brief report: deficiency of a dystrophin-associated glycoprotein (adhalin) in a patient with muscular dystrophy and cardiomyopathy. N Engl J Med 334:362-6, 1996.
45. van der Kooi AJ, de Voogt WG, Barth PG, et al: The heart in limb girdle muscular dystrophy. Heart 79:73-7, 1998.
46. Melacini P, Fanin M, Duggan DJ, et al: Heart involvement in muscular dystrophies due to sarcoglycan gene mutations. Muscle Nerve 22:473-9, 1999.
47. Tsubata S, Bowles KR, Vatta M, et al: Mutations in the human delta-sarcoglycan gene in familial and sporadic dilated cardiomyopathy. J Clin Invest 106:655-62, 2000.
48. Barresi R, Di Blasi C, Negri T, et al: Disruption of heart sarcoglycan complex and severe cardiomyopathy caused by beta sarcoglycan mutations. J Med Genet 37:102-7, 2000.
49. Coral-Vazquez R, Cohn RD, Moore SA, et al: Disruption of the sarcoglycan-sarcospan complex in vascular smooth muscle: A novel mechanism for cardiomyopathy and muscular dystrophy. Cell 98:465-74, 1999.
50. Gnecchi-Ruscone T, Taylor J, Mercuri E, et al: Cardiomyopathy in Duchenne, Becker, and sarcoglycanopathies: A role for coronary dysfunction? Muscle Nerve 22:1549-56, 1999.
51. Cohn RD, Durbeej M, Moore SA, et al: Prevention of cardiomyopathy in mouse models lacking the smooth muscle sarcoglycan-sarcospan complex. J Clin Invest 107:R1-7, 2001.
52. van der Kooi AJ, Ledderhof TM, de Voogt WG, et al: A newly recognized autosomal dominant limb girdle muscular dystrophy with cardiac involvement. Ann Neurol 39:636-42, 1996.

Facioscapulohomeral Muscular Dystrophy

53. A prospective, quantitative study of the natural history of facioscapulohumeral muscular dystrophy (FSHD): Implications for therapeutic trials. The FSH-DY Group. Neurology 48:38-46, 1997.
54. Orrell RW, Tawil R, Forrester J, et al: Definitive molecular diagnosis of facioscapulohumeral dystrophy. Neurology 52:1822-6, 1999.
55. Laforet P, de Toma C, Eymard B, et al: Cardiac involvement in genetically confirmed facioscapulohumeral muscular dystrophy. Neurology 51:1454-6, 1998.

Friedreich Ataxia

56. Lynch DR, Farmer JM, Balcer LJ, et al: Friedreich ataxia: Effects of genetic understanding on clinical evaluation and therapy. Arch Neurol 59:743-7, 2002.
57. Wong A, Yang J, Cavadini P, et al: The Friedreich's ataxia mutation confers cellular sensitivity to oxidant stress which is rescued by chelators of iron and calcium and inhibitors of apoptosis. Hum Mol Genet 8:425-30, 1999.
58. Rotig A, de Lonlay P, Chretien D, et al: Aconitase and mitochondrial iron-sulphur protein deficiency in Friedreich ataxia. Nature Genet 17:215-7, 1997.
59. Lodi R, Rajagopalan B, Blamire AM, et al: Cardiac energetics are abnormal in Friedreich ataxia patients in the absence of cardiac dysfunction and hypertrophy: An in vivo 31P magnetic resonance spectroscopy study. Cardiovasc Res 52:111-9, 2001.
60. Isnard R, Kalotka H, Durr A, et al: Correlation between left ventricular hypertrophy and GAA trinucleotide repeat length in Friedreich's ataxia. Circulation 95:2247-9, 1997.
61. Maione S, Giunta A, Filla A, et al: May age onset be relevant in the occurrence of left ventricular hypertrophy in Friedreich's ataxia? Clin Cardiol 20:141-5, 1997.
62. Hausse AO, Aggoun Y, Bonnet D, et al: Idebenone and reduced cardiac hypertrophy in Friedreich's ataxia. Heart (British Cardiac Society) 87:346-9, 2002.
63. Schulz JB, Dehmer T, Schols L, et al: Oxidative stress in patients with Friedreich ataxia.[comment]. Neurology 55:1719-21, 2000.

Less Common Neuromuscular Diseases Associated with Cardiac Manifestations

64. Bulman DE: Phenotype variation and newcomers in ion channel disorders. Hum Mol Genet 6:1679-85, 1997.
65. Bulman DE, Scoggan KA, van Oene MD, et al: A novel sodium channel mutation in a family with hypokalemic periodic paralysis. Neurology 53:1932-6, 1999.
66. Ptacek LJ: Channelopathies: Ion channel disorders of muscle as a paradigm for paroxysmal disorders of the nervous system. Neuromusc Disord 7:250-5, 1997.
67. Sansone V, Griggs RC, Meola G, et al: Andersen's syndrome: A distinct periodic paralysis. Ann Neurol 42:305-12, 1997.
68. Plaster NM, Tawil R, Tristani-Firouzi M, et al: Mutations in Kir2.1 cause the developmental and episodic electrical phenotypes of Andersen's syndrome. Cell 105:511-9, 2001.
69. Ai T, Fujiwara Y, Tsuji K, et al: Novel KCNJ2 mutation in familial periodic paralysis with ventricular dysrhythmia. Circulation 105:2592-4, 2002.
70. Tristani-Firouzi M, Jensen JL, Donaldson MR, et al: Functional and clinical characterization of KCNJ2 mutations associated with LQT7 (Andersen syndrome). J Clin Invest 110:381-8, 2002.
71. Simon DK, Johns DR: Mitochondrial disorders: Clinical and genetic features. Ann Rev Med 50:111-27, 1999.
72. Santorelli FM, Tessa A, D'Amati G, et al: The emerging concept of mitochondrial cardiomyopathies. Am Heart J 141:E1, 2001.
73. Anan R, Nakagawa M, Miyata M, et al: Cardiac involvement in mitochondrial diseases. A study on 17 patients with documented mitochondrial DNA defects. Circulation 91:955-61, 1995.
74. Akaike M, Kawai H, Yokoi K, et al: Cardiac dysfunction in patients with chronic progressive external ophthalmoplegia. Clin Cardiol 20:239-43, 1997.
75. Stewart H, Wallace A, McGaughran J, et al: Molecular diagnosis of spinal muscular atrophy. Arch Dis Child 78:531-5, 1998.
76. Iannaccone ST, American Spinal Muscular Atrophy Randomized Trials G: Outcome measures for pediatric spinal muscular atrophy. Arch Neurol 59:1445-50, 2002.
77. Hahn AF: Guillain-Barre syndrome. Lancet 352:635-41, 1998.

Acute Cerebrovascular Disease

78. Sakr YL, Ghosn I, Vincent JL: Cardiac manifestations after subarachnoid hemorrhage: A systematic review of the literature. Prog Cardiovasc Dis 45:67-80, 2002.
79. Zaroff JG, Rordorf GA, Newell JB, et al: Cardiac outcome in patients with subarachnoid hemorrhage and electrocardiographic abnormalities. Neurosurg 44:34-9, 1999.
80. Szabo G, Sebening C, Hackert T, et al: Effects of brain death on myocardial function and ischemic tolerance of potential donor hearts. J Heart Lung Transplant 17:921-30, 1998.

CHAPTER 86

Interface Between Renal Disease and Cardiovascular Illness

Peter A. McCullough

The Cardiorenal Intersection

The heart and kidney are inextricably linked in terms of hemodynamic and regulatory functions. In a normal 70-kg man, each kidney weighs about 130 to 170 gm and receives blood flow of 400 ml/min per 100 gm, which is approximately 20 to 25 percent of the cardiac output, allowing the needed flow to maintain glomerular filtration. This flow is several times greater per unit weight of organ than the blood flow through most other organs. Although the oxygen extraction is low, the kidneys account for about 8 percent of the total oxygen consumption of the body. The kidney has a central role in electrolyte balance, volume, and blood pressure regulation. Communication between these two organs occurs at multiple levels, including the sympathetic nervous system, the renin-angiotensin-aldosterone system (RAAS) (Fig. 86–1), antidiuretic hormone, endothelin, and the natriuretic peptides (Fig. 86–2). With the understanding of these systems has come the development of key diagnostic and therapeutic targets in cardiovascular medicine.

The modern epidemics of obesity and hypertension (HTN) in the developed countries are central drivers of a secondary epidemic of type 2 diabetes with combined chronic kidney disease (CKD) and cardiovascular disease (CVD).[1] Among those with diabetes for 25 years or more, the prevalence of diabetic nephropathy in type 1 and type 2 diabetes is 57 and 48 percent, respectively.[2] Approximately half of all cases of end-stage renal disease (ESRD) are due to diabetic nephropathy. With the aging of the general population and cardiovascular care shifting toward the elderly population, an understanding of why decreasing levels of renal function act as a major adverse prognostic factor after a variety of cardiac events is imperative. Considerable evidence shows that CKD accelerates atherosclerosis, myocardial disease, and valvular disease and promotes an array of cardiac arrhythmias.[3]

Chronic Kidney Disease and Cardiovascular Risk

CKD is defined through a range of estimated glomerular filtration rate (eGFR) values by the National Kidney Foundation Kidney Disease Outcomes Quality Initiative (KDOQI) (Fig. 86–3).[4] A common definition for CKD stipulates an eGFR of less than 60 ml/min/1.73 m^2 or the presence of albuminuria, defined as an albumin-to-creatinine ratio greater than 30 mg/gm on a spot urine sample (Fig. 86–4). Although with normative aging (age 20 to 80), the eGFR declines from about 130 to 60 ml/min/1.73 m^2, a variety of pathobiological processes appear to begin when the eGFR drops below 60 ml/min/1.73 m^2. Most studies of cardiovascular outcomes have found that a break point for the development of contrast-induced nephropathy (CIN), restenosis after percutaneous coronary intervention (PCI), recurrent myocardial infarction (MI), diastolic/systolic congestive heart failure (CHF), arrhythmias, and cardiovascular death occurs below an eGFR of 60 ml/min/1.73 m^2, which roughly corresponds to a serum creatinine (Cr) greater than 1.5 mg/dl in the general population.[4-8] Because Cr is a crude indicator of renal function and often underestimates renal dysfunction in women and elderly people, calculated measures of eGFR or creatinine clearance (CrCl) using the Cockcroft-Gault equation or the Modification of Diet in Renal Disease (MDRD) equation are superior methods for the assessment of renal function.[4] The four-variable MDRD equation for CrCl is the preferred method because it does not rely on body weight.[4] This equation is

$$\text{CrCl} = 186.3\ (\text{serum creatinine}^{-1.154}) \times (\text{age}^{-.203})$$

and calculated values are multiplied by 0.742 for women and by 1.21 for blacks.

In addition, microalbuminuria at any level of eGFR is considered to represent CKD and has been thought to occur as the result of hyperfiltration in the kidneys because of diabetes and HTN-related changes in the glomeruli.[9] Several definitions have been proposed for microalbuminuria.[9] The most widely accepted is a random urine albumin/creatinine ratio (ACR) of 30 to 300 mg/gm. An ACR greater than 300 mg/gm is usually considered gross proteinuria. Microalbuminuria as an independent CVD risk factor is covered elsewhere in this text. The Seventh Report of the Joint National Committee on Prevention, Detection, Evaluation, and Treatment of High Blood Pressure (JNC 7) has recognized CKD as an independent cardiovascular risk state.[10] This risk state has a host

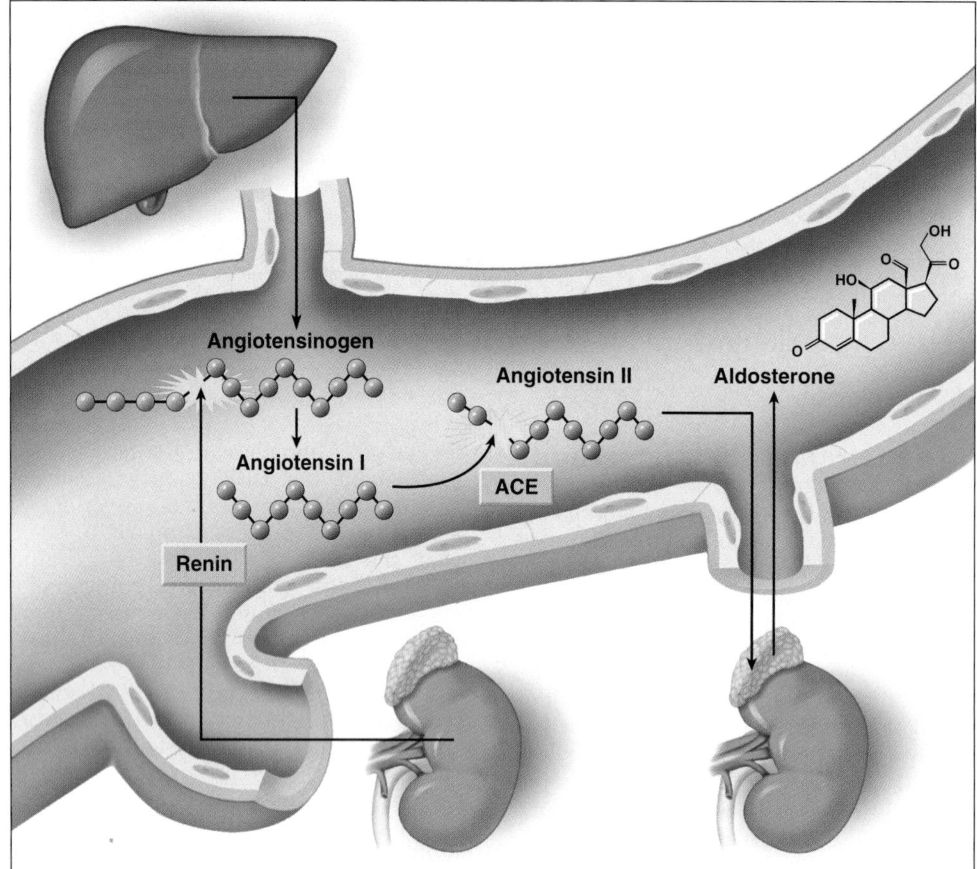

FIGURE 86–1 Angiotensinogen is secreted by the liver and is cleaved by renin, which is secreted into the lumen of renal afferent arterioles by juxtaglomerular cells. Angiotensin I is then converted to angiotensin II by angiotensin-converting enzyme (ACE) primarily in endothelial cells. In the zona glomerulosa of the adrenal cortex, angiotensin II stimulates the production of aldosterone. Aldosterone production is also stimulated by potassium, corticotropin, catecholamines (e.g., norepinephrine), and endothelins. (From Weber KT: Aldosterone in congestive heart failure. N Engl J Med 345:1689, 2001.)

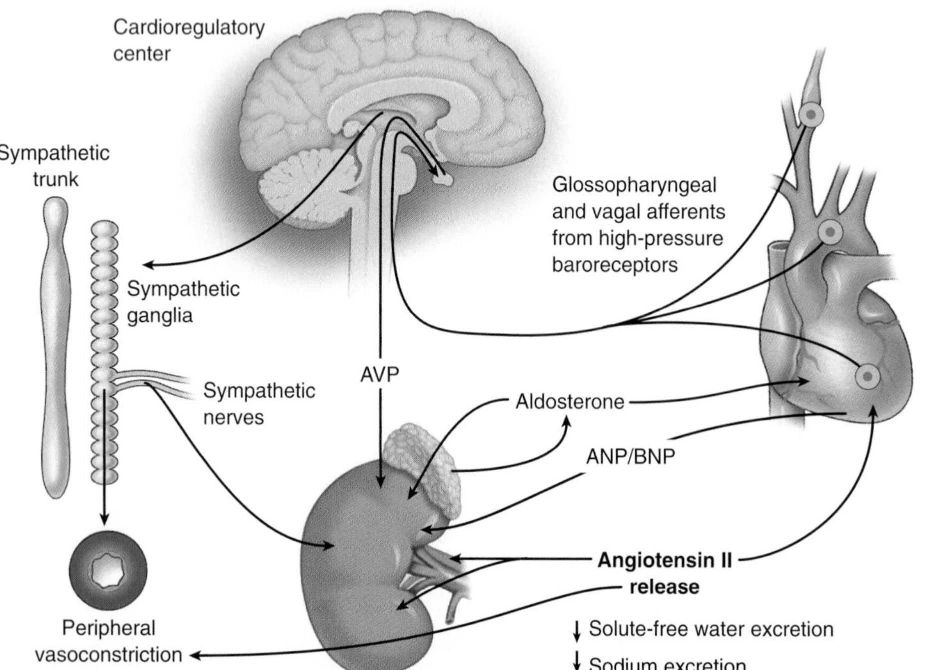

FIGURE 86–2 Major neurohumoral communication systems between the heart and kidney. ANP = A-type natriuretic peptide; AVP = arginine vasopressin; BNP = B-type natriuretic peptide. (Adapted from Schrier RW, Abraham WT: Hormones and hemodynamics in heart failure. N Engl J Med 341:577, 1999.)

of vascular and metabolic abnormalities, which are discussed subsequently (see Fig. 86–4).[11]

Contrast-Induced Nephropathy: Short- and Long-Term Outcomes

The overall risk of CIN, defined as a transient rise in Cr greater than 25 percent above the baseline or an absolute rise greater than 0.5 mg/dl, occurs in approximately 13 percent of nondiabetics and 20 percent of diabetics undergoing PCI (Fig. 86–5).[12] It is critical to understand that the risk of CIN is related in a curvilinear fashion to the eGFR (see Fig. 86–5).[12] Fortunately, among patients undergoing PCI, cases of CIN leading to dialysis are rare (0.5 to 2.0 percent). However, when they occur, they are related to catastrophic outcomes including a 36 percent in-hospital mortality rate and a 2-year survival of only 19 percent.[13] Although not directly attributed to CIN, transient rises in Cr are directly related to longer intensive care unit and hospital ward stays (3 and 4 more days, respectively) after bypass surgery.[14] Even transient rises in Cr translate to differences in adjusted long-term outcomes after PCI (Fig. 86–6).[15]

Rationale for Renal End-Organ Protection for Intervention Patients

End-organ protection for CKD patients at risk (eGFR < 60 ml/min/1.73 m^2) can be thought of in three separate spheres: (1) long-term cardiorenal protection, (2) removal of renal toxins, and (3) prevention measures carried out before PCI. Long-term cardiorenal protection involves two important concepts: blood pressure control to a target of less than 130/80 mm Hg[10] and use of an agent that blocks the RAAS such as an angiotensin-converting enzyme inhibitor (ACEI) or an angiotensin receptor blocker (ARB) as the base of therapy. However, both agents can cause a chronic rise in Cr of more than 25 percent above the baseline in cardiovascular patients.[16] Despite the rise in Cr, studies have shown large benefits of ACEI-ARB agents in reducing new cases of ESRD, CHF, or cardiovascular death.[17-23] These benefits extend to nondiabetics and blacks with CKD.[22,23] Cardiorenal protection is addressed in more detail later in this chapter. Removal of toxins largely refers to discontinuation of nonsteroidal antiinflammatory agents, aminoglycosides, and cyclosporine. These agents all complicate cardiovascular procedures and increase the risk of CIN. Preventive measures taken before PCI include hydration, measures to reduce the direct cellular toxicity of the contrast medium, and measures to reduce the intrarenal vasoconstriction, which occurs uniquely in CKD patients when exposed to iodinated contrast material.[9] On the basis of the totality of evidence to date, if a patient can be carried through a cardiovascular procedure (PCI or bypass surgery) without a rise in Cr, a shorter length of stay and improved long-term survival result.

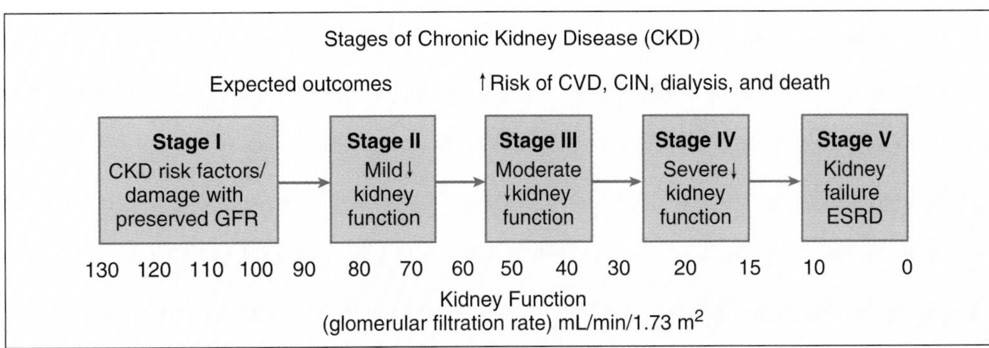

FIGURE 86–3 The classification of chronic kidney disease (CKD) according to the National Kidney Foundation Kidney Disease Outcomes Quality Initiative (KDOQI). Increased rates of adverse events are generally seen below an estimated glomerular filtration rate of 60 ml/min/1.73 m^2. ESRD = end-stage renal disease; GFR = glomerular filtration rate; CIN = contrast-induced nephropathy; CVD = cardiovascular disease. (Adapted from McCullough PA: Why is chronic kidney disease the "spoiler" for cardiovascular outcomes? J Am Coll Cardiol 41:725, 2003.)

Criteria

1. Kidney damage for ≥ 3 months, as defined by structural or functional abnormalities of the kidney, with or without decreased GFR, manifest by *either:*
   - Pathological abnormalities; or
   - Markers of kidney damage, including abnormalities in the composition of the blood or urine, or abnormalities in imaging tests
2. eGFR < 60 mL/min/1.73m^2 for ≥ 3 months, with or without kidney damage

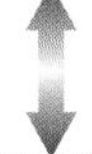

Markers of kidney damage	Findings indicating kidney damage
Proteinuria	Albumin-to-creatinine ratio >30 mg/g
Urine sediment abnormalities	Cellular casts, coarse granular casts, fat
Imaging tests	Abnormalities in kidney size Asymmetry in kidney size or function Irregularities in shape (cysts, scars, mass lesions) Stones Hydronephrosis and other abnormalities of the urinary tract Arterial stenosis and other vascular lesions
Abnormalities in blood or urine composition	Nephrotic syndrome Tubular syndromes (renal tubular acidosis, potassium secretory defects, renal glycosuria, renal phosphaturia, Fanconi's syndrome)

FIGURE 86–4 Diagnostic criteria for chronic kidney disease and kidney damage. eGFR = estimated glomerular filtration rate.

Vascular Pathobiology in Chronic Kidney Disease

There are three core elements in the pathophysiology of CIN: (1) direct toxicity of iodinated contrast material to nephrons, (2) microshowers of atheroemboli to the kidneys, and (3) contrast material- and atheroemboli-induced intrarenal vasoconstriction. Furthermore, as renal function declines, a host of perturbations occur in hemostasis, lipids, endothelial function, protein metabolism, calcium-phosphorus balance, and oxidative stress that are operative in the patient with CKD undergoing PCI (Fig. 86–7).[11,24-26] Direct toxicity to nephrons with iodinated contrast media has been demonstrated and appears to be related to the osmolality of the contrast media.[27] For this reason, low-ionic or nonionic and low-osmolar or isosmolar contrast agents are less nephrotoxic in vitro.

Microshowers of cholesterol emboli are thought to occur in about 50 percent of percutaneous interventions when a guiding catheter is passed through the aorta.[28] Most of these showers are clinically silent. However, in approximately 1 percent of high-risk cases, an acute cholesterol emboli syndrome can develop, manifested by acute renal failure, mesenteric ischemia, decreased microcirculation to the extremities, and, in some cases, embolic stroke (see also Chap. 54). Because acute renal failure occurs after coronary artery bypass surgery with nearly the same risk predictors as in procedures involving contrast media, atheroembolism is considered a common pathogenic feature of both causes of renal failure.[29]

Intrarenal vasoconstriction as a pathological vascular response to contrast media and perhaps as an organ response to cholesterol emboli is a final hypoxic-ischemic injury to the kidney in PCI. Hypoxia triggers activation of the renal sympathetic nervous system and results in further reduction in renal blood flow. When these contrast agents are given to animals, there is disagreement about their direct vasoconstrictor or vasodilator effects in the kidney.[30-32] In completely normal human renal blood vessels, contrast agents probably

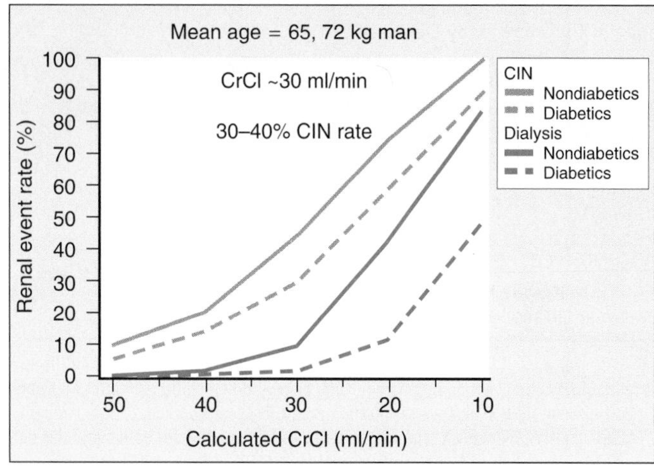

FIGURE 86–5 Validated risk of acute renal failure requiring dialysis after diagnostic angiography and ad hoc angioplasty, assuming a mean contrast dose of 250 ml and a mean age of 65. CrCl = creatinine clearance; CIN = contrast-induced nephropathy. (Data adapted from McCullough PA, Manley HJ: Prediction and prevention of contrast nephropathy. J Interv Cardiol 14:547, 2001.)

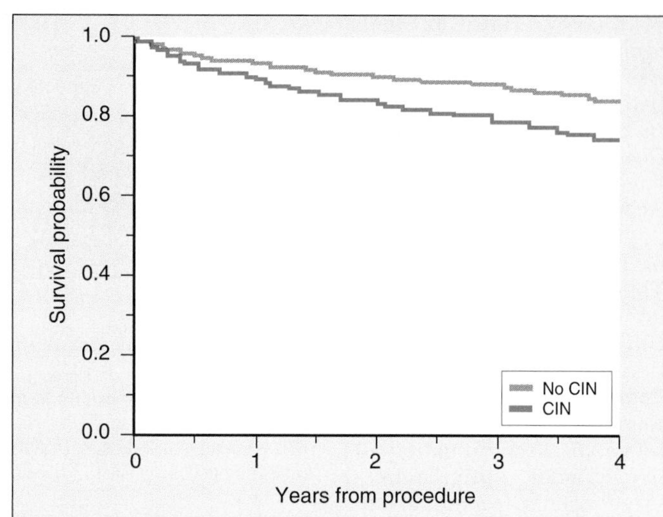

FIGURE 86–6 Adjusted, long-term outcomes in 7586 patients with and without contrast-induced nephropathy (CIN) after angioplasty, $p < 0.0001$. Contrast-induced nephropathy is defined as a 0.5 mg/dl rise in creatinine after percutaneous coronary intervention. (Adapted from Rihal CS, Textor SC, Grill DE, et al: Incidence and prognostic importance of acute renal failure after percutaneous coronary intervention. Circulation 105:2259, 2002.)

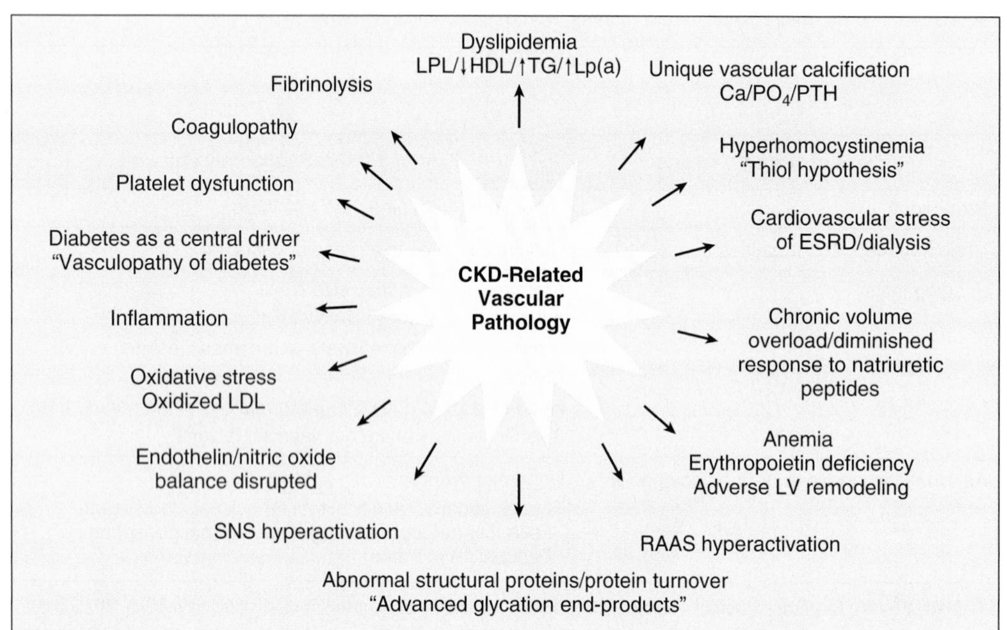

FIGURE 86–7 The pathobiology of the chronic kidney disease state and its effects on the cardiovascular system. Ca = calcium; CKD = chronic kidney disease; ESRD = end-stage renal disease; HDL = high-density lipoprotein; LDL-C = low-density lipoprotein cholesterol; Lp(a) = lipoprotein (a) ; LPL = lipoprotein lipase; LV = left ventricle; NO = nitric oxide; PO_4 = phosphate; PTH = parathyroid hormone; RAAS = renin-angiotensin-aldosterone system; SNS = sympathetic nervous system; TG = triglyceride. (Adapted from McCullough PA: Why is chronic kidney disease the "spoiler" for cardiovascular outcomes? J Am Coll Cardiol 41:725, 2003.)

provoke a vasodilation and an osmotic diuresis. However, when there is vascular disease, endothelial dysfunction, and glomerular injury, the contrast agent and the multifactorial insult of renal hypoxia provoke a vasoconstrictive response and mediate ischemic injury. The most important predictor of CIN is underlying renal dysfunction. The "remnant nephron" theory postulates that after sufficient chronic kidney damage has occurred and the eGFR is reduced to less than 60 ml/min/1.73 m^2, the remaining nephrons must assume the residual filtration load. The residual nephrons also have increased oxygen demands and are more susceptible to ischemic and oxidative injury.

Prevention of Contrast-Induced Nephropathy after Percutaneous Coronary Intervention

A prevention strategy for CIN should be employed for patients with diabetes as well as patients with preexisting CKD (baseline eGFR < 60 ml/min/1.73 m^2). In general, at an eGFR of 30 ml/min/1.73 m^2, the expected rate of contrast nephropathy is 30 to 40 percent and the rates of acute renal failure requiring dialysis are approximately 2 to 8 percent (see Fig. 86–4).[12] There are four basic concepts in contrast nephropathy prevention: (1) hydration, (2) choice and quantity of contrast material, (3) pre-, intra-, and postprocedural end-organ protection with pharmacotherapy, and (4) postprocedural monitoring and expectant care.

Hydration with intravenous normal or half-normal saline is reasonable, starting 3 to 12 hours prior to the procedure at a rate of 1 to 2 ml/kg/hr.[33-36] In those at risk, at least 300 to 500 ml of intravenous hydration should be received before the contrast material is administered. If there are particular concerns regarding volume overload or CHF in individuals in whom clinical assessment of volume status is difficult, a right-heart catheterization may aid management during and after the procedure. The postprocedure hydration target is a urine output of 150 ml/hr. If patients have a diuresis of more than a 150 ml/hr, they should have replacement of extra losses with more intravenous fluid. In general, this strategy calls for hydration orders of normal or half-normal saline at 150 ml/hr for at least 6 hours after the procedure. Achieving adequate urine flow rates in a clinical trial setting reduced the rate of contrast nephropathy by 50 percent.[35]

As discussed previously, two large-scale, double-blind randomized controlled trials indicated that the lower the ionicity and osmolality of the contrast agent, the less renal toxicity is expected; this has now been confirmed. In the Iohexol Cooperative Study, $n = 1196$, iohexol (Omnipaque) was found to be superior to a high-ionic contrast agent (diatrizoate meglumine [Hypaque-76]) in patients with diabetes and baseline CKD.[36] In the Nephrotoxicity in High-Risk Patients Study of Iso-Osmolar and Low-Osmolar Non-Ionic Contrast Media (NEPHRIC), iodixanol (Visipaque), a nonionic, isosmolar contrast agent, proved to be superior to iohexol with lower rates of contrast nephropathy observed.[37] Iodixanol was also demonstrated to be less thrombogenic than other contrast agents in the Contrast Media Utilization in High-Risk Percutaneous Transluminal Coronary Angioplasty (COURT) trial, with a 45 percent reduction in major adverse cardiac events compared with ioxaglate meglumine (Hexabrix); hence, iodixanol is the contrast agent of choice in patients at high renal risk undergoing intervention.[38] Although it is desirable to limit contrast to the smallest volume possible in any setting, there is disagreement about a "safe" contrast limit.[39] The lower the eGFR, the smaller the amount of contrast material needed to cause CIN.[39] In general, it is desirable to limit the contrast medium to less than 100 ml for any procedure.[12,13] If staged procedures are planned, it is advantageous to have more than 10 days between the first and second contrast exposures if contrast nephropathy has occurred with the first procedure.[40]

More than 35 randomized trials have tested various strategies in the prevention of CIN.[12] The majority of these trials were small, underpowered, and did not find the preventive strategy under investigation to be better than placebo. A few lessons have been learned from these trials: (1) diuretics in the form of loop diuretics or mannitol can worsen contrast nephropathy if there is inadequate volume replacement for the diuresis that follows; (2) low-dose or "renal dose" dopamine cannot be achieved despite its popularity in practice, given the counterbalancing forces of intrarenal vasodilation through the dopamine-1 receptor and the vasoconstricting forces of the dopamine-2, alpha, and beta receptors; and (3) renal toxic agents including nonsteroidal antiinflammatory agents, aminoglycosides, and cyclosporine should not be administered in the periprocedural period. There are currently no approved agents for the prevention of CIN.

The most popular strategy at the time of this writing is optimal hydration, iodixanol as the contrast agent of choice, and administration of oral or intravenous *N*-acetylcysteine (NAC), a cytoprotective agent against oxidative injury. In addition, one supportive, double-blind randomized trial of fenoldopam versus placebo demonstrated improved renal blood flow after contrast exposure.[41] However, a large confirmatory trial of fenoldopam failed to demonstrate a protective effect of this agent.[42] Ten trials regarding NAC have now been completed. Five were positive and five were neutral, with an overall edge in favor of NAC (Table 86–1).[43-52] Most operators believe—given the seriousness of CIN, the relative safety of the strategies used, and the evolution of clinical trials shaping our practice—that the combination of hydration, use of iodixanol, and NAC is a reasonable three-pronged approach to minimize CIN and the risk of acute renal failure requiring dialysis in patients at risk.

Postprocedural monitoring is critical in the current era of short stays and outpatient procedures. In general, high-risk patients in the hospital should have hydration started 12 hours before the procedure and continued at least 6 hours

TABLE 86–1 Randomized, Double-Blind, Placebo-Controlled Trials of *N*-Acetylcysteine in the Prevention of Contrast Nephropathy*

Author	Year	*N*	NAC Dose	Contrast Nephropathy Definition	NAC Contrast Nephropathy Rate	Placebo Contrast Nephropathy Rate	*p* Value
Tepel et al[43]	2000	83	600 mg PO b.i.d.	>0.5 mg/dl	1/41 (2.4)	9/42 (21.4)	0.01
Diaz-Sandoval et al[44]	2002	54	600 mg PO b.i.d. (one dose before PCI)	>0.5 mg/dl or >25% rise	2/26 (8.0)	12/28 (45.0)	0.005
Shyu et al[45]	2002	121	400 mg PO b.i.d.	>0.5 mg/dl	2/60 (3.3)	15/61 (24.6)	<0.0001
Kay et al[46]	2003	200	600 mg PO b.i.d.	>25%	4/102 (3.9)	12/98 (12.2)	0.03
Durham et al[47]	2002	79	1200 mg 1 hr before and 3 hr after PCI	>0.5 mg/dl	10/38 (26.3)	9/41 (22.0)	>0.05
Briguori et al[48]	2002	183	600 mg PO b.i.d.	>25%	6/92 (6.5)	10/91 (11.0)	0.22
Allaqaband et al[49]	2002	84	600 mg PO b.i.d.	>0.5 mg/dl	8/45 (17.7)	6/39 (15.3)	0.92
Loutrianakis et al[50]	2003	47	600 mg PO b.i.d.	>0.5 mg/dl >25% rise	6/24 (25.0) 8/24 (33.3)	3/23 (13.0) 2/23 (8.7)	0.20 0.04
RAPPID[51]	2003	80	150 mg/kg over 30 min before and 50 mg/kg over 4 hr after PCI	>0.5 mg/dl or >25% rise	2/41 (4.9)	8/39 (20.5)	0.05
Goldenberg et al[52]	2003	80	600 mg PO t.i.d.	0.5 mg/dl	4/41 (9.8)	3/39 (7.7)	0.52
Total weighted proportions		**1011**	**Various**	**Various**	**45/510 (8.8)**	**85/501 (17.0)**	**0.00001**

*Contrast nephropathy is defined as a rise in creatinine >25% from baseline or an absolute increase >0.5 mg/dl from baseline prior to contrast exposure.
NAC = *N*-acetylcysteine.

afterward. A serum Cr should be measured 24 hours after the procedure. For outpatients, particularly those with eGFR less than 60 ml/min/1.73 m^2, either an overnight stay or discharge to home with 48-hour follow-up and Cr measurement is advised. Individuals in whom severe CIN develops have a rise of Cr greater than 0.5 mg/dl in the first 24 hours after the procedure.[53] Thus, for those who do not have this degree of Cr elevation and an otherwise uneventful course, discharge to home may be considered. Table 86–2 summarizes a strategy for CIN risk assessment and prevention. It is important that CIN risks be discussed in the consent process. For those with eGFR less than 30 ml/min/1.73 m^2, the possibility of dialysis should be mentioned. Lastly, in those with eGFR less than 15 ml/min/1.73 m^2, nephrology consultation is advised with possible planning for dialysis after the procedure.

TABLE 86–2 Ten-Step Checklist for Contrast Nephropathy Risk Stratification and Prevention for Patients at Risk Undergoing Percutaneous Coronary Intervention

Action
1. Calculate eGFR (creatinine clearance)—high risk if <60 ml/min/1.73 m^2
2. Check diabetic status—fivefold higher risk if diabetic
3. Discuss contrast nephropathy risk in informed consent process
4. Discontinue NSAIDs and other renal toxic drugs
5. Nephrology consultation for eGFR <15 ml/min for dialysis planning after PCI
6. Hydration with NS or 0.5 NS 150 ml/hr 3 hr before and 6 hr after procedure
7. Ensure urine flow rate >150 ml/hr after PCI
8. Iodixanol preferred contrast agent
9. Limit contrast volume to <100 ml
10. NAC 600 mg in 30 ml of ginger ale, two doses PO b.i.d. before and 2 doses PO b.i.d. after PCI

eGFR = estimated glomerular filtration rate; NAC = *N*-acetylcysteine; NS = normal saline; NSAID = nonsteroidal antiinflammatory drug; PCI = percutaneous coronary intervention.

CH 86

CKD is the most important factor in predicting adverse short- and long-term outcomes after PCI. The rationale for renal end-organ protection is based on chronic renal protection, avoidance of additive renal insults, and comprehensive CIN prophylaxis. The pathogenesis of CIN goes beyond serum Cr and involves a special vascular pathobiology that interrelates both renal and CVD outcomes.

Renal Disease and Hypertension

The kidney is a central regulator of blood pressure and controls intraglomerular pressure through autoregulation. When glomerular injury is present, a variety of pathways are activated resulting in increased systemic blood pressure (Fig. 86–8). This effect sets up a viscous circle of more glomerular and tubulointerstitial injury and worsened HTN (see Fig. 86–8). A cornerstone of management of combined CKD and CVD is strict blood pressure control (Fig. 86–9). An optimal blood pressure can be defined as less than 120/80 mm Hg, and most patients with CKD and HTN require three or more antihypertensive agents to achieve a goal blood pressure of less than 130/80 mm Hg.[10] Detection and treatment of HTN are outlined elsewhere in this text (see Chaps. 37 and 38). The key life-style issues with CKD and HTN include dietary changes with sodium restriction, weight reduction to a target body mass index less than 25 kg/m^2, and exercise for 60 minutes per day most days of the week. Pharmacological therapy aims for strict blood pressure control with an agent that antagonizes the RAAS often in combined action with a thiazide-type diuretic. Special diagnostic consideration should be given to the possibility of underlying bilateral renal artery stenosis from the clinical clues of poorly controlled blood pressure on more than three agents, abdominal bruits, smoking history, peripheral arterial disease, and a marked change in serum Cr with administration of ACEI.[54] Although renal artery stenosis accounts for less than 3 percent of ESRD cases, it represents a potentially treatable condition. Diagnostic approaches discussed elsewhere in this text should be considered (see Chap. 55).[55]

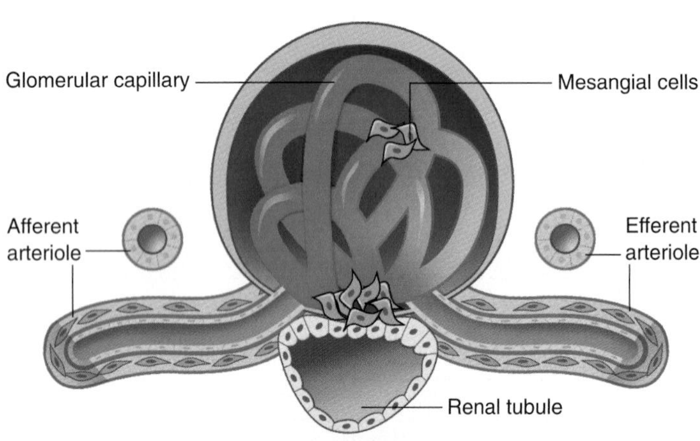

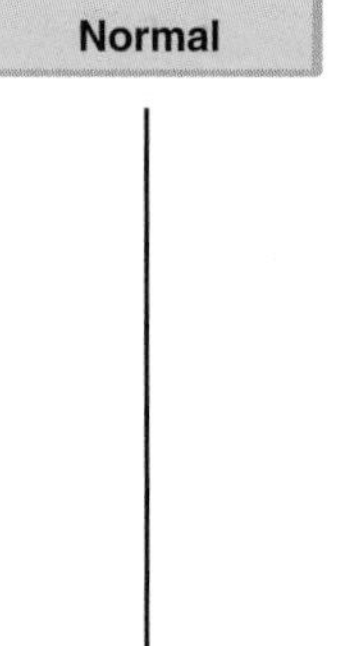

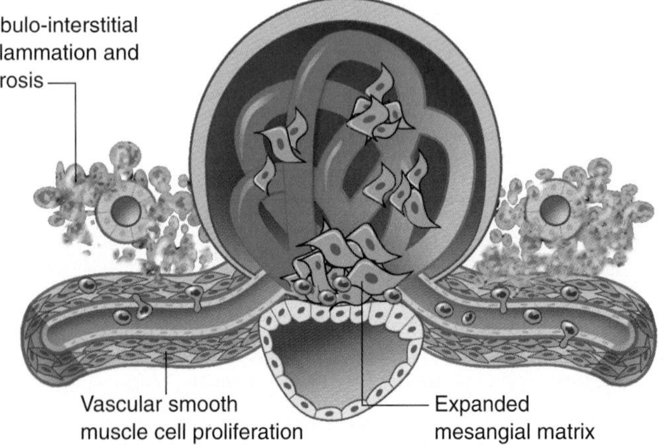

FIGURE 86–8 Pathological changes related to hypertension that occur within the kidney.

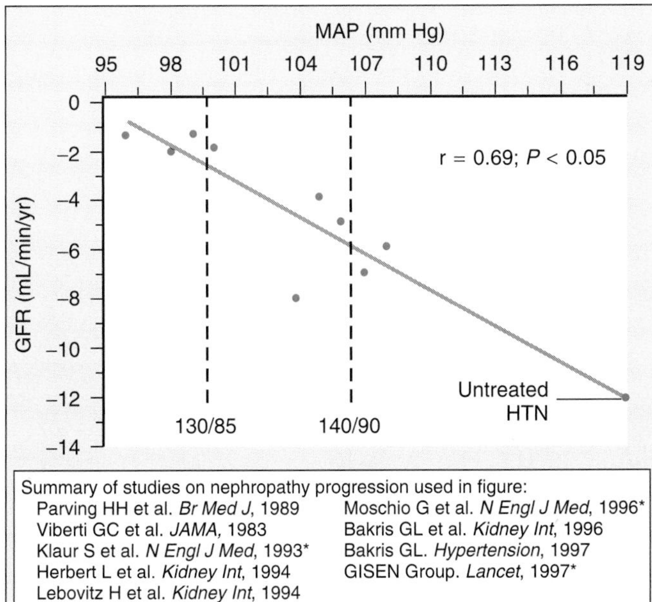

FIGURE 86–9 The influence of systemic blood pressure on the rate of decline in renal function. GFR = glomerular filtration rate; HTN = hypertension; MAP = mean arterial pressure. (Adapted from Bakris GL, Williams M, Dworkin L, et al: Preserving renal function in adults with hypertension and diabetes: A consensus approach. National Kidney Foundation Hypertension and Diabetes Executive Committees Working Group. Am J Kidney Dis 36:646, 2000.)

Diagnosis of Acute Coronary Syndromes in Patients with Chronic Kidney Disease

Multiple studies have found that elderly persons and those with diabetes have higher rates of silent ischemia.[56] Likewise, patients with CKD have shown higher rates of silent ischemia, which cluster with serious arrhythmias and other cardiac events.[57] Hemodialysis patients with ESRD bear considerable hemodynamic stress three times per week during dialysis sessions. Several studies have demonstrated a relationship between ST segment depression and release of cardiac biomarkers (primarily troponin T), before or during dialysis, and poor long-term survival.[57] From a practical perspective, it is important to realize that patients with CKD presenting to the hospital with chest discomfort represent a high-risk group, having a 40 percent cardiac event rate at 30 days.[58] In making the diagnosis of acute myocardial infarction (AMI) in patients with CKD or ESRD, troponin I is the preferred biomarker on the basis of its kinetic profile in patients with renal impairment.[59] The skeletal myopathy of renal disease can elevate creatine kinase, myoglobin, and some troponin T assays, making these tests less desirable. In addition to an elevated biomarker of cardiac injury, supporting evidence of the diagnosis of AMI could be characteristic chest pain, electrocardiographic changes (ST segment elevation or depression, new Q waves), or the identification of a culprit lesion on angiography. Because of the high event rate and prevalence of CVD among patients with CKD, it is advisable to consider admission to the hospital when the presenting symptom is chest discomfort and the eGFR is less than 60 ml/min/1.73 m^2 or the patient has ESRD and is receiving dialysis.[58]

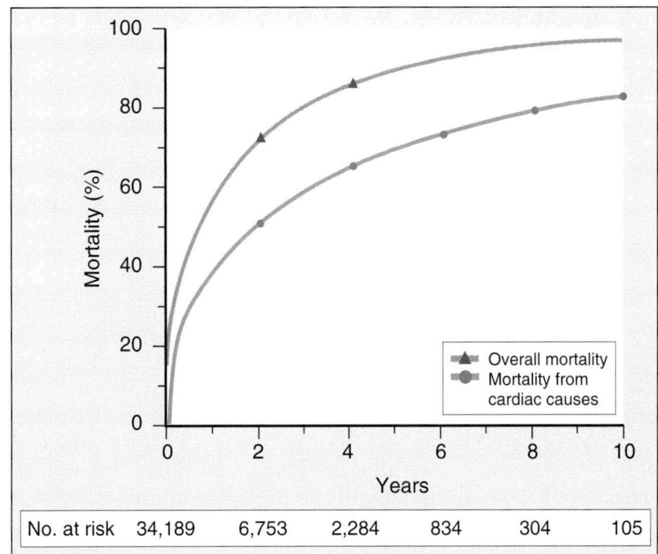

FIGURE 86–10 Cumulative mortality after myocardial infarction in patients with end-stage renal disease from the U.S. Renal Data System. (Adapted from Herzog CA, Ma JZ, Collins AJ: Poor long-term survival after acute myocardial infarction among patients on long-term dialysis. N Engl J Med 339:799, 1998.)

Renal Dysfunction as a Prognostic Factor in Acute Coronary Syndromes

In the last several decades, considerable advances have been made in the diagnosis and treatment of acute coronary syndromes (ACSs) in the general population. These advances include early paramedic response and defibrillation, coronary care units, and pharmacotherapy including antiplatelet agents, antithrombotics, beta receptor–blocking agents, ACEIs, and intravenous thrombolytic agents. Primary angioplasty for ST segment elevation myocardial infarction (STEMI) has become a well-accepted mode of treatment. These advances, however, have not been tested in patients with CKD or ESRD, primarily because these patients have been excluded from randomized treatment trials. Retrospective studies of patients in coronary care units have identified renal dysfunction as the most significant prognostic factor for long-term mortality when adjusting for other clinical factors, including age, gender, and comorbidities.[5-8] In addition, retrospective studies of patients with AMI consistently find renal dysfunction as an independent predictor of death, with a greater impact on mortality than baseline demographics or therapies received.[8] Patients with ESRD have the highest mortality after AMI of any large, chronic disease population (Fig. 86–10).[60]

Reasons for Poor Outcomes in Patients with Renal Dysfunction

Four reasons may explain why patients with renal dysfunction have poor cardiovascular outcomes in a variety of settings: (1) excess comorbidities associated with CKD and ESRD, in particular diabetes and heart failure; (2) therapeutic nihilism; (3) toxicity of therapies; and (4) special biological and pathophysiological factors in renal dysfunction that cause worsened outcomes.[11] In one study by Beattie and coworkers, the comorbidities of patients with STEMI and CKD (mean Cr = 2.7 mg/dl) included older age (mean 70.2 years), diabetes (38.1 percent), and prior heart failure (23.2 percent).[6] Those with ESRD had similar rates of comorbidities including age (mean 64.9 years), diabetes (40.4 percent), and prior heart failure (31.7 percent). This study found that, among the CKD and ESRD groups, there were lower rates of use of reperfusion therapy (thrombolysis or primary angioplasty) and beta blockers, suggesting some contribution to poor outcomes from underutilization of proven therapies (therapeutic nihilism). It is possible that patients with renal dysfunction may present later in their course, have more contraindications, or have other aspects about their presentations that prompt clinicians to use fewer therapies or take a more conservative approach.

Data on the toxicity of treatments for ACSs related to renal dysfunction are often unavailable, primarily because of exclusion of patients with CKD from these trials. The primary defects in thrombosis attributable to uremia are excess thrombin generation and decreased platelet aggregation.[61] Hence, patients with CKD and ESRD can have increased rates of coronary thrombotic events and increased bleeding risks at the same time. In patients with renal dysfunction the risks of bleeding increase with aspirin, unfractionated heparin, low-molecular-weight heparin, thrombolytics, glycoprotein IIb/IIIa receptor antagonists, and thienopyridine antiplatelet agents. The reason is primarily that uremia causes platelet dysfunction in a mechanism that is independent of and therefore additive to pharmacologically induced platelet antagonism or antithrombosis.[61] In patients with renal dysfunction, the best measure of bleeding risk is the bleeding time.[61] Unfortunately, the bleeding time is not a practical test for the ACS patient; consequently, clinicians cannot readily assess the a priori bleeding risk for any given CKD or ESRD patient. However, it is unlikely that bleeding complications account for the large differences seen in mortality between CKD and ESRD and those with preserved renal function with AMI.

The final and most important reason why patients with CKD and ESRD have poor outcomes after ACS is the enhanced vascular pathobiology induced by the chronic renal failure state.[24-26] The processes that contribute to accelerate atherosclerosis include a dyslipidemia characterized by decreased function of lipoprotein lipase, reductions in high-density lipoprotein cholesterol (HDL-C), elevated triglycerides, and normal low-density lipoprotein cholesterol (LDL-C) (see Fig. 86–7). In addition, accelerated vascular calcification is due in part to hypercalcemia, hyperphosphatemia, and elevated parathyroid hormone and is possibly worsened by chronic acidosis and mobilization of calcium from bone. Elevations in homocysteine and other thiols are present when the eGFR drops below 60 ml/min/1.73 m^2, enhancing oxidation of LDL-C and progression of atherosclerotic lesions. Renal dysfunction is a highly inflammatory state, associated with higher rates of plaque rupture and incident CVD events. Lastly, chronic hyperactivation of the sympathetic nervous system and an imbalance between endothelin, a powerful vasoconstrictor, and nitric oxide, a local paracrine vasodilator, may worsen HTN and may augment intravascular wall stress that could further contribute to incident CVD events.

Treatment of Acute Myocardial Infarction in Patients with Renal Dysfunction

The clinician must confront the high-risk populations, those with CKD and ESRD, with little evidence upon which to base treatment decisions in ACS. Therapies that benefit the general population often yield enhanced benefit in patients with CKD and ESRD.[62] A favorable benefit-to-risk ratio has now been demonstrated for aspirin, beta blockers, ACEI, aldosterone receptor antagonists, and statins and is expected for ARBs.[62] Therapies that require dose adjustment on the basis of CrCl include low-molecular-weight heparins and glycoprotein IIb/IIIa antagonists (Table 86–3). Given that the major inputs for bleeding risks include older age, low body weight, and renal dysfunction, Table 86–3 also lists agents that are approved in a weight-adjusted dose form and gives the currently recommended dose adjustments for commonly used antiplatelet and antithrombotic agents.[61] It is possible that greater utilization of such therapies, despite the heightened risk for complications, will attenuate the excess mortality reported in the CKD and ESRD populations. There have been no randomized trials of PCI or bypass surgery in patients with CKD or ESRD. However, in the Bypass Angioplasty Revascularization Investigation (BARI), whether PCI or surgery was used in the management of multivessel coronary disease, CKD and diabetes were associated with worsened long-term survival (Fig. 86–11).[8] Further research is needed into the particular pathogenic mechanisms in the renal failure state that promote plaque rupture, accelerate atherosclerosis, lead to ACS complications, and promote the development of heart failure and arrhythmias.

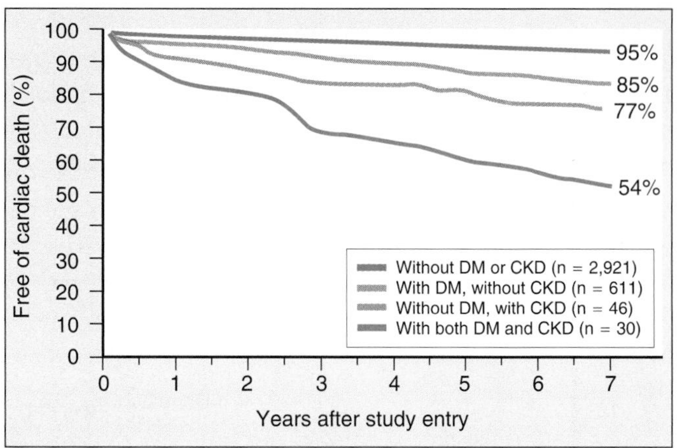

FIGURE 86–11 Freedom from cardiovascular death after angioplasty or bypass surgery in the Bypass Angioplasty Revascularization Investigation (BARI) Trial and Registry, *n* = 3608. CKD = chronic kidney disease; DM = diabetes mellitus. (Adapted from Szczech LA, Best PJ, Crowley E, for the Bypass Angioplasty Revascularization Investigation (BARI) Investigators: Outcomes of patients with chronic renal insufficiency in the bypass angioplasty revascularization investigation. Circulation 105:2253, 2002.)

Chronic Kidney Disease Complicating Congestive Heart Failure

The diagnosis of CHF with concomitant renal failure presents a particular challenge. Patients with CKD, and in particular ESRD, have three key mechanical contributors to CHF: pressure overload (related to HTN), volume overload, and cardiomyopathy. Approximately 20 percent of patients approaching hemodialysis have a diagnosis of CHF.[63] It is unclear how much of this diagnosis can be attributable purely to chronic volume overload from renal failure and how much is due to impaired systolic or diastolic function. Notably, CKD influences the levels of B-type natriuretic peptide (BNP), a diagnostic blood test for CHF. In general, when the eGFR is less than 60 ml/min/1.73 m^2, a higher BNP cut point of 200 pg/ml should be used in the diagnosis of CHF.[64] It is now well recognized that CKD, when it is present in patients with CHF, independently predicts poor outcomes.[65] Again, this excess risk seems to occur at a cut point in eGFR below 60 ml/min/1.73 m^2 (Fig. 86–12).[65] Estimated and actual GFRs clearly can be reduced by decreased renal blood flow related

TABLE 86–3 Recommended Dose Adjustment of Conventional Antithrombotics Used for Acute Coronary Syndromes in Patients with Chronic Kidney Disease and End-Stage Renal Disease

	eGFR (ml/min/1.73 m²)		Creatinine Clearance (ml/min)	
Agent	**60–90 ml/min**	**30–60 ml/min**	**<30 ml/min**	**Dialysis Dependent**
Aspirin	No adjustment needed	No adjustment needed	No adjustment needed	No adjustment needed
Clopidogrel	No adjustment needed	No adjustment needed	No adjustment needed	No adjustment needed
Ticlopidine	No adjustment needed	No adjustment needed	No adjustment needed	No adjustment needed
Heparin	No guidelines	No guidelines	No guidelines	No guidelines
LMWH	No guidelines	No guidelines	Reduced dose by 30%; factor Xa monitoring advocated	No guidelines
Lepirudin	No guidelines	CrCl 45-60 ml/min or SrCr 1.6–2 mg/dl: Reduce bolus to 0.2 mg/kg IV + decrease infusion rate by 50% (0.075 mg/kg/hr IV) CrCl 30-44 ml/min or SrCr 2.1-3 mg/dl: Reduce bolus to 0.2 mg/kg IV + decrease standard initial infusion rate by 70% (0.045 mg/kg/hr IV)	CrCl 15-29 ml/min or SrCr 3.1–6 mg/dl: Reduce bolus to 0.2 mg/kg IV + decrease infusion rate by 85% (0.0225 mg/kg/hr IV) CrCl <15 ml/min or SrCr >6 mg/dl: Reduce bolus to 0.2 mg/kg IV; No infusion	Reduce the bolus dose to 0.2 mg/kg IV; No infusion
Bivalirudin	No guidelines	Reduce infusion dose by 20%	Reduce infusion dose by 60%	Reduce infusion dose by 90%
Argatroban	No dose adjustment	No dose adjustment	No dose adjustment	
Abciximab	No guidelines Monitoring advocated	No guidelines Monitoring advocated	No guidelines Monitoring advocated	No guidelines Monitoring advocated
Eptifibatide	No guidelines	SrCr 2-4 mg/dl: 135 μg/kg IV bolus + 0.5 μg/kg/min IV infusion	SrCr >4.0 mg/dl Contraindicated	No clinical data In vitro data demonstrate clearance
Tirofiban	No dose adjustment	No dose adjustment	0.2 μg/kg/min IV for 30 min, followed by 0.05 μg/kg/min IV	No clinical data In vitro data demonstrate clearance

CrCl = creatinine clearance; eGFR = estimated glomerular filtration rate; LMWH = low-molecular-weight heparin; SrCr = serum creatinine.
Adapted from Sica D: The implications of renal impairment among patients undergoing percutaneous coronary intervention. J Invasive Cardiol 14(Suppl B):30B, 2002.

to low cardiac output. However, multiple studies of patients with class II and III CHF, in whom a low cardiac output state is not present, have shown decreased survival in a graded fashion related to renal impairment (see Fig. 86–12). A leading explanation for this observation is that the anemia that predictably develops when the eGFR drops below 60 ml/min/1.73 m², because of a functional deficiency of erythropoietin alpha, accelerates left ventricular hypertrophy and adverse cardiac remodeling. Small observational studies and randomized trials have suggested that treating patients with CHF, CKD, and anemia with exogenous epoetin alfa and supplemental iron improves symptoms, functional class, and peak oxygen consumption.[24,66] To date, there have been no completed mortality trials utilizing this strategy.

The combination of CHF and CKD presents a challenge to cardiologists with respect to proven treatment options. ACEI, if tolerated, or ARBs, if ACEI is not tolerated, beta blockers, aldosterone antagonists, and loop diuretics are all acceptable combination therapies.[67] Caveats in the use of ACEI and ARBs are the marked elevation in the serum Cr and acute renal failure that are more likely to occur when the patient is volume depleted or in the presence of occult bilateral renal artery stenosis or equivalent (unilateral renal artery stenosis present in a renal transplant recipient).[68] When initiating therapy to block the RAAS, it is advisable to have the systolic blood pressure stable and greater than 90 mm Hg, euvolemia, and a drug regimen without concurrent renal toxic agents. In general, an attempt should be made to use ACEI or ARB in patients down to an eGFR of 15 ml/min/1.73 m².

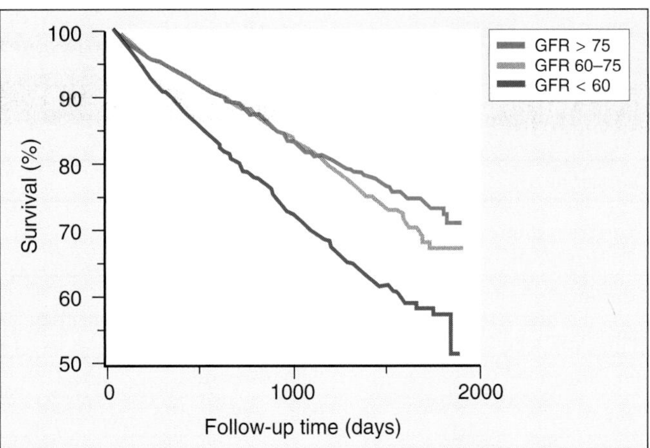

FIGURE 86–12 Kaplan-Meier survival analysis by level of glomerular filtration rate (GFR) as baseline from the Studies of LV Dysfunction (SOLVD) database, which includes patients with functional class I to III congestive heart failure, $n = 6630$. (Adapted from Al-Ahmad A, Rand WM, Manjunath G, et al: Reduced kidney function and anemia as risk factors for mortality in patients with left ventricular dysfunction. J Am Coll Cardiol 38:955, 2001.)

Below this level, case reports suggest a high rate of hyperkalemia and the concern of accelerating the course to ESRD and dialysis.

The management of the patient who is already receiving dialysis and in CHF requires particular care. In general, proven CHF therapies, provided they are tolerated, should be employed along with regular and ad hoc dialysis as needed to control volume overload. In a randomized trial, carvedilol did provide additional benefit in this scenario.[69] In addition, retrospective analysis supports the use of ACEI in patients with ESRD admitted with CHF.[70] Lastly, the acute management of decompensated CHF in patients with impaired eGFR poses a particularly difficult challenge. In fact, an elevated Cr is the single most common reason for the use of positive inotropes or inodilators in hospitalized patients with CHF.[71] There are no published reports of dobutamine leading to long-term favorable outcomes, and in the short term it increases arrhythmias and mortality. Likewise, milrinone has not been shown to reduce mortality, causes arrhythmias, and must be dose adjusted when the eGFR drops below 45 ml/min/1.73 m^2 (Table 86–4).[72] Another option is the use of intravenous BNP (nesiritide), which causes primarily venodilation and natriuresis.[73] Completed studies with nesiritide have evaluated the CKD subgroups and found benefit in CKD equal to that in those with preserved renal function, although the overall effect is modestly better than that with intravenous nitroglycerin.[74] Patients with advanced CHF have reduced renal blood flow, decreased glomerular filtration rate, enhanced proximal reabsorption of water, and an overall reduced capacity of the nephron to excrete water (Fig. 86–13). Furthermore, reduced effective arterial blood volume is a stimulus for antidiuretic hormone release, which plays a dominant role in worsening water retention (see Fig. 86–13). The clinical signs of this deterioration are an elevation in the serum Cr and blood urea nitrogen, hyponatremia, volume retention, and excessive thirst. Treatment efforts should be aimed at improving left ventricular systolic function, often in the hospitalized setting, with the intravenous therapies mentioned previously and discussed in detail elsewhere in this text.

In summary, CKD and CHF present a particularly challenging scenario for clinicians and patients. Frequent monitoring and the combined use of renal and cardioprotective strategies are critical. Future research is needed to confirm anemia correction with erythropoietin as an additional strategy in patients who have a CKD-related anemia. Dialysis patients, despite having volume reduction with mechanical

TABLE 86–4 Recommended Dose Adjustment of Selected Medical Therapy for Hypertension, Dyslipidemia, Heart Failure, and Arrhythmias in Patients with Chronic Kidney Disease and End-Stage Renal Disease

		eGFR (ml/min/1.73 m^2) (CrCl ml/min)			
Drug	**Elimination Route**	***90-60***	***60-30***	***<30***	**Dialysis Dependent**
Central Adrenergic Blockers					
Clonidine	Renal				↓ Dose 50%
Methyldopa	Renal	q.i.d.	q.i.d.	↓ t.i.d.	↓ b.i.d. or qd
Angiotensin-Converting Enzyme Inhibitors (ACEIs)					
Captopril	Renal				↓ Dose 50%
Enalapril	Hepatic			↓ Dose 25%	↓ Dose 50%
Lisinopril	Renal			↓ Dose 25%	↓ Dose 50%
Ramipril	Renal/GI			↓ Dose 75%	↓ Dose 75%
Benazepril	Renal			↓ Dose 25%	↓ Dose 75%
Inotropic Agents					
Digoxin	Renal/nonrenal		↓ Dose 50%	↓ Dose 50%	↓ Dose 75%; change to q.o.d.
Milrinone	Renal		↓ Dose 25%	↓ Dose 50%	↓ Dose 75%
Antiarrhythmics					
Disopyramide	Renal/hepatic	b.i.d.	b.i.d.	↓ qd	↓ q.o.d.
Flecainide	Renal/hepatic				↓ Dose 25–50%
Mexiletine	Renal/hepatic				↓ Dose 50–75%
Procainamide	Renal/hepatic	q.i.d.	↓ t.i.d.	↓ b.i.d.	↓ b.i.d. or qd
Dofetilide	Renal/nonrenal		↓ Dose 50%	↓ Dose 75%	Contraindicated
Beta Blockers					
Atenolol	Renal			↓ Dose 50%	↓ Dose 75%; ↓ q.o.d.
Sotalol	Renal			↓ Dose 50%	↓ Dose 75%
Others					
Verapamil	Hepatic				↓ Dose 50–75%
Hydralazine		q.i.d.	↓ t.i.d	↓ t.i.d.	↓ b.i.d.
Gemfibrozil	Renal			↓ Dose 50%	↓ Dose 75%
Nicotinic acid	Renal/hepatic			↓ Dose 25%	↓ Dose 25%

CrCl = creatinine clearance; eGFR = estimated glomerular filtration rate; GI = gastrointestinal.

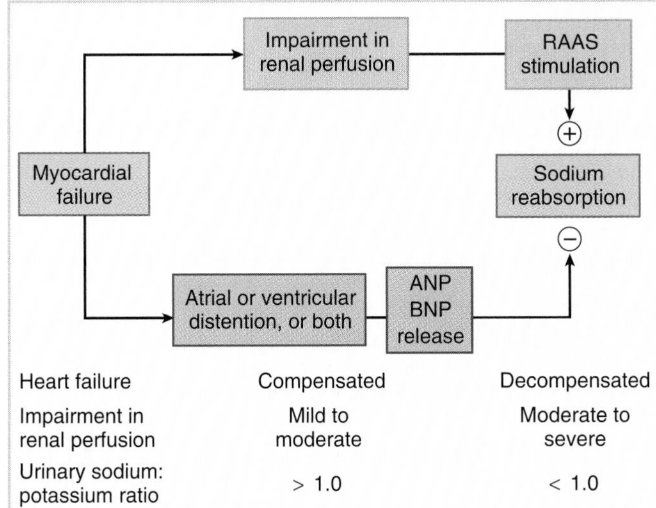

FIGURE 86–13 Pathophysiological processes in combined heart and kidney failure. ANP = A-type natriuretic peptide; BNP = B-type natriuretic peptide; RAAS = renin-angiotensin-aldosterone system. (From Weber KT: Aldosterone in congestive heart failure. N Engl J Med 345:1689, 2001.)

fluid removal, should have medical therapy with ACEIs or ARBs, beta blockers, and additional agents for blood pressure control if needed.

Chronic Kidney Disease and Valvular Heart Disease

Impaired renal function has been linked to mitral annular calcification and to aortic sclerosis. Advanced thickening of the cardiac valves and calcification have been observed in patients with ESRD.[75] Some 80 percent of patients with ESRD have the murmur of aortic sclerosis. Neither of these lesions usually progresses to the point where studies beyond echocardiography are needed. There are no published cases of renal dysfunction being isolated as the cause of valvular disease that required surgical intervention. However, CKD may accelerate degeneration of a tissue valvular prosthesis. Bacterial endocarditis may develop in patients with ESRD who have temporary dialysis access catheters.[76] Endocarditis with common pathogens including *Staphylococcus*, *Streptococcus*, and *Enterococcus*, in the aortic or mitral position, is associated with a mortality rate greater than 50 percent in this setting.[76] It becomes very difficult to treat given the continued need for dialysis access and the delay in surgical placement of permanent arteriovenous shunts or fistulas. Unfortunately, surgical mortality associated with valve replacement in ESRD related to endocarditis is quite high. Infection, and endocarditis in particular, is an increasingly common cause of death in patients with ESRD.

Renal Function and Arrhythmias

Uremia, hyperkalemia, and disorders of calcium-phosphorous balance have all been linked to higher rates of atrial and ventricular arrhythmias.[77] Given a concurrent substrate of left ventricular hypertrophy, left ventricular dilation, CHF, and valvular disease, it is not surprising that higher rates of virtually all arrhythmias have been reported in CKD, including bradyarrhythmias and heart block.[77] Caveats for practical management include dose adjustment for many antiarrhythmic medications including digoxin, sotalol, and procainamide (see Table 86–4). Of concern, CKD, and ESRD in particular, may cause elevated defibrillation thresholds and failure of implantable cardioverter-defibrillators (ICDs).[78] Until this association is better understood, patients receiving ICDs should have frequent surveillance and consideration for noninvasive programmed stimulation for appropriate antitachycardia and defibrillation therapy. Considering the high rates of sudden death in patients with ESRD, clinical trials of prophylactic ICDs in this population are under consideration.

Summary

Recognition has increased over the last decade that patients with CKD have a high risk for CVD. Frequent clinical scenarios in which renal function influences care include CIN, ACS, CHF, valvular disease, and arrhythmias. Results from retrospective studies and clinical trial subgroups form the basis of current recommendations, given the lack of prospective randomized trials in CKD and ESRD. Further study of the adverse metabolic milieu of chronic renal failure is likely to lead to generalizable diagnostic and therapeutic targets for the future management of renal patients with cardiovascular illness.

REFERENCES

Epidemiology and Outcomes

1. Lewis CE, Jacobs DR Jr, McCreath H, et al: Weight gain continues in the 1990s: 10-year trends in weight and overweight from the CARDIA study. Coronary Artery Risk Development in Young Adults. Am J Epidemiol 151:1172, 2000.
2. Bakris GL, Williams M, Dworkin L, et al: Preserving renal function in adults with hypertension and diabetes: A consensus approach. National Kidney Foundation Hypertension and Diabetes Executive Committees Working Group. Am J Kidney Dis 36:646, 2000.
3. McCullough PA: Cardiorenal risk: An important clinical intersection. Rev Cardiovasc Med 3:71, 2002.
4. National Kidney Foundation: Clinical practice guidelines for chronic kidney disease: Evaluation, classification, and stratification. Am J Kidney Dis 2(Suppl 1):S46, 2002.
5. McCullough PA, Soman SS, Shah SS, et al: Risks associated with renal dysfunction in patients in the coronary care unit. J Am Coll Cardiol 36:679, 2000.
6. Beattie JN, Soman SS, Sandberg KR, et al: Determinants of mortality after myocardial infarction in patients with advanced renal dysfunction. Am J Kidney Dis 37:1191, 2001.
7. Chertow GM, Lazarus JM, Christiansen CL, et al: Preoperative renal risk stratification. Circulation 95:878, 1997.
8. Szczech LA, Best PJ, Crowley E, for the Bypass Angioplasty Revascularization Investigation (BARI) Investigators: Outcomes of patients with chronic renal insufficiency in the bypass angioplasty revascularization investigation. Circulation 105:2253, 2002.
9. Keane WF, Eknoyan G: Proteinuria, albuminuria, risk, assessment, detection, elimination (PARADE): A position paper of the National Kidney Foundation. Am J Kidney Dis 33:1004, 1999.
10. Chobanian AV, Bakris GL, Black HR, for the National Heart, Lung, and Blood Institute Joint National Committee on Prevention, Detection, Evaluation, and Treatment of High Blood Pressure; National High Blood Pressure Education Program Coordinating Committee: The Seventh Report of the Joint National Committee on Prevention, Detection, Evaluation, and Treatment of High Blood Pressure: The JNC 7 report. JAMA 289:2560, 2003.
11. McCullough PA: Why is chronic kidney disease the "spoiler" for cardiovascular outcomes? J Am Coll Cardiol 41:725, 2003.
12. McCullough PA, Manley HJ: Prediction and prevention of contrast nephropathy. J Interv Cardiol 14:547, 2001.
13. McCullough PA, Wolyn R, Rocher LL, et al: Acute renal failure after coronary intervention: Incidence, risk factors, and relationship to mortality. Am J Med 103:368, 1997.
14. Mangano CM, Diamondstone LS, Ramsay JG, et al: Renal dysfunction after myocardial revascularization: Risk factors, adverse outcomes, and hospital resource utilization. The Multicenter Study of Perioperative Ischemia Research Group. Ann Intern Med 128:194, 1998.
15. Rihal CS, Textor SC, Grill DE, et al: Incidence and prognostic importance of acute renal failure after percutaneous coronary intervention. Circulation 105:2259, 2002.

Therapy

16. Pitt B, Segal R, Martinez FA, et al: Randomised trial of losartan versus captopril in patients over 65 with heart failure (Evaluation of Losartan in the Elderly Study, ELITE). Lancet 349:747, 1997.
17. Toto R: Angiotensin II subtype 1 receptor blockers and renal function. Arch Intern Med 161:1492, 2001.

18. Brenner BM, Cooper ME, de Zeeuw D, for the RENAAL Study Investigators: Effects of losartan on renal and cardiovascular outcomes in patients with type 2 diabetes and nephropathy. N Engl J Med 345:861, 2001.
19. Lewis EJ, Hunsicker LG, Clarke WR, for the Collaborative Study Group: Renoprotective effect of the angiotensin-receptor antagonist irbesartan in patients with nephropathy due to type 2 diabetes. N Engl J Med 345:851, 2001.
20. Parving HH, Lehnert H, Brochner-Mortensen J, for the Irbesartan in Patients with Type 2 Diabetes and Microalbuminuria Study Group: The effect of irbesartan on the development of diabetic nephropathy in patients with type 2 diabetes. N Engl J Med 345:870, 2001.
21. Dahlof B, Devereux RB, Kjeldsen SE, for the LIFE Study Group: Cardiovascular morbidity and mortality in the Losartan Intervention For Endpoint reduction in hypertension study (LIFE): A randomised trial against atenolol. Lancet 359:995, 2002.
22. Mann JF, Gerstein HC, Pogue J, et al: Renal insufficiency as a predictor of cardiovascular outcomes and the impact of ramipril: The HOPE randomized trial. Ann Intern Med 134:629, 2001.
23. Agodoa LY, Appel L, Bakris GL, for the African American Study of Kidney Disease and Hypertension (AASK) Study Group: Effect of ramipril vs amlodipine on renal outcomes in hypertensive nephrosclerosis: A randomized controlled trial. JAMA 285:2719, 2001.
24. Silverberg DS, Wexler D, Sheps D, et al: The effect of correction of mild anemia in severe, resistant congestive heart failure using subcutaneous erythropoietin and intravenous iron: A randomized controlled study. J Am Coll Cardiol 37:1775, 2001.
25. Friedman AN, Bostom AG, Selhub J, et al: The kidney and homocysteine metabolism. J Am Soc Nephrol 12:2181, 2001.
26. Chertow GM, Burke SK, Raggi P for the Treat to Goal Working Group: Sevelamer attenuates the progression of coronary and aortic calcification in hemodialysis patients. Kidney Int 62:245, 2002.

Percutaneous Coronary Interventions and Contrast-Induced Nephropathy

27. Andersen KJ, Christensen EI, Vik H: Effects of iodinated x-ray contrast media on renal epithelial cells in culture. Invest Radiol 29:955, 1994.
28. Keeley EC, Grines CL: Scraping of aortic debris by coronary guiding catheters: A prospective evaluation of 1,000 cases. J Am Coll Cardiol 32:1861, 1998.
29. Chertow GM, Lazarus JM, Christiansen CL, et al: Preoperative renal risk stratification. Circulation 95:878, 1997.
30. Denton KM, Shweta A, Anderson WP: Preglomerular and postglomerular resistance responses to different levels of sympathetic activation by hypoxia. J Am Soc Nephrol 13:27, 2002.
31. Uder M, Humke U, Pahl M, et al: Nonionic contrast media iohexol and iomeprol decrease renal arterial tone: Comparative studies on human and porcine isolated vascular segments. Invest Radiol 37:440, 2002.
32. Rauch D, Drescher P, Pereira FJ, et al: Comparison of iodinated contrast media–induced renal vasoconstriction in human, rabbit, dog, and pig arteries. Invest Radiol 32:315, 1997.
33. Mueller C, Buerkle G, Buettner HJ, et al: Prevention of contrast media–associated nephropathy: Randomized comparison of 2 hydration regimens in 1620 patients undergoing coronary angioplasty. Arch Intern Med 162:329, 2002.
34. Solomon R, Werner C, Mann D, et al: Effects of saline, mannitol, and furosemide to prevent acute decreases in renal function induced by radiocontrast agents. N Engl J Med 331:1416, 1994.
35. Stevens MA, McCullough PA, Tobin KJ, et al: A prospective randomized trial of prevention measures in patients at high risk for contrast nephropathy: Results of the P.R.I.N.C.E. Study. Prevention of Radiocontrast Induced Nephropathy Clinical Evaluation. J Am Coll Cardiol 33:403, 1999.
36. Rudnick MR, Goldfarb S, Wexler L, et al: Nephrotoxicity of ionic and nonionic contrast media in 1196 patients: A randomized trial. The Iohexol Cooperative Study. Kidney Int 47:254, 1995.
37. Aspelin P, Aubry P, Fransson SG, for the Nephrotoxicity in High-Risk Patients Study of Iso-Osmolar and Low-Osmolar Non-Ionic Contrast Media Study Investigators: Nephrotoxic effects in high-risk patients undergoing angiography. N Engl J Med 348:491, 2003.
38. Davidson CJ, Laskey WK, Hermiller JB, et al: Randomized trial of contrast media utilization in high-risk PTCA: The COURT trial. Circulation 101:2172, 2000.
39. Manske CL, Sprafka JM, Strony JT, Wang Y: Contrast nephropathy in azotemic diabetic patients undergoing coronary angiography. Am J Med 89:615, 1990.
40. Stone GW, Tumlin JA, Madyoon H, et al: Design and rationale of CONTRAST—A prospective, randomized, placebo-controlled trial of fenoldopam mesylate for the prevention of radiocontrast nephropathy. Rev Cardiovasc Med 2(Suppl 1):S31, 2001.
41. Tumlin JA, Wang A, Murray PT, Mathur VS: Fenoldopam mesylate blocks reductions in renal plasma flow after radiocontrast dye infusion: A pilot trial in the prevention of contrast nephropathy. Am Heart J 143:894, 2002.
42. Stone GW, McCullough PA, Tumlin J, et al: A prospective, randomized placebo-controlled multicenter trial evaluating fenoldopam mesylate for the prevention of contrast induced nephropathy: The CONTRAST Trial. J Am Coll Cardiol 41:83A, 2003.
43. Tepel M, van der Giet M, Schwarzfeld C, et al: Prevention of radiographic-contrast-agent-induced reductions in renal function by acetylcysteine. N Engl J Med 343:180, 2000.
44. Diaz-Sandoval LJ, Kosowsky BD, Losordo DW: Acetylcysteine to prevent angiography-related renal tissue injury (the APART trial). Am J Cardiol 89:356, 2002.
45. Shyu KG, Cheng JJ, Kuan P: Acetylcysteine protects against acute renal damage in patients with abnormal renal function undergoing a coronary procedure. J Am Coll Cardiol 40:1383, 2002.
46. Kay J, Chow WH, Chan TM, et al: Acetylcysteine for prevention of acute deterioration of renal function following elective coronary angiography and intervention: A randomized controlled trial. JAMA 289:553, 2003.
47. Durham JD, Caputo C, Dokko J, et al: A randomized controlled trial of *N*-acetylcysteine to prevent contrast nephropathy in cardiac angiography. Kidney Int 62:2202, 2002.
48. Briguori C, Manganelli F, Scarpato P, et al: Acetylcysteine and contrast agent–associated nephrotoxicity. J Am Coll Cardiol 40:298, 2002.
49. Allaqaband S, Tumuluri R, Malik AM, et al: Prospective randomized study of *N*-acetylcysteine, fenoldopam, and saline for prevention of radiocontrast-induced nephropathy. Catheter Cardiovasc Interv 57:279, 2002.
50. Loutrianakis E, Stella D, Hussain A, et al: Randomized comparison of fenoldopam and *N*-acetylcysteine to saline in the prevention of radiocontrast nephropathy. J Am Coll Cardiol 41:327A, 2003.
51. Baker CS, Wragg A, Kumar S, et al: A rapid protocol for the prevention of contrast-induced renal dysfunction (RAPPID Study). J Am Coll Cardiol 41:39A, 2003.
52. Goldenberg I, Jonas M, Matetzki S, et al: Contrast-associated nephropathy and clinical outcome of patients with chronic renal insufficiency undergoing cardiac catheterization: Lack of additive benefit of acetylcysteine to saline infusion. J Am Coll Cardiol 41:537A, 2003.
53. Guitterez N, Diaz A, Timmis GC, et al: Determinants of serum creatinine trajectory in acute contrast nephropathy. J Interv Cardiol 15:349, 2002.
54. Krijnen P, van Jaarsveld BC, Steyerberg EW, et al: A clinical prediction rule for renal artery stenosis. Ann Intern Med 129:705, 1998.

Ischemic Heart Diseases in Patients with Impaired Renal Function

55. Fatica RA, Port FK, Young EW: Incidence trends and mortality in end-stage renal disease attributed to renovascular disease in the United States. Am J Kidney Dis 37:1184, 2001.
56. Conti CR: Silent cardiac ischemia. Curr Opin Cardiol 17:537, 2002.
57. George SK, Singh AK: Current markers of myocardial ischemia and their validity in end-stage renal disease. Curr Opin Nephrol Hypertens 8:719, 1999.
58. McCullough PA, Nowak RM, Foreback C, et al: Emergency evaluation of chest pain in patients with advanced kidney disease. Arch Intern Med 162:2464, 2002.
59. McCullough PA, Nowak RM, Foreback C, et al: Performance of multiple cardiac biomarkers measured in the emergency department in patients with chronic kidney disease and chest pain. Acad Emerg Med 9:1389, 2002.
60. Herzog CA, Ma JZ, Collins AJ: Poor long-term survival after acute myocardial infarction among patients on long-term dialysis. N Engl J Med 339:799, 1998.
61. Sica D: The implications of renal impairment among patients undergoing percutaneous coronary intervention. J Invasive Cardiol 14(Suppl B):30B, 2002.
62. McCullough PA: Acute coronary syndromes in patients with renal failure. Curr Cardiol Rep 5:266, 2003.

Heart Failure in Patients with Kidney Disease

63. Schreiber BD: Congestive heart failure in patients with chronic kidney disease and on dialysis. Am J Med Sci 325:179, 2003.
64. McCullough PA, Duc P, Omland T, for the BNP Multinational Study Investigators: B-type natriuretic peptide and renal function in the diagnosis of heart failure: An analysis from the breathing not properly multinational study. Am J Kidney Dis 41:571, 2003.
65. Al-Ahmad A, Rand WM, Manjunath G, et al: Reduced kidney function and anemia as risk factors for mortality in patients with left ventricular dysfunction. J Am Coll Cardiol 38:955, 2001.
66. Mancini DM, Katz SD, Lang CC, et al: Effect of erythropoietin on exercise capacity in patients with moderate to severe chronic heart failure. Circulation 107:294, 2003.
67. Shlipak MG: Pharmacotherapy for heart failure in patients with renal insufficiency. Ann Intern Med 138:917, 2003.
68. Schoolwerth AC, Sica DA, Ballermann BJ, Wilcox CS for the Council on the Kidney in Cardiovascular Disease and the Council for High Blood Pressure Research of the American Heart Association: Renal considerations in angiotensin converting enzyme inhibitor therapy: A statement for healthcare professionals from the Council on the Kidney in Cardiovascular Disease and the Council for High Blood Pressure Research of the American Heart Association. Circulation 104:1985, 2001.
69. Cice G, Ferrara L, D'Andrea A, et al: Carvedilol increases two-year survival in dialysis patients with dilated cardiomyopathy: A prospective, placebo-controlled trial. J Am Coll Cardiol 41:1438, 2003.
70. McCullough PA, Sandberg KR, Yee J, Hudson MP: Mortality benefit of angiotensin-converting enzyme inhibitors after cardiac events in patients with end-stage renal disease. J Renin Angiotensin Aldosterone Syst 3:188, 2002.
71. Smith GL, Vaccarino V, Kosiborod M, et al: Worsening renal function: What is a clinically meaningful change in creatinine during hospitalization with heart failure? J Card Fail 9:13, 2003.
72. Jain P, Massie BM, Gattis WA, et al: Current medical treatment for the exacerbation of chronic heart failure resulting in hospitalization. Am Heart J 145(2 Suppl):S3, 2003.
73. Keating GM, Goa KL: Nesiritide: A review of its use in acute decompensated heart failure. Drugs 63:47, 2003.
74. Butler J, Emerson C, Peacock WF, et al: The efficacy and safety of B-type natriuretic peptide (nesiritide) in patients with renal insufficiency and acutely decompensated congestive heart failure. Nephrol Dial Transplant 19:391, 2004.

Valvular Heart Disease and Arrhythmias in Patients with Kidney Disease

75. Umana E, Ahmed W, Alpert MA: Valvular and perivalvular abnormalities in end-stage renal disease. Am J Med Sci 325:237, 2003.
76. Manian FA: Vascular and cardiac infections in end-stage renal disease. Am J Med Sci 325:243, 2003.
77. Soman SS, Sandberg KR, Borzak S, et al: The independent association of renal dysfunction and arrhythmias in critically ill patients. Chest 122:669, 2002.
78. Wase A, Basit A, Nazir R, et al: Does chronic renal insufficiency raise defibrillation threshold? [Abstract] Pacing Clin Electrophysiol 25(4, Pt II):594, 2002.

CHAPTER 87

Cardiovascular Manifestations of Autonomic Disorders

Rose Marie Robertson • David Robertson

General Principles

Autonomic control of the cardiovascular system provides second-to-second adjustments of blood pressure and heart rate, allowing humans great flexibility in posture and environment. Normally, autonomic integration of cardiovascular, renal, gastrointestinal, and temperature control adds to the metabolic control directed by the needs of each organ to maintain homeostasis for the entire organism and can even compensate for circumstances of stress or disease. Thus, when the autonomic nervous system fails and this finely tuned cardiovascular control is lost, significant impairment in function results.

Because most autonomic disorders are relatively uncommon, and because many clinicians are unfamiliar with these disorders and their presentation, consultation is usually sought. Since abnormalities in blood pressure, heart rate, or both are prominent features in these patients, and specialists in autonomic function are found in only a few centers, it is the cardiologist who is called upon to provide diagnostic and therapeutic information. In this chapter, we review the current understanding of abnormalities in autonomic cardiovascular control, as well as provide a guide for the consultant cardiologist in arriving at a diagnosis in these circumstances.

Several classification systems exist that can be applied to autonomic disorders, based on whether the disorder is acute or chronic, congenital or acquired, severe or mild, on the etiology (if known), and, in a few cases, on the specific underlying genetic abnormality.[1] Here, we use severity of autonomic impairment as the major feature differentiating these disorders and add the additional factor of the usual circumstances of presentation. This presents a simple approach to differential diagnosis. We also provide the initial approach to therapy for each disorder, recognizing that patients who do not respond adequately may require referral to a center specializing in autonomic dysfunction.

AUTONOMIC CARDIOVASCULAR CONTROL. The autonomic nervous system provides an integrated response by centrally coordinating physiological responses. It may be divided into sympathetic, parasympathetic, and enteric components. We focus on the first two. The effects of autonomic input to the cardiac conduction system,[2] the myocardium itself, and to the coronary and systemic vasculature are discussed in Chapters 19, 27, 37 and 44. Integrated control of blood pressure and heart rate and their modifications by disease are less familiar, and we delineate these in some detail, focusing first on the baroreflex.

BAROREFLEX. The maintenance of blood pressure with postural change in humans is accomplished by a group of reflexes referred to collectively as the *baroreflex*, provided by an integrated complex of neurons whose function reduces the lability of blood pressure. It includes the arterial baroreceptors, with sensory nerve endings within the aortic arch, at the origin of the right subclavian artery, and within the carotid sinuses, as well as the cardiopulmonary receptors (low-pressure receptors) in the walls of the atria and pulmonary artery. At baseline, the baroreflex tonically inhibits sympathetic activity and enhances parasympathetic activity. In the normal healthy human at rest, parasympathetic tone predominates. Additional complexities in the system (e.g., the presence of different populations of sympathetic neurons projecting from the paraventricular nucleus to the spinal cord, some participating in baroreflex-mediated responses, and others with a possible role in nonvasomotor sympathetic control[3]) allow further differentiation of response. However, we focus on the vasomotor aspects of autonomic function.

ARTERIAL BARORECEPTORS. Change in vascular pressure causes a change in the stretch applied to the arterial baroreceptors, and this in turn alters the frequency of discharge of the aortic depressor and carotid sinus nerves, whose first synapse lies within the nucleus tractus solitarii in the brain stem. Baroreceptor function is not the same in all individuals or even in the same individual at different times or in different experimental or disease states. For example, it has been demonstrated that adenoviral-mediated gene transfer of endothelial nitric oxide synthase to carotid sinus adventitia causes sustained, nitric oxide–dependent inhibition of baroreceptor activity and resetting of the baroreceptor function curve to higher pressures, suggesting that nitric oxide levels can modulate baroreceptor function.[4] When blood pressure is altered, afferent information from the baroreceptors is integrated on a beat-to-beat basis and determines efferent sympathetic and parasympathetic activity to minimize fluctuations in arterial pressure. This is accomplished via projections from the nucleus tractus solitarii to those hindbrain nuclei that govern efferent sympathetic activity (the caudal ventrolateral medulla, which projects to the rostral ventrolateral medulla and thus to the intermediolateral columns of the spinal cord) and parasympathetic activity (the nucleus ambiguus and the dorsal motor nucleus of the vagus). For example, when blood pressure rises, activation of the arterial baroreflex, producing an increase in the frequency of firing, leads to a decrease in sympathetic activity and an increase in parasympathetic activity, with the final integrated response being minimal change in blood pressure and heart rate.

In addition to the classic neurotransmitters such as norepinephrine and acetylcholine, cotransmitters such as neuropeptide Y may be released.[5] Studies of animals in which neuropeptide Y is overexpressed demonstrate that this peptide has sympatholytic and hypotensive effects and may have a role in blood pressure regulation. Although the effects of the classic neurotransmitters would seem to predominate, neuropeptide Y may buffer these effects, and in these studies, led to increased longevity.[5]

CARDIOPULMONARY RECEPTORS. Input from cardiopulmonary receptors in the heart and lungs, primarily in response to changes in volume, is also projected via vagal afferents to the nucleus tractus solitarii. These receptors are sensitive to chemical as well as mechanical activation and also provide input to the spinal cord via spinal sympathetic afferents. Stimulation of these receptors produces bradycardia, vasodilation, a resulting fall in blood pressure, and inhibition of vasopressin release. For example, the stimulation of cardiopulmonary receptors by an increase in intracardiac volume produces, via vasopressin and its effect on renal sympathetic nerve activity, an increase in salt and water excretion, an important regulatory mechanism directed at maintaining an optimal central blood volume. The components of the baroreflex are illustrated in Figure 87–1.

POSTURAL RESPONSES. With standing, the blood volume is subjected to gravitational forces that produce pooling of 500 to 800 ml of blood in the capacitance vessels of the lower extremities. Plasma moves to the interstitium (12 to 15 percent of the plasma volume over 20 to 40 minutes),[6] and there is a decrease in venous return and cardiac output.[7,8] This rapid fall in plasma volume with assumption of the upright posture in normal subjects was described in the 1930s by Youmans and associates.[9] The baroreceptor afferent nerves, both arterial and cardiopulmonary, detect reduced stretch and synapse in the nucleus tractus solitarii, and a decrease in parasympathetic tone and increase in sympathetic activity ensue, with the release of norepinephrine and an increase in peripheral resistance. Vasopressin release from the paraventricular nucleus and the supraoptic nucleus is also inhibited by the baroreflex, via the caudal ventrolateral medulla. When intact, this complex of autonomic reflex function protects blood pressure and cerebral perfusion.

Abnormalities of the integrated blood pressure and heart rate control provided by the baroreflex can be caused by dysfunction or failure of any of its separate components, from sensory afferents, to areas of central integration in the brain stem, or efferent effector neurons. The clinical manifestations depend not only on the anatomic sites affected but also on the degree of dysfunction of the components affected. Although there is profound lability of blood pressure and heart rate in patients with complete baroreflex failure, there is a broad range of other disorders that can also produce abnormal blood pressure and heart rate responses.

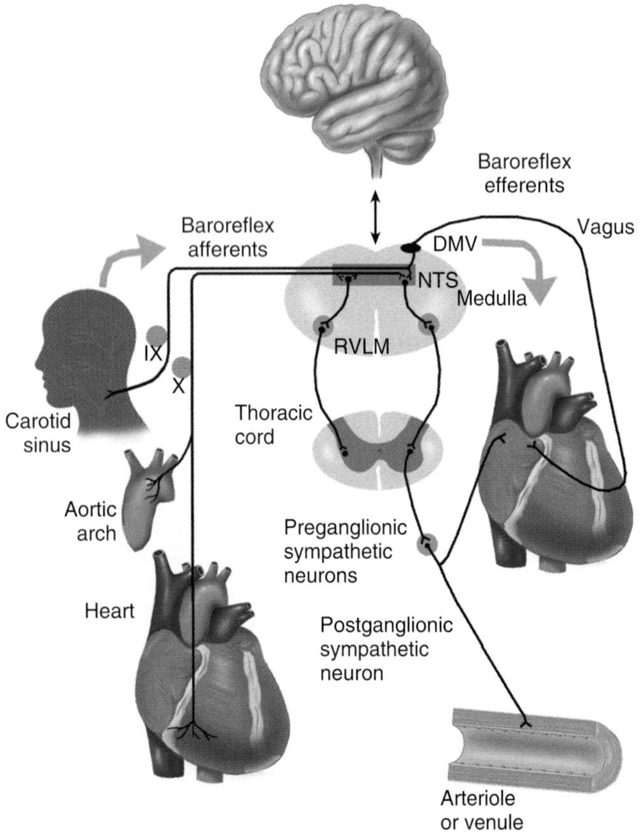

FIGURE 87–1 Components of the baroreflex. DMV = dorsal motor nucleus of the vagus; NTS = nucleus tractus solitarii; RVLM = rostroventrolateral medulla; NE = norepinephrine. (Courtesy of Dr. André Diedrich.)

Autonomic Disorders

Autonomic disorders, also referred to as *dysautonomias*, can be divided according to their effects on blood pressure in the upright posture. The first group includes those that are severe, always causing significant orthostatic hypotension (a fall in blood pressure with standing of more than 20/10 mm Hg, measured with the patient lying quietly and after 5 minutes of quiet standing, or as long as the patient can stand if symptoms limit the duration of standing.). Although these disorders are rare, some can significantly affect longevity, and all are serious.[7,8,10-13] The second group, the mild dysautonomias, are more common but less serious, and orthostatic hypotension is usually absent, though heart rate abnormalities are often prominent.[14-16] Animal models of a number of these disorders have been developed and are useful in studying pathophysiology and therapeutic options.[17] Table 87–1 provides a useful checklist to consider.

SETTINGS. It is also useful to consider the settings in which disorders present. Newly acquired autonomic dysfunction can appear in hospitalized patients and often prompts consultation, either because of new and profound hypotension or hypertension or an inability to discharge the patient due to marked orthostatic hypotension.. However, although patients with disorders that come on gradually over months to years may be referred for outpatient consultation, a subclinical autonomic disorder may also be noticed for the first time during a hospitalization for another disease, unmasked either by that disease or some aspect of its treatment. Chronic disorders often seem acute to the patient, especially if the first manifestation is dramatic, such as syncope, but careful review of the history usually reveals subtle premonitory symptoms. Table 87–2 lists some factors that are likely to worsen symptoms in patients with autonomic dysfunction and thus bring subclinical disorders to attention or, conversely, to improve orthostatic symptoms.[18-27]

TABLE 87–1 Autonomic Disorders Grouped by Severity
Severe dysautonomias—afferent/central dysfunction
Baroreflex failure
Glossopharyngeal neuralgia
Severe dysautonomias—efferent dysfunction
Acquired—symptoms beginning later in life
Multiple system atrophy
Pure autonomic failure
Autoimmune autonomic failure
Autonomic neuropathy (diabetes, amyloid, renal failure associated, vitamin B_{12} deficiency, paraneoplastic syndromes, idiopathic)
Guillain-Barré syndrome
Congenital—symptoms present from birth
Dopamine beta-hydroxylase deficiency
Mild dysautonomias
Postural tachycardia syndrome
Neurally mediated syncope
Norepinephrine transporter deficiency
Medications (norepinephrine transporter blockers)
Bed rest

Factor	Raises Blood Pressure	Lowers Blood Pressure
Intake	Water drinking	Food ingestion
Volume	Hypervolemia	Hypovolemia
Ventilation	Hypoventilation	Hyperventilation
Environment	Cold	Heat
Medications	Sympathomimetics	Vasodilators
Other	—	Infection (even subclinical)

TABLE 87–2 Factors Altering Blood Pressure in Patients with Autonomic Dysfunction

AUTONOMIC TESTING AT THE BEDSIDE. Although there is a wide spectrum of autonomic tests that can be applied to differentiate autonomic disorders, evaluating the sympathetic adrenergic, sympathetic cholinergic, and parasympathetic branches of the autonomic nervous system, a few simple maneuvers at the bedside offer substantial information. Careful measurement of the blood pressure and heart rate in the supine posture should be followed by having the patient stand next to the bed, with support if necessary, with repeat determinations made as soon as the patient complains of symptoms or at 5 minutes. If the patient cannot continue standing for 5 minutes, blood pressure and heart rate should be obtained just prior to sitting. In most healthy individuals, the diastolic blood pressure rises slightly and the systolic pressure falls minimally, if at all. Orthostatic hypotension is defined as a fall of more than 20/10 mm Hg. Heart rate should increase no more than 20 beats/min.

If beat-to-beat heart rate can be obtained via continuous electrocardiographic (ECG) monitoring or an ECG machine set to record continuously for 30 seconds, it may be useful to add a Valsalva maneuver. During continuous recording, the patient blows into a closed system for 12 seconds at 40 mm Hg. A convenient system can be made by attaching the external tube of a 5-ml plastic syringe to the manometer of a sphygmomanometer. Divide the fastest heart rate during the Valsalva maneuver, when increased intrathoracic pressure impedes venous return and leads to a fall in blood pressure, by the slowest heart rate immediately afterward, during the rebound of blood pressure. A ratio of less than 1.4 suggests autonomic impairment. This is most useful if the patient is also instrumented for arterial pressure monitoring, so that the appropriate fall in blood pressure during the Valsalva maneuver can be documented.[28] Patients with congestive heart failure do not have the normal hemodynamic response to the Valsalva maneuver because they are less able to restrict the return of blood to the right atrium, so the maneuver is less helpful in this group. A normal Valsalva maneuver as well as the maneuver in a patient with pure autonomic failure is depicted in Figure 87–2.

Severe Dysautonomias

BAROREFLEX FAILURE. For many years, all patients with abnormalities of autonomic cardiovascular reflex control were considered to have baroreflex failure. And, in the broadest sense, autonomic efferents are a component of the baroreflex arc. However, there is a more specific syndrome of baroreflex failure involving a variety of disorders (surgery,[15] radiation,[29] cerebrovascular accident) affecting afferent neuronal input via the vagus and glossopharyngeal nerves, or damage to brain stem nuclei or interneurons, and we have elucidated its characteristics and distinguished it from the broader group of patients with other forms of

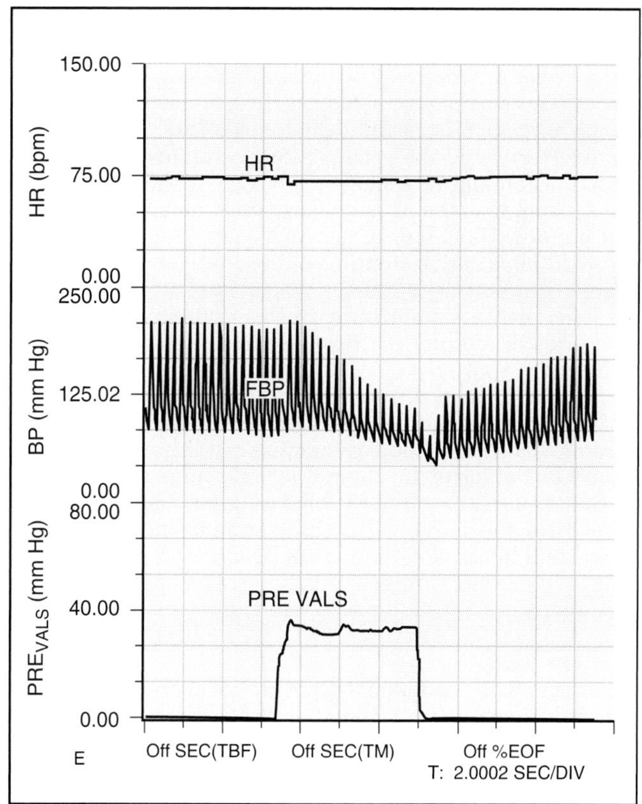

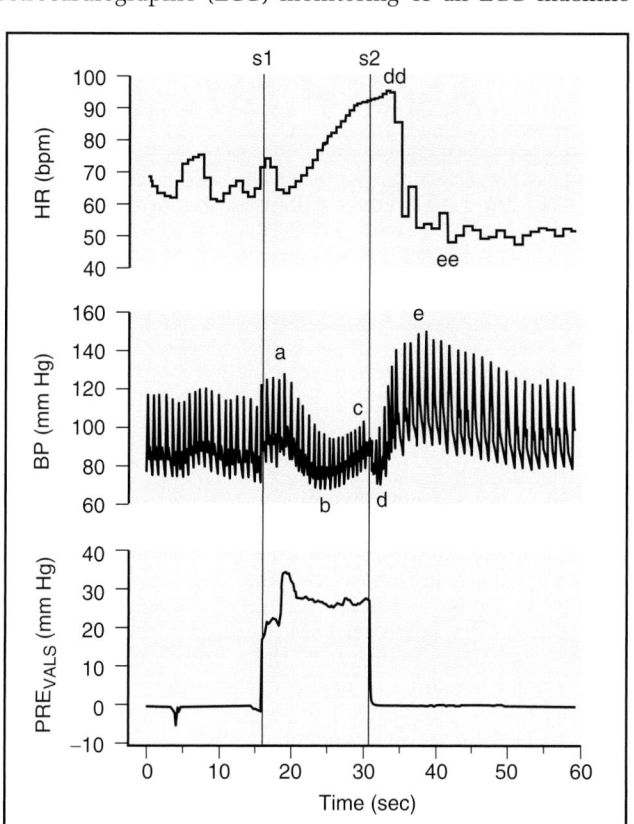

FIGURE 87–2 The Valsalva maneuver in a normal subject **(A)** and in a patient with pure autonomic failure **(B)**. a = increased intrathoracic pressure, beginning of phase 2; b = maximal fall in BP; HR = heart rate; BP = blood pressure; c = return of BP to within 20 mm Hg of baseline, due to sympathetically-mediated peripheral vasoconstriction; d = minimal BP after release of intrathoracic pressure, followed closely by maximal heart rate; e = increased BP as increased venous return is pumped into a vasoconstricted peripheral vascular bed; ee = slowed heart rate due to baroreflex response to the elevated pressure; PRE_{VALS} = pressure against which the subject is blowing with an open glottis; s1 = beginning of phase 1.

autonomic failure.[7] These patients have extremely labile blood pressure with alterations unbuffered by normal control mechanisms. The level of blood pressure at any given moment appears to be dependent on the sum of the input from higher centers on autonomic brain stem nuclei. Our ability to define this syndrome has greatly benefited from identification of a large kindred with an autosomal dominant disorder causing a high incidence of carotid body, glomus jugulare, and glomus vagale tumors, which can cause physical damage to adjacent nerves (glossopharyngeal and vagal).[15] Even if there is minimal impact of the tumors themselves, surgical resection may lead to unavoidable damage of underlying nervous structures, and baroreflex function can be studied in these patients before and after the procedure. This has allowed us to determine that the clinical presentation of baroreflex failure varies over time, with acute baroreflex dysfunction[30,31] appearing much more like pheochromocytoma, with extremely labile blood pressure and heart rate changing in concert (i.e., a rise in blood pressure does not lead to the expected baroreflex-mediated fall in heart rate, but rather heart rate and blood pressure rise and fall together), little or no orthostatic hypotension (presumably because the cortical arousal associated with taking the upright posture leads to increased sympathetic outflow, with its effects on the peripheral vasculature unbuffered), but with more orthostatic hypotension seen later in the course. Figure 87–3 demonstrates the loss of response to changes in carotid baroreceptor stimulation with baroreflex failure.

Some patients undergoing carotid endarterectomy, especially those who have previously had surgery on the other carotid, also develop baroreflex failure acutely, presenting in the postoperative period. Although the proportion is not clearly defined, 9 to 30 percent of carefully studied series of patients exhibit hypertension consistent with this problem,[32-34] and tens of thousands of these procedures are done yearly in the United States.[35] Both the hypertension and hypotension are often difficult to control with usual medical therapy. Although carotid angioplasty and stenting have been proposed as alternative procedures, their long-term outcomes are only now being evaluated. As these procedures also have the potential to affect carotid anatomy, it is not clear that they are likely to avoid the postoperative complications of severe hypertension and its sequelae.

An example of the physiological effect of the loss of baroreflex buffering is demonstrated in Figure 87–4, in which the standard nociceptive stimulus of the cold pressor test, which normally produces a pressor response of 20 to 40 mm Hg, not only has a significantly greater quantitative effect but also leads to a prolonged response in the absence of normal buffering.

In patients with only unilateral involvement, the extent of baroreflex impairment is variable. Although one might assume that preservation of function on the contralateral side would be sufficient for normal or only minimally abnormal baroreflex function, in fact some patients have nearly complete baroreflex failure. This observation led to studies of unilateral and bilateral carotid sinus stimulation, demonstrating that right carotid baroreflex loading was more effective than stimulation of the left carotid and as efficient as bilateral stimulation in modulating the variability of the heart rate and blood pressure.[36,37]

Patients with baroreflex failure are often seen acutely, after surgical intervention, trauma, or stroke (bilateral damage to the nucleus tractus solitarii), and in this setting the hypertension may sometimes be the highest one encounters in contemporary practice (systolic pressures of 200 to 320 mm Hg, with heart rates of 130 to 160 beats/min), with headaches of great severity. Apneic episodes also occur, possibly because of loss of neural afferents conveying information from vascular chemoreceptors. Plasma norepinephrine levels of 1000

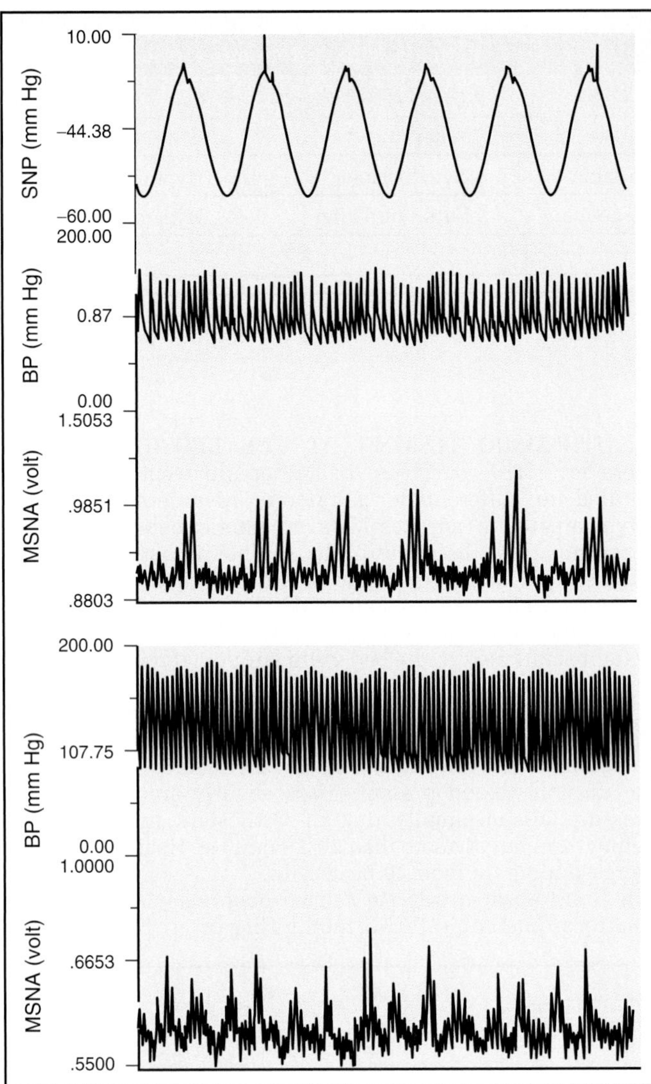

FIGURE 87–3 Effect of carotid sinus stimulation via neck suction in a healthy subject **(top)** and in a patient with chronic baroreflex failure **(bottom)**. **Top,** The effect of bilateral neck suction in a healthy volunteer for sinusoidal carotid sinus stimulation (SNP, period 10 sec) and the blood pressure response (middle trace) modulated by synchronized sympathetic nerve activity (lower trace). **Bottom,** Absent modulation of blood pressure (upper trace) and muscle sympathetic nerve activity (lower trace) by sinusoidal neck suction (period 10 sec) in a patient with baroreflex failure. The timing of carotid sinus stimulation is identical for both panels, although shown only in the top panel. BP = blood pressure; MSNA = muscle sympathetic nerve activity; SNP = sinusoidal neck pressure.

to 3000 pg/ml are not uncommon. Nitroprusside and a centrally acting alpha$_2$-agonist (clonidine) in combination are often needed to control blood pressure over the first 72 hours. Even after the acute phase, patients often continue to suffer from pressor crises, with hot flushing, headache, diaphoresis, and tachycardia, often triggered by minor cortical (anxiety, stress, discomfort, or fear) or other stimuli. Rest, sleep, and sedation may result in very low blood pressures and heart rates.

In these patients, whether the cause was the tumors mentioned earlier, surgery, radiation, trauma, or stroke, we found that the most helpful diagnostic criteria were the depressor response to a small (0.1 to 0.2 mg) dose of clonidine and the absence of heart rate responses to depressor or pressor drug infusions (at a time when stimuli and suppression of endogenous cortical activity, such as mental arithmetic and sedation, respectively, could raise and lower heart rate). These studies

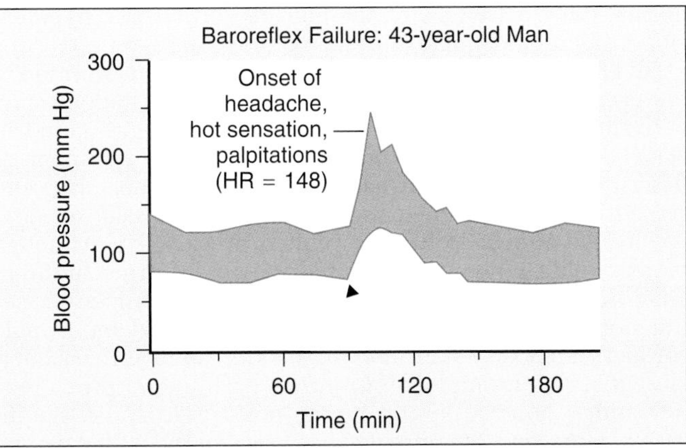

FIGURE 87–4 Response to cold pressor testing in baroreflex failure. The graph shows blood pressure monitoring in a 43-year-old man about 2 weeks after surgical removal of a second carotid body tumor. A 60-second cold pressor test (immersion of the hand in ice water; arrowhead) usually produces a 25- to 50-mm Hg pressor response that resolves within a few minutes. Here, the blood pressure continued to rise after the stimulus was removed and remained elevated above baseline for more than 45 minutes. HR = heart rate (beats/min). HR (trace not shown) peaked at 148, simultaneously with the peak of blood measure.

led to the use of clonidine and methyldopa in the chronic treatment of these patients, usually with good effect.

Chronically, the hallmark of baroreflex failure is labile hypertension and tachycardia, alternating with periods of hypotension and bradycardia. In many patients, low doses of a benzodiazepine aid in preventing cortically induced sympathetic surges, and in some cases, clonidine provides additional benefit in suppressing these surges.

GLOSSOPHARYNGEAL NEURALGIA. In patients who have had recent trauma in the area of the carotid sinus, secondary to causes such as surgery, tumor, or radiation, occasionally an intermittent activation of the glossopharyngeal nerve results. The patient experiences sudden, lancinating pain in the face, neck, or jaw on the affected side, and there is a sudden drop in both blood pressure and heart rate. This may be seen postoperatively and is an unexpected complication in what may be an otherwise benign course. Consultation is often sought for the episodes of hypotension, and the critical historical finding of pain may be overlooked in the focus on the hemodynamics. The episodes are usually self-limited, lasting for minutes, but the hypotension can be severe and symptomatic in itself, especially if the patient is upright. Treatment with yohimbine may ameliorate the episodes, but if all else fails, transection of the nerve may be necessary.[38,39]

MULTIPLE SYSTEM ATROPHY. Multiple system atrophy is a neurodegenerative disorder first described by Shy and Drager in 1960,[40] in which patchy central nervous system lesions are seen, consisting of oligodendroglial cells with cytoplasmic inclusions made up of multilayered fibrils of alpha-synuclein.[41,42] Although several other compounds, such as 14-3-3 proteins and tau, have been suggested to be involved,[43] careful study has shown that lesions can exist without the presence of either.[44] It appears that these inclusions eventually produce cellular degeneration. Patients gradually develop symptoms beginning in their 50s to 60s and exhibit both sympathetic and parasympathetic abnormalities. Autonomic symptoms and findings include impotence, lightheadedness due to orthostatic hypotension,[45] loss of sweating, abnormal pupillary responses,[46] urinary incontinence,[47-49] and respiratory abnormalities such as laryngeal stridor[50] and sleep apnea.[50,51] Urodynamic testing may be helpful in diagnosis in uncertain cases. At the bedside, significant orthostatic hypotension (the upright systolic pressure may fall by as much as 100 mm Hg, and may, in fact, be unobtainable) is accompanied by a minimal rise in heart rate. The fall in blood pressure can cause variable symptoms, with some patients reporting a headache involving the back of the neck,[52] blurring of vision, or a distancing of auditory sensation.

In addition, movement disorders of several forms can be seen in any posture. If there is rigidity, tremor, and bradykinesia, the patient may appear to have Parkinson's syndrome, but the movement generally does not improve with antiparkinsonian medications. A syndrome referred to as *atypical Parkinson's syndrome* has been described as a form of Parkinson's disease, with cell loss and Lewy bodies in autonomic regulatory regions, including the hypothalamus, sympathetic (intermediolateral nucleus of the thoracic cord and sympathetic ganglia), and parasympathetic (dorsal, vagal, and sacral parasympathetic nuclei) systems. Symptoms include orthostatic hypotension, gastrointestinal and urogenital dysfunction, pupillary abnormalities (pupillary control is dependent on both sympathetic and parasympathetic innervation), and disorders of sweating and regulation of temperature.[53] This syndrome may be clinically indistinguishable from multiple system atrophy.

In other patients with multiple system atrophy, the syndrome can be mistaken for spinocerebellar disease because of common symptoms of urinary incontinence and unsteadiness of gait.[54] The autonomic abnormalities, however, especially orthostatic hypotension, help determine that the patient has multiple system atrophy. Magnetic resonance imaging can also be helpful in defining the specific areas involved in multiple system atrophy.[54-56] Plasma catechols in multiple system atrophy show preservation of supine plasma norepinephrine, plasma dihydroxyphenolglycol, and urinary catecholamines.[57] But because the ability of the central nervous system to engage the periphery is impaired, the usual doubling with the upright posture is absent.

Although one might assume that the fall in blood pressure with upright posture is due to reduced arterial resistance, in fact, peripheral vascular resistance is increased in all postures in these patients, and it appears that increased venous compliance is a greater part of the problem.[58] Blood pressure while supine is markedly elevated in more than 50 percent of patients, with low renin levels.[59-62] Although the mechanism of supine hypertension is controversial,[63] studies in some patients suggest that it is due to inappropriately high constitutive catecholamine release.[12]

An additional symptom is a shift in urine production to the night, likely due to pressure diuresis as the low upright pressure during the day is replaced by the high blood pressure seen with the supine posture at night. This then leaves the patient relatively hypovolemic in the morning and worsens orthostatic hypotension.

THERAPEUTIC MANEUVERS. The first line of therapy in these patients is the timing of food and water. It has been demonstrated that food ingestion, particularly of carbohydrates, can lower blood pressure by 30 to 40 mm Hg,[42,60] and this may be helpful in reducing supine hypertension at night. During the day, however, the depressor effect of food ingestion produces an increased need for therapeutic maneuvers with a pressor effect for the periods immediately after meals. Caffeine ingestion of 100 to 250 mg with meals is helpful in some patients,[64] and somatostatin (which must be given by subcutaneous injection) is useful when the depressor effect is severe.[65,66] In contrast to food, drinking water has a significant, dose-dependent pressor effect in patients with autonomic dysfunction, with 16 ounces raising pressure by as much as 100 mm Hg in extreme cases, but routinely by 20 to 40 mm Hg.[21,67-69]

Second, physical maneuvers and exercise are helpful. Patients often have learned some maneuvers on their own to support blood pressure while upright, such as entwining the legs while constricting leg muscles, raising one foot to the seat of a chair, or squatting. Since patients are usually lightheaded with standing, they find it difficult to pursue their usual forms of exercise. Exercise in water is an excellent solution, because water pressure in effect provides compression of the lower extremities. Water temperatures that are excessively warm should be avoided, and care must be taken when emerging from the water. Analogous to standing in water is wearing waist-high garments providing 30 to 40 mm Hg graduated compression over the lower extremities. These should be removed when the patient is supine. Patients often need assistance in putting these garments on if they are tight enough to be effective. Open-crotch models are available. An additional maneuver is elevating the head of the bed 8 to 12 inches at night to reduce nocturia, thus leaving patients less volume depleted when they need to arise in the morning. Nocturia may also be treated with intranasal desmopressin.[67,70,71]

If these maneuvers are inadequate, pharmacological therapy should be instituted. Volume expansion via sodium retention can be produced by fludrocortisone, 0.05 to 0.2 mg orally twice a day. An addition of sodium to the diet is needed to see the full effect of fludrocortisone, and we encourage patients to eat a salty diet or to add 1 gm of salt to breakfast and lunch. A pressor agent is often also needed, and medications such as midodrine (2.5 to 10 mg orally two or three times a day) and yohimbine (5.4 mg orally two or three times a day) have a short enough duration of action to minimize worsening of supine hypertension at night. It is most effective to have patients keep water at the bedside and drink 16 ounces of water with their morning medications (fludrocortisone and a pressor agent) 20 to 30 minutes before arising. The combined pressor effects of the water and the pressor medication reduces the chance that marked orthostatic hypotension will cause a fall when the patient first arises. Anemia is common in patients with severe sympathetic failure, due at least in part to reduced sympathetically mediated erythropoietin release, and treatment with recombinant erythropoietin may be helpful.[72]

Unfortunately, although blood pressure control can be improved in patients with multiple system atrophy, there is currently no therapeutic approach to the overall degenerative neurologic process.[70] Nocturnal stridor is often troublesome in the later stages of the disorder but can be improved by continuous positive-pressure breathing.[73] Since difficulty with ambulation is often compromised more by loss of cell function in brain areas related to movement than by blood pressure, sustained improvement is unlikely. Multiple system atrophy does shorten life, and survival averages 9 years after diagnosis.[63,74] However, the course is variable, and some patients have survived for as long as 14 years. Since patients eventually become bedridden, careful planning with them and their caregivers for measures that maintain quality of life for as long as possible is essential.[59,60,75]

PURE AUTONOMIC FAILURE. In 1925, Bradbury and Eggleston described an "extensive and peculiar disturbance in the functional activity of the vegetative nervous system [accompanied by] idiopathic hypotension."[76] In these patients, with what was later referred to as *pure autonomic failure*, there is no central nervous system abnormality, but dysfunctional peripheral neurons prevent appropriate norepinephrine release. Norepinephrine levels are low in the supine posture and rise only minimally with standing. Autonomic symptoms and findings are as described earlier for multiple system atrophy but with the absence of any central nervous system lesions to produce a movement disorder. Longevity is normal, and control of orthostatic hypotension, using the same therapeutic maneuvers described for multiple system atrophy, is often sufficient to restore patients to most normal daily activities. At the bedside, orthostatic hypotension and an inadequate chronotropic response are seen.

ORTHOSTATIC ANGINA. In some patients, in addition to the symptoms described earlier for multiple system atrophy with the upright posture, or in place of them, chest pain can occur as the signal postural symptom. This symptom as described is indistinguishable from angina pectoris, and since it occurs when the patient stands to undertake an activity, it may appear to be precipitated by exertion. Although patients with pure autonomic failure are not protected from atherosclerosis and coronary artery disease, in many cases this apparent angina occurs in the absence of demonstrable coronary stenosis. With careful history taking, it becomes clear that this form of angina occurs when blood pressure is low and is relieved by the supine posture. It is also significantly worsened by nitroglycerin, especially if the patient remains upright, and appears to be due to severe orthostatic hypotension and inadequate coronary perfusion pressure. It is unclear why this occurs in some patients and not others, but it is important to recognize this pattern of orthostatic angina to provide the appropriate treatment. To determine whether conventional angina is present, supine exercise testing can be used.

AUTOIMMUNE AUTONOMIC FAILURE. In some patients, severe autonomic failure appears to result from immune damage to some aspect of neurons[77-81] and can be modeled by blockade of the N(N)-nicotinic receptor.[82] The findings of autonomic failure may appear suddenly, over days to weeks, or gradually over months to years.[79,83] In some of these patients, antibodies to ganglionic acetylcholine receptors have been demonstrated. When autoimmune autonomic failure appears gradually, it appears clinically indistinguishable from idiopathic pure autonomic failure. However, autoimmune autonomic failure may appear to occur overnight, often in a patient hospitalized for another illness, sometimes infectious in nature. The infection may seem to clear, but as the patient begins to ambulate, orthostatic hypotension can be so severe as to prevent discharge. Autonomic function testing shows postural vital signs with severe orthostatic hypotension and inadequate chronotropic response of heart rate for the degree of hypotension while upright. Autonomic abnormalities of bowel and bladder function are also common, and cholinergic dysfunction is more severe in those with higher antibody titers. Plasma catecholamines show very low norepinephrine levels, which rise only minimally with the upright posture. Although it has been suggested that intravenous gamma globulin may aid in reversing this syndrome,[84] it is not efficacious in all patients. Treatment is identical to that employed in patients with severe pure autonomic failure and multiple system atrophy.

SECONDARY AUTONOMIC NEUROPATHY (DIABETES, AMYLOID, RENAL FAILURE–ASSOCIATED, VITAMIN B_{12} DEFICIENCY, PARANEOPLASTIC SYNDROMES). Autonomic dysfunction is one of the frequent long-term complications of diabetes (see Chap. 51), and diabetes is one example of a number of disorders that lead to peripheral autonomic nerve dysfunction.[85] In patients with diabetes mellitus, both somatic and autonomic (both sympathetic and parasympathetic) neuropathy develop over time,[86,87] and abnormalities of autonomic cardiovascular control have been described both in animal models of diabetes[88,89] and in diabetic patients both with and without orthostatic hypotension.[86,87] In such patients, impairment of autonomic function has independent negative prognostic value,[90] although the underlying basis and extent of the abnormality remain unclear. Jensen-Urstad and associates[86] found a relationship between vascular stiffness, as determined by ultrasound of the carotid artery, and baroreflex sensitivity, suggesting that the abnormality may be caused by changes in the environment of the baroreceptor. Hoeldtke and colleagues[91] have recently demonstrated abnormal sudomotor responses in patients newly diagnosed with type 1 diabetes, especially in the upper body, and believed that this likely represented early sympathetic nerve injury. McDowell and coworkers[88,89] assessed baroreflex function at multiple levels in rabbits rendered diabetic with alloxan, finding normal control of renal sympathetic nerve activity but a selective deficit in baroreflex-mediated bradycardia; they suggested that the abnormal autonomic control seen in diabetics might be due primarily to defective activation of central parasympathetic pathways rather than of parasympathetic withdrawal.[88] This is consistent with studies in streptozotocin-diabetic rats. Gouty and associates[92] used the numbers of c-*Fos*-immunoreactive neurons in the nucleus of the solitary tract to assess function of the afferent limb of the baroreflex and found a reduction at 8 and 16 weeks. These studies strongly suggest that afferent as well as efferent neurons are involved. In humans, it has been clearly demonstrated that rigorous control of glucose provides protection against the microvascular complications of diabetes,[83] and the development of autonomic dysfunction appears to be improved.[83] Indeed, hypoglycemia itself can lead to autonomic dysfunction.[93]

When no obvious cause for peripheral autonomic dysfunction is present, an assessment of renal function and a fat pad biopsy for amyloid[20,94] are appropriate. Antibodies to various aspects of the peripheral autonomic nervous system can also be associated with neoplasms that may be clinically inapparent[81,95] but can still cause neuronal damage.[96] Since there have been reports of the autonomic disorder resolving after removal of the neoplasm, this diagnosis should be sought if antibodies can be demonstrated. In general, patients with this disorder and those with amyloid are poorly responsive to therapeutic measures that are quite effective in other forms of autonomic dysfunction.

GUILLAIN-BARRÉ SYNDROME. Although ascending motor abnormalities are prominent in this rare syndrome, they may be accompanied by autonomic dysfunction as well, which worsens the prognosis.[97,98] If this is the case, there are two aspects of treatment that are affected. While the patient is at bed rest, attention must be paid to potential hypersensitivity to sympathomimetic agents and to the effects of food and water on blood pressure. If autonomic dysfunction persists when the patient is able to assume the upright posture, the treatment of orthostatic hypotension, as in other patients with severe dysautonomias, must be included in the treatment regimen. For some patients, the only autonomic abnormality is orthostatic intolerance secondary to prolonged bed rest that resolves over a few days to weeks as ambulation is undertaken.

DOPAMINE BETA-HYDROXYLASE DEFICIENCY. Dopamine beta-hydroxylase deficiency is a congenital disorder and the first autonomic disorder in which a specific genetic abnormality was identified.[99] These patients lack a functional version of the enzyme that normally converts dopamine to norepinephrine in the vesicle within noradrenergic neurons. The sympathetic cholinergic and parasympathetic systems are normal. Figure 87–5 demonstrates the abnormality in the noradrenergic neuron.

Tyrosine hydroxylase, not dopamine beta-hydroxylase, is the rate-limiting enzyme in the generation of catecholamines. When norepinephrine is not made and cannot exert feedback control on tyrosine hydroxylase, the product just prior to the enzymatic block, in this case dopamine, is present in excess. These patients have two problems: First, they have no norepinephrine to release when sympathetic nerve activity increases, and thus, for example, cannot mount a vasoconstrictor response to upright posture. They have marked orthostatic hypotension (usually a fall in blood pressure to levels < 80 mm Hg systolic), with less heart rate rise than one would

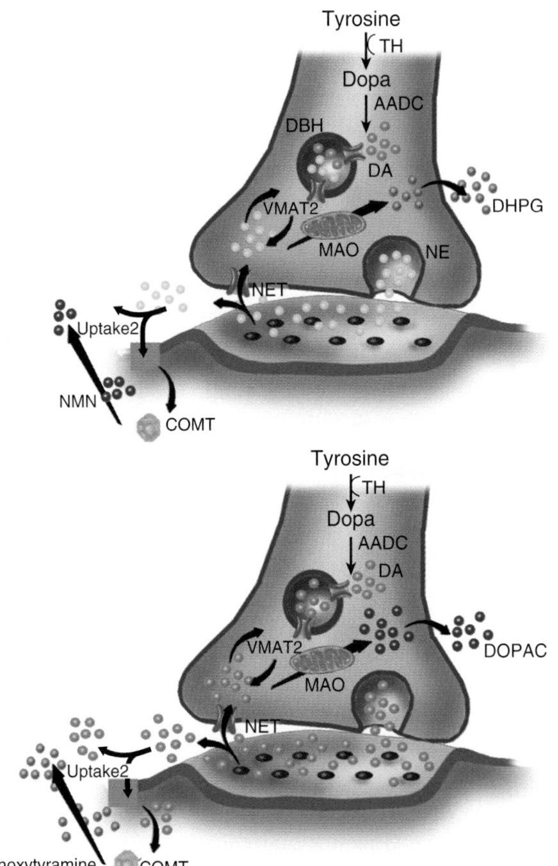

FIGURE 87–5 The enzymatic abnormality in dopamine beta-hydroxylase deficiency. TH = tyrosine hydroxylase; AADC = aromatic acid decarboxylase; DA = dopamine; Dopa = dihydroxyphenylalanine; DBH = dopamine beta-hydroxylase; VMAT2 = vesicular monoamine transporter 2; DHPG = dihydroxyphenylglycol; MAO = monoamine oxidase; NE = norepinephrine; NET = norepinephrine transporter; DOPAC = dihydroxyphenylacetic acid; NMN = normetanephrine; COMT = catechol *O*-methyltransferase. In the absence of functional dopamine beta-hydroxylase, the vesicles in noradrenergic neurons are filled with and release dopamine when the nerve is stimulated.

expect for this fall in blood pressure. Some heart rate rise is seen due to parasympathetic withdrawal. The patient is usually unable to stand quietly for even 60 seconds. Second, since these patients have constitutively higher levels of dopamine, and they release dopamine rather than norepinephrine with sympathetic stimuli, urinary sodium excretion is increased, and patients are slightly volume depleted. In addition, there is ptosis, nasal stuffiness, hyperextensibility of joints, and retrograde ejaculation in men.[100]

Since patients have normal levels of dopa decarboxylase, they are able to convert dihydroxyphenylserine to norepinephrine, and this drug has been used effectively to restore plasma norepinephrine levels and sympathetic responsiveness.[101] It has also been used with some benefit in patients with the more common forms of orthostatic hypotension due to autonomic failure.[102,103]

AUTONOMIC IMPAIRMENT IN CARDIAC DISEASE. Several forms of alteration in autonomic function have been demonstrated in patients with cardiovascular disease.[104-107] For example, increased neurohumoral tone in patients with heart failure has been associated with a worsened prognosis (see Chap. 22); this was the initial motivation for the expanded use of beta blockers in these patients. Of interest is a recent report of studies in a rabbit model of experimental heart failure that demonstrated a beneficial effect of simvastatin on plasma norepinephrine, renal sympathetic nerve activity, and baroreflex function.[108] Although many patients with heart failure are prescribed these agents because of other risk factors or known coronary disease, this suggests that they may have yet another non–lipid-lowering beneficial effect. Studies of autonomic effects in patients without conventional indications for 3-hydroxy-3-methylglutarylcoenzyme A (HMG-CoA) reductase inhibitors should be done.

A recent in vivo study in apolipoprotein E–/– mice, who are genetically dyslipidemic, showed increased blood pressure and heart rate, with decreased circadian rhythm, decreased heart rate variability, and increased blood pressure variability. When treated with rosuvastatin, they demonstrated an improvement in heart rate and blood pressure variability and decreased levels of caveolin 1, an inhibitor of aortic endothelial nitric oxide synthase.[109] It has also been demonstrated in a preliminary study that hypercholesterolemic patients with or without clinical coronary artery disease can improve heart rate variability after treatment with atorvastatin.[110] If confirmed in further studies in humans, this would suggest an additional beneficial effect of HMG-CoA reductase inhibitors in this population.

Mild Dysautonomias

POSTURAL TACHYCARDIA SYNDROME. In recent years, an increasing number of young to middle-aged patients have been recognized to have symptoms on standing, primarily tachycardia and weakness. Many demonstrate excessive sinus tachycardia on standing, according to the criteria of Streeten.[111] Most complain of orthostatic weakness, fatigue, chest discomfort, dizziness, anxiety, and occasionally presyncope or syncope after a period of standing.[112] These symptoms have also been used in the definition of postural tachycardia syndrome (POTS) by Low and coworkers,[112,113] but there is some variability in the inclusion criteria in studies by different investigators. The following criteria are now generally accepted in the clinical and laboratory definition of POTS:

- Orthostatic symptoms of sympathetic activation
- Orthostatic tachycardia (>30 beats/min)
- A fall in blood pressure of <20/10 mm Hg
- Elevated standing plasma norepinephrine (>600 pg/ml)

POTS is not a disease but indeed is a syndrome. Like “anemia” or “fever,” this constellation of symptoms and findings represents the “final common pathway” of likely hundreds of genetic and acquired autonomic and cardiovascular entities. The disorder is not new. It has been recognized for many years and has been reported especially when large groups of young people were evaluated, often in times of war. Many different names have been applied, including *effort syndrome, hyperdynamic beta-adrenergic state, idiopathic hypovolemia, irritable heart, mitral valve prolapse syndrome, neurocirculatory asthenia, orthostatic tachycardia syndrome, soldier's heart, vasoregulatory asthenia,* as well as POTS.

In some cases, specific etiologies have been documented,[57,114-119] and several of these are listed in Table 87–3. We assessed baroreflex function in a group of patients with neuropathic orthostatic intolerance, demonstrating that there is not only alpha- and beta-receptor hypersensitivity but also a reduced baroreflex index (Fig. 87–6).[120]

Because it had been suggested that the tachycardia was an appropriate response to either an effective reduction in blood volume or a circulating vasodilator and that it might represent a healthy autonomic response appropriately maintaining blood pressure and cardiac output, blood flow in the middle cerebral artery has been assessed in these patients during head-up tilt. The more rapid than normal decline in blood velocity in these patients than in matched normal controls confirms that the compensatory response is hemodynamically inadequate.[37,121]

TABLE 87–3 Etiologies of Subsets of Orthostatic Tachycardia

Subset	Cause
Structural	Ehlers-Danlos syndrome
Hypovolemia (absolute)	Channelopathies
Hypovolemia (orthostatic)	Idiopathic
Autoimmune	Anti-NNA3 subunit
Neuropathic	Neuropathic postural tachycardia syndrome
Hyperadrenergic (increased release)	Hyperadrenergia
Hyperadrenergic (decreased clearance)	Norepinephrine transporter deficiency

NNA3 = $N_n\alpha_3$ = the α_3 subunit of the neural nicotinic receptor.

DYNAMIC PLASMA VOLUME CHANGES. Figure 87–7 demonstrates the abnormally increased dynamic plasma volume shifts in a patient with orthostatic intolerance, demonstrating coincident increases in plasma norepinephrine and heart rate and a more gradual rise in dihydroxyphenylglycol, the norepinephrine metabolite.

The magnitude of these changes has important consequences for the study of any orthostatic syndrome, but it has rarely been taken into account. These dynamic changes could either differentially activate cardiopulmonary receptors in patients with orthostatic intolerance or could be quantitatively distinct. Some patients with orthostatic intolerance seem to have both a chronically decreased blood volume (5 to 20 percent) and an excessive dynamic decrease as well.

Treatment is aimed at restoring normal plasma volume and preventing pooling of volume in the periphery, usually beginning with fludrocortisone and compression garments. Additional restraint of beta-mediated tachycardia with beta blockers may be helpful. Often only very low doses of medication are tolerated.

NOREPINEPHRINE TRANSPORTER DEFICIENCY. A rare specific etiology for POTS has been demonstrated to be a mutation in the norepinephrine transporter gene, leading to a higher than 98 percent reduction in the ability to transport released norepinephrine back into the sympathetic nerve ending.[122] The mutant form also exerts a dominant negative effect when it is co-transfected into a heterologous expression system, by causing a conformational disruption interfering with transporter biosynthetic progression and trafficking of not only the mutant transporter but also of the wild-type norepinephrine transporter.[117-119] This results in elevated synaptic levels of the neurotransmitter whenever norepinephrine release is triggered, with resultant excessive heart rate.

MEDICATIONS (NOREPINEPHRINE TRANSPORTER BLOCKERS). Medications such as tricyclic antidepressants produce a syndrome of orthostatic tachycardia and sometimes orthostatic hypotension.[123] Vasodilators may produce a similar effect. A review of the patient's medications for drugs with a potential hemodynamic effect should be a first consideration in evaluating patients with autonomic findings.

BED REST. Studies of normal subjects after a period of bed rest and studies of astronauts during exposure to microgravity have demonstrated the development of orthostatic tachycardia and, in some, an increased propensity to syncope with prolonged (30 minutes) quiet standing.[117,118,124] This resolves completely after normal ambulation is resumed, but symptoms may take several days to weeks to abate, especially if the period of bed rest is long. Gradually increasing periods

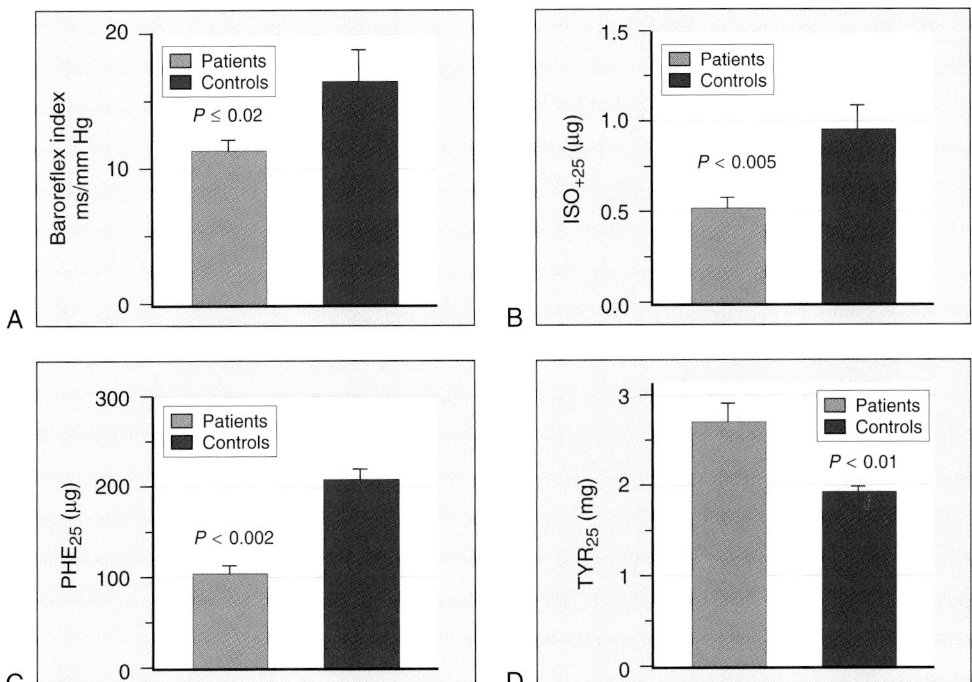

FIGURE 87–6 Pharmacological assessment of adrenergic receptor and baroreflex function in patients with orthostatic intolerance. For each agent (PHE = phenylephrine; ISO = isoproterenol; TYR = tyramine), the dose required to produce a pressor (PHE and TYR) or depressor (ISO) effect of 25 mm Hg is compared with the doses required in age-matched normal control subjects.

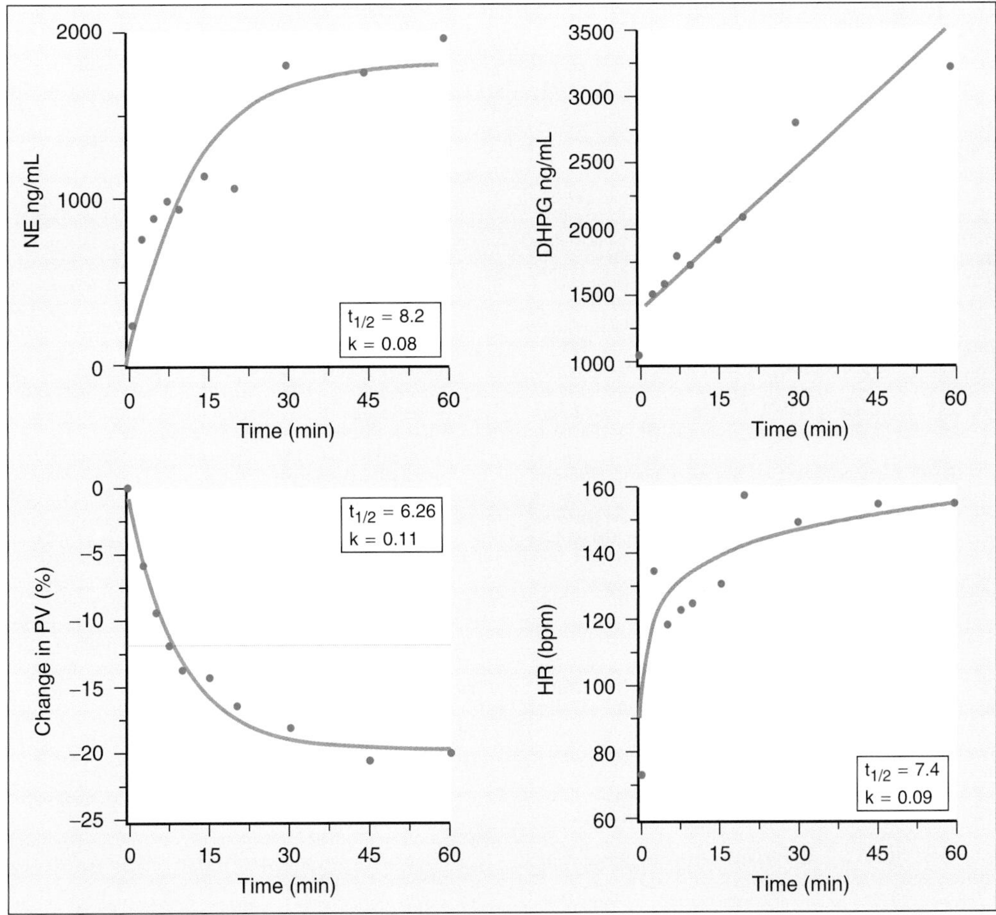

FIGURE 87–7 Effect of assuming the upright posture in a 39-year-old woman with orthostatic intolerance. From the bottom left, going counterclockwise, the PV decreases 20 percent over 45 minutes and is mirrored by an increase in HR. While the dihydroxyphenylglycol (DHPG) rises more gradually, the change in plasma norepinephrine (NE) parallels the change in heart rate.

of seated and then upright posture are usually all that is required, but compression garments may be helpful in situations where resolution is slow.

NEURALLY MEDIATED SYNCOPE. Most patients referred with syncope do not have either the orthostatic hypotension of the severe dysautonomias or the orthostatic tachycardia characteristic of orthostatic intolerance. In fact, between episodes of syncope, their autonomic function testing is entirely normal. After elimination of cardiac causes, most patients with neurally mediated syncope have a relatively benign prognosis, with risk related only to the circumstances in which they might have episodes of syncope. Their evaluation and treatment are covered in Chapter 34.

REFERENCES

General Principles

1. Diedrich, A, Jordan, J, Shannon, JR, et al: Modulation of QT interval during autonomic nervous system blockade in humans. Circulation 106:2238-2243, 2002.
2. Choy, AMJ, Lang, CC, Roden, DM, et al: Abnormalities of the QT interval in primary disorders of autonomic failure. Am Heart J 136:664-671, 1998.
3. Chen QH, Toney GM: Identification and characterization of two functionally distinct groups of spinal cord–projecting paraventricular nucleus neurons with sympathetic-related activity. Neuroscience 118:797-807, 2003.
4. Meyrelles, S, Sharma, R, Mao, H, et al: Modulation of baroreceptor activity by gene transfer of nitric oxide synthase to carotid sinus adventitia. Am J Physiol Regul Integr Comp Physiol 284: R1190-R1198, 2003.
5. Michalkiewicz M, Knestaut K, Bytchkova E, Michalkiewicz T: Hypotension and reduced catecholamines in neuropeptide Y transgenic rats. Hypertension 41:1056-1062, 2003.
6. Jacob G, Ertl AC, Shannon JR, et al: Effect of standing on neurohumoral responses and plasma volume in healthy subjects. J Appl Physiol 84:914-921, 1998.
7. Ketch T, Biaggioni I, Robertson R, Robertson D: Four faces of baroreflex failure: Hypertensive crisis, volatile hypertension, orthostatic tachycardia, and malignant vagotonia. Circulation 105:2518-2523, 2002.
8. Kim CH, Zabetian CP, Cubells JF, et al: Mutations in the dopamine beta-hydroxylase gene are associated with human norepinephrine deficiency. Am J Med Genet 108:140-147, 2002.
9. Youmans J, Akeroyd JJ, Frank H: Changes in the blood and circulation with changes in posture: The effect of exercise and vasodilatation. J Clin Invest 14:739-753, 1935.

Autonomic Disorders

10. Jordan J, Shannon JR, Black BK, et al: Malignant vagotonia due to selective baroreflex failure. Hypertension 30:1072-1077, 1997.
11. Parikh SM, Diedrich A, Biaggioni I, Robertson D: The nature of the autonomic dysfunction in multiple system atrophy. J Neurol Sci 200:1-10, 2002.
12. Shannon JR, Jordan J, Diedrich A, et al: Sympathetically mediated hypertension in autonomic failure. Circulation 101:2710-2715, 2000.
13. Takaya N, Sumiyoshi M, Nakata Y: Prolonged cardiac arrest caused by glossopharyngeal neuralgia. Heart 89:381, 2003.
14. Robertson D: The epidemic of orthostatic tachycardia and orthostatic intolerance. Am J Med Sci 317:75-77, 1999.
15. Shannon JR, Flattem NL, Jordan J, et al: Orthostatic intolerance and tachycardia associated with norepinephrine-transporter deficiency. N Engl J Med 342:541-549, 2000.
16. Mosqueda-Garcia R, Furlan R, Fernandez-Violante R, et al: Sympathetic and baroreceptor reflex function in neurally mediated syncope evoked by tilt. J Clin Invest 99:2736-2744, 1997.
17. Carson RP, Robertson D: Genetic manipulation of noradrenergic neurons. J Pharmacol Exp Ther 301:410-417, 2002.
18. Thomaides T, Bleasdale-Barr K, Chaudhuri KR, et al: Cardiovascular and hormonal responses to liquid food challenge in idiopathic Parkinson's disease, multiple system atrophy, and pure autonomic failure. Neurology 43:900-904, 1993.
19. Robertson D, Biaggioni I, Ertl AC, et al: Orthostatic intolerance: Emerging genetic and environmental etiologies. J Gravit Physio 6:151-154, 1999.
20. Carvalho MJ, van den Meiracker AH, Boomsma F, et al: Diurnal blood pressure variation in progressive autonomic failure. Hypertension 35:892-897, 2000.
21. Cariga P, Mathias CJ: Haemodynamics of the pressor effect of oral water in human sympathetic denervation due to autonomic failure. Clin Sci (Lond) 101:313-319, 2001.
22. Jordan J, Shannon JR, Grogan E, et al: The acute pressor effect of drinking water. J Hypertens 16:S32-S32, 1998.
23. Novak V, Spies JM, Novak P, et al: Hypocapnia and cerebral hypoperfusion in orthostatic intolerance. Stroke 29:1876-1881, 1998.
24. Jordan J, Shannon JR, Pohar B, et al: Contrasting effects of vasodilators on blood pressure and sodium balance in the hypertension of autonomic failure. J Am Soc Nephrol 10:35-42, 1999.
25. Shannon JR, Jordan J, Robertson D: Blood pressure in autonomic failure: Drinks, meals, and other ordeals. Clin Sci (Lond) 94:5, 1998.
26. Jordan J, Shannon JR, Diedrich A, et al: Interaction of carbon dioxide and sympathetic nervous system activity in the regulation of cerebral perfusion in humans. Hypertension 36:383-388, 2000.
27. Jordan J, Tank J, Shannon JR, et al: Baroreflex buffering and susceptibility to vasoactive drugs. Circulation 105:1459-1464, 2002.
28. Goldstein DS, Tack C: Noninvasive detection of sympathetic neurocirculatory failure. Clin Auton Res 10:285-291, 2000.

Severe Dysautonomias

29. Sharabi Y, Dendi R, Holmes C, Goldstein DS: Baroreflex failure as a late sequela of neck irradiation. Hypertension 42:110-116, 2003.
30. Robertson D, Hollister AS, Biaggioni I, et al: The diagnosis and treatment of baroreflex failure. N Engl J Med 329:1449-1455, 1993.
31. Robertson D, Jacob G, Ertl A, et al: Clinical models of cardiovascular regulation after weightlessness. Med Sci Sports Exerc 28(10 Suppl):S80-S84, 1996.
32. Dorman T, Thompson D, Breslow M, et al: Nicardipine versus nitroprusside for breakthrough hypertension following carotid endarterectomy. J Clin Anesth 13:16-19, 2001.
33. Dimakakos P, Antoniou A, Mourikis D, et al: Surgical outcome of carotid artery disease: Analysis of 367 carotid endarterectomies. Int Surg 83:350-354, 1998.
34. Landesberg G, Adam D, Berlatzky Y, Akselrod S: Step baroreflex response in awake patients undergoing carotid surgery: Time-and frequency-domain analysis. Am J Physiol 274:H1590-H1597, 1998.
35. Kresowik T, Bratzler D, Karp H, et al: Multistate utilization, processes, and outcomes of carotid endarterectomy. J Vasc Surg 32:227-234, 2001.
36. Furlan R, Diedrich A, Rimoldi A, et al: Effects of unilateral and bilateral carotid baroreflex stimulation on cardiac and neural sympathetic discharge oscillatory patterns. Circulation 108:717-723, 2003.
37. Jordan J, Shannon JR, Black BK, et al: Evidence for sympathetically-mediated cerebral vasoconstriction in idiopathic orthostatic intolerance. Circulation 98:827-827, 1998.
38. Moretti R, Torre P, Antonello RM, et al: Gabapentin treatment of glossopharyngeal neuralgia: A follow-up of four years of a single case. Eur J Pain 6:403-407, 2002.
39. Ozenci M, Karaoguz R, Conkbayir C, et al: Glossopharyngeal neuralgia with cardiac syncope treated by glossopharyngeal rhizotomy and microvascular decompression. Europace 5:149-152, 2003.
40. Shy G, Drager G: A neurological syndrome associated with orthostatic hypotension. Arch Neurol 2:511-527, 1960.
41. Benarroch EE: New findings on the neuropathology of multiple system atrophy. Auton Neurosci 96:59-62, 2002.
42. Robertson D, Shannon JR, Jordan J, et al: Multiple system atrophy: New developments in pathophysiology and therapy. Parkinsonism Relat Disord 7:257-260, 2001.
43. Abe H, Yagishita S, Amano N, et al: Argyrophilic glial intracytoplasmic inclusions in multiple system atrophy: Immunocytochemical and ultrastructural study. Acta Neuropathol (Berl) 84:273-277, 1992.
44. Giasson BI, Mabon ME, Duda JE, et al: Tau and 14-3-3 in glial cytoplasmic inclusions of multiple system atrophy. Acta Neuropathol (Berl) 106;243-250, 2003.
45. Austin MT, Davis TL, Robertson D, Charles PD: Multiple system atrophy: Clinical presentation and diagnosis. Tenn Med 92:55-57, 1999.
46. Micieli G, Tassorelli C, Martignoni E, et al: Further characterization of autonomic involvement in multiple system atrophy: A pupillometric study. Funct Neurol 10:273-280, 1995.
47. Oertel WH, Bandmann O: Multiple system atrophy. J Neural Transm 56:(Suppl):155-164, 1999.
48. Sakakibara R, Hattori T, Uchiyama T, et al: Urinary dysfunction and orthostatic hypotension in multiple system atrophy: Which is the more common and earlier manifestation? J Neurol Neurosurg Psychiatry 68:65-69, 2000.
49. Beck RO, Betts CD, Fowler CJ: Genitourinary dysfunction in multiple system atrophy: Clinical features and treatment in 62 cases. J Urol 151:1336-1341, 1994.
50. Yamaguchi M, Arai K, Asahina M, Hattori T: Laryngeal stridor in multiple system atrophy. Eur Neurol 49:154-159, 2003.
51. Asahina M, Yamaguchi M, Fukutake T, Hattori T: [Sleep apnea in multiple system atrophy]. Nippon Rinsho 58:1722-1727, 2000.
52. Bleasdale-Barr KM, Mathias CJ: Neck and other muscle pains in autonomic failure: Their association with orthostatic hypotension. J R Soc Med 91:355-359, 1998.
53. Micieli G, Tosi P, Marcheselli S, Cavallini A: Autonomic dysfunction in Parkinson's disease. Neurol Sci 24(Suppl 1):S32-S34, 2003.
54. Lee WY, Jin DK, Oh MR, et al: Frequency analysis and clinical characterization of spinocerebellar ataxia types 1, 2, 3, 6, and 7 in Korean patients. Arch Neurol 60:858-863, 2003.
55. Savoiardo M: Differential diagnosis of Parkinson's disease and atypical parkinsonian disorders by magnetic resonance imaging. Neurol Sci 24(Suppl 1):S35-S37, 2003.
56. Miwa H, Kajimoto Y, Nakanishi I, et al: T2-low signal intensity in the cortex in multiple system atrophy. J Neurol Sci 211:85-88, 2003.
57. Goldstein DS, Holmes C, Sharabi Y, et al: Plasma levels of catechols and metanephrines in neurogenic orthostatic hypotension. Neurology 60:1327-1332, 2003.
58. Smit AA, Halliwill JR, Low PA, Wieling W: Pathophysiological basis of orthostatic hypotension in autonomic failure. J Physiol 519:1-10, 1999.
59. Biaggioni I, Robertson RM: Hypertension in orthostatic hypotension and autonomic dysfunction. Cardiol Clin 20:291-301, 2002.
60. Colosimo C, Pezzella FR: The symptomatic treatment of multiple system atrophy. Eur J Neurol 9:195-199, 2002.
61. Jordan J, Biaggioni I: Diagnosis and treatment of supine hypertension in autonomic failure patients with orthostatic hypotension. J Clin Hypertens (Greenwich) 4:139-145, 2002.
62. Chandler MP, Mathias CJ: Haemodynamic responses during head-up tilt and tilt reversal in two groups with chronic autonomic failure: Pure autonomic failure and multiple system atrophy. J Neurol 249:542-548, 2002.
63. Goldstein DS, Pechnik S, Holmes C, et al: Association between supine hypertension and orthostatic hypotension in autonomic failure. Hypertension 42:136-142, 2003.
64. Onrot J, Goldberg MR, Biaggioni I, et al: Hemodynamic and humoral effects of caffeine in autonomic failure: Therapeutic implications for postprandial hypotension. N Engl J Med 313:549-554, 1985.

65. Hoeldtke RD, Dworkin GE, Gaspar SR, et al: Effect of the somatostatin analogue SMS-201-995 on the adrenergic response to glucose ingestion in patients with postprandial hypotension. Am J Med 86:673-677, 1989.
66. Lamarre-Cliche M, Cusson J: Octreotide for orthostatic hypotension. Can J Clin Pharmacol 213-215, 1999.
67. Mathias C, Young T: Plugging the leak—benefits of the vasopressin-2 agonist, desmopressin in autonomic failure. Clin Auton Res 13:85-87, 2003.
68. Shannon JR, Diedrich A, Biaggioni I, et al: Water drinking as a treatment for orthostatic syndromes. Am J Med 112:355-360, 2002.
69. Jordan J: Acute effect of water on blood pressure: What do we know? Clin Auton Res 12:250-255, 2002.
70. Riley DE: Orthostatic hypotension in multiple system atrophy. Curr Treat Options Neurol 2:225-230, 2000.
71. Sakakibara R, Matsuda S, Uchiyama T, et al: The effect of intranasal desmopressin on nocturnal waking in urination in multiple system atrophy patients with nocturnal polyuria. Clin Auton Res 13:106-108, 2003.
72. Winkler AS, Marsden J, Parton M, et al: Erythropoietin deficiency and anaemia in multiple system atrophy. Mov Disord 16:233-239, 2001.
73. Iranzo A, Santamaria J, Tolosa E: Continuous positive air pressure eliminates nocturnal stridor in multiple system atrophy. Barcelona Multiple System Atrophy Study Group. Lancet 356:1329-1330, 2000.
74. Wenning GK, Geser F: Multiple system atrophy. Rev Neurol (Paris) 159:3S31-3S38, 2003.
75. Gill CE, Khurana RK: Caregiver burden in Shy-Drager syndrome. J Nerv Ment Dis 188:47-50, 2000.
76. Bradbury S, Eggleston C: Postural hypotension: A report of three cases. Am Heart J 1:73-86, 1925.
77. Vernino S, Low PA, Fealey RD, et al: Autoantibodies to ganglionic acetylcholine receptors in autoimmune autonomic neuropathies. N Engl J Med 343:847-855, 2000.
78. Goldstein DS, Holmes C, Dendi R, et al Pandysautonomia associated with impaired ganglionic neurotransmission and circulating antibody to the neuronal nicotinic receptor. Clin Auton Res 12:281-285, 2002.
79. Klein CM, Vernino S, Lennon VA, et al: The spectrum of autoimmune autonomic neuropathies. Ann Neurol 53:752-758, 2003.
80. Low PA, Vernino S, Suarez G: Autonomic dysfunction in peripheral nerve disease. Muscle Nerve 27:646-661, 2003.
81. Vernino S, Adamski J, Kryzer TJ, et al: Neuronal nicotinic ACh receptor antibody in subacute autonomic neuropathy and cancer-related syndromes. Neurology 50:1806-1813, 1998.
82. Jordan J, Shannon JR, Black BK, et al: N(N)-nicotinic blockade as an acute human model of autonomic failure. Hypertension 31:1178-1184, 1998.
83. UK Prospective Study Group: Intensive blood-glucose control with sulphonylureas or insulin compared with conventional treatment and risk of complications in patients with type 2 diabetes (UKPDS 33). Lancet 352:837-853, 1998.
84. Smit AA, Vermeulen M, Koelman JH, Wieling W: Unusual recovery from acute panautonomic neuropathy after immunoglobulin therapy. Mayo Clin Proc 72:333-335, 1997.
85. Vinik AI, Erbas T: Recognizing and treating diabetic autonomic neuropathy. Cleve Clin J Med 68:928-944, 2001.
86. Jensen-Urstad K, Reichard P, Jensen-Urstad M: Decreased heart rate variability in patients with type 1 diabetes mellitus is related to arterial wall stiffness. J Intern Med 245:57-61, 1999.
87. Bernardi L: Clinical evaluation of arterial baroreflex activity in diabetes. Diabetes Nutr Metab 13:331-340, 2000.
88. McDowell T, Chapleau M, Hajduczok G, Abboud FM: Baroreflex dysfunction in diabetes mellitus: I. Selective impairment of parasympathetic control of heart rate. Am J Physiol 266:H235-H243, 1994.
89. McDowell T, Hajduczok G, Abboud F, Chapleau M: Baroreflex dysfunction in diabetes mellitus: II. Site of baroreflex impairment in diabetic rabbits. Am J Physiol 266:H244-H249, 2003.
90. Valensi P, Sachs RN, Harfouche B, et al: Predictive value of cardiac autonomic neuropathy in diabetic patients with or without silent myocardial ischemia. Diabetes Care 24:339-343, 2001.
91. Hoeldtke RD, Bryner KD, Horvath GG, et al: Redistribution of sudomotor responses is an early sign of sympathetic dysfunction in type 1 diabetes. Diabetes 436:436-443, 2001.
92. Gouty S, Regalia J, Helke C: Attenuation of the afferent limb of the baroreceptor reflex in streptozotocin-induced diabetic rats. Auton Neurosci 89:86-95, 2001.
93. Diedrich L, Sandoval D, Davis SN: Hypoglycemia-associated autonomic failure. Clin Auton Res 12:358-365, 2002.
94. Singer W, Opfer-Gehrking TL, McPhee BR, et al: Acetylcholinesterase inhibition: A novel approach in the treatment of neurogenic orthostatic hypotension. J Neurol Neurosurg Psychiatry 74:1294-1298, 2003.
95. Low PA: Autonomic neuropathies. Curr Opin Neurol 15:605-609, 2002.
96. Scaravilli F, An SF, Groves M, Thom M: The neuropathology of paraneoplastic syndromes. Brain Pathol 9:251-260, 1999.
97. Low PA: Autonomic neuropathies. Curr Opin Neurol 7:402-406, 1994.
98. Santiago S, Ferrer T, Espinosa ML: Neurophysiological studies of thin myelinated (A delta) and unmyelinated (C) fibers: Application to peripheral neuropathies. Neurophysiol Clin 30:27-42, 2000.
99. Robertson D, Goldberg MR, Onrot J, et al: Isolated failure of autonomic noradrenergic neurotransmission—evidence for impaired beta-hydroxylation of dopamine. N Engl J Med 314:1494-1497, 1986.
100. Biaggioni I, Goldstein DS, Atkinson T, Robertson D: Dopamine-beta-hydroxylase deficiency in humans. Neurology 40:370-373, 1990.
101. Vincent S, Robertson D: The broader view: Catecholamine abnormalities. Clin Auton Res 12(Suppl 1):I44-I49, 2002.
102. Freeman R, Landsberg L, Young J: The treatment of neurogenic orthostatic hypotension with 3,4-D,L-threo-dihydroxyphenylserine: A randomized, placebo-controlled, crossover trial. Neurology 53:2151-2157, 1999.
103. Kaufmann H, Saadia D, Voustianiouk A, et al: Norepinephrine precursor therapy in neurogenic orthostatic hypotension. Circulation 108:724-728, 2003.
104. Lanfranchi PA, Somers VK: Arterial baroreflex function and cardiovascular variability: Interactions and implications. Am J Physiol Regul Integr Comp Physiol 283:R815-R826, 2002.
105. Gerritsen J, Dekker JM, TenVoorde BJ, et al: Impaired autonomic function is associated with increased mortality, especially in subjects with diabetes, hypertension, or a history of cardiovascular disease: The Hoorn Study. Diabetes Care 24:1793-1798, 2001.
106. Stevens MJ: New imaging techniques for cardiovascular autonomic neuropathy: A window on the heart. Diabetes Technol Ther 3:9-22, 2001.
107. Sleight P: The importance of the autonomic nervous system in health and disease. Aust N Z J Med 27:467-473, 1997.
108. Pliquett R, Cornish K, Peuler J, Zucker I: Simvastatin normalizes autonomic neural control in experimental heart failure. Circulation 107:2493-2498, 2003.
109. Pelat M, Dessy C, Massion P, et al: Rosuvastatin decreases caveolin-1 and improves nitric oxide-dependent heart rate and blood pressure variability in apolipoprotein E-/- mice in vivo. Circulation 107:2480-2486, 2003.
110. Pehlivanidis AN, Athyros VG, Demitriadis DS, et al: Heart rate variability after long-term treatment with atorvastatin in hypercholesterolaemic patients with or without coronary artery disease. Atherosclerosis 157:463-469, 2001.

Mild Dysautonomias

111. Streeten DH: Orthostatic intolerance: A historical introduction to the pathophysiological mechanisms. Am J Med Sci 11:78-87, 1999.
112. Low PA, Schondorf R, Rummans TA: Why do patients have orthostatic symptoms in POTS? Clin Auton Res 11:223-224, 2001.
113. Novak V, Novak P, Opfer-Gehrking TL, et al: Clinical and laboratory indices that enhance the diagnosis of postural tachycardia syndrome. Mayo Clin Proc 73:1141-1150, 1998.
114. Rowe PC, Barron DF, Calkins H, et al: Orthostatic intolerance and chronic fatigue syndrome associated with Ehlers-Danlos syndrome. J Pediatr 135:494-499, 1999.
115. Kuchel O, Leveille J: Idiopathic hypovolemia: A self-perpetuating autonomic dysfunction? Clin Auton Res 8:341-346, 1998.
116. Jacob G, Costa F, Shannon JR, et al: The neuropathic postural tachycardia syndrome. N Engl J Med 343:1008-1014, 2000.
117. Ertl AC, Diedrich A, Biaggioni I: Baroreflex dysfunction induced by microgravity: Potential relevance to postflight orthostatic intolerance. Clin Auton Res 10:269-277, 2000.
118. Ertl AC, Diedrich A, Biaggioni I, et al: Human muscle sympathetic nerve activity and plasma noradrenaline kinetics in space. J Physiol 538:321-329, 2002.
119. Hahn MK, Robertson D, Blakely RD: A mutation in the human norepinephrine transporter gene (SLC6A2) associated with orthostatic intolerance disrupts surface expression of mutant and wild-type transporters. J Neurosci 23:4470-4478, 2003.
120. Jacob G, Shannon JR, Costa F, et al: Abnormal norepinephrine clearance and adrenergic receptor sensitivity in idiopathic orthostatic intolerance. Circulation 99:1706-1712, 1999.
121. Schondorf R, Benoit J, Stein R: Cerebral autoregulation in orthostatic intolerance. Ann N Y Acad Sci 940:514-526, 2001.
122. Robertson D, Flattem N, Tellioglu T, et al: Familial orthostatic tachycardia due to norepinephrine transporter deficiency. Ann N Y Acad Sci 940:527-543, 2001.
123. Schroeder C, Tank J, Boschmann M, et al: Selective norepinephrine reuptake inhibition as a human model of orthostatic intolerance. Circulation 105:347-353, 2002.
124. Convertino VA: G-factor as a tool in basic research: mechanisms of orthostatic tolerance. J Gravit Physiol 6:73-76, 1999.

DISCLOSURE INDEX

The following contributors have indicated that they have a relationship that, in the context of their participation in the writing of a chapter for the seventh edition of *Braunwald's Heart Disease,* could be perceived by some people as a real or apparent conflict of interest, but do not consider that it has influenced the writing of their chapter. Codes for the disclosure information (institution[s] and nature of relationship[s]) are provided below.

Relationship Codes

A—Stock options or bond holdings in a for-profit corporation or self-directed pension plan
B—Research grants
C—Employment (full or part-time)
D—Ownership or partnership
E—Consulting fees or other remuneration received by the contributor or immediate family
F—Nonremunerative positions, such as board member, trustee, or public spokesperson
G—Receipt of royalties
H—"Speaker's bureau"

Institution and Company Codes

001—ARCA Discovery, Inc.
002—Abbott Labs
003—Adelphi, Inc.
004—Aderis Pharmaceuticals, Inc.
005—Actelion
006—Ajinomoto Pharmaceuticals
007—Alexion Pharmaceuticals
008—Alliance Medical
009—Alza
010—American Association for Cancer Research
011—American Cancer Society
012—American College of Cardiology
013—American Heart Association
014—American Society of Echocardiography
015—Amersham Health
016—Amersham, Inc.
017—Arrow
018—Asahi Chemical Company
019—Astra Zeneca, Inc.
020—Avant Immunotherapeutics
021—Aventis
022—Avon Foundation
023—BASF
024—Baxter Pharmaceuticals
025—Bayer
026—Bayer Diagnostics
027—Berkeley Heart Lab
028—Berlex
029—Best Med
030—Beth Israel Deaconess Medical Center
031—Bioheart Scientific
032—Biomarin Pharmaceuticals
033—Biosite, Inc.
034—Blue Cross Blue Shield of Michigan
035—Boeringer Ingelheim
036—Boston Scientific Corporation
037—Bracco
038—Bristol Meyers Squibb, Co.
039—British Biotech
040—Burrill and Company
041—C2R
042—Cardiac Dimensions
043—Cardiofocus
044—Cardiovascular Biosciences
045—Cardiovascular Imaging Solutions
046—Cell Therapeutics
047—Centocor
048—Chiron
049—Churchill Livingstone
050—Columbia University
051—Cordis Corporation
052—Corvas BMS
053—Covalent
054—Cryocor
055—CTI, Inc.
056—Cubist Pharmaceuticals
057—Current Medicine LLC
058—Current Science
059—CV Therapeutics, Inc.
060—CVRx
061—Dade Behring
062—Denver Health Medical Center
063—Discovery East
064—Discovery, Inc.
065—Doris Duke Foundation
066—EBR systems
067—Eli Lilly and Company
068—Encysive
069—Esperion Therapeutics
070—Excerpta Medica
071—Exhale Therapeutics
072—eV3
073—Fondation Leducq (Paris)
074—Fujisawa
075—Genentech
076—Genvec
077—Genzyme
078—Glaxo Smith Kline
079—GMP Companies, Inc.
080—Goldant
081—GSK
082—GTC Therapeutics
083—Guerbet
084—Guidant Corporation
085—Interleukin Genetics
086—Intraluminal
087—Johnson and Johnson
088—Johnson and Johnson—Merck Consumer Pharmaceuticals
089—K-23 National Institute of Health
090—King Pharmaceuticals
091—KOS
092—Lancet International
093—Life Sentry
094—Lippincott
095—MC Communications
096—McGraw Hill
097—McNeil
098—Medical Decision Point
099—Medicines Company
100—Medreviews
101—Medtronic, Inc.
102—Merck & Co., Inc.
103—Merck Frosst/Schering Plough
104—Merck-Schering Plough Corp.
105—Michael Marcus and Associates Science Partners, LLC
106—Micromed
107—Millennium Pharmaceuticals
108—Mitsubishi
109—Molecular Insight Pharmaceuticals
110—Momenta Pharmaceuticals
111—Mylan
112—Myogen, Inc.
113—National Cancer Institute
114—National Heart, Lung and Blood Institute
115—NCME
116—New York University School of Medicine
117—NIH/NCRR Research Resource for Complex Physiologic Signals
118—Nitromed
119—Novartis, Inc.
120—Novonordisk Pharmaceuticals
121—Nuvelo
122—Octagon Corporation
123—Omnisonics
124—Ortho Biotech, Inc.
125—Ortho-Clinical Diagnostics
126—Ortho-McNeil
127—Otsuka
128—Pacific Mountain Affiliate
129—Paion
130—Pfizer, Inc.

131—Pharmacia Diagnostics
132—Pharmacia-Upjohn, Inc.
133—Philips
134—Philips Canada
135—Pierre Fabre
136—Point Biomedical
137—Procter and Gamble
138—Radiant Medical
139—Reliant Pharmaceuticals
140—Restore Medical
141—Rey Institute for Nonlinear Dynamics in Medicine
142—Roche Diagnostics
143—Sankyo
144—Sanofi-Synthelabo, Inc.
145—Sanyo
146—Scientific American Medicine Editorial Board
147—Scios, Inc.
148—Servier
149—Schering Plough Corp.
150—Siemens
151—SmithKline Beecham
152—St. Jude Medical
153—Stanford University
154—Sunol Molecular
155—Takeda
156—Terumo Cardiovascular Systems Corporation
157—Terumo Heart, Inc.
158—Thoratec
159—TJ Martel Foundation
160—Transneuronix
161—TYCO
162—United Therapeutics, Inc.
163—University of Colorado Health Sciences Center
164—University of Wisconsin, Medical School
165—Vasogen
166—Vasogenix
167—Vertex
168—Vicaron
169—Volcano Therapeutics
170—Women's Health Initiative
171—Wyeth
172—ZLB Behring

Contributors

Antman, Elliot, B-033, B-038, B-039, B-047, B-052, B-061, B-067, B-075, B-102, B107, B-142, B-154
Antman, Karen, A-055; B-011, B-022, B-113, B-159; E-019, E-065, E-110, E-146; F-010, F-011, F-092; G-094
Armstrong, William F., E-019, E-152; H-038
Baim, Donald S., E-036
Barsky, Arthur, B-130
Beckman, Joshua A., B-067, B-130; E-038; H-067, H-102, H-119
Beller, George A., B-038
Bonow, Robert O., B-114; E-038, E-090, E-130, E-155
Braunwald, Eugene, B-021, B-038, B-059, B-067, B-107, B-121; E-045, E-073, E-084, E-095, E-110, E-147; F-012, F-116, F-170; G-057, G-096
Bristow, Michael, A-001, A-064, A-112; E-019, E-041, E-042, E-053, E-060, E-077, E-081, E-084, E-102, E-108, E-111, E-119, E-147
Calkins, Hugh, B-080, B-101, B-152; E-080
Cannon, Christopher, B-038, B-102, B-144; F-018, F-019, F-025, F-078, F-099, F-125, F-130, F-167; H-021, H-038, H-047, H-067, H-075, H-102, H-107, H-144
Creager, Mark A., B-028, B-038, B-067, B-130, B-144, B-171; E-003, E-007, E-028, E-038, E-076, E-077, E-091, E-100, E-127, E-130, E-144, E-165; G-058; H-038, H-127, H-144
Dilsizian, Vasken, B-037, B-112, B-133; E-109; H-038, H-074
Douglas, Pamela S., E-012, E-014, E-102, E-119; F-012, F-014
Eagle, Kim A., C-021, C-034, C-130; E-012; F-114
Eisenhauer, Andrew C., B-84, B-101; E-101
Fleisher, Lee A., B-024; E-024
Gaziano, J. Michael, B-023, B-097, B-142, B-171; E-097; H-130
Genest, Jacques, E-019, E-103, E-130; H-019
Goldhaber, Sam, B-019, B-021; E-021, E-025, E-129, E-130, E-137
Gotto, Antonio M., E-019, E-025, E-038, E-102, E-119 E-130, E-139; F-069
Groh, William, B-067, B-084, B-101
Hayes, David, A-084, A-101; B-084, B-101, B-141; H-084, H-101, H-152
Hoffman, Gary, B-047; E-047; H-130, H-171
Isselbacher, Eric M., H-101, H-130
Kabbani, Samer, E-102, E-144; F-102, F-144
Kaplan, Norman, H-002, H-019, H-119, H-130, H-145, H-148
Karchmer, A. W., A-130; B-025, B-074, B-102, B-126, B-168; E-056, E-130, E-168
Klein, Irwin L., B-090, B-142; E-038
Konkle, Barbara A, B-006, B-025, B-046, B-120, B-122, B-171, B-172; E-025, E-078, E-082, E-120, E-171
Krauss, Ronald M., B-102, B-130; E-002, E-019, E-091, E-102, E-130; H-002, H-104
Libby, Peter, B-019, B-025, B-038, B-102, B-107, B-119, B-130, B-143, B-151; E-019, E-020, E-25, E-038, E-085, E-102, E-107, E-119, E-130, E-135, E-143, E-144, E-149, E-151; H-019, H-025, H-038, H-102, H-119, H-130
Linas, Stuart, E-019, E-062; E-102, E-130; H-019, H-102, H-130
Lipshultz, Steve, B-130, B-132, B-142; E-035
Lowes, Brian D, B-089; C-163; E-112; H-081, H-130
Mark, Daniel, B-008, B-101, B-130, B-137
McCullough, Peter A., E-002, E-015, E-033, E-119, E-124, E-147
McLaughlin, Vallerie, B-068, B-112, B-130; E-005, E-071, E-162; H-005, H-162
Miller, John, B-084, B-101; E-084, E-101
Morrow, David, B-021, B-026, B-061, B-107, B-142, B-154
Myerburg, Robert, E-137, E-144; H-028, H-084, H-137
Nabel, Elizabeth, E-036
Naka, Yoshifumi, E-157
Nesto, Richard W., H-081, H-102, H-130
Olgin, Jeffrey, A-101, A-102; E-036, E-101, E-171
Opie, Lionel, F-102
Pasternak, Richard C., E-019, E-038, E-088, E-091, E-102, E-130, E-144; H-038, H-091, H-102, H-104, H-130, H-144
Pennell, Dudley J., B-083, B-150, B-161; D-045; E-008, E-015, E-038, E-108; G-049
Popma, Jeffrey J., B-002, B-036, B-051, B-072, B-084, B-086, B-101, B-138; H-036, H-051, H-101, H-107, H-149
Port, J. David, A-001, A-112; F-013, F-128; G-112; H-019
Priori, Silvia, B-059, B-101, B-130
Pyeritz, Reed E., E-032, E-077, E-102, E-104; H-102, H-104
Rich, Stuart, A-162; C-162
Ridker, Paul M, B-019, B-038, B-119, B-131; E-002
Robertson, David, No information supplied.
Robertson, Rose Marie, No information supplied.
Roden, Dan, B-038; E-009, E-019, E-059, E-077, E-078, E-087; F-066
Rose, Eric, B-017, B-106, B-158
Rosenfield, Kenneth, A-123; B-002, B-036, B-051; E-002, E-036, E-051; H-067
Schwartz, Janice, A-136; E-054, E-140, E-160; G-096
Smallhorn, Jeffrey F., B-134
Sweitzer, Nancy K., B-147; H-078, H-147
Udelson, James E., B-038, B-090, B-127; E-038, E-076, E-090, E-109, E-127; H-038, H-081
Yancy, Clyde W. Jr., B-078, B-118, B-147; E-101; H-078, H-101, H-147
Zipes, Douglas P., A-043; B-101; D-105; E-004, E-040, E-043, E-059, E-077, E-079, E-093, E-101, E-156; F-012

INDEX

Note: Page numbers followed by f and t indicate figures and tables, respectively.